The 5-Minute Clinical Consult

2020

28th EDITION

The 5-Minute Clinical Consult

2020

28th EDITION

Editor-in-Chief

Frank J. Domino, MD
Professor and Director of Predoctoral Education
Department of Family Medicine and Community Health
University of Massachusetts Medical School
Worcester, Massachusetts

Associate Editors

Robert A. Baldor, MD, FAAFP
Professor and Senior Vice-Chairman
Department of Family Medicine and Community Health
University of Massachusetts Medical School
Worcester, Massachusetts

Jeremy Golding, MD, FAAFP
Professor of Family Medicine and Obstetrics & Gynecology
University of Massachusetts Medical School
Quality Officer
Department of Family Medicine and Community Health
University of Massachusetts Memorial Health Care
Hahnemann Family Health Center
Worcester, Massachusetts

Mark B. Stephens, MD
Professor of Family and Community Medicine
Penn State University College of Medicine
State College, Pennsylvania

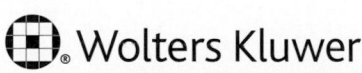 Wolters Kluwer

Philadelphia · Baltimore · New York · London
Buenos Aires · Hong Kong · Sydney · Tokyo

5MinuteConsult

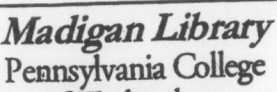
Director, Medical Practice: Brian Brown-Gertner
Digital Product Development Editor: Leanne Vandetty
Editorial Assistant: Brian Convery
Production Project Manager: Bridgett Dougherty
Design Coordinator: Steven Druding
Manufacturing Coordinator: Beth Welsh
Marketing Manager: Rachel Mante Leung
Prepress Vendor: Absolute Service, Inc.

28th edition

Copyright © 2020 Wolters Kluwer

9 8 7 6 5 4 3 2 1

Printed in China

Library of Congress Cataloging-in-Publication Data available from the Publisher upon request.

ISBN-13: 978-1-9751-3641-3

shop.lww.com

Again, I offer this reminder: In the 1600s, Isaac Newton said, "If I have seen further, it is by standing on the shoulder of giants."

Each year for the last 14 years, my mother would ask, "Why haven't you dedicated the book to me?" I would remind her my dedications were to those who had died—the book being a living memorial.

The 2020 edition of The 5-Minute Clinical Consult *is dedicated to Angela Domino, my mom. Education and perseverance were my mother's doctrine in my youth. When young, neither she nor my father was much interested in education, but for her children, this would not be the case. On the advice of my brother's 5th grade teacher, my mother chose to push us to read and always do well in all we did. In my brother's words, she was a 1960s "Tiger Mom." This book would not be in your hands, nor would I have gone on with my education, had it not been for my mother's dedication to encouraging education as the path to your goals and your life.*

Thanks to the power of hospice, I was able to spend time with her prior to her death and thank her, a luxury I did not have with my father.

So, look to your giants and give them your thanks.

FRANK J. DOMINO, MD

PREFACE

> **"If you can't feed a hundred people then feed just one."**
>
> **–MOTHER TERESA**

On my schedule this past week was a 12-year-old boy for his yearly physical. After hearing his mom's concerns and then asking her to leave, we proceeded with the usual promise of confidentiality. 20 minutes into the visit, he disclosed he was cutting . . . and was being bullied at school.

The pressures of practice, the electronic record, the variety of formularies, billing rules, and the like are all contributing to "burnout." Around the country, I hear these complaints and see the sadness and apathy that results.

Yet, every day, we have 10 to 20 opportunities to help others, in ways no pill can. We listen, we encourage, and offer advice, and, most important, we are our patient's advocate. The best evidence on what LDL or A1c level to chase (and again this year, which BP requires treatment) are population-based answers. I use them to guide my patient discussions. The real care we give is helping each person, one at a time. My presence helped my 12-year-old open up and the possibility of preventing a more than superficial cut.

> **"Any man may easily do harm but not every man can do good to another."**
>
> **–PLATO**

Go into every visit knowing you make a difference; feed each one, and do them well. Even if you cannot offer a cure or a solution, we can always do good.

Welcome to the 2020 edition of *The 5-Minute Clinical Consult.* Much of the work delivered by primary care providers focused on helping the patients help themselves to be healthier. Diet, exercise, safety, and prevention are the interventions that provide the greatest number of people with the greatest return on longevity and its enjoyment.

The 5-Minute Clinical Consult is here to assist in fulfilling our role as health care providers. In each patient interaction, in addition to bringing your clinical expertise, remember how your patients view you, as their advocate, someone who prioritizes their well-being unlike anyone else.

Our editorial team has collaborated with hundreds of authors so that you may deliver your patients the best care. Each topic provides you with quick answers you can trust, where and when you need them most, either in print or online at www.5MinuteConsult.com.

This highly organized content online provides you with the following:

- Differential diagnosis support from our expanded collection of algorithms
- Current evidence-based designations highlighted in each topic
- 540+ commonly encountered diseases in print, with an additional 1,500 online topics, including content from *The 5-Minute Pediatric Consult*
- FREE point-of-care CME and CE: 1/2 hour credit for every digital search
- Thousands of images to help support visual diagnosis of all conditions
- Video library of procedures, treatment, and physical therapy
- A to Z drug database from Facts & Comparisons
- Laboratory test interpretation from *Wallach's Interpretation of Diagnostic Tests*
- More than 3,000 patient handouts in English and Spanish
- ICD-10 codes and *DSM-5* criteria; additionally, SNOMED codes are available online.

Our website, www.5MinuteConsult.com, delivers quick answers to your questions. It is an ideal resource for patient care. Integrating *The 5-Minute Clinical Consult* content into your workflow is easy and fast, and our patient education handouts can assist in helping you meet meaningful use compliance.

If you purchased the Premium Edition, your access includes 1-year FREE use of our expanded website; the standard edition includes a free 10-day trial! The site promises an easy-to-use interface, allowing smooth maneuverability between topics, algorithms, images, videos, and patient education materials as well as more than 1,500 online-only topics.

Evidence-based health care is the integration of the best medical information with the values of the patient and your skill as a clinician. We have updated our evidence-based medicine (EBM) content so you can focus on how to best apply it in your practice.

The algorithm section includes both diagnostic and treatment algorithms. This easy-to-use graphic method helps you evaluate an abnormal finding and prioritize treatment. They are also excellent teaching tools, so share them with the learners in your office.

This book and website are a source to solve problems and to help evaluate, diagnose, and treat patients' concerns. Use your knowledge, expressed through your words and actions, to address their anxiety.

The 5-Minute Clinical Consult editorial team values your observations, so please share your thoughts, suggestions, and constructive criticism through our website: www.5MinuteConsult.com.

FRANK J. DOMINO, MD

EVIDENCE-BASED MEDICINE

WHAT IS EVIDENCE-BASED MEDICINE?

Remember when we used to treat every otitis media with antibiotics? These recommendations came about because we applied logical reasoning to observational studies. If bacteria cause an acute otitis media, then antibiotics should help it resolve sooner, with less morbidity. Yet, when rigorously studied (via a systematic review), we found little benefit to this intervention.

The underlying premise of EBM is the evaluation of medical interventions and the literature that supports those interventions, in a systematic fashion. EBM hopes to encourage treatments proven to be effective and safe. And when insufficient data exist, it hopes to inform you on how to safely proceed.

EBM uses end points of real patient outcomes, morbidity, mortality, and risk. It focuses less on intermediate outcomes (bone density) and more on patient conditions (hip fractures).

Implementing EBM requires three components: the best medical evidence, the skill and experience of the provider, and the values of the patients. Should this patient be screened for prostate cancer? It depends on what is known about the test, on what you know of its benefits and harms, your ability to communicate that information, and that patient's informed choice.

This book hopes to address the first EBM component, providing you access to the best information in a quick format. Although not every test or treatment has this level of detail, many of the included interventions here use systematic review literature support.

The language of medical statistics is useful in interpreting the concepts of EBM. Below is a list of these terms, with examples to help take the confusion and mystery out of their use.

Prevalence: *proportion of people* in a population who have a disease (in the United States, 0.3% [3 in 1,000] people >50 years have colon cancer)

Incidence: how many *new cases of a disease* occur in a population during an interval of time; for example, "The estimated incidence of colon cancer in the United States is 104,000 in 2005."

Sensitivity: percentage of people with disease who test positive; for mammography, the sensitivity is 71–96%.

Specificity: percentage of people without disease who test negative; for mammography, the specificity is 94–97%.

Suppose you saw ML, a 53-year-old woman, for a health maintenance visit, ordered a *screening* mammogram, and the report demonstrates an irregular area of microcalcifications. She is waiting in your office to receive her test results, what can you tell her?

Sensitivity and specificity refer to characteristics of people who are *known to have disease* (sensitivity) or those who are *known not to have disease* (specificity). But, what you have is an abnormal test result. To better explain this result to ML, you need the positive predictive value.

Positive predictive value (PPV): percentage of *positive* test results that are truly positive; the PPV for a woman aged 50 to 59 years is approximately 22%. That is to say that only 22% of abnormal screening mammograms in this group truly identified cancer. The other 78% are false positives.

You can tell ML only 1 out of 5 abnormal mammograms correctly identifies cancer; the four are false positives, but the only way to know which mammogram is correct is to do further testing.

The corollary of the PPV is the negative predictive value (NPV), which is the percentage of negative test results that are truly negative.

The PPV and NPV tests are population dependent, whereas the sensitivity and specificity are characteristics of the test and have little to do with the patient in front of you. So when you receive an abnormal lab result, especially a screening test such as mammography, understand their limits based on their PPV and NPV.

Treatment information is a little different. In discerning the statistics of randomized controlled trials of interventions, first consider an example. The Scandinavian Simvastatin Survival Study (4S) (*Lancet.* 1994;344[8934]:1383–1389) found using simvastatin in patients at high risk for heart disease for 5 years resulted in death for 8% of simvastatin patients versus 12% of those on placebo; this results in a relative risk of 0.70, a relative risk reduction of 33%, and a number needed to treat of 25.

There are two ways of considering the benefits of an intervention with respect to a given outcome. The absolute risk reduction is the difference in the percentage of people with the condition before and after the intervention. Thus, if the incidence of myocardial infarction (MI) was 12% for the placebo group and 8% for the simvastatin group, the absolute risk reduction is 4% (12% − 8% = 4%).

The relative risk reduction reflects the improvement in the outcome as a percentage of the original rate and is commonly used to exaggerate the benefit of an intervention. Thus, if the risk of MI were reduced by simvastatin from 12% to 8%, then the relative risk reduction would be 33% (4% / 12% = 33%); 33% sounds better than 4%, but the 4% is the absolute risk reduction and reflects the true outcome.

Absolute risk reduction is usually a better measure of *clinical* significance of an intervention. For instance, in one study, the treatment of mild hypertension has been shown to have relative risk reduction of 40% over 5 years (40% fewer strokes in the treated group). However, the absolute risk reduction was only 1.3%. Because mild hypertension is not strongly associated with strokes, aggressive treatment of mild hypertension yields only a small clinical benefit. Don't confuse relative risk reduction with relative risk.

Absolute (or attributable) risk (AR): the percentage of people in the placebo or intervention group who reach an end point; in the simvastatin study, the absolute risk of death was 8%.

Relative risk (RR): the risk of disease of those treated or exposed to some intervention (i.e., simvastatin) divided by those in the placebo group or who were untreated
  - If RR is <1.0, it reduces risk—the smaller the number, the greater the risk reduction.
  - If RR is >1.0, it increases risk—the greater the number, the greater the risk increase.

Relative risk reduction (RRR): the relative decrease in risk of an end point compared to the percentage of that end point in the placebo group

If you are still confused, just remember that the RRR is an over-estimation of the actual effect.

Number needed to treat (NNT): This is the number of people who need to be treated by an intervention to prevent one adverse outcome. A "good" NNT can be a large number (>100) if risk of serious outcome is great. If the risk of an outcome is not that dangerous, then lower (<25) NNTs are preferred.

The NNT should be compared to a similar statistic, the number needed to harm (NNH). This is the number of people who have to be given treatment before one excess side effect or harm occurs. When the NNT is compared to the NNH, you and the patient can judge whether the benefit of the intervention is great enough to outweigh the risk of harm.

EVIDENCED-BASED GRADING

To help you interpret diagnostic and treatment recommendations within *The 5-Minute Clinical Consult*, we have graded the best information within the text and highlighted this content.

An "A" grade means the reference is from the highest quality resource, such as a systematic review. A *systematic review* is a summary of the medical literature on a given topic that uses strict, explicit methods to perform a thorough search of the literature and then provides a critical appraisal of individual studies, concluding in a recommendation. The most prestigious collection of systematic reviews is from the Cochrane Collaboration (www.cochrane.org).

A "B" grade means the data referenced comes from high-quality randomized controlled trials performed to minimize bias in their outcome. Bias is anything that interferes with the truth; in the medical literature, it is often unintentional, but it is much more common than we appreciate. In short, always assume some degree of bias exist in any research endeavor.

A "C" grade implies the reference used does not meet the A or B requirements; they are often treatments recommended by consensus groups (such as the American Cancer Society). In some cases, they may be the standards of care. But implicit in a group's recommendation is the bias of the author or the group that supports the reference. For example, the American Urological Society's recommendation around screening for prostate cancer may be motivated by their narrow scope and financial benefit. Compare this to the recommendations of the U.S. Preventive Services Task Force (www.ahrq.gov), which recommends against screening for prostate cancer.

BIAS

Bias is anything that interferes with the truth. There are many types of bias that should be considered by the publishers of medical information. Below describes a number of bias types that often affect our care without us knowing it is present.

Publication bias occurs when research is not published; this is often when a study finds data that does *not* support an intervention. The motivation to publish information that "didn't work" is low. It is estimated that up to 40% of all medical research never get published. When you read of an effective intervention, wonder if other studies did not show benefit and went unpublished.

Comparator bias occurs when research compares an intervention to not the standard of care. Knowing a new treatment is more effective than placebo for treating a condition is not helpful if you typically use a drug or procedure. Why not study comparing the new to the standard of care? Sometimes, the new treatment is no better than the current standard. And if a study was done to see if the new is better than the old and not published, you have an example of publication bias.

Selection bias involves choosing study populations that might be different than the average patient or just reporting a just subset of study participants from a study. Either will result in the data being skewed because it can only be applied to small subset of people.

Attrition bias and the concept of intention to treat. Attrition bias is when researchers do not fully acknowledge and address how a study deals with participants who do not adhere to the research protocol or drop out completely. Intention to treat analysis hopes to diminish attrition bias by statistically considering the nonadhering or dropped out patients as unsuccessfully benefiting from the intervention.

Commercial (funder) bias involves who paid for the research being done, and do they have a vested interest in the outcome. If the developer of a new drug does a large study, or a researcher has a personal financial interest in seeing a study succeed, they may consciously or unconsciously alter what is reported in a study. The data may be accurate, but until this is studied by less vested interests, some feel its outcome cannot be clinically applied.

Have you been annoyed how 1 week you learn of a randomized controlled trial that supports a treatment, to be followed the next week with a contradictory article? Statisticians have figured out how to resolve this using something called a systematic review.

A systematic review gathers all the literature on a topic, say using antibiotics to treat otitis media, and combines the data to determine if the sum of all the trials tells a different story than any single trial. The large number of participants in this type of research results in a much more statistically (and clinically) significant conclusion than any single paper. Want more? Check this out: http://community.cochrane.org/about-us/evidence-based-health-care.

A meta-analysis is a quantitative systematic review and demonstrates its outcomes in the form of a forest plot. The bottom line with interpretation of a forest plot is to look for the diamond on the bottom. If it is to LEFT of the vertical line, it means risk of an outcome was reduced by the intervention. If it is fully to the RIGHT, then risk of that outcome was increased. And if the diamond touches the vertical line, it means there was no statistical influence of the intervention on the outcome.

We hope this brief introduction to EBM has been informative, clear, and helpful. If any of the information above seems unclear, or if you have a question, please contact us via www.5MinuteConsult.com.

ACKNOWLEDGMENTS

This is the 28th edition of *The 5-Minute Clinical Consult*, a comprehensive point-of-care tool to assist in the care of patients. From beginning to end, one cannot find a more current and easy-to-use collection of clinically useful content.

Developing and maintaining a book and website of this magnitude requires an equally broad effort from its supporting team. I wish to thank the dedication and tireless efforts of many: director, medical practice, Rebecca Gaertner; digital product development editor, Leanne Vandetty; and publisher, Lisa McAllister.

This 2020 edition is the direct result of the dedication and insights of our associate editors. I wish to thank Drs. Robert Baldor, Jeremy Golding, and Mark Stephens for their hard work and overwhelming commitment to *The 5-Minute Clinical Consult*.

I wish to especially thank my wife, Sylvia, and my daughter, Molly, who have given greatly for this book.

The challenge of completing a book covering this broad spectrum of medicine requires insights and skills far beyond my own. Many thanks to my mentors Bob Baldor and Mark Quirk who have been an enormous support—always there to encourage, reassure, and impart wisdom.

Many in the academic and health care worlds are due thanks for support, insight, and friendship: Daniel Lasser, Alan Chuman, Michele Pugnaire, Karen Rayla, Maryanne Adams, Jennifer Masoud, Phil Fournier, Erik Garcia, Jeff Stovall, Jim Comes, Leah Honor, J. Herb Stevenson, Michael Kidd, Zainab Nawab, Sanjiv and Amita Chopra, Vasilios (Bill) Chrisostomidis, James (Jay) Broadhurst, Danuta Antkowiak, Atreyi Chakrabarti, Joseph Frappier, Kate Peasha, the staff of Shrewsbury Family Medicine, Deb Huchowski, Joyce Paquette, Kate Peasha, Priscila Velez, Fanny Rodriguez, Meghan Plaza, and Angie Dell'Ovo, Mark Powicki, Steve Messineo, Rick Watson and Sara Floros, Frits Pennings, and the faculty and amazing students of the University of Massachusetts Medical School.

Our work is to focus on the care we give. For the care received for my mother, I wish to thank TJ Fitzgerald, Mary C. O'Brien, Brigid Carlson, Amy McKenzie, Melissa Lazar, Ann Rosenberg, Ashraf Elkerm, and the amazing team at MetroWest Homecare & Hospice, especially Bernadette and Melanie.

Medicine is a challenge I have fortunately not had to meet alone. Thanks to my parents, Frank and Angela (Jean); my brother, John, and his family, Marylou, Cate, and Jane; Frank, Mary Anne, Diane, and David Christian; the Diana and Hymie Lipschitz family; and the Bob and Ruth Pabreza family; they are responsible for who I am and my success in life.

I am blessed with the best of friends; without them, I would not be a physician. Thanks to Bob Bacic; Ron Jautz; Richard Onorato; John Horcher; Auguste Turnier; Bob Smith; Paul Saivetz; Bob and Nancy Gallinaro; Drew and Jill Grimes; Louay Toma; Laurie, Alan, Daniel, Jenny, and Matt Bugos; Alan Ehrlich; Andy Jennings; Bill Demianiuk; Mark Steenbergen; John and Kathleen Polanowicz; Phil and Carol Pettine; Mark and Linda Shelton; Steve Bennett; Vicki Triolo; Bob and Laurie Jenal; and Michael Bernatchez.

—FRANK J. DOMINO, MD

CONTRIBUTING AUTHORS

Adil Abdalla, MD
Department of Gastroenterology
CHI Health
Omaha, Nebraska

Thomas L. Abell, MD
Arthur M. Schoen, MD Chair in
    Gastroenterology
Department of Gastroenterology
University of Louisville
Louisville, Kentucky

Ralph Abi-Hachem, MD, MSc
Assistant Professor of Surgery and
    Neurosurgery
Rhinology and Skull Base Surgery
Division of Head and Neck Surgery &
    Communication Sciences
Department of Surgery
Duke University Health System
Durham, North Carolina

Hanadi Abou Dargham, MD
Family Physician, Hospitalist
St. Joseph Medical Center
Stockton, California

George M. Abraham, MD, MPH, FACP
Chief
Department of Medicine
Saint Vincent Hospital
Professor of Medicine
University of Massachusetts Medical
    School
Worcester, Massachusetts

Kevin T. Abraham, MD
University of Massachusetts Worcester
Family Medicine Residency
University of Massachusetts Medical
    School
Worcester, Massachusetts

Mohammed Abunada, MD
General and Colorectal Surgery Senior
    Consultant
Hamad General Hospital
Doha, Qatar

Adel M. Abuzeid, MBBS
Assistant Professor
Department of Surgery
Medical College of Georgia
Augusta, Georgia

Kenneth T. Acha, MD
Resident
University of California Riverside Family
    Medicine Residency Program
Palm Springs, California

Utkarsh H. Acharya, DO
Attending Physician of Immunotherapy
Seattle Cancer Care Alliance
Assistant Professor of Medical Oncology
University of Washington School of
    Medicine
Seattle, Washington

Karla C. Acosta, MD, MPH
San Antonio, Texas

Anne C. Adams, MD[†]
Family Medicine
Cincinnati Health Department
Cincinnati, Ohio

Praphopphat Adhatamsoontra,
    MD, MPH
Graduate Student Researcher
Division of Gastroenterology and Liver
    Disease
George Washington University
School of Medicine and Health Sciences
Washington, DC

Ronald N. Adler, MD, FAAFP
Associate Professor
Department of Family Medicine and
    Community Health
University of Massachusetts Medical
    School
Worcester, Massachusetts

Dayyan M. Adoor, MD[†]
Weill Cornell Medicine-Qatar
Doha, Qatar

Michael T. Aguilar, DO
Tripler Army Medical Center
Honolulu, Hawaii

Faraz Ahmad, MD, MPH[†]
Assistant Clinical Professor
Department of Family Medicine
Ohio State University
Columbus, Ohio

Hiba Ahmad, PharmD[†]
Clinical Oncology Pharmacist II
Department of Women's Health
    (Breast and Gynecology Oncology)
Smilow Cancer Hospital
Yale-New Haven Health
New Haven, Connecticut

Nadir Ahmad, MD, FACS
Division Head
Otolaryngology—Head & Neck Surgery
Director
Head & Neck Cancer Program
Associate Professor
Cooper University Hospital
MD Anderson at Cooper Cancer Center
Cooper Medical School of Rowan
    University
Camden, New Jersey

Sumera R. Ahmad, MD[†]
Assistant Professor of Medicine
Department of Pulmonary, Allergy and
    Critical Care
University of Massachusetts Memorial
    Medical Center and Medical School
Worcester, Massachusetts

Saeed Ahmed, MD
Resident Physician
The Department of Psychiatry and
    Behavioral Sciences
Nassau University Medical Center
East Meadows, New York

Yasir Ahmed, MD
Dallas, Pennsylvania

Yousef Ahmed, MD[†]
Undersea Medical Officer
Naval Special Warfare Group ONE
Coronado, California

Corinne Ainsworth, MD
University of Massachusetts Medical
    School
Worcester, Massachusetts

Gabriel M. Aisenberg, MD
Associate Professor of Medicine
Department of Internal Medicine
University of Texas
John P. and Kathrine G. McGovern
    Medical School
Houston, Texas

Saira Ajmal, MD
Clinical Assistant Professor
Department of Medicine
University of Illinois at Chicago
Division of Infectious Diseases
Advocate Christ Medical Center
Oak Lawn, Illinois

Assim AlAbdulKader, MD, MPH
Chief Resident
Family & Preventive Medicine Residency
 Program
Department of Family Medicine and
 Community Health
University Hospitals Cleveland Medical
 Center
Case Western Reserve University School
 of Medicine
Cleveland, Ohio

Uthman A. Alamoudi, MBBS
Teaching Assistant
Department of Emergency Medicine
King Abdulaziz University
Jeddah, Saudi Arabia

Mustafa Alavi, MD
Oregon Health & Science University
Portland, Oregon

Karla M. Alba, MD
Department of Family & Community
 Medicine
University of Texas Health Science Center
San Antonio, Texas

Peter C. Albertsen, MD, MS
Professor and Program Director
Division of Urology
Department of Surgery
University of Connecticut Health Center
Farmington, Connecticut

Stetson R. Albertson, DO
Traditional Intern
Michigan State University College of
 Osteopathic Medicine Statewide
 Campus System
Beaumont Hospital
Trenton, Michigan

Daniel Albo, MD, PhD
Director, Surgical Oncology Services
Director, Health Services Research
Augusta University
Augusta, Georgia

Pedro Emilio Alcedo, MD[†]
Department of Internal Medicine
McGovern Medical School
University of Texas Health Science Center
 at Houston
Houston, Texas

Rahma Ali Aldhaheri, MD
Research Fellow
Department of Gastroenterology
George Washington University
Washington, DC

Abdul Aleem, MD[†]
Division of Gastroenterology &
 Hepatology
Department of Internal Medicine
Lehigh Valley Health Network
Allentown, Pennsylvania

Andrew G. Alexander, MD[†]
Associate Dean
Clinical Medical Education
University of California, Riverside School
 of Medicine
Riverside, California

Mohamed Ali AlHabash, MD
Hamad General Corporation
Doha, Qatar

Fozia Akhtar Ali, MD
Associate Professor/Clinical
Department of Family & Community
 Medicine
University of Texas Health San Antonio
San Antonio, Texas

Jason B. Alisangco, DO, FAAFP[†]
Sports Medicine Fellow
Fort Belvoir Community Hospital
Fort Belvoir, Virginia

Richard W. Allinson, MD
Associate Professor
Department of Ophthalmology
The Texas A&M University System
Health Sciences Center
College Station, Texas
Senior Staff Physician
Department of Ophthalmology
Baylor Scott & White Clinic
Waco, Texas

Elizabeth R. Allocco, MD[†]
Resident Physician
Department of Obstetrics and Gynecology
University of Massachusetts Medical
 School
Worcester, Massachusetts

Abdulaziz Almedimigh, MBBS[†]
Research Fellow
Department of Medicine
The George Washington University
Washington, DC

Muhannad Almubarak, MD
The University of Alabama at Birmingham
Birmingham, Alabama

AbdulWahid Al-Mulla, MD
Hamad Medical Corporation
Doha, Qatar

Lolwa Al-Obaid, MD
Resident Physician
Department of Internal Medicine
Lahey Hospital & Medical Center
Burlington, Massachusetts

Jowhara Al-Qahtani, MD
General Surgery Resident
Maimonides Medical Center
Brooklyn, New York

Najwan Alsulaimi, MBBS
Medical Research Fellow
Department of Internal Medicine
Division of Gastroenterology
George Washington University School of
 Medicine and Health Sciences
Washington, DC

Melanie Dawn Altizer, MD
Assistant Professor
Department of Obstetrics and Gynecology
Carilion Clinic
Roanoke, Virginia

Roberto S. Amado, MD
Fitchburg Family Medicine Residency
 Program
University of Massachusetts Medical
 School
Worcester, Massachusetts

Pius Ogenyi Ameh, BM, BCh
Fellow West African College of Physicians
Family Medicine Head of Department
Accident and Emergency
Federal Medical Centre
Keffi, Nasarawa State, Nigeria,
 West Africa

Amulya D. Amirneni, MD[†]
Internal Medicine Chief Resident
University of Massachusetts Medical
 School-Baystate Internal Medicine
 Residency Programs
Springfield, Massachusetts

Hafsa Amjed, MD
Resident Physician
Department of Internal Medicine
University of Illinois at Chicago/Advocate
 Christ Medical Center
Oak Lawn, Illinois

Robert C.M. Ander, MD
Resident Physician
Department of Family Medicine
Presence Saint Joseph Hospital
Chicago, Illinois

Craig P. Anderson, DO, MPH[†]
Chief Medical Officer
Pine Bluff Arsenal Occupational Health
    Clinic
Pine Bluff, Arkansas

David L. Anderson, MD[†]
Resident Physician
Department of Family Medicine
Dwight D. Eisenhower Army Medical
    Center
Augusta, Georgia

Garland E. Anderson II, MD
Clinical Professor of Family Medicine
Louisiana State University Health
    Sciences Center-New Orleans
Rural Family Medicine Program, Gratis
Our Lady of the Angels Hospital
Bogalusa, Louisiana

Ellen Anderson Penno, MD, MS
Western Laser Eye Associates
Calgary, Alberta, Canada

Nehman Andry, MD
Associate Professor/Clinical and
    Clerkship Director
Department of Family & Community
    Medicine
University of Texas Health San Antonio–
    Joe R. and Teresa Lozano Long School
    of Medicine
San Antonio, Texas

Tanya E. Anim, MD
Fellow in Women's Health with Obstetrics
    Focus
Florida Hospital Family Medicine
    Residency Program
Winter Park, Florida

Asif Ansari, MD, MRCP, FACP, FASN
Associate Clinical Professor
Texas Tech University of Health Sciences
Odessa, Texas

Shari Anthony, MD
Resident
Department of Family Medicine
Bayfront Family Health Center
St. Petersburg, Florida

Kashif S. Anwar, MD
Physician
Department of Family Medicine
University Hospitals Portage Medical
    Center
Ravenna, Ohio

Yajai Apibunyopas, MD[†]
Research Assistant
Department of Emergency Medicine
University of Missouri-Kansas City
Kansas City, Missouri

Maria F. Arbelaez, MD[†]
Family and Community Medicine Resident
Department of Family and Community
    Medicine
University of Texas at San Antonio
San Antonio, Texas

Edgar Argulian, MD, MPH[†]
Assistant Professor of Medicine
Mount Sinai St. Luke's Hospital
Mount Sinai Heart
Icahn School of Medicine at Mount Sinai
New York, New York

Michael Argyle, DO
Resident
David Grant USAF Medical Center
Travis Air Force Base, California

Katyayini Aribindi, MD
Resident Physician
Department of Internal Medicine
University of Texas Health Science Center
    at Houston
Houston, Texas

Ann M. Aring, MD, FAAFP
Associate Program Director
OhioHealth Riverside Family Medicine
    Residency Program
Adjunct Clinical Professor
The Ohio State University College of
    Medicine
Columbus, Ohio

Forest W. Arnold, DO, MSc
Associate Professor of Medicine
Division of Infectious Diseases
University of Louisville School of Medicine
Louisville, Kentucky

James J. Arnold, DO, FACOFP, FAAFP[†]
Director
Osteopathic Education
Eglin Air Force Base Family Medicine
    Residency
Eglin Air Force Base, Florida

Michael J. Arnold, MD[†]
Assistant Professor
Family Medicine Department
Uniformed Services University of the
    Health Sciences
Bethesda, Maryland

Adriana Arocha, MD
Resident
Department of Family & Community
    Medicine
University of Texas Health Science Center
    School of Medicine
San Antonio, Texas

Maryam Arshad, MD[†]
Emergency Medicine
Houston, Texas

Robert L. Ashley, MD[†]
Eglin Family Medicine Residency
Eglin Air Force Base
Valparaiso, Florida

Hadi Atassi, DO[†]
Internal Medicine Residency Program
Department of Internal Medicine
University of Louisville School of Medicine
Louisville, Kentucky

Kimberly Atianzar, MD[†]
Medical Director
Structural Heart
Medical Director of Structural Imaging
Assistant Professor of Medicine
Department of Cardiology
Medical College of Georgia at Augusta
    University
Augusta, Georgia

Robert R. Atkins, MD
Assistant Professor and Director
East Kentucky Family Medicine Residency
University of Kentucky
Department of Community and Family
    Medicine
Hazard, Kentucky

Maximos Attia, MD, FAAFP
Core Faculty
Guthrie/Robert Packer Hospital Family
    Medicine Residency Program
Clinical Assistant Professor
Geisinger Commonwealth School of
    Medicine
Medical Director
Guthrie Sayre Walk-in Clinic
Medical Director
Guthrie Anti-Coagulation Clinics
Sayre, Pennsylvania

Stephen E. Auciello, MD
Assistant Program Director, Riverside
    Family Medicine
Medical Director, Community Outreach
OhioHealth
Columbus, Ohio

Sudeep K. Aulakh, MD, FACP, FRCPC
Director, Ambulatory Education
Baystate Internal Medicine Residency
Assistant Professor
University of Massachusetts Medical
    School–Baystate
Baystate Health
Springfield, Massachusetts

Alexis C. Aust, MD[†]
Family Medicine Resident
Eglin Air Force Base Family Medicine
    Residency
Eglin Air Force Base, Florida

Swati Avashia, MD, FAAP, FACP, ABIHM
Internal Medicine/Pediatrics
Assistant Professor
Division of Family Medicine
Department of Population Health
Dell Medical School, University of Texas
    at Austin
Austin, Texas

Nida S. Awadallah, MD
Assistant Professor
Department of Family Medicine
University of Colorado
Aurora, Colorado

Javier Ayo, MD
Emergency Medicine Resident
University of Florida College of
    Medicine-Jacksonville
Jacksonville, Florida

Jennifer L. Ayres, PhD
Director of Behavioral Health Services
Dell Medical School Family Medicine
    Residency Program
University of Texas at Austin
Austin, Texas

Sanaa Ayyoub, MD
Department of Endocrinology, Diabetes
    and Metabolism
University of Massachusetts Medical
    School
Worcester, Massachusetts

Holly L. Baab, MD
Associate Director
Family Medicine Residency
Bayfront Health St. Petersburg
St. Petersburg, Florida

Vasilis Babaliaros, MD
Professor of Medicine and Surgery
Emory University School of Medicine
Co-Director, Structural Heart and
    Valve Center
Emory Healthcare
Atlanta, Georgia

Franklyn C. Babb, MD, FAAFP
Associate Professor
Clerkship Director, Family Medicine
Department of Family Medicine
Texas Tech University Health Sciences
    Center School of Medicine
Lubbock, Texas

Megan Babb, DO
Family Medicine
Mercy Medical Group
Folsom, California

Mathura Babu, MD
Hospitalist, Internal Medicine
Deaconess Health System
Clinical Assistant Professor of Medicine
Indiana School of Medicine
Evansville, Indiana

Elisabeth L. Backer, MD
Clinical Associate Professor
Department of Family Medicine
University of Nebraska Medical Center
Omaha, Nebraska

Abdul Moeen Baco, MBchB, FICMS,
    FRCS
Consultant
Orthopaedic and Spinal Surgeon
Spinal Fellowship Program Director
Hamad Medical Corporation
Doha, Qatar

Ambuga Badari, MD
Yuma Regional Medical Center
Yuma, Arizona

Melissa Badowski, PharmD, MPH
Clinical Associate Professor
Department of Pharmacy Practice
University of Illinois at Chicago College of
    Pharmacy
Chicago, Illinois

Christy L. Baggett, DO
Department of Family Medicine
Mayo Clinic Florida
Jacksonville, Florida

Shaun Baker, DO
ENT Resident Physician
Philadelphia College of Osteopathic
    Medicine
Philadelphia, Pennsylvania

Sara Bakhtiar, MBBS[†]
Family Medicine Resident
Creighton University Medical Center
Omaha, Nebraska

Maryse E. Bakouetila, MD
Resident Physician
Department of Family and Community
    Medicine
University of Texas Health San Antonio
San Antonio, Texas

Prakash Balan, JD, MD
Assistant Professor, Cardiovascular
    Medicine
The University of Texas Health Science
Center at Houston
Houston, Texas

Robert A. Baldor, MD, FAAFP
Professor and Senior Vice-Chairman
Department of Family Medicine and
    Community Health
University of Massachusetts Medical
    School
Worcester, Massachusetts

Andrew Baldwin, MD, MPH[†]
Family Medicine Residency Staff
Fort Belvoir Community Hospital
Fort Belvoir, Virginia

Jonathan R. Ballard, MD, MPH, MPhil[†]
Associate Professor
Department of Family and Community
    Medicine
Geisel School of Medicine at Dartmouth
Lebanon, New Hampshire

Kenneth A. Ballou, MD, FAAFP
Assistant Clinical Professor
Department of Family Medicine
University of California at Riverside
    School of Medicine
Riverside, California

Rahul Banerjee, MD[†]
Chief Resident in Quality and Safety
Department of Medicine
Corporal Michael J. Crescenz VA Medical
    Center
Hospital of the University of Pennsylvania
Philadelphia, Pennsylvania

Eric M. Bankert, DO
Primary Care Sports Medicine Fellow
Greenville Health System
Greenville, South Carolina

Purnima Bansal, MD
Family Physician
Greater Lawrence Family Health Center
Nashville, Tennessee

Krishna M. Baradhi, MD
Associate Professor
Department of Internal Medicine and
    Nephrology
University of Oklahoma, School of
    Community Medicine
Tulsa, Oklahoma

Arham K. Barakzai, MD
Resident
Department of Internal Medicine—Crittenton
Wayne State University School of Medicine
Detroit, Michigan

Sarah E. Barker, DO
Resident
Novant Health Family Medicine Residency
    Program
Charlotte, North Carolina

Elise J. Barney, DO[†]
Nephrologist and Clinical Assistant
    Professor of Medicine
Department of Internal Medicine
Arizona College of Osteopathic Medicine
    of Midwestern University
Glendale, Arizona

John P. Barrett, MD, MPH, MS, FAAFP,
    FACPM[†]
COL, MC, USA
Associate Professor
Uniformed Services University of the
    Health Sciences
Bethesda, Maryland

Eesha Salman Bashir, MBBS
Shifa College of Medicine
Islamabad, Pakistan

Khalid Bashir, MD
Division Chief and Assistant Professor
Department of Medicine, Renal Division
Creighton University School of Medicine
Associate Director
CHI Nephrology
CHI Health Clinic
Omaha, Nebraska

Janani Baskaran, MBBS[†]
Internal Medicine
Creighton University
Omaha, Nebraska

Jonathan S. Bassett, MD[†]
Faculty Physician
Eglin Family Medicine Residency
Eglin Air Force Base
Valparaiso, Florida

Erin Bassett-Novoa, MD[†]
Greater Lawrence Family Residency
Lawrence, Massachusetts

Sumana Basu, MD
Primary Care Sports Medicine Fellow
Department of Sports Medicine
Houston Methodist Hospital–Willowbrook
Houston, Texas

Brian P. Bateson, DO
General Surgery Resident
Department of General Surgery
Medical College of Georgia
Augusta, Georgia

Stuart H. Batten, MD[†]
Resident Physician
Womack Family Medicine Residency
Fort Bragg, North Carolina

Jennifer L. Bauer, MD[†]
Second Year Medical Resident
Family Medicine Residency Program
David Grant Medical Center
Fairfield, California

Kay A. Bauman, MD, MPH
Retired Professor
John A. Burns School of Medicine
University of Hawaii
Honolulu, Hawaii

Dennis J. Baumgardner, MD
Clinical Adjunct Professor of Family
    Medicine and Community Health
University of Wisconsin School of
    Medicine and Public Health
Aurora University of Wisconsin Medical
    Group
Aurora Health Care, Inc.
Milwaukee, Wisconsin

Sheryl Beard, MD, FAAFP
Clinical Associate Professor and Senior
    Associate Program Director
University of Kansas School of Medicine–
    Wichita
Family Medicine Residency Program at
    Via Christi
Wichita, Kansas

Patricia Beauzile, MD[†]
Resident Physician
Department of Obstetrics and Gynecology
Virginia Tech Carilion School of Medicine
Roanoke, Virginia

Kenneth Beer, MD[†]
Beer Dermatology
West Palm Beach, Florida

Adriane E. Bell, MD, FAAFP[†]
Assistant Professor
Department of Family Medicine
Uniformed Services University of the
    Health Sciences
Bethesda, Maryland

Hershey S. Bell, MD, MS, FAAFP
Professor
Vice President of Academic Affairs and
    Dean
Lake Erie College of Osteopathic
    Medicine School of Pharmacy
Erie, Pennsylvania and Bradenton, Florida

Pallavi Bellamkonda, MBBS[†]
Assistant Professor
Division of Cardiology
Department of Medicine
Creighton University School of Medicine
Omaha, Nebraska

Paul P. Belliveau, PharmD
Professor of Pharmacy Practice
Massachusetts College of Pharmacy and
    Health Science University
Worcester, Massachusetts

Sunil Shashikumar Bellur, MD[†]
Ophthalmology Resident
Department of Ophthalmology
George Washington University
Washington, DC

Regina Belokovskaya, DO[†]
Endocrinology Fellow
Division of Endocrinology, Diabetes, and
    Bone Diseases
Icahn School of Medicine at Mount Sinai
New York, New York

David A. Belyea, MD, MBA, FACS[†]
Professor and Vice Chair
Department of Ophthalmology
George Washington University School of
    Medicine
Washington, DC

Sheldon Benjamin, MD
Professor of Psychiatry and Neurology
Department of Psychiatry
University of Massachusetts Medical School
Worcester, Massachusetts

Terrell Benold, MD[†]
Assistant Clinical Professor
Dell Medical School, University of Texas
    at Austin
Austin, Texas

Jennifer Bepko, MD[†]
Faculty of Family Medicine
Family Medicine Residency
Davis Grant Medical Center
Travis Air Force Base, California

Jasmine S. Beria, DO, MPH
Department of Internal Medicine
Icahn School of Medicine at Mount Sinai
Mount Sinai St. Luke's and Mount Sinai
    West Hospitals
New York, New York

Jamie L. Berkes, MD
Assistant Professor of Medicine
Medical Director
Liver Transplantation
Loyola University
Maywood, Illinois

Bettina Bernstein, DO[†]
Clinical Assistant Professor of Psychiatry
Philadelphia College of Osteopathic
  Medicine
Philadelphia, Pennsylvania

John F. Bertagnolli Jr., DO[†]
Associate Professor and Director of
  House Call Program
Department of Geriatrics/New Jersey
  Institute for Successful Aging
Rowan University School of Osteopathic
  Medicine
Stratford, New Jersey

Michaela E. Beynon, MD, MA[†]
Obstetrics and Gynecology Resident
Department of Obstetrics and Gynecology
Aultman Hospital
Canton, Ohio

Sanna R. Bhajjan, DO
First Year Resident
Department of Family and Community
  Medicine
University of Texas Health Science Center
San Antonio, Texas

Amit Bhojwani, DO, MBS, MSHM
Chief Resident
Department of Otolaryngology—Head and
  Neck Surgery
Rowan University School of Osteopathic
  Medicine
Stratford, New Jersey

Ghazaleh Bigdeli, MD, FCCP
Pulmonary Rehab Associates
Youngstown, Ohio

Stephanie J. Billings, MD
Family Medicine Doctor
Holyoke Health
Holyoke, Massachusetts

Shawn M. Bishop, MD
Eglin Family Medicine Residency Clinic
Eglin Air Force Base, Florida

James D. Blake, MD[†]
Hoover Family Medicine
Hoover, Alabama

Eric P. Blazar, MD
Assistant Professor of Emergency
  Medicine
Rowan University School of Osteopathic
  Medicine
Vineland, New Jersey

Cameron D. Blegen, MD
Resident Physician
St. John's Family Medicine Residency
University of Minnesota
St. Paul, Minnesota

Lewis S. Blevins Jr., MD
Professor of Neurological Surgery and
  Medicine
Director
California Center for Pituitary Disorders at
  University of California San Francisco
San Francisco, California

Warren A. Bodine, DO, CAQSM
Director of Sports Medicine
Lawrence Family Medicine Residency
Lawrence, Massachusetts

Elise Bognanno, MD
Core Faculty
Beaumont Grosse Pointe Family Medicine
  Residency
St. Clair Shores, Michigan

Kamran Boka, MD
Assistant Professor
Pulmonary Critical Care and Sleep
  Medicine
McGovern Medical School
The University of Texas Health Science
  Center at Houston
Houston, Texas

Kimberly Bombaci, MD
Faculty
Department of Family Medicine and
  Community Health
University of Massachusetts Medical
  School
Worcester, Massachusetts

Diana Bonaccorsi, DO[†]
Clinical Faculty
Department of Family Medicine
Amita Saint Joseph Hospital
Chicago, Illinois

Brandon W. Bonds, MD
West Kendall Baptist Hospital Family
Medicine Residency
Miami, Florida

Katrina A. Booth, MD
Assistant Professor
Division of Gerontology, Geriatrics, and
  Palliative Care
University of Alabama at Birmingham
Birmingham, Alabama

Azra Borogovac, MD
Internal Medicine Resident
University of Massachusetts Medical
  School
Worcester, Massachusetts

Marie L. Borum, MD, EdD, MPH, MACP,
  FACG, AGAF
Professor of Medicine
Director
Division of Gastroenterology and Liver
  Diseases
George Washington University
Washington, DC

Subhasish Bose, MD, FASN
Consultant, Nephrology
Lynchburg Nephrology Associates
Lynchburg, Virginia

Douglas J. Bosin, DO[†]
Special Operations Flight Surgeon
27 Special Operations Support Squadron
  Operational Support Medicine
Cannon Air Force Base
Clovis, New Mexico

Christian Bosquet, MD
Resident Physician
SUNY Downstate Medical Center
Brooklyn, New York

Sandy Botros, MD
Attending Physician
Department of Family Medicine
Community Health Network
Indianapolis, Indiana

Emily Bouley, MD
University of Massachusetts Medical
  School
Worcester, Massachusetts

Matthew J. Brennan, MD
Resident
Georgetown University—Providence
  Hospital Family Medicine Residency
  Program
Washington, DC

P. Clint Bricker, MD[†]
Chief Resident
Family Medicine Residency
Martin Army Community Hospital
Fort Benning, Georgia

Jacob Michael Bright, DO[†]
Captain of Medical Corps, U.S. Army
Family Medicine Residency Program
Dwight D. Eisenhower Army Medical
  Center
Fort Gordon, Georgia

Emma Brooks, MD[†]
Assistant Professor and Assistant
  Director of Inpatient and Maternity
  Services
Department of Family Medicine
Oregon Health & Science University
Portland, Oregon

David T. Broome, MD
Internal Medicine Resident
Clinical Scholars Program (CLIMSCHOP)
Cleveland Clinic Foundation
Cleveland, Ohio

Christine M. Broszko, MD[†]
CPT, USAF, MC
Faculty Physician
Eglin Air Force Base Family Medicine
    Residency
Eglin Air Force Base, Florida

Colin E. Brown, MD
Ophthalmology Resident
Department of Ophthalmology and Visual
    Sciences
University of Nebraska Medical Center
Omaha, Nebraska

Kathryn M. Brown, MD
Assistant Professor of Medicine
Department of Family Medicine and
    Community Health
Minneapolis, Minnesota

M. Ashleigh Brown, DO
Surgical Resident
Department of General Surgery
Augusta University—Medical College of
    Georgia
Augusta, Georgia

Matthew E. Bryant, MD[†]
Family Practice Physician
Dwight D. Eisenhower Army Medical
    Center
Fort Gordon, Georgia

Carl Bryce, MD[†]
Assistant Professor
Offutt Air Force Base Family Medicine
    Residency
University of Nebraska Medical School
Omaha, Nebraska

Christine Bryson, DO
Assistant Professor of Medicine
University of Massachusetts
Medical Director, Teaching Services,
    Hospital Medicine Program
Baystate Medical Center
Springfield, Massachusetts

Merima Bucaj, DO, FAAFP
Program Director
Abrazo Health Network
Family Medicine Residency Program
Phoenix, Arizona

Nitin Budhwar, MD
Associate Professor
Department of Family and Community
    Medicine
University of Texas Southwestern Medical
    Center
Dallas, Texas

Han Q. Bui, MD[†]
Woodbridge, Virginia

Christopher W. Bunt, MD, FAAFP
Associate Professor
Department of Family Medicine
Assistant Dean for Student Affairs
Military Medical Advisor
Medical University of South Carolina
Charleston, South Carolina

Jason A. Burchett, DO[†]
CPT, USAF
Family Medicine Resident
Nellis Air Force Base, Nevada

Jacob M. Burdett, DO
Otolaryngology and Facial Plastics
    Resident
Philadelphia College of Osteopathic
    Medicine
Philadelphia, Pennsylvania

Kristina Burgers, MD, FAAFP[†]
Associate Program Director
Family Medicine Residency
Womack Army Medical Center
Fort Bragg, North Carolina

John R. Burk, MD, FACP
Texas Pulmonary and Critical Care
    Consultants
Sleep Consultants
Fort Worth, Texas

Liam P. Burke, MD
Assistant Professor of Medicine
Department of Family Medicine and
    Community Health
University of Massachusetts Medical
    School
Worcester, Massachusetts

Harold J. Bursztajn, MD
Associate Professor of Psychiatry,
    Part-time
Co-founder, Program in Psychiatry and
    the Law
Beth Israel Deaconess Medical Center
Department of Psychiatry
Harvard Medical School
President
The American Unit of the UNESCO
    Bioethics Chair
Boston, Massachusetts

David C. Bury, DO[†]
Family Medicine Residency Program
Martin Army Community Hospital
Fort Benning, Georgia

Mark M. Butterly, MD
Associate Professor, Pediatrics
Department of Pediatrics
Rosalind Franklin University of Medicine
    and Science
Chicago, Illinois
Vice Chair and Residency Program
    Director, Pediatrics
Advocate Children's Hospital—Oak Lawn
Oak Lawn, Illinois

Nancy Byatt, DO, MBA, FAPM
Assistant Professor of Psychiatry and
    Obstetrics & Gynecology
UMass Memorial Medical Center/UMass
    Medical School
Worcester, Massachusetts

David C. Cadena Jr., MD[†]
Assistant Clinical Professor
Medical Director of PA Clinic
Primary Care Center
University of Texas Health San Antonio
Long School of Medicine
San Antonio, Texas

Stephen D. Cagle Jr., MD
CPT, USAF, MC
Nellis Air Force Base
Las Vegas, Nevada

Daniel Callaway, MD, MPH
Assistant Professor of Pediatrics
Sanford School of Medicine
University of South Dakota
Sioux Falls, South Dakota

Christine Ramos Camacho, MD, MS
Family Medicine Resident
Department of Family and Community
    Medicine
University of Texas Health Science Center
    at San Antonio
San Antonio, Texas

Caroline R. Campbell, MD[†]
Department of General Surgery
Medical College of Georgia at Augusta
    University
Augusta, Georgia

Joanna J. Campodonico, MD, MPH[†]
Phoenix, Arizona

Eduardo Camps-Romero, MD
Assistant Professor
Department of Psychiatry and Behavioral
    Health
Director of Behavioral Health
Department of Humanities Health and
    Society
Florida International University Herbert
    Wertheim College of Medicine
Miami, Florida

Patrick M. Carey, DO[†]
Assistant Professor
Uniformed Services University of the
    Health Sciences
Faculty
Family Medicine Residency
Martin Army Community Hospital
Fort Benning, Georgia

Stephanie A. Carey, MD, MPH
Resident Physician
Department of Family & Community
    Medicine
Penn State Milton S. Hershey Medical
    Center
Hershey, Pennsylvania

Samuel B. Carli, MD
Physician, Internal Medicine
PeaceHealth Southwest Medical Center
Vancouver, Washington

Robert T. Carlisle, MD, MPH[†]
Faculty Physician
Department of Family Medicine
Tripler Army Medical Center
Honolulu, Hawaii

Noel J.M. Carrasco, MD, FAAP[†]
Professor of Pediatrics, Neonatal-
    Perinatal Medicine
A.T. Still University School of Osteopathic
    Medicine
Mesa, Arizona

Dana G. Carroll, PharmD, BCPS, CDE,
    BCGP
Clinical Professor
Department of Family, Internal and Rural
    Medicine
University of Alabama
Pharmacy Practice Department
Auburn University
Tuscaloosa, Alabama

Sarah L. Carroll, DO[†]
Resident
Eglin Family Medicine Residency
Eglin Air Force Base, Florida

Smita Carroll, MD, MBA[†]
Resident Physician
Department of Obstetrics and Gynecology
University of Massachusetts Medical
    School
Worcester, Massachusetts

Kitty Carter-Wicker, MD[†]
Associate Professor
Department of Family Medicine
Morehouse School of Medicine
Atlanta, Georgia

Fernando Casado-Castillo, MD
Resident Physician
Department of Internal Medicine
BronxCare Hospital Center
Bronx, New York

Sara Casey, DO
Assistant Professor
UMass Memorial Health Care
Worcester, Massachusetts

Casandra Cashman, MD, FAAFP
Assistant Director
Community East Family Medicine
    Residency Program
Indianapolis, Indiana

Jean Khara G. Casillan, RN, MD[†]
Resident
Department of Family and Community
    Medicine
University of Texas Health San Antonio
San Antonio, Texas

Abel Casso Dominguez, MD
Cardiology Fellow
Mount Sinai St. Luke's–West
Icahn School of Medicine at Mount Sinai
New York, New York

Adriana M. Castro, MD, DABP
Assistant Professor Community Pediatrics
Department of Family Medicine
West Kendall Baptist Hospital/FIU
Herbert Wertheim School of Medicine
Miami, Florida

Mary Cataletto, MD, FAAP, FCCP
Professor of Clinical Pediatrics
Stony Brook University, School of
    Medicine
Stony Brook, New York
New York University-Winthrop Hospital
Mineola, New York

Jeanne M. Cawse-Lucas, MD
Associate Professor
Theodore J. Phillips Endowed Professor
    of Family Medicine
Department of Family Medicine
University of Washington School of
    Medicine
Seattle, Washington

Jan Cerny, MD, PhD[†]
Associate Professor of Medicine
Department of Medicine
Division of Hematology/Oncology
University of Massachusetts Medical School
Worcester, Massachusetts

Olga Cerón, MD[†]
Staff Ophthalmologist
Reliant Medical Group
Worcester, Massachusetts

Amar R. Chadaga, MD[†]
Clinical Assistant Professor and Associate
    Program Director
Internal Medicine
Advocate Christ Medical Center Program
University of Illinois at Chicago College of
    Medicine
Chicago, Illinois

Sarah Chaffin, MD
Clinical Faculty
Mercy Methodist Family Medicine
    Residency Program
Dignity Health
Sacramento, California

Joumana Chaiban, MD, FACE
Associate Professor of Clinical Medicine
Internal Medicine Residents Research
    Director
Internal Medicine Department
Endocrinology Division
University of Illinois at Chicago/Advocate
    Christ Medical Center
Chicago, Illinois

Cindy J. Chambers, MD, MAS, MPH
Department of Dermatology
UC Davis Health System
Sacramento, California

Ronald G. Chambers Jr., MD, FAAFP[†]
Program Director, DIO, Dignity Health
    Methodist Family Medicine Residency
    Program of Sacramento
Chair, Family Medicine Department
Medical Director, Mercy Family Health Center
    and Mercy Human Trafficking Clinic
Physician Advisor, Human Trafficking
    Response
Chief, South Sacramento Hill Physicians
Sacramento, California

Matthew G. Chan, MD
Assistant Professor of Family Medicine
Oregon Health & Science University
Portland, Oregon

Sangili Chandran, MD, MS(ortho)
Director Primary Care Sports Medicine
Advocate Christ Family Medicine
    Residency Program
Hometown, Illinois

Felix B. Chang Cruz, MD, FAAMA,
    ABIHM
Inpatient Service Director
University of Massachusetts Fitchburg
    Family Medicine Residency Program
University of Massachusetts Health
    Alliance Leominster Hospital
Associate Professor
University of Massachusetts Department
    of Family Medicine and Community
    Health
Academic Hospitalist
University of Massachusetts Memorial
    Medical Group
Leominster, Massachusetts

Jennifer G. Chang, MD[†]
Assistant Professor
Department of Family Medicine
Uniformed Services University of the
    Health Sciences
Bethesda, Maryland

Rowland Chang, MD, MPH
Professor of Preventive Medicine,
    Medicine, and Physical Medicine &
    Rehabilitation
Northwestern University Feinberg School
    of Medicine
Chicago, Illinois

Jason Chao, MD, MS
Professor of Family Medicine and
    Community Health
Case Western Reserve University School
    of Medicine and University Hospitals
    Cleveland Medical Center
Cleveland, Ohio

Justin L. Chapman, MD
Department of Emergency Medicine
University of Massachusetts Medical
    School
Worcester, Massachusetts

Matthew F. Charek, MD
Department of Emergency Medicine
University of Pittsburgh Medical Center
Pittsburgh, Pennsylvania

Kathya M. Chartre, MD[†]
St. Joseph Hospital/University of Illinois
    at Chicago Program Faculty
Department of Family Medicine
Chicago, Illinois

Arka Chatterjee, MD, FACC, FSCAI
Assistant Professor
Division of Cardiovascular Disease
University of Alabama at Birmingham
Birmingham, Alabama

Emily M. Chau, MD, MS
Clinical Instructor of Family and
    Community Medicine
Northeast Ohio Medical University
Rootstown, Ohio

Aqib Chaudhry, MD
University of Massachusetts Medical
    School
Worcester, Massachusetts

Crystal Haydee Chavez, MD
Assistant Professor
Department of Family Medicine and
    Community Medicine
University of Texas Health Science Center
San Antonio, Texas

Tori Chee, MD, MBA[†]
LT, MC, USN
Naval Hospital Jacksonville
Jacksonville, Florida

Amy Chen, MD, PhD
Associate Professor
Department of Neurology
Medical University of South Carolina
Charleston, South Carolina

Byron Chen, MD
UMass Memorial Health Care
Worcester, Massachusetts

Richard J. Chen, MD
Resident Physician
Department of Emergency Medicine
Robert Wood Johnson Medical School
New Brunswick, New Jersey

Anthony M. Cheng, MD
Assistant Physician
Department of Family Medicine
Oregon Health & Science University
Portland, Oregon

Suma Chennubhotla, MD
Department of Internal Medicine
University of Louisville
Louisville, Kentucky

Fairouz L. Chibane, MD[†]
General Surgery Resident
Department of General Surgery
Augusta University Medical Center
Augusta, Georgia

Edwin Y. Choi, MD[†]
Assistant Program Director
Department of Family Medicine
    Residency
Womack Army Medical Center
Fort Bragg, North Carolina

Hiu Ying Joanna Choi, MD
Resident
Department of Family Medicine
Georgetown University Medical Center
Washington, DC

Lea S. Choi, DO[†]
Department of Family Medicine
Womack Army Medical Center
Fort Bragg, North Carolina

Efstathia Choros, MD, CPA
Chief Resident
Hahnemann Family Health Center
Department of Family Medicine and
    Community Health
University of Massachusetts Medical
    School
Worcester, Massachusetts

Monzurul H. Chowdhury, MD
Renal Fellow
Department of Renal Medicine
University of Massachusetts Medical
    School
Worcester, Massachusetts

Vasilios Chrisostomidis, DO
Associate Professor
University of Massachusetts Medical
    School
UMass Memorial Medical Center
Worcester, Massachusetts

Marissa T. Christian, PharmD
Clinical Pharmacy Specialist
Solid Organ Transplant
Department of Pharmacy
Penn State Health
Milton S. Hershey Medical Center
Hershey, Pennsylvania

Bianca K. Chun, MD[†]
Board Certified Family Medicine Physician
Milton, Florida

Connie Y. Chung, MD[†]
Flight Medicine Medical Director
Flight and Operational Medicine Clinic
Eglin Air Force Base, Florida

Erica K. Cichowski, MD
Assistant Professor of Medicine
Creighton University School of Medicine
Program Director
Creighton Internal Medicine Residency
Omaha, Nebraska

Mateo Cindric, MD
Department of Family Medicine
Creighton University Family Medicine
Omaha, Nebraska

Lindsay M. Clarke, MD, MS
George Washington University School of
    Medicine & Health Sciences
Washington, DC

S. Lindsey Clarke, MD, FAAFP[†]
Medical University of South Carolina Area
    Health Education Consortium Professor
    (Greenwood/Family Medicine)
Director of Resident Education and
    Associate Program Director
Self Regional Healthcare
Greenwood, South Carolina

Nanci Swan Claus, DNP, CRNP, CCRN
Instructor of Nursing
The University of Alabama at Birmingham
Birmingham, Alabama

Erik R. Clauson, DO[†]
Staff Physician
Eglin Family Medicine Residency Program
Eglin Air Force Base, Florida
Assistant Professor
Department of Family Medicine
Uniformed Services University of Health
    Sciences
Bethesda, Maryland

Karl T. Clebak, MD, FAAFP[†]
Assistant Professor
Department of Family and Community
    Medicine
Penn State College of Medicine
Hershey, Pennsylvania

George Clement, MD[†]
CPT, MC
Family Medicine Resident
Womack Army Medical Center
Fort Bragg, North Carolina

Roselyn Jan W. Clemente-Fuentes, MD,
    FAAFP[†]
Family Medicine Faculty Physician
Eglin Family Medicine Residency
Eglin Air Force Base, Florida

Lisa Clemons, MD
Blackstock Family Health Center
Austin, Texas

Kara M. Coassolo, MD
Division of Maternal Fetal Medicine
Lehigh Valley Health Network
Allentown, Pennsylvania

Katie Coble, MD[†]
Obstetrical Fellow and Staff Family
    Medicine Physician
Darnall Family Medicine Residency
Fort Hood, Texas

Stephanie N. Cochran, DO
Cardiology Fellow
Largo Medical Center
Largo, Florida

Mark Coelho, MD
Pediatric Resident
UConn Health
Farmington, Connecticut

Mauricio G. Cohen, MD, FACC, FSCAI
Professor of Medicine
Director, Cardiac Catheterization
    Laboratory
University of Miami Miller School of
    Medicine
Miami, Florida

Jason E. Cohn, DO[†]
Department of Otolaryngology, Head and
    Neck, Facial Plastic Surgery
Philadelphia College of Osteopathic
    Medicine
Philadelphia, Pennsylvania

Timothy J. Coker, MD, FAAFP[†]
Assistant Professor
Uniformed Services University of Health
    Sciences
Bethesda, Maryland

David Cole, MD
Resident Physician
Department of Family and Community
    Medicine
Pennsylvania State Health, Milton S.
    Hershey Medical Center
Hershey, Pennsylvania

Brian R. Coleman, MD
Associate Professor
Department of Family Medicine
University of Oklahoma
Oklahoma City, Oklahoma

Sarah Coles, MD
Assistant Professor
Department of Family, Community, and
    Preventive Medicine
University of Arizona College of
    Medicine—Phoenix
Phoenix, Arizona

Irene Coletsos, MD
Cape Cod Hospital
Hyannis, Massachusetts

Charisse Colvin, MD
Psychiatry Resident
John T. Mather Memorial Hospital
Port Jefferson, New York

Jose F. Condado, MD, MS
Medical House Staff
Emory University School of Medicine
Atlanta, Georgia

Stephen J. Conner, MD[†]
Chief of Family Medicine Maternal-
    Newborn Service
Dwight D. Eisenhower Army Medical
    Center
Fort Gordon, Georgia

Stephanie L. Conway, PharmD
Assistant Professor of Pharmacy Practice
Massachusetts College of Pharmacy and
    Health Sciences University
Worcester, Massachusetts

Ronald L. Cook, DO, MBA
Braddock Chairman
Associate Professor
Department of Family Medicine and
    Community Medicine
Texas Tech University Health Sciences
    Center
School of Medicine
Lubbock, Texas

Brandon D. Coons, MD
Resident Physician
Department of Internal Medicine
University of Louisville School of Medicine
Louisville, Kentucky

Jadranko Corak, MD
Associate Professor
Department of Internal Medicine
The University of Texas at Austin Dell
    Medical School
Austin, Texas

Tatiana Cordova, MD[†]
Clinical Assistant Professor
Family and Community Medicine
    Department
University of Texas Health San Antonio
San Antonio, Texas

Jennifer M. Cornwell, DO[†]
Family Practice Physician
Department of Family Medicine
Irwin Army Community Hospital
Fort Riley, Kansas

Glency Sue Marie S. Corominas, MD[†]
Resident
Department of Family Medicine and
    Community Health
University of Texas Health Science Center
    at San Antonio
San Antonio, Texas

Mathew J. Cosenza, DO, RPh
Adena ENT and Allergy
Adena Regional Medical Center
Chillicothe, Ohio

Chloe S. Courchesne, MD
Department of Family and Community
    Medicine
Penn State Hershey Medical Center
Hershey, Pennsylvania

Jennifer M. Courtier, MD
St. Claire Family Medicine Residency
University of Kentucky
Morehead, Kentucky

Erica F. Crannage, PharmD, BCPS,
    BCACP
Associate Professor of Pharmacy Practice
    and Clinical Pharmacist
St. Louis College of Pharmacy/Saint
    Louis University School of Medicine
St. Louis, Missouri

Paul Crawford, MD[†]
COL, USAF, MC
Director of Medical Education and
    Designated Institutional Official
Professor of Family Medicine
99th Medical Group
Mike O'Callaghan Military Medical Center
Nellis Air Force Base, Nevada

Dustin Creech, MD
Air Force Medicine—Scott
Belleville Family Medicine Clinic
Belleville, Illinois

Julie A. Creech, DO[†]
Family Medicine Resident
Eglin Air Force Base Family Medicine
    Residency
Eglin Air Force Base, Florida

Alan Cropp, MD, FCCP
Department of Pulmonary Medicine
St. Elizabeth Hospital Health Center
Youngstown, Ohio

Steven J. Crosby, MA, BSP, RPh, FASCP
Assistant Dean of Student Engagement
    and Success
Assistant Professor of Pharmacy Practice
Massachusetts College of Pharmacy and
    Health Sciences University
Boston, Massachusetts

Jason E. Cross, PharmD[†]
Associate Professor of Pharmacy Practice
Massachusetts College of Pharmacy and
    Health Sciences University
Worcester, Massachusetts
Assistant Director
Pharmacy Residency
Baystate Health Medical Center
Springfield, Massachusetts

Juliana Zamora Cubillos, MD
Resident
Department of Family & Community
    Medicine
University of Texas Health Science Center
    School of Medicine
San Antonio, Texas

Hongyi Cui, MD, PhD
Associate Professor of Surgery
Department of Surgery
University of Massachusetts Medical
    School
Associate Director, Acute Care Surgery
University of Massachusetts Memorial
    Medical Center
Worcester, Massachusetts

Emily M. Culliney, MD, FAAFP[†]
Major, MC, USAF
Assistant Professor of Family Medicine
Uniformed Services University of Health
    Sciences
Department of Family Medicine
Saint Louis University Family Medicine
    Residency Program
Belleville, Illinois

Yulibeth Curbelo Peña, MD
Rehabilitation Department
Vall D'Hebron Hospital
Barcelona, Spain

Yuhamy Curbelo-Peña, MD[†]
Department of General Surgery
Vic University Hospital
Vic, Barcelona, Spain

Cragin D. Currence, MD
General Surgery Resident
Spartanburg Regional Health System
Spartanburg, South Carolina

Alexander CVitan, MD
University of Massachusetts Medical
    School
Worcester, Massachusetts

Tina D'Amato, DO
Attending Family Physician
Charlotte Family Medicine
Charlotte, Vermont

William Dabbs, MD
Assistant Professor and Clerkship
    Director
Department of Family Medicine
University of Tennessee Graduate School
    of Medicine
Knoxville, Tennessee

Adam R. Dahlen, DO
Internal Medicine Residency Program
Southeastern Regional Medical Center
Lumberton, North Carolina

Christine M. Dahlhausen, MD[†]
Department of General Surgery and
    Surgical Oncology
Augusta University Medical Center
Augusta, Georgia

Heather A. Dalton, MD[†]
Assistant Program Director
Faculty Family Medicine Physician
Department of Family Medicine
David Grant Medical Center Family
    Medicine Residency
Travis Air Force Base, California

Paul E. Daniel Jr., MD[†]
Hospitalist
Assistant Professor Family Medicine
University of Massachusetts Memorial
    Healthcare
Worcester, Massachusetts

Lisa M. Dapuzzo-Argiriou, MD[†]
Physician
Department of Obstetrics and
    Gynecology
Practice Leader
Center for Women's Medicine
Lehigh Valley Health Network
Associate Professor
University of South Florida
Allentown, Pennsylvania

Salman S. Dar, MD[†]
Ophthalmology Resident
Department of Ophthalmology
George Washington University
Washington, DC

Akhil Das, MD, FACS
Associate Professor
Department of Urology
Thomas Jefferson University
Philadelphia, Pennsylvania

Samaresh Dasgupta, DO, MHA, FACEP
Inspira Health Network
Director of Emergency Medicine Research
Director of Emergency Department
Elmer Hospital
Clinical Assistant Professor
Department of Emergency Medicine at
    Rowan University
Vineland, New Jersey

Adrian DaSilva-DeAbreu, MD
Fellow
John Ochsner Heart & Vascular Institute
New Orleans, Louisiana

Neha Datta, MD[†]
Psychiatry Resident
Department of Psychiatry
Northwell, Mather Hospital
Port Jefferson, New York

Dawn M. Davis, MD, MPH
Assistant Professor of Family and
    Community Medicine
Saint Louis University School of Medicine
St. Louis, Missouri

Valerie F. Davis Barnabas, MD
Resident
Department of Family and Community
    Medicine
University of Texas Health Science Center
    at San Antonio
San Antonio, Texas

Courtney Dawley, DO
Department of Adult Medicine/Family
    Medicine
Vacaville Medical Center
Vacaville, California

Sondra M. De Antonio, MD
Adjunct Assistant Professor Neurology
Department of Internal Medicine
Rowan University School of Osteopathic
    Medicine
Stratford, New Jersey

Mayralis De Jesús-Cortés, MD, MPH
Family Medicine
MedFirst Primary Care
San Antonio, Texas

Alexei O. DeCastro, MD
Assistant Professor
Director, Medical University of South
    Carolina/Trident Family Medicine
    Residency Program
Chief, Primary Care Sports Medicine
Department of Family Medicine
Health Sports Medicine
Charleston, South Carolina

Timothy Dekker, MD[†]
Resident Physician
Family Medicine Department
Mayo Clinic—Florida
Jacksonville, Florida

Renee F. del Carmen, MD
Department of Family and Community
    Medicine
University of Texas Health San Antonio
San Antonio, Texas

Patrick M. Del Santo, DO
Bayfront Family Medicine Residency
St. Petersburg, Florida

Leah N. Delfinado, MD, FACOG
Residency Program Director
Department of Obstetrics and Gynecology
Advocate Illinois Masonic Medical Center
Chicago, Illinois

Federico Delgado, MD
University of Carabobo
Valencia, Venezuela

Jeanne R. Delgado, MD
Pediatric Resident
Children's National Medical Center
Washington, DC

Konstantinos E. Deligiannidis, MD, MPH,
    FAAFP
Assistant Professor and Director of
    House Calls Education Program
Donald and Barbara Zucker School of
    Medicine at Hofstra/Northwell
Hempstead, New York

Deborah M. DeMarco, MD, FACP
Senior Associate Dean of Clinical Affairs
Associate Dean of Graduate Medical
    Education
University of Massachusetts Medical
    School
Professor of Medicine
Division of Rheumatology
Worcester, Massachusetts

Theodore J. Demetriou, DO
Assistant Professor and Associate
    Vice Chair of Inpatient Medicine
Department of Family and Community
    Medicine
Penn State College of Medicine
Hershey, Pennsylvania

Melissa Dennis, MD
Vice Chairman
Department of Obstetrics and Gynecology
Advocate Illinois Masonic Medical Center
Chicago, Illinois

LeeAnne Denny, MD
Clinical Educator
Banner Good Samaritan Hospital
Phoenix, Arizona

Richard F. DeSouza, MD
Clinical Instructor
Yale School of Medicine
Attending Physician/Hospitalist
Yale-New Haven Hospital
New Haven, Connecticut

Sara M. DeSpain, MD[†]
Chief Resident
Family Medicine Residency
Offutt Air Force Base
University of Nebraska Medical Center
Omaha, Nebraska

Nicholas C. DeStefano, MD[†]
CPT, MC, USA
Chief Resident
Department of Family Medicine
Madigan Army Medical Center
Tacoma, Washington

Harish C. Devineni, MD[†]
Department of Cardiology
East Carolina University/Vidant Medical
    Center
Greenville, North Carolina

Katharine Devin-Holcombe, MD[†]
Department of Emergency Medicine
University of Massachusetts Medical
    School
Worcester, Massachusetts

William W. Dexter, MD, FACSM
Sports Medicine Program
Maine Medical Center
Portland, Maine

Henry DeYoung, MD[†]
Lieutenant, VFA-106 Flight Surgeon
Department of Aviation Medicine
Virginia Beach, Virginia

Manjeet Dhallu, MD
Department of Medicine
Icahn School of Medicine at Mount Sinai
New York, New York
Bronx-Lebanon Hospital Center
Bronx, New York

Luis Diaz-Quintero, MD
Internal Medicine Resident
Department of Medicine
University of Chicago (NorthShore)
    Program
Evanston, Illinois

Daniel R. DiBlasi, DO[†]
Resident
Department of Dermatology
Walter Reed National Military Medical
    Center
Bethesda, Maryland

Aimee Dietle, PharmD
Assistant Professor of Pharmacy Practice
School of Pharmacy
Massachusetts College of Pharmacy and
    Health Sciences University
Worcester, Massachusetts

Andrew Dinh, DO
Department of Family Medicine and
    Community Health
University of Texas Health Science Center
    at San Antonio
San Antonio, Texas

Anh V. Dinh, MD
Resident
Family and Community Medicine
University of Texas at San Antonio
San Antonio, Texas

Bich Hien Dinh, MD
Family Medicine
San Antonio, Texas

Sydney Dittman, MD
University of Colorado Family Medicine
    Residency
Denver, Colorado

Adriel G. Dizon, MD[†]
Family Medicine Resident
Department of Family Medicine
Womack Army Medical Center
Fort Bragg, North Carolina

John M. Doan, DO[†]
USAF, Flight Surgeon
Moody Air Force Base, Georgia

Michael S. Dobson, MD
Resident
Department of Family Medicine
College of Medicine
University of Nebraska Medical Center
Omaha, Nebraska

Kerian L. Dodds, MD
Department of Internal Medicine
George Washington University
Washington, DC

Sarah S. Dolbear, MD[†]
USAF, Flight Surgeon
Moody Air Force Base, Georgia

Lorena C. Dollani, MD
Internal Medicine/Dermatology
Georgetown University Hospital/
    Washington Hospital Center
Washington, DC

Frank J. Domino, MD
Professor and Director of Predoctoral
    Education
Department of Family Medicine and
    Community Health
University of Massachusetts Medical School
Worcester, Massachusetts

Ryan J. Dono, MD
Core Faculty at Lawrence Family
    Medicine Residency
Greater Lawrence Family Health Center
Lawrence, Massachusetts

Malerie Dooling, PharmD, RPh
Clinical Pharmacist
Shields Health Solutions
Quincy, Massachusetts

Nicole A. Doria, MD
George Washington University School of
    Medicine & Health Sciences
Washington, DC

Heather C. Doty, DO
Associate Director
Novant Health Family Medicine Residency
    Program
Huntersville, North Carolina

Cassandra Doucet, MD
Department of Medicine
Vanderbilt University Medical Center
Nashville, Tennessee

Matthew D. Dow, DO
Family Medicine
Dallas, Texas

John Doyle, MD
Resident Psychiatrist
Department of Psychiatry
Zucker School of Medicine at
    Hofstra/Northwell
Hempstead, New York

Drew-Anne Drapala, MD
Resident Physician
Methodist Hospital Family Medicine
    Residency
Sacramento, California

Brynn Dredla, MD
Sleep Medicine Specialist
Neurologist
Departments of Pulmonary Medicine and
    Neurology
Mayo Clinic
Jacksonville, Florida

Scott A. Drummond Jr., DO, DABR[†]
Department of Radiology, Chief
Bassett Army Community Hospital
Fort Wainwright, Alaska

Maurice Duggins, MD
Associate Director
Ascension Via Christi FM Residency
Clinical Associate Professor
Kansas University School of Medicine—
    Wichita
Ascension Via Christi Hospitals
Wichita, Kansas

Whitney A. Dunlap, MD, MS
Assistant Professor of Medicine
University of Massachusetts Medical
    School
Director of Allergy
Division of Pulmonary, Allergy & Critical
    Care Medicine
University of Massachusetts Medical
    School
Worcester, Massachusetts

Angela M. Dunn, DO, MPH[†]
Staff, Family Medicine Residency
Department of Family Medicine
Madigan Army Medical Center
Tacoma, Washington

Noel Dunn, MD[†]
Staff Physician
Madigan Army Medical Center
Tacoma, Washington

Maegen Dupper, MD[†]
Assistant Clinical Professor
Department of Family Medicine
University of California, Riverside School
    of Medicine
Riverside, California

Cheryl Durand, PharmD
Associate Professor
Department of Pharmacy Practice
Massachusetts College of Pharmacy and
    Health Science University
Manchester, New Hampshire

Muhammad Durrani, DO, MS[†]
Department of Emergency Medicine
Inspira Medical Center
Vineland, New Jersey

Alan M. Ehrlich, MD
Assistant Professor of Family Medicine
University of Massachusetts Medical
    School
Worcester, Massachusetts

William G. Elder, PhD
Chair and Clinical Professor
Department of Behavioral and Social
  Sciences
University of Houston
College of Medicine
Houston, Texas

Carrie Lynn Ellis, DVM, MS
Associate Veterinarian
Animal Hospital on Mt. Lookout Square
Cincinnati, Ohio

Robert Ellis, MD
Associate Professor
Department of Family and Community
  Medicine
University of Cincinnati
Cincinnati, Ohio

William S. Ellis, DO[†]
CPT, MC, USAF
Family Physician
Deputy Chief of Medical Staff
Family Health Clinic
Cannon Air Force Base, New Mexico

Pamela Ellsworth, MD
Chief, Division of Urology
Professor of Urology
Nemours Children's Hospital
University of Central Florida College of
  Medicine
Orlando, Florida

Eussra El-Magbri, MD[†]
Resident Physician
Department of Emergency Medicine
University of Pittsburgh Medical Center
  (UPMC)
Pittsburgh, Pennsylvania

Nida (Joy) Emko, MD, FAAFP
Associate Clinical Professor
Department of Family and Community
  Medicine
University of Texas Health San Antonio
San Antonio, Texas

Ngozi N. Emuchay, MD
Internal Medicine
University of Illinois at Chicago/Advocate
  Christ Medical Center
Oak Lawn, Illinois

Benjamin M. Enciso, DO
Medical College of Georgia
Augusta, Georgia

Todd J. Endicott, DO[†]
CDR, MC, USN
Comprehensive Ophthalmologist
Naval Hospital Jacksonville
Jacksonville, Florida

Deborah R. Erlich, MD, MMedEd, FAAFP
Associate Professor
Department of Family Medicine
Family Medicine Clerkship Director
Tufts University School of Medicine
Boston, Massachusetts

Daniel A. Ermann, MD[†]
Internal Medicine Resident
Creighton University Medical Center
Omaha, Nebraska

William A. Fabricius, MD
Hematology-Oncology Fellow
Division of Hematology and Oncology
Department of Medicine
University of Massachusetts Medical School
Worcester, Massachusetts

Stephen C. Fabry, MD
Senior Staff Physician
Lahey Hospital & Medical Center
Associate Clinical Professor of Medicine
Tufts University School of Medicine
Boston, Massachusetts

Donald J. Fahey-Ahrndt, MD
Family Medicine Resident
Department of Family Medicine and
  Community Health
University of Minnesota Medical School
Minneapolis, Minnesota

Cristian P. Fernandez Falcon, MD, DABFM,
  CAQGM, CAQHPM, CMD
Family Medicine Hospital Service (FMHS)
  Medical Director
Assistant Professor, Clinical
Family and Community Medicine
  Department
University of Texas Health San Antonio
San Antonio, Texas

Pang-Yen Fan, MD
Professor of Medicine
Division of Renal Medicine
University of Massachusetts Medical
  School
Worcester, Massachusetts

William G. Farkas, DO, FS[†]
MAJ, MC
Battalion Flight Surgeon
3rd General Support Aviation Battalion
82nd Combat Aviation Brigade
Fort Bragg, North Carolina

Mark A. Farnie, MD
Associate Professor
Department of Pediatrics
McGovern Medical School
The University of Texas Health Science
  Center at Houston
Houston, Texas

Umer Farooq, MD[†]
Medical Director Behavioral Health
  Emergency Service
Department of Psychiatry
Mather Memorial Hospital
NorthWell Health Care
Port Jefferson, New York

Julia S. Fast, DO[†]
Fort Bragg, North Carolina

Aelia Fatima, MD
Resident Physician
Department of Internal Medicine
University of Illinois at Chicago/Advocate
  Christ Medical Center
Oak Lawn, Illinois

Rhonda A. Faulkner, PhD[†]
Director of Behavioral Medicine
Department of Family Medicine
Saint Joseph Hospital
University of Illinois at Chicago College of
  Medicine Master Affiliate
Chicago, Illinois

Kinder Fayssoux, MD
Core Clinical Faculty
Eisenhower Family Medicine Residency
  Program
La Quinta, California

Jeffrey P. Feden, MD, FACEP
Associate Professor, Clinician Educator
Department of Emergency Medicine
The Warren Alpert Medical School of
  Brown University
Providence, Rhode Island

Ryan B. Feeney, PharmD, BCPS, BCGP
Clinical Manager
Department of Pharmacy Services
Temple University Hospital
Philadelphia, Pennsylvania

Matthew Feist, MD[†]
Family Medicine Resident
Naval Hospital Jacksonville
Jacksonville, Florida

Neil Feldman, DPM[†]
Fellow
American College of Foot and Ankle
  Surgeons
Diplomate
American Board of Podiatric Surgery
Central Massachusetts Podiatry, PC
Worcester, Massachusetts

Edward Feller, MD, FACP, FACG
Clinical Professor of Medical Sciences
The Warren Alpert Medical School of
  Brown University
Providence, Rhode Island

James Auteri Ferguson, MD, MPH, CPH
Department of Family Medicine and
    Community Health
Case Western Reserve University
Cleveland, Ohio

Noelia Fernandez, RN
Registered Nurse of Medical
    Emergencies
Hospital de Sant Joan Despí Moises Broggi
Barcelona, Spain

Kelsey C. Ferrell, DO
Resident Physician
Traditional Rotating Internship Residency
    Program
Good Samaritan Regional Medical Center
Corvallis, Oregon

Kathy Ferrer, MD
Assistant Professor of Pediatrics
Division of Infectious Disease, Special
    Immunology Section
Division of Hospitalist Medicine
Global Health Initiative
Children's National Health System
The George Washington University School
    of Medicine and Health Sciences
Washington, DC

William J. Fiden, MD†
Assistant Professor of Family Medicine
Department of Family Medicine-
    Uniformed Services University of the
    Health Sciences
Family Medicine Residency Program
Womack Army Medical Center
Fort Bragg, North Carolina

Scott A. Fields, MD, MHA
Adjunct Associate Professor of Family
    Medicine
Oregon Health & Science University
Portland, Oregon

Matthew J. Filippo, DO
Chief Psychiatry Resident
Department of Psychiatry
Advocate Lutheran General Hospital
Park Ridge, Illinois

Stanley Fineman, MD
Adjunct Associate Professor
Department of Pediatrics
Atlanta Allergy & Asthma
Emory University School of Medicine
Atlanta, Georgia

Jorge Finke, MD

Daniel J. Fisher, MD
Assistant Director of Family Medicine
Community East Family Medicine Residency
Community Health Network
Indianapolis, Indiana

Eric L. Fisher, MD†
Assistant Professor
University of Louisville Glasgow Family
    Medicine Residency
Department of Family and Geriatric
    Medicine
University of Louisville School of Medicine
Glasgow, Kentucky

Theodore B. Flaum, DO, FACOFP
Associate Professor
Department of Osteopathic Manipulative
    Medicine
Attending Physician
Academic Health Care Center
New York Institute of Technology College
    of Osteopathic Medicine
Old Westbury, New York

Joseph A. Florence, MD
Professor and Director of Rural Programs
Department of Family Medicine
East Tennessee State University
James H. Quillen College of Medicine
Johnson City, Tennessee

Emily K. Flores, PharmD, BCPS
Associate Professor
Department of Pharmacy Practice
Gatton College of Pharmacy
Adjunct Faculty
Department of Family Medicine
Quillen College of Medicine
East Tennessee State University
Johnson City, Tennessee

Kendra Flores, MS, CGC
Licensed Genetic Counselor
Christiana Health Care System
Newark, Delaware
Clinical Instructor of Genetics
Thomas Jefferson University
Philadelphia, Pennsylvania

Harry W. Flynn Jr., MD
Professor of Ophthalmology
The J. Donald M. Gass Distinguished
    Chair in Ophthalmology
Bascom Palmer Eye Institute
University of Miami, Miller School of
    Medicine
Miami, Florida

Michael Flynn, MD, MHS
Associate Professor of Obstetrics/
    Gynecology
Department of Obstetrics/Gynecology
University of Massachusetts Medical
    School
Worcester, Massachusetts

Jay Fong, MD†
Assistant Professor
Department of Pediatrics
Division of Gastroenterology, Nutrition,
    and Hepatology
University of Massachusetts Medical
    Center
Worcester, Massachusetts

Heather C. Forkey, MD
Associate Professor of Pediatrics
Division Director, Child Protection
    Program
Director, Foster Children Evaluation
    Service
University of Massachusetts Medical
    School
Worcester, Massachusetts

Angelique S. Forrester, MPH, MD†
Family Medicine Resident
Eglin Air Force Base Family Residency
    Program
Eglin Air Force Base, Florida

Lorna Fountain, MD, FAAFP
Program Director
Family Medicine Residency Program
Bayfront Health St. Petersburg
St. Petersburg, Florida

Phillip Fournier, MD
Professor of Family Medicine and
    Community Health
University of Massachusetts Medical
    School
Worcester, Massachusetts

Robert L. Frachtman, MD
Assistant Clinical Professor of Internal
    Medicine
Dell Medical School, University of Texas
    at Austin
Austin Gastroenterology, PA
Austin, Texas

Mony Fraer, MD, FACP, FASN
Clinical Professor of Internal Medicine
    and Nephrology
University of Iowa Hospital and Clinics
Iowa City, Iowa

David A. Frankel, DO
Resident Physician
Department of Family Medicine
Advocate BroMenn Medical Center
Normal, Illinois

Charles Fredericks, MD
General Surgery Resident
Rush University
Chicago, Illinois

Anna Freitag, MD, FACP, FACE, MACDS
Endocrinology
Trinity Health of New England Medical
  Group
Waterbury, Connecticut

Minjin K. Fromm, MD
Assistant Professor
Department of Orthopedics and Physical
  Rehabilitation
University of Massachusetts Medical
  School
Worcester, Massachusetts

Noah L. Furr, MD†
Resident Physician
Eglin Family Medicine Residency
Eglin Air Force Base, Florida

Steven W. Gale, MD†
Staff Physician
Peterson Air Force Base
Fort Carlson, Colorado

Samuel Galima, DO†
USAF, Flight Surgeon
Kleber Health Clinic
Kaiserslautern, Germany

Rodolfo J. Galindo, MD
Assistant Professor of Medicine
Division of Endocrinology, Diabetes and
  Lipids
Emory University School of Medicine
Medical Chair, Inpatient Diabetes Taskforce
Emory Healthcare System
Atlanta, Georgia

Curtis L. Galke, DO
Assistant Professor
Family and Community Medicine
The University of Texas Health Science
  Center at San Antonio
San Antonio, Texas
Associate Program Director, Family
  Medicine Residency
The University of Texas Health
  Science Center at Antonio—Rio
  Grande Valley-Doctors Hospital at
  Renaissance
Edinburg, Texas

Amy Gallardo, FNP-C
Norfolk, Virginia

Siavash Ganjbakhsh, MD
Resident Physician
Department of Family Medicine
SUNY Downstate Medical Center
Brooklyn, New York

Curtis Gapinski, DO
Air Force Medicine—Kadena
Kadena Air Base, Japan

Luis T. Garcia, MD
Chairman and Residency Program Director
Family Medicine
Amita Saint Joseph Hospital
Chicago, Illinois

Guillermo Garcia-Manero, MD
Department of Leukemia
University of Texas MD Anderson Cancer
  Center
Houston, Texas

Victor Garcia-Rodriguez, MD
Internal Medicine Resident
The University of Texas Health Science
  Center at Houston
Houston, Texas

Loreli Garnica Moya, MD
Department of Family and Community
  Medicine
University of Texas Health San Antonio
San Antonio, Texas

William T. Garrison, PhD†
Professor of Pediatrics
Department of Pediatrics
University of Massachusetts Medical School
Worcester, Massachusetts

Anette Galang Gawelko, DO
Clinical Associate Professor
Department of Family Medicine
Arizona College of Osteopathic Medicine
Midwestern University
Glendale, Arizona

Breanna L. Gawrys, DO†
CPT, USAF
Family Medicine—Obstetrics Physician
Faculty
Scott Air Force Base
St. Louis University Family Medicine
  Residency Program
Belleville, Illinois

John N. Gayk, MD†
Family Medicine Resident
Eglin Air Force Base Family Residency
Eglin Air Force Base, Florida

Brandon Gerard Gaynor, MD
Neurosurgeon
Advocate Medical Group
Oak Lawn, Illinois

Barry C. Gentry, MD†
Naval Hospital Camp Lejeune
Camp Lejeune, North Carolina

Shari L. Gentry, MD†
Naval Hospital Camp Lejeune
Camp Lejeune, North Carolina

Paul George, MD
Assistant Dean for Medical Education
Associate Professor of Family Medicine/
  Associate Professor of Medical Science
The Warren Alpert Medical School of
  Brown University
Providence, Rhode Island

Nicole Gerardo, PharmD
University of Illinois at Chicago College of
  Pharmacy
Chicago, Illinois

Fereshteh Gerayli, MD, FAAFP
Professor of Family Medicine
Johnson City Family Medicine Residency
  Program
James H. Quillen College of Medicine
East Tennessee State University
Johnson City, Tennessee

Anastasia N. Gevas, DO
Internal Medicine
Southeastern Regional Medical Center
Lumberton, North Carolina

Kelli M. Gevas, MD†
Obstetrics/Gynecology Physician
Trinity Mount Carmel Hospital System
Columbus, Ohio

Faraz Ghoddusi, MD†
Resident Physician
Department of Family Medicine
University of Nebraska Medical Center
Omaha, Nebraska

Stacey A. Ghoddusi, MPH
Creighton University
Omaha, Nebraska

Amaninderapal S. Ghotra, MD
Cardiology Fellow
Department of Internal Medicine
Division of Cardiovascular Disease
University of Texas—Houston
Houston, Texas

An-Hoa Giang, MD, MPH
Family Medicine Resident
Department of Family Medicine and
  Community Health
University of Massachusetts
Worcester, Massachusetts

Lawrence M. Gibbs, MD, MSEd, FAAFP
Faculty Physician
Methodist Charlton Family Medicine
  Residency Program
Methodist Charlton Medical Center
Dallas, Texas

Richard Gibson, MD
Bayfront Family Medicine Residency
St. Petersburg, Florida

Marzena Gieniusz, MD
Faculty Attending Physician
Department of Medicine
Division of Geriatric and Palliative
    Medicine
North Shore University Hospital and LIJ
    Medical Center
Northwell Health
Assistant Professor
Donald and Barbara Zucker School of
    Medicine at Hofstra/Northwell
Manhasset, New York

Brittani Gierisch, MD
Family Medicine Resident
University of Texas Health San Antonio
San Antonio, Texas

Bernadatte G. Gilbert, MD
Assistant Professor and Staff Physician
Department of Family and Community
    Medicine
Penn State Health/Penn State College of
    Medicine
Hershey, Pennsylvania

Cameron S. Gilbert, MD[†]
USAF, CSARME Flight Surgeon
Moody Air Force Base, Georgia

Catherine A. Gill, MD, FAAFP[†]
Family Medicine Residency Faculty
Martin Army Community Hospital
Fort Benning, Georgia

Prabhcharan Gill, MD, FRCOG,
    FACOG[†]
Maternal–Fetal Medicine
Aultman Hospital
Director
Aultman OBGYN Residency Program
Chair-Professor
Northeast Ohio Medical University
    (NEOMED) College of Medicine
Canton, Ohio

Bonnie Gillis, MD[†]
CPT, USAF, MC
Family Medicine Resident Physician
96 MDOS
Eglin Air Force Base, Florida

Jared Giordano, MD
Internal Medicine Residency
Alpert Medical School
Brown University
Providence, Rhode Island

Daniel V. Girzadas Jr., MD, RDMS
Director of Faculty Development
Department of Emergency Medicine
Advocate Christ Medical Center
Oak Lawn, Illinois

Joseph B. Gladwell, MD, CPHQ, CPPS[†]
Medical Director of Quality and Safety
Assistant Program Director
Family Medicine
OhioHealth Riverside Methodist Hospital
Columbus, Ohio

Gerald Gleich, MD[†]
Associate Professor
Department of Family Medicine and
    Community Health
University of Massachusetts Medical School
Worcester, Massachusetts

Ankur Goel, MD
Department of General Surgery
Georgia Regents University
Augusta, Georgia

Sujan Gogu, DO[†]
Resident
Department of Family Medicine
The University of Texas Health Science
    Center at San Antonio
San Antonio, Texas

Scott M. Goldberg, MD
Primary Care Sports Medicine Fellow
Department of Family Medicine and
    Community Health
University of Massachusetts Medical School
Worcester, Massachusetts

Jeremy Golding, MD, FAAFP
Professor of Family Medicine and
    Obstetrics & Gynecology
University of Massachusetts Medical
    School
Quality Officer
Department of Family Medicine and
    Community Health
University of Massachusetts Memorial
    Health Care
Hahnemann Family Health Center
Worcester, Massachusetts

Mercedes E. Gonzalez, MD
Clinical Assistant Professor
University of Miami Miller School of
    Medicine
Department of Dermatology
Medical Director
Pediatric Dermatology of Miami
Miami, Florida

Herbert P. Goodheart, MD
Associate Clinical Professor
Department of Dermatology
Mount Sinai College of Medicine in
    New York City
New York, New York
Director of Dermatology
Elmhurst Hospital Center
Queens, New York

Chelsea Gordner, DO, MPH
Assistant Professor
Adult and Pediatric Endocrinology
University of Massachusetts Medical
    School—Baystate
Springfield, Massachusetts

Dónal Kevin Gordon, MD, FAAFP
Executive Director/Program Director
Cedar Rapids Family Medicine Residency
Cedar Rapids, Iowa
Adjunct Clinical Assistant Professor
University of Iowa College of Medicine
Iowa City, Iowa

Fredric D. Gordon, MD[†]
Vice-Chair
Division of Transplantation and
    Hepatobiliary Diseases
Lahey Hospital & Medical Center
Burlington, Massachusetts
Associate Professor in Medicine
Tufts Medical School
Boston, Massachusetts

Miranda Gordon-Zigel, MD
Family Medicine Resident
Department of Family Medicine and
    Community Health
Hospital of the University of Pennsylvania
Philadelphia, Pennsylvania

Emily Gorman, DO[†]
OhioHealth Riverside Department of
    Family Medicine
Columbus, Ohio

Cait Goss, MD
Family Medicine
Department of Family Medicine
Oregon Health and Science University
Portland, Oregon

Edward A. Gotfried, DO, FACOS[†]
Director
New York Institute of Technology Center
    for Global Health
Associate Professor
Department of Osteopathic Manipulative
    Medicine
New York Institute of Technology College
    of Osteopathic Medicine
Old Westbury, New York

Samantha Faryn Gottlieb, DO, MS
New York Institute of Technology College
    of Osteopathic Medicine
Old Westbury, New York

Ginny L. Gottschalk, MD
Assistant Professor and Family Medicine
  Clerkship Director
Department of Family and Community
  Medicine
University of Kentucky College of
  Medicine
Lexington, Kentucky

Jagathi Govindu, MD
Heywood Hospital
Gardner, Massachusetts

Kellen H. Gower, MD[†]
Family Medicine Resident
Bayfront Health Family Medicine
  Residency
St. Petersburg, Florida

Parag Goyal, MD, MSc
Assistant Professor of Medicine
Division of Cardiology
Division of General Internal Medicine
Department of Medicine
Weill Cornell Medical Center
New York, New York

Aaron Grant, MD[†]
Ophthalmologist
Lackland Air Force Base, Texas

Jessica Gray, MD
Attending Physician
UMC Physicians
Adjunct Faculty
Texas Tech Health Sciences Center
  School of Medicine
Lubbock, Texas

Michael J. Gray, MD, MA, MS, ATC
Attending Physician
Emergency Care Center
Harrington Hospital
Southbridge, Massachusetts

Whitney A. Gray, MSN, CRNP[†]
Division of Gerontology, Geriatrics, and
  Palliative Care
The University of Alabama at Birmingham
  Hospital
Birmingham, Alabama

Jonathan Green, MD, MSCI
General Surgery Resident
Department of General Surgery
University of Massachusetts Medical School
Worcester, Massachusetts

Ellen M. Greenblatt, MD[†]
Medical Director
Mount Sinai Fertility
Professor
Department of Obstetrics and Gynecology
University of Toronto
Toronto, Ontario, Canada

Adam B. Greenfest, MD
School of Medicine and Health Sciences
George Washington University
Washington, DC

David A. Greenwald, MD
Director of Clinical Gastroenterology and
  Endoscopy
Mount Sinai Hospital
Professor of Medicine
Icahn School of Medicine at Mount Sinai
New York, New York

Simon B. Griesbach, MD[†]
Assistant Director
Waukesha Family Medicine Residency
  Program
Waukesha, Wisconsin

Charles K. Grigsby, MD
Resident, Surgery
Georgia Regents University
Augusta, Georgia

Andrew E. Grimes, MD
Partner, US Anesthesia Partners
Assistant Professor
Department of Surgery and Perioperative
  Care
Dell Medical School
Austin, Texas

Matthew K. Griswold, MD
Assistant Professor
Department of Emergency Medicine
Hartford Hospital
Hartford, Connecticut

Scott P. Grogan, DO, MBA, FAAFP[†]
Family Medicine Residency Director
Madigan Army Medical Center
Tacoma, Washington

Gena M. Grospe, DO
Department of Family Medicine
Advocate Christ Medical Center
Oak Lawn, Illinois

Esther Guard, DO[†]
Family Medicine Residency Faculty
Eglin Air Force Base, Florida

John A. Guisto, MD
Professor of Clinical Emergency Medicine
Department of Emergency Medicine
University of Arizona College of Medicine
Tucson, Arizona

Padma Priya Gummadi, MBBS
Internal Medicine Resident
Bergan Mercy Hospital
Creighton University
Omaha, Nebraska

Nathan D. Gundacker, MD
Assistant Professor
Division of Infectious Diseases
Department of Medicine
Medical College of Wisconsin
Milwaukee, Wisconsin

Sabrina Gunn, DO
Psychiatry Resident
Grandview Medical Center
Dayton, Ohio

Neena R. Gupta, MD[†]
Associate Professor of Pediatrics
Medical Director
Pediatric Kidney Transplant Program
Department of Pediatrics
University of Massachusetts Children's
  Medical Center
Worcester, Massachusetts

Aaron J. Gustin, DO
Neurosurgery Resident
Advocate Aurora Health Care
Downers Grove, Illinois

Christina S. Gutta, MD
Chief Resident
Bayfront Health Family Medicine
  Residency
St. Petersburg, Florida

Silas Gyimah, MD
Family Medicine Resident
Eisenhower Health
Rancho Mirage, California

Reem Hadi, MD
Family Medicine
The University of Texas Health Science
  Center at San Antonio
San Antonio, Texas

Katherine E. Haga, DO
Family Medicine Resident
Novant Health Family Medicine Residency
  Program
Cornelius, North Carolina

Shanzay Haider, MD
Medicine Resident
Department of Internal Medicine
St. Mary's Hospital
Waterbury, Connecticut

Sean P. Haight, MD[†]
LCDR, MC (Flight Surgeon), USN
Assistant Professor of Military Medicine
Uniformed Services
University of the Health Sciences
Pace, Florida

Shahrad Hakimian, MD
Gastroenterology Fellow
Department of Medicine
Division of Gastroenterology
University of Massachusetts Medical School
Worcester, Massachusetts

Ildiko Halasz, MD
VA Boston Healthcare System
Primary Care Clinic
West Roxbury, Maryland

Cynthia D. Hall, MD[†]
Associate Professor and Fellowship
    Director
Female Pelvic Medicine and
    Reconstructive Surgery
Department of Obstetrics and Gynecology
University of Massachusetts Medical School
Worcester, Massachusetts

Shadi Hamdeh, MD
Department of Internal Medicine
Creighton University School of Medicine
Omaha, Nebraska

Jennifer L. Hamilton, MD, PhD, FAAFP
Assistant Professor
Department of Family, Community, and
    Preventive Medicine
Drexel University College of Medicine
Philadelphia, Pennsylvania

Lynn M. Hamrich, MD, FAAFP
Associate Director of Residency Education
Summa Health System—Akron Campus
    Family Medicine Residency Program
Akron, Ohio
Associate Professor of Family and
    Community Medicine
Northeast Ohio Medical University
    (NEOMED)
Rootstown, Ohio

Ihab Hamzeh, MD, FACC[†]
Associate Program Director
Cardiovascular Medicine Fellowship
Baylor College of Medicine
Houston, Texas

Jessica L. Handel, DO
Associate Program Director
St. Elizabeth Family Medicine Residency
Youngstown, Ohio

Thomas J. Hansen, MD, FAAFP[†]
Chief Academic Officer
Advocate Health Care
Downers Grove, Illinois

Sonali Harchandani, MBBS
Fellow
Department of Hematology/Oncology
University of Massachusetts Medical School
Worcester, Massachusetts

Andrew Harner, MD[†]
General Surgery Resident
Augusta University
Augusta, Georgia

Thomas A. Haroldson, MD[†]
Primary Care Sports Medicine Fellow
Altru Sports Medicine Fellowship
Grand Forks, North Dakota

Chelsea Harris, MD
Family Medicine Resident
Lawrence Family Medicine Residency
Lawrence, Massachusetts

Gabriel T. Harris, MD, FAAFP[†]
Assistant Professor
Department of Family Medicine
Uniformed Services University of Health
    Sciences
Bethesda, Maryland

Lisa M. Harris, DO[†]
Faculty Physician
Womack Army Medical Center
Fort Bragg, North Carolina

Ayesha Hasan, MD
Department of Obstetrics and Gynecology
Akron General Medical Center
Akron, Ohio

Robert M. Hasty, DO, FACOI, FACP
Vice President of Medical Education
Southeastern Health
Associate Dean for Postgraduate Affairs
Campbell University School of
    Osteopathic Medicine
Lumberton, North Carolina

Steven Hatch, MD, MSc[†]
Associate Professor of Medicine
Program Director
Infectious Diseases Fellowship
Department of Internal Medicine
University of Massachusetts Medical
    School
Worcester, Massachusetts

Betul A. Hatipoglu, MD
Clinical Associate Professor of Medicine,
    Staff
Endocrinology & Metabolism Institute
Cleveland Clinic
Cleveland, Ohio

Fern R. Hauck, MD, MS
Spencer P. Bass MD Twenty-First Century
    Professor of Family Medicine
Professor of Public Health Sciences
Department of Family Medicine
University of Virginia Health System
Charlottesville, Virginia

J. Christopher Hawkins, DO
Neurosurgery Resident
Advocate BroMenn Medical Center
Normal, Illinois

Beverly N. Hay, MD
Associate Professor of Pediatrics
Chief, Division of Genetics
University of Massachusetts Medical
    School
UMass Memorial Medical Center
Worcester, Massachusetts

Pamela P. Hayes, MD
Medical Fellow
Department of Hematology and Oncology
Baylor University Medical Center
Dallas, Texas

Kasey Hebert, MD
University of Massachusetts Medical School
Worcester, Massachusetts

Cassandra Heiselman, DO, MPH
Department of Obstetrics and Gynecology
Cleveland Clinic Akron General
Akron, Ohio

Andrew S. Hellenga, MD
Resident Physician
Department of Family and Community
    Medicine
Saint Louis University School of Medicine
St. Louis, Missouri

Irmanie Hemphill, MD, FAAFP
Humanities, Health and Society
Herbert Wertheim College of Medicine
Florida International University
Miami, Florida

Scott T. Henderson, MD
Director, Medical Services
Student Health Center
University of Missouri
Columbia, Missouri

Phillip R. Hendley, MD[†]
Special Operations Flight Surgeon
27th Special Operations Support Squadron
    Operational Support Medicine
Cannon Air Force Base
Clovis, New Mexico

Michelle Henne, MD
Department of Sports Medicine
Orlando Health
Winter Haven, Florida

Alex M. Hennessey, MD
Resident
Department of Urology
University of Connecticut School of
    Medicine
Farmington, Connecticut

Gina Henry, MD
Resident Physician
Department of Family Medicine
Loma Linda University Health Education
    Consortium
Loma Linda, California

Matthew A. Henry, DO[†]
CPT, USAF, MC
Staff Family Physician
Joint Base Langley-Eustis
Hampton, Virginia

Byron C. Hepburn, MD, FAAFP
Professor of Family and Community
    Medicine
University of Texas Health San Antonio
San Antonio, Texas

Jaroslaw T. Hepel, MD
Assistant Professor
Department of Radiation Oncology
Rhode Island Hospital
Brown University
Providence, Rhode Island
Department of Radiation Oncology
Tufts Medical Center, Tufts University
Boston, Massachusetts

Matthew E. Herberg, MD[†]
Chief
Department of Surgery
Associate Professor
Texas A&M College of Medicine
Associate Professor
Uniformed Services University of the
    Health Sciences
Carl R. Darnall Army Medical Center
Fort Hood, Texas

Yasmin Herrera, MD
Instituto Tecnológico de Santo Domingo
Santo Domingo, Dominican Republic

David N. Herrmann, MBBCh
Professor of Neurology and Pathology
University of Rochester
Rochester, New York

Lee J. Herskowitz, DO, MBA, FAAP
Associate Professor and Regional
Director of Medical Education
NW Regional Primary Care Campus
Portland, Oregon
A.T. Still University School of Osteopathic
Medicine Arizona
Mesa, Arizona

Brian Hertz, MD[†]
Internal Medicine
Kaiser Permanente
San Rafael, California

Joseph L. Hesse, MD
Resident Physician
University of Texas Dell Medical School
    Family Medicine Program
Austin, Texas

Jo Marie C. Hewitt, MD
Resident
Department of Family Medicine
Creighton University School of Medicine
Omaha, Nebraska

David L. Heymann, MD, DTMH
Professor of Infectious Disease
    Epidemiology
London School of Hygiene & Tropical
    Medicine
London, England, United Kingdom

Ashley Hicks, PharmD, BCOP
Clinical Oncology Pharmacist
University of Wisconsin Hospital and Clinics
Chicago, Illinois

David G. Hicks, MD
Professor and Director of Surgical
    Pathology
Department of Pathology and Laboratory
    Medicine
University of Rochester Medical Center
Rochester, New York

Scott D. Hines, DO[†]
Family Medicine Resident
Mike O'Callaghan Military Medical Center
Nellis Air Force Base, Nevada

Michael P. Hirsh, MD, FACS, FAAP[†]
Professor of Surgery
Pediatrics, Family Medicine and
    Quantitative Health Sciences
Surgeon-in-Chief
University of Massachusetts Memorial
    Children's Medical Center
Director
Division of Pediatric Surgery and Trauma
Co-Director
Injury Free Coalition for Worcester
Medical Director
John C. Wood II Foundation to Prevent
    Firearm Injury
Founder
Greater Worcester Goods For Guns Gun
    Buyback Program
Medical Director
Worcester Division of Public Health
Worcester, Massachusetts

Crystal L. Hnatko, DO, CAQSM[†]
Adjunct Faculty and Assistant Director of
    Sports Medicine
David Grant Medical Center Family
    Medicine Residency
Travis Air Force Base, California
Orthopedics and Sports Medicine
    Department
Napa-Solano Family Medicine Residency
Kaiser Permanente
Napa-Solano, California

Abigail Weil Hoffman, MD
General Surgery Resident
Georgia Regents University
Augusta, Georgia

Jason J. Hofstede, DO[†]
Resident Family Physician
Eglin Air Force Base Family Medicine
    Residency
Eglin Air Force Base, Florida

Thomas S. Hoke, MD
Primary Care
Sports Medicine Fellow
Maine Medical Center
Portland, Maine

Kathryn Holder, MD
Family Medicine
Vallejo Medical Center
The Permanente Medical Group
Vallejo, California

N. Wilson Holland, MD, FACP
Adjunct Associate Professor of Medicine
Master Clinician Clinical Distinction
Department of Medicine
Emory University School of Medicine
Atlanta, Georgia

Roger P. Holland, MD, PhD[†]
Family Medicine Residency
Dwight D. Eisenhower Army Medical
    Center
Fort Gordon, Georgia

Sarah R. Hollis, MD
Family Medicine Resident
University of Cincinnati
The Christ Hospital Family Medicine
    Residency
Cincinnati, Ohio

Steven B. Holsten Jr., MD
Professor of Surgery
Department of Surgery
The Medical College of Georgia at August
    University
Augusta, Georgia

Cody E. Homistek, DO
Chief Resident
Novant Health Family Medicine
    Residency Program
Cornelius, North Carolina

Laurie Hommema, MD[†]
Program Director
Riverside Family Medicine Residency
OhioHealth Riverside Methodist Hospital
Columbus, Ohio

Amer Homsi, MD
General Surgery Resident
Department of Surgery
The Brooklyn Hospital Center
Brooklyn, New York

J. David Honeycutt, MD, FAAFP[†]
Nellis Family Medicine Residency
Nellis Air Force Base, Nevada

Stanton C. Honig, MD[†]
Clinical Professor of Urology
Director, Men's Health
Clinical Lead, Gender Affirming Surgery
    Program
Department of Urology
Yale School of Medicine
New Haven, Connecticut

Maeve K. Hopkins, MD[†]
Fellow, Maternal–Fetal Medicine
Hospital of the University of Pennsylvania
Philadelphia, Pennsylvania

Michael P. Hopkins, MD, MEd[†]
Professor
Department of Obstetrics and Gynecology
Northeast Ohio Medical University
Aultman Hospital
Canton, Ohio

Muhammad M. Hossain, DO
Family Medicine Resident
Advocate Christ Family Medicine
Hometown, Illinois

Robert W. Hostoffer, DO, LhD, FACOP,
    FAAP, FCCP, FACOI[†]
Associate Professor of Pediatrics
Case Western Reserve University
Program Director of Allergy/Immunology
University Hospital
Cleveland Medical Center
Cleveland, Ohio

James E. Hougas III, MD, FAAFP
Assistant Professor
Faculty
Department of Family Medicine and
    Community Health
St. John's Family Medicine Residency
University of Minnesota Medical School
St. Paul, Minnesota

Steven A. House, MD, FAAFP, FAAHPM
Professor
Department of Family & Geriatric Medicine
University of Louisville
Program Director
Glasgow Family Medicine Residency
    Program
University of Louisville/Glasgow
Glasgow, Kentucky

Alexander P. Houser, DO
Womack Army Medical Center
Fort Bragg, North Carolina

Elizabeth Hoy, MD, MS, MSPH[†]
Psychiatry Resident
Citrus Health Network
Hialeah, Florida

Kattie D. S. Hoy, MD, FAAFP[†]
Associate Program Director
Family Medicine Residency
Eglin Air Force Base, Florida

Amanda Hu, MD, FRCSC
Assistant Professor
Department of Otolaryngology–Head &
Neck Surgery
Drexel University College of Medicine
Philadelphia, Pennsylvania

Chi Huang, MD, SFHM, FACP
Executive Medical Director
General Medicine and Hospital Medicine
    Shared Services
Wake Forest Baptist Health System
Section Chief of Hospital Medicine
Department of Internal Medicine
Associate Professor of Internal Medicine
Wake Forest Medical School
Winston-Salem, North Carolina

Heather J. Hue, MD, MPH[†]
Hematology & Medical Oncology
Boston, Massachusetts

Dennis E. Hughes, DO, FAAFP, FACEP
360 Degree Medicine
Branson, Missouri

Karen A. Hughes, MD, FAAFP[†]
Associate Director
Family Medicine Residency Program
Tupelo, Mississippi

Pamela R. Hughes, MD[†]
Mike O'Callaghan Military Medical Center
Nellis Air Force Base, Nevada

Karen A. Hulbert, MD
Associate Professor
Department of Family & Community
    Medicine
Medical College of Wisconsin
Milwaukee, Wisconsin

Carol H. Hungerford, DO[†]
Family Medicine Resident
Nellis Air Force Base Family Medicine
    Residency
Mike O'Callaghan Federal Medical Center
Nellis Air Force Base, Nevada

Carolina Hurtado, MD
Internal Medicine Resident Physician
Department of Internal Medicine
Icahn School of Medicine at Mount Sinai
Mount Sinai St. Luke's and Mount Sinai
West Hospitals
New York, New York

John C. Huscher, MD
Associate Professor and Associate
    Program Director
Family Medicine Residency, Rural Training
    Track
University of Nebraska Medical School
Norfolk, Nebraska

Alia A. Hussain, MD, BSc (Hons)[†]
Family Medicine
Creighton University Family Medicine
Omaha, Nebarska

Nida Hussain, MD
Family Medicine Resident
Department of Family Medicine and
    Community Health
University of Texas Health Science Center
San Antonio, Texas

Benjamin Hyatt, MD
Gastroenterologist
Middlesex Gastroenterology
Acton, Massachusetts

Brenda W. Iddins, DNP, FNP-BC
University of Alabama at Birmingham
Birmingham, Alabama

Benjamin Ihms, DO
Osteopathic Manipulative Medicine Director
Mountain Vista Medical Center
Faculty Mountain Vista Medical Center
    Family Medicine Residency Program
Mesa, Arizona

Adedapo Iluyomade, MD, MBA
Cardiovascular Disease Fellow
Division of Cardiovascular Medicine
University of Miami Miller School of
    Medicine
Miami, Florida

Rasheen Syeda Imtiaz, MD
Internal Medicine
Dermatology Resident
Department of Dermatology
University of Oklahoma Health Science
    Center
Oklahoma City, Oklahoma

P. Charles Inboriboon, MD, MPH, FACEP
Associate Professor
Department of Emergency Medicine
University of Missouri–Kansas City
    School of Medicine
Kansas City, Missouri

Kimberly Insel, MD, MPH
Director of Fellowship Programs
Department of Family Medicine
St. Anthony Family Medicine Residency
Westminster, Colorado

Jamal Islam, MD, MS[†]
Associate Professor and Assistant
    Director of Residency Program
Department of Family Medicine
University of Texas Medical Branch
Galveston, Texas

Reem Itani, DO
Internal Medicine Residency Program
Southeastern Health
Lumberton, North Carolina

Pablo Hernandez Itriago, MD, MHCM,
    FAAFP[†]
Chief Medical Officer/Assistant
    Professor
Edward M. Kennedy Community Health
    Center
Department of Family Medicine and
    Community Health
University of Massachusetts Medical
    School
Worcester, Massachusetts

Jacqueline R. Ivey-Brown, MD, FACP
Associate Program Director
Internal Medicine Residency Program
University of Illinois at Chicago/Advocate
    Christ Medical Center
Clinical Assistant Professor
University of Illinois at Chicago
Oak Lawn, Illinois

Anna Loyal Jackson, MD
Psychiatry Resident
Department of Psychiatry and Behavioral
    Sciences
Vanderbilt University Medical Center
Nashville, Tennessee

R. Morgan Jackson, DO[†]
Resident
Family Medicine Residency
Martin Army Community Hospital
Fort Benning, Georgia

Tiphany Jackson, MD
Resident Physician
Department of Obstetrics & Gynecology
Advocate Illinois Masonic Medical Center
Chicago, Illinois

Anna James, DO
Honorhealth Family Medicine Residency
Scottsdale, Arizona

Sarah Jamshed, MD
Department of Pathology
University of Massachusetts Medical
    School
Worcester, Massachusetts

Quratulanne H. Jan, MD
Department of Family Medicine
Henry Ford Health System
Southfield, Michigan

Kyu K. Jana, MD
Assistant Professor
University of Texas Medical Branch
Galveston, Texas

David W. Jang, MD
Assistant Professor
Department of Surgery
Division of Head and Neck Surgery &
    Communication Sciences
Duke University
Durham, North Carolina

Adam J. Janicki, MD[†]
Department of Emergency Medicine
The Warren Alpert Medical School of
    Brown University
Providence, Rhode Island

Elizabeth Janopaul-Naylor, MD
Child & Adolescent Psychiatry Fellow
Department of Child & Adolescent
    Psychiatry
New York University School of Medicine
New York, New York

Kyle Jarnagin, MD[†]
Family Medicine Physician
Lackland Air Force Base, Texas

Lisa N. Jarnagin, MB, BCh, BAO
Department of Internal Medicine
Lahey Hospital & Medical Center
Burlington, Massachusetts

Sana Javed, MD
Neurology Specialist
Panama City, Florida

Salmaan A. Jawaid, MD
Advanced Endoscopy Fellow
University of Florida College of Medicine
Gainesville, Florida

Melissa Jefferis, MD, FAAFP
Associate Program Director
Riverside Methodist Hospital Family
    Medicine Residency Program
Columbus, Ohio

Justin Jenkins, DO, MBA[†]
Assistant Professor
Department of Family Medicine
University of Tennessee Graduate School
    of Medicine
Knoxville, Tennessee

Tarang P. Jethwa, MD, MS
Resident Physician
Department of Family Medicine
Mayo Clinic
Jacksonville, Florida

Trisha E. Jethwa, MD[†]
Family Medicine
Mayo Clinic School of Graduate Medical
    Education
Jacksonville, Florida

Zaiba Jetpuri, DO, MBA, CPH, FAAFP
Director of Medical Student Education in
    Family Medicine
Assistant Professor
Department of Family and Community
    Medicine
University of Texas Southwestern Medical
    Center
Dallas, Texas

Aravdeep Jhand, MD
Resident Physician
Department of Internal Medicine
Creighton University School of Medicine
Omaha, Nebraska

Devi Jhaveri, DO, FAAP, FACOP[†]
Associate Program Director
Allergy Immunology Fellowship
University Hospitals of Cleveland
Case Western Reserve University School
    of Medicine Clinical Faculty
Ohio University Heritage College of
    Osteopathic Medicine
Clinical Assistant Professor
Cleveland, Ohio

Amy Jimenez, BS, IBCLC, RLC

Nasheena Jiwa, MD
Chief Resident
Internal Medicine Residency Program
St. Mary's Hospital Yale University School
    of Medicine
Trinity Health of New England
Waterbury, Connecticut

Anub G. John, MD
Interventional Cardiology Fellow
University of Louisville
Louisville, Kentucky

Brett Johnson, DO[†]
Family Medicine
Mike O'Callaghan Federal Medical Center
Nellis Air Force Base
Las Vegas, Nevada

Jessica Johnson, MD, MPH
Clinical Assistant Professor
Department of Family Medicine
Brown University
Thundermist Health Center
Woonsocket and Pawtucket, Rhode Island

Tisha K. Johnson, MD, MPH[†]
Assistant Professor
Department of Preventive Medicine and
    Environmental Health
University of Kentucky College of Public
    Health
Lexington, Kentucky

Helen N. Johnson-Wall, MD
Associate Program Director
Internal Medicine Residency
Departments of Medical Education and
    Hospital Medicine
Southeastern Regional Medical Center
Lumberton, North Carolina
Campbell University School of
    Osteopathic Medicine
Buies Creek, North Carolina

Julie Ann Johnston, MD
Faculty
Lawrence Family Medicine Residency
Lawrence, Massachusetts
Clinical Instructor
Department of Family Medicine
Tufts University School of Medicine
Boston, Massachusetts

Caitlin E. Jones, MD
General Surgery Resident
Department of Surgery
Medical College of Georgia
Augusta, Georgia

Collin R. Jones, MD
Department of Family Medicine
Mayo Clinic Florida
Jacksonville, Florida

Stacy L. Jones, MD, FASA
Vice Chair for Operations
Department of Anesthesiology
The University of Arkansas for Medical
    Sciences
Little Rock, Arkansas

Melody A. Jordahl-lafrato, MD, FAAFP
Assistant Director
Community East Family Medicine
    Residency Program
Indianapolis, Indiana

Seena Mariate Jose, MD
Family Medicine Resident
University of Texas Health San Antonio
San Antonio, Texas

Sherine Jose, DO
Resident
University of Texas Health Science
    Center of San Antonio Family Medicine
    Residency Program
San Antonio, Texas

Gardith Joseph, MD
Internal Medicine
Icahn School of Medicine at Mount Sinai
Mount Sinai Brooklyn
Brooklyn, New York

Greta M. Josephson, DO
Internal Medicine Resident
University of Illinois at Chicago/Advocate
    Christ Hospital
Chicago/Oak Lawn, Illinois

Arjun S. Joshi, MD, FACS, FRCSC
Associate Professor of Surgery
Director Head and Neck Oncology/
    Microvascular Reconstruction
Division of Otolaryngology–Head and
    Neck Surgery
The George Washington University
Washington, DC

Maurice F. Joyce, MD, EdM
Assistant Professor of Surgery (Anesthesia)
Division of Anesthesia
Lifespan Physicians Group
Warren Alpert Medical School of Brown
    University
Providence, Rhode Island

Patrick Wakefield Joyner, MD, MS[†]
OrthoCollier
Department of Sports Medicine &
    Orthopaedic Surgery
Naples, Florida

Albert Juarez Jr., PA-C[†]
Womack Army Medical Center
Fort Bragg, North Carolina

Melida A. Juarez, MD[†]
Fellow
Department of Hospice and Palliative
    Medicine
The University of Texas Health
    San Antonio
San Antonio, Texas

Sandeep S. Jubbal, MD[†]
Assistant Professor of Medicine
Department of Medicine
University of Massachusetts Medical
    School
Worcester, Massachusetts

Alexandra Jubran, DO, MPH
Resident Physician
Department of Family Medicine
Loma Linda University Health Education
    Consortium
Loma Linda, California

Hani Judeh, MD
Assistant Professor
Internal Medicine
Icahn School of Medicine at Mount Sinai
The Mount Sinai Hospital, Mount Sinai
    St. Luke's, and Mount Sinai West
New York, New York

Tya-Mae Y. Julien, MD[†]
Consultant in Gastroenterology/
    Hepatology
Richardson, Texas

Tipsuda Junsanto-Bahri, MD
Chair
Basic Biomedical Sciences
Assistant Professor
Pathology and Internal Medicine
Touro College of Osteopathic Medicine
New York, New York

Natasha S. Kadakia, DO[†]
Resident
Department of Internal Medicine
University of Illinois at Chicago/Advocate
    Christ Hospital
Oak Lawn, Illinois

Jenna Kahn, MD
Radiation Oncology Resident
Department of Radiation Oncology
Virginia Commonwealth University Health
    System
Richmond, Virginia

Michael B. Kalinowski, DO, MS[†]
Internal Medicine Resident
University of Illinois at Chicago/Advocate
    Christ Medical Center
Oak Lawn, Illinois

Dana J. Kamenetsky, MD
Resident Physician
Department of Internal Medicine
Lahey Hospital and Medical Center
Burlington, Massachusetts

Zachariah John Kamla, DO[†]
Resident
Womack Army Medical Center
Fort Bragg, North Carolina

Danby Kang, MD
General Surgery Resident
Rush University
Chicago, Illinois

Dhivya Kannabiran, MD, FACOG
Assistant Professor of Obstetrics and
    Gynecology
University of Massachusetts Medical
    School
Worcester, Massachusetts

Lovella Duru Kanu, MD
Faculty Attending Physician
Family Medicine Residency Program
Advocate Christ Medical Center
Oak Lawn, Illinois

Amar Kapur, DO†
CPT, MC, USA
Medical Director
JBER–Soldier-Centered Medical Home
Fort Richardson, Alaska

Rahul Kapur, MD, CAQSM
Assistant Professor
Family Medicine and Sports Medicine
Department of Family Medicine and
    Community Health
St. John's Family Medicine Residency
    Program
University of Minnesota Sports Medicine
Minneapolis-St. Paul, Minnesota

Atil Y. Kargi, MD
Program Director, J. Maxwell McKenzie
    Fellowship Program
Associate Professor of Medicine
Division of Endocrinology, Diabetes, and
    Metabolism
University of Miami Miller School of
    Medicine
Miami, Florida

Torin W. Karsonovich, DO
Neurological Surgery Resident
Advocate Bromenn Medical Center
Normal, Illinois

Praneeth Katrapati, MD
Resident Physician
Department of Internal Medicine
University of Louisville School of Medicine
Louisville, Kentucky

Prashanth S. Katrapati, MD, FACC
Attending Cardiologist
Department of Cardiology at Providence
    Medical Center
Kansas City, Kansas

Delila Katz, PharmD, BCOP
Pharmacy Specialist
Palliative Care
Division Palliative Care
University of Massachusetts Memorial
    Medical Center
Worcester, Massachusetts

Anubhav Kaul, MD
Associate Professor
Department of Family Medicine
Loma Linda University School of Medicine
Loma Linda, California

Jasleen Kaur, MD
Intern
Tufts University Department of Family
    Medicine
Cambridge Health Alliance
Malden, Massachusetts

Simranjeet Kaur, MD
Creighton University Family Medicine
Omaha, Nebraska

Michael G. Kavan, PhD
Professor of Family Medicine and Psychiatry
Associate Dean for Student Affairs
Creighton University School of Medicine
Omaha, Nebraska

Ryan Kavilaveettil, DO
Internal Medicine Resident
Southeastern Regional Medical Center
Lumberton, North Carolina

Borna Kavousi, MD
Physical Medicine & Rehabilitation
    Residency Program
SUNY Downstate Medical Center
Brooklyn, New York

Omar El Kawkgi, MD
Internal Medicine Resident
Baystate Health
Springfield, Massachusetts

Fatima M. Kazi, MD†
Resident Physician
Department of Internal Medicine
Advocate Christ Medical Center
Oak Lawn, Illinois

Clara M. Keegan, MD
Assistant Professor
Department of Family Medicine
University of Vermont Medical Center
Burlington, Vermont

Jennifer Tickal Keehbauch, MD, FAAFP†
Associate Professor of Family Medicine
University of Vermont Medical Center
Burlington, Vermont

Brian P. Keene, DO†
Resident
Martin Army Community Hospital
Fort Benning, Georgia

Jeremy R. Kenison, DO†
Senior Medical Officer
USN, MC
Marine Corp Base Hawaii
Kaneohe Bay, Hawaii

Anne Marie Kennedy, DO†
Family Medicine Resident Physician
Eglin Family Medicine Clinic
Eglin Air Force Base, Florida

Tara M. Kennedy, MD
Resident
Department of Family and Community
    Medicine
Pennsylvania State College of Medicine
Hershey, Pennsylvania

Casey P. Kernan, DO
Family Medicine Residency
Northwest Washington
Bremerton, Washington

John Kerr, DO
Resident
OhioHealth Doctors Hospital
Department of Otolaryngology
Columbus, Ohio

Robert M. Kershner, MD, MS, FACS
Eye Physician and Surgeon
Refractive and Cataract Surgery
Professor and Chairman
Department of Ophthalmic Medical
    Technology
Palm Beach State College
Palm Beach Gardens, Florida
President and CEO
Eye Laser Consulting
Consultant Specialist
Biophotonics, Pharmaceutical, and
    Ophthalmic Medical Devices
Palm Beach Gardens, Florida

Todd Kettering, DO, FAAFP
Director of Medical Education
Program Director
Family Medicine
Advocate BroMenn Medical Center
Graduate Medical Education
Normal, Illinois

Tarun Kewalramani, MD
Department of Hematology and Oncology
Lahey Hospital & Medical Center
Burlington, Massachusetts

Misbahuddin Khaja, MD
Attending Physician
Assistant Professor of Medicine
Division of Pulmonary and Critical Care
    Medicine
Bronx Care Health System
Icahn School of Medicine at Mount Sinai
Bronx, New York

Anila Khaliq, MD
Faculty & Primary Care
Orange Regional Medical Center
Tuoro College of Osteopathic Medicine
Department of Family Medicine
Middletown Campus, New York

Abid Khan, MD
Resident
Rush University Medical Center
Chicago, Illinois

Ali A. Khan, MD, MPH
Resident Physician
Internal Medicine
George Washington University
Washington, DC

Aruna S. Khan, MD
Family Medicine Resident
Department of Family Medicine
Mayo Clinic
Jacksonville, Florida

Omar Khan, MD, MHS, FAAFP
Physician Leader of Primary Care and
    Community Medicine
Christiana Care Health System
Wilmington, Delaware
Clinical Associate Professor
Department of Family and Community
    Medicine
Sidney Kimmel Medical College/Thomas
    Jefferson University
Philadelphia, Pennsylvania

Rabeea Khan, MD
Assistant Instructor
Department of Ophthalmology
The University of Texas Southwestern
    Medical Center
Dallas, Texas

Sajid Khan, MD[†]
Assistant Professor of Emergency Medicine
University of Missouri–Kansas City
Kansas City, Missouri

Shiva Kheradmand, DO[†]
Traditional Rotating Intern
Largo Medical Center
Largo, Florida

Teresa Khoo, MD
University of California, Riverside
Riverside, California

John Kiel, DO, MPH[†]
Assistant Professor of Emergency
    Medicine
Assistant Professor of Sports Medicine
University of Florida- Jacksonville College
    of Medicine
Jacksonville, Florida

Christopher R. Kieliszak, DO[†]
Fellow
Facial Plastic and Reconstructive Surgery
Mittelman Plastic Surgery Center
Los Altos, California

Barbara M. Kiersz Muller, DO
Family and Osteopathic Medicine
    Physician
Austin Regional Clinic–Far West
Austin, Texas

Christopher Kim, MD

Daniel Y. Kim, MD, FACS
Chairman
Department of Otolaryngology–Head &
    Neck Surgery
University of Massachusetts
Worcester, Massachusetts

Edward Kim, MD
Resident
University of Texas Health Science Center
    San Antonio Family and Community
    Medicine
San Antonio, Texas

Gemma Kim, MD
Associate Clinical Professor
Department of Family Medicine
University of California, Riverside School
    of Medicine
Riverside, California

Tae K. Kim, MD
Associate Clinical Professor
Department of Family Medicine
University of California, Riverside School
    of Medicine
Riverside, California

Walter M. Kim, MD, PhD
Associate Physician/Instructor
Division of Gastroenterology, Hepatology
    and Endoscopy
Brigham and Women's Hospital
Harvard Medical School
Boston, Massachusetts

Brian J. Kimbrell, MD, FACS
Assistant Professor of Surgery
University of Florida
Trauma Medical Director
Medical Director of Critical Care Medicine
Blake Medical Center
Bradenton, Florida

Rebecca M. King, MD
Resident Physician
Family and Community Medicine
Penn State Health Milton S. Hershey
    Medical Center
Hershey, Pennsylvania

Cecilia M. Kipnis, MD, FAAFP[†]
Assistant Program Director
Naval Hospital Jacksonville Family
    Medicine Residency
Naval Hospital Jacksonville
Jacksonville, Florida

Jeffrey T. Kirchner, DO, FAAFP, AAHIVS
Department of Family and Community
    Medicine
Penn Medicine/LG Health
Lancaster General Hospital
Lancaster, Pennsylvania

Kinga Kiszko, DO[†]
Hospice and Palliative Care Fellow
Northwell Health System
Manhasset, New York

Kimberly S. Klapchar, DO
Otolaryngology and Facial Plastic Surgery
    Residency Program
Doctor's Hospital
Columbus, Ohio

Richard T. Klapchar, DO, FOCOO
Program Director
Ohio Health Ear, Nose, & Throat
    Residency
Doctors Hospital
Columbus, Ohio

Gloria J. Klapstein, PhD
Associate Professor
Department of Basic Sciences
Touro University California College of
    Osteopathic Medicine
Vallejo, California

Ann Klega, MD
Woman's Health Director
Florida Hospital Family Medicine
    Residency Program
Winter Park, Florida

Randolph J. Kline, MD[†]
Family Medicine Resident
David Grant Medical Center
Travis Air Force Base, California

Laura K. Klug, PharmD
Assistant Professor
Departments of Pharmacy Practice
School of Pharmacy and Health
    Professions
Department of Family Medicine
School of Medicine
Creighton University
Omaha, Nebraska

Sandra L. Knaur, APRN, BC
Texas Pulmonary and Critical Care
    Consultants of Texas, PA
Fort Worth, Texas

Karin Britta Knutson, MD
Resident Physician
Department of Obstetrics and Gynecology
University of Massachusetts
Worcester, Massachusetts

Sharon L. Koehler, DO, FACS[†]
Assistant Professor, Breast Surgery
Department of Clinical Specialties
New York Institute of Technology
    College of Osteopathic Medicine
Old Westbury, New York

Kimberly Kone, MD[†]
Resident in Family and Community
    Medicine
University of Texas Southwestern Medical
    Center
Dallas, Texas

Scott E. Kopec, MD
Associate Professor of Medicine
Director of Pulmonary and Critical Care
    Fellowship
Associate Director
Internal Medicine Residency
University of Massachusetts Medical School
Worcester, Massachusetts

Rita A. Kostecke, MD
Family Medicine
Fort Bragg, North Carolina

Rajitha Kota, MD, MPH
Family Medicine Resident
Department of Family Medicine
Saint Joseph Hospital
Chicago, Illinois

Adam W. Kowalski, MD[†]
Family Medicine Residency
Carl R. Darnall Army Medical Center
Fort Hood, Texas

Rudolph M. Krafft, MD, FAAFP
Clinical Professor of Family and
    Community Medicine
Northeast Ohio Medical University
Rootstown, Ohio

Robert J. Krause, MD, MPH, CIME[†]
Aerospace and Occupational Medicine
Department Head
Operational and Aviation Medicine
Branch Clinic Oceana
Naval Medical Center
Portsmouth, Maine

Armand Krikorian, MD, FACE, FACP
Program Director, Internal Medicine
University of Illinois at Chicago/Advocate
    Christ Medical Center
Associate Professor of Clinical Medicine
University of Illinois at Chicago
Oak Lawn, Illinois

Mridula Krishnan, MBBS
Department of Internal Medicine
Creighton University
Omaha, Nebraska

Merrill Krolick, DO, FACC, FACP, FSCAI[†]
Director of Cardiac
International Fellowship
Largo Medical Center
Largo, Florida

David C. Krulak, MD, MPH, MBA,
    FAAFP[†]
Physician
United States Navy
Yokosuka, Japan

David W. Kruse, MD
Orthopaedic Specialty Institute
Associate Faculty
Long Beach Memorial Primary Care
    Sports Medicine Fellowship
Orange, California

E. James Kruse, DO
Associate Professor of Surgery
Chief of Surgical Oncology Section
Department of Surgery
Augusta University
Augusta, Georgia

Archana Kudrimoti, MD, MBBS, MPH
Associate Professor
Residency Program Director
Department of Family and Community
    Medicine
University of Kentucky Health Care at
    Turfland
Lexington, Kentucky

Karl A. Kuersteiner, MD[†]
Chief Resident
Department of Family Medicine
Naval Hospital Jacksonville
Jacksonville, Florida

Jeffrey D. Kueter, MD, FAAFP[†]
Col, MC, USAF
Family Medicine Faculty Physician
Eglin Air Force Base Family Medicine
    Residency
Eglin Air Force Base, Florida

Christina N. Kufel, DO, MS
Resident
Obstetrics and Gynecology
Aultman Hospital
Canton, Ohio

Keshav Kukreja, MD[†]
Department of Internal Medicine
University of Texas Health Sciences
    Center at Houston
Houston, Texas

Ajoy Kumar, MD, FAAFP
Chief Medical Officer
Bayfront Health St. Petersburg
St. Petersburg, Florida

Vineet Kumar, MD
Division of Cardiovascular Disease
University of Alabama at Birmingham
    School of Medicine
Birmingham, Alabama

Sabrina E. Kunciw, MD[†]
Family Medicine Physician
121st Combat Support Hospital/Brian
    Allgood Community Hospital
USAG Yongsan, South Korea

Jason Kurland, MD
Associate Professor of Medicine
Division of Renal Medicine
University of Massachusetts Medical School
Worcester, Massachusetts

Daniel B. Kurtz, PhD, BS[†]
Associate Professor and Chair, Biology
Utica College
Utica, New York

Melinda Y. Kwan, DO, MPH
Urgent Care/Family Medicine Physician
Urgent Care Department
Southwest Medical Associates
Las Vegas, Nevada

Kiet T. La, MD
Family Medicine Resident
Bayfront Health St. Petersburg
St. Petersburg, Florida

Rita M. Lahlou, MD, MPH
Assistant Professor
Department of Family Medicine
Oregon Health & Science University
Portland, Oregon

Jeffrey Lai, MD
Department of Emergency Medicine
University of Massachusetts Medical School
Worcester, Massachusetts

John E. Laird, MD, FAAFP, FAAMA[†]
CDR, MC, USN
Assistant Professor
Uniformed Services University of the
    Health Sciences
Department of Family Medicine
Naval Hospital, Guam

R. Aaron Lambert, MD, FAAFP
Associate Professor of Family Medicine
Cabarrus Family Medicine Residency
    Program
Concord, North Carolina

J.E. Lambrecht, MD, PharmD, FACP, FSHM[†]
Assistant Professor
Department of Internal Medicine
Creighton University School of Medicine
Omaha, Nebraska

Stephen K. Lane, MD
Scituate Family Practice
Healthcare South, PC
Scituate, Massachusetts

Michael Lao, MD
Fellow in Men's Health/Infertility/ Andrology
Smith Institute of Urology
Northwell Health
Lake Success, New York

Eduardo Lara-Torre, MD, FACOG
Vice-Chairman for Academic Affairs
Section Chief
Academic Specialists in General Obstetrics and Gynecology
Carilion Clinic
Professor
Departments of Obstetrics and Gynecology and Pediatrics
Virginia Tech Carilion School of Medicine
Roanoke, Virginia

Deborah A. Lardner, DO, DTM&H
Assistant Professor
Department of Family Medicine
Department of Emergency Medicine
New York Institute of Technology College of Osteopathic Medicine
New York Institute of Technology Center for Global Health
Old Westbury, New York

Shane L. Larson, MD[†]
Assistant Professor of Family Medicine
Uniformed Services University of the Health Sciences
Bethesda, Maryland

Tiana M. Larsow, MD, CAQSM
Assistant Professor
Department of Surgery
Frank H. Netter, MD School of Medicine at Quinnipiac University
St. Vincent's Medical Center
Bridgeport, Connecticut

Kristin Yeung Lasseter, MD
Resident Physician
Department of Psychiatry
Dell Medical School at The University of Texas at Austin
Austin, Texas

Linda Lau, MD, FAAFP
Clinical Faculty
Mountain Vista Family Medicine Residency Program
Clinical Faculty
Midwestern University
Arizona College of Osteopathic Medicine
Mesa, Arizona

Julianne Lauring, MD[†]
Assistant Professor of Obstetrics and Gynecology
Department of Obstetrics and Gynecology
Division of Maternal–Fetal Medicine
University of Massachusetts Medical Center
Worcester, Massachusetts

Rebecca Lauters, MD[†]
Family Medicine with Obstetrics Staff
Eglin Air Force Base Family Medicine Residency Program
Eglin Air Force Base, Florida

Justin P. Lavin Jr., MD
Chairman Emeritus
Department of Obstetrics and Gynecology
Cleveland Clinic Akron General
Professor Emeritus
Northeastern Ohio Medical University
Akron, Ohio

Victoria Lawn, DO, MPH
Obstetrics and Gynecology
Lehigh Valley Health Network
Allentown, Pennsylvania

Ashik Lawrence, MD
Resident
East Jefferson General Hospital
Metairie, Louisiana

Kelley V. Lawrence, MD, IBCLC, FAAFP, FABM
Associate Program Director
Novant Health Family Medicine Residency
Cornelius, North Carolina

Lima Lawrence, MD
Endocrine Fellow
Department of Endocrinology and Metabolism Institute
Cleveland Clinic
Cleveland, Ohio

Miles C. Layton, DO[†]
Major, Medical Corps
Officer in Charge
Gastroenterology Clinic
Faculty of Family Medicine Residency
Martin Army Community Hospitals
Fort Benning, Georgia

Thuy Thanh Thi Le, DO
Internal Medicine Resident
Southeastern Regional Medical Center
Lumberton, North Carolina

Eleanor D. Lederer, MD, FASN
Kidney Disease Program
University of Louisville Hospital
Louisville, Kentucky

Andrew G. Lee, MD
Professor of Ophthalmology, Neurology, and Neurosurgery, Institute for Academic Medicine
Full Clinical Member, Research Institute
Chair, Department of Ophthalmology-Blanton Eye Institute
Houston Methodist
Weill Cornell Medical College
Houston, Texas

Bianca Lee, DO, MS
Nassau University Medical Center
Department of Internal Medicine
East Meadow, New York

Daniel T. Lee, MD, MA
Clinical Professor of Family Medicine
David Geffen School of Medicine at University of California Los Angeles
Associate Director
University of California Los Angeles Family Medicine Residency Program
Santa Monica, California

David L. Lee, MD
Resident
Department of Family and Community Medicine
Penn State Health Milton S. Hershey Medical Center
Hershey, Pennsylvania

Hanna J. Lee, MD
Assistant Professor
Division of Endocrinology, Diabetes and Bone Diseases
Icahn School of Medicine at Mount Sinai
New York, New York

Hobart Lee, MD, FAAFP
Assistant Professor
Family Medicine Residency Program Director
Department of Family Medicine
Loma Linda University
Loma Linda, California

Vivian Lee, MD
George Washington University School of Medicine and Health Sciences
Washington, DC

F. Stuart Leeds, MD, MS
Assistant Professor of Family Medicine
Department of Family Medicine
Wright State University Boonshoft School
    of Medicine
Dayton, Ohio

Angelia Leipelt, BA, IBCLC, ICCE, CLE
Lactation Consultant
Dignity Health Methodist Hospital of
    Sacramento
Sacramento, California

Elise Leisinger, DO[†]
CPT, MC
Faculty
Womack Family Medicine Residency
Fort Bragg, North Carolina

Edgar V. Lerma, MD, FACP, FASN,
    FPSN (Hon)[†]
Clinical Professor of Medicine
Section of Nephrology
University of Illinois at Chicago College
    of Medicine/Advocate Christ Medical
    Center
Oak Lawn, Illinois

Maya Leventer-Roberts, MD, MPH
Deputy Director
Clalit Research Institute
Tel Aviv, Israel
Adjunct Assistant Professor, Pediatrics
    and Preventive Medicine
Icahn School of Medicine at Mount Sinai
New York, New York

Jarad Levin, MD
Assistant Professor
Department of Dermatology
Oklahoma University Health Sciences
    Center
Oklahoma City, Oklahoma

Nikki A. Levin, MD, PhD
Associate Professor
Department of Dermatology
University of Massachusetts Medical
    School
Worcester, Massachusetts

Gary I. Levine, MD
Associate Professor
Department of Family Medicine
Brody School of Medicine
East Carolina University
Greenville, North Carolina

Keidren Lewi, MD[†]
Family Medicine Resident
Department of Family Medicine
Creighton University Medical School
Omaha, Nebraska

Brent M. Lewis, MD
Emergency Medicine Resident
Rutgers Robert Wood Johnson Medical
    School
New Brunswick, New Jersey

Douglas P. Lewis, MD, FAAFP
Director
Via Christi Family Medicine Residency
Associate Director
Via Christi Adult Cystic Fibrosis Specialty
    Clinic
Assistant Clinical Professor
Kansas University School of Medicine–
    Wichita
Wichita, Kansas

Jonathan T. Lin, MD
Instructor in Medicine
Division of Nephrology and Hypertension
Weill Cornell Medicine
Nephrologist
The Rogosin Institute
New York, New York

Christopher Lin-Brande, MD[†]
Emergency Services Physician
Osan Air Base, Republic of Korea

Briana Lindberg, MD[†]
Chief Resident
Department of Family Medicine
Womack Army Medical Center
Fort Bragg, North Carolina

Mary S. Lindholm, MD[†]
Associate Professor and Third Year
    Clerkship Director
Department of Family Medicine and
    Community Health
University of Massachusetts Medical School
Worcester, Massachusetts

Chang L. Lipinski, DO[†]
Resident Physician
Department of Family and Community
    Medicine
Penn State Hershey Medical Center
Hershey, Pennsylvania

Melanie J. Lippmann, MD
Associate Professor of Emergency
    Medicine
Brown University
Alpert Medical School
Providence, Rhode Island

Katelin M. Lisenby, PharmD, BCPS
Assistant Clinical Professor of Pharmacy
    Practice
Auburn University Harrison School of
    Pharmacy
Department of Internal, Family, and Rural
    Medicine
University of Alabama College of
    Community Health Sciences
Tuscaloosa, Alabama

Kimberly E. Liu, MD
Assistant Professor
Department of Obstetrics and Gynecology
University of Toronto
Toronto, Ontario, Canada

Samuel Livingston, MD, FAAFP[†]
Faculty Family Physician
Naval Hospital Jacksonville
Jacksonville Family Medicine Residency
    Program
Jacksonville, Florida

Jenifer R. Lloyd, DO, FAAD
Dermatology Program Director
University Hospitals
Richmond Heights Hospital
Case Western Reserve University
Cleveland, Ohio

Vincent Lo, MD, FAAFP
Methodist Family Medicine Residency
Sacramento, California

Derek Lodico, DO[†]
Associate Professor
F. Edward Hebert School of Medicine
Chief Cardiothoracic Anesthesia
Department of Anesthesia, Critical Care,
    and Pain Medicine
Walter Reed National Military Medical
    Center
Bethesda, Maryland

Jayson R. Loeffert, DO[†]
Assistant Professor
Department of Orthopedics and
    Rehabilitation and Family and
    Community Medicine
Penn State Health
Hershey, Pennsylvania

Maria Lombardi, DO
Assistant Professor
Department of Pediatrics
New York Medical College
Valhalla, New York

Marissa A. Lombardo, MD
Cardiovascular Medicine Fellow
Department of Cardiology
New York University Langone Health
New York, New York

David London, MD
The University of Texas Health Science
   Center at Houston
Houston, Texas

Maria Cynthia S. Lopez, MD
Director of Community Medicine
Family Medicine Residency Program
Adventist Health White Memorial
Los Angeles, California

Elida M. Lopez Villa, MD[†]
Department of Family and Community
   Medicine
University of Texas Health Science
   Center at San Antonio
San Antonio, Texas

Anthony Lorusso, MD
Assistant Professor
Family Medicine
University of Massachusetts Medical School
UMass Memorial Medical Center
Worcester, Massachusetts

Bency K. Louidor-Paulynice, MD
Family Medicine
University of Massachusetts Medical
   School
Worcester, Massachusetts

John R. Luksch, DO
Chief Resident
Department of Family Medicine
Rowan University School of Osteopathic
   Medicine
Stratford, New Jersey

Marie Luksch, DO
Obstetrics and Gynecology
Paoli Hospital
Paoli, Pennsylvania

Thanh-Ha Luong, MD
Attending
Hematology & Oncology
BronxCare Health System
Bronx, New York

Alicia G. Lydecker, MD
Assistant Professor
Department of Emergency Medicine
Division of Medical Toxicology
Albany Medical Center
Albany, New York

Ann M. Lynch, PharmD, RPh, AE-C
Professor of Pharmacy Practice
Department of Pharmacy Practice
Massachusetts College of Pharmacy and
   Health Sciences University
Worcester, Massachusetts

Jonathan MacClements, MD, FAAFP
Professor and Assistant Dean of
   Graduate Medical Education
Designated Institutional Official
Dell Medical School, University of Texas
   at Austin
Austin, Texas

Marina MacNamara, MD, MPH
Family Physician
Mission Health
Asheville, North Carolina

Douglas W. MacPherson, MD,
   MSc–CTM, FRCPC[†]
Associate Professor
Department of Pathology and Molecular
   Medicine
Michael G. DeGroote School of Medicine
Hamilton, Ontario, Canada
Department of Medicine (Infectious
   Diseases)
St. Thomas Elgin General Hospital
St. Thomas, Ontario, Canada

Michael Maddaleni, MD
Family Medicine Resident
Department of Family Medicine and
   Community Health
University of Massachusetts Medical
   School
Worcester, Massachusetts

Andrea Madrigrano, MD[†]
Assistant Professor
Department of Surgery
Rush University Medical Center
Chicago, Illinois

Adela S. Magallanes, MD
Resident Physician
Family & Community Medicine
Penn State Milton S. Hershey Medical
   Center
Hershey, Pennsylvania

Michelle Magid, MD, MBA[†]
President
Austin PsychCare PA
Clinical Associate Professor
Department of Psychiatry
University of Texas, Dell Medical School
Austin, Texas

Keri Maher, DO
Hematology/Oncology Fellow
University of Arizona
Tucson, Arizona

Deepali Maheshwari, DO, MPH[†]
Fellow
Female Pelvic Medicine & Reconstructive
   Surgery
Department of Obstetrics & Gynecology
University of Massachusetts Medical
   School
Worcester, Massachusetts

Christina A. Majd, MD
Resident Physician
Department of Family and Community
   Medicine
University of Texas Health Science Center
   at San Antonio
San Antonio, Texas

Maricarmen Malagon-Rogers, MD
Pediatric Nephrologist
Associate Professor of Family Medicine
University of Tennessee Graduate School
   of Medicine
Knoxville, Tennessee

Samir Malkani, MD, MRCP–UK
Professor of Medicine
Diabetes Center of Excellence
University of Massachusetts Medical
   School
Worcester, Massachusetts

Michael A. Malone, MD[†]
Associate Professor
Department of Family and Community
   Medicine
Penn State College of Medicine
Hershey, Pennsylvania

Dejon Maloney, MD[†]
Resident Physician
Family Medicine Residency
Bayfront Health St. Petersburg
St. Petersburg, Florida

Mary Maloney, MD
Professor of Medicine and Director of
   Dermatologic Surgery
University of Massachusetts Medical School
Worcester, Massachusetts

Alison Mancuso, DO, FACOFP
Associate Professor
Vice Chair & Residency Program Director
Department of Family Medicine
Rowan University School of Osteopathic
   Medicine
Stratford, New Jersey

Krishna Manda, MD, MRCP
Renal Medicine
University of Massachusetts Memorial
   Health Care
Worcester, Massachusetts

Yugandhar Manda, MD

Matthew J. Mandell, DO
Internal Medicine Resident Physician
University of Illinois at Chicago College
of Medicine/Advocate Christ Medical
Center
Oak Lawn, Illinois

Megha Manek, MD[†]
Assistant Professor of Family Medicine
and Community Health
Southern Illinois University
Carbondale, Illinois

Eric J. Mao, MD
Assistant Clinical Professor
Department of Internal Medicine
Division of Gastroenterology
University of California, Davis
Sacramento, California

Jessica Marabella, MD
Family Medicine Physician
Chicago, Illinois

Jyothi Margapuri, MD
Geriatrics Fellow
Department of Geriatrics Medicine
University of Massachusetts Medical School
Worcester, Massachusetts

Michelle D. Marieni, MD
Resident Physician
Department of Obstetrics and Gynecology
University of Massachusetts Medical
School
Worcester, Massachusetts

Wendy K. Marsh, MD, MS
Associate Professor
Department of Psychiatry
Director
Bipolar Disorders and Depression
Specialty Clinics
University of Massachusetts Medical
School
Worcester, Massachusetts

Cara Marshall, MD
Associate Program Director
Lawrence Family Medicine Residency
Lawrence, Massachusetts

Christopher A. Marshall, MD
Assistant Professor of Medicine
Division of Gastroenterology
Department of Medicine
University of Massachusetts Medical
School
Worcester, Massachusetts

Michelle Martin, PharmD, FCCP, BCPS,
BCACP
Clinical Pharmacist
University of Illinois at Chicago Hospital
and Health Sciences System
Clinical Associate Professor
University of Illinois at Chicago College of
Pharmacy
Chicago, Illinois

Rafael F. Martin, MD
Professor and Acting Chair
Department of Dermatology
University of Puerto Rico School of
Medicine
San Juan, Puerto Rico

Stephen A. Martin, MD, EdM
Associate Professor
Department of Family Medicine and
Community Health
Barre Family Health Center
University of Massachusetts Medical
School
Barre, Massachusetts

Gustavo Adolfo Martin Small, MD
Family Medicine and Community Health
Resident
Unitat Docent Medicina Familiar y
Comunitaria
Costa de Ponent
Barcelona, Spain

Dennis Martinez, DO
Faculty
Department of Internal Medicine
Advocate Christ Medical Center
Clinical Instructor
University of Illinois at Chicago
Chicago, Illinois

Marni L. Martinez, APRN
Austin Gastroenterology
Austin, Texas

Joseph Marvin, MD
Family and Community Medicine
Penn State Health
Milton S. Hershey Medical Center
Hershey, Pennsylvania

Sandra Marwill, MD, MPH
Staff Physician
Internal Medicine
Edward M. Kennedy Community Health
Center
Framingham, Massachusetts

Haidy Marzouk, MD[†]
Assistant Professor
State University of New York Upstate
Medical Center
Department of Otolaryngology and
Communication Sciences
Syracuse, New York

Jack Masur, MD
George Washington University School of
Medicine & Health Sciences
Washington, DC

Jared H. Mataska, MD
Chief Resident
Department of Family & Community
Medicine
Texas Tech University Health Sciences
Center
Lubbock, Texas

Donnah Mathews, MD
Assistant Professor
Alpert School of Brown University
Medical Director of Clinical Management
Rhode Island Hospital
Chief Compliance Officer
Brown Medicine
Associate Medical Director
Hope Hospice of Rhode Island
Providence, Rhode Island

Samuel E. Mathis, MD[†]
Assistant Professor
Department of Family Medicine
University of Texas Medical Branch
Galveston, Texas

Nidha Mattappally, MD
Department of Obstetrics & Gynecology
University of Massachusetts Medical
School
Worcester, Massachusetts

Kimberly E. Matz, DO
Family Medicine Resident
Department of Graduate Medical Education
Trios Health
Kennewick, Washington

Rebecca N. Matz, MD[†]
MAJ, USAF
Physician
Department of Dermatology
Keesler Air Force Base, Mississippi

Douglas M. Maurer, DO, MPH, FAAFP[†]
Associate Professor of Family Medicine
Uniformed Services University of the
Health Sciences
Bethesda, Maryland
University of Washington School of
Medicine
Seattle, Washington

George Maxted, MD
CPT, USPHS (ret)
Family Medicine and Geriatrics
Associate Clinical Professor
Tufts University School of Medicine
Boston, Massachusetts

Beth K. Mazyck, MD
Associate Professor
Department of Family Medicine and
    Community Health
University of Massachusetts Medical
    School
Worcester, Massachusetts

Thomas Mazzoni, DO, FAOCO, RPh
Clinical Instructor
New York College of Osteopathic
    Medicine
Department of Otolaryngology/Facial
    Plastic Surgery
Saint Barnabas Medical Center/Robert
    Wood Johnson (RWJBarnabas Health)
Livingston, New Jersey

Frank M. Mazzotta, DO
Clinical Instructor
Family and Community Medicine
Thomas Jefferson University Hospital
Philadelphia, Pennsylvania

Andrew McBride, MD, CAQSM
Clinical Instructor
University of Colorado Department of
    Family Medicine
Boulder Community Health
Boulder, Colorado

David B. McCaleb, MD
Chief Resident
Family Medicine Residency
Bayfront Health St. Petersburg
St. Petersburg, Florida

Kelly McCants, MD
Piedmont Heart Institute
Atlanta, Georgia

Jason C. McCarthy, MD[†]
Travis Air Force Base Family Medicine
    Residency
Travis Air Force Base, California

Madeline L. McCarthy, MD, MS
Assistant Professor Pediatrics
Division of Pediatric Emergency Medicine
University of Massachusetts Memorial
    Medical Center
Worcester, Massachusetts

Charles J. McClure, DO[†]
Family Medicine Residency
Madigan Army Medical Center
Tacoma, Washington

Margaret J. McCormick, MS, RN, CNE
Clinical Associate Professor
Towson University
Towson, Maryland

KrisEmily McCrory, MD, FAAFP
Core Faculty
Ellis Family Medicine Residency
Schenectady, New York

Bradley McCullough, DO[†]
Travis Family Medicine Residency
David Grant Medical Center
Travis Air Force Base
Fairfield, California

Sarah C. McCullough, DO[†]
Family Medicine Residency
Eglin Air Force Base, Florida

Andrew J. McDermott, MD, FAAFP[†]
Faculty, Family Medicine Residency
    Program
Naval Hospital Jacksonville
Jacksonville, Florida

Jonathan McDivitt, MD[†]
Cardiologist
United States Naval Ship
    Comfort—T AH 20
Norfolk, Virginia

Ian J. McDowell, DO[†]
Family Medicine Physician
51st Medical Operation Squadron
Osan Air Base, Korea

Jeannette M. McIntyre, MD[†]
Resident
Department of Family Medicine
Naval Hospital Jacksonville
Jacksonville, Florida

Marc W. McKenna, MD
Program Director
Chestnut Hill Family Medicine Residency
Philadelphia, Pennsylvania

J. Andrew McKenzie, MD
General Surgery Resident
Department of Surgery
Medical College of Georgia at Augusta
    University
Augusta, Georgia

Jaine L. McKenzie, MD
General Surgery Resident
Department of Surgery
Medical College of Georgia at Augusta
    University
Augusta, Georgia

Brian McKinnon, MD, MBA, MPH,
    FCPP, FACS
Associate Professor and Vice Chair
Department of Otolaryngology—Head &
    Neck Surgery
Associate Professor
Department of Neurosurgery
Drexel University College of Medicine
Philadelphia, Pennsylvania

Donna-Marie McMahon, DO, FAAP
Associate Professor of Pediatrics
New York Institute of Technology College
    of Osteopathic Medicine
Old Westbury, New York

Vanessa W. McNair, MD, MPH[†]
Assistant Professor of Family Medicine
Jacksonville Family Medicine Residency
Naval Hospital Jacksonville
Jacksonville, Florida

Cody D. Mead, DO, FAAFP[†]
MAJ, MC, USA
Deputy Commander
Clinical Services
Raymond W. Bliss Army Health Center
Fort Huachuca, Arizona

Toussaint L. Mears-Clarke, MD
Faculty Physician
Family Medicine Residency Program
Departments of Family Medicine/
    Obstetrics & Gynecology
Director of Obstetrics Education
Dignity Health Methodist Hospital of
    Sacramento
Sacramento, California

Nolberto Adrián Medina-Gallardo, MD,
    PhD[†]
Digestive and General Surgeon Specialist
Attending of the Department of General
    Surgery
Hospital Universitari de Vic
Consorci Hospitalari de Vic
Vic, Barcelona, Spain

Paavan Mehta, MD
University of Massachusetts Medical
    School
Worcester, Massachusetts

M. Tyler Melson, DO
Cullman Regional Urgent Care Center
Cullman, Alabama

Donna I. Meltzer, MD
Clinical Associate Professor
Department of Family, Population &
    Preventive Medicine
State University of New York Stony Brook
Stony Brook, New York

Megan H. Mendez Miller, DO[†]
Assistant Professor
Department of Family and Community
    Medicine
Penn State Health Milton S. Hershey
    Medical Center
Hershey, Pennsylvania

Caleb J. Mentzer, DO
Assistant Professor
Division of Trauma, Critical Care, & Acute
    Care Surgery
Spartanburg Medical Center
Spartanburg, South Carolina

Marcelle Meseeha, MD
Internal Medicine Hospitalist
Guthrie/Robert Packer Hospital
Sayre, Pennsylvania

Nessa S. Meshkaty, MD
Infectious Disease Department
Baystate Medical Center
Springfield, Massachusetts

Christopher D. Meyering, DO[†]
Fort Knox, Kentucky

Christina Mezzone, DO, MS
Chief Resident
Department of Pediatrics
Maria Fareri Children's Hospital at
    Westchester Medical Center
Valhalla, New York

Alyssa Miceli, DO[†]
Resident Physician
Department of Dermatology
Orange Park Medical Center
Orange Park, Florida

Nicholas J. Michols, DO, ATC[†]
Medical Corps Officer
United States Navy
Norfolk, Virginia

Tracy O. Middleton, DO, FACOFP
Chair and Clinical Professor
Midwestern University
Arizona College of Osteopathic Medicine
Glendale, Arizona

Jeffrey M. Milch, DO[†]
MAJ, MC (Flight Surgeon)
Fox Army Health Center
Redstone Arsenal, Alabama

Mariya Milko, DO, MS
Largo, Florida

Heidi S. Millard, MD
Assistant Clinical Faculty
University of California, Riverside School
    of Medicine
Riverside, California

Kennon Miller, MD
Chief of Urology
Memorial Hospital of Rhode Island
Providence, Rhode Island

Paul G. Millner, MD
Assistant Professor of Medicine
Department of Internal Medicine
CHI Health
Creighton University Medical Center
Omaha, Nebraska

Stacey L. Milunic, MD
Assistant Professor of Family and
    Community Medicine
Penn State College of Medicine
Hershey, Pennsylvania

Jasmit S. Minhas, MD[†]
Resident Physician
Department of Internal Medicine
Lahey Hospital & Medical Center
Burlington, Massachusetts

Osmaan A. Minhas, DO
Urgent Care Physician
Orange Regional Medical Center
Middletown, New York

Suzanne Minor, MD, FAAFP
Clerkship Director
Family Medicine
Assistant Professor
Division of Family Medicine
Department of Humanities, Health, and
    Society
Herbert Wertheim College of Medicine
Florida International University
Miami, Florida

Mark M. Minot, MD, MSEE, PhD, MBA
Core Faculty, Family Medicine Residency
    Program
Eisenhower Health 365 Primary Care
Eisenhower Medical Center
Rancho Mirage, California

Tasaduq Hussain Mir, MD, FAAFP
Assistant Professor
Department of Family & Community
    Medicine
University of Texas Southwestern
    Medical Center
Dallas, Texas

Zeeshan Mirza, MD
Clinical Research Head, Neck and Lung
University of Oklahoma Health Science
    Center
Oklahoma City, Oklahoma

Andrew B. Mitchell, MD
Department of Surgery
Augusta University
Augusta, Georgia

Cory N. Mitchell, MD
Providence Family Medicine—Walla Walla
Walla Walla, Washington

Lauren C. Mitchell, DO[†]
Resident
Family Medicine
David Grant Medical Center
Travis Air Force Base, California

Kriti Mittal, MD, MS, FACP
Assistant Professor
Division of Hematology Oncology
Department of Medicine
University of Massachusetts
Worcester, Massachusetts

Saadia Mohsin, MD
Resident Physician
Family Medicine
Summa Barberton Hospital
Barberton, Ohio

Cesar R. Mojica Vazquez, MD[†]
Chief Resident
Family Medicine
Naval Hospital Jacksonville
Jacksonville, Florida

Tin Ming Timothy Mok, MD
Family Physician
Avera Marshall Regional Medical Center
Marshall, Minnesota

Daniel Molinar, MD
Family Medicine Resident
University of Massachusetts Fitchburg
    Family Medicine
Fitchburg, Massachusetts

Katherine Montag Schafer, PharmD,
    BCACP
Assistant Professor
Department of Family Medicine and
    Community Health
University of Minnesota Medical School
Minneapolis, Minnesota

Jahan Montague, MD[†]
Clinical Associate Professor of Medicine
Director Nephrology Fellowship
University of Massachusetts Medical School
Worcester, Massachusetts

Maria Montanez Villacampa, MD
Assistant Professor/Clinical
University of Texas Health Science San
    Antonio
San Antonio, Texas

Aaron L. Moody, MD[†]
LT, MC, USN
Family Medicine
7th Marine Regiment Medical Officer
Twentynine Palms, California

Judson A. Moore, MD[†]
Pediatric Cardiology Fellow
Department of Pediatrics
Baylor College of Medicine
Houston, Texas

Michael B. Moore, DO[†]
Attending Physician and Medical Director
Baumholder AHC
Department of Family Medicine
Landstuhl Army Medical Center
Landstuhl, Germany

Stephen Morais, MD, MBA, MS
Rheumatology Fellow
Department of Rheumatology
University of Massachusetts Medical
    School
Worcester, Massachusetts

Jonathan Moreira, MD
Hematology and Medical Oncology
Northwestern Medical Group
Chicago, Illinois

Wynne S. Morgan, MD
Assistant Professor of Psychiatry
Division of Child & Adolescent Psychiatry
Department of Psychiatry
University of Massachusetts Medical
    School
Worcester, Massachusetts

Michael G. Morkos, MD, MS[†]
Assistant Professor
Department of Endocrinology, Diabetes,
    and Metabolism
Indiana University
Avon, Indiana

Jesse A. Morse, MD, MBA
Florida Orthopaedic Specialists
Port St. Lucie, Florida

Bassem M. Mostafa Elsawy, MD,
    FAAFP, CMD[†]
Teaching Faculty
Family Medicine, Geriatric Medicine
Methodist Charlton Family Medicine
    Residency Program
Dallas, Texas

Timothy F. Mott, MD[†]
Assistant Professor
Family Medicine
Uniformed Services University of Health
    Sciences
Bethesda, Maryland

Corey Mottesheard, DO
Family Medicine Physician
Davidson, North Carolina

Josiah Moulton, DO
Resident
Scott Air Force Base
Saint Louis University
Belleville, Illinois

Mohammad Ansar Mughal, MD[†]
Community Medicine Associate
University Health System
San Antonio, Texas

Shani I. Muhammad, MD
Family Medicine Physician
Kaiser Permanente Fresno Medical
    Center
Fresno, California

S. Mimi Mukherjee, PharmD, BCPS,
    CDE
Associate Professor of Pharmacy Practice
Massachusetts College of Pharmacy and
    Health Science University
Worcester, Massachusetts
Clinical Pharmacist
Edward M. Kennedy Community Health
    Center
Framingham, Massachusetts

Heidi E. K. Mullen, DO
Midwestern University
Downers Grove, Illinois

Sahil Mullick, MD
Assistant Clinical Professor
Department of Family Medicine
Creighton University Medical Center
Omaha, Nebraska

Ahmed Munir, MBBS[†]
Resident Physician
Department of Internal Medicine
Creighton University Medical Center
Omaha, Nebraska

Amanda B. Murchison, MD
Associate Professor and Residency
    Program Director
Department of Obstetrics and Gynecology
Virginia Tech Carilion School of Medicine
Roanoke, Virginia

Gregory P. Murphy, MD[†]
Assistant Professor of Urologic Surgery
Washington University Medical School
St. Louis, Missouri

Evangelia Murray, MD, MS
University of Massachusetts Medical School
Worcester, Massachusetts

Ghulam Murtaza, MD
Chief Medical Resident
NCH Healthcare System
Naples, Florida

Mark T. Nadeau, MD, MBA[†]
Professor and Program Director
Department of Family and Community
    Medicine
University of Texas Health Science Center
    at San Antonio
San Antonio, Texas

Stuti Nagpal, MD, FAAFP
Assistant Professor
Department of Family and Community
    Medicine
University of Texas Health Science Center
    at San Antonio
San Antonio, Texas

Adithi Naidu, MD, ABFM, CCFP
Family Medicine Physician
Enhanced Care Clinic
Etobicoke, Ontario, Canada

Turya Nair, MD
Assistant Professor and Associate
    Residency Program Director
Department of Family and Community
    Medicine
University of Texas Southwestern
Dallas, Texas

Eddie Nance, MD, MS
Family Medicine Residency Program
Naval Hospital Jacksonville
Jacksonville, Florida

S. Humayun Naqvi, MD, MBA
Internal Medicine Resident
Department of Internal Medicine
University of Texas-McGovern Medical
    School
Houston, Texas

Syed Jaan Naqvi, MD
Ross University School of Medicine
Miramar, Florida

Munima Nasir, MD
Assistant Professor
Department of Family and Community
    Medicine
Penn State Milton S. Hershey Medical
    Center
Penn State Health
Hershey, Pennsylvania

David Navel, MD[†]
Assistant Professor
Department of Family Medicine
Uniformed Services University of the
    Health Sciences
Bethesda, Maryland

Reethu K. Nayak, MD[†]
Family Medicine Resident
Department of Family and Community
    Medicine
University of Texas Health Science Center
    at San Antonio
San Antonio, Texas

Jessica C. Nazzaro, DO
Obstetrics and Gynecology Resident
Aultman Hospital
Canton, Ohio

Chisalu Tessa Nchekwube, MD, MBA
Resident
Department of Family Medicine
Advocate Christ Medical Center
Hometown, Illinois

James G. Nee, MD, FAAFP
Clinical Faculty
Department of Family Medicine
University of Illinois at Chicago
Amita Health Saint Joseph Hospital
Chicago, Illinois

Michael O. Needham, MD[†]
United States Army Health Clinic
    Kaiserslautern
Kaiserslautern, Germany

Nanako Negome-Kapur, PsyD
Primary Care Behaviorist
Hawai'i Pacific Health
Honolulu, Hawaii

Justin Bowen Neisler, MD
St. Anthony North Family Medicine
    Residency
Westminster, Colorado

Vicki R. Nelson, MD, PhD
Clinical Assistant Professor
Department of Family Medicine, Sports
    Medicine
University of South Carolina School of
    Medicine—Greenville
Greenville, South Carolina

Sarah Nester, MD
Family Medicine Resident
Department of Family and Community
    Medicine
University of Kentucky College of
    Medicine
Lexington, Kentucky

Brian E. Neubauer, MD[†]
Assistant Professor of Medicine
Uniformed Services University of the
    Health Sciences
Bethesda, Maryland

Nancy V. Nguyen, DO
Clinical Faculty Physician
Mercy Methodist Family Medicine
    Residency Program
Sacramento, California

Tam T. Nguyen, MD
Clinical Instructor
Department of Family Medicine
Washington Township Medical Group
Fremont, California

Tran K. Nguyen, MD[†]
Department of Family and Community
    Medicine
University of Texas Health San Antonio
San Antonio, Texas

Tu Dan (Kathy) Nguyen, MD
Primary Care Sports Medicine Physician
Clinical Assistant Professor
McGovern Medical School
Memorial Hermann Medical Group
Houston, Texas

Yummy Nguyen, MD[†]
Family Medicine Physician
Naval Hospital Pensacola
Pensacola, Florida

Brian D. Nicholas, MD[†]
Associate Professor
Department of Otolaryngology and
    Communication Sciences
Upstate Medical University
Syracuse, New York

Caitlin A. Nicholson, MD
Resident Physician
Department of Family Medicine and
    Community Health
University of Pennsylvania Health System
Philadelphia, Pennsylvania

Frederick W. Nielson, MD[†]
MAJ, USAF, MC
Medical Director Family Health
Spangdahlem Air Base, Germany

Kathy Niu, MD[†]
Resident
Department of Neurology and Psychiatry
University of Massachusetts Medical
    School
Worcester, Massachusetts

Thomas Noh, MD
Resident
Department of Neurological Surgery
Henry Ford Hospital
Detroit, Michigan

Laura Novak, MD
Associate Director
Summa Barberton Family Medicine
    Residency
Summa Health Systems
Barberton, Ohio

Jonathan M. Novotney, DO[†]
Staff Family Physician
Fort Carson
Colorado Springs, Colorado

Olga L. Nunez, MD
Resident
Department of Family & Community
    Medicine
University of Texas Health San Antonio
San Antonio, Texas

Crystal Nwagwu, MD
Assistant Professor
Department of Family and Community
    Medicine
Baylor College of Medicine
Houston, Texas

Kamala M. Nyamathi, MD[†]
Adjunct Instructor/Clinician Teacher
Department of Family Medicine
Oregon Health & Science University
Portland, Oregon

David T. O'Gurek, MD, FAAFP
Assistant Professor
Department of Family and Community
    Medicine
Temple University School of Medicine
Philadelphia, Pennsylvania

Elisa D. O'Hern, MD[†]
Pediatrician
Madigan Army Medical Center
Joint Base Lewis–McChord
Tacoma, Washington

Justin M. O'Keefe, MD[†]
Chief Resident
Department of Family Medicine
Eglin Air Force Base Hospital
Eglin Air Force Base, Florida

Keith O'Malley, MD, FACS
Professor of Surgery and Interim Director
Division of Trauma, Acute Care Surgery,
    and Surgical Critical Care
Department of Surgery
Medical College of Georgia at Augusta
    University
Augusta, Georgia

Adedotun Anthony Ogunsua, MD, MPH[†]
Cardiovascular Diseases Fellow
Department of Cardiology
University of Massachusetts Medical School
Worcester, Massachusetts

Annie Lee Oh, MD
Assistant Professor of Clinical Medicine
Hematology/Oncology, Department of
  Medicine
The University of Illinois at Chicago
Chicago, Illinois

Arthur Ohannessian, MD
Assistant Clinical Professor
Residency Associate Program Director
David Geffen School of Medicine at
  University of California Los Angeles
Los Angeles, California

Cynthia Y. Ohata, MD
Director of Wellness and Faculty Attending
Advocate Christ Family Medicine Residency
Oak Lawn, Illinois

Smriti Ohri, MD
Assistant Professor and Medical Director
Department of Family Medicine
University of Connecticut Medical School
Farmington, Connecticut

Nneka I. Okafor, MD, MPH
Resident
Department of Family & Community
  Medicine
The University of Texas Health Science
  Center at San Antonio
San Antonio, Texas

Amy Okpaku, DO
Associate Program Director
Family Medicine Residency
Dell Medical School, University of Texas
  at Austin
Austin, Texas

Leann Olansky, MD[†]
Cleveland Clinic
Cleveland, Ohio

Jacqueline L. Olin, MS, PharmD, BCPS,
  CDE, FASHP, FCCP
Professor of Pharmacy
Wingate University School of Pharmacy
Wingate, North Carolina

Christian Olivo Freites, MD
Internal Medicine Resident
Department of Internal Medicine
Mount Sinai St. Luke's–West Hospitals
Icahn School of Medicine at Mount Sinai
New York, New York

Folashade Omole, MD, FAAFP[†]
Professor and Chair
Department of Family Medicine
Morehouse School of Medicine
Atlanta, Georgia

Cherry Onaiwu, MD, MS
Faculty
Department of Internal Medicine
CHI Baylor St. Luke's Health
Houston, Texas

Amy Ondeyka, MD
Clinical Assistant Professor
Department of Emergency Medicine
Rowan University School of Osteopathic
  Medicine
Emergency Medical Service Director
Emergency Medicine Residency Program
Inspira Health Network
Vineland, New Jersey

Cybill Oragwu, MD[†]
Resident Physician
Department of Family and Community
  Medicine
Penn State Milton S. Hershey Medical
  Center
Hershey, Pennsylvania

Cinthya Pena Orbea, MD[†]
Internal Medicine
John H. Stroger Jr. Hospital of Cook County
Chicago, Illinois

Brooke E. Organ, DO[†]
Resident Physician
Eglin Family Medicine Residency
Eglin Air Force Base, Florida

Sean M. Oser, MD, MPH
Associate Professor of Family and
  Community Medicine
Associate Chief Medical Officer
Penn State Health Faculty Practice Division
Penn State College of Medicine
Hershey, Pennsylvania

Tamara K. Oser, MD
Associate Professor
Residency Research Director
Department of Family and Community
  Medicine
Penn State College of Medicine
Hershey, Pennsylvania

Chidinma Osineme, MD
Assistant Professor and Family Medicine–
  Obstetrics Residency Faculty
Virginia Tech Carilion School of Medicine
Edward Via College of Osteopathic
  Medicine
Virginia Tech Carilion
Roanoke, Virginia

Shannon A. Sanchez Oviedo, MD, MS
Novant Health Family Residency Program
Cornelius, North Carolina

Berenice Subero Pablo, MD[†]
Resident Physician
Department of Family Medicine and
  Community Health
Mount Sinai Hospital
Chicago, Illinois

Soraira Pacheco, DO
Resident Physician
Department of Family Medicine
University of Texas Medical Branch
Galveston, Texas

Andrea Padilla, MD
Family and Community Medicine
University of Texas Health Science Center
  at San Antonio
San Antonio, Texas

Kelly Pagidas, MD[†]
Professor of Obstetrics Gynecology and
  Women's Health
Division and Program Director
Reproductive Endocrinology and Infertility
University of Louisville School of Medicine
Louisville, Kentucky

Miguel A. Palacios, MD
Assistant Professor/Clinical
Department of Family and Community
  Medicine
University of Texas Health San Antonio
San Antonio, Texas

Melissa L. Palma, MD
Preventive Medicine Resident
Division of Preventive Medicine
Cook County Health and Hospitals System
Chicago, Illinois

Linda Paniagua, MD[†]
Valley Baptist Medical Center
Brownsville, Texas

Sally-Ann L. Pantin, MD, FAAFP
Associate Program Director
Mayo Clinic Florida Family Medicine
  Residency
Department of Family Medicine
Mayo Clinic School of Graduate Medical
  Education
Jacksonville, Florida

Debra Papa, MD
Assistant Professor
Department of Obstetrics and Gynecology
University of Massachusetts Medical School
UMass Memorial Health Care
Worcester, Massachusetts

Paul M. Papajohn, DO
Resident
Otolaryngology—Head and Neck Surgery
Philadelphia College of Osteopathic
 Medicine
Philadelphia, Pennsylvania

Anupama Parameswaran, MD[†]
Chief Dermatology Resident
University of Massachusetts Medical School
Worcester, Massachusetts

Jon S. Parham, DO, MPH, FAAFP
Associate Professor and Director of
 Preventive Education
Department of Family Medicine
University of Tennessee Graduate School
 of Medicine
Knoxville, Tennessee

Farrah J. Parker, DO
Resident
HonorHealth Osborn Family Medicine
 Residency
Scottsdale, Arizona

Douglas S. Parks, MD
Associate Professor
University of Wyoming
Family Medicine Residency at Cheyenne
Cheyenne, Wyoming

Naomi Parrella, MD, FAAFP, Dipl. ABOM
Assistant Professor and Medical Director
Center for Weight Loss and Lifestyle
 Medicine
Department of Family Medicine
Department of Surgery
Rush University Medical School
Chicago, Illinois

David O. Parrish, MS, MD, FAAFP
Director of Family Medicine Residency
Bayfront Health St. Petersburg
St. Petersburg, Florida
Clinical Associate Professor
University of South Florida College of
 Medicine
Tampa, Florida

Sarah Parrott, DO
Assistant Professor
Division of Primary Care Medicine
Kansas City University of Medicine and
 Biosciences
Kansas City, Missouri

Michael T. Partin, MD
Resident Physician
Department of Family and Community
 Medicine
Penn State Milton S. Hershey Medical
 Center
Hershey, Pennsylvania

Michael Passafaro, DO, DTM&H, FACEP,
 FACOEP
Attending Physician
Department of Emergency Medicine
CarePoint Health
Jersey City, New Jersey

Paul Pastor, MD
Catholic University of Santiago de
 Guayaquil
Guyaquil, Ecuador

Amit B. Patel, DO
Internal Medicine Resident
Advocate Christ Medical Center
Chicago, Illinois

Birju B. Patel, MD, FACP, AGSF[†]
Geriatrician
Emory University School of Medicine
Duluth, Georgia

Krunal Patel, MD
Gastroenterology Fellow
Department of Medicine
University of Massachusetts Medical
 School
Worcester, Massachusetts

Mahesh C. Patel, MD
Associate Professor
Department of Internal Medicine
Division of Infectious Diseases
University of Illinois at Chicago College of
 Medicine
Chicago, Illinois

Manisha J. Patel, MD
Department of Internal Medicine
Lahey Hospital & Medical Center
Burlington, Massachusetts

Nihal K. Patel, MD
Gastroenterology Fellow
Dartmouth Hitchcock Medical Center
Lebanon, New Hampshire

Nupam A. Patel, MD
Resident
Pathology and Laboratory Medicine
University of Cincinnati College of
 Medicine
Cincinnati, Ohio

Rajen H. Patel, MD
Family Medicine Physician
Primary Care Sports Medicine Fellow
Christus Santa Rosa
San Antonio, Texas

Ravin V. Patel, MD
Family Medicine
Department of Family Medicine
Saint Louis University/Belleville Campus
Belleville, Illinois

Rinku J. Patel, DO
Advocate Children's Hospital
Oak Lawn, Illinois

Ruchita Patel, DO
Endocrinologist
Division of Endocrinology, Diabetes, and
 Metabolism
University of Illinois at Chicago/Advocate
 Christ Medical Center
Oak Lawn, Illinois

Samata Pathireddy, MD
Hospitalist, Internal Medicine
Clinical Assistant
Professor of Medicine
Indiana School of Medicine
Deaconess Health System
Evansville, Indiana

Joseph E. Patruno, MD
Associate Clinical Professor
Department of Obstetrics and Gynecology
Lehigh Valley Health Network
University of South Florida—College of
 Medicine
Allentown, Pennsylvania

Emily I. Patton, DO[†]
Flight Surgeon/General Medical Officer
Tucson, Arizona

Jared M. Patton, MD, MS[†]
Senior Medical Officer
Camp Kinser Branch Medical Clinic
United States Navy
Okinawa, Japan

Jill Patton, DO
Program Director and Vice Chair
Department of Medicine
Advocate Lutheran General Hospital
Park Ridge, Illinois

Aaron Patzwahl, MD[†]
Family Medicine Residency
David Grant Medical Center
Travis Air Force Base, California

Charles Pavia, PhD
Associate Professor of Microbiology
Department of Biomedical Sciences
New York Institute of Technology College
 of Osteopathic Medicine
Old Westbury, New York

Gisela M. Lopez Payares, MD
Department of Family and Community
 Medicine
The University of Texas Health Science
 Center at San Antonio
San Antonio, Texas

Jon Payne, MD
Resident
Department of Family Medicine
Methodist Health Systems
Dallas, Texas

Matthew S. Peckham, MD
Resident
Department of Radiology
University of Massachusetts Medical
    School
Worcester, Massachusetts

Randall Pellish, MD
Assistant Professor of Medicine
Department of Medicine
Program Director
Gastroenterology Fellowship
University of Massachusetts Medical
    School
Worcester, Massachusetts

Lauren Penwell-Waines, PhD
Director of Behavioral Science
Novant Health Family Medicine Residency
Cornelius, North Carolina

Brian P. Peppers, DO, PhD
Allergy and Immunology Research Fellow
Department of Allergy and Immunology
University Hospitals Cleveland Medical
    Center
Case Western Reserve University
Cleveland, Ohio

Luis L. Pérez, DO
Program Director
Transitional Year Residency Program
Clinical Associate Professor of Family
    Medicine
Firelands Regional Medical Center
Sandusky, Ohio
Ohio University Heritage College of
    Osteopathic Medicine
Athens, Ohio

Jose L. Perez-Lara, MD
Resident
Department of Internal Medicine
BronxCare Health System
Bronx, New York
Department of Internal Medicine
Icahn School of Medicine at Mount Sinai
New York, New York

T. Ray Perrine, MS, MD, FAAFP[†]
Faculty Attending
Family Medicine Residency Center
North Mississippi Medical Center
Tupelo, Mississippi

Christine S. Persaud, MD, CAQSM
Program Director
Non-Operative Sports Medicine
    Fellowship
Medical Director
Division of Sports Medicine
Primary Care Sports Medicine
Department of Orthopaedic Surgery
SUNY Downstate Medical Center
Brooklyn, New York

Gene Pershwitz, MD
Department of Cardiology
Hartford Hospital
Hartford, Connecticut

Bobby Peters, MD, FAAEM
Assistant Professor
Emergency Department
University of Iowa Hospitals
Iowa City, Iowa

Keith E. Petersen, DO[†]
Associate Program Director
Family Medicine Residency
Madigan Army Medical Center
Tacoma, Washington

Lindsay Petersen, MD
Breast Surgeon
Department of Surgery, Breast Oncology
    Program
Henry Ford Hospital System
Detroit, Michigan

Hugh R. Peterson, MD, FACP
Associate Professor of Medicine
Division of General Internal Medicine,
    Medical Education, and Palliative Care
Department of Medicine
University of Louisville School of Medicine
Louisville, Kentucky

Kelsey E. Phelps, MD[†]
Assistant Professor of Family Medicine
Louisiana State University Rural Family
    Medicine Residency, Bogalusa
Louisiana State University
Bogalusa, Louisiana

Teny Anna Philip, MD
Department of Family & Community
    Medicine
The University of Texas Health Science
    Center at San Antonio
San Antonio, Texas

Shawn F. Phillips, MD, MSPT
Assistant Professor of Family and
    Community Medicine and Orthopedics
    and Rehabilitation
Pennsylvania State University College of
    Medicine/Milton S. Hershey Medical
    Center
Department of Family and Community
    Medicine
Hershey, Pennsylvania

Kantima Phisitkul, MD[†]
Staff Nephrologist
Iowa City VA Health Care System
Iowa City, Iowa

Gregory M. Piech, MD, MPH[†]
Resident
Department of Internal Medicine
The George Washington University
Washington, DC

Jonathan Piercy, MD, FACP
Assistant Professor
Department of Family and Community
    Medicine
University of Kentucky College of Medicine
Lexington, Kentucky

Claudeleedy Pierre, MD[†]
Assistant Professor
Department of Family Medicine and
    Community Health
University of Massachusetts Medical
    School
Worcester, Massachusetts

Anusha B. Pinjala, MBBS
Internal Medicine Resident
Creighton University Medical Center
Omaha, Nebraska

Maria A. Pino, PhD, MS, Rph[†]
Assistant Professor of Pharmacology
Department of Clinical Specialties
New York Institute of Technology College
    of Osteopathic Medicine
Old Westbury, New York

Robert W. Plambeck, MD
Assistant Professor of Medicine
Division of Pulmonary and Critical Care
Creighton University School of Medicine
Omaha, Nebraska

Yahaira Plata, MD, MPH
Obstetrics and Gynecology Physician
    Resident
Department of Obstetrics and Gynecology
Advocate Illinois Masonic Medical Center
Chicago, Illinois

Maria M. Plummer, MD[†]
Associate Professor
Department of Clinical Specialties
Division of Pathology
New York Institute of Technology College
    of Osteopathic Medicine
Old Westbury, New York

Kenneth Polezoes, MD
Family Medicine Resident
Presence Saint Joseph Hospital
Chicago, Illinois

Adriana Polisano, MD
University of Massachusetts Medical
    School
Worcester, Massachusetts

David E. Polzin, MD[†]
Assistant Program Director
US Air Force Regional Hospital Program
Eglin Air Force Base, Florida

Stacy E. Potts, MD, MEd
Associate Professor and Residency
    Program Director
Department of Family Medicine and
    Community Health
University of Massachusetts Medical
    School
Worcester, Massachusetts

James E. Powers, DO, FACEP, FAAEM
Professor of Emergency Medicine
Campbell University School of
    Osteopathic Medicine
Lillington, North Carolina

Faruq Pradhan, MD
Gastroenterology Fellow
Banner University Medical Center
    Phoenix
Phoenix, Arizona

Zachary Prather, MD[†]
Bayne Jones Army Community Hospital
Fort Polk, Louisiana

Amy E. Pratt, DO
Hematology/Oncology Fellow
Department of Medicine, Division of
    Hematology/Oncology
University of Massachusetts Medical
    School
Worcester, Massachusetts

George G.A. Pujalte, MD, FACSM[†]
Senior Associate Consultant
Family Medicine and Sports Medicine
Assistant Professor
Mayo Clinic College of Medicine
Vice-Chair for Academics
Department of Family Medicine
Associate Program Director
Sports Medicine Fellowship Program
Vice-Chair for Communications
American Medical Society for Sports
    Medicine
Team Physician
USA Taekwondo
Jacksonville, Florida

Matthew J. Putty, DO
Neurosurgical Resident
Advocate Health Care System
Normal, Illinois

Natasha J. Pyzocha, DO, FAWM, FAAFP[†]
Flight Surgeon and Family Physician
Department of Family Medicine
DiRaimondo Aviation Clinic
Fort Carson, Colorado

Juan Qiu, MD, PhD
Associate Professor
Department of Family & Community
    Medicine
Pennsylvania State University College of
    Medicine
State College, Pennsylvania

Jeffrey D. Quinlan, MD, FAAFP[†]
Associate Professor and Chairman
Department of Family Medicine
Uniformed Services University of the
    Health Sciences
Bethesda, Maryland

Patricia Martinez Quinones, MD
General Surgery Resident
Medical College of Georgia at Augusta
    University
Augusta, Georgia

Raymundo A. Quintana, MD
Cardiovascular Disease Fellow
Department of Medicine
Emory University School of Medicine
Atlanta, Georgia

Gabriela Quinteros, MD
Northwell Health
Manhasset, New York

Maria G. Quinteros Flores, MD
Palliative Care Fellow
Department of Geriatrics and Palliative
    Care
Northwell Health–Hofstra University
Manhasset, New York

Carla M. Basadre Quiroz, MD
Resident, Family and Community Medicine
Department of Family & Community
    Medicine
The University of Texas Health Science
    Center at San Antonio
San Antonio, Texas

Hannan Qureshi, MD
Resident Surgeon and Postdoctoral
    Research Fellow
Department of Otolaryngology–Head and
    Neck Surgery
University of Washington
Seattle, Washington

Jeremy S. Raab, MD[†]
MAJ, MC, USAF
97th Medical Operations Squadron
Altus Air Force Base, Oklahoma

Naureen Rafiq, MBBS[†]
Associate Professor and Core Faculty
Department of Family Medicine
    Residency Program
Creighton University School of Medicine
Omaha, Nebraska

Rachel Ragosta, MCHS, PA-C,
    CAQ-Hospital, RN
Lecturer
MEDEX Northwest
Department of Family Medicine
University of Washington
Seattle, Washington

Sumrine S. Raja, MD, MSc
Attending Physician
University of Massachusetts Memorial
    Medical Center
Assistant Professor
Department of General Internal Medicine
University of Massachusetts Memorial
    Medical Center
Worcester, Massachusetts

G. Rajashekar, MBBS
Resident
Department of Internal Medicine
Texas Tech University of Health Sciences
    Center at Permian Basin
Odessa, Texas

Deepika Ram, DO
University of Texas Health San Antonio
Department of Family & Community
    Medicine
Lake Erie College of Osteopathic Medicine
San Antonio, Texas

Jyoti Ramakrishna, MD, MPH[†]
Adjunct Associate Professor
Tufts University School of Medicine
Boston, Massachusetts

Kalyanakrishnan Ramakrishnan, MD
Professor
Department of Family and Preventive
    Medicine
University of Oklahoma Health Sciences
    Center
Oklahoma City, Oklahoma

Muthalagu Ramanathan, MD
Associate Professor of Medicine
Co-Director of Blood and Marrow
    Transplant Program
Director of Myelodysplastic Syndrome
    Program
Division of Hematology and Oncology
Department of Medicine
University of Massachusetts Medical School
Worcester, Massachusetts

Sarah Ines Ramirez, MD
Assistant Professor
Family and Community Medicine
Department of Family and Community
    Medicine
Penn State Health/Milton S. Hershey
    Medical Center
Hershey, Pennsylvania

Juan R. Ramos Dominguez, MD, MPH[†]
Resident
Department of Family and Community
    Medicine
University of Texas Health San Antonio
San Antonio, Texas

Alvaro J. Ramos-Rodriguez, MD
Senior Resident
Icahn School of Medicine at Mount
    Sinai West
Department of Internal Medicine
New York, New York

Chandini Rathee, MD
Resident
Novant Health Family Medicine Residency
Charlotte, North Carolina

Abirami Raveendran, MD
Resident Physician
Department of Family Medicine and
    Community Health
University of Massachusetts Medical
    School
Worcester, Massachusetts

Tharani Ravi, MD
Assistant Professor
Department of Family and Community
    Medicine
University of Texas Health San Antonio
San Antonio, Texas

Mohammad A. Razaq, MD[†]
Assistant Professor of Medicine
Division of Hematology/Oncology
University of Oklahoma Health Sciences
    Center
Oklahoma City, Oklahoma

Sean Rea, DO
Southeastern Regional Medical Center
Lumberton, North Carolina

John L. Reagan, MD
Assistant Professor of Medicine
Alpert Medical School of Brown University
Director of Hematology
Lifespan Cancer Institute
Providence, Rhode Island

Narothama Reddy Aeddula, MD, FACP,
    FASN
Consultant Nephrologist
Deaconess Health System
Assistant Clinical Professor
Department of Medicine
Indiana University School of Medicine
Evansville, Indiana

Donovan S. Reed, MD[†]
CPT, USAF, MC
Department of Ophthalmology
Wilford Hall Eye Center
Brooke Army Medical Center
Clinical Instructor of Surgery
Uniformed Services
University of the Health Sciences
Fort Sam Houston, Texas

Grant M. Reed, DO
Family Medicine Physician
St. Margaret's Health
Peru, Illinois

Tyler R. Reese, MD, FAAFP[†]
Faculty of Family Medicine
Department of Family Medicine
Madigan Healthcare System
Tacoma, Washington

Jennifer Reidy, MD, MS, FAAHPM
Chief
Division of Palliative Care
University of Massachusetts Memorial
    Health Care
Assistant Professor
University of Massachusetts Medical School
Worcester, Massachusetts

Shelby M. Reimer, MD
Riverside Methodist Family Medicine
Columbus, Ohio

Sarah Renna, MD
Family Medicine Resident
Creighton University
Department of Family Medicine
Omaha, Nebraska

Caitlyn M. Rerucha, MD[†]
Faculty, Family Medicine Residency
    Program
Carl R. Darnall Army Medical Center
Fort Hood, Texas

Leigh G. Rexius, DO[†]
Resident
Womack Army Medical Center
Fort Bragg, North Carolina

Arlene Reyes, MD[†]
Resident Physician
Department of Family & Community
    Medicine
University of Texas Health San Antonio
San Antonio, Texas

Blair Rhodehouse, DO, ATC[†]
CPT, MC, USA
Womack Army Family Medicine Resident
Fort Bragg, North Carolina

Andrew J. Richardson, MD
Department of Family Medicine
Baylor Scott and White Health
College Station, Texas

John M. Richardson, MD[†]
Family Medicine Resident
Fort Belvoir Family Medicine Residency
Fort Belvoir, Virginia

Sean W. Richardson, DO[†]
Martin Army Community Hospital
Fort Benning, Georgia

Harry Richter III, MD
Associate Professor
Rush University Medical Center
Chicago, Illinois

David L. Riegleman, MD[†]
Family Medicine Resident Physician
Eglin Family Medicine Residency Clinic
Eglin Air Force Base, Florida

Maizal Cuauhtemoc Rivera, FNP
Nurse Practitioner
San Antonio, Texas

Vanessa M. Rivera, MD[†]
Resident Physician
Family Medicine Residency
Carl R. Darnall Army Medical Center
Fort Hood, Texas

Sonia Rivera-Martinez, DO
Associate Professor and Associate
    Medical Director
Department of Family Medicine
New York Institute of Technology College
    of Osteopathic Medicine
Old Westbury, New York

Ramona Roach-Davis, DNP, FNP-BC[†]
Hoover Family Medicine
Hoover, Alabama

Wayne K. Robbins, DO
Ear, Nose, and Throat Associates
Grand Blanc, Michigan

Amanda Roberts, MD

Michele Roberts, MD, PhD
Paxton, Massachusetts

Sean C. Robinson, MD, CAQSM
Assistant Professor
Oregon Health & Science University
Sports & Family Medicine Department
Director of Electives and Sub-internship
Head Team Physician
Lewls and Clark College
Portland, Oregon

Shannon Roche, DO
Family Health Resident
Family Medicine and Community Health
UMass Medical School
Worcester, Massachusetts

Jack Rock, MD
Vice-Chairman of Education
Department of Neurosurgery
Director of Neurosurgery Residency
    Program
Co-Director
Surgical Neuro-Oncology Clinic and
Metastatic Tumor—Brain Program
Director of Skullbase and Pituitary Tumor
    Program
Henry Ford Hospital
Detroit, Michigan

Michelle Rodriguez, MD
Department of Family and Community
    Medicine
University of Texas Health Science Center
    at San Antonio
San Antonio, Texas

Yvo A. Rodriguez, MD[†]
Neurology Resident
Department of Neurology
McGovern Medical School
The University of Texas Health Science
    Center
Houston, Texas

Alexis J. Rogers, MD
University of Nebraska Medical Center
Omaha, Nebraska

Cristhiam Rojas-Hernandez, MD
Assistant Professor
Section of Benign Hematology
University of Texas MD Anderson Cancer
    Center
Houston, Texas

Ashley A. Roselle, DO
Family Medicine Physician
Womack Army Medical Center
Fort Bragg, North Carolina

Noah M. Rosenberg, MD, MBA
Clinical Assistant Professor
Department of Medicine
Tufts University School of Medicine
Boston, Massachusetts

Montiel T. Rosenthal, MD
Professor and Director of Maternity
    Services
Department of Family and Community
    Medicine
University of Cincinnati College of Medicine
Cincinnati, Ohio

David A. Ross, MD, CAQSM[†]
Primary Care Sports Medicine
Ross Medical Group
Miami, Florida

Nicole A. Ross, DO[†]
Resident Physician
Department of Family Medicine
West Kendall Baptist Hospital
Florida International University Herbert
    Wertheim College of Medicine
Miami, Florida

Anthony Rowe, MD
George Washington University
Washington, DC

Sasmit Roy, MD, MBBS
Renal Fellow
Division of Renal Medicine
University of Massachusetts Medical
    School
Worcester, Massachusetts

Lloyd A. Runser, MD, MPH, FAAFP[†]
Associate Program Director
Novant Health Family Medicine Residency
    Clinic
Charlotte, North Carolina
Assistant Clinical Professor
Department of Family Medicine
Campbell University Jerry M. Wallace
    School of Osteopathic Medicine
Lillington, North Carolina
Assistant Clinical Professor
Department of Family Medicine
Edward Via College of Osteopathic
    Medicine (VCOM)
Blacksburg, Virginia

Frances M. Rusnack, DO
New York Institute of Technology College
    of Osteopathic Medicine
Glen Head, New York

Travis C. Russell, MD, FAWM[†]
Core Faculty
Nellis Family Medicine
Nellis Air Force Base
Las Vegas, Nevada

Anthony Russo, MD[†]
Assistant Professor
Department of Family Medicine and
    Community Health
Eastern Virginia Medical School
Norfolk, Virginia

Ashlee N. Russo, MD
Pulmonary and Critical Care Medicine
Pulmonary Rehabilitation Associates
Youngstown, Ohio

Veronica J. Ruston, DO
General Practice Physician
Litchfield Park, Arizona

Jessica A. Ryder, MD
Emergency Medicine Resident
Department of Emergency Medicine
University of Florida College of Medicine,
    Jacksonville
Jacksonville, Florida

Valerie Rygiel, DO
Chief Resident
Family Medicine Residency Program
Advocate Christ Medical Center
Oak Lawn, Illinois

Muhammad Saad, MD
Attending, Primary Care/Preventive
    Medicine
BronxCare Health System
Bronx, New York

Austin C. Saavedra, MD[†]
Resident Physician
Department of Family Medicine
Creighton University School of Medicine
Omaha, Nebraska

Anup Sabharwal, MD, MBA, FACE
Professor of Medicine
Division of Endocrinology, Diabetes, and
    Metabolism
Florida International University
Herbert Wertheim College of Medicine
Miami, Florida

Corey Sadler, MD[†]

Faisal Saeed, MD
Staff Physician
Pulmonary and Critical Care Medicine
HSHS St. John's Hospital
Springfield, Illinois

Sidra Saeed, MD
Resident
Department of Family Medicine and
    Community Health
Southern Illinois University School of
    Medicine
Springfield, Illinois

Joel Saeedi, MD[†]
Resident Physician
Department of Internal Medicine
University of Illinois at Chicago/Advocate
    Christ Medical Center
Oak Lawn, Illinois

Adriana Saenz, MD
Resident
Department of Family and Community
    Medicine
University of Texas Health San Antonio
San Antonio, Texas

Khalid Salaheldin, MD
Resident Psychiatrist
Department of Psychiatry
Zucker School of Medicine at Hofstra/
    Northwell
Hempstead, New York

Brian M. Salata, MD, MS
Resident
Joan and Sanford I. Weill Department of
    Medicine
New York–Presbyterian Hospital/Weill
    Cornell Medical Center
New York, New York

Ruben Salinas Jr., MD, FAAFP[†]
Col, USA
Geriatrics Director
Family Medicine Residency Program
Fort Hood, Texas

Kathryn Samai, PharmD, BCPS
Clinical Pharmacist of Emergency
    Medicine
Department of Pharmaceutical Care
    Services
Sarasota Memorial Healthcare System
Sarasota, Florida

Haroon Samar, MD, MPH[†]
CPT, MC
Battalion Surgeon
Fort Carson, Colorado

Geetha Samuel, MD
Resident
Creighton University School of Medicine
Omaha, Nebraska

Vicente T. San Martin, MD
Endocrinology Fellow
Endocrinology & Metabolism Institute
Cleveland Clinic
Cleveland, Ohio

Adriana S. Sanchez, MD
Family and Community Medicine Resident
University of Texas Health Science Center
    at San Antonio
San Antonio, Texas

Gabriel Sánchez, MD
Psychiatry Resident
Citrus Health Network
Miami, Florida

Gabriela Sanchez-Petitto, MD
Hematology and Medical Oncology Fellow
University of Maryland Marlene and
    Stewart Greenebaum Cancer Center
Baltimore, Maryland

Arthur B. Sanders, MD, MHA
Professor
Department of Emergency Medicine
University of Arizona College of
    Medicine–Tucson
Tucson, Arizona

Marissa G. Sanderson, DO
Resident
Department of Obstetrics and Gynecology
Aultman Hospital
Canton, Ohio

Ivanna Sanoja, MD
Department of Anesthesiology and Pain
    Management
John H. Stroger Jr. Hospital of Cook County
Chicago, Illinois

Yaneidy Santana, MD
BronxCare Health System
Bronx, New York

Andres E. Santayana, MD
Resident Physician
Family Medicine Residency
Bayfront Health St. Petersburg
St. Petersburg, Florida

Adam K. Saperstein, MD[†]
Associate Professor
Department of Family Medicine
F. Edward Hebert School of Medicine
Uniformed Services University of the
    Health Sciences
Bethesda, Maryland

Hatem H. Sarhan, MBBCh[†]
Cardiac Surgery Resident
Department of Cardiothoracic Surgery
Heart Hospital
Hamad Medical Corporation
Doha, Qatar

Albert P. Sarno Jr., MD, MPH
Director, Fetal Cardiology
Maternal–Fetal Medicine
Vice Chairman
Obstetrics/Gynecology
Lehigh Valley Health Network
Allentown, Pennsylvania
Professor of Obstetrics/Gynecology
Morsani College of Medicine
University of South Florida
Tampa, Florida

Luay Sarsam, MD
Department of Cardiovascular Disease
Arnot Ogden Medical Center
Elmira, New York

John A. Saryan, MD
Allergy and Immunology, Asthma Center
Lahey Hospital & Medical Center
Burlington, Massachusetts
Lahey Medical Center, Peabody
Peabody, Massachusetts

Robert T. Sataloff, MD, DMA, FACS[†]
Professor and Chairman
Department of Otolaryngology–Head and
    Neck Surgery
Senior Associate Dean for Clinical
    Academic Specialties
Drexel University College of Medicine
Philadelphia, Pennsylvania

Milan Satcher, MD
Family Medicine Resident
Boston University Medical Campus
Boston, Massachusetts

Shailendra K. Saxena, MD, PhD
Professor of Family Medicine
Department of Family Medicine
School of Medicine
Creighton University Medical Center
Omaha, Nebraska

Durr-e-Shahwaar Sayed, DO
Attending Family Physician
Inspira Medical Group
Glassboro, New Jersey

Payam Sazegar, MD, CCFP†
Clinical Assistant Professor
Department of Family Practice
University of British Columbia Faculty of
  Medicine
Vancouver, British Columbia, Canada

Renata Scalabrin Reis, MD†
Chief Resident
Department of Family and Community
  Medicine
University of Texas Health San Antonio
San Antonio, Texas

Catherine Scarbrough, MD, MSc, FAAFP
Faculty
St. Vincent's East Family Medicine
  Residency Program
Christ Health Center
Birmingham, Alabama

Richard Scharf, DO, FACOO
Program Director Otolaryngology
  Residency Program
St. Barnabas Medical Center
Livingston, New Jersey
Associate Clinical Professor
New York College of Osteopathic
  Medicine
Long Island, New York

Matthew J. Schear, DO†
Fellow
Cornea, External Diseases, & Refractive
  Surgery
Manhattan Eye, Ear, & Throat Hospital
Northwell Health
New York, New York

Jeffrey A. Schievenin, MD†
Faculty Physician
Eglin Air Force Base Family Medicine
  Residency Program
Eglin Air Force Base, Florida

Ashley M. Schinske, MD
Resident
Department of Family Medicine
University of Colorado School of Medicine
Denver, Colorado

Daniel J. Schlegel, MD, MHA
Program Director
Penn State Hershey Family Medicine
  Residency Program
Assistant Professor
Department of Family and Community
  Medicine
Milton S. Hershey Medical Center
Penn State Health Milton S. Hershey
  Medical Center
Hershey, Pennsylvania

Alexander D. Schloe, MD†
Eglin Family Medicine Residency
Eglin Air Force Base
Valparaiso, Florida

Lauren Schneekloth, MD
Resident Physician
Family and Community Medicine
Penn State Health at University Park
State College, Pennsylvania

Benjamin N. Schneider, MD
Assistant Professor of Family Medicine
Assistant Dean of Student Affairs
Undergraduate Medical Education
Oregon Health and Science University
Portland, Oregon

Brian J. Schneider, MD
Sports Medicine Fellow
University of Colorado
Denver, Colorado

Sebastian Schnellbacher, DO, MPH†
Madigan Army Medical Center
Tacoma, Washington

Elizabeth Schofield, MS, LCGC
Lehigh Valley Health Network
Allentown, Pennsylvania

Lisa M. Schroeder, MD†
Assistant Director
Summa Barberton Family Practice
  Residency Program
Northeast Ohio Medical University
Barberton, Ohio

Jennifer B. Schwartz, MD†
Family and Sports Medicine Physician
Beth Israel Deaconess Medical Center
Affiliated Physicians Group
Brookline, Massachusetts

Ingrid U. Scott, MD, MPH†
Jack and Nancy Turner Professor of
  Ophthalmology
Professor of Public Health Sciences
Penn State College of Medicine
Hershey, Pennsylvania

Gail Scully, MD, MPH
Assistant Professor
Division of Infectious Disease
Department of Medicine
University of Massachusetts Medical
  School
Worcester, Massachusetts

Paul E. Seales, MD†
Resident
Department of Family Medicine
Naval Hospital Jacksonville
Jacksonville, Florida

Sajeewane M. Seales, MD, MPH
Resident
Department of Family Medicine
Naval Hospital Jacksonville
Jacksonville, Florida

David P. Sealy, MD
Professor
Medical University of South Carolina
Area Health Education Consortium
  Greenwood
Director
Primary Care Sports Medicine Fellowship
Self Regional Healthcare Sports Medicine
  Center
Greenwood, South Carolina

Stephen C. Sears, DO†
LT, MC (Flight Surgeon), USN
Aviation Medicine Department
United States Naval Hospital Yokosuka
Branch Health Clinic Iwakuni
Marine Corps Air Station
Iwakuni, Japan

Margaret Seaver, MD, MPH
Palliative Medicine Service
Lahey Hospital & Medical Center
Burlington, Massachusetts

L. Michelle Seawright, DO†
Family Medicine Residency
Naval Hospital Camp Lejeune
Camp Lejeune, North Carolina

Sheila M. Seed, PharmD, MPH, RPh
Professor and Interim Chair of Pharmacy
  Practice
Department of Pharmacy Practice
Massachusetts College of Pharmacy and
  Health Science University
School of Pharmacy-Worcester/Manchester
Worcester, Massachusetts

Nicholas E. Seeliger, MD
Family Medicine
Banner Health
San Francisco, California

Amy Seery, MD
Assistant Professor
Department of Family and Community
  Medicine
University of Kansas School of Medicine
Faculty
Via Christi Family Medicine Residency
Wichita, Kansas

Jason M. Seibly, DO, FACOS
Neurosurgeon
Advocate Healthcare Neurological
  Surgery
Residency Program Director
Normal, Illinois

Mohammad Selim, MBBCh
Medicine Resident
Department of Internal Medicine
Creighton University
Omaha, Nebraska

Christopher R. Selinsky, DO
Assistant Program Director
Otolaryngology—Head and Neck Surgery
OhioHealth Doctor's Hospital
Ohio University Heritage College of
  Osteopathic Medicine
Columbus, Ohio

Jarrett Sell, MD, AAHIVS
Associate Professor
Department of Family and Community
  Medicine
Penn State Health Milton S. Hershey
  Medical Center
Hershey, Pennsylvania

Peter J. Sell, DO
Associate Professor
Department of Pediatrics
University of Massachusetts Medical
  School
Worcester, Massachusetts

Maria Lidón Serrano Barragan, MD

Jessica T. Servey, MD, MHPE, FAAFP[†]
Assistant Dean for Faculty Development
Associate Professor
Family Medicine and Medicine
Uniformed Services University of the
  Health Sciences
Bethesda, Maryland

Patricia L. Seymour, MD[†]
Associate Professor
Department of Family Medicine and
  Community Health
University of Massachusetts Medical School
Worcester, Massachusetts

Chirag N. Shah, MD, FACEP
Associate Professor
Department of Emergency Medicine
Rutgers-Robert Wood Johnson Medical
  School
New Brunswick, New Jersey

Hiral Shah, MD, FASGE, FAGA, FACG[†]
Program Director
Gastroenterology Fellowship
Lehigh Valley Health Network
Eastern Pennsylvania Gastroenterology
  and Liver Specialists
Allentown, Pennsylvania

Jay N. Shah, DO, MPH[†]
Assistant Professor of Pediatrics
Division of Gastroenterology, Hepatology
  and Nutrition
University of Texas Health San Antonio
San Antonio, Texas

Nehal R. Shah, MD[†]
Assistant Professor of Medicine
Virginia Commonwealth University
Richmond, Virginia

Prachi Shah, DO
Resident
Family Medicine
Advocate Christ Medical Center
Oak Lawn, Illinois

Samir A. Shah, MD, FACG, FASGE, AGAF
Clinical Professor of Medicine
The Warren Alpert Medical School of
  Brown University
Chief of Gastroenterology
The Miriam Hospital
Gastroenterology Associates
Providence, Rhode Island

Ammar Shahid, MD[†]
Chief Resident
Chestnut Hill Family Practice
Philadelphia, Pennsylvania

Rory M. Shallis, MD
Yale Cancer Center
New Haven, Connecticut

Kevin C. Shannon, MD, MPH, FAAFP
Associate Professor
Department of Family Medicine
Loma Linda University School of Medicine
Loma Linda, California

Denise Sharon, MD, PhD, FAASM[†]
Assistant Professor
Tulane University School of Medicine
New Orleans, Louisiana
Consultant
Pomona Valley Hospital and Medical Center
Adult and Children Sleep Disorders Center
Claremont, California

Victoria R. Sharon, MD, DTMH
Assistant Professor of Dermatology &
  Mohs Surgery Director
Dermatology Inpatient Consultation
University of California, Davis
Davis, California

Karen Sheflin, DO
Assistant Professor
Department of Family Medicine
College of Osteopathic Medicine
New York Institute of Technology
Old Westbury, New York

Paula A. Shelton, MD
Family Medicine
University of Texas Health Science Center
  at San Antonio
San Antonio, Texas

Rameeza Sheriff, MD
Resident Physician
Department of Family and Community
  Medicine
University of Kentucky College of
  Medicine
Lexington, Kentucky

Nicole Shields, MD
Assistant Professor of Family Medicine
DeBusk College of Osteopathic Medicine
Lincoln Memorial University
Harrogate, Tennessee

Jeffrey A. Shih, MD
Assistant Professor of Medicine
Medical Director
Ventricular Assist Device Program
Advanced Heart Failure and Cardiac
  Transplantation
Cardiovascular Medicine
Worcester, Massachusetts

David C. Shin, MD
Sports Medicine Fellow
Long Beach Memorial Primary Care
  Sports Medicine
University of California, Irvine
Irvine, California

Amal Shine, MD
Resident Physician
Department of Internal Medicine
University of Louisville School of Medicine
Louisville, Kentucky

Cassandra Shipp, MD[†]
Department of Family Medicine
Mount Sinai Hospital
Chicago, Illinois

Scott D. Sholem, DO, MS
General Surgery Resident
St. Joseph's Regional Medical Center
Paterson, New Jersey

Jacob C. Shook, DO[†]
Family Medicine Resident
Fort Hood Family Medicine Residency
Fort Hood, Texas

Christiana Shoushtari, MD
Resident Physician
Internal Medicine
Advocate Medical Group
Park Ridge, Illinois

Megan M. Sick, MD[†]
LCDR, MC, USN
Family Medicine-Obstetrics
Naval Hospital Camp Pendleton
Camp Pendleton, California

Irfan H. Siddiqui, MD
Chief Resident and Clinical Instructor
Department of Internal Medicine
Advocate Christ Medical Center/
    University of Illinois at Chicago
Oak Lawn, Illinois

Saima Siddiqui, MD, MSCI
Associate Professor
Department of Family & Community
    Medicine
University of Texas Health Science Center
    at San Antonio
San Antonio, Texas

Julia Siegel, MD
University of Massachusetts Medical School
Worcester, Massachusetts

Karlynn Sievers, MD
Faculty Physician
St. Mary's Family Medicine Residency
    Program
Grand Junction, Colorado

Peter Silberstein, MD, FACP
Professor
School of Medicine
Creighton University
Oncology, Hematology
CHI Health Creighton University Medical
    Center
Omaha, Nebraska

Hugh Silk, MD, MPH, FAAFP
Professor
Department of Family Medicine and
    Community Health
University of Massachusetts Medical
    School
Worcester, Massachusetts

Matthew A. Silva, PharmD, RPh, BCPS
Professor
Department of Pharmacy Practice
Massachusetts College of Pharmacy and
    Health Sciences University
Worcester, Massachusetts

Sabrina L. Silver, DO, CAQSM[†]
Assistant Professor
Department of Family Medicine
Uniformed Services University
Eglin Air Force Base, Florida

Anna L. Silverman, MD
Resident Physician
Department of Internal Medicine
University of California San Diego
San Diego, California

Tiffany A. Moore Simas, MD, MPH, MEd,
    FACOG
Associate Professor
Obstetrics/Gynecology, Pediatrics,
    Psychiatry and Quantitative Health
    Sciences
Vice-Chair
Department of Obstetrics & Gynecology
University of Massachusetts Medical
    School
University of Massachusetts Memorial
    Health Care
Worcester, Massachusetts

LuDane Simmons, MD[†]
Creighton Department of Family Medicine
Outpatient Chief Resident
Omaha, Nebraska

Lauren M. Simon, MD, MPH
Associate Professor
Department of Family Medicine
Loma Linda University School of Medicine
Loma Linda, California

Madhavi Singh, MD[†]
Assistant Professor
Department of Family and Community
    Medicine
Penn State Health
State College, Pennsylvania

Navpreet K. Singh, MD[†]
Sleep Medicine Fellow
Hahnemann University Hospital
Drexel University
Philadelphia, Pennsylvania

Blake D. Singletary, DO[†]
Fellow
Cardiovascular Medicine
Largo Medical Center
Nova Southeastern College of
    Osteopathic Medicine
Largo, Florida

Ana Lucia Siu Chang, MD
Resident Physician
Department of Family Medicine
University of Texas Medical Branch
Galveston, Texas

Losika Sivaganeshan, MD, MPH[†]
Creighton Family Medicine Resident
University of Creighton
Omaha, Nebraska

Kara Sjogren, DO
Baptist Health Kentucky
Madisonville, Kentucky

Nicholas J. Skertich, MD
General Surgery Resident
Department of Surgery
Rush University Medical Center
Chicago, Illinois

Brian G. Skotko, MD, MPP
Emma Campbell Endowed Chair on Down
    Syndrome
Division of Medical Genetics
Massachusetts General Hospital
Boston, Massachusetts

Natalie Slepski, MD, MPH[†]
Flight Surgeon
United States Navy
Washington, DC

Benjamin J. Slocum, DO[†]
Family Medicine Resident
Department of Family Medicine and
    Community Health
University of Massachusetts Medical
    School
Worcester, Massachusetts

Jason C. Sluzevich, MD
Assistant Professor of Dermatology
Mayo Clinic
Jacksonville, Florida

Shaun O. Smart, MD
Assistant Professor of Neurology
Department of Neurology
McGovern School of Medicine
The University of Texas Health Science
    Center
Houston, Texas

Andrew Smith, MD
Assistant Professor
Department of Family Medicine
Tufts University School of Medicine
Boston, Massachusetts

Brandon Smith, MD
University of Massachusetts Medical
    School
Worcester, Massachusetts

Dennis Smith, DO, FAAFP
Program Director
North Mississippi Medical Center Family
    Medicine Residency Program
Tupelo, Mississippi

Kayla J. Smith, MD
Georgia Regents University
Augusta, Georgia

Roxanne Smith, MD, MPH
Family Medicine Residency Director
Advocate Christ Medical Center
Oak Lawn, Illinois

Savannah W. Smith, MD[†]
CPT, MC, USA
Family Medicine Physician
Camp Humphreys, South Korea

John C. Smulian, MD, MPH
Vice Chair
Department of Obstetrics and Gynecology
Chief
Division of Maternal Fetal Medicine
Lehigh Valley Health Network
Allentown, Pennsylvania
Professor
Department of Obstetrics and Gynecology
University of South Florida–Morsani
    College of Medicine
Tampa, Florida

Caroline K. Snowberger, DO
Family Medicine Physician
Christiana Care Hospital
New Castle, Delaware

L. Michael Snyder, MD
Professor
Department of Pathology
University of Massachusetts Medical
    School
Worcester, Massachusetts

Matthew J. Snyder, DO[†]
Associate Program Director
Saint Louis University Family Medicine
    Residency Program
Belleville, Illinois

Leah Soley, MD
Family Medicine
Jacksonville, Florida

D'Ann Somerall, DNP, MAEd, CRNP,
    FNP-BC
Assistant Professor
Family Child and Health Systems
University of Alabama at Birmingham
Birmingham, Alabama

William E. Somerall Jr., MD, MEd
Visiting Associate Professor School of
    Nursing
Adult/Acute Health, Chronic Care &
    Foundations
School of Nursing
University of Alabama at Birmingham
Birmingham, Alabama

Christine Song, DO
Family Medicine
Department of Family Medicine and
    Community Health
University of Texas Health Science Center
    at San Antonio
San Antonio, Texas

Michael Sorrenti, MD
Internal Medicine
University of Illinois at Chicago College
    of Medicine/Advocate Christ Medical
    Center
Chicago, Illinois

Adam J. Sorscher, MD
Associate Professor Community and
    Family Medicine
The Geisel School of Medicine at
    Dartmouth
Lebanon, New Hampshire

Charles M. Sow, MD, MSCR[†]
Associate Professor
Department of Family Medicine
Morehouse School of Medicine
Atlanta, Georgia

Thomas C. Spalla, MD
Director
Ear, Nose, and Throat Facial Plastic Surgery
Cooper University Hospital
Assistant Professor
Cooper Medical School of Rowan
    University
Adjunct Assistant Professor
Drexel University College of Medicine
Department of Otolaryngology–Head &
    Neck Surgery
Adjunct Assistant Professor
MD Anderson Cancer Center
University of Texas
Department of Otolaryngology–Head &
    Neck Surgery
Camden, New Jersey

Mikayla L. Spangler, PharmD
Associate Professor
Department of Pharmacy Practice
School of Pharmacy and Health
    Professions
Department of Family Medicine
Creighton University School of Medicine
Omaha, Nebraska

Dana Sprute, MD, MPH, FAAFP[†]
Associate Professor
Division of Family Medicine
Family Medicine Residency Director
Department of Population Health
University of Texas Austin Dell Medical
    School
Austin, Texas

Jack R. Stacey, MD[†]
LT, MC, USN
Department of Family Medicine
Naval Hospital Jacksonville
Jacksonville, Florida

Misty Stafford, MD
Child and Adolescent Psychiatry Fellow
Department of Psychiatry and Human
    Behavior
Warren Alpert Medical School of Brown
    University
Providence, Rhode Island

Chi Nguyen Stasio, DO
Resident Physician
Department of Family & Community
    Medicine
University of Texas Health San Antonio
San Antonio, Texas

Laura Steadman, EdD, CRNP, MSN, RN[†]
Assistant Professor
School of Nursing
University of Alabama at Birmingham
Birmingham, Alabama

Joseph L. Steele, MPAS, APA-C[†]
Chief of Occupational Health
Department of Preventative Medicine
Reynolds Army Health Clinic
Pine Bluff, Arkansas

Michael C. Stefanowicz, DO
Chief Medical Resident
University of Texas Dell Medical School
Division of Family Medicine
Austin, Texas

Susan L. Steffans, DO
Assistant Professor
Department of Family and Community
    Medicine
A.T. Still University School of Osteopathic
    Medicine in Arizona
Mesa, Arizona

Daniel J. Stein, MD, MPH
Fellow
Division of Gastroenterology
Beth Israel Deaconess Medical Center
Boston, Massachusetts

Anne S. Steiner, MD
Assistant Professor of Ophthalmology
Hofstra Northwell Health School of
    Medicine
Director
Ocular Surface Center
Department of Ophthalmology
Northwell Health System
Great Neck, New York

Kyle B. Stephens, DO, MPH
Identity Medical Group
Ventura, California

Nathaniel Stepp, DO[†]
LCDR, USN
Family Medicine Physician
Family Medicine Residency Staff
Naval Hospital Camp Lejeune
Camp Lejeune, North Carolina

Bernadette M. Stevenson, MD, PhD
Medical Director, Adult Inpatient
    Psychiatry & Partial Hospital Program
Core Faculty Attending, Psychiatry
    Residency Training Program
Advocate Lutheran General Hospital
Park Ridge, Illinois

J. Herbert Stevenson, MD[†]
Director of Sports Medicine
Director Sports Medicine Fellowship
    Program
Associate Professor
University of Massachusetts Medical
    School
University of Massachusetts Department
    of Family and Community Medicine
Joint Appointment
University of Massachusetts Department
    of Orthopedics
Worcester, Massachusetts

James E. Steward, MD
Urology Resident
Thomas Jefferson University Hospitals
Philadelphia, Pennsylvania

Haley Stewart, DO
St. John's Hospital Family Medicine
    Resident
University of Minnesota Department of
    Family Medicine and Community Health
St. Paul, Minnesota

Sheila O. Stille, DMD
Associate Professor and Director of the
    General Practice Residency in Dentistry
Department of Surgical Dentistry
University of Colorado School of Dental
    Medicine
Aurora, Colorado

Tamar Stokelman, MD
Family Medicine Resident
Department of Family Medicine
Methodist Hospital of Sacramento
Sacramento, California

Rachel L. Storey, DO
Family Medicine Resident
Novant Health Family Medicine Residency
    Program
Cornelius, North Carolina

Jeffrey Stovall, MD
Associate Professor
Department of Psychiatry and Behavioral
    Sciences
Vanderbilt University School of Medicine
Nashville, Tennessee

Adam Strosberg, DNP, ARNP-BC
AIDS Healthcare Foundation
Christine E. Lynn College of Nursing
Florida Atlantic University
Boca Raton, Florida

Karyn M. Sullivan, PharmD, MPH
Professor of Pharmacy Practice
Massachusetts College of Pharmacy and
    Health Sciences University
Worcester, Massachusetts

Jeff Sumner, MD
Pediatric Residency Program
MassGeneral Hospital for Children
Boston, Massachusetts

Jennifer E. Svarverud, DO[†]
Family Medicine Resident
Nellis Family Medicine Residency
Nellis Air Force Base, Nevada

Jeff Svec, MD
Chief Resident
Department of Family and Community
    Medicine
University of Texas Health San Antonio
San Antonio, Texas

Sasha Svendsen, MD
Assistant Professor
Pediatrics
University of Massachusetts Medical School
UMass Memorial Medical Center
Worcester, Massachusetts

Jennifer L. Swails, MD[†]
Assistant Professor of Medicine
Residency Program Director
Department of Internal Medicine
McGovern Medical School
The University of Texas Health Science
    Center
Houston, Texas

Farha K. Syed, MD
Resident Physician
Department of Family Medicine
University of Texas Medical Branch Health
Galveston, Texas

Huzaefah Syed, MD
Assistant Professor
Department of Internal Medicine
Division of Rheumatology, Allergy and
    Immunology
Virginia Commonwealth University
Richmond, Virginia

Kirin K. Syed, DO, FACOS
Associate Physician and Co-Director
The Department of Urology Global
    Prostate Cancer Team
Department of Urology
Holy Cross Hospital
Fort Lauderdale, Florida

Michelle E. Szczepanik, MD[†]
Hardin Memorial Hospital
Elizabethtown, Kentucky

Daniel P. Szvarca, MD
Department of Gastroenterology and
    Liver Diseases
George Washington School of Medicine
    and Health Sciences
Washington, DC

Nadeem Tabbara, MD[†]
George Washington University School of
    Medicine and Health Sciences
Washington, DC

Katherine Tadros, DO
Resident
Department of Obstetrics and Gynecology
Advocate Illinois Masonic Medical Center
Chicago, Illinois

Alfonso Tafur, MD, MS[†]
Director
Vascular Medicine
Medical Director
Anticoagulation Clinics
Medical Director
Cardiovascular Research
NorthShore University HealthSystem
Evanston, Illinois

Nicole E. Tafuri, DO[†]
Family Medicine
Eglin Air Force Base Family Medicine
    Residency Program
Eglin Air Force Base, Florida

Amar Talati, DO
Resident Physician
Family Medicine Residency
Bayfront Health St. Petersburg
St. Petersburg, Florida

Asif Talukder, MD
Resident Physician
Department of Surgery
Georgia Regents University
Augusta, Georgia

Alex J. F. Tampio, MD
Otolaryngology Resident
Department of Otolaryngology
State University of New York Upstate
    Medical University
Syracuse, New York

Benjamin T. Tan, DO
Resident Physician
Department of Family Medicine
Mayo Clinic
Jacksonville, Florida

Irene J. Tan, MD, FACR[†]
Professor of Clinical Medicine
Director of Rheumatology Fellowship
    Program
Section of Rheumatology
Lewis Katz School of Medicine at Temple
    University
Philadelphia, Pennsylvania

Kathrine R. Tan, MD, MPH[†]
Chief
Domestic Response Unit, Malaria Branch
Centers for Global Health/Division of
    Parasitic Diseases and Malaria
Centers for Disease Control and
    Prevention
Atlanta, Georgia

Danielle Taylor, DO
Urogynecology Fellow
Department of Obstetrics and Gynecology
Division of Urogynecology and
    Reconstructive Pelvic Surgery
University of Massachusetts Medical
    School
University of Massachusetts Memorial
    Hospital
Worcester, Massachusetts

James L. Taylor, PharmD
Ambulatory Care Manager
North Mississippi Medical Center
Tupelo, Mississippi

Timothy J. Taylor, DO[†]
Instructor
Campbell University College of
    Osteopathic Medicine
Lumberton, North Carolina

Randolph Taylor II, MD
Memorial Family Medicine Residency
Sugar Land, Texas

Sireesha Teegala, MD[†]
Resident
Department of Family and Community
    Medicine
University of Texas Health San Antonio
San Antonio, Texas

Bethany N. Teer, MD[†]
Family Medicine Residency Faculty
Department of Family and Community
    Medicine
Carl R. Darnall Army Medical Center
Fort Hood, Texas

Jordan I. Teitelbaum, DO[†]
Clinical Fellow
Rhinology & Endoscopic Skull Base
    Surgery
Duke University Medical Center
Durham, North Carolina

Jairo J. Tejada-Tejada, MD[†]
Resident
Department of Internal Medicine
BronxCare Health System
Bronx, New York

Yutthapong Temtanakitpaisan, MD
Co-Director
Cardiac Catheterization Laboratory
Division of Cardiology
Bangkok Hospital
Khon Kaen, Thailand

Anna Cecilia S. Tenorio, MD
Academic Chief Resident
Department of Family and Community
    Medicine
University of Texas Health Science Center
    at San Antonio
San Antonio, Texas

Frances A. Tepolt, MD
Resident
St. John's Residency Program
Department of Family Medicine and
    Community Health
University of Minnesota
St. Paul, Minnesota

Stephen M. Testa, MD
Gastroenterology Fellow
The George Washington University Hospital
Washington, DC

Nimmy Thakolkaran, MD
Geriatrics Fellow
Department of Geriatrics
Rush University Medical Center
Chicago, Illinois

Abhishek Thandra, MBBS
Internal Medicine Resident
CHI Health Creighton University Medical
    Center
Omaha, Nebraska

Wesley M. Theurer, DO, MBA, MPH[†]
Program Director
Womack Family Medicine Residency
Fort Bragg, North Carolina

Feba Thomas, MD, MS
Chief Resident
Division of Family Medicine
Department of Population Health
Dell Medical School, University of Texas
    at Austin
Austin, Texas

Chelsea Hayes Thompson, MD[†]
Family Medicine Resident
Naval Hospital Jacksonville
Jacksonville, Florida

Margaret E. Thompson, MD
Associate Professor
Department of Family Medicine
Michigan State University College of
    Human Medicine
Grand Rapids, Michigan

Matthew W. Thompson, MD[†]
Family Medicine Resident
Department of Family Medicine
Womack Army Medical Center
Fort Bragg, North Carolina

Krystal M. Thumann, MD[†]
Family Medicine Resident
Eglin Air Force Base Family Medicine
    Residency
Eglin Air Force Base, Florida

Matthew E. Tick, DO
Resident Physician
Department of Internal Medicine
George Washington University
Washington, DC

Robert J. Tiller, MD, FAAFP
Family Medicine Residency Program
    Director
Associate Professor of Family Medicine
Self Regional Healthcare
Greenwood, South Carolina

Dmitriy Timerman, MD
Resident
Columbia University Medical Center
Department of Dermatology
New York, New York

Kaleigh Timmins, MD
University of Massachusetts Medical School
Worcester, Massachusetts

Jill N. Tirabassi, MD
Assistant Professor
Department of Family Medicine and
    Community Health
University of Massachusetts Medical
    School
Worcester, Massachusetts

Jonathan M. Tisdell, MD[†]
St. Vincent Medical Group Neurology
Worcester, Massachusetts

Adam Z. Tobias, MD, MPH, FACEP
Assistant Professor of Emergency
    Medicine
University of Pittsburgh School of
    Medicine
Pittsburgh, Pennsylvania

Alexander Toirac, MD
Internal Medicine Residency Program
Jackson Memorial Hospital
Miami, Florida

Rachelle E. Toman, MD, PhD
Associate Professor and Residency
    Program Director
Department of Family Medicine
Georgetown University School of
    Medicine
Washington, DC

Sebastian T. Tong, MD, MPH
Assistant Professor
Department of Family Medicine and
    Population Health
Virginia Commonwealth University
Richmond, Virginia

Tiffany Tonismae, MD
Virginia Tech Carilion
Roanoke, Virginia

David Toomey, MD
The Brigham and Women's/Massachusetts
    General Hospital Harvard Affiliated
    Emergency Medicine Residency
Boston, Massachusetts

Moshe S. Torem, MD[†]
Professor of Psychiatry
Northeast Ohio Medical University
Cleveland Clinic Akron General
Akron, Ohio

Veronica A. Torres, MD
Resident Physician
University of Massachusetts Family
    Medicine Residency
Worcester, Massachusetts

John R. Torro, MD
Attending Physician and Faculty
Lawrence Family Medicine Residency
Lawrence, Massachusetts

Theresa A. Townley, MD, MPH[†]
Associate Professor of Internal Medicine
    and Pediatrics
Creighton University School of Medicine
Omaha, Nebraska

Zachary Townsend, DO[†]
Resident Physician
Family Medicine Residency Program
Firelands Regional Medical Center
Sandusky, Ohio

Huy T. Tran, MD[†]
Family Medicine
San Diego, California

Adam N. Treitman, MD
Clinical Assistant Professor of Medicine
Section of Infectious Diseases
University of Illinois at Chicago College of
    Medicine
Advocate Christ Medical Center
Oak Lawn, Illinois

Sophia Margareth Marie Tribie, MD[†]
Resident
Department of Family Medicine
State University of New York Downstate
    Hospital
Brooklyn, New York

Kashyap Trivedi, MD
Hertz and Associates in Gastroenterology
Los Alamitos, California

Zoltan Trizna, MD, PhD
Director
Dermatology and Dermatological Surgery
Austin, Texas

Katherine M. Tromp, PharmD
Associate Professor of Pharmacy Practice
School of Pharmacy
Lake Erie College of Osteopathic
    Medicine
Bradenton, Florida

Caroline Tschibelu, MD
Clinical Content Specialist
Emergency Medicine Department
Robert Wood Johnson University Hospital
New Brunswick, New Jersey

Julia Tse, MD
Family Medicine Resident Physician
Lawrence Family Medicine Residency
Lawrence, Massachusetts

Pamela R. Tsinteris, MD, MPH
Family Physician
Program Director
Controlled Substances and Office Based
    Addiction Treatment Programs
The Family Health Center of Worcester
Instructor
Department of Family Medicine and
    Community Health
University of Massachusetts Medical
    School
Worcester, Massachusetts

Terrence C. Tsui, DO
Primary Care Sports Medicine Fellow
University of Massachusetts
Worcester, Massachusetts

Katherine Tsung, MD
Resident
Psychiatry Residency Program
Mather Hospital
Port Jefferson, New York

Sarah A. Turki, MBBS
Teaching Assistant
Department of Internal Medicine
King Abdulaziz University
Jeddah, Saudi Arabia

Alethea Y. Turner, DO
Associate Program Director
HonorHealth Family Medicine Residency
    Program
Scottsdale, Arizona

Bradley M. Turner, MD, MPH, MHA,
    FCAP, FASCP[†]
Associate Professor
Pathology and Laboratory Medicine
Department of Pathology and Laboratory
    Medicine
Breast and Gynecologic Subspecialty
    Services
Co-Director Breast and Gynecologic
    Pathology Fellowship
University of Rochester Medical Center
School of Medicine and Dentistry
Strong Health Highland Hospital
Board Certified in Anatomic and Clinical
    Pathology
Rochester, New York

Danielle Turrin, DO
Department of Emergency Medicine
Department of Geriatrics and Palliative
    Care
Northwell Health—North Shore University
    Hospital
Manhasset, New York

Kimberly S. Tustison, MD
Assistant Clinical Professor
Department of Women's Health
University of California Riverside School
    of Medicine
Riverside, California

Cheryll Udani, MD
Resident
University of Texas Health Science Center
    at San Antonio
San Antonio, Texas

John K. Uffman, MD, MPH
Pediatric Surgery
Cook Children's Medical Center
Fort Worth, Texas

Katherine S. Upchurch, MD, MACR
Professor of Medicine
University of Massachusetts Medical
    School
Division of Rheumatology
University of Massachusetts Memorial
    Medical Center
Worcester, Massachusetts

Ryan Paul B. Urbi, MD
Wellness Chief Resident
Department of Family and Community
    Medicine
University of Texas Health Science Center
    at San Antonio
San Antonio, Texas

Geraldine N. Urse, DO, FACOFP, MHPEd
Director of Medical Education/DIO
Doctors Hospital
Columbus, Ohio

Sara Usman, MBBS
Dow University of Health Sciences
Karachi, Pakistan

Onameyore Utuama, MD, MPH
Hospitalist
Physicians of Central Florida
Mt. Dora, Florida

Santiago O. Valdes, MD, FAAP
Associate Professor
The Lillie Frank Abercrombie Section of
    Pediatric Cardiology
Texas Children's Hospital
Baylor College of Medicine
Houston, Texas

Carrie Valenta, MD, FACP, FHM
Assistant Professor of Internal Medicine
Division Chief of Academic Hospital
    Medicine
CHI Health Creighton University Medical
    Center
Creighton University School of Medicine
Omaha, Nebraska

Sara L. Valente, MD[†]
University of Connecticut
Farmington, Connecticut

Anne M. Valeri White, DO, FAAFP
Associate Director
Family Medicine Residency
Summa Health, Akron Campus
Akron, Ohio
Associate Professor of Family and
    Community Medicine
Northeast Ohio Medical University
Rootstown, Ohio
Clinical Assistant Professor of Family
    Medicine
Ohio University Heritage College of
    Osteopathic Medicine
Athens, Ohio

Virginia J. Van Duyne, MD
Assistant Professor and Associate
    Residency Director
Department of Family Medicine and
    Community Health
University of Massachusetts Medical School
Worcester, Massachusetts

Mai C. Vang, MD
Family Medicine Residency Program
Dignity Health Methodist Hospital of
    Sacramento
Sacramento, California

Kathleen M. Vazzana, DO, MSc
Pediatric Rheumatology Fellow
Children's National Medical Center
Washington, DC

Nandhini Veeraraghavan, MD, CAQSM,
    FAAFP
Associate Program Director
Family Medicine Residency
St. Luke's Sacred Heart Campus
Allentown, Pennsylvania

Julian Vega, DO[†]
Family Medicine Resident
Martin Army Community Hospital
Fort Benning, Georgia

Crystal Verdick, DO, MS
Resident
Southeastern Regional Medical Center
Department of Internal Medicine
Campbell University School of
    Osteopathic Medicine
Lumberton, North Carolina

Astrud San Antonio Villareal, MD[†]
Chief Resident
Department of Family and Community
    Medicine
University of Texas Southwestern Medical
    Center
Dallas, Texas

Pradeepa P. Vimalachandran, MD, MPH
Rural Health Family Medicine Physician
Oakland Mercy Medical Hospital
Oakland, Nebraska

Conrad H. Vinalon, MD
St. Petersburg, Florida

Alicia H. Vinyard, DO
Assistant Professor of Surgery
Associate Surgery Clerkship Director
Department of Surgical Oncology
Augusta University Medical Center
Augusta, Georgia

Kirsten Vitrikas, MD[†]
Program Director
David Grant Medical Center
Family Medicine Residency
Travis Air Force Base, California

Kendall J. Vogel, DO[†]
Resident
Eglin Air Force Base Family Medicine
    Residency Program
Eglin Air Force Base, Florida

Yongkasem Vorasettakarnkij, MD, MSc[†]
Faculty of Medicine
Department of Medicine
Chulalongkorn University
Cardiac Center
King Chulalongkorn Memorial Hospital
Thai Red Cross Society
Bangkok, Thailand

Audrey C. Voss, DO[†]
Board Certified Family Medicine Physician
Sports Medicine Fellow
San Diego, California

Joseph R. Wagner, MD
Urologic Oncology and Minimally Invasive
    Surgery
Hartford Healthcare Medical Group
Director of Robotic Surgery
Hartford Hospital
Hartford, Connecticut

Jeffrey H. Walden, MD, FAAFP
Assistant Professor of Family Medicine
Department of Family Medicine
University of North Carolina Medical
    School
Cone Health Family Medicine Residency
Greensboro, North Carolina

Leslie A. Waldman, MD, FAAFP
Associate Program Director
Northwest Washington Family Medicine
    Residency
Bremerton, Washington

Thomas A. Waller, MD
Assistant Professor of Family Medicine
Residency Director
Department of Family Medicine
Mayo Clinic Florida
Jacksonville, Florida

Anne Walsh, ANP-BC
Northwell Health Solutions Advanced
    Illness Management
New Hyde Park, New York
Adjunct Clinical Faculty
Hofstra School of Graduate Nursing and
    PA Studies
Family Nurse Practitioner Department
Hempstead, New York

Nathaniel Walsh, MD
Chief Resident, General Surgery
Department of Surgery
Medical College of Georgia
Augusta University
Augusta, Georgia

Kenneth C. Walters, MD
Medical Center at Augusta University
Augusta, Georgia

Eugene Y. Wang, MD
Family Medicine Resident
Novant Health
Cornelius, North Carolina

Samuel C. Wang, MD, FAAFP
Associate Program Director
Memorial Family Medicine Residency
    Program
Sugar Land, Texas

Sicong Wang, MD[†]
Department of Family Medicine
Madigan Army Medical Center
Joint Base Lewis–McChord, Washington

Waiz Wasey, MD
Fellow
Department of Sleep Medicine
Mayo Clinic Florida
Jacksonville, Florida

Caitlin G. Waters, MD
Primary Care Sports Medicine Fellow
Department of Family Medicine and
    Community Health
University of Massachusetts Medical
    School
Worcester, Massachusetts

Lynn Weaver, MD
Resident
Department of Family and Community
    Medicine
Penn State College of Medicine
Hershey, Pennsylvania

Christopher J. Weber, MD[†]
LT, MC, USN
Family Medicine Resident
Department of Family Medicine
Naval Hospital Jacksonville
Jacksonville, Florida

Grant Wei, MD
Associate Professor and Program
    Director
Department of Emergency Medicine
Rutgers Robert Wood Johnson Medical
    School
New Brunswick, New Jersey

Jill T. Wei Doherty, MD
Santa Monica Family Physicians
Saint John's Physician Partners
Santa Monica, California

Travis Weinsheim, DO
Resident Physician
Department of Otolaryngology—Head and
    Neck Surgery
Philadelphia College of Osteopathic
    Medicine
Philadelphia, Pennsylvania

Patrice M. Weiss, MD
Executive Vice President and Chief
    Medical Officer
Carilion Clinic
Professor
Virginia Tech Carilion School of Medicine
Roanoke, Virginia

Jennifer Greene Welch, MD
Associate Professor of Pediatrics
Division of Pediatric Hematology/
    Oncology
Hasbro Children's Hospital
Alpert Medical School of Brown University
Providence, Rhode Island

Maggie C. Wertz, MD[†]
Operational Staff Physician
USAF
Fort Gordon, Georgia

James E. West, MD[†]
Associate Professor for Internal Medicine
Program Director for Internal Medicine
Southeastern Regional Medical Center
Campbell University School of Medicine
Lumberton, North Carolina

Katie L. Westerfield, DO, IBCLC, FAAFP[†]
Assistant Program Director
Martin Army Community Hospital Family
    Medicine Program
Fort Benning, Georgia

Rebecca Wetzel, DO[†]
CPT, MC, USA
Internal Medicine
Walter Reed National Military Medical
    Center
Bethesda, Maryland

Kellie D. Wheeler, MD
Department of Family, Community and
    Preventive Medicine
University of Arizona College of
    Medicine–Phoenix
Phoenix, Arizona

Vernon Wheeler, MD, FAAFP[†]
Assistant Professor
Department of Family and Community
    Medicine
Carl R. Darnall Army Medical Center
Fort Hood, Texas

Ebony B. Whisenant, MD
Assistant Professor of Family Medicine
Department of Humanities, Health and
    Society
Florida International University, Herbert
    Wertheim College of Medicine
Miami, Florida

Cassandra Q. White, MD, FACS
Assistant Professor and Program Director
Surgical Critical Care Fellowship
Department of Surgery
Medical College of Georgia at Augusta
    University
Augusta, Georgia

Christopher White, MD, JD, MHA
Associate Professor and Research
    Division Director
Department of Family and Community
    Medicine
University of Cincinnati College of Medicine
Cincinnati, Ohio

Todd A. Wical, DO[†]
Family Medicine Resident
Department of Primary Care
Martin Army Community Hospital
Fort Benning, Georgia

Marcy Wiemers, MD
Assistant Professor/Clinical
Associate Program Director
University of Texas Health Science Center
    San Antonio Family and Community
    Medicine Residency
San Antonio, Texas

Susanne Wild, MD
Associate Program Director for Academic
    Affairs
Banner University Medical Center
    Phoenix Family Medicine Residency
Clinical Assistant Professor
Department of Family and Community
    Medicine
University of Arizona College of Medicine
Phoenix, Arizona

Tyler J. Willenbrink, MD
Department of Dermatology
Dell Medical School at the University of
    Texas
Austin, Texas

Faren H. Williams, MD, MS[†]
Chief and Clinical Professor, Physical
    Medicine & Rehabilitation
Department of Orthopedics and Physical
    Rehabilitation
University of Massachusetts Medical School
Worcester, Massachusetts

Katherine Williams, MD
Resident, Family Medicine
Summa Health
Akron, Ohio

Amy B. Wilson-LaMothe, PharmD, BCPS
Assistant Professor of Pharmacy Practice
Massachusetts College of Pharmacy and
    Health Sciences University
Worcester, Massachusetts

Norton Winer, MD
Assistant Clinical Professor of Neurology
Case Western Reserve University School
    of Medicine
Cleveland, Ohio

Elisa R. Wing, MD
Resident
Department of Emergency Medicine
Advocate Christ Medical Center
Oak Lawn, Illinois

Robyn Wing, MD, MPH
Assistant Professor of Emergency
    Medicine & Pediatrics
Department of Emergency Medicine
The Warren Alpert Medical School of
    Brown University
Providence, Rhode Island

Fawn J. Winkelman, DO
Elite Medicine and Aesthetic Institute
Clinical Assistant Professor
Department of Osteopathic Family Medicine
Nova Southeastern University of
    Osteopathic Medicine
Boca Raton, Florida

Jay Winner, MD, FAAFP
Family Physician and Founder/Teacher
    Stress Reduction Classes
Sansum Clinic
Santa Barbara, California
Clinical Assistant Professor of Family
    Medicine
University of Southern California School
    of Medicine
Los Angeles, California

Kirsten A. Winnie, MD[†]
Family Medicine Resident
Offutt Air Force Base Family Medicine
    Residency Program
University of Nebraska Medical Center
Omaha, Nebraska

Christopher M. Wise, MD
Division of Rheumatology, Allergy, and
    Immunology
Virginia Commonwealth University Health
    System
Richmond, Virginia

Amy L. Wiser, MD
Assistant Professor
Department of Family Medicine
Oregon Health & Science University
Portland, Oregon

Daniel Wojenski, PharmD, BCOP, BCPS
Northwestern Memorial Hospital
Chicago, Illinois

Katherine F. Wojnowich, MD, CAQSM
Assistant Director, Family Medicine
    Residency
Assistant Director, Sports Medicine
    Fellowship
Family Medicine Residency
Bayfront Health St. Petersburg
St. Petersburg, Florida

Jeffrey D. Wolfrey, MD
Professor and Chair
Department of Family, Community, and
    Preventive Medicine
University of Arizona College of
    Medicine—Phoenix
Phoenix, Arizona

William W. Wong, DO[†]
Assistant Professor of Medicine
Department of Pulmonary and Critical
    Care Medicine
University of Massachusetts Medical
    School
Worcester, Massachusetts

Sundonia J. W. Wonnum, PhD, LCSW[†]
Assistant Professor
Department of Family Medicine
Uniformed Services University of Health
    Sciences
Bethesda, Maryland

J. Andrew Woods, PharmD, BCPS
Associate Professor of Pharmacy
Wingate University School of Pharmacy
Wingate, North Carolina

Anne Worth, DO
Riverside Family Practice
Columbus, Ohio

Barry P. Wright, MD
Hospitalist
Jacksonville, Florida

Taylor Wright, MD
Assistant Professor of Family Medicine
University of Tennessee, Knoxville
Knoxville, Tennessee

Frances Y. Wu, MD, FAAFP
Assistant Professor of Family Medicine
Assistant Director
Robert Wood Johnson Somerset Family
    Medicine Residency
Robert Wood Johnson Medical School
    Rutgers University
Somerville, New Jersey

Kristen M. Wyrick, MD[†]
Assistant Professor of Family Medicine
Uniformed Service University of the
    Health Sciences
Clinical Physician
The Everett Clinic
Marysville, Washington

Kai-Soon "David" Yang, MD
Family Practice
Methodist Charlton Medical Center
Dallas, Texas

Michael Y. Yang, MD
Primary Care Sports Medicine Physician
Departments of Orthopedics
Mercy Philadelphia Hospital
Philadelphia, Pennsylvania

Ahmad H. Yassin, DO, MA, FS[†]
Warrior Transition Unit Attending
Department of Family Medicine
Madigan Army Medical Center
Joint Base Lewis—McChord, Washington

Jennifer Yates, MD
Assistant Professor and Vice Chair
    (Academic Affairs)
Residency Program Director
University of Massachusetts Medical School
UMass Memorial Health Care
Worcester, Massachusetts

Dinesh Yogaratnam, PharmD, BCPS,
    BCCCP
Assistant Professor
School of Pharmacy Worcester/Manchester
Massachusetts College of Pharmacy and
    Health Sciences University
Worcester, Massachusetts

James R. Yon, MD
Department of Trauma and Acute Care
    Surgery
Swedish Medical Center
Englewood, Colorado

Kyung In Yoon, MD
Department of Emergency Medicine
Robert Wood Johnson University Hospital
New Brunswick, New Jersey

D. Harrison Youmans, MD
Director, Primary Care Sports Medicine
Fellowship
Orlando Health Orthopedic Institute/
University of Florida Health
Orlando, Florida

Edward L. Yourtee, MD, FACP
Chief Medical Officer
Parkland Medical Center
Derry, New York

David H. Yun, MD[†]
Family Physician
Okubo Family Health Clinic
Joint Base Lewis–McCord, Washington

Jacqueline L. Yurgil, DO[†]
Family Medicine Physician and Medical
Director
Family Health Clinic
78th Medical Operations Squadron
78th Medical Group
Robins Air Force Base, Georgia

Edlira Yzeiraj, DO, MS
Internal Medicine
Cleveland Clinic
Cleveland, Ohio

Isabel Zacharias, MD
Staff Physician
Department of Gastroenterology
UMass Memorial Medical Center
Worcester, Massachusetts

Christopher A. Zagar, MD, FAAFP
Associate Program Director
Family Medicine Residency Program
Novant Health
Cornelius, North Carolina

Nida Zahra, MD[†]
Assistant Professor and Medical Director
Department of Family and Community
Medicine
University of Texas Southwestern
Medical Center
Dallas, Texas

Jessica R. Zarndt, DO
Department of Family Medicine
UCLA Medical Center, Santa Monica
Santa Monica, California

Steven M. Zeddun, MD[†]
Assistant Professor of Medicine
Division of Gastroenterology and Liver
Diseases
George Washington University
Washington, DC

Peter M. Zhang, MD
Resident
Department of Family Medicine
University of California Riverside
Palm Springs, California

Youhua Zhang, MD, PhD
Associate Professor
Department of Biomedical Sciences
New York Institute of Technology College
of Osteopathic Medicine
Old Westbury, New York

Anna K. Zheng, MD
Assistant Professor, Appointment Pending
University of Massachusetts Memorial
Medical Center
Department of Family Medicine and
Community Health
Edward M. Kennedy Community Health
Center
Worcester, Massachusetts

Keren Zhou, MD
Clinical Fellow
Department of Endocrinology, Diabetes &
Metabolism
Cleveland Clinic
Cleveland, Ohio

Emily Ziady, MD
Clinical Fellow in Pediatrics
Massachusetts General Hospital
Boston, Massachusetts

Erika Zimmons, DO, MS
Assistant Professor
Department of Family Medicine and
Community Health
Division of Geriatric Medicine
University of Massachusetts Medical School
Worcester, Massachusetts

Gennine M. Zinner, RNCS, ANP
Clinical Professor
Massachusetts General Hospital Institute
of Health Professions
Nurse Practitioner
Boston Health Care for the Homeless
Program
Boston, Massachusetts

Patrick M. Zito, DO
Faculty, School of Nursing
Walden University
Minneapolis, Minnesota

Susan L. Zweizig, MD
Professor and Director
Division of Gynecologic Oncology
Department of Obstetrics and Gynecology
University of Massachusetts Medical
School
Worcester, Massachusetts

David Zwillenberg, MD
Professor of Clinical Otolaryngology Head
and Neck Surgery
Professor of Clinical Pediatrics
Department of Pediatrics
Drexel University College of Medicine
Chief, Section of Otolaryngology
St. Christopher's Hospital for Children
Philadelphia, Pennsylvania

Seth Zwillenberg, MD
Professor
Department of Otolaryngology—Head &
Neck Surgery
Drexel University College of Medicine
Philadelphia, Pennsylvania

[†]The views expressed are those of the authors and do not reflect the official policy of the Department of the Army, Department of the Navy, Department of the Air Force, the Department of Defense, or the United States Government.

CONTENTS

Topics

Contents

Diagnosis and Treatment: An Algorithmic Approach

This section contains flowcharts (or algorithms) to help the reader in the diagnosis of clinical signs and symptoms and treatment of a variety of clinical problems. They are organized by the presenting sign, symptom, or diagnosis.

These algorithms were designed to be used as a quick reference and adjunct to the reader's clinical knowledge and impression. They are not an exhaustive review of the management of a problem, nor are they meant to be a complete list of diseases.

ABDOMINAL PAIN, CHRONIC

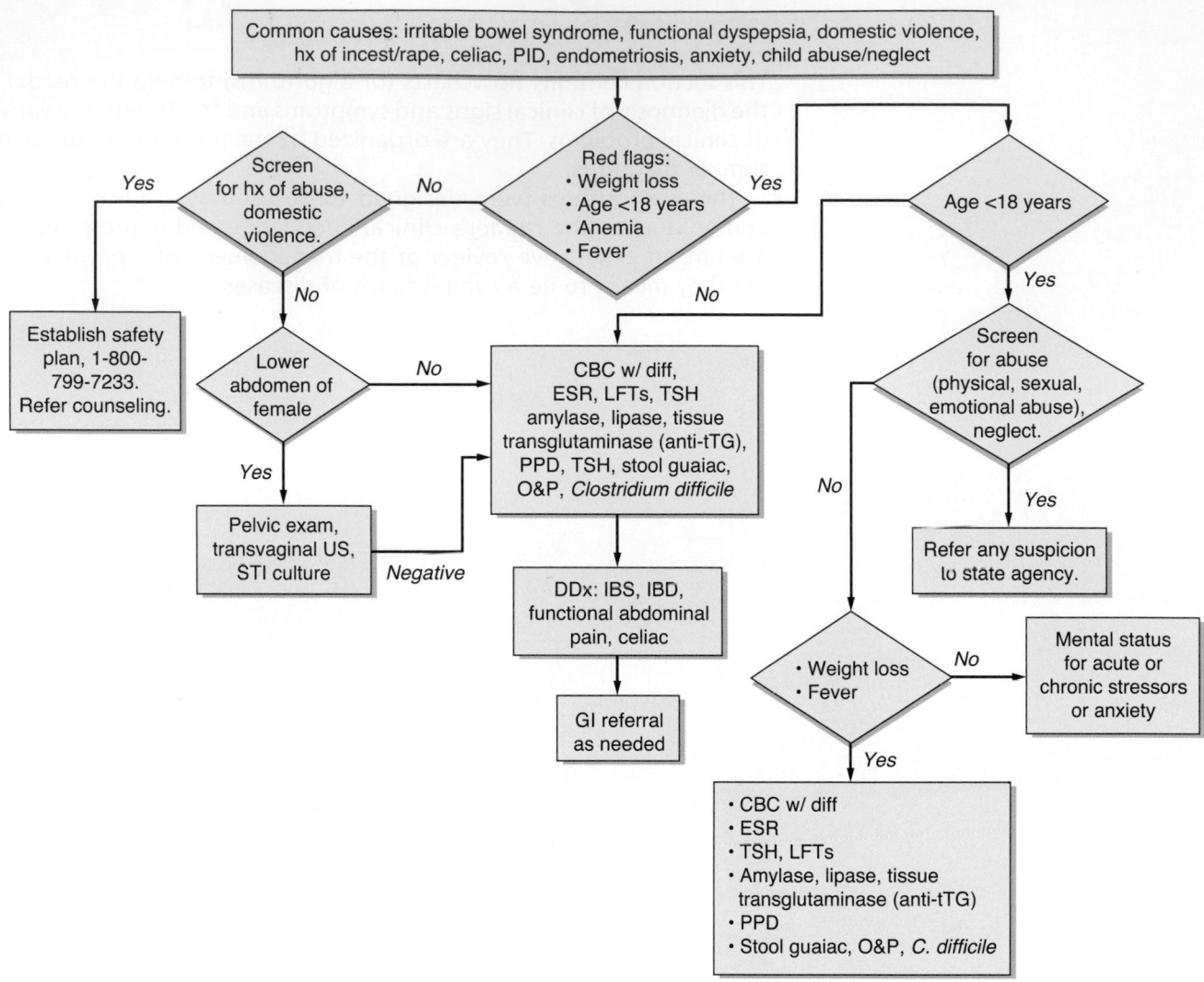

Note: Only check for *C. difficile* if the patient has concomitant diarrhea.

Shadi Hamdeh, MD and Adil Abdalla, MD

Camilleri M. Management of patients with chronic abdominal pain in clinical practice. *Neurogastroenterol Motil.* 2006;18(7):499–506.

ABDOMINAL PAIN, LOWER

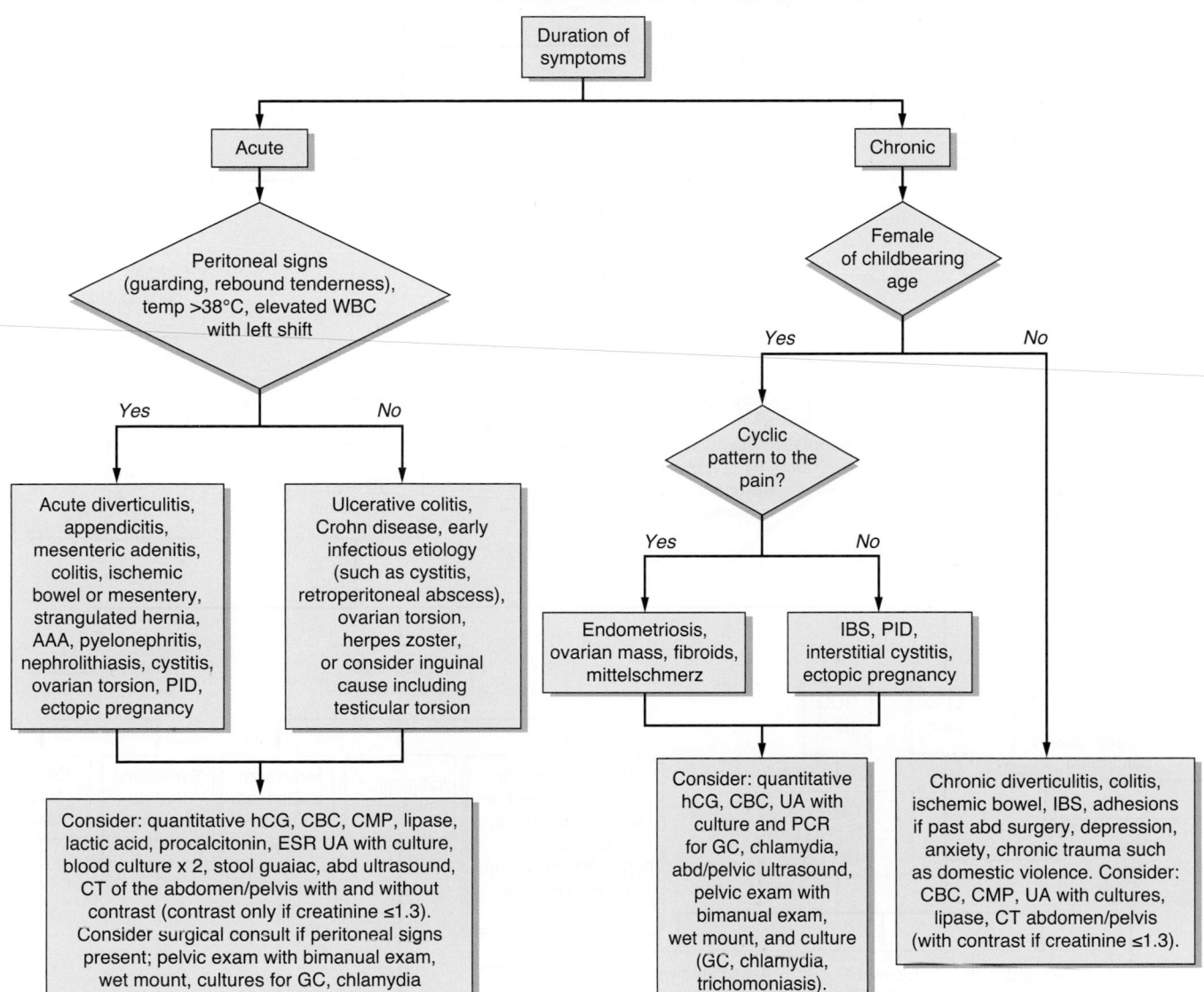

Abdominal abscess, adenitis, aortic aneurysm, appendicitis, inflammatory bowel disease, diverticulitis, ischemic bowel, colitis, pyelonephritis, nephrolithiasis, cystitis, strangulated hernia, ectopic pregnancy, PID, ovarian mass, torsion

Duration of symptoms

Acute

Peritoneal signs (guarding, rebound tenderness), temp >38°C, elevated WBC with left shift

Yes

Acute diverticulitis, appendicitis, mesenteric adenitis, colitis, ischemic bowel or mesentery, strangulated hernia, AAA, pyelonephritis, nephrolithiasis, cystitis, ovarian torsion, PID, ectopic pregnancy

No

Ulcerative colitis, Crohn disease, early infectious etiology (such as cystitis, retroperitoneal abscess), ovarian torsion, herpes zoster, or consider inguinal cause including testicular torsion

Consider: quantitative hCG, CBC, CMP, lipase, lactic acid, procalcitonin, ESR UA with culture, blood culture x 2, stool guaiac, abd ultrasound, CT of the abdomen/pelvis with and without contrast (contrast only if creatinine ≤1.3). Consider surgical consult if peritoneal signs present; pelvic exam with bimanual exam, wet mount, cultures for GC, chlamydia

Chronic

Female of childbearing age

Yes

Cyclic pattern to the pain?

Yes

Endometriosis, ovarian mass, fibroids, mittelschmerz

No

IBS, PID, interstitial cystitis, ectopic pregnancy

Consider: quantitative hCG, CBC, UA with culture and PCR for GC, chlamydia, abd/pelvic ultrasound, pelvic exam with bimanual exam, wet mount, and culture (GC, chlamydia, trichomoniasis).

No

Chronic diverticulitis, colitis, ischemic bowel, IBS, adhesions if past abd surgery, depression, anxiety, chronic trauma such as domestic violence. Consider: CBC, CMP, UA with cultures, lipase, CT abdomen/pelvis (with contrast if creatinine ≤1.3).

Maegen Dupper, MD, Kenneth A. Ballou, MD, FAAFP, and Andrew G. Alexander, MD

Cartwright SL, Knudson MP. Diagnostic imaging of acute abdominal pain in adults. *Am Fam Physician*. 2015;91(7):452–459.

ABDOMINAL PAIN, UPPER

Common causes: GERD, functional dyspepsia, PUD, gastritis, pancreatitis, biliary dysfunction, angina, esophageal/gastric cancer, medications, IBS

Acute severe pain + hypotension?

Yes →

Stabilize patient, US, CT chest/abdomen.

↓

Aortic dissection, AAA, severe acute pancreatitis, perforated viscous

No →

Suspicion of cardiac disease?

Yes →

Cardiac evaluation, cardiac enzymes, ECG

↓

Angina, MI, pericarditis

No →

GI alarm symptoms:

Bleeding: tachycardia, hypotension, hematemesis, hematochezia, melena, fatigue, SOB, drop in hematocrit

Neoplasia: weight loss, age >50 years, family hx of gastroesophageal malignancy, anemia, dysphagia, early satiety

Yes →

Endoscopy

↓

PUD, esophageal/gastric carcinoma

No alarm symptoms

↓

Epigastric pain

Poorly localizable

LUQ pain

RUQ pain

Fever, tenderness

CMP, LFTs, GGT, RUQ US

Pain radiating to back, hx of alcohol abuse, gallstones, recent ERCP, hypertriglyceridemia, hypercalcemia, smoking

Indigestion, bloating

Heartburn, acidic taste in mouth, worse at night

Symptoms that do not resolve with PPI

Cough, fever, CXR

Elevated bilirubin, alkaline phosphatase, fever, jaundice

Elevated AST/ALT, elevated bilirubin, hepatomegaly on US

Associated with meals, +/– elevated WBC/fever, + Murphy sign

Elevated lipase amylase, + imaging

If US is negative, obtain hepatobiliary scintigraphy (HIDA scan).

Splenic abscess, infarct

Cholangitis

Acute hepatitis, Budd-Chiari syndrome

Cholecystitis, biliary colic

Pancreatitis

IBS, PUD, gastroparesis, gastritis, GERD

GERD

Functional dyspepsia, IBS

Pneumonia

Daniel P. Szvarca, MD, Praphopphat Adhatamsoontra, MD, MPH, and Marie L. Borum, MD, EdD, MPH, MACP, FACG, AGAF

Natesan S, Lee J, Volkamer H, et al. Evidence-based medicine approach to abdominal pain. *Emerg Med Clin North Am.* 2016;34(2):165–190.

ACETAMINOPHEN POISONING, TREATMENT

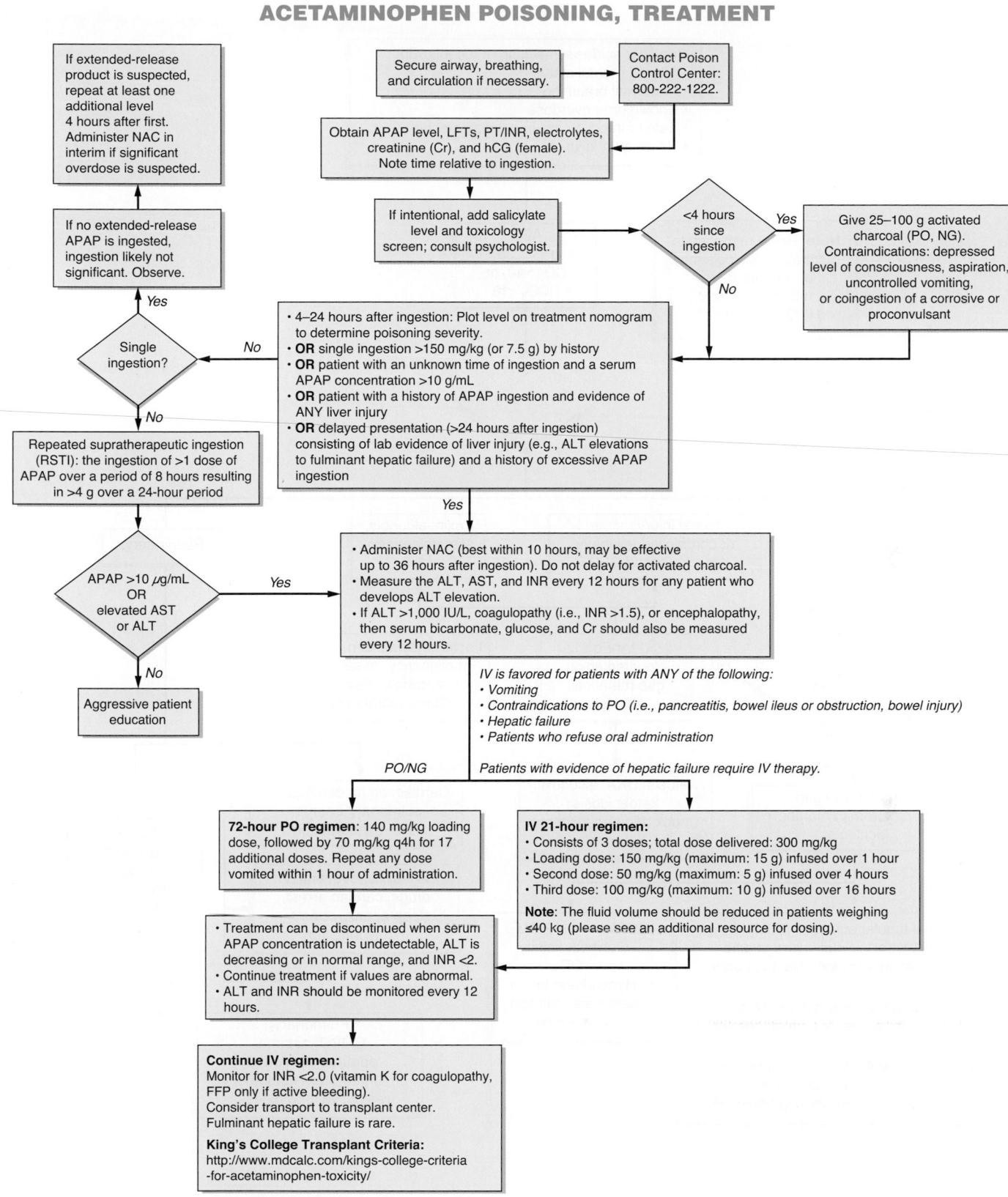

APAP, acetaminophen; NAC, *N*-acetylcysteine.

Marissa T. Christian, PharmD, Ryan B. Feeney, PharmD, and Frank M. Mazzotta, DO

Hodgman MJ, Garrard AR. A review of acetaminophen poisoning. *Crit Care Clin.* 2012;28(4):499–516.

ACIDOSIS

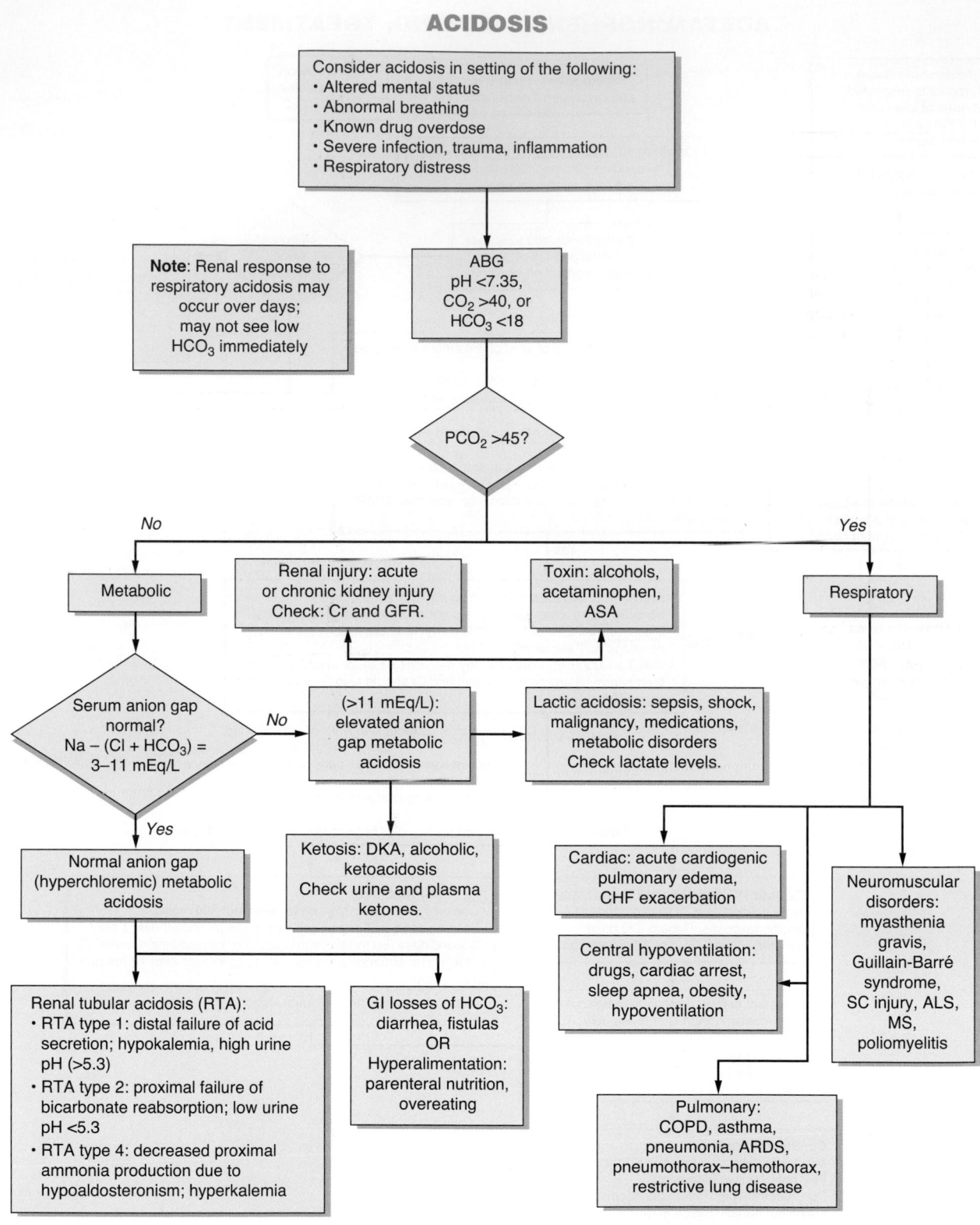

Consider acidosis in setting of the following:
- Altered mental status
- Abnormal breathing
- Known drug overdose
- Severe infection, trauma, inflammation
- Respiratory distress

Note: Renal response to respiratory acidosis may occur over days; may not see low HCO_3 immediately

ABG
pH <7.35, CO_2 >40, or HCO_3 <18

PCO_2 >45?

No — *Yes*

Metabolic

Renal injury: acute or chronic kidney injury Check: Cr and GFR.

Toxin: alcohols, acetaminophen, ASA

Respiratory

Serum anion gap normal?
$Na - (Cl + HCO_3) = 3-11$ mEq/L

No

(>11 mEq/L): elevated anion gap metabolic acidosis

Lactic acidosis: sepsis, shock, malignancy, medications, metabolic disorders Check lactate levels.

Yes

Normal anion gap (hyperchloremic) metabolic acidosis

Ketosis: DKA, alcoholic, ketoacidosis Check urine and plasma ketones.

Cardiac: acute cardiogenic pulmonary edema, CHF exacerbation

Neuromuscular disorders: myasthenia gravis, Guillain-Barré syndrome, SC injury, ALS, MS, poliomyelitis

Renal tubular acidosis (RTA):
- RTA type 1: distal failure of acid secretion; hypokalemia, high urine pH (>5.3)
- RTA type 2: proximal failure of bicarbonate reabsorption; low urine pH <5.3
- RTA type 4: decreased proximal ammonia production due to hypoaldosteronism; hyperkalemia

GI losses of HCO_3: diarrhea, fistulas
OR
Hyperalimentation: parenteral nutrition, overeating

Central hypoventilation: drugs, cardiac arrest, sleep apnea, obesity, hypoventilation

Pulmonary: COPD, asthma, pneumonia, ARDS, pneumothorax–hemothorax, restrictive lung disease

Frank J. Domino, MD

Kaplan LJ, Frangos S. Clinical review: acid-base abnormalities in the intensive care unit—part II. *Crit Care*. 2005;9(2):198–203.

ACNE

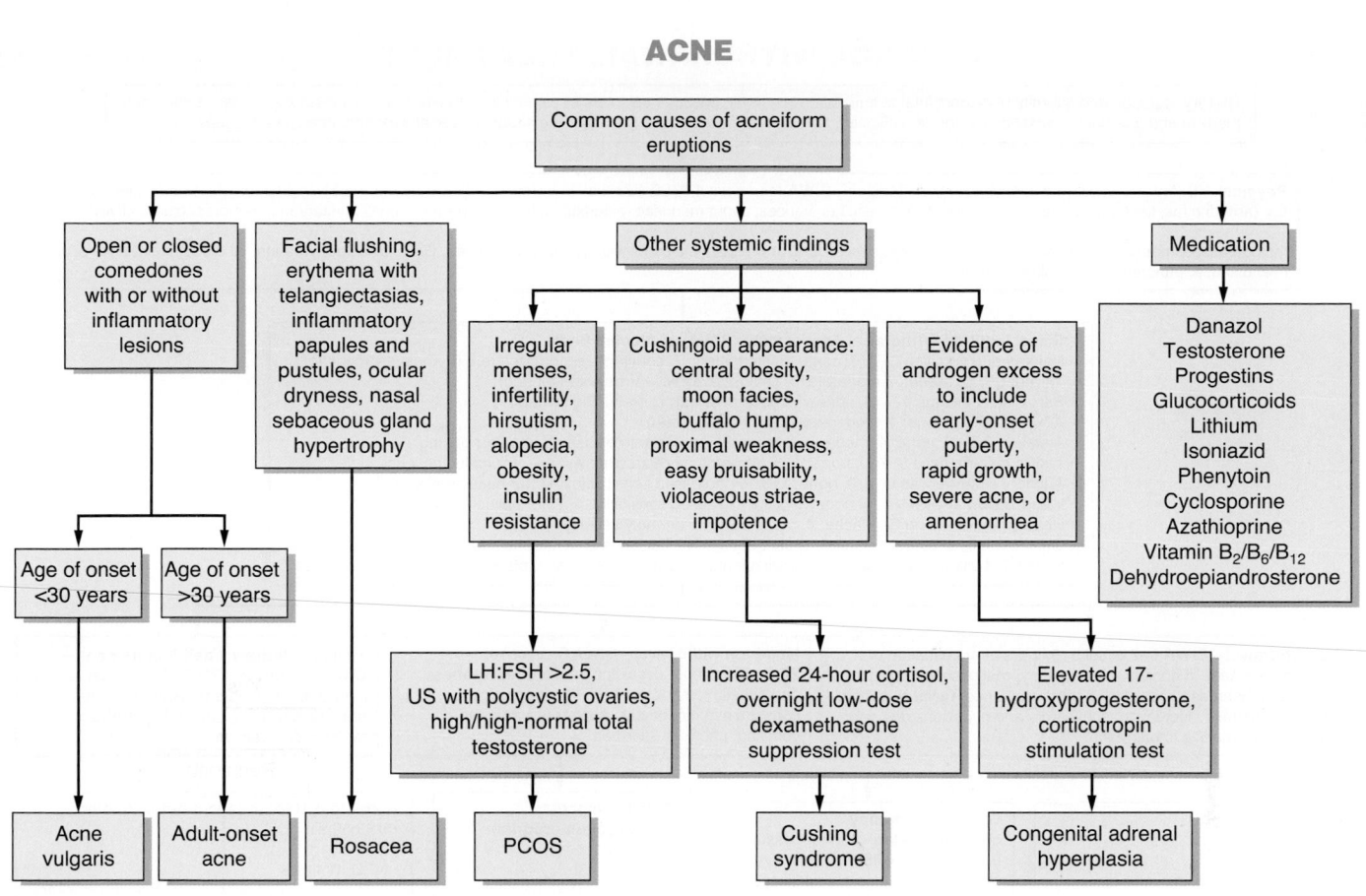

Lloyd A. Runser, MD, MPH, FAAFP

Lolis MS, Bowe WP, Shalita AR. Acne and systemic disease. *Med Clin North Am.* 2009;93(6):1161–1181.

ALCOHOL WITHDRAWAL, TREATMENT

History: duration and quantity of alcohol intake, time since last drink, previous episodes of alcohol withdrawal, concurrent substance use, preexisting medical and psychiatric conditions, prior detoxification admissions, prior seizure activity, living situation, social supports, stressors, triggers

Physical: VS (fever, tachycardia, tachypnea, hypertension), **CIWA** (see below), MSE (arousal, orientation, hallucinations), HEENT (diaphoresis, scleral icterus), CV (arrhythmias, M/R/G), evaluate s/sx of liver failure (ascites, varices, caput medusae, asterixis, palmar erythema), neuro (nystagmus, tremor, seizure activity)

Include assessment of conditions likely to *complicate*, *exacerbate*, or *precipitate* alcohol withdrawal: arrhythmias, CHF, CAD, dehydration, GI bleeding, infections, liver disease, pancreatitis, neurologic deficits.

Clinical Institute Withdrawal Assessment (CIWA) of Alcohol Scale
- Nausea and vomiting 0–7 (0, none; 4, intermittent; 7, constant nausea; frequent dry heaves/vomiting)
- Tremor 0–7 (0, none; 4, moderate; 7, severe; even with arms not extended)
- Paroxysmal sweats 0–7 (0, none; 4, beads of sweat; 7, drenching sweats)
- Anxiety 0–7 (0, none; 4, moderate; 7, acute panic state)
- Agitation 0–7 (0, none; 4, moderately restless; 7, constantly thrashing about or pacing)
- Tactile disturbances 0–7 (0, none; 1–3, for pruritus or paresthesias; 4–7, for hallucinations)
- Auditory disturbances 0–7 (0, none; 1–3, for increased sensitivity; 4–7, for hallucinations)
- Visual disturbances 0–7 (0, none; 1–3, for increased sensitivity; 4–7, for hallucinations)
- Headache 0–7 (0, no headache; 4, moderate; 7, extremely severe)
- Orientation 0–4 (0, fully oriented; 1, cannot do serial additions or is uncertain about date; 2, disoriented to date but within 2 calendar days; 3, disoriented to date by >2 days; 4, disoriented to place or person)

Mild withdrawal—CIWA 0–7 onset 5–8 hours after cessation or significant decrease in consumption: anxiety, restlessness, agitation, mild nausea, decreased appetite, sleep disturbance, facial sweating, mild tremulousness, fluctuating tachycardia and hypertension, possible mild cognitive impairment

Moderate withdrawal—CIWA 8–14 onset 24–72 hours after cessation: marked restlessness and agitation, moderate tremulousness with constant eye movement, diaphoresis, nausea, vomiting, anorexia, diarrhea

Severe withdrawal/delirium tremens— CIWA 15–30 onset 72–96 hours after alcohol cessation: marked tremulousness, fever, drenching sweats, severe hypertension and tachycardia, delirium

Good candidate for outpatient therapy:
- Not pregnant
- No comorbid illnesses requiring hospitalization
- No history of seizures
- Not a suicide risk
- Low risk of delirium tremens
- No history of unsuccessful outpatient detoxification
- Good access to follow-up medical care
- Tolerating oral medication
- Adequate social support available

Outpatient therapy contraindicated: pregnant, history of seizures or withdrawal seizures, chronic or acute comorbid illness requiring inpatient observation, lack of ability to follow-up

High risk of delirium tremens:
- Age >30 years
- Heavy drinking >8 years
- Drinking >100 g ethanol per day
- Random BAC >200 mg/dL
- Elevated MCV
- Cirrhosis

Admit to inpatient detoxification program:
- VS q4h
- CIWA q1–3h
- Institute seizure precautions.
- IV fluids

Admit to ICU for inpatient detoxification:
- VS q30min
- CIWA q1h
- NPO, IV fluids
- Lateral decubitus position, restrain if necessary
- Glucose, sodium, potassium, phosphate, and magnesium replacement as needed

Labs:
- Toxicology screen/EtOH level to assess need for and timing of withdrawal regimen
- CBC, electrolytes, phosphate, magnesium; vitamin B_{12} and folate to be repleted regardless of blood levels
- Amylase/lipase if suspected pancreatitis
- PT, PTT if suspected liver failure

Imaging:
- Head CT if history of trauma, mental status changes greater than expected, or focal neurologic changes
- Consider addition of EEG if focal neurologic signs or prolonged postictal state seizure.

Medications:
- Diazepam 5–20 mg IV q10min until calm and then q1h to maintain light somnolence for duration of delirium

If severe liver disease, severe asthma or respiratory failure, elderly, debilitated, or low serum albumin:
- Lorazepam 1–4 mg IV q10min until calm and then q1h to maintain light somnolence for duration of delirium

Treat as outpatient:
- Thiamine 100 mg once daily for 5 days
- Folic acid 1 g once daily for 5 days
- Evaluate daily until symptoms decrease.
- Assess blood pressure, heart rate, and CIWA-Ar score at each follow-up visit.
- Perform alcohol breath analysis randomly.
- Facilitate entry into a long-term outpatient therapy program (Alcoholics Anonymous).
- **If patient misses an appointment or resumes drinking, refer to addiction specialist or inpatient treatment facility.**

Example outpatient regimen: Fixed diazepam schedule
Day 1: 10 mg q6h
Day 2: 10 mg q8h
Day 3: 10 mg q12h
Day 4/5: 10 mg at bedtime

Symptom-triggered diazepam schedule:
Give dose if CIWA >8.
Day 1: 10 mg q4h PRN
Day 2: 10 mg q6h PRN
Day 3: 10 mg q6h PRN
Days 4/5: 10 mg twice a day PRN

Discharge planning:
- CIWA scores <8–10 for 24 hours
- Begin 1:1 or group therapy.
- Discharge to treatment center, day program, home.
- Facilitate entry into Alcoholics Anonymous.
- Evaluate for outpatient treatment with benzodiazepine.
- Nutrition/social work consultation

Medications:
Nutritional replacement
- Thiamine 100 mg IV/IM or PO once daily for 5 days
- Folic acid 1 g PO once daily for 5 days
Sympatholytic adjunctive therapy (no effect on prevention of withdrawal seizure and should be used with benzodiazepine therapy)
- Atenolol 50–100 mg once daily
- Clonidine 0.2 mg 3 times daily
For hallucinations associated with withdrawal:
- Haloperidol 2–5 mg IM/PO q1–4h max 5 mg/day
- Use only in conjunction with benzodiazepines and with extreme caution because haloperidol may lower seizure threshold.

Medications:
Long-acting benzodiazepines (diazepam) have rapid onset of action and provide smooth treatment course with fewer breakthrough symptoms.
- Diazepam 20 mg PO q1–2h until CIWA <8
  OR
- Diazepam 2–5 mg IV/min—maximum 10–20 mg q1h

Short-acting benzodiazepines (lorazepam) may have lower risk when there is concern about prolonged sedation, for example, elderly patients or those with severe hepatic insufficiency.
- Lorazepam 1–2 mg PO q2–4h until CIWA <8

Umer Farooq, MD and Sana Javed, MD

Muncie HL Jr, Yasinian Y, Oge' L. Outpatient management of alcohol withdrawal syndrome. *Am Fam Physician*. 2013;88(9):589–595.

ALKALINE PHOSPHATASE ELEVATION

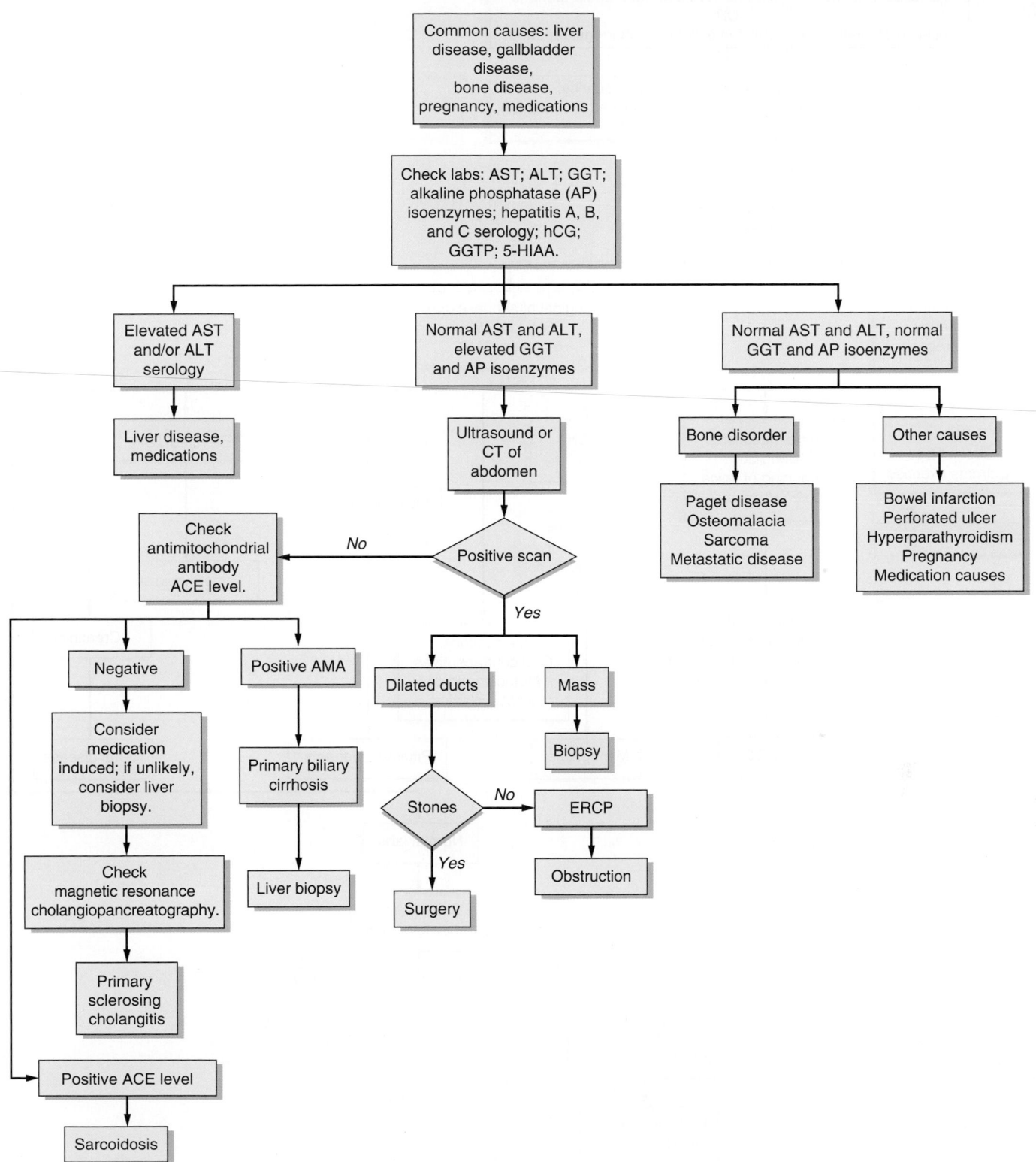

Reem Hadi, MD and Fozia Akhtar Ali, MD

Siddique A, Kowdley KV. Approach to a patient with elevated serum alkaline phosphatase. *Clin Liver Dis*. 2012;16(2):199–229.

AMENORRHEA, SECONDARY

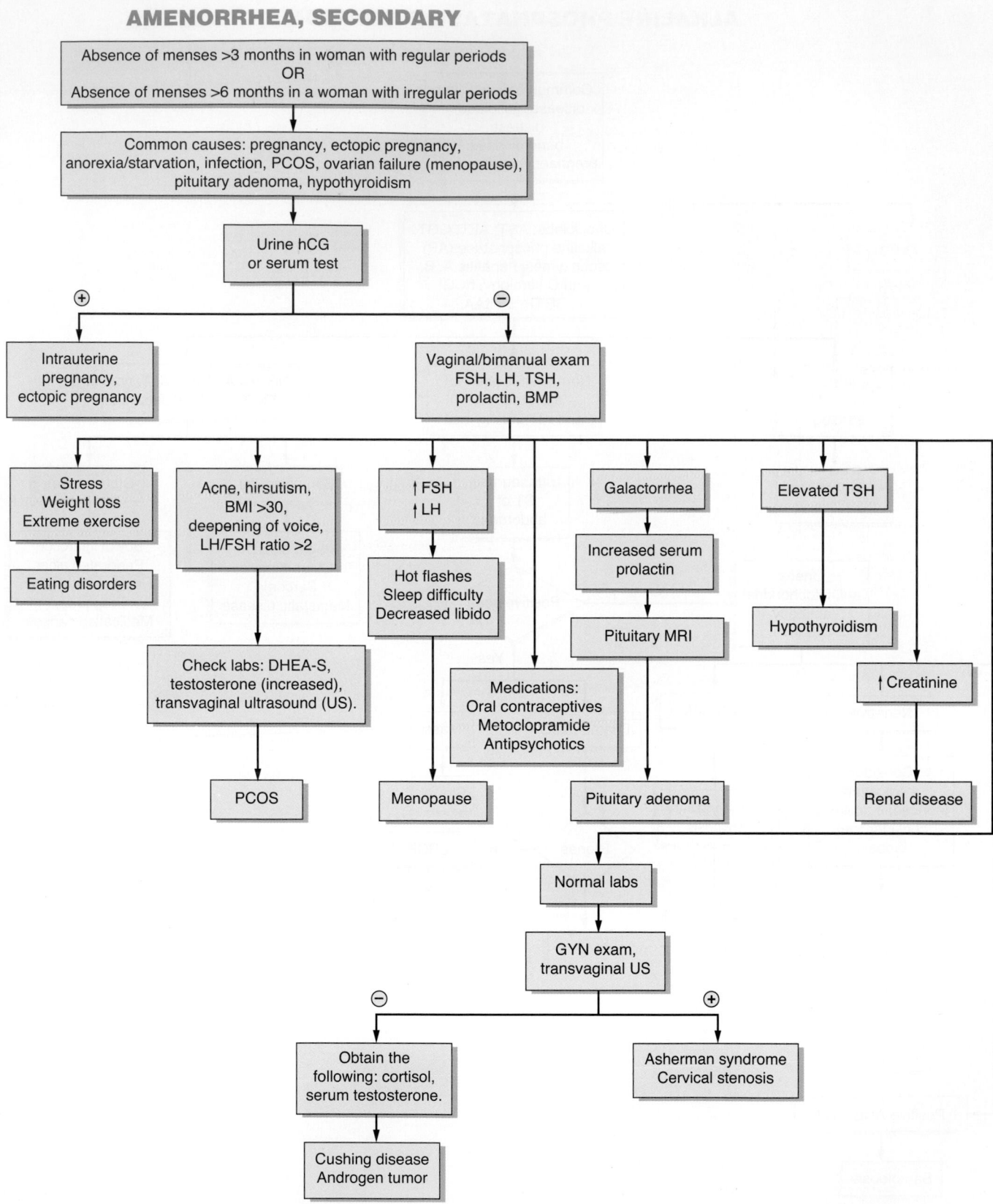

Maria Montanez Villacampa, MD and Fozia Akhtar Ali, MD

Klein DA, Poth MA. Amenorrhea: an approach to diagnosis and management. *Am Fam Physician.* 2013;87(11):781–788.

ANEMIA

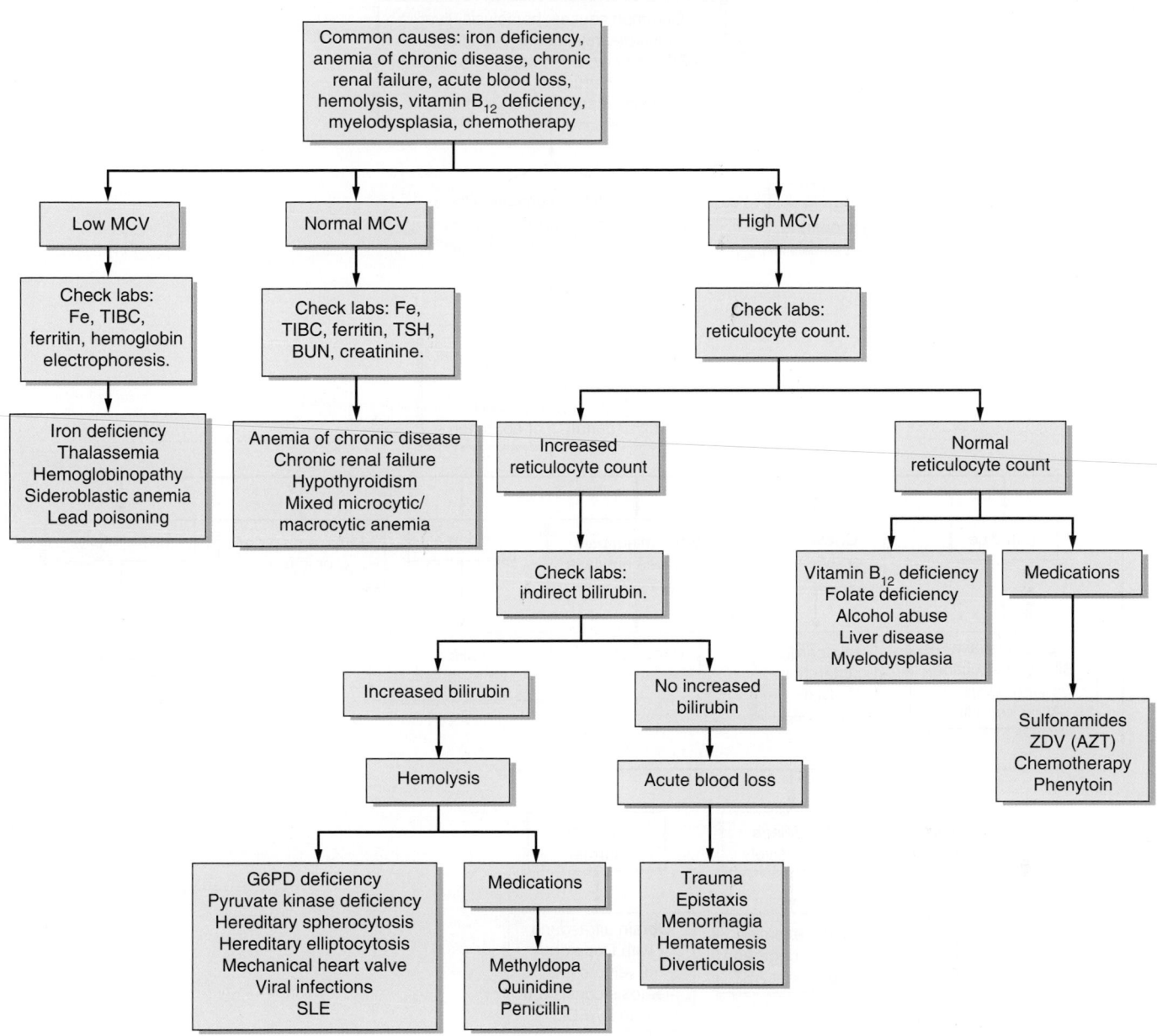

Robert A. Baldor, MD, FAAFP and Alan M. Ehrlich, MD

Smith DL. Anemia in the elderly. *Am Fam Physician.* 2000;62(7):1565–1572.

AST ELEVATION

Common causes: hemolysis, liver disease, myocardial infarction, NAFDL/obesity, CHF, acute renal failure, biliary obstruction, pancreatitis, muscle disorders, medications

EtOH or medication use (ASA, NSAIDs, statins, ACEI, estrogen)

Yes → Attempt to discontinue.

No

Check LFTs. Consider CBC, BUN, creatinine, hepatitis serologies, CPK, amylase, CXR, ultrasound/CT of abdomen.

| Jaundice | Chest pain or dyspnea | Abdominal pain Elevated amylase | Edema | Muscle disorder or injury | Liver toxicity |

| Liver disease Biliary obstruction Hemolysis Viral hepatitis | Myocardial infarction CHF | Pancreatitis | CHF Acute renal failure | | Alcohol Medications |

| Anemia | Exercises aggressively | All tests normal |

| Hemolysis | Limit exercise for 72 degrees and repeat AST. | Obtain ultrasound with Doppler. Evaluate for steatosis consistent with NAFDL. |

| LDL, haptoglobin | | |

Daniel J. Stein, MD, MPH and Stephen K. Lane, MD

Giboney PT. Mildly elevated liver transaminase levels in the asymptomatic patient. *Am Fam Physician.* 2005;71(6):1105–1110.

ASTHMA EXACERBATION, PEDIATRIC ACUTE

Initial evaluation: brief history of present illness, physical exam
Asthma history: emergency department visits, hospital and ICU admissions, home medications, frequency of oral steroid use, history of intubation, rapidly progressive episodes, food allergies
Physical exam: auscultation, use of accessory muscles, ability to speak, heart rate, oxygen saturation, PEF, or FEV_1

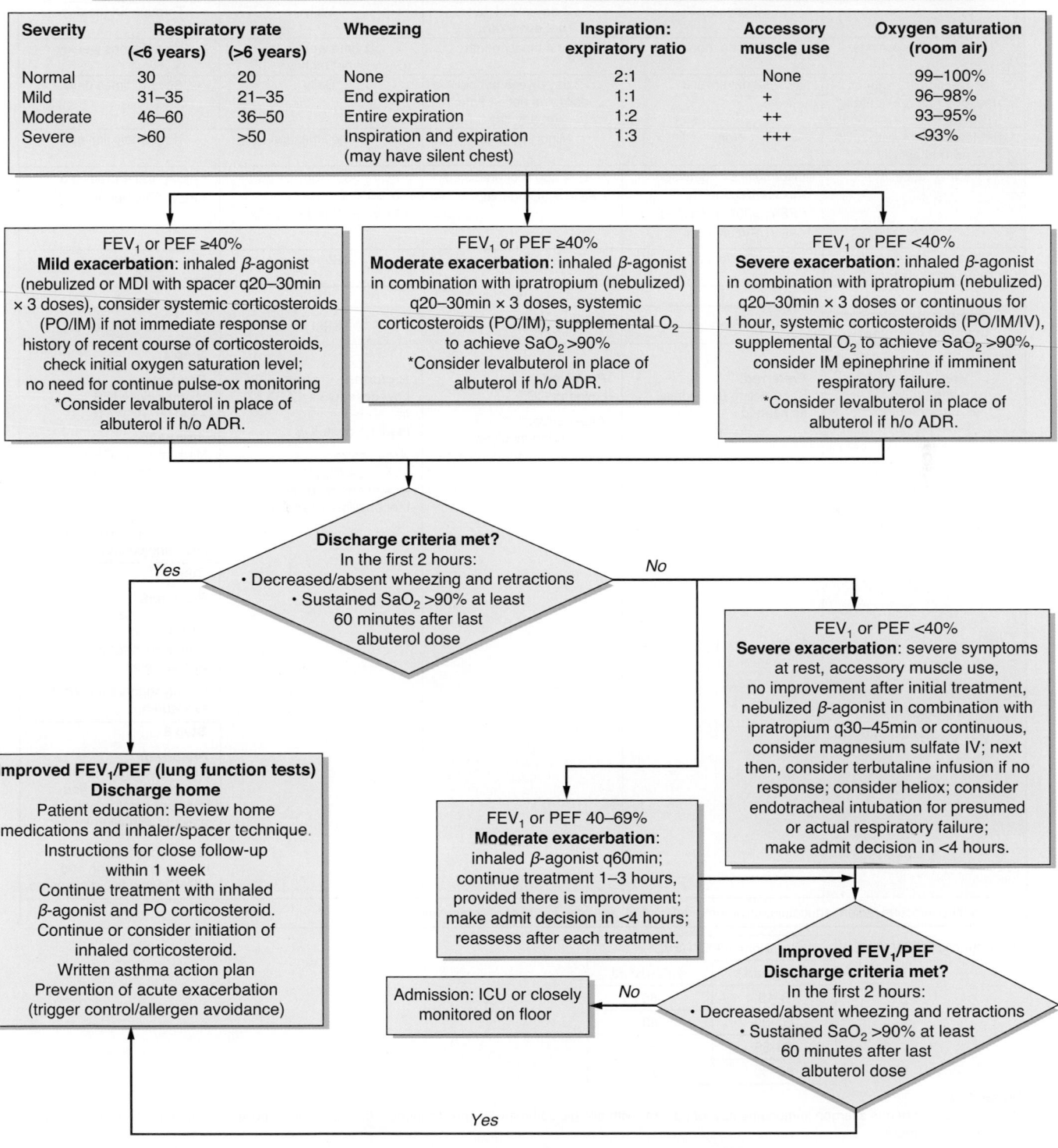

Severity	Respiratory rate (<6 years)	Respiratory rate (>6 years)	Wheezing	Inspiration: expiratory ratio	Accessory muscle use	Oxygen saturation (room air)
Normal	30	20	None	2:1	None	99–100%
Mild	31–35	21–35	End expiration	1:1	+	96–98%
Moderate	46–60	36–50	Entire expiration	1:2	++	93–95%
Severe	>60	>50	Inspiration and expiration (may have silent chest)	1:3	+++	<93%

FEV_1 or PEF ≥40%
Mild exacerbation: inhaled β-agonist (nebulized or MDI with spacer q20–30min × 3 doses), consider systemic corticosteroids (PO/IM) if not immediate response or history of recent course of corticosteroids, check initial oxygen saturation level; no need for continue pulse-ox monitoring
*Consider levalbuterol in place of albuterol if h/o ADR.

FEV_1 or PEF ≥40%
Moderate exacerbation: inhaled β-agonist in combination with ipratropium (nebulized) q20–30min × 3 doses, systemic corticosteroids (PO/IM), supplemental O_2 to achieve SaO_2 >90%
*Consider levalbuterol in place of albuterol if h/o ADR.

FEV_1 or PEF <40%
Severe exacerbation: inhaled β-agonist in combination with ipratropium (nebulized) q20–30min × 3 doses or continuous for 1 hour, systemic corticosteroids (PO/IM/IV), supplemental O_2 to achieve SaO_2 >90%, consider IM epinephrine if imminent respiratory failure.
*Consider levalbuterol in place of albuterol if h/o ADR.

Discharge criteria met?
In the first 2 hours:
• Decreased/absent wheezing and retractions
• Sustained SaO_2 >90% at least 60 minutes after last albuterol dose

Yes → No →

Improved FEV_1/PEF (lung function tests)
Discharge home
Patient education: Review home medications and inhaler/spacer technique.
Instructions for close follow-up within 1 week
Continue treatment with inhaled β-agonist and PO corticosteroid.
Continue or consider initiation of inhaled corticosteroid.
Written asthma action plan
Prevention of acute exacerbation (trigger control/allergen avoidance)

FEV_1 or PEF 40–69%
Moderate exacerbation:
inhaled β-agonist q60min; continue treatment 1–3 hours, provided there is improvement; make admit decision in <4 hours; reassess after each treatment.

FEV_1 or PEF <40%
Severe exacerbation: severe symptoms at rest, accessory muscle use, no improvement after initial treatment, nebulized β-agonist in combination with ipratropium q30–45min or continuous, consider magnesium sulfate IV; next then, consider terbutaline infusion if no response; consider heliox; consider endotracheal intubation for presumed or actual respiratory failure; make admit decision in <4 hours.

Admission: ICU or closely monitored on floor

No →

Improved FEV_1/PEF
Discharge criteria met?
In the first 2 hours:
• Decreased/absent wheezing and retractions
• Sustained SaO_2 >90% at least 60 minutes after last albuterol dose

Yes

Jasmit S. Minhas, MD and John A. Saryan, MD

National Asthma Education and Prevention Program. Expert Panel Report 3 (EPR-3): guidelines for the diagnosis and management of asthma—summary report 2007. *J Allergy Clin Immunol.* 2007;120(5)(Suppl):S94–S138.

ASTHMA, INITIAL TREATMENT

Management of chronic asthma
Classification of asthma severity in youth ≥12 years of age and adults

Components of severity	Intermittent	Mild persistent	Moderate persistent	Severe persistent
Daytime symptoms	≤2 days/week	>2 days/week but not every day	Daily	Throughout the day
Nighttime awakenings	≤2 times/month	3 or 4 times/month	>1 time weekly but not nightly	Often 7 times weekly
Short-acting β_2-agonist use for symptom control	≤2 days/week	>2 days/week but not daily and not >1 time on any day	Daily	Several times daily
Interference with normal activity	None	Minor limitation	Some limitation	Extremely limited
Lung function*	• Normal FEV_1 between exacerbations • FEV_1 >80% predicted • FEV_1/FVC normal	• FEV_1 ≥80% of predicted • FEV_1/FVC normal	• FEV_1 >60% but <80% predicted • FEV_1/FVC reduced 5%	• FEV_1 <60% predicted • FEV_1/FVC reduced >5%
Asthma exacerbations requiring oral steroids	0–1/year	≥2/year	≥2/year	≥2/year

Recommended step for initiating treatment	Step 1	Step 2[†]	Step 3	Step 4, 5, or 6
Preferred and alternative pharmacotherapy based on step	**Preferred:** Short-acting β_2-agonist as needed	**Preferred:** Low-dose ICS **Alternative:** Leukotriene modifier, nedocromil, or theophylline	**Preferred:** Low-dose ICS + LABA or medium-dose ICS **Alternative:** Low-dose ICS + leukotriene modifier, theophylline, or zileuton	**Step 4** **Preferred:** Medium-dose ICS + LABA **Alternative:** Medium-dose ICS + leukotriene modifier, theophylline, or zileuton Identify triggers (cold air, dust, allergic exposures/pets) and control exposures. **Step 5** **Preferred:** High-dose ICS + LABA, and consider omalizumab for patients with allergies Identify triggers and control exposures. **Step 6** **Preferred:** High-dose ICS + LABA + oral corticosteroid, and consider omalizumab for patients with allergies Identify patients at risk for reactions to aspirin and NSAIDs and avoid exposure.

At each step, discuss patient education, environmental control, and management of comorbidities.

*Lung function (FEV_1/FVC):

Normal FEV_1/FVC	
Age (years)	% Predicted
8–19	85
20–39	80
40–59	75
60–80	70

[†]Steps 2–4:
Consider subcutaneous allergen immunotherapy for patients with allergic asthma with specific triggers (i.e., dust mites, pollens, animal danders, etc.) in addition to standard treatment.

Kevin T. Abraham, MD and Claudeleedy Pierre, MD

Elward KS, Pollart SM. Medical therapy for asthma: updates from the NAEPP guidelines. *Am Fam Physician.* 2010;82(10):1242–1251.

ASTHMA, MAINTENANCE

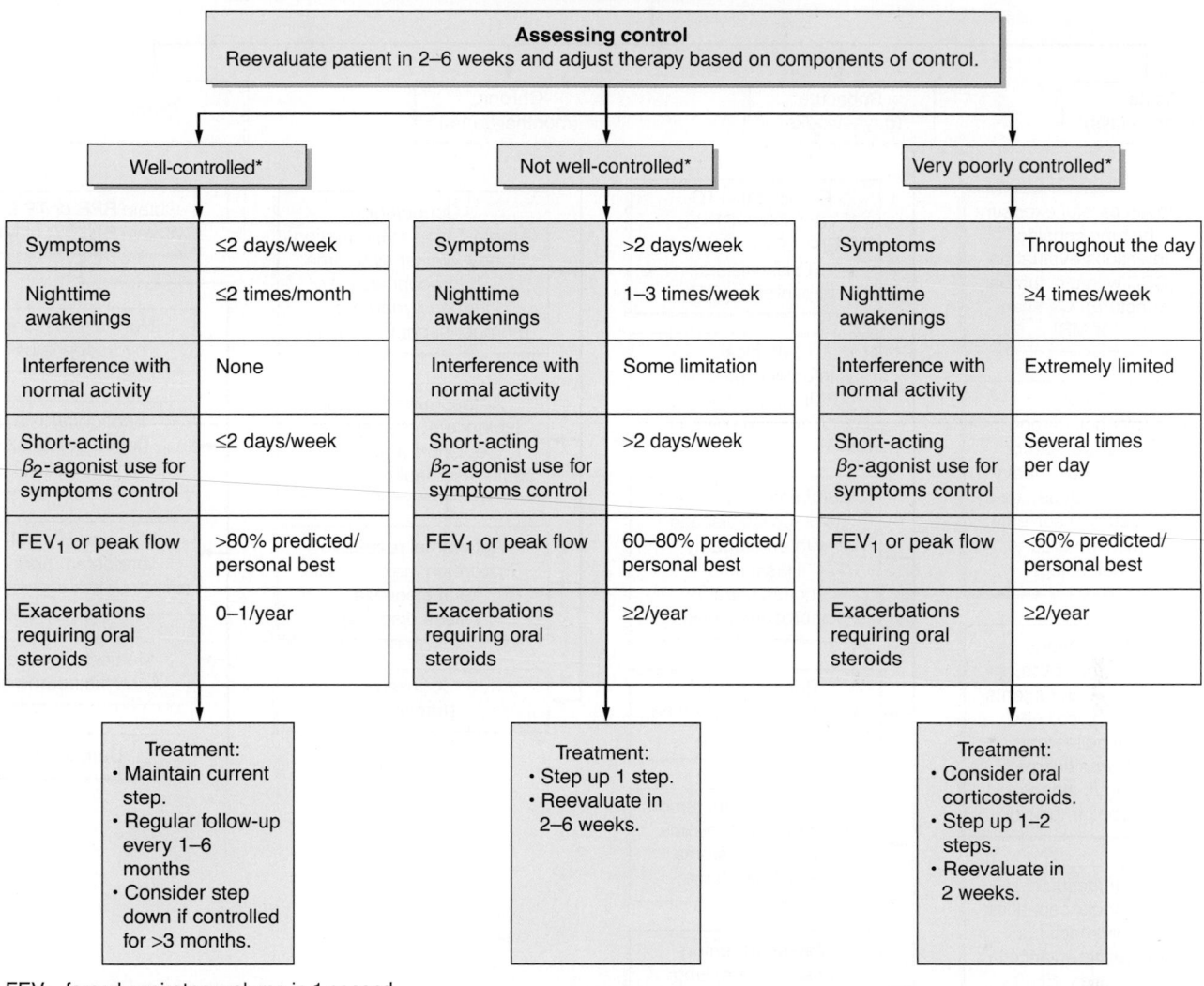

Assessing control
Reevaluate patient in 2–6 weeks and adjust therapy based on components of control.

Well-controlled*

Symptoms	≤2 days/week
Nighttime awakenings	≤2 times/month
Interference with normal activity	None
Short-acting β_2-agonist use for symptoms control	≤2 days/week
FEV$_1$ or peak flow	>80% predicted/ personal best
Exacerbations requiring oral steroids	0–1/year

Treatment:
• Maintain current step.
• Regular follow-up every 1–6 months
• Consider step down if controlled for >3 months.

Not well-controlled*

Symptoms	>2 days/week
Nighttime awakenings	1–3 times/week
Interference with normal activity	Some limitation
Short-acting β_2-agonist use for symptoms control	>2 days/week
FEV$_1$ or peak flow	60–80% predicted/ personal best
Exacerbations requiring oral steroids	≥2/year

Treatment:
• Step up 1 step.
• Reevaluate in 2–6 weeks.

Very poorly controlled*

Symptoms	Throughout the day
Nighttime awakenings	≥4 times/week
Interference with normal activity	Extremely limited
Short-acting β_2-agonist use for symptoms control	Several times per day
FEV$_1$ or peak flow	<60% predicted/ personal best
Exacerbations requiring oral steroids	≥2/year

Treatment:
• Consider oral corticosteroids.
• Step up 1–2 steps.
• Reevaluate in 2 weeks.

FEV$_1$, forced expiratory volume in 1 second.

*Can also be assessed using certified questionnaires in the outpatient setting:

ACT	≥20	16–19	≤15
ACQ	≤0.75	≥1.5	—
ATAQ	0	1–2	3–4

Kevin T. Abraham, MD and Claudeleedy Pierre, MD

Pollart SM, Elward KS. Overview of changes to asthma guidelines: diagnosis and screening. *Am Fam Physician.* 2009;79(9):761–767.

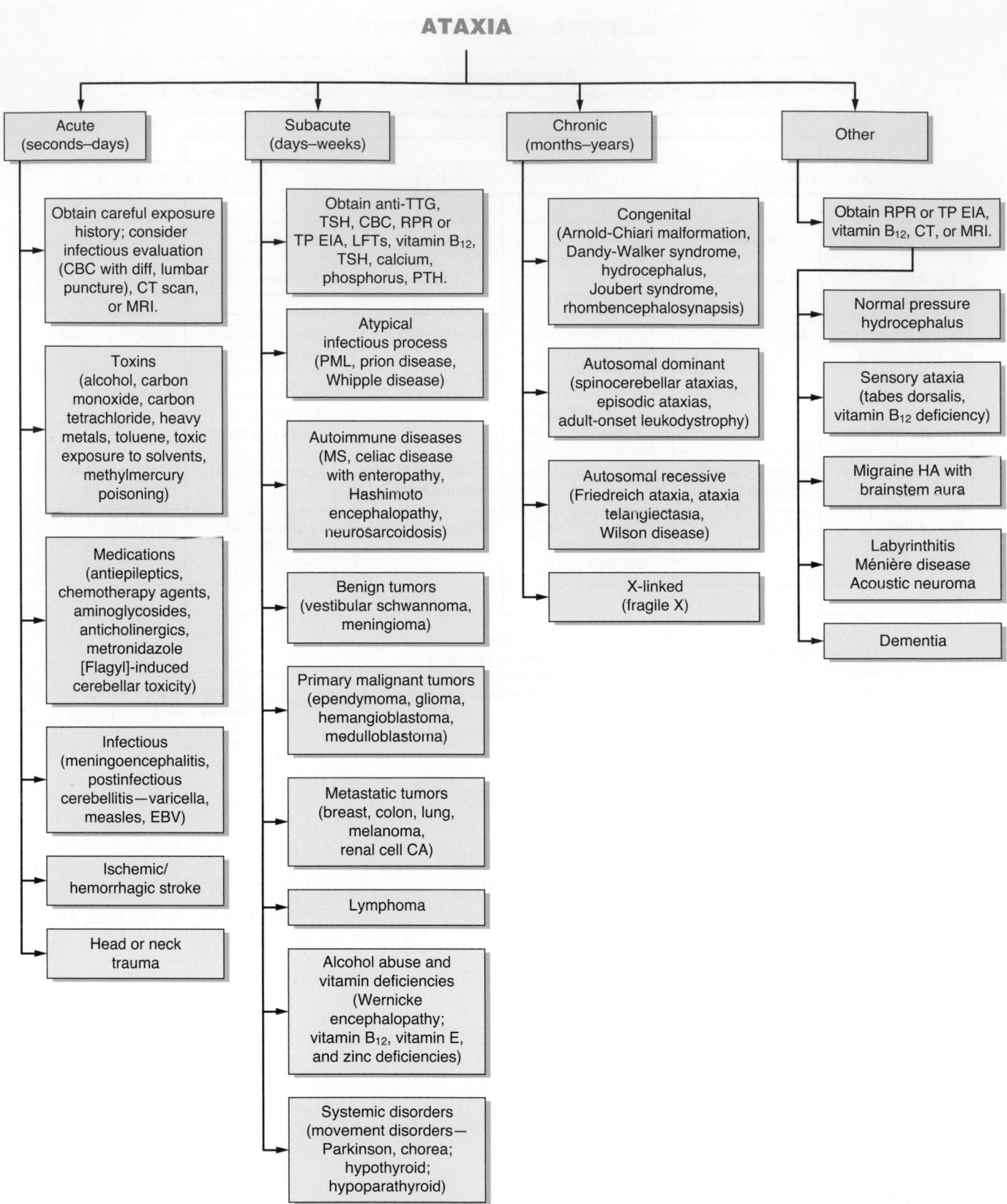

ATAXIA

Acute (seconds–days)

- Obtain careful exposure history; consider infectious evaluation (CBC with diff, lumbar puncture), CT scan, or MRI.
- Toxins (alcohol, carbon monoxide, carbon tetrachloride, heavy metals, toluene, toxic exposure to solvents, methylmercury poisoning)
- Medications (antiepileptics, chemotherapy agents, aminoglycosides, anticholinergics, metronidazole [Flagyl]-induced cerebellar toxicity)
- Infectious (meningoencephalitis, postinfectious cerebellitis—varicella, measles, EBV)
- Ischemic/hemorrhagic stroke
- Head or neck trauma

Subacute (days–weeks)

- Obtain anti-TTG, TSH, CBC, RPR or TP EIA, LFTs, vitamin B_{12}, TSH, calcium, phosphorus, PTH.
- Atypical infectious process (PML, prion disease, Whipple disease)
- Autoimmune diseases (MS, celiac disease with enteropathy, Hashimoto encephalopathy, neurosarcoidosis)
- Benign tumors (vestibular schwannoma, meningioma)
- Primary malignant tumors (ependymoma, glioma, hemangioblastoma, medulloblastoma)
- Metastatic tumors (breast, colon, lung, melanoma, renal cell CA)
- Lymphoma
- Alcohol abuse and vitamin deficiencies (Wernicke encephalopathy; vitamin B_{12}, vitamin E, and zinc deficiencies)
- Systemic disorders (movement disorders—Parkinson, chorea; hypothyroid; hypoparathyroid)

Chronic (months–years)

- Congenital (Arnold-Chiari malformation, Dandy-Walker syndrome, hydrocephalus, Joubert syndrome, rhombencephalosynapsis)
- Autosomal dominant (spinocerebellar ataxias, episodic ataxias, adult-onset leukodystrophy)
- Autosomal recessive (Friedreich ataxia, ataxia telangiectasia, Wilson disease)
- X-linked (fragile X)

Other

- Obtain RPR or TP EIA, vitamin B_{12}, CT, or MRI.
- Normal pressure hydrocephalus
- Sensory ataxia (tabes dorsalis, vitamin B_{12} deficiency)
- Migraine HA with brainstem aura
- Labyrinthitis Ménière disease Acoustic neuroma
- Dementia

Fozia Akhtar Ali, MD and Teny Anna Philip, MD

Brunberg JA; for Expert Panel on Neurologic Imaging. Ataxia. *AJNR Am J Neuroradiol.* 2008;29(7):1420–1422.

AZOTEMIA AND UREMIA

Azotemia is the elevation of blood urea nitrogen (BUN). It can be divided into prerenal, intrinsic renal, and postrenal azotemia based on the cause. This is important because treatments differ. Uremia is essentially symptomatic azotemia and is mostly due to the accumulation of BUN and other toxins or waste products normally filtered by the kidneys. Untreated uremia may progress to seizures, coma, and death.

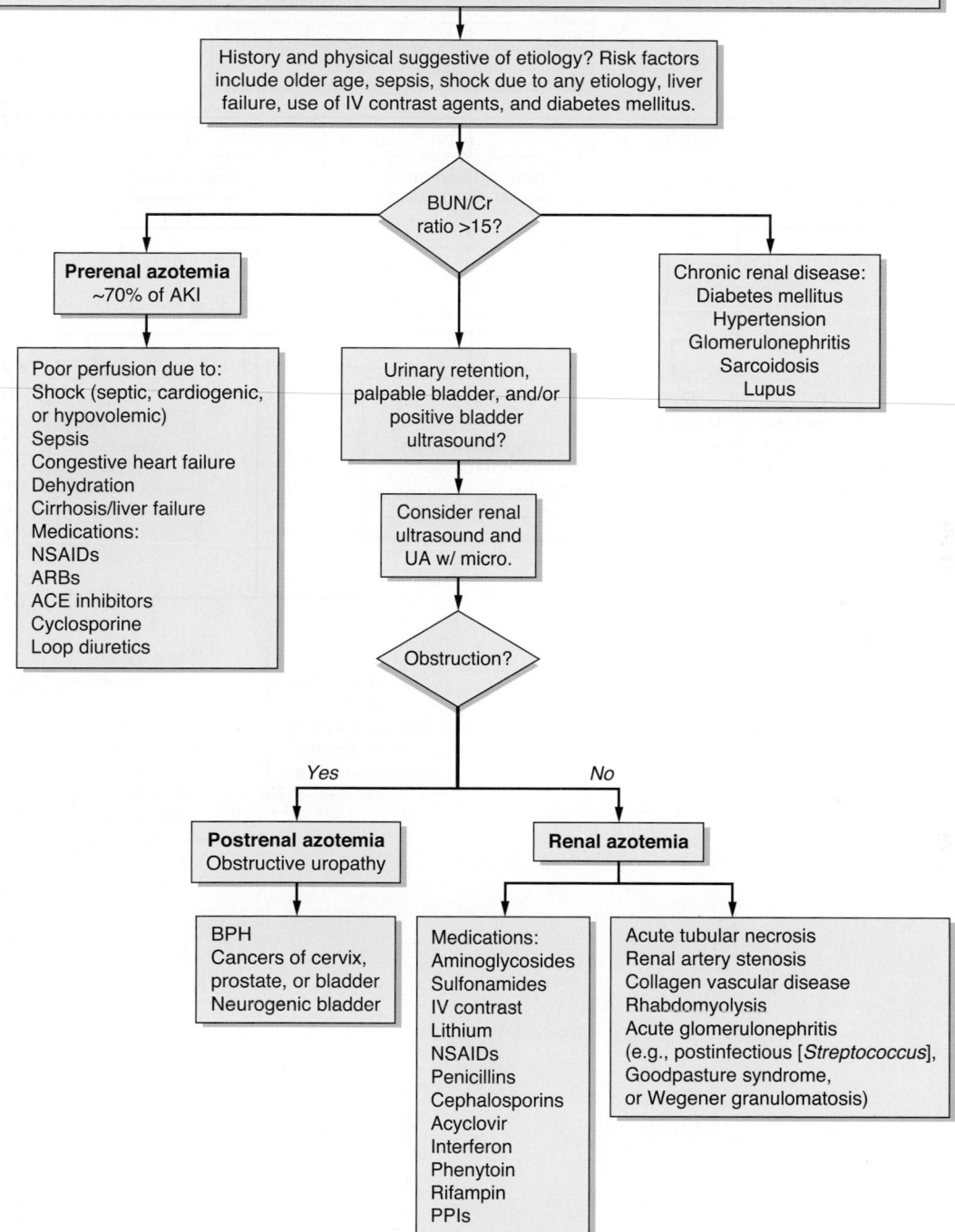

History and physical suggestive of etiology? Risk factors include older age, sepsis, shock due to any etiology, liver failure, use of IV contrast agents, and diabetes mellitus.

BUN/Cr ratio >15?

Prerenal azotemia
~70% of AKI

Poor perfusion due to:
Shock (septic, cardiogenic, or hypovolemic)
Sepsis
Congestive heart failure
Dehydration
Cirrhosis/liver failure
Medications:
NSAIDs
ARBs
ACE inhibitors
Cyclosporine
Loop diuretics

Urinary retention, palpable bladder, and/or positive bladder ultrasound?

Consider renal ultrasound and UA w/ micro.

Obstruction?

Yes   *No*

Chronic renal disease:
Diabetes mellitus
Hypertension
Glomerulonephritis
Sarcoidosis
Lupus

Postrenal azotemia
Obstructive uropathy

Renal azotemia

BPH
Cancers of cervix, prostate, or bladder
Neurogenic bladder

Medications:
Aminoglycosides
Sulfonamides
IV contrast
Lithium
NSAIDs
Penicillins
Cephalosporins
Acyclovir
Interferon
Phenytoin
Rifampin
PPIs

Acute tubular necrosis
Renal artery stenosis
Collagen vascular disease
Rhabdomyolysis
Acute glomerulonephritis
(e.g., postinfectious [*Streptococcus*],
Goodpasture syndrome,
or Wegener granulomatosis)

Steven A. House, MD, FAAFP, FAAHPM

Rahman M, Shad F, Smith MC. Acute kidney injury: a guide to diagnosis and management. *Am Fam Physician*. 2012;86(7):631–639.

CARDIAC ARRHYTHMIAS

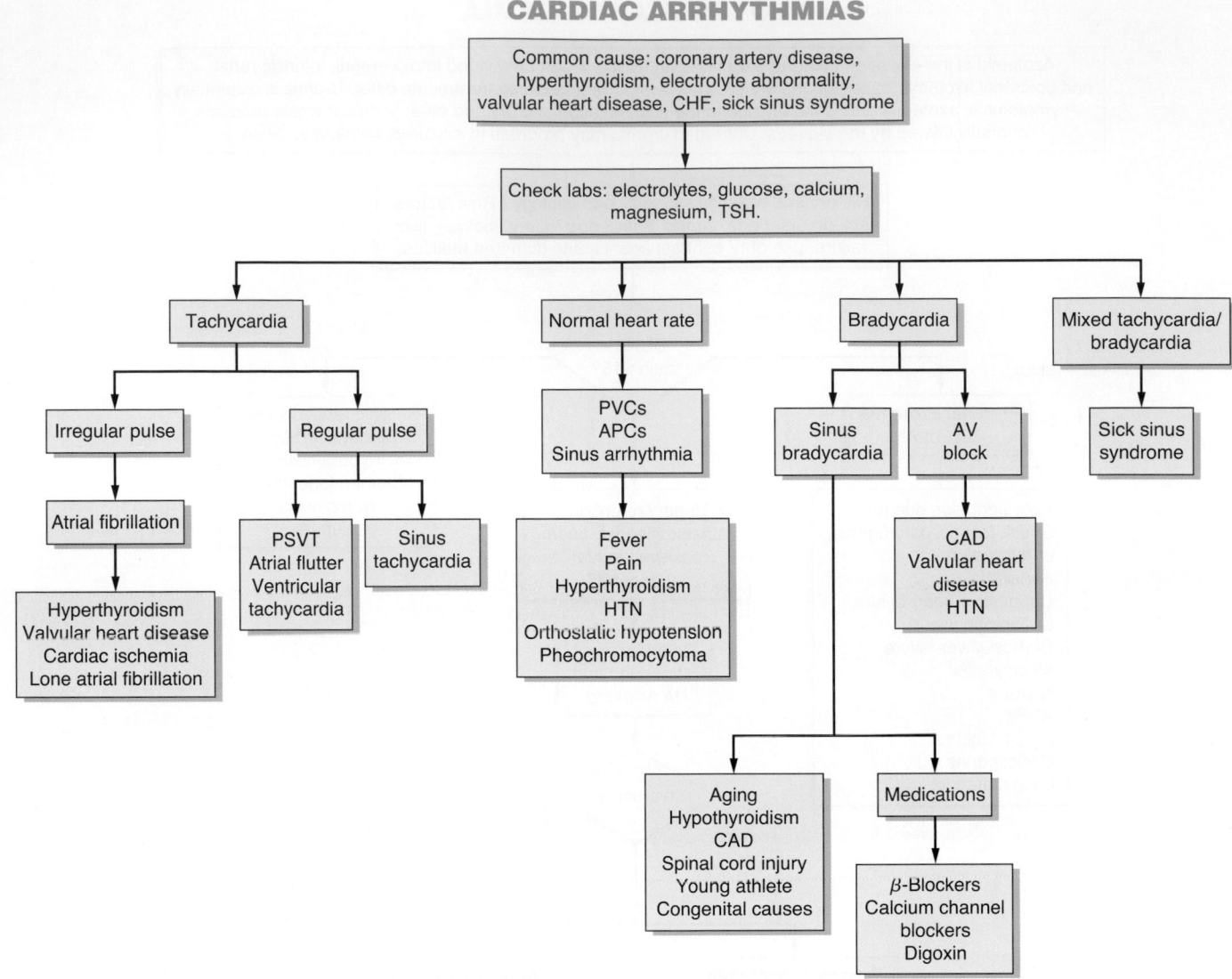

Common cause: coronary artery disease, hyperthyroidism, electrolyte abnormality, valvular heart disease, CHF, sick sinus syndrome

Check labs: electrolytes, glucose, calcium, magnesium, TSH.

Tachycardia

Normal heart rate

Bradycardia

Mixed tachycardia/ bradycardia

Irregular pulse

Regular pulse

PVCs
APCs
Sinus arrhythmia

Sinus bradycardia

AV block

Sick sinus syndrome

Atrial fibrillation

PSVT
Atrial flutter
Ventricular tachycardia

Sinus tachycardia

Fever
Pain
Hyperthyroidism
HTN
Orthostatic hypotension
Pheochromocytoma

CAD
Valvular heart disease
HTN

Hyperthyroidism
Valvular heart disease
Cardiac ischemia
Lone atrial fibrillation

Aging
Hypothyroidism
CAD
Spinal cord injury
Young athlete
Congenital causes

Medications

β-Blockers
Calcium channel blockers
Digoxin

Amaninderapal S. Ghotra, MD, Suma Chennubhotla, MD, and Kelly McCants, MD

Link MS. Clinical practice. Evaluation and initial treatment of supraventricular tachycardia. *N Engl J Med.* 2012;367(15):1438–1448.

CERVICAL HYPEREXTENSION INJURY

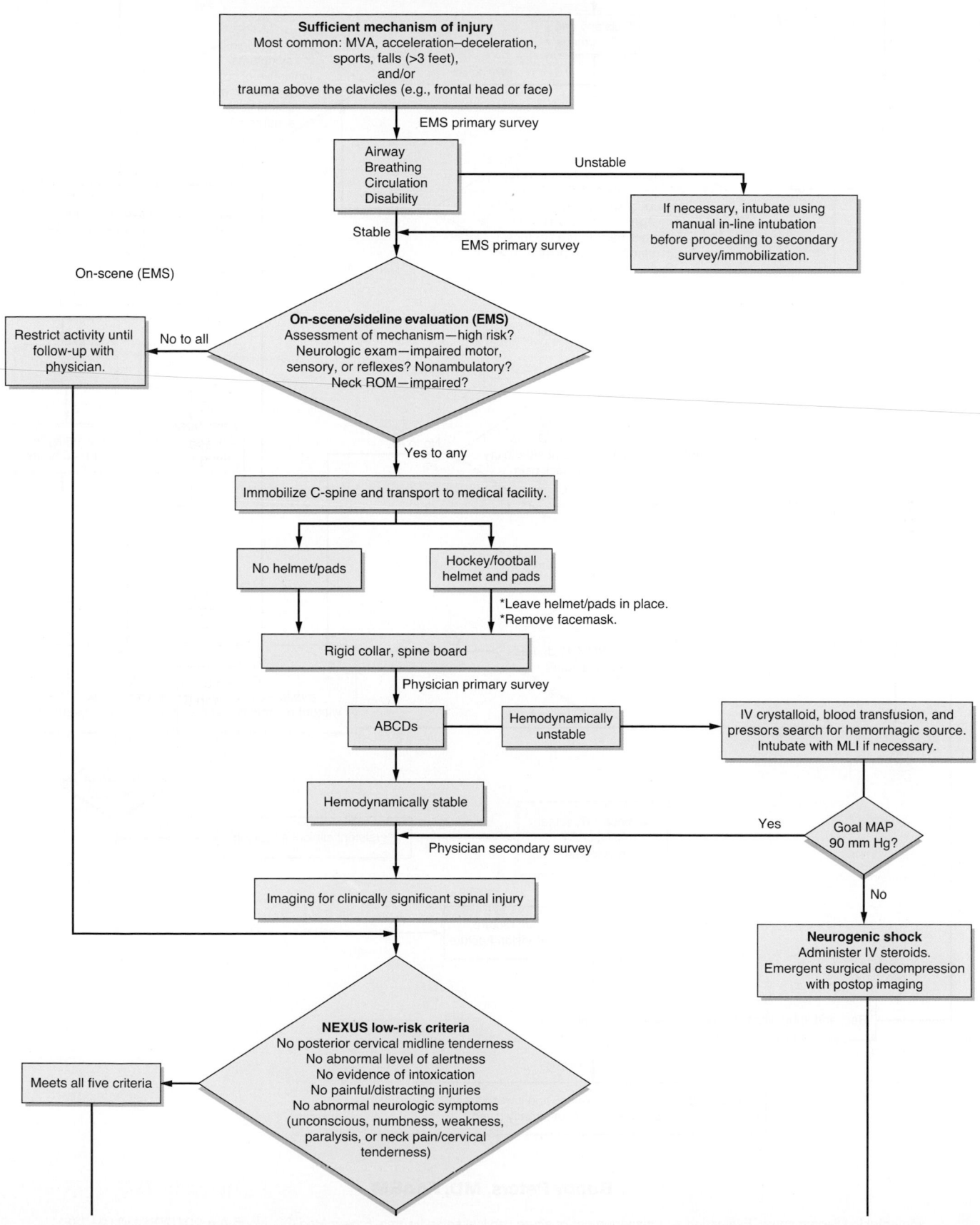

Sufficient mechanism of injury
Most common: MVA, acceleration–deceleration,
sports, falls (>3 feet),
and/or
trauma above the clavicles (e.g., frontal head or face)

EMS primary survey

Airway
Breathing
Circulation
Disability

Unstable

If necessary, intubate using
manual in-line intubation
before proceeding to secondary
survey/immobilization.

Stable ← EMS primary survey

On-scene (EMS)

On-scene/sideline evaluation (EMS)
Assessment of mechanism—high risk?
Neurologic exam—impaired motor,
sensory, or reflexes? Nonambulatory?
Neck ROM—impaired?

No to all

Restrict activity until
follow-up with
physician.

Yes to any

Immobilize C-spine and transport to medical facility.

No helmet/pads

Hockey/football
helmet and pads

*Leave helmet/pads in place.
*Remove facemask.

Rigid collar, spine board

Physician primary survey

ABCDs

Hemodynamically
unstable

IV crystalloid, blood transfusion, and
pressors search for hemorrhagic source.
Intubate with MLI if necessary.

Hemodynamically stable

Goal MAP
90 mm Hg?

Yes

No

Physician secondary survey

Imaging for clinically significant spinal injury

Neurogenic shock
Administer IV steroids.
Emergent surgical decompression
with postop imaging

NEXUS low-risk criteria
No posterior cervical midline tenderness
No abnormal level of alertness
No evidence of intoxication
No painful/distracting injuries
No abnormal neurologic symptoms
(unconscious, numbness, weakness,
paralysis, or neck pain/cervical
tenderness)

Meets all five criteria

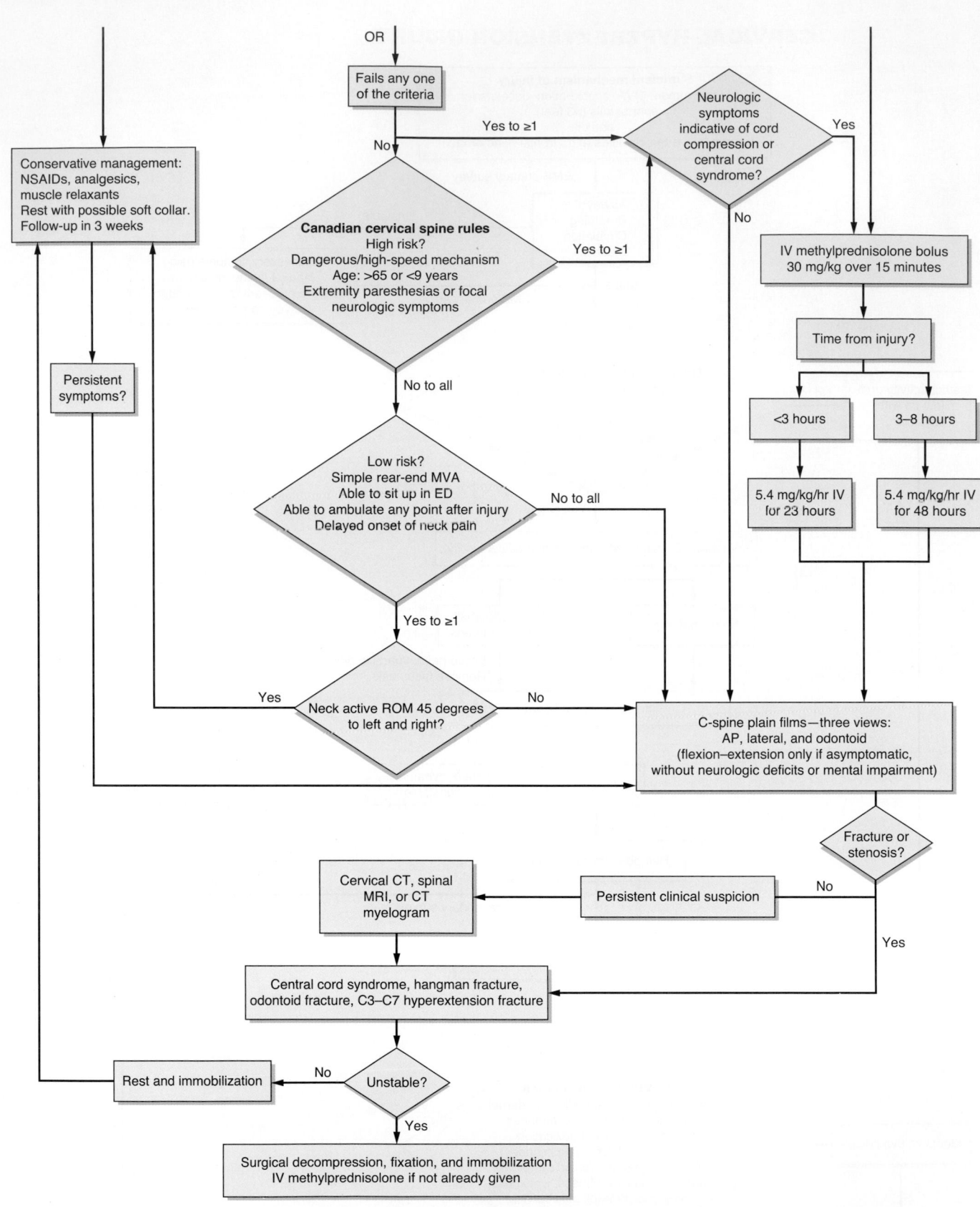

Bobby Peters, MD, FAAEM

Pimentel L, Diegelmann L. Evaluation and management of acute cervical spine trauma. *Emerg Med Clin North Am*. 2010;28(4):719–738.

CHEST PAIN/ACUTE CORONARY SYNDROME

Common DDx: STEMI, NSTEMI/unstable angina, PE, aortic dissection, anxiety, costochondritis, GI-related, domestic violence

ST elevation

ECG, troponin, oxygen, 325 mg ASA STAT, SL NTG q5min × 3, IV NTG if needed for pain and will not delay treatment, MSO$_4$ PRN, heparin, clopidogrel 300 mg, ticagrelor 180 mg, or prasugrel 60 mg

PCI available within 120 minutes

Yes   *No*

PCI

Thrombolytic therapy if not contraindicated or transfer to PCI facility

Successful treatment

No   *Yes*

Consider CABG.

Medical therapy
– ASA 81 mg
– Clopidogrel 75 mg daily for variable time depending on stent, other considerations
– High-intensity statin
– β-Blocker unless CHF or shock
– Cardiac rehabilitation
– Smoking cessation
– ACE inhibitor for patients with reduced EF
– Consider aldosterone antagonist if EF <40%.

No ST elevation

Rule out MI protocol: ECGs and troponin in ER and 3–6 hours later. ASA 325 mg STAT

Risk-stratify for CAD

High risk   **Low risk**

Admit to CCU or telemetry:
– Heparin (UFH or LMWH)
– ASA 81 mg daily
– Nitrates
Consider clopidogrel, β-blocker, ACE inhibitor, statin.

Exercise stress test

Positive

Cardiology evaluation for consideration of cardiac catheterization. If cardiology is unavailable, risk-stratify using TIMI or GRACE to determine next step (early invasive approach vs. medical therapy).

Negative

Review DDx: anxiety, GERD, PE, biliary dysfunction, musculoskeletal pain, domestic violence.

Jeremy Golding, MD, FAAFP

Amsterdam EA, Wenger NK, Brindis RG, et al. 2014 AHA/ACC guideline for the management of patients with non-ST-elevation acute coronary syndromes: executive summary: a report of the American College of Cardiology/American Heart Association Task Force on Practice Guidelines. *Circulation.* 2014;130(25):2354–2394.

CHILD ABUSE

When should you consider abuse?	
Physical abuse	**Sexual abuse**

• When a child makes a disclosure
• When there is no history to explain an injury
• When the history is not consistent with the injury seen
• When key parts of the history change
• Any bruise on a nonambulating child
• Any unreasonable or persistent delay in seeking medical care
	• Child makes a disclosure.
	• Child displays sexualized behaviors.
	  – Doing something with/saying something about private parts
	  – Doing something that looks like sex/talking about sex
	• Child has genital injury or infection.
	• Any pregnancy in child <16 years old

Medical history

- When >5 years old, ask open-ended questions that do not introduce concepts of abusive acts or abuser. For children <5 years old, acquire information away from the child's presence if possible.
- For all children: Listen attentively, BELIEVE them, and thank them for telling you. Reassure them and avoid any anger because the child may misinterpret this as you being angry at them.

1. Obtain a focused injury history (especially timeline).
2. Routine past medical history, including prior traumas, injuries, surgeries, and hospitalizations
3. Family history (bleeding/bruising concerns, bone/fracture concerns, metabolic or genetic issues)
4. Developmental and behavioral health history
5. Social history*: where they live, who they live with (including OTHER CHILDREN in household), substance use/abuse, job loss, other stressors, etc. Consult social worker if able.

*Note: History is the most important part of this entire process.

Physical examination

1. General assessment– child's alertness, demeanor, degree of pain, growth parameters, evidence of neglect (severe caries, diaper dermatitis, neglected wound care, cachexia, etc.)
2. Complete head-to-toe skin examination, looking for bruises, lacerations, burns, bites, etc. This includes oral cavity, ears, external genitalia, and perianal regions. All providers should conduct a thorough examination, even if referring patient to specialist.
3. Complete neurologic examination (including assessment of development and behavioral health).
4. Consider photographs* and/or sketches of physical signs.
5. If sexual abuse suspected, a detailed genital examination should be performed by a trained medical professional (i.e., a child abuse physician). A sexual assault nursing evaluation (SANE) may be warranted as well if event occurred in last 5 days. Postassault lab testing and HIV prophylaxis may also be needed. Please contact your local child abuse team, SANE service, or emergency department for further assistance with management. All providers should conduct a thorough examination, even if referring patient to specialist.

*Only secure cameras should be used to photograph patients. This typically excludes personal cell phones. If forensic photographs are needed, please contact local social services or child abuse team.

Diagnostic testing for suspected child physical abuse

Age ≤6 months	**Age 6–24 months**	**Age >24 months**

1. Child protection team consult
2. Head CT or MRI
3. Skeletal survey
4. Lab evaluation:
  a. AST/ALT
  b. Consider urine toxicology.
5. Ophthalmology consult only if focal neuro exam findings or intracranial blood
 	
If unexplained:
• Bruising—send CBC, PT, and aPTT
• Fractures—send Ca, Mg, phos, alk phos, iPTH, 25-OH vitamin D
	1. Child protection team consult
	2. Skeletal survey
	3. Lab evaluation:
	  a. AST/ALT
	  b. Consider urine toxicology.
	4. Low threshold for head CT or MRI
	
	If unexplained:
	• Bruising—send CBC, PT, and aPTT
	• Fractures—send Ca, Mg, phos, alk phos, iPTH, 25-OH vitamin D
		1. Consider child protection team consult.
		2. If >5 years old, consider history from child.
		3. Consider lab evaluation:
		  a. AST/ALT
		  b. Urine toxicology
		
		If unexplained:
		• Bruising—send CBC, PT, and aPTT
		• Fractures—send Ca, Mg, phos, alk phos, iPTH, 25-OH vitamin D

Management

1. Referral to investigative agencies/child protection agencies according to state-specific mandated reporting laws. State reporting statutes and other resources available from Child Welfare Information Gateway (www.childwelfare.gov). Additional information on child abuse and neglect (COCAN): www2.aap.org/sections/childabuseneglect/
2. Referral to appropriate medical providers (such as a pediatric trauma center)
3. Referral to appropriate behavioral health counselor for trauma symptom screening and education. Early mental health interventions (within the first 30 days following a traumatic event); educational information under resources at the National Child Traumatic Stress Network webpage (http://www.nctsn.org/resources)
4. Medicolegal documentation
5. Safety plan in place prior to discharge with appropriate follow-up plan. This may require coordination with local social services.

Sasha Svendsen, MD and Peter J. Sell, DO

Campbell KA, Olson LM, Keenan HT. Critical elements in the medical evaluation of suspected child physical abuse. *Pediatrics.* 2015;136(1):35–43.

CHRONIC JOINT PAIN AND STIFFNESS

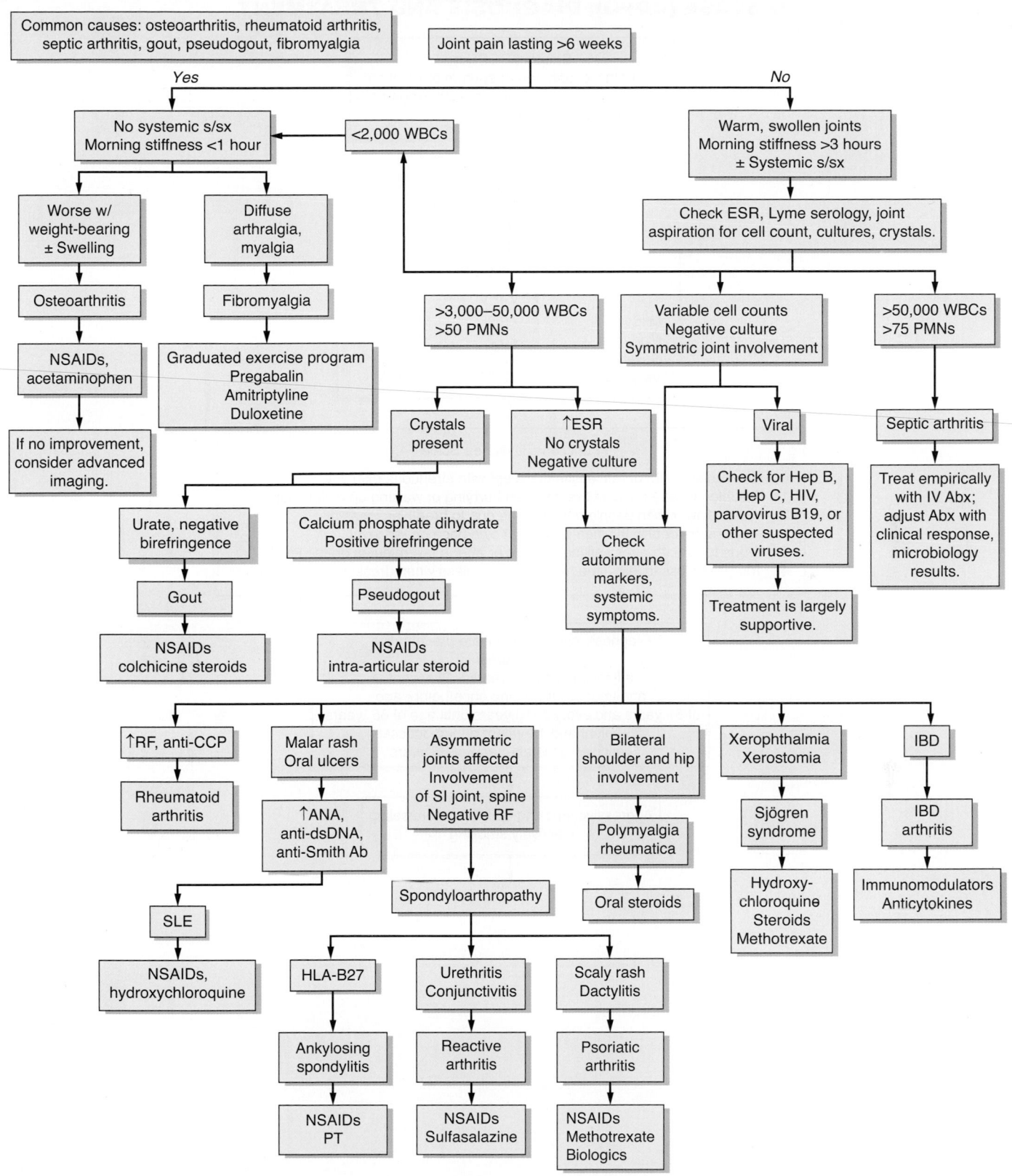

Common causes: osteoarthritis, rheumatoid arthritis, septic arthritis, gout, pseudogout, fibromyalgia

Joint pain lasting >6 weeks

Yes — No systemic s/sx, Morning stiffness <1 hour ← <2,000 WBCs

No — Warm, swollen joints, Morning stiffness >3 hours ± Systemic s/sx

Worse w/ weight-bearing ± Swelling → Osteoarthritis → NSAIDs, acetaminophen → If no improvement, consider advanced imaging.

Diffuse arthralgia, myalgia → Fibromyalgia → Graduated exercise program, Pregabalin, Amitriptyline, Duloxetine

Check ESR, Lyme serology, joint aspiration for cell count, cultures, crystals.

>3,000–50,000 WBCs >50 PMNs

Variable cell counts, Negative culture, Symmetric joint involvement

>50,000 WBCs >75 PMNs

Crystals present

↑ESR No crystals Negative culture

Viral

Septic arthritis

Urate, negative birefringence → Gout → NSAIDs colchicine steroids

Calcium phosphate dihydrate, Positive birefringence → Pseudogout → NSAIDs intra-articular steroid

Check autoimmune markers, systemic symptoms.

Check for Hep B, Hep C, HIV, parvovirus B19, or other suspected viruses. → Treatment is largely supportive.

Treat empirically with IV Abx; adjust Abx with clinical response, microbiology results.

↑RF, anti-CCP → Rheumatoid arthritis

Malar rash, Oral ulcers → ↑ANA, anti-dsDNA, anti-Smith Ab → SLE → NSAIDs, hydroxychloroquine

Asymmetric joints affected, Involvement of SI joint, spine, Negative RF → Spondyloarthropathy

Bilateral shoulder and hip involvement → Polymyalgia rheumatica → Oral steroids

Xerophthalmia, Xerostomia → Sjögren syndrome → Hydroxychloroquine, Steroids, Methotrexate

IBD → IBD arthritis → Immunomodulators, Anticytokines

HLA-B27 → Ankylosing spondylitis → NSAIDs, PT

Urethritis, Conjunctivitis → Reactive arthritis → NSAIDs, Sulfasalazine

Scaly rash, Dactylitis → Psoriatic arthritis → NSAIDs, Methotrexate, Biologics

Scott M. Goldberg, MD and J. Herbert Stevenson, MD

Pujalte GG, Albano-Aluquin SA. Differential diagnosis of polyarticular arthritis. *Am Fam Physician.* 2015;92(1):35–41.

CHRONIC OBSTRUCTIVE PULMONARY DISEASE (COPD), DIAGNOSIS AND TREATMENT

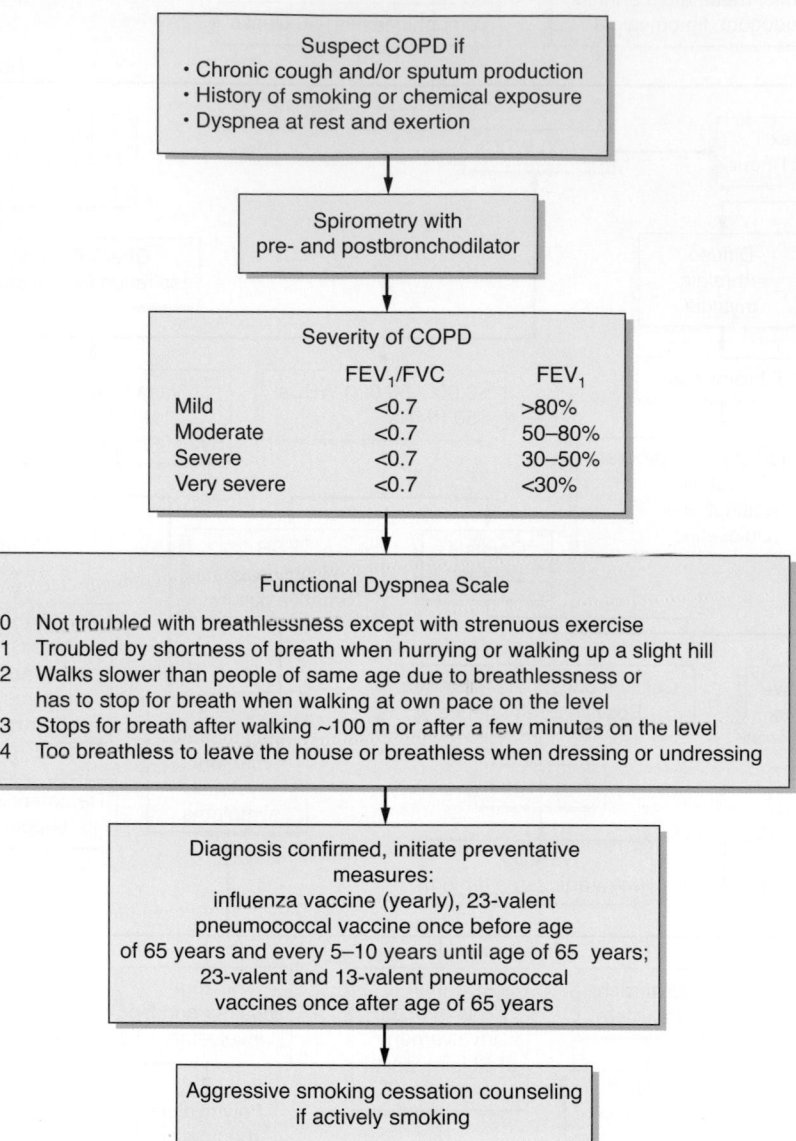

Suspect COPD if
• Chronic cough and/or sputum production
• History of smoking or chemical exposure
• Dyspnea at rest and exertion

Spirometry with
pre- and postbronchodilator

Severity of COPD

	FEV_1/FVC	FEV_1
Mild	<0.7	>80%
Moderate	<0.7	50–80%
Severe	<0.7	30–50%
Very severe	<0.7	<30%

Functional Dyspnea Scale

0 Not troubled with breathlessness except with strenuous exercise
1 Troubled by shortness of breath when hurrying or walking up a slight hill
2 Walks slower than people of same age due to breathlessness or
   has to stop for breath when walking at own pace on the level
3 Stops for breath after walking ~100 m or after a few minutes on the level
4 Too breathless to leave the house or breathless when dressing or undressing

Diagnosis confirmed, initiate preventative
measures:
influenza vaccine (yearly), 23-valent
pneumococcal vaccine once before age
of 65 years and every 5–10 years until age of 65 years;
23-valent and 13-valent pneumococcal
vaccines once after age of 65 years

Aggressive smoking cessation counseling
if actively smoking

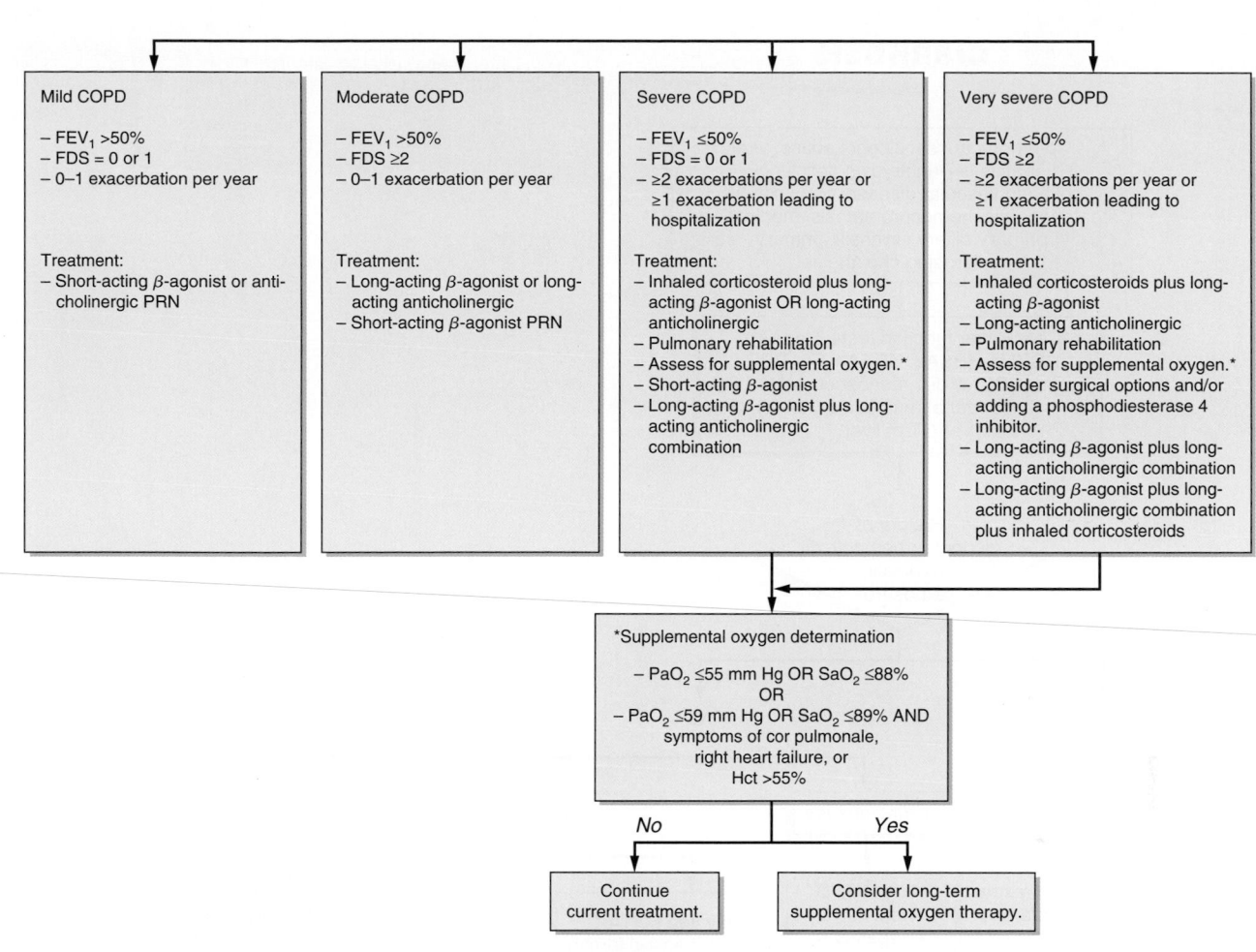

Mild COPD

– FEV_1 >50%
– FDS = 0 or 1
– 0–1 exacerbation per year

Treatment:
– Short-acting β-agonist or anti-cholinergic PRN

Moderate COPD

– FEV_1 >50%
– FDS ≥2
– 0–1 exacerbation per year

Treatment:
– Long-acting β-agonist or long-acting anticholinergic
– Short-acting β-agonist PRN

Severe COPD

– FEV_1 ≤50%
– FDS = 0 or 1
– ≥2 exacerbations per year or ≥1 exacerbation leading to hospitalization

Treatment:
– Inhaled corticosteroid plus long-acting β-agonist OR long-acting anticholinergic
– Pulmonary rehabilitation
– Assess for supplemental oxygen.*
– Short-acting β-agonist
– Long-acting β-agonist plus long-acting anticholinergic combination

Very severe COPD

– FEV_1 ≤50%
– FDS ≥2
– ≥2 exacerbations per year or ≥1 exacerbation leading to hospitalization

Treatment:
– Inhaled corticosteroids plus long-acting β-agonist
– Long-acting anticholinergic
– Pulmonary rehabilitation
– Assess for supplemental oxygen.*
– Consider surgical options and/or adding a phosphodiesterase 4 inhibitor.
– Long-acting β-agonist plus long-acting anticholinergic combination
– Long-acting β-agonist plus long-acting anticholinergic combination plus inhaled corticosteroids

*Supplemental oxygen determination

– PaO_2 ≤55 mm Hg OR SaO_2 ≤88%
OR
– PaO_2 ≤59 mm Hg OR SaO_2 ≤89% AND symptoms of cor pulmonale, right heart failure, or Hct >55%

No

Continue current treatment.

Yes

Consider long-term supplemental oxygen therapy.

William W. Wong, DO and Scott E. Kopec, MD

Global Initiative for Chronic Obstructive Lung Disease. Pocket guide to COPD diagnosis, management and prevention. A guide for health care professionals. 2017 edition. http://www.goldcopd.org/. Accessed July 19, 2017.

CIRRHOSIS

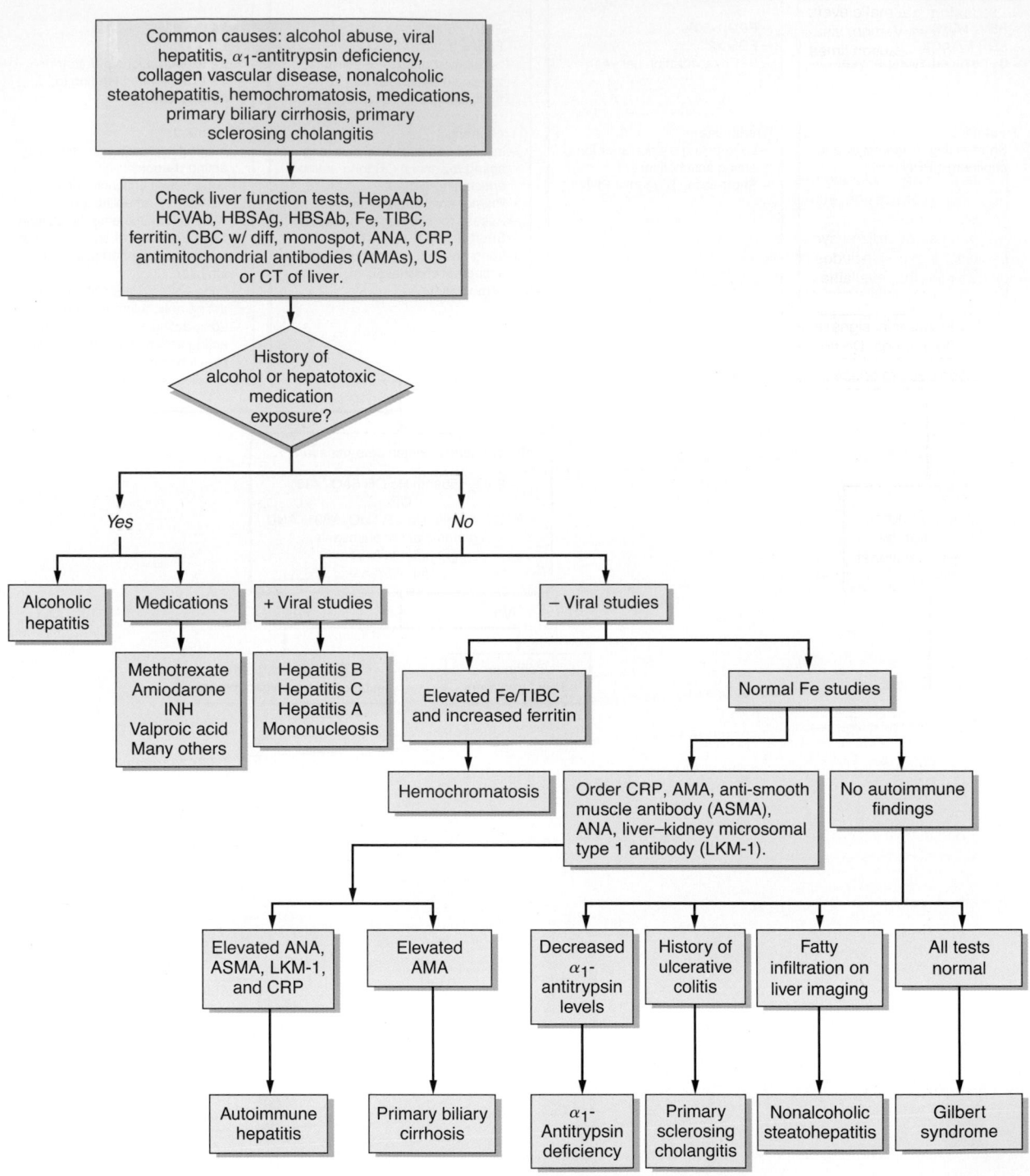

Common causes: alcohol abuse, viral hepatitis, α_1-antitrypsin deficiency, collagen vascular disease, nonalcoholic steatohepatitis, hemochromatosis, medications, primary biliary cirrhosis, primary sclerosing cholangitis

Check liver function tests, HepAAb, HCVAb, HBSAg, HBSAb, Fe, TIBC, ferritin, CBC w/ diff, monospot, ANA, CRP, antimitochondrial antibodies (AMAs), US or CT of liver.

History of alcohol or hepatotoxic medication exposure?

Yes — No

Alcoholic hepatitis

Medications → Methotrexate, Amiodarone, INH, Valproic acid, Many others

+ Viral studies → Hepatitis B, Hepatitis C, Hepatitis A, Mononucleosis

− Viral studies

Elevated Fe/TIBC and increased ferritin → Hemochromatosis

Normal Fe studies

Order CRP, AMA, anti-smooth muscle antibody (ASMA), ANA, liver–kidney microsomal type 1 antibody (LKM-1).

No autoimmune findings

Elevated ANA, ASMA, LKM-1, and CRP → Autoimmune hepatitis

Elevated AMA → Primary biliary cirrhosis

Decreased α_1-antitrypsin levels → α_1-Antitrypsin deficiency

History of ulcerative colitis → Primary sclerosing cholangitis

Fatty infiltration on liver imaging → Nonalcoholic steatohepatitis

All tests normal → Gilbert syndrome

Robert A. Baldor, MD, FAAFP and Alan M. Ehrlich, MD

Porter ML, Dennis BL. Hyperbilirubinemia in the term newborn. *Am Fam Physician.* 2002;65(4):599–606.

CONCUSSION, SIDELINE EVALUATION
Stable, No C-spine injury

Concussion: traumatic event AND change in neurologic function OR one of the following signs/symptoms: **somatic** (HA, nausea/vomiting [N/V], dizziness, vertigo, visual problems, sensitivity to light or sound, numbness/tingling), **cognitive** (LOC, memory problems, feeling "foggy," slower reaction times, confusion), **emotional/behavioral** (i.e., irritability, sadness), **sleep** (i.e., drowsiness)

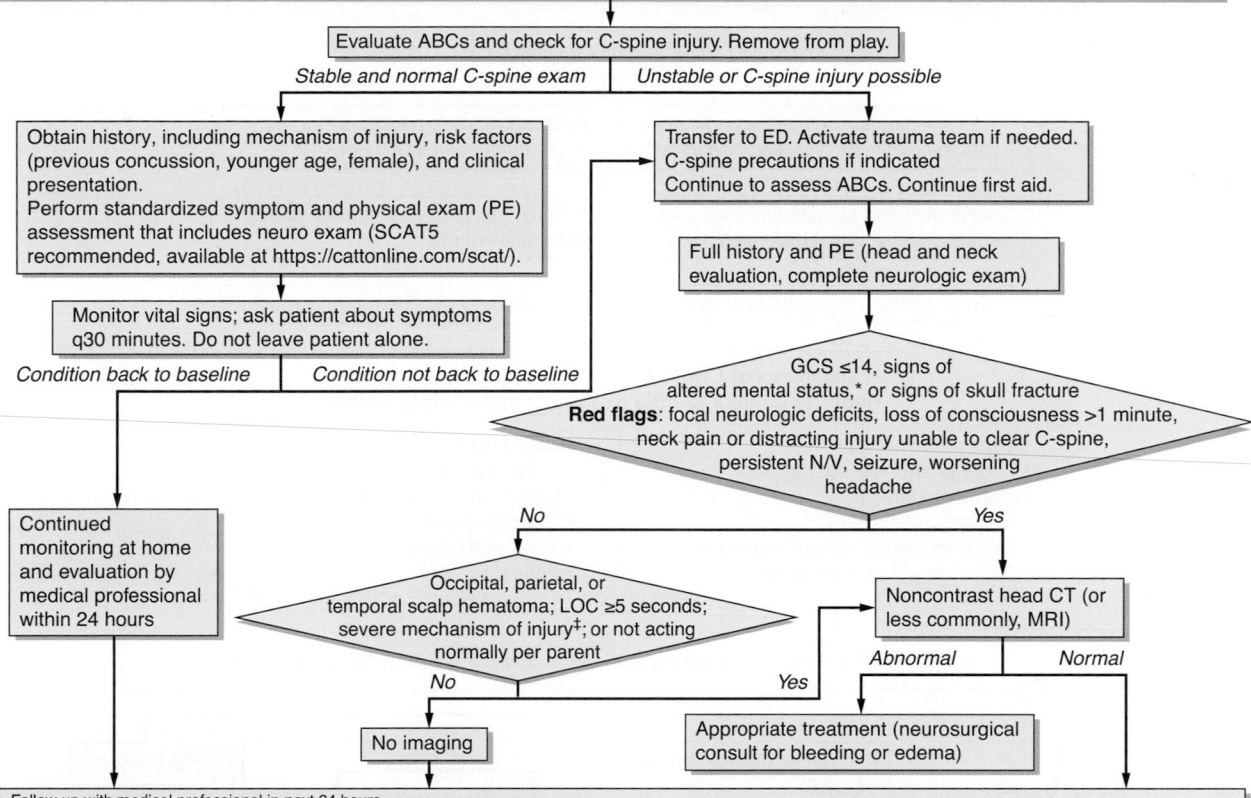

Evaluate ABCs and check for C-spine injury. Remove from play.

Stable and normal C-spine exam | *Unstable or C-spine injury possible*

Obtain history, including mechanism of injury, risk factors (previous concussion, younger age, female), and clinical presentation.
Perform standardized symptom and physical exam (PE) assessment that includes neuro exam (SCAT5 recommended, available at https://cattonline.com/scat/).

Transfer to ED. Activate trauma team if needed.
C-spine precautions if indicated
Continue to assess ABCs. Continue first aid.

Full history and PE (head and neck evaluation, complete neurologic exam)

Monitor vital signs; ask patient about symptoms q30 minutes. Do not leave patient alone.

Condition back to baseline | *Condition not back to baseline*

GCS ≤14, signs of altered mental status,* or signs of skull fracture
Red flags: focal neurologic deficits, loss of consciousness >1 minute, neck pain or distracting injury unable to clear C-spine, persistent N/V, seizure, worsening headache

No | *Yes*

Continued monitoring at home and evaluation by medical professional within 24 hours

Occipital, parietal, or temporal scalp hematoma; LOC ≥5 seconds; severe mechanism of injury‡; or not acting normally per parent

No | *Yes*

Noncontrast head CT (or less commonly, MRI)

Abnormal | *Normal*

No imaging

Appropriate treatment (neurosurgical consult for bleeding or edema)

A. Follow up with medical professional in next 24 hours.
  • History and PE (including complete neurologic exam and symptom checklist)
  • Patient should undergo physical and cognitive rest while symptoms persist.
  • If at neurologic baseline, review Return to Play protocol.
  • If not at neurologic baseline, consider ED evaluation or neuroimaging, close follow-up, and symptomatic treatment.
B. Consider neuropsych testing (paper-and-pencil, ImPACT, CogState, HeadMinder, ANAM, etc.).
  • The ideal timing, frequency, and type of neuropsych testing have not been determined.
  • Most concussions can be managed appropriately without the use of neuropsych testing.
  • Neuropsych testing may be most helpful for high-risk athletes, those with prior concussions, and those who may downplay symptoms in an effort to return to play sooner.
C. Return to Learn protocol
  • Once the patient can tolerate visual and auditory stimuli for 30–45 minutes, they may return to school.
  • Academic adjustments such as a limited course load, reduced testing, or shortened classes may be necessary while recovering.
D. Return to Play protocol
  • No athlete may return to play the same day. All school-aged athletes must return to school fully before they can return to play. Patient should not be on any medications to treat concussion symptoms before returning to play.
  • Once asymptomatic at a stage for 24 hours, may move on to next stage; if symptoms arise, must take a 24-hour period of complete rest before dropping back one stage and starting from there.
  • Most athletes should return no sooner than 6 days after concussion.
      o Stage 1: no activity (complete physical AND cognitive rest; cognitive rest includes no driving.)
      o Stage 2: light aerobic exercise (walking, swimming, or stationary cycling at <70% max HR)
      o Stage 3: sport-specific exercise (sport-specific drills such as skating or running; no head impact activities)
      o Stage 4: noncontact training drills (progression to more complex training drills such as passing; may start progressive resistance training)
      o Stage 5: full contact practice
      o Stage 6: return to game play
  • For children of younger age or those that took >7–10 days for initial symptoms resolution, consider waiting 1 week in between steps rather than 24 hours.
E. Symptom management: If concussive symptoms (typically HA, sleep, cognitive, and mood disturbances) are persistent and interfering with function, consider symptomatic treatment.
  • In the acute setting, ASA and NSAIDs should be used with caution due to increased risk of intracranial bleeding. Acetaminophen and physical modalities are OK.
  • If HA persists for a few days, consider typical abortive treatment. There is no established role for pharmacotherapy in the acute treatment of concussion-induced sleep, cognitive, or mood disturbances.
  • If symptoms persist beyond a few weeks, consider referral to specialist (neurology, sports medicine, etc.). Multidisciplinary approach is often needed.
  • If symptoms do not resolve despite appropriate evaluation and treatment, consider terminating athletic season or athletic career (no clear guidelines have been established; this decision should be made on a case-by-case basis).

*Signs of altered mental status: agitation, somnolence, repetitive questioning, or slow response to verbal communication.
‡Severe mechanism of injury: motor vehicle crash with patient ejection, death of another passenger, or rollover; pedestrian or bicyclist without helmet struck by motorized vehicle; falls of >3 feet for patients <2 years old or >5 feet for patients ≥2 years old; or head struck by high-impact object.

Frank J. Domino, MD and Kaleigh Timmins, MD

Harmon KG, Drezner JA, Gammons M, et al. American Medical Society for Sports Medicine position statement: concussion in sport. *Br J Sports Med.* 2013;47(1):15–26.

CONGESTIVE HEART FAILURE: DIFFERENTIAL DIAGNOSIS

Common causes: CAD, MI, valvular disease, arrhythmia, idiopathic cardiomyopathy, pulmonary HTN, renal disease, medication noncompliance

Diagnosis made clinically

History: exercise intolerance, dyspnea on exertion or at rest, cough, orthopnea, paroxysmal nocturnal dyspnea, chest discomfort, fatigue, weight gain

Exam: elevated jugular venous pressure, rales, S_3/S_4 gallop, hepatojugular reflux, increased abdominal distention, pallor, lower extremity edema

Testing: chest x-ray, ECG, troponin, echo, BNP, BMP, LFTs, TSH, UA, uric acid

Diagnosis of CHF: Framingham Diagnostic Criteria
Requires 2 major criteria or 1 major and 2 minor criteria

Major criteria
- Acute pulmonary edema
- Cardiomegaly
- Hepatojugular reflux
- Elevated jugular venous pressure
- Paroxysmal nocturnal dyspnea
- Rales
- S_3

Minor criteria
- Ankle edema
- Dyspnea on exertion
- Hepatomegaly
- Nocturnal cough
- Pleural effusion
- Tachycardia to >120 bpm

97% and 89% sensitive for systolic and diastolic heart failure (HF), respectively

BNP <500

Alternative diagnosis:
- COPD
- Asthma
- Lung disease
- Pulmonary embolus

LVEF <50% (systolic HF)

LVEF >50% (diastolic HF)

BNP >500

CHF

Ischemic
- History of CAD/MI
- Positive stress test
- CAD on cardiac catheterization
- Troponin elevation

Evaluate for causes of CHF.
- Ischemic: CAD/MI
- Nonischemic: HTN, idiopathic CM, valvular disease, HOCM, arrhythmia, myocarditis/pericarditis, collagen vascular disease
- Due to volume: medication noncompliance, renal failure

Cardiac catheterization unless contraindicated

Nonischemic cardiomyopathy

Idiopathic cardiomyopathy

Other: HTN, thyrotoxicosis, alcoholism, chemotherapy induced, cocaine, autoimmune, collagen vascular disease, infiltrative (amyloid, hemochromatosis), obstructive sleep apnea

Tachycardia mediated (atrial fibrillation/flutter, SVT, frequent PVCs)

Valvular disease cardiomyopathy

Viral mediated (coxsackievirus, adenovirus, HIV, EBV)

Frank J. Domino, MD

King M, Kingery J, Casey B. Diagnosis and evaluation of heart failure. *Am Fam Physician.* 2012;85(12):1161–1168.

CONSTIPATION, DIAGNOSIS AND TREATMENT (ADULT)

Functional constipation
(Rome IV criteria)
- 2 of the following for 12 weeks in past 6 months:
  - <3 stools per week
  - For 25% of time, any of the following:
    - Hard stools
    - Straining
    - Manual assist
    - Sense of incomplete evacuation
    - Sense of anorectal blockade
- Rare loose stools without laxative use
- Does NOT meet criteria for IBS

Common causes: primary—functional, slow transit, pelvic floor dysfunction; secondary—IBS, diabetes mellitus, hypothyroidism, hypercalcemia, pregnancy, obstruction, medication side effect

↓

History and physical:
Diet, fluid intake, exercise, Rome IV criteria, digital rectal exam, abdominal exam, neurologic exam

↓

Red flags:
Unintentional weight loss, hematochezia, family Hx IBD or colon cancer, positive fecal occult, anemia, new onset in age >50 years, change in stool size, neurologic findings → *Yes* → Colonoscopy

No

↓

Colonoscopy → Anemia

Consider medication effect: Adjust and/or begin with empiric treatment. ← *Yes* ← Medication Hx: anticholinergics, opiates, calcium channel blockers, antidepressants, antacids → *No* → Diagnostic testing: CBC, glucose, creatinine, calcium, TSH → *Positive* → Anemia / Hypothyroidism / Hypercalcemia / Diabetes mellitus

Negative

↓

Empiric treatment:
Increase exercise and water intake;
trial of 25–35 g/day of fiber (inulin up to 6 g/day, psyllium up to 10 g/day, etc.); increase exercise and water intake (2 L/day).

↓

Symptoms improved? → *No* → Add polyethylene glycol and/or stimulant laxative.

Yes

↓

Continue therapy.

Add polyethylene glycol and/or stimulant laxative. ↓

Symptoms improved? → *Yes* → Continue therapy.

→ *No* → Treatment failure → Anorectal manometry with balloon expulsion

Partial

Anorectal manometry with balloon expulsion → Normal ARM → Consider colonic transit time. → Add adjunctive agents such as lubiprostone and linaclotide.

Anorectal manometry with balloon expulsion → Abnormal ARM → Pelvic floor dysfunction → Biofeedback. Consider MRI/defecography and surgical referral.

Daniel J. Stein, MD, MPH and Stephen K. Lane, MD

Lacy BE, Mearin F, Chang L, et al. Bowel disorders. *Gastroenterology*. 2016;150(6):1393–1407.e5.

CONSTIPATION, TREATMENT (PEDIATRIC)

*Red flags:
Constipation <1 month
No meconium in 48 hours
Family history of Hirschsprung disease
Ribbon stools
Blood in the stools without anal fissures
Failure to thrive
Fever
Bilious vomiting
Abnormal thyroid gland
Severe abdominal distention
Perianal fistula
Abnormal position of anus
Absent anal or cremasteric reflex
Decreased lower extremity tone
Tuft of hair on spine
Sacral dimple
Gluteal cleft deviation
Extreme fear during anal inspection
Anal scars

Rome III Criteria (≥2 criteria):
≤2 defecations per week
At least one episode of incontinence per week after toilet training
History of excessive stool retention
History of painful/hard bowel movements
Presence of a large fecal mass
History of large diameter stools that may obstruct the toilet

↓

Careful history and physical exam; digital rectal exam is not required for diagnosis.

↓

Are red flags present?

Yes →

Obtain based on symptoms: CBC, TSH, calcium, glucose, creatinine, tissue transglutaminase (tTG), and endomysium antibody (EMA).

↓

Differential diagnosis:
Celiac disease
Hypothyroidism
Hypercalcemia
Hypokalemia
Diabetes mellitus
Drugs/toxins—opiates, anticholinergics, antidepressants, chemotherapy, heavy metals
Vitamin D intoxication
Botulism
Cystic fibrosis
Hirschsprung disease
Anal achalasia
Colonic inertia
Anal malformations
Pelvic mass
Spinal cord abnormalities
Abnormal abdominal musculature
Pseudoobstruction
Multiple endocrine neoplasia type 2B

↓

Refer for specialty evaluation.

No →

Functional constipation

↓

Fecal impaction?

Yes →

First line: polyethylene glycol 3350 1.0–1.5 g/kg/day for 3–6 days

Second line: enemas daily for 3–6 days

No →

Maintenance therapy:
First line: PEG 0.4 g/kg/day adjusted for one to two soft bowel movements per day

Lactulose is acceptable if PEG is not available.

↓

Dietary changes/family education:
– High-fiber diet (1–5 years: 14 g/day; 5–13 years: 17–25 g/day; >13 years: 25–31 g/day). Increase fiber gradually to minimize flatulence.
– Add fiber gummies (inulin) up to 15 g BID as tolerated.
– Limit caffeine and milk products (<16 oz/milk/day).
– If symptoms persist, add: <6 months—sorbitol-containing juices, >6 months—lactulose (1–3 mL/kg/day to max 60 mL/day), or polyethylene glycol 3350 (0.5–1.0 g/kg/day to max 17 g/day).

Bethany N. Teer, MD

Tabbers MM, DiLorenzo C, Berger MY, et al. Evaluation and treatment of functional constipation in infants and children: evidence-based recommendations from ESPGHAN and NASPGHAN. *J Pediatr Gastroenterol Nutr.* 2014;58(2):258–274.

CONTRACEPTION

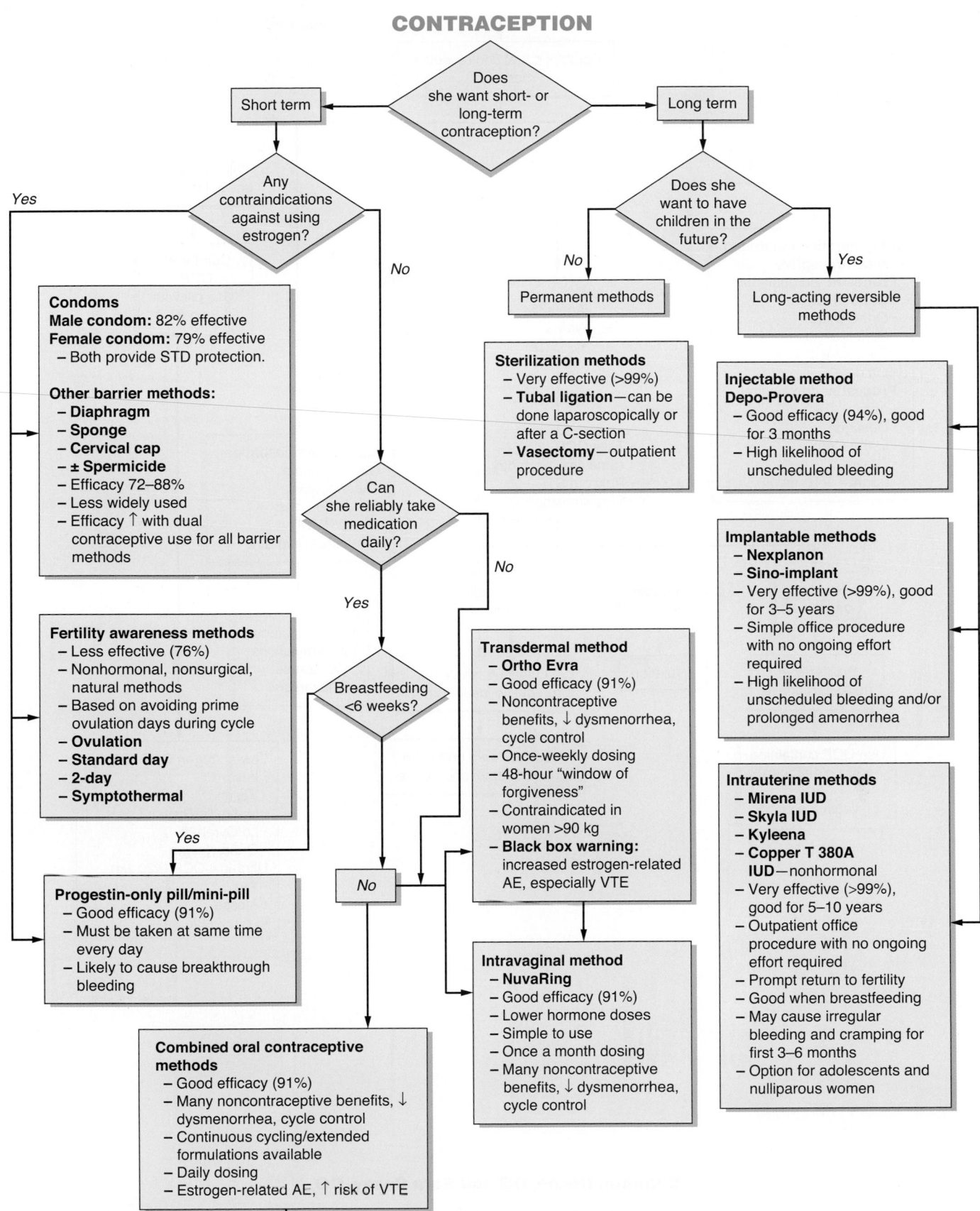

Does she want short- or long-term contraception?

Short term — **Any contraindications against using estrogen?**

Yes →

Condoms
Male condom: 82% effective
Female condom: 79% effective
– Both provide STD protection.

Other barrier methods:
– **Diaphragm**
– **Sponge**
– **Cervical cap**
– **± Spermicide**
– Efficacy 72–88%
– Less widely used
– Efficacy ↑ with dual contraceptive use for all barrier methods

Fertility awareness methods
– Less effective (76%)
– Nonhormonal, nonsurgical, natural methods
– Based on avoiding prime ovulation days during cycle
– **Ovulation**
– **Standard day**
– **2-day**
– **Symptothermal**

Progestin-only pill/mini-pill
– Good efficacy (91%)
– Must be taken at same time every day
– Likely to cause breakthrough bleeding

No →

Can she reliably take medication daily?

Yes → **Breastfeeding <6 weeks?**

Yes → (Progestin-only pill/mini-pill)

No →

Combined oral contraceptive methods
– Good efficacy (91%)
– Many noncontraceptive benefits, ↓ dysmenorrhea, cycle control
– Continuous cycling/extended formulations available
– Daily dosing
– Estrogen-related AE, ↑ risk of VTE

No →

Transdermal method
– **Ortho Evra**
– Good efficacy (91%)
– Noncontraceptive benefits, ↓ dysmenorrhea, cycle control
– Once-weekly dosing
– 48-hour "window of forgiveness"
– Contraindicated in women >90 kg
– **Black box warning:** increased estrogen-related AE, especially VTE

Intravaginal method
– **NuvaRing**
– Good efficacy (91%)
– Lower hormone doses
– Simple to use
– Once a month dosing
– Many noncontraceptive benefits, ↓ dysmenorrhea, cycle control

Long term — **Does she want to have children in the future?**

No → **Permanent methods**

Sterilization methods
– Very effective (>99%)
– **Tubal ligation**—can be done laparoscopically or after a C-section
– **Vasectomy**—outpatient procedure

Yes → **Long-acting reversible methods**

Injectable method
Depo-Provera
– Good efficacy (94%), good for 3 months
– High likelihood of unscheduled bleeding

Implantable methods
– **Nexplanon**
– **Sino-implant**
– Very effective (>99%), good for 3–5 years
– Simple office procedure with no ongoing effort required
– High likelihood of unscheduled bleeding and/or prolonged amenorrhea

Intrauterine methods
– **Mirena IUD**
– **Skyla IUD**
– **Kyleena**
– **Copper T 380A IUD**—nonhormonal
– Very effective (>99%), good for 5–10 years
– Outpatient office procedure with no ongoing effort required
– Prompt return to fertility
– Good when breastfeeding
– May cause irregular bleeding and cramping for first 3–6 months
– Option for adolescents and nulliparous women

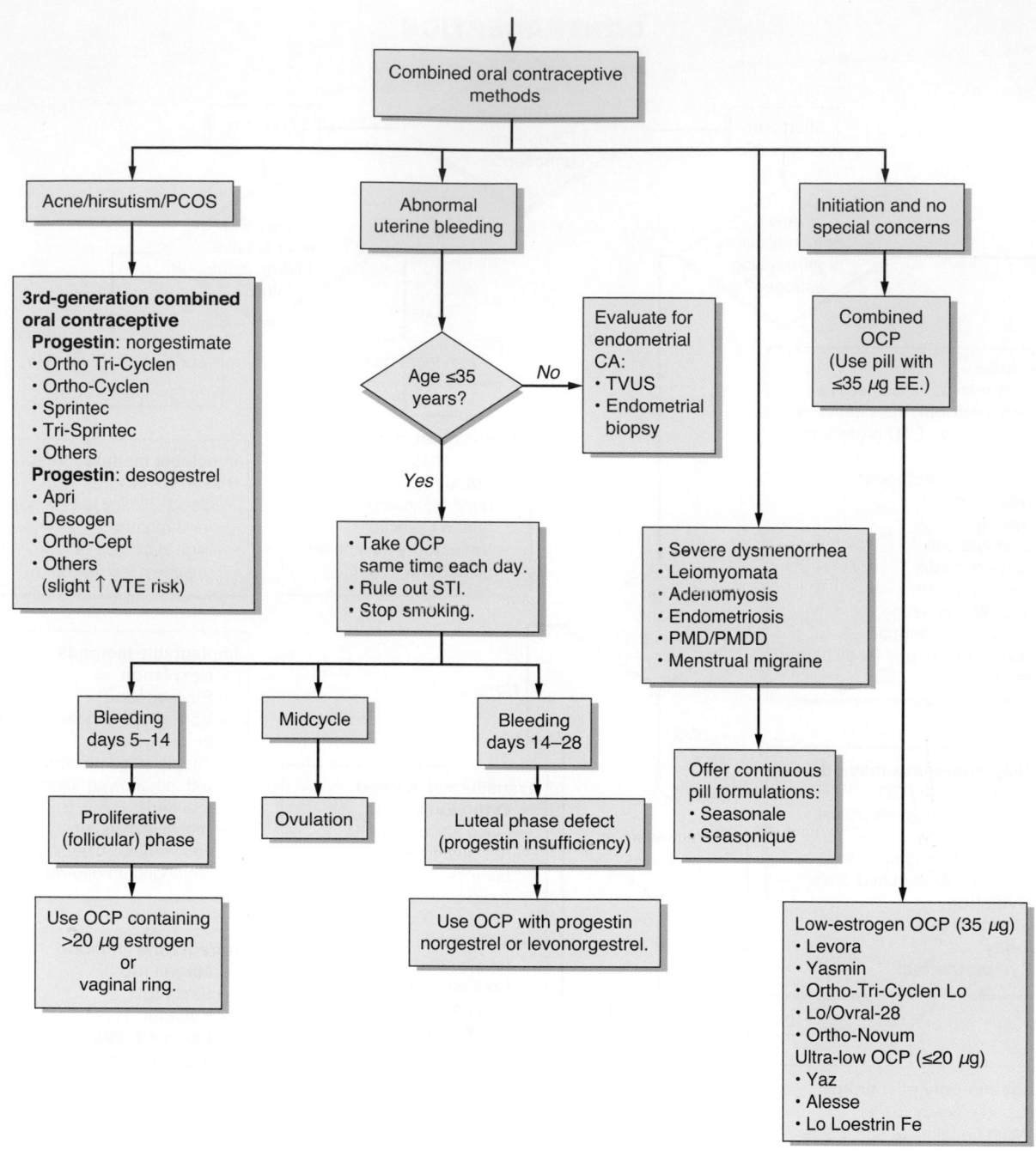

Combined oral contraceptive methods

Acne/hirsutism/PCOS

3rd-generation combined oral contraceptive
Progestin: norgestimate
- Ortho Tri-Cyclen
- Ortho-Cyclen
- Sprintec
- Tri-Sprintec
- Others

Progestin: desogestrel
- Apri
- Desogen
- Ortho-Cept
- Others
(slight ↑ VTE risk)

Abnormal uterine bleeding

Age ≤35 years? — *No* →

Evaluate for endometrial CA:
- TVUS
- Endometrial biopsy

Yes

- Take OCP same time each day.
- Rule out STI.
- Stop smoking.

Bleeding days 5–14

Proliferative (follicular) phase

Use OCP containing >20 μg estrogen or vaginal ring.

Midcycle

Ovulation

Bleeding days 14–28

Luteal phase defect (progestin insufficiency)

Use OCP with progestin norgestrel or levonorgestrel.

Initiation and no special concerns

Combined OCP (Use pill with ≤35 μg EE.)

- Severe dysmenorrhea
- Leiomyomata
- Adenomyosis
- Endometriosis
- PMD/PMDD
- Menstrual migraine

Offer continuous pill formulations:
- Seasonale
- Seasonique

Low-estrogen OCP (35 μg)
- Levora
- Yasmin
- Ortho-Tri-Cyclen Lo
- Lo/Ovral-28
- Ortho-Novum
Ultra-low OCP (≤20 μg)
- Yaz
- Alesse
- Lo Loestrin Fe

Shannon Roche, DO and Sara Casey, DO

Division of Reproductive Health, National Center for Chronic Disease Prevention and Health Promotion, Centers for Disease Control and Prevention. U.S. selected practice recommendations for contraceptive use, 2013: adapted from the World Health Organization selected practice recommendations for contraceptive use, 2nd edition. *MMWR Recomm Rep.* 2013;62(RR-05):1–60.

DEEP VENOUS THROMBOSIS, DIAGNOSIS AND TREATMENT

Determine Wells score

• Active cancer	+1
• Calf swelling >3 cm	+1
• Collateral superficial veins	+1
• Pitting edema	+1
• Previous DVT	+1
• Pain along venous system	+1
• Paralysis or recent immobilization (cast)	+1
• Recently bedridden for >3 days or general anesthesia	+1
• Recent diagnosis of DVT	+1

  • ≤1 DVT unlikely
  • ≥2 DVT likely

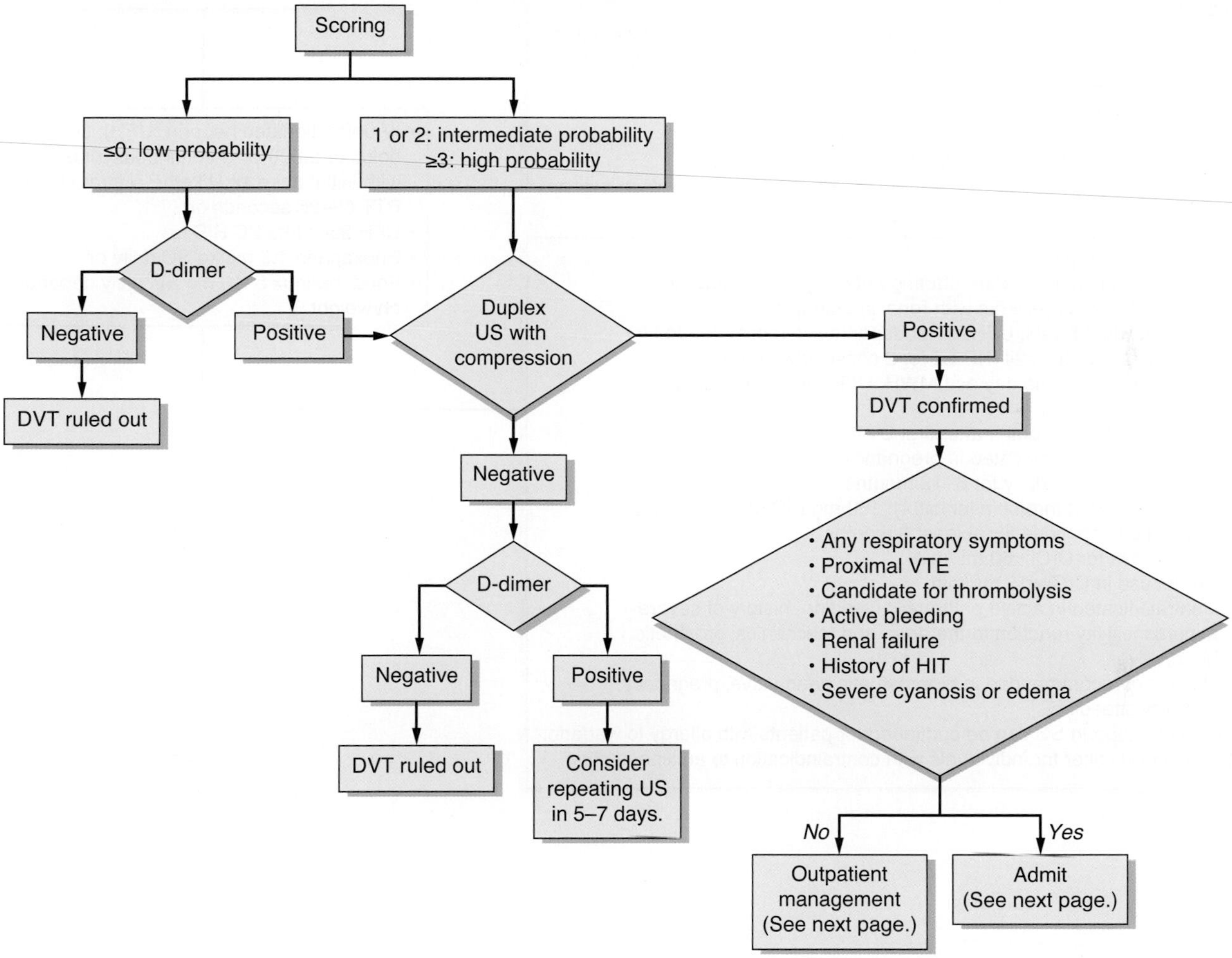

Scoring

≤0: low probability

1 or 2: intermediate probability
≥3: high probability

D-dimer

Negative

DVT ruled out

Positive

Duplex US with compression

Positive

DVT confirmed

Negative

D-dimer

Negative

DVT ruled out

Positive

Consider repeating US in 5–7 days.

• Any respiratory symptoms
• Proximal VTE
• Candidate for thrombolysis
• Active bleeding
• Renal failure
• History of HIT
• Severe cyanosis or edema

No

Outpatient management
(See next page.)

Yes

Admit
(See next page.)

Treatment

```
        ┌─────────────┐                                    ┌─────────────┐
        │  Outpatient  │                                   │  Inpatient   │
        │  management  │                                   │  management  │
        └─────────────┘                                    │  indications │
              │                                             └─────────────┘
              ▼                                                   │
```

Low-molecular-weight heparin (LMWH):
- Enoxaparin 1 mg/kg SC BID or
- Dalteparin 200 IU/kg SC daily for patients with cancer
- LMWH is the preferred treatment in pregnancy.

Rivaroxaban (factor Xa inhibitor):
- 15 mg BID with food for 3 weeks followed by 20 mg daily for 6–12 months
- Contraindicated in patients with active pathologic bleeding or history of severe hypersensitivity reaction to the drug
- Avoid in patients with CrCl <30 mL/min.
- Use is not recommended in pregnancy or breastfeeding.
- Current use is limited due to cost and lack of reversal agent.

Maintenance therapy
- Hypercoagulation test before starting anticoagulation therapy
- UFH is preferred in patients with renal impairment.
- Treatment with LMWH, UFH, or fondaparinux is recommended for at least 5 days AND until INR ≥2 for 2 consecutive days.
- Start warfarin on same day as LMWH, UFH, and fondaparinux.
  - Goal INR 2–3
  - Continue for 3–6 months after first DVT.
  - Warfarin is contraindicated in pregnancy.
- Rivaroxaban 20 mg daily for 6–12 months
- Dabigatran (direct thrombin inhibitor): 150 mg BID after 7–10 days of LMWH and continue for at least 6 months
  - Adjust dose for CrCl <50 mL/min.
  - Do not use in CrCl <15 mL/min.
  - Contraindicated in active pathologic bleeding, history of severe hypersensitivity reaction to the drug, and mechanical prosthetic heart valve
  - Use is not recommended in bioprosthetic heart valve, pregnancy, and breastfeeding.
- LMWH or heparin SC can be continued for patients with allergy to warfarin.
- Consider IVC filter for individuals with contraindication to anticoagulation.

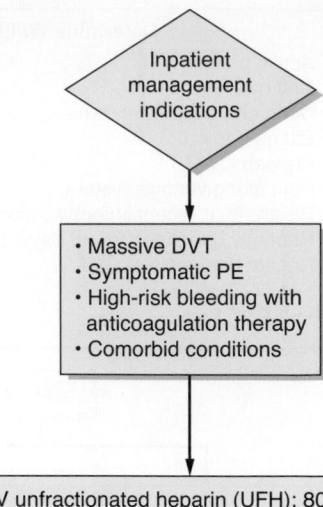

- Massive DVT
- Symptomatic PE
- High-risk bleeding with anticoagulation therapy
- Comorbid conditions

- IV unfractionated heparin (UFH): 80 U/kg bolus or 5,000 U → continuous infusion with initial dose 18 U/kg/hr → titrate to goal PTT 60–85 seconds or
- UFH 250 U/kg SC BID or
- Enoxaparin 1.5 mg/kg SC daily or
- Fondaparinux 5–10 mg SC daily depending on weight

Bency K. Louidor-Paulynice, MD

Wells P, Forgie M, Rodger M. Treatment of venous thromboembolism. *JAMA.* 2014;311(7):717–728.

DEHYDRATION, PEDIATRIC

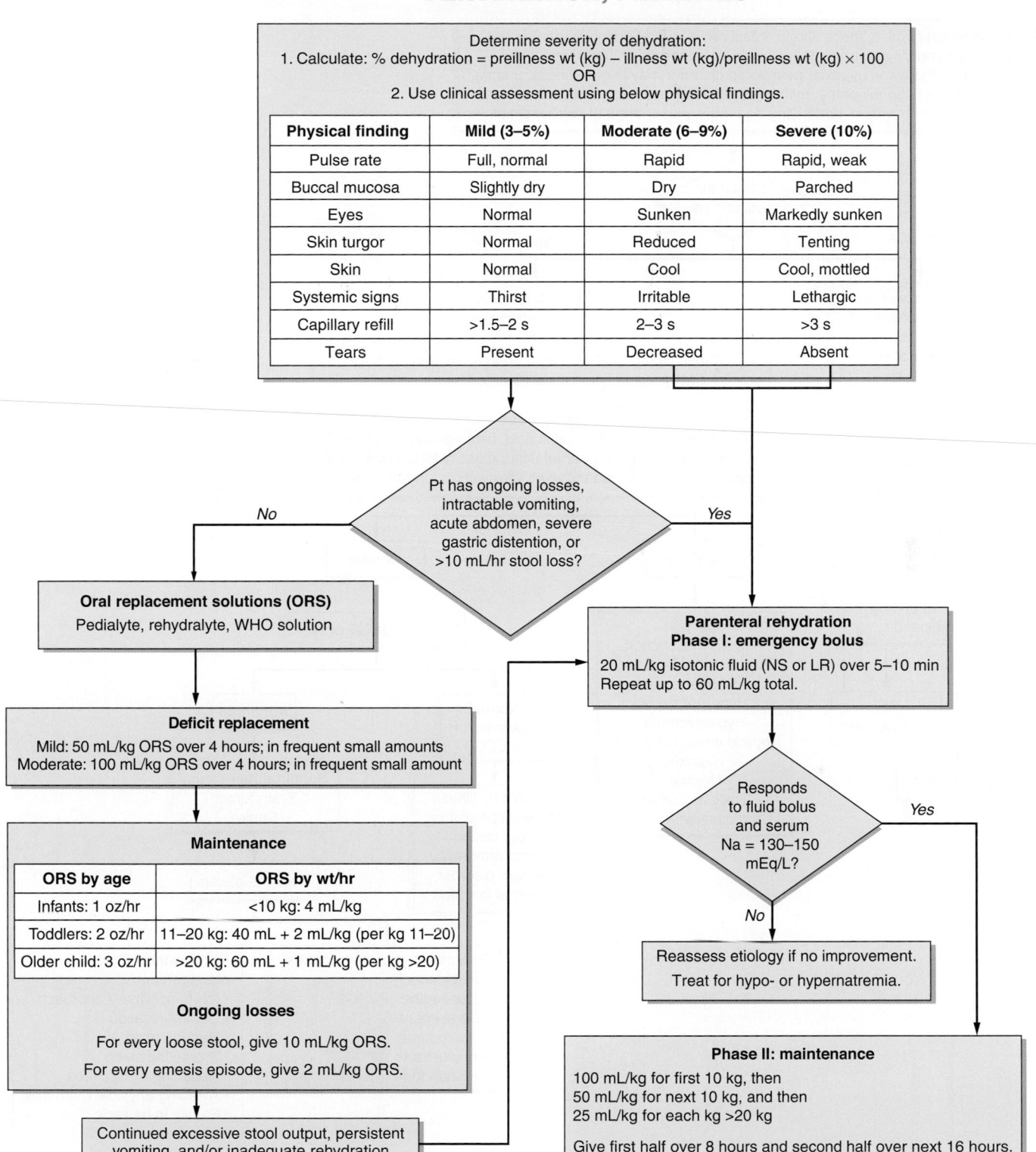

Determine severity of dehydration:
1. Calculate: % dehydration = preillness wt (kg) − illness wt (kg)/preillness wt (kg) × 100
OR
2. Use clinical assessment using below physical findings.

Physical finding	Mild (3–5%)	Moderate (6–9%)	Severe (10%)
Pulse rate	Full, normal	Rapid	Rapid, weak
Buccal mucosa	Slightly dry	Dry	Parched
Eyes	Normal	Sunken	Markedly sunken
Skin turgor	Normal	Reduced	Tenting
Skin	Normal	Cool	Cool, mottled
Systemic signs	Thirst	Irritable	Lethargic
Capillary refill	>1.5–2 s	2–3 s	>3 s
Tears	Present	Decreased	Absent

Pt has ongoing losses, intractable vomiting, acute abdomen, severe gastric distention, or >10 mL/hr stool loss?

No → **Oral replacement solutions (ORS)**
Pedialyte, rehydralyte, WHO solution

Yes → **Parenteral rehydration**
Phase I: emergency bolus
20 mL/kg isotonic fluid (NS or LR) over 5–10 min
Repeat up to 60 mL/kg total.

Deficit replacement
Mild: 50 mL/kg ORS over 4 hours; in frequent small amounts
Moderate: 100 mL/kg ORS over 4 hours; in frequent small amount

Responds to fluid bolus and serum Na = 130–150 mEq/L?

Maintenance

ORS by age	ORS by wt/hr
Infants: 1 oz/hr	<10 kg: 4 mL/kg
Toddlers: 2 oz/hr	11–20 kg: 40 mL + 2 mL/kg (per kg 11–20)
Older child: 3 oz/hr	>20 kg: 60 mL + 1 mL/kg (per kg >20)

Ongoing losses

For every loose stool, give 10 mL/kg ORS.

For every emesis episode, give 2 mL/kg ORS.

No → Reassess etiology if no improvement.
Treat for hypo- or hypernatremia.

Yes → **Phase II: maintenance**
100 mL/kg for first 10 kg, then
50 mL/kg for next 10 kg, and then
25 mL/kg for each kg >20 kg

Give first half over 8 hours and second half over next 16 hours.

Continued excessive stool output, persistent vomiting, and/or inadequate rehydration

L. Michelle Seawright, DO and Nathaniel Stepp, DO

Canavan A, Arant BS Jr. Diagnosis and management of dehydration in children. *Am Fam Physician*. 2009;80(7):692–696.

DELIRIUM

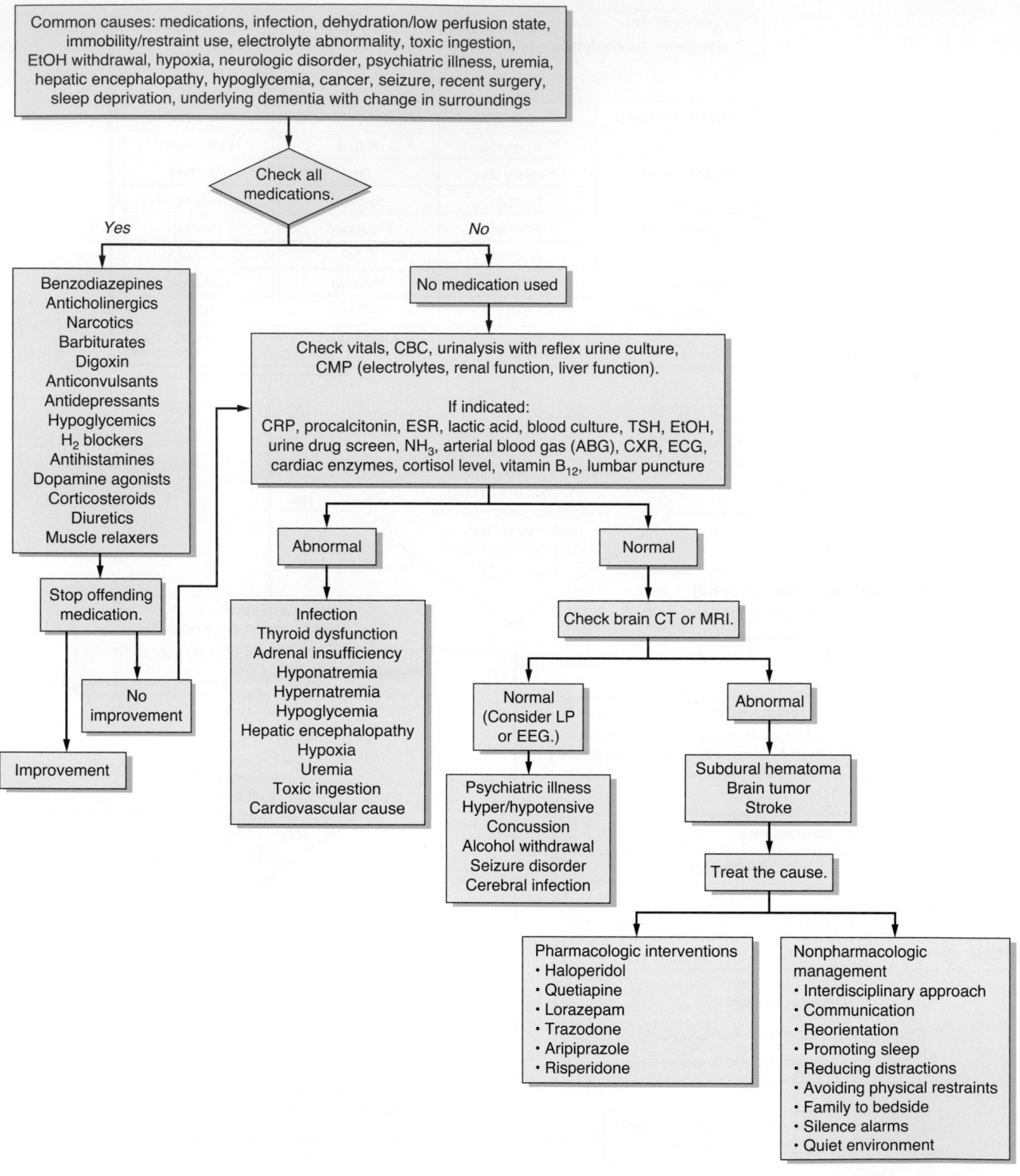

Kellen H. Gower, MD and Holly L. Baab, MD

Kalish VB, Gillham JE, Unwin BK. Delirium in older persons: evaluation and management. *Am Fam Physician*. 2014;90(3):150–158.

DEMENTIA

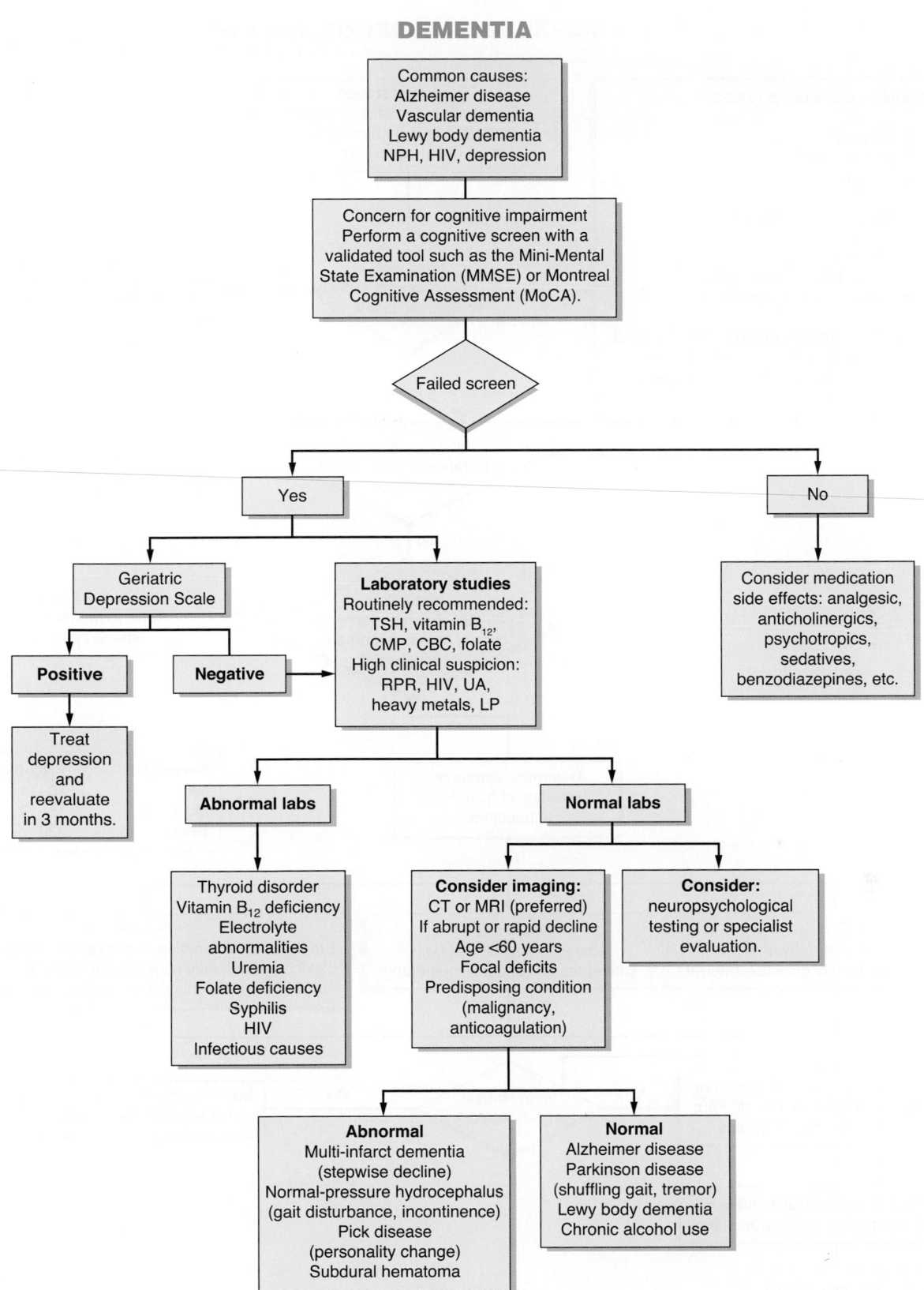

Common causes:
Alzheimer disease
Vascular dementia
Lewy body dementia
NPH, HIV, depression

Concern for cognitive impairment
Perform a cognitive screen with a
validated tool such as the Mini-Mental
State Examination (MMSE) or Montreal
Cognitive Assessment (MoCA).

Failed screen

Yes

No

Geriatric
Depression Scale

Consider medication
side effects: analgesic,
anticholinergics,
psychotropics,
sedatives,
benzodiazepines, etc.

Positive

Negative

Laboratory studies
Routinely recommended:
TSH, vitamin B_{12},
CMP, CBC, folate
High clinical suspicion:
RPR, HIV, UA,
heavy metals, LP

Treat
depression
and
reevaluate
in 3 months.

Abnormal labs

Normal labs

Thyroid disorder
Vitamin B_{12} deficiency
Electrolyte
abnormalities
Uremia
Folate deficiency
Syphilis
HIV
Infectious causes

Consider imaging:
CT or MRI (preferred)
If abrupt or rapid decline
Age <60 years
Focal deficits
Predisposing condition
(malignancy,
anticoagulation)

Consider:
neuropsychological
testing or specialist
evaluation.

Abnormal
Multi-infarct dementia
(stepwise decline)
Normal-pressure hydrocephalus
(gait disturbance, incontinence)
Pick disease
(personality change)
Subdural hematoma

Normal
Alzheimer disease
Parkinson disease
(shuffling gait, tremor)
Lewy body dementia
Chronic alcohol use

Robert A. Baldor, MD, FAAFP

Simmons BB, Hartmann B, Dejoseph D. Evaluation of suspected dementia. *Am Fam Physician.* 2011;84(8):895–902.

DEPRESSIVE EPISODE, MAJOR

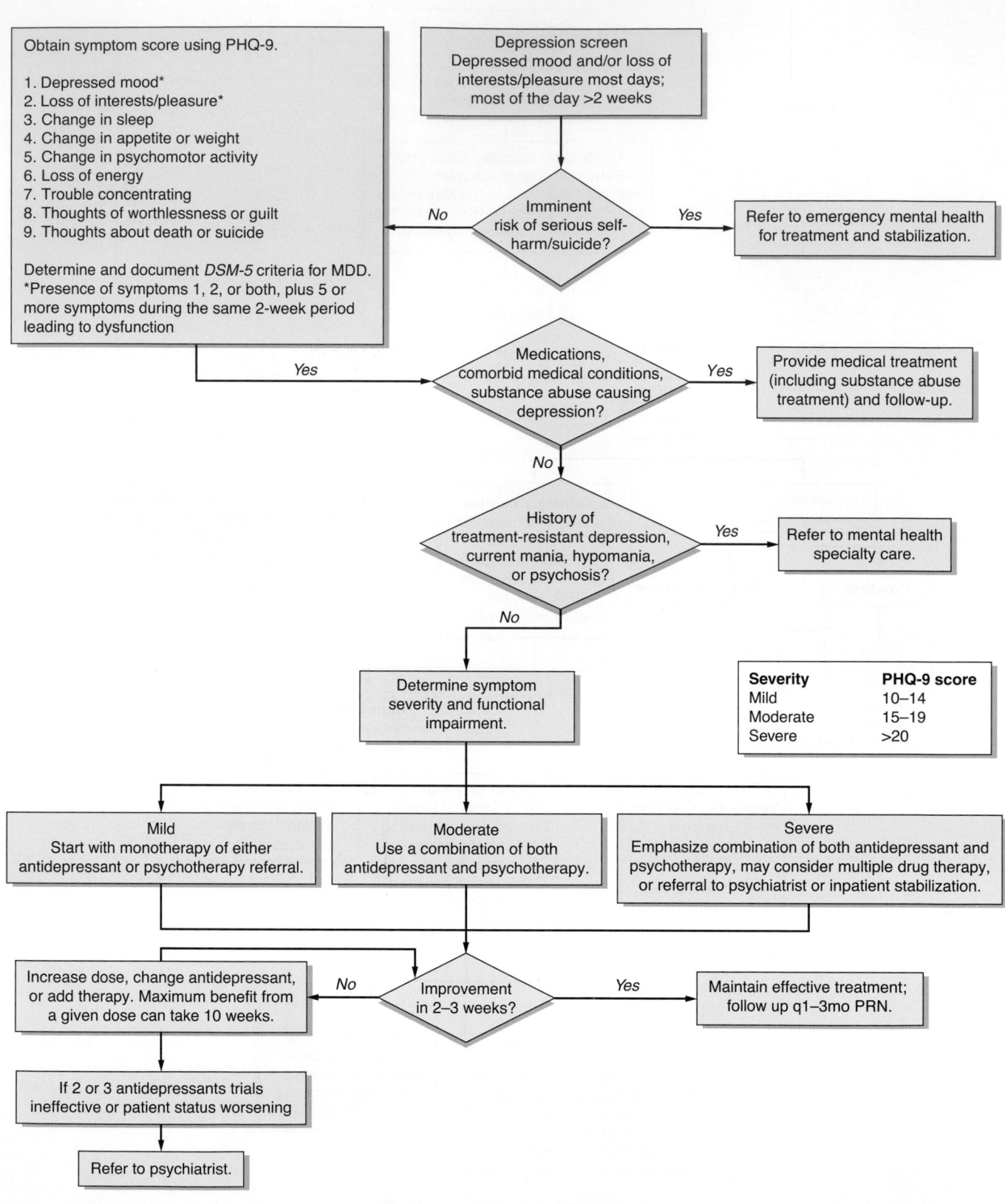

Obtain symptom score using PHQ-9.

1. Depressed mood*
2. Loss of interests/pleasure*
3. Change in sleep
4. Change in appetite or weight
5. Change in psychomotor activity
6. Loss of energy
7. Trouble concentrating
8. Thoughts of worthlessness or guilt
9. Thoughts about death or suicide

Determine and document *DSM-5* criteria for MDD.
*Presence of symptoms 1, 2, or both, plus 5 or more symptoms during the same 2-week period leading to dysfunction

Depression screen
Depressed mood and/or loss of interests/pleasure most days; most of the day >2 weeks

Imminent risk of serious self-harm/suicide? — No / Yes

Refer to emergency mental health for treatment and stabilization.

Medications, comorbid medical conditions, substance abuse causing depression? — Yes / No

Provide medical treatment (including substance abuse treatment) and follow-up.

History of treatment-resistant depression, current mania, hypomania, or psychosis? — Yes / No

Refer to mental health specialty care.

Determine symptom severity and functional impairment.

Severity	PHQ-9 score
Mild	10–14
Moderate	15–19
Severe	>20

Mild
Start with monotherapy of either antidepressant or psychotherapy referral.

Moderate
Use a combination of both antidepressant and psychotherapy.

Severe
Emphasize combination of both antidepressant and psychotherapy, may consider multiple drug therapy, or referral to psychiatrist or inpatient stabilization.

Improvement in 2–3 weeks? — No / Yes

Increase dose, change antidepressant, or add therapy. Maximum benefit from a given dose can take 10 weeks.

Maintain effective treatment; follow up q1–3mo PRN.

If 2 or 3 antidepressants trials ineffective or patient status worsening

Refer to psychiatrist.

Wendy K. Marsh, MD, MSc

U.S. Department of Veterans Affairs, U.S. Department of Defense. *VA/DoD Clinical Practice Guideline for Management of Major Depressive Disorder.* Washington, DC: U.S. Department of Veterans Affairs, U.S. Department of Defense; 2016.

DIABETIC KETOACIDOSIS (DKA), TREATMENT

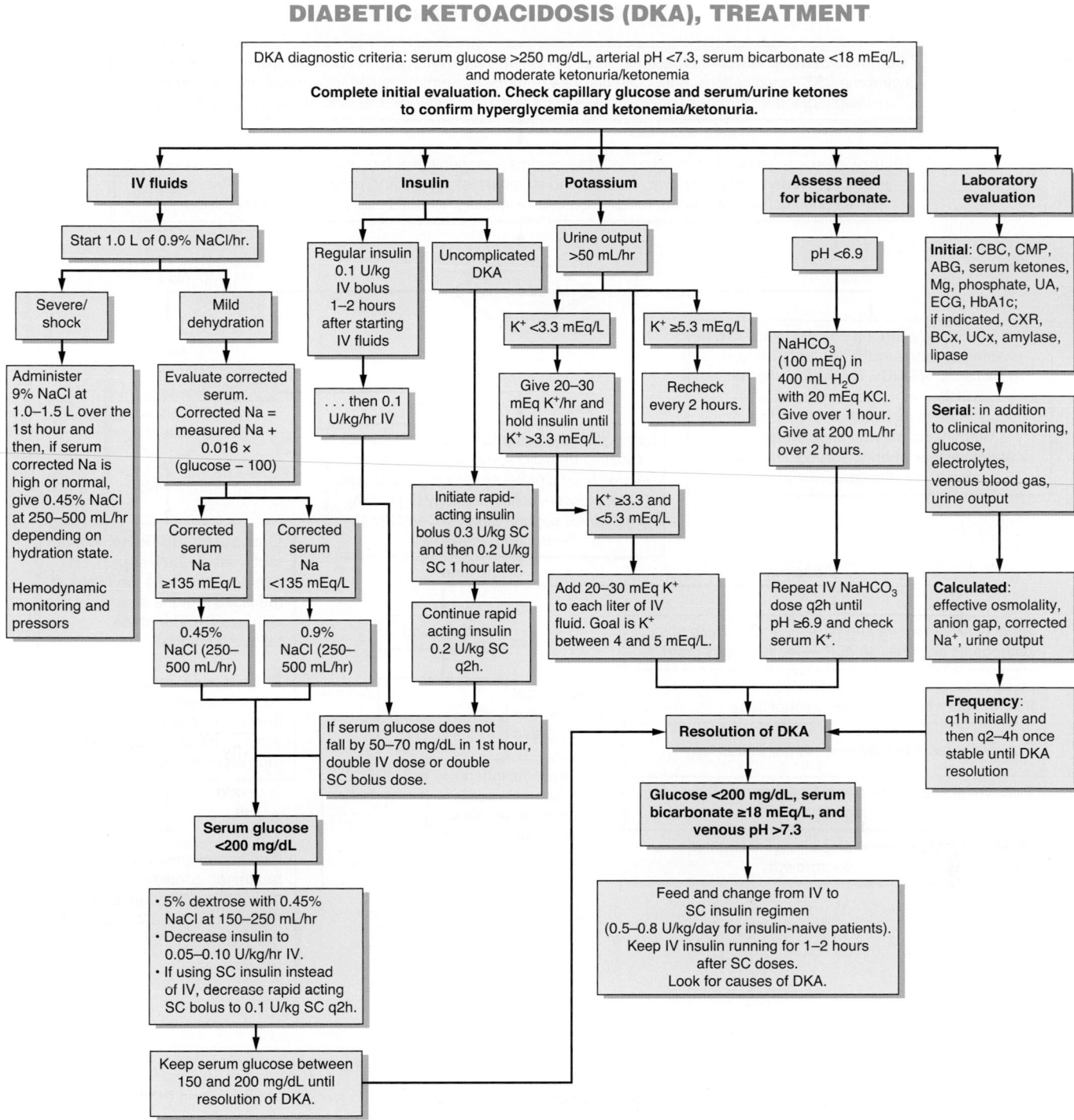

DKA diagnostic criteria: serum glucose >250 mg/dL, arterial pH <7.3, serum bicarbonate <18 mEq/L, and moderate ketonuria/ketonemia
Complete initial evaluation. Check capillary glucose and serum/urine ketones to confirm hyperglycemia and ketonemia/ketonuria.

IV fluids

Start 1.0 L of 0.9% NaCl/hr.

Severe/ shock

Administer 9% NaCl at 1.0–1.5 L over the 1st hour and then, if serum corrected Na is high or normal, give 0.45% NaCl at 250–500 mL/hr depending on hydration state.

Hemodynamic monitoring and pressors

Mild dehydration

Evaluate corrected serum. Corrected Na = measured Na + 0.016 × (glucose − 100)

Corrected serum Na ≥135 mEq/L

Corrected serum Na <135 mEq/L

0.45% NaCl (250–500 mL/hr)

0.9% NaCl (250–500 mL/hr)

Insulin

Regular insulin 0.1 U/kg IV bolus 1–2 hours after starting IV fluids

. . . then 0.1 U/kg/hr IV

Uncomplicated DKA

Initiate rapid-acting insulin bolus 0.3 U/kg SC and then 0.2 U/kg SC 1 hour later.

Continue rapid acting insulin 0.2 U/kg SC q2h.

If serum glucose does not fall by 50–70 mg/dL in 1st hour, double IV dose or double SC bolus dose.

Serum glucose <200 mg/dL

• 5% dextrose with 0.45% NaCl at 150–250 mL/hr
• Decrease insulin to 0.05–0.10 U/kg/hr IV.
• If using SC insulin instead of IV, decrease rapid acting SC bolus to 0.1 U/kg SC q2h.

Keep serum glucose between 150 and 200 mg/dL until resolution of DKA.

Potassium

Urine output >50 mL/hr

K^+ <3.3 mEq/L

Give 20–30 mEq K^+/hr and hold insulin until K^+ >3.3 mEq/L.

K^+ ≥3.3 and <5.3 mEq/L

Add 20–30 mEq K^+ to each liter of IV fluid. Goal is K^+ between 4 and 5 mEq/L.

K^+ ≥5.3 mEq/L

Recheck every 2 hours.

Assess need for bicarbonate.

pH <6.9

$NaHCO_3$ (100 mEq) in 400 mL H_2O with 20 mEq KCl. Give over 1 hour. Give at 200 mL/hr over 2 hours.

Repeat IV $NaHCO_3$ dose q2h until pH ≥6.9 and check serum K^+.

Laboratory evaluation

Initial: CBC, CMP, ABG, serum ketones, Mg, phosphate, UA, ECG, HbA1c; if indicated, CXR, BCx, UCx, amylase, lipase

Serial: in addition to clinical monitoring, glucose, electrolytes, venous blood gas, urine output

Calculated: effective osmolality, anion gap, corrected Na^+, urine output

Frequency: q1h initially and then q2–4h once stable until DKA resolution

Resolution of DKA

Glucose <200 mg/dL, serum bicarbonate ≥18 mEq/L, and venous pH >7.3

Feed and change from IV to SC insulin regimen (0.5–0.8 U/kg/day for insulin-naive patients). Keep IV insulin running for 1–2 hours after SC doses. Look for causes of DKA.

Emily Bouley, MD and Frank J. Domino, MD

Westerberg DP. Diabetic ketoacidosis: evaluation and treatment. *Am Fam Physician.* 2013;87(5):337–346.

DIARRHEA, CHRONIC

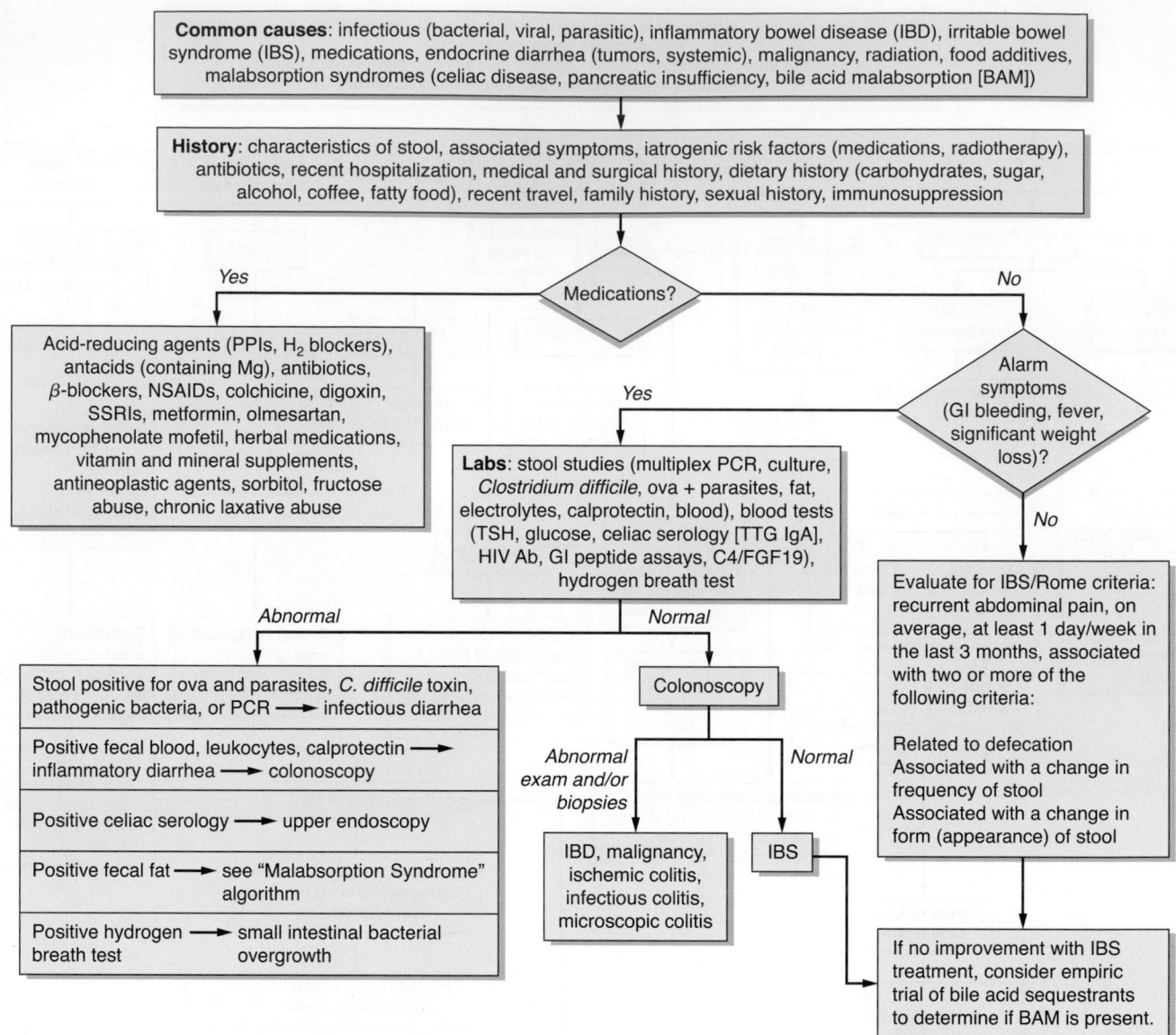

Common causes: infectious (bacterial, viral, parasitic), inflammatory bowel disease (IBD), irritable bowel syndrome (IBS), medications, endocrine diarrhea (tumors, systemic), malignancy, radiation, food additives, malabsorption syndromes (celiac disease, pancreatic insufficiency, bile acid malabsorption [BAM])

History: characteristics of stool, associated symptoms, iatrogenic risk factors (medications, radiotherapy), antibiotics, recent hospitalization, medical and surgical history, dietary history (carbohydrates, sugar, alcohol, coffee, fatty food), recent travel, family history, sexual history, immunosuppression

Medications?

Yes →

Acid-reducing agents (PPIs, H₂ blockers), antacids (containing Mg), antibiotics, β-blockers, NSAIDs, colchicine, digoxin, SSRIs, metformin, olmesartan, mycophenolate mofetil, herbal medications, vitamin and mineral supplements, antineoplastic agents, sorbitol, fructose abuse, chronic laxative abuse

No →

Alarm symptoms (GI bleeding, fever, significant weight loss)?

No ↓

Yes →

Labs: stool studies (multiplex PCR, culture, *Clostridium difficile*, ova + parasites, fat, electrolytes, calprotectin, blood), blood tests (TSH, glucose, celiac serology [TTG IgA], HIV Ab, GI peptide assays, C4/FGF19), hydrogen breath test

Abnormal

Stool positive for ova and parasites, *C. difficile* toxin, pathogenic bacteria, or PCR ⟶ infectious diarrhea

Positive fecal blood, leukocytes, calprotectin ⟶ inflammatory diarrhea ⟶ colonoscopy

Positive celiac serology ⟶ upper endoscopy

Positive fecal fat ⟶ see "Malabsorption Syndrome" algorithm

Positive hydrogen breath test ⟶ small intestinal bacterial overgrowth

Normal

Colonoscopy

Abnormal exam and/or biopsies

IBD, malignancy, ischemic colitis, infectious colitis, microscopic colitis

Normal

IBS

Evaluate for IBS/Rome criteria: recurrent abdominal pain, on average, at least 1 day/week in the last 3 months, associated with two or more of the following criteria:

Related to defecation
Associated with a change in frequency of stool
Associated with a change in form (appearance) of stool

If no improvement with IBS treatment, consider empiric trial of bile acid sequestrants to determine if BAM is present.

Jack Masur, MD and Marie L. Borum, MD, EdD, MPH, MACP, FACG, AGAF

Schiller LR. Evaluation of chronic diarrhea and irritable bowel syndrome with diarrhea in adults in the era of precision medicine. *Am J Gastroenterol.* 2018;113(5):660–669.

DIZZINESS

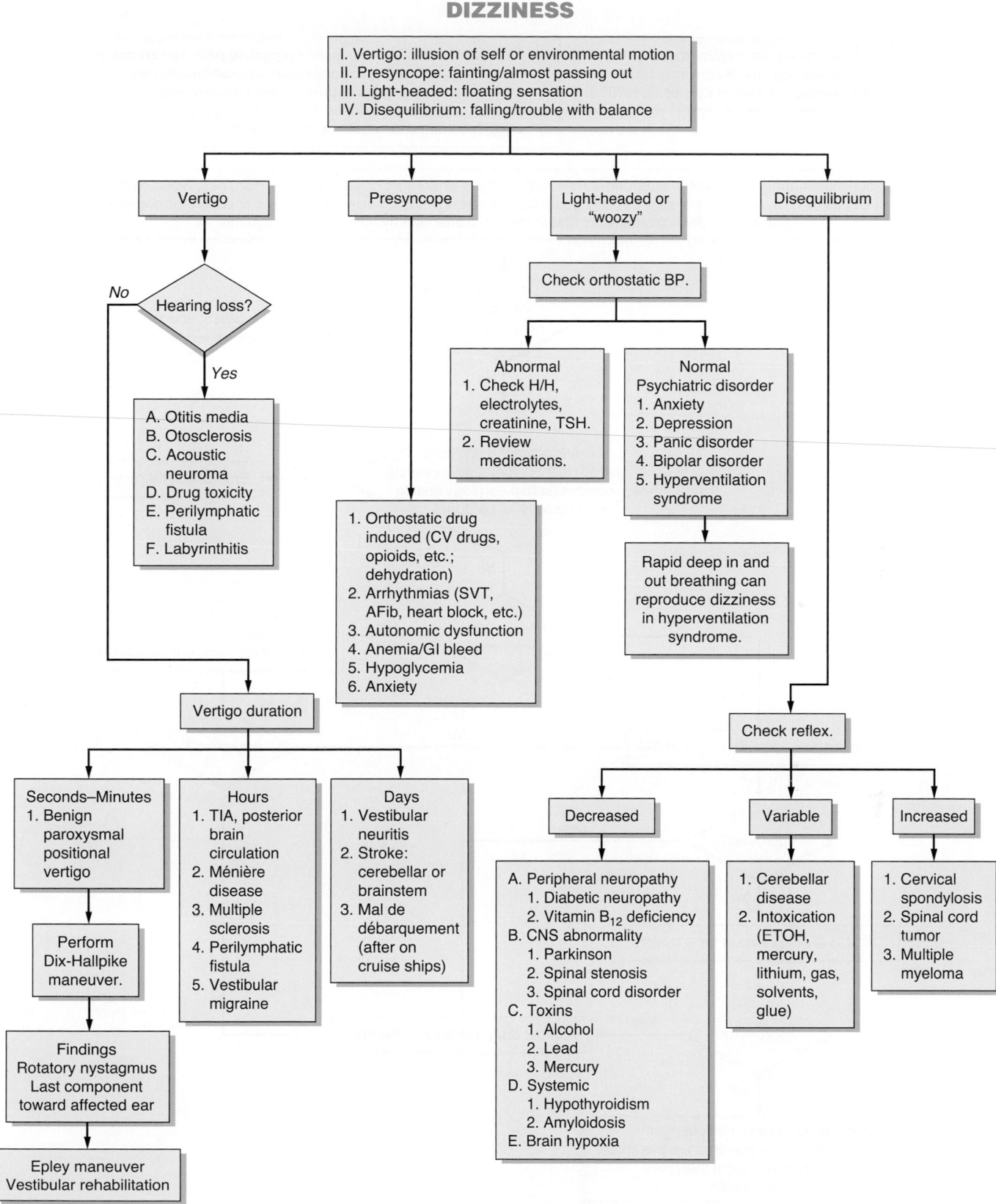

I. Vertigo: illusion of self or environmental motion
II. Presyncope: fainting/almost passing out
III. Light-headed: floating sensation
IV. Disequilibrium: falling/trouble with balance

Vertigo

Hearing loss? — No

Yes

A. Otitis media
B. Otosclerosis
C. Acoustic neuroma
D. Drug toxicity
E. Perilymphatic fistula
F. Labyrinthitis

Vertigo duration

Seconds–Minutes
1. Benign paroxysmal positional vertigo

Perform Dix-Hallpike maneuver.

Findings
Rotatory nystagmus
Last component toward affected ear

Epley maneuver
Vestibular rehabilitation

Hours
1. TIA, posterior brain circulation
2. Ménière disease
3. Multiple sclerosis
4. Perilymphatic fistula
5. Vestibular migraine

Days
1. Vestibular neuritis
2. Stroke: cerebellar or brainstem
3. Mal de débarquement (after on cruise ships)

Presyncope

1. Orthostatic drug induced (CV drugs, opioids, etc.; dehydration)
2. Arrhythmias (SVT, AFib, heart block, etc.)
3. Autonomic dysfunction
4. Anemia/GI bleed
5. Hypoglycemia
6. Anxiety

Light-headed or "woozy"

Check orthostatic BP.

Abnormal
1. Check H/H, electrolytes, creatinine, TSH.
2. Review medications.

Normal
Psychiatric disorder
1. Anxiety
2. Depression
3. Panic disorder
4. Bipolar disorder
5. Hyperventilation syndrome

Rapid deep in and out breathing can reproduce dizziness in hyperventilation syndrome.

Disequilibrium

Check reflex.

Decreased
A. Peripheral neuropathy
  1. Diabetic neuropathy
  2. Vitamin B_{12} deficiency
B. CNS abnormality
  1. Parkinson
  2. Spinal stenosis
  3. Spinal cord disorder
C. Toxins
  1. Alcohol
  2. Lead
  3. Mercury
D. Systemic
  1. Hypothyroidism
  2. Amyloidosis
E. Brain hypoxia

Variable
1. Cerebellar disease
2. Intoxication (ETOH, mercury, lithium, gas, solvents, glue)

Increased
1. Cervical spondylosis
2. Spinal cord tumor
3. Multiple myeloma

Jamal Islam, MD, MS

Post RE, Dickerson LM. Dizziness: a diagnostic approach. *Am Fam Physician*. 2010;82(4):361–369.

DYSPEPSIA

Common causes: peptic ulcer (<10%), gastroesophageal cancer (<1%), gastroparesis, functional dyspepsia (>70%)

Main forms of functional dyspepsia: **epigastric pain syndrome** (intermittent pain/burning in epigastrium at least weekly) and **postprandial distress syndrome** (at least several episodes weekly of bothersome fullness after meals or early satiety). The two syndromes may both be present in the same patient.

GI red flags: onset at age 55 years or later (lower threshold in areas where gastric cancer is common, e.g., Southeast Asia), overt GI bleeding, dysphagia, persistent vomiting, unintentional weight loss, family hx of gastric or esophageal cancer, palpable abdominal/epigastric mass, abnormal adenopathy, iron deficiency anemia

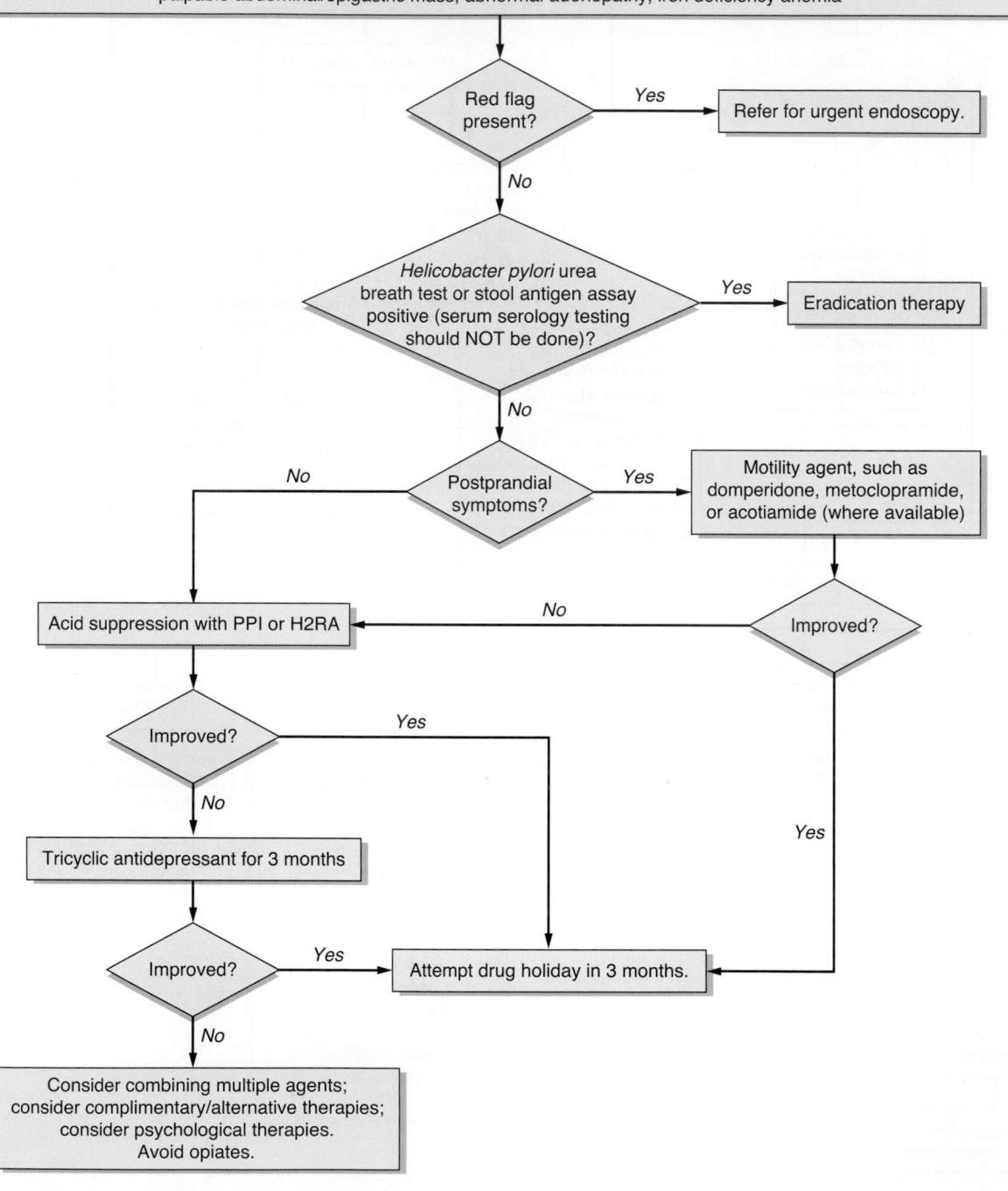

Jennifer L. Hamilton, MD, PhD, FAAFP

Talley NJ, Ford AC. Functional dyspepsia. *N Engl J Med.* 2015;373(19):1853–1863.

DYSPHAGIA

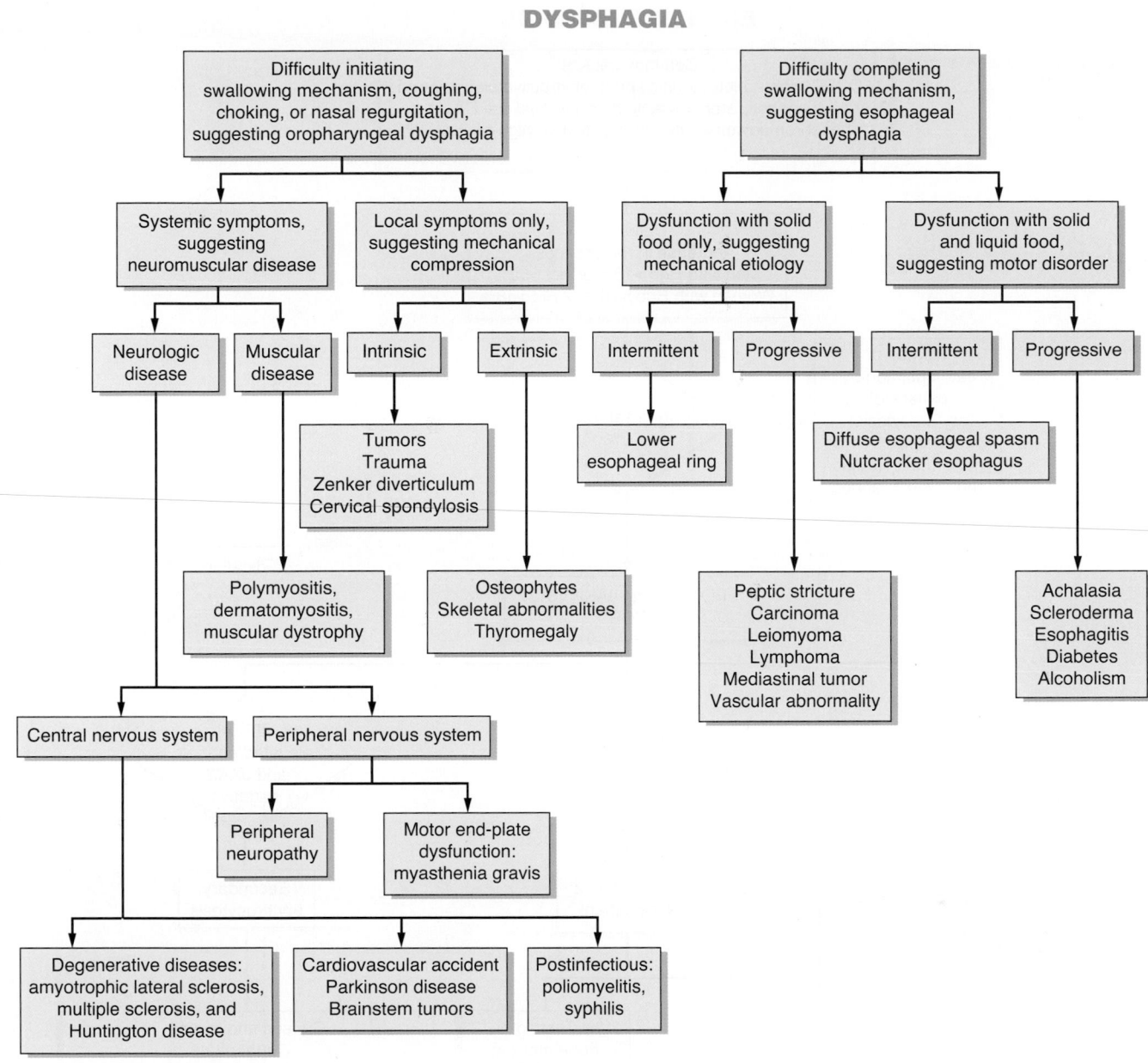

Shari Anthony, MD and Maria Cynthia S. Lopez, MD

Malagelada JR, Bazzoli F, Boeckxstaens G, et al. World Gastroenterology Organisation global guidelines: dysphagia—global guidelines and cascades update September 2014. *J Clin Gastroenterol.* 2015;49(5):370–378.

ERYTHROCYTOSIS

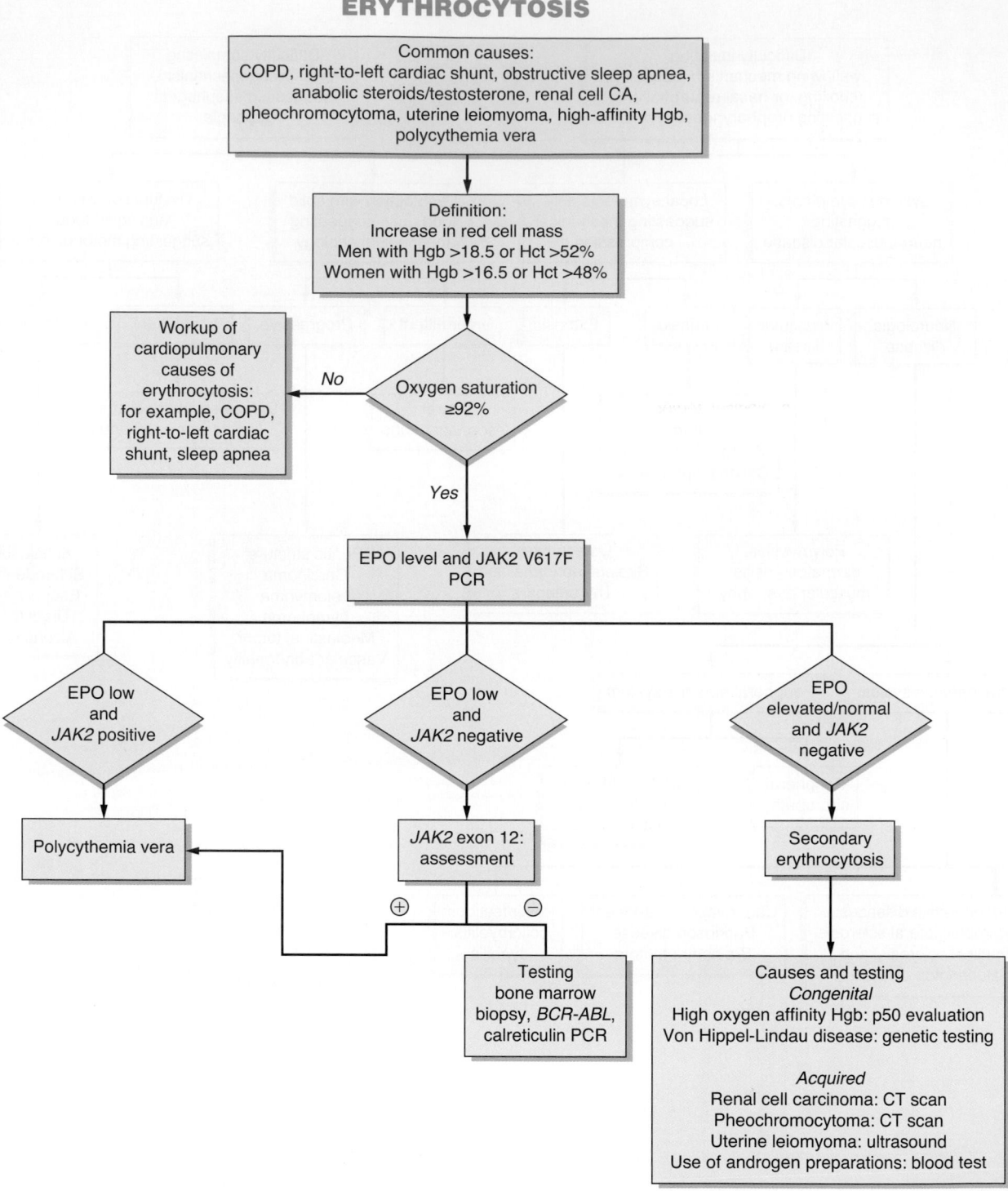

Common causes:
COPD, right-to-left cardiac shunt, obstructive sleep apnea, anabolic steroids/testosterone, renal cell CA, pheochromocytoma, uterine leiomyoma, high-affinity Hgb, polycythemia vera

Definition:
Increase in red cell mass
Men with Hgb >18.5 or Hct >52%
Women with Hgb >16.5 or Hct >48%

Oxygen saturation ≥92%

No → Workup of cardiopulmonary causes of erythrocytosis: for example, COPD, right-to-left cardiac shunt, sleep apnea

Yes

EPO level and JAK2 V617F PCR

EPO low and *JAK2* positive

EPO low and *JAK2* negative

EPO elevated/normal and *JAK2* negative

Polycythemia vera

JAK2 exon 12: assessment

Secondary erythrocytosis

⊕   ⊖

Testing bone marrow biopsy, *BCR-ABL*, calreticulin PCR

Causes and testing
Congenital
High oxygen affinity Hgb: p50 evaluation
Von Hippel-Lindau disease: genetic testing

Acquired
Renal cell carcinoma: CT scan
Pheochromocytoma: CT scan
Uterine leiomyoma: ultrasound
Use of androgen preparations: blood test

Manisha J. Patel, MD and Tarun Kewalramani, MD

Patnaik MM, Tefferi A. The complete evaluation of erythrocytosis: congenital and acquired. *Leukemia.* 2009;23(5):834–844.

FATIGUE

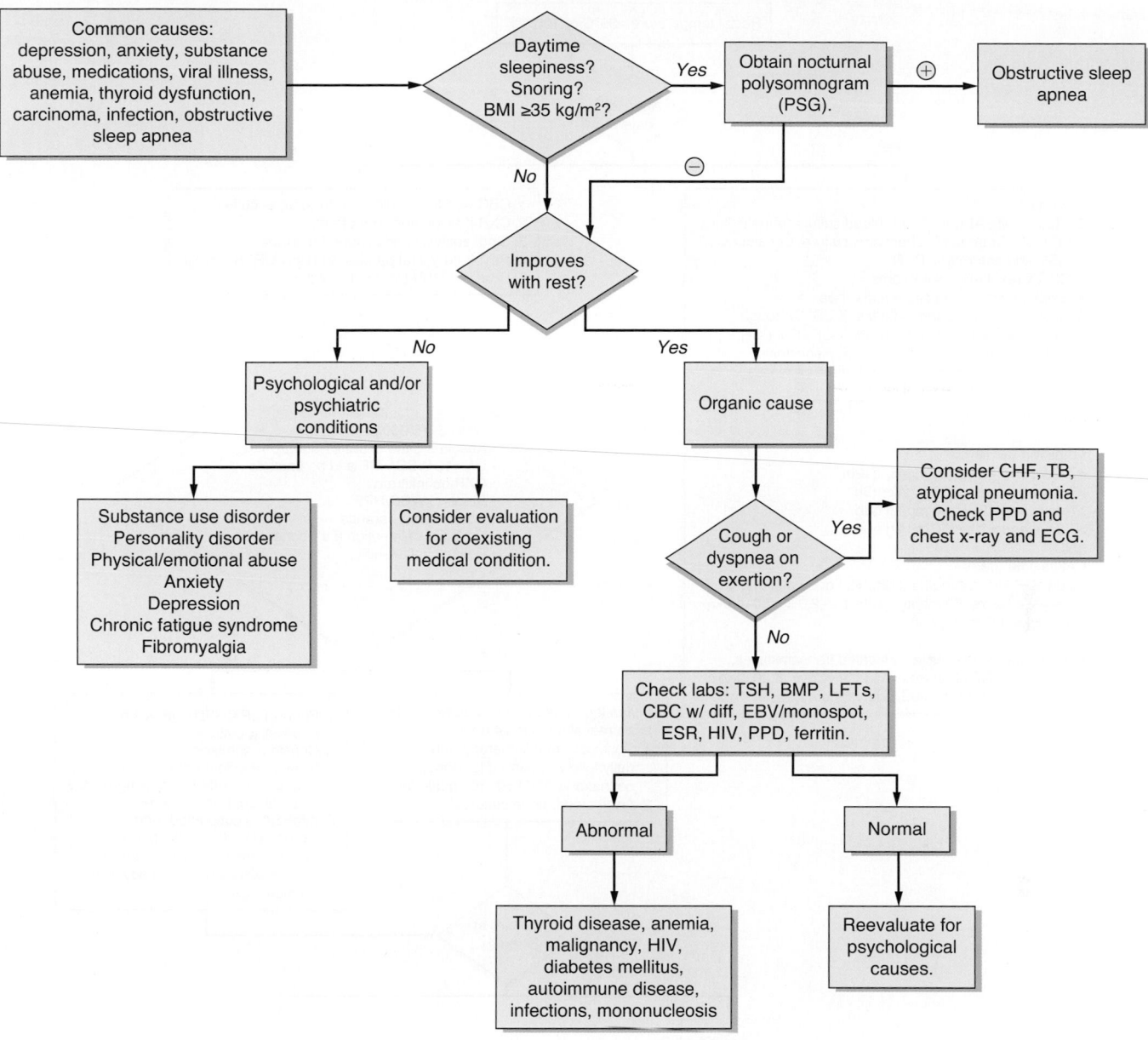

Paavan Mehta, MD and Frank J. Domino, MD

Rosenthal TC, Majeroni BA, Pretorius R, et al. Fatigue: an overview. *Am Fam Physician*. 2008;78(10):1173–1179.

FEVER IN THE FIRST 3 MONTHS OF LIFE

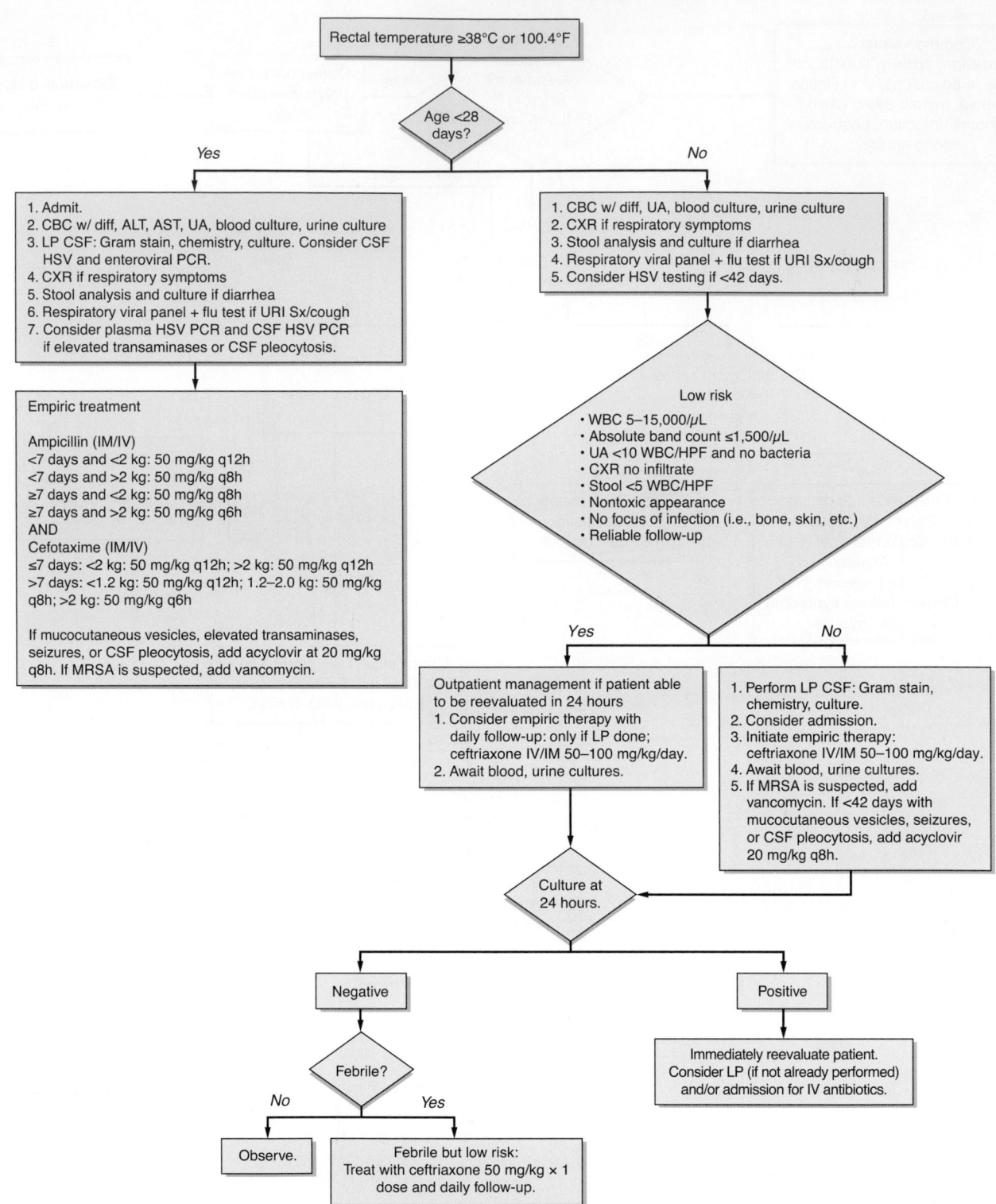

Robyn Wing, MD, MPH and Madeline L. McCarthy, MD, MS

Byington CL, Reynolds CC, Korgenski K, et al. Costs and infant outcomes after implementation of a care process model for febrile infants. *Pediatrics.* 2012;130(1):e16–e24.

FEVER OF UNKNOWN ORIGIN

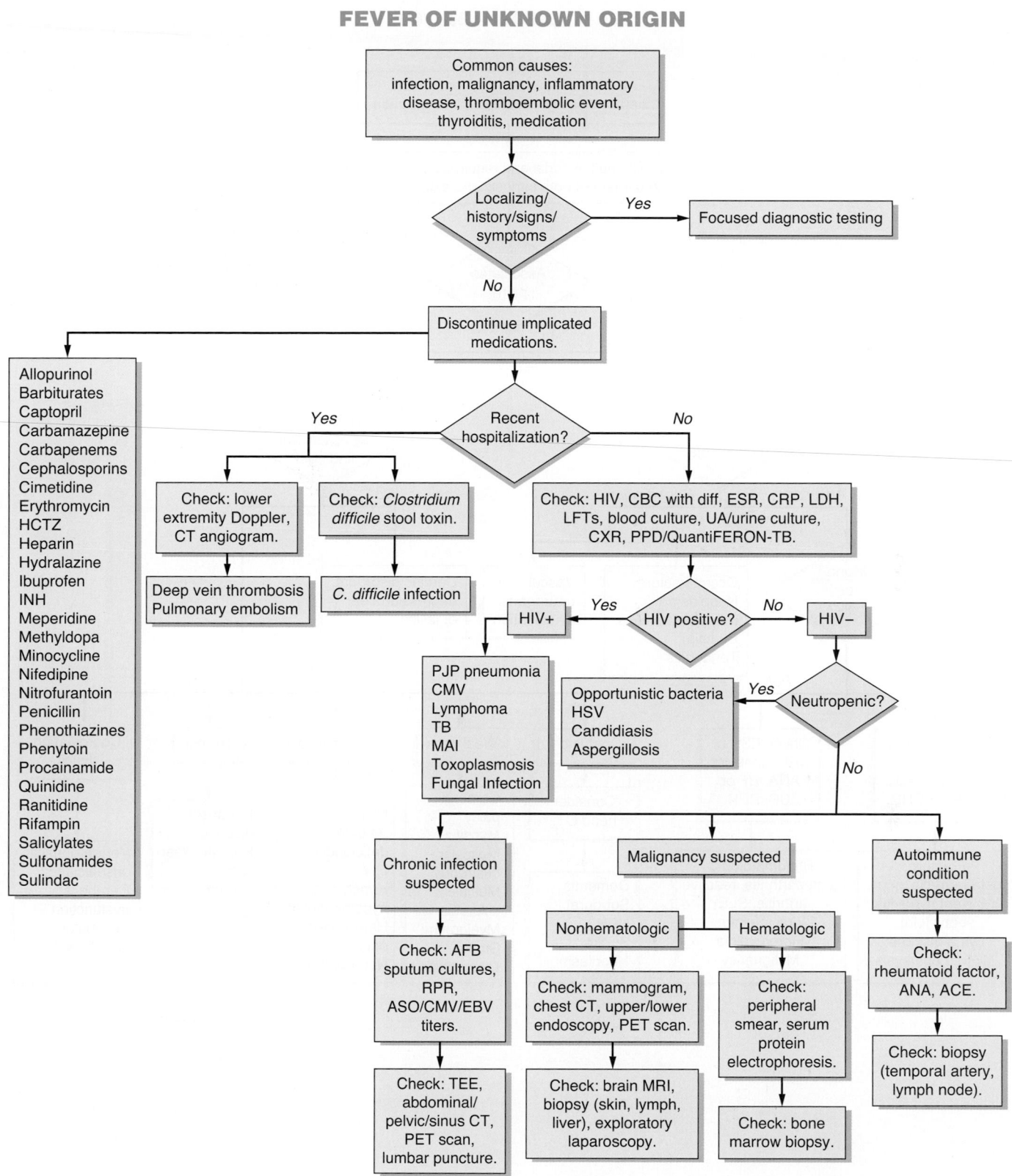

Rachelle E. Toman, MD, PhD, Matthew J. Brenan, MD, and Hiu Ying Joanna Choi, MD

Hersch EC, Oh RC. Prolonged febrile illness and fever of unknown origin in adults. *Am Fam Physician.* 2014;90(2):91–96.

GAIT DISTURBANCE

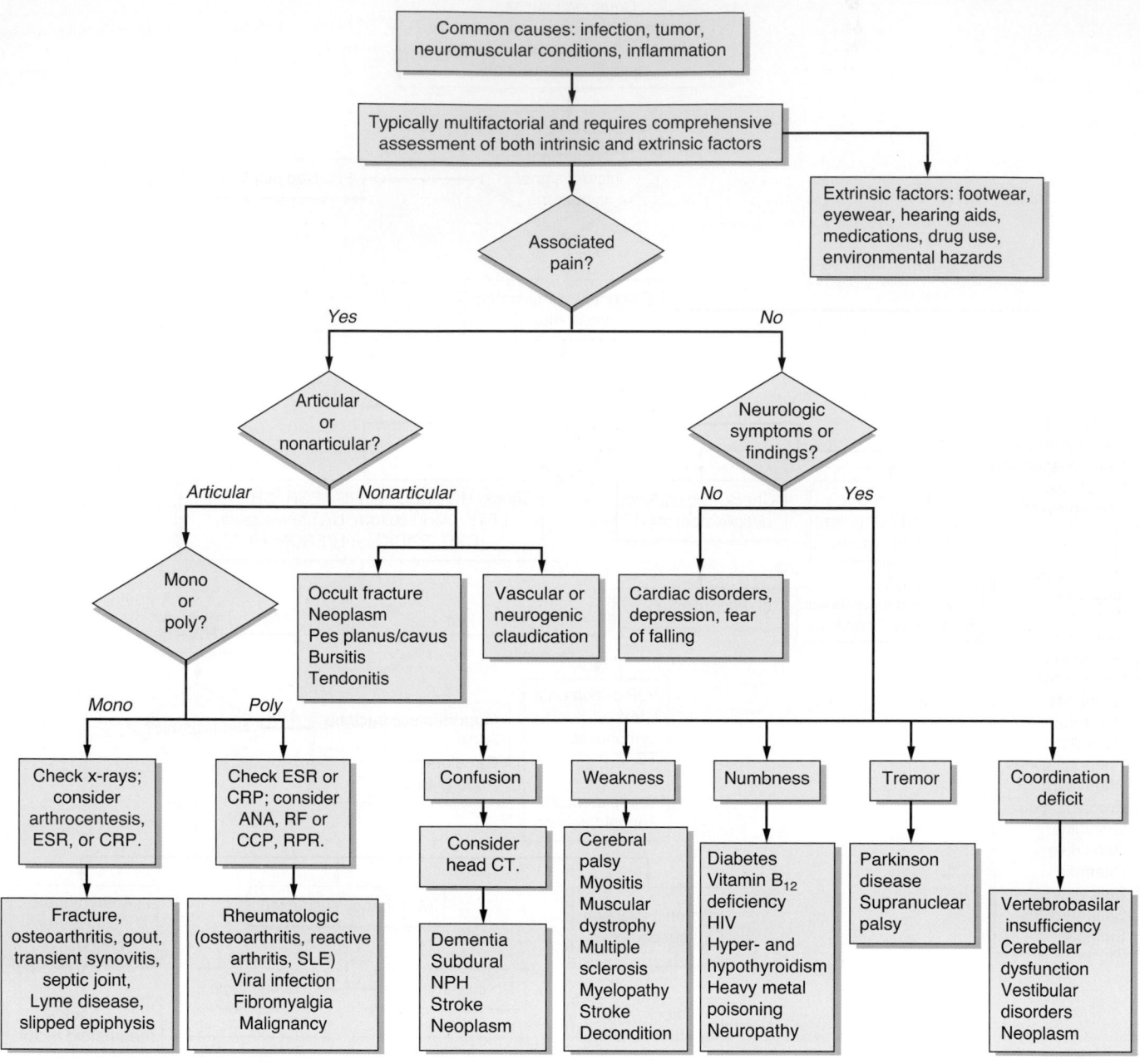

David T. O'Gurek, MD, FAAFP

Salzman B. Gait and balance disorders in older adults. *Am Fam Physician.* 2010;82(1):61–68.

GASTROESOPHAGEAL REFLUX DISEASE (GERD), DIAGNOSIS AND TREATMENT

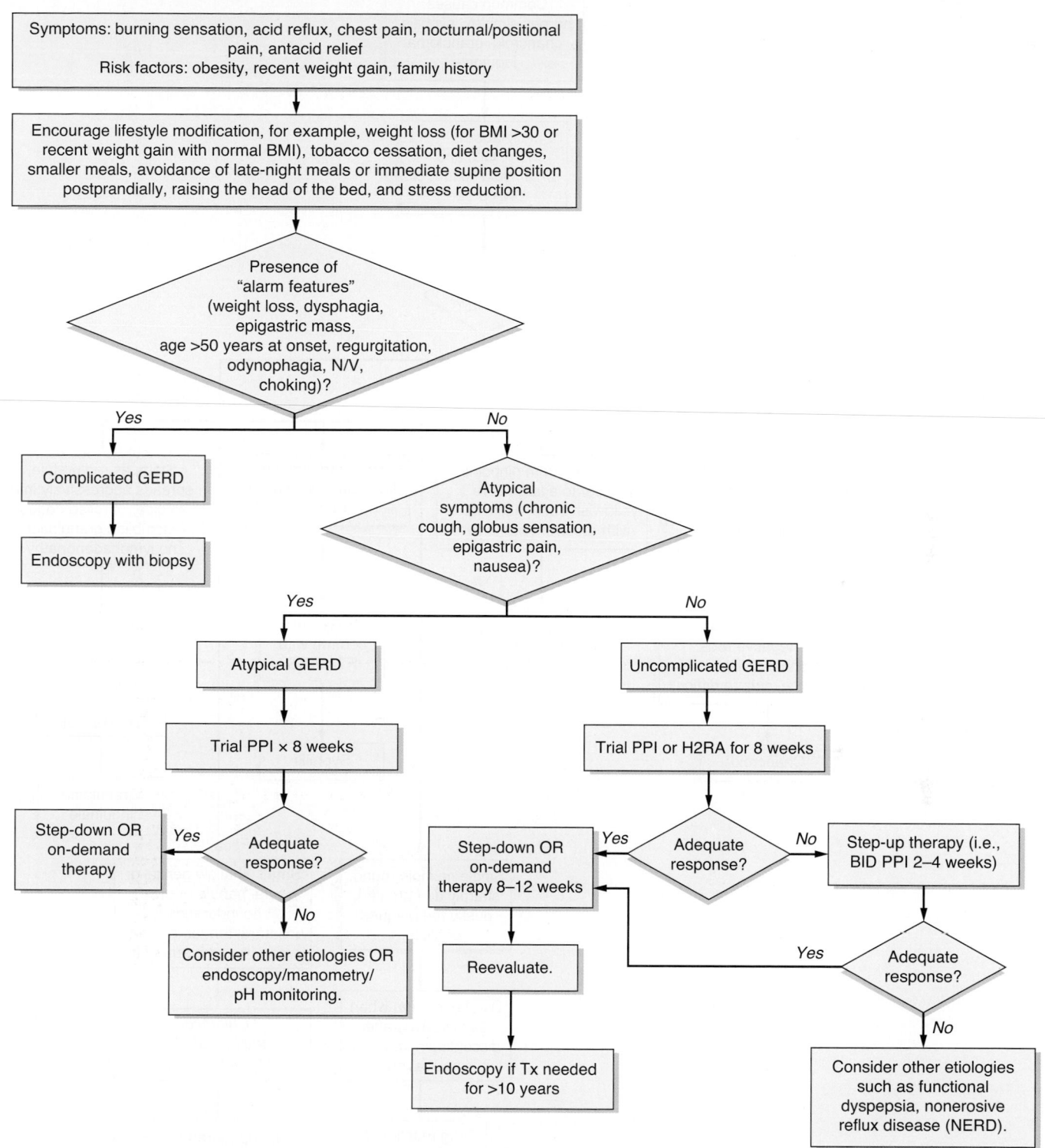

Hadi Atassi, DO and Thomas L. Abell, MD

Katz PO, Gerson LB, Vela MF. Guidelines for the diagnosis and management of gastroesophageal reflux disease. *Am J Gastroenterol.* 2013;108(3):308–329; quiz 329..

GENITAL ULCERS

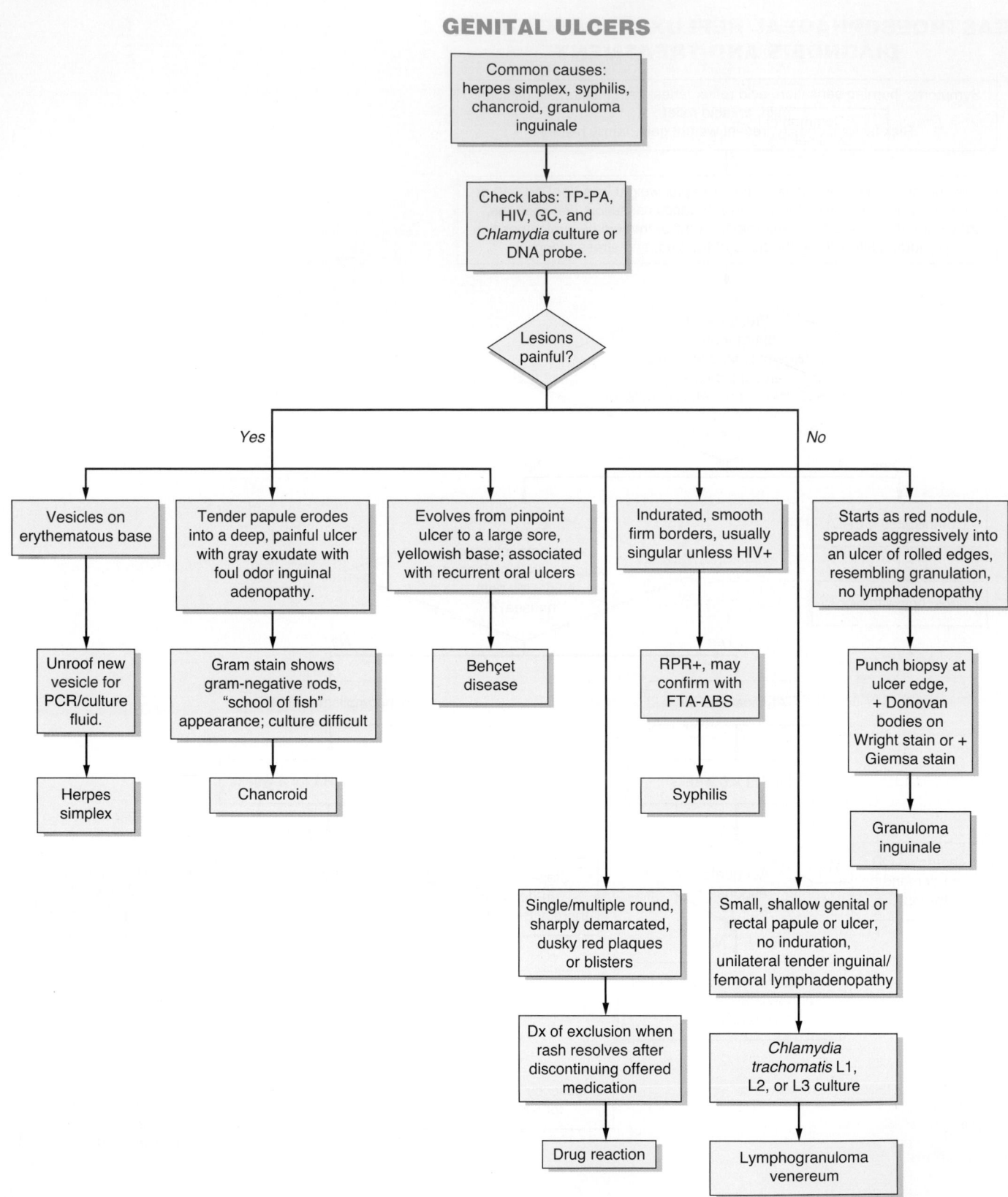

Chidinma Osineme, MD

Roett MA, Mayor MT, Uduhiri KA. Diagnosis and management of genital ulcers. *Am Fam Physician.* 2012;85(3):254–262.

GRANULOCYTOSIS (LEUKOCYTOSIS)

WBC $>11.0 \times 10^9$/L

Common causes: infection, inflammation, drugs (steroid/lithium/β-agonists, G-CSF, GM-CSF, etc.), stress, smoking, asplenia/hyposplenism, stress, pregnancy, myeloproliferative disorder, leukemia/lymphoma

Repeat CBC.
Order manual smear.

Leukocytosis confirmed? — No → No further workup necessary

Yes

Leukocytosis explained by additional pertinent history and/or physical examination? — Yes →

No

Patient presents with weight loss, fatigue, fevers, night sweats, splenomegaly, lymphadenopathy, bruising? Abnormal red blood cell (RBC) and platelet count? Risk of or history of prior malignancy? — Yes →

Consider malignancy.
Review peripheral blood smear.
Hematology/oncology consultation
Bone marrow biopsy and flow cytometry, cytogenetics or molecular testing on bone marrow or peripheral blood

No

Determine affected cell line.

LYMPHOCYTOSIS
($>4,500$/mm^3 [4.5×10^9/L])

PLEOMORPHIC (REACTIVE)

MONOMORPHIC
Suspect lymphoproliferative disorder.

Look for:
Infections (viral, pertussis)
Hypersensitivity
Consider:
Immunization
Contact history
Chest x-ray
Viral panels

MONOCYTOSIS
(>880/mm^3 [0.88×10^9/L])
Look for:
Chronic infection (EBV, fungal, protozoal, rickettsial)
Autoimmune
Splenectomy
Myelodysplastic syndrome
Consider:
Contact, travel, medical history
Monospot test, PPD, ESR, CRP, ANA

If persistent

INCREASED BLASTS

BASOPHILIA
(>100/mm^3 [0.1×10^9/L])
Rare: Suspect MPN.
Consider:
Karyotyping
BCR-ABL1
JAK-2 V617F

EOSINOPHILIA
(>500/mm^3 [0.5×10^9])
Look for reactive etiology:
Allergic conditions
Eosinophilic esophagitis
Drug reaction
Dermatologic conditions
Parasitic infections
Consider:
Drug, travel history
Full skin exam and biopsy if indicated
Allergy/immunology testing
Stool for ova and parasites
Upper GI endoscopy

If negative, rule out myeloproliferative neoplasm, Hodgkin lymphoma.
Consider:
FISH/PCR for PDGFRA mutation

NEUTROPHILIA
($>7,000$/mm^3 [7×10^9/L])

WBC $>50,000$: malignant

WBC $<50,000$: leukemoid reaction

Look for:
Infection
Chronic inflammation
Stressors
Medications (including GM-CSF)
Splenectomy
Cigarette smoking
Leukoerythroblastic reaction
Consider:
Medical, surgical drug, contact, social history
ESR, CRP, ANA
Blood smear review for nucleated RBCs
Blood culture, lumbar puncture
Additional system-specific studies

Hematology/oncology consult
Bone marrow biopsy
Flow cytometry, cytogenetics, and molecular analysis of bone marrow or peripheral blood

Sarah Jamshed, MD and L. Michael Snyder, MD

George TI. Malignant or benign leukocytosis. *Hematology Am Soc Hematol Educ Program.* 2012;2012:475–484.

HEADACHE, CHRONIC

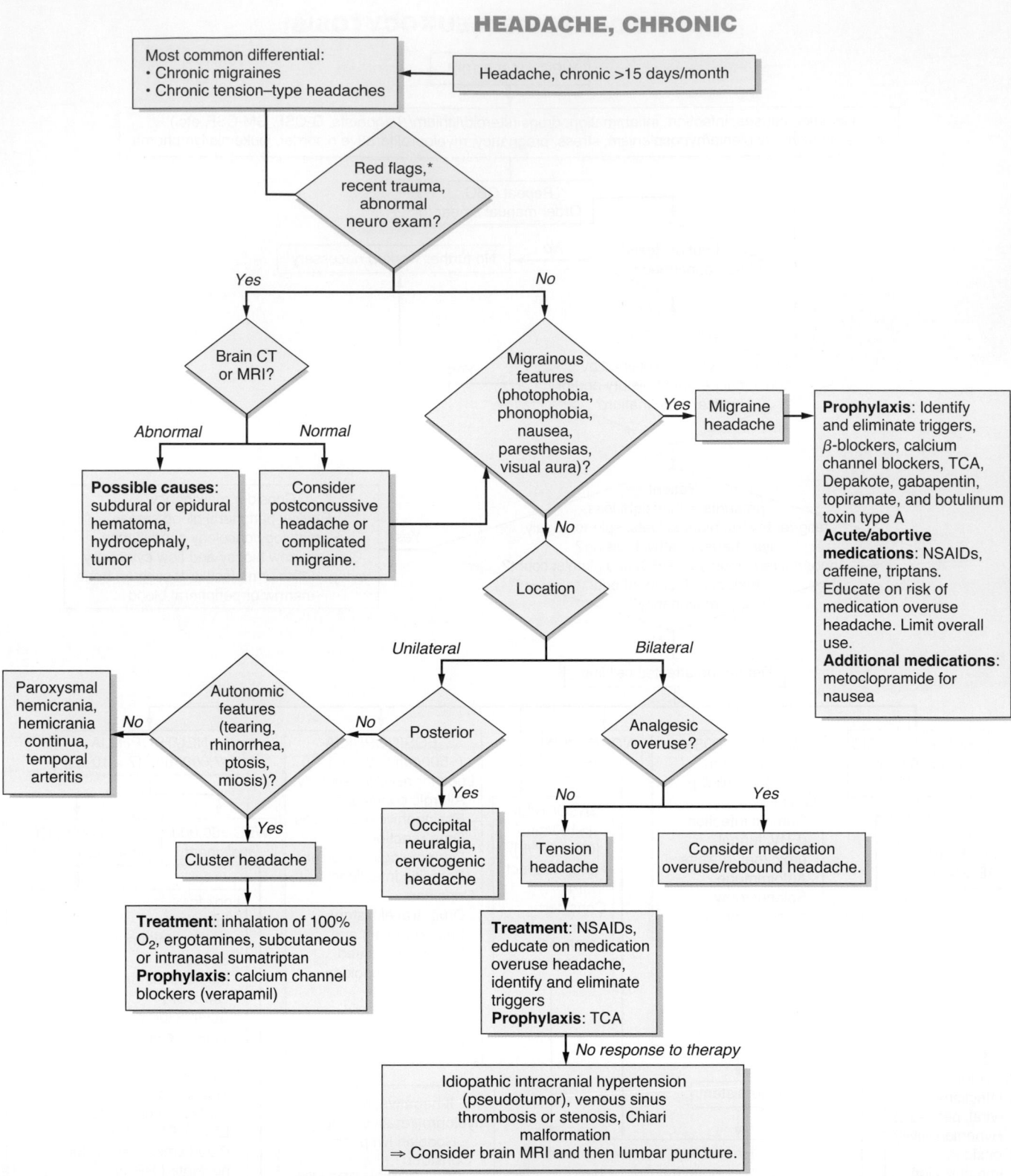

Headache, chronic >15 days/month

Most common differential:
• Chronic migraines
• Chronic tension–type headaches

Red flags,* recent trauma, abnormal neuro exam?

Yes → Brain CT or MRI?
- *Abnormal* → **Possible causes**: subdural or epidural hematoma, hydrocephaly, tumor
- *Normal* → Consider postconcussive headache or complicated migraine.

No → Migrainous features (photophobia, phonophobia, nausea, paresthesias, visual aura)?
- *Yes* → Migraine headache → **Prophylaxis**: Identify and eliminate triggers, β-blockers, calcium channel blockers, TCA, Depakote, gabapentin, topiramate, and botulinum toxin type A **Acute/abortive medications**: NSAIDs, caffeine, triptans. Educate on risk of medication overuse headache. Limit overall use. **Additional medications**: metoclopramide for nausea
- *No* → Location

Location
- *Unilateral* → Posterior
  - Autonomic features (tearing, rhinorrhea, ptosis, miosis)?
    - *No* → Paroxysmal hemicrania, hemicrania continua, temporal arteritis
    - *Yes* → Cluster headache → **Treatment**: inhalation of 100% O₂, ergotamines, subcutaneous or intranasal sumatriptan **Prophylaxis**: calcium channel blockers (verapamil)
  - *Yes* → Occipital neuralgia, cervicogenic headache
- *Bilateral* → Analgesic overuse?
  - *No* → Tension headache → **Treatment**: NSAIDs, educate on medication overuse headache, identify and eliminate triggers **Prophylaxis**: TCA
    - *No response to therapy* → Idiopathic intracranial hypertension (pseudotumor), venous sinus thrombosis or stenosis, Chiari malformation ⇒ Consider brain MRI and then lumbar puncture.
  - *Yes* → Consider medication overuse/rebound headache.

*Red flags include onset of headache after age 50 years, altered mental status (including confusion, personality changes), papilledema, report of "worst headache of my life," and focal neurologic deficits such as weakness or ataxia headaches that worsen with positional change, headaches that worsen with Valsalva, and headaches associated with unexplained fever, chills, or weight loss.

Frank J. Domino, MD and Alexander CVitan, MD

Yancey JR, Sheridan R, Koren KG. Chronic daily headache: diagnosis and management. *Am Fam Physician.* 2014;89(8):642–648.

HEART MURMUR

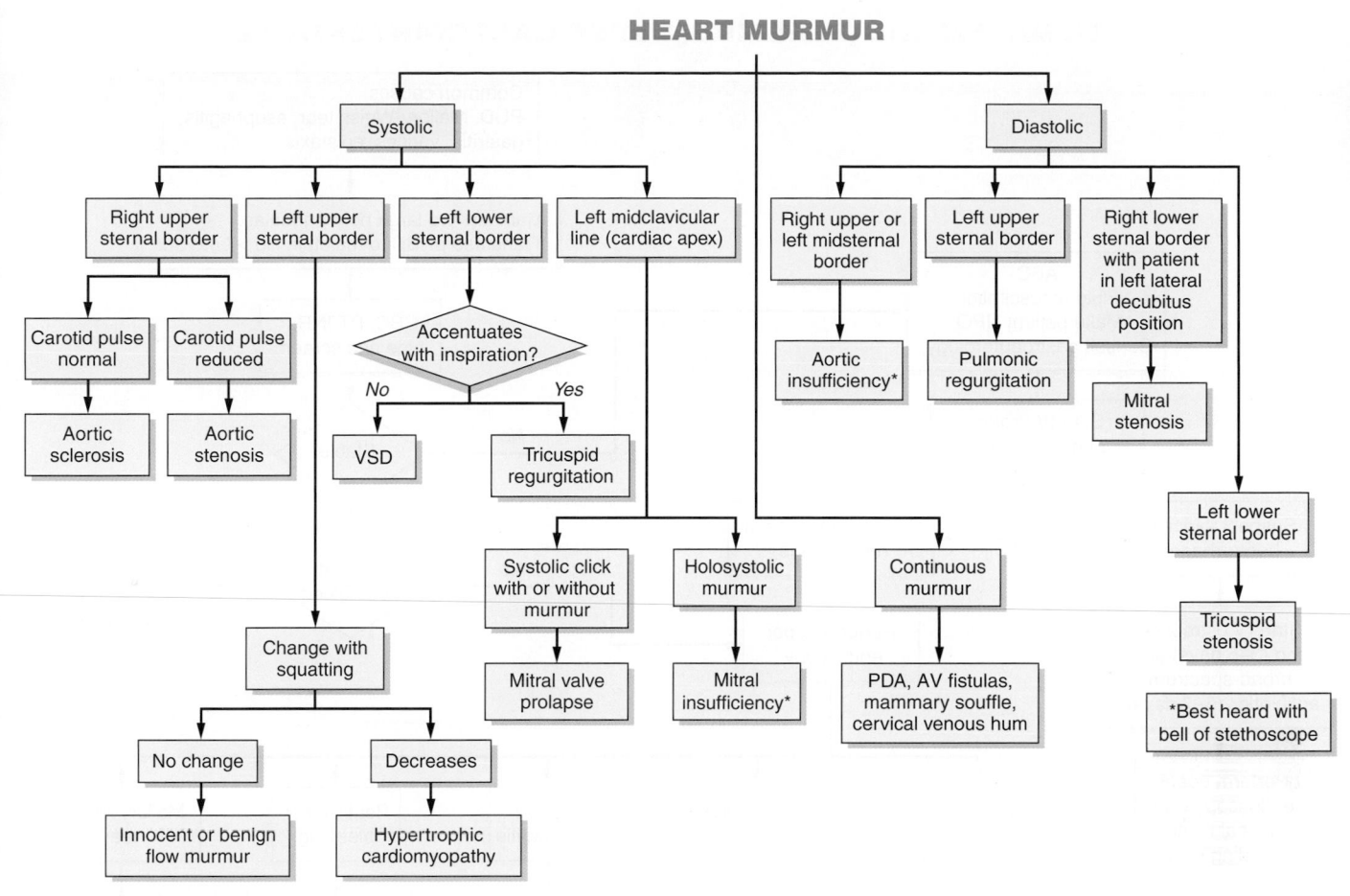

Michael Argyle, DO and Brett Johnson, DO

Bonow RO, Carabello BA, Chatterjee K, et al. 2008 Focused update incorporated into the ACC/AHA 2006 guidelines for the management of patients with valvular heart disease: a report of the American College of Cardiology/American Heart Association Task Force on Practice Guidelines (writing committee to revise the 1998 Guidelines for the Management of Patients With Valvular Heart Disease): endorsed by the Society of Cardiovascular Anesthesiologists, Society for Cardiovascular Angiography and Interventions, and Society of Thoracic Surgeons. *Circulation.* 2008;118(15):e523–e661.

HEMATEMESIS (BLEEDING, UPPER GASTROINTESTINAL)

Common causes:
PUD, Mallory-Weiss tear, esophagitis, gastritis, varices, epistaxis

Maintain two large bore cannulas.
Transfuse pRBC to maintain Hb >7 mg/dL.

CBC, PT/INR, type and screen

Stable — No

Stable — Yes

Recent nose bleed — Yes → Epistaxis

Recent nose bleed — No

ABC
Fluid resuscitation
Make patient NPO.
Consult gastroenterology.

Start IV proton pump inhibitor.

Suspect variceal hemorrhage.

Suspect nonvariceal hemorrhage.

Perform upper endoscopy.

Start IV octreotide drip (3–5 days) and broad-spectrum antibiotics (5–7 days).

Perform upper endoscopy with variceal ligation banding within 6–24 hours.

Has the bleeding stopped?

Yes → Start prophylactic nonselective β-blocker after octreotide complete.

Repeat endoscopy in 1–2 weeks and reband as needed.

No → Sengstaken-Blakemore tube

Consider emergent transjugular intrahepatic portosystemic shunt or surgery depending on local expertise.

No source identified
Consider repeat endoscopy and push enteroscopy.

Arteriovenous malformation, Dieulafoy ulcer
Endoscopic therapy with epinephrine, thermocoagulation, or clipping

Erosive esophagitis
Continue proton pump inhibitor therapy.

Peptic ulcer bleeding
Endoscopic therapy with epinephrine, thermocoagulation, and/or clips

Has the bleeding stopped?

Yes → Continue proton pump inhibitor therapy; eradicate *Helicobacter pylori* infection if present, and consider discontinuing NSAIDs/aspirin if possible.

No → Reattempt upper endoscopy; otherwise, consider arteriography with embolization or surgery.

Mallory-Weiss tear
Antiemetic and proton pump inhibitor; endoscopic treatment only if active bleeding

Lolwa Al-Obaid, MD, Lisa N. Jarnagin, MBBCh, BAO, and Stephen C. Fabry, MD

Wilkins T, Khan N, Nabh A, et al. Diagnosis and management of upper gastrointestinal bleeding. *Am Fam Physician.* 2012;85(5):469–476.

HEMATURIA

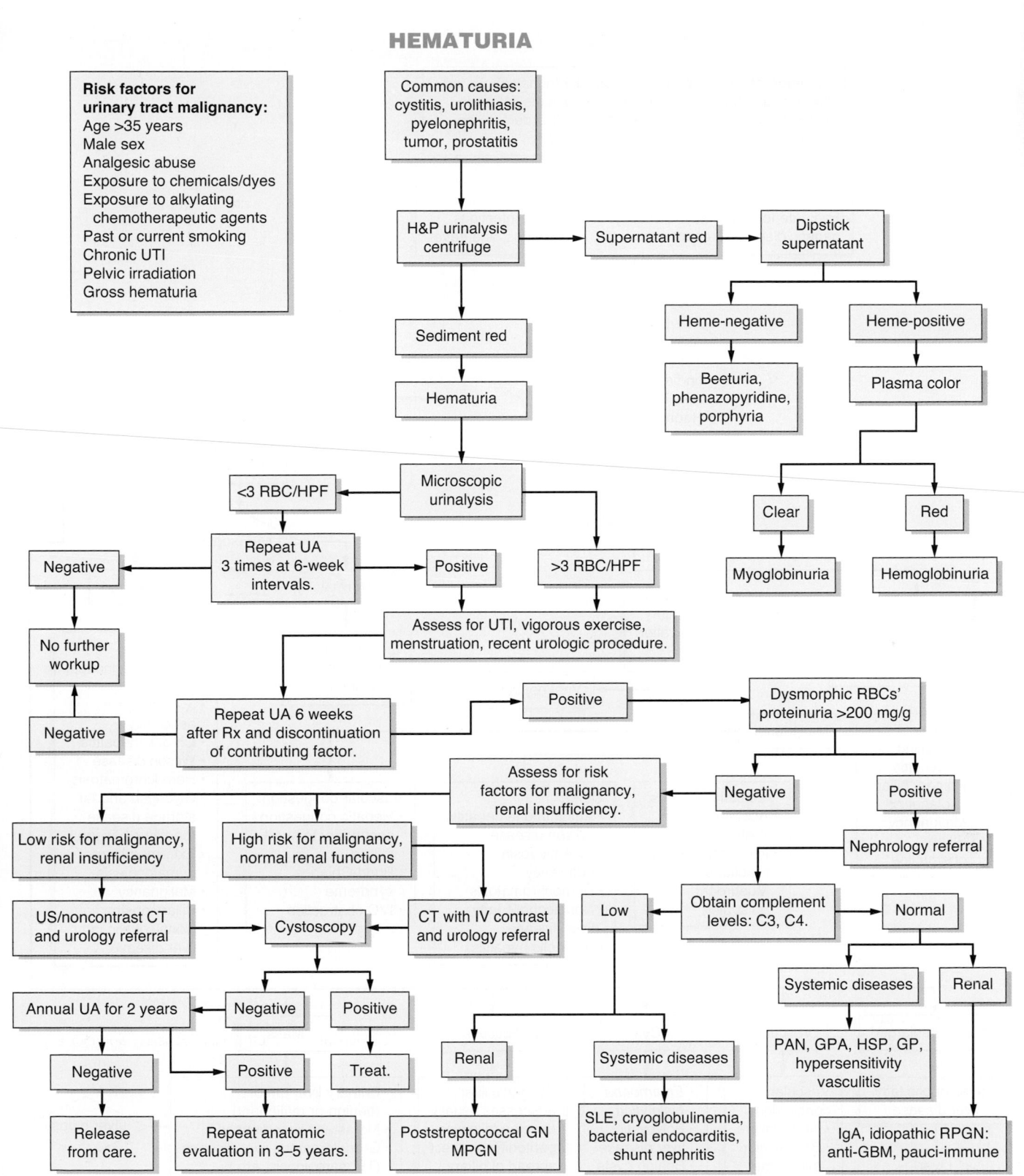

Risk factors for urinary tract malignancy:
Age >35 years
Male sex
Analgesic abuse
Exposure to chemicals/dyes
Exposure to alkylating chemotherapeutic agents
Past or current smoking
Chronic UTI
Pelvic irradiation
Gross hematuria

Krishna Manda, MD, MRCP and Jagathi Govindu, MD

Sharp VJ, Barnes KT, Erickson BA. Assessment of asymptomatic microscopic hematuria in adults. *Am Fam Physician*. 2013;88(11):747–754.

HEPATOMEGALY

Common causes: liver disease, obesity (nonalcoholic fatty liver disease and steatohepatitis), neoplasms, infection, vascular disease, fat/glycogen storage disorders, biliary disease, toxins, and metabolic disturbances

History:
Evaluate for heart failure, obesity, alcohol use, infections, genetic diseases, recent exposures, medications, and travel.

Initial labs:
- ALT/AST
- Total bilirubin (indirect/direct)
- Alkaline phosphatase
- Hepatitis serologies

Normal → Imaging: CT, ultrasound → Abnormal

Normal

Liver biopsy

Normal → Liver is normal; reevaluate in 6 months.

Abnormal → Consider the following diagnoses:
- Cirrhosis
- α_1-Antitrypsin deficiency
- Chronic hepatitis
- Wilson disease
- Hemochromatosis
- Glycogen and fat storage disease (pediatric patients)
- Extramedullary hematopoiesis
- Malignancy
- Biliary obstruction
- Nonalcoholic fatty liver disease

Abnormal

Cholestatic injury: predominant elevation of bilirubin and alkaline phosphatase

- Primary sclerosing cholangitis
- Primary biliary cholangitis
- Malignancy
- Biliary obstruction

Hepatocellular injury: predominant elevation of ALT and AST

Viral hepatitis

Malignancy

Medications/toxins:
- Acetaminophen
- Statins
- Idiosyncratic drug reactions
- Mushroom poisoning

Other:
- Autoimmune hepatitis
- Wilson disease
- α_1-Antitrypsin deficiency
- Hemochromatosis
- Nonalcoholic fatty liver disease
- Alcoholic hepatitis

Vascular congestion:
- Hepatic congestion secondary to heart failure
- Budd-Chiari syndrome
- IVC obstruction

Uniformly enlarged

Nonalcoholic fatty liver disease

Liver biopsy +/− fibrosure

Vascular

Vascular congestion:
- Heart failure
- Budd-Chiari syndrome
- IVC obstruction

Cyst

- *Entamoeba histolytica*
- Polycystic liver disease
- Benign cysts

Abscess

Pyogenic liver abscesses usually develop following peritonitis or direct spread of biliary infection.

Mass

- Primary liver tumor (benign or malignant)
- Metastatic liver disease
- Granulomatous liver disease (TB, sarcoidosis, etc.)

Liver biopsy

Daniel P. Szvarca, MD and Marie L. Borum, MD, EdD, MPH, MACP, FACG, AGAF

Kwo PY, Cohen SM, Lim JK. ACG clinical guideline: evaluation of abnormal liver chemistries. *Am J Gastroenterol.* 2017;112(1):18–35.

HYPERBILIRUBINEMIA AND JAUNDICE

Jaundice: a yellow discoloration of skin, sclera, and mucous membranes by bilirubin, a bile pigment formed by the breakdown of heme rings; detected when the serum bilirubin level >3 mg/dL. Bilirubin is a product of hemoglobin breakdown in the spleen. Heme is converted to unconjugated bilirubin, bound to albumin, and then sent to the liver where it is then conjugated.

Common causes: Gilbert syndrome, hemolysis, hepatitis, and choledocholithiasis

CBC w/ diff, LFTs: ALT, AST, serum alkaline phosphatase (AP), total bilirubin (TB) and direct bilirubin (DB), haptoglobin, hepatitis serologies, amylase, lipase, hCG, urinalysis with urine bilirubin; US or CT

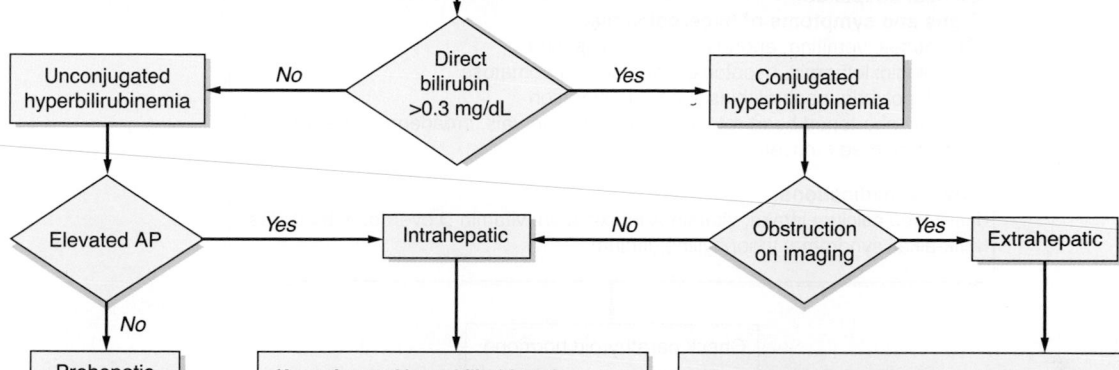

Prehepatic

- **Hemolytic anemia**
- **Reabsorption of large hematoma**

Labs: anemia, possible reticulocytosis, mild TB elevation (5 mg/dL), increased indirect bilirubin, normal DB levels, and negative urine bilirubin. All other LFTs are normal.

Unconjugated hyperbilirubinemia

○ **Gilbert syndrome**: mild defect in UDP glucuronosyltransferase (UGT, responsible for conjugation of bilirubin)
○ **Crigler-Najjar syndrome**: more severe defect in UGT, usually presents during infancy

Conjugated hyperbilirubinemia

○ **Dubin-Johnson syndrome**: defective secretion of conjugated bilirubin
○ **Rotor syndrome**

Both conjugated and unconjugated hepatocellular injury:

○ **Hepatitis**: viral, alcohol, or autoimmune insult leading to inflammation that impedes or prevents transport/secretion of conjugated bilirubin
○ **Medication/drug**: acetaminophen
○ **Cirrhosis**
○ **Congestive heart failure:** Hypoxia/anoxia of hepatocytes leads to cellular injury.

Intrahepatic cholestasis (no elevated LFTs, [primarily AP], US shows normal sized bile ducts)

Other:
○ **Medication/drug induced**
○ **Total parenteral nutrition (TPN)**
○ **Sepsis**
○ **Sarcoidosis**
○ **Pregnancy**

Extrahepatic cholestasis (labs: elevated TB and DB, elevated AP, and positive urine bilirubin. US shows dilated bile duct[s].)

- **Choledocholithiasis**
- **Chronic pancreatitis**: alcohol
- **Cholangitis**: fever, pain and jaundice, altered mental status, sepsis
- **Biliary structure**: history of surgical/invasive procedure
- **Primary biliary cirrhosis**
- **Primary sclerosing cholangitis**
- **Biliary tract tumor/cholangiocarcinoma**: hepatomegaly, weight loss, abdominal pain
- **Pancreatic tumor**: painless jaundice, palpable gallbladder (rare)

Krunal Patel, MD and Isabel Zacharias, MD

Roche SP, Kobos R. Jaundice in the adult patient. *Am Fam Physician*. 2004;69(2):299–304.

HYPERCALCEMIA

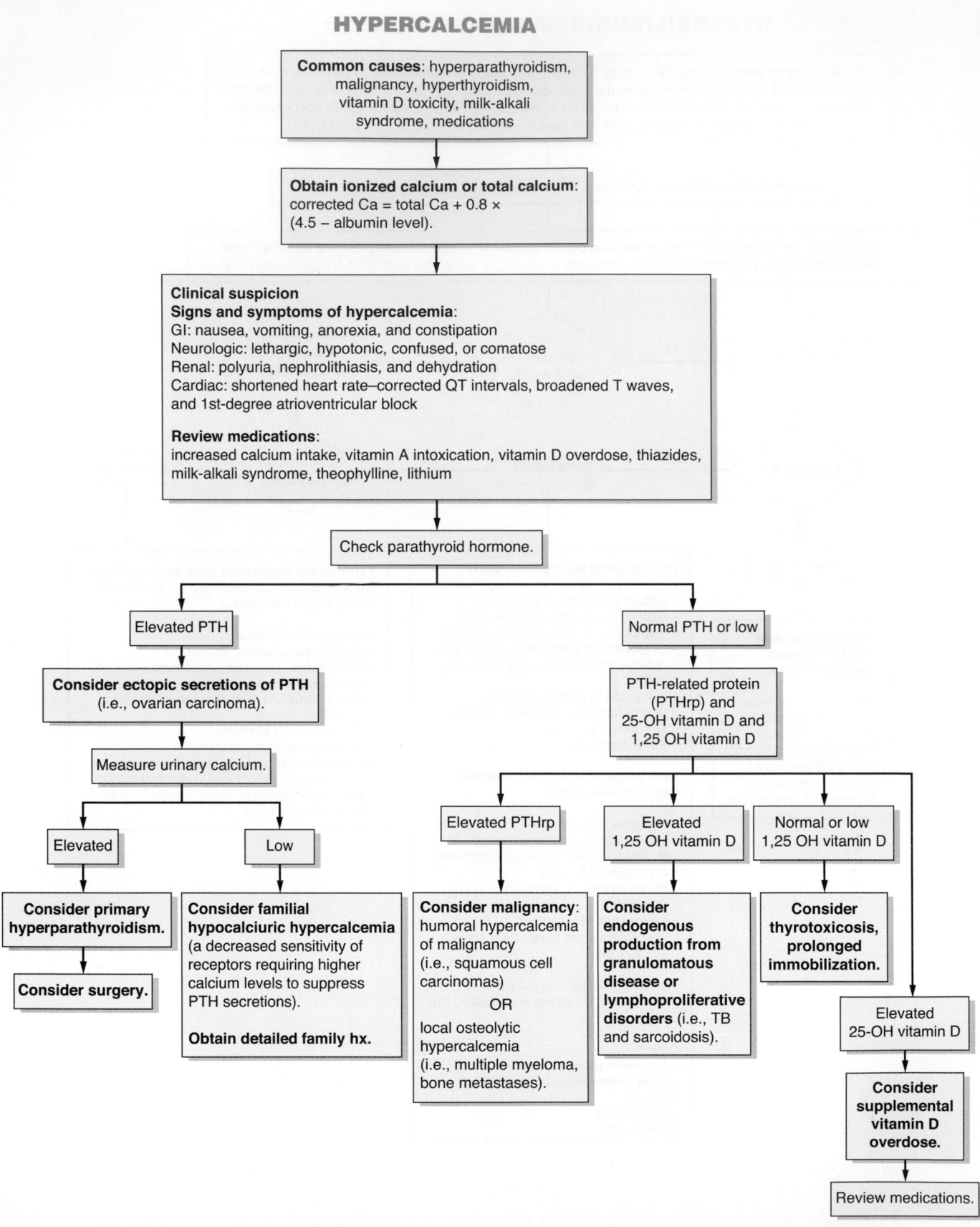

Common causes: hyperparathyroidism, malignancy, hyperthyroidism, vitamin D toxicity, milk-alkali syndrome, medications

Obtain ionized calcium or total calcium: corrected Ca = total Ca + 0.8 × (4.5 − albumin level).

Clinical suspicion
Signs and symptoms of hypercalcemia:
GI: nausea, vomiting, anorexia, and constipation
Neurologic: lethargic, hypotonic, confused, or comatose
Renal: polyuria, nephrolithiasis, and dehydration
Cardiac: shortened heart rate–corrected QT intervals, broadened T waves, and 1st-degree atrioventricular block

Review medications:
increased calcium intake, vitamin A intoxication, vitamin D overdose, thiazides, milk-alkali syndrome, theophylline, lithium

Check parathyroid hormone.

Elevated PTH

Consider ectopic secretions of PTH (i.e., ovarian carcinoma).

Measure urinary calcium.

Elevated

Low

Consider primary hyperparathyroidism.

Consider surgery.

Consider familial hypocalciuric hypercalcemia (a decreased sensitivity of receptors requiring higher calcium levels to suppress PTH secretions).

Obtain detailed family hx.

Normal PTH or low

PTH-related protein (PTHrp) and 25-OH vitamin D and 1,25 OH vitamin D

Elevated PTHrp

Elevated 1,25 OH vitamin D

Normal or low 1,25 OH vitamin D

Consider malignancy: humoral hypercalcemia of malignancy (i.e., squamous cell carcinomas)

OR

local osteolytic hypercalcemia (i.e., multiple myeloma, bone metastases).

Consider endogenous production from granulomatous disease or lymphoproliferative disorders (i.e., TB and sarcoidosis).

Consider thyrotoxicosis, prolonged immobilization.

Elevated 25-OH vitamin D

Consider supplemental vitamin D overdose.

Review medications.

Deborah A. Lardner, DO, DTM&H and Michael Passafaro, DO, DTM&H, FACEP, FACOEP

Kacprowicz RF, Lloyd JD. Electrolyte complications of malignancy. *Emerg Med Clin North Am.* 2009;27(2):257–269.

HYPERKALEMIA

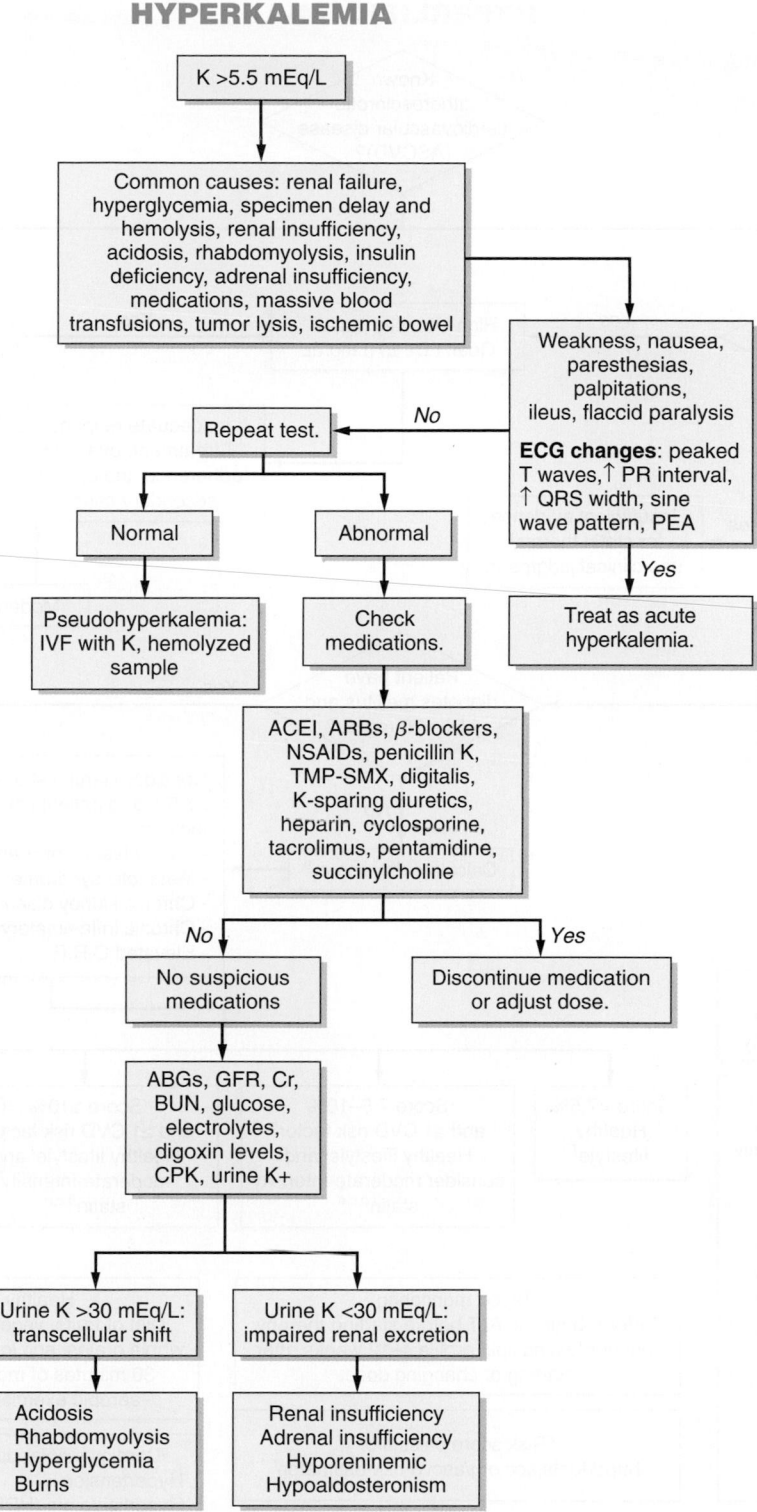

Frank J. Domino, MD

Kovesdy CP. Management of hyperkalemia: an update for the internist. *Am J Med.* 2015;128(12):1281–1287.

HYPERLIPIDEMIA

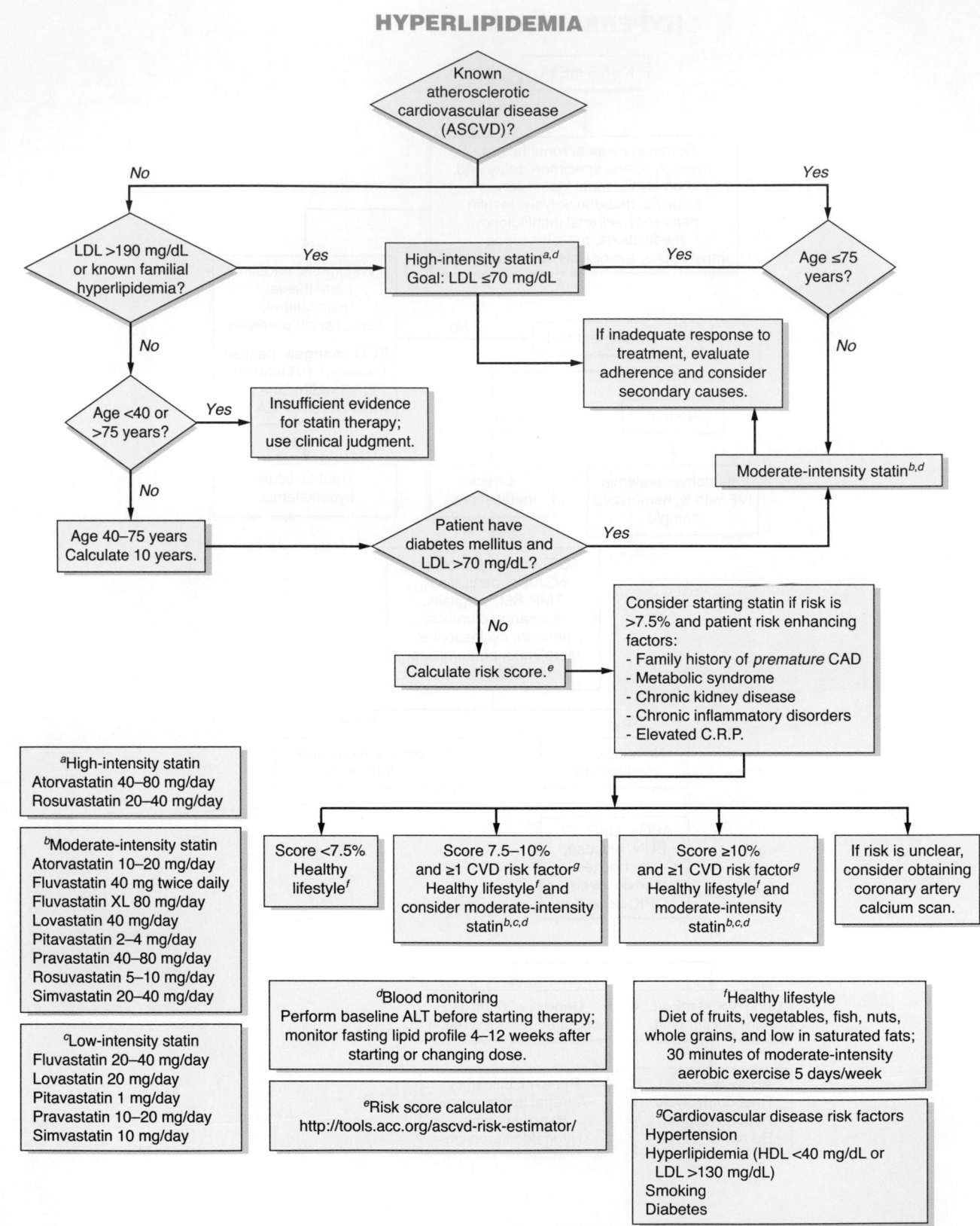

Jason E. Cross, PharmD, Dinesh Yogaratnam, PharmD, BCPS, BCCCP, and Sudeep K. Aulakh, MD, FACP, FRCPC

Grundy SM, Stone NJ, Bailey AL, et al. 2018 AHA/ACC/AACVPR/AAPA/ABC/ACPM/ADA/AGS/APhA/ASPC/NLA/PCNA guideline on the management of blood cholesterol [published online ahead of print November 10, 2018]. *Circulation*. doi:10.1161/CIR.0000000000000625.

HYPERNATREMIA

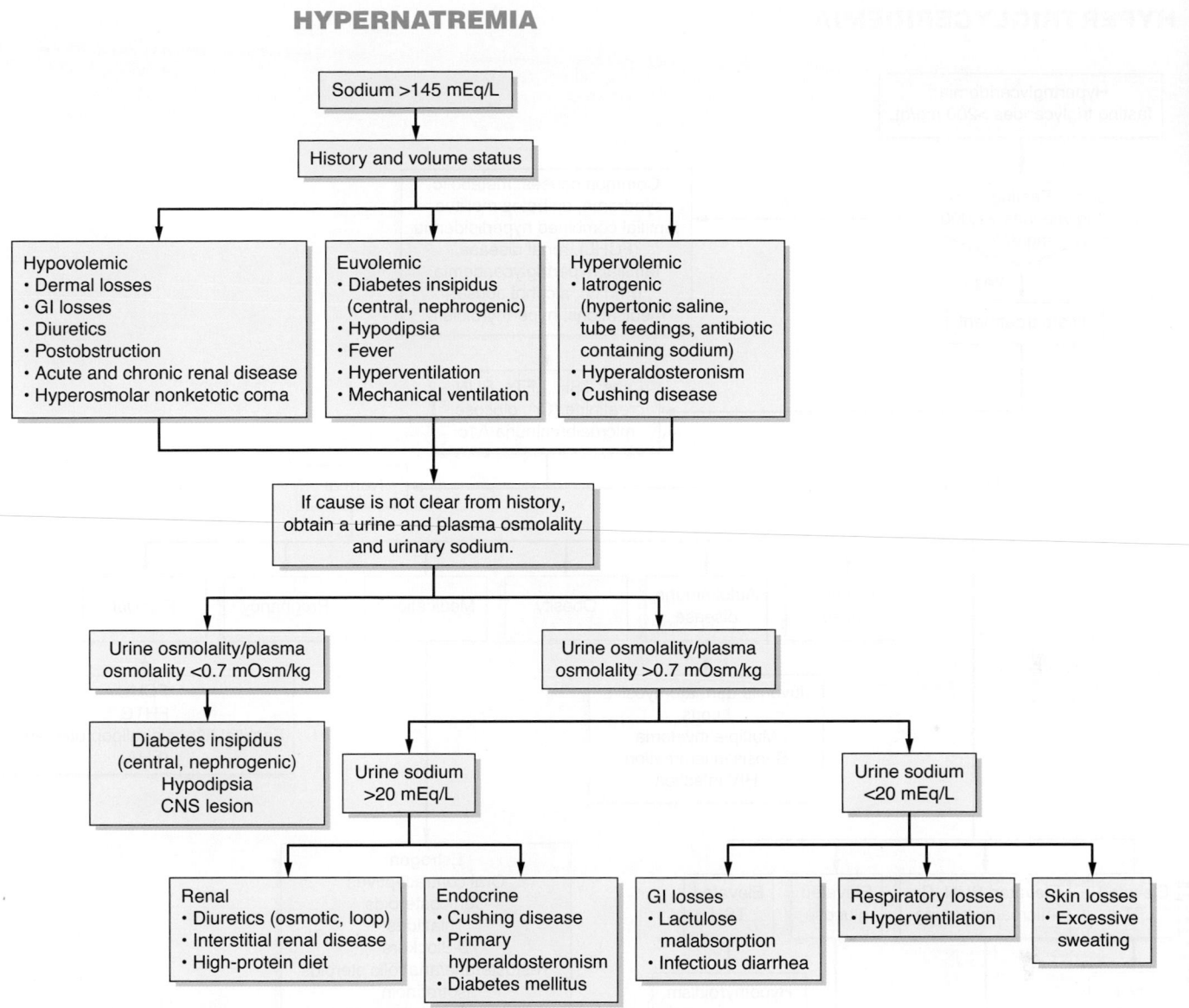

Timothy J. Coker, MD, FAAFP

Braun MM, Barstow CH, Pyzocha NJ. Diagnosis and management of sodium disorders: hyponatremia and hypernatremia. *Am Fam Physician.* 2015;91(5):299–307.

HYPERTRIGLYCERIDEMIA

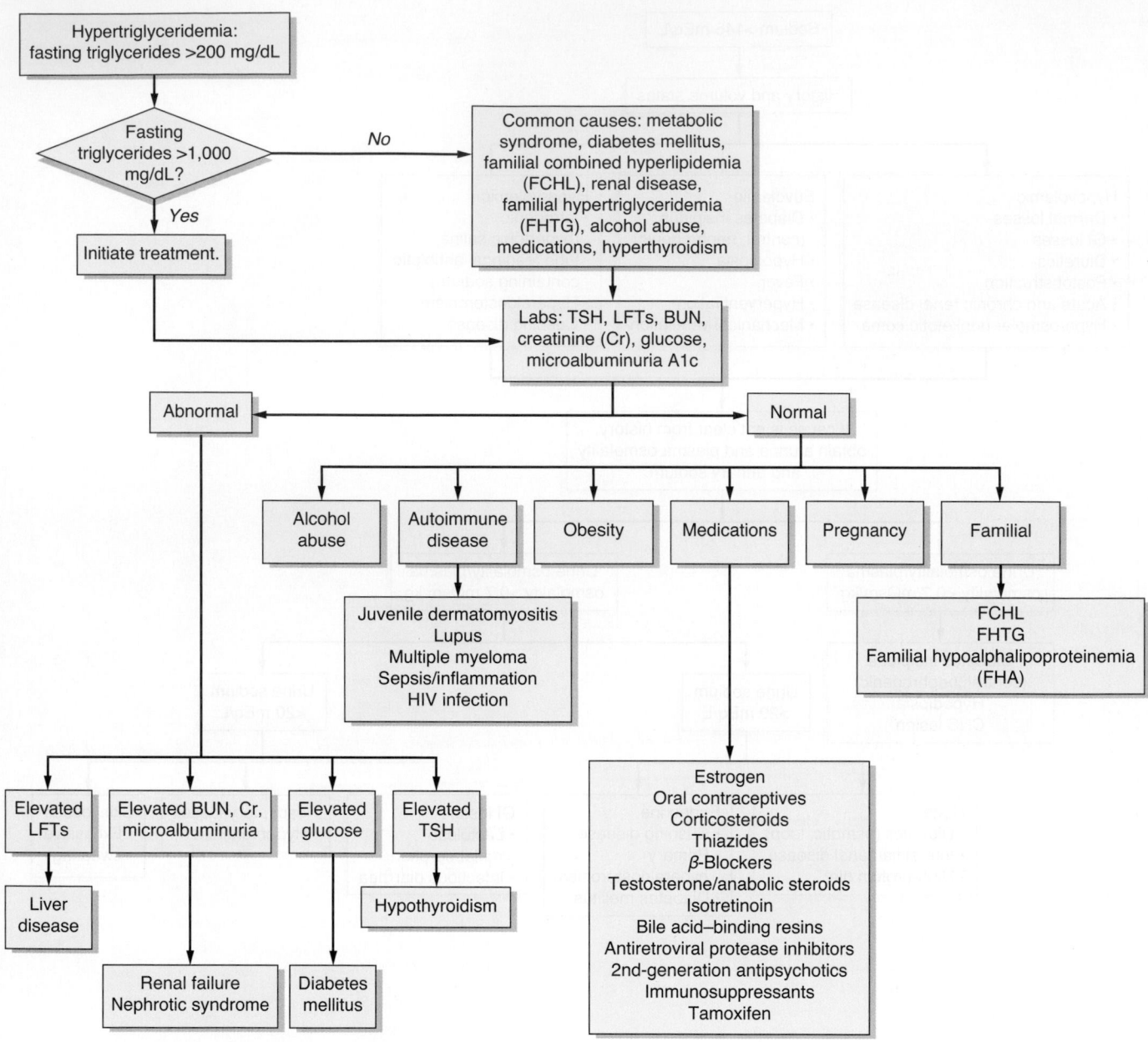

Steven W. Gale, MD and Timothy J. Coker, MD, FAAFP

Berglund L, Brunzell JD, Goldberg AC, et al; for Endocrine Society. Evaluation and treatment of hypertriglyceridemia: an Endocrine Society clinical practice guideline. *J Clin Endocrinol Metab.* 2012;97(9):2969–2989.

HYPOALBUMINEMIA

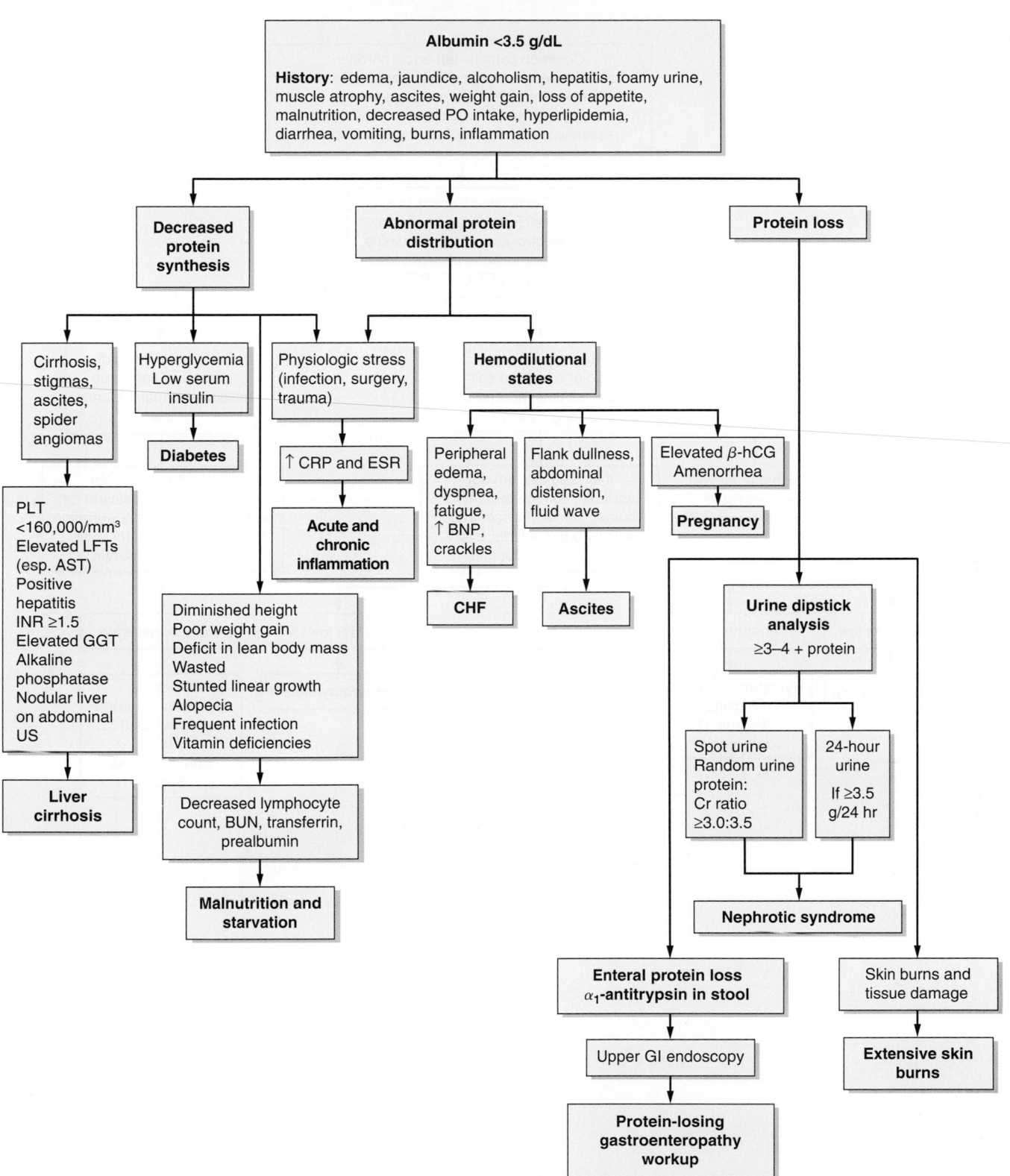

Jon Payne, MD and Lawrence M. Gibbs, MD, MSEd, FAAFP

Gatta A, Verardo A, Bolognesi M. Hypoalbuminemia. *Intern Emerg Med.* 2012;7(Suppl 3):S193–S199.

HYPOCALCEMIA

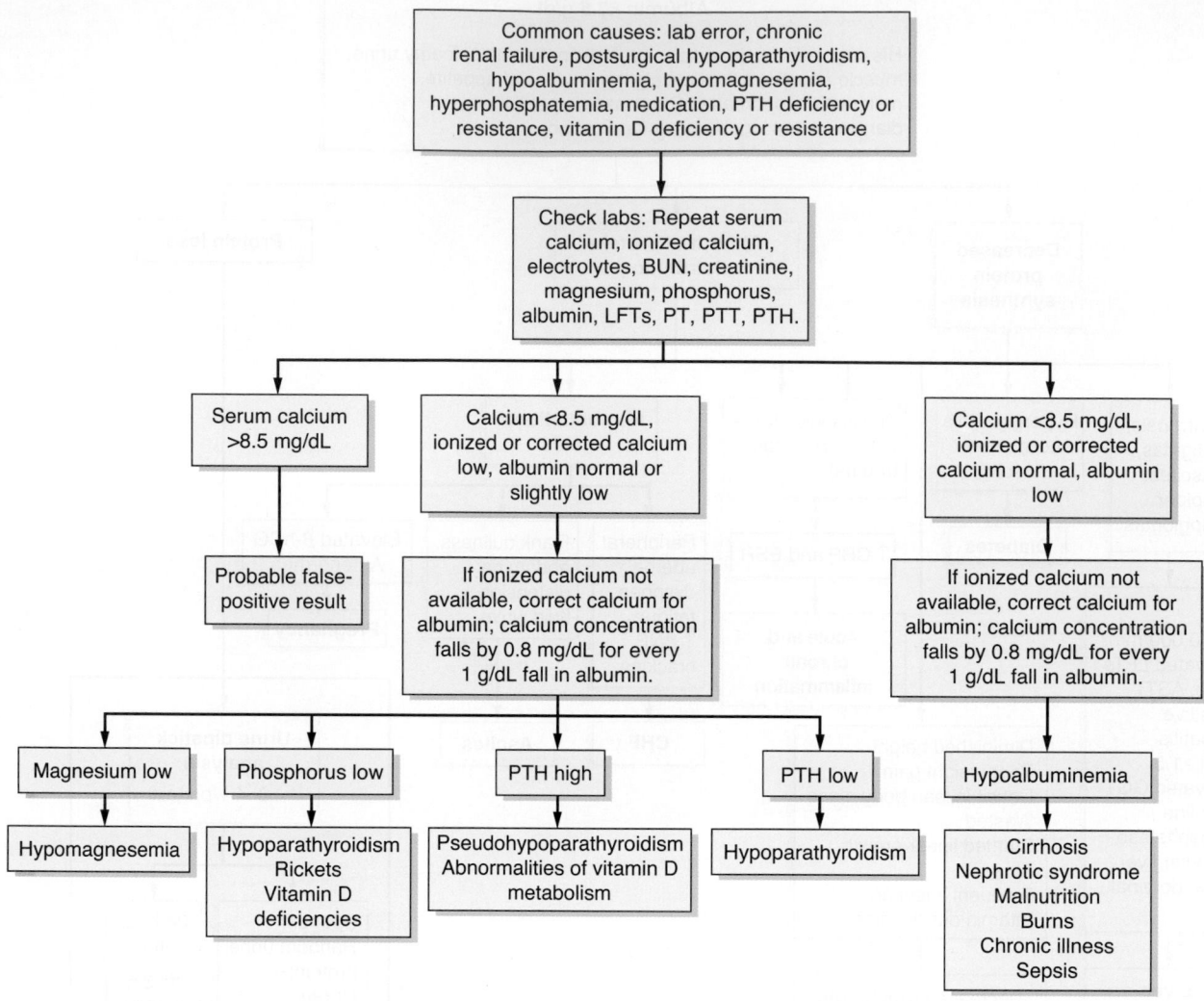

Timothy J. Coker, MD, FAAFP

Michels TC, Kelly KM. Parathyroid disorders. *Am Fam Physician*. 2013;88(4):249–257.

HYPOGLYCEMIA

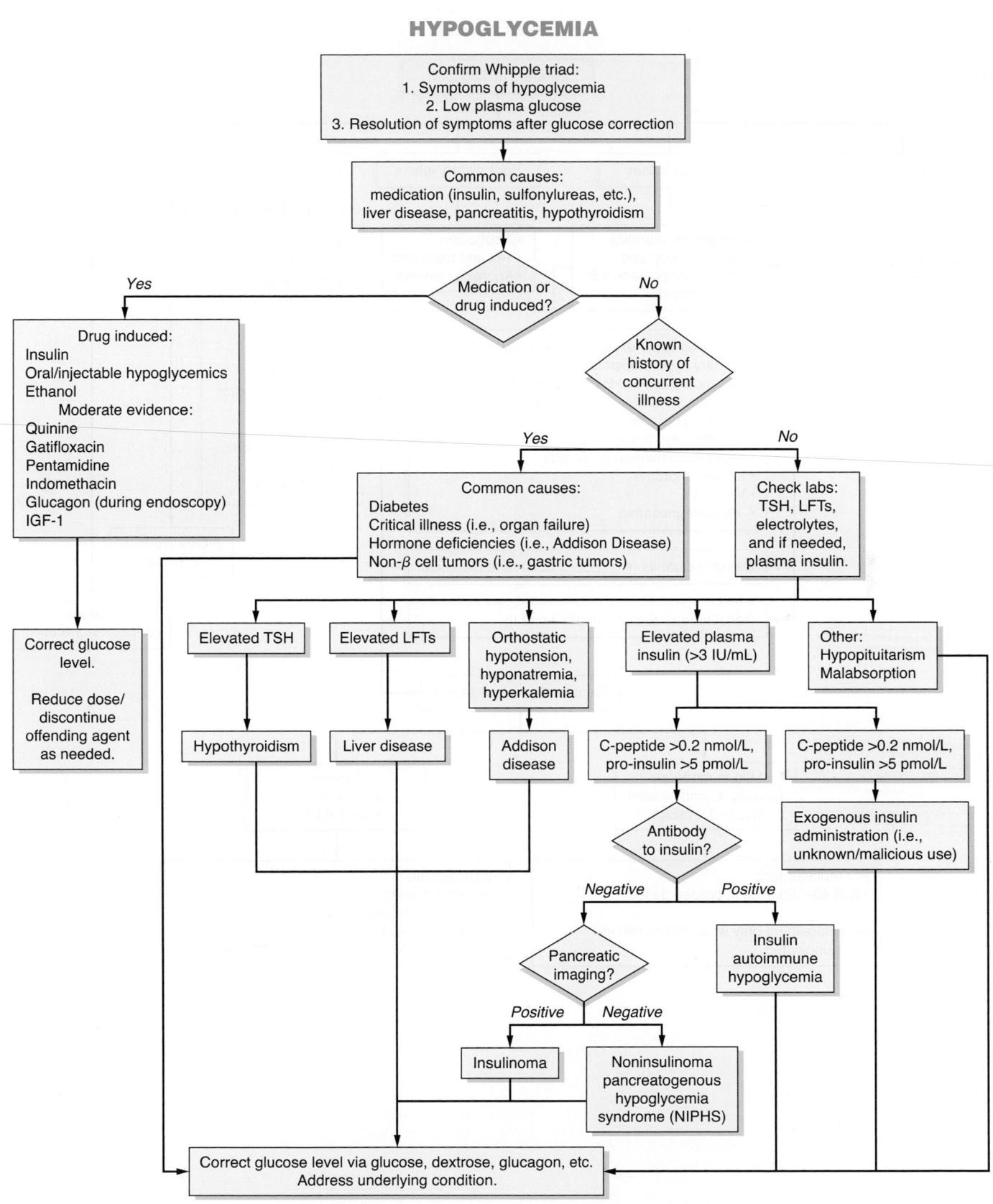

Aimee Dietle, PharmD and Stephanie J. Billings, MD

Kandaswamy L, Raghavan R, Pappachan JM. Spontaneous hypoglycemia: diagnostic evaluation and management. *Endocrine*. 2016;53(1):47–57.

HYPOKALEMIA

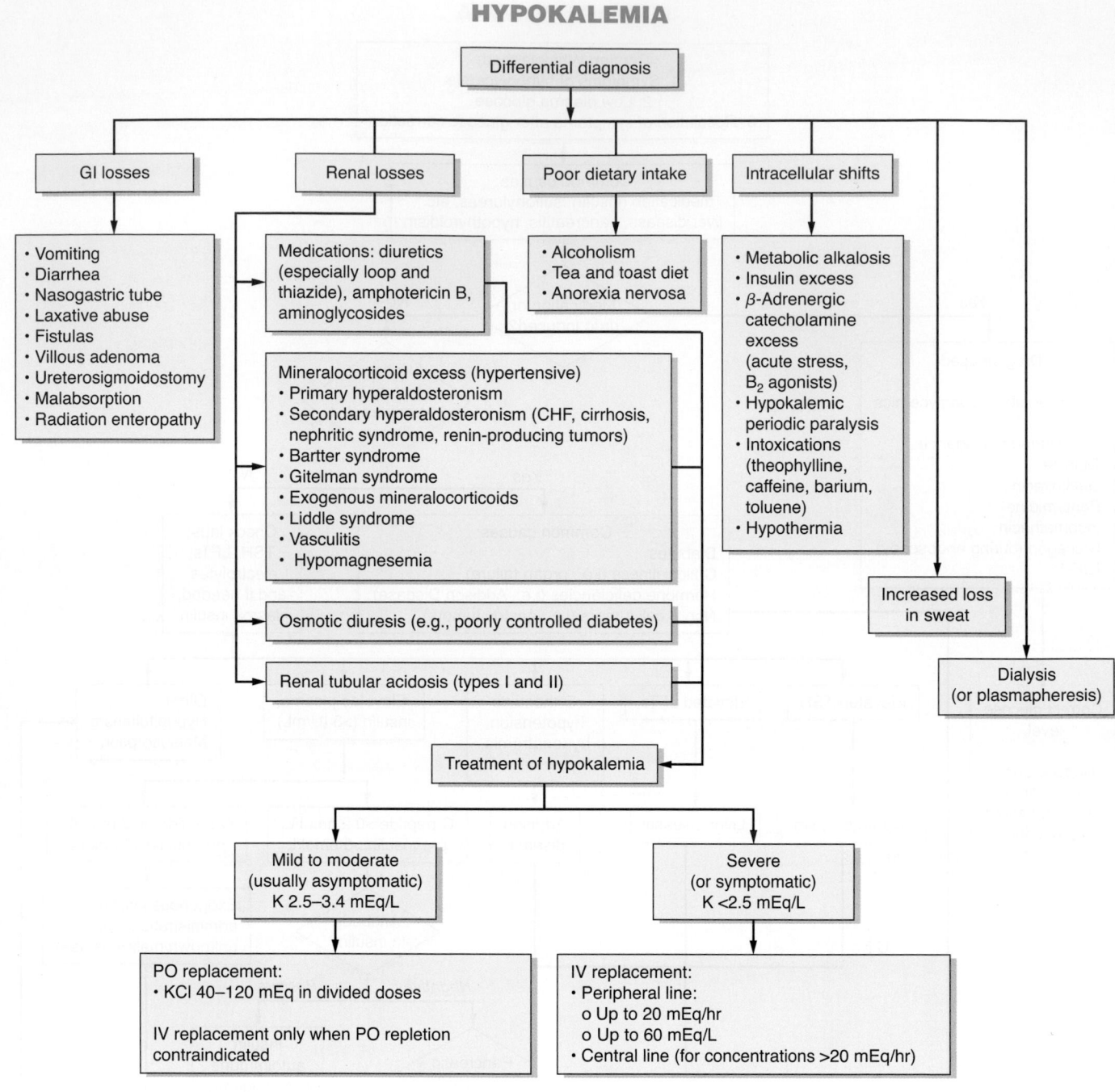

Abirami Raveendran, MD and Kimberly Bombaci, MD

Medford-Davis L, Rafique Z. Derangements of potassium. *Emerg Med Clin North Am.* 2014;32(2):329–347.

HYPONATREMIA

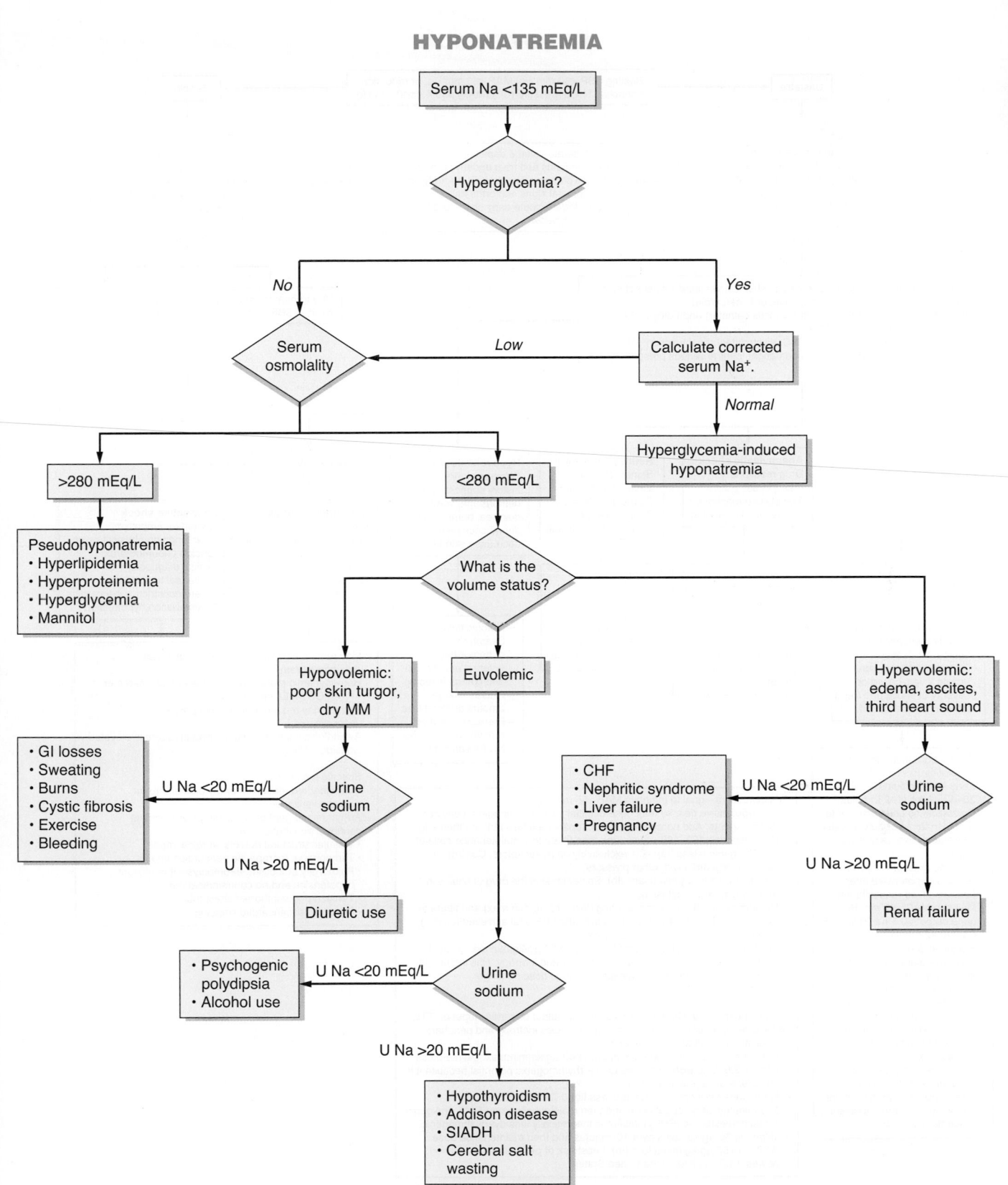

Aqib Chaudhry, MD and Frank J. Domino, MD

Lien YH, Shapiro JI. Hyponatremia: clinical diagnosis and management. *Am J Med.* 2007;120(8):653–658.

HYPOTENSION

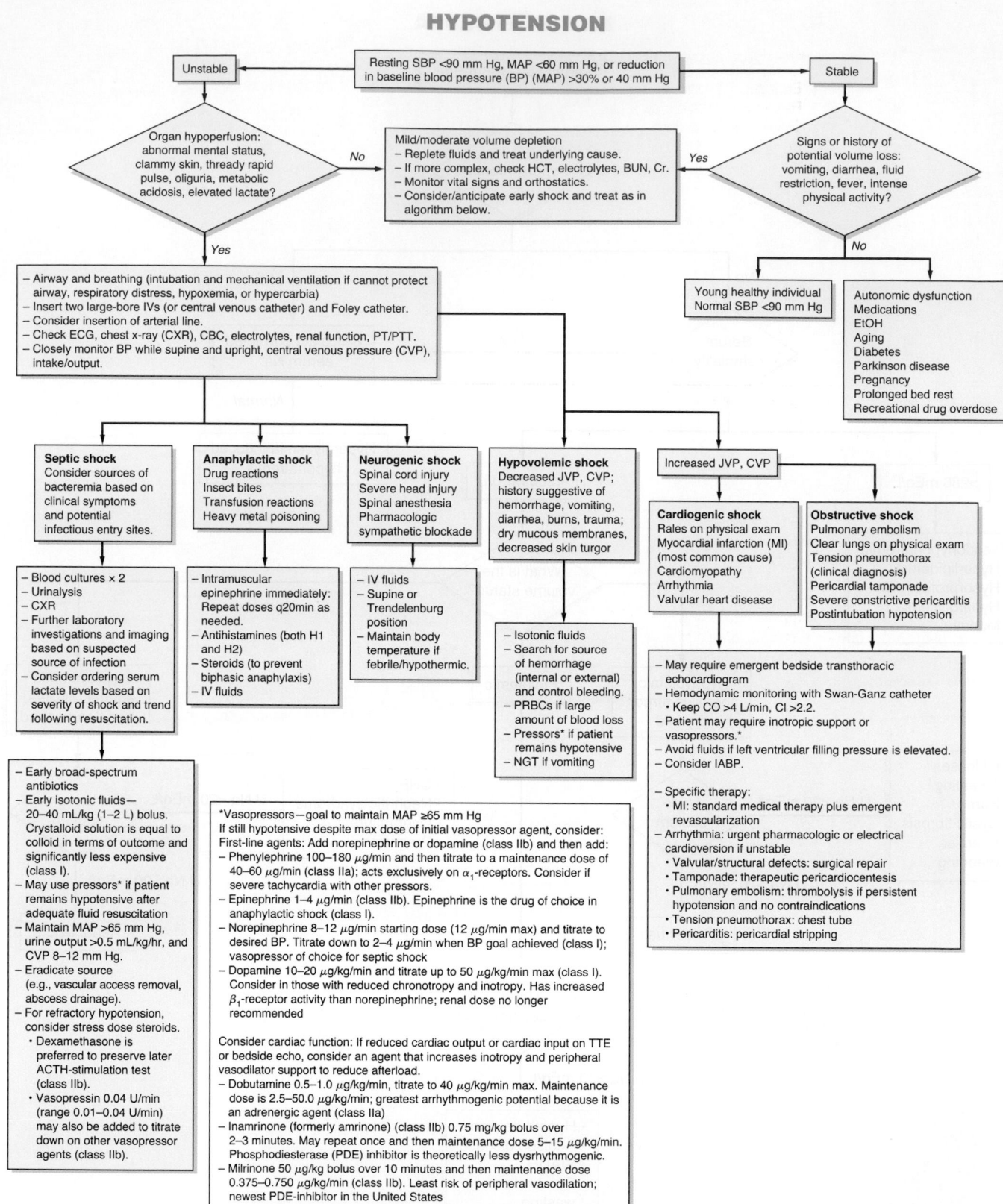

Amar Talati, DO and David O. Parrish, MS, MD, FAAFP

Mouncey PR, Osborn TM, Power GS, et al; for ProMISe Trial Investigators. Trial of early, goal-directed resuscitation for septic shock. *N Engl J Med.* 2015;372(14):1301–1311.

INFERTILITY

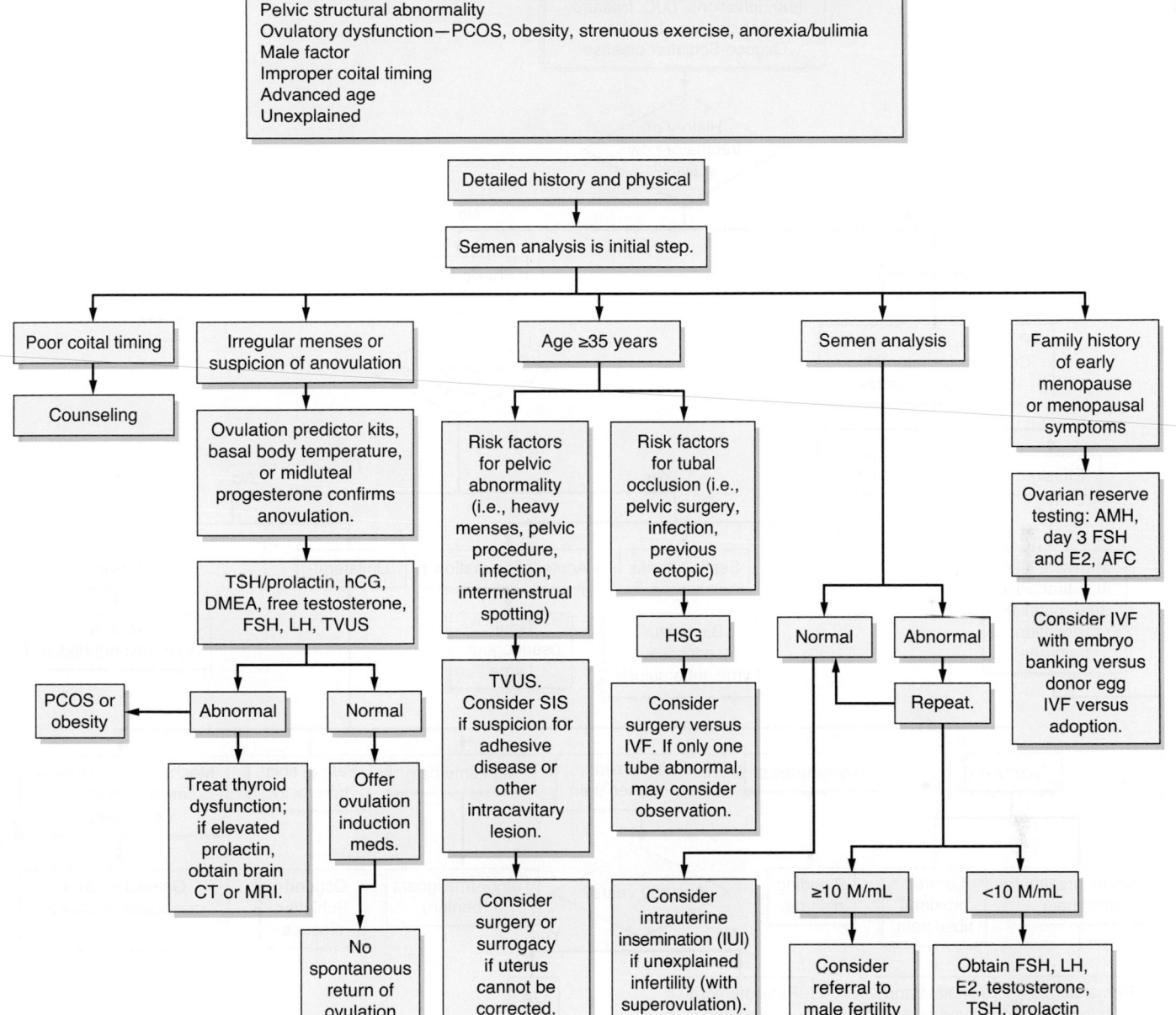

Common causes
Endocrine disorders—thyroid disease, polycystic ovarian syndrome (PCOS)
Pelvic structural abnormality
Ovulatory dysfunction—PCOS, obesity, strenuous exercise, anorexia/bulimia
Male factor
Improper coital timing
Advanced age
Unexplained

Detailed history and physical

Semen analysis is initial step.

Poor coital timing
Counseling

Irregular menses or suspicion of anovulation
Ovulation predictor kits, basal body temperature, or midluteal progesterone confirms anovulation.

TSH/prolactin, hCG, DMEA, free testosterone, FSH, LH, TVUS

PCOS or obesity ← Abnormal | Normal

Treat thyroid dysfunction; if elevated prolactin, obtain brain CT or MRI.

Offer ovulation induction meds.

No spontaneous return of ovulation

Age ≥35 years

Risk factors for pelvic abnormality (i.e., heavy menses, pelvic procedure, infection, intermenstrual spotting)

TVUS. Consider SIS if suspicion for adhesive disease or other intracavitary lesion.

Consider surgery or surrogacy if uterus cannot be corrected.

Risk factors for tubal occlusion (i.e., pelvic surgery, infection, previous ectopic)

HSG

Consider surgery versus IVF. If only one tube abnormal, may consider observation.

Consider intrauterine insemination (IUI) if unexplained infertility (with superovulation).

Semen analysis

Normal | Abnormal

Repeat.

≥10 M/mL

Consider referral to male fertility specialist versus IUI.

<10 M/mL

Obtain FSH, LH, E2, testosterone, TSH, prolactin karyotype, CF testing, Y chromosome microdeletion, and consider referral to male fertility specialist; can consider donor sperm versus IVF with ICS

Family history of early menopause or menopausal symptoms

Ovarian reserve testing: AMH, day 3 FSH and E2, AFC

Consider IVF with embryo banking versus donor egg IVF versus adoption.

TVUS = transvaginal ultrasound; HSG = hysterosalpingogram; SIS = saline-infused ultrasound

Frank J. Domino, MD

Practice Committee of the American Society for Reproductive Medicine. Diagnostic evaluation of the infertile female: a committee opinion. *Fertil Steril.* 2015;103(6):e44–e50.

KNEE PAIN

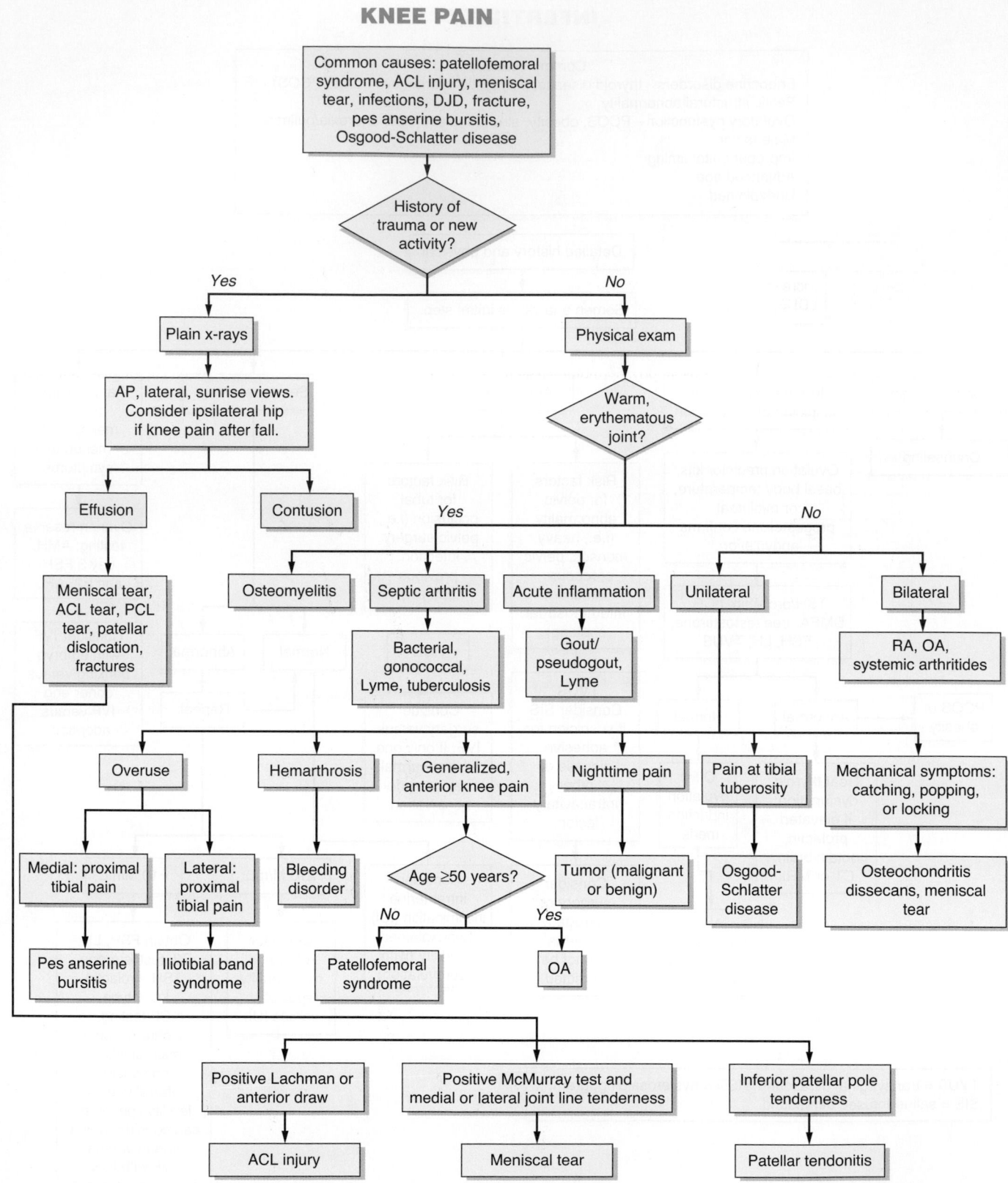

Alexei O. DeCastro, MD

Calmbach WL, Hutchens M. Evaluation of patients presenting with knee pain: part I. History, physical examination, radiographs, and laboratory tests. *Am Fam Physician.* 2003;68(5):907–912.

LACTATE DEHYDROGENASE ELEVATION

Common causes: MI, PE, CHF, hepatitis, muscular diseases, pancreatitis, anemia, hypothyroidism, malignancy

↓

Check LDH isoenzymes, types 1–5.

LDH1 > LDH2 → Acute MI

Increased LDH2, LDH3, and LDH4
- **LDH2 ≤18**
  - **LDH4 ≤29** → Pneumonia
  - **LDH4 >29** → Malignancy
- **LDH2 >18**
  - **Total LDH ≤95** → CHF
  - **Total LDH >95**
    - **LDH1 <24**
      - **LDH4 <22** → Malignancy
      - **LDH4 >22** → CHF
    - **LDH1 >24** → CHF

Increased LDH5 → Musculoskeletal disorder (i.e., dystrophy, dermatomyositis)

Increased LDH5 and anemia → Anemia of chronic disease

LDH4/LDH5 <1.05 → Hepatic disease

Other → Check amylase, haptoglobin, and TSH.
- **Elevated LDH4 and amylase** → Pancreatitis
- **Decreased haptoglobin** → Hemolysis
- **Increased TSH** → Hypothyroidism

Curtis L. Galke, DO

Lossos IS, Breuer R, Intrator O, et al. Differential diagnosis of pleural effusion by lactate dehydrogenase isoenzyme analysis. *Chest.* 1997;111(3):648–651.

LOW BACK PAIN, CHRONIC

Common causes: radiculitis, SI joint dysfunction, trauma, trochanteric bursitis, piriformis syndrome, osteoporosis, osteoarthritis, pars interarticularis fracture, ankylosing spondylitis, epidural abscess, malignancy, varicella zoster virus (postherpetic neuralgia), abdominal aortic aneurysm

↓

Pain >3 months

↓

Abnormal gait, bowel/bladder incontinence, acute urinary retention, bilateral sciatica, IV drug abuse, history of malignancy, pain worse when supine, saddle anesthesia, progressive neurologic symptoms, recent infection

Yes → Urgent imaging (CT or MRI) and neurosurgical referral

No ↓

Fever or concern of infection?

No →

Yes ↓

MRI or CT scan

Negative → Nonpharmacotherapy (left box)

Positive → Neurosurgical referral

Hx of trauma? *No* → No need for imaging

Yes ↓

Plain x-rays *Positive* → Neurosurgical referral

Negative →

Nonpharmacotherapy: structured exercise, multidisciplinary rehab, weight loss, acupuncture, spinal manipulation therapy, progressive relaxation, cognitive-behavioral therapy

Pharmacotherapy: NSAIDs, skeletal muscle relaxants (i.e., carisoprodol, tizanidine, cyclobenzaprine), antidepressants (i.e., duloxetine), anticonvulsants (i.e., topiramate), Botox, tramadol, other opioids

↓

No improvement: Consider surgical or psychiatry referral.

Nonpharmacotherapy: structured exercise, multidisciplinary rehab, weight loss, acupuncture, spinal manipulation therapy, progressive relaxation, cognitive-behavioral therapy

Pharmacotherapy: NSAIDs, skeletal muscle relaxants (i.e., carisoprodol, tizanidine, cyclobenzaprine), antidepressants (i.e., duloxetine), anticonvulsants (i.e., topiramate), Botox, tramadol, other opioids

Kiet T. La, MD and Holly L. Baab, MD

Herndon CM, Zoberi KS, Gardner BJ. Common questions about chronic low back pain. *Am Fam Physician*. 2015;91(10):708–714.

LYMPHADENOPATHY

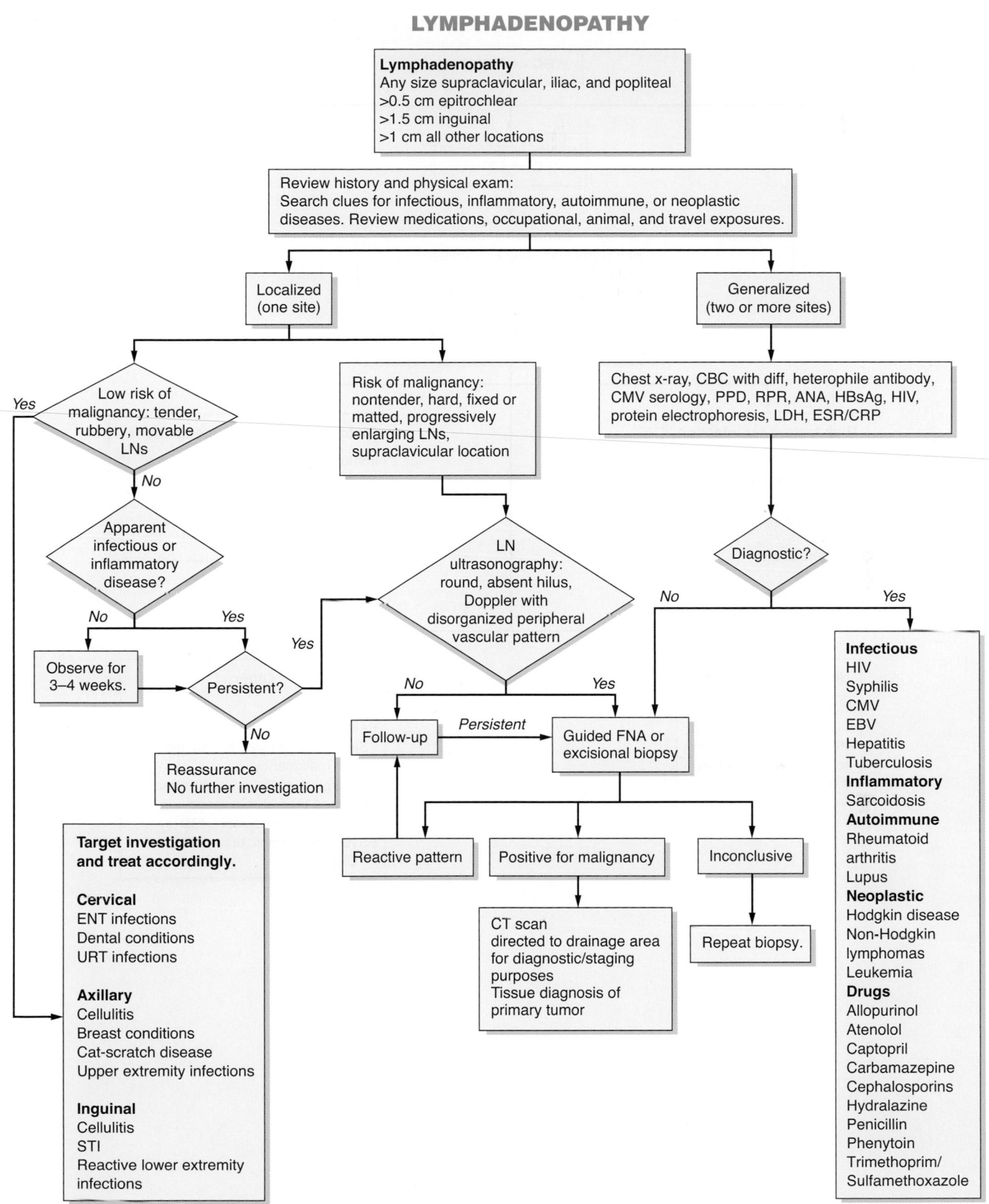

Lymphadenopathy
Any size supraclavicular, iliac, and popliteal
>0.5 cm epitrochlear
>1.5 cm inguinal
>1 cm all other locations

Review history and physical exam:
Search clues for infectious, inflammatory, autoimmune, or neoplastic diseases. Review medications, occupational, animal, and travel exposures.

Localized (one site)

Generalized (two or more sites)

Low risk of malignancy: tender, rubbery, movable LNs

Risk of malignancy: nontender, hard, fixed or matted, progressively enlarging LNs, supraclavicular location

Chest x-ray, CBC with diff, heterophile antibody, CMV serology, PPD, RPR, ANA, HBsAg, HIV, protein electrophoresis, LDH, ESR/CRP

Apparent infectious or inflammatory disease?

LN ultrasonography: round, absent hilus, Doppler with disorganized peripheral vascular pattern

Diagnostic?

No *Yes*

Observe for 3–4 weeks.

Persistent?

No

No *Yes*

Follow-up

Persistent

Guided FNA or excisional biopsy

Reassurance
No further investigation

Reactive pattern

Positive for malignancy

Inconclusive

CT scan
directed to drainage area for diagnostic/staging purposes
Tissue diagnosis of primary tumor

Repeat biopsy.

Target investigation and treat accordingly.

Cervical
ENT infections
Dental conditions
URT infections

Axillary
Cellulitis
Breast conditions
Cat-scratch disease
Upper extremity infections

Inguinal
Cellulitis
STI
Reactive lower extremity infections

Infectious
HIV
Syphilis
CMV
EBV
Hepatitis
Tuberculosis
Inflammatory
Sarcoidosis
Autoimmune
Rheumatoid arthritis
Lupus
Neoplastic
Hodgkin disease
Non-Hodgkin lymphomas
Leukemia
Drugs
Allopurinol
Atenolol
Captopril
Carbamazepine
Cephalosporins
Hydralazine
Penicillin
Phenytoin
Trimethoprim/Sulfamethoxazole

Pamela R. Hughes, MD and Jonathan S. Bassett, MD

Mohseni S, Shojaiefard A, Khorgami Z, et al. Peripheral lymphadenopathy: approach and diagnostic tools. *Iran J Med Sci.* 2014;39(Suppl 2):158–170.

LYMPHOPENIA OR LYMPHOCYTOPENIA

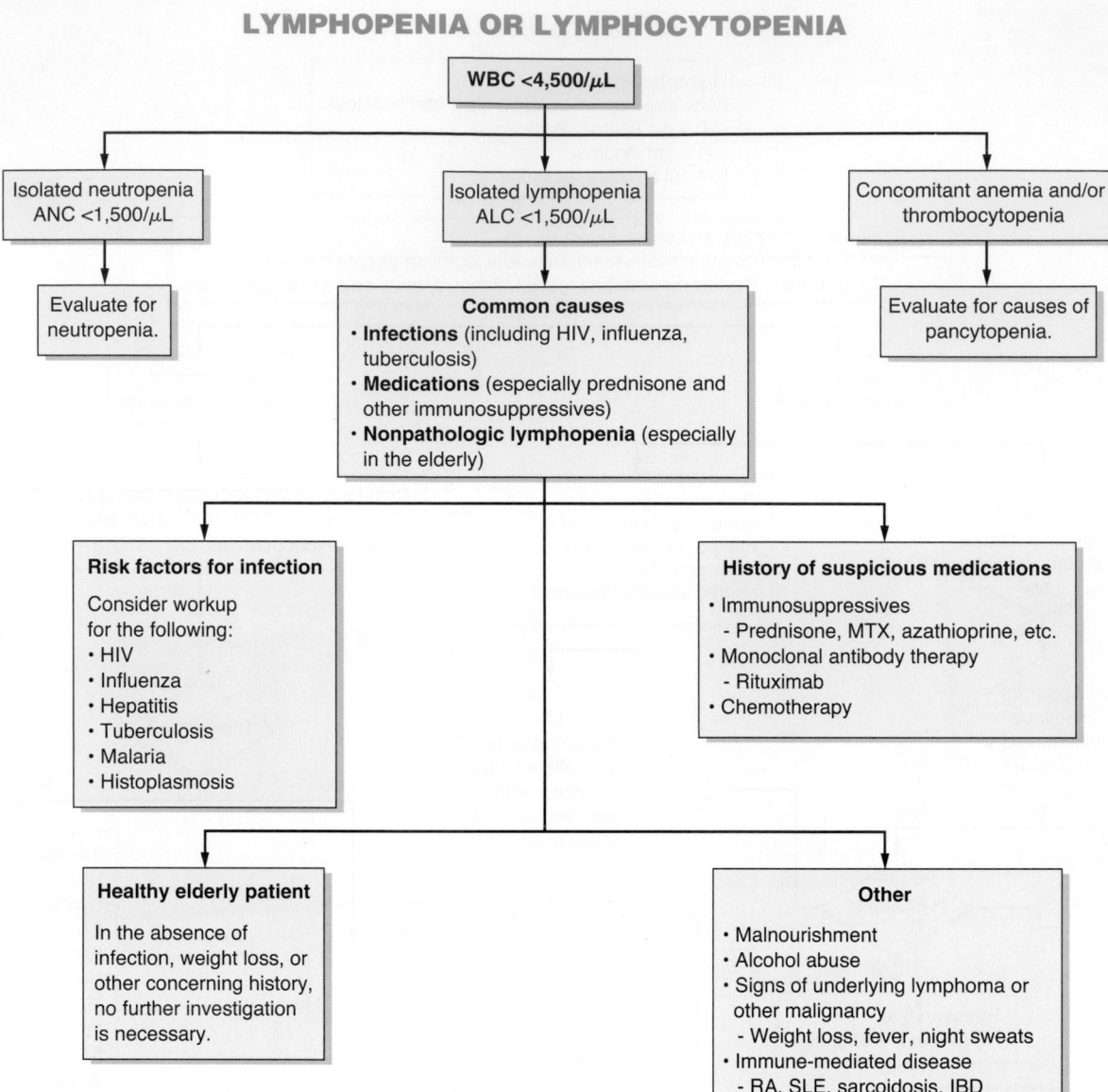

WBC <4,500/μL

Isolated neutropenia
ANC <1,500/μL

Evaluate for neutropenia.

Isolated lymphopenia
ALC <1,500/μL

Common causes
- **Infections** (including HIV, influenza, tuberculosis)
- **Medications** (especially prednisone and other immunosuppressives)
- **Nonpathologic lymphopenia** (especially in the elderly)

Concomitant anemia and/or thrombocytopenia

Evaluate for causes of pancytopenia.

Risk factors for infection

Consider workup for the following:
- HIV
- Influenza
- Hepatitis
- Tuberculosis
- Malaria
- Histoplasmosis

History of suspicious medications
- Immunosuppressives
  - Prednisone, MTX, azathioprine, etc.
- Monoclonal antibody therapy
  - Rituximab
- Chemotherapy

Healthy elderly patient

In the absence of infection, weight loss, or other concerning history, no further investigation is necessary.

Other
- Malnourishment
- Alcohol abuse
- Signs of underlying lymphoma or other malignancy
  - Weight loss, fever, night sweats
- Immune-mediated disease
  - RA, SLE, sarcoidosis, IBD
- Systemic, chronic disorders
  - CKD, CHF

Andrew Smith, MD and Erin Bassett-Novoa, MD

Brass D, McKay P, Scott F. Investigating an incidental finding of lymphopenia. *BMJ.* 2014;348:g1721.

MENOPAUSE, EVALUATION AND MANAGEMENT PART I

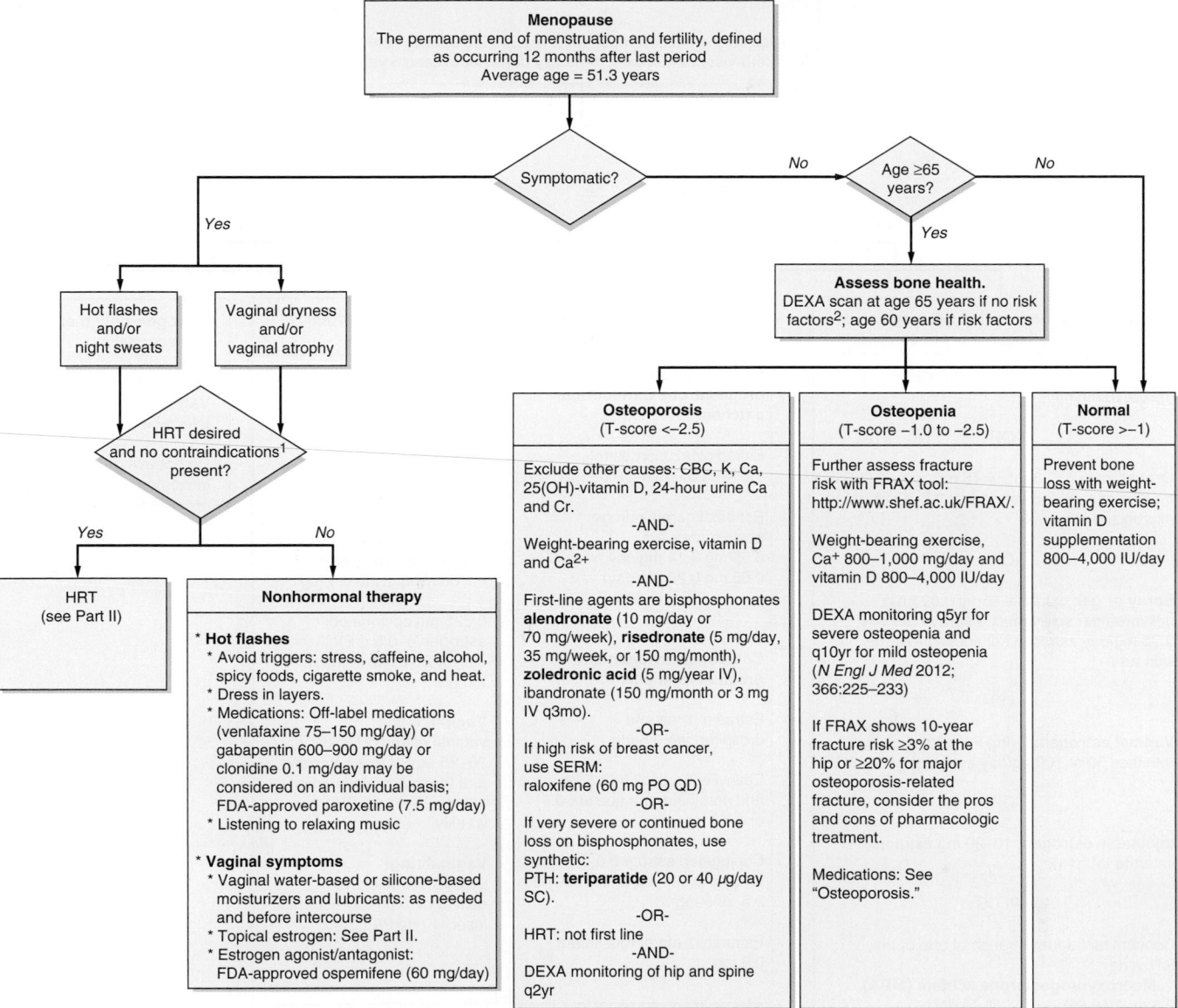

Menopause
The permanent end of menstruation and fertility, defined as occurring 12 months after last period
Average age = 51.3 years

Symptomatic?

Yes

Hot flashes and/or night sweats

Vaginal dryness and/or vaginal atrophy

HRT desired and no contraindications[1] present?

Yes | *No*

HRT (see Part II)

Nonhormonal therapy

* **Hot flashes**
  * Avoid triggers: stress, caffeine, alcohol, spicy foods, cigarette smoke, and heat.
  * Dress in layers.
  * Medications: Off-label medications (venlafaxine 75–150 mg/day) or gabapentin 600–900 mg/day or clonidine 0.1 mg/day may be considered on an individual basis; FDA-approved paroxetine (7.5 mg/day)
  * Listening to relaxing music

* **Vaginal symptoms**
  * Vaginal water-based or silicone-based moisturizers and lubricants: as needed and before intercourse
  * Topical estrogen: See Part II.
  * Estrogen agonist/antagonist: FDA-approved ospemifene (60 mg/day)

No → Age ≥65 years? → *No*

Yes

Assess bone health.
DEXA scan at age 65 years if no risk factors[2]; age 60 years if risk factors

Osteoporosis
(T-score <–2.5)

Exclude other causes: CBC, K, Ca, 25(OH)-vitamin D, 24-hour urine Ca and Cr.
-AND-
Weight-bearing exercise, vitamin D and Ca^{2+}
-AND-
First-line agents are bisphosphonates **alendronate** (10 mg/day or 70 mg/week), **risedronate** (5 mg/day, 35 mg/week, or 150 mg/month), **zoledronic acid** (5 mg/year IV), ibandronate (150 mg/month or 3 mg IV q3mo).
-OR-
If high risk of breast cancer, use SERM: raloxifene (60 mg PO QD)
-OR-
If very severe or continued bone loss on bisphosphonates, use synthetic: PTH: **teriparatide** (20 or 40 µg/day SC).
-OR-
HRT: not first line
-AND-
DEXA monitoring of hip and spine q2yr

Osteopenia
(T-score –1.0 to –2.5)

Further assess fracture risk with FRAX tool: http://www.shef.ac.uk/FRAX/.

Weight-bearing exercise, Ca^+ 800–1,000 mg/day and vitamin D 800–4,000 IU/day

DEXA monitoring q5yr for severe osteopenia and q10yr for mild osteopenia (*N Engl J Med* 2012; 366:225–233)

If FRAX shows 10-year fracture risk ≥3% at the hip or ≥20% for major osteoporosis-related fracture, consider the pros and cons of pharmacologic treatment.

Medications: See "Osteoporosis."

Normal
(T-score >–1)

Prevent bone loss with weight-bearing exercise; vitamin D supplementation 800–4,000 IU/day

PART II

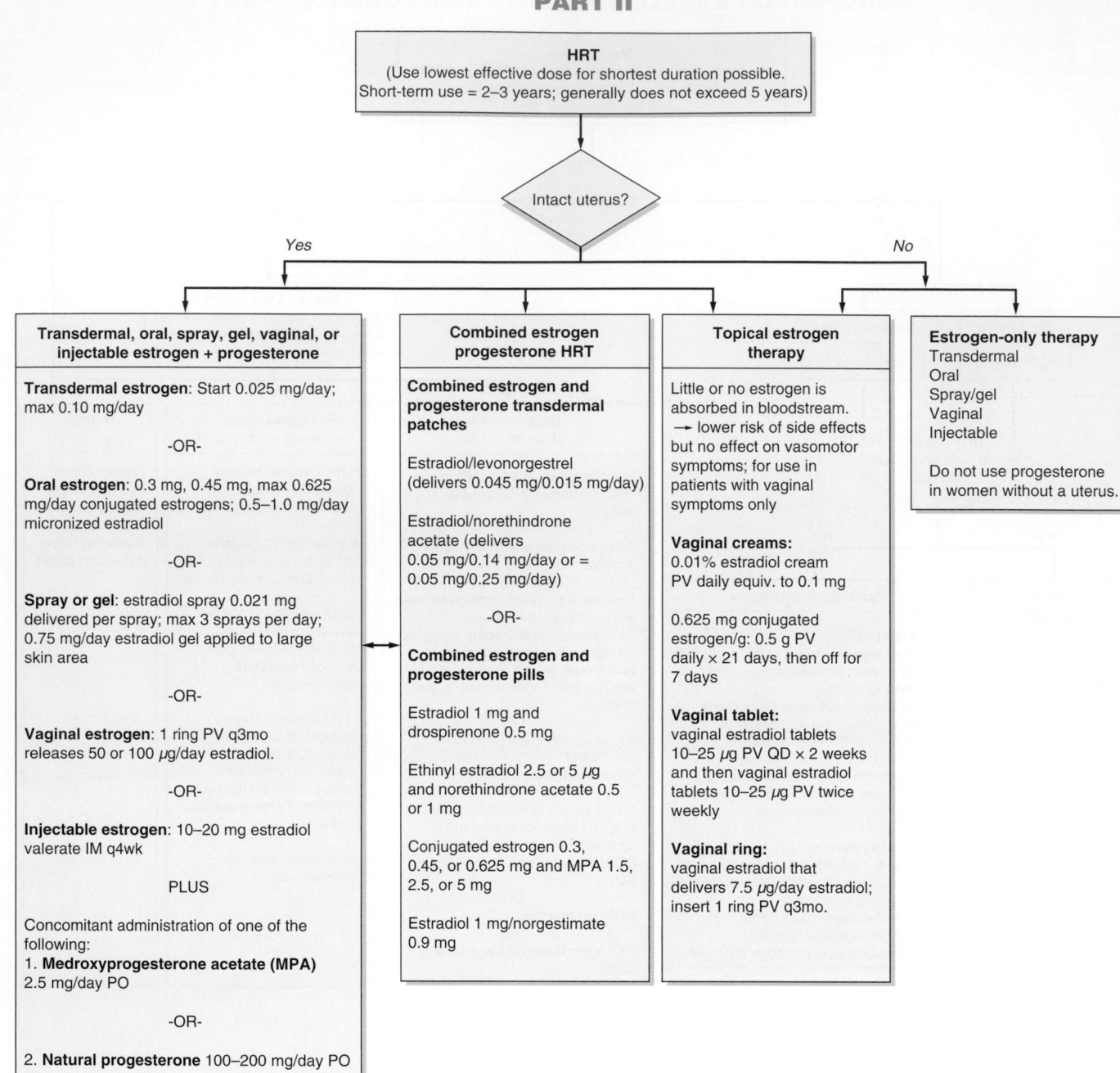

HRT
(Use lowest effective dose for shortest duration possible.
Short-term use = 2–3 years; generally does not exceed 5 years)

Intact uterus?

Yes   *No*

Transdermal, oral, spray, gel, vaginal, or injectable estrogen + progesterone

Transdermal estrogen: Start 0.025 mg/day; max 0.10 mg/day

-OR-

Oral estrogen: 0.3 mg, 0.45 mg, max 0.625 mg/day conjugated estrogens; 0.5–1.0 mg/day micronized estradiol

-OR-

Spray or gel: estradiol spray 0.021 mg delivered per spray; max 3 sprays per day; 0.75 mg/day estradiol gel applied to large skin area

-OR-

Vaginal estrogen: 1 ring PV q3mo releases 50 or 100 µg/day estradiol.

-OR-

Injectable estrogen: 10–20 mg estradiol valerate IM q4wk

PLUS

Concomitant administration of one of the following:
1. **Medroxyprogesterone acetate (MPA)** 2.5 mg/day PO

-OR-

2. **Natural progesterone** 100–200 mg/day PO

Combined estrogen progesterone HRT

Combined estrogen and progesterone transdermal patches

Estradiol/levonorgestrel (delivers 0.045 mg/0.015 mg/day)

Estradiol/norethindrone acetate (delivers 0.05 mg/0.14 mg/day or = 0.05 mg/0.25 mg/day)

-OR-

Combined estrogen and progesterone pills

Estradiol 1 mg and drospirenone 0.5 mg

Ethinyl estradiol 2.5 or 5 µg and norethindrone acetate 0.5 or 1 mg

Conjugated estrogen 0.3, 0.45, or 0.625 mg and MPA 1.5, 2.5, or 5 mg

Estradiol 1 mg/norgestimate 0.9 mg

Topical estrogen therapy

Little or no estrogen is absorbed in bloodstream.
→ lower risk of side effects but no effect on vasomotor symptoms; for use in patients with vaginal symptoms only

Vaginal creams:
0.01% estradiol cream PV daily equiv. to 0.1 mg

0.625 mg conjugated estrogen/g: 0.5 g PV daily × 21 days, then off for 7 days

Vaginal tablet:
vaginal estradiol tablets 10–25 µg PV QD × 2 weeks and then vaginal estradiol tablets 10–25 µg PV twice weekly

Vaginal ring:
vaginal estradiol that delivers 7.5 µg/day estradiol; insert 1 ring PV q3mo.

Estrogen-only therapy
Transdermal
Oral
Spray/gel
Vaginal
Injectable

Do not use progesterone in women without a uterus.

Kelly Pagidas, MD

ACOG Practice Bulletin No. 141: management of menopausal symptoms. *Obstet Gynecol.* 2014;123(1):202–216.

MIGRAINE, TREATMENT

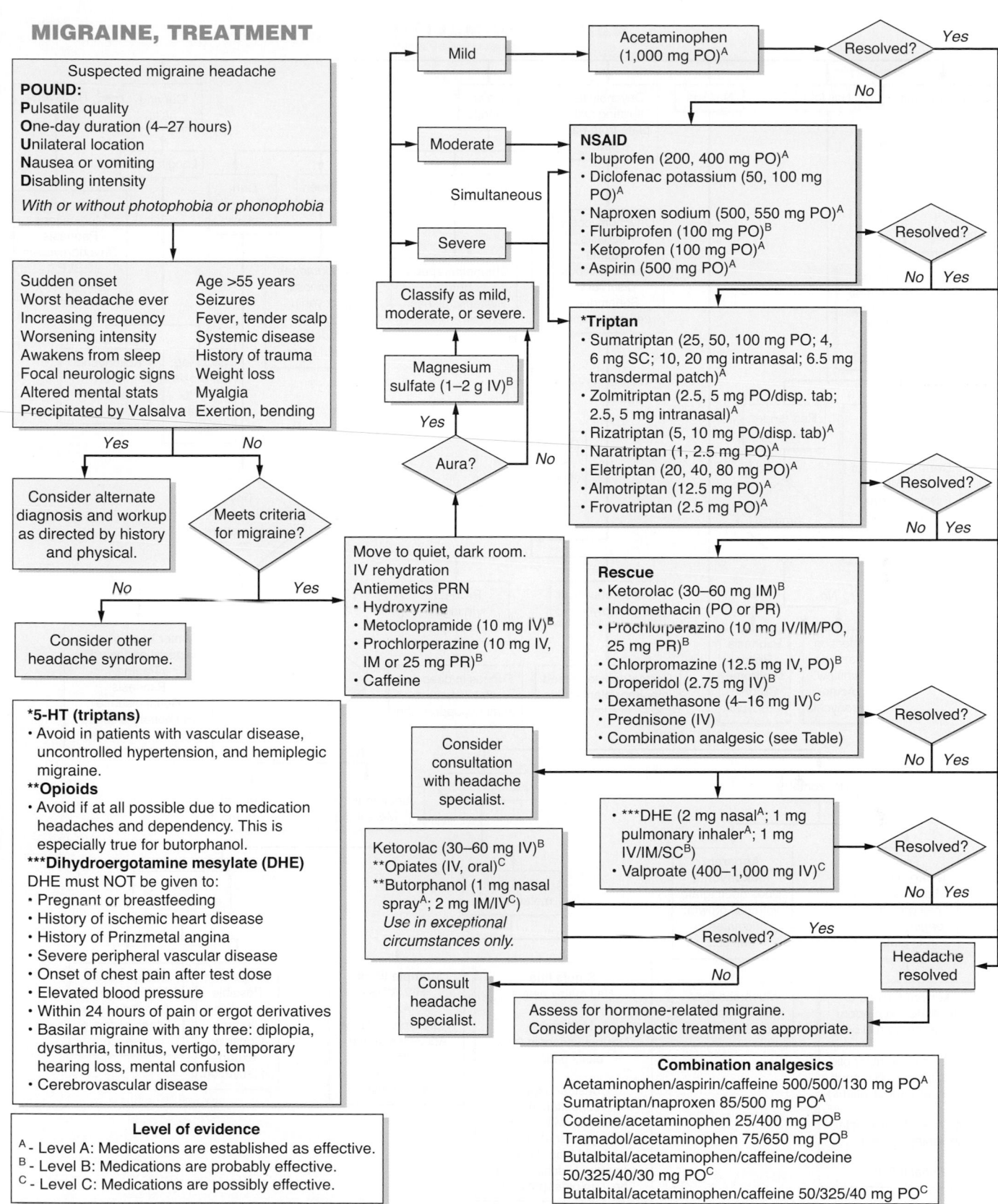

Suspected migraine headache

POUND:
Pulsatile quality
One-day duration (4–27 hours)
Unilateral location
Nausea or vomiting
Disabling intensity

With or without photophobia or phonophobia

Sudden onset · Age >55 years
Worst headache ever · Seizures
Increasing frequency · Fever, tender scalp
Worsening intensity · Systemic disease
Awakens from sleep · History of trauma
Focal neurologic signs · Weight loss
Altered mental stats · Myalgia
Precipitated by Valsalva · Exertion, bending

Yes / No

Consider alternate diagnosis and workup as directed by history and physical.

Meets criteria for migraine?

No / Yes

Consider other headache syndrome.

Mild → Acetaminophen (1,000 mg PO)[A] → Resolved? Yes / No

Moderate

Simultaneous

Severe

Classify as mild, moderate, or severe.

Magnesium sulfate (1–2 g IV)[B]

Aura? Yes / No

Move to quiet, dark room.
IV rehydration
Antiemetics PRN
· Hydroxyzine
· Metoclopramide (10 mg IV)[B]
· Prochlorperazine (10 mg IV, IM or 25 mg PR)[B]
· Caffeine

NSAID
· Ibuprofen (200, 400 mg PO)[A]
· Diclofenac potassium (50, 100 mg PO)[A]
· Naproxen sodium (500, 550 mg PO)[A]
· Flurbiprofen (100 mg PO)[B]
· Ketoprofen (100 mg PO)[A]
· Aspirin (500 mg PO)[A]

Resolved? No / Yes

***Triptan**
· Sumatriptan (25, 50, 100 mg PO; 4, 6 mg SC; 10, 20 mg intranasal; 6.5 mg transdermal patch)[A]
· Zolmitriptan (2.5, 5 mg PO/disp. tab; 2.5, 5 mg intranasal)[A]
· Rizatriptan (5, 10 mg PO/disp. tab)[A]
· Naratriptan (1, 2.5 mg PO)[A]
· Eletriptan (20, 40, 80 mg PO)[A]
· Almotriptan (12.5 mg PO)[A]
· Frovatriptan (2.5 mg PO)[A]

Resolved? No / Yes

Rescue
· Ketorolac (30–60 mg IM)[B]
· Indomethacin (PO or PR)
· Prochlorperazine (10 mg IV/IM/PO, 25 mg PR)[B]
· Chlorpromazine (12.5 mg IV, PO)[B]
· Droperidol (2.75 mg IV)[B]
· Dexamethasone (4–16 mg IV)[C]
· Prednisone (IV)
· Combination analgesic (see Table)

Resolved? No / Yes

Consider consultation with headache specialist.

Ketorolac (30–60 mg IV)[B]
**Opiates (IV, oral)[C]
**Butorphanol (1 mg nasal spray[A]; 2 mg IM/IV[C])
Use in exceptional circumstances only.

· ***DHE (2 mg nasal[A]; 1 mg pulmonary inhaler[A]; 1 mg IV/IM/SC[B])
· Valproate (400–1,000 mg IV)[C]

Resolved? No / Yes

Resolved? Yes / No

Headache resolved

Consult headache specialist.

Assess for hormone-related migraine. Consider prophylactic treatment as appropriate.

***5-HT (triptans)**
· Avoid in patients with vascular disease, uncontrolled hypertension, and hemiplegic migraine.

****Opioids**
· Avoid if at all possible due to medication headaches and dependency. This is especially true for butorphanol.

*****Dihydroergotamine mesylate (DHE)**
DHE must NOT be given to:
· Pregnant or breastfeeding
· History of ischemic heart disease
· History of Prinzmetal angina
· Severe peripheral vascular disease
· Onset of chest pain after test dose
· Elevated blood pressure
· Within 24 hours of pain or ergot derivatives
· Basilar migraine with any three: diplopia, dysarthria, tinnitus, vertigo, temporary hearing loss, mental confusion
· Cerebrovascular disease

Level of evidence
[A] - Level A: Medications are established as effective.
[B] - Level B: Medications are probably effective.
[C] - Level C: Medications are possibly effective.

Combination analgesics
Acetaminophen/aspirin/caffeine 500/500/130 mg PO[A]
Sumatriptan/naproxen 85/500 mg PO[A]
Codeine/acetaminophen 25/400 mg PO[B]
Tramadol/acetaminophen 75/650 mg PO[B]
Butalbital/acetaminophen/caffeine/codeine 50/325/40/30 mg PO[C]
Butalbital/acetaminophen/caffeine 50/325/40 mg PO[C]

Matthew A. Henry, DO, Sarah C. McCullough, DO, and Sabrina L. Silver, DO, CAQSM

Marmura MJ, Silberstein SD, Schwedt TJ. The acute treatment of migraine in adults: the American Headache Society evidence assessment of migraine pharmacotherapies. *Headache.* 2015;55(1):3–20.

NAIL ABNORMALITIES

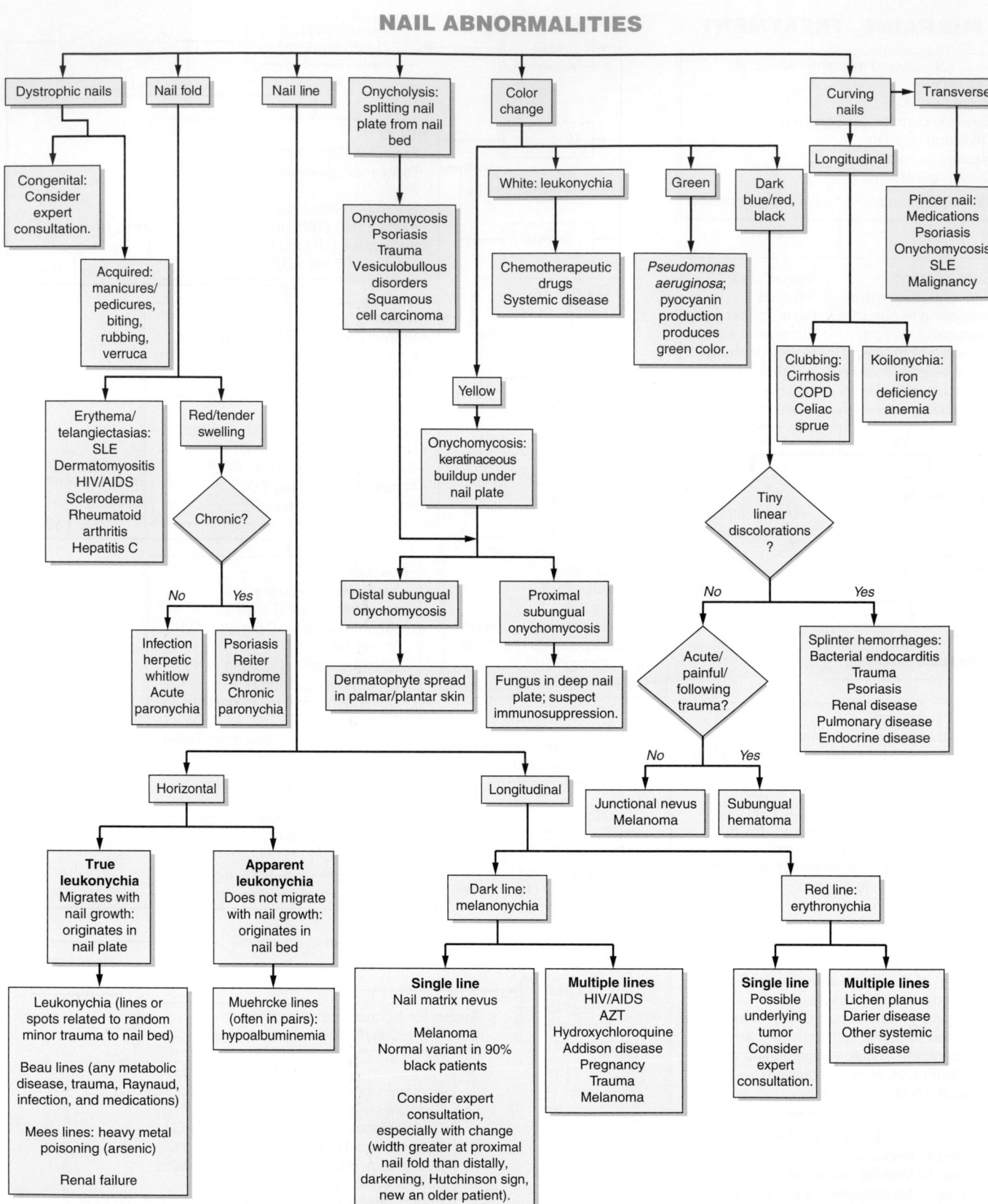

Natasha J. Pyzocha, DO, FAWM, FAAFP, Douglas M. Maurer, DO, MPH, FAAFP, and Amanda Roberts, MD

Tully AS, Trayes KP, Studdiford JS. Evaluation of nail abnormalities. *Am Fam Physician.* 2012;85(8):779–787.

NEUTROPENIA

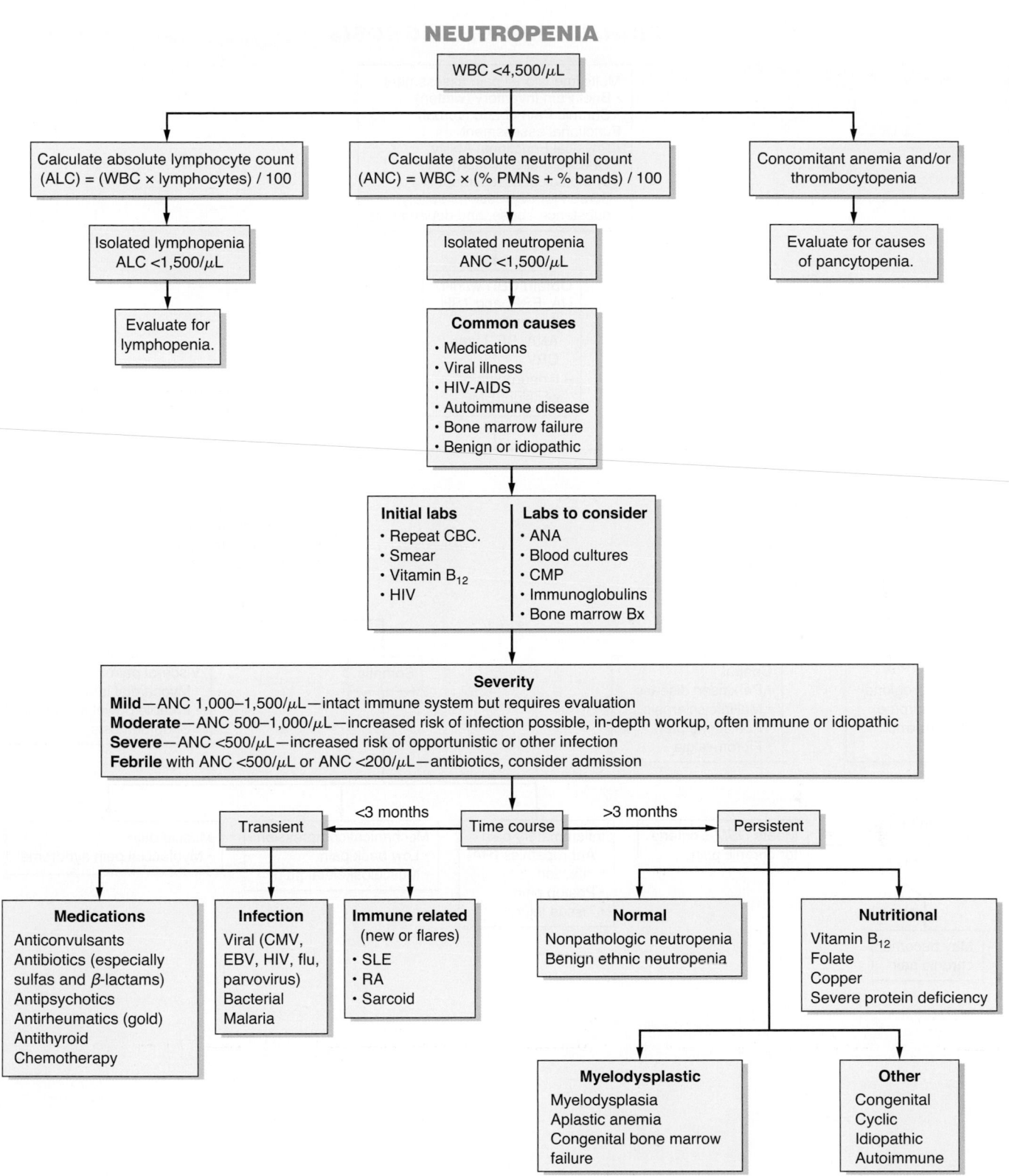

WBC <4,500/μL

Calculate absolute lymphocyte count (ALC) = (WBC × lymphocytes) / 100

Calculate absolute neutrophil count (ANC) = WBC × (% PMNs + % bands) / 100

Concomitant anemia and/or thrombocytopenia

Isolated lymphopenia ALC <1,500/μL

Isolated neutropenia ANC <1,500/μL

Evaluate for causes of pancytopenia.

Evaluate for lymphopenia.

Common causes
- Medications
- Viral illness
- HIV-AIDS
- Autoimmune disease
- Bone marrow failure
- Benign or idiopathic

Initial labs
- Repeat CBC.
- Smear
- Vitamin B$_{12}$
- HIV

Labs to consider
- ANA
- Blood cultures
- CMP
- Immunoglobulins
- Bone marrow Bx

Severity
Mild—ANC 1,000–1,500/μL—intact immune system but requires evaluation
Moderate—ANC 500–1,000/μL—increased risk of infection possible, in-depth workup, often immune or idiopathic
Severe—ANC <500/μL—increased risk of opportunistic or other infection
Febrile with ANC <500/μL or ANC <200/μL—antibiotics, consider admission

Transient ←<3 months— Time course —>3 months→ Persistent

Medications
Anticonvulsants
Antibiotics (especially sulfas and β-lactams)
Antipsychotics
Antirheumatics (gold)
Antithyroid
Chemotherapy

Infection
Viral (CMV, EBV, HIV, flu, parvovirus)
Bacterial
Malaria

Immune related
(new or flares)
- SLE
- RA
- Sarcoid

Normal
Nonpathologic neutropenia
Benign ethnic neutropenia

Nutritional
Vitamin B$_{12}$
Folate
Copper
Severe protein deficiency

Myelodysplastic
Myelodysplasia
Aplastic anemia
Congenital bone marrow failure

Other
Congenital
Cyclic
Idiopathic
Autoimmune

Andrew Smith, MD and Erin Bassett-Novoa, MD

Newburger PE, Dale DC. Evaluation and management of patients with isolated neutropenia. *Semin Hematol.* 2013;50(3):198–206.

PAIN, CHRONIC, DIAGNOSIS

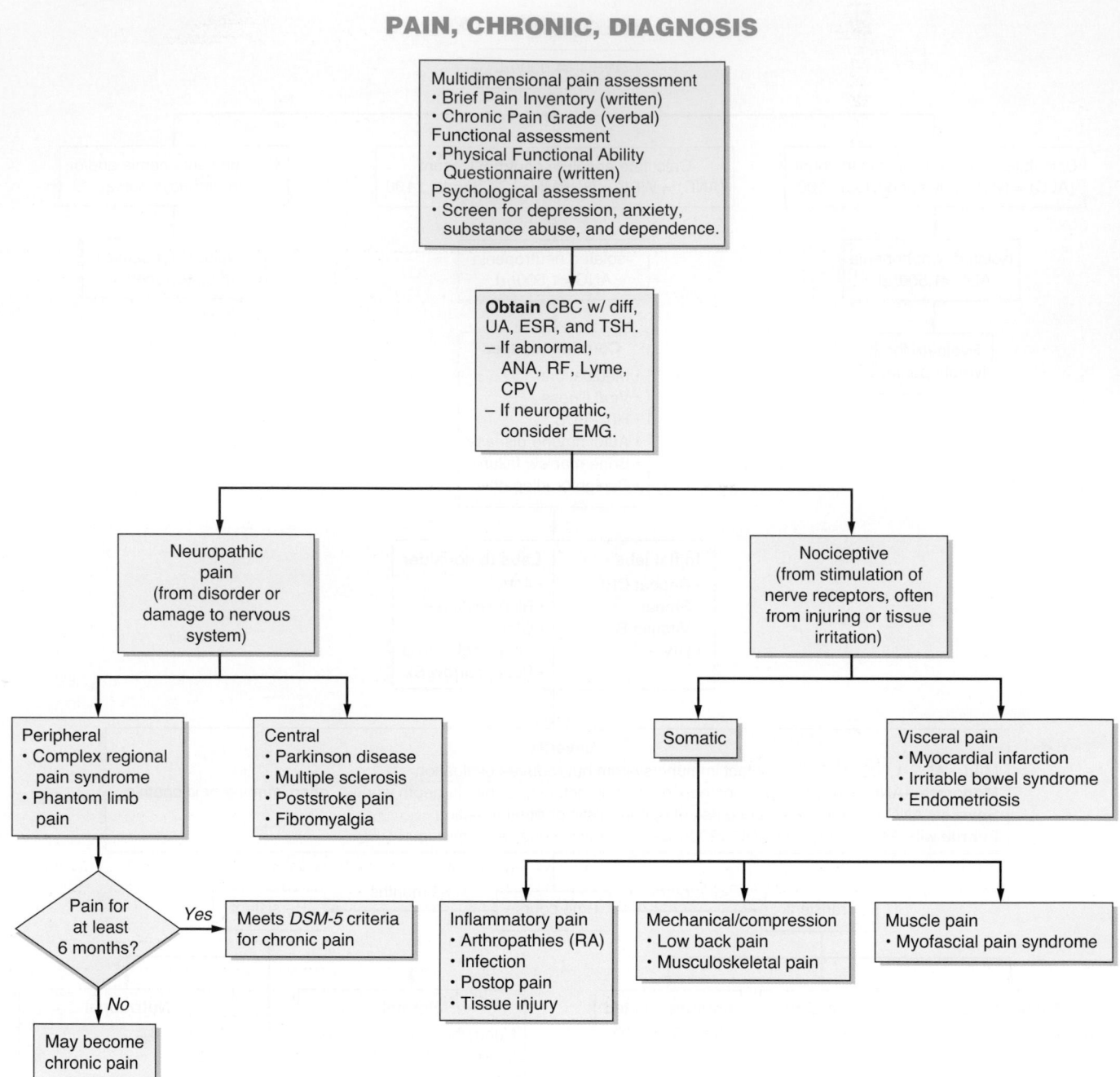

Ashik Lawrence, MD, Anubhav Kaul, MD, and Margaret Seaver, MD, MPH

Institute for Clinical Systems Improvement. *Health Care Guideline: Assessment and Management of Chronic Pain*. 5th ed. Bloomington, MN: Institute for Clinical Systems Improvement; 2011.

PALPABLE BREAST MASS

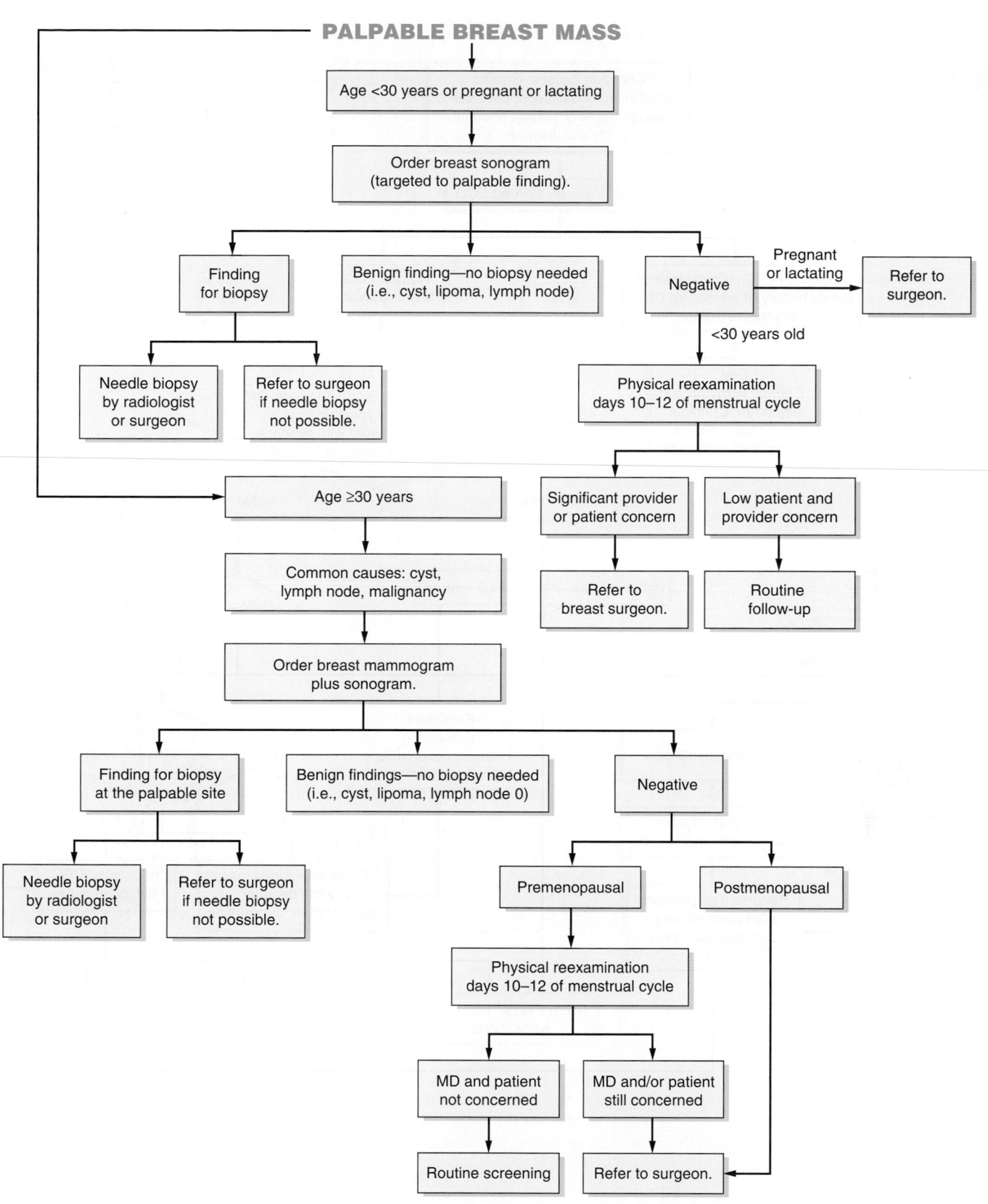

Lindsay Petersen, MD and Andrea Madrigrano, MD

Salzman B, Fleegle S, Tully AS. Common breast problems. *Am Fam Physician.* 2012;86(4):343–349.

PALPITATIONS

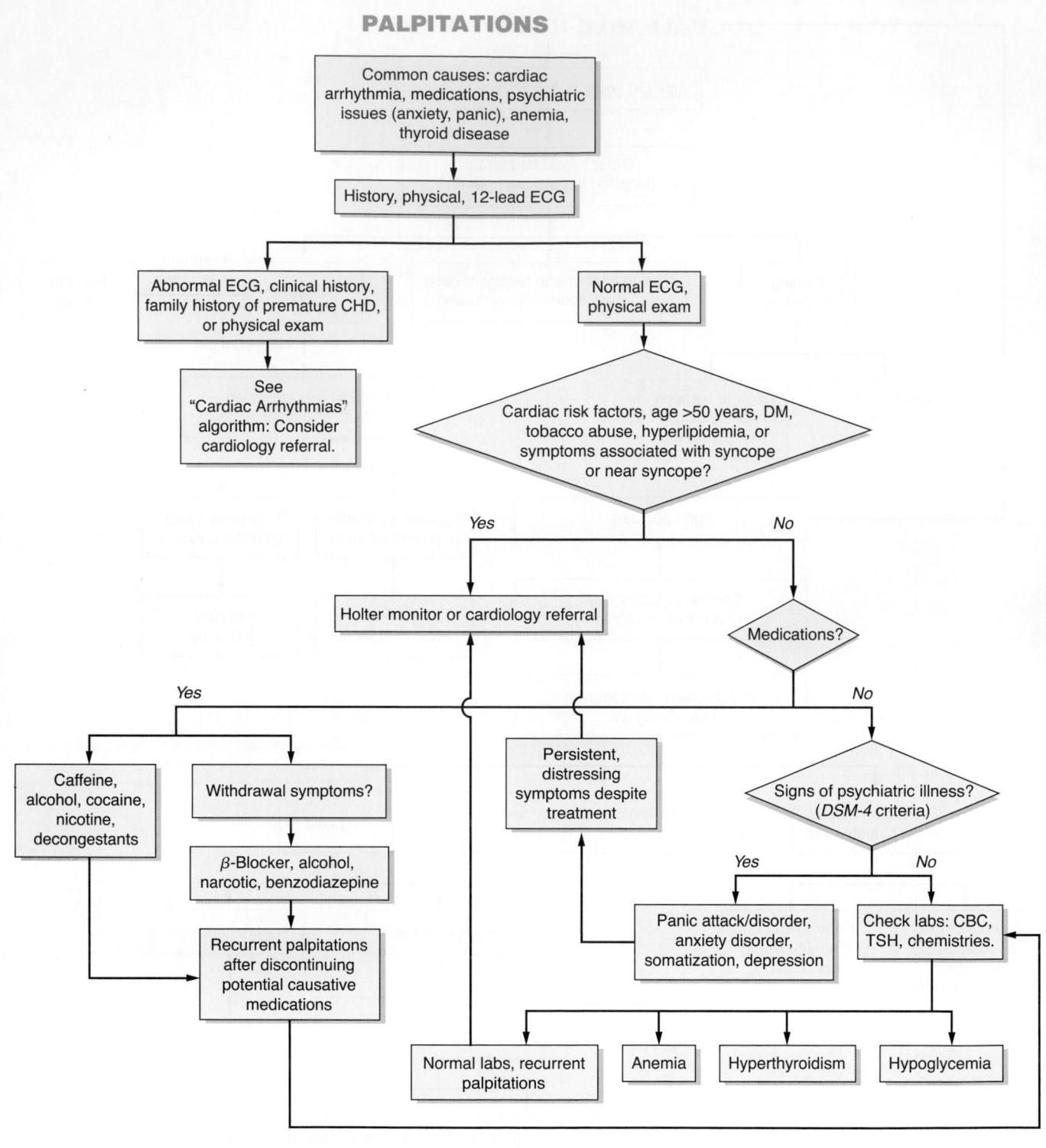

Common causes: cardiac arrhythmia, medications, psychiatric issues (anxiety, panic), anemia, thyroid disease

History, physical, 12-lead ECG

Abnormal ECG, clinical history, family history of premature CHD, or physical exam

Normal ECG, physical exam

See "Cardiac Arrhythmias" algorithm: Consider cardiology referral.

Cardiac risk factors, age >50 years, DM, tobacco abuse, hyperlipidemia, or symptoms associated with syncope or near syncope?

Yes

No

Holter monitor or cardiology referral

Medications?

Yes

No

Caffeine, alcohol, cocaine, nicotine, decongestants

Withdrawal symptoms?

Persistent, distressing symptoms despite treatment

Signs of psychiatric illness? (*DSM-4* criteria)

Yes

No

β-Blocker, alcohol, narcotic, benzodiazepine

Recurrent palpitations after discontinuing potential causative medications

Panic attack/disorder, anxiety disorder, somatization, depression

Check labs: CBC, TSH, chemistries.

Normal labs, recurrent palpitations

Anemia

Hyperthyroidism

Hypoglycemia

Frank J. Domino, MD

Wexler RK, Pleister A, Raman S. Outpatient approach to palpitations. *Am Fam Physician.* 2011;84(1):63–69.

PAP, NORMAL AND ABNORMAL IN NONPREGNANT WOMEN AGES 25 YEARS AND OLDER

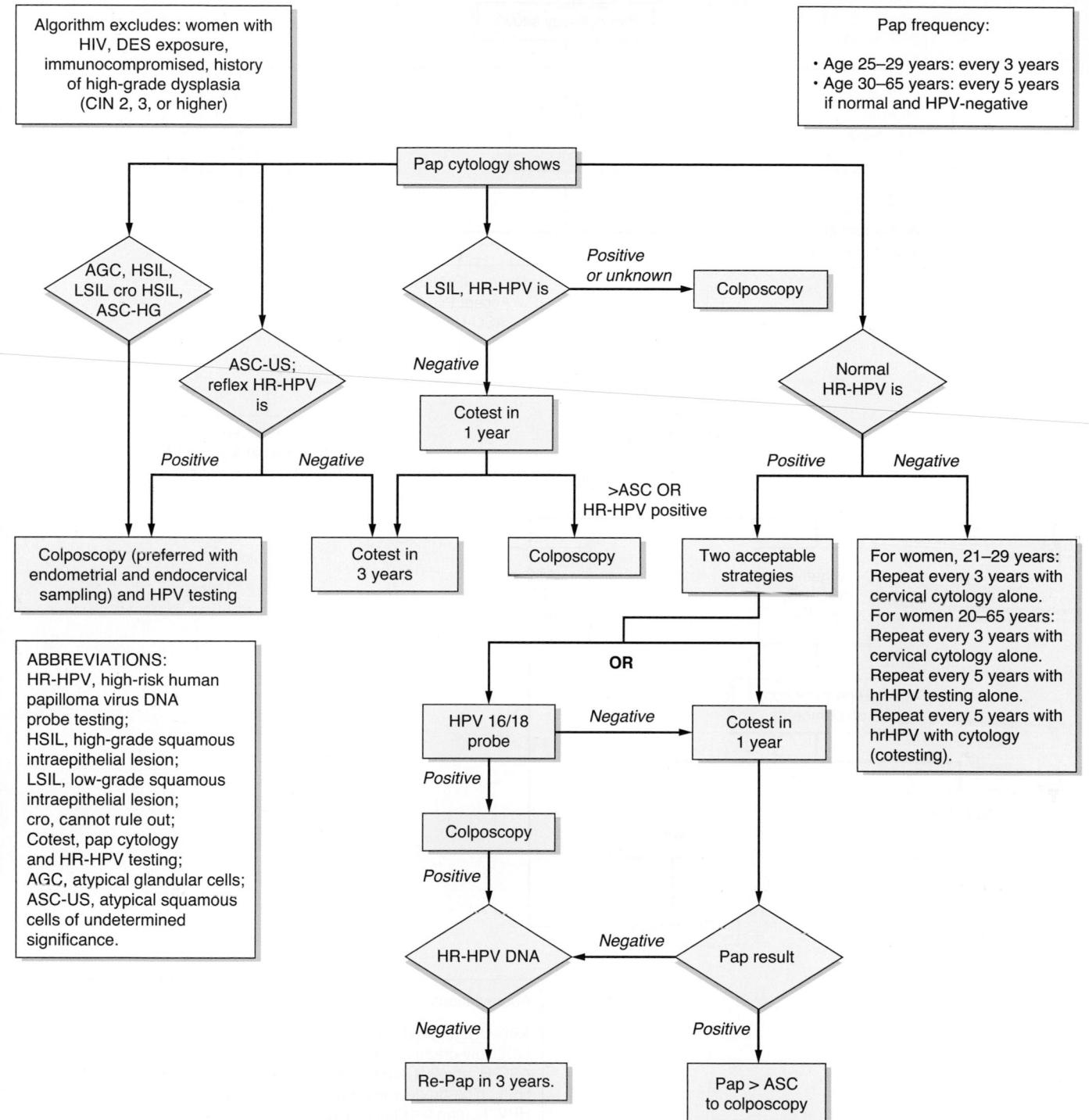

Algorithm excludes: women with HIV, DES exposure, immunocompromised, history of high-grade dysplasia (CIN 2, 3, or higher)

Pap frequency:
- Age 25–29 years: every 3 years
- Age 30–65 years: every 5 years if normal and HPV-negative

Pap cytology shows

AGC, HSIL, LSIL cro HSIL, ASC-HG

LSIL, HR-HPV is
→ Positive or unknown → Colposcopy

ASC-US; reflex HR-HPV is

Negative

Normal HR-HPV is

Positive — Negative

Cotest in 1 year

Colposcopy (preferred with endometrial and endocervical sampling) and HPV testing

Cotest in 3 years

>ASC OR HR-HPV positive

Colposcopy

Two acceptable strategies

For women, 21–29 years: Repeat every 3 years with cervical cytology alone.
For women 20–65 years: Repeat every 3 years with cervical cytology alone. Repeat every 5 years with hrHPV testing alone. Repeat every 5 years with hrHPV with cytology (cotesting).

ABBREVIATIONS:
HR-HPV, high-risk human papilloma virus DNA probe testing;
HSIL, high-grade squamous intraepithelial lesion;
LSIL, low-grade squamous intraepithelial lesion;
cro, cannot rule out;
Cotest, pap cytology and HR-HPV testing;
AGC, atypical glandular cells;
ASC-US, atypical squamous cells of undetermined significance.

OR

HPV 16/18 probe — Negative → Cotest in 1 year

Positive

Colposcopy

Positive

HR-HPV DNA ← Negative — Pap result

Negative

Re-Pap in 3 years.

Positive

Pap > ASC to colposcopy

Paul Pastor, MD

Adapted from American Society for Colposcopy and Cervical Pathology. Algorithms: updated consensus guidelines for managing abnormal cervical cancer screening tests and cancer precursors. http://www.asccp.org/Portals/9/docs/Algorithms%207.30.13.pdf. Accessed 2015.

PAP, NORMAL AND ABNORMAL IN WOMEN AGES 21–24 YEARS

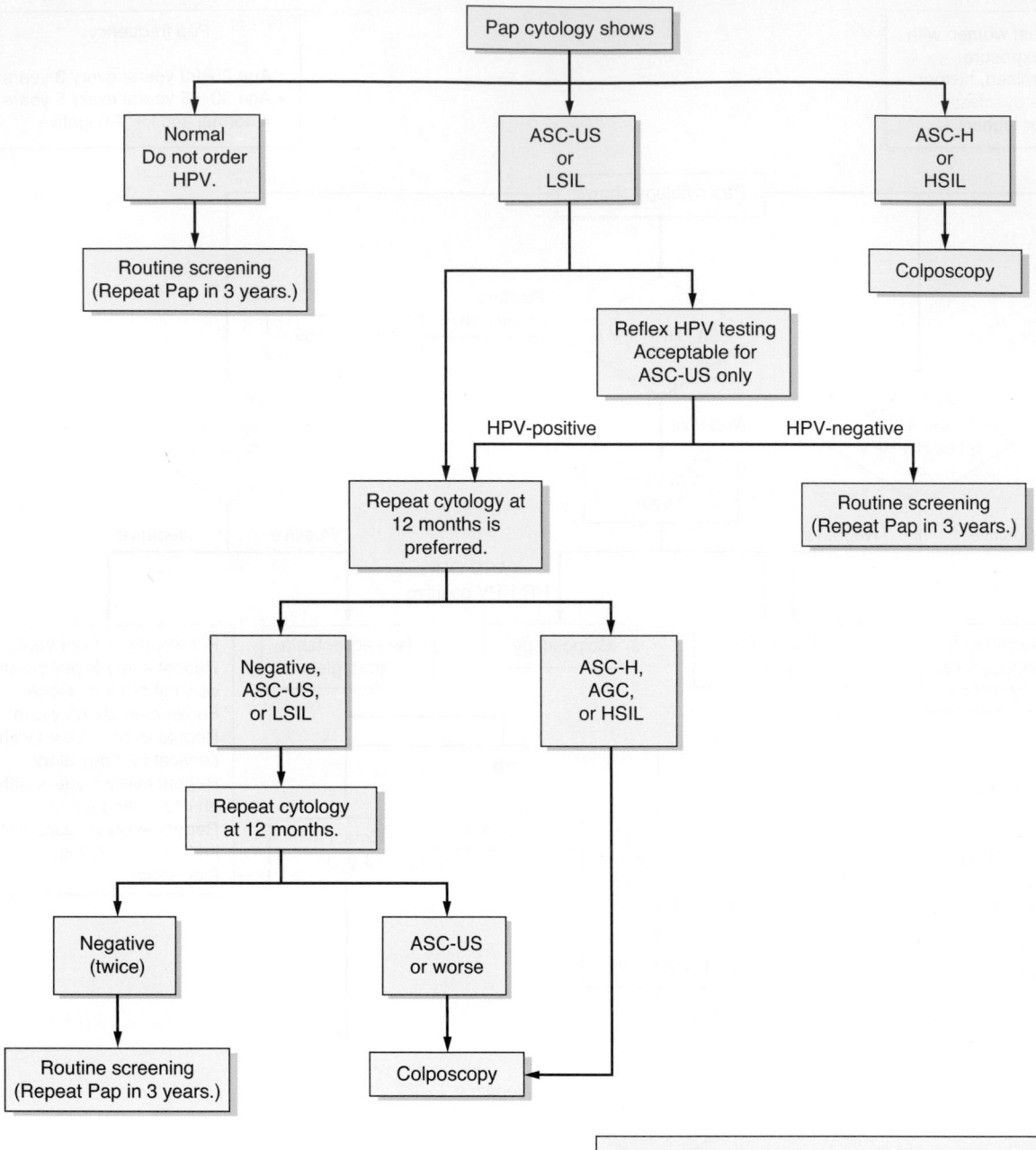

Abbreviations

ASC-US: atypical squamous cells of undetermined significance
LSIL: low-grade squamous intraepithelial lesion
ASC-H: atypical squamous cells, cannot rule out high-grade SIL
HSIL: high-grade squamous intraepithelial lesion
HPV: human papillomavirus
AGC: atypical glandular cells

Susan L. Steffans, DO

Massad LS, Einstein MH, Huh WK, et al. 2012 updated consensus guidelines for the management of abnormal cervical cancer screening tests and cancer precursors. *J Low Genit Tract Dis.* 2013;17(5 Suppl 1):S1–S27.

PARKINSON DISEASE, TREATMENT

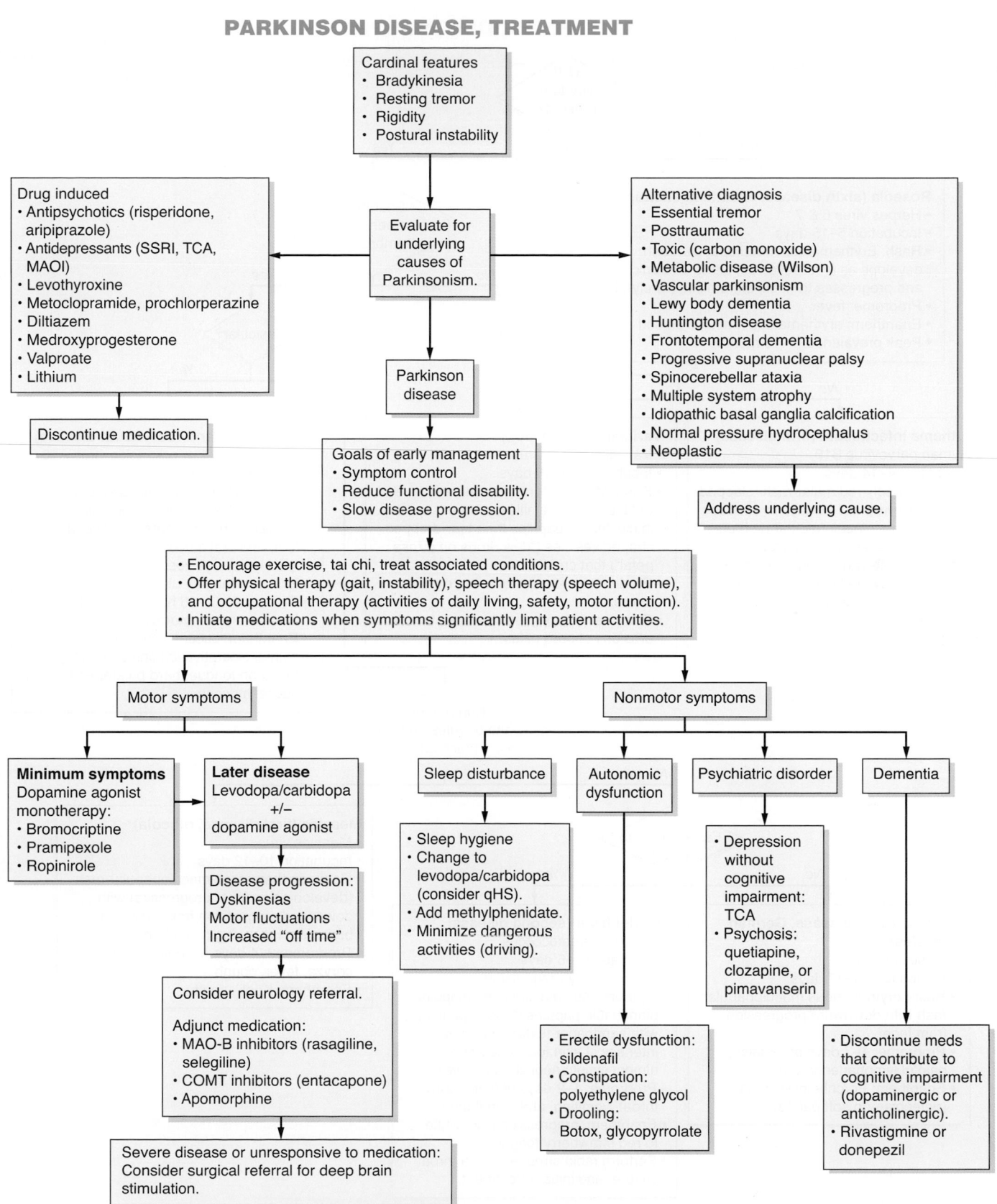

Cardinal features
- Bradykinesia
- Resting tremor
- Rigidity
- Postural instability

Evaluate for underlying causes of Parkinsonism.

Drug induced
- Antipsychotics (risperidone, aripiprazole)
- Antidepressants (SSRI, TCA, MAOI)
- Levothyroxine
- Metoclopramide, prochlorperazine
- Diltiazem
- Medroxyprogesterone
- Valproate
- Lithium

Discontinue medication.

Alternative diagnosis
- Essential tremor
- Posttraumatic
- Toxic (carbon monoxide)
- Metabolic disease (Wilson)
- Vascular parkinsonism
- Lewy body dementia
- Huntington disease
- Frontotemporal dementia
- Progressive supranuclear palsy
- Spinocerebellar ataxia
- Multiple system atrophy
- Idiopathic basal ganglia calcification
- Normal pressure hydrocephalus
- Neoplastic

Address underlying cause.

Parkinson disease

Goals of early management
- Symptom control
- Reduce functional disability.
- Slow disease progression.

- Encourage exercise, tai chi, treat associated conditions.
- Offer physical therapy (gait, instability), speech therapy (speech volume), and occupational therapy (activities of daily living, safety, motor function).
- Initiate medications when symptoms significantly limit patient activities.

Motor symptoms

Nonmotor symptoms

Minimum symptoms
Dopamine agonist monotherapy:
- Bromocriptine
- Pramipexole
- Ropinirole

Later disease
Levodopa/carbidopa +/– dopamine agonist

Disease progression:
Dyskinesias
Motor fluctuations
Increased "off time"

Consider neurology referral.

Adjunct medication:
- MAO-B inhibitors (rasagiline, selegiline)
- COMT inhibitors (entacapone)
- Apomorphine

Severe disease or unresponsive to medication: Consider surgical referral for deep brain stimulation.

Sleep disturbance
- Sleep hygiene
- Change to levodopa/carbidopa (consider qHS).
- Add methylphenidate.
- Minimize dangerous activities (driving).

Autonomic dysfunction
- Erectile dysfunction: sildenafil
- Constipation: polyethylene glycol
- Drooling: Botox, glycopyrrolate

Psychiatric disorder
- Depression without cognitive impairment: TCA
- Psychosis: quetiapine, clozapine, or pimavanserin

Dementia
- Discontinue meds that contribute to cognitive impairment (dopaminergic or anticholinergic).
- Rivastigmine or donepezil

Sarah Coles, MD and William Dabbs, MD

Gazewood JD, Richards DR, Clebak K. Parkinson disease: an update. *Am Fam Physician*. 2013;87(4):267–273.

PEDIATRIC EXANTHEMS, DIAGNOSTIC

URI symptoms present?

No →

Roseola (sixth disease, exanthem subitum)
- Herpes virus 6 & 7
- Incubation 5–15 days
- Rash: Erythematous maculopapular rash develops as fever resolves; starts on trunk and progresses to neck, extremities (rarely), face
- Prodrome: fever
- Enanthem: erythematous macules on soft palate
- Peak prevalence: 7–13 months

Yes →

Enanthem (involvement of mucous membranes)?

No → Vesicular?

No →

Erythema infectiosum (fifth disease)
- Human parvovirus B19
- Incubation 4–14 days
- Rash: intensely red malar rash "slapped cheek" followed in 1–2 days by reticular erythematous maculopapular rash on trunk, extremities, and buttocks; recrudescence can last up to months.
- Prodrome: generally mild, may have 1–4 days of headache, chills, URI symptoms
- Enanthem: none

Yes →

Varicella (chickenpox)
- Varicella zoster virus
- Incubation 14–16 days
- Rash: Macules form on trunk and spread to face and extremities; progress quickly in clusters to papules then tear-dropped shaped vesicles ("dew drops on a rose petal") that crust over or umbilicate
- Prodrome: 1–2 days of fever, malaise, anorexia
- Enanthem: Rarely, vesicles can lead to erosions of hard palate.

Yes → Vesicular?

No / **Yes →**

Coxsackie (hand-foot-mouth disease)
- Enterovirus 71 or coxsackie virus A16
- Incubation 3–6 days
- Rash: erythematous macules and papules ~2–3 mm found on palmar surface of hand, plantar surface of feet, and oral mucosa; progresses quickly through vesicular phase to form central gray ulcer
- Prodrome: 12–36 hours of cough, fever, malaise, anorexia, abdominal pain
- Enanthem: occurs with exanthem as painful ulcerative lesions commonly found on tongue, hard palate, and buccal mucosa

Koplik spots (white papules on buccal mucosa)?

No →

Fast-spreading rash?

No →

Rubella (third disease, German measles)
- Rubella virus
- Incubation 14–17 days
- Rash: erythematous maculopapular rash with downward progression from face
- Prodrome: 1–7 days of malaise, painful lymphadenopathy
- Enanthem: Forchheimer spots (petechiae on soft palate)

Yes →

Scarlet fever (second disease)
- Group A streptococcus
- Incubation 1–5 days
- Rash: rapidly progressing erythematous macules and pinpoint, blanchable papules ("goose pimples") with sandpaper texture, greatest intensity at skin folds occurring almost simultaneously with fever
- Prodrome: 1–2 days of fever, sore throat, vomiting, abdominal pain
- Enanthem: progression from white to red strawberry tongue
- Perform rapid strep testing, a throat culture, and initiate treatment.

Yes →

Measles (first disease, rubeola)
- Measles virus
- Incubation 10–12 days
- Rash: erythematous maculopapular rash (developing as fever progresses) with downward progression from face and brownish hue during resolution
- Prodrome: 3–4 days of conjunctivitis, coryza, fever, cough
- Enanthem: Koplik spots

Phillip Fournier, MD

Dyer JA. Childhood viral exanthems. *Pediatr Ann.* 2007;36(1):21–29.

PELVIC PAIN

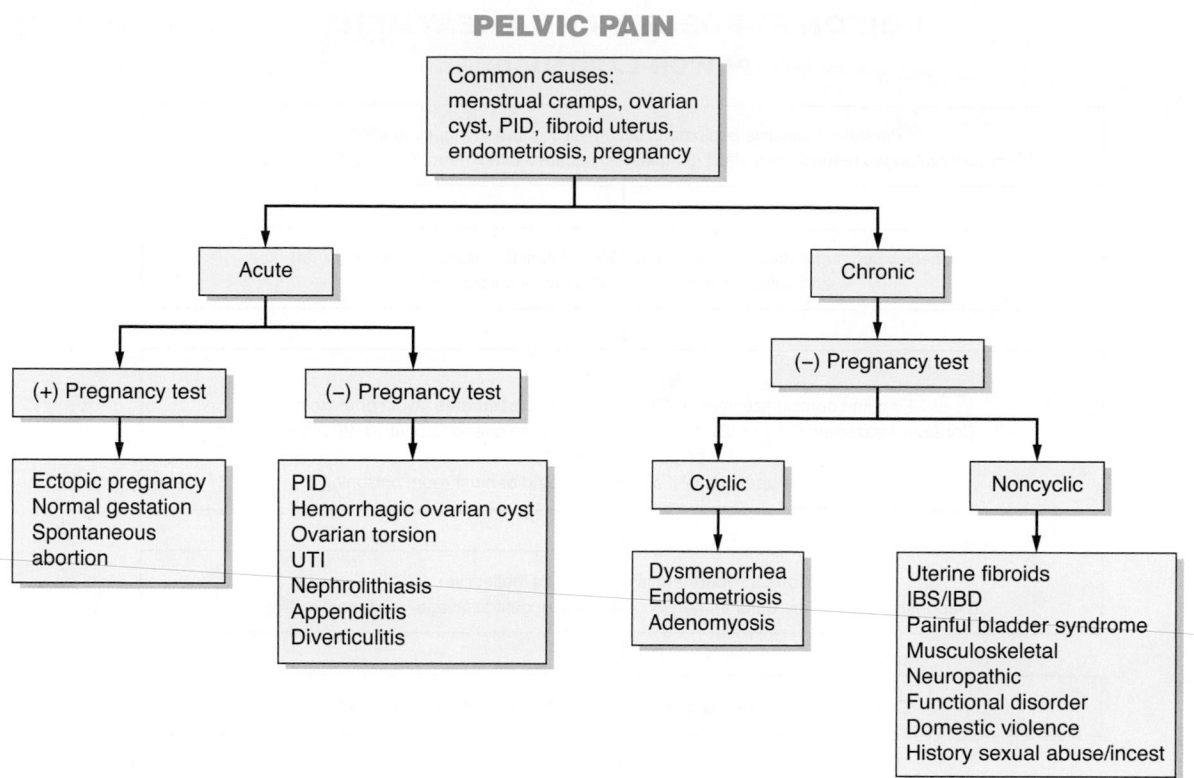

Common causes: menstrual cramps, ovarian cyst, PID, fibroid uterus, endometriosis, pregnancy

Acute

- (+) Pregnancy test
  - Ectopic pregnancy
  - Normal gestation
  - Spontaneous abortion
- (−) Pregnancy test
  - PID
  - Hemorrhagic ovarian cyst
  - Ovarian torsion
  - UTI
  - Nephrolithiasis
  - Appendicitis
  - Diverticulitis

Chronic

- (−) Pregnancy test
  - Cyclic
    - Dysmenorrhea
    - Endometriosis
    - Adenomyosis
  - Noncyclic
    - Uterine fibroids
    - IBS/IBD
    - Painful bladder syndrome
    - Musculoskeletal
    - Neuropathic
    - Functional disorder
    - Domestic violence
    - History sexual abuse/incest

Frank J. Domino, MD

Howard FM. Chronic pelvic pain. *Obstet Gynecol.* 2003;101(3):594–611.

POISON EXPOSURE AND TREATMENT
POISON EXPOSURE

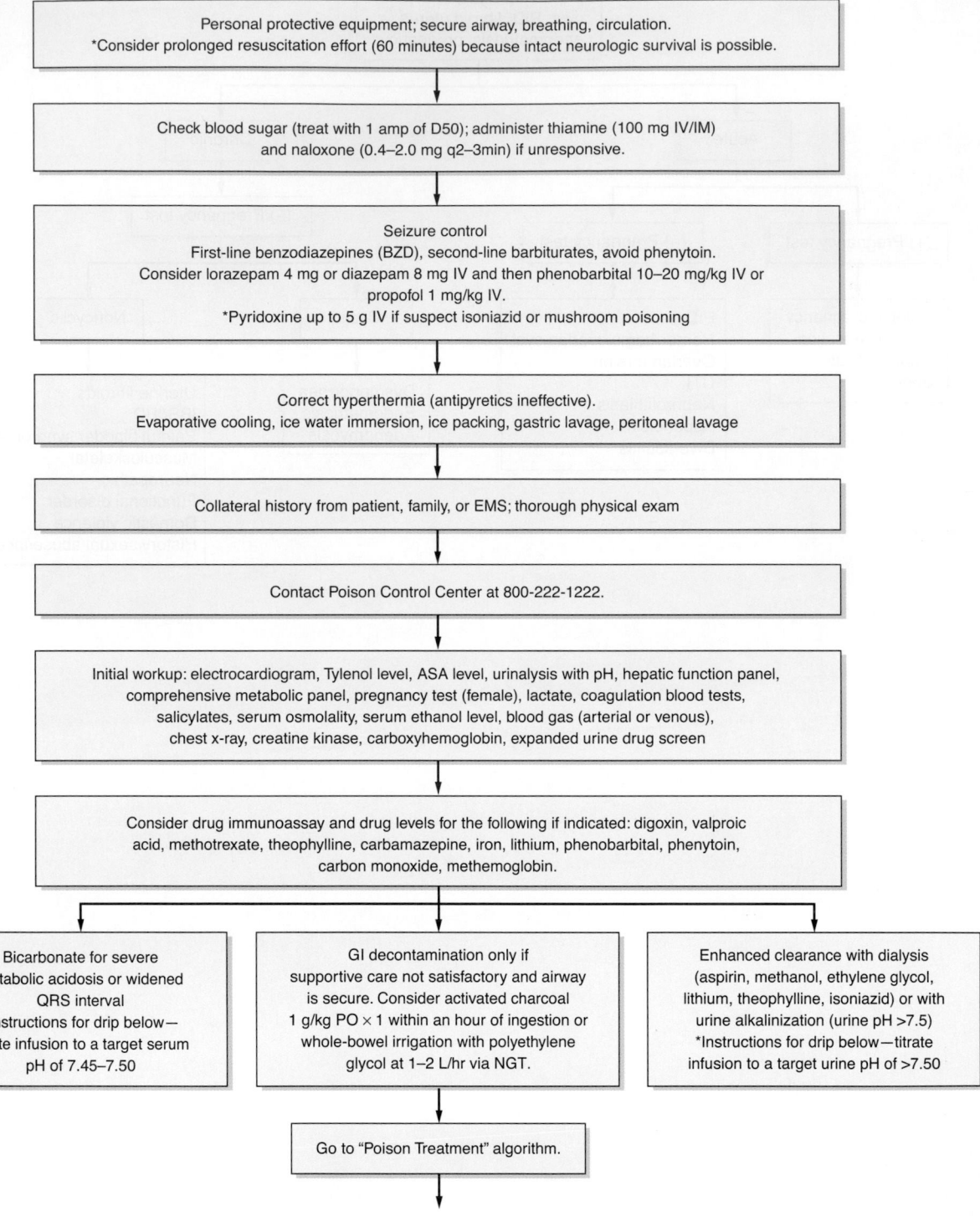

Personal protective equipment; secure airway, breathing, circulation.
*Consider prolonged resuscitation effort (60 minutes) because intact neurologic survival is possible.

Check blood sugar (treat with 1 amp of D50); administer thiamine (100 mg IV/IM)
and naloxone (0.4–2.0 mg q2–3min) if unresponsive.

Seizure control
First-line benzodiazepines (BZD), second-line barbiturates, avoid phenytoin.
Consider lorazepam 4 mg or diazepam 8 mg IV and then phenobarbital 10–20 mg/kg IV or
propofol 1 mg/kg IV.
*Pyridoxine up to 5 g IV if suspect isoniazid or mushroom poisoning

Correct hyperthermia (antipyretics ineffective).
Evaporative cooling, ice water immersion, ice packing, gastric lavage, peritoneal lavage

Collateral history from patient, family, or EMS; thorough physical exam

Contact Poison Control Center at 800-222-1222.

Initial workup: electrocardiogram, Tylenol level, ASA level, urinalysis with pH, hepatic function panel,
comprehensive metabolic panel, pregnancy test (female), lactate, coagulation blood tests,
salicylates, serum osmolality, serum ethanol level, blood gas (arterial or venous),
chest x-ray, creatine kinase, carboxyhemoglobin, expanded urine drug screen

Consider drug immunoassay and drug levels for the following if indicated: digoxin, valproic
acid, methotrexate, theophylline, carbamazepine, iron, lithium, phenobarbital, phenytoin,
carbon monoxide, methemoglobin.

Bicarbonate for severe
metabolic acidosis or widened
QRS interval
*Instructions for drip below—
titrate infusion to a target serum
pH of 7.45–7.50

GI decontamination only if
supportive care not satisfactory and airway
is secure. Consider activated charcoal
1 g/kg PO × 1 within an hour of ingestion or
whole-bowel irrigation with polyethylene
glycol at 1–2 L/hr via NGT.

Enhanced clearance with dialysis
(aspirin, methanol, ethylene glycol,
lithium, theophylline, isoniazid) or with
urine alkalinization (urine pH >7.5)
*Instructions for drip below—titrate
infusion to a target urine pH of >7.50

Go to "Poison Treatment" algorithm.

POISON TREATMENT

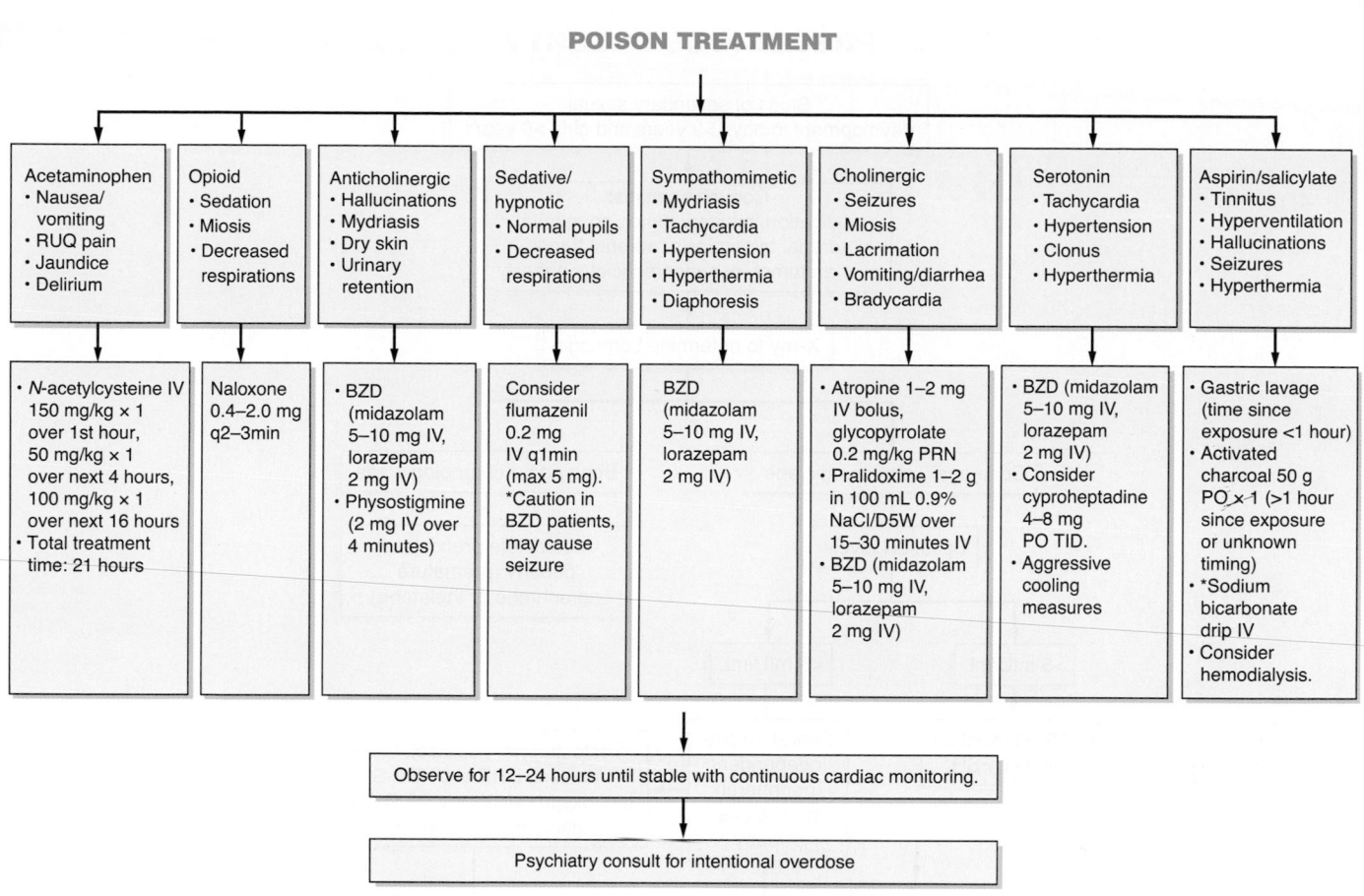

Acetaminophen
- Nausea/vomiting
- RUQ pain
- Jaundice
- Delirium

↓

- *N*-acetylcysteine IV 150 mg/kg × 1 over 1st hour, 50 mg/kg × 1 over next 4 hours, 100 mg/kg × 1 over next 16 hours
- Total treatment time: 21 hours

Opioid
- Sedation
- Miosis
- Decreased respirations

↓

- Naloxone 0.4–2.0 mg q2–3min

Anticholinergic
- Hallucinations
- Mydriasis
- Dry skin
- Urinary retention

↓

- BZD (midazolam 5–10 mg IV, lorazepam 2 mg IV)
- Physostigmine (2 mg IV over 4 minutes)

Sedative/hypnotic
- Normal pupils
- Decreased respirations

↓

- Consider flumazenil 0.2 mg IV q1min (max 5 mg). *Caution in BZD patients, may cause seizure

Sympathomimetic
- Mydriasis
- Tachycardia
- Hypertension
- Hyperthermia
- Diaphoresis

↓

- BZD (midazolam 5–10 mg IV, lorazepam 2 mg IV)

Cholinergic
- Seizures
- Miosis
- Lacrimation
- Vomiting/diarrhea
- Bradycardia

↓

- Atropine 1–2 mg IV bolus, glycopyrrolate 0.2 mg/kg PRN
- Pralidoxime 1–2 g in 100 mL 0.9% NaCl/D5W over 15–30 minutes IV
- BZD (midazolam 5–10 mg IV, lorazepam 2 mg IV)

Serotonin
- Tachycardia
- Hypertension
- Clonus
- Hyperthermia

↓

- BZD (midazolam 5–10 mg IV, lorazepam 2 mg IV)
- Consider cyproheptadine 4–8 mg PO TID.
- Aggressive cooling measures

Aspirin/salicylate
- Tinnitus
- Hyperventilation
- Hallucinations
- Seizures
- Hyperthermia

↓

- Gastric lavage (time since exposure <1 hour)
- Activated charcoal 50 g PO × 1 (>1 hour since exposure or unknown timing)
- *Sodium bicarbonate drip IV
- Consider hemodialysis.

↓

Observe for 12–24 hours until stable with continuous cardiac monitoring.

↓

Psychiatry consult for intentional overdose

*To mix a bicarbonate drip: 150 mEq (3 amps) $NaHCO_3$ in 1 L of D5W and then start at a rate of 150–200 mL/hr

Pediatric dosing (adult doses in algorithm)
- Activated charcoal (0.5–1.0 g/kg PO)
- Atropine (0.02 mg/kg IV)
- Bicarbonate (1–2 mEq/kg IV*)
- Chlorpromazine (not recommended)
- Cyproheptadine (0.25 mg/kg/day divided BID or TID)
- Dextrose (2.5 mL/kg of 10% or 1 mL/kg of 25% IV)
- Flumazenil (5 μg/kg IV)
- Glycopyrrolate (4 μg/kg IV)

- Lorazepam (0.05–0.10 mg/kg IV)
- Midazolam (0.1 mg/kg IV)
- Phenobarbital (10–20 mg/kg IV)
- Physostigmine (10–30 μg/kg IV)
- Polyethylene glycol (250–500 mL/hr PO/NG)
- Pralidoxime (20–40 mg/kg IV)
- Pyridoxine (same as adults)
- Naloxone (0.1 mg/kg IV q2–3min)
- Thiamine (not routinely given)

Justin L. Chapman, MD

Frithsen IL, Simpson WM Jr. Recognition and management of acute medication poisoning. *Am Fam Physician.* 2010;81(3):316–323.

PRECOCIOUS PUBERTY

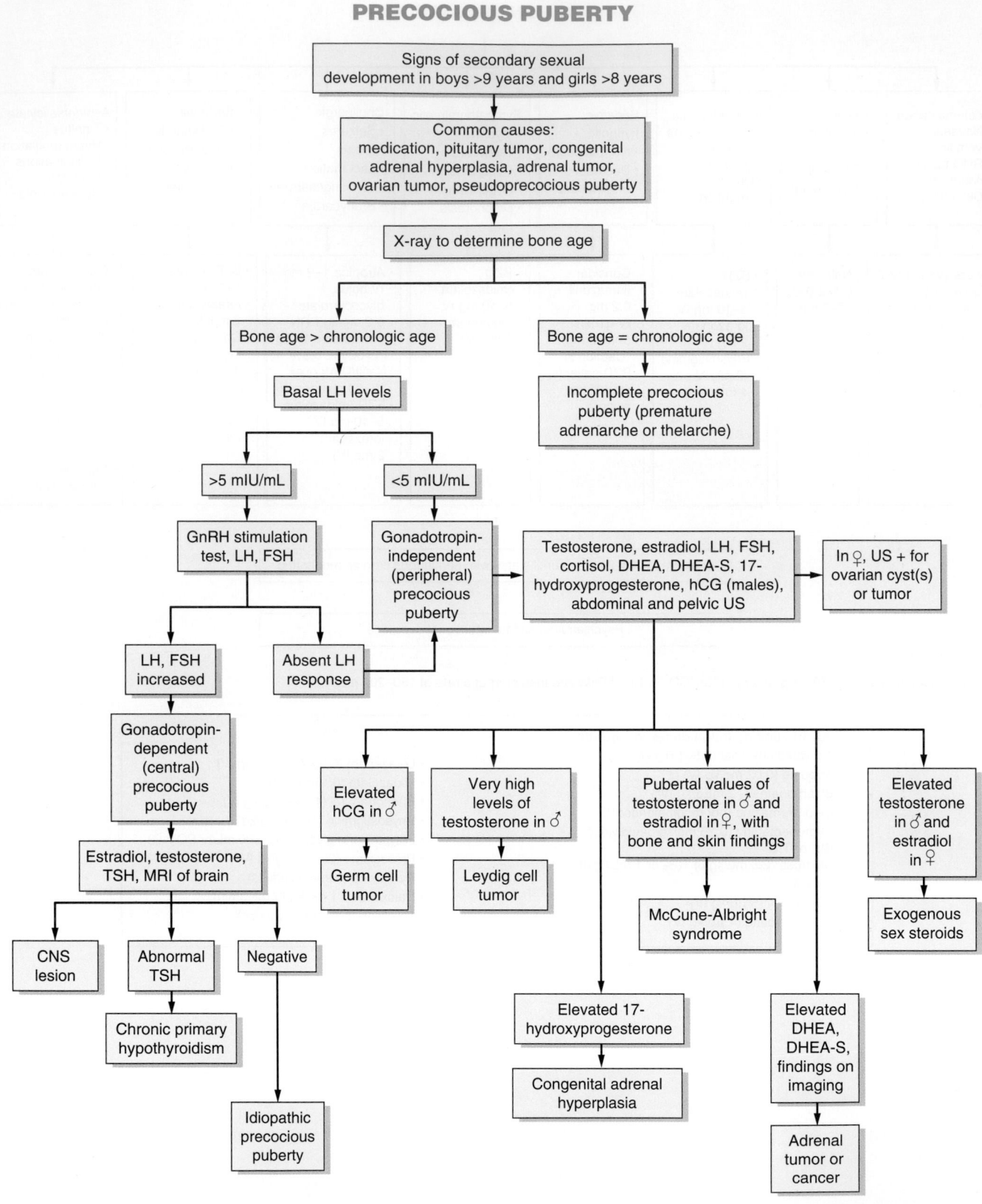

Nicole Shields, MD

Berberoğlu M. Precocious puberty and normal variant puberty: definition, etiology, diagnosis and current management. *J Clin Res Pediatr Endocrinol.* 2009;1(4):164–174.

PREOPERATIVE EVALUATION OF NONCARDIAC SURGICAL PATIENT

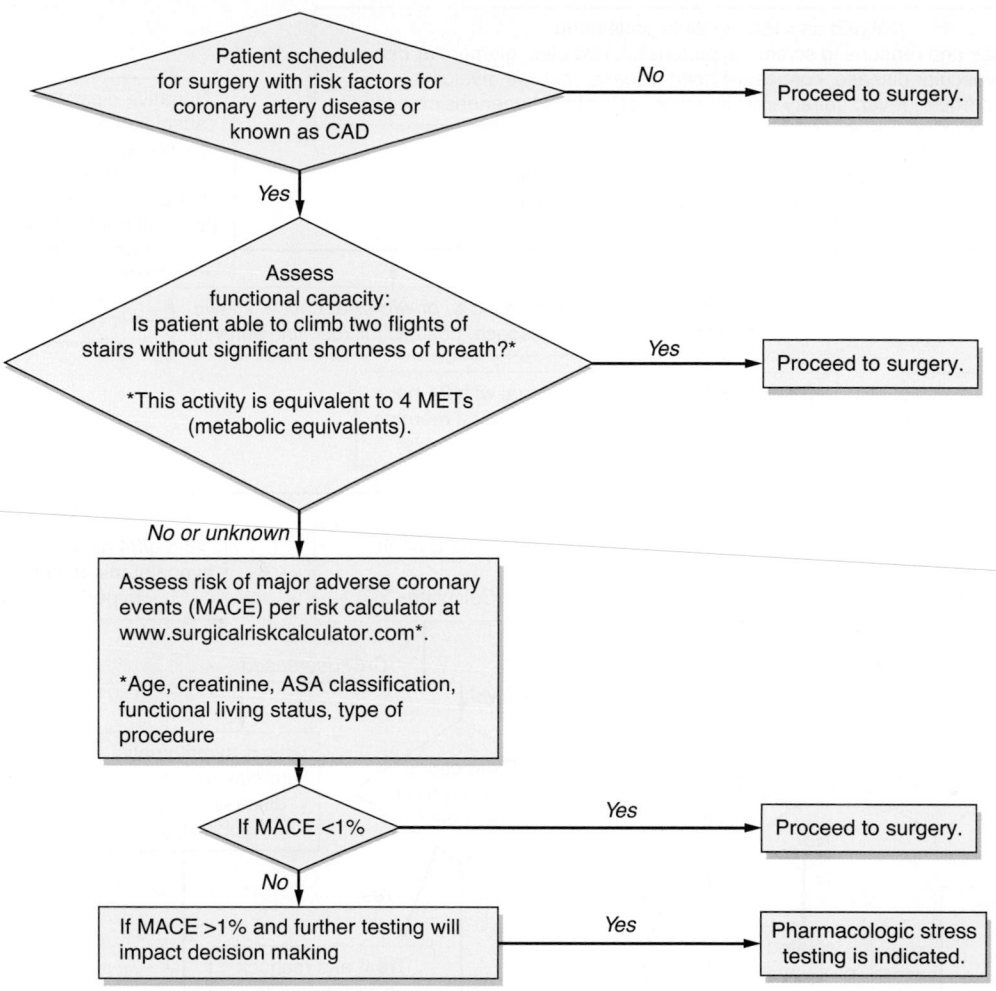

Andrew E. Grimes, MD and Stacy L. Jones, MD, FASA

Ghadimi K, Thompson A. Update on perioperative care of the cardiac patient for noncardiac surgery. *Curr Opin Anaesthesiol.* 2015;28(3):342–348.

PROTEINURIA

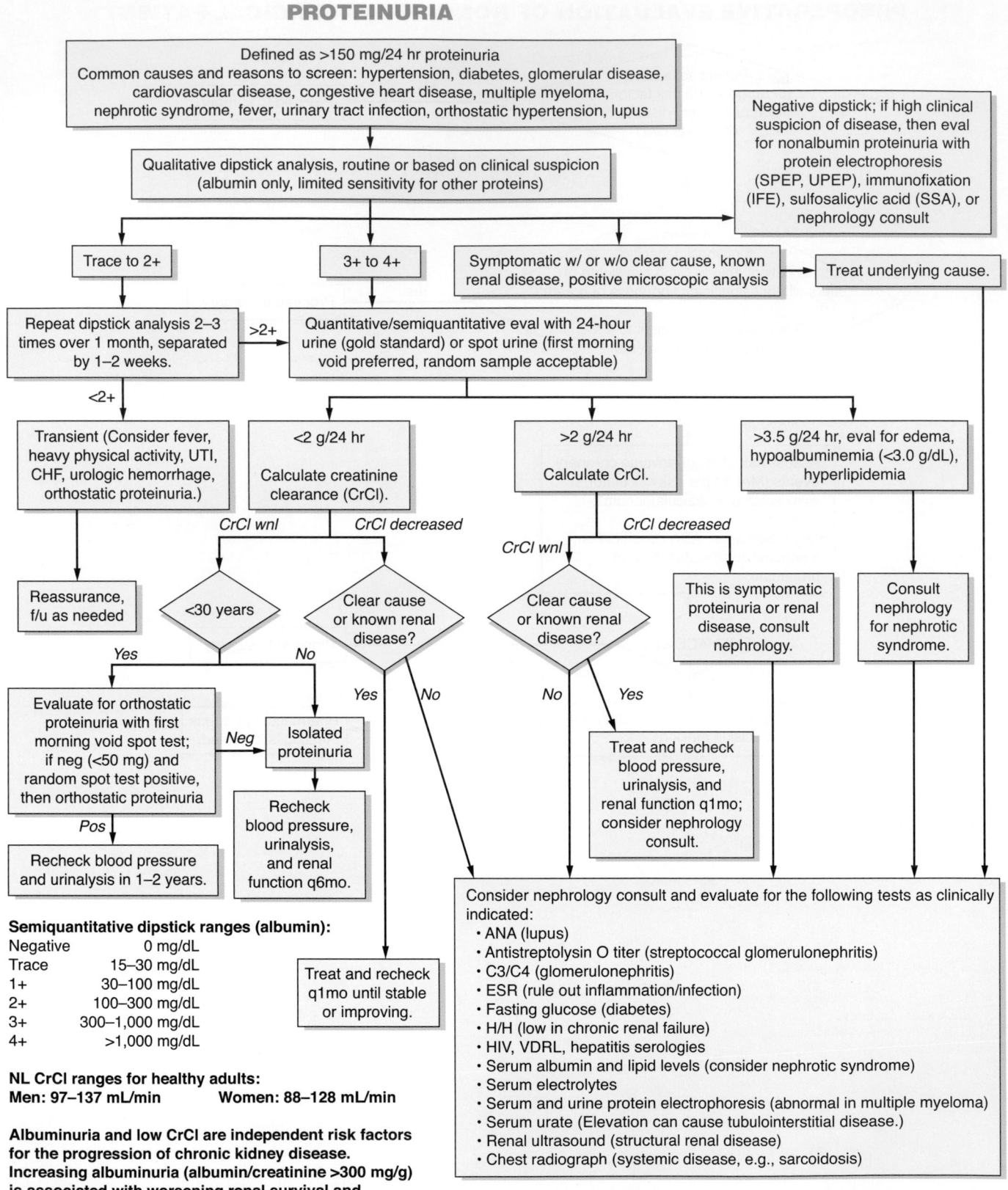

Semiquantitative dipstick ranges (albumin):

Negative	0 mg/dL
Trace	15–30 mg/dL
1+	30–100 mg/dL
2+	100–300 mg/dL
3+	300–1,000 mg/dL
4+	>1,000 mg/dL

NL CrCl ranges for healthy adults:
Men: 97–137 mL/min   Women: 88–128 mL/min

Albuminuria and low CrCl are independent risk factors for the progression of chronic kidney disease. Increasing albuminuria (albumin/creatinine >300 mg/g) is associated with worsening renal survival and should be referred to a nephrologist.

Consider nephrology consult and evaluate for the following tests as clinically indicated:
- ANA (lupus)
- Antistreptolysin O titer (streptococcal glomerulonephritis)
- C3/C4 (glomerulonephritis)
- ESR (rule out inflammation/infection)
- Fasting glucose (diabetes)
- H/H (low in chronic renal failure)
- HIV, VDRL, hepatitis serologies
- Serum albumin and lipid levels (consider nephrotic syndrome)
- Serum electrolytes
- Serum and urine protein electrophoresis (abnormal in multiple myeloma)
- Serum urate (Elevation can cause tubulointerstitial disease.)
- Renal ultrasound (structural renal disease)
- Chest radiograph (systemic disease, e.g., sarcoidosis)

John N. Gayk, MD, Shawn M. Bishop, MD, and Jeffrey A. Schievenin, MD

Sperati JC, Fine DM. Evaluation of proteinuria. BMJ Best Practice Monogram 875. http://us.bestpractice.bmj.com/bestpractice/monograph/875.html. Updated November 2017. Accessed July 18, 2018.

PULMONARY EMBOLISM, DIAGNOSIS

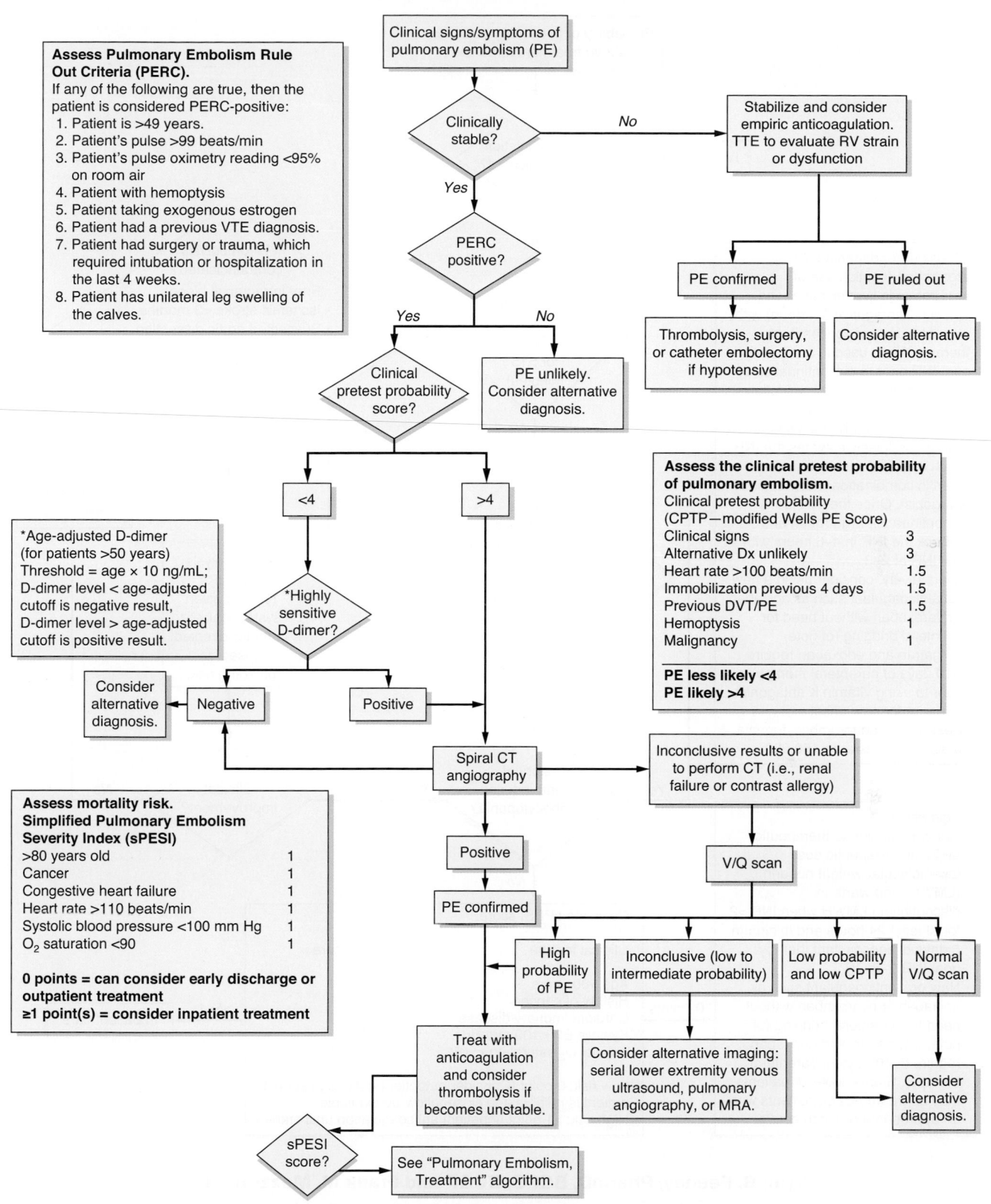

Assess Pulmonary Embolism Rule Out Criteria (PERC).
If any of the following are true, then the patient is considered PERC-positive:
1. Patient is >49 years.
2. Patient's pulse >99 beats/min
3. Patient's pulse oximetry reading <95% on room air
4. Patient with hemoptysis
5. Patient taking exogenous estrogen
6. Patient had a previous VTE diagnosis.
7. Patient had surgery or trauma, which required intubation or hospitalization in the last 4 weeks.
8. Patient has unilateral leg swelling of the calves.

Clinical signs/symptoms of pulmonary embolism (PE)

Clinically stable? — *No* → Stabilize and consider empiric anticoagulation. TTE to evaluate RV strain or dysfunction

Yes

PERC positive?

PE confirmed → Thrombolysis, surgery, or catheter embolectomy if hypotensive

PE ruled out → Consider alternative diagnosis.

Yes — Clinical pretest probability score?

No — PE unlikely. Consider alternative diagnosis.

Assess the clinical pretest probability of pulmonary embolism.
Clinical pretest probability
(CPTP—modified Wells PE Score)

Clinical signs	3
Alternative Dx unlikely	3
Heart rate >100 beats/min	1.5
Immobilization previous 4 days	1.5
Previous DVT/PE	1.5
Hemoptysis	1
Malignancy	1

PE less likely <4
PE likely >4

<4   >4

*Age-adjusted D-dimer (for patients >50 years)
Threshold = age × 10 ng/mL;
D-dimer level < age-adjusted cutoff is negative result,
D-dimer level > age-adjusted cutoff is positive result.

*Highly sensitive D-dimer?

Consider alternative diagnosis. ← Negative   Positive →

Assess mortality risk.
Simplified Pulmonary Embolism Severity Index (sPESI)

>80 years old	1
Cancer	1
Congestive heart failure	1
Heart rate >110 beats/min	1
Systolic blood pressure <100 mm Hg	1
O$_2$ saturation <90	1

0 points = can consider early discharge or outpatient treatment
≥1 point(s) = consider inpatient treatment

Spiral CT angiography → Inconclusive results or unable to perform CT (i.e., renal failure or contrast allergy)

Positive

PE confirmed

V/Q scan

High probability of PE | Inconclusive (low to intermediate probability) | Low probability and low CPTP | Normal V/Q scan

Treat with anticoagulation and consider thrombolysis if becomes unstable.

Consider alternative imaging: serial lower extremity venous ultrasound, pulmonary angiography, or MRA.

Consider alternative diagnosis.

sPESI score? → See "Pulmonary Embolism, Treatment" algorithm.

Jon Payne, MD and Lawrence M. Gibbs, MD, MSEd, FAAFP

van der Hulle T, Dronkers CE, Klok FA, et al. Recent developments in the diagnosis and treatment of pulmonary embolism. *J Intern Med.* 2016;279(1):16–29.

PULMONARY EMBOLISM, TREATMENT

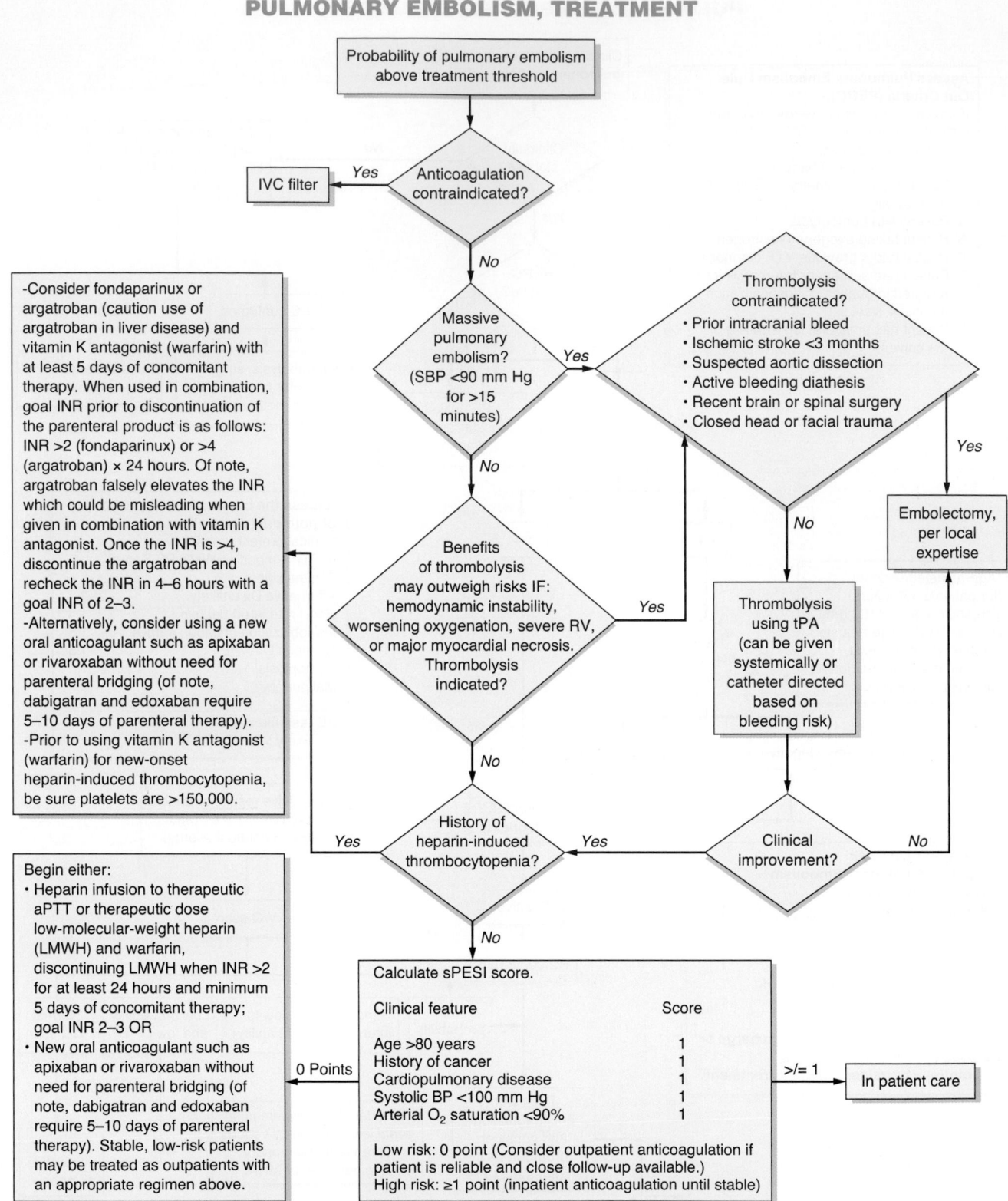

Ryan B. Feeney, PharmD, BCPS, BCGP and Frank M. Mazzotta, DO

Jaff MR, McMurtry MS, Archer SL, et al; for American Heart Association Council on Cardiopulmonary, Critical Care, Perioperative and Resuscitation; American Heart Association Council on Peripheral Vascular Disease; American Heart Association Council on Arteriosclerosis, Thrombosis and Vascular Biology. Management of massive and submassive pulmonary embolism, iliofemoral deep vein thrombosis, and chronic thromboembolic pulmonary hypertension: a scientific statement from the American Heart Association. *Circulation.* 2011;123(16):1788–1830.

RASH

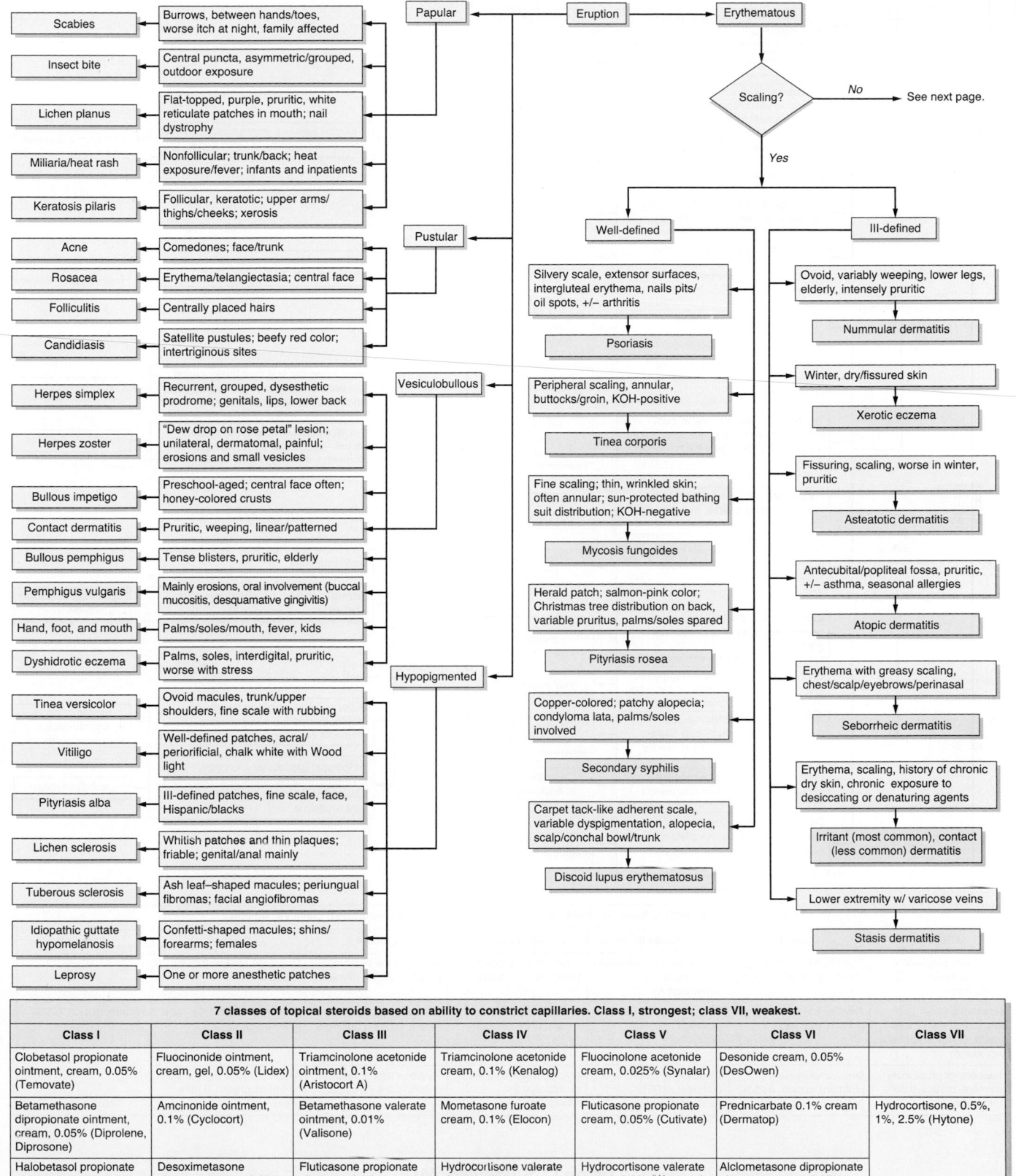

7 classes of topical steroids based on ability to constrict capillaries. Class I, strongest; class VII, weakest.						
Class I	**Class II**	**Class III**	**Class IV**	**Class V**	**Class VI**	**Class VII**
Clobetasol propionate ointment, cream, 0.05% (Temovate)	Fluocinonide ointment, cream, gel, 0.05% (Lidex)	Triamcinolone acetonide ointment, 0.1% (Aristocort A)	Triamcinolone acetonide cream, 0.1% (Kenalog)	Fluocinolone acetonide cream, 0.025% (Synalar)	Desonide cream, 0.05% (DesOwen)	
Betamethasone dipropionate ointment, cream, 0.05% (Diprolene, Diprosone)	Amcinonide ointment, 0.1% (Cyclocort)	Betamethasone valerate ointment, 0.01% (Valisone)	Mometasone furoate cream, 0.1% (Elocon)	Fluticasone propionate cream, 0.05% (Cutivate)	Prednicarbate 0.1% cream (Dermatop)	Hydrocortisone, 0.5%, 1%, 2.5% (Hytone)
Halobetasol propionate ointment, cream, 0.05% (Ultravate)	Desoximetasone ointment, cream, 0.25%; gel, 0.05% (Topicort)	Fluticasone propionate ointment, 0.05% (Cutivate)	Hydrocortisone valerate ointment, 0.2% (Westcort)	Hydrocortisone valerate cream, 0.2% (Westcort)	Alclometasone dipropionate ointment, cream, 0.05% (Aclovate)	

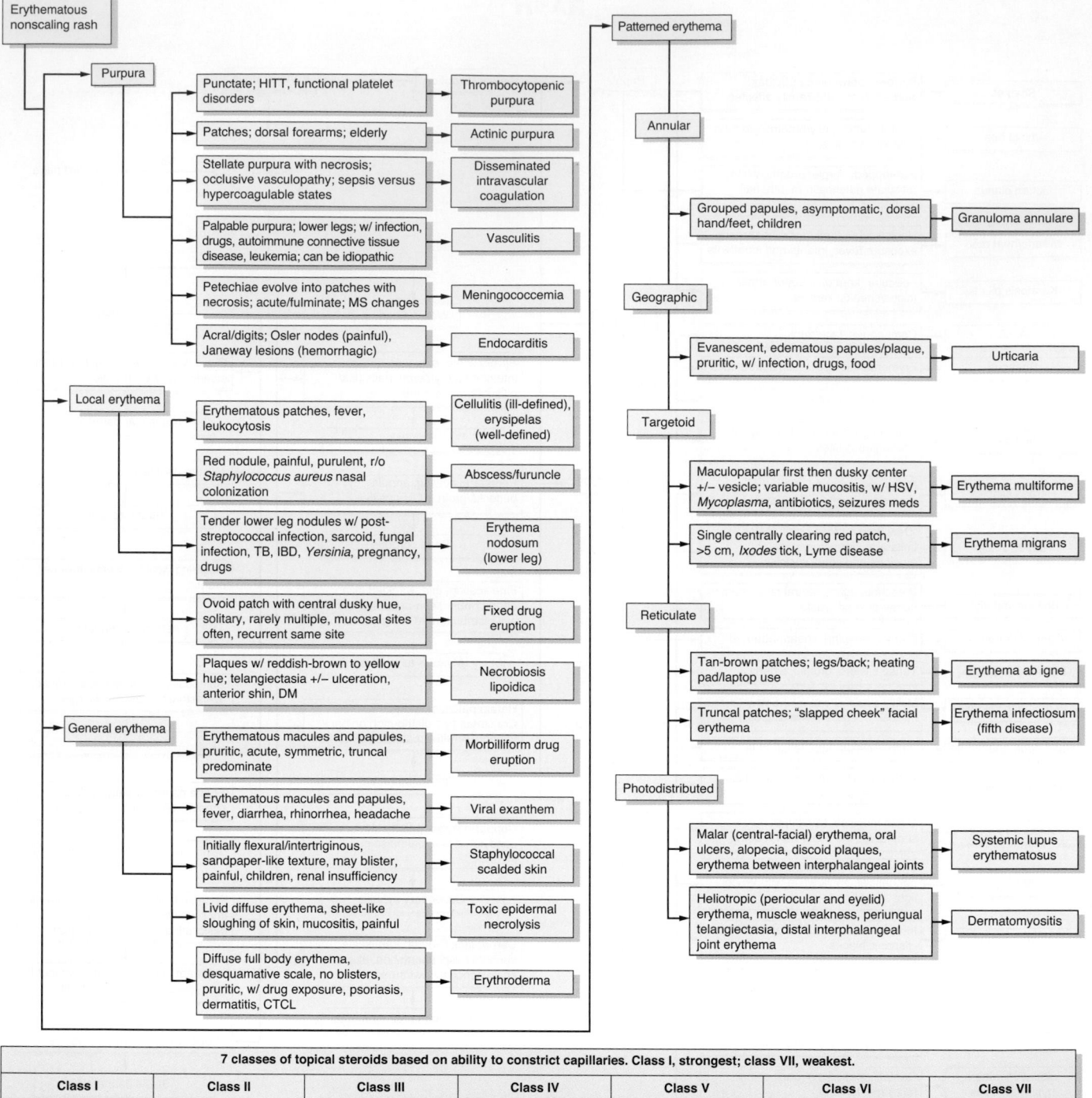

7 classes of topical steroids based on ability to constrict capillaries. Class I, strongest; class VII, weakest.						
Class I	**Class II**	**Class III**	**Class IV**	**Class V**	**Class VI**	**Class VII**
Clobetasol propionate ointment, cream, 0.05% (Temovate)	Fluocinonide ointment, cream, gel 0.05% (Lidex)	Triamcinolone acetonide ointment, 0.1% (Aristocort A)	Triamcinolone acetonide cream, 0.1% (Kenalog)	Fluocinolone acetonide cream, 0.025% (Synalar)	Desonide cream, 0.05% (DesOwen)	
Betamethasone dipropionate ointment, cream, 0.05% (Diprolene, Diprosone)	Amcinonide ointment, 0.1% (Cyclocort)	Betamethasone valerate ointment, 0.01% (Valisone)	Mometasone furoate cream, 0.1% (Elocon)	Fluticasone propionate cream, 0.05% (Cutivate)	Prednicarbate 0.1% cream (Dermatop)	Hydrocortisone, 0.5%, 1%, 2.5% (Hytone)
Halobetasol propionate ointment, cream, 0.05% (Ultravate)	Desoximetasone ointment, cream, 0.25%; gel, 0.05% (Topicort)	Fluticasone propionate ointment, 0.05% (Cutivate)	Hydrocortisone valerate ointment, 0.2% (Westcort)	Hydrocortisone valerate cream, 0.2% (Westcort)	Alclometasone dipropionate ointment, cream, 0.05% (Aclovate)	

Jason C. Sluzevich, MD

Wolf R, Parish LC. Advances in dermatologic diagnosis, Part II. *Clin Dermatol.* 2011;29(5):481–482.

RECTAL BLEEDING AND HEMATOCHEZIA

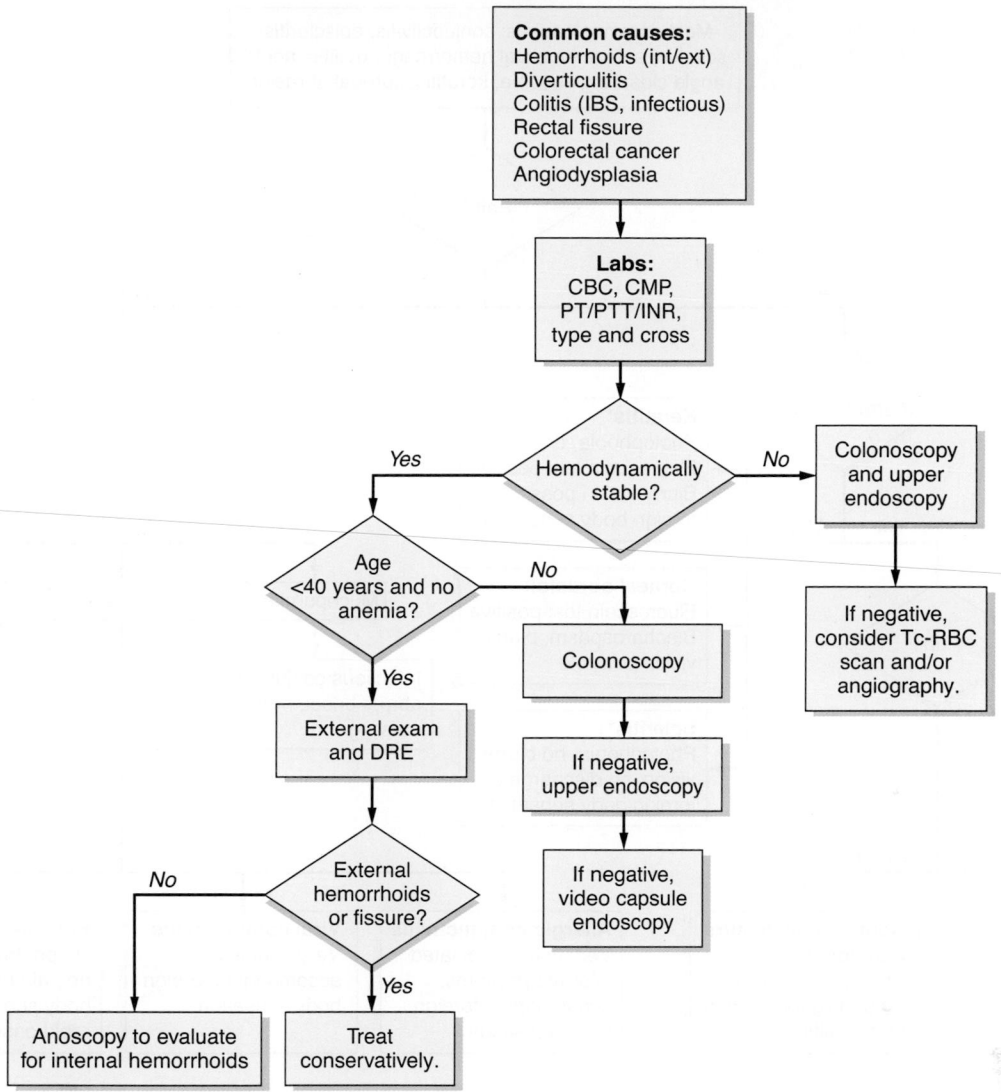

Common causes:
Hemorrhoids (int/ext)
Diverticulitis
Colitis (IBS, infectious)
Rectal fissure
Colorectal cancer
Angiodysplasia

Labs:
CBC, CMP,
PT/PTT/INR,
type and cross

Hemodynamically stable?

Yes / *No*

Colonoscopy and upper endoscopy

If negative, consider Tc-RBC scan and/or angiography.

Age <40 years and no anemia?

No

Colonoscopy

If negative, upper endoscopy

If negative, video capsule endoscopy

Yes

External exam and DRE

External hemorrhoids or fissure?

No

Anoscopy to evaluate for internal hemorrhoids

Yes

Treat conservatively.

Mohammad Ansar Mughal, MD

Hoedema RE, Luchtefeld MA. The management of lower gastrointestinal hemorrhage. *Dis Colon Rectum.* 2005;48(11):2010–2024.

RED EYE

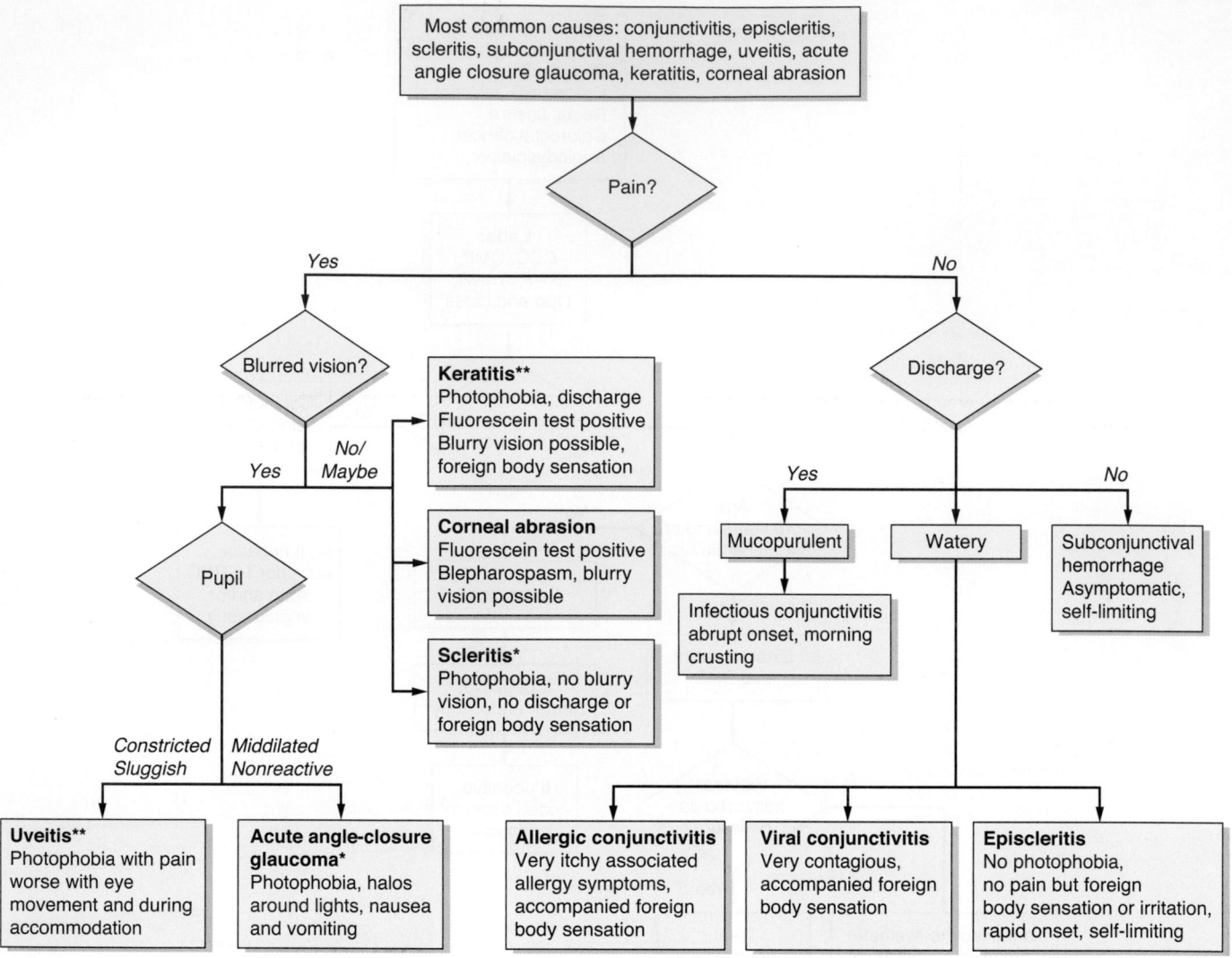

Most common causes: conjunctivitis, episcleritis, scleritis, subconjunctival hemorrhage, uveitis, acute angle closure glaucoma, keratitis, corneal abrasion

Pain?

Yes — *No*

Blurred vision?

Yes — *No/Maybe*

Keratitis**
Photophobia, discharge
Fluorescein test positive
Blurry vision possible,
foreign body sensation

Corneal abrasion
Fluorescein test positive
Blepharospasm, blurry
vision possible

Scleritis*
Photophobia, no blurry
vision, no discharge or
foreign body sensation

Pupil

Constricted Sluggish — *Middilated Nonreactive*

Uveitis**
Photophobia with pain
worse with eye
movement and during
accommodation

**Acute angle-closure
glaucoma***
Photophobia, halos
around lights, nausea
and vomiting

Discharge?

Yes — *No*

Mucopurulent — **Watery**

Infectious conjunctivitis
abrupt onset, morning
crusting

**Subconjunctival
hemorrhage**
Asymptomatic,
self-limiting

Allergic conjunctivitis
Very itchy associated
allergy symptoms,
accompanied foreign
body sensation

Viral conjunctivitis
Very contagious,
accompanied foreign
body sensation

Episcleritis
No photophobia,
no pain but foreign
body sensation or irritation,
rapid onset, self-limiting

*Urgent ophthalmology consultation.
**Consultation within 24 hours.

Drew-Anne Drapala, MD and Vincent Lo, MD, FAAFP

Cronau H, Kankanala RR, Mauger T. Diagnosis and management of red eye in primary care. *Am Fam Physician.* 2010;81(2):137–144.

SALICYLATE POISONING, ACUTE, TREATMENT

Assess airway, breathing, and circulation (ABC).
Provide appropriate ABC management. Avoid intubation unless patient is unable to protect airway. Intubation may increase acidosis and result in cardiovascular collapse.

Early toxicity: tachypnea, hyperpnea, nausea, vomiting, tinnitus, vertigo
Late toxicity: hyperthermia, hypotension, altered mental status

Does the patient exhibit signs of severe toxicity (altered mental status/coma, seizure, pulmonary edema, or need for endotracheal intubation and mechanical ventilation)?

No → **History and physical**
Obtain careful history of ingestion (time, reported ingestion, coingestants, etc.) and perform thorough physical exam for hemodynamic instability, alterations in respiratory pattern, and changes in mental status.

Yes → **Initiate emergent hemodialysis.**
Begin volume resuscitation and alkalinization using 150 mEq (3 amps) $NaHCO_3$ + 40 mEq KCl in 1 L D5W unless prohibited by cerebral/pulmonary edema. Administer 25 g (1 amp) D50 for altered mental status. Do not delay treatment for diagnostic studies.

Note: Volume resuscitation and alkalinization are the mainstays of therapy and should be given to all symptomatic patients unless pulmonary or cerebral edema is present. Respiratory alkalosis (pH >7.5) is NOT a contraindication to therapy. Do not delay for charcoal or diagnostic studies.

Is the patient asymptomatic, stable, and known to have ingested <150 mg/kg?

No → **Initial treatment**
1. Early volume resuscitation with isotonic saline
2. Urinary alkalinization using 150 mEq (3 amps) $NaHCO_3$ + 40 mEq KCl mixed in 1 L D5W, infused at 2–3 mL/kg/hr
3. Administer first-dose activated charcoal at 1 g/kg (max 50 g) ONLY if patient is alert, cooperative, has bowel sounds on exam, and can tolerate. Consider additional doses of 50 g q4h for two more doses if patient continues to meet the aforementioned criteria.

Yes → **Evaluation/observation**
Obtain first salicylate level, noting time since ingestion occurred.

ASA detectable?

No → Recheck if within 2 hours of presentation. Discharge after 6 hours observation if patient remains asymptomatic and levels are nondetectable.

Yes → Recheck levels q2h until persistently within therapeutic range, trending down, or nondetectable. Routinely reassess for changes in clinical status and initiate treatment if indicated.

Obtain diagnostic studies.
Labs: salicylate level (note time since ingestion), ABG/VBG, basic electrolytes, BUN, creatinine, LFTs, coags, lactate, UA. Obtain tox screen if polysubstance overdose suspected.
Imaging: chest radiograph (to evaluate for pulmonary edema). Consider head CT for altered mental status to evaluate for cerebral edema or alternative causes of mental status changes.

Presence of salicylate level >90 mg/dL, arterial pH <7.3, pulmonary or cerebral edema, renal failure, or has patient deteriorated?

No → **Maintenance therapy and evaluation**
1. Continue bicarbonate infusion to maintain urine output of 1–2 mL/kg/hr.
2. Measure urine pH hourly and titrate infusion to goal pH of 7.5–8.0.
3. Measure serum K hourly and replete if <4.5 mEq/L.
4. Measure ABG or VBG hourly and decrease rate of bicarbonate drip if serum pH exceeds 7.6.
5. Measure serum salicylate level q2h until salicylate level begins to decline and acid–base status is normal.

Disposition
Treatment should be continued with frequent clinical assessment for improvement. Treatment and testing may be stopped ONLY when patient is asymptomatic, acid–base status is stable, AND salicylate level has fallen into therapeutic range (10–30 mg/dL).

Yes → Initiate hemodialysis.

Alicia G. Lydecker, MD and Matthew K. Griswold, MD

Juurlink DN, Gosselin S, Kielstein JT, et al; for EXTRIP Workgroup. Extracorporeal treatment for salicylate poisoning: systematic review and recommendations from the EXTRIP workgroup. *Ann Emerg Med.* 2015;66(2):165–181.

SEIZURE, NEW ONSET

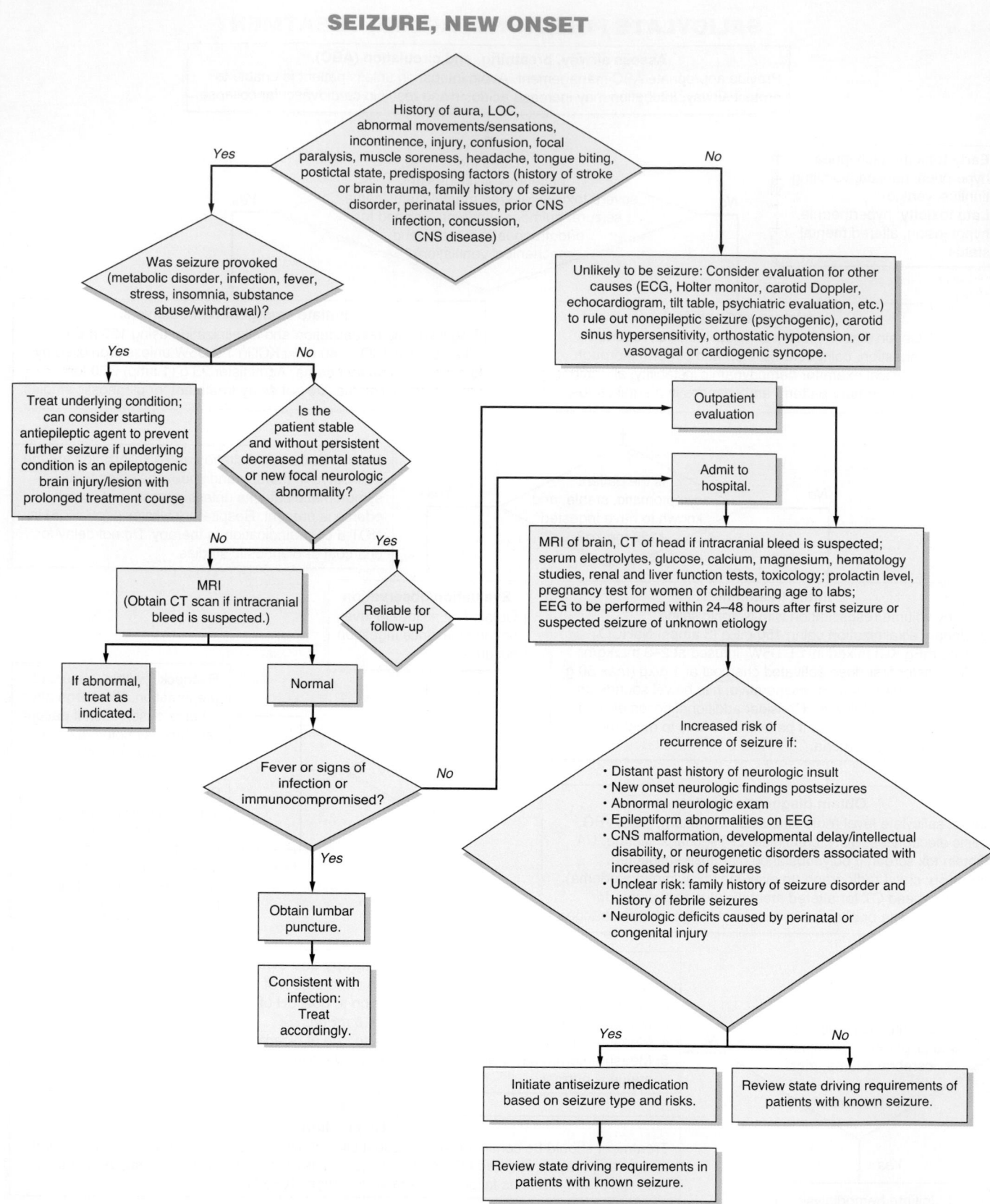

History of aura, LOC, abnormal movements/sensations, incontinence, injury, confusion, focal paralysis, muscle soreness, headache, tongue biting, postictal state, predisposing factors (history of stroke or brain trauma, family history of seizure disorder, perinatal issues, prior CNS infection, concussion, CNS disease)

Yes → Was seizure provoked (metabolic disorder, infection, fever, stress, insomnia, substance abuse/withdrawal)?

No → Unlikely to be seizure: Consider evaluation for other causes (ECG, Holter monitor, carotid Doppler, echocardiogram, tilt table, psychiatric evaluation, etc.) to rule out nonepileptic seizure (psychogenic), carotid sinus hypersensitivity, orthostatic hypotension, or vasovagal or cardiogenic syncope.

Yes → Treat underlying condition; can consider starting antiepileptic agent to prevent further seizure if underlying condition is an epileptogenic brain injury/lesion with prolonged treatment course

No → Is the patient stable and without persistent decreased mental status or new focal neurologic abnormality?

No → MRI (Obtain CT scan if intracranial bleed is suspected.)
- If abnormal, treat as indicated.
- Normal

Yes → Reliable for follow-up
- Outpatient evaluation
- Admit to hospital.

MRI of brain, CT of head if intracranial bleed is suspected; serum electrolytes, glucose, calcium, magnesium, hematology studies, renal and liver function tests, toxicology; prolactin level, pregnancy test for women of childbearing age to labs; EEG to be performed within 24–48 hours after first seizure or suspected seizure of unknown etiology

Fever or signs of infection or immunocompromised?

No →

Yes → Obtain lumbar puncture. → Consistent with infection: Treat accordingly.

Increased risk of recurrence of seizure if:
- Distant past history of neurologic insult
- New onset neurologic findings postseizures
- Abnormal neurologic exam
- Epileptiform abnormalities on EEG
- CNS malformation, developmental delay/intellectual disability, or neurogenetic disorders associated with increased risk of seizures
- Unclear risk: family history of seizure disorder and history of febrile seizures
- Neurologic deficits caused by perinatal or congenital injury

Yes → Initiate antiseizure medication based on seizure type and risks. → Review state driving requirements in patients with known seizure.

No → Review state driving requirements of patients with known seizure.

Andrew S. Hellenga, MD and Matthew J. Snyder, DO

Wilden JA, Cohen-Gadol AA. Evaluation of first nonfebrile seizures. *Am Fam Physician*. 2012;86(4):334–340.

SHOULDER PAIN, TREATMENT

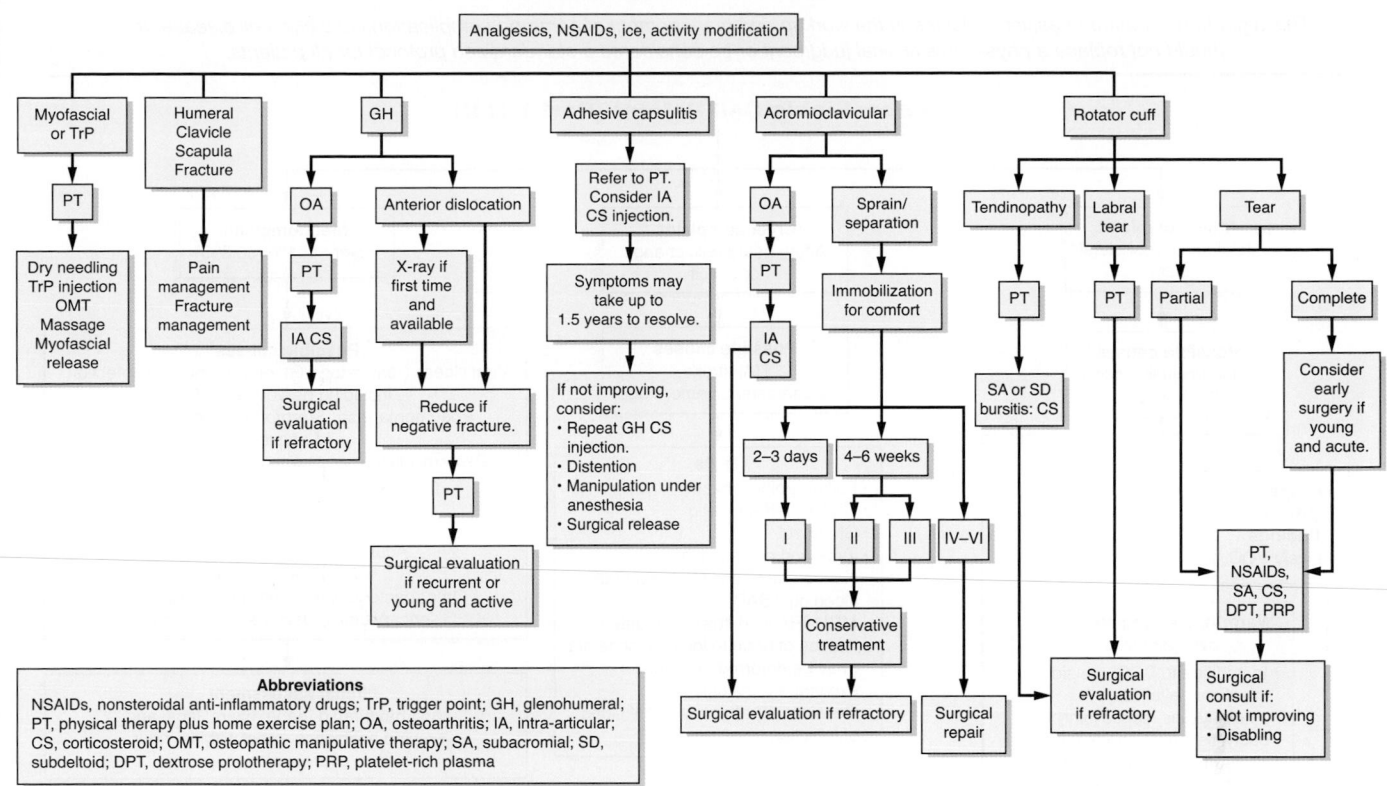

Abbreviations

NSAIDs, nonsteroidal anti-inflammatory drugs; TrP, trigger point; GH, glenohumeral; PT, physical therapy plus home exercise plan; OA, osteoarthritis; IA, intra-articular; CS, corticosteroid; OMT, osteopathic manipulative therapy; SA, subacromial; SD, subdeltoid; DPT, dextrose prolotherapy; PRP, platelet-rich plasma

Shane L. Larson, MD, Blair Rhodehouse, DO, ATC, and Adriel G. Dizon, MD

Cotter EJ, Hannon CP, Christian D, et al. Comprehensive examination of the athlete's shoulder. *Sports Health*. 2018;10(4):366–375.

SICKLE CELL ANEMIA, ACUTE, EVALUATION AND MANAGEMENT

This algorithm is meant to assist clinicians in the workup and management of common complications of sickle cell disease. It should not replace a physician's clinical judgment or be considered a standardized protocol for all patients.

Known Sickle Cell Patient (Part I of II)

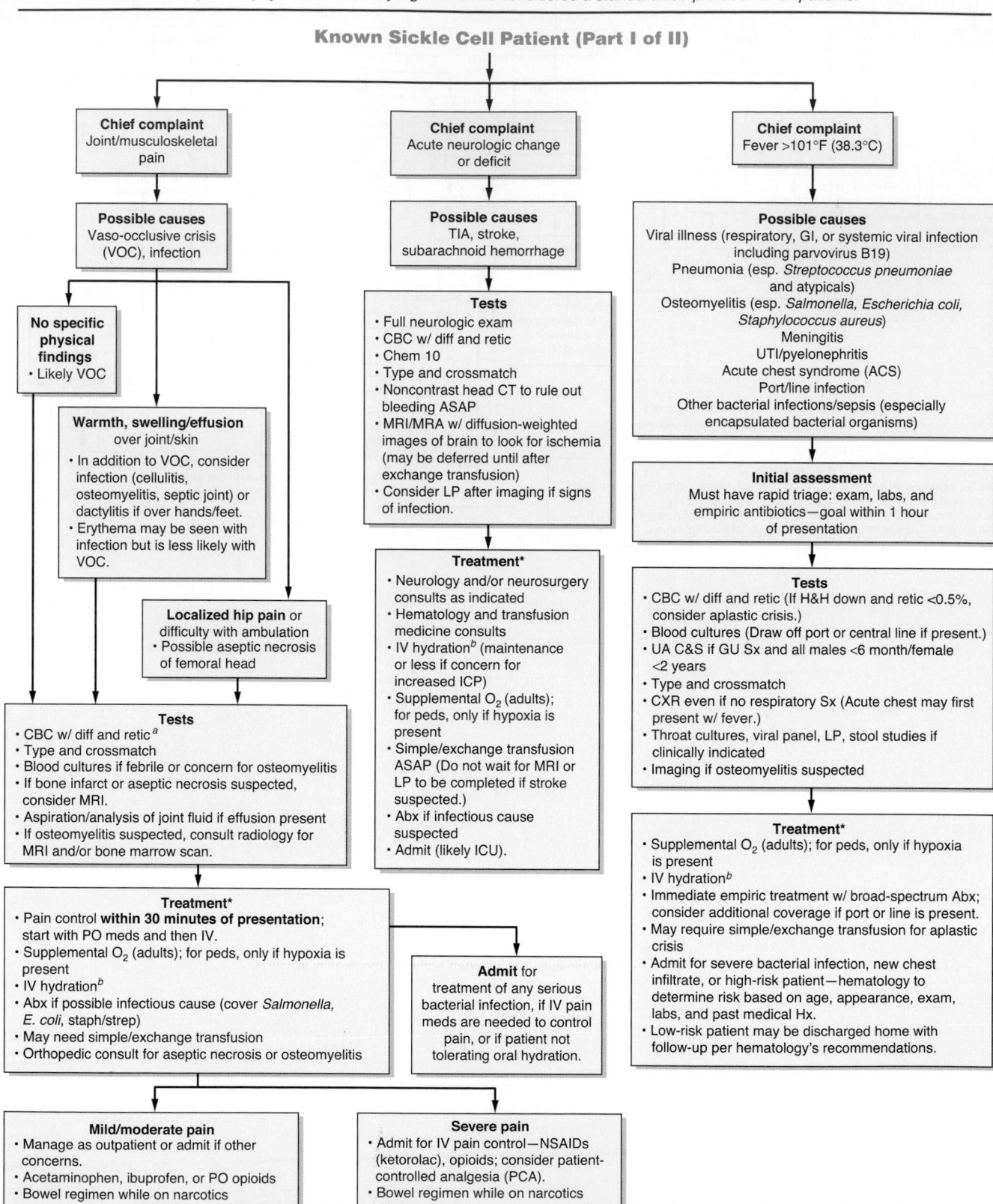

Chief complaint
Joint/musculoskeletal pain

Possible causes
Vaso-occlusive crisis (VOC), infection

No specific physical findings
· Likely VOC

Warmth, swelling/effusion over joint/skin
· In addition to VOC, consider infection (cellulitis, osteomyelitis, septic joint) or dactylitis if over hands/feet.
· Erythema may be seen with infection but is less likely with VOC.

Localized hip pain or difficulty with ambulation
· Possible aseptic necrosis of femoral head

Tests
· CBC w/ diff and retic[a]
· Type and crossmatch
· Blood cultures if febrile or concern for osteomyelitis
· If bone infarct or aseptic necrosis suspected, consider MRI.
· Aspiration/analysis of joint fluid if effusion present
· If osteomyelitis suspected, consult radiology for MRI and/or bone marrow scan.

Treatment*
· Pain control **within 30 minutes of presentation;** start with PO meds and then IV.
· Supplemental O_2 (adults); for peds, only if hypoxia is present
· IV hydration[b]
· Abx if possible infectious cause (cover *Salmonella, E. coli,* staph/strep)
· May need simple/exchange transfusion
· Orthopedic consult for aseptic necrosis or osteomyelitis

Mild/moderate pain
· Manage as outpatient or admit if other concerns.
· Acetaminophen, ibuprofen, or PO opioids
· Bowel regimen while on narcotics

Severe pain
· Admit for IV pain control—NSAIDs (ketorolac), opioids; consider patient-controlled analgesia (PCA).
· Bowel regimen while on narcotics

Chief complaint
Acute neurologic change or deficit

Possible causes
TIA, stroke, subarachnoid hemorrhage

Tests
· Full neurologic exam
· CBC w/ diff and retic
· Chem 10
· Type and crossmatch
· Noncontrast head CT to rule out bleeding ASAP
· MRI/MRA w/ diffusion-weighted images of brain to look for ischemia (may be deferred until after exchange transfusion)
· Consider LP after imaging if signs of infection.

Treatment*
· Neurology and/or neurosurgery consults as indicated
· Hematology and transfusion medicine consults
· IV hydration[b] (maintenance or less if concern for increased ICP)
· Supplemental O_2 (adults); for peds, only if hypoxia is present
· Simple/exchange transfusion ASAP (Do not wait for MRI or LP to be completed if stroke suspected.)
· Abx if infectious cause suspected
· Admit (likely ICU).

Admit for treatment of any serious bacterial infection, if IV pain meds are needed to control pain, or if patient not tolerating oral hydration.

Chief complaint
Fever >101°F (38.3°C)

Possible causes
Viral illness (respiratory, GI, or systemic viral infection including parvovirus B19)
Pneumonia (esp. *Streptococcus pneumoniae* and atypicals)
Osteomyelitis (esp. *Salmonella, Escherichia coli, Staphylococcus aureus*)
Meningitis
UTI/pyelonephritis
Acute chest syndrome (ACS)
Port/line infection
Other bacterial infections/sepsis (especially encapsulated bacterial organisms)

Initial assessment
Must have rapid triage: exam, labs, and empiric antibiotics—goal within 1 hour of presentation

Tests
· CBC w/ diff and retic (If H&H down and retic <0.5%, consider aplastic crisis.)
· Blood cultures (Draw off port or central line if present.)
· UA C&S if GU Sx and all males <6 month/female <2 years
· Type and crossmatch
· CXR even if no respiratory Sx (Acute chest may first present w/ fever.)
· Throat cultures, viral panel, LP, stool studies if clinically indicated
· Imaging if osteomyelitis suspected

Treatment*
· Supplemental O_2 (adults); for peds, only if hypoxia is present
· IV hydration[b]
· Immediate empiric treatment w/ broad-spectrum Abx; consider additional coverage if port or line is present.
· May require simple/exchange transfusion for aplastic crisis
· Admit for severe bacterial infection, new chest infiltrate, or high-risk patient—hematology to determine risk based on age, appearance, exam, labs, and past medical Hx.
· Low-risk patient may be discharged home with follow-up per hematology's recommendations.

Known Sickle Cell Patient (Part II of II)

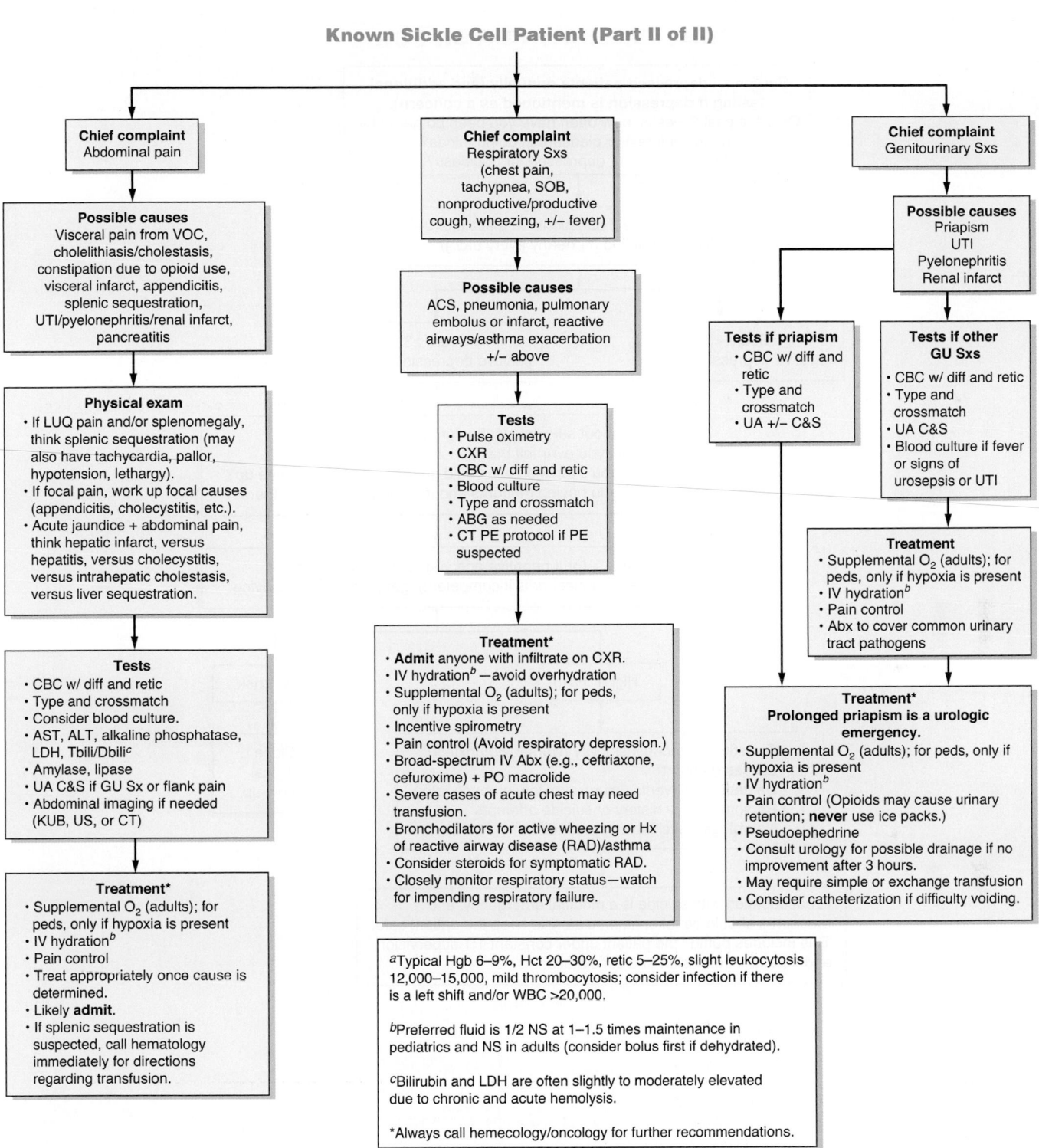

Chief complaint
Abdominal pain

Possible causes
Visceral pain from VOC, cholelithiasis/cholestasis, constipation due to opioid use, visceral infarct, appendicitis, splenic sequestration, UTI/pyelonephritis/renal infarct, pancreatitis

Physical exam
- If LUQ pain and/or splenomegaly, think splenic sequestration (may also have tachycardia, pallor, hypotension, lethargy).
- If focal pain, work up focal causes (appendicitis, cholecystitis, etc.).
- Acute jaundice + abdominal pain, think hepatic infarct, versus hepatitis, versus cholecystitis, versus intrahepatic cholestasis, versus liver sequestration.

Tests
- CBC w/ diff and retic
- Type and crossmatch
- Consider blood culture.
- AST, ALT, alkaline phosphatase, LDH, Tbili/Dbili[c]
- Amylase, lipase
- UA C&S if GU Sx or flank pain
- Abdominal imaging if needed (KUB, US, or CT)

Treatment*
- Supplemental O_2 (adults); for peds, only if hypoxia is present
- IV hydration[b]
- Pain control
- Treat appropriately once cause is determined.
- Likely **admit**.
- If splenic sequestration is suspected, call hematology immediately for directions regarding transfusion.

Chief complaint
Respiratory Sxs (chest pain, tachypnea, SOB, nonproductive/productive cough, wheezing, +/– fever)

Possible causes
ACS, pneumonia, pulmonary embolus or infarct, reactive airways/asthma exacerbation +/– above

Tests
- Pulse oximetry
- CXR
- CBC w/ diff and retic
- Blood culture
- Type and crossmatch
- ABG as needed
- CT PE protocol if PE suspected

Treatment*
- **Admit** anyone with infiltrate on CXR.
- IV hydration[b] —avoid overhydration
- Supplemental O_2 (adults); for peds, only if hypoxia is present
- Incentive spirometry
- Pain control (Avoid respiratory depression.)
- Broad-spectrum IV Abx (e.g., ceftriaxone, cefuroxime) + PO macrolide
- Severe cases of acute chest may need transfusion.
- Bronchodilators for active wheezing or Hx of reactive airway disease (RAD)/asthma
- Consider steroids for symptomatic RAD.
- Closely monitor respiratory status—watch for impending respiratory failure.

Chief complaint
Genitourinary Sxs

Possible causes
Priapism
UTI
Pyelonephritis
Renal infarct

Tests if priapism
- CBC w/ diff and retic
- Type and crossmatch
- UA +/– C&S

Tests if other GU Sxs
- CBC w/ diff and retic
- Type and crossmatch
- UA C&S
- Blood culture if fever or signs of urosepsis or UTI

Treatment
- Supplemental O_2 (adults); for peds, only if hypoxia is present
- IV hydration[b]
- Pain control
- Abx to cover common urinary tract pathogens

Treatment*
Prolonged priapism is a urologic emergency.
- Supplemental O_2 (adults); for peds, only if hypoxia is present
- IV hydration[b]
- Pain control (Opioids may cause urinary retention; **never** use ice packs.)
- Pseudoephedrine
- Consult urology for possible drainage if no improvement after 3 hours.
- May require simple or exchange transfusion
- Consider catheterization if difficulty voiding.

[a]Typical Hgb 6–9%, Hct 20–30%, retic 5–25%, slight leukocytosis 12,000–15,000, mild thrombocytosis; consider infection if there is a left shift and/or WBC >20,000.

[b]Preferred fluid is 1/2 NS at 1–1.5 times maintenance in pediatrics and NS in adults (consider bolus first if dehydrated).

[c]Bilirubin and LDH are often slightly to moderately elevated due to chronic and acute hemolysis.

*Always call hemecology/oncology for further recommendations.

Efstathia Choros, MD, CPA and Paul E. Daniel Jr., MD

New England Pediatric Sickle Cell Consortium. Clinical practice guidelines. http://www.nepscc.org/nepscc.html. Accessed November 25, 2016.

SUICIDE, EVALUATING RISK FOR

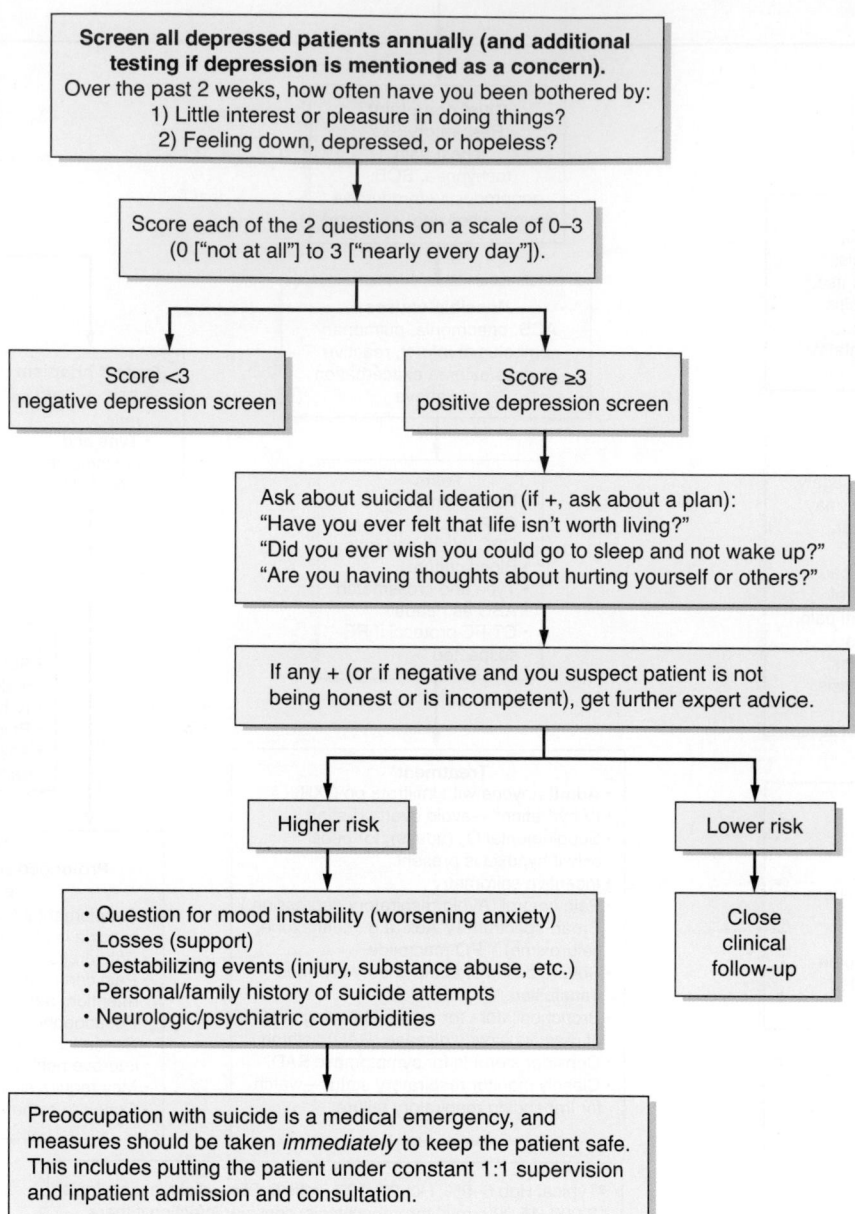

Screen all depressed patients annually (and additional testing if depression is mentioned as a concern).
Over the past 2 weeks, how often have you been bothered by:
1) Little interest or pleasure in doing things?
2) Feeling down, depressed, or hopeless?

Score each of the 2 questions on a scale of 0–3 (0 ["not at all"] to 3 ["nearly every day"]).

Score <3 negative depression screen

Score ≥3 positive depression screen

Ask about suicidal ideation (if +, ask about a plan):
"Have you ever felt that life isn't worth living?"
"Did you ever wish you could go to sleep and not wake up?"
"Are you having thoughts about hurting yourself or others?"

If any + (or if negative and you suspect patient is not being honest or is incompetent), get further expert advice.

Higher risk

Lower risk

• Question for mood instability (worsening anxiety)
• Losses (support)
• Destabilizing events (injury, substance abuse, etc.)
• Personal/family history of suicide attempts
• Neurologic/psychiatric comorbidities

Close clinical follow-up

Preoccupation with suicide is a medical emergency, and measures should be taken *immediately* to keep the patient safe. This includes putting the patient under constant 1:1 supervision and inpatient admission and consultation.

Irene Coletsos, MD and Harold J. Bursztajn, MD

Posner K, Oquendo MA, Gould M, et al. Columbia Classification Algorithm of Suicide Assessment (C-CASA): classification of suicidal events in the FDA's pediatric suicidal risk analysis of antidepressants. *Am J Psychiatry.* 2007;164(7):1035–1043.

SYNCOPE

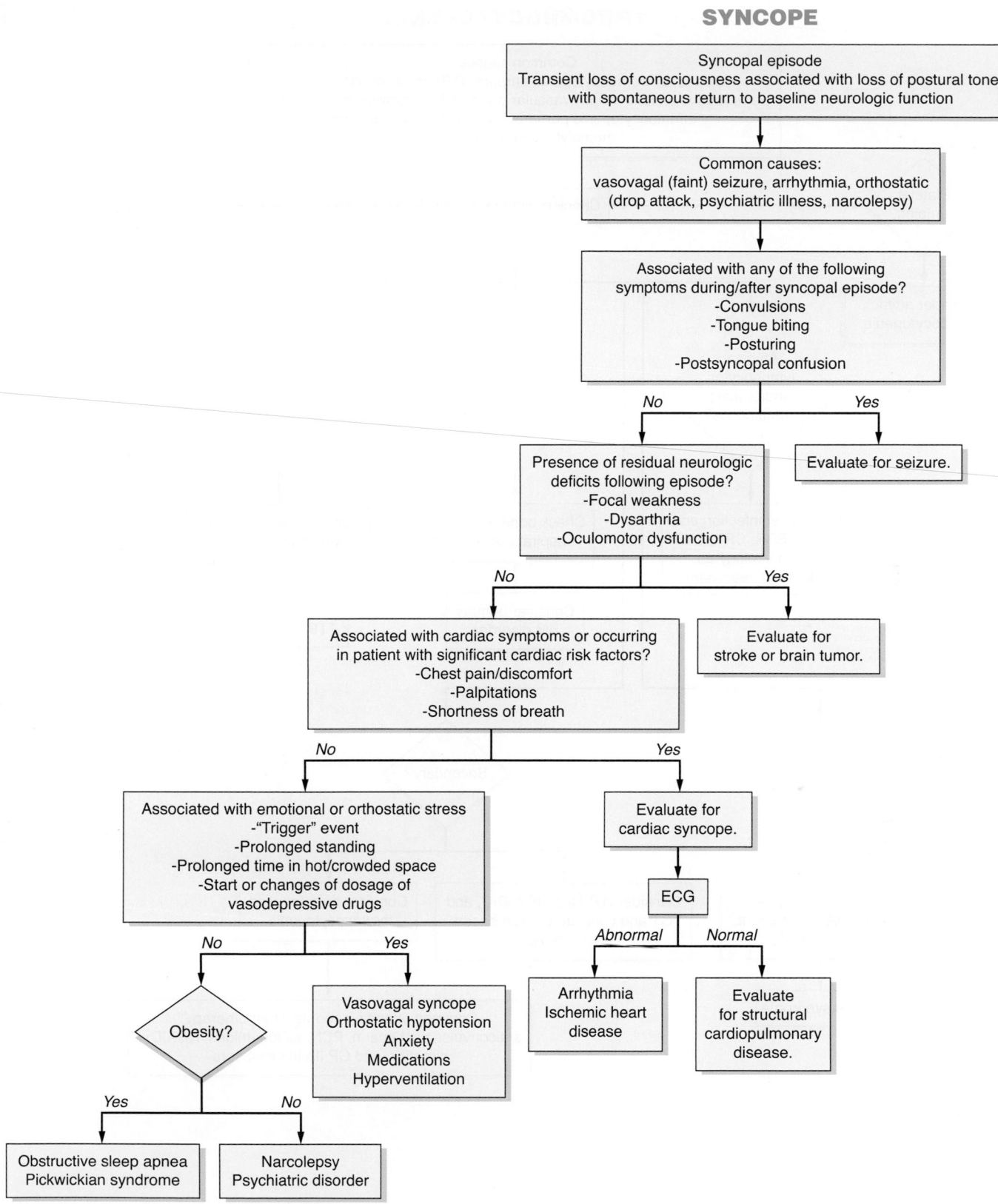

David Toomey, MD and Frank J. Domino, MD

Runser LA, Gauer RL, Houser A. Syncope: evaluation and differential diagnosis. *Am Fam Physician*. 2017;95(5):303–312.

THROMBOCYTOPENIA

Common causes:
idiopathic thrombocytopenic purpura (ITP), medications, DIC, pernicious anemia, collagen vascular disease, hypersplenism, thrombotic thrombocytopenic purpura (TTP), ICU patient/sepsis hemolytic uremic syndrome

Check peripheral smear.

Platelet clumping?
→ Consider artifact thrombocytopenia.

Giant platelets?
→ Consider hereditary thrombocytopenia.

Atypical lymphocytes and/or toxic granulations?
→ Consider infection and check ESR, CRP, CXR, and virology as deemed necessary.

Blasts, nucleated RBCs, or Pelger-Huet?
→ Check bone marrow aspirate or Bx.
→ Consider primary BM disorder.

Are there schistocytes?
→ Check LDH, bilirubin, haptoglobin, coags, D-dimer, and fibrinogen.
→ TTP/HUS or DIC

Spherocytes?
→ Confirm hemolysis: positive DAT, retic count, LDH, and nili.
→ Evans syndrome

Secondary?
→ Consider ITP, HIV, HCV, DIC, and GT and continue workup based on history.
→ Consider drug-induced thrombocytopenia.
→ Common offending agents: chemotherapy, anticonvulsants, heparin, PCN, sulfonamides, NSAIDs, diuretics, and GP IIb/IIIa inhibitors

Nupam A. Patel, MD and Samuel B. Carli, MD

Reese JA, Li X, Hauben M, et al. Identifying drugs that cause acute thrombocytopenia: an analysis using 3 distinct methods. *Blood*. 2010;116(12):2127–2133.

TINNITUS

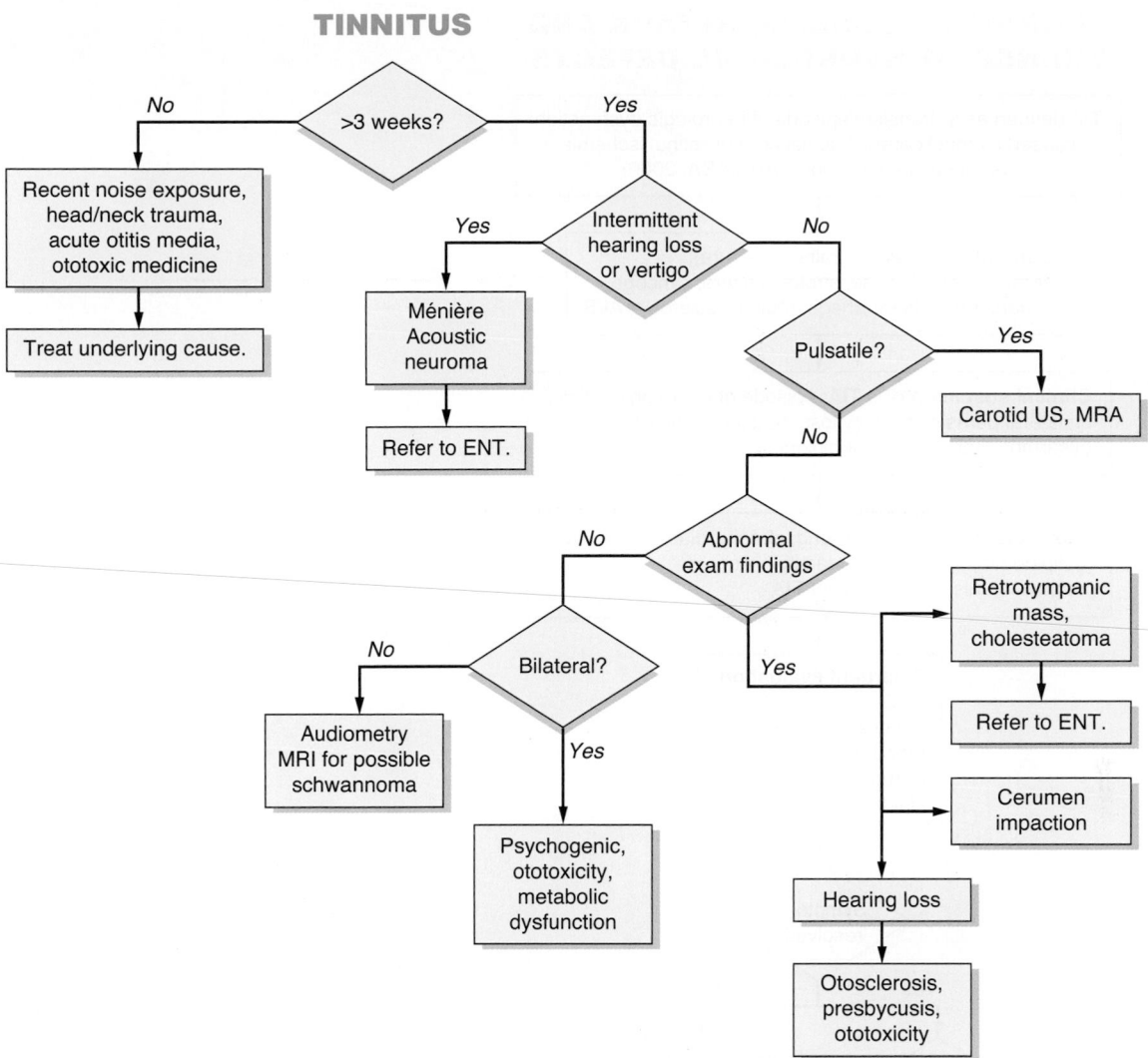

Shannon Roche, DO and Sara Casey, DO

Yew KS. Diagnostic approach to patients with tinnitus. *Am Fam Physician*. 2014;89(2):106–113.

TRANSIENT ISCHEMIC ATTACK AND TRANSIENT NEUROLOGIC DEFECTS

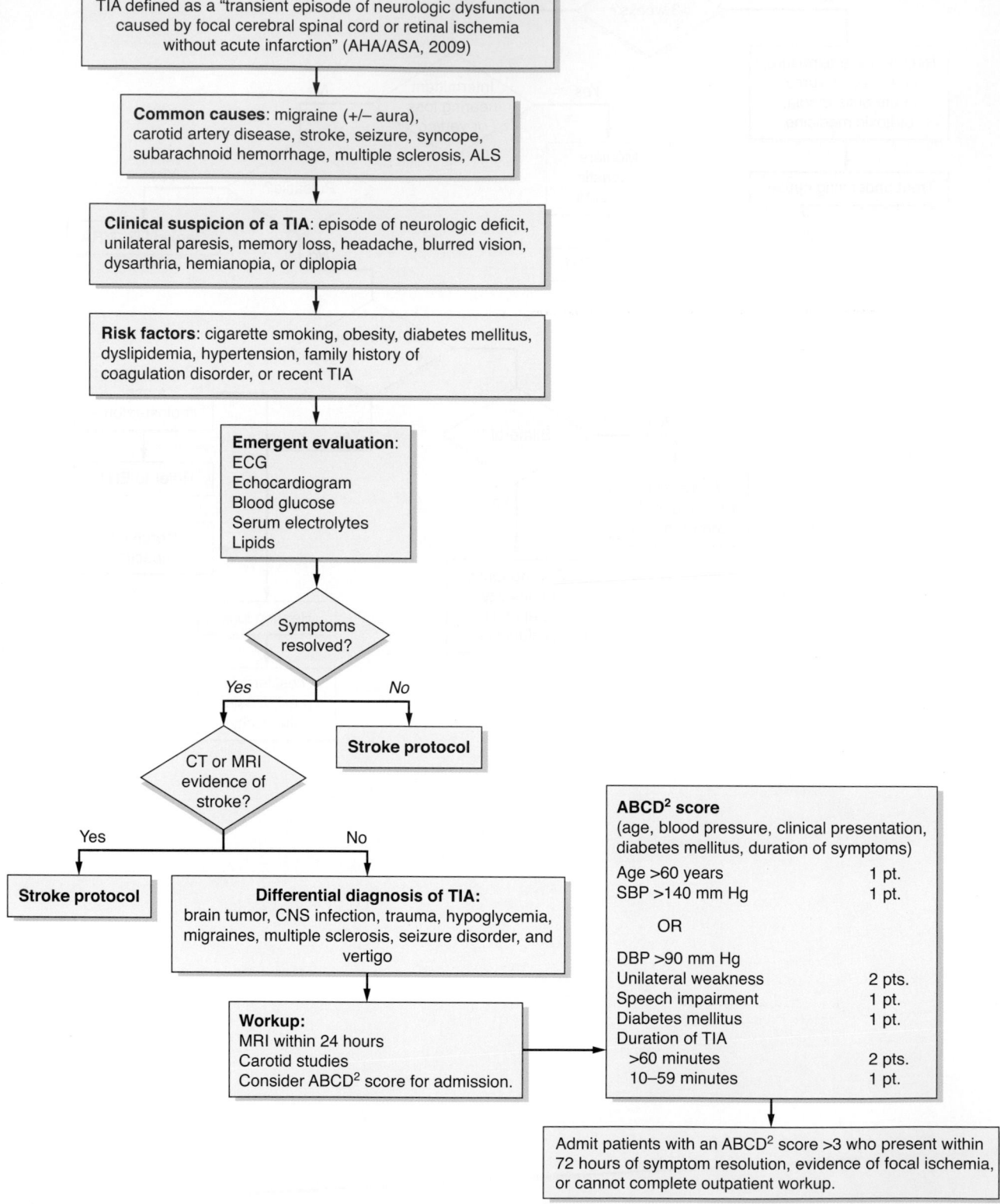

TIA defined as a "transient episode of neurologic dysfunction caused by focal cerebral spinal cord or retinal ischemia without acute infarction" (AHA/ASA, 2009)

Common causes: migraine (+/– aura), carotid artery disease, stroke, seizure, syncope, subarachnoid hemorrhage, multiple sclerosis, ALS

Clinical suspicion of a TIA: episode of neurologic deficit, unilateral paresis, memory loss, headache, blurred vision, dysarthria, hemianopia, or diplopia

Risk factors: cigarette smoking, obesity, diabetes mellitus, dyslipidemia, hypertension, family history of coagulation disorder, or recent TIA

Emergent evaluation:
ECG
Echocardiogram
Blood glucose
Serum electrolytes
Lipids

Symptoms resolved?

Yes — *No*

Stroke protocol

CT or MRI evidence of stroke?

Yes — No

Stroke protocol

Differential diagnosis of TIA: brain tumor, CNS infection, trauma, hypoglycemia, migraines, multiple sclerosis, seizure disorder, and vertigo

Workup:
MRI within 24 hours
Carotid studies
Consider ABCD^2 score for admission.

ABCD^2 score
(age, blood pressure, clinical presentation, diabetes mellitus, duration of symptoms)

Age >60 years	1 pt.
SBP >140 mm Hg	1 pt.
OR	
DBP >90 mm Hg	
Unilateral weakness	2 pts.
Speech impairment	1 pt.
Diabetes mellitus	1 pt.
Duration of TIA	
>60 minutes	2 pts.
10–59 minutes	1 pt.

Admit patients with an ABCD^2 score >3 who present within 72 hours of symptom resolution, evidence of focal ischemia, or cannot complete outpatient workup.

Deborah A. Lardner, DO, DTM&H and Michael Passafaro, DO, DTM&H, FACEP, FACOEP

Simmons BB, Cirignano B, Gadegbeku AB. Transient ischemic attack: part I. Diagnosis and evaluation. *Am Fam Physician.* 2012;86(6):521–526.

TREMOR

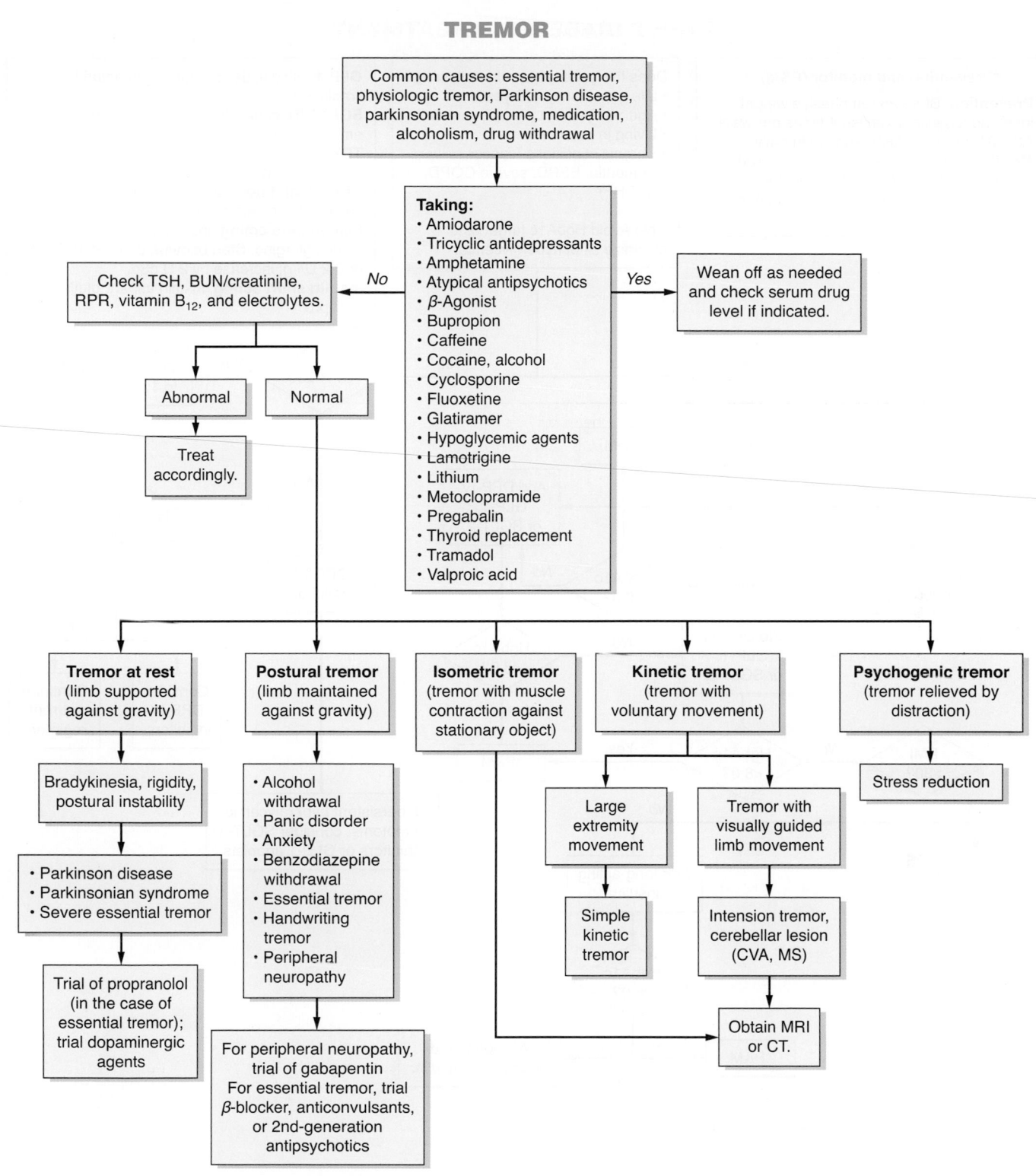

Common causes: essential tremor, physiologic tremor, Parkinson disease, parkinsonian syndrome, medication, alcoholism, drug withdrawal

Taking:
- Amiodarone
- Tricyclic antidepressants
- Amphetamine
- Atypical antipsychotics
- β-Agonist
- Bupropion
- Caffeine
- Cocaine, alcohol
- Cyclosporine
- Fluoxetine
- Glatiramer
- Hypoglycemic agents
- Lamotrigine
- Lithium
- Metoclopramide
- Pregabalin
- Thyroid replacement
- Tramadol
- Valproic acid

No → Check TSH, BUN/creatinine, RPR, vitamin B₁₂, and electrolytes.

Yes → Wean off as needed and check serum drug level if indicated.

Abnormal → Treat accordingly.

Normal

Tremor at rest (limb supported against gravity)

Bradykinesia, rigidity, postural instability

- Parkinson disease
- Parkinsonian syndrome
- Severe essential tremor

Trial of propranolol (in the case of essential tremor); trial dopaminergic agents

Postural tremor (limb maintained against gravity)

- Alcohol withdrawal
- Panic disorder
- Anxiety
- Benzodiazepine withdrawal
- Essential tremor
- Handwriting tremor
- Peripheral neuropathy

For peripheral neuropathy, trial of gabapentin
For essential tremor, trial β-blocker, anticonvulsants, or 2nd-generation antipsychotics

Isometric tremor (tremor with muscle contraction against stationary object)

Kinetic tremor (tremor with voluntary movement)

Large extremity movement → Simple kinetic tremor

Tremor with visually guided limb movement → Intension tremor, cerebellar lesion (CVA, MS)

Obtain MRI or CT.

Psychogenic tremor (tremor relieved by distraction)

Stress reduction

Malerie Dooling, PharmD, RPh, Steven J. Crosby, MA, BSP, RPh, FASCP, and Ildiko Halasz, MD

Crawford P, Zimmerman EE. Differentiation and diagnosis of tremor. *Am Fam Physician*. 2011;83(6):697–702.

TYPE 2 DIABETES, TREATMENT

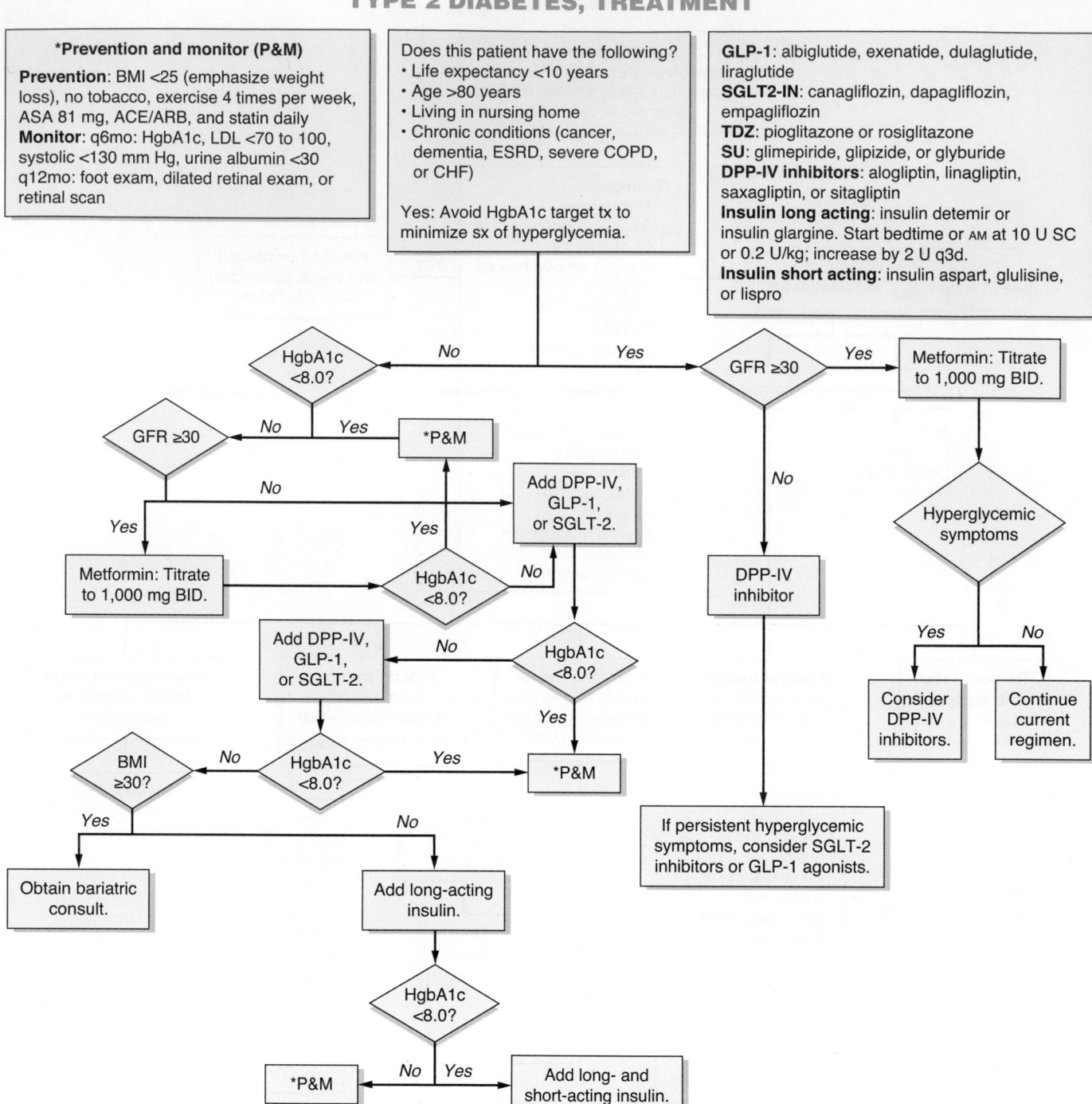

*Prevention and monitor (P&M)

Prevention: BMI <25 (emphasize weight loss), no tobacco, exercise 4 times per week, ASA 81 mg, ACE/ARB, and statin daily
Monitor: q6mo: HgbA1c, LDL <70 to 100, systolic <130 mm Hg, urine albumin <30 q12mo: foot exam, dilated retinal exam, or retinal scan

Does this patient have the following?
• Life expectancy <10 years
• Age >80 years
• Living in nursing home
• Chronic conditions (cancer, dementia, ESRD, severe COPD, or CHF)

Yes: Avoid HgbA1c target tx to minimize sx of hyperglycemia.

GLP-1: albiglutide, exenatide, dulaglutide, liraglutide
SGLT2-IN: canagliflozin, dapagliflozin, empagliflozin
TDZ: pioglitazone or rosiglitazone
SU: glimepiride, glipizide, or glyburide
DPP-IV inhibitors: alogliptin, linagliptin, saxagliptin, or sitagliptin
Insulin long acting: insulin detemir or insulin glargine. Start bedtime or AM at 10 U SC or 0.2 U/kg; increase by 2 U q3d.
Insulin short acting: insulin aspart, glulisine, or lispro

Frank J. Domino, MD and Jasleen Kaur, MD

Qaseem A, Wilt TJ, Kansagara D, et al. Hemoglobin A1c targets for glycemic control with pharmacologic therapy for nonpregnant adults with type 2 diabetes mellitus: a guidance statement updated from the American College of Physicians. *Ann Intern Med.* 2018;168(8):569–576.

VAGINAL BLEEDING, ABNORMAL

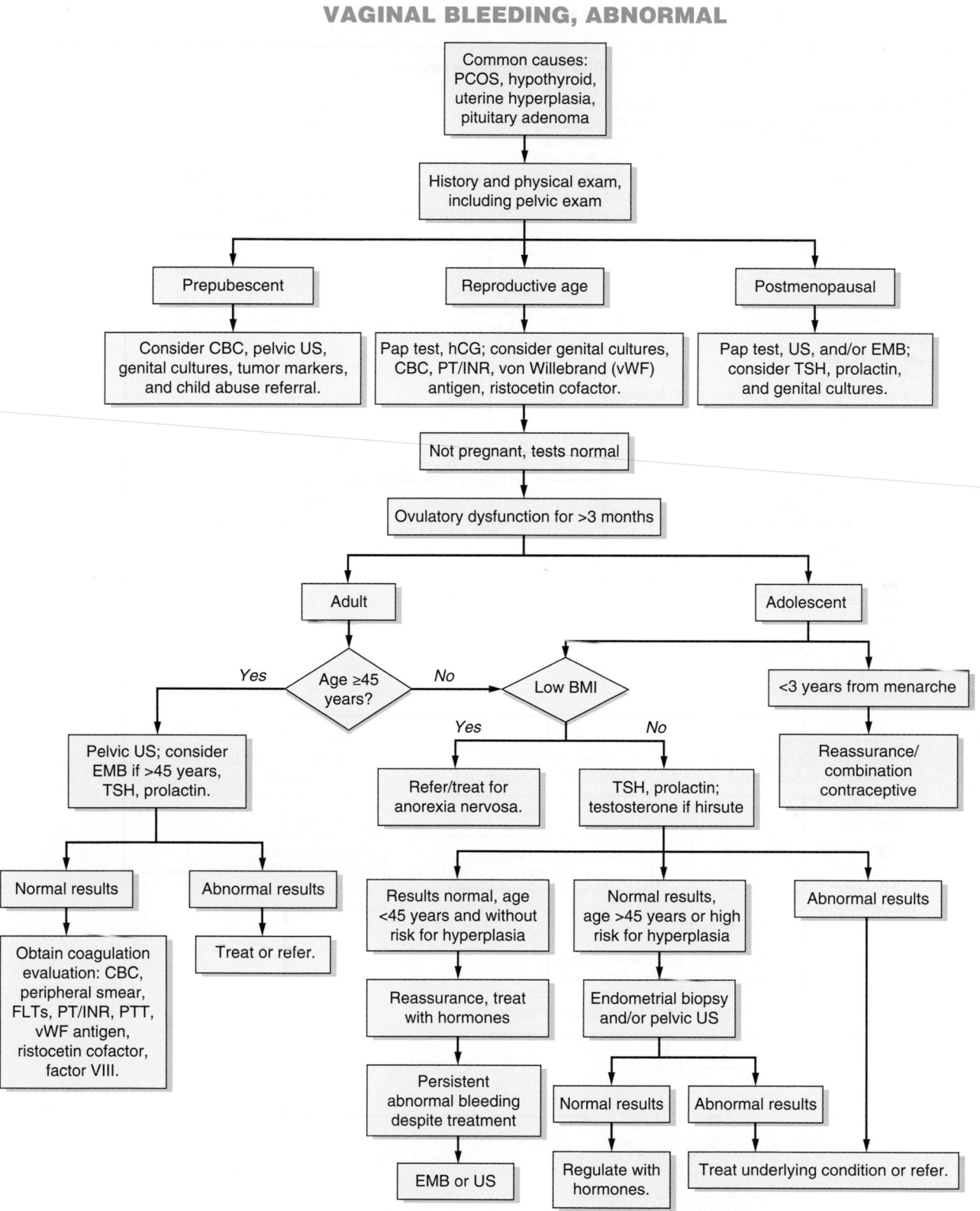

Common causes: PCOS, hypothyroid, uterine hyperplasia, pituitary adenoma

History and physical exam, including pelvic exam

Prepubescent
Consider CBC, pelvic US, genital cultures, tumor markers, and child abuse referral.

Reproductive age
Pap test, hCG; consider genital cultures, CBC, PT/INR, von Willebrand (vWF) antigen, ristocetin cofactor.

Postmenopausal
Pap test, US, and/or EMB; consider TSH, prolactin, and genital cultures.

Not pregnant, tests normal

Ovulatory dysfunction for >3 months

Adult

Adolescent

Age ≥45 years? — *Yes* / *No*

Low BMI — *Yes* / *No*

<3 years from menarche

Reassurance/ combination contraceptive

Pelvic US; consider EMB if >45 years, TSH, prolactin.

Refer/treat for anorexia nervosa.

TSH, prolactin; testosterone if hirsute

Normal results

Abnormal results

Results normal, age <45 years and without risk for hyperplasia

Normal results, age >45 years or high risk for hyperplasia

Abnormal results

Obtain coagulation evaluation: CBC, peripheral smear, FLTs, PT/INR, PTT, vWF antigen, ristocetin cofactor, factor VIII.

Treat or refer.

Reassurance, treat with hormones

Endometrial biopsy and/or pelvic US

Persistent abnormal bleeding despite treatment

Normal results

Abnormal results

EMB or US

Regulate with hormones.

Treat underlying condition or refer.

Ann Klega, MD, Tanya E. Anim, MD, and Jennifer Tickal Keehbauch, MD, FAAFP

Munro MG, Critchley HO, Broder MS, et al; for FIGO Working Group on Menstrual Disorders. FIGO classification system (PALM-COEIN) for causes of abnormal uterine bleeding in nongravid women of reproductive age. *Int J Gynaecol Obstet.* 2011;113(1):3–13.

VITAMIN D DEFICIENCY

Risk factors/common causes:

- Age >65 years
- Insufficient sunlight exposure (homebound, veiled)
- Renal disease
- Liver disease
- Depression

- Dark skin
- Insufficient dietary intake
- GI malabsorption
- Obesity (BMI >30)
- Immigrants to colder climates
- Chronic use of glucocorticoids
- Periosteal bone pain (e.g., sternum, tibia)

- GI malabsorption (celiac, cystic fibrosis, inflammatory bowel disease)
- Pregnancy
- Medications: anticonvulsants, antiretroviral, and glucocorticoids
- Gastrectomy or extensive bowel surgery

Significant risk factors?

No → Low suspicion for vitamin D deficiency

Yes

Requirements:
<1 year old: 400 IU/day
>1 year old: 600 IU/day
To reach levels >30 ng/mL, may require 1,000 IU/day
Obese children: 2–3 times more vitamin D for their age group
Maintenance dose:
0–6 months: 1,000–2,000 IU/day
6 months–1 year: 1,500–2,000 IU/day
1–3 years: 2,500–4,000 IU/day
4–8 years: 3,000–4,000 IU/day
>8 years: 4,000 IU/day
Vitamin D deficiency:
0–1 year: 2,000 IU/day for 6 weeks or 50,000 IU weekly for 6 weeks followed by maintenance 400–1,000 IU/day
1–18 years: 2,000 IU/day for 6 weeks or 50,000 IU weekly for 6 weeks followed by maintenance 600–1,000 IU/day

Age <18 years?

Yes ←   → No

Lab: serum 25-hydroxyvitamin D concentration

Level <20 ng/mL (vitamin D deficiency)

Level <21–29 ng/mL (vitamin D insufficiency)

Level >30 ng/mL normal

Treatment

Start 50,000 IU D2 once a week for 8–12 weeks and then begin 2,000–4,000 IU vitamin D per day.

Treatment

2,000–4,000 IU vitamin D per day

Maintenance

Supplement with 600–4,000 IU of vitamin D per day.

After 6 months, consider repeating serum 25-hydroxyvitamin D level.

Recheck serum 25-hydroxyvitamin D concentration.

Level <20 ng/mL?

No →

Yes

Consult endocrinology if no malabsorptive disease.

Gisela M. Lopez Payares, MD, Carla M. Basadre Quiroz, MD, and Fozia Akhtar Ali, MD

Holick MF, Binkley NC, Bischoff-Ferrari HA, et al. Evaluation, treatment, and prevention of vitamin D deficiency: an Endocrine Society clinical practice guideline. *J Clin Endocrinol Metab.* 2011;96(7):1911–1930.

WEIGHT LOSS, UNINTENTIONAL

Weight loss, unintentional, >5% over last 6 months

Common causes: hyperthyroid, TB, celiac disease, cancer, dentition

Adequate food intake? 25–30 kcal/kg/day

Yes

Increased expenditure

Fever
Sweats
Tachycardia
Tremors

TSH
Glucose
PPD
CBC with diff
ESR/CRP
HIV

Endocrine
Hyperthyroidism
Diabetes
Infectious
HIV
Tuberculosis
Chronic disease
Cardiac
Pulmonary
Renal
Malignancy
(lymphoma,
leukemia, and
solid tumor)
**Increased
activity level**

Increased loss

Chronic diarrhea/ loose stools

Malabsorption

• Anti-transglutaminase
• Antiendomysium
• Fecal fat study
• Stool O&P
• Upper GI endoscopy
• Colonoscopy
If all negative,
check the following:
• Upper GI/barium
follow-through
• Endoscopic capsule

Celiac disease
Pancreatic insufficiency
Giardia
Inflammatory bowel disease
Whipple disease
GI resections or bypasses

No

Food available?

Yes

Difficulty ingesting food?

Loss of appetite?

Psych?

Mood instability
Distorted body image

Depression
Anxiety
Bulimia
Anorexia

Drugs?

Polypharmacy
Fluoxetine
Alcohol
Amphetamines
Cocaine
Opiates
Topiramate

No

Social evaluation

Financial issues
Inability to obtain
preferred foods

Oral?

Poorly
fitting
dentures
Poor
dentition
Periodontal
disease
Xerostomia

GI?

Dysphagia
Odynophagia
Vomiting
Abdominal pain
Distention
Constipation

Upper GI endoscopy
Esophageal
manometry
Upper GI series
Occult fecal blood
Barium enema
Colonoscopy

Cancer
Peptic stricture
Caustic stricture
Esophageal diverticula
Extrinsic compression
Gastric volvulus
Inflammatory bowel disease

Neuro?

Memory
loss
Cognitive
impairment
Sensory/motor
deficit

CNS
imaging

Dementia
Alzheimer
Parkinson
Stroke

Crystal Nwagwu, MD and Fozia Akhtar Ali, MD

Gaddey HL, Holder K. Unintentional weight loss in older adults. *Am Fam Physician*. 2014;89(9):718–722.

ABNORMAL (DYSFUNCTIONAL) UTERINE BLEEDING

Rebecca Lauters, MD • Corey Sadler, MD

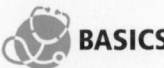

BASICS

DESCRIPTION
- Abnormal uterine bleeding (AUB) is irregular menstrual bleeding (usually heavy, prolonged, or frequent); it is a diagnosis of exclusion after establishment of normal anatomy and the absence of other medical illnesses and pregnancy.
- May be acute or chronic (occurring >6 months)
- The International Federation of Gynecology and Obstetrics (FIGO) revised the terminology system and now uses AUB rather than dysfunctional uterine bleeding (DUB).
- Commonly associated with anovulation

EPIDEMIOLOGY
Adolescent and perimenopausal women are affected most often.

Incidence
5% of reproductive-aged women will see a doctor in any given year for AUB.

Prevalence
10–30% of reproductive-aged women have AUB.

ETIOLOGY AND PATHOPHYSIOLOGY
- Anovulation accounts for 90% of AUB.
  - Loss of cyclic endometrial stimulation
  - Elevated estrogen levels stimulate endometrial growth.
  - No organized progesterone withdrawal bleeding
  - Endometrium eventually outgrows blood supply, breaks down, and sloughs from uterus.
  - 6–10% will have polycystic ovarian syndrome (PCOS).
- Adolescent AUB is usually due to an immature hypothalamic-pituitary-ovarian (HPO) axis that leads to anovulatory cycles.
- The mnemonic PALM-COEIN was developed as the new nomenclature to describe AUB in reproductive-aged women.
- PALM describes structural causes of AUB, and COEIN describes nonstructural causes of AUB.
  - PALM: polyp, adenomyosis, leiomyoma, and malignancy and/or hyperplasia
  - COEIN: coagulopathy, ovulatory disorders, endometrial, iatrogenic, and not yet classified
  - Reproductive pathology and structural disorders
    o Uterus: leiomyomas, endometritis, hyperplasia, polyps, trauma
    o Adnexa: salpingitis, functional ovarian cysts
    o Cervix: cervicitis, polyps, STIs, trauma
    o Vagina: trauma, foreign body
    o Vulva: lichen sclerosus, STIs
- Malignancy of the vagina, cervix, uterus, and ovaries
- Systemic diseases
  - Hematologic disorders (e.g., von Willebrand disease, thrombocytopenia)
- Diseases causing anovulation
  - Hyperthyroidism/hypothyroidism
  - Adrenal disorders
  - Pituitary disease (prolactinoma)
  - PCOS
  - Eating disorders
- Medications (iatrogenic causes)
  - Anticoagulants
  - Steroids
  - Tamoxifen
  - Hormonal medications: intrauterine devices (IUDs)
  - Selective serotonin reuptake inhibitors (SSRIs)
  - Antipsychotic medications
  - Postmenopausal hormone therapy

- Other causes of AUB not defined in PALM-COEIN
  - Pregnancy: ectopic pregnancy, threatened or incomplete abortion, or hydatidiform mole
  - Advanced or fulminant liver disease
  - Chronic renal disease
  - Inflammatory bowel disease
  - Excessive weight gain
  - Increased exercise

Genetics
Unclear but can include inherited disorders of hemostasis

RISK FACTORS
Risk factors for endometrial cancer (which can cause AUB)
- Age >40 years
- Obesity
- PCOS
- Diabetes mellitus
- Nulliparity
- Early menarche or late menopause (>55 years of age)
- Hypertension
- Chronic anovulation or infertility
- Unopposed estrogen therapy
- History of breast cancer or endometrial hyperplasia
- Tamoxifen use
- Family history: gynecologic, breast, or colon cancer
- Thyroid disease

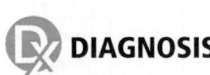

DIAGNOSIS

HISTORY
- Menstrual history
  - Onset, severity (quantified by pad/tampon use, presence and size of clots), timing of bleeding (unpredictable or episodic)
  - Menorrhagia with onset of menarche is suggestive of a coagulation disorder.
  - Menopausal status
  - Association with other factors (e.g., coitus, contraception, weight loss/gain)
- Gynecologic history: gravidity and parity, STI history, previous Pap smear results
- Review of systems (Exclude symptoms of pregnancy and of bleeding disorders, stress, exercise, recent weight change, visual changes, headaches, galactorrhea.)
- Medication history: Evaluate for use of aspirin, anticoagulants, hormones, and herbal supplements (1,2).

ALERT
Postmenopausal bleeding is any bleeding that occurs >1 year after the last menstrual period; cancer must always be ruled out (2)[C].

PHYSICAL EXAM
Discover anatomic or organic causes of AUB.
- Evaluate for
  - Body mass index (obesity)
  - Pallor, vital signs (anemia)
  - Visual field defects (pituitary lesion)
  - Hirsutism or acne (hyperandrogenism)
  - Goiter (thyroid dysfunction)
  - Galactorrhea (hyperprolactinemia)
  - Purpura, ecchymosis (bleeding disorders)
- Pelvic exam
  - Evaluate for uterine irregularities and Tanner stage.
  - Check for foreign bodies.
  - Rule out rectal or urinary tract bleeding.
  - Include Pap smear and tests for STIs (2)[C].

Pediatric Considerations
Premenarchal children with vaginal bleeding should be evaluated for foreign bodies, physical/sexual abuse, possible infections, and signs of precocious puberty.

DIFFERENTIAL DIAGNOSIS
See "Etiology and Pathophysiology."

DIAGNOSTIC TESTS & INTERPRETATION

Initial Tests (lab, imaging)
- Everyone: urine human chorionic gonadotropin (hCG; rule out pregnancy and/or hydatidiform mole) and complete blood count (CBC) (1)
  - For acute bleeding, a type and cross should be obtained (3)[C].
- If disorder of hemostasis is suspected, a partial thromboplastin time (PTT), prothrombin time (PT), activated partial thromboplastin time (aPTT), and fibrinogen level are appropriate (3)[C].
- If anovulation is suspected: thyroid-stimulating hormone (TSH) level, prolactin level (1)
- Consider other tests based on differential diagnosis.
  - Follicle-stimulating hormone (FSH) level to evaluate for hypo- or hypergonadotropism
  - 17-Hydroxyprogesterone if congenital adrenal hyperplasia is suspected
  - Testosterone and/or dehydroepiandrosterone sulfate (DHEA-S) if PCOS
  - Screening for STI
- Endometrial biopsy (EMB) should be performed as part of the initial evaluation for postmenopausal uterine bleeding and in premenopausal women with risk factors for endometrial carcinoma. Medical management can be initiated in premenopausal women with low risk for malignancy (1)[A].
- TVUS in postmenopausal AUB
  - Postmenopausal endometrial thickness (ET) <4 mm does not require endometrial sampling unless bleeding is persistent or recurrent, whereas ET >4 mm should prompt further evaluation.
  - ET <3 mm: 99.7% negative predictive value (NPV)
  - ET <5 mm: 99.6% NPV for ruling out endometrial cancer (4)
  - Incidentally found endometrial measurement >4 mm without associated bleeding in postmenopausal women should not trigger evaluation; however, assessment based on individual risk factors is appropriate.
- TVUS, sonohysterography, and hysteroscopy may be similarly effective in detection of intrauterine pathology in premenopausal women with AUB (1)[A].
- If normal findings following imaging in patients without known risk factors for endometrial carcinoma, a biopsy should be performed if not done so previously (2)[C].

Diagnostic Procedures/Other
- Pap smear to screen for cervical cancer if age >21 years (2)[C]
- EMB should be performed in
  - Women age >35 years with AUB to rule out cancer or premalignancy
  - Postmenopausal women with ET ≥5 mm
  - Women aged 18 to 35 years with AUB and risk factors for endometrial cancer (see "Risk Factors")
  - Perform on or after day 18 of cycle, if known; secretory endometrium confirms ovulation occurred.
- Dilation and curettage (D&C)
  - Perform if bleeding is heavy, uncontrolled, or if emergent medical management has failed.
  - Perform if unable to perform EMB in office (2)[C].
- Hysteroscopy if another intrauterine lesion is suspected

Test Interpretation

Pap smear could reveal carcinoma or inflammation indicative of cervicitis. Most EMBs show proliferative or dyssynchronous endometrium (suggesting anovulation) but can show simple or complex hyperplasia without atypia, hyperplasia with atypia, or endometrial adenocarcinoma.

TREATMENT

Attempt to rule out other causes of bleeding prior to instituting therapy.

GENERAL MEASURES

NSAIDs (naproxen sodium 500 mg BID, mefenamic acid 500 mg TID, ibuprofen 600 to 1,200 mg/day) (1)[B]

- Decreases amount of blood loss and pain compared with placebo, with no one NSAID clearly superior

MEDICATION

First Line

- Acute, emergent, nonovulatory bleeding
  - Conjugated equine estrogen (Premarin): 25 mg IV q4h (max 6 doses) or 2.5 mg PO q6h should control bleeding in 12 to 24 hours (5)[A].
  - D&C if no response after 2 to 4 doses of Premarin or sooner if bleeding >1 pad per hour (2)[C]
  - Then change to oral contraceptive pill (OCP) or progestin for cycle regulation, that is, IUD (6)[A]
- Acute, nonemergent, nonovulatory bleeding
  - Combination OCP with ≥30 μg estrogen given as a taper. An example of a tapered dose: 4 pills per day for 4 days; 3 pills per day for 3 days; 2 pills per day for 2 days, daily for 3 weeks then 1 week off, then cycle on OCP for at least 3 months
- Nonacute, nonovulatory bleeding (ranked in order based on decision analysis as best option based on efficacy, cost, side effects, and consumer acceptability) (6)[A]
  - Levonorgestrel IUD (Mirena) is the most effective form of progesterone delivery and is not inferior to surgical management.
  - Progestins: medroxyprogesterone acetate (Provera) 10 mg/day for 5 to 10 days each month. Daily progesterone for 21 days per cycle results in significantly less blood loss.
  - OCPs: 20 to 35 μg estrogen plus progesterone
- Do not use estrogen if contraindications, such as suspicion for endometrial hyperplasia or carcinoma, history of deep vein thrombosis (DVT), migraine with aura, or the presence of smoking in women >35 years of age (relative contraindication), are present.
- Precautions
  - Failed medical treatment requires further workup.
  - Consider DVT prophylaxis when treating with high-dose estrogens (2)[C].

Second Line

- Leuprolide (varying doses and duration of action); gonadotropin-releasing hormone (GnRH) agonist
- Danazol (200 to 400 mg/day for a maximum of 9 months) more effective than NSAIDs but limited by androgenic side effects and cost. It has been replaced by GnRH agonists.
- Antifibrinolytics such as tranexamic acid (Lysteda) 650 mg, 2 tablets TID (max 5 days during menstruation) (1)[A]
- Metformin or clomifene (Clomid) alone or in combination in women with PCOS who desire ovulation and pregnancy

ISSUES FOR REFERRAL

- If an obvious cause for vaginal bleeding is not found in a pediatric patient, refer to a pediatric endocrinologist or gynecologist.
- Patients with persistent bleeding despite medical treatment require reevaluation and possible referral.

ADDITIONAL THERAPIES

- Antiemetics if treating with high-dose estrogen or progesterone (2)[C]
- Iron supplementation with vitamin C if anemia (usually iron deficiency) is identified

SURGERY/OTHER PROCEDURES

- Hysterectomy in cases of endometrial cancer or if medical therapy fails or if other uterine pathology is found
- Endometrial ablation, less expensive than hysterectomy and associated with high patient satisfaction; failure of primary medical treatment is not necessary (1,5)[A].
  - This is a permanent procedure and should be avoided in patients who desire continued fertility.
- Uterine artery embolization if bleeding is refractory to medications or confirmed fibroids

ADMISSION, INPATIENT, AND NURSING CONSIDERATIONS

- Significant hemorrhage causing acute anemia with signs of hemodynamic instability; with acute bleeding, replace volume with crystalloid and blood, as necessary (1)[A].
- Pad counts and clot size can be helpful to determine and monitor amount of bleeding.
- Discharge criteria
  - Hemodynamic stability
  - Control of vaginal bleeding (2)[C]

ONGOING CARE

FOLLOW-UP RECOMMENDATIONS

- Once stable from acute management, recommend follow-up evaluation in 4 to 6 months for further evaluation (6).
- Routine follow-up with a primary care or OB/GYN provider

Patient Monitoring

Women treated with estrogen or OCPs should keep a menstrual diary to document bleeding patterns and their relation to therapy.

DIET

No restrictions, although a 5% reduction in weight can induce ovulation in anovulation caused by PCOS

PATIENT EDUCATION

Explain possible/likely etiologies.

- Answer all questions, especially those related to cancer and fertility.
- https://www.acog.org/Patients
- https://www.uptodate.com (patient education)

PROGNOSIS

- Varies with pathophysiologic process
- Most anovulatory cycles can be treated with medical therapy and do not require surgical intervention.

COMPLICATIONS

- Iron deficiency anemia
- Uterine cancer in cases of prolonged unopposed estrogen stimulation

REFERENCES

1. Sweet MG, Schmidt-Dalton TA, Weiss PM, et al. Evaluation and management of abnormal uterine bleeding in premenopausal women. *Am Fam Physician*. 2012;85(1):35–43.
2. Committee on Practice Bulletins—Gynecology. Practice Bulletin No. 128: diagnosis of abnormal uterine bleeding in reproductive-aged women. *Obstet Gynecol*. 2012;120(1):197–206.
3. American College of Obstetricians and Gynecologists. ACOG Committee Opinion No. 557: management of acute abnormal uterine bleeding in nonpregnant reproductive-aged women. *Obstet Gynecol*. 2013;121(4):891–896.
4. Wong AS, Lao TT, Cheung CW, et al. Reappraisal of endometrial thickness for the detection of endometrial cancer in postmenopausal bleeding: a retrospective cohort study. *BJOG*. 2016;123(3):439–446.
5. Bradley L, Gueye N. The medical management of abnormal uterine bleeding in reproductive-aged women. *Am J Obstet Gynecol*. 2016;214(1):31–44.
6. Whitaker L, Critchley H. Abnormal uterine bleeding. *Best Pract Res Clin Obstet Gynaecol*. 2016;34:54–65.

ADDITIONAL READING

- Goldstein SR, Lumsden MA. Abnormal uterine bleeding in perimenopause. *Climacteric*. 2017;20(5):414–420.
- Lethaby A, Cooke I, Rees M. Progesterone or progestogen-releasing intrauterine systems for heavy menstrual bleeding. *Cochrane Database Syst Rev*. 2005;(4):CD002126.
- Lethaby A, Irvine G, Cameron I. Cyclical progestogens for heavy menstrual bleeding. *Cochrane Database Syst Rev*. 2008;(1):CD001016.
- Matteson KA, Rahn DD, Wheeler TL II, et al; for Society of Gynecologic Surgeons Systematic Review Group. Nonsurgical management of heavy menstrual bleeding: a systematic review. *Obstet Gynecol*. 2013;121(3):632–643.
- Matthews ML. Abnormal uterine bleeding in reproductive-aged women. *Obstet Gynecol Clin North Am*. 2015;42(1):103–115.

SEE ALSO

- Dysmenorrhea; Menorrhagia (Heavy Menstrual Bleeding)
- Algorithm: Abnormal Uterine Bleeding

CODES

ICD10

- N93.9 Abnormal uterine and vaginal bleeding, unspecified
- N93.8 Other specified abnormal uterine and vaginal bleeding
- N91.2 Amenorrhea, unspecified

CLINICAL PEARLS

- AUB is irregular bleeding that occurs in the absence of pregnancy or pathology, making it a diagnosis of exclusion.
- Anovulation accounts for 90% of AUB.
- An EMB should be performed in all women >35 years of age with AUB to rule out cancer or premalignancy, and it should be considered in women aged 18 to 35 years with AUB and risk factors for endometrial cancer.
- It is appropriate to initiate medical therapy in females <35 years of age with no apparent risk of endometrial cancer prior to performing an EMB.

ABNORMAL PAP AND CERVICAL DYSPLASIA

Tharani Ravi, MD • Fozia Akhtar Ali, MD • Jeremy Golding, MD, FAAFP

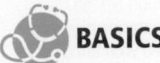 **BASICS**

DESCRIPTION

- Cervical dysplasia: premalignant cervical disease that is also called cervical intraepithelial neoplasia (CIN); precancerous epithelial changes in the transformation zone of the uterine cervix almost always associated with human papillomavirus (HPV) infections
- CIN encompasses a range of histologic diagnoses.
  - CIN I: mild dysplasia; low-grade lesion; cellular changes are limited to the lower 1/3 of the squamous epithelium.
  - CIN II: moderate dysplasia; high-grade lesion; cellular changes are limited to the lower 2/3 of the squamous epithelium.
  - CIN III or carcinoma in situ: severe dysplasia; high-grade lesion; cellular changes involve the full thickness of the squamous epithelium.
- System(s) affected: reproductive

Pediatric Considerations

Only 0.1% of cervical cancers occur before age 20 years. Screening women age <21 years (regardless of sexual history) does not reduce cervical cancer incidence and mortality compared with beginning screening at age 21 years. Screenings of adolescents lead to unnecessary evaluation and overtreatment of cervical lesions, which are highly likely to spontaneously regress.

Geriatric Considerations

- Women age >65 years who have had adequate prior screening and no history of CIN II+ in the last 20 years should not be screened for cervical cancer. Adequate prior screening is defined as three consecutive, negative cytology results or two consecutive, negative HPV-positive cytology "contesting" results within 10 years before cessation of screening (with the most recent test within the last 5 years).
- Routine screening should continue for at least 20 years after spontaneous regression or appropriate management of a high-grade precancerous lesion, even if this extends screening past the age 65 years.

Pregnancy Considerations

- Squamous intraepithelial lesions can progress during pregnancy but often regress postpartum.
- Colposcopy only to exclude the presence of invasive cancer in high-risk women
- Endocervical curettage is contraindicated during pregnancy.
- Unless cancer is identified or suspected, treatment of CIN is contraindicated during pregnancy.

EPIDEMIOLOGY

Cervical cancer is the fourth most common type of cancer in women worldwide. It is the second leading cause of cancer death in women aged 20 to 39 years (1). However, in the United States, due to improved screening practices, cervical cancer has dropped to 14th place in the list of most common cancers. Incidence of CIN III peaks between ages 25 and 29 years; invasive disease peaks 15 years later. Cervical cancer most commonly occurs in women aged 35 to 44 years. >15% of cervical cancer cases occur in women >65 years of age (occurs in those who did not get regular screening).

Incidence

- In United States: In 2018, approximately 13,240 new cases of invasive cervical cancer will be diagnosed and 4,170 women will die from the disease (1).
- The incidence of cervical cancer in the United States has decreased by >50% in the past 40 years because of widespread cervical cancer screening tests.

Prevalence

- In 2015, there were an estimated 257,524 women living with cervical cancer in the United States.
- In 2013 to 2014, the estimated prevalence of CIN II among 21- to 24-year-olds was 732/100,000 screened women in the United States (2).

ETIOLOGY AND PATHOPHYSIOLOGY

HPV DNA is found in virtually all cervical carcinomas and precursor lesions worldwide. HPV is so common that most sexually active men and women will get at least one type of HPV at some point in their lives.

- High-risk HPV types: 16, 18, 31, 33, 35, 45, 52, and 58 are common oncogenic virus types for cervical cancer.
- HPV 16 and 18 are associated with ~70% of all cervical cancers.
- Most HPV infections are transient, becoming undetectable within 1 to 2 years. Persistent infections are what place women at significant risk for developing precancerous lesions. Compared to younger women, women age >30 years are less likely to clear a new HPV infection.
- Low-risk types: HPV viral types 6, 11, 42, 43, and 44 are considered common low-risk types and may cause genital warts. HPV 6 and 11 (cause 90% of benign anogenital warts) can lead to low-grade squamous intraepithelial lesion (LSIL) and CIN I.

RISK FACTORS

- Previous or current HPV infection
- HIV infection and other immunosuppressive conditions
- In utero exposure to diethylstilbestrol
- Previous treatment of a high-grade precancerous lesion or cervical cancer
- Cigarette smoking
- Early age at first coitus (<20 years) and multiple sexual partners
- Some correlation with low socioeconomic status, high parity, oral contraceptive use, and poor nutrition

GENERAL PREVENTION

- Immunization: Immunization decreases high-risk HPV infections and cervical pathology for at least 5 to 7 years but has not yet been shown to decrease cervical cancer.
  - Ideally, HPV immunization of girls, boys, and women should be initiated prior to first intercourse. Per the Advisory Committee on Immunization Practices (ACIP), offer HPV vaccine to adolescents 11 to 12 years of age.
  - Gardasil 9: approved in December 2014 for use in females and males ages 9 to 26 years and in 2018 for ages 27 to 45 years; reduces dysplasia due to HPV types 16 and 18 (75% of cervical cancer), types 6 and 11 (anogenital warts), and protection against five additional HPV types which cause approximately 25% of CIN II+ lesions
  - Vaccine schedule: if vaccine begun before 15th birthday: 2 doses only 6 to 12 months apart
  - If vaccine begun on or after 15th birthday: 3 doses at 0, 2, and 6 months
  - Immunocompromising conditions: 3 doses needed
- Safe sex practices: condom use
- Screening
  - Pap smear has been the main screening test for cervical cellular pathology, with or without cotesting for HPV. A 2017 draft recommendation on cervical screening from the U.S. Preventive Services Task Force recommends either cytology testing at 3-year intervals or primary HPV testing at 5-year intervals for women 30 to 65 years of age.
  - Clinicians will need to choose whether to adopt an HPV-only approach or a cotesting approach (3)[B].
  - Screening recommendations by age and source (see algorithm "Pap, Normal and Abnormal in Nonpregnant Women Ages 25 Years and Older" and separate algorithm "Pap, Normal and Abnormal in Women Ages 21–24 Years")
    ○ <21 years: Do not screen (4)[A] (USPSTF/ASCCP/ACS/ASCP/ACOG).
  - Frequency of screening recommendation: USPSTF/ASCCP/ACS/ASCP generally agree by age and screen.
    ○ 21 to 29 years: Screen with cytology (Pap smear) every 3 years (4)[A]. Do not screen with HPV testing alone or combined with cytology (4).
    ○ 30 to 65 years: Screen with cytology every 3 years (acceptable) or cotesting (cytology/HPV testing) every 5 years (preferred).
    ○ >65 years (who have had adequate prior screening and are not high risk): Do not screen (4).
- Special circumstances: women after hysterectomy with removal of the cervix and with no history of CIN II+: Do not screen (4)[A]. Women with history of CIN II+ should continue screening until 20 years following their diagnosis of CIN II+.
- HIV-positive women: Screen every 3 years in those who have had three consecutive normal annual Pap tests and every 3 years cotesting in women ages 30 years and older.

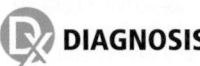 **DIAGNOSIS**

HISTORY

Usually asymptomatic until there is invasive disease. Patients may present with vaginal discharge, abnormal vaginal bleeding, postcoital bleeding, pelvic pain, cervical mass, or bladder obstruction.

PHYSICAL EXAM

Pelvic exam occasionally reveals external HPV lesions. Examine for exophytic or ulcerative cervical lesions, with or without bleeding.

DIFFERENTIAL DIAGNOSIS

Acute or chronic cervicitis; cervical glandular hyperplasia; cervical polyp; cervical fibroid; HPV infection; invasive cervical malignancy; uterine malignancy

DIAGNOSTIC TESTS & INTERPRETATION

- Current evidence indicates no clinically important differences between conventional cytology and liquid-based cytology in detecting cervical cancer precursors. Conventional Pap smear involves a cervical sample plated on a microscope slide with fixative. ThinPrep is a liquid-based collection and thin-layer preparation.
- To ensure an adequate sample of both the ecto- and endocervix, use a cytobrush and an extended tip spatula.
- Sensitivity of conventional Pap smear ranges from 30% to 70% for lesser cervical abnormalities. For detection of CIN II or higher, sensitivity was higher (44–99%) and had narrower specificity (91–98%) (5). Pap smears done routinely at recommended intervals increase the sensitivity further.
- The sensitivity and specificity of using HPV and Pap testing together (cotesting) for dysplasia is near 100% and 92.5%, respectively. Cotesting leads to earlier diagnosis of CIN III+ and cancer than does cytology alone, but it is likely that testing for high-risk HPV without cytology will become the dominant strategy, particularly for poorly screened or unscreened populations (6)[A].

- Cytology report component: specimen type (conventional Pap smear or liquid based), adequacy (presence of endocervical cells), and categorization (negative for intraepithelial lesion or malignancy or epithelial cell abnormality; i.e., squamous/glandular)
- Bethesda 2014 system (cytologic grading) epithelial cell abnormalities
  - Squamous cell
    - Atypical squamous cells (ASC) (of undetermined significance [ASC-US], cannot exclude high-grade squamous intraepithelial lesion or HSIL [ASC-H])
    - HPV, mild dysplasia, CIN I
    - Moderate/severe dysplasia CIS, CIN II, and CIN III
  - Glandular cell
    - AGCs (atypical glandular cells)
      - AGCs: not otherwise specified
      - AGCs: favor neoplasia
    - AIS (adenocarcinoma in situ)
    - Adenocarcinoma

Diagnostic Procedures/Other
Some algorithms differ for women age 21 to 24 years; see "ASCCP guidelines" (7) and algorithm "Pap, Normal and Abnormal in Women Ages 21–24 Years"; below recommendations for ages as noted

- HPV positive, cytology negative (30 years of age and older)
  - Option 1: HPV DNA typing: If HPV 16 or 18 positive, proceed to colposcopy; if negative, repeat cotesting at 1 year.
  - Option 2: Repeat cotesting at 1 year: If ASC or HPV positive, proceed to colposcopy; if negative, repeat cotesting at 3 years.
- ASC-US: (>24 years of age)
  - Option 1: HPV testing (preferred)
    - If HPV positive, proceed to colposcopy (7)[B].
    - If HPV negative, repeat cotesting at 3 years (7)[B].
  - Option 2: Repeat cytology at 1 year (acceptable) (7).
    - If repeat cytology ASC or greater, proceed to colposcopy.
    - If repeat cytology is negative, proceed to routine screening in 3 years.
- ASC-H: colposcopy required
- LSIL: (>24 years of age)
  - LSIL with negative HPV test: Repeat cotesting at 1 year (preferred).
    - If repeat cotesting is negative, repeat cotesting in 3 years.
    - If cotesting is positive, proceed to colposcopy.
  - LSIL with no HPV test or positive HPV test: Proceed to colposcopy.
  - LSIL in pregnancy: colposcopy preferred, but it is acceptable to defer colposcopy to postpartum (7)
- HSIL: loop electrosurgical excision procedure (LEEP) or colposcopy (7)[B]
- AGCs: colposcopy with endocervical sampling and endometrial sampling (if 35 years or older or at risk for endometrial neoplasia) (7)[A]
- Atypical endometrial cells: endometrial and endo-cervical sampling
  - If negative, perform colposcopy.
- Women with no lesion on colposcopy or CIN I (preceded by "lesser abnormalities" such as ASC-US, LSIL, HPV 16+, HPV 18+, and persistent HPV)
  - Follow-up without treatment: cotesting at 12 months
  - If both HPV and cytology are negative, age-appropriate retesting 3 years later
  - If either positive, proceed to colposcopy. If persistent CIN I for at least 2 years, proceed to treatment with ablative or excisional methods.
- Ages 21 to 24 years: Management is slightly different than above; see "ASCCP guidelines" (7) or algorithm "Pap, Normal and Abnormal in Women Ages 21–24 Years."
- Age >30 years: If cytology is negative but HPV is positive, repeat cotesting at 1 year is acceptable.

Test Interpretation
Atypical squamous or columnar cells, coarse nuclear material, increased nuclear diameter, koilocytosis (HPV hallmark)

 TREATMENT

ASCCP guidelines: Evidence-based management algorithms guide Pap smear and postcolposcopic diagnostics and therapeutics are available online at http://www.asccp.org/asccp-guidelines (7).

GENERAL MEASURES
Office evaluation and observation; promote smoking cessation; promote protected intercourse; promote immunization.

MEDICATION
- Infective/reactive Pap smear: Treat trichomoniasis, symptomatic *Candida*, or shift in flora suggestive of bacterial vaginosis found on Pap smear results.
- Condyloma acuminatum treatment options: See chapter "Condylomata Acuminata."

SURGERY/OTHER PROCEDURES
- Persistent CIN I, II, or III: ablative or excisional methods. If inadequate colposcopy for CIN II or III or recurrent CIN II or III, diagnostic excisional procedure is done. For AIS, hysterectomy is preferred.
- Cryotherapy, laser ablation, LEEP/large loop excision of transition zone, or cold-knife conization are all effective but require different training and with different side effects for patient. If cervical malignancy, see "Cervical Malignancy."

 ONGOING CARE

FOLLOW-UP RECOMMENDATIONS
After treatment (excision or ablation) of CIN II or III, women may reenter routine screening only after negative cotesting between 12 and 24 months. Screening should be continued for 20 years.

DIET
Promote increased intake of antioxidant-rich foods.

PATIENT EDUCATION
HPV vaccination, smoking cessation, protected intercourse, regular screening with Pap smear per guidelines

PROGNOSIS
- Progression of CIN to invasive cervical cancer is slow, and the likelihood of regression is high: Up to 43% of CIN II and 32% of CIN III lesions may regress. CIN III has a 30% probability of becoming invasive cancer over a 30-year period, although only about 1% if treated (3).
- CIN III becomes invasive: Lesions discovered early are amenable to treatment with excellent results and few recurrences.
- 1- and 5-year relative survival rates for cervical cancer patients are 87% and 68%, respectively. The 5-year survival rate for patients diagnosed with localized disease is 91% (3).

COMPLICATIONS
Aggressive cervical surgery may be associated with cervical stenosis, cervical incompetence, and scarring affecting cervical dilatation in labor.

REFERENCES

1. Siegel RL, Miller KD, Jemal A. Cancer statistics, 2018. *CA Cancer J Clin*. 2018;68(1):7–30.
2. Markowitz LE, Gee J, Chesson H, et al. Ten years of human papillomavirus vaccination in the United States. *Acad Pediatr*. 2018;18(Suppl 2):S3–S10.
3. Ogilvie GS, van Niekerk D, Krajden M, et al. Effect of screening with primary cervical HPV testing vs cytology testing on high-grade cervical intraepithelial neoplasia at 48 months: the HPV FOCAL randomized clinical trial. *JAMA*. 2018;320(1):43–52.
4. Moyer VA; for U.S. Preventive Services Task Force. Screening for cervical cancer: U.S. Preventive Services Task Force recommendation statement. *Ann Intern Med*. 2012;156(12):880–891.
5. Naucler P, Ryd W, Törnberg S, et al. Human papillomavirus and Papanicolaou tests to screen for cervical cancer. *N Engl J Med*. 2007;357(16):1589–1597.
6. Melnikow J, Henderson JT, Burda BU, et al. *Screening for Cervical Cancer With High-Risk Human Papillomavirus Testing: A Systematic Evidence Review for the U.S. Preventive Services Task Force*. Rockville, MD: Agency for Healthcare Research and Quality; 2018. Report No. 17-05231-EF-1.
7. Massad LS, Einstein MH, Huh WK, et al. 2012 updated consensus guidelines for the management of abnormal cervical cancer screening tests and cancer precursors. *J Low Genit Tract Dis*. 2013;17(5 Suppl 1):S1–S27.

ADDITIONAL READING

American Society for Colposcopy and Cervical Pathology. Management guidelines. http://www.asccp.org/asccp-guidelines. Accessed January 5, 2018.

 SEE ALSO

- Cervical Malignancy; Condylomata Acuminata; Trichomoniasis; Vulvovaginitis, Prepubescent
- Algorithms: Pap, Normal and Abnormal in Nonpregnant Women Ages 25 Years and Older; Pap, Normal and Abnormal in Women Ages 21–24 Years

 CODES

ICD10
- R87.619 Unspecified abnormal cytological findings in specimens from cervix uteri
- N87.9 Dysplasia of cervix uteri, unspecified
- N87.1 Moderate cervical dysplasia

CLINICAL PEARLS

- HPV is present in virtually all cervical cancers (99.7%), but most HPV infections are transient.
- Vaccine should be offered prior to onset of any sexual activity for maximum effectiveness but may be offered up to age 45 years (88% protective in women age 27 to 45 years against warts, squamous intraepithelial lesion, and cancer).
- Know and adhere to recognized screening guidelines to avoid the harms of overscreening.
- Optimal screening strategy is in evolution. HPV primary with cytology-secondary strategies will likely supplant current guidelines in near future.

ACETAMINOPHEN POISONING

Luis T. Garcia, MD • Kenneth Polezoes, MD

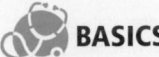

BASICS

DESCRIPTION
- A disorder characterized by hepatic necrosis following large ingestions of acetaminophen. Although patients can be asymptomatic, common presenting symptoms include nausea, vomiting, diaphoresis, malaise, jaundice, confusion, somnolence, coma, and potentially death. A clinical hallmark is the onset of symptoms within 24 hours of ingestion of acetaminophen only or combination acetaminophen products. Ingestion should be treated before symptoms develop if at all possible.
- Acetaminophen poisoning is most often encountered following large, single ingestions of acetaminophen-containing medications. Toxic doses are typically >10 g in adults and >200 rng/kg in children. Poisoning also occurs after acute and chronic ingestions of lesser amounts in individuals who regularly abuse alcohol, are chronically malnourished, or take medications that affect hepatic acetaminophen metabolism.
- Therapeutic adult doses are 0.5 to 1.0 g q4–6h to a maximum of 4 g/day. Therapeutic pediatric doses are 10 to 15 mg/kg q4–6h, not to exceed 5 doses in 24 hours.
- System(s) affected: gastrointestinal, cardiovascular, renal/urologic, CNS
  - Multisystem organ failure can occur.
- Synonym(s): paracetamol poisoning

Geriatric Considerations
Increased risk of hepatic damage in frail elderly patients due to decreased hepatic metabolism and coingestion of other hepatotoxic medications. Keep dose of acetaminophen ≤3,000 mg/day in seniors and patients with liver disease and/or alcohol abuse disorders.

Pediatric Considerations
Hepatic damage after ingestion of toxic acetaminophen doses can be less in young children, potentially due to larger glutathione stores.

Pregnancy Considerations
Increased incidence of spontaneous abortion, especially with overdose at early gestational age. Incidence of spontaneous abortion or fetal death appears to be increased when *N*-acetylcysteine (NAC) treatment is delayed. IV NAC is generally preferred in pregnancy due to greater bioavailability.

EPIDEMIOLOGY
- Predominant age: children and adults
- Predominant sex: no reported association
- Intentional versus unintentional ingestion (52% vs. 48%)

Incidence
The annual reported incidence of acetaminophen overdosing increased from 2 (95% CI 0.2–7.2) cases per 10,000 patients in 2005 to 3.4 (95% CI 1.1–8.8) in 2010.

Prevalence
- >38,000 hospitalizations per year for acetaminophen-related poisonings in the United States, nearly 1/2 were unintentional (mostly involving opioid–acetaminophen combinations).
- <1% of hospitalizations in patients <18 years had coexistent liver toxicity.

ETIOLOGY AND PATHOPHYSIOLOGY
- Accidental or intentional ingestion of acetaminophen or combination medications containing acetaminophen
- 96% of ingested acetaminophen is metabolized in the liver, only 2–4% is excreted unchanged in the urine. When taken in therapeutic doses, 90–95% of hepatic metabolism results in the formation of benign metabolites. 5–10% of hepatic metabolism is by oxidation through the cytochrome P450 enzyme system (CYP 3A4 and CYP 2E1), resulting in the formation of the toxic metabolite *N*-acetyl-*p*-benzoquinone imine (NAPQI). NAPQI is rapidly conjugated with glutathione to form a nontoxic metabolite. Metabolites are excreted in the urine with a small amount of unchanged drug. Hepatocellular damage occurs when toxic doses of acetaminophen saturate the glucuronidation and sulfation pathways with production of excessive NAPQI. Available glutathione stores become depleted, NAPQI accumulates, and hepatocellular damage occurs.

RISK FACTORS
- Concurrent poisoning with other substances
- Psychiatric illness, history of suicide attempts
- Regular ingestion of large amounts of alcohol
- Possible risk related to previous weight loss surgery

GENERAL PREVENTION
- Poison Control: 1-800-222-1222 for any questions
- FDA labeling guidance: http://www.fda.gov/Drugs /GuidanceComplianceRegulatoryInformation /Guidances/default.htm

DIAGNOSIS

- May initially be asymptomatic, particularly with history of ingestion in preceding 8 hours. Signs and symptoms of poisoning are related to liver toxicity and develop over the first 24 hours following large ingestions; may last up to 8 days
- Symptoms may develop gradually following long-term ingestion of near maximal-therapeutic amounts of acetaminophen. Such patients may present in varying stages, without a history of toxic ingestion.
- Severe symptoms indicate large ingestions or coingestants.
  - Stage 1: first 24 hours after ingestion:
    - Nausea and anorexia
    - Vomiting
    - Diaphoresis
  - Stage 2: days 2 to 3 following ingestion
    - Right upper quadrant pain
    - Typically less nausea, vomiting, diaphoresis, and malaise than in stage 1
  - Stage 3: days 3 to 4 following ingestion
    - Nausea, vomiting, and malaise reappear.
    - Severe poisonings may result in jaundice, confusion, somnolence, and coma.
  - Stage 4: 5 or more days after ingestion
    - Possible deterioration due to multiorgan failure and death. Symptoms resolve over time in survivors.
- Fulminant hepatic failure occurs in <1% of adults and is very rare in children <6 years of age.
- An unexplained rise in liver function tests (LFTs) with negative acetaminophen levels might suggest stage 3 toxicity.

HISTORY
Ingestion or suspected ingestion of acetaminophen-containing product

DIFFERENTIAL DIAGNOSIS
- Consider presence of coingestants, especially alcohol, opiates, and aspirin.
- Other ingested toxins that produce severe acute hepatic injury, including the mushroom *Amanita phalloides* and products containing yellow phosphorus or carbon tetrachloride

DIAGNOSTIC TESTS & INTERPRETATION
Initial Tests (labs, imaging)
- Draw plasma acetaminophen levels on all patients ≥4 hours after ingestion (levels prior to 4 hours are not helpful). Draw additional levels at 6 and 8 hours if extended release form.
- Alanine transaminase (ALT), aspartate transaminase (AST), prothrombin time (PT)/international normalized ratio (INR), bilirubin, lactate dehydrogenase (LDH)
- Electrolytes, glucose, BUN, creatinine
- Pregnancy screen in females (urine or serum)
- Urinalysis
- Consider arterial blood gas (ABG).
- Screen for suspected coingestants (aspirin, iron, etc.), especially if suicide gesture/attempt.
- With toxic ingestions, AST (serum glutamic-oxaloacetic transaminase), ALT (serum glutamic-pyruvic transaminase), and bilirubin levels begin to rise in stage 2 and peak in stage 3.
- With severe poisonings, PT/INR rise in parallel with LFT changes.
- Improvement in ALT with therapy is an encouraging clinical sign.
- Laboratory abnormalities usually resolve by stage 4.
- Renal function abnormalities are common in patients with hepatotoxicity.
- Evidence of damage to pancreas and heart may present following severe poisonings.
- Anion-gap metabolic acidosis due to accumulation of 5-oxoproline may rarely be seen.
- Diseases or toxic substances that damage the liver (particularly alcohol) may alter laboratory results.
- No specific imaging required

Follow-Up Tests & Special Considerations
During recovery, liver tests should normalize.

Test Interpretation
Centrilobular hepatic necrosis

TREATMENT

- Contact a regional/local poison control center for recommendations. In the United States: (800) 222-1222
- Give NAC when plasma acetaminophen concentrations measured ≥4 hours after ingestion are in the "possible risk" or higher levels on the Rumack-Matthew nomogram. This corresponds to acetaminophen levels >150 μg/mL (993 μmol/L), >75 μg/mL (497 μmol/L), and >37 μg/mL (244 μmol/L) at 4, 8, and 12 hours after ingestion, respectively. See http://www.ars-informatica.ca /toxicity_nomogram.php?calc=acetamin.

- Consideration: The nomogram does not help determining the need for NAC for sustained-release products or chronic ingestions. If a sustained-released product has been ingested, obtain two serum acetaminophen levels 4 to 6 hours apart. Treat if either level is above the possible toxicity line. For chronic toxicity or those patients who present 24 hours postingestion, treat based on clinical effects, LFTs, and the acetaminophen level.
- Start NAC within 8 hours of ingestion for maximal hepatic protection. Patients presenting near 8 hours should empirically receive NAC while waiting for labs.
- All patients with acetaminophen liver injury (even after 8 hours) should receive NAC.
- NAC therapy may be effective up to ≥36 hours after ingestion.
- Give single-dose activated charcoal within 1 to 2 hours (and possibly up to 4 hours) of ingestion (especially in cases of coingestants) (1,2)[C].

ALERT
Never delay NAC administration for use of activated charcoal.

- Ipecac and gastric lavage are no longer recommended for routine use at home or in health care facilities.

MEDICATION
First Line
- Initiate acetylcysteine (NAC, Mucomyst) within 8 hours of ingestion whenever possible; single-dose activated charcoal (1 g/kg PO) may be effective if given within 1 to 2 hours of ingestion especially if other substances concomitantly ingested. *Never delay oral NAC for activated charcoal.*
- Acetylcysteine may be given PO or IV, depending on situation and availability:
  - IV loading dose of acetylcysteine (Acetadote, Cetylev) 150 mg/kg over 60 minutes followed by an infusion of 50 mg/kg over 4 hours (12.5 mg/kg/hr); this is followed by an infusion of 100 mg/kg over the next 16 hours (6.25 mg/kg/hr) (20-hour regimen).
  - Oral loading dose of 140 mg/kg, followed by 70 mg/kg q4h for 17 additional doses (72-hour regimen)
  - No treatment regimen has been shown to be superior over the other (1)[A].
- Contraindications: medication allergies
- Precautions:
  - Oral NAC may cause significant nausea and vomiting due to its sulfur content; consider nasogastric tube.
  - Nausea can be treated with metoclopramide (Reglan), 1 to 2 mg/kg IV, or ondansetron (Zofran), 0.15 mg/kg IV (for age >4 years, usually 4 mg/dose).
  - IV NAC (Acetadote) may cause anaphylactoid reactions, (3–6%) including rash, bronchospasm, pruritus, angioedema, tachycardia, or hypotension (higher rates seen in asthmatics and those with atopy) (3)[C].
- Reactions usually occur with loading dose. To prevent this, slow or temporarily stop the infusion; may concurrently treat with antihistamines
- Failure rates of NAC of 3–7% have been observed (3)[C].

Second Line
- Oral racemethionine (methionine)
- In massive ingestions (e.g., levels >1,000 mg/L, acidosis, coma/hypotension), hemodialysis may improve survival (4)[C].
- In January 2016, acetylcysteine (Acetadote, Cetylev), an effervescent lemon mint–flavored NAC tablet, was approved by the FDA. Tablets come in strengths of 500 mg and 2.5 g.

ISSUES FOR REFERRAL
- Behavioral health evaluation for intentional ingestions
- Child abuse reporting if neglect led to overdose

ADMISSION, INPATIENT, AND NURSING CONSIDERATIONS
- Toxic and intentional ingestions
- Increased LFTs, acidosis on ABG, elevated creatinine, or other signs of target organ damage merit admission.
- Age- and weight-appropriate IV hydration

 ## ONGOING CARE

FOLLOW-UP RECOMMENDATIONS
- Evaluate all patients at a health care facility.
- Evaluate patients with evidence of organ failure, increased LFTs, or coagulopathy for emergency liver transplant (ELT) at a transplant center.
- Restrict activity if hepatic damage is significant.
- Outpatient management is adequate for nontoxic accidental ingestions.

Patient Monitoring
Ask about ingestion by others (i.e., suicide pacts).

DIET
No special diet, except with severe hepatic damage

PATIENT EDUCATION
- Counsel patients to avoid acetaminophen (Tylenol, others) or other forms of acetaminophen, particularly if using combination product(s) containing acetaminophen.
- Educate parents/caregivers during well-child visits.
- Anticipatory guidance for caregivers, family, and cohabitants of potentially suicidal patients
- Educate patients on long-term acetaminophen therapy.

PROGNOSIS
- Complete recovery with early therapy
- <1% of adult patients develop hepatic failure. King criteria (pH <7.3, PT >100 s [INR >65], creatinine >3.4 mg/dL [>300 μmol/L]) is associated with a poor prognosis and possible need for liver transplant (5)[C]. Early referral increases the chance for transplant success.
- Hepatic failure is very rare in children <6 years of age.

COMPLICATIONS
Rare following recovery from acute poisoning

REFERENCES
1. Chiew AL, Gluud C, Brok J, et al. Interventions for paracetamol (acetaminophen) overdose. *Cochrane Database Syst Rev.* 2018;(2):CD003328.
2. Spiller HA, Winter ML, Klein-Schwartz W, et al. Efficacy of activated charcoal administered more than four hours after acetaminophen overdose. *J Emerg Med.* 2006;30(1):1–5.
3. Chiew AL, Isbister GK, Duffull SB, et al. Evidence for the changing regimens of acetylcysteine. *Br J Clin Pharmacol.* 2016;81(3):471–481.
4. Gosselin S, Juurlink DN, Kielstein JT, et al; for EXTRIP Workgroup. Extracorporeal treatment for acetaminophen poisoning: recommendations from the EXTRIP workgroup. *Clin Toxicol (Phila).* 2014;52(8):856–867.
5. McPhail MJ, Farne H, Senvar N, et al. Ability of King's College Criteria and model for end-stage liver disease scores to predict mortality of patients with acute liver failure: a meta-analysis. *Clin Gastroenterol Hepatol.* 2016;14(4):516.e5–525.e5.

ADDITIONAL READING
- Major JM, Zhou EH, Wong HL, et al. Trends in rates of acetaminophen-related adverse events in the United States. *Pharmacoepidemiol Drug Saf.* 2016;25(5):590–598.
- Mund ME, Quarcoo D, Gyo C, et al. Paracetamol as a toxic substance for children: aspects of legislation in selected countries. *J Occup Med Toxicol.* 2015;10:43.
- Serper M, Wolf MS, Parikh NA, et al. Risk factors, clinical presentation, and outcomes in overdose with acetaminophen alone or with combination products: results from the Acute Liver Failure Study Group. *J Clin Gastroenterol.* 2016;50(1):85–91.

 ## CODES

ICD10
- T39.1X4A Poisoning by 4-Aminophenol derivatives, undetermined, init
- K71.10 Toxic liver disease with hepatic necrosis, without coma
- T39.1X1A Poisoning by 4-Aminophenol derivatives, accidental, init

CLINICAL PEARLS
- Consult with Poison Control center for management recommendations (800) 222-1222 in United States.
- Give NAC when plasma acetaminophen concentrations (measured ≥4 hours after ingestion) are in the "possible risk" or higher levels. This corresponds to acetaminophen levels >150 μg/mL (993 μmol/L), >75 μg/mL (497 μmol/L), and >37 μg/mL (265 μmol/L) at 4, 8, and 12 hours after ingestion, respectively.
- Start NAC within 8 hours of ingestion for best chance of hepatic protection. Patients presenting near 8 hours should empirically receive NAC while waiting for labs.
- All patients with acetaminophen liver injury (even after 8 hours) should receive NAC.
- To enhance palatability, dilute oral NAC with a beverage of choice. Serve in a cup with lid and straw.
- For extended release acetaminophen, some authorities recommend following plasma levels at 4, 6, and 8 hours after ingestion. Start NAC if any level is elevated.

ACNE ROSACEA

Daniel R. DiBlasi, DO • Shane L. Larson, MD

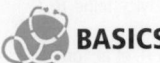 **BASICS**

DESCRIPTION
- Rosacea is a chronic condition characterized by recurrent episodes of facial flushing, erythema (due to dilatation of small blood vessels in the face), papules, pustules, and telangiectasia (due to increased reactivity of capillaries) in a symmetric, central facial distribution; sometimes associated with ocular symptoms (ocular rosacea)
- Four subtypes:
  - Erythematotelangiectatic rosacea (ETR)
  - Papulopustular rosacea (PPR)
  - Phymatous rosacea
  - Ocular rosacea
- System(s) affected: skin/exocrine
- Synonym(s): rosacea

Geriatric Considerations
- Chronic inflammatory dermatosis with middle-age onset
- Effects of aging might increase the side effects associated with oral isotretinoin used for treatment (at present, data are insufficient due to lack of clinical studies in elderly patients ≥65 years).

EPIDEMIOLOGY
Prevalence
- Predominant age of onset: 30 to 50 years
- Predominant sex: female > male. However, males are at greater risk for progression to later stages.
- More common in Fitzpatrick skin types I and II

ETIOLOGY AND PATHOPHYSIOLOGY
- No proven cause
- Possibilities include the following:
  - Thyroid and sex hormone disturbance
  - Alcohol, coffee, tea, spiced food overindulgence (unproven)
  - Demodex follicular parasite (suspected)
  - Exposure to cold, heat
  - Emotional stress
  - Dysfunction of the GI tract (possible association with *Helicobacter pylori*)

Genetics
- People of Northern European and Celtic background commonly afflicted
- Associated with three human leukocyte antigen (HLA) alleles: HLA-DRB1, HLA-DQB1, and HLA-DQA1 (MHC class II)

RISK FACTORS
- Exposure to spicy foods, hot drinks
- Environmental factors: sun, wind, cold, heat

GENERAL PREVENTION
No preventive measures known

COMMONLY ASSOCIATED CONDITIONS
- Seborrheic dermatitis of scalp and eyelids
- Keratitis with photophobia, lacrimation, visual disturbance
- Corneal lesions
- Blepharitis
- Uveitis

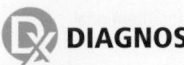 **DIAGNOSIS**

HISTORY
- Usually have a history of episodic flushing with increases in skin temperature in response to heat stimulus in mouth (hot liquids), spicy foods, alcohol, sun exposure
- Acne may have preceded onset of rosacea by years; nevertheless, rosacea usually arises de novo without preceding history of acne or seborrhea.
- Excessive facial warmth and redness are the predominant presenting complaints. Itching is generally absent.

PHYSICAL EXAM
- Rosacea has four subtypes:
  - The rosacea diathesis: episodic erythema, "flushing and blushing"
  - Progression from one subtype to another is hypothetical.
  - ETR: persistent erythema with telangiectases
  - PPR: persistent erythema, telangiectases, papules, pustules
  - Phymatous: persistent deep erythema, dense telangiectases, papules, pustules, nodules; rarely persistent "solid" edema of the central part of the face (phymatous)
- Facial erythema, particularly on cheeks, nose, and chin. At times, entire face may be involved.
- Inflammatory papules are prominent; pustules and telangiectasia may be present.
- Comedones are absent (unlike acne vulgaris).
- Women usually have lesions on the chin and cheeks, whereas the nose is commonly involved in men.
- Ocular findings (mild dryness and irritation with blepharitis, conjunctival injection, burning, stinging, tearing, eyelid inflammation, swelling, and redness) are present in 50% of patients.

DIFFERENTIAL DIAGNOSIS
- Drug eruptions (iodides and bromides)
- Granulomas of the skin
- Cutaneous lupus erythematosus
- Carcinoid syndrome
- Acne vulgaris
- Seborrheic dermatitis
- Steroid rosacea (abuse)
- Systemic lupus erythematosus
- Lupus pernio (sarcoidosis)

DIAGNOSTIC TESTS & INTERPRETATION
- Diagnosis is based on physical exam findings.
- A recent change in classification has been proposed based on the phenotype that reflects the clinical presentation and to better focus treatment options, which are targeted to address the main clinical presentation (1).

Test Interpretation
Histology of affected skin may reveal:
- Inflammation around hypertrophied sebaceous glands, producing papules, pustules, and cysts
- Absence of comedones and blocked ducts
- Vascular dilatation and dermal lymphocytic infiltrate
- Granulomatous inflammation

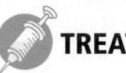 **TREATMENT**

GENERAL MEASURES
- Proper skin care and photoprotection are important components of management plan (1)[B]. Use of mild, nondrying soap is recommended; local skin irritants should be avoided.
- Avoidance of triggers
- Reassurance that rosacea is completely unrelated to poor hygiene
- Treat psychological stress if present.
- Topical steroids should not be used because they may aggravate rosacea.
- Avoid oil-based cosmetics:
  - Others are acceptable and may help women tolerate symptoms.
- Electrodesiccation or chemical sclerosis of permanently dilated blood vessels
- Possible evolving laser therapy
- Support physical fitness.

MEDICATION
First Line
- Topical metronidazole preparations once (1% formulation) or twice (0.75% formulations) daily for 7 to 12 weeks was significantly more effective than placebo in patients with moderate to severe rosacea. A rosacea treatment system (cleanser, metronidazole 0.75% gel, hydrating complexion corrector, and sunscreen SPF 30) may offer superior efficacy and tolerability to metronidazole (2)[A].
- Azelaic acid (Finacea) is very effective as initial therapy; azelaic acid topical alone is effective for maintenance (3)[B].
- Topical ivermectin 1% cream (2)[A]
  - Recently found to be more effective than metronidazole for treatment of PPR
- Topical brimonidine tartrate 0.5% gel is effective in reducing erythema associated with ETR (4)[A].
  - α_2-Adrenergic receptor agonist; potent vasoconstrictor

- Oxymetazoline 1% cream, an α_{1A}-adrenergic receptor agonist recently approved for the treatment of persistent erythema associated with rosacea in adults (5)[B]
- Doxycycline 40-mg dose is at least as effective as 100-mg dose and has a correspondingly lower risk of adverse effects but is much more expensive (6)[A].
- Precautions: Tetracyclines may cause photosensitivity; sunscreen is recommended.
- Significant possible interactions:
  - Tetracyclines: Avoid concurrent administration with antacids, dairy products, or iron.
  - Broad-spectrum antibiotics: may reduce the effectiveness of oral contraceptives; however, this finding has only been associated with rifampin; consider adding barrier method.

Second Line
- Topical erythromycin
- Topical clindamycin (lotion preferred)
  - Can be used in combination with benzoyl peroxide; commercial topical combinations are available.
- Possible use of calcineurin inhibitors (tacrolimus 0.1%; pimecrolimus 1%). Pimecrolimus 1% is effective to treat mild to moderate inflammatory rosacea.
- Permethrin 5% cream; similar efficacy compared to metronidazole for severe cases, oral isotretinoin at 0.3 mg/kg for a minimum of 3 months

Pediatric Considerations
Tetracyclines: not for use in children <8 years

Pregnancy Considerations
- Tetracyclines: not for use during pregnancy
- Isotretinoin: teratogenic; not for use during pregnancy or in women of reproductive age who are not using reliable contraception; requires registration with iPLEDGE program

ADDITIONAL THERAPIES
Cyclosporine 0.05% ophthalmic emulsion may be more effective than artificial tears for ocular rosacea.

SURGERY/OTHER PROCEDURES
Laser treatment is an option for progressive telangiectasias or rhinophyma.
- Pulsed dye laser (585 nm or 595 nm) is effective in treating telangiectases and erythema.
- CO_2 fractional ablative laser can be used to treat rhinophyma.

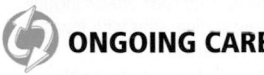 **ONGOING CARE**

FOLLOW-UP RECOMMENDATIONS
Outpatient treatment

Patient Monitoring
- Occasional and as needed
- Close follow-up and laboratory assessment for patients using isotretinoin per prescribing instructions and iPLEDGE program guidance
- Consider ophthalmology evaluation in patients with ocular symptoms.

DIET
Avoid alcohol and hot drinks of any type.

PROGNOSIS
- Slowly progressive
- Subsides spontaneously (sometimes)

COMPLICATIONS
- Rhinophyma (dilated follicles and thickened bulbous skin on nose), especially in men
- Conjunctivitis
- Blepharitis
- Keratitis
- Visual deterioration

REFERENCES

1. Schaller M, Almeida LM, Bewley A, et al. Rosacea treatment update: recommendations from the global ROSacea COnsensus (ROSCO) panel. *Br J Dermatol.* 2017;176(2):465–471.
2. van Zuuren EJ, Fedorowicz Z, Carter B, et al. Interventions for rosacea. *Cochrane Database Syst Rev.* 2015;(4):CD003262.
3. Thiboutot DM, Fleischer AB, Del Rosso JQ, et al. A multicenter study of topical azelaic acid 15% gel in combination with oral doxycycline as initial therapy and azelaic acid 15% gel as maintenance monotherapy. *J Drugs Dermatol.* 2009;8(7):639–648.
4. Fowler J Jr, Jackson M, Moore A, et al. Efficacy and safety of once-daily topical brimonidine tartrate gel 0.5% for the treatment of moderate to severe facial erythema of rosacea: results of two randomized, double-blind, and vehicle-controlled pivotal studies. *J Drugs Dermatol.* 2013;12(6):650–656.
5. Oxymetazoline cream (Rhofade) for rosacea. *Med Lett Drugs Ther.* 2017;59(1521):84–86.
6. Del Rosso JQ, Webster GF, Jackson M, et al. Two randomized phase III clinical trials evaluating anti-inflammatory dose doxycycline (40-mg doxycycline, USP capsules) administered once daily for treatment of rosacea. *J Am Acad Dermatol.* 2007;56(5):791–802.

ADDITIONAL READING

- Kim MB, Kim GW, Park HJ, et al. Pimecrolimus 1% cream for the treatment of rosacea. *J Dermatol.* 2011;38(12):1135–1139.
- Koçak M, Yağli S, Vahapoğlu G, et al. Permethrin 5% cream versus metronidazole 0.75% gel for the treatment of papulopustular rosacea. A randomized double-blind placebo-controlled study. *Dermatology.* 2002;205(3):265–270.
- Leyden JJ. Efficacy of a novel rosacea treatment system: an investigator-blind, randomized, parallel-group study. *J Drugs Dermatol.* 2011;10(10): 1179–1185.
- Liu RH, Smith MK, Basta SA, et al. Azelaic acid in the treatment of papulopustular rosacea: a systematic review of randomized controlled trials. *Arch Dermatol.* 2006;142(8):1047–1052.
- Mikkelsen CS, Holmgren HR, Kjellman P, et al. Rosacea: a clinical review. *Dermatol Reports.* 2016;8(1):6387.

 SEE ALSO

- Acne Vulgaris; Blepharitis; Dermatitis, Seborrheic; Lupus Erythematosus, Discoid; Uveitis
- Algorithm: Acne

 CODES

ICD10
- L71.9 Rosacea, unspecified
- L71.8 Other rosacea

CLINICAL PEARLS

- Rosacea usually arises de novo without any preceding history of acne or seborrhea.
- Rosacea may cause chronic eye symptoms, including blepharitis.
- Avoid alcohol, sun exposure, and hot drinks.
- Medication treatment resembles that of acne vulgaris, with oral and topical antibiotics.

ACNE VULGARIS

Gary I. Levine, MD

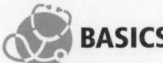 **BASICS**

DESCRIPTION

- Acne vulgaris is a disorder of the pilosebaceous units. It is a chronic inflammatory dermatosis notable for open/closed comedones, papules, pustules, nodules.
- Systems affected: skin/exocrine

Geriatric Considerations
Favre-Racouchot syndrome: comedones on face and head due to sun exposure

Pregnancy Considerations
- May result in a flare or remission of acne
- Typically improves in 1st trimester; may worsen in 3rd trimester
- Topical benzoyl peroxide, azelaic acid, erythromycin or clindamycin, and oral erythromycin or cephalexin can be used in pregnancy; use topical agents when possible.
- Isotretinoin is teratogenic; pregnancy Category X
- Avoid topical tretinoin and adapalene because they may cause retinoid embryopathy; class C
- Contraindicated: isotretinoin, tazarotene, tetracycline, doxycycline, minocycline

Pediatric Considerations
- Neonatal acne (neonatal cephalic pustulosis)
  - Newborn to 8 weeks; lesions limited to face; usually self-limited, may respond to topical ketoconazole 2% cream (1,2)
- Infantile acne
  - Newborn to 1 year; lesions on face, neck, back, and chest; topical/systemic Rx (1)
- Early to middle childhood acne
  - 1 to 7 years; rare; consider hyperandrogenism (1).
- Preadolescent acne
  - 7 to 12 years; common, 47% of children, usually due to adrenal awakening, comedonal lesions
- Do not use tetracyclines in those <8 years of age (1); other therapies similar to adolescent acne

EPIDEMIOLOGY
- Predominant age: early to late puberty, may persist in 20–40% of affected individuals into 4th decade
- Predominant sex
  - Male > female (adolescence)
  - Female > male (adult)

Prevalence
- 80–95% of adolescents affected. A smaller percentage will seek medical advice.
- 8% of adults aged 25 to 34 years; 3% at 35 to 44 years
- African Americans 37%, Caucasians 24%

ETIOLOGY AND PATHOPHYSIOLOGY
- Androgens (testosterone and dehydroepiandrosterone sulfate [DHEA-S]) stimulate sebum production/qualitative sebum changes and proliferation of keratinocytes in hair follicles (3).
- Keratin plug obstructs follicle os, causing sebum accumulation and follicular distention.
- *Propionibacterium acnes*, an anaerobe, colonizes and proliferates within a biofilm in the plugged follicle.
- *P. acnes* promote proinflammatory mediators, causing inflammation of follicle and dermis.

Genetics
- Familial association in 50%
- If a family history exists, the acne may be more severe and occur earlier.

RISK FACTORS
- Increased endogenous androgenic effect
- Oily cosmetics, cocoa butter

- Rubbing or occluding skin surface (e.g., sports equipment such as helmets and shoulder pads), telephone, or hands against the skin
- Polyvinyl chloride, chlorinated hydrocarbons, cutting oil, tars
- Numerous drugs, including androgenic steroids (e.g., steroid abuse, some birth control pills), lithium, phenytoin
- Endocrine disorders: polycystic ovarian syndrome, Cushing syndrome, congenital adrenal hyperplasia, androgen-secreting tumors, acromegaly
- Stress
- High-glycemic load and possibly high-dairy diets may exacerbate acne (3).
- Severe acne may worsen with smoking.

COMMONLY ASSOCIATED CONDITIONS
- Acne fulminans, pyoderma faciale
- Acne conglobata, hidradenitis suppurativa
- Pomade acne
- SAPHO syndrome (synovitis, acne, pustulosis, hyperostosis, and osteitis)
- Pyogenic arthritis, pyoderma gangrenosum, and acne (PAPA) and seborrhea, acne, hirsutism, and alopecia (SAHA) syndromes
- Behçet syndrome, Apert syndrome
- Dark-skinned patients: 50% keloidal scarring and 50% acne hyperpigmented macules

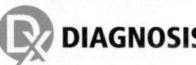 **DIAGNOSIS**

HISTORY
- Ask about duration, medications, cleansing products, stress, smoking, exposures, diet, and family history.
- Females may worsen 1 week prior to menses.

PHYSICAL EXAM
- Closed comedones (whiteheads)
- Open comedones (blackheads)
- Nodules or papules
- Pustules ("cysts")
- Scars: ice pick, rolling, boxcar, atrophic macules, hypertrophic, depressed, sinus tracts
- Consistent grading is useful; no specific universal grading system is recommended per guidelines (4).
- Grading system (American Academy of Dermatology, 1990) (3)
  - Mild: few papules/pustules; no nodules
  - Moderate: some papules/pustules; few nodules
  - Severe: numerous papules/pustules/nodules
  - Very severe: acne conglobata, acne fulminans, acne inversa
- Most common areas affected are face, chest, back, and upper arms (areas of greatest concentration of sebaceous glands) (3).
- Adult female—mandibular and perioral lesion location

DIFFERENTIAL DIAGNOSIS
- Folliculitis: gram-negative and gram-positive
- Acne (rosacea, cosmetica, steroid induced)
- Perioral dermatitis
- Chloracne
- Pseudofolliculitis barbae
- Drug eruption
- Verruca vulgaris and plana
- Keratosis pilaris
- Molluscum contagiosum
- Sarcoidosis
- Seborrheic dermatitis
- Miliaria
- Lupus erythematosus

DIAGNOSTIC TESTS & INTERPRETATION
Initial Tests (lab, imaging)
Only indicated if additional signs of androgen excess; if so, test for free and total testosterone and DHEA-S and consider LH and FSH (PCOS).

 **TREATMENT**

- Comedonal (grade 1): keratolytic agent (see as follows for specific agents)
- Mild inflammatory acne (grade 2): benzoyl peroxide or topical retinoid or benzoyl peroxide +/− topical antibiotic +/− topical retinoid
- Moderate inflammatory acne (grade 3): Add systemic antibiotic to grade 2 regimen.
- Severe inflammatory acne (grade 4): as in grade 3, or isotretinoin
- Topical retinoid plus a topical antimicrobial agent is first line treatment for more than mild disease.
- Topical retinoid + antibiotic (topical or PO) is better than either alone for mild/moderate acne.
- Topical retinoids are first-line agents for maintenance. Avoid long-term antibiotics for maintenance.
- Avoid topical antibiotics as monotherapy (4)[A].
- Can use isotretinoin for treatment of resistant moderate acne (4)
- Recommended vehicle type
  - Dry or sensitive skin: cream, lotion, or ointment
  - Oily skin, humid weather: gel, solution, or wash
  - Hair-bearing areas: lotion, hydrogel, or foam
- Apply topical agents to entire affected area, not just visible lesions.
- Mild soap daily to control oiliness; avoid abrasives.
- Avoid drying agents with keratolytic agents.
- Gentle cleanser and noncomedogenic moisturizer help decrease irritation.
- Oil-free, noncomedogenic sunscreens
- Stress management if acne flares with stress

MEDICATION

ALERT
Most prescription branded topical medications are very expensive, costing from $100 to several hundred dollars per tube.

- Keratolytic agents (α-hydroxy acids, salicylic acid, topical retinoids, azelaic acid) (side effects include dryness, erythema, and scaling; start with lower strength, increase as tolerated)
- Tretinoin (Retin-A, Retin-A Micro, Avita, Atralin) varying strengths and formulations: Apply at bedtime; wash skin; let skin dry 30 minutes before application.
  - Retin-A Micro, Atralin, and Avita are less irritating and stable with BP.
  - May cause an initial flare of lesions; may be eased by every other day application for first 2 to 4 weeks
  - Avoid in pregnant and lactating women.
  - Cost varies based on formulation—$50 to $150 per tube for generic.
- Adapalene (Differin): 0.1%, apply topically at night.
  - Effective; less irritation than tretinoin or tazarotene
  - May be combined with benzoyl peroxide (Epiduo)—very effective in skin of color
  - First FDA-approved over-the-counter (OTC) retinoid *much* less expensive than other Rx retinoids ($10 to $15 per tube)
- Tazarotene (Tazorac): Apply at bedtime.
  - Most effective and most irritating; teratogenic

- Azelaic acid (Azelex, Finevin): 20% topically, BID
  - Keratinolytic, antibacterial, anti-inflammatory
  - Reduces postinflammatory hyperpigmentation in dark-skinned individuals
  - Side effects: erythema, dryness, scaling, hypopigmentation
  - Effective in postadolescent acne
  - 20% Rx >$400 per tube
  - OTC 10% and 15% formulations cost $10 to $40 per tube.
- Salicylic acid: 2%, less effective and less irritating than tretinoin
- α-Hydroxy acids: available OTC
- Topical antibiotics and anti-inflammatories
  - Topical benzoyl peroxide
    - 2.5% as effective as stronger preparations
    - Gel penetrates better into follicles.
    - When used with tretinoin, apply benzoyl peroxide in morning and tretinoin at night.
    - Side effects: irritation; may bleach clothes; photosensitivity
- Topical antibiotics: Do not use as monotherapy (4)[A].
  - Erythromycin 2%
  - Clindamycin 1%
  - Metronidazole gel or cream: Apply once daily.
  - Azelaic acid (Azelex, Finevin): 20% cream: enhanced effect and decreased risk of resistance when used with zinc and benzoyl peroxide
  - Benzoyl peroxide-erythromycin (Benzamycin): especially effective with azelaic acid
  - Benzoyl peroxide-clindamycin (BenzaClin, DUAC, Clindoxyl)
  - Benzoyl peroxide-salicylic acid (Cleanse & Treat, Inova): similar in effectiveness to benzoyl peroxide-clindamycin
  - Sodium sulfacetamide (Sulfacet-R, Novacet, Klaron): useful in acne with seborrheic dermatitis or rosacea
  - Dapsone (Aczone) 5% gel: useful in adult females with inflammatory acne; may cause yellow/orange skin discoloration when mixed with BP; very rare methemoglobinemia
- Oral antibiotics: use for shortest possible period, generally needs 8 to 12 weeks of therapy, reevaluate for discontinuation at 12 to 16 weeks duration (4); indicated when acne is more severe, trunk involvement, unresponsive to topical agents, or at greater risk for scarring (5)[A]
  - Tetracycline: 500 to 1,000 mg/day divided BID; high dose initially, taper in 6 months, less effective than doxycycline or minocycline (4), side effects: photosensitivity, esophagitis
  - Minocycline: 100 to 200 mg/day, divided daily— BID; side effects include photosensitivity, urticaria, gray-blue skin, vertigo, hepatitis, lupus.
  - Doxycycline: 20 to 200 mg/day, divided daily— BID; side effects include photosensitivity.
  - Erythromycin: 500 to 1,000 mg/day; divided BID–QID; decreasing effectiveness as a result of increasing P. acnes resistance
  - Trimethoprim-sulfamethoxazole (Bactrim DS, Septra DS): 1 daily or BID
  - Azithromycin (Zithromax): 500 mg 3 days/week × 1 month and then 250 mg every other day × 2 months
- Oral retinoids
  - Isotretinoin: 0.5 to 1.0 mg/kg/day divided BID to maximum 2 mg/kg/day divided BID for very severe disease; 60–90% cure rate; usually given for 12 to 20 weeks; maximum cumulative dose = 120 to 150 mg/kg; 20% of patients relapse and require retreatment (3)[A], 0.25 to 0.40 mg/kg/day in moderately severe acne
    - Side effects: teratogenic, pancreatitis, excessive drying of skin, hypertriglyceridemia, hepatitis,

blood dyscrasias, hyperostosis, premature epiphyseal closure, night blindness, erythema multiforme, Stevens-Johnson syndrome, suicidal ideation, psychosis
  - Avoid tetracyclines or vitamin A preparations during isotretinoin therapy due to risk of pseudotumor cerebri.
  - Monitor for pregnancy, psychiatric/mood changes, complete blood count (CBC), lipids, glucose, and liver function tests at baseline and every month.
  - Patient and provider must be registered and adhere to manufacturer's iPLEDGE program (www.ipledgeprogram.com), two forms of effective contraception required.
- Medications for women only
  - FDA-approved oral contraceptives (in order of possible effectiveness) (6)[B]
    - Drospirenone/ethinyl estradiol (Yaz), or drospirenone/ethinyl estradiol/levomefolate (Beyaz) > norgestimate/ethinyl estradiol (Ortho Tri-Cyclen) > norethindrone acetate/ethinyl estradiol (Estrostep)
    - Most combined contraceptives also effective; may take months to become effective
- Spironolactone (Aldactone); 25 to 200 mg/day; antiandrogen; reduces sebum production, not FDA-approved for acne Rx

ISSUES FOR REFERRAL
Consider referral/consultation to dermatologist.
- Refractory lesions despite appropriate therapy
- Consideration of isotretinoin therapy
- Management of acne scars

ADDITIONAL THERAPIES
- Acne hyperpigmented macules
  - Topical hydroquinones (1.5–10%)
  - Azelaic acid (20%) topically
  - Topical retinoids
  - Corticosteroids: low dose, suppresses adrenal androgens
  - Dapsone 5% gel (Aczone): topical, anti-inflammatory; use in patients >12 years.
  - Sunscreen for prevention
- Light-based treatments (lack high quality evidence of effectiveness)
  - Ultraviolet A/ultraviolet B (UVA/UVB), blue or blue/red light; pulse dye, KTP, or infrared laser
  - Photodynamic therapy for 30 to 60 minutes with 5-aminolevulinic acid for three sessions is effective for inflammatory lesions.
    - Greatest use when used as adjunct to medications or if can't tolerate medications

SURGERY/OTHER PROCEDURES
- Comedo extraction after incising the layer of epithelium over closed comedo
- Inject large cystic lesions with 0.05 to 0.30 mL triamcinolone (Kenalog 2 to 5 mg/mL); use 30-gauge needle, inject through pore, slightly distend cyst.
- Acne scar treatment: retinoids, steroid injections, cryosurgery, electrodessication, micro-/dermabrasion, chemical peels, laser resurfacing, pulsed dye laser, microneedling, fillers, punch elevation

COMPLEMENTARY & ALTERNATIVE MEDICINE
- Evidence suggests tea tree oil, seaweed extract, Kampo formulations, Ayurvedic formulations, rose extract, basil extract, epigallocatechin gallate, barberry extract, gluconolactone solution, and green tea extract may be useful (4).
- Limited data on use of dermocosmetics for acne Rx

 ONGOING CARE

FOLLOW-UP RECOMMENDATIONS
Use oral or topical antibiotics for 3 months; taper as inflammatory lesions resolve.

DIET
Data suggests that high-glycemic index foods and milk may influence acne (4)[B].

PATIENT EDUCATION
- There may be a worsening of acne during first 2 weeks of treatment.
- Results are typically seen after a minimum of 4 weeks of treatment.

PROGNOSIS
Gradual improvement over time (usually within 8 to 12 weeks after beginning therapy)

COMPLICATIONS
- Acne conglobata: severe confluent inflammatory acne with systemic symptoms
- Facial scarring and psychological distress, including anxiety, depression, and suicidal ideation (3)
- Postinflammatory hyperpigmentation, keloids, and scars are more common in skin of color.

REFERENCES

1. Admani S, Barrio VR. Evaluation and treatment of acne from infancy to preadolescence. *Dermatol Ther*. 2013;26(6):462–466.
2. Picardo M, Eichenfield LF, Tan J. Acne and rosacea. *Dermatol Ther (Heidelb)*. 2017;7(Suppl 1):43–52.
3. Dawson AL, Dellavalle RP. Acne vulgaris. *BMJ*. 2013;346:f2634.
4. Zaenglein AL, Pathy AL, Schlosser BJ, et al. Guidelines of care for the management of acne vulgaris. *J Am Acad Dermatol*. 2016;74(5):945.e33–973.e33.
5. Del Rosso JQ, Kim G. Optimizing use of oral antibiotics in acne vulgaris. *Dermatol Clin*. 2009;27(1):33–42.
6. Lortscher D, Admani S, Satur N, et al. Hormonal contraceptives and acne: a retrospective analysis of 2147 patients. *J Drugs Dermatol*. 2016;15(6):670–674.

ADDITIONAL READING

Nguyen HL, Tollefson MM. Endocrine disorders and hormonal therapy for adolescent acne. *Curr Opin Pediatr*. 2017;29(4):455–465.

 SEE ALSO

- Acne Rosacea
- Algorithm: Acne

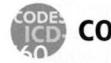 **CODES**

ICD10
- L70.0 Acne vulgaris
- L70.4 Infantile acne
- L70.1 Acne conglobata

CLINICAL PEARLS

- Full results for changes in therapy take 8 to 12 weeks.
- Decrease topical frequency to every day or to every other day for irritation.
- Use benzoyl peroxide every time a topical or oral antibiotic is used.

ACUTE CORONARY SYNDROMES: NSTE-ACS (UNSTABLE ANGINA AND NSTEMI)

Aravdeep Jhand, MBBS • Harish C. Devineni, MD • Gene Pershwitz, MD

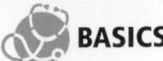

BASICS

DESCRIPTION
- Unstable angina (UA) and non–ST-segment elevation myocardial infarction (NSTEMI) are acute coronary syndromes without ST-segment elevation (NSTE-ACS).
- NSTEMI is defined by the rise and fall of cardiac biomarkers (preferably troponin) with at least one value above the 99th percentile upper reference limit and accompanied by one of the following: symptoms of ischemia, new ST-segment/T-wave changes, development of pathologic Q waves on ECG, or imaging evidence of loss of viable myocardium or new regional wall motion abnormality (1).
- UA is defined by the presence of clinical symptoms of cardiac ischemia (new-onset anginal chest pain, or change in typical anginal pattern, or development of angina at rest, or change in typical anginal equivalent), without myocardial necrosis as evidenced by normal cardiac biomarkers of injury (troponin). ECG changes, such as ST-segment depression or T-wave inversions, may be present (1).

EPIDEMIOLOGY
Incidence
- Estimated annual incidence of new and recurrent MI is 605,000 and 200,000, respectively (2).
- In United States, average age at first MI is 65.6 years for males and 72.0 years for females (2).
- Incidence of MI is higher in blacks across all age groups as compared to the white population (2).

Prevalence
- An estimated 16.5 million Americans ≥20 years have coronary artery disease (CAD) with the overall prevalence of MI being 3.0% (3.8% for males and 2.3% for females) (2).
- Mortality
  - CAD is the leading cause of death in adults in the United States with overall age-adjusted mortality of 98.8/100,000 (2).
  - Death rate is higher in men as compared to women and in blacks as compared to whites (2).

ETIOLOGY AND PATHOPHYSIOLOGY
- NSTE-ACS occurs primarily due to a sudden decrease in myocardial blood flow due to acute plaque rupture or plaque erosions leading to partially occluding thrombosis.
- Other mechanisms include:
  - Dynamic obstruction triggered by intense spasm of a coronary artery (Prinzmetal angina or coronary vasospasm induced by cocaine or methamphetamine)
  - Increased myocardial oxygen demand resulting in supply–demand mismatch, microcirculatory dysfunction without epicardial coronary obstruction
  - Less common causes include coronary arterial inflammation, dissection/rupture, thromboembolism.

RISK FACTORS
- Traditional/classic
  - Age (strongest risk factor), male gender, prior MI, hypertension, tobacco use, diabetes mellitus (DM), dyslipidemia, and family history of premature CAD (Premature CAD is defined as age of onset prior to 55 years in males and <65 years in females.)
- Novel/emerging risk factors
  - Sedentary lifestyle, overweight/obesity (metabolic syndrome), inflammation (psoriasis, rheumatoid arthritis), psychosocial factors (anxiety/depression), chronic kidney disease (CKD), obstructive sleep apnea, higher intake of red meat, radiation exposure

GENERAL PREVENTION
- Smoking cessation, healthy diet, weight control, physical activity
- Risk factor control: diabetes and blood pressure control, lipid-lowering therapy (statins), daily aspirin (in select patients)

COMMONLY ASSOCIATED CONDITIONS
- Vascular disease (cerebrovascular and peripheral vascular disease, aneurysms, erectile dysfunction)
- Other forms of heart disease (heart failure, valvular disease, high-output states)
- Disease related to underlying risk factors: COPD and thrombophilic disorders

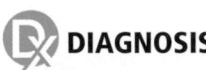

DIAGNOSIS

HISTORY
- Chest heaviness/tightness lasting ≥10 minutes; occurs with or without exertion, may increase in frequency. Pain or discomfort is typically retrosternal and can radiate to the neck, jaw, interscapular area, upper extremities, or epigastrium.
- Pain is typically described as a pressure, tightness, heaviness, squeezing, or fullness.
- Associated symptoms of palpitations, dyspnea, nausea, diaphoresis, light-headedness, syncope, or dysphoria can occur.
- Patients especially elderly, diabetics, and women can present without chest pain with symptoms such as dyspnea, diaphoresis, and extreme fatigue which represent "anginal equivalents."
- Risk factors for CAD
- Use of cocaine or amphetamines

PHYSICAL EXAM
- General: abnormal vital signs including tachycardia or bradycardia, hypertension or hypotension, widened pulse pressure, tachypnea, fever, transverse ear crease, poor dental hygiene, stigmata of tobacco use
- Cardiovascular: dysrhythmia, jugular venous distention (JVD), new murmur, rub or gallop, diminished peripheral pulses, carotid bruits
- Respiratory: tachypnea, ↑ work of breathing, crackles
- Neurologic: fatigue, weakness, altered mental status
- Musculoskeletal: Sharp pain reproducible with movement or palpation is unlikely to be cardiac.
- Skin: cool skin, pallor, diaphoresis, signs of dyslipidemia (xanthomas, xanthelasma)

DIFFERENTIAL DIAGNOSIS
- Cardiac: aortic dissection, myocarditis, pericarditis, pericardial effusion/tamponade, heart failure, hypertensive emergency, stress cardiomyopathy (Takotsubo), dysrhythmia, and mitral valve disease
- Pulmonary: pulmonary embolism, pneumothorax, pneumonia, pleuritis, bronchitis
- Panic disorder and anxiety disorders
- Musculoskeletal pain: costochondritis, rib fracture
- GI: gastroesophageal reflux disease (GERD), esophageal spasm, esophagitis, esophageal rupture or perforation, hiatal hernia, penetrating or perforating peptic ulcer, biliary or pancreatic pain

DIAGNOSTIC TESTS & INTERPRETATION
Initial Tests (lab, imaging)
- 12-lead ECG (3)[C]: should be obtained within 10 minutes of presentation; applies to both UA and NSTEMI
  - New ST-segment depression ≥0.5 mm in two or more contiguous leads and/or T-wave inversions ≥1 mm in two or more contiguous leads with prominent R wave or R/S ratio >1
  - ST depression and/or tall R wave in V_1/V_2 with upright T waves may indicate transmural STEMI of posterior wall. ECG with posterior leads (V_7–V_9) should be performed.
  - If initial ECG is nondiagnostic but symptoms persist with suspicion for ACS, perform serial ECGs at 15- to 30-minute intervals.
- CBC, BMP, and serum biomarker (negative by definition in UA)
  - Troponin concentration rises 3 to 6 hours after onset of ischemic symptoms but can be delayed up to 8 to 12 hours (troponin T is not specific in patients with renal dysfunction).
  - Ultra-high sensitive troponins have a higher sensitivity than standard assays, but further validation is required.
  - With contemporary troponin assays, older cardiac markers of injury-like LDH, CK-MB, and myoglobin are less specific and have limited utility in the routine management of ACS (3)[A]. CK-MB has been shown to have better specificity than troponins in post-PCI MI.
  - Patients with negative biomarkers within 6 hours of the onset of symptoms should have biomarkers remeasured 8 to 12 hours from onset of symptoms.
- CXR, CT with contrast to exclude other etiologies
- Transthoracic echocardiography is recommended to assess for regional wall motion abnormalities, systolic function, and to exclude alternate etiologies.

Follow-Up Tests & Special Considerations
- Fasting lipid profile, preferably within 24 hours
- Activated partial thromboplastin time (aPTT)
- Urine drug screen in selected patients
- Other lab tests: B-type natriuretic peptide or N-terminal pro–B-type natriuretic peptide; increases with MI and may not indicate heart failure

Diagnostic Procedures/Other
- For low- to intermediate-risk patients with resolution of symptoms and nondiagnostic ECG with negative biomarkers, consider noninvasive cardiac testing with standard exercise treadmill test (3)[A], stress echocardiography, or nuclear stress study (3)[B].
- Alternatively, coronary CTA can be performed as well to exclude NSTE-ACS (3)[A].

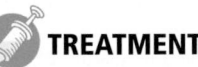

TREATMENT

GENERAL MEASURES
- Risk stratify using TIMI or GRACE score to select use of early invasive approach (coronary angiography within 24 hours of admission) versus ischemia-guided therapy (3)[A]
  - Urgent invasive management for very high-risk patients, such as those with hemodynamic instability or cardiogenic shock, recurrent or ongoing chest pain refractory to medical therapy, life-threatening arrhythmias or cardiac arrest, mechanical complications, acute heart failure, and recurrent dynamic ST-T wave changes (3)[A]

- Bed/chair rest with continuous ECG monitoring, maintain O₂ saturation >90%, and tight BP control
- Avoid continuation of NSAIDs.
- Deep vein thrombosis prophylaxis
- Smoking cessation
- Correction of electrolyte abnormalities (K and Mg)

MEDICATION

First Line

- Antiplatelet therapy: Dual antiplatelet therapy is recommended for all patients with NSTE-ACS.
- Aspirin, nonenteric coated, initial dose of 162 to 325 mg chewed or crushed for all patients; decreases mortality and morbidity (3)[A]
- Maintenance dose of 75 to 100 mg/day indefinitely
- P2Y12 inhibitors:
  – Should be given at the time of diagnosis unless invasive approach is planned in a very high–bleeding-risk patient (3)[B]
  – Ticagrelor, loading dose 180 mg PO, followed by 90 mg PO twice daily; avoid in patients with 2nd- and 3rd-degree heart block (3)[B] OR
  – Prasugrel 60 mg PO, followed by 10 mg PO daily. Reserved for post-PCI patients treated with coronary stents; contraindicated in patients ≥75 years or those with history of CVA/TIA (3)[B] OR
  – Clopidogrel, loading dose 300 to 600 mg PO, followed by 75 mg PO daily. Use with caution in patients with thrombocytopenia and CKD.
  – Patients unable to take aspirin should receive loading and maintenance dose of a P2Y12 inhibitor (3)[B].
  – GP IIb/IIIa inhibitors: Add eptifibatide or tirofiban in select high-risk patients (persistent chest pain, large thrombus burden on angiography) after PCI (3)[B].
- Nitroglycerin sublingual 0.4 mg every 5 minutes for total of 3 doses and then assess need for IV nitroglycerin. Avoid if hypotension or if used PDE (−) within the 24 to 48 hours.
- Morphine sulfate 1 to 5 mg IV in patients with continuous ischemic chest pain, with increments of 2 to 8 mg repeated at 5- to 30-minute intervals (3)[B]
- Oral β-blocker therapy should be initiated within 24 hours in patients without signs of heart failure, cardiogenic shock, or other contraindications. Recommended dose is metoprolol tartrate 25 to 50 mg every 6 to 12 hours or atenolol 25 to 50 mg twice daily. IV therapy may be considered in patients with severe ischemia (1,3)[A].
- In patients with concomitant ACS, stabilized heart failure, and reduced systolic function (LVEF <40%), the recommended β-blockers are metoprolol succinate, carvedilol, and bisoprolol (3)[C].
- Lipid-lowering therapy: Initiate or continue high-intensity statin therapy (preferred due to nonlipid benefit on vascular function) with atorvastatin 80 mg daily or rosuvastatin 20 to 40 mg daily (3)[A]. Ezetimibe, omega-3 fatty acids, PCSK9 inhibitors, and/or fibrates can be considered in statin-intolerant patients.
- ACE inhibitor (ACEi) is recommended in all patients with ACS particularly in the presence of diabetes, LV dysfunction, or heart failure (3)[A].
- Aldosterone antagonist (spironolactone or eplerenone) is recommended in NSTEMI for patients without significant renal dysfunction or hyperkalemia who are on a therapeutic dose of ACEi/ARB and β-blocker and have LVEF ≤40%, DM, or heart failure (3)[A].
- Antithrombotic therapy: Initiate anticoagulant: enoxaparin or unfractionated heparin (UFH), fondaparinux, or bivalirudin. Bivalirudin has been associated with a lower bleeding risk.

Second Line

- Nondihydropyridine calcium channel blocker (CCB) (verapamil or diltiazem) to reduce myocardial oxygen demand when β-blockers are contraindicated if normal EF (3)[C]. Use oral long-acting CCB only after β-blockers and nitrates have been fully used (3)[C]. Long-acting CCBs are recommended in treatment of patients with coronary artery spasm (3)[C]. Avoid in patients with heart block (3)[B].
- Long-term nitrate therapy for recurrent angina/ischemia or heart failure
- Sublingual nitroglycerin at discharge
- Ranolazine indicated in treatment of chronic angina not responsive to other meds; 500 to 1,000 mg, twice a day (3)[A]
- Benzodiazepines in patients with cocaine/methamphetamine intoxication. Avoid β-blockers in cocaine or methamphetamine users.

ISSUES FOR REFERRAL

- Cardiology consultation is appropriate for NSTE-ACS.
- Patients will need close follow-up with a cardiologist.
- Referral to exercise-based cardiac rehabilitation program prior to hospital discharge (3)[B]

SURGERY/OTHER PROCEDURES

- Coronary reperfusion
  – PCI with stent placement
  – CABG surgery
- Intra-aortic balloon pump for patients with refractory symptoms/shock

ADMISSION, INPATIENT, AND NURSING CONSIDERATIONS

- Admit patients with risk factors who present with chest pain and suspected NSTE-ACS.
- Considerations in special populations
  – Older population (≥75 years)
    ○ Benefit of early invasive management in elderly ≥ young population (3)[A]
    ○ Pharmacotherapy should be individualized based on weight and renal function.
  – Pregnancy
    ○ Specific risk factors for ACS in pregnancy include advanced maternal age, gestational diabetes, and preeclampsia/eclampsia.
    ○ Spontaneous coronary artery dissection and thromboembolism should be considered in evaluation of pregnant women with ACS.
    ○ ACEi, ARBs, and statins are contraindicated.

 ONGOING CARE

FOLLOW-UP RECOMMENDATIONS

- It is reasonable in patients with suspected ACS (low risk) who have normal serial ECGs and cardiac troponins to have a treadmill ECG (3)[A], stress myocardial perfusion imaging, or stress echocardiography before or within 72 hours after discharge (3)[B].
- Follow up 2 to 6 weeks (low risk) and 14 days (high risk).
- All patients with reduced EF need reevaluation for ICD placement for primary prevention >40 days to 3 months (postrevascularization) after discharge.

DIET

Diet relationship to CAD is complex; low-sodium and low-saturated fat diets often recommended

PATIENT EDUCATION

Education on diet, exercise, smoking cessation, and lifestyle modification. It is safe to resume exercise, sexual activity within 2 weeks in asymptomatic patients after outpatient reevaluation.

- Recommend pneumococcal and influenza vaccination.

PROGNOSIS

UA/NSTEMI patients have lower in-hospital mortality than those with STEMI but a similar or worse long-term outcome.

COMPLICATIONS

Cardiogenic shock, heart failure, mitral regurgitation, ventricular aneurysm, dysrhythmia, acute pulmonary embolism, acute thromboembolic stroke, pericarditis/Dressler syndrome, depression (increases mortality risk)

REFERENCES

1. Anderson JL, Adams CD, Antman EM, et al; for American College of Cardiology Foundation/American Heart Association Task Force on Practice Guidelines. 2012 ACCF/AHA focused update incorporated into the ACCF/AHA 2007 guidelines for the management of patients with unstable angina/non–ST-elevation myocardial infarction: a report of the American College of Cardiology Foundation/American Heart Association Task Force on Practice Guidelines. *Circulation.* 2013;127(23):e663–e828.
2. Benjamin EJ, Virani SS, Callaway CW, et al; for American Heart Association Council on Epidemiology and Prevention Statistics Committee and Stroke Statistics Subcommittee. Heart disease and stroke statistics—2018 update: a report from the American Heart Association. *Circulation.* 2018;137(12):e67–e492.
3. Amsterdam EA, Wenger NK, Brindis RG, et al. 2014 AHA/ACC guideline for the management of patients with non–ST-elevation acute coronary syndromes: a report of the American College of Cardiology/American Heart Association Task Force on Practice Guidelines. *J Am Coll Cardiol.* 2014;64(24):e139–e228.

ADDITIONAL READING

Hoenig MR, Aroney CN, Scott IA. Early invasive versus conservative strategies for unstable angina and non-ST elevation myocardial infarction in the stent era. *Cochrane Database Syst Rev.* 2010;(3):CD004815.

CODES

ICD10

- I24.9 Acute ischemic heart disease, unspecified
- I20.0 Unstable angina
- I21.4 Non-ST elevation (NSTEMI) myocardial infarction

CLINICAL PEARLS

- Discontinue NSAIDs, nonselective or selective cyclooxygenase (COX)-2 agents, except for ASA, due to increased risks of mortality, reinfarction, hypertension, heart failure, and myocardial rupture.
- Discontinue clopidogrel or prasugrel or ticagrelor 5 to 7 days before elective CABG.
- Do not use nitrate products in patients who recently used a phosphodiesterase 5 inhibitor (24 hours of sildenafil or vardenafil, or 48 hours of tadalafil).
- Duration of antithrombotic therapy after NSTEMI depends on type of stent received and medications administered.
- Avoid β-blockers in cocaine or methamphetamine user.

ACUTE CORONARY SYNDROMES: STEMI

Adedotun Anthony Ogunsua, MD, MPH • Kimberly Atianzar, MD • Yutthapong Temtanakitpaisan, MD

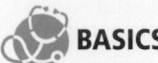
BASICS

DESCRIPTION
Acute myocardial infarction (AMI) is the rapid development of myocardial necrosis resulting from a sustained and complete absence of blood flow to a portion of the myocardium. ST-segment elevation myocardial infarction (STEMI) occurs when coronary blood flow ceases, usually following complete athero-thrombotic occlusion of a large coronary artery, resulting in transmural ischemia. This is accompanied by release of serum cardiac biomarkers and ST-segment elevation on an electrocardiogram (ECG).

EPIDEMIOLOGY
Incidence
There are >650,000 cases of AMI reported annually in the United States. Early revascularization and AMI management has improved mortality, with a 30-day survival of 95%.

Prevalence
- Leading cause of morbidity and mortality in the United States
- ~7.5 million people in the United States are affected by AMI.
- Prevalence increases with age and is higher in men (5.5%) compared to women (2.9%).

ETIOLOGY AND PATHOPHYSIOLOGY
- Atherosclerotic coronary artery disease (CAD):
  - Atherosclerotic lesions can be fibrotic, calcified, or lipid laden. Thin-capped atheromas are more likely to rupture, causing atherothrombotic occlusion.
- Nonatherosclerotic causes:
  - Embolism from either infective vegetations, or thrombi originating within the right atrium across the foramen ovale ("paradoxical"), from the left atrium or from within the left ventricle
  - Spontaneous coronary artery dissection: prevalent in fibromuscular dysplasia (FMD) and in young women
  - Mechanical or iatrogenic obstruction: chest trauma, dissection of the aorta and/or coronary arteries
  - Coronary artery spasm from increased vasomotor tone; anginal variant
  - Arteritis and other etiologies: hematologic causes (disseminated intravascular coagulation [DIC], severe anemia), aortic stenosis, cocaine, IV drug use, severe burns, prolonged hypotension

RISK FACTORS
Advancing age, hypertension, tobacco use, diabetes mellitus, dyslipidemia, family history of premature onset of CAD, sedentary lifestyle

GENERAL PREVENTION
Smoking cessation/abstinence; healthy diet; weight loss/control; regular physical activity and exercise; control of hypertension, hyperlipidemia, and diabetes mellitus

COMMONLY ASSOCIATED CONDITIONS
Abdominal aortic aneurysm, cerebrovascular disease, atherosclerotic peripheral vascular disease

DIAGNOSIS

HISTORY
- Symptoms:
  - Classically, sudden onset of chest heaviness/tightness, with or without exertion, lasting minutes to hours
  - Pain/discomfort radiating to neck, jaw, interscapular area, upper extremities, and/or epigastrium
  - Patients with inferior MI may present primarily with abdominal discomfort.
- Previous history of myocardial ischemia (stable or unstable angina, AMI, coronary bypass surgery, or percutaneous coronary intervention [PCI])
- Assess risk factors for CAD, history of bleeding, non-cardiac surgery, family history of premature CAD.
- Medications: Ask if recent use of phosphodiesterase type 5 inhibitors (if recent use, avoid concomitant nitrates).
- Tobacco, alcohol, and/or drug abuse (especially cocaine)

PHYSICAL EXAM
- General: restlessness, agitation, hypothermia, fever
- Neurologic: dizziness, syncope, fatigue, asthenia, disorientation (especially in the elderly)
- Cardiovascular (CV): dysrhythmia, hypotension, widened pulse pressure, S_3 and S_4, jugular venous distention (JVD)
- Respiratory: dyspnea, tachypnea, crackles, rales
- GI: abdominal pain, nausea, vomiting, hiccups
- Musculoskeletal: pain in neck, back, shoulders, or upper limbs
- Skin: cool skin, pallor, diaphoresis

Geriatric and Gender Considerations
- Elderly patients may have an atypical presentation, including silent or unrecognized MI. They may often present with syncope, weakness, shortness of breath, unexplained nausea, epigastric pain, altered mental status, or delirium.
- Women present with "atypical" symptoms such as fatigue, dyspnea, and malaise.
- Patients with diabetes mellitus may have fewer and less dramatic chest symptoms.

DIFFERENTIAL DIAGNOSIS
Unstable angina, aortic dissection, pulmonary embolism (PE), perforating gastric ulcer, pericarditis, dysrhythmias, gastroesophageal reflux disease (GERD), esophageal spasm, biliary/pancreatic pain, hyperventilation syndrome

DIAGNOSTIC TESTS & INTERPRETATION
Initial Tests (lab, imaging)
- 12-lead ECG:
  - ≥1 mm ST elevation in a regional pattern, involving at least two contiguous leads, with or without abnormal Q waves
  - STEMI of posterior wall: ST depression ± tall R waves in V_1–V_2
  - Absence of Q waves represents partial or transient occlusion or early infarction.
  - Consider right-sided and posterior chest leads if inferior MI pattern (examine V_3R, V_4R, V_7–V_9).
  - In the setting of ventricular pacing or a prior bundle branch block, the Sgarbossa criteria may be helpful.
- 2-Dimensional transthoracic echocardiography is useful in evaluating regional wall motion in MI and left ventricular function.
  - Useful in assessing mechanical complications and mural thrombus
- Once diagnosis is suspected, emergent coronary angiography with PCI is preferred.

Follow-Up Tests & Special Considerations
- Serum biomarkers
  - Troponin I and T (cTnI, cTnT) rise 3 to 6 hours after onset of ischemic symptoms.
  - Elevations in cTnI persist for 7 to 10 days, whereas cTnT elevations persist for 10 to 14 days after MI.
  - Myoglobin fraction of creatine kinase-MB (CK-MB) rises 3 to 4 hours after onset of myocardial injury; peaks at 12 to 24 hours and remains elevated for 2 to 3 days; CK-MB adds little diagnostic value in assessment of possible ACS to troponin testing.
- Other pertinent labs: fasting lipid profile, complete blood count (CBC), electrolytes, magnesium, BUN, serum creatinine, glucose, hemoglobin A1C, international normalized ratio (INR) if anticoagulation is contemplated, brain natriuretic peptide (BNP)
- Gender and minorities considerations
  - It is important to note that women and minorities receive less treatment compared with men and Caucasians.

Pregnancy Considerations
Pregnant patients presenting with STEMI will need discussion of risks and benefits of invasive coronary angiography with radiation exposure to fetus. Management should otherwise be the same as in nonpregnant patients.

Diagnostic Procedures/Other
- High-quality portable chest x-ray; transthoracic and/or transesophageal echocardiography; chest computed tomography angiography (CTA) scan may occasionally be of value acutely in equivocal presentations to evaluate for alternative diagnoses (aortic dissection, PE, ventricular aneurysm).
- Coronary angiography is the definitive test.

ALERT
Patients with chronic kidney disease need special attention to amount of contrast media used. Reduced volume of contrast and use of low or isosmolar contrast media may lower risk of progression of renal impairment.

TREATMENT

GENERAL MEASURES
- See "Medication" for ED management.
- Following emergent revascularization, admit the patient to the coronary care unit (CCU) or a telemetry unit with continuous ECG monitoring and bed rest, and use:
  - Anxiolytics, if needed; stool softeners
  - Antiarrhythmics as needed for unstable dysrhythmia
  - Deep vein thrombosis (DVT) prophylaxis
  - Dual antiplatelet therapy (DAPT) with continuation of aspirin 81 mg/day with clopidogrel 75 mg/day or prasugrel 10 mg/day or ticagrelor 90 mg twice daily
  - β-Blocker (BB), ACE inhibitors (or ARB if ACE intolerant), lipid-lowering therapy including high intensity statins
  - Tight BP control, progressively increased physical activity, smoking cessation/abstinence

MEDICATION
Medication recommendations are based on the 2013 ACC/AHA focused guideline updates (1,2).

First Line
(*While awaiting revascularization*)

- Supplemental oxygen 2 to 4 L/min for patients with oxygen saturation <90% or respiratory distress
- Nitroglycerin (NTG) sublingual 0.4 mg q5min for a total of 3 doses, followed by nitroglycerin IV if ongoing pain and/or hypertension and/or management of pulmonary congestion if no contraindications exist such as systolic <90 mm Hg or >30 mm Hg below baseline, right ventricle (RV) infarct, use of sildenafil or vardenafil within 24 hours or within 48 hours of tadalafil
- Morphine sulfate 4 to 8 mg IV with 2 to 8 mg IV repeated at 5- to 15-minute intervals to relieve pain, anxiety, or pulmonary congestion
- Antiplatelet agents:
  - Aspirin (ASA), non–enteric-coated, initial dose 162 to 325 mg chewed (1)[A]
  - A loading dose of a P2Y12 inhibitor is recommended for patients with STEMI for whom PCI is planned. Prasugrel or ticagrelor is preferred.
    - Prasugrel 60 mg loading dose should be given as soon as possible for primary PCI. Prasugrel is contraindicated in patients with previous stroke/transient ischemic attack. Do not recommend in patients aged >75 years or lower body weight (<60 kg).
    - Ticagrelor 180 mg loading dose. Ticagrelor may cause transient dyspnea.
    - Clopidogrel 600 mg loading dose should be given if neither prasugrel nor ticagrelor is available.
    - Cangrelor may be considered in patients not pretreated with oral P2Y12 receptor inhibitors at the time of PCI or in those who are unable to take oral agents.
    - Duration of DAPT is recommended for 12 months after PCI. In patients who are at high risk of severe bleeding complications, a P2Y12 inhibitor may be discontinued after 6 months.
- Anticoagulation therapy:
  - Unfractionated heparin (UFH) 50- to 70-U/kg IV bolus
  - Enoxaparin 0.5-mg/kg IV bolus
  - Bivalirudin 0.75-mg/kg IV bolus and then 1.75-mg/kg/hr infusion for up to 4 hours after procedure
- PCI versus fibrinolysis: Goal is to keep total ischemic time within 120 minutes. Door to needle time should be within 30 minutes or door to balloon time within 90 minutes.
  - Coronary reperfusion therapy
    - Primary PCI (balloon angioplasty, coronary stents) in the following:
      - Symptom onset of ≤12 hours
      - Symptom onset of ≤12 hours and contraindication to fibrinolytic therapy irrespective of time delay
      - Cardiogenic shock or acute severe heart failure (HF) irrespective of time delay from onset of MI
      - Evidence of ongoing ischemia 12 to 24 hours after symptom onset
    - Radial access is recommended over femoral access.
  - Procedural considerations
    - Routine aspiration thrombectomy no longer recommended prior to PCI because usefulness and safety are not fully established (3)[C]
    - PCI of infarct-related artery (IRA) is indicated.
    - Routine revascularization of non-IRA lesions in cardiogenic shock is not recommended during primary PCI (4)[B].

- Fibrinolysis
  - If presenting to a hospital without PCI capability and cannot be transferred to a PCI-capable facility to undergo PCI within 120 minutes of first medical contact
  - If no contraindications, administer within 12 to 24 hours of symptom onset, if there is evidence of ongoing ischemia.
    - Alteplase (tPA): 15-mg IV bolus, followed by 0.75 mg/kg (up to 50 mg) IV over 30 minutes and then 0.5 mg/kg (up to 35 mg) over 60 minutes; maximum 100 mg over 90 minutes
    - Reteplase (rPA): 10 units IV bolus; give second bolus 30 minutes apart.
    - Tenecteplase (TNK-tPA): 30- to 50-mg (based on weight) IV bolus. Recommend to reduce to half dose in patients ≥75 years of age.
  - Adjunctive antiplatelet therapy with fibrinolysis
    - Aspirin: 162- to 325-mg loading dose followed by 81 mg daily indefinitely
    - Clopidogrel (300-mg loading dose for patients <75 years of age, 75-mg dose for patients >75 years of age). Clopidogrel 75 mg daily should be continued for at least 14 days and up to 1 year.
  - Adjunctive anticoagulation therapy with fibrinolysis
    - Use anticoagulants (UFH, enoxaparin, or fondaparinux) as ancillary therapy to reperfusion therapy for minimum of 48 hours and preferably duration of admission (up to 8 days) or until revascularization, if performed.
      □ Glycoprotein IIb/IIIa receptor antagonists at time of primary PCI in selected patients if there is no reflow or thrombotic complications (abciximab, eptifibatide, or tirofiban)
      □ IV BB should be considered at the time of presentation, if no contraindications exist (signs of congestive heart failure [CHF], low output state) and SBP >120 mm Hg.
- ACE inhibitors should be initiated orally within 24 hours of STEMI in patients with anterior infarction, HF, diabetes, or ejection fraction (EF) ≤0.40 unless contraindicated.
- High-intensity statin therapy should be started as early as possible.
- Mineralocorticoid receptor antagonist (spironolactone, eplerenone) is recommended in patients with EF <40% and HF or diabetes, who are already receiving an ACE inhibitor and a BB, if there is no renal failure or hyperkalemia.

Second Line
Long-acting nondihydropyridine calcium channel blocker (CCB) when BB is ineffective or contraindicated and EF is normal; do not use immediate-release nifedipine.

SURGERY/OTHER PROCEDURES
Urgent coronary artery bypass graft (CABG) surgery is indicated in patients with STEMI and coronary anatomy not amenable to PCI who have ongoing or recurrent ischemia, cardiogenic shock, severe HF, or other high-risk features.

ADMISSION, INPATIENT, AND NURSING CONSIDERATIONS
- All STEMI patients should be admitted to a CCU or an intensive cardiac care unit for evaluation and treatment.
- Transfer high-risk patients who receive fibrinolytic therapy as primary reperfusion therapy at a non–PCI-capable facility to a PCI-capable facility as soon as possible.
- Right ventricular infarction may need fluid resuscitation for hypotension.

 ONGOING CARE

FOLLOW-UP RECOMMENDATIONS
Emphasize medication adherence. Identify high-risk patients for implantable cardioverter defibrillator (ICD) placement (especially those with an EF <30%). Consider an exercise-based cardiac rehabilitation program. Encourage smoking cessation.

DIET
Low-fat/healthy-fat diet: reduced intake of saturated fats (to <7% of total calories) (but dairy fats are not likely associated with CAD), eliminate *trans* fatty acids (to <1% of total calories). Impact of low-cholesterol diet remains uncertain. Mediterranean diet is healthy.

PATIENT EDUCATION
May resume sexual activity 1 or more weeks after uncomplicated MI or 6 to 8 weeks after CABG; smoking cessation and low-fat diet

COMPLICATIONS
HF, myocardial wall rupture, left ventricular aneurysm, pericarditis, dysrhythmias, acute mitral regurgitation, and depression (common)

REFERENCES

1. O'Gara PT, Kushner FG, Ascheim DD, et al; for CF/AHA Task Force. 2013 ACCF/AHA guideline for the management of ST-elevation myocardial infarction: executive summary: a report of the American College of Cardiology Foundation/American Heart Association Task Force on Practice Guidelines. *Circulation*. 2013;127(4):529–555.
2. Ibánez B, James S, Agewall S, et al. 2017 ESC guidelines for the management of acute myocardial infarction in patients presenting with ST-segment elevation. *Rev Esp Cardiol (Engl Ed)*. 2017;70(12):1082.
3. Levine GN, Bates ER, Blankenship JC, et al. 2015 ACC/AHA/SCAI focused update on primary percutaneous coronary intervention for patients with ST-elevation myocardial infarction: an update of the 2011 ACCF/AHA/SCAI guideline for percutaneous coronary intervention and the 2013 ACCF/AHA guideline for the management of ST-elevation myocardial infarction. *J Am Coll Cardiol*. 2016;67(10):1235–1250.
4. Neumann FJ, Sousa-Uva M, Ahlsson A, et al. 2018 ESC/EACTS guidelines on myocardial revascularization [published online ahead of print August 25, 2018]. *Eur Heart J*. doi:10.1093/eurheartj/ehy394.

 CODES

ICD10
- I24.9 Acute ischemic heart disease, unspecified
- I21.3 ST elevation (STEMI) myocardial infarction of unspecified site
- I25.10 Athscl heart disease of native coronary artery w/o ang pctrs

CLINICAL PEARLS

For elective surgeries in patients on DAPT, it is recommended to wait until completion of mandatory regimen and continue ASA perioperatively.

ACUTE KIDNEY INJURY

Jason Kurland, MD

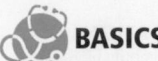 **BASICS**

DESCRIPTION
Abrupt loss of kidney function, defined as a rise in serum creatinine (SCr) of ≥0.3 mg/dL within 48 hours; a 50% increase in SCr within 7 days or urine output of <0.5 mL/kg/hr for >6 hours, resulting in retention of nitrogenous waste as well as electrolyte, acid–base, and volume homeostasis abnormalities (1)

EPIDEMIOLOGY
Incidence
5% of hospital and 30% of ICU admissions have acute kidney injury (AKI). 25% of patients develop AKI while in the hospital; 50% of these cases are iatrogenic. Developing AKI as an inpatient is associated with >4-fold increased risk of death (2).

ETIOLOGY AND PATHOPHYSIOLOGY
Three categories: prerenal, intrarenal, and postrenal

- Prerenal (reduced renal perfusion, typically reversible)
  - Hypotension, volume depletion (GI losses, excessive sweating, diuretics, hemorrhage); renal artery stenosis/embolism; burns; heart/liver failure
  - Decreased renal perfusion (often due to hypovolemia) leads to a decrease in glomerular filtration rate (GFR), which (if prolonged or severe) can progress to ischemic acute tubular necrosis (ATN).
- Intrarenal (intrinsic kidney injury, often from prolonged or severe renal hypoperfusion)
  - ATN (from prolonged prerenal azotemia, radiographic contrast material, aminoglycosides, NSAIDs, or other nephrotoxic substances), glomerulonephritis (GN), acute interstitial nephritis (AIN; drug induced), arteriolar insults, vasculitis, accelerated hypertension, cholesterol embolization (following an intra-arterial procedure), intrarenal deposition/sludging (uric acid nephropathy and multiple myeloma [Bence Jones proteins])
- Postrenal (obstruction of the collecting system)
  - Extrinsic compression (e.g., benign prostatic hypertrophy [BPH], carcinoma, pregnancy); intrinsic obstruction (e.g., calculus, tumor, clot, stricture, sloughed papillae); decreased function (e.g., neurogenic bladder), leading to obstruction of the urinary collection system

Genetics
No known genetic pattern

RISK FACTORS
- Chronic kidney disease (CKD)
- Comorbid conditions (e.g., diabetes mellitus, hypertension, heart failure, liver failure)
- Advanced age
- Radiocontrast material exposure (intravascular)
- Medications that impair autoregulation of GFR (NSAIDs, ACEI/ARB, cyclosporine/tacrolimus)
- Nephrotoxic medications (e.g., aminoglycoside antibiotics, platinum-based chemotherapy)

- Hypovolemia (e.g., diuretics, hemorrhage, GI losses)
- Sepsis, surgery, rhabdomyolysis
- Solitary kidney (risk in nephrolithiasis)
- BPH; malignancy (e.g., multiple myeloma)

COMMONLY ASSOCIATED CONDITIONS
Hyperkalemia, hyperphosphatemia, hypercalcemia, hyperuricemia, hydronephrosis, BPH, nephrolithiasis, congestive heart failure (CHF), uremic pericarditis, cirrhosis, CKD, malignant hypertension, vasculitis, drug reactions, sepsis, severe trauma, burns, transfusion reactions, recent chemotherapy, rhabdomyolysis, internal bleeding, dehydration

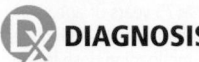 **DIAGNOSIS**

HISTORY
- Ascertain changes in PO intake, urine output, and body weight.
- Thorough medication history
- Prerenal: thirst, orthostatic symptoms
- Intrarenal: nephrotoxic medications, radiocontrast material, other toxins
- Livedo reticularis, SC nodules, and ischemic digits despite good pulses suggest atheroembolization.
- Flank pain may suggest renal artery or vein occlusion.
- Postrenal: Colicky flank pain that radiates to the groin suggests ureteric obstruction such as a stone; nocturia, frequency, and hesitancy suggest prostatic disease; suprapubic and flank pain are usually secondary to distension of the bladder and collecting system; anticholinergic drugs inhibit bladder emptying.
- Uremic symptoms: lethargy, nausea/vomiting, anorexia, pruritus, restless legs, sleep disturbance, hiccups

PHYSICAL EXAM
- Uremic signs: altered sensorium, seizures, asterixis, myoclonus, pericardial friction rub, peripheral neuropathies
- Prerenal signs: tachycardia, decreased jugular venous pressure (JVP), orthostatic hypotension, dry mucous membranes, decreased skin turgor; comorbid stigmata of sepsis, liver disease, or heart failure
- Intrinsic renal signs: pruritic rash, livedo reticularis, SC nodules, ischemic digits despite good pulses
- Postrenal signs: suprapubic distension, flank pain, enlarged prostate

DIAGNOSTIC TESTS & INTERPRETATION
Initial Tests (lab, imaging)
- Compare to baseline renal function (creatinine [Cr]/GFR)
- Urinalysis: dipstick for blood and protein; microscopy for cells, casts, and crystals
- Sterile pyuria (especially WBC casts) suggests AIN; triad of fever, rash, and eosinophilia present in 10% of cases

- Proteinuria, hematuria, and edema, often with nephritic urine sediment (RBCs and RBC casts), suggest GN or vasculitis.
- Casts: transparent hyaline casts—prerenal etiology; pigmented granular/muddy brown casts—ATN; WBC casts—AIN; RBC casts—GN
- Urine eosinophils: ≥1% eosinophils suggest AIN (poor sensitivity).
- Urine electrolytes in an oliguric state
  - $FENa = [(U_{Na} \times P_{Cr}) / (P_{Na} \times U_{Cr})] \times 100$
  - $FENa <1\%$, likely prerenal; >2%, likely intrarenal
  - If patient on diuretics, use FE_{urea} instead of FE_{Na}: $FE_{urea} = [(U_{urea} \times P_{Cr}) / (P_{BUN} \times U_{urea})] \times 100$; $FE_{urea} <35\%$ suggests prerenal etiology.
- CBC, BUN, SCr, electrolytes (including Ca/Mg/P); consider arterial or venous blood gas (ABG/VBG).
- BUN/Cr ratio not reliable in distinguishing prerenal azotemia from AKI (3)[B]
- Common lab abnormalities in AKI
  - Increased: K^+, phosphate, Mg, uric acid
  - Decreased: Hgb, Na, Ca
- Calculate creatinine clearance (CrCl) to ensure appropriate medication dosing.
- Imaging:
  - Renal ultrasound (US): first line; excludes postrenal causes; identifies kidney size, hydronephrosis, and nephrolithiasis
  - Doppler-flow renal US: evaluates for renal artery stenosis/thrombosis; operator dependent
  - Abdominal x-ray (kidney, ureter, bladder [KUB]): identifies calcification, renal calculi, kidney size
- Novel biomarkers such as urinary IL-18, neutrophil gelatinase-associated lipocalin (NGAL), kidney injury molecule-1 (KIM-1), plasma cystatin C, TIMP-2, and *IGFBP7* under investigation (4)[C]

Follow-Up Tests & Special Considerations
- Consider CK (rhabdomyolysis) and immunologic testing (if GN or vasculitis suspected).
- Advanced imaging if initial tests unrevealing
  - Prerenal: US as effective as CT for obstruction
  - Noncontrast helical CT: most sensitive test for nephrolithiasis
  - Radionuclide renal scan: evaluates renal perfusion, function (GFR), and presence of obstructive uropathy and extravasation
  - MRI: acute tubulointerstitial nephritis with increased T2-weighted signal. Gadolinium contrast is contraindicated if GFR <30 mL/min due to risk of nephrogenic systemic fibrosis.

Diagnostic Procedures/Other
Cystoscopy with retrograde pyelogram evaluates for bladder tumor, hydronephrosis, obstruction, and upper tract abnormalities without risk of contrast nephropathy.

Test Interpretation
Kidney biopsy: last resort if patient does not respond to therapy or if diagnosis remains unclear; most useful to evaluate intrinsic AKI of unclear cause (AIN, GN, vasculitis, or renal transplant rejection)

TREATMENT

GENERAL MEASURES
Identify and correct prerenal and postrenal causes.
- Stop nephrotoxic drugs and renally dose others.
- Strictly monitor intake/output and daily weight.
- Optimize cardiac output to maintain renal perfusion.
- Optimize nutrition and treat any infections.
- Indications for renal replacement therapy (RRT): volume overload, severe or progressive hyperkalemia, or severe metabolic acidosis refractory to medical management; advanced uremic complications (pericarditis, encephalopathy, bleeding diathesis)

MEDICATION
First Line
- Find and treat the underlying cause.
- Prevent fluid overload, and correct electrolyte imbalances—particularly hyperkalemia.
  – If patient is oliguric and not volume overloaded, a monitored fluid challenge may help.
- Furosemide is ineffective in preventing and treating AKI but can (judiciously) be used to manage volume overload and/or hyperkalemia. Furosemide stress test may predict the likelihood of progressive AKI, need for RRT, and mortality (4)[B].
- Dopamine, natriuretic peptides, insulin-like growth factor, and thyroxine have no benefit in the treatment of AKI.
- Fenoldopam, a dopamine agonist, has been equivocal in decreasing risk of RRT and mortality in AKI; not currently recommended (1)[C]
- Hyperkalemia with ECG changes: Give IV calcium gluconate, isotonic sodium bicarbonate (only if acidemic, and avoid use of hypertonic "amps" of $NaHCO_3$), glucose with insulin, and/or high-dose nebulized albuterol (to drive K^+ into cells); Kayexalate and/or furosemide (to increase K^+ excretion); hemodialysis if severe/refractory
- Fluid restriction may be required for oliguric patients to prevent worsening hyponatremia.
- Metabolic acidosis (particularly pH <7.2): Sodium bicarbonate can be given (judiciously); be aware of volume overload, hypocalcemia, and hypokalemia.
- Effective strategies for AKI prevention: isotonic IVF, once-daily dosing of aminoglycosides; use of lipid formulations of amphotericin B, use of iso-osmolar nonionic contrast media
- Risk of contrast-induced AKI reduced by avoidance of hypovolemia: isotonic saline 1 mL/kg/hr morning of procedure and continued until next morning or isotonic $NaHCO_3$ 3 mL/kg/hr × 1 hour before and 1 mL/kg/hr × 6 hours after contrast administration; N-acetylcysteine not of benefit

Second Line
- Tamsulosin or other selective α-blockers for bladder outlet obstruction secondary to BPH
- Dihydropyridine calcium channel blockers may have a protective effect in posttransplant ATN.

ISSUES FOR REFERRAL
- Consider nephrology consultation.
- Urology consults for obstructive nephropathy

SURGERY/OTHER PROCEDURES
- Relieve obstruction by retrograde ureteral catheters/percutaneous nephrostomy.
- Hemodialysis catheter placement

COMPLEMENTARY & ALTERNATIVE MEDICINE
Many herbal and dietary supplements are potentially nephrotoxic (aristolochic acid, ochratoxin A, Djenkol bean, impila, orellanine, cat's claw).

ADMISSION, INPATIENT, AND NURSING CONSIDERATIONS
- Most patients require admission.
- Treat life-threatening complications: hyperkalemia, metabolic acidosis, volume overload, and advanced uremia.
- If hypovolemic, give isotonic IV fluids.
- Monitor fluid balance and daily weights.
- Consider catheter to quantify urine output.
- Stabilize renal function and ensure treatment plan prior to discharge.
- Dialysis if necessary

 ONGOING CARE

FOLLOW-UP RECOMMENDATIONS
Nephrology follow-up if persistent renal impairment and/or proteinuria

DIET
- Total caloric intake of 20 to 30 kcal/kg/day (1)
- Restrict Na^+ to 2 g/day (unless hypovolemic).
- Consider K^+ restriction (2 to 3 g/day) if hyperkalemic.
- If hyperphosphatemic, consider use of phosphate binders, although no evidence of benefit in AKI.
- Avoid magnesium- and aluminum-containing compounds.

PATIENT EDUCATION
Keep well-hydrated. Avoid nephrotoxic drugs, such as NSAIDs and aminoglycosides.

PROGNOSIS
- Depending on the cause, comorbid conditions, and age of patient, mortality ranges from 5% to 80%.
- In cases of prerenal and postrenal AKI, short duration of AKI correlates with good rates of recovery. Intrarenal etiologies take longer to recover.
- Even with complete recovery from AKI, affected patients are at higher subsequent risk of developing CKD and ESRD.
- Among patients who require RRT for AKI, recovery more likely with higher baseline eGFR, AKI from ATN due to sepsis or surgery; recovery less likely with preexisting heart failure (5)

COMPLICATIONS
Death, sepsis, infection, seizures, paralysis, peripheral edema, CHF, arrhythmias, uremic pericarditis, bleeding, hypotension, anemia, hyperkalemia, uremia

REFERENCES
1. International Society of Nephrology. Summary of recommendation statements. *Kidney Int Suppl (2011)*. 2012;2(1):8–12.
2. Wang HE, Muntner P, Chertow GM, et al. Acute kidney injury and mortality in hospitalized patients. *Am J Nephrol*. 2012;35(4):349–355.
3. Manoeuvrier G, Bach-Ngohou K, Batard E, et al. Diagnostic performance of serum blood urea nitrogen to creatinine ratio for distinguishing prerenal from intrinsic acute kidney injury in the emergency department. *BMC Nephrol*. 2017;18(1):173.
4. Koyner JL, Davison DL, Brasha-Mitchell E, et al. Furosemide stress test and biomarkers for the prediction of AKI severity. *J Am Soc Nephrol*. 2015;26(8):2023–2031.
5. Hickson LJ, Chaudhary S, Williams AW, et al. Predictors of outpatient kidney function recovery among patients who initiate hemodialysis in the hospital. *Am J Kidney Dis*. 2015;65(4):592–602.

ADDITIONAL READING
- ACT Investigators. Acetylcysteine for prevention of renal outcomes in patients undergoing coronary and peripheral vascular angiography: main results from the randomized Acetylcysteine for Contrast-Induced Nephropathy Trial (ACT). *Circulation*. 2011;124(11):1250–1259.
- Coca SG, Singanamala S, Parikh CR. Chronic kidney disease after acute kidney injury: a systematic review and meta-analysis. *Kidney Int*. 2012;81(5):442–448.
- McCullough PA, Kellum JA, Haase M, et al. Pathophysiology of the cardiorenal syndromes: executive summary from the eleventh consensus conference of the Acute Dialysis Quality Initiative (ADQI). *Contrib Nephrol*. 2013;182:82–98.
- Singh NP, Prakash A. Nephrotoxic potential of herbal drugs. *JIMSA*. 2011;24(2):79–81.

 SEE ALSO

- Glomerulonephritis, Acute; Hepatorenal Syndrome; Hyperkalemia; Prostatic Hyperplasia, Benign (BPH); Chronic Kidney Disease; Reye Syndrome; Rhabdomyolysis; Sepsis
- Algorithm: Anuria or Oliguria

 CODES

ICD10
- N17.9 Acute kidney failure, unspecified
- N17.0 Acute kidney failure with tubular necrosis
- N00.9 Acute nephritic syndrome with unsp morphologic changes

CLINICAL PEARLS
- Three categories of AKI:
  – Prerenal: decreased renal perfusion (often from hypovolemia) leading to a decrease in GFR; reversible
  – Intrarenal: intrinsic kidney damage; ATN most common due to ischemic/nephrotoxic injury
  – Postrenal: extrinsic/intrinsic obstruction of the urinary collection system
- Indications for emergent hemodialysis: severe hyperkalemia, metabolic acidosis, or volume overload refractory to conservative therapy; uremic pericarditis, encephalopathy, or neuropathy; and selected alcohol and drug intoxications
- Management of ATN is supportive; no specific treatments are proven to effectively hasten recovery.

ADENOMYOSIS

Bradley M. Turner, MD, MPH, MHA, FCAP, FASCP

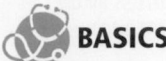

BASICS

DESCRIPTION
- Benign invasion of the endometrium into the myometrium, producing a diffusely enlarged uterus
- Microscopically, there are ectopic, nonneoplastic endometrial glands and stroma surrounded by hypertrophic and hyperplastic myometrium.
- Can be either diffuse or focal, depending on the extent of myometrial invasion
- In some cases, it may manifest as a circumscribed myometrial mass referred to as an adenomyoma.
- Most commonly affects the posterior wall of the uterus
- Typically associated with the uterus; however, the term "adenomyosis" can also be applied to benign hyperplastic changes in the bile ducts, gallbladder, and ampulla of Vater.

EPIDEMIOLOGY
- Most frequently presents in the 4th and 5th decades
- Wide variation among racial and ethnic groups and among different geographic regions

Incidence
- Variability in the criteria used for diagnosis makes an accurate determination of true incidence difficult.
- Depending on the criteria used for diagnosis, the incidence has been estimated as between 5% and 50%.
- The incidence has been reported to be higher (35–50%) in women presenting with pelvic pain and infertility.

Prevalence
- As with incidence, an accurate determination of prevalence is difficult due to the variability in the criteria used for diagnosis.
- Depending on the criteria used for diagnosis, the prevalence has been reported to vary from 5% to 70%, with the mean frequency of adenomyosis at hysterectomy given as approximately 20–30%.

ETIOLOGY AND PATHOPHYSIOLOGY
- Adenomyosis has been described as an abnormal ingrowth and invagination of the basal endometrium into the inner layer of the myometrium (junctional zone [JZ]).
- The exact mechanism regarding how this occurs and is maintained is not clear and likely to be multifactorial.
- Sex steroid hormone aberrations, inflammation, altered cell proliferation, and neuroangiogenesis are likely key pathogenic mechanisms of pain, bleeding, and infertility in adenomyosis.
- In women with adenomyosis, the JZ may represent a region of morphologic dysfunction and structural weakness, with varying susceptibility to invagination of endometrial stromal cells.
- Increased uterine pressure associated with pregnancy, leiomyomas, or other pathology may modulate the JZ environment, making it more susceptible to invagination of endometrial stromal cells.
- Other theories for pathogenesis include the following:
  - *Metaplasia theory*: metaplasia of myometrial smooth muscle cells
  - *Müllerian remnants theory*: de novo development from müllerian rests in the myometrium
  - *Tissue remodeling theory*: ectopic endometrial tissue arising secondary to tissue remodeling associated with uterine trauma either physiologic (e.g., during menstruation, childbirth, or spontaneous abortion) or iatrogenic (e.g., during uterine surgery)
  - *Multipotential perivascular theory*: Multipotential perivascular stem cells may be associated with increased angiogenesis and pathophysiologic vascular remodeling, leading to vascular smooth muscle hypertrophy, proliferation, or migration.
  - *Epithelial–mesenchymal transition theory*: Increased estrogen concentrations may enhance endometrial tissue growth, angiogenesis, and invagination into the JZ.
  - *Hyperproliferation of uterine smooth muscle cell theory*: Activation of the MAPK/ERK pathway has been associated with hyperproliferative uterine smooth cells in women with adenomyosis.
  - *Mast cell activation theory*: Nerve growth factor, a mast cell–derived mediator, can be used as an indicator for the severity of adenomyosis. This and other mast cell–derived mediators may contribute to the differentiation and development of the myometrium and maintenance of adenomyosis.

Genetics
- DNA microarray and proteomics analysis have identified specific genes that are differentially expressed in adenomyosis and matched eutopic endometrium.
- Data suggest that genetic and epigenetic abnormalities contribute to the pathogenesis of adenomyosis.

RISK FACTORS
- Age >35 years, however, the disease may cause dysmenorrhea and chronic pelvic pain in women of younger age, including adolescents. Reports suggest that early-stage adenomyosis might present a different clinical phenotype compared to late-stage disease.
- Multiparity
- Tamoxifen treatment
- Other possible risk factors:
  - Previous uterine surgery (Studies have been inconsistent.)
  - Smoking (Studies have been inconsistent.)

COMMONLY ASSOCIATED CONDITIONS
- Leiomyomas (uterine fibroids)
- Endometriosis
- Endometrial polyps
- Urinary tract dysfunction

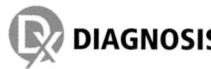

DIAGNOSIS

Pelvic pain, dysmenorrhea, and an enlarged uterus are the usual cues that prompt imaging by ultrasound or MRI; endometrial or uterine biopsies may be indicated in some cases.

HISTORY
- Presenting symptoms are nonspecific and the patient is often asymptomatic.
- Symptoms often include (1,2,3) the following:
  - Menorrhagia
  - Dysmenorrhea
  - Chronic pelvic pain
  - Abnormal uterine bleeding
- Urinary tract symptoms (e.g., stress urinary incontinence, urgency, daytime frequency, and urge urinary incontinence) have been associated with an increased incidence of adenomyosis; however, data are limited (4).

PHYSICAL EXAM
Uterus may be enlarged and tender.

DIFFERENTIAL DIAGNOSIS
- Pregnancy
- Benign uterine tumors
- Malignant uterine tumors
- Metastatic disease

DIAGNOSTIC TESTS & INTERPRETATION

Initial Tests (lab, imaging)
- Transvaginal ultrasound (TVUS) is the imaging method of choice for initial evaluation of suspected adenomyosis (2,3)[A].
- TVUS can be either two- or three-dimensional (2)[A].
- Three-dimensional TVUS can provide JZ thickness.
- TVUS has a sensitivity of 72–82.5% and a specificity of 81–84.6% (3)[A].
- TVUS is less sensitive than MRI in differentiating adenomyosis from leiomyoma (2)[A].
- TVUS with power color flow Doppler can be used to differentiate adenomyosis from leiomyoma (2,3)[B] depending on the operator (2)[C].
- Although MRI is more sensitive (3)[A] than TVUS, the higher cost of the procedure limits its use as a first-line diagnostic tool.
- MRI has a sensitivity of 77–93% and a specificity of 67–99% (3)[A].
- Leiomyomas are associated with adenomyosis in 36–50% of cases, making MRI an ideal imaging method (3)[A].
- MRI should be considered when TVUS cannot provide a definitive diagnosis.

Diagnostic Procedures/Other
- Uterine biopsy with histologic interpretation
- Uterine-sparing operative treatment (USOT) with histologic interpretation
- Hysterectomy with histologic interpretation

Test Interpretation
- The two-dimensional sonographic markers of adenomyosis include the following (2,3)[A]:
  - Uterine enlargement (with no visualized leiomyoma)
  - Cystic anechoic spaces or lakes in the myometrium
  - Uterine wall thickening
  - Subendometrial echogenic linear striations
  - Heterogeneous echo texture
  - Obscure endometrial/myometrial border
  - Thickening of the transition zone
- With three-dimensional TVUS, a JZ maximum (JZ max) ≥8 mm and a JZ max − JZ minimum (JZ min) ≥4 mm have been reported as significantly more associated with adenomyosis than two-dimensional features (2)[B].
- Features of adenomyosis on MRI include low-intensity widening of the JZ on T2-weighted images, which corresponds to smooth muscle hyperplasia and thickening of the JZ (2,3)[A].
- Three objective parameters have been identified for an MRI diagnosis of adenomyosis:
  - Thickening of the JZ to at least 8 to 12 mm (2)[B]
  - JZ max/total myometrium >40% (2)[B]
  - JZ max − JZ min >5 mm (2)[B]

- Histologic interpretation has traditionally been considered the most practicable way to establish a definitive diagnosis of adenomyosis (3)[C].
- Pathologic interpretation of uterine biopsy:
  - Presence of endometrial glands and stromal elements within the myometrium
  - Often difficult to definitively diagnose adenomyosis due to sampling bias and/or biopsy artifact (1)[A]
- Pathologic interpretation of USOT and hysterectomy:
  - In morcellated specimens, diagnostic difficulty arises due to modification of the spatial arrangement of the tissue, leading to difficulty in referencing the surface. Sampling bias can also be an issue (1)[A].
  - Even in cases where the surface is accurately referenced, criteria vary among pathologists regarding the depth of invasion, which "definitively" defines adenomyosis (1,3)[A].

 TREATMENT

- The mainstay of treatment has been surgical therapy.
- Medical therapy shows promise in certain patients.

MEDICATION
Continuous use of oral contraceptive pills, high-dose progestins, and selective progesterone receptor modulators can temporarily improve the symptoms. Moreover, use of a levonorgestrel-releasing intrauterine device, danazol, aromatase inhibitors, and GnRHa may temporarily induce regression of AD (5)[A].

ADDITIONAL THERAPIES
Immunomodulators of angiogenesis may offer future options for medical treatment of adenomyosis.

SURGERY/OTHER PROCEDURES
- Hysterectomy is curative.
- USOT might be considered for women who wish to preserve fertility or do not wish to have a hysterectomy.
- USOT **excisional** techniques (1)[B]:
  - Complete excision (adenomyomectomy)
  - Cytoreduction (partial adenomyomectomy)
- USOT **nonexcisional** techniques (1)[B]:
  - Laparoscopic techniques including electrocoagulation, uterine artery ligation
  - Hysteroscopic techniques including endometrial ablation, endomyometrial resection
  - MRI or ultrasound-guided high-frequency ultrasound ablation (high-intensity focused ultrasound [HIFU])
  - Uterine artery embolization (UAE)
  - Other reported techniques include the following: alcohol instillation (cystic adenomyosis), radiofrequency ablation (focal adenomyosis), microwave ablation, and thermoablation (diffuse adenomyosis).
- Of the nonexcisional techniques, HIFU and UAE seem to offer the most encouraging results (1)[C].
- Increasing percentages of necrosis after UAE may be an important factor associated with decreased recurrence of symptoms.
- A systemic review of USOT for adenomyosis in reproductive-aged women suggests that USOT may possibly improve fertility, although the best method of surgery is yet to be seen (6)[A].

 ONGOING CARE

PATIENT EDUCATION
Adenomyosis, PubMed health, at https://www.ncbi.nlm.nih.gov/pubmedhealth/?term=adenomyosis

PROGNOSIS
- Adenomyosis is a benign proliferation of endometrial tissue.
- Symptoms usually resolve after menopause.
- Hysterectomy is curative.
- Additional studies are still needed to determine the impact of untreated adenomyosis and USOT on fertility and reproductive outcomes.
- Additional studies are still needed to clarify the role of medical treatment in women with adenomyosis.
- A consensus on the criterion for diagnosing adenomyosis needs to be reached.

COMPLICATIONS
- Anemia from blood loss associated with heavy periods
- Patients with adenomyosis have been reported to be at increased risk for malignant disease; however, to date, there has not been sufficient morphologic, genetic, or epigenetic evidence to substantiate the malignant transformation of adenomyosis.

REFERENCES
1. Taran FA, Stewart EA, Brucker S. Adenomyosis: epidemiology, risk factors, clinical phenotype and surgical and interventional alternatives to hysterectomy. *Geburtshilfe Frauenheilkd*. 2013;73(9):924–931.
2. Exacoustos C, Manganaro L, Zupi E. Imaging for the evaluation of endometriosis and adenomyosis. *Best Pract Res Clin Obstet Gynaecol*. 2014;28(5):655–681.
3. Shwayder J, Sakhel K. Imaging for uterine myomas and adenomyosis. *J Minim Invasive Gynecol*. 2014;21(3):362–376.
4. Ekin M, Cengiz H, Öztürk E, et al. Genitourinary symptoms in patients with adenomyosis. *Int Urogynecol J*. 2013;24(3):509–512.
5. Pontis A, D'Alterio MN, Pirarba S, et al. Adenomyosis: a systematic review of medical treatment. *Gynecol Endocrinol*. 2016;32(9):696–700.
6. Younes G, Tulandi T. Conservative surgery for adenomyosis and results: a systematic review. *J Minim Invasive Gynecol*. 2018;25(2):265–276.

ADDITIONAL READING
- Bae SH, Kim MD, Kim GM, et al. Uterine artery embolization for adenomyosis: percentage of necrosis predicts midterm clinical recurrence. *J Vasc Interv Radiol*. 2015;26(9):1290.e2–1296.e2.
- Champaneria R, Abedin P, Daniels J, et al. Ultrasound scan and magnetic resonance imaging for the diagnosis of adenomyosis: systematic review comparing test accuracy. *Acta Obstet Gynecol Scand*. 2010;89(11):1374–1384.
- Dong X, Yang Z. High-intensity focused ultrasound ablation of uterine localized adenomyosis. *Curr Opin Obstet Gynecol*. 2010;22(4):326–330.
- Dueholm M. Uterine adenomyosis and infertility, review of reproductive outcome after in vitro fertilization and surgery. *Acta Obstet Gynecol Scand*. 2017;96(6):715–726.
- Ekin M, Cengiz H, Ayağ ME, et al. Effects of the levonorgestrel-releasing intrauterine system on urinary symptoms in patients with adenomyosis. *Eur J Obstet Gynecol Reprod Biol*. 2013;170(2):517–520.
- Grimbizis GF, Mikos T, Tarlatzis B. Uterus-sparing operative treatment for adenomyosis. *Fertil Steril*. 2014;101(2):472–487.
- Hirata T, Izumi G, Takamura M, et al. Efficacy of dienogest in the treatment of symptomatic adenomyosis: a pilot study. *Gynecol Endocrinol*. 2014;30(10):726–729.
- Koike N, Tsunemi T, Uekuri C, et al. Pathogenesis and malignant transformation of adenomyosis (review). *Oncol Rep*. 2013;29(3):861–867.
- Maheshwari A, Gurunath S, Fatima F, et al. Adenomyosis and subfertility: a systematic review of prevalence, diagnosis, treatment and fertility outcomes. *Hum Reprod Update*. 2012;18(4):374–392.
- Popovic M, Puchner S, Berzaczy D, et al. Uterine artery embolization for the treatment of adenomyosis: a review. *J Vasc Interv Radiol*. 2011;22(7):901–909.
- Streuli I, Santulli P, Chouzenoux S, et al. Activation of the MAPK/ERK cell-signaling pathway in uterine smooth muscle cells of women with adenomyosis. *Reprod Sci*. 2015;22(12):1549–1560.
- Vannuccini S, Tosti C, Carmona F, et al. Pathogenesis of adenomyosis: an update on molecular mechanisms. *Reprod Biomed Online*. 2017;35(5):592–601.
- Verit FF, Yucel O. Endometriosis, leiomyoma and adenomyosis: the risk of gynecologic malignancy. *Asian Pac J Cancer Prev*. 2013;14(10):5589–5597.
- Weiss G, Maseelall P, Schott LL, et al. Adenomyosis a variant, not a disease? Evidence from hysterectomized menopausal women in the Study of Women's Health Across the Nation (SWAN). *Fertil Steril*. 2009;91(1):201–206.

 CODES

ICD10
N80.0 Endometriosis of uterus

CLINICAL PEARLS
- Adenomyosis is often asymptomatic.
- Both TVUS and MRI are very accurate for the diagnosis of adenomyosis.
- MRI is more sensitive than TVUS, particularly in differentiating adenomyosis from leiomyoma. Differentiation of adenomyosis from leiomyoma is critical because the former is often treated with hysterectomy, whereas the latter is often treated with uterine conservation.
- Various medical and surgical therapeutic options, including uterine-sparing operative techniques, are available for adenomyosis.
- Hysterectomy is curative.

ADHESIVE CAPSULITIS (FROZEN SHOULDER)

Berenice Subero Pablo, MD • Cassandra Shipp, MD • George G.A. Pujalte, MD, FACSM

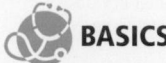 BASICS

DESCRIPTION

- Frozen shoulder or adhesive capsulitis (AC):
  - Presents as progressive painful restriction in range of movement of the glenohumeral (GH) joint (1)
  - Resolution ranges from complete to varying degrees of limitation for active and passive shoulder movements (1).
  - Unlike early disease (typically painful), late AC can present as pain-free restricted motion.
- Subtypes:
  - Primary AC:
    - Idiopathic
    - Usually associated with diabetes mellitus (DM) (1)
    - Typically resolves in 9 to 18 months (2)
  - Secondary AC:
    - Typically due to prolonged immobilization
    - Most commonly as complication of rotator cuff impingement syndrome (rotator cuff tendonitis) that remains incompletely treated
    - Sometimes called "shoulder-hand-syndrome" which is a complex regional pain syndrome (or reflex sympathetic dystrophy), if it is characterized by shoulder pain, diffuse swelling, and decreased range of motion (ROM) (2)
- Clinical course:
  - Phase 1 (2 to 9 months): painful phase. Pain is constant. Diagnosis may be difficult if restricted movement is not present in early disease.
  - Phase 2 (4 to 12 months): stiffening or freezing phase. Movement becomes restricted, especially during external rotation.
  - Phase 3 (12 to 42 months): resolution or thawing phase; gradual return to normal shoulder mobility (2)

EPIDEMIOLOGY

- Incidence: 2.4/1,000 people per year (2)
- Prevalence: 2–5% in the general population, 10–20% among diabetics (2)

ETIOLOGY AND PATHOPHYSIOLOGY

Underlying fundamental processes:
- Idiopathic
- Inflammation: Mast cells, T cells, B cells, and macrophages have been identified histologically, suggesting an inflammatory process.
- Angiogenesis
- Scarring: Fibroblasts and myofibroblasts have been identified histologically. Capsular contracture reduces the joint volume to 3 to 4 mL compared to the normal 10 to 15 mL.

Genetics
No predisposition identified

RISK FACTORS

- Shoulder immobilization; often due to impingement syndrome (most significant risk factor)
- Increasing age (1)
- Female gender (1)
- Diabetes (1)
- Thyroid disease (1)
- Atherosclerotic cardiovascular disease (ASCVD): cerebrovascular accident (CVA)/myocardial infarction (MI)/hyperlipidemia (2)
- Antiretroviral medication use
- Parkinson disease
- Trauma/surgery (1)
- Prior history of AC in contralateral shoulder

GENERAL PREVENTION

- Active lifestyle, while avoiding shoulder injury
- Control of diabetes, atherosclerotic disease, thyroid, and autoimmune conditions

COMMONLY ASSOCIATED CONDITIONS

DM, autoimmune disorders, Parkinson disease, highly active antiretroviral therapy (HAART) use, CVA/MI, cervical disc disease, hyperthyroidism (1)

 DIAGNOSIS

HISTORY

- Identify possible risk factors.
- Progressive and worsening stiffness of the GH joint
- Majority will have diffuse shoulder pain, especially at the beginning of the disease.
- On the late phase of the disease, stiffness becomes predominant.

PHYSICAL EXAM

- Limitation in both active and passive ROM
- Capsular pattern of restriction is demonstrated, with external rotation most affected, followed by abduction, and then flexion (1).
- Pain with rotator cuff impingement tests
- Inability to reach overhead or back pocket
- Scapular substitution frequently accompanies active shoulder movement.
- Injection test can be helpful in differentiating AC from subacromial pathologies such as rotator cuff tendinopathy (which should improve with injection of local anesthetics, in contrast to AC). This should only be done if the diagnosis is still uncertain after a thorough history and physical.

DIFFERENTIAL DIAGNOSIS

- Rotator cuff strain/tear/impingement syndrome
- GH or acromioclavicular joint osteoarthritis (OA)
- Cervical strain/radiculopathy/OA
- Subacromial bursitis
- Parsonage-Turner syndrome: brachial plexus inflammation secondary to a trigger, such as an infection, trauma, or autoimmune condition
- Myofascial pain syndrome
- Calcific tendonitis
- Fracture
- Shoulder subluxation/dislocation
- Bony neoplasm/metastasis

DIAGNOSTIC TESTS & INTERPRETATION

Initial Tests (lab, imaging)

- No labs are required for idiopathic AC. Blood tests can be used to check for associated/related conditions, such as diabetes, thyroid disease, a stroke, autoimmune diseases, and, in rare cases, Parkinson disease (e.g., thyroid-stimulating hormone, hemoglobin A1C, erythrocyte sedimentation rate).
- Imaging
  - Plain radiographs of the affected shoulder (posteroanterior, external rotation, axillary, and supraspinatus outlet views)
    - Preferred initial tests
    - In most cases, will be negative
    - Used primarily to rule out other pathologies such as GH OA, fractures, dislocation, or tumors (2)
  - Magnetic resonance imaging (MRI)
    - Not indicated unless there is a concomitant pathology in the shoulder or neurologic deficit
    - May show thickening of the joint capsule and the coracohumeral ligament along with edema and increased joint fluid (2)
  - Ultrasound (US)
    - Indications similar to those for MRI
    - Selection depends on individual cases and clinician's preference.
    - Can also reveal joint capsule thickening and increased joint fluid
    - Doppler can show increased vascularity around the intra-articular portion of the biceps tendon and coracohumeral ligament.

TREATMENT

- In most cases, self-limited
- Manage patient expectations; resolution often takes 18 months of medication and rehabilitation (2).

MEDICATION

- Pain management
  – Acetaminophen or nonsteroidal anti-inflammatory drugs (NSAIDs) are first line of treatment.
- Glucocorticoid injections:
  – Can be beneficial especially when administered at the beginning of the disease
  – A short course of physical therapy after an injection, for 4 to 6 weeks, can improve pain and ROM (3).
  – Injection may be diluted with a local anesthetic like lidocaine. Triamcinolone 20 to 40 mg or methylprednisolone 20 to 40 mg can be used.

ADDITIONAL THERAPIES

- Exercise and physical therapy:
  – Gentle ROM exercises should be offered to every patient.
  – Exercises should be performed daily and as tolerated. A structured plan should be given to the patient (4).
  – Physical therapy has been found to be beneficial especially in phases 2 and 3 of AC. Best data supports its use in conjunction with other treatment, like corticosteroids (5).
- Laser has been suggested as a possible treatment, particularly for pain relief; not enough evidence for support

SURGERY/OTHER PROCEDURES

- Should be reserved for patients who do not respond to conservative measures for at least 1 year
- Some of the most common procedures include manipulation under anesthesia, arthroscopic capsular release, distension arthrogram, among others (2).

 ONGOING CARE

FOLLOW-UP RECOMMENDATIONS

- After establishing a diagnosis, assess the need for pain control and start the patient on NSAIDs, in combination with a gentle exercise program.
- Follow up in 3 to 4 weeks: if no significant improvement, may consider intra-articular corticosteroid injections (5)

- Physical therapy should also be considered because it can hasten the rate of recovery and increase ROM (5).
- For secondary AC, consider evaluation by a multidisciplinary team.
- If no improvement, consider surgical intervention (2).

PATIENT EDUCATION

- Patient education is important; explain prognosis and ensure compliance with treatment.
- Climbing the wall: Face a wall and place the hand from the affected shoulder flat on the surface of the wall; use the fingers to "climb" the wall; pause 30 seconds every few inches. Repeat the exercise after turning the torso 90 degrees to wall (abduction).
- In case of secondary AC, address the importance of treating underlying causes.

PROGNOSIS

- Recovery is dependent on onset of treatment, symptoms, and comorbidities in patient.
- Variable duration, lasting 1 to 3 years without intervention (1)
- Patients with idiopathic frozen shoulder have a good rate of recovery (6).

REFERENCES

1. Zreik NH, Malik RA, Charalambous CP. Adhesive capsulitis of the shoulder and diabetes: a meta-analysis of prevalence. *Muscles Ligaments Tendons J*. 2016;6(1):26–34.
2. Rangan A, Goodchild L, Gibson J, et al. Frozen shoulder. *Shoulder Elbow*. 2015;7(4):299–307.
3. Page MJ, Green S, Kramer S, et al. Manual therapy and exercise for adhesive capsulitis (frozen shoulder). *Cochrane Database Syst Rev*. 2014;(8):CD011275.
4. Jain TK, Sharma NK. The effectiveness of physiotherapeutic interventions in treatment of frozen shoulder/adhesive capsulitis: a systematic review. *J Back Musculoskelet Rehabil*. 2014;27(3):247–273.
5. Russel S, Jariwala A, Conlon R, et al. A blinded, randomized, controlled trial assessing conservative management strategies for frozen shoulder. *J Shoulder Elbow Surg*. 2014;23(4):500–507.
6. Vastamäki H, Kettunen J, Vastamäki M. The natural history of idiopathic frozen shoulder: a 2- to 27-year follow up study. *Clin Orthop Relat Res*. 2012;470(4):1133–1143.

 CODES

ICD10

- M75.00 Adhesive capsulitis of unspecified shoulder
- M75.01 Adhesive capsulitis of right shoulder
- M75.02 Adhesive capsulitis of left shoulder

CLINICAL PEARLS

- Frozen shoulder or AC is generally a self-limiting global restriction in ROM of the shoulder joint. Up to 50% will have permanent inability to externally rotate the shoulder.
- Natural course consists of a painful phase, freezing phase, and thawing phase. It occurs mostly in older women; total prevalence is 2–5% of the general population and roughly 10–20% of the diabetic population.
- Most common physical exam finding is diminished ability to externally rotate the shoulder. Other signs include pain on provocation of subacromial space and inability to reach overhead or for back pocket.
- Plain x-rays are the preferred initial imaging modality. MRI and US are done only if there is concomitant pathology or neurologic deficit.
- Treatment includes pain control with NSAIDs or acetaminophen, glucocorticoid therapy (injections or short course of oral steroids), physical therapy, or surgery.
- Resolution of symptoms often takes 18 or more months.

ADOPTION, INTERNATIONAL

R. Aaron Lambert, MD, FAAFP

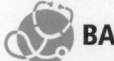 **BASICS**

DESCRIPTION

- Although international adoptions have decreased in the past 10 years, they still represent a significant portion of ~136,000 yearly U.S. adoptions.
- Diverse birth countries, disease exposures, and unknown health histories require special attention.
- Multidisciplinary teams are often necessary for appropriate care. Many adoptive parents seek advice regarding adoption health needs from their primary care provider.

EPIDEMIOLOGY

Incidence

- 4,714 children were adopted internationally in 2017. This number has decreased every year since 2004.
- 5% of current U.S. adoptions are international.
- In 2017, the most common countries of origin for internationally adopted children were China, Ethiopia, Russia, South Korea, and Ukraine.
- In 2017, 47% of internationally adopted children were <5 years, 36% were ages 5 to 12 years, and 16% were ≥13 years. An equal number of boys and girls are adopted internationally (1).

RISK FACTORS

- Unknown birth, medical, and vaccination histories
- Possible in utero or postnatal toxin exposure
- Inadequate nutrition (before or after birth)
- Exposures to infectious diseases not commonly seen in the United States (2)
- Overcrowded or institutionalized living situations (e.g., orphanages)
- History of neglect, deprivation, or abuse
- Potential risks associated with foreign travel for the adopting family (3)

GENERAL PREVENTION

- A state department physician must examine the child in their native country before immigration to the United States. This is a limited examination targeted at identifying diseases excluding visa qualification.
- Children should be examined by a physician within 2 weeks of arrival in the United States (3).
- A follow-up visit 4 to 6 weeks after their postadoption appointment is also recommended.
- Screen for hearing, vision, growth, and developmental delay.
- A travel medicine visit is encouraged for family members who are traveling to the adopted child's country of origin (3).
- A preadoption visit can help clarify medical diagnoses, review available medical records (including photos and/or video) to confirm/refute specific diagnoses (2).

COMMONLY ASSOCIATED CONDITIONS

- 80% of international adoptees have medical or developmental issues, 20% of these are severe (4).
- Infectious diseases:
  - Hepatitis A/B/C
  - Intestinal parasites
  - Tuberculosis (TB), primarily latent
  - Syphilis, including inadequately treated
  - HIV
  - *Helicobacter pylori*
- Emotional or behavioral problems
- Developmental delay
- Fetal alcohol syndrome
- Feeding difficulties, malnutrition, rickets
- Anemia
- Congenital anomalies (e.g., cleft lip/palate, orthopedic deformities)
- Prematurity or low birth weight
- Inadequate immunizations
- Lead poisoning
- Sensorineural and conductive hearing loss
- Strabismus, blindness

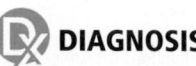 **DIAGNOSIS**

HISTORY

- Medical records are often limited or difficult to access.
- Review immunization records carefully. Records that are "too perfect" should raise suspicion.
  - Some vaccinations (e.g., *Haemophilus influenzae* type B [Hib], pneumococcal, varicella) are not routine in other countries.
- Birth/prenatal history, including exposures
- Available family history
- Documented history of emotional or nutritional deprivation, or physical or sexual abuse
- Time (if any) spent in orphanage or other institution
- Growth charts are critical. The first sign of malnutrition is failure to gain weight, followed by slowed linear growth, and a lag in head circumference.
- Review or observe (as able) data regarding developmental milestones, behavior, attachment, parent stress, and parent–child interactions.

PHYSICAL EXAM

- This may be the child's first comprehensive exam; be sensitive to cues the child is providing and use a translator as necessary.
- Comprehensive physical exam. Highlight:
  - Growth parameters
  - General appearance; presence of features suggestive of genetic disorder, syndromes, or congenital defects
  - Skin—infection or signs of prior abuse (4)
  - Genitalia—signs of abuse or ritual cutting

- Neurologic—sensorimotor skills, coordination, reflexes
- Oral exam: tooth development and signs of decay
- Assess development using a validated instrument, the date of birth may be unknown (2). Assess development at each visit to identify delay and potential need for additional services. 50–90% of internationally adopted children are delayed on adoption; most have normal cognition at long-term follow-up.

DIAGNOSTIC TESTS & INTERPRETATION

- Developmental screening
- Hearing and vision screening

Initial Tests (lab, imaging)

- Based on history and physical exam (2)[C],(3,5)[A]:
  - Hepatitis A (Hep A IgM, Hep A IgG)
  - Hepatitis B (HBsAg, HBsAb, HBcAb)
  - Hepatitis C (enzyme immunoassay [EIA])
  - HIV 1 and 2 antibody testing/ELISA
  - Syphilis: nontreponemal (RPR, VDRL, or ART) and treponemal (MHA-TP, FTA-ABS, or TPPA)
  - Tuberculin skin test (TST) in all ages or interferon-γ release assay ages ≥5 years
  - Three stool specimens for ova and parasites, specific request for *Giardia intestinalis* and *Cryptosporidium* species testing of one sample
  - CBC with indices and differential
  - Blood lead concentration for ages ≤6 years
  - Thyroid-stimulating hormone (TSH)
  - Urinalysis
  - Hemoglobinopathy/blood disorder screen: sickle cell, thalassemia, glucose-6-phosphate dehydrogenase (G6PD) deficiency
- Consider:
  - Antibody titers depending on veracity of immunization records (6)[C]
  - Stool cultures for bacterial pathogens (diarrhea) (2)[C]
  - *H. pylori* testing (dyspepsia, abdominal pain, or anemia)
  - Ca^{++}, PO_4, alkaline phosphate, and 25-hydroxyvitamin D level (rickets) (2)[C]
  - >12 months of age: for Chagas disease via *Trypanosoma cruzi*, serologic testing in adoptees from endemic countries (Mexico, Central and South America)
  - >24 months of age: Review CBC for eosinophilia to consider lymphatic filariasis in children from sub-Saharan Africa, Egypt, Southern Asia, Western Pacific Islands, the NE coast of Brazil, Guyana, Haiti, and the Dominican Republic (5)[A].

Follow-Up Tests & Special Considerations

> **ALERT**
> If initially negative, repeat HIV, Hep B, Hep C, and TB testing is recommended at 6 months; negative tests may represent a "window" period or be falsely negative due to malnutrition (in the case of TST).

- HIV: Confirm antibody positive in children <18 months with DNA PCR (may represent maternal antibody) (3)[A].

- Hep C: Confirm positive tests with recombinant immunoblot assay (RIBA) and/or HCV RNA PCR; an initial positive in children <18 months may be due to maternal antibody, repeat after 18 months of age.
- Positive TST (TB): Do *not* attribute to bacillus Calmette-Guérin (BCG) vaccine. Evaluate for active disease; treat latent TB infection (LTBI).
- Test for intestinal parasites if GI symptoms persist.
- Eosinophilia >450 cells/mm³ with negative stool ova and parasites: serologic testing for *Schistosoma*; add *Strongyloides* for adoptees from sub-Saharan African, Latin American, and Southeast Asian countries (2)[C].
- Behavioral concerns may first present during adolescence, even for children adopted in infancy.
- For children with history of treated congenital syphilis, follow with ophthalmologic, audiologic, neurologic, and developmental screening.

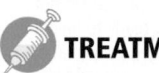

TREATMENT

GENERAL MEASURES
- Regular diet for children who arrive malnourished
- Monitor linear growth.
- Consider early intervention for children with suspected delays.
- Involve parents in local and online support groups.
- Postadoption depression may occur in parents.

MEDICATION
- Immunizations: Catch up vaccines per CDC schedule (http://www.cdc.gov/vaccines/schedules/).
  - No further Hep B vaccine if HBsAg positive, HBsAb and HBcAb positive, or HBsAb positive and HBV vaccine given appropriately
  - MMR for vaccination for mumps and rubella, even if measles antibodies present (6)[C]
- Possible approaches (5)[A]:
  - Repeating questionable vaccinations negates the need to obtain serologic tests.
  - To minimize/avoid vaccine administration, check antibody titers—infants 6 to 12 months: polio; diphtheria; children, >1 year: Hep A; MMR; varicella (6)[C]
- Ensure adoptive parents, caretakers, and household members are up-to-date with Tdap, Hep A/B, and measles vaccines (3)[A],(4)[C].

ISSUES FOR REFERRAL
- Time referrals and elective procedures to allow adjustment to new home (2)[C]
- Individual or family counseling may help adjustment.
- Internationally adopted children may exhibit self-stimulating behaviors (e.g., rocking, head banging) related to prior sensory deprivation. These behaviors typically decrease with time, and no treatment is necessary if the child is otherwise developing normally. If in doubt, refer to developmental pediatrics or occupational therapy.
  - If a child continues to have disruptive behaviors, or would rather self-soothe than seek nurturing human interaction, consider intervention.
  - Persistent behavioral issues in the parent–child interactions merit further evaluation.

- Refer to pediatric ophthalmology for strabismus (seen in 10–25% of previously institutionalized adoptees).
- Refer to audiology and/or ENT for concerns, questionable screening results, or if slow to acquire language skills.
- No longer hearing one's native language slows speech development. Speech therapy helps children from non–English-speaking countries.
- Pediatric dental evaluation by 12 months of age; sooner if signs of dental pathology is present (2)[C]

 ONGOING CARE

FOLLOW-UP RECOMMENDATIONS
Patient Monitoring
- Regular well-child visits, particularly within first months of entry into the United States
- Close monitoring of developmental milestones, behavior, and attachment

DIET
- Regular diet, with specific attention to known nutritional deficiencies within country of origin (http://adoptionnutrition.org)
- Up to 68% of international adoptees fall >2 standard deviations below the mean for one or more growth parameters; most begin to follow an appropriate growth curve (<2 deviations from the mean) within 9 to 12 months of arrival to the United States

PATIENT EDUCATION
- Allow ad lib access to healthy foods to promote self-regulatory eating behaviors.
- Toileting: Some children may not be trained yet; others may regress in their new home. Time, positive reinforcement, and avoiding punishment often resolve this issue as the child adjusts to new surroundings.
- Sleeping: Children must learn to trust their new home and parents. Avoid aggressive sleep rules. Parents should be present physically and emotionally to establish safety and promote bedtime ritual.
- Language: Adoptive family should learn key phrases in the child's native language prior to adoption. When using translator services, be careful to avoid perception of translator use equating to potential return to native country.
- Adopted children may grieve lost family, relationships, and culture; encourage parents to acknowledge this and openly work through it. Provide counseling if needed.
- Encourage families to learn about the child's culture and ethnicity of origin (4).

PROGNOSIS
- Recovery from developmental delay correlates with time spent in institutional setting.
  - Risk of long-term developmental, behavioral, or academic problems increases with adoption age.
  - Rate of recovery exceeds rate of normal development (3).
- Children may regress in previously acquired skills (2).
- A desire to search for biologic family is common in adolescence (4).
- American Academy of Pediatrics' Council on Foster Care, Adoption, and Kinship Care (http://www2.aap.org/sections/adoption/index.html)

REFERENCES
1. U.S. Department of State, Bureau of Consular Affairs. Intercountry adoption. https://travel.state.gov/content/adoptionsabroad/en.html. Accessed July 25, 2018.
2. Jones VF; and Committee on Early Childhood, Adoption, and Dependent Care. Comprehensive health evaluation of the newly adopted child. *Pediatrics*. 2012;129(1):e214–e223.
3. Centers for Disease Control and Prevention. *CDC Health Information for International Travel 2014*. New York, NY: Oxford University Press; 2014.
4. Barratt MS. International adoption. *Pediatr Rev*. 2013;34(3):145–146.
5. American Academy of Pediatrics. Medical evaluation of internationally adopted children for infectious diseases. In: Pickering LK, ed. *Red Book: 2012 Report of the Committee on Infectious Diseases*. 29th ed. Elk Grove Village, IL: American Academy of Pediatrics; 2012:239–240.
6. Feja KN, Tolan RW Jr. Infections related to international travel and adoption. *Adv Pediatr*. 2013;60(1):107–139.

ADDITIONAL READING
- Dawood F, Serwint JR. International adoption. *Pediatr Rev*. 2008;29(8):292–294.
- National Center for Immunization and Respiratory Diseases. General recommendations on immunization—recommendations of the Advisory Committee on Immunization Practices (ACIP). *MMWR Recomm Rep*. 2011;60(2):1–64.

 CODES

ICD10
- Z02.82 Encounter for adoption services
- Z62.821 Parent-adopted child conflict

CLINICAL PEARLS
- Internationally adopted children may exhibit self-stimulating behaviors (e.g., rocking, head banging) that usually decrease over time. Refer to developmental or occupational specialist when concerns persist.
- A preadoption visit can identify medical concerns and prepare resources prior to a child's arrival.
- Initial labs for internationally adopted children include Hep A/B/C, HIV 1/2, CBC, TSH, lead, G6PD deficiency, hemoglobin electrophoresis, PPD/TST (or IGRA ages ≥5 years), ova and parasites (three stool specimens, including single specimen for *Giardia* and *Cryptosporidium* antigens), and urinalysis.
- If initially negative, repeat HIV, Hep B/C, and TST at 6 months.
- Catch up immunizations per CDC schedule (http://www.cdc.gov/vaccines/schedules/).
- Ensure that appropriate immunizations are up-to-date for adoptive family and caretakers.

ADVANCE CARE PLANNING

Christopher Lin-Brande, MD • Heather A. Dalton, MD

 BASICS

DESCRIPTION

- Advance care planning (ACP) allows patients to have a voice in the decisions that affect their care after they lose the ability to do so for themselves.
- There are several methods addressing uncertainty of goals of care as patients age:
  - Advance directives, living wills (LW), heath care durable powers of attorney (DPOA), physician/medical orders for life-sustaining treatment (POLST/MOLST), and facilitated conversations with family and significant others
- ACP is an important aspect of patient-centered care as the population ages and individuals lose decision-making capacity.
- It can be challenging to interpret patient wishes in the context of individual illness circumstances, negotiate conflicts in decisions, and to help patients determine what is in their best interest based on personal values.
- Definitions
  - Advance directives (1): written instructions to guide decision making in the event a patient is unable to provide informed consent
    - LW and DPOA usually only take effect if the patient has been determined to lack capacity to decide care for him or herself; otherwise, patient preference takes precedence (even if contradictory to a LW).
  - LW: a patient's written instructions of his or her wishes regarding medical care
    - Each state has specific legal requirements. Certain states do not recognize LW but have other "medical directive" forms. LW and medical directives can take effect immediately (e.g., when a patient is diagnosed with a terminal illness) or when a patient can no longer make decisions for him or herself.
    - LW have direct treatment instructions.
    - Challenges of LW include lack of standardization, potential completion too far in advance of use, and narrow scope.
    - LW do not expire but they can be revised.
    - The LW is NOT a medical directive, so it cannot prevent life-sustaining treatment in an emergent situation (as a POLST can [see below]).

- DPOA: a written document designating a surrogate decision maker in the event a patient cannot speak for him or herself
  - A health care proxy (HCP) speaks on behalf of the patient to make decisions aligned as closely as possible to the patient's wishes. Ideally, this is someone the patient knows well and trusts and who has had discussions with the patient about his or her values.
  - If multiple HCP are named, disagreements about who speaks for the patient must be resolved before a decision can be made.
  - If there is a conflict between an LW provision and an HCP decision, different states have varying rules regarding precedence. In some states, the DPOA supersedes the LW; in other states, the most recently executed document is legally binding.
- POLST/MOLST: a medical directive, which (unlike LW) directs point of care decision making by EMS for patients in advanced stages of illness
  - Designed to minimize confusion in emergent situations, these are adjunctive documents to LW and DPOA that provide clear instruction regarding resuscitation, intubation, and treatment
  - These documents are portable and follow a patient across different care settings. Given their simplicity, POLST/MOLST is more likely to be followed than LW, which can be difficult to locate.
  - Although EMS may be concerned about the legal implications of withholding life-sustaining treatment, POLST forms provide legal protection if patient wishes are followed.
  - Patients with POLST documents have fewer unwanted interventions.
- Nursing home residents and patients with dementia often do not have capacity to complete legal documents related to LW and DPOA.
- ACP should be completed while patients are able to make decisions about their future care.
- There are no guidelines for when to initiate discussions about ACP; age 65 years may be an appropriate time for a realistic conversation prior to the onset of dementia or other incapacitating illness.
  - Each conversation must be individualized.

Pediatric Considerations
- Pediatric ACP (pACP) is less common.
- For children with serious acute or terminal illness, it is a difficult (but important) part of treatment.
  - Provider fears about increasing parental distress when discussing pACP are unfounded.
  - pACP may unburden parents from difficult decisions and is associated with increased positive emotions, understanding of the patient's illness, and provider rapport.

 TREATMENT

- Suggested discussion points:
  - All adult patients:
    - Discuss basic medical decision making.
    - Assess willingness to engage in ACP. Do not force patients if they are not ready to have this potentially emotionally charged conversation.
    - Ask patients to identify who they would like to make decisions for them if they were unable to do so.
    - Encourage patients to inform trusted family or friends about new diagnoses or changes in health.
    - Discuss what values are most important to patients.
    - Document decisions concisely and clearly.
  - Any patient with a chronic or terminal illness:
    - Discuss the natural course of disease progression, including time course and end-of-life expectations.
  - "Elderly patients":
    - Consider routine discussions of ACP at ~age 65 years. The exact age is less important. It is crucial to speak with patients while they still have decision-making capacity. Discussions should be repeated regularly to ensure patient preferences have not changed.
    - Refer patients to legal services for AD/DPOA.
    - Complete POLST forms in clinic.
  - Any change in clinical status (including frequent ER visits or hospitalizations):
    - Changes in functional statuses should prompt a discussion about prognosis and future wishes. Hospitalizations are important milestones to discuss recovery or decline.
    - Consider palliative care services.
    - Consider support services to prevent caregiver burnout.

- At the end of life, if it is the patient's desire, it is important to engage hospice services in a timely manner.
  – ACP discussions are often complicated by social, familial, cultural, and medical factors. It is important to be sensitive to each patient's individual context.
    ○ African Americans are less likely than whites to complete AD.
    ○ Preference for life-sustaining treatment, religious beliefs, and mistrust of the medical community contribute to this difference.
  – Do not force the conversation if a patient is resistant or unprepared to discuss ACP.
    ○ Motivational interviewing can be used to gauge interest and readiness to discuss ACP.
    ○ Addressing implications for friends and family who may be burdened with decision making may help promote ACP conversations.
  – The first time ACP is brought up often serves as an introduction to the topic and an opportunity for the patient to consider options. Subsequent visits can address specific scenarios and choices (2).
  – Avoid medical jargon (CPR, mechanical ventilation, parenteral nutrition, etc.) when addressing options. Patients may not understand the severity of illness or the implications of advanced life-saving interventions.

 ONGOING CARE

Reimbursement: The Centers for Medicare & Medicaid Services reimburses physicians for ACP discussions.
- Current CPT codes are 99497 for the first 30 minutes of discussion and completion of forms and 99498 for each additional 30 minutes (3).
- There are no limits to the number of times ACP can be reported in a given period of time.
- An advance directive does not have to be completed in order to bill for services.
- No specific diagnosis is required for the ACP codes.

FOLLOW-UP RECOMMENDATIONS
Patient Monitoring
- There are no specific guidelines for how often a LW or DPOA discussion should be revisited after completion.
- When there is a new diagnosis or a significant change in clinical status, have the patient consider how it would affect his or her ACP decision making.
- Have patients display POLST/MOLST forms prominently for ease of visibility to EMS.

PATIENT EDUCATION
- See references for links to: The National Hospice and Palliative Care Organization, Aging with Dignity, National Healthcare Decisions Day, and the American Bar Association have resources to help patients.
- Online platforms such as MyDirectives allow patients to specify their wishes electronically.
- DeathWise is a nonprofit organization with worksheets patients can use for the health, financial, care of body, and service components of ACP.

COMPLICATIONS
- Often LW, DPOA, and POLST are completed, but physicians do not have access to them. Electronic health records are a convenient place to store documents, but they may be difficult to retrieve.
  – Any ACP form should be part of the medical record with open access (if possible) to facilitate appropriate decision making.
  – Medical bracelets or other devices are often used to notify EMS of patient directives.
- Emergency rooms are vulnerable to uncertainty about what interventions patients want if they cannot communicate for themselves and guiding documents aren't readily available.
  – POLST forms can help avoid confusion.
- There is often misunderstanding on the part of both doctors and patients regarding do not resuscitate (DNR) and do not intubate (DNI) orders.
  – DNR/DNI orders can be reversed or should not be honored in certain situations.
  – DNR/DNI in a person with a chronic progressive illness does not necessarily mean DNR/DNI for an acute reversible process.
  – The prognosis for successful resuscitation on a hospital ward is approximately 14%; it is 50–80% for patients undergoing surgery.

REFERENCES
1. American Association of Retired Persons. Advance directive forms by state. http://www.aarp.org/home-family/caregiving/free-printable-advance-directives/. Accessed August 1, 2018.
2. Spoelhof GD, Elliott B. Implementing advance directives in office practice. *Am Fam Physician*. 2012;85(5):461–466.
3. Centers for Medicare and Medicaid Services. Frequently asked questions about billing the physician fee schedule for advance care planning services. https://www.cms.gov/Medicare/Medicare-fee-for-service-Payment/PhysicianFeeSched/downloads/FAQ-Advance-Care-Planning.pdf. Accessed August 1, 2018.

ADDITIONAL READING
- Aging with Dignity. Five wishes. https://www.agingwithdignity.org/. Accessed August 1, 2018.
- American Bar Association. Toolkit for health care advance planning. https://www.americanbar.org/groups/law_aging/resources/health_care_decision_making/consumer_s_toolkit_for_health_care_advance_planning.html. Accessed August 1, 2018.
- DeathWise: http://deathwise.wpengine.com/.
- Heyland DK. Engaging seriously ill older patients in advance care planning. https://psnet.ahrq.gov/webmm/case/404/engaging-seriously-ill-older-patients-in-advance-care-planning. Published April 2017. Accessed August 1, 2018.
- My Directives: https://www.mydirectives.com/.
- National Healthcare Decisions Day: https://www.nhdd.org/.
- National Hospice and Palliative Care Organization, CaringInfo: http://www.caringinfo.org/i4a/pages/index.cfm?pageid=1.
- Pearlman RA, Tonelli M, Braddock C III, et al. Advance care planning & advance directives. https://depts.washington.edu/bioethx/topics/adcare.html. Updated March 11, 2014. Accessed August 1, 2018.

 ## CODES

ICD10
- Z71.89 Other specified counseling
- Z51.5 Encounter for palliative care
- Z66 Do not resuscitate

CLINICAL PEARLS
- ACP is an important and underutilized element of compassionate and comprehensive patient-centered care.
- The primary barriers to discussing advanced directives from the patient perspective include lack of knowledge, fear of burdening family, and a desire for physicians to initiate the discussion.
- The primary barriers to discussing advanced directives from the physician perspective include discomfort with the topic, lack of emotional support, lack of reimbursement, and lack of time to fully address the topic.
- Fewer unwanted interventions occur in the emergency room and inpatient setting when ACP is actively reviewed and wishes documented/conveyed appropriately.

ALCOHOL USE DISORDER (AUD)

Gennine M. Zinner, RNCS, ANP

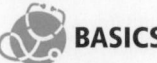 **BASICS**

DESCRIPTION

- Any pattern of alcohol use causing significant physical, mental, or social dysfunction; key features are tolerance, withdrawal, and persistent use despite problems.
- Alcohol abuse: maladaptive pattern of alcohol use manifested by ≥1 of:
  - Failure to fulfill obligations at work, school, or home
  - Recurrent use in hazardous situations
  - Recurrent alcohol-related legal problems
  - Continued use despite related social or interpersonal problems
- Alcohol dependence: maladaptive pattern of use manifested by ≥3 of the following:
  - Tolerance
  - Withdrawal
  - Using more than intended
  - Persistent desire or attempts to cut down/stop
  - Significant amount of time obtaining, using, or recovering from alcohol
  - Social, occupational, or recreational activities sacrificed for alcohol use
  - Continued use despite physical or psychological problems
- National Institute on Alcohol Abuse and Alcoholism criteria for "at-risk" drinking: men: >14 drinks a week or >4 per occasion; women: >7 drinks a week or >3 per occasion
- Women experience harmful effects at lower levels of alcohol consumption and are less likely to report problems related to drinking.
- System(s) affected: nervous, gastrointestinal (GI)
- Synonym(s): alcoholism; alcohol abuse; alcohol dependence

Geriatric Considerations
- Common and underdiagnosed in elderly; less likely to report problem; may exacerbate normal age-related cognitive deficits and disabilities
- Multiple drug interactions
- Signs and symptoms may be different or attributed to chronic medical problem or dementia.
- Common assessment tools may be inappropriate.

Pediatric Considerations
- Children of alcoholics are at increased risk for problem drinking.
- 2.5% of adolescents have alcohol use disorder (AUD); 13.4% of youth age 12 to 20 years report binge drinking in the past month; negative effect on maturation and normal brain development
- Early onset drinkers (those who start drinking before age 21 years) are 4 times more likely to develop a problem than those who begin after age 21 years.
- Depression, suicidal or disorderly behavior, family disruption, violence or destruction of property, poor school or work performance, sexual promiscuity, social immaturity, lack of interests, isolation, moodiness

Pregnancy Considerations
- Women should abstain during conception and throughout pregnancy.
- 10–50% of children born to women who are heavy drinkers will have fetal alcohol syndrome.

EPIDEMIOLOGY
- Predominant age: 18 to 25 years, but all ages affected
- Predominant sex: male > female (3:1)

Prevalence
- 27% of Americans age 18 years or older reported they engaged in binge drinking in the past month; 7% reported they engaged in heavy alcohol use in the past month.
- 15 million adults (6%) age >18 years has AUD.

ETIOLOGY AND PATHOPHYSIOLOGY
- Multifactorial: genetic, environment, psychosocial
- Alcohol is a CNS depressant, facilitating γ-aminobutyric acid (GABA) inhibition and blocking N-methyl-D-aspartate receptors.

Genetics
50–60% of risk is genetic.

RISK FACTORS
- Family history
- Depression (40% with comorbid alcohol abuse)
- Anxiety
- Tobacco use; other substance abuse
- Male gender; lower socioeconomic status
- Unemployment
- Poor self-esteem—seeking peer/social approval
- Family dysfunction or childhood trauma
- Posttraumatic stress disorder
- Antisocial personality disorder
- Bipolar disorder
- Eating disorders
- Criminal behavior

GENERAL PREVENTION
Counsel with family history and risk factors.

COMMONLY ASSOCIATED CONDITIONS
- Cardiomyopathy, atrial fibrillation
- Hypertension
- Peptic ulcer disease/gastritis
- Cirrhosis, fatty liver, cholelithiasis
- Hepatitis
- Diabetes mellitus
- Pancreatitis
- Malnutrition
- Upper GI malignancies
- Peripheral neuropathy, seizures
- Abuse and violence
- Trauma (falls, motor vehicle accidents [MVAs])
- Behavioral disorders (depression, bipolar, schizophrenia): >50% of patients with these disorders have a comorbid substance abuse problem.

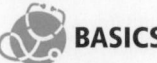 **DIAGNOSIS**

HISTORY
- Thorough behavioral history
  - Anxiety, depression, insomnia
  - Psychological and social dysfunction, marital, or relationship problems
  - Social isolation/withdrawal
  - Domestic violence
  - Alcohol-related legal problems
  - Repeated attempts to stop/reduce drinking
  - Loss of interest in nondrinking activities
  - Employment problems (tardiness, absenteeism, decreased productivity, interpersonal problems, frequent job loss)
  - Blackouts
  - Complaints about alcohol-related behavior
  - Frequent trauma, MVAs, ED visits

- Physical symptoms
  - Anorexia
  - Nausea, vomiting, abdominal pain
  - Palpitations
  - Headache
  - Impotence
  - Menstrual irregularities
  - Infertility

PHYSICAL EXAM
- Physical exam may be completely normal.
- General: fever, agitation, diaphoresis
- Head/eyes/ears/nose/throat: plethoric face, rhinophyma, poor oral hygiene, oropharyngeal malignancies
- Cardiovascular: hypertension, dilated cardiomyopathy, tachycardia, arrhythmias
- Respiratory: aspiration pneumonia
- GI: stigmata of chronic liver disease, peptic ulcer disease, pancreatitis, esophageal malignancies, esophageal varices
- Genitourinary: testicular atrophy
- Musculoskeletal: poorly healed fractures, myopathy, osteopenia, osteoporosis, bone marrow suppression
- Neurologic: tremors, cognitive deficits (e.g., memory impairment), peripheral neuropathy, Wernicke-Korsakoff syndrome (from severe acute deficiency of thiamine: Korsakoff psychosis is a chronic neurologic sequela of Wernicke encephalopathy)
- Endocrine/metabolic: hyperlipidemias, cushingoid appearance, gynecomastia
- Dermatologic: burns (e.g., cigarettes), bruises, poor hygiene, palmar erythema, spider telangiectasias, caput medusae, jaundice

DIFFERENTIAL DIAGNOSIS
- Other substance use disorders
- Depression, dementia
- Cerebellar ataxia; cerebrovascular accident (CVA)
- Benign essential tremor; seizure disorder
- Hypoglycemia; diabetic ketoacidosis
- Viral hepatitis

DIAGNOSTIC TESTS & INTERPRETATION
Screening

- CAGE questionnaire: (Cut down, Annoyed, Guilty, and Eye opener): >2 "yes" answers is 74–89% sensitive, 79–95% specific for AUD; less sensitive for white women, college students, elderly; not an appropriate tool for less severe forms of alcohol abuse
- Single question for unhealthy use: "How many times in the last year have you had X or more drinks in 1 day?" (X = 5 for men, 4 for women); 81.8% sensitive, 79% specific for AUDs (1)[C]
- Alcohol Use Disorders Identification Test (AUDIT): 10 items, if >4: 70–92% sensitive, better in populations with low incidence of alcoholism: https://www.nams.sg/helpseekers/alcohol/self-assessment-tool/Pages/default.aspx

Initial Tests (lab, imaging)
- CBC; liver function tests (LFTs); electrolytes; BUN/creatinine; lipid panel; thiamine; folate; hepatitis A, B, and C serology
- Amylase, lipase (if GI symptoms present)
- Serum levels increased in chronic abuse:
  - AST/ALT ratio >2.0
  - γ-Glutamyl transferase (GGT)
  - Carbohydrate-deficient transferrin
  - Elevated mean corpuscular volume (MCV)

– ↑ Prothrombin time
– Uric acid
– ↑ Triglycerides and cholesterol (total)
- Often decreased
  – Calcium, magnesium, potassium, phosphorus
  – BUN
  – Hemoglobin, hematocrit, platelet count
  – Serum protein, albumin
  – Thiamine, folate
- Blood alcohol concentration warning levels
  – >100 mg/dL in outpatient setting
  – >150 mg/dL without obvious signs of intoxication
  – >300 mg/dL at any time
- CAT scan or MRI of brain: cortical atrophy, lesions in thalamic nucleus, and basal forebrain
- Abdominal ultrasound (US): ascites, periportal fibrosis, fatty infiltration, inflammation

Test Interpretation
- Liver: inflammation or fatty infiltration (alcoholic hepatitis), periportal fibrosis (Alcoholic cirrhosis occurs in only 10–20% of alcoholics.)
- Gastric mucosa: inflammation, ulceration
- Pancreas: inflammation, liquefaction necrosis
- Heart: dilated cardiomyopathy
- Immune system: decreased granulocytes
- Endocrine organs: elevated cortisol levels, testicular atrophy, decreased female hormones
- Brain: cortical atrophy, enlarged ventricles

 TREATMENT

- For management of acute withdrawal, please see "Alcohol Withdrawal."
- http://www.aafp.org/afp/2005/0201/p495.html

GENERAL MEASURES
- Brief interventions and counseling by clinicians have proven efficacy for problem drinking (2)[B].
- Treat comorbid problems (sleep, anxiety, etc.), but do not prescribe medications with cross tolerance to alcohol (benzodiazepines).
- Group programs and/or 12-step programs shown to have benefit in helping patients accept treatment
- Consider referring patients with alcohol dependence to an addiction specialist or treatment program.

MEDICATION
First Line
- Adjuncts to withdrawal regimens:
  – Naltrexone: 50 to 100 mg/day PO or 380 mg IM once every 4 weeks; opiate antagonist reduces craving and likelihood of relapse and decreases number of heavy drinking days in recalcitrant alcohol abusers (IM route may enhance compliance and efficacy) (3,4)[B].
  – Acamprosate (Campral): 666 mg PO TID after withdrawal completed; reduces relapse risk. If helpful, use for 1 year (3,4)[B].
  – Topiramate (Topamax): 25 to 300 mg/day PO or divided BID; may enhance abstinence (5)[B] (off-label FDA use)
- Supplements for all
  – Thiamine: 100 mg/day (first dose IV prior to glucose to avoid Wernicke encephalopathy)
  – Folic acid: 1 mg/day
  – Multivitamin: daily
- Contraindications
  – Naltrexone: pregnancy, acute hepatitis, hepatic failure
  – Monitor LFTs.

- Precautions: organic pain, organic brain syndromes
- Significant possible interactions: alcohol, sedatives, hypnotics, naltrexone, and narcotics

ALERT
Treat acute symptoms if in alcohol withdrawal; give thiamine 100 mg/day with first dose prior to glucose.

Second Line
- Disulfiram: 250 to 500 mg/day PO; unproven efficacy; may provide psychological deterrent; most effective if used with close supervision (4)[A]
- Baclofen: Low dose (30 to 60 mg/day) has a more tolerable side effect profile and is possibly more efficacious than higher doses (>60 mg/day) (6)[A].
- Selective serotonin reuptake inhibitors may be beneficial if comorbid depression exists (3)[A].

ISSUES FOR REFERRAL
Addiction specialist, 12-step or long-term program, behavioral health professional

ADMISSION, INPATIENT, AND NURSING CONSIDERATIONS
- Assess medical and psychiatric comorbidities.
  – CIWA >8: a 10-item scale used in the assessment and management of alcohol withdrawal
- Correct electrolyte imbalances, acidosis, and hypovolemia (treat if in alcohol withdrawal).
- Thiamine: 100 mg IM, followed by 100 mg PO; folic acid: 1 mg/day
- Benzodiazepines used to lower risk of alcohol withdrawal, seizures

 ONGOING CARE

FOLLOW-UP RECOMMENDATIONS
Patient Monitoring
- Outpatient detoxification: daily visits (not recommended for patients with heavy alcohol abuse)
- Early outpatient rehabilitation: weekly visits
- Detoxification alone is not sufficient.

PATIENT EDUCATION
- Center for Substance Abuse Treatment: (800) 662-HELP or https://www.samhsa.gov/find-help
- Alcoholics Anonymous: http://www.aa.org/
- Rational Recovery: https://rational.org/index.php?id=1
- Secular Organizations for Sobriety: http://www.centerforinquiry.net/sos
- Alcohol Answers: http://www.alcoholanswers.org/: an evidence-based web site for those seeking credible information on alcohol dependence and online support forums

PROGNOSIS
- Chronic relapsing disease; mortality rate more than twice general population, death 10 to 15 years earlier
- Abstinence benefits: survival, mental health, family, employment
- 12-step programs, cognitive behavior, and motivational therapies are often effective during 1st year following treatment.

COMPLICATIONS
- Psychosocial complications (family, employment, etc.)
- Cirrhosis (women sooner than men)
- GI malignancies
- Neuropathy, dementia, Wernicke-Korsakoff syndrome
- Stroke; ketoacidosis; infections
- Adult respiratory distress syndrome
- Depression; suicide; trauma

REFERENCES
1. Smith PC, Schmidt SM, Allensworth-Davies D, et al. Primary care validation of a single-question alcohol screening test. *J Gen Intern Med*. 2009;24(7):783–788.
2. Kaner EF, Beyer FR, Muirhead C, et al. Effectiveness of brief alcohol interventions in primary care populations. *Cochrane Database Syst Rev*. 2018;(2):CD004148.
3. Miller PM, Book SW, Stewart SH. Medical treatment of alcohol dependence: a systematic review. *Int J Psychiatry Med*. 2011;42(3):227–266.
4. Jonas DE, Amick HR, Feltner C, et al. *Pharmacotherapy for Adults with Alcohol-Use Disorders in Outpatient Settings. Comparative Effectiveness Review No. 134.* Rockville, MD: Agency for Healthcare Research and Quality; 2016. AHRQ Publication No. 14-EHC029-EF.
5. Müller CA, Geisel O, Banas R, et al. Current pharmacological treatment approaches for alcohol dependence. *Expert Opin Pharmacother*. 2014;15(4):471–481.
6. Pierce M, Sutterland A, Beraha EM, et al. Efficacy, tolerability, and safety of low-dose and high-dose baclofen in the treatment of alcohol dependence: a systematic review and meta-analysis. *Eur Neuropsychopharmacol*. 2018;28(7):795–806.

ADDITIONAL READING
National Institute on Alcohol Abuse and Alcoholism. Helping patients who drink too much: a clinician's guide. http://www.niaaa.nih.gov/guide. Accessed August 19, 2018.

 SEE ALSO

Alcohol Withdrawal; Substance Use Disorders

CODES
ICD10
- F10.10 Alcohol abuse, uncomplicated
- F10.20 Alcohol dependence, uncomplicated
- F10.239 Alcohol dependence with withdrawal, unspecified

CLINICAL PEARLS
- CAGE questionnaire: >2 "yes" answers is 74–89% sensitive, 79–95% specific for AUD; less sensitive for white women, college students, elderly; not an appropriate tool for less severe forms of alcohol abuse
- Single question for unhealthy use screening: "How many times in the last year have you had X or more drinks in 1 day?" (X = 5 for men, 4 for women); 81.8% sensitive, 79% specific for AUDs
- National Institute on Alcohol Abuse and Alcoholism criteria for "at-risk" drinking: men >14 drinks a week or >4 per occasion; women: >7 drinks a week or >3 per occasion

ALCOHOL WITHDRAWAL
Sebastian T. Tong, MD, MPH

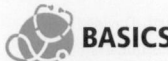 **BASICS**

DESCRIPTION
Alcohol withdrawal syndrome (AWS) is a spectrum of symptoms that results from abrupt cessation or reduction in alcohol intake, which has previously been heavy or prolonged. Symptoms generally start 6 to 24 hours after the last drink.

EPIDEMIOLOGY
- 15.1 million Americans meet diagnostic criteria for alcohol use disorder (AUD). Approximately 50% of those with AUD have experienced AWS in their lifetime.
- 8% of those admitted to the hospital are at risk for AWS.
- Higher prevalence in men, whites, Native Americans, younger and unmarried adults, and those with lower socioeconomic status

ETIOLOGY AND PATHOPHYSIOLOGY
- Consumption of alcohol potentiates the effect of the inhibitory neurotransmitter γ-aminobutyric acid (GABA). With chronic alcohol ingestion, this repeated stimulation downregulates the inhibitory effects of GABA.
- Concurrently, alcohol ingestion inhibits the stimulatory effect of glutamate on the CNS, with chronic alcohol use upregulating excitatory NMDA glutamate receptors.
- When alcohol is abruptly stopped, the combined effect of a downregulated inhibitory neurotransmitter system (GABA modulated) and upregulated excitatory neurotransmitter system (glutamate modulated) results in brain hyperexcitability when no longer suppressed by alcohol; clinically seen as AWS

Genetics
Some evidence for a genetic basis of AUD

RISK FACTORS
- High tolerance, prolonged use, high quantities
- Previous alcohol withdrawal episodes, detoxifications, alcohol withdrawal seizures, and delirium tremens (DTs)
- Serious medical problems
- Concomitant benzodiazepine (BZD) use

Geriatric Considerations
Elderly with AUD are more susceptible to withdrawal, and chronic comorbid conditions place them at higher risk of complications from withdrawal; use of short-acting medications preferred for management

Pregnancy Considerations
Hospitalization or inpatient detoxification is usually required for treatment of acute alcohol withdrawal.

GENERAL PREVENTION
- Routinely screen all adults for alcohol misuse (1)[B].
- Screen with the CAGE or similar questionnaire.
  - Feeling the need to **C**ut down
  - **A**nnoyed by criticism about alcohol use
  - **G**uilt about drinking/behaviors while intoxicated
  - "**E**ye opener" to quell withdrawal symptoms
  - Useful to detect problematic alcohol use; positive screen is ≥2 "yes" responses.
- Three-question AUDIT-C screening test is also useful to identify problem drinking.

COMMONLY ASSOCIATED CONDITIONS
- General: poor nutrition, electrolyte abnormalities (hyponatremia, hypomagnesemia, hypophosphatemia), thiamine deficiency, dehydration
- GI: hepatitis, cirrhosis, esophageal varices, GI bleed
- Heme: splenomegaly, thrombocytopenia, macrocytic anemia

- Cardiovascular: cardiomyopathy, hypertension, atrial fibrillation, other arrhythmias, stroke
- CNS: trauma, seizure disorder, generalized atrophy, Wernicke-Korsakoff syndrome
- Peripheral nervous system: neuropathy, myopathy
- Pulmonary: aspiration pneumonitis or pneumonia; increased risk of anaerobic infections
- Psychiatric: depression, posttraumatic stress disorder, bipolar disease, polysubstance use disorder

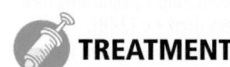 **DIAGNOSIS**

- *Diagnostic and Statistical Manual of Mental Disorders* AWS criteria are diagnosed when ≥2 of the following present within a few hours to several days after the cessation or reduction of heavy and prolonged alcohol ingestion (2)[C]:
  - Autonomic hyperactivity (sweating, tachycardia)
  - Increased hand tremor
  - Insomnia
  - Psychomotor agitation
  - Anxiety
  - Nausea or vomiting
  - Generalized tonic–clonic seizures
  - Transient visual, auditory, or tactile hallucinations or illusions
- Criteria for DTs include ≥2 of the criteria for AWS and disturbances in orientation, memory, attention, awareness, visuospatial ability, or perception.
- These should cause clinically significant distress or impair functioning and not be secondary to an underlying medical condition or mental disorder.
- AWS can be divided into stages based on time of onset and severity:
  - Minor withdrawal: onset 6 to 8 hours after cessation
    - Mild anxiety, restlessness, and agitation
    - Mild nausea/GI upset and decreased appetite
    - Sleep disturbance
    - Sweating
    - Mild tremulousness
    - Fluctuating tachycardia and hypertension
  - Major withdrawal: onset 24 to 72 hours after cessation
    - Marked restlessness and agitation
    - Moderate tremulousness with constant eye movements
    - Diaphoresis
    - Nightmares
    - Nausea, vomiting, diarrhea, anorexia
    - Marked tachycardia and hypertension
    - Alcoholic hallucinosis (auditory, tactile, or visual) may have mild confusion but can be reoriented.
  - DTs: onset 72 to 96 hours after cessation
    - Fever
    - Severe hypertension, tachycardia
    - Delirium
    - Drenching sweats
    - Marked tremors
    - Persistent hallucinations
  - Alcohol withdrawal–associated seizures are often brief, generalized tonic–clonic seizures, and typically occur 6 to 48 hours after last drink.

HISTORY
Essential historical information should be as follows:
- Duration and quantity of alcohol intake, time since last drink
- Previous episodes/symptoms of alcohol withdrawal, prior admissions for medically managed withdrawal
- Concurrent substance use

- Preexisting medical and psychiatric conditions, prior seizure activity
- Social history: living situation, social support, stressors, and triggers

PHYSICAL EXAM
Should include assessment of conditions likely to complicate or that are exacerbated by AWS
- Cardiovascular: arrhythmias, heart failure, coronary artery disease
- GI: GI bleed, liver disease, pancreatitis
- Neuro: oculomotor dysfunction, gait ataxia, neuropathy
- Psych: orientation, memory (may be complicated by hepatic encephalopathy)
- General: hand tremor (six to eight cycles per second), infections

DIFFERENTIAL DIAGNOSIS
- Cocaine intoxication
- Opioid, marijuana, and amphetamine withdrawal
- Anticholinergic drug toxicity
- Neuroleptic malignant syndrome
- ICU delirium
- Liver failure
- Sepsis, CNS infection, or hemorrhage
- Mania, psychosis
- Thyroid crisis

DIAGNOSTIC TESTS & INTERPRETATION
Initial Tests (lab, imaging)
- Blood alcohol level, urine drug screen
- CBC; comprehensive metabolic panel
- CNS imaging if acute mental status changes
- If first seizure, full neurologic workup, including EEG, brain imaging, and lumbar puncture

TREATMENT

GENERAL MEASURES
The goal is to prevent and treat withdrawal symptoms (e.g., seizures, DTs, cardiovascular events). This is done primarily with BZDs, which reduce the duration of symptoms and raise the seizure threshold.
- Exclude other medical and psychiatric causes.
- Provide a quiet, protective environment.
- The Clinical Institute Withdrawal Assessment of Alcohol Scale, Revised (CIWA-Ar) is useful for determining medication dosing and frequency of evaluation for AWS. Severity of symptoms are rated on a scale from 0 to 7, with 0 being without symptoms and 7 being the maximum score (except orientation and clouding of sensorium, scale 0 to 4).
  - Nausea and vomiting
  - Tactile disturbances
  - Tremor
  - Auditory disturbances
  - Paroxysmal sweats
  - Visual disturbances
  - Anxiety
  - Headache or fullness in head
  - Agitation
  - Orientation and clouding of sensorium
- The maximum CIWA-Ar score achievable is 67.
  - Mild withdrawal = score <8: likely resolve without medication
  - Moderate withdrawal = 8 to 14: often require management with medication
  - Severe withdrawal = >15: are associated with the highest risk of seizures and development of DTs
- Frequent reevaluation with CIWA-Ar score is crucial.

MEDICATION

First Line

- BZD monotherapy remains the treatment of choice (3)[A]; it is associated with fewer complications compared with neuroleptics (4)[A].
- BZD should be chosen by the following considerations:
  - Agents with rapid onset control agitation more quickly (e.g., IV diazepam [Valium]).
  - Long-acting BZDs (diazepam, chlordiazepoxide [Librium]) are more effective at preventing breakthrough seizures and delirium management.
  - Short-acting BZDs (lorazepam [Ativan], oxazepam [Serax]) are preferable when prolonged sedation is a concern (e.g., elderly patients or other serious concomitant medical illness) and preferable when severe hepatic insufficiency may impair metabolism (4)[A].
- BZD dosages will vary by patients.
- Can use symptom-triggered or fixed-schedule regimens
  - Symptom-triggered regimens have been found to require less BZD amounts and reduce hospitalization.
  - Fixed-schedule regimens more appropriate if nursing staff do not have training for symptom triggered, if patient with severe coronary artery disease, or if history of past withdrawal seizures
- Symptom-triggered regimen: Administer one of the following medications every hour when CIWA-Ar ≥8:
  - Chlordiazepoxide 50 to 100 mg PO
  - Diazepam 10 to 20 mg PO
  - Oxazepam 30 to 60 mg PO
  - Lorazepam 2 to 4 mg PO
- Fixed-schedule regimen: Administer one of the following medications every 6 hours:
  - Chlordiazepoxide 50 mg PO for 4 doses and then 25 mg PO for 8 doses
  - Diazepam 10 mg PO for 4 doses and then 5 mg PO for 8 doses
  - Lorazepam 2 mg PO for 4 doses and then 1 mg PO for 8 doses
  - Important to monitor closely and provide additional BZDs if CIWA-Ar ≥8
- Thiamine: 50 to 100 mg daily IV or IM for at least 3 days (4)[C]
  - Do not administer IV glucose before giving thiamine because this may precipitate Wernicke encephalopathy and Korsakoff psychosis.

Second Line

- β-Blockers (e.g., atenolol or propranolol) and α₂-agonists (e.g., clonidine) help to control hypertension and tachycardia and can be used with BZDs. Not used as monotherapy, due to their inability to prevent DTs and seizures; may worsen underlying delirium
- Carbamazepine: not recommended as first-line therapy; associated with reduced incidence of seizures but more studies are needed
- If the patient exhibits significant agitation and alcoholic hallucinosis, an antipsychotic (3,5)[C] (haloperidol [Haldol]) can be used, but this requires close observation because it lowers the seizure threshold.
- Neuroleptic agents are not recommended as monotherapy due to their association with increased mortality, longer duration of delirium, and complications when compared with sedative agents (6)[A].

ADDITIONAL THERAPIES

Peripheral neuropathy and cerebellar dysfunction merit physical therapy evaluation.

ADMISSION, INPATIENT, AND NURSING CONSIDERATIONS

Criteria for inpatient admission:
- CIWA-Ar score >15 or severe withdrawal
- Concurrent acute illness requiring inpatient care
- Laboratory abnormalities (e.g., electrolyte imbalance)
- Poor ability to follow up or no reliable social support
- Pregnancy
- History of severe withdrawal symptoms
- History of withdrawal seizures or DTs
- Concurrent psychiatric illness

 ONGOING CARE

FOLLOW-UP RECOMMENDATIONS

- Managing alcohol withdrawal is only first step toward treating patient's underlying AUD.
- Discharge arrangements should include:
  - Development of plan to engage patient in further treatment
  - Transition to outpatient substance use counseling, peer support groups, and/or residential treatment facility
  - Prescription of available medication-assisted treatment such as acamprosate (Campral), naltrexone (ReVia, Vivitrol), or disulfiram (Antabuse)
- Acamprosate (666 mg PO TID): glutamate and GABA modulator indicated to reduce cravings
  - Contraindications: renal impairment (CrCl <30 mL/min)
- Naltrexone (50 mg/day PO; 380 mg IM every 4 weeks): opiate receptor antagonist, theorized to attenuate pleasurable effects of alcohol and reduce craving. Initiate therapy after patient is opioid free for at least 7 days.
  - Contraindications: acute hepatitis/liver failure, concomitant opioid therapy
- Disulfiram (250 mg/day PO): irreversibly inhibits aldehyde dehydrogenase, blocking alcohol metabolism, leading to an accumulation of acetaldehyde
  - Second-line option due to limited evidence of efficacy for relapse prevention
  - Contraindications: concomitant use of metronidazole and ethanol-containing products, psychosis, severe myocardial disease, and coronary occlusion

Patient Monitoring

Frequent follow-up to monitor for relapse

PATIENT EDUCATION

- Alcoholics Anonymous: http://www.aa.org/
- SMART Recovery (Self-Management and Recovery Training): http://www.smartrecovery.org/ (not spiritually based)
- National Institute on Alcohol Abuse and Alcoholism: http://www.niaaa.nih.gov/guide/
- FamilyDoctor.Org: alcoholism (Spanish resources available)

PROGNOSIS

Mortality from severe withdrawal (DTs) is 1–5%.

COMPLICATIONS

Occurs more frequently in individuals who have prior episodes of withdrawal or concurrent illnesses

REFERENCES

1. Moyer VA; for Preventive Services Task Force. Screening and behavioral counseling interventions in primary care to reduce alcohol misuse: U.S. Preventive Services Task Force recommendation statement. *Ann Intern Med*. 2013;159(3):210–218.
2. American Psychiatric Association. *Diagnostic and Statistical Manual of Mental Disorders*. 5th ed. Arlington, VA: American Psychiatric Association; 2013.
3. Amato L, Minozzi S, Vecchi S, et al. Benzodiazepines for alcohol withdrawal. *Cochrane Database Syst Rev*. 2010;(3):CD005063.
4. Amato L, Minozzi S, Davoli M. Efficacy and safety of pharmacological interventions for the treatment of the alcohol withdrawal syndrome. *Cochrane Database Syst Rev*. 2011;(6):CD008537.
5. Minozzi S, Amato L, Vecchi S, et al. Anticonvulsants for alcohol withdrawal. *Cochrane Database Syst Rev*. 2010;(3):CD005064.
6. Mayo-Smith MF, Beecher LH, Fischer TL, et al; for Working Group on the Management of Alcohol Withdrawal Delirium, Practice Guidelines Committee, American Society of Addiction Medicine. Management of alcohol withdrawal delirium. An evidence-based practice guideline. *Arch Intern Med*. 2004;164(13):1405–1412.

ADDITIONAL READING

- Muncie HL Jr, Yasinian Y, Oge' L. Outpatient management of alcohol withdrawal syndrome. *Am Fam Physician*. 2013;88(9):589–595.
- Sarff M, Gold JA. Alcohol withdrawal syndromes in the intensive care unit. *Crit Care Med*. 2010;38(Suppl 9):S494–S501.

 SEE ALSO

Substance Use Disorders

 CODES

ICD10

- F10.239 Alcohol dependence with withdrawal, unspecified
- F10.230 Alcohol dependence with withdrawal, uncomplicated
- F10.231 Alcohol dependence with withdrawal delirium

CLINICAL PEARLS

- Any BZD dose should be patient specific, sufficient to achieve and maintains a "light somnolence" (e.g., sleeping but easily arousable), and should be tapered off carefully even after AWS resolves to prevent BZD withdrawal.
- Administer thiamine before patient receives glucose, so as not to precipitate Wernicke encephalopathy.
- Avoid administering diazepam and lorazepam intramuscularly because of erratic absorption.
- Managing AWS is the first step toward treating AUD. Ensure patient has outpatient follow-up to continue treatment.

ALOPECIA

Anastasia N. Gevas, DO • Kelli M. Gevas, MD

 BASICS

DESCRIPTION

- Alopecia: absence of hair from areas where it normally grows
  - Anagen phase: growing hairs, 90% scalp hair follicles at any time, lasts 2 to 6 years
  - Catagen phase: regression of follicle, <1% follicles, lasts 3 weeks
  - Telogen phase: Resting phase lasts 2 to 3 months; 50 to 150 telogen hairs shed per day.
- Classified as scarring (cicatricial), nonscarring, or structural
- Scarring (cicatricial) alopecia
  - Inflammatory disorders leading to permanent hair loss and follicle destruction
  - Includes lymphocytic, neutrophilic, and mixed subtypes
- Nonscarring alopecia
  - Lack of inflammation, no destruction of follicle
  - Includes focal, patterned, and diffuse hair loss such as androgenic alopecia, alopecia areata (AA), telogen effluvium, anagen effluvium, syphilitic hair loss
- Structural hair disorders
  - Brittle or fragile hair from abnormal hair formation or external insult

EPIDEMIOLOGY

- Androgenic alopecia: onset in males between 20 and 25 years of age; onset in females prior to 40 years of age, affecting as many as 70% of women >65 years of age
- AA: onset usually prior to 30 years of age; men and women are equally affected; well-documented genetic predisposition

Incidence

Incidence greatest in Caucasians, followed by Asians, African Americans, and Native Americans; in females, 13% premenopausal, with as many as 70% females >65 years of age

Prevalence

- Androgenic alopecia: in males, 30% Caucasian by 30 years of age, 50% by 50 years of age, and 80% by 70 years of age
- AA: 1/1,000 with lifetime risk of 1–2%
- Scarring alopecia: rare, 3–7% of all hair disorder patients

ETIOLOGY AND PATHOPHYSIOLOGY

- Scarring (cicatricial) alopecia
  - Slick smooth scalp without follicles evident
  - Inflammatory disorders leading to permanent destruction of the follicle; it is not known what causes inflammation to develop.
  - Three major subtypes based on type of inflammation: lymphocytic, neutrophilic, and mixed
  - Primary scarring includes discoid lupus, lichen planopilaris, dissecting cellulitis of scalp, primary fibrosing, among others.
  - Secondary scarring from infection, neoplasm, radiation, surgery, and other physical trauma, including tinea capitis
  - Central centrifugal cicatricial alopecia most common form of scarring hair loss in African American women; etiology unknown but likely secondary to hair care practices

- Nonscarring alopecia
  - Focal alopecia
  - AA
    - Patchy hair loss, usually autoimmune in etiology, T cell–mediated inflammation resulting in premature transition to catagen then telogen phases
    - May occur with hair loss in other areas of the body (alopecia totalis [entire scalp]), alopecia universalis (rapid loss of all body hair)
    - Nail disease frequently seen
    - High psychiatric comorbidity (1)
  - Alopecia syphilitica: "moth-eaten" appearance, secondary syphilis
  - Postoperative, pressure-induced alopecia: from long periods of pressure on one area of scalp
  - Temporal triangular alopecia: congenital patch of hair loss in temporal area, unilateral or bilateral
  - Traction alopecia: patchy, due to physical stressor of braids, ponytails, hair weaves
- Pattern hair loss
  - Androgenic alopecia: hair transitions from terminal to vellus hairs
  - Male pattern hair loss: androgen-mediated hair loss in specific distribution; bitemporal, vertex occurs where androgen sensitive hairs are located on scalp. This is a predominantly hereditary condition (2).
    - Increased androgen receptors, increased 5-α reductase leads to increased testosterone conversion in follicle to dihydrotestosterone (DHT). This leads to decreased follicle size and vellus hair (2).
    - Norwood Hamilton classification type I to VII
    - Female pattern hair loss: thinning on frontal and vertex areas (Ludwig classification, grade I to III). Females with low levels of aromatase have more testosterone available for conversion to DHT (3). This carries an unclear inheritance pattern (2).
    - Polycystic ovarian syndrome, adrenal hyperplasia, and pituitary hyperplasia all lead to androgen changes and can result in alopecia.
  - Drugs (testosterone, progesterone, danazol, adrenocorticosteroids, anabolic steroids)
- Trichotillomania: intentional pulling of hair from scalp; may present in variety of patterns
- Diffuse alopecia
  - Telogen effluvium: sudden shift of many follicles from anagen to telogen phase resulting in decreased hair density but not bald areas
    - May follow major stressors, including childbirth, injury, illness; occurs 2 to 3 months after event
    - Can be chronic with ongoing illness, including SLE, renal failure, IBS, HIV, thyroid disease, pituitary dysfunction
    - Adding or changing medications (oral contraceptives, anticoagulants, anticonvulsants, SSRIs, retinoids, β-blockers, ACE inhibitors, colchicine, cholesterol-lowering medications, etc.)
    - Malnutrition from malabsorption, eating disorders; poor diet can contribute.
  - Anagen effluvium
    - Interruption of the anagen phase without transition to telogen phase; days to weeks after inciting event
    - Chemotherapy is most common trigger.
    - Radiation, poisoning, and medications can also trigger.

- Structural hair disorders
  - Multiple inherited hair disorders including Menkes disease, monilethrix, and so forth. These result in the formation of abnormal hairs that are weakened.
  - May also result from chemical or heat damaging from hair processing treatments

Genetics

- Family history of early patterned hair loss is common in androgenic alopecia, also in AA.
- Rare structural hair disorders may be inherited.

RISK FACTORS

- Genetic predisposition
- Chronic illness including autoimmune disease, infections, cancer
- Physiologic stress including pregnancy and childbirth
- Poor nutrition
- Medication, chemotherapy, radiation
- Hair chemical treatments, braids, weaves/extensions

GENERAL PREVENTION

Minimize risk factors where possible.

COMMONLY ASSOCIATED CONDITIONS

- See "Etiology and Pathophysiology."
- Vitiligo—4.1% patients with AA; may be the result of similar autoimmune pathways (4)

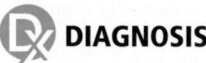 **DIAGNOSIS**

HISTORY

- Description of hair loss problem: rate of loss, duration, location, degree of hair loss, other symptoms including pruritus, infection, hair care, and treatments
- Medications
- Medical illness including chronic disease, recent illness, surgeries, pregnancy, thyroid disorder, iron deficiency, poisonings, exposures
- Psychological stress
- Dietary history and weight changes
- Family history of hair loss or autoimmune disorders

PHYSICAL EXAM

- Pattern of hair loss
  - Generalized, patterned, focal
  - Assess hair density, vellus versus terminal hairs, broken hair.
- Scalp scaling, inflammation, papules, pustules
- Presence of follicular ostia to determine class of alopecia
- Hair pull test
  - Pinch 25 to 50 hairs between thumb and forefinger and exert slow, gentle traction while sliding fingers up.
    - Normal: 1 to 2 dislodge
    - Abnormal: ≥6 hairs dislodged
    - Broken hairs (structural disorder)
    - Broken-off hair at the borders patch that are easily removable (in AA)
- Hair loss at other sites, nail disorders, skin changes
- Clinical signs of thyroid disease, lupus, or other diseases
- Clinical signs of virilization: acne, hirsutism, acanthosis nigricans, truncal obesity

DIFFERENTIAL DIAGNOSIS

Search for type of alopecia and then for reversible causes.

DIAGNOSTIC TESTS & INTERPRETATION
Initial Tests (lab, imaging)
- No testing may be indicated depending on clinical appearance.
- Nonandrogenic alopecia
  - TSH, CBC, ferritin
  - Consider: LFT, BMP, zinc, VDRL, ANA, prolactin all depending on clinical history and exam
- Androgenic alopecia: especially in females
  - Consider free testosterone and dehydroepiandrosterone sulfate.

Diagnostic Procedures/Other
- Light hair-pull test: Pull on 25 to 50 hairs; ≥6 hairs dislodged is consistent with shedding (effluvium, AA).
- Direct microscopic exam of the hair shaft
  - Anagen hairs: elongated, distorted bulb with root sheath attached
  - Telogen hairs: rounded bulb, no root sheath
  - Exclamation point hairs: club-shaped root with thinner proximal shaft (AA)
  - Broken and distorted hairs may be associated with multiple hair dystrophies.
- Biopsy: most important in scarring alopecia
- Ultraviolet light fluorescence and potassium hydroxide prep (to rule out tinea capitis)

TREATMENT
GENERAL MEASURES
- Consider potential harms and benefits to the patient prior to treatment. Many will gain an improved quality of life that is of benefit (2)[A].
- Stop any possible medication causes if possible; this will often resolve telogen effluvium (5)[C].
- Treat underlying medical causes (e.g., thyroid disorder, syphilis).
- Traction alopecia: Change hair care practices; education
- Trichotillomania: often requires psychological intervention to induce behavior change

MEDICATION
- Nonscarring
- **Androgenic alopecia**: Treatment must be continued indefinitely; can use in combination
  - Minoxidil (Rogaine): 2% topical solution (1 mL BID) for women, 5% topical solution (1 mL BID) or foam (daily) for men; works in 60% of cases (3)[A]
    - Unclear mechanism of action; appears to prolong anagen phase
    - Adverse effects: skin irritation, hypertrichosis of face/hands, tachycardia; category C in pregnancy (3)[A]
  - Finasteride (Propecia): 1 mg/day for men and women (off-label) (6)[A]; 30–50% improvement in males, poor data in females (2)[A]
    - 5-α reductase inhibitor, reduces DHT in system, increases total and anagen hairs, slows transition of terminal to vellus hairs
    - Works best on vertex, least in anterior, temporal areas
    - Adverse effects: loss of libido, gynecomastia, depression. Caution in liver disease; absolutely no use or contact during pregnancy, category X, reliable contraception required in female use (6)[A]
  - Spironolactone (Aldactone): 100 to 200 mg/day (off-label) (3)[C]
    - Aldosterone antagonist, antiandrogen; blocks the effect of androgens, decreasing testosterone production
    - Adverse effects: dose dependent, hyperkalemia, menstrual irregularity, fatigue; category D in pregnancy

- Ketoconazole: decreases DHT levels at follicle, works best with minoxidil in female androgenic alopecia (6)[A]
- Combination: Finasteride + minoxidil has superior efficacy to monotherapy (2)[A].
- **AA**: no FDA-approved treatment; high rate of spontaneous remission in patchy AA. Treatments all focus on symptom management rather than etiology.
- Intralesional steroids
  - Triamcinolone: 2.5 to 5.0 mg/mL (3)[C]
    - First line if <50% scalp involved
    - Inject 0.1 mL into deep dermal layer at 0.5 to 1.0 cm intervals with 1/2 in 30-gauge needle, every 4 to 6 weeks; maximum 20 mg per session (1)[C]
    - Adverse effects: local burning, pruritus, skin atrophy
  - Topical steroids: very limited evidence for efficacy
  - Betamethasone: 0.1% foam shows limited hair regrowth (1)[C].
    - Adverse effects: folliculitis, high relapse rate after discontinuation
  - Systemic glucocorticoids: Use in extensive, multifocal AA; may induce regrowth but requires long-term monthly treatment to maintain growth (1)[B]
    - Adverse effects: hyperglycemia, adrenal insufficiency, osteoporosis, cataracts, obesity
    - Psychiatric: SSRIs, psychiatric care, support groups
  - PUVA light therapy + prednisone: moderate effectiveness in diffuse AA
  - Tinea capitis: See "Tinea (Capitis, Corporis, Cruris)."

SURGERY/OTHER PROCEDURES
- Hair transplantation
- Wigs, hairpieces, extensions
- Surgical: graft transplantation, flap transplantation, or excision of the scarred area; used primarily in scarring alopecia
- Platelet-rich plasma: has been shown to restore dormant hair follicles and stimulate new hair growth
- Laser therapies to promote growth: lacks evidence

COMPLEMENTARY & ALTERNATIVE MEDICINE
- Many herbal medications are available; no clear evidence at this time
- Volumizing shampoos can help remaining hair look fuller.

ONGOING CARE
DIET
If nutritional deficit noted, supplementation may be necessary.

PATIENT EDUCATION
National Alopecia Areata Foundation: www.naaf.org

PROGNOSIS
- Androgenic alopecia: Prognosis depends on response to treatment.
- AA: often regrows within 1 year even without treatment. Recurrence common. 10% have severe, chronic form; poor prognosis more likely with long duration, extensive hair loss, autoimmune disease, nail involvement, and young age
- Telogen effluvium: maximum shedding 3 months after the inciting event and recovery following correction of the cause. Usually subsides in 3 to 6 months but takes 12 to 18 months for cosmetically significant regrowth; rarely, permanent hair loss, usually with long-term illness

- Anagen effluvium: Shedding begins days to a few weeks after the inciting event, with recovery following correction of the cause; rarely, permanent hair loss
- Traction alopecia: excellent prognosis with behavior modification
- Cicatricial alopecia: hair follicles permanently damaged; prognosis depends on type of alopecia and available treatments.
- Tinea capitis: excellent prognosis with treatment

REFERENCES
1. Alkhalifah A. Alopecia areata update. *Dermatol Clin.* 2013;31(1):93–108.
2. Blumeyer A, Tosti A, Messenger A, et al; for European Dermatology Forum. Evidence-based (S3) guideline for the treatment of androgenic alopecia in women and in men. *J Dtsch Dermatol Ges.* 2011;9(Suppl 6):S1–S57.
3. Rathnayake D, Sinclair R. Innovative use of spironolactone as an antiandrogen in the treatment of female pattern hair loss. *Dermatol Clin.* 2010;28(3):611–618.
4. Kumar S, Mittal J, Mahajan B. Colocalization of vitiligo and alopecia areata: coincidence or consequence? *Int J Trichology.* 2013;5(1):50–52.
5. Harrison S, Bergfeld W. Diffuse hair loss: its triggers and management. *Cleve Clin J Med.* 2009;76(6):361–367.
6. Atanaskova Mesinkovska N, Bergfeld WF. Hair: what is new in diagnosis and management? Female pattern hair loss update: diagnosis and treatment. *Dermatol Clin.* 2013;31(1):119–127.

ADDITIONAL READING
Otberg N. Primary cicatricial alopecias. *Dermatol Clin.* 2013;31(1):155–166.

SEE ALSO
- Hyperthyroidism; Lichen Planus; Lupus Erythematosus, Systemic (SLE); Polycystic Ovarian Syndrome (PCOS); Syphilis; Tinea (Capitis, Corporis, Cruris)
- Algorithm: Alopecia

CODES
ICD10
- L65.9 Nonscarring hair loss, unspecified
- L64.9 Androgenic alopecia, unspecified
- L63.9 Alopecia areata, unspecified

CLINICAL PEARLS
- History and physical are necessary in determining type of alopecia for appropriate treatment.
- Treatment of underlying medical condition or removal of triggering medication will often resolve hair loss.
- Educating the patient about the nature of the condition and expectations is key to care.
- Alopecia can affect the psychological condition of the patient, and it may be necessary to address this in any type of hair loss.

ALTITUDE ILLNESS

Douglas J. Bosin, DO • Phillip R. Hendley, MD • William S. Ellis, DO

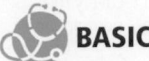 **BASICS**

DESCRIPTION
- A spectrum of medical problems ranging from mild discomfort to fatal illness that occur on ascent to higher altitudes as a direct result of inadequate acclimatization
- Categories of altitude: intermediate, 1,520 to 2,440 m; high, 2,440 to 4,270 m; very high, 4,270 to 5,490 m; and extreme, >5,490 m
- Altitude illness can affect anyone, including experienced and fit individuals. For most, it is an unpleasant but self-limiting syndrome that will not require medical intervention (1).
- Acute mountain sickness (AMS): Symptoms associated with a physiologic response to a hypobaric, hypoxic environment. Onset usually occurs within 6 to 12 hours after ascending >2,500 m. Neurologic symptoms predominate, ranging from mild/moderate headache and malaise to severe impairment.
- High-altitude pulmonary edema (HAPE): noncardiogenic pulmonary edema; typically after 2 or more days at altitudes >3,000 m, rare between 2,500 and 3,000 m
- High-altitude cerebral edema (HACE): a potentially fatal neurologic syndrome considered to be the end stage of AMS; onset after at least 2 days at altitudes >4,000 m
- System(s) affected: nervous/pulmonary (2)
- Synonym(s): mountain sickness

Geriatric Considerations
- Risk does not increase with age.
- Age alone should not preclude travel to high altitude; allow extra time to acclimate.
- Worsening of preexisting medical problems referred to as altitude-exacerbated conditions

Pediatric Considerations
- Altitude illness seems to have the same incidence in children as in adults; diagnosis may be delayed in younger children.
- Any child who experiences behavioral symptoms after recent ascent should be presumed to be suffering from altitude illness.

Pregnancy Considerations
- The risk during pregnancy is unknown.
- No evidence suggests that exposure to high altitudes (1,500 to 3,500 m) poses a risk to a pregnancy.
- It may be prudent to advise a low-altitude dwelling for any pregnant woman experiencing complications.

EPIDEMIOLOGY
Most epidemiologic studies are limited to relatively homogeneous male populations.

Incidence
- AMS: 10–25% of unacclimatized persons who ascend to 2,500 m; 50–85% at altitudes of 4,500 to 5,500 m
- HAPE/HACE: 0.5–1.0% of unacclimatized persons with 2 or more days of exposure at altitudes exceeding 3,000 m. Risk increases with rate of ascent (2).

ETIOLOGY AND PATHOPHYSIOLOGY
- Individuals with a prior history of AMS, HACE, or HAPE are at a higher risk of recurrent AMS.
- Hypobaric hypoxia and hypoxemia are the pathophysiologic precursors to altitude illness.
- Symptoms of AMS may be the result of cerebral swelling, either through vasodilatation induced by hypoxia or through cerebral edema.
- Other mechanisms include impaired cerebral autoregulation, release of vasogenic mediators, and alteration of the blood–brain barrier.
- HAPE is a noncardiogenic pulmonary edema characterized by exaggerated pulmonary hypertension leading to vascular leakage through overperfusion, stress failure, or both.

RISK FACTORS
- Failure to acclimatize at a lower altitude
- Ascent rate >300 to 500 m/day
- Extreme altitude
- Increased duration at high altitude
- Higher altitude during sleep cycle
- Prior history of altitude illness
- Cardiac congenital abnormalities
- Female gender
- History of migraines (3)
- Younger age (<46 years)

GENERAL PREVENTION
- General guidelines
  - Preacclimatization protects against altitude illness.
  - >2,500 m, do not ascend faster than 500 m/day; rest every 3 to 4 days (2).
  - Lower sleeping elevation: "Climb high and sleep low" for anyone going >3,500 m.
  - Avoid heavy exertion for the first 1 to 3 days at altitude.
  - Avoid respiratory depressants (alcohol and sedatives).
  - Preascent physical conditioning is not preventive but does increase odds of summiting.
- Drug prophylaxis
  - Acetazolamide, dexamethasone, and ibuprofen (see "Treatment")
  - For prevention of HAPE only (if at risk):
    ○ Consider nifedipine, β-agonists, and tadalafil (see "Treatment").

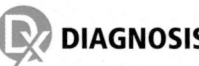 **DIAGNOSIS**

HISTORY
- AMS, mild to moderate symptoms
  - Headache, plus at least one of:
    ○ Anorexia
    ○ Nausea or vomiting
    ○ Dizziness or light-headedness
    ○ Insomnia
- AMS, severe symptoms
  - Increased headache
  - Irritability
  - Marked fatigue

- Dyspnea with exertion
- Nausea and vomiting
- HAPE (Lake Louise diagnostic criteria)
  ○ At least two of the following: dyspnea at rest, cough, weakness, decreased exercise performance, chest tightness, congestion
  ○ *AND* at least two of crackles or wheezing in at least one lung field, central cyanosis, tachycardia, tachypnea (Note: Fatigue may be a sign of pulmonary edema.)
- HACE symptoms: mental status changes (irrational behavior, lethargy, obtundation, coma)
  ○ May progress to ataxia and confusion (2)

PHYSICAL EXAM
- HAPE
  - Lung crackles or wheezing
  - Central cyanosis
  - Tachycardia
  - Tachypnea
- HACE
  - Abnormal mental status exam (behavioral change, lethargy, obtundation, coma)
  - Truncal ataxia
  - Papilledema, retinal hemorrhage, cranial nerve palsies
  - Focal neurologic deficits (rare)

DIFFERENTIAL DIAGNOSIS
- Onset of symptoms >3 days at a given altitude, the absence of headache, or the lack of rapid response to oxygen or descent suggests an alternative diagnosis.
- AMS/HACE
  - Subarachnoid hemorrhage, CNS mass, cerebrovascular accident
  - Migraine headache
  - Dehydration
  - Ingestion of toxins, drugs, or alcohol
  - Carbon monoxide exposure
  - CNS infection
  - Acute psychosis
- HAPE
  - Pneumonia
  - Cardiogenic pulmonary edema
  - Spontaneous pneumothorax
  - Pulmonary embolism
  - Asthma
  - Bronchitis
  - Myocardial infarction
  - Hyperventilation syndrome

DIAGNOSTIC TESTS & INTERPRETATION
Initial Tests (lab, imaging)
- AMS: Laboratory studies are nonspecific and rarely required for diagnosis.
- HAPE: severe hypoxemia demonstrated with oximetry or blood gas analysis
- Chest radiographs usually show patchy infiltrates. Clear lung fields suggest an alternate diagnosis.
- ECG may show sinus tachycardia or right-sided heart strain (1).

TREATMENT

GENERAL MEASURES
- Individuals without previous altitude exposure should adhere to acclimatization guidelines.
- Early recognition is important.
- Stop ascent, acclimatize at the same altitude, and/or descend if symptoms do not abate over 24 hours. Definitive treatment is to descend to a lower altitude. Dramatic improvement accompanies even modest reductions in altitude.
- Oxygen helps relieve symptoms. Give continuously by cannula or mask, and titrate to SaO_2 >90% (1).
- Given that most high-altitude travel is recreational and acetazolamide has side effects, prophylaxis is not generally recommended in children (4).
- AMS
  - Acetazolamide reduces mild to moderate symptoms of AMS (see "Medication").
  - Dexamethasone may also be effective in treating moderate AMS (see "Medication").
- HAPE
  - Oxygen therapy
  - Minimize exertion and keep patient warm.
  - Immediate descent or evacuation to a lower altitude
  - Portable hyperbaric therapy (2 to 15 psi using Gamow bag or Chamberlite) is an effective and practical alternative when descent is not possible.
  - Nifedipine (see "Medication")
- HACE
  - Immediate descent
  - Supplemental oxygen (highest flow available; maintain SaO_2 >90%)
  - Dexamethasone (see "Medication")
  - Portable hyperbaric therapy if available and unable to descend

MEDICATION
First Line
- Oxygen: 2 to 15 L/min to maintain SaO_2 >90% until symptoms improve
- Acetazolamide: If patient has a history of problems at altitude and/or plans to ascend >500 m/day above 2,500 m, consider therapy for primary prevention. Avoid in patients with a sulfonamide allergy.
  - Primary prevention of AMS: 125 to 250 mg PO BID starting 8 to 24 hours before ascent and continued for 2 days at a stable altitude; not recommended for children as a preventive medication (5)[A]
  - Treatment of AMS: 250 mg PO BID until symptoms resolve; pediatric dose: 2.5 mg/kg q12h (4)
- Dexamethasone: may significantly reduce the incidence and severity of AMS. Adverse side effects are rare (5)[A].
  - Prevention of AMS: 2 mg PO q6h or 4 mg PO q12h, starting 1 day before ascent and discontinued cautiously after 2 days at maximum altitude. Do not use for pediatric prevention (4).
  - Treatment of AMS: 4 mg PO/IV/IM q6h; pediatric dose: 0.15 mg/kg dose q6h (4)
  - Treatment of HACE: 8 mg PO/IV/IM initially and then 4 mg q6h; pediatric dose: 0.15 mg/kg dose q6h (4)

- Nifedipine (reduces pulmonary arterial pressure) (1)
  - Prevention of HAPE: 30 mg extended-release PO BID starting 1 day prior to ascent and continued for 2 days at maximum altitude
  - Treatment of HAPE: 30 mg extended-release PO q12h (likely unnecessary if oxygen is available)
- Tadalafil: Consider for the prevention of HAPE (1).
  - Prevention HAPE: 10 mg PO BID 1 day prior to ascent in HAPE susceptible individual
- Adjunct therapy
  - Salmeterol
    - Prevention and possible treatment of HAPE: 125 μg inhaled BID starting 1 day before ascent and continued for 2 days at maximum altitude
    - Recommended as adjunct to nifedipine
  - NSAIDs: possible benefit in AMS prevention and treatment of headache
    - Aspirin: 325 mg PO q4h for total 3 doses
    - Ibuprofen: 400 to 600 mg PO q8h
  - Antiemetics
    - Prochlorperazine: 10 mg PO/IM q6–8h
    - Promethazine: 25 to 50 mg PO/IM/PR q6h
- Other trialed therapies
  - Furosemide: previously studied for treatment of AMS or HACE, 20 to 80 mg PO/IV q12h for a total of 2 doses. Currently out of favor; not recommended for prophylaxis; not established for use in HAPE
  - Hypertonic saline/mannitol: No evidence supports use.

ADMISSION, INPATIENT, AND NURSING CONSIDERATIONS
Outpatient treatment for mild cases

ONGOING CARE

FOLLOW-UP RECOMMENDATIONS
Patient Monitoring
- For mild cases, no follow-up is needed.
- For more severe cases, follow until symptoms subside.

PATIENT EDUCATION
Counsel patients about the risks of high-altitude travel and how to recognize symptoms of high-altitude illness.

PROGNOSIS
Most cases of mild to moderate AMS are self-limiting and do not require medical intervention. Patients may resume ascent once the symptoms subside. HAPE and HACE respond well to descent, evacuation, and/or pharmacologic treatment if identified early.

COMPLICATIONS
High-altitude retinal hemorrhage, can cause visual changes, is usually asymptomatic.

REFERENCES

1. Davis C, Hackett P. Advances in the prevention and treatment of high altitude illness. *Emerg Med Clin North Am.* 2017;35(2):241–260.
2. Bärtsch P, Swenson ER. Clinical practice: acute high-altitude illnesses. *N Engl J Med.* 2013;368(24):2294–2302.
3. Richalet JP, Larmignat P, Poitrine E, et al. Physiological risk factors for severe high-altitude illness: a prospective cohort study. *Am J Respir Crit Care Med.* 2012;185(2):192–198.
4. Garlick V, O'Connor A, Shubkin CD. High-altitude illness in the pediatric population: a review of the literature on prevention and treatment. *Curr Opin Pediatr.* 2017;29(4):503–509.
5. Sridharan K, Sivaramakrishnan G. Pharmacological interventions for preventing acute mountain sickness: a network meta-analysis and trial sequential analysis of randomized clinical trials. *Ann Med.* 2018;50(2):147–155.

ADDITIONAL READING

- Imray C, Booth A, Wright A, et al. Acute altitude illnesses. *BMJ.* 2011;343:d4943.
- Luks AM, McIntosh SE, Grissom CK, et al. Wilderness Medical Society practice guidelines for the prevention and treatment of acute altitude illness: 2014 update. *Wilderness Environ Med.* 2014;25(Suppl 4):S4–S14.

CODES

ICD10
- T70.20XA Unspecified effects of high altitude, initial encounter
- T70.20XD Unspecified effects of high altitude, subsequent encounter
- T70.20XS Unspecified effects of high altitude, sequela

CLINICAL PEARLS
- Slow ascent and timely descent are important in the prevention and treatment of high-altitude illnesses.
- Lack of symptom resolution with appropriate descent suggests an alternative diagnosis.
- High-flow oxygen, followed by oxygen titrated to maintain SaO_2 >90%, is the first-line treatment for all patients with more than mild altitude illness.

ALZHEIMER DISEASE

John P. Barrett, MD, MPH, MS, FAAFP, FACPM

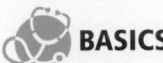

BASICS

DESCRIPTION
- Alzheimer disease (AD) is the most common cause of dementia: 60–80% of those afflicted with dementia.
- AD is a progressive, irreversible, degenerative neurologic disease that results in neuron death.
- AD is the sixth leading cause of death in the United States (1).
- People ≥65 years with new AD live 4 to 8 years on average.
- AD is underdiagnosed (~50%), and many people diagnosed with AD are unaware of diagnosis (>50%).
- Economic burden in 2018: >$277 billion, projected at $1.1 trillion by 2050 (1)
- Dementia should be distinguished from:
  – Age-related cognitive decline: lifelong process of changes in mental ability and memory; highly variable and part of normal aging
  – Mild cognitive impairment (MCI): greater impairment than cognitive decline with individual and/or friends—family able to note impairment
    ○ MCI: People are generally able to live independently from a cognitive perspective.
    ○ MCI: affects 15–20% of those ≥65 years, with 32–38% developing dementia within 5 years
- AD diagnostic classification:
  – Preclinical AD: research settings only at this time; no cognitive symptoms, AD biomarkers present
  – MCI due to AD: if AD biomarkers present and not attributed to other causes; impairment often only in memory; no major social/occupational deficits
  – Dementia due to AD:
    ○ Early stage: memory impairment beyond MCI
    ○ Middle stage: impairment in communication and response to environment
    ○ Late stage: lose ability to appropriately recognize and respond to environment
- System affected: nervous
- Synonym(s): presenile dementia; senile dementia of the Alzheimer type

Geriatric Considerations
- "Welcome to Medicare" preventive visit (first 12 months of enrollment) and Medicare Annual Wellness Visit both require assessment of cognitive function.
- Even though the U.S. Preventive Services Task Force has a grade I (insufficient evidence) recommendation on asymptomatic routine screening for dementia
- Advanced care planning: Medicare reimbursable

EPIDEMIOLOGY
- Predominant age: >65 years
- Incidence: females = males
- Prevalence: females > males, due to longer average lifespan in women

Incidence
New cases of AD in the United States: 484,000/year (1)
- 65 to 75 years: 2 new cases per 1,000 people
- 75 to 84: 11 new cases per 1,000 people
- ≥85: 37 new cases per 1,000 people

Prevalence
>5.7 million in United States; ~44 million worldwide
- 14.4 million in United States by 2050
- 1 in 10 of those ≥65 years have AD dementia.
- 32% of those ≥85 years have AD dementia.
- ~200,000 in United States with early-onset AD (<65 years)

ETIOLOGY AND PATHOPHYSIOLOGY
- Progressive, irreversible disease where cognitive impairment worsens over time
- Caused by β-amyloid plaques outside of neurons and τ protein tangles inside of neurons, resulting in loss of connections between neurons and cell death
- Age, genetics, systemic disease, lifestyle behaviors, and other factors may influence AD progression.

Genetics
- Autosomal dominant: <5% of AD, usually early onset (<65 years)
- Familial inheritance AD (nonautosomal dominant): 15–25% of AD, may be early- or late-age onset
- Sporadic, idiopathic: most of AD

RISK FACTORS
- Nonmodifiable risk factors (1,2,3):
  – Age
  – Gender (due to longer lifespan in women)
  – Family history
  – Genetic mutations
  – APOE-e4 gene variant: e4 heterozygous 2- to 3-fold risk; homozygous 10-fold risk (vs. e2 or e3)
- Cardiovascular disease–related risk factors (1,2):
  – Hypertension (HTN) (especially in midlife years)
  – Obesity
  – Diabetes and impaired glucose processing
  – Hyperlipidemia
  – Tobacco use
  – Unhealthy diet
  – Lack of physical activity/exercise
  – Cerebrovascular (stroke) risks and injury
- Other potentially modifiable risk factors (1,2):
  – Less years of formal education (<8th grade)
  – Lack of continuous brain activity—learning
  – Traumatic brain injuries: repetitive mild and moderate/severe
  – Lack of social engagement
  – Late-life depression
  – Poor quality and inadequate sleep
  – Hearing and vision deficits
  – High alcohol consumption
  – Possible environmental factors (e.g., pollution)

GENERAL PREVENTION
- Slowing/preventing cognitive decline, MCI, and AD are the top interest and concern of Americans ≥50 years.
- Evidence suggests that HTN management, increased physical activity, cognitive training may delay/prevent cognitive decline, MCI, and AD (2)[B].
- NSAIDs, estrogen, and vitamin E do NOT delay AD onset; insufficient evidence for statins (2)[A]
- Healthy lifestyle (e.g., exercise, sleep), potentially modifiable risk factors, may prevent or delay AD at the individual and population health level (2)[B].
- Actions to avert delirium during hospitalizations
- Treat psychiatric conditions (e.g., depression).
- Numerous medication can cause decreased cognition and delirium in the elderly.

COMMONLY ASSOCIATED CONDITIONS
- Down syndrome
- Depression

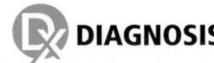

DIAGNOSIS

Diagnosis of dementia is straightforward. Diagnosis of the specific dementia–type cause may not be straightforward and requires a thorough history,

examination, cognitive testing, and potentially other diagnostic tests.
- 2000 *DSM-IV-TR* criteria widely in use: progressive impairment in ≥2 areas of memory, executive function, attention, language, or visuospatial skills AND significant interference in ability to function in work, home, or social interactions
- 2013 *DSM-5* uses term "neurocognitive disorder" instead of dementia and requires impairment in one or more cognitive areas sufficient to disrupt independent living (4):
  – Complex attention, executive function, learning and memory, language, perceptual motor, social cognition

HISTORY
- Include informant: family member, caregiver, or friend.
- Alzheimer's Association 10 signs (1,3):
  – Memory loss that disrupts daily life
  – Difficulty completing familiar tasks
  – Challenges in planning and problem-solving
  – New problems with words in speaking or writing
  – Trouble with visual images or spatial relationships
  – Changes in mood or personality
  – Misplacing things, losing ability to retrace steps
  – Decreased or poor judgment
  – Withdrawal from work or social activities
  – Confusion with time and place

PHYSICAL EXAM
- Exam to rule out other causes of dementia or delirium
- Noncognitive portions of physical exam often normal for age except in late stage AD (2,3,4)
- Vital signs, cardiovascular exam
- Speech and language, vision and hearing
- Neuro: gait, balance, reflexes, muscle strength and tone, tremor, abnormal movements (akathisia, bradykinesia/dyskinesia)
- Late stage: skin lesions, nutrition–hydration status
- Brief cognitive testing: for example, Mini-Cog, Montreal Cognitive Assessment (MoCA), Mini-Mental State Examination (MMSE, under copyright, fee for use)
- Assess depression: for example, PHQ-9, Geriatric Depression Scale (GDS).
- Functional assessment: instrumental activities of daily living (IADLs), Functional Activities Questionnaire (FAQ)

DIFFERENTIAL DIAGNOSIS
- Other dementias (most common):
  – Vascular (large and microvessel, mixed)
  – Mixed type (with AD)
  – Frontotemporal lobar degeneration
  – Dementia with Lewy bodies
  – Parkinson
  – Normal pressure hydrocephalus
  – Creutzfeldt-Jakob
  – Huntington
  – Wernicke-Korsakoff
- Metabolic: hyper/hypothyroid, vitamin-nutrient deficiency, uremia/renal, hepatic, hyponatremia
- Autoimmune: vasculitis, end-stage multiple sclerosis
- Infectious: HIV, syphilis, Lyme disease, VZV, prion
- Depression
- Brain tumor: primary or metastatic
- Subdural hematoma (usually acute presentation)
- Medications, drug–alcohol reactions/addiction

DIAGNOSTIC TESTS & INTERPRETATION
Specialty referral and possible neuropsychological testing for atypical symptoms, young age, unclear presentation, or if resources available and need to determine level of independent decision making (5)

Initial Tests (lab, imaging)

- To help rule out other causes of dementia (3,5)[A]
  - CBC
  - Chemistry panel: electrolytes, BUN, serum creatinine, glucose, LFTs, serum calcium
  - Thyroid function, lipid panel, folate, and vitamin B₁₂
  - Special considerations: ESR, VDRL or RPR, HIV
- Imaging (biomarkers): Different standards exist; may help determine cause of dementia (2,3,5)[A]
  - Consider MRI or computed tomography (CT) scan if
    - Cognitive decline is recent and rapid, age <65 years, history of stroke atypical presentation
    - Concern for cancer, bleeding risk
  - Single photon emission CT (SPECT) and positron emission tomography (PET): only if diagnostic uncertainty after CT or MRI; *insufficient evidence to use alone*

Follow-Up Tests & Special Considerations

- Consider genetic testing for concern about autosomal dominant and familial AD.
- CSF biomarker testing not currently indicated in routine clinical use, although extensive study in research settings

Test Interpretation

Labs, neuropsychiatric testing, and imaging help exclude treatable and atypical causes of dementia.

 TREATMENT

GENERAL MEASURES

- Optimize treatment of risk factors and associated comorbid conditions (e.g., hearing and vision loss).
- Assess environment for safety/security; avoid sudden changes to environment.
- Advanced care planning is critical early, before individual loses ability for independent decisions.
- Assess caregiver support and burnout.

ALERT

American Geriatrics Society recommends "Don't prescribe cholinesterase inhibitors (ChEIs) for dementia without periodic assessment for perceived cognitive benefits and adverse gastrointestinal effects" in their Choosing Wisely statement.

MEDICATION

First Line

- ChEIs (2,3,6)[A]
  - Best in mild to moderate disease; *may* be effective in Lewy body dementia
  - Equally effective; all have potential for GI and other side effects, such as bradycardia/syncope.
  - When used for at least 6 months, it provide mild benefit in cognition and behavior.
  - Try different ChEI if no benefit.
  - Donepezil (Aricept): Start at 5 mg/day PO; may increase to 10 mg/day after 1 month, may increase to 23 mg/day after 3 months if needed
  - Orally disintegrating tablets; generic available
  - Caution with digoxin or β-blockers (Donepezil may prolong PR interval.)
  - Rivastigmine (Exelon): Start at 1.5 mg PO BID and increase by 1.5 mg BID every 2 weeks; maintenance 6 to 12 mg/day total
  - Capsule, solution, or patch (reduced side effects)
  - Galantamine (Razadyne): Start at 4 mg BID for 4 weeks and then increase by 4 mg BID every month with goal of 16 to 24 mg/day dose.
  - Tablets, solution, extended-release (ER) capsule, and transdermal formulations

- Vitamin E—2,000 IU/day supplementation was found to slow decline in one study.
- Memantine, a N-methyl-D-aspartate (NMDA) receptor antagonist for moderate to severe AD
  - Monotherapy or in combination with acetylcholinesterase inhibitors (2,3,6)[A]
  - Memantine immediate release: 5 mg/day; titrate up to 10 mg BID, adding 5 mg/day every week PRN.
  - Memantine extended release: 7 mg/day up to 28 mg/day, adding 7 mg/day every week PRN
- Neuropsychiatric symptoms: assessment and treatment for delirium, environmental modification, sleep hygiene, exercise, cognitive interventions, hearing/vision aids, and if necessary for moderate to severe symptoms, consider second-line care (2,3,6)[A]

Second Line

- For moderate to severe depression: SSRIs preferred
- Insomnia: Medications have little efficacy for sleep in AD (2,3,6)[A].
  - Avoid diphenhydramine and antihistamines in elderly due to negative side effects.
  - If using low-dose risperidone, trazodone, or sleep aid (e.g., zolpidem), use caution and lowest dose possible in elderly.
- Moderate agitation, anxiety/restlessness: first-line care; may consider low-dose risperidone or SSRIs (citalopram) (2)[B]
- Risperidone at low dose for severe psychosis and safety concern; treatment not usually required (2)[A]
- Precautions
  - Avoid anticholinergic drugs when possible.
  - Benzodiazepines may produce paradoxical excitation or daytime drowsiness.
  - Triazolam (Halcion) can produce confusion, memory loss, and psychotic behavior.
  - Donepezil: caution with anticholinergics, sick sinus syndrome, and history of peptic ulcers

ISSUES FOR REFERRAL

- Consider geriatric psychiatry referral for AD patients with behavioral symptoms requiring psychotropic medications.
- Support groups for patient and family: Alzheimer's Association: http://www.alz.org/

ADDITIONAL THERAPIES

- Exercise to reduce restlessness.
- Cognitive stimulation therapy
- Occupational, music, aroma, and pet therapy

COMPLEMENTARY & ALTERNATIVE MEDICINE

- In general, herbals and supplement therapies have questionable to no efficacy in AD.
- Exercise, cognitive interventions, environmental therapies have benefit in AD and continue to be assessed.

 ONGOING CARE

FOLLOW-UP RECOMMENDATIONS

Patient Monitoring

- Review all health conditions and medications, including OTCs, vitamins, and supplements.
- Recommend:
  - Healthy lifestyle: exercise, nutrition, sleep, being socially and intellectually active
  - Cognitive training/stimulation
- Inform about products advertised (with unproven benefit) to improve brain health, such as some medications, nutritional supplements, and brain games.
- Until dose stable, frequently assess medication side effects and effectiveness (ChEIs/memantine).

- Late AD may require skilled care placement.
- National Highway Traffic Safety Administration's safe driving assessment: https://www.nhtsa.gov/older-drivers/driving-safely-while-aging-gracefully

PATIENT EDUCATION

- Alzheimer's Association: http://www.alz.org/
- Explain progressive nature of the disease.
- Early advanced care planning, such as advanced directives, financial planning, caregiver support

PROGNOSIS

Average survival from diagnosis is 4 to 8 years, and initial diagnosis is often delayed.

COMPLICATIONS

- Behavioral: hostility, agitation, wandering, falls
- Infections, inadequate nutrition/hydration, drug toxicity
- "Sundowning," depression (1/3 of patients), suicide

REFERENCES

1. Alzheimer's Association. 2018 Alzheimer's disease facts and figures. *Alzheimers Dement*. 2018;14(3):367–429.
2. Livingston G, Sommerlad A, Orgeta V, et al. Dementia prevention, intervention, and care. *Lancet*. 2017;390(10113):2673–2734.
3. Scheltens P, Blennow K, Breteler MM, et al. Alzheimer's disease. *Lancet*. 2016;388(10043):505–517.
4. American Psychiatric Association. *Diagnostic and Statistical Manual of Mental Disorders*. 5th ed. Arlington, VA: American Psychiatric Association; 2013.
5. Ferrari C, Nacmias B, Sorbi S. The diagnosis of dementias: a practical tool not to miss rare causes. *Neurol Sci*. 2018;39(4):615–627.
6. Szeto J, Lewis S. Current treatment options for Alzheimer's disease and Parkinson's disease dementia. *Curr Neuropharmacol*. 2016;14(4):326–338.

ADDITIONAL READING

The Gerontological Society of America. KAER tool kit: 4-step process to detecting cognitive impairment and earlier diagnosis of dementia. https://www.geron.org/images/gsa/kaer/kaertoolkitsummary.pdf. Accessed December 26, 2018.

 SEE ALSO

Depression; Delirium; Hypothyroidism, Adult; Substance Use Disorders

 CODES

ICD10

- G30.9 Alzheimer's disease, unspecified
- G30.0 Alzheimer's disease with early onset
- G30.1 Alzheimer's disease with late onset

CLINICAL PEARLS

- AD is very common, >32% in those >85 years, and greatly underdiagnosed.
- Imaging not needed for diagnosis for typical of AD
- Early diagnosis allows advance care planning (e.g., advanced directives) and caregiver support planning: Encourage caregivers to join Alzheimer's Association.
- Atypical antipsychotic medications increase mortality.

AMENORRHEA
Thomas A. Waller, MD • Sally-Ann L. Pantin, MD, FAAFP

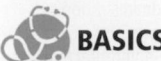 **BASICS**

DESCRIPTION
- Primary amenorrhea
  - No menses by age 13 years with absence of secondary sexual characteristics OR
  - No menses by age 15 years with normal secondary characteristics
- Secondary amenorrhea: cessation of menses for 3 months if previously normal menstruation or 6 months if a history of irregular cycles
- System(s) affected: endocrine/metabolic; reproductive

Pregnancy Considerations
Pregnancy is by far the most common cause of secondary amenorrhea.

EPIDEMIOLOGY
Prevalence
- Primary amenorrhea: <1% of female population
- Secondary amenorrhea: 3–5% of female population
- No evidence for race and ethnicity affecting prevalence

ETIOLOGY AND PATHOPHYSIOLOGY
Absence of menses that can be temporary or permanent due to dysfunction of the hypothalamus, pituitary, uterus, ovaries, or vagina

ETIOLOGY
- Primary amenorrhea
  - Gonadal dysgenesis (e.g., Turner syndrome [45,X]) or failure (e.g., autoimmune, idiopathic)
  - Anatomic abnormalities (e.g., müllerian agenesis, imperforate hymen, transverse vaginal septum)
  - Hypothalamic–pituitary abnormalities
    - Functional hypothalamic amenorrhea (reduced GnRH secretion, e.g., weight loss/anorexia nervosa)
    - Constitutional delay of puberty
    - Central lesions (tumors, hypophysitis, granulomas)
    - Pituitary dysfunction (hyperprolactinemia, abnormal follicle-stimulating hormone [FSH], luteinizing hormone [LH], or GnRH)
    - Thyroid dysfunction
  - Polycystic ovarian syndrome (PCOS)
  - Androgen insensitivity syndrome
- Secondary amenorrhea
  - Pregnancy
  - Hypothalamic dysfunction (reduced GnRH secretion)
    - Functional hypothalamic amenorrhea (stress, anorexia nervosa, and/or excessive exercise)
    - Hypothalamic tumors
    - Severe systemic illness (e.g., diabetes mellitus type 1 or celiac disease)
  - Pituitary disease (e.g., hyperprolactinemia, Sheehan syndrome, Cushing syndrome)
  - Thyroid disease
  - PCOS
  - Ovarian disorders (e.g., premature ovarian failure [due to chemotherapy, radiation, fragile X syndrome] or ovarian tumors)
  - Uterine disorders (e.g., intrauterine adhesions [Asherman syndrome])
- Pathophysiology varies, depending on etiology.

Genetics
May occur with Turner syndrome or testicular feminization

RISK FACTORS
- Obesity
- Excessive exercise (commonly associated "female athlete triad")
- Eating disorders
- Malnutrition
- Anovulatory disorders
- Stress
- Treatment with antipsychotic medications

GENERAL PREVENTION
Maintenance of proper body mass index (BMI) and healthy lifestyle with respect to food and exercise

COMMONLY ASSOCIATED CONDITIONS
- Premature ovarian failure may be associated with autoimmune abnormalities (autoimmune thyroiditis, type 1 diabetes).
- PCOS is associated with insulin resistance and obesity.
- Decreased exposure to estrogen may increase risk for osteopenia or osteoporosis.

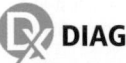 **DIAGNOSIS**

HISTORY
- Review of systems, including weight change, symptoms of pregnancy or menopause, virilizing changes, cyclic pelvic pain, galactorrhea, headaches, vision changes, fatigue, palpitations, polyuria/polydipsia
- Growth and pubertal development history, including age of breast development, pubertal growth spurt, and adrenarche (early sexual maturation)
- History of chronic illness, trauma, surgery, medications, prior chemotherapy or radiation
- Psychiatric history
- Social history, including diet and exercise history, drug abuse, and sexual history
- Family history of delayed or absent puberty

PHYSICAL EXAM
- General appearance
- Vital signs, height, weight, growth percentile and BMI, hypotension, bradycardia, hypothermia (anorexia nervosa)
- HEENT exam: evidence of dental erosions, trauma to palate (bulimia), visual field defect, funduscopic changes, cranial nerve findings (prolactinoma), webbed neck (Turner syndrome), thyromegaly
- Skin exam: evidence of androgen excess (acne, hirsutism), acanthosis nigricans (PCOS), fine downy hair on body (anorexia nervosa), striae
- Breast: state of development, evidence of galactorrhea (prolactinoma), shield chest (Turner syndrome)
- Pelvic exam: presence or absence of pubic hair (if sparse: androgen insensitivity or deficiency); clitoromegaly (androgen excess); distention or bulging of external vagina (imperforate hymen); thin, pale vaginal mucosa without rugae (estrogen deficiency and ovarian failure); presence of cervical mucus (evidence for estrogen production); blind vaginal pouch (müllerian agenesis, androgen insensitivity syndrome); ovarian enlargement (tumors, PCOS, autoimmune oophoritis)

DIAGNOSTIC TESTS & INTERPRETATION
Initial Tests (lab, imaging)
- Primary amenorrhea
  - Serum human chorionic gonadotropin (hCG), prolactin (PRL), thyroid-stimulating hormone (TSH), and FSH
  - If no breast development:
    - FSH low suggests primary hypothalamic or pituitary etiology.
    - FSH elevated suggests gonadal failure, and karyotype analysis should be performed.
  - If breast development has occurred, evaluate for anatomic abnormalities. If uterus is absent or abnormal, perform karyotype analysis, testosterone level, and dehydroepiandrosterone sulfate (DHEA-S).
- Secondary amenorrhea
  - Serum hCG, PRL, TSH, and FSH
    - If PRL >100 ng/mL suggests empty sella syndrome or pituitary adenoma; perform MRI for evaluation.
    - If PRL <100 ng/mL: Evaluate for other etiologies, of which medications are most common.
  - To determine endogenous estrogen production, perform a progestin challenge (see "Treatment"): If withdrawal bleed, likely chronic anovulation (most commonly PCOS). If no withdrawal bleed, perform estrogen and progestin challenge (see "Treatment"):
    - If no bleed: Consider outflow tract obstruction.
    - If bleed occurs: Check FSH/LH: elevated in premature ovarian failure; decreased in pituitary tumors, eating disorders, chronic illness.
- If there is evidence for hyperandrogenism, measure total testosterone, DHEA-S, and 17-OH progesterone levels. Initiate evaluation for androgen-secreting tumor if testosterone >200 ng/dL.
- Imaging is not generally indicated as a first approach.
- US may show ovarian cysts (PCOS), presence or absence of uterus, and endometrial thickness (consider MRI if unable to tolerate US probe).

Follow-Up Tests & Special Considerations
- Women <30 years with ovarian failure (see below) should have karyotype analysis and be investigated for premutations of *FMR1* gene (fragile X syndrome) and for adrenal antibodies.
- If absence of uterus or foreshortened vagina, karyotype analysis should also be performed.
- Laparoscopy: diagnosis of streak ovaries (Turner syndrome) or polycystic ovaries
- Hysterosalpingogram: Rule out Asherman syndrome and other etiologies of outflow obstruction.

Diagnostic Procedures/Other
- If constitutional delay is suspected, obtain bone age.
- If hypothalamic amenorrhea from functional suppression is suspected, consider dual energy x-ray absorptiometry (DEXA) scan to assess bone loss (1).

TREATMENT

GENERAL MEASURES
Identify and correct underlying pathology if possible.

MEDICATION
- Progesterone challenge and replacement: medroxy-progesterone (Provera): 10 mg/day for 10 days will result in withdrawal bleed within 7 days of last dose if hypothalamic–pituitary–gonadal axis is intact (i.e., amenorrhea is a consequence of anovulation and lack of progesterone), although experts disagree (2).
- Estrogen replacement: Cycling with a combination oral contraceptive (containing 35 or 50 μg of estrogen) or conjugated estrogen (Premarin) 0.625 mg for 25 days with progesterone added as above for the last 10 days will result in a withdrawal bleed if the uterus and lower genital tract are normal (hypothalamic-pituitary axis pathologic).
- Use of hormonal therapies will not correct the underlying problem. Other drugs might be required to treat specific conditions (e.g., bromocriptine for hyperprolactinemia).
- Use of hormonal replacement therapy is not recommended for long-term management of amenorrhea in older women.
  – May be safe for symptom management in young women
  – Give to maintain secondary sex characteristics and to prevent osteoporosis in adolescents and young women (3)[A].
- Combination estrogen/progesterone contraceptives (oral contraceptive pills [OCPs], patch, ring) replace estrogen and prevent pregnancy.
  – Have a positive effect on bone mineral density in oligo-/amenorrheic women but not in functional hypothalamic amenorrhea (4)[A]
  – Can decrease hirsutism in PCOS
- Calcium supplementation: 1,500 mg/day if cause is hypoestrogenism
- Because PCOS is related to insulin resistance, metformin (Glucophage) has been used (start at 500 mg BID) to correct metabolic abnormalities, improve ovulation, and restore normal menstrual patterns. Of note, treatment with metformin has shown an increase in clinical pregnancy rates but not in live birth rates (5)[A].
- Functional hypothalamic amenorrhea appears to improve with administration of exogenous leptin (still under investigation) (6)[C].
- Contraindications to estrogen administration
  – Pregnancy, thromboembolic disease, previous myocardial infarction or cerebrovascular accident, estrogen-dependent malignancy, severe hepatic impairment or disease
- Precautions
  – Patients with amenorrhea who desire pregnancy should not be given hormone replacement therapy but should receive treatment for infertility based on the specific cause.

ISSUES FOR REFERRAL
Many causes of amenorrhea require referral to specialists in ob/gyn, endocrine, surgery, and/or psychiatry.

SURGERY/OTHER PROCEDURES
- Hymenectomy for primary amenorrhea if due to imperforate hymen
- Lysis of adhesions in Asherman syndrome is often effective in restoring regular menses and fertility.
- If karyotype is XY, gonads must be removed due to increased risk of tumors.
- Patients with congenital short vagina can undergo surgery to create a functioning vagina.

ONGOING CARE

FOLLOW-UP RECOMMENDATIONS
If excessive exercise is suspected, activity level should be reduced by 25–50%.

Patient Monitoring
- Depends on the cause and treatment chosen
- If hormonal replacement is used, discontinue after 6 months to assess spontaneous resumption of menses.

DIET
- Correct overweight or underweight by dietary management and behavior modification.
- If PCOS is the etiology, a weight-loss diet will help restore ovulation.

PATIENT EDUCATION
- Educate on the circumstances and complications of her condition and its underlying etiology.
- Specific educational resources are helpful (e.g., prenatal classes and menopause support groups).
- Discuss the expected duration of amenorrhea (temporary or permanent), effect on fertility, and the long-term sequelae of untreated amenorrhea (e.g., osteoporosis, vaginal dryness).
- Appropriate contraceptive advice should be given because fertility returns before menses.
- Additional support may be needed if the amenorrhea is associated with a reduction in, or loss of, fertility.

PROGNOSIS
Reflects the underlying cause. In functional hypothalamic amenorrhea, one study demonstrated 83% reversal rate in presence of obvious contributing factor.

COMPLICATIONS
- Estrogen-deficiency symptoms (e.g., hot flashes, vaginal dryness) and osteoporosis in prolonged hypoestrogenic amenorrhea
- Increased risk of endometrial cancer in patients whose amenorrhea is secondary to anovulation with estrogen excess (obesity, PCOS)
- Premature ovarian failure may increase cardiovascular risk.

REFERENCES

1. Gordon CM. Clinical practice. Functional hypothalamic amenorrhea. *N Engl J Med*. 2010;363(4):365–371.
2. Klein DA, Poth MA. Amenorrhea: an approach to diagnosis and management. *Am Fam Physician*. 2013;87(11):781–788.
3. Marjoribanks J, Farquhar C, Roberts H, et al. Long term hormone therapy for perimenopausal and postmenopausal women. *Cochrane Database Syst Rev*. 2012;(7):CD004143.
4. Liu SL, Lebrun CM. Effect of oral contraceptives and hormone replacement therapy on bone mineral density in premenopausal and perimenopausal women: a systematic review. *Br J Sports Med*. 2006;40(1):11–24.
5. Tang T, Lord JM, Norman RJ, et al. Insulin-sensitising drugs (metformin, rosiglitazone, pioglitazone, D-chiro-inositol) for women with polycystic ovary syndrome, oligo amenorrhoea and subfertility. *Cochrane Database Syst Rev*. 2012;(5):CD003053.
6. Chou SH, Chamberland JP, Liu X, et al. Leptin is an effective treatment for hypothalamic amenorrhea. *Proc Natl Acad Sci U S A*. 2011;108(16):6585–6590.

ADDITIONAL READING

- Practice Committee of American Society for Reproductive Medicine. Current evaluation of amenorrhea. *Fertil Steril*. 2008;90(Suppl 5):S219–S225.
- Santoro N. Update in hyper- and hypogonadotropic amenorrhea. *J Clin Endocrinol Metab*. 2011;96(11):3281–3288.

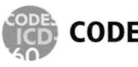 SEE ALSO

- Hyperthyroidism; Hypothyroidism, Adult; Osteoporosis and Osteopenia
- Algorithms: Amenorrhea, Primary (Absence of Menarche by Age 16 Years); Amenorrhea, Secondary; Delayed Puberty

CODES

ICD10
- N91.2 Amenorrhea, unspecified
- N91.0 Primary amenorrhea
- N91.1 Secondary amenorrhea

CLINICAL PEARLS

- First evaluate whether amenorrhea is primary or secondary and exclude pregnancy. TSH and PRL are usual first blood tests.
- Progestin challenge may cause withdrawal bleed in women with intact hypothalamic–pituitary–gonadal axis.

ANAL FISSURE

Anne Walsh, ANP-BC • Kashyap Trivedi, MD

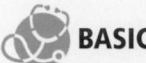 **BASICS**

DESCRIPTION
Anal fissure (fissure in ano): longitudinal tear in the lining of the anal canal distal to the dentate line, most commonly at the posterior midline; characterized by a knifelike tearing sensation on defecation, often associated with bright red blood per rectum. This common benign anorectal condition is often confused with hemorrhoids; may be acute (<8 weeks) or chronic (>8 weeks) in duration

EPIDEMIOLOGY
- Affects all ages. Common in infants 6 to 24 months; not common in older children, suspect abuse, or trauma; elderly less common due to lower resting pressure in the anal canal
- Sex: male = female; women more likely to get anterior midline fissures (25%) versus men (8%)

Incidence
Exact incidence is unknown (1). Patients often treat with home remedies and do not seek medical care.

Prevalence
- 80% of infants, usually self-limited
- 10–20% of adults, most of whom do not seek medical advice.

ALERT
- Lateral fissure: Rule out infectious disease.
- Atypical fissure: Rule out Crohn disease.

ETIOLOGY AND PATHOPHYSIOLOGY
High-resting pressure within the anal canal (usually as a result of constipation/straining) leads to ischemia of the anoderm, resulting in splitting of the anal mucosa during defecation and spasm of the exposed internal sphincter.

Genetics
None known

RISK FACTORS
- Constipation (25% of patients)
- Diarrhea (6% of patients)
- Passage of hard or large-caliber stool
- High-resting pressure of internal anal sphincter (prolonged sitting, obesity)
- Trauma (sexual activity or abuse, foreign body, childbirth, mountain biking)
- Prior anal surgery with scarring/stenosis
- Inflammatory bowel disease (Crohn disease)
- Infection (chlamydia, syphilis, herpes, tuberculosis)

GENERAL PREVENTION
All measures to prevent constipation; avoid straining and prolonged sitting on toilet.

COMMONLY ASSOCIATED CONDITIONS
Constipation, irritable bowel syndrome, Crohn disease, tuberculosis, leukemia, and HIV

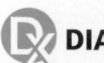 **DIAGNOSIS**

HISTORY
- Severe, sharp rectal pain, often with and following defecation but can be continuous; some patients will see bright red blood on the stool or when wiping.
- Occasionally, anal pruritus or perianal irritation

PHYSICAL EXAM
- Gentle spreading of the buttocks with close inspection of the anal verge will reveal a smooth-edged tear in the anodermal tissue, typically posterior midline, occasionally anterior midline, rarely eccentric to midline. Digital rectal exam and anoscopy are painful and can be deferred if inspection confirms the diagnosis.
- Minimal edema, erythema, or bleeding may be seen.
- Chronic fissures may demonstrate rolled edges, exposed muscle fibers, hypertrophic papillae at proximal end, and a sentinel pile (tag) at distal end.

DIFFERENTIAL DIAGNOSIS
- Thrombosed external hemorrhoid: swollen, painful mass at anal verge
- Perirectal abscess: tender, warm erythematous induration or fluctuance
- Perianal fistula: abnormal communication between rectum and perianal epithelium with feculent or purulent drainage
- Pruritus ani: shallow excoriations rather than true fissure

DIAGNOSTIC TESTS & INTERPRETATION
Diagnostic Procedures/Other
- Avoid anoscopy/sigmoidoscopy initially unless necessary for other diagnoses or for chronic fissures.
- Due to pain, some patients may require exam under anesthesia in order to confirm the diagnosis.

 TREATMENT

The goal of treatment is to avoid repeated tearing of the anal mucosa with resultant spasm of the internal anal sphincter by decreasing the patient's high sphincter tone and addressing its underlying cause.

GENERAL MEASURES
- Wash area gently with warm water; consume high-fiber diet, increase fluids, add daily fiber supplement; avoid constipation, maintain healthy weight.
- Medical therapy for chronic fissures usually initiated in a stepwise manner: nitrates, calcium channel blockers, botulinum toxin

MEDICATION
First Line
Acute fissures—50% heal spontaneously with supportive measures (1)[B].
- Fiber supplements (e.g., psyllium, methylcellulose, inulin) daily and increase fluid intake
- Osmotic laxatives as needed (polyethylene glycol)
- Topical analgesics (2% lidocaine gel or 3% cream) 2 to 3 times daily for pain control
- Topical lubricants/emollients (Balneol cream, petroleum jelly) for comfort with defecation
- Topical hydrocortisone 1% cream short term for inflammation/pruritus
- Sitz baths (sit in plain warm water bath for 10 to 20 minutes) 2 to 3 times daily after bowel movements

Second Line
Chronic fissures—will not heal without treatment (2)[A]:
- Chemical sphincterotomy
  - Topical nitroglycerin 0.2–0.4% ointment applied BID; nitroglycerin 0.4% ointment available commercially (Rectiv): marginally but significantly better than placebo in healing (48.6% vs. 37%); late recurrence common (50%) (2)[A]; reduces resting anal pressure through the release of nitric oxide. Headache, hypotension, dizziness are major side effects (20–30%).
  - Topical calcium channel blockers (nifedipine 0.2–0.3% gel, diltiazem 2% ointment), applied 2 to 4 times per day, relax the internal sphincter muscle, thereby reducing the resting anal pressure no better than nitrates for healing but fewer side effects consider as first-line treatment (1)[A]. Oral calcium channel blockers confer lower healing rates, more side effects, and equal rates of recurrence (3)[A].
  - Botulinum toxin 4 mL (20 units) injected into the internal sphincter muscle: no better than topical nitrates for healing but fewer side effects; inhibits the release of acetylcholine from nerve endings to inhibit muscle spasm (4)[B]

ISSUES FOR REFERRAL

- Late recurrence is common (50%), particularly if the underlying issue remains untreated (constipation, irritable bowel).
- Medical therapy usually tried for 90 to 120 days prior to colorectal surgery referral. Select patients with chronic fissure may be referred directly for surgical therapy due to proven superior healing rates (1)[A].

ADDITIONAL THERAPIES

Anococcygeal support (modified toilet seat) may offer some advantage in chronic fissures to avoid surgery.

SURGERY/OTHER PROCEDURES

- Surgery typically reserved for failure of medical therapy
- Lateral internal sphincterectomy (LIS) involves division of the internal sphincter muscle and is the surgical procedure of choice (95% healing) (1)[A].
  - Risk for fecal or flatus incontinence: up to 45% short term, up to 6–8% long term
  - Open and closed techniques have similar results and are equally acceptable (1)[A].
  - May be repeated for recurrent fissures with similar outcomes (1)[C]
  - Not typically performed on women of childbearing potential due to increased risk of fecal incontinence with or without subsequent obstetrical injury (1)
- Anocutaneous flap safe alternative to LIS with less incontinence but lower healing rates (1)[B]
- Botulinum toxin injections also first-line treatment; less effective (60–80% healing) than surgery but fewer complications (4)[C]
  - Risk for fecal or flatus incontinence: 18% short term, no long term
  - May be repeated as needed with same efficacy; lower doses as effective as higher doses with lower rates of complications, including incontinence and recurrence (5)[A]
  - Higher doses combined with fissurectomy may be as effective as surgical sphincterotomy (6)[C].
- Controlled pneumatic balloon dilation may be used by gastroenterologists if surgical referral not available; should not be used first line as benefits are not well documented. Uncontrolled manual dilation is no longer recommended (5)[C].

 ONGOING CARE

DIET

High fiber (>25 g/day; augment with daily fiber supplements); increase fluid intake, decrease caffeine.

PATIENT EDUCATION

- Avoid prolonged sitting or straining during bowel movements; drink plenty of fluids; avoid constipation; lose weight if obese.
- Avoid use of triple antibiotic ointment and long-term use of steroid creams to anal area.
- Use a finger cot or glove when applying nitroglycerin ointment, and apply first dose before bedtime to minimize side effects.
- Topical medications should be applied directly to anal verge; no need to insert rectally
- Alternative medicine therapies (hibiscus extract, clove oil, anal self-massage) need further study before they can be recommended as first-line treatment.

PROGNOSIS

Most acute fissures heal within 6 weeks with conservative therapy. Medical therapy is less likely to be successful for chronic anal fissures (40% failure rate).

COMPLICATIONS

- Chronic fissure is a complication of nonhealing acute fissure.
- Recurrence is a common complication especially when underlying cause is not addressed.
- Abscess and fistula formation are less common complications.
- Fecal and flatus incontinence are primarily associated with surgery (5–45% postoperative), which may become permanent (up to 8% long term, primarily to flatus).

REFERENCES

1. Stewart DB Sr, Gaertner W, Glasgow S, et al. Clinical practice guideline for the management of anal fissures. *Dis Colon Rectum.* 2017;60(1):7–14.
2. Altomare DF, Binda GA, Canuti S, et al. The management of patients with primary chronic anal fissure: a position paper. *Tech Coloproctol.* 2011;15(2):135–141.
3. Sahebally SM, Ahmed K, Cerneveciute R, et al. Oral versus topical calcium channel blockers for chronic anal fissure—a systematic review and meta-analysis of randomized controlled trials. *Int J Surg.* 2017;44:87–93.
4. Wald A, Bharucha AE, Cosman BC, et al. ACG clinical guideline: management of benign anorectal disorders. *Am J Gastroenterol.* 2014;109(8): 1141–1157.
5. Lin JX, Krishna S, Su'a B, et al. Optimal dosing of botulinum toxin for treatment of chronic anal fissure: a systematic review and meta-analysis. *Dis Colon Rectum.* 2016;59(9):886–894.
6. Barnes TG, Zafrani Z, Abdelrazeq AS. Fissurectomy combined with high-dose botulinum toxin is a safe and effective treatment for chronic anal fissure and a promising alternative to surgical sphincterotomy. *Dis Colon Rectum.* 2015;58(10):967–973.

ADDITIONAL READING

- Fargo MV, Latimer KM. Evaluation and management of common anorectal conditions. *Am Fam Physician.* 2012;85(6):624–630.
- Gee T, Hisham RB, Jabar MF, et al. Ano-coccygeal support in the treatment of idiopathic chronic posterior anal fissure: a prospective non-randomised controlled pilot trial. *Tech Coloproctol.* 2013;17(2):181–186.
- Sinha R, Kaiser AM. Efficacy of management algorithm for reducing need for sphincterotomy in chronic anal fissures. *Colorectal Dis.* 2012;14(6):760–764.
- Sugerman DT. JAMA patient page. Anal fissure. *JAMA.* 2014;311(11):1171.
- Yiannakopoulou E. Botulinum toxin and anal fissure: efficacy and safety systematic review. *Int J Colorectal Dis.* 2012;27(1):1–9.

 CODES

ICD10

- K60.2 Anal fissure, unspecified
- K60.0 Acute anal fissure
- K60.1 Chronic anal fissure

CLINICAL PEARLS

- Avoid anoscopy or sigmoidoscopy initially unless necessary for other diagnoses.
- Best chance to prevent recurrence is to treat the underlying cause (e.g., chronic constipation).
- No medical therapy approaches the cure rate of surgery for chronic fissure.

ANEMIA, APLASTIC

Muthalagu Ramanathan, MD • Jan Cerny, MD, PhD

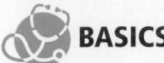
BASICS

DESCRIPTION
- Pancytopenia due to hypocellular bone marrow without the presence of infiltrates or fibrosis; classified as acquired (much more common) and congenital
- Acquired aplastic anemia: insidious onset; due to exogenous insult triggering an autoimmune reaction; often responsive to immunosuppression
- Congenital forms: rare, mostly present in childhood (exception is atypical presentation of Fanconi syndrome in adults; 30s for males and 40s for females)
- The occurrence of specific mutations in genes of the telomere complex in acquired aplastic anemia has blurred the distinction between the congenital and acquired forms.
- System(s) affected: heme/lymphatic/immunologic
- Synonym(s): hypoplastic anemia; panmyelophthisis; refractory anemia; aleukia hemorrhagica; toxic paralytic anemia

ALERT
- Early intervention for aplastic anemia greatly improves the chances of treatment success.
- Hematopoietic growth factors require close monitoring in newly diagnosed patients.

Geriatric Considerations
The elderly are often exposed to large numbers of drugs and therefore may be more susceptible to acquired aplastic anemia.

Pediatric Considerations
- Congenital forms of aplastic anemia require different treatment regimens than acquired forms.
- Acquired aplastic anemia is seen in children exposed to ionizing radiation or treated with cytotoxic chemotherapeutic agents.

Pregnancy Considerations
- Pregnancy is a real but rare cause of aplastic anemia. Symptoms may resolve after delivery and with termination.
- Complications in pregnancy can occur from low platelet counts and paroxysmal nocturnal hemoglobinuria-associated aplastic anemia.

EPIDEMIOLOGY
- Predominant age (1): biphasic 15 to 25 years (more common) and >60 years
- Predominant sex: male = female

Incidence
- 2 to 3 new cases per million per year in Europe and North America
- The incidence is 3-fold higher in Thailand and China versus the Western world.

ETIOLOGY AND PATHOPHYSIOLOGY
- Idiopathic (~70% of the cases)
- Drugs: phenylbutazone, chloramphenicol, sulfonamides, gold, cytotoxic drugs, antiepileptics (felbamate, carbamazepine, valproic acid, phenytoin)
- Viral: HIV, Epstein-Barr virus (EBV), nontypeable postinfectious hepatitis (not A, B, or C), parvovirus B19 (mostly in the immunocompromised), atypical mycobacterium
- Toxic exposure (benzene, pesticides, arsenic)
- Radiation exposure
- Immune disorders (systemic lupus erythematosus, eosinophilic fasciitis, graft versus host disease)
- Pregnancy (rare)

- Congenital (Fanconi anemia, dyskeratosis congenita, Shwachman-Diamond syndrome, amegakaryocytic thrombocytopenia)
- The immune hypothesis: activation of T cells with associated cytokine production leading to destruction or injury of hematopoietic stem cells. This leads to a hypocellular bone marrow without marrow fibrosis.
- The activation of T cells likely occurs because of both genetic and environmental factors. Exposure to specific environmental precipitants, diverse host, genetic risk factors, and individual differences in characteristics of immune response likely account for variations in its clinical manifestations and patterns of responsiveness to treatment.
- Telomerase deficiency leads to short telomeres. This leads to impaired regenerative capacity and hence a reduction in marrow progenitors and qualitative deficiency in the repair capacity of hematopoietic tissue.
- Reduction of natural killer cells in the bone marrow
- A somatic mutation of the *PIGA* gene underlies the clonal disease paroxysmal nocturnal hemoglobinuria (PNH): There is direct evidence that the expansion of the *PIGA* mutant clone results from Darwinian selection exerted by a glycosylphosphatidylinositol (GPI)-specific autoimmune attack (2).

Genetics
- Telomerase mutations found in a small number of patients with acquired and congenital forms. These mutations render carriers more susceptible to environmental insults.
- Mutations in genes called TERC and TERT were found in pedigrees of adults with acquired aplastic anemia who lacked the physical abnormalities or a family history typical of inherited forms of bone marrow failure. These genes encode for the RNA component of telomerase.
- HLA-DR2 incidence in aplastic anemia is twice that in the normal population.

RISK FACTORS
- Treatment with high-dose radiation or chemotherapy
- Exposure to toxic chemicals
- Use of certain medications
- Certain blood diseases, autoimmune disorders, and serious infections
- Tumors of thymus (red cell aplasia)
- Pregnancy, rarely

GENERAL PREVENTION
- Avoid possible toxic industrial agents.
- Use safety measures when working with radiation.

DIAGNOSIS

HISTORY
- Solvent and radiation history; family, environmental, travel, and infectious disease history
- Patients are often asymptomatic but may have frequent infections, fatigue, shortness of breath, headache, or bleeding/bruising.

PHYSICAL EXAM
- Mucosal hemorrhage, petechiae
- Pallor
- Fever
- Hemorrhage, menorrhagia, occult stool blood, melena, epistaxis
- Dyspnea

- Palpitations
- Progressive weakness
- Retinal flame hemorrhages
- Systolic ejection murmur
- Weight loss
- Signs of congenital aplastic anemia
  - Short stature
  - Microcephaly
  - Nail dystrophy
  - Abnormal thumbs
  - Oral leukoplakia
  - Hyperpigmentation (café au lait spots) or hypopigmentation

DIFFERENTIAL DIAGNOSIS
Includes other causes of bone marrow failure and pancytopenia
- Hypoplastic MDS
- Marrow replacement
  - Acute lymphoblastic leukemia
  - Lymphoma
  - Hairy cell leukemia (increased reticulin and infiltration of hairy cells)
  - Large granular lymphocyte leukemia
  - Fibrosis
- Megaloblastic hematopoiesis
  - Folate deficiency
  - Vitamin B_{12} deficiency
- Paroxysmal nocturnal hemoglobinuria, hemolytic anemia (dark urine), pancytopenia, and venous thrombosis (classically hepatic veins)
- Systemic lupus erythematosus
- Prolonged starvation or anorexia nervosa (Bone marrow is gelatinous with loss of fat cells and increased ground substance.)
- Transient erythroblastopenia of childhood
- Drug-induced agranulocytosis that may be reversible on withdrawal of drug
- Overwhelming infection
  - HIV with myelodysplasia
  - Viral hemophagocytic syndrome

DIAGNOSTIC TESTS & INTERPRETATION
Screening tests to exclude other etiologies
- CBC and absolute reticulocyte count
- Blood smear exam
- Cytogenetic studies to exclude MDS and of peripheral lymphocytes if <35 years of age to exclude Fanconi anemia
- Liver function test
- Viral serology: hepatitis A, B, C; EBV; cytomegalovirus (CMV); HIV
- Vitamin B_{12} and folate levels
- Autoantibody screening antinuclear antibody (ANA) and anti-DNA
- Flow cytometry looking for GPI, negative neutrophils, and RBCs for detecting paroxysmal nocturnal hemoglobinuria
- Fetal hemoglobin in children
- Red cell adenosine deaminase (pure red cell aplasia)
- Cytogenetic analysis of bone marrow

Initial Tests (lab, imaging)
- CBC: pancytopenia, anemia (usually normocytic), leukopenia, neutropenia, thrombocytopenia
- Decreased absolute number of reticulocytes
- Increased serum iron secondary to transfusion
- Normal total iron-binding capacity (TIBC)
- High mean corpuscular volume (MCV) >104

- CD 34+ cells decreased in blood and marrow
- Urinalysis: hematuria
- Abnormal liver function tests (hepatitis)
- Increased fetal hemoglobin (Fanconi)
- Increased chromosomal breaks under specialized conditions (Fanconi)
- Molecular determination of abnormal gene (Fanconi)
- CT of thymus region if thymoma-associated RBC aplasia suspected
- Radiographs of radius and thumbs (if congenital anemia suspected)
- Renal ultrasound (to rule out congenital anemia or malignant hematologic disorder)
- Chest x-ray to exclude infections such as mycobacterial infection

Diagnostic Procedures/Other
Bone marrow aspiration and biopsy

Test Interpretation
- Normochromic RBC
- Bone marrow
  - Decreased cellularity (<10%): no fibrosis, no malignant cells or dysplastic cells seen
  - Decreased megakaryocytes
  - Decreased myeloid precursors
  - Decreased erythroid precursors
  - Prominent fat spaces and marrow stroma, polyclonal plasma cells

TREATMENT

Early treatment increases the chance of success. Two major options: immunosuppressive therapy (3) and hematopoietic stem cell transplantation. Treatment decisions are based on age of the patient, severity of disease, and availability of a human leukocyte antigen (HLA)–matched sibling donor for transplantation.

GENERAL MEASURES
- Supportive measures: RBC and platelet transfusions. Use only irradiated leukocyte-reduced or CMV-negative blood especially if patient is a candidate for hematopoietic stem cell transplantation.
- Antibiotics, antifungals, antivirals when appropriate, especially if absolute neutrophil count (ANC) <100 cells/μL
- Oxygen therapy for severe anemia
- Good oral hygiene
- Control menorrhagia with norethisterone or oral contraceptive pills.
- Avoid/discontinue causative agents/isolation if necessary.
- HLA testing on all patients and their immediate families
- Transfusion support (judiciously prescribed RBCs for severe anemia; platelets for severe thrombocytopenia)
  - Transfuse when
    - Hb <7 g/dL or if Hb <8 g/dL and symptomatic ± congestive heart failure (CHF)
    - Platelet count is <10 × 109 or if <20 × 109 with fever/bleeding

MEDICATION
First Line
- Corticosteroids (methylprednisolone) are often given with immunosuppressive regimens.
- Immunosuppressive therapy (3)
  - A combination of antithymocyte globulin (ATG) plus cyclosporine. ATG eliminates lymphocytes, and cyclosporine blocks T-cell function.

- ATG
  - Horse serum containing polyclonal antibodies against human T cells
  - First-choice treatment for patients >40 years of age and for younger patients without a compatible donor. Consider in patients 30 to 40 years of age.
  - May be used as a single agent but has better response in combination with cyclosporine
- Cyclosporine following initial ATG therapy for minimum of 6 months (3)
  - Monitor through blood levels. Normal values for assays vary.
  - Note: Relapses may occur after the initial response to the immunosuppressive therapy if cyclosporine is discontinued too early. Restarting cyclosporine can lead to a response in up to 25% of patients.
- Granulocyte-colony stimulating factor (G-CSF)
  - May be used in conjunction with ATG and cyclosporine
  - Shows faster neutrophil recovery, but survival is not improved
  - Treatment is costly and is disputed in two randomized trials.
- Stem cell transplant: matched sibling allogeneic stem cell transplant for age <20 years and ANC <500 or age 20 to 40 years and ANC <200

Second Line
- Rabbit ATG + cyclosporine
- Campath
- Androgen such as danazol (4) can be used in a subset of patients who have anemia as a predominant feature.
- Matched unrelated donor stem cell transplant
- Eltrombopag (5)
- In trials: thrombopoietin (TPO) receptor agonists (5)

SURGERY/OTHER PROCEDURES
- First-line hematopoietic stem cell transplantation is recommended for patients with an HLA-identical donor and severe aplastic anemia when age <20 years and ANC <500 or age 20 to 40 years and ANC <200. Consider in patients 40 to 50 years of age in good general medical condition.
- Patients >40 years of age have higher rates of graft versus host disease and graft rejection.
- Unrelated donor transplants should be considered for patients age <40 years without HLA-matched sibling donor who fail first-line immunosuppressive therapy.
- Thymectomy for thymoma

ADMISSION, INPATIENT, AND NURSING CONSIDERATIONS
If neutropenic, use antiseptic mouthwash such as chlorhexidine.

ONGOING CARE

DIET
If neutropenic, avoid foods that can expose patient to bacteria, such as uncooked foods. https://www.lls.org/managing-your-cancer/diet-guidelines-for-immunosuppressed-patients

PATIENT EDUCATION
- Stay away from people who are sick; avoid large crowds.
- Wash your hands often.
- Brush and floss your teeth; get regular dental care to reduce risk of infections.

- Pneumonia vaccine and annual flu shot
- Printed patient information available from Aplastic Anemia and MDS International Foundation, Inc., 800-747-2828. Web site: http://www.aamds.org/aplastic

PROGNOSIS
- Hematopoietic stem cell transplantation with HLA-matched sibling
  - Age <16 years, 91% at 5 years
  - Age >16 years, 70–80% at 5 years
- Immunosuppressive therapy using ATG and cyclosporine: overall survival of 75%; 90% among responders at 5 years

COMPLICATIONS
- Infection (fungal, sepsis)
- Graft versus host disease in bone marrow transplant recipients (acute 18%; chronic 26%)
- Side effects of immunosuppressant medications
- Hemorrhage
- Transfusion hemosiderosis
- Transfusion hepatitis
- Heart failure
- Development of secondary cancer: leukemia or myelodysplasia (15–19% risk at 6 to 10 years)
- Refractory pancytopenia

REFERENCES

1. Brodsky RA, Jones RJ. Aplastic anaemia. *Lancet*. 2005;365(9471):1647–1656.
2. Luzatto L, Risitano AM. Advances in understanding the pathogenesis of acquired aplastic anemia. *Br J Haematol*. 2018;182(6):758–776.
3. Scheinberg P, Young NS. How I treat acquired aplastic anemia. *Blood*. 2012;120(6):1185–1196.
4. Jaime-Pérez JC, Colunga-Pedraza PR, Gómez-Ramírez CD, et al. Danazol as first-line therapy for aplastic anemia. *Ann Hematol*. 2011;90(5):523–527.
5. Desmond R, Townsley DM, Dunbar C, et al. Eltrombopag in aplastic anemia. *Semin Hematol*. 2015;52(1):31–37.

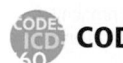

SEE ALSO

- Lupus Erythematosus, Systemic (SLE); Myelodysplastic Syndromes (MDS)
- Algorithm: Anemia

CODES

ICD10
- D61.9 Aplastic anemia, unspecified
- D61.89 Oth aplastic anemias and other bone marrow failure syndromes
- D61.01 Constitutional (pure) red blood cell aplasia

CLINICAL PEARLS

- Acquired aplastic anemia has an insidious onset and is caused by an exogenous insult triggering an autoimmune reaction. This form is usually responsive to immunosuppressive therapy.
- Immunosuppressive therapy using ATG and cyclosporine: overall survival of 75%; 90% among responders at 5 years

ANEMIA, CHRONIC DISEASE

Christopher Lin-Brande, MD • Jason C. McCarthy, MD

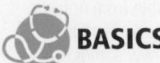 **BASICS**

DESCRIPTION
- Otherwise known as anemia of chronic inflammation
- During chronic systemic infection, inflammation, or malignancy, the production of proinflammatory mediators causes inhibition of erythropoiesis as well as the imbalance in iron homeostasis (1).
- Anemia of chronic disease (ACD) is characterized as a normocytic, normochromic, hypoproliferative anemia and classically has low serum iron levels, elevated ferritin levels, and elevated total iron-binding capacity (TIBC) (1,2).
- Anemia is typically mild to moderate with hemoglobin (Hgb) rarely <8 g/dL.

EPIDEMIOLOGY
Prevalence
ACD is the second most common anemia after iron deficiency anemia (IDA) due to the aging population and the high prevalence of chronic infections and inflammatory disorders in the United States.

ETIOLOGY AND PATHOPHYSIOLOGY
- Production of red blood cells is decreased as a result of functional iron deficiency.
- In general, the severity of the anemia will correspond with the severity of the underlying disease (1).
- Proinflammatory cytokines such as interleukins (IL), tumor necrosis factor (TNF), bone morphogenic proteins (BMP), and interferons (IFN) create changes in iron homeostasis in several ways (1):
  - Dysregulating iron homeostasis
  - Diminishing proliferation as well as differentiation of red blood cell progenitor cells
  - Blunting the erythropoietic response
  - Increasing erythrocyte phagocytosis and apoptosis
- Iron overload and the proinflammatory cytokines IL-1, IL-6, and BMP6 increase the production of the iron-regulating hormone hepcidin in hepatocytes, macrophages, and enterocytes (1).
  - Hepcidin binds to ferroportin causing internalization and degradation, preventing efflux of iron from stores in macrophages and hepatocytes, stopping iron absorption by duodenal enterocytes.
    - This results in low serum iron levels and inhibited erythropoiesis known as iron-restricted erythropoiesis.
  - As a result, iron delivery to erythroid progenitor cells within bone marrow is reduced and erythropoiesis is diminished, causing anemia.
- Erythropoietin (EPO) production and the response to EPO by erythroid bone marrow is suppressed by proinflammatory cytokines such as IL-1, TNF-α, and IFN-γ (1).
- Inflammatory cytokines may also cause erythrophagocytosis and oxidative damage, reducing RBC survival.

COMMONLY ASSOCIATED CONDITIONS
- Chronic systemic diseases
  - Rheumatoid arthritis (RA), systemic lupus erythematosus (SLE), sarcoidosis, temporal arteritis, inflammatory bowel disease (IBD), systemic inflammatory response syndrome (SIRS)
- Hepatic disease or failure
- Congestive heart failure or coronary artery disease
- Chronic kidney disease (CKD)

- Acute or chronic infections
  - Viral
    - HIV, HCV
  - Bacterial
    - Abscess, subacute bacterial endocarditis, tuberculosis, osteomyelitis
  - Fungal
  - Parasitic
- Malignancies
- Cytokine dysregulation (anemia of aging)
- Hypometabolic states
  - Protein malnutrition, thyroid disease, panhypopituitarism, diabetes mellitus, Addison disease

 DIAGNOSIS

HISTORY
- ACD is often discovered incidentally on routine CBC with differential.
- ACD presents with the underlying causative infectious, inflammatory, or malignant process without any source of occult bleeding; often, patients will have mild and vague anemia symptoms, such as fatigue, light-headedness, and palpitations (1).
- Those with a cardiovascular condition may experience symptoms of angina, shortness of breath, and reduced exercise capacity with even a moderate Hgb level (10 to 11 g/dL).

PHYSICAL EXAM
Physical exam findings are associated with the underlying condition.

DIFFERENTIAL DIAGNOSIS
- IDA
- Anemia of CKD
- Drug-induced marrow suppression or hemolysis
- Endocrine disorders
- Thalassemia
- Sideroblastic anemia
- Dilutional anemia

DIAGNOSTIC TESTS & INTERPRETATION
Initial Tests (lab, imaging)
- Hgb/Hct, mean corpuscular volume (MCV), reticulocyte count, ferritin, B$_{12}$/folate, serum iron, TIBC
- Hgb (1)
  - Typically, <13 g/dL in males or <12 g/dL in females
  - An Hgb of <8 g/dL suggests a concurrent secondary cause for the anemia.
- MCV
  - Usually normal (80 to 100 fL), but microcytosis may be present with concurrent iron deficiency or long-standing disease (<25% of cases)
- RBC morphology
  - Normocytic and normochromic
  - Increased protoporphyrin levels
- Serum ferritin
  - Nonspecific acute phase reactant
  - Normal or slightly elevated (30 to 200 μg/L)
  - In CKD, ferritin can reach 800 μg/L.
  - Serum ferritin levels <30 μg/L suggest coexisting iron deficiency
- Serum iron levels
  - Low due to increased retention and decreased release from stores
  - <50
- TIBC
  - Extremely low
  - <300

- Absolute reticulocyte count
  - Inappropriately low (reticulocyte index, 20,000 to 25,000/mL) due to reduced erythropoiesis
- Serum B$_{12}$ and folate
  - Diminished due to decreased absorption or lacking in diet

	IDA	ACD	IDA + ACD
Iron	Low	Low	Low
Reticulocyte count	Low	Low	Low
Transferrin, TIBC	High	Low	Normal/high
Transferrin saturation	Low	Normal	Low
Ferritin	Low	Normal/high	Normal
sTfR index	High	Low/normal	High
Hepcidin	Low	High	Normal
EPO	High	Normal/high	High
Inflammatory markers	Normal	High	High

Diagnostic Procedures/Other
- Traditional gold standard: bone marrow biopsy with Prussian blue stainable iron combined with anemia, hypoferremia, and low TSAT (1)
  - Staining is qualitative and may not be accurate.
- Reticulocyte Hgb concentration <28 pg (2)
- Soluble transferrin receptor (sTfR) and the sTfR/log ferritin index
  - Ratio reflects erythropoiesis within bone marrow and differentiates among ACD, IDA, and ACD + IDA.
    - However, sTfR alone may have greater clinical value than the sTfR index because transferrin is not affected by chronic disease/inflammation, unlike ferritin.
- Functional test: supplemental iron increase H/H in IDA and little effect on ACD
- Although a known cause of anemia may be present, iron, B$_{12}$, and folate deficiencies should be ruled out.

TREATMENT

GENERAL MEASURES
- Primary management should focus on the underlying cause of ACD (1).
  - Treatment of the primary disease will generally restore Hgb back to baseline.
- In cases where primary treatment is not possible (e.g., terminal cancer, end-stage renal disease), additional treatment can be considered.
  - The two main forms of treatment are erythropoietin-stimulating agents (ESAs) and transfusions.
  - ACD is frequently responsive to ESAs (epoetin-α, darbepoetin) in pharmacologic doses (3).
  - Replete iron to maximize ESA effectiveness.
  - Transfusion should only be initiated in severe anemia or acute symptoms.
- Currently, no target Hgb exists, but treatment to Hgb >13 g/dL is associated with adverse outcomes (1).
- Coexisting B$_{12}$ or folate deficiency should be considered and corrected in severe cases of anemia.
  - Reduced dietary intake of nutrients is common among patients who are chronically ill.
  - Patients who regularly undergo hemodialysis will often lose these during treatment.

MEDICATION

- ESAs
  - Specifically approved for CKD, but there is evidence that they may also have applications in RA, IBD, HIV, and cancer
  - Indication for ESA therapy is an Hgb <10 g/dL (3)[C].
  - ESAs do not improve symptoms or outcomes in mild anemia of CHF.
  - Do not use in certain cancers: breast, cervical, head and neck, lymphoid, and non–small cell lung cancers. Do not administer to patients with active malignancy not receiving curative therapy.
- Epoetin-α (1,3,4)
  - Indications
    - Hgb <10 g/dL
    - Fatigue or exertional intolerance
    - CKD (eGFR <60 mL/min)
    - Anemia due to IBD, RA, hepatitis C
    - Chemotherapy in patients with specific malignancies (palliative therapy)
  - Dosing and schedule
    - Lowest effective dose to maintain an Hgb level generally between 10 and 12 g/dL (1,3,4)
    - CKD associated: Start 50 to 100 U/kg SC/IV 3 times per week.
  - Patients with cancer who are undergoing chemotherapy: 150 U/kg SC 3 times per week or 40,000 U once a week
  - Adverse effects:
    - Increased risk of cardiovascular complications, mortality, and thromboembolism
    - Pure red cell aplasia (decrease in Hgb, low reticulocyte count, normal WBC and platelets)
    - Risk of tumor progression in certain cancer patients
- Darbepoetin-α
  - Long-acting, molecularly modified EPO preparation with a half-life 3 to 4 times longer than recombinant human EPO, reducing the frequency of injections to weekly or biweekly
  - Dosing and schedule
    - Administer SC/IV q1–2wk; hold if Hgb >12 g/dL; IV route is preferred in hemodialysis patients.
  - Adverse effects
    - Similar to EPO
- Epoetin-α or darbepoetin-α dose adjustments
  - Follow FDA-approved labeling.
  - Treatment beyond 6 to 8 weeks without appropriate rise of Hgb (>1 to 2 g/dL) is not recommended.

ADDITIONAL THERAPIES

- Iron (3)
  - Indications
    - Coexisting iron deficiency
    - Resistance to EPO
  - Forms
    - Oral: ferrous sulfate. Poorly tolerated (GI side effects); incomplete absorption (due to hepcidin)
    - Intravenous: ferric gluconate, iron sucrose, iron dextran (potential allergic and anaphylactoid reactions), ferumoxytol
  - Adverse effects
    - May stimulate hepcidin production and exacerbate iron restriction
  - Benefits
    - Relatively safe
    - Inexpensive
    - May decrease ESA requirements (DRIVE study)
- Transfusions
  - 1 to 2 U packed red blood cells (1)
  - Indications
    - Life-threatening/severe anemia: A "restrictive threshold" of Hgb 7 to 8 g/dL to guide transfusion in asymptomatic patients should be used (5)[A].
    - Patients with underlying cardiac or pulmonary disease, active ACS, elderly patients, or patients with acute bleeding or hemorrhagic shock may require transfusion at Hgb of higher threshold (>10 g/dL).
    - Symptomatic anemia (chest pain, SOB, reduced exercise capacity) and/or ECG changes
    - Lack of response to medical therapy
  - Possible adverse effects
    - Infection (HIV, hepatitis)
    - Volume overload
    - Transfusion reaction
  - Specific benefits
    - Rapid correction of anemia
  - When an infection occurs during EPO therapy, it is best to cease EPO therapy and rely on transfusion therapy instead until the infection is properly treated.
- Future directions (1)
  - Antihepcidin antibodies, hepcidin-production inhibitors
  - Anti-BMP, anti–IL-6 antibodies
  - Ferroportin stabilizers
  - Vitamin D (lowers hepcidin)
  - Heparin (impairs hepcidin transcription)

 ONGOING CARE

FOLLOW-UP RECOMMENDATIONS
Referral to a hematologist is not always warranted.

Patient Monitoring
- Hgb should not be increased >11 to 12 g/dL because normalization of Hgb has been associated with higher mortality (4).
- Baseline and periodic monitoring of transferrin saturation and ferritin levels every 3 months may be of value (3).

PATIENT EDUCATION
Patients receiving medical therapy should be advised about the following possible risks:
- Mortality, cardiovascular complications, thromboembolism, progression of cancer

PROGNOSIS
ACD does not typically progress.

COMPLICATIONS
- Adverse effects of ACD:
  - Mortality
  - Cardiovascular complications
  - Symptoms affecting daily life
- Adverse effects of ESAs:
  - Heightened risk of mortality and/or cardiovascular complications in CKD patients
  - Heightened risk of mortality and/or tumor progression in cancer patients
  - Elevated risk of thromboembolism

REFERENCES

1. Gangat N, Wolanskyj AP. Anemia of chronic disease. Semin Hematol. 2013;50(3):232–238.
2. Thomas DW, Hinchliffe RF, Briggs C, et al; for British Committee for Standards in Haematology. Guidelines for the laboratory diagnosis of functional iron deficiency. Br J Haematol. 2013;161(5):639–648.
3. Kidney Disease: Improving Global Outcomes Anemia Work Group. KDIGO clinical practice guideline for anemia in chronic kidney disease. Kidney Inter Suppl. 2012;2(4):279–335.
4. Babitt JL, Lin HY. Mechanisms of anemia in CKD. J Am Soc Nephrol. 2012;23(10):1631–1634.
5. Carson JL, Carless PA, Hebert PC. Transfusion thresholds and other strategies for guiding allogeneic red blood cell transfusion. Cochrane Database Syst Rev. 2012;(4):CD002042.

ADDITIONAL READING

- Besarab A, Bolton WK, Browne JK, et al. The effects of normal as compared with low hematocrit values in patients with cardiac disease who are receiving hemodialysis and epoetin. N Engl J Med. 1998;339(9):584–590.
- Fishbane S, Schiller B, Locatelli F, et al; for EMERALD Study Groups. Peginesatide in patients with anemia undergoing hemodialysis. N Engl J Med. 2013;368(4):307–319.
- Macdougall IC, Provenzano R, Sharma A, et al; for PEARL Study Groups. Peginesatide for anemia in patients with chronic kidney disease not receiving dialysis. N Engl J Med. 2013;368(4):320–332.
- Pfeffer MA, Burdmann EA, Chen CY, et al; for TREAT Investigators. A trial of darbepoetin alfa in type 2 diabetes and chronic kidney disease. N Engl J Med. 2009;361(21):2019–2032.
- Singh AK, Szczech L, Tang KL, et al; for CHOIR Investigators. Correction of anemia with epoetin alfa in chronic kidney disease. N Engl J Med. 2006;355(20):2085–2098.
- Swedberg K, Young JB, Anand IS, et al; for RED-HF Committees and Investigators. Treatment of anemia with darbepoetin alfa in systolic heart failure. N Engl J Med. 2013;368(13):1210–1219.

 SEE ALSO

Anemia, Iron Deficiency; Iron Studies; Microcytic Anemia

 CODES

ICD10
- D63.8 Anemia in other chronic diseases classified elsewhere
- D63.0 Anemia in neoplastic disease
- D63.1 Anemia in chronic kidney disease

CLINICAL PEARLS
- ACD is the second most common anemia seen clinically.
- One of the most common diagnostic problems is making the distinction between ACD, IDA, and combined ACD + IDA.
  - Iron level is usually nondiagnostic.
  - Use markers such as transferrin/TIBC, TSAT, and ferritin to distinguish. New markers are under development (hepcidin, sTfR, sTfR index).
- IV iron should be given to all patients treated with ESAs.
- Hgb should be kept in low to normal range.

ANEMIA, IRON DEFICIENCY

Deborah R. Erlich, MD, MMedEd, FAAFP

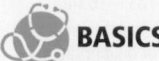 **BASICS**

DESCRIPTION
- Low serum iron associated with low hemoglobin (Hgb) or microcytic, hypochromic red blood cells (RBCs)
- Because normal Hgb varies with age and sex, anemia is defined as Hgb level 2 standard deviations below normal for age and sex (1).
- Onset acute (rapid blood loss) or chronic (slow blood loss, deficient iron intake, or poor absorption)
- Both low Hgb per RBC and fewer RBC in total lead to blood oxygen deficiency, which can have serious systemic consequences.
- System(s) affected: hematologic, lymphatic, immunologic, cardiac, and gastrointestinal systems

Geriatric Considerations
Iron deficiency anemia (IDA) is associated with increased hospitalization, morbidity, and mortality in older adults (2).

Pediatric Considerations
Risks for IDA in children include low birth weight, history of prematurity, lead exposure, low income status, and immigrant status. Additionally, infants who drink cow's milk before 12 months of age have a higher risk for IDA. The U.S. Preventive Services Task Force (USPSTF) did not find sufficient evidence for screening low-risk infants, the Centers for Disease Control (CDC) recommends screening high-risk infants at 6 to 12 months, and the AAP recommends universal screening at 12 months (1)[B].

Pregnancy Considerations
- The USPSTF did not find sufficient evidence for screening pregnant women for IDA; the CDC recommends screening women for anemia at the first prenatal visit and giving low-dose iron to all pregnant women, whereas the American College of Obstetricians and Gynecologists (ACOG) recommends screening all pregnant women for IDA and treating those with IDA.
- Iron supplements are recommended during pregnancy to improve maternal hematologic indexes, although significant clinical outcomes have not been proven (3)[A].

EPIDEMIOLOGY
- Iron deficiency is the most common nutritional deficiency in the world (4,5), and IDA is the most common cause of anemia (50%) (4).
- Predominant age: all ages but especially toddlers and menstruating and pregnant women
- Predominant sex: female
- Predominant race: Mexican American and black females (4)
- Common in both developing and developed countries

Incidence
- Adults: men 2%, women 15–20% annually
- Infants and toddlers: 3–5% annually
- Pregnant patients: may be as high as 20% (1)

Prevalence
2 billion people worldwide (5)
- Infants and children age <12 years: 4–7%
- Men: 2–5%
- Menstruating women: 30% (5)

ETIOLOGY AND PATHOPHYSIOLOGY
Depletion of iron stores leads to decrease in both reticulocyte count and production of Hgb. Causes:
- Blood loss (menses, GI bleeding, trauma)
- Poor iron intake
- Poor iron absorption (e.g., atrophic gastritis, post-gastrectomy, celiac disease)
- Increased demand for iron (e.g., infancy, adolescence, pregnancy, breastfeeding)

RISK FACTORS
- Premenopausal woman
- Frequent blood donor
- Pregnancy/lactation, young maternal age
- Strict vegan diet
- Use of NSAIDs
- Hospitalized with frequent blood draws
- Living in or visiting countries with endemic hookworm infection

GENERAL PREVENTION
- Consider screening asymptomatic pregnant women and high-risk children at 1 year of age (guidelines vary) (1)[C].
- Supplementation in asymptomatic children aged 6 to 12 months if at risk for IDA (e.g., malnutrition, abuse, cow's milk <12 months) (1,3)
- Iron- and vitamin C–rich diet for menstruating women
- Iron 30 mg/day for asymptomatic pregnant women (3)

COMMONLY ASSOCIATED CONDITIONS
- GI tract malignancy, peptic ulcer disease (PUD), Helicobacter pylori infection, irritable bowel disease
- Hookworm or other parasitic infestations
- Hypermetrorrhagia
- Pregnancy
- Obesity treated with gastric bypass surgery
- Malnutrition
- Medications such as NSAIDs or antacids

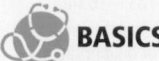 **DIAGNOSIS**

HISTORY
- Asymptomatic in most cases
- Weakness, fatigue, and/or malaise
- Exertional dyspnea
- Angina with coronary artery disease
- Headaches or inability to concentrate
- Melena
- Pica

PHYSICAL EXAM
- Pallor (skin, conjunctivae, sublingual)
- Tachycardia, tachypnea
- Cool extremities
- Brittle nails/hair
- Signs of heart failure

DIFFERENTIAL DIAGNOSIS
- GI bleeding (e.g., gastritis, PUD, carcinoma, varices, celiac disease)
- Chronic intravascular hemolysis (e.g., paroxysmal nocturnal hemoglobinuria, malfunctioning prosthetic valve)
- Defective iron usage (e.g., thalassemia trait, sideroblastosis, G6PD deficiency)
- Defective iron reutilization (e.g., infection, inflammation, cancer, hypothyroid, chronic diseases)
- Hypoproliferation (e.g., decreased erythropoietin from hypothyroidism, renal failure)
- Other anemias such as anemia of chronic disease, thalassemia, lead poisoning

DIAGNOSTIC TESTS & INTERPRETATION
Initial Tests (lab, imaging)
- Test with signs and symptoms of anemia, and fully evaluate if iron deficiency is confirmed (1,5).
- Hgb (to define anemia):
  - <13 g in men and <12 g in women (5)
  - Hgb 2 standard deviations below normal for age and sex (1)
  - Patients with comorbidities (e.g., chronic hypoxemia, smokers, high altitudes) may be anemic at higher Hgb levels.
- Mean corpuscular volume (MCV): <80 Fl
  - MCV may be low normal in mild anemia or hidden by large cells (reticulocytes, macrocytes).
- Ferritin is most sensitive and specific for diagnosing iron deficiency as cause of anemia (5):
  - <15 μg/L diagnoses IDA (<30 μg/L likely) (1).
  - >100 μg/L rules out iron deficiency.
- Iron studies:
  - Decreased: ferritin, serum iron, transferrin saturation
  - Increased: total iron-binding capacity (TIBC), transferrin
- Red cell distribution width (RDW) increases with a mixed population of cells (e.g., mixed IDA and vitamin B_{12} deficiency).
- CBC with differential, peripheral smear, reticulocyte count, and index
  - Peripheral smear usually shows hypochromia and microcytosis but may be normal, and reticulocyte production index is low (1).
- Consider testing for G6PD deficiency.
- Evaluate for thalassemia.
  - Very low MCV <80, elevated Hgb A2 or Hgb F, family history, and especially high or high normal RBC count
  - Microcytosis with ovalocytosis and unresponsive to iron suggests the thalassemia trait.
- IgA antiendomysial antibodies (IgA anti-EmA) and/or IgA antitissue transglutaminase (IgA anti-TTG) for celiac disease
- TSH for hypothyroidism
- An empiric trial of iron at 3 mg/kg/day may help diagnose decreased iron stores in children; reticulocytes become elevated in 7 to 10 days or Hgb increases >1 g/dL weekly, indicating iron deficiency.
- Drugs that may alter lab results:
  - Iron supplements or multivitamin–mineral preparations that contain iron
- Disorders that may alter lab results:
  - Elevated ferritin: acute inflammation, acute or chronic liver disease, Hodgkin disease, acute leukemia, solid tumors, fever, renal dialysis
  - Elevated Hgb: smoking, chronic hypoxemia, high altitude

Diagnostic Procedures/Other
- Stool guaiac
- Stool for ova and parasites if at risk
- Colonoscopy and endoscopy to evaluate for bleeding sites and colorectal and gastric carcinoma for:
  - Premenopausal women with negative GYN workup and/or lack of response to iron
  - Men and postmenopausal women (1)[C]
- Bone marrow aspiration rarely performed

TREATMENT

GENERAL MEASURES
- Search for underlying cause and correct.
- Avoid transfusions, except in rare cases.

MEDICATION
- Elemental iron 100 to 200 mg/day for adults (whether pregnant or not) (3,5)[C]
- Elemental iron 3 to 6 mg/kg/day for children (5)
- Ferrous sulfate 325 mg TID, ferrous gluconate 300 mg 1 to 3 tablets BID–TID, or ferrous fumarate 324 mg 1 tablet BID on an empty stomach 1 hour before meals (1)[C]
- Constipation will occur in ~1/4 of patients. Consider a stool softener along with iron.
  - Medications that reduce gastric acid secretion such as proton pump inhibitors and H_2 antagonists reduce iron absorption (1).
  - Special oral iron formulations (e.g., enteric-coated iron) are expensive and reduce symptoms only to the degree that they reduce the delivery of iron.
- IV iron is indicated for patients who cannot tolerate the side effects of oral replacement (e.g., pregnant women or patients with GI disorders) or for patients who do not sufficiently respond to oral replacement. Other indications for IV iron: bariatric surgery status, heavy uterine bleeding, malabsorption, inflammatory bowel disease, ongoing/severe losses
- Outside of the United States, IV iron is becoming first line ahead of oral iron for its superiority in efficacy and toxicity.
- IV iron formulations available in the United States:
  - Low-molecular-weight iron dextran 1,000 mg over 1 hour
  - Ferumoxytol 510 mg over 3 minutes
  - Ferric carboxymaltose 750 mg over 15 minutes
- Liquid iron preparations (used for children) can also be used in adults when tablets are not absorbed or low tolerance requires a dose reduction.
  - Continued bleeding and untreated hypothyroidism are causes for "failure to respond" to iron.
  - Formula to determine elemental iron needed: elemental iron (mg) = dose (mL) = 0.0442 (desired Hgb − observed Hgb) × LBW + (0.26 × LBW)
    - Desired Hgb = target Hgb in g/dL
    - Observed Hgb = current Hgb in g/dL
    - LBW = lean body weight in kg
    - For males: LBW = 50 kg + 2.3 kg for each inch of height >5 feet
    - For females: LBW = 45.5 kg + 2.3 kg for each inch of height >5 feet
    - Normal Hgb (males and females)
      - >15 kg (33 lb) . . . 14.8 g/dL
      - <15 kg (33 lb) . . . 12.0 g/dL
- Relative contraindications for oral iron:
  - Tetracycline
  - Allopurinol
  - Antacids
  - Penicillamine
  - Fluoroquinolones
  - Vitamin E
- Consider parenteral iron for patients with an Hgb level <6 g/dL, malabsorption, chronic kidney disease, or failure to respond to higher oral doses with concomitant vitamin C (5).
- Issues for parenteral iron formulations:
  - Give test dose for iron dextran prior to first dose to avoid anaphylaxis; ferric gluconate or iron sucrose may be safer alternative. Dimercaprol increases risk of nephrotoxicity.
  - Dosing is product dependent; refer to individual product for suggested dosing.

- Precautions
  - Iron may cause dark stools and constipation.
  - Iron overdose is highly toxic; absorption is limited to 1 to 2 mg daily (5); keep tablets and liquids out of reach of small children.
- Blood transfusion for severe acute blood loss or severely symptomatic patients (e.g., demand ischemia due to anemia). Hgb threshold varies by risk factors and clinical scenario. Pregnant women with Hgb <6 should be transfused (1)[C].

ISSUES FOR REFERRAL
- Men and postmenopausal women with IDA (Test for colon cancer.)
- Pregnant women with Hgb level <9 g/dL
- Men or nonpregnant women with an Hgb level <6 g/dL
- Failure to respond to a 4- to 6-week trial of oral iron

 ONGOING CARE

FOLLOW-UP RECOMMENDATIONS
Patient Monitoring
- Monitor patients every 3 months after Hgb normalizes for a year and then yearly (1)[C].
- Hgb increases 1 g/dL every 3 to 4 weeks.
- Iron stores may take up to 4 weeks to correct after Hgb normalizes.

DIET
- Iron-rich foods include red meat; poultry; fish (all heme iron sources, best absorbed); and iron-fortified breads/cereals, lentils, beans, dark green vegetables, and raisins (all non-heme iron sources, less well absorbed) (6).
- Foods and beverages containing ascorbic acid (vitamin C) enhance iron absorption when taken simultaneously (5).
- Avoid milk or dairy products within 2 hours of iron tablet ingestion.
- Limit milk to 16 oz/day (adults).
- Limit tea, coffee, and caffeinated beverages.
- Increase fluid and dietary fiber to decrease likelihood of constipation.
- Limit foods with high levels of chemicals (phytates and polyphenols).

PATIENT EDUCATION
- http://familydoctor.org/familydoctor/en/diseases-conditions/anemia.html
- http://patient.info/pdf/4392.pdf

PROGNOSIS
- IDA can be resolved with iron therapy if the underlying cause is discovered and appropriately treated.
- Treat coexisting subclinical hypothyroidism and IDA together. Failure to treat hypothyroidism results in poor response to iron therapy.

COMPLICATIONS
- Hidden bleeding, particularly a bleeding malignancy
- Ischemic events or heart failure, especially in elderly
- Poor growth, failure to thrive, motor and cognitive developmental delay in children (4)

REFERENCES
1. Short MW, Domagalski JE. Iron deficiency anemia: evaluation and management. *Am Fam Physician.* 2013;87(2):98–104.
2. Goodnough LT, Schrier SL. Evaluation and management of anemia in the elderly. *Am J Hematol.* 2014;89(1):88–96.
3. McDonagh M, Cantor A, Bougatsos C, et al. *Routine Iron Supplementation and Screening for Iron Deficiency Anemia in Pregnant Women: A Systematic Review to Update the U.S. Preventive Services Task Force Recommendation. Evidence Syntheses No. 123.* Rockville, MD: Agency for Healthcare Research and Quality; 2015.
4. Centers for Disease Control and Prevention. Iron deficiency—United States, 1999–2000. *MMWR Morb Mortal Wkly Rep.* 2002;51(40):897–899.
5. Camaschella C. Iron-deficiency anemia. *N Engl J Med.* 2015;372(19):1832–1843.
6. National Institutes of Health Office of Dietary Supplements. Iron: fact sheet for health professionals. https://ods.od.nih.gov/factsheets/Iron-HealthProfessional/. Accessed June 29, 2018.

ADDITIONAL READING
- Auerbach M, Deloughery T. Single-dose intravenous iron for iron deficiency: a new paradigm. *Hematology Am Soc Hematol Educ Program.* 2016;2016(1):57–66.
- Chertow GM, Mason PD, Vaage-Nilsen O, et al. On the relative safety of parenteral iron formulations. *Nephrol Dial Transplant.* 2004;19(6):1571–1575.
- Johnson-Wimbley TD, Graham DY. Diagnosis and management of iron deficiency anemia in the 21st century. *Therap Adv Gastroenterol.* 2011;4(3):177–184.
- Murphy MF, Wallington TB, Kelsey P, et al; for British Committee for Standards in Haematology, Blood Transfusion Task Force. Guidelines for the clinical use of red cell transfusions. *Br J Haematol.* 2001;113(1):24–31.
- Murray-Kolb LE, Beard JL. Iron deficiency and child and maternal health. *Am J Clin Nutr.* 2009;89(3):946S–950S.
- USPSTF Recommendations. Iron Deficiency Anemia in Pregnant Women: Screening and Supplementation. Released September 2015. Accessed June 29, 2018.
- World Health Organization. *Guideline: Intermittent Iron and Folic Acid Supplementation in Menstruating Women.* Geneva, Switzerland: World Health Organization; 2011.

 SEE ALSO

Algorithm: Anemia

CODES

ICD10
- D50.9 Iron deficiency anemia, unspecified
- D62 Acute posthemorrhagic anemia
- D50.0 Iron deficiency anemia secondary to blood loss (chronic)

CLINICAL PEARLS
- IDA due to poor dietary iron intake is the most common anemia.
- Blood loss and reduced iron stores due to poor utilization or malabsorption are risk factors for IDA.
- Premenopausal women and children are at the greatest risk for IDA.
- Cow's milk should not be given to children aged <12 months.
- Oral iron supplementation is the standard first-line treatment for IDA.

ANEMIA, SICKLE CELL
Tipsuda Junsanto-Bahri, MD

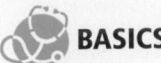 **BASICS**

DESCRIPTION
- Hereditary, hemoglobinopathy marked by chronic hemolytic anemia, acute episodes of painful "crises," and increased susceptibility to infections
- The heterozygous condition (Hb AS), sickle cell trait, is usually asymptomatic without anemia.
- Synonym(s): sickle cell disease (SCD); Hb SS disease

Pediatric Considerations
- Sequestration crises and hand–foot syndrome seen typically in infants/young children
- Strokes occur mainly in childhood.
- Adolescence/young adulthood
  - Frequency of complications and organ/tissue damage increases with age.
  - Psychological complications: body image, interrupted schooling, restriction of activities; stigma of disease; low self-esteem

Pregnancy Considerations
- Complicated, especially during 3rd trimester and delivery
  - Fetal mortality 35–40%. Fetal survival is >90% if the fetus reaches the 3rd trimester.
  - High prevalence of small for gestational age (SGA) babies
- Increased risk of thrombosis, preterm delivery, pain, toxemia, infection, pulmonary infarction, and phlebitis
- Partial exchange transfusion in 3rd trimester may reduce maternal morbidity and fetal mortality but is controversial.
- Chronic transfusions have been effective in diminishing pain episodes in pregnant women. However, this method should be used with caution due to risk of alloimmunization.

EPIDEMIOLOGY
Prevalence
- ~90,000 Americans have sickle cell anemia (SCA), and 3.5 million people in the United States have sickle cell trait.
- The condition affects mainly people of African descent. Hispanic, Middle Eastern, and Asian Indian ancestry may also be affected.

ETIOLOGY AND PATHOPHYSIOLOGY
- Hemoglobin S (HbS) results from the substitution of the amino acid valine for glutamic acid at the sixth position of the β-globin chain.
- HbS polymerizes in the RBC in the deoxygenated state, resulting in RBC sickling.
- Sickle RBCs are inflexible, causes increased blood viscosity, stasis, obstruction of small arterioles and capillaries, and ischemia.
- Chronic anemia; crises
  - Vaso-occlusive crisis: tissue ischemia and necrosis; progressive organ failure/tissue damage from repeated episodes
  - Hand–foot syndrome: Vessel occlusion/ischemia affects small blood vessels in hands or feet.
  - Aplastic crisis: suppression of RBC production by severe infection (e.g., parvoviral and other viral infections)
  - Suppression of RBC production
  - Hyperhemolytic crisis: accelerated hemolysis with reticulocytosis; increased RBC fragility/shortened lifespan
  - Sequestration crisis: splenic sequestration of blood (only in young children as spleen is later lost to autoinfarction)

- Susceptibility to infection: impaired/absent splenic function leading to decreased ability to clear infection; defect in alternate pathway of complement activation
- Increased RBC destruction causes decreased hemoglobin levels and results in anemia and fatigue.
- Sickle cells exhibit increased adhesion and decreased ability to maneuver through small vessels, leading to vaso-occlusion.

Genetics
- Autosomal recessive. Homozygous condition, Hb SS; heterozygous condition, Hb AS
- The heterozygote condition can also be combined with other hemoglobinopathies: Sickle cell hemoglobin C (HbSC) disease and Sβ + thalassemia are clinically similar to the heterozygous condition, whereas Sβ thalassemia is clinically similar to the homozygous condition.

RISK FACTORS
- Vaso-occlusive crisis ("painful crisis"): hypoxia, dehydration, fever, infection, acidosis, cold, anesthesia, strenuous physical exercise, smoking
- Aplastic crisis (suppression of RBC production): severe infections, human parvovirus B19 infection, folic acid deficiency
- Hyperhemolytic crisis (accelerated hemolysis with reticulocytosis): acute bacterial infections, exposure to oxidant

GENERAL PREVENTION
- Prevention of crises
  - Avoid hypoxia, dehydration, cold, infection, fever, acidosis, and anesthesia.
  - Prompt management of fever, infections, pain
  - Hydration
  - Avoid alcohol and smoking.
  - Avoid high-altitude areas.
- Minimizing trauma: Aseptic technique is imperative.

 DIAGNOSIS

Diagnosis is often made by newborn screening programs.

HISTORY
- Often asymptomatic in early months of life due to presence of fetal hemoglobin
- In those >6 months of age, earliest symptoms are irritability and painful swelling of the hands and feet (hand–foot syndrome); may also see pneumococcal sepsis or meningitis, severe anemia and acute splenic enlargement (splenic sequestration), acute chest syndrome, pallor, jaundice, or splenomegaly
- Manifestations in older children include anemia, severe or recurrent musculoskeletal or abdominal pain, aplastic crisis, acute chest syndrome, splenomegaly or splenic sequestration, and cholelithiasis.
- Painful crises in bones, joints, abdomen, back, and viscera account for 90% of all hospital admissions.
- Acute chest syndrome: tachycardia, fever, bilateral infiltrates caused by pulmonary infarctions

PHYSICAL EXAM
Fever, pale skin and nail beds, mild jaundice

DIFFERENTIAL DIAGNOSIS
Anemia: other hemoglobinopathies

DIAGNOSTIC TESTS & INTERPRETATION
Initial Tests (lab, imaging)
- Screening test: Sickledex test/Hb electrophoresis (diagnostic test of choice); SCA (FS pattern)
  - 80–100% Hb S, variable amounts of Hb F, and no Hb A1
  - Sickle cell trait (FS pattern): 30–45% Hb S, 50–70% Hb A1, minimal Hb F
- Hemoglobin ~5 to 10 g/dL; RBC indices: mean corpuscular volume (MCV) normal to increased; mean corpuscular hemoglobin concentration (MCHC) increased; reticulocytes 3–15%
- Leukocytosis; bands in absence of infection, platelets elevated; peripheral smear: sickled RBCs, nucleated RBCs, Howell-Jolly bodies
- Serum bilirubin mildly elevated (2 to 4 mg/dL); ferritin very elevated in multiply transfused patients; serum lactate dehydrogenase (LDH) elevated
- Fecal/urinary urobilinogen high
- Haptoglobin absent or very low
- Urine analysis: hemoglobinuria, hematuria (sickle cell trait may have painless hematuria), increased albuminuria (Monitor for progressive kidney disease.)
- Imaging depends on clinical circumstances.
  - Bone scan to rule out osteomyelitis
  - CT/MRI to rule out CVA; high index of suspicion required for any acute neurologic symptoms other than mild headache
  - Chest x-ray: may show enlarged heart; diffuse alveolar infiltrates in acute chest syndrome
  - Transcranial Doppler: Start at age 2 years; repeat yearly. Transcranial Doppler ultrasound identifies children age 2 to 16 years at higher risk of stroke; may be normal in clinically silent strokes
  - ECG to detect pulmonary hypertension and echocardiogram every other year from age 15 years and older

Test Interpretation
Hyposplenism due to autosplenectomy is common; hypoxia/infarction in multiple organs

 TREATMENT

GENERAL MEASURES
- Painful crises: hydration, analgesics; oxygen regardless of whether the patient is hypoxic
- Retinal evaluation starting at school age to detect proliferative sickle retinopathy (1)[A]
- Occupational therapy, cognitive and behavioral therapies, support groups
- All standard childhood vaccinations should be administered accordingly.
- Special immunizations
  - Influenza vaccine yearly
  - Conjugated pneumococcal vaccine (PCV13) at ages 2, 4, and 6 months; booster at 12 to 15 months
  - Patients <5 years of age with incomplete vaccination history should receive catch-up doses accordingly.
  - Adults age ≥19 years who have functional asplenia and have not received pneumococcal vaccination should receive 1 dose PCV13, followed by administration of PPSV23 at least 8 weeks later (1)[A].
- Meningococcal vaccine:
  - 6 weeks old: Hib-MenCY at ages 2, 4, 6, and 12 months
  - 9 months old: 2 doses of MCV4 separated by 3 months
  - ≥2 years of age: 2 doses of MCV4-D-CRM separated by 2 months; boosters recommended every 5 years

MEDICATION

First Line

- Prophylactic penicillins indicated in infants and children starting at 2 months: A dose of 125 mg BID is recommended for children <5 years. A dose of 250 mg BID is recommended for children >5 years. Amoxicillin 20 mg/kg/day is an alternative to penicillin; if high risk remains, continue until puberty (2)[A].
- Supplemental oxygen
- Painful crises (mild, outpatient)
  – Nonopioid analgesics (ibuprofen)
- Painful crises (severe, hospitalized)
  – Parenteral opioids (e.g., morphine on fixed schedule); patient-controlled analgesia (PCA) pump may be useful (1)[A]. Patients given strong opioids in the acute care setting should be safely monitored. Alternative to morphine as well as intranasal or transmucosal routes for rapid onset may be considered (3)[B].
- Hydroxyurea for prevention of painful acute chest syndrome, vaso-occlusive episodes, and very severe anemia. Increases fetal hemoglobin concentration. Adults: Start 15 mg/kg/day single daily dose; children: 20 mg/kg/day; titrate upward every 8 weeks (max dose of 35 mg/kg/day). Monitor blood counts (avoid severe neutropenia, thrombocytopenia) (1)[A].
- Acute chest syndrome: Patients may deteriorate quickly; monitor patients with vaso-occlusive crisis with incentive spirometry. Treat with aggressive management with oxygen, analgesics, antibiotics, and simple or exchange transfusion (1)[A].
- Empiric antibiotics to cover *Mycoplasma pneumoniae* and *Chlamydia pneumoniae* (cephalosporins or azithromycin) (1)[A]. If osteomyelitis, cover for *Staphylococcus aureus* and *Salmonella* (e.g., ciprofloxacin).
- Precautions: Avoid high-dose estrogen oral contraceptives; consider Depo-Provera. G-CSF use is contraindicated as it may lead to vaso-occlusive episodes and multiorgan failure.

Second Line

Folic acid: 0 to 6 months: 0.1 mg/day; 6 to 12 months: 0.25 mg/day; 1 to 2 years: 0.5 mg/day; >2 years of age: 1 mg/day

ADDITIONAL THERAPIES

Transfusions and additional therapies (4)[A]

- Transfusion for aplastic crises, severe complications (i.e., CVA), prophylactically before surgery, and treatment for acute chest syndrome; prophylactic transfusions for primary or secondary stroke prevention in children
- Preoperative transfusions have been shown to reduce the risk of perioperative complications.
- Avoid blood hyperviscosity.
- Consider chelation with deferasirox, an oral agent, if the patient is multiply transfused (after age 2 years). Red cell exchange transfusion minimizes risk of iron overload.

SURGERY/OTHER PROCEDURES

- Targeted fetal hemoglobin induction treatment (5)[A]
- Hematopoietic stem cell transplant (HSCT): curative, but with significant morbidity and mortality; limited to individuals <16 years old
- Gene therapy, where autologous hematopoietic cells treated with lentiviral vector encoding a therapeutic HBB gene, may be considered in the future (6)[C].

ADMISSION, INPATIENT, AND NURSING CONSIDERATIONS

- Admission criteria/initial stabilization: severe pain, suspected infection or sepsis, evidence of acute chest syndrome
- The preferred maintenance IV fluid is 1/2 NS because NS may theoretically increase the risk of sickling.

 ONGOING CARE

FOLLOW-UP RECOMMENDATIONS

Patient Monitoring

- Treat infections early. Parents/patients: Any temperature of ≥101°F (38.3°C) requires immediate medical attention.
- Monitor for hepatitis C and hemosiderosis in patients who receive chronic transfusions.
- Periodic eye evaluations: starting age 10 years to detect proliferative sickle retinopathy; rescreen 1 to 2 year intervals (2)[A].
- Biannual examination for hepatic, renal, and pulmonary dysfunction
- Neuroimaging screening for risk of stroke: transcranial Doppler beginning at age 2 years and continuing up to age 16 years
- Baseline pulmonary evaluation at each visit to assess for wheezing, shortness of breath, or cough (indicators of disease severity and pulmonary hypertension). Echocardiography for symptomatic patients; right heart catheterization for diagnosis
- Consider venous thromboembolism (VTE) prophylaxis because there is an increased incidence of thromboembolism.

DIET

- Folic acid supplementation; avoid alcohol (leads to dehydration); maintain hydration.
- Multivitamin without iron is recommended because there is high incidence of vitamin D deficiency and decreased bone marrow density in SCD patients.

PATIENT EDUCATION

- SickleCellKids.org—education Web site for children with sickle cell anemia: http://www.sicklecelldisease.org
- American Sickle Cell Anemia Association: http://www.ascaa.org

PROGNOSIS

- Anemia occurs in infancy; sickle cell crises at 1 to 2 years of age; some children die in their 1st year.
- In adulthood, fewer crises but more complications. Median age of death is 42 years for men and 48 years for women. Complications are mentioned below.

COMPLICATIONS

- Alloimmunization, bone infarct and osteomyelitis, aseptic necrosis of femoral head
- CVA (peak age 6 to 7 years), impaired mental development, even without history of stroke
- Cholelithiasis/abnormal liver function
- Chronic leg ulcers, poor wound healing
- Impotence, priapism, hematuria/hyposthenuria, renal complications (proteinuria)
- Retinopathy, splenic infarction (by age 10 years)
- Acute chest syndrome (infection/infarction) leading to chronic pulmonary disease
- Infections (pneumonia, osteomyelitis, meningitis, pyelonephritis); sepsis (leading cause of morbidity and mortality)
- Hemosiderosis (secondary to multiple transfusions)
- Substance abuse related to chronic opioid use

REFERENCES

1. Yawn BP, Buchanan GR, Afenyi-Annan AN, et al. Management of sickle cell disease: summary of the 2014 evidence-based report by expert panel members. *JAMA*. 2014;312(10):1033–1048.
2. Cober MP, Phelps SJ. Penicillin prophylaxis in children with sickle cell disease. *J Pediatr Pharmacol Ther*. 2010;15(3):152–159.
3. Telfer P, Bahal N, Lo A, et al. Management of acute painful crisis in sickle cell disease—a reevaluation of the use of opioids in adult patients. *Br J Hematol*. 2014;166(2):157–164.
4. Chou ST. Transfusion therapy for sickle cell disease: a balancing act. *Hematology Am Soc Hematol Educ Program*. 2013;2013:439–446.
5. Manwani D, Frenette PS. Vaso-occlusion in sickle cell disease: pathophysiology and novel targeted therapies. *Blood*. 2013;122(24):3892–3898.
6. Ribeil JA, Hacein-Bey-Abina S, Payen E, et al. Gene therapy in a patient with sickle cell disease. *N Eng J Med*. 2017;376(9):848–855.

ADDITIONAL READING

- Costa VM, Viana MB, Aguilar RA. Pregnancy in patients with sickle cell disease: maternal and perinatal outcomes. *J Matern Fetal Neonatal Med*. 2015;28(6):685–689.
- Machado RF, Farber HW. Pulmonary hypertension associated with chronic hemolytic anemia and other blood disorders. *Clin Chest Med*. 2013;34(4):739–752.
- Naik RP, Streiff MB, Lanzkron S. Sickle cell disease and venous thromboembolism: what the anticoagulation expert needs to know. *J Thromb Thrombolysis*. 2013;35(3):352–358.
- Sandu MK, Cohen A. Aging in sickle cell disease: co-morbidities and new issues in management. *Hemoglobin*. 2015;39(4):221–224.

 SEE ALSO

Algorithm: Anemia

CODES

ICD10

- D57.1 Sickle-cell disease without crisis
- D57.3 Sickle-cell trait
- D57.00 Hb-SS disease with crisis, unspecified

CLINICAL PEARLS

- >90,000 Americans have SCA (~1 in 375 African Americans).
- The preferred maintenance IV fluid is 1/2 NS because NS may theoretically increase the risk of sickling.
- Painful crises in bones, joints, abdomen, back, and viscera account for 90% of all hospital admissions.
- Acute chest syndrome: tachycardia, fever, bilateral infiltrates caused by pulmonary infarctions

ANEURYSM OF THE ABDOMINAL AORTA

Katyayini Aribindi, MD • Adrian DaSilva-DeAbreu, MD • Raymundo A. Quintana, MD

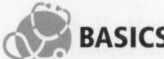 **BASICS**

DESCRIPTION

- There are two types of aneurysms: true and false. A true aneurysm involves all three vessel wall layers. False aneurysms or pseudoaneurysms occur when the intimal and medial layers are disrupted, and the dilated segment is surrounded by the adventitia only, and possibly a perivascular clot. Ruptures are usually higher with false aneurysms due to poor support of the aneurysmal wall.
- Abdominal aortic aneurysm (AAA) is the most common true aneurysm. False aneurysms of the abdominal aorta are usually due to trauma or infection.
- The average diameter of the infrarenal aorta is 2.0 cm; an aortic diameter of ≥3.0 cm is considered aneurysmal.
- In men, AAA diameters are predictive of clinical events. In women, aneurysms are still defined as >3.0 cm, but the aortic scaling index (ASI; diameter [cm] / body surface area [m^2]) is more predictive of clinical events.
- System(s) affected: cardiovascular; neurologic; heme/lymphatic/immunologic
- Synonym(s): aortic aneurysms; AAA

Geriatric Considerations
Incidence of AAA, risk of rupture, and operative morbidity and mortality all rise with age.

Pediatric Considerations
Rare in children; may be associated with umbilical artery catheters, connective tissue diseases, arteritides, or congenital abnormalities

EPIDEMIOLOGY

- Estimated prevalence of AAA in developed countries is 2–8%. Age-related increase is seen more with men than women.
- Ultrasound studies show that 4–8% of older men have an occult AAA.
- 90% of all AAA >4 cm are related to atherosclerotic disease, with the vast majority located infrarenally.
- Predominant sex: male > female

Incidence
- >10,000 deaths per year in United States
- 3.9–7.2% males >50 years
- 1.0–1.3% females >50 years

Prevalence
- Roughly 1 million U.S. individuals have an AAA, with the prevalence increasing in age for men and women.
- The prevalence of AAA-associated mortality has decreased by 50% since the 1990s, likely due to the decline in cigarette smoking, increased screening for AAA detection, and early interventions.
- With the increasing life expectancy in developed countries, the prevalence of AAA is expected to increase, but the decreased prevalence of smoking will have the opposite effect.

ETIOLOGY AND PATHOPHYSIOLOGY

- AAAs are caused by degradations of abnormal production of elastin and collagen, the structural components of the aortic wall.
- There are many causes of aortic aneurysms: inflammation, degenerative disorders, vasculitis, infections,

and trauma. However, the vast majority of AAA are caused by inflammation with atherosclerosis as the inciting factor.
- B-cell and T-cell lymphocytes, macrophages, inflammatory cytokines, and matrix metalloproteinases degrade elastin and collagen, thus decreasing the aortic wall strength, leading to a decreased ability to accommodate the pulsatile flow.
- Histopathology shows elastin and collagen destruction, decreased vascular smooth muscle, ingrowth of new blood vessels, and subsequent inflammation.
- Although most aortic aneurysms are caused by inflammatory or degenerative destruction of elastin and collagen, infections, trauma, and connective tissues disorders can also degrade elastin and collagen, leading to similar presentations.

Genetics
- Familial aggregations exist: Aneurysms may develop at an earlier age.
- ~10% of AAA are familial, with a prevalence of 13% among affected families.
- Marfan syndrome
- Ehlers-Danlos syndrome
- Polycystic kidney disease
- Tuberous sclerosis
- Gene associations:
  - ANRIL: antisense RNA regulating cyclin-dependent kinase inhibitors
  - DAB2: cell growth and survival inhibitor
  - LRP1: low-density lipoprotein receptor–related protein 1, plasma receptor in vascular smooth muscle, and macrophage endocytosis
  - IL-6R and IL-1RN: part of the interleukin family contributing to IL-1 inhibition

RISK FACTORS
Older age, male sex, Caucasian race, family history, smoking, hypertension (HTN), hyperlipidemia, atherosclerosis, peripheral aneurysms, obesity

GENERAL PREVENTION
- Address cardiovascular disease risk factors.
- Follow screening guidelines: U.S. screening for detection of AAA in male patients, 65 to 75 years, who have ever smoked.

COMMONLY ASSOCIATED CONDITIONS
- HTN, myocardial infarction (MI), heart failure, carotid artery atherosclerosis, and/or lower extremity peripheral arterial disease
- Screening for thoracic aneurysm should also be considered.
- 20% of patients with AAA have concurrent thoracic aneurysm (1).

DIAGNOSIS

- Asymptomatic AAA (majority)
  - USPSTF recommends a one-time screen for an AAA by abdominal ultrasonography for men aged 65 to 75 years with a smoking history (2)[A].
  - Selective screening for AAAs in nonsmoker men aged 65 to 75 years can be offered based on personal or family history and patient's preferences (2)[A].
  - Current recommendations are against routine screening for women, regardless of smoking history.

- Symptomatic: The triad of shock, pulsatile mass, and abdominal pain always suggest rupture of AAA, and immediate surgical evaluation is recommended (1)[A].
  - Hemodynamically stable patients (shock is absent as the rupture is contained) may undergo a CT abdomen with IV contrast for evaluation of an AAA.
  - Unstable patients (rupture is uncontained) undergo a focused bedside ultrasound and surgical repair if AAA is present.
- Unusual presentations:
  - Primary aortoenteric fistula: erosion/rupture of AAA into duodenum
  - Aortocaval fistula: erosion/rupture of AAA into vena cava or left renal vein: 3–6%
  - Inflammatory aneurysm: encasement by thick inflammatory rind; can cause chronic abdominal pain, weight loss, and elevated ESR. Surrounding viscera may be densely adherent.

HISTORY
- Abdominal, back, or flank pain; AAA risk factors, hypotension if presenting in an emergency situation
- Found on routine screening if presenting in an outpatient setting

PHYSICAL EXAM
- Pulsatile supraumbilical mass
- In one study, sensitivity varied based on abdominal girth and size of aneurysm. However, the sensitivity was 100% of aneurysms >5.0 cm when the girth was <100 cm. The sensitivity and specificity varied from 23% to 68% and 75% to 91%, respectively (3).
- Encroachment by aneurysm
  - Vertebral body erosion, gastric outlet obstruction, ureteral obstruction
  - Lower extremity ischemia secondary to embolization of mural thrombus
- Rupture leads to tachycardia, hypotension, evidence of shock and anemia, and possible flank contusion (Grey Turner sign).

DIFFERENTIAL DIAGNOSIS
- Other abdominal masses
- Other causes of abdominal or back pain (e.g., peptic ulcer disease, renal colic, diverticulitis, appendicitis, incarcerated hernia, bowel obstruction, GI hemorrhage, arthritis, metastatic disease, MI)

DIAGNOSTIC TESTS & INTERPRETATION
Initial Tests (lab, imaging)
- If rupturing AAA is considered: complete blood chemistry (chemistries, PT/INR, PTT, type and cross), ECG
- Ultrasound: simplest and least expensive diagnostic procedure with a high sensitivity (94–100%) and specificity (98–100%) (1)[A]
- Surveillance of asymptomatic aneurysm
  - 2.6 to 2.9 cm: Screen at 5-year intervals.
  - 3.0 to 3.9 cm: Screen at 3-year intervals.
  - 4.0 to 5.4 cm: Screen every 6 to 12 months.
- CT scans are preferred preoperative study (caution with IV contrast in renal failure) (1).
- MRI/MRA can visualize AAA but is often not possible in emergent situations.
- Aortography does not define outer dimensions of aneurysm.
- Abdominal x-rays can be diagnostic if calcifications exist; not a diagnostic tool of choice

Follow-Up Tests & Special Considerations

- Evaluation for coronary artery disease is appropriate prior to elective AAA repair, including stress test, echocardiography, and ECG if appropriate.
- If AAA was discovered at any location, then full assessment of entire aorta, including thoracic aorta and aortic valve, is recommended (1)[C].

Diagnostic Procedures/Other

ALERT

Use clinical judgment: Patients with known AAA having abdominal or back pain symptoms may be rupturing despite a negative CT scan.

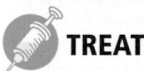 TREATMENT

GENERAL MEASURES

- Treat atherosclerotic risk factors: HTN, dyslipidemia, diabetes mellitus, and smoking (2)[A].
- Smoking was associated with a 0.35 mm/year AAA growth, twice as fast as AAA growth in nonsmokers, and is the most important AAA outcome predictor (1).
- Emergent treatment in unstable or symptomatic patients requires immediate vascular surgery consultation, adequate IV access and resuscitation, type and cross for multiple units, and rapid bedside ultrasound (1).
- Less acute treatment of AAA/prevention of rupture is elective repair and risk factor modification.

MEDICATION

- β-Blockers, aspirin, and statins theoretically reduce the rate of growth of AAAs by decreasing shear wall stress, inflammation, and prevention of an intraluminal mural thrombus. However, there are conflicting RCT and meta-analysis trials. Because concomitant atherosclerosis is often a precipitating factor in AAAs, their use is recommended for reduced mortality in patients with coronary artery disease or its equivalents (4)[A].
- The use of ACE inhibitors has shown to be inconclusive with regard to growth of AAA; however, studies do indicate a decreased rate of AAA rupture (4)[A].
- Doxycycline and roxithromycin, previously theorized to decreased wall inflammation, have not been shown to have any effect on AAA (5).

SURGERY/OTHER PROCEDURES

Current recommendations are the following:
- Elective
  - 5.5-cm diameter is threshold for repair in "average" patient (1)[A].
  - Younger, low-risk patients with long-life expectancy may prefer early repair.
  - Saccular aneurysms should be considered for elective repair (1)[C].
  - Women or AAA with high risk of rupture: Consider elective repair at 4.5 to 5.0 cm.
    - Consider delayed repair in high-risk patients.
    - 5% perioperative mortality for open elective repair (1)
- High risk of rupture
  - Expansion >0.5 cm/year
  - Smoking/COPD severe/steroids
  - Family history; multiple relatives
  - HTN if poorly controlled
  - Shape nonfusiform
- High-risk patients for elective repair
  - Risk factors for open repair include age >75 years, COPD, chronic kidney disease with Cr >1.75, and suprarenal clamp site.

- The leading cause of early mortality after AAA repair is coronary artery disease, with open AAA repair being much higher risk than endovascular AAA repair (1)[A].
- The RCT IMPROVE trial showed a similar 30-day mortality for patients with ruptured AAA who underwent endovascular repair versus open repair (35.4% vs. 37.4%); 1-year follow-up all cause mortality between the two groups (41.1% vs. 45.1%) (5)[A]
- Although difficult to quantify, perioperative morbidity rates are lower for EVAR, suggesting that an EVAR is preferable in patients with a ruptured AAA with poor prognostic factors for an open repair, such as SBP <80, age >80 years, Cr >1.3 on admission, ischemic heart disease, female sex, and hemoglobin <9.0 on admission (2,5)[A].
- Contraindications for AAA endovascular repair are an aortic neck >32 mm and a ruptured AAA with aortic neck length <7 mm. In these patients, an open AAA repair is performed due to anatomical constrictions.

ADMISSION, INPATIENT, AND NURSING CONSIDERATIONS

Risk of abdominal compartment syndrome after repair, 4–12%; usually associated with large fluid resuscitation

 ONGOING CARE

FOLLOW-UP RECOMMENDATIONS

Patient Monitoring

- May do a CT scan 5 years after an open repair for possible late aortic dilatation or pseudoaneurysm (2)[C]
- Follow-up imaging should be tailored to patient. Once renal function stabilizes postoperatively, a CT can be performed to evaluate the endograft (2)[C].
- Aggressive risk factor modification always recommended postoperatively (2)[A]

DIET

Low-fat, low-salt, and low-caffeine diet; nutrition optimized prior to elective repair

PATIENT EDUCATION

Smoking cessation, aerobic exercise

PROGNOSIS

- Naturally progressive disorder, expands at an average rate of 0.3 to 0.4 cm per year. A fast expansion is considered >0.6 cm per year and should be evaluated for operative management.
- Possibility of rupture increases with an aneurysm diameter of >5.5 cm or a fast rate of expansion (>0.5 cm over a 6-month period), continued cigarette use, female sex, recent surgery, uncontrolled HTN, and aneurysm couture.

COMPLICATIONS

- Emergent AAA repair and elective AAA repair have similar complications, with a higher incidence in emergent AAA repair.
- Complications include MI, respiratory failure, and acute kidney injury in the early period.
- Late complications such as aortic graft infection, aortoenteric fistula, and graft occlusion have similar rates between emergent and elective repair.
- Ischemic bowel and abdominal compartment syndrome are complications usually after a ruptured open AAA repair given the massive blood loss, increased operative time, and magnitude of fluid resuscitation.

REFERENCES

1. Chaikof EL, Dalman RL, Eskandari MK, et al. The Society for Vascular Surgery practice guidelines on the care of patients with an abdominal aortic aneurysm. *J Vasc Surg*. 2018;67(1):2.e2–77.e2.
2. LeFevre ML; for U.S. Preventive Services Task Force. Screening for abdominal aortic aneurysm: U.S. Preventive Services Task Force recommendation statement. *Ann Intern Med*. 2014;161(4):281–290.
3. Fink HA, Lederle FA, Roth CS, et al. The accuracy of physical examination to detect abdominal aortic aneurysm. *Arch Intern Med*. 2000;160(6):833–836.
4. Guessous I, Periard D, Lorenzetti D, et al. The efficacy of pharmacotherapy for decreasing the expansion rate of abdominal aortic aneurysms: a systematic review and meta-analysis. *PLoS One*. 2008;3(3):e1895.
5. Braithwaite B, Cheshire NJ, Greenhalgh RM, et al; for IMPROVE Trial Investigators. Endovascular strategy or open repair for ruptured abdominal aortic aneurysm: one-year outcomes from the IMPROVE randomized trial. *Eur Heart J*. 2015;36(31):2061–2069.

ADDITIONAL READING

- Aggarwal S, Qamar A, Sharma V, et al. Abdominal aortic aneurysm: a comprehensive review. *Exp Clin Cardiol*. 2011;16(1):11–15.
- Kuivaniemi H, Ryer EJ, Elmore JR, et al. Understanding the pathogenesis of abdominal aortic aneurysms. *Expert Rev Cardiovasc Ther*. 2015;13(9):975–987.
- Mussa FF. Screening for abdominal aortic aneurysm. *J Vasc Surg*. 2015;62(3):774–778.
- Sweeting MJ, Thompson SG, Brown LC, et al; for RESCAN Collaborators. Meta-analysis of individual patient data to examine factors affecting growth and rupture of small abdominal aortic aneurysms. *Br J Surg*. 2012;99(5):655–665.

 SEE ALSO

Aortic Dissection; Arteritis, Temporal; Ehlers-Danlos Syndrome; Marfan Syndrome; Polyarteritis Nodosa; Turner Syndrome

 CODES

ICD10

- I71.4 Abdominal aortic aneurysm, without rupture
- I71.3 Abdominal aortic aneurysm, ruptured

CLINICAL PEARLS

- Males with a smoking history aged 65 to 75 years should undergo a one-time screening abdominal ultrasound to evaluate for an AAA.
- Larger AAAs should be screened more often, with elective repair with AAA >5.5 cm or an expansion of >0.5 cm every 6 months.
- Patients with a ruptured AAA present in shock, with abdominal pain and a pulsatile mass. A bedside ultrasound should be done quickly to evaluate for an AAA, or an emergent CT scan can be performed if the patient is hemodynamically stable.
- AAA are treated either open or endovascularly as an elective or emergent procedure. 30-day and 1-year mortality between the two methods remain the same; however, there is increased mortality with an emergent AAA repair.
- Patients require aggressive risk factor modification, especially smoking cessation.

ANGIOEDEMA

Kathryn M. Brown, MD • Haley Stewart, DO • Katherine Montag Schafer, PharmD, BCACP

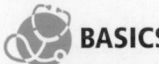 BASICS

DESCRIPTION
- Angioedema (AE) is acute, localized swelling of skin, mucosa, and submucosa caused by extravasation of fluid into the affected tissues.
- AE develops in minutes to hours and resolves in hours to days but can be life-threatening if the upper airway is involved.
- Two major classifications of AE exist:
  - Histamine- or immune-mediated AE (HIAE) with urticarial
  - Bradykinin-mediated AE without urticaria; both with unique subtypes
- Synonym(s): angioneurotic edema; Quincke edema

EPIDEMIOLOGY
- Predominant age
  - HIAE or idiopathic AE (IAE): any age
  - Hereditary AE (HAE): age of onset infancy to 2nd decade of life
  - Acquired AE (AAE): often patients >40 years
- Predominant gender: male = female (except HAE with normal compliment: women > men)

Prevalence
- AE occurs in 15% of the population over a lifetime.
- AE: 0.1–2.2% of patients receiving angiotensin-converting enzyme (ACE) inhibitors: African Americans have a 4 to 5 times greater risk of ACE inhibitor–induced AE than Caucasians.
- HAE: 1:10,000 to 50,000 population in the United States

ETIOLOGY AND PATHOPHYSIOLOGY
- HIAE with urticarial (1):
  - Allergy to food (shellfish, nuts, eggs, milk, wheat soy), latex, venom, or medication (aspirin, NSAIDs, antibiotics, narcotics, and OCPs)
  - Acute and chronic spontaneous urticaria
  - Other urticarial/AE syndromes: cold urticaria, urticarial vasculitis, exercise-induced urticaria or anaphylaxis, episodic eosinophilia with AE, vibration-induced urticaria
  - IAE
- Bradykinin-mediated AE without urticarial (1):
  - Attacks are triggered by prolonged mechanical pressure, cold, heat, trauma, emotional stress, menses, illness, and inflammation.
  - HAE due to C1 INH deficiency
    - Type I: the most common form, caused by decreased production of C1 esterase inhibitor (C1 INH)
    - Type II: functionally impaired C1 INH
  - HAE with normal C1 INH levels
    - Formerly type III HAE
    - Involves mutations in coagulation factor XII gene, often estrogen dependent, associated with estrogen administration
  - AAE with C1 INH deficiency
    - Rare condition
    - Associated with lymphoproliferative disorders, autoimmune diseases (e.g., lupus)
    - Type I: lack of anti–C1 INH autoantibody
    - Type II: presence of anti–C1 INH autoantibody

- AE due to medications
  - ACE inhibitors
  - Dipeptidyl peptidase-4 inhibitors
  - Direct renin inhibitor
  - IAE

Genetics
- HAE types I and II are autosomal dominant, whereas HAE with normal C1 INH is dominant X-linked.
- HAE occurs in 25% of patients as a result of spontaneous genetic mutations.

RISK FACTORS
- Consuming medications and foods that can cause allergic reactions
- Preexisting diagnosis of HAE or AAE
- Positive family history

GENERAL PREVENTION
- Avoid known triggers.
- Do not use ACE inhibitors in type I or II HAE.

COMMONLY ASSOCIATED CONDITIONS
- Quincke disease (AE of the uvula)
- Urticaria

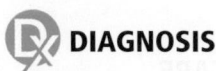 DIAGNOSIS

HISTORY
- Acute, typically asymmetric, swelling with onset in minutes to hours (2)
- In comparison with urticaria, AE typically is nonpruritic, but it can cause a painful, burning sensation (2).
- Recent exposure to food allergens or medications (2)
- Identify potential triggers such as environmental exposure or trauma (2).
- Family history of AE (2)
- Recent infection, history of autoimmune disease, or malignancy (3)

PHYSICAL EXAM
- Vitals: Symptoms of hypotension, tachycardia, and tachypnea indicate systemic involvement and increased severity (3).
- Tense, nonpitting skin swelling that is skin colored or slightly erythematous (2)
- Commonly affects the mucus membranes of the face including periorbital, lips, tongue, or larynx but can involve any part of the body (2)
- Evaluate for involvement of oropharynx or symptoms such as stridor (3).
- GI tract involvement is more common in HAE and AAE and may manifest as intermittent, unexplained abdominal pain (2).
- May be accompanied by hives and itching (1)

ALERT
- Select history and exam findings increase the likelihood for early intubation and tracheostomy, including involvement of the anterior tongue, base of the tongue or larynx, stridor within 4 hours of onset of symptoms, and drooling (1)[C].
- Patients with HAE or bradykinin-mediated AE are at higher risk for intubation, tracheostomy, and death, although these complications can occur with any subtype (3)[C].

DIFFERENTIAL DIAGNOSIS
Urticaria; anaphylaxis; contact dermatitis; food/drug allergy; erysipelas; connective tissue disease: systemic lupus erythematosus, dermatomyositis; lymphedema; insect bite reaction; diffuse subcutaneous infiltrative process (4)[C]

DIAGNOSTIC TESTS & INTERPRETATION
Initial Tests (lab, imaging)
- Initial diagnosis should be based on history and clinical assessment alone (3)[C].
- Laboratory testing includes CBC, ESR, complement testing (C4, C1 INH, C1 INH function), allergy testing, and screening for paraproteinemia (1,2)[C].
- For emergent management, C4 and tryptase levels may assist in diagnosis of HAE and AE associated with anaphylaxis (3)[C].
- Complement testing assists in distinguishing between various types of HAE and AAE (1)[C]:
  - Low serum C4 is a sensitive but nonspecific screening test for hereditary and acquired C1 INH deficiency.
  - If C4 is normal, determine C1 INH level and function and recheck C4 during an acute attack.
  - If C4 level and C1 INH level and function are still normal, consider other causes (i.e., medications or HAE type III) of AE.
  - If C4 level, C1 INH level, and C1 INH function are low, these indicate HAE type I.
  - HAE type II is characterized by low C4 and low C1 INH function, but C1 INH level can be normal or elevated.
- For recurrent AE with urticaria, complement levels should be obtained in addition to allergy testing for potential triggers (1)[C].
- Abdominal radiographs and CT scan can demonstrate GI AE or ileus (1)[C].
- C1 INH deficiency may occur in association with internal malignancy, so AE rarely can be a paraneoplastic disease. Imaging (CT scan, radiography, etc.) would be done as part of a neoplastic workup for patients with AAE (1)[C].

Follow-Up Tests & Special Considerations
If C4 and C1q antigen are low (as in AAE), neoplastic and autoimmune workup is warranted. CBC, a peripheral smear, protein electrophoresis, immunophenotyping of lymphocytes, and imaging studies are often undertaken to rule out hematologic malignancies or cancer (2)[C].

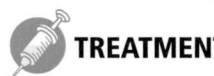 TREATMENT

GENERAL MEASURES
- Intubation if airway is threatened (3)[C]
- Eliminate suspected trigger (2)[C].
- Volume replacement is essential for patients who are unstable or refractory to initial therapy (3)[C].

MEDICATION

First Line

- If AE presenting with signs of anaphylaxis (hypotension, respiratory compromise): epinephrine 1:1,000; 0.1 mg/kg (maximum 0.3 mg for children, 0.5 mg for adults) intramuscularly q5–15min (3,5)[C]
- If cause of AE is unknown:
  – Epinephrine, if airway involvement
  – H_1 antagonist (IV diphenhydramine, adult: 25 to 50 mg, children: 1 mg/kg, maximum 50 mg). In older adults, side effects can include delirium, urinary retention, constipation, and increased ocular pressure (3,5)[C].
  – H_2 antagonists (IV ranitidine, adult: 50 mg, children: 1 mg/kg, maximum 50 mg) (3,5)[C]
  – Corticosteroids (IV hydrocortisone, adult: 200 mg, children: maximum 100 mg; or IV methylprednisolone, adult: 50 to 100 mg, children: 1 mg/kg, maximum 50 mg) (3,5)[C]
- HIAE acute treatment: H_1 antagonist, H_2 antagonist, corticosteroids, and epinephrine, if airway involvement (3,5)[C]
  – If time critical, IV therapy preferred
  – If time is not critical, can consider 2nd-generation (nonsedating) H_1 antagonist
- HAE acute treatment:
  – H_1 antagonists, corticosteroids, and epinephrine are ineffective and not recommended (6)[C].
  – GI involvement: analgesics and antiemetics for pain and nausea (3)[C]
  – Ruconest (recombinant human C1 INH): Trained adult and adolescent (13 to 17 years of age) patients may self-administer via slow IV injection (over 5 minutes). Dosing: 50 U/kg (maximum 4,200 U) if <84 kg and 4,200 IU if ≥84 kg. Maximum of 2 doses in 24 hours. Serious adverse reaction: anaphylaxis (1)[C]
  – Berinert (human plasma-derived [pd] C1 INH [pdC1 INH]): Trained adult and adolescent patients may self-administer via peripheral vein IV infusion (4 mL/min). Dosing: 20 U/kg. *Do not shake* (will denature the protein). Serious adverse reaction: anaphylaxis (1)[C]
  – Ecallantide (Kalbitor): labeled for use in those ≥12 years. Dosing: 30 mg subcutaneously (SC) with three separate 10 mg/mL injections in the abdomen, thigh, or upper arm, and a second 30-mg dose may be repeated within 24 hours if needed. Injection-site rotation is not necessary but must be 2 inches away from attack site. Serious adverse reaction: anaphylaxis; unlike previous agents, required administration in health care setting (1)[C]
  – Icatibant (Firazyr): Adult patients may self-administer via slow SC injection (over 30 seconds). Dosing: 30 mg in the abdomen, thigh, or upper arm. Subsequent doses of 30 mg may be repeated in 6-hour intervals (max 90 mg/24 hours) (1)[C].
- AAE acute treatment:
  – H_1 antagonists, corticosteroids, and epinephrine are ineffective and not recommended (6)[C].
  – Off-label uses: C1 INH replacement, ecallantide, icatibant (1,6)[C]
  – Associated improvement, possible remission, through treatment of underlying disease (6)[C]

- IAE, recurrent, acute treatment:
  – H_1 antagonists, corticosteroids, and epinephrine may be effective (1,2)[C].
  – Anecdotal, off-label uses: C1 INH replacement, ecallantide, icatibant (1)[C]
- HAE prophylaxis:
  – All patients are eligible for short-term prophylaxis during periods where known exposure to trigger is expected (e.g., dental work, invasive medical or surgical procedures) (6)[C].
    ○ Off-label use: Cinryze (IV pdC1 INH concentrate), androgens (danazol)
  – During these exposures, should ensure access to acute treatment modalities (6)[C]
  – In patients not managed successfully with acute treatment, can consider use of long-term prophylactic agent (6)[C]
    ○ FDA-approved therapies: Cinryze (IV pdC1 INH concentrate), Haegarda (SC pdC1 INH concentrate), lanadelumab (Takhzyro), androgens (danazol)

Second Line

HAE acute treatment: FFP can be considered if first-line treatments unavailable; however, can potentially worsen attack, so caution is required (6)[C]

ISSUES FOR REFERRAL

Patients presenting with first episode of AE with a positive family history or recurrent AE will benefit from management from allergy/immunology specialist for diagnosis, treatment selection, education, and formation of emergency and procedural action plans (3)[C].

SURGERY/OTHER PROCEDURES

Tracheostomy if progressive laryngeal edema prevents endotracheal intubation

ADMISSION, INPATIENT, AND NURSING CONSIDERATIONS

Need for admission is based on severity of airway involvement. Ishoo criteria can be used for risk stratification. All patients with respiratory distress or in need of airway support will benefit from treatment in an intensive care unit (3)[C].

ONGOING CARE

FOLLOW-UP RECOMMENDATIONS

Patient Monitoring

- Diagnostic workup if symptoms are severe, persistent, or recurrent
- For those with recurrent AE, specialty management is recommended.

DIET

Avoid identified food allergens.

PATIENT EDUCATION

Educate on avoidance of known triggers, types of treatment, when to seek emergency care, and wearing medical alert bracelet.

PROGNOSIS

- AE symptoms often resolve in hours to 2 to 4 days. If airway is compromised, AE can be life-threatening.
- Patients with HAE have an average of 20 attacks per year; each may last 3 to 5 days. Prophylaxis can decrease the frequency of events and number of missed days of school or work.

COMPLICATIONS

Anaphylaxis

REFERENCES

1. LoVerde D, Files DC, Krishnaswamy G. Angioedema. *Crit Care Med*. 2017;45(4):725–735.
2. Temiño VM, Peebles RS Jr. The spectrum and treatment of angioedema. *Am J Med*. 2008;121(4):282–286.
3. Bernstein JA, Cremonesi P, Hoffmann TK, et al. Angioedema in the emergency department: a practical guide to differential diagnosis and management. *Int J Emerg Med*. 2017;10(1):15.
4. Radonjic-Hoesli S, Hofmeier KS, Micaletto S, et al. Urticaria and angioedema: an update on classification and pathogenesis. *Clin Rev Allergy Immunol*. 2018;54(1):88–101.
5. Simons FE, Ardusso LR, Bilò MB, et al; for World Allergy Organization. World Allergy Organization anaphylaxis guidelines: summary. *J Allergy Clin Immunol*. 2011;127(3):587–593.
6. Zuraw BL, Bernstein JA, Lang DM, et al; for American Academy of Allergy, Asthma and Immunology, American College of Allergy, Asthma and Immunology. A focused parameter update: hereditary angioedema, acquired C1 inhibitor deficiency, and angiotensin-converting enzyme inhibitor-associated angioedema. *J Allergy Clin Immunol*. 2013;131(6):1491–1493.

SEE ALSO

Anaphylaxis; Urticaria

CODES

ICD10

- T78.3XXA Angioneurotic edema, initial encounter
- D84.1 Defects in the complement system

CLINICAL PEARLS

- AE is an acute, localized swelling of skin, mucosa, and submucosa caused by extravasation of fluid into the affected tissues.
- Onset is in minutes to hours and often resolves in hours to days, but it can be life-threatening if the upper airway is involved.
- There are two major classifications of AE: HIAE and bradykinin-mediated AE (subtypes include HAE and AAE). IAE can be of either type.
- HIAE is more likely to be associated with urticaria and responsive to H_1 antagonists, corticosteroids, and epinephrine.
- Any recurrent AE requires specialist management.
- Patients with a history of HIAE should be prescribed an epinephrine autoinjector.

ANKLE FRACTURES

Jeffrey P. Feden, MD, FACEP

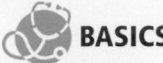

BASICS

- Bones: tibia, fibula, talus
- Mortise: tibial plafond, medial and lateral malleolus
- Ligaments: syndesmotic, lateral collateral, and medial collateral (deltoid) ligament

DESCRIPTION

- Two common classification systems help describe fractures (but do not always predict fracture stability).
  - Danis-Weber system: based on level of the fibular fracture in relationship to the ankle joint
    - Type A (30%): below ankle joint; usually stable
    - Type B (63%): at the level of the ankle joint; may be stable or unstable
    - Type C (7%): above ankle joint; usually unstable
  - Lauge-Hansen (LH): based on foot position and direction of applied force relative to the tibia
    - Supination-adduction (SA)
    - Supination-external rotation (SER): most common (40–75% of fractures)
    - Pronation-abduction (PA)
    - Pronation-external rotation (PER)
- Stability-based classification
  - Stable
    - Isolated lateral malleolar fractures (Weber A/B) without talar shift and with negative stress test
    - Isolated nondisplaced medial malleolar fractures
  - Unstable
    - Bi- or trimalleolar fractures
    - High fibular fractures (Weber C) or lateral malleolar fracture with medial injury and positive stress test
    - Lateral malleolar fracture with talar shift/tilt (bimalleolar equivalent)
    - Displaced medial malleolar fractures
- Pilon fracture: tibial plafond fracture due to axial loading (unstable)
- Maisonneuve: fracture of proximal 1/3 of fibula associated with ankle fracture (unstable); high risk of peroneal nerve injury

Pediatric Considerations

- Ankle fractures are more common than sprains in children compared to adults because ligaments are stronger than physis.
- Talar dome: osteochondral fracture of talar dome; suspect in child with nonhealing ankle "sprain" or recurrent effusions.
- Tillaux: isolated Salter-Harris III of distal tibia with growth plate involvement
- Triplane fracture: Salter-Harris IV with fracture lines oriented in multiple planes: 2-, 3-, and 4-part variants

EPIDEMIOLOGY

- Ankle fractures are responsible for 9% of all adult and 5% of all pediatric fractures.
- Peak incidence: females 45 to 64 years; males 8 to 15 years (average is 46 years)

Incidence

107 to 184 per 100,000 people per year

ETIOLOGY AND PATHOPHYSIOLOGY

- Most common: falls (38%), inversion injury (32%), sports related (10%)
- Plantar flexion (joint less stable in this position)
- Axial loading: tibial plafond or pilon fracture

RISK FACTORS

- Age, fall, fracture history, polypharmacy, intoxication
- Obesity, sedentary lifestyle
- Sports, physical activity
- History of smoking or diabetes
- Alcohol or slippery surfaces

GENERAL PREVENTION

- Nonslip, flat, protective shoes
- Fall precautions in elderly

COMMONLY ASSOCIATED CONDITIONS

- Most ankle fractures are isolated injuries, but 5% have associated fractures, usually in ipsilateral lower limb.
- Ligamentous or cartilage injury (sprains)
- Ankle or subtalar dislocation
- Other axial loading or shearing injuries (i.e., vertebral compression or contralateral pelvic fractures)

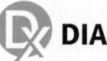

DIAGNOSIS

HISTORY

- Location of pain, timing, and mechanism of injury (key historical element is exact mechanism)
- Weight-bearing status after injury
- History of ankle injury or surgery
- Tetanus status
- Assess for safety and fall risk (especially in elderly).

PHYSICAL EXAM

- Examine skin integrity (open vs. closed fracture).
- Assess point of maximal tenderness.
- Assess neurovascular status and ability to bear weight.
- Consider associated injuries.
- Assess ankle stability: anterior drawer test for the anterior talofibular ligament (ATFL), talar tilt test for lateral and medial ligaments, squeeze test and external rotation stress test for the tibiofibular syndesmosis.

DIFFERENTIAL DIAGNOSIS

- Ankle sprain
- Other fractures: talus, 5th metatarsal, calcaneus

DIAGNOSTIC TESTS & INTERPRETATION

- Plain radiographs: first line for suspected fractures based on pretest probability (Ottawa Rules)
- Ottawa Ankle Rules (OAR): Overall sensitivity of 98% in adults increases to 99.6% if applied within the first 48 hours after trauma (1)[A].
- OAR obtain films in patients aged 18 to 55 years if:
  - Tenderness at the posterior edge of distal 6 cm of tibia or tip of the medial malleolus, *or*
  - Tenderness at the posterior edge or distal 6 cm of fibula or tip of the lateral malleolus, *or*
  - Inability to bear weight both immediately and in the ED for four steps, *or*
  - Tenderness at navicular or 5th metatarsal (Ottawa Foot Rules)

- If initial x-ray is normal, but severe symptoms persist past 48 to 72 hours, obtain repeat x-rays.
- In children >1 year old, OAR sensitivity is 98.5%.
- OAR not valid for intoxicated patients, those with multiple injuries, or sensory deficits (neuropathy)
- Three standard views
  - Anteroposterior (AP)
  - Lateral: Talar dome/distal tibia incongruity indicates instability.
  - Mortise (15- to 25-degree internal rotation view): symmetry of mortise; space between the medial malleolus and talus should be ≤4 mm.
  - Additional stress view may demonstrate instability: increased medial clear space with manual external rotation

Pediatric Considerations

- Consider tenderness over distal fibula with normal films as Salter-Harris I.
- Stress views unnecessary in children and may cause physeal damage.
- Salter-Harris V often missed, diagnosed when leg length discrepancy or angular deformity after Salter-Harris I; rare, 1% of fractures

Follow-Up Tests & Special Considerations

- CT recommended for operative planning in trimalleolar, Tillaux, triplane, pilon fractures, or fractures with intra-articular involvement
- MRI not routinely indicated; does not increase sensitivity for detecting complex ankle fractures
  - MRI useful for chronic instability, osteochondral lesions, occult fractures, and unexpected stiffness in children

Diagnostic Procedures/Other

- Ultrasound for soft tissue injury associated with displaced fractures
- Bone scan or MRI for stress fracture

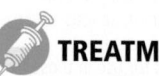

TREATMENT

GENERAL MEASURES

- Immobilize in temporary cast/splint and protect with crutches/non–weight-bearing.
  - 1 to 2 weeks to allow decreased swelling, if not open or irreducible fracture (2)[C]
- Ice and elevate the extremity; pain due to swelling best controlled with elevation
  - Compression stockings offer no benefit for swelling (3)[A].
- Closed ankle fractures—must determine stability
  - Stable = nonoperative
  - Unstable = surgery
  - Lateral shift of talus ≥2 mm or displacement of either malleolus by 2 to 3 mm = surgery (2)[C]
  - In adults with displaced fractures: insufficient evidence if surgery or nonoperative management produces superior long-term outcomes (4)[A]
- Stable syndesmosis injury = nonoperative
- Fracture dislocations: urgent reduction
  - Do not wait for imaging if neurovascular compromise or obvious deformity.
  - Flex hip and knee 90 degrees for easier reduction.
  - Postreduction: neurovascular exam and x-rays

MEDICATION

First Line

- NSAIDs and/or acetaminophen for pain
- Initial IM pain injection (i.e., ketorolac, ≥50-kg adult: 60 mg or 30 mg q6h, max 120 mg daily; children 2 to 16 years old, <50 kg or age of ≥65 years: 1 mg/kg, 30 mg, or 15 mg q6h, max 60 mg daily)
- For suspected open fractures: tetanus booster, broad-spectrum cephalosporin and aminoglycoside within 3 hours postinjury (2)[C]
- Intra-articular or hematoma block

Second Line

Opioid analgesics as adjunctive therapy

ISSUES FOR REFERRAL

- Consultation for neurovascular compromise, tenting of skin or open fracture, displaced or unstable fracture, compartment syndrome
- All other fractures: Follow up within 1 week and remain non–weight-bearing. Consult orthopedics if not comfortable with routine fracture management.

ADDITIONAL THERAPIES

- Nonoperative = cast immobilization
  - No difference in type of immobilization (Air-Stirrup, cast, orthosis) (3)[A]
  - Initially non–weight-bearing with crutches and then advance to 50% with crutches; full weight-bearing after 6 weeks postinjury
  - If removable cast, gentle range of motion exercises at 4 weeks
- Open ankle fractures (2%)
  - Remove gross debris/contamination in ED.
  - Duration of optimal antibiotic therapy controversial
  - Surgical emergency; best if repaired within 24 hours

SURGERY/OTHER PROCEDURES

- Surgical options
  - Open reduction and internal fixation (ORIF); preferred in athletes and unstable fractures
  - External fixation may be preferred in extreme tissue injury or comminuted fractures; may have more malunion compared to ORIF but no difference in wound complications
- Timing of surgery
  - Immediately if neurovascular compromise, open fracture, unsuccessful reduction, tissue necrosis (2)[C]
  - Otherwise delay >5 days postinjury because inflammation can affect wound healing (2)[C].
- Length of recovery is usually 6 to 8 weeks.

Pediatric Considerations

- Salter-Harris I and II = nonoperative
  - Distal tibia: long leg cast for 4 to 6 weeks and then short leg cast for 2 to 3 weeks (5)[C]
  - Distal fibula: posterior splint or ankle brace 3 to 4 weeks, weight-bearing; if displaced, then short leg cast 4 to 6 weeks, non–weight-bearing (5)[C]
  - Limit reduction attempts because of potential injury to growth plate (5,6)[C].
  - Reduction not recommended if presenting ≥1 week postinjury (5)[C]
  - Intra-articular displacement of ≥2 mm in child with >2 years growth remaining = ORIF (6)[C]

- Salter-Harris III and IV:
  - Distal tibia: if >2 mm displacement = ORIF (6)[C]
  - Distal fibula: rare, usually stable after tibial reduction (6)[C]
  - Tillaux and triplane: ORIF if displaced ≥2 mm (5,6)[C]

Geriatric Considerations

- Higher surgical risk due to age/comorbidities
- Osteoporosis increases risk of implant/fixation failure (4)[A].
- Risks from surgery/anesthesia: wound healing problems, pulmonary embolism, mortality, amputation, reoperation

ADMISSION, INPATIENT, AND NURSING CONSIDERATIONS

- Admit if:
  - Emergency surgery required
  - Patient nonadherent, lacks social support, unable to maintain non–weight-bearing status, or has significant associated injuries
  - Concerning mechanism of injury (i.e., syncope, myocardial infarction, head injury)
- Nursing: non–weight-bearing; maintain splint/cast; apply ice; keep leg elevated; pain control; assist ADLs.
- Discharge criteria:
  - Ambulates with walker or crutches
  - Medical workup (if needed) completed
  - Orthopedic follow-up arranged

 ONGOING CARE

FOLLOW-UP RECOMMENDATIONS

Patient Monitoring

- Orthopedic follow-up: serial x-rays
  - In children, sclerotic lines on x-ray (Parker-Harris growth arrest lines) indicate growth disturbance (5)[C].
- Immobilize for 4 to 6 weeks and then progressive activity, weight-bearing, with removable splint or boot (3)[A].
- Physical therapy referral: no difference in outcomes between stretching, manual therapy, exercise program (3)[A]

DIET

NPO if surgery is being considered

PATIENT EDUCATION

- Ice and elevate for 2 to 3 weeks; use crutches/cane as instructed; splint/cast care (avoid getting wet, etc.)
- Notify physician if swelling increases, paresthesias, pain, or change in color of extremity.

PROGNOSIS

- Good results can be achieved without surgery if fracture is stable.
  - Most return to activity within 3 to 4 months.
- Most athletes return to preinjury activity levels.
- Increasing age, *not* injury severity, is associated with worsening mobility after fracture.

COMPLICATIONS

- Displaced fracture or instability
- Delayed union, malunion, or nonunion (0.9–1.9%)
- Postsurgical wound problems: loss of fixation, further surgery, amputation
- Deep venous thrombosis
- Complex regional pain syndrome, extensor retinaculum syndrome in children (5)[C]
- Infection (osteomyelitis)
- Posttraumatic arthritis, degenerative joint disease, growth arrest in children

REFERENCES

1. Polzer H, Kanz KG, Prall WC, et al. Diagnosis and treatment of acute ankle injuries: development of an evidence-based algorithm. *Orthop Rev (Pavia)*. 2012;4(1):e5.
2. Mandi DM. Ankle fractures. *Clin Podiatr Med Surg*. 2012;29(2):155–186.
3. Lin CW, Donkers NA, Refshauge KM, et al. Rehabilitation for ankle fractures in adults. *Cochrane Database Syst Rev*. 2012;(11):CD005595.
4. Donken CC, Al-Khateeb H, Verhofstad MH, et al. Surgical versus conservative interventions for treating ankle fractures in adults. *Cochrane Database Syst Rev*. 2012;(8):CD008470.
5. Parrino A, Lee MC. Ankle fractures in children. *Curr Orthop Pract*. 2013;24:617–624.
6. Kay RM, Matthys GA. Pediatric ankle fractures: evaluation and treatment. *J Am Acad Orthop Surg*. 2001;9(4):268–278.

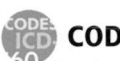 CODES

ICD10

- S82.899A Oth fracture of unsp lower leg, init for clos fx
- S82.899B Oth fracture of unsp lower leg, init for opn fx type I/2
- S82.56XA Nondisp fx of medial malleolus of unsp tibia, init

CLINICAL PEARLS

- OAR are nearly 100% sensitive in determining the need for x-rays.
- Assess neurovascular status, ability to bear weight, and associated injuries.
- Assess joint above/below to avoid overlooking extent of injury (i.e., Maisonneuve).
- Normal x-rays with point tenderness suggest Salter-Harris type I fractures in children.
- Assessment of fracture stability (using classification systems) often dictates conservative versus operative management.

ANKYLOSING SPONDYLITIS

Benjamin J. Slocum, DO • Virginia J. Van Duyne, MD

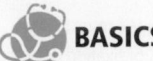 **BASICS**

DESCRIPTION

- Ankylosing spondylitis (AS) is an axial inflammatory spondyloarthropathy (axSpA) characterized by evidence of sacroiliitis on plain radiography.
- System(s) affected: musculoskeletal; eyes; cardiac; neurologic; pulmonary
- Synonym(s): Marie-Strümpell disease; "bamboo spine"

EPIDEMIOLOGY

- Onset usually in early 20s; rarely occurs after age 40 years
- Male > female (approximately 2 to 3:1)

Incidence

Age- and gender-adjusted rate of 6.3 to 7.3/100,000 person-years

Prevalence

~0.55% for AS and ~1.4% for all axSpA in the United States (1)

ETIOLOGY AND PATHOPHYSIOLOGY

- Autoinflammation at sites of bacterial exposure (e.g., intestines) or mechanical stress in genetically susceptible individuals (2)
- Inflammation at the insertion of tendons, ligaments, and fasciae to bone (enthesopathy) causes erosion, remodeling, and new bone formation.
- Inflammation-independent pathways of bony changes have also been hypothesized (2).

Genetics

- 80–90% of patients with AS are *HLA-B27*–positive.
- Other genetic associations include endoplasmic reticulum aminopeptidase 1 (*ERAP1*), interleukin-23 receptor (*IL23R*), and gene deserts on chromosome *2p15* and *21q22* (2).

RISK FACTORS

- HLA-B27
  - 1–8% of HLA-B27–positive adults have AS.
- Positive family history
  - HLA-B27–positive child of a parent with AS has a 10–30% risk of developing the disease.

COMMONLY ASSOCIATED CONDITIONS

- Peripheral arthritis (30%)
- Enthesopathy (29%): Achilles tendonitis, plantar fasciitis
- Uveitis (23%)
- Psoriasis (10%)
- Dactylitis "sausage digit" (6%)
- Inflammatory bowel disease (IBD) (4%) (3)[A]
- Peripheral spondyloarthritis (SpA): psoriatic arthritis, reactive arthritis, IBD-related arthritis, juvenile idiopathic arthritis
- Aortitis and cardiac conduction defects

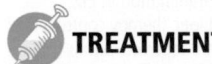 **DIAGNOSIS**

HISTORY

- Inflammatory back pain
  - Insidious onset
  - Duration >3 months
  - Morning stiffness in spine lasting >1 hour
  - Nighttime awakenings secondary to back pain
  - Pain and stiffness increase at rest and improve with activity.
- Alternating buttock/hip pain is common.

- Constitutional symptoms (fatigue, weight loss, low-grade fever) are common.
- Inspirational chest pain due to enthesitis at costochondral junction and diminished chest wall expansion
- Other symptoms associated with enthesopathy (Achilles pain, plantar fascia pain), dactylitis (oligoarthritis), iritis (painful red eye, photophobia, vision changes)

PHYSICAL EXAM

- Sacroiliac joint tenderness, loss of lumbar lordosis, and cervical spine rotation
- Diminished range of motion in the lumbar spine in all three planes of motion
- Modified Wright-Schober test for lumbar spine flexion:
  - Mark patient's back over the L5 spinous process (or at dimples of Venus) and measure 10 cm above and 5 cm below this point. Normal is at least 5 cm of expansion between these two marks on maximal forward flexion.
- Thoracocervical kyphosis (usually after at least 10 years of symptoms)
- Occiput–wall distance increased (distance between occiput and wall when standing with back flat against a vertical surface; zero is normal)
- Respiratory excursion of chest wall
  - Normal is >5 cm of maximal respiratory excursion of chest wall measured at 4th intercostal space; <2.5 cm is consistent with AS.
- Tenderness of insertional sites—Achilles, plantar fascia
- Peripheral oligoarthritis/dactylitis seen mostly with peripheral SpA
- Cauda equina syndrome rarely occurs in late disease.
- Extra-articular manifestations: uveitis, psoriasis, IBD
- Aortic regurgitation murmur (1%)

DIFFERENTIAL DIAGNOSIS

- Nonradiographic axSpA (features of AS with evidence of sacroiliitis on MRI but not on plain radiographs—can progress to AS); other SpA
- Osteoarthritis of the axial spine
- Diffuse idiopathic skeletal hyperostosis (DISH)
- Osteitis condensans ilii: benign sclerotic changes in the iliac portion of the SI joint after pregnancy
- Infectious arthritis or discitis, unilateral sacroiliitis: tuberculosis, brucellosis, bacterial infection (particularly in IV drug users)

DIAGNOSTIC TESTS & INTERPRETATION

- Up to 10% of Caucasian population and 4% of African American population are HLA-B27–positive. Genetic testing is not necessary as part of initial evaluation, particularly with a consistent history and exam.
- ESR and C-reactive protein (CRP) may be mildly elevated or normal; if high, correlates with disease activity and prognosis
- Absence of rheumatoid factor
- Mild normochromic anemia (15%)
- Synovial fluid: mild leukocytosis
- SI joints: Oblique projection is preferred.
  - X-ray changes may not be apparent for up to 10 years after disease onset. MRI is more sensitive; increased signal from the bone and bone marrow suggests osteitis and edema.
  - Sequential radiographic changes over time: widening of SI joint, erosions, sclerosis on both sides of joint not extending >1 cm from articular surface, and (lastly) ankyloses

- Spine: lateral view preferred
  - Early plain radiograph changes: "shiny corners" due to osteitis and sclerosis at site of annulus fibrosus attachments to the corners of vertebral bodies with "squaring" due to erosion and remodeling of vertebral body; contrast-enhanced MRI is more sensitive for detecting early changes.
  - Late changes: ossification of annulus fibrosis resulting in bony bridging between vertebral bodies (syndesmophytes) giving classic "bamboo spine" appearance; ankylosis of apophyseal joints, ossification of spinal ligaments, and/or spondylodiscitis also occurs.
- Peripheral joints
  - Asymmetric pericapsular ossification, sclerosis, loss of joint space, and erosions may occur.

Diagnostic Procedures/Other

Screening for cardiac conduction defects with ECG and for valvular heart disease with echocardiograms not recommended but may consider if symptomatic

Test Interpretation

- Erosive changes and new bone formation at bony attachment of the tendons and ligaments result in ossification of periarticular soft tissues.
- Synovial hypertrophy and pannus formation, mononuclear cell infiltrate into subsynovium and subchondral bone marrow inflammation in the SI joint with erosions, followed by granulation tissue formation, and finally obliteration of joint space by fusion of joint and sclerosis of para-articular bone

TREATMENT

GENERAL MEASURES

- Symptom control, maintaining spinal flexibility and normal posture, reducing functional limitations, maintain work ability, and decreased disease complications are primary treatment goals.
- Aggressive physical therapy is the most important nonpharmacologic management.
- Posture training and spinal range of motion exercises are essential.
- Firm bed; sleep in supine position without a pillow.
- Breathing exercises 2 to 3 times per day
- Smoking cessation

MEDICATION

First Line

- Nonsteroidal anti-inflammatory drugs (NSAIDs) are first-line pharmacologic agent for pain and stiffness in AS (4)[A].
- NSAIDs provide rapid and dramatic symptomatic relief, which may aid in diagnosis. No single NSAID preferred. Higher doses tend to be more efficacious.
- NSAIDS may be effective in slowing radiographic disease progression, and this may be best achieved by continuous rather than on demand use (4)[A].
- Precautions
  - Consider CVD, GI, and renal risks of NSAIDs. Use with caution in patients with a bleeding diathesis or on anticoagulants.
  - Consider GI prophylaxis (PPIs or misoprostol) while on NSAIDs in patients with hx of PUD, gastritis, or age >60 years.
- Injection of intra-articular corticosteroids into SI joints and prostheses can provide transient relief, but systemic corticosteroids are not recommended (5)[C].

Pregnancy Considerations
Infants exposed to NSAIDs in 1st trimester may have a higher incidence of cardiac malformations.

Second Line
- Biologic agents: tumor necrosis factor (TNF)-α antagonists
  - Recommended for active disease after lack of response to at least two different NSAIDs over 1 month (5)[C]
  - FDA-approved agents for AS include etanercept (recombinant TNF receptor fusion protein), infliximab (chimeric monoclonal IgG1 antibody to TNF-α), adalimumab (fully humanized IgG1 monoclonal antibody to TNF-α), and golimumab (human IgG1 kappa monoclonal antibody to TNF-α).
  - Approved agents improve pain, function, and symptoms of AS as compared to placebo (6)[A].
  - No definitive evidence for TNF-α blockers with regard to disease remission, prevention of radiologic progression, or prevention of extra-articular manifestations
  - Monoclonal TNF-α blockers are preferred when IBD is involved (5)[C].
  - Further investigation as to the effectiveness of TNF blocker therapy with NSAIDs is needed.
- Precautions with TNF-α blockers
  - Anti-TNFs increase the risk of serious bacterial, mycobacterial, fungal, opportunistic, and viral infections. Screen for tuberculosis and hepatitis B.
  - Monitor for reactivation of tuberculosis and invasive fungal infections, such as histoplasmosis, in all patients, especially those who travel to (or residents in) endemic areas.
  - Lymphomas, nonmelanoma skin cancers, and other malignancies have been reported in patients receiving anti-TNFs.
  - Immunizations (especially live vaccines) should be updated before initiating anti-TNFs; live vaccines are contraindicated once patients receive anti-TNFs.
- Disease-modifying antirheumatic drugs (DMARDs), such as methotrexate and sulfasalazine, are ineffective for axial disease; sulfasalazine may be effective for peripheral arthritis; this class may be considered in patients with contraindications to TNF agents (5)[C].

ISSUES FOR REFERRAL
- Physical therapy can assist with treatment plan (including home regimens).
- Coordinate care with a rheumatologist for diagnosis, monitoring, and management (anti-TNF therapy).
- Management of aortic regurgitation, uveitis, spinal fractures, pulmonary fibrosis, hip joint involvement, renal amyloidosis, and cauda equina syndrome may require referral to appropriate specialty.

ADDITIONAL THERAPIES
Bisphosphonate medications if osteopenia or osteoporosis is present

SURGERY/OTHER PROCEDURES
- Evaluate for C-spine ankylosis/instability before intubation in patients with AS undergoing surgery.
- Total hip replacement with advanced hip arthritis (5)[C]
- Vertebral osteotomy can improve posture for patients with severe cervical or thoracolumbar flexion.

ONGOING CARE

FOLLOW-UP RECOMMENDATIONS
Patient Monitoring
- Monitor posture and range of motion with 6- to 12-month visits; increase frequency if higher disease activity.
- Bath Ankylosing Spondylitis Disease Activity Index (BASDAI) or Ankylosing Spondylitis Disease Activity Score (ASDAS) can be used to measure disease activity.
- Fall prevention/evaluation
- Regular-interval monitoring of CRP or ESR
- Screening for osteopenia/osteoporosis with dual energy x-ray absorptiometry scan

PATIENT EDUCATION
- Maintain physical activity and posture.
- Swimming, tai chi, and walking are excellent activities.
- Avoid trauma/contact sports.
- Appropriate ergonomic modification of workplace
- Counsel about risk of spinal fracture.
- MedicAlert bracelet (helpful if intubation required)
- Arthritis Foundation: http://www.arthritis.org
- Spondylitis Association of America: http://www.spondylitis.org

PROGNOSIS
- Extent and rapidity of progression of ankylosis are highly variable.
- Progressive limitation of spinal mobility necessitates lifestyle modification.

COMPLICATIONS
- MSK/spine
  - Osteoporosis (13%); 10% higher risk of nonvertebral fracture in AS patients
  - Spinal fusion causing kyphosis
  - Cervical spine fracture or subluxation carries high mortality rate; fracture can occur at any level of ankylosed spine.
  - Cauda equina syndrome (rare)
- Pulmonary: restrictive lung disease, upper lobe fibrosis (rare)
- Cardiac: conduction defects at atrioventricular (AV) node, aortic insufficiency, aortitis, pericarditis (extremely rare)
- Eye: uveitis and cataracts
- Renal: IgA nephropathy, amyloidosis (<1%)
- GI: microscopic, subclinical ileal, and colonic mucosal ulcerations in up to 50% of patients, mostly asymptomatic

REFERENCES

1. Reveille JD, Weisman MH. The epidemiology of back pain, axial spondyloarthritis and HLA-B27 in the United States. *Am J Med Sci.* 2013;345(6):431–436.
2. Dougados M, Baeten D. Spondyloarthritis. *Lancet.* 2011;377(9783):2127–2137.
3. de Winter JJ, van Mens LJ, van der Heijde D, et al. Prevalence of peripheral and extra-articular disease in ankylosing spondylitis versus non-radiographic axial spondyloarthritis: a meta-analysis. *Arthritis Res Ther.* 2016;18:196.
4. Kroon FP, van der Burg LR, Ramiro S, et al. Nonsteroidal anti-inflammatory drugs (NSAIDs) for axial spondyloarthritis (ankylosing spondylitis and non-radiographic axial spondyloarthritis). *Cochrane Database Syst Rev.* 2015;(7):CD010952.
5. Ward MM, Deodhar A, Akl EA, et al. American College of Rheumatology/Spondylitis Association of America/Spondyloarthritis Research and Treatment Network 2015 recommendations for the treatment of ankylosing spondylitis and nonradiographic axial spondyloarthritis. *Arthritis Rheumatol.* 2016;68(2):282–298.
6. Maxwell LJ, Zochling J, Boonen A, et al. TNF-alpha inhibitors for ankylosing spondylitis. *Cochrane Database of Syst Rev.* 2015;(4):CD005468.

ADDITIONAL READING

- Adams K, Bombardier C, van der Heijde DM. Safety of pain therapy during pregnancy and lactation in patients with inflammatory arthritis: a systematic literature review. *J Rheumatol Suppl.* 2012;90:59–61.
- Garg N, van den Bosch F, Deodhar A. The concept of spondyloarthritis: where are we now? *Best Pract Res Clin Rheumatol.* 2014;28(5):663–672.
- Gensler L, Inman R, Deodhar A. The "knowns" and "unknowns" of biologic therapy in ankylosing spondylitis. *Am J Med Sci.* 2012;343(5):360–363.
- Sieper J. Treatment challenges in axial spondylarthritis and future directions. *Curr Rheumatol Rep.* 2013;15(9):356. doi:10.1007/s11926-013-0356-9.
- Sieper J, Rudwaleit M, Baraliakos X, et al. The Assessment of SpondyloArthritis International Society (ASAS) handbook: a guide to assess spondyloarthritis. *Ann Rheum Dis.* 2009;68(Suppl 2):ii1–ii44.
- van der Heijde D, Ramiro S, Landewé R, et al. 2016 Update of the ASAS-EULAR management recommendations for axial spondyloarthritis. *Ann Rheum Dis.* 2017;76(6):978–991.

 SEE ALSO

Arthritis, Psoriatic; Arthritis, Rheumatoid (RA); Crohn Disease; Reactive Arthritis (Reiter Syndrome); Ulcerative Colitis

 CODES

ICD10
- M45.9 Ankylosing spondylitis of unspecified sites in spine
- M08.1 Juvenile ankylosing spondylitis
- M45.8 Ankylosing spondylitis sacral and sacrococcygeal region

CLINICAL PEARLS
- Diagnosis of AS is suggested by a history of inflammatory back pain, pain when supine and lasting over an hour on movement, evidence of limited chest wall expansion, restricted spinal movements in all planes, radiographic evidence of sacroiliitis, and a therapeutic response to NSAIDs.
- HLA-B27 testing supports the diagnosis if clinical features are not definitive.
- MRI is more sensitive at detecting SI joint inflammation than plain radiography.
- Physical therapy is important in helping to maintain posture and mobility.
- NSAIDs and TNF-α blockers are the mainstays of pharmacologic treatment of AS.

ANOREXIA NERVOSA

Umer Farooq, MD • Katherine Tsung, MD

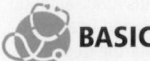 **BASICS**

DESCRIPTION

- Restriction of energy intake leading to significantly low weight in the context of age, sex, developmental trajectory, and physical health, with intense fear of weight gain and body image disturbance. Significantly, low weight is defined as weight that is less than minimally normal/expected.
- *Diagnostic and Statistical Manual of Mental Disorders*, 5th edition (*DSM-5*), divides anorexia into two types:
  - Restricting type: not engaged in binge eating or purging behaviors for last 3 months
  - Binge eating/purging type: regularly engages in binge eating or purging behaviors (last 3 months)
- System(s) affected: cardiovascular, endocrine, metabolic, gastrointestinal, nervous, reproductive
- Severity of anorexia nervosa (AN) is based on BMI (per *DSM-5*):
  - Mild: BMI $\geq$17 kg/m^2
  - Moderate: BMI 16.00 to 16.99 kg/m^2
  - Severe: BMI 15.00 to 15.99 kg/m^2
  - Extreme: BMI <15 kg/m^2

EPIDEMIOLOGY

- Predominant age: 13 to 20 years
- Predominant sex: female > male (10:1 female-to-male ratio)

Incidence

8 to 19 women/2 men per 100,000 per year

Prevalence

- 0.9% in women (0.3% in young females)
- 0.3% in men (higher in gay and bisexual men)

ETIOLOGY AND PATHOPHYSIOLOGY

- Complex relationship among genetic, biologic, environmental, psychological, and social factors that result in the development of this disorder
- Subsequent malnutrition may lead to multiorgan damage.
- Serotonin, norepinephrine, and dopamine neuronal systems are implicated.

Genetics

- There is evidence of higher concordance rates in monozygotic than in dizygotic twins.
- First-degree female relative with eating disorder increases risk 6- to 10-fold.
- One genome-wide significant locus identified for AN on chromosome 12

RISK FACTORS

- Female gender
- Adolescence
- Body dissatisfaction
- Perfectionism
- Negative self-evaluation
- Academic pressure
- Severe life stressors
- Participation in sports or artistic activities that emphasize leanness or involve subjective scoring: ballet, running, wrestling, figure skating, gymnastics, cheerleading, weight lifting
- Type 1 diabetes mellitus
- Family history of substance abuse, affective disorders, or eating disorder

GENERAL PREVENTION

Prevention programs can reduce risk factors and future onset of eating disorders.

- Target adolescents and young women 15 years of age or older.
- Encourage realistic and healthy weight management strategies and attitudes.
- Promote self-esteem.
- Reduce focus on thin as ideal.
- Decrease co-occurring anxiety/depressive symptoms and improve stress management.

COMMONLY ASSOCIATED CONDITIONS

- Mood disorder—major depressive disorder
- Anxiety disorders—social phobia, obsessive-compulsive disorder, posttraumatic stress disorder
- Substance use disorder
- High rates of cluster C personality disorders

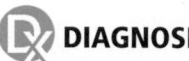 **DIAGNOSIS**

HISTORY

- Onset may be insidious or stress related.
- Patient unlikely to self-identify problem (lack of insight into the illness); corroborate with parent/relative.
- Restriction of energy intake relative to requirement, leading to significantly low body weight in the context of age, sex, developmental trajectory, and physical health
- Fear of weight gain and/or distorted body image
- Report feeling fat even when emaciated
- Preoccupation with body size, weight control
- Elaborate food preparation and eating rituals.
- Other possible signs and symptoms:
  - Extensive exercise
  - Amenorrhea (primary or secondary)
  - Weakness, fatigue, cognitive impairment
  - Cold intolerance
  - Constipation, bloating, early satiety
  - Growth arrest, delayed puberty
  - History of fractures (decreased bone density)
- Screening
  - Clinician-administered eating disorder screen for primary care to identify patients with eating disorders
    - Are you satisfied with your eating patterns? (No is abnormal.)
    - Do you ever eat in secret? (Yes is abnormal.)
    - Does your weight affect the way you feel about yourself? (Yes is abnormal.)
    - Have any members of your family suffered with an eating disorder? (Yes is abnormal.)
    - Do you currently suffer with or have you ever suffered in the past with an eating disorder? (Yes is abnormal.)

PHYSICAL EXAM

- May be normal
- Abnormal vital signs: hypothermia, bradycardia, orthostatic hypotension
- Body weight <85% of expected
- Cardiac: dysrhythmias, midsystolic click from mitral valve prolapse
- Skin/extremities: dry skin; lanugo hair on extremities, face, and trunk; hair loss; edema
- Neurologic and abdominal exams: to rule out other causes of weight loss and vomiting
- Gynecologic: amenorrhea

DIFFERENTIAL DIAGNOSIS

- Hyperthyroidism, adrenal insufficiency
- Inflammatory bowel disease, malabsorption
- Immunodeficiency, chronic infections
- Uncontrolled diabetes
- CNS lesion
- Bulimia, body dysmorphic disorder
- Depressive disorders with loss of appetite
- Anxiety disorder, food phobia
- Conversion disorder

DIAGNOSTIC TESTS & INTERPRETATION

- Psychological self-report screening tests may be helpful, but diagnosis is based on meeting the *DSM-5* criteria.
- Most findings are related directly to starvation and/or dehydration. All findings may be within normal limits.
- Screening tools:
  - SCOFF questionnaire (1)[B]
  - Eating Disorder Screen for Primary Care

Initial Tests (lab, imaging)

- CBC: anemia, leukopenia, thrombocytopenia
- Low-serum luteinizing hormone, follicle-stimulating hormone; low-serum testosterone in men
- Thyroid function tests: low thyroid-stimulating hormone with normal T$_3$/T$_4$
- Liver function tests: abnormal liver enzymes
- Chem 7: altered BUN, creatinine clearance; electrolyte disturbances
- Hypoglycemia, hypercholesterolemia, hypercortisolemia, hypophosphatemia
- Low vitamin D and hypocalcemia
- 12-Lead electrocardiogram to assess for prolonged QT interval
- If underweight for >6 months: dual energy x-ray absorptiometry of bone to assess for diminished bone density

Test Interpretation

- Osteoporosis/osteopenia, pathologic fractures
- Sick euthyroid syndrome, dehydration
- Cardiac impairment
- AN may exist concurrently with chronic medical disorders.

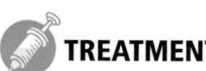 **TREATMENT**

GENERAL MEASURES

- Initial treatment goal geared to weight restoration; most managed as outpatients (OPs)
- OP treatment:
  - Interdisciplinary team (primary care physician, mental health provider, dietitian)
  - Average weekly weight gain goal: 0.5 to 1.0 kg, with stepwise increase in calories
  - Cognitive-behavioral therapy (CBT), interpersonal psychotherapy, motivational interviewing, family-based therapy
  - Focus on health, not weight gain alone.
  - Build trust and a treatment alliance.
  - Involve the patient in establishing diet and exercise goals.
  - Challenge fear of uncontrolled weight gain; help the patient to recognize feelings that lead to disordered eating.
  - In chronic cases, goal may be to achieve a safe weight rather than a healthy weight.

- Inpatient treatment:
  - If possible, admit to a specialized eating disorders unit.
  - Monitor vital signs, electrolytes, cardiac function, edema, and weight gain.
  - Assess risk for refeeding syndrome (metabolic shift from a catabolic to anabolic state). Treat by slowing nutritional intake and aggressively correcting electrolyte imbalances.
  - Initial supervised meals may be necessary.
  - Stepwise increase in activity
  - Tube feeding or total parenteral nutrition is used only as a last resort.
  - Supportive symptomatic care as needed
- Psychotherapy (e.g., CBT or family therapy) should be offered (2,3)[A].
- CBT has demonstrated effectiveness as a means of improving treatment adherence and minimizing dropout among patients with AN (4)[A].

MEDICATION

First Line
- No medications are available that effectively treat patients with AN, but pharmacotherapy may be used as an adjuvant to CBTs (5)[A].
- If medications are used, start with low doses due to increased risk for adverse effects.
- SSRIs may:
  - Help to prevent relapse after weight gain
  - Treat comorbid depression or obsessive-compulsive disorder
  - Use of atypical antipsychotics is being studied with mixed findings to date. Olanzapine is potentially beneficial as an adjuvant treatment of underweight individuals in the inpatient settings.
- Attend to black box warnings concerning antidepressants.
- The antidepressant bupropion should be avoided because it is associated with a higher incidence of seizures.

Second Line
- Management of osteopenia:
  - Primary treatment is weight gain.
  - Elemental calcium 1,200 to 1,500 mg/day plus vitamin D 800 IU/day
  - No indication for bisphosphonates in AN
  - Weak evidence for use of hormone-replacement therapy
- Psyllium (Metamucil) preparations to prevent constipation

ISSUES FOR REFERRAL
Patients with AN require an interdisciplinary team (primary care physician, mental health provider, nutritionist). An important step in management is to arrange OP mental health therapist.

ADMISSION, INPATIENT, AND NURSING CONSIDERATIONS
- Suggested physiologic values to admit: heart rate <40 beats/min, BP <90/60 mm Hg, symptomatic hypoglycemia, temperature <97.0°F (36.1°C), dehydration, other cardiovascular abnormalities, weight <75% of expected, rapid weight loss, lack of improvement while in OP therapy
- Suggested psychological indications: poor motivation/insight, lack of cooperation with OP treatment, inability to eat, need for nasogastric feeding, suicidal intent or plan, severe coexisting psychiatric disease, problematic family environment
- Suggested lab indications: potassium <3 mmol/L, prolonged QTC (>0.499 ms), urine specific gravity >1.03 or <1.01

Pediatric Considerations
- Children often present with nausea, abdominal pain, fullness, and inability to swallow.

- Additional indications for hospitalization: heart rate <50 beats/min, orthostatic BP, hypokalemia or hypophosphatemia, rapid weight loss even if weight not <75% below normal
- Children and adolescents should be offered family-based therapy and treatment.

Geriatric Considerations
Late-onset AN (>50 years of age) may be a long-term disease or triggered by death of loved one, marital discord, or divorce.
- Has a high comorbidity with depression
- Always consider other organic causes of weight loss.
- Discharge when medically stable. Arrange OP appointment with mental health provider and primary care provider.

 ONGOING CARE

FOLLOW-UP RECOMMENDATIONS
- Close follow-up until patient demonstrates forward progress in care plan
- Family and individual therapy is extremely important for long-term benefits/outcomes.
- CBT is helpful for the treatment of AN and may aid in the prevention of relapse.
- Emphasize importance of moderate activity for health, not thinness.

Patient Monitoring
- Level of exercise activity
- Weigh weekly until stable and then monthly.
- Depression, suicidal ideation

DIET
- Dietary consultation while patient is hospitalized
- Nutritional education programs

PATIENT EDUCATION
- Provide patients and families with information about the diagnosis and its natural history, health risks, and treatment strategies.
- http://www.mayoclinic.org/diseases-conditions /anorexia/home/ovc-20179508
- National Alliance on Mental Illness: http://www .nami.org/Learn-More/Mental-Health-Conditions /Eating-Disorders

PROGNOSIS
- Prognosis: ~50% recover, 30% improve, 20% are chronically ill.
- Outcomes in men are likely better than in women.
- Mortality: 5–18% (annual mortality rate of 5 per 1,000 person-years)

ALERT
High risk of suicide (approximately 1 in 5 individuals with AN who died had committed suicide) (6)[A]

COMPLICATIONS
- Refeeding syndrome
- Cardiac arrhythmia, cardiac arrest
- Cardiomyopathy, congestive heart failure
- Delayed gastric emptying, necrotizing colitis
- Seizures, Wernicke encephalopathy, peripheral neuropathy, cognitive deficits
- Osteopenia, osteoporosis

Pregnancy Considerations
- Fertility may be affected.
- Behaviors may persist, decrease, or recur during pregnancy and the postpartum interval.
- Increased risk for preterm labor, operative delivery, and infants with low birth weight; anemia, genitourinary infections, and labor induction should be managed as high risk.

REFERENCES

1. Cotton MA, Ball C, Robinson P. Four simple questions can help screen for eating disorders. *J Gen Intern Med*. 2003;18(1):53–56.
2. Hay PJ, Claudino AM, Touyz S, et al. Individual psychological therapy in the outpatient treatment of adults with anorexia nervosa. *Cochrane Database Syst Rev*. 2015;(7):CD003909.
3. Bulik CM, Berkman ND, Brownley KA, et al. Anorexia nervosa treatment: a systematic review of randomized controlled trials. *Int J Eat Disord*. 2007;40(4):310–320.
4. Galsworthy-Francis L, Allan S. Cognitive behavioural therapy for anorexia nervosa: a systematic review. *Clin Psychol Rev*. 2014;34(1):54–72.
5. Claudino AM, Hay P, Lima MS, et al. Antidepressants for anorexia nervosa. *Cochrane Database Syst Rev*. 2006;(1):CD004365.
6. Arcelus J, Mitchell AJ, Wales J, et al. Mortality rates in patients with anorexia nervosa and other eating disorders. A meta-analysis of 36 studies. *Arch Gen Psychiatry*. 2011;68(7):724–731.

ADDITIONAL READING
- American Psychiatric Association. *Practice Guideline for the Treatment of Patients with Eating Disorders*. 3rd ed. Arlington, VA: American Psychiatric Association; 2006.
- Dalle Grave R. Eating disorders: progress and challenges. *Eur J Intern Med*. 2011;22(2):153–160.
- National Collaborating Centre for Mental Health. *Eating Disorders: Core Interventions in the Treatment and Management of Anorexia Nervosa, Bulimia Nervosa and Related Eating Disorders*. Leicester, United Kingdom: British Psychological Society; 2004.

 SEE ALSO

- Amenorrhea; Bulimia Nervosa; Osteoporosis and Osteopenia
- Algorithm: Weight Loss, Unintentional

 CODES

ICD10
- F50.00 Anorexia nervosa, unspecified
- F50.01 Anorexia nervosa, restricting type
- F50.02 Anorexia nervosa, binge eating/purging type

CLINICAL PEARLS
- "Are you satisfied with your eating patterns?" and/or "Do you worry that you have lost control over how you eat?" may help to screen those with an eating problem.
- Assess for suicide risk.
- Studies have shown patients with AN will not accept medications unless combined with psychotherapy.
- To care for a patient with AN, an interdisciplinary team that includes a medical provider, a dietitian, and a behavioral health professional is the most accepted approach.
- Family analysis is necessary for the patients with AN to determine what kind of therapy would be most helpful.
- 3 months amenorrhea is no longer a criteria needed for the diagnosis of AN.

ANTIPHOSPHOLIPID ANTIBODY SYNDROME
Krishna M. Baradhi, MD • Narothama Reddy Aeddula, MD, FACP, FASN

BASICS

DESCRIPTION
Antiphospholipid antibody syndrome (APS) is a systemic autoantibody-mediated thrombophilic disorder characterized by recurrent arterial or venous thrombosis and/or recurrent fetal loss in the presence of persistent antiphospholipid antibodies (APAs) as evidenced by lupus anticoagulant (LAC), anticardiolipin antibodies (aCL), and/or anti–β_2 glycoprotein-I (GPI) antibody. The APAs enhance clot formation by interacting with phospholipid-binding plasma proteins. The resulting APS can cause morbidity and mortality in both pregnant and nonpregnant individuals:
- Types of APS (based on clinical presentation)
  - Primary: no underlying condition evident
  - Secondary: most commonly associated with autoimmune diseases like systemic lupus erythematosus (SLE); transient APAs have been linked to certain infections, drugs, and malignancies.
  - Catastrophic APS (CAPS) a.k.a. Asherson syndrome (<1%)
    - Most severe form of disease; characterized by thrombotic microangiopathy and associated with multiorgan failure
    - High mortality if treatment is delayed

Pregnancy Considerations
- Complications include maternal venous thromboembolism, stroke, fetal demise, preeclampsia and placental insufficiency, fetal growth retardation, miscarriage, and preterm birth.
- Triple antibody positivity is considered the most noteworthy risk factor.
- Low-dose aspirin and low-molecular-weight heparin (LMWH) or unfractionated heparin are the drugs of choice in pregnancy.
- Prophylactic-dose heparin is recommended in the postpartum period (unless patient is on therapeutic anticoagulation) given high risk of thrombosis during this time. With adequate treatment, >70% of patients with APS deliver viable infants.

EPIDEMIOLOGY
- The prevalence of APAs increases with age but is not necessarily associated with a higher risk of thrombosis.
- For APS, female > male

Incidence
- Incidence of APS is around 5 new cases per 100,000 persons per year.
- In patients with positive APAs without prior risk of thrombosis, the annual incident risk of thrombosis is 0–3.8%. This risk is increased to 5.3% in those with triple positivity. 10–15% of recurrent abortions are attributable to APS.

Prevalence
Prevalence around 40 to 50 cases per 100,000 persons per year. APAs are present in 1–5% of the general population and in ~40% of those with SLE. A higher prevalence is seen in those with venous thromboembolism and stroke.

ETIOLOGY AND PATHOPHYSIOLOGY
- Anti–β_2-GP1 antibodies play a central role in the pathogenesis of APS. The procoagulant effect is mediated by various possible mechanisms:
  - Endothelial effects: inhibition of prostacyclin production and loss of annexin V cellular shield
  - Platelet activation resulting in adhesion and aggregation

- Interference of innate anticoagulant pathways (such as inhibition of protein C)
  - Complement activation
- Pregnancy-related complications are also a result of autoantibody-mediated effects:
  - Interference with expression of trophoblastic adhesion molecules resulting in abnormal placentation and placental thrombosis
- Proposed mechanisms: excess production of natural antibodies, molecular mimicry due to infections, exposure of phospholipid antigens during platelet activation, cardiolipin peroxidation, and genetic predisposition
- A "second hit" by environmental factors is often required to manifest APS.

Genetics
Most cases of APS are acquired. There are a few studies of familial occurrence of aCL and LAC. A valine 247/leucine polymorphism in β_2-GP1 could be a genetic risk for the presence of anti–β_2-GP1 antibodies and APS.

RISK FACTORS
- Age >55 years in males, >65 years in females
- Cardiovascular risk factors (hypertension [HTN], hyperlipidemia, diabetes, obesity, smoking, combined oral contraceptive use)
- Underlying autoimmune disease (SLE, rheumatoid arthritis, collagen vascular disease, Sjögren syndrome, idiopathic thrombocytopenic purpura, Behçet syndrome)
- Positive APAs
- Surgery, immobilization, pregnancy

GENERAL PREVENTION
Risk factor modification: Control HTN and diabetes; smoking cessation; avoidance of oral contraceptives in high-risk patients; start thromboprophylaxis in established cases; preconception assessment

COMMONLY ASSOCIATED CONDITIONS
- Autoimmune diseases: SLE (most common), scleroderma, Sjögren syndrome, dermatomyositis, and rheumatoid arthritis
- Malignancy
- Infections: viral, bacterial, parasitic, and rickettsial
- Certain drugs associated with APA production without increased risk of thrombosis: phenothiazines, hydralazine, procainamide, and phenytoin
- Hemolysis, elevated liver enzymes, and low platelet count in association with pregnancy (HELLP) syndrome
- Sneddon syndrome (APS variant syndrome with livedo reticularis, HTN, and stroke)

DIAGNOSIS

Sapporo criteria (also called Sydney criteria), revised 2006:
- At least one of the following clinical criteria:
  - Vascular thrombosis
    - ≥1 clinical episodes of arterial, venous, or small vessel thrombosis, occurring within any tissue or organ and confirmed by unequivocal imaging studies or histopathology without associated inflammation in the vessel wall
    - Superficial venous thrombosis does not meet the criteria for APS.

- Complications of pregnancy (any one of the following):
  - ≥3 consecutive spontaneous abortions before the 10th week of pregnancy, unexplained by maternal/paternal chromosomal abnormalities or maternal anatomic/hormonal causes
  - ≥1 unexplained deaths of morphologically normal fetuses (documented by ultrasonography or by direct examination) at ≥10th week of gestation
  - ≥1 premature births of morphologically normal newborn babies at ≤34th week of pregnancy due to severe preeclampsia, eclampsia, or placental insufficiency
- AND the presence of at least one of three laboratory findings (confirmed on ≥2 occasions at least 12 weeks apart):
  - LAC detected in blood
  - Anticardiolipin IgG and/or IgM antibodies present at moderate or high levels in the blood (>40 GPL or MPL or >99th percentile) via a standardized ELISA
  - Anti–β_2-GP1 IgG and/or IgM antibodies in blood at a titer >99th percentile by standardized ELISA

HISTORY
- History of VTE or arterial thrombosis (stroke, MI)
- History of recurrent fetal loss or other obstetric complications
- Bleeding from thrombocytopenia if severe or acquired factor II deficiency
- Personal or family history of autoimmune disease

PHYSICAL EXAM
- Signs of venous thrombosis in extremities
- Skin manifestations, including a vasculitic rash in the form of palpable purpura or livedo reticularis, superficial thrombophlebitis, or lower extremity ulcers
- Livedo reticularis
- Cardiac murmurs
- Focal neurologic or cognitive deficits

DIFFERENTIAL DIAGNOSIS
- Thrombophilic conditions
  - Inherited: deficiency of protein C, protein S, antithrombin III; mutation of factor V Leiden, prothrombin gene mutation
  - Acquired: neoplastic and myeloproliferative disorders, hyperviscosity syndromes, nephrotic syndrome
- Embolic disease secondary to atrial fibrillation, LV dysfunction, endocarditis, cholesterol emboli
- Disseminated intravascular coagulation
- Heparin-induced thrombocytopenia
- Behçet syndrome
- CAPS: hemolytic-uremic syndrome, TTP, or malignant HTN

DIAGNOSTIC TESTS & INTERPRETATION
- LAC assay and IgG and IGM aCL by ELISA and anti–β_2-GP1 IgG and IgM antibodies are diagnostic tests of choice.
- The LAC assay combines at least two out of three screening tests (prolongation of aPTT, dilute Russell viper venom time [dRVVT], and kaolin clotting) with two confirmatory tests.
- A weakly positive LAC result should be considered clinically important (1).
- Anti–β_2-GP1 antibodies are important in the pathogenesis of thrombosis. A positive LAC assay recognizes antibodies against β_2-GP1 and prothrombin.

- Although testing for antibodies to phosphatidyl-serine and prothrombin can help to assess the risk of thrombosis, routine evaluation for prothrombin antibodies is not recommended.
- The clinical significance of other autoantibodies (annexin V, phosphatidic acid, and phosphatidylinositol) remains unclear.
- The utility of β_2-GP1 anti-domain I antibodies is being evaluated thoroughly for its diagnostic and risk stratification value.

Initial Tests (lab, imaging)
- CBC, PT/INR, aPTT, LAC, aCL, anti–β_2-GP1 antibodies (2)[B]
- Prevalence of APAs in SLE ranges from 11% to 87%; hence, it is important to screen for SLE.
- Imaging is based on clinical picture, suspected sites of thrombosis, and organ involvement.

Follow-Up Tests & Special Considerations
- The results of LAC are difficult to interpret in patients treated with warfarin. Unfractionated heparin or LMWH and fondaparinux do not affect the LAC assay.
- Repeat testing at 12 weeks for persistence of APA.

Diagnostic Procedures/Other
Biopsy of the affected organ system may be necessary to distinguish from vasculitis.

Test Interpretation
Usual finding is thrombosis and minimal vascular or perivascular inflammation:
- Acute changes: capillary congestion and noninflammatory fibrin thrombi
- Chronic changes: ischemic hypoperfusion, atrophy, and fibrosis

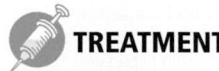 TREATMENT

MEDICATION
First Line
- Primary thromboprophylaxis: is controversial in patients with APAs and no clinical symptoms (3)[B]. Low-dose aspirin or heparin is indicated only in patients with high risk of thrombosis.
- Secondary thromboprophylaxis: All symptomatic, nonpregnant patients with APS need indefinite anticoagulation. The target INR depends on the severity and type of thrombosis:
  – Venous thrombosis (first episode): warfarin with target INR of 2.0 to 3.0 (3)[B]
  – Arterial thrombosis or recurrent venous thrombosis despite anticoagulation: warfarin with target INR 3.0 to 4.0
  – LMWH and fondaparinux are alternatives.
- Direct oral anticoagulants (DOACs) such as rivaroxaban, apixaban, and dabigatran; all have been approved for treatment of DVT/PE; however, studies in APS are lacking; a prospective randomized trial in 2016 of warfarin versus rivaroxaban in patients with thrombotic APS showed increase in endogenous thrombin potential in patients who switched to rivaroxaban. The 15th International Congress on Antiphospholipid Antibodies Task Force published in 2017 concluded that there is insufficient evidence to recommend DOACs in APS. DOACs may be alternatives to warfarin in patients intolerant to warfarin.
  – Rituximab may be an option in severe cases, possibly in those with thrombotic microangiopathy (4,5)[B].
- Danaparoid, fondaparinux, and argatroban can be considered in heparin-induced thrombocytopenia.

- Statins can decrease proinflammatory and pro-thrombotic state in APS but not recommended in the absence of hyperlipidemia.
- Hydroxychloroquine can be added in recalcitrant APS.
- Eculizumab may be useful in refractory cases.
- Vitamin D deficiency/insufficiency should be corrected in all APA-positive patients, but its role in APS needs further study.
- Low-dose aspirin is superior to low-dose aspirin with low-dose warfarin due to decreased bleeding risk with no differences in number of thrombosis (6).
- CAPS: Anticoagulants and high-dose steroids may suffice in less severe cases. Aggressive treatment with either IVIG or plasma exchange is often required in severe cases. These measures have improved survival up to 66%.
- Treatment in pregnancy:
  – Patients with APAs and no prior thrombotic events should not receive thromboprophylaxis during pregnancy.
  – For women with no prior history of thrombosis and ≥2 early miscarriages, treat with either 81 mg ASA alone or in combination with unfractionated heparin (5,000 to 10,000 units SC q12h) or LMWH (prophylactic dose). In those with a previous late pregnancy loss (>10 weeks' gestation) or preterm (<34 weeks) delivery due to severe preeclampsia, a combination of ASA and heparin is recommended.
  – Preconception assessment and treatment with low-dose aspirin, vitamin D, and folate should be offered in selected patients.
  – In those with a history of thrombosis, low-dose ASA plus either therapeutic low-dose heparin (dosed every 8 to 12 hours to maintain mid-interval aPTT or factor Xa levels) or LMWH (therapeutic dose)
  – Refractory cases: Up to 30% of patients have recurrent pregnancy loss despite the use of ASA and heparin. There is no role for warfarin due to risk of teratogenicity. Such cases are best managed in consultation with a maternal–fetal medicine specialist.

SURGERY/OTHER PROCEDURES
Patients with thrombosis may require thrombectomy or an IVC filter, when anticoagulation is contraindicated.

 ONGOING CARE

FOLLOW-UP RECOMMENDATIONS
Patient Monitoring
- Standard guidelines for monitoring to maintain INR at therapeutic goal on warfarin therapy
- Close monitoring is required during pregnancy.

DIET
Heart-healthy diet. Patients on warfarin should avoid foods rich in vitamin K (kale, spinach, sprouts, greens).

PATIENT EDUCATION
- Compliance with warfarin therapy to keep INR at goal
- Awareness of drug and diet interactions with warfarin
- Avoid oral hormonal contraceptives.

PROGNOSIS
- Pulmonary HTN, neurologic involvement, myocardial ischemia, nephropathy, gangrene of extremities, and CAPS are associated with a worse prognosis.
- 30% risk of recurrent thrombosis in the absence of adequate anticoagulation

COMPLICATIONS
- Pregnancy complications and pulmonary HTN are associated with higher morbidity and mortality.
- Thrombotic complications are the common cause of death.

REFERENCES
1. Bertolaccini ML, Amengual O, Andreoli L, et al. 14th International Congress on Antiphospholipid Antibodies Task Force. Report on antiphospholipid syndrome laboratory diagnostics and trends. *Autoimmun Rev.* 2014;13(9):917–930.
2. Giannakopoulos B, Passam F, Ioannou Y, et al. How we diagnose the antiphospholipid syndrome. *Blood.* 2009;113(5):985–994.
3. Lim W, Crowther MA, Eikelboom JW. Management of antiphospholipid antibody syndrome: a systematic review. *JAMA.* 2006;295(9):1050–1057.
4. Arachchillage DJ, Cohen H. Use of new oral anticoagulants in antiphospholipid syndrome. *Curr Rheumatol Rep.* 2013;15(6):331.
5. Erkan D, Aguiar CL, Andrade D, et al. 14th International Congress on Antiphospholipid Antibodies: task force report on antiphospholipid syndrome treatment trends. *Autoimmun Rev.* 2014;13(6):685–696.
6. Cuadrado MJ, Bertolaccini ML, Seed PT, et al. Low-dose aspirin vs low-dose aspirin plus low-intensity warfarin in thromboprophylaxis: a prospective, multicentre, randomized, open, controlled trial in patients positive for antiphospholipid antibodies (ALIWAPAS). *Rheumatology (Oxford).* 2014;53(2):275–284.

ADDITIONAL READING
- Andrade D, Cervera R, Cohen H, et al. 15th International Congress on Antiphospholipid Antibodies Task Force on antiphospholipd syndrome treatment trends report. In: Erkan D, Lockshin M, eds. *Antiphospholipid Syndrome.* New York, NY: Springer International; 2017:317.
- Cohen H, Hunt BJ, Efthymiou M, et al. Rivaroxaban versus warfarin to treat patients with thrombotic antiphospholipid syndrome, with or without systemic lupus erythematosus (RAPS): a randomised, controlled, open-label, phase 2/3, non-inferiority trial. *Lancet Haematol.* 2016;3(9):e426–e436.
- Committee on Practice Bulletins—Obstetrics, American College of Obstetricians and Gynecologists. Practice Bulletin no. 132: antiphospholipid syndrome. *Obstet Gynecol.* 2012;120(6):1514–1521.

 CODES

ICD10
- D68.61 Antiphospholipid syndrome
- D68.69 Other thrombophilia
- D68.62 Lupus anticoagulant syndrome

CLINICAL PEARLS
- APS is a multisystem autoimmune disorder with recurrent arterial/venous thrombosis and fetal loss and positive APAs.
- Both clinical and laboratory criteria are required for diagnosis. The latter must be confirmed on two separate occasions at least 12 weeks apart.
- Thrombotic manifestations of APS require lifelong anticoagulation.

ANXIETY (GENERALIZED ANXIETY DISORDER)

Rhonda A. Faulkner, PhD • Diana Bonaccorsi, DO

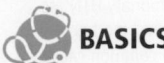 **BASICS**

DESCRIPTION
- A condition characterized by persistent, excessive, and difficult-to-control worry associated with significant symptoms of motor tension, autonomic hyperactivity, and/or disturbances of sleep or concentration
- System(s) affected: nervous (increased sympathetic tone and catecholamine release); secondary effects on other symptoms such as cardiac (tachycardia), pulmonary (dyspnea), and GI (nausea, irregular bowels)

EPIDEMIOLOGY
Prevalence
- 12-month prevalence rate: 1.8%
- Lifetime prevalence rate in United States 5.1–11.9%
- Elderly prevalence as high as 7–10%
- Onset can occur any time in life but is typically during adulthood; median age of onset in the United States is 31 years.
- Predominant sex: female > male (2:1)
- Generally recurrent and chronic in nature; gradual in onset; fluctuates in severity; complete remission less likely (1)

ETIOLOGY AND PATHOPHYSIOLOGY
- May be mediated by abnormalities of neurotransmitter systems (i.e., serotonin, norepinephrine, and γ-aminobutyric acid [GABA])
- Associated with altered regional brain function (increased activity in the amygdala and prefrontal cortex)

Genetics
- Strongly linked to depression in heritability studies
- A variant of the serotonin transporter gene (*5HT1A*) or other genes may contribute to both conditions.

RISK FACTORS
- Adverse life events
- Family history
- Chronic physical illness
- Lack of social support
- Poverty
- Comorbid psychiatric disorders (2)

GENERAL PREVENTION
- Physical activity and cardiorespiratory fitness are associated with decreased generalized anxiety and depression.
- Cognitive-behavioral therapy (CBT) and parental intervention in children with early anxiety may protect against the development of GAD (2).

COMMONLY ASSOCIATED CONDITIONS
- Major depressive disorder (>60%), dysthymia, bipolar disorder, schizophrenia
- Alcohol/drug abuse
- Cigarette smoking in adolescence
- Panic disorder, agoraphobia, simple phobia, social anxiety disorder, anorexia nervosa, posttraumatic stress disorder (PTSD), obsessive-compulsive disorder (OCD), ADHD
- Somatoform and pain disorders

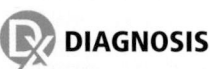 **DIAGNOSIS**

HISTORY
- Diagnosis is primarily made through history taking. Pathologic anxiety must be distinguished from normal anxiety reactions.

- *DSM-5* criteria are as follows:
  - Symptoms of excessive anxiety and worry must occur more often than not for at least 6 months.
  - Patient finds it difficult to control the worry.
  - At least three additional criteria are required for diagnosis of GAD in adults; only one is required in children.
    - Restlessness or feeling keyed up or on edge
    - Easily fatigued
    - Difficulty concentrating or mind going blank
    - Irritability
    - Muscle tension
    - Sleep disturbances (difficulty falling or staying asleep)
  - Persistent worry must cause significant distress or impairment in social, occupational, or other areas of functioning.
  - Focus of anxiety and worry is not consistent with or limited to the occurrence of other types of psychiatric disorders and is not directly related to PTSD.
  - Symptoms are not the result of a substance, another medical condition, or other *DSM-5* diagnosis.

PHYSICAL EXAM
Useful for identifying other differential diagnosis (see below). No specific physical findings in GAD, but patient may exhibit irritability, bitten nails, tremor, or clammy hands.

DIFFERENTIAL DIAGNOSIS
- Cardiovascular: ischemic heart disease, valvular heart disease (mitral valve prolapse), cardiomyopathies, arrhythmias, congestive heart failure
- Respiratory: asthma, chronic obstructive pulmonary disease, pulmonary embolism
- CNS: stroke, seizures, dementia, migraine, vestibular dysfunction, neoplasms
- Metabolic and hormonal: hyper- or hypothyroidism, pheochromocytoma, adrenal insufficiency, Cushing syndrome, hypokalemia, hypoglycemia, hyperparathyroidism
- Drug-induced anxiety: alcohol, sympathomimetics (cocaine, amphetamine, caffeine), corticosteroids, herbals (ginseng)
- Withdrawal: alcohol, sedative-hypnotics
- Psychiatric: other disorders (e.g., panic disorder, OCD, PTSD, social phobia, adjustment disorder, and somatization disorder)

DIAGNOSTIC TESTS & INTERPRETATION
Initial Tests (lab, imaging)
- Laboratory tests are normal. Initial tests may include thyroid-stimulating hormone, CBC, basic metabolic panel, urine drug screen, and ECG.
- GAD-2: two-question self-reporting scale (22% positive predictive value [PPV]/78% negative predictive value [NPV])
- PHQ-4 provides a very brief screen for both anxiety and depression (2).

Diagnostic Procedures/Other
Psychological testing
- GAD-7: five additional questions; provides more detailed information for treatment (29% PPV/71% NPV); also may be indicative of panic disorder (GAD-7: 29% PPV/71% NPV)
- Hamilton Anxiety Scale (HAM-A), Anxiety Disorders Interview Schedule (ADIS-IV)
- In pediatric populations: ADIS-IV Parent and Child Version, Multidimensional Anxiety Scale for Children (MASC), Screen for Child Anxiety Related Emotional Disorders (SCARED)

 TREATMENT

GENERAL MEASURES
- Assess for suicidality given increased risk.
- Identify and treat coexisting substance abuse and other psychiatric conditions.
- Psychoeducation recommended for all patients in addition to physical exercise and mindfulness-based stress reduction approaches
- Start early because delayed treatment may result in poorer clinical outcomes compared with patients treated within 1 year of symptom onset.
- Consider utilizing self-reported measures at each visit to quantify the level of anxiety as well as to track severity and treatment response (i.e., GAD-7).
- Remission may not occur until 4 to 6 months into treatment. Treat for at least 12 months.
- Persistence with therapy necessary to achieve maximum benefit and ensure sustained improvement
- Psychotherapeutic approaches
  - Psychological treatments are effective in treating GAD: number needed to treat (NNT) = 2 (3)[A].
  - CBT: most well-studied psychological treatment; may improve comorbid conditions such as depression; treatment of choice when available (2)[A]
  - Relaxation/mindfulness training (2)[A]
  - Psychodynamic psychotherapy: Treatment is focused on patient discovering and verbalizing unconscious conflicts (2)[C].

MEDICATION
First Line
- SSRI and SNRI antidepressants have demonstrated efficacy, are well-tolerated, do not cause abuse/dependence, and treat comorbid depression. Data to compare between agents are limited (4)[A].
- Medication selection based on side-effect profile, drug-drug interactions, and/or patient treatment history/preference
- In general, with SSRIs/SNRIs, start at the lowest available dose, up-titrate every 2 to 4 weeks, and use highest tolerated FDA-approved dose for at least 4 to 6 weeks before deeming ineffective. Then, consider switching to a different SSRI/SNRI.
- Switching between medications without adequate dose or duration of therapy can lead to ineffective treatment.
- Taper all doses gradually to discontinue.
- Common side effects of SSRIs may include nausea, diarrhea, insomnia, agitation or sedation, drug interactions, weight gain, and sexual side effects (decreased libido, delayed orgasm).
- Common side effects of SNRIs may include nausea, dizziness, insomnia, sedation, constipation, sweating, and some may cause blood pressure elevation.
  - SSRIs: escitalopram (Lexapro): initially 10 mg/day; may titrate to a maximum of 20 mg/day
  - Sertraline (Zoloft): initially 25 mg/day; may titrate by 25 to 50 mg/day qwk to a maximum of 200 mg/day
  - Paroxetine (Paxil): initially 10 to 20 mg/day; may titrate by 10 mg/day qwk to a maximum of 50 mg/day (no added benefit >20 mg/day)
  - Fluoxetine (Prozac) and citalopram (Celexa) likely have efficacy for GAD but do not have FDA indications.

- SNRIs
  - Duloxetine (Cymbalta): initially 30 mg/day; may titrate by 30 mg/day qwk to a maximum of 120 mg/day; doses >60 mg/day rarely more effective
  - Venlafaxine XR (Effexor XR): initially 37.5 to 75.0 mg; may titrate up by 75 mg every 4 days to a maximum of 225 mg/day

Second Line
- Benzodiazepines: efficacious in the short term but less effective long term, risk for dependence and abuse (4)[A]
  - Clonazepam (Klonopin): 0.25 mg BID; may increase to 4 mg/day divided BID
  - Diazepam (Valium): 2 to 5 mg BID–QID; may increase to a maximum of 40 mg/day
  - Lorazepam (Ativan): 0.5 mg BID–TID; may increase to 6 mg/day divided TID
  - Alprazolam (Xanax): 0.25 mg TID; may increase to 4 mg/day
- Hydroxyzine (Vistaril, Atarax): CNS depressant, antihistamine, anticholinergic; decreased risk of dependence compared with benzodiazepines: usual dose: 50 to 100 mg PO QID; limit use in the elderly (3)[B].
- Azapirones: buspirone (BuSpar): less risk of dependence, although may be less effective; 15 mg/day divided BID–TID initially; maximum of 60 mg/day divided BID–TID (4)[A]
- Pregabalin (Lyrica): decreases anxiety scores and reduces relapse at 75 to 300 mg BID; may cause less sexual dysfunction and sleep disruption than SSRIs. Taper to discontinue; has rapid onset of action (4)[A]
- Quetiapine (Seroquel): optimal dose 150 mg/day. 2nd-generation antipsychotic. Efficacious but less well tolerated than SSRIs (5)[A]. Consider using as augmentation.

Geriatric Considerations
- Avoid TCAs and long-acting benzodiazepines; benzodiazepines may cause delirium.
- Pregabalin may cause dizziness and somnolence.

Pediatric Considerations
- CBT is first-line treatment for pediatric patients with mild to moderate GAD.
- CBT in combination with SSRI is first-line treatment with severe GAD in pediatric population.
- Black box warning (SSRIs): Antidepressants increase the risk of suicidal thinking and behavior in children, adolescents, and young adults.
- However, studies have also shown increase in suicide attempts in adolescents after SSRI discontinuation.
- SSRIs and SNRIs have all been shown to be effective in pediatric population.
- SSRIs are first-line choice among medications because they are associated with greater side effect tolerance among children and adolescents.
- Anxiety and ADHD often co-occur. Treat the more debilitating first and consider using nonstimulating medications.

Pregnancy Considerations
- Buspirone: Category B: secreted in breast milk; inadequate studies to assess risk
- Benzodiazepines: Category D: may cause lethargy and weight loss in nursing infants; avoid breastfeeding if the mother is taking chronically or in high doses.
- SSRIs: If possible, taper and discontinue. After 20 weeks' gestation, there is increased risk of pulmonary hypertension; mild transient neonatal

syndrome of CNS; and motor, respiratory, and GI signs. Studies regarding risk of autism show mixed results. Most are Category C, with the exception of:
  - Paroxetine: Category D: conflicting evidence regarding the risk of congenital cardiac defects and other congenital anomalies in the 1st trimester
  - Hydroxyzine: Category C: Case reports of neonatal withdrawal exist.

ALERT
Precautions

- Benzodiazepines: age >65 years, respiratory disease/sleep apnea, contraindicated with narrow-angle glaucoma, precaution with open-angle glaucoma; sudden discontinuation increases seizure risk. Long-term use has potential for tolerance and dependence; use with caution in patients with history of substance abuse.
- Buspirone: hepatic and/or renal dysfunction; monoamine oxidase inhibitor (MAOI) treatment
- SSRIs: Use caution in those with comorbid bipolar disorder; may increase risk of serotonin syndrome, especially in combination with other serotonergic drugs

ISSUES FOR REFERRAL
Concomitant depression, refractory anxiety, or other comorbidities may warrant a psychiatric evaluation in light of increased suicide risk.

COMPLEMENTARY & ALTERNATIVE MEDICINE
- Patients frequently engage in complementary and alternative medicine (CAM); providers should be familiar with common therapies.
- Probable benefit but more study needed on several complementary therapies including acupuncture, yoga, massage, tai chi, and aromatherapy (5)[A]
- Kava: some evidence for benefit over placebo in mild to moderate anxiety, but concern regarding potential hepatotoxicity. Safety is potentially affected by manufacturing quality, plant part used, dose, and interactions with other substances (5)[A].
- Strong evidence to support regular physical activity to relieve anxiety symptoms (5)[A]
- Small study showed possible benefit from repetitive transcranial magnetic stimulation (rTMS) to the right dorsal lateral prefrontal cortex for pharmacotherapy treatment refractory patients.

ADMISSION, INPATIENT, AND NURSING CONSIDERATIONS
Patients at risk for suicide should be treated as inpatients; may be considered as well for patients with substantial interference in daily function

ONGOING CARE

FOLLOW-UP RECOMMENDATIONS
Patient Monitoring
- Follow up within 2 to 4 weeks from starting new medications.
- Medications should be continued past the initial period of response and recommend continued treatment for 12 months.
- Monitor mental status on benzodiazepines and avoid drug dependence or abrupt discontinuation.
- Monitor all patients for suicidal ideation but especially those on SSRIs and SNRIs.

DIET
- Limit caffeine intake.
- Avoid alcohol (drug interactions, high rate of abuse, potential for increased anxiety) and nicotine.

PATIENT EDUCATION
- Regular exercise may be beneficial for both anxiety and comorbid conditions.
- Psychoeducation regarding normal versus pathologic anxiety, the fight or flight response, and the physiology of anxiety can be extremely helpful.

PROGNOSIS
- Probability of recovery is approximately 40–60%, but relapse is common.
- Comorbid psychiatric disorders and poor relationships with spouse or family make relapse more likely.

REFERENCES

1. Ruscio A, Hallion L, Lim C, et al. Cross-sectional comparison of the epidemiology of DSM-5 generalized anxiety disorder across the globe. *JAMA Psychiatry*. 2017;74(5):465–475.
2. Patel G, Fancher TL. In the clinic. Generalized anxiety disorder. *Ann Intern Med*. 2013;159(11):ITC6-1–ITC6-12.
3. Cuijpers P, Sijbrandij M, Koole S, et al. Psychological treatment of generalized anxiety disorder: a meta-analysis. *Clin Psychol Rev*. 2014;34(2):130–140.
4. Huh J, Goebert D, Takeshita J, et al. Treatment of generalized anxiety disorder: a comprehensive review of the literature for psychopharmacologic alternatives to newer antidepressants and benzodiazepines. *Prim Care Companion CNS Disord*. 2011;13(2):PCC.08r00709.
5. Sarris J, Moylan S, Camfield DA, et al. Complementary medicine, exercise, meditation, diet, and lifestyle modification for anxiety disorders: a review of current evidence. *Evid Based Complement Alternat Med*. 2012;2012:809653.

 SEE ALSO

Algorithms: Anxiety; Depressive Episode, Major

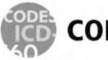 **CODES**

ICD10
- F41.9 Anxiety disorder, unspecified
- F41.1 Generalized anxiety disorder
- F41.8 Other specified anxiety disorders

CLINICAL PEARLS
- Psychiatric comorbidities, especially depression, are extremely common with GAD; patients are at increased risk for suicidality.
- CBT and SSRIs (possibly in combination) are the treatments of choice.
- Start medication at low doses, with careful titration to full therapeutic dosing, helps minimize side effects while maximizing efficacy.
- Benzodiazepines may be used initially but should be tapered and withdrawn if possible.
- CAM use is common, and certain therapies may be effective.

AORTIC VALVULAR STENOSIS

Jeremy Golding, MD, FAAFP

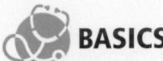 BASICS

DESCRIPTION

Aortic stenosis (AS) is a narrowing of the aortic valve area causing obstruction to left ventricular (LV) outflow. The disease has a long asymptomatic latency period, but development of severe obstruction or onset of symptoms such as syncope, angina, and congestive heart failure (CHF) are associated with a high mortality rate without surgical intervention.

EPIDEMIOLOGY

AS is the most common primary valve disease leading to surgery or catheter intervention in Europe and North America, with a growing prevalence due to the aging population (1). Cause by age at presentation:

- <30 years: congenital
- 30 to 65 years: congenital or rheumatic fever (RF)
- >65 years: degenerative calcification of aortic valve

Prevalence

- Affects 1.3% of population 65 to 74 years old, 2.4% 75 to 84 years old, 4% >84 years old
- Bicuspid aortic valve: 1–2% of population. Bicuspid aortic valve predisposes to development of AS at an earlier age.

ETIOLOGY AND PATHOPHYSIOLOGY

- Progressive aortic leaflet thickening and calcification results in LV outflow obstruction. Obstruction causes increased afterload and, over time, decreased cardiac output.
- Increase in LV systolic pressure is required to preserve cardiac output; this leads to development of concentric LV hypertrophy (LVH). The compensatory LVH preserves ejection fraction but adversely affects heart functioning.
  - LVH impairs coronary blood flow during diastole by compression of coronary arteries and reduced capillary ingrowth into hypertrophied muscle.
  - LVH results in diastolic dysfunction by reducing ventricular compliance.
- Diastolic dysfunction necessitates stronger left atrial (LA) contraction to augment preload and maintain stroke volume. Loss of LA contraction by atrial fibrillation can induce acute deterioration.
- Diastolic dysfunction may persist after relief of AS due to the presence of interstitial fibrosis.
- Angina: increased myocardial demand due to higher LV pressure. Myocardial supply is compromised due to LVH.
- Syncope (exertional): can be multifactorial from inability to augment cardiac output due to the fixed obstruction to LV outflow; arrhythmias; or most commonly, abnormal baroreceptor response resulting in failure to appropriately augment blood pressure
- Heart failure: Eventually, LVH cannot compensate for increasing afterload resulting in high LV pressure and volume, which are accompanied by an increase in LA and pulmonary pressures.
- Degenerative calcific changes to aortic valve (2)
  - Mechanism involves mechanical stress to valve leaflets as well as atherosclerotic changes to the valve tissue. Bicuspid valves are at higher risk for mechanical stress.
  - Early lesions: subendothelial accumulation of oxidized LDL and macrophages and T lymphocytes (inflammatory response)

- Disease progression: Fibroblasts undergo transformation into osteoblasts; protein production of osteopontin, osteocalcin, and bone morphogenic protein-2 (BMP-2), which modulates calcification of leaflets
- Congenital: unicuspid valve, bicuspid valve, tricuspid valve with fusion of commissures, hypoplastic annulus
- RF: chronic scarring with fusion of commissures

RISK FACTORS

- Congenital unicommissural valve or bicuspid valve
  - Unicommissural valve: Most cases were detected during childhood.
  - Bicuspid valve: predisposes to the development of AS earlier in adulthood (4th to 5th decade) compared to tricuspid valve (6th to 8th decade)
- RF
  - Prevalence of chronic rheumatic valvular disease has declined significantly in the United States.
  - Most cases are associated with mitral valve disease.
- Degenerative calcific changes
  - Most common cause of acquired AS in the United States
  - Risk factors are similar to that of coronary artery disease (CAD) and include the following: hypercholesterolemia, hypertension, smoking, male gender, age, and diabetes mellitus.

COMMONLY ASSOCIATED CONDITIONS

- CAD (50% of patients)
- Hypertension (40% of patients): results in "double-loaded" left ventricle (dual source of increased afterload as a result of obstruction from AS and hypertension)
- Aortic insufficiency (common in calcified bicuspid valves and rheumatic disease)
- Mitral valve disease: 95% of patients with AS from RF also have mitral valve disease.
- LV dysfunction and CHF
- Acquired von Willebrand disease: Impaired platelet function and decreased vWF results in bleeding (ecchymosis and epistaxis) in 20% of AS patients. Severity of coagulopathy is directly related to severity of AS.
- Gastrointestinal arteriovenous malformations (AVMs)
- Cerebral or systemic embolic events due to calcium emboli

℞ DIAGNOSIS

HISTORY

- Primary symptoms: angina, syncope, and heart failure. Angina is the most frequent symptom. Syncope is often exertional. Heart failure symptoms include fatigue, exertional dyspnea, orthopnea, paroxysmal nocturnal dyspnea, and shortness of breath.
- Palpitations
- Neurologic events (transient ischemic attack or cerebrovascular accident) secondary to embolization
- Geriatric patients may have subtle symptoms such as fatigue and exertional dyspnea.
- Note: Symptoms do not always correlate with valve area (severity of AS) but most commonly occur when aortic valve area is <1 cm², jet velocity is >4.0 m/s, or the mean transvalvular gradient is ≥40 mm Hg.

PHYSICAL EXAM

- Auscultation
  - Harsh, systolic crescendo–decrescendo murmur is best heard at 2nd right sternal border and radiates into the carotid arteries. Peak of murmur correlates with severity of stenosis; later peaking murmur suggests greater severity.
  - High-pitched blowing diastolic murmur suggests associated aortic insufficiency.
  - Paradoxically split S_2 or absent A_2. Note: Normally split S_2 reliably excludes severe AS.
  - S_4 due to stiffening of the left ventricle
- Other associated signs include *pulsus parvus et tardus*: decreased and delayed carotid upstroke. LV heave; findings of CHF: pulmonary and/or lower extremity edema

DIFFERENTIAL DIAGNOSIS

- Mitral regurgitation: High-frequency, pansystolic murmur, best heard at the apex, often radiates to the axilla.
- Hypertrophic obstructive cardiomyopathy: also systolic crescendo–decrescendo murmur but best heard at left sternal border and may radiate into axilla. Murmur intensity increases by changing from squatting to standing and/or by Valsalva maneuver.
- Discrete fixed subaortic stenosis: 50–65% has associated cardiac deformity (patent ductus arteriosus [PDA], ventricular septal defect [VSD], aortic coarctation).
- Aortic supravalvular stenosis: Williams syndrome, homozygous familial hypercholesterolemia

DIAGNOSTIC TESTS & INTERPRETATION

Initial Tests (lab, imaging)

- Chest x-ray (CXR)
  - May be normal in compensated, isolated valvular AS
  - Boot-shaped heart reflective of concentric hypertrophy
  - Poststenotic dilatation of ascending aorta and calcification of aortic valve (seen on lateral PA CXR)
- ECG: often normal ECG (ECG is nondiagnostic), or may show LVH, LA enlargement, and nonspecific ST- and T-wave abnormalities
- Echo indications
  - Initial workup
    - Doppler echocardiogram: primary test in the diagnosis and evaluation of AS (1)[A]
    - Assesses valve anatomy and severity of disease
    - Assesses LV wall thickness, size, and function, and pulmonary artery pressure
  - In known AS and changing signs/symptoms
  - In known AS and pregnancy due to hemodynamic changes of pregnancy
- Echo findings
  - Aortic valve thickening, calcification
  - Decreased aortic valve excursion
  - Reduced aortic valve area
  - Transvalvular gradient across aortic valve
  - LVH and diastolic dysfunction
  - LV ejection fraction
  - Wall-motion abnormalities suggesting CAD
  - Evaluate for concomitant aortic insufficiency or mitral valve disease.
- AS severity based on echo values (2)
  - Stage A (at risk): bicuspid aortic valve, sclerosis, or other congenital abnormality; mean pressure gradient: 0 mm Hg; jet vel. <2 m/s
  - Stage B (progressive): bicuspid or trileaflet valve
    - Mild: mean pressure gradient: <20 mm Hg; jet vel. 2.0 to 2.9 m/s
    - Moderate: mean pressure gradient: 20 to 40 mm Hg; jet vel. 3.0 to 3.9 m/s

- Stage C (asymptomatic severe AS):
  - C1 (without LV dysfunction): AVA ≤1.0 or AVAi ≤0.6 cm²/m²; mean pressure gradient: 40 to 60 mm Hg; jet vel. ≥4 to 5 m/s
  - C2 (with LV dysfunction): AVA ≤1.0 or AVAi ≤0.6 cm²/m²; mean pressure gradient: ≥40 mm Hg; jet vel. ≥4 m/s
- Stage D (symptomatic severe AS):
  - D1 (high gradient): AVA ≤1.0 cm²; mean pressure gradient: >40 mm Hg; jet vel. >4 m/s
  - D2 (low flow/low gradient with reduced EF <50%): AVA ≤1.0 cm²; mean pressure gradient: <40 mm Hg; jet vel. <4 m/s
  - D3 (low gradient, normal EF ≥50% or paradoxical low-flow severe AS): AVA ≤1.0 cm²; AVAi ≤0.6 cm²/m² and stroke volume index <35 mL/m²; mean pressure gradient: <40 mm Hg; jet vel. <4 m/s

Diagnostic Procedures/Other
- Exercise stress testing
  - Asymptomatic patients with severe AS: helpful to uncover subtle symptoms or changes, abnormal BP (increase <20 mm Hg), and ECG changes (ST depressions). 1/3 of patients develop symptoms with exercise testing; STOP testing at this point.
  - Symptomatic patients: DO NOT perform exercise stress testing because it may induce hypotension or ventricular tachycardia.
  - CHF patients: Dobutamine stress echocardiography is reasonable to evaluate patients with low-flow/low-gradient AS and LV dysfunction.
- Cardiac catheterization
  - Perform prior to aortic valve replacement (AVR) in patients with suspected CAD. Determines need for coronary artery bypass graft (CABG). If unambiguous diagnosis of AS, perform only coronary angiography.
  - Can also use if noninvasive testing is inconclusive or if there is discrepancy between severity of symptoms and findings on echo
  - Measures transvalvular flow and transvalvular pressure gradient, which facilitates calculation of effective valve area
  - Hemodynamic measurements with infusion of dobutamine can be useful for evaluation of patients with low-flow/low-gradient AS and LV dysfunction.

Test Interpretation
- Aortic valve: nodular calcification on valve cusps (initially at bases), cusp rigidity, cusp thickening, and fibrosis
- LVH, myocardial interstitial fibrosis
- 50% incidence of concomitant CAD

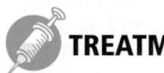

TREATMENT

MEDICATION
- No effective medical therapy for severe or symptomatic AS
- Prevention: currently no recommended medical therapy. Statins have been thought to slow progression if initiated during mild disease. However, this has not been supported by large, randomized controlled trials.
- Antibiotic prophylaxis against recurrent RF is indicated for patients with rheumatic AS (penicillin G 1,200,000 U IM q4wk; duration varies with age and history of carditis).

- Antibiotic prophylaxis is no longer indicated for prevention of infective endocarditis.
- Comorbidities: hypertension: angiotensin-converting enzyme (ACE) inhibitors, start with low dose and increase cautiously. Be cautious of vasodilators, which may cause hypotension.

SURGERY/OTHER PROCEDURES
- AVR is recommended for most symptomatic patients with evidence of significant AS on echocardiography (3).
- Indications for AVR surgery:
  - Symptomatic and severe high-gradient AS by history or exercise testing (2)[B] when surgical risk is low or intermediate
  - Asymptomatic, severe AS and LVEF <50% (2)[B]
  - Severe AS (stage C or D) when undergoing other cardiac surgery (2)[B]
- AVR surgery is reasonable in patients who are:
  - Asymptomatic with severe AS (C1) with jet vel. ≥5 m/s and low surgical risk, decreased exercise tolerance, or have an exercise fall in blood pressure (2)[B]
  - Symptomatic stage D2, with a low-dose dobutamine stress with jet vel. ≥4.0 m/s or mean pressure gradient ≥40 mm Hg with ≤1.0 cm² at any dobutamine dose (2)[B]
  - Symptomatic stage D3 with LVEF >50% if clinical and hemodynamic data support valve obstruction as likely cause of symptoms (2)[C]
  - Stage B who are undergoing other cardiac surgery, or asymptomatic stage C1 with rapid disease progression and low surgical risk (2)[C]

ALERT
Note: If the aortic valve area is >1.5 cm² and the gradient is <15 mm Hg, there is no benefit from AVR.

- Transcatheter AVR (TAVR) offers a less invasive option for some patients (1).
  - For those who are high at surgical risk and considered inoperable, TAVR has demonstrated superiority to medical therapy.
  - For those who are high at surgical risk, TAVR has demonstrated noninferiority to surgical AVR (1).
  - For those who are intermediate at surgical risk, TAVR may emerge as a reasonable alternative to surgical risk, although this indication has not yet been approved in the United States.
  - Valve-in-valve TAVR can be considered in high-risk patients with failed surgically implanted bioprosthetic valves.
- Percutaneous balloon valvuloplasty may have role in palliation or as a bridge to valve replacement in hemodynamically unstable or high-risk patients but is not recommended as an alternative to valve replacement.

ONGOING CARE

FOLLOW-UP RECOMMENDATIONS
- Advise patients to immediately report symptoms referable to AS.
- Asymptomatic patients: yearly history and physical
- Serial ECHO: yearly for severe AS, every 1 to 2 years for moderate AS, every 3 to 5 years for mild AS

PATIENT EDUCATION
Physical activity limitations
- Asymptomatic mild AS: no restrictions
- Asymptomatic moderate to severe AS: Avoid strenuous exercise. Consider exercise stress test prior to starting exercise program.

PROGNOSIS
- Although survival in asymptomatic patients is comparable to that in age- and sex-matched control patients, it decreases rapidly after symptoms appear (3).
- 25% mortality per year in symptomatic patients who do not undergo valve replacement; average survival is 2 to 3 years without AVR surgery.
- Median survival in symptomatic AS: heart failure: 2 years; syncope: 3 years; angina: 5 years
- Perisurgical mortality: AVR surgery has 4% mortality rate; AVR + CABG has 6.8% mortality rate.
- Adverse postoperative prognostic factors: age, heart failure New York Heart Association (NYHA) class III/IV, cerebrovascular disease, renal dysfunction, CAD

REFERENCES
1. Baumgartner H, Falk V, Bax JJ, et al; for ESC Scientific Document Group. 2017 ESC/EACTS guidelines for the management of valvular heart disease. Eur Heart J. 2017;38(36):2739–2791.
2. Nishimura RA, Otto CM, Bonow RO, et al. 2017 AHA/ACC focused update of the 2014 AHA/ACC guideline for the management of patients with valvular heart disease: a report of the American College of Cardiology/American Heart Association Task Force on Clinical Practice Guidelines. Circulation. 2017;135(25):e1159–e1195.
3. Grimard BH, Safford RE, Burns EL. Aortic stenosis: diagnosis and treatment. Am Fam Physician. 2016;93(5):371–378.

CODES

ICD10
- I35.0 Nonrheumatic aortic (valve) stenosis
- I06.0 Rheumatic aortic stenosis
- Q23.0 Congenital stenosis of aortic valve

CLINICAL PEARLS
- AS is diagnosed on physical exam by a systolic crescendo–decrescendo murmur and delayed and diminished pulses.
- Symptomatic AS most commonly presents as angina, syncope, and heart failure.
- Symptomatic AS has a very poor prognosis, unless treated with surgical intervention.

APPENDICITIS, ACUTE

Cragin D. Currence, MD • Caleb J. Mentzer, DO

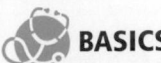 **BASICS**

DESCRIPTION
- Acute inflammation of the appendix
- Arising from the base of the cecum in right lower quadrant (RLQ), the appendix can be anterior, posterior, medial, or lateral to the cecum as well as in the pelvis. Vascular supply provided by appendicular artery, a branch of the ileocolic artery; nerve supply derived from the superior mesenteric plexus
- Most common cause of acute surgical abdomen

EPIDEMIOLOGY
- Predominant age: 10 to 30 years; rare in infancy
- Predominant sex: slight male predominance
  - Ages 10 to 30 years: male > female (3:2)
  - Age >30 years: male = female

Incidence
- 1 case per 1,000 people per year
- Lifetime incidence 1 in every 15 people (7%)

Pregnancy Considerations
- Most common extrauterine surgical emergency
- Incidence similar in pregnancy
- Higher rate of perforation; more likely to present with peritonitis

ETIOLOGY AND PATHOPHYSIOLOGY
Obstruction of the appendiceal lumen is thought to lead to distention, ischemia, and bacterial overgrowth. Without intervention, appendicitis can lead to perforation and subsequent abscess formation or generalized peritonitis. Causes of obstruction:
- Fecaliths (most common)
- Lymphoid tissue hyperplasia (in children)
- Vegetable, fruit seeds, and other foreign bodies
- Intestinal worms (ascarids)
- Strictures, fibrosis, neoplasms

Genetics
First-degree relative with history of appendicitis increases risk; no direct genetic link has been found.

RISK FACTORS
Adolescent males, familial tendency, intra-abdominal tumors

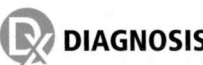 **DIAGNOSIS**

- Diagnosis relies on history and physical examination with supporting laboratory studies and imaging.
- Scoring systems
  - Modified Alvarado Scoring System (MASS): The use of MASS in the diagnosis of acute appendicitis improves diagnostic accuracy and reduces negative appendectomy and complication rates.
  - Supplement MASS in female patients with additional investigations (e.g., abdominal ultrasound or laparoscopy).
  - Migratory right iliac fossa pain (1 point)
  - Nausea/vomiting (1 point)
  - Anorexia (1 point)

- Tenderness in right iliac fossa (2 points)
- Rebound tenderness in right iliac fossa (1 point)
- Elevated temperature (1 point)
- Leukocytosis (2 points)
- A MASS score >7 suggests appendicitis without the need for further imaging.
- A cutoff point of 6 for the MASS score yields higher sensitivity but is also associated with a higher negative appendectomy rate (normal appendix).
- Pediatric Appendicitis Score—helps predict the likelihood of acute appendicitis (diagnosis is still clinical)

HISTORY
- Classic history is vague periumbilical pain, followed by anorexia, nausea, and vomiting. Over the next 4 to 48 hours, pain migrates to the RLQ.
- Only 50% of patients present with a classic history.
- Pain before vomiting (~100% sensitive), abdominal pain (~100%), pain migration (50%)
- Anorexia (~100%), nausea (90%), vomiting (75%), obstipation
- Atypical symptoms and pain suggest a retrocecal or pelvic appendix.

PHYSICAL EXAM
- Fever; temperature >100.4°F (may be absent); tachycardia
- RLQ tenderness; maximal tenderness at McBurney point (1/3 the distance from the anterior superior iliac spine to the umbilicus)
- Voluntary and involuntary guarding
- Rovsing sign: RLQ pain with palpation of left lower quadrant
- Psoas sign: pain with right thigh extension (retrocecal appendix)
- Obturator sign: pain with internal rotation of flexed right thigh (pelvic appendix); local and suprapubic pain on rectal exam (pelvic appendix)
- Pelvic and rectal exams are helpful to assess other causes of lower abdominal pain (e.g., pelvic inflammatory disease, prostatitis).
- Serial exams can be useful in indeterminate cases.

DIFFERENTIAL DIAGNOSIS
- GI
  - Gastroenteritis, inflammatory bowel disease
  - Diverticulitis, ileitis
  - Cholecystitis, pancreatitis
  - Intussusception, volvulus
- Gynecologic
  - Pelvic inflammatory disease, ectopic pregnancy
  - Ovarian cyst, ovarian torsion, tubo-ovarian abscess
  - Endometriosis
  - Ruptured graafian follicle
- Urologic
  - Testicular torsion, epididymitis
  - Kidney stones, prostatitis, cystitis, pyelonephritis
- Systemic
  - Diabetic ketoacidosis
  - Henoch-Schönlein purpura
  - Sickle cell crisis
  - Porphyria

- Other
  - Acute mesenteric lymphadenitis
  - No organic pathologic condition
  - Hernias
  - Psoas abscess
  - Rectus sheath hematoma
  - Epiploic appendagitis
  - Pneumonia (basilar)

Pediatric Considerations
- Decreased diagnostic accuracy of history and physical exam
- Higher fever; more vomiting and diarrhea

Pregnancy Considerations
- Appendicitis is more difficult to diagnose in pregnancy.
- Normal inflammatory response is suppressed.
- Appendix displaced out of pelvis by gravid uterus

Geriatric Considerations
Decreased diagnostic accuracy, more likely to be atypical presentation

DIAGNOSTIC TESTS & INTERPRETATION

Initial Tests (lab, imaging)
- Leukocytosis: WBC >10,000/mm³ (70%)
- Polymorphonuclear predominance—"left shift" (>90%)
- Urinalysis: hematuria, pyuria (30%)
- Human chorionic gonadotropin (hCG) (If positive, rule out ectopic pregnancy.)
- C-reactive protein: nonspecific inflammatory marker; when paired with an elevated WBC, increases predictive value for appendicitis
- Drugs may alter lab results: antibiotics, steroids
- Imaging if the diagnosis is not clear; helps to detect complications (abscess, perforation)
- Plain films: minimal utility, nonspecific findings, may visualize fecalith
- CT with contrast: sensitivity 91–98%; specificity 95–99%; imaging modality of choice. Consider radiation dose, particularly in young patients.
- Ultrasound: alternative in pregnancy, children, and women with suspected gynecologic pathology. Sensitivity and specificity vary skill of the ultrasonographer. Increasing use adult populations, with positive predictive value approaching 100% in some studies (1)[B]. Can rule in appendicitis but cannot reliably exclude the diagnosis. An effective strategy is to start with ultrasound and, if negative, obtain a CT scan if suspicion warrants.
- MRI: increasing use in pregnant patients. May help in patients with contrast allergies renal failure. Limitations include cost, availability, and time required to complete study.
- Radioisotope-labeled WBC scans: may be used in patients with indeterminate CT scans and suspected appendicitis as an alternative to observation or surgery. Limitations include availability and time required to complete study.

Diagnostic Procedures/Other

Exploratory laparotomy/laparoscopy. Acceptable appendectomy rates vary based on age and gender and may be higher for females of childbearing age than males.

Test Interpretation

- Acute appendiceal inflammation, local vascular congestion, obstruction
- Gangrene, perforation with abscess (15–30%)
- Fecalith

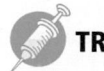

TREATMENT

GENERAL MEASURES

- Surgery (appendectomy) has been the standard of care for acute, uncomplicated appendicitis. There is growing evidence for medical management in select cases—antibiotic therapy, with appendectomy reserved for those who do not respond to treatment (2).
- Delay in surgery for complicated appendicitis is associated with increased complications and cost (3)[A].

MEDICATION

First Line

- Uncomplicated acute appendicitis: perioperative dose of antibiotic: single dose of cefoxitin or ampicillin/sulbactam (Unasyn) or cefazolin plus metronidazole
- Nonoperative antibiotic of choice: ertapenem for 3 days followed by 7 days PO levofloxacin and metronidazole (4)[B]
- Gangrenous or perforating appendicitis
  - Broadened antibiotic coverage for aerobic and anaerobic enteric pathogens
  - Piperacillin and tazobactam (Zosyn) or ticarcillin and clavulanate (Timentin) or a 3rd-generation cephalosporin plus metronidazole are initial options.
  - Adjust dosage and choice of antibiotic based on intraoperative cultures.
  - Continue antibiotics for at least 7 days postoperatively or until patient becomes afebrile with normal WBC count.

Second Line

- Uncomplicated acute appendicitis: clindamycin plus one of the following: ciprofloxacin, levofloxacin, gentamicin, or aztreonam
- In the case of acute appendicitis complicated by abscess formation or phlegmon in pediatric patients, some studies show initial conservative management with antibiotics alone to carry fewer risks and complications than emergent appendectomy.
- Gangrenous or perforated appendicitis: ciprofloxacin or levofloxacin plus metronidazole or monotherapy with a carbapenem (imipenem and cilastatin, meropenem, ertapenem)

ISSUES FOR REFERRAL

All cases of appendicitis require emergent surgical consultation.

SURGERY/OTHER PROCEDURES

- The American College of Surgeons, Society for Surgery of the Alimentary Tract, and others recommend surgery as the treatment of choice.
- Antibiotic treatment might be used as an alternative in specific patients or if surgery is contraindicated.
- Nonoperative management with antibiotics with up to a reported 39% recurrence rate at 5 years for uncomplicated acute appendicitis (4)[B]

ADMISSION, INPATIENT, AND NURSING CONSIDERATIONS

- Admit all patients with appendicitis.
- Fluid resuscitation with normal saline (NS) or lactated Ringer (LR) solution
- Correct fluid and electrolyte deficits.
- Discharge when tolerating oral intake, return of bowel function, afebrile, normal WBC.

ONGOING CARE

FOLLOW-UP RECOMMENDATIONS

- Return to work in 1 to 2 weeks is typically following most cases of uncomplicated appendicitis.
- Restrict activity for 4 to 6 weeks after surgery: no heavy lifting (>10 lb) or strenuous physical activity.
- If managed nonoperatively and patient is >40 years, consider colonoscopy to rule out malignancy.

PATIENT EDUCATION

Postoperative warning signs:

- Anorexia, nausea, vomiting
- Abdominal pain, fever, chills
- Signs/symptoms of wound infection

PROGNOSIS

- Generally uncomplicated course in young adults with unruptured appendicitis
- Extremes of age and appendiceal rupture increase morbidity and mortality.
- Morbidity rates
  - Nonperforated appendicitis: 3%
  - Perforated appendicitis: 47%
- Mortality rates
  - Unruptured appendicitis: 0.1%
  - Ruptured appendicitis: 3%
  - Patients >60 years of age make up 50% of total deaths from appendicitis.
  - Older patients with ruptured appendix: 15%

Pediatric Considerations

- Rupture earlier
- Rupture rate: 15–60%

Pregnancy Considerations

- Rupture rate: 40%
- Fetal mortality rate: 2–8.5%

Geriatric Considerations

Rupture rate: 67–90%

COMPLICATIONS

- Wound infection, intra-abdominal abscess; lower rate with antibiotic prophylaxis (5)[A], intestinal fistulas
- Intestinal obstruction, paralytic ileus, incisional hernia
- Liver abscess (rare), pyelophlebitis
- Stump appendicitis: recurrence of appendicitis at appendiceal stump after appendectomy; incidence 0.15% (6)[B]

REFERENCES

1. Benedetto G, Ferrer Puchol MD, Llavata Solaz A. Suspicion of acute appendicitis in adults. The value of ultrasound in our hospital. *Radiologia*. 2019;61(1):51–59.
2. Flum DR. Clinical practice. Acute appendicitis—appendectomy or the "antibiotics first" strategy. *N Engl J Med*. 2015;372(20):1937–1943.
3. Symer MM, Abelson JS, Sedrakyan A, et al. Early operative management of complicated appendicitis is associated with improved surgical outcomes in adults. *Am J Surg*. 2018;216(3):431–437.
4. Salminen P, Tuominen R, Paajanen H, et al. Five-year follow-up of antibiotic therapy for uncomplicated acute appendicitis in the APPAC randomized clinical trial. *JAMA*. 2018;320(12):1259–1265.
5. Wilms IM, de Hoog DE, de Visser DC, et al. Appendectomy versus antibiotic treatment for acute appendicitis. *Cochrane Database Syst Rev*. 2011;(11):CD008359.
6. Dikicier E, Altintoprak F, Ozdemir K, et al. Stump appendicitis: a retrospective review of 3130 consecutive appendectomy cases. *World J Emerg Surg*. 2018;13:22.

ADDITIONAL READING

Bhangu A, Søreide K, Di Saverio S, et al. Acute appendicitis: modern understanding of pathogenesis, diagnosis, and management. *Lancet*. 2015;386(10000):1278–1287.

SEE ALSO

Algorithm: Abdominal Rigidity

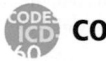

CODES

ICD10

- K35.80 Unspecified acute appendicitis
- K35.2 Acute appendicitis with generalized peritonitis
- K35.3 Acute appendicitis with localized peritonitis

CLINICAL PEARLS

- Anorexia with periumbilical pain localizing to RLQ is the classic history for acute appendicitis.
- Diagnosis is more challenging in children, pregnant patients, and the elderly due to varying symptoms and signs.
- In equivocal cases, CT is the diagnostic test of choice. Ultrasound and MRI are alternatives.
- Acute appendicitis is the most common surgical emergency during pregnancy.

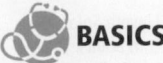

BASICS

DESCRIPTION

Pretravel consultations assess trip plans to determine potential health hazards, discuss risks and methods for prevention, provide immunizations for vaccine-preventable disease and medications for prophylaxis and/or self-treatment, and provide education to mitigate risks associated with international travel.

EPIDEMIOLOGY

Incidence

Illness and injury are common during travel. Specific incidence is difficult to ascertain. There were 1.2 billion international tourist travel arrivals in 2015 (CDC).

RISK FACTORS

Risks vary by destination, length of the trip, planned activities, age, and health status of the traveler.

- Traveler details
  - Past medical history (age, gender, medical conditions, allergies, medications)
    - Flying is contraindicated within 3 weeks of a myocardial infarction and within 10 days of a thoracic or abdominal surgery.
    - If preexisting eustachian tube dysfunction, use of a vasoconstricting nasal spray immediately before air travel may help lessen the likelihood of otitis or barotrauma (1).
  - Special conditions (pregnancy, breastfeeding, disability or handicap, immunocompromised state, older age)
    - Flying is not recommended after the 36th week of pregnancy. Many airlines require a provider letter if flying after this time.
  - Immunization history
  - Prior travel experience (previous malaria prophylaxis, experience with altitude, illnesses related to prior travel)
- Trip details
  - Itinerary (countries/specific regions, rural or urban; side trips)
  - Timing (length, season, time until departure)
  - Reason for travel
  - Special activities (disaster relief, medical care, high altitude or climbing, diving, cruise ship, rafting, cycling, extreme sports)

GENERAL PREVENTION

- Routine vaccinations
  - *Haemophilus influenzae* type b
  - Hepatitis B
  - Influenza
  - Measles, mumps, rubella—more common in countries without routine childhood immunizations
  - Meningococcal—outbreaks common in sub-Saharan Africa especially during the dry season (December through June). Saudi Arabia requires the quadrivalent vaccine for Hajj pilgrims (2).
  - Pneumococcal
  - Polio
  - Rotavirus—common in developing countries
  - Tetanus, diphtheria, pertussis
  - Varicella—more common in countries without routine childhood immunizations
  - Zoster—stress may trigger reactivation.
  - Human papillomavirus (HPV)—sexual activity during travel may lead to HPV infection.
- Travel-specific vaccinations (destination dependent)
  - Cholera (not available in the United States)
  - Hepatitis A—often recommended regardless of destination
  - Japanese encephalitis
  - Rabies—if immunoglobulin would be difficult to obtain, consider vaccination to simplify postexposure prophylaxis.
  - Tick-borne encephalitis (not available in United States)
  - Typhoid—highest risk in India, Pakistan, and Bangladesh. Do not give oral vaccine to immunocompromised patients or those who have taken antibiotics in the previous 72 hours (2).
  - Yellow fever—highest risk in sub-Saharan Africa and the Amazon regions of South America. Vaccination is not considered valid until 10 days after administration (2).
- Malaria prophylaxis
  - Based on destination, types of planned activities, and patient preferences. CDC has up-to-date recommendations.
  - Chloroquine-sensitive malaria (2,3)
    - Chloroquine—begin 1 to 2 weeks prior to travel, continue 4 weeks after leaving malaria-endemic area; may increase QTc interval (particularly if given with other QTc-prolonging drugs)
      - Adult dose: 300 mg base (500 mg salt) orally once weekly
      - Pediatric dose: 5 mg/kg base (8.3 mg/kg salt) orally once weekly (up to 300 mg base per dose)
    - Hydroxychloroquine—begin 1 to 2 weeks prior to travel, continue for 4 weeks after leaving malaria-endemic area; dosed weekly
      - Adult dose: 310 mg base (400 mg salt) orally once weekly
      - Pediatric dose: 5 mg/kg base (6.5 mg/kg salt) orally once weekly (up to 310 mg base per dose)
  - Chloroquine-resistant malaria (2,3)
    - Atovaquone/proguanil—begin 1 to 2 days before travel and continue for 1 week after leaving malaria-endemic area.
      - Adult dose: 250 mg/100 mg atovaquone/proguanil PO daily
      - Pediatric dose: Tablets contain 62.5 mg/25 mg atovaquone/proguanil hydrochloride.
        - 5 to 8 kg: 1/2 pediatric tablet daily
        - 8 to 10 kg: 3/4 pediatric tablet daily
        - 10 to 20 kg: 1 pediatric tablet daily
        - 20 to 30 kg: 2 pediatric tablets daily
        - 30 to 40 kg: 3 pediatric tablets daily
        - >40 kg: 1 adult tablet daily
    - Doxycycline—begin 1 to 2 days before travel and continue for 4 weeks after leaving malaria-endemic area.
      - Adult dose: 100 mg orally daily
      - Pediatric dose: ≥8 years old 2.2 mg/kg up to adult dose of 100 mg daily
    - Mefloquine—begin ≥2 weeks before travel and continue for 4 weeks after leaving malaria-endemic area; has a number of drug interactions
      - Adult dose: 228 mg base (250 mg salt) orally once weekly
      - Pediatric dose
        - ≤9 kg: 4.6 mg/kg base (5 mg/kg salt) orally once weekly
        - >9 to 19 kg: 1/4 tablet once weekly
        - >19 to 30 kg: 1/2 tablet once weekly
        - >30 to 45 kg: 3/4 tablet once weekly
        - >45 kg: 1 tablet once weekly
- Protection against mosquitoes and ticks
  - Avoid areas of known outbreaks of communicable disease. Refer to the CDC travelers' health Web site for updates.
  - Avoid peak exposure times and places.
    - Mosquitoes may bite at any time of the day.
    - Peak biting activity for vectors of some diseases (such as dengue, Zika, and chikungunya) is during daylight hours (1).
    - Peak biting activity for vectors of other diseases (such as malaria, West Nile, and Japanese encephalitis) are most active in twilight periods (dawn and dusk) or after dark.
  - Wear appropriate clothing: Minimize exposed skin.
  - Check for ticks.
  - Bed nets
  - Insecticides and repellants—reapply regularly.
    - DEET
    - Picaridin
    - Oil of lemon eucalyptus
    - IR3535
    - 2-Undecanone
- Traveler's diarrhea
  - Symptoms range from mild abdominal cramping and urgent loose stools to severe abdominal pain, fever, vomiting, and bloody diarrhea.
  - Approximately 80–90% bacterial, 5–8% viral, 10% protozoal (1)
  - Length—bacterial causes last 3 to 7 days if untreated. Viral lasts 2 to 3 days. Protozoal can last weeks to months if not treated.
  - High-risk areas include Asia, Middle East, Africa, Mexico, and Central and South America (2).
  - Intermediate-risk areas include countries in Eastern Europe, South Africa, and some of the Caribbean islands (2).
  - Strategies to minimize diarrhea (2)
    - Wash hands or use sanitizer prior to eating.
    - Avoid raw or undercooked meat, fish, or shellfish, salads, uncooked vegetables, unpasteurized fruit juices, or unpasteurized milk or milk products.

○ Avoid unpeeled raw fruit. Peel it yourself if possible.

○ Tap water may be unsafe for drinking, making ice, preparing food, washing dishes, or brushing teeth; use sealed bottled water if possible.

– For high-risk patients—bismuth subsalicylate reduces incidence of travelers' diarrhea by 50%; 2 oz of liquid or two chewable tablets 4 times per day (not recommended for children <3 years) (2)

– Antibiotic options for diarrhea self-treatment
  ○ Ciprofloxacin 500 mg q12h × 2 doses
  ○ Azithromycin 500 mg daily for 1 to 3 days

– Adjunct medications
  ○ Loperamide
    ▪ 4 mg initially followed by 2 mg after each loose stool (max 16 mg/day)
    ▪ Pediatric dose
    ▪ Not recommended for children <6 years
    ▪ 6 to 8 years—2 mg initial dose, followed by 1 mg after each loose stool (max 4 mg/day)
    ▪ 9 to 11 years—2 mg after initial dose, followed by 1 mg after each loose stool (max 6 mg/day)
    ▪ ≥12 years: Refer to adult dosing.
  ○ Diphenoxylate
    ▪ 5 mg (2 tablets) 3 or 4 times per day until control achieved (max 20 mg/day)
    ▪ Pediatric dose: not recommended for children <2 years; 0.3 to 0.4 mg/kg/day in 4 divided doses

• Altitude illness
  – Acute mountain sickness (AMS)—most common. Typically presents with headache starting 2 to 12 hours after arrival. Other symptoms include fatigue, loss of appetite, nausea, and vomiting; usually resolves within 24 to 48 hours of acclimatization (2)
  – High-altitude cerebral edema (HACE)—severe progression of AMS. Lethargy, drowsiness, confusion, ataxia; requires immediate descent (2)
  – High-altitude pulmonary edema (HAPE)—can occur by itself or with AMS and HACE. Symptoms begin with shortness of breath on exertion and progress to shortness of breath at rest, weakness, and cough. Supplemental oxygen and immediate descent. HACE and HAPE can be fatal (2).
  – Preventive measures
    ○ Ascend gradually—from low altitude to <9,000 feet in 1 day. >9,000 feet, don't climb >1,600 feet per day. Plan an extra day for acclimatization every 3,300 feet (2).
    ○ In first 48 hours, avoid alcohol and only perform mild exercise.
  – Preventive medications
    ○ Recommended for those at high risk for AMS (based on rate of ascent or history of HACE or HAPE): Consider for those at moderate risk.
    ○ Acetazolamide—dose: 125 mg BID (250 mg BID if >100 kg); pediatric dose: 2.5 mg/kg q12h (2)

○ Dexamethasone—usually reserved for treatment; dose: 2 mg q6h or 4 mg q12h; should not be used for prophylaxis in pediatric patients (2)
○ Nifedipine—for prevention of HAPE only; dose: 30 mg SR q12h or 20 mg SR q8h (2)
○ Tadalafil—useful for prevention of HAPE only; dose: 10 mg BID (2)

• Jet lag
  – Before travel, adjust sleep cycle (and possibly meal times) 1 to 2 hours earlier or later (depending on direction of travel) for several days prior to departure.
  – Drink plenty of water to remain hydrated.
  – Optimize sunlight exposure to destination.
  – Sedative hypnotics (nonbenzodiazepine), such as zolpidem, can be useful.
  – If using benzodiazepines, use short-acting agents, such as temazepam.

• Motion sickness
  – High-risk individuals
    ○ Children ages 2 to 12 years
    ○ Women, especially when pregnant, menstruating, or on hormones
    ○ People who get migraines, especially during a migraine
    ○ Some medications
  – Prevention strategies
    ○ Avoidance of known triggers
    ○ Strategic positioning (front of car, overwing of aircraft)
    ○ Treatment
      ▪ Dimenhydrinate dose: pediatric dose: 1.0 to 1.5 mg/kg 1 hour before travel and every 6 hours during the trip
      ▪ Diphenhydramine: pediatric dose: 0.5 to 1.0 mg/kg per dose up to 25 mg 1 hour before travel and every 6 hours during the trip
      ▪ Scopolamine—transdermal patch to hairless area behind ear at least 4 hours prior to exposure and every 3 days as needed

• Environmental hazards
  – Avoid walking barefoot (parasites can enter skin).
  – Avoid swimming in freshwater where there is a risk for schistosomiasis or leptospirosis.
  – Use sunscreen.
  – If scuba diving, avoid flying or altitude exposure >2,000 feet (2).
    ○ ≥12 hours after surfacing from nondecompression dive
    ○ ≥18 hours after repetitive dives or multiple days of diving
    ○ 24 to 28 hours after a dive that required decompression stops

• Other information
  – Avoid contact with animals because bites and scratches may transmit rabies.
  – Discuss risks such as traffic accidents, alcohol misuse, personal assault, robbery, and water safety.
  – Check hotels or other sleeping locations for bed bugs on bedding and furniture.

– Consider travel insurance (including coverage for evacuation).
– Hand carry medications and supplies.
– Include medications to manage exacerbations or complications of existing chronic diseases.
– Avoid areas with known outbreaks of communicable disease. Reference the CDC Travelers' Health Web site before travel.
– The Department of State's Smart Traveler Enrollment Program provides destination-specific travel alerts.

REFERENCES

1. Bagshaw M, DeVoll J, Jennings R, et al. Medical guidelines for airline passengers: Aerospace Medical Association. https://www.asma.org/asma/media/asma/Travel-Publications/paxguidelines.pdf. Accessed December 11, 2018.

2. Brunette GW, Kozarsky PE, Cohen NJ, et al. *CDC Yellow Book 2018: Health Information for International Travel*. New York, NY: Oxford University Press; 2018.

3. Sanford C, McConnell A, Osborn J. The pretravel consultation. *Am Fam Physician*. 2016;94(8): 620–627.

ADDITIONAL READING

• Centers for Disease Control and Prevention. Travelers' health. http://www.cdc.gov/travel/. Accessed November 20, 2018.
• Freedman DO, Chen LH, Kozarsky PE. Medical considerations before international travel. *N Engl J Med*. 2016;375(3):247–260.
• Sanford CA, Pottinger PS, Jong EC. *The Travel and Tropical Medicine Manual*. 5th ed. St. Louis, MO: Elsevier; 2017.
• Travel.State.Gov: http://www.travel.state.gov/content/travel.html
• World Travel and Tourism Council: http://www.wttc.org

 CODES

ICD10
• Z71.9 Counseling, unspecified
• Z71.89 Other specified counseling

CLINICAL PEARLS

• The CDC Travelers' Health Web site is a useful point-of-care tool for destination-specific travel advice (https://wwwnc.cdc.gov/travel/).
• To allow adequate time for vaccine response and necessary pretrip medications, patients should seek advice several weeks prior to anticipated travel.

ARTERITIS, TEMPORAL

Chloe S. Courchesne, MD • Karl T. Clebak, MD, FAAFP • Munima Nasir, MD

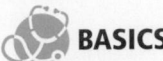 **BASICS**

DESCRIPTION
- Technically termed giant cell arteritis (GCA)
- A chronic, generalized, cellular, and humoral immune-mediated vasculitis of large- and medium-sized vessels, predominantly affecting the cranial arteries originating from the aortic arch, although vascular involvement may be widespread. Inflammation of the aorta is observed in 50% of cases.
- Frequent features include fatigue, headaches, jaw claudication, loss of vision, scalp tenderness, polymyalgia rheumatica (PMR), and aortic arch syndrome (decreased or absent peripheral pulses, discrepancies of blood pressure, arterial bruits).
- Considered medical emergency due to risk of permanent vision loss if not treated

EPIDEMIOLOGY
- Most common form of systemic vasculitis affecting persons ≥50 years old
- Typically occurs ages 70 to 80 years (80% of cases)
- Women are affected about 2 times as often as men.
- Most common vasculitis in individuals of Northern European descent (Scandinavian countries)
- Rare in Asians and African Americans

Incidence
- Prevalence in individuals >50 years: 1 in 500
- Cyclic incidence: peaking every 5 to 7 years

ETIOLOGY AND PATHOPHYSIOLOGY
- The exact etiology of GCA remains unknown, although current theory suggests that advanced age, ethnicity, and specific genetic predisposition lead to a maladaptive response to endothelial injury, intimal hyperplasia, and ultimately vascular stenosis.
- Temporal arteritis (TA) is a chronic, systemic vasculitis primarily affecting the elastic lamina of medium- and large-sized arteries. Histopathology of affected arteries is marked by transmural inflammation of the intima, media, and adventitia, as well as patchy infiltration by lymphocytes, macrophages, and multinucleated giant cells. Mural hyperplasia can result in arterial luminal narrowing, resulting in subsequent distal ischemia.
- Current theory regarding the etiology of TA is that a maladaptive response to endothelial injury leads to an inappropriate activation of T-cell–mediated immunity via immature antigen-presenting cells. The subsequent release of cytokines within the arterial vessel wall can attract macrophages and multinucleated giant cells, which form granulomatous infiltrates and give diseased vessels their characteristic histology. This also leads to an oligoclonal expansion of T-cells directed against antigens in or near the elastic lamina. Ultimately, this cascade results in vessel wall damage, intimal hyperplasia, and eventual stenotic occlusion.

- In recent years, GCA and PMR have increasingly been considered to be closely related conditions.
- Varicella zoster virus has been proposed as possible immune trigger for GCA; however, this has not been substantiated, and adjunctive treatment with antivirals remains controversial.

Genetics
The gene for *HLA-DRB1–04* has been identified as a risk factor for TA, and polymorphisms of *ICAM-1* and *PTPN-22* have also been implicated.

RISK FACTORS
- Increasing age >70 years is the greatest risk factor.
- Genetic predisposition
- Environmental factors influence susceptibility.
- History of smoking
- Early menopause (<43 years) and lower BMI at menopause in women 50 to 69 years old

COMMONLY ASSOCIATED CONDITIONS
Population studies have shown 40–60% of patients diagnosed with GCA also have PMR symptoms, and 16–21% of patient with PMR have GCA.

 DIAGNOSIS

HISTORY
- Most common presenting symptom is headache (2/3 of patients).
- Constitutional symptoms (fever, fatigue, weight loss)
- Any visual disturbances (amaurosis fugax, diplopia)
- Vision loss (20% of patients); unilateral is most common, often proceeds to bilateral if untreated.
- Jaw claudication (presence of symptom significantly increases likelihood of a positive biopsy)
- Scalp tenderness or sensitivity
- Claudication of upper extremities or tongue
- Symptoms of PMR (shoulder and hip girdle pain and stiffness)
- Distal extremity swelling/edema
- Upper respiratory symptoms

PHYSICAL EXAM
- Temporal artery abnormalities (beading, prominence, tenderness)
- Typically appear "ill"
- Decreased peripheral pulses in the presence of large vessel diseases
- Funduscopic exam shows pale and edema of the optic disc, scattered cotton wool patches, and small hemorrhages.
- Unlike other forms of vasculitis, GCA rarely involves the skin, kidneys, and lungs.
- Bruits supraclavicular, axillary, supra-orbital

DIFFERENTIAL DIAGNOSIS
- Migraines
- Herpes zoster
- Other vasculitis (Takayasu arteritis, Wegner, PAN)
- Other rheumatologic condition (RA, PMR, MCTD)

DIAGNOSTIC TESTS & INTERPRETATION
- American College of Rheumatology classification criteria are as follows:
  – Age >70 years
  – New localized headache
  – Temporal artery abnormality (tenderness to palpation, decreased or absent pulses)
  – ESR >50 mm/hr
  – Abnormal temporal artery biopsy showing vasculitis with predominance of mononuclear cell infiltration or granulomatous inflammation
- ACR criteria may lack sensitivity.

Initial Tests (lab, imaging)
- ESR >50 mm/hr (86% sensitivity), although non-specific (27%); infrequently, may be normal
- C-reactive protein (CRP) >2.45 mg/dL is a more sensitive marker of inflammation (97% sensitivity) and is associated with increased odds of a positive biopsy result.
- A normal ESR and/or CRP renders the diagnosis of GCA unlikely.
- Platelet count $>400 \times 10^3$
- Acute-phase reactants (fibrinogen, interleukin-6) are frequently elevated but very nonspecific and reserved for diagnostically difficult cases.
- Mild anemia: very nonspecific but may be associated with a lower rate of ischemic complications
- Color Doppler US of the temporal artery may identify vascular occlusion, stenosis, or edema ("halo sign"); it is low cost and noninvasive but also very operator dependent and does not significantly improve on the clinical exam. It may aid in the diagnosis of larger vessel involvement.
- Atherosclerotic disease with carotid intima-media thickness >0.9 mm may mimic halo sign.
- MRI and MRA may be beneficial in diagnosis (78% sensitive, 90% specific) if performed within 5 days of steroids.
- Positron emission tomography (PET), like MRI/MRA and color Doppler, may be useful in diagnostically difficult cases to quantify the inflammatory burden and early in the course of disease, as the metabolic changes occur prior to structural vascular damage, but it also lacks studies to support its use.

Follow-Up Tests & Special Considerations
- Development of aortic aneurysms (late and potentially serious complication of GCA) can lead to aortic dissection.
- Due to the risk of irreversible vision loss, treatment with high-dose steroids should be started on strong clinical suspicion of TA, prior to the temporal biopsy being done.

Diagnostic Procedures/Other
- Gold standard diagnostic study: histopathologic examination of the temporal artery biopsy specimen
- Overall sensitivity is 87%.
- The temporal artery is chosen because of its accessibility in the systemic disease; alternatively, facial artery or other cranial arteries may be used.
- Length of biopsy specimen should be at least 2 cm to avoid false-negative results because skip lesions may occur.
- Diagnostic yield of biopsy may be increased if procedure is coupled with imaging (high-resolution MRI or color Doppler US).
- Bilateral temporal artery biopsy should not be performed, unless the initial histopathology is negative and the suspicion for GCA remains high.
- May be negative in up to 42% of patients with GCA, especially in large vessel disease, and a negative biopsy alone should not dictate treatment
- Biopsy results are not affected by prior glucocorticoids, so treatment should not be delayed.

Test Interpretation
- Inflammation of the arterial wall, with fragmentation and disruption of the internal elastic lamina
- Multinucleated giant cells are found in <50% of cases and are not specific for the disease.
- TA occurs in three histologic patterns: classic, atypical, and healed.

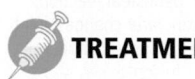

TREATMENT

MEDICATION
First Line
Glucocorticoids:
- The typical dose of prednisone is between 40 and 60 mg/day (or 1 mg/kg/day), and the dose may be titrated up to relieve symptoms. Steroids should not be in the form of alternate day therapy because this is more likely to lead to a relapse of vasculitis (1)[A].
- IV steroids indicated if vision loss has been noted, otherwise PO steroids are equally as effective (1)[C]
- Given risk of irreversible vision loss, immediate steroid therapy should be initiated prior to confirmation by biopsy.
- The initial dose of steroids is continued for 2 to 4 weeks and slowly tapered over 9 to 12 months. Tapering may require ≥2 years (1)[A]. Assess for relapse during taper by monitoring symptoms, ESR, CRP.
- Tocilizumab 162 mg SQ weekly or biweekly in addition to prednisone may be superior to prednisone alone (2)[B].
- It has been suggested that low-dose aspirin might be effective for patients with GCA (3)[B].

Second Line
- Methotrexate as an adjunct to glucocorticoid therapy may have a modest effect in decreasing the relapse rate of TA (4)[A].
- Cyclophosphamide have shown some benefit in patients who have not adequately responded to glucocorticoids (5)[A].
- Therapies directed at TNF as adjunct to steroids have not shown significant benefit (1)[B].

ONGOING CARE

FOLLOW-UP RECOMMENDATIONS
Sun avoidance and protection of the head and the face from photodamage may eventually prove to be important preventive measures for TA.

Patient Monitoring
- TA is typically self-limited and lasts several months or years.
- Overall, TA does not seem to decrease longevity. Nevertheless, it may lead to serious complications such as visual loss, which occurs in about 15–20% of patients.
- Another complication of GCA is the development of aortic aneurysms, usually affecting the ascending aorta. Yearly, chest x-rays may be useful to identify this problem (6)[C].
- About 50% of the patients with GCA will eventually develop PMR (stiffness of shoulder and hip girdle).

DIET
Calcium (due to steroid therapy) and vitamin D supplementation

PATIENT EDUCATION
- Consequences of discontinuing steroids abruptly (adrenal insufficiency, disease relapse)
- Risks of long-term steroid use (infection, hyperglycemia, weight gain, impaired wound healing, osteoporosis, hypertension)
- Possibility of relapse and importance of reporting new headaches and vision changes to provider immediately

PROGNOSIS
- Life expectancy is not affected by the disease unless severe aortitis is present.
- Once vision loss has occurred, it is unlikely to be recovered, but treatment resolves the other symptoms and prevents future vision loss and stroke.
- In most patients, glucocorticoid therapy can eventually be discontinued without complications. In a few patients, however, the disease is chronic, and prednisone must be continued for years.
- Disease relapse is a distinct possibility.

COMPLICATIONS
- Vision loss with delayed diagnosis
- Glucocorticoid-related toxicity

REFERENCES

1. Borchers AT, Gershwin ME. Giant cell arteritis: a review of classification, pathophysiology, geoepidemiology and treatment. *Autoimmun Rev*. 2012;11(6–7):A544–A554.
2. Stone JH, Tuckwell K, Dimonaco S, et al. Trial of tocilizumab in giant-cell arteritis. *N Eng J Med*. 2017;377(4):317–328.
3. Lee MS, Smith SD, Galor A, et al. Antiplatelet and anticoagulant therapy in patients with giant cell arteritis. *Arthritis Rheum*. 2006;54(10):3306–3309.
4. Mahr AD, Jover JA, Spiera RF, et al. Adjunctive methotrexate for treatment of giant cell arteritis: an individual patient data meta-analysis. *Arthritis Rheum*. 2007;56(8):2789–2797.
5. Quartuccio L, Maset M, De Maglio G, et al. Role of oral cyclophosphamide in the treatment of giant cell arteritis. *Rheumatology (Oxford)*. 2012;51(9):1677–1686.
6. Tomasson G, Peloquin C, Mohammad A, et al. Risk for cardiovascular disease early and late after a diagnosis of giant-cell arteritis: a cohort study. *Ann Intern Med*. 2014;160(2):73–80.

ADDITIONAL READING

- De Miguel E, Beltran LM, Monjo I, et al. Atherosclerosis as a potential pitfall in the diagnosis of giant cell arteritis. *Rheumatology (Oxford)*. 2018;57(2):318–321.
- Ing EB, Ing R, Liu X, et al. Does herpes zoster predispose to giant cell arteritis: a geo-epidemiologic study. *Clin Ophthalmol*. 2018;12:113–118.
- Larsson K, Mellstrom D, Nordborg E, et al. Early menopause, low body mass index, and smoking are independent risk factors for developing giant cell arteritis. *Ann Rheum Dis*. 2006;65(4):529–532.
- Mukhtyar C, Guillevin L, Cid MC, et al; for European Vasculitis Study Group. EULAR recommendations for the management of large vessel vasculitis. *Ann Rheum Dis*. 2009;68(3):318–323.
- Salvarani C, Cantini F, Hunder GG. Polymyalgia rheumatic and giant-cell arteritis. *Lancet*. 2008;372(9634):234–245.

 SEE ALSO

Depression; Fibromyalgia; Headache, Cluster; Headache, Tension; Polymyalgia Rheumatica; Polymyositis/Dermatomyositis

 CODES

ICD10
- M31.6 Other giant cell arteritis
- M31.5 Giant cell arteritis with polymyalgia rheumatica

CLINICAL PEARLS
- Due to the risk of irreversible vision loss, treatment with high-dose steroids (prednisone 60 mg/day) should be started immediately in patients suspected of TA.
- Temporal artery biopsy is the gold standard for diagnosis. Temporal artery biopsy is not likely to be affected by a few weeks of treatment.
- Treatment consists of a very slow steroid taper. Bone protection therapy and low-dose aspirin should be considered.
- Normal ESR level = value of age/2 for men and age + 10/2 for women
- Patients on corticosteroids should be placed on therapy to minimize osteoporosis, unless there are contraindications.

ARTHRITIS, JUVENILE IDIOPATHIC

Donna-Marie McMahon, DO, FAAP • Kathleen M. Vazzana, DO, MSc

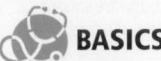

BASICS

DESCRIPTION
- Juvenile idiopathic arthritis (JIA) is the most common chronic pediatric rheumatologic disease.
- JIA is associated with significant disability.
  – Age of onset: <16 years of age
  – Common symptoms: joint swelling, restricted range of motion, warmth, redness, pain
  – Often ≥6 weeks of symptoms prior to diagnosis
- Seven (International League of Associations for Rheumatology [ILAR]) subtypes determined by clinical characteristics in first 6 months of illness (1):
  – Systemic: 10%; preceded by febrile onset of ≥2 weeks with rash, serositis, hepatosplenomegaly, or lymphadenopathy (1)
  – Polyarticular rheumatoid factor (RF) (+): 2–7%; ≥5 joints involvement (1); large and small joints; RF positive on two tests ≥3 months apart (2)
  – Polyarticular RF (−): 10–30%; ≥5 (large and small) joints involved (1); RF negative (2)
  – Oligoarticular: 30–60%; involvement of 1 to 4 joints; risk for chronic uveitis in antinuclear antibodies (ANA) (+) females (1) and axial skeletal involvement in older boys (2). Types: (i) persistent (40%): knee, ankle, elbow; (ii) extended type (20%): >4 joints after first 6 months
  – Psoriatic arthritis: 5%; arthritis with psoriasis or arthritis with >2 of the following: dactylitis, nail changes (pitting), psoriasis in first-degree relative (1)
  – Enthesitis-related arthritis: 1–11%; arthritis and enthesitis or one of them plus at least two of the following: sacroiliac or lumbosacral pain, Reiter syndrome or acute anterior uveitis in first-degree relative, acute symptomatic anterior uveitis, human leukocyte antigen (HLA)-B27 (+), history of ankylosing spondylitis, sacroiliitis with inflammatory bowel disease, onset of arthritis in male >6 years old (1)[C]
  – Undifferentiated arthritis (11–21%): presents with overlapping symptoms in ≥2 categories above or arthritis that does not fulfill above categories (2)
- Systems affected: musculoskeletal, hematologic, lymphatic, immunologic, dermatologic, ophthalmologic, gastrointestinal
- Synonyms: juvenile chronic arthritis; juvenile arthritis; juvenile rheumatoid arthritis (JRA); Still disease (2)

EPIDEMIOLOGY
- Male = female (1); onset: throughout childhood; 54% of cases occur in children 0 to 5 years.
- Polyarticular RF (+): female > male, 3:1 (2); onset: late childhood or adolescence (1)
- Polyarticular RF (−): female > male, 3:1; onset: early peak, 2 to 4 years; late peak, 6 to 12 years (2)
- Oligoarticular: female > male, 5:1; onset: 2 to 4 years (2)
- Psoriatic: female > male, 1:0.95 (2); onset: early peak, 2 to 3 years; late peak, 10 to 12 years (1)
- Enthesis: female > male, 1:7; onset: early peak, 2 to 4 years; late peak, 6 to 12 years (2)
- Affected patients have an increased risk of developing cancer, although short-term risk is low.

Incidence
2 to 20/100,000 children <16 years in developed nations

Prevalence
16 to 150/100,000 children <16 years in developed nations (1)

ETIOLOGY AND PATHOPHYSIOLOGY
- Humoral and cellular immunodysregulation. T lymphocytes play a key role.
- Genetic predisposition; IL2RA/CD25 and VTCN1 implicated as genetic loci
- Environmental triggers, possibly infectious
  – Rubella or parvovirus B19 (3)
  – Heat shock proteins (3)
- Immunoglobulin or complement deficiency

Genetics
- HLA class I (A, B, C) and II (DR, DP, DQ) alleles
- HLA-A2 = early onset oligoarthritis in females
- HLA class II increases risk of systemic and oligoarticular JIA.
- HLA-B27 increases risk of enthesitis-related arthritis.
- HLA-DR4 is associated with polyarthritis RF (+) (3)[C].

RISK FACTORS
Female gender 3:1

GENERAL PREVENTION
None identified

COMMONLY ASSOCIATED CONDITIONS
Other autoimmune disorders, chronic anterior uveitis (iridocyclitis), nutritional impairment, growth issues (3)[C]

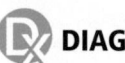

DIAGNOSIS

Clinical criteria: age of onset <16 years and >6 weeks duration of objective arthritis (swelling or restricted range of motion of a joint with heat, pain, or tenderness and no other form of childhood arthritis) in ≥1 joints

HISTORY
- Arthralgias, fever, fatigue, malaise, myalgias, weight loss, morning stiffness, rash
- Limp, if lower extremity involvement
- Arthritis for ≥6 weeks

PHYSICAL EXAM
- Arthritis: swelling, effusion, loss of musculoskeletal landmarks, limited range of motion, tenderness, pain with motion, warmth
- Rash, rheumatoid nodules (uncommon), lymphadenopathy, hepato- or splenomegaly, enthesis, dactylitis (mainly in psoriatic type)

DIFFERENTIAL DIAGNOSIS
- Legg-Calvé-Perthes, toxic synovitis, growing pains, Perthes disease
- Septic arthritis, osteomyelitis, viral infection, mycoplasmal infection, Lyme disease
- Reactive arthritis: postinfectious, rheumatic fever, Reiter syndrome
- Inflammatory bowel disease
- Hemoglobinopathies, hemarthrosis, rickets
- Leukemia (particularly acute lymphocytic leukemia), bone tumors (osteoid osteoma), neuroblastoma
- Vasculitis, Henoch-Schönlein purpura, Kawasaki disease

- Systemic lupus erythematosus, dermatomyositis, mixed connective tissue disease, sarcoidosis, systemic sclerosis, collagen disorders
- Farber disease
- Accidental or nonaccidental trauma

DIAGNOSTIC TESTS & INTERPRETATION
Initial Tests (lab, imaging)
- CBC: Leukocyte count is normal or elevated (systemic); lymphopenia, reactive thrombocytosis, anemia; liver function test (LFT; hepatic involvement) and renal function studies (prior to therapy with nephrotoxic drugs)
- Joint-fluid aspiration/analysis to exclude infection
- ESR and C-reactive protein typically elevated; C-reactive protein often disproportionately high
- Myeloid-related proteins (MRP 8/14) associated with flares
- ANA-positive patients have increased risk of uveitis; ANA positive in up to 70% with oligoarticular JIA
- RF (+): 2–10% (usually polyarticular); poor prognosis
- HLA-B27 positive: enthesitis-related arthritis
- Diagnostic radiography, MRI, ultrasound, and CT; no one modality has superior diagnostic value (4)[A].
- Radiograph of affected joint(s): early radiographic changes: soft tissue swelling, periosteal reaction, juxta-articular demineralization; later changes: joint space loss, articular surface erosions, subchondral cyst formation, sclerosis, joint fusion
- If orthopnea, obtain ECG to rule out pericarditis.
- Radionuclide scans: for infection/malignancy
- CT is best for bony abnormalities. MRI can assess synovial hypertrophy and cartilage degeneration; MRI more sensitive to monitor disease activity and clinical responsiveness to treatment in peripheral joints

Follow-Up Tests & Special Considerations
Use pediatric (not adult) controls when interpreting results of dual energy x-ray absorptiometry.

Diagnostic Procedures/Other
Ultrasound: Assess for inflammation (4)[A].

Synovial biopsy: if synovial fluid cannot be aspirated or if infection is suspected in spite of negative synovial fluid culture

Test Interpretation
Synovial biopsy → synovial cells hyperplasia, hyperemia, infiltration of small lymphocytes, and mononuclear cells

TREATMENT

GENERAL MEASURES
- Goal is to control active disease, minimize extra-articular manifestations, and achieve clinical remission.
- All patients require regular (every 3 to 4 months for oligoarticular JIA and in ANA-positive patients) ophthalmic exams to uncover asymptomatic eye disease, particularly for the first 3 years following diagnosis.
- Moist heat or electric blanket for morning stiffness
- Splints for contractures
- Aerobic exercise: weight-bearing or aquatic therapy to improve functional capacity

MEDICATION

First Line

- ≤4 joints
- NSAIDs: adequate in ~50%; symptoms often improve within days; full efficacy 2 to 3 months
- Drugs for children include:
  - Ibuprofen: 30 to 50 mg/kg/day, divided QID; max dose 2,400 mg/day
  - Naproxen: 10 to 15 mg/kg/day, divided BID; max dose 1,250 mg/day
  - Tolmetin sodium: 20 mg/kg/day, TID or QID; max dose 30 mg/kg/day
  - Diclofenac: 2 to 3 mg/kg, divided TID; max dose 50 mg TID
  - Indomethacin: 1 to 2 mg/kg/day, divided BID to QID; max dose of 4 mg/kg/day or 200 mg/day
  - NSAIDs are contraindicated if known allergy.
  - Precautions: may worsen bleeding diatheses; use caution in renal insufficiency and hypovolemic states; take with food.
  - Significant drug interactions: may lower serum levels of anticonvulsants and blunt the effect of loop diuretics; NSAIDs may increase serum methotrexate levels.
- Intra-articular long-acting corticosteroids: immediately effective; improve synovitis, joint damage, contractures, prevent leg length discrepancy (4)[B]
  - Indication: patients with oligoarthritis who fail a 2-month NSAID trial or with poor prognosis (2)
  - Triamcinolone hexacetonide
- ≥5 joints
  - If high disease activity or a failed 1 to 2 months NSAID trial → methotrexate (5)[C]

Second Line

- 30–40% of patients require addition of disease-modifying antirheumatic drugs (DMARDs): methotrexate, sulfasalazine, leflunomide, and tumor necrosis factor (TNF) antagonists (etanercept, infliximab, adalimumab); newer biologic therapies, including IL-1 and IL-6 receptor antagonists, are currently under investigation.
- Methotrexate: 10 mg/m²/week PO or SC
  - Plateau of efficacy reached with 15 mg/m²/week; further increase in dosage is not associated with therapeutic benefit.
- Sulfasalazine: oligoarticular and HLA-B27 spondyloarthritis
- Etanercept: 0.8 mg/kg (max of 50 mg/dose) given SC q1wk or 0.4 mg/kg SC twice a week (max of 25 mg/dose)
- Infliximab: 5 mg/kg q6–8wk
- Adalimumab: if weight 15 kg to <30 kg, 20 mg SC q2wk; if weight ≥30 kg, 40 mg SC q2wk
- Rituximab: monoclonal antibody; National Health Service (NHS) England guidelines recommend for polyarticular RF+ who have failed two TNF-α inhibitors (4).
- Tocilizumab: now included in the NHS England guidelines for RF-pJIA who have failed two TNF-α inhibitors (4)
- Anakinra: IL-1 receptor antagonist is being used as monotherapy or in combination with other treatments (6).
- Begin treatment with TNF-α inhibitors in children with a history of arthritis in ≤4 joints and significant active arthritis despite treatment with methotrexate or arthritis in ≥5 joints and any active arthritis following an adequate trial of methotrexate (6)[C].

- Begin treatment with anakinra in children with systemic arthritis and active fever whose treatment requires a second medication, in addition to systemic glucocorticoids (6).
- Analgesics, including narcotics for pain control

ISSUES FOR REFERRAL

- Pediatric rheumatologist for management of JIA
- Orthopedics as needed for articular complications
- Ophthalmology: to evaluate for uveitis
- Physical therapy to maintain range of motion, improve muscle strength, and prevent deformities
- Occupational therapy to maintain and improve appropriate age-related functional activities
- Behavioral health if difficulty coping with disease

SURGERY/OTHER PROCEDURES

- Total hip and/or knee replacement for severe disease
- Soft tissue release if splinting/traction unsuccessful
- Correct limb length or angular deformities
- Synovectomy is rarely performed.

ADMISSION, INPATIENT, AND NURSING CONSIDERATIONS

- Admit if:
  - Patient unable to ambulate
  - Signs/symptoms of pericarditis
  - Persistent fever or diagnostic confusion to facilitate evaluation and workup
  - Need for surgery
- Discharge when fever, swelling, and serositis resolved.

 ONGOING CARE

FOLLOW-UP RECOMMENDATIONS

Patient Monitoring

Determined by medication and disease activity

- NSAIDs: periodic CBC, urinalysis, LFTs, renal function tests
- Aspirin and/or other salicylates: transaminase and salicylate levels weekly for 1 month and then every 3 to 4 months
- Methotrexate: monthly LFTs, CBC, BUN, creatinine

DIET

Regular diet. Ensure adequate calcium, iron, protein, and caloric intake.

PATIENT EDUCATION

- Psychosocial needs; school issues; behavioral strategies for dealing with pain and noncompliance; available health care resources; support groups
- http://www.rheumatology.org/I-Am-A/Patient-Caregiver

PROGNOSIS

- 50–60% of patients will ultimately achieve remission.
- Functional ability depends on adequacy of therapy (disease control, maintaining muscle and joint function).
- Poor prognosis: patients with active disease at 6 months; polyarticular disease; extended pauciarticular disease course; female gender; RF (+); ANA (+); persistent morning stiffness; rapid appearance of erosions; hip involvement

COMPLICATIONS

- Blindness, band keratopathy, glaucoma, short stature, micrognathia if temporomandibular joint involvement, debilitating joint disease, disseminated intravascular coagulation, hemolytic anemia
- NSAIDs: peptic ulcer, GI hemorrhage, CNS reactions, renal disease, leukopenia
- DMARDs: bone marrow suppression, hepatitis, renal disease, dermatitis, mouth ulcers, retinal toxicity (antimalarials; rare)
- TNF antagonists: higher risk of infection
- Osteoporosis, avascular necrosis
- Methotrexate: Folate supplementation decreases hepatic/GI symptoms; may reduce stomatitis
- Macrophage activation syndrome: decreased blood cell precursors secondary to histiocyte degradation of marrow

REFERENCES

1. Giancane G, Alongi A, Ravelli A. Update on the pathogenesis and treatment of juvenile idiopathic arthritis. *Curr Opin Rheumatol*. 2017;29(5):523–529.
2. Prakken B, Albani S, Martini A. Juvenile idiopathic arthritis. *Lancet*. 2011;377(9783):2138–2149.
3. Collado P, Vojinovic J, Nieto JC, et al; for Omeract Ultrasound Pediatric Group. Toward standardized musculoskeletal ultrasound in pediatric rheumatology: normal age-related ultrasound findings. *Arthritis Care Res (Hoboken)*. 2016;68(3):348–356.
4. Webb K, Wedderburn L. Advances in the treatment of polyarticular juvenile idiopathic arthritis. *Curr Opin Rheumatol*. 2015;27(5):505–510.
5. Beukelman T, Patkar NM, Saag KG, et al. 2011 American College of Rheumatology recommendations for the treatment of juvenile idiopathic arthritis: initiation and safety monitoring of therapeutic agents for the treatment of arthritis and systemic features. *Arthritis Care Res (Hoboken)*. 2011;63(4):465–482.
6. Grevich S, Shenoi S. Update on the management of systemic juvenile idiopathic arthritis and role of IL-1 and IL-6 inhibition. *Adolesc Health Med Ther*. 2017;8:125–135.

ADDITIONAL READING

Shenoi S. Juvenile idiopathic arthritis—changing times, changing terms, changing treatments. *Pediatr Rev*. 2017;38(5):221–232.

CODES

ICD10

- M08.90 Juvenile arthritis, unspecified, unspecified site
- M08.80 Other juvenile arthritis, unspecified site
- M08.00 Unsp juvenile rheumatoid arthritis of unspecified site

CLINICAL PEARLS

- JIA is the most common form of arthritis in children.
- Consider JIA in any child presenting with a limp.
- High-titer RF correlates with disease severity; prognosis worse if positive RF titers
- DMARDs improve JIA-associated symptoms.

ARTHRITIS, PSORIATIC

Lorena C. Dollani, MD • Nikki A. Levin, MD, PhD

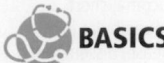

BASICS

A chronic, destructive, seronegative arthropathy most common in patients with long-standing psoriasis

DESCRIPTION
- Psoriatic arthritis (PsA) is a seronegative spondylo-arthropathy characterized by inflammatory arthritis and enthesitis.
- Five patterns of arthritis in PsA:
  - Asymmetric oligoarthritis: <5 joints
  - Distal interphalangeal (DIP) joint predominant: osteoarthritis-like, associated with nail psoriasis
  - Symmetric polyarthritis: may be indistinguishable from rheumatoid arthritis (RA)—typically milder
  - Spondyloarthritis: asymmetric and discontinuous, unlike ankylosing spondylitis (AS)
  - Arthritis mutilans: destructive, resorptive arthritis; produces "opera-glass" or "telescoping" digit
- Psoriasis may be limited in extent.
  - Course of arthritis and extent of psoriasis do not correlate.
  - Other extra-articular features, such as iritis, are less common.
  - Damaging joint disease may occur in 40–60%. Characteristic radiologic changes include "pencil-in-cup" deformity and periostitis.
- Rheumatoid factor (RF) and anti–cyclic citrullinated peptide (anti-CCP) antibody are usually negative. HLA-B27 may be positive.

EPIDEMIOLOGY
- Peak onset age: 30 to 50 years
- Predominant gender: female = male
- Polyarthritis is more common in women.
- Spondylitis in up to 25%, more common in males
- Psoriasis precedes arthritis in most patients by an average of 12 years. Arthritis preceding psoriasis occurs in up to 15% of patients, usually children. Arthritis and psoriasis may present simultaneously.
- Psoriasis occurs in 2–3% of the U.S. population; 6–42% will develop PsA (1).

Prevalence
Prevalence: 1 to 2/1,000 population (1)

ETIOLOGY AND PATHOPHYSIOLOGY
- CD4+/CD8+ T cells; tumor necrosis factor α (TNF-α); interleukins 1 (IL-1), 6, 8, and 10; and matrix metalloproteases present in synovial fluid
- Osteoclast precursor cell upregulation
- Unknown. Probably multifactorial: immunologic, genetic, environmental factors

Genetics
- 30–40% concordance in identical twins
- HLA-B27 in 15–50% with PsA (spondylitis pattern) versus 90% in AS
- Other HLA associations in PsA: HLA-B7, HLA-B38, HLA-B39, HLA-Cw6

RISK FACTORS
- Psoriasis
- Family history of PsA

GENERAL PREVENTION
No known prevention strategies; unknown whether early treatment of psoriasis prevents onset of PsA

COMMONLY ASSOCIATED CONDITIONS
Psoriasis

DIAGNOSIS

- A history of inflammatory arthritis, dactylitis, or enthesitis in patients with existing psoriasis is usually adequate to establish the diagnosis; often difficult to differentiate from other inflammatory arthropathies
- Classification of PsA (CASPAR) criteria (91% sensitivity; 99% specificity) are validated to screen patients for PsA. Inflammatory articular disease (joint, spine, or entheseal) with ≥3 points from the following five categories:
  - Evidence of current psoriasis, a personal or family history of psoriasis (2 points)
  - Typical psoriatic nail dystrophy, including ony-cholysis, pitting, and hyperkeratosis (1 point)
  - Negative RF (ELISA preferred) (1 point)
  - Current or prior history of dactylitis (1 point)
  - Radiologic evidence of new bone formation (excluding osteophyte formation) on plain radio-graphs of the hand or foot (1 point)

HISTORY
History and physical exam are often adequate to establish the diagnosis of PsA.
- (Generally) long-standing history of psoriasis
- Morning stiffness of hands, feet, or low back for >30 minutes
- Pain of involved joints
- Swelling or redness of peripheral joints
- Low back or buttock pain
- Ankle or heel pain
- Dactylitis or uniform swelling of an entire digit

PHYSICAL EXAM
- Affected peripheral joints may have overlying erythema, warmth, and swelling.
  - Synovitis
  - Dactylitis
  - Swelling of tendons (e.g., Achilles tendon) and tenderness at insertion sites (e.g., calcaneus)
  - Limited range of motion of axial skeleton
  - Pain with stress of the sacroiliac joint

- Well-demarcated pink-to-red erythematous plaques with a white silvery scale; common locations include scalp, ears, trunk, buttocks, gluteal cleft, elbows and forearms, knees and legs, and palms and soles.
- Nails may be dystrophic with pits, oil spots, crumbling, leukonychia, and red lunulae.

DIFFERENTIAL DIAGNOSIS
- Reactive arthritis
- Psoriasis and RA
- Psoriasis and osteoarthritis
- Psoriasis and polyarticular gout
- Psoriasis and AS

DIAGNOSTIC TESTS & INTERPRETATION
Initial Tests (lab, imaging)
- Serum RF (usually negative)
- Anti-CCP (usually negative)
- Antinuclear antibodies (usually negative)
- Acute-phase reactants (ESR and C-reactive protein) may be elevated.
- HLA-B27 is noted in 50–70% with axial disease and <15% with peripheral disease.
- Baseline radiographs of affected joints
- Plain radiographs may aid diagnosis, assess joint damage, disease progression, and response to therapy.
- Juxta-articular new bone formation (periostitis) and marginal joint erosions that progress centrally ("pencil-in-cup" erosions) are characteristic radio-graphic features.

Follow-Up Tests & Special Considerations
Follow-up radiographs; interval based on severity

Diagnostic Procedures/Other
Diagnosis is typically clinical.

Test Interpretation
Biopsy of skin or synovium is not usually required.

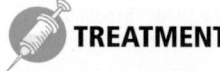

TREATMENT

GENERAL MEASURES
Physical therapy and/or occupational therapy typically benefit all stages of disease.
- Treatment algorithms for PsA are based on severity of joint symptoms, extent of structural damage, and severity of psoriasis.
- Patients with moderate to severe arthritis should be started on disease-modifying antirheumatic drugs (DMARDs) to reduce or prevent joint damage and preserve joint integrity and function.
- In addition to pharmacotherapy, patients should be educated on lifestyle modifications such as smoking cessation, weight reduction, joint protection, physical activity, exercise, and stress coping mechanisms (2).

First Line

- NSAIDs to control symptoms of mild disease. Intermittent intra-articular glucocorticoid injections may help.
- There are no systematic trials of NSAIDs for PsA. NSAIDs doses are directed toward suppressing mild inflammation. Selection is based on patient preference and dosing convenience. Sample NSAIDs include ibuprofen 400 to 800 mg PO TID–QID, naproxen 250 to 500 mg PO BID–TID, diclofenac 100 to 150 mg QD, indomethacin 100 to 150 mg QD.
- Monotherapy is as effective as combination therapy ($\geq$2 drugs from the following: analgesics, NSAIDs, opioids, opioid-like drugs, and neuromodulators [antidepressants, anticonvulsants, and muscle relaxants]) for adults (3)[A].

Second Line

- Recommended DMARDs include sulfasalazine, leflunomide, methotrexate; no evidence to support the use of combination DMARD therapy
- Initial dosing regimens for DMARDs: sulfasalazine (2 to 3 g/day PO divided in BID dosing), leflunomide (loading dose of 100 mg/day PO for 3 days and then 20 mg/day PO), methotrexate (1 test dose of 2.5 to 5.0 mg PO to assess for significant bone marrow suppression and then 15 to 25 mg once weekly), azathioprine (0.5 mg/kg/day, with a max dose of 2.5 mg/kg/day if no signs of cytopenia at lower doses)
- Avoid systemic corticosteroids if possible (may help when used short term for severe flares while initiating a biologic agent).
- Consider anti–TNF-α therapy in patients who do not respond to at least one standard DMARD or in patients with poor prognosis, even if they have not failed a standard DMARD (4)[A].
- Dosing regimens for biologics: adalimumab (40 mg SC q2wk), etanercept (50 mg SC weekly), golimumab (50 mg SC monthly), infliximab (5 mg/kg at 0, 2, and 6 weeks, q8wk afterward); certolizumab pegol 200 mg every 2 week; for maintenance dosing or 400 mg every 4 weeks
- Anti–interleukin-17 agents include:
  - Ixekizumab 80 mg q2wk (5)
  - Secukinumab 150 mg weekly from 0 to 4 weeks and then monthly (5)
- Anti–interleukin-12/interleukin-23 agents include:
  - Ustekinumab is currently dosed at 45 or 90 mg (depending on weight) at 0, 4, and 12 weeks and then q12wk thereafter (3).
- PDE4 inhibitors include:
  - Apremilast 30 mg PO BID (5)
- JAK 1 and JAK 3 inhibitors include:
  - Tofacitinib citrate dosed at 5 mg PO BID immediate release or 11 mg once daily extended release (1)
- Selective T-cell costimulation blocker:
  - Abatacept dosed at 125 mg once weekly SC or according to body weight. Following the initial IV infusion (using the weight-based dosing), repeat IV infusion (using the same weight-based dosing) q2wk and q4wk after the initial infusion, and q4wk thereafter (1).

- Above medications are FDA-approved for PsA.
- Do not use anti-TNF agents in the setting of active infection (including TB and hepatitis B). Do not use anti-TNF agents with concurrent live vaccinations, with New York Heart Association classes III to IV congestive heart failure, with malignancy, or in patients with a history of demyelinating disease.
- Do not use ustekinumab in patients with active infection, mycobacterial or *Salmonella* infection, with concurrent live vaccinations, including bacillus Calmette-Guérin vaccination or with history of malignancy.

Pregnancy Considerations

- Avoid teratogenic medications (e.g., methotrexate, leflunomide) during pregnancy.
- Adalimumab, etanercept, golimumab, infliximab, ustekinumab, and certolizumab pegol, secukinumab, are currently listed as Category B medications. Apremilast, abatacept, tofacitinib citrate, ixekizumab are listed as pregnancy Category C medication.

ISSUES FOR REFERRAL

- Rheumatology
- Dermatology

SURGERY/OTHER PROCEDURES

Joint fusion or replacement for advanced destruction

ONGOING CARE

FOLLOW-UP RECOMMENDATIONS

Epidemiologic data suggest a relationship between psoriasis, metabolic syndrome, myocardial infarction, and stroke. Control of weight, blood pressure, lipids, and glucose is recommended (2).

PATIENT EDUCATION

- PsA is not contagious.
- National Psoriasis Foundation: http://www.psoriasis.org/i-have-psoriatic-arthritis
- Arthritis Foundation: http://www.arthritis.org/about-arthritis/types/psoriatic-arthritis/
- American College of Rheumatology: https://www.rheumatology.org

PROGNOSIS

- Course is typically insidious with chronic joint disease and recurring/remitting skin disease.
- Prognosis is more favorable than for RA (except for patients who develop arthritis mutilans).

COMPLICATIONS

- Chronicity
- Disability
- Psychosocial impact of psoriasis

REFERENCES

1. Ritchlin CT, Colbert RA, Gladman DD. Psoriatic arthritis. *N Engl J Med.* 2017;376(10):957–970.
2. Ahmed N, Prior JA, Chen Y, et al. Prevalence of cardiovascular-related comorbidity in ankylosing spondylitis, psoriatic arthritis and psoriasis in primary care: a matched retrospective cohort study. *Clin Rheumatol.* 2016;35(12):3069–3073.
3. Gossec L, Smolen JS, Ramiro S, et al. European League Against Rheumatism (EULAR) recommendations for the management of psoriatic arthritis with pharmacological therapies: 2015 update. *Ann Rheum Dis.* 2016;75(3):499–510.
4. Coates LC, Kavanaugh A, Mease PJ, et al. Group for Research and Assessment of Psoriasis and Psoriatic Arthritis 2015 treatment recommendations for psoriatic arthritis. *Arthritis Rheumatol.* 2016;68(5):1060–1071.
5. Ash Z, Gaujoux-Viala C, Gossec L, et al. A systematic literature review of drug therapies for the treatment of psoriatic arthritis: current evidence and meta-analysis informing the EULAR recommendations for the management of psoriatic arthritis. *Ann Rheum Dis.* 2012;71(3):319–326.

ADDITIONAL READING

- Donahue KE, Jonas D, Hansen RA, et al. *Drug Therapy for Psoriatic Arthritis in Adults: Update of a 2007 Report.* Rockville, MD: Agency for Healthcare Research and Quality; 2012.
- Kavanaugh A, Mease PJ, Gomez-Reino JJ, et al. Treatment of psoriatic arthritis in a phase 3 randomised, placebo-controlled trial with apremilast, an oral phosphodiesterase 4 inhibitor. *Ann Rheum Dis.* 2014;73(6):1020–1026.
- Landewé R, Braun J, Deodhar A, et al. Efficacy of certolizumab pegol on signs and symptoms of axial spondyloarthritis including ankylosing spondylitis: 24-week results of a double-blind randomised placebo-controlled phase 3 study. *Ann Rheum Dis.* 2014;73(1):39–47.
- Tillett W, McHugh N. Treatment algorithms for early psoriatic arthritis: do they depend on disease phenotype? *Curr Rheumatol Rep.* 2012;14(4):334–342.

 ## CODES

ICD10

- L40.50 Arthropathic psoriasis, unspecified
- L40.51 Distal interphalangeal psoriatic arthropathy
- L40.53 Psoriatic spondylitis

CLINICAL PEARLS

- One in four patients with psoriasis develops PsA.
- The severity of psoriasis often correlates with the likelihood of developing arthritis. The severity of psoriasis does not correlate with severity of arthritis.
- Commonly overlooked locations of psoriasis include scalp, ears, umbilicus, and gluteal cleft.
- Osteoarthritis and polyarticular gout may mimic or coexist with PsA.
- The polyarticular pattern of PsA mimics RA. The presence of both enthesitis and psoriasis helps differentiate PsA from RA.
- Axial skeletal involvement in PsA is asymmetric and discontinuous.

ARTHRITIS, RHEUMATOID (RA)

Mariya Milko, DO, MS

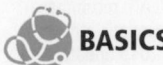 **BASICS**

DESCRIPTION

- Chronic systemic autoimmune inflammatory disease with symmetric polyarthritis and synovitis
- Progressive chronic inflammation leads to large and small joint destruction, deformity, decline in functional status, and premature morbidity/mortality.
- System(s) affected: musculoskeletal, skin, hematologic, lymphatic, immunologic, muscular, renal, cardiovascular, neurologic, pulmonary

Geriatric Considerations
Decreased medication tolerance; increased incidence of hydroxychloroquine-associated maculopathy and sulfasalazine-induced nausea/vomiting, NSAID-induced gastric ulcers, and corticosteroid-induced diabetes and osteoporosis

Pregnancy Considerations
- Use effective contraception in patients taking disease-modifying antirheumatic drugs (DMARDs).
- Methotrexate, leflunomide, cyclophosphamide, and cyclosporine are teratogenic. Sulfasalazine and hydroxychloroquine are safe to use during pregnancy and breastfeeding.
- 50–80% of patients improve during pregnancy because of immunologic tolerance. Most relapse in 6 months after delivery. First episode may occur in pregnancy or postpartum.

EPIDEMIOLOGY
Incidence
- 25 to 30/100,000 for males
- 50 to 60/100,000 for females
- Peak age at onset is 35 to 50 years.

Prevalence
1% of the U.S. population

ETIOLOGY AND PATHOPHYSIOLOGY
- An insult (e.g., infection, smoking, trauma) precipitates an autoimmune reaction activating antibody-complement complexes, resulting in endothelial activation, synovial hypertrophy, and joint inflammation/damage.
- Pathogenesis is mediated by abnormal B- and T-cell interactions and cytokine overproduction (TNF, interleukin-6 [IL-6]).
- Multifactorial disease with genetic, host (hormonal, immunologic), and environmental (socioeconomic, smoking) factors

Genetics
- Rheumatoid arthritis (RA) is 50% attributable to genetic causes. HLA-DR4 is a shared epitope in >50% of cases.
- Monozygotic twin concordance is 15–20%, suggesting nongenetic factors also contribute.
- Individuals with HLA-DR4 and DRB1, and mutations in STAT4, CD40+ have increased relative risk.

RISK FACTORS
- First-degree relatives have 2- to 3-fold increased risk.
- Smokers have elevated relative risk. Smoking is associated with an increased risk of developing anticitrullinated protein antibody (ACPA)-positive antibodies.
- Pregnancy and breastfeeding lowers risk up to 50%.
- Women affected 3:1; difference diminishes with age.

COMMONLY ASSOCIATED CONDITIONS
Accelerated atherosclerosis, pericarditis, amyloidosis, Felty syndrome (RA, splenomegaly, neutropenia), interstitial lung disease, pulmonary nodules, rheumatoid nodules, vasculitis, lymphomas, carpal tunnel syndrome

DIAGNOSIS

HISTORY
- Symmetric polyarthritis—most commonly of hands and feet
- Constitutional symptoms: fatigue, malaise, weight loss, low-grade fevers (1)
- Articular symptoms: tender/swollen joints, early morning stiffness (at least 60 minutes), and difficulty with activities of daily living (ADL) (1)
- Extra-articular involvement: skin, pulmonary, cardiovascular, ocular symptoms; onset is typically insidious. Patients rarely present with abrupt onset of symptoms and extra-articular manifestations (1).

PHYSICAL EXAM
- Evaluate for swollen, boggy, or tender joints with pain and decreased ROM; usually symmetric
  - Small joints: metacarpophalangeal (MCP), leading to Boutonnière and swan-neck deformities, carpal bones of wrist, 2nd to 5th metatarsophalangeal (MTP), and thumb interphalangeal (IP) joints
  - Large joints: Shoulders, elbows, hips, knees, and ankles will show evidence of effusions.
- Joint deformity, nodules, and fusion are late findings.
- Extra-articular findings:
  - Splenomegaly, lymphadenopathy, subcutaneous nodules, peripheral neuropathy, and atlantoaxial joint instability. Axial migration of dens into foramen magnum may be associated with occipital headaches.
  - Cardiovascular mortality increased with RA—evaluate rhythm, presence of murmurs (valvular dysfunction), and for pericardial effusion.
  - Pulmonary disease typically manifests as pleural effusion and fibrosis (dullness, rales).

DIFFERENTIAL DIAGNOSIS
Sjögren syndrome, systemic lupus erythematosus, systemic sclerosis, adult Still disease, psoriatic arthritis, polymyalgia rheumatica (older), seronegative polyarthritis, erosive osteoarthritis, crystal arthropathy, septic arthritis, chronic Lyme disease, viral-induced arthritis (parvovirus B19, Chikungunya virus, hepatitis C [with cryoglobulinemia]), occult malignancy, vasculitis (Behçet syndrome), inflammatory bowel disease, RS3PE hemochromatosis, sarcoidosis

DIAGNOSTIC TESTS & INTERPRETATION
Initial Tests (lab, imaging)
- CBC: Mild anemia and thrombocytosis are common and relate to disease activity (1)[A].
- ESR and C-reactive protein (CRP) are nonspecific markers used to assess disease activity (1)[A].
- Rheumatoid factor (RF): >1:80 in 70–80% of patients with RA (most commonly IgM Ab) (1)[A]
- Anticyclic citrullinated peptide antibodies (anti-CCP antibodies); specificity >90% (1)[A]
- Antinuclear antibody: present in 20–30%
- Electrolytes, creatinine, liver function, and urinalysis to assess comorbid states, establish baseline, and to assist with medication management (2)[A]
- Radiographs help establish diagnosis and monitor progression (1)[A].
- Plain film radiographs are preferred for RA:
  - Initial radiographs of the hands, wrists, and feet
  - Hallmark is a lack of bony remodeling and symmetric joint space narrowing.
  - Earliest pattern of erosions is loss of cortical distinctness, followed by dot-dash pattern of cortical bone loss. Marginal erosions at cortical bone within joint capsule not covered by cartilage result in "mouse-ear" erosions.
- MRI of hands and wrists (erosions, pannus, synovitis)
- Ultrasound can assess synovial thickening/erosions.
- Diagnostic criteria: 2010 ACR/EULAR criteria (1)[A]
  - ≥1 joint with definitive clinical synovitis not explained by another disease plus either:
    ○ Presence of ≥2 typical periarticular erosions
    ○ Score of ≥6 on following:
      ■ Joint involvement (0 to 5)
        □ 1 medium to large joint: 0
        □ 2 to 10 medium to large joints: 1
        □ 1 to 3 small joints: 2 (DIP, 1st MCP, and 1st MTP joints are excluded from assessment.)
        □ 4 to 10 small joints: 3
        □ >10 joints (>1 small joint): 5
      ■ Serology score (0 to 3)
        □ Negative RF and ACPA: 0
        □ Low positive RF or low positive ACPA: 2
        □ High positive RF or high positive ACPA: 3
      ■ Acute-phase reactants score (0 to 2)
        □ Normal CRP and normal ESR: 0
        □ Abnormal CRP or ESR: 1
      ■ Duration of symptoms score (0 to 1)
        □ <6 weeks: 0
        □ ≥6 weeks: 1
      ■ Patients with a score of <6/10 do not meet RA criteria. Reevaluate these patients over time.

Diagnostic Procedures/Other
- Joint aspiration (if needed) to exclude crystal arthropathy and septic arthritis
- Synovial fluid analysis:
  - Gram stain, cell count, culture, crystal analysis, and overall appearance
  - Yellowish-white, turbid, poor viscosity in RA
  - WBC increased (3,500 to 50,000 cells/mm³)
  - Protein: ~4.2 g/dL (42 g/L)
  - Serum-synovial glucose difference ≥30 mg/dL (≥1.67 mmol/L)

TREATMENT

GENERAL MEASURES
- Goal is to achieve remission/minimize disease activity, prevent structural damage, and prevent disability (3)[A].
- Early, aggressive treatment prevents structural damage and disability (3)[A].
- Periodic evaluation of disease activity and extent of synovitis can establish severity of disease (3)[A].
- Disease activity measures include the Disease Activity Score (DAS28) score (https://www.nras.org.uk/the-das28-score) and the RAPID 3 score (3)[A].
- Treatment is based on severity of disease (3)[A].

MEDICATION
- Early DMARD therapy to slow disease progression and induce remission is standard of care (3)[A].
- Nonbiologic DMARDs:
  - Start within 3 months of diagnosis.
  - Initial therapy with a nonbiologic DMARD-greater convenience, lower toxicity, quicker onset
  - Methotrexate is the first-line DMARD in patients with active RA; start with 7.5 to 25.0 mg/week PO. Titrate to optimal dosage within 4 to 8 weeks. DMARD with the most predictable benefit. Folic acid 1 mg PO daily reduces toxicity. Monitor CBC, renal and liver function every month for 3 months and then every 3 months; contraindicated in renal and hepatic diseases, pregnancy, and breastfeeding
  - Sulfasalazine: 500 mg/day, increase to 2 g/day over 1 month; max: 2 to 3 g/day; 6-month trial. Monotherapy for low disease activity. Monitor CBC, liver enzymes every 2 weeks for 3 month, then every month for 3 months, and then every 3 months. Screen for G6PD deficiency.
  - Leflunomide (Arava): loading dose 100 mg/day × 3 days and then 10 to 20 mg/day. GI side effects and potentially teratogenic; contraindicated in pregnancy. Monitor CBC, LFTs, and phosphate monthly for the first 6 months. Stop use if ALT >3 times upper limit normal.
  - Hydroxychloroquine (Plaquenil) 400 mg QHS for 2 to 3 months and then 200 mg QHS; 6-month trial. Usually used to treat milder forms or in combination with other DMARDs. Ophthalmologic exam every 6 to 12 months due to potential maculopathy. Adjust dose in renal insufficiency.
  - Minocycline (100 mg BID), antibiotic with anti-inflammatory properties; used in mild disease
- Biologic DMARDs:
  - TNF inhibitors: IV infliximab (Remicade), SC adalimumab (Humira), and SC etanercept (Enbrel). No evidence that one is superior; certolizumab pegol (Cimzia) and golimumab (Simponi), approved in moderate to severe disease
  - Janus kinase (JAK) inhibitor: tofacitinib citrate (Xeljanz), used for moderate to severe disease in adults that failed methotrexate
  - IL-6 receptor antagonist: tocilizumab (Actemra) for moderate to severe active RA that failed DMARD therapy. Sarilumab (Kevzara), newly FDA-approved for treatment of moderate to severe RA in patients with an inadequate response or intolerance to anti-TNF therapy; need to monitor CBS for neutropenia (4)[A]

- Abatacept (Orencia) and anakinra (Kineret) no longer considered cost-effective or efficacious treatment for RA
- Rituximab (Rituxan): A chimeric monoclonal antibody that targets CD20 on B cells. It is recommended with or without methotrexate for active moderate to severe RA with inadequate response to other DMARDs or failed anti-TNF agent.
- All biologics can be used in combination with a DMARD or steroids (3)[A].
- In patients with history of lymphoproliferative disorders, rituximab is preferred to TNF inhibitor (3)[A].
- In patients with skin cancer, DMARD are preferred to biologic agents (3)[A].
- In patients with CHF, combo DMARD therapy, a non-TNF biologic, or tofacitinib is recommended over a TNF inhibitor (3)[A].
- Check purified protein derivative (PPD) and screen for hepatitis prior to treatment.
- Ensure vaccinations (pneumococcal, HPV, hepatitis B, influenza, varicella zoster) are up-to-date.
- Treating flare-ups:
  - Intra-articular steroids: if disease is well controlled after ruling out intra-articular infection
  - Repository corticotropin injection, an ACTH analogue (Acthar gel)

ADDITIONAL THERAPIES
Symptomatic therapy in addition to DMARDs:
- NSAIDs: naproxen (500 mg BID) or ibuprofen (800 mg TID) for symptomatic relief. If poor response to initial NSAID after 2 weeks, try alternative NSAID.
- If still poor response, prednisone (5 to 30 mg/day)
- Capsaicin cream: 3 to 4 times/day as needed
- Physical therapy to minimize loss of joint function

SURGERY/OTHER PROCEDURES
- Consider synovectomy, tendon reconstruction, joint fusion, and joint replacement to prevent disability.
- Flexion/extension films of cervical spine prior to any surgery due to high risk of atlantoaxial joint instability and subluxation
- Ultrasound-guided synovial biopsy to evaluate for number of synovial sublining macrophages is a novel technique for evaluating efficacy of treatment. Reduction in number of synovial macrophages correlates with a decrease in disease activity and therefore a good response to treatment (5)[B].

 ONGOING CARE

FOLLOW-UP RECOMMENDATIONS
Encourage full activity as tolerated. Avoid heavy work or exercise during active (flare) phases. Emphasize exercise, mobility, and reduction of joint stress.

Patient Monitoring
DAS28 questionnaire helps monitor disease activity, and Health Assessment Questionnaire (HAQ) helps evaluate functional status.

PROGNOSIS
- Poor prognostic findings
  - Persistent moderate to severe disease; early or advanced age at disease onset
  - Many affected joints; positive MCP squeeze test, and PIP and MCP symmetric involvement
- 50% cannot function in their primary jobs within 10 years of onset.

REFERENCES
1. Aletaha D, Neogi T, Silman AJ, et al. 2010 Rheumatoid arthritis classification criteria: an American College of Rheumatology/European League Against Rheumatism collaborative initiative. *Arthritis Rheum.* 2010;62(9):2569–2581.
2. Singh JA, Furst DE, Bharat A, et al. 2012 Update of the 2008 American College of Rheumatology recommendations for the use of disease-modifying antirheumatic drugs and biologic agents in the treatment of rheumatoid arthritis. *Arthritis Care Res (Hoboken).* 2012;64(5):625–639.
3. Singh JA, Saag KG, Bridges SL Jr, et al. 2015 American College of Rheumatology guideline for the treatment of rheumatoid arthritis. *Arthritis Rheumatol.* 2016;68(1):1–26.
4. Fleischmann R, van Adelsberg J, Lin Y, et al. Sarilumab and nonbiologic disease-modifying anti-rheumatic drugs in patients with active rheumatoid arthritis and inadequate response or intolerance to tumor necrosis factor inhibitors. *Arthritis Rheumatol.* 2017;69(2):277–290.
5. Mandelin AM II, Homan P, Shaffer AM, et al. Transcriptional profiling of synovial macrophages using minimally invasive ultrasound-guided synovial biopsies in rheumatoid arthritis. *Arthritis Rheumatol.* 2018;70(6):841–854.

ADDITIONAL READING
Pincus T, Yazici Y, Bergman MJ. RAPID3, an index to assess and monitor patients with rheumatoid arthritis, without formal joint counts: similar results to DAS28 and CDAI in clinical trials and clinical care. *Rheum Dis Clin North Am.* 2009;35(4):773–778.

CODES

ICD10
- M06.9 Rheumatoid arthritis, unspecified
- M05.60 Rheu arthritis of unsp site w involv of organs and systems
- M05.30 Rheumatoid heart disease w rheumatoid arthritis of unsp site

CLINICAL PEARLS
- Early diagnosis is important to improve outcomes and functional status.
- Plain films are the initial imaging modality of choice.
- Early treatment with DMARDs slows disease progression and improves the chance for remission.
- Methotrexate is the first-line DMARD in patients with active RA.

ARTHRITIS, SEPTIC
Jeffrey P. Feden, MD, FACEP

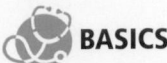 **BASICS**

DESCRIPTION
- Infection due to bacterial invasion of the joint space
- Systems affected: musculoskeletal
- Synonyms: suppurative arthritis; infectious arthritis; pyarthrosis; pyogenic arthritis; bacterial arthritis

EPIDEMIOLOGY
- May occur at any age; incidence is higher in very young and in the elderly.
- Prevalence: 27% of patients presenting with monoarticular arthritis have nongonococcal septic arthritis (1).
- Gender differences:
  - Gonococcal: female > male
  - Nongonococcal: male > female

ETIOLOGY AND PATHOPHYSIOLOGY
- Multiple pathogens
- Nongonococcal:
  - *Staphylococcus aureus* (most common in adults)
    - MRSA risk increased in elderly, intravenous drug users (IVDU), postsurgical
  - *Streptococcus* spp. (second most common in adults)
  - Gram-negative rods (GNR): IVDU, trauma, extremes of age, immunosuppressed
- *Neisseria gonorrhoeae* (most common in young, sexually active adults)
- Other: rickettsial (e.g., Lyme), fungal, mycobacterial
- Risk by specific age (2):
  - <1 month: *S. aureus*, group B streptococcus (GBS), GNR
  - 1 month to 4 years: *S. aureus*, *Streptococcus pneumoniae*, *Neisseria meningitidis*
  - 16 to 40 years: *N. meningitidis*, *S. aureus*
  - >40 years: *S. aureus*
- Specific high-risk groups:
  - Rheumatoid arthritis (RA): *S. aureus*
  - IVDU: *S. aureus*, GNR, opportunistic pathogens
  - Neonates: GBS
  - Immunocompromised: gram-negative bacilli, fungi
  - Trauma patients with open injuries: mixed flora
- Pathogenesis:
  - Hematogenous spread (most common)
  - Direct inoculation by microorganisms secondary to trauma or iatrogenesis (e.g., joint surgery)
  - Adjacent spread (e.g., osteomyelitis)
- Pathophysiology:
  - Microorganisms initially enter through synovial membrane and spread to the synovial fluid.
  - Resulting inflammatory response releases cytokines and destructive proteases leading to systemic symptoms and joint damage.

RISK FACTORS
- Age >80 years
- Low socioeconomic status, alcoholism
- Cellulitis and skin ulcers
- Violation of joint capsule
  - Prior orthopedic surgery
  - Intra-articular steroid injection
  - Trauma
- History of previous joint disease
  - Inflammatory arthritis (RA: 10-fold increased risk)
  - Osteoarthritis
  - Crystal arthritides
- Systemic illness
  - Diabetes mellitus, liver disease, HIV, malignancy, end-stage renal disease/hemodialysis, immuno-suppression, sickle cell anemia
- Risks for hematogenous spread
  - IVDU, severe sepsis/systemic infection

GENERAL PREVENTION
- Prompt treatment of skin and soft tissue infections.
- Control risk factors.
- Immunization (*S. pneumoniae*, *N. meningitidis*)

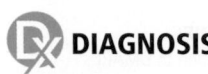 **DIAGNOSIS**

HISTORY
- Typically presents with a combination of joint pain, swelling, warmth, and decreased range of motion
- Nongonococcal arthritis: mostly monoarticular (80%)
  - Typically large joints (knee in 50% of cases)
  - Most patients report fever.
  - IV drug users may develop infection in axial joints (e.g., sternoclavicular joint).
  - Prosthetic joints may show minimal findings and present with draining sinus over the joint.
  - Patients on chronic immunosuppressive drugs and those receiving steroid joint injections may have atypical presentations (no fever or joint pain).
- Pediatric considerations
  - Infants may refuse to move limb (can be mistaken as neurologic problem).
  - Hip pain may be referred to knee and/or thigh.
- Gonococcal arthritis
  - Bacteremic phase: migratory polyarthritis, tenosynovitis, high fever, chills, pustules (dermatitis–arthritis syndrome)
  - Localized phase: monoarticular, low-grade fever

PHYSICAL EXAM
- Physical exam has poor sensitivity and specificity for septic arthritis. Common findings include:
  - Limited range of motion
  - Joint effusion and tenderness
  - Erythema and warmth over affected joint
  - Pain with passive range of motion
- Hip and shoulder involvement may reveal severe pain with range of motion and less obvious swelling.
- Infants with septic hip arthritis maintain the joint in flexion external rotation.

DIFFERENTIAL DIAGNOSIS
- Crystal arthritis: gout, pseudogout, calcium oxalate, cholesterol
- Infectious arthritis: fungi, spirochetes, rheumatic fever, HIV, viral
- Inflammatory arthritis: RA, spondyloarthropathy, systemic lupus erythematosus, sarcoidosis
- Osteoarthritis
- Trauma: meniscal tear, fracture, hemarthrosis
- Other: bursitis, cellulitis, tendinitis

DIAGNOSTIC TESTS & INTERPRETATION
Initial Tests (lab, imaging)
- Synovial fluid analysis is the gold standard:
  - Obtain prior to antibiotic therapy when possible.
  - Include Gram stain, culture, cell count/differential, and crystal analysis.
  - Use blood culture bottles to increase yield.
  - Gram stain (positive in 50%); culture (positive in 50–70%)
  - >50,000 WBCs/HPF with >90% polymorpho-nuclear leukocytes is suggestive; *synovial WBC (sWBC) count alone is insufficient to rule in or rule out septic arthritis* (2)[A].
  - Crystals (e.g., urate or calcium pyrophosphate) *do not exclude concurrent infectious arthritis.*
  - Prosthetic joint: WBC count is unreliable; a lower number of sWBCs may indicate infection.
- Serum tests:
  - WBC count alone is neither sensitive nor specific.
  - ESR >15 mm/hr has sensitivity up to 94% but poor specificity (3)[B].
  - CRP >20 mg/L has sensitivity of 92% (3)[B].
  - Synovial lactate is a potential biomarker (4)[A].
  - Blood cultures are positive in 50% of cases.
- Other tests:
  - Disseminated gonococcus: culture blood, cervix, urine, urethra, pharynx in addition to joint fluid
  - Suspected Lyme arthritis: must send serum titers
- Pediatrics: No single lab test distinguishes septic arthritis from transient synovitis.
  - The combination of fever, non–weight-bearing, and elevated ESR and CRP is suspicious; synovial fluid should be obtained.
- Imaging helps to identify effusion but does not differentiate septic from other forms of arthritis.
  - Plain films:
    - Nondiagnostic for septic arthritis; useful for trauma, soft tissue swelling, osteoarthritis, or osteopenia

○ May show nonspecific inflammatory arthritic changes (i.e., erosions, joint destruction, or joint space loss)
– Ultrasound:
  ○ Guides arthrocentesis
  ○ Recommended for aspiration of the hip
– MRI:
  ○ Highly sensitive for effusion; may help distinguish between transient synovitis and septic arthritis in children
– Other imaging techniques:
  ○ CT is not routinely indicated.
  ○ Bone scans are not performed unless there is suspicion for osteomyelitis.

Diagnostic Procedures/Other
Arthrocentesis in all suspected cases (prior to starting antibiotics). Avoid contaminated tissue (e.g., overlying cellulitis) when performing arthrocentesis.

Test Interpretation
Synovial biopsy shows polymorphonuclear leukocytes and (possibly) the causative organism.

 TREATMENT

GENERAL MEASURES
• Admit for parenteral antibiotics and monitoring. Begin antibiotics immediately after arthrocentesis.
• Drainage of purulent material is *required* if:
  – Pediatric: Surgical drainage and irrigation is recommended if hip is involved due to high risk of avascular necrosis.
  – Prosthetic joint: antibiotics and consult with orthopedics for consideration of revision arthroplasty, resection arthroplasty, or débridement
• Antibiotic therapy for total of 4 to 6 weeks in most cases
  – Exception: gonococcal (2 to 3 weeks)
• Intra-articular antibiotics are not recommended.

MEDICATION
First Line
• Initial antibiotic choice is guided by Gram stain or the most likely organism based on age, clinical history, and risk factors.
• Nongonococcal (5)[C]:
  – Gram-positive cocci:
    ○ Vancomycin 15 to 20 mg/kg 2 to 3 times daily or linezolid 600 mg twice daily
  – Gram-negative bacilli:
    ○ Cefepime 2 g twice daily or ceftriaxone 2 g daily or ceftazidime 2 g 3 times daily or cefotaxime 2 g 3 times daily
    ○ For cephalosporin allergy: Consider treatment with ciprofloxacin 400 mg 3 times daily.

– Negative Gram stain:
  ○ Vancomycin 15 to 20 mg/kg 2 to 3 times daily plus 3rd-generation cephalosporin until cultures and susceptibilities return
– Duration of therapy: typically 2 weeks of IV and an additional 2 to 4 weeks PO while monitoring therapeutic response
• Gonococcal:
  – Ceftriaxone 1 g IV/IM daily for 7 to 14 days (and at least 24 to 48 hours after symptoms resolve)
  – May require concurrent drainage of affected joint
  – Concomitant treatment for *Chlamydia* (doxycycline 100 mg twice daily or azithromycin 1 g daily)
• Other considerations:
  – Narrow antibiotic therapy based on culture results.
  – Consider *Salmonella* in pediatric patients with a history of sickle cell disease: 3rd-generation cephalosporin helpful in this instance
  – Lyme arthritis: doxycycline 100 mg PO twice daily or amoxicillin 500 mg PO 3 times daily for 28 days if no neurologic involvement, otherwise ceftriaxone 2 g IV daily

ISSUES FOR REFERRAL
• Infectious disease and orthopedic consultations
• Consult ID specialist for IVDU and immunosuppression; prosthetic joint infection best managed with orthopedic consultation

SURGERY/OTHER PROCEDURES
• Consider drainage in all cases—particularly shoulder, hip, and prosthetic joints.
• Other treatment options include repeat needle aspiration, arthroscopy, or arthrotomy.

 ONGOING CARE

FOLLOW-UP RECOMMENDATIONS
Patient Monitoring
• Can monitor synovial fluid to verify decreasing WBC and sterile fluid after initial treatment
• If no improvement within 24 hours, reevaluate and consider arthroscopy.
• Follow up at 1 week and 1 month after stopping antibiotics to exclude relapse.

PROGNOSIS
• Early treatment improves functional outcome.
• Delayed recognition/treatment is associated with higher morbidity and mortality.
• Elderly, concurrent RA, *S. aureus* infections, and infection of hip and shoulder also increase risk of poor outcome.

COMPLICATIONS
• Mortality estimated at 11% (1)
• Limited joint range of motion, ankylosis
• Secondary osteoarthritis
• Flail, fused, or dislocated joint
• Sepsis, septic necrosis
• Sinus formation
• Osteomyelitis, postinfectious synovitis
• Limb length discrepancy (in children)

REFERENCES

1. Mathews CJ, Weston VC, Jones A, et al. Bacterial septic arthritis in adults. *Lancet*. 2010;375(9717): 846–855.
2. Margaretten ME, Kohlwes J, Moore D, et al. Does this adult patient have septic arthritis? *JAMA*. 2007;297(13):1478–1488.
3. Hariharan P, Kabrhel C. Sensitivity of erythrocyte sedimentation rate and C-reactive protein for the exclusion of septic arthritis in emergency department patients. *J Emerg Med*. 2011;40(4):428–431.
4. Carpenter CR, Schuur JD, Everett WW, et al. Evidence-based diagnostics: adult septic arthritis. *Acad Emerg Med*. 2011;18(8):781–796.
5. Madruga Dias J, Costa MM, Pereira da Silva JA, et al. Septic arthritis: patients with or without isolated infectious agents have similar characteristics. *Infection*. 2014;42(2):385–391.

 CODES

ICD10
• M00.9 Pyogenic arthritis, unspecified
• M00.20 Other streptococcal arthritis, unspecified joint
• M00.00 Staphylococcal arthritis, unspecified joint

CLINICAL PEARLS
• Arthrocentesis and synovial fluid analysis are mandatory in cases of suspected septic arthritis.
• Gram stain has variable sensitivity in septic arthritis. sWBC count is generally >50,000/HPF but is unreliable as a sole diagnostic feature.
• Early IV antibiotics and (if necessary) drainage of infected joints are critical to successful management.
• Crystalline disease may coexist with septic arthritis.
• Initial antibiotic therapy is guided by arthrocentesis results (Gram stain), age, and patient-specific risk factors.

ARTHROPOD BITES AND STINGS

James E. Powers, DO, FACEP, FAAEM

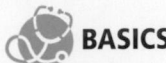 **BASICS**

DESCRIPTION

- Arthropods are the largest division of the animal kingdom. Two classes, insects and arachnids, have the greatest impact on human health.
- Arthropods affect humans by inoculating poison, microorganisms, or irritative substances through a bite or sting; by invading tissue, or by contact allergy to their skin, hairs, or secretions.
- Transmission of infectious microorganisms during feeding is of the greatest concern.
- Sequelae of bites, stings, or contact include:
  - Local redness with itch, pain, and swelling: common, usually immediate and transient
  - Large local reactions that increase over 24 to 48 hours
  - Systemic reactions with anaphylaxis, neurotoxicity, organ damage, or other systemic toxin effects
  - Tissue necrosis or secondary infection
  - Infectious disease transmission: Presentation may be delayed weeks to years.

EPIDEMIOLOGY

Incidence
28,087 cases of arthropod exposures were reported in 2015. This is a small fraction of arthropod encounters.

Prevalence
Widespread, with regional and seasonal variations

ETIOLOGY AND PATHOPHYSIOLOGY

- Arthropods: four medically important classes
  - Insects: *Hymenoptera* (bees, wasps, hornets, fire ants), mosquitoes, bed bugs, flies, lice, fleas, beetles, caterpillars, and moths
  - Arachnids: spiders, scorpions, mites, and ticks
  - Chilopods: centipedes
  - Diplopods: millipedes
- Four general categories of pathophysiologic effects: toxic, allergic, infectious, and traumatic
  - Toxic effects of venom: local (tissue inflammation or destruction) versus systemic (neurotoxic or organ damage)
  - Allergic: Antigens in saliva or venom may cause local inflammation. Exaggerated immune responses may result in anaphylaxis or serum sickness.
  - Trauma: Mechanical injury from biting or stinging causes pain, swelling, and portal of entry for bacteria and secondary infection. Retention of arthropod parts can cause a granulomatous reaction.
  - Infection: Arthropods transmit bacterial, viral, and protozoal diseases.

Genetics
Family history of atopy may be a factor in the development of more severe allergic reactions.

RISK FACTORS

- Previous sensitization
- Although most arthropod contact is inadvertent, certain activities, occupations, and travel exposures increase risk.
- Greater risk for adverse outcome in young, elderly, immunocompromised, and those with chronic or poorly controlled cardiac or respiratory disease
- Increased risk of anaphylaxis in patients with mastocytosis

GENERAL PREVENTION

- Avoid common arthropod habitats.
- Insect repellents (not effective for bees, spiders, scorpions, caterpillars, bed bugs, fleas, ants)
  - N,N-diethyl-meta-toluamide (DEET)
    - Most effective broad-spectrum repellent against biting arthropods (1,2)[A]
    - Formulations with higher concentrations (20–50%) are first-line choice in areas of endemic arthropod-borne diseases (2)[A].
    - Concentrations >30% have longer duration of action.
    - Safe for children >6 months of age and pregnant and lactating women (2)[B]
  - Icaridin (formerly known as *picaridin*)
    - 20% spray comparable to 20% DEET for mosquito protection (2)[A]
  - P-menthane-3,8-diol (PMD; lemon eucalyptus extract)
    - 30% concentrations give 4 to 5 hours of protection against mosquitoes and ticks (1)[A]
  - IR3535: less effective in most studies; not appropriate for malaria-endemic regions (1)[B]
- Barrier methods: clothing, bed nets
  - Use of light-colored pants, long-sleeved shirts, and hats may reduce arthropod impact.
  - Permethrin: synthetic insecticide derived from chrysanthemum plant. Do not apply directly to skin. Permethrin-impregnated clothing provides good protection against arthropods.
  - Mosquito nets: advised for all travelers to disease-endemic areas at risk from biting arthropods. Permethrin-treated nets may offer additional protection (2)[B].
- Desensitization 75–95% effective for *Hymenoptera*-specific venom
  - Skin tests to determine sensitivity
  - Refer to allergist/immunologist.
- Fire ant control (but not elimination) possible
  - Baits; sprays, dusts, aerosols; biologic agents
- Risk of tick-borne diseases may be decreased by prompt removal of ticks within 24 hours of attachment.

DIAGNOSIS

HISTORY

- Sudden onset of pain or itching with visualization of arthropod
- Many cases unknown to patient or asymptomatic initially (bed bugs, lice, scabies, ticks). Consider in patients presenting with localized erythema, urticaria, wheals, papules, pruritus, or bullae.
- May identify insect by its habitat or by remnants brought by patient
- History of prior exposure useful but not always available or reliable
- Travel, occupational, social, and recreational history

PHYSICAL EXAM

- If stinger is still present in skin, remove by flicking or scraping away from skin.
- Anaphylaxis is a clinical diagnosis. Signs and symptoms include (3)[A]:
  - Erythema, urticaria, angioedema
  - Itching/edema of lips, tongue, uvula; drooling
  - Respiratory distress, wheeze, repetitive cough, stridor, dysphonia
  - Hypotension, dysrhythmia, syncope, chest pain
- If anaphylaxis not present, exam focuses on the sting or bite itself. Common findings include local erythema, swelling, wheals, urticaria, papules, or bullae; excoriations from scratching
- Thorough exam to look for arthropod infestation (lice, scabies) or attached ticks. Body lice usually found in seams of clothing; skin scraping to identify scabies
- Signs of secondary bacterial infection after 24 to 48 hours: increasing erythema, pain, fever, lymphangitis, or abscess

DIFFERENTIAL DIAGNOSIS

- Urticaria and localized dermatologic reactions:
  - Contact dermatitis, drug eruption, mastocytosis, bullous diseases, dermatitis herpetiformis, tinea, eczema, vasculitis, pityriasis, erythema multiforme, viral exanthem, cellulitis, abscess, impetigo, folliculitis, erysipelas, necrotizing fasciitis
- Anaphylactic-type reactions
  - Cardiac, hemorrhagic, or septic shock; acute respiratory failure, asthma; angioedema, urticarial vasculitis; flushing syndromes (catecholamines, vasoactive peptides); syncope
  - Differential diagnosis of the acute abdomen should include black widow spider bite.

DIAGNOSTIC TESTS & INTERPRETATION

Initial Tests (lab, imaging)
Seldom needed; basic lab parameters usually normal

Follow-Up Tests & Special Considerations

- Severe envenomations may affect organ function and require monitoring of lab values (CBC, comprehensive metabolic panel, prothrombin time/international normalized ratio).
- Potential arthropod-borne diseases:
  - Ticks: Lyme disease, Rocky Mountain spotted fever, relapsing fever, anaplasmosis, babesiosis, tularemia; ehrlichiosis, Powassan disease; Heartland virus (HRTV); Bourbon virus
  - Flies: tularemia, leishmaniasis, African trypanosomiasis, bartonellosis, loiasis
  - Fleas: plague, tularemia, murine typhus
  - Chigger mites: scrub typhus
  - Body lice: epidemic typhus, relapsing fever
  - Kissing bugs: Chagas disease
  - Mosquitoes: malaria, yellow fever, dengue fever, West Nile virus, equine encephalitis, chikungunya, Zika virus
- With history of anaphylaxis, significant systemic symptoms, progressively severe reactions, refer to allergist for formal testing (3)[B].

Diagnostic Procedures/Other
Skin and immunologic tests available to identify specific allergens

TREATMENT

Most studies are retrospective or based on clinical observations.

ALERT
- Rapid anaphylaxis is severe and potentially life-threatening. Most deaths due to anaphylaxis occur within 30 to 60 minutes of sting.
- Give epinephrine as soon as diagnosis of anaphylaxis is suspected. Delay is associated with increasing rates of fatality (3,4)[A].
- Antihistamines and steroids do not replace epinephrine and are never initial therapy in anaphylaxis; no direct outcome data regarding their effectiveness in anaphylaxis available (3)[A]
- Airway management critical for angioedema

GENERAL MEASURES
Management directed at relieving itching, pain, and swelling; local wound care, ice compress, analgesics

MEDICATION
First Line
- For arthropod bites/stings with anaphylaxis
  - Expert opinion consensus (3)[C]
  - Epinephrine: most important: IM injection in midanterolateral thigh
    - IM injection: epinephrine 1:1,000 (1 mg/mL): adult: 0.3 to 0.5 mg per dose; pediatric: Give 0.01 mg/kg to a maximum dose of 0.3 mg per dose, can repeat every 5 to 15 minutes to total of three injections (3,4)[A].
  - Oxygen up to 100%, as needed
  - IV fluids: Establish 1 to 2 large-bore IV lines. Normal saline bolus 1 to 2 L IV; repeat as needed (pediatrics 20 to 30 mL/kg) (4)[A].
  - H_1 antagonists: diphenhydramine 25 to 50 mg IV (pediatrics 1 to 2 mg/kg) (3)[A]
  - H_2 antihistamines: ranitidine 50 mg IV (4)[A]
  - β_2 Agonists: albuterol for bronchospasm nebulized 2.5 to 5.0 mg in 3 mL (4)[A]
  - *Corticosteroids: 2012 Cochrane review showed no benefit in acute anaphylaxis (4)[A]. May be of benefit in preventing biphasic allergic reactions (4)[C]*; prednisone, methylprednisolone *frequently used*
- Arthropod bites/stings without anaphylaxis
  - Tetanus booster, as indicated
  - Oral antihistamines may be helpful.
    - Diphenhydramine adults: 25 to 50 mg PO/IV/IM every 4 to 6 hours. Pediatrics: 1 to 2 mg/kg to a max dose of 50 mg PO/IV/IM; daily maximum dose of 300 mg for adults and pediatrics
    - Cetirizine adults: 5 to 10 mg PO daily; pediatrics: 6 to 23 months—2.5 mg PO daily; 2 to 5 years—5 mg PO daily; 6 years and older—5 to 10 mg PO daily
    - H_2 blockers: ranitidine adults: 150 mg PO 1 to 2 times daily as needed; pediatrics: 2 to 4 mg PO 1 to 2 times daily as needed
  - Oral steroids: Consider short course for severe pruritus or local reactions; prednisone or prednisolone 1 to 2 mg/kg once daily
  - Consider topical steroid cream or ointment for 3 to 5 days.
    - OTC 1% hydrocortisone
    - May consider higher potency such as triamcinolone 0.1%, fluocinolone 0.025%
  - Wound care: antibiotics only if infection

- Other specific therapies:
  - Scorpion stings: Treat excess catecholamine release (nitroprusside, prazosin, β-blockers). Atropine for hypersalivation (4). Only one FDA-approved scorpion antivenom in United States. Use only in consultation with toxicologist. Black widow bites: Treat muscle spasms with benzodiazepines and opioid analgesics (4). Antivenom: for severe symptoms only (5)[B]; available but should be administered in conjunction with toxicologist
  - Consult poison control hotline for questions regarding management: 1-800-222-1222.
  - Fire ants: characteristically cause sterile pustules; leave intact—do not open or drain.
  - Brown recluse spider: pain control, supportive treatment; surgical consult if débridement needed
  - Ticks: early removal
  - Pediculosis: head, pubic, and body lice
    - First line: permethrin 1% topical lotion
    - Alternatives: Pyrethrins, ivermectin orally shown to be effective but not FDA-approved for pediculosis.
    - Repeat treatment in 7 to 10 days.
  - *Sarcoptes scabiei* scabies
    - Permethrin 5% cream is drug of choice: Apply to entire body. Wash off after 8 to 14 hours. Repeat in 1 week.
    - Ivermectin: 200 μg/kg PO once; repeat in 2 weeks shown to be effective but not FDA-approved for scabies.

ISSUES FOR REFERRAL
Patients with history of anaphylaxis, severe systemic symptoms, or progressively severe reactions benefit from consultation with allergy/immunology.

SURGERY/OTHER PROCEDURES
Débridement and delayed skin grafting may be needed for severe brown recluse spider and other bites.

COMPLEMENTARY & ALTERNATIVE MEDICINE
- Cool compresses
- Calamine lotion not shown to have benefit.
- A paste of 3 tsp of baking soda and 1 tsp water may help salve bites.

ADMISSION, INPATIENT, AND NURSING CONSIDERATIONS
Anaphylaxis, vascular instability, neuromuscular events, pain, GI symptoms, renal damage/failure

 ONGOING CARE

FOLLOW-UP RECOMMENDATIONS
- Venom immunotherapy is the cornerstone of treatment for *Hymenoptera*; 80–98% effective (3)[A]
- Provide epinephrine for patient self-administration if history of anaphylaxis (3)[A]. Consider "med-alert" identifiers.

Patient Monitoring
- Monitor for delayed effects, including infectious diseases from arthropod bites.
- Serum sickness reactions, vasculitis (rare)

PATIENT EDUCATION
Arthropod avoidance and preventive measures

PROGNOSIS
- Excellent for local reactions
- For systemic reactions, best response with early intervention to prevent cardiorespiratory collapse

COMPLICATIONS
- Scarring
- Secondary bacterial infection
- Arthropod-associated infectious diseases
- Psychological effects, phobias

REFERENCES
1. Alpern JD, Dunlop SJ, Dolan BJ, et al. Personal protection measures against mosquitoes, ticks, and other arthropods. *Med Clin North Am*. 2016;100(2):303–316.
2. Moore SJ, Mordue Luntz AJ, Logan JG. Insect bite prevention. *Infect Dis Clin North Am*. 2012;26(3):655–673.
3. Lieberman P, Nicklas RA, Randolph C, et al. Anaphylaxis—a practice parameter update 2015. *Ann Allergy Asthma Immunol*. 2015;115(5): 341–384.
4. Singer E, Zodda D. Allergy and anaphylaxis: principles of acute emergency management. *Emerg Med Pract*. 2015;17(8):1–20.
5. Erickson TB, Cheema N. Arthropod envenomation in North America. *Emerg Med Clin North Am*. 2017;35(2):355–375.

ADDITIONAL READING
- Centers for Disease Control and Prevention. FAQ. Insect repellent use & safety. http://www.cdc.gov/westnile/faq/repellent.html. Accessed December 12, 2018.
- Centers for Disease Control and Prevention. Parasites: lice. https://www.cdc.gov/parasites/lice/head/treatment.html. Accessed December 12, 2018.
- Centers for Disease Control and Prevention. Parasites: scabies. https://www.cdc.gov/parasites/scabies/health_professionals/meds.html. Accessed December 22, 2018.
- Centers for Disease Control and Prevention. Protection against mosquitoes, ticks, & other arthropods. https://wwwnc.cdc.gov/travel/yellowbook/2018/the-pre-travel-consultation/protection-against-mosquitoes-ticks-other-arthropods. Accessed December 12, 2018.
- Juckett G. Arthropod bites. *Am Fam Physician*. 2013;88(12):841–847.
- Rosenberg R, Lindsey NP, Fischer M, et al. Vital signs: trends in reported vectorborne disease cases—United States and territories, 2004–2016. *MMWR Morb Mortal Wkly Rep*. 2018;67(17): 496–501.

 CODES

ICD10
- T63.481A Toxic effect of venom of arthropod, accidental, init
- T63.301A Toxic effect of unsp spider venom, accidental, init
- T63.484A Toxic effect of venom of oth arthropod, undetermined, init

CLINICAL PEARLS
- Urgent administration of epinephrine is the key to successful treatment of anaphylaxis.
- Local treatment and symptom management are sufficient in most insect bites and stings.
- Tick-borne illness is on the rise in the United Stings.

ASCITES
Daniel J. Stein, MD, MPH • Stephen K. Lane, MD

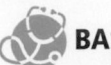 **BASICS**

DESCRIPTION
- Accumulation of fluid in the peritoneal cavity; may occur in conditions that cause generalized edema
- Men generally have no fluid in peritoneal cavity; women may have up to 20 mL depending on menstrual phase.

EPIDEMIOLOGY
- Children: most commonly associated with nephrotic syndrome and malignancy
- Adults: cirrhosis (81%), cancer (10%), heart failure (3%), other (6%)

Incidence
~50–60% of cirrhotic patients develop ascites within 10 years (1).

Prevalence
10% of patients with cirrhosis have ascites.

ETIOLOGY AND PATHOPHYSIOLOGY
- Portal hypertension versus nonportal hypertension causes
  - Cannot reliably establish/confirm etiology without paracentesis
  - Serum-ascites albumin gradient (SAAG): (serum albumin level: ascites albumin level) helps to differentiate causes
- High portal pressure (SAAG ≥1.1)
  - Cirrhosis
  - Hepatitis (alcoholic, viral, autoimmune, medications)
  - Acute liver failure
  - Liver malignancy (primary or metastatic)
  - Elevated right-sided filling pressures from heart failure or constrictive pericarditis
  - Hepatic venous thrombosis (Budd-Chiari syndrome)
  - Portal vein thrombosis
- Normal portal pressure (SAAG <1.1)
  - Peritoneal carcinomatosis
  - Tuberculosis
  - Severe hypoalbuminemia (nephrotic syndrome; severe enteropathy with protein loss)
  - Meigs syndrome (ovarian cancer)
  - Lymphatic leak (chylous ascites)
  - Pancreatitis
  - Inflammatory (vasculitis, lupus serositis, sarcoidosis)
  - Other infections (parasitic, fungal)
  - Hemoperitoneum (trauma or ectopic pregnancy)
- Pathophysiology is best described for portal hypertensive (typically cirrhotic) ascites.
  - Reduced renal and carotid perfusion activates systemic vasoconstrictors and antinatriuretic mechanisms. This stimulates the sympathetic nervous system and renin-angiotensin-aldosterone system to retain sodium and water.
  - Most ascites is due to portal hypertension, with preferentially dilated splanchnic vasculature causing systemic hypotension.

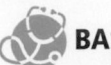 **DIAGNOSIS**

HISTORY
- Address risk factors (e.g., EtOH use, TB exposure, prior malignancies, sexual partners, transfusion history, metabolic syndrome, increased risk of non-alcoholic steatohepatitis progressing to cirrhosis).

- Progressive abdominal distention may be painful.
- Weight gain, dyspnea/orthopnea, edema, early satiety, nausea
- Patients with spontaneous bacterial peritonitis (SBP) may present with fever, abdominal tenderness, and altered mentation.
- Individuals with underlying malignancy may present with weight loss.

PHYSICAL EXAM
- Abdominal distention with flank/shifting dullness is the most sensitive (83%) and specific (56%) exam finding; requires >1,500 mL of fluid to detect
- Edema (penile/scrotal, pedal), pleural effusion, rales
- Stigmata of cirrhosis (palmar erythema, spider angiomata, dilated abdominal wall collateral veins)
- Other signs of advanced liver disease: jaundice, muscle wasting, gynecomastia, leukonychia
- Signs of underlying malignancy: cachexia; umbilical (Virchow) node suggests upper abdominal malignancy.

DIAGNOSTIC TESTS & INTERPRETATION
Initial Tests (lab, imaging)
- Diagnostic paracentesis for fluid analysis to determine etiology and rule out infection in all patients with ascites requiring hospital admission and in any new-onset or new-to-treatment patients (1)[C]
  - Paracentesis complication rate is 1% (despite high rates of coexisting coagulation abnormalities).
  - Routine attempts to correct platelet or coagulation defects not needed prior to paracentesis (1)[B]
  - Ascitic fluid analysis (1)[C]:
    ○ Cell count and differential:
      ▪ Polymorphonuclear (PMN) leukocytes ≥250 cells/mm³ suggest infection.
    ○ Albumin to calculate SAAG:
      ▪ <1.1 g indicates a low portal pressure exudative process (i.e., inflammatory, biliary/pancreatic, carcinomatosis, TB).
      ▪ ≥1.1 g indicates portal hypertensive/transudative process (cirrhosis, CHF, constrictive pericarditis, thrombosis).
    ○ Total protein (low in cirrhosis, nephrotic disease and high in cardiac ascites)
  - Other tests (based on clinical scenario) (1)[C]:
    ○ Bacterial gram stain/culture if infection suspected (Cirrhotic patients with ascites can fail to mount fever or leukocytosis.)
      ▪ Fluid cultures are traditionally positive in 50–90% of cases of SBP.
      ▪ Yield is improved if inoculated to blood culture bottles at bedside and if fluid is obtained before first dose of antibiotics.
    ○ Amylase (suspicion for bowel perforation, choledocholithiasis, or pancreatitis)
    ○ Triglyceride if fluid appears milky
    ○ Cytology if concern for malignancy (less sensitive in the absence of carcinomatosis)
    ○ Lactate dehydrogenase (LDH): An ascitic fluid–to–serum LDH ratio >1.0 can indicate infection, perforation, or tumor.
    ○ Carcinoembryonic antigen and alkaline phosphatase (elevated in viscous perforation)
- Mycobacterial culture/PCR for suspicion of TB
- BUN/creatinine, electrolytes (renal function)
  - Brain natriuretic peptide (heart failure)
  - Liver function tests and hepatitis serologies (hepatitis)

- Abdominal ultrasound (US) can confirm ascites; highly sensitive, cost-effective, involves no radiation
- Portal US Doppler can detect thrombosis or cirrhosis.
- CT scan for intra-abdominal pathology (malignancy)
- MRI preferred for evaluation of liver disease or confirmation of portal vein thrombosis

Diagnostic Procedures/Other
Laparoscopy: if imaging and paracentesis are nondiagnostic
- Allows for direct visualization and biopsy of peritoneum, liver, and intra-abdominal lymph nodes
- Preferred for evaluating suspected peritoneal tuberculosis or malignancies

Test Interpretation
Cytology may reveal malignant cells: adenocarcinoma (ovary, breast, GI tract) or primary peritoneal carcinoma (most commonly associated with ascites).

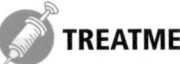 **TREATMENT**

For all patients:
- Daily weight
- Restrict dietary sodium to ≤2 g/day if the cause is due to portal hypertension (high SAAG) (1)[A].
- Water restriction (1.0 to 1.5 L/day) only necessary if serum sodium <120 to 125 mEq/L (1)[C]
- If creatinine >2.0 mg/dL, then decrease diuretic doses.
- Avoid alcohol and ensure adequate nutrition if liver disease (1)[A].
- Baclofen may be used to reduce alcohol craving/consumption (1)[C] in EtOH cirrhosis.

MEDICATION

ALERT
- Care with diuresis; aggressive diuresis can induce prerenal acute kidney injury, encephalopathy, and hyponatremia. Monitor creatinine and electrolytes closely. Serum creatinine >2 mg/dL or serum sodium <120 mmol/L warrants withdrawal of diuretics.
- Avoid NSAIDs (can exacerbate oliguria/azotemia).
- ACE inhibitors and angiotensin receptor blockers (ARBs) may be harmful in patients with cirrhosis/ascites due to an increased risk of hypotension and renal failure (1)[C]. Avoid in refractory ascites (1)[B].
- Consider discontinuing β-blockers in patients with refractory ascites, worsening hypotension, or azotemia (1)[B].

First Line
- Sodium restriction and diuretics are the mainstay of treatment for patients with elevated portal pressures (1)[A]; other causes (e.g., carcinomatosis) are less likely to respond to medical therapy.
  - Spironolactone 100 to 400 mg daily PO; typical initial dose is 100 to 200 mg given in AM.
    ○ Diuretic of choice due to antialdosterone effects; can be used as single agent in minimal ascites. Monitor for hyperkalemia (1)[B].
  - Furosemide 40 to 160 mg daily PO; typical initial dose is 40 mg given in AM.
    ○ Antinatriuretic effect helps achieve negative sodium balance.
    ○ Preferred in combination with spironolactone rather than as monotherapy (1)[B]

- Add-on therapies for patients with severe asthma, when patients persist with symptoms despite optimized treatment with high-dose controller medications (ICS + LABA)
  - Anticholinergic agents, tiotropium (long-acting muscarinic antagonist [LAMA]) (1)[B] or ipratropium (short-acting muscarinic antagonist [SAMA])
  - Anti-immunoglobulin E (anti-IgE) (omalizumab) treatment (1)[A]
  - Leukotriene receptor antagonist (LTRA) (montelukast, pranlukast, zafirlukast) (1)[B]
  - Chromones (nedocromil sodium, sodium cromoglicate) (1)[A]
- Initial recommended controllers by patient's presenting symptoms (1):
  - No controller recommended (1) when:
    - Typical symptoms or need for SABA <2 times per month, no waking up from sleep in last month, no risk factor for exacerbations, no exacerbation in the past year
  - Low-dose ICS (1) when:
    - Infrequent asthma symptoms but patient has presence of >1 risk factors for exacerbation
  - Low-dose ICS (1)[B] when:
    - Typical symptoms or need for SABA 2 times per month/week or patient wakes up from sleep
  - Low-dose ICS (1)[A] when:
    - Symptoms recurs or need for SABA >2 times per week; alternative treatment—LTRA or theophylline
  - Medium- to high-dose ICS (1)[A] or low-dose ICS/LABA (1)[A] when:
    - Symptoms recurs most of the day, patient wakes up from sleep >1 a week, presence of risk factors for asthma exacerbation
  - Short course of oral corticosteroids (OCS) plus regular controller treatment—high-dose ICS or moderate-dose ICS/LABA (budesonide/formoterol; beclomethasone/formoterol) when:
    - Severe uncontrolled asthma or acute exacerbation
  - Stepwise approach for asthma treatment (1):
    - Step 1: as needed reliever inhaler:
      - First: inhaled SABA (1)[A]; alternatives: low-dose ICS (1)[B]
    - Step 2: low-dose controller + as needed reliever:
      - First: low-dose ICS + SABA; alternatives for controllers: second: LTRA; third: low-dose ICS/LABA
    - Step 3: one or two controllers + as needed reliever:
      - First (adults/adolescents): low-dose ICS/LABA + SABA or ICS/formoterol as both controller + reliever; first (ages 6 to 11 years) and second alternative (adults/adolescents): moderate-dose ICS + SABA; third: low-dose ICS + LTRA versus low-dose sustained-release theophylline
    - Step 4: two or more controllers + as needed reliever:
      - First (adults/adolescents): low-dose ICS/formoterol as both controller + reliever OR moderate-dose ICS/LABA + SABA; first (ages 6 to 11 years): referral to specialist; alternative: second: LAMA, sustained-release theophylline or LTRA as add-on therapy
    - Step 5: referral to specialist and add-on therapy (i.e., LAMA, anti-IgE, anti-IL5)
- Combination therapy with a LABA + ICS resulted in fewer asthma exacerbations than treatment with ICS alone (3).

Pediatric Considerations
- Theophylline should not be used in children.
- Tiotropium is not indicated in children <12 years.

Pregnancy Considerations
- Do not use bronchial provocation test nor step down controller treatment until after delivery.
- Asthma symptoms tend to worsen in 1/3 of patients, 1/3 improves, and 1/3 remains unchanged (1).
- Exacerbations are common in 2nd trimester.
- Poorly controlled asthma results in low birth weight, increased prematurity, and perinatal mortality.
- All short-acting agents (SABA) are pregnancy Category C as well as ICS.
- ICS prevents asthma exacerbation during pregnancy.
- Cessation of ICS during pregnancy is a significant risk factor for exacerbation.
- Montelukast and zafirlukast are Category B but are not studied extensively in pregnancy.

Geriatric Considerations
- Underdiagnosed due to comorbidities; electrocardiogram (ECG), echocardiogram, and measurement of plasma brain natriuretic peptide (BNP) may be helpful in diagnosis.
- Management challenges due to comorbidities (like arthritis) and due to polypharmacy

ISSUES FOR REFERRAL
- Specialized testing (e.g., bronchoprovocation)
- Specialized treatments (e.g., immunotherapy, anti-IgE therapy)
- Poorly controlled asthma, frequent exacerbation, or multiple ED visits
- Occupational asthma if suspected, refer for consultation due to legal implications (1)[A].

ADDITIONAL THERAPIES
- Exercise-induced bronchoconstriction (EIB): Pharmacotherapy show to reduce symptoms, SABA prior exercise, or LTRA/chromones.
- Athletes: Limit exertion in extreme cold or pollution.
- Allergen immunotherapy when clear relationship between symptoms and exposure to an unavoidable allergen
- Bronchial thermoplasty involves treatment of the airway.
- Management of acute exacerbation of asthma
  - Outpatient:
    - Mild: speak in full sentence, HR <120 bpm, oxygen saturation 90–95%, and peak flow >50% of predicted can be managed as outpatient in clinic; should start SABA and prednisolone; if symptoms resolve within 1 hour, could be discharge home with close follow-up
    - Severe symptoms: not able to speak in full sentence, HR >120 bpm, oxygen saturation <90%, peak flow <50% predicted, drowsy, confused, or silent chest; transfer to inpatient facility.
  - Treatment for severe:
    - Oxygen: to maintain saturation 93–95%
    - SABA: within 1 hour of arrival, initially around the clock followed by on demand
    - Systemic steroids: Oral is as effective as IV. 50 mg prednisolone (morning dose) or 200 mg hydrocortisone divided in doses. Duration should be 5 to 7 days.
    - Epinephrine: only when asthma is associated with angioedema or anaphylaxis
    - Avoid sedative.
    - Careful respiratory monitoring including vital signs, pulse oximetry, response and duration of response to SABA, and when possible, an objective measure of lung function such as PEF or FEV_1
    - Asthma education

- Discharge criteria
  - Minimal or absent asthma symptoms
  - Hypoxia has resolved.
  - FEV_1 or PEF ≥70% predicted or personal best
  - Bronchodilator response sustained ≥60 minutes

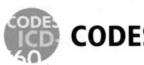 ## ONGOING CARE

FOLLOW-UP RECOMMENDATIONS
- Identify triggers and control exposures.
- Consider stepping down treatment once symptoms are controlled for 3 months and patient is at low risk for exacerbation.

PATIENT EDUCATION
- American Academy of Allergy, Asthma & Immunology: 800-822-2762 or http://www.aaaai.org/
- American Lung Association: 800-586-4872 or http://www.lung.org/
- Asthma and Allergy Foundation of America: 800-727-8462 or http://www.aafa.org/

PROGNOSIS
Prognosis is good for male patients, nonsmokers, and children with mild disease.

COMPLICATIONS
- Atelectasis
- Pneumonia
- Air leak syndromes: pneumomediastinum, pneumothorax
- Medication-specific side effects/adverse effects/interactions
- Respiratory failure
- Death: ~50% of asthma deaths occur in the elderly (age >65 years), and mortality is increasing in that population.

REFERENCES
1. Global Initiative for Asthma. 2018 GINA report, global strategy for asthma management and prevention. http://ginasthma.org/2018-gina-report-global-strategy-for-asthma-management-and-prevention/. Accessed October 28, 2018.
2. National Heart, Lung, and Blood Institute. *National Asthma Education and Prevention Program: Expert Panel Report 3: Guidelines for the Diagnosis and Management of Asthma*. Washington, DC: National Institutes of Health; 2007. NIH Publication No. 07-4051.
3. Busse WW, Bateman ED, Caplan AL, et al. Combined analysis of asthma safety trials of long-acting β_2-agonists. *N Engl J Med*. 2018;378(26): 2497–2505.

CODES

ICD10
- J45.909 Unspecified asthma, uncomplicated
- J45.901 Unspecified asthma with (acute) exacerbation
- J45.20 Mild intermittent asthma, uncomplicated

CLINICAL PEARLS
- SABA is the most effective rescue therapy for acute asthma symptoms.
- Holding chambers should be used by all.
- ICSs are the preferred long-term control therapy for patients of all ages.

ATELECTASIS

Keshav Kukreja, MD • Adrian DaSilva-DeAbreu, MD • Raymundo A. Quintana, MD

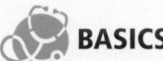

BASICS

DESCRIPTION
- Atelectasis is defined as the incomplete expansion of lung tissue due to collapse or closure. The loss of lung volume and function leads to impaired airway mucus clearance.
- Broadly categorized as:
  - Obstructive: airway blockage
  - Nonobstructive: loss of contact between the parietal and visceral pleurae, replacement of lung tissue by scarring or infiltrative disease, surfactant dysfunction, and parenchymal compression
- Symptoms depend on the rate of collapse, the amount of lung involved, and whether the patient has underlying lung disease and/or comorbidities.
- Reduced respiratory gas exchange can cause hypoxemia.

EPIDEMIOLOGY
- Mean age is 60 years, but all ages are susceptible.
- Male = female; no racial or socioeconomic predilection

Incidence
- Rounded atelectasis can be seen in up to 65–70% of asbestos workers.
- Lobar atelectasis is variable based on the collateral ventilation and number of lobes involved.

Prevalence
Postoperative atelectasis, especially after major cardiovascular or gastrointestinal (GI) procedures; can be seen in up to 90% of patients

ETIOLOGY AND PATHOPHYSIOLOGY
- Obstructive (resorptive) atelectasis is caused by intrinsic airway blockage and is the most common variety. It can be caused by luminal blockage (i.e., foreign body, mucus plug, asthma, cystic fibrosis, trauma, mass lesion) or airway wall abnormality (i.e., congenital malformation and emphysema).
  - Distal to the obstruction, alveolar air is rapidly reabsorbed into the deoxygenated venous system, causing complete collapse of the alveolar tissue.
  - Fraction of inspired oxygen (FiO_2): Compared to the rapid dissociation of O_2 distal to the obstruction, the 79% atmospheric nitrogen in atmospheric dissociates more slowly from the alveoli. This prevents collapse by maintaining positive pressure inside the alveoli. However, with increased FiO_2, the concentration of nitrogen is decreased, allowing rapid development of atelectasis at the onset of obstruction.
  - The patency and function of the collateral ventilatory systems in each lobe (pores of Kohn, canals of Lambert, and fenestrations of Boren) depends on multiple patient factors including age, underlying lung disease, and FiO_2.
  - In patients with emphysema, the fenestra of Boren become enlarged, which acts as a compensatory mechanism and can lead to a delay in atelectasis despite an obstructing lesion or mass.
- Nonobstructive atelectasis
  - Passive atelectasis (i.e., during a pleural effusion or pneumothorax) is due to pleural membrane separation of the visceral and parietal layers.
  - Compression atelectasis occurs with space-occupying lesions, cardiomegaly, abscess, or significant lymphadenopathy.
    - Increased chest wall pressure compresses the alveoli, leading to diminished functional residual capacity (FRC) or resting lung volume.

- Adhesive atelectasis in the setting of acute respiratory distress syndrome (ARDS), radiation, smoke inhalation, or uremia. The underlying surfactant dysfunction causes increased surface tension and alveoli collapse.
  - Cicatrization represents pleural or parenchymal scarring and is common in granulomatous disease (i.e., sarcoidosis), toxic or radiation exposure, and drug-induced fibrosis (i.e., amiodarone, cyclophosphamide).
  - Replacement atelectasis: diffuse tumor (i.e., bronchioalveolar cell carcinoma) manifestation resulting in complete lobar collapse
- Rounded atelectasis is a distinct form of atelectasis seen in patients with asbestos exposure as a result of their significant pleural disease.
- Others
  - Hypoxemia from a pulmonary embolus
  - Muscular weakness: due to anesthesia side-effect, or in neuromuscular diseases with respiratory muscle involvement

Pediatric Considerations
Children are at a higher risk of developing atelectasis due to their less developed collateral ventilation and compensatory mechanisms.

RISK FACTORS
- Critical care and prolonged immobilization
- General anesthesia (including long-acting muscle relaxants, postoperative epidural anesthesia)
- Positive fluid balance
- Massive blood transfusion (≥4 units)
- Nasogastric tube placement
- Hypothermia
- Mechanical ventilation with high tidal volume (Vt >10 mL/kg) and plateau pressure (>30 cm H_2O)
- Patient risk factors for postoperative atelectasis:
  - Age >60 years and <6 years
  - Chronic obstructive pulmonary disease (COPD)
  - Obstructive sleep apnea
  - Congestive heart failure (CHF)
  - Alcohol abuse, smoking
  - Pulmonary hypertension
  - Albumin <3.5 g/dL
  - Hemoglobin <10 g/dL
  - BMI >27 kg/m² (weak evidence)
  - ASA class II+ functional dependence in activities of daily living (ADLs)
  - Surgical procedures: cardiothoracic, vascular, upper GI, neurosurgical, oromaxillofacial, and ENT
  - Often a precursor to more serious pulmonary complications postoperatively (1)
- Right middle lobe syndrome (Brock syndrome): wedge-shaped density extending inferiorly and anteriorly from the hilum. Best seen on lateral chest radiography; no consistent clinical definition

GENERAL PREVENTION
- Early mobilization, deep breathing exercises, coughing, and frequent changes in body position
- Preoperative physical therapy lowered rates of atelectasis, pneumonia, and length of stay (LOS) in patients undergoing elective cardiac surgery. However, there was no change in other postoperative pulmonary complications or mortality (2)[A]. Furthermore, large RCTs are needed before conclusions can be drawn regarding the efficacy of chest physiotherapy and incentive spirometry (IS).

- Mechanical ventilation settings with high Vt (Vt >10 mL/kg) and plateau pressures (>30 cm H_2O) and without positive end-expiratory pressure (PEEP) are associated with postoperative pulmonary complications (i.e., pneumonia, respiratory failure):
  - Minimize ventilator-induced injury by employing low Vt and plateau pressures at sufficient PEEP.
  - Ensure lower FiO_2 during anesthetic induction and intraoperatively to prevent nitrogen washout.
- Continuous positive airway pressure (CPAP) during anesthesia induction and reversal of anesthesia-induced atelectasis after intubation by a recruitment maneuver may decrease postoperative pulmonary complications (3)[C].

COMMONLY ASSOCIATED CONDITIONS
- Obstructive lung diseases (COPD and asthma)
- Trauma
- ARDS, neonatal RDS, pulmonary edema, pulmonary embolism, pneumonia, pleural effusion, pneumothorax
- Respiratory syncytial virus (RSV), bronchiolitis
- Bronchial stenosis, pulmonic valve disease, and pulmonary hypertension
- Neuromuscular disorders (muscular dystrophy, spinal muscular atrophy, spinal cord injury, and Guillain-Barré syndrome) and cystic fibrosis

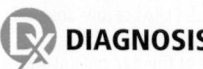

DIAGNOSIS

HISTORY
- Frequently asymptomatic
- Tachypnea and sudden-onset dyspnea
- Nonproductive cough
- Pleuritic pain on affected side
- History of smoking, COPD, pulmonary insufficiency, exposure to radiation, asbestos, or other air pollutants

PHYSICAL EXAM
- Signs of hypoxia or cyanosis
- Tracheal or precordial impulse displacement toward the affected side; dullness to percussion
- Bronchial breathing in patent airway
- Wheezing or absent breath sounds in occluded airway
- Diminished chest expansion

DIFFERENTIAL DIAGNOSIS
See "Etiology and Pathophysiology."

DIAGNOSTIC TESTS & INTERPRETATION
Initial Tests (lab, imaging)
- CBC and respiratory Gram stain, culture, and viral panel if infection suspected
- ABG: Despite hypoxemia, $PaCO_2$ level is usually normal or low.
- Chest x-ray (CXR), PA, and lateral
  - Displaced hilum, mediastinal shift toward the side of atelectatic lung, volume loss in ipsilateral hemithorax, raised diaphragm
  - Crowding of the ribs and silhouetting of the diaphragm or heart border
  - Compensatory hyperlucency of remaining lobes of affected lung and compensatory hyperinflation in unaffected lung
  - Lobar collapse
  - Wedge-shaped densities: obstructive atelectasis

- Small, linear bands (Fleischner lines) often at lung bases: discoid (subsegmental or plate) atelectasis
- Direct signs: displacement of fissures and opacification of the collapsed lobe. Right upper lobe collapse may display the inverted "S sign of Golden," representing neoplastic shift of the minor fissure.
- Air bronchograms: Pleural fluid or air may indicate compressive atelectasis.
- Adhesive atelectasis may present as a diffuse reticular granular pattern, which can progress to a pulmonary edema pattern and to bilateral opacification in severe cases.
- Pleural-based round density: round atelectasis
- Complete atelectasis of entire lung: opacification of the entire hemithorax and a shift of the mediastinum to atelectatic lung

Follow-Up Tests & Special Considerations

- Chest CT or MRI may be indicated to visualize airway and mediastinal structures and identify cause of atelectasis in unclear cases.
- Pulmonary function tests (PFTs) can help identify obstructive or restrictive disease and decreased respiratory muscle pressures.
- Hypoalbuminemia (albumin <3.5 g/L) is a powerful marker of increased risk for postoperative pulmonary complications, including atelectasis.

Diagnostic Procedures/Other

Flexible fiber-optic bronchoscopy can be considered in unexplained or refractory cases.

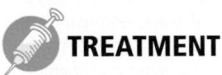

TREATMENT

GENERAL MEASURES

- Identify and treat the underlying etiology.
- PEEP for prevention following surgery or general anesthesia (3)[C]
- Lay on unaffected side, encourage frequent coughing, deep breathing exercises, and early mobility.
- IS every hour while awake
  - Frequently used despite lack of evidence for IS preventing postoperative pulmonary complications after coronary artery bypass grafting (CABG) (4)[A]
- Mechanical ventilate with PEEP in severe respiratory distress or hypoxemia:
  - Lower Vt (6 mL/kg) and lower plateau pressures (<30 mm Hg) associated with reduced mortality
  - PEEP 15 to 20 mL may be necessary to maintain arterial O_2 saturation in surfactant-impaired lung regions.

MEDICATION

First Line

Pharmacotherapy should address underlying etiology:

- Antibiotics for infection
- Chemotherapy or radiation for malignancy
- Inhalers and steroids for asthma
- Effective analgesia to permit deep inspiration and coughing
- Mucolytics can be considered to promote airway clearance (i.e., N-acetylcysteine and saline).

Pediatric Considerations

- Dornase alfa may be effective clearing mucinous secretions in refractory mucous plugging in children (used in cystic fibrosis).
- Chest physiotherapy (i.e., percussion, drainage, deep insufflation, and saline lavage) is the most commonly utilized therapy in the inpatient setting.

- Other physically stimulating modalities (mechanical insufflation-exsufflation, intrapulmonary percussive ventilation, intermittent positive pressure breathing) may have utility in patients with neuromuscular disease and cystic fibrosis to enhance mucus clearance.
- Applying continuous distending pressure has shown some benefit in the treatment of preterm infants with RDS and has the potential to reduce lung damage particularly if used early (5)[A].
- In obstructive atelectasis, bronchoscopy remains controversial. However, in the presence of a mucus plug or cast, bronchoscopy may be beneficial.

Second Line

Fiber-optic bronchoscopy to improve airway clearance has been efficacious in several studies; however, there is debate regarding its efficacy in the treatment of atelectasis. It may be beneficial in those with unsuccessful attempts or contraindications to chest physiotherapy (i.e., chest wall trauma).

SURGERY/OTHER PROCEDURES

Appropriate surgical resection for underlying disease (i.e., tumor, severe lymphadenopathy)

> **ALERT**
> The association between postoperative atelectasis and fever is likely coincidental rather than causal.

ADMISSION, INPATIENT, AND NURSING CONSIDERATIONS

Ensure adequate oxygenation (may start with 100% FiO_2 then taper) and humidification. Note: if obstructive atelectasis is suspected, then judiciously increase FiO_2 to prevent nitrogen washout, which can hasten atelectasis.

ONGOING CARE

FOLLOW-UP RECOMMENDATIONS

Patient Monitoring

- Frequency/adequacy of monitoring will vary by underlying cause and concurrent comorbidities.
- For uncomplicated cases of atelectasis associated (i.e., those associated with asthma or infection), outpatient monitoring may be appropriate.

PATIENT EDUCATION

Maximize mobility as tolerated and encourage frequent coughing and deep breathing exercises. Seek further treatment or return to ED for worsening symptoms or shortness of breath.

PROGNOSIS

- Postoperative atelectasis usually spontaneous resolves within 24 hours but can persist for days.
- Resolution of lobar atelectasis due to endobronchial obstruction depends on treatment of underlying disease or malignancy.
- Surgical intervention is indicated only for resectable etiologies (i.e., tumor) or if atelectasis is severe and causes chronic infections and bronchiectasis.

COMPLICATIONS

- Pneumonia or other pulmonary infections
- Acute atelectasis: hypoxemia, respiratory failure, postobstructive drowning of the lung
- Chronic atelectasis: bronchiectasis, pleural effusion, empyema

REFERENCES

1. Restrepo RD, Braverman J. Current challenges in the recognition, prevention and treatment of perioperative pulmonary atelectasis. *Expert Rev Respir Med*. 2015;9(1):97–107.
2. Hulzebos EH, Smit Y, Helders PP, et al. Preoperative physical therapy for elective cardiac surgery patients. *Cochrane Database Syst Rev*. 2012;(11):CD010118.
3. Baltieri L, Santos LA, Rasera I Jr, et al. Use of positive pressure in the bariatric surgery and effects on pulmonary function and prevalence of atelectasis: randomized and blinded clinical trial. *Arq Bras Cir Dig*. 2014;27(Suppl 1):26–30.
4. Freitas ER, Soares BG, Cardoso JR, et al. Incentive spirometry for preventing pulmonary complications after coronary artery bypass graft. *Cochrane Database Syst Rev*. 2012;(9):CD004466.
5. Ho JJ, Henderson-Smart DJ, Davis PG. Early versus delayed initiation of continuous distending pressure for respiratory distress syndrome in preterm infants. *Cochrane Database Syst Rev*. 2002;(2):CD002975.

ADDITIONAL READING

- Brower RG. Consequences of bed rest. *Crit Care Med*. 2009;37(Suppl 10):S422–S428.
- Guimarães MM, El Dib R, Smith AF, et al. Incentive spirometry for prevention of postoperative pulmonary complications in upper abdominal surgery. *Cochrane Database Syst Rev*. 2009;(3):CD006058.
- Mavros MN, Velmahos GC, Falagas ME. Atelectasis as a cause of postoperative fever: where is the clinical evidence? *Chest*. 2011;140(2):418–424.
- Tusman G, Böhm SH, Warner DO, et al. Atelectasis and perioperative pulmonary complications in high-risk patients. *Curr Opin Anaesthesiol*. 2012;25(1):1–10.
- Wu KH, Lin CF, Huang CJ, et al. Rigid ventilation bronchoscopy under general anesthesia for treatment of pediatric pulmonary atelectasis caused by pneumonia: a review of 33 cases. *Int Surg*. 2006;91(5):291–294.

 CODES

ICD10
J98.11 Atelectasis

CLINICAL PEARLS

- Low serum albumin (<3.5 g/L) is a strong predictor of postoperative pulmonary complications, including atelectasis.
- Anesthesia-induced atelectasis occurs in almost all anesthetized patients but can be reduced by employing PEEP intraoperatively or when reversing anesthesia.
- Early mobilization, coughing, deep breathing exercises, and treating the underlying cause are the mainstays of therapy.
- Bronchogenic carcinoma can present as atelectasis and must be excluded in all patients >35 years.
- In complete atelectasis of an entire lung, the mediastinal ipsilateral shift separates atelectasis from massive pleural effusion.
- No strong clinical evidence supports atelectasis as an early cause of postoperative fever.

ATRIAL FIBRILLATION AND ATRIAL FLUTTER

Bianca Lee, DO, MS • Youhua Zhang, MD, PhD

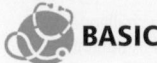 **BASICS**

This topic covers both atrial fibrillation (AFib) and atrial flutter (AFlut).

DESCRIPTION
- AFib: paroxysmal or continuous supraventricular tachyarrhythmia characterized by rapid, uncoordinated atrial electrical activity and an irregularly irregular ventricular response. In most patients, the ventricular rate is rapid because the atrioventricular (AV) node is bombarded with very frequent atrial electrical impulses (400 to 600 bpm).
- AFlut: paroxysmal or continuous supraventricular tachyarrhythmia with rapid but organized atrial electrical activity. The atrial rate is typically between 250 and 350 bpm and is often manifested as "saw-tooth" flutter (F) waves on the ECG, particularly in the inferior leads and V_1. AFlut commonly occurs with 2:1 or 3:1 AV block, so the ventricular response may be regular and typically at a rate of 150 bpm.
- AFib and AFlut are related arrhythmias, sometimes seen in the same patient. Distinguishing the two is important because there may be implications for management.
- Clinical classifications:
  - Paroxysmal: self-terminating episodes, usually <7 days
  - Persistent: sustained >7 days, usually requiring pharmacologic or DC cardioversion to restore sinus rhythm
  - Permanent: Sinus rhythm cannot be restored or maintained.
  - Nonvalvular AFib: absence of rheumatic mitral stenosis, a mechanical or bioprosthetic heart valve or mitral valve repair
- Lone AFib occurs in patients <60 years (with possible genetic predisposition) who have no clinical or echocardiographic evidence of cardiovascular disease, including hypertension (HTN).

EPIDEMIOLOGY
- Incidence/prevalence increases significantly with age.
- Young patients with AFib, particularly lone AFib, are most commonly males.

Incidence
- AFib: from <0.1%/year <40 years to >1.5%/year >80 years
- Lifetime risk: 25% for those ≥40 years
- AFlut is less common.

Prevalence
- Estimated at 0.4–1% in general population, with 2.7 million patients in America
- Increase with age, up to 8% in those ≥80 years

ETIOLOGY AND PATHOPHYSIOLOGY
- Cardiac: HTN, ischemic heart disease, heart failure, valvular heart disease, cardiomyopathy, pericarditis, and infiltrative heart disease
- Pulmonary: pulmonary embolism (PE), chronic obstructive pulmonary disease (COPD), obstructive sleep apnea, pneumonia
- Ingestion: ethanol, caffeine
- Endocrine: hyperthyroidism, diabetes
- Obesity
- Postoperative: cardiac, pulmonary, or esophageal
- Idiopathic: lone AFib
- Patients with paroxysmal episodes are usually associated with premature atrial beats and/or bursts of tachycardia, originating in pulmonary vein ostia or other sites.

- Many patients with AFib are thought to have some degree of atrial fibrosis or scarring. This is often subclinical and usually not detectable with current cardiac imaging techniques but plays an important role in the pathogenesis of the arrhythmia.
- Autonomic (vagal and sympathetic) tone may play a role in triggering the arrhythmia.
- The presence of AFib is associated with electrical and structural remodeling processes that promote arrhythmia maintenance in the atria, termed "AFib begets AFib."

Genetics
Familial forms are rare but do exist. There are ongoing efforts to identify the genetic underpinnings of such cases.

RISK FACTORS
Age, HTN, and obesity are the most important risk factors for both AFib and AFlut.

GENERAL PREVENTION
Adequate control of HTN may prevent development of AFib due to hypertensive heart disease and is the most significant modifiable risk factor for AFib. Weight reduction may decrease the risk of AFib in obese patients. Ethanol consumption may trigger AFib in some.

COMMONLY ASSOCIATED CONDITIONS
HTN and other cardiac diseases

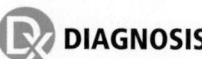 **DIAGNOSIS**

HISTORY
Symptoms vary from none to mild (palpitations, lightheadedness, fatigue, poor exercise capacity) to severe (angina, dyspnea, syncope).

PHYSICAL EXAM
- AFib: irregularly irregular heart rate and pulse, frequently tachycardiac, pulse deficit
- AFlut: similar to AFib but may have regular pulse

DIFFERENTIAL DIAGNOSIS
- Multifocal atrial tachycardia
- Sinus tachycardia with frequent atrial premature beats
- Paroxysmal supraventricular tachycardia (Wolff-Parkinson-White [WPW], atrioventricular nodal reentry tachycardia [AVNRT])

DIAGNOSTIC TESTS & INTERPRETATION
- Although screening with ECG can detect asymptomatic cases of AFib, the USPSTF notes that it has not been shown to detect more cases than screening focused on pulse palpation. Also, treatments for AFib reduce the risk of stroke and all-cause mortality and increase the risk of bleeding, but trials have not assessed whether treatment of screen-detected asymptomatic older adults results in better health outcomes than treatment after detection by usual care or after symptoms develop (1)[A].
- The ECG is diagnostic, with findings of low-amplitude fibrillatory waves without discrete P waves and an irregularly irregular pattern of QRS complexes. There is often tachycardia in the absence of heart rate–controlling medications (2).
- AFlut: The ECG is diagnostic. Saw-tooth F waves are the classic sign, generally best seen in the inferior leads, although ventricular rate may need to be slowed to see the waves. QRS complexes may be regular or irregular; there is usually tachycardia (2).
- Ambulatory rhythm monitoring (e.g., telemetry, Holter monitoring, event recorders) is helpful in diagnosing suspected paroxysmal AFib or AFlut and monitoring for recurrence (2)[C].

Initial Tests (lab, imaging)
TSH, electrolytes, CBC, 2D transthoracic echocardiogram, PT/INR (if anticoagulation is contemplated); digoxin level (if appropriate)

Follow-Up Tests & Special Considerations
- Occasional Holter monitoring and/or exercise stress testing to assess for adequacy of rate and/or rhythm control
- Chest x-ray (CXR) for cardiopulmonary disease
- ECG for signs of cardiac hypertrophy, ischemia, and/or other arrhythmias
- Transesophageal echocardiogram to detect left atrial appendage thrombus if cardioversion is planned
- Sleep study may be useful if sleep apnea is suspected.

Test Interpretation
Evaluate for presence of atrial dilatation and fibrosis, atrial thrombus (especially in atrial appendage), valvular/rheumatic disease, cardiomyopathy.

 **TREATMENT**

MEDICATION
- Two primary issues in the management of AFib and/or AFlut: decisions on heart rate control (control ventricular rate while allowing AFib to continue) or rhythm control (terminate AFib and restore normal sinus rhythm) and decision to anticoagulate or not
- Anticoagulation therapy to prevent thromboembolism (primarily stroke) reduces risk of stroke by about 2/3. Several calculators exist for estimating yearly risk of thromboembolic event (ATRIA, CHADS2, CHA2DS2VASc). If risk is sufficiently low, or risk of bleeding is high, no anticoagulation may be indicated. Clinical judgment and patient preference remain important.
- AHA/ACC anticoagulation guidelines (the same for AFib and AFlut) (2,3)[C]:
  - CHA2DS2VASc scoring (**C**HF [1 point], **H**TN [1 point], **A**ge ≥75 years [2 points], **D**M [1 point], prior **S**troke or transient ischemic attack [TIA] [2 points], **V**ascular disease [1 point], **A**ge 65 to 74 years [1 point], female **S**ex **c**ategory [1 point]). CHA_2DS_2VASc is the recommended stroke risk assessment for patients with nonvalvular AFib (2)[B].
    - In patients with nonvalvular AFib and a CHA_2DS_2VASc score of 0, antithrombotic therapy may be omitted (2)[B].
    - In patients with nonvalvular AFib and a CHA_2DS_2VASc score of 1, no antithrombotic therapy or oral anticoagulant or aspirin is recommended (2)[C].
  - Unless contraindicated, patients with nonvalvular AFib with any high-risk factors for stroke (prior TIA/cerebrovascular accident [CVA]/thromboembolism) or a CHA_2DS_2VASc score ≥2 should receive oral anticoagulants. The following oral anticoagulants include warfarin with maintenance of an INR of 2.0 to 3.0 (2)[A], dabigatran (2)[B], rivaroxaban (2)[B], or apixaban (2)[B]. Patients with mechanical valves should maintain an INR of 2.0 to 3.0 or 2.5 to 3.5 dependent on the type and location of the prosthesis (2)[B]. For patients with AFib and mitral stenosis, a target INR range of 2.0 to 3.0 is recommended (3)[B].

– Dabigatran (Pradaxa), a direct thrombin inhibitor, and apixaban (Eliquis) and rivaroxaban (Xarelto), factor Xa inhibitors, can be alternatives to warfarin for the prevention of first and recurrent stroke in patients with nonvalvular AFib (4)[C]. The selection of an antithrombotic should be individualized (2)[B]; consider the risks of each agent, cost, patient preference, and tolerability (2)[C].

ALERT
Renal function should be evaluated prior to initiation of direct thrombin or factor Xa inhibitors (2)[B]. Dosing of such agents may in fact need individualized adjustment. Specific reversal agents for severe bleeding now available:

- Idarucizumab (Praxbind) for dabigatran
- Coagulation factor Xa (recombinant), inactivated-zhzo (Andexxa) for apixaban and rivaroxaban
  - Anticoagulation recommendations are independent of AFib pattern (paroxysmal, persistent, and permanent) (2,3)[B], although ongoing efforts to better understand who may be at greater and lesser risk of thromboembolism continue. Four classes of medications are available to achieve ventricular rate control: β-blockers (i.e., metoprolol), nondihydropyridine calcium channel blockers (i.e., verapamil, diltiazem), digoxin, and amiodarone. Optimal target for ventricular rate has not been firmly established, but there is evidence that aggressive control of the ventricular rate (<80 bpm) offers no benefit beyond more modest rate control (i.e., resting heart rate <110 bpm) (2)[B].
- Preventing rapid ventricular response (RVR) rates using AV nodal blocking medications is also often effective at controlling a patient's symptoms associated with AFib or AFlut. Patients in whom rate control cannot be achieved or who continue to have persistent symptoms despite reasonable heart rate control may require attempts at restoration of sinus rhythm.
- Ventricular rate control can often be difficult to achieve in AFlut due to the more organized nature of the atrial electrical activity. For this reason, conversion to sinus rhythm is often the preferred strategy for symptomatic patients, and catheter ablation is also considered as a first-line treatment in recurrent AFlut (2).
- Restoration of sinus rhythm using electrical or pharmacologic cardioversion may significantly reduce the symptom burden of AFib or AFlut in many patients and may also be useful for controlling ventricular rate. Cardioversion does not impact the long-term risk/benefit ratio of anticoagulation:
  - Cardioversion is most often performed electrically but may also be achieved using antiarrhythmic drug therapy in some instances, by experienced clinicians (2)[A].
  - If duration of AFib is >48 hours or unknown, anticoagulate for ≥3 weeks before cardioversion to reduce the risk of stroke. Alternatively, once anticoagulation is established, a transesophageal echo may be performed to exclude the presence of left atrial thrombus, allowing cardioversion to proceed. After cardioversion, anticoagulation should be continued for ≥4 weeks in all patients in whom duration of AFib/AFlut is >48 hours, as the postcardioversion period is a time of increased stroke risk (2,3)[B].
- Randomized clinical trials (AFFIRM and RACE) comparing the outcomes of rate versus rhythm control found no difference in morbidity, mortality, and stroke rates in patients assigned to one therapy or the other (2).

ISSUES FOR REFERRAL
Management of AFib or AFlut refractory to standard medical therapy (i.e., unable to achieve adequate rate control with medication or development of significant bradycardia with treatment) may require the use of more aggressive treatments. These may include pacemaker implantation (to allow for more intensive pharmacologic blocking of the AV node) or an ablation procedure. AFlut in particular is often very amenable to ablation; thus, consideration should be given to early expert referral in appropriate patients. Antiarrhythmic drug therapy can often be very effective but should be prescribed by experienced practitioners.

SURGERY/OTHER PROCEDURES
- Electrophysiologic study and ablation may be considered for patients with either AFib or AFlut. In the case of AFlut, ablation is a procedure generally viewed as a first-line therapy due to its high rate of success in appropriate candidates. Ablation of AFib is a much more complex procedure with a more variable success rate. Thus, it is typically reserved for drug-refractory patients.
- Cardiac surgery (e.g., the maze procedure, ligation of the left atrial appendage) may be considered in patients planning to undergo cardiac surgery for other reasons.
- A left atrial appendage closure device WATCHMAN may be useful in those at increased risk of stroke and systemic embolism that seek a nonpharmacologic approach to anticoagulation.

ADMISSION, INPATIENT, AND NURSING CONSIDERATIONS
- Patients with significant symptoms, RVR, AFib/AFlut triggered by an acute process (e.g., MI, CHF, PE), or in whom antiarrhythmic therapy is being started likely require admission to the hospital for a period of stabilization.
- Outpatient management is reasonable for low-risk patients with controlled ventricular rates.
- Acute therapy for symptomatic patients with AFib or AFlut:
  - IV β- or nondihydropyridine calcium channel blockers for control of ventricular rate in patients without preexcitation (2)[B]
- Commonly used therapies in the acute setting include (2):
  - Metoprolol tartrate: 2.5 to 5.0 mg IV bolus over 2 minutes; up to 3 doses
  - Diltiazem: 0.25 mg/kg IV bolus over 2 minutes and then 5 to 15 mg/hr
  - Some patients will be far more responsive to one class of agents than another. For this reason, if rate control is difficult to achieve, switching drug classes may be useful.
- Urgent cardioversion should be performed in hemodynamically unstable patients (2)[B]. It is somewhat unusual for AFib or AFlut alone to cause marked hemodynamic insult; thus, the possibility of a concurrent process should be considered in this setting.
- Consider the initiation of PO anticoagulation therapy. Bridging therapy with heparin/LMWH is generally not necessary for patients being started on warfarin.

 ONGOING CARE

Many patients may benefit from elective expert consultation. In patients with no significant symptoms, if ventricular rate control or sinus rhythm is easily achieved and the choice of thromboembolic prevention is clear, management in a primary care setting may be appropriate.

FOLLOW-UP RECOMMENDATIONS
Patient Monitoring
Adequate anticoagulation levels (if warfarin is employed) should be determined at least weekly during initiation and monthly when stable (2)[A]. Ventricular rate control should be assessed on a regular basis.

DIET
Patients on warfarin should attempt to consume a stable amount of vitamin K.

PROGNOSIS
Yearly risk of stroke in untreated nonvalvular AFib has declined and now lies between 4% and 5% per year.

- Anticoagulation reduces the annual embolic stroke rate by about 2/3 for most patients. AFib and AFlut may increase morbidity and mortality, but the overall prognosis is a function of underlying heart disease and adherence with therapy. Reported risk of anticoagulation varies but lies between 1% and 4% per year for major hemorrhage.

COMPLICATIONS
- Embolic stroke
- Peripheral arterial embolization
- Bleeding with anticoagulation
- Tachycardia-induced cardiomyopathy with prolonged periods of inadequate rate control

REFERENCES

1. Jonas DE, Kahwati LC, Yun JDY, et al. Screening for atrial fibrillation with electrocardiography: evidence report and systematic review for the US Preventive Services Task Force. *JAMA.* 2018;320(5):485–498.
2. January CT, Wann LS, Alpert JS, et al; for ACC/AHA Task Force Members. 2014 AHA/ACC/HRS guideline for the management of patients with atrial fibrillation: executive summary: a report of the American College of Cardiology/American Heart Association Task Force on practice guidelines and the Heart Rhythm Society. *Circulation.* 2014;130(23):2071–2104.
3. You JJ, Singer DE, Howard PA, et al. Antithrombotic therapy for atrial fibrillation: Antithrombotic Therapy and Prevention of Thrombosis, 9th ed: American College of Chest Physicians evidence-based clinical practice guidelines. *Chest.* 2012;141(Suppl 2):e531S–e575S.
4. Nishimura RA, Otto CM, Bonow RO, et al. 2017 AHA/ACC focused update of the 2014 AHA/ACC guideline for the management of patients with valvular heart disease: a report of the American College of Cardiology/American Heart Association Task Force on clinical practice guidelines. *Circulation.* 2017;135(25):e1159–e1195.

CODES

ICD10
- I48.91 Unspecified atrial fibrillation
- I48.92 Unspecified atrial flutter
- I48.0 Paroxysmal atrial fibrillation

CLINICAL PEARLS
- Primary decision in persistent AFib is rate control or rhythm control. Younger patients often do better with a rhythm control strategy, whereas older patients often do well with rate control. Decision is complex.
- Whether to anticoagulate or not is based on risk of thromboembolism regardless of AFib pattern.

ATRIAL SEPTAL DEFECT

Edlira Yzeiraj, DO, MS • Edward A. Gotfried, DO, FACOS

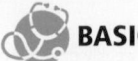 **BASICS**

DESCRIPTION
- Anatomy
  - Opening in the atrial septum allowing flow of blood between the two atria
  - Patent foramen ovale is also an open communication between the atria, but it is not considered an ASD because no septal tissue is missing.
- Types (by location in the interatrial septum) (1)
  - Classified based on their different anatomic location and abnormal embryogenesis: secundum ASD, primum ASD, sinus venosus ASD, coronary sinus ASD
  - 70%: Ostium secundum defect occurs in the fossa ovalis region.
  - 15–20%: Ostium primum defect occurs in the inferior septum; often associated with cleft mitral valve and failure of endocardial cushion development
  - 5–10%: Sinus venosus defect occurs in the superior-posterior septum near the orifice of the superior vena cava; usually associated with partial anomalous right upper pulmonary venous return
  - <1%: coronary sinus defect: Part of the entire common wall between the coronary sinus and the LA is absent.
- Hemodynamic effects
  - Left-to-right shunting in late ventricular systole and early diastole
  - Degree depends on size of the defect and relative pressures of the two ventricles.
  - Causes excessive blood flow through the right-sided circulation, ultimately leading to reactive pulmonary hypertension and heart failure
- Systems affected: cardiovascular; pulmonary

Pediatric Considerations
- Most cases of ASD are detected and corrected in the pediatric population.
- The smaller the defect and the younger the child, the greater the chance of spontaneous closure.

EPIDEMIOLOGY
Incidence
- Predominant age: present from birth, may be diagnosed at any age
- Slight female predominance (2)
- No race predilection
- 2/1,000 live births

Prevalence
ASDs account for 13% of congenital heart disorders.

ETIOLOGY AND PATHOPHYSIOLOGY
- Flow across ASD usually left-to-right shunt because of higher left-sided pressures:
  - Minimal right-to-left shunting in early ventricular systole, especially during inspiration
  - Increased right-sided pressure/pulmonary hypertension can cause reversal of shunt flow (Eisenmenger syndrome) with resulting cyanosis and clubbing.
- Symptoms typically occur due to right ventricular and pulmonary vascular volume overload and right-sided heart failure.

Genetics
- Most cases are spontaneous.
- 5% with chromosomal abnormalities; other rare mutations exist.
- 25% prevalence in Down syndrome

RISK FACTORS
- Other congenital heart defects
- Family history (~7–10% recurrence)
- Thalidomide, alcohol exposure in utero, smoking, maternal age >35 years, and elevated blood glucose have been associated with increased risk (2).

COMMONLY ASSOCIATED CONDITIONS
- ASDs may occur as a component of other complex cardiac structural defects.
- Important to exclude anomalous pulmonary venous return
- Occasionally can indicate underlying genetic syndromes, for example, Holt-Oram (ASD present in 66%), Ellis-van Creveld, VACTERL syndrome, or Noonan syndrome.
- Overall, ~70% isolated (1)

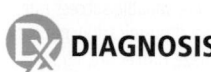 **DIAGNOSIS**

HISTORY
- Most ASDs are small and do not cause symptoms in infancy and childhood and are often found on routine physical examination when a cardiac murmur is detected incidentally.
- Infants with large ASDs may present with right-sided heart failure (more advanced, only 10% at diagnosis), recurrent respiratory infections, or failure to thrive.
- Should be considered in children with other congenital heart defects, Down syndrome
- In uncorrected defects, most people become symptomatic by age 40 years. Common symptoms in adults include atrial arrhythmias (the most frequent presenting symptom), exercise intolerance, dyspnea, and fatigue.

PHYSICAL EXAM
- Signs vary according to extent of shunting.
- Cardiac auscultation
  - *Fixed, widely split S_2 (key physical finding)*
  - May also have
    - Systolic ejection murmur (pulmonic flow murmur)
    - Low-pitched diastolic rumble (tricuspid flow murmur)
    - Diastolic murmur (pulmonic regurgitation)
    - Systolic murmur (mitral regurgitation)
- Right ventricular heave
- Palpable pulmonary artery pulse at left upper sternal border
- If heart failure has developed, may hear a fourth heart sound (right-sided)
- Signs of Eisenmenger syndrome:
  - Cyanosis and clubbing
  - Jugular venous distention and edema

DIFFERENTIAL DIAGNOSIS
- Other congenital heart disease
- Right bundle branch block (for widely split S_2)

DIAGNOSTIC TESTS & INTERPRETATION
Initial Tests (lab, imaging)
- Echocardiography is the test of choice (1)[C].
- Generally start with transthoracic Doppler imaging of the entire atrial septum (sensitivity is ~89% for secundum, ~100% for primum, and ~44% of sinus venosus ASDs), with progression to trans-esophageal echocardiography (TEE) if transthoracic echocardiography (TTE) is nondiagnostic.

- Patients with right ventricular overload by TTE but an otherwise negative study should have further testing.
- Oximetry: Cyanosis may suggest Eisenmenger syndrome (right-to-left shunting).
- ECG is not typically diagnostic, but findings may include the following:
  - Right axis deviation
  - Right atrial enlargement (tall P in inferior leads)
  - Right ventricular conduction delay
  - Q wave in lead V_1
  - Right bundle branch block
  - Leftward axis, inverted P wave in lead III (sinus venosus)
  - Leftward axis (ostium primum)

Follow-Up Tests & Special Considerations
- Bubble contrast enhancement may be helpful.
- TEE may be required to define ASD morphology and to locate the pulmonary veins; often used prior to percutaneous closure. TEE has excellent sensitivity and specificity.

Diagnostic Procedures/Other
- Cardiac catheterization (1)[C]
  - Demonstrates right ventricle enlargement, location/fraction of the shunt, size of the ASD, any valvular disease, and overall anatomy
  - Used to assess pulmonary vascular resistance if pulmonary hypertension is suspected, particularly if surgery is planned
  - Generally not used in young patients for initial diagnosis, more often reserved for use when
    - Part of a planned interventional closure
    - Evaluating other disease simultaneously (e.g., coronary artery disease)
    - Visualization by other methods insufficient
- Cardiac magnetic resonance: a noninvasive follow-up to echo that allows viewing the defect/pulmonary veins and measurement of shunt fraction and right ventricular function—particularly useful for sinus venosus defects (2)
- Exercise testing: useful to quantify symptoms not consistent with clinical findings or to document change over time (1)[C]
- Chest x-ray: may demonstrate right ventricular and pulmonary artery enlargement, increased pulmonary vascular markings
- Cardiac CT scans can also define ASDs but with significant radiation exposure.

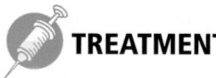 **TREATMENT**

GENERAL MEASURES
- 75% of small secundum ASDs (<8 mm) will close spontaneously by 18 months of age; however, close follow-up is warranted (2).
- The likelihood of spontaneous closure is mainly determined by defect diameter: >10 mm at time of diagnosis is unlikely to spontaneously close (3).
- Primum and sinus venosus defects do not generally close and generally require surgical closure (2).

MEDICATION
First Line
- Treatment of secondary atrial fibrillation/supraventricular tachycardia with anticoagulation and cardioversion, followed by anticoagulation with maintenance of sinus rhythm if possible, or rate control if this fails (1)[A]

- Pulmonary vasodilator therapy may be considered for adults with progressive/severe pulmonary vascular disease (1)[B].
- Treatment of heart failure (diuretics, oxygen, digoxin, etc.)

Second Line
- Antibiotic prophylaxis is NOT recommended for unrepaired/isolated ASDs.
- The American Heart Association (AHA) recommends antibiotic prophylaxis against infective endocarditis during dental procedures for 6 months after the repair in patients whom a device or prosthetic material is used.
  - In patients with repaired ASD who have a residual defect at or adjacent to the device, prophylaxis is recommended indefinitely.
  - If prophylaxis is indicated, for dental procedures, amoxicillin 2 g (adults) or 50 mg/kg (children). Other options include cephalosporins (e.g., ceftriaxone 1 g [adults] or 50 mg/kg [children] IM or IV) or clindamycin 600 mg PO (adults) or 20 mg/kg PO (children) or azithromycin 500 mg PO (adults) or 15 mg/kg (children) in patients who are penicillin-sensitive (4)[B].
- To prevent thrombus formation after device deployment, aspirin alone or a combination of aspirin and clopidogrel 75 mg for at least 6 months is recommended (5).

SURGERY/OTHER PROCEDURES
- The majority of small secundum defects, <6 mm, close spontaneously by 2 years of age, and some as late as 5 years. Closure is generally indicated in children with:
  - Defect >8 mm (unlikely to close) in children >2 years of age (to allow time for spontaneous closure, even though uncommon)
  - Defects of any size in a child >5 years with related symptoms
- Closure for secundum defects is not recommended in asymptomatic patients before 2 years of age given the possibility of spontaneous closure.
- In adults, secundum closure via percutaneous transcatheter device or surgery to reduce subsequent morbidity and mortality, if:
  - Right side heart enlargement regardless of symptoms (1)[B]
  - Pulmonary systemic flow ratio is 2:1 (or >1.5:1 and <21 years old according to the AHA).
  - Symptoms such as documented orthodeoxia/platypnea or paradoxical embolism (1)[C]
- Surgical repair is standard for a sinus venosus, coronary sinus, or primum ASD (1,2)[B]. These defects rarely close spontaneously and are not considered amenable to percutaneous closure.
- Percutaneous closure is considered the treatment of choice of secundum ASD in adults (6)[A]. It is safe and effective with satisfactory long-term clinical follow-up. In addition, the use of closure device does not significantly affect aortic or mitral valve function (6)[B].
- Secundum ASDs that are suitable for percutaneous closure should be ~35 mm in stretched balloon diameter and should have a sufficient rim of surrounding atrial tissue.
- Closure is not indicated for patients who have developed irreversible severe pulmonary hypertension without continued shunting or those who never develop symptoms and have an ASD <5 mm (1)[B].

- Overall, closing small asymptomatic secundum ASDs is controversial and not often done.
- Maze procedure may be considered before or after closure for patients with intermittent or chronic atrial tachyarrhythmias (1)[C].

ONGOING CARE

FOLLOW-UP RECOMMENDATIONS
Echocardiography can be used to monitor both repaired and unrepaired ASDs.

Patient Monitoring
- In otherwise asymptomatic healthy children, follow up until defect has closed or become negligible in size.
- Appropriate evaluation and management for atrial tachyarrhythmias in patients with long-term follow-up (1)[C]
- If ASD repaired as an adult, periodic long-term follow-up is indicated (1)[C].
- ASDs repaired in childhood generally do not have late complications.
- In female patients with unrepaired ASD and Eisenmenger syndrome, pregnancy is not recommended due to increased risk of maternal and fetal mortality (1)[C].
- Pregnancy is well tolerated in patients with repaired ASD and small unrepaired ASDs (1)[A].
- Scuba diving and high-altitude travel must be approached with caution in patients with unrepaired ASDs; consultation is recommended.

PATIENT EDUCATION
For patient education materials on this topic, consult the following:
- AHA: http://www.heart.org
- Mayo Clinic information: http://www.mayoclinic.com/health/atrial-septal-defect/DS00628

PROGNOSIS
- ASD closure in asymptomatic or minimally symptomatic adults reduces morbidity but not mortality (7).
- ASD closure before age 25 years in symptomatic adults reduces morbidity and likely also mortality.
- ASD repair deferred until after adolescence may not decrease long-term risk of future atrial arrhythmias.
- Up to 50% mortality by age 50 years in untreated symptomatic patients with large defects

COMPLICATIONS
- Unrepaired: congestive heart failure, stroke, pulmonary hypertension/Eisenmenger syndrome, atrial arrhythmias, increased infection risk (pulmonary, cerebral abscess, infective endocarditis)
- Surgically repaired: late-onset arrhythmias 10 to 20 years after surgery (5%), perioperative atrial tachyarrhythmias in 10–13% of patients
- Device closure: device embolization (1%), cardiac perforation, thrombus formation, endocarditis, supraventricular arrhythmias, and device erosions

REFERENCES

1. Warnes CA, Williams RG, Bashore TM, et al. ACC/AHA 2008 guidelines for the management of adults with congenital heart disease: a report of the American College of Cardiology/American Heart Association Task Force on Practice Guidelines (writing committee to develop guidelines on the management of adults with congenital heart disease). Developed in collaboration with the American Society of Echocardiography, Heart Rhythm Society, International Society for Adult Congenital Heart Disease, Society for Cardiovascular Angiography and Interventions, and Society of Thoracic Surgeons. *J Am Coll Cardiol.* 2008;52(23):e143–e263.
2. Geva T, Martins JD, Wald RM. Atrial septal defects. *Lancet.* 2014;383(9932):1921–1932.
3. Hanslik A, Pospisil U, Salzer-Muhar U, et al. Predictors of spontaneous closure of isolated secundum atrial septal defect in children: a longitudinal study. *Pediatrics.* 2006;118(4):1560–1565.
4. Nishimura RA, Carabello BA, Faxon DP, et al. ACC/AHA 2008 guideline update on valvular heart disease: focused update on infective endocarditis: a report of the American College of Cardiology/American Heart Association Task Force on Practice Guidelines: endorsed by the Society of Cardiovascular Anesthesiologists, Society for Cardiovascular Angiography and Interventions, and Society of Thoracic Surgeons. *Circulation.* 2008;118(8):887–896.
5. Inglessis I, Landzberg MJ. Interventional catheterization in adult congenital heart disease. *Circulation.* 2007;115(12):1622–1633.
6. Scacciatella P, Marra S, Pullara A, et al. Percutaneous closure of atrial septal defect in adults: very long-term clinical outcome and effects on aortic and mitral valve function. *J Invasive Cardiol.* 2015;27(1):65–69.
7. Attie F, Rosas M, Granados N, et al. Surgical treatment for secundum atrial septal defects in patients >40 years old. A randomized clinical trial. *J Am Coll Cardiol.* 2001;38(7):2035–2042.

SEE ALSO

Aortic Valvular Stenosis; Coarctation of the Aorta; Patent Ductus Arteriosus; Pulmonary Valve Stenosis; Tetralogy of Fallot; Ventricular Septal Defect

CODES

ICD10
- Q21.1 Atrial septal defect
- Q21.2 Atrioventricular septal defect

CLINICAL PEARLS

- ASD is often missed due to subtle clinical presentation.
- Ideally, hemodynamically significant ASDs should be closed in early childhood, although some benefit from closure is present in older patients.
- Many ASDs can be treated by catheter-directed percutaneous closure rather than open-heart surgery.
- Routine endocarditis prophylaxis is not recommended for unrepaired ASDs.
- Generally, symptomatic and hemodynamically significant ASDs are repaired; management of asymptomatic small ASDs is unclear.
- Patent foramen ovales, unlike large ASDs, are very common and generally require no treatment in asymptomatic individuals.

ATTENTION DEFICIT/HYPERACTIVITY DISORDER, ADULT

Amal Shine, MD • Anub G. John, MD • Hugh R. Peterson, MD, FACP

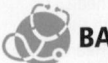 **BASICS**

- Adult attention deficit hyperactivity disorder (adult ADHD) is a psychiatric condition resulting in inattention and/or hyperactivity or impulsivity. It is typically associated with a combination of low self-esteem, dysfunctional or unstable social relationships, and impaired academic/job performance.
- Adult ADHD has been shown to affect a significant portion of the adult population; 30–60% of patients diagnosed with ADHD as a child will continue to meet criteria as adults.
- During transition from pediatric to adult care, poor control of high-risk behaviors during a hiatus of ADHD treatment can lead to increased morbidity.

DESCRIPTION
- Symptoms include difficulty concentrating, impulsivity, and hyperactivity/overactivity. Impairment in executive functioning and emotional dysregulation are common features.
- The three main types of ADHD are (i) hyperactivity-impulsivity predominant, (ii) inattentive predominant, and (iii) combined.

EPIDEMIOLOGY
Prevalence
ADHD affects approximately 4.4–5.2% of adults between 18 and 44 years of age (1).

RISK FACTORS
- ADHD has a strong genetic component, with heritability of approximately 0.8, suggesting that genetic factors would account for about 65% of phenotypic variance (2).
- Studies have shown that the risk of ADHD is increased among offsprings of mothers who smoked or had obesity and diabetes during pregnancy. Risk is also increased in those who had lead exposure in childhood. It is unknown whether these associations are causal.
- Premature birth; very low birth weight; and extreme neglect, abuse, or social deprivation also increase the risk as do certain infections during pregnancy, at birth, and in early childhood.
- ADHD is more commonly diagnosed among adult males than females, with an odds ratio of 1.6:1.0 (1); however, some studies have shown that this is due to the less overt symptoms in females.

COMMONLY ASSOCIATED CONDITIONS
- Substance use and substance abuse disorders
- Mood disorders
- Anxiety disorders
- Intellectual disabilities
- Obsessive-compulsive disorder (OCD)
- Tic disorders

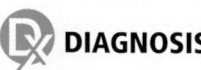 **DIAGNOSIS**

- Diagnosis is made from patient's history and detailing patient's current level of functioning in at least two different settings (e.g., work and home).
- It is important to gather history of patient's childhood and school performance. Several inattentive or hyperactive-impulsive symptoms should be present prior to age 12 years.

HISTORY
- History of childhood ADHD symptoms before age 12 years
- *DSM-5* criteria for adults ≥17 years include ≥5 hyperactivity/impulsivity symptoms and/or ≥5 inattentive symptoms. These symptoms must be present for ≥6 months (1).
- Symptoms must result in maladaptive behavior that impairs the patient's function.
- There must be clear evidence of impaired function due to inattention/hyperactivity in ≥2 settings (e.g., home and work).
- These symptoms must not be related to a psychotic episode or mood disorder and must not be better explained by another *DSM* diagnosis. However, *DSM-5* allows a comorbid diagnosis with autism spectrum disorder.
- Reports of symptoms from adult patients are likely to be less accurate than reports from others. Specifically, symptoms regarding problems with employment (e.g., job dismissal), domestic life (e.g., strained relationships with one's spouse and children), and social activities (e.g., friendship breakups). Therefore, the *DSM-5* recommends obtaining history from a friend or family member with long-term knowledge of the patient (2).
- Personal and family history of cardiac disease or sudden death should be documented.
- History of exposure to lead or other toxins
- History of thyroid disease
- History of medication or substances including anticonvulsants, steroids, antihistamines, nicotine, and caffeine that have side effects that impact attentiveness and mimic ADHD symptoms

PHYSICAL EXAM
- Physical exam is key to ruling out other medical conditions.
- Focus on thyroid and neurologic examinations; look for findings suggestive of substance abuse.
- Record BP and baseline weight; monitor if starting medical treatment.

DIFFERENTIAL DIAGNOSIS
Hearing impairment; hyperthyroid/hypothyroid; sleep deprivation; sleep apnea; phenylketonuria; OCD; lead toxicity; substance abuse (3)[A]

DIAGNOSTIC TESTS & INTERPRETATION
- Adult ADHD screening tools: Retrospective scales include the Childhood Symptom Scale and the Wender Utah Rating Scale; current symptom scales include the Adult ADHD Rating Scale IV, Adult Self Report Scale Symptom Checklist, and the Connor Adult Rating Scale (1). These scales can take 5 to 20 minutes to complete.
- Provider/patient screening checklist
  – https://add.org/wp-content/uploads/2015/03/adhd-questionnaire-ASRS111.pdf
  – https://med.nyu.edu/psych/sites/default/files/psych/psych_adhd_screener_0.pdf
- Developments in imaging techniques have revealed structural and functional brain differences between individuals with and without ADHD, but there is no evidence for clinical utility (1).

Initial Tests (lab, imaging)
- Thyroid-stimulating hormone (TSH)
- Rapid plasma reagin (RPR) or venereal disease research laboratory (VDRL) test
- ECG with concerns for cardiac disease in patient or family history
- Serum lead levels (pending history)

Follow-Up Tests & Special Considerations
- Liver function test monitoring (with atomoxetine)
- A history of childhood behaviors is helpful, but adult patients often don't accurately recall childhood symptomology.
- Inquire about family history of ADHD, family and personal substance abuse, and tic disorders to facilitate formulation of an accurate diagnosis and recognition of high-risk behaviors.
- Caution against stimulant use in pregnancy because of high risk of low fetal birth weight and preterm birth. Risks and benefits of treatment must be discussed in detail with patient and preferably with her spouse (4)[B].
- Caution against use of stimulants in adult patients with cardiac history.

ALERT
Mood disorders, generalized anxiety disorders, and substance abuse can also coexist with adult ADHD; treating both the ADHD and comorbid conditions will improve the patient's prognosis.

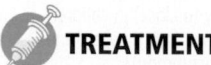 **TREATMENT**

- Most of the research and medication trials have been performed in children.
- There is increasing evidence that stimulants and nonstimulants used in children are also effective in adults (3)[A].

ALERT
Because stimulant medication may induce dependency, substance abuse, and diversion, it is necessary to do pill counts, screen urine for drugs, monitor behavior, and query prescription databases. Misuse of amphetamines may cause sudden death and serious cardiovascular adverse events.

GENERAL MEASURES
When substance abuse is not present, stimulants are first-line treatment for ADHD and highly efficacious. There are multiple formulations of stimulants, and patients may require trials of different dosages, formulations, and medications before an optimal response in symptoms and functions is achieved. Non-stimulants are useful when there is abuse potential, comorbid conditions, or poor response to stimulants.

MEDICATION
- Psychotropic medications play a large part in the treatment of ADHD symptoms. Medications should be titrated slowly to effective dose to avoid side effects.
- Stimulants are more effective than antidepressants or nonstimulants, but up to 30% discontinue medications because of side effects.

- Stimulants can be grouped into those related to methylphenidate and those related to amphetamine. Both groups include both short- and long-acting preparations. Recent evidence suggests that adherence and persistence rates improve in those using long-acting agents (1).
- Antidepressants studied for ADHD include bupropion, which has been shown to have a medium effect compared with stimulants (3)[A].

First Line

- Stimulants: methylphenidate (Concerta, Ritalin), dexmethylphenidate (Focalin), dextroamphetamine/amphetamine (Adderall), dextroamphetamine (Dexedrine), lisdexamfetamine (Vyvanse)
  - Methylphenidate preparations are available in short acting, intermediate acting, long acting, and patch formulations.
  - Ritalin LA may be used for patients naive to stimulants. It can be started at 20 mg daily and dose titrated by 10 mg increments weekly to symptoms response; max dose of 60 mg/day
  - Concerta ER is another option in adults up to 65 years of age. Starting dose of 18 mg/day; adjust in increments of 18 mg weekly until symptoms improve. Max dose 72 mg/day; also has an oral osmotic release to decrease abuse potential
  - Amphetamines also come in immediate-release preparations and sustained-release preparations.
  - Dextroamphetamine is commonly used (half-life of 4 to 6 hours) with an initial dose of 5 mg BID; titrate up by 5 mg weekly to maximum of 20 mg BID.
  - Dextroamphetamine/amphetamine (Adderall) is a 75%/25% mix that also comes in an extended-release form. Initial dosing can be started at 5 mg BID for short acting or 20 mg daily for long acting and increased by 5 mg/week for short acting and 10 mg/week long acting to a maximum of 40 to 60 mg total daily.
  - Lisdexamfetamine (Vyvanse) is an extended-release stimulant that is a prodrug requiring metabolization to active component, dextroamphetamine.
  - Common side effects of stimulants include hypertension (HTN), tachycardia, insomnia, weight loss, stomach upset, increased anxiety/irritability, or worsening of tics (3)[A].
- Nonstimulants:
  - Atomoxetine (Strattera) has been shown effective in adults with ADHD when compared to placebo (5)[B]. It may be given as a single dose or split dose and has low abuse potential, making it a better choice over a stimulant medication for patients with substance abuse history. Onset of effect may take up to 4 weeks. Atomoxetine may be particularly useful when anxiety, mood or tics co-occur with ADHD. Also, there are rare cases of liver damage associated with these medications. Monitor for increased suicidal thinking.
  - Antidepressants: best used for those at high risk or with history of substance abuse disorder. Bupropion (Wellbutrin) is an antidepressant effective in adults with ADHD symptoms, especially if they have comorbid depression (4)[A].

- Tricyclic antidepressants (desipramine and nortriptyline) have also shown to be effective in ADHD (1).
- α_2-Agonists (guanfacine, clonidine) have been found to be effective in children and adolescents; however, their efficacy, safety, and tolerability have not been studied extensively in adults (6)[C]. These may be used with comorbid tics and/or disruptive behavior disorders.
- Combining stimulants with a nonstimulant medication such as atomoxetine, guanfacine, or clonidine has shown positive effects among patients who are resistant to stimulants alone.

ISSUES FOR REFERRAL

Patients with comorbid conditions may need referral for diagnosis and treatment. Consider cardiology consult for patients with known cardiac issues who may require stimulant treatment. Consider referral to obstetrician experienced in high-risk pregnancies when treating pregnant women with ADHD.

ADDITIONAL THERAPIES

- Cognitive-behavioral therapy (CBT) can be useful in conjunction with medication to help patient modify and cope with symptoms. CBT helps reduce impairments resulting from executive dysfunction (EDF) that is not optimally ameliorated with medication (1).
- Among adults with ADHD and EDFs, addition of memantine as an adjunct to extended-release methylphenidate was associated with improved executive functioning, supporting the need for further research.

COMPLEMENTARY & ALTERNATIVE MEDICINE

Vitamin–mineral supplementation is an area of active research that holds promise for improved ADHD treatment.

ONGOING CARE

Transfer from pediatric to adult care must be closely coordinated to avoid hiatus in treatment.

- Support groups (e.g., www.chadd.org and www.add.org) assist the newly diagnosed adult by providing education, treatment options, available resources, and peer support.

FOLLOW-UP RECOMMENDATIONS

- Close follow-up of medication as dose is titrated
- Continue to monitor for medication side effects.
- Repeat screening checklists to quantify benefit of interventions as needed.
- Reinforce behavioral change (e.g., self-initiated through CBT), which is essential goal of long-term management.

REFERENCES

1. Young JL, Goodman DW. Adult attention-deficit/hyperactivity disorder diagnosis, management, and treatment in the DSM-5 era. *Prim Care Companion CNS Disord*. 2016;18(6). doi:10.4088/PCC.16r02000.
2. Volkow ND, Swanson JM. Clinical practice: adult attention deficit–hyperactivity disorder. *N Engl J Med*. 2013;369(20):1935–1944.
3. Castells X, Ramos-Quiroga JA, Bosch R, et al. Amphetamines for attention deficit hyperactivity disorder (ADHD) in adults. *Cochrane Database Syst Rev*. 2011;(6):CD007813.
4. Verbeeck W, Tuinier S, Bekkering GE. Antidepressants in the treatment of adult attention-deficit hyperactivity disorder: a systematic review. *Adv Ther*. 2009;26(2):170–184.
5. Asherson P, Bushe C, Saylor K, et al. Efficacy of atomoxetine in adults with attention deficit hyperactivity disorder: an integrated analysis of the complete database of multicenter placebo-controlled trials. *J Psychopharmacol*. 2014;28(9):837–846.
6. Hirota T, Schwartz S, Correll CU. Alpha-2 agonists for attention-deficit/hyperactivity disorder in youth: a systematic review and meta-analysis of monotherapy and add-on trials to stimulant therapy. *J Am Acad Child Adolesc Psychiatry*. 2014;53(2):153–173.

ADDITIONAL READING

American Psychiatric Association. *Diagnostic and Statistical Manual of Mental Disorders*. 5th ed. Arlington, VA: American Psychiatric Association; 2013.

 CODES

ICD10

- F90.9 Attention-deficit hyperactivity disorder, unspecified type
- F90.1 Attn-defct hyperactivity disorder, predom hyperactive type
- F90.0 Attn-defct hyperactivity disorder, predom inattentive type

CLINICAL PEARLS

- Adult ADHD results in inattention, easy distractibility, hyperactivity, and impulsive behavior; it is associated with low self-esteem, problematic interpersonal relationships, and difficulty meeting academic and job expectations.
- Psychotropic medications plus cognitive behavioral treatments are the cornerstone of management.
- Substance abuse is a common comorbidity; recommend use of nonstimulant medication in those at high risk

ATTENTION DEFICIT/HYPERACTIVITY DISORDER, PEDIATRIC

Laura Novak, MD • Katherine Williams, MD

BASICS

DESCRIPTION
- Attention deficit hyperactivity disorder (ADHD) is a neurodevelopmental disorder that manifests in early childhood characterized by distractibility, impulsivity, hyperactivity, and/or inattention.
- Three subsets: predominantly hyperactivity impulsive (ADHD-HI), predominantly inattentive (ADHD-I), or combined (ADHD-C)
- System(s) affected: nervous
- Synonym(s): attention deficit disorder; hyperactivity

EPIDEMIOLOGY
- Predominant age: onset <12 years; lasts into adolescence and adulthood; 50% meet diagnostic criteria by age 4 years.
- Predominant sex: male > female (2:1); ADHD-I is more common in girls.

Prevalence
5–11% of children 4 to 17 years

ETIOLOGY AND PATHOPHYSIOLOGY
Not definitive

Genetics
Familial pattern

RISK FACTORS
- Family history
- Medical causes (affecting brain development)
- Environmental causes (toxins such as lead, fetal alcohol, and nutritional deficiencies)

COMMONLY ASSOCIATED CONDITIONS
- Depression (in up to 1/3 of cases)
- Oppositional defiant disorder
- Conduct disorder
- Anxiety disorder
- Learning disabilities

DIAGNOSIS

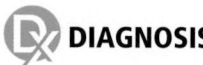

- American Academy of Pediatrics (AAP) guidelines recommend *DSM-5* criteria to establish diagnosis (1)[C].
- *DSM-5* criteria for children <17 years: ≥6 inattention criteria and/or ≥6 hyperactivity/impulsivity criteria. Symptoms must occur often, be present before age of 12 years, for >6 months, be noticed in ≥2 settings (e.g., home, school), reduce quality of social or scholastic functioning, be excessive for development level of child, and are not better explained by or occur with another mental disorder (e.g., mood, anxiety, or personality disorder) (2)[C].
- Inattention
  - Careless mistakes in tasks
  - Difficulty sustaining attention or in organizing
  - Does not seem to listen
  - Doesn't follow through or finish tasks
  - Avoids tasks that require sustained mental effort
  - Loses things
  - Forgetful in daily activities
  - Distracted by external stimuli
  - Forgetful

- Hyperactivity/impulsivity
  - Fidgets
  - Difficulty remaining seated
  - Runs/climbs excessively or inappropriately; difficulty playing quietly
  - Acts as if "driven by a motor" or seeming to always be "on the go"
  - Talks excessively
  - Blurts out answers before question is complete
  - Has difficulty waiting turn
  - Interrupts others
- Children undergoing extreme stress (parent's divorce, illness, homelessness, abuse) may demonstrate ADHD behaviors secondary to stress (1)[C]. This can be assessed using the American Academy of Child and Adolescent Psychiatry (AACAP) screening tool.
- If diagnostic behaviors are noted in only one setting, explore the stressors in that setting.
- The diagnostic behaviors are more noticeable in tasks that require concentration or boredom tolerance.

HISTORY
- Birth and development history
- Psychosocial evaluation of home environment
- School performance and school absences
- Psychiatric history or history of comorbid disorder(s)
- Cardiac history

PHYSICAL EXAM
- Baseline weight for future monitoring
- Note any soft neurologic signs, such as tics, clumsiness, mixed handedness.
- Assess hearing and vision.

DIFFERENTIAL DIAGNOSIS
- Activity level appropriate for age
- Dysfunctional family situation
- Learning disability (e.g., dyslexia)
- Hearing/vision/language disorder
- Autism spectrum disorders
- Oppositional/defiant disorder or conduct disorder
- Tourette syndrome: motor and verbal tics
- Absence seizures (ADHD-I only)
- Lead poisoning
- Sequelae of central nervous system infection/trauma
- Medication
- Sleep disorder

DIAGNOSTIC TESTS & INTERPRETATION
- Behavior rating scales completed by parents, caregivers, and teachers prior to initiation of therapy and then repeated after therapy
- Forms are available from the ADHD toolkit at http://www.nichq.org/adhd.html (Vanderbilt Assessment Scales).
- Testing for learning disability through the school

Initial Tests (lab, imaging)
Rarely needed. Consider lead.

Diagnostic Procedures/Other
- EEG is rarely needed.
- ECG prior to stating stimulant medication if positive family history of premature CV disease

TREATMENT

GENERAL MEASURES
- Parent/school/patient education
- Work closely with teacher.
- Behavioral therapy/environmental changes
- Regular physical activity 60 min/day
- Mindfulness meditation may help stress and mood.

MEDICATION
- 2011 AAP guideline recommends: ages 4 to 5 years—behavioral interventions
- Ages 6 to 17 behavioral interventions plus stimulant medications (3)[A]
- Stimulant choice should be based on cost, formulary, convenience, and duration. A second type of stimulant should be tried if the first treatment fails. All stimulant capsules can be opened and sprinkled (Note: Concerta is a pill).

First Line
Stimulant:
- Methylphenidate
  - Short acting—duration of action (DOA) 2 to 4 hours
    ○ Ritalin, Methylin: initial 2.5 mg BID before breakfast and lunch; increase by 5 q3–7d to max dose of 60 mg/day (divided BID/TID).
  - Intermediate acting—DOA 3 to 8 hours
    ○ Ritalin XR: 20 mg once in AM; increase by 10 mg weekly up to max dose of 40 to 60 mg.
    ○ Metadate ER: 10 mg BID; increase by 10 mg weekly to max dose of 40 to 60 mg.
  - Long acting—DOA 8 to 12 hours
    ○ Metadate CD: 20 mg in AM; increase by 10 to 20 mg weekly to max dose of 40 to 60 mg.
    ○ Quillivant XR: 20 mg in AM; increase 10 to 20 mg weekly to max dose of 40 to 60 mg.
    ○ Ritalin LA: 10 to 20 mg in AM; increase 10 mg weekly to max dose of 40 to 60 mg.
    ○ Concerta: 18 to 36 mg in AM; increase by 18 mg weekly to max dose of 54 to 72 mg.
    ○ Daytrana transdermal patch: 10-mg patch on (hip area) 2 hours before effect is needed; patch removed 9 hours after application; increase to next higher patch weekly until max dose 30-mg patch.
- Dexmethylphenidate
  - Focalin: DOA 4 to 6 hours; initial: 2.5 mg BID; increase by 2.5 mg weekly up to max dose of 20 mg/day.
  - Focalin XR: DOA 12 hours; initial: 5 mg in AM; increase by 5 mg weekly up to max dose of 30 mg/day.
- Dextroamphetamine SR DOA 8 to 12 hours
  - 5 mg BID; increase by 5 mg weekly to max dose of 40 mg daily.
- Dextroamphetamine/amphetamine mixed salts
  - Short acting—DOA 4 to 5 hours
    ○ Adderall: 2.5 mg daily or BID; increase by 5 mg weekly to a max divided dose of 40 mg daily.
  - Long acting—DOA 10 to 12 hours
    ○ Adderall XR: 5 mg in AM; increase by 5 mg weekly until max dose of 30 mg/day.
- Lisdexamfetamine (prodrug)—DOA 10 to 12 hours
  - Vyvanse: 30 mg in AM; increase by 10 mg weekly up to a max dose of 70 mg/day.

ALERT
Screen by history +/− ECG for cardiac disease before starting stimulant medication (2)[C].

- Precautions:
  - If not responding, check compliance and consider another diagnosis.
  - Some children experience withdrawal (tearfulness, agitation) after a missed dose or when medication wears off. A small, short-acting dose at 4 PM may help to prevent this.
  - Stimulants are drugs of abuse and should be monitored carefully.
  - Drug holidays are not recommended but may be tried in weight loss or ADHD-I.
- Common adverse effects:
  - Anorexia, insomnia, GI effects, and headache
- Significant possible interactions: may increase levels of anticonvulsants, SSRIs, tricyclics, and warfarin
- High-caffeine energy drinks, albuterol inhalers, and decongestants may increase side effects.
- The FDA reports permanent skin discoloration with Daytrana patches.

Pregnancy Considerations
Medications are Category C: caution in pregnancy

Second Line
Nonstimulant:

- SNRI
  - Atomoxetine (Strattera):
    - ≤70 kg: 0.5 mg/kg/day initial; increase after a minimum of 3 days to target dose of 1.2 mg/kg/day; maximum of 1.4 mg/kg/day
    - >70 kg: 40 mg daily; increase after minimum of 3 days to target dose of 80 mg/day; dose may be increased to maximum of 100 mg/day after additional 2 to 4 weeks.
- α_2-Agonist
  - Modest efficacy, high side effects. Consider consultation before use.
    - Clonidine XR (Kapvay): 0.1 mg once daily at bedtime; increase by 0.1 mg weekly; doses should be taken twice daily with equal or higher split dosage given at HS; maximum of 0.4 mg/day; taper when discontinued.
    - Guanfacine XR (Intuniv): 1 mg daily; increase by 1 mg weekly until 1 to 4 mg daily; taper when discontinued.

ALERT
Atomoxetine carries a "black box" warning regarding potential exacerbation of suicidality (similar to SSRIs). Close follow-up is recommended.

- Associated with hepatic injury in a small number of cases; check liver enzymes if symptoms develop.
- Interacts with paroxetine (Paxil), fluoxetine (Prozac), and quinidine

ISSUES FOR REFERRAL
Consider referral for children <6 years if there are additional mental health, developmental issues, or poor response to treatment.

COMPLEMENTARY & ALTERNATIVE MEDICINE
- Surveys have shown that parents of children with ADHD use herbals and complementary treatments frequently (20–60%) but very limited evidence to support any intervention.
- If nutritional deficiency is suspected, assess and replace deficits.

 ONGOING CARE

FOLLOW-UP RECOMMENDATIONS
Patient Monitoring
- Parent/teacher rating scales
- Office visits to monitor side effects and efficacy: End points are improved grades, rating scales, family interactions, and peer interactions.
- Monitor growth (especially weight) and BP.

DIET
- There is "insufficient evidence to suggest that dietary interventions reduce the symptoms of ADHD" (2)[C].
- The AAP recommends that a trial of a preservative-free food coloring–free diet is a reasonable intervention (3)[B].

PATIENT EDUCATION
- Excellent reference: http://www.parentsmedguide.org
- Teachers reference: Teachers Nations Resource Center on ADHD
- Key points for parents:
  - Find things the child is good at and emphasize these; reinforce good behavior; give one task at a time; stop behavior with quiet discipline; coordinate homework with teachers; and have external organization tools—charts, schedules, tokens.
  - Develop an individualized education plan (IEP) with the school.
- Support groups:
  - Children and Adults with Attention Deficit Disorder (CHADD): http://www.chadd.org
  - Attention Deficit Disorder Warehouse: http://www.addwarehouse.com
  - The Center for Parent Information and Resources (CPIR): https://www.parentcenterhub.org

PROGNOSIS
- May last into adulthood; plan for a transition at age 17 years.
- Relative deficits in academic and social functioning may persist into late adolescence/adulthood.
- Encourage career choices that allow autonomy and mobility.

COMPLICATIONS
- Untreated ADHD can lead to failing in school, parental abuse, social isolation, and poor self-esteem.
- Possible withdrawal when medication wears off
- Monitor growth with stimulant use. If appetite is poor, eat before the medication is given and after it wears off. Consider a shorter duration medication.

- There is an increased risk of substance abuse which may decrease with treatment of ADHD.
- There is an increased incidence of automobile accidents and injuries, which decreases with medication.

REFERENCES
1. American Psychiatric Association. *Diagnostic and Statistical Manual of Mental Disorders*. 5th ed. Arlington, VA: American Psychiatric Association; 2013.
2. Wolraich M, Brown L, Brown RT, et al; for Subcommittee on Attention-Deficit/Hyperactivity Disorder, Steering Committee on Quality Improvement and Management. ADHD: clinical practice guideline for the diagnosis, evaluation, and treatment of attention-deficit/hyperactivity disorder in children and adolescents. *Pediatrics*. 2011;128(5):1007–1022.
3. Sinn N. Nutritional and dietary influences on attention deficit hyperactivity disorder. *Nutr Rev*. 2008;66(10):558–568.

ADDITIONAL READING
- Felt BT, Biermann B, Christner JG, et al. Diagnosis and management of ADHD in children. *Am Fam Physician*. 2014;90(7):456–464.
- Laforett DR, Murray DW, Kollins SH. Psychosocial treatments for preschool-aged children with attention-deficit hyperactivity disorder. *Dev Disabl Res Rev*. 2008;14(4):300–310.
- Millichap JG, Yee MM. The diet factor in attention-deficit/hyperactivity disorder. *Pediatrics*. 2012;129(2):330–337.

 CODES

ICD10
- F90.9 Attention-deficit hyperactivity disorder, unspecified type
- F90.0 Attn-defct hyperactivity disorder, predom inattentive type
- F90.1 Attn-defct hyperactivity disorder, predom hyperactive type

CLINICAL PEARLS
- AAP recommends behavioral interventions for age 4 to 5 years and behavioral interventions plus stimulant medications as first-line treatment for age 6 to 17 years.
- Children undergoing extreme stress (parent's divorce, illness, homelessness, abuse) may demonstrate ADHD behaviors secondary to stress.
- Parents may also have ADHD and may have difficulty helping the child with organization.

ATYPICAL MOLE (DYSPLASTIC NEVUS) SYNDROME

Simranjeet Kaur, MD • Sahil Mullick, MD

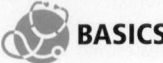

BASICS

Atypical mole syndrome (AMS), also known as dysplastic nevi syndrome (DNS), B-K mole syndrome, Clark nevi syndrome, or familial atypical multiple mole melanoma (FAMMM) syndrome, is a condition characterized by a large number of pigmented nevi with architectural disorder, which arise sporadically or by inheritance and are associated with an increased risk of melanoma.

DESCRIPTION

There is no consensus on criteria for AMS.

- Elevated total body nevi count, including clinically atypical nevi, is usually >50 and often >100.
  - Larger number in hereditary AMS versus sporadic atypical nevi (as few as <10)
- Increased risk of melanoma
  - Up to 90% occurrence by age 80 years in certain high-risk individuals
  - Earlier onset than in sporadic melanoma
  - More arise de novo than from an existing nevus
  - Higher risk for appearance at unusual sites (e.g., scalp, eyes, and sun-protected areas)
- Median age of diagnosis for melanoma in AMS is 10 to 20 years earlier than the general population, with documented cases of melanoma as early as in the 2nd and 3rd decades of life.

EPIDEMIOLOGY

Incidence
Uncertain due to phenotype variability, limited data

Prevalence
Affects between 2% and 8% of fair-skinned adults as well as those with high exposure to ultraviolet radiation

ETIOLOGY AND PATHOPHYSIOLOGY

- Cyclin-dependent kinase inhibitor 2A (*CDKN2A*) mutations have been observed in familial DNS and multiple melanomas. The *CDKN2A* gene on 9p21 encodes for the proteins p16 and p14. p16 binds to CDK4/6 and is a negative cell-cycle regulator via inhibition of the CDK–cyclin D interaction needed for cell cycle progression from G1 to S. p14 functions by stabilizing the tumor-suppressor protein p53 in the G1 phase of the cell cycle.
- Familial cases of germline *CDKN2A* mutations are transmitted in an autosomal dominant fashion.
- No clear somatic mutation patterns in sporadic cases

Genetics
CDKN2A gene mutation is observed in 25–40% of hereditary cases, with autosomal dominant inheritance but variable expressivity and incomplete penetrance.

RISK FACTORS
Family history of melanoma or multiple nevi, sun exposure, neonatal blue-light phototherapy, history of painful sunburns

GENERAL PREVENTION
- Primary prevention with sun avoidance, sun protection
- Secondary prevention of melanoma with routine skin exams, biopsy of suspect lesions, and environmental risk mitigation as above

COMMONLY ASSOCIATED CONDITIONS
- Malignant melanoma, including ocular melanoma
- Ocular nevi
- Pancreatic cancer in *CDKN2A* mutation

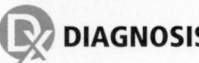

DIAGNOSIS

AMS is a clinical diagnosis with various classifications schemes proposed. Although not widely accepted, diagnostic criteria, as defined by the NIH, require the three features of (i) malignant melanoma in ≥1 first- or second-degree relatives; (ii) numerous melanocytic nevi (frequently >50), some of which are clinically atypical; and (iii) nevi that have certain histologic features (1).

HISTORY
- Changing lesions: bleeding, scaling, size, texture, nonhealing, hyper- or hypopigmentation
- Large number of nevi
- Congenital nevi
- Sun exposure
- Prior skin biopsies
- Prior melanoma
- Immunosuppression (e.g., AIDS, chemotherapy, pancreatic cancer)
- First- or second-degree relatives with:
  - AMS
  - Melanoma
  - Pancreatic cancer

PHYSICAL EXAM
- Full-body skin exams
- Goal to distinguish melanoma from AMS
- ABCDE mnemonic for skins lesions concerning for melanoma: Asymmetry, Border irregularity, Color variegation, Diameter >6 mm, and Evolving lesion
  - Atypical mole (AM) is often defined as ≥5 mm and at least two other features.
  - Melanoma typically has several characteristics of ABCDEs, with increased specificity for melanoma if lesion diameter is >6 mm.
- "Ugly duckling sign" (2)[B]:
  - Melanoma screening strategy for increasing accuracy of diagnosis of melanoma by identifying malignant nevi straying from the predominant nevus pattern when numerous atypical nevi are present
- Most common features of AM on dermoscopy include (3)[C]:
  - Reticular pattern most common
  - Uniform pigmentation most common followed by multifocal hypo/hyperpigmentation
  - Homogenous brown globules
  - Pigmentation with central heterogeneity and abrupt termination

- Dermatoscopic features more suggestive of melanoma include (4)[C]:
  - Depigmented areas
  - Whitish veil
  - Homogenous areas distributed irregularly, in multiple areas, or >25% of total lesion
  - ≥4 colors

DIFFERENTIAL DIAGNOSIS
- Common nevus: acquired or congenital
- Melanoma
- Seborrheic keratosis
- Dermatofibroma
- Lentigo
- Pigmented actinic keratosis
- Pigmented basal cell carcinoma
- Blue rubber bleb nevus syndrome

DIAGNOSTIC TESTS & INTERPRETATION
Diagnosis is first suspected with history and physical exam and then confirmed by biopsy and histopathology.

Initial Tests (lab, imaging)
- Dermoscopy can be used for a more detailed exam of nevus to aid in distinguishing between benign and malignant lesions as well as for further classification to any of the 11 subtypes.
- Genetic testing is available for *CDKN2A* mutations, but it is not recommended outside of research studies because results cannot be adequately used for management or surveillance (5)[C].
- When the total nevus count is high and following each nevus is impractical, total body photography may aid in the evaluation of evolving nevi as well as in documenting new nevi (6)[C].

Diagnostic Procedures/Other
- Biopsy is recommended for any lesion where melanoma cannot be excluded.
- Biopsy entails full-thickness biopsy of the entire lesion with a narrow 1- to 3-mm margin of normal skin down to fat for adequate depth assessment (7)[C].
  - Excisional biopsy, elliptical or punch excision, provides the most accurate diagnosis and should be performed when possible.
  - Scoop shave biopsy can also be used, but care must be taken to not transect the lesion.
- Reexcision of mild to moderately dysplastic nevi with positive margins may not change pathologic diagnosis, but for severely dysplastic nevi, consider reexcision, with surgical margins of 2 to 5 mm (6)[C].

Test Interpretation
"Dysplastic nevus" is a term more accurately reserved as a histologic diagnosis. Features may include melanocyte proliferation in the dermoepidermal junction extending through at least three rete ridges in a specific pattern, fusing of rete ridges, dermal fibrosis, neovascularization, and interstitial lymphocytic inflammation (6)[C].

TREATMENT

MEDICATION

No medications have been shown to treat AMS (6)[C].

ISSUES FOR REFERRAL

- Dermatologist for routine skin exam for those patients at high risk for melanoma
- Ophthalmologic exams for ocular nevi/melanoma screening/papilledema
- Oncology or specialized genetics study group involvement if strong family predisposition to pancreatic cancer

ADDITIONAL THERAPIES

- Topical chemo- and immunotherapies have been unsuccessfully attempted to treat AMs (6)[C].
- Laser treatment should be avoided because it is both unsafe and ineffective for melanocytic nevi (6)[C].

SURGERY/OTHER PROCEDURES

Surgical excision of all atypical nevi is not recommended because most melanomas in AMS appear de novo on healthy skin and the procedure leads to both poor cosmetic outcomes and a false sense of security. Lesions suspicious for melanoma should be biopsied or removed surgically.

 ONGOING CARE

FOLLOW-UP RECOMMENDATIONS

Close follow-up with a dermatologist or other physician experienced with assessment of atypical nevi:

- Total body skin exam (including nails, scalp, genital area, and oral mucosa) every 6 months initially, starting at puberty; may be reduced to annually once nevi are stable
- Dermoscopic evaluation for suspected lesions
- Ocular exam for those with familial AMS
- Excision of suspected lesions
- Total body photography at baseline

Patient Monitoring

Monthly self-exams of skin

PATIENT EDUCATION

For young adults with fair skin, counsel to minimize exposure to ultraviolet radiation to reduce risk of skin cancer (USPSTF grade B).

- Fair skin: light eye, hair, or skin color, freckles
- Educate on sun avoidance, proper application of sunscreen, use of protective clothing (e.g., hats), avoidance of tanning booths and sunburns.
- Teach "ABCDE" mnemonic + "ugly duckling sign" to assess nevi and identify potential melanomas.
- Provide instruction on skin self-exam techniques.
- A sample listing of patient-centric review sources on this topic are as follows:
  – American Academy of Dermatology (https://www .verywellhealth.com/the-abcdes-of-skin -cancer-514388)
  – Skin Cancer Foundation (https://www.skincancer .org/skin-cancer-information/atypical-moles)
  – Melanoma Research Foundation (https://www .melanoma.org/understand-melanoma/what-is -melanoma)

PROGNOSIS

- Most AM either regress or do not change.
- Multiple classification schemes have been developed over the years to delineate risk of melanoma in patients with AMS. Individuals with a family history of melanoma are at greatest risk. The Rigel classification system can be applied in the clinical setting. Points are assigned based on incidence of melanoma, with 1 point given for a personal history with melanoma and 2 points for each family member with melanoma (modified nuclear family consisting of first-degree relatives plus grandparents and uncles/aunts) and stratified as follows:
  – Score = 0, Rigel group 0, 6% 25-year accumulated risk for melanoma
  – Score = 1, Rigel group 1, 10% risk
  – Score = 2, Rigel group 2, 15% risk
  – Score ≥3, Rigel group 3, 50% risk
- The CDKN2A mutation has also been associated with a 60–90% risk of melanoma by age 80 years and a 17% risk for pancreatic cancer by age 75 years.

COMPLICATIONS

- Malignant melanoma
- Poor cosmetic outcomes from biopsy

REFERENCES

1. Goldsmith LA, Askin FB, Chang AE, et al. Diagnosis and treatment of early melanoma: NIH consensus development panel on early melanoma. JAMA. 1992;268(10):1314–1319.
2. Gaudy-Marqueste C, Wazaefi Y, Bruneu Y, et al. Ugly duckling sign as a major factor of efficiency in melanoma detection. JAMA Dermatol. 2017;153(4):279–284.
3. Hofmann-Wellenhof R, Blum A, Wolf IH, et al. Dermoscopic classification of atypical melanocytic nevi (Clark nevi). Arch Dermatol. 2001;137(12):1575–1580.
4. Salopek TG, Kopf AW, Stefanato CM, et al. Differentiation of atypical moles (dysplastic nevi) from early melanomas by dermoscopy. Dermatol Clin. 2001;19(2):337–345.
5. Kefford R, Bishop JN, Tucker M, et al; for Melanoma Genetics Consortium. Genetic testing for melanoma. Lancet Oncol. 2002;3(11):653–654.
6. Duffy K, Grossman D. The dysplastic nevus: from historical perspective to management in the modern era: part I. Historical, histologic, and clinical aspects. J Am Acad Dermatol. 2012;67(1):1.e1–1.e18.
7. Strazzula L, Vedak P, Hoang MP, et al. The utility of re-excising mildly and moderately dysplastic nevi: a retrospective analysis. J Am Acad Dermatol. 2014;71(6):1071–1076.

ADDITIONAL READING

- Csoma Z, Tóth-Molnár E, Balogh K, et al. Neonatal blue light phototherapy and melanocytic nevi: a twin study. Pediatrics. 2011;128(4):e856–e864.
- Czajkowski R, Placek W, Drewa G, et al. FAMMM syndrome: pathogenesis and management. Dermatol Surg. 2004;30(2, Pt 2):291–296.
- Duffy K, Grossman D. The dysplastic nevus: from historical perspective to management in the modern era: part II. Molecular aspects and clinical management. J Am Acad Dermatol. 2012;67(1):19.e1–19.e12, quiz 31–32.

- Farber MJ, Heilman ER, Friedman RJ. Dysplastic nevi. Dermatol Clin. 2012;30(3):389–404.
- Friedman RJ, Farber MJ, Warycha MA, et al. The "dysplastic" nevus. Clin Dermatol. 2009;27(1):103–115.
- Gandini S, Sera F, Cattaruzza MS, et al. Meta-analysis of risk factors for cutaneous melanoma: I. Common and atypical naevi. Eur J Cancer. 2005;41(1):28–44.
- Matichard E, Le Hénanff A, Sanders A, et al. Effect of neonatal phototherapy on melanocytic nevus count in children. Arch Dermatol. 2006;142(12):1599–1604.
- Mize DE, Bishop M, Reese E, et al. Familial atypical multiple mole melanoma syndrome. In: Riegert-Johnson DL, Boardman LA, Hefferon T, et al, eds. Cancer Syndromes. Bethesda, MD: National Center for Biotechnology Information; 2009.
- Moloney FJ, Guitera P, Coates E, et al. Detection of primary melanoma in individuals at extreme high risk: a prospective 5-year follow-up study. JAMA Dermatol. 2014;150(8):819–827.
- Naeyaert JM, Brochez L. Clinical practice. Dysplastic nevi. N Engl J Med. 2003;349(23):2233–2240.
- Newton JA, Bataille V, Griffiths K, et al. How common is the atypical mole syndrome phenotype in apparently sporadic melanoma? J Am Acad Dermatol. 1993;29(6):989–996.
- Perkins A, Duffy RL. Atypical moles: diagnosis and management. Am Fam Physician. 2015;91(11):762–767.
- Rigel DS, Rivers JK, Friedman RJ, et al. Risk gradient for malignant melanoma in individuals with dysplastic naevi. Lancet. 1988;1(8581):352–353.
- Robson ME, Storm CD, Weitzel J, et al. American Society of Clinical Oncology policy statement update: genetic and genomic testing for cancer susceptibility. J Clin Oncol. 2010;28(5):893–901.
- Silva JH, Sá BC, Avila AL, et al. Atypical mole syndrome and dysplastic nevi: identification of populations at risk for developing melanoma—review article. Clinics (Sao Paulo). 2011;66(3):493–499.
- Slade J, Marghoob AA, Salopek TG, et al. Atypical mole syndrome: risk factor for cutaneous malignant melanoma and implications for management. J Am Acad Dermatol. 1995;32(3):479–494.

 CODES

ICD10

- D22.9 Melanocytic nevi, unspecified
- D22.4 Melanocytic nevi of scalp and neck
- D22.30 Melanocytic nevi of unspecified part of face

CLINICAL PEARLS

- In describing nevi, "atypical" is a clinical term, whereas "dysplastic" is a histologic term.
- Melanoma in AMS tends to arise from healthy skin despite a large number of atypical nevi.
- ~20% of individuals with familial AMS will develop pancreatic cancer by age 75 years.
- Patients with AMS tend to produce neoplasms in unusual sites such as the scalp, eyes, and sun-protected areas (e.g., gluteal folds).

AUTISM SPECTRUM DISORDERS

Richard Gibson, MD • Holly L. Baab, MD

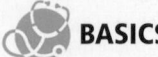

BASICS

DESCRIPTION

- Group of neurodevelopmental disorders of early childhood characterized by (i) persistent deficits in social communication and interaction and (ii) restricted, repetitive patterns of behavior, interests, or activities
- *DSM-5*: umbrella term autism spectrum disorder (ASD), which encompasses a group of pervasive developmental disorders with designations for varying severities and associated symptoms
- ASD combines former diagnoses, including autistic disorder, childhood disintegrative disorder, Asperger disorder, pervasive developmental disorder not otherwise specified (PDD-NOS), early infantile autism, childhood autism, Kanner autism, high-functioning autism, and atypical autism; many of which are still used by ICD-10 coding.
- Although symptoms must be present in the early development period, they may not be apparent until social demands exceed capacity.
- Symptoms must cause functional impairment.
- Severity levels
  – Level 1: requiring support
  – Level 2: requiring substantial support
  – Level 3: requiring very substantial support
- Specifiers for associated symptoms include with catatonia; intellectual impairment; language impairment; known medical or genetic condition; and neurodevelopmental, mental, or behavioral disorders.
- Important to distinguish ASD from similar symptoms that could be better explained by intellectual disability or global developmental delay

EPIDEMIOLOGY

- Incidence: estimated 1 in every 110 children in the United States diagnosed per year
- Predominant age: onset in early childhood
- Predominant sex: male > female (4:1)

Pediatric Considerations

Symptom onset can often be seen in children <3 years of age but may not become apparent until social demands exceed capacity.

Prevalence

- According to the Centers for Disease Control and Prevention (CDC) in 2014, an estimated prevalence of 1 in every 59 children between the ages of 3 and 17 years carried a diagnosis of ASD.
- This has been a steady increase since 2000 when the CDC reported the prevalence to be 1 in 150.
- Systematic literature reviews suggest changes in prevalence can be largely accounted for by changes in definition and increased awareness.

ETIOLOGY AND PATHOPHYSIOLOGY

- No single cause has been identified.
- General consensus: A genetic abnormality leads to altered neurologic development.
- No scientific evidence relating vaccines, such as vaccines for measles, mumps, rubella (MMR) or thimerosal causing ASDs
- Pathophysiology is not fully understood.

Genetics

- Genetic concordance: A 2009 Swedish population-based cohort study of 2 million subjects showed a cumulative risk of 59% for monozygotic twins.

- Rate in siblings: The American College of Medical Genetics and Genomics practice guidelines lists the risk of siblings of children diagnosed with ASD without an identifiable cause to be:
  – 7% if the affected child is female
  – 4% if the affected child is male
  – >30% if there are two or more affected children

RISK FACTORS

- Male sex
- Family history
- Advanced paternal age
- Very low birth weight
- Maternal use of selective serotonin reuptake inhibitors (SSRIs) or valproate during pregnancy
- Note: Epidemiologic evidence does not support an association between immunizations and ASD.

GENERAL PREVENTION

- Screening for early intervention is associated with improved prognosis.
- Routine screening for ASD with a validated tool is recommended at 18- and 24-month well-child visits to assist with early detection.

COMMONLY ASSOCIATED CONDITIONS

- Intellectual disability
- ADHD, anxiety, depression, or obsessive behavior
- Motor impairments including hypotonia, apraxia, toe walking, or gross motor delays
- Phenylketonuria (PKU), tuberous sclerosis, fragile X syndrome, Angelman syndrome, and fetal alcohol syndrome (rare)
- Seizures (increased risk if severe mental retardation)
- Sleep issues: insomnia, circadian rhythm sleep–wake disorder, sleep-related movement disorder
- Chronic constipation, diarrhea, abdominal pain

DIAGNOSIS

HISTORY

- Listen to parents' concerns and test early if they or you have suspicion of a neurodevelopmental disorder
- Impairment in social-emotional reciprocity
  – Failure of normal back-and-forth conversations
  – Unable to develop peer relationships
  – Reduced sharing of interests, emotions, or affect
  – Failure to initiate or respond to social interaction
- Deficits in nonverbal communication
  – Abnormalities in eye contact or body language
  – Deficits in understanding and use of gestures
  – Lack of facial expression and nonverbal communication
- Deficits in developing, maintaining, and understanding relationships
  – Difficulties adjusting behavior to suit various social contexts
  – Difficulties in sharing imaginative play or in making friends
  – Absence of interest in peers
- Repetitive and stereotyped patterns of behavior
  – Stereotyped or repetitive motor movements, use of objects, or speech
  – Insistence on sameness, inflexible adherence to routines, or ritualized patterns of behavior
  – Highly restricted, fixated interests that are abnormal in intensity or focus
  – Hyper- or hyporeactivity to sensory input or unusual interest in sensory aspects of the environment
- Prenatal, neonatal, and developmental history

- Seizure disorder
- Family history of autism, genetic disorders, learning disabilities, psychiatric illness, neurologic disorders, or mental retardation
- Commonly associated with sleep disorders

PHYSICAL EXAM

- Measurement of growth parameters including height, weight, and head circumference because macrocephaly is present in 25% of ASD
- Vision and hearing assessment
- Speech, language, and communication assessments
- Developmental and sensorimotor testing
- Neurologic exam, including muscle tone and reflexes
- Examination for dysmorphic features consistent with genetic disorders such as fragile X syndrome and Angelman syndrome
- Wood lamp skin exam to rule out tuberous sclerosis

DIFFERENTIAL DIAGNOSIS

- Other mental and CNS disorders
- Obsessive-compulsive disorder
- Elective mutism
- Language disorder/hearing impairment
- Intellectual disability/global developmental delay
- Stereotyped movement disorder
- Severe early deprivation/reactive attachment disorder
- Anxiety disorder
- Social communication disorder
- Developmental language disorder

DIAGNOSTIC TESTS & INTERPRETATION

- The Modified Checklist for Autism in Toddlers (M-CHAT) is the most commonly used test to screen for ASDs in 16 to 30 months of age (https://m-chat.org/) (1)[B].
- The Modified Checklist for Autism in Toddlers Revised, Follow-up (M-CHAT-R/F) shows improved PPV and lower false-positive rate in children aged 16 to 30 months (http://mchatscreen.com/mchat-rf/) (1)[B].
- Screening Tool for Autism in Two-Year-Olds (STAT) shows promising evidence as level 2 screening to detect 2-year-olds with autism with other developmental disorders (1)[B].
- Social Communication Questionnaire (SCQ) (formerly Autism Screening Questionnaire)—used with children age 4+ years (1)[B]

Initial Tests (lab, imaging)

- Chromosomal microarray (CMA), DNA analysis, and karyotype testing (2)[B]
- Lead and PKU screening
- Metabolic testing if signs of lethargy, limited endurance, unusual habits, hypotonia, recurrent vomiting and dehydration, developmental regression, or specific food intolerance
- Consider MRI if focal neurologic symptoms.

Follow-Up Tests & Special Considerations

- Children with ASD have the same general health care needs as other children and should receive the same preventative care and screening.
- Follow-up appointments and testing recommended as indicated for comorbidities
- Consider additional hearing tests such as audiometry and brainstem auditory evoked response (BAER) or consultation to audiology.

- Comprehensive speech and language evaluation
- Consider genetics consult.
- Evaluation by multidisciplinary team: includes a psychiatrist, neurologist, psychologist, and other autism specialists
- Intellectual level needs to be established and monitored
- Tests used to follow autism are the following:
  – Autism Behavior Checklist (ABC)
  – Gilliam Autism Rating Scale (GARS)
  – Childhood Autism Rating Scale (CARS)
  – Autism Diagnostic Interview-Revised (ADI-R)
  – Autism Diagnostic Observation Schedule-Generic (ADOS-G) Imaging

Diagnostic Procedures/Other
EEG if displaying signs or symptoms suggestive of seizures

 ## TREATMENT

GENERAL MEASURES
- Early intensive behavioral intervention (EIBI) involving treatment for at least 25 hours per week to address social communication, language, play skills, and maladaptive behavior leads to improvement in cognitive ability, language, and adaptive skills (3)[A].
- Cognitive-behavioral therapy (CBT) has been shown to substantially reduce anxiety in older children with ASD who have average to above-average IQ (3)[A].
- Targeted play therapy has led to improvements in early social communication skills (4)[A].
- Programs designed for training and education of parents improve language skills and decrease disruptive behavior in children with ASD (4)[A].
- Core features of a successful education program (4)[A]
  – High staff–student ratio 1:2
  – Individualized programming
  – Specialized teacher training with ongoing evaluation of teachers and programs
  – 25 hours a week minimum of specialized services
  – A structured routine environment
  – Ongoing program evaluation and adjustment with routine functional analysis of individual child behavioral problems
  – Family involvement

MEDICATION
- Autism behavior issues should be managed with maximal behavioral management.
- No true first-line medical therapy; medications used to treat targeted symptoms

First Line
- Currently, the only FDA-approved psychotropic medications for ASD are risperidone and aripiprazole. Risperidone (approved age >5 years; oral; initial dose: 0.01 mg/kg/dose for 2 days and then 0.02 mg/kg/dose once daily; max 0.06 mg/kg/dose) has shown short-term efficacy for treatment for irritability, repetitious behaviors, and social withdrawal (4)[B]. Aripiprazole (approved ages 6 to 17 years; oral; initial dose: 2 mg daily for 2 days, then 5 mg daily for 2 days, and then 10 mg daily; max 30 mg/day) has shown efficacy for treating short-term irritability, hyperactivity, and repetitive movements (5)[A].
- Stimulants (such as methylphenidate) have been efficacious in treating concomitant symptoms of ADHD such as impulsivity, hyperactivity, and inattention; however, the magnitude of response is less than in typically developing children, and adverse effects are more frequent (5)[A].

- SSRIs have limited evidence for autism. It has shown help in reducing ritualistic behavior and improving mood and language skills; initial choice for anxiety and depressive mood (5)[A]
- Melatonin used for patients with concomitant sleep disorders has shown mixed efficacy (5)[A].

ISSUES FOR REFERRAL
- Refer early to
  – Early learning for evaluation of behavior and language, genetic counseling, and audiology
- Consider referrals to psychiatry, ophthalmology, otolaryngology, neurology, and nutrition.
- Refer family members to parent support groups and respite programs.

COMPLEMENTARY & ALTERNATIVE MEDICINE
- Medications such as secretin, IVIG, chelation therapy, vitamin B_6, and magnesium have shown no benefit in ASD and may carry significant risks (6)[A].
- Therapies such as auditory integration therapy, facilitated communication, gluten- or casein-free diets, and hyperbaric oxygen have shown no benefit (6)[A].
- Therapies such as music, massage, therapeutic horseback riding, and other pet therapies would merit further review (6)[A].

 ## ONGOING CARE

FOLLOW-UP RECOMMENDATIONS
Patient Monitoring
- Constant monitoring by caregivers
- Reevaluation every 6 to 12 months by physician for seizures, sleep and nutritional problems, and to follow-up prescribed medical management
- Intellectual and language testing every 2 years in childhood

DIET
- There is insufficient evidence for recommendations of any certain dietary modifications for ASD.
- Gluten- or casein-free diets have shown no benefit across several randomized clinical trials (6)[A].

PATIENT EDUCATION
- Refer parents to the partners in policymaking course (https://partnersonlinecourses.com/) to learn how to advocate for their child and themselves.
- Economic costs
  – An additional $17,000 to $21,000 is an estimated cost for raising an ASD child.
  – Due to caretaker burden, family earnings are found to be 28% less among families with ASD compared to children without health conditions.

PROGNOSIS
- Prognosis influenced by IQ, early intervention, strength of early language skills, and psychiatric comorbidities
- The general expected course is for a lifelong need for supervised structured care; however, some patients will develop gainful employment, independent living, and social relationships.

COMPLICATIONS
- Increasing incidents of seizure disorders in up to 1 in 4 children
- Increased risk for physical and sexual abuse
- With pica, increased risk of lead poisoning
- Increased risk for GI symptoms, including weight abnormalities and abnormal stool patterns

REFERENCES
1. Zwaigenbaum L, Bauman ML, Fein D, et al. Early screening of autism spectrum disorders: recommendations for practice and research. *Pediatrics*. 2015;136(Suppl 1):S41–S59.
2. Battaglia A, Carey JC. Etiologic yield of autism spectrum disorders: a prospective study. *Am J Med Genet C Semin Med Genet*. 2006;142C(1):3–7.
3. Maglione MA, Gans D, Das L, et al; for Technical Expert Panel, HRSA Autism Intervention Research–Behavioral (AIR-B) Network. Nonmedical interventions for children with ASD: recommended guidelines and further research needs. *Pediatrics*. 2012;130(Suppl 2):S169–S178.
4. Weitlauf AS, McPheeters ML, Peters B, et al. *Therapies for Children with Autism Spectrum Disorder: Behavioral Interventions Update*. Rockville, MD: Agency for Healthcare Research and Quality; 2014. AHRQ Report No. 14-EHC036-EF.
5. Parikh MS, Kolevzon A, Hollander E. Psychopharmacology of aggression in children and adolescents with autism: a critical review of efficacy and tolerability. *J Child Adolesc Psychopharmacol*. 2008;18(2):157–158.
6. Levy SE, Hyman SL. Complementary and alternative medicine treatments for children with autism spectrum disorders. *Child Adolesc Psychiatr Clin N Am*. 2008;17(4):803–820.

ADDITIONAL READING
- Myers SM, Johnson CP; for American Academy of Pediatrics Council on Children with Disabilities. Management of children with autism spectrum disorders. *Pediatrics*. 2007;120(5):1162–1182.
- Sanchack K, Thomas C. Autism spectrum disorder: primary care principles. *Am Fam Physician*. 2016;94(12):972–979.

 ## SEE ALSO

Algorithm: Intellectual Disability

 ## CODES

ICD10
- F84.0 Autistic disorder
- F84.5 Asperger's syndrome
- F84.3 Other childhood disintegrative disorder

CLINICAL PEARLS
ALARM mnemonic from the American Academy of Pediatrics (AAP)
- **A**SD is prevalent (screen ALL children between 18 and 24 months).
- **L**isten to parents when they feel something is wrong.
- **A**ct early: Screen all children who fall behind in language and social developmental milestones (use early learning to help with evaluation).
- **R**efer to multidisciplinary teams (speech and language evaluation, genetic screening, social support groups).
- **M**onitor support for patient and families.

BABESIOSIS

Frederick W. Nielson, MD

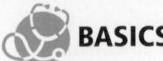

BASICS

DESCRIPTION
- Rare tick-borne hemolytic disease caused by intraerythrocytic protozoan parasites of the genus *Babesia*
- Infrequently reported outside the United States
  - Sporadic cases have been reported from
    - France, Italy, the United Kingdom, Ireland, the former Soviet Union, Mexico (1)
    - China, Italy, and Turkey have reported a reemergence of cases.
  - In the United States, infections have been reported in many states. The most endemic areas are:
    - Islands off the coast of Massachusetts (including Nantucket and Martha's Vineyard)
    - New York (including Long Island, Shelter Island, and Fire Island); Connecticut
    - Asymptomatic infection common in these areas (1)
- Incubation period varies from 5 to 33 days:
  - Most patients do not recall specific tick exposure.
  - After transfusion of infected blood, the incubation period can be up to 9 weeks (1).
- System(s) affected: cardiovascular, gastrointestinal, hemic/lymphatic/immunologic, musculoskeletal, nervous, pulmonary, renal/urologic

Pediatric Considerations
Transplacental and perinatal transmission rarely reported (1,2)

Geriatric Considerations
- Morbidity and mortality higher in patients >60 years
- Cases more common in patients >70 years who have medical comorbidities

EPIDEMIOLOGY
Babesiosis affects patients of all ages. Most patients present in their 40s or 50s (1).

Incidence
- Cases reported to the CDC appear to be on the rise from 911 in 2012 to 1,744 in 2014.
- Prevalence is difficult to estimate due to lack of surveillance and asymptomatic infections.
- Transfusion-associated babesiosis and transplacental/perinatal transmission have been reported (1).
- In patients at high risk for tick-borne diseases, seroconversion data show antibodies to *Babesia microti* in 7 of 671 individuals (1%) (1).

ETIOLOGY AND PATHOPHYSIOLOGY
- *B. microti* (in the United States) and *Babesia divergens* and *Babesia bovis* (in Europe) cause most human infections (1). *B. divergens* and a new strain *Babesia duncani* appear to be more virulent. Other species identified in case reports. All share morphologic, antigenic, and genetic characteristics (1).
- Ixodid (hard-bodied) ticks, particularly *Ixodes dammini* (*Ixodes scapularis*: deer tick) and *Ixodes ricinus*, are the primary vectors.

- The white-footed mouse is the primary reservoir.
- Infection is passed to humans through the saliva of a nymphal-stage tick during a blood meal. Sporozoites introduced at the time of the bite enter red blood cells and form merozoites through binary fission (classic morphology on blood smear). Humans are a dead-end host for *B. microti*.

RISK FACTORS
- Residing in endemic areas
- Asplenia
- Immunocompromised state

GENERAL PREVENTION
- Avoid endemic regions during the peak transmission months of May to September (1).
- Appropriate insect repellent is advised during outdoor activities, especially in wooded or grassy areas:
  - 10–35% N,N-diethyl-meta-toluamide (DEET) provides adequate protection (1).
- Early removal of ticks—daily skin checks
- Examine pets for ticks; flea/tick control for pets

COMMONLY ASSOCIATED CONDITIONS
- Coinfection with *Borrelia burgdorferi* and *B. microti*, particularly in endemic areas (1). Coinfection rates may be as high as ~27%.
- Coinfection with *Ehrlichia* (1)

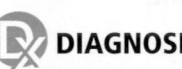

DIAGNOSIS

HISTORY
- The tick must remain attached for at least 24 hours before the transmission of *B. microti* occurs (1).
- Travel/exposure history
- Comorbidities (immunosuppression, chronic disease)
- Fever (68–89%), fatigue (78–79%), chills (39–68%), sweats (41–56%), headache (32–75%), myalgia (32–37%), anorexia (24–25%), cough (17–23%), arthralgias (17–32%), nausea (9–22%). Other symptoms reported by case reports include abdominal pain, vomiting, diarrhea, and emotional lability.

PHYSICAL EXAM
- High fever (up to 40°C [104°F])
- Hemodynamic instability (shock in extremely ill)
- Hepatomegaly and splenomegaly (mild if noted)
- Rash (uncommon)
- CNS involvement includes headache, photophobia, neck and back stiffness, altered sensorium, and emotional lability
- Jaundice and dark urine may develop later in course of illness.

DIFFERENTIAL DIAGNOSIS
- Bacterial sepsis
- Hepatitis
- Lyme disease; ehrlichiosis
- Leishmaniasis
- Malaria
- HIV; EBV
- HELLP syndrome (in pregnancy)

DIAGNOSTIC TESTS & INTERPRETATION

Initial Tests (lab, imaging)
- Diagnosis requires a high index of clinical suspicion. Nonspecific laboratory clues include evidence of mild to severe hemolytic anemia, normal to slightly depressed leukocyte count (1), elevated LDH or transaminase level, elevated BUN and Cr, proteinuria with hemoglobinuria (1,2).
- Definitive diagnosis is made by blood smear.
  - Wright- or Giemsa-stained peripheral blood smear demonstrates intraerythrocytic parasites (2)[B].
  - Dividing "cross-like" tetrads of merozoites (Maltese cross) are pathognomonic (2).
  - Serial blood smears may be required (low parasite load early in the illness) (2).
  - Can be confused with *Plasmodium falciparum* on peripheral smear
- If blood smears are negative but suspicion remains, IgM serologies through indirect immunofluorescent antibody testing (IFAT) for *B. microti* antigen:
  - Positive titer results vary by lab. Titers of >1:64 or a 4-fold increase from baseline are consistent with *B. microti* infection (3). Titers may be >1:1,024 in acute infection (2)[B]. Titers often elevated 8 to 12 months and can persist for years.
  - In New England, seroprevalence is 0.5–16% (3).
- Detection of *B. microti* by polymerase chain reaction (PCR) is more sensitive and equally specific in acute cases. PCR can also be used to monitor disease progression (2)[B]. Newer real-time PCR tests have a sensitivity and specificity approaching 100%.
- If lab tests are inconclusive and infection is strongly suspected, inoculation of laboratory animals with patient blood can reveal *B. microti* organisms in the blood of the animal within 2 to 4 weeks (2).

Follow-Up Tests & Special Considerations
Monitoring intraerythrocytic parasitemia helps guide treatment (4)[C].

Diagnostic Procedures/Other
Based on blood smear, history, and epidemiologic information (2)

TREATMENT

GENERAL MEASURES
- In areas endemic for Lyme disease and ehrlichiosis, consider adding doxycycline (Vibramycin) 100 mg BID PO to empirically treat coinfection until serologic testing is complete (1)[C].
- Drug resistance has emerged in severely immunocompromised patients (2).
- Consider treating asymptomatic patients if parasitemia persists for >3 months; otherwise, do not treat in absence of symptoms (1),(4)[C].

MEDICATION
First Line
- Mild to moderate infection with *B. microti*: 7 to 10 days of atovaquone 750 mg PO BID plus azithromycin 500 to 1,000 mg/day PO on day 1, followed by 250 mg/day. Pediatrics: atovaquone 20 mg/kg (max 750 mg) BID and azithromycin 10 mg/kg (max 500 mg) on day 1 and then 5 mg/kg (max 250 mg) (4)[B]. For severe *B. microti* infection: oral quinine 650 mg TID or QID plus oral clindamycin 600 mg TID for 7 to 10 days. Pediatrics: clindamycin 7 to 10 mg/kg (max 600 mg) TID or QID and quinine 8 mg/kg (max 650 mg) TID. IV formulations can be used (4)[C].
- Persistent or relapsing babesiosis: Treat for 6 weeks, including 2 weeks after *Babesia* is no longer detected on blood smear (5)[B].

Second Line
- Combination of quinine sulfate 650 mg PO TID and clindamycin 600 mg PO TID or 1.2 g parenterally BID for 7 to 10 days is the most commonly used treatment. Pediatric: quinine 8 mg/kg (max 650 mg) every 6 to 8 hours for 7 to 10 days and clindamycin 7 to 10 mg/kg (max 600 mg) PO q6–8h for 7 to 10 days. Some experts prefer this regimen for severe infections (4)[C].
- Other drugs including tetracycline, primaquine, sulfadiazine (Microsulfon), and sulfadoxine/pyrimethamine (Fansidar) have been evaluated. Results vary. Pentamidine (Pentam) is moderately effective in diminishing symptoms and decreasing parasitemia (1)[C].

ALERT
Clindamycin can lead to *Clostridium difficile*–associated diarrhea.

ISSUES FOR REFERRAL
Severe disease: Consider consultation with hematology and infectious disease for exchange transfusion in extremely ill patients (blood parasitemia >10%, massive hemolysis, and asplenia) (2)[C].

 ONGOING CARE

FOLLOW-UP RECOMMENDATIONS
- If left untreated, silent babesiosis may persist for months or years (2).
- Of 139 hospitalized cases from 1982 to 1993:
  - 9 patients (7%) died.
  - 25% were admitted to the ICU.
  - 25% hospitalized for >14 days
- Alkaline phosphatase levels >125 U/L, WBC counts >5 × 10⁹/L, history of cardiac abnormality, history of splenectomy, presence of heart murmur, and parasitemia of 4% or higher are associated with disease severity.

Patient Monitoring
The need for monitoring depends on disease severity. Severe infections: Follow hematocrit and parasitemia levels until clinical improvement, and parasitemia is <5%. Mild to moderate: Expect clinical improvement within 48 hours and complete resolution within 3 months (4)[C].

COMPLICATIONS
- Many remain asymptomatic.
- Complications in hospitalized patients: CHF (12%), DIC (18%), ARDS (21%), renal failure (6%), coma/lethargy (9%), death (9%)
- Other reported complications include neutropenia and myocardial infarction.
- In asplenic patients, warm autoimmune hemolytic anemia has been reported.

REFERENCES
1. Mylonakis E. When to suspect and how to monitor babesiosis. *Am Fam Physician*. 2001;63(10):1969–1974.
2. Vannier E, Krause PJ. Human babesiosis. *N Engl J Med*. 2012;366(25):2397–2407.
3. Vannier EG, Diuk-Wasser MA, Ben Mamoun C, et al. Babesiosis. *Infect Dis Clin North Am*. 2015;29(2):357–370.
4. Wormser GP, Dattwyler RJ, Shapiro ED, et al. The clinical assessment, treatment, and prevention of Lyme disease, human granulocytic anaplasmosis, and babesiosis: clinical practice guidelines by the Infectious Diseases Society of America. *Clin Infect Dis*. 2006;43(9):1089–1134.
5. Krause PJ, Gewurz BE, Hill D, et al. Persistent and relapsing babesiosis in immunocompromised patients. *Clin Infect Dis*. 2008;46(3):370–376.

ADDITIONAL READING
- Curcio SR, Tria LP, Gucwa AL. Seroprevalence of *Babesia microti* in individuals with Lyme disease. *Vector Borne Zoonotic Dis*. 2016;16(12):737–743.
- Lempereur L, Beck R, Fonseca I, et al. Guidelines for the detection of Babesia and Theileria parasites. *Vector Borne Zoonotic Dis*. 2017;17(1):51–65.
- Mosqueda J, Olvera-Ramirez A, Aguilar-Tipacamu G, et al. Current advances in detection and treatment of babesiosis. *Curr Med Chem*. 2012;19(10):1504–1518.
- Teal AE, Habura A, Ennis J, et al. A new real-time PCR assay for improved detection of the parasite *Babesia microti*. *J Clin Microbiol*. 2012;50(3):903–908.
- White DJ, Talarico J, Chang HG, et al. Human babesiosis in New York state: review of 139 hospitalized cases and analysis of prognostic factors. *Arch Intern Med*. 1998;158(19):2149–2154.
- Woolley AE, Montgomery MW, Savage WJ, et al. Post-babesiosis warm autoimmune hemolytic anemia. *N Engl J Med*. 2017;376(10):939–946.

 CODES

ICD10
B60.0 Babesiosis

CLINICAL PEARLS
- Ticks must remain in place for 24 hours to transmit infection—encourage daily "tick checks" if people are exposed in high-risk areas.
- Most patients do not recall tick exposure, and incubation can last up to a month.
- Left untreated, silent babesial infection may persist for months or years.
- First-line treatment for mild or moderate disease is atovaquone plus azithromycin.
- Patients with mild-to-moderate disease should show clinical improvement within 48 hours after starting therapy. Symptoms should fully resolve in 3 months.
- Coinfection with *B. burgdorferi* and *Ehrlichia* species is common in endemic areas. In areas endemic for Lyme disease and ehrlichiosis, consider adding doxycycline until serologic testing is completed.

BACK PAIN, LOW

Michael Maddaleni, MD • J. Herbert Stevenson, MD

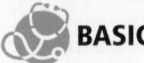

BASICS

DESCRIPTION
- Low back pain (LBP) is extremely common and includes a wide range of symptoms involving the lumbosacral spine and pelvic girdle.
- Characterized by duration or associated symptoms
- Duration (1)[A]
  - Acute (<6 weeks)
  - Subacute (>6 weeks but <3 months)
  - Chronic (>3 months)
- Associated symptoms (1)[A]
  - Localized/nonspecific "mechanical" LBP
  - Back pain with lower extremity symptoms
  - Systemic and visceral symptoms
- A specific cause is not found for most patients with LBP. Most cases resolve in 4 to 6 weeks.
- Rule out "red" flag symptoms indicating the need for immediate intervention.
- System(s) affected: musculoskeletal, neurologic
- Synonym(s): lumbago, lumbar sprain/strain, low back syndrome

EPIDEMIOLOGY
Incidence
- 1-year incidence for first episode: 6.3–15.3% (2)
- 1-year incidence for *any* episode: 1.5%–36% (2)
- A very common primary care complaint (1)

Prevalence
- Lifetime prevalence: 84% (1)
- Global point prevalence: 9% (1)
- Chronic point prevalence in United States: 13.1%
- Predominant sex: male = female
- Age: The highest incidence is in the 3rd decade (20 to 29 years); overall prevalence increases with age until age 65 years and then declines (1).

ETIOLOGY AND PATHOPHYSIOLOGY
LBP can be commonly due to muscle spasm/tension. Estimated 39% of chronic LBP due to disk degeneration. 30% estimated to be from facet joint syndrome. Other possibilities include sacroiliac injuries/degeneration and spinal stenosis. Age-related degenerative changes of the lumbosacral spine and atrophy of supporting musculature may contribute as well (2)[A].

RISK FACTORS
- Age (1)[A]
- Activity (lifting, sudden twisting, bending) (1)[A]
- Obesity (1)[A]
- Sedentary lifestyle (1)[A]
- Physically strenuous work (1)[A]
- Psychosocial factors—anxiety, depression, stress (1)[A]
- Genetic factors (2)
- Heavy operating equipment (2)
- Poor flexibility (2)
- Smoking (1)[A]

GENERAL PREVENTION
- Maintain normal weight (1)[A].
- Adequate physical fitness and activity (1)[A]
- Stress reduction (1)[A]
- Proper lifting technique and good posture
- Smoking cessation
- There is insufficient evidence to recommend for or against routine preventive measures in adults.

DIAGNOSIS

HISTORY
- Onset of pain (sudden or gradual) (1)
- Pain from spinal structures (musculature, ligaments, facet joints and disks) can refer to the thigh region but rarely below the knee. However, facet pain most commonly radiates to sacroiliac joint/PSIS region (1).
- Sacroiliac pain often refers to the thigh and can radiate below the knee (1).
- Irritation, impingement, or compression of lumbar nerve roots often results in more leg pain than back pain (1).
- Pain from the L1–L3 nerve roots radiates to the hip and/or thigh, whereas pain from the L4–S1 nerve roots radiates below the knee.
- Red flags
  - Recent trauma
  - Neurologic deficits
    ○ Bowel/bladder incontinence or urinary retention
    ○ Saddle anesthesia
    ○ Weakness, falls
  - Night pain, sweats, fever, weight loss
  - Age >70 years with or without trauma
  - Age >50 years with minor trauma
  - History of cancer
  - Osteoporosis
  - Immunosuppression, prolonged glucocorticoid use
- Yellow flags (predicting poor long-term prognosis):
  - Lack of social support
  - Unsupportive work environment
  - Depression and/or anxiety
  - Abuse of alcohol or other substances
  - History of physical or sexual abuse
  - Excessive mobility in spine or other joints (2)
  - Fear of reinjury, movement, or pain (2)
  - Low expectation of recovery (2)
  - Passive coping style (2)
- Pain can be provoked with motion: flexion–extension, side-bending rotation, sitting, standing, and lifting. Pain often relieved with rest.
- Radicular pain may radiate to buttocks, thighs, and lower legs.

Pediatric Considerations
Back pain is not normal in children and must be carefully evaluated. Trauma from high impact or hyperextension sports would be the leading cause requiring further evaluation.

PHYSICAL EXAM
- Observe gait, positioning, and facial expressions.
- Test lumbar spine range of motion.
- Evaluate for point tenderness or muscle spasm.
- Evaluate for signs of muscle atrophy.
- Complete thorough physical exam to assess for wide differential (full differential listed in subsequent section).
  - Completely evaluate reflexes, strength, pulses, sensation.
  - Slump test: Have patient sit on table and slump shoulders forward. Then have patient touch chin to chest and attempt to have them extend one leg at a time. Do this while continually reassessing for symptom reproduction; can be indicative of disk herniation
  - Straight leg test: Raise the patient's leg straight while the patient is lying down. Keep the knee straight. For more specificity, dorsiflex ankle while lifting leg. This can also evaluate for herniated disk.
  - Evaluate for saddle anesthesia, anal wink reflex.
  - Straight leg test
  - FABER and FADIR test of hips bilaterally
  - Evaluate for psychological distress that may be contributing.
  - Stork test: Stand on one leg with opposite hip held in flexion. Extend back. Pain in lumbosacral area is a positive test—consider spondylolisthesis versus facet OA.
  - Waddell sign—overreaction to physical exam, widespread tenderness—may indicate psychological component/underlying depression

DIFFERENTIAL DIAGNOSIS
- Localized/nonspecific "mechanical" LBP (87%) (1)[A]
  - Lumbar strain/sprain (70%)
  - Disk/facet degeneration (10%)
  - Osteoporotic compression fracture (4%)
  - Spondylolisthesis (2%)
  - Severe scoliosis, kyphosis
  - Asymmetric transitional vertebrae (<1%)
  - Traumatic fracture (<1%)
- Back pain with lower extremity symptoms (7%) (1)[A]
  - Disk herniation (4%)
  - Spinal stenosis (3%)
- Systemic and visceral symptoms (1)[A]
  - Neoplasia (0.7%)
    ○ Multiple myeloma; metastatic carcinoma
    ○ Lymphoma/leukemia
    ○ Spinal cord tumors, retroperitoneal tumors
  - Infection (0.01%)
    ○ Osteomyelitis
    ○ Septic discitis
    ○ Paraspinous abscess; epidural abscess
    ○ Shingles
  - Inflammatory disease (0.03%)
    ○ Ankylosing spondylitis, psoriatic spondylitis
    ○ Reactive arthritis
    ○ Inflammatory bowel disease
  - Visceral disease (0.05%)
    ○ Prostatitis
    ○ Endometriosis
    ○ Chronic pelvic inflammatory disease
    ○ Nephrolithiasis, pyelonephritis
    ○ Perinephric abscess
    ○ Aortic aneurysm
    ○ Pancreatitis; cholecystitis
    ○ Penetrating ulcer
  - Other
    ○ Osteochondrosis
    ○ Paget disease
    ○ Cauda equina syndrome

DIAGNOSTIC TESTS & INTERPRETATION
Initial Tests (lab, imaging)
- No clinical benefit of routine imaging (2)
  - Imaging only recommended for progressive, severe neurologic deficits or in the setting of "red flags" (2)
  - Significant amount of false positives; evidence of possible herniated disk material seen in 20–76% of asymptomatic patients on CT, MRI, myelography (2)
- X-ray of the lumbar spine (1,3)[A]
  - Not recommended for initial presentation without red flags. Defer films for 6 weeks, unless there is a history of acute trauma (fall, etc.) or high risk of disease.
  - Useful to evaluate bony etiology (e.g., fracture)

- MRI of the lumbar spine (1,3)[A] for patients presenting with neurologic deficits, failure to improve with 6 weeks of conservative treatment, or if there is a strong suspicion of cancer or cauda equina syndrome
  - Useful for suspected herniated disk, nerve root compression, or metastatic disease
- CT scan of the lumbar spine (1,3)[A]
  - Appropriate alternative to MRI for patient with pacemaker, metallic hardware, or other contraindication to MRI
- Labs are unnecessary with initial presentation if no related red flags, signs, or symptoms (1,3)[A].
- If infection or bone marrow neoplasm is suspected, consider (1,3)[A]
  - Complete blood count (CBC) with differential
  - Erythrocyte sedimentation rate (ESR)
  - C-reactive protein (CRP) level

Diagnostic Procedures/Other
Neurosurgical consult for acute neurologic deficits or suspected cauda equina syndrome (1)[A]

 TREATMENT

The primary goal is to provide supportive care and allow return to functional activity. Patients should be aware of alarm symptoms to prompt a return visit.

MEDICATION

First Line
- Physical therapy
- Patient education
  - Reassure patients that pain is usually self-limited; treatment should relieve pain and improve function.
  - Encouraging activity as tolerated leads to quicker recovery.
  - Early intervention with formal physical therapy (2)
- Medications (1,3)[A]
  - Acetaminophen 325 to 650 mg PO q4–6h PRN pain (max 4 g/day)
  - NSAIDs
    ○ Ibuprofen 400 to 600 mg PO 3 to 4 times daily (max 3,200 mg/day)
    ○ Naproxen 250 to 500 mg PO q12h (max 1,500 mg/day)
  - Manual medicine (4)[A], osteopathic manipulative treatments (OMT): myofascial, counterstrain, bilateral ligamentous techniques as well as muscle energy, if tolerated
- Obstetric considerations (5)[B]
  - Use medications cautiously in pregnancy—benefit must clearly outweigh risk.
- OMT and chiropractic care may be used in a multidisciplinary approach; may be used in the general population as well as the obstetric patient

Second Line
- Second-line therapy for moderate to severe pain (1,3)[A]
  - Cyclobenzaprine 5 to 10 mg PO up to TID PRN (max 30 mg/day)
  - Tizanidine 2 mg PO up to TID PRN
  - Opioid use (≤4 days, maximum) for LBP is clinical judgment; however, studies show opioids in the setting of LBP do not have a significantly better effect than NSAIDs plus placebo or placebo alone (4)[A].
  - Recent practice shows that physicians will prescribe Valium in people already taking naproxen—recent study shows that adding Valium to a naproxen regimen does not improve disability or pain scores.

- Other treatments (1,3)[A]
  - Antidepressants (1,3)[A]
    ○ Tricyclic antidepressants (amitriptyline, nortriptyline, desipramine) have been shown in randomized trials to provide a small pain reduction in patients. No clear evidence that SSRIs are more effective than placebo in cases of chronic LBP. Treatment of concurrent depression may have positive effect on LBP.
- Injections (5)[A]
  - Facet: Therapeutic facet joint nerve blocks in the lumbar spine and lumbar intra-articular injections have all shown benefit.
  - Epidural: provide short-term relief of persistent pain associated with documented radicular symptoms caused by herniated disk (1,3,5)[A]
  - Lumbar radiofrequency: Recent RCT showed no clinically significant improvement of LBP when radiofrequency was done with exercise program versus exercise program alone (6).

Geriatric Considerations
- Older persons taking nonselective NSAIDs should use a proton pump inhibitor or misoprostol for gastrointestinal protection.
- Patients taking a COX-2 selective inhibitor with aspirin should use a proton pump inhibitor or misoprostol for gastrointestinal protection.
- Age-related decline in cytochrome P450 function and polypharmacy (common in elderly patients) increases risk for adverse medication reactions.

COMPLEMENTARY & ALTERNATIVE MEDICINE
- Recent guideline updates suggest not recommending acupuncture.
- Yoga can help with chronic LBP (1,3)[A].

 ONGOING CARE

FOLLOW-UP RECOMMENDATIONS
- Regular exercise to manage weight and control symptoms (3)[A]
- Educate patients regarding chronicity, recurrence, and red flags (3)[A].

Patient Monitoring
- Reassurance is important. Follow up within 2 to 4 weeks of initial presentation to monitor progress. Most patients spontaneously improve.
  - Assess severity and quality of pain, range of motion, and other historical features (red flags).
- Reevaluate for organic causes if no adequate improvement.

COMPLICATIONS
- Regular NSAID use can increase risk of gastrointestinal toxicity and nephrotoxicity (1)[A].
- Acetaminophen has potential hepatotoxicity (1)[A].
- Centrally acting skeletal muscle relaxants and opioid agonists carry the risk for sedation, confusion, dependence, and abuse (1)[A].

REFERENCES
1. Golob AL, Wipf JE. Low back pain. *Med Clin North Am*. 2014;98(3):405–428.
2. Delitto A, George SZ, Van Dillen LR, et al; for Orthopaedic Section of the American Physical Therapy Association. Low back pain. *J Orthop Sports Phys Ther*. 2012;42(4):A1–A57.

3. Chaparro LE, Furlan AD, Deshpande A, et al. Opioids compared with placebo or other treatments for chronic low back pain: an update of the Cochrane Review. *Spine (Phila Pa 1976)*. 2014;39(7):556–563.
4. Friedman BW, Dym AA, Davitt M, et al. Naproxen with cyclobenzaprine, oxycodone/acetaminophen, or placebo for treating acute low back pain: a randomized clinical trial. *JAMA*. 2015;314(15):1572–1580.
5. Manchikanti L, Kaye AD, Boswell MV, et al. A systematic review and best evidence synthesis of the effectiveness of therapeutic facet joint interventions in managing chronic spinal pain. *Pain Physician*. 2015;18(4):E535–E582.
6. Kapural L, Provenzano D, Narouze S. RE: Juch JNS, et al. Effect of radiofrequency denervation on pain intensity among patients with chronic low back pain: the mint randomized clinical trials. JAMA 2017;318(1):68–81. *Neuromodulation*. 2017;20(8):844.

ADDITIONAL READING
- Andronis L, Kinghorn P, Qiao S, et al. Cost-effectiveness of non-invasive and non-pharmacological interventions for low back pain: a systematic literature review. *Appl Health Econ Health Policy*. 2017;15(2):173–201.
- de Leon-Casasola OA. Opioids for chronic pain: new evidence, new strategies, safe prescribing. *Am J Med*. 2013;126(3 Suppl 1):S3–S11.
- Friedman BW, Irizarry E, Solorzano C, et al. Diazepam is no better than placebo when added to naproxen for acute low back pain. *Ann Emerg Med*. 2017;70(2):169–176.e1.
- George JW, Skaggs CD, Thompson PA, et al. A randomized controlled trial comparing a multimodal intervention and standard obstetrics care for low back and pelvic pain in pregnancy. *Am J Obstet Gynecol*. 2013;208(4):295.e1–295.e7.

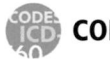 **SEE ALSO**

Algorithm: Low Back Pain, Acute

CODES

ICD10
- M54.5 Low back pain
- G89.29 Other chronic pain
- M53.3 Sacrococcygeal disorders, not elsewhere classified

CLINICAL PEARLS
- LBP is one of the most common complaints in primary care. Most cases resolve spontaneously within 4 to 12 weeks of onset.
- Assess for red flag symptoms in every patient, such as bowel/bladder incontinence, history of cancer, or recent trauma.
- Labs and imaging studies are unnecessary for most cases of back pain if no red flag symptoms are present. Symptoms typically will resolve in 6 weeks or less.
- In the absence of red flags, physical activity as tolerated speeds recovery.
- Early intervention with formal physical therapy can reduce symptoms, strengthen musculature, and speed up recovery.

BACTERIURIA, ASYMPTOMATIC

Onameyore Utuama, MD, MPH • Pius Ogenyi Ameh, BM, BCh • Kitty Carter-Wicker, MD

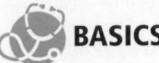 BASICS

DESCRIPTION
Asymptomatic bacteriuria (ASB) is specific bacterial growth $\geq 10^5$ CFU/mL in one and two consecutive midstream urine samples for men and women, respectively >18 years. This definition applies to individuals with no clinical symptoms (1).

EPIDEMIOLOGY
Incidence
- Premenopausal females: 1–5%
- Pregnancy: 2–10%
- Older females and males: 4–19%
- Institutionalized older population: 15–50%

Prevalence
- Variable, increased with age, female gender, sexual activity, and presence of genitourinary (GU) abnormalities
- Pregnancy: 2–10%
- Short- and long-term indwelling catheter 9–23% and 100%, respectively
- Long-term care residents in women 25–50% and men 15–40%

ETIOLOGY AND PATHOPHYSIOLOGY
- Microbiology is similar to that of other UTI, with bacteria originating from periurethral area, vagina, or gut.
- Organisms are less virulent in ASB than those causing UTI.
- The most common organism is *Escherichia coli.* Other common organisms are *Klebsiella pneumoniae, Enterobacter, Proteus mirabilis, Staphylococcus aureus,* group B *Streptococcus* (GBS), and *Enterococcus.*

Genetics
Genetic variations that reduce toll-like receptor-4 function (*TLR4*) have been associated with ASB by lowering innate immune response and delaying bacterial clearance.

RISK FACTORS
- Pregnancy
- Older age
- Female gender

- Sexual activity, use of diaphragm with spermicide
- GU abnormalities: neurogenic bladder, urinary retention, urinary catheter use (indwelling, intermittent, or condom catheter)
- Institutionalized elderly population
- Diabetes mellitus
- Immunocompromised status
- Spinal cord injuries or functional impairment
- Hemodialysis

COMMONLY ASSOCIATED CONDITIONS
Depends on the risk factors

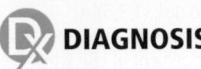 DIAGNOSIS

HISTORY
- Asymptomatic
- Lack of symptoms attributable to UTI such as fever, acute dysuria (<1 week), new or worsening urinary urgency/frequency/incontinence, or acute gross hematuria

PHYSICAL EXAM
- Afebrile
- No suprapubic and costovertebral angle tenderness

DIFFERENTIAL DIAGNOSIS
- UTI
- Uncomplicated cystitis
- Contaminated urine specimen

DIAGNOSTIC TESTS & INTERPRETATION
Initial Tests (lab, imaging)
- Urinalysis (UA):
  - The presence of pyuria, leukocyte esterase, and nitrite in ASB is common.
- Urine culture
- Screening urine culture in asymptomatic patients is indicated in only two conditions:
  - Pregnancy: screening between 12 and 16 weeks' gestation or at first prenatal visit if later (1)[A]
  - Prior to transurethral resection of prostate (TURP) (1)[A] or any urologic interventions when mucosal bleeding is anticipated (1)[C]
- Screening for ASB in men and nonpregnant women is not recommended.

Follow-Up Tests & Special Considerations
- Noncontaminated urine specimen should be used for urine culture.
- In pregnancy, periodic screening urine culture should be done after ASB treatment (1)[A] but not required in GBS bacteriuria (2,3)[C].

Test Interpretation
- Patient with significant bacteriuria with or without pyuria and without symptoms referable to UTI should be diagnosed as ASB per Infectious Diseases Society of America.
  - Significant bacteriuria is defined based on type of urine specimen, sex, and the amount of bacteria.
  - By midstream, clean catch specimen
    ○ Male: >100,000 CFU/mL of single bacteria species
    ○ Female: the same criteria as male but needs two positive consecutive specimens
    ○ By catheterized specimen male and female: >100 CFU/mL of one bacterial species; required one-time collection only
- The presence of pyuria or leukocyte esterase is common but not a marker of infection.
- Positive nitrite is an indicator of the presence of bacteriuria but cannot differentiate UTI from ASB or poor collection technique.

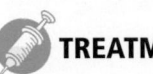 TREATMENT

GENERAL MEASURES

ALERT
- Antibiotic treatment of ASB is indicated in only two conditions:
  - Pregnancy (1)[A]
    ○ Rationale: Treatment prevents up to 70% of pregnant women from developing acute pyelonephritis, which reduces the risk of low birth weight and preterm delivery that are perinatal complications (1,3,4).
  - Prior to TURP (1)[A]
    ○ Rationale: Antibiotic treatment can effectively prevent postprocedure bacteremia and sepsis.

- Treatment of ASB in other conditions (nonpregnant women, diabetic women, indwelling catheter, patients with spinal cord injury, or the elderly living in the community) does not provide any known clinical benefit, does not reduce the risk of symptomatic infection nor improve morbidity or mortality. It increases health care cost, adverse drug side effects, development of resistant organisms, and reinfection rate (1).
- Inadequate evidence to guide management in nonurologic procedure and solid organ transplant (1)

MEDICATION

- Pregnancy
  - Intrapartum antibiotic prophylaxis with IV penicillin or clindamycin (penicillin allergy) is recommended for women with GBS bacteriuria occurring at any stage of pregnancy and of any colony count to prevent GBS disease in the newborn (3)[C].
  - No consensus on choice of antibiotics and duration of treatment in pregnancy; however, the cure rate is higher for the 4 to 7 days of treatment than 1-day treatment (1)[A].
  - Choice of antibiotics should be guided by bacterial pathogen, local resistance rate, adverse effects, and comorbidities of patients (1).
  - Common oral antibiotics (FDA-B) that have been used
    - Nitrofurantoin 100 mg BID for 5 days (low level of resistance, may cause hemolysis in glucose-6-phosphate dehydrogenase deficiency)
    - Amoxicillin/clavulanate 500/125 mg BID for 5 to 7 days
    - Cefuroxime 250 mg BID for 5 days
    - Cephalexin 500 mg BID for 5 days
    - Fosfomycin 3 g for 1 single dose (not effective when glomerular filtration rate is <30 mL/min, may be used in highly resistant bacteria such as methicillin-resistant S. aureus [MRSA], vancomycin-resistant enterococci [VRE], and extended-spectrum β-lactamase [ESBL]-producing organism bacteria) (5)
  - Avoid trimethoprim in 1st trimester and near term. Avoid sulfa after 32 weeks' gestation.
  - Contraindicated: fluoroquinolones (FDA-C), tetracyclines (FDA-D)
- Prior to invasive urologic interventions
  - Initiate antibiotic the night before or immediately before the procedure (1)[A].
  - Antibiotic should be continued until the indwelling catheter is removed postprocedure (1)[B].

ONGOING CARE

FOLLOW-UP RECOMMENDATIONS

No consensus on screening frequency of ASB in pregnancy, but monthly screening of urine culture after ASB treatment is recommended except GBS (1,3).

Patient Monitoring

Development of any signs/symptoms of UTI should warrant antibiotic treatment.

DIET

Daily cranberry juice or cranberry capsules twice daily may reduce the frequency of ASB during pregnancy, but it has not been confirmed in large study (6) (see "Additional Reading").

PATIENT EDUCATION

Patient should seek medical attention when UTI symptoms develop.

COMPLICATIONS

- Late pregnancy pyelonephritis occurs in 20–35% of women with untreated bacteriuria (20- to 30-fold higher than women with negative initial screening urine cultures or in whom bacteriuria was treated). Pyelonephritis is associated with premature delivery and worse fetal outcomes (infant with group B streptococcal infections, low-birth-weight infant). Antimicrobial treatment will decrease the risk of subsequent pyelonephritis from 20–35% to 1–4% and the risk of having a low-birth-weight baby from 15% to 5%.
- If bacteriuria remains untreated in patients who undergo traumatic urologic procedures, up to 60% develop bacteremia after the procedure and 5–10% progress to severe sepsis/septic shock.

REFERENCES

1. Nicolle LE, Bradley S, Colgan R, et al. Infectious Diseases Society of America guidelines for the diagnosis and treatment of asymptomatic bacteriuria in adults. *Clin Infect Dis*. 2005;40(5):643–654.
2. Zolotor AJ, Carlough MC. Update on prenatal care. *Am Fam Physician*. 2014;89(3):199–208.
3. Nicolle LE. Asymptomatic bacteriuria. *Curr Opin Infect Dis*. 2014;27(1):90–96.
4. Kalinderi K, Delkos D, Kalinderis M, et al. Urinary tract infection during pregnancy: current concepts on a common multifaceted problem. *J Obstet Gynaecol*. 2018;38(4):448–453.
5. Keating GM. Fosfomycin trometamol: a review of its use as a single-dose oral treatment for patients with acute lower urinary tract infections and pregnant women with asymptomatic bacteriuria. *Drugs*. 2013;73(17):1951–1966.
6. Wing DA, Rumney PJ, Hindra S, et al. Pilot study to evaluate compliance and tolerability of cranberry capsules for the prevention of asymptomatic bacteriuria. *J Altern Complement Med*. 2015;21(11):700–706.

ADDITIONAL READING

- Köves B, Cai T, Veeratterapillay R, et al. Benefits and harms of treatment of asymptomatic bacteriuria: a systematic review and meta-analysis by the European Association of Urology Urological Infection Guidelines Panel. *Eur Urol*. 2017;72(6):865–868.
- Wing DA, Rumney PJ, Preslicka CW, et al. Daily cranberry juice for the prevention of asymptomatic bacteriuria in pregnancy: a randomized, controlled pilot study. *J Urol*. 2008;180(4):1367–1372.

CODES

ICD10

- N39.0 Urinary tract infection, site not specified
- B96.20 Unsp Escherichia coli as the cause of diseases classd elswhr
- B96.1 Klebsiella pneumoniae as the cause of diseases classd elswhr

CLINICAL PEARLS

- ASB is a common and benign disorder for which treatment is not indicated in most patients.
- The presence of pyuria, leukocyte esterase, and nitrite is common in ASB and not an indication for antimicrobial treatment.
- Antibiotic treatment is indicated for ASB in pregnancy, patients who require TURP, or any urologic interventions with mucosal bleeding.
- Treatment of ASB in other conditions does not decrease the frequency of UTI or improve outcome.
- Overtreatment of ASB may result in negative consequences such as antimicrobial resistance, adverse drug reaction, and unnecessary cost.

BALANITIS, PHIMOSIS, AND PARAPHIMOSIS
John M. Doan, DO • Sarah S. Dolbear, MD

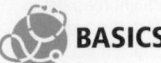 **BASICS**

DESCRIPTION
- Balanitis:
  - An inflammation of the glans penis
  - Posthitis is an inflammation of the foreskin.
  - Balanitis xerotica obliterans (BXO) is lichen sclerosus of the glans penis (uncommon).
- Phimosis and paraphimosis:
  - Phimosis: tightness of the distal penile foreskin that prevents it from being drawn back from over the glans
  - Paraphimosis: constriction by foreskin of an uncircumcised penis, preventing the foreskin from returning to its position over the glans; occurs after the retracted foreskin becomes swollen and engorged; a urologic emergency
- System(s) affected: renal/urologic; reproductive; skin/exocrine

ALERT
- Recurrent infection and irritations (condom catheters) can lead to phimosis.
- Recurrent balanitis, either chemical or infectious, can lead to an acquired phimosis.
- Inappropriate forced reduction of a physiologic foreskin can lead to chronic scarring and acquired phimosis; unfortunately, many times done due to instructions from health care providers
- Paraphimosis is a pediatric emergency; if left untreated, can lead to necrosis and autoamputation

EPIDEMIOLOGY
- Balanitis: predominant age: adult; predominant gender: male only
- Phimosis/paraphimosis: predominant age: infancy and adolescence; unusual in adults; risk returns in geriatrics; predominant sex: male only

Incidence
Balanitis: will affect 3–11% of males

Prevalence
Phimosis: in the United States: 8% of boys age 6 years and 1% of men >16 years of age (1)

ETIOLOGY AND PATHOPHYSIOLOGY
- Balanitis:
  - Allergic reaction (condom latex, contraceptive jelly)
  - Infections (*Candida albicans, Borrelia vincentii,* streptococci, *Trichomonas,* HPV)
  - Fixed-drug eruption (sulfa, tetracycline)
  - Plasma cell infiltration (Zoon balanitis)
  - Autodigestion by activated pancreatic transplant exocrine enzymes
- Phimosis:
  - Physiologic: present at birth; resolves spontaneously during the first 2 to 3 years of life through nocturnal erections, which slowly dilate the phimotic ring
  - Acquired: recurrent inflammation, trauma, or infections of the foreskin

- Paraphimosis:
  - Often iatrogenically or inadvertently induced by the foreskin not being pulled back over the glans after voiding, cleaning, cystoscopy, or catheter insertion

Geriatric Considerations
Condom catheters can predispose to balanitis.

Pediatric Considerations
Oral antibiotics predispose male infants to *Candida balanitis*. Inappropriate care of physiologic phimosis can lead to acquired phimosis by repeated forced reduction of the foreskin.

RISK FACTORS
- Balanitis:
  - Presence of foreskin
  - Morbid obesity
  - Poor hygiene
  - Diabetes; probably most common
  - Nursing home environment
  - Condom catheters
  - Chemical irritants
  - Edematous conditions: CHF, nephrosis
- Phimosis:
  - Poor hygiene
  - Diabetes by repeated balanitis
  - Frequent diaper rash in infants
  - Recurrent posthitis
- Paraphimosis:
  - Presence of foreskin
  - Inexperienced health care provider (leaving foreskin retracted after catheter placement)
  - Poor education about care of the foreskin

GENERAL PREVENTION
- Balanitis:
  - Proper hygiene and avoidance of allergens
  - Circumcision
- Phimosis/paraphimosis:
  - If the patient is uncircumcised, appropriate hygiene and care of the foreskin are necessary to prevent phimosis and paraphimosis.

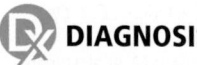 **DIAGNOSIS**

HISTORY
- Balanitis:
  - Pain
  - Drainage
  - Dysuria
  - Odor
  - Ballooning of foreskin with voiding
  - Redness
- Phimosis:
  - Painful erections
  - Recurrent balanitis
  - Foreskin balloons when voiding
  - Inability to retract foreskin at appropriate age

- Paraphimosis:
  - Uncircumcised
  - Pain
  - Drainage
  - Voiding difficulty

PHYSICAL EXAM
- Balanitis:
  - Erythema
  - Tenderness
  - Edema
  - Discharge
  - Ulceration
  - Plaque
- Phimosis:
  - Foreskin will not retract.
  - Secondary balanitis
  - Physiologic phimosis—preputial orifice appears normal and healthy.
  - Pathologic phimosis—preputial orifice has fine white fibrous ring of scar.
- Paraphimosis:
  - Edema of prepuce and glans
  - Drainage
  - Ulceration

DIFFERENTIAL DIAGNOSIS
- Balanitis:
  - Leukoplakia
  - Lichen planus
  - Psoriasis
  - Reiter syndrome
  - Lichen sclerosus et atrophicus
  - Erythroplasia of Queyrat
  - BXO: atrophic changes at end of foreskin; can form band that prevents retraction
- Phimosis/paraphimosis:
  - Penile lymphedema, which can be related to insect bites, trauma, or allergic reactions
  - Penile tourniquet syndrome: foreign body around penis, most commonly hair
  - Anasarca

DIAGNOSTIC TESTS & INTERPRETATION

Initial Tests (lab, imaging)
- Microbiology culture
- Wet mount
- Serology for syphilis
- Serum glucose; ESR (if concerns about Reiter syndrome)
- STD testing
- HIV testing
- Gram stain

Diagnostic Procedures/Other
Biopsy, if persistent

Pathologic Findings
Plasma cells infiltration with Zoon balanitis

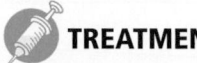 **TREATMENT**

GENERAL MEASURES
- Consider circumcision for recurrent balanitis and paraphimosis.
- Warm compresses or sitz baths
- Local hygiene

MEDICATION
- Balanitis:
  - Antifungal:
    - Clotrimazole (Lotrimin) 1% BID
    - Nystatin (Mycostatin) BID–QID
    - Fluconazole: 150 mg PO single dose
- Antibacterial:
  - Bacitracin QID
  - Neomycin–polymyxin B–bacitracin (Neosporin) QID
  - If cellulitis, cephalosporin or sulfa drug PO or parenteral:
    - Dermatitis: topical steroids QID
    - Zoon balanitis: topical steroids QID
- Phimosis:
  - 0.05% fluticasone propionate daily for 4 to 8 weeks with gradual traction placed on foreskin (2)[B]
  - 1% pimecrolimus BID for 4 to 6 weeks; not for use in children <2 years (3)[C]
- Paraphimosis:
  - Manual reduction, if possible (should be done with the patient sedated). Place the middle and index fingers of both hands on the engorged skin proximal to the glans. Place both thumbs on glans and, with gentle pressure, push on the glans and pull on the foreskin to attempt reduction. If unsuccessful, a dorsal slit will be necessary, with eventual circumcision after the edema resolves.
- Osmotic agents: granulated sugar placed on edematous tissue for several hours to reduce edema
- Puncture technique: Multiple punctures of foreskin with a 21-gauge needle will allow edematous fluid to escape and thus allow reduction.
- Dorsal slit; done by surgeon or urologist
- BXO:
  - 0.05% betamethasone BID
  - 0.1% tacrolimus BID

ISSUES FOR REFERRAL
Recurrent infections or development of meatal stenosis

SURGERY/OTHER PROCEDURES
- Balanitis and phimosis: Consider circumcision as preventive measure.
- For paraphimosis:
  - Represents a true surgical emergency to avoid necrosis of glans
  - Dorsal slit with delayed circumcision, if reduction is not possible
  - Operative exploration if the possibility of penile tourniquet syndrome cannot be eliminated. Hair removal cream can be applied if a hair is thought to be the cause of the tourniquet.

ADMISSION, INPATIENT, AND NURSING CONSIDERATIONS
- Admission criteria/initial stabilization
  - Uncontrolled diabetes
  - Sepsis
- Appropriate hygiene if condom catheters are used
- Discharge on resolution of problem

 ONGOING CARE

FOLLOW-UP RECOMMENDATIONS
Patient Monitoring
Balanitis:
- Every 1 to 2 weeks until etiology has been established
- Persistent balanitis may require biopsy to rule out malignancy or BXO.
- Evaluation for resolution of phimosis

DIET
Weight reduction, if obese

PATIENT EDUCATION
- Need for appropriate hygiene
- Appropriate foreskin care
- Avoidance of known allergens
- No sexual activity for 2 to 3 weeks after circumcision

PROGNOSIS
Should resolve with appropriate treatment

COMPLICATIONS
- Meatal stenosis
- Premalignant changes from chronic irritation
- UTIs
- Acquired phimosis
- Unreducible paraphimosis can lead to gangrene.
- Posthitis (inflammation of the prepuce)

REFERENCES
1. Oster J. Further fate of the foreskin. Incidence of preputial adhesions, phimosis, and smegma among Danish schoolboys. *Arch Dis Child.* 1968;43(228):200–203.
2. Zavras N, Christianakis E, Mpourikas D, et al. Conservative treatment of phimosis with fluticasone proprionate 0.05%: a clinical study in 1185 boys. *J Pediatr Urol.* 2009;5(3):181–185.
3. Georgala S, Gregoriou S, Georgala C, et al. Pimecrolimus 1% cream in non-specific inflammatory recurrent balanitis. *Dermatology.* 2007;215(3):209–212.

ADDITIONAL READING
- Hollowood AD, Sibley GN. Non-painful paraphimosis causing partial amputation. *Br J Urol.* 1997;80(6):958.
- Kiss A, Csontai A, Pirót L, et al. The response of balanitis xerotica obliterans to local steroid application compared with placebo in children. *J Urol.* 2001;165(1):219–220.
- Palmer LS, Palmer JS. The efficacy of topical betamethasone for treating phimosis: a comparison of two treatment regimens. *Urology.* 2008;72(1):68–71.
- Pandher BS, Rustin MH, Kaisary AV. Treatment of balanitis xerotica obliterans with topical tacrolimus. *J Urol.* 2003;170(3):923.
- Stary A, Soeltz-Szoets J, Ziegler C, et al. Comparison of the efficacy and safety of oral fluconazole and topical clotrimazole in patients with candida balanitis. *Genitourin Med.* 1996;72(2):98–102.

 SEE ALSO

Reactive Arthritis (Reiter Syndrome)

 CODES

ICD10
- N48.1 Balanitis
- N47.1 Phimosis
- N48.0 Leukoplakia of penis

CLINICAL PEARLS
- Balanitis is an inflammation of the glans penis. Posthitis is an inflammation of the foreskin. BXO is lichen sclerosus of the glans penis.
- With recurrent infections and a plaque, a biopsy should be done to rule out BXO or malignancy.
- If there is a true phimosis that interferes with appropriate hygiene, treat the phimosis with steroids or circumcision to help with hygiene.

BARRETT ESOPHAGUS

Daniel J. Stein, MD, MPH

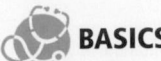 **BASICS**

DESCRIPTION
- Metaplasia of the distal esophageal mucosa from native stratified squamous epithelium to abnormal columnar (intestinalized) epithelium, likely as a consequence of chronic GERD
- Predisposes to the development of adenocarcinoma of the esophagus

EPIDEMIOLOGY
- Predominant age >50 years, more common in men
- Estimated to be present in 1–2% of adult population
- Very rare in pediatric population

Incidence
- 10–15% of patients undergoing endoscopy for evaluation of reflux symptoms
- Esophageal adenocarcinoma (EAC) incidence is rising in the United States (1); 6-fold increase (to 2.5 cases per 100,000) since 1970s
- Annual incidence of adenocarcinoma in all Barrett patients estimated at 0.5% per year
- Attributed to changes in smoking and obesity rather than reclassification or overdiagnosis

Prevalence
Difficult to ascertain, may be as many as 1.5 to 2 million adults in the United States (extrapolated from a 1.6% prevalence in Swedish general population)

ETIOLOGY AND PATHOPHYSIOLOGY
- Chronic gastric reflux injures the esophageal mucosa, triggering columnar metaplasia. Refluxed bile acids likely induce differentiation in gastroesophageal junction (GEJ) cells.
- Columnar cells in the esophagus have higher malignant potential than squamous cells. Activation of *CDX2* gene and overexpression of HER2/neu (ERBB2) oncogene promotes carcinogenesis.
- Elevated levels of COX-2, a mediator of inflammation and regulator of epithelial cell growth, are associated with Barrett esophagus (BE) (1).
- Classic progression: normal epithelium → esophagitis/reflux exposure → metaplasia (BE) → dysplasia (low- or high-grade) → adenocarcinoma

Genetics
- Familial predisposition to GERD and BE with multiple genetic markers have been identified.
- Acquired genetic changes lead to adenocarcinoma and are being investigated as biomarkers for risk stratification and early detection.

RISK FACTORS
- Chronic reflux (>5 years)
- Hiatal hernia
- Age >50 years
- Male gender
- White ethnicity—incidence in white males is much higher than white women and African American men
- Smoking history
- Intra-abdominal obesity
- Family history—at least one first-degree relative with BE or EAC

GENERAL PREVENTION
Weight loss, smoking cessation, robust intake of fruits and vegetables, and moderate wine consumption may decrease risk of BE and lower progression to esophageal cancer (1)[C].

COMMONLY ASSOCIATED CONDITIONS
GERD, obesity, hiatal hernia

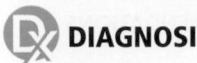 **DIAGNOSIS**

HISTORY
- Assess underlying risk factors.
- Common GERD symptoms: heartburn, regurgitation
- Atypical symptoms include chest pain, odynophagia, chronic cough, water brash, globus sensation, laryngitis, or wheezing.
- Symptoms suggestive of complicated GERD or cancer include weight loss, anorexia, dysphagia, odynophagia, hematemesis, or melena.

ALERT
BE often not symptomatic; up to 50% of EAC and BE patients do not report GERD.

PHYSICAL EXAM
No findings on physical exam are specific for BE.

DIFFERENTIAL DIAGNOSIS
- Erosive esophagitis
- Uncomplicated GERD
- Hiatal hernia

DIAGNOSTIC TESTS & INTERPRETATION
Endoscopy with multiple biopsies demonstrating intestinal metaplasia extending ≥1 cm proximal to the GEJ is required to diagnose BE.
- Gastric cardia–type epithelium on pathology does not have clear malignant significance and may reflect sampling error.
- Specialized intestinal metaplasia at the GEJ: unclear significance, cancer risk difficult to assess with varying definitions of GEJ landmarks

ALERT
- Endoscopic screening is controversial and has not been prospectively studied. Consider screening for men with chronic GERD (>5 years) and/or frequent GERD symptoms with two or more risk factors: age >50 years, white ethnicity, central obesity, smoking history, family history of BE or EAC (ACG), or patients with multiple risk factors (1,2)[B].
- Screening for BE in the general population with GERD is *not* routinely recommended (1,2)[C].

Initial Tests (lab, imaging)
None
- *Helicobacter pylori* testing is *not* indicated. Meta-analyses show an inverse relationship between *H. pylori* infections and BE, which may be related to decreased acid production.
- No current biomarkers are effective for diagnosis; some under investigation for risk stratification (1)[B]

Diagnostic Procedures/Other
- Endoscopy: Visual identification of columnar epithelium (reddish, velvety appearance) replacing squamous epithelium (pale, glossy appearance) of the distal esophagus is standard for diagnosis/ monitoring.

- Biopsies are needed to confirm the diagnosis.
- Classify disease extent: long segment (≥3 cm) versus short segment (<3 cm).
- The Prague grading system used to describe BE using the squamocolumnar junction and GEJ. "C" represents circumferential extent of the columnar changes. "M" indicates the maximal proximal extent of columnar mucosa.
- Advanced imaging techniques, such as narrow band imaging (NBI) and confocal laser endomicroscopy, may help identify dysplasia (not in routine use).
- Systematic endoscopic biopsies confirm diagnosis:
  - Seattle protocol: four-quadrant biopsies at regular intervals with biopsies of visible mucosal irregularities; more time-consuming but higher diagnostic yield than random biopsies (1)[A]
  - Capsule endoscopy has lower sensitivity than conventional endoscopy.

Test Interpretation
- Specialized intestinal metaplasia (also called specialized columnar epithelium) is diagnostic (3)[C].
- Diagnosis of dysplasia (and grade) should be confirmed by two gastrointestinal pathologists before treatment. Benign BE is established by a single pathologist report (3)[C].
- Cardia-type columnar epithelium may predispose to malignancy (unclear risk); International Consensus Group recommends defining BE by the presence of columnar mucosa in the esophagus (noting if intestinal metaplasia is present) (3)[C].
- If screening endoscopy reveals erosive esophagitis, repeat endoscopy after 8 to 12 weeks of proton pump inhibitor (PPI) therapy to exclude underlying BE; defer biopsies until healing occurs (2)[C].

 TREATMENT

MEDICATION
- The goal of medical therapy is to control GERD and reduce esophagitis.
- Neither suppression of gastric acid production via high-dose PPIs nor reduction in esophageal acid exposure via antireflux surgery induces regression of BE. These therapies may, however, decrease progression/cancer risk (1)[A],(4)[B].

First Line
- Unlike the stepwise management of GERD without evidence of BE, all patients with BE should be treated with a daily PPI.
- Dose PPIs 30 to 60 minutes before a meal (ideally, the first meal of the day).
- Patients should remain on lifetime PPI therapy. If GERD symptoms were initially present, PPI should be increased until symptoms are controlled (2)[A].

ALERT
Titrate PPI therapy to symptoms; routine pH monitoring is *not* recommended (1)[C]. In patients with symptoms uncontrolled on PPI, manage according to current standards for treatment of uncontrolled GERD.

ISSUES FOR REFERRAL
- Most patients with low-grade dysplasia (except those who do not desire intervention) and all those with high-grade dysplasia or intramucosal carcinoma should be referred for endoscopic eradication of their Barrett.

- Initiate PPI therapy prior to endoscopy to reduce reactive esophagitis/atypia (2)[C].
- Refer patients considering esophagectomy (rare) to a high-volume institution.

ADDITIONAL THERAPIES

- Aspirin combined with high dose twice daily PPI may reduce progression to dysplasia (not yet routinely recommended).
  - COX-2 selective inhibitor celecoxib use not shown to affect progression of Barrett dysplasia to adenocarcinoma (1)[A]
  - Consider low-dose aspirin in patients with BE and risk factors for cardiovascular disease (1)[C].
- Statins, alone or in combination with aspirin or NSAIDs, may be effective in chemoprevention but are not yet routinely recommended (1)[B].
- No dysplasia: No other therapy is generally indicated; continue regular surveillance assuming good overall patient health (3,5)[C].
- Treatment of dysplasia:
  - Low-grade dysplasia: Refer for a discussion of endoscopic therapy (usually radiofrequency ablation or cryotherapy) to reduce the risk of progression to adenocarcinoma (3,5)[C].
  - High grade dysplasia: Refer for endoscopic mucosal resection and/or endoscopic therapy to prevent progression to adenocarcinoma unless unable to tolerate the procedure (3,5)[C].
  - Intramucosal carcinoma: endoscopic resection if possible, followed by ablation of remaining Barrett, with surgery as a backup (6)[C]
  - More advanced carcinoma: Refer to oncology and surgery to discuss resection.
  - Indeterminate grade dysplasia should have a re-evaluation with biopsies on increased PPI dosage.
  - Endoscopic eradication is successful in >90% of patients but often requires multiple sessions (5).
  - Patients with ablation need ongoing surveillance.

ALERT

Endoscopic eradication not recommended for most BE without dysplasia; therapy should be individualized. Continue surveillance in these patients.

SURGERY/OTHER PROCEDURES

Antireflux surgery such as fundoplication may control GERD symptoms but have not been shown to reverse BE, decrease risk of cancer, or be superior to medical therapy (1)[A].

ALERT

Antireflux surgery does not appear to decrease risk of esophageal cancer.

- Esophagectomy is definitive and can be offered as an alternative to endoscopic eradication therapy for high-grade dysplasia (1)[B] or in patients for whom endoscopic treatment has failed. Morbidity and mortality are higher than with endoscopic treatment.
  - Preferred for patients with evidence of submucosal invasion (stage T1SM2 or higher) or T1a patients with poor differentiation, lymphovascular invasion, or incomplete endoscopic mucosal resection
  - Added benefit of lymph node removal
  - Mortality rate: <5% in patients with high-grade dysplasia who are otherwise healthy
  - Serious postoperative complications: 30–50%
  - Should ideally be performed by an experienced surgeon in a high-volume center (1)[A]

COMPLEMENTARY & ALTERNATIVE MEDICINE

A prospective study of 339 men and women with BE found those taking either a multivitamin, vitamin C, or vitamin E once a day were less likely to develop EAC.

Geriatric Considerations

Surveillance or no treatment may be preferable to endoscopic eradication therapy or esophagectomy in patients who are poor operative candidates. Discontinue surveillance in patients who are not candidates for treatment.

 ONGOING CARE

FOLLOW-UP RECOMMENDATIONS

- Surveillance (to detect high-grade dysplasia or early carcinoma), although controversial, is recommended in patients with histologically confirmed BE, especially for those in high-risk groups.
- Surveillance intervals depend on grade of dysplasia (1)[C].
- Patients diagnosed with BE on initial exam do not require endoscopy in 1 year (2)[C].
- No dysplasia: Survey every 3 to 5 years.
  - Discontinue surveillance if life expectancy is ≤5 years (3)[C].
- Low-grade dysplasia: Survey every 6 to 12 months (2,3,5)[C].
  - Routine surveillance if patients have confirmed absence of low-grade dysplasia after two consecutive endoscopies (3)[C]
- Indefinite for dysplasia: Repeat after 3 to 6 months of increased acid suppression, and if unchanged, survey every 12 months (3)[C].
- High-grade dysplasia without eradication therapy: Survey every 3 months; with eradication therapy: Survey every 3 months for 4, then every 6 months twice, and then every 12 months (1,2)[C].

ALERT

Adherence to recommended surveillance protocols may improve rates of dysplasia and cancer detection.

- Continue surveillance even if the patient has had endoscopic ablation therapy, antireflux surgery, or esophagectomy.

DIET

Avoid foods that trigger reflux: caffeine, alcohol, chocolate, peppermint, carbonated drinks, garlic, onions, spicy foods, fatty foods, citrus, and tomato-based products.

PATIENT EDUCATION

- Lifestyle modifications: smoking cessation, weight loss, avoid supine position after meals, avoid tight-fitting clothes, elevate head of bed
- No evidence that treating GERD reverses BE or necessarily prevents esophageal cancer.

PROGNOSIS

Annual incidence of esophageal cancer in patients with BE is estimated 0.12–0.6% per year (5):

- Low-grade dysplasia: may be transient; cancer risk 0.7–0.8% per year (5)
- High-grade dysplasia: cancer risk 5–9% per year (2,5)
- Promising areas for future research include the use of biomarkers for risk stratification, chemoprevention of neoplastic progression, capsule endoscopy for screening, and the use of vitamins and antioxidants for prevention and treatment.

COMPLICATIONS

Same as GERD: stricture, bleeding, ulceration

REFERENCES

1. Spechler SJ, Sharma P, Souza RF, et al; for American Gastroenterological Association. American Gastroenterological Association medical position statement on the management of Barrett's esophagus. *Gastroenterology*. 2011;140(3):1084–1091.
2. Shaheen NJ, Falk GW, Iyer PG, et al. ACG clinical guideline: diagnosis and management of Barrett's esophagus. *Am J Gastroenterol*. 2016;111(1):30–51.
3. Bennett C, Moayyedi P, Corley DA, et al; for BOB CAT Consortium. BOB CAT: a large-scale review and Delphi consensus for management of Barrett's esophagus with no dysplasia, indefinite for, or low-grade dysplasia. *Am J Gastroenterol*. 2015;110(5):662–683.
4. Singh S, Garg SK, Singh PP, et al. Acid-suppressive medications and risk of oesophageal adenocarcinoma in patients with Barrett's oesophagus: a systematic review and meta-analysis. *Gut*. 2014;63(8):1229–1237.
5. Evans JA, Early DS, Fukami N, et al; for Standards of Practice Committee of the American Society for Gastrointestinal Endoscopy. The role of endoscopy in Barrett's esophagus and other premalignant conditions of the esophagus. *Gastrointest Endosc*. 2012;76(6):1087–1094.
6. Wani S, Qumseya B, Sultan S, et al; for Standards of Practice Committee. Endoscopic eradication therapy for patients with Barrett's esophagus–associated dysplasia and intramucosal cancer. *Gastrointest Endosc*. 2018;87(4):907–931.e9.

ADDITIONAL READING

- Dunbar KB, Spechler SJ. Controversies in Barrett esophagus. *Mayo Clin Proc*. 2014;89(7):973–984.
- Zimmerman TG. Common questions about Barrett esophagus. *Am Fam Physician*. 2014;89(2):92–98.

 CODES

ICD10

- K22.70 Barrett's esophagus without dysplasia
- K22.719 Barrett's esophagus with dysplasia, unspecified
- K22.710 Barrett's esophagus with low grade dysplasia

CLINICAL PEARLS

- The incidence of esophageal cancer is rising faster than any other major malignancy. BE is a precursor to esophageal carcinoma.
- The highest incidence of BE is in white males >50 years of age.
- Endoscopic eradication therapy is preferred for dysplasia with or without submucosal invasion.
- Esophagectomy is generally limited to patients with invasive carcinoma or those failing to respond to endoscopic therapy.

BASAL CELL CARCINOMA
William G. Farkas, DO, FS

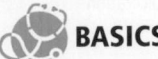 BASICS

DESCRIPTION
Basal cell carcinoma (BCC) is the most common cancer, originating from the basal cell layer of the skin appendages.
- Rarely metastasizes but capable of local tissue destruction

Geriatric Considerations
Greater frequency in geriatric patients (Ages 55 to 75 years have 100 times the incidence when compared with those aged <20 years.)

Pediatric Considerations
- Rare in children, but childhood radiation treatment is contributory, as are frequent or severe sunburns
- The Centers for Disease Control and Prevention recommends against using tanning beds and lamps in their guidelines for cancer prevention in school-age children.

EPIDEMIOLOGY
Worldwide, the most common form of cancer

Incidence
- Incidence in the United States: 2 million cases each year; 2.5 times more common than squamous cell carcinoma (SCC); Australia has highest incidence in the world.
- White people have a 1 in 5 chance of developing BCC during their lifetime.
- Predominant age: generally >40 years, although incidence increasing in younger populations
- Predominant sex: male > female (2:1 ratio)

ETIOLOGY AND PATHOPHYSIOLOGY
- UV-induced inflammation and cyclooxygenase activation in skin
- In chromosome 9q22, mutation of PTCH1 (patched homolog 1), a tumor-suppressor gene that inhibits the hedgehog signaling pathway
- UV-induced mutations of the TP53 (tumor protein 53), a tumor-suppressor gene
- Activation of BCL2, an antiapoptosis proto-oncogene

Genetics
- Several genetic conditions increase the risk of developing BCC:
  - Albinism (recessive alleles)
  - Xeroderma pigmentosum (autosomal recessive)
  - Bazex syndrome (rare, X-linked dominant)
  - Nevoid BCC syndrome/Gorlin syndrome (rare, autosomal dominant)
  - Cytochrome P450 CYP2D6 and glutathione S-transferase detoxifying enzyme gene mutations (especially in truncal BCC, marked by clusters of BCCs and a younger age of onset)
  - Mutations in the tumor suppressor gene Patched, or activated mutations in Smoothened, resulting in upregulation of hedgehog pathway signaling

RISK FACTORS
- Chronic sun exposure (UV radiation); most common in the following phenotypes:
  - Light complexion: skin type I (burns but does not tan) and skin type II (usually burns, sometimes tans)
  - Red or blond hair
  - Blue or green eyes
- Tendency to sunburn
- Male sex, although increasing risk in women due to lifestyle changes, such as tanning beds
- History of nonmelanoma skin cancer

- Family history of skin cancer
- Chronic immunosuppression: transplant recipients (10 times higher incidence), patients with HIV, or lymphomas
- No significant association between age and recurrence rate, according to most studies

GENERAL PREVENTION
- Use broad-spectrum sunscreens of at least SPF 30 daily and reapply after swimming or sweating.
- Avoid overexposure to the sun by seeking shade between 10 AM and 4 PM and wearing wide-brimmed hats and long-sleeved shirts.
- The American Cancer Society recommends cancer-related checkups every 3 years in patients 20 to 40 years old and yearly in patients >40 years.

COMMONLY ASSOCIATED CONDITIONS
- Cosmetic disfigurement because head and neck most often affected
- Loss of vision with orbital involvement
- Loss of nerve function due to perineural spread or extensive and deep invasion
- Ulcerating neoplasms are prone to infections.

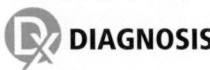 DIAGNOSIS

HISTORY
Exposure to risk factors, family history

PHYSICAL EXAM
- 80% on face and neck, 20% on trunk and lower limbs (mostly women)
- Nodular: most common (50–80%); presents as pinkish, pearly papule, plaque, or nodule, often with telangiectatic vessels, ulceration, and a rolled periphery, usually on the head or neck (1)
  - Pigmented: presents as a translucent papule with "floating pigment"; more commonly seen in darker skin types; may give a blue, brown, or black appearance and be confused with melanoma (1)
- Superficial: 10–30%; light red, scaly plaque resembling eczema or psoriasis but with thin, rolled borders and central clearing, usually on trunk or extremities; least invasive of BCC subtypes (1)
- Morpheaform: 5–10%; resembles plaque with poorly defined borders; most common on head or neck (1)

DIFFERENTIAL DIAGNOSIS
- Sebaceous hyperplasia
- Epidermal inclusion cyst
- Intradermal nevi (pigmented and nonpigmented)
- Molluscum contagiosum
- SCC
- Nummular dermatitis
- Psoriasis
- Melanoma (pigmented lesions)
- Atypical fibroxanthoma
- Rare adnexal neoplasms

DIAGNOSTIC TESTS & INTERPRETATION
Diagnostic Procedures/Other
- Clinical diagnosis and histologic subtype are confirmed through skin biopsy and pathologic examination (2).
- Shave biopsy is typically sufficient; however, punch biopsy is more useful to assess depth of tumor and perineural invasion.
- If a genetic disorder is suspected, additional tests may be needed to confirm it.

Test Interpretation
- Nodular BCC
  - Extending from the epidermis are nodular aggregates of basaloid cells.
  - Tumor cells are uniform; rarely have mitotic figures; large, oval, hyperchromatic nuclei with little cytoplasm, surrounded by a peripheral palisade
  - Early lesions are usually connected to the epidermis, unlike late lesions.
  - Increased mucin in dermal stroma
    - Cleft formation (retraction artifact) common between BCC "nests" and stroma due to mucin shrinkage during fixation and staining
- Superficial BCC
  - Appear as buds of basaloid cells attached to undersurface of epidermis
  - Peripheral palisading
- Morpheaform BCC
  - Thin cords and strands of basaloid cells; embedded in dense, fibrous, scar-like stroma
  - Less peripheral palisading and retraction, greater subclinical involvement
- Infiltrating BCC
  - Like morpheaform BCC but no scar-like stroma and thicker, more spiky, irregular strands
  - Less peripheral palisading and retraction, greater subclinical involvement
- Micronodular BCC
  - Small, nodular aggregates of tumor cells
  - Less retraction artifact and higher subclinical involvement than nodular BCC

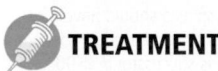 TREATMENT

MEDICATION
- May be especially useful in those who cannot tolerate surgical procedures and in those who refuse to have surgery as well as for low-risk superficial and/or nodular BCC
- 5-Fluorouracil (5-FU) cream inhibits thymidylate synthetase, interrupting DNA synthesis for superficial lesions in low-risk areas; primary treatment only; 5% applied BID for 3 to 10 weeks.
- Imiquimod (Aldara) cream approved for treatment of low-risk superficial BCC; daily dosing for 6 to 12 weeks; 80% clearance rate (2)[A]
- 5-FU is reserved for superficial BCC (2); however, with nodular BCC, imiquimod has been shown to have 5-year clearance rates ranging between 75% and 85% (3)[A].
- Topical treatment failure may yield skip lesions that yield false-negative margins, making Mohs and excisional surgery potentially less effective.
- Emerging therapies:
  - Vismodegib, a sonic hedgehog pathway inhibitor; for patients with advanced BCC when other options are exhausted; not considered appropriate therapy for low-risk tumors (4)[B]; also beneficial for multiple BCC and BCC nevus syndrome (4)[A]. Demonstrated success with this has led to research on other hedgehog inhibitor compounds, including sonidegib, which is approved for treatment of locally advanced BCC or those who are not candidates for surgery or RT (3).
  - Intralesional injection: Efficacy for small (<1 cm) nodular and superficial BCCs varies from 67% to 94% based on the type of agent used (2)[C].
  - Ingenol mebutate: derived from the plant *Euphorbia peplus*; in one trial, 63% of lesions, significant histologic cure rates were seen 85 days after treatment, but long-term studies need to be conducted (3)[A].

– Laser therapy: Evidence for monotherapy is currently lacking in randomized controlled trials, but anecdotal evidence supports treatment for superficial BCC; in one RCT in which it was used as a pretreatment to photodynamic therapy (PDT), 1-year recurrence rates ranged from 1% to 8%, depending on the laser form used (3)[A]; one retrospective study with superpulsed carbon dioxide therapy for superficial and nodular BCC showed no recurrence in 3-year follow-up (2)[B].

ADDITIONAL THERAPIES

- Radiation therapy
  – Useful for patients, typically older, who cannot or will not undergo surgery
  – Used following surgery, particularly if margins of tumor were not cleared
  – Cure rate is ~90%.
  – Tumors that recur in areas previously treated with radiation are harder to treat, and the area is more difficult to reconstruct.
  – Local treatment
  – Recurrence rates are 7–8%.
- PDT
  – Methyl aminolevulinate and 5-aminolevulinic acid, photosensitizers, are activated by specific wavelengths of light, creating singlet oxygen radicals that destroy local tissue (no damage to surrounding or deep tissues).
  – Decades old, well studied form of treatment currently approved in Canada, Europe, Australia, and New Zealand; off-label treatment for BCC in the United States (3)
  – Useful in areas where tissue preservation is cosmetically or functionally important; considered inferior to surgical excision in terms of efficacy (5)
  – When examining 5-year recurrence rates, may be equivalent to cryotherapy
  – More favorable for superficial versus nodular BCC (3)[A]

SURGERY/OTHER PROCEDURES

- Surgical excision is first-line treatment (4)[A]; specific treatment selection varies with extent and location of lesion as well as tumor border demarcation.
- High-risk areas
  – Inner canthus, nasolabial sulcus, philtrum, preauricular area, retroauricular sulcus, lip, temple, "mask areas" of the face (5)[C]
- Curettage and electrodesiccation
  – If nodular lesion <1 cm, in low-risk area, not deeply invasive
  – Avoid in the hair-bearing areas due to risk of the tumor extending down follicular structures.
  – 5-year cure rate of 91–97%; recurrence as high as 27% for high-risk lesions (2)
- Excision with postoperative margin assessment
  – Treatment of choice for low-risk lesions <2 cm in diameter
  – Goal is 4-mm margin.
  – 5-year cure rate of 98%
- Cryosurgery
  – Reserved for nodular and superficial BCC, not indicated for tumors with depth exceeding 3 mm
  – Contraindicated in hair-bearing areas and over the lower extremities (2)
  – Typically for tumors with low risk of recurrence
  – May want pre- and posttreatment biopsies (5)[C]
  – Mean recurrence rates are approximately 1%.

- Mohs surgery
  – Preferred microsurgically controlled surgical treatment for lesions in high-risk areas, recurrent lesions, and lesions exhibiting an aggressive growth pattern (5)[A]
  – 5-year recurrence rate of 2.5% (2)[A]
  – Requires referral to appropriately trained dermatologic surgeon

ADMISSION, INPATIENT, AND NURSING CONSIDERATIONS

Outpatient, unless extensive lesion

 ONGOING CARE

FOLLOW-UP RECOMMENDATIONS

- Seek shade, especially between 10 AM and 4 PM.
- Oral retinoids may prevent the development of new BCCs in patients with Gorlin syndrome, renal transplant recipients, and patients with severe actinic damage.

Patient Monitoring

- Every 6 to 12 months for first 5 years and then annually for life
- Increased risk of other skin cancers
- Recurrence:
  – Local: Follow NCCN 2018 guidelines for primary treatment.
  – Regional: surgery and/or radiation therapy
  – Metastatic: multidisciplinary tumor board consultation

PATIENT EDUCATION

- Teach patient-appropriate sun-avoidance techniques.
- Monthly skin self-exam
- Educate patients concerning adequate vitamin D intake. Use broad-spectrum UVA/UVB sunscreen SPF 15 or higher.
- Keep newborns out of the sun. Apply sunscreen to babies 6 months or older.

PROGNOSIS

- Proper treatment yields 90–95% cure.
- Most recurrences happen within 5 years. 56% of primary high-risk BCC are reported to recur >5 years postoperatively.
- Development of new BCCs: Many patients (30–50%) will develop a new lesion within 5 years.

COMPLICATIONS

- Local recurrence and spread
- Usually, recurrences will appear within 5 years.
- Metastasis: rare (<0.1%) but metastatic disease usually fatal within 8 months

REFERENCES

1. Cameron MC, Lee E, Hibler B, et al. Basal cell carcinoma: part 1 [published online ahead of print May 18, 2018]. *J Am Acad Dermatol*. doi:10.1016/j.jaad.2018.03.060.
2. Cameron MC, Lee E, Hibler B, et al. Basal cell carcinoma, part II: contemporary approaches to diagnosis, treatment, and prevention [published online ahead of print May 18, 2018]. *J Am Acad Dermatol*. doi:10.1016/j.jaad.2018.02.083.
3. Lanoue J, Goldenberg G. Basal cell carcinoma: a comprehensive review of existing and emerging nonsurgical therapies. *J Clin Aesthet Dermatol*. 2016;9(5):26–36.
4. Amaral T, Garbe C. Non-melanoma skin cancer: new and future synthetic drug treatments. *Expert Opin Pharmacother*. 2017;18(7):689–699.
5. Clark CM, Furniss M, Mackay-Wiggan JM. Basal cell carcinoma: an evidence-based treatment update. *Am J Clin Dermatol*. 2014;15(3):197–216.

ADDITIONAL READING

- Connolly KL, Nehal KS, Disa JJ. Evidence-based medicine: cutaneous facial malignancies: nonmelanoma skin cancer. *Plast Reconstr Surg*. 2017;139(1):181e–190e.
- Dzubow L, Goldberg LH, Lebwohl M, et al. *Basal Cell Carcinoma Prevention Guidelines*. New York, NY: The Skin Cancer Foundation; 2018. http://www.skincancer.org/skin-cancer-information/basal-cell-carcinoma/bcc-prevention-guidelines. Accessed July 22, 2018.
- Feller L, Khammissa RA, Kramer B, et al. Basal cell carcinoma, squamous cell carcinoma and melanoma of the head and face. *Head Face Med*. 2016;12:11.
- Kundu RV, Patterson S. Dermatologic conditions in skin of color: part I. Special considerations for common skin disorders. *Am Fam Physician*. 2013;87(12):850–856.
- Marghoob AA, Usatine RP, Jaimes N. Dermoscopy for the family physician. *Am Fam Physician*. 2013;88(7):441–450.
- National Comprehensive Cancer Network. *NCCN Clinical Practice Guidelines in Oncology: Basal Cell Skin Cancer, Version I.2018*. https://www.nccn.org/professionals/physician_gls/pdf/nmsc.pdf. Published October 3, 2016. Accessed July 22, 2018.

 CODES

ICD10

- C44.91 Basal cell carcinoma of skin, unspecified
- C44.31 Basal cell carcinoma of skin of other and unspecified parts of face
- C44.41 Basal cell carcinoma of skin of scalp and neck

CLINICAL PEARLS

- BCC is the most common cancer, originating from the basal cell layer of the skin appendages.
- Nodular: pearly papule, plaque, or nodule often with telangiectatic vessels, ulceration, and a rolled periphery, usually on face
- Pigmented: presents as a translucent papule with "floating pigment"; more commonly seen in darker skin types
- Superficial: scaly papule or plaque with atrophic center, ringed by translucent micropapules, usually on trunk or extremities; more common in men
- Morpheaform: firm, smooth, flesh-colored, scar-like papule or plaque with ill-defined borders
- Use diagnostic keys above to differentiate between BCC and cutaneous SCC. SCC arises from actinic keratosis in 60% of cases and generally presents as an asymptomatic hyperkeratotic lesion. If unsure, biopsy or refer to a specialist.
- Some hyperpigmented BCCs may appear similar to melanoma. Remember the ABCDEs of melanoma recognition: **A**symmetry, **B**order irregularities, **C**olor variability, **D**iameter >6 mm, **E**nlargement. If unsure, refer to a specialist.
- The USPSTF concludes insufficient evidence and recommends for or against routine total body skin exams for melanoma, BCC, or SCC. Exams should be based on risk factors, including exposure and family and prior medical history. All patients should receive education about risks and self-exam.

BED BUGS

Fawn J. Winkelman, DO • Adam Strosberg, DNP, ARNP-BC

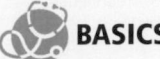

BASICS

DESCRIPTION
- Nocturnal obligate blood parasites residing in furniture and bedding
- 5 to 7 mm oval, reddish brown, flat, wingless

EPIDEMIOLOGY
Incidence
- Bed bug infestations increasing and difficult to treat, more so than cockroaches, termites, and ants (1)
- Resurgence due to changes in pesticide, increased travel, use of secondhand furniture, and high turnover rates of hotel guests

Prevalence
- Infestations are increasing across the United States.
- Bed bugs have increased 10–30% in public places (schools, hospitals, hotels/motels, aircraft) over the past decade (2).
- The global population of bed bugs (*Cimex lectularius* and *Cimex hemipterus*, family Cimicidae) has undergone a significant resurgence since the late 1990s. This is likely due to an increase in global travel, trade, and the number of insecticide-resistant bed bugs. The global bed bug population is estimated to be increasing by 100–500% annually (3).

ETIOLOGY AND PATHOPHYSIOLOGY
- Insect family Cimicidae
- Three species bite humans: *C. lectularius*, *C. hemipterus*, and *Leptocimex boueti* (2)[B].
- Most prevalent species is *C. lectularius* (2)[B].
- Found in tropical and temperate climates
- Hide in crevices of mattresses, box springs, headboards, and baseboards
- Infestations occur in hotels/motels, hospitals, cinemas, vehicles, aircraft, and homes.

- Unlike other infestations, they are not associated with hygienic deficiencies.
- Reactions range from an absent or minimal response to the typical pruritic, erythematous maculopapular rash. Less commonly, there is an urticarial or anaphylactoid response.
- Skin reactions are due to host immunologic response to parasite salivary proteins.
- Urticarial reactions are mediated via immunoglobulin (Ig) G antibody response to salivary proteins (4)[B].
- Bullous reactions caused by an IgE-mediated hypersensitivity to nitrophorin in bug saliva (4)[B]
- Bugs are attracted to body warmth and exhaled carbon dioxide (5).
- Bites do not transmit other known pathogens.

GENERAL PREVENTION
- Traps typically use carbon dioxide and heat to attract and trap bugs but can be cost prohibitive (6)[B].
- Vector control: Vacuum regularly, reduce clutter, seal cracks in walls, inspect luggage and clothing.
- Launder all bedding and clothing in >130°F (50°C) for 2 hours or place in 20°F (−5°C) or cooler environment for at least 5 days.
- If present in the home, eradicate using professional extermination services. Some pest control companies use canines to detect live bed bugs and eggs based on pheromones from the bed bugs (6)[B].

RISK FACTORS
- Immunocompromised
- High hotel turnover
- Secondhand furniture in home

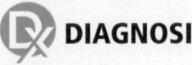

DIAGNOSIS

HISTORY
- Recent travel
- Bed bug sighting; blood specks on sheets
- New skin lesions in the morning
- Intense pruritus, pain, or burning

PHYSICAL EXAM
- Characteristic lesions are erythematous pruritic papules in an irregular linear pattern.
- Found on body surfaces exposed during sleeping such as face, neck, arms, legs, and shoulders
- May appear hours to days after being bitten
- Patients are usually asymptomatic but may present with papular urticaria, diffuse urticaria, bullous lesions, and/or anaphylactoid symptoms.

DIFFERENTIAL DIAGNOSIS
- Urticaria; insect or spider bite; scabies
- Dermatitis herpetiformis

DIAGNOSTIC TESTS & INTERPRETATION
Initial Tests (lab, imaging)
- Skin scraping with mineral oil preparation
- Skin biopsy

Test Interpretation
- Skin scraping is negative with mineral oil, which helps to exclude scabies.
- Skin biopsy shows nonspecific perivascular eosinophilic infiltrate consistent with arthropod bite reaction.

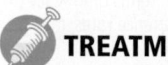

TREATMENT

GENERAL MEASURES
- Self-limited and resolves within 1 to 2 weeks
- Treat symptomatically.
- Avoid and control bed bugs.

MEDICATION

First Line

- Disease is self-limited; treat symptoms.
- Oral antihistamines (i.e., diphenhydramine, hydroxyzine)
- Topical antipruritics (i.e., pramoxine/calamine ointment or doxepin cream)
- Topical low- to midpotency corticosteroids for 2 weeks (i.e., hydrocortisone, triamcinolone)
- Systemic corticosteroids (severe cases)

ADDITIONAL THERAPIES

- If secondarily infected, use topical or oral antibiotics against *Staphylococcus* and *Streptococcus* spp. (i.e., cephalexin, tetracycline, doxycycline, clindamycin, topical mupirocin).
- Epinephrine for anaphylaxis
- Professional extermination may be necessary.
- The CDC recommends a comprehensive integrated pest management program—remove clutter, seal cracks, heat treatment, vacuum, and nonchemical pesticides.
- New approaches (more research necessary) include xenointoxication (oral arthropodicidal agent) toxic to the bed bugs.

 ONGOING CARE

FOLLOW-UP RECOMMENDATIONS

- Not necessary as disease is self-limited
- May need specific care in extreme cases or if anaphylactoid reactions

PATIENT EDUCATION

- Avoid scratching to prevent superinfection.
- Inspect bedding, furniture, and luggage regularly.
- CDC: www.cdc.gov/parasites/bedbugs/
- EPA: http://www2.epa.gov/bedbugs

- Myth 1: *Bed bugs are invisible*. They are nocturnal and hide during the daytime. Adult bugs are ~1/4-inch long, and eggs are the size of a pin head.
- Myth 2: *Bed bugs reproduce rapidly*. Their life cycle is 4 to 5 weeks, longer than the house fly.
- Myth 3: *Bed bugs can live without feeding*. Bugs can live 3 to 5 months without a blood meal.
- Tips to prevent and control bed bugs
  - Ensure infestation is bed bugs (not fleas, other insects, and/or ticks).
  - Regularly wash and heat dry your clothing and bedding, especially if it touches the floor.
  - EPA tips: https://www.epa.gov/bedbugs/top-ten-tips-prevent-or-control-bed-bugs

COMPLICATIONS

- Bed bug dermatitis, allergic reactions, asthma exacerbations, anaphylaxis
- Significant psychological distress (insomnia, depression, anxiety, delusional parasitosis) (4)
- Secondary bacterial infections
- Transmission of blood-borne diseases (rare)

REFERENCES

1. Woloski JR, Burman D, Adebona O. Mite and bed bug infections. *Prim Care*. 2018;45(3):409–421.
2. Studdiford JS, Conniff KM, Trayes KP, et al. Bedbug infestation. *Am Fam Physician*. 2012;86(7): 653–658.
3. Lai O, Ho D, Glick S, et al. Bed bugs and possible transmission of human pathogens: a systematic review. *Arch Dermatol Res*. 2016;308(8):531–538.
4. Williams K, Willis MS. Bedbugs in the 21st century: the reemergence of an old foe. *Lab Med*. 2012;43(5):141–148.
5. Vaidyanathan R, Feldlaufer MF. Bed bug detection: current technologies and future directions. *Am J Trop Med Hyg*. 2013;88(4):619–625.
6. Ogg B. Bed bug myths—rely on research for facts. *The Nebline*. 2012;347–348.

ADDITIONAL READING

- Lancaster Extension Education Center: http://lancaster.unl.edu/pest/bugs.shtml
- National Pesticide Information Center: http://npic.orst.edu/

 CODES

ICD10

- S00.96XA Insect bite (nonvenomous) of unspecified part of head, initial encounter
- S10.96XA Insect bite of unspecified part of neck, initial encounter
- S40.269A Insect bite (nonvenomous) of unspecified shoulder, initial encounter

CLINICAL PEARLS

- 90% of infestations occur within 3 feet of beds.
- Wash bedding/clothing regularly in hot water and vacuum carpet daily or steam clean daily.
- Inspect furniture, bedding, and luggage regularly.
- Bed bug have become resistant to over-the-counter (OTC) products (permethrin, cyfluthrin, bifenthrin, and deltamethrin or fluvalinate and esfenvalerate).

BEHAVIORAL PROBLEMS, PEDIATRIC

William G. Elder, PhD • Ginny L. Gottschalk, MD

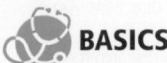 **BASICS**

DESCRIPTION

Behavior that disrupts at least one area of psychosocial functioning. Commonly reported behavioral problems are as follows:

- Noncompliance: active or passive refusal to do as requested by parent or other authority figure
- Temper tantrums: loss of internal control provoked by overtiredness, physical discomfort, or fear that leads to crying, whining, breath holding, or in extreme cases, aggressive behavior
- Sleep problems: sleep patterns that are distressing to caregivers or child; difficulty going to sleep or staying asleep at night, nightmares, and night terrors
- Nocturnal enuresis: enuresis that occurs only at night in children >5 years of age with no medical problems
  - Primary: children who have never been dry at night
  - Secondary: children dry at night for at least 6 months
- Functional encopresis: repeated involuntary fecal soiling that is not caused by organic defect or illness
- Problem eating: "picky eating," difficult mealtime behaviors
- Normative sexual behaviors: developmentally appropriate behaviors in children in the absence of abuse
- Thumb-sucking: an innate reflex that is self-soothing; may be protective against sudden infant death. If persists, past eruption of primary teeth can affect teeth alignment and mouth shape.

EPIDEMIOLOGY

- Noncompliance issues: may manifest as children develop autonomy; males have a modestly greater likelihood of being noncompliant; decreases with age
- Temper tantrums: 87% of 18- to 24-month-old children; 91% of 30- to 36-month-old children; 59% of 3.5- to 4-year-old children; in children with severe tantrums, 52% have other behavioral/emotional problems (1).
- Sleep problems
  - Night waking in 25–50% of infants 6 to 12 months; bedtime refusal in 10–30% of toddlers
  - Nightmares in 10–50% of preschoolers; peaks between ages 6 and 10 years
  - Night terrors in 1–6.5% early childhood; peaks between ages 4 and 12 years
  - Sleepwalking frequently in 3–5%; peaks between ages 4 and 8 years (2)
- Nocturnal enuresis
  - At least 20% of children in the 1st grade wet the bed occasionally; 4% wet ≥2 times per week.
  - At 10 years of age, 7% in boys, 3% in girls (3)
- Functional encopresis
  - Rare before age 3 years, most common in 5- to 10-year-olds; more common in boys (4)
- Problem eating
  - Prevalence peaks at 50% at 24 months of age; no relation to sex/ethnicity/income (5)
- Normative sexual behaviors
  - Rare in infancy, except hand to genital contact
  - Increased in 3- to 5-year-olds; less observed in >5-year-olds because more covert
- Thumb-sucking: decreases with age; most children spontaneously stop between 2 and 4 years.

COMMONLY ASSOCIATED CONDITIONS

- Noncompliance: If exceeds what seems normative, rule out depression, compulsive patterns, adjustment disorder, inappropriate discipline.
- Temper tantrums: difficult child temperament, stress
- Sleep problems: often with inconsistent bedtime routine or sleep schedule, stimulating bedtime environment; can be associated with hyperactive behavior, poor impulse control, and poor attention in young children (2). Acute or chronic anxiety is associated with insomnia. Long-acting stimulant medications disturb sleep quality.
- Enuresis: secondary often with medical problems, especially constipation, and frequent behavior problems, especially ADHD and autism
- Functional encopresis: enuresis, UTIs, ADHD
- Normative sexual behaviors: family stressors such as separation or divorce

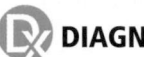 **DIAGNOSIS**

HISTORY

- Noncompliance: complete history from caregivers and teachers, if applicable; direct observation of child or child–caregiver interaction
  - Criteria: problematic for at least some adults, leading to difficult interactions for at least 6 months
  - Reduces child's ability to take part in structured activities
  - Creates stressful relationships with compliant children
  - Disrupts academic progress; places child at risk for physical injury
- Temper tantrums: history, with focus on development, family functioning, or violence; may consist of stiffening limbs and arching back, dropping to floor, shouting, screaming, crying, pushing/pulling, stamping, hitting, kicking, throwing, or running away (1)
- Sleep disorders: screening questions about sleep during well-child visit, such as the Bedtime problems, Excessive daytime sleepiness, Awakenings during the night, Regularity and duration of sleep, and Snoring (BEARS) screen; bedtime routine (2)
- Nocturnal enuresis: severity, onset, and duration; dry overnight previously; daytime wetting or any associated genitourinary symptoms; family history of enuresis; medical and psychosocial history; constipation; child and caregiver's motivation for treatment; voiding diary
- Problem eating: review of child's diet, growth curves, nutritional needs, and caregiver's response to behavior (5)
- Normative sexual behaviors: When was behavior first noticed? Any recent changes or stressors in family? Behavior solitary or with another; if with another, what age? Changes in frequency or nature of behaviors; occurs at home, daycare, school? Is behavior disruptive, intrusive, or coercive? (See "Child Sexual Behavior Inventory" in the following discussion.)

PHYSICAL EXAM

- Nocturnal enuresis
  - Physical exam of abdomen for enlarged bladder, kidneys, or fecal masses; rectal exam if history of constipation; back for spinal dysraphism seen in dimpling or hair tufts
  - Neurologic exam: Focus on lower extremities.
  - Genitourinary exam
    - Males: meatal stenosis, hypospadias, epispadias, phimosis

- Females: vulvitis, vaginitis, labial adhesions, ureterocele at introitus; wide vaginal orifice with scar or healed laceration may be evidence of abuse.
- Functional encopresis
  - Height and weight; abdominal exam for masses or tenderness; rectal exam for tone, size of rectal vault, fecal impaction, masses, fissures, hemorrhoids; back for signs of spinal dysraphism seen in dimpling or hair tufts

DIFFERENTIAL DIAGNOSIS

Temper tantrums: disruptive mood dysregulation disorder (DMDD)—distinguishable because of baseline irritable mood between outbursts and older age (6 to 18 years)

DIAGNOSTIC TESTS & INTERPRETATION

Initial Tests (lab, imaging)

- For nocturnal enuresis: urinalysis (dipstick test OK); if abnormal, consider urine culture.
  - For secondary enuresis: serum glucose, creatinine, TSH
  - Urinary tract imaging and urodynamic studies if significant daytime symptoms with history or diagnosis of UTI or history of structural renal abnormalities
- For functional encopresis: TSH for hypothyroidism or celiac disease if poor growth or family history; urinalysis and culture if enuresis or features of UTI (4)
  - Spine imaging if evidence of spinal dysraphism or if both encopresis and daytime enuresis; barium enema if suspect Hirschsprung disease

Follow-Up Tests & Special Considerations

Sleep disorders: Sleep studies may be performed in children if there is a history of snoring and/or observed apnea spells to rule out obstructive sleep apnea (OSA); daytime ADHD-type symptoms may be present (2).

Diagnostic Procedures/Other

- Pediatric symptom checklist: https://brightfutures.org/mentalhealth/pdf/professionals/ped_sympton_chklst.pdf
- National Initiative for Children's Healthcare Quality (NICHQ) Vanderbilt Assessment (ADHD screen): http://www.myadhd.com/vanderbiltparent6175.html
- Child Sexual Behavior Inventory: completed by female caregiver to assist with differentiation of normative versus abnormal behaviors particularly those related to sexual abuse: https://www.nctsn.org/measures/child-sexual-behavior-inventory

 TREATMENT

GENERAL MEASURES

- Educate caregiver about specific behavioral problem.
- Parent management training programs and techniques are effective for many child behavior problems.
- Noncompliance: In the case of extreme child disobedience, consider parent training programs. Child may need to be formally screened for ADHD, obsessive-compulsive disorder (OCD), oppositional defiant disorder (ODD), or conduct disorder (CD).
- Temper tantrums: Remind caregiver this is a normal aspect of early childhood.
  - Educate caregiver that tantrums are not attention seeking, although they may reveal that the child needs more attention from caregiver. This attention should be developmentally appropriate and not occur when the child is tantruming but at other times and prior to the tantrum.
  - If tantrum is set off by external factors, such as hunger or overtiredness, then correct.

- Other methods for dealing with a tantrum include one of the following:
  - Ignore the tantrum; remove the child and place him or her in time-out (1 minute for each year of age); hold/restrain child until calmed down; provide child with clear, firm, and consistent instructions as well as enough time to obey.
- Sleep problems: Intervention consists largely of education of the caregiver who may need a road-map for dealing with this difficult and distressing problem. Developmental stages; environmental factors and cues; caregiver emotions and reactions; and child fears, stress, and habits are all important factors in sleep onset and maintenance that should be explored and explained to the caregiver.
- Specific recommendations may also consist of other interventions including the following (2)[A]:
  - Graduated extinction: Caregiver ignores cries for specified period; can check at a fixed time or increasing intervals
  - Fading: gradual decrease in direct contact with the child as child falls asleep; goal is for the caregiver to exit the room and allow child to fall asleep independently.
  - Consider the "5S intervention" for settling problems in toddlers (used to comfort infants in nurseries): swaddling, sucking, shushing, stomach/side position, and swinging.
  - If fearful, preferred routines or inert sprays or glitter spread by the child (while avoiding the eyes) may help the child feel more secure.
- Nocturnal enuresis
  - Bed-wetting alarm: first-line therapy for caregivers who can overcome objection of having their sleep disturbed; about 2/3 of children respond while using the alarm; if enuresis recurs after use, it will often resolve with a second trial.
  - Decrease fluids an hour before bedtime.
  - Not as effective as bed-wetting alarm but evidence for other behavioral intervention, including positive reinforcement (small reward for each dry night) or responsibility training (if developmentally able, child is responsible for changing or washing sheets), encouraging daily bowel movements, and frequent bladder emptying during the day (3)[A]
- Functional encopresis
  - First disimpaction: PO with polyethylene glycol solution or mineral oil; if unsuccessful, manual mineral oil enemas
  - Maintenance therapy
    - Medical: osmotics, such as polyethylene glycol, fiber, lactulose; stimulants, such as senna or bisacodyl
    - Behavior modification: toileting after meals for 10 minutes 2 to 3 times a day, star charts, and rewards (4)[C]
- Problem eating
  - Avoid punishment, prodding, or rewards. Offer a variety of healthy foods at every meal; limit milk to 24 oz per day and decrease juice (5)[C]. Food characteristics such a texture affect acceptance, and interaction with foods prior to tasting may increase acceptance (6)[C].
- Normative sexual behavior: No treatment needed; caregivers may need encouragement not to punish or admonish child and to use gentle distraction to redirect behavior when in public setting.
- Thumb-sucking: Recommendations to caregivers include praising children when not sucking their thumb, offer alternatives that are soothing (e.g., stuffed toys), provide reminders or negative reinforcement in the form of a bandage around or bitters on the thumb (5)[C].

MEDICATION

Most pediatric behavioral issues respond well to nonpharmacologic therapy:

- Sleep disorders
  - Insufficient efficacy data exist to recommend routine psychopharmacology. As in adults, cognitive-behavioral therapy and/or sleep hygiene should be first-line treatment.
  - For certain delayed sleep-onset disorders, after behavioral methods are exhausted, melatonin 0.5 to 10.0 mg PO can be tried while behavior modification is continued. Sleep latency is likely to be reduced. However, this is not approved by the FDA for children. Expect rebound insomnia. Daytime exposure to bright or sunlight should be assured before treatment.
- Nocturnal enuresis
  - First line: Desmopressin can decrease urine output to reduce enuresis episodes. Expect fewer episodes, not full cessation. Not before age 6 years; begin with 0.2 mg tablet nightly 1 hour before bedtime; titrate to 0.6 mg. Consider use for special occasions (sleepovers). However, use is questionable because its effects do not persist posttreatment. Intranasal formulations can cause severe hyponatremia, resulting in seizures and death in children (3).
  - Second line: Anticholinergic agent (e.g., oxybutynin) works as control, not cure; oxybutynin 5 mg before bedtime
  - Third line: Tricyclic antidepressants (e.g., imipramine) have been compared solely or in combination with desmopressin interventions, with similar outcomes to desmopressin (e.g., one fewer wet night in 7-night period). Effects are inferior to alarms, are short term, and do not sustain posttreatment (3)[A].
  - Behavioral interventions are more likely to sustain and should be first-line treatment.

ISSUES FOR REFERRAL

- A patient who exhibits self-injurious behaviors, slow recovery time from tantrums, more tantrums in the home than outside the home, or more aggressive behaviors toward others may require referral to a psychologist or psychiatrist.
- Children with chronic insomnia or anxiety that interferes with sleep should be referred to a psychologist or psychiatrist.
- With enuresis and OSA symptoms, refer for sleep studies because surgical correction of airway obstruction often improves or cures enuresis and daytime wetting.
- Must distinguish sexual behavior problems: Developmentally inappropriate behaviors—greater frequency or earlier age than expected—becomes a preoccupation, recurs after adult intervention/corrective efforts. If abuse is not suspected, consider referral to a child psychologist. If abuse is suspected, must report to child protective services.
- If disimpaction by either manual or medical methods is unsuccessful, consult gastroenterology or general surgery. Patients who show no improvement after 6 months of maintenance medical therapy should be referred to gastroenterology (4).
- Thumb-sucking resistant to behavioral intervention and threatening oral development may be evaluated by a pediatric dentist for use of habit-breaking dental appliances (5)[C].

COMPLEMENTARY & ALTERNATIVE MEDICINE

Nocturnal enuresis

- Traditional Chinese medicine with Suo Quan Wan capsule in combination with desmopressin had higher complete response rate and lower relapse rate (7)[C].

 ONGOING CARE

DIET

Nutrition is very important in behavioral issues. Avoiding high-sugar foods and caffeine and providing balanced meals have been shown to decrease aggressive and noncompliant behaviors in children.

PATIENT EDUCATION

- Yale Parenting Center, Kazdin Method Sessions Webinars: http://yaleparentingcenter.yale.edu/kazdin-method-sessions
- See *Parent Training Programs: Insight for Practitioners* at: http://www.cdc.gov/violenceprevention/pdf/Parent_Training_Brief-a.pdf
- *The Happiest Baby Guide to Great Sleep: Simple Solutions for Kids from Birth to 5 Years*. Harvey Karp, MD New York, HarperCollins Publishers 2012, 384 pp.

REFERENCES

1. Potegal M, Davidson RJ. Temper tantrums in young children: 1. Behavioral composition. *J Dev Behav Pediatr.* 2003;24(3):140–147.
2. Bhargava S. Diagnosis and management of common sleep problems in children. *Pediatr Rev.* 2011;32(3):91–99.
3. Robson WL. Clinical practice. Evaluation and management of enuresis. *N Engl J Med.* 2009;360(14):1429–1436.
4. Har AF, Croffie JM. Encopresis. *Pediatr Rev.* 2010;31(9):368–374.
5. Nasir A, Nasir L. Counseling on early childhood concerns: sleep issues, thumb-sucking, picky eating, school readiness, and oral health. *Am Fam Physician.* 2015;92(4):274–278.
6. McCrickerd K, Forde CG. Sensory influences on food intake control: moving beyond palatability. *Obes Rev.* 2016;17(1):18–29.
7. Ma Y, Liu X, Shen Y. Effect of traditional Chinese and Western medicine on nocturnal enuresis in children and indicators of treatment success: randomized controlled trial. *Pediatr Int.* 2017;59(11):1183–1188.

 CODES

ICD10

- F91.9 Conduct disorder, unspecified
- F91.1 Conduct disorder, childhood-onset type
- F91.2 Conduct disorder, adolescent-onset type

CLINICAL PEARLS

- Well-child visits provide opportunities for systematic screening for these common conditions.
- Noncompliance: In extreme child disobedience, child may need to be screened for ADHD, OCD, ODD, or CD.
- Self-injurious behaviors, slow recovery time from tantrums, more tantrums in the home than outside the home, or more aggressive behaviors toward others may require referral to a psychologist or psychiatrist.
- Parental education, including a review of age-appropriate discipline, is a key component of treatment.

BELL PALSY

Assim AlAbdulKader, MD, MPH • Jason Chao, MD, MS

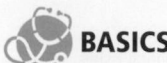 **BASICS**

DESCRIPTION
An acute, usually unilateral, peripheral facial nerve palsy of unknown etiology. Herpes-mediated viral inflammatory/immune mechanism is the likely cause of most cases, causing subsequent swelling and compression of cranial nerve VII (facial) and the associated vasa nervorum.

EPIDEMIOLOGY
- Affects 0.002% of the population annually
- No race, geographic, or gender predominance
- Median age of onset is 40 years but affects all ages.
- Accounts for about half of all cases of unilateral facial paralysis
- Occurs with equal frequency on the left and right sides of the face
- Most patients recover, but as many as 30% are left with facial disfigurement and pain.

Incidence
- 25 to 30 cases per 100,000 people in the United States per year
- Lowest in children ≤10 years of age; highest in adults ≥70 years of age
- Higher among pregnant women (3 times the risk)

Prevalence
Affects 40,000 Americans every year

ETIOLOGY AND PATHOPHYSIOLOGY
- Results from damage to the facial cranial nerve (VII)
- Exact pathogenesis is still controversial; infective, immune, and ischemic mechanisms are potential contributors.
- The most likely cause is activation of latent herpes virus (herpes simplex virus [HSV] type 1 and herpes zoster virus) in cranial nerve ganglia.
- Inflammation of cranial nerve VII causes swelling and subsequent compression and possibly demyelination of both the nerve and the associated vasa nervorum.
- Ischemia from arteriosclerosis associated with diabetes mellitus

Genetics
May be associated with a genetic predisposition, but it remains unclear, which factors are inherited

RISK FACTORS
- Pregnancy, especially in the 3rd trimester or in the 1st postpartum week
- Immunocompromised status
- Diabetes mellitus, possibly secondary to microvascular ischemia
- Age >30 years
- Exposure to cold temperatures
- Upper respiratory infection (e.g., coryza, influenza)
- Chronic hypertension (HTN)
- Obesity
- Migraine headache

COMMONLY ASSOCIATED CONDITIONS
- HSV
- Herpes zoster virus
- Lyme disease
- Diabetes mellitus
- HTN
- Ramsay-Hunt syndrome
- Sjögren syndrome
- Sarcoidosis
- Eclampsia
- Amyloidosis

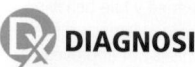 **DIAGNOSIS**

HISTORY
- Time course of the illness: rapid onset of sudden unilateral lower motor neuron-type facial weakness
- Peak of symptoms occur within 72 hours.
- Predisposing factors: history of Bell palsy, recent viral infection, tick bite, trauma, new medications, HTN, diabetes mellitus
- Associated symptoms (in 50–60% of cases):
  - Mastoid or postauricular pain
  - Hyperacusis: increased sensitivity to sounds (nerve to the stapedius muscle)
  - Dysgeusia: alteration of taste on the ipsilateral anterior 2/3 of the tongue (chorda tympani branch of the facial nerve)
  - Numbness on the ipsilateral side of the face
  - Skin rash (suggestive of herpes zoster, Lyme disease, or sarcoid)
  - Decreased lacrimation or salivation (parasympathetic effects)

PHYSICAL EXAM
- Neurologic
  - Flaccid paralysis of muscles on the affected side, including the forehead
    - Impaired ability to raise the ipsilateral eyebrow
    - Impaired closure of the ipsilateral eye
    - Impaired ability to smile, grin, or purse the lips
    - Bell phenomenon: upward diversion of the eye with attempted closure of the lid
  - Determine if the weakness is caused by either a central (upper motor neuron) or peripheral (lower motor neuron) lesion.
  - In contrast to low motor neuron lesions, the forehead muscles are usually spared in upper motor neuron lesions.
  - Patients may complain of numbness, but no deficit is present on sensory testing.
  - Examine for involvement of other cranial nerves.
- Head, ears, eyes, nose, and throat
  - Carefully examine to exclude a space-occupying lesion.
  - Perform pneumatic otoscopic exam.
- Skin: Examine for erythema migrans (Lyme disease) and vesicular rash (herpes zoster virus).

DIFFERENTIAL DIAGNOSIS
- Misdiagnosis is not uncommon (10.8%).
- Facial cranial nerve palsy etiologies include:
  - Congenital causes: genetic syndromes, birth-related trauma, developmental hypoplasia of facial muscles
  - Acquired causes: infective (herpes zoster virus, Lyme, TB, HIV), inflammatory (vasculitis, sarcoidosis, autoimmune), neoplastic (benign, malignant), cerebrovascular (stroke, aneurysm), and traumatic

- Clinical approach based on facial palsy pattern (1)[B]:
  - Recurrent, ipsilateral palsy: neoplasm of the nerve (schwannoma) or adjacent structures (parotid, temporal bone, or cerebellopontine angle [CPA])
  - Bilateral palsy: neurologic (Guillain-Barré syndrome) or associated with neoplasm (lymphoma, disseminated carcinomatosis, malignant pachymeningitis); rare: cryptococcal meningitis associated with HIV, autoimmune (MS, myasthenia gravis), sarcoid, Wegener
  - Palsy at birth: segmental developmental palsy (associated with synkinesis, recovers spontaneously)
  - Facial palsy syndromes: Ramsay-Hunt (rash in the ear [zoster oticus] and/or mouth caused by VZV); Melkersson-Rosenthal (orofacial edema, recurrent facial palsy, and fissured tongue); Heerfordt-Waldenström (parotid enlargement, anterior uveitis, facial palsy, and fever)

DIAGNOSTIC TESTS & INTERPRETATION
Bell palsy is a clinical diagnosis. It is not recommended to obtain routine lab testing or diagnostic imaging in new-onset Bell palsy (2)[C]. However, further testing may be considered in:
- Atypical presentation of facial palsy
- Recurrent facial palsy
- Slowly progressive disease >3 weeks
- Lack of improvement after months

Initial Tests (lab, imaging)
- Blood glucose level (if diabetes a consideration)
- CBC, CRP/ESR to rule out inflammatory process
- Lyme serology: ELISA or IFA, followed by Western blot for IgM, IgG for *Borrelia burgdorferi*
- Consider rapid plasma reagin (RPR) test.
- Consider HIV test.
- Consider titers for VZV, rubella, cytomegalovirus, hepatitis A, hepatitis B, and hepatitis C.
- Salivary polymerase chain reaction (PCR) for HSV-1 or herpes zoster virus (mostly for research purposes)

Follow-Up Tests & Special Considerations
- Trauma: facial radiographs to evaluate for fractures
- Contrast-enhanced CT: to evaluate for stroke and/or temporal bone fracture
- Gadolinium-enhanced MRI: to evaluate for brain and/or parotid neoplasms
- Invasive diagnostic procedures are not indicated because biopsy could further damage the nerve.

Diagnostic Procedures/Other
- Electromyography (EMG)
- Nerve Conduction Study (NCS)
- Parotid gland biopsy: considered if no recovery with negative imaging at 7 months

Test Interpretation
Test results mainly help determine prognosis and surgical planning, if indicated.

TREATMENT

GENERAL MEASURES

- Artificial tears should be used to lubricate the cornea.
- The ipsilateral eye should be patched and taped shut at night to avoid drying and infection.

MEDICATION

- Corticosteroids decrease inflammation and limit nerve damage, thereby increase the number of patients who make full recovery and reduce disabling sequelae.
- Antiviral agents are less likely to produce full recovery than corticosteroids.
- The combination of corticosteroids and antivirals is more effective than corticosteroids alone for complete recovery (NNT = 15) and for resolution of excessive tear production and motor dyskinesis (NNT = 12) (3)[B].
- The use of antivirals alone is not recommended (3)[A].
- Corticosteroids:
  - Recommended in all Bell palsy cases (4,5)[A]
  - Should be started within 72 hours of symptoms onset
  - Prednisone 50 mg PO daily for 10 days, or prednisone 60 mg PO daily for the first 5 days, and then tapering dose (by 10 mg/day) the next 5 days. Both regimens are equally effective (5)[A].
  - Precautions: Use with discretion in patients with peptic ulcer disease and diabetes.
  - Contraindications: documented hypersensitivity, preexisting infections (TB, systemic mycosis)
- Antivirals:
  - Agents that target HSV-1 and VZV
  - Should not be used alone (3)[A], rather in combination with steroids (3)[B]
  - Valacyclovir has a higher bioavailability than acyclovir.
  - Valacyclovir 1,000 mg PO TID for 7 days
  - Precautions: Use with discretion in patients with chronic kidney disease.
  - Contraindications: documented hypersensitivity

Pregnancy Considerations
Steroids should be used cautiously during pregnancy; consult with an obstetrician. Acyclovir and valacyclovir are considered category B drugs in pregnancy by the U.S. FDA.

ISSUES FOR REFERRAL
Patients should be referred to a facial nerve specialist when they experience worsening neurologic findings at any point, ocular symptoms developing at any point, or incomplete recovery at 3 months after onset of initial symptoms (2)[C].

ADDITIONAL THERAPIES
- Physical therapy: insufficient evidence that physical therapy combined with drug treatment has positive effect on grade and time of recovery compared with drug treatment only (2,6)[C]
- Electrostimulation and mirror biofeedback rehabilitation have limited evidence of effect.

- Acupuncture with strong stimulation has shown some therapeutic promise but no clear recommendations (2)[B].
- Routine use of eye-protective measures for patients with incomplete eye closure is recommended (4)[A].

SURGERY/OTHER PROCEDURES
- Surgical treatment of Bell palsy remains controversial and is reserved for intractable cases.
- There is insufficient evidence to decide whether surgical intervention is beneficial or harmful in the management of Bell palsy (2)[B].
- In those cases where surgical intervention is performed, cranial nerve XII is surgically decompressed at the entrance to the meatal foramen where the labyrinthine segment and geniculate ganglion reside.
- Decompression surgery should not be performed >14 days after the onset of paralysis because severe degeneration of the facial nerve is likely irreversible after 2 to 3 weeks.

 ONGOING CARE

FOLLOW-UP RECOMMENDATIONS
Patient Monitoring
- Patients should start steroid treatment immediately and be followed for 12 months.
- Patients who do not recover complete facial nerve function should be referred to an ophthalmologist for tarsorrhaphy.

PATIENT EDUCATION
FamilyDoctor.org from AAFP: https://familydoctor.org /condition/bells-palsy

PROGNOSIS
- Most patients achieve complete spontaneous recovery within 2 weeks. >80% recover within 3 months.
- 85% of untreated patients will experience the first signs of recovery within 3 weeks of onset.
- 16% are left with a partial palsy, motor synkinesis, and autonomic synkinesis.
- 5% experience severe sequelae, and a small number of patients experience permanent facial weakness and dysfunction.
- Poor prognostic factors include the following:
  - Age >60 years
  - History of recurrence
  - Complete facial weakness
  - HTN
  - Ramsay Hunt syndrome
- The Sunnybrook and House-Brackmann facial grading systems are clinical prognostic models that identify Bell palsy patients at risk for nonrecovery at 12 months.
- Treatment with corticosteroids and the Sunnybrook score are significant factors for predicting nonrecovery at 1 month.
- Patients with no improvement or progression of symptoms should be referred to ENT (4)[A] and may require neuroimaging to rule out neoplasms (4)[A].

COMPLICATIONS
- Corneal abrasion or ulceration
- Steroid-induced hyperglycemia, psychological disturbances; avascular necrosis of the hips, knees, and/or shoulders
- Steroid use can unmask subclinical infection (e.g., TB).

REFERENCES
1. Hohman MH, Hadlock TA. Etiology, diagnosis, and management of facial palsy: 2000 patients at a facial nerve center. *Laryngoscope*. 2014;124(7):E283–E293.
2. Baugh RF, Basura GJ, Ishii LE, et al. Clinical practice guideline: Bell's palsy. *Otolaryngol Head Neck Surg*. 2013;149(Suppl 3):S1–S27.
3. Gagyor I, Madhok VB, Daly F, et al. Antiviral treatment for Bell's palsy (idiopathic facial paralysis). *Cochrane Database Syst Rev*. 2015;(11):CD001869.
4. de Almeida JR, Guyatt GH, Sud S, et al; and Bell Palsy Working Group, Canadian Society of Otolaryngology—Head and Neck Surgery and Canadian Neurological Sciences Federation. Management of Bell palsy: clinical practice guideline. *CMAJ*. 2014;186(12):917–922.
5. Salinas RA, Alvarez G, Daly F, et al. Corticosteroids for Bell's palsy (idiopathic facial paralysis). *Cochrane Database Syst Rev*. 2010;(3):CD001942.
6. Ferreira M, Marques EE, Duarte JA, et al. Physical therapy with drug treatment in Bell palsy: a focused review. *Am J Phys Med Rehabil*. 2015;94(4):331–340.

 SEE ALSO

Amyloidosis; Diabetes Mellitus, Type 1; Diabetes Mellitus, Type 2; Herpes Simplex; Herpes Zoster (Shingles); Lyme Disease; Sarcoidosis; Sjögren Syndrome

 CODES

ICD10
G51.0 Bell's palsy

CLINICAL PEARLS
- Do not obtain routine labs or diagnostic imaging in a typical new-onset Bell palsy.
- Look closely at the voluntary movement on the upper part of the face on the affected side; in Bell palsy, all of the muscles are involved (weak or paralyzed), whereas in a stroke, the upper muscles are spared (because of bilateral innervation).
- Initiate steroids immediately following the onset of symptoms.
- Protect the affected eye with lubrication and taping.
- In areas with endemic Lyme disease, Bell palsy should be considered due to Lyme disease until proven otherwise.

BIPOLAR I DISORDER

Wendy K. Marsh, MD, MSc

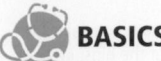 **BASICS**

DESCRIPTION

- Bipolar I (BP-I) is an episodic mood disorder of at least one manic or mixed (mania and depression) episode that causes marked impairment, psychosis, and/or hospitalization; major depressive episodes are not required but usually occur.
- Symptoms are not caused by a substance or general medical condition.

Geriatric Considerations
New onset in older patients (>50 years of age) requires a workup for organic or chemically induced pathology.

Pediatric Considerations
Diagnosis less well defined. For example, mood elevation symptoms overlap with those of ADHD.

Pregnancy Considerations
- Pregnancy does not reduce risk of mood episodes.
- Need to weigh risk of exposure to mood episode to that of medication
- Avoid divalproex due to high teratogenicity risk.
- Postpartum carries high risk of severe acute episode with psychosis and/or infanticidal ideation.

EPIDEMIOLOGY
Onset usually between 15 and 30 years of age

Prevalence
- 1.0–1.6% lifetime prevalence
- Equal among men and women (manic episodes more common in men; depressive episodes more common in women)
- Equal among races; however, clinicians tend to diagnose schizoaffective in African Americans with BP-I.

ETIOLOGY AND PATHOPHYSIOLOGY
Genetic predisposition and major life stressors can trigger initial and subsequent episodes:
- Dysregulation of biogenic amines or neurotransmitters (particularly serotonin, norepinephrine, and dopamine)
- MRI findings suggest abnormalities in prefrontal cortical areas, striatum, and amygdala that predate illness onset (1)[C].

Genetics
- Monozygotic twin concordance 40–70%
- Dizygotic twin concordance 5–25%
- 50% have at least one parent with a mood disorder.
- First-degree relatives are 7 times more likely to develop BP-I than the general population.

RISK FACTORS
Genetics, major life stressors, or substance abuse

GENERAL PREVENTION
No known way to prevent onset, but treatment adherence and education can help to prevent relapses.

COMMONLY ASSOCIATED CONDITIONS
Substance abuse (60%), ADHD, anxiety disorders, and eating disorders

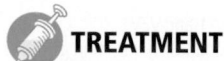 **DIAGNOSIS**

- The diagnosis of BP-I requires at least one manic or mixed episode (simultaneous mania and depression). Although a depressive episode is not necessary for the diagnosis, 80–90% of people with BP-I also experience depression.
- Manic episode, *DSM-5* criteria (2)
  – Distinct period of abnormally and persistently elevated, expansive, or irritable mood plus increased activity or energy for at least 1 week (or any duration if hospitalization is necessary)
  – During the period of mood disturbance, three or more of the "DIG FAST" symptoms must persist (four if the mood is only irritable) and must be present to a significant degree.
    ○ Distractibility
    ○ Insomnia, decreased need for sleep
    ○ Grandiosity or inflated self-esteem
    ○ Flight of ideas or racing thoughts
    ○ Agitation or increase in goal-directed activity
    ○ Speech pressured/more talkative than usual
    ○ Taking risks: excessive involvement in pleasurable activities that have a high potential for painful consequences (e.g., financial or sexual)
  – Mixed specifier: when three or more symptoms of opposite mood pole are present during primary mood episode, for example, mania with mixed features (of depression)

HISTORY
- Collateral information makes diagnostics more complete and is often necessary for a clear history.
- History: safety concerns (e.g., Suicidal/homicidal ideation? Safety plan? Psychosis present?), physical well-being (e.g., Number of hours of sleep? Weight change? Substance abuse?), personal history (e.g., Talkative? Risky driving? Excessive spending? Credit card debt? Promiscuity? Other risk-taking behavior? Legal trouble?)

PHYSICAL EXAM
- Mental status exam in acute mania
  – General appearance: bright clothing, excessive makeup, disorganized or discombobulated, psychomotor agitation
  – Speech: pressured, difficult to interrupt
  – Mood/affect: euphoria, irritability, expansive, labile
  – Thought process: flight of ideas (streams of thought occur to patient at rapid rate), easily distracted
  – Thought content: grandiosity, paranoia, hyperreligious
  – Perceptual abnormalities: 3/4 of manic patients experience delusions, grandiose, or paranoia.
  – Suicidal/homicidal ideation: aggression toward self or others; suicidal ideation is common with mixed episode.
  – Insight/judgment: poor/impaired
- See "Bipolar II Disorder" for an example of a mental status exam in depression.
- With mixed episodes, patients may exhibit a combination of manic and depressive mental states.

DIFFERENTIAL DIAGNOSIS
- Other psychiatric considerations: unipolar depression ± psychotic features, schizophrenia, schizoaffective disorder, personality disorders (particularly antisocial, borderline, histrionic, and narcissistic), ADD ± hyperactivity, substance-induced mood disorder
- Medical considerations: epilepsy (e.g., temporal lobe), brain tumor, infection (e.g., AIDS, syphilis), stroke, endocrine (e.g., thyroid) disease, multiple sclerosis
- In children, consider ADHD and ODD.

DIAGNOSTIC TESTS & INTERPRETATION
- BP-I is a clinical diagnosis.
- The Mood Disorder Questionnaire is a self-assessment screen for bipolar disorders (sensitivity 73%, specificity 90%) (3).
- Patient Health Questionnaire-9 helps to determine the presence and severity of a depressive episode.

Initial Tests (lab, imaging)
- TSH, CBC, BMP, LFTs, RPR, HIV, ESR
- Drug/alcohol screen with each presentation
- Dementia workup if new onset in elderly
- Consider brain imaging (CT, MRI) with initial onset of mania to rule out organic cause (e.g., tumor, infection, or stroke), especially with onset in elderly and if psychosis is present.

Diagnostic Procedures/Other
Consider EEG if presentation suggests temporal lobe epilepsy (hyperreligiosity, hypergraphia).

TREATMENT

GENERAL MEASURES
- Ensure safety.
- Psychotherapy for depression (e.g., cognitive-behavioral therapy, social rhythm, interpersonal) in conjunction with medications
- Regular daily schedule, exercise, a healthy diet, and sobriety
- Stress reduction
- Patient and family education

MEDICATION
- Acute mania
  – First line
    ○ Lithium monotherapy (see lithium)
    ○ Atypical: quetiapine, risperidone, aripiprazole, ziprasidone, asenapine, or olanzapine* monotherapy (see atypicals)
    ○ Divalproex (see antiseizure)
    ○ Lithium or divalproex plus atypical
  – Second line
    ○ Haloperidol
    ○ Paliperidone
    ○ Lithium plus divalproex
    ○ Lithium or divalproex plus haloperidol
    ○ Carbamazepine
- Acute bipolar depression
  – First line
    ○ Quetiapine monotherapy (see atypicals)
    ○ Lamotrigine (see antiseizure)
    ○ Lurasidone monotherapy (see atypicals)
    ○ Lurasidone or quetiapine adjunctive to lithium or divalproex

– Second line
  ○ Lithium
  ○ Olanzapine* (see atypicals) + SSRI/fluoxetine
  ○ Divalproex
  ○ Two drug combination of above of different classes (i.e., not two atypicals)
- *Side effects concerns: Weight gain, metabolic syndrome, and extrapyramidal symptoms (EPS) warrant vigilance and monitoring by the clinician.
- Treatment mood stabilizer(s) or other psychotropic medications. When combining, use different classes (e.g., an atypical antipsychotic and/or an antiseizure medication and/or lithium) (3,4)[A].
  – Lithium (Lithobid, Eskalith, generic): dosing: 600 to 1,200 mg/day divided BID–QID; start 600 to 900 mg/day divided BID–TID, titrate based on blood levels. *Warning*: caution in kidney and heart disease; use can lead to diabetes insipidus or thyroid disease. Caution with diuretics or ACE inhibitors; dehydration can lead to toxicity (seizures, encephalopathy, arrhythmias). Pregnancy Category D (Ebstein anomaly). *Monitor*: Check ECG >40 years, TSH, BUN, creatinine, electrolytes at baseline and every 6 months; check level 5 to 7 days after initiation or dose change, then every 2 weeks × 3, and then every 3 months (goal: 0.8 to 1.2 mmol/L).
- Antiseizure medications
  – Divalproex sodium, valproic acid (Depakote, Depakene, generic): dosing: Start 250 to 500 mg BID–TID; maximum 60 mg/kg/day. Black box warnings: hepatotoxicity, pancreatitis, thrombocytopenia, pregnancy Category D. Monitor CBC and LFTs at baseline and every 6 months; check level 5 days after initiation and dose changes (goal: 50 to 125 μg/mL).
  – Carbamazepine (Equetro, Tegretol, generic): dosing: 800 to 1,200 mg/day PO divided BID–QID; start 100 to 200 mg PO BID and titrate to lowest effective dose. *Warning*: Do not use with tricyclic antidepressant (TCA) or within 14 days of an MAOI. Caution in kidney/heart disease; risk of aplastic anemia/agranulocytosis, enzyme inducer; pregnancy Category D. Monitor CBC and LFTs at baseline and every 3 to 6 months; check level 4 to 5 days after initiation and dose changes (goal: 4 to 12 μg/mL).
  – Lamotrigine (Lamictal, generic): dosing: 200 to 400 mg/day; start 25 mg/day for 2 weeks, then 50 mg/day for 2 weeks, then 100 mg/day for 1 week, and then 150 mg/day. (Note: Use different dosing if adjunct to valproate.) *Warning*: Titrate slowly (risk of Stevens-Johnson syndrome); caution with kidney/liver/heart disease; pregnancy Category C
  – Oxcarbazepine (Trileptal) dosing: 300 mg PO QD. Titrate to 1,800 to 2,400/day max.
- Atypical antipsychotics
  – Side effects: orthostatic hypotension, metabolic side effects (glucose and lipid dysregulation, weight gain), tardive dyskinesia, neuroleptic malignant syndrome (NMS), prolactinemia (except aripiprazole [Abilify]), increased risk of death in elderly with dementia-related psychosis, pregnancy Category C
  – Monitor LFTs, lipids, glucose at baseline, 3 months and annually; check for EPS with Abnormal Involuntary Movement Scale (AIMS) and assess weight (with abdominal circumference) at baseline; at 4, 8, and 12 weeks; and then every 3 to 6 months; monitor for orthostatic hypotension 3 to 5 days after starting or changing dose.
  – Aripiprazole (Abilify): dosing: 15 to 30 mg/day; less likely to cause metabolic side effects

– Asenapine: dosing: 5 to 10 mg sublingual BID
– Cariprazine: dosing: 1.5 mg/day only for depression; 3 to 6 mg/day mood elevation
– Lurasidone: dosing: 20 to 60 mg/day; FDA-approved for bipolar depression
– Olanzapine (Zyprexa, Zydis, generic): dosing: 5 to 20 mg/day; most likely to cause metabolic side effects (weight gain, diabetes)
– Paliperidone dosing: 6 mg every morning; may cause agranulocytosis, cardiac arrhythmias
– Quetiapine (Seroquel, Seroquel XR, generic): dosing: in mania, 200 to 400 mg BID; in bipolar depression, 50 to 300 mg QHS; XR dosing 50 to 400 mg QHS
– Risperidone (Risperdal, Risperdal Consta, generic): dosing: 1 to 6 mg/day divided QD–QID; IM preparation available (q2wk)
– Ziprasidone (Geodon): dosing: 40 to 80 mg BID; less likely to cause metabolic side effects. Caution: QTc prolongation (>500 ms) has been associated with use (0.06%). Consider ECG at baseline.
- Unipolar antidepressants
  – There is inadequate information to recommend in bipolar disorder. If used (e.g., for anxiety), antimanic agent is essential.
- Avoid
  – TCAs and serotonin norepinephrine reuptake inhibitor (SNRI); increases mood cycling risk

ISSUES FOR REFERRAL
- Refer to psychiatry, depends on knowledge level of the doctor, stability of patient.
- Patients benefit from a multidisciplinary team, including a primary care physician, psychiatrist, and therapist.

ADDITIONAL THERAPIES
- Electroconvulsive therapy can be helpful in acute or treatment-resistant mania and depression.
- Modest evidence supports transcranial magnetic stimulation, vagus nerve stimulation, ketamine infusion, sleep deprivation, and hormone therapy (e.g., thyroid) in bipolar depression.
- Blue-blocking glasses or dark therapy for mania

ADMISSION, INPATIENT, AND NURSING CONSIDERATIONS
- Admit if dangerous to self or others.
- To admit involuntarily, the patient must have a psychiatric diagnosis (e.g., BP-I) and present a danger to self or others, or the mental disease must be inhibiting the person from obtaining basic needs (e.g., food, clothing).
- Nursing: Alert staff to potentially dangerous or agitated patients. Acute suicidal threats need continuous observation.
- Discharge criteria determined by safety

 ONGOING CARE

FOLLOW-UP RECOMMENDATIONS
- Regularly scheduled visits support adherence with treatment.
- Frequent communication among primary care doctor, psychiatrist, and therapist

Patient Monitoring
Mood charts are helpful to monitor symptoms.

PATIENT EDUCATION
- National Alliance on Mental Illness (NAMI): http://www.nami.org/
- National Institutes of Mental Health (NIMH): http://www.nimh.nih.gov/index.shtml

- Depression and Bipolar Support Alliance (DBSA): http://www.dbsalliance.org

PROGNOSIS
- Frequency and severity of episodes are related to medication adherence, consistency with therapy, quality of sleep, and support systems.
- 40–50% of patients experience another manic episode within 2 years of first episode.
- 25–50% attempt suicide, and 15% die by suicide.
- Substance abuse, unemployment, psychosis, depression, and male gender are associated with a worse prognosis.

REFERENCES
1. American Psychiatric Association. *Diagnostic and Statistical Manual of Mental Disorders*. 5th ed. Arlington, VA: American Psychiatric Association; 2013.
2. Ostacher MJ, Tandon R, Suppes T. Florida Best Practice Psychotherapeutic Medication Guidelines for Adults with Bipolar Disorder: a novel, practical, patient-centered guide for clinicians. *J Clin Psychiatry*. 2016;77(7):920–926.
3. Yatham LN, Kennedy SH, Parikh SV, et al. Canadian Network for Mood and Anxiety Treatments (CANMAT) and International Society for Bipolar Disorders (ISBD) collaborative update of CANMAT guidelines for the management of patients with bipolar disorder: update 2013. *Bipolar Disord*. 2013;15(1):1–44.

ADDITIONAL READING
- Canadian Network for Mood and Anxiety Treatments: http://canmat.org/
- Licht RW. A new BALANCE in bipolar I disorder. *Lancet*. 2010;375(9712):350–352.

 SEE ALSO

Algorithm: Depressive Episode, Major

 CODES

ICD10
- F31.9 Bipolar disorder, unspecified
- F31.10 Bipolar disorder, current episode manic without psychotic features, unspecified
- F31.30 Bipolar disord, crnt epsd depress, mild or mod severt, unsp

CLINICAL PEARLS
- BP-I is characterized by at least one manic or mixed episode that causes marked impairment; major depressive episodes usually occur but are not necessary.
- 25–50% of BP-I patients attempt suicide, and 15% die by suicide.
- There is no known way to prevent BP-I, but treatment adherence and education helps reduce further episodes.
- Goal of treatment is to decrease the intensity, length, and frequency of episodes as well as greater mood stability between episodes.

BIPOLAR II DISORDER

Wendy K. Marsh, MD, MSc

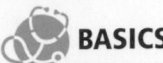 **BASICS**

DESCRIPTION

Bipolar II (BP-II) is a mood disorder characterized by at least one episode of major depression (with or without psychosis) and at least one episode of hypomania, a nonsevere mood elevation.

Geriatric Considerations

New onset in older patients (>50 years) requires a workup for organic or chemically induced pathology.

Pediatric Considerations

Diagnosis less well defined

Pregnancy Considerations

- Pregnancy does not reduce risk of mood episodes.
- Need to weigh risk of exposure to mood episode to that of medication
- Avoid divalproex due to high teratogenicity risk.
- Postpartum caries high risk of severe acute episode with psychosis and/or infanticidal ideation.

EPIDEMIOLOGY

Onset usually between 15 and 30 years of age

Prevalence

- 0.5–1.1% lifetime prevalence
- More common in women

ETIOLOGY AND PATHOPHYSIOLOGY

Dysregulation of biogenic amines or neurotransmitters (particularly serotonin, norepinephrine, and dopamine)

Genetics

Heritability estimate: >77%

RISK FACTORS

Genetics, major life stressors, or substance abuse

GENERAL PREVENTION

No known way to prevent onset, but treatment adherence and education can help to prevent further episodes.

COMMONLY ASSOCIATED CONDITIONS

Substance abuse or dependence, ADHD, anxiety disorders, and eating disorders

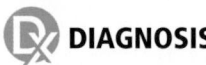 **DIAGNOSIS**

- *DSM-5* criteria: one hypomanic episode and at least one major depressive episode. The symptoms cause unequivocal change in functioning noticed by others but not severe enough to cause marked impairment (1)[C].
- Hypomania is a distinct period of persistently elevated, expansive, or irritable mood, different from usual euthymic mood, including increase in activity or energy lasting at least 4 days:
  - The episode must include at least three of the "DIG FAST" symptoms *plus increased energy* below (four if the mood is only irritable):
    ○ Distractibility
    ○ Insomnia, decreased need for sleep
    ○ Grandiosity or inflated self-esteem
    ○ Flight of ideas or racing thoughts
    ○ Agitation or increase in goal-directed activity (socially, at work or school, or sexually)
    ○ Speech pressured/more talkative than usual
    ○ Taking risks: excessive involvement in pleasurable activities that have high potential for painful consequences (e.g., sexual or financial)

- Major depression
  - Depressed mood or diminished interest and four or more of the "SIG E CAPS" symptoms are present during the same 2-week period:
    ○ Sleep disturbance (e.g., trouble falling asleep, early-morning awakening)
    ○ Interest: loss or anhedonia
    ○ Guilt (or feelings of worthlessness)
    ○ Energy, loss of
    ○ Concentration, loss of
    ○ Appetite changes, increase or decrease
    ○ Psychomotor changes (retardation or agitation)
    ○ Suicidal/homicidal thoughts
  - Rapid cycling is ≥4 mood episodes in 12 months (major depression or hypomania).
  - Mixed specifier: when three or more symptoms of opposite mood pole are present during primary mood episode, for example, hypomania with mixed features (of depression)
- Note: If symptoms have *ever* met criteria for a full manic episode or hospitalization was necessary secondary to manic/mixed symptoms or psychosis was present, then the diagnosis is BP-I.

HISTORY

- Collateral information makes diagnostics more complete and is often necessary for a clear history.
- History: safety concerns (e.g., Suicidal/homicidal ideation? Safety plan? Psychosis present?), physical well-being (e.g., Number of hours of sleep? Substance abuse?), personal history (e.g., Risky driving? Excessive spending? Credit card debt? Promiscuity? Other risk-taking behavior? Legal trouble?)

PHYSICAL EXAM

- Mental status exam in hypomania
  - General appearance: usually appropriately dressed, with psychomotor agitation
  - Speech: may be pressured, talkative, difficult to interrupt
  - Mood/affect: euphoria, irritability/congruent, or expansive
  - Thought process: may be easily distracted, difficulty concentrating on one task
  - Thought content: usually positive, with "big" plans
  - Perceptual abnormalities: none
  - Suicidal/homicidal ideation: low incidence of homicidal or suicidal ideation
  - Insight/judgment: usually stable/may be impaired by their distractibility
- Mental status exam in acute depression
  - General appearance: unkempt, psychomotor retardation, poor eye contact
  - Speech: low, soft, monotone
  - Mood/affect: sad, depressed/congruent, flat
  - Thought process: ruminating thoughts, generalized slowing
  - Thought content: preoccupied with negative or nihilistic ideas
  - Perceptual abnormalities: 15% of depressed patients experience hallucinations or delusions.
  - Suicidal/homicidal ideation: Suicidal ideation is very common.
  - Insight/judgment: often impaired

DIFFERENTIAL DIAGNOSIS

- Other psychiatric considerations
  - BP-I disorder, unipolar depression, personality disorders (particularly borderline, antisocial, and narcissistic), ADD with hyperactivity, substance-induced mood disorder

- Medical considerations
  - Epilepsy (e.g., temporal lobe), brain tumor, infection (e.g., AIDS, syphilis), stroke, endocrine (e.g., thyroid disease), multiple sclerosis

DIAGNOSTIC TESTS & INTERPRETATION

- BP-II is a clinical diagnosis.
- Mood Disorder Questionnaire, self-assessment screen for BP, sensitivity 73%, specificity 90%
- Hypomania Checklist-32 distinguishes between BP-II and unipolar depression (sensitivity 80%, specificity 51%) (2)[B].
- Patient Health Questionnaire-9 helps to determine the presence and severity of depression.

Initial Tests (lab, imaging)

- Rule out organic causes of mood disorder during initial episode.
- Drug/alcohol screen is prudent with each presentation.
- Dementia workup if new onset in elderly
- With initial presentation: Consider CBC, chem 7, TSH, LFTs, ANA, RPR, HIV, and ESR.
- Consider brain imaging (CT, MRI) with initial onset of hypomania to rule out organic cause, especially with onset in the elderly.

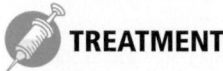 **TREATMENT**

GENERAL MEASURES

- Ensure safety.
- Psychotherapy (e.g., CBT, social rhythm, interpersonal, family focused) in conjunction with medications
- Regular daily schedule, exercise, a healthy diet, and sobriety have been shown to help.
- Stress reduction
- Patient and family education
- Refer to psychiatrist

MEDICATION

- Acute mood elevation
  - First line
    ○ Lithium monotherapy (see lithium)
    ○ Atypical: quetiapine, risperidone, aripiprazole, ziprasidone, asenapine, or, olanzapine monotherapy (see atypicals)
    ○ Divalproex (see antiseizure)
    ○ Lithium or divalproex plus atypical
  - Second line
    ○ Haloperidol
    ○ Paliperidone
    ○ Lithium plus divalproex
    ○ Lithium or divalproex plus haloperidol
    ○ Carbamazepine
- Acute bipolar depression
  - First line
    ○ Quetiapine monotherapy (see atypicals)
    ○ Lamotrigine (see antiseizure)
    ○ Lurasidone monotherapy (see atypicals)
    ○ Lurasidone or quetiapine adjunctive to lithium or divalproex
  - Second line
    ○ Lithium
    ○ Olanzapine (see atypicals) + SSRI/fluoxetine
    ○ Divalproex
    ○ Two drug combination of above of different classes (i.e., not two atypicals)
- Side effects concerns: Weight gain, metabolic syndrome, and extrapyramidal symptoms (EPS) warrant vigilance and monitoring by the clinician.

- Treatment mood stabilizer(s) or other psychotropic medications. When combining, use different classes (e.g., an atypical antipsychotic and/or an antiseizure medication and/or lithium) (2,3)[A].
- Lithium (Lithobid, Eskalith, generic): dosing: 600 to 1,200 mg/day divided BID–QID; start 600 to 900 mg/day divided BID–TID, titrate based on blood levels. *Warning*: caution in kidney and heart disease; use can lead to diabetes insipidus or thyroid disease. Caution with diuretics or ACE inhibitors; dehydration can lead to toxicity (seizures, encephalopathy, arrhythmias). Pregnancy Category D (Ebstein anomaly). *Monitor*: Check ECG >40 years, TSH, BUN, creatine, electrolytes at baseline and every 6 months; check level 5 to 7 days after initiation or dose change, then every 2 weeks × 3, and then every 3 months (goal: 0.8 to 1.2 mmol/L).
- Antiseizure medications
  - Divalproex sodium, valproic acid (Depakote, Depakene, generic): dosing: Start 250 to 500 mg BID–TID; maximum 60 mg/kg/day. Black box warnings: hepatotoxicity, pancreatitis, thrombocytopenia, pregnancy Category D. Monitor CBC and LFTs at baseline and every 6 months; check level 5 days after initiation and dose changes (goal: 50 to 125 μg/mL).
  - Carbamazepine (Equetro, Tegretol, generic): dosing: 800 to 1,200 mg/day PO divided BID–QID; start 100 to 200 mg PO BID and titrate to lowest effective dose. *Warning*: Do not use with tricyclic antidepressants (TCAs) or within 14 days of monoamine oxidase inhibitor (MAOI). Caution in kidney/heart disease; risk of aplastic anemia/agranulocytosis, enzyme inducer; pregnancy Category D. Monitor CBC and LFTs at baseline and every 3 to 6 months; check level 4 to 5 days after initiation and dose changes (goal: 4 to 12 μg/mL).
  - Lamotrigine (Lamictal, generic): dosing: 200 to 400 mg/day; start 25 mg/day for 2 weeks, then 50 mg/day for 2 weeks, then 100 mg/day for 1 week, and then 150 mg/day. (Note: Use different dosing if adjunct to valproate.) *Warning*: Titrate slowly (risk of Stevens-Johnson syndrome); caution with kidney/liver/heart disease; pregnancy Category C
  - Oxcarbazepine (Trileptal) dosing: 300 mg PO QD. Titrate to 1,800 to 2,400/day max.
- Atypical antipsychotics
  - Side effects: orthostatic hypotension, metabolic side effects (glucose and lipid dysregulation, weight gain), tardive dyskinesia, neuroleptic malignant syndrome (NMS), prolactinemia (except Abilify), increased risk of death in elderly with dementia-related psychosis, pregnancy Category C
  - Monitor LFTs, lipids, glucose at baseline, 3 months and annually; check for EPS with Abnormal Involuntary Movement Scale (AIMS), and assess weight (with abdominal circumference) at baseline; at 4, 8, and 12 weeks; and then every 3 to 6 months; monitor for orthostatic hypotension 3 to 5 days after starting or changing dose.
  - Aripiprazole (Abilify): dosing: 15 to 30 mg/day; less likely to cause metabolic side effects

  - Asenapine: dosing: 5 to 10 mg sublingual BID
  - Cariprazine: dosing: 1.5 mg/day only for depression; 3 to 6 mg/day mood elevation
  - Lurasidone: dosing: 20 to 60 mg/day; FDA-approved for bipolar depression
  - Olanzapine (Zyprexa, Zydis, generic): dosing: 5 to 20 mg/day; most likely to cause metabolic side effects (weight gain, diabetes)
  - Paliperidone: dosing 6 mg every morning; may cause agranulocytosis, cardiac arrhythmias
  - Quetiapine (Seroquel, Seroquel XR, generic): dosing: in mania, 200 to 400 mg BID; in bipolar depression, 50 to 300 mg QHS; XR dosing 50 to 400 mg QHS
  - Risperidone (Risperdal, Risperdal Consta, generic): dosing: 1 to 6 mg/day divided QD–QID; IM preparation available (q2wk)
  - Ziprasidone (Geodon): dosing: 40 to 80 mg BID; less likely to cause metabolic side effects. Caution: QTc prolongation (>500 ms) has been associated with use (0.06%). Consider ECG at baseline.
- Unipolar antidepressants
  - There is inadequate information to recommend in bipolar disorder. If used (e.g., for anxiety), antimanic agent is essential.
- Avoid
  - TCAs and serotonin-norepinephrine reuptake inhibitor (SNRI); increases mood cycling risk

ISSUES FOR REFERRAL
- Refer to psychiatry, depends on knowledge level of the doctor, stability of patient.
- Patients benefit from a multidisciplinary team, including a primary care physician, psychiatrist, and therapist.

ADDITIONAL THERAPIES
- Electroconvulsive therapy can be helpful in acute or treatment-resistant mania and depression.
- Modest evidence supports transcranial magnetic stimulation, vagus nerve stimulation, ketamine infusion, sleep deprivation, and hormone therapy (e.g., thyroid) in bipolar depression.
- Blue-blocking glasses or dark therapy for mania

ADMISSION, INPATIENT, AND NURSING CONSIDERATIONS
- Admit if dangerous to self or others.
- To admit involuntarily, the patient must have a psychiatric diagnosis (e.g., BP-I) and present a danger to self or others, or the mental disease must be inhibiting the person from obtaining basic needs (e.g., food, clothing).
- Nursing: Alert staff to potentially dangerous or agitated patients. Acute suicidal threats need continuous observation.
- Discharge criteria determined by safety

 ONGOING CARE

FOLLOW-UP RECOMMENDATIONS
- Regularly scheduled visits support adherence with treatment.
- Frequent communication among primary care doctor, psychiatrist, and therapist

Patient Monitoring
Mood charts are helpful to monitor symptoms.

PATIENT EDUCATION
- National Alliance on Mental Illness (NAMI): http://www.nami.org/
- National Institute of Mental Health (NIMH): http://www.nimh.nih.gov/index.shtml
- Depression and Bipolar Support Alliance (DBSA): http://www.dbsalliance.org

PROGNOSIS
- Frequency and severity of episodes are related to medication adherence, consistency with therapy, quality of sleep, and support systems.
- 40–50% of patients experience another manic episode within 2 years of first episode.
- 25–50% attempt suicide and 15% die by suicide.
- Substance abuse, unemployment, psychosis, depression, and male gender are associated with a worse prognosis.

REFERENCES
1. American Psychiatric Association. *Diagnostic and Statistical Manual of Mental Disorders*. 5th ed. Arlington, VA: American Psychiatric Association; 2013.
2. Ostacher MJ, Tandon R, Suppes T. Florida best practice psychotherapeutic medication guidelines for adults with bipolar disorder: a novel, practical, patient-centered guide for clinicians. *J Clin Psychiatry*. 2016;77(7):920–926.
3. Yatham LN, Kennedy SH, Parikh SV, et al. Canadian Network for Mood and Anxiety Treatments (CANMAT) and International Society for Bipolar Disorders (ISBD) collaborative update of CANMAT guidelines for the management of patients with bipolar disorder: update 2013. *Bipolar Disord*. 2013;15(1):1–44.

 SEE ALSO

Algorithm: Depressive Episode, Major

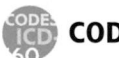 **CODES**

ICD10
F31.81 Bipolar II disorder

CLINICAL PEARLS
- BP-II is characterized by at least one episode of major depression and one episode of hypomania.
- Patients may not recognize symptoms and or decline treatment during a hypomanic episode; they may enjoy the elevated mood and productivity.
- Patients with BP-II are at great risk of both attempting and completing suicide.

BITES, ANIMAL AND HUMAN

Kathryn Samai, PharmD, BCPS • Brian J. Kimbrell, MD, FACS

 BASICS

DESCRIPTION

- Animal bite rates vary by species: dogs (60–90%), cats (5–20%), rodents (2–3%), humans (2–3%), and (rarely) other animals, including snakes
- System(s) affected: potentially any

Pediatric Considerations
Young children are more likely to sustain bites and have bites that include the face, upper extremity, or trunk.

EPIDEMIOLOGY

- All ages but children > adults
- Dog bites, male > female; cat bites, female > male

Incidence
- 3 to 6 million animal bites per year in the United States (1)
- Account for 1% of all injury-related ED visits
- 1–2% will require hospital admission, and 20 to 35 victims die from dog bite complications annually.

ETIOLOGY AND PATHOPHYSIOLOGY

- Most dog bites are from a domestic pet known to the victim.
- Most (~90%) cat bites are provoked.
- Dog bites are most commonly associated with pit bull terriers and German shepherds.
- Human bite wounds are typically incurred by striking another in the mouth with a clenched fist.
- Human bites also occur incidentally (e.g., paronychia due to nail biting, thumb sucking, or nonmalicious gentle bites to the face, breasts, or genital areas).
- Animal bites can cause tears, punctures, scratches, avulsions, or crush injuries.
- Contamination by oral flora leads to infection.

RISK FACTORS

- Older, male dogs are more likely to bite.
- Clenched-fist human bites are frequently associated with the use of alcohol or drugs.
- Patients presenting >8 hours following the bite are at greater risk of infection.

GENERAL PREVENTION

- Instruct children and adults about animal hazards.
- Enforce animal control laws.
- Educate dog owners.

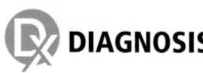 **DIAGNOSIS**

HISTORY

- Detailed history of the incident (provoked or unprovoked); type/breed of animal; vaccine status
- Site of the bite
- Geographic setting
- Underlying medical history

PHYSICAL EXAM

- Dog bites
  - Hands and face most common site of injury in adults and children, respectively
  - More likely to have associated crush injury
- Cat bites
  - Predominantly involve the hands, followed by lower extremities, face, and trunk
- Human bites
  - Intentional bite: semicircular or oval area of erythema and bruising, with/without break in skin
  - Clenched-fist injury: small wounds over the metacarpophalangeal joints from striking the fist against another's teeth
- Signs of wound infection include fever, erythema, swelling, tenderness, purulent drainage, and lymphangitis.

ALERT
Cat bites (often puncture wounds) are twice as likely to become infected as are dog bites (with higher risks of osteomyelitis, tenosynovitis, and septic arthritis).

Pediatric Considerations
Human bite marks on a child with an intercanine distance >3 cm, are likely from an adult and should raise concerns about child abuse.

DIAGNOSTIC TESTS & INTERPRETATION
Initial Tests (lab, imaging)
- Gram stain and culture any wound drainage
  - If wound fails to heal, culture for atypical pathogens (fungi, *Nocardia*, and mycobacteria); keep bacterial cultures for 7 to 10 days (some pathogens are slow-growing).
- 85% of bite wounds will yield a positive culture; most are polymicrobial with an average of five pathogens.
- Obtain aerobic and anaerobic blood cultures before starting antibiotics if bacteremia is suspected.
- Recent antibiotic therapy may alter culture results.

ALERT
If bite wound is near a bone or joint, obtain a plain radiograph to check for bone injury (this film is also helpful for later comparison if osteomyelitis is suspected) (2).

- Radiographs to check for fractures in clenched-fist injuries

Follow-Up Tests & Special Considerations
- Plain radiograph and/or MRI for suspected osteomyelitis.
- CT scan for severe skull bites. Ultrasound can detect abscess formation.

Diagnostic Procedures/Other
Surgical exploration may be needed to determine the extent of injuries or to drain deep infections (e.g., tendon sheath), especially in serious hand wounds.

Test Interpretation
- Dog bites (3,4)
  - *Pasteurella* species present in 50% of bites
  - Viridans streptococci, *Staphylococcus aureus, Staphylococcus intermedius, Bacteroides, Capnocytophaga canimorsus, Fusobacterium*
- Cat bites (4)
  - *Pasteurella* species in 75% of bites
  - *Streptococcus* spp. (including *Streptococcus pyogenes*), *Staphylococcus* spp. (including methicillin-resistant *S. aureus* [MRSA]), *Fusobacterium* spp., *Bacteroides* spp., *Porphyromonas* spp., *Moraxella* spp.
- Human bites
  - *Streptococcus* spp., *S. aureus, Eikenella corrodens* (29%), and various anaerobic bacteria (e.g., *Fusobacterium, Peptostreptococcus, Prevotella,* and *Porphyromonas* spp.)
  - Although rare, case reports suggest transmission of viruses (hepatitis, HIV, and herpes simplex).
- Reptile bites
  - *Pseudomonas aeruginosa, Proteus* spp., *Salmonella, Bacteroides fragilis,* and *Clostridium* species
- Rodent bites
  - *Streptobacillus moniliformis* or *Spirillum minus,* which causes rat-bite fever
- Monkey bites
  - All monkey bites can transmit rabies, and bites of a macaque monkey may transmit herpes B virus, which is potentially fatal.
- Ungulate (hooved animals) bites
  - Pigs are the most likely to bite; commonly polymicrobial infections (*Staphylococcus* and *Streptococcus* spp, *Haemophilus influenzae, Pasteurella, Actinobacillus* and *Flavobacterium* species)
  - Other ungulates are more like to cause injury by kicking or crushing.

ALERT
Asplenic patients and those with underlying hepatic disease are at risk for bacteremia and fatal sepsis after dog bites infected with *C. canimorsus*.

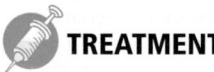 **TREATMENT**

GENERAL MEASURES
- Complete and submit bite report per local policy.
- Elevate the injured extremity to prevent swelling.
- Contact local health department to determine rabies prevalence in biting species (highest in bats).
- Snake bite: If venomous, transport for appropriate evaluation and antivenom. Be sure patient is stable for transport; assess coagulation and renal status.
- Monkey bite: Contact CDC; consider an antiviral, such as valacyclovir, active against herpes B virus.

MEDICATION

- Determine need for antirabies therapy: rabies immunoglobulin and human diploid cell rabies vaccine for those bitten by wild animals (primary vector in the United States is bat or raccoon), rabid pets, unvaccinated pets, or in situations where the animal cannot be quarantined for 10 days.

ALERT
Refer to State and Local Rabies Consultation (https://www.cdc.gov/rabies/resources/contacts.html).

- Tetanus toxoid (Td) for previously immunized with >10 years since their last dose (2)[C]; tetanus, diphtheria, and pertussis (Tdap) preferred to Td (2)[C]
- Anti-HBs negative patients bitten by HBsAg-positive individuals should receive both hepatitis B immunoglobulin (HBIG) and hepatitis B vaccine.
- HIV postexposure prophylaxis is generally not recommended for human bites, unless there is significant blood exposure to broken skin.
- Preemptive antibiotics recommended only for human bites and high-risk wounds (deep puncture, crush injury, venous or lymphatic compromise, hands or near joint, face or genital area, immunocompromised hosts, requiring surgical repair, asplenic, advanced liver, edema)
- For preemptive therapy and for empiric treatment of established infection, amoxicillin and clavulanate is first-line antibiotic (2)[B].
  - Duration of therapy: preemptive, 3 to 5 days; treatment of cellulitis/skin abscess, 5 to 10 days
  - Adults: amoxicillin and clavulanate 875/125 mg PO BID
  - Children: <3 months: 30 mg/kg/day PO q12h; ≥3 months and <40 kg: 25 to 45 mg/kg/day q12h; >40 kg, use adult dosing
- Alternative regimens
  - Adults: clindamycin (300 mg PO TID) plus either trimethoprim-sulfamethoxazole (TMP-SMX; 1 DS tablet PO BID) or ciprofloxacin (500 to 750 mg PO BID)
  - Children: clindamycin 25 to 30 mg/kg/day PO in 3 divided doses to a maximum of 300 mg per dose plus TMP-SMX (8 to 10 mg/kg/day of trimethoprim) PO in 2 divided doses
- Avoid 1st-generation cephalosporins (e.g., cephalexin), penicillinase-resistant penicillins (e.g., dicloxacillin), macrolides (e.g., erythromycin), and clindamycin (when not administered with another agent) because they lack activity against *Pasteurella multocida* (dog/cat bites) and *E. corrodens* (human bites).

Pregnancy Considerations
- Pregnant women who cannot take penicillins or cephalosporin due to severe allergy
  - Azithromycin 250 to 500 mg PO every day
- Observe closely and note potential increased risk of treatment failure.

ALERT
Consider community-acquired MRSA as possible pathogen (from human skin or colonized pet). If high suspicion, doxycycline or TMP-SMX provide good coverage.

ISSUES FOR REFERRAL
- Deep wounds to the hand and face should be referred to a hand surgeon or plastic surgeon.
- Bites from primates or unusual species of animals should be referred to infectious disease specialist.

SURGERY/OTHER PROCEDURES
- Copious irrigation of the wound with normal saline via a catheter tip to reduce risk of infection
- Débride devitalized tissue.
- Débridement of puncture wounds is not advised.
- Consider primary closure if the wound is clean after irrigation, the bite is <12 hours old, and in bites to the face (cosmesis).
- Infected wounds and those at high risk for infection (cat bites, human bites, bites to the hand, crush injuries, presentation >12 hours from injury) should be left open.
- Delayed primary closure in 3 to 5 days is an option for infected wounds.
- Splint injured hand.
- Large, gaping wounds should be reapproximated with widely spaced sutures or adhesive strips.

ADMISSION, INPATIENT, AND NURSING CONSIDERATIONS
Patients with deep or severe wound infections, systemic infections requiring IV therapy, and the immunocompromised:
- Adults: ampicillin and sulbactam 1.5 to 3.0 g IV q6h *or* piperacillin and tazobactam 3.375 g IV q6h. Alternative: ciprofloxacin 400 mg IV q12h or levofloxacin 750 mg IV every day with metronidazole 500 mg IV q8h (2)
- Children: ampicillin and sulbactam 200 mg/kg/day (dosed on ampicillin component) IV given in 4 divided doses to maximum of 3 g per dose
- Discharge pending clinical improvement.

 ONGOING CARE

FOLLOW-UP RECOMMENDATIONS
Patient Monitoring
- Recheck for infection in 24 to 48 hours.
- Daily follow-up for infections to ensure resolution
- Base revisions of antibiotic therapy on culture results and clinical response.

PATIENT EDUCATION
Educate parents how to avoid animal bites.

PROGNOSIS
Wounds should improve and close over 7 to 10 days.

COMPLICATIONS
- Septic arthritis
- Osteomyelitis
- Extensive soft tissue injuries with scarring
- Hemorrhage
- Gas gangrene
- Sepsis
- Meningitis
- Endocarditis
- Posttraumatic stress disorder
- Death

REFERENCES

1. Aziz H, Rhee P, Pandit V, et al. The current concepts in management of animal (dog, cat, snake, scorpion) and human bite wounds. *J Trauma Acute Care Surg*. 2015;78(3):641–648.
2. Stevens DL, Bisno AL, Chambers HF, et al. Practice guidelines for the diagnosis and management of skin and soft tissue infections: 2014 update by the Infectious Disease Society of America. *Clin Infect Dis*. 2014;59(2):e10–e52.
3. Bini JK, Cohn SM, Acosta SM, et al; for TRISAT Clinical Trials Group. Mortality, mauling, and maiming by vicious dogs. *Ann Surg*. 2011;253(4):791–797.
4. Abrahamian FM, Goldstein EJ. Microbiology of animal bite wound infections. *Clin Microbiol Rev*. 2011;24(2):231–246.

ADDITIONAL READING
- Okonkwo U, Changulani M, Moonot P. Animal bites: practical tips for effective management. *J Emerg Nurs*. 2008;34(3):225–226.
- World Health Organization. Animal bites. http://www.who.int/news-room/fact-sheets/detail/animal-bites. Accessed October 4, 2018.

 SEE ALSO

Bartonella Infections; Cellulitis; Rabies; Snake Envenomation

CODES

ICD10
- S61.459A Open bite of unspecified hand, initial encounter
- S01.85XA Open bite of other part of head, initial encounter
- S20.97XA Other superficial bite of unspecified parts of thorax, initial encounter

CLINICAL PEARLS
- Cleanse, débride, and culture.
- Antibiotic prophylaxis is recommended for human bites and high-risk wounds.
- Consider rabies and tetanus vaccination.
- Adjust antibiotic choice and duration of therapy based on culture results and clinical improvement.
- Animal and human bites require close follow-up to monitor for infection.

BLADDER CANCER

Margaret E. Thompson, MD

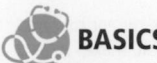 BASICS

DESCRIPTION
- Primary malignant neoplasms arising in the urinary bladder
- Most common type is transitional cell carcinoma (90%).
- Other types include adenocarcinoma, small cell carcinoma, and squamous cell carcinoma.
- Rhabdomyosarcoma of the bladder may occur in children.

EPIDEMIOLOGY
Incidence
- Increases with age (median age at diagnosis is 73 years) (1)
- More common in Caucasians than in Asians or African Americans
- Male > female (4:1); but in smokers, risk is 1:1.
- 34.3/100,000 men per year (1)
- 8.3/100,000 women per year (1)
- 19.5/100,000 men and women per year (1)

Prevalence
In 2015, 708,444 cases in the United States (1)

ETIOLOGY AND PATHOPHYSIOLOGY
Unknown, other than related to risk factors:
- 70–80% is nonmuscle invasive (in lamina propria or mucosa):
  – Usually highly differentiated with long survival
  – Initial event seems to be the activation of an oncogene on chromosome 9 in superficial cancers.
- 20% of tumors are muscle invasive (deeper than lamina propria) at presentation:
  – Tend to be high grade with worse prognosis
  – Associated with other chromosome deletions

Genetics
Hereditary transmission is unlikely, although transitional cell carcinoma pathophysiology is related to oncogenes. The GSTM1-null genotype may be associated with increased risk.

RISK FACTORS
- Smoking is the single greatest risk factor (increases risk 4-fold) and increases risk equally for men and women (2).
- Use of pioglitazone for >1 year may be associated with an increased risk of bladder cancer. The risk seems to increase with duration of therapy and may also be present with other thiazolidinediones.
- Other risk factors:
  – Occupational carcinogens in dye, rubber, paint, plastics, metal, carbon black dust, and automotive exhaust
  – Schistosomiasis in Mediterranean (squamous cell) cancer
  – Arsenic in well water
  – History of pelvic irradiation
  – Chronic lower UTI
  – Chronic indwelling urinary catheter
  – Cyclophosphamide exposure
  – High-fat diet
  – Coffee consumption associated with reduced risk (RR 0.83; 95% CI 0.73–0.94)

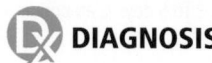 ALERT
Any patient who smokes and presents with microscopic or gross hematuria or irritative voiding symptoms such as urgency and frequency not clearly due to UTI should be evaluated by cystoscopy for the presence of a bladder neoplasm.

GENERAL PREVENTION
- Avoid smoking and other risk factors.
- Counseling of individuals with occupational exposure
- The U.S. Preventive Services Task Force has concluded that there is insufficient evidence to determine the balance between risk and harm of screening for bladder cancer (3).

DIAGNOSIS

HISTORY
- Painless hematuria is the most common symptom.
- Urinary symptoms (frequency, urgency)
- Abdominal or pelvic pain in advanced disease
- Exposures (see "Risk Factors")

PHYSICAL EXAM
Normal in early cases, pelvic or abdominal mass in advanced disease, wasting in systemic disease

DIFFERENTIAL DIAGNOSIS
- Other urinary tract neoplasms
- UTI
- Prostatism
- Bladder instability
- Interstitial cystitis
- Urolithiasis
- Interstitial nephritis
- Papillary urothelial hyperplasia

DIAGNOSTIC TESTS & INTERPRETATION
Initial Tests (lab, imaging)
- Urinalysis is the initial test in patients presenting with gross hematuria or urinary symptoms such as frequency, urgency, and dysuria.
- Urine cytology (Consult your local lab for volume needed and proper fixative/handling.)
- Cystoscopy with biopsy is the gold standard for at-risk patients with painless hematuria.
- CT or MRI prior to resection of suspected muscle-invasive cancer may be helpful in staging.
- Macroscopic hematuria (55% sensitivity, positive predictive value [PPV] 0.22 for urologic cancer)

Follow-Up Tests & Special Considerations
- Urine cytology: 54% sensitivity overall (lower in less advanced tumors), 94% specific
- Other urine markers (of little clinical benefit):
  – Nuclear matrix protein-22 (NMP22): 67% sensitive, 78% specific
  – Bladder tumor–associated antigen stat: 70% sensitive, 75% specific, may be falsely positive in inflammatory conditions
  – Fluorescence in situ hybridization (FISH) assay: 69% sensitive, 78% specific (PPV 27.1, negative predictive value 95.3) for all tumors, more sensitive and specific for higher grade
  – *FGFR3* mutation has high specificity (99.9%) but low sensitivity (34.5%); PPV 95.2%

- Bottom line: None of the urine markers is sensitive enough to rule out bladder cancer on its own.
- Liver function tests, alkaline phosphatase if metastasis suspected
- Done for staging and to evaluate extent of disease but not for diagnosis itself:
  – CT urogram replacing IVP to image upper tracts if there is a suspicion of disease there
  – Diffusion-weighted MRI and multidimensional CT scan are undergoing study for use in diagnosis and staging of bladder tumors.
  – For invasive disease, metastatic workup should include chest x-ray.
  – Bone scan should be performed if the patient has bone pain or if alkaline phosphatase is elevated.
- Urologic CT scan (abdomen, pelvis, with and without contrast) or MRI (40–98% accurate), with MRI slightly more accurate, is recommended if metastasis is suspected.
- Regular cystoscopy (initiated at 3 months postprocedure) is indicated after transurethral resection of bladder tumor (TURBT) and intravesical chemotherapy for superficial bladder cancers. Urinary biomarkers should not be routinely used for follow-up.

Diagnostic Procedures/Other
- Cystoscopy with biopsy is the gold standard for diagnosis, but one study showed that 33% of patients had residual tumor after TURBT.
- Using photodynamic diagnosis (PDD; employing a photosensitizing agent in the bladder that is taken up by tumor cells and visualized using a particular wavelength of light, which is changed to a different wavelength by the photosensitizing agent) has been shown to increase detection and identification of cancerous superficial tumors when compared with plain white light cystoscopy. A recent meta-analysis shows that this increases the likelihood of total resection.

Test Interpretation
- Characterized as superficial (nonmuscle invasive) or invasive (muscle invasive)
- 70–80% present as superficial lesion.
- Superficial lesions
  – Carcinoma in situ: flat lesion, high grade
  – Ta: noninvasive papillary carcinoma
  – T1: extends into submucosa, lamina propria
- Invasive cancer
  – T2: invasion into muscle
    ○ pT2a: invasion into superficial muscle
    ○ pT2b: invasion into deep muscle
  – T3: invasion into perivesical fat
    ○ pT3a: microscopic
    ○ pT3b: macroscopic
  – T4: invasion into adjacent organs
    ○ aT4a: invades prostate, uterus, or vagina
    ○ aT4b: invades abdominal or pelvic wall
- N1–N3: invades lymph nodes
- M: metastasis to bone or soft tissue

TREATMENT

For nonmuscle-invasive bladder cancer, the treatment is generally removal via cystoscopic surgery (see earlier discussion on PDD). For muscle-invasive cancer, a radical cystectomy with pelvic lymphadenectomy is preferred.

MEDICATION

First Line

- A recent meta-analysis demonstrated neoadjuvant chemotherapy using platinum-based combination chemotherapy (with ≥1 of doxorubicin/epirubicin, methotrexate, or vinblastine), but not platinum alone, confers a significant survival advantage in patients with invasive bladder cancer, with an increase in survival at 5 years from 45% (without neoadjuvant treatment) to 50% (with treatment) (combined hazard ratio 0.86; 95% CI 0.77–0.95).
- Intravesical bacillus Calmette-Guérin (BCG) after TURBT in high-grade lesions has been shown to decrease recurrence in Ta and T1 tumors (4)[A]. Urinary biomarkers may have some utility in tracking response to BCG.

Second Line

- Chemotherapy is the first-line treatment for metastatic bladder cancer:
  - Methotrexate, vinblastine, doxorubicin, cisplatin is the preferred regimen.
- A recent review showed that gemcitabine plus cisplatin may be better tolerated and result in equivalent survival to methotrexate, vinblastine, doxorubicin, cisplatin, making it a possible first choice in metastatic bladder cancer.

ISSUES FOR REFERRAL

Patients with microscopic or gross hematuria not otherwise explained or resolving should be referred to a urologist for cystoscopy.

ADDITIONAL THERAPIES

Radiotherapy:

- In the United States, used for patients with muscle-invasive cancer who are not surgical candidates
- Preoperative (radical cystectomy) radiotherapy also an option
- Treatment of choice for muscle-invasive cancer in some European and Canadian centers:
  - 65 to 70 Gy over 6 to 7 weeks is standard.

SURGERY/OTHER PROCEDURES

- Surgery is definitive therapy for superficial and invasive cancer:
  - Superficial cancer: TURBT sometimes followed by intravesical therapy
- Invasive cancer
  - Radical cystectomy for invasive disease that is confined to the bladder is more effective than radical radiotherapy. There is insufficient evidence to recommend one form of urinary diversion over another (5).
  - Currently under trial is a trimodal therapy implementing transurethral resection, radiotherapy, and radiosensitizing chemotherapy (6).

ADMISSION, INPATIENT, AND NURSING CONSIDERATIONS

Need for surgery or intensive therapy

 ONGOING CARE

FOLLOW-UP RECOMMENDATIONS

- Superficial cancers
  - Urine cytology alone has not been shown to be sufficient for follow-up.
  - Cystoscopy every 3 months for 18 to 24 months, every 6 months for the next 2 years and then annually
- Follow-up for invasive cancers depends on the approach to treatment.
- Patients treated with BCG require lifelong follow-up.

DIET

Continue adequate fluid intake.

PATIENT EDUCATION

Smoking cessation

PROGNOSIS

- 5-year relative survival rates (1)
  - Overall survival: 77.3%
    - In situ: 95.7%
    - Localized: 70.1%
    - Regional metastasis: 35.2%
    - Distant metastasis: 5.0%
- Superficial bladder cancer
  - BCG treatment prevents recurrence versus TURBT alone; difference 30%, NNT 3.3
  - BCG prevents progression versus TURBT alone; difference 8%
- Invasive cancer
  - T2 disease: Radical cystectomy results in 60–75% 5-year survival.
  - T3 or T4 disease: Radical cystectomy results in 20–40% 5-year survival.
  - Neoadjuvant chemotherapy with cystectomy has led to varying degrees of increased survival.
  - Radiation with chemotherapy has led to varying degrees of increased survival.
- Metastatic cancer:
  - Methotrexate, vinblastine, doxorubicin, cisplatin resulted in mean survival of 12.5 months.

COMPLICATIONS

- Superficial bladder cancer
  - Local symptoms
    - Dysuria, frequency, nocturia, pain, passing debris in urine
    - Bacterial cystitis
    - Perforation
  - General symptoms
    - Flulike symptoms
    - Systemic infection
- Invasive cancer
  - Symptoms related to definitive treatment, including incontinence, bleeding
  - Patients with neobladder at risk for azotemia and metabolic acidosis

REFERENCES

1. National Cancer Institute. Cancer stat facts: bladder cancer. http://seer.cancer.gov/statfacts/html/urinb.html. Accessed July 13, 2018.
2. Freedman ND, Silverman DT, Hollenbeck AR, et al. Association between smoking and risk of bladder cancer among men and women. *JAMA*. 2011;306(7):737–745.
3. U.S. Preventive Services Task Force. Bladder cancer in adults: screening. http://www.uspreventiveservicestaskforce.org/Page/Topic/recommendation-summary/bladder-cancer-in-adults-screening. Accessed December 6, 2016.
4. Shelley MD, Court JB, Kynaston H, et al. Intravesical bacillus Calmette-Guerin versus mitomycin C for Ta and T1 bladder cancer. *Cochrane Database Syst Rev*. 2003;(3):CD003231.
5. Cody JD, Nabi G, Dublin N, et al. Urinary diversion and bladder reconstruction/replacement using intestinal segments for intractable incontinence or following cystectomy. *Cochrane Database Syst Rev*. 2012;(2):CD003306.
6. Kamat AM, Hahn NM, Efstathiou JA, et al. Bladder cancer. *Lancet*. 2016;388(10061):2796–2810.

ADDITIONAL READING

- Msaouel P, Koutsilieris M. Diagnostic value of circulating tumor cell detection in bladder and urothelial cancer: systematic review and meta-analysis. *BMC Cancer*. 2011;11:336.
- Sharma S, Ksheersagar P, Sharma P. Diagnosis and treatment of bladder cancer. *Am Fam Physician*. 2009;80(7):717–723.
- Zhu Z, Shen Z, Lu Y, et al. Increased risk of bladder cancer with pioglitazone therapy in patients with diabetes: a meta-analysis. *Diabetes Res Clin Pract*. 2012;98(1):159–163.

 SEE ALSO

- Hematuria
- Algorithm: Hematuria

 CODES

ICD10

- C67.9 Malignant neoplasm of bladder, unspecified
- C67.4 Malignant neoplasm of posterior wall of bladder
- C67.3 Malignant neoplasm of anterior wall of bladder

CLINICAL PEARLS

- Painless hematuria should be evaluated with cystoscopy.
- Be aware of potential link between pioglitazone treatment and risk for bladder cancer.
- The U.S. Preventive Services Task Force recommends against routine screening for bladder cancer.

BORDERLINE PERSONALITY DISORDER

William G. Elder, PhD • Robert R. Atkins, MD

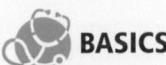

BASICS

DESCRIPTION
A psychiatric disorder that begins no later than adolescence or early adulthood, borderline personality disorder (BPD) is a consistent and pervasive pattern of unstable and reactive moods and sense of self, impulsivity, and volatile interpersonal relationships (1):
- Common behaviors and variations:
  - Self-mutilation: pinching, scratching, cutting
  - Suicide: ideation, history of attempts, plans
  - Splitting: idealizing then devaluing others
  - Presentation of helplessness or victimization
  - High utilization of emergency department and resultant inpatient hospitalizations for psychiatric treatment
- High rate of associated mental disorders
- Typically display little insight into behavior

Geriatric Considerations
Illness (both acute and chronic) may exacerbate BPD and may lead to intense feelings of fear and helplessness.

Pediatric Considerations
Diagnosis is rarely made in children. Axis I disorders and general medical conditions (GMCs) are more probable.

Pregnancy Considerations
Physical, emotional, and social concerns may transiently mimic symptoms of BPD: Consider delay in diagnosis until pregnancy completed. Pregnancy may also induce stress or increased fears, resulting in escalation of borderline behaviors.

EPIDEMIOLOGY
Predominant age: onset no later than adolescence or early adulthood (may go undiagnosed for years)

Prevalence
- General population: 0.5–5.9% of U.S. population
- May be over represented in primary care
- 10% of all psychiatric outpatients and between 15% and 25% of patients in psychiatry inpatient settings have BPD (2).

ETIOLOGY AND PATHOPHYSIOLOGY
Undetermined but generally accepted that BPD is due to a combination of the following:
- Hereditary temperamental traits
- Environment (i.e., history of childhood sexual and/ or physical abuse, history of childhood neglect, ongoing conflict in home)
- Neurobiologic research suggests that stress exerts damaging effects on the brain, specifically the hippocampus (2). Other findings demonstrate heightened activity in brain circuits involved in the experience of negative emotions and reduced activation that normally suppresses negative emotion once it is generated.

Genetics
First-degree relatives are at greater risk for this disorder (undetermined if due to genetic or psychosocial factors).

RISK FACTORS
- Genetic factors contribute; however, no specific genes have yet been identified.
- Childhood sexual and/or physical abuse and neglect

- Disrupted family life
- Physical illness and external social factors may exacerbate BPD.

GENERAL PREVENTION
- Tends to be a multigenerational problem
- Children, caregivers, and significant others should have some time and activities away from the borderline individual, which may protect them.

COMMONLY ASSOCIATED CONDITIONS
Other psychiatric disorders, including:
- Co-occurring personality disorders, frequent
- Mood disorders, common
- Anxiety disorders, common
- Substance-related disorders, common
- Eating disorders, common
- Posttraumatic stress disorder, common
- BPD does not appear to be independently associated with increased risk of violence.

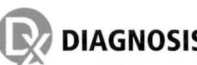

DIAGNOSIS

- The comprehensive evaluation should identify
  - Comorbid conditions
  - Functional impairments
  - Adaptive/maladaptive coping styles
  - Psychosocial stressors
  - Patient strengths; needs/goals
- Initial assessment should focus on risk factors:
  - Establish treatment agreement with patient and outline treatment goals.
  - Assess suicide ideation and self-harm behavior.
  - Assess for psychosis.
  - Hospitalization is necessary if patient presents a threat of harm to self or others.

HISTORY
- Clinic visits for problems that do not have biologic findings
- Conflicts with medical staff members
- Idealizing or unexplained anger at physician
- History of unrealistic expectations of physician (e.g., "I know you can take care of me." "You're the best, unlike my last provider.")
- Obtain collateral information (i.e., from family, partner) about patient behaviors.
- History of interpersonal difficulties, affective instability, and impulsivity
- History of self-injurious behavior, possibly with suicidal threats or attempts

PHYSICAL EXAM
- BPD patients should have a thorough physical examination to help lower suspicion of organic disease (especially thyroid disease) (1,2).
- Often, physical examination reveals no gross abnormalities other than related to scarring from self-mutilation.

DIFFERENTIAL DIAGNOSIS
- Mood disorders:
  - Look at baseline behaviors when considering BPD versus mood disorder.
  - BPD symptoms increase the likelihood of misdiagnosing bipolar disorder.

- In particular, disruptive mood dysregulation disorder, a new diagnosis appearing in *DSM-5* and characterized by severe recurrent temper outbursts manifesting verbally or behaviorally and grossly out of proportion to the situation, may appear quite similar to the acting out and intense emotions seen in BPD. Look for other symptoms characteristic of BPD to differentiate (1).
- Psychotic disorder:
  - With BPD, typically only occurs under intense stress and is characterized as "micropsychotic"
- Other PD:
  - Thoughts, feelings, and behavior will differentiate BPD from other PDs.
- GMC:
  - Traits may emerge due to the effect of a GMC on the CNS.
- Substance use

DIAGNOSTIC TESTS & INTERPRETATION
- Consider age of onset. To meet criteria for BPD, borderline pattern will be present from adolescence or early adulthood.
- Formal psychological testing
- Rule out personality change due to a GMC (1)[C]:
  - Traits may emerge due to the effect of a GMC on the CNS.
- Rule out symptoms related to substance use.
- If symptoms begin later than early adulthood or are related to trauma (e.g., after a head injury), a GMC, or substance use, then consider other diagnoses.

Diagnostic Procedures/Other
According to *DSM-5* criteria, patient must meet at least five of the following criteria (1)[C]:
- Attempt to avoid abandonment
- Volatile interpersonal relationships
- Identity disturbance
- Impulsive behavior:
  - In ≥2 areas
  - Impulsive behavior is self-damaging.
- Suicidal or self-mutilating behavior
- Mood instability
- Feeling empty
- Is unable to control anger or finds it difficult
- Paranoid or dissociative when under stress
- With advent of *DSM-5*, an alternative model is being promulgated that may come to define the diagnosis as impairments in personality functioning AND the presence of pathologic traits. Attention to these features may ultimately enhance provider understanding, diagnosis, and treatment of patients with personality dysfunction.
  - Criteria regarding personality functioning refer to impairments of self-functioning (i.e., identity or self-direction) AND interpersonal functioning (i.e., empathy or intimacy).
  - Pathologic personality traits refer to characteristics in the domains of negative affectivity (i.e., emotional liability, anxiousness, separation insecurity, depressivity), disinhibition (i.e., impulsivity, risk taking), OR antagonism (1).

TREATMENT

- Outpatient psychotherapy for BPD is the preferred treatment (2)[B]:
  – Dialectical behavior therapy (DBT) combines cognitive behavioral techniques for emotional regulation and reality testing with concepts of distress tolerance, acceptance, and self-awareness.
    ○ Following a dialectal process, therapists are tough-minded allies, who validate feelings and are unconditionally accepting while also reminding patients to accept their dire level of emotional dysfunction and to apply better alternative behaviors.
    ○ DBT may be done individually and in groups.
- Schema-focused therapy (SFT) shows promise as a comprehensive treatment for BPD with high acceptance and high remission rates. However, treatment may last 3 years with twice weekly sessions (3)[B].
- Also consider CBT or transference-focused (psychodynamic) psychotherapy.
- Patient may need to be placed on suicide watch.
- Brief inpatient hospitalizations are ineffective in changing Axis II disorder behaviors:
  – Hospitalizations should be limited and of short duration to adjust medications, implement psychotherapy for crisis intervention, and to stabilize patients from psychosocial stressors.
- Extended inpatient hospitalization should be considered for the following reasons:
  – Persistent/severe suicidal ideation or risk to others
  – Comorbid substance use and/or nonadherence to outpatient or partial hospitalization treatments
  – Comorbid Axis I disorders that may increase threat to life for the patient (i.e., eating disorders, mood disorders)

GENERAL MEASURES

- Patients with BPD require more medical care and increased "intentionality" by the provider. Therefore, it is important to be aware of which patients in your practice have BPD and to limit this number if demands exceed practice resources.
- Focus on patient management rather than on "fixing" behaviors:
  – Schedule consistent appointment follow-ups to relieve patient anxiety.
  – Meet with and rely on treatment team to avoid splitting of team by patient and to provide opportunity to discuss patient issues.
  – Treatment is usually most effective when both medications and psychotherapy are used simultaneously.

MEDICATION

- Although no specific medications are approved by the FDA to treat BPD, American Psychiatric Association (APA) guidelines recommend pharmacotherapy to manage symptoms (2)[A],(4)[B].
- Treat Axis I disorders.
- Consider high rate of self-harm and suicidal behavior when prescribing (2)[A].
- APA guideline recommendations (4)[B]:
  – Affective dysregulation: mood stabilizers, SSRIs, and monoamine oxidase inhibitors (MAOIs)
  – Impulsive-behavioral control: SSRIs and mood stabilizers
  – Cognitive-perceptual symptoms: antipsychotics on a short-term basis

- With more neurobiologic causes considered in relation to BPD, SSRIs are having a less prominent roles with more emphasis on mood stabilizers and atypical antipsychotics, but research is uncertain and inconclusive (4)[B].

ISSUES FOR REFERRAL

- If hospitalized, consider for suicide risk, mood or anxiety disorders, or substance-related disorders.
- Urgency for scheduled follow-up depends on community resources (e.g., outpatient day programs for suicidal patients; substance abuse programs):
  – With increased risk for self-harm or self-defeating behaviors and low community resources, the patient can/will have increased need for frequent visits.

ADDITIONAL THERAPIES

Consider referring patient for specialized mental health behavioral services, including partial hospital therapy.

COMPLEMENTARY & ALTERNATIVE MEDICINE

Omega-3 fatty acid dietary supplementation has shown beneficial effects (2)[B].

ADMISSION, INPATIENT, AND NURSING CONSIDERATIONS

Admit for inpatient services immediately in presence of psychosis or threat of injury to self or others; include police, as necessary, for safety measures.

- Assess suicidal ideation.
- Consider trial of antipsychotic medications for psychosis.
- Nurses can be instrumental in managing and calling patients, potentially relieving patient stress.
- Patient should not present risk of harm to self or others and have a safety plan.
- Follow-up should be scheduled with a mental health specialist and primary care provider.

ONGOING CARE

FOLLOW-UP RECOMMENDATIONS

- Schedule visits that are short, more frequent, and focused to relieve patients' anxiety about relationships with their physician/provider and to help reduce risk of provider burnout.
- Maintain open lines of communication with mental health professionals providing psychological support.
- Emphasize importance of healthy lifestyle modifications (i.e., exercise, rest, diet).

Patient Monitoring

Monitor for suicidal or other self-harm behaviors.

PATIENT EDUCATION

Include patients in the diagnosis so they can make sense of their disease process and participate in the treatment strategy.

PROGNOSIS

- Borderline behaviors may decrease with age and over time.
- Patients in treatment improve at a rate of 7 times compared with following natural course.

- Treatment is complex and takes time.
- Medical focus includes patient management and caring for medical and Axis I disorders.

REFERENCES

1. American Psychiatric Association. *Diagnostic and Statistical Manual of Mental Disorders*. 5th ed. Arlington, VA: American Psychiatric Association; 2013.
2. Leichsenring F, Leibing E, Kruse J, et al. Borderline personality disorder. *Lancet*. 2011;377(9759): 74–84.
3. Bateman A, O'Connell J, Lorenzeni N, et al. A randomised controlled trial of mentalization-based treatment versus structured clinical management for patients with comorbid borderline personality disorder and antisocial personality disorder. *BMC Psychiatry*. 2016;16:304.
4. Stoffers JM, Lieb K. Pharmacotherapy for borderline personality disorder—current evidence and recent trends. *Curr Psychiatry Rep*. 2015;17(1):534.

ADDITIONAL READING

Elder W. Personality disorders. In: South-Paul J, Matheny S, Lewis E, eds. *Current Diagnosis & Treatment in Family Medicine*. 4th ed. New York, NY: McGraw Hill Professional; 2015:618–625.

CODES

ICD10
F60.3 Borderline personality disorder

CLINICAL PEARLS

- BPD may be discerned by the impropriety of reactions to situations others find or minor.
- View BPD as a chronic condition with waxing and waning features. It is important to adjust medications/treatments as clinically appropriate when symptoms change.
- If there are problems with the patient disrespecting the physician or support staff, clear guidelines should be established with the treatment team and then with the patient.
- When considering terminating care, the patient may improve if empathetically confronted about certain behaviors and is given clear guidelines on how to behave in the clinic. It is the patient's job to follow the guidelines, and it is you and your team's job to enforce the guidelines. Designate a case management nurse or well-trained support staff person who can be the primary contact person for the patient.
- Have an agenda when you visit with BPD patients. Be cordial—they deserve the same professionalism any patient gets. Have and identify one to two issues to be discussed per clinic visit. Frequently scheduled visits can help with this.
- Regularly scheduled psychotherapy improves medical care by becoming the "home" for mental health treatment, leaving the physician to focus on the patient's immediate medical issues.

BRAIN INJURY, TRAUMATIC

Caleb J. Mentzer, DO • James R. Yon, MD

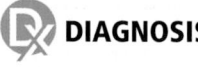 BASICS

DESCRIPTION
- Traumatic brain injury (TBI) is defined as an alteration in brain function or other evidence of brain pathology, caused by an external force.
- System(s) affected: neurologic; psychiatric; cardiovascular; endocrine/metabolic; gastrointestinal
- Synonym(s): head injury, concussion

EPIDEMIOLOGY

Incidence
- 2.2 million ED visits and 280,000 hospitalizations per year
- 50,000 deaths per year; ~30% of all injury-related deaths
- Incidence in males twice that of females with 4-fold risk of fatal trauma

Prevalence
- Predominant age: 0 to 4 years, 15 to 19 years, and >65 years
- Predominant gender: male > female (2:1)

ETIOLOGY AND PATHOPHYSIOLOGY
- Falls (40%)
- Motor vehicle accidents (14%)
- Assault (10%)
- Child abuse (24% of TBI age ≤2 years)
- Recreational activities (21% of pediatric TBI, peak seasons spring/summer; peak ages 10 to 14 years)
- Primary insult: direct mechanical damage
- Secondary insult: actuation of complex cellular and molecular cascades that promote cerebral edema, ischemia, and apoptotic cell death

RISK FACTORS
Alcohol and drug use, prior/recurrent head injury, contact sports, seizure disorder, ADHD, male sex, luteal phase of female menstrual cycle

Geriatric Considerations
Subdural hematomas are common after a fall or blow in elderly; symptoms may be subtle and not present until days after trauma. Many elderly patients are on antiplatelet or anticoagulation therapy.

GENERAL PREVENTION
- Safety education
- Seat belts; bicycle and motorcycle helmets
- Protective headgear for contact sports

Pediatric Considerations
Child abuse: Consider if dropped or fell <4 feet (e.g., off bed, couch), suspicious history, significant injury present, or any retinal hemorrhages.

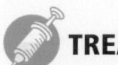 DIAGNOSIS

HISTORY
- Loss of consciousness (LOC), headache, vomiting, amnesia
- Epidural hemorrhage from blunt trauma: 30% with a "lucid interval" (initial LOC followed by recovery of consciousness and then LOC recurs and persists)

PHYSICAL EXAM
- Neurologic and cognitive testing is important.
- Repeat neurologic exams every 30 minutes until 2 hours after Glasgow Coma Scale (GCS) reaches 15, then hourly for 4 hours, and then every 2 hours.
- Evidence of increased intracranial pressure (ICP) (elevated BP, decreased pulse rate, or slow/irregular breathing [Cushing triad]—only 30% have all three)
- Decorticate or decerebrate posturing
- Signs of basilar skull fracture: raccoon eyes, Battle sign, hemotympanum, CSF rhinorrhea or otorrhea

DIFFERENTIAL DIAGNOSIS
Other causes of altered mental status (e.g., toxicologic, infectious, metabolic, vascular)

DIAGNOSTIC TESTS & INTERPRETATION

Initial Tests (lab, imaging)
- Mild TBI and concussions cognitive screening tests
  - Sports Concussion Assessment Tool 3 (SCAT3)
  - Child SCAT3
  - Concussion Recognition Tool (CRT)
  - Standardized Assessment of Concussion (SAC)
  - King-Devick Test
  - Balance Error Scoring System (BESS)
- Evaluate for coagulopathy.
- Type and screen for possible surgical intervention.
- Perform drug and alcohol screening.
- CT, noncontrast, is the study of choice to review bone windows, tissue windows, and subdural space.
- NEXUS II study demonstrated that if all eight clinical criteria are absent, there is a low likelihood of significant TBI:
  - Evidence of significant skull fracture (depressed, basilar, or diastatic)
  - Altered level of alertness
  - Neurologic deficit
  - Persistent vomiting
  - Presence of scalp hematoma
  - Abnormal behavior
  - Coagulopathy
  - Age >65 years

Follow-Up Tests & Special Considerations
Blast-related TBI: much higher rates of postconcussive syndrome, PTSD, depression, and chronic pain. Chronic impairment is strongly correlated with psychological factors; return to battlefield guidelines similar to return to play (RTP) in sports (see "General Measures") (1)[A]

Pediatric Considerations
Skull radiographs are not indicated unless abuse is suspected in which case they can detect fractures not seen under CT; no return to activity until they are asymptomatic and return to school should precede return to sport/physical activity (2)[A]

Diagnostic Procedures/Other
CSF rhinorrhea
- Contains glucose; nasal mucus does not.
- Check for the double halo sign: If nasal discharge contains CSF and blood, two rings appear when placed on filter paper—a central ring followed by a paler ring.

TREATMENT

GENERAL MEASURES
- Acute management depends on injury severity. Most patients need no interventions.
- Immediate goal: Determine who needs further therapy, imaging studies (CT), and hospitalization to prevent further injury.
- For the mildly injured patient
  - Early education is beneficial for recovery (3)[A].
  - RTP
    ○ Never RTP on same day.
    ○ Strict guidelines for graduated return to cognitive and physical activity when there are no evident signs or symptoms (physical, cognitive, emotional, or behavioral) on neuropsychological and clinical evaluation (2)[A]
- For the moderate to severely injured patient
  - Avoid hypotension or hypoxia. Head injury causes increased ICP secondary to edema, and cerebral perfusion pressure (CPP) should be maintained between 60 and 70 mm Hg (4)[A].
  - 30-degree head elevation decreases ICP and improves CPP.
  - Hyperventilation (hypocapnia)
    ○ Use should be limited to patients with impending herniation while preparing for definitive treatment or intraoperatively; risk of worsening cerebral ischemia and organ damage (4,5)[A]
    ○ Addition of tromethamine can offset deleterious effects and lead to better outcomes (5)[A].
  - Mild systematic hypothermia lowers ICP but leads to increased rates of pneumonia. Selective brain cooling may also decrease ICP with improved outcomes at 2 years postinjury (5)[A].
- Seizure prophylaxis
  - Does not change morbidity or mortality. Consider phenytoin or levetiracetam for 1 week postinjury or longer for patients with early seizures, dural-penetrating injuries, multiple contusions, and/or subdural hematomas requiring evacuation (6)[A].

MEDICATION

First Line
- Pain
  - Morphine: 1 to 2 mg IV PRN, with caution, because it can depress mental status, further altering serial neurologic evaluations

ALERT
Bolus doses increase ICP and decrease CPP (7)[A].

- Increased ICP
  - Hypertonic saline: 2 mL/kg IV decreases ICP without adverse hemodynamic status; preferred agent (4,7)[A]
  - Mannitol: 0.25 to 2.00 g/kg (0.25 to 1.00 g/kg in children) given over 30 to 60 minutes in patients with adequate renal function. Prophylactic use is associated with worse outcomes (7)[A].
- Sedation
  - Propofol: preferred due to short duration of action. Avoid high doses to prevent propofol infusion syndrome. When combined with morphine, it can also effectively decrease ICP and decrease use of other meds (7)[A].
  - Midazolam: similar sedating effect to propofol but may cause hypotension (7)[A]

- Seizures
  - Phenytoin (Dilantin): 15 mg/kg IV (1 mg/kg/min IV, not to exceed 50 mg/min). Stop infusion if QT interval increases by >50%.

ALERT
Avoid corticosteroid use because it increases mortality rates and risk of developing late seizures (7)[A]. Avoid barbiturates due to risk of hypotension (7)[A].

ISSUES FOR REFERRAL
Consult neurosurgery for:
- All penetrating head trauma
- All abnormal head CTs

ADDITIONAL THERAPIES
- Emerging therapies with limited but promising evidence: coma arousal therapy: amantadine, zolpidem, and levodopa/carbidopa; postcoma therapy: bromocriptine
- Mixed results for therapeutic hypothermia with defined physiologic parameters (8)[A]
- Increased evidence for continuous hyperosmolar therapy improving survival (9)[A]

SURGERY/OTHER PROCEDURES
- Early evacuation of trauma-related intracranial hematoma decreases mortality especially with GCS <6 and CT evidence of hematoma, cerebral swelling, or herniation.
- Decompressive craniectomy reduces ICP especially when a large bone flap is removed; ONLY for adults and ONLY with GCS >6 (5)[A]
- Hyperbaric oxygen temporarily lowers ICP and improves mortality, but evidence is conflicting about outcomes at 6 to 12 months postinjury (5)[A].
- CSF drainage reduces ICP but has not been demonstrated to have long-term benefit (5)[A].
- CSF leakage often resolves in 24 hours with bed rest, but if not, may require surgical repair (4)[A].

COMPLEMENTARY & ALTERNATIVE MEDICINE
Music therapy in conjunction with multimodal stimulation improves awareness in comatose TBI patients (8)[B].

ADMISSION, INPATIENT, AND NURSING CONSIDERATIONS
- Abnormal GCS or CT
- Clinical evidence of basilar skull fracture
- Persistent neurologic deficits (e.g., confusion, somnolence)
- Patient with no competent adult at home for observation
- Possibly admit: LOC, amnesia, patients on anticoagulants with negative CT
- ABCs take priority over head injury.
- C-spine immobilization should be considered in all head trauma.
- Use normal saline for resuscitation fluid.
- Discharge criteria: normal CT with return to normal mental status and responsible adult to observe patient at home (see "Patient Monitoring")

ONGOING CARE

FOLLOW-UP RECOMMENDATIONS
- Schedule regular follow-up within a week to determine return to activities.
- Rehabilitation indicated following a significant acute injury. Set realistic goals.
- For patients on anticoagulants, net benefit to restarting therapy after discharge despite increased bleeding risk

Patient Monitoring
Patient should be discharged to the care of a competent adult with clear instructions on signs and symptoms that warrant immediate evaluation (e.g., changing mental status, worsening headache, focal findings, or any signs of distress). Patients should be monitored but not awakened from sleep.

DIET
As tolerated, monitor for signs of nausea.

PATIENT EDUCATION
Proper counseling, symptomatic management, and gradual return to normal activities are essential.

PROGNOSIS
- Gradual improvement may continue for years.
- 30–50% of severe head injuries may be fatal.
- Predicting outcome is difficult; many with even minor to moderate injuries have moderate to severe disability at 1 year, whereas prolonged coma may be followed by satisfactory outcome.
- Patients may have new-onset seizures over 2 years following trauma.
- Poor prognostic factors: low GCS on admission, nonreactive pupils, old age, comorbidity, midline shift

COMPLICATIONS
- Chronic subdural hematoma, which may follow even "mild" head injury, especially in the elderly; often presents with headache and decreased mentation
- Delayed hematomas and hydrocephalus
- Emotional disturbances and psychiatric disorders resulting from head injury may be refractory to treatment.
- Seizures: seen in 50% of penetrating head injuries, 20% of severe closed head injuries, and <5% of head injuries overall. Hematomas increase risk of epilepsy.
- Postconcussion syndrome can follow mild head injury without LOC and includes headaches, dizziness, fatigue, and subtle cognitive or affective changes.
- Second-impact syndrome occurs when the CNS loses autoregulation. An individual with a minor head injury is returned to a contact sport, and, following even minor trauma (e.g., whiplash), the patient loses consciousness and may quickly herniate, with a 50% mortality. A similar syndrome of malignant edema can occur in children with even a single injury.
- Increased risk for Alzheimer disease, Parkinson disease, and other brain disorders whose prevalence increases with age

REFERENCES

1. Rosenfeld JV, McFarlane AC, Bragge P, et al. Blast-related traumatic brain injury. *Lancet Neurol*. 2013;12(9):882–893.
2. McCrory P, Meeuwisse WH, Aubry M, et al. Consensus statement on concussion in sport: the 4th International Conference on Concussion in Sport held in Zurich, November 2012. *Br J Sports Med*. 2013;47(5):250–258.
3. Nygren-de Boussard C, Holm LW, Cancelliere C, et al. Nonsurgical interventions after mild traumatic brain injury: a systematic review. Results of the International Collaboration on Mild Traumatic Brain Injury Prognosis. *Arch Phys Med Rehabil*. 2014;95(Suppl 3):S257–S264.
4. Tsang KK, Whitfield PC. Traumatic brain injury: review of current management strategies. *Br J Oral Maxillofac Surg*. 2012;50(4):298–308.
5. Meyer MJ, Megyesi J, Meythaler J, et al. Acute management of acquired brain injury part I: an evidence-based review of non-pharmacological interventions. *Brain Inj*. 2010;24(5):694–705.
6. Agrawal A, Timothy J, Pandit L, et al. Post-traumatic epilepsy: an overview. *Clin Neurol Neurosurg*. 2006;108(5):433–439.
7. Meyer MJ, Megyesi J, Meythaler J, et al. Acute management of acquired brain injury part II: an evidence-based review of pharmacological interventions. *Brain Inj*. 2010;24(5):706–721.
8. Crossley S, Reid J, McLatchie R, et al. A systematic review of therapeutic hypothermia for adult patients following traumatic brain injury. *Crit Care*. 2014;18(2):R75.
9. Asehnoune K, Lasocki S, Seguin P, et al; for ATLANREA group, COBI group. Association between continuous hyperosmolar therapy and survival in patients with traumatic brain injury—a multicentre prospective cohort study and systematic review. *Crit Care*. 2017;21(1):328.

CODES

ICD10
- S06.9X0A Unsp intracranial injury w/o loss of consciousness, init
- S06.5X0A Traum subdr hem w/o loss of consciousness, init
- S06.6X0A Traum subrac hem w/o loss of consciousness, init

CLINICAL PEARLS

- TBI involves two distinct phases: the primary mechanical insult and secondary dysregulation of the cerebrovascular system with cerebral edema, ischemia, and cell-mediated death.
- Indications for imaging include evidence of skull fracture, altered consciousness, neurologic deficit, persistent vomiting, scalp hematoma, abnormal behavior, coagulopathy, age >65 years.
- Strict criteria exist for patients to return to normal sport activity following head injury to avoid the second-impact syndrome, which has 50% mortality.

BREAST ABSCESS

Shannon A. Sanchez Oviedo, MD, MS • Kelley V. Lawrence, MD, IBCLC, FAAFP, FABM •
Lloyd A. Runser, MD, MPH, FAAFP

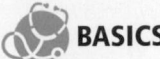

BASICS

DESCRIPTION
- Localized accumulation of infected fluid within the breast parenchyma
- Can be associated with lactation or fistulous tracts secondary to squamous epithelial neoplasm or duct occlusion
- System(s) affected: skin/exocrine, immune
- Synonym(s): mammary abscess; peripheral breast abscess; subareolar abscess; puerperal abscess

Pregnancy Considerations
Most commonly associated with postpartum lactation

EPIDEMIOLOGY
- Predominantly reproductive age and perimenopausal
  - Puerperal abscess: lactational
  - Subareolar abscess: perimenopause to postmenopause (1)
- Predominant sex: female
- Higher incidence in African American women, diabetics, smokers

Incidence
- Ranges from 0.4% to 11% of breastfeeding women; the Academy of Breastfeeding Medicine cites 3% (1,2).
- Puerperal abscess has highest incidence within 6 weeks postpartum and while weaning from breastfeeding (2).

ETIOLOGY AND PATHOPHYSIOLOGY
- Puerperal abscesses:
  - Insufficient treatment of mastitis
  - Unattended postpartum engorgement
  - Plugged lactiferous duct causing stasis, leading to microbial growth and secondary abscess formation
- Subareolar abscess: associated with squamous metaplasia of the lactiferous duct epithelium, keratin plugs, ductal ectasia, fistula formation (1)
- Microbiology
  - *Staphylococcus aureus* is most common cause.
  - Less common causes
    - *Streptococcus pyogenes, Escherichia coli, Bacteroides*
    - *Corynebacterium*
    - *Pseudomonas*
    - *Proteus*
  - Methicillin-resistant *S. aureus* (MRSA) is a significant cause.

RISK FACTORS
- Maternal age >30 (3)
- Primiparous (3)
- Gestational age ≥41 weeks (3)
- Puerperal mastitis
  - Up to 11% progression to abscess (4)
  - Most often due to inadequate therapy
  - Risk factors (stasis):
    - Infrequent or missed feeds
    - Poor latch (1)
    - Damage or irritation of the nipple
    - Suboptimal use of breast pump
    - Illness in mother or baby
    - Rapid weaning; plugged duct
    - Mother employed outside the home (4)
    - Breastfeeding difficulties identified by in-hospital lactation consultant (4)
- General risk factors
  - Smoking
  - Diabetes
  - Obesity
  - Rheumatoid arthritis
- Medically related risk factors
  - Steroids
  - Silicone/paraffin implant
  - Lumpectomy with radiation
  - Inadequate antibiotics to treat mastitis
  - Topical antifungal medication used for mastitis
- Nipple retraction
- Nipple piercing (mastitis, subareolar abscess)
- Higher recurrence rate if polymicrobial abscess

GENERAL PREVENTION
- Frequent breast emptying with on-demand feeding and/or pumping to prevent mastitis
- Early treatment of mastitis with milk expression, antibiotics, and compresses
- Smoking cessation to minimize occurrence/recurrence

COMMONLY ASSOCIATED CONDITIONS
Lactation, weaning

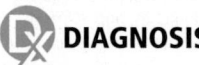

DIAGNOSIS

HISTORY
- Tender breast lump, usually unilateral
- Breastfeeding, weaning, returning to work
- Perimenopausal/postmenopausal
- Systemic malaise (usually less than with mastitis)

- Localized erythema, edema, and pain
- Fever, nausea, vomiting
- Spontaneous nipple drainage
- Prior beast infection
- Diabetes

PHYSICAL EXAM
- Fever, tachycardia, (not always present)
- Erythema of overlying skin
- Tenderness, fluctuance on palpation
- Induration (4)
- Local edema
- Draining pus or skin ulceration
- Nipple and/or skin retraction
- Regional lymphadenopathy
- Puerperal abscesses are generally peripheral; nonlactational abscesses are more commonly found in periareolar/subareolar region (4).

DIFFERENTIAL DIAGNOSIS
- Engorgement
- Plugged milk duct
- Galactocele (sometimes referred to as a milk lake)
- Fibrocystic breasts
- Fat necrosis
- Tuberculosis (may be associated with HIV infection)
- Sarcoid; granulomatous mastitis
- Syphilis
- Foreign body reactions (e.g., to silicone and paraffin)
- Mammary duct ectasia
- Carcinoma (inflammatory or primary squamous cell)

DIAGNOSTIC TESTS & INTERPRETATION
- Ultrasound (US) helps identify fluid collection (5).
- CBC (leukocytosis), elevated ESR
- Culture and sensitivity of expressed breast milk or infected aspirate to identify pathogen (usually *Staphylococcus* or *Streptococcus*)
- MRSA is an increasingly important pathogen in both lactational and nonlactational abscesses.
- Other bacteria:
  - Nonlactational abscess and recurrent abscesses associated with anaerobic bacteria
    - *E. coli, Proteus*; mixed bacteria less common
- Mammogram to rule out carcinoma (generally not during acute phase)

Diagnostic Procedures/Other
Aspiration for culture (does not exclude carcinoma); cytology (particularly in nonlactating patient)

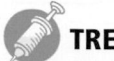 **TREATMENT**

GENERAL MEASURES

- Cold and/or warm compresses for pain control
- Continue to breastfeed or express milk to drain the affected breast.
- Antibiotic treatment without puerperal abscess drainage is ineffective (3)[A].

MEDICATION

Combination of antibiotics and drainage for cure

First Line

- NSAIDs for analgesia and/or antipyresis
- Optimal antibiotic first-line treatment for *mastitis* includes dicloxacillin 500 mg q6h or 1st-generation cephalosporin; clindamycin if penicillin allergic
- Breast abscess first-line treatment includes empiric antibiotics to cover community-acquired MRSA.
- Nonsevere infection:
  - TMP-SMZ DS 1 to 2 PO BID for 10 to 14 days
  - Clindamycin 300 to 450 mg PO QID as alternative for penicillin allergic and if concern for anaerobes (1)[C]
  - *Contraindications*: antibiotic allergy
- In severe infections, vancomycin as an inpatient may be necessary (6)[C].
  - Dose (30 mg/kg) IV in 2 divided doses every 24 hours until culture results are available
- Daptomycin can be used as an alternative to vancomycin due to once daily infusion (outpatient), allowing breastfeeding mothers to feed and pump frequently at home (6)[C].
  - Dose (4 mg/kg) IV every 24 hours may be necessary until culture results are available.
  - Modify antibiotics based on culture and sensitivity (1)[A].

SURGERY/OTHER PROCEDURES

Drain all abscesses and treat with antibiotics (1)[A].

- Aspiration with or without US guidance for abscesses <3 cm (1)[B] (Serial aspirations may be necessary.)
- Consider US-guided percutaneous catheter placement if abscess >3 cm (1)[B].
- Consider incision and drainage (I&D) if abscess is >5 cm, recurrent, or chronic (1)[B].
- Biopsy all nonpuerperal abscesses to rule out carcinoma; remove all fistulous tracts in nonlactating patients as well (1)[C].

COMPLEMENTARY & ALTERNATIVE MEDICINE

- Lecithin supplementation
- Acupuncture may help with breast engorgement and prevention of breast abscess.
- Breast lymphatic massage may ease engorgement.
- Judicious use of cabbage leaves applied over affected area (to decrease inflammation and milk production)

ADMISSION, INPATIENT, AND NURSING CONSIDERATIONS

- Outpatient, unless systemically immunocompromised, septic, or requiring inpatient antibiotic treatment
- Hospital-grade breast pump should be made available to patient from time of admission.

 ONGOING CARE

FOLLOW-UP RECOMMENDATIONS

Patient Monitoring

Ensure complete resolution to exclude carcinoma.

PATIENT EDUCATION

- Wound care, rest, breast milk emptying
- Continue with breastfeeding or pumping (if breastfeeding is not possible due to location of abscess) to prevent engorgement.

PROGNOSIS

- Drained abscess heals from inside out (in 8 to 10 days).
- Subareolar abscesses frequently recur, even after I&D and antibiotics; may require surgical removal of ducts

COMPLICATIONS

- Fistula: mammary duct or milk fistula
- Poor cosmetic outcome
- Early cessation of breastfeeding (2)

REFERENCES

1. Lam E, Chan T, Wiseman SM. Breast abscess: evidence based management recommendations. *Expert Rev Anti Infect Ther*. 2014;12(7):753–762.
2. Amir L; for Academy of Breastfeeding Medicine Protocol Committee. ABM clinical protocol #4: mastitis, revised March 2014. *Breastfeed Med*. 2014;9(5):239–243.
3. Irusen H, Rohwer AC, Steyn DW, et al. Treatments for breast abscesses in breastfeeding women. *Cochrane Database Syst Rev*. 2015;(8):CD010490.
4. Branch-Elliman W, Golen TH, Gold HS, et al. Risk factors for *Staphylococcus aureus* postpartum breast abscess. *Clin Infect Dis*. 2012;54(1):71–77.
5. Jari I, Naum AG, Ursaru M, et al. Breast infections: diagnosis with ultrasound and mammography. *Rev Med Chir Soc Med Nat Iasi*. 2015;119(2):419–424.
6. Stevens DL, Bisno AL, Chambers HF, et al; for Infectious Diseases Society of America. Practice guidelines for the diagnosis and management of skin and soft tissue infections: 2014 update by the Infectious Diseases Society of America. *Clin Infect Dis*. 2014;59(2):e10–e52.

ADDITIONAL READING

Chandika AB, Gakwaya AM, Kiguli-Malwadde E, et al. Ultrasound guided needle aspiration versus surgical drainage in the management of breast abscesses: a Ugandan experience. *BMC Res Notes*. 2012;5:12.

 CODES

ICD10

- N61 Inflammatory disorders of breast
- O91.13 Abscess of breast associated with lactation
- O91.12 Abscess of breast associated with the puerperium

CLINICAL PEARLS

- 0.4–11% of cases of puerperal mastitis go on to abscess (most often due to inadequate therapy for mastitis).
- Risk factors for mastitis result from milk stasis (poor milk transfer, infrequent feeds, missing feeds, weaning) (1,2).
- Treat abscesses not associated with lactation with antibiotics that cover anaerobic bacteria and work up for malignancy.
- The treatment of choice for most breast abscesses is the combination of antibiotics and aspiration.
- US-guided aspiration of breast abscess is preferred to I&D in most cases due to better cosmesis and faster recovery.
- Continue to empty the breast (feeding, pumping, or expression of breast milk) with lactation-associated breast infections.

BREAST CANCER
Fairouz L. Chibane, MD • Alicia H. Vinyard, DO

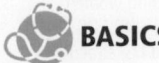 **BASICS**

DESCRIPTION
- Malignant neoplasm of cells native to the breast—epithelial, glandular, or stroma
- Types: ductal carcinoma in situ (DCIS), infiltrating ductal carcinoma, infiltrating lobular carcinoma, Paget disease, phyllodes tumor, inflammatory breast cancer (BC), angiosarcoma
- Molecular subtypes: luminal A (HR+/HER2−), triple negative (HR−/HER2−), luminal B (HR+/HER2+), HER2-enriched (HR−/HER2+)

EPIDEMIOLOGY
Incidence
- Estimated new female BC cases for in situ 63,410; invasive 252,710 in 2017
- Estimated new male BC cases 2,470
- Estimated deaths 2017 females 40,610; males 460
- Most commonly diagnosed cancer (CA) and the second most common cause of CA death for U.S. women

Prevalence
- >3.5 million U.S. women with a history of BC were alive on January 1, 2016 (1).

ETIOLOGY AND PATHOPHYSIOLOGY
- Genes such as *BRCA1* and *BRCA2* function as tumor suppressor genes, and mutation leads to cell cycle progression and limitations in DNA repair (2).
- Mutations in estrogen/progesterone induce cyclin D1 and *c-Myc* expression, leading to cell cycle progression.
- Additional tumors (33%) may cross talk with estrogen receptors and epidermal growth factors receptors (EGFR), leading to similar abnormal cellular replication.

Genetics
- Criteria for additional risk evaluation/gene testing in affected individual (2)[A]
  - BC at age ≤50 years
  - BC at any age and ≥1 family member with BC ≤50 years of age or ovarian/fallopian tube/primary peritoneal CA any age or ≥2 family members with BC or pancreatic CA any age or population at increased risk (e.g., Ashkenazi Jew with BC or ovarian CA at any age)
  - Triple-negative BC (ER−, PR−, HER2−)
  - Two BC primaries in single patient
  - Ovarian/fallopian tube/primary peritoneal CA
  - 1+ family member with BC and CA of thyroid, adrenal cortex, endometrium, pancreas, CNS, diffuse gastric, aggressive prostate (Gleason >7), leukemia, lymphoma, sarcoma, dermatologic manifestations, and/or macrocephaly, GI hamartomas
  - Male BC
  - Known BC *susceptibility gene* mutation in family
- Criteria for additional risk evaluation/gene testing in unaffected BC individual
  - First- or second-degree relative with BC ≤45 years of age
  - ≥2 breast primaries in one individual or ≥1 ovarian/fallopian tube/primary peritoneal CA from same side of family or ≥2 w/ breast primaries on same side of family
  - 1+ family member with BC and CA of thyroid, adrenal cortex, endometrium, pancreas, CNS, diffuse gastric, aggressive prostate, leukemia, lymphoma, sarcoma, dermatologic manifestations, and/or macrocephaly, GI hamartomas

- Ashkenazi Jewish with BC/ovary CA at any age
- Male BC
- Known BC *susceptibility gene* mutation in family
- *BRCA1* and *BRCA2* are inherited in an autosomal fashion and account for 5–10% of female and 5–20% male CAs; 15–20% familial BCs
  - Mutations higher in Ashkenazi Jewish descent (2%)
  - Mutation in *BRCA* raises risk to 45–65% from 7% at age 70 years.
- Other BC associated genes: ATM, BARD1, BRIP, CDH1, PTEN, STK11, CHEK2, p53, ERBB2, DIRAS3, NBN, RAD50, RAD51
- Syndromes associated with BC: Cowden syndrome (PTEN), Li-Fraumeni syndrome (TP53), ataxia-telangiectasia (ATM), and Peutz-Jeghers (STK11)

RISK FACTORS
- Risk calculator: http://www.cancer.gov/bcrisktool/
- Relative risk (RR) >4.0: age >65 years, biopsy confirmed atypical hyperplasia, *BRCA* mutation, DCIS, LCIS, personal history of early onset BC (<40 years), two or more first-degree relatives diagnosed at an early age
- RR 2.1 to 4.0: personal history of BC (40+ years), postmenopausal, radiation history, one first-degree relative of BC
- RR 1.1 to 2.0: EtOH, Ashkenazi Jewish, DES exposure, early menarche (<12 years), late menopause (>55 years), high socioeconomic status, first pregnancy >30 years, proliferative breast disease without atypia (fibroadenoma or ductal hyperplasia), dense breasts (>50%), never breastfed, no full-term pregnancies, obesity, personal history of endometrial or ovarian CA, HRT long term, recent OCP use, height (tall)
- 20–25% lifetime risk should receive an annual MRI beginning at age 30 years: *BRCA* mutation, first-degree relative with *BRCA* mutation, history of radiation age 10 to 30 years, Li-Fraumeni or Cowden syndrome or first-degree relative with the same
- 15–20% lifetime risk: personal history of BC, DCIS, LCIS, atypical ductal hyperplasia, atypical lobular hyperplasia, dense or unevenly dense breasts

GENERAL PREVENTION
- Maintain healthy weight—obesity increases BC risk, physical activity, and healthy diet are key.
- Limit EtOH—moderate alcohol use increases risk of BC.
- Breast self-exams (BSE): ACS no longer recommend monthly structured BSE but support self-awareness.
- Clinical breast exam (CBE):
  - USPSTF: insufficient evidence to assess clinical benefits and harms (3)[A]
  - ACS: no clear benefit or structured guidelines in average-risk women (1)
- Mammography:
  - USPSTF: women biennial mammogram at age 50 to 74 years (3)[B]
  - ACS: women annual mammograms starting at age 45 years and transition to biennial mammograms at age 55 years (1)

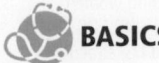 **DIAGNOSIS**

HISTORY
- Painless lump in breast or axilla, breast pain, heaviness
- Swelling, thickening, redness, or dimpling of the skin (sign of advanced BC)
- Nipple discharge (bloody), erosion, or retraction
- Abnormal findings or calcifications on screening mammography

PHYSICAL EXAM
- Visualize breasts with patient sitting and supine for skin dimpling, peau d'orange, asymmetry.
- Palpation of breast and regional lymph node exam: supraclavicular, infraclavicular, axillary

DIFFERENTIAL DIAGNOSIS
- Benign breast disease: fibrocystic disease, fibroadenoma, intraductal papilloma (bloody nipple discharge), duct ectasia, cyst, sclerosing adenosis, fat necrosis (serial/parallel [s/p] breast trauma)
- Infection: abscess, cellulitis, mastitis

DIAGNOSTIC TESTS & INTERPRETATION
Initial Tests (lab, imaging)
- All newly diagnosed BC should be offered multidisciplinary care: history and physical, pathology review, ER/PR and HER2 status determination, genetic counseling if high risk, fertility counseling if indicated; assess for clinically palpable nodes and obtain ultrasound (U/S) and core needle biopsy.
- Calcifications on screening mammography needs to be evaluated with diagnostic mammogram (Dx MMG) and stereotactic guided biopsy. Palpable masses on exam should be evaluated with Dx MMG and US ± biopsy.
- Mammography BI-RADS: Breast Imaging–Reporting and Data System is a quality assurance (QA) method published by the American Radiology Society. BI-RADS interpretation: 0: incomplete (need additional imaging); 1: negative; 2: benign; 3: probably benign; 4: suspicious; 5: highly suggestive of malignancy; 6: known biopsy—proven malignancy
- Palpable mass ≥30 years: Obtain Dx MMG and US to determine cystic versus solid.
  - If BI-RADS 1 to 3, then get US ± biopsy.
  - If BI-RADS 4 to 6, then get core needle biopsy ± surgical excision.
- Palpable mass <30 years: Obtain US ± Dx MMG ± biopsy; if low clinical suspicion, may observe for 1 to 2 menstrual cycles for resolution
- Spontaneous, reproducible nipple discharge: Obtain Dx MMG ± US.
  - If negative, then get ductogram or MRI ± surgical excision.
- Asymmetric thickening/nodularity ≥30 years: Obtain Dx MMG+ US ± biopsy.
- Asymmetric thickening/nodularity <30 years: Obtain US ± Dx MMG ± biopsy.
- Skin changes, peau d'orange: Obtain Dx MMG ± US ± biopsy for underlying mass, if no mass, then perform punch biopsy of skin change.
- Palpable lymph nodes: Obtain CT chest, abdomen/pelvis and bone scan.

Follow-Up Tests & Special Considerations
- Consider additional studies only if signs and symptoms warrant.
- Advanced disease (stage IIIA or higher)
  - Chest diagnostic CT, abdominal ± pelvis CT, FDG positron emission tomography (PET)/CT scan, bone scan or sodium fluoride PET/CT if FDG-PET/CT indeterminate
- Most common metastasis: lungs, liver, bone, brain
- Bone scan: localized pain, elevated alkaline phosphate
- Abdominal ± pelvis CT: abdominal symptoms, elevated alkaline phosphate, abnormal LFTs
- Chest imaging: pulmonary symptoms
- MRI: CNS/spinal cord symptoms

Diagnostic Procedures/Other
- Primary tumor: FNA, US-guided core needle biopsy, stereotactic-guided core needle biopsy; MRI-guided biopsies for abnormalities only visualized on breast MRI
- Axillary lymph nodes: US of axilla during workup and core-needle biopsy or FNA if suspicious, otherwise, excise during sentinel lymph node biopsy.
- Distant disease on staging scans: Obtain biopsy to confirm metastatic disease.
- Postbiopsy may get inflammatory changes/hematoma/bruising and reactive lymph nodes.

Test Interpretation
- Ductal/lobular/other: tumor size, inflammatory component, invasive/noninvasive, margins, nodal involvement
- Tumor receptor status: ER, PR, HER2 assay. Positive receptor status allows for targeted therapies.

 TREATMENT

MEDICATION
- Neoadjuvant chemotherapy: Premenopausal women should be counseled on potential effect of chemotherapy on fertility; refer to fertility expert.
  - Locally advanced (positive lymph nodes), inoperable advanced BC (stage III)
  - Early operable BC for breast conservation surgery
  - Triple negative BC and tumor size >0.5 cm
  - HER 2 (+) tumors ≥2 cm
- Consider 21-gene PT-PCR assay in ER/PR(+) tumors with (−) nodes to potentially assess risk of recurrence; not validated to predict chemotherapy response; can determine if chemotherapy indicated in the adjuvant setting
- Cytotoxic therapy: anthracyclines, taxanes, alkylating agents, antimetabolites
  - Higher risk patients with nonmetastatic operable tumors
  - Patients with high risk of recurrence after local treatment (s/p surgery ± radiation)
  - Online tool to estimate recurrence risk and benefits of adjuvant chemotherapy (https://adjuvantonline.com/)
  - Monitor cardiac toxicity via ECG, especially with anthracycline.
- Dose-dense chemotherapy demonstrates overall survival advantage in early BC (4)[A].
- Anti-HER2/neu antibody (e.g., trastuzumab with or without pertuzumab) in HER2/neu-positive patients; given with other chemotherapy agents in the neoadjuvant or adjuvant setting

ADDITIONAL THERAPIES
- Radiation Therapy (RT)
  - Upon completion of surgery ± chemotherapy, whole breast radiation should be offered for patients undergoing breast conservation therapy (BCT) prior to starting endocrine therapy.
  - Mastectomy alone versus lumpectomy + RT overall survival is similar (5).
  - Postmastectomy RT is offered if tumor >5 cm, ≥4 lymph nodes are involved, chest wall/skin involvement, unable to obtain clear margins.
  - Side effects may include skin hyperpigmentation, skin thickening/fibrosis, loss of breast volume, and chronic pain.
- Secondary prevention
  - ASA use at least once per week may be associated with as much as a 50% reduction in death from BC; chemoprevention/hormone therapy for patients age ≥35 years
  - Risk reduction for ER-positive tumors

- Hormone therapy for ER-positive tumors
  - SERM (tamoxifen, raloxifene, and toremifene): premenopausal at diagnosis: 5-year treatment and consider for additional 5 years; avoid during lactation, pregnancy, or with history of deep venous thrombosis/pulmonary embolism.
  - Aromatase inhibitors (anastrozole, letrozole, and exemestane): postmenopausal women, 5-year treatment following endocrine therapy for 4.5 to 6 years, or endocrine therapy for up to 10 years
  - Ovarian ablation or suppression with luteinizing hormone–releasing hormone agonists: premenopausal women
- Advanced disease
  - Hormone therapy and cytotoxic therapy
  - Bisphosphonates to decrease skeletal complications
  - Antivascular endothelial growth factor antibody
  - Anti-HER2/neu antibody in select HER2/neu-positive patients

Pregnancy Considerations
- Treatment varies on trimester.
- Surgical: mastectomy or breast conservation: mastectomy preferred due to limitations of radiation during pregnancy. BCT can be offered in 3rd trimester.
- SLNB: safe to use with lymphoscintigraphy
- Chemotherapy: appropriate in 2nd and 3rd trimesters; trastuzumab contraindicated
- RT: Avoid until after delivery.

SURGERY/OTHER PROCEDURES
- Breast-conserving therapy (lumpectomy), offered if negative margins can be achieved and the patient will also receive adjuvant RT
- Mastectomy indicated for multifocal disease, large tumor to breast size ratio, inflammatory BC, T₄ disease, contraindication to RT, patient preference
- Evaluation of axillary nodes: preop US and biopsy for all patients with clinically suspicious axillary nodes. If biopsy is positive, an axillary node dissection should be performed. If negative, an SLNB at the time of surgery should be performed. Patients with clinically negative axillary nodes should undergo an SLNB at the time of surgery regardless lumpectomy versus mastectomy.
- Secondary prevention
  - Risk-reducing mastectomy and bilateral salpingo-oophorectomy for BC and ovary CA genetic mutations (i.e., *BRCA1* and *BRCA2* mutations)

ADMISSION, INPATIENT, AND NURSING CONSIDERATIONS
- Mastectomy
  - Complications: seroma, hematoma, cellulitis, chest wall/axilla/arm pain
- Axillary dissection
  - Complications: lymphedema—avoid having BP and blood draws/IV taken on side of surgery
  - Important to have patient see occupational therapist pre/postop for exercises to improve ROM and strategies to reduce lymphedema

 ONGOING CARE

FOLLOW-UP RECOMMENDATIONS
- Every 4 to 6 months for 5 years and then annually
- No evidence to support the use of routine CBC, LFTs, "tumor markers," bone scan, CXR, liver US, CT scans, MRI, PET
- Mammogram performed 6 months postradiation and then annually

- Annual gynecologic exam for women on endocrine therapy; bone mineral density at baseline and follow-up for women on aromatase inhibitors or with ovarian failure secondary to treatment

REFERENCES
1. American Cancer Society. *Breast Cancer Facts & Figures 2017–2018*. Atlanta, GA: American Cancer Society; 2017. http://www.cancer.org. Accessed August 21, 2018.
2. National Comprehensive Cancer Network. NCCN guidelines: breast cancer (Version 2.2016) © 2016. http://www.nccn.org. Accessed September 4, 2017.
3. U.S. Preventative Services Task Force. Final update summary: breast cancer: screening. https://www.uspreventiveservicestaskforce.org/Page/Document/UpdateSummaryFinal/breast-cancer-screening1. Accessed August 21, 2018.
4. Lyman GH, Barron RL, Natoli JL, et al. Systematic review of efficacy of dose-dense versus non-dose-dense chemotherapy in breast cancer, non-Hodgkin lymphoma, and non-small cell lung cancer. *Crit Rev Oncol Hematol*. 2012;81(3):296–308.
5. Onitilo AA, Engel JM, Stankowski RV, et al. Survival comparisons for breast conserving surgery and mastectomy revisited: community experience and the role of radiation therapy. *Clin Med Res*. 2015;13(2):65–73.

ADDITIONAL READING
- Giuliano AE, Hunt KK, Ballman KV, et al. Axillary dissection vs no axillary dissection in women with invasive breast cancer and sentinel node metastasis: a randomized clinical trial. *JAMA*. 2011;305(6):569–575.
- Rothwell PM, Wilson M, Price JF, et al. Effect of daily aspirin on risk of cancer metastasis: a study of incident cancers during randomised controlled trials. *Lancet*. 2012;379(9826):1591–1601.

 CODES

ICD10
- C50.919 Malignant neoplasm of unsp site of unspecified female breast
- D05.90 Unspecified type of carcinoma in situ of unspecified breast
- Z12.31 Encntr screen mammogram for malignant neoplasm of breast

CLINICAL PEARLS
- BC is most common CA death in U.S. women; lifetime risk of 1 in 8
- High alcohol use, high body mass index (BMI), and physical inactivity are modifiable risk factors.
- Pursue/refer all abnormal breast physical examination/imaging findings.
- If patient ≥30 years of age with palpable mass, obtain Dx MMG; if <30 years of age, obtain US.
- Normal mammography does not exclude possibility of CA with a palpable mass.

BREASTFEEDING

Angelia Leipelt, BA, IBCLC, ICCE, CLE • Ronald G. Chambers Jr., MD, FAAFP

 BASICS

- Breastfeeding is the natural process of feeding human milk directly from the breast.
- Breast milk is the preferred nutritional source and the normal and physiologic way to feed all newborns and infants.
- Breast milk contains >200 active components which provide nutrition, fight pathogens, promote healthy gut microbiome, and aid in maturity of immune system.
- The American Academy of Pediatrics (AAP), the American Academy of Family Physicians (AAFP), American Congress of Obstetricians and Gynecologists (ACOG), WHO, and other medical organizations recommend exclusive breastfeeding for 6 months, with continuation of breastfeeding for ≥1 year as desired by mother and infant (1)[A].

DESCRIPTION
- Maternal benefits (as compared with mothers who do not breastfeed) include the following:
  - Rapid involution/decreased postpartum bleeding (due to oxytocin release)
  - Association of decreased risk of postpartum depression and increased bonding
  - Associated postpartum weight loss
  - Decreased risk of breast cancer and association of decreased risk of pre- and postmenopausal ovarian cancer, decreased risk of type 2 diabetes, hypertension, hyperlipidemia, rheumatoid arthritis, and cardiovascular disease
  - Decreased risk of prematurity due to child spacing
  - Increased bone density
  - Convenience and economic savings
  - Association of longer continuation in work/school activities
- Infant benefits (as compared with children who are formula-fed) include the following (1):
  - Ideal food: easily digestible, nutrients well absorbed, less constipation
  - Lower rates of virtually all infections via maternal antibody protection
    - Fewer respiratory and GI infections
    - Decreased incidence of otitis media
    - Decreased risk of bacterial meningitis, pneumonia, and sepsis
    - Decreased incidence of necrotizing enterocolitis
    - Decreased risk of ear infections
  - Decreased incidence of obesity and type 1 and 2 diabetes
  - Decreased incidence of allergies, clinical asthma, and atopic dermatitis in childhood
  - Decreased risk of developing celiac disease and inflammatory bowel disease
  - Decreased risk of childhood leukemia
  - Decreased risk of sudden infant death syndrome (SIDS) and decreased mortality
  - Enhanced neurodevelopmental performance
  - Increased attachment between mother and baby
  - Decreased child abuse
  - Decreases the risk of urinary tract infection

EPIDEMIOLOGY
Incidence
- According to CDC's Breastfeeding Scorecard, U.S. breastfeeding rates are on the rise in 2016: any breastfeeding: 81.1% (however, differs among different sociodemographic and culture) (2)
- Breastfeeding at 6 months: 51.8%
- Breastfeeding at 12 months: 30.7%

- Exclusive breastfeeding at 3 months: 44.4%
- Exclusive breastfeeding at 6 months: 22.3%

ETIOLOGY AND PATHOPHYSIOLOGY
- The mechanism of milk production is based on several hormones: Prolactin triggers milk production and oxytocin releases milk based on supply and demand (3). Endocrine control system triggers making of colostrum at 5 months' gestation.
- Alveoli make milk in response to hormone prolactin. Sucking stimulates secretion of prolactin, which triggers milk production.
- Stimulation of areola causes secretion of oxytocin. Oxytocin is responsible for let-down reflex when myoepithelial cells contract and milk is ejected into milk ducts (3).
- Endocrine/metabolic: Cystic fibrosis, diabetes, galactosemia, phenylketonuria, and thyroid dysfunction may cause delayed lactation or decreased milk.

GENERAL PREVENTION
- Most vaccinations can be given to breastfeeding mothers. The CDC recommends that the diphtheria-tetanus-acellular pertussis, hepatitis B, inactivated influenza virus (as opposed to live attenuated), mumps, measles, rubella (MMR), and inactivated polio and varicella vaccines can be given. The CDC recommends avoiding the yellow fever or smallpox vaccine in breastfeeding mothers (4).
- The inactivated influenza virus is preferred to the live attenuated virus in women with infants' age 6 to 23 months, regardless of whether these infants are being breastfed (4).
- Protective measures include breastfed infants who are more easily aroused than formula-fed infants, triggering a mechanism for the protective effect of breastfeeding against SIDS (5).

 DIAGNOSIS

PHYSICAL EXAM
Examine breasts, ideally during pregnancy, looking for scars, lumps, or flat/inverted nipples. Confirm history of infertility, endocrine disorders, breast and hormonal pathology, overall health and psychosocial concerns, perinatal complications, and previous breastfeeding problem.

ALERT
A breast lump should be followed to complete resolution or worked up if present and not just attributed to changes from lactation.

 TREATMENT

GENERAL MEASURES
Breastfeeding initiation
- Initiate breastfeeding immediately after birth, ideally placing the infant on mother's chest skin-to-skin *in first hour* (1,5)[A].
- Mother placed in a comfortable position, usually sitting or leaning back, with baby naked on mom's naked chest allowing baby to move toward breast
- As baby opens wide, bring baby close, tucking baby in "belly to belly." Line baby's nose to nipple, baby tilts its head back with wide open mouth, bring baby close as baby latches to ensure baby's gum takes in more of the areola. •
- Baby's lips are flanged, rounded cheeks, no clicking or popping sounds, and absence of nipple pain when latched.

- Feed baby on demand, practice rooming in, watch for hunger cues and cluster feeding.
- Feed baby 2 to 8 times for first 24 hours and 8 to 15 times per 24 hours, feeding 10 or more minutes, emptying and alternating breasts.
- Observation of a nursing session by an experienced physician, nurse, or IBCLC
- Avoid supplementation with formula or water and/or artificial nipples unless medically indicated.
- Contraindications to breastfeeding are few (WHO) (1).
  - Maternal HIV (in industrialized world) or human T-cell leukemia virus (HTLV) infection
  - Active untreated tuberculosis
  - Active herpes simplex virus (HSV) lesions on the breast*
  - Substances of abuse without evaluation
  - Review medications that will pass into human milk.
  - Infants with galactosemia or maple syrup urine disease should not be fed with breast milk. Infants with phenylketonuria may be fed breast milk under close observation.
  - Mothers who develop varicella 5 days before through 2 days after delivery*
  - Mothers acutely infected with influenza H1N1 until afebrile*
  - Maternal hepatitis is *not* a contraindication.
  - *Expressed milk be used

ISSUES FOR REFERRAL
- Refer to trained physician, nurse, or IBCLC for inpatient and/or outpatient teaching.
- Frequent follow-up if having problems with latching, sore nipples, breast pain, over active let down, over supply inadequate milk production

COMPLEMENTARY & ALTERNATIVE MEDICINE
Galactagogues
- Metoclopramide, domperidone, oxytocin, fenugreek, goat's rue, and milk thistle have mixed results in improving milk production, but efficacy and safety data are lacking in literature.

 ONGOING CARE

FOLLOW-UP RECOMMENDATIONS
See mother and baby within a few days of hospital discharge, especially if first time breastfeeding.
- Risk factors for suboptimal initiation
  - Breast surgery, especially reduction surgery, prior to pregnancy may disrupt breast milk production.
  - Severe postpartum hemorrhage may lead to Sheehan syndrome, associated with difficulty breastfeeding due to poor milk production.
  - Other factors: delivery mode, duration of labor, gestational age, maternal infection, parity, culture, mother–baby separation, maternal anxiety, use of artificial nipple, and non–breast milk fluids

Patient Monitoring
- Monitor maternal breast milk supply concerns.
- Monitor infant's weight, behavior, and output closely. Consider using breast milk–specific weight-loss nomograms in assessment (newbornweight.org).
- Supplementation with infant formula should be considered if infant has lost ≥10% of birth weight and is recommended if signs of dehydration such as decreased urine output are present.
- Supplementation without persistent breast stimulation with frequent feedings or breast pump use will decrease milk production and decrease breastfeeding success.

B

DIET

- For mothers:
  - Drink plenty of fluids to satisfy thirst and optimal hydration.
  - Breastfeeding mothers may require ~500 more calories per day.
  - Gassy foods can cause baby to be fussy.
  - Limit caffeine to <300 mg/day.
  - Alcohol should be avoided. Possible long-term effects of alcohol in maternal milk remain unknown. If alcohol is used, limit intake to no more than 0.5 (in United States, one drink contains ~14 g of pure alcohol, which is found in 12 oz of beer [~5% alcohol], 5 oz of wine [~12% alcohol], or 1.5 oz of distilled spirits [~40% alcohol]). Intake over this level may impair the milk ejection reflex.
- Continue prenatal vitamin supplements.
- For infants:
  - In 2008, the AAP increased its recommended daily intake of vitamin D for infants from 200 to 400 IU. For exclusively breastfed babies, this will require taking a vitamin supplement, such as Poly-Vi-Sol or Vi-Daylin vitamin drops, 0.5 mL/day, beginning in the first few days of life (1).
  - In 2010, the AAP recommended adding supplementation for breastfed infants with oral iron 1 mg/kg/day beginning at age 4 months.
    - Preterm infants fed by human milk should receive an iron supplement of 2 mg/kg/day by 1 month of age, and this should be continued until the infant is weaned to iron-fortified formula or begins eating complementary foods that supply the 2 mg/kg of iron.
    - Fluoride supplement is unnecessary until 6 months of age (1).

PATIENT EDUCATION

- Primary care–initiated interventions and support measures to normalize breastfeeding have been shown to be successful with respect to child and maternal health outcomes.
  - U.S. Preventive Services Task Force (USPSTF) recommends structured breastfeeding education and behavioral counseling programs to promote breastfeeding.
    - Regular promotion of the advantages of breastfeeding/risks of not breastfeeding (5)[A]
    - Emphasize importance of exclusive breastfeeding for first 4 weeks of life to allow adequate buildup of sufficient milk supply.
- Milk usually transitions to mature milk about postpartum day 3 to 5.
- Frequent nursing (8 to 12 feedings per 24 hours by day 2)
- Baby should have 6 to 8 wet diapers per day and 3 to 4 bowel movements per day by day 6 to 8.
- Signs of adequate nursing
  - Baby feeding on demand
  - Proper latching and positioning, nipples intact
  - Hard breasts become soft after feeding.
  - Baby satisfied; appropriate weight gain (average 1 oz/day in first few months)
- Weaning
  - Solid food may be introduced at 4 months with continuation of breastfeeding.
  - Mothers returning to work/school should be introduced to alternative feeding methods 1 to 2 weeks prior. Initiate pumping to supply expressed breast milk.
- Family planning
  - Lactational amenorrhea method (LAM): Breastfeeding may be used as effective birth control option if (i) infant is <6 months old, (ii) infant is exclusively breastfeeding, and (iii) mother is amenorrheic.

- Other options include barrier methods, implants, Depo-Provera, PO contraception, and intrauterine devices (IUDs). ACOG recommends that progesterone-only pills be used 2 to 3 weeks postpartum, and that Depo-Provera, IUDs, combined OCPs, and Implanon can be used 6 weeks postpartum. However, ACOG recommends delaying use of combined OCPs until after 6 weeks postpartum when lactation is well established.
  - Monitor for changes in milk supply after starting a contraceptive.

COMPLICATIONS

- Breast milk jaundice should be considered if jaundice persists for >1 week in an otherwise healthy, well-hydrated newborn. It peaks at 10 to 14 days.
- Plugged duct
  - Mother is well except for sore lump in one or both breasts and is without fever.
  - Use moist, hot packs on lump prior to, and during, nursing; more frequent nursing on affected side
- Mastitis (see "Mastitis")
  - Sore lump in one or both breasts plus maternal fever and/or redness on skin overlying lump
  - Use moist, hot packs on lump prior to, and during, nursing.
  - Antibiotics covering for *Staphylococcus aureus* (most common organism)
  - Other possible sources of fever should be ruled out, that is, endometritis and pyelonephritis.
  - Mother should get increased rest; use acetaminophen (Tylenol) PRN.
  - Fever should resolve within 48 hours or consider changing antibiotics. Lump should resolve. If it continues, an abscess may be present, requiring surgical drainage.
- Milk supply inadequate
  - Check infant weight gain.
  - Review signs of adequate supply; technique, frequency, and duration of nursing
  - Check to see if mother has been supplementing with formula, thereby decreasing her own milk production.
  - Review health concerns for causes of low milk supply.
- Sore nipples
  - Check technique and improve latch-on.
  - Baby should be taken off the breast by breaking the suction with a finger in the mouth.
  - Air-dry nipples after each nursing and/or coat with expressed breast milk.
  - Use lanolin cream to help in healing.
  - Do not wash nipples with soap and water.
  - Check for signs of thrush in baby and on mother's nipple. If affected, treat both.
  - Check for evidence of ankyloglossia (tongue tie) in the infant. Correction of ankyloglossia may lead to decreased nipple soreness and improved breastfeeding.
  - Nipple bleb (a blister on the nipple that can be filled with serous fluid or another fluid) due to improper positioning. Moist heat and improve latching techniques.
- Flat or inverted nipples
  - When stimulated, inverted nipples will retract inward, flat nipples remain flat; check for this on initial prenatal physical.
  - Nipple shells, a doughnut-shaped insert, can be worn inside the bra during the last month of pregnancy to force the nipple gently through the center opening of the shell.
- Engorgement
  - Develops after milk first comes in (day 3 or 4 postpartum), resolves within a day or 2
  - Signs are warm, hard, sore breasts.
    - To resolve, offer baby more frequent nursing; breastfeed long enough to empty breasts.
    - Pump to relieve discomfort.
    - Explore reasons for ongoing problems.

REFERENCES

1. Johnston M, Landers S, Noble L, et al. Breastfeeding and the use of human milk. *Pediatrics*. 2012;129(3):e827–e841.
2. Centers for Disease Control and Prevention. *Breastfeeding Report Card—United States, 2014*. Atlanta, GA: Centers for Disease Control and Prevention; 2014. http://www.cdc.gov/breastfeeding/pdf/2014breastfeedingreportcard.pdf. Accessed September 30, 2017.
3. Sinusas K, Gagliardi A. Initial management of breastfeeding. *Am Fam Physician*. 2001;64(6): 981–988.
4. Centers for Disease Control and Prevention. *Breastfeeding Vaccinations*. Atlanta, GA: Centers for Disease Control and Prevention; 2010. http://www.cdc.gov/breastfeeding/recommendations/vaccinations.htm. Accessed September 30, 2017.
5. American College of Obstetricians and Gynecologists Women's Health Care Physicians; Committee on Health Care for Underserved Women. Committee Opinion No. 570: breastfeeding in underserved women: increasing initiation and continuation of breastfeeding. *Obstet Gynecol*. 2013;122(2, Pt 1): 423–428.

ADDITIONAL READING

- American Academy of Pediatrics, American College of Obstetricians and Gynecologists. *Breastfeeding Handbook for Physicians*. 2nd ed. Elk Grove Village, IL: American Academy of Pediatrics; 2014.
- Bibbins-Domingo K, Grossman DC, Curry SJ, et al; for U.S. Preventive Services Task Force. Primary care interventions to support breastfeeding: US Preventive Service Task Force. *JAMA*. 2016;316(16):1688–1693.
- Philipp BL, Bunik M, Chantry CJ, et al. ABM Clinical Protocol #7: Model Breastfeeding Policy (Revision 2010). *Breastfeed Med*. 2010;5(4):173–177.
- Wagner CL, Greer FR, Bhatia JJ, et al. Prevention of rickets and vitamin D deficiency in infants, children, and adolescents. *Pediatrics*. 2008;122(5):1142–1152.
- Websites/books:
  - Baby Friendly USA at www.babyfriendly.org
  - La Leche League at www.llli.org
  - World Health Organization, United Nations Children's Fund. *Protecting, Promoting and Supporting Breastfeeding: The Special Role of Maternity Services. A Joint WHO/UNICEF Statement*. Geneva, Switzerland: World Health Organization; 1989. http://www.unicef.org/newsline/tenstps.htm

 ## CODES

ICD10

Z39.1 Encounter for care and examination of lactating mother

CLINICAL PEARLS

- Women who do not receive support are at risk for shorter durations of breastfeeding.
- Virtually all mothers can breastfeed, provided they have accurate information, and the support of their family, the health care system, and society at large.
- Breast milk is the optimal food for infants, with myriad health benefits for mothers and children.
- USPSTF recommends regular, structured education during pregnancy to promote breastfeeding.

BRONCHIECTASIS
Sumera R. Ahmad, MD • Scott E. Kopec, MD

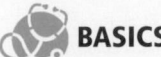 **BASICS**

DESCRIPTION
- Bronchiectasis is an irreversible dilatation of ≥1 airways accompanied by recurrent transmural bronchial infection/inflammation and chronic mucopurulent sputum production.
- Generally classified into cystic fibrosis (CF) and noncystic fibrosis (non-CF) bronchiectasis

EPIDEMIOLOGY
- Predominant age: most commonly presents in 6th decade of life
- Predominant sex: female > male (1)

Incidence
Incidence has decreased in the United States for two reasons:
- Widespread childhood vaccination against pertussis
- Effective treatment of childhood respiratory infections with antibiotics

Prevalence
- In the United States, prevalence estimated to be 52.3/100,000
- Prevalence increased substantially with age from 4.2/100,000 persons aged 18 to 34 years to 271.8/100,000 among those aged ≥75 years (1).

ETIOLOGY AND PATHOPHYSIOLOGY
- CF bronchiectasis: bronchiectasis due to CF
- Non-CF bronchiectasis
  - Most cases are idiopathic.
  - Most commonly associated with non-CF bronchiectasis is childhood infection.
- Vicious circle hypothesis: Transmural infection, generally by bacterial organisms, causes inflammation and obstruction of airways. Damaged airways and dysfunctional cilia foster bacterial colonization, which leads to further inflammation and obstruction.

RISK FACTORS
- Nontuberculous mycobacterial infection is both a cause and a complication of non-CF bronchiectasis.
- Severe respiratory infection in childhood (measles, adenovirus, influenza, pertussis, or bronchiolitis)
- Systemic diseases (e.g., rheumatoid arthritis and inflammatory bowel disease)
- Chronic rhinosinusitis
- Recurrent pneumonia
- Aspirated foreign body
- Immunodeficiency
- Congenital abnormalities

GENERAL PREVENTION
- Routine immunizations against pertussis, measles, *Haemophilus influenzae* type B, influenza, and pneumococcal pneumonia
- Genetic counseling if congenital condition is etiology
- Smoking cessation

COMMONLY ASSOCIATED CONDITIONS
- Mucociliary clearance defects
  - Primary ciliary dyskinesia
  - Young syndrome (secondary ciliary dyskinesia)
  - Kartagener syndrome
- Other congenital conditions
  - α_1-Antitrypsin deficiency
  - Marfan syndrome
  - Cartilage deficiency (Williams-Campbell syndrome)
- Chronic obstructive pulmonary disease
- Pulmonary fibrosis, causing traction bronchiectasis

- Postinfectious conditions
  - Bacteria (*H. influenzae* and *Pseudomonas aeruginosa*)
  - Mycobacterial infections (tuberculosis [TB] and *Mycobacterium avium* complex [MAC])
  - Whooping cough
  - *Aspergillus* species
  - Viral (HIV, adenovirus, measles, influenza virus)
- Immunodeficient conditions
  - Primary: hypogammaglobulinemia
  - Secondary: allergic bronchopulmonary aspergillosis (ABPA), posttransplantation
  - Sequelae of toxic inhalation or aspiration (e.g., chlorine, luminal foreign body)
- Rheumatic/chronic inflammatory conditions
  - Rheumatoid arthritis
  - Sjögren syndrome
  - Systemic lupus erythematosus
  - Inflammatory bowel disease
- Miscellaneous
  - Yellow nail syndrome

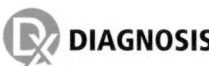 **DIAGNOSIS**

- Typical symptoms include chronic productive cough, wheezing, and dyspnea.
- Symptoms are often accompanied by repeated respiratory infections.
- Once diagnosed, investigate etiology.

HISTORY
- Any predisposing factors (congenital, infectious, and/or exposure related)
- Immunization history

PHYSICAL EXAM
Symptoms are commonly present for many years and include the following:
- Chronic cough (90%)
- Sputum: may be copious and purulent (90%)
- Rhinosinusitis (60–70%)
- Fatigue: may be a dominant symptom (70%)
- Dyspnea (75%)
- Chest pain: may be pleuritic (20–30%)
- Hemoptysis (20–30%)
- Wheezing (20%)
- Bibasilar crackles (60%)
- Rhonchi (44%)
- Digital clubbing (3%)

DIFFERENTIAL DIAGNOSIS
- CF
- Chronic obstructive pulmonary disease
- Asthma
- Chronic bronchitis
- Pulmonary TB
- ABPA

DIAGNOSTIC TESTS & INTERPRETATION
- Spirometry
  - Moderate airflow obstruction and hyperresponsive airways
  - Forced expiratory volume in the 1st second of expiration (FEV_1): <80% predicted and FEV_1/FVC <0.7
  - Special tests
  - Ciliary biopsy by electron microscopy
- Sputum culture
  - *H. influenzae*, nontypeable form (42%)
  - *P. aeruginosa* (18%)

- Cultures may also be positive for *Streptococcus pneumoniae*, *Moraxella catarrhalis*, MAC, and *Aspergillus*.
  - Screen for TB and non-TB in selected individuals.
  - Of all isolates, 30–40% will show no growth.
- Special tests
  - Sweat test for CF
  - Purified protein derivative (PPD) test for TB
  - Skin test for *Aspergillus*
  - HIV
  - Serum immunoglobulins to test for humoral immunodeficiency
  - Protein electrophoresis to test for α_1-antitrypsin deficiency
  - Barium swallow to look for abnormalities of deglutition, achalasia, esophageal hypomotility
  - pH probe to characterize reflux
  - Screening tests for rheumatologic diseases
- Chest radiograph
  - Nonspecific; increased lung markings or may appear normal
- Chest computed tomography (CT)
  - Noncontrast high-resolution chest CT is the most important diagnostic tool.
  - Bronchi are dilated and do not taper, resulting in "tram track sign"; parallel opacities seen on scan
  - Varicose constrictions and balloon cysts may be seen.
  - For focal bronchiectasis, rule out endobronchial obstruction.
  - For exclusively upper lobe bronchiectasis, consider CF and ABPA.

Diagnostic Procedures/Other
- Bronchoscopy may be used to obtain cultures and evacuate sputum.
- Bronchoscopy for hemoptysis
- Bronchoscopy may be useful to rule out airway-obstructing lesions with focal bronchiectasis.

Test Interpretation
Bronchoscopy findings include the following:
- Dilatation of airways and purulent secretions
- Thickened bronchial walls with necrosis of bronchial mucosa
- Peribronchial scarring

 TREATMENT

- Treat underlying conditions.
- Recognize an acute exacerbation with four out of nine criteria.
  - Change in sputum production
  - Increased dyspnea
  - Increased cough
  - Fever
  - Increased wheezing
  - Malaise, fatigue, lethargy
  - Reduced pulmonary function
  - Radiographic changes
  - Changes in chest sounds
- Non-CF bronchiectasis: Determine cause of exacerbations; promote good bronchopulmonary hygiene via daily airway clearance.
- Consider surgical resection of damaged lung for focal disease that is refractory to medical management.
- Medical management: Reduce morbidity by controlling symptoms and preventing disease progression.
- Patients with non-CF bronchiectasis may not respond to CF treatment regimens in the same way as patients with CF do.

MEDICATION
- Insufficient evidence exists to support efficacy of short-course antibiotics in adults and children with bronchiectasis (2).
- Frequent exacerbations may be treated with prolonged and aerosolized antibiotics (3,4).
- Role of mucolytics, anti-inflammatory agents, and bronchodilators is still unclear.

First Line
- Antibiotics
  - Potentially useful in acute exacerbations
  - Limited evidence supports quinolones over β-lactams for hospitalized patients.
  - Chronic therapy decreases sputum production, number of exacerbations, and hospitalizations, but there is a risk of emergence of resistance to antibiotics (5,6).
  - Use of inhaled antibiotics can be considered for selected individuals with gram-negative organisms. Caution needs to be taken with airway and systemic adverse effects noted with inhaled tobramycin and aztreonam (4).
  - Patients may require twice the usual dose and longer treatment for 14 days (10 to 21 days) for an acute exacerbation.
  - Sputum culture and sensitivity should direct therapy; antibiotic selection is complicated by a wide range of pathogens and resistant organisms.
  - Should be administered IV in cases of severe infection (4)
    - Ciprofloxacin: 750 mg PO q12h for adults
    - Amoxicillin clavulanate (Augmentin): 500 mg PO q8–12h; pediatric: base dosing on amoxicillin content
    - Trimethoprim/sulfamethoxazole (SMX): 160 mg trimethoprim/800 mg SMX PO q12h; pediatric: ≥2 months, 8 mg/kg trimethoprim and 40 mg/kg SMX PO/24 hours, administered in 2 divided doses q12h
    - Doxycycline and cefaclor given PO are also effective.
    - Nebulized aminoglycosides (tobramycin): 300 mg by aerosol BID
    - Macrolides: appear to have immunomodulatory benefits
- Chronic use of azithromycin as an oral macrolide for 6 to 12 months in non-CF bronchiectasis has been shown to reduce exacerbations; needs caution with respect to cardiovascular deaths, where it is a QTc-prolonging medication
- All patients considered for chronic therapy with azithromycin should be screened for non-TB mycobacterium infection prior (4).
- Bronchodilators
  - Chronic use of β_2-agonists (e.g., albuterol) reverses airflow obstruction (2).
- Inhaled corticosteroids
  - Inhaled corticosteroids may improve lung function, but the effect is small (6).
    - Fluticasone propionate: 110 to 220 μg inhaled BID
  - Use of combination of long-acting bronchodilator with inhaled corticosteroid may reduce dyspnea, wheeze, and cough (6).
    - Budesonide 160 μg/formoterol 4.5 μg 2 puffs inhaled BID

Second Line
Other broad-spectrum antimicrobials, including those with antipseudomonal coverage

ADDITIONAL THERAPIES
Sputum clearance techniques, including chest physiotherapy (percussion and postural drainage) and pulmonary rehabilitation (improves exercise tolerance)

SURGERY/OTHER PROCEDURES
- Surgery if area of bronchiectasis is localized and symptoms remain intolerable despite medical therapy or if disease is life-threatening (3)
- Surgery effectively improves symptoms in 80% of these cases.

ADMISSION, INPATIENT, AND NURSING CONSIDERATIONS
Bronchiectasis can present as life-threatening massive hemoptysis. In this situation, in addition to airway protection and resuscitation, bronchial artery embolization or surgical intervention is necessary to control bleeding (2).

 ONGOING CARE

Long-term outpatient treatment recommendations for bronchiectasis in children and adults (3):
- Children and adults with CF and non–CF-related bronchiectasis should be treated by comprehensive interdisciplinary chronic disease management programs.
- In children, aim to achieve normal growth and development.
- Patients with primary and secondary immune deficiencies should be under joint care with a clinical immunologist.
- Patient with CF should be referred to a CF center.
- Patient should be informed of the various techniques for airway clearance.
- Nebulized saline or hypertonic saline (7% saline) use prior to airway clearance techniques can help augment sputum production (3)[B].
- Whereas nebulized dornase and high-dose anti-inflammatory agents such as ibuprofen have some benefit in CF-related bronchiectasis, there is no role of such agents in non–CF-related bronchiectasis. In fact, nebulized dornase in adults can be harmful with more frequent exacerbations and decline in lung function.
- Pulmonary rehabilitation should be offered to patients with symptoms of breathlessness affecting activities of daily living (3)[B].
- In situation of an acute exacerbation, use and modify antibiotics as per sputum microbiology.
- Consider suitability of long-term antibiotics for patients with recurrent exacerbations.
- Noninvasive ventilation can improve quality of life in patients with chronic respiratory failure and can reduce hospitalizations.
- Consider lung transplant evaluation in patients with declining respiratory status and FEV₁ <30%. However, because non-CF bronchiectasis has significantly lower mortality hazard compared to CF-related bronchiectasis, separate referral and listing criteria should be considered (7).

FOLLOW-UP RECOMMENDATIONS
Regular exercise is recommended.

Patient Monitoring
- Serial spirometry at least annually (3)
- Chest CTs to monitor progression of disease may be indicated with some conditions such as bronchiectasis with MAC infections.
- Routine microbiologic sputum analysis

PATIENT EDUCATION
http://www.lungusa.org/

PROGNOSIS
- Mortality rate (death due directly to bronchiectasis) is 10.6–29.7% (7).
- *Pseudomonas* infection, low body mass index, and advanced age are associated with poorer prognosis (5).

COMPLICATIONS
- Hemoptysis
- Recurrent pulmonary infections
- Pulmonary hypertension
- Cor pulmonale
- Lung abscess

REFERENCES
1. Weycker D, Edelsberg J, Oster G, et al. Prevalence and economic burden of bronchiectasis. *Clin Pulm Med*. 2005;12(4):205–209.
2. Wurzel D, Marchant JM, Yerkovich ST, et al. Short courses of antibiotics for children and adults with bronchiectasis. *Cochrane Database Syst Rev*. 2011;(6):CD008695.
3. Pasteur MC, Bilton D, Hill AT; for British Thoracic Society Non-CF Bronchiectasis Guideline Group. British Thoracic Society guideline for non-CF bronchiectasis. *Thorax*. 2010;65(Suppl 1):i1–i58.
4. O'Donnell AE. Bronchiectasis: which antibiotics to use and when? *Curr Opin Pulm Med*. 2015;21(3):272–277.
5. Hnin K, Nguyen C, Carson KV, et al. Prolonged antibiotics for non-cystic fibrosis bronchiectasis in children and adults. *Cochrane Database Syst Rev*. 2015;(8):CD001392.
6. Welsh EJ, Evans DJ, Fowler SJ, et al. Interventions for bronchiectasis: an overview of Cochrane systematic reviews. *Cochrane Database Syst Rev*. 2015;(7):CD010337.
7. Hayes D Jr, Kopp BT, Tobias JD, et al. Survival in patients with advanced non-cystic fibrosis bronchiectasis versus cystic fibrosis on the waitlist for lung transplantation. *Lung*. 2015;193(6):933–938.

ADDITIONAL READING
Kaehne A, Milan SJ, Felix LM, et al. Head-to-head trials of antibiotics for bronchiectasis. *Cochrane Database Syst Rev*. 2018;(9):CD012590.

CODES

ICD10
- J47.9 Bronchiectasis, uncomplicated
- J47.1 Bronchiectasis with (acute) exacerbation
- J47.0 Bronchiectasis with acute lower respiratory infection

CLINICAL PEARLS
- Symptoms of bronchiectasis include chronic productive cough, wheezing, and dyspnea often accompanied by repeated respiratory infections.
- A chest x-ray has poor sensitivity and specificity for the diagnosis; a noncontrast high-resolution chest CT is the most important diagnostic tool.
- Current practice guidelines recommend treating acute exacerbations with a 14-day course of antibiotics. Frequent exacerbations may be treated with prolonged and aerosolized antibiotics.

BRONCHIOLITIS
Dennis E. Hughes, DO, FAAFP, FACEP

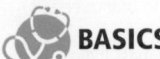 **BASICS**

DESCRIPTION
- Inflammation and obstruction of small airways and reactive airways generally affecting infants and young children—upper respiratory infection (URI) prodrome followed by increased respiratory effort, crackles, and wheezing
- Usual course: insidious, acute, progressive
- Leading cause of hospitalizations in infants and children in most Western countries
- Predominant age: newborn—2 years (peak age <6 months). Neonates are not protected despite transfer of maternal antibody.
- Predominant sex: male > female

EPIDEMIOLOGY
Incidence
- There is a 21–25% prevalence of bronchiolitis (<12 months of age, 13% 12 to 24 months) in the United States and it accounts for ~$1.7B in health care cost in United States. Incidence is estimated at 3.2/1,000. Almost 100% of children experience RSV infection by two seasons.
- Usually seasonal (October to May in the Northern Hemisphere) and often occurs in epidemics—in subtropical regions, RSV is endemic year-round
- Responsible for 18.8% (90,000 annually) of all pediatric hospitalizations (excluding live births) in children <2 years
- Incidence increasing since 1980 (with concomitant increase in relative rate of hospitalization from 2002 to 2007); of those <12 months with condition, the hospitalization rate ~2–3%

ETIOLOGY AND PATHOPHYSIOLOGY
RSV accounts for 70–85% of all cases (children <12 months of age), but rhinovirus, parainfluenza virus, adenovirus, influenza virus, *Mycoplasma pneumoniae*, and *Chlamydophila pneumoniae* have all been implicated:
- Infection results in necrosis and lysis of epithelial cells and subsequent release of inflammatory mediators.
- Edema and mucus secretion, which combined with accumulating necrotic debris and loss of cilia clearance, result in airflow obstruction.
- Ventilation–perfusion mismatching resulting in hypoxia
- Air trapping is caused by dynamic airways narrowing during expiration, which increases work of breathing.
- Bronchospasm appears to play little or no role.

RISK FACTORS
- Secondhand cigarette smoke
- Low birth weight, premature birth
- Immunodeficiency
- Formula feeding (little or no breastfeeding)
- Contact with infected person (primary mode of spread)
- Children in daycare environment
- Congenital cardiopulmonary disease
- <12 weeks of age

GENERAL PREVENTION
- Hand washing or use of alcohol-based hand rubs (preferred)—this simple exercise has been estimated to have the largest impact on prevention of transmission.
- Contact isolation of infected babies
- Persons with colds should keep contact with infants to a minimum.
- Breastfeeding of infants has been associated with reduced morbidity of disease.
- Palivizumab (Synagis), a monoclonal product, administered monthly, October to May, 15 mg/kg IM; used for RSV prevention ONLY in high-risk patients (see American Academy of Pediatrics [AAP] recommendations)

Pediatric Considerations
Prior infection does not seem to confer subsequent immunity.

COMMONLY ASSOCIATED CONDITIONS
- Upper respiratory congestion
- Conjunctivitis
- Pharyngitis
- Otitis media
- Diarrhea

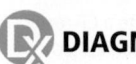 **DIAGNOSIS**

History and physical examination should be the basis for the diagnosis of bronchiolitis; ancillary testing only indicated if clinical picture is unclear (no single of group of tests confirmatory for bronchiolitis)

HISTORY
- Irritability
- Anorexia
- Fever
- Noisy breathing (due to rhinorrhea)
- Cough
- Grunting
- Cyanosis
- Apnea
- Vomiting

PHYSICAL EXAM
- Tachypnea
- Retractions (increased work of breathing)
- Rhinorrhea
- Wheezing
- Upper respiratory findings: pharyngitis, conjunctivitis, otitis

DIFFERENTIAL DIAGNOSIS
- Other pulmonary infections such as pertussis, croup, or bacterial pneumonia
- Aspiration
- Vascular ring
- Foreign body
- Asthma
- Heart failure
- Gastroesophageal reflux
- Cystic fibrosis

DIAGNOSTIC TESTS & INTERPRETATION
Laboratory and other ancillary testing (including chest x-ray) are not required if clinical diagnosis is bronchiolitis. Recent meta-analysis found no single history or physical factor that predicted air-space disease on chest radiograph (1)[B].

Initial Tests (lab, imaging)
- Arterial oxygen saturation by pulse oximetry. Results need to be interpreted in clinical context. Transient hypoxemia is a common phenomenon in healthy infants (2); capnography not found to aid in prediction of disease severity or need for hospitalization
- Rapid respiratory viral antigen testing is not necessary during RSV season because the disease is managed symptomatically but may be useful for epidemiologic, hospital cohorting, or in the very young to reduce unnecessary other workup; also indicated in infants admitted while receiving palivizumab prophylaxis (if positive, prophylaxis may be discontinued)
- The AAP does not recommend routine RSV testing in infants and children with bronchiolitis.
- Chest x-ray findings are variable and may include atelectasis, peribronchial cuffing, hyperinflation, and perihilar infiltrates.

 TREATMENT

The cornerstone of therapy is supportive to include upper airway suctioning, prevention of significant and prolonged hypoxia, and dehydration. The other interventions noted have historically varying effect on the course of the illness despite numerous studies. Recent clinical practice guidelines do not support the routine use of corticosteroids, bronchodilators, or epinephrine. Parental education and support is vital (2)[A].

MEDICATION
First Line
- Humidified oxygen for hypoxia of <90% (many feel that transient pulse oximetry in 85–90% range during sleeping in clinically well-appearing infant may be observed) (2)[C]
- Nebulized hypertonic saline (3%) can be effective in reducing LOS in hospitalized patients but not recommended use in the ED (more recent literature review shows some signal of benefit) (2,3)[B].
- Antibiotics only if secondary bacterial infection present (rare); not indicated for routine use (2)[B]
- Positive-pressure ventilation (PPV) in the form of continuous positive airway pressure (CPAP) can be used in cases of respiratory failure. There is limited clinical evidence other than observational studies (4)[C].
- High-flow nasal cannula oxygen widely used in various settings to improve oxygen saturation with resultant reduction in end-tidal CO_2 ($ETCO_2$) and respiratory rate, but overall effectiveness remains unproven to date (4)[C]. (A prospective, randomized, multicenter trial is ongoing in Australia and New Zealand.)

ADDITIONAL THERAPIES

- Ribavirin and palivizumab for patients at high risk (for prophylaxis per CDC/AAP guidelines) (5)[A]
- Heliox therapy (70% helium and 30% oxygen) may be of benefit early in moderate to severe bronchiolitis to reduce degree of respiratory distress due to air flow restriction, but Cochrane Review found little evidence of sustained benefit at 24 hours (6)[A].
- Although not routinely recommended, inhaled β-agonists (albuterol) can be effective in selected cases (particularly in patients with a history of bronchospasm). Many clinicians will attempt an empiric trial of bronchodilators in a primary presentation to judge the clinical response (some argue that this condition maybe asthma equivalent).

ADMISSION, INPATIENT, AND NURSING CONSIDERATIONS

- Bronchiolitis can be associated with apnea in children <6 weeks of age.
- Respiratory rate >45 breaths/min with respiratory distress or apnea
- Hypoxia is common, so clinical criteria are more helpful (pulse oximetry <94% used by many as cutoff).
- Ill or toxic appearance
- Underlying heart condition, respiratory condition, or immune suppression
- High risk for apnea (age <30 days, preterm birth [<37 weeks])
- Dehydrated or unable to feed (<50% of normal intake suggested as threshold for hospitalization consideration)
- Uncertain home care
- Use of respiratory distress assessment instrument may aid in determining admission. The five best predictors of admission, age, respiratory rate, heart rate, oxygen saturation, and duration of symptoms, were recently incorporated into a scoring instrument.
- Supplemental oxygen for pulse oximetry <94% on room air if clinically indicated (i.e., retractions, increased WOB, etc.). AAP recommends O_2 saturation >90% if infant otherwise well.
- IV fluids indicated only if tachypnea precludes oral feeding; weight-based maintenance rate plus insensible losses
- Discharge criteria
  - Normal respiratory rate and no oxygen requirement: Recent small studies suggest that after a period of observation, children can be safely discharged on home oxygen with home health follow-up. Despite reassuring appearance, the clinical course is unpredictable, so follow-up and parental education is important.

 ## ONGOING CARE

FOLLOW-UP RECOMMENDATIONS
Patient Monitoring
- Hospitalization is usually required only if oxygen is a requirement or unable to feed/drink.
- For a hospitalized patient, monitor as needed depending on the severity of the infection.
- If the patient is receiving home care, follow daily by telephone call for 2 to 4 days; the patient may need frequent office visits.

PATIENT EDUCATION
- American Academy of Pediatrics: http://www.aap.org
- American Academy of Family Physicians: http://www.familydoctor.org

PROGNOSIS
- Recovery time is variable. 40% can have symptoms at 14 days and 10% at 4 weeks.
- Mortality statistics differ but probably <1%.
- High-risk infants (bronchopulmonary dysplasia, congenital heart disease) may have a prolonged course.

COMPLICATIONS
- Bacterial superinfection
- Bronchiolitis obliterans
- Apnea
- Respiratory failure
- Death
- Increased incidence of development of reactive airway disease (asthma)

REFERENCES

1. Chao JH, Lin RC, Marneni S, et al. Predictors of airspace disease on chest x-ray in emergency department patients with bronchiolitis: a systematic review and meta-analysis. *Acad Emerg Med*. 2016;23(10):1107–1118.
2. Ralston SL, Lieberthal AS, Meissner HC, et al. Ralston SL, Lieberthal AS, Meissner HC, et al. Clinical practice guideline: the diagnosis, management, and prevention of bronchiolitis. Pediatrics. 2014;134(5):e1474–e1502. *Pediatrics*. 2015;136(4):782.
3. Baron J, El-Chaar G. Hypertonic saline for the treatment of bronchiolitis in infants and young children: a critical review of the literature. *J Pediatr Pharmacol Ther*. 2016;21(1):7–26.
4. Øymar K, Skjerven HO, Mikalsen IB. Acute bronchiolitis in infants, a review. *Scand J Trauma Resucs Emerg Med*. 2014;22:23.
5. Pickering LK, Kimberlin DW, Long SS, eds. *Red Book: 2012 Report of the Committee on Infectious Diseases*. 29th ed. Elk Grove Village, IL: American Academy of Pediatrics; 2012.
6. Liet JM, Ducruet T, Gupta V, et al. Heliox inhalation therapy for bronchiolitis in infants. *Cochrane Database Syst Rev*. 2015;(9):CD006915.

ADDITIONAL READING

Smith DK, Seales S, Budzik C. Respiratory syncytial virus bronchiolitis in children. *Am Fam Physician*. 2017;95(2):94–99.

CODES

ICD10
- J21.9 Acute bronchiolitis, unspecified
- J21.0 Acute bronchiolitis due to respiratory syncytial virus
- J21.8 Acute bronchiolitis due to other specified organisms

CLINICAL PEARLS

- Bronchiolitis is the leading cause of hospitalizations in infants and children—especially <3 months of age.
- Diagnosis is a clinical one of children in the first 2 years of life, associated with rhinorrhea, cough, labored breathing, and irritability.
- RSV causes the majority of bronchiolitis.
- Parental education and support is essential.
- Nasal and upper airway suctioning mainstay of treatment

BRONCHITIS, ACUTE

Ashlee N. Russo, MD • Alan Cropp, MD, FCCP • Ghazaleh Bigdeli, MD, FCCP

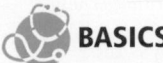

BASICS

DESCRIPTION
- Inflammation of trachea, bronchi, and bronchioles resulting from a respiratory tract infection or chemical irritant (1)
- Cough, the predominant symptom, may last as long as 3 weeks (2,3).
- Generally self-limited, with complete healing and full return of function (2)
- Most infections are viral if no underlying cardiopulmonary disease is present (2).
- Synonym(s): tracheobronchitis

Geriatric Considerations
Can be serious, particularly if part of influenza, with underlying COPD or CHF (3)

Pediatric Considerations
- Usually occurs in association with other conditions of upper and lower respiratory tract (trachea usually involved)
- If repeated attacks occur, child should be evaluated for anomalies of the respiratory tract, immune deficiencies, or for asthma.
- Acute bronchitis caused by RSV may be fatal.
- Antitussive medication not indicated in patients age <6 years (2)

EPIDEMIOLOGY
- Predominant age: all ages
- Predominant gender: male = female

Incidence
- ~5% of adults per year
- Common cause of infection in children

Prevalence
Results in 10 to 12 million office visits per year

ETIOLOGY AND PATHOPHYSIOLOGY
- Viral infections such as adenovirus, influenza A and B, parainfluenza virus, coxsackievirus, RSV, rhinovirus, coronavirus (types 1 to 3), herpes simplex virus, metapneumovirus (2)
- Bacterial infections, such as *Chlamydia pneumoniae*, *Mycoplasma*, *Bordetella pertussis*, *Haemophilus influenzae*, *Streptococcus pneumoniae*, *Moraxella catarrhalis*, and *Mycobacterium tuberculosis* (2)
- Secondary bacterial infection as part of an acute upper respiratory infection
- Possible fungal infections
- Chemical irritants
- Acute bronchitis causes an injury to the epithelial surfaces, resulting in an increase in mucus production and thickening of the bronchiole wall (1).

Genetics
No known genetic pattern

RISK FACTORS
- Infants
- Elderly
- Air pollutants
- Smoking
- Secondhand smoke
- Environmental changes
- Chronic bronchopulmonary diseases
- Chronic sinusitis
- Tracheostomy or endobronchial intubation
- Bronchopulmonary allergy
- Hypertrophied tonsils and adenoids in children
- Immunosuppression
  – Immunoglobulin deficiency
  – HIV infection
  – Alcoholism
- Gastroesophageal reflux disease (GERD)

GENERAL PREVENTION
- Avoid smoking and secondhand smoke.
- Control underlying risk factors (i.e., asthma, sinusitis, and reflux).
- Avoid exposure, especially daycare.
- Pneumovax, influenza immunization

COMMONLY ASSOCIATED CONDITIONS
- Allergic rhinitis
- Sinusitis
- Pharyngitis
- Epiglottitis (rare but can be rapidly fatal)
- Coryza
- Croup
- Influenza
- Pneumonia
- Asthma
- COPD/emphysema
- GERD

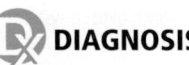

DIAGNOSIS

HISTORY
- Onset of cough for >5 days and no evidence of pneumonia, asthma, exacerbation of COPD (3)
- Cough is initially dry and nonproductive, then productive; later, mucopurulent sputum, which may indicate secondary infection
- Cough lasts >5 days (1).
- Dyspnea, wheeze, and fatigue may occur.
- Possible contact with others who have respiratory infections (1)
- Fever may suggest pneumonia or influenza infection (1).

PHYSICAL EXAM
- Fever
- Tachypnea
- Pharynx injected
- Rhonchi, wheezing
- No evidence of pulmonary consolidation

DIFFERENTIAL DIAGNOSIS
- Common cold
- Acute sinusitis
- Bronchopneumonia
- Influenza
- Bacterial tracheitis
- Bronchiectasis
- Asthma
- Reactive airways dysfunction syndrome (RADS)
- Allergy
- Eosinophilic pneumonitis
- Aspiration
- Retained foreign body
- Inhalation injury
- Cystic fibrosis
- Bronchogenic carcinoma
- Heart failure
- GERD
- Chronic cough

DIAGNOSTIC TESTS & INTERPRETATION
Initial Tests (lab, imaging)
- None normally needed; diagnosis is based on history and physical exam showing no postnasal drip or rales (1,3).
- For a complicated picture, consider the following:
  – CBC with differential
  – Sputum culture/sensitivity if CXR is abnormal (3)
  – Influenza titers (if appropriate for time of year) (1)
  – Viral panel
- No testing needed unless concerned about pneumonia
- Pulse oximetry if underlying pulmonary disease is present
- CXR
  – Lungs normal, if uncomplicated
  – Helps to rule out other diseases (pneumonia) or complications

Follow-Up Tests & Special Considerations
- Arterial blood gases: hypoxemia (rarely)
- Pulmonary function tests (seldom needed during acute stages): increased residual volume, decreased maximal expiratory rate (2)
- Sputum culture in those patients intubated or with tracheostomy

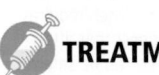

TREATMENT

GENERAL MEASURES
- Outpatient treatment unless elderly or complicated by severe underlying disease
- Rest
- Stop smoking and avoid secondhand smoke.
- Steam inhalations
- Vaporizers
- Adequate hydration
- Antitussives
- Antibiotics are usually not recommended (1,3,4)[A].
- Treat associated illnesses (e.g., GERD).

MEDICATION

ALERT
Antibiotics are not recommended (1,3)[A] unless a treatable pathogen has been identified or significant comorbidities are present. This should be explained to patients who likely expect an antibiotic to be prescribed (3)[B].

First Line
- Supportive; increased fluids (Cough results in increased fluid loss.)
- Antipyretic analgesic such as aspirin, acetaminophen, or ibuprofen
- Decongestants if accompanied by sinus condition
- Cough suppressant for troublesome cough (not with COPD); honey, benzonatate (Tessalon), guaifenesin with codeine or dextromethorphan; not indicated in children age <6 years (2)[C]
- Mucolytic agents are not recommended (3)[B].
- Inhaled β-agonist (e.g., albuterol) or in combination with high-dose inhaled corticosteroids for cough with bronchospasm in those with known airflow obstruction (2,5)[B]
- If influenza is highly suspected and symptom onset is <48 hours: oseltamivir (Tamiflu) or zanamivir (Relenza) (2)[B]
- Antibiotics ONLY if a treatable cause (i.e., pertussis) is identified (2)[A].
  - Clarithromycin (Biaxin): 500 mg q12h or azithromycin (Zithromax) Z-Pak for atypical or pertussis infection (1)[A]
  - In patients with acute bronchitis of a suspected bacterial cause, azithromycin tends to be more effective in terms of lower incidence of treatment failure and adverse events than amoxicillin or amoxicillin-clavulanic acid (6)[B].
    - Doxycycline: 100 mg/day × 10 days if *Moraxella*, *Chlamydia*, or *Mycoplasma* suspected
    - Quinolone for more serious infections or other antibiotic failure or in elderly or patients with multiple comorbidities
- Contraindication(s): Doxycycline and quinolones should not be used during pregnancy or in children.
- Precautions:
  - Multiple antibiotics have the potential to interfere with the effectiveness of oral contraceptives.
  - Antibiotic use can be associated with *Clostridium difficile* infections.
  - Cough and cold preparations should not be used in children <6 years (2)[B].

Second Line
Other antibiotics if indicated by sputum culture

ISSUES FOR REFERRAL
- Complications such as pneumonia or respiratory failure
- Comorbidities such as COPD
- Cough lasting >3 months

ADDITIONAL THERAPIES
- Antipyretic for fever (e.g., acetaminophen, or ibuprofen)
- Inhaled β-agonist (e.g., albuterol) or in combination with high-dose inhaled corticosteroids for cough with bronchospasm (2)[B]
- Oral corticosteroids probably not indicated (2)[C]

COMPLEMENTARY & ALTERNATIVE MEDICINE
Throat lozenges for pharyngitis

ADMISSION, INPATIENT, AND NURSING CONSIDERATIONS
- Hypoxia—may require supplemental oxygen
- Respiratory failure that may require CPAP/bilevel ventilation
- Severe bronchospasm
- Exacerbation of underlying disease
- Bronchodilators if patient is bronchospastic
- IV fluids may be helpful if patient is dehydrated.
- Ensure patient comfort and monitor for signs of deterioration, especially if underlying lung disease exists.
- May need to follow oxygen saturation in patients with underlying lung disease
- Discharge criteria: improvement in symptoms and comorbidities

 ## ONGOING CARE

FOLLOW-UP RECOMMENDATIONS
- Usually a self-limited disease not requiring follow-up
- Cough may linger for several weeks.
- In children, if recurrent, need to consider other diagnoses, such as asthma (4)

Patient Monitoring
- Oximetry until no longer hypoxemic
- Recheck for chronicity.

DIET
Increased fluids (3 to 4 L/day) while febrile

PATIENT EDUCATION
- For patient education materials favorably reviewed on this topic, contact the American Lung Association: 1740 Broadway, New York, NY 10019 (212) 315-8700; www.lungusa.org
- American Academy of Family Physicians: www.familydoctor.org

PROGNOSIS
- Usual: complete resolution
- Can be serious in the elderly or debilitated
- Cough may persist for several weeks after an initial improvement.
- Postbronchitic reactive airways disease (rare)
- Bronchiolitis obliterans and organizing pneumonia (rare)

COMPLICATIONS
- Superinfection such as bronchopneumonia
- Bronchiectasis
- Hemoptysis
- Acute respiratory failure
- Chronic cough

REFERENCES
1. Wenzel RP, Fowler AA III. Clinical practice. Acute bronchitis. *N Engl J Med*. 2006;355(20): 2125–2130.
2. Albert RH. Diagnosis and treatment of acute bronchitis. *Am Fam Physician*. 2010;82(11): 1345–1350.
3. Braman SS. Chronic cough due to acute bronchitis: ACCP evidence-based clinical practice guidelines. *Chest*. 2006;129(Suppl 1):95S–103S.
4. Gonzales R, Anderer T, McCulloch CE, et al. A cluster randomized trial of decision support strategies for reducing antibiotic use in acute bronchitis. *JAMA Intern Med*. 2013;173(4):267–273.
5. Becker L, Hom J, Villasis-Keever M, et al. Beta2-agonists for acute cough or a clinical diagnosis of acute bronchitis. *Cochrane Database Syst Rev*. 2015;(9):CD001726.
6. Panpanich R, Lerttrakarnnon P, Laopaiboon M. Azithromycin for acute lower respiratory tract infections. *Cochrane Database Syst Rev*. 2008;(1): CD001954.

 ## SEE ALSO

- Asthma; Chronic Obstructive Pulmonary Disease and Emphysema
- Algorithm: Cough, Chronic

 ## CODES

ICD10
- J20.9 Acute bronchitis, unspecified
- J68.0 Bronchitis and pneumonitis due to chemicals, gases, fumes and vapors
- B97.0 Adenovirus as the cause of diseases classified elsewhere

CLINICAL PEARLS
- Acute bronchitis is a common and generally self-limited disease.
- It usually does not require treatment with antibiotics. This needs to be explained to patients who expect antibiotics to be prescribed.
- Cough may linger for several weeks.
- Recurrent or seasonal episodes may suggest another disease process, such as asthma.
- Fever is uncommon and should prompt investigation for pneumonia or influenza.

BULIMIA NERVOSA

Umer Farooq, MD • Neha Datta, MD

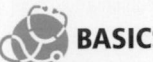 **BASICS**

DESCRIPTION
- Binge eating is characterized by eating, in a discrete period of time (within 2-hour period), an amount of food that is definitely larger than most people would eat during a similar period of time and a sense of lack of control over eating during the episode, followed by recurrent inappropriate compensatory behavior to prevent weight gain, such as self-induced vomiting, misuse of laxatives, excessive exercise, and so forth.
- Binge eating and inappropriate compensatory behaviors both occur once a week for 3 months.
- *DSM-5* classifies bulimia nervosa severity as the following:
  - Mild: 1 to 3 episodes of inappropriate compensatory behaviors per week
  - Moderate: 4 to 7 episodes of inappropriate compensatory behaviors per week
  - Severe: 8 to 13 episodes of inappropriate compensatory behaviors per week
  - Extreme: 14 or more episodes of inappropriate compensatory behaviors per week
- System(s) affected: oropharyngeal, endocrine/metabolic, gastrointestinal, dermatologic, cardiovascular, pulmonary, psychiatric

EPIDEMIOLOGY
- Predominant age: adolescents and young adults
- Mean age of onset: 18 to 21 years
- Predominant sex: female > male (13:1)

Incidence
28.8 women, 0.8 men per 100,000 per year

Prevalence
- More prevalent than anorexia nervosa
- 1.5% in women age 16 to 35 years
- 0.5% in young men

ETIOLOGY AND PATHOPHYSIOLOGY
- Combination of biologic, psychological, environmental, and social factors. Unique contribution of any specific factor remains unclear.
- Strong evidence of serotonergic dysregulation in bulimia nervosa
- Substantial literature shows genetic evidence for bulimia nervosa.
- Multiple studies demonstrate altered brain function and structure in bulimia nervosa.

RISK FACTORS
- Female gender
- History of obesity and dieting
- Body dissatisfaction: critical comments about weight, body shape, or eating: low self-esteem
- Severe life stressor
- Perfectionist or obsessive thinking
- Poor impulse control, substance abuse
- Environment stressing high achievement, physical fitness (e.g., armed forces, ballet, cheerleading, gymnastics, or modeling): perceived pressure to be thin
- Family history of substance abuse, affective disorders, eating disorder, or obesity
- Type 1 diabetes
- Childhood trauma (sexual abuse)

GENERAL PREVENTION
- Prevention programs can reduce risk factors and future onset of eating disorders.
- Target adolescents and young women ≥15 years.

- Realistic and healthy weight management strategies and attitudes
- Decrease body dissatisfaction and promote self-esteem.
- Reduce focus on thin as ideal.
- Decrease anxiety/depressive symptoms and improve stress management.

COMMONLY ASSOCIATED CONDITIONS
- Major depression and dysthymia
- Anxiety disorders
- Substance use disorder
- Bipolar disorder
- Obsessive-compulsive disorder
- Borderline personality disorder

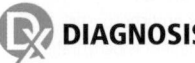 **DIAGNOSIS**

HISTORY
- Patients unlikely to self-identify binge eating or purging behaviors; corroborate with parent/relative.
- Unhappiness and/or preoccupation with weight and diet attempts
- Pattern of binge eating and compensatory behaviors
  - Binge is context specific (usually within 2-hour period, they will eat what would be an unusually large amount for most people).
  - Vomiting (often with little effort)
  - Vigorous aerobic exercise
  - Distress/shame related to loss of control
- Depressed mood and self-depreciation following the binges
- Other possible signs and symptoms
  - Requesting weight loss help and mildly underweight to overweight
  - Diet pill, diuretic, laxative, ipecac, and thyroid medication use/abuse, frequent fluctuations in weight
  - Menstrual disturbance
  - Fatigue and lethargy
  - Abdominal pain, bloating, constipation, diarrhea, rectal prolapse
  - Sore throat and thermal tooth sensitivity
  - Omission/underdosing insulin in diabetes patients
- Screening
  - Clinician administered eating-disorder screen for primary care to identify patients with eating disorders.
    - Are you satisfied with your eating patterns? (No is abnormal.)
    - Do you ever eat in secret? (Yes is abnormal.)
    - Does your weight affect the way you feel about yourself? (Yes is abnormal.)
    - Have any members of your family suffered with an eating disorder? (Yes is abnormal.)
    - Do you currently suffer with or have you ever suffered in the past with an eating disorder? (Yes is abnormal.)

PHYSICAL EXAM
- Often normal
- Tachycardia
- Erosion of dental enamel
- Perimylolysis, cheilosis, gingivitis
- Sialadenosis (parotid gland swelling and/or asymptomatic, noninflammatory parotid gland enlargement)
- Epigastric tenderness to palpation
- Calluses, abrasions, bruising on hand, thumb (Russell sign)
- Peripheral edema

DIFFERENTIAL DIAGNOSIS
- Anorexia, binge eating/purging type
- Major depressive disorder
- Addison disease
- Celiac disease
- Diabetes mellitus
- Hyperthyroidism, hypothyroidism
- Hyperpituitarism
- Hypothalamic brain tumor
- Kleine-Levin syndrome
- Body dysmorphic disorder
- Borderline personality disorder

DIAGNOSTIC TESTS & INTERPRETATION
All lab results may be within normal limits and are not necessary for diagnosis.
- Psychological self-report screening tests may be helpful, but diagnosis is based on meeting the *DSM-5* criteria:
  - SCOFF Questionnaire (1)[B]
  - Primary Care Evaluation of Mental Disorders Patient Health Questionnaire

Initial Tests (lab, imaging)
- Blood work, CBC, CMP, and LFTs
  - Hypokalemia, hypochloremia
  - Hypomagnesemia, hyponatremia, hypocalcemia, hypophosphatemia, hypoglycemia
  - Serum amylase levels and alkalosis
  - Elevated BUN
- Urinalysis
  - Increased urine specific gravity

Diagnostic Procedures/Other
- Pregnancy test
- Electrocardiogram: bradycardia or arrhythmias, conduction defects, depressed ST segment due to hypokalemia

Test Interpretation
- Esophagitis
- Acute pancreatitis
- Cardiomyopathy and muscle weakness due to ipecac abuse
- Melanosis coli and cathartic colon syndrome
- Delayed or arrested skeletal growth
- Stress fracture and/or osteopenia/osteoporosis
- Irreversible dental erosions

 TREATMENT

Cognitive-behavioral therapy (CBT) should be considered as first-line treatment (2,3)[A].

GENERAL MEASURES
- Multidisciplinary team
  - Primary care physician, behavioral health provider, nutritionist
- Build trust; increase motivation for change.
- Assess psychological and nutritional status.
- Consider evidence-based self-help program.
- CBT for bulimia nervosa (2,3)[A]
  - Sixteen to twenty 50-minute appointments
  - Involve patient in establishing goals.
  - Self-monitoring of food intake, frequency of binges/purges, related antecedents, consequences, thoughts, and emotions
  - Self-monitoring of weight once per week
  - Educate about ineffectiveness of purging for weight control and adverse outcomes.

– Establish prescribed eating plan to develop regular eating habits and realistic weight goal.
– Gradually introduce feared foods into diet and challenge fear of loss of control.
– Problem-solve how to cope with triggers.
– Decrease ruminations about calories, weight, and purging.
– Establish relapse prevention plan.
– Gradual laxative withdrawal
- Interpersonal therapy
– May act more slowly than CBT
- Transdiagnostic CBT
- Dialectical behavior therapy
- Family therapy for adolescents
- Nutritional education, relaxation techniques
- Educate patient to brush teeth and use baking soda to rinse mouth after vomiting.

ALERT
Contraindications to treating bulimia nervosa with CBT (4)[B] are

- Medical instability
- Severe major depression
- Substance use disorder
- Suicidal ideation or behavior
- Psychosis

MEDICATION
First Line
- Selective serotonin reuptake inhibitors (SSRIs) (5)[A], (6)[B], particularly fluoxetine (Prozac) titrated to 60 mg/day, are effective in reducing symptoms with relatively few side effects. Higher doses than standard doses for depression are often needed.
  – Combination of medication and CBT has been shown to have added benefit over medication or therapy alone.
- To prevent relapse, maintain antidepressant at full therapeutic dose for at least 1 year.
- Avoid bupropion: contraindicated due to its association with seizures in patients who purge
- Precautions
  – Serious toxicity following overdose is common.
  – Patients may vomit medications.

Second Line
- Select different SSRI (citalopram, fluvoxamine, and sertraline).
- Ondansetron (Zofran) 4 to 8 mg TID between meals can help prevent vomiting.
- The anticonvulsant topiramate may have some usefulness in helping to diminish binge-purge episodes in bulimic patients. Additionally, bright light therapy in certain controlled trials has reduced binge-purge frequency in bulimia nervosa patients.
- Psyllium (Metamucil) preparations, 1 tbsp QHS with glass of water, can prevent constipation during laxative withdrawal.

ISSUES FOR REFERRAL
Patients with bulimia require a multidisciplinary team, including a primary care physician, behavioral health provider, and a nutritionist. Important part of treatment is to arrange mental health therapist for psychotherapy.

ADDITIONAL THERAPIES
Most patients can be treated as outpatients.

COMPLEMENTARY & ALTERNATIVE MEDICINE
Bright light therapy may help.

ADMISSION, INPATIENT, AND NURSING CONSIDERATIONS
If possible, admit to a specialized eating disorders unit.
- Supervised meals and bathroom privileges
- Monitor weight and physical activity.
- Monitor electrolytes.
- Gradually shift control to patients as they demonstrate improvement.
- Hospitalize if severe malnutrition.
- Admission to inpatient general guidelines:
  – Syncope
  – Potassium <3.0
  – Esophageal tears
  – Cardiac arrhythmias
  – Hypothermia
  – Suicide risk
  – Intractable vomiting
  – Hematemesis
  – Failure to response outpatient treatment

 ONGOING CARE

FOLLOW-UP RECOMMENDATIONS
Patient Monitoring
- Binge-purge activity, including antecedents and consequences, level of exercise activity
- Self-esteem, comfort with body and self
- Ruminations and depressive symptoms
- Repeat any abnormal lab values weekly or monthly until stable.

DIET
- Balanced diet, normal eating pattern
- Nutritional rehabilitation aims to restore a structured and consistent meal pattern: three meals and two snacks per day

PATIENT EDUCATION
https://www.nami.org/Learn-More/Mental-Health-Conditions/Eating-Disorders/Overview

PROGNOSIS
- After effective CBT
  – In the short term, 50% of treated individuals do not meet criteria for diagnosis.
  – In the long term (2 to 10 years), 70% may be asymptomatic.
  – Symptomatic individuals may demonstrate remissions, relapses, subclinical, or other eating disorder–related behaviors.
- Untreated
  – Likely to remain chronic/relapsing problem
- Greater weight fluctuations, other impulsive behaviors, childhood obesity, low self-esteem, family history of alcohol abuse, psychiatric comorbidity, and personality disorder diagnoses (e.g., avoidant personality disorder) may predict poor prognosis.
- Mortality rate: 0.4%. The death rate for bulimia nervosa is much lower than that for anorexia nervosa. Patients who remain in remission for >1 year have a better long-term outcome.

COMPLICATIONS
- Substance use disorder
- Osteopenia/osteoporosis
- Stress fracture
- Gastric dilatation
- Boerhaave syndrome
- Mallory-Weiss tears
- Pseudo-Bartter syndrome

- Spontaneous pneumomediastinum
- Potassium depletion, cardiac arrhythmia, cardiac arrest
- Suicide

Pregnancy Considerations
Maternal and fetal problems if pregnant
- Binging/purging behaviors may persist, increase, or decrease with pregnancy.
- Increased risk for preterm delivery, operative delivery, and infants with low birth weight should be managed as high risk.

REFERENCES
1. Cotton MA, Ball C, Robinson P. Four simple questions can help screen for eating disorders. *J Gen Intern Med*. 2003;18(1):53–56.
2. Hay PP, Bacaltchuk J, Stefano S, et al. Psychological treatments for bulimia nervosa and binging. *Cochrane Database Syst Rev*. 2009;(4):CD000562.
3. Shapiro JR, Berkman ND, Brownley KA, et al. Bulimia nervosa treatment: a systematic review of randomized controlled trials. *Int J Eat Disord*. 2007;40(4):321–336.
4. Cooper Z, Fairburn C. Cognitive behavior therapy for bulimia nervosa. In: Grilo C, Mitchell J, eds. *The Treatment of Eating Disorders*. New York, NY: The Guilford Press; 2010:243–270.
5. Bacaltchuk J, Hay P, Trefiglio R. Antidepressants versus psychological treatments and their combination for bulimia nervosa. *Cochrane Database Syst Rev*. 2001;(4):CD003385.
6. Bellini M, Merli M. Current drug treatment of patients with bulimia nervosa and binge-eating disorder: selective serotonin reuptake inhibitors versus mood stabilizers. *Int J Psychiatry Clin Pract*. 2004;8(4):235–243.

ADDITIONAL READING
- American Psychiatric Association. *Practice Guideline for the Treatment of Patients with Eating Disorders*. 3rd ed. Washington, DC: American Psychiatric Association; 2006. http://www.psychiatry.org/. Accessed November 28, 2017.
- National Institute for Health and Care Excellence. *Eating Disorders: Core Interventions in the Treatment and Management of Anorexia Nervosa, Bulimia Nervosa and Related Eating Disorders (NICE Guidelines)*. London, United Kingdom: National Institute for Health and Clinical Excellence; 2004. http://www.nice.org.uk. Accessed November 28, 2017.

 CODES

ICD10
F50.2 Bulimia nervosa

CLINICAL PEARLS
- Asking "Are you satisfied with your eating patterns?" and/or "Do you worry that you have lost control over how much you eat?" may help to screen for an eating problem.
- Consider multidisciplinary team approach with PCP, behavioral health provider, and nutritionist.
- SSRIs, particularly fluoxetine (60 mg daily), may be helpful as a first step or as an adjunctive treatment with CBT.
- Pharmacotherapy alone is reasonable if specialized nutritional rehabilitation and psychotherapy are not available.

BUNION (HALLUX VALGUS)

Jennifer G. Chang, MD

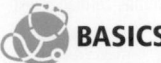 **BASICS**

DESCRIPTION
- Lateral deviation of the great toe ("Hallux abducto valgus" derives from the Latin for "big toe askew.")
- Associated medial deviation of the 1st metatarsal, leading to a medial prominence of the 1st metatarsophalangeal (MTP) joint (also known as "bunion")
- Progressive subluxation of the 1st MTP joint in later stages
- System(s) affected: musculoskeletal/skin

EPIDEMIOLOGY
- Predominant age: more common in adults
  - Estimated 23% in adults aged 18 to 65 years
  - Estimated 35.7% in elderly >65 years
- Predominant sex: female > male by ~2:1

Prevalence
- Prevalence increases with age particularly in females.
- Juvenile hallux valgus
  - More common in girls (>80% of cases)
- Commonly bilateral

ETIOLOGY AND PATHOPHYSIOLOGY
Multifactorial. Contributing factors include the following:
- Valgus deviation of the hallux promotes varus position of the 1st metatarsal.
- Medial MTP joint capsule stretches and attenuates, whereas the lateral capsule contracts.
- Metatarsal head moves medially, shifting the sesamoid bones to a more lateral position.
- Extensor hallucis longus deviates laterally.
- Lateral and plantar migration of abductor hallucis moves the great toe into plantar flexion and lateral pronation.
- Medial collateral ligament stretches and eventually ruptures, decreasing stability and causing progressive subluxation of the 1st MTP joint.

RISK FACTORS
- Genetic predisposition
- Abnormal biomechanics (i.e., flexible flat feet)
- Foot deformities: joint laxity, hindfoot pronation, Achilles tendon tightness, pes planus (fallen arches), metatarsus primus varus
- Amputation of 2nd toe
- Inflammatory joint disease
- Neuromuscular disorders (cerebral palsy, stroke)
- Improper footwear (high heels; narrow toe box)

GENERAL PREVENTION
Proper footwear may decrease the progression of the disease.

COMMONLY ASSOCIATED CONDITIONS
- Medial bursitis of the 1st MTP joint (most common)
- Hammertoe deformity of the 2nd phalanx
- Plantar callus
- Metatarsalgia
- Degeneration of 1st metatarsal head cartilage
- Pronated feet; ankle equinus
- Onychocryptosis (ingrown toenail)
- Entrapment of the medial dorsal cutaneous nerve
- Synovitis of the MTP joint

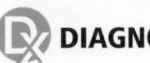 **DIAGNOSIS**

- Based on clinical exam
- Radiographs are used for staging.

HISTORY
- Painful MTP joint (most common symptom in adults)
- Abnormal position of great toe
- Enlargement of the MTP joint medially (patients complain of a "bump")
- Shoes do not fit properly.
- Pain with ambulation
- Skin irritation, blister, or callus at the 1st MTP

PHYSICAL EXAM
- Observe gait; may be antalgic due to pain
- Medial prominence at the MTP joint
- Skin changes: erythema, blistering, callus or ulceration at the MTP joint
- Great toe over- or underriding the 2nd toe
- Examine the entire 1st metatarsal and toe for:
  - 1st MTP range of motion
  - 1st tarsometatarsal (TMT) mobility
  - Neurovascular integrity
  - Degenerative osteoarthritis

DIFFERENTIAL DIAGNOSIS
- Trauma
  - Turf toe; sesamoiditis; stress fracture
- Infection
  - Osteomyelitis; septic arthritis
- Joint disorder
  - Osteoarthritis; rheumatoid arthritis; pseudogout; gout
- Tendon disorder
  - Tendinosis; tenosynovitis; tendon rupture
- Other
  - Bursitis; ganglion cyst; foreign body granuloma

DIAGNOSTIC TESTS & INTERPRETATION
- Weight-bearing AP and lateral radiographs (sesamoid view optional) to assess:
  - Joint congruency and degenerative changes
  - Lateral sesamoid bone displacement
  - Rounded 1st metatarsal head
  - Longer 1st metatarsal

- Radiographic parameters:
  - Hallux valgus angle (HVA): Long axis of the 1st MT and proximal phalanx is normally <15 degrees.
  - Intermetatarsal angle (IMA): Between long axis of 1st and 2nd metatarsal is normally <9 degrees.
  - Distal metatarsal articular angle (DMAA): Between 1st metatarsal long axis and line through base of distal articular cap is normally <15 degrees.
  - Hallux valgus interphalangeus: Between long axis of distal phalanx and proximal phalanx is normally <10 degrees.

 TREATMENT

- Primary indication for treatment is pain.
- There are conservative (nonoperative) and surgical approaches.
- Only surgical approaches can correct the hallux valgus deformity.
- Surgical treatment is generally more effective in improving pain but has attendant risks.

GENERAL MEASURES
Nonoperative treatment options may improve symptoms and delay the progression of hallux valgus deformity, although high-quality evidence is limited:
- Proper fitting footwear: low-heeled, wide-toe shoes to decrease stress on MTP joint (i.e., wide toe box)
- Orthotics: correct foot alignment (pes planus and overpronation). Improving gait may prevent bunion formation and reduce pressure on the MTP.
- Night splinting: in theory, stabilizes and balances soft tissue structures around the MTP. Limited evidence shows improvement in degree of angulation in mild hallux valgus.
- Manual and manipulative therapy (MMT) stretches contracted soft tissue.
- Foot exercises and stretching may improve intrinsic foot muscle strength and increase range of motion.
- Pads/spacers: Pads decrease friction on the MTP joint. A toe spacer in the 1st interdigital space may reduce pain (1)[C].

MEDICATION
- Topical and oral medications (NSAIDs) can be used to relieve pain and swelling. Other topical options include capsaicin cream.
- Corticosteroid injections may improve pain (rarely used).

ADDITIONAL THERAPIES
Custom orthoses are a safe intervention that may decrease pain at 6 and 12 months compared with no treatment; however, this improvement is less than that seen with surgical intervention (2)[B].

SURGERY/OTHER PROCEDURES

- Surgery is indicated for patients with severe pain, dysfunction, or persistent symptoms that do not abate with conservative therapy.
- >100 different surgical techniques exist to treat hallux valgus.
  - No technique is proven superior; no universally accepted standard exists for procedure selection.
  - Minimally-invasive techniques are gaining popularity.
  - Choice of technique depends on disease severity, radiographic findings, and patient/surgeon-specific factors:
    ○ Arthrodesis: fusion of the 1st MTP joint; used for severe and/or recurrent hallux valgus; fusion of the 1st TMT joint (modified Lapidus) is considered for TMT joint hypermobility.
    ○ Arthroplasty: removing the joint or replacing it with a prosthesis; high revision rates
    ○ Exostectomy/bunionectomy: removing the medial bony prominence of the MTP joint
    ○ Soft tissue realignment: alters the function of surrounding ligaments and tendons; used for minor deformities or as an adjunct to bony correction techniques
    ○ Osteotomy and realignment: various techniques; can correct large deformities, but evidence of long-term outcome is lacking (3)[C]
    ○ Mini-tight rope procedure: use of a FiberWire to correct the misalignment of the deformity
- Some patients may have little to no improvement in symptoms despite interventions. Providers should establish realistic expectations prior to surgery.
- In pediatric patients, surgery should generally be delayed until skeletal maturity (4)[C].

COMPLEMENTARY & ALTERNATIVE MEDICINE

Marigold ointment may reduce pain and soft tissue swelling related to bunion.

 ONGOING CARE

FOLLOW-UP RECOMMENDATIONS

- Postoperative treatment includes physical therapy, physiotherapy, supportive footwear, continuous passive motion, or manual manipulation.
- Time until full weight-bearing depends on the surgical procedure.

PROGNOSIS

Patient outcome varies depending on biomechanical factors, severity of the deformity, and treatment modality used. The radiologic HA angle predicts surgical outcomes. Patients with an HA angle <37 degrees have a higher chance of having the deformity successfully corrected with surgery compared with patients with an HA angle >37 degrees (5)[B].

COMPLICATIONS

- Risks associated with surgery include infection, persistent pain, and poor cosmetic result.
- Additional risks vary with the surgical procedure.
- Other complications may include:
  - Early swelling
  - Hallux varus
  - Recurrence of bunion
  - Metatarsal fracture
  - Decreased sensation over the 1st metatarsal or phalanx

REFERENCES

1. Tehraninasr A, Saeedi H, Forogh B, et al. Effects of insole with toe-separator and night splint on patients with painful hallux valgus: a comparative study. *Prosthet Orthot Int.* 2008;32(1):79–83.
2. Torkki M, Malmivaara A, Seitsalo S, et al. Surgery vs orthosis vs watchful waiting for hallux valgus: a randomized controlled trial. *JAMA.* 2001;285(19):2474–2480.
3. Choi JH, Zide JR, Coleman SC, et al. Prospective study of treatment of adult primary hallux valgus with scarf osteotomy and soft tissue realignment. *Foot Ankle Int.* 2013;34(5):684–690.
4. Chell J, Dhar S. Pediatric hallux valgus. *Foot Ankle Clin.* 2014;19(2):235–243.
5. Deenik AR, de Visser E, Louwerens JW, et al. Hallux valgus angle as main predictor for correction of hallux valgus. *BMC Musculoskelet Disord.* 2008;9:70.

ADDITIONAL READING

- Dayton P, Sedberry S, Feilmeier M. Complications of metatarsal suture techniques for bunion correction: a systematic review of the literature. *J Foot Ankle Surg.* 2015;54(2):230–232.
- Dux K, Smith N, Rottier FJ. Outcome after metatarsal osteotomy for hallux valgus: a study of postoperative foot function using revised foot function index short form. *J Foot Ankle Surg.* 2013;52(4):422–425.

- Fraissler L, Konrads C, Hoberg M, et al. Treatment of hallux valgus deformity. *EFFORT Open Rev.* 2016;1(8):295–302.
- Hecht PJ, Lin TJ. Hallux valgus. *Med Clin North Am.* 2014;98(2):227–232.
- Holmes GB Jr, Hsu AR. Correction of intermetatarsal angle in hallux valgus using small suture button device. *Foot Ankle Int.* 2013;34(4):543–549.
- Khan MT. The podiatric treatment of hallux abducto valgus and its associated condition, bunion, with Tagetes patula. *J Pharm Pharmacol.* 1996;48(7):768–770.
- Maffulli NI, Longo UG, Marinozzi AN, et al. Hallux valgus: effectiveness and safety of minimally invasive surgery. A systematic review. *Br Med Bull.* 2011;97:149–167.
- Nix S, Smith M, Vicenzino B. Prevalence of hallux valgus in the general population: a systematic review and meta-analysis. *J Foot Ankle Res.* 2010;3:21.
- Nix SE, Vicenzino BT, Collins NJ, et al. Characteristics of foot structure and footwear associated with hallux valgus: a systematic review. *Osteoarthritis Cartilage.* 2012;20(10):1059–1074.
- Perera AM, Mason L, Stephens MM. The pathogenesis of hallux valgus. *J Bone Joint Surg Am.* 2011;93(17):1650–1661.
- Smith SE, Landorf KB, Butterworth PA, et al. Scarf versus chevron osteotomy for the correction of 1–2 intermetatarsal angle in hallux valgus: a systematic review and meta-analysis. *J Foot Ankle Surg.* 2012;51(4):437–444.
- Trnka HJ, Krenn S, Schuh R. Minimally invasive hallux valgus surgery: a critical review of the evidence. *Int Orthop.* 2013;37(9):1731–1735.

 CODES

ICD10

- M20.10 Hallux valgus (acquired), unspecified foot
- M20.11 Hallux valgus (acquired), right foot
- M20.12 Hallux valgus (acquired), left foot

CLINICAL PEARLS

- Avoid footwear with high heels, pointed toe boxes, or inadequate toe space to reduce development or progression of bunions.
- Surgery generally results in superior outcomes for pain relief in appropriately selected patients.
- No single surgical method has shown to be superior for long-term pain relief.
- Establish realistic expectations prior to surgery to improve patient satisfaction with surgical outcomes.

BURNS

Caleb J. Mentzer, DO • Cragin D. Currence, MD • James R. Yon, MD

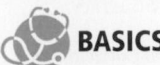

BASICS

DESCRIPTION
- Tissue injuries caused by application of heat, chemicals, electricity, or irradiation
- Extent of injury (depth of burn) is a result of intensity and duration of exposure.
  - 1st degree involves superficial layers of epidermis.
  - 2nd degree involves varying amounts of epidermis (with blister formation) and part of the dermis.
  - 3rd degree involves destruction of all skin elements (full thickness) with coagulation of subdermal plexus.
- System(s) affected: endocrine/metabolic, pulmonary, skin/exocrine

Geriatric Considerations
- Prognosis is worse for severe burns.
- Patients >60 years of age account for 11% of all burns.

Pediatric Considerations
Consider child abuse or neglect when dealing with hot water burns in children; abuse accounts for 15% of pediatric burns. Special concerns are sharply demarcated wounds, immersion injuries, and suspect stories. Involve child welfare services early.

EPIDEMIOLOGY
- Predominant age: 30 years; 13% infants; 11% >60 years of age
- Predominant gender: Males account for 70%.

Incidence
Per year in the United States
- 1.2 to 2.0 million burns; 700,000 emergency room visits; 45,000 to 50,000 hospitalizations; 3,900 deaths owing to burn-related complications
- In children: 250,000 burns; 15,000 hospitalizations; 1,100 deaths
- Estimated total cost of $2 billion annually for burn care
- House fires cause 75% of deaths.
- Burn deaths decreasing nationally due to improved prevention and treatment
- Increase in burns from the illegal production of methamphetamines. Patients can present with a combination of chemical burn, thermal burn, and explosion injury.

ETIOLOGY AND PATHOPHYSIOLOGY
- Open flame and hot liquid are the most common causes of burns (heat usually ≥45°C): flame burns more common in adults; scald burns are more common in children.
- Caustic chemicals or acids (may show little signs or symptoms for the first few days)
- Electricity (may have significant injury with very little damage to overlying skin)
- Excess sun exposure

RISK FACTORS
- Water heaters set too high
- Workplace exposure to chemicals, electricity, or irradiation
- Young children and older adults with thin skin are more susceptible to injury.

- Carelessness with burning cigarettes: related to 18% of fatal fires in 2006
- Inadequate or faulty electrical wiring
- Lack of smoke detectors: Lacking or nonfunctioning smoke alarms are implicated in 63% of residential fires.
- Arson: cause of 12.4% of fires that resulted in fatalities in 2012

GENERAL PREVENTION
Home safety education should be a key mechanism for injury prevention.
- Families educated on home safety were more likely to have safe hot water temperatures.
- Safety education results in more families having functioning smoke alarms and increased use of fireguards.

COMMONLY ASSOCIATED CONDITIONS
Smoke inhalation syndrome
- May involve thermal burn to respiratory mucosa (e.g., trachea, bronchi) as well as carbon monoxide inhalation
- Occurs within 72 hours of burn
- Should be suspected in all burns occurring in an enclosed space or exposure to explosions

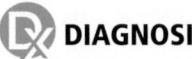

DIAGNOSIS

HISTORY
- History of source of burn
- In children or elderly: Check for consistency between the history and the burn's physical characteristics.

PHYSICAL EXAM
- 1st degree: erythema of involved tissue, skin blanches with pressure; skin may be tender.
- 2nd degree: Skin is red and blistered; skin is very tender.
- 3rd degree: Burned skin is tough and leathery; skin is nontender.
- Rule of 9s
  - Each upper extremity: adult and child 9%
  - Each lower extremity: adult 18%; child 14%
  - Anterior trunk: adult and child 18%
  - Posterior trunk: adult and child 18%
  - Head and neck: adult 10%; child 18%
- Quick estimate: The surface area of the patient's hand (palmar surface plus fingers) is 1% of the body surface area (BSA).
- Careful documentation of extent of burn and the estimated depth of burn
- Check for any signs suggestive of potential airway involvement: singed nasal hair, facial burns, carbonaceous sputum, progressive hoarseness, inflamed oropharynx, circumferential burns around the neck, tachypnea.

DIAGNOSTIC TESTS & INTERPRETATION
- Children: glucose (hypoglycemia may occur in children because of limited glycogen storage)
- Smoke inhalation: arterial blood gas, carboxyhemoglobin
- Electrical burns: ECG, urine myoglobin, creatine kinase isoenzymes

Initial Tests (lab, imaging)
- Labs: hematocrit; type and crossmatching; electrolytes, including BUN and creatinine; urinalysis
- Imaging: chest radiograph; xenon scan is useful in suspected smoke inhalation.

Diagnostic Procedures/Other
Bronchoscopy may be necessary in smoke inhalation to evaluate lower respiratory tract (1)[A].

TREATMENT

- Prehospital care
  - Remove the patient from the source of burn.
  - Extinguish and remove all burning clothing.
  - Room-temperature water may be poured onto burn but only in the first 15 minutes following burn exposure.
  - Wrap patient to prevent hypothermia.
  - All patients to receive 100% oxygen via face mask
- Hospitalization for all serious burns
  - 2nd-degree burns >10% of BSA
  - Any 3rd-degree burn
  - Burns of hands, feet, face, or perineum
  - Electrical or lightning burns
  - Inhalation injury
  - Chemical burns
  - Circumferential burn
- Transfer to burn center for (2)[C]
  - 2nd- and 3rd-degree burns >10% of BSA in patients <10 years and >50 years of age
  - 2nd-degree burns >20% of BSA and full-thickness burns >5% BSA in any age range
  - 3rd-degree burns in any age group
  - Burns of hands, feet, face, or perineum
  - Electrical or lightning burns
  - Inhalation injury
  - Chemical burns
  - Circumferential burn
  - Burns in patients with additional trauma (fractures, etc.) in which the burn is the more severe injury; otherwise, send to trauma center for stabilization
  - Burn injuries in patients with preexisting medical conditions that could affect management, mortality, or recovery

GENERAL MEASURES
- Based on depth of burns and accurate estimate of total BSA involved (rule of 9s)
- Tetanus prophylaxis (if not current)
- Remove all rings, watches, and other items from injured extremities to avoid tourniquet effect.
- Remove clothing and cover all burned areas with dry sheets.
- Flush area of chemical burn (for ~2 hours).
- For all major burns, use 100% oxygen administration; consider early intubation.
- Do not apply ice to burn site.
- Nasogastric tube (high risk of paralytic ileus)
- Foley catheter
- Analgesia
- ECG monitoring in first 24 hours following electrical burn

- Whirlpool hydrotherapy followed by silver sulfadiazine (Silvadene) occlusive dressings in severe burns
- Daily or BID cleansing with dressing changes
- Burn fluid resuscitation
  - Calculate fluid resuscitation from time of burn, not from time treatment begins.
  - 2 to 4 mL lactated Ringer × body weight (kg) × % BSA burn (1/2 given in first 8 hours, in second 8 hours, and in third 8 hours); in children, this is given in addition to maintenance fluids and is adjusted according to urine output and vital signs. Protocol-based resuscitation leads to superior outcomes.
  - Colloid solutions are not recommended during the first 12 to 24 hours of resuscitation (3)[A].
  - Other: Use of biologic membranes or skin substitutes may be indicated for burn coverage.
- Inhalation injury
  - Intubation, ventilation with positive end-expiratory pressure assistance. Employ lung protective ventilation strategies.
  - Hyperbaric oxygen treatment may be useful in patients with carbon monoxide levels >25%; patients with coma, focal neurologic deficit, ischemic ECG changes; and pregnant patients.
  - Prophylactic antibiotics and steroids are not indicated (4)[C].

MEDICATION

First Line

- IV morphine or hydromorphone (Dilaudid) for severe pain
- Oral analgesics, such as acetaminophen (Tylenol) with codeine, acetaminophen with oxycodone (Percocet), or acetaminophen with hydrocodone (Lortab) for moderate pain
- Silver sulfadiazine (Silvadene): Apply topically to burn site (can cause leukopenia). Do not use in sulfa-allergic patients, women who are pregnant/breastfeeding, or infants (<2 months).
- Neosporin or bacitracin ointment: Apply to facial burns.
- Mupirocin: has potent inhibitory activity against methicillin-resistant *Staphylococcus aureus* (MRSA)
- Acticoat A.B. (a dressing consisting of two sheets of high-density polyethylene mesh coated with nanocrystalline silver) has a more controlled, prolonged release of silver, allowing less frequent dressing changes.
- Electrical burn with myoglobinuria will require alkalinization of urine and mannitol.
- Consider H_2 blockers (e.g., famotidine) or proton pump inhibitors (e.g., lansoprazole, pantoprazole) for stress ulcer prophylaxis in severely burned patients.
- Tetanus toxoid/tetanus immunoglobulin
- There is no clear indication for prophylactic systemic antibiotics.
- Use of negative pressure wound therapy may result in a low-protease environment with higher levels of angiogenic factor (vascular endothelial growth factor [VEGF]) during wound healing, leading to more chaotic, hyperkeratinized, thickened epidermis when compared with a standard hydrocolloid dressing.

Second Line

- Mafenide (Sulfamylon) for full-thickness burn, best against *Pseudomonas* (caution: metabolic acidosis, painful)
- Silver nitrate 0.5% (messy, leeches electrolytes from burn, causes water toxicity)

- Povidone-iodine (Betadine) may result in iodine absorption from burn and "tan eschar," makes débridement more difficult.
- Travase (enzymatic débridement)

SURGERY/OTHER PROCEDURES

- Escharotomy may be necessary in constricting circumferential burns of extremities or chest due to compartment syndrome.
- Tangential excision with split-thickness skin grafts: Early excision of burns results in a significant reduction in mortality (excluding patients with inhalational injury) and a significant decrease in hospital length of stay (5)[B].
- Various dressings (e.g., biosynthetic, biologic) are available to help reduce the number of dressing changes and promote healing.

ONGOING CARE

FOLLOW-UP RECOMMENDATIONS

Early mobilization is the goal.

DIET

- High-protein, high-calorie diet when bowel function resumes
- Nasogastric tube feedings may be required in early postburn period.
- Total parenteral nutrition if NPO is expected for >5 days
- Early initiation of enteral nutrition in the first 24 hours of admission results in shorter intensive care unit (ICU) stay and lower wound infection rates.

PATIENT EDUCATION

- Use of sunscreen: Skin grafts or newly epithelialized skin is highly sensitive to sun exposure and thermal extremes.
- Prevent access to electrical cords/outlets.
- Isolate household chemicals.
- Use low-temperature setting for water heater (<54°C).
- Household smoke detectors with special emphasis on maintenance
- Family/household evacuation plan
- Proper storage and use of flammable substances
- Burn management: http://www.aafp.org/afp/2000/1101/p2029.html
- Burn prevention: http://www.aafp.org/afp/2000/1101/p2032.html

PROGNOSIS

- 1st-degree burn: complete resolution
- 2nd-degree burn: epithelialization in 10 to 14 days (deep 2nd-degree burns probably will require skin graft)
- 3rd-degree burn: no potential for reepithelialization; skin graft is required.
- Baux score (sum of age and TBSA burned) and Denver 2 score (pulmonary score ranging 0 to 3, using PaO_2/FiO_2 cutoffs of 100, 175, and 250, renal score (0 to 3, using creatinine cutoffs of 1.8, 2.5, and 5.0 mg/dL), hepatic score (0 to 3, using bilirubin cutoffs of 2, 4, and 8 mg/dL), and cardiac score (0 to 3, based on number and dosage of inotropes) can be used to estimate mortality (6)[B].
- Length of hospital stay and need for ICU care depend on extent of burn, smoke inhalation, comorbidities, and age.

- Burn size is correlated to complications; >60% TBSA burned in children and >40% in adults are at increased risk for mortality and morbidity (6)[B].
- A 50% survival rate can be expected with a 62% burn in patients aged 0 to 14 years, 63% burn in patients aged 15 to 40 years, 38% burn in patients aged 40 to 65 years, and 25% burn in patients >65 years of age.
- 90% of survivors can be expected to return to an occupation comparable to their preburn employment.

COMPLICATIONS

- Gastroduodenal ulceration (Curling ulcer)
- Marjolin ulcer: malignant squamous cell carcinoma developing in old burn site
- Signs of infection: discoloration, green fat, edema, eschar separation, and conversion of 2nd-degree to 3rd-degree wound
- Biopsy is the best way to diagnose wound infection.
- Burn wound sepsis: most commonly *S. aureus* (including MRSA), vancomycin-resistant enterococci, and gram-negative organisms
- Pneumonia
- Decreased mobility with possibility of future flexion contractures
- Hypertrophic scarring common with burns

REFERENCES

1. Dries DJ, Endorf FW. Inhalation injury: epidemiology, pathology, treatment strategies. *Scand J Trauma Resusc Emerg Med*. 2013;21:31.
2. Bezuhly M, Fish JS. Acute burn care. *Plast Reconstr Surg*. 2012;130(2):349e–358e.
3. Perel P, Roberts I, Ker K. Colloids versus crystalloids for fluid resuscitation in critically ill patients. *Cochrane Database Syst Rev*. 2013;(2):CD000567.
4. ISBI Practice Guidelines Committee, Steering Subcommittee, Advisory Subcommittee. ISBI practice guidelines for burn care. *Burns*. 2016;42(5):953–1021.
5. Ong YS, Samuel M, Song C. Meta-analysis of early excision of burns. *Burns*. 2006;32(2):145–150.
6. Jeschke MG, Pinto R, Kraft R, et al; and Inflammation and the Host Response to Injury Collaborative Research Program. Morbidity and survival probability in burn patients in modern burn care. *Crit Care Med*. 2015;43(4):808–815.

 CODES

ICD10

- T30.0 Burn of unspecified body region, unspecified degree
- T30.4 Corrosion of unspecified body region, unspecified degree

CLINICAL PEARLS

- 1st degree: erythema of involved tissue; skin blanches with pressure. Skin may be tender.
- 2nd degree: Skin is red and blistered. Skin is very tender.
- 3rd degree: Burned skin is tough and leathery. Skin is not tender.

BURSITIS, PES ANSERINE (PES ANSERINE SYNDROME)
Jennifer B. Schwartz, MD

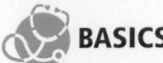 **BASICS**

DESCRIPTION
- The pes anserinus ("goosefoot") is the combined insertion of the sartorius, gracilis, and semitendinosus (SGT) tendons on the anteromedial tibia.
- The pes anserine muscles help flex the knee and resist valgus stress.
- The pes anserine bursa lies deep to the SGT tendons and superficial to the tibial attachment of the medial collateral ligament.
- *Pes anserine syndrome* is due to irritation of the bursa and/or tendons in this area.

EPIDEMIOLOGY
Incidence
Inflammation of the pes anserine bursa is detected in up to 2.5% of MRI studies of patients with knee pain. The overall incidence is likely higher.

ETIOLOGY AND PATHOPHYSIOLOGY
Pes anserine bursitis occurs due to:
- Overuse injury
- Excessive valgus and rotary stresses
- Mechanical forces and degenerative changes
- Direct trauma

RISK FACTORS
- Obesity
- Age, female gender
- Pes planus; genu valgum
- Knee joint laxity/ligamentous injury
- Long-distance running, hill running; change in mileage
- Swimming ("breaststroker's knee"); cycling
- Sports with side-to-side (cutting) activity (soccer, basketball, racquet sports)

COMMONLY ASSOCIATED CONDITIONS
- Osteoarthritis (OA)
- Knee pain due to OA is often associated with pes anserine bursitis, both of which may need specific treatment.
- Higher grades of OA associated with a thicker pes anserine bursa and larger area of bursitis (1)[C]
- Valgus knee deformity
- Obesity
- Diabetes mellitus (questionable association)

 DIAGNOSIS

HISTORY
- Medial knee pain is the most common complaint.
- Pain is located 4 to 6 cm distal to the medial joint line on the anteromedial aspect of the tibia.
- Pain exacerbated by knee flexion:
  - Going up or down stairs
  - Getting out of a chair

PHYSICAL EXAM
- Common findings include:
  - Tenderness to palpation at the pes anserine insertion
    - 30% of asymptomatic patients will have tenderness to deep palpation in this area.
  - Pain worsens with flexion of the knee against resistance.
  - Localized swelling of the pes anserine insertion
- Findings that suggest an alternative diagnosis: joint effusion, tenderness directly over the joint line, erythema or warmth, locking of the knee, systemic signs such as fever or pain with passive knee movement

DIFFERENTIAL DIAGNOSIS
- Medial collateral ligament injury
- Medial meniscal injury
- Medial plica syndrome
- Medial compartment OA
- Semimembranosus bursitis
- Popliteal/meniscal cyst
- Tibial stress fracture
- Septic arthritis

DIAGNOSTIC TESTS & INTERPRETATION
Initial Tests (lab, imaging)
- Primarily a clinical diagnosis
- Lab work not indicated
- Imaging is not indicated unless there is concern for bony injury/fracture, ligamentous injury, or meniscal tear.

Follow-Up Tests & Special Considerations
- Ultrasound (US)
  - Can demonstrate focal edema within the pes anserine bursa but has poor correlation with clinical findings
  - Many patients with the clinical diagnosis of pes anserine bursitis have no morphologic changes of the pes anserine complex on US.
- MRI: can demonstrate inflammation of the bursa and delineate the pes anserine bursa from other structures. T2-weighted axial images are best on MRI.
  - No large studies have evaluated the correlation between the clinical diagnosis of pes anserine bursitis and radiographic evidence of pes anserine pathology on MRI.
  - May see fluid in the pes bursa on MRI in 5% of asymptomatic patients

TREATMENT

Pes anserine bursitis is often self-limited. Conservative therapy is most common:
- Relative rest and activity modification to avoid offending movements (especially knee flexion)
- Ice to the affected area
- Physical therapy for knee strengthening and range of motion activities (2)[C]
- NSAIDs for pain control
- Corticosteroid injection
- Weight loss to improve biomechanical forces at the knee
- Extracorporeal shock wave therapy (3)[C]

MEDICATION
First Line
NSAIDs, such as ibuprofen (800 mg PO TID) or naproxen (500 mg PO BID), are common first-line therapy.

Second Line

- Corticosteroid injection combined with local anesthetic provides relief in many patients.
  - Inject at the point of maximal tenderness using standard aseptic technique.
  - ~2 mL of anesthetic (i.e., 1% lidocaine) and 1 mL of steroid (i.e., 40 mg of methylprednisolone) is injected into the bursa using a small (e.g., 25-gauge, 1-inch) needle.
  - Insert needle perpendicular to the skin until bone is felt and then withdraw slightly before injecting.
  - Avoid injecting directly into the tendon (4)[C].
- US-guided injection is superior to blind injection (5)[C].
- Platelet-rich plasma injections also provide pain relief (6)[C].

ADDITIONAL THERAPIES

- Hamstring and Achilles stretching
- Quadriceps strengthening—particularly of the vastus medialis (terminal 30 degrees of knee extension)
- Adductor strengthening

SURGERY/OTHER PROCEDURES

- No role for surgery in routine isolated cases
- Drainage or removal of bursa may be used in severe/refractory cases.

 ONGOING CARE

Home exercise program focusing on flexibility and strengthening

DIET

Consider dietary changes as part of a comprehensive weight-loss program if obesity is a contributing factor.

PROGNOSIS

Most cases of pes anserine syndrome respond to conservative therapy. Recurrence is common, and multiple treatments may be required.

REFERENCES

1. Uysal F, Akbal A, Gökmen F, et al. Prevalence of pes anserine bursitis in symptomatic osteoarthritis patients: an ultrasonographic prospective study. *Clin Rheumatol*. 2015;34(3):529–533.
2. Sarifakioglu B, Afsar SI, Yalbuzdag SA, et al. Comparison of the efficacy of physical therapy and corticosteroid injection in the treatment of pes anserine tendino-bursitis. *J Phys Ther Sci*. 2016;28(7):1993–1997.
3. Khosrawi S, Taheri P, Ketabi M. Investigating the effect of extracorporeal shock wave therapy on reducing chronic pain in patients with pes anserine bursitis: a randomized, clinical-controlled trial. *Adv Biomed Res*. 2017;6:70.
4. Stephens MB, Beutler AI, O'Connor FG. Musculoskeletal injections: a review of the evidence. *Am Fam Physician*. 2008;78(8):971–976.
5. Finnoff JT, Nutz DJ, Henning PT, et al. Accuracy of ultrasound-guided versus unguided pes anserinus bursa injections. *PM R*. 2010;2(8):732–739.
6. Rowicki K, Płomiński J, Bachta A. Evaluation of the effectiveness of platelet rich plasma in treatment of chronic pes anserinus pain syndrome. *Ortop Traumatol Rehabil*. 2014;16(3):307–318.

ADDITIONAL READING

- Alvarez-Nemegyei J. Risk factors for pes anserinus tendinitis/bursitis syndrome: a case control study. *J Clin Rheumatol*. 2007;13(2):63–65.
- Chatra PS. Bursae around the knee joints. *Indian J Radiol Imaging*. 2012;22(1):27–30.
- Rennie WJ, Saifuddin A. Pes anserine bursitis: incidence in symptomatic knees and clinical presentation. *Skeletal Radiol*. 2005;34(7):395–398.
- Wittich CM, Ficalora RD, Mason TG, et al. Musculoskeletal injection. *Mayo Clin Proc*. 2009;84(9): 831–836; quiz 837.

 CODES

ICD10

- M70.50 Other bursitis of knee, unspecified knee
- M70.51 Other bursitis of knee, right knee
- M70.52 Other bursitis of knee, left knee

CLINICAL PEARLS

- Consider pes anserine syndrome in patients presenting with medial knee pain.
- Pes anserine syndrome is relatively common in athletes and in older, obese patients with OA.
- Tenderness over the insertion of the pes anserine tendon on the medial aspect of the tibia 4 to 6 cm distal to the joint line is common in asymptomatic patients as well—correlation of the entire clinical picture is necessary for accurate diagnosis.
- Consider pes anserine syndrome in patients who have persistent symptoms associated with medial-sided OA.
- Treatment is typically conservative. A local steroid/anesthetic injection may provide pain relief and enhance rehabilitation.

CANDIDIASIS, MUCOCUTANEOUS

Karlynn Sievers, MD • Sheila O. Stille, DMD

BASICS

DESCRIPTION
- Heterogeneous mucocutaneous disorder caused by infection with common commensal *Candida* species
- Characterized by superficial infection of the skin, mucous membranes, and nails
- >20 *Candida* species cause infection in humans. *Candida albicans is most common*, at 80% of isolates.
- Candidiasis affects:
  - Aerodigestive system
    - Oropharyngeal candidiasis (thrush): mouth, pharynx (1)
    - Angular cheilitis: corner of the mouth
    - Esophageal candidiasis
    - Gastritis and/or ulcers, associated with thrush; alimental or perianal
  - Other systems
    - Candida vulvovaginitis: vaginal mucosa and/or vulvar skin
    - Candidal balanitis: glans of the penis
    - Candidal paronychia: nail bed or nail folds
    - Folliculitis
    - Interdigital candidiasis: webs of the digits
    - Candidal diaper dermatitis and intertrigo (within skin folds)
- *Synonym(s): monilia; thrush; yeast; intertrigo*

ALERT
Vaginal antifungal creams and suppositories can weaken condoms and diaphragms.

Pregnancy Considerations
- Vaginal candidiasis is common during pregnancy.
- Extend topical treatment during pregnancy by several days (typically a full 7-day course).
- Vaginal yeast infection at birth increases the risk of newborn thrush but is of no overall harm to baby.

EPIDEMIOLOGY
- Common in the United States; particularly with immunodeficiency and/or uncontrolled diabetes
- Age considerations
  - Infants and seniors: thrush and cutaneous infections (infant diaper rash)
  - Women of childbearing age: vaginitis
  - Prepubertal or postmenopausal: yeast vaginitis
  - Predominant sex: female > male

Incidence
Unknown—mucocutaneous candidiasis is common in immunocompetent patients. Complication rates are low.

Prevalence
Candida species are normal flora of oral cavity, pharynx, esophagus, and GI tract that are present in >70% of the U.S. population.

ETIOLOGY AND PATHOPHYSIOLOGY
C. albicans (responsible for 80–92% vulvovaginal and 70–80% oral isolates). Altered cell–mediated immunity against *Candida* species (either transient or chronic) increases susceptibility to infection (2).

Genetics
Chronic mucocutaneous candidiasis is a heterogeneous, genetic syndrome with infection of skin, nails, hair, and mucous membranes; typically presents in infancy

RISK FACTORS
- Immune suppression (antineoplastic treatments, transplant patients, cellular immune defects) (2)
- Malignant diseases
- AIDS or hematologic/immune disorders (neutropenia)
- Corticosteroid use
- Smoking and alcoholism
- Hyposalivation (Sjögren disease, drug-induced xerostomia, radiotherapy) (2)
- Broad-spectrum antibiotic therapy
- Douches, chemical irritants, and concurrent vaginitides alter vaginal pH and predispose patients to candidal vaginitis.
- Denture wear, poor oral hygiene
- Birth control pills, intrauterine devices
- Endocrine alterations (DM, pregnancy, renal failure, hypothyroidism)
- Uncircumcised men at higher risk for balanitis

GENERAL PREVENTION
- Use antibiotics and steroids judiciously; rinse mouth after inhaled steroid use (1).
- Avoid douching.
- Treat other vaginal infections.
- Minimize perineal moisture (wear cotton underwear; frequent diaper changes).
- Clean dentures often; use well-fitting dentures and remove during sleep.
- Optimize glycemic control in diabetics.
- Preventive regimens during cancer treatments (2)
- Treat with HAART in HIV-infected patients.
- Antifungal prophylaxis against oral candidiasis is not recommended in HIV-infected adults unless patients have frequent or severe recurrences (2).

COMMONLY ASSOCIATED CONDITIONS
- HIV
- Leukopenia
- Diabetes mellitus
- Cancer and other immunosuppressive conditions

DIAGNOSIS

HISTORY
- Infants/children
  - Oral: adherent white patches on oral mucosae or on the tongue that do not wipe away easily
  - Perineal: erythematous rash with characteristic satellite lesions; painful if skin layer eroded. 40–75% of diaper rashes >3 days are *C. albicans* (2).
  - Angular cheilitis: painful fissures at mouth corners
- Adults
  - Vulvovaginal lesions; whitish "curd-like" discharge; pruritus; burning
  - Balanitis: erythema, erosions, scaling; dysuria
- Immunocompromised hosts
  - Oral: white, raised, painless, distinct patches; red, slightly raised patches/petechiae

- Esophagitis: dysphagia, odynophagia, retrosternal pain; usually concomitant thrush
- GI symptoms: abdominal pain
- Folliculitis: follicular pustules

PHYSICAL EXAM
- Infants/children
  - Oral: white, raised, distinct patches within the mouth; when wiped off, reveals red base
  - Perineal: erythematous maculopapular rash with satellite pustules or papules
  - Angular cheilitis: tender fissures in mouth corners, often cracked and bleeding
- Adults
  - Vulvovaginal: thick, whitish, cottage cheese–like discharge; vagina or perineum erythema
  - Balanitis: erythema, linear erosions, scaling
  - Interdigital: redness, excoriation at base and web spaces of fingers and/or toes, possible maceration
- Immunocompromised hosts
  - Oral: white, raised, nontender, distinct patches; red, slightly raised patches; thick, dark-brownish coating; deep fissures
  - Esophagitis: Often, oral thrush is visible.
  - Folliculitis: follicular pustules
  - Interdigital: redness, excoriations at base of fingers and/or toes, often maceration

DIFFERENTIAL DIAGNOSIS
- For oral candidiasis
  - Leukoplakia; lichen planus; geographic tongue
  - Herpes simplex; erythema multiforme
  - Pemphigus
- Baby formula or breast milk can mimic thrush— easier to remove than thrush (no red base when wiped away).
- Hairy leukoplakia: does not rub off; dorsum and lateral margins of tongue
- Angular cheilitis from vitamin B or iron deficiency, staphylococcal infection, or edentulous overclosure
- Bacterial vaginosis and *Trichomonas vaginalis* tend to have more odor, itch, and a different discharge.

DIAGNOSTIC TESTS & INTERPRETATION
Initial Tests (lab, imaging)
- 10% KOH slide preparation: mycelia (hyphae) or pseudomycelia (pseudohyphae) yeast forms; few WBC or 15–30% NaOH (3,4)[A]
- Associated with normal vaginal pH (<4.5)
- Barium swallow: cobblestone appearance, fistulas, or dilatation (denervation)

Diagnostic Procedures/Other
- If first-line treatment fails, obtain samples for culture.
- Sabouraud dextrose agar for fungal growth (3)[A]
- Biopsy of hyperplastic candidiasis (3)[A]
- Esophagitis may require endoscopy with biopsy (if suspicious for cancer).
- HIV-seropositive patients with thrush and dysphagia relieved by antifungal have *Candida* esophagitis.

Test Interpretation
Biopsy: epithelial parakeratosis with polymorphonuclear leukocytes in superficial layers; periodic acid–Schiff staining reveals candidal hyphae (3,4)[A].

TREATMENT

GENERAL MEASURES
Screen for immunodeficiency (diabetes, HIV, autoimmune disease).

MEDICATION

First Line
- Vaginal (choose 1)
  - Miconazole (Monistat) 2% cream: one applicator or 200 mg (one suppository), intravaginally QHS for 7 days
  - Clotrimazole (Gyne-Lotrimin, Mycelex): intravaginal suppository (100 mg QHS for 7 days; 200 mg QHS for 3 days; 500 mg daily for 1 day) or 2% cream (one applicator QHS for 3 days)
  - Fluconazole 150 mg PO single dose
- Oropharyngeal
  - Mild disease
    - Clotrimazole (Mycelex): oral 10-mg troche; 20 minutes 5 times daily for 7 to 14 days
    - Nystatin suspension: 100,000 U/mL swish and swallow 400,000 to 600,000 U 4 times per day
    - Nystatin pastilles: 200,000 U each, QID daily for 7 to 14 days (4)[A]
    - Denture wearers
      - Nystatin ointment: 100,000 U/g under denture and corners of mouth for 3 weeks
      - Remove dentures at night; clean 2 times weekly with diluted (1:20) bleach.
  - Moderate to severe disease
    - Fluconazole: 200 mg load and then 100 to 200 mg (>14 days of age: 6 mg/kg × 1 dose and then 3 mg/kg q24h × 7 to 14 days [max 100 mg/day])
- Esophagitis
  - Fluconazole: PO 400 mg load and then 200 to 400 mg/day for 14 to 21 days or IV 400 mg (6 mg/kg) daily if oral therapy not tolerated

Pregnancy Considerations
2% miconazole cream, intravaginally, for 7 days in uncomplicated candidiasis; systemic amphotericin B for invasive candidiasis in pregnancy

Second Line
- Vaginal
  - Terconazole (Terazol): 0.4% cream (one applicator QHS for 7 days of induction therapy); 0.8% cream/80-mg suppositories (one applicator or one suppository QHS for 3 days)
  - For recurrent cases (≥4 symptomatic episodes in 1 year): induction therapy with 10 to 14 days of topical or oral azole and then fluconazole 150 mg once per week for 6 months (4)[A]
    - In HIV patients: Concerns with this regimen include emergence of drug resistance (5)[A].
- Oropharyngeal
  - Miconazole oral gel (20 mg/mL): QID, swish and swallow.
  - Itraconazole (Sporanox) suspension: 200 mg (20 mL) daily; swish and swallow for 7 to 14 days.
  - Posaconazole (Noxafil) oral suspension: 400 mg BID for 3 days and then 400 mg daily for up to 28 days
  - Amphotericin B (Fungizone) oral suspension (100 mg/mL): 1 mL QID daily, swish and swallow; use between meals.
- Esophagitis
  - Amphotericin B (variable dosing) IV dose of 0.3 to 0.7 mg/kg daily or an echinocandin should be used for patients who cannot tolerate oral therapy.

- For refractory disease:
  - Itraconazole (Sporanox) oral solution: 200 mg daily
  - Posaconazole (Noxafil) oral suspension: 400 mg BID
  - Voriconazole (Vfend) 100 to 200 mg q12h PO or IV for 14 to 21 days (4)[A]
- Continue treatments for 2 days after infection gone:
  - Contraindications
    - Ketoconazole, itraconazole, or nystatin (if swallowed): severe hepatotoxicity
    - Amphotericin B: can cause nephrotoxicity
  - Precautions
    - Miconazole: can potentiate the effect of warfarin but drug of choice in pregnancy
    - Fluconazole: renal excretion: rare; hepatotoxicity: resistance frequent
    - Itraconazole: Doubling the dosage results in ~3-fold increase in itraconazole plasma concentrations.
- Possible interactions (rarely seen with creams, lotions, or suppositories)
  - Fluconazole
    - Rifampin: decreased fluconazole concentrations
    - Tolbutamide: decreased concentrations
    - Warfarin, phenytoin, cyclosporine: altered metabolism; check levels.
  - Itraconazole: potent CYP3A4 inhibitor. Carefully assess all coadministered medications.
  - Work in progress for a vaccine in patients with chronic mucocutaneous candidiasis (3)[A]

ISSUES FOR REFERRAL
- Evaluate patients, without obvious reasons, with recurrent superficial candidal infections, for immunodeficiency (5)[A].
- GI candidiasis

ADDITIONAL THERAPIES
- For infants with thrush: Boil pacifiers and bottle nipples; assess mother's breasts/nipples for Candida infection.
- For denture-related candidiasis: Disinfect dentures (using soak solution of benzoic acid, 0.12% chlorhexidine gluconate, 1:20 NaOCl or alkalize proteases) and treat orally.

COMPLEMENTARY & ALTERNATIVE MEDICINE
Probiotics: Lactobacillus and Bifidobacterium may inhibit Candida spp.

ADMISSION, INPATIENT, AND NURSING CONSIDERATIONS
Proper oral hygiene. Protocols for brushing, denture care, and oral cavity moistening reduce oral candidiasis.

ONGOING CARE

FOLLOW-UP RECOMMENDATIONS

Patient Monitoring
Immunocompromised persons benefit from regular evaluation and screening.

DIET
Active culture yogurt or other live lactobacillus may decrease colonization; indeterminate evidence

PATIENT EDUCATION
- Advise patients at risk for recurrence about potential for overgrowth with antibacterial therapy.
- "Azole" medications are pregnancy Category C.
- Polyene medications are pregnancy Category B; however, only give orally when benefits outweigh risks.

PROGNOSIS
- Benign prognosis in immunocompetent patients
- For immunosuppressed persons, Candida may become an AIDS-defining illness with significant morbidity.

COMPLICATIONS
In HIV patients, moderate immunosuppression (e.g., CD4 200 to 500 cells/mm³) may be associated with chronic candidiasis (5)[A]. With more severe immunosuppression (e.g., CD4 <100 cells/mm³), esophagitis or systemic fungal infections are possible.

REFERENCES
1. Dekhuijzen PNR, Batsiou M, Bjermer L, et al. Incidence of oral thrush in patients with COPD prescribed inhaled corticosteroids: effect of drug, dose, and device. Respir Med. 2016;120:54–63.
2. Coronado-Castellote L, Jiménez-Soriano Y. Clinical and microbiological diagnosis of oral candidiasis. J Clin Exp Dent. 2013;5(5):e279–e286.
3. Hani U, Shivakumar HG, Vaghela R, et al. Candidiasis: a fungal infection—current challenges and progress in prevention and treatment. Infect Disord Drug Targets. 2015;15(1):42–52.
4. Martins N, Ferreira IC, Barros L, et al. Candidasis: predisposing factors, prevention, diagnosis and alternative treatment. Mycopathologia. 2014;177(5–6):223–240.
5. Wang X, van der Veerdonk FL, Netea MG. Basic genetics and immunology of Candida infections. Infect Dis Clin North Am. 2016;30(1):85–102.

ADDITIONAL READING
- Glenny AM, Gibson F, Auld E, et al. The development of evidence-based guidelines on mouth care for children, teenagers and young adults treated for cancer. Eur J Cancer. 2010;46(8):1399–1412.
- Kumar S, Bansal A, Chakrabarti A, et al. Evaluation of efficacy of probiotics in prevention of Candida colonization in a PICU—a randomized controlled trial. Crit Care Med. 2013;41(2):565–572.

SEE ALSO

Candidiasis, Invasive; HIV/AIDS

CODES

ICD10
- B37.9 Candidiasis, unspecified
- B37.0 Candidal stomatitis
- B37.49 Other urogenital candidiasis

CLINICAL PEARLS
- Candidiasis is typically a clinical diagnosis. KOH preparations are a simple confirmatory office test. Culture and biopsy are rarely needed.
- Person-to-person transmission is rare.
- If tongue pain continues after treatment, consider burning mouth syndrome. Obtain a biopsy if there is concern for oral cancer.
- Oral antifungal medications are hepatically metabolized and may have serious side effects.

CARBON MONOXIDE POISONING

Henry DeYoung, MD • Natalie Slepski, MD, MPH • Robert J. Krause, MD, MPH, CIME

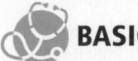 **BASICS**

DESCRIPTION
- Carbon monoxide (CO) is an odorless, tasteless, colorless gas produced during the incomplete combustion of carbon-based compounds. If inhaled, CO may cause nonspecific symptoms and is potentially fatal.
  - CO inhalation leads to displacement of oxygen from binding sites on hemoglobin to form carboxy hemoglobin (COHb).
  - The formation of COHb leads to tissue hypoxia from decreased oxygen carrying capacity and a left shift of the oxyhemoglobin dissociation curve.
  - CO binds to mitochondrial cytochrome oxidase, impairing adenosine triphosphate (ATP) production. It also binds to myoglobin, affecting muscle function.
- System(s) affected: cardiovascular, pulmonary, musculoskeletal, nervous

Pregnancy Considerations
Tissue hypoxia due to CO poisoning may cause significant fetal abnormalities because CO has a stronger affinity and a longer half-life when bound to fetal hemoglobin. The fetus is therefore susceptible to adverse outcomes even if the mother is unaffected.

EPIDEMIOLOGY
Incidence
CO poisoning is the third leading cause of poisoning death in the United States.
- Accounts for 50,000 ER visits annually (16 cases per 100,000 population); 1–3% are fatal.
- Approximately 15,000 intentional poisoning occur per year, accounting for 2/3 reported deaths (10-fold higher than unintentional poisonings).
- Vague symptoms may cause patients to not seek care, leading to underdiagnosis.

ETIOLOGY AND PATHOPHYSIOLOGY
- CO is rapidly absorbed through the lungs, binding hemoglobin with 210 to 240 times the affinity of oxygen. This stabilizes hemoglobin in the relaxed high affinity state (R state), reducing oxygen-carrying capacity and delivery, leading to left shift of the oxyhemoglobin dissociation curve.
- CO inactivates cytochrome oxidase. This leads to decreased ATP production, especially in tissues with high metabolic demands (brain, heart). The electron transport chain continues, generating superoxide radicals, leading to further damage.
- Increased peroxynitrite production contributes to impaired mitochondrial function and hypoxia.
- CO displaces NO from platelets, leading to platelet activation and aggregation. Oxidative stress, lipid peroxidation, and apoptosis are additional effects.
- Proteases released from neutrophil degranulation interact with xanthine hydrogenase forming xanthine oxidase. This inhibits endogenous defense against oxidative stress.
- Brain hypoxia leads to excitatory amino acid production and increased nitrite levels, resulting in further ischemia.
- CO also promotes the release of NO which can lead to profound hypotension.

RISK FACTORS
- Alcohol and tobacco use
- Closed or improperly ventilated spaces
- Fires and fire-related injuries
- High-risk vocations: coal miners, auto mechanics, paint stripping, work in the solvent industry
- Exposure to exhaust from motor vehicles, faulty furnaces, stoves, generator use (power outages and storms), and other fuel burning devices
- If exposed, infants, elderly patients, and patients with comorbid conditions such as cardiovascular disease, anemia, and chronic respiratory conditions have increased risk for poor outcomes.
- Increased endogenous CO production occurs in patients with hemolytic anemia.

GENERAL PREVENTION
- Appropriate ventilation around fuel-burning devices
- Installation of in-home CO monitors or alarms
- Postexposure determination of CO source to limit future exposures and/or eliminate source
- Public policy to ensure building code safety

COMMONLY ASSOCIATED CONDITIONS
- CO and cyanide poisoning often occur simultaneously after smoke inhalation and have synergistic effects.
- Intentional poisoning often occurs in the context of coingestion of other substances (~40%).
- Up to 50–75% of fire-related injuries have a component of CO poisoning.

DIAGNOSIS

- Clinical triad of (i) relevant symptoms, (ii) history of CO exposure, (iii) elevated COHb levels (1)
- An elevated carboxyhemoglobin level of >3% in a nonsmoker and >10% in smokers confirms exposure. The COHb level does not correlate with the severity of the illness or long-term prognosis but is necessary for the diagnosis (1,2,3,4).
- Older pulse oximeters do not differentiate COHb from oxyhemoglobin, with normal oximeter readings in a hypoxic patient (3). Eight-wavelength CO oximeters can detect CO exposure but cannot reliably make a definitive diagnosis of CO poisoning (1,2).

HISTORY
- The diagnosis of CO poisoning is dependent on duration and mechanism of exposure. No single symptom is sensitive or specific. A high index of suspicion is necessary.
- Common symptoms include
  - Headache (84% of patients)
  - Confusions/impaired judgment
  - Dizziness
  - Nausea/vomiting
  - Fatigue
  - Chest pain and shortness of breath
- Patients may also present with visual disturbances, seizures, syncope, arrhythmias, and loss of consciousness.
- Long-term (subacute) exposure defined as >24 hours and occurs with repeated exposure to low concentrations of CO. Symptoms include chronic fatigue, emotional distress, memory deficits, difficulty working, sleep disturbances, vertigo, neuropathy, recurrent infections, polycythemia, paresthesia, abdominal pain, and diarrhea.
- Exclude pregnancy in all female patients.

PHYSICAL EXAM
- Findings vary. Patients often report confusion or have altered mental status.
- Classically described "cherry red" skin coloring of lips and skin is rare (<1% of cases).
- Examine for signs of burns (enclosed space fires) or other secondary injuries.
- Full neurologic and mental status examinations; confusion/CNS depression, ataxia, visual field defects, papilledema, and nystagmus
- Respiratory depression or tachypnea, and cyanosis
- Tachycardia, hypotension, cardiac dysrhythmias

DIFFERENTIAL DIAGNOSIS
- Cyanide toxicity (also coexistent)
- Methylene chloride (dichloromethane) inhalation or ingestion
- Viral syndromes
- Behavioral disorders (major depressive disorder)
- Other causes of mental status changes:
  - Infections (meningitis or encephalitis)
  - Metabolic causes (hypoglycemia)
  - Alcohol intoxication, opiates, acetylsalicylic acid (ASA) overdose
  - Trauma
  - CNS lesions

DIAGNOSTIC TESTS & INTERPRETATION
Initial Tests (lab, imaging)
- Diagnosis requires a recent history of CO exposure, consistent symptoms, and demonstration of an elevated COHb level.
- Noninvasive COHb measurement should not be used to diagnose CO poisoning (2)[A].
- Arterial or venous blood gas is recommended:
  - COHb levels of >3% in nonsmokers, >10% in smokers. COHb may be low despite significant poisoning (e.g., treatment with O_2 or significant time elapses before the level is drawn).
  - Significant metabolic acidosis; anion gap >16
  - Elevated lactate confers worse prognosis.
  - PaO_2 tends to be normal because O_2 dissolved in blood is not affected by CO.
- Basic labs: serum chemistries, CBC
- ECG in all patients
  - Cardiac enzymes in patients with moderate or severe poisoning. If elevated, there is an increased risk of mortality. Important for (2)[B]:
    ○ Patients ≥65 years
    ○ Patients with cardiac risk factors or anemia
    ○ Symptoms suggestive of cardiac ischemia
- Pregnancy test in all women of childbearing age
- Toxicology screen
- CK to evaluate for rhabdomyolysis
- Head CT/MRI scan can help to rule out other neurologic causes; may also show infarction due to hypoxia/ischemia. Long-term white matter hyperintensities and hippocampal atrophy also occur.

Follow-Up Tests & Special Considerations
- Consider CO poisoning in younger patients with chest pain or symptoms suggestive of ischemia.
- Consider the diagnosis in afebrile patients with vague or "flulike" symptoms. CO poisoning and the flu are both common during the winter time.

- Patients may present as a group (coworkers, family members, school children) with similar symptoms.
- Patients with intentional poisoning should undergo behavioral evaluation when stable.
- Implement suicide precautions if appropriate.

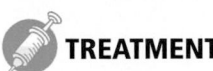

TREATMENT

GENERAL MEASURES
- Prompt removal from the CO source
- Supportive care as necessary
- Intubation and mechanical ventilation may be necessary for severe intoxication, particularly if the patient is unable to protect their airway or if there are signs of respiratory failure.
- Poison Control: 800-222-1222 (United States)

MEDICATION
100% oxygen via nonrebreathing reservoir facemask until COHb is normal (<3%) and patient is asymptomatic, regardless of oxygen saturation or PO$_2$ (1) [C],(2,4)[A]

ADDITIONAL THERAPIES
- The efficacy of hyperbaric oxygen (HBO$_2$) remains controversial; unclear whether HBO$_2$ reduces the incidence of adverse neurologic outcomes compared to normobaric oxygen (NBO$_2$) alone (2,4,5)[A]
- NBO$_2$ and HBO$_2$ reduce the elimination half-life of COHb to ~85 minutes and 20 minutes, respectively (1).
- If HBO$_2$ is unavailable, administer NBO$_2$ until CO has normalized and symptoms have resolved (2,4,5)[A].
- HBO$_2$ therapy may reduce permanent neurologic deficit by reversing inflammatory response and mitochondrial dysfunction (1)[C].
- Optimal HBO$_2$ protocols are unclear (4)[C].
- HBO$_2$ currently recommended for:
  - Age >36 years (4)[C]
  - Exposure >24 hours (4)[C]
  - Levels >25% (1,4)[C]
  - Loss of consciousness (1,4)[C]
  - Abnormal neurologic or psychiatric signs (1)[C]
  - Cardiovascular dysfunction (1)[C]
  - Severe acidosis (1,4)[C]
- Empirically treat patients for cyanide poisoning who present with CO poisoning from a house fire, if the pH is <7.20 or plasma lactate is >10 mmol/L (1,4)[C].
- HBO$_2$ not as likely to be helpful if >24 hours has elapsed since exposure
- Expert consensus favors HBO$_2$ therapy for pregnant women (4)[C].

ADMISSION, INPATIENT, AND NURSING CONSIDERATIONS
- Patients whose symptoms do not improve after 4 to 5 hours of 100% O$_2$ should be transported to the nearest HBO$_2$ facility. Hospitalize patients with severe poisoning, ECG or laboratory evidence of end-organ damage, and those with concerning medical or social factors.
- Admit unconscious patients with CO poisoning to ICU.
- Patients with accidental poisoning and mild symptoms that resolve in the ED can be safely discharged.

 ## ONGOING CARE

FOLLOW-UP RECOMMENDATIONS
- All patients treated for acute CO poisoning should follow up in 1 to 2 months after discharge (1,4).
- If there are behavioral or cognitive concerns, pursue neuropsychological evaluation, particularly following intentional CO poisoning.
- Long-term cognitive, psychiatric, speech, occupational, and physical rehab may be necessary.

Patient Monitoring
Repeat measurement of COHb levels with arterial blood gases.

PATIENT EDUCATION
- Professional installation and maintenance of combustion devices
- Consumer Product Safety Commission hotline 1-800-638-2772
- CO detector in bedrooms and by potential CO sources
- Annual furnace inspections (6)[B]
- Avoid use of combustion engines indoors; periodic furnace inspection
- www.cdc.gov/co/default.htm

PROGNOSIS
Although most patients completely recover, chronic neuropsychiatric impairment is described in 12–68% of patients.

COMPLICATIONS
- High-activity metabolic tissues are at higher risk.
- Cardiac:
  - Myocardial infarction (acute and long term)
  - Demand ischemia
  - Reduced left ventricular function
  - Dysrhythmia (prolonged QT)
- Pulmonary:
  - Inhalation injury
  - Pulmonary edema
  - Pneumonia (aspiration)
  - Acute respiratory failure
- Neurologic:
  - Anoxic encephalopathy
  - Vestibular and motor deficits
  - Hippocampal atrophy
  - Cognitive dysfunction
  - Delayed posthypoxic leukoencephalopathy
  - Diffuse brain atrophy
  - Parkinsonism
- Behavioral:
  - Depression, anxiety
  - Irritability, moodiness, and violence

Geriatric Considerations
Increased number of comorbid leading to possibility of complications and worse outcomes

REFERENCES
1. Rose JJ, Wang L, Xu Q, et al. Carbon monoxide poisoning: pathogenesis, management, and future directions of therapy. Am J Respir Crit Care Med. 2017;195(5):596–606.
2. Wolf SJ, Maloney GE, Shih RD, et al; for American College of Emergency Physicians Clinical Policies Subcommittee (Writing Committee) on Carbon Monoxide Poisoning. Clinical policy: critical issues in the evaluation and management of adult patients presenting to the emergency department with acute carbon monoxide poisoning. Ann Emerg Med. 2017;69(1):98–107e6.
3. Weaver LK. Clinical practice. Carbon monoxide poisoning. N Engl J Med. 2009;360(12):1217–1225.
4. Hampson NB, Piantadosi CA, Thom SR, et al. Practice recommendations in the diagnosis, management, and prevention of carbon monoxide poisoning. Am J Respir Crit Care Med. 2012;186(11):1095–1101.
5. Buckley NA, Juurlink DN, Isbister G, et al. Hyperbaric oxygen for carbon monoxide poisoning. Cochrane Database Syst Rev. 2011;(4):CD002041.
6. Rupert DJ, Poehlman JA, Damon SA, et al. Risk and protective behaviours for residential carbon monoxide poisoning. Inj Prev. 2013;19(2):119–123.

ADDITIONAL READING
- Centers for Disease Control and Prevention: http://www.cdc.gov/co
- Centers for Disease Control and Prevention. Carbon monoxide poisoning after a disaster. http://www.cdc.gov/disasters/carbonmonoxide.html. Accessed October 2, 2017.
- Jung JW, Lee JH. Serum lactate as a predictor of neurologic outcome in emergency department patients with acute carbon monoxide poisoning [published online ahead of print July 24, 2018]. Am J Emerg Med. doi:10.1016/j.ajem.2018.07.046.
- Sircar K, Clower J, Shin MK, et al. Carbon monoxide poisoning deaths in the United States, 1999 to 2012. Am J Emerg Med. 2015;33(9):1140–1145.

 ## CODES

ICD10
- T58.91XA Toxic effect of carb monx from unsp source, acc, init
- T58.8X1A Toxic effect of carb monx from oth source, accidental, init
- T58.01XA Toxic effect of carb monx from mtr veh exhaust, acc, init

CLINICAL PEARLS
- CO poisoning warrants a high index of suspicion, especially in patients exposed to fire; during the winter months, in young patients with chest pain; and when patients present as a group.
- Noninvasive CO oximeters are not reliable for the diagnosis of CO poisoning.
- If CO poisoning is suspected, remove individuals from the source and immediately administer 100% oxygen.
- Although not required, consider HBO$_2$ for the treatment of CO poisoning if it is available.

CARDIOMYOPATHY

Yousef Ahmed, MD • Henry DeYoung, MD • Derek Lodico, DO

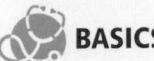 **BASICS**

DESCRIPTION

- Cardiomyopathies are myocardial diseases which result in structural and functional heart abnormalities in the absence of coronary artery disease, congenital heart disease, valvular disease, or hypertension which could sufficiently explain the clinical myocardial dysfunction (1).
- Current classification scheme attempt to differentiate between myocardial diseases confined to the myocardium (primary) and those due to systemic disorders (secondary). Specific causes of myocardial dysfunction due to other cardiovascular disorders are considered a third, separate category (1).
- Classification of cardiomyopathies
  - Primary (mainly involves the myocardium)
    ○ Genetic
      ■ Hypertrophic cardiomyopathy (HCM)
      ■ Arrhythmogenic right ventricular cardiomyopathy/dysplasia (ARVC/D)
      ■ Left ventricular (LV) noncompaction (LVNC)
      ■ Glycogen storage (Danon type, PRKAG2)
      ■ Conduction defects
      ■ Mitochondrial myopathies
      ■ Ion channel disorders: long QT syndrome (LQTS), Brugada syndrome, short QT syndrome, and catecholaminergic polymorphic ventricular tachycardia (CPVT)
    ○ Mixed (genetic and nongenetic)
      ■ Dilated cardiomyopathy (DCM)
      ■ Restrictive (nonhypertrophied and nondilated)
    ○ Acquired
      ■ Myocarditis, stress cardiomyopathy, peripartum, tachycardia induced, infants of type 1 diabetic mothers
  - Secondary (multiorgan involvement; see list below)
    ○ Specific: ischemic, valvular, hypertensive, and congenital heart disease
- Patients with end-stage cardiomyopathy have stage D heart failure or severe symptoms at rest refractory to standard medical therapy.
- Systems affected: cardiovascular, renal, hepatic, and pulmonary

Pediatric Considerations
Progressive course and early diagnosis may alter disease course. Causes: DCM, HCM, RCM, LVNC in childhood, endocrine, uremic, nutritional

Pregnancy Considerations
Peripartum cardiomyopathy (PPCM) may occur in peripartum women well before and up to months after delivery.

EPIDEMIOLOGY
Predominant age: Ischemic cardiomyopathy is the most common etiology; predominantly in patients aged >50 years. Consider uncommon causes in young. In the young, HCM is the most common cause of sudden cardiac death and important underlying cause of heart failure disability.

Incidence
DCM: 5 to 8 new cases per 100,000 population annually

Prevalence
- DCM: roughly 1:2,500; third most common cause of heart failure and most common reason for heart transplantation

- HCM: at least 1:500 of the adult population
- RCM: more commonly seen in the tropics

ETIOLOGY AND PATHOPHYSIOLOGY
- HCM: hypertrophied, nondilated left ventricle without other systemic or cardiac disease which could produce wall thickening
- ARVC/D: involves the right ventricle with progressive loss of myocytes and fatty/fibrofatty tissue replacement; can be associated with myocarditis (adenovirus or enterovirus)
- LVNC: congenital cardiomyopathies with "spongy" appearance of the LV myocardium
- LQTS: most common ion channelopathy with prolonged ventricular repolarization and QTc
- DCM: Ventricular chamber enlargement and systolic dysfunction with normal LV wall thickness result in progressive heart failure and further complications; strong genetic component with infectious and toxic etiologies
- RCM: normal/decreased ventricular volume with restrictive physiology, biatrial enlargement, and impaired ventricular filling
- Myocarditis: acute or chronic inflammation of the myocardium produced by toxins, drugs, or infectious causes
- PPCM: a form of DCM with LV systolic dysfunction and heart failure of unknown etiology
- Stress cardiomyopathies: triggered by profound psychological stress resulting in acute but rapidly reversible LV systolic dysfunction
- Endocrine: diabetes mellitus, hyperthyroidism, hypothyroidism, hyperparathyroidism, pheochromocytoma, acromegaly
- Nutritional deficiencies: beriberi, pellagra, scurvy, selenium, carnitine, kwashiorkor
- Autoimmune/collagen: systemic lupus erythematosus, dermatomyositis, rheumatoid arthritis, scleroderma, polyarteritis nodosa
- Infectious causes
  - Viral (e.g., HIV, coxsackievirus, adenovirus)
  - Bacterial and mycobacterial (e.g., diphtheria, rheumatic fever)
  - Parasitic (e.g., toxoplasmosis, *Trypanosoma cruzi*)
- Infiltrative (2): amyloidosis, Gaucher disease, Hurler disease, Hunter disease, Fabry disease
- Storage: hemochromatosis, glycogen storage disease (type II, Pompe), Niemann-Pick disease
- Neuromuscular/neurologic: Duchenne and Emery-Dreifuss muscular dystrophies, Friedreich ataxia, myotonic dystrophy, neurofibromatosis, tuberous sclerosis
- Toxic: alcohol, drugs and chemotherapy (anthracyclines, cyclophosphamide, trastuzumab [Herceptin]), radiation, heavy metal, chemical agents
- Inflammatory (granulomatous): sarcoidosis
- Idiopathic
- Endomyocardial: endomyocardial fibrosis, hypereosinophilic syndrome (Loeffler endocarditis)

Genetics
Autosomal dominant HCM is the most common form of primary genetic cardiomyopathy, which is commonly caused by many mutations that encode contractile proteins of the cardiac sarcomere. Genetic causes of DCM are less common, accounting for 1/3 cases, with mostly autosomal dominant inheritance. LVNC and ARVC are also inherited in an autosomal dominant fashion in addition to LQTS and other ion-channel disorders.

RISK FACTORS
- Hypertension
- Hyperlipidemia
- Obesity
- Coronary artery disease
- Diabetes mellitus
- Smoking
- Physical inactivity
- Excessive alcohol intake
- Dietary sodium
- Obstructive sleep apnea
- Chemotherapy

GENERAL PREVENTION
Reduce salt and water intake, and perform home blood pressure (BP) and daily weight measurements.

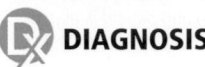 **DIAGNOSIS**

HISTORY
- Dyspnea at rest or with exertion
- Paroxysmal nocturnal dyspnea
- Orthopnea
- Postprandial dyspnea
- Right upper quadrant pain or bloating
- Fatigue
- Syncope
- Edema

PHYSICAL EXAM
- Tachypnea
- Cheyne-Stokes breathing
- Low pulse pressure
- Cool extremities
- Jugular venous distention
- Bibasilar rales
- Tachycardia
- Displaced point of maximal impulse (PMI)
- S_3 gallop
- Blowing systolic murmur
- Hepatosplenomegaly
- Ascites
- Edema

DIFFERENTIAL DIAGNOSIS
- Severe pulmonary disease
- Primary pulmonary hypertension
- Recurrent pulmonary embolism
- Constrictive pericarditis
- Some advanced forms of malignancy
- Anemia

DIAGNOSTIC TESTS & INTERPRETATION
- ECG: LV hypertrophy, interventricular conduction delay, atrial fibrillation, evidence of prior Q-wave infarction
- Hyponatremia
- Prerenal azotemia
- Anemia
- Mild elevation in troponin
- Elevated B-type natriuretic peptide (BNP) or pro-BNP
- Mild hyperbilirubinemia
- Elevated liver function tests
- Elevated uric acid

Initial Tests (lab, imaging)

- ECG
- Chest radiograph
  - Cardiomegaly
  - Increased vascular markings to the upper lobes
  - Pleural effusions may or may not be present.
- Echocardiography
  - In DCM, four-chamber enlargement and global hypokinesis are present.
  - In HCM, severe LV hypertrophy is present.
  - Segmental contraction abnormalities of the LV are indicative of previous localized myocardial infarction.
- Cardiac MRI
  - May be useful to characterize certain nonischemic cardiomyopathies
- Stress myocardial perfusion imaging (MPI)
  - Recommended in those with new-onset LV dysfunction or when ischemia is suspected

Diagnostic Procedures/Other
Cardiac catheterization

- Helpful to rule out ischemic heart disease
- Characterize hemodynamic severity
- Pulmonary artery catheters may be reasonable in patients with refractory heart failure to help guide management.

TREATMENT

See "Heart Failure, Chronic" for detailed treatment protocols.

GENERAL MEASURES
- Reduction of filling pressures
- Treatment of electrolyte disturbances

MEDICATION
First Line
- Systolic failure syndromes
  - Either an ACE inhibitor or an ARB is equally effective and should be considered in all patients; initiate at low doses and titrate as tolerated to target doses (3)[A].
  - Sacubitril/valsartan (Entresto), a combination drug containing a neprilysin inhibitor and valsartan (ARNI), was approved in 2015 for the treatment of systolic heart failure (ejection fraction [EF] <40%) as an alternative to an ACE/ARB (4)[A].
  - In patients who have been stable on an ACE or ARB, morbidity and mortality may be further reduced (all-cause mortality reduction approximately NNT 33 over 2 years treatment) by replacement with an ARNI (4)[A], with careful monitoring needed for hypotension and angioedema.
  - Loop diuretics
    ○ May need to be given IV initially and then orally as patient stabilizes
  - Furosemide, 40 to 120 mg/day or TID (3)[A]
  - β-Blockers
    ○ Use with caution in acutely decompensated or low-cardiac output states.
    ○ Initiate with low doses and titrate as tolerated.
  - Metoprolol succinate, 12.5 to 200 mg/day; carvedilol, 3.125 to 25 mg BID; or bisoprolol, 1.25 to 10 mg/day (3)[A]
  - Patients with New York Heart Association (NYHA) II to IV heart failure, EF <35%, on standard therapy: aldosterone antagonists: spironolactone or eplerenone (3)[A]

- Digoxin, 0.125 to 0.250 mg/day for symptomatic patients on standard therapy (3)[B]
- Combination hydralazine/isosorbide dinitrate is first-line treatment in African American patients with classes III and IV symptoms already on standard therapy and for all patients with reduced EF and symptoms incompletely responsive to ACE inhibitor and β-blocker (3)[A].
  ○ Contraindications
    ▪ β-Blockers: low cardiac output, 2nd- or 3rd-degree heart block
    ▪ Avoid use of diltiazem and verapamil in patients with systolic dysfunction.
    ▪ Aldosterone antagonists: oliguria, anuria, renal dysfunction
    ▪ Loop diuretics: hypokalemia, hypomagnesemia
    ▪ ACE inhibitors: pregnancy, angioedema
    ▪ ARNIs: patients currently on an ACE inhibitor or who have taken one in the past 36 hours, patients with a history of angioedema
- Precautions
  - In patients with chronic kidney disease, digoxin dosage should be ≤0.125 mg/day and drug levels followed carefully to avoid toxicity.
  - Closely monitor electrolytes.
  - ACE inhibitors and ARNIs: Initiate with care if BP is low.
  - β-Blockers: Avoid in patients with evidence of poor tissue perfusion; they may further depress systolic function.
  - Milrinone, dobutamine: long-term use associated with increased mortality
- Medications to avoid
  - NSAIDs
  - Glitazones
  - Cilostazol

Second Line
- Inotropic therapy (e.g., dobutamine or milrinone) for cardiogenic shock and support prior to surgery or cardiac transplantation (3)[B]
- Continuous inotrope infusion may be considered in stage D outpatients for symptom control in those who are not eligible for transplantation or mechanical circulatory support (3)[B].

ISSUES FOR REFERRAL
Management by a heart failure team improves outcomes and facilitates early transplant referral.

ADDITIONAL THERAPIES
- Prophylactic implantable cardioverter-defibrillator (ICD) should be considered for patients with a left ventricular ejection fraction (LVEF) <35% and mild to moderate symptoms (3)[A].
- Cardiac resynchronization therapy (CRT) is recommended and should be considered for patients in sinus rhythm with a QRS >150 ms, LVEF <35%, in functional class (FC) I to III, and ambulatory FC IV patients (3)[A].
- Patients with severe, refractory heart failure with no reasonable expectation of improvement should not be considered for an ICD. Palliative care is a reasonable option in such patients.
- Consideration of an LV assist device as "permanent" or destination therapy or cardiac transplantation is reasonable in selected stage D patients.

ONGOING CARE

DIET
Low fat, low salt, fluid restriction

PROGNOSIS
~20–40% of patients in NYHA FC IV die within 1 year. With a transplant, 1-year survival is as high as 94%.

COMPLICATIONS
Worsening congestive heart failure syncope, renal failure, arrhythmias, or sudden death

REFERENCES

1. Maron BJ, Towbin JA, Thiene G, et al. Contemporary definitions and classification of the cardiomyopathies: an American Heart Association Scientific Statement from the Council on Clinical Cardiology, Heart Failure and Transplantation Committee; Quality of Care and Outcomes Research and Functional Genomics and Translational Biology Interdisciplinary Working Groups; and Council on Epidemiology and Prevention. *Circulation*. 2006;113(14):1807–1816.
2. Seward JB, Casaclang-Verzosa G. Infiltrative cardiovascular diseases: cardiomyopathies that look alike. *J Am Coll Cardiol*. 2010;55(17):1769–1779.
3. Yancy CW, Jessup M, Bozkurt B, et al. 2017 ACC/AHA/HFSA focused update of the 2013 ACCF/AHA guideline for the management of heart failure: a report of the American College of Cardiology/American Heart Association Task Force on Clinical Practice Guidelines and the Heart Failure Society of America. *Circulation*. 2017;136(6):e137–e161.
4. McMurray JJ, Packer M, Desai AS, et al; for PARADIGM-HF Investigators and Committees. Angiotensin-neprilysin inhibition versus enalapril in heart failure. *N Engl J Med*. 2014;371(11):993–1004.

 SEE ALSO

- Alcohol Use Disorder (AUD); Alcohol Withdrawal; Amyloidosis; Diabetes Mellitus, Type 1; Diabetes Mellitus, Type 2; Hypertension, Essential; Hypertrophic Cardiomyopathy; Hypothyroidism, Adult; Protein–Energy Malnutrition; Rheumatic Fever; Sarcoidosis
- Algorithm: Congestive Heart Failure: Differential Diagnosis

CODES

ICD10
- I42.9 Cardiomyopathy, unspecified
- I42.0 Dilated cardiomyopathy
- I42.5 Other restrictive cardiomyopathy

CLINICAL PEARLS
- Cardiomyopathy represents the end-stage of a large number of disease processes involving the heart muscle.
- Ischemic, hypertensive, postviral, familial, alcoholic, and incessant tachycardia-induced are the most common cardiomyopathy varieties seen in the United States.
- Core therapy for heart failure applies salt restriction, diuretics, ACE inhibitors, β-blockers, digoxin, and electrical treatments, such as cardiac resynchronization and implantable defibrillators, as appropriate.

CAROTID SINUS HYPERSENSITIVITY

Amal Shine, MD • Anub G. John, MD • Hugh R. Peterson, MD, FACP

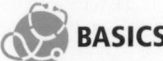 **BASICS**

DESCRIPTION

- The carotid sinus, located at the bifurcation of the internal and external carotid arteries, contains baroreceptors that are responsive to increases or decreases in arterial pressure. It plays a central role in blood pressure (BP) homeostasis.
- An endogenous increase in BP or external pressure applied to a carotid sinus causes an increase in the baroreceptor firing rate and activates vagal efferents and/or inhibits the sympathetic discharge to the heart and blood vessels, resulting in a slowing of the heart rate and/or drop in BP.
- In carotid sinus hypersensitivity (CSH), stimulation of one or both carotid sinuses causes an exaggerated baroreceptor response that can result in dizziness or syncope.
- CSH is defined as asystole for at least 3 seconds and/or a drop in systolic BP of at least 50 mm Hg during carotid sinus massage (CSM).
- CSH is generally divided into three subtypes, based on response to CSM:
  - Cardioinhibitory (70–75%): asystole for at least 3 seconds
  - Vasodepressor (5–10%): fall in systolic BP of at least 50 mm Hg
  - Mixed (20–25%): combination of the first 2 subtypes
- Carotid sinus syndrome (CSS) typically (but not consistently) refers to CSH *with syncope and may be classified as*:
  - Spontaneous CSS: syncope after accidental mechanical manipulation (trigger) of the carotid sinuses (e.g., shaving, tight collars, or tumors)
  - Induced CSS: syncope diagnosed by CSM, although no mechanical trigger is found

EPIDEMIOLOGY

- Disease of elderly; virtually unknown in people aged <50 years
- More prevalent in males by ratio of 4:1
- Typical patient is an older man, usually with a history of coronary artery disease (CAD) and hypertension (HTN), with right CSH > left CSH.
- CSH may be a cause of the symptoms in 30% of elderly patients with unexplained syncope (1).
- CSH was also present in 35% of community-dwelling older individuals without any symptoms of syncope, falls or drop attacks (2).

ETIOLOGY AND PATHOPHYSIOLOGY

- The exact mechanism of CSH remains unknown. Changes in any part of the reflex arc or the target organs may give rise to this condition, or it may be a part of a generalized autonomic disorder associated with autonomic dysregulation.
- Associated with resting sympathetic overactivity and increased baroreflex sensitivity (2)

- Bradycardia and asystole seen in cardioinhibitory and mixed CSH subtypes appear to be mediated by vagal efferents, whereas vasodilatation and arterial hypotension in the vasodepressor and mixed subtypes are attributed to decrease sympathetic tone.
- Symptomatic CSH has been shown to be associated with impaired cerebral autoregulation, and in asymptomatic CSH, it was found to be normal (2).
- Atherosclerosis may diminish carotid sinus compliance, resulting in a reduction in afferent impulse traffic in the baroreflex pathway (3).
- CSH is often idiopathic but can be caused by:
  - Carotid body tumors
  - Inflammatory and malignant lymph nodes in the neck
  - Extensive scarring from prior neck surgery in the area of the carotid sinus
  - Metastatic cancer

RISK FACTORS

- Male gender
- Advanced age
- CAD
- HTN
- DM

COMMONLY ASSOCIATED CONDITIONS

- Sick sinus syndrome
- Atrioventricular block
- CAD
- HTN
- Orthostatic hypotension
- Vasovagal syncope
- Alzheimer disease
- Parkinson disease

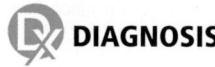 **DIAGNOSIS**

HISTORY

- Recurrent syncope: usually sudden, unexplained, of short duration, seemingly spontaneous, and with complete recovery, although fractures and other injuries may occur
- Unexplained falls: Evidence of a causal relationship is suggested between falls and the cardioinhibitory subgroup.
- Dizziness: manifests as transient light-headedness or presyncope but not usually as true vertigo; associated more with vasodepressor and mixed subtypes
- Syncope may be associated with prodrome or retrograde amnesia.
- Causative or exacerbating factors
  - Any CSM-like maneuver such as shaving, wearing tight collars, or turning one's head sharply
  - Neck tumors, extensive neck scarring secondary to radical dissection or radiation fibrosis, and neck trauma

- Certain medications can potentiate symptoms associated with CSH:
  - Digoxin or β-blockers (especially with cardioinhibitory subtype)
  - Physostigmine, morphine, methacholine: increase vagal sensitivity and may predispose to cardioinhibitory subtype of CSH

PHYSICAL EXAM

Normal unless carotid baroreceptor is stimulated and then
- Bradycardia
- Hypotension
- Pallor
- Diaphoresis

DIFFERENTIAL DIAGNOSIS

- Neurocardiogenic syncope
- Postural hypotension
- Situational syncope
- Postural tachycardia syndrome (POTS)
- Primary autonomic insufficiency
- Hypovolemia
- Dysrhythmias
- Sick sinus syndrome
- Cerebrovascular insufficiency
- Other causes of syncope (e.g., metabolic, psychogenic)
- ECG may demonstrate sinus pause(s) or atrial-ventricular block.
- Carotid duplex scan to rule out carotid stenosis in presence of a bruit (see the following section)

DIAGNOSTIC TESTS & INTERPRETATION

Diagnostic Procedures/Other

CSM is indicated in patients >40 years of age with syncope of unknown etiology after a negative initial evaluation (4)[B]. Commonly accepted technique for accurate diagnosis involves the following steps:

- Patient in supine for 5 minutes with continuous BP monitoring and ECG (on footplate-type tilt table for increased diagnostic accuracy); baseline BP and ECG are recorded.
- For 5 to 10 seconds, apply firm longitudinal massage over the right carotid sinus (between the superior border of the thyroid and the angle of the mandible) at the site of maximal pulsation:
  - Note that light pressure over the carotid sinus will not reliably produce a hypersensitivity response.
  - Record symptoms, BP, and note ECG changes.
  - Discontinue if asystole ≥3 seconds.
- Positive response defined per criteria is listed above (asystole ≥3 seconds and/or drop in BP ≥50 mm Hg), although specificity of the CSM technique increases if reproduction of a patient's syncope is demonstrated during a test (4)[B]. If nondiagnostic, apply pressure to the left carotid sinus while the patient remains supine; if still nondiagnostic, repeat in 70-degree head-up tilt (first on the right and then, if necessary, the left), allowing time for hemodynamic adjustment to the head-up position.

- Evidence behind the testing strategy
  - Right side first: Up to 66% with CSH have positive response on the right; if a positive right response, no need to repeat test on the left side
  - 30% of CSM exams are found to be nondiagnostic in the supine position but diagnostic in the 70-degree position (1).
  - Positive predictive value increases from 77% to 96% with a specificity of 93% by also performing CSM in 60- to 70-degree tilt position (5).
- Absolute contraindications for CSM testing
  - Carotid bruit present: must examine via carotid ultrasound with Doppler first:
    ○ No testing if >70% stenosis
    ○ Supine only testing if 50–70% stenosis
  - Myocardial infarction, transient ischemic attack, or stroke within the past 3 months
- Relative contraindications to CSM testing
  - History of ventricular tachycardia or ventricular fibrillation
  - False-positive results with CSM are relatively common in the elderly. Care should be taken to exclude other causes of syncope.
- Neurologic and cardiovascular complications have been reported during CSM. Cardiovascular complications (primarily arrhythmia) are extremely rare. Transient neurologic symptoms and signs occur in up to 0.9% of patients. Persistent neurologic deficits are extremely rare following CSM. Correctly performed CSM should be considered a safe, low-risk procedure (3)[C].

 TREATMENT

GENERAL MEASURES
- No treatment is required for asymptomatic individuals.
- High-dietary salt intake and increased fluid intake may be helpful to maintain intravascular volume in patients with vasodepressor subtype and absence of other cardiovascular disease.

MEDICATION
First Line
No single agent has demonstrated long-term effectiveness for treatment of recurrent and symptomatic CSH.

Second Line
- Fludrocortisone or midodrine may be used to improve orthostatic symptoms in patients with vasodepressor subtype (not approved by FDA for this indication). However, fludrocortisone causes sodium and water retention and should be used with caution in elderly patients with heart disease. An adverse effect with midodrine is that it increases mean ambulatory BP (3)[C].
- Atropine may be used in the acute setting in patients with cardioinhibitory subtype with bradycardia.
- Some evidence of benefit from sertraline and fluoxetine in patients unresponsive to pacemakers (3)[C]

SURGERY/OTHER PROCEDURES
- Permanent pacing: treatment of choice for patients with cardioinhibitory and mixed type CSH with recurrent syncope; based on 2012 ACCF/AHA/HRS Focused Update Incorporated into the ACCF/AHA/HRS 2008 Guidelines for Device-Based Therapy in CSH (6)[C]:
  - Class I indication: Permanent pacing is indicated for recurrent syncope caused by spontaneously occurring carotid sinus stimulation and carotid sinus pressure that induces ventricular asystole of >3 seconds.
  - Class IIa indication: Permanent pacing is reasonable for syncope without clear, provocative events and with a hypersensitive cardioinhibitory response of 3 seconds or longer.
  - Class IIb indication: Permanent pacing may be considered for significantly symptomatic neurocardiogenic syncope associated with bradycardia documented spontaneously or at the time of tilt-table testing.
  - Class III indication: Permanent pacing is not indicated for a hypersensitive cardioinhibitory response to carotid sinus stimulation without symptoms or with vague symptoms.
- Permanent pacing may reduce the frequency of symptoms but may not completely eliminate them.
- Surgery for patients with CSH secondary to mass effect from tumor burden
- Carotid sinus denervation by surgery or radiation therapy is no longer recommended because of the high rate of complications.

 ONGOING CARE

PATIENT EDUCATION
- Avoid precipitating maneuvers (as described above) that place pressure on the neck, such as tight collars and neckties.
- With syncope, restrict driving or other potentially hazardous activities until the patient is cleared by the physician (4).
- Avoid precipitating medications like vasodilators and those temporally related to symptoms.
- Teach patient to assume supine position if prodromal symptoms or presyncope occurs.
- Explain diagnosis, provide reassurance, and explain risk of recurrence.

PROGNOSIS
- The presence of CSH has not been demonstrated to confer an independent mortality risk.
- Untreated CSS patients have a syncope recurrence rate as high as 62% within 4 years.
- Patients with cardioinhibitory CSH who received a pacemaker had a significant reduction in their mean number of falls, from 9.3 to 4.1 falls in a 1-year follow-up period (3).

REFERENCES
1. Parry SW, Richardson DA, O'Shea D, et al. Diagnosis of carotid sinus hypersensitivity in older adults: carotid sinus massage in the upright position is essential. *Heart*. 2000;83(1):22–23.
2. Tan MP, Chadwick TJ, Kerr SR, et al. Symptomatic presentation of carotid sinus hypersensitivity is associated with impaired cerebral autoregulation. *J Am Heart Assoc*. 2014;3(3):e000514.
3. Seifer C. Carotid sinus syndrome. *Cardiol Clin*. 2013;31(1):111–121.
4. Moya A, Sutton R, Ammirati F, et al; for European Heart Rhythm Association, Heart Failure Association, Heart Rhythm Society. Guidelines for the diagnosis and management of syncope (version 2009): The task force for the diagnosis and management of syncope of the European Society of Cardiology (ESC). *Eur Heart J*. 2009;30(21):2631–2671.
5. Kapoor JR. Carotid sinus hypersensitivity: a diagnostic pearl. *J Am Coll Cardiol*. 2009;54(17):1633.
6. Epstein AE, DiMarco JP, Ellenbogen KA, et al. 2012 ACCF/AHA/HRS focused update incorporated into the ACCF/AHA/HRS 2008 guidelines for device-based therapy of cardiac rhythm abnormalities: a report of the American College of Cardiology Foundation/American Heart Association Task Force on Practice Guidelines and the Heart Rhythm Society. *J Am Coll Cardiol*. 2013;61(3):e6–e75.

ADDITIONAL READING
Moore A, Watts M, Sheehy T, et al. Treatment of vasodepressor carotid sinus syndrome with midodrine: a randomized, controlled pilot study. *J Am Geriatr Soc*. 2005;53(1):114–118.

 SEE ALSO

Syncope

 CODES

ICD10
G90.01 Carotid sinus syncope

CLINICAL PEARLS
- Consider CSH as a potential cause for syncope, dizziness, or unexplained falls, especially in the elderly.
- Diagnose CSH via CSM (using firm pressure for 5 to 10 seconds), producing asystole of at least 3 seconds and/or a drop in systolic BP of at least 50 mm Hg. (See contraindications discussed earlier before undertaking CSM as a diagnostic maneuver.)
- Remember to auscultate for carotid artery bruit prior to considering CSM.
- Consider dual-chamber pacemaker in patients with recurrent syncope and cardioinhibitory or mixed CSH subtypes.
- The finding of CSH does not exclude other causes of syncope.

CAROTID STENOSIS

Naureen Rafiq, MBBS • Austin C. Saavedra, MD

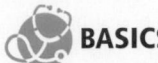

BASICS

Carotid stenosis may be caused by atherosclerosis, intimal fibroplasia, vasculitis, adventitial cysts, or vascular tumors; atherosclerosis is the most common etiology.

DESCRIPTION

- Narrowing of the carotid artery lumen is typically due to atherosclerotic changes in the vessel wall. Atherosclerotic plaques are responsible for 90% of extracranial carotid lesions and up to 30% of all ischemic strokes.
- A "hemodynamically significant" carotid stenosis produces a drop in pressure or a reduction in flow. It corresponds approximately to a 60–99% diameter-reducing stenosis.
- Carotid lesions are classified by the following:
  - Symptom status
    - Asymptomatic: tend to be homogenous and stable
    - Symptomatic: tend to be heterogeneous and unstable; present with stroke or transient cerebral ischemic attack
  - Degree of stenosis
    - High grade: 80–99% stenosis
    - Moderate grade: 50–79% stenosis
    - Low grade: <50% stenosis

EPIDEMIOLOGY

More common in men and with increasing age (see "Risk Factors")

Incidence

Unclear (Asymptomatic patients often go undiagnosed.)

Prevalence

- Moderate stenosis
  - Age <50 years: men 0.2%, women 0%
  - Age >80 years: men 7.5%, women 5%
- Severe stenosis
  - Age <50 years: men 0.1%, women 0%
  - Age >80 years: men 3.1%, women 0.9%

ETIOLOGY AND PATHOPHYSIOLOGY

- Atherosclerosis begins during adolescence, consistently at the carotid bifurcation. The carotid bulb has unique blood flow dynamics. Hemodynamic disturbances cause endothelial injury and dysfunction. Plaque formation in vessel wall results and stenosis then ensues.
- Initial cause is not well understood, but certain risk factors are frequently present (see "Risk Factors"). Tensile stress on the vessel wall, turbulence, and arterial wall shear stress seem to be involved.

Genetics

- Increased incidence among family members
- Genetically linked factors
  - Diabetes mellitus (DM), race, hypertension (HTN), family history, obesity
  - In a recent single nucleotide polymorphism study, the following genes were strongly associated with worse carotid plaque: *TNFSF4*, *PPARA*, *TLR4*, *ITGA2*, and *HABP2*.

RISK FACTORS

- Nonmodifiable factors: advanced age (>65 years old), male sex, family history, coronary artery disease (CAD), peripheral artery disease, aortic aneurysmal disease, congenital arteriopathies
- Modifiable factors: smoking, diet, dyslipidemia, physical inactivity, obesity, HTN, DM
- Possible factors: *Chlamydia pneumoniae* and *Cytomegalovirus*

GENERAL PREVENTION

- Antihypertensive treatment to maintain BP <140/90 mm Hg (Systolic BP of 150 mm Hg is target in elderly.)
- Smoking cessation to reduce the risk of atherosclerosis progression and stroke
- Lipid control: regression of carotid atherosclerotic lesions seen with statin therapy

COMMONLY ASSOCIATED CONDITIONS

- Transient ischemic attack (TIA)/stroke
- CAD/myocardial infarction (MI)
- Peripheral vascular disease (PVD)
- HTN
- DM
- Hyperlipidemia

DIAGNOSIS

Screening for carotid stenosis is not recommended. However, in the setting of symptoms suggestive of stroke or TIA, workup for this condition may be indicated.

HISTORY

- Identification of modifiable and nonmodifiable comorbidities (see "Risk Factors")
- History of cerebral ischemic event
- Stroke, TIA, amaurosis fugax (monocular blindness), aphasia
- CAD/MI
- Peripheral arterial disease
- Review of systems, with focus on risk factors for
  - Cardiovascular disease
  - Stroke (HTN and arrhythmias)

PHYSICAL EXAM

- Lateralizing neurologic deficits: contralateral motor and/or sensory deficit
- Amaurosis fugax: ipsilateral transient visual obscuration from retinal ischemia
- Visual field defect
- Dysarthria, aphasia (in the case of dominant hemisphere involvement, usually left)
- Carotid bruit (low sensitivity and specificity)

DIFFERENTIAL DIAGNOSIS

- Aortic valve stenosis
- Aortic arch atherosclerosis
- Arrhythmia with cardiogenic embolization
- Migraine
- Brain tumor
- Metabolic disturbances
- Functional/psychological deficit
- Seizure

DIAGNOSTIC TESTS & INTERPRETATION

Initial Tests (lab, imaging)

Workup for suspected TIA/stroke may include the following:

- CBC with differential
- Basic metabolic panel
- ESR (if temporal arteritis a consideration)
- Glucose/hemoglobin A1c
- Fasting lipid profile
- Duplex ultrasonography is the recommended initial diagnostic test in asymptomatic patients with known or suspected carotid stenosis.
- Duplex ultrasound (US) identifies ≥50% stenosis, with 98% sensitivity and 88% specificity.

Follow-Up Tests & Special Considerations

- Proceed to imaging if there is suggestion of stenosis from history or physical exam.
- Other noninvasive imaging techniques can add detail to duplex results:
  - CT angiography
    - 88% sensitivity and 100% specificity
    - Requires IV contrast with risk for subsequent renal morbidity
  - MR angiography
    - 95% sensitivity and 90% specificity
    - Evaluates cerebral circulation (extracranial and intracranial) as well as aortic arch and common carotid artery
    - The presence of unstable plaque can be determined if the following characteristics are seen:
      - Presence of thin/ruptured fibrous cap
      - Presence of lipid-rich necrotic core
      - Tends to overestimate degree of stenosis

Diagnostic Procedures/Other

Cerebral angiography is the traditional gold standard for diagnosis:

- Delineates the anatomy pertaining to aortic arch and proximal vessels
- The procedure is invasive and has multiple risks:
  - Contrast-induced renal dysfunction (1–5% complication rate)
  - Thromboembolic-related complications (1–2.6% complication rate) and neurologic complications
  - Should be used only when other tests are not conclusive

Test Interpretation

- Stenosis consistently occurs at the carotid bifurcation, with plaque formation most often at the level of the proximal internal carotid artery:
  - Plaque is thickest at the carotid bifurcation.
  - Plaque occupies the intima and inner media and avoids outer media and adventitia.
- Plaque histology
  - Homogenous (stable) plaques seldom hemorrhage or ulcerate:
    - Fatty streak and fibrous tissue deposition
    - Diffuse intimal thickening
  - Heterogenous (unstable) plaques may hemorrhage or ulcerate:
    - Presence of lipid-laden macrophages, necrotic debris, cholesterol crystals
    - Ulcerated plaques
  - Soft and gelatinous clots with platelets, fibrin, and red and white blood cells

TREATMENT

Smoking cessation, BP control, blood glucose control, antiplatelet medication, and statin medication are the primary treatments for both asymptomatic and symptomatic carotid stenosis.

GENERAL MEASURES

- Lifestyle modifications: dietary control and weight loss, exercise of 30 min/day at least 5 days/week
- Patients should be advised to quit smoking and offered smoking cessation intervention to reduce the risk of atherosclerotic progression and stroke.
- Control of HTN with antihypertensive agents to maintain BP <140/90 mm Hg; <150/90 mm Hg in the elderly. In carefully selected individuals, tighter blood pressure control might reduce cerebrovascular events, but this remains uncertain.

MEDICATION

- Antihypertensive treatment (<140/90 mm Hg), <150/90 mm Hg in the elderly
- Diet, smoking cessation, and exercise are useful adjuncts to therapy.
- Statin initiation is recommended; choose moderate- to high-intensity statin therapy for anti-inflammatory benefit.
- A comprehensive program that includes tight control of HTN with ACEI or ARB treatment reduces the risk in individuals with diabetes. Stroke prevention benefit of intensive glucose lowering therapy has not been established (1)[A].
- Aspirin: 75 to 325 mg/day
- If patient has sustained TIA or ischemic stroke, antiplatelet therapy with
  - Aspirin alone (75 to 325 mg/day) or
  - Clopidogrel alone (75 mg/day), or
  - Aspirin plus extended-release dipyridamole (25 and 200 mg BID, respectively)
  - A combination of clopidogrel plus aspirin is NOT recommended within 3 months post-TIA or CVA.

ISSUES FOR REFERRAL

- For acute symptomatic stroke, order imaging and contact neurology.
- For known carotid stenosis, some suggest duplex imaging every 6 months if stenosis is >50% and patient is a surgical candidate.

SURGERY/OTHER PROCEDURES

- Symptomatic carotid stenosis (history of ischemia ipsilateral to stenosis)
  - Carotid endarterectomy (CEA) is of some benefit in 50–69% symptomatic stenosis, highly beneficial for those with 70–99% stenosis without near occlusion and has no benefit in people with carotid near-occlusion (2)[A].
  - CEA is recommended for patients with a life expectancy of at least 5 years. The anticipated rate of perioperative stroke or mortality must be <6% (3)[B].
  - Treatment with aspirin (81 to 325 mg/day) is recommended for all patients who are having CEA. Aspirin should be started prior to surgery and continued for at least 3 months postsurgery but may be continued indefinitely (3)[B].
  - Carotid artery stenting (CAS) provides similar long-term outcomes as CEA (4)[A]. Age should be considered when planning a carotid intervention.
    - CAS has an increased risk of adverse cerebrovascular events in the elderly compared to the young but similar mortality risk. CEA is associated with similar neurologic outcomes in the elderly and young, at the expense of increased mortality (5)[A].
    - CAS is suggested in selected patients with neck anatomy unfavorable for arterial surgery and those with comorbid conditions that greatly increase the risk of anesthesia and surgery.
    - Dual antiplatelet therapy with aspirin (81 to 325 mg/day) plus clopidogrel (75 mg/day) is recommended for 30 days post-CAS.
- Asymptomatic patients
  - As compared with CAS, CEA is the preferred option for the management of asymptomatic carotid stenosis if a surgical option is chosen. CAS has the potential for increased risks of periprocedural stroke and periprocedural death (6)[A].
  - The advantage of surgical compared with medical therapy has decreased with contemporary medical management. It is not possible to make an evidence-based recommendation for or against surgical therapy with current literature (1)[A].

ADMISSION, INPATIENT, AND NURSING CONSIDERATIONS

- Any patient with presentation of acute symptomatic carotid stenosis should be hospitalized for further diagnostic workup and appropriate therapy.
- Rapid evaluation for symptoms compatible with TIA should be obtained in the emergency department (ED) or inpatient setting.
- Discharge criteria: 24 to 48 hours post-CEA, if ambulating, taking adequate PO intake, and neurologically intact

 ONGOING CARE

FOLLOW-UP RECOMMENDATIONS

Patient Monitoring

- Duplex at 2 to 6 weeks postoperatively
- Duplex every 6 to 12 months
- Reoperative CEA or CAS is reasonable, if there is rapidly progressive restenosis.
- Patients with any of the following: renal failure, heart failure, diabetes, and age >80 years have a high readmission rate following CEA; thus, intensive medical therapy and rigorous follow-up is recommended.

DIET

Heart-healthy diet low in saturated fat, no transfat

PATIENT EDUCATION

For patient education materials on this topic, consult the following:

- American Heart Association: http://www.heart.org
- Mayo Clinic Information: http://www.mayoclinic.org/diseases-conditions/carotid-artery-disease/basics/definition/con-20030206

COMPLICATIONS

- Untreated: TIA/stroke (risk of ipsilateral stroke approximately 1.68% per year)
- Postoperative (status post CEA)
  - Perioperative (within 30 days)
    - Stroke/death, cranial nerve injury, hemorrhage, hemodynamic instability, MI
  - Late (>30 days postop)
    - Recurrent stenosis, false aneurysm at surgical site

REFERENCES

1. Meschia JF, Bushnell C, Boden-Albala B, et al; and American Heart Association Stroke Council, Council on Cardiovascular and Stroke Nursing, Council on Clinical Cardiology, Council on Functional Genomics and Translational Biology, Council on Hypertension. Guidelines for the primary prevention of stroke: a statement for healthcare professionals from the American Heart Association/American Stroke Association. *Stroke*. 2014;45(12):3754–3832.
2. Orrapin S, Rerkasem K. Carotid endarterectomy for symptomatic carotid stenosis. *Cochrane Database Syst Rev*. 2017;(6):CD001081.
3. Chaturvedi S, Bruno A, Feasby T, et al. Carotid endarterectomy—an evidence-based review: report of the Therapeutics and Technology Assessment Subcommittee of the American Academy of Neurology. *Neurology*. 2005;65(6):794–801.
4. Bonati LH, Lyrer P, Ederle J, et al. Percutaneous transluminal balloon angioplasty and stenting for carotid artery stenosis. *Cochrane Database Syst Rev*. 2012;(9):CD000515.
5. Antoniou GA, Georgiadis GS, Georgakarakos EI, et al. Meta-analysis and meta-regression analysis of outcomes of carotid endarterectomy and stenting in the elderly. *JAMA Surg*. 2013;148(12):1140–1152.
6. Moresoli P, Habib B, Reynier P, et al. Carotid stenting versus endarterectomy for asymptomatic carotid artery stenosis: a systematic review and meta-analysis. *Stroke*. 2017;48(8):2150–2157.

ADDITIONAL READING

- Go C, Avgerinos ED, Chaer RA, et al. Long-term clinical outcomes and cardiovascular events after carotid endarterectomy. *Ann Vasc Surg*. 2015;29(6):1265–1271.
- Jonas DE, Feltner C, Amick HR, et al. Screening for asymptomatic carotid artery stenosis: a systematic review and meta-analysis for the U.S. Preventive Services Task Force. *Ann Intern Med*. 2014;161(5):336–346.
- Paraskevas KI, Mikhailidis DP, Veith FJ. Comparison of the five 2011 guidelines for the treatment of carotid stenosis. *J Vasc Surg*. 2012;55(5):1504–1508.
- Rundek T, Sacco R. Risk factor management to prevent first stroke. *Neurol Clin*. 2008;26(4):1007–1045.

 SEE ALSO

Algorithms: Stroke; Transient Ischemic Attack and Transient Neurologic Defects

 CODES

ICD10

- I65.29 Occlusion and stenosis of unspecified carotid artery
- I65.21 Occlusion and stenosis of right carotid artery
- I65.22 Occlusion and stenosis of left carotid artery

CLINICAL PEARLS

- Atherosclerosis is responsible for 90% of all cases of carotid artery stenosis.
- Duplex US is the best initial imaging modality.
- Antiplatelet therapy and aggressive treatment of vascular risk factors are the mainstays of medical therapy.
- Compared with CEA, CAS increases the risk of any stroke and decreases the risk of MI. For every 1,000 patients opting for stenting rather than endarterectomy, 19 more patients would have strokes and 10 fewer would have MIs.

CARPAL TUNNEL SYNDROME

Frances A. Tepolt, MD • Rahul Kapur, MD, CAQSM

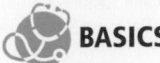 **BASICS**

DESCRIPTION
- Symptomatic compression neuropathy of the median nerve
- Increased pressure within the carpal tunnel leads to compression of the median nerve and characteristic motor-sensory findings.
- The dorsal aspect of the carpal tunnel is composed of the carpal bones. The transverse carpal ligament defines the palmar boundary:
  - The carpal tunnel contains nine flexor tendons and the median nerve.
- Symptoms most commonly affect the dominant hand; >50% of patients will experience bilateral symptoms.
- System(s) affected: musculoskeletal, nervous

ALERT
Increased incidence during pregnancy (up to 20–45%)

EPIDEMIOLOGY
- Predominant age: 40 to 60 years
- Predominant sex: female > male (3:1 to 10:1)

Incidence
- Two peaks: late 50s (women), late 70s (both genders)
- Incidence up to 276/100,000 has been reported.
- Incidence increases with age.

Prevalence
- 9% in women and 6% in men; 50 cases per 1,000 individuals per year in United States
- 14% in diabetics without neuropathy and 30% in patients with diabetic neuropathy
- Rising prevalence may be the result of increasing lifespan and increasing prevalence of diabetes.
- Most expensive upper extremity musculoskeletal disorder; >$2 billion per year
- Median time lost by U.S. workers with carpal tunnel syndrome (CTS) = 28 days

ETIOLOGY AND PATHOPHYSIOLOGY
- Combination of mechanical trauma, inflammation, increased pressure, and ischemic injury to the median nerve within the carpal tunnel
- Acute CTS caused by rapid and sustained pressure in carpal tunnel, usually secondary to trauma, may require urgent surgical decompression.
- Distal radius fractures and volar lunate dislocations increase risk.
- Chronic CTS divided into four categories:
  - Idiopathic: combination of edema and fibrous hypertrophy without inflammation
  - Anatomic: persistent median artery, ganglion cyst, infection, space-occupying lesion in carpal tunnel
  - Systemic: associated with conditions such as obesity, diabetes, hypothyroidism, rheumatoid arthritis, amyloidosis, scleroderma, renal failure, and drug toxicity
  - Exertional: repetitive use of hands and wrists, repeated palmar impact, use of vibratory tools. Repetitive use is an objective cause of CTS.

Genetics
Unknown; however, a familial type has been reported.

RISK FACTORS
- Prolonged postures in extremes of wrist flexion and extension including activities such as gardening, cycling, or tennis; repetitive exposure to vibration
- Typing is NOT a risk factor.
- Alterations of fluid balance: pregnancy, rheumatoid arthritis, obesity, renal failure, hypothyroidism, congestive heart failure
- CTS is the most common neuropathy in patients with rheumatoid arthritis.
- Neuropathic factors: diabetes, alcoholism, vitamin deficiency, or exposure to toxins

GENERAL PREVENTION
There is no known prevention for CTS. It is recommended to take occasional (e.g., hourly) breaks when doing repetitive work involving hands or if prolonged occupational exposure to vibratory tools.

COMMONLY ASSOCIATED CONDITIONS
- Diabetes, obesity; pregnancy; hypothyroidism
- Osteoarthritis of small joints of hand and wrist
- Hyperparathyroidism, hypocalcemia

 DIAGNOSIS

HISTORY
- Nocturnal pain, numbness, and tingling of the thumb, index, long, and radial portion of the ring fingers; patients may not localize and alternatively describe the entire hand as being affected.
- Hand weakness during tasks as opening jars is often noted early in the disorder.
- Atypical presentation involves paresthesias in radial digits, with pain radiating proximally along median nerve to elbow and sometimes the shoulder.
- Symptoms characteristically are relieved by shaking or rubbing the hands.
- During waking hours, symptoms occur when driving, talking on the phone, and occasionally when using the hands for repetitive maneuvers.
- Presence of predisposing factors, such as diabetes, obesity, acromegaly, pregnancy, or occupational exposure

PHYSICAL EXAM
- Durkan compression test: Direct compression of median nerve at carpal tunnel for 30 seconds elicits symptoms (87% sensitivity; 90% specificity).
- Positive Phalen sign: Holding the wrist in fully flexed position for 60 seconds precipitates paresthesias (68% sensitivity; 73% specificity).
- Positive Tinel sign: Tapping over the palmar surface of the wrist proximal to the carpal tunnel may produce an electric sensation along the distribution of the median nerve (50% sensitivity; 77% specificity).
- Loss of two-point discrimination
- Wasting of thenar musculature is a late sign, poorly associated with ruling out CTS.

DIFFERENTIAL DIAGNOSIS
- Cervical spondylosis (carpal tunnel may also occur with cervical spine disease; "double crush")
- Generalized peripheral neuropathy
- Brachial plexopathy, in particular upper trunk
- CNS disorders (multiple sclerosis, cerebral infarction)
- Thoracic outlet syndrome
- Pronator syndrome
- Anterior interosseous syndrome
- Musculoskeletal disorders of the wrist:
  - Trauma or distal radius fracture
  - Degenerative joint disease
  - Rheumatoid arthritis
  - Ganglion cyst
- Scleroderma

DIAGNOSTIC TESTS & INTERPRETATION
- No laboratory test is diagnostic.
  - Normal serum thyrotropin (thyroid-stimulating hormone [TSH]) and normal serum chemistries help exclude secondary conditions associated with CTS.
- Special tests
  - Electrodiagnostic studies
    ○ Sensitivity 85%; specificity 95%
    ○ Most useful with low pretest probability and suspicion of alternate peripheral neuropathy, radiculopathy, or "double-crush" phenomenon with compression at multiple locations
    ○ Nerve conduction studies compare latency and amplitude of median nerve signals across the carpal tunnel.
    ○ The most sensitive indicator is median sensory distal latency, which is prolonged in CTS.
- Standard radiographs of the wrist evaluate bony anatomy and degenerative joint disease but are not necessary to diagnose CTS.
- Ultrasound—rapid, noninvasive, painless modality; sensitivity 82%; specificity 92%; hypoechoic median nerve cross-sectional area >10 mm
- Magnetic resonance imaging is of limited benefit.

 TREATMENT

GENERAL MEASURES
- Splinting the wrist in a neutral position while sleeping may provide significant symptom relief and may lead to the avoidance of surgery, particularly in mildly symptomatic patients:
  - Limited evidence indicates that night splints are more effective than no treatment in the short term; insufficient evidence to recommend a specific splint design or wearing schedule (1)[A]
  - American Academy of Orthopaedic Surgeons (AAOS) guidelines indicate immobilization (brace/splint/orthosis) improves outcomes in patients treated nonoperatively.
- Strong evidence supports the splinting, and corticosteroid injection are effective versus placebo injection in the short term, although long-term benefits have not been shown (2)[A].
- Manual therapy was shown to have similar efficacy to surgery for improving self-reported function, symptom severity, and grip force at 3, 6, and 12 months (3)[B].

MEDICATION

First Line

NSAIDs, such as ibuprofen or naproxen sodium, are commonly used. There is insufficient evidence to determine their routine efficacy:

- Contraindications: GI intolerance
- Precautions: GI side effects of NSAIDs may preclude their use in selected patients.

Second Line

- Local steroid injection: Methylprednisolone injections are more effective than systemic steroids or placebo at 1 and 3 months and more effective than splinting at 6 months.
- Response to injections helps confirm diagnosis of CTS and predicts a better response to surgery.
- Injection using landmarks with only 75% accuracy in one recent study (4)[B]
- Side effects include reduction of collagen and proteoglycan synthesis, limiting tenocytes, and reducing mechanical strength of tendon, leading to further degeneration and risk for rupture.
- Oral steroids may provide a short-term improvement (2 to 8 weeks) in symptoms.
- The long-term risks of even a short course of steroids should be balanced with the limited potential benefit of symptom improvement.

ISSUES FOR REFERRAL

Preoperative electrodiagnostic studies are generally obtained prior to any surgical intervention.

SURGERY/OTHER PROCEDURES

- Completely dividing the transverse carpal ligament provides symptom relief in >95% of patients.
- Surgical decompression is an outpatient procedure performed under local or regional anesthesia.
- Incisional healing generally takes 2 weeks; an additional 2 weeks may be required before using the affected hand for tasks requiring strength.
- Complete resolution of numbness in 93.8% of patients with severe CTS by EMG at follow-up of 9.3 years (5)[B]
- Recent randomized, controlled studies indicate that surgery leads to better functional improvements at 1 year compared with nonoperative management.
- Open versus endoscopic surgical procedures produce similar outcomes at 6 months. The approach should be based on surgeon and patient preference.
- Risk of transient nerve injuries is higher with endoscopic release (6)[A].

COMPLEMENTARY & ALTERNATIVE MEDICINE

No trial data support the use of vitamin B_6 in the prevention or treatment of CTS.

ADMISSION, INPATIENT, AND NURSING CONSIDERATIONS

Outpatient

 ONGOING CARE

FOLLOW-UP RECOMMENDATIONS

Patient Monitoring

- Patients treated nonoperatively (splinting, injections) require follow-up over 4 to 12 weeks to ensure adequate progress.
- There is only limited, low-quality evidence to suggest that rehabilitation exercises such as wrist immobilization, ice therapy, and multimodal hand rehabilitation are beneficial.
- 7–20% of patients treated surgically may experience recurrence.

PATIENT EDUCATION

American Society for Surgery of the Hand: http://www.assh.org/Public/HandConditions/Pages/CarpalTunnelSyndrome.aspx

PROGNOSIS

- Patients with severe CTS may not recover completely after surgical release. Paresthesias and weakness may persist, but night symptoms generally resolve.
- If untreated, more severe cases of CTS can lead to numbness and weakness in the hand, atrophy of the thenar muscles, and permanent loss of median nerve function.

COMPLICATIONS

- Postoperative infection (rare)
- Injury to the median nerve or its recurrent (motor) branch

REFERENCES

1. Page MJ, Massy-Westropp N, O'Connor D, et al. Splinting for carpal tunnel syndrome. *Cochrane Database Syst Rev*. 2012;(7):CD010003.
2. Huisstede BM, Randsdorp MS, van den Brink J, et al. Effectiveness of oral pain medication and corticosteroid injections for carpal tunnel syndrome: a systematic review. *Arch Phys Med Rehabil*. 2018;99(8):1609–1622.e10.
3. Fernández-de-Las-Peñas C, Cleland J, Palacios-Ceña M, et al. The effectiveness of manual therapy versus surgery on self-reported function, cervical range of motion, and pinch grip force in carpal tunnel syndrome: a randomized clinical trial. *J Orthop Sports Phys Ther*. 2017;47(3):151–161.
4. Green DP, MacKay BJ, Seiler SJ, et al. Accuracy of carpal tunnel injection: a prospective evaluation of 756 patients [published online ahead of print July 1, 2018]. *Hand (N Y)*. doi:10.1177/1558944718787330.
5. Tang CQY, Lai SWH, Tay SC. Long-term outcome of carpal tunnel release surgery in patients with severe carpal tunnel syndrome. *Bone Joint J*. 2017;99-B(10):1348–1353.
6. Sayegh ET, Strauch RJ. Open versus endoscopic carpal tunnel release: a meta-analysis of randomized controlled trials. *Clin Orthop Relat Res*. 2015;473(3):1120–1132.

ADDITIONAL READING

- Calandruccio JH, Thompson NB. Carpal tunnel syndrome: making evidence-based treatment decisions. *Orthop Clin North Am*. 2018;49(2):223–229.
- Graham B, Peljovich AE, Afra R, et al. The American Academy of Orthopaedic Surgeons evidence-based clinical practice guideline on: management of carpal tunnel syndrome. *J Bone Joint Surg Am*. 2016;98(20):1750–1754.
- Hermiz SJ, Kalliainen LK. Evidence-based medicine: current evidence in the diagnosis and management of carpal tunnel syndrome. *Plast Reconstr Surg*. 2017;140(1):120e–129e.
- Middleton SD, Anakwe RE. Carpal tunnel syndrome. *BMJ*. 2014;349:g6437.
- Paryavi E, Zimmerman RM, Means KR Jr. Endoscopic compared with open operative treatment of carpal tunnel syndrome. *JBJS Rev*. 2016;4(6). doi:10.2106/JBJS.RVW.15.00071.
- Vasiliadis HS, Georgoulas P, Shrier I, et al. Endoscopic release for carpal tunnel syndrome. *Cochrane Database Syst Rev*. 2014;(1):CD008265.

 SEE ALSO

- Arthritis, Rheumatoid (RA); Hypoparathyroidism; Lupus Erythematosus, Systemic (SLE); Scleroderma
- Algorithms: Carpal Tunnel Syndrome; Pain in Upper Extremity

 CODES

ICD10

- G56.00 Carpal tunnel syndrome, unspecified upper limb
- G56.01 Carpal tunnel syndrome, right upper limb
- G56.02 Carpal tunnel syndrome, left upper limb

CLINICAL PEARLS

- Paresthesias associated with CTS are characteristically confined to the thumb, index, long, and radial 1/2 of the ring fingers of the affected hand.
- Thenar atrophy is a late finding, indicating severe nerve damage.
- The Durkan (carpal compression) test is superior to Tinel sign (tapping on median nerve over carpal tunnel) and Phalen maneuver (holding wrists in flexion) for the clinical diagnosis of CTS.
- Ultrasound is sensitive and specific for diagnosis.
- Steroid injections offer short-term relief, but clinical outcomes at 1 year are no different than placebo.
- Surgical release of the carpal tunnel is >90% effective long-term.

CATARACT
Yasir Ahmed, MD • Ingrid U. Scott, MD, MPH

 BASICS

DESCRIPTION
- A cataract is any opacity or discoloration of the lens, localized or generalized; the term is usually reserved for changes that affect visual acuity (1,2).
- Etymology: from Latin *cataractes*, for "waterfall"; named after foamy appearance of opacity
- Leading cause of blindness worldwide, estimated 20 million people (1,2)
- Types include the following:
  - Age related: 90% of total
  - Metabolic (diabetes via accelerated sorbitol pathway, hypocalcemia, Wilson disease)
  - Congenital (1/250 newborns; 10–38% of childhood blindness)
  - Systemic disease associated (myotonic dystrophy, atopic dermatitis [AD])
  - Secondary to associated eye disease, so-called complicated (e.g., uveitis associated with juvenile rheumatoid arthritis or sarcoid, tumor such as melanoma or retinoblastoma)
  - Traumatic (e.g., heat, electric shock, radiation, concussion, perforating eye injuries, intraocular foreign body)
  - Toxic/nutritional (e.g., corticosteroids)
- Morphologic classification:
  - Nuclear: exaggeration of normal aging changes of *central* lens nucleus, often associated with myopia due to increased refractive index of lens (Some elderly patients consequently may be able to read again *without spectacles*, so-called second sight of the aged.)
  - Cortical: outer portion of lens; may involve anterior, posterior, or equatorial cortex; radial, spoke-like opacities
  - Subcapsular: Posterior subcapsular cataract has more profound effect on vision than nuclear or cortical cataract; patients particularly troubled under conditions of miosis; near vision frequently impaired more than distance vision
- System(s) affected: nervous

Geriatric Considerations
Some degree of cataract formation is expected in all people >70 years of age.

Pediatric Considerations
See Congenital cataract; may present as leukocoria

Pregnancy Considerations
See Congenital cataract (i.e., medications, metabolic dysfunction, intrauterine infection, and malnutrition).

EPIDEMIOLOGY
Incidence
- ~48% of the 37 million cases of blindness worldwide result from cataracts (1,2).
- Leading cause of treatable blindness and vision loss in developing countries (1,2)
- Predominant age: depends on type of cataract
- Predominant sex: male > female

Prevalence
- Cataract type and prevalence are highly variable based on population demographic.
- An estimated 50% of people 65 to 74 years of age and 70% of people >75 years of age have age-related cataract.

ETIOLOGY AND PATHOPHYSIOLOGY
- Age-related cataract:
  - Continual addition of layers of lens fibers throughout life creates hard, dehydrated lens nucleus that impairs vision (nuclear cataract).
  - Aging alters biochemical and osmotic balance required for lens clarity; outer lens layers hydrate and become opaque, adversely affecting vision.
- Congenital:
  - Usually unknown etiology
  - Drugs (corticosteroids in 1st trimester, sulfonamides)
  - Metabolic (diabetes in mother, galactosemia in fetus)
  - Intrauterine infection during 1st trimester (e.g., rubella, herpes, mumps)
  - Maternal malnutrition
- Other cataract types:
  - Common feature is a biochemical/osmotic imbalance that disrupts lens clarity.
  - Local changes in lens protein distribution lead to light scattering (lens opacity).

Genetics
- Congenital (e.g., chromosomal disorders [Down syndrome])
- Genetics of age-related cataract are not yet established but likely multifactorial contribution.

RISK FACTORS
- Aging
- Cigarette smoking
- Ultraviolet (UV) sunlight exposure
- Diabetes
- Prolonged high-dose steroids
- Positive family history
- Alcohol

GENERAL PREVENTION
- Use of UV protective glasses
- Avoidance of tobacco products
- Effective control of diabetes
- Care with high-dose, long-term steroid use (systemic therapy > inhaled treatment)
- Protective methods using pharmaceutical intervention (e.g., antioxidants, acetylsalicylic acid [ASA], hormone replacement therapy [HRT]) show no proven benefit to date.

COMMONLY ASSOCIATED CONDITIONS
- Diabetes (especially with poor glucose control)
- Myotonic dystrophy (90% of patients develop visually innocuous change in 3rd decade; becomes disabling in 5th decade)
- AD (10% of patients with severe AD develop cataracts in 2nd to 4th decades; often bilateral)
- Neurofibromatosis type 2

- Associated ocular disease or "secondary cataract" (e.g., chronic anterior uveitis, acute [or repetitive] angle-closure glaucoma or high myopia)
- Drug induced (e.g., steroids, chlorpromazine)
- Trauma

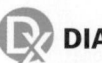 **DIAGNOSIS**

HISTORY
- Age-related cataract:
  - Decreased visual acuity, blurred vision, distortion, or "ghosting" of images (1,2)
  - Problems with visual acuity in any lighting condition
  - Falls or accidents; injuries (e.g., hip fracture)
- Congenital: often asymptomatic; leukocoria; parents notice child's visual inattention or strabismus.
- Other types of cataract:
  - May also present with decreased visual acuity
  - Appropriate clinical history or signs to help with diagnosis

PHYSICAL EXAM
- Visual acuity assessment for all cataracts
- Age-related cataract: lens opacity on eye examination
- Congenital:
  - Lens opacity present at birth or within 3 months of birth
  - Leukocoria (white pupil), strabismus, nystagmus, signs of associated syndrome (as with Down or rubella syndrome)
  - *Note*: must always rule out ocular tumor; early diagnosis and treatment of retinoblastoma may be lifesaving.
- Other types of cataract: may present with decreased visual acuity associated with characteristic physical findings (e.g., metabolic, trauma)

DIFFERENTIAL DIAGNOSIS
- An opaque-appearing eye may be due to opacities of the cornea (e.g., scarring, edema, calcification), lens opacities, tumor, or retinal detachment. Biomicroscopic examination (slit lamp) or careful ophthalmoscopic exam should provide diagnosis.
- In the elderly, visual impairment is often due to multiple factors such as cataract and macular degeneration, both contributing to visual loss.
- Age-related cataract is significant if symptoms and ophthalmic exam support cataract as a major cause of vision impairment.
- Congenital lens opacity in the absence of other ocular pathology may cause severe amblyopia.
- *Note*: Cataract *does not* produce a relative afferent pupillary reaction defect. Abnormal pupillary reactions mandate further evaluation for other pathology.

DIAGNOSTIC TESTS & INTERPRETATION
- Visual quality assessment: Glare testing, contrast sensitivity is sometimes indicated.
- Retinal/macular function assessment: potential acuity meter testing
- Workup of underlying process

Test Interpretation
Consistent with lens changes found in the type of cataract; however, diagnosis is made by clinical examination.

TREATMENT
- Outpatient (usually)
- ~1.64 million cataract extractions in the United States yearly (3,4)

GENERAL MEASURES
Eye protection from UV light

MEDICATION
There are currently no medications to prevent or slow the progression of cataracts.

ISSUES FOR REFERRAL
If patient has cataract and symptoms do not seem to support recommended surgery, a second opinion by another ophthalmologist may be indicated.

SURGERY/OTHER PROCEDURES
- Age-related cataract:
  - Surgical removal is indicated if visual impairment–producing symptoms are distressing to the patient, interfering with lifestyle or occupation, or posing a risk for fall or injury (3,4)[A].
  - Because significant cataract may develop gradually, the patient may not be aware of how it has changed his or her lifestyle. Physician may note a significant cataract, and patient reports "no problems." Thus, evaluation requires effective physician–patient exchange of information.
  - Preoperative evaluation: by the primary care physician:
    ○ Patients on anticoagulants may need to be temporarily discontinued 1 to 2 weeks before surgery if possible (but not always necessary, thus need to discuss with ophthalmologist).
    ○ Patients who have ever taken an α-blocker such as tamsulosin (Flomax) should alert their ophthalmologist (increased risk of intraoperative floppy iris syndrome [IFIS] even in patients who no longer use these drugs).
  - Anesthesia: usually regional injection or topical with sedation and monitoring of vital signs
  - Surgical technique: cataract extraction via phacoemulsification through small incisions created by blade or laser, followed by implantation of a prosthetic intraocular lens; lenses have power calculated based on size of the eye and curvature of cornea usually to correct for distance vision; surgery performed on one (usually worse) eye, with contralateral surgery after recovery and if deemed necessary; generally takes <1 hour depending on surgical technique

- Postoperative care: usually protective eye shield as directed, topical antibiotic, NSAIDs, and steroid ophthalmic medications; keeping eye protected, avoid lifting or bending over for a few weeks.
- Congenital cataract:
  - Treatment is surgical removal of cataract. Newborns may require surgery within days to reduce risk of severe amblyopia. Use of lens implants is controversial because the eyes are growing.
  - Postoperative care: long-term patching program for good eye to combat amblyopia; refractive correction of operative eye, with multiple repeat examinations; challenging for physician and parents

ONGOING CARE

FOLLOW-UP RECOMMENDATIONS
Patient Monitoring
- As cataract progresses, an ophthalmologist may change spectacle correction to maintain vision. When this is no longer successful and interferes with patient's activities of daily living, surgery is indicated.
- Following surgery, spectacle correction may be required to maximize near and/or far visual acuity. Refraction is usually prescribed several weeks after surgery.

PATIENT EDUCATION
Medline Plus on cataracts at: https://www.nlm.nih.gov/medlineplus/cataract.html

PROGNOSIS
- Ocular prognosis is good after cataract removal if no prior or coexisting ocular disease: 94.3% of otherwise healthy eyes achieve best corrected visual acuity of 20/40 or better. Success rates are lower with comorbidities such as diabetes and glaucoma (5).
- In congenital cataracts, prognosis often is poorer because of the high risk of amblyopia.

COMPLICATIONS
- Vary widely from delay in visual recovery or protracted visual discomfort to blindness and loss of eye
- Nearly all reported complications occur rarely (<2% of eyes) except for posterior capsule opacification (14.7–42.7% of eyes, usually treated with Nd:YAG laser capsulotomy in office with a rate of 4–25.3%) (6)[B].
- Poor preoperative visual acuity is related to surgical complications.

REFERENCES
1. Asbell PA, Dualan I, Mindel J, et al. Age-related cataract. *Lancet.* 2005;365(9459):599–609.
2. Abraham AG, Condon NG, West Gower E. The new epidemiology of cataract. *Ophthalmol Clin North Am.* 2006;19(4):415–425.
3. Riaz Y, Mehta JS, Wormald R, et al. Surgical interventions for age-related cataract. *Cochrane Database Syst Rev.* 2006;(4):CD001323.
4. Fedorowicz Z, Lawrence D, Gutierrez P. Day care versus in-patient surgery for age-related cataract. *Cochrane Database Syst Rev.* 2005;(1):CD004242.
5. Biber JM, Sandoval HP, Trivedi RH, et al. Comparison of the incidence and visual significance of posterior capsule opacification between multifocal spherical, monofocal spherical, and monofocal aspheric intraocular lenses. *J Cataract Refract Surg.* 2009;35(7):1234–1238.
6. Lundström M, Barry P, Henry Y, et al. Visual outcome of cataract surgery; study from the European Registry of Quality Outcomes for Cataract and Refractive Surgery. *J Cataract Refract Surg.* 2013;39(5):673–679.

SEE ALSO
- Floppy Iris Syndrome
- Algorithm: Cataracts

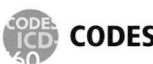

CODES

ICD10
- H26.9 Unspecified cataract
- H25.9 Unspecified age-related cataract
- Q12.0 Congenital cataract

CLINICAL PEARLS
- Cataracts are the leading cause of blindness worldwide; 90% are age-related.
- Primary indication for cataract surgery is visual impairment leading to significant lifestyle changes for the patient.
- For congenital cataracts, must always rule out ocular tumor because early diagnosis and treatment of retinoblastoma may be lifesaving.
- Before prescribing an α-blocker for an older adult with hypertension or a prostate or urinary retention problem, consider whether the patient has cataracts (due to increased risk of IFIS).

CELIAC DISEASE
Zachariah John Kamla, DO • Lloyd A. Runser, MD, MPH, FAAFP

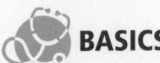 **BASICS**

DESCRIPTION
- An immune-mediated reaction to dietary gluten (found in wheat, barley, rye) primarily affecting the small intestine in genetically predisposed individuals
- Presentations
  - Typical
    - Diarrheal illness characterized by villous atrophy with symptoms of malabsorption (steatorrhea, weight loss, vitamin deficiencies, anemia); resolves with a gluten-free diet (GFD)
    - <50% of adults present with gastrointestinal (GI) symptoms.
  - Atypical
    - Minor GI symptoms, with a myriad of extraintestinal manifestations (e.g., anemia, LFTs, dental enamel defects, neurologic symptoms, infertility)
  - Asymptomatic (silent) disease
    - Found when screening first-degree relatives
    - Positive laboratory tests and genetics, without signs/symptoms; normal histology on biopsy
- System(s) affected: GI
- Synonym(s): celiac sprue; gluten enteropathy

EPIDEMIOLOGY
Incidence
- 1 to 13/100,000 worldwide (1)
- 6.5/100,000 in United States (2)
- Primarily affects those of Northern European ancestry
- Predominant sex: female > male (3:2)

Prevalence
- 0.7% in the United States; an estimated 3 million Americans have celiac disease (3).
- 8 to 204/100,000 worldwide and (1)

ETIOLOGY AND PATHOPHYSIOLOGY
Sensitivity to gluten, specifically gliadin protein fraction. Tissue transglutaminase (tTG) modification of the gliadin protein leads to immunologic cross-reactivity, inflammation, and tissue damage (villous atrophy) with subsequent GI symptoms and malabsorption.

Genetics
Homogenicity for *HLA-DQ2/DQ8* increases risk of celiac disease and enteropathy-associated T-cell lymphoma.

RISK FACTORS
- First-degree relatives: 5–20% incidence (1)
- Second-degree relatives

Pediatric Considerations
No other risk factors (e.g., grain processing, genetically modified organisms, hygiene and illness during childhood, breastfeeding, time of introduction of solid foods, pollution, tobacco use, and medication) explain why some susceptible individuals develop celiac, whereas others do not (4).

COMMONLY ASSOCIATED CONDITIONS
- *Dermatitis herpetiformis*: 85% of patients have celiac disease. All patients should follow GFD (1).
- Secondary lactase deficiency
- Osteopenia and osteoporosis
- Thyroid disease: Hashimoto thyroiditis
- Type 1 diabetes: 3–10% of patients with type 1 diabetes also have celiac disease (1).

- Symptomatic iron deficiency: 10–15% have celiac disease.
- Elevated AST and ALT (with no direct cause)
- Hyposplenism
- Irritable bowel syndrome (IBS)
- Restless leg syndrome
- Celiac disease is associated with increased risk for adenocarcinoma and lymphoma of the small bowel.
  - The risk of lymphoproliferative malignancies depends on small intestinal histopathology.
  - Little to no increased risk in latent celiac disease (seropositive but normal biopsy)
- Associated autoimmune conditions (type 1 diabetes, autoimmune thyroiditis, primary biliary cirrhosis, autoimmune hepatitis, psoriasis, Sjögren disease)
- Associated genetic conditions (Down syndrome, IgA deficiency, Turner syndrome, Williams syndrome)

Pregnancy Considerations
- Prevalence of celiac disease: 2.5 to 3.5 times higher in women with unexplained infertility
- Up to 19% of men with celiac disease have androgen resistance. Semen quality and likelihood of pregnancy increase with GFD.
- Higher rates of low birth weight, prematurity, spontaneous abortions, intrauterine growth restriction, and stillbirths

Pediatric Considerations
Children with celiac disease at higher risk for type 1 diabetes, Down syndrome, Turner syndrome, Williams syndrome, IgA deficiency, and autoimmune thyroid disease (5)[C]

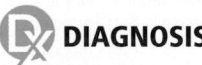 **DIAGNOSIS**

HISTORY
- Diarrhea, cramping are the most common GI symptoms.
- Steatorrhea (fatty stools)
- Abdominal pain or distension
- Nausea, vomiting, flatulence
- Weight loss, weakness, fatigue
- Delayed puberty
- Iron deficiency anemia
- Recurrent aphthous stomatitis
- Dental enamel hyperplasia
- Muscle cramps
- Bone or joint pain
- Anxiety, depression
- Tingling numbness in hands, feet
- Migraines
- In children, malabsorption may manifest as failure to thrive, short stature, or chronic fatigue (5).
- Anorexia
- Constipation or encopresis

PHYSICAL EXAM
Often normal; look for specific findings with:
- Oropharynx: aphthous stomatitis
- Skin: dermatitis herpetiformis (symmetric erythematous papules and blisters on elbows, knees, buttocks, and back), signs of anemia
- Abdomen: distention

DIFFERENTIAL DIAGNOSIS
- Gluten allergy–type II allergic reaction with signs of anaphylaxis
- Nonceliac gluten sensitivity—GI symptoms and/or systemic symptoms improved by GFD but without biomarkers characteristic of celiac disease
- Short bowel syndrome, small intestinal bacterial overgrowth
- Lactose intolerance; dyspepsia
- Gastroesophageal reflux disease (GERD)
- Pancreatic exocrine insufficiency
- Crohn disease; Whipple disease
- Tropical sprue; hypogammaglobulinemia
- Intestinal lymphoma; microscopic colitis
- Autoimmune enteropathy; HIV enteropathy
- Acute enteritis; radiation enteritis
- Eosinophilic gastroenteritis; giardiasis
- IBS

DIAGNOSTIC TESTS & INTERPRETATION
Initial Tests (lab, imaging)
- Do not base diagnosis solely on serology in adults. Patients with symptoms highly suggestive of celiac disease or those with positive serologies should undergo endoscopy for small bowel biopsy while on a gluten-containing diet. *Tissue biopsy is the gold standard for diagnosis.*
- IgA anti-tTG is the preferred serologic test in patients >2 years (1)[C].
- Total serum IgA to screen for IgA deficiency

ALERT
Positive IgA tTG has high sensitivity and specificity (sensitivity, 95–98%; specificity, 95%) if on normal (non–gluten-free) diet for at least 4 weeks.

- IgA-deficient patients have false-negative IgA anti-tTG antibodies.
- IgA deficiency is 10 to 15 times more prevalent in patients with celiac disease.
- The tTG antibody test is the preferred test (over the deamidated gliadin peptide [DGP] antibody).

Follow-Up Tests & Special Considerations
- If patient is IgA deficient OR if IgA anti-tTG are negative, follow up with anti-DGP IgA and IgG.
  - Sensitivity, 94%; specificity, 99% (~anti-tTG)
- Do not use HLA DQ serotyping for initial diagnosis. Consider if discrepant serology–histology results in patients unable to test on GFD and children with Down syndrome (1)[C].
- Consider bone mineral density testing at the time of diagnosis and after 1 year (if osteopenia/osteoporosis on initial testing) or 2 years (if normal initially and patient still symptomatic or nonadherent to diet).

Pediatric Considerations
- Test symptomatic pediatric patients with IgA and IgA anti-tTG antibodies.
- Periodic monitoring with IgA anti-tTG Ab can assess dietary adherence.
- Negative serology cannot rule out CD.
- Consider HLA for high-risk children with negative serology.
- Limit IgA antiendomysial antibodies to patients with illnesses that increase false-positive tTG Ab, such as type I diabetes or autoimmune liver disease.

Diagnostic Procedures/Other

- Endoscopy with a minimum of four biopsies of distal duodenum and two of duodenal bulb at time of initial evaluation correctly diagnose 95% of children (1)[C].
- Video capsule endoscopy is a promising alternative with a sensitivity and specificity of 80% and 95%; particularly helpful if antibody screening and clinical picture are consistent with celiac disease despite nondiagnostic duodenal biopsies

Test Interpretation

Small-bowel biopsy

- Villous atrophy, hyperplasia and lengthening of crypts, infiltration of plasma cells, and intraepithelial lymphocytosis in lamina propria
- Villous atrophy also caused by Crohn disease, radiation enteritis, giardia, and other food intolerances

 TREATMENT

GENERAL MEASURES

- GFD.
  - Rice, corn, and nut flour are safe and palatable substitutes (1)[C].
  - Grains: uncontaminated oats, rice, corn, tapioca, quinoa, amaranth, sorghum
- Levels of IgA antigliadin normalize with gluten abstinence.
- *Lifelong* abstinence is required; immune response to gluten will recur with resumption of gluten intake.

MEDICATION

First Line

Usually no medications. GFD is primary treatment.

Second Line

- In refractory disease, consult with GI for consideration of choice, dosing, and duration of second-line agents:
  - Steroids (prednisone (1)[C] or budesonide (1)[B])
  - Azathioprine (used with caution; use may lead to lymphoma) (1)[C]
  - Cyclosporine
  - Infliximab
  - Cladribine
- Depending on disease severity, patients may develop nutritional deficiencies that require appropriate supplementation.

ISSUES FOR REFERRAL

- Additional nutritional support with qualified dietitian
- Refractory celiac disease
- Child with positive celiac serology

COMPLEMENTARY & ALTERNATIVE MEDICINE

Many alternative therapies are under development. Future treatment may include predigestion of gluten with peptidase, tight junction blockade, transglutaminase 2 or HLA DQ2/DQ8 blockers, and induction of immune tolerance (4).

 ONGOING CARE

FOLLOW-UP RECOMMENDATIONS

- Consultation with registered dietitian
- Screen for osteoporosis and treat accordingly.
- Follow-up with GI at 3 to 6 months for serology and 12 months for repeat biopsy if indicated

Patient Monitoring

- Repeat EGD if no clinical response to GFD or relapse in symptoms (1)[C].
- Follow anti-tTG IgA or deaminated antigliadin antibodies as a measure of response/compliance with diet (vs. antigliadin IgA or IgG).

DIET

- Remove gluten: wheat, rye, barley, and products with gluten additives (processed food/meat, medications, hygiene products).
- Dietary change is challenging (especially identifying sources of "hidden" gluten) and should be coordinated with a skilled registered dietitian.

PATIENT EDUCATION

- Discuss how to recognize gluten in various products.
- Highlight potential complications and outcomes of failing to follow a GFD.
- Support groups and self-education
- Celiac Disease Foundation: https://www.celiac.org/; Quick start GFD guide for celiac disease and non-celiac gluten sensitivity. http://celiac.org/wp-content/uploads/2013/12/quick-start-guide.pdf
- National Celiac Association: https://nationalceliac.org/
- Beyond Celiac: https://www.beyondceliac.org/

PROGNOSIS

- Good prognosis if adherent to GFD
- Patients should see improvement within 7 days of dietary modification.
- Symptoms usually resolve in 4 to 6 weeks.
- It is unknown whether strict dietary adherence decreases cancer risk.

COMPLICATIONS

- Malignancy: Untreated and refractory patients have increased cancer risk, but successful treatment decreases risk to population baseline (1)[C].
- Refractory disease (rare ~1–2% of all patients)
  - May respond to prednisone
  - May need total parenteral nutrition
- Osteoporosis
- Dehydration
- Electrolyte depletion

REFERENCES

1. Rubio-Tapia A, Hill ID, Kelly CP, et al; for American College of Gastroenterology. ACG clinical guidelines: diagnosis and management of celiac disease. *Am J Gastroenterol*. 2013;108(5):656–677.
2. Riddle MS, Murray JA, Porter CK. The incidence and risk of celiac disease in a healthy US adult population. *Am J Gastroenterol*. 2012;107(8):1248–1255.
3. Rubio-Tapia A, Ludvigsson JF, Brantner TL, et al. The prevalence of celiac disease in the United States. *Am J Gastroenterol*. 2012;107(10):1538–1544.
4. Freeman H. Celiac disease: a disorder emerging from antiquity, its evolving classification and risk, and potential new treatment paradigms. *Gut Liver*. 2015;9(1):28–37.
5. Snyder J, Butzner JD, DeFelice AR, et al. Evidence-informed expert recommendations for the management of celiac disease in children. *Pediatrics*. 2016;138(3):e20153147.

ADDITIONAL READING

- Green PH, Lebwohl B, Greywoode R. Celiac disease. *J Allergy Clin Immunol*. 2015;135(5):1099–1106.
- Husby S, Koletzko S, Korponay-Szabó IR, et al; for ESPGHAN Working Group on Coeliac Disease Diagnosis, ESPGHAN Gastroenterology Committee, European Society for Pediatric Gastroenterology, Hepatology, and Nutrition. European Society for Pediatric Gastroenterology, Hepatology, and Nutrition guidelines for the diagnosis of coeliac disease. *J Pediatr Gastroenterol Nutr*. 2012;54(1):136–160.
- Pinto-Sánchez MI, Verdu EF, Liu E, et al. Gluten introduction to infant feeding and risk of celiac disease: systematic review and meta-analysis. *J Pediatr*. 2016;168:132.e3–143.e3.

 SEE ALSO

Algorithms: Diarrhea, Chronic; Malabsorption Syndrome

 CODES

ICD10

K90.0 Celiac disease

CLINICAL PEARLS

- Screen for celiac disease in patients with nonspecific GI symptoms, presumed IBS, dermatitis herpetiformis, unexplained transaminitis, or unexplained iron deficiency anemia.
- Test total IgA levels along with IgA anti-tTG antibodies in patients >2 years of age. Positive serology is not definitive.
- Diagnostic testing must be completed while on a gluten-containing diet.
- Endoscopic biopsy is the gold standard for diagnosis.
- Standard of treatment is a GFD. Patient symptoms should improve in 7 days if fully compliant.

CELLULITIS

Lynn Weaver, MD • Karl T. Clebak, MD, FAAFP • Jarrett Sell, MD, AAHIVS

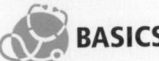

BASICS

A common global health burden with >650,000 admissions per year in the United States alone (1)

DESCRIPTION

- An acute bacterial infection of the dermis and subcutaneous (SC) tissue
- Types and locations:
  - Periorbital cellulitis: bacterial infection of the eyelid and surrounding tissues (anterior compartment)
  - Orbital cellulitis: infection of the eye posterior to the septum; sinusitis is most common risk factor.
  - Facial cellulitis: preceded by upper respiratory infection or otitis media
  - Buccal cellulitis: infection of cheek in children associated with bacteremia (common before *Haemophilus influenzae* type B vaccine)
  - Peritonsillar cellulitis: common in children; associated with fever, sore throat, and "hot potato" speech
  - Abdominal wall cellulitis: common in morbidly obese patients
  - Perianal cellulitis: sharply demarcated, bright, perianal erythema
  - Necrotizing cellulitis: gas-producing bacteria in the lower extremities; more common in diabetics

EPIDEMIOLOGY

- Predominant sex: male = female
- Seasonality increased hospitalizations for cellulitis in the summer with fewer in the winter months (2).

Incidence

200/100,000 patient/years

Prevalence

- The exact prevalence is uncertain because cellulitis is common and not reportable. It affects all age groups and all races; however, certain types of cellulitis/microorganisms occur in certain populations.
- In the United States, ~14.5 million annual cases of cellulitis account for $3.7 billion in ambulatory costs (1).

ETIOLOGY AND PATHOPHYSIOLOGY

Cellulitis is caused by bacterial penetration through a break in the skin. Hyaluronidase mediates SC spread.

- Microbiology
  - β-Hemolytic streptococci (groups A, B, C, G, and F), *Staphylococcus aureus*, including MRSA, and gram-negative aerobic bacilli are most common.
  - *S. aureus* seen in periorbital and orbital cellulitis and IV drug users
  - *Pseudomonas aeruginosa* seen in diabetics and other immunocompromised patients
  - *H. influenza* causes buccal cellulitis.
  - Clostridia and non–spore-forming anaerobes: necrotizing cellulitis (crepitant/gangrenous)
  - *Streptococcus agalactiae*: cellulitis following lymph node dissection
  - *Pasteurella multocida* and *Capnocytophaga canimorsus*: cellulitis preceded by bites
  - *Streptococcus iniae*: immunocompromised hosts
  - Rare causes: *Mycobacterium*, fungal (mucormycosis, aspergillosis, syphilis)

Genetics

No genetic pattern

RISK FACTORS

- Disruption of skin barrier: trauma, infection, insect bites, injection drug use, body piercing
- Inflammation: eczema or radiation therapy
- Edema due to venous insufficiency; lymphatic obstruction due to surgery or congestive heart failure (CHF)
- Elderly, diabetes, hypertension, obesity
- Recurrent cellulitis:
  - Cellulitis recurrence score (predicts recurrence of lower extremity cellulitis based on presence of lymphedema, chronic venous insufficiency, peripheral vascular disease, and deep venous thrombosis) (3)[A]
  - Recurrent cellulitis is seen in immunocompromised patients (HIV/AIDS), steroids and TNF-α inhibitor therapy, diabetes, hypertension, cancer, peripheral arterial or venous diseases, chronic kidney disease, dialysis, IV or SC drug use (3).

GENERAL PREVENTION

- Good skin hygiene
- Support stockings to decrease edema
- Maintain tight glycemic control and proper foot care in diabetic patients.

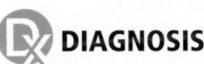

DIAGNOSIS

Primarily a clinical diagnosis

HISTORY

- Previous trauma, surgery, animal/human bites, dermatitis, and fungal infection are portals of entry for bacterial pathogens.
- Pain, itching, and/or burning
- Fever, chills, and malaise

PHYSICAL EXAM

- Localized pain and tenderness with erythema, induration, swelling, and warmth
- Regional lymphadenopathy
- Purulent drainage (from abscesses)
- Orbital cellulitis: proptosis, globe displacement, limitation of ocular movements, vision loss, diplopia
- Facial cellulitis: malaise, anorexia, vomiting, pruritus, burning, anterior neck swelling

DIFFERENTIAL DIAGNOSIS

Toxic shock syndrome, venous stasis dermatitis (commonly mistaken as cellulitis), bursitis, acute dermatitis or intertrigo, herpes zoster or herpetic whitlow, deep vein thrombosis or thrombophlebitis, acute gout or pseudogout, necrotizing fasciitis or myositis, gas gangrene, osteomyelitis, erythema chronicum migrans or malignancy, drug reaction, sunburn, or insect stings

DIAGNOSTIC TESTS & INTERPRETATION

Initial Tests (lab, imaging)

- If there are signs of systemic disease (fever, heart rate >100 bpm, or systolic blood pressure <90 mm Hg): blood cultures, CPK, CRP. Consider serum lactate levels.
- WBC has 84% specificity and 43% sensitivity; CRP has a sensitivity of 67% and specificity of 95% (PPV 95% and NPV 68%).
- Aspirates from point of maximum inflammation are more sensitive (45% positive culture) than aspirates from leading edge (5% positive culture).
- Blood cultures: pathogens isolated in <5% of patients. Blood cultures in children are more likely to show a contaminant than true positive.
- Swab open cellulitis wounds for culture.
- Plain radiographs, CT, and MRI are useful if osteomyelitis, fracture, necrotizing fasciitis, retained foreign body.
- MRI and ultrasound are most useful for evaluation of potential underlying abscesses.
- Gallium-67 scintigraphy helps detect cellulitis superimposed on chronic limb lymphedema.

Diagnostic Procedures/Other

Consider lumbar puncture in children with *H. influenzae* type B or if meningeal signs and facial cellulitis.

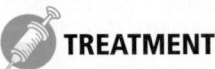

TREATMENT

GENERAL MEASURES

- Immobilize/elevate involved limb to reduce swelling.
- Sterile saline dressings or cool aluminum acetate compresses for pain relief
- Edema: compression stocking, pneumatic pumps; diuretic therapy for CHF patients
- Mark the area of cellulitis to monitor progression.
- Tetanus immunization if needed, particularly if there is an open (traumatic) wound

MEDICATION

First Line

- Target treatment if known pathogen and/or with certain exposures (animal bites)
- Empiric antibiotic selection:
  - Nonpurulent cellulitis
    - With nonpurulent drainage, target treatment toward β-hemolytic streptococci and MSSA.
    - Outpatient: treatment duration of 5 to 10 days (4)[C]
      - Oral: for mild cellulitis
      - Cephalexin 500 mg PO q6h; children: 25 to 50 mg/kg/day in 3 to 4 doses
      - Dicloxacillin 500 mg PO q6h; children: 25 to 50 mg/kg/day in 4 doses
      - Clindamycin 300 to 450 mg PO q6–8h; children: 20 to 30 mg/kg/day in 4 doses
      - IV: for rapidly progressing cellulitis
      - Cefazolin 1 to 2 g IV q8h; children: 100 mg/kg/day IV in 2 to 4 divided doses
      - Oxacillin 2 g IV q4h; children: 150 to 200 mg/kg/day IV in 4 to 6 doses
      - Nafcillin 2 g IV q4h; children: 150 to 200 mg/kg/day IV in 4 to 6 doses
      - Clindamycin 600 to 900 mg IV q8h; children: 25 to 40 mg/kg/day IV in 3 to 4 doses

- Purulent cellulitis (probable CA-MRSA)
  - Culture purulent wounds and follow up in 48 hrs.
  - Incise and drain abscesses and start empiric antibiotic therapy. Modify based on culture results; tailor duration based on clinical response (5)[C]:
    - Oral
      - Clindamycin 300 to 450 mg PO; children: 40 mg/kg/day in 3 to 4 doses
      - Trimethoprim-sulfamethoxazole (TMP-SMX) 1 DS tab PO BID; children: dose based on TMP at 8 to 12 mg/kg/day divided in 2 doses
      - Doxycycline 100 mg PO BID; children >8 years of age: ≤45 kg: 4 mg/kg/day divided in 2 doses; >45 kg: 100 mg PO BID
      - Minocycline 200 mg PO once and then 100 mg PO BID; children >8 years old: 4 mg/kg PO once and then 4 mg/kg PO BID
      - Linezolid 600 mg PO BID; children <12 years: 10 mg/kg/dose (max 600 mg/dose) PO TID; ≥12 years: 600 mg PO BID
      - Tedizolid 200 mg PO once daily; children: Dosing is not established.
    - IV
      - Vancomycin 15 to 20 mg/kg/dose IV every 8 to 12 hours
      - Daptomycin 4 mg/kg/dose IV once daily; if bacteremia is present or suspected: 6 mg/kg IV once daily
      - Linezolid 600 mg IV BID
      - Tedizolid 200 mg IV once daily
      - Ceftaroline 600 mg IV q12h
      - Tigecycline 100 mg IV once, thereafter 50 mg IV q12h
- Necrotizing cellulitis: requires broad-spectrum coverage to cover clostridial and anaerobic species: ampicillin-sulbactam 1.5 to 3.0 g q6–8h IV or piperacillin-tazobactam 3.37 g q6–8h IV plus ciprofloxacin 400 mg q12h IV plus clindamycin 600 to 900 mg q8h IV; have a low threshold for consultation, intensive care, and emergent surgical consultation
- Freshwater exposure: penicillinase-resistant: penicillin plus gentamicin or fluoroquinolone; salt water exposure: doxycycline 200 mg IV in 2 divided doses
- Bites: The combination of amoxicillin and clavulanic acid is recommended for human and dog bites. Ticarcillin and clavulanic acid or the combination of a 3rd-generation cephalosporin (i.e., ceftriaxone) plus metronidazole provides adequate parenteral therapy for animal or human bites. If allergic to penicillin, use fluoroquinolone plus metronidazole.
- Facial cellulitis in adults: ceftriaxone IV
- Diabetic foot infection:
  - Mild/moderate: cephalexin or cephalexin plus doxycycline or TMP-SMX plus amoxicillin clavulanate
  - Severe: ampicillin/sulbactam or imipenem/cilastatin or meropenem; alternative: combinations of targeting anaerobes as well as gram-positive and gram-negative aerobes
- If severe infection, toxicity, immunocompromised patients, or worsening infection despite empirical therapy, admit for empiric antibiotic therapy covering MRSA.

- Recurrent streptococcal cellulitis: penicillin 250 mg BID, or if penicillin-allergic, use erythromycin 250 mg BID
- Dalbavancin, a 2nd-generation lipoglycopeptide antibiotic with MRSA coverage, can be used to treat cellulitis and be administered rarely as once a week (5)[C].

Pediatric Considerations
Avoid doxycycline in children ≤8 years old and during pregnancy.

Second Line
Mild infection
- Penicillin allergy: erythromycin 500 mg PO q6h
- Cephalexin remains a cost-effective therapy for outpatient management of cellulitis at current estimated MRSA levels.

SURGERY/OTHER PROCEDURES
- Débridement for gas and purulent matter
- Intubation or tracheotomy may be needed for cellulitis of the head or neck.

ADMISSION, INPATIENT, AND NURSING CONSIDERATIONS
- Severe infection, suspicion of deeper or rapidly spreading infection, tissue necrosis, or severe pain
- Marked systemic toxicity or worsening symptoms that do not resolve after 24 to 48 hours of therapy
- Patients with underlying risk factors or severe comorbidities
- Patients not improved with initial outpatient management

 ONGOING CARE

FOLLOW-UP RECOMMENDATIONS
Patient Monitoring
- Repeat relevant labs (blood culture, CBC, potentially lumbar puncture) if patient is toxic or not improving.
- Cutaneous inflammation may worsen in the first 24 hours due to release of bacterial antigens. Symptomatic improvement usually occurs in 24 to 48 hours, but visible improvement may take 72 hours.

DIET
Glucose control in diabetics

PATIENT EDUCATION
Good skin hygiene

PROGNOSIS
With adequate antibiotic treatment, prognosis is good.
- Low-dose penicillin prophylaxis in patients with recurrent cellulitis decreases recurrence (6)[B].
- Older age, higher BMI, and diabetes mellitus are factors that have been shown to lower early response to antibiotics.

COMPLICATIONS
- Local abscess or bacteremia, sepsis
- Superinfection with gram-negative organisms
- Lymphangitis, especially if recurrent
- Thrombophlebitis or venous thrombosis
- Bacterial meningitis
- Gangrene

REFERENCES
1. Raff A, Kroshinsky D. Cellulitis: a review. *JAMA*. 2016;316(3):325–337.
2. Peterson RA, Polgreen LA, Cavanaugh JE, et al. Increasing incidence, cost, and seasonality in patients hospitalized for cellulitis. *Open Forum Infect Dis*. 2017;4(1):ofx008.
3. Tay EY, Fook-Chong S, Oh CC, et al. Cellulitis recurrence score: a tool for predicting recurrence of lower limb cellulitis. *J Am Acad Dermatol*. 2015;72(1):140–145.
4. Stevens DL, Bisno AL, Chambers HF, et al. Practice guidelines for the diagnosis and management of skin and soft tissue infections: 2014 update by the Infectious Diseases Society of America. *Clin Infect Dis*. 2014;59(2):147–159.
5. Bender S, Oakden K. New developments and treatment options of cellulitis in the hospital. In: Conrad K, ed. *Clinical Approaches to Hospital Medicine: Advances, Updates and Controversies*. Cham, Switzerland: Springer; 2018:77–87.
6. Thomas KS, Crook AM, Nunn AJ, et al; for U.K. Dermatology Clinical Trials Network's PATCH I Trial Team. Penicillin to prevent recurrent leg cellulitis. *N Engl J Med*. 2013;368(18):1695–1703.

ADDITIONAL READING
- Liu C, Bayer A, Cosgrove SE, et al. Clinical practice guidelines by the Infectious Diseases Society of America for the treatment of methicillin-resistant *Staphylococcus aureus* infections in adults and children: executive summary. *Clin Infect Dis*. 2011;52(3):285–292.
- Obaitan I, Dwyer R, Lipworth AD, et al. Failure of antibiotics in cellulitis trials: a systematic review and meta-analysis. *Am J Emerg Med*. 2016;34(8): 1645–1652.
- Oh CC, Ko HC, Lee HY, et al. Antibiotic prophylaxis for preventing recurrent cellulitis: a systematic review and meta-analysis. *J Infect*. 2014;69(1):26–34.

 CODES

ICD10
- L03.90 Cellulitis, unspecified
- H05.019 Cellulitis of unspecified orbit
- L03.211 Cellulitis of face

CLINICAL PEARLS
- *S. aureus* and group A *Streptococcus* are the most common organisms causing cellulitis.
- Consider MRSA if cellulitis does not respond to antibiotics within 48 hours or if purulence present.
- Rapid expansion of infected area with red/purple discoloration and severe pain may suggest necrotizing fasciitis, requiring urgent surgical evaluation.
- Venous stasis dermatitis can easily mimic cellulitis and may lead to improper use of antibiotics.

CELLULITIS, ORBITAL
Robert T. Carlisle, MD, MPH

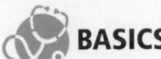 **BASICS**

DESCRIPTION
- Acute, severe, vision-threatening infection of orbital contents posterior to orbital septum. Preseptal (previously referred to as periorbital) cellulitis is anterior to the septum. Distinguishing location determines the appropriate workup and treatment.
- Synonym(s): postseptal cellulitis

ALERT
- Differentiating orbital from preseptal cellulitis is the critical diagnostic step. Preseptal cellulitis can be identified by exam or, if needed, by CT scan.
- Both preseptal and orbital cellulitis present with a red, swollen painful eye or eyelid.
- Diplopia, proptosis, vision loss, and fever suggest orbital involvement.
- Contrast CT is the imaging method of choice and must be done for suspicion of orbital cellulitis.
- Treat with immediate IV antibiotics, hospital admission, and ophthalmology referral.
- Monitor frequently for vision loss, cavernous sinus thrombosis, abscess, and meningitis.

EPIDEMIOLOGY
- No difference in frequency between genders in adults
- More common in children; mean age of surgical cases: 10.1 years; medical pediatric cases: 6.1 years
- Much less common than preseptal cellulitis

Incidence
Orbital cellulitis has declined since *Haemophilus influenzae* type b (Hib) vaccine was introduced. Haemophilus is no longer the leading cause of orbital cellulitis (1,2)[B].

ETIOLOGY AND PATHOPHYSIOLOGY
- Sinusitis is classically associated with orbital cellulitis. Local skin conditions are typically associated with preseptal cellulitis.
- The ethmoid sinus is separated from the orbit by the lamina papyracea ("layer of paper"), a thin bony separation, and is often the source of contiguous spread of infection to the orbit.
- The orbital septum is a connective tissue barrier that extends from the skull into the lid and separates the preseptal from the orbital space.
- Cellulitis in the closed bony orbit causes proptosis, globe displacement, orbital apex syndrome (mass effect on the cranial nerves), optic nerve compression, and vision loss.
- Cultures of surgical specimens in adults often grow multiple organisms. In over 1/3 of cases, no pathogen is recovered (3)[B].
- Most common organisms (1,2)[C]:
  - *Staphylococcus aureus, Streptococcus pneumoniae, Streptococcus anginosus*

- Less common organisms:
  - *Moraxella catarrhalis, H. influenzae*, group A β-hemolytic *Streptococcus, Pseudomonas aeruginosa*, anaerobes, phycomycosis (mucormycosis), aspergillosis, *Mycobacterium tuberculosis, Mycobacterium avium* complex, trichinosis, *Echinococcus*
- There are increasing cases of methicillin-resistant *S. aureus* (MRSA).

Genetics
No known genetic predisposition

RISK FACTORS
- Sinusitis present in 80–90% of cases (1)[C]
- Orbital trauma, retained orbital FB, ophthalmic surgery
- Dental, periorbital, skin, or intracranial infection; acute dacryocystitis (inflammation of the lacrimal sac) and acute dacryoadenitis (inflammation of the lacrimal gland)
- Atopy and HSV can lead to recurrent episodes (2).
- Immunosuppressed patients are at increased risk of adverse outcomes.

GENERAL PREVENTION
- Routine Hib vaccination
- Appropriate treatment of bacterial sinusitis
- Proper wound care and perioperative monitoring of orbital surgery and trauma
- Avoid trauma to the sinus and orbital regions.
- High index of suspicion in febrile patients presenting with periocular pain, swelling, and erythema

COMMONLY ASSOCIATED CONDITIONS
- Trauma and intraorbital FB
- Preseptal cellulitis
- Adverse outcomes of orbital apex syndrome, vision loss, ophthalmoplegia, abscess, meningitis, or cavernous sinus thrombosis

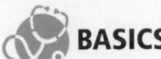 **DIAGNOSIS**

HISTORY
- Complaints of acute onset red, swollen, tender eye or eyelid, and pain with eye movements
- History of surgery, trauma, sinus or upper respiratory infection, dental infection
- Malaise, fever, stiff neck, mental status changes
- Specific signs of orbital cellulitis include:
  - Proptosis, double vision, ophthalmoplegia, vision loss (or decreased field of vision), pain with eye movement, decreased color vision

ALERT
- Septic appearance, mental status changes, contralateral cranial nerve palsy, or bilateral orbital cellulitis may indicate CNS involvement.
- MRSA orbital cellulitis may present without associated upper respiratory infection.

PHYSICAL EXAM
Vital signs
- Assess visual acuity (with glasses if required).
- Lid exam and palpation of the orbit
- Pupillary reflex for afferent pupillary defect
- Extraocular movements; assess for pain with eye movement—if present, concerning for orbital cellulitis.
- Red desaturation: Patient views red object with one eye and compares to the other; reduced red color may indicate optic nerve involvement.
- Confrontation visual field testing

DIFFERENTIAL DIAGNOSIS
- Preseptal cellulitis
  - Eyelid erythema with or without conjunctival erythema, afebrile, no pain on eye movement, no diplopia, normal eye exam, vision intact
- Metastatic tumors and autoimmune inflammation may masquerade as orbital cellulitis in rare cases; usually present with painless slow onset of symptoms
- Idiopathic orbital inflammatory disease (orbital pseudotumor) (1)[C]
  - Afebrile, normal WBCs; usually subacute, may have pain, responds to steroids after ruling out orbital cellulitis
- Orbital foreign body
- Arteriovenous fistula (carotid-cavernous fistula)
  - Spontaneous or due to trauma; bruit may be present; insidious, subacute onset
- Cavernous sinus thrombosis
  - Signs of orbital cellulitis with cranial nerves III, IV, V, and VI findings; often bilateral and acute
  - Severely ill
- Acute thyroid orbitopathy
  - Afebrile; possible signs of thyroid disease
  - Bilateral orbital involvement
- Orbital tumor
  - Rhabdomyosarcoma, acute lymphoblastic leukemia, or metastatic tumors
  - Unilateral
  - Slow onset
- Trauma, insect bite, ruptured dermoid cyst
- Clinical signs help distinguish preseptal from orbital cellulitis. Preseptal infection causes erythema, induration, and tenderness of the eyelid and/or periorbital tissues, and patients rarely show signs of systemic illness. Local skin trauma, lacerations, or bug bites can be seen. Extraocular movements and visual acuity are intact.
- Orbital cellulitis also presents with complaints of a red, swollen, painful eye or eyelid. It also results in proptosis, conjunctival edema, ophthalmoplegia (diminished ocular movement), or decreased visual acuity.

DIAGNOSTIC TESTS & INTERPRETATION
- CBC with differential, C-reactive protein, ESR
- Swab cultures of eye secretions or nasopharyngeal aspirates are often contaminated by normal flora but may identify causative organism(s).

- Cultures from orbital and sinus abscesses at the time of surgery more often yield positive results but should be limited to cases where invasive procedures are indicated. Cultures from sinus aspirates and abscesses may grow multiple organisms.
- Blood cultures (usually negative) should be obtained prior to initiation of antibiotic therapy in ill-appearing or febrile patients.

Initial Tests (lab, imaging)
- CT scan of orbits and sinuses with axial and coronal views, with and without contrast, is imaging modality of choice (4)[C]. US and MRI are alternatives.
  - Thin section (2 mm) CT, coronal and axial views with bone windows to differentiate preseptal from orbital cellulitis, confirm extension into orbit, detect coexisting sinus disease, identify orbital or subperiosteal abscesses requiring surgery
  - Deviation of medial rectus indicates intraorbital involvement.
- MRI offers superior soft tissue resolution for identification of cavernous sinus thrombosis but is less effective for bone imaging.
- US is used to rule out orbital myositis, locate FBs or abscesses, and follow progression of drained abscess.

Follow-Up Tests & Special Considerations
- Frequent eye exam and vital signs (q4h)
- Identify associated conditions, such as meningitis or orbital abscess.

Diagnostic Procedures/Other
Consult ophthalmology for slit lamp and dilated funduscopic exam; proptosis, color vision, automated visual field; and need for surgery.

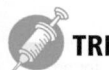 **TREATMENT**

Admit patients with orbital cellulitis for monitoring and treatment with broad-spectrum IV antibiotics (1).

MEDICATION
- Empiric antibiotic therapy to cover pathogens associated with acute sinusitis (*S. pneumoniae*, *H. influenzae*, *M. catarrhalis*, *Streptococcus pyogenes*) as well as for *S. aureus*, *S. anginosus*, and anaerobes
- Modify IV antibiotic treatment when culture and sensitivity results are available. Duration of IV therapy is usually a week. Additional PO therapy depends on response.
- PO antibiotic therapy for 2 to 3 weeks or longer (3 to 6 weeks) is recommended for patients with severe sinusitis and bony destruction.

First Line
- Ampicillin/sulbactam (Unasyn) or ceftriaxone plus metronidazole or clindamycin if anaerobic infection is suspected (3)
  - Ampicillin/sulbactam: 3 g IV q6h for adult; 200 to 300 mg/kg/day divided q6h for children
  - Ceftriaxone: 1 to 2 g IV q12h for adults or 100 mg/kg/day divided BID in children with maximum 4 g/day
  - Clindamycin: 600 mg IV q8h for adults; 20 to 40 mg/kg/day IV q6–8h for children (5)
  - Metronidazole: 500 mg IV q8h for adult; 30 to 35 mg/kg/day divided q8h for children

- Vancomycin: 1 g IV q12h for adults; 40 mg/kg/day IV divided q8–12h, max daily dose 2 g for children (3)

ADDITIONAL THERAPIES
- Steroid use is controversial (1)[C].
- PO steroids as an adjunct to IV antibiotics for orbital cellulitis may speed resolution of inflammation (6)[C].
- Topical erythromycin or nonmedicated ophthalmic ointment protects the cornea from exposure in cases with severe proptosis.
- PO antibiotics for ≥2 weeks are traditionally recommended following IV treatment.
- Children may be treated with amoxicillin/clavulanate 20 to 40 mg/kg/day divided TID or in adults 250 to 500 mg TID.

ISSUES FOR REFERRAL
Always admit to the hospital and consult with ophthalmology. Consider consultation with ID and ENT for orbital cellulitis; neurology/neurosurgery if intracranial spread is suspected

SURGERY/OTHER PROCEDURES
- IV antibiotic therapy is the initial therapy.
- Surgical intervention warranted for visual loss, complete ophthalmoplegia, well-defined large abscess (>10 mm) on presentation or no clinical improvement after 24 to 48 hours of antibiotic therapy
- Trauma cases may need débridement or FB removal.
- Orbital abscess may need surgical drainage.
- Surgical drainage with 4 to 8 weeks of antibiotics is the treatment of choice for brain abscess.
- Surgical interventions may include external ethmoidectomy, endoscopic ethmoidectomy, uncinectomy, antrostomy, and subperiosteal drainage.

ADMISSION, INPATIENT, AND NURSING CONSIDERATIONS
Patients with orbital cellulitis should be admitted for IV antibiotics and serial eye exams to evaluate progression of infection or involvement of optic nerve.
- Follow temperature, WBC, visual acuity, pupillary reflex, ocular motility, and proptosis.
- Repeat CT scan, or surgical intervention, may be required for worsening orbital cellulitis cases.

 ONGOING CARE

FOLLOW-UP RECOMMENDATIONS
Patient Monitoring
Serial visual acuity testing and slit lamp exams

PATIENT EDUCATION
- Maintain proper hand washing and good skin hygiene.
- Avoid skin or lid trauma.

COMPLICATIONS
- Vision loss, CNS involvement, and death
- Permanent vision loss
  - Corneal exposure
  - Optic neuritis
  - Endophthalmitis
  - Septic uveitis or retinitis
  - Exudative retinal detachment
  - Retinal artery or vein occlusions
  - Globe rupture
  - Orbital compartment syndrome
- CNS complications
  - Intracranial abscess, meningitis, cavernous sinus thrombosis (2)[B]

REFERENCES

1. Chadha NK. An evidence-based staging system for orbital infections from acute rhinosinusitis. *Laryngoscope*. 2012;122(Suppl 4):S95–S96.
2. Hauser A, Fogarasi S. Periorbital and orbital cellulitis. *Pediatr Rev*. 2010;31(6):242–249.
3. Seltz LB, Smith J, Durairaj VD, et al. Microbiology and antibiotic management of orbital cellulitis. *Pediatrics*. 2011;127(3):e566–e572.
4. Mahalingam-Dhingra A, Lander L, Preciado DA, et al. Orbital and periorbital infections: a national perspective. *Arch Otolaryngol Head Neck Surg*. 2011;137(8):769–773.
5. Bedwell J, Bauman NM. Management of pediatric orbital cellulitis and abscess. *Curr Opin Otolaryngol Head Neck Surg*. 2011;19(6):467–473.
6. Pushker N, Tejwani LK, Bajaj MS, et al. Role of oral corticosteroids in orbital cellulitis. *Am J Ophthalmol*. 2013;156(1):178.e1–183.e1.

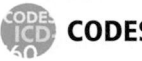 **CODES**

ICD10
- H05.019 Cellulitis of unspecified orbit
- H05.011 Cellulitis of right orbit
- H05.012 Cellulitis of left orbit

CLINICAL PEARLS
- Septal cellulitis presents with diplopia, proptosis, vision loss, and fever versus preseptal cellulitis, eyelid erythema with or without conjunctival erythema, afebrile, no diplopia, normal eye exam, vision intact.
- Most orbital cellulitis cases result from sinusitis.
- MRSA orbital cellulitis may present without an associated upper respiratory infection.
- CT of orbits and sinuses with axial and coronal views with and without contrast is diagnostic modality of choice for suspected cases of orbital cellulitis.
- Patients with orbital cellulitis must be admitted to the hospital for visual monitoring and IV antibiotic therapy.
- Older age (>10 years) and diplopia predict need for surgical intervention in children.
- Ophthalmoplegia, mental status changes, contralateral cranial nerve palsy, or bilateral orbital cellulitis raise suspicion for intracranial involvement.

CELLULITIS, PERIORBITAL
Fozia Akhtar Ali, MD

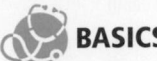 **BASICS**

DESCRIPTION
- An acute bacterial infection of the skin and subcutaneous tissue anterior to the orbital septum; does not involve the orbital structures (globe, fat, and ocular muscles)
- Synonym(s): preseptal cellulitis

ALERT
It is essential to distinguish periorbital cellulitis from orbital cellulitis. Orbital cellulitis is a potentially life-threatening condition. *Orbital cellulitis is posterior to the orbital septum; symptoms include restricted eye movement, pain with eye movement, proptosis, and vision changes.*

EPIDEMIOLOGY
- Occurs more commonly in children; mean age 21 months
- 3 times more common than orbital cellulitis (1)[C]

Incidence
Increased incidence in the winter months (due to increased cases of sinusitis) (1)[C]

ETIOLOGY AND PATHOPHYSIOLOGY
- The anatomy of the eyelid distinguishes periorbital (preseptal) from orbital cellulitis:
  - A connective tissue sheet (orbital septum) extends from the orbital bones to the margins of the upper and lower eyelids; it acts as a barrier to infection of deeper orbital structures.
  - Infection of tissues anterior to the orbital septum is periorbital (preseptal) cellulitis.
  - Infection deep to the orbital septum is orbital (postseptal) cellulitis.
- Periorbital cellulitis typically arises from a contiguous infection of soft tissues of the face.
  - Sinusitis (via lamina papyracea) extension
  - Local trauma; insect or animal bites
  - Foreign bodies
  - Dental abscess extension
  - Hematogenous seeding
- Common organisms (1)[C]
  - *Staphylococcus aureus*, typically MSSA (MRSA is increasing.)
  - *Staphylococcus epidermidis*
  - *Streptococcus pyogenes*
- Atypical organisms
  - *Acinetobacter* sp.; *Nocardia brasiliensis*
  - *Bacillus anthracis*; *Pseudomonas aeruginosa*
  - *Neisseria gonorrhoeae*; *Proteus* sp.
  - *Pasteurella multocida*; *Mycobacterium tuberculosis*; *Trichophyton* sp. (ringworm)
- Since vaccine introduction, the incidence of *Haemophilus influenzae* disease has decrease (should still be suspected in unimmunized or partially immunized patients).

Genetics
No known genetic predisposition

RISK FACTORS
- Contiguous spread from upper respiratory infection
- Acute sinusitis
- Conjunctivitis
- Blepharitis
- Dental infection
- Local skin trauma/puncture wound
- Insect bite
- Bacteremia

GENERAL PREVENTION
- Avoid trauma around the eyes.
- Avoid swimming in fresh or salt water with facial skin abrasions.
- Routine vaccination: particularly *H. influenzae* type B and *Streptococcus pneumoniae*

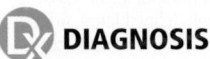 **DIAGNOSIS**

HISTORY
- Induration, erythema, warmth, and/or tenderness of periorbital soft tissue, usually with normal vision and normal eye movements
- Chemosis (conjunctival swelling), proptosis; pain with extraocular eye movements can occur in severe cases of periorbital cellulitis and are concerning for orbital cellulitis.
- Fever (not always present)

ALERT
Pain with eye movement, fever, and conjunctival swelling raise the suspicion for orbital cellulitis.

PHYSICAL EXAM
- Vital signs and general appearance (Patients with orbital cellulitis often appear systemically ill.)
- Inspect eyes and surrounding structures—lids, lashes, conjunctiva, and skin.
- Erythema, swelling, and tenderness of lids without orbital congestion
  - Violaceous discoloration of eyelid is more commonly associated with *H. influenzae*.
- Evaluate for skin break down.
- Look for vesicles to rule out herpetic infection.
- Inspect nasal vaults and palpate sinuses for signs of acute sinusitis.
- Examine oral cavity for dental abscesses.
- Test ocular motility and visual acuity.

DIFFERENTIAL DIAGNOSIS
- Orbital cellulitis
  - Orbital cellulitis may have the same signs and symptoms as periorbital cellulitis, with fever, proptosis, chemosis, ophthalmoplegia, decreased visual acuity, pain with ocular movement.
- Abscess
- Dacryocystitis
- Hordeolum (stye)
- Allergic inflammation
- Orbital or periorbital trauma
- Idiopathic inflammation from orbital pseudotumor
- Orbital myositis
- Rapidly progressive tumors
  - Rhabdomyosarcoma
  - Retinoblastoma
  - Lymphoma
- Leukemia

DIAGNOSTIC TESTS & INTERPRETATION
Initial Tests (lab, imaging)
- CBC with differential
- Blood cultures (low yield) (2)[C]
- Wound culture of purulent drainage (if present)
- Imaging is indicated if there is suspicion for orbital cellulitis (marked eyelid swelling, fever, and leukocytosis or failure to improve on appropriate antibiotics within 24 to 48 hours).
- CT to evaluate the extent of infection and detect orbital inflammation or abscess:
  - CT with contrast, thin sections (2 mm); coronal and axial views with bone windows
  - The classic sign of orbital cellulitis on CT scan is bulging of the medial rectus.

Follow-Up Tests & Special Considerations
- Children with periorbital or orbital cellulitis often have underlying sinusitis.
- If a child is febrile, <15 months old, and appears toxic, admit for blood cultures, antibiotic therapy, and consider lumbar puncture.

TREATMENT

MEDICATION

- Treat periorbital cellulitis with oral antibiotics and ensure close follow-up.
- Empiric antibiotic treatment should cover the most likely organisms (*Staphylococcus* and *Streptococcus*).
- Observe local prevalence of MRSA to determine need for coverage.
- No evidence that IV antibiotics are more effective than PO in reducing recovery time or preventing secondary complications in simple periorbital cellulitis (1)[C]
- No evidence for steroid use

First Line

- Uncomplicated posttraumatic periorbital cellulitis
  - Usually due to skin flora, including *Staphylococcus* and *Streptococcus*
  - Cephalexin 500 mg PO q6h or dicloxacillin 500 mg PO q6h
  - Clindamycin 300 mg PO TID, doxycycline 100 mg PO BID, or trimethoprim-sulfamethoxazole (TMP-SMX) 1 to 2 DS tablets PO q12h if MRSA is suspected
- Extension from sinusitis
  - Amoxicillin-clavulanate 875 mg PO BID
  - 3rd-generation cephalosporin (e.g., cefdinir 300 mg PO BID)
- Dental abscess
  - Amoxicillin-clavulanate 875 mg PO BID or clindamycin 300 mg PO TID
- Bacteremic cellulitis
  - May be associated with meningitis
  - Ceftriaxone 1 g IV q24h plus vancomycin 15 mg/kg/dose IV q8–12h or clindamycin 600 to 900 mg IV q8h to cover MRSA
  - Duration of therapy: A 10- to 14-day course is usually sufficient. Follow patients treated with oral antibiotics for presumed periorbital cellulitis closely (daily follow-up until improvement occurs) for response to antibiotics and possible progression to orbital cellulitis. If symptoms do not improve within 24 hours, reevaluate for IV antibiotic therapy.

ISSUES FOR REFERRAL

Consult ENT and ophthalmology if there is concern for orbital cellulitis or if patients do not respond quickly to first-line treatment (3).

SURGERY/OTHER PROCEDURES

- Usually not indicated in uncomplicated cases
- If there is an abscess or potential compromise of critical structures, orbital surgery is indicated.
- Diplopia is the strongest clinical predictor for surgery.

ADMISSION, INPATIENT, AND NURSING CONSIDERATIONS

- If the patient is stable and there are no systemic signs of toxicity, mild cases in adults and children >1 year of age can be safely managed on an outpatient basis.
- Consider hospitalization and IV antibiotics:
  - If patient appears systemically ill
  - Children <1 year of age (3,4)[C]
  - Patients not immunized against *S. pneumoniae* or *H. influenzae*
  - If patients do not improve or deteriorate within 24 hours of oral antibiotics
  - High suspicion for orbital cellulitis (eyelid swelling with reduced vision, diplopia, abnormal light reflexes, or proptosis)
- No strict guidelines indicate when to switch from parenteral to PO therapy. In general, a switch from IV to oral antibiotics is reasonable once eyelid edema and erythema have significantly improved.
- A 10- to 14-day course of antibiotics is indicated.

 ONGOING CARE

FOLLOW-UP RECOMMENDATIONS

Patient Monitoring

Follow for signs of orbital involvement, including decreased visual acuity or painful/limited ocular motility.

PATIENT EDUCATION

- Maintain good skin hygiene.
- Avoid skin trauma.
- Report early skin changes (swelling, redness, and pain) if recurrent after a course of therapy.

PROGNOSIS

- With timely treatment, patients do well.
- Recurrent periorbital cellulitis occurs with ≥3 periorbital infections in 1 year with at least 1 month of in between episodes; must be differentiated from treatment failure due to antibiotic resistance (1)[C]

COMPLICATIONS

- Orbital cellulitis; orbital abscess formation
- Scarring
- Vision loss
- Cavernous sinus thrombosis
- Osteomyelitis

REFERENCES

1. Hauser A, Fogarasi S. Periorbital and orbital cellulitis. *Pediatr Rev*. 2010;31(6):242–249.
2. Baring DE, Hilmi OJ. An evidence based review of periorbital cellulitis. *Clin Otolaryngol*. 2011;36(1):57–64.
3. Upile NS, Munir N, Leong SC, et al. Who should manage acute periorbital cellulitis in children? *Int J Pediatr Otorhinolaryngol*. 2012;76(8):1073–1077.
4. Georgakopoulos CD, Eliopoulou MI, Stasinos S, et al. Periorbital and orbital cellulitis: a 10-year review of hospitalized children. *Eur J Ophthalmol*. 2010;20(6):1066–1072.

ADDITIONAL READING

- Ekhlassi T, Becker N. Preseptal and orbital cellulitis. *Dis Mon*. 2017;63(2):30–32.
- Mahalingam-Dhingra A, Lander L, Preciado DA, et al. Orbital and periorbital infections: a national perspective. *Arch Otolaryngol Head Neck Surg*. 2011;137(8):769–773.

 CODES

ICD10
L03.211 Cellulitis of face

CLINICAL PEARLS

- Periorbital (preseptal) and orbital (postseptal) cellulitis occur most commonly in children.
- CT scan of sinuses and orbits can differentiate periorbital cellulitis from orbital cellulitis.
- Orbital cellulitis typically has fever, pain with eye movement, diplopia, and/or proptosis.
- Prompt imaging is necessary if there is a concern for orbital cellulitis.

CEREBRAL PALSY

Christina Mezzone, DO, MS • Maria Lombardi, DO

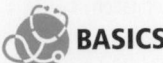 **BASICS**

DESCRIPTION

Cerebral palsy (CP) is a group of clinical syndromes characterized by motor and postural dysfunction due to permanent and nonprogressive disruptions in the developing brain. Motor impairment resulting in activity limitation is necessary for this diagnosis. CP is classified by the nature of the movement disorder and its functional severity. Individuals with this disorder are affected with secondary musculoskeletal and neurologic problems (intellectual, sensory, speech and language impairment, and seizures).

EPIDEMIOLOGY

Incidence
- Overall, 1.5 to 2.5/1,000 live births
- Incidence increases as gestational age (GA) at birth decreases:
  - 146/1,000 for GA of 22 to 27 weeks
  - 62/1,000 for GA of 28 to 31 weeks
  - 7/1,000 for GA of 32 to 36 weeks
  - 1/1,000 for GA of 37+ weeks

Prevalence
3 to 4/1,000 of the population

ETIOLOGY AND PATHOPHYSIOLOGY
- Multifactorial; CP results from static injury or lesions in the developing brain, occurring prenatally, perinatally, or postnatally.
- Neuropathology linked to GA at time of brain insult
- Cytokines, free radicals, and inflammatory response are likely contributing factors.
- Etiology is most likely multifactorial and depends on timing of brain insult: prenatally, perinatally, or postnatally (see "Risk Factors").
- Spastic CP is most common, usually related to premature birth, with either periventricular leukomalacia or germinal matrix hemorrhage.
- Dystonic or athetotic CP, often resulting from kernicterus, is now rare due to improved management of hyperbilirubinemia.

Genetics
There are reports of associations between CP and polymorphisms of certain genes: thrombophilic, cytokines, and apolipoprotein E.

RISK FACTORS
- Prenatal: congenital anomalies, multiple gestation, in utero stroke, intrauterine infection (cytomegalovirus [CMV], varicella), intrauterine growth retardation (IUGR), clinical and histologic chorioamnionitis, antepartum bleeding, maternal factors (cognitive impairment, seizure disorders, hyperthyroidism), abnormal fetal position (e.g., breech)
- Perinatal: preterm birth, low-birth weight, periventricular leukomalacia, perinatal hypoxia/asphyxia, intracranial hemorrhage/intraventricular hemorrhage, neonatal seizure or stroke, hyperbilirubinemia
- Postnatal: traumatic brain injury or stroke, sepsis, meningitis, encephalitis, asphyxia, and progressive hydrocephalus

GENERAL PREVENTION
- Treating mothers with magnesium sulfate during preterm delivery is neuroprotective for fetus and may reduce the risk of CP. Effect on term fetus is unknown.

- Improved management of hyperbilirubinemia with decrease in kernicterus has greatly reduced dyskinetic CP.
- Prevention or reduction of chorioamnionitis and premature births

COMMONLY ASSOCIATED CONDITIONS
- Seizure disorder (22–40%)
- Intellectual impairment (23–44%)
- Behavioral problems
- Speech and language impairment (42–81%)
  - May have an impact on expressive and/or receptive language
  - May be nonverbal
- Sensory impairments
  - Hearing deficits
  - Visual (62–71%): poor visual acuity, strabismus (50%), or hemianopsia
- Feeding impairment, swallowing dysfunction, and aspiration: when severe, may require gastrostomy feedings
- Poor dentition, excessive drooling
- GI conditions: constipation (59%), vomiting (22%), gastroesophageal reflux
- Decreased linear growth and weight abnormalities (under- and overweight)
- Osteopenia
- Bowel and bladder incontinence
- Orthopedic: contractures, hip subluxation/dislocation, scoliosis (60%)

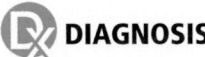 **DIAGNOSIS**

- A clinical diagnosis including
  - Delayed motor milestones
  - Abnormal tone
  - Abnormal neurologic exam suggesting a cerebral etiology for motor dysfunction
  - Absence of regression (not losing function)
  - Absence of underlying syndromes or alternative explanation for etiology
- Although the pathologic lesion is static, clinical presentation may change as the infant grows and develops.
- Accurate early diagnosis remains difficult. Neurologic abnormalities observed in the first 1 to 2 years of life may resolve; be cautious of diagnosing CP before age 2 years.
- Serial exams are often required for a definitive diagnosis.

HISTORY
- Presentation: concerns over movements or delayed motor development
- Ask about
  - Prenatal, perinatal, and postnatal risk factors
  - Neurobehavioral signs
    - Poor feeding/frequent vomiting
    - Irritability
  - Timing of motor milestones: Delay in milestones is not sensitive or specific until after 6 months of age.
  - Abnormal spontaneous general movements
  - Asymmetry of movements such as early hand preference
- Regression of motor skills does not occur with CP.

PHYSICAL EXAM
- Assess for more than one type of neurologic impairment:
  - Spasticity: increased tone/reflexes/clonus
  - Dyskinesia: abnormal movements
  - Hypotonia: decreased tone
  - Ataxia: abnormal balance/coordination
- Areas of exam
  - Tone: may be increased or decreased
  - Trunk and head control: often poor but may be advanced due to high tone
  - Reduced strength and motor control
  - Persistence of primitive reflexes
  - Asymmetry of movement or reflexes
  - Decreased joint range of motion and contractures
  - Brisk deep tendon reflexes
  - Clonus
  - Delayed motor milestones: serial exams most effective
  - Gait abnormalities: scissoring, toe walking
- CP is classified by the following:
  - Muscle tone or movement disorder
    - Spasticity
      - Unilateral: hemiplegic
      - Bilateral: diplegic (lower extremity [LE] > upper extremity [UE] involvement) or quadriplegic (UE ≥ LE involvement)
    - Dystonia: hypertonia and reduced movement
    - Choreoathetosis: irregular spasmodic involuntary movements of the limbs or facial muscles
    - Ataxia: loss of orderly muscular coordination
  - Motor function severity
    - The Gross Motor Function Classification System (GMFCS) scores I to V are the following:
      - Score of I: ambulates without limitation
      - Score of II: ambulates without assistive devices but some limitation
      - Score of III: ambulates with assistive mobility devices
      - Score of IV: self-mobility limited, but technology can help
      - Score of V: self-mobility severely limited, even with technology
    - The Manual Ability Classification System (MACS) can be used to assess UE and fine motor function.

DIFFERENTIAL DIAGNOSIS
Benign congenital hypotonia, brachial plexus injury, familial spastic paraplegia, dopa-responsive dystonia, transient toe-walking, muscular dystrophy, metabolic disorders (e.g., glutaric aciduria type 1), mitochondrial disorders, genetic disorders (e.g., Rett syndrome)

DIAGNOSTIC TESTS & INTERPRETATION
CP is a clinical diagnosis based on history, physical, and risk factors. Laboratory testing is not needed to make diagnosis but can help exclude other etiologies.
- Testing for metabolic and genetic syndromes (1)[C]
  - Not routinely obtained in the evaluation for CP
  - Considered if no specific etiology is identified by neuroimaging or there are atypical features in clinical presentation
  - Detection of certain brain malformations may warrant genetic or metabolic testing to identify syndromes.
- Screening for coagulopathies: Diagnostic testing for coagulopathies should be considered in children with hemiplegic CP with cerebral infarction identified on neuroimaging (1)[C].

Initial Tests (lab, imaging)

- Neuroimaging is not essential, but it is recommended in children with CP for whom the etiology has not been established (1)[C].
- MRI is preferred to CT if need to determine etiology and timing of a brain insult (1)[C].
- Abnormalities found in 80–90% of patients: brain malformation, cerebral infarction, intraventricular or other intracranial hemorrhage, periventricular leukomalacia, ventricular enlargement, or other CSF space abnormalities

Diagnostic Procedures/Other

- The Communication Function Classification System has recently been developed as another means of assessing verbal performance.
- International Classification of Functioning, Disability and Health for CP have been newly developed to standardize functional assessments.
- Screening for comorbid conditions: developmental delay/intellectual impairment, vision/hearing impairments, speech and language disorders, feeding/swallowing dysfunction, or seizures
- Electroencephalograms (EEGs) should only be obtained if there is a history of suspected seizures.

Test Interpretation

Perinatal brain injury may include the following:
- White matter damage
  - Most common in premature infants
  - Periventricular leukomalacia: gliosis with or without focal necrosis with resulting cysts and scarring; may be multiple lesions of various ages. Necrosis can lead to cysts/scarring.
  - Germinal matrix hemorrhage: may lead to intraventricular hemorrhage
- Gray matter damage: more common in term infants; cortical infarcts, focal neuronal damage, myelination abnormalities

 **TREATMENT**

Focuses on control of symptoms; treatments reduce spasticity to prevent painful contractures, manage comorbid conditions, and optimize functionality and quality of life.

GENERAL MEASURES

- Early intervention programs for preterm infants influences motor and cognitive outcomes (2)[A].
- Referral to early intervention for children ages 0 to 3 years is essential.
- Various therapy modalities enhance functioning:
  - Physical therapy to improve posture stability and gait, motor strength and control, and prevent contractures
  - Occupational therapy to increase functional activities of daily living and other fine motor skills
  - Speech therapy for verbal and nonverbal speech and to aid in feeding
- Equipment optimizes participation in activities:
  - Orthotic splinting (ankle–foot orthosis) maintains functional positioning and prevents contractures.
  - Spinal bracing (body jacket) may slow down scoliosis.
  - Augmentative communication with pictures, switches, or computer systems for nonverbal individuals
  - Therapeutic and functional electrical stimulation decreases activity limitation in gait.
  - Use of adaptive equipment such as crutches, walkers, gait trainers, and wheelchairs for mobility and standers for weight-bearing

MEDICATION

First Line

- Diazepam (3)[A]
  - Short-term treatment for generalized spasticity; insufficient evidence on motor function
  - A γ-aminobutyric acid-A ($GABA_A$) agonist that facilitates CNS inhibition at spinal and supraspinal levels to reduce spasticity
  - Adverse effects: ataxia and drowsiness
  - Adult dose: 2 to 12 mg/dose PO q6–12h
  - Pediatric dose (<12 years and <15 kg): <8.5 kg: 0.5 to 1.0 mg HS; 8.5 to 15.0 kg: 1 to 2 mg HS; children 5 to 16 years of age and ≥15 kg: 1.25 mg TID
- Botulinum toxin type A (3)[A]
  - Acts at neuromuscular junction to inhibit the release of acetylcholine to reduce tone
  - Injected directly into muscles of interest for localized spasticity; insufficient evidence on motor function
  - Higher functional benefit when combined with occupational therapy
  - Lasts for 12 to 16 weeks following injection

Second Line

- Baclofen (3)[A]
  - $GABA_B$ agonist, facilitates presynaptic inhibition of mono- and polysynaptic reflexes
  - Adverse effects: drowsiness and sedation
  - Abrupt withdrawal symptoms: spasticity, hallucinations, seizures, confusion, hyperthermia
  - Adults: Initial dose is 5 mg TID; increase dosage every 3 days to an average maintenance dose of 20 mg TID, 80 mg/day maximum.
  - Pediatric dose (>2 years): initial 10 to 15 mg/day. Titrate to effective dose (maximum 40 mg/day). <8 years old: 60 mg/day maximum; >8 years old: 60 mg/day maximum
- Intrathecal baclofen (baclofen pump) (4)[A]
  - Continuous intrathecal route allows greater maximal response with smaller dosage to reduce spasticity.
  - May help ambulatory individuals with gait but no improvement seen in nonambulatory patients
  - Adverse effects: infection, catheter malfunction, CSF leakage

ADDITIONAL THERAPIES

- Multidisciplinary care including ophthalmology; neurology; orthopedics; physiatry along with physical, occupational, and speech therapists
- A primary care "medical home" that coordinates medical and community services, provides support for the patient and the patient's family

SURGERY/OTHER PROCEDURES

- Dorsal root rhizotomy selectively cuts dorsal rootlets from L1–S2. Best for patients with normal intelligence with spastic diplegia. Decreases spasticity in lower limbs when done in conjunction with physiotherapy but associated with adverse effects. Evidence is lacking as to long-term outcomes.
- Surgical treatment of joint dislocations/subluxation, scoliosis management, tendon lengthening, gastrostomy

COMPLEMENTARY & ALTERNATIVE MEDICINE

- Therapeutic horse riding or hippotherapy improves postural control and balance.
- Aquatherapy improves gross motor function in patients with various motor severities (5)[B].

 ONGOING CARE

PROGNOSIS

Reduced lifespan strongly associated with level of functional impairment and intellectual disability

REFERENCES

1. Ashwal S, Russman BS, Blasco PA, et al; for the Quality Standards Subcommittee of the American Academy of Neurology, Practice Committee of the Child Neurology Society. Practice parameter: diagnostic assessment of the child with cerebral palsy: report of the Quality Standards Subcommittee of the American Academy of Neurology and the Practice Committee of the Child Neurology Society. *Neurology*. 2004;62(6):851–863.
2. Spittle A, Orton J, Anderson P, et al. Early developmental intervention programmes post-hospital discharge to prevent motor and cognitive impairments in preterm infants. *Cochrane Database Syst Rev*. 2012;(12):CD005495.
3. Delgado MR, Hirtz D, Aisen M, et al; and the Quality Standards Subcommittee of the American Academy of Neurology, Practice Committee of the Child Neurology Society. Practice parameter: pharmacologic treatment of spasticity in children and adolescents with cerebral palsy (an evidence-based review): report of the Quality Standards Subcommittee of the American Academy of Neurology and the Practice Committee of the Child Neurology Society. *Neurology*. 2010;74(4):336–343.
4. Pin TW, McCartney L, Lewis J, et al. Use of intrathecal baclofen therapy in ambulant children and adolescents with spasticity and dystonia of cerebral origin: a systematic review. *Dev Med Child Neurol*. 2011;53(10):885–895.
5. Lai CJ, Liu WY, Yang TF, et al. Pediatric aquatic therapy on motor function and enjoyment in children diagnosed with cerebral palsy of various motor severities. *J Child Neurol*. 2015;30(2):200–208.

ADDITIONAL READING

- Himpens E, Van den Broeck C, Oostra A, et al. Prevalence, type, distribution, and severity of cerebral palsy in relation to gestational age: a meta-analytic review. *Dev Med Child Neurol*. 2008;50(5):334–340.
- Nguyen TM, Crowther CA, Wilkinson D, et al. Magnesium sulphate for women at term for neuroprotection of the fetus. *Cochrane Database Syst Rev*. 2013;(2):CD009395.
- O'Shea TM. Diagnosis, treatment, and prevention of cerebral palsy. *Clin Obstet Gynecol*. 2008;51(4):816–828.

 CODES

ICD10

- G80.9 Cerebral palsy, unspecified
- G80.1 Spastic diplegic cerebral palsy
- G80.2 Spastic hemiplegic cerebral palsy

CLINICAL PEARLS

- Management should focus on maximizing functioning and quality of life using multidisciplinary team approach.
- Regression of motor skills does not occur with CP.

CERVICAL HYPEREXTENSION INJURIES

Shane L. Larson, MD • Rita A. Kostecke, MD

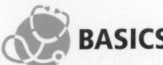 **BASICS**

DESCRIPTION
- Class of neck injuries typically seen in rapid, forceful extension of the cervical spine
- Flexion–extension injuries ("whiplash") are usually from motor vehicle accidents (MVAs).
- Other causes include falls, violence, or sports (1).
- May involve:
  - Injury to vertebral and paravertebral structures: fractures, dislocations, ligamentous tears, and disc disruption/subluxation
  - Spinal cord injury (SCI): traumatic central cord syndrome (CCS) secondary to cord compression or vascular insult, SCI without radiologic abnormality (SCIWORA)
  - Blunt cerebrovascular injury (BCVI): vertebral artery or carotid artery dissection
  - Soft tissue injury: cervical strain/sprain (i.e., whiplash), cervical stingers (see "Brachial Plexopathy")

EPIDEMIOLOGY
- Predominant age: SCI average age of injury 43 years, CCS average age 53 years
- Trauma and sports injuries are more common in young adults (average age 29 years).
- About 78% of new SCI cases are male (1).

Incidence
In the United States
- Cervical fractures: 2 to 5/100 blunt trauma patients
- CCS: 4/100,000 people/year
- BCVI: estimated 1/1,000 of hospitalized trauma patients; incidence increased with cervical spine or thoracic injury.
- Cervical strain: 3 to 4/1,000 people/year
- Whiplash is the most common injury in MVAs and accounts for 28% of all ED visits for MVAs.
- Incidence of whiplash is 70 to 328/100,000 with rates highest in 20- to 24-year-old females.
- 2–6% of patients with blunt trauma have SCI.
- The incidence of traumatic SCI is approximately 54 cases per million population per year (1).

ETIOLOGY AND PATHOPHYSIOLOGY
Blunt trauma due to MVAs, falls, sports injuries, and violence (primarily gunshot wounds)

RISK FACTORS
- Whiplash: initial injury, no seat belt use, female gender
- Chronic pain and/or disability: litigation, previous neck pain or injury, female gender, report of headache/low back pain at onset, low education level (2)[C]
- Fractures: osteoporosis, conditions predisposing to spinal rigidity, such as ankylosing spondylitis or other spondyloarthropathies
- CCS: preexisting spinal stenosis present in >50%
  - Acquired: prior trauma, spondylosis
  - Congenital: Klippel-Feil syndrome (congenital fusion of any two cervical vertebrae)

GENERAL PREVENTION
Seat belts, use of proper safety equipment, rule changes for sports activities, and proper technique in sports activities can prevent or minimize injury.

COMMONLY ASSOCIATED CONDITIONS
Closed head injuries, whiplash-associated disorders (WAD), SCI, soft tissue trauma

 DIAGNOSIS

HISTORY
Usually acute presentation with mechanism of cervical hyperextension and complaints of neck pain, stiffness, or headaches ± neurologic symptoms; include Glasgow Coma Scale (GCS).

PHYSICAL EXAM
- External signs of trauma on the head and neck such as abrasions, lacerations, or contusions provide clues to mechanism and associated injuries.
- Presence, severity, and location of neck tenderness help localize involved structure(s):
  - Posterior, midline bony tenderness raises concern for underlying fracture.
  - Paraspinal or lateral soft tissue tenderness suggests muscular/ligamentous injury.
  - Anterior tenderness concerning for vascular injury
- Carotid bruit suggests carotid dissection.
- Neurologic exam: Paresthesias, weakness suggests SCI or stroke secondary to BCVI:
  - CCS often presents as
    - Distal > proximal symptom distribution, upper extremity > lower extremity
    - Extremity weakness/paralysis predominates.
    - Variable sensory changes below level of lesion (including paresthesias and dysesthesia)
    - Bladder/bowel incontinence may occur.

DIFFERENTIAL DIAGNOSIS
- Acute or chronic disc pathology (herniation or internal disruption)
- Osteoarthritis
- Cervical radiculopathy
- For CCS
  - Bell cruciate palsy
  - Bilateral brachial plexus injuries
  - Carotid or vertebral artery dissection

DIAGNOSTIC TESTS & INTERPRETATION
Initial Tests (lab, imaging)
- Low-risk patients can be cleared clinically (without imaging) using either the Canadian C-Spine Rule (CCR) or the National Emergency X-Ray Utilization Study (NEXUS) criteria (3)[B]:
  - CCR: Stable, ≥16-year-old patient with acute head and neck trauma and no history of cervical spine disease/surgery can be cleared if all of the following conditions are met:
    - GCS ≥15
    - No dangerous mechanism or extremity paresthesias
    - Age <65 years
    - At least one "low-risk factor" (i.e., simple rear-end MVA, ambulation at the accident scene, no midline cervical tenderness, delayed onset of neck pain, or sitting at the time of exam)

  - NEXUS: clinically clear if all of the following:
    - No posterior, midline C-spine tenderness
    - No evidence of intoxication
    - Normal level of alertness
    - No focal/neurologic deficits
    - No distracting injury
  - Reported sensitivity/specificity: CCR (90–100%/1–77%), NEXUS (83–100%/13–46%) (4)[B]
- In patients with high-risk mechanism or concerning historical/physical exam, recommend imaging based on the suspected injury and level of clinical suspicion:
  - Plain radiographs: in some patients who cannot be cleared clinically but are still in low-suspicion category: sensitivity for C-spine injury 39%:
    - Dynamic: flexion–extension; only if asymptomatic and no neurologic deficits or mental impairment, poor identification of ligamentous injury, limited diagnostic value
  - Axial CT from occiput to T1 with coronal and sagittal reconstructions has replaced plain radiography as the test of choice for cases with moderate to high clinical suspicion of C-spine injury, given high sensitivity (90–100%).
  - MRI: test of choice in CCS with direct visualization of traumatic cord lesions (edema or hematomyelia), soft tissue compressing cord, and/or stenosis of canal; detects ligamentous injury and abnormalities of intervertebral discs and soft tissues; MRI is less helpful for fractures.
  - CT angiography: visualization of cervical and cerebral vascular structures to detect BCVI, sensitivity approaches 100% when a ≥16-slice CT scanner is used. MR angiography is an alternative, although sensitivity of 47–50% limits utility.

Test Interpretation
- CCS: thought to be due to white matter axonal disruption of the lateral column, particularly the corticospinal tracts
- BCVI: intimal disruption, leading to thrombosis and embolization
- Acute cervical strain/sprain: Models suggest myofascial tearing, edema, and inflammation.

Geriatric Considerations
- Degenerative changes of the C-spine may be confused with acute traumatic change; osteopenia may limit fracture visualization on x-ray—CT is more accurate.
- Degenerative disease and osteopenia increase risk of upper cervical spine injuries (even with low-velocity trauma).

Pediatric Considerations
SCIWORA: high incidence at <9 years accounting for up to 50% of pediatric cervical spine injuries. MRI helps detect injury.

 TREATMENT

GENERAL MEASURES
- Whiplash, WAD
  - Limited or no benefit to cervical collar. If provided, use for <72 hours.
  - No advantage to engaging early multiprofessional intervention (e.g., pain management and psychology) (4)[C]

– No outcome differences with physical therapy (PT) versus passive (immobilization, rest) treatment; advance activity levels as tolerated.

– No preferred treatment approach in absence of fracture

• Fractures

– Stability determined by imaging

– Decompression and stabilization are indicated for:
  ○ Incomplete SCIs with spinal canal compromise
  ○ Clinical deterioration or failure to improve despite conservative management

– Hangman fracture: traumatic spondylolisthesis of C2 with bilateral fractures through C2 pedicles, often with anterior subluxation of C2 over C3; can be unstable:
  ○ Managed with halo vest immobilization for 12 weeks until flexion–extension films normal

– Odontoid fractures: treat according to type:
  ○ I: through apex; usually stable; external immobilization with a cervical collar (less often halo vest) for up to 12 weeks
  ○ II: most common, at base of dens, usually unstable; nonunion rates of up to 67% with halo immobilization alone, especially with dens displacement >6 mm or age >50 years
  ○ III: through C2 body, usually stable; immobilization in halo or cervical collar for 12 to 20 weeks

– Hyperextension teardrop fractures
  ○ If stable, rigid collar or cervicothoracic brace for 8 to 14 weeks
  ○ If unstable, halo brace for up to 3 months

• CCS: neck immobilization with cervical collar, PT/occupational therapy (OT)

• Cervical strain: no difference in outcomes with active (PT) versus passive (immobilization, rest) treatment; may use soft cervical collar for 10 days for symptomatic relief and then mobilize and increase activity as tolerated; no clear EBM guidelines

MEDICATION

• Fractures: pain control with analgesics

• CCS: Within 8 hours of injury, consider methylprednisolone 30 mg/kg IV over 15 minutes and then continuous infusion 5.4 mg/kg/hr IV for 23 hours. Further improvement in motor function recovery may be seen if infusion is continued for 48 hours, especially if initial bolus administration is delayed after injury (5,6)[A].

• BCVI: Anticoagulation with IV heparin, followed by warfarin therapy for 3 to 6 months and then long-term antiplatelet therapy; antiplatelet agent as sole initial therapy in patients with contraindications to anticoagulation

• Cervical strain: NSAIDs or acetaminophen. There is little benefit to adding cyclobenzaprine for acute cervical strain.

ISSUES FOR REFERRAL

• If cervical spine injury is suspected, immobilize patient and send to ED for evaluation and clearance.

• Emergent consultation from a spine surgeon for any concern for unstable fracture or SCI

SURGERY/OTHER PROCEDURES

• Fractures

– Hangman fracture: surgical fixation for excessive angulation or subluxation, disruption of intervertebral disc space, or failure to obtain alignment with external orthosis

– Odontoid fractures
  ○ Type II: Early surgical stabilization is recommended in setting of age >50 years, dens displacement >5 mm, and specific fracture patterns.
  ○ Type III: Surgical intervention is often reserved for cases of nonunion/malunion after trial of external immobilization.

• CCS: Surgical decompression/fixation is indicated in setting of unstable injury, herniated disc, or when neurologic function deteriorates.

• BCVI: Surgical and/or angiographic intervention may be required if there is evidence of pseudoaneurysm, total occlusion, or transection of the vessel.

ADMISSION, INPATIENT, AND NURSING CONSIDERATIONS

• Varies by injury; clinical judgment, imaging findings, concomitant injuries, and need for operative intervention

• Advanced Trauma Life Support protocol with backboard and collar

 ## ONGOING CARE

FOLLOW-UP RECOMMENDATIONS

Patient Monitoring

Follow patients with known injuries using serial imaging under the care of a specialist.

PATIENT EDUCATION

ThinkFirst Foundation: http://www.thinkfirst.org

PROGNOSIS

• Presenting neurologic status is the most important factor in determining prognosis.

• Fractures

– Hangman fracture: 93–100% fusion rate after 8 to 14 weeks external immobilization

– Odontoid fracture, fusion rate by type: type I, ~100% with external immobilization alone; type II, nonunion rates of up to 67% with halo immobilization alone, especially with dens displacement >6 mm or age >50 years; type III, 85% with external immobilization, 100% with surgical fixation

• BCVI: Patients have fewer neurologic sequelae with early diagnosis and antithrombotic therapy.

• CCS

– Spontaneous recovery of motor function in >50% over several weeks. Younger patients are more likely to regain function.

– Leg, bowel, and bladder functions return first, followed by upper extremities.

• WAD: Prognostic factors for development of late whiplash syndrome (>6 months of symptoms affecting normal activity) include increased initial pain intensity, pain-related disability, and cold hyperalgesia.

COMPLICATIONS

• Fractures: instability or malunion/nonunion necessitating second operation, reactions, and infection related to orthosis

• BCVI: embolic ischemic events and pseudoaneurysm formation

REFERENCES

1. National Spinal Cord Injury Statistical Center. *Spinal Cord Injury: Facts and Figures at a Glance*. Birmingham, AL: National Spinal Cord Injury Statistical Center; 2017.
2. Walton DM, Macdermid JC, Giorgianni AA, et al. Risk factors for persistent problems following acute whiplash injury: update of a systematic review and meta-analysis. *J Orthop Sports Phys Ther*. 2013;43(2):31–43.
3. Stiell IG, Clement CM, McKnight RD, et al. The Canadian C-spine rule versus the NEXUS low-risk criteria in patients with trauma. *N Engl J Med*. 2003;349(26):2510–2518.
4. Michaleff ZA, Maher CG, Verhagen AP, et al. Accuracy of the Canadian C-spine rule and NEXUS to screen for clinically important cervical spine injury in patients following blunt trauma: a systematic review. *CMAJ*. 2012;184(16):E867–E876.
5. Jull G, Kenardy J, Hendrikz J, et al. Management of acute whiplash: a randomized controlled trial of multidisciplinary stratified treatments. *Pain*. 2013;154(9):1798–1806.
6. Bracken MB. Steroids for acute spinal cord injury. *Cochrane Database Syst Rev*. 2012;(1):CD001046.

ADDITIONAL READING

• Franz RW, Willette PA, Wood MJ, et al. A systematic review and meta-analysis of diagnostic screening criteria for blunt cerebrovascular injuries. *J Am Coll Surg*. 2012;214(3):313–327.
• Puvanesarajah V, Qureshi R, Cancienne JM, et al. Traumatic sports-related cervical spine injuries. *Clin Spine Surg*. 2017;30(2):50–56.
• Siasios I, Fountas K, Dimopoulos V, et al. The role of steroid administration in the management of dysphagia in anterior cervical procedures. *Neurosurg Rev*. 2018;41(1):47–53.
• Song KJ, Lee SK, Ko JH, et al. The clinical efficiency of short-term steroid treatment in multilevel anterior cervical arthrodesis. *Spine J*. 2014;14(12):2954–2958.

 ## CODES

ICD10

• S13.4XXA Sprain of ligaments of cervical spine, initial encounter
• S13.101A Dislocation of unspecified cervical vertebrae, init encntr
• S14.109A Unsp injury at unsp level of cervical spinal cord, init

CLINICAL PEARLS

• Use NEXUS or CCR to determine need for imaging in every patient with a potential neck injury.
• Always perform imaging if clinical judgment suggests the need to do so.
• Inquire about preexisting cervical spine conditions, especially in the elderly, because this may increase risk of injury or change radiographic interpretation.
• Suspect SCI until fully cleared through exam and imaging.
• Consider BCVI when neurologic deficits are inconsistent with level of known injury or in the setting of a significant mechanism of injury.

CERVICAL MALIGNANCY

Olga L. Nunez, MD • Jean Khara G. Casillan, RN, MD • Stuti Nagpal, MD, FAAFP

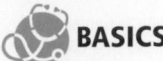 BASICS

DESCRIPTION
- Most cervical cancers begin in the transformation zone.
- 60–75% are from squamous epithelium and 25–40% are glandular.

EPIDEMIOLOGY

Incidence
- Cervical cancer is the second most common malignancy in women worldwide and the most common gynecologic cancer.
- The disease has a bimodal distribution, with the highest risk among women aged 40 to 59 years and >70 years. However, in recent years, there has been an increase in incidence in women aged 30 to 35 years.

Prevalence
- In 2018, the American Cancer Society (ACS) estimates 13,240 new cases of invasive cancer and 4,170 deaths in the United States.
- In the United States, Hispanic women are at highest risk followed by African Americans, Asians, and whites. American Indians and Alaskan natives have the lowest risk, perhaps attributed to low screening rates.

ETIOLOGY AND PATHOPHYSIOLOGY
- Human papillomavirus (HPV) infection is the most important etiologic factor. Infection with serotypes 16 and 18 account for 70% of all cervical cancer.
- Persistent HPV infection promotes coding errors in the cell cycle, resulting in dysplastic changes to the endocervical cellular lining. In addition, HPV activates E6 and E7 oncogenic proteins, which in turn inactivate p53 and Rb tumor suppressor genes.
- Tumor growth is via lymphatic and hematogenous spread (Halstedian growth).

RISK FACTORS
- Persistent HPV infection is the primary risk factor for developing cervical cancer.
- HPV infection has high prevalence with nearly 80 million people infected in the United States and 14 million new cases each year worldwide.
- Other risk factors include:
  - Lack of or decreased access to health care and ability to obtain regular Pap smears
  - Early coitarche
  - Multiple sexual partners
  - Unprotected sex
  - A history of sexually transmitted diseases (STDs)
  - Low socioeconomic status
  - Obesity (increases the risk for adenocarcinoma type)
  - High parity (>3 full-term deliveries)
  - Cigarette smoking (doubles the risk)
  - Immunosuppression (HIV/AIDS, chemotherapy)
  - Diethylstilbestrol (DES) exposure in utero

GENERAL PREVENTION
- Education on vaccination, safe sex practices, and smoking cessation are the cornerstone of prevention.
- HPV vaccines protect against the most common HPV strains associated with cervical cancer development, 16 and 18, as well the strains responsible for warts (6 and 11).
- There are three kind of FDA-approved vaccines, Gardasil 4, Gardasil 9, and Cervarix.

- Vaccination is recommended for:
  - Girl and boys ages 11 or 12 years, respectively, in 2 doses with 6 to 12 months apart
  - Children ≥14 years should receive 3 doses over the course of 6 months.
  - Immunocompromised patients ages 9 through 26 years, men who have sex with men, and the LGBTQ community
  - Women ages 9 through age 26 years
  - Men ages 9 through age 21 years
- Routine screening with Pap smear (or HPV testing) is virtually the only way to identify premalignant lesions and possibly prevent progression to cancer. Screening has the potential to prevent up to 80% of cervical cancer worldwide.
- Current guidelines from the American College of Obstetricians and Gynecologists (ACOG) and the American Society for Colposcopy and Cervical Pathology (ASCCP) screening should be performed as follows:
  - Cytology alone every 3 years between 21 and 29 years of age (1)[A]
  - Cytology plus HPV testing every 5 years after 30 years (1)[A]. The International Federation of Gynecology and Obstetrics (FIGO) recommends visual inspection with acetic acid (VIA) or Lugol iodine (VILI) as alternatives to Pap smears in resource-poor settings (2)[C].
- Despite HPV vaccination, cervical cancer screening will remain the main preventive measure for both vaccinated and unvaccinated women.

COMMONLY ASSOCIATED CONDITIONS
- Condyloma acuminata
- Preinvasive/invasive lesions of the vulva, vagina, oral and oropharyngeal cancers

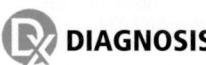 DIAGNOSIS

HISTORY
- Patient with HPV infection may be asymptomatic. The most common symptom is postcoital vaginal bleeding. Other symptoms are intermenstrual or postmenopausal bleeding and vaginal discharge.
- Less common symptoms include low back pain with radiation down posterior leg, lower extremity edema, vesicovaginal and rectovaginal fistula, and urinary symptoms.

PHYSICAL EXAM
- Thorough pelvic exam is essential:
  - Many patients have a normal exam, especially with microinvasive disease.
  - Lesions may be exophytic, endophytic, polypoid, papillary, ulcerative, or necrotic.
  - May have watery, purulent, or bloody discharge
- Bimanual and rectovaginal examination should be performed to evaluate uterine size; vaginal wall; rectovaginal septum; and parametrial, uterosacral, and pelvic sidewall involvement.
- Enlarged supraclavicular or inguinal lymphadenopathy, lower extremity edema, ascites, or decreased breath sounds with lung auscultation may indicate metastases or advanced disease.

DIFFERENTIAL DIAGNOSIS
- Marked cervicitis and erosion
- Glandular hyperplasia
- Sexually transmitted infections
- Cervical condyloma, leiomyoma, or polyp
- Metastasis from endometrial carcinoma or gestational trophoblastic neoplasia

DIAGNOSTIC TESTS & INTERPRETATION

Initial Tests (lab, imaging)
- Colposcopy with directed biopsies and/or biopsy of gross lesions are the definitive means of diagnosis.
- CBC may show anemia.
- Urinalysis may show hematuria.
- In advanced disease, BUN, creatinine, and liver function tests (LFTs) may be helpful.
- CT scan of the chest, abdomen, and pelvis and/or a positron emission tomography (PET) scan for metastatic workup
- Apart from chest x-ray (CXR) and intravenous pyelogram (IVP), imaging does not alter tumor stage.
- MRI may be helpful in evaluating parametrial involvement in patients who are surgical candidates or for radiation treatment planning.

Follow-Up Tests & Special Considerations
- Exam under anesthesia may be helpful in determining clinical stage, disease extent, and suitability for surgery.
- Endocervical curettage and cervical conization as indicated to determine depth of invasion and presence of lymphovascular involvement
- Cystoscopy to evaluate bladder invasion
- Proctoscopy for invasion into rectum

Test Interpretation
- Majority of cases are invasive squamous cell types arising from the ectocervix.
- Adenocarcinomas arise from endocervical mucus-producing glandular cells. Often, a "bulky," "barrel-shaped" cervix is present on exam.
- Other cell types include rare mixed cell types, neuroendocrine tumors, sarcomas, lymphomas, and melanomas.

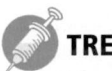 TREATMENT

GENERAL MEASURES
Improve nutritional state, correct anemia (Hb <12 g/dL), and treat pelvic infections.

MEDICATION
- Chemoradiation with cisplatin-containing regimen has superior survival over pelvic and extended-field radiation alone.
- Neoadjuvant chemotherapy may improve survival for early and locally advanced tumors, but more data are needed (3)[A].
- Adjuvant chemotherapy after chemoradiation may improve progression-free survival in patients who receive primary chemoradiation for stages IIB to IVA tumors. The OUTBACK trial will further investigate these findings (http://www.clinicaltrials.gov).
- The addition of the antiangiogenesis drug bevacizumab to standard combination chemotherapy (cisplatin/topotecan or cisplatin/paclitaxel) for recurrent, persistent, or metastatic disease has been shown to improve overall survival (4)[A].

ISSUES FOR REFERRAL
Multidisciplinary management of patients as needed and in a timely fashion

ADDITIONAL THERAPIES
- Chemoradiation (without surgery) is the first-line therapy for tumors stage IIB and higher (gross lesions with obvious parametrial involvement) and for most bulky stage IB2 tumors.

- Combination of external beam pelvic radiation and brachytherapy is usually employed.
- If para-aortic lymph node metastases are suspected, extended-field radiation or lymph node dissection prior to radiation therapy may be performed.

SURGERY/OTHER PROCEDURES

- Surgical management is an option for patients with early-stage tumors.
- Removal of precursor lesions (cervical intraepithelial neoplasia [CIN]) by loop electrosurgical excision procedure (LEEP), cold knife conization, laser ablation, or cryotherapy. Stage IA1 (lesions with <3-mm invasion from basement membrane) without lymphovascular space invasion: option of conization or simple extrafascial hysterectomy
- Stage IA2 (lesions with >3-mm but <5-mm invasion from basement membrane): option of radical hysterectomy with lymph node dissection or radiation depending on clinical setting. Robotic radical hysterectomy (RRH) has demonstrated to be superior to laparoscopic radical hysterectomy and open radical hysterectomy in intraoperative blood loss, length of hospital stay, and intraoperative and postoperative complications; RRH can be regarded as a safe and effective therapeutic procedure for the management of cervical cancer (5).
- Stages IA2 to IB1: Fertility-sparing radical trachelectomy may be considered in selected patients.
- Stages IB1 to IIA (gross lesions without obvious parametrial involvement): option of radical hysterectomy with lymph node sampling or primary chemoradiation with brachytherapy and teletherapy, depending on clinical setting. In stage IB, when comparing adjuvant radiotherapy with no adjuvant radiotherapy, there is no significant difference in survival at 5 years between women who received radiation and those who received no further treatment (risk ratio [RR] = 0.8, 95% confidence interval [CI] 0.3–2.4). However, women who received radiation had a significantly lower risk of disease progression at 5 years (RR 0.6, 95% CI 0.4–0.9) (6).
- Stage IVA (lesions limited to central metastasis to the bladder and/or rectum): Primary pelvic exenteration may be feasible.
- Stage IVB disease is treated with goal of palliation. Early referral to palliative care should be made.

Pregnancy Considerations

- Management is guided by consideration of stage of lesion, gestational age, and maternal assessment of risks and benefits from treatment.
- Abnormal cytology is best followed up by colposcopy with directed biopsies.
- In pregnant women diagnosed with cervical cancer before 16 weeks of gestation, treatment should be started immediately.
- In pregnant women with early stages (IA1, IA2, IB) diagnosed after 16 weeks of gestation, treatment may be delayed to allow for fetal maturity.
- In pregnant women with advance disease (stage IB2) diagnosed after 16 weeks, treatment may be based on gestational age at the time of diagnosis. Microinvasive carcinoma: conization or trachelectomy. If depth of invasion ≤3 mm, follow up at the 6-week postpartum visit.
- Invasive carcinoma requires definitive therapy, with timing determined by maternal preference, stage of disease, and gestational age at the time of diagnosis.

ADMISSION, INPATIENT, AND NURSING CONSIDERATIONS

- Signs of active bleeding
- Urinary symptoms
- Dehydration
- Complications from surgery, chemotherapy, or radiation
- Active vaginal bleeding can be controlled with timely vaginal packing and radiation therapy.
- Recognition of ureteral blockage, hydronephrosis, urosepsis, and timely intervention
- Discharge criteria based on multidisciplinary assessment

 ONGOING CARE

FOLLOW-UP RECOMMENDATIONS
Patient Monitoring

- With completion of definitive therapy and based on individual risk factors, patients are evaluated with physical/pelvic examinations:
  - Every 3 to 6 months for 2 years
  - Every 6 to 12 months until the 5th year
  - Yearly thereafter
- Pap smears may be performed yearly but have a low sensitivity for detecting recurrence.
- CT and PET scan are useful in locating metastasis when recurrence is suspected.
- Signs of recurrence include vaginal bleeding, unexplained weight loss, leg edema, and pelvic or thigh pain.

PATIENT EDUCATION

- ACOG at http://www.acog.org
- The Society of Gynecologic Oncology at http://www.sgo.org and the Foundation for Women's Cancer at http://www.foundationforwomenscancer.org
- American Cancer Society at http://www.cancer.org and the National Cancer Institute at http://www.cancer.gov

PROGNOSIS

- If detected early, invasive cervical cancer can be treated successfully.
- The 5-year survival rate for early stage (stage 1A, in which the cancer has minimal spread to the inside of the cervix) is estimated at 92%.
- An elevated squamous cell carcinoma antigen (SCC-Ag) serum levels estimated by ELISA technique can be used to predict the clinical response to neoadjuvant chemotherapy and residual disease. Persistently elevated SCC-Ag level at 2 to 3 months after RT had a significantly higher incidence of treatment failure.
- Serum SCC-Ag levels are also useful for monitoring treatment efficacy, disease progression, recurrence, and poor prognosis in SCCs. The combination of clinical pelvic examination and SCC-Ag levels provides useful information for the further need of treatment.

COMPLICATIONS

- Loss of ovarian function from radiotherapy or indication for bilateral oophorectomy
- Hemorrhage
- Pelvic infection
- Genitourinary fistula
- Bladder dysfunction
- Sexual dysfunction
- Ureteral obstruction with renal failure
- Bowel obstruction
- Pulmonary embolism
- Lower extremity lymphedema

REFERENCES

1. Committee on Practice Bulletins—Gynecology. ACOG Practice Bulletin Number 131: screening for cervical cancer. *Obstet Gynecol.* 2012;120(5):1222–1238.
2. International Federation of Gynecology and Obstetrics. Global guidance for cervical cancer prevention and control. http://www.rho.org/files/FIGO_cervical_cancer_guidelines_2009.pdf. Accessed January 4, 2018.
3. Rydzewska L, Tierney J, Vale CL, et al. Neoadjuvant chemotherapy plus surgery versus surgery for cervical cancer. *Cochrane Database Syst Rev.* 2012;(12):CD007406.
4. Tewari KS, Sill MW, Penson RT, et al. Bevacizumab for advanced cervical cancer: final overall survival and adverse event analysis of a randomised, controlled, open-label, phase 3 trial (Gynecologic Oncology Group 240). *Lancet.* 2017;390(10103):1654–1663.
5. Jin YM, Liu SS, Chen J, et al. Robotic radical hysterectomy is superior to laparoscopic radical hysterectomy and open radical hysterectomy in the treatment of cervical cancer. *PLoS One.* 2018;13(3):e0193033.
6. Rogers L, Siu SS, Luesley D, et al. Radiotherapy and chemoradiation after surgery for early cervical cancer. *Cochrane Database Syst Rev.* 2012;(5):CD007583.

ADDITIONAL READING

- Martin-Hirsch PP, Paraskevaidis E, Bryant A, et al. Surgery for cervical intraepithelial neoplasia. *Cochrane Database Syst Rev.* 2013;(12):CD001318.
- National Comprehensive Cancer Network. NCCN guidelines: cervical cancer. http://www.nccn.org/professionals/physician_gls/pdf/cervical.pdf. Accessed January 4, 2017.
- Scarinci IC, Garcia FA, Kobetz E, et al. Cervical cancer prevention: new tools and old barriers. *Cancer.* 2010;116(11):2531–2542.

 SEE ALSO

Abnormal Pap and Cervical Dysplasia

 CODES

ICD10

- C53.9 Malignant neoplasm of cervix uteri, unspecified
- C53.0 Malignant neoplasm of endocervix
- C53.1 Malignant neoplasm of exocervix

CLINICAL PEARLS

- Cervical cancer is the second most common malignancy in women worldwide. Improving access to screening is likely to have the greatest impact in reduction of the burden of disease.
- Women with cervical cancer may be asymptomatic and have a normal physical exam.
- Surgical management is an option for patients with early-stage tumors.
- Chemoradiation is the first-line therapy for higher stage tumors.

CHICKENPOX (VARICELLA ZOSTER)

Andrew J. Richardson, MD

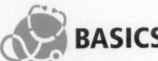

BASICS

DESCRIPTION

- Common, highly contagious, generalized exanthem characterized by crops of pruritic vesicles on the skin and mucous membranes following exposure to varicella-zoster virus (VZV)
- VZV is spread by respiratory (airborne) droplets and direct contact with vesicles.
- VZV establishes latency in the dorsal root ganglia; reactivation results in zoster (shingles).
- Outbreaks tend to occur late winter through early spring in temperate climates.
- Usual incubation period is 14 to 16 days (range: 10 to 21 days). Patients are infectious from ~48 hours before appearance of vesicles until the final lesions have crusted. Historically, most people acquired chickenpox during childhood and develop lifelong immunity. Varicella is currently part of recommended primary vaccination schedule.
- System(s) affected: nervous, skin/exocrine
- Synonym(s): varicella

EPIDEMIOLOGY

- Predominant age: peak incidence 3 to 9 years but may occur at any age
- Predominant gender: male = female

Incidence

- Decreasing incidence since routine vaccination; estimated 3.5 million cases annually prior to vaccine, with an incidence of 8–9% in children age 1 to 9 years
- Reported U.S. varicella cases: 1991: 147,076; 2015: 8,953 cases (1,2)
- Prior to vaccine, ~100 deaths per year were reported in the US; in 2015, there were 6 reported deaths (2).
- U.S. rates: 1994, prior to vaccine: 136/100,000 persons; 2013 to 2014: <0.001/100,000 persons
- Rates of varicella in the United States dropped after vaccine introduction until mid-2000s when they plateaued; second dose of vaccine recommended in 2006, and rates have again declined
- In developing countries, varicella is still associated with a severe disease burden.
- Susceptible (immunologically naive) individuals exposed to varicella are at risk to develop disease and are also potentially infectious for 21 days.

ETIOLOGY AND PATHOPHYSIOLOGY

- Skin lesions are histologically identical to herpes simplex virus.
- In fatal cases, intranuclear inclusions are found in vascular endothelium and most organs.
- VZV is a double-stranded DNA virus of the α-Herpesviridae subfamily.
- Humans are primary disease reservoir.

RISK FACTORS

- No history of prior varicella infection or immunization
- Immunocompromised (especially children with leukemia/lymphoma in remission or receiving high-dose corticosteroids)
- Pregnancy

Geriatric Considerations

- Infection is more severe in adults.
- Reactivation of latent infection causes zoster (shingles).
- The CDC recommends vaccinating all immunocompetent adults with the herpes zoster vaccine.
- Two forms of the vaccine are available. The recombinant zoster vaccine is currently preferred over the live attenuated vaccine.
- The recombinant zoster vaccine is administered as a 2-dose series separated by 2 to 6 months and can be given as early as age 50 years. This vaccine can be given to patients with a history of shingles or who have already had a dose of the live attenuated zoster vaccine (https://www.cdc.gov/vaccines/vpd/shingles/hcp/shingrix/recommendations.html).
- The live attenuated zoster vaccine can still be used as a single-dose vaccine for patients ≥60 years but should not be used in patients who are immunocompromised, such as those with HIV, on chronic steroid therapy, on chemotherapy, or those who have cancers affecting the bone marrow or lymphatic system (lymphoma, leukemia, etc.)
- Primary viral pneumonia is the most common cause of death from varicella.

Pediatric Considerations

- Neonates born to mothers who develop chickenpox from 5 days before to 2 days after delivery are at risk for serious disease and should receive varicella-zoster immune globulin (VZIG).
- Newborns are at highest risk for severe disease during the 1st month of life, especially if mother is seronegative.
- Delivery prior to 28 weeks increases risk.
- Varicella bullosa is seen mainly in children <2 years. Lesions appear as bullae instead of vesicles. The clinical course is otherwise similar.
- Septic complications and encephalitis are the most common causes of death from zoster in children.
- Avoid aspirin/acetylsalicylic acid in children because of link to Reye syndrome.

Pregnancy Considerations

- 25% risk of transplacental infection after maternal infection
- Congenital malformations are seen in 2% of patients when the fetus is infected during the 1st or 2nd trimester, characterized by limb atrophy, cutaneous scarring, and occasional CNS and eye manifestations.
- Morbidity (e.g., pneumonia) is increased in women infected during pregnancy.

GENERAL PREVENTION

- Isolate hospitalized patients.
- When indicated, administer passive immunization using VZIG within 96 hours (can be as long as up to 10 days) after exposure. VZIG recommended for:
  – Patients exposed to chickenpox or shingles who are immunocompromised, newborns of mothers with onset of chickenpox <5 days before delivery or <2 days after delivery, premature infants (<28 weeks) exposed in neonatal period either whose mothers are not immune, or babies who weigh <1,000 g regardless of maternal immunity

- Active immunization prevents or reduces the severity of varicella if given within 72 hours of exposure.
- Active immunization: varicella virus vaccine (Varivax): live attenuated vaccine recommended by ACIP for immunization of healthy patients ≥12 months who have not had chickenpox
  – 12 months to 12 years: initial dose 0.5 mL SC at age 12 to 15 months; second dose at age 4 to 6 years. Single dose is 85–94% effective in preventing severe disease. The 2-dose regimen is 96–98% effective. Breakthrough disease generally has <50 lesions, shorter duration, and lower fever incidence (3)[A].
  – ≥13 years: two 0.5 mL SC doses 4 to 8 weeks apart, seroconversion rates 78–82% after 1 dose, 99% after 2 doses; adult efficacy in lower end of this range
  – 2014 U.S. estimate: 91% one or more-dose vaccine coverage for children 19 to 35 months (4)
  – Vaccine side effects are pain and redness at the vaccine site (19% of children; 24% of teens and adults). 1 in 10 develops fever. 1 in 25 will develop a mild varicella-like rash up to 1 month after vaccination.
  – Vaccine contraindications
    ○ Severe allergic reaction (e.g., anaphylaxis) to a previous dose or vaccine component
    ○ Severe immunodeficiency (e.g., HIV patients with very low CD4 counts, chemotherapy, congenital immunodeficiency, long-term immunosuppressive therapy)
    ○ Pregnancy
- MMRV vaccine, combines the measles, mumps, and rubella vaccine with varicella, is equally effective. There are rare reports of an increased risk of febrile seizures 5 to 12 days after vaccination in 1/2,300 to 2,600 patients.
- May be considered for a subset of HIV-positive children in CDC class I with CD4 >25%
  – Vaccine recipients who develop a rash should avoid contact with immunocompromised people, pregnant women who have never had chickenpox, and their newborns.
  – Allow at least 3 months between doses 1 and 2 in children needing catch-up vaccination.

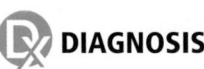

DIAGNOSIS

HISTORY

- Prodromal symptoms: fever, malaise, anorexia, mild headache
- Malaise, muscle aches, arthralgias, and headache are more common in adults.
- Subclinical in ~4% of cases
- Characteristic rash

PHYSICAL EXAM

- Characteristic rash: crops of vesicles on erythematous bases ("dew drops on a rose petal")
- Lesions erupt in successive crops.

- Progress from macule to papule to vesicle and then begin to crust
- Pruritic rash is present in various stages of development.
- Lesions may be present on mucous membranes, both oral and vaginal.

DIFFERENTIAL DIAGNOSIS
- Herpes simplex: herpes zoster
- Smallpox
- Impetigo
- Coxsackievirus infection
- Scabies
- Dermatitis herpetiformis
- Drug rash
- Rickettsial pox infection

DIAGNOSTIC TESTS & INTERPRETATION
The diagnosis of chickenpox is primarily clinical. Testing is generally reserved for complicated cases or epidemiologic studies.

Initial Tests (lab, imaging)
- VZV polymerase chain reaction (PCR) is the current method of choice (best is fluid from intact vesicle).
- Leukocyte count varies; marked leukocytosis suggests secondary infection.
- Multinucleated giant cells on Tzanck smear from vesicle scrapings
- Isolate virus from human tissue culture.

Follow-Up Tests & Special Considerations
- Serologies show acute (IgM) or prior (IgG) infection.
- Visualization by electron microscopy, tissue culture (costly), and various methods of acute and convalescent sera collection: latex agglutination (most available), enzyme immunoassay, indirect immunofluorescence antibody, fluorescent antibody to membrane assay, or PCR assay, which can detect wild from vaccine viral strains
- Vaccine-modified cases can be more difficult to diagnose; PCR testing of skin lesions is most sensitive and specific for diagnosing varicella, especially in vaccinated persons.

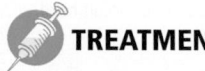 TREATMENT

Generally outpatient, except for complicated cases

GENERAL MEASURES
- Supportive/symptomatic treatment
- Antihistamines and/or oatmeal baths for itch
- Acetaminophen and/or ibuprofen for pain and fever
- Clipping nails can help prevent scarring or secondary infection from excessive itching.

MEDICATION
First Line
- Supportive: antipyretics for fever; avoid aspirin in children.
- Local and/or systemic antipruritic agents for itching

- VZIG available for passive immunization for:
  - Immunocompromised patients, newborn infants of mothers who have signs and symptoms of varicella at the time of delivery; premature infants born at 28 weeks or more whose mothers do not have evidence of immunity to varicella; premature infants <28 weeks' gestation or who weigh <1,000 g regardless of maternal immunity
  - Give VZIG within 96 hours after exposure (5).
- Acyclovir: decreases duration of fever and shortens time of viral shedding; recommended for adolescents, adults, and high-risk patients; most beneficial if initiated early in the disease (≤24 hours)
  - 2- to 16-year-old patients: 20 mg/kg/dose (max 800 mg/dose) QID for 5 days
  - Adults: 800 mg 5 times daily for 5 days
- Contraindication
  - Hypersensitivity to the drug
- Precautions
  - Renal insufficiency with acyclovir
  - Concurrent administration of probenecid increases half-life; increased effects with zidovudine (e.g., drowsiness, lethargy)

Second Line
- Famciclovir: 500 mg TID for 7 to 10 days (adults)
- Valacyclovir: 1 g TID for 7 to 10 days (adults)

 ONGOING CARE

FOLLOW-UP RECOMMENDATIONS
Patient Monitoring
- Not needed in mild cases. Intensive supportive care may be required in the setting of complications.
- Activity as tolerated. Children may return to school when lesions have completely scabbed.

DIET
No special diet

PATIENT EDUCATION
- In otherwise healthy children, chickenpox is rarely serious and the recovery is almost always complete.
- Native chickenpox typically confers lifelong immunity.
- A second attack is rare, but subclinical infection can occur; occasionally, after vaccination in children
- Latent infection may recur years later as herpes zoster in adults (and sometimes in children).
- Fatalities are rare.

COMPLICATIONS
- Although only 2% of cases are reported after 2nd decade, 35% of deaths occur in this age group.
- Secondary bacterial infection: cellulitis, abscess, erysipelas, sepsis, septic arthritis/osteomyelitis, or staphylococcal pyomyositis
- Pneumonia: 20–30% of adults with chickenpox have lung involvement; 1/400 is hospitalized.
- Encephalitis (the most common CNS complication)
- Meningitis; Reye syndrome
- Purpura, thrombocytopenia
- Glomerulonephritis; arthritis; hepatitis

REFERENCES
1. Centers for Disease Control and Prevention. Summary of notifiable diseases: United States, 2009. *MMWR Morb Mortal Wkly Rep.* 2011;58(53):1–100.
2. Centers for Disease Control and Prevention. National notifiable infectious diseases and conditions: United States. https://wonder.cdc.gov/nndss/static/2016/annual/2016-table2o.html. Accessed October 20, 2018.
3. Marin M, Güris D, Chaves SS, et al; for Advisory Committee on Immunization Practices, Centers for Disease Control and Prevention. Prevention of varicella: recommendations of the Advisory Committee on Immunization Practices (ACIP). *MMWR Recomm Rep.* 2007;56(RR-4):1–40.
4. Hill HA, Elam-Evans L, Yankey D, et al. National, state, and selected local area vaccination coverage among children aged 19-35 months—United States, 2014. *MMWR Morb Mortal Wkly Rep.* 2015;64(33):889–896.
5. Centers for Disease Control and Prevention. Updated recommendations for use of VariZIG—United States, 2013. *MMWR Morb Mortal Wkly Rep.* 2013;62(28):574–576.

ADDITIONAL READING
- Dooling KL, Guo A, Patel M, et al. Recommendations of the Advisory Committee on Immunization Practices for use of herpes zoster vaccines. *MMWR Morb Mortal Wkly Rep.* 2018;67(3):103–108.
- Laing KJ, Ouwendijk WJD, Koelle DM, et al. Immunobiology of varicella-zoster virus infections. *J Infect Dis.* 2018;218(Suppl 2):S68–S74.

 SEE ALSO

Herpes Zoster (Shingles)

CODES

ICD10
- B01.9 Varicella without complication
- B02.9 Zoster without complications
- P35.8 Other congenital viral diseases

CLINICAL PEARLS
- Varicella zoster infection is more likely to produce serious illness in adults than in children.
- Introduction of the varicella vaccine has reduced morbidity and mortality. Currently, 2 doses of vaccine are recommended.
- Recombinant herpes zoster vaccine is recommended for immunocompetent persons ≥50 years of age to decrease chance of shingles.

CHILD ABUSE

Karen A. Hulbert, MD

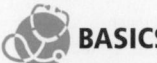 **BASICS**

DESCRIPTION

- Types of abuse: neglect (most common and highest mortality), physical abuse, emotional/psychological abuse, sexual abuse
- Neglect includes physical (e.g., failure to provide necessary food or shelter or lack of appropriate supervision), medical (e.g., failure to provide necessary medical or mental health treatment), educational (e.g., failure to educate a child or attend to special education needs), and emotional (e.g., inattention to a child's emotional needs, failure to provide psychological care, or permitting the child to use alcohol or other drugs).
- System(s) affected: gastrointestinal (GI), endocrine/metabolic, musculoskeletal, nervous, renal, reproductive, skin/exocrine, psychiatric
- Synonym(s): suspected nonaccidental trauma; child maltreatment; child neglect

EPIDEMIOLOGY

Incidence

- The National Incidence Study (NIS) estimates the incidence of neglect in the United States using estimates from child protective services (CPS) statistics and other sources. Most recent *NIS-4* (published 2010) looked at data from 2004 to 2009.
- Using the stringent "harm standard" definition, >1.25 million children experience maltreatment (1 in 58).
- Using the "endangerment standard," 3 million children experienced maltreatment (1 child in 25).

Prevalence

Children's Bureau report for federal fiscal year (FFY) 2015 (1):

- CPS agencies received an estimated 4.0 million referrals (national referral rate of 53.2 referrals per 1,000 children).
- Approximately 3.4 million children received either an investigation or alternative response. Of those investigated, 9.2 per 1,000 children were found to be victims of abuse or neglect.
- The overall rate of child fatalities was 2.25 deaths per 100,000 children in the national population.
- The majority of perpetrators were parents—one or both parents maltreated 91.6% of victims.
- Types of maltreatment:
  - 75.3% neglect
  - 17.2% physical abuse
  - 8.4% sexual abuse

RISK FACTORS

- African American children had the highest rates of victimization at 14.5 per 1,000 children (1).
- Children in the age group of birth to 1 year had the highest rate of victimization (1).
- Slightly more than one half of the child victims were girls and 48.6% were boys.
  - Risk of physical abuse increases with age.
  - Risk of fatal abuse is more common in those <3 years (74.8% of children who died were <3 years old).
- Poverty, drug abuse, lower educational status, parental history of abuse, mentally ill parent/maternal depression, poor support network, and domestic violence:
  - Child abuse is 4.9 times more likely in family with spouse abuse.
  - Children in households with unrelated adults, 50 times more likely to die of inflicted injuries
  - Adults who were abused as children are at higher risk of becoming abusers than those not abused.

GENERAL PREVENTION

- Know your patients and document their family situations; have increased suspicion to screen for risk factors at prenatal, postnatal, and pediatric visits.
- Physicians can educate parents on range of normal behaviors to expect in infants and children:
  - Anticipatory guidance on ways to handle crying infants; methods of discipline for toddlers
- Train first responders—teachers, childcare workers—to look for signs of abuse.
- Some studies suggest developing screening tools to identify high-risk families early and offer interventions such as early childhood home visitation programs.

COMMONLY ASSOCIATED CONDITIONS

- Failure to thrive
- Prematurity
- Developmental deficits
- Poor school performance
- Poor social skills
- Low self-esteem, depression

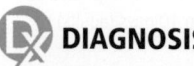 **DIAGNOSIS**

- Relatively minor injuries, frenulum tears, or bruising in precruising infants may be the first indications of child physical abuse; these minor, suspicious injuries have been termed "sentinel injuries" (2)[B].
- In a retrospective study of infants who were definitely abused, 27.5% had a sentinel injury (80% had a bruise), and in 41.9% of those cases, the parent reported that a medical provider was aware of the injury (2)[B].
- Patients may present with seemingly unrelated complaints; multiple studies have documented repeated visits (to the PCP, to the emergency department [ED]) before child abuse is suspected.
- Infants with injuries caused by child abuse often present with vague complaints; important to have high index of suspicion when evaluating infants for fussiness
- Documentation
  - The medical record is an important piece of evidence for investigation and litigation (3)[C].
  - Critical elements include the following (3)[C]:
    - Brief statement of child's disclosure or caregiver's explanation, including any alternate explanations offered
    - Time the incident occurred and date/time of disclosure
    - Whether witnesses were present
    - Developmental abilities of child
    - Objective medical findings
- DO NOT use terms such as "rule out," "R/O," and "alleged." They may cause ambiguity; clearly state physician opinion (3)[C].
- The child should be separated from the parent for the interview if at all possible.
- Any description of abuse given by the child should be recorded word for word using quotation marks in the child's own language and attributed to the child.
- The child should not be rewarded after a disclosure (e.g., "Tell me what happened and you can go back to your mom . . . ").
- Remember this is a medical interview and physician is obtaining information needed for diagnostic and treatment decisions.
- Documentation should include disposition of patient and record any report made to CPS (3)[C].

HISTORY

- History of a sentinel injury should prompt consideration of abuse; it may be the first and only abusive injury; there may be escalating and repeated violence instead of a single event of momentary loss of control (2)[B].
- Use nonjudgmental, open-ended questions (ask: who, what, when, and where; NEVER why).
- Use quotes whenever possible.
- Document past medical and developmental history, child's temperament, and family interactions.
- Suggestive of intentional trauma
  - No explanation or vague explanation
  - Important detail of explanation changes dramatically.
  - Explanation is inconsistent with pattern, age, or severity.
  - Explanation is inconsistent with child's physical or developmental abilities.
  - Different witnesses provide different history.
  - Considerable delay in seeking treatment
- Nonspecific symptoms of abuse:
  - Behavior changes; self-destructive behavior
  - Anxiety and/or depression
  - Sleep disturbances, night terrors
  - School problems

PHYSICAL EXAM

- Explain what the exam will involve and why procedures are needed. Examine child in a comfortable setting.
- Allow child to choose who will be in the room.
- Use appropriate positions to examine the anal and genital areas of children.
- General assessment for signs of physical abuse, neglect, and self-injurious behaviors
- Thorough physical exam
  - Skin, head, eyes, ears, nose, and mouth
  - Chest/abdomen
  - Genital (consider exam under sedation) or refer to ED
  - Extremities, with focus on inner arms and legs
  - Growth data
- Maintain high index of suspicion for occult head, chest, and abdominal trauma.
- Physical abuse
  - Skin markings (e.g., lacerations, burns, ecchymoses, linear/shaped contusions, bites)
  - Immersion injuries with clearly distinguished outlines (e.g., from boiling water)
  - Oral trauma (e.g., torn frenulum, loose teeth)
  - Ear trauma (e.g., signs of ear pulling)
  - Eye trauma (e.g., hyphema, hemorrhage)
  - Head/abdominal blunt trauma
  - Fractures
- Sexual abuse
  - Unexplained penile, vaginal, hymenal, perianal, or anal injuries/bleeding/discharge
  - Pregnancy or STIs
  - Sperm is a definitive finding of child abuse.
- Neglect
  - Child may be low weight for height, unclean, unkempt.
  - Rashes
  - Fearful or too trusting
  - Clinging to or avoiding caregiver
  - Flat or balding occiput
  - Abnormal development or growth parameters
- Measurements, photographs, and careful descriptions are critical for accurate diagnosis.
- Collaboration with specialist and child abuse assessment team

C

DIFFERENTIAL DIAGNOSIS

- Physical trauma
  - Accidental injury; toxic ingestion
  - Bleeding disorders (e.g., classic hemophilia)
  - Metabolic or congenital conditions
  - Conditions with skin manifestations (e.g., mongolian spots, Henoch-Schönlein purpura, meningococcemia, erythema multiforme, hypersensitivity, car seat burns, staphylococcal scalded skin syndrome, chickenpox, impetigo)
  - Cultural practices (e.g., cupping, coining)
- Neglect
  - Endocrinopathies (e.g., diabetes mellitus)
  - Constitutional
  - GI (clefts, malabsorption, irritable bowel)
  - Seizure disorder
  - Sudden infant death syndrome (SIDS)
- Skeletal trauma
  - Obstetrical trauma
  - Nutritional (scurvy, rickets)
  - Infection (congenital syphilis, osteomyelitis)
  - Osteogenesis imperfecta

DIAGNOSTIC TESTS & INTERPRETATION

Initial Tests (lab, imaging)

- Directed by history and physical exam:
  - Urinalysis (e.g., abdominal/flank/back/genital trauma), urine DNA probe for STIs
  - CBC, bleeding, abdominal trauma
  - Electrolytes, creatinine, BUN, glucose
  - Liver and pancreatic function tests (e.g., abdominal trauma)
  - Guaiac stool (abdominal trauma)
- In cases of suspected neglect:
  - Stool exam, calorie count, purified protein derivative and anergy panel, sweat test, lead and zinc levels
- In cases of suspected sexual abuse:
  - STI testing: gonorrhea, chlamydia, *Trichomonas*; also consider HIV, herpes simplex virus (HSV), hepatitis panel, syphilis.
  - The American Academy of Pediatrics (AAP) recommends the use of NAATs when evaluating children and adolescents for *Chlamydia trachomatis* and *Neisseria gonorrhoeae*.
  - Serum pregnancy test
- Skeletal survey is a mainstay of child abuse evaluation; 22 radiographs. It is recommended for:
  - Infants <6 months with bruising, regardless of pattern (given rarity of accidental bruising in young nonmobile infants)
  - Children with bruising attributed to abuse or domestic violence
  - Children <12 months with bruising on the cheek, eye area, ear, neck, upper arm, upper leg, hand, foot, torso, buttocks, or genital area
  - All children with fractures and children with suspicious injuries <2 years:
    - Consider bone scan for acute rib fractures and subtle long bone fractures.
  - Intracranial and extracranial injury:
    - CT scan of head
    - Consider MRI of head/neck for better dating of injuries, looking at subtle findings, intercerebral edema, or hemorrhage.
  - Intra-abdominal injuries:
    - CT scan of abdomen

Follow-Up Tests & Special Considerations

- Bruising is a common presenting feature:
  - Bruising in babies who are not independently mobile is very uncommon (<1%).

- Patterns suggestive of abuse
  - Bruises seen away from bony prominences
  - Bruises to face, back, abdomen, arms, buttocks, ears, hands
  - Multiple bruises in clusters or uniform shape
  - Patterned injuries (such as bite marks or the imprint of an object like a belt or cord) should be considered inflicted until proven otherwise.
- Red flags
  - History that is inconsistent with the injury
  - No explanation offered for the injury or injury blamed on sibling or another child
  - History that is inconsistent with the child's developmental level
- Sexual abuse
  - Consider whether child should be triaged to facility such as children's hospital where collection of forensic samples can be performed.

Test Interpretation

- Spiral fractures in nonambulatory patients (Children who are not walking or cruising should not have bruising or fractures from "falls.")
- Chip or bucket-handle fractures
- Epiphyseal/metaphyseal rib fractures in infants
- Rupture of liver/spleen in abdominal blunt trauma
- Retinal hemorrhages in shaken baby syndrome
- Recent literature notes a greater risk of abuse with skull and femur fractures, unexplained injuries, and a delay in seeking care.

 TREATMENT

GENERAL MEASURES

- If diagnosed with STI, treat promptly.
- If HIV exposure possible, consider prophylaxis.

MEDICATION

First Line

Antibiotics as indicated for STIs

> **ALERT**
> Emergency contraception reduces rate of pregnancy after sexual assault:

- Levonorgestrel (Plan B): single dose of 1.5 mg or two 0.75-mg doses taken together or 12 hours apart; effective up to 72 hours
- Ulipristal (Ella): 30-mg single dose as soon as possible; effective up to 120 hours

ISSUES FOR REFERRAL

Responding to possible abuse, consider:

- The child's safety; is the child at imminent risk or additional harm if sent back to environment where possible perpetrator has access to child?
- Health professionals report *suspected* abuse/neglect.
- Child's mental health
  - Need for a physical exam and need for forensic collection; consider referral to ER.

ADMISSION, INPATIENT, AND NURSING CONSIDERATIONS

Admission if:

- Moderate to severe injuries or unstable
- Acute psychological trauma
- Safety of child outside the hospital cannot be guaranteed.

 ONGOING CARE

FOLLOW-UP RECOMMENDATIONS

As clinically indicated

Patient Monitoring

- Monitor injury healing over time.
- Follow up assessment for STIs that may not present acutely (e.g., HPV).

PROGNOSIS

Without intervention, child abuse is often a chronic and escalating phenomenon.

COMPLICATIONS

Sexual, physical, and emotional abuse in childhood are risk factors for poorer adult mental and physical health; includes maltreatment and depressive disorder, drug use, suicide attempts, and risky sexual behaviors

REFERENCES

1. Children's Bureau. Child maltreatment 2015. https://www.acf.hhs.gov/programs/cb/resource/child-maltreatment-2015. Accessed November 14, 2017.
2. Sheets LK, Leach ME, Koszewski IJ, et al. Sentinel injuries in infants evaluated for child physical abuse. *Pediatrics*. 2013;131(4):701–707.
3. Jackson AM, Rucker A, Hinds T, et al. Let the record speak: medicolegal documentation in cases of child maltreatment. *Clin Ped Emerg Med*. 2006;7(3):181–185.

ADDITIONAL READING

- American Academy of Pediatrics. Child abuse and neglect. https://www.aap.org/en-us/advocacy-and-policy/aap-health-initiatives/resilience/Pages/Child-Abuse-and-Neglect.aspx. Accessed November 14, 2017.
- Centers for Disease Control and Prevention. Violence prevention: child abuse and neglect prevention. https://www.cdc.gov/violenceprevention/childabuseandneglect/index.html. Accessed December 26, 2018.

 CODES

ICD10

- T74.12XA Child physical abuse, confirmed, initial encounter
- T74.32XA Child psychological abuse, confirmed, initial encounter
- T74.22XA Child sexual abuse, confirmed, initial encounter

CLINICAL PEARLS

- When a bruise is present, it should be considered as potentially sentinel for physical abuse if no plausible explanation is given.
- High index of suspicion is important for prevention and recognition of abuse. Vague complaints and repeated visits to the office and/or ED should prompt further investigation.
- Neglect is the most common and lethal form of abuse and should be aggressively reported.
- Detailed exam with documentation is key.
- Mandated reporting is required for *suspected* child abuse and neglect; the physician does not have to prove abuse before reporting.
- National hotline: 800.4.A.CHILD (800.422.4453)
- National resources: https://www.childwelfare.gov/pubs/reslist/tollfree/

CHLAMYDIA INFECTION (SEXUALLY TRANSMITTED)

Casandra Cashman, MD, FAAFP

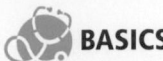 **BASICS**

DESCRIPTION

- *Chlamydia trachomatis* is an intracellular membrane-bound prokaryotic organism. Chlamydia derives from the Greek word for "cloak."
- Chlamydia is the most common bacterial sexually transmitted infection (STI) in the United States (1)[A].
- Transmitted through vaginal, anal, or oral sex; transmitted vertically during vaginal delivery
- Most cases are asymptomatic, especially in females. Untreated disease can lead to pelvic inflammatory disease (PID), ectopic pregnancy, and infertility.
- System(s) affected: reproductive

Pregnancy Considerations
Perinatal acquisition may result in neonatal pneumonia and/or conjunctivitis.

EPIDEMIOLOGY

Incidence
- Mandatory reporting started in 1985; there has generally been a steady increase in incidence since.
- ~1.6 million *reported* cases in 2016. Increasing incidence reflects broader screening, improved testing, and better reporting (rather than a large increase in disease burden) (1).
- Swedish new variant of *C. trachomatis* (nvCT) first reported in 2006; often produces false-negative tests; largely confined to Nordic countries

Prevalence
- 497/100,000 people in the United States in 2016 (1)
- Young females, ethnic minorities most affected
- Highest prevalence ages 20 to 24 years
- Predominant sex: females > males. Females have 2 times higher reported incidence and prevalence than males. This likely reflects increased testing in females. Increasing use of highly sensitive nucleic acid amplification test (NAAT) urine screening may increase identification in males.
- Infection rates ~6 times higher in blacks than whites. Rates are higher in larger urban areas.
- Highest male prevalence in heterosexual adolescents
- Estimated to affect ~2% of young sexually active individuals in the United States

ETIOLOGY AND PATHOPHYSIOLOGY
C. trachomatis serotypes D to K associated with genital tract infections. Chlamydia is an obligate intracellular organism. Chlamydia has biphasic life cycle. Exists extracellularly as elementary body (EB) that is metabolically inactive and infectious. Once taken up by host cell (typically columnar epithelium of the genital tract), the EB prevents lysosomal phagocytosis and transforms to reticulate body (RB) which requires energy from host cell to synthesize RNA, DNA, and proteins. After taking up host cell residence, EB are released and are capable of infecting neighboring cells or spreading the infection through sexual contact.

RISK FACTORS
Risk correlates with:
- Number of lifetime sexual partners and number of concurrent sexual partners
- No use of barrier contraception during intercourse
- Black/Hispanic/Native American and Alaskan Native ethnicity
- Men who have sex with men (MSM) may be at higher risk for rectal and pharyngeal chlamydia than other groups; consider testing with NAAT when appropriate (2)[B].

GENERAL PREVENTION
- Screen populations with prevalence >5% at least annually (1)[A].
- Screening recommended if new or >1 sex partner in past 6 months; attending an adolescent clinic, family planning clinic, STD or abortion clinic, or attending a jail or other detention center clinic. Screen if rectal pain, discharge or tenesmus, testicular pain; test all individuals with urethral or cervical discharge.
- All sexually active women ≤25 years of age should be screened at least yearly. Repeat testing in ~3 months is recommended for those who screen positive because reinfection rate is high regardless of whether the sexual partner is treated (3)[A].
- Consider screening sexually active men ≤25 years of age particularly in high-risk populations.
- Screen high-risk MSM annually with genital and extragenital screening (4)[A].
- NAAT is the preferred screening test in all circumstances except child sexual abuse involving boys or rectal/oropharyngeal testing in prepubescent girls. For these situations, culture and susceptibility testing is preferred (4)[A].
- Acceptable to screen women for chlamydia on same day as intrauterine device (IUD) insertion—treat if positive (no need to remove IUD in this circumstance) (5)[B]

COMMONLY ASSOCIATED CONDITIONS
- Females
  - PID: ~10% develop PID within 12 months if untreated.
  - Infertility, ectopic pregnancy
  - Chronic pelvic pain
  - Urethral syndrome (dysuria, frequency, and pyuria in the absence of infection)
  - Arthritis (less common)
  - Spontaneous abortion
- Males
  - Epididymitis and nongonococcal urethritis
  - Reiter syndrome (HLA-B27)
  - Proctitis
- Neonates
  - Inclusion conjunctivitis (occurs in ~40% of exposed neonates)
  - Otitis media
  - Pneumonia
  - Pharyngitis
- Diseases caused by other chlamydial species
  - Lymphogranuloma venereum (LGV): *C. trachomatis* serotypes L1 to L3
  - Trachoma: *C. trachomatis* serotypes A to C

 DIAGNOSIS

Many patients are asymptomatic.

Pregnancy Considerations
- Test all patients at first prenatal visit.
- Obtain repeat testing 3 to 4 weeks after treatment for all pregnant patients with confirmed chlamydial infection. Test again 3 months after.
- Repeat screening in 3rd trimester in high-risk patients (3)[A].

HISTORY
- Complete sexual history, including number of sex partners (lifetime and past year), prior history of STIs, use of barrier protection, commercial sex work, oral or anal receptive intercourse, and partner fidelity
- In females, the most common symptoms are:
  - Mucopurulent vaginal discharge, dysuria (urethral syndrome), bartholinitis, abdominopelvic pain (endometritis, salpingitis/PID), right upper quadrant pain (Fitz-Hugh–Curtis syndrome)
- In males, the most common symptoms are:
  - Dysuria, urethral discharge (urethritis), scrotal pain (epididymitis), rectal pain or discharge (proctitis), acute arthritis (Reiter syndrome)

PHYSICAL EXAM
- Men and women: external genitalia (rash, lesions), urethral discharge, inguinal lymphadenopathy, pharyngeal exudate, and perianal lesions
- Women: cervix (discharge, motion tenderness), bimanual examination for cervical motion tenderness, uterine, ovarian/adnexal tenderness or mass
- LGV (*C. trachomatis* serovars L1, L2, or L3): Primary lesion is a small papule that may ulcerate at the site of transmission after an incubation period of 3 to 30 days. Unilateral tender lymphadenopathy. With rectal transmission, LGV causes an invasive proctocolitis.

DIFFERENTIAL DIAGNOSIS
- *Neisseria gonorrhoeae*: urethritis, proctitis, epididymitis, cervicitis, PID, Bartholin abscess
- *Mycoplasma* or *Ureaplasma urealyticum*: urethritis, epididymitis, Reiter disease, PID
- *C. trachomatis* (serotypes L1 to L3): LGV, proctitis
- Trichomoniasis

DIAGNOSTIC TESTS & INTERPRETATION
Initial Tests (lab, imaging)
- NAAT: sensitivity >95%; specificity >99%
- Urine test is as sensitive as cervical swab.
- Self-collected vaginal swabs are effective.
- Lab result may remain positive for 3 weeks after successful treatment.
- Test for concurrent STIs, including gonorrhea, HIV, and syphilis; perform cervical cancer (Pap smear) screening according to recommended guidelines.

Follow-Up Tests & Special Considerations
See "Patient Monitoring."

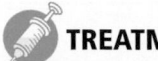 **TREATMENT**

GENERAL MEASURES
- Offer patients concurrent testing for gonorrhea, HIV (after counseling and consent), and possibly syphilis. Ensure women are up to date with recommended cervical cancer screening.
- Consider treating gonorrhea empirically.
- Test and treat all partners (most recent partner and all partners within the past 60 days).

MEDICATION
First Line
- http://www.cdc.gov/std/tg2015/chlamydia.htm
- Treatment of chlamydial urethritis, cervicitis (including sexual partners of infected persons)
- Azithromycin 1 g PO single dose or
- Doxycycline 100 mg PO BID for 7 days
- First-line PID treatment (outpatient)
  – Ceftriaxone 250 mg IM × 1 *plus* doxycycline 100 mg PO for 14 days with or without metronidazole 500 mg PO BID for 14 days *or*
  – Cefoxitin 2 g IM × 1 with probenecid 1 g PO × 1 *plus* doxycycline 100 mg PO for 14 days with or without metronidazole 500 mg PO BID for 14 days
- Azithromycin and ceftriaxone may be given simultaneously in the office to treat both chlamydia and gonorrhea. This reduces nonadherence (2)[A].
- Asymptomatic rectal chlamydia can be treated with doxycycline 100 mg BID × 7 days. Azithromycin 1 g for 1 day is slightly less effective but can also be used, especially if compliance or medication availability is an issue (6)[A].

ALERT
Use azithromycin with caution in patients with known QT prolongation, hypokalemia, hypomagnesemia, bradycardia, or who are currently treated with antiarrhythmics.

Pregnancy Considerations
- Tetracyclines (doxycycline) and quinolones (ofloxacin, levofloxacin) are contraindicated in pregnant women.
- Consider the following:
  – Azithromycin 1 g PO *or*
  – Amoxicillin 500 mg PO TID for 7 days (3)[A] *or*
  – Erythromycin base 500 mg PO QID for 7 days

ALERT
Tetracyclines and quinolones are contraindicated in young children:
- <45 kg: erythromycin base or ethinyl succinate 500 mg/kg/day PO QID for 14 days
- >45 kg but <8 years: azithromycin 1 g PO once
- >8 years: adult regimen
- Rule out sexual abuse in children with chlamydial infections.

Second Line
For chlamydial urethritis/cervicitis
- Erythromycin base 500 mg PO QID for 7 days OR erythromycin ethylsuccinate 800 mg PO QID for 7 days
- Levofloxacin 500 mg PO daily for 7 days or ofloxacin 300 mg PO BID for 7 days

ADDITIONAL THERAPIES
Patient-delivered partner therapy (PDPT) or expedited partner therapy (EPT): Provide medications or prescriptions to take to sexual partners of persons infected with STIs without clinical assessment.
- EPT reduces recurrence more effectively than traditional partner referral.
- http://www.cdc.gov/std/ept/legal/

ADMISSION, INPATIENT, AND NURSING CONSIDERATIONS
- Inpatient treatment of PID: pregnancy, lack of response or intolerance to oral medicines, suspicion of poor compliance, severe clinical illness, pelvic abscess, and possible need for surgical intervention
- Otherwise, treat PID as outpatient unless moderately or severely ill.

 ONGOING CARE

FOLLOW-UP RECOMMENDATIONS
Abstain from sexual contact for at least 7 days after treatment (single-dose treatment) or until completion of the full course of other antibiotics.

Patient Monitoring
- Test of cure not routinely recommended except in pregnancy. Do not repeat NAAT <3 weeks after testing; may be falsely positive due to nonviable organisms
- Test of cure in 3 to 4 weeks in pregnancy as well as test for reinfection in 3 months.
- Consider rescreening higher risk pregnant women in 3rd trimester even if initial screening negative.
- Test for reinfection (not cure) 3 months after treatment or, if not possible, then at next presentation to medical care if within 12 months.
- Sexual partners should be treated.

PATIENT EDUCATION
- Counsel regarding safe sexual practices, barrier protection, and abstinence.
- Complete antibiotic course (patient and partners).

PROGNOSIS
Prognosis is good following therapy.

COMPLICATIONS
- Both sexes: Chlamydial infection enhances transmission of and susceptibility to HIV.
- Females: tubal infertility (most common cause of acquired infertility), tubal (ectopic) pregnancy, chronic pelvic pain
  – Annual screening of sexually active women would prevent 61% of chlamydia-related PID.
- Males: transient oligospermia and postepididymitis urethral stricture (rare)

REFERENCES
1. Centers for Disease Control and Prevention. 2016 sexually transmitted disease surveillance. http://www.cdc.gov/std/stats16/chlamydia.htm. Accessed June 29, 2018.
2. Pinsky L, Chiarilli DB, Klausner JD, et al. Rates of asymptomatic nonurethral gonorrhea and chlamydia in a population of university men who have sex with men. *J Am Coll Health*. 2012;60(6): 481–484.
3. Centers for Disease Control and Prevention. 2015 sexually transmitted diseases treatment guidelines. http://www.cdc.gov/std/tg2015/chlamydia.htm. Accessed June 29, 2018.
4. Centers for Disease Control and Prevention. Recommendations for the laboratory-based detection of *Chlamydia trachomatis* and *Neisseria gonorrhoeae*—2014. http://www.cdc.gov/mmwr/preview/mmwrhtml/rr6302a1.htm. Accessed June 29, 2018.
5. Sufrin CB, Postlethwaite D, Armstrong MA, et al. *Neisseria gonorrhea* and *Chlamydia trachomatis* screening at intrauterine device insertion and pelvic inflammatory disease. *Obstet Gynecol*. 2012;120(6):1314–1321.
6. Elgalib A, Alexander S, Tong CY, et al. Seven days of doxycycline is an effective treatment for asymptomatic rectal *Chlamydia trachomatis* infection. *Int J STD AIDS*. 2011;22(8):474–477.

ADDITIONAL READING
- Drummond F, Ryder N, Wand H, et al. Is azithromycin adequate treatment for asymptomatic rectal chlamydia? *Int J STD AIDS*. 2011;22(8):478–480.
- Price MJ, Ades AE, De Angelis D, et al. Risk of pelvic inflammatory disease following *Chlamydia trachomatis* infection: analysis of prospective studies with a multistate model. *Am J Epidemiol*. 2013;178(3):484–492.
- Won H, Ramachandran P, Steece R, et al. Is there evidence of the new variant *Chlamydia trachomatis* in the United States? *Sex Transm Dis*. 2013;40(5):352–353.

 SEE ALSO

Cervicitis, Ectropion, and True Erosion; Epididymitis; Gonococcal Infections; HIV/AIDS; Pelvic Inflammatory Disease (PID); Syphilis; Urethritis

 CODES

ICD10
- A56.8 Sexually transmitted chlamydial infection of other sites
- A56.01 Chlamydial cystitis and urethritis
- A56.02 Chlamydial vulvovaginitis

CLINICAL PEARLS
- *C. trachomatis* is common in young sexually active individuals. Annual screening is recommended in sexually active women 25 years of age and younger and in other individuals with known risk factors.
- To prevent recurrence, treat patients and their partners concurrently.
- Test of cure is only recommended for pregnant patients 3 to 4 weeks after treatment for an identified chlamydia infection. Test for reinfection 3 months afterward. Repeat screens in 3rd trimester for high-risk patients regardless of initial test results.

CHOLELITHIASIS
Hongyi Cui, MD, PhD

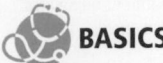 **BASICS**

DESCRIPTION
- The presence of cholesterol, pigment, or mixed stones (calculi) within the gallbladder
- Synonym(s): gallstones

Pediatric Considerations
- Uncommon in children <10 years
- Most gallstones in children are pigment stones associated with blood dyscrasias.

EPIDEMIOLOGY
Incidence
- Increased in Native Americans and Hispanics
- Increases with age ~1–3% per year; peaks at 7th decade
- 2% of the U.S. population develops gallstones annually.

Prevalence
- 8–10% of the U.S. population with gallstones
- 20% >65 years of age
- Female > male (2 to 3:1)

ETIOLOGY AND PATHOPHYSIOLOGY
- Gallstone formation is a complex process mediated by genetic, metabolic, immune, and environmental factors. Gallbladder sludge (a mixture of cholesterol crystals, calcium bilirubinate granules, and mucin gel matrix) serves as the nidus for gallstone formation.
- Bile supersaturated with cholesterol (cholesterol stones) precipitates as microcrystals that aggregate and expand. Stone formation is enhanced by biliary stasis or impaired gallbladder motility.
- Decrease in bile phospholipid (lecithin) or decreased bile salt secretion
- Excess unconjugated bilirubin in patients with hemolytic diseases; passage of excess bile salt into the colon with subsequent absorption of excess unconjugated bilirubin in patients with inflammatory bowel disease (IBD) or after distal ileal resection (black or pigment stones)
- Hydrolysis of conjugated bilirubin or phospholipid by bacteria in patients with biliary tract infection or stricture (brown stones or primary bile duct stones; rare in the Western world and common in Asia)

RISK FACTORS
- Age peaks in patients 60 to 80 years of age.
- Female gender, pregnancy, multiparity, obesity, and metabolic syndrome
- Caucasian, Hispanic, or Native American descent
- High-fat diet rich in cholesterol
- Cholestasis or impaired gallbladder motility in association with prolonged fasting, long-term total parenteral nutrition (TPN), following vagotomy, long-term somatostatin therapy, and rapid weight loss
- Hereditary (p.D19H variant for the hepatic canalicular cholesterol transporter ABCG5/ABG8)
- Short gut syndrome, terminal ileal resection, IBD
- Hemolytic disorders (hereditary spherocytosis, sickle cell anemia, etc.), cirrhosis (black/pigment stones)
- Medications (birth control pills, estrogen replacement therapy at high doses, and long-term corticosteroid or cytostatic therapy)
- Viral hepatitis, biliary tract infection, and stricture (promotes intraductal formation of pigment stones)

GENERAL PREVENTION
- Ursodiol (Actigall) taken during rapid weight loss prevents gallstone formation.
- Regular exercise and dietary modification may reduce the incidence of gallstone formation.
- Lipid-lowering drugs (statins) may prevent cholesterol stone formation by reducing bile cholesterol saturation.

COMMONLY ASSOCIATED CONDITIONS
90% of people with gallbladder carcinoma have gallstones and chronic cholecystitis.

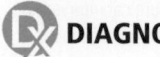 **DIAGNOSIS**

HISTORY
- Mostly asymptomatic (80%): 2% become symptomatic each year. Over their lifetime, <50% of patients with gallstones develop symptoms.
- Episodic right upper quadrant or epigastric pain lasting >15 minutes and sometimes radiating to the back (biliary colic—due to transient cystic duct obstruction)
- Pain is usually postprandial.
- Pain sometimes awakens patients from sleep.
- Most patients develop recurrent symptoms after a first episode of biliary colic.
- Other symptoms include nausea, vomiting, indigestion or bloating sensation, and fatty food intolerance.

PHYSICAL EXAM
- Physical exam is *usually normal* in patients with cholelithiasis in the absence of an acute attack.
- Epigastric and/or right upper quadrant tenderness (Murphy sign) is a traditional physical finding associated with acute cholecystitis. Murphy sign has limited sensitivity and specificity.
- Charcot triad: fever, jaundice, right upper quadrant pain
- Reynolds pentad: fever, jaundice, right upper quadrant pain, hemodynamic instability, mental status changes; classically associated with ascending cholangitis
- Flank and periumbilical ecchymoses (Cullen sign and Grey Turner sign) in patients with acute hemorrhagic pancreatitis
- Courvoisier sign: palpable mass in the right upper quadrant in patient with obstructive jaundice most commonly due to malignant tumors within the biliary tree or pancreas

DIFFERENTIAL DIAGNOSIS
- Peptic ulcer diseases and gastritis
- Hepatitis
- Pancreatitis
- Cholangitis
- Gallbladder cancer
- Gallbladder polyps
- Acalculous cholecystitis
- Biliary dyskinesia
- Choledocholithiasis

DIAGNOSTIC TESTS & INTERPRETATION
No laboratory study is specific for cholelithiasis.

Initial Tests (lab, imaging)
- Leukocytosis and elevated C-reactive protein level are associated with acute calculus cholecystitis.
- Ultrasound (US) is the preferred imaging modality. US detects gallstones in 97–98% of patients.

- Thickening of the gallbladder wall (≥5 mm), pericholecystic fluid, and direct tenderness when the probe is pushed against the gallbladder (sonographic Murphy sign) are associated with acute cholecystitis.
- CT scan has no advantage over US except for detecting distal common bile duct (CBD) stones.
- MR cholangiopancreatography (MRCP) is reserved for cases of suspected CBD stones. However, MRCP has no therapeutic value, and preoperative MRCP is not more cost-effective than initial cholecystectomy with cholangiography in the diagnosis of patients with suspected CBD stones.
- Endoscopic US is as sensitive as endoscopic retrograde cholangiopancreatography (ERCP) for detection of CBD stones in patients with gallstone pancreatitis (GP).
- Hepatobiliary iminodiacetic acid (HIDA) scan is useful in diagnosing acute cholecystitis secondary to cystic duct obstruction. It is also useful in differentiating acalculous cholecystitis from other causes of abdominal pain. False-positive tests can result from a fasting state, insufficient resistance of the sphincter of Oddi, and gallbladder agenesis.
- Cholecystokinin (CCK)-HIDA is specifically used to diagnose gallbladder dysmotility (biliary dyskinesia).
- 10–30% of gallstones are radiopaque calcium or pigment-containing gallstones (visible on plain x-ray). A "porcelain gallbladder" is a calcified gallbladder (also visible by x-ray) that is associated with chronic cholecystitis and gallbladder cancer.

Test Interpretation
- Pure cholesterol stones are white or slightly yellow.
- Pigment stones may be black or brown. Black stones contain polymerized calcium bilirubinate, most often secondary to cirrhosis or hemolysis; these almost always form within the gallbladder.
- Brown stones are associated with biliary tract infection, caused by bile stasis, and as such may form either in the bile ducts or gallbladder.

 TREATMENT

GENERAL MEASURES
- Treat symptomatic cholelithiasis.
- Conservative therapy is preferred during pregnancy; surgery in the 2nd trimester if necessary
- Prophylactic cholecystectomy for patients with calcified (porcelain) gallbladder (risk for gallbladder cancer), patients with large stones (≥3 cm), patients with sickle cell disease, patients planning an organ transplant, and patients with recurrent pancreatitis due to microlithiasis
- In morbidly obese patients, cholecystectomy may be performed in combination with bariatric procedures to reduce subsequent stone-related comorbidities.
- Prophylactic cholecystectomy is recommended for gallstones discovered incidentally during open abdominal surgery.

Geriatric Considerations
Gallstones are more common in the elderly. Age alone should not alter the therapeutic plan.

MEDICATION

First Line

- Analgesics for pain relief
  - NSAIDs are the first-choice treatment for pain control which is equivalent to opioid therapy.
  - Opioids are an option for patients who cannot tolerate or fail to respond to NSAIDs.
- Antibiotics for patients with acute cholecystitis
- Prophylactic antibiotics in low-risk patients do not prevent infections during laparoscopic cholecystectomy (LC) (1)[A].

ISSUES FOR REFERRAL

Patients with retained or recurrent bile duct stones following cholecystectomy should be referred for ERCP.

SURGERY/OTHER PROCEDURES

- Surgery should be considered for patients who have symptomatic cholelithiasis or gallstone-related complications (e.g., cholecystitis) or in asymptomatic patients with immune suppression, calcified gallbladder, or family history of gallbladder cancer.
- Open and LC have similar mortality and complication rates. LC offers less pain and quicker recovery and is the current gold-standard treatment.
- In well-selected patients, single-incision LC (SILC) and robotic LC are treatments for symptomatic cholelithiasis. SILC has not been shown to be superior to conventional multiport LC in terms of pain and risk of complications (2)[A]. Natural orifice transluminal endoscopic surgery (NOTES) is investigational. Surgery-related complications include CBD injury (0.2%), right hepatic duct/artery injury, retained stones, duct leak, biloma formation, and bile duct stricture. Bile spillage during LC has been shown to be a risk factor for surgical site infection.
  - Conversion to open procedure is based on clinical judgment. Male gender, previous upper abdominal surgery, thickened gallbladder wall, and acute cholecystitis increase the likelihood of need to convert to an open procedure.
  - In 10–15% of patients with symptomatic cholelithiasis, CBD stones are detected by intraoperative cholangiogram (IOC). CBD stone(s) can be removed by laparoscopic CBD exploration or postoperative ERCP.
  - IOC helps delineate bile duct anatomy when dissection is difficult. Routine use of IOC is controversial and may be associated with decreased incidence and severity of bile duct injury.
- Early LC (<24 hours after diagnosis of biliary colic) decreases hospital stay and operating time (3)[A].
- For patients with acute cholecystitis, early LC (<7 days of clinical presentation) is safe and may shorten the total hospital stay versus delayed LC (>6 weeks after index admission with acute cholecystitis) (4)[A].
- Percutaneous cholecystostomy (PC) is used for high-risk patients with cholecystitis or gallbladder empyema. Interval cholecystectomy is recommended.
- Symptomatic patients who are not candidates for surgery or those who have small gallstones (5 mm or smaller) in a functioning gallbladder with a patent cystic duct are candidates for oral dissolution therapy (ursodiol [Actigall]). The recurrence rate is >50% once medication is discontinued.

- Extracorporeal shock wave lithotripsy is a noninvasive therapeutic alternative for symptomatic patients who are not candidates for surgery. It helps break down large bile duct stones before ERCP. Complications include biliary pancreatitis, hepatic hematoma, incomplete ductal stone clearance, and recurrence.

ADMISSION, INPATIENT, AND NURSING CONSIDERATIONS

For patients with symptomatic cholelithiasis, LC is typically an outpatient procedure. For patients with complications (i.e., cholecystitis, cholangitis, pancreatitis), inpatient care is necessary.

- Acute phase: NPO, IV fluids, and antibiotics
- Adequate pain control with narcotics and/or NSAIDs

 ONGOING CARE

FOLLOW-UP RECOMMENDATIONS

Patient Monitoring

- Follow for signs of symptomatic cholelithiasis.
- Follow patients on oral dissolution agents with serial liver enzymes, serum cholesterol, and imaging.

DIET

A low-fat diet may help.

PATIENT EDUCATION

- Change in lifestyle (e.g., regular exercise) and dietary modification (low-fat diet and reduction of total caloric intake) reduce gallstone-related hospitalizations.
- Patients with asymptomatic gallstones should be educated about the typical symptoms of biliary colic and gallstone-related complications.

PROGNOSIS

- <50% of patients with gallstones become symptomatic.
- Cholecystectomy-related mortality is <0.5% in elective cases and 3–5% in emergency cases; morbidity is <10% in elective cases and 30–40% in emergency cases.
- ~10–15% of patients have associated choledocholithiasis.
- After cholecystectomy, stones may recur within the biliary tree in patients with associated risk factors.

COMPLICATIONS

- Acute cholecystitis (90–95% secondary to gallstones)
- GP; ERCP ± sphincterotomy of no clear benefit in patients with mild GP but reduces complications in those with severe GP (5)[A]
- CBD stones with obstructive jaundice and acute cholangitis. In patients undergoing ERCP for CBD stones, early LC reduces the risk of recurrent biliary events (6)[B].
- Biliary-enteric fistula and gallstone ileus
- Bouveret syndrome is a variant of gallstone ileus where the gallstone lodges in the duodenum or pylorus causing a gastric outlet obstruction.
- Gallbladder cancer
- Mirizzi syndrome (extrinsic bile duct obstruction caused by gallstones lodged in gallbladder or cystic duct)

REFERENCES

1. Sanabria A, Dominguez LC, Valdivieso E, et al. Antibiotic prophylaxis for patients undergoing elective laparoscopic cholecystectomy. *Cochrane Database Syst Rev.* 2010;(12):CD005265.

2. Gurusamy KS, Vaughan J, Rossi M, et al. Fewer-than-four ports versus four ports for laparoscopic cholecystectomy. *Cochrane Database Syst Rev.* 2014;(2):CD007109.

3. Gurusamy KS, Koti R, Fusai G, et al. Early versus delayed laparoscopic cholecystectomy for uncomplicated biliary colic. *Cochrane Database Syst Rev.* 2013;(6):CD007196.

4. Gurusamy KS, Davidson C, Gluud C, et al. Early versus delayed laparoscopic cholecystectomy for people with acute cholecystitis. *Cochrane Database Syst Rev.* 2013;(6):CD005440.

5. Burstow MJ, Yunus RM, Hossain MB, et al. Meta-analysis of early endoscopic retrograde cholangiopancreatography (ERCP) ± endoscopic sphincterotomy (ES) versus conservative management for gallstone pancreatitis (GSP). *Surg Laparosc Endosc Percutan Tech.* 2015;25(3):185–203.

6. Huang RJ, Barakat MT, Girotra M, et al. Practice patterns for cholecystectomy after endoscopic retrograde cholangiopancreatography for patients with choledocholithiasis. *Gastroenterology.* 2017;153(3):762.e2–771.e2.

ADDITIONAL READING

- Brown LM, Rogers SJ, Cello JP, et al. Cost-effective treatment of patients with symptomatic cholelithiasis and possible common bile duct stones. *J Am Coll Surg.* 2011;212(6):1049.e1–1060.e7.
- Keus F, Gooszen HG, van Laarhoven CJ. Open, small-incision, or laparoscopic cholecystectomy for patients with symptomatic cholecystolithiasis. An overview of Cochrane Hepato-Biliary Group reviews. *Cochrane Database Syst Rev.* 2010;(1):CD008318.
- Peponis T, Eskesen TG, Mesar T, et al. Bile spillage as a risk factor for surgical site infection after laparoscopic cholecystectomy: a prospective study of 1,001 patients. *J Am Coll Surg.* 2018;226(6):1030–1035.

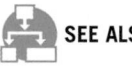 **SEE ALSO**

Cholangitis, Acute; Choledocholithiasis

 CODES

ICD10

- K80.20 Calculus of gallbladder w/o cholecystitis w/o obstruction
- K80.21 Calculus of gallbladder w/o cholecystitis with obstruction
- K80.01 Calculus of gallbladder w acute cholecystitis w obstruction

CLINICAL PEARLS

- Most patients with gallstones are asymptomatic.
- Transabdominal US is the imaging modality of choice for the diagnosis of cholelithiasis (sensitivity, 97%; specificity, 95%).
- LC is the preferred surgical procedure for symptomatic cholelithiasis.
- Acute acalculous cholecystitis is associated with bile stasis and gallbladder ischemia.
- Prophylactic cholecystectomy is not indicated in patients with asymptomatic gallstones.

CHRONIC COUGH

Jacqueline L. Olin, MS, PharmD, BCPS, CDE, FASHP, FCCP • Brian Hertz, MD •
J. Andrew Woods, PharmD, BCPS

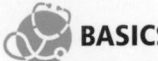 BASICS

DESCRIPTION
- Chronic cough is defined as a cough that persists for >8 weeks in adults.
- In children, chronic cough is often defined as a cough of >4 weeks in duration.
- Subacute cough describes a cough lasting 3 to 8 weeks.
- Patients present because of fear of the causative illness (e.g., cancer), annoyance, self-consciousness, and hoarseness.
- System(s) affected: gastrointestinal (GI), pulmonary

EPIDEMIOLOGY
- Predominant age: all age groups
- Predominant sex: male = female, with females more likely to seek out medical attention

Incidence
Persistent unexplained cough occurs in up to 10% of patients presenting with chronic cough and up to 46% referred to specialty cough clinics (1).

Prevalence
Chronic cough is one of the most common reasons for primary care visits.

ETIOLOGY AND PATHOPHYSIOLOGY
Varies with findings and disorders implicated
- Often multiple etiologies, but most are related to bronchial irritation. Frequent etiologies (account for >90% of cases) in nonsmokers include the following:
  - Upper airway cough syndrome (UACS) and other upper airway abnormalities, including allergic and vasomotor rhinitis syndromes
  - Chronic rhinitis with postnasal drip (allergic, nonallergic, chronic sinusitis, etc.)
  - Postviral cough
  - Asthma
  - Gastroesophageal reflux disease (GERD)
- Other causes:
  - ACE inhibitors
  - Chronic smoking or exposure to smoke or pollutants
  - Aspiration
  - Bronchiectasis
  - Infections (e.g., pertussis, tuberculosis)
  - Nonasthmatic eosinophilic bronchitis (NAEB)
  - Cystic fibrosis
  - Sleep apnea
  - Restrictive lung diseases
  - Neoplasms: bronchogenic or laryngeal
  - Psychogenic (habit cough)

- Cough hypersensitivity syndrome defines a syndrome of cough with characteristic trigger symptoms not adequately explained by other medical conditions.
- Etiologies of chronic cough in young children differ from those in older children and adults with asthma, protracted bacterial bronchitis, and UACS as most common causes (2,3).

RISK FACTORS
Although various conditions may contribute to chronic cough, the main causes include smoking and pulmonary diseases.

COMMONLY ASSOCIATED CONDITIONS
Patients with UACS, asthma, and GERD may present with chronic cough as the only symptom and not the usual symptoms associated with the diagnoses.

 DIAGNOSIS

HISTORY
- Patient's age, associated signs/symptoms, medical history, medication history (i.e., ACE inhibitors), environmental and occupational exposures, potential for aspiration, and smoking history may make some causes more likely.
- The character of cough or description of sputum quality is rarely helpful in predicting the underlying cause.
- Cough diaries have not correlated well with objective measures.
- Hemoptysis or signs of systemic illness preclude empiric therapy.

PHYSICAL EXAM
- Signs and symptoms are variable and related to the underlying cause; usually, a nonproductive cough with no other signs or symptoms
- Possible signs and symptoms of UACS, sinusitis, GERD, congestive heart failure, chronic stressors
- Absence of additional signs/symptoms of a particular condition not necessarily helpful
  - For example, 5% of patients with GERD have no other signs or symptoms and sometimes have poor response to empiric proton pump inhibitor (PPI) trials.

DIAGNOSTIC TESTS & INTERPRETATION
- Evaluation often starts with empiric therapy directed at likely underlying etiology and/or simple testing such as a chest x-ray (CXR).
- Extensive testing only if indicated by the history and physical

Pediatric Considerations
Children with chronic cough not responsive to an inhaled β-agonist and without overt stressors should undergo spirometry (if age-appropriate) and foreign body evaluation (CXR).

Initial Tests (lab, imaging)
- Evaluation will be dictated by findings in the comprehensive history and physical.
- Evaluation of peak flow may be indicated.
- If considering neoplasm, heart failure, or infectious etiologies, CXR or B-type natriuretic peptide (BNP) may be indicated.
- In cases of failure to respond to initial trial of empiric therapy, CXR may also be beneficial.

Follow-Up Tests & Special Considerations
- Examples:
  - If considering chronic obstructive pulmonary disease (COPD), asthma, or restrictive lung disease: spirometry
  - If suspicious of cystic fibrosis: sweat chloride testing
  - If suspicious of hypereosinophilic syndrome, tuberculosis, or malignancy: sputum for eosinophils and cytology
- If abnormal CXR, suspected neoplasm, or underlying pulmonary disorder, consider a chest CT.
- Consider pulmonary consultation.
- Consider specialist cough clinic.
- Refer to gastroenterologist for endoscopy.

Diagnostic Procedures/Other
If diagnosis suggested and inadequate response to initial measures, other procedures can be considered:
- Pulmonary function testing
- Purified protein derivative (PPD) skin testing
- Allergen testing
- 24-hour esophageal pH monitor
- Bronchoscopy, if history of hemoptysis or smoking with normal CXR
- Endoscopic or video fluoroscopic swallow evaluation or barium esophagram
- Sinus CT
- Ambulatory cough monitoring and cough challenge with citric acid, capsaicin, or other bronchodilator (at specialized cough clinic)
- Echocardiogram

Test Interpretation
Specific to underlying cause

 TREATMENT

GENERAL MEASURES
- With chronic cough, empiric treatment should be directed at the most common causes as clinically indicated (UACS, asthma, GERD) (1,3)[C].
- Empiric trial of nasal steroids and/or antihistamines should be considered if allergic symptoms or postnasal drip is present.

- With concomitant complaints of heartburn and regurgitation, GERD should be considered as a potential etiology (3)[C].
- In patients with cough associated with the common cold, nonsedating antihistamines were not found to be effective in reducing cough (1,3)[C]. Many patients will have resolution of cough after smoking cessation.
- When indicated, ACE inhibitor therapy should be switched in patients in whom intolerable cough occurs. It may take several days or weeks for cough to resolve after stopping ACE inhibitor therapy.
- Empirically treat postnasal drip and GERD.
- Empiric PPI are not recommended in children or adults in the absence of a GERD diagnosis (3)[C].
- Multimodality speech pathology therapy had a positive benefit on cough severity in some adults (1)[C].
- Attempt maximal therapy for single most likely cause for several weeks and then search for coexistent etiologies.

MEDICATION
- Treatments (nasal steroids, classic antihistamines, antacids, bronchodilators, inhaled corticosteroids, PPIs, antibiotics) should be directed at the specific cause of cough.
- If history and physical exam suggest GERD, may want to trial empiric PPI therapy prior to further diagnostic testing
- The FDA issued a public health advisory stating that OTC cough and cold medicines, including antitussives, expectorants, nasal decongestants, antihistamines, or combinations, should not be given to children <2 years. Subsequently, manufacturers have changed labeling to state "do not use" in children <4 years. In 2017, the FDA issued a contraindication to codeine for cough treatment in children <12 years.
- Routine empiric treatment of children with chronic cough with leukotriene receptor antagonists lacks evidence and cannot be recommended.

First Line
In adults:
- Nasal steroids: fluticasone, budesonide, others, 1 spray BID for those with allergic rhinitis symptoms or postnasal drip or an empiric trial of PPI (omeprazole, others) once a day

Second Line
- A peripherally acting antitussive agent has been used:
  – In patients >10 years, benzonatate (Tessalon Perles) 100 to 200 mg PO TID as needed (maximum 600 mg/day)
- Gabapentin was evaluated in a randomized, double-blind, placebo-controlled trial of patients with refractory chronic cough. Gabapentin demonstrated improved cough-specific quality of life compared to placebo. Nausea and fatigue occurred in 31%. A therapeutic trial with a risk-benefit assessment at 6 months is suggested (1)[C].

- A comparative effectiveness review of 49 studies with common opioid and nonanesthetic antitussives stated there is some efficiency for treating cough in adults, but evidence is limited (4)[C].
- Studies evaluating inhaled corticosteroid use in chronic cough for patients without additional indication such as asthma did not show consistent benefits (1)[C].

ISSUES FOR REFERRAL
Patients with chronic cough may benefit from evaluation by pulmonary, gastroenterology, ear/nose/throat (ENT), and/or allergy specialists. Consider specialist cough clinic.

SURGERY/OTHER PROCEDURES
Fundoplication may be effective for cough secondary to refractory GERD.

 ONGOING CARE

FOLLOW-UP RECOMMENDATIONS
Consider stepwise withdrawal of medications after resolution of cough.

Patient Monitoring
Frequent follow-up is necessary to assess the effectiveness of treatment.

DIET
Dietary modification: Patients with GERD may benefit by avoiding ethanol, caffeine, nicotine, citrus, tomatoes, chocolate, and fatty foods.

PATIENT EDUCATION
- Reassure patient that most cases of chronic cough are not life-threatening and that the condition can usually be managed effectively.
- Counsel that several weeks to a month may be needed for significant reduction or elimination of cough.
- Prepare the patient for the possibility of multiple diagnostic tests and therapeutic regimens because the treatment is very often empiric.

PROGNOSIS
- >80% of patients can be effectively diagnosed and treated using a systematic approach.
- Cough from any cause may take weeks to months until resolution, and resolution depends greatly on efficacy of treatment directed at underlying etiology.

COMPLICATIONS
- Cardiovascular: arrhythmias, syncope
- Stress urinary incontinence
- Abdominal and intercostal muscle strain
- GI: emesis, hemorrhage, herniation
- Neurologic: dizziness, headache, seizures
- Respiratory: pneumothorax, laryngeal, or tracheobronchial trauma

- Skin: petechiae, purpura, disruption of surgical wounds
- Medication side effects
- Other: negative impact on quality of life

REFERENCES
1. Gibson P, Wang G, McGarvey L, et al; and CHEST Expert Cough Panel. Treatment of unexplained chronic cough: CHEST guideline and expert panel report. Chest. 2016;149(1):27–44.
2. Chang AB, Oppenheimer JJ, Weinberger M, et al; and CHEST Expert Cough Panel. Etiologies of chronic cough in pediatric cohorts: CHEST guideline and expert panel report. Chest. 2017;152(3):607–617.
3. Michaudet C, Malaty J. Chronic cough: evaluation and management. Am Fam Physician. 2017;96(9):575–580.
4. Yancy WS Jr, McCrory DC, Coeytaux RR, et al. Efficacy and tolerability of treatments for chronic cough: a systematic review and meta-analysis. Chest. 2013;144(6):1827–1838.

 SEE ALSO

- Asthma; Bronchiectasis; Eosinophilic Pneumonias; Gastroesophageal Reflux Disease; Laryngeal Cancer; Lung, Primary Malignancies; Pertussis; Pulmonary Edema; Rhinitis, Allergic; Sinusitis; Tuberculosis
- Algorithm: Cough, Chronic

 CODES

ICD10
- R05 Cough
- J44.9 Chronic obstructive pulmonary disease, unspecified
- J41.0 Simple chronic bronchitis

CLINICAL PEARLS
- Chronic cough is defined as a cough that persists for >8 weeks in adults.
- In patients with chronic cough, most frequent etiologies include a history of smoking, asthma, UACS, and GERD.
- The FDA issued a public health advisory stating that OTC cough and cold medicines should not be given to children <2 years. OTC cough expectorant and suppressant product labels state "do not use" in children <4 years. Codeine is contraindicated for cough treatment in children <12 years.

CHRONIC KIDNEY DISEASE

Crystal Verdick, DO, MS • James E. West, MD

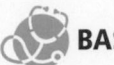 **BASICS**

Chronic kidney disease (CKD) is defined as structural or functional abnormalities of the kidney for ≥3 months, as determined by either pathologic abnormalities or markers of damage—including abnormalities in blood or urine tests, histology, imaging studies, or history of kidney transplant—*or a GFR <60 mL/min/1.73 m² for ≥3 months.*

DESCRIPTION
- In 2012, Kidney Disease: Improving Global Outcomes (KDIGO) classified CKD in six categories by GFR estimation (in mL/min/1.73 m²):
  - G1: kidney damage with normal or increased GFR ≥90
  - G2: mild ↓ GFR 60 to 89
  - G3a: mild to moderate ↓ GFR 45 to 59
  - G3b: moderate to severe ↓ GFR 30 to 44
  - G4: severe ↓ GFR 15 to 29
  - G5: kidney failure: GFR <15 or dialysis
- CKD per albumin-to-creatinine ratio (ACR) category:
  - A1: normal to mildly increased: <30 mg/g or <3 mg/mmol
  - A2: moderately increased: 30 to 300 mg/g or 3 to 30 mg/mmol
  - A3: severely increased: >300 mg/g or >30 mg/mmol
- Risk of progression depends on comorbid conditions.
- System(s) affected: renal/urinary, cardiovascular, skeletal, endocrine, metabolic, hematologic, lymphatic, immune, neurologic
- Synonym(s): chronic renal failure; chronic renal insufficiency

Geriatric Considerations
GFR normally decreases with age, despite normal creatinine (Cr). Adjust renally cleared drugs for GFR in the elderly.

Pediatric Considerations
CKD definition is not applicable for children <2 years because of lower GFR even when corrected for body surface area. Calculated GFR based on serum Cr is used in this age group.

Pregnancy Considerations
Renal function in CKD may deteriorate during pregnancy. Cr >1.5 and hypertension (HTN) are major risk factors for worsening renal function.
- Increased risk of premature labor, preeclampsia
- ACE inhibitors (ACE-Is) and angiotensin receptor blockers (ARBs) are contraindicated due to teratogenicity. Use diuretics with caution.

EPIDEMIOLOGY
- African Americans are 3.6 times more likely to develop CKD than Caucasians.
- Predominant sex: similar in both sexes; however, incidence rate of end-stage renal disease (ESRD) is 1.6 times higher in males than females.

Incidence
Estimated annual incidence of 1,700/1 million population

Prevalence
Overall prevalence of CKD is 14.2%. Unadjusted prevalence/incidence rates of ESRD (stage 5) are 1,752 and 362.4/1 million, respectively. Numbers do not reflect the burden of earlier stages of CKD (stages 1 to 4), which are estimated to affect 13.1% of the population nationwide or 26.3 million in the United States.

ETIOLOGY AND PATHOPHYSIOLOGY
Progressive destruction of kidney nephrons; GFR will drop gradually, and plasma Cr values will approximately double, with 50% reduction in GFR and 75% loss of functioning nephrons mass. Hyperkalemia usually develops when GFR falls to <20 to 25 mL/min. Anemia develops from decreased renal synthesis of erythropoietin.
- Renal parenchymal/glomerular
  - Nephritic: hematuria, RBC casts, HTN, variable proteinuria
    - Focal proliferative: IgA nephropathy, systemic lupus erythematosus (SLE), Henoch-Schönlein purpura, Alport syndrome, proliferative glomerulonephritis, crescenteric glomerulonephritis
    - Diffuse proliferative: membranoproliferative glomerulonephritis, SLE, cryoglobulinemia, rapidly progressive glomerulonephritis (RPGN), Goodpasture syndrome
  - Nephrotic: proteinuria (>3.5 g/day), hypoalbuminemia, hyperlipidemia, and edema
    - Minimal change disease, membranous nephropathy, focal segmental glomerulosclerosis
    - Amyloidosis, diabetic nephropathy
- Vascular: HTN, thrombotic microangiopathies, vasculitis (Wegener), scleroderma
- Interstitial tubular: infections, obstruction, toxins, allergic interstitial nephritis, multiple myeloma, connective tissue disease, cystic disease
- Postrenal: obstruction (benign prostatic hyperplasia [BPH]), neoplasm, neurogenic bladder

Genetics
- Alport syndrome, Fabry disease, sickle cell anemia, SLE, and autosomal dominant polycystic kidney disease can lead to CKD.
- Polymorphisms in gene that encodes for podocyte nonmuscle myosin IIA are more common in African Americans than Caucasians and appear to increase risk for nondiabetic ESRD.

RISK FACTORS
- Type 1 or 2 diabetes mellitus (DM); most common
- Age >60 years
- Cardiovascular disease (CVD) (e.g., HTN [common], renal artery stenosis, atheroemboli)
- Previous kidney transplant
- Urinary tract obstruction (e.g., BPH)
- Autoimmune disease, vasculitis/connective tissue disorder
- Family history of CKD
- Nephrotoxic drugs (lithium, salicylate, high-dose or chronic NSAIDs, sulfonamide)
- Congenital anomalies, obstructive uropathy, renal aplasia/hypoplasia/dysplasia, reflux nephropathy
- Hyperlipidemia
- Low income/education/ethnic minority status
- Obesity/smoking/heroin use
- Chronic infection (hepatitis B, hepatitis C, HIV)

GENERAL PREVENTION
- Treat reversible causes: hypovolemia, infections, diuretics, drugs (NSAIDs, aminoglycosides, IV contrast).
- Treat risk factors: DM, HTN, hyperlipidemia, smoking, and obesity; adjust medication doses to prevent renal toxicity.

COMMONLY ASSOCIATED CONDITIONS
HTN, DM, CVD

 DIAGNOSIS

HISTORY
Patients with CKD stages 1 to 3 are usually asymptomatic; can present with
- Oliguria, nocturia, polyuria, hematuria, change in urinary frequency
- Bone disease
- Edema, HTN, dyspnea
- Fatigue, depression, weakness
- Pruritus, ecchymosis
- Metallic taste in mouth, anorexia, nausea, vomiting
- Hyperlipidemia, claudication, restless legs
- Erectile dysfunction, decrease libido, amenorrhea

PHYSICAL EXAM
- Volume status (pallor, BP/orthostatic; edema; jugular venous distention; weight)
- Skin: sallow complexion, uremic frost
- Ammonia-like odor (uremic fetor)
- Cardiovascular: Assess for murmurs, bruits, pericarditis.
- Chest: pleural effusion
- Rectal: enlarged prostate
- CNS: asterixis, confusion, seizures, coma, peripheral neuropathy

DIAGNOSTIC TESTS & INTERPRETATION
Initial Tests (lab, imaging)
- GFR can be estimated using the Modification of Diet in Renal Disease (MDRD) and Chronic Kidney Disease-Epidemiology Collaboration (CKD-EPI) equations. A recent meta-analysis found that MDRD has greater accuracy at GFR 60, whereas the CKD-EPI is more accurate at GFR >60 (1)[A].
- Cr clearance (CrCl) can be calculated using Cockcroft-Gault formula to determine medication adjustments.
- Urine analysis to assess for evidence of damage
  - Urine microscopy: WBC casts in pyelonephritis, RBC casts in glomerulonephritis/vasculitis
  - Urine electrolytes: sodium, Cr, urea (if on loop diuretics)
  - Albuminuria is more sensitive than proteinuria at detecting disease (2)[B]. Meta-analyses link CVD mortality with albuminuria (2)[A].
    - Report as a ratio of albumin concentration to Cr concentration (mg/mmol or mg/g)
- Ultrasound (initial imaging test of choice): small, echogenic kidneys; may see obstruction (e.g., hydronephrosis); cysts; kidneys may be enlarged with HIV and diabetic nephropathy.
- Doppler ultrasound to assess for renovascular disease, thrombosis
- Noncontrast CT scan: obstruction, calculi, cysts, neoplasm, renal artery stenosis
- MRI/MRA: Avoid gadolinium because of the risk of nephrogenic systemic fibrosis.
- Renal arteriogram for renal artery stenosis can be therapeutic (angioplasty or stenting).
- Renal scan to screen for differential function between kidneys
- Retrograde pyelogram: if strong suspicion for obstruction despite negative finding on ultrasound

Follow-Up Tests & Special Considerations
- Additional evaluation may be indicated to assess for complications or cause, as clinically indicated:
  - Hematology: normochromic, normocytic anemia; increased bleeding time

- Chemistry: elevated BUN, Cr, hyperkalemia, metabolic acidosis, increased PTH, HLD, hyperphosphatemia, decreased 25-(OH) vitamin D, hypocalcemia, decreased albumin
- Serology: antinuclear antibody (ANA); double-stranded DNA, antineutrophil cytoplasmic antibody; complements (C3, C4, CH50); anti-glomerular basement membrane (GBM) antibodies; hepatitis B, C; and HIV screening
- Serum and urine immunoelectrophoresis
- Follow-up tests and monitoring:
  - Monitoring the parameters with frequency based on GFR and risk of progression:
    ○ Urine albumin and GFR at least annually
    ○ Hb: clinically indicated for GFR ≥60, annually for 30 to 59, twice per year for <30 (3)[B]
    ○ Calcium, phosphate, PTH, alkaline phosphate actively beginning at CKD stage G3a (4)[C]
    ○ 25(OH)D (calcidiol) levels with repeated testing determined by baseline values and therapeutic interventions (4)[C]
  - Therapeutic decisions should be based on trends rather than on a single laboratory value, taking into account all available CKD-MBD assessments (4)[C].

ALERT
Drugs that may alter lab result:

- Cimetidine: inhibits Cr tubular secretion
- Trimethoprim: inhibits Cr and K^+ secretion and may cause/worsen hyperkalemia
- Cefoxitin and flucytosine: increases serum Cr
- Diltiazem and verapamil (like ACE/ARBs) have significant antiproteinuric effects in patients with CKD.

Diagnostic Procedures/Other
Biopsy: hematuria, proteinuria, acute/progressive renal failure, nephritic or nephrotic syndrome

 ## TREATMENT

GENERAL MEASURES
- Lowering salt intake to <2 g/day of sodium in adults, unless contraindicated (5)[C]
- Minimize radiocontrast exposure; prehydrate; N-acetylcysteine use is controversial. Avoid nephrotoxins (NSAIDs, aminoglycosides, etc.).
- Encourage smoking cessation, encourage weight loss (if applicable), and limit alcohol consumption (5)[C].
- Protein restriction to 0.8 kg/kg/day is recommended in CKD G4 to G5 (2)[B]. CKD at risk of progression should avoid dietary protein >1.3 g/kg/day to avoid accelerating progression (2)[B].

MEDICATION
- HTN: Goal in adults is BP <130/80 mm Hg if urine albumin excretion is ≥30 mg/24 hr and <140/90 mm Hg if urine albumin excretion is <30 mg/24 hr. Goal in children is <90th percentile for age, sex, weight (5)[B].
  - ACE-I or ARB recommended for diabetic and nondiabetic adults with albumin excretion >30 mg/24 hr based on evidence of reductions in proteinuria, improved CVD outcomes, and decreased progression of CKD (5)[A]. Monitor potassium and serum Cr (tolerate up to 30% rise unless hyperkalemia develops).
  - Additional antihypertensive agents should be selected based on the type of CKD and comorbid factors.
- Secondary hyperparathyroidism
  - For GFR <45, monitor for hyperphosphatemia, hypocalcemia, and vitamin D deficiency if intact PTH is elevated beyond lab normals (2)[C].
  - Cinacalcet, paricalcitol (decrease PTH levels)

- Hyperphosphatemia: Maintain phosphate according to reference lab normals (2)[C]. Recommended serum phosphate maintenance levels for CKD patients:
  - Stages 3 to 5 CKD (not on dialysis): Restrict dietary phosphate to 800 to 1,000 mg/day.
    ○ Calcium-containing phosphate binders (with meals): calcium carbonate, calcium acetate (risk of hypercalcemia)
    ○ Noncalcium phosphate binders (with meals): sevelamer, lanthanum
    ○ Vitamin D: inactive vitamin D 25 (ergocalciferol or cholecalciferol), calcitriol (active vitamin D 1,25 [OH]): Vitamin D may increase absorption of phosphate by intestines and should not be started until serum phosphate concentration is controlled.
- Anemia: Hb <13 g/dL in adult males or <12 g/dL in adult females. Treat with iron replacement therapy with or without erythropoietin-stimulating agents (ESAs) (3)[B]. Consider ESA if Hb >9 g/dL and <10 g/dL. ESA initiation not recommended for Hb >10 g/dL. If using ESA, goal Hb range 10 to 11 g/dL, not to exceed 11.5 g/dL (3)[B].
- Hyperlipidemia: Statins with low-density lipoprotein (LDL) goal is similar to coronary heart disease patients (LDL <70 to 100).
- Glycemic control: Target for HbA1c should be adjusted based on risk of hypoglycemia, comorbid conditions, and life expectancy (2)[B]. HbA1c may be falsely low in patients with decreased RBC; glucose logs may be more accurate reflection of glycemic control (2)[C]. Metformin use should be reviewed for GFR between 30 and 44 and discontinued if GFR <30 mL/min/1.73 m² (2)[C].
- Metabolic acidosis: Start treatment when bicarbonate <22 mEq/L with goal to maintain in normal range (2)[C].

ISSUES FOR REFERRAL
- Nephrology consult: GFR <15: immediate
- GFR 15 to 29: urgent
- GFR 30 to 59: nonurgent referral
- GFR 60 to 89: not required unless with comorbidities
- Renal replacement: Prepare for dialysis or transplant when GFR <30 mL/min/1.73 m².

SURGERY/OTHER PROCEDURES
Placement of dialysis access or transplantation

ADMISSION, INPATIENT, AND NURSING CONSIDERATIONS
Uremia: nausea/vomiting, fluid overload, pericarditis, uremic encephalopathy, resistant HTN, hyperkalemia, metabolic acidosis, hyperphosphatemia

 ## ONGOING CARE

DIET
Nutrition consult for CKD diet (2)[C]

PATIENT EDUCATION
- Annual influenza vaccine unless contraindicated (2)
- Polyvalent pneumococcal vaccine if GFR <30 mL/min/1.73 m² and those at high risk of pneumococcal infection (2)
- Hepatitis B vaccine with serologic confirmation if high risk of CKD progression and GFR <30 mL/min/1.73 m² (2)
- National Kidney Federation patient Web site at: http://www.kidney.org/patients

PROGNOSIS
Risk of progression and complications is based on cause, GFR category, albuminuria category, and comorbid conditions (2)[B]. Progression defined as decline in GFR category with 25% decrease in GFR from baseline (2). Rapid progression is decrease in GFR by >5 mL/min/1.73 m²/year (2). Patients with CKD gradually progress to ESRD, with bad prognoses. 5-year survival rate for U.S. patients on dialysis is ~35%.

COMPLICATIONS
HTN, anemia, secondary hyperparathyroidism, renal osteodystrophy, sleep disturbances, infections, malnutrition, electrolyte imbalances, platelet dysfunction/bleeding, pseudogout, gout, metabolic calcification, sexual dysfunction

REFERENCES

1. Earley A, Miskulin D, Lamb EJ, et al. Estimating equations for glomerular filtration rate in the era of creatinine standardization: a systematic review. *Ann Intern Med*. 2012;156(11):785–795.
2. Kidney Disease: Improving Global Outcomes (KDIGO) CKD Work Group. KDIGO 2012 clinical practice guideline for the evaluation and management of chronic kidney disease. *Kidney Int Suppl*. 2013;3(1):1–150.
3. Kidney Disease: Improving Global Outcomes (KDIGO) Anemia Work Group. KDIGO clinical practice guideline for anemia in chronic kidney disease. *Kidney Int Suppl*. 2012;2(4):279–335.
4. Kidney Disease: Improving Global Outcomes (KDIGO) CKD–MBD Work Group. KDIGO 2017 clinical practice guideline update for the diagnosis, evaluation, prevention, and treatment of chronic kidney disease-mineral and bone disorder (CKD–MBD). *Kidney Int Suppl*. 2017;7(1):1–59.
5. Kidney Disease: Improving Global Outcomes (KDIGO) Blood Pressure Work Group. KDIGO clinical practice guideline for the management of blood pressure in chronic kidney disease. *Kidney Int Suppl*. 2012;2(5):337–414.

 ## SEE ALSO

- Hydronephrosis; Nephrotic Syndrome; Polycystic Kidney Disease; Proteinuria
- Algorithm: Anuria or Oliguria

 ## CODES

ICD10
- N18.9 Chronic kidney disease, unspecified
- Q63.9 Congenital malformation of kidney, unspecified
- N18.3 Chronic kidney disease, stage 3 (moderate)

CLINICAL PEARLS

- CKD is defined based on >3 months of kidney functional or structural abnormalities and classified based on GFR and albuminuria.
- ACE-I and ARB are first line for HTN treatment in CKD with albuminuria.
- Care should be taken in prescribing medication in CKD due to reduced renal clearance of certain medications.
- Consider nonurgent nephrologist referral for GFR ≤59 and urgent nephrologist referral for GFR ≤29.

CHRONIC OBSTRUCTIVE PULMONARY DISEASE AND EMPHYSEMA

Dennis Martinez, DO • Aelia Fatima, MD • Amit B. Patel, DO

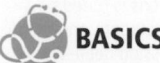 BASICS

DESCRIPTION
- The Global Initiative for Chronic Obstructive Lung Disease (GOLD) describes COPD in the following words: COPD is a common, preventable, and treatable disease that is characterized by persistent respiratory symptoms and airflow limitation that is due to airway and/or alveolar abnormalities usually caused by significant exposure to noxious particles or gases. The chronic airflow limitation that characterizes COPD is caused by a mixture of small airways disease (e.g., obstructive bronchiolitis) and parenchymal destruction (emphysema), the relative contributions of which vary from person to person. Chronic inflammation causes structural changes, small airways narrowing, and destruction of lung parenchyma. A loss of small airways may contribute to airflow limitation and mucociliary dysfunction, a characteristic feature of the disease (1).
- This new definition no longer includes the terms "emphysema" and "chronic bronchitis."
- Third leading cause of death in the United States (2)
- Projected to be the third leading cause of death globally by 2020 (3); 3.2 million deaths worldwide (3)

EPIDEMIOLOGY
Incidence
The incidence of COPD is 8.9/1,000 person-years (4).

Prevalence
The prevalence of COPD is 4.7% (4).

ETIOLOGY AND PATHOPHYSIOLOGY
Exposure to noxious gasses or particles (see "Risk Factors") leading to the following pathologic processes in the lung:
- Impaired gas (carbon dioxide and oxygen) exchange
- Persistent airway obstruction
- Destruction of lung parenchyma

Genetics
- Genetics may contribute to host response to noxious gasses or particles.
- Antiprotease deficiency (due to α_1-antitrypsin deficiency) is an inherited, rare disorder due to two autosomal codominant alleles.

RISK FACTORS
- Smoking: including passive smoking and water pipe. Marijuana may also contribute (1,2,3).
- Severe pneumonia early in life including viral (5)
- Aging
- Lower level of education and poverty (5)
- Asthma (1)
- Indoor pollution (especially indoor biomass cooking worldwide) (5)
- Occupational organic or inorganic dusts (5)

GENERAL PREVENTION
- Avoidance of smoking is the most important preventive measure.
- Early detection through pulmonary function tests (PFTs) in high-risk patients may be useful in preserving remaining lung function.

COMMONLY ASSOCIATED CONDITIONS
- Pulmonary: lung cancer, chronic respiratory failure, acute bronchitis, sleep apnea, pulmonary hypertension (HTN), asthma
- Cardiac: coronary artery disease, arrhythmia
- Ear/nose/throat (ENT): chronic sinusitis, laryngeal carcinoma
- Miscellaneous: malnutrition, osteoporosis, muscle dysfunction, depression

 DIAGNOSIS

HISTORY
- Discuss patient's use of tobacco and cannabis.
- Consider indoor pollution and occupational exposures (5).
- Symptoms: exertional dyspnea, chronic cough, sputum production
- Review possible causes of exacerbation (e.g., cold weather, recent exposure to URI, PNA, contact with flu, noncompliance with medications).
- Exacerbation: increased frequency of sputum production, change in sputum color, frequency and/or amount, fevers, wheezing, chest tightness/pain

PHYSICAL EXAM
- Prolonged expiration, wheezing
- Barrel chest, diminished breath sounds, distant heart sounds
- Accessory muscle use, pursed lip breathing, cyanosis
- Cachexia
- Clubbing not typical for COPD, however may indicate another process (e.g., lung cancer)

DIFFERENTIAL DIAGNOSIS
- Asthma (including occupational)
- Bronchiectasis
- Lung cancer
- Acute bronchitis
- Normal aging of lungs
- Chronic pulmonary embolism
- Sleep apnea
- Primary alveolar hypoventilation
- Chronic sinusitis
- Reactive airways dysfunction syndrome (RADS)
- Congestive heart failure (CHF)
- Bronchiolitis obliterans
- Gastroesophageal reflux disease
- Cystic fibrosis

DIAGNOSTIC TESTS & INTERPRETATION
Spirometry (the most reliable/objective measurement of airflow obstruction) (1,2,3)[A]

Initial Tests (lab, imaging)
- Spirometry (see "Diagnostic Procedures/Other")
- Arterial blood gases (ABGs) may show hypercapnia and hypoxia.
- May see polycythemia, reflecting chronic hypoxia
- Imaging important to rule out other conditions
- Emphysema CXR: hyperinflation, flat diaphragms, and possibly bullous changes

Follow-Up Tests & Special Considerations
- Pulse oximetry to assess need for oxygen
- α_1-Antitrypsin screening for those with COPD age <45 years, have a blood relative with this disease, or spirometry out of proportion to tobacco use
- Chest CT may show parenchymal destruction and bullae.

Diagnostic Procedures/Other
- Pulmonary function testing without/with bronchodilator (2,3)[A]
  – Decreased postbronchodilator FEV_1:FVC ratio <0.7. This is the diagnostic criteria for airway obstruction; repeat spirometry recommended if between 0.6 and 0.8 (1)
  – Reduced FEV_1
  – Normal or decreased FVC
  – Normal or increased total lung capacity
  – Increased residual volume and functional residual capacity
  – Diffusing capacity is normal or reduced.
  – Typically not bronchodilator responsive (change in FEV_1 or FVC of 12% or greater and change in volume of 200 mL or greater)
- Staging: GOLD criteria for airflow limitation (1)
  – Stage 1: FEV_1 ≥80% predicted
  – Stage 2: FEV_1 50–80% predicted
  – Stage 3: FEV_1 30–50% predicted
  – Stage 4: FEV_1 <30% predicted or FEV_1 <50% predicted plus chronic respiratory failure
  – FEV_1 was previously used to grade severity; however, it was found to correlate poorly with patients' functional capacity and risk for exacerbation (1).
- Symptom assessment:
  – COPD Assessment Tool (CAT)
  – Modified Medical Research Council (mMRC) questionnaire

Test Interpretation
- The ABCD assessment tool incorporates severity of patient's symptoms and exacerbation history.
- Group A: low risk, less symptoms: 0 to 1 exacerbation per year and no prior hospitalization for exacerbation; and CAT score <10 or mMRC grade 0 to 1
- Group B: low risk, more symptoms: 0 to 1 exacerbation per year and no prior hospitalization for exacerbation; and CAT score ≥10 or mMRC grade ≥2
- Group C: high risk, less symptoms: ≥2 exacerbations per year or ≥1 hospitalization for exacerbation; and CAT score <10 or mMRC grade 0 to 1
- Group D: high risk, more symptoms: ≥2 exacerbations per year or ≥1 hospitalization for exacerbation; and CAT score ≥10 or mMRC grade ≥2

TREATMENT

GENERAL MEASURES
- Smoking cessation: This is the most important intervention to decrease risk (2,3)[A].
- Medications help reduce symptoms and exacerbations (2).
- Home oxygen: may improve survival; should be initiated at partial pressure of arterial oxygen (PaO_2) ≤55 mm Hg or pulse oximetry trends ≤88% (2)[A], or if PaO_2 between 55 and 60 mm Hg and evidence of erythrocytosis or cor pulmonale

- Influenza and pneumococcal immunizations (3)[B]
- Pulmonary rehabilitation
- NPPV may improve hospitalization-free survival in selected patients after recent hospitalization.

MEDICATION

Treatment is based on a combination of PFTs (GOLD criteria), symptoms (mMRC Dyspnea Scale or CAT), and risk of exacerbation (BODE index).

First Line

- Minimally symptomatic, low risk of exacerbation (Category A):
  - First line: a short-acting bronchodilator to use as a rescue drug (2)
  - Short-acting β-agonists: albuterol, levalbuterol
  - Short-acting muscarinic antagonists: ipratropium, oxitropium
- More symptomatic, low risk of exacerbation (Category B)
  - First line: regular use of long-acting bronchodilator in addition to as needed short-acting bronchodilator
  - Second line: If uncontrolled symptoms with a single long-acting agent, then use combined long-acting β-agonists (LABA)–long-acting muscarinic antagonists (LAMA) rather than steroids.
  - LABA: formoterol, arformoterol, salmeterol
  - LAMA: tiotropium, aclidinium, umeclidinium, glycopyrrolate
- Minimally symptomatic, high risk of exacerbation (Category C)
  - First line: LAMA
  - Second line:
    - LAMA-LABA combination
    - LABA and inhaled corticosteroid (ICS)
- More symptomatic, high risk of exacerbation (Category D)
  - First line: LAMA-LABA combination
  - Second line: can add triple therapy with LAMA-LABA and ICS therapy
    - PD4 inhibitor (roflumilast) if FEV_1 <50% and chronic bronchitis. Chronic macrolide therapy if active smoker or recently stopped smoking; theophylline not preferred due to side effects

Second Line

As above

ALERT

Precautions

- β-Agonists: sinus tachycardia, arrhythmias in susceptible patients; can consider levalbuterol
- Anticholinergics: minimal systemic absorption in inhaled form; urinary retention possible
- ICS: increased risk of pneumonia; oral candidiasis
- Corticosteroids: weight gain, diabetes, adrenal suppression, osteoporosis, infection (pneumonia)
- Macrolides: Long-term use can possibly lead to bacterial resistance and hearing impairment.
- Theophylline: arrhythmia, CNS symptoms, nausea, vomiting

ISSUES FOR REFERRAL

Severe exacerbation, frequent hospitalizations, age <40 years, rapid progression, weight loss, severe disease, or surgical evaluation

ADDITIONAL THERAPIES

- Advanced therapies (surgical/bronchoscopic) for select patients
- Palliative care for select patients
- Acute COPD exacerbations: Mild to moderate exacerbations can be treated with short-acting bronchodilators and possibly short courses of steroids and/or antibiotics (5 to 7 days). Severe exacerbations require inpatient admission (see below).

SURGERY/OTHER PROCEDURES

- Lung reduction surgery (selected cases)
- Bronchoscopic lung reduction procedures (selected cases)
- Surgical bullectomy
- Lung transplantation (selected cases)

ADMISSION, INPATIENT, AND NURSING CONSIDERATIONS

- Severe acute exacerbation: Maintain oxygenation, short-acting inhaled β-agonists/inhaled anticholinergic agents, and oral or IV corticosteroids prednisone (up to 1 mg/kg/day commonly 40 mg/day for 5 days) (6)[A]. Antibiotics for moderate/severe exacerbations with increased sputum volume or sputum purulence; optimal antibiotic therapy has not been determined (1)[B]; noninvasive positive pressure ventilation if necessary
- May lead to acute or acute on chronic respiratory failure requiring ICU admission and intubation
- Prior to discharge: Assess proper inhaler use, prescribe proper maintenance inhalers, and ensure understanding; assess need for home oxygen.

ALERT

If not already in place, have patient delineate an advance directive. Progressive nature of disease and severity of treatment methods (ventilation, etc.) make revisiting patient preferences beneficial.

 ONGOING CARE

FOLLOW-UP RECOMMENDATIONS

- May taper or stop oral steroids as outpatient
- Pulmonary rehabilitation for exertional dyspnea (2)[A]

Patient Monitoring

Follow-up should be initially within 4-week period and a 12-week period after an exacerbation; paying attention to symptoms, medication compliance, and the need for O_2 in 4 weeks and in addition to the above repeating spirometry in 12 weeks

DIET

Referral for nutritional support indicated in malnourished patients

PATIENT EDUCATION

American Lung Association: www.lung.org/lung-disease/copd/

PROGNOSIS

- Symptoms, exacerbation history, comorbidities, and postbronchodilator FEV_1 are the most important predictors of prognosis (1).
- Supplemental O_2, when indicated, is shown to increase survival (may only need at night) (2)[A].
- Smoking cessation improves prognosis (3).

- For severe upper lobe disease and poor control or poor postrehabilitation exercise capacity, lung volume reduction surgery may be considered.
- For very severe disease unresponsive to all interventions, patient may be candidate for lung transplant.

COMPLICATIONS

- Malnutrition, poor sleep quality, infections, secondary polycythemia
- Acute or chronic respiratory failure, bullous lung disease, pneumothorax
- Arrhythmias, cor pulmonale, pulmonary HTN

REFERENCES

1. Global Initiative for Chronic Obstructive Lung Disease. Global strategy for the diagnosis, management, and prevention of chronic obstructive pulmonary disease: 2018 report. www.goldcopd.org. Accessed September 25, 2018.
2. Qaseem A, Wilt TJ, Weinberger SE, et al; for American College of Physicians, American College of Chest Physicians, American Thoracic Society, European Respiratory Society. Diagnosis and management of stable chronic obstructive pulmonary disease: a clinical practice guideline update from the American College of Physicians, American College of Chest Physicians, American Thoracic Society, and European Respiratory Society. *Ann Intern Med*. 2011;155(3):179–191.
3. Vestbo J, Hurd SS, Agustí AG, et al. Global strategy for the diagnosis, management, and prevention of chronic obstructive pulmonary disease: GOLD executive summary. *Am J Respir Crit Care Med*. 2013;187(4):347–365.
4. Terzikhan N, Verhamme KM, Hofman A, et al. Prevalence and incidence of COPD in smokers and non-smokers: the Rotterdam Study. *Eur J Epidemiol*. 2016;31(8):785–792.
5. Lamprecht B, McBurnie MA, Vollmer WM, et al; for BOLD Collaborative Research Group. COPD in never smokers: results from the population-based burden of obstructive lung disease study. *Chest*. 2011;139(4):752–763.
6. Leuppi JD, Schuetz P, Bingisser R, et al. Short-term vs conventional glucocorticoid therapy in acute exacerbations of chronic obstructive pulmonary disease: the REDUCE randomized clinical trial. *JAMA*. 2013;309(21):2223–2231.

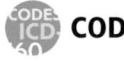 **SEE ALSO**

Bronchitis, Acute

CODES

ICD10

- J44.9 Chronic obstructive pulmonary disease, unspecified
- J43.9 Emphysema, unspecified
- J42 Unspecified chronic bronchitis

CLINICAL PEARLS

- Consider screening PFTs on any high-risk patient.
- Overnight oximetry if daytime SaO_2 is borderline
- Influenza/pneumococcal vaccines should be current.
- Advance directive before patient is seriously ill.

CHRONIC PAIN MANAGEMENT: AN EVIDENCE-BASED APPROACH

Jennifer Reidy, MD, MS, FAAHPM • Delila Katz, PharmD, BCOP

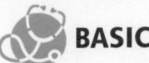 BASICS

- Chronic pain is typically defined as pain persisting beyond the time anticipated for normal tissue healing, usually >3 months.
- Over time, neuroplastic changes in the CNS transform pain into a chronic disease. Pain levels typically exceed the pathology observed on exam or imaging.
- Pain experience is inherently related to emotional, psychological, and cognitive factors.
- An epidemic of undertreated pain coexists with an epidemic of prescription drug abuse in the United States.
- Use an evidence-based, systems-based practice to safely and effectively prescribe opioid medications only when indicated for chronic, nonmalignant pain.

EPIDEMIOLOGY

Incidence
- Incidence is rising, but exact rate is unclear.
- The annual economic cost of chronic pain in the United States is estimated at $560 to $635 billion (1).

Prevalence
In the United States, an estimated 50 million adults live with chronic pain. Individuals reporting severe pain are more likely to have impaired health status, use more health care, and suffer more disability (1).

ALERT
Caution: Opioid-related overdoses are at an all-time high. From 2000 to 2016, over half a million people died from drug overdoses (http://www.cdc.gov/drugoverdose/index.html).

ETIOLOGY AND PATHOPHYSIOLOGY
- With intense, repeated, or prolonged stimulation of damaged or inflamed tissues, the threshold for activating primary afferent pain fibers is lowered, the frequency of firing is higher, and there is increased response to noxious and/or normal stimuli (peripheral and central sensitization). The amygdala, prefrontal cortex, and cortex relay emotions related to the pain experience, and these areas undergo structural and functional changes over time.
- Patients often have an identifiable etiology (most commonly musculoskeletal problems or headache), but pain levels are often worse than observable tissue injury. Many patients have no obvious source of chronic pain.

Genetics
Current research suggests a genetic polymorphism in opioid receptors; may affect patient's response and/or side effects to individual opioids

RISK FACTORS
- Traumatic: motor vehicle accidents, repetitive motion injuries, sports injuries, work-related injuries, and falls
- Postsurgical: especially back surgeries, amputations, and thoracotomies
- Psychiatric comorbidities: substance abuse, depression, posttraumatic stress disorder (PTSD), personality disorders
- Aging: increased incidence with age but should not be considered a "normal" part of aging

GENERAL PREVENTION
- Prevent work-related injuries through the use of ergonomic workplace design.
- Exercise and physical therapy help prevent work-related low back pain.
- Varicella vaccine and rapid treatment of shingles to lower risk of postherpetic neuralgia
- Tight glycemic control for diabetic patients, prevention of alcohol abuse, smoking cessation

COMMONLY ASSOCIATED CONDITIONS
Any chronic disease and/or its treatment can cause chronic pain, including diabetes, cardiovascular disease, HIV, progressive neurologic conditions, lung disease, cirrhosis, autoimmune disease, cancer, renal failure, depression, and mental illness.

 DIAGNOSIS

Two general categories of pain:
- Nociceptive pain (two types)
  - *Somatic*: skin, bone, soft tissue disease; described as well localized, sharp, stabbing, aching
  - *Visceral*: visceral inflammation/injury; described as poorly localized, dull, aching; may refer to sites remote from lesion; can wax and wane
- Neuropathic pain: damaged peripheral or central nerves; described as burning, tingling, and/or numbness
  - Sympathetically mediated pain: Peripheral nerve injury can cause severe burning pain, swelling of the affected limb, and focal changes in sweat production and skin appearance (e.g., complex regional pain syndrome).

HISTORY
- Pain history: location, onset, intensity, duration, quality, temporal pattern, exacerbating agents, alleviators, prior treatments
- Assess and document how pain affects patient's functioning and quality of life and what they expect from treatment.
- Screen for personal or family history of substance abuse (including tobacco addiction), mental health conditions, domestic violence, or sexual abuse.
- Standardized tools: pain severity—Brief Pain Inventory (short form); mood—Patient Health Questionnaire-9 (PHQ-9); substance abuse—Screener and Opioid Assessment for Patients with Pain (SOAPP), multiple versions
- Stratify patients for risks of chronic opioid therapy and need for increased monitoring; a positive screen does not automatically exclude patients from opioid therapy.

PHYSICAL EXAM
Exam is guided by history and includes functional and behavioral assessments.

DIFFERENTIAL DIAGNOSIS
- Multiple medical and surgical conditions can lead to chronic pain.
- Aberrant drug-taking behaviors:
  - Inadequate analgesia ("pseudoaddiction"), disease progression, opioid-resistant pain, opioid-induced hyperalgesia, addiction, opioid tolerance, self-medication of nonpain symptoms, criminal intent (diversion)

DIAGNOSTIC TESTS & INTERPRETATION
Base testing on history, exam, and differential diagnosis.

Initial Tests (lab, imaging)
- Urine drug screen: qualitative analysis for drugs of abuse and quantitative analysis for individual drugs (e.g., as part of prescription opioid contract)
- Most tests are immunoassays, which detect morphine and heroin but often not other opioids. Laboratory-based chromatography/spectrometry can identify specific drugs.

Follow-Up Tests & Special Considerations
For chronic opioid therapy, order random urine drug screens.

Diagnostic Procedures/Other
- Consider interventional pain clinic for complex injections and nerve blocks, which can be diagnostic.
- If complex regional pain syndrome is suspected, a sympathetic block can be diagnostic and possibly prevent chronic pain.

TREATMENT
- Goals of treatment are to restore function and decrease pain while balancing risks and benefits of therapies.
- Interdisciplinary teams offer the most effective approach to treating the physical, emotional, and behavioral aspects of chronic pain. These multidisciplinary teams include the patient, family, primary care doctor, nurse, pain management specialist, pharmacist, psychologist, psychiatrist, physical and occupational therapists, physiatrist, complementary medicine practitioners, social worker, and an addiction medicine specialist.
- Treatment should always include nonpharmacologic therapies such as exercise, cognitive-behavioral therapy (CBT), patient and family education, yoga, massage, relaxation techniques, support groups, meditation, and acupuncture.
- For complex regional pain syndrome refer to pain management specialist (if available), and start treatment for neuropathic pain (if not contraindicated) in order to minimize risk of chronic pain.

GENERAL MEASURES
Keep a pain and function diary to record pain and activity level and medication use.

MEDICATION
- Always begin with exercise, physical therapy, CBT, and self-management skills. Use sequential time-limited trials of medications, start at low doses, and gradually increase until effect or dose-limiting side effects are reached. Use rational polypharmacy (e.g., an opioid + neuropathic agent) if indicated and consult with pain specialists as available and as necessary.
- For mild to moderate chronic pain
  - Acetaminophen: daily dose not to exceed total 4 g in healthy adults and 2 g in the elderly or those with hepatic disease or active or past history of alcohol use
  - NSAIDs: Use COX-2 selective inhibitors with caution because of cardiac risks (may have less gastric risk). If high cardiac risk, consider nonselective COX inhibitor (such as naproxen) with or without gastric prophylaxis (depending on ulcer risk). Caution: Combinations can lead to serious acetaminophen or NSAID toxicities if patients exceed recommended doses.

- Tramadol: an opioid analgesic with weak serotonin-norepinephrine reuptake inhibitor (SNRI), may be helpful in neuropathic pain but has ceiling dose and risk of seizures (initial dose 50 mg q6h PRN, ceiling dose 400 mg/day or 300 mg/day for older adults).
- Topical agents: NSAIDs (diclofenac gel 1–3% BID), lidocaine (4% gel OTC is less effective but more affordable than 5% patch), ketamine 0.5–10% BID–QID, capsaicin 0.035–0.1% QD–QID
- For neuropathic pain
  - Classes of medications include (i) tricyclic antidepressants (desipramine [25 to 100 mg QD but start with 10 mg QD in frail elderly] and nortriptyline [25 to 100 mg QD but start with 10 mg QD in frail elderly] have fewer side effects), (ii) SNRI antidepressants (duloxetine 30-60 mg BID), (iii) anticonvulsants (α2-δ ligands, gabapentin [initial dose 300 mg/day and titrate to max of 3,600 mg/day in 3 divided doses] and pregabalin [100 to 300 mg/day in 2 to 3 divided doses]); and (iv) last line is opioids, including tramadol; example: combination of nortriptyline + gabapentin
  - See "Diagnosis."
- For moderate to severe chronic pain
  - Morphine, oxycodone, hydromorphone, oxymorphone, fentanyl. Check opioid equianalgesic table (https://www.cms.gov/Medicare/Prescription-Drug-Coverage/PrescriptionDrugCovContra/Downloads/Opioid-Morphine-EQ-Conversion-Factors-Aug-2017.pdf) or dosing by route of administration.
  - No evidence supports any of these opioids as superior or having improved side effect profile.
  - In patients with chronic back pain, aberrant medication-taking behaviors range from 5% to 24%.
    - Avoid morphine in patients with renal insufficiency.
    - Methadone should only be prescribed by experienced providers. Methadone has many drug interactions and can contribute to potentially fatal cardiac arrhythmias.
  - Once stable dose of opioids is established, change to sustained-release formulations if pain is constant or frequent; short-acting formulations for breakthrough/episodic pain only
  - Common side effects: constipation: Senna should be prescribed at time opioids are started and importance of regular bowel movements emphasized; also nausea, sedation, mental status changes, and pruritus
  - Coprescribe nasal naloxone for at-risk patients on chronic opioids (see "Ongoing Care") (2)[C].

ALERT
Patients on chronic opioid therapy must agree to monitoring. Use universal precautions and systems-based practice, including written agreements, random urine drug screens (testing for drugs of abuse and specifically for the drug prescribed), pill/patch counts, and other measures (see "Ongoing Care").

SURGERY/OTHER PROCEDURES
Consider interventional procedures, including joint injections, nerve blocks, spinal cord stimulation, and intrathecal medication among others, as needed.

COMPLEMENTARY & ALTERNATIVE MEDICINE
- Acupuncture works well for chronic neck and back pain and fibromyalgia.
- Exercise works well in low back pain and fibromyalgia.
- For adults with chronic low back pain, consider mindfulness-based stress reduction (MBSR) or CBT, (3)[A].
- Mind–body interventions: yoga, tai chi, hypnosis, progressive muscle relaxation, meditation
- Yoga as effective as standard physical therapy for moderate to severe chronic low back pain (2)[A]

 ## ONGOING CARE

FOLLOW-UP RECOMMENDATIONS
Patient Monitoring
- It can be difficult to identify appropriate pain relief–seeking behavior from inappropriate drug seeking
- Maintain a nonjudgmental approach.
- Assess and document benefits, pain levels, functioning, and quality of life.
- *Universal precautions* as a systems-based approach:
  - Informed consent for opioid therapy
  - Written agreement between patient and clinician
  - One prescriber and one pharmacy
  - No after-hours prescriptions or early refills
  - Mandatory police reporting for medication thefts
  - Random urine drug tests, pill/patch counts
  - Continue with physical therapy, counseling, psychiatric medications, and necessary treatments.
  - Participate in state's prescription drug monitoring program: http://www.cdc.gov/drugoverdose/pdmp/.
  - Taper and discontinue medications (5% dose reduction per week) if patient does not benefit, if side effects outweigh benefits. If medications are abused or diverted, more rapid taper is appropriate. If addiction is suspected, always offer treatment for substance abuse.
  - Patients on long-term opioid therapy may see improvement in pain, function, and quality of life with voluntary dose reductions (4)[A].
- Nasal naloxone
  - For patients at increased risk of overdose: history of overdose, history of substance use disorder, concurrent benzodiazepine use, high opioid doses
  - Naloxone kit: two 1 mg/mL prefilled syringes with intranasal mucosal atomization device; takes effect in 2 to 5 minutes, lasts 30 to 90 minutes

PATIENT EDUCATION
American Chronic Pain Association: https://theacpa.org

COMPLICATIONS
- Rate of addiction in chronic pain patients ~3–19%
- Definitions
  - Addiction: chronic biopsychological disease characterized by impaired control over drug use, compulsive use, and continued use despite harm
  - Physical dependence: withdrawal syndrome produced by abrupt cessation or rapid dose reduction
  - Tolerance: state of adaptation when a drug induces changes that diminish its effects over time
  - Diversion: selling drugs or giving them to persons other than for whom they are prescribed

REFERENCES
1. Institute of Medicine, Committee on Advancing Pain Research, Care, and Education. *Relieving Pain in America: A Blueprint for Transforming Prevention, Care, Education, and Research*. Washington, DC: National Academies Press; 2011.
2. Saper RB, Lemaster C, Delitto A, et al. Yoga, physical therapy, or education for chronic low back pain: a randomized noninferiority trial. *Ann Intern Med*. 2017;167(2):85–94.
3. Cherkin DC, Sherman KJ, Balderson BH, et al. Effect of mindfulness-based stress reduction vs cognitive behavioral therapy or usual care on back pain and functional limitations in adults with chronic low back pain: a randomized clinical trial. *JAMA*. 2016;315(12):1240–1249.
4. Frank JW, Lovejoy TI, Becker WC, et al. Patient outcomes in dose reduction or discontinuation of long-term opioid therapy: a systematic review. *Ann Intern Med*. 2017;167(3):181–191.

ADDITIONAL READING
- Bohnert ASB, Guy GP Jr, Losby JL. Opioid prescribing in the United States before and after the Centers for Disease Control and Prevention's 2016 opioid guideline. *Ann Intern Med*. 2018;169(6):367–375.
- Reisfield GM, Goldberger BA, Berthoff RL. Choosing the right laboratory: a review of clinical and forensic toxicology services for urine drug testing in pain management. *J Opioid Manag*. 2015;11(1):37–44.
- SCOPE of Pain (Safe and Competent Opioid Prescribing Education)—free online modules from Boston University School of Medicine: https://www.scopeofpain.com.

 ## CODES

ICD10
- G89.29 Other chronic pain
- G89.21 Chronic pain due to trauma
- G89.28 Other chronic postprocedural pain

CLINICAL PEARLS
- Start with the presumption that a patient's pain is *real*, even if pathophysiologic evidence is initially lacking.
- Emphasize that a pain-free life may not be possible—better function and quality of life are shared goals.
- Use a multidisciplinary approach with nonpharmacologic therapies, exercise, self-management and thoughtful medication use with clear goals, expectations, and documentation of care plan.
- Universal precautions are a systems-based for opioid prescription in cases of chronic pain.

CIRRHOSIS OF THE LIVER

Liam P. Burke, MD • Anna K. Zheng, MD

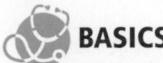 BASICS

DESCRIPTION

A chronic hepatocellular disease with inflammation, necrosis, and fibrosis potentially leading to liver failure and/or cancer

EPIDEMIOLOGY

- Predominant age at diagnosis: 40 to 60 years old
- Predominant sex: male > female; more women with cirrhosis from alcohol abuse
- Liver disease and cirrhosis are the 9th leading cause of death among U.S. adult males; 12th overall

ETIOLOGY AND PATHOPHYSIOLOGY

- Chronic hepatitis C virus (HCV) (26%)
- Alcohol abuse (21%)
- Nonalcoholic steatohepatitis (NASH)/obesity (~10%)
- Hepatitis B virus (HBV) plus hepatitis D infection (15%)
- Other: hemochromatosis, autoimmune hepatitis, primary biliary cirrhosis, secondary biliary cirrhosis, biliary atresia, idiopathic biliary fibrosis, primary sclerosing cholangitis, Wilson disease, α_1-antitrypsin deficiency, granulomatous disease (e.g., sarcoidosis); drug-induced liver disease (e.g., methotrexate, α-methyldopa, amiodarone); venous outflow obstruction (e.g., Budd-Chiari syndrome, veno-occlusive disease); chronic right-sided heart failure; tricuspid regurgitation; and rare genetic, metabolic, and infectious causes
- Hepatocellular injury results in cellular hyperplasia (regenerating nodules), fibrous changes, and angiogenesis. Distortions in blood flow result in portal hypertension.

Genetics

Hemochromatosis, Wilson disease, and α_1-antitrypsin deficiency in adults are associated with cirrhosis.

RISK FACTORS

Alcohol abuse, intravenous drug abuse, obesity

GENERAL PREVENTION

- Mitigate risk factors (e.g., alcohol abuse); >80% of chronic liver disease is preventable.
- Limit alcohol consumption and advise weight loss in overweight or obese patients.

COMMONLY ASSOCIATED CONDITIONS

HCV, alcohol and drug abuse, diabetes, depression, obesity

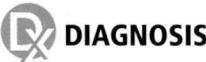 DIAGNOSIS

HISTORY

- Review risk factors (alcohol abuse, viral hepatitis, family history of primary liver cancer, other liver disease, or autoimmune disease).
- Symptoms
  - Fatigue, malaise, weakness
  - Anorexia, weight loss (weight gain if ascites/edema)
  - Right upper abdominal pain
  - Bruising, bleeding, hematemesis, hematochezia, melena
  - Tea-colored urine, clay-colored stools
  - Edema, abdominal swelling/bloating, pruritus
  - Bruising, bleeding, hematemesis, hematochezia, melena
  - Absent/irregular menses, chronic anovulation
  - Diminished libido, erectile dysfunction
  - Night blindness

PHYSICAL EXAM

Physical exam may be normal until end-stage disease.

- Skin changes: spider angiomas, palmar erythema, jaundice, scleral icterus, ecchymoses, caput medusa, hyperpigmentation, decreased body hair, facial telangiectasias
- Hepatomegaly (small, fibrotic liver when end-stage disease)
- Splenomegaly (if portal hypertension)
- Abdominal fluid wave, shifting dullness (ascites)
- Gynecomastia
- Dupuytren contractures
- Pretibial, presacral pitting edema, and clubbing (especially in hepatopulmonary syndrome)
- Asterixis, mental status changes
- Muscle wasting, weakness
- Fetor hepaticus (in severe portosystemic shunting)

DIFFERENTIAL DIAGNOSIS

Steatohepatitis, other causes of portal hypertension (e.g., portal vein thrombosis, lymphoma); metastatic or multifocal cancer in the liver; vascular congestion (e.g., cardiac cirrhosis); acute alcoholic hepatitis

DIAGNOSTIC TESTS & INTERPRETATION

Initial Tests (lab, imaging)

- Aspartate aminotransferase/alanine aminotransferase (AST/ALT): mildly elevated, typically AST > ALT; enzymes may normalize as cirrhosis progresses.
- Elevated alkaline phosphatase (ALP), γ-glutamyl transpeptidase (GGT), and total/direct bilirubin
- Anemia from hemolysis, folate deficiency, and/or splenomegaly
- Thrombocytopenia (<110; 95% specific for cirrhosis)
- Impaired synthetic liver function denoted by hypoalbuminemia, low cholesterol, prolonged prothrombin time (PT), international normalized ratio (INR), and partial thromboplastin time (PTT); coagulopathy of vitamin K–dependent clotting factors (II, VII, IX, X)
- Progressive cirrhosis indicated by hyperammonemia, elevated BUN, hyperkalemia, and hyponatremia
- Abdominal ultrasound q6–12mo to screen for hepatocellular carcinoma (HCC)
- Doppler ultrasound to assess liver parenchyma and hepatic/portal veins

Follow-Up Tests & Special Considerations

Consider:

- Hepatitis serologies
- Serum ethanol and GGT if alcohol abuse suspected
- Antimitochondrial antibody to screen for primary biliary cirrhosis
- Anti-smooth muscle and antinuclear antibodies to screen for chronic active (autoimmune) hepatitis
- Transferrin saturation (>50%) and ferritin (markedly increased) to screen for hemochromatosis; if abnormal, check hemochromatosis (HFE) genetics/mutation analysis.
- α_1-Antitrypsin phenotype screen
- Ceruloplasmin to screen for Wilson disease; if low, check copper excretion (serum copper plus 24-hour urine copper).
- α-Fetoprotein level to screen for HCC

Diagnostic Procedures/Other

- Liver biopsy: required for definitive diagnosis, percutaneous if INR <1.5 and no ascites; otherwise, transjugular; serologic testing gaining use as a surrogate for biopsy
- Ultrasound-based elastography: noninvasive alternative to liver biopsy, increasing availability; evaluates fibrosis
- Endoscopy if esophageal varices/portal hypertensive gastropathy are a concern
- Magnetic resonance elastography: most accurate noninvasive method in obese and/or nonalcoholic fatty liver disease (NAFLD) (1)[A]

Test Interpretation

Fibrous bands and regenerative nodules are classic biopsy features of cirrhosis. Other histologic patterns:

- Alcoholic liver disease: steatosis, polymorphonuclear (PMN) leukocyte infiltrate, ballooning degeneration of hepatocytes, Mallory bodies, giant mitochondria
- HBV/HCV: periportal lymphocytic inflammation
- NASH: same as alcoholic liver disease; steatosis may "burn-out" in advanced disease.
- Biliary cirrhosis: PMN infiltrate in wall of bile ducts, inflammation increased in portal spaces, progressive loss of bile ducts in portal spaces
- Hemochromatosis: intrahepatic iron stores increased via iron stain or weighted biopsy tissue
- α_1-Antitrypsin deficiency: positive periodic acid–Schiff bodies in hepatocytes

 TREATMENT

Outpatient care except for major GI bleeding, altered mental status, sepsis/infection, rapid hepatic decompensation, or renal failure

GENERAL MEASURES

- Abstain from alcohol, drugs, hepatotoxic medications, and hepatotoxic herbs (2)[B].
- Pneumococcal, hepatitis A/B, and influenza vaccines
- Weight loss, exercise, and control of lipids/glucose (2)[B]

MEDICATION

First Line

Treat the underlying cause first (note prescribing precautions in decompensated cirrhosis).

- HCV: Goal is to eradicate viral RNA in serum. Latest therapies are genotype dependent. Typical regimens with or without cirrhosis include sofosbivir-ledipasivir and elbasivir-grazoprevir for up to 12 weeks duration. Pegylated interferon (PEG-IFN) is no longer first line.
- HBV: In compensated cirrhosis with viremia, goal of treatment is to reduce HCC risk and decompensation with 48-week therapy. If decompensated, indefinite therapy recommended. Entecavir 0.5 to 1.0 mg PO daily, tenofovir 300 mg PO daily, and telbivudine 600 mg PO daily are first line. Adefovir 10 mg PO daily second line; PEG-IFN α-2a 180 μg SC weekly for 48 weeks in compensated cirrhosis if not contraindicated; lamivudine not recommended as first-line agent due to resistance (3)[B]
- NAFLD: weight loss of 7–10% to improve histopathogic features. Improved fitness and/or >150 min/week of physical activity improves metabolic and hepatic indices (2)[B].

- Alcoholic hepatitis: Treat alcohol withdrawal; Maddrey discriminant function score for risk stratification; >32 indicates poor prognosis, patients may benefit from prednisolone 40 mg/day for 28 days with 2 to 4 week; taper to reduce short-term mortality; pentoxifylline for patients who cannot tolerate steroids
- Hereditary hemochromatosis: phlebotomy every 1 to 2 weeks as tolerated to goal serum ferritin of 50 to 100 µg/L and then 2 to 6 times per year as needed
- Primary biliary cirrhosis: ursodeoxycholic acid (ursodiol) 13 to 15 mg/kg PO divided BID–QID with food (3)[A]; bile acid sequestrants are first-line therapy for pruritus: cholestyramine 4 to 8 g PO BID; antihistamines; rifampicin 150 to 300 mg PO BID or naltrexone 50 mg/day can be used for pruritus if ursodiol is ineffective. Evaluate and treat for malabsorption, fat-soluble vitamin deficiencies, metabolic bone disease, hypercholesterolemia, hypothyroidism, and anemia.
- Wilson disease: initial treatment with penicillamine 1,000 to 1,500 mg/day PO BID–QID or trientine 750 to 1,500 mg/day PO BID–TID on empty stomach. Trientine 750 to 1,500 mg/day PO BID–TID is better tolerated. After 1 year, zinc acetate 150 mg/day PO BID–TID for maintenance; zinc for presymptomatic, pregnant, and pediatric populations
- Autoimmune (chronic active) hepatitis: Treat if AST or ALT >10 times ULN, or if either >5 times ULN and γ globulins >2 times ULN with prednisolone 30 to 60 mg/day initially, maintenance 5 to 20 mg/day with or without azathioprine (Imuran) 0.5 to 1.0 mg/kg; adjust to keep transaminase levels normal. The combination is preferred. Discontinue maintenance after at least 24 months of treatment if AST and ALT are normal.
- Esophageal varices: for primary prophylaxis of variceal bleed, propranolol >40 mg, carvedilol 6.25 mg or nadolol 40 mg PO daily, to lower portal pressure by 20 mm Hg, systolic pressure from 90 to 100 mm Hg, and pulse rate by 25%; PPI also indicated for portal hypertensive gastropathy
- Ascites/edema: low-sodium (<2 g/day) diet and spironolactone 100 to 400 mg/day with or without furosemide 40 to 160 mg/day PO; torsemide may substitute for furosemide. If serum sodium <120 mmol/L, then 1.0 to 1.5 L/day water restriction. If new onset, rule out SBP. If history of SBP, consider SBP prophylaxis (TMP-SMX DS daily, norfloxacin 400 mg PO daily).
- Encephalopathy: lactulose 15 to 45 mL BID; titrate to induce 2 to 3 loose bowel movements daily. Combination therapy with rifaximin (550 mg PO BID) is recommended regimen to prevent recurrent hepatic encephalopathy (4)[B].
- Pruritus: ursodiol, cholestyramine, or antihistamines (e.g., hydroxyzine)
- Renal insufficiency: Stop NSAIDs, diuretics, and nephrotoxic drugs; normalize electrolytes; and hospitalize for plasma expansion or dialysis.
- Prophylactic antibiotics for invasive procedures, GI bleeding, or history of spontaneous bacterial peritonitis
- Proton pump inhibitor for esophageal varices requiring banding or portal hypertensive gastropathy

ISSUES FOR REFERRAL
Evaluate for liver transplant at onset of complications (ascites, variceal bleeding, encephalopathy), jaundice, or liver lesion suggestive of HCC and/or when evidence of hepatic dysfunction develops (Child-Turcotte-Pugh >7 and Model for End-Stage Liver Disease [MELD] >10).

SURGERY/OTHER PROCEDURES
- Varices: endoscopic ligation, 4 to 6 treatments (if acute bleed, use pre-esophagogastroduodenoscopy [EGD] octreotide as vasoconstrictor); transjugular intrahepatic shunt (TIPS) second-line or salvage therapy for acute bleed
- Ascites: if tense, therapeutic paracentesis every 2 weeks PRN; caution if pedal edema absent.
- Fulminant hepatic failure: liver transplantation
- HCC: curable if small with radiofrequency ablation or resection and transplant

COMPLEMENTARY & ALTERNATIVE MEDICINE
- Zinc sulfate 220 mg BID may improve dysgeusia and appetite; adjunct for hepatic encephalopathy
- Milk thistle may lower transaminases and improve symptoms.
- Danshen and huangqi injections may promote improvement; further studies needed

ADMISSION, INPATIENT, AND NURSING CONSIDERATIONS
Major GI bleeding, altered mental status, sepsis/infection, rapidly progressing hepatic decompensation, renal failure

 ## ONGOING CARE

FOLLOW-UP RECOMMENDATIONS
Regular physical conditioning may help with fatigue.

Patient Monitoring
- Once stable, monitor liver enzymes, platelets, and PT q6–12mo.
- Patients >55 years with chronic HBV or HCV, elevated INR, or low platelets are at highest risk for HCC; serial α-fetoprotein and liver ultrasound screening q6–12mo in patients with cirrhosis
- MRI best follow-up test for HCC if α-fetoprotein elevated and/or liver mass found on ultrasound
- Endoscopy at diagnosis and every 3 years (compensated) and every 1 year (decompensated) to screen for varices

DIET
Protein (1.0 to 1.5 g/kg body weight), high fiber, daily multivitamin (without iron), sodium restriction (<2 g/day), combined with fluid restriction, essential if ascites/edema

PATIENT EDUCATION
- Educate about when to seek emergency care (e.g., hematemesis, altered mental status).
- Drug, alcohol and smoking cessation (no cannabis)
- Update required immunizations; HCV transmission precautions

PROGNOSIS
- 5 to 20 years of asymptomatic disease from time of initial diagnosis
- After onset of complications, death typically within 5 years without transplant
  - 5% per year develop HCC.
  - 50% of cirrhotics develop ascites over 10 years; 50% 5-year survival after ascites develop.
  - Acute variceal bleeding is the most common fatal complication; 30% mortality
  - Median survival after complications (ascites, variceal bleeding, encephalopathy) is 1.5 years.
  - With transplant, 85% survive 1 year; after transplant, ~5% annual mortality
- <25% of eligible patients receive a transplant because of donor organ shortage.

COMPLICATIONS
Ascites, edema, infections, encephalopathy, GI bleeding, esophageal varices, gastropathy, colopathy, hepatorenal syndrome, hepatopulmonary syndrome, HCC, fulminant hepatic failure, complications after transplant (e.g., surgical, rejection, infections)

REFERENCES
1. Singh S, Venkatesh SK, Wang Z, et al. Diagnostic performance of magnetic resonance elastography in staging liver fibrosis: a systematic review and meta-analysis of individual participant data. *Clin Gastroenterol Hepatol*. 2015;13(3):440–451.e6.
2. Hart CL, Morrison DS, Batty GD, et al. Effect of body mass index and alcohol consumption on liver disease: analysis of data from two prospective cohort studies. *BMJ*. 2010;340:c1240.
3. Batirel A, Guclu E, Arslan F, et al. Comparable efficacy of tenofovir versus entecavir and predictors of response in treatment-naïve patients with chronic hepatitis B: a multicenter real-life study. *Int J Infect Dis*. 2014;28:153–159.
4. Sharma BC, Sharma P, Lunia MK, et al. A randomized, double-blind, controlled trial comparing rifaximin plus lactulose with lactulose alone in treatment of overt hepatic encephalopathy. *Am J Gastroenterol*. 2013;108(9):1458–1463.

ADDITIONAL READING
- Chalasani N, Younossi Z, Lavine JE, et al. The diagnosis and management of nonalcoholic fatty liver disease: practice guidance from the American Association for the Study of Liver Diseases. *Hepatology*. 2018;67(1):328–357.
- Chou R, Wasson N. Blood tests to diagnose fibrosis or cirrhosis in patients with chronic hepatitis C virus infection: a systematic review. *Ann Intern Med*. 2013;158(11):807–820.
- Nierhoff J, Chávez Ortiz AA, Herrmann E, et al. The efficiency of acoustic radiation force impulse imaging for the staging of liver fibrosis: a meta-analysis. *Eur Radiol*. 2013;23(11):3040–3053.

 ## SEE ALSO

Algorithm: Cirrhosis

 ## CODES

ICD10
- K74.60 Unspecified cirrhosis of liver
- K70.30 Alcoholic cirrhosis of liver without ascites
- K74.69 Other cirrhosis of liver

CLINICAL PEARLS
- 80% of chronic liver disease that leads to cirrhosis is preventable (primarily alcohol abuse).
- After diagnosis of cirrhosis, abdominal ultrasound every 6 months for early detection of HCC
- Update necessary immunizations and treat underlying cause (HCV, alcohol abuse, etc.).

CLOSTRIDIUM DIFFICILE INFECTION
Sally-Ann L. Pantin, MD, FAAFP • Thomas A. Waller, MD

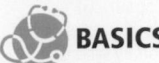 **BASICS**

DESCRIPTION
- A gram-positive, spore-forming anaerobic bacillus that releases toxins to produce clinical disease
- Infection caused by *Clostridium difficile* is frequently associated with antibiotic use, hospitalization, residence at long-term care facilities, and age.
- Severity of infection can range from diarrhea to pancolitis, perforation, and death.
- System(s) affected: gastrointestinal
- Synonyms(s): *C. difficile*–associated disease or diarrhea (CDAD); *C. difficile* infection; *C. difficile* colitis; *C. diff*

EPIDEMIOLOGY
Incidence
- *C. difficile* is a common hospital-acquired infection. The incidence is rising (1).
- There are ~15 new cases per 1,000 clinical discharges; higher with increased age (2)
- Rates of complications are also increasing (1).

Prevalence
- *C. difficile* causes ~25% of all cases of antibiotic-associated diarrhea.
- Prevalence of community-acquired *C. difficile* infection is increasing. Up to 40% of patients require hospitalization (2).
- *C. difficile* is a commensurate organism in 2–5% of the adult U.S. population.

ETIOLOGY AND PATHOPHYSIOLOGY
- *C. difficile* is an anaerobic toxin-producing, gram-positive bacillus bacteria existing in vegetative and spore forms.
- Spores can survive for months in harsh conditions and outside of the body.
- Spread by fecal–oral contact. Acid-resistant spores pass through stomach to reside mostly in the colon.
- Colonic colonization causes disruptions in barrier functions of the normal microbiome (2).
- *C. difficile* is noninvasive. Toxins mediate disease:
  - Toxins A (enterotoxin) and B (cytotoxin) attract neutrophils and monocytes, de-grading colonic epithelial cells and causing clinical disease.
- The hypervirulent strain BI/NAP1/027 of *C. difficile* produces a much more virulent form of disease. It is associated with higher rates of colectomy and death.

Genetics
No known genetic factors

RISK FACTORS
- Host risk factors
  - Age >65 years
  - Hospitalization or long-term health care facility
  - Comorbidities, including inflammatory bowel disease, immunosuppression, chronic liver disease, and end-stage renal disease
  - Enteral feeding
  - Previous *C. difficile* infection

- Factors that disrupt normal colonic microbiota:
  - Exposure to antibiotics (including perioperative prophylaxis) increases risk for *C. difficile* infection.
  - Commonly implicated antibiotics: ampicillin, amoxicillin, clindamycin (most common), cephalo-sporins, and fluoroquinolones
  - Chronic acid suppression may allow more bacteria to reach the colon (2).
- Recurrence from prior infection
  - Recurrence rates are ~20%; recurrence more likely with each additional episode (2)
- Can colonize ileum in patients with prior colectomy
- Community-acquired *C. difficile* infections (no over-night admission in >12 weeks) are more frequent in patients without other risk factors (younger, no recent antibiotic exposure).

Geriatric Considerations
C. difficile is the most common cause of acute diarrheal illness in long-term care facilities. Elderly patients often have multiple risk factors (comorbid disease, antibiotic exposure, medication use).

Pediatric Considerations
- Neonates have a higher rate of *C. difficile* colonization (25–80%) but are generally less symptomatic than adults (possibly due to immature toxin receptors).
- Frequently serve as carrier for infection in adults

GENERAL PREVENTION
- Antibiotic stewardship program decreases the incidence of *C. difficile* infection.
- 2010 Society for Healthcare Epidemiology of America (SHEA)/Infectious Diseases Society of America (IDSA) guidelines for prevention (3):
  - For health care workers, patients, and visitors:
    - Contact precautions, including gloves and gowns, on entry to room
    - Alcohol-based hand sanitizers are not effective. Hand washing with soap and water before and after patient interaction is recommended.
    - Accommodate patients with *C. difficile* infection in private rooms, if possible.
  - Environmental cleaning and disinfection
    - Disinfect with hypochlorite or other spore-killing solution.
    - Identify and reduce environmental sources of *C. difficile*, including the use of nondisposable rectal thermometers.
  - Antimicrobial restrictions
    - Minimize the frequency and duration of antibi-otic therapy. Use particular care when prescrib-ing commonly implicated antibiotics.

COMMONLY ASSOCIATED CONDITIONS
Pseudomembranous colitis, toxic megacolon, sepsis, colonic perforation

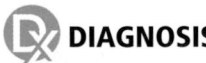 **DIAGNOSIS**

HISTORY
- Age and underlying comorbidities
- Recent antibiotic use
- Diarrhea (defined as >3 stools in 24 hours) that is watery, foul-smelling, and sometimes bloody (1)

- Fever (<10%), anorexia, nausea
- Recent hospitalization or stay at nursing facility

PHYSICAL EXAM
- Mild or moderate: cramping and lower abdominal pain
- Severe: fever, nausea/vomiting, dehydration
- Severe, complicated: shock, peritonitis, ileus

DIFFERENTIAL DIAGNOSIS
- Acute abdomen
- Antibiotic-associated diarrhea
- Inflammatory bowel disease
- Enteric infections
- Foodborne illness

DIAGNOSTIC TESTS & INTERPRETATION
Initial Tests (lab, imaging)
- The optimal diagnostic test is unclear (4).
- *C. difficile* can be identified by polymerase chain reaction (PCR)-based testing; rapid, highly sensitive, and highly specific (2)[B]
- *C. difficile* can be identified by immunoassays or nucleic acid amplification test (NAAT):
  - Glutamate dehydrogenase (GDH) antigen, in both toxic and nontoxic strains of *C. difficile* (sensitivity, 85–95%; specificity, 89–99%)
  - Toxins (A/B or A); rapid, inexpensive, easy to use (sensitivity 63–94%)
- Stool culture is the most sensitive; non–toxin-producing strains are also detected.
- Repeat testing during the same episode of diarrhea is not recommended. Stool carriage persists for 3 to 6 weeks after successful treatment (2)[A].
- Routine radiologic examination is not recommended in the absence of signs of systemic disease or clinical suspicion for complicated/severe disease.
  - Plain films may show thumbprinting and colonic distension.
  - CT may show mucosal thickening, colonic wall thickening, pericolonic inflammation, or signs of complicated infection in severe cases (i.e., extra-luminal air).

Diagnostic Procedures/Other
Endoscopy can evaluate for presence of pseudomem-branes and exclude other conditions.
- Although not all patients with *C. difficile* infection have pseudomembranes, their presence is pathognomonic.
- Flexible sigmoidoscopy may miss 15–20% of pseudomembranes (from the proximal colon).

Test Interpretation
SHEA/IDSA guidelines (3)
- Mild or moderate disease: leukocytosis with white blood cell (WBC) count <15,000 cells/μL and a serum creatinine level <1.5× the premorbid level
- Severe, uncomplicated disease: leukocytosis with WBC count >15,000 cells/μL or a serum creatinine level >1.5× the premorbid level
- Severe, complicated disease: hypotension, sepsis, markedly elevated WBC count, and imaging findings of complicated disease

TREATMENT

GENERAL MEASURES
- Antimotility agents are contraindicated.
- Avoid indiscriminate use of antibiotics.
- Proton pump inhibitors are associated with recurrent infection but have not been shown to be causal.
- Discontinue offending antibiotic, whenever possible.

MEDICATION

First Line
- Mild or moderate infection (4)[A]
  - Vancomycin 125 mg given QID for 10 days
  - Fidaxomicin 200 mg given BID for 10 days
  - If above agents are unavailable: metronidazole, 500 mg 3 times per day PO for 10 days
  - If patient is unable to take oral medications, then intravenous (IV) metronidazole or intraluminal (PO) vancomycin can be used.
- Severe infection (4)[A]
  - Enteral vancomycin is first-line therapy in patients with severe *C. difficile* infection:
    ◦ 125 mg PO QID for 10 to 14 days
    ◦ Fidaxomicin 200 mg given BID for 10 days
    ◦ Vancomycin retention enema if unable to take PO or if there is evidence of poor gastrointestinal motility
- Severe, complicated infection—consider surgical and critical care consultation (4)[A].
  - VAN 500 mg PO QID or by nasogastric tube. If ileus, consider adding rectal instillation of VAN and
  - Intravenously administered metronidazole (500 mg every 8 hours)
- First recurrence
  - If a standard regimen was used for the initial episode, use vancomycin taper: 125 mg QID for 10 to 14 days, BID for a week, once per day for a week, and then every 2 or 3 days for 2 to 8 weeks or
  - Fidaxomicin 200 mg given BID for 10 days if VAN was used for the initial episode
- Second recurrence
  - Vancomycin taper and/or pulse: vancomycin 125 mg PO QID for 10 to 14 days, then 125 mg PO BID for 7 days, then 125 mg PO once daily for 7 days, and then 125 mg PO every 2 to 3 days for 2 to 8 weeks:
    ◦ Pulse dosing every 2 to 3 days allows spores to germinate and then be killed or
  - Vancomycin 125 mg PO QID for 10 days followed by rifaximin 400 mg 3 times daily for 20 days, OR
  - Fidaxomicin 200 mg given BID for 10 days, or
  - Fecal microbiota transplantation

ALERT
When using vancomycin to treat *C. difficile* infection, use oral or rectal formulations. IV formulations (not excreted into the colonic lumen) are ineffective.

Second Line
- Oral metronidazole
- 500 mg PO 3 times daily for 10 to 14 days
- Vancomycin: for patients who cannot tolerate or have failed metronidazole therapy and for pregnancy

- Fecal transplant: stool from healthy, screened donor. Administered via either rectal or oral route. Highly effective for recurrent infections (80–90% cure rate) after offending antibiotic stopped; recipient gut flora transformed in as few as 3 days following fecal transplantation (5)[A].

SURGERY/OTHER PROCEDURES
- Severe abdominal pain or signs of hemodynamic instability in the setting of known infection should prompt surgical and critical care consultation.
- Perforation of the colon (4)[A]

ALERT
BI/NAP1/027 strain is commonly associated with fulminant colitis, often requiring surgical intervention in younger patients with severe disease.

COMPLEMENTARY & ALTERNATIVE MEDICINE
- Adjunctive IV immunoglobulin (IVIG) has shown promise; more data needed before routine use
- Probiotics *Lactobacillus acidophilus* and *Saccharomyces boulardii* have inhibitory effects on *C. difficile* and can help prevent *C. difficile* infection.
- Other investigational treatments:
  - Newer antibiotics (rifalazil, tolevamer, and ramoplanin)
  - Monoclonal antibodies to modulate toxin effects
  - Vaccine form of *C. difficile* antitoxin antibody

ADMISSION, INPATIENT, AND NURSING CONSIDERATIONS
- Admission criteria/initial stabilization
  - Hypovolemia
  - Inability to keep up with enteric losses
  - Hematochezia
  - Electrolyte disturbances
- IV fluids to maintain volume status
- Discharge criteria
  - Decreased diarrhea severity and frequency
  - Tolerating oral diet and medications

ONGOING CARE

FOLLOW-UP RECOMMENDATIONS
Do not repeat testing for toxins because patients may shed for weeks following an acute infection.

Patient Monitoring
- Relapses of colitis occur in 15–30%.
- Relapses typically occur 2 to 10 days after discontinuing antibiotics.

DIET
- Regular diet
- NPO if severe colitis and surgical evaluation pending

PATIENT EDUCATION
Educate patients about *C. difficile* transmission, the importance of hand washing and not relying on alcohol-based sanitizers, and the appropriate use of antibiotics.

PROGNOSIS
- Most patients improve with conservative management and oral antibiotics.
- 1–3% of patients develop severe/fulminant colitis requiring emergency colectomy.

REFERENCES
1. Khanna S, Pardi DS. *Clostridium difficile* infection: management strategies for a difficult disease. *Therap Adv Gastroenterol*. 2014;7(2):72–86.
2. Leffler DA, Lamont JT. *Clostridium difficile* infection. *N Engl J Med*. 2015;372(16):1539–1548.
3. Cohen SH, Gerding DN, Johnson S, et al; for Society for Healthcare Epidemiology of America, Infectious Diseases Society of America. Clinical practice guidelines for *Clostridium difficile* infection in adults: 2010 update by the Society for Healthcare Epidemiology of America (SHEA) and the Infectious Diseases Society of America (IDSA). *Infect Control Hosp Epidemiol*. 2010;31(5):431–455.
4. Debast SB, Bauer MP, Kuijper EJ; and European Society of Clinical Microbiology and Infectious Diseases. European Society of Clinical Microbiology and Infectious Diseases: update of the treatment guidance document for *Clostridium difficile* infection. *Clin Microbiol Infect*. 2014;20(Suppl 2):1–26.
5. Shankar V, Hamilton MJ, Khoruts A, et al. Species and genus level resolution analysis of gut microbiota in *Clostridium difficile* patients following fecal microbiota transplantation. *Microbiome*. 2014;2:13.

ADDITIONAL READING
- Johnston BC, Ma SS, Goldenberg JZ, et al. Probiotics for the prevention of *Clostridium difficile*-associated diarrhea: a systematic review and meta-analysis. *Ann Intern Med*. 2012;157(12):878–888.
- McCollum DL, Rodriguez JM. Detection, treatment, and prevention of *Clostridium difficile* infection. *Clin Gastroenterol Hepatol*. 2012;10(6):581–592.
- McDonald LC, Gerding DN, Johnson S, et al. Clinical practice guidelines for *Clostridium difficile* infection in adults and children: 2017 update by the Infectious Diseases Society of America (IDSA) and Society for Healthcare Epidemiology of America (SHEA). *Clin Infect Dis*. 2018;66(7):e1–e48.
- Paknikar R, Pekow J. Fecal microbiota transplantation for the management of *Clostridium difficile* infection [published online ahead of print October 9, 2018]. *Surg Infect (Larchmt)*. doi:10.1089/sur.2018.221.

CODES

ICD10
A04.7 Enterocolitis due to Clostridium difficile

CLINICAL PEARLS
- *C. difficile* is spread by fecal–oral contact.
- Alcohol-based hand sanitizers are ineffective against *C. difficile*. Wash hands with soap and water.
- Testing and treatment of asymptomatic patients is not recommended.
- *C. difficile* and organismal by-products (e.g., toxin) are identifiable from stool samples.
- Patients may shed organism or toxin for weeks after treatment. Repeat toxin assays following treatment are not helpful.
- Vancomycin or fidaxomicin is now considered first line.

COLIC, INFANTILE

Daniel T. Lee, MD, MA • Arthur Ohannessian, MD

 BASICS

DESCRIPTION
- Colic is defined as excessive crying in an otherwise healthy baby.
- A commonly used criteria is the Wessel criteria or the Rule of Three, when crying lasts for:
  - >3 hr/day
  - >3 days/week
  - Persists >3 weeks
- Many clinicians do not strictly adhere to the criterion of persistence for >3 weeks because few parents or clinicians will wait that long before evaluation or intervention.
- Some clinicians feel that colic represents the extreme end of the spectrum of normal crying, whereas most feel that colic is a distinct clinical entity.

EPIDEMIOLOGY
Incidence
- Predominant age group is between 2 weeks and 4 months of age.
- Equal predominance among males and females

Prevalence
Wide range between 8% and 40% of infants, however, more likely affects between 10% and 25% of infants

Pediatric Considerations
This is a problem during infancy.

ETIOLOGY AND PATHOPHYSIOLOGY
The cause is unknown. Factors that may play a role include the following:
- Infant gastroesophageal reflux disease
- Allergy to cow's milk, soy milk, or breast milk protein
- Fruit juice intolerance
- Swallowing air during the process of crying, feeding, or sucking
- Overfeeding or feeding too quickly; underfeeding has also been proposed.
- Inadequate burping after feeding
- Family tension and/or stess
- Parental anxiety, depression, and/or fatigue
- Parent–infant interaction mismatch
- Infant's inability to console him- or herself when dealing with stimuli
- Possible early manifestation of childhood migraine
- Increases in the gut hormone motilin, causing hyperperistalsis
- Functional lactose overload (i.e., breast milk that has a lower lipid content can have faster transit time in the intestine, leading to more lactose fermentation in the gut and hence gas and distension)
- Alterations in fecal microflora
- Tobacco smoke exposure
- Prenatal exposure to maternal smoking or nicotine replacement therapy

RISK FACTORS
- Physiologic predispositions in an infant may play a role, but no definitive risk factors have been established.
- Emerging data suggest maternal smoking or exposure to nicotine replacement therapy during pregnancy is associated with higher incidence of infantile colic.
- Infants with a maternal history of migraine headaches are twice as likely to have colic.

GENERAL PREVENTION
Colic is generally not preventable.

 DIAGNOSIS

HISTORY
- Evaluation for Wessel criteria: Crying lasts for >3 hr/day, >3 days/week, and persists >3 weeks.
- Episodes usually have a clear beginning and end.
- The crying is generally spontaneous, without preceding events triggering the episodes.
- The crying is typically different from normal crying. Colicky crying may be louder, more turbulent, variable in pitch, and appears more like screaming.
- The infant may be difficult to soothe or console despite all of the parents' efforts.
- The infant acts normally when not colicky.
- Assess the support system of caregivers and families, including coping skills.

PHYSICAL EXAM
- A comprehensive physical exam is normal.
- Because excessive crying may be a risk factor for abuse, be sure to examine the child carefully for signs of shaken baby syndrome or other types of child abuse.

DIFFERENTIAL DIAGNOSIS
Any organic cause for excessive or qualitatively different crying in infants such as:
- Infectious causes such as meningitis, sepsis, otitis media, or UTI
- Gastrointestinal causes such as gastroesophageal reflux disease, intussusception, lactose intolerance, constipation, anal fissure, or strangulated hernia
- Trauma, which includes foreign bodies, corneal abrasion, occult fracture, digit or penile hair tourniquet syndrome, or child abuse

DIAGNOSTIC TESTS & INTERPRETATION
Initial Tests (lab, imaging)
Infantile colic is a clinical diagnosis. No testing is typically performed unless clinical symptoms imply other causes (UTI, weight loss, etc.).

Diagnostic Procedures/Other
A thorough history and physical exam should be performed to rule out other causes. Otherwise, no diagnostic procedures or imaging are indicated.

 TREATMENT

GENERAL MEASURES
- Soothe by holding and rocking the baby (1)[B].
- Use a pacifier (1)[B].
- Use of gentle rhythmic motion (e.g., strollers, infant swings, car rides) (1)[B]
- Place near white noise (e.g., vacuum cleaner, clothes dryer, white noise machine) (1)[B].
- Crib vibrators or car ride simulators have not proven to be helpful (1)[B].
- Increased carrying or use of infant carrier has not been shown to improve colic (1)[B].
- Burping does not significantly lower colic events.
- Employ the 5 Ss (need to be done concurrently):
  - Swaddling: tight wrapping with blanket; may be especially beneficial in infants <8 weeks old (2)[B]
  - Side: laying baby on side
  - Shushing: loud white noise
  - Swinging: rhythmic, jiggle motion
  - Sucking: on a nipple, finger, or pacifier

MEDICATION
- No medication has been found to be universally beneficial in treating infantile colic. Probiotics are safe and effective. Their use is discussed in the "Complementary & Alternative Medicine" section.
- Dicyclomine (Bentyl) has been proven beneficial, but the potential serious adverse effects, such as apnea, seizures, and syncope, have precluded its use. Furthermore, the manufacturer has made the medication contraindicated for infants <6 months (3)[B].
- Simethicone has not been shown to be beneficial (3)[B].
- Omeprazole has not been shown to be beneficial.

ISSUES FOR REFERRAL
Excessive vomiting, poor weight gain, recurrent respiratory diseases, or bloody stools should prompt referral to a specialist.

COMPLEMENTARY & ALTERNATIVE MEDICINE
- Recent data from a large randomized controlled study involving nine neonatal units in Italy found that prophylactic use of *Lactobacillus reuteri* was beneficial. At 3 months of age, the mean duration of crying time (38 vs. 71 minutes; $p < .01$), the mean number of regurgitations per day (2.9 vs. 4.6; $p < .01$), and the mean number of evacuations per day (4.2 vs. 3.6; $p < .01$) for the *L. reuteri* DSM 17938 and placebo groups, respectively, were significantly different (4)[A]. A possible mechanism of action for this intervention may be related to the fact that colic in infants is associated with low-grade systemic inflammation. Thus, specific bacterial species beyond conventional probiotics may have anti-inflammatory properties that may help to modulate microbiota and alleviate colic-related inflammation.

- However, the effect of *L. reuteri* has not been as robust in infants already diagnosed with colic. A placebo-controlled study of 50 infants given *L. reuteri* had significantly reduced median daily crying times throughout the study (370 to 35 min/day vs. 300 to 90 min/day in placebo group). However, weight gain, stooling frequency, and incidence of regurgitation were similar in both groups (5)[B].
- *L. reuteri* is available as over-the-counter drops; however, it is not regulated by the FDA.
- Anecdotal evidence that car rides, both real and simulated, can be effective. You can find a 10-hour recording of a simulated car ride at the following link: https://www.youtube.com/watch?v=8KAXmIe-T_4.
- Providing "white noise," such as running a vacuum cleaner, clothes dryer, white noise generator, or infant sound machine. Avoid excessively loud and/or prolonged noise to minimize potential adverse effects on hearing or auditory development.
- Herbal teas and supplements may help but are not recommended because of limited, inconclusive evidence.
  - Herbal teas containing mixtures of chamomile, vervain, licorice, and balm-mint used up to TID may be beneficial. However, the study used high dosages, raising clinical concerns that this therapy may impair needed milk consumption in infants and be impractical to administer. In addition, preparations used in the study may not be commercially available in the United States.
  - There is evidence supporting the effectiveness of different preparations of fennel, such as oils, teas and herbal compounds, in treating infantile colic (6)[A].
- A home-based intervention focusing on reducing infant stimulation and synchronizing infant sleep-wake cycles with the environment, as well as parental support, has been shown to be effective.
- Use of music may help.
- Chiropractic treatment has shown no benefit over placebo.
- Infant massage has not been shown to be helpful.

 ## ONGOING CARE

FOLLOW-UP RECOMMENDATIONS
Frequent outpatient visits as needed for parental reassurance, education, and monitoring and to ensure the health of the infant and parents

Patient Monitoring
Follow for proper feeding, growth, and development.

DIET
- If breastfeeding:
  - Continue breastfeeding; switching to formula unlikely to help
  - Possible therapeutic benefit from eliminating milk products, eggs, wheat, nuts, soy, and/or fish from the maternal diet of breastfeeding mothers (1)[B]

- If formula feeding:
  - Feeding the infant in a vertical position using a curved bottle or bottle with collapsible bag may help to reduce air swallowing.
  - If no intervention or dietary change has been effective, consider a 1-week trial of hypoallergenic formulas such as whey hydrolysate (e.g., Good Start) or casein hydrolysate (e.g., Alimentum, Nutramigen, Pregestimil) (1)[B],(3)[C].
  - Adding fiber to formula also has not been shown to be helpful (1)[B].
- Supplementing with sucrose solution may be helpful, but the effect may be short-lived (<1 hour) (1,3)[B].
- Switching to soy protein formula is unlikely to be helpful.
- Despite the proposed mechanism of functional lactose overload, use of lactase enzymes in formula or breast milk or given directly to the infant has no therapeutic benefit (1)[B].

PATIENT EDUCATION
- Reassure parents that colic is not the result of bad parenting, and advise parents about having proper rest breaks, adequate sleep, and help in caring for the infant.
- Explain the spectrum of crying behavior.
- Avoid over- or underfeeding.
- Instruct parents regarding beneficial feeding techniques such as improved bottles (low air, curved) and sufficient burping after feeding.
- Information for parents of colicky infants can be found at the following link from the American Academy of Family Physician: https://www.aafp.org/afp/2004/0815/p741.html

PROGNOSIS
- Usually subsides by 3 to 6 months of age, often on its own
- Despite apparent abdominal pain, colicky infants eat well and gain weight normally.
- A few studies indicate temper tantrums may be more common among formerly colicky infants as studied in toddlers up to 4 years old.
- Colic has no bearing on the baby's intelligence or future development.

COMPLICATIONS
- Colic is self-limiting, and there is no proven untoward lasting effects to the infant.
- Possible associations with increased risk/incidence of postpartum depression among either or both parents, child abuse, caregiver burnout, and early cessation of breastfeeding

REFERENCES

1. Johnson JD, Cocker K, Chang E. Infantile colic: recognition and treatment. *Am Fam Physician*. 2015;92(7):577–582.
2. van Sleuwen BE, L'hoir MP, Engelberts AC, et al. Comparison of behavior modification with and without swaddling as interventions for excessive crying. *J Pediatr*. 2006;149(4):512–517.
3. Wade S, Kilgour T. Extracts from "clinical evidence": infantile colic. *BMJ*. 2001;323(7310):437–440.
4. Indrio F, Di Mauro A, Riezzo G, et al. Prophylactic use of a probiotic in the prevention of colic, regurgitation, and functional constipation: a randomized clinical trial. *JAMA Pediatr*. 2014;168(3):228–233.
5. Savino F, Cordisco L, Tarasco V, et al. *Lactobacillus reuteri* DSM 17938 in infantile colic: a randomized, double-blind, placebo-controlled trial. *Pediatrics*. 2010;126(3):e526–e533.
6. Anheyer D, Frawley J, Koch AK, et al. Herbal medicines for gastrointestinal disorders in children and adolescents: a systematic review. *Pediatrics*. 2017;139(6).

ADDITIONAL READING

- Anabrees J, Indrio F, Paes B, et al. Probiotics for infantile colic: a systematic review. *BMC Pediatr*. 2013;13:186.
- Gelfand AA, Thomas KC, Goadsby PJ. Before the headache: infant colic as an early life expression of migraine. *Neurology*. 2012;79(13):1392–1396.
- Johnson JD, Cocker K, Chang E. Infantile colic: recognition and treatment. *Am Fam Physician*. 2015;92(7):577–582.
- Savino F, Pelle E, Palumeri E, et al. *Lactobacillus reuteri* (American Type Culture Collection Strain 55730) versus simethicone in the treatment of infantile colic: a prospective randomized study. *Pediatrics*. 2007;119(1):e124–e130.

 ## CODES

ICD10
R10.83 Colic

CLINICAL PEARLS

- Colic is defined as excessive crying in an otherwise healthy baby (3 hr/day, 3 day/week, persists >3 weeks).
- Excessive crying may be a risk factor for shaken baby syndrome or other forms of child abuse.
- Usually subsides spontaneously by 3 to 6 months of age
- Provide advice, support, and reassurance to parents.
- Prevent caregiver burnout by advising parents to get proper rest breaks, sleep, and help in caring for the infant.
- Employ the 5 Ss (need to be done concurrently):
  - Swaddling: tight wrapping with blanket
  - Side: laying baby on side
  - Shushing: loud white noise
  - Swinging: rhythmic, jiggle motion
  - Sucking: on a nipple, finger, or pacifier

COLITIS, ISCHEMIC

Praphopphat Adhatamsoontra, MD, MPH • Nicole A. Doria, MD •
Marie L. Borum, MD, EdD, MPH, MACP, FACG, AGAF

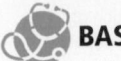

BASICS

Ischemic colitis (IC) results from decreased blood flow to the colon with resultant inflammation and tissue damage.

DESCRIPTION

- More common in the elderly; can affect patients of all ages
- Patients present in several ways:
  - *Nonacute IC* from a chronic process with irreversible ischemic injury
  - *Acute IC*—self-limited transient mucosal ischemia
- IC is self-limited and reversible in 80% of patients:
  - 20% of patients progress to full-thickness necrosis requiring surgical intervention.
- Most commonly, ischemia is related to a nonocclusive reduction in blood flow.
- Presentation varies, but patients with acute IC typically present with localized abdominal pain and tenderness. Frequent loose, bloody stools may be seen within 12 to 24 hours of onset.
- Laboratory and radiographic findings are nonspecific and must be correlated with clinical presentation.
- Colonoscopy is the gold standard for diagnosis of IC.
- In the absence of complications, most patients recover with supportive care including IV fluids, bowel rest, and clinical monitoring.

EPIDEMIOLOGY

- Men and women are at equal risk.
- Evidence of IC seen in 1 of every 100 endoscopies

Geriatric Considerations

Rare in patients <60 years old. 70 years is the average age at diagnosis.

Incidence

- 4.5 to 44 cases per 100,000 in the general population
- 1 of every 2,000 hospital admissions
- True incidence may be underestimated due to nonspecific clinical manifestations.

Prevalence

19 cases per 100,000 in the general population

ETIOLOGY AND PATHOPHYSIOLOGY

- Local hypoperfusion in the colon compromises the ability to meet metabolic demands. Reperfusion injury may also play a role.
- Most commonly, an acute, self-limited process
- The colon is perfused by both the superior and inferior mesenteric arteries (SMAs and IMAs) and branches of the internal iliac arteries. Occlusion of branches of the SMA or IMA rarely leads to ischemic consequences due to extensive collateral circulation.
- Watershed areas of the colon (splenic flexure and rectosigmoid junction) are most susceptible to ischemic damage. Blood is carried by narrow branches of the SMA and IMA to these areas, putting them at increased risk for ischemia. The splenic flexure is supplied by the terminal branches of the SMA, and the rectosigmoid junction is supplied by the terminal branches of the IMA.

- Left colon is more commonly affected than the right.
- The rectum is often spared because of additional blood supply from the internal iliac arteries.
- Poor perfusion may result from systemic disease, local vascular compromise, and anatomic or functional changes in the colon itself. An occlusion of large vessels is usually not identified.
  - Hypoperfusion from shock, trauma
  - Embolic occlusion of mesenteric vessels
  - Hypercoagulable states, vasculitis
  - Sickle cell disease
  - Arterial thrombosis; venous thrombosis
  - Mechanical obstruction of the colon (e.g., tumor, adhesions, hernia, volvulus, prolapse, diverticulitis)
  - Surgical complications
  - Medications (intestinally active vasoconstrictive substances, medications that induce hypotension and thus, hypoperfusion)
  - Cocaine abuse
  - Aortic dissection
  - Strenuous physical activity (e.g., long-distance running)
- Repeated episodes of ischemia and inflammation may result in chronic colonic ischemia, possible stricture formation, recurrent bacteremia, and sepsis. These patients may have unresolving areas of colitis and require segmental colonic resection.

RISK FACTORS

- Age >60 years (90% of patients)
- Smoking (most common cause of recurrent IC) (1)
- Hypertension, diabetes mellitus (1)
- Rheumatologic disorders/vasculitis
- Cerebrovascular disease, ischemic heart disease (1)
- Recent abdominal surgery
- Constipation-inducing medications (1)
- History of vascular surgery (1)
- History of ileostomy
- Chronic obstructive pulmonary disease
- Hypoalbuminemia; hemodialysis
- Hypercoagulability, oral contraceptive (1)
- AAA repair (IMA ligation) (1)
- IBS (1)

DIAGNOSIS

- Diagnosis is based on history, risk factors, and physical examination (2)[A].
- Laboratory values and radiographic findings are usually nonspecific (2)[A].
- Colonoscopy is diagnostic (2)[A].

HISTORY

- Abdominal pain is the most common symptom (3).
- Symptoms vary depending on severity (4)[A].
- Sudden-onset, mild to moderate abdominal pain with tenderness over the affected segment of bowel (4)[A]
- Sudden urge to defecate followed by passage of either bright red or maroon stool (4)[A]
- Lower GI bleeding is rarely heavy (2)[A].
- Loose, bloody bowel movements may occur, typically within 12 to 24 hours of abdominal pain onset (4)[A].

PHYSICAL EXAM

- Individual signs and symptoms are poorly predictive of IC (5)[A].
- Vital signs: hypotension; tachycardia
- Tenderness over the involved segment of bowel (4)[A]
- Abdominal distention with vomiting (due to an associated ileus) (2)[A]
- In the uncommon setting of transmural ischemia, patients may develop peritoneal signs such as rebound and guarding (6)[A].

DIFFERENTIAL DIAGNOSIS

- Infectious colitis (6)[A]
- Inflammatory bowel disease (ulcerative colitis, Crohn disease) (6)[A]
- Colon cancer (6)[A]; diverticulitis (6)[A]
- Pseudomembranous colitis (5)[A]

DIAGNOSTIC TESTS & INTERPRETATION

- Depends on clinical presentation, extent of colonic involvement, transmural involvement, acuity (2)[A]
- CT scan is the initial diagnostic test for patients with nonspecific abdominal pain (5)[A].
- Colonoscopy most sensitive for diagnosis (2)[A].
- Radiographic tests and laboratory values are otherwise nonspecific (5)[A].

Initial Tests (lab, imaging)

- The following lab markers of ischemia are not specific to IC but can help determine disease severity (5)[A]:
  - CBC (leukocytosis) (5)[A]
  - BMP, ABG (signs of metabolic acidosis) (5)[A]
  - Lactate, LDH, CPK, amylase (5)[A]
  - Alkaline phosphatase (5)[A]
  - Albumin (4)[B]
- Abdominal plain film should be obtained to look for:
  - 20% of patients show signs of IC such as thumbprinting and mural thickening; may predict worse prognosis (6)[A]
  - Bowel perforation and pneumoperitoneum (6)[A]
- Abdominal CT scan with contrast if suspected IC (2)[A]:
  - The most common CT findings are thickening of the colonic wall and pericolonic fat stranding (4).
  - Other common CT findings include hyperdense mucosa, submucosal edema, and mesenteric inflammation (2)[A].
  - Pneumatosis, pneumoperitoneum, and free peritoneal fluid suggest advanced ischemia (2)[A].

Follow-Up Tests & Special Considerations

- Stool cultures, fecal leukocytes, stool ova, and parasites to rule out infection (5)[A]
- Patients undergoing aortic surgery may benefit from postoperative colonoscopy within 2 to 3 days to look for signs of IC (4)[A].
- Cardiac workup including electrocardiogram, Holter monitoring, or transthoracic echocardiogram to exclude cardiogenic embolism as indicated (5)[A]
- Drug and toxicology screening (4)[A]

Diagnostic Procedures/Other

- Colonoscopy is gold standard; sigmoidoscopy used to evaluate postoperative left sided ischemia (2)[A]
- Cyanotic hemorrhagic tissue and edematous mucosa suggest ischemia (4)[A].
  - Segmental distribution (watershed), hemorrhagic nodules, and rectal sparing (4)[A]
  - "Colon single-stripe sign" is a single line of erythema, with a 75% histopathologic yield (4)[A].
  - Routine biopsy no longer advised, as results are typically nonspecific (2)[A]
- In cases of isolated right colon ischemia, noninvasive vascular imaging studies are recommended to evaluate acute SMA occlusion (4)[A].

Test Interpretation

- Fulminant gangrenous IC seen in 15% of cases requires surgical intervention (2)[A].
- Acute transient IC seen in 85% of cases requires clinical evaluation for further workup (2)[A].
- Biopsied specimens reveal mucosal infarction and ghost cells, which show normal cellular outlines but lack intracellular contents (2)[A].

 TREATMENT

- Treatment depends on disease severity (2)[A].
- Continuous clinical monitoring, including vital signs and serial abdominal exams (6)[A]
- In the absence of colonic necrosis or perforation, most patients respond to supportive care (1)[A]:
  - Bowel rest (4)[A]
  - IV fluids to maintain hemodynamic stability (4)[A]
  - Broad-spectrum antibiotics covering aerobic and anaerobic bacteria to avoid bacterial translocation secondary to colonic mucosal damage (4)[A]
    - Ciprofloxacin 400 mg IV BID or 500 mg PO BID
    - Metronidazole 500 mg PO/IV TID
  - Avoid intestinally active vasoconstrictive medications (4)[A].
  - Avoid systemic corticosteroids—may worsen ischemia and increase risk of perforation (2)[A].
  - If ileus is present, place nasogastric tube (2)[A].
- If radiographic abnormalities present, serial abdominal x-rays help follow improvement (4)[A]
- If signs of clinical deterioration are present despite supportive care (increased abdominal pain, peritoneal signs, persistent diarrhea, bleeding, or sepsis), consider surgery (2)[A].

MEDICATION

- Broad-spectrum antibiotics (i.e., metronidazole, ciprofloxacin) (4)[A]
- If cardiac workup reveals CHF or cardiac arrhythmias, initiate appropriate medical treatment (4)[A].

SURGERY/OTHER PROCEDURES

- 20% of patients require surgical intervention (3)[A].
- Pneumatosis intestinalis, portal vein air, or free peritoneal air are indications for urgent surgery (2)[A].
- Surgery may be indicated for:
  - Peritoneal signs, increased abdominal tenderness, new-onset shock, lactic acidosis, or acute renal failure (2)[A]
  - Diarrhea, lower GI bleeding, or exudative colitis persisting past 14 days (2)[A]
- Most common surgical intervention is colectomy with end ileostomy (5)[A].
  - Cholecystectomy may prevent resuscitation-related acute acalculous cholecystitis (2)[A].

 ONGOING CARE

DIET

- Bowel rest until symptoms resolve
- Parenteral nutrition for patients needing prolonged bowel rest who have contraindications to surgery

PROGNOSIS

- In most patients, IC symptoms resolve in 24 to 48 hours.
- Radiographic or endoscopic resolution within 2 weeks
- Right-sided IC is the most significant predictor of outcome. Patients with right-sided IC have a 2-fold increase in mortality and a 4-fold increase in morbidity (4).
- Secondary cardiovascular prevention minimizes recurrence.
- Male gender, low hemoglobin, low serum albumin, high BUN, and presence of metabolic acidosis are poor prognostic factors (1).
- Chronic kidney disease, COPD, long-term care facilities increase mortality in IC (1).

COMPLICATIONS

20–30% of patients develop chronic IC, with persistent diarrhea or stricture formation requiring surgery.

REFERENCES

1. Brandt LJ, Feuerstadt P, Longstreth GF, et al. ACG clinical guideline: epidemiology, risk factors, patterns of presentation, diagnosis, and management of colon ischemia (CI). *Am J Gastroenterol.* 2015;110(1):18–45.
2. Moszkowicz D, Mariani A, Trésallet C, et al. Ischemic colitis: the ABCs of diagnosis and surgical management. *J Visc Surg.* 2013;150(1):19–28.
3. Yadav S, Dave M, Edakkanambeth Varayil J, et al. A population-based study of incidence, risk factors, clinical spectrum, and outcomes of ischemic colitis. *Clin Gastroenterol Hepatol.* 2015;13(4): 731.e6–738.e6, quiz e41.
4. Feuerstadt P, Brandt LJ. Update on colon ischemia: recent insights and advances. *Curr Gastroenterol Rep.* 2015;17(12):45.
5. Theodoropoulou A, Koutroubakis IE. Ischemic colitis: clinical practice in diagnosis and treatment. *World J Gastroenterol.* 2008;14(48):7302–7308.
6. Sun MY, Maykel JA. Ischemic colitis. *Clin Colon Rectal Surg.* 2007;20(1):5–12.

ADDITIONAL READING

- Cosse C, Sabbagh C, Browet F, et al. Serum value of procalcitonin as a marker of intestinal damages: type, extension, and prognosis. *Surg Endosc.* 2015;29(11):3132–3139.
- Iacobellis F, Berritto D, Somma F, et al. Magnetic resonance imaging: a new tool for diagnosis of acute ischemic colitis? *World J Gastroenterol.* 2012;18(13):1496–1501.
- Joo HH, Jo HJ, Jung TD, et al. Adipose-derived stem cells on the healing of ischemic colitis: a therapeutic effect by angiogenesis. *Int J Colorectal Dis.* 2012;27(11):1437–1443.
- O'Neill S, Yalamarthi S. Systematic review of the management of ischaemic colitis. *Colorectal Dis.* 2012;14(11):e751–e763. doi:10.1111/j.1463-1318 .2012.03171.x.
- Yoon SY, Jung SA, Na SK, et al. What's the clinical features of colitis in elderly people in long-term care facilities? *Intest Res.* 2015;13(2):128–134.

 CODES

ICD10

- K55.9 Vascular disorder of intestine, unspecified
- K55.0 Acute vascular disorders of intestine
- K55.1 Chronic vascular disorders of intestine

CLINICAL PEARLS

- Suspect IC in patients with multiple risk factors who present with abdominal pain and loose bloody stools.
- Colonoscopy is the diagnostic gold standard.
- Most often, IC is self-limited, responding well to conservative management with IV fluids, bowel rest, and empiric broad-spectrum antibiotics.
- Peritoneal signs or lack of clinical improvement suggests more extensive ischemia and need for surgical intervention.
- Right-sided IC is associated with higher morbidity and mortality.

C

COLON CANCER

Jaine L. McKenzie, MD • Asif Talukder, MD • Daniel Albo, MD, PhD

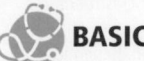 **BASICS**

DESCRIPTION
- Colon and rectal cancers (CRC) are often grouped together but are two distinct clinical entities that differ in their prognosis, presentation, staging, and management.
- CRC is the second leading cause of cancer deaths and is the third most common cancer in men and women in the United States.
- Screening for colon cancer reduces the incidence of and mortality from colon cancer.

EPIDEMIOLOGY
Incidence
- 93,090 new cases of colon cancer in 2015
- 49,700 deaths from CRC combined were estimated in the United States in 2015 (1).
- Incidence is equal between men and women.

Prevalence
- The lifetime risk for developing colon cancer in the United States is about 1 in 21 (4.8%).
- Incidence and death rates have been declining due to improved screening, prevention, and treatment.

ETIOLOGY AND PATHOPHYSIOLOGY
- Progression from the first abnormal cells to the appearance of colon cancer usually occurs over 10 to 15 years, a disease characteristic that contributes to the effectiveness of prevention.
- High-risk polyp findings include multiple polyps, villous polyps, and larger polyps.
- Hyperplastic polyps are less likely to evolve into CRC.
- Multiple genetic and environmental factors have been linked to the development of CRC.

Genetics
- <10% of CRC cases are linked to an inherited gene.
  - APC, a tumor suppressor gene, is altered in familial adenomatous polyposis (FAP).
  - Genes encoding DNA mismatch repair (MMR) enzymes are implicated in hereditary nonpolyposis colon cancer (HNPCC): MLH1, MSH2, MSH6, PMS1, PMS2, and others.
  - STK11, a tumor suppressor gene, is altered in Peutz-Jeghers syndrome.
- Sporadic cases of CRC have been linked to oncogenes: Kras, c-Myc, c-Src, HER-2/neu, and others.

RISK FACTORS
- Age: >90% of people diagnosed with colon cancer are >50 years of age.
- Personal history of colorectal polyps
  - Risk increases with multiple polyps, villous polyps, larger polyps, and presence of dysplasia.
- Personal history of cancer
  - 30% increase in risk of developing metachronous (new primary tumors unrelated to the patients' previous cancers) colon cancer
  - 2–4% incidence of local recurrence with colon cancer, 3–5% incidence of synchronous colon cancer
- History of inflammatory bowel disease (IBD)
  - Prevalence of CRC in ulcerative colitis and Crohn disease is ~3%, with a cumulative risk of CRC of 2% at 10 years, 8% at 20 years, and 18% at 30 years.
- Family history of CRC
  - Having a single first-degree relative with a history of CRC increases risk 1.7-fold.
  - Risk is more than double for those who have a history of CRC or polyps in:
    - Any first-degree relative <60 years of age
    - ≥2 first-degree relatives, regardless of age

- Inherited syndromes
  - HNPCC (formerly Lynch syndrome)
    - Often develops at young age (Average age at diagnosis of CRC is 44 years.)
    - Lifetime risk of CRC is 52–69%.
    - Accounts for ~2% of all CRCs
  - FAP
    - Affected individuals develop hundreds to thousands of polyps in colon and rectum.
    - CRC usually present by age 40 years
    - Accounts for <1% of CRCs
  - Peutz-Jeghers syndrome
    - Individuals may have hyperpigmented mucocutaneous lesions (mouth, hands, feet) and large polyps in GI tract.
    - 81–93% risk for CRC and increased risk for other cancers
- Race and ethnicity
  - African Americans have the highest CRC incidence and mortality rates in the United States. It is unclear whether this is biologic or due to lower rates of access to screening.
  - Colonoscopy is underutilized, particularly in minorities.
  - Several different gene mutations have been identified among Ashkenazi Jews.
- Lifestyle factors that increase risk
  - Smoking, obesity, diet high in fat and low in fiber

GENERAL PREVENTION
- Optimal screening method for colon cancer is unclear. Stool-based testing such as guaiac fecal occult blood test (gFOBT) and fecal immunochemical test (FIT) or FIT-DNA tests are less invasive, but endoscopic testing such as flexible sigmoidoscopy or colonoscopy offers ability to provide intervention if polyp discovered.
- Lifestyle factors that may reduce risk:
  - Low-fat, high-fiber diet (rich in fruits and vegetables)
  - Supplementation with vitamin D, calcium, folate, and fiber may lower CRC risk; more research is needed to understand how diet affects risks of CRC.

ALERT
The U.S. Preventive Services Task Force (USPSTF) strongly recommends screening adults, beginning at age 50 years and continuing until age 75 years and gives this an "A" grade, meaning screening's benefits far outweigh its harms.

- Screening methods include
  - Colonoscopy every 10 years
  - Flexible sigmoidoscopy every 5 to 10 years (2)[C]
  - FIT annually (1)[C]
  - Fecal occult blood testing annually (1)[A]
  - Stool DNA (sDNA) test every 3 years (2)[C]
  - Note: The USPSTF does not recommend barium enema as a screening test and concludes the evidence is insufficient to assess the benefits and harms of CT colonography and sDNA testing as screening modalities for CRC. The USPSTF also recommends AGAINST routine screening for CRC in adults 76 to 85 years of age but acknowledges there may be considerations that support screening in certain patients and recommends AGAINST screening those age >85 years.
- American Cancer Society recommends screening with colonoscopy every 10 years. For those patients refusing colonoscopy, an alternative cancer detection tests method is recommended.

- Screening in high-risk groups:
  - The American College of Gastroenterology recommends screening African American patients starting at age 45 years.
  - People with a history of polyps need frequent colonoscopy screening, depending on risk.
  - People who have a first-degree relative or two second-degree relatives with CRC or adenomatous polyps before age 60 years should begin colonoscopy at age 40 or 10 years younger than the age of relative at cancer diagnosis, whichever is earlier.
  - People with IBD should have regular surveillance colonoscopy with biopsies to detect dysplasia; guidelines generally indicate starting surveillance by 8 to 10 years of onset of symptoms followed by surveillance every 1 to 2 years.
  - Genetic testing may be appropriate for individuals with a strong family history of CRC or polyps:
    - Family members of a person affected by HNPCC should start colonoscopy surveillance at age 25 years.
    - Individuals with suspected FAP should have yearly flexible sigmoidoscopy beginning at age 10 to 12 years; those who test positive for the gene linked to FAP may consider colectomy.

 DIAGNOSIS

HISTORY
- Most patients with colon cancer are asymptomatic.
- Microcytic anemia in men of any age and postmenopausal women is CRC until proven otherwise; evaluation must include diagnostic colonoscopy.
- Symptoms may indicate advanced disease. Common presenting symptoms include:
  - Abdominal pain or cramping
  - Change in bowel habits (constipation, diarrhea, narrowing of stool)
  - Rectal bleeding, dark stools, or blood in stool
  - Weakness or fatigue
  - Unintentional weight loss
- Other presentations may include symptoms due to the presence of metastatic lesions (lymph nodes, liver, lung, peritoneum), fever of unknown origin, and *Streptococcus bovis* or *Clostridium septicum* sepsis.

PHYSICAL EXAM
- Signs of anemia
- Weight loss
- Palpable abdominal mass (late presentation)
- Must include digital rectal exam

DIFFERENTIAL DIAGNOSIS
- >95% of colon cancers are adenocarcinomas. Other colonic tumors include carcinoid tumors, lymphomas, and Kaposi sarcoma in HIV.
- Many conditions can mimic CRC, including other cancers, hemorrhoids, IBD, infection, and extrinsic masses (i.e., cysts, abscesses).

DIAGNOSTIC TESTS & INTERPRETATION
Initial Tests (lab, imaging)
- Should any screening method identify an increased risk, colonoscopy must be performed because it can be both diagnostic and therapeutic.
- For confirmed colorectal cancer, obtain:
  - CBC, ferritin to evaluate iron deficiency anemia
  - CEA, LFTs

Follow-Up Tests & Special Considerations

- If CT chest, abdomen, and pelvis to evaluate presence of metastatic disease
- Intraoperative US may be used to evaluate solid organs (e.g., the liver) after tumor resection.
- In selected cases, positron emission tomography (PET) may be used to detect metastatic disease.
- Biopsy is usually performed (most often during colonoscopy) if cancer is suspected.
- CT-guided biopsy may be needed to evaluate a suspected tumor or metastasis.
- Staging of colon cancer
  - The American Joint Committee on Cancer (AJCC) TNM staging is preferred.
    - Stage 0: limited to the mucosa (carcinoma in situ or intramucosal carcinoma) (Tis, N0, M0)
    - Stage I: invades mucosa (T1) or muscularis propria (T2); no invasion of lymph nodes or distant sites (T1, N0, M0 or T2, N0, M0)
    - Stage IIA: invades pericolorectal tissues; no lymph nodes or distant sites (T3, N0, M0)
    - Stage IIB: penetrates to surface of visceral peritoneum; no lymph nodes or distant sites (T4a, N0, M0)
    - Stage IIC: directly invades or adherent to other organs or structures (T4b, N0, M0)
    - Stage IIIA: invades submucosa or muscularis propria with spread to 1 to 3 lymph nodes; no distant sites (T1, N1, M0 or T2, N1, M0)
    - Stage IIIB: invades pericolorectal tissues or surface of visceral peritoneum + spread to 1 to 3 lymph nodes; no distant sites (T3, N1, M0 or T4a, N1, M0)
    - Stage IIIC: invades pericolorectal tissues or peritoneum or other organs and to ≥4 nearby lymph nodes; no distant sites (any T3 or T4, N2, M0)
    - Stage IVA: any level of invasion with spread to one organ or site (any T, any N, M1a)
    - Stage IVB: any level of invasion with spread to more than one organ or site or peritoneum (any T, any N, M1b)

TREATMENT

- Colon cancer is typically treated with surgery and chemotherapy.
- Data suggest multidisciplinary communication among providers of colon cancer patients can improve cancer survival.

SURGERY/OTHER PROCEDURES

- Surgery is the primary treatment for localized colon cancer.
  - Minimally invasive (i.e., laparoscopic) surgery has fewer complications, less blood loss, shorter hospital stay, less time to bowel movement, and lower 30-day mortality when compared to open surgery with equivalent oncologic outcomes. This approach allows patients to have less pain and faster recovery. For health systems, decreased length of stay and fewer complications improve the cost of care (3).
  - There are no significant differences between minimally invasive and open colorectal surgery in long-term survival and recurrence rates (3).
- Radiation therapy is most often used for peritoneal cancers; it may also be used to relieve symptoms.

ADDITIONAL THERAPIES

Adjuvant chemotherapy is most clearly beneficial for stage III (node-positive) disease, in which improvements of 30% can be achieved in both disease recurrence and overall survival, compared with untreated controls.

Chemotherapeutic regimens for metastatic disease may extend overall survival from 6 months to 2 years (2)[B].

- First-line therapy includes combination chemotherapy with oxaliplatin, irinotecan, fluorouracil, leucovorin, and capecitabine.
- Targeted therapies may be used alongside first-line agents or alone if first-line agents are ineffective.
- Bevacizumab (Avastin) is a monoclonal antibody that targets vascular endothelial growth factor (VEGF); inhibits angiogenesis
- Cetuximab (Erbitux) and panitumumab (Vectibix) are monoclonal antibodies that target epidermal growth factor receptor (EGFR).
- Aflibercept and regorafenib are newer agents with actions on VEGF.

ONGOING CARE

FOLLOW-UP RECOMMENDATIONS

Patient Monitoring

- Risk of recurrence is greatest in the first 2 to 4 years after treatment; 80% occur in first 2.5 years from date of surgery.
- H&P and CEA should be performed every 3 to 6 months for 5 years.
- Annual CT scan of chest, abdomen, and pelvis for 3 years
- Surveillance colonoscopy 1 year after initial surgery. Subsequent colonoscopies should generally be every 5 years if findings are normal.
- In obstructive colon cancer precluding from preoperative colonoscopy, recommend colonoscopy within 3 to 6 months after surgery to detect synchronous cancer and complete resection of precancerous polyps.
- CEA is used to detect recurrences after resection of primary colon cancer. CEA levels decrease and normalize within 4 to 6 weeks after surgery. Persistent elevation of CEA levels can suggest incomplete resection or occult metastasis. Elevated CEA should raise suspicion for recurrent disease, and adjustments of routine surveillance program should be undertaken (4,5).

PROGNOSIS

5-year relative survival rate after surgical resection alone (6):

- Stage I: 85–95%
- Stage II: 60–80%
- Stage III: 30–60%
- Stage IV: 25–40% following resection of hepatic metastases with clear margins

COMPLICATIONS

- Surgery: pain, deep vein thrombosis (DVT), anatomic leaks, wound infection, incisional hernia. Incidence complications are lower with minimally invasive (i.e., laparoscopic) approach.
- Chemotherapy: hair loss, nausea, vomiting, bruising, fatigue, increased risk for infections
- Radiation therapy: skin irritation, nausea, rectal pain, incontinence, bladder irritation, fatigue, and sexual problems

PATIENT EDUCATION

- NIH: colorectal cancer: http://www.nlm.nih.gov/medlineplus/colorectalcancer.html
- NCI: colorectal cancer: http://www.cancer.gov/types/colorectal
- AAFP: colorectal cancer: http://www.aafp.org/afp/2015/0115/p93-s1.html

REFERENCES

1. Siegel RL, Miller KD, Jemal A. Cancer statistics, 2015. *CA Cancer J Clin*. 2015;65(1):5–29.
2. Brenner H, Kloor M, Pox CP. Colorectal cancer. *Lancet*. 2014;383(9927):1490–1502.
3. Wang CL, Qu G, Xu HW. The short- and long-term outcomes of laparoscopic versus open surgery for colorectal cancer: a meta-analysis. *Int J Colorectal Dis*. 2014;29(3):309–320.
4. Kahi CJ, Boland CR, Dominitz JA, et al. Colonoscopy surveillance after colorectal cancer resection: recommendations of the US Multi-Society Task Force on colorectal cancer. *Gastroenterology*. 2016;150(3):758.e11–768.e11.
5. Meyerhardt JA, Mangu PB, Flynn PJ, et al. Follow-up care, surveillance protocol, and secondary prevention measures for survivors of colorectal cancer: American Society of Clinical Oncology clinical practice guideline endorsement. *J Clin Oncol*. 2013;31(35):4465–4470.
6. Labianca R, Nordlinger B, Beretta GD, et al. Primary colon cancer: ESMO Clinical Practice Guidelines for diagnosis, adjuvant treatment and follow-up. *Ann Oncol*. 2010;21(Suppl 5):v70–v77.

ADDITIONAL READING

- Benson AB III, Venook AP, Bekaii-Saab T, et al. Colon cancer, version 3.2014. *J Natl Compr Canc Netw*. 2014;12(7):1028–1059.
- Enewold L, Horner MJ, Shriver CD, et al. Socioeconomic disparities in colorectal cancer mortality in the United States, 1990–2007. *J Community Health*. 2014;39(4):760–766.
- Marshall CL, Balentine CJ, Robinson CN, et al. A multidisciplinary cancer center maximizes surgeons' impact. *J Surg Res*. 2011;171(1):15–22.
- Marshall CL, Chen GJ, Robinson CN, et al. Establishment of a minimally invasive surgery program leads to decreased inpatient cost of care in veterans with colon cancer. *Am J Surg*. 2010;200(5):632–635.
- Zauber AG, Winawer SJ, O'Brien MJ, et al. Colonoscopic polypectomy and long-term prevention of colorectal-cancer deaths. *N Engl J Med*. 2012;366(8):687–696.

CODES

ICD10

- C18.9 Malignant neoplasm of colon, unspecified
- C18.2 Malignant neoplasm of ascending colon
- C18.8 Malignant neoplasm of overlapping sites of colon

CLINICAL PEARLS

- Microcytic anemia in men of all ages and postmenopausal women is CRC until proven otherwise.
- Colon cancer screening decreases mortality from colon cancer, but optimal screening method is unclear.
- Colonoscopy offers ability for diagnosis of colon cancer and intervention if polyp is discovered.
- Multidisciplinary communication in the treatment of colorectal cancer patients improves outcomes.
- Minimally invasive surgery leads to less pain and faster recovery for patients with equivalent oncologic outcomes.

COLONIC POLYPS

Marcelle Meseeha, MD • Maximos Attia, MD, FAAFP

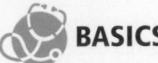 **BASICS**

DESCRIPTION
- Intraluminal colonic tissue growth; most commonly sporadic or part of polyposis syndromes
- Size classification:
  - Diminutive ≤5 mm, small 6 to 9 mm, large ≥10 mm
- Morphologic classification:
  - Depressed, flat, sessile, or pedunculated
- Clinical significance:
  - >95% of colon adenocarcinoma arise from polyps.

EPIDEMIOLOGY
Colorectal polyps are more common in non-Caucasian men in Western countries.

Incidence
Incidence increases with age.

Prevalence
- 15–20% of all adults
- 30% of U.S. population >50 years
- 6% of children
- 12% of children with lower GI bleed

ETIOLOGY AND PATHOPHYSIOLOGY
- Mucosal
  - Neoplastic
    - Adenomatous polyps (tubular >80%, villous 5–15%, tubulovillous 5–15%)
    - Serrated polyps
    - Sessile serrated polyps are common, more in proximal colon, with low malignant potential if no dysplasia and significant malignant potential if dysplastic.
    - Traditional serrated adenoma is uncommon, more often noted in distal colon, with significant malignant potential.
  - Nonneoplastic polyps (hyperplastic, juvenile polyps, hamartomas, inflammatory pseudopolyps)
    - Hyperplastic polyps are very common, more in distal colon, with very low malignant potential.
    - Juvenile polyps are common in childhood, benign hamartomas, more in rectosigmoid, and not premalignant.
- Submucosal (lipomas, lymphoid aggregates, carcinoids)

Genetics
- Inactivation of tumor suppressor genes as adenomatous polyposis coli (APC) or mismatch repair genes *(MLH1)* causes polyps to grow into cancer.
- Familial adenomatous polyposis (FAP) is autosomal dominant. By age 40 years, almost all patients develop colorectal cancer (CRC).
- MUTYH-associated polyposis (MAP) is autosomal recessive caused by biallelic mutations in *MUTYH* gene.
- Juvenile polyposis syndrome (JPS) is autosomal dominant. 50–60% of patients have a mutation in the *SMAD4* or *BMPR1A* gene. By age 35 years, 20% of patients develop CRC.

RISK FACTORS
- Family history of intestinal polyposis, polyps, or CRC
- Advancing age; male
- High-fat, low-fiber diet; tobacco use
- Excessive alcohol intake: >8 drinks a week
- Inflammatory bowel disease is associated with a decreased prevalence of colon polyps (but with higher risk of colon cancer).

GENERAL PREVENTION
- Low-fat, high-fiber diet
- Avoid smoking.
- Decrease alcohol intake.
- Use of NSAIDs and calcium is associated with decreased incidence and recurrence of polyps.
- No lower rates of CRC with azathioprine, 6-mercaptopurine, folate, calcium, multivitamins, or statins

COMMONLY ASSOCIATED CONDITIONS
Hereditary polyposis syndromes:
- Adenomatous
  - FAP
    - Classic (CFAP)
    - Attenuated (AFAP)
  - MAP
  - FAP variants:
    - Gardner syndrome
    - Turcot syndrome
- Hamartomatous
  - Peutz-Jeghers syndrome (PJS)
  - JPS
  - Familial juvenile polyposis
  - Cowden syndrome

ALERT
JPS imposes a higher risk of CRC, although juvenile polyps are not premalignant.

 DIAGNOSIS

HISTORY
- Generally asymptomatic
- Painless rectal bleeding, bright or dark red, mixed with stools, dripping, or on wiping
- Diarrhea or mucous stool
- Abdominal pain
- Constipation
- Chronic bleeding, resulting in iron deficiency anemia
- McKittrick-Wheelock syndrome; large hypersecretory rectosigmoid villous adenoma, resulting in persistent severe diarrhea, electrolyte disorder, dehydration, and prerenal acute renal failure
- Social and family history

PHYSICAL EXAM
- Usually normal
- Rectal polyps noted as prolapsed or palpated on digital rectal examination (DRE)
- Fecal occult blood test (FOBT) by DRE is less effective than FOBT by stool passed spontaneously.

DIAGNOSTIC TESTS & INTERPRETATION
Initial Tests (lab, imaging)
- CBC; anemia with chronic bleeding
- Basic metabolic panel; electrolyte disorder with hypersecretory adenomas
- FOBT, insensitive screening test, because small polyps don't usually bleed:
  - Guaiac (gFOBT)—uses a chemical indicator with color change in presence of blood
  - Immunochemical (iFOBT or fecal immunochemical test [FIT])—uses antibodies against human hemoglobin
- Stool DNA test is more sensitive and less specific than FIT.

Diagnostic Procedures/Other
- Colonoscopy is the gold standard test for detection of polyps and allows for concurrent polypectomy; not a perfect screening test, with increased miss rate with right-sided colon polyps, smaller polyp size, low quality of colon prep, less endoscopist experience
- Computed tomographic colonography (CTC) is less sensitive with flat polyps and requires excellent bowel preparation.
- Double-contrast barium enema
- Colon capsule endoscopy
- Enhanced optical technologies can potentially differentiate between neoplastic and nonneoplastic colonic lesions (1)[A].
- Enhanced optical technologies include:
  - Narrowed spectrum endoscopy (narrow-band imaging [NBI])
  - Image-enhanced endoscopy (i-scan)
  - Fujinon intelligent chromoendoscopy (FICE)
  - Confocal laser endomicroscopy (CLE)
- Patients with >10 colorectal adenomas should undergo genetic testing for APC and MUTYH (2)[C].

Test Interpretation
- Tubular adenoma
  - Gross: tends to be polypoid
  - Micro: dysplastic epithelium, tubular architecture
- Villous adenoma:
  - Gross: tends to be sessile
  - Micro: dysplastic epithelium, fingerlike projections
- Tubulovillous adenomas have a combination of tubular and villous architecture.
- Hyperplastic polyps are composed of hyperplastic colonic mucosa
- Hamartomatous polyps include muscularis mucosa.
- Juvenile polyp
  - Gross: pedunculated, smooth red mass, 1 to 3 cm (3)

TREATMENT

SURGERY/OTHER PROCEDURES

- Colonic polypectomy; diagnostic, therapeutic:
  - Snare polypectomy with electrocautery for pedunculated polyps
  - Endoscopic mucosal resection for sessile polyps
  - Endoscopic submucosal dissection
- Colorectal surgery; prophylactic in FAP and MAP and when there are numerous polyps or persistent bleeding (2,3)[C]:
  - Total colectomy ileorectal anastomosis
  - Proctocolectomy ileal pouch anal anastomosis
- Chemoprevention: NSAIDs and calcium may reduce incidence and recurrence of polyps in patients with FAP and MAP (4)[A].

 ## ONGOING CARE

FOLLOW-UP RECOMMENDATIONS
Follow-up colonoscopy in:

- 10 years if no polyps or distal small hyperplastic polyps (<10 mm) (5)[B]
- 5 to 10 years if 1 to 2 small tubular adenomas (<10 mm) (5)[B]
- 3 years if 3 to 10 adenomas if any polyp ≥ 6 mm (5)[B] or if all polyps <6 mm (5)[C]
- <3 years if >10 adenomas (5)[B]
- 3 years if one or more adenomas ≥10 mm (5)[A]
- 3 years if one or more adenomas with villous features of any size or with HGD (5)[B]
- 5 years if sessile serrated polyp(s) <10 mm with no dysplasia (5)[C]
- 3 years if sessile serrated polyp(s) ≥10 mm or with dysplasia or traditional serrated adenoma (5)[C]
- 1 year if serrated polyposis syndrome (5)[B]

Patient Monitoring
- Colonoscopy for CRC screening starts at age 50 years and earlier for at-risk patients.
- American Cancer Society (ACS) recommends that people at average risk of CRC start screening at age 45 years through age of 75 years, may extend to 85 years, based on life expectancy and overall health.
- Stop screening if life expectancy is <10 years.
- In CFAP and AFAP, screen for extracolonic manifestations: thyroid cancer, desmoid tumors, and gastroduodenal polyposis (every 6 months to 5 years) (2)[C].
- In families, lifetime screening for mutation carriers (2)[C]:
  - In CFAP: with sigmoidoscopy or colonoscopy, every 1 to 2 years starting at age of 10 to 11 years
  - In AFAP and MAP: with colonoscopy, every 1 to 2 years starting at age of 18 to 20 years

- After colorectal surgery, surveillance of the rectum (every 6 to 12 months) or pouch (every 6 months to 5 years) is indicated (2)[C].
- First-degree relatives of patients with JPS require screening by colonoscopy and upper endoscopy after age 12 years (3)[C].

DIET
Low-fat, high-fiber diet (insufficient evidence)

PATIENT EDUCATION
Importance of colonoscopy as a screening tool

PROGNOSIS
- Regression or no change in size, more with small hyperplastic polyps and with patients on NSAIDs
- Recurrence: Juvenile polyps recur in 45% of children with multiple polyps and 17% with solitary polyps (3).
- Risk factors for colon cancer (6)[A]:
  - Polyp pathology
    - Adenomatous
    - Serrated
    - With high-grade dysplasia
    - With >25% villous histology
    - Polyp size >1 cm in diameter
    - Polyps located in proximal colon
    - More than three polyps
- Recurrence rates <10% postpolypectomy

COMPLICATIONS
- Polyps: progression to cancer
- Polypectomy: bleeding 2–11%, perforation 0–1%, higher with endoscopic submucosal dissection
- Colonoscopy: complications related to anesthesia and procedure itself

REFERENCES

1. Wanders LK, East JE, Uitentuis SE, et al. Diagnostic performance of narrowed spectrum endoscopy, autofluorescence imaging, and confocal laser endomicroscopy for optical diagnosis of colonic polyps: a meta-analysis. *Lancet Oncol*. 2013;14(13):1337–1347.
2. Stoffel EM, Mangu PB, Limburg PJ; for American Society of Clinical Oncology. Hereditary colorectal cancer syndromes: American Society of Clinical Oncology clinical practice guideline endorsement of the familial risk-colorectal cancer: European Society for Medical Oncology clinical practice guidelines. *J Oncol Pract*. 2015;11(3):e437–e441.
3. Thakkar K, Fishman DS, Gilger MA. Colorectal polyps in childhood. *Curr Opin Pediatr*. 2012;24(5):632–637.
4. Johnson CC, Hayes RB, Schoen RE, et al. Nonsteroidal anti-inflammatory drug use and colorectal polyps in the prostate, lung, colorectal, and ovarian cancer screening trial. *Am J Gastroenterol*. 2010;105(12):2646–2655.
5. Lieberman DA, Rex DK, Winawer SJ, et al. Guidelines for colonoscopy surveillance after screening and polypectomy: a consensus update by the US Multi-Society Task Force on Colorectal Cancer. *Gastroenterology*. 2012;143(3):844–857.
6. Gao Q, Tsoi KK, Hirai HW, et al. Serrated polyps and the risk of synchronous colorectal advanced neoplasia: a systematic review and meta-analysis. *Am J Gastroenterol*. 2015;110(4):501–509.

ADDITIONAL READING

- Ashraf I, Paracha SR, Arif M, et al. Digital rectal examination versus spontaneous passage of stool for fecal occult blood testing. *South Med J*. 2012;105(7):357–361.
- Cooper K, Squires H, Carroll C, et al. Chemoprevention of colorectal cancer: systematic review and economic evaluation. *Health Technol Assess*. 2010;14(32):1–206.
- Rex DK, Boland CR, Dominitz JA, et al. Colorectal cancer screening: recommendations for physicians and patients from the U.S. Multi-Society Task Force on Colorectal Cancer. *Gastroeneterology*. 2017;153(1):307–323.

 ## SEE ALSO

Colon Cancer; Rectal Cancer

 ## CODES

ICD10
- K63.5 Polyp of colon
- D12.6 Benign neoplasm of colon, unspecified
- K51.40 Inflammatory polyps of colon without complications

CLINICAL PEARLS

- Colonoscopy is the gold standard for diagnosing polyps.
- Biopsy small hyperplastic polyps to differentiate adenomatous and serrated polyps.
- Use of NSAIDs and calcium is associated with decreased incidence and recurrence of polyps.
- The progression from normal mucosa to polyp to carcinoma takes years to develop.

COMPLEMENTARY AND ALTERNATIVE MEDICINE

Paul Crawford, MD

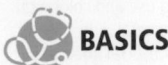 **BASICS**

DESCRIPTION

- Complementary and alternative medicine (CAM) are medical and health care systems, practices, and products that are not currently considered as part of conventional Western medicine.
- The National Center for Health Statistics (NCHS) reports nonvitamin, nonmineral dietary supplements, chiropractic or osteopathic manipulation, yoga, and massage therapy to be the most common complementary health approaches.
- Medical professionals who incorporate CAM into their medical practice often refer to this as a model of "integrative medicine."
- Definitions and additional terms
  - *Complementary medicine* is used in conjunction with conventional medicine to address a health concern, for example, massage plus physical therapy for low back pain or medication plus osteopathic manipulation for recurrent headaches.
  - *Alternative medicine* is used in place of conventional medicine to promote healing of conditions not fully explained by the conventional biomedical model or for which the effectiveness of therapy is not yet established by clinical research.
  - *Integrative medicine* is the combination of allopathic medicine with CAM and may be provided to the patient by a single licensed medical professional trained in CAM or by a group of diverse health care providers.
  - *Holistic* is a descriptive term for a practitioner's approach to patient care. Holistic care assesses the emotional, spiritual, mental, and physical state of wellness of the patient and works to provide comprehensive care. A holistic practice may include practitioners of different disciplines to address multiple aspects of wellness or illness.
- *Biologically* based therapies: diets, herbals, vitamins, supplements, flower essences
- Manipulative and body-based methods
  - Massage therapy is manipulation of soft tissues using knowledge of anatomy and physiology to restore function, promote relaxation, and relieve pain. There are different types of massage.
  - Osteopathic manipulative medicine (OMM) includes indirect techniques (e.g., muscle energy, myofascial release, osteopathy in the cranial field, and strain–counterstrain approach) and direct action techniques (high-velocity thrusts).
  - Craniosacral therapy is a gentle release of bony and fascial restrictions in the craniosacral system (cranium, sacrum, spinal cord, meninges, cerebrospinal fluid).
  - Chiropractic therapy focuses on imbalances in the musculoskeletal and nervous system to treat back, neck, and joint pain. Doctors of chiropractic (DCs) complete 4 to 5 years of intensive training in anatomy, physiology, and manipulation.

- Mind–body medicine
  - Meditation is a practice of detachment in which a person sits quietly, generally focusing on the breath, while releasing thoughts from the mind with the intention to center the self, restore balance, and enhance well-being. Mindfulness meditation involves making oneself aware of the most immediate of activities in order to gain control over actions and anxiety.
  - Spiritual practices (e.g., prayer)
  - Yoga is an exercise of mindfulness, meditation, strength, and balance, composed of *asanas* (postures) and *pranayamas* (focused breathing).
  - Aromatherapy uses highly concentrated plant extracts to stimulate healing. Aromatic oils are rubbed on the skin, aerosolized, or used in compresses.
  - Relaxation techniques include breathing exercises, progressive muscle relaxation, and guided imagery.
  - *Tai chi* and *qi gong* are Chinese exercise systems that combine meditation, regulated breathing, and flowing dance-like movements to enhance and balance *chi* (*qi*)—life force energy.
- Alternative medical systems
  - Traditional Chinese medicine incorporates Chinese herbs and acupuncture. Acupuncture is the practice of regulating *chi* by inserting thin needles at specific points along meridian pathways of the body. In this model, *Chi* energy movement is responsible for animating and protecting the body; relieving pain; and regulating cellular blood flow, oxygen delivery, and nourishment.
  - Ayurvedic medicine originated in India and is one of the world's oldest medical systems. It uses healing modalities and herbs to integrate and balance the body, mind, and spirit.
  - Homeopathy proposes that dilute quantities of an offending agent can stimulate innate immunity. In general, homeopathic remedies are considered safe and unlikely to cause serious adverse reactions. Only three states license homeopathic providers.
  - Naturopathy includes herbs, vitamins, supplements, dietary counseling, homeopathic remedies, manipulative therapies, acupuncture, and hydrotherapy. 4-year doctoral training programs are available. 20 states/territories have licensing laws for naturopathic practitioners.
- Energy therapies
  - *Reiki*, which means "source energy," is a healing practice from Japan. Laying hands lightly on the patient or holding the hands just above the body, the *Reiki* practitioner facilitates spiritual and physical healing by stimulating life force energy.

- Common reasons patients choose CAM
  - Additive therapy to address issues not covered by conventional medical treatment
  - Conventional medicine has been unsuccessful in fully addressing ailment.
  - Preventive health care
  - Desire for a holistic/natural approach to well-being
  - Preference for noninvasive treatment options
  - Concern about medication side effects
  - Desire to include spiritual support into healing
  - Cultural or familial belief system more aligned with "natural" solutions not provided for or supported by the standard allopathic model of health care

EPIDEMIOLOGY

- All ages use CAM; most prevalent among adults aged 30 to 69 years
- Gender ratio: female > male
- College graduates and residents of western states are more likely to use CAM.
- Cancer survivors are more likely than the general population to use CAM.
- Six most used CAM therapies:
  - Nonvitamin, nonmineral dietary supplements (18%)
  - Chiropractic and osteopathic manipulation (8.5%)
  - Yoga (8%)
  - Massage (7%)
  - Meditation (4%)
  - Special diets (3%)

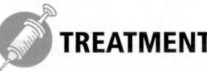 **TREATMENT**

- Variable evidence supports safety and efficacy of:
  - Meditation for lowering BP
  - Acupuncture for chronic low back pain (1)[B]
  - Spinal manipulative therapy for prophylactic treatment of headaches
  - Ginger for nausea, including that associated with chemotherapy
  - Manipulation, massage, and mobilization for acute low back and posterior neck pain
  - Massage therapy to promote weight gain in preterm infants
  - Saffron (*Crocus sativus L.*) reduces depressive symptoms in mothers with mild postpartum depression.
  - Massage (30 minutes × 3) during labor shortens the second stage and reduces pain.
  - Acupuncture for chemotherapy-induced nausea and vomiting
  - Tai chi for improving balance and decreasing the risk of and fear of falling in elderly
  - Mind–body techniques for migraines, chronic pain, and insomnia
  - Cognitive-behavioral therapy is highly effective for the treatment of insomnia (2)[A].

– Homeopathic remedy for the treatment of chemotherapy-induced stomatitis in children
– Riboflavin for migraine prophylaxis
– Horse chestnut seed extract to improve lower leg venous tone, pain, and edema
– Glucosamine for osteoarthritis and knee pain
– Yoga and meditation appear to improve endothelial function in patients with CAD and can have potential beneficial effects on depressive disorders.
– Yoga throughout pregnancy shortens labor by 140 to 190 minutes.
– Exercise in both preconception and early pregnancy reduces chance of gestational diabetes mellitus.
– Exercise has a small to moderate effect in reducing symptoms in persons with diagnosed anxiety disorders.
– Breast stimulation in late pregnancy increases successful induction of labor (NNT 3.2) and reduces postpartum hemorrhage (NNT 19).
– Oral probiotics in preterm infants to decrease necrotizing enterocolitis and reduce mortality (3)[A]
– Oral probiotics to prevent URIs in children and influenza in the elderly
– Oral probiotics to shorten the duration of acute and antibiotic-associated diarrhea and as prophylaxis for traveler's diarrhea
– Vitamin D 800 IU/day may reduce falls and fractures in the elderly.
– *Acupuncture* for recurrent headache
– *Ginkgo biloba* extract EGb 761 improves cognition in patients with dementia (4)[A].
– Cupping reduces chronic low back pain.
• Evidence supports safety, but evidence regarding efficacy is inconclusive:
– *Homeopathy* for induction and augmentation of labor
– Chondroitin sulfate is ineffective for osteoarthritis.
– *Sterile water injections* do not reduce labor pain.
– Fish oil might be an effective treatment for hypertriglyceridemia.
– Omega-3 fatty acids may reduce inflammation and anxiety in young healthy adults.
– *Dietary fat reduction* for certain types of cancer
– *Mind–body techniques* for metastatic cancer
– *Copper and magnetic bracelets* for pain
– *Vitamin D levels* >30 ng/mL correlate with lower risk of some cancers. Adequate vitamin D intake may decrease atopy and asthma symptoms.
• Evidence supports efficacy, but evidence regarding safety is inconclusive or poor:
– St. John's wort extract for short-term treatment of depression in adults
– Licorice for gastritis
– Goldenseal

• Evidence indicates serious risk:
– Black cohosh, blue cohosh, and evening primrose oil are unsafe to induce labor.
– Delay in seeking medical care or replacement of curative conventional treatment
– Use of toxic herbs or substances
– Known herb–drug interactions

ONGOING CARE

PATIENT EDUCATION
The National Center for Complementary and Integrative Health (https://nccih.nih.gov/)

COMPLICATIONS

ALERT
Ginkgo, goldenseal, and St. John's wort account for most reported herb–drug interactions.

• Herbs with possible adverse effects
– Serious adverse events from herbal remedies are uncommon.
– Some ethnic medicines, as those prescribed by practitioners of Ayurveda or traditional Chinese medicine, may intentionally contain heavy metals or other toxic substances. These are usually listed by their pharmacopeial names, for example, Qian Dan = lead oxide.
– Bitter orange (*Citrus sinensis*): sympathomimetic; increases heart rate (HR), BP
– Black cohosh (*Actaea racemosa*) reduces effectiveness of statins.
– California poppy (*Eschscholzia californica*): may cause respiratory depression, drowsiness; contains opioids
– Cascara sagrada (*Frangula purshiana*): depletes serum potassium
– Chaparral (*Larrea tridentata*): hepatotoxic
– Ephedra (*Ephedra spp.*): sympathomimetic; increases HR, BP; insomnia, gastric distress
– Ginkgo (*Ginkgo biloba*): extravasation, increased bleeding time
– Goldenseal (*Hydrastis canadensis*) interferes with nearly all prescription drugs.
– Guarana (*Paullinia cupana*): tachycardia, hypertension; contains caffeine
– Kava (*Piper methysticum*): decreases use of niacin; possibly hepatotoxic
– Licorice (*Glycyrrhiza spp.*): Long-term use depletes serum potassium
– Lily of the valley (*Convallaria majalis*): contains cardiac glycosides
– Poke root (*Phytolacca species*): strong gastric irritant; may cause sedation
– Senna (*Cassia senna*): depletes serum potassium
– Snakeroot (*Aristolochia spp.*): nephrotoxic

– St. John's wort (*Hypericum perforatum*): numerous drug interactions; induces CYP(3A4) pathway, speeding metabolism of cyclosporine, tacrolimus, warfarin, protease inhibitors, theophylline, venlafaxine, digoxin, and oral contraceptives
– Wormwood (*Artemisia absinthium*): elevates serotonin level, may raise BP
– Yohimbe (*Pausinystalia yohimbe*): elevates BP

Geriatric Considerations
Ginkgo biloba commonly interacts with warfarin (Coumadin).

Pediatric Considerations
Iron is a leading cause of accidental poisoning in children <6 years of age. Minerals (i.e., potassium, calcium, magnesium, zinc, copper, and selenium) may cause toxicity.

• Vitamin A is the most common cause of hypervitaminosis.
• β-Carotene has a limited potential for overdose.

REFERENCES

1. Vickers AJ, Vertosick EA, Lewith G, et al; for Acupuncture Trialists' Collaboration. Acupuncture for chronic pain: update of an individual patient data meta-analysis. *J Pain.* 2018;19(5):455–474.
2. Kligler B, Teets R, Quick M. Complementary/integrative therapies that work: a review of the evidence. *Am Fam Physician.* 2016;94(5):369–374.
3. Alfaleh K, Anabrees J, Bassler D, et al. Probiotics for prevention of necrotizing enterocolitis in preterm infants. *Cochrane Database Syst Rev.* 2011;(3):CD005496.
4. Asher GN, Corbett AH, Hawke RL. Common herbal dietary supplement-drug interactions. *Am Fam Physician.* 2017;96(2):101–107.

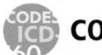 ## CODES

ICD10
Z76.89 Persons encountering health services in other specified circumstances

CLINICAL PEARLS

• Oral probiotics reduce respiratory and diarrheal infections and reduce mortality in preterm infants.
• Acupuncture is effective for back pain, headaches, and knee pain.
• Cognitive-behavioral therapy reduces insomnia.
• Yoga and breast stimulation shorten labor.
• Ginkgo, goldenseal, and St. John's wort account for most of the herb–drug interactions reported in the medical literature.

COMPLEX REGIONAL PAIN SYNDROME

Dennis E. Hughes, DO, FAAFP, FACEP

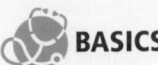 **BASICS**

DESCRIPTION
- Complex regional pain syndrome (CRPS) is a pain syndrome that can be chronic and debilitating. It is divided into two subtypes and can have significant physical and psychosocial short- and long-term disability. Most cases are a result of a physical insult to an extremity such as trauma or surgery.
  – Type I: no nerve injury (reflex sympathetic dystrophy [RSD])
  – Type II: associated with a demonstrable nerve injury (causalgia)
- Synonym(s): traumatic erythromelalgia; Weir Mitchell causalgia; causalgia; RSD; posttraumatic neuralgia; sympathetically maintained pain

EPIDEMIOLOGY
- Incidence of 5.46 to 26.2/100,000 for type I and 0.82/100,000 for type II in United States (1,2)
- Peak age 50 to 70 years
- Predominant gender: female > male (3:1, 60–81%), favoring postmenopausal
- Recent studies found 3.8% occurrence after wrist fracture and 7% occurrence after intra-articular ankle fracture—both independent strong risk for CRPS (3)[B].
- More prevalent in patients that report higher than usual expected pain in early phases of trauma. Latency depends on normal injury recovery time—prolonged pain after injury hints at diagnosis (3).

ETIOLOGY AND PATHOPHYSIOLOGY
- Poorly understood activation of abnormal sympathetic reflex that lowers pain threshold
  – Increased excitability of nociceptive neurons in the spinal cord; "central sensitization"
  – Exaggerated responses to normally nonpainful stimuli (hyperalgesia, allodynia)
- Type II is associated with physical injury to nerve.
- Emerging information reveals CNS changes (functional, anatomic, biochemical) in addition to spinal level changes. Increased levels of immunomodulators suggest autoimmune component (2).

Genetics
No known genetic pattern

RISK FACTORS
- Minor or severe trauma (upper extremity fracture noted in 44%)
- Surgery (particularly carpal tunnel release)
- Lacerations
- Burns
- Frostbite
- Casting/immobilization after extremity injury

- Penetrating injury
- Polymyalgia rheumatica
- Myocardial infarction (MI)
- Cerebral vascular accident

GENERAL PREVENTION
- Early mobilization after fracture, stroke, and MI has proven benefit in reducing incidence of CRPS.
- One study of wrist fractures found that addition of 500 mg/day of vitamin C lowered rates of CRPS.
- There is evidence that limiting use of tourniquets, liberal regional anesthetic use, and ensuring adequate perioperative analgesia can reduce the incidence of CRPS-I.

COMMONLY ASSOCIATED CONDITIONS
- Serious injury to bone and soft tissue
- Herpes zoster
- Postherpetic neuralgia results from partial or complete damage to afferent nerve pathways.
- Pain occurs in dermatomes as a sequela of herpes zoster.
- Signal exists for patients having comorbid painful conditions or psychiatric diagnosis at increased risk of developing CPRS.

 DIAGNOSIS

Unprovoked pain is the hallmark of the condition, and the diagnosis of CRPS is excluded by the existence of conditions that would otherwise account for the degree of symptoms. Budapest clinical diagnostic criteria can aid in establishing diagnosis (4).

HISTORY
- Continuing pain, which is disproportionate to any inciting event
- One reported symptom in three of the four following categories:
  – Sensory: hyperalgesia and/or allodynia
  – Vasomotor: skin, temperature, color asymmetry
  – Sudomotor/edema: edema, sweating changes, or sweating asymmetry
  – Motor/trophic: decreased range of motion or motor dysfunction and/or trophic changes (hair, nail, skin) (3)

PHYSICAL EXAM
At least one sign at evaluation in two of the following:
- Sensory: hyperalgesia (to pinprick) or allodynia (to light touch, pressure, or joint movement)
- Vasomotor: evidence of temperature, skin, color asymmetry
- Sudomotor/edema: evidence of edema or sweating changes or asymmetry
- Motor/trophic: decreased range of motion; motor dysfunction; or trophic changes in hair, nails, skin (3)

DIFFERENTIAL DIAGNOSIS
- Infection
- Hypertrophic scar
- Bone fragments
- Neuroma
- CNS tumor or syrinx
- Deep vein thrombosis or thrombophlebitis
- Thoracic outlet syndrome

DIAGNOSTIC TESTS & INTERPRETATION

Initial Tests (lab, imaging)
- CBC
- Erythrocyte sedimentation rate (ESR)
- Plain radiographs may show patchy demineralization within 3 to 6 weeks of onset of CRPS that are more pronounced than would be seen from disuse alone.
- Three-phase bone scanning has varying sensitivity but is most accurate for support of the diagnosis when there is diffuse activity (especially on phase 3).
- Bone density

Diagnostic Procedures/Other
- Electromyelography (EMG) shows nerve injury with type II CRPS.
- Sudomotor function testing (resting sweat testing, resting skin temperature, quantitative sudomotor axon reflex testing; all related to increased autonomic activity of the affected limb)

Test Interpretation
- Partial or complete damage to afferent nerve pathways and probably reorganized central pain pathways
- Nerves most commonly involved are median and sciatic.
- Atrophy in affected muscles
- Incomplete nerve plexus lesion

 TREATMENT

GENERAL MEASURES
Discourage maladaptive behaviors (pain medication seeking, secondary gain). Principal of functional restoration is a stepwise and multidisciplinary approach.

MEDICATION

First Line
- NSAIDs recommended early in course but mixed support in literature
- The following have literature support of either limited or suggestive benefit in treatment of CRPS-I:
  – Corticosteroids (prednisone 30 mg/day × 2 to 12 weeks with taper) are the only class of drugs

that have direct clinical trial support early in the course. A recent retrospective case review found that patients showed significant improvement with various measurable physical parameters after treatment with prednisolone (30 mg starting dose tapering by 5 mg every 3 days for a total of 3 weeks treatment) (4)[C].

– Gabapentin 600 to 1,800 mg/day for 8 weeks following diagnosis
– 50% DMSO cream applied to affected extremity up to 5 times daily
– N-Acetylcysteine 600 mg TID
– Bisphosphonates (alendronate) at 40 mg/day (however, optimal dose uncertain)
– Nifedipine 20 mg/day showed benefit early in the course of the condition.

- Although many have advocated the use of tricyclic antidepressants in the treatment of CRPS, there is no credible evidence of improvement of pain. They may be helpful in controlling depressive symptoms that develop with disease progression (1)[B].

ISSUES FOR REFERRAL

- After 2 months of the illness, psychological evaluation generally is indicated to identify and treat any comorbid conditions.
- Physical therapy and occupational therapy early for guided motor and mirror therapy (1)

ADDITIONAL THERAPIES

Type I

- Physical and occupational therapy (beneficial to the overall prognosis for recovery) and should be initiated early in the course of treatment
  – "Mirror therapy" has shown good results.
- Transcutaneous nerve stimulation
- Psychotherapy
- Use of subdissociative (0.2 to 0.5 mg/kg) infusions of ketamine has shown some promise, but effects seem to be time limited; systemic literature review failed to find and high-quality support for ketamine treatment (5)[C]

SURGERY/OTHER PROCEDURES

- Type II responds more favorably to nerve-directed treatment.
  – Sympathetic blocks
  – Cervicothoracic or lumbar sympathectomies have little data to support their use and should be used judiciously and after all other therapies have failed.
- Anesthetic blockade (chemical or surgical) of sympathetic nerve function
  – Transient relief suggests that chemical or surgical sympathectomy will be helpful.
  – Little in the way of quality clinical trials exist to support local sympathetic blockage as the gold standard of therapy.

- IV regional sympathetic block with guanethidine or reserpine by pain specialist or anesthetist
- Transcutaneous electric nerve stimulation (controversial)
- Inject myofascial painful trigger points.
- Dorsal root ganglion (DRG) stimulation higher rate of success than spinal cord stimulation in recent comparative study; more specific target as DRG home of soma of sensory neurons (2)
- Intrathecal analgesia
- Amputation as a last resort in severe cases, with patients reporting improved quality of life
- Single case study of topical 5% lidocaine revealed significant pain reduction and improved range of motion and function (6).

COMPLEMENTARY & ALTERNATIVE MEDICINE

- Vitamin C (500 mg/day) may help to prevent CRPS in those with wrist fracture.
- Briskly rub the affected part several times per day.
- Acupuncture
- Hypnosis can be suggested.
- Relaxation training (alternate muscle relaxing and contracting)
- Biofeedback
- Whirlpool baths

ADMISSION, INPATIENT, AND NURSING CONSIDERATIONS

Only for proposed surgical therapy

 ## ONGOING CARE

FOLLOW-UP RECOMMENDATIONS

Weekly, to monitor progress and initiate additional modalities as needed

PATIENT EDUCATION

- Stress need to remain active physically.
- Instruct carefully about any prescribed medications.
- Reflex Sympathetic Dystrophy Syndrome Association: http://rsds.org/; 203-877-3790
- American RSD Hope Group: http://www.rsdhope .org; 207-583-4589

PROGNOSIS

Most improve with early treatment, but symptoms may be lifelong if there is limited response to initial treatments.

COMPLICATIONS

- Depression
- Disability
- Opioid dependence

REFERENCES

1. Lo JC, Cavazos J, Burnett C. Management of complex regional pain syndrome. *Proc (Bayl Univ Med Cent)*. 2017;30(3):286–288.
2. Tajerian M, Clark JD. New concepts in complex regional pain syndrome. *Hand Clin*. 2016;32(1):41–49.
3. Pons T, Shipton EA, Williman J, et al. Potential risk factors for the onset of complex regional pain syndrome type 1: a systematic literature review. *Anesthesiol Res Pract*. 2015;2015:956539.
4. Birklein F, Dimova V. Complex regional pain syndrome up-to-date. *Pain Rep*. 2017;2(26):e624.
5. Connolly SB, Prager JP, Harden RN. A systematic review of ketamine for complex regional pain syndrome. *Pain Med*. 2015;16(5):943–969.
6. Hanlan AR, Mah-Jones D, Mills PB. Early adjunct treatment with topical lidocaine results in improved pain and function in a patient with complex regional pain syndrome. *Pain Physician*. 2014;17(5):E629–E635.

ADDITIONAL READING

Goh EL, Chidambaram S, Ma D. Complex regional pain syndrome: a recent update. *Burns Trauma*. 2017;5:2.

 ## CODES

ICD10

- G90.50 Complex regional pain syndrome I, unspecified
- G90.519 Complex regional pain syndrome I of unspecified upper limb
- G90.529 Complex regional pain syndrome I of unspecified lower limb

CLINICAL PEARLS

- A pain syndrome disproportioned to injury
- Pain control and early mobility are the key to recovery.
- Avoid use of opiate analgesics.
- Use a multidisciplinary approach.

CONDYLOMATA ACUMINATA

Caroline R. Campbell, MD • M. Ashleigh Brown, DO • E. James Kruse, DO

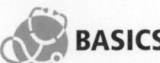 **BASICS**

DESCRIPTION
- Condylomata acuminata are soft, skin-colored, fleshy lesions (commonly called genital warts) that are caused by human papillomavirus (HPV):
  – Warts appear singly or in groups (a single wart is a "condyloma"; multiple warts are "condylomas" or "condylomata"); small or large; typically appear on the anogenital skin (penis, scrotum, introitus, vulva, perianal area); and may occur in the anogenital tract (vagina, cervix, rectum, urethra, anus); also conjunctival, nasal, oral, and laryngeal warts
- System(s) affected: skin/exocrine, reproductive, occasionally respiratory
- HIV considerations:
  – Treatment of external genital warts should not be different for HIV-infected persons (1).
  – Lesions may be larger or more numerous (1).
  – May not respond as well to therapy as immunocompetent persons (1)

Pediatric Considerations
- Consider sexual abuse if seen in children, although children can be infected by other means (e.g., transfer from wart on another child's hand or prolonged latency period) (2).
- American Academy of Pediatrics recommends all school-aged children who present with lesions be evaluated for abuse and screened for other STDs (2).

Pregnancy Considerations
- Warts often grow larger during pregnancy and regress spontaneously after delivery.
- Neonatal infection is thought to occur through vertical transmission. Incidence remains controversial. Cesarean section is not absolutely indicated for maternal condylomata (3).
- Cervical infection has been found to be a risk factor for preterm birth (3).
- Few documented cases of laryngeal papillomas due to HPV transmission at the time of delivery. Although rare, the condition is life-threatening.
- HPV vaccination is contraindicated in pregnancy.
- Treatment during pregnancy is somewhat controversial but may include topical trichloroacetic acid (TCA), cryotherapy, electrocautery, or surgical excision.
- The safety of imiquimod, sinecatechins, podophyllin, and podofilox during pregnancy has not been established (3).

EPIDEMIOLOGY
- HPV types 6 and 11 associated with 90% of condylomata acuminata. Types 16, 18, 31, 33, and 35 may be found in warts and may be associated with high-grade intraepithelial dysplasia in immunocompromised states such as HIV.
- Highly contagious; incubation period may be from 1 to 8 months. Initial infections may very well go unrecognized, so a "new" outbreak may be a relapse of an infection acquired years prior.
- Predominant age: 15 to 30 years
- Predominant sex: 1:1 male to female
- Most infections are transient and clear spontaneously within 2 years.

Incidence
One study population demonstrated that from 2007 to 2010, with the introduction of HPV vaccines, the incidence of genital warts decreased 35% (from 0.94% per year to 0.61% per year) in females <21 years and decreased 19% in males <21 years.

Prevalence
- Most common viral sexually transmitted infection (STI) in the United States. Most sexually active men and women will have acquired a genital HPV infection, usually asymptomatic, at some time.
- Estimated 6.2 million Americans become infected with genital HPV each year.
- Peak prevalence in ages 17 to 33 years
- 10–20% of sexually active women may be actively infected with HPV. Studies in men suggest a similar prevalence.
- Pregnancy and immunosuppression favor recurrence and increased growth of lesions.

ETIOLOGY AND PATHOPHYSIOLOGY
HPV is a circular, double-stranded DNA molecule. There are >120 HPV subtypes. HPV types that cause genital warts do not cause anogenital cancers.

RISK FACTORS
- Usually acquired by unprotected sexual activity
  – Young adults and adolescents
  – Multiple sexual partners; short interval between meeting new sex partner and first intercourse
  – Not using protective barriers
  – Young age of commencing sexual activity
  – History of other STI
- Immunosuppression (particularly HIV)
- Cigarette smoking
- Use of oral contraceptives
- Radiation therapy

GENERAL PREVENTION
- Sexual abstinence or monogamy
- HPV vaccination is for prevention of HPV infections and HPV-associated cancers. This vaccine is targeted to adolescents before the period of their greatest risk for exposure to HPV. The vaccine does not treat previous infections:
  – A 2-dose schedule (0, 6 to 12 months) will have efficacy equivalent to a 3-dose schedule (0, 1 to 2, 6 months) if the HPV vaccination series is initiated before the 15th birthday (4).
  – The 9-valent HPV (9vHPV; Gardasil 9) vaccine protects against the two most common HPV serotypes (types 6 and 11, which cause most anogenital warts) and the two most cancer-promoting types (16 and 18) as well as 31, 33, 45, 52, and 58 (4).
  – Quadrivalent HPV (4vHPV) and 9vHPV vaccines (Gardasil and Gardasil 9) are licensed for use in females and males aged 9 through 45 years (5).
  – The Advisory Committee on Immunization Practices (ACIP) has recommended routine vaccination at age 11 or 12 years for females since 2006 and since 2011 for males (4).
- Use of condoms is partially effective, although warts may be easily spread by lesions not covered by a condom (e.g., 40% of infected men have scrotal warts).
- Abstinence until treatment completed

COMMONLY ASSOCIATED CONDITIONS
- >90% of cervical cancer associated with HPV types 16, 18, 31, 33, and 35
- 60% of oropharyngeal and anogenital squamous cell carcinomas are associated with HPV.
- STIs (e.g., gonorrhea, syphilis, chlamydia), AIDS

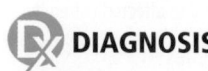 **DIAGNOSIS**

HISTORY
- Explore sexual history, contraception use, and other lifestyle topics.
- Most warts are asymptomatic but symptoms include
  – Pruritus, burning, redness, pain, bleeding
  – Vaginal discharge
  – Large warts may cause obstructive symptoms in the anus (with defecation) or vaginal canal (with intercourse or childbirth).

PHYSICAL EXAM
- Lesions often have a typical rough, warty appearance with multiple fingerlike projections but may be soft, sessile, and smooth.
- Large lesions are cauliflower-like and may grow to >10 cm.
- Most common sites: penis, vaginal introitus, and perianal region
- May be seen anywhere on the anogenital epithelium or in the anogenital tract
- Warts often occur in clusters.
- Bleeding or irritation of the lesions may be noted.

DIFFERENTIAL DIAGNOSIS
- Condylomata lata (flat warts of syphilis)
- Lichen planus
- Normal sebaceous glands
- Seborrheic keratosis
- Molluscum contagiosum
- Keratomas, micropapillomatosis
- Scabies
- Crohn disease
- Skin tags
- Melanocytic nevi
- Vulvar intraepithelial neoplasia
- Squamous cell carcinoma

DIAGNOSTIC TESTS & INTERPRETATION
- Diagnosis is usually clinical, made by unaided visual examination of the lesions.
- Biopsy
- Acetowhitening test: Subclinical lesions can be visualized by applying moistened gauze soaked with 5% acetic acid (vinegar) to the affected area for 5 minutes. Using a 10× hand lens or colposcope, warts appear as tiny white papules. A shiny white appearance of the skin represents foci of epithelial hyperplasia (subclinical infection), but because of low specificity, the CDC recommends against routine use of this test to screen for HPV mucosal infection.

Initial Tests (lab, imaging)
- Usually not required for diagnosis
- Serologic tests for syphilis may be helpful to rule out condylomata lata.
- Other testing for STIs
- Pap smear may be indicated.

Follow-Up Tests & Special Considerations

Because squamous cell carcinoma may resemble or coexist with condylomata, biopsy may be considered for lesions refractory to therapy.

Diagnostic Procedures/Other

- Biopsy with highly specialized identification techniques, such as HPV DNA detected through polymerase chain reaction, is rarely useful.
- Colposcopy, antroscopy, anoscopy, and urethroscopy may be required to detect anogenital tract lesions.
- Screening men who have sex with men (MSM) with anal Pap smears is controversial.

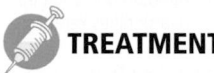

TREATMENT

GENERAL MEASURES

- Approximately, 30% resolve spontaneously in 4 months.
- Change therapy if no improvement after three treatments, clearance not complete after six treatments, or therapy's duration or dosage exceeds manufacturer's recommendations.
- Appropriate screening/counseling of partners

MEDICATION

First Line

- No single therapy for genital warts is ideal for all patients or clearly superior to other therapies.
- Recommendations for external genital warts, patient applied:
  - Podofilox (Condylox) (3)[A]: antimitotic action; apply 0.5% solution or gel to warts twice daily (allowing to dry) for 3 consecutive days at home followed by 4 days of no therapy; may repeat up to 4 total cycles; maximum of 0.5 mL/day or area <10 cm^2
  - Imiquimod (Aldara) (3)[A]: immune enhancer; self-treatment with a 5% cream applied once daily at bedtime 3 times weekly until warts resolve for up to 16 weeks. Wash off with soap and water 6 to 10 hours after application. Imiquimod has been noted to weaken condoms and diaphragms; therefore, patients should refrain from sexual contact while the cream is on the skin.
  - Sinecatechins (Veregen): immune enhancer and antioxidant, extract from green tea; apply a 0.5-cm strand of ointment 3 times daily for up to 16 weeks. Do not wash off after.
- Recommendations for external genital warts, provider applied:
  - Cryotherapy: liquid nitrogen applied to warts for two bursts of approximately 10 seconds (or whatever time is needed to freeze the wart without extension significantly deep or lateral to the wart) with thawing in between; usually requires 2 to 3 weekly sessions (3)[A]
  - Podophyllin 10–25% in tincture of benzoin. Apply directly to warts, air-dry in office before coming into contact with clothes. Wash off in 1 to 4 hours. Repeat every 7 days in office until gone (3)[A].
  - TCA: 80% solution. Apply only to warts; powder/talc to remove unreacted acid. Repeat in office at weekly intervals; ideal for isolated lesions in pregnancy (3)[A]
- Recommendations for exophytic cervical warts: biopsy to exclude high-grade squamous intraepithelial lesion (SIL) (3)[A]
- Recommendations for vaginal warts: cryotherapy or TCA or bichloroacetic acid (BCA) 80–90% (3)[A]

- Recommendations for urethral meatus warts: cryotherapy or podophyllin 10–25% in compound tincture of benzoin (3)[A]
- Recommendations for anal warts: cryotherapy, TCA or BCA 80–90%, or surgery; specialty consultation for intra-anal warts (3)[A]

Pregnancy Considerations

Cryotherapy, surgery, or TCA; medications contraindicated in pregnancy: podophyllin, podophyllotoxin, sinecatechins, interferon, and imiquimod (3)[C]

Second Line

Intralesional interferon, photodynamic therapy, topical cidofovir (3)[A]

SURGERY/OTHER PROCEDURES

- Larger warts may require surgical excision, laser treatment, or electrocoagulation (including infrared therapy):
  - Precaution: Laser treatment may create smoke plumes that contain HPV. CDC recommendation is for the use of a smoke evacuator no <2 inches from the surgical site. Masks are recommended; N95 the most efficacious (6)
- Intraurethral, external (penile and perianal), anal, and oral lesions can be treated with fulgurating CO_2 laser. Oral or external penile/perianal lesions can also be treated with electrocautery or surgery.

ONGOING CARE

FOLLOW-UP RECOMMENDATIONS

No restrictions, except for sexual contact

Patient Monitoring

- Patients should be seen every 1 to 2 weeks until lesions resolve.
- Patients should follow up 3 months after completion of treatment.
- Persistent warts require biopsy.
- Sexual partners require monitoring.

PATIENT EDUCATION

- Provide information on HPV, STI prevention, and condom use.
- Explain to patients that it is difficult to know how or when a person acquired an HPV infection; a diagnosis in one partner does not prove sexual infidelity in the other partner.
- Emphasize the need for women to follow recommendations for regular Pap smears.

PROGNOSIS

- Asymptomatic infection persists indefinitely.
- Treatment has not clearly been shown to decrease transmissible infectivity.
- Warts may clear with treatment or resolve spontaneously. However, recurrences are frequent, particularly in the first 3 months, and may necessitate repeated treatments.

COMPLICATIONS

- Cervical dysplasia (probably does not occur with type 6 or 11, which cause most warts)
- Malignant change: Progression of condylomata to cancer rarely, if ever, occurs, although squamous cell carcinoma may coexist in larger warts.
- Urethral, vaginal, or anal obstruction from treatment
- The prevalence of high-grade dysplasia and cancer in anal canal is higher in HIV-positive than in HIV-negative patients, probably because of increased HPV activity.

REFERENCES

1. Gormley RH, Kovarik CL. Human papillomavirus-related genital disease in the immunocompromised host: part II. *J Am Acad Dermatol*. 2012;66(6): 883.e1–883.e17, quiz 899–900.
2. Unger ER, Fajman NN, Maloney EM, et al. Anogenital human papillomavirus in sexually abused and nonabused children: a multicenter study. *Pediatrics*. 2011;128(3):e658–e665.
3. Workowski KA, Bolan GA; for Centers for Disease Control and Prevention. Sexually transmitted diseases treatment guidelines, 2015. *MMWR Recomm Rep*. 2015;64(RR-03):1–137.
4. Meites E, Kempe A, Markowitz LE. Use of a 2-dose schedule for human papillomavirus vaccination—updated recommendations of the Advisory Committee on Immunization Practices. *MMWR Morb Mortal Wkly Rep*. 2016;65(49):1405–1408.
5. U.S. Food and Drug Administration. FDA approves expanded use of Gardasil 9 to include individuals 27 through 45 years old. https://www.fda.gov /NewsEvents/Newsroom/PressAnnouncements /ucm622715.htm. Accessed December 12, 2018.
6. Bryant C, Gorman R, Stewart J, et al. *NIOSH Health Hazard Evaluation Report*. Bryn Mawr, PA: National Institute for Occupational Safety and Health; 1988. HETA 85-126-1932.

ADDITIONAL READING

- Bauer HM, Wright G, Chow J. Evidence of human papillomavirus vaccine effectiveness in reducing genital warts: an analysis of California public family planning administrative claims data, 2007–2010. *Am J Public Health*. 2012;102(5):833–835.
- Giuliano AR, Palefsky JM, Goldstone S, et al. Efficacy of quadrivalent HPV vaccine against HPV infection and disease in males. *N Engl J Med*. 2011;364(5):401–411.
- Gormley RH, Kovarik CL. Human papillomavirus-related genital disease in the immunocompromised host: part I. *J Am Acad Dermatol*. 2012;66(6): 867.e1–867.e14, quiz 881–882.
- Yanofsky V, Patel R, Goldenberg G. Genital warts: a comprehensive review. *J Clin Aesthet Dermatol*. 2012;5(6):25–36.

CODES

ICD10
A63.0 Anogenital (venereal) warts

CLINICAL PEARLS

- Condylomata acuminata are soft, skin-colored, fleshy lesions caused by HPV subtypes 6, 11, 16, 18, 31, 33, and 35.
- The majority of sexually active men and women will have acquired a genital HPV infection, usually asymptomatic, at some time.
- No single therapy for genital warts is ideal for all patients or clearly superior to other therapies.
- 9vHPV vaccine is effective in preventing HPV infection, particularly if administered prior to the onset of engaging in sexual activity. Gardasil is approved and recommended for use in males and females aged 9 to 45 years.

CONJUNCTIVITIS, ACUTE

Frances Y. Wu, MD, FAAFP

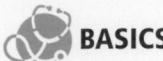 **BASICS**

DESCRIPTION
- Inflammation of the bulbar and/or palpebral conjunctiva of <4 weeks' duration
- System(s) affected: nervous, skin/exocrine
- Synonym(s): pink eye

Geriatric Considerations
- Suspect autoimmune, systemic, or irritative process.
- If purulent, risk of bacterial cause increases with age, with age >65 years and bilateral lid adherence risk for bacterial infection is >70%.

Pediatric Considerations
- Neonatal conjunctivitis may be gonococcal, chlamydial, irritative, or related to dacryocystitis.
- Pediatric ER study; 78% positive bacterial culture, mostly *Haemophilus influenzae*; 13% no growth; other studies showed >50% adenovirus.
- Children <5 years 7 times more likely have bacterial involvement than older children or mid aged adults.
- Despite lack of evidence, daycare regulations may require a child with presumed conjunctivitis to be treated with a topical antibiotic before returning (1)[A].

EPIDEMIOLOGY
- Predominant age
  - Pediatric: viral, bacterial
  - Adult: viral, bacterial, allergic
- Predominant sex: male = female

Incidence
1–2% of ambulatory office visits, up to 3% of ER visits

ETIOLOGY AND PATHOPHYSIOLOGY
- Viral
  - Adenovirus (common cold), coxsackievirus (implicated in recent hemorrhagic conjunctivitis epidemics in Asia and Middle East)
  - Enterovirus (acute hemorrhagic conjunctivitis)
  - Herpes simplex
  - Herpes zoster or varicella
  - Measles, mumps, or influenza
- Bacterial
  - *Staphylococcus aureus* or *Staphylococcus epidermidis*
  - *Streptococcus pneumoniae*
  - *H. influenzae* (children)
  - *Pseudomonas* spp. or anaerobes (contact lens users)
  - *Acanthamoeba*-contaminated contact lens solution may cause keratitis (rare; ~30 cases per year in United States).
  - *Neisseria gonorrhoeae* and *Neisseria meningitidis*
  - *Chlamydia trachomatis*: gradual onset 1 to 4 weeks
  - *Escherichia coli* neonatal conjunctivitis reported rarely, and tuberculosis reported in treatment resistant cases
- Allergic
  - Hay fever, seasonal allergies, atopy
- Nonspecific
  - Irritative: topical medications, wind, dry eye, UV light exposure, smoke
  - Autoimmune: Sjögren syndrome, pemphigoid, Wegener granulomatosis
  - Rare: *Rickettsia*, fungal, parasitic, tuberculosis, syphilis, Kawasaki disease, chikungunya, Graves disease, gout, carcinoid, sarcoid, psoriasis, Stevens-Johnson syndrome, Reiter syndrome

RISK FACTORS
- History of contact with infected persons
- Sexually transmitted disease (STD) contact: gonococcal, chlamydial, syphilis, or herpes
- Contact lenses: pseudomonal or acanthamoeba keratitis
- Epidemic bacterial (streptococcal) conjunctivitis reported in school settings

GENERAL PREVENTION
- Wash hands frequently.
- Eyedropper technique: while eye is closed and head back, several drops over nasal canthus and then open eyes to allow liquid to enter. Never touch tip of dropper to skin or eye.

COMMONLY ASSOCIATED CONDITIONS
- Viral infection (e.g., common cold)
- Possible sexually transmitted infection

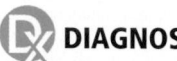 **DIAGNOSIS**

HISTORY

> **ALERT**
> Red flag: Any decrease in visual acuity is not consistent with conjunctivitis alone; must document normal vision for diagnosis of isolated conjunctivitis

- Viral: contact or travel
  - May start with one eye and then both
  - If herpetic, recurrences or vesicles on skin
- Bacterial: difficult to distinguish from viral, unless contact lens user. Assume bacterial in contact lens wearer unless cultures are negative. If recent STD, suspect chlamydia or gonococcus.
- Allergic: itching, atopy, seasonal, dander
- Irritative: feels dry, exposure to wind, tear-film deficit may persist 30 days after acute conjunctivitis, chemicals, or drug: atropine, aminoglycosides, iodide, phenylephrine, antivirals, bisphosphonates, retinoids, topiramate, chamomile, COX-2 inhibitors
- Foreign body: Redness may persist 24 hours after removal.

PHYSICAL EXAM
- General: common to all types of conjunctivitis
  - Red eye, conjunctival injection
  - Foreign body sensation
  - Eyelid sticking or crusting, discharge
  - Normal visual acuity and pupillary reactivity
- Viral
  - Palpable preauricular lymphadenopathy may be present.
  - Hemorrhagic coxsackievirus-related epidemics were reported.
  - Severe viral: herpes simplex or zoster:
    - Burning sensation, rarely itching
    - Unilateral, herpetic skin vesicles in zoster
    - Palpable preauricular node
- Bacterial (non-STD): may be epidemic
  - Mild pruritus, discharge mild to heavy
  - Conjunctival chemosis/edema
  - If contact lens user, must rule out pseudomonal (or other bacterial) keratitis
- Bacterial: gonococcal (or meningococcal) hyperacute infection
  - Rapid onset 12 to 24 hours
  - Severe purulent discharge
  - Chemosis/conjunctival/eyelid edema
  - Rapid growth of superior corneal ulceration

- Preauricular adenopathy
- Signs of STDs (chlamydia, GC, HIV, etc.)
- Allergic
  - Itching predominant, chemosis, edema
  - Seasonal or dander allergies
- Nonspecific irritative
  - Dry eyes, intermittent redness, chemical/drug exposure
  - Foreign body: may have redness and discharge 24 hours after removal
- Must document normal visual acuity
- Cornea should be clear and without fluorescein uptake. Cloudy or ulcerated cornea signifies keratitis; consult ophthalmologist.
- Recommend fluorescein exam: Evert lid to inspect for foreign bodies.
- Skin: Look for herpetic vesicles, nits on lashes (lice), scaliness (seborrhea), or styes.
- Limbal flush at corneal margin if uveitis
- If pupil is irregular (i.e., penetrating foreign body), emergent referral is warranted.
- Discharge but no conjunctival injection: blepharitis

DIFFERENTIAL DIAGNOSIS
- Uveitis (iritis, iridocyclitis, choroiditis): limbal flush (red band at corneal margin), hazy anterior chamber, and decreased visual acuity
- Penetrating ocular trauma: emergently hospitalize
- Acute glaucoma (emergency): headache, corneal clouding, poor visual acuity
- Corneal ulcer, keratitis, or foreign body: lesions or tear-film deficits on fluorescein exam
- Dacryocystitis: tenderness and swelling over tear sac (below medial canthus)
- Scleritis and episcleritis: red injected vessels radially oriented, sectoral (pie wedge), nodularity of sclera
- Pingueculitis: inflammation of a yellow nodular or wedge-like area of chronic conjunctival degeneration (pinguecula)
- Ophthalmia neonatorum: neonates in the first 2 days of life (gonococcal; 5 to 12 days of life): chlamydial, herpes simplex virus (HSV), very rare *Neisseria meningitides*. Consider specialty consultation for required systemic therapy; rare report of *E. coli* found on culture
- Blepharitis: Lid margins are inflamed producing itching, scale, or discharge but no conjunctival injection.

DIAGNOSTIC TESTS & INTERPRETATION
- Usually not needed initially for most common causes
- Culture swab if STD is suspected, very severe symptoms, patient is a contact lens user, or if resistant to prior treatment.
- Viral swab (10-minute test) for adenovirus is costly, requires six passes to acquire sample, and may not be tolerated by children.

Diagnostic Procedures/Other
- Fluorescein exam for corneal ulcer or abrasion
- Remove small, superficial foreign bodies with irrigation or moistened swab.
- Refer cases of prolonged symptoms to confirm diagnosis and exclude need for biopsy.

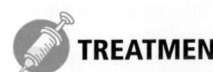 **TREATMENT**

GENERAL MEASURES
- Viral conjunctivitis does not require antibiotics and resolves spontaneously.
- Clean external eyelid with wet cloth up to QID.

- Stop use of contact lenses while eye is red.
- Eye patching is not beneficial.

MEDICATION

First Line
- Viral (nonherpetic)
  - Artificial tears for symptomatic relief
  - Vasoconstrictor/antihistamine (e.g., naphazoline/pheniramine) QID for severe itching
  - May consider topical antibiotic (see bacterial below) if return to daycare requires treatment
- Viral (herpetic) (ophthalmology consultation)
  - Ganciclovir gel: 0.15%, 5 times per day for 7 days (2)[B]
  - Acyclovir: PO 400 mg 5 times per day for HSV; 800 mg for zoster for 7 days
- Bacterial (nonsexually transmitted): 3 days of cool compresses before starting antibiotic is associated with no adverse effects and reduces unnecessary antibiotic use.
  - After 3 days, consider topical antibiotics (NNT 7 at day 6) (immediate antibiotics shortened course by only 3 days in children): Bacitracin ophthalmic ointment: Apply 3 to 4 times per day for 5 to 7 days.
  - Polymyxin B-trimethoprim solution 1 gtt 6 times per day for 5 to 7 days
  - Erythromycin ophthalmic ointment: 1/2 inch 2 to 4 times per day for 5 days
  - Sodium sulfacetamide (Bleph-10) (10% solution): 2 drops q4h (while awake) for 5 days
  - Tobramycin or gentamicin: 0.3% ophthalmic drops/ointment q4h (drops) to q8h (ointment) for 7 days
- Bacterial (gonococcal)
  - Neonates: Hospitalize for IV therapy.
  - Adults: ceftriaxone: 1 g IM as single dose and topical bacitracin ophthalmic ointment 1/2 inch QID. Neonates 25 to 50 mg/kg IV or IM, not to exceed 125 mg, as a single dose. Chlamydia in neonates requires oral erythromycin: 50 mg/kg/day divided q6h PO for 14 days, max 3 g/day.
- Allergic and atopic over-the-counter (OTC) medications are efficacious, no evidence favoring one over another, but cost ranges from $15 to $300 (3)[A].
  - Ketotifen (Zaditor, Alaway, and other generics OTC): 0.25% 1 drop 2 times per day
  - Ketorolac (Acular): 0.1% 1 drop 4 times per day
  - Cetirizine (Zerviate): 24% 1 drop 2 times per day
  - Olopatadine (Pataday, Patanol): 0.1% 1 drop 2 times per day or 0.2% 1 drop daily
  - Cromolyn (Opticrom): 4% 1 drop 4 times per day
  - Azelastine (Astelin): 0.05% 1 drop 2 times per day
  - Nedocromil (Alocril): 2% 1 drop 2 times per day
  - Alcaftadine (Lastacaft): 0.25% 1 drop daily
  - Emedastine (Emadine): 0.05% 1 drop 2 times per day
  - Epinastine (Elestat): 0.05% 2 times per day
  - Bepotastine (Bepreve): 1.5% 1 drop 2 times per day
  - Lodoxamide tromethamine (Alomide): 0.1% 1 drop 4 times per day
  - Oral nonsedating antihistamines (cetirizine [Zyrtec] 10 mg/day, fexofenadine [Allegra] 60 mg BID, etc.) may treat nasal symptoms but cause ocular drying; oral antihistamine (e.g., diphenhydramine 25 mg TID) in severe cases of itching
- Contraindications: steroids *not* beneficial in treatment of bacterial keratitis (4)[A]. Topical immune modulators (tacrolimus, cyclosporine) should be reserved for specialist use only in the most difficult cases.

- Precautions
  - Do not allow dropper to touch the eye.
  - Case reports of eye irritation from gentamicin in infants, moxifloxacin in adults, sulfacetamide in allergic individuals
  - Vasoconstrictor/antihistamine: rebound vasodilation after prolonged use

Second Line
- Viral and allergic: numerous OTC products
- Bacterial: second line (quinolones used as postoperative or for known resistant organisms)
  - Ofloxacin: 0.3% 1 gtt QID for 7 days
  - Ciprofloxacin: 0.3% 1 gtt QID for 7 days
  - Levofloxacin: 0.3% 1 gtt QID for 7 days
  - Gatifloxacin: 0.3% 1 gtt TID for 7 days
  - Moxifloxacin: 0.5% 1 gtt TID for 7 days
  - Besifloxacin: 0.6% 1 gtt TID for 7 days
  - Azithromycin: 1.5% BID for 3 days

ISSUES FOR REFERRAL
- Refer to ophthalmology for any significantly decreased visual acuity, herpetic keratitis, or contact lens–related conjunctivitis or immunocompromised (HIV).
- Refer for symptoms or worsening over 7 days (concern for severe adenoviral keratitis) (5).

COMPLEMENTARY & ALTERNATIVE MEDICINE
- Usually benign and self-limited; saline flushes, cool compresses, and similar treatments help.
- Mandarin orange yogurt showed improvement over 2 weeks for allergic conjunctivitis in a small study.

ADMISSION, INPATIENT, AND NURSING CONSIDERATIONS
- Acute gonococcal conjunctivitis (or very rare case of meningococcal conjunctivitis) requires inpatient treatment with ceftriaxone 50 mg/kg IV everyday (pediatric), 1 g IM for one (adult) along with ophthalmologic consultation.
- Admission criteria/initial stabilization
  - Penetrating ocular trauma, gonococcal conjunctivitis

 ONGOING CARE

FOLLOW-UP RECOMMENDATIONS
- If not resolved within 5 to 7 days, reconsider diagnosis or consult specialist; some epidemic keratoconjunctivitis and other adenoviral conjunctivitis typically last 1 to 2 weeks.
- Children may be excluded from school until eye is no longer red, depending on school policy. Allergic conjunctivitis should return to school with doctor's note.

PATIENT EDUCATION
- No contacts until eyes are fully healed (~1 week).
- Discard current contacts.
- Discard eye makeup, especially mascara.
- Cool, moist compresses can ease irritation and itch.

PROGNOSIS
- Viral: 5 to 10 days of symptoms for pharyngitis with conjunctivitis, 2 weeks with adenovirus
- Herpes simplex: 2 to 3 weeks of symptoms
- Most common bacterial—*H. influenzae*, *Staphylococcus*, *Streptococcus*: self-limited; 74–80% resolution within 7 days, whether treated or not

COMPLICATIONS
- Corneal scars with herpes simplex
- Lid scars or entropion with varicella zoster and chlamydia
- Corneal ulcers or perforation, very rapid with gonococcal
- Hypopyon: pus in anterior chamber
- Chlamydial neonatal (ophthalmic): could have concomitant pneumonia
- Otitis media may follow *H. influenzae* conjunctivitis.
- Very rarely *N. meningitidis* conjunctivitis may be followed by meningitis.

REFERENCES
1. Steeples L, Mercieca K. Acute conjunctivitis in primary care: antibiotics and placebo associated with small increase in the proportion cured by 7 days compared with no treatment. *Evid Based Med*. 2012;17(6):177–178.
2. Wilhelmus KR. Antiviral treatment and other therapeutic interventions for herpes simplex virus epithelial keratitis. *Cochrane Database Syst Rev*. 2015;(1):CD002898.
3. Castillo M, Scott NW, Mustafa MZ, et al. Topical antihistamines and mast cell stabilisers for treating seasonal and perennial allergic conjunctivitis. *Cochrane Database Syst Rev*. 2015;(6):CD009566.
4. Herretes S, Wang X, Reyes JM. Topical corticosteroids as adjunctive therapy for bacterial keratitis. *Cochrane Database Syst Rev*. 2014;(10):CD005430.
5. Mammas IN, Theodoridou M, Kramvis A, et al. Paediatric virology: a rapidly increasing educational challenge. *Exp Ther Med*. 2017;13(2):364–377.

ADDITIONAL READING
Watson S, Cabrera-Aguas M, Khoo P. Common eye infections. *Aust Prescr*. 2018;41(3):67–72.

 SEE ALSO

- Rhinitis, Allergic
- Algorithm: Eye Pain

 CODES

ICD10
- H10.30 Unspecified acute conjunctivitis, unspecified eye
- H10.33 Unspecified acute conjunctivitis, bilateral
- H10.32 Unspecified acute conjunctivitis, left eye

CLINICAL PEARLS
- Conjunctivitis does *not* cause decreased acuity or photophobia. If visual acuity is decreased, consider more serious ophthalmic disorders.
- Culture discharge in all *contact lens wearer*. Consider referral and discard current lenses until eyes are fully healed.
- Antibiotics are of no value in viral conjunctivitis (most cases of infectious conjunctivitis).
- Cool compresses for 3 days before using any antibiotic is appropriate for treating conjunctivitis in healthy adults and children >1 month.

CONSTIPATION

S. Mimi Mukherjee, PharmD, BCPS, CDE • Sandra Marwill, MD, MPH

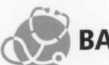 **BASICS**

Unsatisfactory defecation characterized by infrequent stools, difficult stool passage, or both. Characteristics include <3 bowel movements a week, hard stools, excessive straining, prolonged time spent on the toilet, a sense of incomplete evacuation, and abdominal discomfort/bloating.

DESCRIPTION
- System(s) affected: gastrointestinal (GI)
- Synonym(s): obstipation

Geriatric Considerations
Colorectal neoplasms may be associated with constipation; new-onset constipation after age 50 years is a "red flag." Use warm water enemas (instead of sodium phosphate enemas) for impaction in geriatric patients. Sodium phosphate enemas have been associated with fatalities and severe electrolyte disturbances (1).

Pediatric Considerations
Consider Hirschsprung disease (absence of colonic ganglion cells) in cases of pediatric constipation. Hirschsprung disease accounts for 25% of all newborn intestinal obstructions and can present as milder cases diagnosed in older children with chronic constipation, abdominal distension, and decreased growth. Hirschsprung has a 5:1 male-to-female ratio and is associated with inherited conditions (e.g., Down syndrome).

Pregnancy Considerations
Avoid misoprostol.

EPIDEMIOLOGY
- More pronounced in children and elderly
- Predominant sex: female > male (2:1)
- Nonwhites > whites

Incidence
- 5 million office visits annually
- 100,000 hospitalizations

Prevalence
- 16% of adults >18 years, rising to 33% of adults >60 years of age
- 3% of pediatric visits relate to constipation.

ETIOLOGY AND PATHOPHYSIOLOGY
- As food leaves the stomach, the ileocecal valve relaxes (gastroileal reflex), and chyme enters the colon (1 to 2 L/day) from the small intestine. In the colon, sodium is actively absorbed in exchange for potassium and bicarbonate. Water follows the osmotic gradient. Peristaltic contractions move chyme through the colon into the rectum. Chyme is converted into feces (200 to 250 mL).
- Normal transit time is 4 hours to reach the cecum and 12 hours to reach the distal colon.
- Defecation reflexively follows as stool reaches the rectal vault. This reflex can be inhibited by voluntarily contracting the external sphincter or facilitated by straining to contract the abdominal muscles while voluntarily relaxing the anal sphincter. Rectal distention initiates the defecation reflex. The urge to defecate occurs with an increase in rectal pressure. Distention of the stomach also initiates rectal contractions and a desire to defecate (gastrocolic reflex).
- Primary and secondary defecation disorders result from delay in colonic transit, altered rectal motor activity, and structural or functional problems with pelvic floor muscles (including paradoxical contractions, diminished sphincter relaxation, and/or poor propulsion).

Genetics
Unknown but may be familial

RISK FACTORS
- Very young and very old
- Polypharmacy
- Sedentary lifestyle or condition
- Improper diet and inadequate fluid intake

GENERAL PREVENTION
High-fiber diet, adequate fluids, exercise, and training to "obey the urge" to defecate

COMMONLY ASSOCIATED CONDITIONS
- General debilitation (disease or aging)
- Dehydration
- Hypothyroidism
- Hypokalemia
- Hypercalcemia
- Nursing home resident

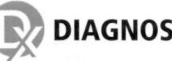 **DIAGNOSIS**

ALERT
Red flags:

- New onset after age of 50 years
- Hematochezia/melena
- Unintentional weight loss
- Family history of colon cancer
- Anemia
- Neurologic defects

HISTORY
- Assess onset of symptoms, number of bowel movements per week, straining, completeness of evacuation, and use of manual manipulation.
- Identify red flags; evaluate diet, lifestyle, prescription, and OTC medication use; identify reversible causes; ask about history of sexual abuse, opioid use.
- Bristol Stool Form Scale—seven categories of consistency (2)
- A diary of dietary intake and bowel patterns helps to measure treatment response.
- Rome III criteria:
  - At least two of the following for 12 weeks in the previous 6 months:
    - <3 stools per week
    - Straining at least 1/4 of the time
    - Hard stools at least 1/4 of time
    - Need for manual assist at least 1/4 of time
    - Sense of incomplete evacuation at least 1/4 of time
    - Sense of anorectal blockade at least 1/4 of time
  - Loose stools rarely seen without use of laxatives
  - Frequent constipation but does not meet irritable bowel syndrome (IBS) criteria
  - Although there can be overlap, the history of primary constipation differs from constipation-predominant IBS.
    - In primary constipation, pain and bloating are relieved by adequate defecation. In IBS, pain and bloating predominate and are not readily relieved by defecation.
- Bowel Function Index—for opioid-induced constipation (OIC) score of 0 to 100, mean of three variables; ease of defecation, completeness of emptying, patient's rating of constipation severity

PHYSICAL EXAM
- Vital signs
- Abdominal exam, previous surgical scars, hypoactive bowel sounds, tenderness, and masses
- Gynecologic exam: Evaluate for masses and rectocele.
- Digital rectal exam: Evaluate for masses, pain, stool, fissures, and hemorrhoids; assess sphincter tone.
- Neurologic exam

DIFFERENTIAL DIAGNOSIS
- Primary constipation (primary problem is within the GI tract) has four subtypes.
  - Normal colonic transit time most common subtype; can be difficult to differentiate from constipation-predominant IBS
  - Slow colonic transit time
  - Pelvic floor/anal sphincter dysfunction
  - Combination pelvic floor/anal sphincter dysfunction and slow transit
- Secondary constipation (outside the GI tract)
  - Endocrine dysfunction (diabetes mellitus, hypothyroid)
  - Metabolic disorder (increased calcium, decreased potassium)
  - Mechanical (obstruction, rectocele)
  - Pregnancy
  - Neurologic disorders (Hirschsprung, multiple sclerosis, spinal cord injuries, Parkinson disease)
- Congenital
  - Hirschsprung disease/syndrome
  - Hypoganglionosis
  - Congenital dilation of the colon
  - Small left colon syndrome
- Medication effect
  - Opioids
  - Antidepressants
  - Antipsychotics
  - Antacids (calcium, aluminum)
  - Nondihydropyridine calcium channel blockers, especially verapamil
  - Iron and multivitamins with iron
  - Diuretics
  - Overuse of antidiarrheal medications

DIAGNOSTIC TESTS & INTERPRETATION
Identify red flags, secondary causes, and reversible conditions. If none present, go to first-line treatment.

Initial Tests (lab, imaging)
- CBC to screen for iron deficiency anemia
- Consider tox screen if illicit opioid use is suspected.
- Calcium, glucose, and thyroid function testing (TSH) based on history and exam. If red flags are present, refer for sigmoid/colonoscopy.

Follow-Up Tests & Special Considerations
For patients with pelvic floor dysfunction or exam abnormalities (e.g., rectocele) and/or patients who are refractory to initial treatment, refer to an experienced subspecialist. A physical therapist experienced in biofeedback can also be very helpful.

Diagnostic Procedures/Other
- Anorectal manometry (ARM)
- Balloon expulsion testing (BET)
- Scintigraphy
- MRI
- Defecography
- Colonic marker studies

Test Interpretation
- ARM and BET recommended for all refractory cases
- If ARM and BET are negative, scintigraphy may help evaluate transit time. Some recommend biofeedback prior to scintigraphy.

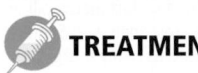

TREATMENT

Address immediate concerns:
- Bloating/discomfort/straining: osmotic agents
- Postoperative, after childbirth, hemorrhoids, fissures: stool softener to aid defecation
- If impacted: manual disimpaction and then treat any underlying conditions

GENERAL MEASURES
In patients with no known secondary causes, conservative nonpharmacologic treatment is recommended.
- Eliminate medications that cause constipation.
- Increase fluid intake.
- Increase soluble fiber in diet.
- Encourage regular defecation attempts after eating.
- Regular exercise
- Enemas if other methods fail (avoid sodium phosphate enemas in geriatric patients) (1)[B]

MEDICATION
Nonprescription medications are first line. If patient goals are not reached, advance to prescription medications.

First Line
Bulking agents (accompanied by adequate fluids):
- Hydrophilic colloids (bulk-forming agents)
  – Psyllium (Konsyl, Metamucil, Perdiem Fiber): 1 tbsp in 8-oz liquid PO daily up to TID
  – Methylcellulose (Citrucel): 1 tbsp in 8-oz liquid PO daily up to TID
  – Polycarbophil (Mitrolan, FiberCon): 2 caplets with 8-oz liquid PO up to QID
- Stool softeners
  – Docusate sodium (Colace): 50 to 100 mg PO TID
- Osmotic laxatives
  – Polyethylene glycol (PEG) (MiraLAX) 17 g/day PO dissolved in 4 to 8 oz of beverage (current evidence shows PEG to be superior to lactulose) (3)[B]
  – Lactulose (Chronulac, Enulose) 15 to 60 mL PO QHS (flatulence, bloating, cramping)
  – Sorbitol: 15 to 60 mL PO QHS (as effective as lactulose)
  – Magnesium salts (milk of magnesia): 15 to 30 mL PO once daily; avoid in renal insufficiency.

Second Line
- Stimulants (irritate bowel, causing muscle contraction; usually combined with a softener; work in 8 to 12 hours)
  – Senna/docusate (Senokot-S, Ex-lax, Peri-Colace): 1 to 2 tablets or 15 to 30 mL PO at bedtime
  – Bisacodyl (Dulcolax, Correctol): 1 to 3 tablets PO daily
- Lubricants (soften stool and facilitate passage of the feces by its lubricating oily effects)
  – Mineral oil (15 to 45 mL/day)
  – Short-term use only; can bind fat-soluble vitamins, with the potential for deficiencies; may similarly decrease absorption of some drugs
  – Avoid in those at risk for aspiration (lipoid pneumonia).
- Suppositories
  – Osmotic: sodium phosphate
  – Lubricant: glycerin
  – Stimulatory: bisacodyl
  – Enemas: saline (Fleet enema)

- Lubiprostone (Amitiza): a selective chloride channel activator; 24 μg PO BID
- Guanylate cyclase-C agonists (adult use only)
  – Linaclotide (Linzess): dose: 145 μg PO once daily; can use lower dose 72 μg once daily
  – Plecanatide (Trulance): dose: 3 mg PO once daily
- Peripherally acting μ-opioid receptor antagonists, indicated for OIC. Try laxatives first; lubiprostone also approved for OIC
  – Methylnaltrexone (Relistor): dose: 38 to <62 kg: 8 mg; 62 to 114 kg: 12 mg SC every other day PRN
  – Naloxegol (Movantik): dose: 12.5 to 25.0 mg PO daily; discontinue other laxatives for 3 days when initiating naloxegol; avoid in patients on strong CYP3A4 inhibitors due to increased naloxegol levels and risk of opioid withdrawal.
  – Naldemedine (Symproic): dose: 0.2 mg PO daily; monitor for opioid withdrawal in patients on strong CYP3A4 inhibitors or P-gp inhibitors.
- Prokinetic agents (partial 5-HT4 agonists) have been withdrawn due to cardiac side effects; only available in IND protocols: tegaserod (Zelnorm), cisapride (Propulsid)
- Other agents not approved by the FDA:
  – Misoprostol (Cytotec): a prostaglandin that increases colonic motility
  – Colchicine: neurogenic stimulation to increase colonic motility

ADDITIONAL THERAPIES
- Other nonpharmacologic therapies include biofeedback, a first-line recommendation for patients with refractory constipation due to functional conditions involving dyssynergic defecation or inadequate propulsive force.
- Behavior therapy
- Acupuncture: initial randomized trial effective at 20 weeks; longer term trials needed (4)[B]

SURGERY/OTHER PROCEDURES
Surgery rarely indicated; sometimes required for anatomic findings (rectocele or enterocoele)

ADMISSION, INPATIENT, AND NURSING CONSIDERATIONS
- Toxic megacolon
- Manual disimpaction occasionally required in chronic refractory cases

 ONGOING CARE

FOLLOW-UP RECOMMENDATIONS
Encourage exercise and physical activity.

Patient Monitoring
If functional constipation persists, revisit secondary causes.

DIET
Increase soluble fiber (bloating and gas can be problematic with insoluble fiber):
- Gradually increase intake to 25 g/day over a 6-week period.
- Oat bran (hard outer layer of cereal grains)
- Peas; onions; lentils; beans; seeds; nuts; and fruits, including bananas, apples, and strawberries
- Encourage liberal intake of fluids.

PATIENT EDUCATION
- Occasional mild constipation is normal.
- Bowel training: The best time to move bowels is in the morning, after eating breakfast, when the normal bowel transit and defecation reflexes are functioning.

PROGNOSIS
- Occasional constipation responds well to simple measures.
- Habitual constipation can be a lifelong nuisance.
- Patients with neurologic compromise can suffer from obstipation, impaction, and toxic megacolon.
- No evidence for laxative dependence or harm from stimulant use; melanosis coli may develop but is a benign condition.

COMPLICATIONS
- Volvulus
- Toxic megacolon
- Acquired megacolon in severe, long-standing cases
- Fluid and electrolyte depletion: laxative abuse
- Rectal ulceration (stercoral ulcer) related to recurrent fecal impaction
- Anal fissures

REFERENCES
1. Ori Y, Rozen-Zvi B, Chagnac A, et al. Fatalities and severe metabolic disorders associated with the use of sodium phosphate enemas: a single center's experience. *Arch Intern Med*. 2012;172(3): 263–265.
2. Lewis SJ, Heaton KW. Stool form scale as a useful guide to intestinal transit time. *Scand J Gastroenterol*. 1997;32(9):920–924.
3. Lee-Robichaud H, Thomas K, Morgan J, et al. Lactulose versus polyethylene glycol for chronic constipation. *Cochrane Database Syst Rev*. 2010;(7):CD007570.
4. Liu Z, Yan S, Wu J, et al. Acupuncture for chronic severe functional constipation: a randomized trial. *Ann Intern Med*. 2016;165(11):761–769.

ADDITIONAL READING
- Ford AC, Moayyedi P, Lacy BE, et al. American College of Gastroenterology monograph on the management of irritable bowel syndrome and chronic idiopathic constipation. *Am J Gastroenterol*. 2014;109(Suppl 1):S2–S26.
- Shah BJ, Rughwani N, Rose S. In the clinic. Constipation. *Ann Intern Med*. 2015;162(7):ITC1.

 CODES

ICD10
- K59.00 Constipation, unspecified
- K59.01 Slow transit constipation
- K59.09 Other constipation

CLINICAL PEARLS
- Constipation (especially with normal transit time) is common. Reversible risk factors include inadequate hydration, sedentary lifestyle, poor dietary habits, and medication side effects.
- Red flags: onset >50 years, hematochezia/melena, unintentional weight loss, anemia, neurologic defects
- Osmotic agents (PEG) are most clinically effective.

C

CONTRACEPTION

Gena M. Grospe, DO • Roxanne Smith, MD, MPH

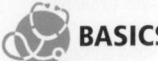 **BASICS**

DESCRIPTION
- Medications or procedures that control timing of pregnancies and prevent unintended pregnancies
- Contraception options are divided into two major categories: hormonal and nonhormonal.
- The most effective methods of contraception are vasectomy, female sterilization, and the long-acting reversible contraceptives (LARCs).

EPIDEMIOLOGY
Incidence
- The estimated prevalence of contraception use among women age 15 to 44 years is 61% in the United States (1).
- 49% of all pregnancies in the United States are unintended, and half of these occur in women using a form of reversible contraception.
- 43% of all unintended pregnancies in the United States result in termination.
- The most commonly used methods were the pill (16.0%), female sterilization (15.5%), condoms (9.4%), and LARCs (7.2%).

RISK FACTORS
Unintended pregnancy: higher rates among women ages 18 to 24 and >40 years, unmarried/cohabitating women, women with less than a college education, and minority women

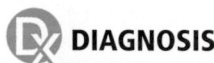 **DIAGNOSIS**

HISTORY
- Review past medical, family, social, obstetric, and gynecologic histories including menstrual history, prior experience with contraceptives, and prior sexually transmitted diseases (STDs).
- Screen for hypertension.
- In family history of thrombophilia, testing can be considered before initiation of estrogen-containing contraception, especially if specific defect is known.
- Contraindications: See CDC medical eligibility criteria (MEC) (2).
  - Estrogen-progestin contraceptives
    - Absolute: age ≥35 years and smoking ≥15 cigarettes per day, <21 days postpartum, SBP ≥160 mm Hg or DBP ≥100 mm Hg, multiple CAD risk factors, current/prior venous thromboembolism (VTE), thrombophilia, long-standing/complicated diabetes, ischemic heart disease, stroke, complicated valvular disease, systemic lupus, migraine with aura, breast cancer, severe cirrhosis, solid organ transplant, hepatocellular adenoma, or malignant hepatoma
    - Relative: age ≥35 years and smoking <15 cigarettes per day, breastfeeding <42 days postpartum, SBP 140 to 159 mm Hg or DBP 90 to 99 mm Hg (or well-controlled on medications), symptomatic cholelithiasis, certain anticonvulsants, bariatric surgery, migraines without aura but ≥35 years, or breast cancer history in remission >5 years
  - Progestin-only (pill/Depo/implant)
    - Absolute: current breast cancer
    - Relative: bariatric surgery, ischemic heart disease, history of stroke, lupus, migraine with aura, severe cirrhosis, certain anticonvulsants, hepatocellular adenoma, or malignant hepatoma

- Levonorgestrel—intrauterine device (IUD)
  - Absolute: immediate postseptic abortion, postpartum sepsis, gestational trophoblastic disease, current breast cancer, distorted uterine cavity. The following are absolute contraindications for initiation but not continuation of method: cervical/endometrial cancer, unexplained vaginal bleeding, current pelvic inflammatory disease (PID), purulent cervicitis, gonorrhea/chlamydia infection, pelvic tuberculosis (TB).
  - Relative: ischemic heart disease, lupus, severe cirrhosis, hepatocellular adenoma or malignant hepatoma, increased risk of STDs, solid organ transplant
- IUD–copper ("ParaGard")
  - Absolute: same as levonorgestrel-IUD except use in cancer of breast, possibly cervix OK
  - Relative: severe thrombocytopenia, increased risk of STDs, solid organ transplant

DIAGNOSTIC TESTS & INTERPRETATION
- A negative pregnancy test (urine or serum) is advised prior to initiating contraception.
- Consider testing for gonorrhea and chlamydia prior to IUD insertion especially if age <25 years or multiple sexual partners. Testing can be done at time of insertion if symptomatic infection is ruled out.
- Perform Pap smear if otherwise indicated.

 TREATMENT

GENERAL MEASURES
- Method(s) should be selected based on patient preference, effectiveness, need for STD prevention, side effects, and contraindications.
- General categories included hormonal and nonhormonal methods.
  - Nonhormonal methods include condoms, diaphragm, cervical cap, copper IUD, vasectomy, female sterilization, fertility awareness, sponge, spermicides, and abstinence.
  - Hormonal methods include oral contraceptives, patch, ring, injectables, IUDs, and implants.

MEDICATION
- Estrogen-progestin contraceptives
  - Mechanism of action: suppression of ovulation, thickening cervical mucus, and endometrial changes that interfere with transport of sperm to egg and with implantation
  - Efficacy: failure rate of about 9% with typical use and 0.3% with perfect use at 1 year (3)
  - Side effects: nausea, bloating, headaches, mastalgia, depression, acne, and hirsutism
  - Side effect management: Breakthrough bleeding is usually self-limiting after 3 months; if persists, change pill. Amenorrhea: Rule out pregnancy.
  - Combined oral contraceptives (COCs): pill
    - All COCs contain the same type of estrogen (ethinyl estradiol) but differ in the amount of estrogen (range of 10 to 50 μg) and the type of progestin.
    - VTE risk is highest with those containing 50 μg estrogen. Newer 3rd-generation progestins (norgestimate and desogestrel) are less androgenic but have increased rate of VTE (4).
    - Start with a pill that contains an average amount of estrogen (30 to 35 μg).
    - Dosing: Most pills have a 21/7 regimen (21 active days and 7 placebo); alternatively, can take active pills continuously with four yearly scheduled withdrawal bleeds

  - Initiation: recommended: quick start (begin pill on the day medication is obtained)
  - Alternative: 1st day start (begin the pill on the 1st day of menses) or Sunday start (begin pill on first Sunday). If OCs are prescribed with Sunday or 1st-day-of-menses start, as many as 25% of women do not start.
- Weekly hormonal patch (Ortho Evra, Xulane):
  - Releases 20 μg/day ethinyl estradiol and 150 μg/day norelgestromin
  - Applied transdermally and changed weekly
  - Produces higher serum estrogen levels than oral 20-μg pill and may be associated with a slightly increased risk of blood clot
  - Patch may cause local skin irritation; reduced efficacy in women >90 kg
- Vaginal contraceptive ring (NuvaRing):
  - Flexible polymer ring with 15 μg/day of ethinyl estradiol and 120 μg/day of etonogestrel absorbed via vaginal wall
  - Insert into vagina for 3 weeks/cycle or use continuous cycling for 4 weeks, then replace immediately with a new ring (off-label).
  - Although systemic exposure to estrogen is about 50% of exposure with COCs, the risk of blood clots is about the same.
- Progestin-only birth control
  - Mechanism of action: thickening cervical mucus and thinning endometrial lining
  - Progestin-only pill (Micronor)
    - Efficacy: failure rate of about 0.3% with perfect use, 9% with typical use at 1 year (3)
    - Can be used in women with contraindication to estrogen, including breastfeeding women after 6 weeks postpartum
    - Dosing: 1 pill at the same time daily, no placebo days
    - Side effects: irregular bleeding
  - Injectable contraceptive (medroxyprogesterone acetate) "Depo-Provera"
    - Efficacy: failure rate of 0.2% with perfect use, 6% with typical use at 1 year (3)
    - Dosing: 150 mg IM or Depo-SubQ Provera 104 mg SC, both are given every 3 months. Contraceptive levels of hormone persist for up to 4 months (2- to 4-week margin of safety).
    - Side effects include irregular bleeding, weight gain (average of 5 lb/year of use), and amenorrhea.
- LARCs: IUDs and implantable devices
  - Mirena (52-mg levonorgestrel-releasing IUD):
    - Mechanism of action: sterile inflammatory reaction due to foreign body that is toxic to sperm and ova, thickens cervical mucus, endometrial decidualization and glandular atrophy, inhibiting sperm-egg binding, partial inhibition of ovarian follicular development, and ovulation
    - Efficacy: failure rate of 0.2% with both perfect and typical use at 1 year (3)
    - Dosing: releases 20 μg/day (very low serum levels) initially and subsequently reduces to 10 μg/day
    - Approved for use up to 5 years; has been used off-label for up to 7 years
    - Safe in nulliparous women/teenagers
    - Can be inserted immediately postpartum or immediately following dilation and curettage for miscarriage or abortion; these are associated with higher rates of expulsion compared to delayed placement (6 to 10 weeks).
    - Side effects: irregular menstrual spotting for the first 3 to 6 months that usually resolves after 6 months of use; may see absence of menses after 1 year

○ Side effect management: Consider NSAIDs, COCs, or progestin-only pills for spotting and cramps.
○ Can reduce heavy bleeding in menorrhagia
- Liletta (52-mg levonorgestrel-releasing IUD):
  ○ Releases 18.6 μg/day initially; approved for 3 years, at which time it releases 12.6 μg/day
- Kyleena (19.5-mg levonorgestrel-releasing IUD):
  ○ Releases 17.5 μg/day for the 1st year, down to 7.5 μg/day. Approved for 5 years. Smaller insertion tube with 3.8 mm diameter offers potential for easier insertion in nulliparous women.
- Skyla (13.5-mg levonorgestrel-releasing IUD):
  ○ Releases 14 μg/day initially, down to 5 μg/day. Approved for 3 years. Smaller insertion tube (3.8 mm diameter); more bleeding days than Mirena
- ParaGard (copper IUD):
  ○ Mechanism of action: In addition to sterile inflammatory reaction due to foreign body, free copper and copper salts enhance the cytotoxic inflammatory reaction—toxic to sperm and ova.
  ○ Efficacy: failure rate of 0.6% with perfect use, 0.8% with typical use at 1 year (3)
  ○ Approved for up to 10 years
  ○ Same insertion timing as levonorgestrel-IUD
  ○ Side effects: increased menstrual bleeding and cramping
- Nexplanon (etonogestrel implant):
  ○ Mechanism of action: thickening cervical mucus and thinning endometrial lining
  ○ Efficacy: failure rate of 0.05% with perfect use, 0.3% with typical use at 1 year
  ○ Dosing: 40 mm × 2 mm semirigid plastic rod containing 68 mg of etonogestrel; initially releases 60 to 70 μg/day, down to 25 to 30 μg/day at the end of the 3rd year
  ○ Effective for up to 3 years
  ○ Inserted only by certified providers
  ○ Side effects: menstrual irregularities (common in first 6 to 12 months, may persist for 3 years)
- Emergency contraception: should be initiated as soon as possible post-unprotected intercourse. Copper IUD is the most effective, followed by ulipristal, levonorgestrel, and Yuzpe method (least effective) (5)[A].
  - Copper-bearing IUD (ParaGard): Insert up to 5 days after intercourse; failure rate of 0.04–0.19%
  - Ulipristal acetate (Ella): 30 mg once; selective progesterone modulator, effective up to 5 days after unprotected intercourse with minimal decline in efficacy; about 2% failure rate
  - Levonorgestrel: 1.5 mg taken as two 0.75-mg tablets (Plan B) or one 1.5-mg tablet (Plan B One-Step). Failure rate: 1.1–2.4%. Less nausea than "Yuzpe regimen." Available over the counter; may be less expensive if prescribed. Most effective within 72 hours, efficacy declines with time. Likely ineffective for women with BMI >30. Estradiol/levonorgestrel (Preven, Lo Ovral, Ogestrel): "Yuzpe regimen" 50 μg/0.25 mg, 2 tablets q12h (4 tablets total). Any OC may be used as long as the dose of estrogen component ≥100 μg/dose. Failure rate: 3.2%. *Note:* Antiemetic should be given 1 to 2 hours before each dose.

ADDITIONAL THERAPIES
- Male condoms: failure rate of 2% with perfect use, 18% with typical use at 1 year (3)
- Spermicides: All contain nonoxynol-9; may alter vaginal flora and mucosal barrier. Failure rate: 28% with typical use at 1 year (3)
- Sponge (Today Sponge): Soft foam disk contains nonoxynol-9. Moisten with water before use; effective for 24 hours; must leave in for 6 hours after use; less effective in parous women. Failure rate: 12–24% with typical use (3)

- Diaphragm: latex or silicone dome-shaped device with flexible spring-activated rim, works by preventing sperm from entering cervix; used with spermicides. Failure rate: 12% with typical use, 6% with perfect use at 1 year (3)

SURGERY/OTHER PROCEDURES
Permanent sterilization
- Female: tubal ligation. Failure rate: 0.5% at 1 year (3)
- Male: vasectomy. Less complicated than female. Failure rate: 0.15% at 1 year (3)

COMPLEMENTARY & ALTERNATIVE MEDICINE
- Fertility awareness methods: calendar method, cervical mucus method, temperature method. Low cost but generally not as effective as other methods. Failure rate: 24% at 1 year with typical use (3)
- Withdrawal method: Male withdraws from vagina before ejaculation. Failure if not timed accurately. Failure rate: 22% at 1 year with typical use (3)
- Lactational amenorrhea method: Breastfeeding is effective contraception only if the infant is <6 months old, the infant is exclusively breast-feeding, and the mother has not resumed regular menses. Failure rate: 7% at 1 year with typical use

Pediatric Considerations
- AAP and ACOG recommend LARCs as first-line agents for use in sexually active adolescents.
- Contraception counseling should include anticipated adverse effects, need to use condoms for STD prevention, and indications for emergency contraception (including options and how to obtain).

 ONGOING CARE

FOLLOW-UP RECOMMENDATIONS
Patient Monitoring
- Pelvic exam, Pap smear, and STI testing per guidelines and routine follow-up 2 to 3 months postinitiation of all methods to assess tolerance
- Check for IUD strings 1 month after insertion; spontaneous expulsion rate highest in the 1st month
- BP check within 3 months of initiation in patients on estrogen-containing methods

DIET
St. John's wort may alter estrogen levels, reducing efficacy or causing breakthrough bleeding.

PATIENT EDUCATION
- Diaphragm: device inspected prior to each use, 1 tablespoon of spermicide in hollow of the dome, diaphragm is inserted into the vagina. If placed >6 hours prior to intercourse, need additional applicator of spermicide. Position must be checked postintercourse, and additional spermicide applied prior to each new episode of intercourse. Diaphragm should remain in place for at least 6 hours after the last episode of intercourse to maximize effectiveness.
- Male condoms: New condom is placed on the penis before genital contact, remains intact until the penis is withdrawn; new condom with every act of intercourse
- IUD: Patient should monitor presence of the string monthly following menses.
- OCP: Pill should be taken at the same time each day. Backup birth control method is needed for the first 7 days with quick start and Sunday start methods.

COMPLICATIONS
- Estrogen-progestin contraceptives:
  - Serious (requires discontinuation): stroke, thromboembolism, hypertension, myocardial infarction, and cholestatic jaundice
  - Overall 4-fold increased risk of VTE compared to nonusers, comparable to the 4-fold increased risk during pregnancy, but absolute risk is low (4)
- Injectable contraceptive:
  - Potential for decreased bone mineral density (BMD) if used for ≥2 years. Mostly recovers after discontinuation. Consider calcium/vitamin D supplementation if prolonged use.
- Nexplanon: insertion site reaction including pain, bleeding, paresthesias, and infection
- IUDs:
  - PID: Treat without removal unless serious infection or failure to respond to therapy.
  - Uterine perforation
  - Absolute risk of ectopic pregnancy is reduced with IUD, but if pregnancy does occur, there is a higher risk that it will be ectopic.
- Sponge and diaphragm: rarely associated with toxic shock syndrome

REFERENCES
1. Daniels K, Daugherty J, Jones J. *Current Contraceptive Status among Women Aged 15–44: United States, 2011–2013.* Hyattsville, MD: National Center for Health Statistics; 2014. NCHS Data Brief, No. 173.
2. Centers for Disease Control and Prevention. US Medical Eligibility Criteria (US MEC) for Contraceptive Use, 2016. https://www.cdc.gov/reproductive health/contraception/mmwr/mec/summary.html. Accessed September 23, 2018.
3. Trussell J. Contraceptive failure in the United States. *Contraception.* 2011;83(5):397–404.
4. de Bastos M, Stegeman BH, Rosendaal FR, et al. Combined oral contraceptives: venous thrombosis. *Cochrane Database Syst Rev.* 2014;(3):CD010813.
5. American College of Obstetricians and Gynecologists. Practice Bulletin No. 152: emergency contraception. *Obstet Gynecol.* 2015;126(3):e1–e11.

ADDITIONAL READING
"CDC Contraception" Available as chart and app for smartphone

 CODES

ICD10
- Z30.9 Encounter for contraceptive management, unspecified
- Z30.41 Encounter for surveillance of contraceptive pills
- Z30.431 Encounter for routine checking of intrauterine contracep dev

CLINICAL PEARLS
- Hormonal and IUD contraceptives may be initiated immediately if the likelihood of preexisting pregnancy is low.
- LARC methods provide high efficacy and convenience for patients.
- All patients should be counseled on emergency contraception options.

COR PULMONALE

Marissa A. Lombardo, MD • Parag Goyal, MD, MSc

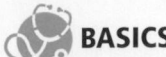 **BASICS**

DESCRIPTION

- The term "cor pulmonale" derives from the Latin *cor* (heart) and *pulmonale* (lungs). Hence, cor pulmonale is a cardiac complication of primary pulmonary disease.
- Acute or chronic pulmonary processes can lead to increased right-sided cardiac pressures. Resultant pulmonary hypertension (PH) subsequently induces structural alterations and/or impairs right ventricle (RV) function.
- PH is defined by a mean pulmonary artery pressure (mPAP) ≥25 mm Hg at rest measured by right heart catheterization.
- PH may be secondary to abnormalities of the pulmonary system, including disorders of the lung parenchyma, pulmonary circulation, chest wall, and/or ventilatory mechanisms. The pathophysiologic mechanisms of pulmonary arterial hypertension (WHO Group I) and PH secondary to pulmonary processes are biologically and clinically distinct. Therefore, for the purposes of this review, pulmonary arterial hypertension (WHO Group I) will not be considered as a cause of cor pulmonale.
- Cor pulmonale may occur in acute or chronic setting.
  - Acute: rapid increase of pulmonary arterial pressure resulting in RV overload, dysfunction, and potential cardiovascular collapse
  - Chronic: progressive hypertrophy and dilation of the RV over months to years, leading to dysfunction and potential failure

EPIDEMIOLOGY

- ~6–7% of all types of adult heart disease in United States. Globally, the incidence of cor pulmonale is widely variable due to air pollution, tobacco use, and toxic exposure.
- An estimated 10–30% of heart failure admissions in the United States are the result of cor pulmonale, most commonly related to chronic obstructive pulmonary disease (COPD).

Incidence

Difficult to assess: Best estimate is 1/10,000 to 3/10,000 per year.

Prevalence

Difficult to assess: Best estimate is 2/1,000 to 6/1,000.

ETIOLOGY AND PATHOPHYSIOLOGY

- Acute: A sudden event, such as large pulmonary embolism (PE), increases resistance to blood flow in the pulmonary vasculature, causing a quick and significant increase of pressure proximal to the right ventricular outflow tract. The RV may not be able to generate adequate force to overcome this pressure, leading to low RV cardiac output, which ultimately leads to a decreased left ventricle (LV) cardiac output. Increased RV pressures in conjunction with a low cardiac output may cause coronary ischemia, further impairing cardiac output and potentially causing complete cardiovascular collapse.
- Chronic: a disorder of the pulmonary system leading to chronic hypoxia, which results in progressive vasoconstriction of the pulmonary vasculature. Over time, the pulmonary arterial system hypertrophies and intrinsic vasoactive mechanisms (mediated by nitric oxide, cyclooxygenase, and endothelin) become dysregulated, leading to an increase in pulmonary vasculature resistance.

- Increased pulmonary vascular resistance yields PH. PH transmits increased pressures and volumes to the thin-walled, low-pressure RV causing maladaptive remodeling (concentric hypertrophy, followed by eccentric dilation), which is frequently associated with tricuspid regurgitation and subsequent impairment in RV systolic and diastolic function.
- Indicators for the presence of PH in these patients may include a disproportionally low diffusing capacity of the lungs for carbon monoxide (DLCO) and an elevated pCO_2.
- Pulmonary disorders
  - Lung parenchymal disease: COPD (most common), interstitial lung disease (ILD), and pulmonary fibrosis
  - Pulmonary circulation: thromboembolic disease (associated with WHO Group IV PH)
  - Chest wall: severe obesity, kyphoscoliosis
  - Ventilation: obstructive sleep apnea (OSA) and obesity hypoventilatory syndrome; neuromuscular diseases such as Guillain-Barré syndrome, muscular dystrophy, myasthenia gravis, spinal cord injuries
- Left ventricular failure is not considered a cause of cor pulmonale.

RISK FACTORS

- Acute cor pulmonale (most commonly caused by PE)
- Chronic cor pulmonale (most commonly caused by underlying pulmonary disorder)
  - Risk factors associated with pulmonary disorders
    - Tobacco use (COPD)
    - Occupational exposures (ILD)
    - Hypercoagulable state (chronic thromboembolic disease)
    - Obesity, age (chest wall/ventilatory abnormalities)

GENERAL PREVENTION

Management of underlying pulmonary disorders, including aggressive correction of hypoxia and acidosis, which may contribute to worsening PH

COMMONLY ASSOCIATED CONDITIONS

PH, defined as the presence of a resting mPAP >25 mm Hg

DIAGNOSIS

HISTORY

- Dyspnea is the most common symptom. Although nonspecific, dyspnea may be present at rest, with exertion, or manifests as paroxysmal nocturnal dyspnea.
- Other pulmonary symptoms: pleuritic chest pain, cough, hemoptysis
- General heart failure symptoms: fatigue, lethargy, syncope; exertional angina less likely
- Right-sided heart failure symptoms: anorexia, early satiety, digital cyanosis, clubbing, right upper quadrant discomfort (hepatic congestion), lower extremity edema
- Hoarseness secondary to compression of the left recurrent laryngeal nerve by enlarged pulmonary vessels
- Cardiovascular collapse, shock, and/or cardiac arrest may occur in acute or advanced chronic setting.

PHYSICAL EXAM

- Peripheral edema is the most common sign of right-sided heart failure, although it is nonspecific.
- General: pallor, diaphoresis, clubbing, cyanosis, tachypnea

- Neck: jugular venous distention, with prominent *a*-wave
- Lungs: tachypnea, wheezing
- Heart
  - Increased intensity of pulmonic component of second heart sound (P_2)
  - Splitting of S_2 over the cardiac apex with inspiration
  - Audible right-sided S_3 or S_4
  - RV heave
  - Pansystolic murmur heard best at right midsternal border increasing with inspiration, consistent with tricuspid regurgitation (typically a late sign)
- Abdomen: hepatomegaly
- Extremities: clubbing, cyanosis, bilateral lower extremity edema, may also signs of deep vein thrombosis (DVT) such as tenderness or unilateral swelling

DIFFERENTIAL DIAGNOSIS

Other causes of right-sided failure:

- Left-sided heart failure
- WHO Groups I, II, and V PH
- Right-sided intrinsic cardiomyopathy

DIAGNOSTIC TESTS & INTERPRETATION

- 2D echocardiogram (1)[C]
  - Initial diagnostic test of choice
  - Elevated pulmonary arterial pressures
  - Right ventricular hypertrophy
  - Bulging of the interventricular septum into the LV with systole
  - Flattening of the interventricular or interatrial septum
  - Dilation and hypokinesis of the RV
  - Tricuspid regurgitation
  - Dilation of the right atrium
  - Acute thromboembolic pulmonary disease as evidenced by right ventricular hypokinesis with sparing of the apex (McConnell sign)
  - Echocardiography can over- or underestimate the pulmonary arterial pressures depending on image quality or operator. Pulmonary arterial pressures should therefore be verified by right heart catheterization.
- MRI
  - If echocardiography is inconclusive or as a substitute
  - Most accurate modality for diagnosing emphysema and ILD
  - Can assess cardiac pressures, size, function, myocardial mass, and viability
- Right heart catheterization (1)[C]
  - Gold standard for diagnosis of PH and therefore critical for diagnosis of cor pulmonale
  - Elevated central venous pressure (CVP)
  - Mean PAP ≥25 mm Hg at rest

Initial Tests (lab, imaging)

- CBC may show signs of polycythemia due to chronic hypoxia.
- Basic metabolic panel (BMP) may demonstrate elevated creatinine secondary to poor cardiac output.
- Liver function tests (LFTs) may be abnormal due to proximal hepatic congestion or poor distal cardiac output secondary to RV failure.
- Brain natriuretic peptide (BNP) and cardiac troponin can be elevated secondary to right ventricular strain.
- D-dimer may be positive as evidence of underlying thromboembolic pulmonary disease.
- Arterial blood gas may show hypercapnia due to COPD or hypoxemia due to ILD.

- Arterial blood gases of COPD patients show a decreased PaO_2 with normal or increased $PaCO_2$.
- ECG often shows signs of right-sided enlargement.
  - Right axis deviation
  - An R/S wave ratio >1 in V_1
  - Right ventricular hypertrophy (R wave in V_1 and V_2 with S waves in V_5 and V_6)
  - Right atrial enlargement as evidenced by P pulmonale (increased amplitude of P wave in leads II, III, and avF with a "tent-like" appearance)
  - Incomplete or complete right bundle branch block
  - $S_1S_2S_3$ pattern or $S_1Q_3T_3$ inverted pattern
- Chest x-ray
  - Cardiomegaly
  - Enlargement of the central pulmonary arteries and reduced size of peripheral vessels (oligemia)
  - Reduced retrosternal space due to right ventricular enlargement on lateral views
  - Enlargement of the right atrium resulting in prominence of the right heart border
  - Evidence of COPD, ILD, and structural disease (i.e., kyphosis)
  - Evidence of PE (Westermark sign, Fleischner sign, and Hampton hump)
- Spiral computed tomography (CT) scan of chest
  - Diagnosis of acute PE
  - Diagnosis of COPD and ILD
- Ventilation/perfusion (V/Q) scan
  - High specificity and sensitivity for acute and chronic thromboembolic disease
  - Screening method of choice for chronic thromboembolic PH because of its higher sensitivity compared with CT pulmonary angiogram
  - May be used for diagnosis of acute thromboembolic disease if contraindication to chest spiral CT
  - Diagnosis of chronic thromboembolic disease (WHO Group IV PH) may warrant confirmation by pulmonary angiography.
- Pulmonary angiography
  - Gold standard in diagnosis of chronic thromboembolic pulmonary disease
- Polysomnography
  - Gold standard for diagnosis of OSA
- Pulmonary function tests (PFTs)
  - DLCO: A decrease in lung volume combined with decreased diffusion capacity for carbon monoxide may indicate ILD. COPD is associated with a decreased DLCO.
  - Obstructive or restrictive ventilatory defects (ILD, chest wall abnormalities, and COPD)

TREATMENT

Reduce symptoms, improve quality of life, and increase survival. Reduce disease burden via oxygenation, preservation of cardiac function, and attenuation of PH.

GENERAL MEASURES
- Treat underlying disease (2)[A].
  - For underlying pulmonary disease, long-acting bronchodilators, long-acting antimuscarinic agents, and/or inhaled corticosteroids may be beneficial for long-term disease management.
  - For underlying chronic thromboembolic disease, anticoagulation may be indicated.

- Supportive therapy as necessary
  - Continuous positive airway pressure/bilevel positive airway pressure may be used for hypoxia/sleep disorders.
  - Ventilation using positive-pressure masks, negative-pressure body suits, or mechanical ventilation is suggested for patients with neuromuscular disease.
  - Phlebotomy may be indicated for severe polycythemia or signs and symptoms of hyperviscosity (hematocrit >55%).

MEDICATION
- Oxygen (3)[A]
  - Long-term continuous oxygen therapy improves the survival of hypoxemic patients with COPD and cor pulmonale.
  - All patients with PH whose PaO_2 is consistently <55 mm Hg or saturation ≤88% at rest, during sleep, or with ambulation should be prescribed oxygen to keep O_2 >92 mm Hg.
  - Exposure to high altitude should be avoided. Supplemental oxygen should be used during altitude exposure or air travel as needed to maintain oxygen saturations >91%.
- Preservation of cardiac function (4)[B]
  - Inotropes: Dobutamine and milrinone may improve cardiac output.
  - Diuretics: decrease RV filling pressures and reduce peripheral edema secondary to RHF
    - Excessive volume depletion should be avoided.
    - Monitor closely for metabolic alkalosis because this may suppress ventilatory drive and contribute to hypoxia.
- Ameliorate PH (1,4)[C].
  - Treatment of underlying disease is hallmark of management.
  - When refractory to traditional medical treatment, advanced therapies may be beneficial, although evidence is lacking.
  - For chronic thromboembolic–associated PH (WHO Group IV), riociguat and macitentan may be used.

ISSUES FOR REFERRAL
Patients with cor pulmonale should be referred to a specialized center for expert consultation.

SURGERY/OTHER PROCEDURES
- Endarterectomy for chronic thromboembolic disease (WHO Group IV)
- Lung volume reduction surgery (LVRS) is a surgical option that may be beneficial for patients with advanced upper-lobe predominant emphysema who have poor disease control despite maximal medical therapy (5).
- Moderate to severe disease refractory to medication may require lung and/or heart transplantation.

 ONGOING CARE

DIET
Salt and fluid restriction

PATIENT EDUCATION
- Smoking cessation and avoidance of exposure to secondary smoke is strongly recommended.
- Level of physical activity should be discussed with physician.
- Pregnancy should be avoided.

PROGNOSIS
Patients with cor pulmonale resulting from COPD have a greater likelihood of dying than do similar patients with COPD alone. In patients with COPD and mild disease (PAP 20 to 35 mm Hg), 5-year survival is 50%.

REFERENCES
1. Seeger W, Adir Y, Barberà JA, et al. Pulmonary hypertension in chronic lung diseases. *J Am Coll Cardiol.* 2013;62(Suppl 25):D109–D116.
2. Simonneau G, Gatzoulis MA, Adatia I, et al. Updated clinical classification of pulmonary hypertension. *J Am Coll Cardiol.* 2013;62(Suppl 25):D34–D41.
3. Galiè N, Humbert M, Vachiery JL, et al. 2015 ESC/ERS guidelines for the diagnosis and treatment of pulmonary hypertension: The Joint Task Force for the Diagnosis and Treatment of Pulmonary Hypertension of the European Society of Cardiology (ESC) and the European Respiratory Society (ERS): endorsed by: Association for European Paediatric and Congenital Cardiology (AEPC), International Society for Heart and Lung Transplantation (ISHLT). *Eur Heart J.* 2016;37(1):67–119.
4. Taichman DB, Ornelas J, Chung L, et al. Pharmacologic therapy for pulmonary arterial hypertension in adults: CHEST guideline and expert panel report. *Chest.* 2014;146(2):449–475.
5. DeCamp M, Lipson D, Krasna M, et al. The evaluation and preparation of the patient for lung volume reduction surgery. *Proc Am Thorac Soc.* 2008;5(4):427–431.

 SEE ALSO

- Chronic Obstructive Pulmonary Disease and Emphysema; Pulmonary Arterial Hypertension; Pulmonary Embolism
- Algorithm: Congestive Heart Failure: Differential Diagnosis

 CODES

ICD10
- I27.81 Cor pulmonale (chronic)
- I26.09 Other pulmonary embolism with acute cor pulmonale

CLINICAL PEARLS
- Treatment of cor pulmonale requires treatment of the underlying disease. Therefore, accurate diagnosis of primary pulmonary disease is critical to clinical management and treatment therapy.
- Continuous, long-term oxygen therapy improves life expectancy and quality of life in cor pulmonale.
- Referral of patients with cor pulmonale to a specialized center is strongly recommended.

CORNEAL ABRASION AND ULCERATION

Sophia Margareth Marie Tribie, MD • Christine S. Persaud, MD, CAQSM

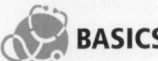

BASICS

DESCRIPTION
- Corneal abrasions: result from cutting, scratching, or abrading the thin, protective, clear coat of the exposed anterior portion of the ocular epithelium. These injuries cause pain, tearing, photophobia, foreign body sensation, and a gritty feeling (1).
- Corneal ulceration: break in the epithelial layer of the cornea leading to exposure of the underlying corneal stroma, which results in a corneal ulcer. Superficial ulcers, limited to loss of the corneal epithelium, are the most common form of ulceration (2).
- Corneal abrasion and ulceration can both lead to impaired vision from scarring.

EPIDEMIOLOGY

Incidence
- Corneal abrasions are commonly seen in primary care. Eye-related diagnoses make up 8% of total ER visits. Of those eye-related visits, 45% are corneal abrasions. Abrasions are the third leading cause of red eye, following conjunctivitis and subconjunctival hemorrhage (3).
- Associated with significant morbidity and loss of productivity

ETIOLOGY AND PATHOPHYSIOLOGY
- Corneal abrasions are most often caused by mechanical trauma but may also result from foreign bodies: sand and dust, contact lenses wear, or chemical and flash burns.
- Corneal ulceration: Contact lenses use, HIV, trauma, ocular surface disease, and ocular surgery increase the incidence. Edema plays a major role in epithelial defect. Edema can lead to trauma, ischemia, and increased intraocular pressure. Excessive fluid disrupts the normal architecture of the epithelial layer (4).
- Causes of ulcerations include the following:
  - Infection with gram-positive organisms ~29–53% (*Staphylococcus aureus* and coagulase-negative *Streptococcus* are common ones.)
  - Infection with gram-negative organisms ~47–50% (*Pseudomonas* being most common, followed by *Serratia marcescens*, *Proteus mirabilis*, and gram-negative enteric bacilli)
  - Herpes simplex with bacterial superinfection
  - Varicella virus

- Corneal abrasion and eye surgery (cataract, eye transplant)
  - Autoimmune disorder: Sjögren, rheumatoid arthritis, inflammatory bowel disease
- Increased risk of corneal ulceration in HIV and diabetes mellitus (DM) patients and immunocompromised such as cancer
- Eyelid abnormalities (chronic blepharitis, entropion)
- Nutritional deficiencies (vitamin A and protein undernutrition)
- Dry eyes/bullous keratopathy/mucous membrane pemphigoid

RISK FACTORS
- History of trauma (direct blunt trauma, chemical burn, radiation exposure, etc.)
- Contact lenses wear
- Male gender
- Age: 20 to 34 years old
- Job (construction, manufacturing)
- Lack of eye protection

GENERAL PREVENTION
Protective eyewear during work (auto mechanics, metal workers, miners, etc.) and during sports

COMMONLY ASSOCIATED CONDITIONS
- Vitamin A deficiency is associated with corneal ulcers.
- Neuropathy of cranial nerve (CN) V
- DM, thyroid dysfunction, immunocompromised states, connective tissue disease

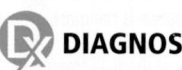

DIAGNOSIS

HISTORY
Corneal abrasion is a clinical diagnosis. It includes a history of recent ocular trauma and acute pain. Other symptoms include photophobia, pain with extraocular muscle movement, eye twitching, excessive tearing, blepharospasm, foreign body sensation, gritty feeling, blurred or decreased vision, nausea, and headache.

PHYSICAL EXAM
- Gross examination of the anatomy: eyelids, surface of the eye, pupils, and extraocular muscles
- Snellen chart
- Tonometry

- Penlight
- Blepharospasm: fluorescein stain
- Wood lamp (5)

DIFFERENTIAL DIAGNOSIS
- Corneal abrasion
  - Acute angle-closure glaucoma
    ○ Conjunctivitis
  - Infective keratitis
    ○ Uveitis
    ○ Keratoconjunctivitis (3,5)
- Corneal ulceration
  - Herpes zoster
    ○ Herpes zoster ophthalmicus

DIAGNOSTIC TESTS & INTERPRETATION

Initial Tests (lab, imaging)
- Ulcer culture
- Pretreatment with topical antibiotics may alter culture results.

Diagnostic Procedures/Other
- Slit lamp and fluorescein dye to identify and evaluate corneal abrasions
- Trauma/foreign body has geographic shape; if due to contact lenses, several punctate lesions (5)
- Document visual acuity.

Test Interpretation
Scraping culture/staining identifies bacteria, yeast, or intranuclear inclusions to help narrow diagnosis.

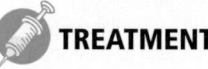

TREATMENT

GENERAL MEASURES
- Most uncomplicated corneal abrasions heal in 24 to 48 hours.
- May not require follow-up if lesion is <4 mm, uncomplicated abrasion, normal vision, and resolving symptoms
- But untreated abrasions can lead to corneal ulceration
- Do not rinse with tap or bottled water because it may contain microorganisms such as acanthamoeba instead rinse with a saline solution or multipurpose contact lenses solutions.
- Patching not recommended
  - Does not reduce pain
  - Delays healing (4)[A]

MEDICATION

- Treatment guidelines: pain control, infection prevention, and daily symptom monitoring
- Oral analgesic: narcotics, acetaminophen, NSAIDs
- Topical anesthetics include proparacaine hydrochloride 0.1–0.5%, tetracaine hydrochloride 1%.
  - Proparacaine may be less cytotoxic than tetracaine (4)[B].
  - Topical anesthetics should be avoided after initial examination because they can retard healing and cause corneal damage.

First Line

- Ophthalmic NSAIDs: Diclofenac 0.1% one drop QID helps relieve moderate pain:
  - Alternatives include ketorolac 0.5% one drop QID and bromfenac 0.09%.
  - Caution: Ophthalmic NSAIDs may rarely cause corneal melting and perforation.
  - Caution in patients with bleeding tendency
- Ophthalmic antibiotics may help prevent further infection and ulceration of corneal abrasions (6)[C].
- Some ophthalmic antibiotics include bacitracin 500 IU BID or QID, ofloxacin/ciprofloxacin 0.3%, gentamicin 0.3%, erythromycin 0.5%, polymyxin B/trimethoprim (Polytrim), and tobramycin 0.3%.
- Anti-pseudomonas antibiotics should be used, especially if patient wears contact lenses, and this latter should be discontinued until healing and completion of treatment.
- Large corneal abrasions (>4 mm) or very painful abrasions should be treated with a combination of topical antibiotic and topical NSAID.
- Fungal keratitis is treated with a protracted course of topical antifungal agents (by ophthalmologist).
- Herpetic keratitis should be referred promptly to ophthalmologist and treated initially with trifluridine:
  - Vidarabine and acyclovir are alternatives.

ISSUES FOR REFERRAL

- Indications for referral include:
  - Chemical burn
  - Evidence of corneal ulcer or infiltrate
  - Failure to heal after 3 to 4 days

- Inability to remove a foreign body
- Increase size of abrasion after 24 hours
- Penetrating injury
- Presence of hyphema (blood) or hypopyon (pus)
- Rust ring
- Vision loss of >20/40
- Worsening symptoms or improvement after 24 hours (5)
  - Immediate ophthalmology consultation for corneal ulceration for culture and initiation of treatment

 ONGOING CARE

FOLLOW-UP RECOMMENDATIONS

Patient Monitoring

- Most uncomplicated corneal abrasions heal in 24 to 48 hours.
- Follow-up not necessary for small (<4 mm), uncomplicated abrasions, normal vision, and resolving symptoms
- Lesions >4 mm, decreased vision, and abrasions due to contact lenses need follow-up within 24 hours (3)[C].

PATIENT EDUCATION

Prevention of abrasions and proper handling of contact lenses can prevent recurrence of corneal ulcers.

PROGNOSIS

- Corneal abrasions heal within 24 to 72 hours.
- Ophthalmology consult with penetrating eye injury

COMPLICATIONS

- Recurrence
- Scarring of the cornea
- Loss of vision

REFERENCES

1. Wilson SA, Last A. Management of corneal abrasions. *Am Fam Physician*. 2004;70(1):123–128.
2. Belknap EB. Corneal emergencies. *Top Companion Anim Med*. 2015;30(3):74–80.
3. Wipperman JL, Dorsch JN. Evaluation and management of corneal abrasions. *Am Fam Physician*. 2013;87(2):114–120.
4. Malafa MM, Coleman JE, Bowman RW, et al. Perioperative corneal abrasion: updated guidelines for prevention and management. *Plast Reconstr Surg*. 2016;137(5):790e–798e.
5. Pflipsen M, Massaquoi M, Wolf S. Evaluation of the painful eye. *Am Fam Physician*. 2016;93(12): 991–998.
6. Fraser S. Corneal abrasion. *Clin Ophthalmol*. 2010;4:387–390.

 CODES

ICD10

- S05.00XA Inj conjunctiva and corneal abrasion w/o fb, unsp eye, init
- H16.009 Unspecified corneal ulcer, unspecified eye
- H16.049 Marginal corneal ulcer, unspecified eye

CLINICAL PEARLS

- Contact lenses use should be discontinued until corneal abrasion or ulcer is healed and pain is fully resolved.
- Eye patching is not recommended.
- Prescribe topical and/or oral analgesic medication for symptom relief, and consider ophthalmic antibiotics.
- Prompt referral to an ophthalmologist should be made with suspicion of an ulcer, recurrence of abrasion, retained foreign body, viral keratitis, significant visual loss, or lack of improvement despite therapy.
- Protective eyewear should be used at all times during work (e.g., miners, woodworkers, landscapers, metal worker) and certain sports (e.g., hockey, racquetball, lacrosse).
- Healing can take 2 to 3 days for small abrasion (4 mm) for larger one may take 4 to 5 days.
- Treatment usually involves frequent topical antimicrobials application (e.g., every 1 to 2 hours).

C

CORNS AND CALLUSES

Sangili Chandran, MD, MS(ortho) • Valerie Rygiel, DO

 BASICS

DESCRIPTION

- A callus (tyloma) is a diffuse area of hyperkeratosis, usually without a distinct border.
  - Typically, the result of exposure to repetitive forces, including friction and mechanical pressure; tend to occur on the palms of hands and soles of feet (1)
- A corn (heloma) is a circumscribed hyperkeratotic lesion with a central conical core of keratin that causes pain and inflammation. The conical core in a corn is a thickening of the stratum corneum.
- Hard corn or heloma durum (more common): often on toe surfaces, especially 5th toe (proximal inter-phalangeal [PIP] joint)
- Soft corn or heloma molle: commonly in the interdigital space (1)
- Digital corns are also known as clavi or heloma durum.
- Intractable plantar keratosis is usually located under a metatarsal head (1st and 5th most common), is typically more difficult to resolve, and often is resistant to usual conservative treatments.

EPIDEMIOLOGY

Corns and calluses have the largest prevalence of all foot disorders.

Incidence

- Incidence of corns and calluses increases with age.
- Less common in pediatric patients
- Women affected more often than men
- Blacks report corns and calluses 30% more often than whites.

Prevalence

- 9.2 million Americans
- ~38/1,000 people affected

ETIOLOGY AND PATHOPHYSIOLOGY

Increased activity of keratinocytes in superficial layer of skin leads to hyperkeratosis. This is a normal response to excess friction, pressure, or stress.

- Calluses typically arise from repetitive friction, motion, or pressure to skin. The increased pressure is often secondary to a metatarsal deformity (long metatarsal or plantarflexed metatarsal) or another bone spur or deformity.
- Hard corns are an extreme form of callus with a keratin-based core; often found on the digital surfaces and commonly linked to bony protrusions, causing skin to rub against shoe surfaces
- Soft corns arise from increased moisture from perspiration leading to skin maceration, along with mechanical irritation, especially between toes.

Genetics

No true genetic basis was identified because most corns and calluses are due to mechanical stressors on the foot/hands.

RISK FACTORS

- Extrinsic factors producing pressure, friction, and local stress
  - Ill-fitting shoes or walking barefoot
  - Not using socks/gloves
  - Activities that increase stress applied to skin of hands or feet (manual labor, running, walking, sports)
- Intrinsic factors
  - Bony prominences: bunions, hammertoes, mallet deformities, deformed metatarsals
  - Motor or sensory neuropathy such as secondary to diabetes

GENERAL PREVENTION

External irritation and pressure are by far the most common cause of calluses and corns. General measures to reduce friction or pressure on the skin are recommended to reduce incidence of callus formation. Examples include wearing shoes that fit well and using socks and gloves.

Geriatric Considerations

In elderly patients, especially those with neurologic or vascular compromise, skin breakdown from calluses/corns may lead to increased risk of infection/ulceration. 30% of foot ulcers in the elderly arise from eroded hyperkeratosis. Regular foot exams are emphasized for these patients as well as diabetic patients (2).

COMMONLY ASSOCIATED CONDITIONS

- Foot ulcers: especially noted in diabetic patients or patients with neuropathy or vascular compromise
- Infection: look for warning signs including
  - Increasing size, redness, pain, or swelling
  - Purulent drainage
  - Fever
  - Change in color of fingers or toes
- Signs of gangrene (color change, coolness)

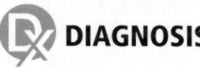 **DIAGNOSIS**

- Most commonly a clinical diagnosis based on visualization of the lesion
- Examination of footwear may also provide clues.

HISTORY

- Careful history can usually pinpoint cause.
- Ask about neurologic and vascular history and diabetes. These may be risk factors for progression of corns/calluses to frank ulcerations and infection.

PHYSICAL EXAM

- Calluses
  - Thickening of skin without distinct borders
  - Often on feet, hands; especially over palms of hands, soles of feet
  - Colors range from white to gray-yellow, brown, red.
  - May be painless or tender
  - May throb or burn
- Corns
  - Hard corns
    - Commonly on feet: dorsum of toes or 5th PIP joint
    - Varied texture: dry, waxy, and transparent to a hornlike mass

- ○ Distinct borders
- ○ Often painful
- – Soft corns
  - ○ Commonly between toes, especially between 4th and 5th digits at the base of the web space
  - ○ Often yellowed, macerated appearance
  - ○ Often extremely painful

DIFFERENTIAL DIAGNOSIS
- Plantar warts (typically a loss of skin lines within the wart), which are viral in nature
- Porokeratoses (blocked sweat gland)
- Underlying ulceration of skin, with or without infection (important to rule out especially with diabetic patients)

DIAGNOSTIC TESTS & INTERPRETATION
Initial Tests (lab, imaging)
- Radiographs may be warranted if no external cause is found. Look for abnormalities in foot structure, bone spurs.
- Use of metallic radiographic marker and weight-bearing films often highlights the relationship between the callus and bony prominence.

Diagnostic Procedures/Other
Biopsy with microscopic evaluation in rare cases

Test Interpretation
Abnormal accumulation of keratin in epidermis, stratum corneum

 # TREATMENT

GENERAL MEASURES
- Most therapy for corns and calluses can be done as self-care in the home (1).
- Use bandages, soft foam padding, or silicone sleeve over the affected area to decrease friction on the skin and promote healing with digital clavi.
- Use socks or gloves regularly.
- Padding to off-load bony prominences
- Low-heeled shoes; soft upper with deep and wide toe box
- Avoidance of activities that contribute to painful lesions
- Prefabricated or custom orthotics

MEDICATION
- Keratolytic agents, such as urea or ammonium lactate, can be applied safely.
- Intralesional bleomycin injections have shown improvement in size and pain of warts.

- In office débridement of affected tissue and use of protective padding
- Use sandpaper discs or pumice stones over hard, thickened areas of skin; can be done safely at home

Geriatric Considerations
Use of salicylic acid corn plasters can cause skin breakdown and ulceration in patients with thin, atrophic skin; diabetes; and those with vascular compromise. The skin surrounding the callus will often turn white and can become quite painful. Sometimes, the acids are weak enough to not penetrate the thick skin, but they can burn the adjacent skin, making the condition worse. Aggressive use of pumice stones can also lead to skin breakdown, especially surrounding the callus.

ISSUES FOR REFERRAL
- May benefit from referral to podiatrist if use of topical agents and shoe changes are ineffective
- Abnormalities in foot structure may require surgical treatment.
- Diabetic, vascular, and neuropathic patients may benefit from referral to podiatrist for regular foot exams to prevent infection or ulceration.

SURGERY/OTHER PROCEDURES
- Surgical treatment to areas of protruding bone where corns and calluses form
- Rebalancing of foot pressure through functional foot orthotics
- Shaving or cutting off hardened area of skin using a chisel or 15-blade scalpel. For corns, remove keratin core and place pad over area during healing.

COMPLEMENTARY & ALTERNATIVE MEDICINE
- May benefit from urea-based lotions, creams, or ointments
- Warm water/Epsom salt soaks

ADMISSION, INPATIENT, AND NURSING CONSIDERATIONS
- Admission usually not necessary, unless progression to ulcerated lesion with signs of severe infection, gangrene
- May require aggressive débridement in operating room if an abscess or deep-space infection is suspected. Deep-space infections can develop where an abscess can penetrate into tendon sheaths and/or deep compartments within the foot or hand, potentially leading to rapid sepsis. Vascular status must be assessed and vascular referral considered.
- Nursing
  - Wound care, dressing changes for infected lesions

 # ONGOING CARE

PATIENT EDUCATION
- General information: http://www.mayoclinic.org/diseases-conditions/corns-and-calluses/basics/definition/con-20014462
- American Podiatric Medical Association: http://www.apma.org

PROGNOSIS
Complete cure is possible once factors causing pressure or injury are eliminated.

COMPLICATIONS
Ulceration, infection

REFERENCES
1. Freeman DB. Corns and calluses resulting from mechanical hyperkeratosis. *Am Fam Physician*. 2002;65(11):2277–2280.
2. Pinzur MS, Slovenkai MP, Trepman E, et al; for Diabetes Committee of American Orthopaedic Foot and Ankle Society. Guidelines for diabetic foot care: recommendations endorsed by the Diabetes Committee of the American Orthopaedic Foot and Ankle Society. *Foot Ankle Int*. 2005;26(1):113–119.

ADDITIONAL READING
- American College of Foot and Ankle Surgeons: http://www.acfas.org/
- Theodosat A. Skin diseases of the lower extremities in the elderly. *Dermatol Clin*. 2004;22(1):13–21.

 # CODES

ICD10
L84 Corns and callosities

CLINICAL PEARLS
Most therapy for corns and calluses can be done as self-care in the home using padding over the affected area to decrease friction or pressure. However, if simple home care is not helpful, then removal of the lesions is often immediately curative.

C

CORONARY ARTERY DISEASE AND STABLE ANGINA

Blake D. Singletary, DO • Merrill Krolick, DO, FACC, FACP, FSCAI

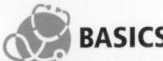 **BASICS**

DESCRIPTION

- Coronary artery disease (CAD) refers to the atherosclerotic narrowing of the epicardial coronary arteries. It may manifest insidiously as angina pectoris or as an acute coronary syndrome (ACS).
- Stable angina is a chest discomfort due to myocardial ischemia that is predictably reproducible at a certain level of exertion or emotional stress.
- The spectrum of ACS includes unstable angina (UA), non–ST elevation myocardial infarction (NSTEMI), and ST elevation myocardial infarction (STEMI). See chapters on ACS for further information.
- Definitions
  - Typical angina: exhibits three classical characteristics: (i) substernal chest pressure, pressure or heaviness that may radiate to the jaw, back, or arms and generally lasts from 2 to 15 minutes; (ii) occurs at a certain level of myocardial oxygen demand from exertion, emotional stress, or increased sympathetic tone; and (iii) relieved with rest or sublingual nitroglycerin
  - Atypical angina: exhibits two of the above typical characteristics
  - Noncardiac chest pain: exhibits ≤1 of the above typical characteristics
  - Anginal equivalent: Patients may present without chest discomfort but with nonspecific symptoms such as dyspnea, diaphoresis, fatigue, belching, nausea, light-headedness, or indigestion that occur with exertion or stress. Patients with diabetes mellitus, women, and the elderly may present with more atypical features as compared to the general population.
  - UA: anginal symptoms that are new or more frequent, more severe or occurring with lessening degrees of myocardial demand; it is considered ACS but does not present with cardiac biomarker elevation. (See "Acute Coronary Syndromes: NSTE-ACS (Unstable Angina and NSTEMI)" chapter.)
  - NSTEMI: elevation of cardiac biomarker (troponin) with either anginal symptoms, ischemic ECG changes other than ST elevation, or both. (See "Acute Coronary Syndromes: NSTE-ACS (Unstable Angina and NSTEMI)" chapter.)
  - STEMI: presents with typical symptoms as mentioned above with ST elevations noted on ECG; generally caused by acute plaque rupture and complete obstruction of culprit vessel and may present prior to laboratory detection of troponin. (See "Acute Coronary Syndromes: STEMI" chapter.)
- Canadian Cardiovascular Society grading scale:
  - Class I: Angina does not limit ordinary physical activity, occurring only with strenuous or prolonged exertion (7 to 8 metabolic equivalents [METs]).
  - Class II: Angina causes slight limitation of ordinary activity. It occurs when walking rapidly, uphill, or >2 blocks; climbing >1 flight of stairs; or with emotional stress (5 to 6 METs).
  - Class III: Angina causes marked limitation of ordinary physical activity. It occurs when walking 1 to 2 blocks or climbing one flight of stairs (3 to 4 METs).
  - Class IV: Angina occurs with any physical activity and may occur at rest (1 to 2 METs).

Geriatric Considerations
- The elderly may present with atypical symptoms.
- Physical limitations may delay recognition of angina until it occurs with minimal exertion or at rest.
- Maintain a high degree of suspicion during evaluation of dyspnea and other nonspecific complaints.

- Geriatric patients may be very sensitive to the side effects of medications used to treat angina.

EPIDEMIOLOGY
- CAD is the leading cause of death for adults both in the United States and worldwide.
- CAD is responsible for about 1 in every 3 deaths in the United States alone.
- The cost of CAD in the United States was $555 billion in 2016 and is expected to rise to $1.1 trillion by 2035.
- ~80% of CAD is preventable with a healthy lifestyle.

Incidence
In the United States, the lifetime risk of a 40-year-old developing CAD is 49% for men and 32% for women.

Prevalence
In the United States, 28.4 million people carry a diagnosis of CAD, whereas 7.12 million have angina pectoris (1).

ETIOLOGY AND PATHOPHYSIOLOGY
- Anginal symptoms occur during times of myocardial ischemia caused by a mismatch between coronary perfusion and myocardial oxygen demand.
- Atherosclerotic narrowing of the coronary arteries is the most common etiology of angina, but it may also occur in those with significant aortic stenosis, pulmonary hypertension, hypertrophic cardiomyopathy, coronary spasm, or volume overload.
- Sensory nerves from the heart enter the spinal cord at levels C7–T4, causing diffuse referred pain/discomfort in the associated dermatomes.

RISK FACTORS
- Traditional risk factors: hypertension, ↓ HDL, ↑ LDL, smoking, diabetes, premature CAD in first-degree relatives (men <55 years old; women <65 years old), age (>45 years for men; >55 years for women)
- Nontraditional risk factors: obesity, sedentary lifestyle, chronic inflammation, abnormal ankle-brachial indices, renal disease

GENERAL PREVENTION
- Smoking cessation
- Regular aerobic exercise program
- Weight loss for obese patients (goal BMI <25 kg/m²)
- BP control (goal <140/90 mm Hg; consider <130/80 mm Hg for those with 10-year ASCVD risk ≥10%) (2)[C]
- Diabetes management
- Statin therapy for those with diabetes age 40 to 75 years and those with 10-year risk ≥7.5–10% (recommendations vary)
- Low-dose aspirin may be considered in those with 10-year risk ≥10% and without aspirin-use risks.

COMMONLY ASSOCIATED CONDITIONS
Hyperlipidemia, peripheral vascular disease, cerebrovascular disease, hypertension, obesity, diabetes

DIAGNOSIS

HISTORY
- Careful history is important to elicit symptoms.
- Pain may be described with a clenched fist over the center of the chest (Levine sign).
- Discomfort is usually not affected by position or deep inspiration.
- Episodes of angina are generally of the same character and in the same location.
- Recent decrease in level of physical activity may be due to worsening anginal symptoms.

- Dyspnea on exertion may present as the only symptom. Atypical symptoms are more likely in women, the elderly, and diabetic patients.
- May present with symptoms similar to gastric reflux or GI upset (indigestion, nausea, diaphoresis)

PHYSICAL EXAM
- Normal cardiac exam does not exclude the diagnosis of angina or CAD.
- Cardiac exam may reveal dysrhythmias, heart murmurs indicative of valvular disease, gallops, or signs of congestive heart failure.
- Evidence of peripheral vascular disease (diminished pulses, bruits, abdominal aortic aneurysm [AAA]) may or may not be noted.

DIFFERENTIAL DIAGNOSIS
- Vascular: aortic dissection, pericarditis, myocarditis, myocardial infarction (MI), vasospasm
- Pulmonary: pleuritis, pulmonary embolism, pneumothorax
- Gastroesophageal: gastric reflux, esophageal spasm, peptic ulcer
- Musculoskeletal: costochondritis, arthritis, muscle strain, rib fracture
- Other: anxiety, psychosomatic, cocaine abuse

DIAGNOSTIC TESTS & INTERPRETATION
Initial Tests (lab, imaging)
- Serial cardiac troponins for those presenting acutely with symptoms
- CBC, lipid profile, HgbA1c for risk stratification (1)[C]
- Basic metabolic panel to rule out electrolyte abnormalities and assess renal function
- ECG
  - Should be obtained unless there is a noncardiac cause of the chest pain (1)[C]
  - Frequently unremarkable between anginal episodes; may show signs of myocardial ischemia during symptomatic episodes, evidence of old MI
  - Left bundle branch block or ventricular pacing makes interpretation for ischemia unreliable.
- Chest x-ray may exclude other causes of pain (1)[C].

Follow-Up Tests & Special Considerations
- Goal is to detect high-risk coronary lesions where intervention would improve long-term mortality or alleviate anginal symptoms.
- Stress testing is most helpful for patients at intermediate risk of CAD.
  - Exercise testing for those who can physically exercise (≥5 METs) (1)[A]
    - Standard exercise ECG for those with normal baseline ECG
    - Exercise stress testing with echo or perfusion imaging for those with abnormal baseline ECG or in premenopausal women
  - In patients who cannot tolerate exercise, consider pharmacologic stress testing (1)[A].
- Echocardiogram should be obtained in patients with a new or loud (≥III/VI) murmur, evidence of MI, symptoms of heart failure, concern for hypertrophic cardiomyopathy or pericardial effusion, and in those with new arrhythmias (1)[A].
- Echocardiogram can be considered in patients with hypertension or diabetes and abnormal ECG (1).
- CT coronary angiography or cardiac MRI can be considered as a supplement/alternative to stress testing in patients with continued symptoms despite negative stress testing, inconclusive stress testing, or need for better anatomic definition of disease (1)[A].

Diagnostic Procedures/Other

- Cardiac catheterization with coronary angiography is the gold standard for confirmation and delineation of coronary disease and direction of interventional therapy or surgery. It is indicated if noninvasive testing suggests a high-risk lesion or if patient fails to respond to appropriate medical management.
- Significant CAD is defined as ≥50% stenosis of the left main coronary artery or ≥70% stenosis of other major coronary arteries by angiography.
- Borderline lesions may be assessed with a pressure wire. Fractional flow reserve (FFR) of ≤0.8 demonstrates a hemodynamically significant lesion.

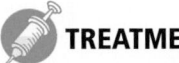

TREATMENT

GENERAL MEASURES

- BP control goal for most patients with significant CAD: <130/80 mm Hg (2)[A].
- Smoking cessation goal: complete cessation, no exposure to secondhand smoke or e-cigarettes
- Physical activity goal: 30 to 60 minutes of moderate aerobic activity, at least 5 (preferably 7) days/week
- Weight management goal: BMI 18.5 to 24.9 kg/m²; waist circumference <35 inches (women) or <40 inches (men)
- Individualize glycemic control goals in diabetics: Avoid hypoglycemic episodes.

MEDICATION

First Line

- β-Blockers: decrease myocardial oxygen demand by lowering heart rate, BP, and contractility
  - Improve mortality in patients with MI or heart failure and should be used as initial therapy (1)[A]
  - Can improve symptoms of angina
  - Metoprolol (25 to 400 mg daily [succinate] or divided BID [tartrate]) or carvedilol (3.125 to 25 mg BID). Adjust doses according to clinical response. Maintain resting heart rate 50 to 60 bpm.
  - Side effects: bradycardia, fatigue, and sexual dysfunction predominantly in men
- Calcium channel blockers (CCBs): cause arterial vasodilation, decreased myocardial oxygen demand, and improved coronary blood flow. Similar effectiveness to β-blockers; may be used instead of, or in addition to β-blockers (1)[A]. Only long-acting CCBs should be used:
  - Dihydropyridine CCBs: Nifedipine (30 to 90 mg/day), amlodipine (5 to 10 mg/day), or felodipine (2.5 to 10 mg/day) work predominantly on arterial vasodilation and can improve coronary blood flow.
  - Nondihydropyridine CCBs: Diltiazem (120 to 480 mg/day) or verapamil (120 to 480 mg/day) also have negative inotropic effects and should not be used in those with EF <40% because they may precipitate heart failure. Side effects include constipation and peripheral edema.
- Nitrates: dilate systemic veins and arteries (including coronary vessels) and cause decreased preload. At higher doses, they decrease BP.
  - Sublingual nitroglycerin (0.4 mg every 5 minutes for up to 3 doses) used for acute anginal episodes (1)[A]
  - Long-acting nitrates such as isosorbide mononitrate (30 to 240 mg daily [extended release]) can be used for angina prophylaxis.
  - Side effects include headache and hypotension but tend to improve with continued usage.
  - Contraindicated with concomitant PDE5 inhibitor use (e.g., sildenafil)
- Lipid-lowering agents:
  - High-intensity statin therapy is indicated for all patients with CAD regardless of lipid levels.

- Statin therapy should also be encouraged for those with high CAD risk (lifetime ASCVD risk ≥7.5–10%, <75 to 80 years. Evidence is sparse for statins in primary prevention after 75 years.).
  - Atorvastatin (40 to 80 mg/day) and rosuvastatin (20 to 40 mg/day) are high-intensity statins.
  - Statins reduce risk of MI and revascularization need. Side effects include myalgias, transaminitis, rhabdomyolysis (rare), and impaired glucose tolerance.
  - Ezetimibe added to statin therapy, little evidence for improved clinical outcomes.
  - Evolocumab and possibly other PCSK-9 inhibitors further reduces LDL levels when used in combination with statins for high-risk patients and may reduce cardiovascular events in highly selected patients but are very expensive. Clinical trials are ongoing.
- Antiplatelets: decrease risk of thrombosis
  - Aspirin (75 to 162 mg/day) decreases risk of first MI and reduces adverse cardiovascular events in those with stable angina (1)[A].
  - Clopidogrel (75 mg/day) may be used in patients with contraindications to aspirin (1)[A].
  - Dual antiplatelet therapy with aspirin + clopidogrel, prasugrel, or ticagrelor is indicated after MI or percutaneous coronary intervention (PCI) (use prasugrel only after PCI. Do not use in patient with CVA history).
- Angiotensin-converting enzyme inhibitors (ACEIs): act on the renin-angiotensin-aldosterone system to reduce BP and afterload. They also have effects on cardiac remodeling after MI.
  - ACEIs such as lisinopril (5 to 40 mg/day) and enalapril (2.5 to 20.0 mg BID) have been shown to reduce both cardiovascular death and MI in patients with CAD and left ventricular systolic dysfunction (1)[A].
  - Angiotensin receptor blockers such as candesartan (4 to 32 mg daily) may be used in patients intolerant to ACEIs.
  - Side effects include cough (ACEIs predominantly), hyperkalemia, and angioedema.

Second Line

Ranolazine (500 to 1,000 mg BID) decreases calcium overload in myocytes, acting as an antianginal/anti-ischemic agent.

- Does not affect heart rate or BP
- Use as adjunctive therapy when symptoms persist despite optimal doses of other antianginals
- Side effects can include nausea, constipation, dizziness, QT prolongation, and headache.

SURGERY/OTHER PROCEDURES

- Revascularization should be considered when noninvasive testing suggests a high-risk lesion. It can also be performed if optimal medical therapy is inadequate to control symptoms.
- PCI with balloon angioplasty and/or stent placement (with drug-eluting or bare-metal stent) is performed for significant lesions. Additional techniques include laser therapy and atherectomy.
- Current literature does not definitively show that PCI decreases mortality or risk of MI versus aggressive medical management in those with stable angina.
- Coronary artery bypass graft (CABG) is preferred over PCI for those with severe left main coronary stenosis, significant lesions in ≥3 major coronary arteries, and for lesions not amenable to PCI.

COMPLEMENTARY & ALTERNATIVE MEDICINE

Relaxation/stress reduction therapy for angina

ONGOING CARE

FOLLOW-UP RECOMMENDATIONS

- Lifestyle modifications should be aggressively stressed at every visit.
- Patients should be followed clinically; routine stress testing is not necessary for asymptomatic patients.

Patient Monitoring

Frequent follow-up after initial event: every 4 to 6 months in first year and then 1 to 2 times per year

DIET

- Reduced intake of trans-fatty acids (1)[C]
- Adherence to dietary modification for comorbid conditions (diabetes, heart failure, hypertension)

PROGNOSIS

Variable; depends on severity of symptoms, extent of CAD, and left ventricular function

COMPLICATIONS

ACS, arrhythmia, cardiac arrest, heart failure

REFERENCES

1. Fihn SD, Gardin JM, Abrams J, et al. 2012 ACCF/AHA/ACP/AATS/PCNA/SCAI/STS guideline for the diagnosis and management of patients with stable ischemic heart disease: a report of the American College of Cardiology Foundation/American Heart Association Task Force on Practice Guidelines, and the American College of Physicians, American Association for Thoracic Surgery, Preventive Cardiovascular Nurses Association, Society for Cardiovascular Angiography and Interventions, and Society of Thoracic Surgeons. *J Am Coll Cardiol.* 2012;60(24):e44–e164.
2. Whelton PK, Carey RM, Aronow WS, et al. 2017 ACC/AHA/AAPA/ABC/ACPM/AGS/APhA/ASH/ASPC/NMA/PCNA guideline for the prevention, detection, evaluation, and management of high blood pressure in adults: a report of the American College of Cardiology/American Heart Association Task Force on Clinical Practice Guidelines. *J Am Coll Cardiol.* 2018;71(19):e127–e248.

SEE ALSO

Algorithm: Chest Pain/Acute Coronary Syndrome

CODES

ICD10

- I25.119 Athscl heart disease of native cor art w unsp ang pctrs
- I25.118 Athscl heart disease of native cor art w oth ang pctrs
- I20.9 Angina pectoris, unspecified

CLINICAL PEARLS

- Maximize antianginal therapy: Combine β-blockers, CCBs, and nitrates as tolerated, along with high-intensity statin therapy.
- Lifestyle changes and optimal medical therapy must be emphasized to prevent progression of atherosclerosis and to control contributing risk factors.

COSTOCHONDRITIS

Smriti Ohri, MD • Scott A. Fields, MD, MHA

 BASICS

DESCRIPTION
- Anterior chest wall pain and tenderness of the costochondral and costosternal regions, most often affecting the 2nd to the 5th costal cartilages
- System(s) affected: musculoskeletal
- Synonym(s): costosternal syndrome; parasternal chondrodynia; anterior chest wall syndrome

EPIDEMIOLOGY
- Predominant age: 20 to 40 years
- Predominant gender: female

Incidence
- 30% emergency room visits for chest pain
- 13% primary care visits for chest pain

ETIOLOGY AND PATHOPHYSIOLOGY
Although not fully understood, inflammation can be caused by pulling from adjoining muscles at costochondral or costosternal regions.

RISK FACTORS
- Unusual physical activity or upper extremity overuse
- Recent trauma (including motor vehicle accident, domestic violence) or new-onset physical activity
- Recent upper respiratory infection (URI) with coughing

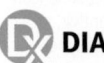 **DIAGNOSIS**

- Pain is usually sharp, achy, or pressure-like, involving multiple (and mostly unilateral 2nd to 5th) costal cartilages.
- Exacerbated by upper body movements and exertional activities
- Reproduced by palpation of the affected cartilage segments
- Chest tightness is often associated with the pain.

HISTORY
- A complete and thorough history (including a cardiac risk factor evaluation) is mandatory for the diagnosis.
- Social history: careful screening and evaluation for domestic violence and substance abuse

PHYSICAL EXAM
- A thorough cardiopulmonary exam to exclude other conditions presenting with chest pain
  - Cardiac rhythm; murmurs; gallops, rubs
  - Adventitious lung sounds—rales, rhonchi, wheezes, rubs
- Tenderness over the costochondral junctions is necessary to establish the diagnosis but does not completely exclude other causes of chest pain.
- If swelling or redness of costal cartilage is present, the presentation is often termed Tietze syndrome.
- Movement of upper extremity of the same side may reproduce the pain.
- Abdominal exam: tenderness, masses, organomegaly

Pediatric Considerations
- Consider psychogenic chest pain in children who perceive family discord.
- Consider slipping rib syndrome in children with chronic chest and abdominal pain (1).

Geriatric Considerations
Consider herpes zoster in elderly patients.

DIFFERENTIAL DIAGNOSIS
- Cardiac
  - Coronary artery disease (CAD)
  - Cardiac contusion from trauma
  - Aortic aneurysm
  - Pericarditis
  - Myocarditis
- Gastrointestinal
  - Gastroesophageal reflux
  - Peptic esophagitis
  - Esophageal spasm
  - Cholecystitis
- Musculoskeletal (1)
  - Fibromyalgia
  - Slipping rib syndrome
  - Costovertebral arthritis
  - Painful xiphoid syndrome
  - Rib trauma
  - Ankylosing spondylitis
- Psychogenic
  - Panic attacks
  - Hyperventilation
- Respiratory
  - Asthma
  - Pulmonary embolism
  - Pneumonia
  - Chronic cough
  - Pneumothorax
- Other
  - Domestic violence and abuse
  - Herpes zoster
  - Spinal tumor
  - Metastatic cancer
  - Substance abuse (cocaine)

DIAGNOSTIC TESTS & INTERPRETATION
- Primarily a clinical diagnosis
- Laboratory exams and imaging to rule out other diagnoses
- ESR is inconsistently elevated.

Initial Tests (lab, imaging)
Imaging is not indicated for the diagnosis of costochondritis.

Diagnostic Procedures/Other
- None indicated for the diagnosis of costochondritis
- Consider ECG in patients age >35 years and for patients with history of or at risk for CAD (2)[C].
- Consider chest x-ray in patients with appropriate cardiopulmonary symptoms (2)[C].
- Consider CT imaging if high suspicion of infectious or neoplastic process (2)[C].
- Consider spiral CT for pulmonary embolism and D-dimer if history or risk factors are present.

Test Interpretation
Costochondral joint inflammation

TREATMENT
Reassurance of benign nature of condition and potential for long, slow recovery from pain

GENERAL MEASURES
- Rest and heat (or ice) massage
- Stretching exercises
- Minimize symptom-provoking activities (e.g., reduce frequency or intensity of exercise/work activity).

MEDICATION
- Pain relief with NSAIDs (ibuprofen, naproxen, or diclofenac), acetaminophen or other analgesics
- Use of skeletal muscle relaxants may be beneficial if associated with muscle spasm.

ISSUES FOR REFERRAL
- Consider referral to physical therapy for pain reduction and improvement in function (3)[B].
- Refractory cases of costochondritis can be treated with local injections of combined lidocaine/corticosteroid into costochondral areas; rarely necessary (2)[C]

COMPLEMENTARY & ALTERNATIVE MEDICINE
Limited data but may be safely tried if patient interested
- Chiropractic manipulation; exercise prescription
- Dry needling by properly trained providers (4)[C]
- Acupuncture (5)[C]
- Massage

ADMISSION, INPATIENT, AND NURSING CONSIDERATIONS
Only if differential diagnosis is unclear and cardiac or other serious etiology of chest pain is being considered

ONGOING CARE

FOLLOW-UP RECOMMENDATIONS
Follow-up within 1 week if diagnosis is unclear or symptoms do not abate with conservative treatment

PATIENT EDUCATION
- Educate regarding the self-limited (although potentially recurrent) nature of the illness.
- Instruct patient on proper physical activity regimens to avoid overuse syndromes.
- Avoid sudden, significant changes in activity.

PROGNOSIS
- Self-limited illness lasts for weeks to months and usually abates by 1 year: sometimes chronic particularly in adolescents
- Often recurs

COMPLICATIONS
Incomplete attention to differential diagnosis or overly aggressive interventions to ensure a more life-threatening diagnosis is not missed

REFERENCES
1. Ayloo A, Cvengros T, Marella S. Evaluation and treatment of musculoskeletal chest pain. *Prim Care*. 2013;40(4):863–887, viii.
2. Proulx AM, Zryd TW. Costochondritis: diagnosis and treatment. *Am Fam Physician*. 2009;80(6): 617–620.
3. Zaruba RA, Wilson E. Impairment based examination and treatment of costochondritis: a case series. *Int J Sports Phys Ther*. 2017;12(3): 458–467.
4. Westrick RB, Zylstra E, Issa T, et al. Evaluation and treatment of musculoskeletal chest wall pain in a military athlete. *Int J Sports Phys Ther*. 2012;7(3):323–332.
5. Lin K, Tung C. Integrating acupuncture for the management of costochondritis in adolescents. *Med Acupunct*. 2017;29(5):327–330.

CODES

ICD10
M94.0 Chondrocostal junction syndrome [Tietze]

CLINICAL PEARLS
- A common disorder, accounting for up to 30% of all cases of chest pain
- Diagnosis is primarily clinical. Lab and other testing is done to exclude other conditions based on patient risk.
- Self-limited (potentially recurrent) condition. Activity modification helps prevent recurrence.

COUNSELING TYPES
William T. Garrison, PhD

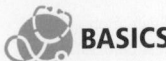 **BASICS**

DESCRIPTION

- Psychotherapeutic and counseling interventions play an important role in the management of chronic and acute-onset diseases and disorders. They are typically the primary initial mode of evaluation and/or treatment for most mild to moderate psychiatric disorders that reach criteria using the *DSM-5* (1) or *ICD-10* (2) diagnostic classification systems. It should be noted that the *DSM* system has recently been revised with significant changes in several disorder categories and their criteria. Treatment and successful control of either medical or psychological conditions require some form of professional counseling experience. Best outcomes occur when they are employed by a skilled practitioner. However, psychotherapy differs from generic counseling, which can take many forms and is delivered commonly in nonmedical settings, with mixed results.
- Counseling approaches are usually tailored to the specific presenting problem or issue and serve educational and emotional support functions. Typically, such counseling in medical settings will be time-limited and problem-focused and often not intended to lead to major medical symptom relief or major behavioral changes.
- The goals of psychotherapy range from increasing individual psychological insight and motivation for change to reduction of interpersonal conflict in the marriage or family, reduction of chronic or acute emotional suffering, and reversal of dysfunctional or habitual behaviors. There are several general types of psychotherapy, starting with individual, marital, or family approaches. In addition, a number of psychological theories guide various methods and treatment philosophies. The following is a brief overview of commonly used psychotherapeutic and counseling methods.
  - Psychodynamic therapy: Unconscious conflict manifests as patient's symptoms/problem behaviors:
    ○ Short term (4 to 6 months) and long term (≥1 year)
    ○ Focus is on increasing insight of underlying conflict or processes to initiate symptomatic change.
    ○ Therapist actively helps patient identify patterns of behavior stemming from existence of an unconscious conflict or motivations that may not be accurately perceived.
  - Cognitive-behavioral therapy (CBT): Patterns of thoughts and behaviors can lead to development and/or maintenance of symptoms. Thought patterns may not accurately reflect reality and may lead to psychological distress:
    ○ Therapy aims at modifying thought patterns by increasing cognitive flexibility and changing dysfunctional behavioral patterns.
    ○ Encourages patient self-monitoring of symptoms and the precursors or results of maladaptive behavior

  ○ Uses therapist-assisted challenges to patient's basic beliefs/assumptions
  ○ May use *exposure*, a procedure derived from basic learning theories, which encourages gradual steps toward change
  ○ Can be offered in group or individual formats
  ○ Therapist's role is suggestive and supportive.
  - Dialectical behavior therapy (DBT): Techniques such as social skills training, mindfulness, and problem solving are used to modulate impulse control and affect management:
    ○ Derivative of CBT
    ○ Originally used in treatment of patients with self-destructive behaviors (e.g., cutting, suicide attempts)
    ○ Seeks to change rigid patterns of cognitions and behaviors that have been maladaptive
    ○ Uses both individual and group treatment modalities
    ○ Therapist takes an active role in interpretation and support.
  - Interpersonal psychotherapy: Interpersonal relationships in a patient's life are linked to symptoms. Therapy seeks to alleviate symptoms and improve social adjustment through exploration of patient's relationships and experiences. Focus is on one of four potential problem areas:
    ○ Grief
    ○ Interpersonal role disputes
    ○ Role transitions
    ○ Interpersonal deficits: Therapist works with the patient in resolving the problematic interpersonal issues to facilitate change in symptoms.
  - Family therapy: focuses on the family as a unit of intervention
    ○ Uses psychoeducation to increase patient's and family's insight
    ○ Teaches communication and problem-solving skills
  - Motivational interviewing: focuses on motivation as a key to successful change process
    ○ Short term and problem focused
    ○ Focuses on identifying discrepancies between goals and behavior
    ○ "5 A's" model is a brief counseling framework developed specifically for physicians to effect behavioral change in patients:
      ▪ Assess for a problem.
      ▪ Advise making a change.
      ▪ Agree on action to be taken.
      ▪ Assist with self-care support to make the change.
      ▪ Arrange follow-up to support the change.
  - Counseling (heterogeneous treatment)
    ○ Often focuses on situational factors maintaining symptoms
    ○ Often encourages the use of community resources
  - Behavioral therapy: relatively nontheoretical approach to behavioral change or symptom reduction/eradication through application of principles of stimulus and response

Pediatric Considerations

- Important distinctions are made between psychotherapy and counseling for children/teens compared to adults/couples.
- The focus of evaluation must include attention to parent and family processes and factors. Interventions typically include interactions and sessions with parents as well as collateral work with teachers and other school personnel.
- Younger children will often be evaluated and diagnosed through behavioral descriptions provided by parents and other adults who know them well as well as through direct observation and/or play techniques. Children of all ages should be screened using behavioral checklists that are norm-referenced for age.
- Any child or teenager who requests counseling should be interviewed initially by the primary care provider and referred appropriately. Most referrals will be in response to parental request, however.
- Psychotherapeutic interventions with the strongest empirical basis with children include behavior therapy/modification, CBT, and family/parenting therapy. Play therapy has the least empirical support, and insight-oriented therapies appear to be more effective with older children (>11 years).
- There is controversy regarding the efficacy of psychopharmacologic treatment in preadolescents, although clear benefits have been demonstrated in some studies. Treatment guidelines for mild to moderate depressed mood and/or anxiety disorders typically recommend pediatric CBT initially, and studies have typically supported this approach in preteen and milder cases.

EPIDEMIOLOGY

- ~18.8 million adults suffer from clinical depression, and 20 million suffer from a diagnosable anxiety disorder.
- One in four Americans report seeking some form of mental health treatment in their adult life. This includes generic counseling in nonmedical settings such as work, clergy, or school settings and also includes visits to primary care providers. It is estimated that between 3.5% and 5% of adults in the United States actually participate in formal mental health psychotherapy annually.
- Public health experts report that the majority of those adults with diagnosable psychiatric disorders, however, do not receive professional mental health services. This is due to multiple factors, including failure to identify, noncompliance with psychiatric referral, regional shortages of providers, economic barriers, and excessive time duration from referral to available service.
- A large study conducted between 1987 and 1997 concluded that the percentage of adults in psychotherapy remained relatively stable over that decade, the use of psychopharmacology doubled, and older adults (aged 55 to 64 years) increasingly sought psychotherapy services. In that same study, it was found that psychotherapy duration (number of sessions) decreased substantially and about 1/3 of psychotherapy patients only attended one or two sessions.

RISK FACTORS

The need for psychotherapy or counseling services is directly and indirectly associated with a host of socioeconomic and biogenetic factors, including the general effects of poverty, family or marital dysfunction, life stressors, medical diseases or conditions, and individual biologic predisposition to mental health disorders.

GENERAL PREVENTION

It is generally assumed that early identification and intervention of child and adolescent psychopathology increases the likelihood of reducing the risk for adult psychopathology, but this has not been sufficiently validated in all categories of psychological disorders. Data support such claims in disorders such as childhood ADHD, anxiety disorders, and habit disorders of childhood, however.

 TREATMENT

GENERAL MEASURES

There is evidence of a "dose effect" in psychotherapy outcomes research, with some investigators suggesting that 6 to 8 sessions are necessary to yield positive initial effects and upward of 15 to 20 sessions for longer term, sustainable therapeutic effects. This dose effect may not be applicable to counseling services with primarily informational or emotional/supportive functions. Also, long-term therapy should be evaluated at 6- to 12-month intervals to determine efficacy.

MEDICATION

- Psychotherapy is most likely to be accompanied by use of pharmaceutical adjuncts in moderate to severe cases of psychological dysfunction that do not respond to other therapies or in cases of extremely poor quality of life or high risk. The most common examples are in cases of clinical depression or anxiety that clearly incapacitates the patient or significantly reduces his or her quality of life. Patients at risk for suicide or who represent a danger to others are also candidates for acute psychopharmacotherapy. Studies suggest that verbal and behaviorally oriented therapies can add efficacy to medication treatment in both depression and anxiety.
- There is controversy in the research field regarding the efficacy of medication alone versus psychotherapy alone versus combined treatments. The most recent consensus has been that combined treatments in moderate to severe psychological dysfunction are most likely to render positive short-term results and increase the likelihood that such effects can be sustained over time.

ADDITIONAL THERAPIES

- Anxiety disorders
  - Panic disorder with and without agoraphobia: CBT, psychodynamic therapy
  - Generalized anxiety disorder: CBT
  - Obsessive-compulsive disorder: CBT
  - Posttraumatic stress disorder: CBT
  - Specific phobia: CBT
  - Social phobia: CBT
- Mood disorders
  - Unipolar depression: CBT, interpersonal therapy, psychodynamic therapy
  - Bipolar disorder: family therapy, interpersonal therapy, CBT
  - Schizophrenia: psychodynamic therapy, family therapy, CBT
- Eating disorders
  - Binge eating disorder: CBT, interpersonal therapy
  - Bulimia nervosa: CBT, interpersonal therapy
- Personality disorders
  - Borderline: DBT, CBT
- Substance-use disorders
  - Alcohol: counseling, CBT, motivational interviewing
  - Cocaine: CBT, counseling
  - Heroin: CBT, counseling
  - Smoking: 5 A's
- Somatoform disorders:
  - Hypochondriasis: CBT
  - Body dysmorphic disorder: CBT

COMPLEMENTARY & ALTERNATIVE MEDICINE

A host of nonempirically based psychological and nutritional therapies can be found outside of mainstream medicine and psychological science. Very little or no evidence exists to support such experimental therapies, but all have the considerable power of the placebo effect fueling their anecdotal supports or claims. Placebo effects are also thought to be powerfully enhanced by the use of ingested or applied substances that create real physiologic, although not therapeutic, changes in the patient. If it makes them feel different, they are more likely to believe it helps.

 ONGOING CARE

FOLLOW-UP RECOMMENDATIONS

Patient Monitoring

There is evidence of a "dose effect" in psychotherapy outcomes research, with some investigators suggesting that 6 to 8 sessions are necessary to yield positive initial effects and upward of 15 to 20 sessions for longer term, sustainable therapeutic effects. This dose effect may not be applicable to counseling services with primarily informational or emotional/supportive functions. Because many patients cease attendance to psychotherapy sessions after one or a few sessions, most interventions of this type cannot be accurately evaluated by the referring provider. Long-term therapy should also be evaluated for effectiveness at regular periods.

REFERENCES

1. American Psychiatric Association. *Diagnostic and Statistical Manual of Mental Disorders*. 5th ed. Arlington, VA: American Psychiatric Association; 2013.
2. World Health Organization. *The ICD-10 Classification of Mental and Behavioural Disorders: Clinical Descriptions and Diagnostic Guidelines*. Geneva, Switzerland: World Health Organization; 1992.

ADDITIONAL READING

- Bortolotti B, Menchetti M, Bellini F, et al. Psychological interventions for major depression in primary care: a meta-analytic review of randomized controlled trials. *Gen Hosp Psychiatry*. 2008;30(4): 293–302.
- Eddy KT, Dutra L, Bradley R, et al. A multidimensional meta-analysis of psychotherapy and pharmacotherapy for obsessive-compulsive disorder. *Clin Psychol Rev*. 2004;24(8):1011–1030.
- Furukawa TA, Watanabe N, Churchill R. Combined psychotherapy plus antidepressants for panic disorder with or without agoraphobia. *Cochrane Database Syst Rev*. 2007;(1):CD004364.
- Hunot V, Churchill R, Silva de Lima M, et al. Psychological therapies for generalised anxiety disorder. *Cochrane Database Syst Rev*. 2007;(1):CD001848.

 CODES

ICD10

- Z71.9 Counseling, unspecified
- Z71.89 Other specified counseling
- Z63.9 Problem related to primary support group, unspecified

CLINICAL PEARLS

- Combined medication and psychotherapeutic treatments in moderate to severe psychological dysfunction are most likely to render positive short-term results and increase the likelihood such effects can be sustained over time.
- Relapse is common over time and/or as treatments are discontinued.
- Children <10 years may benefit significantly from counseling or psychotherapy alone for symptom relief.
- Older children and those with more severe symptoms typically require psychopharmacologic options in concert with counseling or verbal therapy approaches.

CROHN DISEASE

Eric J. Mao, MD • Samir A. Shah, MD, FACG, FASGE, AGAF

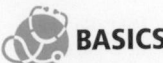

BASICS

DESCRIPTION
A chronic, relapsing inflammatory GI tract disorder, most commonly involving the terminal ileum (80%)

- Hallmark features of Crohn disease (CD)
  - Transmural inflammation resulting in fibrotic, strictures, fistulae, fissures, or abscesses
  - Noncaseating granulomas (30%)
  - Skip lesions: segmental disease distribution interspersed with normal mucosa; can also be continuous, mimicking ulcerative colitis (UC)
  - Diverse presentations: ileitis (1/3), ileocolitis (1/3); isolated colitis (1/3)
- Early disease
  - Ulcerations: focal lesions with surrounding edema, resembling aphthous ulcers
  - Perianal disease (pain, anal fissures, perirectal abscess) may precede intestinal disease.
  - May present as wasting illness or anorexia
- Developed disease
  - Mucosal cobblestoning; luminal stenosis; creeping fat; fissures between mucosal folds result in strictures or fistulae.

EPIDEMIOLOGY
Incidence
- 8 to 15 cases per 100,000 North American adults; incidence rising in North America and Western Europe
- Bimodal age distribution: Predominant age is 15 to 25 years, with a second smaller peak at 50 to 70 years.
- Women slightly more affected than men; increased incidence in northern climates
- Increased risk in whites versus nonwhites: 2- to 5-fold
- Increased risk in Ashkenazi Jews: 3- to 5-fold

Prevalence
U.S. adults: 100 to 200 cases per 100,000

ETIOLOGY AND PATHOPHYSIOLOGY
- General: Clinical manifestations result from activation of inflammatory cells and subsequent tissue injury.
- Mechanism of diarrhea: excess fluid secretion and impaired absorption; bile salt malabsorption in inflamed ileum; steatorrhea; bacterial overgrowth
- Multifactorial: Genetics, environmental triggers, commensal microbial antigens, and immunologic abnormalities result in inflammation and tissue injury.

Genetics
- 15% of CD patients have a first-degree relative with inflammatory bowel disease (IBD); first-degree relative of an IBD patient has 3- to 30-fold increased risk of developing IBD by age 28 years; >200 genes associated with IBD; >71 CD genes
- Mutations in susceptibility loci
  - Ileal CD: IBD1 gene, NOD2
  - Early-onset CD (age ≤15 years): 5q31–33 (IBD5), 21q22, and 20q13
  - Extraintestinal manifestations of CD: mutations in HLA-A2, HLA-DR1, HLA-DQw5
  - Others: IL-10, IL-23 receptors, ATG16L1, IRGM
- Associated genetic syndromes: Turner and Hermansky-Pudlak syndromes, glycogen storage disease type 1b

RISK FACTORS
- Environmental factors
  - Cigarette smoking doubles the risk of CD; tobacco cessation reduces flares and relapses.

- Dietary factors: higher incidence if diet high in refined sugars, animal fat, protein (meat, fish)
- *Salmonella* or *Campylobacter* increases risk of developing IBD.
- *Clostridium difficile* infection may trigger flare and make treatment more difficult.
- Immunologic abnormalities: an aggressive immune response against commensal enteric bacteria
  - Tumor necrosis factor (TNF): upregulation of inflammatory Th1 cytokines

COMMONLY ASSOCIATED CONDITIONS
- Extraintestinal manifestations
  - Arthritis (20%): seronegative, small and large joints; ankylosing spondylitis (AS) and sacroiliitis (SI)
  - Skin disorders (10%): erythema nodosum, pyoderma gangrenosum, psoriasis
  - Ocular disease (5%): uveitis, iritis, episcleritis
  - Kidney stones: calcium oxalate stones (from steatorrhea and diarrhea) or uric acid stones (from dehydration and metabolic acidosis)
  - Fat-soluble vitamin deficiency (A, D, E, K)
  - Osteopenia and osteoporosis; hypocalcemia
  - Hypercoagulability: venous thromboembolism prophylaxis essential in hospitalized patients
  - Gallstones: cholesterol stones resulting from impaired bile acid reabsorption
  - Primary sclerosing cholangitis (5%): more common in men with UC; asymptomatic, elevated alkaline phosphatase as marker; increased colon cancer risk (annual colonoscopy)
  - Autoimmune hemolytic anemia
- Conditions associated with increased disease activity
  - Peripheral arthropathy (not SI and AS)
  - Episcleritis (not uveitis)
  - SI, AS, and uveitis are associated with HLA-B27.
  - Oral aphthous ulcers and erythema nodosum
  - Other complications: GI bleed, toxic megacolon, bowel perforation, peritonitis, malignancy, rectovaginal fistula

DIAGNOSIS

HISTORY
Hallmarks: fatigue, fever, weight loss, prolonged diarrhea, perianal disease, crampy abdominal pain (+/− bleeding). Children may present with failure to thrive.

- Factors exacerbating CD: concurrent infection, smoking, NSAIDs, antibiotics, stress

PHYSICAL EXAM
Presentation varies with location of disease.
- General: signs of sepsis/disease activity (fever, tachycardia, hypotension) or wasting/malnutrition
- Abdominal: focal or diffuse tenderness, distension, rebound/guarding, rectal bleeding, palpable mass
- Perianal: fistulae, fissures
- Skin: erythema nodosum; psoriasis

DIFFERENTIAL DIAGNOSIS
- Acute, severe abdominal pain: perforated viscus, pancreatitis, appendicitis, diverticulitis, bowel obstruction, kidney stones, ovarian torsion
- Chronic diarrhea with crampy pain (colitis like): UC, radiation colitis, infection, drugs, ischemia, microscopic colitis, IBD, celiac disease, malignancy (lymphoma, carcinoma), carcinoid
- Wasting illness: malabsorption, malignancy

DIAGNOSTIC TESTS & INTERPRETATION
Initial Tests (lab, imaging)
- CBC, serum chemistries, LFTs, erythrocyte sedimentation rate, C-reactive protein, serum iron, vitamin B_{12}, vitamin D-25 OH, stool calprotectin
- If diarrhea, stool specimen for routine culture, *C. difficile*, and ova and parasites
- With severe flares, KUB to rule out toxic megacolon
- Ileocolonoscopy provides the greatest diagnostic sensitivity and specificity; biopsy normal and abnormal mucosa (1)[C]
- Upper endoscopy for patients with upper GI signs or symptoms (1)[C]
  - Signs of upper GI CD: antral narrowing, segmental stricturing, inflammatory mucosa
- Small bowel: sensitivity of CT or magnetic resonance enterography (MRE) better than small bowel follow through. MRE has no radiation exposure (important in younger patients). Capsule endoscopy allows small bowel visualization but no biopsy (2)[A].
  - Signs of small bowel disease: narrowed lumen with nodularity (string sign); cobblestone appearance, fistula and abscess formation, bowel loop separation (transmural inflammation)
- Perianal disease: endoscopic ultrasound (EUS) or MRI pelvis with exam under anesthesia
- Contraindications to endoscopy: perforated viscus, recent myocardial infarction, severe diverticulitis, toxic megacolon, or intolerance of bowel preparation
- In most cases, unprepared limited sigmoidoscopy allows adequate visualization to assess severity, extent, aspirate stool for *C. difficile*, obtain biopsies to assess histologic severity, and exclude other disorders (e.g., cytomegalovirus).

Follow-Up Tests & Special Considerations
Evidence of complications
- Stricture: obstructive signs—nausea, vomiting, pain, weight loss, diarrhea, or inability to pass gas/feces
- Abscess/phlegmon: localized abdominal peritonitis with fever and abdominal pain; diffuse peritonitis suggests perforation or abscess rupture (may be masked by steroids, opiates).
- Fistula:
  - Enteroenteric: asymptomatic or a palpable, commonly indolent, abdominal mass
  - Enterovesical: pneumaturia, recurrent UTI
  - Retroperitoneal: psoas abscess, ureteral obstruction
  - Enterovaginal: vaginal passage of gas or feces; clear, nonfeculent drainage from ileal fistula (may be misdiagnosed as primary vaginal infection)

Diagnostic Procedures/Other
How to distinguish CD from UC
- CD: small bowel disease, rectal sparing; skip lesions; granulomas, perianal disease, and/or fistulae; no gross bleeding: RLQ pain is common.
- UC: continuous involvement including the rectum; loss of vascularity, friable tissue; LLQ pain; typically only affects colon; rectal bleeding common

ALERT
CD can mimic UC with continuous bowel involvement; 10–15% of cases are difficult to differentiate.

TREATMENT

- Disease severity: Crohn Disease Activity Index (CDAI)
  - Asymptomatic: spontaneous, after medical/surgical intervention, or while on steroids (CDAI <150)
  - Mild to moderate CD: ambulatory patients able to tolerate PO intake without dehydration, obstruction, or >10% weight loss; no abdominal tenderness, toxicity, or mass (CDAI 150 to 220)
  - Moderate to severe CD: patients who have failed initial treatment or who continue to have mild symptoms such as fever, weight loss, and abdominal pain (CDAI 220 to 450)
  - Severe: persistent symptoms despite therapy with glucocorticoids and/or biologics or fulminant disease (peritonitis, cachexia, intestinal obstruction, abscess) (CDAI >450)
  - Step-up approach: Begin treatment with milder therapy (5-ASA, antibiotics) followed by more aggressive agents (steroids, immunomodulators, anti-TNF agents) as needed.
  - Top-down approach: early management with immunomodulators and/or anti-TNF agents before patients receive steroids, become steroid dependent, or require surgery

GENERAL MEASURES

- Oral lesions: triamcinolone acetonide in benzocaine and carboxymethyl cellulose or topical sucralfate for aphthous ulcers, cheilitis, and/or granulomatous sialadenitis
- Gastroduodenal CD: no clinical trials; slow-release mesalamine for superficial disease. Case reports show success of anti-TNF therapies; symptomatic relief possible from proton pump inhibitors, H_2 receptor blockers, and/or sucralfate
- Ileitis: Supplemental fat-soluble vitamins, iron, vitamin B_{12}, folate, and calcium may be necessary.
- Treatment toxicity: pancreatitis, bone marrow toxicity, lymphoma, nonmelanoma skin cancer, infections (TB, histoplasmosis, others), malignancy

MEDICATION

First Line

- Asymptomatic with minimal endoscopic disease: observation alone
- Mild CD
  - 5-Aminosalicylates have minimal role in CD management; used for colonic CD without deep ulcerations or fibrostenosing disease
  - Antibiotics not more effective than placebo (1)[C]
  - Glucocorticoid therapy: controlled ileal release budesonide (9 mg/day for 8 to 16 weeks and then discontinued over 2- to 4-week taper) for distal ileum and/or right colon involvement (3)[A]
  - Adjunctive therapy: antidiarrheals (loperamide); bile acid–binding resin (cholestyramine 4 to 12 g/day); probiotics (either alone or in combination may reduce inflammation/symptoms in acute CD)
  - Induction/maintenance: 5-ASA is not recommended (3)[C]. Controlled ileal release budesonide, 9 mg/day, is effective for induction and maintenance for up to 4 months (1)[C].
- Moderate to severe CD
  - Induction: anti-TNF as initial induction agent to avoid corticosteroids; controlled-release budesonide (for isolated, moderate ileitis) or prednisone 40 to 60 mg/day for short-term to alleviate symptoms (1)[C]
  - Maintenance: no role for mesalamine. If steroids required for induction, use biologic (anti-TNF agent) (3)[B] or immunomodulator (3)[B] for maintenance.
  - Except for budesonide, do not use steroids for maintenance (1)[A].

- Severe CD: immunomodulators, anti-TNF ± steroids
  - Thiopurines: azathioprine or 6-mercaptopurine (6MP) for maintenance but not induction (1)[C]: Check thiopurine methyltransferase (TPMT) and LFTs prior to initiation; CBC/LFTs q2–3mo
  - Methotrexate: effective for induction and maintenance of steroid-dependent CD (1)[C]
    ○ Folic acid 1 mg/day; follow LFT, CBC.
  - Anti-TNF: infliximab, adalimumab, certolizumab pegol for induction and maintenance of remission (1)[A]
    ○ Check for evidence of TB and HBV infection prior to initiation of anti-TNF therapy.
    ○ Avoid live vaccines.
    ○ Monitoring: CBC, LFT, drug levels
- Combination therapy: anti-TNF and immunomodulator
  - Immunomodulator can be added as adjunctive therapy or to reduce immunogenicity against biologic.
  - Azathioprine + infliximab is more effective than either alone if no previous therapy with either.
  - Rare complication: hepatosplenic T-cell lymphoma (fatal, seen in young males) with thiopurines only
- Antiadhesion molecules: prevent inflammatory cells from entering GI tract
  - Vedolizumab: gut-specific, used in anti-TNF failures or anti-TNF naïve patients as induction and maintenance; given IV, no risk of progressive multifocal leukoencephalopathy (PML) (1)[B].
  - Natalizumab: non–gut-specific, used for induction and maintenance (1)[B]; PML risk (1/1,000); can minimize risk by testing for John Cunningham (JC) virus antibody; avoid risk of PML now with vedolizumab.
- Anti–IL-12 and anti–IL-23 monoclonal antibody: ustekinumab efficacious in induction and maintenance of remission in anti-TNF naïve and anti-TNF failures. Excellent safety profile; monitor CBC and LFTs.
- Therapeutic drug monitoring: Optimize biologics to avoid side effects. Measure trough levels of drug, and if drug not present, assess for antibody to the drug. If low or absent drug level and no antibodies, increase dose or frequency. If no drugs and high antibody levels, switch agents. If drug present and no antibodies, switch treatment if active disease (4)[C].
- New/investigational therapies:
  - JAK1 kinase selective inhibitor, anti–IL-23 agents, and sphingosine-1-phosphate receptor modulator

 ONGOING CARE

FOLLOW-UP RECOMMENDATIONS

Patient Monitoring

Vaccinations

- Check titers; avoid live vaccines (MMR, varicella, Zostavax) in patients on immunosuppressive therapy (steroids, 6MP, azathioprine, methotrexate, or biologics).
- Regardless of immunosuppression: HPV, influenza, pneumococcal, meningococcal, hepatitis A, B; Tdap; Shingrix for those 50 years or older
- Cancer prevention
  - Colonoscopy with targeted biopsies every 1 to 3 years after 8 to 10 years of CD with colonic involvement; consider chromoendoscopy if available (5)[C].
  - Annual PAP smears if immunocompromised
  - Annual skin exam if immunocompromised

- Bone health
  - Calcium and vitamin D supplementation with each course of corticosteroids or if vitamin D deficient
  - Bone density assessment if previous steroid use, maternal history of osteoporosis, malnourished, amenorrheic, postmenopausal

PATIENT EDUCATION

Crohn and Colitis Foundation: (800) 932-2423; http://www.crohnscolitisfoundation.org

COMPLICATIONS

- Peritonitis: bowel rest and antibiotic therapy (7 to 10 days parenteral antibiotics, followed by 2- to 4-week course of PO ciprofloxacin and metronidazole); surgery as indicated
  - Consider holding steroids which masks sepsis.
- Abscess: antibiotics, percutaneous drainage, or surgery with resection of affected segments
- Small bowel obstruction: IV hydration, nasogastric (NG) tube for decompression, total parenteral nutrition (TPN) for malnutrition, resolution typically in 24 to 48 hours; surgery for nonresponders

REFERENCES

1. Lichtenstein GR, Loftus EV, Isaacs KL, et al. ACG clinical guideline: management of Crohn's disease in adults. *Am J Gastroenterol*. 2018;113(4):481–517.
2. Baumgart DC, Sandborn WJ. Crohn's disease. *Lancet*. 2012;380(9853):1590–1605.
3. Talley NJ, Abreu MT, Achkar JP, et al; for American College of Gastroenterology IBD Task Force. An evidence-based systematic review on medical therapies for inflammatory bowel disease. *Am J Gastroenterol*. 2011;106(Suppl 1):S2–S26.
4. Feuerstein JD, Nguyen GC, Kupfer SS, et al. American Gastroenterological Association Institute guideline on therapeutic drug monitoring in inflammatory bowel disease. *Gastroenterology*. 2017;153(3):827–834.
5. Laine L, Kaltenbach T, Barkun A, et al. SCENIC international consensus statement on surveillance and management of dysplasia in inflammatory bowel disease. *Gastroenterology*. 2015;148(3): 639.e28–651.e28.

 CODES

ICD10

- K50.919 Crohn's disease, unspecified, with unspecified complications
- K50.00 Crohn's disease of small intestine without complications
- K50.10 Crohn's disease of large intestine without complications

CLINICAL PEARLS

- Cigarette smoking doubles the risk of CD; tobacco cessation reduces flares and need for surgery.
- MRE allows assessment of luminal and extraluminal CD without radiation exposure.
- Assess for TB and HBV infection prior to initiating anti-TNF therapy.
- Test for *C. difficile* infection when evaluating diarrhea in all CD patients.
- Hospitalized CD patients require deep vein thrombosis prophylaxis.
- Anti-TNF therapy effective in delaying or preventing postoperative recurrence in CD

CROUP (LARYNGOTRACHEOBRONCHITIS)

Ryan Paul B. Urbi, MD • Olga L. Nunez, MD • Mark T. Nadeau, MD, MBA

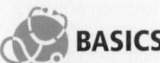 **BASICS**

DESCRIPTION

- Croup is a subacute viral illness frequently preceded by 24 to 72 hours of symptoms such as nonspecific cough, coryza, rhinorrhea, fever with an abrupt onset of seal-like barking cough, and inspiratory stridor. Symptoms are worse at night and can rapidly fluctuate depending on whether the child is calm or agitated.
- The term *croup* is used to refer to viral laryngo-tracheitis or laryngotracheobronchitis (LTB). It is sometimes used for LTB with pneumonitis, bacterial tracheitis, or spasmodic croup.
- Spasmodic croup is a noninfectious form with sudden resolution that is usually self-limiting; it is treated like croup and resolves with mist therapy at home.

EPIDEMIOLOGY

- Croup is the most common cause of upper airway obstruction or stridor in children.
- Predominant age
  - Ranges from 6 months to 6 years
  - Most commonly seen in children among 6 months to 3 years with a peak around the 2nd year of life
- Predominant sex: male > female (1.5:1)
- Timing
  - Possible during any time of year but is most common during the fall and winter
  - Human parainfluenza 1 and respiratory syncytial virus (RSV) are the most common viral causes.

Incidence

- Six cases per year per 100 children <6 years old
- 1.5–6% of cases require hospitalization.
- 2–6% of those require intubation. 60% of barking cough resolved within 48 hours, and only 2% have symptoms persisting for longer than 5 nights.

ETIOLOGY AND PATHOPHYSIOLOGY

- Subglottic region/larynx is entirely encircled by the cricoid cartilage.
- Inflammatory edema and subglottic mucus production decrease airway radius.
- Small children have small airways with more compliant walls.
- Negative-pressure inspiration pulls airway walls closer together.
- The anatomically small airway is more susceptible to compromise and narrowing caused by the combined edema, mucus secretions, and increased compliance. Small decrease in airway radius causes significant increase in resistance (Poiseuille law: resistance proportional to $1/\text{radius}^4$).
- Typically caused by viruses that initially infect oro-pharyngeal mucosa and then migrate inferiorly
- Parainfluenza virus
  - Most common pathogen: 75% of cases
  - Type 1 is the most common, causing 18% of all cases of croup.
  - Types 2, 3, and 4 are also common.
  - Type 3 may cause a particularly severe illness.
- Other viruses: RSV, paramyxovirus, influenza virus type A or B, adenovirus, rhinovirus, enteroviruses (coxsackie and echo), reovirus, measles virus where vaccination not common, and metapneumovirus
- *Haemophilus influenzae* type B now rare with routine immunization
- May have bacterial cause: *Mycoplasma pneumoniae* has been reported.

GENERAL PREVENTION

There is not a specific vaccine for croup, but seasonal influenza shots may contribute to decreased risk.

COMMONLY ASSOCIATED CONDITIONS

- If recurrent (>2 episodes in a year) or during first 90 days of life, consider host factors.
- Underlying anatomic abnormality (e.g., subglottic stenosis)
  - In one study, found to be present in 59% of children with recurrent croup
- Paradoxical vocal cord dysfunction
- Gastroesophageal reflux disease
- Neonatal intubation

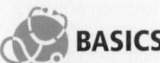 **DIAGNOSIS**

- Croup is a clinical diagnosis; lab tests and imaging serve only ancillary purposes. Most children who present with acute onset of barky cough, inspiratory stridor, hoarseness, and chest wall indrawing have croup.
- Classic "seal-like" barking, spasmodic cough
- May have biphasic stridor
- Low to moderate grade fever
- Upper respiratory infection prodrome lasting 1 to 7 days
- Severity usually is determined by clinical observation for signs of respiratory effort: nasal flaring, retractions, tripoding, sniffing position, abdominal breathing, and tachypnea; later symptoms: hypoxia/cyanosis or fatigue
- Westley croup severity score is most useful for research purposes.
- Westley croup score looks at five clinical features: level of consciousness, cyanosis, stridor, air entry, and retractions (≤2 mild; 3 to 7 moderate; ≥8 severe).
  - Level of consciousness: normal, including sleep = 0; disoriented = 5
  - Cyanosis: none = 0; with agitation = 4; at rest = 5
  - Stridor: none = 0; with agitation = 1; at rest = 2
  - Air entry: normal = 0; decreased = 1; markedly decreased = 2
  - Retractions: none = 0; mild = 1; moderate = 2; severe = 2
- No change in stridor with positioning
- Nontender larynx
- Inflamed subglottic region with normal-appearing supraglottic region
- Differentiate from epiglottitis: non–toxic-appearing, normal voice, no drooling, is coughing (1).

PHYSICAL EXAM

Pulse oximetry often is normal because there is no disturbance of alveolar gas exchange.

- Overall appearance: Is the child comfortable or struggling?
- Work of breathing: labored or comfortable?
- Sound of breathing and voice: hoarse, stridor, inspiratory wheezing, short sentences?
- Observed/subjective tidal volume: sufficient for child's size?
  - Assessment of the severity of croup
    ○ Mild (0 to 2 Westley): occasional barking cough; no audible stridor at rest, and either mild or no suprasternal or intercostal retractions

○ Moderate (3 to 5 Westley): frequent A cough, easily audible stridor at rest, and suprasternal and sternal retractions at rest but little or no agitation
○ Severe (6 to 11 Westley): frequent barking cough, prominent inspiratory and, occasionally, expiratory stridor, marked sternal retractions, and agitation and distress
○ Impending respiratory failure (12 to 17 Westley): barking cough (often not prominent), audible stridor at rest (occasionally hard to hear), sternal retractions (may not be marked), lethargy or decreased level of consciousness, and often dusky appearance in the absence of supplemental oxygen (2)

ALERT

Decreased breath sounds and respiratory effort may indicate the child is progressing into respiratory failure and less able to mount an effort to move air. Even though there may be less obvious sign of distress, clinicians should not miss the clinically deteriorating patient.

DIFFERENTIAL DIAGNOSIS

In order of decreasing frequency:

- Upper respiratory infection, including classic LTB
- Foreign body aspiration: toddler to 4 years of age; often requires high index of suspicion
- Bacterial tracheitis; similar to epiglottitis, acute septic onset
- Retropharyngeal or peritonsillar abscess: similar septic appearance with dysphonia
- Allergic reaction (acute angioneurotic edema) includes spasmodic croup with classic nocturnal exacerbations.
- Epiglottitis: associated with rapid onset, high fever, dysphonia, drooling, and prototypical posture of extended chin and leaning forward; *H. influenzae* being replaced by strep and staph organisms
- Subglottic stenosis
- Trauma
- Airway anomalies (e.g., tracheo-/laryngomalacia)
- Other anatomic obstructions: subglottic hemangioma, subglottic cyst

DIAGNOSTIC TESTS & INTERPRETATION

- LTB, LTBP, and LT are clinical diagnosis and usually do not require confirmatory testing.
- If imaging were to be done, posteroanterior and lateral neck films will show funnel-shaped subglottic region with normal epiglottis: "steeple," "hourglass," or "pencil point" sign (present in 40–60% of children with LTB).
- CT may be more sensitive for defining obstruction in an unclear case.
- Patient should be monitored during imaging, airway obstruction may occur rapidly.
- Also evaluate radiographs for:
  - Retropharyngeal abscess: dimensions of the posterior pharynx (should be same AP width as a contingent vertebral body)
  - Epiglottitis: thumb sign: appearance of a thumb pointing posteriorly, respectively
- Blood work may not be required. WBC counts may be mildly elevated with a predominance of lympho-cytes; an elevated WBC shift to the left (bandemia) would suggest etiology other than LTB, most likely bacterial. Examples of this would be epiglottitis, bacterial tracheitis, and retropharyngeal abscess.

- Microbiologic studies might be used to identify viral strains and specific bacteriologic species in severe presentations or to track epidemiology. *H. influenzae* and diphtheria as etiologic agents are rarely seen in industrialized countries in the pharynx as the result of immunization practices.
- Rapid antigen or viral culture tests are available in many centers.
  - Guide isolation precautions, not management.

Test Interpretation
- Inflammatory reaction of respiratory mucosa
- Loss of epithelial cells
- Thick mucoid secretions

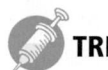 **TREATMENT**

GENERAL MEASURES
- Symptomatic treatment
- Minimize lab tests, imaging, and procedures that upset the child; agitation worsens tachypnea and can be more detrimental than accepting a clinical diagnosis.
- ECG monitoring and pulse oximetry
- Pulse oximetry not as sensitive as frequent clinical checks in identifying worsening disease

MEDICATION
First Line
- Well established in the literature; the cornerstones of treatment are immediate nebulized epinephrine and oral dexamethasone.
- Racemic or L-epinephrine (equal efficacy and side effect profiles; L-epinephrine is used for most other hospital purposes and is less expensive) (2)[A].
  - Reserved for more severe cases with stridor at rest
  - Racemic epinephrine: 0.05 mL/kg/dose (max 0.5 mL) of 2.25% solution nebulized in normal saline to total volume of 3 mL
  - L-epinephrine: 0.5 mL/kg/dose (max 5 mL) of a 1:1,000 dilution nebulized
  - Onset in 1 to 5 minutes, duration of 2 hours
  - Repeat as necessary if side effects are tolerated.
  - Observe child for 2 hours to ensure no recurrence after epinephrine wears off.
- Corticosteroids
  - Dexamethasone (least expensive, easiest), 0.15 to 0.60 mg/kg; higher doses have been traditional care, but studies have shown 0.15 mg/kg has equal efficacy (3)[B]. Single dose; IV/IM/PO has proven equal efficacy.
  - Randomized controlled trials show this begins to improve symptoms within 30 minutes (4)[A]; full effect by 4 hours
  - Other steroids (betamethasone, budesonide (5)[A], prednisolone) are beneficial; there may be minimal superiority of dexamethasone; also, dexamethasone carries benefit of single-dose administration (6)[A].
- Antibiotics are not indicated because this is a viral illness.
- Oxygen as needed
- Humidified air shows no clinical benefit.

Second Line
Oseltamivir for influenza A

SURGERY/OTHER PROCEDURES
Intubation rarely is required; tube 0.5 to 1.0 mm smaller than normal
- After trial of medical management, intubation may be required for fatigue caused by work of breathing or obstruction.

ADMISSION, INPATIENT, AND NURSING CONSIDERATIONS
- Outpatient care in mild cases
- Admit patients who do not respond to therapy or have recurrent stridor at rest after epinephrine wears off. Also admit those who have oxygen requirement, pneumonia, or other serious conditions.
- In most cases, observation in the ED after medical management is sufficient.
- Discharge criteria
  - >2 hours since last epinephrine
  - No stridor at rest, no difficulty breathing
  - Child able to tolerate liquids PO
  - No underlying medical condition
  - Caretakers able to assess changes to clinical picture and reaccess medical care

 ONGOING CARE

FOLLOW-UP RECOMMENDATIONS
Patient Monitoring
Most children with croup do not require specific follow-up; should consider PCP follow-up if patient had stridor for >1 week.

DIET
- Liquid diet is most comfortable for the patient and better tolerated.
- Cold liquids are often more soothing.
- Frequent small feedings with increased fluids for mild cases

PATIENT EDUCATION
- Croup is usually a self-limited and mild disease, but some children will need more intense medical care in the hospital.
- Generally, be calming and keep your child comfortable. Keep the child cool by dressing lightly and use antipyretics if they are febrile.
- Keep the child well hydrated with ample cool liquids or popsicles.
- Keep the patient quiet; crying may exacerbate symptoms.
- Educate parents about when to seek emergency care if symptoms worsen.
- Provide emotional support and reassurance for the patient.
- Absolute need for medical care:
  - Respiratory distress; rapid breathing; working hard to breathe; prominent chest or neck muscles with each breath
  - The child becomes restless or agitated.
  - The child looks unusually pale.
  - High temperature (fever) lasts longer than 1 to 2 days.
- Emergency ambulance if the child is:
  - Blue (cyanosis)
  - Lethargic
  - Struggling to breathe
  - Drooling and unable to swallow

PROGNOSIS
- Prognosis is generally good. The few cases that are severe respond to intensive respiratory management.
- Recurrence is rare in viral-mediated disease.
- If croup recurs, consider an anatomic, allergic, or obstructive etiology.

COMPLICATIONS
- Rare
- Subglottic stenosis in intubated patients
- Bacterial tracheitis
- Cardiopulmonary arrest
- Pneumonia

REFERENCES
1. Abedi GR, Prill MM, Langley GE, et al. Estimates of parainfluenza virus-associated hospitalizations and cost among children aged less than 5 years in the United States, 1998–2010. *J Pediatric Infect Dis Soc.* 2016;5(1):7–13.
2. Bjornson CL, Johnson DW. Croup in children. *CMAJ.* 2013;185(15):1317–1323.
3. Cherry JD. Clinical practice. Croup. *N Engl J Med.* 2008;358(4):384–391.
4. Gardner HG, Powell KR, Roden VJ, et al. The evaluation of racemic epinephrine in the treatment of infectious croup. *Pediatrics.* 1973;52(1):52–55.
5. Narayan S, Funkhouser E. Inpatient hospitalizations for croup. *Hosp Pediatr.* 2014;4(2):88–92.
6. Toward Optimized Practice Working Group for Croup. *Diagnosis and Management of Croup.* Edmonton, AB: Toward Optimized Practice Working Group for Croup; 2008. http://www.topalbertadoctors.org. Accessed December 14, 2016.

ADDITIONAL READING
Zoorob R, Sidani M, Murray J. Croup: an overview. *Am Fam Physician.* 2011;83(9):1067–1073.

 CODES

ICD10
- J05.0 Acute obstructive laryngitis [croup]
- J20.9 Acute bronchitis, unspecified
- J38.5 Laryngeal spasm

CLINICAL PEARLS
- LT and LTB outbreaks are most common in fall and winter time for population aged 6 months to 3 years. Symptoms often occur at night.
- Recurrent episodes should be followed up with a search for anatomic or allergic etiology.
- Foundation of treatment is oxygen, oral/IM steroids, and nebulized epinephrine.
- Consider other diagnoses in acute presentations with toxic appearance: epiglottitis, abscess, bacterial tracheitis.
- Be aware of severity should the child become less noisy; less air movement can be sign of respiratory failure.
- Croup is a clinical diagnosis, thus medical management and stabilization of the patient take priority over lab testing or radiographic images.

CRYPTORCHIDISM
Pamela Ellsworth, MD

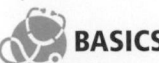 BASICS

DESCRIPTION
- Incomplete or improper descent of one or both testicles; also called *undescended testes* (1)
- Normally, descent is in the 7th to 8th month of gestation. The cryptorchid testis may be palpable or nonpalpable.
- Types of cryptorchidism
  - Abdominal: located inside the internal ring
  - Canalicular: located between the internal and external rings
  - Ectopic: located outside the normal path of testicular descent from abdominal cavity to scrotum; may be ectopic to perineum, femoral canal, superficial inguinal pouch (most common), suprapubic area, or opposite hemiscrotum
  - Retractile: fully descended testis that moves freely between the scrotum and the groin
  - Iatrogenic: Previously descended testis becomes undescended secondary to scar tissue after inguinal surgery, such as an inguinal hernia repair or hydrocelectomy.
  - Also may be referred to as palpable versus nonpalpable (1)
- System(s) affected: reproductive
- Synonym(s): undescended testes (UDT)

EPIDEMIOLOGY
Incidence
- Predominant age: premature newborns
- Predominant sex: male only

Prevalence
- In the United States, cryptorchidism occurs in 1–3% of full-term and 15–30% of premature newborn males (2).
- Spontaneous testicular descent occurs by age 1 to 3 months in 50–70% of full-term males with cryptorchidism.
- Descent at 6 to 9 months of age is rare (1).

ETIOLOGY AND PATHOPHYSIOLOGY
- Not fully known
- May involve alterations in
  - Mechanical factors (gubernaculum, length of vas deferens and testicular vessels, groin anatomy, epididymis, cremasteric muscles, and abdominal pressure), hormonal factors (gonadotropin, testosterone, dihydrotestosterone, and müllerian-inhibiting substance [MIS]), and neural factors (ilioinguinal nerve and genitofemoral nerve)
  - Major regulators of testicular descent from intra-abdominal location into the bottom of the scrotum are the Leydig cell–derived hormones, testosterone, and insulin-like growth factor 3 (IGF-3).
  - Mutations in the gene for IGF-3 and in the androgen receptor gene have been evaluated as possible causes of cryptorchidism as well as chromosomal alterations (1).
  - Environmental factors acting as endocrine disruptors of testicular descent also may contribute to the etiology of cryptorchidism.
- Risk of ascent may be as high as 32% in retractile testis.

Genetics
Occurrence of UDT in siblings as well as fathers suggests a genetic etiology.

RISK FACTORS
- Family history of cryptorchidism: highest risk if brother had UDT, followed by uncle and then father
- Low birth weight, prematurity, and small for gestational age are associated with a substantial increase in incidence of cryptorchidism (1). Retractile testes are at increased risk for ascent.

COMMONLY ASSOCIATED CONDITIONS
- Inguinal hernia/hydrocele
- Abnormalities of vas deferens and epididymis
- Intersex abnormalities
- Hypogonadotropic hypogonadism
- Germinal cell aplasia
- Prune-belly syndrome
- Meningomyelocele
- Hypospadias
- Wilms tumor
- Prader-Willi syndrome
- Kallmann syndrome
- Cystic fibrosis

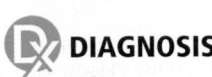 DIAGNOSIS

HISTORY
- ≥1 testicles in a site other than the scrotum
- May be an isolated defect or associated with other congenital anomalies

PHYSICAL EXAM
- Performed with warm hands, with child in sitting, standing, and squatting position
- A Valsalva maneuver and applied pressure to lower abdomen may help to identify the testes, especially a gliding testis.
- Failure to palpate a testis after repeated exams suggests an intra-abdominal or atrophic testis.
- An enlarged contralateral testis in the presence of a nonpalpable testis suggests testicular atrophy/absence.
- Testes should be palpated for quality and position at each recommended well-child visit (1)[B].

DIFFERENTIAL DIAGNOSIS
- Retractile testis (hypermobile testis), a normally descended testis that ascends into the inguinal canal because of an active cremasteric reflex (more common in males 4 to 6 years of age)
- Atrophic testis: may occur as a result of neonatal torsion
- Vanished testis may be the result of a lack of development or in utero torsion.

DIAGNOSTIC TESTS & INTERPRETATION
Initial Tests (lab, imaging)
- In phenotypic male newborn with bilateral, nonpalpable UDTs, hormone levels are helpful to determine whether the testes are present and should be evaluated for possible disorder of sexual development (1)[A].
  - Luteinizing hormone (LH)
  - Follicle-stimulating hormone (FSH)
  - MIS
  - Testosterone
  - Serum electrolytes
  - Karyotype
- If bilateral nonpalpable testes and presenting >3 months of age, a human chorionic gonadotropin (hCG) stimulation test to determine presence or absence of testicular tissue (hCG 2,000 IU/day for 3 days, and check testosterone before and after stimulation) as well as gonadotropins—to say testes are absent—needs negative stimulation test and elevated gonadotropins (3).
- Ultrasound or other imaging modalities should not be performed in the evaluation of boys with cryptorchidism prior to referral to a specialist because they are rarely needed in decision making (1)[B].

Follow-Up Tests & Special Considerations
In newborns and children <6 months of age, periodic examination to determine if testis is palpable and descended prior to considering further intervention (1)

Pediatric Considerations
In the absence of spontaneous testicular descent by 6 months of age (gestational age adjusted), infant should be referred to appropriate specialist, and surgery should be performed within 1 year (1)[B].
- In children with retractile testes, examination should be performed at least yearly to rule out subsequent ascent (1)[B].
- In boys 11 to 30 months of age with unilateral nonpalpable UDT, if the contralateral descended testis is 19 to 20 mm or greater in length measured by caliper, there is a greater likelihood of a vanished/atrophic testis (4)[B].

Diagnostic Procedures/Other
Laparoscopy is useful in a child with nonpalpable cryptorchidism to confirm testicular absence or presence accurately and to determine the feasibility of performing a standard orchidopexy.

Test Interpretation
Higher incidence of carcinoma in UDT and alterations in spermatogenesis. Histologic changes occur by 1.5 years of age and include smaller seminiferous tubules, fewer spermatogonia, and more peritubular tissue (5).

TREATMENT

GENERAL MEASURES
- Rule out retractile testis.
- Appropriate health care: outpatient until surgery is performed
- Administration of chorionic gonadotropin may cause testicular descent in some boys. Reports of efficacy are inconsistent. American Urological Association (AUA) guidelines on cryptorchidism do not recommend use of hormonal therapy to induce testicular descent due to low response rate and lack of evidence for long-term efficacy (1).

MEDICATION
Medical therapy is not indicated in the United States per the AUA guidelines on cryptorchidism 2014 (1).

ISSUES FOR REFERRAL
- ≥1 testes not descended by 6 months age (1)[B]
- Bilateral nonpalpable UDT (1)
- Newly diagnosed cryptorchidism after 6 months of age (1)[B]

SURGERY/OTHER PROCEDURES
- Reasons to consider: avoids torsion, averts trauma, decreases but does not eliminate risk of malignancy, and prevents further alterations in spermatogenesis
- In the absence of spontaneous testicular descent by 6 months of age (gestational age–adjusted), surgery should be performed within 1 year (1)[B].
- Prepubertal orchiopexy decreases risk of testicular cancer and results in 2- to 6-fold reduction in relative risk compared to postpubertal orchiopexy (1).
- Laparoscopy/abdominal exploration is performed first if testis is nonpalpable.
- If palpable, an inguinal approach is usually performed. If low-lying, a single incision scrotal approach can also be considered but may increase the risk of hernia.

 ONGOING CARE

FOLLOW-UP RECOMMENDATIONS
- Initial follow-up within 1 month of surgery and periodically thereafter to assess testicular size/growth
- Patients with retractile testes should be examined at least annually to monitor for secondary ascent until testis is no longer retractile (1)[B].

Patient Monitoring
- Patients should be followed after surgery to evaluate testicular growth.
- Testicular tumors occur mainly during or after puberty; thus, these children should be taught self-examination when they are older.

DIET
No restrictions

PATIENT EDUCATION
Discuss with parents about causes, available treatments, and possible effects on patient's reproductive potential and also increased risk for testicular cancer and need for regular self-examination.

PROGNOSIS
- Disorder is usually corrected with medical or surgical therapy; however, there are possible lifelong consequences.
- If testicle is absent or orchiectomy is required, may consider placement of testicular prosthesis.
- Early orchidopexy may decrease risk of testicular damage and risk of malignancy.

COMPLICATIONS
- Paternity rates are similar to the general population for men with a unilateral UDT; however, are lower (33–65%) for men with bilateral UDT
- Abnormalities also have been identified in the contralateral descended testis, although less severe.

REFERENCES
1. Kolon TF, Herndon CDA, Baker LA, et al. Evaluation and treatment of cryptorchidism. https://www.auanet.org/education/guidelines/cryptorchidism.cfm. Accessed October 3, 2017.
2. Sijstermans K, Hack WW, Meijer RW, et al. The frequency of undescended testis from birth to adulthood: a review. *Int J Androl*. 2008;31(1):1–11.
3. Docimo SG, Silver RI, Cromie W. The undescended testicle: diagnosis and management. *Am Fam Physician*. 2000;62(9):2037–2044, 2047–2048.
4. Braga LH, Kim S, Farrokhyar F, et al. Is there an optimal contralateral testicular cut-off size that predicts monorchism in boys with nonpalpable testicles? *J Pediatr Urol*. 2014;10(4):693–698.
5. Park KH, Lee JH, Han JJ, et al. Histological evidences suggest recommending orchiopexy within the first year of life for children with unilateral inguinal cryptorchid testis. *Int J Urol*. 2007;14(7):616–621.

ADDITIONAL READING
- Agarwal PK, Diaz M, Elder JS. Retractile testis—is it really a normal variant? *J Urol*. 2006;175(4):1496–1499.
- Al-Mandil M, Khoury AE, El-Hout Y, et al. Potential complications with the prescrotal approach for the palpable undescended testis? A comparison of single prescrotal incision to the traditional inguinal approach. *J Urol*. 2008;180(2):686–689.
- Braga LH, Lorenzo AJ. Cryptorchidism: a practical review for all community healthcare providers. *Can Urol Assoc J*. 2017;11(1–2 Suppl 1):S26–S32.
- Cortes D, Thorup JM, Visfeldt J. Cryptorchidism: aspects of fertility and neoplasms. A study including data of 1,335 consecutive boys who underwent testicular biopsy simultaneously with surgery for cryptorchidism. *Horm Res*. 2001;55(1):21–27.
- Fantasia J, Aidlen J, Lathrop W, et al. Undescended testes: a clinical and surgical review. *Urol Nurs*. 2015;35(3):117–126.

- Foresta C, Zuccarello D, Garolla A, et al. Role of hormones, genes, and environment in human cryptorchidism. *Endocr Rev*. 2008;29(5):560–580.
- Hutson JM, Balic A, Nation T, et al. Cryptorchidism. *Semin Pediatr Surg*. 2010;19(3):215–224.
- Kollin C, Hesser U, Ritźen EM, et al. Testicular growth from birth to two years of age, and the effect of orchidopexy at age nine months: a randomized, controlled study. *Acta Paediatr*. 2006;95(3):318–324.
- Lee PA. Fertility after cryptorchidism: epidemiology and other outcome studies. *Urology*. 2005;66(2):427–431.
- Na SW, Kim SO, Hwang EC, et al. Single scrotal incision orchiopexy for children with palpable low-lying undescended testis: early outcome of a prospective randomized controlled study. *Korean J Urol*. 2011;52(9):637–641.
- Pettersson A, Richiardi L, Nordenskjold A, et al. Age at surgery for undescended testis and risk of testicular cancer. *N Engl J Med*. 2007;356(18):1835–1841.
- Walsh TJ, Dall'Era MA, Croughan MS, et al. Prepubertal orchiopexy for cryptorchidism may be associated with lower risk of testicular cancer. *J Urol*. 2007;178(4, Pt 1):1440–1446.
- Wilkerson ML, Bartone FF, Fox L, et al. Fertility potential: a comparison of intra-abdominal and intracanalicular testes by age groups in children. *Horm Res*. 2001;55(1):18–20.
- Wood HM, Elder JS. Cryptorchidism and testicular cancer: separating fact from fiction. *J Urol*. 2009;181(2):452–461.

 CODES

ICD10
- Q53.9 Undescended testicle, unspecified
- Q53.10 Unspecified undescended testicle, unilateral
- Q53.20 Undescended testicle, unspecified, bilateral

CLINICAL PEARLS
- If testicular descent does not occur by 6 months of age, it is unlikely to occur. Therefore, refer patients to a specialist if a testis has not descended by 6 months of age.
- Children with bilateral, nonpalpable UDT require laboratory evaluation to determine if viable testicular tissue is present and to rule out disorder of sexual differentiation.
- Radiologic imaging has no role in the initial evaluation of cryptorchidism.
- The risk of infertility is increased with bilateral UDT.

CUSHING DISEASE AND CUSHING SYNDROME

Linda Paniagua, MD

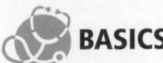

BASICS

DESCRIPTION

- Clinical abnormalities associated with chronic exposure to excessive amounts of cortisol (the major adrenocorticoid)
- Cushing syndrome is defined as excessive corticosteroid exposure from exogenous sources (medications) or endogenous sources (pituitary, adrenal, pulmonary, etc.) or tumor. Exogenous intake of steroids is the primary cause of Cushing syndrome.
- Cushing disease is defined as glucocorticoid excess due to excessive adrenocorticotropic hormone (ACTH) secretion from a pituitary tumor, the most common cause of primary Cushing syndrome.
- System(s) affected: endocrine/metabolic, musculoskeletal, skin/exocrine, cardiovascular; neuropsychiatric

Pediatric Considerations

- Rare in infancy and childhood
- Cushing disease accounts for approximately 75% of all cases of Cushing syndrome in children >7 years.
- In children <7 years, adrenal causes of Cushing syndrome (adenoma, carcinoma, or bilateral hyperplasia) are more common.
- Most common presenting symptom is lack of growth consistent with the weight gain.

Pregnancy Considerations

- Pregnancy may exacerbate disease.
- Cortisol levels increase in normal pregnancy states.

EPIDEMIOLOGY

Incidence

Uncommon: 0.7 to 2.4/1 million per year

Prevalence

2–5% prevalence reported in difficult-to-control diabetics with obesity and hypertension (HTN)

ETIOLOGY AND PATHOPHYSIOLOGY

- Syndrome: excessive corticosteroid exposure from exogenous sources (medications) or endogenous sources (pituitary, adrenal, pulmonary, etc.) or tumor
- Disease: pituitary tumor causing excess ACTH (corticotropin)
- General population
  - Exogenous glucocorticoids
  - Endogenous ACTH–dependent hypercortisolism: 80–85%
    - ACTH-secreting pituitary tumor: 75%
    - Ectopic ACTH production (e.g., small cell carcinoma of lung, bronchial carcinoid): 20%
  - Endogenous ACTH–independent hypercortisolism: 15–20%
    - Adrenal adenoma
    - Adrenal carcinoma
    - Macronodular or micronodular hyperplasia
- Pediatric/adolescent
  - Adrenal hyperplasia secondary to McCune-Albright syndrome: mean age 1.2 years
  - Adrenocortical tumors: mean age 4.5 years
  - Ectopic ACTH syndrome: mean age 10.1 years
  - Primary pigmented nodular adrenocortical disease: mean age 13.0 years
  - Cushing disease: mean age 14.1 years

- Pregnancy
  - Pituitary-dependent Cushing syndrome: 33%
  - Adrenal causes: 40–50%
  - ACTH-independent adrenal hyperplasia: 3%

Genetics

- Multiple endocrine neoplasia
- Carney complex (an inherited multiple neoplasia syndrome)
- McCune-Albright syndrome (mutation of *GNAS1* gene)
- Familial isolated pituitary adenomas (mutations in the aryl hydrocarbon receptor–interacting protein gene)

RISK FACTORS

- Prevalent sex: female > male (3:1)
- Most often occurs between the ages of 25 and 40 years
- Prolonged use of corticosteroids

GENERAL PREVENTION

Avoid corticosteroid exposure, when possible.

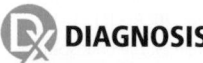

DIAGNOSIS

HISTORY

- Weight gain: 95%
- Decreased libido: 90%
- Menstrual irregularity: 80%
- Depression/emotional lability: 50–80%
- Easy bruising: 95%
- Diabetes or glucose intolerance: 90%

PHYSICAL EXAM

- Obesity (usually central): 95%
- Facial plethora: 90%
- Moon face (facial adiposity): 90%
- Thin skin: 85%
- HTN: 75%
- Skeletal growth retardation in children (epiphyseal plates remain open): 70–80%
- Hirsutism: 75%
- Proximal muscle weakness: 90%
- Purple striae on the skin
- Increased adipose tissue in neck and trunk
- Acne

DIFFERENTIAL DIAGNOSIS

- Obesity
- Diabetes mellitus
- HTN
- Metabolic syndrome X
- Polycystic ovarian disease
- Pseudo-Cushing (e.g., alcoholism, physical stress, severe major depression)

DIAGNOSTIC TESTS & INTERPRETATION

Initial Tests (lab, imaging)

- 2008 Endocrine Society guidelines (1)[C] recommend against widespread testing for Cushing syndrome except with the following:
  - Adrenal incidentaloma
  - Multiple progressive features suggestive of Cushing syndrome
  - Unusual features for their age such as osteoporosis and HTN
  - Abnormal growth (children)

- Late-night salivary cortisol, 24-hour urinary free cortisol, or low-dose dexamethasone suppression testing
  - Elevated late-night salivary cortisol: Obtain at least two measurements. Cortisol secretion is highest in the morning and lowest between 11 PM and midnight. The nadir of serum cortisol is maintained in pseudo-Cushing (e.g., obesity, alcoholism, depression) but not in Cushing syndrome. Sensitivity and specificity are >90–95% (2)[B].
  - 24-hour urinary free cortisol level: Obtain ≥2 samples to rule out intermittent hypercortisolism if results are normal and suspicion is high. Also measure 24-hour urinary creatinine excretion to verify adequacy of collection. Results may be falsely low if glomerular filtration rate <30 mL/min. Overall sensitivity and specificity varies, 90–97% and 85–99%, respectively (2)[B]. Avoid drinking excessive amounts of water due to risk of false-positive values. False-positive values can be seen in the presence of pseudo-Cushing states.
  - Low-dose dexamethasone suppression testing: Dexamethasone 1 mg is given between 11 PM and midnight, and fasting plasma cortisol is measured between 8 and 9 AM the following morning. A serum cortisol level <1.89 μg/dL excludes Cushing syndrome, but specificity is limited. The presence of pseudo-Cushing states (depression, obesity, etc.), hepatic or renal disease, or any drug that induces cytochrome P450 enzymes may cause a false result.
- High-dose dexamethasone suppression test may be useful when baseline ACTH levels are indeterminate:
  - 8 mg overnight dexamethasone suppression test: 8 mg of oral dexamethasone is given at 11 PM, with measurement of an 8-AM cortisol level the next day. A baseline 8-AM cortisol measurement is also obtained the morning prior to ingesting dexamethasone. Suppression of serum cortisol level to <50% of baseline is suggestive of a pituitary source of ACTH rather than ectopic ACTH or primary adrenal disease. Sensitivity and specificity are 95% and 100%, respectively (3)[B].
- If the initial results are positive or if clinical suspicion is high, perform additional studies to confirm diagnosis. Other tests to consider include the following:
  - Awake midnight plasma cortisol: Obtain samples on three consecutive nights. A late-evening serum cortisol >7.5 μg/dL has a sensitivity of 99% and specificity of 100% (4)[B]. Persistently elevated serum cortisol implies Cushing syndrome; nadir of serum cortisol is maintained in obese patients but not in Cushing.
  - Corticotropin-releasing hormone (CRH) after dexamethasone: used to distinguish Cushing syndrome from pseudo-Cushing syndrome. Dexamethasone 0.5 mg is given q9h for 48 hours starting at noon. CRH (1 μg/kg) is given 2 hours after the last dose of dexamethasone. Plasma cortisol is >1.4 μg/dL 15 minutes after CRH in patients with Cushing syndrome but not in those with pseudo-Cushing.
- Pituitary MRI scan if pituitary tumor is suspected
- Abdominal CT scan if adrenal disease is suspected

- Chest CT scan if ectopic ACTH secretion is suspected
- Octreotide scintigraphy to look for occult ACTH-secreting tumor
- Dual energy x-ray absorptiometry to evaluate for osteoporosis

ALERT
- Antiepileptic drugs, progesterone, oral contraceptives (withdraw estrogen-containing drugs 9 weeks before testing), rifampin, and spironolactone may cause a false-positive dexamethasone suppression test.
- Pregnancy (1)[C]: Urine free cortisol is recommended instead of dexamethasone testing in the initial evaluation of pregnant women. Only urine free cortisol in the 2nd or 3rd trimester >3 times the upper limit of normal can be taken to indicate Cushing syndrome.
- Epilepsy (1)[C]: best to use measured cortisol from saliva and urine instead of serum cortisol after dexamethasone. No data to guide length of time needed after withdrawal of such medication to allow dexamethasone metabolism to return to normal; such medication change may not be clinically possible.

Follow-Up Tests & Special Considerations
- Once the diagnosis of Cushing syndrome is confirmed, localization is the next step:
  - ACTH level: elevated in ACTH-dependent Cushing syndrome (e.g., pituitary and ectopic tumor) and low in ACTH-independent Cushing syndrome (e.g., adrenal tumors and exogenous glucocorticoids)
  - High-dose dexamethasone suppression testing: used to distinguish between an ACTH-secreting pituitary tumor and ectopic ACTH-secreting tumors. 0.5 mg dexamethasone is given q9h for 8 doses, with serum cortisol measured at 2 and 9 hours after last dose (sensitivity 79%, specificity 74%) (3)[B].
- Diagnosis of Cushing syndrome is complicated by the nonspecificity and high prevalence of clinical symptoms in patients without the disorder and involves a variety of tests of variable sensitivity and specificity. Efficient screening and confirmatory procedures are essential before considering therapy.

Diagnostic Procedures/Other
Diagnostic procedure depends on clinical judgment. Inferior petrosal sinus sampling with CRH stimulation can be considered if ACTH-dependent tumor is suspected but not localized.

Test Interpretation
- Thyroid function suppressed
- HTN
- Dyslipidemia
- Polycystic ovarian syndrome/hyperandrogenism
- Oligomenorrhea/hypogonadism
- Myopathy/cutaneous wasting
- Neuropsychiatric problems
- Ipsilateral adrenal gland hyperplasia and contralateral adrenal gland atrophy
- Hypercoagulable state
- Osteoporosis
- Nephrolithiasis
- Growth hormone reduced

 TREATMENT

MEDICATION
- Drugs usually not effective for primary long-term treatment; used in preparation for surgery or as adjunctive treatment after surgery, pituitary radiotherapy, or both
- Metyrapone, ketoconazole, and mitotane all lower cortisol by directly inhibiting synthesis and secretion in the adrenal gland. Replacement glucocorticoid therapy is often required. As initial treatment, remission rates up to 85% (5)[C].
- Etomidate also inhibits the adrenals and is the only medical treatment available for severe hypercortisolism who are not immediate surgical candidates and who cannot take oral medication.
- Mifepristone is a potent glucocorticoid receptor antagonist. It is FDA-approved to control hyperglycemia in adults with endogenous Cushing syndrome who have type 2 diabetes or glucose intolerance secondary to hypercortisolism that has not responded to (or who are not candidates for) surgery.
- Pasireotide is a somatostatin receptor ligand with affinity for somatostatin receptor 5. It was approved by the FDA in 2012 for the treatment of Cushing disease when surgery is not successful or cannot be performed.
- Cabergoline is a dopamine agonist that has shown some promise in small studies but still remains off-label use.

SURGERY/OTHER PROCEDURES
- Transsphenoidal surgery
  - Primary treatment for Cushing disease due to remission range of 95–90% (6)[C]
  - Resection of the ACTH-producing ectopic tumor
- Adrenal surgery
  - For unilateral adrenal adenomas, laparoscopic surgery is the treatment of choice.
  - For nodular hyperplasia, bilateral adrenalectomy is usually recommended.
  - For patients with Cushing disease, bilateral laparoscopic adrenalectomy can be considered if the patient has persistent disease even after pituitary surgery and radiotherapy.
- Radiotherapy and stereotactic radiosurgery (SRS) can be used to treat persistent hypercortisolism after transsphenoidal surgery in Cushing disease.
- Fractionated radiotherapy
  - Rates of remission range from 59% to 84%.
  - Its related complications of hypopituitarism have limited its usefulness.
- SRS
- Rates of remission range from 17% to 83%.
- Can be used as primary treatment without resection in patients with cavernous sinus tumors

 ONGOING CARE

PATIENT EDUCATION
- Teaching regarding diet and monitoring daily weight, early treatment of infections, emotional lability
- National Adrenal Disease Foundation. Great Neck, NY 11021; 519-407-4992

PROGNOSIS
- Guardedly favorable prognosis with surgery for Cushing disease; generally chronic course with cyclic exacerbations and rare remissions
- Better prognosis following surgery for benign adrenal tumors; long-term recurrence rate is 20%.

- Poor with small cell carcinoma of the lung producing ectopic hormone; neuroendocrine tumors (bronchial carcinoid) have much better prognosis.

COMPLICATIONS
- Osteoporosis
- Increased susceptibility to infections
- Metastases of malignant tumors
- Increased cardiovascular risk even after treatment
- Lifelong glucocorticoid dependence following treatment with bilateral adrenalectomy
- Nelson syndrome (pituitary tumor) after treatment with bilateral adrenalectomy (can occur in 8–38% of patients)

REFERENCES
1. Nieman LK, Biller BM, Findling JW, et al. The diagnosis of Cushing's syndrome: an Endocrine Society clinical practice guideline. *J Clin Endocrinol Metab*. 2008;93(5):1526–1540.
2. Putignano P, Toja P, Dubini A, et al. Midnight salivary cortisol versus urinary free and midnight serum cortisol as screening tests for Cushing's syndrome. *J Clin Endocrinol Metab*. 2003;88(9):4153–4157.
3. Aytug S, Laws ER Jr, Vance ML. Assessment of the utility of the high-dose dexamethasone suppression test in confirming the diagnosis of Cushing disease. *Endocr Pract*. 2012;18(2):152–157.
4. Isidori AM, Kaltsas GA, Pozza C, et al. The ectopic adrenocorticotropin syndrome: clinical features, diagnosis, management, and long-term follow-up. *J Clin Endocrinol Metab*. 2006;91(2):371–377.
5. Nieman LK, Ilias I. Evaluation and treatment of Cushing's syndrome. *Am J Med*. 2005;118(12):1340–1346.
6. Biller BM, Grossman AB, Stewart PM, et al. Treatment of adrenocorticotropin-dependent Cushing's syndrome: a consensus statement. *J Clin Endocrinol Metab*. 2008;93(7):2454–2462.

 SEE ALSO

Algorithm: Cushing Syndrome

 CODES

ICD10
- E24.9 Cushing's syndrome, unspecified
- E24.0 Pituitary-dependent Cushing's disease
- E24.2 Drug-induced Cushing's syndrome

CLINICAL PEARLS
- Cushing disease is due to excessive ACTH secretion from a pituitary tumor, resulting in corticosteroid excess.
- Cushing syndrome is due to excessive corticosteroid exposure from exogenous sources (medications) or endogenous sources (pituitary, adrenal, pulmonary, etc.) or tumor.
- Depression, alcoholism, medications, eating disorders, and other conditions can cause mild clinical and laboratory findings similar to those in Cushing syndrome (pseudo-Cushing syndrome).

C

CUTANEOUS DRUG REACTIONS

David H. Yun, MD • Jonathan M. Novotney, DO • Sicong Wang, MD

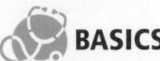 **BASICS**

DESCRIPTION
- An adverse cutaneous reaction in response to administration of a drug. Rashes are the most common form of adverse drug reaction (ADR).
- Severity can range from mild eruptions that resolve within 24 hours after the removal of the inciting agent, to severe skin damage with multiorgan involvement.
- Morbilliform and urticarial eruptions are the most common, accounting for approximately 94% of cutaneous drug reactions.
- Approximately 2% are severe and life-threatening.

EPIDEMIOLOGY
- All ages affected
- Immunosuppressed individuals at increased risk
- Patients with AIDS are 8.7 times more likely to develop cutaneous drug reactions compared to general population.
- Increased likelihood of severe cutaneous and systemic reactions in geriatric population; unclear if due to polypharmacy or change in drug metabolism
- Difficult to distinguish from viral exanthems in pediatric patients

Incidence
In the United States, incidence of 1–3% in hospitalized patients; estimated 1/1,000 hospitalized patients has had a severe cutaneous reaction.

ETIOLOGY AND PATHOPHYSIOLOGY
Two classifications of ADR:
- Predictable (type A): dose dependent, known pharmacologic effect of drug, and drug–drug interaction
- Unpredictable (type B): drug intolerance, drug idiosyncrasy secondary to abnormality in metabolism, drug allergy, and drug pseudoallergy
- Immunologically mediated reaction: immunoglobulin (Ig) E–mediated reaction (type I hypersensitivity), cytotoxic/IgG/IgM induced (type II), immune complex reactions (type III), and delayed-type hypersensitivity (type IV) with T cells, eosinophils, neutrophils, and monocytes
- >700 drugs are known to cause cutaneous drug reactions.
  - Morbilliform/urticarial/exfoliative erythroderma: penicillins, cephalosporins, sulfonamides, tetracyclines, ibuprofen, naproxen, allopurinol, acetylsalicylic acid, radiocontrast media (1)
  - Acneiform: OCPs, corticosteroids, iodinated compounds, hydantoins, lithium
  - Fixed drug eruptions: NSAIDs, sulfonamides, tetracycline, barbiturates, salicylates, OCPs
  - Acute generalized exanthematous pustulosis (AGEP): penicillins, cephalosporins, macrolides, calcium channel blockers, antimalarials, carbamazepine, acetaminophen, terbinafine, nystatin, vancomycin
  - Drug rash with eosinophilia and systemic symptoms (DRESS) syndrome: anticonvulsants, sulfonamides, dapsone, minocycline, allopurinol
  - Erythema multiforme/Stevens-Johnson syndrome (SJS)/toxic epidermal necrolysis (TEN): >100 drugs reported. Most common include sulfonamides, cephalosporins, NSAIDs, barbiturates, hydantoins, anticonvulsants tetracycline, terbinafine, allopurinol.
  - Lichenoid: thiazides, NSAIDs, gold, ACE inhibitors, proton pump inhibitors, antimalarials, sildenafil
  - Photosensitivity: doxycycline, thiazides, sulfonylureas, quinolones, sulfonamides, NSAIDs
  - Hypersensitivity vasculitis: hydralazine, penicillins, cephalosporins, thiazides, gold, sulfonamides, NSAIDs, propylthiouracil
  - Sweet syndrome (acute febrile neutrophilic dermatosis): sulfa drugs, granulocyte colony-stimulating factor (G-CSF), granulocyte-macrophage colony-stimulating factor (GM-CSF), diazepam, minocycline, nitrofurantoin, captopril, penicillamine

Genetics
Genetics may play a role because certain HLA antigens have been associated with increased predisposition to specific drug eruptions:
- HLA-B*5801, HLA-B*5701, and HLA-B*1502 have been linked to allopurinol-induced and carbamazepine-induced SJS/TEN, respectively.
- HLA-DQB1*0301 allele found in 66% of patients of erythema multiforme compared with 31% of control subjects
- HLA class I antigens, such as HLA-A2, HLA-B12, and HLA-B22, have been linked to TEN and fixed drug eruptions, respectively.
- CYP2C9*3 variants linked to phenytoin-induced SJS/TEN

RISK FACTORS
Previous drug reaction, polypharmacy, concurrent infection, immunocompromised, disorders of metabolism, and certain genetic HLA haplotypes

GENERAL PREVENTION
Always ask patients about prior adverse drug events. Be aware of medications with higher incidence of reactions as well as drug–drug reaction.

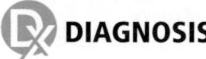 **DIAGNOSIS**

HISTORY
- Any new medication within the preceding 6 weeks (oral, parenteral, and topical agents, including over-the-counter drugs, vitamins, and herbal remedies)
- Consider other etiologies: unrelated acute or chronic urticaria, bacterial infections, viral exanthems, or underlying skin disease including cutaneous lymphoma.

PHYSICAL EXAM
May present as a number of different eruption types, including, but not limited to the following:
- Morbilliform eruptions (exanthems)
  - Most frequent cutaneous reaction (75–95%); difficult to distinguish from viral exanthem; often secondary to an antibiotic
  - Starts on trunk as pruritic red macules and papules, then extends symmetrically to extremities in confluent fashion, sparing face, palms, soles, and mucous membranes
  - Onset usually 7 to 21 days after drug initiation (2)
- Urticaria
  - Pruritic erythematous wheals distributed anywhere on the body, including mucous membranes
  - Lesions can vary in size and shape (e.g., round oval, rhomboid) and may change over time.
  - Angioedema, a related manifestation, may appear as asymmetric soft tissue swelling which can compromise airway and be life-threatening.
  - Individual lesions usually fade within 24 hours, but new lesions may develop.
- Acneiform eruptions
  - Folliculocentric, monomorphous pustules typically involving the face, trunk, and proximal extremities, can also present in areas atypical of acne vulgaris such as forearms and legs.
  - Distinguished from acne vulgaris by absence of comedones
- Fixed drug eruptions
  - Solitary/few, sharply demarcated, round and/or oval erythematous plaques with dusky center that may leave postinflammatory hyperpigmentation; occur on skin or on mucous membrane
  - Appear shortly after drug exposure and recur in identical location after reexposure; some patients have a refractory period during which the drug fails to activate lesions.
  - Onset usually 30 minutes to 8 hours after administration of drug
- AGEP
  - Rapidly appearing multiple nonfollicular sterile pustules on erythematous background typically involving intertriginous areas
  - Usually resolves within 1 to 3 days after removal of offending drug leaving a desquamation pattern
  - AGEP often causes fever and marked leukocytosis with neutrophilia and/or eosinophilia.
- DRESS syndrome
  - Drug-induced, multiorgan inflammatory response which may be life-threatening
  - Presentation can involve cutaneous eruptions (typically pruritic erythematous papules and patchy erythematous macules), fever, eosinophilia (most cases but not all), hepatic dysfunction, renal dysfunction, and lymphadenopathy.
  - Onset usually 2 to 8 weeks after drug exposure
  - Symptoms and organ involvement may worsen after discontinuation of offending agent and persist for months.
  - Mucosal involvement rare (3)
- Erythema multiforme
  - Acute, immune-mediated, mucocutaneous condition
  - Most commonly associated with herpes simplex virus (HSV) and other viral/bacterial etiologies (i.e., Mycoplasma); less likely secondary to drug exposure (<10% of cases)
  - Palpable classic target lesions and/or two-zone atypical target lesions with localized erythema
  - Most commonly distributed symmetrically on extensor surfaces of acral extremities; may involve mucus membrane (25–60%)
- SJS/TEN
  - Classification and distinction between SJS and TEN determined by affected body surface area (BSA)
    ○ SJS: <10% BSA; SJS–TEN overlap: 10–30% BSA; TEN: >30% BSA
  - TEN strongly associated with drug intake (>95%); SJS less strongly associated (~50%)
  - Onset is usually 4 to 28 days but as delayed as 8 weeks after starting offending drug: flat atypical two-zone target lesions and erythematous macules that are truncal and generalized with mucosal involvement
  - May develop confluent areas of bullae, erosions, and necrosis; significant risk for infection and sepsis
  - SJS: 1–5% mortality; TEN: 25–35% mortality
- Lichenoid eruptions
  - Eruption of violaceous, pruritic polygonal papules symmetrically distributed favoring extensor surfaces/sun-exposed areas

– Time frame of onset varies depending on causative medication.

– Chronic lesions persist for weeks/months after the drug discontinued.

- Photosensitivity reaction
  – Phototoxic reactions: usually occur within minutes to hours after sunlight exposure with exaggerated sunburn reaction
  – Photoallergic reactions: more pruritic than painful; photodistributed sparing scalp, submental, and periorbital areas
- Hypersensitivity vasculitis
  – Nonblanching petechiae/palpable purpura which commonly present on lower extremities
  – Onset usually 7 to 21 days after drug exposure
  – Biopsy shows inflammation and necrosis of vessel walls.
  – Renal, hepatic, pulmonary, GI, and CNS involvement possible but uncommon
- Sweet syndrome
  – Fever; neutrophilia; tender, edematous violaceous papules; plaques; or nodules, with or without pustules/vesicles that spontaneously resolve
  – Classically seen in young women after a mild respiratory illness or GI infection
- Exfoliative dermatitis/erythroderma
  – Severe end-stage dermatosis that develops from other drug reactions; commonly associated with systemic manifestations such as fever and chills
  – Generalized erythema with exfoliation and/or fine desquamation of large confluent areas
  – Increased risk of secondary infection and insensible fluid and temperature loss with hemodynamic instability

DIFFERENTIAL DIAGNOSIS
- Viral exanthem: Presence of fever, lymphocytosis, and other systemic findings may help in narrowing differential.
- Primary dermatosis (e.g., pustular psoriasis): Correlation of drug withdrawal to rash resolution may clarify diagnosis; skin biopsy is helpful.
- Bacterial infection: Cultures of pustules may distinguish primary infection from AGEP and acneiform eruptions.

DIAGNOSTIC TESTS & INTERPRETATION
Initial Tests (lab, imaging)
Selection of initial tests should be guided by clinical history and physical exam findings. CBC with differential; significant eosinophilia may be seen in DRESS and other drug-induced allergic reactions. LFT, urinalysis, and serum creatinine to assess for internal organ involvement; chest x-ray if suspected vasculitis

Diagnostic Procedures/Other
- Special tests depend on suspected mechanism:
  – Type I: skin/intradermal testing, radioallergosorbent test (RAST)
  – Type II: direct/indirect Coombs test
  – Type III: ESR, C-reactive protein, ANA, complement components, cryoglobulin assays
  – Type IV: patch testing, lymphocyte proliferation assay (investigational)
  – Anaphylaxis/nonimmunologic mast and basophil cell reaction: plasma histamine, serum tryptase levels, 24-hour urine N-methylhistamine
- Cultures useful in excluding infectious etiology; skin biopsy is nonspecific but useful in characterizing an eruption and excluding primary skin pathologies.
- Develop a timeline documenting the onset and duration of all drugs, dosages, and onset of cutaneous eruption (1)[A].

Test Interpretation
- Nonspecific histologic findings are superficial epidermal and dermal infiltrates composed variably of lymphocytes, neutrophils, and eosinophils.
- SJS/TEN: partial or full-thickness necrosis of the epidermis necrotic keratinocytes, vacuolization leading to subepidermal blister at basal membrane zone

TREATMENT
GENERAL MEASURES
- Monitor for signs of impending cardiovascular collapse: Anaphylactic reactions, DRESS, SJS/TEN, extensive bullous reactions, and generalized erythroderma may require inpatient treatment.
- Do not rechallenge with drugs causing urticaria, bullae, angioedema, DRESS, anaphylaxis, or erythema multiforme.

MEDICATION
- Immediate withdrawal of offending drug. Depending on the type of eruption, symptomatic treatment may be useful, but most require no additional therapy except cessation of offending agent.
- Anaphylaxis or widespread urticaria: epinephrine 0.1 to 0.5 mg (1:1,000 [1 mg/mL] solution) IM in the mid-outer thigh every 5 to 15 min; prednisone PO 1 mg/kg in tapering doses may be given for severe refractory cases.
- Acute urticaria (<6 weeks) and chronic urticaria (>6 weeks): 2nd-generation antihistamines (preferred, less sedating): cetirizine 10 to 20 mg daily, loratadine 10 to 20 mg daily, fexofenadine 180 mg daily. H$_2$ antagonists: ranitidine 150 mg BID
- Erythema multiforme
  – Treatment is generally supportive with management of suspected underlying infection.
  – Recurrent, HSV associated: prophylaxis with acyclovir 400 mg BID, valacyclovir 500 mg BID, or famciclovir 250 mg BID (4)[C]
  – "Magic mouthwash" and oral antiseptic helpful for mucosal erosions. Consider ophthalmology consult for severe ocular involvement (4)[C].
- SJS/TEN: Treatment is supportive. Consult with a dermatologist, ophthalmologist, and gynecologist as applicable. Systemic corticosteroid use remains controversial. Consider IVIG 2 to 3 g/kg for severe disease, although limited studies have not shown survival benefits in adults. In pediatric SJS/TEN patients, IVIG and systemic glucocorticoids appear to improve outcome; varied success rates reported with use of antitumor necrosis factor-α agents, cyclosporine, cyclophosphamide, and plasmapheresis. Avoid débridement and consider using detached epidermis as natural biologic dressing to minimize risk for hypertrophic scars (5)[C].
- DRESS: prompt removal of offending drug and supportive measures; high-potency topical steroids for rash; systemic steroids with severe organ involvement; appropriate supportive multidisciplinary care guided by organ involvement (6)[C]

ONGOING CARE
FOLLOW-UP RECOMMENDATIONS
Patient Monitoring
- For urticarial, bullous, DRESS, or erythema multiforme spectrum lesions, close follow-up is needed; may even require hospitalization if suspicious for life-threatening type including SJS/TEN and DRESS
- Patients with anaphylaxis/angioedema should be given EpiPens to be kept at home, work, and in the car for secondary prevention and a Med-Alert

bracelet; label the patient's medical record with the agent and reaction.
- If the patient needs to take the inciting drug (e.g., antibiotic) in the future, induction of drug tolerance or graded challenge procedures may be necessary.

PROGNOSIS
- Majority of cases are self-limiting upon removal of offending drug.
- Eruptions generally begin fading within days after removing offending agent. With morbilliform eruptions, eruption may spread distally even when agent is removed, resolving over time.
- Anaphylaxis, angioedema, DRESS, SJS/TEN, and bullous reactions are potentially fatal.
- Severity-of-illness score for toxic epidermal necrolysis (SCORTEN), a prognostic scoring system, can be used to guide management of hospitalized patients of SJS/TEN; also, may be helpful when discussing prognosis

COMPLICATIONS
Anaphylaxis, bone marrow suppression, hepatitis (dapsone, hydantoin), renal failure, psychological trauma, sepsis, and pulmonary and thyroid toxicity

REFERENCES

1. Joint Task Force on Practice Parameters, American Academy of Allergy, Asthma and Immunology, American College of Allergy, Asthma and Immunology, et al. Drug allergy: an updated practice parameter. *Ann Allergy Asthma Immunol.* 2010;105(4):259–273.
2. Ahmed AM, Pritchard S, Reichenberg J. A review of cutaneous drug eruptions. *Clin Geriatr Med.* 2013;29(2):527–545.
3. Cacoub P, Musette P, Descamps V, et al. The DRESS syndrome: a literature review. *Am J Med.* 2011;124(7):588–597.
4. Sokumbi O, Wetter DA. Clinical features, diagnosis, and treatment of erythema multiforme: a review for the practicing dermatologist. *Int J Dermatol.* 2012;51(8):889–902.
5. Dodiuk-Gad RP, Chung WH, Valeyrie-Allanore L, et al. Stevens-Johnson syndrome and toxic epidermal necrolysis: an update. *Am J Clin Dermatol.* 2015;16(6):475–493.
6. Hoetzenecker W, Nägeli M, Mehra ET, et al. Adverse cutaneous drug eruptions: current understanding. *Semin Immunopathol.* 2016;38(1):75–86.

CODES
ICD10
- L27.1 Loc skin eruption due to drugs and meds taken internally
- L50.0 Allergic urticaria
- R21 Rash and other nonspecific skin eruption

CLINICAL PEARLS
- Virtually, any drug can cause a rash; antibiotics are the most common culprits that cause cutaneous drug reactions.
- Focus on drug history with new suspicious skin eruptions.
- Usually self-limited after withdrawal of offending agent
- Symptoms such as tongue swelling/angioedema, skin necrosis, blisters, high fever, dyspnea, and mucous membrane erosions signify more severe drug reactions.
- Useful resources: Drug Eruption Reference Manual by Jerome Litt; www.drugeruptiondata.com

CYSTIC FIBROSIS

Fozia Akhtar Ali, MD • Reethu K. Nayak, MD

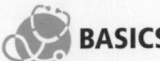

BASICS

DESCRIPTION
- Cystic fibrosis (CF) is an autosomal recessive genetic mutation (*CFTR* gene) that most prominently affects the pulmonary and pancreatic systems.
- The gastrointestinal (GI), endocrine, and reproductive systems as well as the liver, sinuses, and skin can all be involved.
- Initially a pediatric disease, CF has become a chronic pediatric and adult medical condition as improvements in medical care have led to a dramatic increase in long-term survival, resulting in adults living with the disease outnumbering children in 2014 (1)[A].

EPIDEMIOLOGY
CF is the most common lethal inherited disease in Caucasians and is found in every racial group.

Incidence
Number of infants born with CF in relation to the total number of live births in the United States
- 1 in 3,000 Caucasians
- 1 in 4,000 to 10,000 Latin Americans
- 1 in 15,000 to 20,000 African Americans
- 1 in 30,000 Asian Americans

Prevalence
30,000 patients with CF living in the United States

ETIOLOGY AND PATHOPHYSIOLOGY
- Primary defect is abnormal function of an epithelial chloride channel protein encoded by the *CFTR* gene on chromosome band 7q31.2. Abnormal CFTR function leads to abnormally viscous secretions that alter organ function.
- The lungs: Obstruction, infection, and inflammation negatively affect lung growth, structure, and function.
  - Decreased mucociliary clearance
  - Infection is accompanied by an intense neutrophilic response.
  - Degradation of supporting tissues causes bronchiectasis and eventual failure.

Genetics
CFTR gene (CF transmembrane conductance regulator): >1,500 mutations exist that can cause varying severity of phenotypic CF, all of which are recessively inherited. Most common is loss of the phenylalanine residue at 508th position (deltaF508), which accounts for 8.7% of affected alleles in the CF population in the United States. *G551D* mutation accounts for 4.3% of affected alleles.

RISK FACTORS
- CF is a single-gene disorder. The severity of the phenotype can be affected by the specific CFTR mutation (most predictive of pancreatic disease), other modifier genes (CFTM1 for meconium ileus), gastroesophageal reflux disease (GERD), severe respiratory virus infection, and environmental factors such as tobacco smoke exposure.
- Preconception counseling
  - American Congress of Obstetricians and Gynecologists (ACOG) recommends preconception or early (1st/2nd trimester) genetic analysis for all North American couples planning a pregnancy, with appropriate counseling to identified carriers and genetic analysis of siblings of known CF patients.
  - Universal newborn screening (NBS) has been integral in early diagnosis (64% of new CF diagnosis in 2014 were found by NBS). Patients diagnosed prior to onset of symptoms have better lung function and nutritional outcomes and should receive referral and early intervention services by an accredited regional CF center.

COMMONLY ASSOCIATED CONDITIONS
- CF-related diabetes (CFRD)
  - May present as steady decline in weight, lung function, or increased frequency of exacerbation
  - Leading comorbid complication (20.7%)
  - Result of progressive insulin deficiency
  - Early screening and treatment may improve reduced survival found in CFRD.
- Upper respiratory
  - Rhinosinusitis is seen in up to 100% of patients with CF.
  - Nasal polyps are seen in up to 86% of patients.
- The GI tract
  - Pancreatic exocrine insufficiency (85–90%)
  - Malabsorption of fat, protein, and fat-soluble vitamins (A, D, E, and K)
  - Hepatobiliary disease (12.6%)
  - Focal biliary cirrhosis
  - Cholelithiasis
  - Meconium ileus at birth (10–15%)
  - Distal intestinal obstruction syndrome (DIOS): intestinal blockage that typically occurs in older children and adults (5.3%) (1)[A]
  - GERD (32.7%) (1)[A]
- Endocrine
  - Bone mineral disease (16.6%) (1)[A]
  - Joint disease (3.0%) (1)[A]
  - Hypogonadism
  - Frequent low testosterone levels in men
  - Menstrual irregularities are common.
- Reproductive organs
  - Congenital bilateral absence of the vas deferens: obstructive azoospermia in 98% of males
- Depression (12.8%) (1)[A]

Pregnancy Considerations
- Pulmonary disease may worsen during pregnancy.
- CF may cause increased incidence of preterm delivery, IUGR, and cesarean section (2)[A].
- Advances in fertility treatments now allow men with CF to father children (1)[A].

DIAGNOSIS

HISTORY
- Routine prenatal ultrasonography indicates hyperechogenic bowel.
  - The risk is highest if there is evidence of meconium peritonitis (scattered calcifications are seen throughout the fetal peritoneum), bowel dilatation, or absent gallbladder. Parents should be offered prenatal CF carrier screening if any of these findings are present.
- Suspect with failure to thrive, steatorrhea, and recurrent respiratory problems.
  - Chronic/recurrent respiratory symptoms, including airway obstruction and infections
  - Persistent infiltrates on chest x-rays (CXRs)
  - Hypochloremic metabolic acidosis
- History during neonatal period
  - Meconium ileus (20%) (generally considered pathognomonic for CF)
  - Prolonged jaundice
- History during infancy
  - Failure to thrive
  - Chronic diarrhea
  - Anasarca/hypoproteinemia
  - Pseudotumor cerebri (vitamin A deficiency)
  - Hemolytic anemia (vitamin E deficiency)

- History during childhood
  - Recurrent endobronchial infection
  - Bronchiectasis
  - Chronic pansinusitis
  - Steatorrhea
  - Poor growth
  - DIOS
  - Allergic bronchopulmonary aspergillosis (ABPA)
- History for adolescence and adulthood (7% diagnosed >18 years old) (3)[A]
  - Recurrent endobronchial infection
  - Bronchiectasis
  - ABPA
  - Chronic sinusitis
  - Hemoptysis
  - Pancreatitis
  - Portal hypertension
  - Azoospermia
  - Delayed puberty

PHYSICAL EXAM
- Respiratory
  - Rhonchi and/or crackles
  - Hyperresonance on percussion
  - Nasal polyps
- GI: hepatosplenomegaly when cirrhosis present
- Other: digital clubbing, growth retardation, and pubertal delay

DIFFERENTIAL DIAGNOSIS
- Immunologic
  - Severe combined immunodeficiency
- Pulmonary
  - Difficult-to-manage asthma
  - COPD
  - Recurrent pneumonia
  - Chronic/recurrent sinusitis
  - Primary ciliary dyskinesia
- GI
  - Celiac disease
  - Protein-losing enteropathy
  - Pancreatitis of unknown etiology
  - Shwachman-Diamond syndrome

DIAGNOSTIC TESTS & INTERPRETATION

Initial Tests (lab, imaging)
- NBS tests blood levels of immunoreactive trypsin (IRT) (1)[A].
- The diagnosis of CF requires clinical symptoms consistent with CF in at least one organ system or positive NBS test or history of CF in sibling AND evidence of CFTR dysfunction (elevated sweat chloride, presence of two disease-causing mutations in CFTR, or abnormal nasal potential difference).
- Sweat test (gold standard)
  - Sweat chloride
    - >60 mmol/L (on two occasions) is positive for CF.
    - <40 mmol/L is normal.
  - CFTR mutation analysis
  - Limited panel testing: Allele-specific polymerase chain reaction (PCR) identifies >90% of mutations; finite chance of false-negative finding. Full-sequence testing is more costly and time consuming.
  - Nasal potential difference (when sweat test and DNA testing inconclusive)
  - CXR

Follow-Up Tests & Special Considerations
To further investigate the presence of CF-related complications, these tests are generally ordered:
- Sputum culture (common CF organisms)
- Pulmonary function tests (PFTs)

- 72-hour fecal fat, stool elastase
- Oral glucose tolerance test (OGTT) annually after age 10 years
- Head CT: Abnormal sinus CT findings are nearly universal in CF and may include mucosal thickening, intraluminal sinus polyps, and sinus effusions.
- Chest CT (not routine): useful when unusual findings noted on CXR

Diagnostic Procedures/Other
- Flexible bronchoscopy
- Bronchoalveolar lavage

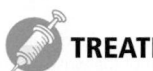

TREATMENT

GENERAL MEASURES
- Cystic Fibrosis Foundation guidelines call for yearly evaluation:
  - Four office visits, four respiratory cultures, PFTs q6mo, and at least one evaluation by a multidisciplinary team, including dietitian, GI, and social worker
  - PFT goals: >75% predicted for adults, >100% predicted for children <18 years old
  - Annual screening for ABPA for patients >6 years with total serum IgE concentration
  - Annual influenza vaccination for all CF patients age >6 months
  - Screen all adults for osteoporosis with a DEXA scan.
  - Annual measurement of fat-soluble vitamins to rule out vitamin deficiencies
  - Annual LFTs
  - Decrease exposure to tobacco smoke.
- All patients should be followed in a CF center (accredited sites are listed at https://www.cff.org/).
- Infant care:
  - Monthly visits for first 6 months of life and then every 2 months until 1 year of life
  - Fecal elastase testing and salt supplementation after diagnosis
  - Consider palivizumab for RSV prophylaxis in infants with CF <2 years (4)[A].

MEDICATION
- Pathogens for pulmonary infections: methicillin-resistant *Staphylococcus aureus* (MRSA) and methicillin-sensitive *S. aureus* (MSSA), *Stenotrophomonas maltophilia*, *Pseudomonas aeruginosa*, *Burkholderia cepacia*, nontuberculous mycobacteria (NTM)
  - Antibiotics for acute pulmonary infections should be prescribed according to most likely pathogen; most antibiotic courses are for 2 weeks.
- Pulmonary infections:
  - Antibiotics, oral
    o *S. aureus*: Bactrim (MRSA), doxycycline (MRSA) or cephalexin
    o *P. aeruginosa*: fluoroquinolones
  - Antibiotics, inhaled
    o Tobi (tobramycin): for *P. aeruginosa*, nebulizer twice daily for 28 days; stop for 28 days and then resume use (5)[A].
    o Colistin (more commonly used in Europe)
    o Cayston (aerosolized aztreonam) (5)[A]
  - Antibiotics, IV
    o *S. aureus*: cefazolin or nafcillin
    o MRSA: vancomycin or linezolid
    o *P. aeruginosa*: Zosyn or ceftazidime plus aminoglycoside (tobramycin)
    o Dual therapy synergistic (5)[A]
- Medications recommended for chronic use in pulmonary disease:
  - Recombinant human DNAse (dornase alfa) (5)[A]
  - Hypertonic saline

  - High-dose ibuprofen in patients 6 to 17 years old with FEV$_1$ ≥60 PPV
  - Inhaled tobramycin or aztreonam in *P. aeruginosa*-positive patients
  - Azithromycin in *P. aeruginosa*-positive patients
  - Ivacaftor (VX770) and lumacaftor: CFTR potentiators approved in 2015 for patients with two copies of the F508del mutation. This vastly increases the number of people with CF eligible for this therapy (>50%) (1)[A].
- Inhaled steroids are not recommended for chronic use in the absence of asthma or ABPA.
- Insufficient evidence to recommend for or against chronic use: inhaled β-agonist, inhaled anticholinergics, leukotriene modifiers, inhaled colistin
  - Pancreatic enzymes (87.3%) (1)[A]
    o Often combined with H$_2$ blocker or PPI to increase effectiveness
  - Fat-soluble vitamin supplementation (A, D, E, and K)
  - Liver disease (cholestasis)
    o Ursodeoxycholic acid has not been proven effective.

ADDITIONAL THERAPIES
- High-frequency chest wall oscillation vest is the most widely used airway clearance technique.
- Aerobic exercise is used as an adjunct therapy for airway clearance.
  - CF-related bone disease: Consider bisphosphonate therapy.

SURGERY/OTHER PROCEDURES
- Timing for lung transplantation (bilateral) is polyfactorial (6)[A].
- 5-year posttransplant survival is up to 62%.
- Liver transplantation is reserved for progressive liver failure ± portal hypertension with GI bleeding.
- Nasal polypectomy in 4.5% of CF patients (1)[A]

ADMISSION, INPATIENT, AND NURSING CONSIDERATIONS
- Pulmonary exacerbation (most common reason for admission)
- Bowel obstruction (due to DIOS, previously known as meconium ileus equivalent [MIE])
- Pancreatitis (in pancreatic-sufficient patients)
- CF exacerbations should always be admitted on contact precautions and private rooms.
- Nasal cannula oxygen when the patient is hypoxemic (SaO$_2$ <90%)
- Increased salt loss increases risk of hyponatremic hypochloremic dehydration.
- Cautious use of IV fluids with worsening lung disease
- Nursing assignments should involve only one CF patient per nurse for isolation purposes.

ONGOING CARE

FOLLOW-UP RECOMMENDATIONS
- Upon discharge for a pulmonary exacerbation, follow-up with CF provider within 2 to 4 weeks.
- Routine clinic visits every 3 months, with airway cultures and pulmonary function testing
- Annual comprehensive nutritional evaluation (4)[A]

DIET
High-calorie, high-fat diet titrated to specific BMI goals established by the Cystic Fibrosis Foundation nutrition guidelines. If not meeting nutritional goals, dietitian, pancreatic enzyme, oral or tube supplemental feeding should be considered if indicated.

PATIENT EDUCATION
Cystic Fibrosis Foundation: https://www.cff.org

PROGNOSIS
- Median survival is 39.3 years.
- Progression of lung disease usually determines length of survival.

REFERENCES
1. Cystic Fibrosis Foundation. *Patient Registry: Annual Data Report to the Center Directors 2013*. Bethesda, MD: Cystic Fibrosis Foundation; 2014.
2. Grigoriadis C, Tympa A, Theodoraki K. Cystic fibrosis and pregnancy: counseling, obstetrical management and perinatal outcome. *Invest Clin*. 2015;56(1):66–73.
3. Gilljam M, Ellis L, Corey M, et al. Clinical manifestations of cystic fibrosis among patients with diagnosis in adulthood. *Chest*. 2004;126(4):1215–1224.
4. Borowitz D, Robinson KA, Rosenfeld M, et al; for Cystic Fibrosis Foundation. Cystic Fibrosis Foundation evidence-based guidelines for management of infants with cystic fibrosis. *J Pediatr*. 2009;155(Suppl 6):S73–S93.
5. Mogayzel PJ Jr, Naureckas ET, Robinson KA, et al; for Pulmonary Clinical Practice Guidelines Committee. Cystic fibrosis pulmonary guidelines. Chronic medications for maintenance of lung health. *Am J Respir Crit Care Med*. 2013;187(7):680–689.
6. Weill D, Benden C, Corris PA, et al. A consensus document for the selection of lung transplant candidates: 2014—an update from the Pulmonary Transplantation Council of the International Society for Heart and Lung Transplantation. *J Heart Lung Transplant*. 2015;34(1):1–15.

ADDITIONAL READING
- Conwell LS, Chang AB. Bisphosphonates for osteoporosis in people with cystic fibrosis. *Cochrane Database Syst Rev*. 2014;(3):CD002010.
- Mall MA, Boucher RC. Pathophysiology of cystic fibrosis lung disease. In: Mall MA, Elborn JS, eds. *Cystic Fibrosis*. Vol 64. Sheffield, United Kingdom: European Respiratory Monograph; 2014:1–13.
- Farrell PM, White TB, Ren CL, et al. Diagnosis of cystic fibrosis: consensus guidelines from the Cystic Fibrosis Foundation. *J Pediatr*. 2017;181S:S4–S15.e1.

CODES

ICD10
- E84.9 Cystic fibrosis, unspecified
- E84.11 Meconium ileus in cystic fibrosis
- E84.0 Cystic fibrosis with pulmonary manifestations

CLINICAL PEARLS
- Meconium ileus is virtually pathognomonic for CF.
- When sweat test is equivocal, CFTR genetic testing is diagnostic.
- CF must be considered in *any* child with chronic diarrhea, especially if associated with poor growth or failure to thrive.
- All children with nasal polyps, digital clubbing, or bronchiectasis should be evaluated.
- A rapid decline in pulmonary function suggests the acquisition of resistant organisms (e.g., *B. cepacia*), CFRD, ABPA, or GERD.

DE QUERVAIN TENOSYNOVITIS

Caitlin G. Waters, MD • J. Herbert Stevenson, MD

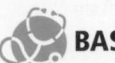

BASICS

DESCRIPTION

- First identified in 1895 by Fritz De Quervain, de Quervain tenosynovitis is a painful condition due to stenosis of the tendon sheath in the 1st dorsal compartment of the radial aspect of the wrist.
- Caused by repetitive motion of the extensor pollicis brevis (EPB) and abductor pollicis longus (APL) over the radial styloid with resultant irritation of the surrounding tendon sheath

EPIDEMIOLOGY

- The predominant age range is 30 to 50 years.
- Women are affected more commonly than men (1).
- With new occupational and professional demands, the prevalence of this condition is increasing gradually.

Incidence

- The overall incidence of de Quervain tenosynovitis is 0.9/1,000 person-years.
- For patients age >40 years, the incidence is 1.4/1,000 person-years compared with 0.6/1,000 person-years for those <20 years.
- Women have an incidence rate ratio of 2.8/1,000 person-years compared with 0.6/1,000 person-years in men.
- The incidence ratio rate of de Quervain tenosynovitis is 1.3/1,000 person-years in blacks and 0.8/1,000 person-years in whites (1).

ETIOLOGY AND PATHOPHYSIOLOGY

- Repetitive motions of the wrist and/or thumb result in microtrauma and thickening of the tendons (EPB, APL) and surrounding tendon sheath.
- EPB and APL movement is resisted as they glide over the radial styloid causing pain with movements of the thumb and wrist.

RISK FACTORS

- Women age 30 to 50 years
- Pregnancy (primarily 3rd trimester and postpartum)
- African American
- Systemic diseases (e.g., rheumatoid arthritis)
- Participation in activities that include repetitive motion or forceful grasping with thumb and wrist deviation such as golf, fly fishing, racquet sports, rowing, or bicycling, video gaming, and more recently text messaging
- Repetitive movements with the hand/thumb requiring forceful grasping with wrist involving ulnar/radial deviation; dental hygienists, musicians, carpenters, assembly workers, and machine operators

GENERAL PREVENTION

Avoid overuse or repetitive movements of the wrist and/or thumb associated with forceful grasping and ulnar/radial deviation.

DIAGNOSIS

HISTORY

- Repetitive motion activity; overuse of wrist or thumb
- Gradually worsening pain along the radial aspect of the thumb and wrist with certain movements, particularly ulnar deviation of the wrist
- Pregnancy
- Sports, leisure, and occupational history
- Trauma (rare)

PHYSICAL EXAM

- Pain over the radial styloid exacerbated when patients move the thumb or make a fist
- Crepitus with movement of the thumb
- Swelling over the radial styloid and base of the thumb
- Decreased range of motion of the thumb
- Pain over the 1st dorsal compartment on resisted thumb abduction or extension
- Tenderness may extend proximally or distally along the tendons with palpation or stress.
- Finkelstein test: The examiner grasps the affected thumb and deviates the hand sharply in the ulnar direction. A positive test occurs when there is pain along the distal radius.
- Eickhoff test: Patient grasps a flexed thumb, and the examiner deviates the wrist in an ulnar direction.
- Finkelstein test is more sensitive for determining tenosynovitis of the APL and EPB tendons (2)[A].

DIFFERENTIAL DIAGNOSIS

- Scaphoid fracture
- Scapholunate ligament tear
- Dorsal wrist ganglion
- Osteoarthritis of the 1st carpometacarpal (CMC) joint
- Flexor carpi radialis tendonitis
- Infectious tenosynovitis
- Tendonitis of the wrist extensors
- Intersection syndrome
- Trigger thumb

DIAGNOSTIC TESTS & INTERPRETATION

Initial Tests (lab, imaging)

- Primarily a clinical diagnosis
- Radiographs of the wrist to rule out other pathology, such as CMC arthritis, if the diagnosis is in question
- MRI is the imaging test of choice to rule out coexisting soft tissue injury or wrist joint pathology.

Follow-Up Tests & Special Considerations

Ultrasound can help to detect anatomic variations in the 1st dorsal extensor compartment of the wrist and target corticosteroid injections (3,4).

Test Interpretation

Inflamed and thickened retinacular sheath of the tendon

TREATMENT

- Most cases of de Quervain syndrome are self-limited.
- Rest and NSAIDs (2)[A]
- Ice (15 to 20 minutes 5 to 6 times a day)
- Immobilization with a thumb spica splint (2)[A]
- Occupational therapy
- Corticosteroid injection (ultrasound guided)
- Consider surgery if conservative measures fail >6 months.

GENERAL MEASURES

- If full relief is not achieved, a corticosteroid injection of the tendon sheath can improve symptoms.
- Anatomic variation, including two tendon sheaths in the 1st compartment or the EPB tendon traveling in a separate compartment may complicate treatment. Ultrasound can distinguish these variants and improve anatomic accuracy of injections (3).
- Surgical release may be indicated after 3 to 6 months of conservative treatment if symptoms persist. Surgery is highly effective and has a relatively low rate of complications.

MEDICATION

First Line

Splinting, rest, and NSAIDs

Second Line

- Corticosteroid injection of the tendon sheath has shown significant cure rates. Additional injections are sometimes required.
- Corticosteroid injection plus immobilization is more effective than immobilization alone (5)[B].
- Percutaneous tenotomy and/or injection of platelet-rich plasma are newer techniques that show promise for treatment of de Quervain tenosynovitis.

ISSUES FOR REFERRAL

Referral to a hand surgeon is indicated if there is no improvement with conservative therapy.

ADDITIONAL THERAPIES

- Hand therapy, along with iontophoresis/phonophoresis, may help improve outcomes in persistent cases.
- Patients may use thumb-stretching exercises as part of their rehabilitation.

SURGERY/OTHER PROCEDURES

- Indicated for patients who have failed conservative treatment
- Endoscopic release may provide earlier relief, fewer superficial radial nerve complications, and greater patient satisfaction with resultant scar compared to open release (5)[B].

ADMISSION, INPATIENT, AND NURSING CONSIDERATIONS

Hospitalization for care associated with surgical treatment

ONGOING CARE

FOLLOW-UP RECOMMENDATIONS

- Additional corticosteroid injection may be performed at 4 to 6 weeks if symptoms persist. Caution with repeat steroid injections.
- Avoid repetitive motions and activities that cause pain.

DIET

As tolerated

PATIENT EDUCATION

Activity modification: Avoid repetitive movement of the wrist/thumb and forceful grasping.

PROGNOSIS

- Extremely good with conservative treatment
- Complete resolution can take up to 1 year.
- 95% success rates have been shown with conservative therapy >1 year.
- Up to 1/3 of patients will have persistent symptoms.

COMPLICATIONS

- Most complications are secondary to treatment. These include GI, renal, and hepatic injury secondary to NSAID use.
- Nerve damage may occur during surgery.
- Hypopigmentation, fat atrophy, bleeding, infection, and tendon rupture have been reported as potential adverse events from corticosteroid injection. Ultrasound guidance reduces the rate of complications.
- If not appropriately treated, thumb flexibility may be lost due to fibrosis.

REFERENCES

1. Wolf JM, Sturdivant RX, Owens BD. Incidence of de Quervain's tenosynovitis in a young, active population. *J Hand Surg Am*. 2009;34(1):112–115.
2. Huisstede BM, Coert JH, Fridén J, et al; for European HANDGUIDE Group. Consensus on a multidisciplinary treatment guideline for de Quervain disease: results from the European HANDGUIDE study. *Phys Ther*. 2014;94(8):1095–1110.
3. Lee KH, Kang CN, Lee BG, et al. Ultrasonographic evaluation of the first extensor compartment of the wrist in de Quervain's disease. *J Orthop Sci*. 2014;19(1):49–54.
4. Di Sante L, Martino M, Manganiello I, et al. Ultrasound-guided corticosteroid injection for the treatment of de Quervain's tenosynovitis. *Am J Phys Med Rehabil*. 2013;92(7):637–638.
5. Kang HJ, Koh IH, Jang JW, et al. Endoscopic versus open release in patients with de Quervain's tenosynovitis: a randomised trial. *Bone Joint J*. 2013;95-B(7):947–951.

ADDITIONAL READING

- Ali M, Asim M, Danish SH, et al. Frequency of de Quervain's tenosynovitis and its association with SMS texting. *Muscles Ligaments Tendons J*. 2014;4(1):74–78.
- Ashraf MO, Devadoss VG. Systematic review and meta-analysis on steroid injection therapy for de Quervain's tenosynovitis in adults. *Eur J Orthop Surg Traumatol*. 2014;24(2):149–157.
- Cavaleri R, Schabrun SM, Te M, et al. Hand therapy versus corticosteroid injections in the treatment of de Quervain's disease: a systematic review and meta-analysis. *J Hand Ther*. 2016;29(1):3–11.
- Goel R, Abzug JM. de Quervain's tenosynovitis: a review of the rehabilitative options. *Hand (N Y)*. 2015;10(1):1–5.
- Kume K, Amano K, Yamada S, et al. In de Quervain's with a separate EPB compartment, ultrasound-guided steroid injection is more effective than a clinical injection technique: a prospective open-label study. *J Hand Surg Eur Vol*. 2012;37(6):523–527.
- Kwon BC, Choi SJ, Koh SH, et al. Sonographic identification of the intracompartmental septum in de Quervain's disease. *Clin Orthop Relat Res*. 2010;468(8):2129–2134.

- Orlandi D, Corazza A, Fabbro E, et al. Ultrasound-guided percutaneous injection to treat de Quervain's disease using three different techniques: a randomized controlled trial. *Eur Radiol*. 2015;25(5):1512–1519.
- Pagonis T, Ditsios K, Toli P, et al. Improved corticosteroid treatment of recalcitrant de Quervain tenosynovitis with a novel 4-point injection technique. *Am J Sports Med*. 2011;39(2):398–403.
- Peters-Veluthamaningal C, van der Windt DA, Winters JC, et al. Corticosteroid injection for de Quervain's tenosynovitis. *Cochrane Database Syst Rev*. 2009;(3):CD005616.
- Rousset P, Vuillemin-Bodaghi V, Laredo JD, et al. Anatomic variations in the first extensor compartment of the wrist: accuracy of US. *Radiology*. 2010;257(2):427–433.
- Scheller A, Schuh R, Hönle W, et al. Long-term results of surgical release of de Quervain's stenosing tenosynovitis. *Int Orthop*. 2009;33(5):1301–1303.

SEE ALSO

Algorithm: Pain in Upper Extremity

CODES

ICD10
M65.4 Radial styloid tenosynovitis [de Quervain]

CLINICAL PEARLS

- Repetitive movements of the wrist and thumb, and activities that require forceful grasping are the most common causes of de Quervain tenosynovitis.
- Initial treatment is typically conservative.
- Corticosteroid injections are helpful and have lower complication rates if done under ultrasound guidance.
- Combined orthosis/corticosteroid injection approaches are more effective than either intervention alone.
- Surgery is helpful for recalcitrant cases.

DEEP VEIN THROMBOPHLEBITIS

Jaine L. McKenzie, MD • Patricia Martinez Quinones, MD • Keith O'Malley, MD, FACS

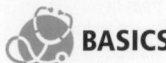 ## BASICS

DESCRIPTION
- Development of blood clot within the deep veins, usually accompanied by inflammation of the vessel wall
- Major clinical consequences are embolization (usually to the lung), recurrent thrombosis, and postphlebitic syndrome.

EPIDEMIOLOGY
- Age- and gender-adjusted incidence of venous thromboembolism (VTE) is 100 times higher in the hospital than in the community. Almost half of all VTEs occur either during or soon after discharge from a hospital stay or surgery.
- Of patients with VTE, 20% complicated with pulmonary embolism (PE). The 28-day deep venous thrombosis (DVT) fatality rate is 5.4%; at 1 year, 20%; at 3 years, 29%.

Incidence
- In the United States, VTE incidence is 50.4/100,000 person per year.
- Increased incidence in Caucasian and African American populations and with aging
- Most common site: lower extremity DVT
- Incidence in pregnancy: ~0.5 to 3/1,000 (1)
- 1–5% of central venous catheters are complicated by thrombosis (2).

Prevalence
- Variable; depends on medical condition or procedure
- At time of DVT diagnosis, as many as 40% of patients also have asymptomatic PE; conversely, 30% of patients diagnosed with PE do not a have demonstrable source.
- Present in 11% of patients with acquired brain injury entering neurorehabilitation

ETIOLOGY AND PATHOPHYSIOLOGY
Factors involved may include venous stasis, endothelial injury, and hypercoagulability (Virchow triad).

Genetics
- Factor V Leiden, the most common thrombophilia, is found in 5% of the population and in 10–65% of all VTE events and increases VTE risk 3- to 6-fold.
- Prothrombin G20210A is found in 3% of Caucasians; increases the risk of thrombosis ~3-fold

RISK FACTORS
- Acquired: previous DVT, cancer, immobilization, trauma, obesity, recent major surgery, medications (oral contraceptives, estrogens, tamoxifen), obesity, smoking, antiphospholipid syndrome, acute infectious process, thrombocytosis, pregnancy/puerperium, central venous catheters
- Hereditary: deficiencies of protein C, protein S, or antithrombin III; factor V Leiden R506Q, prothrombin G20210A mutation, dysfibrinogenemia, elevated factor VIII activity, hyperhomocysteinemia

GENERAL PREVENTION
- Mechanical thromboprophylaxis is recommended in patients with high bleeding risk and as adjunct to pharmacologic thromboprophylaxis.
- For acutely ill and for critically ill hospitalized patients at increased risk of thrombosis, low-molecular-weight heparin (LMWH), low-dose unfractionated heparin, or fondaparinux are recommended (3)[C].

- For most patients, prolonged secondary prophylaxis is not recommended.
- In patients undergoing major abdominal surgery for malignancy, LMWH for up to 4 weeks after surgery have been shown to decrease the incidence of VTE without increased bleeding.

 ## DIAGNOSIS

HISTORY
- Higher clinical suspicion in patient with risk factors (see "Risk Factors" section)
- DVT is classified as provoked or idiopathic based on underlying risk factors.
- Clinical assessment of bleeding risk (bleeding with previous history of anticoagulation, history of liver disease, recent surgeries, history of GI bleed) is important prior to initiating treatment.
- Modified Wells criteria, a validated clinical prediction rule, is useful to determine pretest probability of having a DVT.
  - Active cancer (+1 point)
  - Calf swelling >3 cm compared to other leg (+1 point)
  - Collateral superficial veins (+1 point)
  - Pitting edema to symptomatic leg (+1 point)
  - Previous documented DVT (+1 point)
  - Swelling of entire leg (+1 point)
  - Localized tenderness along deep venous system (+1 point)
  - Paralysis, paresis, or recent cast immobilization of lower extremities (+1 point)
  - Recently bedridden >3 days or major surgery in past 4 weeks (+1 point)
  - Alternative diagnosis at least as likely (−2 points)
- Interpretation: Score of 0, DVT unlikely. Score of 1 to 2, moderate risk. Score of ≥3, DVT likely. D-dimer testing and/or ultrasound should follow based on Wells criteria score.

PHYSICAL EXAM
- Symptoms may present as pain, swelling, or discoloration but may be nonspecific or absent.
- Resistance to dorsiflexion of the foot (Homan sign) is unreliable and nonspecific.
- Edema, due to swelling of collateral veins, is the most specific symptom.
- Uncommonly, patients may have phlegmasia alba dolens ("milk leg") or phlegmasia cerulean dolens due to arterial occlusion secondary to extensive DVTs.

DIFFERENTIAL DIAGNOSIS
Cellulitis, fracture, ruptured synovial cyst (Baker cyst), lymphedema, muscle strain/tear, extrinsic compression of vein (e.g., by tumor/enlarged lymph nodes), compartment syndrome, and localized allergic reaction

DIAGNOSTIC TESTS & INTERPRETATION
Initial Tests (lab, imaging)
- Routine laboratory testing (CBC, metabolic panel, coagulation studies) is not useful for diagnosis.
- D-dimer (sensitive but not specific; has high negative predictive value [NPV]), indicated in patients with low pretest probability of DVT or PE but not indicated high pretest probability patients; false positives in liver disease, inflammation, malignancy, trauma, pregnancy, and recent surgery
- Patients with a prior DVT and those with malignancy have higher rates of VTE, which decreases the NPV of Wells criteria.

- Compression ultrasound (CUS): first-line imaging for DVT due to noninvasive nature and ease of use
- In patients with suspected DVT, the diagnosis process should be guided by the assessment of the pretest probability.
  - Low pretest probability: high-sensitivity D-dimer assay sufficient to exclude DVT if negative. If positive, follow with CUS.
  - Moderate to high pretest probability: CUS initial test; if positive CUS, then treat DVT. If negative, no further testing is necessary; if continued concern, may repeat CUS in 24 hours
- Other imaging modalities, such as CT venography and magnetic resonance venography, are rarely used but may be better than CUS for demonstrating new from old thrombosis.
- Contrast venography and impedance plethysmography are now rarely used.

Follow-Up Tests & Special Considerations
- In young patients and/or those of concern or with idiopathic/recurrent VTE, consider thrombophilia testing (factor V Leiden mutation, prothrombin G20210A genetic assay, ATIII functional assay, protein C functional assay, protein S antigen and functional assay and free S, phospholipid-dependent tests and anticardiolipin antibodies, lupus anticoagulant [drawn before initiation of heparin]).
- Risk of an underlying malignancy is more likely if recurrent VTE, risk 3.2 (95% CI 2.0–4.8). Unprovoked VTE, 4.6 times higher (vs. secondary); upper extremity DVT, not catheter associated; odds ratio (OR) 1.8, abdominal DVT; OR 2.2 (4), bilateral lower extremity DVT, OR 2.1 (4)

TREATMENT

MEDICATION
Consider starting therapy even before diagnosis confirmation in patients with high pretest probability and acceptable risk of bleeding.
- Anticoagulation is mainstay of therapy. Patients with PE or proximal DVT, long-term therapy (at least 3 months) is recommended. Duration of therapy after 3 months is case-by-case basis.
- Indefinite anticoagulation is considered if there is low risk of bleeding, if index event is unprovoked PE, and/or if D-dimer is positive 1 month after stopping anticoagulation (5).
- Direct oral anticoagulants (dabigatran, rivaroxaban, apixaban, or edoxaban) recommended instead of vitamin K antagonists for the first 3 months of treatment in patients with lower extremity DVT or PE and no cancer (4)[B]
- Use and choice of anticoagulation should be considered based on patient's history, bleeding risk, cost, and ease of compliance.

First Line
- Unfractionated heparin
  - IV drip: initial dose of 80 U/kg followed by continuous infusion of 18 U/kg/hr. Target aPTT ratio >1.5 times control. Monitor aPTT every 6 hours and adjust infusion rate accordingly until two successive values are within therapeutic range.
- LMWH
  - Enoxaparin (Lovenox): 1 mg/kg/dose SC q12h or 1.5 mg/kg daily
  - Dalteparin (Fragmin): 200 U/kg SC q24h

- Direct and indirect factor Xa inhibitors
  - Fondaparinux (Arixtra): 5 mg (body weight <50 kg), 7.5 mg (body weight = 50 to 100 kg), or 10 mg (body weight >100 kg) SC once daily
  - Rivaroxaban (Xarelto): 15 mg PO twice daily with food for the first 3 weeks then 20 mg PO every day
  - Apixaban (Eliquis): 10 mg PO twice daily for 1 week followed by 2.5 to 5.0 mg PO twice daily
  - Edoxaban (Savaysa): 60 mg PO daily (>60 kg), 30 mg PO daily (≤60 kg)
- Thrombin inhibitors
  - Dabigatran (Pradaxa): 150 mg PO twice daily for creatinine clearance >30 mL/min
- Vitamin K antagonists
  - Warfarin (Coumadin): Start with 2 to 5 mg/day. Adjust to a target INR of 2 to 3; overlap with parenteral anticoagulant for minimum of 5 days until therapeutic INR sustained ≥24 hours.
- Adverse effects
  - All anticoagulants increase risk of bleeding.
  - Heparin and LMWH can also cause heparin-induced thrombocytopenia (HIT) (LMWH has lower risk) and injection site irritation.
  - Warfarin is teratogenic.
  - Dosage adjustments may be required for patients with decreased creatinine clearance.

Second Line
Heparin can be given by intermittent SC self-injection.

Pregnancy Considerations
- Warfarin (Coumadin) is a teratogen. It is contraindicated in pregnancy but is safe during breastfeeding.
- LMWH are recommended over unfractionated heparin for treatment of acute DVT and PE in pregnancy (1)[B].
- Enoxaparin, dalteparin, fondaparinux, and apixaban are pregnancy Category B.
- Dabigatran, rivaroxaban, edoxaban are pregnancy Category C.

SURGERY/OTHER PROCEDURES
- In selected patients with proximal DVT (acute iliofemoral DVT <14 days, good functional status, >1 year of life expectancy), may consider catheter-directed thrombolysis/open thrombectomy (6)
- Thrombolysis (systemic or catheter directed) reduces incidence of postthrombotic syndrome (PTS) after a proximal (iliofemoral or femoral) DVT by one-third.
- Thrombectomy is recommended in patients with limb-threatening ischemia due to iliofemoral venous outflow obstruction (6).
- IVC filter
  - Not routinely inserted in patients with acute DVT
  - May be considered in patients with DVT or PE with absolute contraindication to anticoagulation or recurrent embolism despite adequate anticoagulation
  - Special considerations can be given to patients who are chronically immobile, such as spinal cord injury patients.

ADMISSION, INPATIENT, AND NURSING CONSIDERATIONS
- In patients with acute PE, if the following criteria are met, then hospital admission is not necessary. Patients who meet these critera but are admitted may be discharged early (<5 days of inpatient treatment) (4):
  - Patient is clinically stable with good cardiopulmonary reserve.
  - No recent bleeding, severe renal or liver disease, or severe thrombocytopenia <70,000
  - Expected to be compliant
  - Patient feels well enough to be treated at home.

- Admission for respiratory distress, elevated cardiac biomarkers, right ventricular dysfunction, candidate for thrombolysis, active bleeding, renal failure, phlegmasia alba dolens, phlegmasia cerulea dolens, history of HIT
- In medically stable and properly anticoagulated patients, overlap of anticoagulation and warfarin monitoring may be done as an outpatient.
- Limb elevation and graduated compression stockings for symptomatic relief

ONGOING CARE

FOLLOW-UP RECOMMENDATIONS
- Resumption of normal activity with avoidance of prolonged immobility
- Compression stockings not routinely recommended for prevention of PTS after acute DVT (4)[B] but can be used for patients who already present with symptoms of PTS

Patient Monitoring
- Monitor platelet count while on heparin, LMWH, and fondaparinux for HIT.
- An anti-Xa activity level may help guide LMWH titration of therapy.
- Investigate significant bleeding (e.g., hematuria or GI hemorrhage) because anticoagulant therapy may unmask a preexisting lesion (e.g., cancer, peptic ulcer disease, or arteriovenous [AV] malformation).

PATIENT EDUCATION
Dietary habits should be discussed when warfarin is initiated to ensure that intake of vitamin K–rich foods is monitored.

PROGNOSIS
- 20% of untreated proximal (iliofemoral, femoral, or popliteal) lower extremity DVTs progress to PE, and 10–20% of those are fatal. However, with anticoagulant therapy, mortality is decreased 5- to 10-fold.
- DVT confined to the infrapopliteal veins has a small risk of embolization but can propagate proximally.
- Up to 75% of patients with symptomatic DVT present with PTS after 5 to 10 years.

COMPLICATIONS
PE (fatal in 10–20%), arterial embolism (paradoxical embolization) with AV shunting, chronic venous insufficiency, PTS, treatment-induced hemorrhage, soft tissue ischemia associated with massive clot and high venous pressures; phlegmasia cerulea dolens (rare but a surgical emergency)

REFERENCES
1. Dresang L, Fontaine P, Leeman L, et al. Venous thromboembolism during pregnancy. *Am Fam Physician*. 2008;77(12):1709–1716.
2. Baumann Kreuziger LB, Jaffray J, Carrier M. Epidemiology, diagnosis, prevention and treatment of catheter-related thrombosis in children and adults. *Thromb Res*. 2017;157:64–71.
3. Holbrook A, Schulman S, Witt DM, et al. Evidence-based management of anticoagulant therapy: antithrombotic therapy and prevention of thrombosis, 9th ed: American College of Chest Physicians evidence-based clinical practice guidelines. *Chest*. 2012;141(Suppl 2):e152S–e184S.
4. Kearon C, Akl EA, Ornelas J, et al. Antithrombotic therapy for VTE disease: CHEST guideline and expert panel report. *Chest*. 2016;149(2):315–352.
5. Kearon C, Akl E. Duration of anticoagulant therapy for deep vein thrombosis and pulmonary embolism. *Blood*. 2014;123(12):1794–1801.
6. Meissner M, Gloviczki P, Comerota A, et al; for Society for Vascular Surgery, American Venous Forum. Early thrombus removal strategies for acute deep venous thrombosis: clinical practice guidelines of the Society for Vascular Surgery and the American Venous Forum. *J Vasc Surg*. 2012;55(5):1449–1462.

ADDITIONAL READING
- Agnelli G, Buller HR, Cohen A, et al; for AMPLIFY Investigators. Oral apixaban for the treatment of acute venous thromboembolism. *N Eng J Med*. 2013;369(9):799–808.
- Kyrle PA, Rosendaal FR, Eichinger S. Risk assessment for recurrent venous thrombosis. *Lancet*. 2010;376(9757):2032–2039.
- Lyman GH, Khorana A, Kuderer N, et al; for American Society of Clinical Oncology Clinical Practice. Venous thromboembolism prophylaxis and treatment in patients with cancer: American Society of Clinical Oncology clinical practice guideline update. *J Clin Oncol*. 2013;31(17):2189–2204.
- Palareti G, Cosmi B, Legnani C, et al; for DULCIS (D-dimer and ULtrasonography in Combination Italian Study) Investigators. D-dimer to guide the duration of anticoagulation in patients with venous thromboembolism: a management study. *Blood*. 2014;124(2):196–203.
- Prins MH, Lensing AW, Bauersachs R, et al; for EINSTEIN Investigators. Oral rivaroxaban versus standard therapy for the treatment of symptomatic venous thromboembolism: a pooled analysis of the EINSTEIN-DVT and PE randomized studies. *Thromb J*. 2013;11(1):21.
- Watson L, Broderick C, Armon MP. Thrombolysis for acute deep vein thrombosis. *Cochrane Database Syst Rev*. 2016;(11):CD002783.

SEE ALSO

Antithrombin Deficiency; Factor V Leiden; Protein C Deficiency; Protein S Deficiency; Prothrombin 20210 (Mutation); Pulmonary Embolism

CODES

ICD10
- I80.209 Phlbts and thombophlb of unsp deep vessels of unsp low extrm
- I80.299 Phlebitis and thombophlb of deep vessels of unsp low extrm
- I80.10 Phlebitis and thrombophlebitis of unspecified femoral vein

CLINICAL PEARLS
- Many cases of VTE are asymptomatic.
- At time of DVT diagnosis, as many as 40% of patients also have asymptomatic PE.
- Wells criteria are useful to determine the pretest probability of a DVT, but follow-up testing and/or imaging should be done if moderate to high probability.
- Choice of anticoagulant therapy should be individualized based on patient's history and compliance.

DEHYDRATION

Tu Dan (Kathy) Nguyen, MD

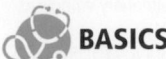 **BASICS**

DESCRIPTION

- A state of negative fluid balance; strictly defined as free water deficiency
- The two types of dehydration:
  - Water loss
  - Salt and water loss (combination of dehydration and hypovolemia)

EPIDEMIOLOGY

- Responsible for 10% of all pediatric hospitalizations in the United States
- Gastroenteritis, one of its leading causes, accounts to 13/1,000 children <5 years of age annually in the United States.

Incidence

- More than half a million hospital admissions annually in the United States for dehydration
- Of hospitalized older persons, 8% are dehydrated (1).
- Worldwide, ~3 to 5 billion cases of acute gastroenteritis occur each year in children <5 years of age, resulting in nearly 2 million deaths.

ETIOLOGY AND PATHOPHYSIOLOGY

- Negative fluid balance occurs when ongoing fluid losses exceed fluid intake.
- Fluid losses can be insensible (sweat, respiration), obligate (urine, stool), or abnormal (diarrhea, vomiting, osmotic diuresis in diabetic ketoacidosis).
- Negative fluid balance can lead to severe intravascular volume depletion (hypovolemia) and end-organ damage from inadequate perfusion.
- The elderly are at increased risk as kidney function, urine concentration, thirst sensation, aldosterone secretion, release of vasopressin, and renin activity are all significantly lowered with age.
- Decreased intake
- Increased output: vomiting, diarrheal illnesses, sweating, frequent urination
- "Third spacing" of fluids: effusions, ascites, capillary leaks from burns, or sepsis

Genetics

Some causes of dehydration have a genetic component (diabetes), whereas others do not (gastroenteritis).

RISK FACTORS

- Children <5 years of age at highest risk
- Elderly
- Decreased cognition
- Lack of access to water such as in critically sick intubated patients

GENERAL PREVENTION

- Patient/parent education on early signs of dehydration
- Universal precautions (including hand hygiene)

Geriatric Considerations

Systematically assessing risk factors helps with early prevention and management of dehydration in the elderly, especially those in long-term care facilities.

Clinical Finding	Mild	Moderate	Severe
Dehydration: children	5–10%	10–15%	>15%
Dehydration: adults	3–5%	5–10%	>10%
General condition: infants	Thirsty, alert, restless	Lethargic/drowsy	Limp, cold, cyanotic extremities, may be comatose
General condition: older children	Thirsty, alert, restless	Alert, postural dizziness	Apprehensive, cold, cyanotic extremities, muscle cramps
Quality of radial pulse	Normal	Thready/weak	Feeble or impalpable
Quality of respiration	Normal	Deep	Deep and rapid/tachypnea
BP	Normal	Normal to low	Low (shock)
Skin turgor	Normal skin turgor	Reduced skin turgor, cool skin	Skin tenting, cool, mottled, acrocyanotic skin
Eyes	Normal	Sunken	Very sunken
Tears	Present	Absent	Absent
Mucous membranes	Moist	Dry	Very dry
Urine output	Normal	Reduced	None passed in many hours
Anterior fontanelle	Normal	Sunken	Markedly sunken

COMMONLY ASSOCIATED CONDITIONS

- Hypo-/hypernatremia
- Hypokalemia
- Hypovolemic shock
- Renal failure

 DIAGNOSIS

Calculate percent dehydration = (preillness weight − illness weight)/preillness weight × 100. Supplement this along with the ongoing fluid loss.

HISTORY

- Fever
- Intake (including description and amount)
- Diarrhea (including duration, frequency, consistency, ± mucus/blood)
- Vomiting (including duration, frequency, consistency, ± bilious/nonbilious)
- Urination pattern
- Sick contacts
- Medication history (e.g., diuretics, laxatives)

PHYSICAL EXAM

- The most useful signs for identifying dehydration in children are prolonged capillary refill time, abnormal skin turgor, and abnormal respiratory pattern.
- Vitals: pulse, BP, temperature
- Orthostatic vital signs: Take BP and heart rate (HR) while supine, sitting, and standing.
  - Systolic BP decrease of 20 mm Hg, diastolic BP decrease by 10 mm Hg, or HR increase by 20 bpm suggests hypovolemia (2).
- Weight loss: <5%, 10%, or >15%
- Mental status
- Head: sunken anterior fontanelle (for infants)
- Eyes: sunken, ± tear production
- Mucous membranes: tacky, dry, or parched
- Capillary refill: ranges from brisk to >3 seconds
- Darker urine color

DIFFERENTIAL DIAGNOSIS

- Decreased intake: ineffective breastfeeding, inadequate thirst response, anorexia, malabsorption, metabolic disorder, obtunded state
- Excessive losses: gastroenteritis, diarrhea, febrile illness, diabetic ketoacidosis, hyperglycemia, hyperosmolar hyperglycemic state, diabetes insipidus, intestinal obstruction, sepsis

DIAGNOSTIC TESTS & INTERPRETATION

Initial Tests (lab, imaging)

- For mild dehydration: generally not necessary
- For moderate to severe dehydration
  - Electrolytes, BUN, creatinine, and glucose
  - Urinalysis (specific gravity, hematuria, glucosuria)
- Imaging does not play a role in the diagnosis of dehydration, unless the specific condition causing the dehydration requires imaging.
- In adults, inferior vena cava collapsibility is a surrogate marker for volume status.

Pediatric Considerations

Infants and the elderly may not concentrate urine maximally, making urine specific gravity less helpful.

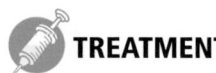 **TREATMENT**

MEDICATION

First Line

- Oral rehydration is the first-line treatment in dehydrated children. If this is unsuccessful, use IV rehydration. If IV unobtainable, nasogastric (NG) or intraosseous (IO) rehydration can be considered (3).
- Oral rehydration is the first-line treatment in dehydrated adults as long as they can tolerate fluids. Have a lower threshold for IV rehydration if needed.

- If the patient is experiencing excessive vomiting, consider using an antiemetic.
- Ondansetron (PO/IV) may be effective in decreasing the rate of vomiting, improving the success rate of oral hydration, preventing the need for IV hydration, and preventing the need for hospital admission (4,5).
- Other antiemetics can be used.

Second Line
- Loperamide may reduce the duration of diarrhea compared with placebo in children with mild to moderate dehydration (two randomized controlled trials [RCTs] yes, one RCT no).
- In children ages 3 to 12 years with mild diarrhea and minimal dehydration, loperamide decreases diarrhea duration and frequency when used with oral rehydration.

Pediatric Considerations
Given a higher risk for serious adverse events, loperamide is not indicated for children <3 years of age with acute diarrhea.

ISSUES FOR REFERRAL
- For severe dehydration, critical care referral and ICU-level care may be warranted.
- Surgical consultation for acute abdominal issues

SURGERY/OTHER PROCEDURES
For specific underlying causes of dehydration, such as intestinal obstruction or appendicitis

ADMISSION, INPATIENT, AND NURSING CONSIDERATIONS
- Intractable vomiting/diarrhea
- Electrolyte abnormalities
- Hemodynamic instability
- Inability to tolerate oral rehydration therapy (ORT)
- Stabilize airway, breathing, circulation.
- If mild dehydration, try ORT.
- If excessive vomiting/severe dehydration with shock, start IV access and IV fluids immediately.
- IV fluids
  - Stage I
    ○ For moderate to severe dehydration in children: isotonic saline or Ringer lactate solution bolus of 10 to 20 mL/kg; may repeat up to 60 mL/kg; if still hemodynamically unstable, consider colloid replacement (blood, albumin, fresh frozen plasma) and address other causes for shock.
    ○ For moderate to severe hypovolemia in adults: isotonic saline or Ringer lactate 20 mL/kg/hr until normal state of consciousness returns/vital signs stabilize. Also consider colloid replacement if continued fluids required beyond 3 L.
  - Stage II: Replace fluid deficit along with maintenance over 48 hours; fluid deficit = preillness weight − illness weight
  - An alternative IV treatment option for moderate (10%) dehydration in children
    ○ Bolus with NS/LR at 20 mL/kg for 1 hour
    ○ Replete fluid deficit with D5 1/2 NS + 20 mEq KCl/L at 10 mL/kg for 8 hours (hours 2 to 9).
    ○ Replete 1.5 for maintenance fluids with D5 1/4 NS + 20 mEq/L of KCl for 16 hours (hours 10 to 24).

- An alternative to IV fluids is hypodermoclysis, the SC infusion of fluids into the body (adults).
  - Indications: hydration of patients with mild to moderate dehydration who do not tolerate oral intake because of cognitive impairment, severe dysphagia, advanced terminal illness, or intractable vomiting. It is also indicated to prevent dehydration, especially in frail elderly residents living in long-term care settings who reject the oral route for any reason; useful technique for patients with difficult IV access
  - Contraindications: severe dehydration or shock, patients with coagulopathy or receiving full anticoagulation, patients with severe generalized edema (anasarca) or congestive heart failure, and those with fluid overload (6)
- Strict inputs and outputs: oral and IV input and output of urine and stool, which may include weighing wet diapers
- Discharge criteria
  - Input > output
  - Underlying etiology treated and improving

ONGOING CARE

FOLLOW-UP RECOMMENDATIONS
Activity as tolerated
- If mild to moderate dehydration, the patient may be mobile without restrictions, although watch for orthostasis/falls.
- If moderate to severe dehydration, bed rest

Patient Monitoring
Ongoing surveillance for recurrence

DIET
- Bland food bananas, rice, applesauce, toast (BRAT) diet
- If diarrhea, lactose-free feeds may reduce the duration of diarrhea in children with mild to severe dehydration, compared with lactose-containing feeds.
- Small frequent sips of room temperature liquids
- Oral rehydration solutions are available commercially.
- Continue breastfeeding ad lib.

PATIENT EDUCATION
- Patients should seek medical care if they (or their child) feel faint or dizzy when rising from a sitting or lying position, becomes lethargic and/or confused, or complains of a rapid HR.
- Patients should call their physician if they are unable to keep down any fluids, vomiting has been going on >24 hours in an adult or >12 hours in a child, diarrhea has lasted >2 days in an adult/child, or an infant/child is much less active than usual or is very irritable.
- http://www.mayoclinic.org/diseases-conditions/dehydration/basics/definition/con-20030056

PROGNOSIS
Self-limited if treated early; potentially fatal if untreated and persistent

COMPLICATIONS
- Seizures
- Renal failure
- Cardiovascular arrest

REFERENCES

1. Thomas DR, Cote TR, Lawhorne L, et al; for Dehydration Council. Understanding clinical dehydration and its treatment. *J Am Med Dir Assoc.* 2008;9(5):292–301.
2. Lanier JB, Mote MB, Clay EC. Evaluation and management of orthostatic hypotension. *Am Fam Physician.* 2011;84(5):527–536.
3. Rouhani S, Meloney L, Ahn R, et al. Alternative rehydration methods: a systematic review and lessons for resource-limited care. *Pediatrics.* 2011;127(3):e748–e757.
4. Colletti JE, Brown KM, Sharieff GQ, et al. The management of children with gastroenteritis and dehydration in the emergency department. *J Emerg Med.* 2010;38(5):686–698.
5. Carter B, Fedorowicz Z. Antiemetic treatment for acute gastroenteritis in children: an updated Cochrane systematic review with meta-analysis and mixed treatment comparison in a Bayesian framework. *BMJ Open.* 2012;2(4):e000622.
6. Lopez JH, Reyes-Ortiz CA. Subcutaneous hydration by hypodermoclysis. *Rev Clin Gerontol.* 2010;20(2):105–113.

 SEE ALSO

Oral Rehydration

 CODES

ICD10
- E86.0 Dehydration
- E87.1 Hypo-osmolality and hyponatremia
- E86.1 Hypovolemia

CLINICAL PEARLS
- Dehydration is the result of a negative fluid balance and is a common cause of hospitalization in both children and the elderly.
- Begin by assessing the level of dehydration, determining the underlying cause, and calculating necessary replacement.
- Treatment is directed at restoring fluid balance via oral rehydration (first line) therapy or IV fluids and treating underlying causes.

D

DELIRIUM

Whitney A. Gray, MSN, CRNP • Katrina A. Booth, MD

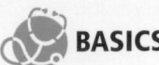

BASICS

DESCRIPTION
- A temporary neurologic complication of illness and/or medication(s), especially common in older patients, manifested by new confusion and impaired attention
- A medical emergency requiring immediate evaluation to decrease morbidity and mortality
- System(s) affected: neurologic
- Synonym(s): acute confusional state, altered mental status, organic brain syndrome, acute mental status change, encephalopathy

EPIDEMIOLOGY
- Predominant age: older persons
- Predominant sex: male = female

Incidence
- >50% in older ICU patients
- 11–51% in postoperative patients
- 10–40% in hospitalized older patients

Prevalence
- 8–17% in older ED patients
- 14% in older postacute care patients

ETIOLOGY AND PATHOPHYSIOLOGY
- Multifactorial: believed to result from a decline in physiologic reserves with aging, resulting in a vulnerability to new stressors
- Neuropathophysiology is not clearly defined; cholinergic deficiency, dopamine excess, and neuroinflammation are leading hypotheses.
- Often interaction between predisposing and precipitating risk factors
- With more predisposing factors (i.e., frail patients), fewer precipitating factors needed to cause delirium
- If few predisposing factors (e.g., very robust patients), more precipitating factors needed to cause delirium
- Multicomponent approach addressing contributing factors can reduce incidence and complications.

RISK FACTORS
- Predisposing risk factors
  - Advanced age, >70 years
  - Preexisting cognitive impairment
  - Functional impairment
  - Dehydration; high BUN:creatinine ratio
  - History of alcohol abuse
  - Malnutrition
  - Hearing or vision impairment
  - Multiple comorbidities
- Precipitating risk factors
  - Severe illness in any organ system(s)
  - Medical devices (urinary catheter, restraints)
  - Polypharmacy (≥5 medications)
  - Specific medications, especially benzodiazepines, opioids meperidine, and anticholinergics diphenhydramine, high-dose neuroleptics
  - Pain
  - Any iatrogenic event
  - Surgery
  - Sleep deprivation

GENERAL PREVENTION
Follow treatment approach.

COMMONLY ASSOCIATED CONDITIONS
Multiple but most common are the following:
- New medicine or medicine changes
- Infections (especially lung, urine, and blood stream, but consider meningitis as well)

- Toxic metabolic (especially low sodium, elevated calcium, renal failure, and hepatic failure)
- Heart attack or stroke
- Alcohol or drug withdrawal
- Preexisting cognitive impairment increases risk.

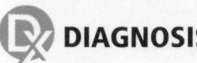

DIAGNOSIS

Diagnosis is made using a careful history, behavioral observation, and cognitive assessment.
- *DSM-5* diagnostic criteria include (1):
  - Disturbance in attention and awareness
  - Change in cognition not due to dementia
  - Onset over short (hours to days) period and fluctuates during course of day
  - Evidence from history, exam, or lab that disturbance is caused by physiologic consequence of medical condition, intoxicating substance, medication use, or more than one cause.
- The Confusion Assessment Method (CAM) is the most well validated and tested clinical tool and has been adapted for ICU setting in adults (CAM-ICU) and children (pediatric CAM-ICU [pCAM-ICU]) (2)[B].

ALERT
- Key diagnostic features of the CAM
  - Acute change in mental status that fluctuates
  - Abnormal attention and either disorganized thinking or altered level of consciousness
- Several nondiagnostic symptoms may be present:
  - Short- and long-term memory problems
  - Sleep–wake cycle disturbances
  - Hallucinations and/or delusions
  - Emotional lability
  - Tremors and asterixis
- Subtypes based on level of consciousness
  - Hyperactive delirium (15%): Patients are loud, agitated, restless, and disruptive.
  - Hypoactive delirium (20%): quietly confused; sleepy; may sit and not eat, drink, or move
  - Mixed delirium (50%): features of both hyperactive and hypoactive delirium
  - Normal consciousness delirium (15%): still displays disorganized thinking, along with acute onset, inattention, and fluctuating mental status
  - Subsyndromal delirium (23%): some delirium symptoms but does not progress to full delirium

HISTORY
- Time course of mental status changes
- Recent medication changes
- Symptoms of infection
- New neurologic signs
- Abrupt change in functional ability

PHYSICAL EXAM
- Comprehensive cardiorespiratory exam is essential.
- Focal neurologic signs are usually absent.
- Mini-Mental State Examination (MMSE) is the most well-known and studied cognitive screen, but it may not be the most appropriate in an acute care setting; shorter cognitive screens have been studied in delirious patients (i.e., Short Blessed Test [SBT], Brief Alzheimer Screen [BAS], and Ottawa 3DY) and may be helpful if performed serially over time. Most patients will perform poorly if delirium is present; dementia cannot be diagnosed when delirium is present.
- GI/GU exam for constipation/urinary retention

DIFFERENTIAL DIAGNOSIS
- Depression (disturbance of mood, normal level of consciousness, fluctuates weeks to months)
- Dementia (insidious onset, memory problems, normal level of consciousness, fluctuates days to weeks)
- Psychosis (rarely sudden onset in older adults)
- Seizure disorders (i.e., nonconvulsive status epilepticus)

DIAGNOSTIC TESTS & INTERPRETATION
Initial Tests (lab, imaging)
- Guided by history and physical exam
  - CBC with differential
  - Comprehensive metabolic panel (CMP)
  - Urinalysis, urine culture, blood culture
  - Medication levels digoxin, theophylline, antiepileptics where applicable
- Chest radiograph for most
- ECG as necessary
- Others, if indicated by history and exam

Follow-Up Tests & Special Considerations
- If lab tests listed above do not indicate a precipitator of delirium, consider
  - Arterial blood gases
  - Troponin
  - Toxicology screen
  - Ammonia
  - Thyroid-stimulating hormone
  - Thiamine
- Noncontrast-enhanced head CT scan if
  - Unclear diagnosis
  - Recent fall
  - Receiving anticoagulants
  - New focal neurologic signs
  - Ruling out mass before lumbar puncture

Diagnostic Procedures/Other
- Lumbar puncture (rarely necessary)
  - Perform if clinical suspicion of a CNS bleed, malignancy-related syndrome, or infection is high.
- EEG (rarely necessary)
  - Consider after above evaluation if cause remains unclear or suspicion of seizure activity.

TREATMENT

- The best treatment is prevention (3)[A].
- Addressing six risk factors (i.e., cognitive impairment, sleep deprivation, dehydration, immobility, vision impairment, and hearing impairment) in at-risk hospitalized patients can reduce the incidence of delirium by 33%.
- Principles: Maintain safety, identify causes, and manage symptoms.
- Stabilize vital signs and ensure immediate evaluation.

GENERAL MEASURES
- Postoperative patients should be monitored for
  - Myocardial infarction/ischemia
  - Infection (i.e., pneumonia, UTI)
  - Pulmonary embolism
  - Urinary or stool retention (attempt catheter removal by postoperative day 2)
  - Anemia/bleeding
- Anesthesia route (general vs. epidural) does not affect the risk of delirium.
- ICU sedation-avoidance of benzodiazepines may reduce risk (4)[B].

- Multifactorial treatment: Identify contributing factors and provide preemptive care to avoid iatrogenic problems, with special attention to
  - CNS oxygen delivery (attempt to attain):
    - SaO_2 >90% with goal of SaO_2 >95%
    - Systolic BP <2/3 of baseline or >90 mm Hg
    - Hematocrit >30%
  - Fluid/electrolyte balance
    - Sodium, potassium, and glucose normal (glucose <300 mg/dL in diabetics)
    - Treat fluid overload or dehydration.
- Treat pain
  - Schedule acetaminophen (650 mg TID–QID) if constant pain; avoid if LFT elevation noted.
  - Opioids morphine, oxycodone may be used for breakthrough pain.

ALERT
- Avoid meperidine (Demerol).
- Eliminate unnecessary medications.
  - Investigate new symptoms as potential medication side effects (i.e., Beers medications).
- Regulate bowel/bladder function.
  - Bowel movement at least every 48 hours
  - Screen for urinary retention.
- Prevent major hospital-acquired problems.
  - Use a pressure-reducing mattress.
  - Avoid urinary catheters.
  - Encourage incentive spirometry.
  - Venous thromboembolism (VTE) prophylaxis if bedfast
  - Early mobilization
  - Environmental stimulation
    - Glasses and hearing aids
    - Clock and calendar
    - Soft lighting
    - Music and television, if desired
  - Sleep
    - Quiet environment
    - Soft music
    - Therapeutic massage
- Restraints increase risk of delirium and falls/injury.
  - Use as a last resort for patients at risk for self-injury or risk for injuring caregivers. Remove as soon as possible.

MEDICATION
- Nonpharmacologic approaches are preferred for initial treatment, but medication may be needed for agitation and injurious behaviors, especially in the ICU setting (5)[C].
- Medications treat the symptoms and do not address the underlying cause.
- No medication is FDA-approved for delirium.
- Medications should not be used as prophylaxis (6)[A].

First Line
- Antipsychotics (in alphabetical order)
  - Aripiprazole (Abilify) 2 to 5 mg PO daily to BID
  - Haloperidol (Haldol): initially, 0.25 to 0.50 mg PO/IM; reevaluate and potentially redose hourly until symptoms controlled and then use effective dose up to QID PRN. Critical care guidelines do not support use of antipsychotics for prevention of ICU delirium (4)[B].
  - Olanzapine (Zyprexa) 2.5 to 5.0 mg PO daily to BID
  - Quetiapine (Seroquel) 12.5 to 25.0 mg PO BID–TID
  - Risperidone (Risperdal) 0.25 to 0.50 mg PO daily
- Contraindications: Avoid haloperidol in patients with parkinsonism or Parkinson disease.
- Precautions: Antipsychotics may cause extrapyramidal effects and increase fall risk.
- Antipsychotics may prolong the QT interval. Aripiprazole (Abilify) has minimal or no QT prolonging effect.

- Nonbenzodiazepines, such as dexmedetomidine are preferred for sedation in ICU patients (5)[C]. The primary adverse effects of this medication include hypotension and bradycardia. Some studies have also found use of clonidine as an oral bridge off of dexmedetomidine.
- Melatonin and melatonin agonists are gaining interest as sleep aids in ICU patients.

Second Line
- Benzodiazepines should generally be avoided except in alcohol withdrawal, if patient taking a benzodiazepine regularly at baseline, or antipsychotic is contraindicated. Benzodiazepines can cause delirium. Lorazepam (Ativan): initially, 0.25 to 0.50 mg PO/IM/IV TID–QID PRN; may need to adjust to effect (caution in impaired liver and renal function)
- Cholinesterase inhibitors should be avoided. Multiple trials demonstrate adverse events with cholinesterase inhibitors in the management of delirium; evidence does not support their use.

ISSUES FOR REFERRAL
Geriatric, psychiatric, or neurologic consultation is helpful if delirium is not easily explainable or resolving after full evaluation. Interprofessional team approach is best.

ADDITIONAL THERAPIES
Early mobilization is critical.
- Out of bed several hours daily starting on hospital day 2 (or postoperative day 1) if no contraindications

ADMISSION, INPATIENT, AND NURSING CONSIDERATIONS
- Cognitive engagement is key.
- New delirium is a medical emergency and requires admission, except in the setting of hospice care.
- IV fluids as needed for dehydration
- Monitor for the development of delirium.
- Assessment of precipitants/contributing factors (infection, pain, constipation, urinary retention)
- Reorient; maintain day/night orientation.
- Skin care and turning regimen for immobile patients
- Maintain and encourage mobility.
- Encourage family presence and participation.
- Discharge criteria
  - Resolution of precipitating factor(s)
  - Safe discharge site if delirium is slow to resolve

 ONGOING CARE

FOLLOW-UP RECOMMENDATIONS
- If delirium at discharge, often needs postacute facility care and ongoing assessment for resolution
- If no delirium at discharge, follow up with primary care physician in 1 to 2 weeks.

Patient Monitoring
- Evaluate and assess mental status daily.
- Continued evaluation for precipitating cause(s)

DIET
- Liberalize diet to increase oral intake.
- Nutritional supplements if oral intake is poor
- Consider temporary nasogastric tube if unable to eat and bowels are working.

PROGNOSIS
- May take weeks/months to fully resolve
- Usually improves with treatment of underlying condition(s); can lead to chronic cognitive impairment
- Delirium increases a person's 1-year mortality risk.

COMPLICATIONS
- Falls and functional decline
- Pressure ulcers and malnutrition

- Future cognitive dysfunction
- Higher risk for institutionalization
- Death

REFERENCES
1. American Psychiatric Association. *Diagnostic and Statistical Manual of Mental Disorders*. 5th ed. Arlington, VA: American Psychiatric Association; 2013.
2. van Eijk MM, van Marum RJ, Klijn IA, et al. Comparison of delirium assessment tools in a mixed intensive care unit. *Crit Care Med*. 2009;37(6):1881–1885.
3. Reston JT, Schoelles KM. In-facility delirium prevention programs as a patient safety strategy: a systematic review. *Ann Intern Med*. 2013;158(5, Pt 2):375–380.
4. Kalabalik J, Brunetti L, El-Srougy R. Intensive care unit delirium: a review of the literature. *J Pharm Pract*. 2014;27(2):195–207.
5. Barr J, Fraser GL, Puntillo K, et al. Clinical practice guidelines for the management of pain, agitation, and delirium in adult patients in the intensive care unit. *Crit Care Med*. 2013;41(1):263–306.
6. Neufeld KJ, Yue J, Robinson TN, et al. Antipsychotics medication for prevention and treatment of delirium in hospitalized adults: a systematic review and meta-analysis. *J Am Geriatr Soc*. 2016;64(4):705–714.

ADDITIONAL READING
- American Geriatrics Society Expert Panel on Postoperative Delirium in Older Adults. American Geriatrics Society abstracted clinical practice guideline for postoperative delirium in older adults. *J Am Geriatr Soc*. 2015;63(1):142–150.
- National Clinical Guideline Centre. *Delirium: Diagnosis, Prevention, and Management*. London, United Kingdom: National Clinical Guideline Centre; 2010.
- Quinlan N, Marcantonio ER, Inouye SK, et al. Vulnerability: the crossroads of frailty and delirium. *J Am Geriatr Soc*. 2011;59(Suppl 2):S262–S268.

 SEE ALSO

- Dementia; Depression; Substance Use Disorders
- Algorithm: Delirium

CODES

ICD10
- R41.0 Disorientation, unspecified
- F19.931 Oth psychoactive substance use, unsp w withdrawal delirium
- F10.231 Alcohol dependence with withdrawal delirium

CLINICAL PEARLS
- The CAM criteria for delirium are acute onset of fluctuating mental status, inattention, and either disorganized thinking or altered level of consciousness.
- Hypoactive subtype of delirium can easily be missed.
- Primary treatment for delirium is to identify and treat the underlying causes.
- Nonpharmacologic measures are preferable over pharmacologics.
- Delirium may not resolve as soon as the treatable contributors resolve; may take weeks or months

DEMENTIA

Umer Farooq, MD • John Doyle, MD

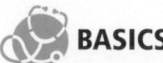 **BASICS**

DESCRIPTION

- *DSM-5* classifies dementias under neurocognitive disorders (major and mild).
- Evidence of cognitive decline from previous level of performance in one of cognitive domains (attention, executive function perceptual-motor, social cognition and memory). The cognitive deficits interfere significantly with ADLs (for major only) and do not occur exclusively in the context of delirium or any other mental disorder.
- *DSM-5* specifies the cause of neurocognitive decline secondary to the following:
  - Alzheimer dementia (AD)
    - Progressive cognitive decline; most common age >65 years
  - Vascular dementia (VaD)
    - Usually correlated with a cerebrovascular event and/or cerebrovascular disease
    - Stepwise deterioration with periods of clinical plateaus
  - Lewy body dementia
    - Fluctuating cognition associated with parkinsonism, hallucinations and delusions, gait difficulties, and falls
  - Frontotemporal dementia
    - Language difficulties, personality changes, and behavioral disturbances
  - Creutzfeldt-Jakob disease (CJD)
    - Very rare; rapid onset
  - HIV dementia
  - Substance-/medication-induced neurocognitive disorder

EPIDEMIOLOGY

Prevalence

- In patients age ≥65 years
  - AD: 5–10% (age 65 to 70 years); 25% (≥70 years)
  - VaD: 0.2% (age 65 to 70 years); up to 16% (≥70 years)
  - Other: 13%
- Estimated 5.4 million Americans had AD in 2010.
  - 5 million >65 years of age; 200,000 <65 years
  - Prevalence expected to double by 2030

ETIOLOGY AND PATHOPHYSIOLOGY

- AD: involves β-amyloid protein accumulation and/or neurofibrillary tangles (NFTs), synaptic dysfunction, neurodegeneration, and eventual neuronal loss
- Age, genetics, systemic disease, smoking, and other host factors may influence the β-amyloid accumulation and/or the pace of progression toward the clinical manifestations of AD.
- VaD: cerebral atherosclerosis/emboli with clinical/subclinical infarcts

Genetics

- AD: positive family history in 50%, but 90% AD is sporadic: *APOE4* increases risk but full role unclear.
- Familial/autosomal dominant AD accounts for <5% AD: amyloid precursor protein (APP), presenilin-1 (PSEN-1), and presenilin-2 (PSEN-2).

RISK FACTORS

- Age; sex: female > male
- Genetic predisposition
- Hypertension: AD; VaD
- Hypercholesterolemia: AD; VaD

- Diabetes: VaD
- Cigarette smoking: VaD
- Endocrine/metabolic abnormalities: hypothyroidism, Cushing syndrome; thiamine and vitamin B_{12} deficiency
- Chronic alcoholism, other drugs
- Lower educational status
- Head injury early in life
- Sedentary lifestyle

GENERAL PREVENTION

- Treat reversible causes of dementia, such as drug-induced, alcohol-induced, and vitamin deficiencies.
- Treat hypertension, hypercholesterolemia, and diabetes.
- No evidence for statins (or any other specific medication) to prevent onset of dementia (1)[A]
- BP control and low-dose aspirin may prevent or lessen cognitive decline in VaD.

COMMONLY ASSOCIATED CONDITIONS

- Anxiety and major depression
- Psychosis (delusions; delusions of persecution are common)
- Delirium
- Behavioral disturbances (agitation, aggression)
- Sleep disturbances

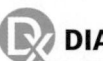 **DIAGNOSIS**

HISTORY

Probable diagnosis AD (2):

- Age between 40 and 90 years (usually >65 years)
- Progressive cognitive decline of insidious onset
- No disturbances of consciousness
- Deficits in areas of cognition
- No other explainable cause of symptoms
- Specifically rule out thyroid disease, vitamin deficiency (B_{12}), grief reaction, and depression.
- Supportive factors: family history of dementia

PHYSICAL EXAM

- Often normal physical
- No disturbances of consciousness
- Cognitive decline demonstrated by standardized instruments, including the following:
  - Mini-Mental State Examination (MMSE)
  - Montreal Cognitive Assessment (MoCA) test
  - ADAS-Cog
  - Clock drawing test
  - Use caution in relying solely on cognition scores, especially in those with learning difficulty, language barriers, or similar limitations.

DIFFERENTIAL DIAGNOSIS

- Major depression
- Medication side effect
- Chronic alcohol use
- Delirium
- Subdural hematoma
- Normal pressure hydrocephalus
- Brain tumor
- Thyroid disease
- Parkinson disease
- Vitamin B_{12} deficiency
- Toxins (aromatic hydrocarbons, solvents, heavy metals, marijuana, opiates, sedative-hypnotics)

DIAGNOSTIC TESTS & INTERPRETATION

Initial Tests (lab, imaging)

- Used to rule out causes
  - CBC, CMP
  - Thyroid-stimulating hormone
  - Vitamin B_{12} level
- Select patients
  - HIV, rapid plasma reagin (RPR)
  - Erythrocyte sedimentation rate (ESR)
  - Folate
  - Heavy metal and toxicology screen
- Research studies with cerebrospinal fluid (CSF) biomarkers in patient with confirmed AD have shown decreased amyloid beta (1 to 42) and increased τ and p-τ levels, which are specific features of AD, and CSF τ proteins are increased in CJD (3)[A].
- Neuroimaging (CT/MRI of brain): cerebral atrophy
  - Early age of onset (<65 years), rapid progression, focal neurologic deficits, cerebrovascular disease risk, or atypical symptoms: neuroimaging (MRI/CT) to rule out other causes
  - Important findings
    - AD: diffuse cerebral atrophy starting in association areas, hippocampus, amygdala
    - VaD: old infarcts, including lacunar

Diagnostic Procedures/Other

PET scan not routinely recommended; has been approved to differentiate between Alzheimer disease and frontotemporal dementia

Test Interpretation

AD

- NFTs: abnormally phosphorylated τ protein
- Senile plaques: APP derivatives
- Microvascular amyloid

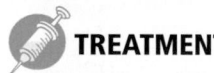 **TREATMENT**

GENERAL MEASURES

- Daily schedules and written directions
- Emphasis on nutrition, personal hygiene, accident-proofing the home, safety issues, sleep hygiene, and supervision
- Socialization (adult daycare)
- Sensory stimulation (display of clocks and calendars) in the early to middle stages
- Discussion with the family concerning support and advance directives

MEDICATION

- Cognitive dysfunction
- Medications for AD (4)[A] show a small improvement in some cognitive measures, but it remains unclear if the improvement is clinically significant.
- Cognitive dysfunction, mild
  - Cholinesterase inhibitors: donepezil (Aricept), 5 to 10 mg/day; rivastigmine (Exelon), 1.5 to 6.0 mg BID, transdermal system 4.6 mg/24 hr and 9.5 mg/24 hr; galantamine (Razadyne), 4 to 12 mg BID, extended release 8 to 24 mg/day
    - Adverse events: nausea, vomiting, diarrhea, anorexia, nightmares, bradycardia/syncope
    - Galantamine warning: associated with mortality in patients with mild cognitive impairment in clinical trial
    - It is suggested to consider cholinesterase inhibitor for patients with mild to moderate dementia (MMSE 10 to 26).

- The patients with moderate to advanced dementia (MMSE <17), recommendations are to add memantine (10 mg BID) to a cholinesterase inhibitor, or using memantine alone in patients who do not tolerate or benefit from a cholinesterase inhibitor.
- In patients with severe dementia (MMSE <10), it is suggested continuing memantine. However, in advanced dementia, medications can be discontinued to maximize quality of life and patient comfort.
- Start drug with lowest acquisition cost; also consider adverse event profile, adherence, medical comorbidity, drug interactions, and dosing profiles.

- Cognitive dysfunction, moderate to severe
  - Cholinesterase inhibitors OR
  - Memantine (Namenda), 5 to 20 mg/day
    - Adverse events: dizziness, confusion, headache, constipation OR
    - Combination cholinesterase inhibitor and memantine
- Commonly associated conditions
  - Psychosis and agitation/aggressive behavior:
    - Look for precipitating factors (infection, pain, depression, medications).
    - Nonpharmacologic therapies (behavioral interventions, music therapy, etc.) are preferred as first-line treatment.
    - Mood stabilizers (valproic acid, carbamazepine) have been used, although evidence is lacking.
    - For moderate/severe symptoms; antipsychotics: Initiate low doses, risperidone 0.25 to 1.00 mg/day; olanzapine 1.25 to 5.00 mg/day; quetiapine 12.5 to 50.0 mg/day; aripiprazole 5 mg/day; ziprasidone 20 mg/day
    - Atypical antipsychotic, quetiapine, is often first line due to decreased extrapyramidal side effect.
    - Novel antipsychotic, pimavanserin (selective 5-HT2A receptor inverse agonist) has shown to effectively treat Parkinson disease psychosis with minimal risk of worsening motor function associated with other treatment (5)[B].

ALERT
Black box warning on antipsychotics due to increased mortality in elderly with dementia

- Depression and insomnia
  - Depression:
    - Selective serotonin reuptake inhibitors (SSRIs): Initiate low doses, citalopram (Celexa) 10 mg/day; escitalopram (Lexapro) 5 mg/day; sertraline (Zoloft) 25 mg/day.
    - Adverse events: nausea, vomiting, agitation, parkinsonian effects, sexual dysfunction, hyponatremia
    - Venlafaxine, mirtazapine, and bupropion are also useful.
  - Sleep disturbances:
    - Low-dose antidepressants (e.g., Remeron) have significant sedative properties at 7.5 mg or 15 mg.
    - Trazodone 25 to 100 mg is frequently used because of better side effect profile.
  - Psychosis and agitation/aggressive behavior:
    - Some data for SSRIs
    - Benzodiazepines if agitation with anxiety; in elderly, use PRN.

Geriatric Considerations
Initiate pharmacotherapy at low doses and titrate slowly up if necessary.

- Benzodiazepines are potentially inappropriate for older adults, yet their use persists.

ALERT
Benzodiazepine use is associated with increased fall risk (6)[A].

- Watch decreased renal function and hepatic metabolism.

ISSUES FOR REFERRAL
Neuropsychiatric evaluation particularly helpful in early stages or mild cognitive impairment

ADDITIONAL THERAPIES
Behavioral modification
- Socialization, such as adult daycare, to prevent isolation and depression
- Sleep hygiene program as alternative to pharmaceuticals for sleep disturbance
- Scheduled toileting to prevent incontinence

COMPLEMENTARY & ALTERNATIVE MEDICINE
- Vitamin E is no longer recommended due to lack of evidence.
- Ginkgo biloba is not recommended due to lack of evidence.
- NSAIDs, selegiline, and estrogen lack efficacy and safety data.

ADMISSION, INPATIENT, AND NURSING CONSIDERATIONS
- Worsening physical health issues
- Psychiatry admission may be required because of safety concerns (self-harm/harm to others), self-neglect, aggressive behaviors, or other behavioral issues.

 ONGOING CARE

FOLLOW-UP RECOMMENDATIONS
Patient Monitoring
- Progression of cognitive impairment by use of standardized tool (e.g., MMSE, ADAS-Cog)
- Development of behavioral problems: sleep, depression, psychosis
- Adverse events of pharmacotherapy
- Nutritional status
- Caregiver evaluation of stress

PATIENT EDUCATION
- Long-term issues: safety, management of finances, medical decision making, possible placement; legal guardianship, if necessary
- Advance directives
- National Institute on Aging. About Alzheimer disease: other dementias: http://www.nia.nih.gov/alzheimers/topics/other-dementias

PROGNOSIS
- AD: usually steady progression leading to profound cognitive impairment:
  - Average survival of AD is about 10 years.
- VaD: incrementally worsening dementia, but cognitive improvement is unlikely
- Secondary dementias: Treatment of the underlying condition may lead to improvement; commonly seen with normal pressure hydrocephalus, hypothyroidism, and brain tumors

COMPLICATIONS
- Wandering
- Delirium
- Sundowner syndrome is common in older people (who are sedated) and also in people who have dementia (adverse reaction to small dose of psychoactive substances).

- Falls with injury
  - Hip fracture
  - Head trauma/hematomas
- Neglect and abuse
- Caregiver burnout

REFERENCES

1. McGuinness B, Craig D, Bullock R, et al. Statins for the prevention of dementia. *Cochrane Database Syst Rev.* 2009;(2):CD003160.
2. Blass DM, Rabins PV. In the clinic. Dementia. *Ann Intern Med.* 2008;148(7):ITC4-1–ITC4-16.
3. van Harten AC, Kester MI, Visser PJ, et al. Tau and p-tau as CSF biomarkers in dementia: a meta-analysis. *Clin Chem Lab Med.* 2011;49(3):353–366.
4. Birks J. Cholinesterase inhibitors for Alzheimer's disease. *Cochrane Database Syst Rev.* 2006;(1):CD005593.
5. Cummings J, Isaacson S, Mills R, et al. Pimavanserin for patients with Parkinson's disease psychosis: a randomised, placebo-controlled phase 3 trial. *Lancet.* 2014;383(9916):533–540.
6. Seppala LJ, Wermelink AMAT, de Vries M, et al; for EUGMS Task and Finish Group on Fall-Risk-Increasing Drugs. Fall-risk-increasing drugs: a systematic review and meta-analysis: II. Psychotropics. *J Am Med Dir Assoc.* 2018;19(4):371.e11–371.e17.

ADDITIONAL READING

Lyketsos CG, Colenda CC, Beck C, et al; for Task Force of American Association for Geriatric Psychiatry. Position statement of the American Association for Geriatric Psychiatry regarding principles of care for patients with dementia resulting from Alzheimer disease. *Am J Geriatr Psychiatry.* 2006;14(7):561–572.

 SEE ALSO

Algorithm: Dementia

 CODES

ICD10
- F03 Unspecified dementia
- G30.9 Alzheimer's disease, unspecified
- F01.50 Vascular dementia without behavioral disturbance

CLINICAL PEARLS

- Medications for AD show a small, statistically significant improvement in some cognitive measures, but it remains unclear if the improvement is clinically significant.
- Do not forget the role of adult protective services in case of elderly abuse—elder abuse hotline: 800-922-2275.
- A particular concern in nursing homes relates to the use of physical restraints and antipsychotic medication, which are regulated by Omnibus Budget Reconciliation Act of 1987.

DEMENTIA, VASCULAR
Birju B. Patel, MD, FACP, AGSF • N. Wilson Holland, MD, FACP

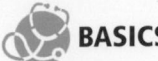

BASICS

Vascular dementia is a heterogeneous disorder caused by the sequel of cerebrovascular disease that manifests in cognitive impairment affecting memory, thinking, language, behavior, and judgment.

DESCRIPTION
- Vascular dementia (previously known as multi-infarct dementia) was first mentioned by Thomas Willis in 1672. Later, it was further described in the late 19th century by Binswanger and Alzheimer as a separate entity from dementia paralytica caused by neurosyphilis. This concept has evolved tremendously since the advent of neuroimaging modalities.
- Synonym(s): vascular cognitive impairment (VCI); vascular cognitive disorder (VCD); arteriosclerotic dementia; poststroke dementia; senile dementia due to hardening of the arteries; Binswanger disease. *Diagnostic and Statistical Manual of Mental Disorders* (*DSM-5*) categorizes vascular dementia as mild or major VCD.

EPIDEMIOLOGY
Second most common cause of dementia after Alzheimer dementia in the elderly and it frequently overlaps with Alzheimer

Incidence
About 6 to 12 cases per 1,000/person age >70 years
- Incidence of vascular dementia is declining in high-income countries in the past several decades likely due to better management of vascular risks.

Prevalence
- ~1.2–4.2% in those age >65 years
- 14–32% prevalence of dementia after a stroke

ETIOLOGY AND PATHOPHYSIOLOGY
On autopsy of those with dementia, many have significant vascular pathology that is present, but this is not necessarily correlated clinically with vascular dementia. No set pathologic criteria exist for the diagnosis of vascular dementia such as those that exist for Alzheimer dementia. Pathology includes the following:
- Large vessel disease: cognitive impairment that follows a stroke
- Small vessel disease: includes white matter changes (leukoaraiosis), subcortical infarcts, and incomplete infarction. This is usually the most common cause of multi-infarct dementia.
- Subcortical ischemic vascular disease: due to small vessel involvement within cerebral white matter, brainstem, and basal ganglia. Lacunar infarcts and deep white matter changes are typically included in this category.
- Noninfarct ischemic changes and atrophy
- Transient ischemic attack (TIA)/stroke
- Vascular, demographic, genetic factors
- Vascular disease (i.e., hypertension [HTN], peripheral vascular disease [PVD], atrial fibrillation, hyperlipidemia, diabetes) (1)[B],(2)[C]

Genetics
- Cerebral autosomal dominant arteriopathy with subcortical infarcts and leukoencephalopathy (CADASIL) is caused by a mutation in the *NOTCH3* gene on chromosome 19 that results in leukoencephalopathy and subcortical infarcts. This is clinically manifested in recurrent strokes, migraine with aura, and vascular dementia.
- *Apolipoprotein E* gene type: Those with ApoE4 subtypes are at higher risk of developing both vascular and Alzheimer dementia.
- Amyloid precursor protein (APP) gene: leads to a form of vascular dementia called heritable cerebral hemorrhage with amyloidosis

RISK FACTORS
- Age
- Previous stroke
- Smoking
- Diabetes (especially with frequent hypoglycemia)
- HTN
- Atrial fibrillation
- PVD
- Hyperlipidemia
- Metabolic syndrome
- Coronary atherosclerotic heart disease
- Previous myocardial infarction (3)[C]

GENERAL PREVENTION
- Optimization and aggressive treatment of vascular risk factors, such as HTN, diabetes, and hyperlipidemia
- HTN is the single most modifiable risk factor and treatment for it must be optimized.
- Smoking is associated with white matter changes on imaging, which may be associated with small vessel disease and vascular dementia progression.
- Lifestyle modification: weight loss, physical activity, smoking cessation
- Medication management for vascular risk reduction: aspirin usage, statin therapy for hyperlipidemia, antihypertensive therapy (4)[B]

COMMONLY ASSOCIATED CONDITIONS
- CADASIL
- Cerebral amyloid angiopathy (CAA) causes ischemic white matter damage due to amyloid deposition in penetrating cortical vessels.

DIAGNOSIS

Differentiation between Alzheimer dementia and vascular dementia can be difficult, and significant overlap is seen in the clinical presentation of these two dementias. The diagnosis of vascular dementia is a clinical diagnosis.

HISTORY
- Gradual, stepwise progression is typical.
- Ask about onset and progression of cognitive impairment and the specific cognitive domains involved.
- Ask about vascular risk factors and previous attempts to control these risk factors.
- Ask about medication compliance.
- Ask about urinary incontinence and gait disturbances. Abnormal gait and falls are strong predictors of development of vascular dementia, particularly unsteady, frontal, and hemiparetic types of gait.
- Look for early symptoms, including difficulty performing cognitive tasks, memory, mood, and assessment of instrumental activities of daily living (IADLs).
- History may include TIAs, cerebrovascular accidents (CVAs), coronary atherosclerotic heart disease, atrial fibrillation, hyperlipidemia, and/or PVD.

PHYSICAL EXAM
- Screen for HTN. Average daily BP and not office BP is associated with progression of cerebrovascular disease and cognitive decline in the elderly.
- Focal neurologic deficits may be present.
- Gait assessment is important, especially looking at gait initiation, gait speed, and balance (5,6).
- Check for carotid bruits as well as abdominal bruits and assess for presence of PVD.
- Check body mass index and waist circumference.
- Do a thorough cardiac evaluation that includes looking for arrhythmias (i.e., atrial fibrillation).

DIFFERENTIAL DIAGNOSIS
- Alzheimer dementia
- Depression
- Drug intoxication
- CNS tumors
- Hypothyroidism
- Vitamin B_{12} deficiency

DIAGNOSTIC TESTS & INTERPRETATION
- Cognitive testing, such as Saint Louis University Mental Status (SLUMS) and Montreal Cognitive Assessment (MoCA), provides more definitive information in terms of cognitive deficits, especially executive function, which may be lost earlier in vascular dementia. The Mini-Mental State Examination is not sensitive in distinguishing Alzheimer dementia from vascular dementia because it does not have good measures of executive function.
- Neuropsychological testing may also be beneficial, especially in evaluating multiple cognitive domains and their specific involvements and deficits.

Initial Tests (lab, imaging)
As appropriate, consider CBC, comprehensive metabolic profile, lipid panel, thyroid function, hemoglobin A1C, and vitamin B_{12}.
- Imaging is used in conjunction with history and physical examination to support a clinical diagnosis of vascular dementia.
- Cognitive deficits observed clinically do not always have to correlate with findings found on neuroimaging studies.
- MRI is best in terms of evaluation of subtle subcortical deficits.
- White matter changes and specific location of these changes can be associated with executive dysfunction and episodic memory impairment.

TREATMENT

Prevention is the real key to treatment:
- Control of risk factors, including HTN, hyperlipidemia, and diabetes
- Avoidance of tobacco and smoking cessation
- Healthy, low-cholesterol diet

MEDICATION
- Clinical evidence for use of acetylcholinesterase inhibitors and memantine reveals limited benefit in vascular dementia but may slow cognitive decline in patients with mixed Alzheimer and vascular dementia (7)[B].
- Controlling BP with any antihypertensive medications, treatment of dyslipidemia (e.g., statins), and treatment of diabetes are very important.
- Selective serotonin reuptake inhibitors (SSRIs) may be of benefit for agitation and psychosis in vascular dementia.

ADDITIONAL THERAPIES
- Limit alcohol drink intake to ≤1/day in women and 2/day in men.
- Heavy sustained alcohol use contributes to HTN.
- Preventing new CVAs is key in managing vascular dementia; aspirin and other anti-platelet agents such as clopidogrel may be useful if no contraindications.

SURGERY/OTHER PROCEDURES
Patients with symptomatic carotid artery stenosis should be referred to a vascular surgeon to be evaluated for carotid endarterectomy. Carotid endarterectomy is recommended over carotid artery stenting in patients >70 years of age if perioperative morbidity/mortality are <6%.

COMPLEMENTARY & ALTERNATIVE MEDICINE
Ginkgo biloba should be avoided due to increased risk of bleeding, especially in CAA.

ADMISSION, INPATIENT, AND NURSING CONSIDERATIONS
- Remain sensitive to functional assessment and avoidance of pressure ulcers after CVAs.
- Avoid Foley catheter usage unless necessary due to increased risk of infection.
- Nonpharmacologic approaches to behavior management should be attempted prior to medication usage.
- Providing optimal sensory input to patients with cognitive impairment is important during hospitalizations to avoid delirium and confusion. Patients should be given frequent cues to keep them oriented to place and time. They should be informed of any changes in the daily schedule of activities and evaluations. Family and caregivers should be encouraged to be with patients with dementia as much as possible to further help them from becoming confused during hospitalization. Recreational, physical, occupational, and music therapy can be beneficial during hospitalization in avoiding delirium and preventing functional decline.

- Emphasis must be placed on screening for, and optimizing, the mood of the patient. Depression is very common in older patients, especially those who have had strokes and have become hospitalized. Depression can present as "pseudodementia" with worsening confusion during hospitalization and is a treatable condition.

ONGOING CARE

Vascular dementia is a condition that should be followed with multiple visits in the office setting with goals of optimizing cardiovascular risk profiles for patients. Future planning and advanced directives should be addressed early. Family and caregiver evaluation and burden should also be evaluated.

FOLLOW-UP RECOMMENDATIONS
Perform regular follow-up with a primary care provider or geriatrician for risk factor modification and education on importance of regular physical and mental exercises as tolerated.

Patient Monitoring
Appropriate evaluation and diagnosis of this condition, need for future planning, optimizing vascular risk factors, lifestyle modification counseling, therapeutic interventions

DIET
- The American Heart Association diet and Dietary Approaches to Stop Hypertension (DASH) diet is recommended for optimal BP and cardiovascular risk factor control.
- Low-fat, decreased concentrated sweets and carbohydrates, especially in those with metabolic syndrome

PATIENT EDUCATION
- Lifestyle modification is important in vascular risk reduction (smoking cessation, exercise counseling, dietary counseling, weight-loss counseling).
- Optimizing vascular risk factors via medications (i.e., HTN, diabetes, atrial fibrillation, PVD, heart disease)
- Avoiding smoking, including secondhand smoke
- Home BP monitoring and glucometer testing of blood sugars if HTN, impaired glucose tolerance, and/or diabetes is present

PROGNOSIS
- Lost cognitive abilities that persist after initial recovery of deficits from stroke do not usually return. Some individuals can have intermittent periods of self-reported improvement in cognitive function.
- Risk factors for progression of cognitive and functional impairment poststroke include age, prestroke cognitive abilities, depression, polypharmacy, and decreased cerebral perfusion during acute stroke.

COMPLICATIONS
- Physical disability from stroke
- Severe cognitive impairment
- Death

REFERENCES

1. Kalaria RN. The pathology and pathophysiology of vascular dementia. *Neuropharmacology*. 2018;134(Pt B):226–239.
2. Dichgans M, Leys D. Vascular cognitive impairment. *Circ Res*. 2017;120(3):573–591.
3. Sundbøll J, Horváth-Puhó E, Adelborg K, et al. Higher risk of vascular dementia in myocardial infarction survivors. *Circulation*. 2018;137(6):567–577.
4. White WB, Wolfson L, Wakefield DB, et al. Average daily blood pressure, not office blood pressure, is associated with progression of cerebrovascular disease and cognitive decline in older people. *Circulation*. 2011;124(21):2312–2319.
5. Montero-Odasso M, Verghese J, Beauchet O, et al. Gait and cognition: a complementary approach to understanding brain function and the risk of falling. *J Am Geriatr Soc*. 2012;60(11):2127–2136.
6. Verghese J, Lipton RB, Hall CB, et al. Abnormality of gait as a predictor of non-Alzheimer's dementia. *N Engl J Med*. 2002;347(22):1761–1768.
7. Kavirajan H, Schneider LS. Efficacy and adverse effects of cholinesterase inhibitors and memantine in vascular dementia: a meta-analysis of randomised controlled trials. *Lancet Neurol*. 2007;6(9):782–792.

ADDITIONAL READING

Eizaguirre NO, Rementeria GP, González-Torres M, et al. Updates in vascular dementia. *Heart Mind*. 2017;1(1):22–35.

SEE ALSO

Alzheimer Disease; Depression; Mild Cognitive Impairment

CODES

ICD10
- F01.50 Vascular dementia without behavioral disturbance
- F01.51 Vascular dementia with behavioral disturbance

CLINICAL PEARLS

- Executive dysfunction and gait abnormalities are often seen early and are more pronounced in vascular dementia as opposed to Alzheimer dementia.
- Memory is relatively preserved in vascular dementia when compared with Alzheimer dementia in the early stages of this disease.
- Stepwise progression, as opposed to progressive decline in Alzheimer dementia, is typical.
- Considerable overlap exists between vascular dementia and Alzheimer dementia in clinical practice, and classification into one of these categories is often difficult. Patients can have mixed etiologies as well.

DENTAL INFECTION

Sheila O. Stille, DMD • Karlynn Sievers, MD

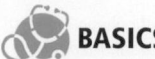

BASICS

DESCRIPTION
- Pain ± swelling in the head and neck region from infection of the teeth and/or supporting structures; if left untreated, can lead to serious and potentially life-threatening illnesses
- Assume any head and neck infection or swelling to be odontogenic in origin until proven otherwise.
- System(s) affected: oropharynx, throat, dental, gastrointestinal
- Synonym(s): odontogenic infections, dental abscess

EPIDEMIOLOGY
- 18% of 5- to 19-year-olds have untreated dental caries.
- 28% of individuals age >20 years have untreated dental caries (1).
- Rates are higher in Hispanic (21.7%) and black (23%) children/teens (1)[A].
- 92% of adults 20 to 64 years have had dental caries.
- 25% of children 5 to 17 years account for 80% of caries in the United States.
- 17% of adults age >64 years are edentulous (1).

ETIOLOGY AND PATHOPHYSIOLOGY
- Dental caries is the most common worldwide chronic disease.
- Caries or trauma can lead to death of the tooth pulp, which can lead to infection and/or abscess of adjacent tissues via direct or hematogenous bacterial colonization.
- Caries (tooth decay; "cavity") represent a contagious bacterial infection causing demineralization and destruction of the tooth tissue (enamel, dentin, and cementum).
- *Streptococcus mutans* is transmitted to newly dentate infants by caregivers.
- Acidic secretions from *S. mutans* are implicated in early caries.
- Often there is polymicrobial mix of anaerobes in dental abscess (viridans streptococci and *Streptococcus anginosus*).
- Anaerobes, including peptostreptococci, *Bacteroides*, *Prevotella*, and *Fusobacterium*, have also been implicated; lactobacilli not seen in healthy subjects but common in patients with extensive caries (2)
- Preventable with good oral hygiene, low-cariogenic diet, access to fluoride, and professional dental care
- Fluoride has dramatically decreased dental caries.

RISK FACTORS
- Low socioeconomic status
- Parent and/or sibling with history of caries or existing untreated dental caries (especially in past 12 months)
- Previous dental caries
- Poor access to dental/health care; lack of dental insurance
- Fear of dentist
- Poor oral hygiene
- Poor nutrition, including diet containing high level of sugary foods and drinks
- Trauma to the teeth or jaw
- Inadequate access to and use of fluoride
- Gingival recession (increased risk of root caries)
- Physical and mental disabilities
- Decreased salivary flow (e.g., use of anticholinergic medications, immunologic diseases, radiation therapy to head and neck)

GENERAL PREVENTION
- Most dental problems can be avoided through flossing/use of interdental brushes; brushing with fluoride toothpaste, systemic fluoride (fluoridated bottled water; fluoride supplements for high-risk patients and in nonfluoridated areas); fluoride varnish for moderate- to high-risk patients and all children age <6 years; regular dental cleanings (1,3).
- Prevent transmission of *S. mutans* from mother/caregiver to infant by improving maternal dentition, chlorhexidine gluconate rinses, and use of xylitol products for mother especially during first 2 years of a child's life. Avoid smoking, which is linked to severe periodontal disease (2).
- Good control of systemic diseases (e.g., diabetes)
- Fluoride varnish provided by dental or medical primary care providers twice per year (2,3)

COMMONLY ASSOCIATED CONDITIONS
- Extensive caries, crowding, multiple missing teeth
- Periapical and periodontal abscess
- Soft tissue cellulitis
- Periodontitis (deep inflammation ± infection of gingiva, alveolar bone support, and ligaments)

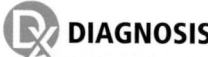

DIAGNOSIS

HISTORY
- Pain of involved tooth; can be referred to ears, jaw, cheek, neck, or sinuses; unexplained headaches
- Hot/cold sensitivity
- Pain can be unprovoked, intermittent, and/or constant.

- Pain with biting or chewing
- Trismus (inability to open mouth)
- Bleeding or purulent drainage from gingival tissues
- When severe infection (systemic)
  – Fever
  – Difficulty breathing or swallowing
  – Raspy voice
  – Mental status changes
- Evaluate children <4 years with stiff neck, sore throat, and dysphagia for retropharyngeal abscess.

PHYSICAL EXAM
- Gingival edema and erythema
- Cheek (extraoral) or vestibular (intraoral) swelling
- Fluctuant mass at involved site
- Suppuration of gingival margin
- Submandibular or cervical lymphadenopathy
- Severe (systemic) infection may present with dysphagia, fever, and signs of airway compromise.

DIFFERENTIAL DIAGNOSIS
- Bacterial or viral pharyngitis
- Pericoronitis (inflammation ± infection of gum flap over mandibular last molar, typically 3rd molars)
- Otitis media or externa
- Sinusitis
- Headache/migraine
- Viral (HSV1, herpangina, hand-foot-mouth disease) or aphthous stomatitis
- Temporomandibular joint (TMJ) dysfunction (myofascial pain, ± internal derangement of TMJ)
- Parotitis
- Jaw pain can be anginal equivalent, especially in women and especially lower left side of the jaw.

DIAGNOSTIC TESTS & INTERPRETATION
Initial Tests (lab, imaging)
- No initial labs needed, unless patient looks acutely ill.
- If acutely ill
  – Consider CBC with differential.
  – If abscess present, aspirate pus and culture for aerobes and anaerobes (4).
  – Typically polymicrobial infections with anaerobic gram-negative rods and anaerobic gram-positive cocci (4)
- Individual films of suspected teeth, including root apices; test with palpation, percussion, and cold sensitivity.
- Panoramic film or CT scan of the teeth and jaw to evaluate the extent of infection

Follow-Up Tests & Special Considerations
- Panoramic radiograph, particularly if trismus present
- CT scan can be helpful if facial swelling extends below inferior border of mandible or into infraorbital space. This helps to locate for potential incision and drainage by oral and maxillofacial surgeon or ENT.

 TREATMENT
- Isolated pain (no swelling or systemic signs of infection) does not warrant antibiotic use.
- If localized, consider incision and drainage.
- Appropriate pain control: Anti-inflammatory agents are first line; short-course opioids in some cases (5)[A]
- Refer to oral health provider for definitive treatment: root canal, extraction, gum therapy (4).
- If infection is severe (systemic symptoms), consider hospitalization with IV antibiotics until stable. May need intraoral or extraoral incision and drainage; definitive treatment (extraction or root canal therapy) necessary to prevent progression or recurrence

GENERAL MEASURES
- Ibuprofen 600 to 800 mg (pediatrics: 10 mg/kg) q6h or acetaminophen 650 to 1,000 mg (pediatrics: 10 to 15 mg/kg) q4–6h PRN for pain
- For more severe pain, consider acetaminophen with ibuprofen (synergistic effect) + short course of opioids.
- Local nerve block with long-acting anesthetic (bupivacaine); avoid penetrating infection to avoid tracking infection.

MEDICATION
First Line
- Amoxicillin: 500 mg TID for 7 to 10 days; in children, 40 to 60 mg/kg/day divided TID
- If penicillin allergic, use clindamycin 300 mg PO TID for 7 days.

Second Line
If long-standing infection or no response to first-line treatment
- Clindamycin: 300 mg PO TID for 7 to 10 days
- Amoxicillin/clavulanic acid (500 mg/125 mg), 1 tablet PO TID for 7 days
- If severe infection, consider IV antibiotics (ampicillin-sulbactam, cefoxitin, cefotetan).
- Consider double coverage with metronidazole 500 mg PO TID for 7 days for better bone penetration and good anaerobic coverage. Do not use metronidazole alone; will increase development of resistant strains; can be used with amoxicillin or clindamycin

ISSUES FOR REFERRAL
Consult an oral health provider, and ensure definitive follow-up.

SURGERY/OTHER PROCEDURES
- Incise and drain large, fluctuant abscesses.
- Root canal or extraction is definitive treatment.

ADMISSION, INPATIENT, AND NURSING CONSIDERATIONS
Criteria for hospital admission: swelling involving deep spaces of the neck, floor of the mouth, or infraorbital region; deviation of the airway; unstable vital signs; fever (>101°F); chills; raspy voice; confusion or delirium; or evidence of invasive infection or cellulitis
- Ensure secure airway.
- IV fluid resuscitation if necessary
- Ensure good oral hygiene.
- Rinse or swab mouth with chlorhexidine gluconate BID.
- Use warm saltwater rinses several times per day, especially after incision and drainage; ice packs to decrease swelling and encourage drainage
- Discharge patient when
  – Airway not compromised
  – Abscess and sepsis eliminated
  – Able to take PO intake and ambulate

 ONGOING CARE

Educate regarding proper oral hygiene, need for follow-up dental care, and potential medical complications that arise due to lack of dental care.

FOLLOW-UP RECOMMENDATIONS
- Follow up with oral health provider within 24 hours.
- Ensure adequate PO intake, including protein.

DIET
- Maintain a healthy diet; bacteria thrive on refined sugar and starch.
- Avoid sugary foods that stick between the teeth.
- Avoid the use of sugary/carbonated drinks throughout day; water as beverage of choice between meals

Pediatric Considerations
In children, limit the frequency of sugary drinks and advise against sleeping with a bottle; fluoride varnish twice a year (more for higher risk children) for children age <6 years (3)

PATIENT EDUCATION
- Control caries and periodontal disease.
- Biannual dental visits at a minimum
  – Limit the frequency of sugar/carbonated drinks and sugary or sticky foods.
- In young children, avoid sleeping with a bottle to decrease the chance of dental caries.
- Brush twice daily and use floss/interdental brush daily.

PROGNOSIS
Prognosis is excellent with proper treatment.

COMPLICATIONS
- Ludwig angina
- Retropharyngeal and mediastinal infection
- Osteomyelitis
- Endocarditis/cardiac tamponade
- Submental infection
- Submandibular infection
- Can cause unstable diabetes in diabetics/worsen preexisting heart disease
- Brain abscess/death

REFERENCES
1. National Center for Health Statistics. *Health, United States, 2016: With Chartbook on Long-term Trends in Health.* Hyattsville, MD: 2017. https://www.cdc.gov/nchs/data/hus/hus16.pdf. Accessed August 31, 2017.
2. Chaffee BW, Gansky SA, Weintraub JA, et al. Maternal oral bacterial levels predict early childhood caries development. *J Dent Res.* 2014;93(3):238–244.
3. Chou R, Cantor A, Zakher B, et al. Preventing dental caries in children <5 years: systematic review updating USPSTF recommendation. *Pediatrics.* 2013;132(2):332–350.
4. Robertson D, Smith AJ. The microbiology of the acute dental abscess. *J Med Microbiol.* 2009;58(Pt 2):155–162.
5. Bali RK, Sharma P, Gaba S, et al. A review of complications of odontogenic infections. *Natl J Maxillofac Surg.* 2015;6(2):136–143.

ADDITIONAL READING
- Clark MB, Douglass AB, Maier R, et al. *Smiles for Life: A National Oral Health Curriculum.* 3rd ed. Leawood, KS: Society of Teachers of Family Medicine; 2010. http://www.smilesforlifeoralhealth.com/buildcontent.aspx?tut=555&pagekey=62948&cbreceipt=0. Accessed December 12, 2018.
- Flynn TR. What are the antibiotics of choice for odontogenic infections, and how long should the treatment course last? *Oral Maxillofac Surg Clin North Am.* 2011;23(4):519–536.
- Lockhart PB, ed. *Oral Medicine and Medically Complex Patients.* 6th ed. New York, NY: Wiley; 2013.
- Stephens MB, Wiedemer JP, Kushner GM. Dental problems in primary care. *Am Fam Physician.* 2018;98(11):654–660.
- U.S. Preventive Services Task Force. Dental caries in children from birth through age 5 years: screening. http://www.uspreventiveservicestaskforce.org/Page/Topic/recommendation-summary/dental-caries-in-children-from-birth-through-age-5-years-screening. Accessed December 12, 2018.

 CODES

ICD10
- K02.9 Dental caries, unspecified
- K04.7 Periapical abscess without sinus
- K12.2 Cellulitis and abscess of mouth

CLINICAL PEARLS
- Do not ignore tooth pain.
- Treat patients with facial swelling aggressively because infections can spread quickly, leading to significant morbidity or even death.
- Prevention (oral hygiene, fluoride, dental visits) is the key to avoiding odontogenic infections.

DEPRESSION

Naureen Rafiq, MBBS • Michael G. Kavan, PhD

BASICS

DESCRIPTION

- A primary mood disorder characterized by a sustained feeling of sadness and/or decreased interest in all or most activities once enjoyed (anhedonia), which represents a change from previous functioning
- Variants: disruptive mood dysregulation disorder, major depressive disorder (MDD), persistent depressive disorder (dysthymia), premenstrual dysphoric disorder, substance/medication-induced depressive disorder, depressive disorder due to another medical condition, other specified depressive disorder, unspecified depressive disorder

EPIDEMIOLOGY

Incidence
In United States, 8.1% of adults aged ≥20 years experienced depression in a given 2-week period between 2013 and 2016 (1).

Prevalence
- 19.2% lifetime risk of having MDD (2)
- Patients can relapse; risk decreases with longer remission periods but increases with severe or multiple episodes and episodes at a younger age.
- Predominant age
  – Low risk before early teens but highest prevalence in teens and young adults
- Predominant gender
  – Females > males (2:1)

ETIOLOGY AND PATHOPHYSIOLOGY
There are diverse theories on the pathophysiology of depression.

- *Monoamine-deficiency hypothesis*: symptoms related to decreased levels of norepinephrine (dullness and lethargy) and serotonin (irritability, hostility, and suicidal ideation) in multiple regions of the brain; other neurotransmitters involved include dopamine, acetylcholine, γ-aminobutyric acid (GABA), glutamate.
- *Stress/hypothalamic–pituitary–adrenal axis*: Abnormalities in cortisol response lead to depression; elevated cortisol levels can be associated with depression, but cortisol tests are not indicated for diagnosis.
- Depression as inflammatory disorder: Proinflammatory marker levels are reported to be elevated in depressed patients. Examples of these markers are C-reactive protein (CRP), interleukin (IL)-6, IL-1, and tumor necrosis factor-α (TNF-α).
- Hormones and depression: Reduction in thyroid hormone, estrogen levels, and elevation in vasopressin has been seen in people with depression.
- Other areas of research interest: abnormal circadian rhythms; impaired synthesis/metabolism of neurotransmitters
- Environmental factors and learned behavior may affect neurotransmitters and/or have an independent influence on depression.

Genetics
Multiple gene loci place a person at increased risk when faced with environmental stressor; twin studies suggest 37% concordance (3).

RISK FACTORS
- Female > male (2:1)
- Severity of first episode
- Persistent sleep disturbances

- Presence of chronic disease(s), recent myocardial infarction (MI), cardiovascular accident (CVA)
- Strong family history (depression, bipolar, suicide, substance abuse), spouse with depression
- Childhood trauma/maltreatment
- Substance abuse and dependence, domestic abuse/violence
- Losses, stressors, unemployment
- Single, divorced, or unhappily married

COMMONLY ASSOCIATED CONDITIONS
- Bipolar disorder, cyclothymic disorder, grief reaction, anxiety disorders, somatoform disorders, schizophrenia/schizoaffective disorders
- Medical comorbidity
- Substance abuse

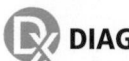

DIAGNOSIS

HISTORY
DSM-5 requires all of the following criteria for MDD:

- Criterion A: ≥5 of the following symptoms present nearly every day during the same 2-week period, with at least 1 of the 5 being either depressed mood or loss of interest or pleasure:
  – Depressed mood most of the day by subjective report or observation from other people
  – Markedly diminished interest or pleasure in all activities most of the day by subjective report or observation from other people
  – Decreased or increased appetite or significant weight loss without dieting or weight gain
  – Insomnia or hypersomnia
  – Fatigue or energy loss
  – Agitation, restlessness, or slowed speech or body movements observable by others
  – Worthlessness, excessive/inappropriate guilty feelings
  – Diminished thinking/concentration, poor memory, indecisiveness
  – Recurrent thoughts of death, suicidal ideations, or suicide attempt or a specific plan for committing suicide
- Criterion B: Symptoms cause significant social, occupational, or functional distress or impairment.
- Criterion C: symptoms not attributable to substance effects or other medical conditions

Geriatric Considerations
- Difficult to diagnose due to medical comorbidity
- Can present as memory difficulties
- Can be the initial presentation of irreversible dementia
- Geriatric Depression Scale (GDS 15) improves rate of diagnosis in primary care setting (4,5)[A].

Pediatric Considerations
- Can present as irritable or angry rather than sad or dejected
- Failure to make expected weight gains can substitute weight loss symptom above.
- Frequent absences from school or a sudden and remarkable drop in grades
- Frequent complaints of physical illnesses (e.g., headaches)

PHYSICAL EXAM
Complete exam to look for evidence of contributing medical or neurologic disorders: psychiatric affect, attention, cognition, memory.

DIFFERENTIAL DIAGNOSIS
- Psychiatric: depressed phase of bipolar disorder—inquire if prior mania, family or personal history of bipolar disorder, prior agitation, or excitement with antidepressant medication. If positive, monitor carefully for mood elevation or destabilization, adjustment disorder, and bereavement.
- Neurologic or degenerative CNS diseases, dementias
- Medical comorbidity: adrenal disease, thyroid disorders, diabetes, metabolic abnormalities (hypercalcemia), liver/renal failure, malignancy, chronic fatigue syndrome, fibromyalgia, lupus
- Nutritional: pernicious anemia, pellagra
- Medications/substances: abuse, side effects, overdose, intoxication, dependence, withdrawal

DIAGNOSTIC TESTS & INTERPRETATION
- A clinical diagnosis made by eliciting personal, family, social, and psychosocial factors
- The Patient Health Questionnaire-9 (PHQ-9) is a brief screening test valid for diagnosis of MDD in primary care settings (5)[A].
- Other validated scales include Beck Depression Inventory, Zung, GDS 15, and so forth, which are also useful to track response to treatment over time (5)[A].
- Rule out metabolic disorders with TSH, CBC, and comprehensive metabolic panel (CMP).
- Urine drug screen if symptoms suggest intoxication

TREATMENT

American Psychiatric Association (APA) 2010 guidelines recommend phasic approach: acute phase (first 3 months), continuation phase (4 to 9 months), and maintenance (9 months until discontinuation) (6)[A].

- Acute phase
  – Full evaluation, including risk to self and others, with selection of appropriate treatment setting (hospitalization for those at risk of harm to self or others or so incapacitated as to be unable to take care of themselves and/or who have no support system to assist with treatment)
  – Goal should be symptom remission, with intervention based on clinical picture, including patient's preference, availability of services.
  – For mild to moderate depression, psychotherapies (individual, interpersonal, or cognitive-behavioral therapy [CBT]) and/or medication are recommended.
  – For refractory/severe depression, medication is indicated.
  – For patients not responding to medication alone, CBT should be added.
  – Continue to increase dosage q3–4wk until symptoms in remission. Full medication effect is complete in 4 to 6 weeks. Augmentation with second medication may be necessary.
  – See within 2 to 4 weeks of starting medication and q2wk until improvement and then monthly to monitor medication changes.
  – ≥6 visits recommended for monitoring (younger patients, those at high suicide risk, see within 1st week, and follow frequently)
- Continuation/maintenance phase
  – Regular visits to monitor for relapse, q3–6mo if stable; depression rating scales should be used.
  – Once remission achieved, dosage should be continued for at least 6 to 9 months to reduce relapse; CBT is also effective in reducing relapse (visits typically q2wk).
  – Medications should be tapered gradually (weeks to months).

ISSUES FOR REFERRAL
- Refer immediately for active suicidal ideation, severe self-neglect, and significant risk of self-harm.
- Failed response to medication, suspected bipolar or personality disorder

MEDICATION
- Effectiveness comparable between/within classes; selection should be based on provider familiarity and patient characteristics/preferences (7)[A].
- Selective serotonin reuptake inhibitors (SSRIs) and tricyclic antidepressants (TCAs) are effective, but TCAs are second line due to side effects and lethality in overdose.

First Line
- SSRIs* (starting dose; usual dose)
  - Fluoxetine (Prozac): 20 mg/day; 20 to 60 mg/day; FDA-approved for teens
  - Sertraline (Zoloft): 50 mg/day; 50 to 200 mg/day
  - Paroxetine (Paxil): 10 mg/day; 20 to 50 mg/day
  - Paroxetine CR (Paxil CR): 12.5 mg/day; 25.0 to 62.5 mg/day
  - Citalopram (Celexa): 20 mg/day; 20 to 40 mg/day (higher doses not advised; ECG monitoring for doses >40 mg/day due to increased risk of QTc prolongation)
  - Escitalopram (Lexapro): 10 mg/day; 10 to 20 mg/day
  - Precautions: Abrupt discontinuation may result in withdrawal symptoms (i.e., dizziness, nausea, headache, paresthesia).
  - Fluoxetine, paroxetine may raise serum levels of other drugs.
  - Common side effects: sexual dysfunction (20%), nausea, GI upset, dizziness, insomnia, headache; typically resolve in the 1st week
  - *Lower starting doses for elderly, adolescents, those with comorbid conditions, panic disorder, significant anxiety, or hepatic conditions
  - Paroxetine is Category D for pregnancy with increased risk of teratogenicity in 1st trimester.
- Others (starting dose; usual dose)
  - Venlafaxine (Effexor, Effexor XR): 37.5 mg/day; 300 mg/day
  - Bupropion XL (Wellbutrin XL): 150 mg/day; 300 to 450 mg/day (precautions: powers seizure threshold at doses >450 mg/day)
  - Duloxetine (Cymbalta): 30 mg/day; 60 to 120 mg/day
  - Desvenlafaxine (Pristiq): 50 to 100 mg/day
  - Vilazodone (Viibryd): Start 10 mg/day; usual target 40 mg/day
  - Vortioxetine (Trintellix): Start 5 mg/day; target dose 20 mg/day
  - Levomilnacipran (Fetzima): Start 20 mg/day; target dose 40 to 120 mg/day

Second Line
- TCAs (starting dose; usual dose)
  - Amitriptyline (Elavil): 25 to 50 mg/day; 100 to 300 mg/day
  - Nortriptyline (Pamelor): 25 mg/day; 50 to 150 mg/day
  - Doxepin (Sinequan): 25 to 50 mg/day; 100 to 300 mg/day
  - Imipramine (Tofranil, Tofranil-PM): 25 to 50 mg/day; 100 to 300 mg/day
  - Desipramine (Norpramin): 25 to 50 mg/day; 100 to 300 mg/day
  - Precautions: advanced age, glaucoma, benign prostatic hyperplasia, hyperthyroidism, cardiovascular disease, liver disease, monoamine oxidase inhibitor (MAOI) treatment, potential for fatal overdose, arrhythmia, worsening glycemic control, SSRIs recommended for patients with diabetes (6)[A]

- Common side effects: dry mouth, blurred vision, constipation, urinary retention, tachycardia, confusion/delirium; elderly particularly susceptible
- α_2-Antagonists (sedating, appetite stimulant) (starting dose; usual dose)
  - Mirtazapine (Remeron): 15 mg/day; 15 to 45 mg/day
- Atypical antipsychotics
  - Adjunctive treatment: aripiprazole or quetiapine
  - Treatment-resistant depression (TRD): olanzapine
  - Significant side effects: dyslipidemia, hypertriglyceridemia, glucose dysregulation, diabetes mellitus, hyperprolactinemia, tardive dyskinesia, neuroleptic malignant syndrome, QTc prolongation (8)[A]
  - Recommended for depression with psychotic features; consult with psychiatrist and consider carefully before starting (6)[A].
- Significant potential interactions
  - TCAs: amphetamines, barbiturates, clonidine, epinephrine, ethanol, norepinephrine
  - All antidepressants: Allow 14-day washout period before starting MAOIs.
  - MAOIs: not recommended in primary care. Significant drug and food interactions; limit use.

ALERT
- Black box warning: increased risk of suicidality in children, adolescents, and young adults up to age 25 years who are treated with antidepressants. Although this has not been extended to adults, suicide risk assessments are warranted for all patients.
- Serotonin syndrome—a rare but potentially lethal complication from rapid increase in dose or new addition of medication with serotonergic effects
- Tapering allows for the detection of recurring symptoms and minimizes discontinuation syndromes.
- Caution with personal or family history of bipolar disorder: Antidepressants can precipitate mania.

Pregnancy Considerations
SSRIs: fluoxetine, sertraline, and bupropion considered safe in pregnancy (paroxetine, Category D; other SSRIs, Category C)

ADDITIONAL THERAPIES
- CBT is a type of psychotherapy that focuses on how persons perceive a situation and helping them to change their unhelpful thinking and behavior, which leads to enduring improvement in their mood and functioning. It is focused on the present, is limited in duration, and is problem-solving oriented.
- Electroconvulsive therapy (ECT) for refractory cases
- Repetitive transcranial magnetic stimulation (rTMS) may be helpful for TRD (8)[A].

COMPLEMENTARY & ALTERNATIVE MEDICINE
Used in mild depression but *not* regulated by FDA nor recommended by APA
- Hypericum perforatum (St. John's wort): multiple drug interactions; not safe in pregnancy
- Data do not support S-adenosyl-l-methionine (SAMe) or acupuncture.

ONGOING CARE

PATIENT EDUCATION
- Depression is a common medical illness, not a character defect.
- Emphasize the need for long-term treatment and follow-up, which includes lifestyle changes.
- Recommend exercise, good sleep hygiene, nutrition, and decreased use of tobacco and alcohol.

PROGNOSIS
- 70% show significant improvement.
- Of patients with a single depressive episode, 50% will relapse over their lifetime.

COMPLICATIONS
- Suicide
- Substance misuse
- Weight gain

REFERENCES
1. Brody DJ, Pratt LA, Hughes JP. *Prevalence of Depression among Adults Aged 20 and Over: United States, 2013–2016.* Hyattsville, MD: National Center for Health Statistics; 2018. NCHS Data Brief No. 303.
2. Kessler RC, Bromet EJ. The epidemiology of depression across cultures. *Annu Rev Public Health.* 2013;34:119–138.
3. Flint J, Kendler KS. The genetics of major depression. *Neuron.* 2014;81(3):484–503.
4. Mitchell AJ, Bird V, Rizzo M, et al. Diagnostic validity and added value of the Geriatric Depression Scale for depression in primary care: a meta-analysis of GDS30 and GDS15. *J Affect Disord.* 2010;125(1–3):10–17.
5. Deneke DE, Schultz H, Fluent TE. Screening for depression in the primary care population. *Prim Care.* 2014;41(2):399–420.
6. American Psychiatric Association. Practice guideline for the treatment of patients with major depressive disorder. www.psychiatryonline.com /pracGuide/pracGuideTopic_7.aspx. Accessed September 21, 2016.
7. Arroll B, Elley CR, Fishman T, et al. Antidepressants versus placebo for depression in primary care. *Cochrane Database Syst Rev.* 2009;(3):CD007954.
8. McIntyre RS, Filteau MJ, Martin L, et al. Treatment-resistant depression: definitions, review of the evidence, and algorithmic approach. *J Affect Disord.* 2014;156:1–7.

 SEE ALSO

Algorithms: Depressed Mood Associated with Medical Illness; Depressive Episode, Major

 CODES

ICD10
- F32.9 Major depressive disorder, single episode, unspecified
- F33.9 Major depressive disorder, recurrent, unspecified
- F34.1 Dysthymic disorder

CLINICAL PEARLS
- Therapeutic alliance is important to treatment success.
- Given the high recurrence rates, long-term treatment is often necessary.

DEPRESSION, ADOLESCENT

Joseph B. Gladwell, MD, CPHQ, CPPS • Sabrina Gunn, DO

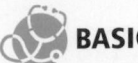 **BASICS**

DESCRIPTION
- *DSM-5* depressive disorders include disruptive mood dysregulations disorder (DMDD), major depressive disorder (MDD), persistent depressive disorder, premenstrual dysphoric disorder, substance/medication-induced depressive disorder, and other nonspecific depression. This chapter focuses on MDD.
- MDD is a primary mood disorder characterized by sadness and/or irritable mood with impairment of functioning; abnormal psychological development; and a loss of self-worth, energy, and interest in typically pleasurable activities.
- DMDD is characterized by having severe, recurrent outbursts along with persistent irritability and anger.
- Persistent depressive disorder is characterized by a depressed mood for most days lasting at least 1 year in a child/adolescent.
- Adolescents with depression are likely to suffer broad functional impairment across social, academic, family, and occupational domains, along with a high incidence of relapse and a high risk for substance abuse and other psychiatric comorbidity.

EPIDEMIOLOGY
Incidence
During adolescence, the cumulative probability of depression ranges from 5% to 20% (1).

Prevalence
- MDD: 6–12% of adolescents; twice as common in females
- DMDD: 2–5%; more prominent in males (2)

ETIOLOGY AND PATHOPHYSIOLOGY
- Unclear; low levels of neurotransmitters (serotonin, norepinephrine) may produce symptoms; decreased functioning of the dopamine system also contributes.
- External factors may affect neurotransmitters independently.
- Hormonal changes during puberty

Genetics
- Offspring of parents with depression have 3 to 4 times increased rates of depression compared with offspring of parents without mood disorder (1).
- Family studies indicate that anxiety in childhood tends to precede adolescent depression (1).

RISK FACTORS
- Increased 3 to 6 times if first-degree relative has a major affective disorder; 3 to 4 times in offspring of parents with depression
- Prior depressive episodes
- History of low self-esteem, anxiety disorders, attention deficit hyperactivity disorder (ADHD), and/or learning disabilities
- Increased screen time (3)
- Female gender
- Low socioeconomic status
- General stressors: adverse life events, difficulties with peers, loss of a loved one, academic difficulties, abuse, chronic illness, and tobacco abuse

GENERAL PREVENTION
Insufficient evidence for universal depression prevention programs (psychological and social)
- Some evidence indicates that child and adolescent mental health can be improved by successfully treating maternal depression (1)[A].
- Agency for Healthcare Research and Quality (AHRQ) recommends the screening of adolescents (12 to 18 years of age) for MDD when systems are in place to ensure accurate diagnosis, appropriate treatment, and follow-up.

COMMONLY ASSOCIATED CONDITIONS
- 2/3 of adolescents with depression have at least one comorbid psychiatric disorder.
- 20% meet the criteria for generalized anxiety disorder.
- Also associated with behavioral disorders, substance abuse, eating disorders

 DIAGNOSIS

HISTORY
- Adolescents may present with medically unexplained somatic complaints (fatigue, irritability, headache).
- Based on *DSM-5* criteria, ≥5 of the following symptoms have been present during the same 2-week period and represent a change from previous functioning: At least one of the symptoms is either depressed mood or loss of interest or pleasure (2):
  – Criterion A
    ○ Depressed mood most of the day, nearly every day, either subjective report or observation by others (feelings of sadness, emptiness, hopelessness; in children, can be irritability)
    ○ Markedly diminished interest or pleasure in all activities most of the day, nearly every day
    ○ Significant weight loss when not dieting or weight gain (>5% body weight in 1 month)
    ○ Insomnia or hypersomnia
    ○ Psychomotor agitation or retardation nearly every day
    ○ Fatigue or loss of energy
    ○ Feelings of worthlessness or excessive or inappropriate feelings of guilt nearly every day
    ○ Diminished ability to think or concentrate, or indecisiveness, nearly every day
    ○ Recurrent thoughts of death, recurrent suicidal ideation, or attempt
  – Criterion B. Symptoms cause clinically significant distress or impairment in social, occupational, or other important areas of functioning.
  – Criterion C. Episode is not attributable to substances' effects or other medical conditions.
  – Criterion D. Episode is not better explained by a schizoaffective, schizophreniform, or delusional disorder.
  – Criterion E. There has never been a manic or hypomanic episode.

PHYSICAL EXAM
- Psychomotor retardation/agitation may be present.
- Clinicians should carefully assess patients for signs of self-injury (such as wrist lacerations) or abuse.

DIFFERENTIAL DIAGNOSIS
- Normal bereavement
- Substance-induced mood disorder
- Bipolar disorder
- Adjustment disorder with depressed mood
- Mood disorder secondary to a medical condition (thyroid, anemia, vitamin deficiency, diabetes)
- Organic CNS diseases
- Malignancy
- Infectious mononucleosis or other viral diseases
- ADHD, posttraumatic stress disorder (PTSD), eating disorders, and anxiety disorders
- Sleep disorder
- Sadness

DIAGNOSTIC TESTS & INTERPRETATION
Initial Tests (lab, imaging)
May be used to rule out other diagnoses (i.e., CBC, TSH, glucose, mono spot, and urine drug)

Follow-Up Tests & Special Considerations
None with sufficient sensitivity/specificity for diagnosis

Diagnostic Procedures/Other
- Depression is primarily diagnosed after a formal interview, with supporting information from caregivers and teachers.
- Standardized tests are useful as screening tools and to monitor response to treatment but should not be used as the sole basis for diagnosis:
  – Beck Depression Inventory II (BDI-II): ages 13 to 18 years (1)[A]
  – Child Depression Inventory 2 (CDI2): ages 7 to 17 years
  – Center for Epidemiologic Studies Depression Scale for Children (CES-DC): ages 6 to 17 years
  – Patient Health Questionnaire-9 (PHQ-9): ages 13 to 17 years with ideal cut point of 11 or higher (instead of 10 used for adults)
- The USPSTF recommends screening for MDD in adolescents ages 12 to 18 years but states that current evidence is insufficient to assess benefits and harms for screening children aged 11 years or younger (4)[B].

 TREATMENT

GENERAL MEASURES
- Active support and monitoring with short validated scales should be used in mild cases for 6 to 8 weeks.
- Psychotherapy and/or medication should be considered if active support and monitoring do to improve symptoms (5)[A].

- Treatment should include psychoeducation, supportive management, and family and school involvement (6)[C].
- Initial management should include treatment planning and ensuring that the patient and family are comfortable with the plan (6)[C].
- A Cochrane review showed that there was no significant difference between remission rates for adolescents treated with cognitive-behavioral therapy (CBT) versus medication or combination therapy immediately postintervention (5)[A].
- A multitreatment meta-analysis showed that combined fluoxetine/CBT had higher efficacy than monotherapies, but other selective serotonin reuptake inhibitors (SSRIs), such as sertraline and escitalopram, were better tolerated (6)[A].

MEDICATION

First Line

- Fluoxetine: for depression in age >8 years. Starting dose 10 mg/day; effective dose 10 to 60 mg/day. The most studied SSRI and with the most favorable effectiveness and safety data has the longest half-life of the SSRIs and is not generally associated with withdrawal symptoms between doses or on discontinuation (5)[A].
- Escitalopram: for depression in age >12 years. Starting dose of 5 mg/day; effective dose of 10 to 20 mg/day (5)[A]
- Citalopram: for depression in age >12 years. Starting dose of 10 mg/day; effective dose of 10 to 40 mg/day (5)[A]
- Sertraline: for depression in age >12 years. Starting dose of 25 mg/day; effective dose of 50 to 200 mg/day (5)[A]
- Can titrate dose every 1 to 2 weeks if no significant adverse effects emerge (headaches, GI upset, insomnia, agitation, behavior activation, suicidal thoughts) (5)[A]
- SSRI black box warning to monitor for worsening condition, behavior changes, and suicidal thoughts (5)[A]
- Antidepressant treatment should be continued for 6 to 12 months at full therapeutic dose after the resolution of symptoms at the same dosage (5)[C].
- Given their rates of increased drug metabolism, adolescents may be at higher risk for withdrawal symptoms from SSRIs than adults; if these are present, twice-daily dosing may be considered (6)[A].
- All other SSRIs except fluoxetine should be slowly tapered when discontinued (5)[A].

Pediatric Considerations

- Tricyclic antidepressants (TCAs) have not been proven to be effective in adolescents and should not be used (5)[A].
- Paroxetine (SSRI): Avoid use due to short half-life, associated withdrawal symptoms, and higher association with suicidal ideation.

ISSUES FOR REFERRAL

- Collaborative care interventions between mental health and primary care have a greater improvement in depressive symptoms after 12 months (5)[B].
- Primary care providers should provide initial treatment of pediatric depression. Refer to a child psychiatrist for severe, recurrent, or treatment-resistant depression or if the patient has comorbidities.

COMPLEMENTARY & ALTERNATIVE MEDICINE

- Physical exercise and light therapy may have a mild to moderate effect (7)[B].
- St. John's wort, acupuncture, S-adenosylmethionine, and 5-hydroxytryptophan have not been shown to have an effect or have inadequate studies to support use in adolescent depression.

ADMISSION, INPATIENT, AND NURSING CONSIDERATIONS

If severely depressed, psychotic, suicidal, or homicidal, one-on-one supervision may be needed.

 ## ONGOING CARE

FOLLOW-UP RECOMMENDATIONS

Patient Monitoring

- Systematic and regular tracking of goals and outcomes from treatment should be performed, including assessment of depressive symptoms and functioning in home, school, and peer settings (5)[A].
- Diagnosis and initial treatment should be reassessed if no improvement is noted after 6 to 8 weeks of treatment (5)[A].
- The goal of treatment should be sustained symptom remission and restoration of full function.
- Educate patients and family members about the causes, symptoms, course and treatments of depression, risks of treatments, and risk of no treatment.

PROGNOSIS

- 60–90% of episodes remit within 1 year.
- 50–70% of remissions develop subsequent depressive episodes within 5 years.
- Depression in adolescence predicts mental health disorders in adult life, psychosocial difficulties, and ill health (2)[A].
- Parental depression at baseline significantly affects intervention effects.

COMPLICATIONS

- Treatment-induced mania, aggression, or lack of improvement in symptoms
- School failure/refusal
- 1/3 of adolescents with suicidal ideation go on to make an attempt (3)[C].

REFERENCES

1. Thapar A, Collishaw S, Pine DS, et al. Depression in adolescence. *Lancet.* 2012;379(9820):1056–1067.
2. American Psychiatric Association. *Diagnostic and Statistical Manual of Mental Disorders.* 5th ed. Arlington, VA: American Psychiatric Association; 2013.
3. Liu M, Wu L, Yao S. Dose-response association of screen time-based sedentary behaviour in children and adolescents and depression: a meta-analysis of observational studies. *Br J Sports Med.* 2016;50(20):1252–1258.
4. Siu AL; for U.S. Preventive Services Task Force. Screening for depression in children and adolescents: U.S. Preventive Services Task Force recommendation statement. *Ann Intern Med.* 2016;164(5):360–366.
5. Cheung AH, Zuckerbrot RA, Jensen PS, et al. Guidelines for Adolescent Depression in Primary Care (GLAD-PC): part II. Treatment and ongoing management. *Pediatrics.* 2018;141(3):e20174082.
6. Nock MK, Green JG, Hwang I, et al. Prevalence, correlates, and treatment of lifetime suicidal behavior among adolescents: results from the National Comorbidity Survey Replication Adolescent Supplement. *JAMA Psychiatry.* 2013;70(3):300–310.
7. Larun L, Nordheim LV, Ekeland E, et al. Exercise in prevention and treatment of anxiety and depression among children and young people. *Cochrane Database Syst Rev.* 2006;(3):CD004691.

ADDITIONAL READING

LeFevre ML; for U.S. Preventive Services Task Force. Screening for suicide risk in adolescents, adults, and older adults in primary care: U.S. Preventive Services Task Force recommendation statement. *Ann Intern Med.* 2014;160(10):719–726.

 ## CODES

ICD10

- F32.9 Major depressive disorder, single episode, unspecified
- F33.9 Major depressive disorder, recurrent, unspecified
- F32.8 Other recurrent depressive disorders

CLINICAL PEARLS

- Adolescent depression is underdiagnosed and often presents with irritability and anhedonia.
- Fluoxetine is the most studied FDA-approved for treatment of adolescent depression.
- Escitalopram, citalopram, and sertraline are also FDA-approved antidepressants.
- CBT combined with fluoxetine is efficacious for adolescents with major depression.
- Paroxetine and TCAs should not be used to treat adolescent depression.
- Referral to a child psychiatrist is appropriate for complex cases or treatment-resistant depression.
- Monitor all adolescents with depression for suicidality, especially during the 1st month of treatment with an antidepressant.

DEPRESSION, GERIATRIC

Fozia Akhtar Ali, MD • Nneka I. Okafor, MD, MPH

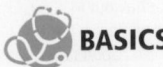

BASICS

DESCRIPTION
Depression is a primary mood disorder characterized by a depressed mood and/or a markedly decreased interest or pleasure in normally enjoyable activities most of the day, almost every day for at least 2 weeks, and causing significant distress or impairment in daily functioning with at least four other symptoms of depression.

EPIDEMIOLOGY
Prevalence rates among the elderly vary largely depending on the specific diagnostic instruments used and their current health and/or home environment:
- 2–10% of community-dwelling elderly
- 5–10% seen in primary care clinics
- 10–37% of hospitalized elderly patients
- 12–27% of nursing home residents

ETIOLOGY AND PATHOPHYSIOLOGY
- Significant gaps exist in the understanding of the underlying pathophysiology.
- Ongoing research has identified several possible mechanisms, including the following:
  - Monoamine transmission and associated transcriptional and translational activity
- Epigenetic mechanisms and resilience factors
- Neurotrophins, neurogenesis, neuroimmune systems, and neuroendocrine systems
- Depression appears to be a complex interaction between heritable and environmental factors.

RISK FACTORS
- General
  - Female sex
  - Lower socioeconomic status
  - Widowed, divorced, or separated marital status
  - Chronic physical health condition(s)
  - History of mental health problems
  - Family history of depression
  - Death of a loved one
  - Caregiving
  - Social isolation
  - Functional/cognitive impairment
  - Lack/loss of social support
  - Significant loss of independence
  - Uncontrolled or chronic pain
  - Insomnia/sleep disturbance
- Prevalence of depression in medical illness
  - Stroke (22–50%)
  - Cancer (18–50%)
  - Myocardial infarction (15–45%)
  - Parkinson disease (10–39%)
  - Rheumatoid arthritis (13%)
  - Diabetes mellitus (5–11%)
  - Alzheimer dementia (5–15%)
- Suicide
  - Suicide is the 11th leading cause of death in the United States for all ages.
  - Elderly account for 24% of all completed suicides.
  - Suicide rates are highest for males aged >85 years (rate 55/100,000).

DIAGNOSIS

HISTORY
- Depressed mood most of the day, nearly every day, and/or loss of interest/pleasure in life for at least 2 weeks
- Other common symptoms include the following:
  - Feeling hopeless, helpless, or worthless
  - Insomnia and loss of appetite/weight (alternatively, hypersomnia with increased appetite/weight in atypical depression)
  - Fatigue and loss of energy
  - Somatic symptoms (headaches, chronic pain)
  - Neglect of personal responsibility or care
  - Psychomotor retardation or agitation
  - Diminished concentration, indecisiveness
  - Thoughts of death or suicide
- Screening with "SIGECAPS"
  - **S**leep: changes in sleep habits from baseline, including excessive sleep, early waking, or inability to fall asleep
  - **I**nterest: loss of interest in previously enjoyable activities (anhedonia)
  - **G**uilt: excessive or inappropriate guilt that may or may not focus on a specific problem or circumstance
  - **E**nergy: perceived lack of energy
  - **C**oncentration: inability to concentrate on specific tasks
  - **A**ppetite: increase/decrease in appetite
  - **P**sychomotor: restlessness and agitation or the perception that everyday activities are too strenuous to manage
  - **S**uicidality: desire to end life or hurt oneself, harmful thoughts directed internally, recurrent thoughts of death or thoughts of homicidality

PHYSICAL EXAM
Mental status exam, thorough neurologic exam, and general physical exam to rule out other conditions

DIFFERENTIAL DIAGNOSIS
Concurrent medical conditions, cognitive disorders, and medications may cause symptoms that mimic depression:
- Medical conditions: hypothyroidism, vitamin B_{12} or folate deficiency, liver or renal failure, cancers, stroke, sleep disorders, electrolyte imbalances, Cushing disease, chronic fatigue syndrome
- Dementia and neurodegenerative disorders
- Delirium
- Medication induced: interferon-α, β_2-blockers, isotretinoin, benzodiazepines, glucocorticoids, levodopa, clonidine, H_2 blockers, baclofen, varenicline, metoclopramide, reserpine
- Psychiatric disorders: adjustment disorder with depressed mood, grief reaction, bipolar disorder, dysthymic disorder, anxiety disorders, substance abuse–related mood disorders, psychotic disorders

DIAGNOSTIC TESTS & INTERPRETATION
Initial Tests (lab, imaging)
Initial laboratory evaluation is done primarily to rule out potential medical factors that could be causing symptoms.
- Thyroid-stimulating hormone (hypothyroidism)
- CBC with differential (anemia, infection)
- Vitamin B_{12}, folic acid (deficiencies)
- Urinalysis (urinary tract infection, glucosuria)
- Comprehensive metabolic panel (uremia, hypo- or hyperglycemia, hypo- or hypernatremia, hypercalcemia, liver failure)
- Urine drug screen
- 24-hour urine-free cortisol (Cushing disease)

Follow-Up Tests & Special Considerations
Additional testing for possible confounding medical and cognitive disorders, as warranted; may consider a sleep study for patients with decreased energy, sleep disturbances, changes in concentration, or psychomotor activity

Diagnostic Procedures/Other
Validated screening tools and rating scales:
- Geriatric Depression Scale: 15- or 30-point scales
- Patient Health Questionnaire (PHQ-2 and PHQ-9)
- Hamilton Depression Rating Scale
- Beck Depression Inventory
- Cornell Scale for Depression in Dementia (1)[A]

TREATMENT

Although response alone, usually interpreted as a 50% reduction in symptoms, can be clinically meaningful, the goal is to treat patients to the point of remission (i.e., essentially the absence of depressive symptoms).

GENERAL MEASURES
- Lifestyle modifications:
  - Increase physical activity.
  - Improve nutrition.
  - Encourage social interactions.
  - Exercise: may be beneficial for depression in the elderly population (2)[A]
- Psychotherapy: Studies do show some benefit in depressed elderly patients (3)[B]:
  - Cognitive-behavioral therapy
  - Problem-solving therapy
  - Interpersonal therapy
  - Psychodynamic psychotherapy

MEDICATION
- Typically, more conservative initial dosing and titration of antidepressants in the elderly, starting with 1/2 of the usual initiation dose and increasing within 2 to 4 weeks, as tolerated
- Continue titrating dose every 2 to 4 weeks, as appropriate, to reach an adequate treatment dose.

First Line
- SSRIs have been found to be effective in treating depression in the elderly and are considered first line in pharmacotherapy for depression (2)[A].
- No single SSRI clearly outperforms others in the class; choice of medication often reflects side effect profile or practitioner familiarity (4)[A]:
  - Citalopram: Start at 10 mg/day; treatment range 10 to 20 mg/day
  - Sertraline: Start at 25 to 50 mg/day; treatment range 50 to 200 mg/day
  - Escitalopram: Start at 10 mg/day; treatment range 10 to 20 mg/day

– Fluoxetine: Start at 10 mg/day; treatment range 20 to 60 mg/day
– Paroxetine: Start at 10 mg/day; treatment range 20 to 40 mg/day
- SSRIs should not be used concomitantly with monoamine oxidase inhibitors (MAOIs).
- Common side effects—increased risk of falls, nausea, diarrhea, sexual dysfunction

Second Line
Atypical antidepressants: more effective than placebo in treatment of depression in the elderly, although additional studies are needed to better delineate patient factors that determine response:

- Bupropion (sustained/twice a day and extended/once daily available): Start at 150 mg/day. Increase dose in 3 to 4 days. Treatment range 300 to 450 mg/day. Avoid in patients with elevated seizure risk, tremors, or anxiety (5)[A].
- Venlafaxine (immediate- and extended-release available): Start at 37.5 mg/day extended release and titrate weekly. Treatment range 150 to 225 mg/day; may be associated with elevated BP at higher doses (5)[C].
- Duloxetine: Start at 20 to 30 mg/day. Treatment range 60 to 120 mg/day. Also, duloxetine may be associated with elevated BP (5)[A].
- Mirtazapine: Start at 7.5 to 15.0 mg nightly. Treatment range 30 to 45 mg/day; can produce problems with dry mouth, weight gain, sedation, and cognitive dysfunction (5)[A]
- Desvenlafaxine: 50 mg/day in AM; higher doses do not confer additional benefit; 50 mg every other day if CrCl <30 mL/min (5)[A]

ISSUES FOR REFERRAL
Depression with suicidal ideation, psychotic depression, bipolar disorder, comorbid substance abuse issues, polypharmacy, severe or refractory illness

ADDITIONAL THERAPIES
- For patients who have not responded to initial SSRI trial:
  – Switch to a different SSRI medication, switch to an atypical antidepressant, or augment initial antidepressant with bupropion.
- 2nd-generation antipsychotic agents (5)[C]:
  – Aripiprazole: 2 to 5 mg/day. Treatment range 5 to 15 mg/day; can produce sedation, weight gain, increased cholesterol levels
  – Should only be used for augmentation in conjunction with other antidepressant medications
- Tricyclic antidepressants (TCAs):
  – Nortriptyline: 25 to 50 mg nightly. Treatment range 75 to 150 mg nightly; can produce anticholinergic effects, weight gain, increase risk of falls (5)[C]
  – TCAs have been shown to be effective in treating depression in the elderly. However, they are difficult for elderly patients to tolerate due to side effect profile and are potentially lethal in overdose, limiting their use as initial treatment agents (6)[A].
- MAOIs also appear more effective than placebo in the treatment of depression in the elderly. They are not used frequently in clinical practice due to potential side effects and necessary dietary restrictions (6)[A].
- Although not FDA-approved, buspirone, lithium, or triiodothyronine is sometimes used off-label to augment a primary antidepressant.

- Evidence for benefit of antidepressants in the treatment of depression in patients with dementia is equivocal. Consideration should be made for a limited trial with close monitoring for symptom improvement or side effects and used only in patients with severe symptoms.
- Electroconvulsive therapy (ECT): has been shown to produce remission of depressive symptoms in the elderly. It should be considered as an initial option for patients with severe or psychotic depression.

COMPLEMENTARY & ALTERNATIVE MEDICINES
- Acupuncture: equally beneficial as counseling
- St. John's wort may have minimal benefit and has numerous drug interactions.
- Tryptophan and hydroxytryptophan: 150 to 300 mg/day; possible efficacy, additional investigation required

ADMISSION, INPATIENT, AND NURSING CONSIDERATIONS
Inpatient care is indicated in cases of imminent safety risk (e.g., acutely suicidal patients) or for those patients unable to care adequately for themselves due to depression.

 ## ONGOING CARE

FOLLOW-UP RECOMMENDATIONS
Due to the delay of benefit following initiation of antidepressant therapy, it is necessary to ensure open communication with the patient to prevent premature discontinuation of therapy. An adequate explanation of potential side effects with instructions to call the office before discontinuing therapy is imperative.

Patient Monitoring
- A patient with severe depression who exhibits suicidality will require admission to an appropriate facility.
- Monitor for worsening anxiety symptoms or increase in suicidality especially in the week following initiation of antidepressants.

DIET
No dietary restrictions are necessary, except for patients taking MAOIs, which necessitates dietary restriction of foods high in tyramine (i.e., certain cheeses and wines).

PATIENT EDUCATION
- Depression is a treatable illness.
- Medications may need to be taken for at least 2 to 4 weeks before any beneficial effect is noted and may take 6 to 8 weeks to reach maximum efficacy.
- Depression is often a recurring illness.
- National Suicide Prevention Lifeline at 1-800-273-TALK (8255) is a free, 24-hour hotline available to anyone in suicidal crisis or emotional distress. Calls will be routed to the nearest crisis center.

PROGNOSIS
- Treatment outcomes in the elderly may be worse than in the general population, possibly mediated by physical comorbidities and other factors.
- Depending on the population studied and specific clinical measures used, estimates vary for initial clinical response and remission (between 30% and 70%).

COMPLICATIONS
- Impairment in social, occupational, or interpersonal functioning
- Difficulty performing activities of daily living and self-care
- Increase in medical services utilization and increased costs of care
- Increase risk of suicide

REFERENCES
1. Blake H, Mo P, Malik S, et al. How effective are physical activity interventions for alleviating depressive symptoms in older people? A systematic review. *Clin Rehabil*. 2009;23(10):873–887.
2. Wilson KC, Mottram PG, Vassilas CA. Psychotherapeutic treatments for older depressed people. *Cochrane Database Syst Rev*. 2008;(1):CD004853.
3. Wilson K, Mottram P, Sivanranthan A, et al. Antidepressant versus placebo for depressed elderly. *Cochrane Database Syst Rev*. 2001;(2):CD000561.
4. Ruhé HG, Huyser J, Swinkels JA, et al. Switching antidepressants after a first selective serotonin reuptake inhibitor in major depressive disorder: a systematic review. *J Clin Psychiatry*. 2006;67(12):1836–1855.
5. Nelson JC, Delucchi K, Schneider LS. Efficacy of second generation antidepressants in late-life depression: a meta-analysis of the evidence. *Am J Geriatr Psychiatry*. 2008;16(7):558–567.
6. Taylor WD. Clinical practice. Depression in the elderly. *N Engl J Med*. 2014;371(13):1228–1236.

 ### SEE ALSO

Algorithms: Depressed Mood Associated with Medical Illness; Depressive Episode, Major

 ### CODES

ICD10
- F32.9 Major depressive disorder, single episode, unspecified
- F03 Unspecified dementia
- F43.21 Adjustment disorder with depressed mood

CLINICAL PEARLS
- Depression is not a normal part of aging.
- Depression in the elderly may be difficult to diagnose precisely due to medical and cognitive comorbidities.
- Depression may present primarily with cognitive dysfunction, and this may improve with treatment of the depression.
- SSRIs are considered first-line therapy for safety and tolerability. A full remission may take upward of 12 weeks of treatment. Long-term treatment may be needed to prevent recurrence.
- A multidisciplinary approach to the treatment of depression is often the most efficacious.

DEPRESSION, POSTPARTUM

Misty Stafford, MD • Nancy Byatt, DO, MBA, FAPM

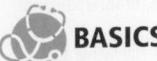 **BASICS**

DESCRIPTION
- Major depressive disorder (MDD) that recurs or has its onset in the postpartum period
- May also occur in mothers adopting a baby or in fathers
- Postpartum depression (PPD) is similar to nonpregnancy depression (sleep disorders, anhedonia, psychomotor changes, etc.); it most often has its onset within the first 12 weeks postpartum yet can occur within 1 year after delivery.
- Different than postpartum "blues" (sadness and emotional lability), which is experienced by 30–70% of women and has an onset and resolution within first 10 days postpartum

EPIDEMIOLOGY
Incidence
14.5% of women have a new episode of major or minor depression during postpartum period (1).

Prevalence
- >50% of women with PPD enter pregnancy depressed or have an onset during pregnancy (2).
- As many as 19.2% women suffer from depression within 3 months postpartum period (3).

ETIOLOGY AND PATHOPHYSIOLOGY
- May be related to sensitivity in hormonal fluctuations, including estrogen; progesterone; and other gonadal hormones as well as neuroactive steroids; cytokines; hypothalamic-pituitary-adrenal (HPA) axis hormones; altered fatty acid, oxytocin, and arginine vasopressin levels; and genetic and epigenetic factors
- Multifactorial including biologic–genetic predisposition in terms of neurobiologic deficit, destabilizing effects of hormone withdrawal at birth, inflammation, and psychosocial stressors

RISK FACTORS
- Previous episodes of PPD
- History of MDD
- MDD during pregnancy
- Anxiety during pregnancy
- History of premenstrual dysphoria
- Family history of depression
- Unwanted pregnancy
- Socioeconomic stress
- Low self-esteem
- Young maternal age
- Alcohol abuse
- Marital conflict
- Multiple births
- African Americans and Hispanics may have higher rates of PPD.
- Postpartum pain, sleep disturbance, and fatigue
- Recent immigrant status
- Increased stressful life events
- History of childhood sexual abuse
- Decision to decrease antidepressants during pregnancy
- Intimate partner violence (4)
- Prepregnancy diabetes

GENERAL PREVENTION
- Universal screening during pregnancy to allow for detection and treatment
- Screen using Edinburgh Postnatal Depression Scale during pregnancy and postpartum year.
- Postnatal visits, psychotherapy, and/or psychoeducation for high-risk women
- For women with depression during pregnancy, psychotherapy or treatment with antidepressants during pregnancy may prevent PPD.
- Depression care manager who provides education, routine telephone contact, and follow-up to engage women in treatment

COMMONLY ASSOCIATED CONDITIONS
- Bipolar mood disorder
- Depressive disorder not otherwise specified
- Dysthymic disorder
- Cyclothymic disorder
- MDD

 DIAGNOSIS

HISTORY
- Increased/decreased sleep
- Decreased interest in formerly compelling or pleasurable activities
- Guilt, low self-esteem
- Decreased energy
- Decreased concentration
- Increased/decreased appetite
- Psychomotor agitation or retardation
- Suicidal ideation

DIFFERENTIAL DIAGNOSIS
- Baby blues: not a psychiatric disorder; mood lability resolves within days.
- Postpartum psychosis: a psychiatric emergency
- Postpartum anxiety/panic disorder
- Postpartum obsessive-compulsive disorder
- Hypothyroidism
- Postpartum thyroiditis: can occur in up to 5.7% of patients in the United States and can present as depression (5)

DIAGNOSTIC TESTS & INTERPRETATION
Initial Tests (lab, imaging)
Thyroid-stimulating hormone (TSH), B_{12}, folate, and Vitamin D

Diagnostic Procedures/Other
- Edinburgh Postnatal Depression Scale is a validated screening tool.
- The Patient Health Questionnaire-9 (PHQ-9) is a validated commonly used screening tool.
- Edinburgh Postnatal Depression Scale (partner version): to be completed by mother's partner to obtain his/her view of mother's depression

 TREATMENT

GENERAL MEASURES
- Outpatient individual psychotherapy in combination with pharmacotherapy
- Interpersonal psychotherapy and cognitive-behavioral therapy

- Strongly consider pharmacotherapy when symptoms are moderate or severe.
- Assess suicidal ideation.
- Assess homicidal ideation and thoughts of harming baby.
- Thoughts of harming the baby require immediate hospitalization.
- Visiting nurse services can provide direct observations of the mother regarding safety concerns and mother–child bonding.

MEDICATION
First Line
- For nonbreastfeeding women, selection of antidepressants is similar to nonpostpartum patients.
- Selective serotonin reuptake inhibitors (SSRIs) are generally effective and safe:
  - Fluoxetine (Prozac): 20 to 80 mg/day PO (most activating of all SSRIs)
  - Sertraline (Zoloft): 50 to 200 mg/day PO (mildly sedating)
  - Paroxetine (Paxil): 20 to 60 mg/day PO (sedating)
  - Citalopram (Celexa): 20 to 40 mg/day PO (FDA recommendation)
  - Escitalopram (Lexapro): 10 to 20 mg/day PO
- Tricyclic antidepressants (TCAs) are effective and less expensive yet also are lethal in overdose and have unfavorable side effects:
  - Avoid TCAs in mothers with a history of suicidal ideation.
- Bupropion (Wellbutrin): 150 to 450 mg/day PO in patients with depression plus psychomotor retardation and hypersomnia and with weight gain. Bupropion is less likely to cause weight gain or sexual dysfunction and is highly activating.
- Mirtazapine (Remeron): 15 to 45 mg/day PO at bedtime; may assist with sleep restoration and weight gain; no sexual dysfunction
- Serotonin-norepinephrine reuptake inhibitors (SNRIs)
  - Venlafaxine (Effexor XR): a dual-action antidepressant that blocks the reuptake of serotonin in doses of up to 150 mg/day and then blocks the reuptake of norepinephrine in doses of 150 to 450 mg/day PO
  - Duloxetine (Cymbalta): more balanced serotonin/norepinephrine reuptake throughout dosing; 40 to 60 mg/day PO (doses >60 mg have not been demonstrated to be more effective)
  - Desvenlafaxine (Pristiq): 50 mg/day PO
- Bipolar disorder requires treatment with mood stabilizer.
- Among breastfeeding mothers
  - Breastfeeding should generally not preclude treatment with antidepressants.
  - SSRIs and some other antidepressants are considered a reasonable option during breastfeeding.
  - All antidepressants are excreted in breast milk but are generally compatible with lactation.
  - Paroxetine and sertraline have lower translactal passage.
  - SSRIs and nortriptyline have a better safety profile.
  - Translactal passage is greater with fluoxetine and citalopram (4)[B].
  - Start with low doses and increase slowly. Monitor infant for adverse side effects.

– Continuing an efficacious medication is preferred over switching antidepressants to avoid exposing the mother and infant to the risks of untreated PPD (4)[B].
– Breastfeeding women need additional education and support regarding the risks and benefits of use of antidepressants during breastfeeding.
– Consider negative effects of untreated PPD on infant and child development.
– Discussions of the treatment options with the patient and her partner when possible. Take into account the patient's personal psychiatric history and previous response to treatment, the risks of no treatment or undertreatment, available data about the safety of medications during breastfeeding, and her individual expectations and treatment preferences.
– For further information: http://toxnet.nlm.nih.gov/

Second Line
Consider switching to a different antidepressant or augmentation if patient has a lack of response. Electroconvulsive therapy (ECT) is an option for depressed postpartum women who do not respond to antidepressant medications, have severe or psychotic symptoms, cannot tolerate antidepressant medications, are actively engaged in suicidal self-destructive behaviors, or have a previous history of response to ECT (5)[B].

ISSUES FOR REFERRAL
• Obtain psychiatric consultation for patients with psychotic symptoms.
• Strongly consider immediate hospitalization if delusions or hallucinations are present.
• Hospitalization is indicated if mother's ability to care for self and/or infant is significantly compromised.

ADDITIONAL THERAPIES
• Psychoeducation, including providing reading material for the patient and family
• Psychotherapy: Interpersonal psychotherapy, cognitive-behavioral therapy, and psychodynamic psychotherapy have shown to be effective.

COMPLEMENTARY & ALTERNATIVE MEDICINE
• Breastfeeding has been associated with reduced stress and improved maternal mood.
• Infant massage, infant sleep intervention, exercise, and bright light therapy may be beneficial (5)[B].

ADMISSION, INPATIENT, AND NURSING CONSIDERATIONS

ALERT
Obtain psychiatric consultation for patients with psychotic symptoms. If delusions or hallucinations are present, strongly consider immediate hospitalization. The psychotic mother should *not* be left alone with the baby.

• Admission criteria/initial stabilization: presence of suicidal or homicidal ideation and/or psychotic symptoms and/or thoughts of harming baby and/or inability to care for self or infant, severe weight loss
• Discharge criteria
– Absence of suicidal or homicidal ideation and/or psychotic symptoms and/or thoughts of harming the baby
– Mother must be able to care for self and infant.

ONGOING CARE

FOLLOW-UP RECOMMENDATIONS
Patient Monitoring
• Collaborative care approach, including primary care visits and case manager follow-ups
• Consultation with the infant's doctor, particularly if the mother is breastfeeding while taking psychotropic medications

DIET
• Good nutrition and hydration, especially when breastfeeding
• Mixed evidence to support the addition of multivitamin with minerals and omega-3 fatty acids

PATIENT EDUCATION
• *This Isn't What I Expected: Overcoming Postpartum Depression*, by Karen R. Kleiman and Valerie Davis Raskin
• *Down Came the Rain: My Journey Through Postpartum Depression*, by Brooke Shields, 2005
• *Behind the Smile: My Journey Out of Postpartum Depression*, by Marie Osmond, Marcia Wilkie, and Judith Moore, 2001
• Web resources
– Postpartum Support International: http://www.postpartum.net/
– La Leche League: http://www.llli.org/
– http://www.womensmentalhealth.org/
– http://www.motherisk.org/
– http://www.step-ppd.com/

PROGNOSIS
• Treatment of maternal depression to remission has been shown to have a positive impact on children's mental health.
• Some patients, particularly those with undertreated or undiagnosed depression, may develop chronic depression requiring long-term treatment.
• Untreated maternal depression is linked to impaired mother–infant bonding and cognitive and language development delay in infants and children (6).
• Postpartum psychosis is associated with tragic outcomes such as maternal suicide and infanticide.

COMPLICATIONS
• Suicide
• Self-injurious behavior
• Psychosis
• Neglect of baby
• Harm to the baby
• Preterm and low-birth-weight baby

REFERENCES

1. Stuart-Parrigon K, Stuart S. Perinatal depression: an update and overview. *Curr Psychiatry Rep.* 2014;16(9):468.
2. Wisner KL, Sit DK, McShea MC, et al. Onset timing, thoughts of self-harm, and diagnoses in postpartum women with screen-positive depression findings. *JAMA Psychiatry.* 2013;70(5):490–498.
3. Bobo WV, Yawn PB. Concise review for physicians and other clinicians: postpartum depression. *Mayo Clin Proc.* 2014;89(6):835–844.
4. Gavin NI, Gaynes BN, Lohr KN, et al. Perinatal depression: a systematic review of prevalence and incidence. *Obstet Gynecol.* 2005;106(5, Pt 1):1071–1083.
5. Pearlstein T, Howard M, Salisbury A, et al. Postpartum depression. *Am J Obstet Gynecol.* 2009;200(4):357–364.
6. Fitelson E, Kim S, Baker AS, et al. Treatment of postpartum depression: clinical, psychological and pharmacological options. *Int J Womens Health.* 2010;3:1–14.

ADDITIONAL READING

• Edinburgh Postnatal Depression Scale: https://pesnc.org/wp-content/uploads/EPDS.pdf
• Gjerdingen D, Katon W, Rich DE. Stepped care treatment of postpartum depression: a primary care-based management model. *Womens Health Issues.* 2008;18(1):44–52.
• Harrington AR, Greene-Harrington CC. Healthy Start screens for depression among urban pregnant, postpartum and interconceptional women. *J Natl Med Assoc.* 2007;99(3):226–231.
• Hirst KP, Moutier CY. Postpartum major depression. *Am Fam Physician.* 2010;82(8):926–933.
• Howard LM, Boath E, Henshaw C. Antidepressant prevention of postnatal depression. *PLoS Med.* 2006;3(10):e389.
• Kendall-Tackett K. A new paradigm for depression in new mothers: the central role of inflammation and how breastfeeding and anti-inflammatory treatments protect maternal mental health. *Int Breastfeed J.* 2007;2:6.
• Musters C, McDonald E, Jones I. Management of postnatal depression. *BMJ.* 2008;337:a736.
• Ng RC, Hirata CK, Yeung W, et al. Pharmacologic treatment for postpartum depression: a systematic review. *Pharmacotherapy.* 2010;30(9):928–941.
• Sit DK, Wisner KL. Identification of postpartum depression. *Clin Obstet Gynecol.* 2009;52(3):456–468.
• Tammentie T, Tarkka MT, Astedt-Kurki P, et al. Family dynamics and postnatal depression. *J Psychiatr Ment Health Nurs.* 2004;11(2):141–149.

CODES

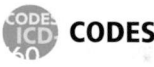

ICD10
• F53 Puerperal psychosis
• O90.6 Postpartum mood disturbance

CLINICAL PEARLS

• PPD is a common, debilitating medical condition that impairs a mother's ability to function and interact with her infant and family.
• Universal screening for depression is recommended during the 1st and 3rd trimester and at regular intervals during the postpartum period.
• Early diagnosis and treatment are vital because untreated PPD can lead to developmental difficulties for the infant and prolonged disability and suffering for the mother.
• Breastfeeding is recommended for maternal and child health. Several medication options for treating depression in mothers are safe for breastfeeding infants.
• Treatment with antidepressants should be individualized for breastfeeding mothers (4)[B].

DEPRESSION, TREATMENT RESISTANT
Michelle Magid, MD, MBA • Kristin Y. Lasseter, MD

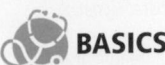

BASICS

DESCRIPTION
- Major depressive disorder (MDD) that has failed to respond to ≥2 adequate trials of antidepressant therapy in ≥2 different classes
- Antidepressant therapy must be given for 6 weeks at standard doses before being considered a failure.

EPIDEMIOLOGY
- Depression affects >16 million people in the United States and >350 million people worldwide.
- 16% lifetime risk of MDD, with majority onset before the age of 30 years
- Approximately 1/3 of patients with MDD will develop treatment-resistant depression.

ETIOLOGY AND PATHOPHYSIOLOGY
- Unclear. Low levels of neurotransmitters (serotonin, norepinephrine, dopamine) have been indicated.
- Serotonin has been linked to irritability, hostility, and suicidal ideation.
- Norepinephrine has been linked to low energy.
- Dopamine may play a role in low motivation and depression with psychotic features.
- Environmental stressors such as abuse and neglect may affect neurotransmission.
- Inflammation and oxidative stress in the brain can contribute to treatment-resistant depression.

Genetics
A genetic abnormality in the serotonin transporter gene (5-HTTLPR) may increase risk for treatment-resistant depression.

RISK FACTORS
- Severity of disease
- Mislabeling bipolar patients as depressed
- Comorbid medical disease (including chronic pain)
- Comorbid personality disorder
- Comorbid anxiety disorder
- Comorbid substance use disorder
- Familial predisposition to poor response to antidepressants

GENERAL PREVENTION
- Medication adherence in combination with psychotherapy
- Maintenance electroconvulsive therapy (ECT) may prevent relapse.

COMMONLY ASSOCIATED CONDITIONS
- Suicide
- Bipolar disorder
- Substance use disorders
- Anxiety disorders
- Dysthymia
- Eating disorders
- Somatic symptom disorders

DIAGNOSIS

HISTORY
- Symptoms are the same as in MDD. However, patients do not respond to standard form of treatment.
- Important to screen for suicidality in treatment-resistant depression
- Screening with SIGECAPS
  - Sleep: too much or too little
  - Interest: inability to enjoy activities
  - Guilt: excessive and uncontrollable
  - Energy: poor
  - Concentration: inability to focus on tasks
  - Appetite: too much or too little
  - Psychomotor changes: restlessness/agitation or slowing/lethargy noted by others
  - Suicidality: desire to end life or feeling hopeless

PHYSICAL EXAM
Mental status exam may reveal poor hygiene, limited eye contact, poor relatedness, restricted affect, tearfulness, weight loss or gain, psychomotor retardation or agitation.

DIFFERENTIAL DIAGNOSIS
- Bipolar disorder
- Persistent depressive disorder
- Posttraumatic stress disorder
- Dementia
- Early-stage Parkinson disease
- Personality disorder
- Medical illness such as malignancy, thyroid disease, HIV
- Substance use disorders

DIAGNOSTIC TESTS & INTERPRETATION
Initial Tests (lab, imaging)
Used to rule out medical factors that could be causing/contributing to treatment resistance
- CBC
- Complete metabolic profile, including liver tests, calcium, and glucose
- Urine drug screen
- Thyroid-stimulating hormone (TSH)
- Vitamin D level (25-OH vitamin D)
- Vitamin B_{12}
- Folate
- Urinalysis
- FSH, LH if applicable
- HCG, if applicable
- Testosterone, if applicable
- CT or MRI of the brain if neurologic disease, tumor, or dementia is suspected

Follow-Up Tests & Special Considerations
Delirium and dementia often look like depression.

Diagnostic Procedures/Other
- Depression is a clinical diagnosis.
- Validated depression rating scales to assist
  - Beck Depression Inventory
  - Hamilton Depression Rating Scale
  - Patient Health Questionnaire 9 (PHQ-9)
  - Edinburgh Postnatal Depression Scale if pregnant or postpartum

TREATMENT

MEDICATION
First Line
- Please see "Depression" topic. When those fail, augmentation and combination strategies are as follows:
  - Antidepressants in combination
    - Citalopram (start 20 mg/day; max dose 40 mg/day) + bupropion (start 100 mg BID; max dose 450 mg total) (1)[B]
    - Tricyclic antidepressants (TCAs) and selective serotonin reuptake inhibitors (SSRIs) may be used in combination. Proceed with caution due to risk of serotonin syndrome; citalopram (start 20 mg/day; max dose 40 mg/day) + nortriptyline (start 50 mg at bedtime; max dose 150 mg at bedtime)
  - Antidepressants + antipsychotics
    - Citalopram (start 20 mg/day; max dose 40 mg/day) + aripiprazole (start 2 mg/day; up to 20 mg/day, different mechanism of action at higher doses) OR + risperidone (start 0.5 to 1.0 mg at bedtime; max dose 6 mg/day) OR + quetiapine (start 25 mg at bedtime; titrate to 100 to 300 mg at bedtime; max dose 600 mg/day) (1)[A]
    - Olanzapine/fluoxetine combination (start 3 mg/25 mg to 12 mg/50 mg at bedtime) (1)[A]
  - Antidepressant + lithium
    - TCA: nortriptyline (start 50 mg at bedtime; max dose 150 mg at bedtime) + lithium (start 300 mg at bedtime; max dose 900 mg BID) (2)[A]
    - SSRI: citalopram (start 20 mg/day; max dose 40 mg QD) + lithium (start 300 mg at bedtime; max dose 900 mg BID) (1)[A]
- In all combinations, citalopram (Celexa) can be replaced with other SSRIs such as fluoxetine (Prozac) 20 to 80 mg/day, sertraline (Zoloft) 50 to 200 mg/day, and escitalopram (Lexapro) 10 to 20 mg/day or with serotonin-norepinephrine reuptake inhibitors (SNRIs) duloxetine (Cymbalta) 30 to 120 mg/day, venlafaxine XR (Effexor XR) 75 to 225 mg/day, or desvenlafaxine (Pristiq) 50 to 100 mg/day, or with a noradrenergic and specific serotonergic antidepressant (NaSSA) mirtazapine (Remeron) 15 to 45 mg at bedtime.
- Maximum doses for medication in treatment-resistant cases may be higher than in treatment-responsive cases.

Second Line

- Citalopram (start 20 mg/day; max dose 40 mg/day) + triiodothyronine (T^3) (12.5 to 50.0 μg/day) (1)[B]
- Citalopram (start 20 mg/day; max dose 40 mg/day) + buspirone (start 7.5 mg twice a day; max dose 30 mg twice a day) (1)[B]
- Citalopram (start 20 mg/day; max dose 40 mg/day) + lisdexamfetamine (Vyvanse) (20 to 50 mg every morning) (1)[B]
- Antidepressant in combination with therapy, particularly, cognitive-behavioral therapy (CBT) (3)[A]
- Monoamine oxidase inhibitor (MAOI)
  - Tranylcypromine (Parnate): Start 10 mg BID and increase 10 mg/day every 1 to 3 weeks; max dose 60 mg/day
  - Selegiline transdermal (Emsam patch): Apply 6-mg patch daily and increase 3 mg/day; max dose 12 mg/day
  - Side-effect profile (e.g., hypertensive crisis), drug–drug interactions, and dietary restrictions make MAOIs less appealing. Patch version does not require dietary restrictions at lower doses.
  - High risk of serotonin syndrome if combined with another antidepressant. 2-week washout period is advised.

ISSUES FOR REFERRAL
Treatment-resistant depression should be managed in consultation with a psychiatrist.

ADDITIONAL THERAPIES
- First line
  - ECT: brief administration of electrical stimulation to the brain via superficial electrode placement
    ○ Safe and cost-effective option for treatment-resistant and life-threatening depression, with a 66.6% response rate (4)[A]
    ○ Known to rapidly relieve suicidality, psychotic depression, and catatonia
    ○ Cognitive side effects during treatment can occur but are more likely with bilateral lead placement
    ○ Three types of lead placements
      ▪ Right unilateral
      ▪ Bitemporal
      ▪ Bifrontal
- Second line
  - Deep brain stimulation (DBS): surgical implantation of intracranial electrodes, connected to an impulse generator implanted in the chest wall:
    ○ Reserved for those who have failed medications, psychotherapy, and ECT
    ○ Preliminary data is promising, showing 40–70% response rate and 35% remission rate. Further trials are being done (2)[B].

- Transcranial magnetic stimulation (TMS): noninvasive brain stimulation technique that is generally safe
  ○ Currently, only FDA-approved for less severe forms of the illness (2)[B]
- Vagus nerve stimulation (VNS): surgical implantation of electrodes onto left vagus nerve
  ○ Its use in treatment-resistant depression has become limited in recent years (2)[B].
- Ketamine (0.5 mg/kg single-dose infusion): Studies show evidence of rapid improvement in mood and suicidal thinking (1)[B].
  ○ Not FDA-approved for treatment of depression
  ○ The effects of ketamine appear temporary, disappearing after days to weeks (2,5)[B].

ADMISSION, INPATIENT, AND NURSING CONSIDERATIONS
- Inpatient care is indicated for severely depressed, psychotic, catatonic, or suicidal patients.
- Discharge criteria: symptoms improving, no longer suicidal, psychosocial stressors addressed

 ONGOING CARE

FOLLOW-UP RECOMMENDATIONS
- Frequent visits (i.e., every month)
- During follow-up, evaluate side effects, dosage, and effectiveness of medication as well as need for referral to ECT.
- Patients who have responded to ECT may need maintenance treatments (q3–12wk) to prevent relapse.
- Combination of lithium/nortriptyline after ECT appears to be as effective as maintenance ECT in reducing relapse.

DIET
Patients on MAOIs need dietary restriction.

PATIENT EDUCATION
- Educate patients that depression is a medical illness, not a character defect.
- Review signs and symptoms of worsening depression and when patient needs to come in for further evaluation.
- Discuss safety plan to address suicidal thoughts.

PROGNOSIS
With medication adherence, close follow-up, improved social support, and psychotherapy, prognosis improves.

COMPLICATIONS
- Suicide
- Disability
- Poor quality of life

REFERENCES

1. McIntyre RS, Filteau MJ, Martin L, et al. Treatment-resistant depression: definitions, review of the evidence, and algorithmic approach. *J Affect Disord.* 2014;156:1–7.
2. Holtzheimer PE. Advances in the management of treatment-resistant depression. *Focus (Am Psychiatr Publ).* 2010;8(4):488–500.
3. Wiles NJ, Thomas L, Turner N, et al. Long-term effectiveness and cost-effectiveness of cognitive behavioural therapy as an adjunct to pharmacotherapy for treatment-resistant depression in primary care: follow-up of the CoBalT randomised controlled trial. *Lancet Psychiatry.* 2016;3(2):137–144.
4. Ross EL, Zivin K, Maixner DF. Cost-effectiveness of electroconvulsive therapy vs pharmacotherapy/psychotherapy for treatment-resistant depression in the United States. *JAMA Psychiatry.* 2018;75(7):713–722.
5. Caddy C, Giaroli G, White TP, et al. Ketamine as the prototype glutamatergic antidepressant: pharmacodynamic actions, and a systematic review and meta-analysis of efficacy. *Ther Adv Psychopharmacol.* 2014;4(2):75–99.

 CODES

ICD10
- F32.9 Major depressive disorder, single episode, unspecified
- F33.9 Major depressive disorder, recurrent, unspecified

CLINICAL PEARLS
- Treatment-resistant depression is common, affecting 1/3 of those with MDD.
- Combination and augmentation strategies with antidepressants, antipsychotics, therapy, and mood stabilizers can be helpful.
- ECT should be considered in severe and life-threatening cases.

DERMATITIS HERPETIFORMIS

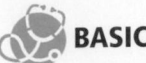

Abdul Aleem, MD • Hiral Shah, MD, FASGE, FAGA, FACG

BASICS

DESCRIPTION
- Dermatitis herpetiformis (DH) presents as a chronic, relapsing, polymorphous, intensely pruritic, erythematous papulovesicular eruption with symmetrical distribution primarily involving extensor skin surfaces of the elbows, knees, buttocks, back, and scalp.
- DH is an autoimmune disease associated with gluten sensitivity with genetic, environmental, and immunologic influences.
- DH is distinguished from other bullous diseases by characteristic histologic and immunologic findings as well as associated gluten-sensitive enteropathy (GSE).
- System(s) affected: skin
- Synonym(s): Duhring disease, Duhring-Brocq disease

EPIDEMIOLOGY
- Occurs most frequently in those of Northern European origin
- Rare in persons of Asian or African American origin
- Predominant age: most common in 4th and 5th decades but may present at any age
- Childhood DH is rare in most countries, although an Italian study showed 27% of patients were age of <10 years and 36% age of <20 years.
- Predominant gender: adults: male > female (1.5:1 in the United States, 2:1 worldwide); children: female > male

Incidence
1/100,000 persons per year in the United States

Prevalence
11/100,000 persons in the U.S. population; as high as 39/100,000 persons worldwide

ETIOLOGY AND PATHOPHYSIOLOGY
- Evidence suggests that epidermal transglutaminase (eTG) 3, a keratinocyte enzyme involved in cell envelope formation and maintenance, is the autoantigen in DH.
- eTG is highly homologous with tissue transglutaminase (tTG), which is the antigenic target in celiac disease and GSE.
- The initiating event for DH is presumed to be the interaction of wheat peptides with tTGs, which results in the formation of an autoantigen with high affinity for particular class II major histocompatibility complex (MHC) molecules.
- Presentation of the autoantigen leads to activation of T cells and the humoral immune system.
- IgA antibodies against tTG cross-react with eTG and result in IgA-eTG immune complexes that are deposited in the papillary dermis. Subsequent activation of complement and recruitment of neutrophils to the area result in inflammation and microabscesses.
- Skin eruption may be delayed up to 5 to 6 weeks after exposure to gluten.
- Gluten applied directly to the skin does not result in the eruption, whereas gluten taken by mouth or rectum does. This implies necessary processing by the GI system.
- Thought to be immune complex–mediated disease

Genetics
- High association with human leukocyte antigen (HLA)-DQ2 (95%), with remaining patients being positive for DQ8, DR4, or DR3
- Strong association with combination of alleles DQA1*0501 and DQB1*0201/0202, DRB1*03 and DRB1*05/07, *or* DQA1*0301 and DQB1*0302

RISK FACTORS
- GSE: >90% of those with DH will have GSE, which may be asymptomatic.
- Family history of DH or celiac disease

GENERAL PREVENTION
Gluten-free diet (GFD) results in improvement of DH and reduces dependence on medical therapy. GFD also may reduce the risk of lymphomas associated with DH.

COMMONLY ASSOCIATED CONDITIONS
- Hypothyroidism is the most common condition associated with DH.
- GSE, gluten ataxia
- Gastric atrophy, hypochlorhydria, pernicious anemia
- GI lymphoma, non-Hodgkin lymphoma
- Hyperthyroidism, thyroid nodules, thyroid cancer
- IgA nephropathy
- Autoimmune disorders, including systemic lupus erythematosus, dermatomyositis, Sjögren syndrome, rheumatoid arthritis, sarcoidosis, Raynaud phenomenon, insulin-dependent diabetes mellitus, myasthenia gravis, Addison disease, vitiligo, alopecia areata, primary biliary cirrhosis, and psoriasis

DIAGNOSIS

Diagnosis of DH involves a clinicopathologic correlation among clinical presentation, histologic and direct immunofluorescence (DIF) evaluation, serology, and response to therapy or dietary restriction.

HISTORY
- Waxing and waning, intensely pruritic eruption with papules and tiny vesicles
- Eruption may worsen with gluten intake.
- GI symptoms may be absent or may not be reported until prompted.

PHYSICAL EXAM
- The classic lesions of DH are described as symmetric, grouped, erythematous papules and vesicles.
- More commonly presents with erosions, excoriations, lichenification, hypopigmentation, and/or hyperpigmentation secondary to scratching and healing of old lesions
- Areas involved include extensor surfaces of elbows (90%), knees (30%), shoulders, buttocks, and sacrum. The scalp is also frequently affected. Oral lesions are rare.
- In children, purpura may be visible on digits and palmoplantar surfaces.
- Adults with associated enteropathy are most often asymptomatic, with about 20% experiencing steatorrhea and <10% with findings of bloating, diarrhea, or malabsorption.
- Children with associated enteropathy may present with abdominal pain, diarrhea, iron deficiency, and reduced growth rate.

DIFFERENTIAL DIAGNOSIS
- In adults
  - Bullous pemphigoid: linear deposition of C3 and IgG at the basement membrane zone
  - Linear IgA disease: homogeneous and linear deposition of IgA at the basement membrane zone, absence of GSE
  - Prurigo nodularis
  - Urticaria: wheals, angioedema, dermal edema
  - Erythema multiforme

- In children
  - Atopic dermatitis: face and flexural areas
  - Scabies: interdigital areas, axillae, genital region
  - Papular urticaria: dermal edema
  - Impetigo

DIAGNOSTIC TESTS & INTERPRETATION
Initial Tests (lab, imaging)
- Serum IgA tTG antibodies: Detection of tTG antibodies was noted to be up to 95% sensitive and >90% specific for DH in patients on unrestricted diets (1,2)[A].
- Serum IgA eTG antibodies: Antibodies to eTG, the primary autoantigen in DH, were shown to be more sensitive than antibodies to tTG in the diagnosis of patients with DH on unrestricted diets (95% vs. 79%) but is not widely available in all labs (1,2)[A].
- Serum IgA endomysial antibodies (EMA): Antibodies to EMA have a sensitivity between 50% and 100% and a specificity close to 100% in patients on unrestricted diets but is more expensive, time-consuming, and operator-dependent than tTG (2).

Follow-Up Tests & Special Considerations
- Serologic assessment of anti-tTG and anti-eTG correlate with intestinal involvement of disease and in conjunction with anti-EMA may be useful in monitoring major deviations from GFD (1,2).
- Genetic testing for haplotypes HLA-DQ2 and HLA-DQ8 can also be offered to patients to determine genetic susceptibility, to screen patients with high risk of CD, or if the diagnosis is not clear (1).

Diagnostic Procedures/Other
- The gold standard test to establish a diagnosis of DH is DIF of the perilesional skin that demonstrate characteristic granular IgA deposits in dermal papillae and/or basement membrane (1,2)[A]. It is this key diagnostic feature that differentiates this blistering skin condition from all other dermatologic diseases (3).
- DIF has a sensitivity and specificity of close to 100% (1).
- In patients with high suspicion for DH with a negative DIF, another perilesional skin biopsy should be obtained from a different site (1).
- Histopathology of these lesions with routine staining reveals neutrophilic microabscesses in the tips of the dermal papillae and may show subepidermal blistering (1,2).

TREATMENT

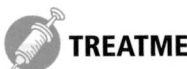

GENERAL MEASURES
- GFD is the mainstay of treatment in DH and can lead to complete resolution of symptoms (1,2)[A].
- Typically requires 18 to 24 months of strict adherence to GFD prior to resolution of skin lesions without any additional treatment
- Lesions can recur within 12 weeks of reintroduction of gluten.

MEDICATION
- Despite being on GFD, the lesions of DH take several months to clear, and active lesions warrant additional treatment (3).
- Medications are useful for immediate symptom management but should only be used as an adjunct to dietary modification (2).

First Line
- Dapsone is approved by the FDA for use in DH and is the most widely used medication (2,4)[A].

- Initial dosing of 25 to 50 mg/day on a strict GFD typically results in improvement of symptoms within 24 to 48 hours (1,3)[C].
- It is recommended to use minimum effective dose with slow titration based on patient's response and tolerability. Average maintenance dose is 1 mg/kg/day (50 to 150 mg/day) and can be increased up to 200 mg to obtain better symptom control.
- Minor outbreaks on the face and scalp are common even with treatment; not ideal for long-term use in DH
- Dapsone works by inhibiting neutrophil recruitment and IL-8 release, inhibiting the respiratory burst of neutrophils, and protecting cells from neutrophil-mediated injury, thereby suppressing the skin reaction. It has no role in preventing IgA deposition or mitigating the immune reaction in the gut (2,4).
- Precautions
  – Common side effects include nausea, vomiting, headache, dizziness, weakness, and hemolysis.
  – A drop in hemoglobin of 1 to 2 g is characteristic with dapsone 100 mg/day.
  – G6PD deficiency increases severity of hemolytic stress. Dapsone should be avoided, if possible, in those who are G6PD-deficient.
  – Dose-related methemoglobinemia may occur with doses >100 mg/day. Cimetidine may reduce the severity of this side effect.
  – Risk of distal motor neuropathy

ALERT
- Monitor for potentially fatal dapsone-induced sulfone syndrome: fever, jaundice and hepatic necrosis, exfoliative dermatitis, lymphadenopathy, methemoglobinemia, and hemolytic anemia.
- Can occur 48 hours or 6 months after treatment, most often 5 weeks after initiation

Pediatric Considerations
- <2 years: Dosing is not established.
- >2 years: 0.5 to 1.0 mg/kg/day

Pregnancy Considerations
- Category C: Safety during pregnancy is not established.
- Secreted in breast milk and will produce hemolytic anemia in infants
- Adherence to a strict GFD 6 to 12 months before conception should be considered with the hope of eliminating need for dapsone during pregnancy.

Second Line
- High-potency topical steroids can be used acutely to control symptoms until dapsone becomes effective (1)[C].
- Sulfapyridine (1 to 2 g/day) is FDA-approved for use in DH and is thought to be the active metabolite in sulfasalazine (2 to 4 g/day) (2,5)[B]. Common side effects include nausea, vomiting, and anorexia. Enteric-coated form may reduce side effects. Other side effects include agranulocytosis, hypersensitivity reactions, hemolytic anemia, proteinuria, and crystalluria (2,5).
- Topical steroids and 3rd-generation antihistamines can be used to provide relief from symptoms of pruritus and itching.

ISSUES FOR REFERRAL
Over time, the management of DH warrants an interdisciplinary treatment that includes providing a referral to dermatologist, gastroenterologist, and registered dietitian (1,2).

ADDITIONAL THERAPIES
A single case report described topical dapsone therapy as potential alternative treatment or as an adjunct to oral dapsone to decrease systemic exposure and risk of severe side effects. However, it has not been studied extensively (6)[C].

ONGOING CARE

FOLLOW-UP RECOMMENDATIONS
Patient Monitoring
- Every 6 to 12 months by physician and dietitian to evaluate GFD adherence and recurrence of symptoms
- Adherence to GFD can be monitored with serologic levels of anti-tTG, anti-eTG, and EMA levels (1).
- Patients on dapsone require lab monitoring weekly for the 1st month, biweekly for 2 months, and then every 3 months for the duration of medication use (1,5).

DIET
- Grains that should be avoided: wheat (includes spelt, kamut, semolina, and triticale), rye, and barley (including malt)
- Safe grains (gluten-free): rice, amaranth, buckwheat, corn, millet, quinoa, sorghum, teff (an Ethiopian cereal grain), and oats
- Care should be taken to avoid gluten-free grains that are contaminated with sources of gluten during processing such as oats.
- Sources of gluten-free starches that can be used as flour alternatives
  – Cereal grains: amaranth, buckwheat, corn, millet, quinoa, sorghum, teff, rice (white, brown, wild, basmati, jasmine), and Montina
  – Tubers: arrowroot, jicama, taro, potato, and tapioca
  – Legumes: chickpeas, lentils, kidney beans, navy beans, pea beans, peanuts, and soybeans
  – Nuts: almonds, walnuts, pistachios, chestnuts, hazelnuts, and cashews
  – Seeds: sunflower, flax, and pumpkin

PATIENT EDUCATION
- Patients started on dapsone should be made aware of potential hemolytic anemia and the signs associated with methemoglobinemia.
- American Academy of Dermatology, 930 N. Meacham Road, P.O. Box 4014, Schaumberg, IL 60168-4014; (708) 330-0230
- The University of Chicago Celiac Disease Center, 5841 S. Maryland Ave., Mail Code 4069, Chicago, IL 60637; (773) 702-7593; www.celiacdisease.net or http://www.cureceliacdisease.org/
- Gluten Intolerance Group of North America, 31214-124 Ave. SE, Auburn, WA 98092; (206) 246-6652; fax (206) 246-6531; https://www.gluten.org/
- The Celiac Disease Foundation, 13251 Ventura Blvd., #1, Studio City, CA 9160; (818) 990-2354; fax (818) 990-2379

PROGNOSIS
- DH is a chronic disease with excellent prognosis, provided strict adherence to a GFD is maintained.
- 10- to 15-year survival rates do not seem to differ from general population.
- Remission in 10–15%
- Skin disease responds readily to dapsone. Occasional new lesions (2 to 3 per week) are to be expected and are not an indication for altering daily dosage.
- Strict adherence to a GFD improves clinical symptoms and decreases dapsone requirement. GFD is the only sustainable method of eliminating cutaneous and GI disease.
- Risk of lymphoma may be decreased in those who maintain a GFD.

COMPLICATIONS
- Majority of complications are associated with GSE.
- Malnutrition, weight loss, nutritional deficiencies (folate, vitamin B_{12}, iron)
- Abdominal pain, dyspepsia
- Osteoporosis, dental abnormalities

- Autoimmune diseases
- Lymphomas

REFERENCES
1. Antiga E, Caproni M. The diagnosis and treatment of dermatitis herpetiformis. *Clin Cosmet Investig Dermatol*. 2015;8:257–265.
2. Bolotin D, Petronic-Rosic V. Dermatitis herpetiformis. Part II. Diagnosis, management, and prognosis. *J Am Acad Dermatol*. 2011;64(6):1027–1034.
3. Reunala T, Salmi TT, Hervonen K. Dermatitis herpetiformis: pathognomonic transglutaminase IgA deposits in the skin and excellent prognosis on a gluten-free diet. *Acta Derm Venereol*. 2015;95(8):917–922.
4. Wozel G, Blasum C. Dapsone in dermatology and beyond. *Arch Dermatol Res*. 2014;306(2):103–124.
5. Willsteed E, Lee M, Wong LC, et al. Sulfasalazine and dermatitis herpetiformis. *Australas J Dermatol*. 2005;46(2):101–103.
6. Handler MZ, Chacon AH, Shiman MI, et al. Letter to the editor: application of dapsone 5% gel in a patient with dermatitis herpetiformis. *J Dermatol Case Rep*. 2012;6(4):132–133.

ADDITIONAL READING
- Bolotin D, Petronic-Rosic V. Dermatitis herpetiformis. Part I. Epidemiology, pathogenesis, and clinical presentation. *J Am Acad Dermatol*. 2011;64(6):1017–1026.
- Cardones AR, Hall RP III. Management of dermatitis herpetiformis. *Immunol Allergy Clin North Am*. 2012;32(2):275–281.
- Cardones AR, Hall RP III. Pathophysiology of dermatitis herpetiformis: a model for cutaneous manifestations of gastrointestinal inflammation. *Immunol Allergy Clin North Am*. 2012;32(2):263–274.
- Kárpáti S. An exception within the group of autoimmune blistering diseases: dermatitis herpetiformis, the gluten-sensitive dermopathy. *Immunol Allergy Clin North Am*. 2012;32(2):255–262.
- Paek SY, Steinberg SM, Katz SI. Remission in dermatitis herpetiformis: a cohort study. *Arch Dermatol*. 2011;147(3):301–305.

SEE ALSO

- Celiac Disease
- Algorithm: Rash

CODES

ICD10
L13.0 Dermatitis herpetiformis

CLINICAL PEARLS

- DH is a chronic, relapsing, intensely pruritic rash that often presents with erosions, excoriations, lichenification, and pigmentary changes secondary to scratching and healing of old papulovesicular lesions.
- Strong association with GSE
- Diagnosis established with perilesional skin biopsy showing DIF demonstrating granular IgA deposits in the dermal papillae
- Serologic levels of IgA transglutaminase aid in diagnosis and monitoring of deviations from GFD.
- Mainstay of treatment is a GFD with dapsone used primarily for short-term symptom relief.

DERMATITIS, ATOPIC
Dennis E. Hughes, DO, FAAFP, FACEP

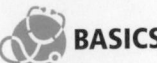

BASICS

DESCRIPTION
- A chronic, relapsing, pruritic eczematous condition affecting characteristic sites
- Early onset cases have coexisting allergen sensitization more often than late onset.
- Clinical phenotypical presentation is highly variable, suggesting multifactorial pathophysiology.
- May have significant effect on quality of life for patient and family—similar to that of psoriasis

EPIDEMIOLOGY
- 45% of all cases begin in the first 6 months of life with 95% onset prior to age 5 years.
- 70% of affected children will have a spontaneous remission before adolescence.
- Incidence on the rise for the past 3 decades in industrialized countries; overall, affects ~15% of children at some time (United States)
- Also, may have late-onset dermatitis in adults or relapse of childhood condition—primarily hand eczema
- Asians and blacks are affected more often than whites.
- 60% if one parent is affected; rises to 80% if both parents are affected

ETIOLOGY AND PATHOPHYSIOLOGY
- Two main hypothesis: immunologic with unbalanced immune response and/or skin barrier dysfunction (1)
- Alteration in stratum corneum results in transepidermal water loss and defect in barrier function.
- Epidermal adhesion is reduced either as a result of (i) genetic mutation resulting in altered epidermal proteins or (ii) defect in immune regulation causing an altered inflammatory response.
- Interleukin-31 (IL-31) upregulation is thought to be a major factor in pruritus mediated by cytokines and neuropeptides rather than histamine excess.

Genetics
- Recent discovery of association between atopic dermatitis (AD) and mutation in the filaggrin gene (*FLG*), which codes for a skin barrier protein (2)
- Both epidermal and immune coding likely involved

RISK FACTORS
- "Itch–scratch cycle" (stimulates histamine release)
- Skin infections
- Emotional stress
- Irritating clothes and chemicals
- Excessively hot or cold climate
- Food allergy in children (in some cases). Studies of breastfeeding conveying decreased risk versus increased risk are mixed in conclusion (3)[C].

- Exposure to tobacco smoke
- Family history of atopy
  - Asthma
  - Allergic rhinitis

COMMONLY ASSOCIATED CONDITIONS
- Food sensitivity/allergy in many cases
- Asthma
- Allergic rhinitis
- Hyper-IgE syndrome (Job syndrome)
  - AD
  - Elevated IgE
  - Recurrent pyodermas
  - Decreased chemotaxis of mononuclear cells

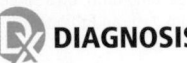

DIAGNOSIS

HISTORY
- Presence of major symptoms, including relapsing of condition, family history, typical distribution, and morphology necessary to make diagnosis of AD
- Upward of 33% report associated mood and sleep disruption.

PHYSICAL EXAM
Primarily skin manifestations
- Distribution of lesions
  - Infants: trunk, face, and flexural surfaces; diaper-sparing
  - Children: antecubital and popliteal fossae
  - Adults: hands, feet, face, neck, upper chest, and genital areas
- Morphology of lesions
  - Infants: erythema and papules; may develop oozing, crusting vesicles
  - Children and adults: Lichenification and scaling are typical with chronic eczema as a result of persistent scratching and rubbing (lichenification rare in infants).
- Associated signs
  - Facial erythema, mild to moderate
  - Perioral pallor
  - Infraorbital fold (Dennie sign/Morgan line)— atopic pleat
  - Dry skin progressing to ichthyosis
  - Increased palmar linear markings
  - Pityriasis alba (hypopigmented asymptomatic areas on face and shoulders)
  - Keratosis pilaris

DIFFERENTIAL DIAGNOSIS
- Photosensitivity rashes
- Contact dermatitis (especially if only the face is involved)
- Scabies

- Seborrheic dermatitis (especially in infants)
- Psoriasis or lichen simplex chronicus if only localized disease is present in adults
- Rare conditions of infancy
  - Histiocytosis X
  - Wiskott–Aldrich syndrome
  - Ataxia-telangiectasia syndrome
- Ichthyosis vulgaris

DIAGNOSTIC TESTS & INTERPRETATION
Initial Tests (lab, imaging)
- No test is diagnostic.
- Serum IgE levels are elevated in as many as 80% of affected individuals, but test is not routinely ordered.
- Eosinophilia tends to correlate with disease severity.
- Scoring atopic dermatitis (SCORAD) is scoring system for AD comprising scores for area, intensity, and subjective symptoms.

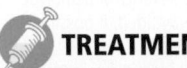

TREATMENT

GENERAL MEASURES
- Minimize flare-ups and control the duration and intensity of flare-up.
- Avoid agents that may cause irritation (e.g., wool, perfumes).
- Minimize sweating.
- Lukewarm (not hot) bathing
- Minimize use of soap (superfatted soaps best).
- Sun exposure may be helpful.
- Humidify the house.
- Avoid excessive contact with water.
- Avoid lotions that contain alcohol.
- If very resistant to treatment, search for a coexisting contact dermatitis.

Pediatric Considerations
Chronic potent fluorinated corticosteroid use may cause striae, hypopigmentation, or atrophy, especially in children.

MEDICATION
First Line
- Frequent systemic lubrication with thick emollient creams (e.g., Eucerin, Vaseline) over moist skin is the mainstay of treatment before any other intervention is considered (1)[A].
- Infants and children: 0.5–1% topical hydrocortisone creams or ointments (use the "fingertip unit [FTU]" dosing) (1)[C]
- Adults: higher potency topical corticosteroids in areas other than face and skin folds

- Short-course, higher potency corticosteroids for flares; then, return to the lowest potency (creams preferred) that will control dermatitis.
- Antihistamines for pruritus (e.g., hydroxyzine 10 to 25 mg at bedtime and as needed)

Second Line
- Topical immunomodulators (tacrolimus or pimecrolimus) for episodic use for children >2 years. There is a black box warning from the FDA regarding potential cancer risk.
- Plastic occlusion in combination with topical medication to promote absorption
- For severe AD, consider systemic steroids for 1 to 2 weeks (e.g., prednisone 2 mg/kg/day PO [max 80 mg/day] initially, tapered over 7 to 14 days).
- Topical tricyclic doxepin, as a 5% cream, may decrease pruritus.
- Modified Goeckerman regimen (tar and ultraviolet light)
- Low-dose methotrexate was established as effective treatment in adults, and recent review suggests it is safe for children and adolescents (4)[B].
- Dupilumab, a biologic that targets mediators of inflammation (IL-22, IL-17, IFN-γ), has completed phase III trials and is awaiting approval (5).

ISSUES FOR REFERRAL
- Ophthalmology evaluation for persistent vernal conjunctivitis
- If using topical steroids around eyes for extended periods, ophthalmology follow-up for cataract evaluation

ADDITIONAL THERAPIES
- Methods to reduce house mite allergens (micropore filters on heating, ventilation, and air-conditioning systems; impermeable mattress covers)
- Behavioral relaxation therapy to reduce scratching
- Bleach baths may reduce staph colonization, but definitive evidence for benefit in the condition is lacking. Recommend 1/2 cup of standard 6% household bleach for a full tub of water and soak for 5 to 10 minutes, blotting skin dry upon leaving the bath.

COMPLEMENTARY & ALTERNATIVE MEDICINE
- Evening primrose oil (includes high content of fatty acids)
  – May decrease prostaglandin synthesis
  – May promote conversion of linoleic acid to omega-6 fatty acid
- Probiotics may reduce the severity of the condition, thus reducing medication use.

 ONGOING CARE

FOLLOW-UP RECOMMENDATIONS
Patient Monitoring
Evaluate to ensure that secondary bacterial or fungal infection does not develop as a result of disruption of the skin barrier. Most patients with AD are colonized by *Staphylococcus*. There is a little evidence for the routine use of antimicrobial interventions to reduce skin bacteria, but treatment of clinical infection with coverage for *Staphylococcus* is recommended.

DIET
- Trials of elimination may find certain "triggers" in some patients.
- Breastfeeding in conjunction with maternal hypoallergenic diets may decrease the severity in some infants (varying opinions).

PATIENT EDUCATION
- http://www.aad.org/skin-conditions/dermatology-a-to-z/atopic-dermatitis
- National Eczema Association: www.nationaleczema.org

PROGNOSIS
- Chronic disease
- Declines with increasing age
- 90% of patients have spontaneous resolution by puberty.
- Localized eczema (e.g., chronic hand or foot dermatitis, eyelid dermatitis, or lichen simplex chronicus) may continue in some adults.

COMPLICATIONS
- Cataracts are more common in patients with AD.
- Skin infections (usually *Staphylococcus aureus*); sometimes subclinical
- Eczema herpeticum
  – Generalized vesiculopustular eruption caused by infection with herpes simplex or vaccinia virus
  – Causes acute illness requiring hospitalization
- Atrophy and/or striae if fluorinated corticosteroids are used on face or skin folds
- Systemic absorption may occur if large areas of skin are treated, particularly if high-potency medications and occlusion are combined.

REFERENCES
1. Thomsen SF. Atopic dermatitis: natural history, diagnosis, and treatment. *ISRN Allergy*. 2014;2014:354250.
2. Wollenberg A, Seba A, Antal AS. Immunological and molecular targets of atopic dermatitis treatment. *Br J Dermatol*. 2014;170(Suppl 1):7–11.
3. Lin HP, Chiang BL, Yu HH, et al. The influence of breastfeeding in breast-fed infants with atopic dermatitis [published online ahead of print June 29, 2017]. *J Microbiol Immunol Infect*. doi:10.1016/j.jmii.2017.06.004.
4. Deo M, Yung A, Hill S, et al. Methotrexate for treatment of atopic dermatitis in children and adolescents. *Int J Dermatol*. 2014;53(8):1037–1041.
5. D'Erme AM, Romanelli M, Chiricozzi A. Spotlight on dupilumab in the treatment of atopic dermatitis: design, development, and potential place in therapy. *Drug Des Devel Ther*. 2017;11:1473–1480.

ADDITIONAL READING
- Boguniewicz M, Leung DY. Recent insights into atopic dermatitis and implications for management of infectious complications. *J Allergy Clin Immunol*. 2010;125(1):4–13.
- Lifschitz C. The impact of atopic dermatitis on quality of life. *Ann Nutr Metab*. 2015;66(Suppl 1):34–40.

 SEE ALSO

Algorithm: Rash

 CODES

ICD10
- L20.9 Atopic dermatitis, unspecified
- L20.89 Other atopic dermatitis
- L20.83 Infantile (acute) (chronic) eczema

CLINICAL PEARLS
- Institute early and proactive treatment to reduce inflammation. Use the lowest potency topical steroid that controls symptoms.
- Monitor for secondary bacterial infection.
- Frequent systemic lubrication with thick emollient creams (e.g., Eucerin, Vaseline) over moist skin is the mainstay of treatment before any other intervention is considered.

DERMATITIS, CONTACT

Anne Walsh, ANP-BC • Konstantinos E. Deligiannidis, MD, MPH, FAAFP

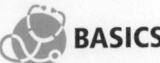

BASICS

DESCRIPTION
- A cutaneous reaction to an external substance
- Each type has a different mechanism, whereas the clinical presentation is the same (1).
- Primary irritant dermatitis (ID) is a result of direct damage to the stratum corneum by chemicals or physical agents that occurs faster than the skin is able to repair itself, which results in an inflammatory nonimmunologic cutaneous reaction. Prior sensitization is not required (2). ID occurs immediately or within 48 hours of exposure (3).
- Allergic contact dermatitis (ACD) affects only individuals previously sensitized to a substance. It represents a delayed hypersensitivity reaction, requiring several hours or days for the cascade of cellular immunity to manifest itself (2,3).
- System(s) affected: skin/exocrine
- Synonym(s): dermatitis venenata

EPIDEMIOLOGY
Common

Incidence
Occupational contact dermatitis accounts for up to 70% of occupational skin disease occurrences and affects 20.5/100,000 workers per year in one Australian study.

Prevalence
- Florists, hairdressers, cooks, beauticians, and metal-working machine operators have the highest incidence (3).
- Predominant sex: male = female
  - Variations due to differences in exposure to offending agents as well as normal cutaneous variations between males and females (eccrine and sebaceous gland function and hair distribution)

Geriatric Considerations
Increased incidence of ID secondary to skin dryness

Pediatric Considerations
Increased incidence of positive patch testing due to better delayed hypersensitivity reactions (4)

ETIOLOGY AND PATHOPHYSIOLOGY
Hypersensitivity reaction to a substance generating cellular immunity response (5)
- Plants
  - Urushiol (allergen): poison ivy, poison oak, poison sumac
  - Primary contact: plant (roots/stems/leaves)
  - Secondary contact: clothes/fingernails (not blister fluid—the established eruption is not itself contagious or transmissible)

- Chemicals
  - Nickel: jewelry, zippers, hooks, and watches (6)
  - Potassium dichromate: tanning agent in leather
  - Paraphenylenediamine: hair dyes, fur dyes, and industrial chemicals
  - Turpentine: cleaning agents, polishes, and waxes
  - Soaps and detergents
- Topical medicines
  - Neomycin: topical antibiotics
  - Thimerosal (Merthiolate): preservative in topical medications
  - Anesthetics: benzocaine
  - Parabens: preservative in topical medications
  - Formalin: cosmetics, shampoos, and nail enamel

Genetics
Increased frequency of ACD in families with allergies

RISK FACTORS
- Occupation
- Hobbies
- Travel
- Cosmetics
- Jewelry

GENERAL PREVENTION
- Avoid causative agents.
- Use of protective gloves (with cotton lining) may be helpful.

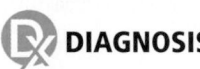

DIAGNOSIS

HISTORY
- Itchy rash
- Assess for prior exposure to irritating substance.

PHYSICAL EXAM
- Acute
  - Papules, vesicles, bullae with surrounding erythema
  - Crusting and oozing
  - Pruritus
- Chronic
  - Erythematous base
  - Thickening with lichenification
  - Scaling
  - Fissuring
- Distribution
  - Where epidermis is thinner (eyelids, genitalia)
  - Areas of contact with offending agent (e.g., nail polish)
  - Palms and soles relatively more resistant, although hand dermatitis is common
  - Deeper skin folds spared
  - Linear arrays of lesions
  - Lesions with sharp borders and sharp angles are pathognomonic.
  - Well-demarcated area with a papulovesicular rash

DIFFERENTIAL DIAGNOSIS
- Based on clinical impression
  - Appearance, periodicity, and localization
- Groups of vesicles
  - Herpes simplex
- Diffuse bullous or vesicular lesions
  - Bullous pemphigoid
- Photodistribution
  - Phototoxic/allergic reaction to systemic allergen
- Eyelids
  - Seborrheic dermatitis
- Scaly eczematous lesions
  - Atopic dermatitis
  - Nummular eczema
  - Lichen simplex chronicus
  - Stasis dermatitis
  - Xerosis
- Id reaction (see separate chapter)

DIAGNOSTIC TESTS & INTERPRETATION
Diagnostic Procedures/Other
Consider patch tests for suspected allergic trigger (systemic corticosteroids or recent, aggressive use of topical steroids may alter results).

Test Interpretation
- Intercellular edema
- Bullae

TREATMENT

GENERAL MEASURES
- Remove offending agent:
  - Avoidance
  - Work modification
  - Protective clothing
  - Barrier creams, especially high-lipid content moisturizing creams (e.g., Keri lotion, petrolatum, coconut oil)
- Topical soaks with cool tap water, Burow solution (1:40 dilution), saline (1 tsp/pt water), or silver nitrate solution
- Lukewarm water baths
- Aveeno oatmeal baths
- Emollients (white petrolatum, Eucerin)

MEDICATION
First Line
- Topical medications (6)[A]
  - Lotion of zinc oxide, talc, menthol 0.15% (Gold Bond), phenol 0.5%
  - Corticosteroids for ACD as well as ID
    - High-potency steroids: fluocinonide (Lidex) 0.05% gel, cream, or ointment TID–QID
    - Use high-potency steroids only for a short time and then switch to low- or medium-potency steroid cream or ointment.
    - Caution regarding face/skin folds: Use lower potency steroids, and avoid prolonged usage. Switch to lower potency topical steroid once the acute phase is resolved.

- Calamine lotion for symptomatic relief
- Topical antibiotics for secondary infection (bacitracin, erythromycin)
- Systemic
  - Antihistamine
    - Hydroxyzine: 25 to 50 mg PO QID, especially useful for itching
    - Diphenhydramine: 25 to 50 mg PO QID
    - Cetirizine: 10 mg PO BID–TID
- Corticosteroids
  - Prednisone: Taper starting at 60 to 80 mg/day PO, over 10 to 14 days, occasionally 21 days.
  - Used for moderate to severe cases, particularly involving face or genitals
  - Little published evidence to compare appropriate length of treatment, but clinical experience suggests that short courses of therapy (i.e., 5 to 7 days) are not adequate to prevent rebound dermatitis.
  - Treatment for up to 21 days for severe/extensive rash resulting from exposure to potent allergens like urushiol (e.g., poison ivy) is commonly recommended to prevent reemergence of dermatitis upon taper (rebound), although 14 days is usually adequate.
  - May use burst dose of steroids for up to 5 days for less persistent immunogens or less severe dermatitis
- Antibiotics for secondary skin infections
  - Dicloxacillin: 250 to 500 mg PO QID for 7 to 10 days
  - Amoxicillin-clavulanate (Augmentin): 500 mg PO BID for 7 to 10 days
  - Erythromycin: 250 mg PO QID in penicillin-allergic patients
  - Trimethoprim-sulfamethoxazole (Bactrim DS): 160 mg/800 mg (1 tablet) PO BID for 7 to 10 days (suspected resistant *Staphylococcus aureus*)
- Precautions
  - Antihistamines may cause drowsiness.
  - Prolonged use of potent topical steroids may cause local skin effects (atrophy, stria, telangiectasia).
  - Use tapering dose of oral steroids if using >5 days.

Second Line
Other topical or systemic antibiotics, depending on organisms and sensitivity

Pregnancy Considerations
Usual caution with medications

ISSUES FOR REFERRAL
May need referral to a dermatologist or allergist if refractory to conventional treatment

COMPLEMENTARY & ALTERNATIVE MEDICINE
The use of complementary and alternative treatment is a supplement and not an alternative to conventional treatment.

ADMISSION, INPATIENT, AND NURSING CONSIDERATIONS
Rarely needs hospital admission

 ONGOING CARE

FOLLOW-UP RECOMMENDATIONS
Stay active, but avoid overheating.

Patient Monitoring
- As necessary for recurrence
- Patch testing for etiology after resolved

DIET
No special diet

PATIENT EDUCATION
- Avoidance of irritating substance
- Cleaning of secondary sources (nails, clothes)
- Fallacy of blister fluid spreading disease

PROGNOSIS
- Self-limited
- Benign
- 55% of patients still had contact dermatitis at 2 years after diagnosis (3).
- Improvement in rash less likely for those who remain in the same or similar profession (3)
- Increased length of exposure and atopy are poor prognostic indicators (3).

COMPLICATIONS
- Generalized eruption secondary to autosensitization
- Secondary bacterial infection

REFERENCES
1. Sultan TA, Hatem AMA. Management of contact dermatitis. *J Dermatol Dermatol Surg*. 2015;19(2):86–91.
2. Tan CH, Rasool S, Johnston GA. Contact dermatitis: allergic and irritant. *Clin Dermatol*. 2014;32(1):116–124.
3. Ahmed S. Contact dermatitis. *Innovait*. 2015;8(11):653.
4. Admani S, Jacob SE. Allergic contact dermatitis in children: review of the past decade. *Curr Allergy Asthma Rep*. 2014;14(4):421.
5. Martin SF. Contact dermatitis: from pathomechanisms to immunotoxicology. *Exp Dermatol*. 2012;21(5):382–389.
6. Usatine RP, Riojas M. Diagnosis and management of contact dermatitis. *Am Fam Physician*. 2010;82(3):249–255.

ADDITIONAL READING
Pelletier JL, Perez C, Jacob SE. Contact dermatitis in pediatrics. *Pediatr Ann*. 2016;45(8):e287–e292.

 SEE ALSO

Algorithm: Rash

 CODES

ICD10
- L25.9 Unspecified contact dermatitis, unspecified cause
- L23.9 Allergic contact dermatitis, unspecified cause
- L25.5 Unspecified contact dermatitis due to plants, except food

CLINICAL PEARLS
- Commonly occurs on hands and face
- Anyone exposed to irritants or allergic substances is predisposed to contact dermatitis, especially in occupations that have high exposure to chemicals.
- The most common allergens causing contact dermatitis are plants of the *Toxicodendron* genus (poison ivy, poison oak, poison sumac).
- Poison-ivy dermatitis typically requires 10 to 14 days (occasionally more) of topical or oral steroid therapy to prevent recurrent eruption.
- Worldwide, nickel is the number one patch-tested allergen causing ACD.
- The usual treatment for contact dermatitis is avoidance of the allergen or irritating substance and temporary use of topical steroids.
- A contact dermatitis eruption presents in a nondermatomal geographic fashion due to the skin being in contact with an external source.

DERMATITIS, DIAPER
Dennis E. Hughes, DO, FAAFP, FACEP

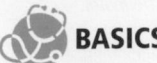 **BASICS**

DESCRIPTION
- Diaper dermatitis is a rash occurring under the covered area of a diaper. It is usually initially a contact dermatitis.
- System(s) affected: skin/exocrine
- Synonym(s): diaper rash; nappy rash; napkin dermatitis

Geriatric Considerations
Incontinence is a significant cofactor.

EPIDEMIOLOGY
Incidence
- The most common dermatitis found in infancy
- Peak incidence: 7 to 12 months of age and then decreases
- Lower incidence reported in breastfed babies due to lower pH, urease, protease, and lipase activity.

Prevalence
Prevalence has been variably reported from 4–35% in the first 2 years of life. Upward of 75% of infants will have episodes of varying duration and severity in United States.

ETIOLOGY AND PATHOPHYSIOLOGY
- Immature infant skin with histologic, biochemical, functional differences compared to mature skin (1)
- Wet skin is central in the development of diaper dermatitis, as prolonged contact with urine or feces results in susceptibility to chemical, enzymatic, and physical injury; wet skin is also penetrated more easily.
- Fecal proteases and lipases are irritants.
- Superhydrase urease enzyme found in the stratum corneum liberates ammonia from cutaneous bacteria.
- Fecal lipase and protease activity is increased by acceleration of GI transit; thus, a higher incidence of irritant diaper dermatitis is observed in babies who have had diarrhea in the previous 48 hours.
- Once the skin is compromised, secondary infection by *Candida albicans* is common. 40–75% of diaper rashes that last >3 days are colonized with *C. albicans*.
- Bacteria may play a role in diaper dermatitis through reduction of fecal pH and resulting activation of enzymes.
- Allergy is exceedingly rare as a cause in infants.

RISK FACTORS
- Infrequent diaper changes
- Improper laundering (cloth diapers)
- Family history of dermatitis
- Hot, humid weather
- Recent treatment with oral antibiotics
- Diarrhea (>3 stools per day increases risk)
- Dye allergy
- Eczema may increase risk.

GENERAL PREVENTION
Attention to hygiene during bouts of diarrhea

COMMONLY ASSOCIATED CONDITIONS
- Contact (allergic or irritant) dermatitis
- Seborrheic dermatitis
- Psoriasis
- Candidiasis
- Atopic dermatitis

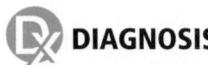 **DIAGNOSIS**

HISTORY
- Onset, duration, and change in the nature of the rash
- Presence of rashes outside the diaper area
- Associated scratching or crying
- Contact with infants with a similar rash
- Recent illness, diarrhea, or antibiotic use
- Fever
- Pustular drainage
- Lymphangitis

PHYSICAL EXAM
- Mild forms consist of shiny erythema ± scale.
- Margins are not always evident.
- Moderate cases have areas of papules, vesicles, and small superficial erosions.
- It can progress to well-demarcated ulcerated nodules that measure ≥1 cm in diameter.
- It is found on the prominent parts of the buttocks, medial thighs, mons pubis, and scrotum.
- Skin folds are spared or involved last.
- *Tidemark dermatitis* refers to the bandlike form of erythema of irritated diaper margins.
- Diaper dermatitis can cause an id reaction (autoeczematous) outside the diaper area.

DIFFERENTIAL DIAGNOSIS
- Contact dermatitis
- Seborrheic dermatitis
- Candidiasis
- Atopic dermatitis
- Scabies
- Acrodermatitis enteropathica
- Letterer-Siwe disease
- Congenital syphilis
- Child abuse
- Streptococcal infection
- Kawasaki disease
- Biotin deficiency
- Psoriasis
- HIV infection

DIAGNOSTIC TESTS & INTERPRETATION
Initial Tests (lab, imaging)
Rarely needed

Follow-Up Tests & Special Considerations
- Consider a culture of lesions or a potassium hydroxide (KOH) preparation.
- The finding of anemia in association with hepatosplenomegaly and the appropriate rash may suggest a diagnosis of Langerhans cell histiocytosis or congenital syphilis.
- Finding mites, ova, or feces on a mineral oil preparation of a burrow scraping can confirm the diagnosis of scabies.

Test Interpretation
- Biopsy is rare.
- Histology may reveal acute, subacute, or chronic spongiotic dermatitis.

 TREATMENT

Prevention is the key to treatment of this condition.

GENERAL MEASURES
- Expose the buttocks to air as much as possible.
- Use mild, slightly acidic cleanser with water; no rubbing and pat dry.
- Avoid impermeable waterproof pants during treatment (day or night); they keep the skin wet and subject to rash or infection.

- Change diapers frequently, even at night, if the rash is extensive.
- Superabsorbable diapers are beneficial because they wick urine away from skin and still allow air to permeate (2)[C].
- Discontinue using baby lotion, powder, ointment, or baby oil (except zinc oxide).
- Use of appropriately formulated baby wipes (fragrance free) is safe and as effective as water (3)[B].
- Apply zinc oxide ointment or other barrier cream to the rash at the earliest sign and BID or TID (e.g., Desitin or Balmex). Thereafter, apply to clean, thoroughly dried skin (4)[C].
- Cornstarch can reduce friction. Talc powders that do not enhance the growth of yeast can provide protection against frictional injury in diaper dermatitis but do not form a continuous lipid barrier layer over the skin and obstruct the skin pores. These treatments are not recommended.

MEDICATION

First Line

- For a pure contact dermatitis, a low-potency topical steroid (hydrocortisone 0.5–1% TID for 3 to 5 days) and removal of the offending agent (urine, feces) should suffice.
- If candidiasis is suspected or diaper rash persists, use an antifungal such as miconazole nitrate 2% cream, miconazole powder, econazole (Spectazole), clotrimazole (Lotrimin), or ketoconazole (Nizoral) cream at each diaper change.
- If inflammation is prominent, consider a very low-potency steroid cream such as hydrocortisone 0.5–1% TID along with an antifungal cream ± a combination product such as clioquinol–hydrocortisone (Vioform–Hydrocortisone) cream.
- If a secondary bacterial infection is suspected, use an antistaphylococcal oral antibiotic or mupirocin (Bactroban) ointment topically.
- Precautions: Avoid high- or moderate-potency steroids often found in combination of steroid antifungal mixtures—these should never be used in the diaper area.

Second Line

- Sucralfate paste for resistant cases
- Recent study suggests that use of hydrocolloid dressings can speed healing of rash.

ISSUES FOR REFERRAL

Consider if a systemic disease such as Langerhans cell histiocytosis, acrodermatitis enteropathica, or HIV infection is suspected.

ADMISSION, INPATIENT, AND NURSING CONSIDERATIONS

- Admission criteria/initial stabilization
  - Febrile neonates
  - Recalcitrant rash suggestive of immunodeficiency
  - Toxic-appearing infants
- Assist first-time parents with hygiene education.

 ONGOING CARE

FOLLOW-UP RECOMMENDATIONS

Patient Monitoring

Recheck weekly until clear and then at times of recurrence.

PATIENT EDUCATION

Patient education is vital to the treatment and prevention of recurrent cases.

PROGNOSIS

- Quick, complete clearing with appropriate treatment
- Secondary candidal infections may last a few weeks after treatment has begun.

COMPLICATIONS

- Secondary bacterial infection (Consider community-acquired methicillin-resistant *Staphylococcus aureus* [MRSA] in pustular dermatitis that does not respond to normal therapy.)
- Rare complication is inoculation with group A β-hemolytic *Streptococcus* resulting in necrotizing fasciitis.
- Secondary yeast infection

REFERENCES

1. Stamatas GN, Tierney NK. Diaper dermatitis: etiology, manifestations, prevention, and management. *Pediatr Dermatol.* 2014;31(1):1–7.
2. Erasala GN, Romain C, Merlay I. Diaper area and disposable diapers. *Curr Probl Dermatol.* 2011;40:83–89.
3. Lavender T, Furber C, Campbell M, et al. Effect on skin hydration of using baby wipes to clean the napkin area of newborn babies: assessor-blinded randomised controlled equivalence trial. *BMC Pediatr.* 2012;12:59.
4. Humphrey S, Bergman JN, Au S. Practical management strategies for diaper dermatitis. *Skin Therapy Lett.* 2006;11(7):1–6.

ADDITIONAL READING

Qiao XP, Ge YZ. Clinical effect of hydrocolloid dressings in prevention and treatment of infant diaper rash. *Exp Ther Med.* 2016;12(6):3665–3669.

 SEE ALSO

Algorithm: Rash

 CODES

ICD10

- L22 Diaper dermatitis
- B37.2 Candidiasis of skin and nail

CLINICAL PEARLS

- Hygiene is the main preventative measure.
- Look for secondary infection in persistent cases.

DERMATITIS, SEBORRHEIC

Juan Qiu, MD, PhD

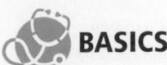 **BASICS**

DESCRIPTION
Chronic, superficial, recurrent inflammatory rash affecting sebum-rich, hairy regions of the body, especially the scalp, eyebrows, and face

EPIDEMIOLOGY
Incidence
- Predominant age: infancy, adolescence, and adulthood
- Predominant sex: male > female

Prevalence
Seborrheic dermatitis: 3–5%

ETIOLOGY AND PATHOPHYSIOLOGY
- Skin surface yeasts *Malassezia* may be a contributing factor (1).
- Genetic and environmental factors: Flares are common with stress/illness.
- Parallels increased sebaceous gland activity in infancy and adolescence or as a result of some acnegenic drugs.
- Seborrheic dermatitis is more common in immunosuppressed patients, suggesting that immune mechanisms are implicated in the pathogenesis of the disease, although the mechanisms are not well defined (1).

Genetics
Positive family history; no genetic marker is identified to date.

RISK FACTORS
- Parkinson disease, epilepsy, traumatic brain and spinal cord injury, Down syndrome (1)
- AIDS, lymphoma, organ transplantation (1)
- Emotional stress (1)
- Medications may flare/induce seborrheic dermatitis: buspirone, chlorpromazine, ethionamide, griseofulvin, haloperidol, interferon-α, methyldopa, psoralen, IL-2 (1)

GENERAL PREVENTION
Seborrheic skin should be washed more often than usual.

COMMONLY ASSOCIATED CONDITIONS
- Parkinson disease
- AIDS

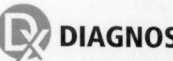 **DIAGNOSIS**

Diagnosis of seborrheic dermatitis usually can be made by history and physical exam.

HISTORY
- Intermittent active phases manifest with burning, scaling, and itching, alternating with inactive periods; activity is increased in winter and early spring, with remissions commonly occurring in summer.
- Infants
  - Cradle cap: greasy scaling of scalp, sometimes with associated mild erythema
  - Diaper and/or axillary rash
  - Age at onset typically ~1 month
  - Usually resolves by 8 to 12 months
- Adults
  - Red, greasy, scaling rash in most locations consisting of patches and plaques with indistinct margins
  - Red, smooth, glazed appearance in skin folds
  - Minimal pruritus
  - Chronic waxing and waning course
  - Bilateral and symmetric
  - Most commonly located in hairy skin areas: scalp and scalp margins, eyebrows and eyelid margins, nasolabial folds, ears and retroauricular folds, presternal area, middle to upper back, buttock crease, inguinal area, genitals, and armpits

PHYSICAL EXAM
- Scalp appearance varies from mild, patchy scaling to widespread, thick, adherent crusts. Plaques are rare.
- Seborrheic dermatitis can spread onto the forehead, the posterior part of the neck, and the postauricular skin, as in psoriasis.
- Skin lesions manifest as brawny or greasy scaling over red, inflamed skin.
- Hypopigmentation is seen in African Americans.
- Infectious eczematoid dermatitis, with oozing and crusting, suggests secondary infection.
- Seborrheic blepharitis may occur independently.

DIFFERENTIAL DIAGNOSIS
- Atopic dermatitis: Distinction may be difficult in infants.
- Psoriasis
  - Usually, knees, elbows, and nails are involved.
  - Scalp psoriasis will be more sharply demarcated than seborrhea, with crusted, infiltrated plaques rather than mild scaling and erythema.

- Candida
- Tinea cruris/capitis: Suspect these when usual medications fail or hair loss occurs.
- Eczema of auricle/otitis externa
- Rosacea
- Discoid lupus erythematosus: Skin biopsy will be beneficial.
- Histiocytosis X: may appear as seborrheic-type eruption
- Dandruff: scalp only, noninflammatory

DIAGNOSTIC TESTS & INTERPRETATION
Diagnostic Procedures/Other
Consider biopsy if
- Usual therapies fail.
- Petechiae are noted.
- Histiocytosis X is suspected.
- Fungal cultures in refractory cases or when pustules and alopecia are present

Test Interpretation
Nonspecific changes
- Hyperkeratosis, acanthosis, accentuated rete ridges, focal spongiosis, and parakeratosis are characteristic.
- Parakeratotic scale around hair follicles and mild superficial inflammatory lymphocytic infiltrate

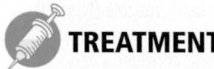 **TREATMENT**

GENERAL MEASURES
- Increase frequency of shampooing.
- Sunlight in moderate doses may be helpful.
- Cradle cap
  - Frequent shampooing with a mild, nonmedicated shampoo
  - Remove thick scale by applying warm mineral oil and then wash off 1 hour later with a mild soap and a soft-bristle toothbrush or terrycloth washcloth
- Adults: Wash all affected areas with antiseborrheic shampoos. Start with over-the-counter products (selenium sulfide) and increase to more potent preparations (containing coal tar, sulfur, or salicylic acid) if no improvement is noted.
- For dense scalp scaling, 10% liquor carbonic detergents in Nivea oil may be used at bedtime, covering the head with a shower cap. This should be done nightly for 1 to 3 weeks.

MEDICATION

First Line

- Cradle cap: Use a coal tar shampoo or ketoconazole (Nizoral) shampoo if the nonmedicated shampoo is ineffective.
- Adults
  - Topical antifungal agents
    - Ketoconazole or miconazole 2% shampoo twice a week for clearance and then once a week or every other week for maintenance (1,2,3)[A]
    - Ketoconazole (Nizoral) and sertaconazole 2% cream may be used to clear scales in other areas (1,2,3)[A].
    - Ciclopirox 1% shampoo twice weekly (1,2,3)[A]
  - Topical corticosteroids
    - Begin with 1% hydrocortisone and advance to more potent (fluorinated) steroid preparations, as needed (1,2,3)[A].
      - Avoid continuous use of the more potent steroids to reduce the risk of skin atrophy, hypopigmentation, or systemic absorption (especially in infants and children).
      - Precautions: Fluorinated corticosteroids and higher concentrations of hydrocortisone (e.g., 2.5%) may cause atrophy or striae if used on the face or on skin folds.
  - Other topical agents
    - Coal tar 1% shampoo twice a week
    - Selenium sulfide 2.5% shampoo twice a week
    - Zinc pyrithione 1% shampoo twice a week
    - Lithium gluconate/succinate 8% ointment/gel twice a week (4)[A]
- Once controlled, washing with zinc soaps or selenium lotion with periodic use of steroid cream may help to maintain remission.

Second Line

- Calcineurin inhibitors
  - Pimecrolimus 1% cream BID (4)[A]
  - Tacrolimus 0.1% ointment (4)[A]
- Systemic antifungal therapy
  - Data are limited.
  - For moderate to severe seborrheic dermatitis
    - Ketoconazole: 200 mg/day (5)[A]
    - Itraconazole: 200 mg/day (5)[A]
    - Daily regimen for 1 to 2 months followed by twice-weekly dosing for chronic treatment
    - Monitor potential hepatotoxic effects.
- Low-molecular-weight hyaluronic acid
  - Hyaluronic acid sodium salt gel 0.2% BID (6)[B]

ISSUES FOR REFERRAL

No response to first-line therapy and concerns regarding systemic illness (e.g., HIV)

 ONGOING CARE

FOLLOW-UP RECOMMENDATIONS

Patient Monitoring

Every 2 to 12 weeks, as necessary, depending on disease severity and degree of patient sophistication

PATIENT EDUCATION

http://familydoctor.org/familydoctor/en/diseases-conditions/seborrheic-dermatitis.html

PROGNOSIS

- In infants, seborrheic dermatitis usually remits after 6 to 8 months.
- In adults, seborrheic dermatitis is usually chronic and unpredictable, with exacerbations and remissions. Disease is usually easily controlled with shampoos and topical steroids.

COMPLICATIONS

- Skin atrophy/striae are possible from fluorinated corticosteroids, especially if used on the face.
- Glaucoma can result from use of fluorinated steroids around the eyes.
- Photosensitivity is caused occasionally by tars.
- Herpes keratitis is a rare complication of herpes simplex: Instruct patient to stop eyelid steroids if herpes simplex develops.

REFERENCES

1. Borda LJ, Wikramanayake TC. Seborrheic dermatitis and dandruff: a comprehensive review. *J Clin Investig Dermatol.* 2015;3(2). doi:10.13188 /2373-1044.1000019.
2. Clark GW, Pope SM, Jaboori KA. Diagnosis and treatment of seborrheic dermatitis. *Am Fam Physician.* 2015;91(3):185–190.
3. Okokon EO, Verbeek JH, Ruotsalainen JH, et al. Topical antifungals for seborrhoeic dermatitis. *Cochrane Database Syst Rev.* 2015;(5):CD008138.
4. Kastarinen H, Oksanen T, Okokon EO, et al. Topical anti-inflammatory agents for seborrhoeic dermatitis of the face or scalp. *Cochrane Database Syst Rev.* 2014;(5):CD009446.
5. Gupta AK, Richardson M, Paquet M. Systematic review of oral treatments for seborrheic dermatitis. *J Eur Acad Dermatol Venereol.* 2014;28(1):16–26.
6. Schlesinger T, Rowland Powell C. Efficacy and safety of a low molecular weight hyaluronic acid topical gel in the treatment of facial seborrheic dermatitis final report. *J Clin Aesthet Dermatol.* 2014;7(5):15–18.

ADDITIONAL READING

- Dessinioti C, Katsambas A. Seborrheic dermatitis: etiology, risk factors, and treatments: facts and controversies. *Clin Dermatol.* 2013;31(4):343–351.
- Hay RJ. Malassezia, dandruff and seborrhoeic dermatitis: an overview. *Br J Dermatol.* 2011;165(Suppl 2):2–8.
- Kim GK, Rosso JD. Topical pimecrolimus 1% cream in the treatment of seborrheic dermatitis. *J Clin Aesthet Dermatol.* 2013;6(2):29–35.
- Stefanaki I, Katsambas A. Therapeutic update on seborrheic dermatitis. *Skin Therapy Lett.* 2010;15(5):1–4.

 SEE ALSO

Algorithm: Rash

 CODES

ICD10

- L21.9 Seborrheic dermatitis, unspecified
- L21.1 Seborrheic infantile dermatitis
- L21.0 Seborrhea capitis

CLINICAL PEARLS

- Search for an underlying systemic disease in a patient who is unresponsive to usual therapy.
- In adults, seborrheic dermatitis is usually chronic and unpredictable, with exacerbations and remissions. Disease is usually easily controlled with shampoos and topical steroids.

DERMATITIS, STASIS

Joseph A. Florence, MD • Fereshteh Gerayli, MD, FAAFP

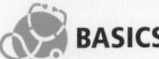

BASICS

DESCRIPTION
- Chronic, eczematous, erythema, scaling, and noninflammatory edema of the lower extremities accompanied by cycle of scratching, excoriations, weeping, crusting, and inflammation in patients with chronic venous insufficiency (CVI), due to impaired circulation and other factors (nutritional edema)
- Clinical skin manifestation of CVI usually appears late in the disease.
- May present as a solitary lesion; can be associated with venous leg ulcer, which is located on the medial or lateral side of the ankle
- System(s) affected: skin/exocrine
- Synonym(s): gravitational eczema; varicose eczema; venous dermatitis

EPIDEMIOLOGY
Incidence
- In the United States: common in patients age >50 years (6–7%)
- Predominant age: adult, geriatric
- Predominant sex: female > male

Geriatric Considerations
Common in this age group:
- Estimated to affect 15 to 20 million patients age >50 years in the United States

ETIOLOGY AND PATHOPHYSIOLOGY
- Incompetence of perforating veins, superficial venous thrombosis from varicose veins, and deep vein thrombosis (DVT) can each contribute to CVI leading to venous hypertension (HTN) and cutaneous inflammation. This can be a pathway to venous leg ulcer.
- Deposition of fibrin around capillaries
- Microvascular abnormalities
- Ischemia
- Continuous presence of edema in ankles, usually present because of venous valve incompetency (varicose veins)
- Weakness of venous walls in lower extremities
- Trauma to edematous, eczematized skin
- Itch may be caused by inflammatory mediators (from mast cells, monocytes, macrophages, or neutrophils) liberated in the microcirculation and endothelium.
- Abnormal leukocyte–endothelium interaction is proposed to be a major factor.
- A cascade of biochemical events leads to ulceration.

Genetics
Familial link probable

RISK FACTORS
- Atopy
- Chronic edema
- Old age
- Obesity
- Previous DVT
- Previous pregnancy
- Prolonged standing
- Secondary infection
- Superimposition of itch–scratch cycle
- Trauma
- Low-protein diet

- Genetic propensity
- Tight garments that constrict the thigh
- Vein stripping
- Vein harvesting for coronary artery bypass graft surgery
- Previous cellulitis

GENERAL PREVENTION
- Use compression stockings to avoid recurrence of edema and to mobilize the interstitial lymphatic fluid from the region of stasis dermatitis and also following DVT.
- Topical lubricants twice a day to prevent fissuring and itching

COMMONLY ASSOCIATED CONDITIONS
- Varicose veins
- Venous insufficiency
- Other eczematous disease
- Hyperhomocysteinemia
- Venous HTN

DIAGNOSIS

HISTORY
- Itching, pain, and burning may precede skin signs, which are aggravated during evening hours.
- Insidious onset
- Usually bilateral
- Description may include aching/heavy legs.
- Erythema, scaling, edema of lower extremities
- Noninflammatory edema preceded the skin eruption and ulceration.
- Edema initially develops around the ankle.

PHYSICAL EXAM
- Evaluation of the lower extremities characteristically reveals:
  - Bilateral scaly, eczematous patches, papules, and/or plaques
  - Violaceous (sometimes brown), erythematous lesions due to deoxygenation of venous blood (postinflammatory hyperpigmentation and hemosiderin deposition within the cutaneous tissue)
- Distribution: medial aspect of ankle, with frequent extension onto the foot and lower leg, occasionally lateral side of ankle
- Brawny induration
- Stasis ulcers (frequently accompany stasis dermatitis) secondary to minor trauma
- Excoriations
- Weeping, crusting, inflammation of the skin
- Varicosities are often associated with ulcers.
- Clinical inspection reveals swelling and warmth.
- Skin changes are more common in the lower 1/3 of the extremity and medially.
- Early signs include prominent superficial veins and pitting ankle edema.
- May present as a solitary lesion mimicking a neoplasm

DIFFERENTIAL DIAGNOSIS
- Other eczematous diseases:
  - Atopic dermatitis
  - Uremic dermatitis
  - Contact dermatitis (due to topical agents used to self-treat)

  - Neurodermatitis
  - Arterial insufficiency
  - Sickle cell disease causing skin ulceration
  - Cellulitis
  - Erysipelas
- Tinea dermatophyte infection
- Pretibial myxedema
- Nummular eczema
- Lichen simplex chronicus
- Xerosis
- Asteatotic eczema
- Amyopathic dermatomyositis

DIAGNOSTIC TESTS & INTERPRETATION
Initial Tests (lab, imaging)
Duplex ultrasound imaging is helpful in diagnosis.

Diagnostic Procedures/Other
- Rule out arterial insufficiency. Check peripheral pulses; ankle brachial pressure index (ABPI or ABI)
- Check for diabetes.

Test Interpretation
- ABPI <0.8 is suggestive of arterial insufficiency.
- ABPI can be elevated, >1.2 in diabetic patients and others with distal small vessel calcifications.
- Arterial duplex ultrasound and angiography are the gold standards.

TREATMENT

GENERAL MEASURES
Primary role of treatment is to reverse effects of venous HTN. Appropriate health care:
- Outpatient:
  - Reduce edema:
    - Leg elevation: legs above the level of heart for 30 minutes, 3 to 4 times daily. Avoid prolonged dependent position.
    - Compression therapy: This is the mainstay of treatment of venous stasis ± ulcers. Compression bandages can be safely applied in patients with ABI of 0.8 to 1.2.
    - Elastic bandage wraps: Ace bandages or Unna paste boot (zinc gelatin) or compression stockings
    - Graduated elastic compression of 30 to 40 mm Hg at the ankle improves ulcer healing rate and may prevent ulcer recurrence (1)[A].
    - Compression bandages containing both elastic and inelastic components (mixed component systems) are as effective as four-layer bandages, are easier to apply, and have less slippage and associated with favorable quality of life outcomes.
    - High compression is contraindicated in arterial insufficiency.
    - Pneumatic compression devices are beneficial, especially in nonambulatory patients and those with a component of arterial insufficiency (2)[B].
- Improvement of lipodermatosclerosis:
  - Activity:
    - Avoid standing still.
    - Stay active and exercise regularly.
    - Elevate foot of bed unless contraindicated.

- Inpatient, for endovascular radiofrequency ablation, vein stripping, sclerotherapy, or skin grafts.
  - Venous ulcer treatment: Treat infection: Débride the ulcer base of necrotic tissue (surgical necrotomy if possible, or enzymatic débridement with collagenase).
    - Autolytic: Modern wound dressings (hydrogel, hydrocolloids, alginate, foam bandages, plain nonadherent dressing) are better than traditional wet to dry dressing because they maintain moist wound environment, with less tissue damage on removal, and less frequent changing requirement (2)[A]. However, there is no difference in healing rate of venous stasis ulcers by use of hydrocolloid dressing versus simple nonadherent dressing when used beneath compression.
    - Biologic: Topical application of granulocyte-macrophage colony-stimulating factor promotes healing of ulcers (insufficient evidence).
    - Mechanical: wet to dry dressings, hydrotherapy, and irrigation
    - Surgical: modifying cause of venous HTN (by venous ligation, valvuloplasty, and endoscopic perforator vein surgery); treat ulcer by graft.

MEDICATION

First Line
- Pentoxifylline 400 mg TID is effective in treating venous leg ulcer.
- The use of low-dose aspirin because adjuvant treatment for venous leg ulcers is not supported (3)[A].
- In light of increasing bacterial resistance to antibiotics, current guidelines recommend the use of antibacterial preparations only for clinical infection (cellulitis, increased pain, warmth, malodorous exudate), not for bacterial colonization (4)[A].
- If secondary infection, treat with PO antibiotics for *Staphylococcus* or *Streptococcus* organisms (e.g., dicloxacillin 250 mg QID, cephalexin 500 mg BID, or levofloxacin 500 mg daily).
- If MRSA suspected, clindamycin 300 mg QID, doxycycline 100 mg BID, TMP/SMX or IV vancomycin
- There is no reliable evidence on the effectiveness of topical antiseptics such as povidone-iodine, peroxide-based preparations, mupirocin, chlorhexidine (4)[A].
- Uncomplicated stasis dermatitis can be treated with short courses (about 2 weeks) of topical steroids (2)[B] (topical triamcinolone 0.1% cream/ointment BID).
- Topical antipruritic: pramoxine, camphor, menthol, and doxepin
- Topical anesthetic (lidocaine/prilocaine) may reduce pain during débridement.
- Systemic steroids for severe cases
- Silver sulfadiazine (SSD) has a positive effect in wound healing (2)[A].

Second Line
- Consider antibiotics on basis of culture results of exudate from infected ulcer craters.
- Lubricants when dermatitis is quiescent
- Chronic stasis dermatitis can be treated with topical emollients (e.g., white petroleum, lanolin).
- Antipruritic medications (e.g., diphenhydramine, cetirizine hydrochloride)
- Hydrocolloid or a foam dressing may reduce ulcer pain; no evidence that ibuprofen dressings offer pain relief

ISSUES FOR REFERRAL
Consider referral for:
- Nonhealing ulcer
- Arterial insufficiency
- Uncertain diagnosis
- Rheumatoid arthritis
- Patch testing to evaluate for contact dermatitis
- Associated disease (e.g., symptomatic varicose veins)

ADDITIONAL THERAPIES
If the patient is on amlodipine, consider discontinuing.

SURGERY/OTHER PROCEDURES
Sclerotherapy and surgery may be required for associated disease.

 ONGOING CARE

FOLLOW-UP RECOMMENDATIONS
Patient Monitoring
- If Unna boot compression is used: Cut off and reapply boot once a week. Unna boots reduce edema by compression and prevent scratching.
- Regular use of high-compression stockings reduces chance of recurrent venous ulcer (5)[A].

DIET
Lose weight, if overweight.

PATIENT EDUCATION
- Encourage staying active to keep circulation and leg muscles in good condition. Walking is ideal.
- Keep legs elevated while sitting or lying.
- Do not wear girdles, garters, or pantyhose with tight elastic tops.
- Do not scratch.
- Avoid leg injury.
- Elevate foot of bed with 2- to 4-inch blocks.
- Apply compression stockings prior to getting out of bed when less edema is present. Regular use of high-compression stockings may prevent recurrence of venous ulcers.

PROGNOSIS
- Chronic course with intermittent exacerbations and remissions
- The healing process for ulceration is often prolonged and may take months.

COMPLICATIONS
- Sensations of itching, pain, and burning have negative impact on the quality of life.
- Secondary bacterial infection
- DVT
- Bleeding at dermatitis sites
- Squamous cell carcinoma in edges of long-standing stasis ulcers
- Scarring, which in turn leads to further compromise to blood flow and increased likelihood of minor trauma

REFERENCES
1. O'Meara S, Cullum N, Nelson EA, et al. Compression for venous leg ulcers. *Cochrane Database Syst Rev.* 2012;(11):CD000265.
2. Evidence-based (S3) guidelines for diagnostics and treatment of venous leg ulcers. *J Eur Acad Dermatol Venereol.* 2016;30(11):1843–1875.
3. Jull A, Wadham A, Bullen C, et al. Low dose aspirin as adjuvant treatment for venous leg ulceration: pragmatic, randomised, double blind, placebo controlled trial (Aspirin4VLU). *BMJ.* 2017;359:j5157.
4. O'Meara S, Al-Kurdi D, Ologun Y, et al. Antibiotics and antiseptics for venous leg ulcers. *Cochrane Database Syst Rev.* 2014;(1):CD003557.
5. Nelson EA, Bell-Syer SE. Compression for preventing recurrence of venous ulcers. *Cochrane Database Syst Rev.* 2012;(8):CD002303.

ADDITIONAL READING
- Coleridge-Smith PD. Leg ulcer treatment. *J Vasc Surg.* 2009;49(3):804–808.
- Coleridge-Smith P, Labropoulos N, Partsch H, et al. Duplex ultrasound investigation of the veins in chronic venous disease of the lower limbs—UIP consensus document. Part I. Basic principles. *Eur J Vasc Endovasc Surg.* 2006;31(1):83–92.
- Collins L, Seraj S. Diagnosis and treatment of venous ulcers. *Am Fam Physician.* 2010;81(8):989–996.
- Partsch H, Flour M, Smith P; for International Compression Club. Indications for compression therapy in venous and lymphatic disease consensus based on experimental data and scientific evidence. Under the auspices of the IUP. *Int Angiol.* 2008;27(3):193–219.
- Sippel K, Mayer D, Ballmer B, et al. Evidence that venous hypertension causes stasis dermatitis. *Phlebology.* 2011;26(8):361–365.

 SEE ALSO

- Varicose Veins
- Algorithm: Rash

 CODES

ICD10
- I83.10 Varicose veins of unsp lower extremity with inflammation
- I83.11 Varicose veins of right lower extremity with inflammation
- I83.12 Varicose veins of left lower extremity with inflammation

CLINICAL PEARLS
- Treatment of edema associated with stasis dermatitis via elevation and/or compression stockings or bandages is essential for optimal results.
- Pentoxifylline may improve venous ulcer healing.
- No difference in healing rate of venous stasis ulcers by use of hydrocolloid dressing versus simple nonadherent dressing when used beneath compression. Decision about the dressing should be based on local cost and patient or physician's preferences.
- Mild topical corticosteroids reduce inflammation and itching; however, these may potentiate infection; high-potency topical corticosteroids should be avoided due to increased risk of atrophy and ulceration.

D

DIABETES MELLITUS, TYPE 1

David T. Broome, MD • Vicente T. San Martin, MD • Betul A. Hatipoglu, MD

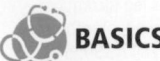 **BASICS**

DESCRIPTION
- Type 1 diabetes mellitus (T1DM) is a chronic disease caused by insulin deficiency following β-cell destruction.
- Results in hyperglycemia and end-organ complications
- Features include:
  - Usually rapid onset
  - Absolute insulin dependence
  - Polyphagia, polydipsia, polyuria, and nocturia
  - Ketosis
  - Body habitus: usually normal or thin physique
- System(s) affected: endocrine/metabolic, cardiovascular, neurologic, renal, ocular

Pregnancy Considerations
- T1DM confers maternal and fetal risk (spontaneous abortion, fetal anomalies, preeclampsia, fetal demise, macrosomia, neonatal hypoglycemia, and neonatal hyperbilirubinemia) (1).
- Preconception counseling should address importance of glycemic control as close to normal as safely possible (goal A1c <6.5%) to reduce congenital anomalies (1).
- Glycemic targets during pregnancy: fasting <95 mg/dL, and either 1-hour postprandial <140 mg/dL, or 2-hour postprandial <120 mg/dL
- Dilated eye examinations should occur before pregnancy or in the 1st trimester and then patients should be monitored every trimester and 1-year postpartum (1).
- Women with T1DM have an increased risk of hypoglycemia in the 1st trimester and have decreased hypoglycemia awareness.
- Pregnancy is a ketogenic state, and women are at risk for diabetic ketoacidosis (DKA).
- Women with T1DM should be prescribed low-dose aspirin 60 to 150 mg/day (81 mg/day) (1).

EPIDEMIOLOGY
- Age of presentation is bimodal: at 4 to 6 years of age and at 10 to 14 years of age (early puberty) (2).
- No gender difference in overall incidence (3)

Incidence
- In the United States, incidence in non-Hispanic white children/adolescents is 23.6/100,000. Prevalence is 2.55/1,000 in non-Hispanic white children/adolescents (4).
- Substantially lower rates in other racial and ethnic groups

Pediatric Considerations
In infants and toddlers, symptoms of T1DM may be subtle or masquerade as an intercurrent illness and thus are frequently misinterpreted or ignored.

ETIOLOGY AND PATHOPHYSIOLOGY
Pathogenesis
- There are two main categories of T1DM: immune-mediated and idiopathic diabetes (1):
  - Immune-mediated diabetes: cellular-mediated autoimmune destruction of β cells of the pancreas (markers: autoantibodies to insulin, GAD65, tyrosine phosphatases IA-2 and IA-2β, including zinc transporter 8 autoantibody [ZnT8A]) (1)

- Idiopathic diabetes: no known etiology. Patients have permanent insulinopenia and are prone to ketoacidosis but have no evidence of autoimmunity (1).
- At least one autoantibody is present in 85–90% of individuals (1).

Genetics
- The disease has strong HLA associations, with linkage to the DQA and DQB genes, and it is influenced by the DRB genes (HLA-DQA1, HLA-DQB1, and DLA-DRB1) (1).
- The major susceptibility locus maps to the HLA class II genes at 6p21 (accounting for 30–50% of genetic T1DM), but there are >40 loci (5).

RISK FACTORS
- HLA variations account for ~40% of the genetic risk for T1DM (5).
- Risk factors: viral infections, vitamin D deficiency, perinatal factors (maternal age, history of preeclampsia, neonatal jaundice), high birth weight for gestational age, and lower gestational age at birth (1)
- Increased susceptibility to T1DM is inheritable:
  - Only 15% of newly diagnosed patients have a positive family history of T1DM.
  - T1DM in monozygous twins with long-term follow-up is >50%.
  - Among first-degree relatives, siblings are at a higher risk (5–10% risk by age 20 years) than offspring.
  - Offspring of diabetic fathers are at a higher risk (~12%) than offspring of diabetic mothers (~6%) (5).

COMMONLY ASSOCIATED CONDITIONS
- Autoimmune diseases, such as celiac disease, vitamin B_{12} deficiency, autoimmune gastritis, vitiligo, and Hashimoto hypothyroidism
- T1DM can also be seen as part of autoimmune polyendocrine syndromes.

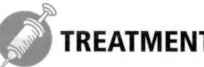 **DIAGNOSIS**

HISTORY
- New-onset polyuria and polydipsia (1)[C]
  - Polyuria may present as nocturia, bed-wetting, or incontinence in a previously continent child.
  - Polyuria may be difficult to appreciate in diaper-clad children.
- Polyuria occurs when serum glucose concentration rises >180 mg/dL (10 mmol/L); weight loss
- Increased fatigue, lethargy, muscle cramps
- Ketosis/DKA leads to abdominal discomfort, nausea.
- Vision changes, such as blurriness (5)
- Silent (asymptomatic) incidental discovery

DIFFERENTIAL DIAGNOSIS
- Type 2 diabetes
- Monogenic diabetes considered when:
  - Diabetes diagnosed before 6 months of age
  - Strong family history of diabetes without classic features of type 2 diabetes
  - Mild fasting hyperglycemia
  - Nonobese diabetic child with negative autoantibodies

- Secondary diabetes
  - Pancreatic disease (chronic pancreatitis, cystic fibrosis, hereditary hemochromatosis)
  - Endocrine-associated diabetes: acromegaly, Cushing syndrome, pheochromocytoma, glucagonoma, neuroendocrine tumors
  - Drug- or chemical-induced glucose intolerance: glucocorticosteroids, HIV protease inhibitors, atypical antipsychotics, tacrolimus, cyclosporine
- Acute poisonings (Salicylate poisoning can mimic DKA.)

DIAGNOSTIC TESTS & INTERPRETATION
Initial Tests (lab, imaging)
- Criteria for the diagnosis of diabetes (1)[C]:
  - Fasting (>8 hours) glucose ≥126 mg/dL (7.0 mmol/L) on more than one occasion
  - Random glucose of ≥200 mg/dL (11.1 mmol/L) in a patient with classic symptoms of hyperglycemia
  - Oral glucose tolerance test (OGTT): plasma glucose ≥200 mg/dL 2 hours after a glucose load of 1.75 g/kg (max dose 75 g)
  - Glycated hemoglobin (HbA1c) level ≥6.5%
- Other tests to consider:
  - Urinalysis for glucose, ketones, and albuminuria (urine albumin:creatinine ratio)
  - Pancreatic autoantibodies
    ○ Islet cell, IAA, GAD, IA2A, and ZnT8A
  - Serum β-hydroxybutyrate (BHB) and urine ketones
- C-peptide insulin level if needed to differentiate from type 2 diabetes because low or no C-peptide indicates insulinopenia

Test Interpretation
- If one of the aforementioned criteria is met, a diagnosis of diabetes can be made.
- In the absence of unequivocal hyperglycemia, results should be confirmed by repeat testing.

TREATMENT

GENERAL MEASURES
- Insulin is the mainstay of therapy (1).
- Education regarding matching of mealtime insulin dose to carbohydrate intake, premeal blood glucose level, and anticipated activity (1)
  - Before meals, strive for blood glucose levels in range of 90 to 130 mg/dL (5.0 to 7.2 mmol/L).
  - Bedtime/overnight: 90 to 150 mg/dL (5.0 to 8.3 mmol/L)
  - A1c goal: <7.5% across all pediatric age groups
  - A1c <7.0% is reasonable if achieved without excessive hypoglycemia.
- Very tight control might be dangerous in young children due to risk of repeated hypoglycemia.
- Adult A1c goal: <7.0% (1)[B]
  - A1c <6.5% reasonable in select individuals (1)[C]
  - Less stringent A1c goals (such as <8%) may be appropriate for elderly patients and other special populations (1)[B].

MEDICATION
- Most people with T1DM should be treated with multiple daily injections (MDI) of prandial insulin and basal insulin, or continuous subcutaneous insulin infusion (CSII) (1)[A].

- Most individuals with T1DM should use rapid-acting insulin analogs to reduce hypoglycemia risk (1)[A].
- Types of insulin (1)[C]:
  – Long-acting insulin analogs: insulin glargine, insulin detemir, and insulin degludec. These should not be mixed with other insulins in the same syringe.
  – Very rapid-acting insulin analogs: insulin lispro, insulin aspart, and insulin glulisine
  – Intermediate-acting insulin (NPH) can be mixed with other insulins.
  – Short-acting (regular) insulin

First Line
- Flexible intensive insulin therapy is the gold standard.
- MDI or CSII has equal efficacy (1)[B].
- Total initial dose is 0.2 to 0.4 units/kg/day for insulin-naive patients (up to 1.0 unit/kg/day in puberty).
- ~50% of total dose given as basal insulin, with the rest as bolus insulin
- MDI regimen (1)[A]:
  – Basal, long-acting insulin once or twice a day
  – Prandial, short-acting insulin based on number of carbohydrate portions (e.g., 1:10, meaning 1 U of insulin for every 10 g of carbohydrates)
  – Correctional short-acting mealtime insulin based on premeal blood glucose level and sensitivity factor (e.g., 1 U for every 50 mg/dL over 150 mg/dL, where 50 mg/dL is the sensitivity factor)
- CSII regimen:
  – CSII and continuous glucose monitoring (CGM) should be encouraged when there is active patient/family participation (1).

Second Line
- Twice-daily injections with NPH along with regular or rapid-acting insulin (not physiologic, but lower cost and fewer injections)
- Pramlintide: delays gastric emptying, blunts pancreatic secretion of glucagon, and enhances satiety
- Pancreatic and islet transplantation have been shown to normalize glucose levels but require lifelong immunosuppression; reserved for simultaneous renal transplantation, recurrent DKA, or severe hyperglycemia (1)
- Investigational agents (not yet FDA-approved): metformin, GLP-1 receptor agonists, DPP-4 inhibitors, and SGLT-2 inhibitors (1)

ADMISSION, INPATIENT, AND NURSING CONSIDERATIONS
Newly diagnosed patients with T1DM may require hospitalization during initiation of insulin therapy, especially if presenting in DKA.

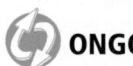 ONGOING CARE

FOLLOW-UP RECOMMENDATIONS
Regular aerobic exercise with care to avoid hypoglycemia

Patient Monitoring
- Blood pressure (BP) checks at every routine visit with a goal of systolic pressure of <130 mm Hg and diastolic of <80 mm Hg (1)[C]
- Daily home blood glucose monitoring with home blood glucose meter: Blood tests should be done at least 4 to 6 times daily (more frequently in pump patients) for optimal monitoring.

- Comprehensive foot exam at least annually
- Quarterly measurement of HbA1c
- For patients of all ages with diabetes and atherosclerotic cardiovascular disease (ASCVD), high-intensity statin therapy should be added to lifestyle therapy (1)[A].
- For patients with diabetes age 40 to 75 years (1)[A] and >75 years (1)[B] without ASCVD, use moderate-intensity statin in addition to lifestyle therapy (1).
- Annual screenings (1)[C]:
  – Albuminuria for earliest signs of possible nephropathy (urine albumin:creatinine ratio)
  – Initial dilated comprehensive eye exam within 5 years of diagnosis and then annually
  – Monofilament testing with pinprick, temperature, and vibration sensation for screening of peripheral neuropathy 5 years after diagnosis and then annually
  – Annual influenza vaccine in patients ≥6 months of age
  – Pneumococcal pneumonia with 13-valent pneumococcal conjugate vaccine (PCV13) is recommended for children before age 2 years. People with diabetes ages 2 to 64 years should also receive 23-valent pneumococcal polysaccharide vaccines (PPSV23). At age >65 years, regardless of vaccine history, additional PPSV23 is recommended (1)[C].
  – Hepatitis B vaccination to unvaccinated adults aged 19 to 59 years. Consider administering 3-dose series of hepatitis B vaccine to unvaccinated adults with diabetes ages ≥60 years (1)[C].

DIET
- American Diabetes Association diet: http://www.diabetes.org/food-and-fitness/food/
- Carbohydrate counting using insulin-to-carbohydrate ratio with all meals and snacks allows patient flexibility in eating.

PROGNOSIS
- Initial remission or honeymoon phase with decreased insulin needs and easier control, usually 3 to 6 months
- Current prognosis for reduced life expectancy:
  – Increasing longevity and quality of life with careful blood glucose monitoring, improvement in insulin delivery regimens, and appropriate glycemic control

COMPLICATIONS
- Microvascular disease (retinopathy, nephropathy, neuropathy)
- Hyperlipidemia
- Macrovascular disease (coronary and cerebral artery disease)
- Chronic foot ulcers/amputations
- Hypoglycemia
- DKA
- Excessive weight gain
- Increased risk for preeclampsia and preterm delivery
- Driving mishaps—recommend checking glucose before driving.
- Psychological problems of chronic disease

REFERENCES
1. American Diabetes Association. 8. Pharmacologic approaches to glycemic treatment: *Standards of Medical Care in Diabetes—2018*. *Diabetes Care*. 2018;41(Suppl 1):S73–S85.
2. Felner EI, Klitz W, Ham M, et al. Genetic interaction among three genomic regions creates distinct contributions to early- and late-onset type 1 diabetes mellitus. *Pediatr Diabetes*. 2005;6(4):213–220.
3. Dabelea D, Mayer-Davis EJ, Saydah S, et al; for SEARCH for Diabetes in Youth Study. Prevalence of type 1 and type 2 diabetes among children and adolescents from 2001 to 2009. *JAMA*. 2014;311(17):1778–1786.
4. Bell RA, Mayer-Davis EJ, Beyer JW, et al; and SEARCH for Diabetes in Youth Study Group. Diabetes in non-Hispanic white youth: prevalence, incidence, and clinical characteristics: the SEARCH for Diabetes in Youth Study. *Diabetes Care*. 2009;32(Suppl 2):S102–S111.
5. Steck AK, Rewers MJ. Genetics of type 1 diabetes. *Clin Chem*. 2011;57(2):176–185.

ADDITIONAL READING
- Mayer-Davis EJ, Lawrence JM, Dabelea D, et al; and SEARCH for Diabetes in Youth Study. Incidence trends of type 1 and type 2 diabetes among youths, 2002–2012. *N Engl J Med*. 2017;376(15):1419–1429.
- Miller KM, Foster NC, Beck RW, et al; for T1D Exchange Clinic Network. Current state of type 1 diabetes treatment in the U.S.: updated data from the T1D Exchange clinic registry. *Diabetes Care*. 2015;38(6):971–978.

CODES

ICD10
- E10.9 Type 1 diabetes mellitus without complications
- E10.8 Type 1 diabetes mellitus with unspecified complications
- E10.69 Type 1 diabetes mellitus with other specified complication

CLINICAL PEARLS
- The age of presentation of T1DM is bimodal: one peak at 4 to 6 years of age and a second peak at 10 to 14 years of age (early puberty).
- At least one autoantibody is present in 85–90% of individuals when fasting hyperglycemia is initially detected. Starting at puberty, preconception counseling should be incorporated into routine diabetes care for all girls of childbearing potential.
- Therapy with MDI or CSII and the use of a multidisciplinary team care approach are associated with improved glycemic control, resulting in better long-term outcomes.
- Adult A1c goal is <7.0%; less stringent A1c goals may be appropriate for elderly patients and other special populations.

DIABETES MELLITUS, TYPE 2
Sanaa Ayyoub, MD • Samir Malkani, MD, MRCP–UK

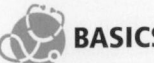 **BASICS**

DESCRIPTION
Diabetes mellitus (DM) type 2 is due to a progressive insulin secretory defect in the setting of insulin resistance.

Geriatric Considerations
Monitor elderly for hypoglycemia; adjust doses for renal/hepatic dysfunction and cognitive function; less aggressive glucose targets than in younger patients

Pediatric Considerations
Incidence is increasing and parallels obesity epidemic.

Pregnancy Considerations
Diet, metformin, glyburide, and insulin are all options for treatment of gestational diabetes.

EPIDEMIOLOGY

Incidence
1.5 million new cases in the United States each year

Prevalence
Estimated 30.3 million Americans (9.4% of the population); 90–95% are likely type 2.

ETIOLOGY AND PATHOPHYSIOLOGY
- Peripheral insulin resistance and/or defective insulin secretion with increased hepatic gluconeogenesis
- Genetic factors: usually polygenic; rarely monogenic (e.g., peroxisome proliferator-activated receptor (*PPAR*) γ and insulin gene mutations)
- Obesity (body mass index [BMI] $\geq$25 kg/m²) and visceral adiposity
- Gut microbiome changes
- Drug or chemical induced (e.g., glucocorticoids, highly active antiretroviral therapy [HAART], atypical antipsychotics, organ transplant immunosuppressants)

Genetics
- Genome-wide association studies show many common variants confer small causal effect; 50% concordance in monozygotic twins
- Family history is strongly predictive of risk.

RISK FACTORS
- Parental history of type 2 diabetes
- Gestational diabetes or history of baby with birth weight $\geq$4 kg (9 lb)
- Polycystic ovarian syndrome (PCOS)
- Hypertriglyceridemia or low high-density lipoprotein (HDL)—marker for insulin resistance
- Ethnicity: African American, Latino, Native American, Asian, and Pacific Islander
- Sedentary lifestyle, visceral obesity
- Use of thiazides, antipsychotics, glucocorticoids, and statins

GENERAL PREVENTION
- Maintenance of normal weight, or weight loss of 7% body weight, decrease intake of carbohydrates and overall calories. Moderate-intensity exercise and resistance training. Exercise 150 min/week.
- Use of metformin, α-glucosidase inhibitors, thiazolidinediones (TZDs), and glucagon-like peptide-1 receptor agonist (GLP-1 RA) in select patients with prediabetes (1)[A]

COMMONLY ASSOCIATED CONDITIONS
Hypertension, dyslipidemia, metabolic syndrome, fatty liver disease, infertility, PCOS, acanthosis nigricans, hemochromatosis

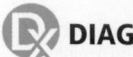 **DIAGNOSIS**

HISTORY
Polyuria, polydipsia, polyphagia, weight loss, weakness, fatigue, blurry vision, neuropathy, and frequent infections

PHYSICAL EXAM
BMI, funduscopic exam, oral exam, cardiopulmonary exam, abdominal exam for hepatomegaly, focused neurologic exam, and diabetic foot exam

DIFFERENTIAL DIAGNOSIS
- Type 1 DM—low or absent insulin C-peptide, positive β-cell autoantibodies, ketosis
- DM is one of the features of Cushing syndrome, acromegaly, and glucagonoma.

DIAGNOSTIC TESTS & INTERPRETATION
Initial Tests (lab, imaging)
Criteria for diagnosis (1)[A]
- HbA1c $\geq$6.5% *or*
- Hyperglycemic symptoms and random plasma glucose $\geq$200 mg/dL (11.1 mmol/L) *or*
- Fasting plasma glucose (FPG) $\geq$126 mg/dL (7.0 mmol/L) *or*
- 2-hour plasma glucose $\geq$200 mg/dL (11.1 mmol/L) during oral glucose tolerance test (OGTT) with 75-g glucose load
- If equivocal, repeat with a different test on the same sample or a repeat test in a separate sample.

Follow-Up Tests & Special Considerations
Screen patients with history of gestational diabetes for persistent diabetes/prediabetes with OGTT 6 to 12 weeks postpartum and every 3 years thereafter.

 TREATMENT

Tight control of type 2 diabetes prevents long-term microvascular complications, but benefits on macrovascular outcomes are not as apparent (2). Individuals likely to benefit from a more aggressive target (below) are those without preexisting DM complications, with recent diagnoses of DM, and with long life expectancy. Most medications have NOT been shown to improve long-term outcomes.
- Use patient-centered approach (individualized).
- Cornerstone of therapy is lifestyle modification, with diet and exercise and control of cardiovascular risk factors (particularly blood pressure [BP] and lipids).
- A1c targets—ADA recommendations (these are NOT universally accepted as not fully evidence based) (1)[C]. ACP targets differ (3)[C].
  - A1c <7.0: for those with a long life expectancy, no cardiovascular disease (CVD), diagnosed DM for a short duration, and no history of hypoglycemia
  - A1c <8.0%: for those with a limited life expectancy, advanced micro- or macrovascular complications, extensive comorbidities, and a history of severe hypoglycemia or long-standing DM in whom the general goal is difficult to attain
  - Many experts recognize more liberal targets (2,3).
  - ADA guidelines—preprandial glucose of 80 to 130 mg/dL and peak postprandial glucose of <180 mg/dL (1)[C]

- Use drugs from different classes for complementary action and limit side effects. Use monotherapy with metformin (if not contraindicated), but if A1c is $\geq$9%, start with dual therapy; if A1c $\geq$10%, BG 300 mg/dL, and patient is symptomatic, consider adding injectable therapy with insulin with/without GLP-1 analog (1)[A].
- Always consider side effect profile, CV benefit, and cost.

GENERAL MEASURES
- Diabetic foot exam at every visit
- Nephropathy: annual urine microalbumin-to-creatinine ratio and plasma creatinine (eGFR)
- Retinopathy: annual diabetic eye exam
- If 40 to 75 years old, begin a statin—moderate to high intensity based on atherosclerotic CVD (ASCVD) risk.
- If >50 years old, low-dose aspirin if at least one additional CV risk factor and low risk for GI bleeding
- Hypertension: goal BP <140/80 mm Hg (Tighter control may be considered on individual basis.)
- Pneumococcal (PPSV23) for all adults and pneumococcal conjugate vaccine (PCV13) for patients >65 years (and some younger—see CDC) and annual influenza vaccine

MEDICATION
Monotherapy
- Metformin
  - Reduces hepatic glucose production and has multiple other mechanisms of action
  - Preferred as first line due to high efficacy in lowering glucose, good safety profile, low risk of hypoglycemia, and low cost; also promotes weight loss
  - Some studies suggest CVD benefit; dosage: 500 to 2,000 mg in divided doses or extended release QD or BID (1)[A]
  - Avoid metformin in renal insufficiency with eGFR <30, prior to radiocontrast agent use, surgery, and severe acute illnesses (e.g., liver disease, cardiogenic shock, pancreatitis, hypoxia) due to risk of lactic acidosis.
  - Caution with acute heart failure, alcohol abuse, elderly; associated with GI side effects, vitamin B$_{12}$ deficiency (Monitor levels yearly.)
  - Can be used in CKD patients with eGFR $\geq$45; reduce dose to $\leq$1,000 mg with close monitoring in patients with eGFR 30 to 45 (2)[A].
  - About 10% of patients on metformin develop diarrhea. For these patients and other patients who have contraindications to metformin use, a different agent can be used as monotherapy.

ADDITIONAL THERAPIES
- General principles
  - If HbA1c not at goal, add second agent. Start with dual therapy when initial HbA1c >9%.
  - If patient has CAD, heart failure, or CKD, consider drugs shown to improve outcomes with these conditions.
  - Consideration should be given to drug-specific side effects (such as weight gain, hypoglycemia).
  - Cost of drug is an important consideration.
  - Choose regimen with patient input to optimize adherence (mode of administration, complexity).
- GLP-1 RA (incretins)
  - Stimulate glucose-dependent insulin secretion.
  - Promote weight loss, no risk of hypoglycemia; some improve CV outcomes (2).

- Small risk of acute pancreatitis. Caution with use in CKD ≥ stage 4. May exacerbate gastroparesis. Injectable drugs, insulin dose may need reduction; relatively expensive
- Should not be used in patients with personal history/family history of medullary thyroid cancer or multiple endocrine neoplasia (MEN) type 2 (black box warning)
- Exenatide (Byetta): 5 to 10 μg SC BID within 60 minutes before meals and at least 6 hours apart or exenatide ER (Bydureon) 2 mg/week
- Liraglutide (Victoza): 0.6 to 1.8 mg/day; reduced composite endpoint of cardiovascular death, nonfatal MI or nonfatal stroke (2)[A]
- Dulaglutide (Trulicity): 0.75 to 1.50 mg weekly
- Lixisenatide (Adlyxin): uptitration to 20 μg SC QD; available in combination (insulin glargine/lixisenatide)—15 to 60 U SC QD
- Semaglutide (Ozempic): 0.25 to 1.00 mg weekly; improved cardiovascular outcomes (2)[A]
- SGLT2 inhibitors
  - Inhibit renal glucose reabsorption
  - Cause weight loss, no hypoglycemia risk
  - Reduced heart failure risk and cardiovascular mortality (2)[A]
  - Empagliflozin and canagliflozin may offer renal benefits.
  - Increase occurrence of genital mycotic infections and UTI. Increased risk of euglycemic diabetic ketoacidosis (DKA); relatively expensive
  - Do not initiate therapy if eGFR <45.
  - Canagliflozin (Invokana): 100 to 300 mg daily; increased risk for lower limb amputation
  - Dapagliflozin (Farxiga): 5 to 10 mg daily
  - Empagliflozin (Jardiance): 10 to 25 mg daily
- Dipeptidyl peptidase-4 (DPP-4) inhibitors
  - Inhibit the enzyme DPP-4 which deactivates endogenous incretins GLP-1 and GIP
  - Minimal risk for hypoglycemia; reduce dose in renal impairment with exception of linagliptin.
  - Weight neutral
  - Alogliptin and saxagliptin are associated with heart failure, but sitagliptin is not.
  - Clinical evidence shows no CV risk reduction (4).
  - Sitagliptin (Januvia): 100 mg/day
  - Saxagliptin (Onglyza): 2.5 or 5.0 mg daily
  - Linagliptin (Tradjenta): 5 mg/day
  - Alogliptin (Nesina): 25 mg/day
- Sulfonylureas
  - Stimulate pancreatic β-cell production of insulin
  - Caution with renal or liver disease, sulfa allergy, creatinine clearance <50 mL/min
  - May cause modest weight gain, hypoglycemia
  - Low cost; widely available
  - Systematic reviews show increased risk with respect to all-cause mortality (2)[B].
  - Glipizide (Glucotrol): 2.5 to 40.0 mg/day; dosage >10 mg/day given BID before meals
  - Glipizide extended-release: 5 to 20 mg/day
  - Glyburide (DiaBeta, Glynase, Micronase): 1.25 to 20.00 mg/day, Glynase: 0.75 to 12.00 mg/day
  - Glimepiride (Amaryl): 1 to 8 mg/day
- TZD
  - Increases insulin sensitivity; activates PPARs to increase glucose utilization
  - Pioglitazone reduces triglycerides (4); low cost
  - Obtain baseline liver function tests (LFTs). Use with caution if history of heart failure.
  - Increased risk of fractures and low bone mass
  - Rosiglitazone (Avandia): 4 to 8 mg/day
    ○ Increased risk of myocardial infarction (4)[C]
  - Pioglitazone (Actos): 15 to 45 mg/day

- Insulin
  - Activates insulin receptors, increases glucose disposal, inhibits hepatic glucose production
  - Potent glucose lowering effect; safe
  - Consider as initial therapy in those with A1c >10%, catabolic symptoms, ketosis.
  - Use as additional therapy if A1c not at goal after dual/triple therapy and GLP1-RA has been tried.
  - Can cause weight gain. High hypoglycemia risk. High cost. NPH and regular insulin are more affordable, safe, and effective.
  - Analogs have lower hypoglycemia risk than NPH and regular insulin.
  - Neutral effects on CV outcomes
  - Start with basal insulin at dose 0.1 to 0.3 U/kg/day. Titrate up to achieve desired blood glucose readings. Add mealtime (rapid/short acting) insulin if fasting glucose is at goal, but postmeal glucose is high. Mealtime starting dose can be 4 U or 10% of basal dose.
  - Rapid-acting analogs—lispro (Humalog), aspart (Novolog), glulisine (Apidra): duration of action 3 to 5 hours; ultrarapid (Fiasp) quicker onset
  - Inhaled insulin (Afrezza): duration of action 4.5 hours
  - Short-acting insulin—human regular (Humulin R/Novolin R/ReliOn R): duration of action 6 to 8 hours
  - Intermediate-acting insulin—human NPH (Humulin N/Novolin N/ReliOn N): duration of action 13 to 20 hours. Human regular U-500 (Humulin R U-500): duration of action 6 to 10 hours
  - Basal insulin analogs—glargine U-100 (Lantus, Basaglar): duration of action 22 to 24 hours; U-300 (Toujeo): duration of action 36 hours; detemir (Levemir): duration of action 21.5 hours. Degludec U-100, U-200 (Tresiba): duration of action 42 hours, does not need to be injected at same time each day
  - Premixed insulin products—NPH/regular 70/30 (Novolin 70/30, Humulin 70/30), 70/30 and 50/50 aspart mix (Novolog mix), 75/25 and 50/50 lispro mix (Humalog mix)
  - Mixed insulin must be taken with meals.
- Amylinomimetic
  - Delays gastric emptying, blunts pancreatic secretion of glucagon, and enhances satiety (1)
  - Causes weight loss and lower insulin doses
  - Pramlintide (Symlin): 60 to 120 μg SC premeal
  - Reduce prandial insulin by 50%.
- α-Glucosidase inhibitors
  - Inhibit intestinal α-glucosidase, slow intestinal carbohydrate digestions/absorption (1)
  - Avoid in renal insufficiency and bowel diseases.
  - Take at beginning of meals to decrease postprandial hyperglycemia.
  - Acarbose (Precose): 25 to 100 mg TID
  - Miglitol (Glyset): 25 to 100 mg TID
- Meglitinides
  - Mechanism similar to SU
  - Take at beginning of meals.
  - Repaglinide (Prandin): 0.5 to 4.0 mg TID
  - Nateglinide (Starlix): 60 to 120 mg TID
- Bile acid sequestrants
  - Colesevelam: 3.75 g/day or 1.875 g BID
- Dopamine-2 agonists
  - Bromocriptine (Cycloset) 1.6 to 4.8 mg PO every AM; mechanism of action uncertain
- Combination therapy
  - Many formulations combine two drugs with complimentary mechanisms of action.
  - Oral combination drugs: metformin with SGLT2 inhibitor, DPP-4 inhibitor, SU, TZD
  - Injectables: basal insulin with GLP analog

SURGERY/OTHER PROCEDURES
For patients with BMI >35 kg/m², consider bariatric surgery (1)[A].

 ONGOING CARE

FOLLOW-UP RECOMMENDATIONS
Patient Monitoring
A1c twice a year for patients with well-controlled blood glucose and quarterly for patients with hyperglycemia or recent changes in therapy

PATIENT EDUCATION
Diabetes self-management education

PROGNOSIS
Normal lifespan with prevention of complications

COMPLICATIONS
- Emergencies: hyperosmolar coma, DKA
- ASCVD, peripheral vascular disease, stroke, foot ulcers, Charcot joints
- Microvascular: peripheral neuropathy, proliferative retinopathy, erectile dysfunction, and diabetic CKD
- Ophthalmic: blindness, cataracts, glaucoma
- GI: nonalcoholic fatty liver disease, gastroparesis
- Neurologic: autonomic dysfunction, insensate feet

REFERENCES

1. American Diabetes Association. Standards of medical care. Diabetes Care. 2019;42(Suppl 1):S1–S193.
2. Davies MJ, D'Alessio DA, Fradkin J, et al. Management of hyperglycemia in type 2 diabetes, 2018. A consensus report by the American Diabetes Association (ADA) and the European Association for the Study of Diabetes (EASD). Diabetes Care. 2018;41(12):2669–2701.
3. Qaseem A, Wilt TJ, Kansagara D, et al; for Clinical Guidelines Committee of the American College of Physicians. Hemoglobin A1c targets for glycemic control with pharmacologic therapy for nonpregnant adults with type 2 diabetes mellitus: a guidance statement update from the American College of Physicians. Ann Intern Med. 2018;168(8):569–576.
4. Carbone S, Dixon DL, Buckley LF, et al. Glucose-lowering therapies for cardiovascular risk reduction in type 2 diabetes mellitus: state-of-the-art review. Mayo Clin Proc. 2018;93(11):1629–1647.

 SEE ALSO

- Diabetes Mellitus, Type 1; Diabetic Ketoacidosis; Hypertension, Essential
- Algorithm: Type 2 Diabetes, Treatment

 CODES

ICD10
- E11.9 Type 2 diabetes mellitus without complications
- E11.319 Type 2 diabetes mellitus with unspecified diabetic retinopathy without macular edema
- E11.21 Type 2 diabetes mellitus with nephropathy

CLINICAL PEARLS

Individualize A1c targets based on life expectancy, preexisting DM complications, comorbidities, and individual patient preferences and values. Hypoglycemia poses more short-term danger than hyperglycemia. Exercise, diet, BP control, and CV risk reduction with statins are the cornerstones of DM treatment.

DIABETIC KETOACIDOSIS
Melanie J. Lippmann, MD

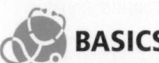 **BASICS**

DESCRIPTION
- A life-threatening medical emergency in diabetics secondary to insulin deficiency and characterized by hyperglycemia, ketosis, metabolic acidosis, electrolyte disturbances, and marked dehydration
- System(s) affected: endocrine/metabolic

EPIDEMIOLOGY
Incidence
- In the United States: 46 episodes per 10,000 diabetics; 2/100 patient-years of type 1 diabetes mellitus (DM) (1)
- Predominant age: 19 to 44 years (56%) and 45 to 65 years (24%); only 18% are <20 years.

ETIOLOGY AND PATHOPHYSIOLOGY
A deficiency of insulin, exacerbated by an increase in counterregulatory hormones (e.g., catecholamines, cortisol, glucagon, and growth hormone) leading to a hyperglycemic crisis, osmotic diuresis, ketosis with metabolic acidosis, and frequently accompanied by electrolyte disturbances
- Noncompliance/insufficient insulin: 25%
- Infection: 30–40%
- First presentation of DM: 10–25%
- Myocardial infarction (MI): 5–7%
- No cause identified: 10–30%
- Medications (corticosteroids, sympathomimetics, atypical antipsychotics)
- Illicit drugs (cocaine)
- Trauma
- Surgery
- Emotional stress
- Pregnancy
- Cerebrovascular accident (CVA)

RISK FACTORS
- Type 1 > type 2 DM
- Younger patients at higher risk

GENERAL PREVENTION
- Close monitoring of glucose during periods of stress, infection, illness, and trauma
- Careful insulin control and regular monitoring of blood glucose levels
- "Sick day" management instructions

COMMONLY ASSOCIATED CONDITIONS
Complications of chronic (and poorly controlled) DM such as nephropathy, neuropathy, and retinopathy

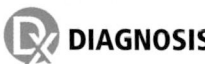 **DIAGNOSIS**

HISTORY
- Recent illness, injury, or surgery
- Changes in diet or medications
- Missed insulin doses/noncompliance
- Insulin pump failure
- Weight loss in patients recently diagnosed with type 1 DM
- Polyuria, nocturia, polydipsia
- Hyperphagia
- Generalized weakness
- Malaise, fatigue, lethargy
- Anorexia or increased appetite
- Nausea, vomiting
- Abdominal pain
- Decreased perspiration
- Fever

PHYSICAL EXAM
- Hypotension
- Tachycardia
- Fever or hypothermia
- Tachypnea, hyperpnea, Kussmaul respirations
- Fruity odor of ketotic breath (acetone smell)
- Decreased reflexes
- Abdominal tenderness, decreased bowel sounds
- Dry mucous membranes, poor skin turgor, dehydration
- Altered mental status
- Coma

DIFFERENTIAL DIAGNOSIS
- Hyperosmolar hyperglycemic crisis
- Alcoholic ketoacidosis
- Starvation ketosis
- Toxic ingestions (e.g., salicylates, methanol)
- Lactic acidosis
- Uremia/chronic renal failure
- Sepsis
- Acute pancreatitis

DIAGNOSTIC TESTS & INTERPRETATION
Initial Tests (lab, imaging)

ALERT
- Diagnostic criteria (1)[C]:
  - Hyperglycemia (glucose usually 250 to 800 mg/dL) as rapidly assessed on fingerstick glucose testing and confirmed on serum chemistry
  - Low HCO_3 (usually ≤18 mEq/L)
  - Metabolic acidosis on arterial blood gases (ABGs) (pH <7.3)
  - Anion gap = serum sodium − (serum chloride + bicarbonate); >10 mmol
- Other important labs:
  - Serum ketosis: Check β-hydroxybutyrate (β-HB) instead of ketones to evaluate ketosis (2)[B]. β-HB is the predominant ketone produced and is preferred over serum ketones. β-HB >3 mg/dL is abnormal and should be decreased to <1.5 mg/dL within 12 to 24 hours (3)[B].
  - Urine ketosis (urinalysis [UA]) may only identify acetoacetate and not β-HB.
  - Increased creatinine and BUN: Markedly increased serum ketones may cross-react and cause a falsely high serum creatinine.
  - Pseudohyponatremia: Hyperglycemia or hypertriglyceridemia may cause an artificially low sodium concentration. The measured sodium is suppressed by 1.6 mg/dL for every 100 mg/dL of glucose >100 mg/dL.
  - Decreased calculated total body K^+: Severe acidosis gives an artificially high K^+ level.
  - Increased serum osmolality (mOsm/kg) = [2 × serum Na (mEq/L) + glucose (mg/dL)/18 + BUN (mg/dL)/2.8]; if calculated osmolality <320 mOsm/kg, consider etiologies other than diabetic ketoacidosis (DKA).
  - Elevated base deficit
  - HbA1c (glycosylated hemoglobin) helps assess long-term history of diabetic control.
  - Glycosuria
  - Hyperamylasemia, hyperlipasemia
  - Hypertriglyceridemia/hypercholesterolemia
- CBC, electrolytes, BUN, creatinine
- Serum β-HB or ketones
- ABG; venous blood gases (VBGs) may also be used (VBG pH correlates with 0.03 lower than ABG pH).
- Urine and blood cultures if concern for infection
- Troponin if concern for cardiac ischemia
- Other Tests
  - ECG
    - Frequently shows sinus tachycardia (nonspecific)
    - Changes consistent with electrolyte abnormalities
    - Ischemia/MI as a precipitating factor
  - Chest x-ray to rule out possible infectious etiology
  - Consider lumbar puncture if concern for meningitis.
  - Head CT scan if suspected CVA or cerebral edema

Diagnostic Procedures/Other
Only if surgical disease is the underlying precipitant (e.g., appendicitis, cholecystitis)

 TREATMENT

- Oxygen and airway management, as needed
- Establish IV access.
- Cardiac monitoring
- Start isotonic crystalloid solution (e.g., 0.9% saline, or lactated ringers bolus).

GENERAL MEASURES
- All, but mild cases require inpatient management.
- Severe DKA requires an ICU setting.
- Goals
  - Fluid resuscitation
  - Insulin therapy to normalize serum glucose
  - Resolution of anion gap acidosis and ketosis
  - Correction of electrolytes
- Identify and treat the precipitating cause (e.g., insulin noncompliance, infection, MI).
- Laboratory testing during management:
  - Serum glucose q1–2h until stable
  - Electrolytes, phosphorus, and venous pH q2–6h

MEDICATION
First Line
- Insulin (1)[C]
  - Optional initial bolus 0.1 U/kg IV and then continuous infusion at 0.1 U/kg/hr (do not use initial insulin bolus in children)
  - If without bolus, 0.14 U/kg/hr continuous infusion
  - Aim for rate of serum glucose decline of 100 mg/dL/hr
  - When glucose 200 mg/dL, reduce infusion to 0.02 to 0.05 U/kg/hr IV or give rapid-acting insulin at 0.1 U/kg SC q2h; goal glucose is 150 to 200 mg/dL.
  - Overlap and continue IV insulin infusion for 1 to 2 hours after SC insulin is initiated.
- IV fluids to correct dehydration: Start with 0.9% NaCl bolus, calculate corrected sodium; if serum Na^+ is high, consider 0.45% NaCl to replace free fluid loss or when adding potassium replacement.
  - When glucose is 200 mg/dL, change to 5% dextrose with 0.45% NaCl at 150 to 250 mL/hr.

- Potassium: falsely elevated due to acidosis; when K^+ ≤5.2 mg/dL and if urine output is adequate, start replacement with 20 to 30 mEq/L of K^+ in 1 L IV fluids (1).
  - Hold insulin if K^+ ≤3.3 mg/dL; give IV potassium 20 to 30 mEq/hr with fluids until >3.3 mg/dL to prevent cardiac arrhythmia (class III).
  - For each 0.1 unit of pH, serum K^+ will change by ~0.6 mEq in opposite direction.
- Phosphorus: Routine replacement may lead to hypocalcemia; if very low (<1.0), give 20 to 30 mEq/L of K-Phos in fluids.
- Sodium bicarbonate: no demonstrable benefit with a pH >7.0 (2)[B]; rehydration usually leads to resolution of acidosis although some guidelines recommend its use with pH <6.9 or in patients with life-threatening hyperkalemia; however, there is evidence that it may increase cerebral edema, especially in children (3)[A].
- Magnesium: If Mg ≤1.8 mg/dL and the patient is symptomatic, consider replacement.
- Precautions
  - If the patient is on an insulin pump, it should be stopped.
  - If glucose does not fall by 10% in first hour, give regular insulin 0.14 U/kg IV bolus and then continuous infusion at previous rate.
  - If using bicarbonate, add 100 mmol or 2 ampules of sodium bicarbonate to 400 mL isotonic solution with 20 mEq KCL >200 mL/hr for 2 hours until venous pH is >7.0 and then stop infusion (1).

Second Line
Insulin, SC or IM: Load with 0.3 U/kg SC, followed by 0.1 U/kg/hr; space dosing to q2h once glucose <250 mg/dL; in uncomplicated DKA, may be safe and cost-effective (4)[B]

Pediatric Considerations
- Children with moderate to severe DKA should be transferred to the nearest pediatric critical care hospital.
- Cerebral edema is a rare complication (~1%) but has a mortality of 20–50%:
  - Diagnostic criteria exist for diagnosis; CT may rule out alternative diagnoses.
  - Treat with IV bolus of mannitol 1 g/kg in 20% solution, reduce IV fluid rate, and consider hypertonic 3% saline (5).

Geriatric Considerations
Must be careful with impaired renal function or congestive heart failure when correcting fluid and electrolyte abnormalities

Pregnancy Considerations
- Pregnancy itself is diabetogenic and also results in a compensated respiratory alkalosis (HCO_3 19 to 20 mEq/L) with theoretically reduced buffering capacity.
- Pregnant women are more susceptible to DKA.
- Euglycemic DKA
- Increased risk of preeclampsia and fetal death
- β-Tocolytics and corticosteroids can trigger DKA.
- Perinatal death: 9–35%

ADMISSION, INPATIENT, AND NURSING CONSIDERATIONS
- ADA admission guidelines: blood glucose >250 mg/dL; pH <7.3; HCO_3 ≤15 mEq/L; ketones in urine; ICU setting for severe DKA (6)
- IV fluids
  - 1.0 to 1.5 L over the first hour, then, if serum corrected Na is high or normal, give 0.45% NaCl at 250 to 500 mL/hr depending on hydration state.
  - Switch to 5% dextrose in 0.45% saline at maintenance rate when serum glucose <200 mg/dL; maintain blood glucose between 150 and 250 mg/dL.
  - Overly rapid correction of fluid balance may precipitate cerebral edema (2)[C]; if the blood glucose level is falling too rapidly, consider using a 10% dextrose solution instead.

Pediatric Considerations
Bolus 10 to 20 mL/kg initially; 4-hour fluid total should be <50 mL/kg to reduce chance of cerebral edema.

- Discharge criteria
  - Discharge when DKA has resolved: anion gap <12, glucose <200 mg/dL; pH >7.3; bicarbonate >18 mEq/L; additionally, patients must be tolerating PO intake and able to resume home medication regimen
  - Underlying precipitant (e.g., infection) must be identified and treated.

 ONGOING CARE

FOLLOW-UP RECOMMENDATIONS
Patient Monitoring
- Monitor mental status, vital signs, and urine output q30–60min until improved and then q2–4h.
- Monitor blood sugar q1h until <200 mg/dL and then q2–6h.
- Monitor electrolytes, BUN, venous pH, and creatinine q2–4h.

DIET
- NPO initially
- Advance to preketotic diet when nausea and vomiting are controlled.
- Avoid foods with high glycemic index (e.g., soft drinks, fruit juice, white bread, added sugar, etc.).

PROGNOSIS
- DKA accounts for 16% of all diabetes-related fatalities
- Overall DKA mortality of 0.5–2%
- In children <10 years of age, DKA causes 70% of diabetes-related fatalities.

COMPLICATIONS
- Cerebral edema (most common cause of death in children with DKA)
- Pulmonary edema
- Vascular thrombosis
- Hypokalemia
- Hypophosphatemia
- Cardiac dysrhythmia (secondary to hypokalemia or acidosis)
- MI, myocardial injury

- Acute gastric dilatation
- Late hypoglycemia (secondary to treatment)
- Erosive gastritis
- Infection, mucormycosis
- Respiratory distress

REFERENCES
1. Kitabchi AE, Umpierrez GE, Miles JM, et al. Hyperglycemic crises in adult patients with diabetes. *Diabetes Care.* 2009;32(7):1335–1343.
2. Agus MS, Wolfsdorf JI. Diabetic ketoacidosis in children. *Pediatr Clin North Am.* 2005;52(4):1147–1163.
3. Chua HR, Schneider A, Bellomo R. Bicarbonate in diabetic ketoacidosis—a systematic review. *Ann Intensive Care.* 2011;1(1):23.
4. Umpierrez GE, Latif K, Stoever J, et al. Efficacy of subcutaneous insulin lispro versus continuous intravenous insulin for the treatment of patients with diabetic ketoacidosis. *Am J Med.* 2004;117(5):291–296.
5. Watts W, Edge JA. How can cerebral edema during treatment of diabetic ketoacidosis be avoided? *Pediatr Diabetes.* 2014;15(4):271–276.
6. American Diabetes Association. Hospital admission guidelines for diabetes. *Diabetes Care.* 2004;27(Suppl 1):S103.

ADDITIONAL READING
- American Diabetes Association. Standards of medical care in diabetes—2013. *Diabetes Care.* 2013;36(Suppl 1):S11–S66.
- Sheikh-Ali M, Karon BS, Basu A, et al. Can serum beta-hydroxybutyrate be used to diagnose diabetic ketoacidosis? *Diabetes Care.* 2008;31(4):643–647.

 SEE ALSO

- Diabetes Mellitus, Type 1
- Algorithm: Diabetic Ketoacidosis (DKA), Treatment

 CODES

ICD10
- E10.10 Type 1 diabetes mellitus with ketoacidosis without coma
- E13.10 Oth diabetes mellitus with ketoacidosis without coma
- E10.11 Type 1 diabetes mellitus with ketoacidosis with coma

CLINICAL PEARLS
- Admit if blood glucose >250 mg/dL, pH <7.3, HCO_3 ≤15 mEq/L, and ketones in urine.
- Potassium is falsely elevated due to acidosis; start replacement when K^+ ≤5.2 mg/dL and urine output is adequate.

DIABETIC POLYNEUROPATHY

Samir Malkani, MD, MRCP–UK

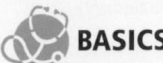

BASICS

DESCRIPTION
Peripheral nerve dysfunction seen in diabetes; several patterns described (1):
- Symmetric polyneuropathy
  - Distal sensory or sensorimotor
- Mononeuropathy, radiculopathy, and polyradiculopathy
  - Cranial neuropathy
  - Focal limb or truncal neuropathy
  - Radiculoplexus neuropathy (diabetic amyotrophy)
- Acute painful small fiber neuropathy
- Autonomic neuropathies
- Chronic inflammatory demyelinating polyneuropathy (CIDP)

EPIDEMIOLOGY
Prevalence
- Generalized polyneuropathy
  - 10% at diabetes diagnosis
  - 50% at 10 years
  - Cross-sectional prevalence: 15% by symptoms; 50% by nerve conduction
- Autonomic neuropathy: 16.7% in a United Kingdom study

ETIOLOGY AND PATHOPHYSIOLOGY
- Metabolic derangement due to hyperglycemia
  - Aldose reductase converts excess glucose to sorbitol, which causes nerve damage.
  - Nonenzymatic glycation of neural proteins and lipids forms damaging advanced glycosylation end products.
  - Protein kinase C activation causes vascular endothelial changes.
  - Oxidative stress from excessive production of reactive oxygen species
  - Cyclooxygenase-2 and poly (ADP-ribose) polymerase activation
- Vasculopathy causing nerve ischemia: predominant factor in mononeuropathies

RISK FACTORS
- Poor glycemic control
- Duration of diabetes
- Hypertension
- Hyperlipidemia
- Tobacco and alcohol consumption

GENERAL PREVENTION
- Maintenance of normal blood sugar
- Exercise and appropriate diet

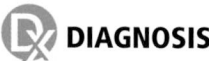

DIAGNOSIS

HISTORY
- Most common form (typical): symmetric distal sensory or sensorimotor polyneuropathy
  - Distressing numbness, tingling, pain of legs/feet, usually worse at night; allodynia; hyperalgesia
  - Often silent sensory loss, patient unaware
  - Ataxia due to proprioceptive loss
  - Neuropathic foot ulcers due to analgesia and repetitive injury
  - Neuropathic degeneration of foot joints

- Hands involved late
- Distal muscle involvement, usually mild
- Symmetric proximal polyneuropathy
  - Proximal leg weakness and wasting
  - Muscles of shoulder girdle rarely involved
  - Pain and sensory changes less prominent
- Focal cranial or limb mononeuropathy
  - May involve 3rd, 4th, 6th, or 7th cranial nerve
  - Femoral, sciatic, or peroneal neuropathy: weakness or pain in nerve distribution
  - Any major peripheral nerve can be involved.
- Truncal neuropathies: painful radiculopathy over dermatomes
- Lumbar radiculoplexus neuropathy (diabetic amyotrophy)
  - Unilateral hip, thigh pain
  - Pelvic girdle and thigh weakness with atrophy
  - Recovery over months
- Diabetic autonomic neuropathy
  - GI: nocturnal diarrhea, sometimes alternating with constipation; gastroparesis with postprandial fullness; nausea and vomiting
  - Cardiovascular: postural dizziness, exercise intolerance
  - Urogenital: urinary hesitancy, overflow incontinence; erectile dysfunction; vaginal dryness; sexual dysfunction
  - Sudomotor: anhidrosis or hyperhidrosis; gustatory sweating of head and upper body
- CIDP: progressive, severe motor loss
- Diabetic cachexia: painful small fiber neuropathy with prominent weight loss and depression

PHYSICAL EXAM
- Symmetric distal polyneuropathy
  - "Stocking-and-glove" distal sensory loss
  - Large-fiber neuropathy: loss of perception of vibration and light touch (10-g monofilament)
  - Small fiber involvement: loss of temperature and pinprick
  - Absent ankle reflexes
  - Wasting, weakness of small muscles in foot; changes to arch of foot or clawing of toes
  - With small fiber involvement, there may be lack of objective sensory deficit despite pain.
- Symmetric proximal polyneuropathy
  - Proximal leg, arm wasting, and weakness
  - Loss of patellar reflexes
- Focal cranial or limb mononeuropathy
  - 3rd cranial nerve palsy: painful ophthalmoplegia and ptosis; preserved pupillary reflexes (in contrast to compressive palsies)
  - 6th cranial nerve: lateral gaze palsy
  - Femoral neuropathy: weakness of lower leg extension, hip flexion, quadriceps wasting, absent patellar reflex, sensory loss in anterior thigh
  - Sciatic neuropathy: pain or sensory loss in back of thigh and leg; weakness of hamstrings, lower leg muscles
  - Peroneal neuropathy: foot drop
- Truncal neuropathies: sensory loss along dermatome
- Lumbar radiculoplexopathy (amyotrophy)
  - Weakness and wasting pelvic girdle and thigh
  - Sensory loss in L2–L3
  - Absent patellar reflex

- Autonomic neuropathy
  - Cardiovascular: resting tachycardia; orthostatic hypotension
  - Gastroparesis: postprandial distension; gastric splash
- CIDP: motor weakness

DIFFERENTIAL DIAGNOSIS
- Uremic polyneuropathy
- Drug induced
  - Antineoplastic drugs: cisplatin, vincristine
  - Isoniazid
  - Amiodarone
- Toxic
  - Chronic arsenic poisoning
  - *n*-Hexane, methyl-*n*-butyl ketone
- Nutritional deficiency
  - Usually associated with alcoholism
- Paraneoplastic polyneuropathy
- Hypothyroidism

DIAGNOSTIC TESTS & INTERPRETATION
Initial Tests (lab, imaging)
- Fasting plasma glucose, 2-hour glucose tolerance test or hemoglobin A1c for diagnosis and to assess glycemic control; may occur in "prediabetes"
- Serum vitamin B_{12}
- Thyroid function
- Creatinine and BUN
- Syphilis testing
- Serum protein electrophoresis
- 25-OH Vitamin D
- In mononeuropathy/mononeuritis multiplex, test for vasculitis, paraproteinemia, and sarcoid
- In radiculopathy or mononeuropathy, imaging studies to exclude compressive lesions

Diagnostic Procedures/Other
- Bedside testing of vibration perception with 128-Hz tuning fork, monofilament perception of 10-g filament
- Quantitative sensory testing for vibratory and thermal thresholds
  - Standardized measures for assessing severity and risk of foot ulceration
- Electromyogram nerve conduction velocity
  - Useful to confirm mononeuropathy and entrapment syndromes
  - Sensitive but nonspecific index of presence and severity of diabetic polyneuropathy
  - In small unmyelinated fiber painful neuropathy, test may be normal.
- Lumbar puncture
  - In CIDP, elevation of spinal fluid protein
- Skin biopsy with epidermal nerve fiber density
  - Enables direct study of small nerve fibers that are difficult to assess electrophysiologically
- Corneal confocal microscopy
  - Noninvasive approach based on examination of corneal innervation

Test Interpretation
- In nerve biopsy of peripheral nerve, wallerian degeneration, focal axonal swellings containing neurofilaments, axonal atrophy, and demyelination are seen.

- Thick neural capillary basement membrane and endothelial proliferation
- Obliterative microvascular lesions and perivascular inflammation

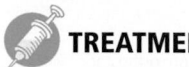 **TREATMENT**

GENERAL MEASURES
- Maintain blood glucose close to normal.
- Provide appropriate footwear to prevent pressure damage to insensate feet.

MEDICATION

First Line
Management of pain and sensory neuropathy
- Calcium channel modulators: gabapentin (2,3)[A] (off-label)
  - Binds Ca^{2+} channel–associated protein α_2-δ; inhibits neurotransmitter release
  - Dose range 300 to 1,200 mg TID, NNT ~4 to 8
  - Reduce dose in renal insufficiency.
  - Adverse effects: dizziness, fatigue, edema
- Calcium channel modulators: pregabalin (2,4)[A]
  - Binds same calcium channel as gabapentin
  - Linear pharmacokinetics and quicker onset of action compared to gabapentin
  - Usual dose: 150 to 600 mg/day, NNT ~4 to 8
  - Adverse effects are dizziness and edema.
- Duloxetine (2,4)[A]
  - Selective serotonin and norepinephrine reuptake inhibitor
  - Usual dose is 30 to 60 mg/day; NNT ~4 to 9
  - Adverse effects are nausea and dizziness.
- Tricyclic antidepressants (TCA) (2,4)[A] (off-label)
  - Analgesia may be related to effects on sodium channels; NNT ~2 to 5, NNH ~3 to 16
  - Amitriptyline 25 to 150 mg at bedtime
  - Nortriptyline (25 to 150 mg); desipramine (25 to 200 mg) less sedating than amitriptyline but limited trial data
    - Anticholinergic effects and cardiac arrhythmias may occur.
- Management of autonomic neuropathy
  - Orthostatic hypotension
    - Fludrocortisone (off-label)
    - Midodrine (off-label)
  - Gastroparesis
    - Metoclopramide or domperidone
    - Erythromycin (off-label)
  - Diabetic diarrhea
    - Loperamide
    - Clonidine (off-label)
    - Octreotide (off-label)
    - Antibiotics for bacterial overgrowth
  - Hyperhidrosis
    - Propantheline (off-label)

Geriatric Considerations
Anticholinergic effects of TCAs may cause urinary retention and cardiac arrhythmias.

Second Line
- Antidepressants
  - Venlafaxine (2,4)[A] (75 to 225 mg daily) (off-label), NNT ~2 to 5
    - Serotonin-norepinephrine reuptake inhibitor

- Anticonvulsants
  - Carbamazepine (2)[C] (off-label)
    - Blocks sodium channels
    - Dose 100 to 800 mg/day
- Topical therapies
  - Capsaicin 0.075% cream applied TID
    - Depletes C fibers in skin of substance P
    - Limited data on efficacy
  - Lidocaine (2)[C] 5% (700 mg) patches applied daily to feet (off-label):
    - Causes sodium channel blockade
- Opiate analgesia
  - Tramadol (2)[B] (off-label): 100 to 400 mg/day, NNT ~3 to 9
    - Binds opiate receptors; also inhibits reuptake of norepinephrine and serotonin; fewer opiate side effects
  - Tapentadol (2)[B]
    - Binds to μ-opiate receptor and inhibits norepinephrine uptake

ISSUES FOR REFERRAL
If CIDP is suspected, refer to neurologist for investigation and treatment.

ADDITIONAL THERAPIES
- Transcutaneous electrical nerve stimulation
- Percutaneous nerve stimulation
- Electrical spinal cord stimulation
- Actovegin, dextromethorphan with quinidine
- C-peptide

SURGERY/OTHER PROCEDURES
Electrical spinal cord stimulation

COMPLEMENTARY & ALTERNATIVE MEDICINE
Acupuncture, Reiki, electromagnetic field treatment: no convincing trial data

 ONGOING CARE

PROGNOSIS
- Generalized symmetric polyneuropathies
  - Usually slow, chronic progression
  - Insensitive but painless foot as pain lessens
- Focal neuropathies
  - Recovery over months to years

COMPLICATIONS
- Claw foot deformity
- Neurotropic ulceration
  - Painless ulcers on weight-bearing area
  - Callus formation is a precursor to ulceration.
- Neuropathic arthropathy
  - Results in complete disorganization of joint structure in foot, Charcot joint

REFERENCES
1. Pop-Busui R, Boulton AJ, Feldman EL, et al. Diabetic neuropathy: a position statement by the American Diabetes Association. *Diabetes Care*. 2017;40(1):136–154.
2. Iqbal Z, Azmi S, Yadav R, et al. Diabetic peripheral neuropathy: epidemiology, diagnosis, and pharmacotherapy. *Clin Ther*. 2018;40(6):828–849.
3. Moore A, Derry S, Wiffen P. Gabapentin for chronic neuropathic pain. *JAMA*. 2018;319(8):818–819.
4. Waldfogel JM, Nesbit SA, Dy SM, et al. Pharmacotherapy for diabetic peripheral neuropathy pain and quality of life: a systematic review. *Neurology*. 2017;88(20):1958–1967.

ADDITIONAL READING
- Cooper TE, Chen J, Wiffen PJ, et al. Morphine for chronic neuropathic pain in adults. *Cochrane Database Syst Rev*. 2017;(5):CD011669.
- Finnerup NB, Attal N, Haroutounian S, et al. Pharmacotherapy for neuropathic pain in adults: a systematic review and meta-analysis. *Lancet Neurol*. 2015;14(2):162–173.
- Vinik AI. Clinical practice. Diabetic sensory and motor neuropathy. *N Engl J Med*. 2016;374(15):1455–1464.
- Vinik AI, Camacho PM, Davidson JA, et al; for Task Force to Develop an AACE Position Statement on Autonomic Testing. American Association of Clinical Endocrinologists and American College of Endocrinology position statement on testing for autonomic and somatic nerve dysfunction. *Endocr Pract*. 2017;23(12):1472–1478.
- Ziegler D, Fonseca V. From guideline to patient: a review of recent recommendations for pharmacotherapy of painful diabetic neuropathy. *J Diabetes Complications*. 2015;29(1):146–156.

 SEE ALSO

Diabetes Mellitus, Type 1; Diabetes Mellitus, Type 2

 CODES

ICD10
- E10.42 Type 1 diabetes mellitus with diabetic polyneuropathy
- E11.42 Type 2 diabetes mellitus with diabetic polyneuropathy
- E13.42 Oth diabetes mellitus with diabetic polyneuropathy

CLINICAL PEARLS
- Occasionally, when glycemic control improves dramatically, as can occur when treatment for diabetes is initiated, there may be a worsening of neuropathy symptoms (described as treatment-induced neuropathy). Symptoms usually stabilize and gradually improve as glycemic control is maintained.
- It is common to combine agents with different mechanisms of action in the management of neuropathic pain. Topical therapies can be combined with systemic therapies. There is limited evidence-based data to support combination therapy.

DIARRHEA, ACUTE

Rahma Ali Aldhaheri, MD • Stephen M. Testa, MD • Marie L. Borum, MD, EdD, MPH, MACP, FACG, AGAF

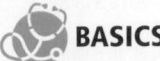 **BASICS**

DESCRIPTION
- An abnormal increase in stool water content, volume, or frequency (≥3 in 24 hours) for <14 days duration
- Acute viral diarrhea (50–70%)
  - Most common cause of infectious diarrhea; noninflammatory (watery)
  - Frequently presents with associated nausea and/or vomiting
  - Symptoms usually develop after an incubation period of ~1 day and last for 1 to 3 days; typically self-limited
- Bacterial diarrhea (15–20%)
  - Most common infectious cause of inflammatory (bloody) diarrhea
  - Incubation period variable; diarrhea caused by preformed enterotoxin presents within 1 to 6 hours of contaminated food ingestion, whereas bacterial infection typically presents within 1 to 3 days.
  - Symptoms usually resolve in 1 to 7 days; antibiotic use attenuates length and/or severity of disease.
  - Suspect when concurrent illness in others who have shared potentially contaminated food.
  - Suspect *Clostridium difficile* in patients with recent antibiotic use or hospitalization.
- Protozoal infections (10–15%)
  - Typically cause noninflammatory (watery) diarrhea
  - Long incubation period and prolonged disease course, symptoms develop approximately 7 days after exposure and commonly last >7 days
  - Suspect when outbreaks of watery diarrhea in areas with contaminated water or food supply.
- Traveler's diarrhea (TD) typically begins 3 to 7 days after arrival in foreign location and resolves within 5 days; rapid onset, generally self-limited

EPIDEMIOLOGY
- In developing countries, acute diarrhea is more common in children; no age predilection in developed countries
- Acute diarrhea accounts for >128,000 U.S. hospital admissions and ~1.5 million annual deaths worldwide (1).

Prevalence
- Second leading cause of death in children <5 years and seventh leading cause of death among all ages worldwide
- Affects 11% of the general population
- Rotavirus and adenovirus most common in children <2 years, bacteria are more common in children >2 years
- In developing world, acute diarrhea is largely due to contaminated food and water (1).

ETIOLOGY AND PATHOPHYSIOLOGY
- Bacterial
  - *Escherichia coli*
  - *Salmonella, Shigella, Campylobacter jejuni*
  - *Vibrio parahaemolyticus, Vibrio cholerae*
  - *Yersinia enterocolitica*
  - *C. difficile*
  - *Staphylococcus aureus*
  - *Bacillus cereus*
  - *Clostridium perfringens*
  - *Listeria monocytogenes*
- Viral
  - *Rotavirus* and *Norovirus* (most common)
  - Adenovirus
  - Astrovirus
  - Cytomegalovirus (in immunocompromised)
- Protozoal
  - *Giardia lamblia*
  - *Entamoeba histolytica*
  - *Cryptosporidium*
  - *Isospora belli*
  - *Cyclospora, Microspora*
- Pathophysiology (1)
  - Noninflammatory: most commonly viral; increased intestinal secretions without disruption of intestinal mucosa; watery
  - Inflammatory: generally invasive or toxin-producing bacteria; disrupts mucosal integrity with subsequent tissue invasion/damage; bloody stools
- Viral diarrhea: changes in small intestine cell morphology, including villous shortening, increased number of crypt cells, and increased cellularity of the lamina propria
- Bacterial diarrhea: Bacterial invasion of colonic wall leads to mucosal hyperemia, edema, and leukocytic infiltration.

RISK FACTORS
- Travel to developing countries
- Failure to observe food/water precautions
- Immunocompromised host
- Antibiotic use
- Proton pump inhibitor (PPI) use
- Daycare exposure
- Fecal-oral sexual contact
- Nursing home residence
- Pregnancy (12-fold increase for listeriosis) (1)

GENERAL PREVENTION
- Frequent hand washing; hand washing promotion may reduce incidence of diarrhea by approximately 30%.
- Proper food and water precautions, particularly during foreign travel—"boil it, peel it, cook it, or forget it"
- Avoid undercooked meat, raw fish, unpasteurized milk.
- Rotavirus vaccine (for infants)
- Typhoid fever and cholera vaccine (for travel to endemic areas)
- TD prophylaxis
  - Pretravel counseling on high-risk food/beverage
    - Consider daily prophylaxis with bismuth subsalicylate (BSS) in all travelers (can reduce the risk of TD by up to 60%); usual dosing of 2 tablets (262 mg each) or 2 oz (60 mL) liquid formulation 4 times daily
    - Antibiotic prophylaxis should not be routinely used.
    - IDSA recommends chemoprophylaxis with fluoroquinolones: norfloxacin 400 mg/day or ciprofloxacin 500 mg orally once or twice daily. Fluoroquinolones are not recommended for prophylaxis by the International Society of Travel Medicine, which advocates the use of rifaximin 200 mg once or twice daily (2)[C]
    - Probiotics, prebiotics, and synbiotics have unclear benefit as prophylaxis.

COMMONLY ASSOCIATED CONDITIONS
- Inflammatory bowel disease (IBD)
- Immunocompromised (HIV, malignancy, chemotherapy)

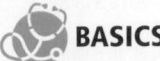 **DIAGNOSIS**

HISTORY
- Duration of symptoms <14 days
- Historical clues for dehydration: orthostatic hypotension, dizziness, increased thirst, decreased urinary output, or altered mental status
- Description of stool—characteristics and output
  - Frequency; quantity; consistency; character: presence of mucus, blood, or fat; floating
  - *Giardia* associated with pale, greasy stools
- Weight loss
- Associated symptoms: change in appetite, abdominal pain or bloating, nausea/vomiting, or fever
- Recent hospitalization or antibiotic use
- Travel history
- Ingestion of raw or undercooked meat, raw seafood, unpasteurized milk
- Sick contacts
- Immunocompromised state
- Pregnancy
- Daycare exposure
- Sexual history (e.g., men who have sex with men [MSM], fecal-oral contact, HIV)
- Nursing home residence

PHYSICAL EXAM
- Assess degree of dehydration (1); ill-appearing, dry mucous membranes, tachycardia, orthostatic hypotension, decreased skin turgor, delayed capillary refill, altered mental status
- Fever is more suggestive of inflammatory diarrhea.
- Abdomen: Assess for tenderness, distention, rigidity.
- Rectum: blood, tenderness, stool consistency

Geriatric Considerations
Fecal impaction or obstructing neoplasm can cause overflow diarrhea with chronic constipation.

DIFFERENTIAL DIAGNOSIS
- IBD
- Malabsorption
- Medications (cholinergic agents, magnesium-containing antacids, chemotherapy, antibiotics)
- *C. difficile* colitis secondary to antibiotic use
- Diverticulitis, ischemic colitis
- Spastic (irritable) colon
- Fecal impaction
- Endocrinopathies: thyroid disease
- Neoplasia

DIAGNOSTIC TESTS & INTERPRETATION
Initial Tests (lab, imaging)
- Reserve laboratory testing for patients with persistent fever, moderate-severe disease characterized by passage of ≥6 stools per day, duration of >72 hours, dysentery, profuse watery diarrhea, immunosuppression, or if suspected outbreak (3)[C].
- CBC
  - Leukocytosis, anemia (blood loss), eosinophilia (parasite infection), thrombocytopenia (hemolytic-uremic syndrome [HUS])
- Serum electrolytes
- BUN and creatinine may elevate with volume depletion.
- Nonanion gap metabolic acidosis
- Stool sample
  - Occult blood (IBD, bowel ischemia, and certain bacterial infections)
  - Fecal leukocytes

- Stool ova and parasites
- Stool culture: For bloody diarrhea, consider *Salmonella*, *Shigella*, *Campylobacter*, *E. coli* 0157:H7, *Y. enterocolitica*, *E. histolytica*.
- *C. difficile* toxin (especially IBD, recently hospitalized or recent antibiotic use) (4)[C]
- *Giardia* ELISA >90% sensitive in at-risk population
- Abdominal radiographs (flat plate and upright) if severe abdominal pain or concern for obstruction
- Abdominal CT scan is preferred to evaluate intra-abdominal disease (5)[C].

Diagnostic Procedures/Other
- Consider sigmoidoscopy or colonoscopy in patients with persistent diarrhea, when there is no clear diagnosis after routine blood and stool tests, and if empiric or supportive therapy is ineffective.
- Consider colonoscopy in immunocompromised patients to evaluate for CMV colitis.
- Colonoscopy helps to distinguish infectious diarrhea from IBD, ischemic colitis, cancer, or other noninfectious etiologies (5)[C].

TREATMENT

GENERAL MEASURES
- Oral rehydration and electrolyte management are key to successful treatment.
- Oral intake, as tolerated—"if the gut works, use it"
- Balanced electrolyte rehydration solutions recommended in elderly and profuse, watery TD (3)[C]
- IV fluids if patient cannot tolerate oral rehydration or presents with severe dehydration

MEDICATION
First Line
- Consider empiric antibiotics (fluoroquinolones or macrolides) in patients with signs and symptoms of systemic infection, severe disease, or clear cases of TD (3)[C].
  - Fever; bloody diarrhea; fecal leukocytes
  - Immunocompromised host
  - Signs of severe volume depletion
  - Symptoms >1 week
- Tailor antibiotics to stool culture results (3)[C].
  - *Giardia*: metronidazole 250 mg PO TID for 5 to 7 days, tinidazole 2 g PO once
  - *E. histolytica*: metronidazole 500 to 750 mg PO TID for 7 to 10 days, tinidazole 2 g PO daily for 3 to 5 days
  - *Shigella*: ciprofloxacin 500 mg PO BID for 3 to 5 days or ceftriaxone 1 to 2 g IM/IV daily for 5 days
  - *Campylobacter*: azithromycin 500 mg PO daily for 3 to 5 days or erythromycin 500 mg PO QID for 5 days
  - *C. difficile*: vancomycin 125 to 500 mg PO QID for 10 to 14 days, or fidaxomicin 200 mg PO BID for 10 days; consider fecal microbiota transplant in recurrent mild to moderate *C. difficile* infections.
  - TD: ciprofloxacin 500 mg PO BID for 1 to 3 days, azithromycin (if suspicion of quinolone-resistant pathogens) 500 mg PO daily or 1 g PO daily for 1 to 3 days, rifaximin 200 mg PO TID for 3 days; combined with loperamide 4 mg PO initial dose, followed by 2 mg after each episode of diarrhea for maximum of 8 mg daily; loperamide or BSS may be used alone in cases of mild TD (2)[C].
- General considerations
  - Antibiotics are not recommended in *Salmonella* infections unless caused by *Salmonella typhosa* or if the patient is febrile or immunocompromised.
  - Avoid antibiotics in patients with *E. coli* 0157:H7 due to risk for HUS.

- Antibiotics are not indicated for foodborne toxigenic diarrhea.
- Avoid antimotility agents (e.g., loperamide) in patients with febrile or bloody diarrhea (especially, *E. coli* 0157:H7) or antibiotic-associated colitis.
- Antimotility agents used in combination with antibiotics may speed recovery from TD.
- Antibiotics are not recommended for the treatment of mild TD (2)[C].
- *C. difficile* infections in IBD patients: Initially treat with vancomycin or fidaxomicin; consider fecal microbiota transplant in patients with recurrent *C. difficile* infections (4)[C].
- Significant medication interactions
  - Salicylate absorption from BSS can cause toxicity in patients already taking aspirin-containing compounds and may alter anticoagulation control in patients taking warfarin.
  - Avoid alcoholic beverages with metronidazole due to the possibility of a disulfiram reaction.

COMPLEMENTARY & ALTERNATIVE MEDICINE
- BSS may help control rate of diarrhea stools (3,6)[C].
- Probiotics are recommended for prevention of antibiotic-associated diarrhea and *C. difficile* infection recurrence and to treat acute infectious diarrhea in setting of symptomatic IBS (6)[C].
- Probiotic use >10^{10}/g may help in patients with antibiotic-associated diarrhea (2)[A].
- Probiotic strains *Lactobacillus rhamnosus GG* (LGG) and *Saccharomyces boulardii* most effective; may reduce duration by up to 1 day
- Avoid probiotics in immunocompromised patients (2)[A].
- Zinc supplementation can decrease diarrhea duration in children 6 months to 5 years of age who reside in countries with a high prevalence of zinc deficiency or who have signs of malnutrition (IDSA, 2017).

ADMISSION, INPATIENT, AND NURSING CONSIDERATIONS
Outpatient management, except for patients who are severely ill with signs of volume depletion

ONGOING CARE

DIET
- Early oral refeeding is encouraged. Regular diets are as effective as restricted diets.
- The traditional bananas, rice, applesauce, toast (BRAT) diet has little evidence-based support (despite heavy clinical use) and may result in suboptimal nutrition.
- During periods of active diarrhea, coffee, alcohol, dairy products, fruits, vegetables, red meats, and heavily seasoned foods may exacerbate symptoms.

PATIENT EDUCATION
See "General Prevention."

PROGNOSIS
Acute diarrhea is rarely life-threatening if adequate hydration is maintained.

COMPLICATIONS
- Volume depletion, shock, sepsis
- Anemia
- Hemolytic uremic syndrome with *E. coli* 0157:H7
- Guillain-Barré syndrome with *C. jejuni*
- Reactive arthritis with *Salmonella*, *Shigella*, and *Yersinia*
- Functional bowel disorders (e.g., postinfectious irritable bowel syndrome [PI-IBS])

REFERENCES

1. Barr W, Smith A. Acute diarrhea. *Am Fam Physician*. 2014;89(3):180–189.
2. Riddle MS, Connor BA, Beeching NJ, et al. Guidelines for the prevention and treatment of travelers' diarrhea: a graded expert panel report. *J Travel Med*. 2017;24(Suppl 1):S57–S74.
3. Riddle MS, DuPont HL, Connor BA. ACG clinical guideline: diagnosis, treatment, and prevention of acute diarrheal infections in adults. *Am J Gastroenterol*. 2016;111(5):602–622.
4. Khanna S, Shin A, Kelly CP. Management of *Clostridium difficile* infection in inflammatory bowel disease: expert review from the Clinical Practice Updates Committee of the AGA Institute. *Clin Gastroenterol Hepatol*. 2017;15(2):166–174.
5. DuPont HL. Acute infectious diarrhea in immuno-competent adults. *N Engl J Med*. 2014;370(16): 1532–1540.
6. Wilkins T, Sequoia J. Probiotics for gastrointestinal conditions: a summary of the evidence. *Am Fam Physician*. 2017;96(3):170–178.

ADDITIONAL READING

- Chapman BC, Moore HB, Overbey DM, et al. Fecal microbiota transplant in patients with *Clostridium difficile* infection: a systematic review. *J Trauma Acute Care Surg*. 2016;81(4):756–764.
- Islam S. Clinical uses of probiotics. *Medicine (Baltimore)*. 2016;95(5):e2658.
- Santos VS, Marques DP, Martins-Filho PR, et al. Effectiveness of rotavirus vaccines against rotavirus infection and hospitalization in Latin America: systematic review and meta-analysis. *Infect Dis Poverty*. 2016;5(1):83.
- World Health Organization. The top 10 causes of death in the world, May 2018. http://www.who .int/mediacentre/factsheets/fs310/en/. Accessed September 8, 2018.

SEE ALSO

Botulism; Cholera; Food Poisoning, Bacterial

CODES

ICD10
- R19.7 Diarrhea, unspecified
- A09 Infectious gastroenteritis and colitis, unspecified
- A08.4 Viral intestinal infection, unspecified

CLINICAL PEARLS
- Viruses are the most common causes of acute diarrheal illness in the United States.
- Oral rehydration is the most important and effective treatment for acute diarrhea.
- Routine stool culture is not recommended, unless patients present with bloody diarrhea, fever, severe dehydration, signs of inflammatory disease, persistent symptoms >7 days, or have a history of immunosuppression.
- Start empiric antibiotics in patients who are severely ill or immunocompromised.

D

DIARRHEA, CHRONIC

Sarah A. Turki, MBBS • Stephen M. Testa, MD • Marie L. Borum, MD, EdD, MPH, MACP, FACG, AGAF

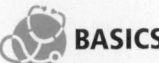 **BASICS**

DESCRIPTION
- An increase in frequency of defecation, urgency, or decrease in stool consistency (typically >3 loose stools per day) for >4 weeks (1,2)
  - Abnormal stool form is the most important defining factor; frequent defecation with normal consistency is termed pseudodiarrhea (2).
- Etiologies include osmotic, secretory, malabsorptive, inflammatory, infectious, and hypermotility.
- Infectious causes of chronic diarrhea are uncommon in immunocompetent patients. Parasitic etiologies are more common than bacterial.

EPIDEMIOLOGY
Prevalence
Varies by etiology; overall, ~3–5% of the population in developed countries is affected (2)

ETIOLOGY AND PATHOPHYSIOLOGY
Chronic diarrhea is typically the result of disturbances in luminal water and electrolyte balance within the intestine.
- Osmotic (fecal osmotic gap >75 mOsm/kg) (2)
  - Carbohydrate malabsorption
    - Disaccharides, including lactose
    - Monosaccharides, including fructose
    - Polyols, including sorbitol, xylitol, sucralose, and saccharin (common sugar substitutes)—cannot be metabolized and create an osmotic gradient.
  - Magnesium, phosphate, and sulfate overload
- Secretory (fecal osmotic gap <50 mOsm/kg) (2,3)
  - Stimulant laxative ingestion
  - Postcholecystectomy
    - Excessive intestinal bile salts cause choleretic diarrhea; often resolves in 6 to 12 months
  - Ileal bile acid malabsorption
  - Ileal resection of <100 cm leads to choleretic diarrhea due to excessive colonic bile salts.
  - Disordered motility
    - Postvagotomy
    - Diabetic autonomic neuropathy
    - Hyperthyroidism
  - Neuroendocrine tumors
    - VIPoma
    - Gastrinoma
    - Somatostatinoma
    - Carcinoid syndrome
  - Metastatic medullary carcinoma of the thyroid
  - Adrenal insufficiency
  - Noninvasive infection: giardiasis, cryptosporidiosis
  - Microscopic colitis (lymphocytic or collagenous)
  - Protein-losing enteropathy
  - Idiopathic secretory diarrhea
- Malabsorption (2,3)
  - Celiac disease
  - Whipple disease
  - Giardiasis
  - Chronic mesenteric ischemia
  - Lymphatic obstruction
  - Short bowel syndrome: Ileal resection of >100 cm leads to insufficient bile salt concentrations in the duodenum for optimal fat absorption, leading to fat and fat-soluble vitamin malabsorption.
  - Small intestinal bacterial overgrowth
  - Pancreatic exocrine insufficiency (cystic fibrosis [CF], chronic pancreatitis)
  - Inadequate bile acid production/secretion

- Inflammatory (2,3)
  - Ulcerative colitis; Crohn disease
  - Microscopic colitis (lymphocytic or collagenous)
  - Vasculitis; radiation enterocolitis
  - Eosinophilic enterocolitis
  - Invasive or inflammatory infections: *Clostridium difficile*, *Entamoeba histolytica*, cytomegalovirus, tuberculosis
- Hypermotility (normal fecal osmotic gap) (1,2)
  - Irritable bowel syndrome (IBS)
  - Functional diarrhea
- Drugs (2,3)
  - Adverse effect of >700 drugs, most commonly: NSAIDs, PPIs, colchicine, metformin, digoxin, SSRIs, β-blockers
  - Factitious diarrhea: excessive laxative use
- Herbal products: St. John's wort, echinacea, garlic, saw palmetto, ginseng, cranberry extract, *Aloe vera*
- Infectious (2)
  - Bacterial: *C. difficile*, *Mycobacterium avium-intracellulare*
  - Viral: cytomegalovirus
  - Parasitic: *Giardia lamblia*, *Cryptosporidium*, *Isospora*, *E. histolytica*
  - Helminthic: *Strongyloides*
- Food allergies (2)

Genetics
- Celiac disease is associated with HLA-DQ2 and HLA-DQ8 haplotypes on major histocompatibility complex (MHC) class II antigen-presenting cells (4).
- Inflammatory bowel disease (IBD) is polygenic (5).
- CF is caused by a mutation in the CF transmembrane conductance regulator (CFTR), resulting in abnormal exocrine gland secretions.

RISK FACTORS
- Osmotic
  - Excess ingestion of nonabsorbable carbohydrates
  - Lactose intolerance
  - Celiac disease
- Secretory (2)
  - Postsurgical: extensive small bowel resection/ileal surgery, vagotomy, bile acid malabsorption
  - History of neuroendocrine disease
  - History of stimulant laxative abuse
  - Dysmotility syndromes
- Malabsorptive
  - CF
  - Chronic alcohol abuse
  - Chronic pancreatitis/pancreatic insufficiency
  - Celiac disease
  - Medications (e.g., orlistat, acarbose)
- Inflammatory
  - IBD
  - NSAID use
  - Thoracoabdominal radiation
  - HIV/AIDS
  - Antibiotic use
  - Immunosuppressant therapy
- Hypermotility
  - Psychosocial stress
  - Preceding infection
- Genetic predisposition

ALERT
Diabetes mellitus and/or prior cholecystectomy both cause secretory and osmotic diarrhea.

GENERAL PREVENTION
Varies by etiology; treat the underlying cause.

COMMONLY ASSOCIATED CONDITIONS
- Extraintestinal manifestations of IBD include arthralgias, aphthous stomatitis, uveitis/episcleritis, erythema nodosum, pyoderma gangrenosum, perianal fistulas, rectal fissures, ankylosing spondylitis, and primary sclerosing cholangitis.
- Celiac disease is associated with dermatitis herpetiformis, type 1 diabetes, other autoimmune disorders, and IgA deficiency.
- Many patients with IBS have behavioral comorbidities.
- Latex-food allergy syndrome: associated allergies to latex and banana, avocado, kiwi, and walnut (2)

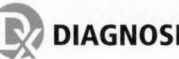 **DIAGNOSIS**

HISTORY
- Detailed history of symptoms (1,2):
  - Onset, pattern, and frequency of stooling
  - Stool volume and quality (including presence of blood or mucus)
  - Presence of nocturnal symptoms
  - Travel history
  - Antibiotic exposure
  - Dietary patterns
  - Current medications
  - Family history
- Determine aggravating or alleviating factors; changes with oral intake or improvement with selective food avoidance (e.g., dairy products)
- Unintentional weight loss
- Skin changes (rashes, hives), arthritis, ocular problems, heat intolerance, polyuria/polydipsia, headache, fever, flushing, alcohol intake
- Food allergies are rare, occurring in only 1–2% of adults. Consider in patients with hives (2).
- Flatus and bloating are predominant features of carbohydrate malabsorption (2).
- Prior surgery or radiation therapy (3)
- History of systemic illness: endocrine, immunologic
- IBS or functional diarrhea by Rome IV criteria (3):
  - IBS: recurrent abdominal pain at least 1 day/week for past 3 months (symptoms >6 months); ≥2 of:
    - Related to defecation
    - Associated with change in frequency of stool
    - Associated with change in form of stool
  - Functional diarrhea: ≥25% loose or watery stools without prominent abdominal pain or bloating for >3 months (symptoms >6 months)

PHYSICAL EXAM
- General: volume depletion, nutritional status, recent weight loss (2)
- Skin: flushing (carcinoid), erythema nodosum (IBD), pyoderma gangrenosum (IBD), ecchymoses (vitamin K deficiency), dermatitis herpetiformis (celiac disease), hyperpigmentation (Addison disease) (1,2)
- HEENT: iritis/uveitis (IBD), lid lag (hyperthyroid)
- Neck: goiter (hyperthyroid), lymphadenopathy (Whipple disease)
- Cardiovascular: tachycardia (hyperthyroid), heart murmur (carcinoid syndrome) (3)
- Pulmonary: wheezing (carcinoid)
- Abdomen: hyperactive bowel sounds (IBD), abdominal distension (IBD/IBS), diffuse tenderness (IBD/IBS)
- Anorectal: anorectal fistulas (IBD), anal fissures (IBD)
- Extremities: arthritis (IBD)
- Neurologic: tremor (hyperthyroid)

DIFFERENTIAL DIAGNOSIS
See "Etiology and Pathophysiology," "Commonly Associated Conditions," and "Risk Factors."

DIAGNOSTIC TESTS & INTERPRETATION

Initial Tests (lab, imaging)

Test patients with alarm symptoms (bleeding, weight loss) or persistent symptoms and no identifiable cause.

- Blood: CBC, electrolytes (Mg, P, Ca), total protein, albumin, thyroid-stimulating hormone, free T_4, erythrocyte sedimentation rate, C-reactive protein, IgA anti–tissue transglutaminase (TTG), iron studies (2,3)
- Stool: WBCs or fecal calprotectin (preferred), culture, ova and parasites, *Giardia* stool antigen, *C. difficile* toxin, electrolytes (fecal osmotic gap), occult blood, qualitative fecal fat (Sudan stain) (2)
- CT to evaluate for chronic pancreatitis or malignancy if evidence of malabsorption (1,2)
- CT or MR enterography for small bowel imaging when Crohn disease is suspected (2)

Follow-Up Tests & Special Considerations

- Celiac disease: antiendomysial antibody IgA, anti-TTG IgA, antigliadin (AGA) IgA, serum IgA (10% of celiac patients have IgA deficiency—may cause false-negative results) (4)[A]
- Chronic pancreatic insufficiency: fecal elastase and chymotrypsin (2)[C]
- Protein-losing enteropathy: fecal α_1-antitrypsin (2)[C]
- Microscopic colitis: mucosal biopsy from colon (3)[C]
- Carbohydrate malabsorption: fecal pH ($<$7.0) and hydrogen breath test
- Small bowel overgrowth: hydrogen breath test
- Recent hospitalization or antibiotics: *C. difficile* toxin
- HIV ELISA, *Isospora/Cryptosporidium* stains (2)[C]
- Consider testing for protozoa, atypical infections, *Strongyloides*, and tropical sprue in travelers and migrants of endemic areas (2)[C].
- Allergy testing (2)[C]
- Laxative abuse: stool osmolality, osmotic gap (3)[C]
- Neuroendocrine tumor (1,3)[C]
  - Serum: chromogranin A, VIP, gastrin, calcitonin
  - Urine: 5-HIAA, histamine

Diagnostic Procedures/Other

- Ileocolonoscopy with biopsies: IBD, microscopic colitis, CMV colitis, and colorectal neoplasia (6)[A]
- Flexible sigmoidoscopy: especially if pregnant, with comorbidities, or if left-sided symptoms predominate (tenesmus and urgency) (6)[A]
- Esophagogastroduodenoscopy (EGD) with small bowel biopsies if malabsorption is suspected:
  - Celiac, *Giardia* infection, Crohn disease, eosinophilic gastroenteropathy, Whipple disease, intestinal amyloid, pancreatic insufficiency (6)[A]
- Capsule endoscopy if further evaluation of small bowel is needed (6)[C]
- Upper GI series with small bowel follow-through
- CT or magnetic resonance (MR) enterography (1,2)

Test Interpretation

- Celiac disease: Marsh classification:
  - Intraepithelial lymphocytosis, crypt hyperplasia, villous atrophy (4)
- Crohn disease: cobblestoning, linear ulcerations, skip lesions, noncaseating granulomas
- Ulcerative colitis: crypt abscesses, superficial inflammation (6)
- Lymphocytic colitis: increased intraepithelial lymphocytes, increased inflammatory cells within the lamina propria, normal mucosal architecture (6)
- Melanosis coli suggests laxative abuse (2).

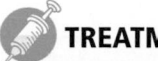 TREATMENT

GENERAL MEASURES

- Volume resuscitation if necessary
- Electrolyte replacement if indicated
- If stable, treatment is generally outpatient (2)[C].

MEDICATION

First Line

- Based on underlying cause:
  - Lactose intolerance: lactose-free diet
  - Cholecystectomy or ileal resection: cholestyramine or colestipol 2 to 16 g/day PO divided BID
  - Diabetes: glucose control
  - Hyperthyroidism: methimazole 5 to 20 mg/day PO, propylthiouracil (PTU) 100 to 150 mg/day PO divided; thyroid ablation
  - *C. difficile*: vancomycin 125 mg PO q6h or metronidazole (Flagyl) 500 mg PO q8h or fidaxomicin 200 mg PO BID
  - *G. lamblia*: metronidazole 250 mg PO q8h, nitazoxanide 500 mg PO q12h (2)[A]
  - Whipple disease: ceftriaxone 2 g IV for 14 days then trimethoprim and sulfamethoxazole (Bactrim DS) 160/800 mg PO BID for 1 to 2 years
  - Small intestinal bacterial overgrowth: rifaximin 550 mg PO BID, fluoroquinolones 250 to 750 mg PO BID, metronidazole 500 mg PO q6–8h, penicillins
  - Pancreatic insufficiency: enzyme replacement
  - HIV/AIDS: antiretroviral therapy
  - Microscopic colitis: budesonide 9 mg/day PO, mesalamine 800 mg PO TID, Bismuth subsalicylate (Pepto-Bismol) 786 mg PO TID
  - IBD: 5-aminosalicylic acid (5-ASA), corticosteroids (short-term only), antibiotics (short-term only), immunomodulators (6-mercaptopurine [6-MP], azathioprine, methotrexate), anti-TNF therapy (infliximab, adalimumab, certolizumab) (5)[A]
  - Neuroendocrine tumor: octreotide 100 to 600 g/day SC (2)[C]
  - Celiac disease: gluten-free diet (wheat/barley/rye avoidance) (4)[A]
  - IBS diarrhea predominant: rifaximin 550 mg PO BID, alosetron 0.5 to 1.0 mg PO BID, peppermint oil, eluxadoline 100 mg PO BID (2)[C]
- Symptom relief (2)[C]:
  - Loperamide 4 to 8 mg/day PO divided
  - Diphenoxylate-atropine 1 to 2 tabs PO BID–QID
  - Fiber supplementation
  - Bismuth subsalicylate 525 to 1,050 mg every 0.5 to 1 hour; max dose 4,200 mg/day (2)[C]

SURGERY/OTHER PROCEDURES

- Resection of neuroendocrine tumors
- Intestinal resection for medically refractory IBD
- Fecal transplant for recurrent *C. difficile* infection

COMPLEMENTARY & ALTERNATIVE MEDICINE

Many homeopathic and naturopathic formulations are available; most have not been evaluated by the FDA.

 ONGOING CARE

DIET

Avoid gluten-containing foods, nonabsorbable carbohydrates, lactose-containing products, and food allergens depending on etiology of diarrhea.

- Low FODMAP (fermentable oligosaccharides, disaccharides, monosaccharides, and polyols) diet helps symptoms in up to 75% of IBS patients (2).

PATIENT EDUCATION

- Wide variation in "normal" bowel habits
- Restrict colon stimulants.
- Base specific education and dietary changes on underlying etiology.

PROGNOSIS

Varies according to etiology

COMPLICATIONS

- Fluid and electrolyte abnormalities (1)
- Malnutrition (1); anemia (1)
- Malignancy (colon cancer in IBD, small bowel cancer in celiac disease and Crohn disease, lymphoma with IBD therapies) (5)
- Infection with immunomodulator, biologic, and corticosteroid therapies for IBD (5)

REFERENCES

1. Schiller LR. Definitions, pathophysiology, and evaluation of chronic diarrhoea. *Best Pract Res Clin Gastroenterol.* 2012;26(5):551–562.
2. Schiller LR, Pardi DS, Sellin JH. Chronic diarrhea: diagnosis and management. *Clin Gastroenterol Hepatol.* 2017;15(2):182–193.e3.
3. Schiller LR. Evaluation of chronic diarrhea and irritable bowel syndrome with diarrhea in adults in the era of precision medicine. *Am J Gastroenterol.* 2018;113(5):660–669.
4. Rubio-Tapia A, Hill ID, Kelly CP, et al. ACG clinical guidelines: diagnosis and management of celiac disease. *Am J Gastroenterol.* 2013;108(5):656–677.
5. Talley NJ, Abreu MT, Achkar JP, et al. An evidence-based systematic review on medical therapies for inflammatory bowel disease. *Am J Gastroenterol.* 2011;106(Suppl 1):S2–S26.
6. Shen B, Khan K, Ikenberry SO, et al; for ASGE Standards of Practice Committee. The role of endoscopy in the management of patients with diarrhea. *Gastrointest Endosc.* 2010;71(6):887–892.

ADDITIONAL READING

- Camilleri M, Sellin JH, Barrett KE. Pathophysiology, evaluation, and management of chronic watery diarrhea. *Gastroenterology.* 2017;152(3):515–532.e2.
- Ford AC, Lacy BE, Talley NJ. Irritable bowel syndrome. *N Engl J Med.* 2017;376(26):2566–2578.
- Lacy BE, Mearin F, Chang L, et al. Bowel disorders. *Gastroenterology.* 2016;150(6):1393–1407.

 SEE ALSO

Algorithm: Diarrhea, Chronic

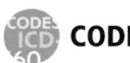 CODES

ICD10

K52.9 Noninfective gastroenteritis and colitis, unspecified

CLINICAL PEARLS

- A comprehensive medical history guides the appropriate workup and avoids unnecessary testing.
- Consider IBS, IBD, malabsorption syndromes (e.g., lactose intolerance), celiac disease, over-the-counter medications, herbal products, and chronic infections (immunocompromised) in differential diagnosis.
- Treatment is based on the underlying cause.

DIFFUSE INTERSTITIAL LUNG DISEASE

J. Andrew Woods, PharmD, BCPS • Jacqueline L. Olin, MS, PharmD, BCPS, CDE, FASHP, FCCP • Brian Hertz, MD

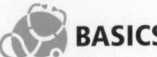 **BASICS**

DESCRIPTION

- Interstitial lung diseases (ILDs) represent a diverse group of chronic progressive lung diseases associated with alveolar inflammation and/or potentially irreversible pulmonary fibrosis.
- >200 individual diseases may present with similar characteristics, making ILD difficult to classify.
- A classification scheme proposed by the American Thoracic Society and European Respiratory Society includes these subtypes:
  - Known causes (environmental, occupational, or drug-associated disease)
  - Systemic disorders (e.g., sarcoidosis, Wegener granulomatosis, collagen vascular disease)
  - Rare lung diseases (e.g., pulmonary histiocytosis, lymphangioleiomyomatosis)
  - Idiopathic interstitial pneumonias (IIPs)
- Based on clinical, radiologic, and histologic features, IIPs are further subclassified into the following diagnoses (1):
  - Major IIPs, including idiopathic pulmonary fibrosis (IPF), nonspecific interstitial pneumonia (NSIP), respiratory bronchiolitis-associated ILD (cryptogenic organizing pneumonia [COP], etc.)
  - Rare IIPs
  - Unclassifiable IIPs
- Classification of IIPs and relationships between the subtypes are difficult to classify due to mixed patterns of injury.

Pediatric Considerations
ILD in infants and children represents a heterogeneous group of respiratory disorders. Diseases result from a variety of processes involving genetic factors and inflammatory or fibrotic responses, and processes are distinct from those that cause ILD in adults (2). Some diseases result from developmental disorders and growth abnormalities in infancy (2). After common causes are excluded, referral of infants to a subspecialist is recommended (2).

EPIDEMIOLOGY

Incidence
- Exact incidence and prevalence are difficult to determine because of differences in case definitions and procedures used in diagnosis.
- Cited incidence of IPF in the United States: 16.3 to 17.4/100,000 and pediatric ILD 1.32/1,000,000

Prevalence
Cited prevalence of IPF in the United States: 42.7 to 63 cases/100,000 in the general population and pediatric ILD of 3.6/1 million

ETIOLOGY AND PATHOPHYSIOLOGY

- Alveolar inflammation may progress into irreversible fibrosis.
- Varying degrees of ventilatory dysfunction occur among the ILD subtypes.
- ILD associated with collagen vascular disease and systemic connective disorders can manifest involvement of skin, joints, muscular, and ocular systems.
- Some types of ILD are associated with specific exposures:
  - Medications (amiodarone, antibiotics [especially nitrofurantoin], chemotherapy agents, gold, illicit drugs)

  - Inorganic dusts (silicates, asbestos, talc, mica, coal dust, graphite)
  - Organic dusts (moldy hay, inhalation of fungi, bacteria, animal proteins)
  - Metals (tin, aluminum, cobalt, iron, barium)
  - Gases, fumes, vapors, aerosols

Genetics
Some subtypes of ILD may be associated with specific predisposing genes and environmental exposures; however, the role of genetic factors is unknown.

RISK FACTORS
- Environmental or occupational exposure to inorganic or organic dusts
- 66–75% of patients with ILD have a history of smoking.
- Due to diversity of diseases, age is not a reliable predictor of pathology:
  - Most patients with connective tissue disease–related pathology and inherited subtypes present between ages 20 and 40 years
  - Median age of patients with IPF is 66 years. Studies of clinical predictors of survival including age, ethnicity, and smoking status have been inconsistent.

COMMONLY ASSOCIATED CONDITIONS
Many systemic disorders and primary diseases are associated with ILD. A partial list includes the following:
- Collagen vascular disease
- Sarcoidosis
- Amyloidosis
- Goodpasture syndrome
- Churg-Strauss syndrome
- Wegener granulomatosis

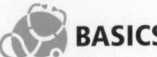 **DIAGNOSIS**

- Accurate diagnosis is imperative because treatment choices and prognosis can vary with pathogenesis.
- Diagnosis of IPF requires exclusion of other known ILD causes, the presence of a UIP pattern on high-resolution computed tomography (HRCT), and/or surgical lung biopsy pattern (2).

HISTORY
- Symptoms may include progressive exertional dyspnea and nonproductive cough.
- Patients may also present with hemoptysis or fatigue.
- Obtaining a history of illness duration (acute vs. chronic), potential environmental/occupational exposures, travel, medical conditions (including systemic diseases), and medication reconciliation is important in assessing the cause of the ILD.
- Some cases of lung disease may occur weeks to years after discontinuation of an offending agent.

PHYSICAL EXAM
Physical findings are usually nonspecific. Some common features include the following:
- Crackles (typically present on auscultation of lung bases on posterior axillary line)
- Rales
- Inspiratory "squeaks"
- Clubbing of the digits and cyanosis in advanced disease

DIFFERENTIAL DIAGNOSIS
- Acute pulmonary edema
- Diffuse hemorrhage
- Atypical pneumonia
- Diffuse bronchoalveolar cell carcinoma or lymphatic spread of tumor

DIAGNOSTIC TESTS & INTERPRETATION

Initial Tests (lab, imaging)
- O₂ saturation
- Peak expiratory flow rate
- CBC with differential, comprehensive metabolic profile
- CRP or sedimentation rate
- Chest x-ray (CXR): most commonly reticular pattern, less commonly nodular or mixed patterns

Follow-Up Tests & Special Considerations
HRCT of the chest is the most useful tool for distinguishing among ILD subclasses, especially if normal CXRs:
- If indicated, arterial blood gas (ABG), hypersensitivity pneumonitis panel, plasma ACE inhibitor concentration (sarcoidosis)
- If a systemic disorder is suspected, consider antinuclear antibody (ANA), rheumatoid factor (RF), erythrocyte sedimentation rate (ESR), and antineutrophil cytoplasmic antibodies (ANCA).

Diagnostic Procedures/Other
- Pulmonary function test (PFT; spirometry, lung volumes, carbon monoxide diffusing capacity)
  - Commonly demonstrates a restrictive defect (decreased vital capacity and total lung capacity)
  - Forced vital capacity (FVC) has been shown to decline 100 to 200 mL/year in the placebo arm of IPF patients in clinical trials.
- Bronchoscopy
  - Bronchoalveolar lavage (BAL) cellular analysis studies may be useful in distinguishing subtypes (including sarcoidosis, hypersensitivity pneumonitis, cancer). If performed, the BAL target site should be chosen based on the HRCT finding.
  - Bronchoscopic transbronchial lung biopsy may help diagnose sarcoidosis and, on occasion, is sufficiently supportive of other ILD diagnoses.
- Thoracoscopic surgery for lung biopsy has the greatest diagnostic specificity for ILDs but is less frequently used given improved specificity of HRCT may be indicated if a diagnosis cannot be determined from transbronchial biopsy or HRCT

Test Interpretation
- Diagnostic classifications of IIPs are based on histopathologic patterns seen on lung biopsy.
- Major histologies include an inflammation and fibrotic and granulomatous patterns.
- Characteristic changes on HRCT may help to distinguish between the following subtypes:
  - Reticulonodular, ground glass opacities, and, in later stages, honeycombing may be seen.
  - Associated hilar and mediastinal adenopathy are characteristic of stage I and II sarcoidosis.
- No specific test is the gold standard, which emphasizes the importance of a multidisciplinary consensus for diagnosis with clinical, radiologic, and pathologic findings.

TREATMENT

- Evidence does not support the routine use of any specific therapy for ILD in general, especially IPF (2,3).
- No survival benefit of home oxygen use in ILD
- Corticosteroids have a role in some ILD subtypes.
- Current evidence does not clearly support routine use of noncorticosteroid anti-inflammatory agents for IPF, including cyclosporine, colchicines, cyclophosphamide, cytokines, sildenafil, dual endothelin receptor antagonists (bosentan, macitentan), etanercept, methotrexate, or interferon.
- Clinical trials have indicated that anticoagulation (warfarin), ambrisentan, imatinib, and the combination of prednisone, azathioprine, and N-acetylcysteine are ineffective, potentially harmful, and therefore not recommended in the treatment of IPF (3)[A].
- Recombinant human thrombomodulin improved 3-month survival in the setting of acute exacerbation of IPF in a small historical control study.

GENERAL MEASURES

- Avoid/minimize offending environmental/occupational exposures/medications.
- Smoking cessation
- Supplemental oxygen, if indicated

MEDICATION

First Line

- Corticosteroids are most effective for certain ILDs, especially exacerbations of sarcoidosis, NSIP, COP, and hypersensitivity pneumonitis. However, response rates have been variable across and within subtypes. The optimal dose and duration of therapy are unknown.
- Common starting dose of prednisone is 0.5 to 1.0 mg/kg/day for 4 to 12 weeks with potential up-titration based on patient response.
- Two antifibrotic agents approved for IPF exhibited modest slowing of FVC decline over 52 weeks compared to placebo. Both decreased all-cause mortality rates. It is not clear if FVC is the most conclusive meaningful efficacy variable for IPF.
  - Pirfenidone (Esbriet) decreased the rate of decline in FVC compared to placebo. Secondary trial findings include a significant improvement in progression-free survival, and pooled analysis reveals a significant reduction in all-cause death and death from IPF (4). Pirfenidone has been shown to reduce respiratory-related hospitalizations in IPF (5). The most common adverse effects are GI related (nausea, vomiting, anorexia, weight loss, GERD, and dyspepsia), rash, insomnia, dizziness, fatigue, and aminotransferase elevation. Most AEs are mild to moderate in nature and do not result in pirfenidone discontinuation. Pirfenidone is not recommended for patients with severe liver impairment or ESRD (4)[A].

  - Pirfenidone is titrated over 2 weeks to 801 mg PO 3 times daily with food.
  - Nintedanib (Ofev) reduced the annual rate of decline in FVC, and fewer acute exacerbations occurred compared to placebo. The most common adverse effects are GI upset (nausea, vomiting, diarrhea, abdominal pain), anorexia, aminotransferase elevation, and hypertension. It is not recommended in moderate to severe liver impairment and can cause birth defects (6)[A].
  - Nintedanib is given at 150 mg PO twice daily with food.
  - Adding pirfenidone to nintedanib may convey a synergistic effect but could be limited by GI upset (7). Further investigation is warranted.

Second Line

- The addition of tacrolimus to corticosteroids (with cyclosporine, cyclophosphamide, or no additional therapy) may improve event-free survival in patients with ILD complicated with polymyositis or dermatomyositis.
- Several second-line agents have been used in Wegener granulomatosis:
  - Cyclophosphamide is commonly used in treatment of Wegener granulomatosis. It is given 1.5 to 2.0 mg/kg/day PO for 3 to 6 months.
  - Methotrexate has been used in treatment of mild Wegener granulomatosis in combination with corticosteroids. A studied dosing regimen consisted of an initial dose of 0.3 mg/kg (max dose of 15 mg) once weekly, with 2.5 mg titration each week (max dose of 25 mg/week).
  - Other second-line agents that have been studied include mycophenolate, mofetil, and rituximab.

SURGERY/OTHER PROCEDURES

- Single- or double-lung transplantation may be a treatment of last resort. Lung transplant among selected IPF patients has demonstrated median survival of 4.5 years (6)[A]. Some ILDs associated with systemic disease may recur in the recipient lung.
- Alveolar type II cell intratracheal transplantation may benefit patients with moderate to progressive IPF.
- Clinical trials to assess the safety and efficacy of allogeneic human mesenchymal stem cell infusion in patients with mild to moderate IPF are ongoing.

ONGOING CARE

FOLLOW-UP RECOMMENDATIONS
Follow-up testing should include PFTs, cardiopulmonary stress test, pulse oximetry, and CXR.

PATIENT EDUCATION
National Heart, Lung, and Blood Institute: http://www.nhlbi.nih.gov/health/health-topics/topics/ipf/

PROGNOSIS
IPF confers the worst prognosis (median survival of 2.5 to 3 years). A clinical prediction model to estimate the risk of death from ILD has been described (ILD-GAP model). Other subtypes, including hypersensitivity pneumonitis, NSIP, and COP, have a good prognosis.

COMPLICATIONS
- Cor pulmonale
- Pneumothorax
- Progressive respiratory failure

REFERENCES

1. Kurland G, Deterding RR, Hagood JS, et al; for American Thoracic Society Committee on Childhood Interstitial Lung Disease (chILD) and the chILD Research Network. An official American Thoracic Society clinical practice guideline: classification, evaluation, and management of childhood interstitial lung disease in infancy. Am J Respir Crit Care Med. 2013;188(3):376–394.
2. Raghu G, Collard HR, Egan JJ, et al; for ATS/ERS/JRS/ALAT Committee on Idiopathic Pulmonary Fibrosis. An official ATS/ERS/JRS/ALAT statement: idiopathic pulmonary fibrosis: evidence-based guidelines for diagnosis and management. Am J Respir Crit Care Med. 2011;183(6):788–824.
3. Raghu G, Rochwerg B, Zhang Y, et al; for American Thoracic Society, European Respiratory Society, Japanese Respiratory Society, Latin American Thoracic Association. An official ATS/ERS/JRS/ALAT clinical practice guideline: treatment of idiopathic pulmonary fibrosis. An update of the 2011 clinical practice guideline. Am J Respir Crit Care Med. 2015;192(2):e3–e19.
4. King TE Jr, Bradford WZ, Castro-Bernardini S, et al. A phase 3 trial of pirfenidone in patients with idiopathic pulmonary fibrosis. N Engl J Med. 2014;370(22):2083–2092.
5. Ley B, Swigris J, Day BM, et al. Pirfenidone reduces respiratory-related hospitalizations in idiopathic pulmonary fibrosis. Am J Respir Crit Care Med. 2017;196(6):756–761.
6. Richeldi L, du Bois RM, Raghu G, et al; for INPULSIS Trial Investigators. Efficacy and safety of nintedanib in idiopathic pulmonary fibrosis. N Engl J Med. 2014;370(22):2071–2082.
7. Vancheri C, Kreuter M, Richeldi L, et al; for INJOURNEY Trial Investigators. Nintedanib with add-on pirfenidone in idiopathic pulmonary fibrosis. Results of the INJOURNEY trial. Am J Respir Crit Care Med. 2018;197(3):356–363.

CODES

ICD10
- J84.9 Interstitial pulmonary disease, unspecified
- J84.10 Pulmonary fibrosis, unspecified
- J84.111 Idiopathic interstitial pneumonia, not otherwise specified

CLINICAL PEARLS

- ILD differs from chronic obstructive pulmonary disease (COPD); anatomically, ILD involves the lung parenchyma (i.e., alveoli), and COPD involves both airways and alveoli.
- In some cases, avoiding or minimizing offending environmental/occupational exposures, medications, and smoking may alter disease severity.

DIVERTICULAR DISEASE

Andrew Harner, MD • Brian P. Bateson, DO • Steven B. Holsten Jr., MD

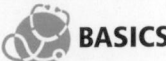

BASICS

DESCRIPTION
Diverticulum (single) or diverticula (multiple) are outpouchings in the colonic wall. Diverticular disease is a spectrum of diseases impacting the entire GI tract (except the rectum):
- Asymptomatic diverticulosis: common incidental finding on routine colonoscopy
- Symptomatic diverticulosis: also known as symptomatic uncomplicated diverticular disease (SUDD); recurrent abdominal pain attributed to diverticulosis without colitis or diverticulitis (1)
- Acute diverticulitis: diverticular disease with associated inflammation and/or infection
  - Uncomplicated diverticulitis: left lower quadrant (LLQ) pain, tenderness, leukocytosis but no peritoneal signs or systemic toxicity
  - Complicated diverticulitis: secondary abscess formation, bowel obstruction or perforation, peritonitis, fistula, or stricture
- Diverticular bleeding
  - Accounts for >40% of lower GI bleeds and 30% of cases of hematochezia in general
  - Bleeding more common with right-sided diverticula

EPIDEMIOLOGY
Incidence
- Diverticular disease accounts for ~300,000 hospitalizations per year in the United States.
- Diverticulitis occurs in 1–2% of the general population and in 4% of patients with diverticulosis over the course of their lifetime (1).
- Diverticular bleeding occurs in 3–5% of patients with diverticulosis.

Prevalence
- Prevalence of diverticulosis and the number of diverticula increase with age.
  - Diverticulosis occurs in 20% of those age 40 years, 60% of those age 60 years, and 70% by the age of 80 years.
  - Incidence increased from 62 to 75/100,000 from 1998 to 2005; large increase in patients <45 years of age—mostly due to changes in diet
- Male = female overall; more common in men <65 years of age and more common in women >65 years

ETIOLOGY AND PATHOPHYSIOLOGY
Diverticula form at points of weakness along the intestinal wall where small blood vessels (vasa recta) penetrate through the muscular layer of the colon.
- Age-related degeneration of the mucosal wall; increased intraluminal pressure from dense, fiber-depleted stools; and abnormal colonic motility contribute to diverticulosis.
- Most right-sided diverticula are true diverticula (involves all layers of the colonic wall).
- Most left-sided diverticula are pseudodiverticula (outpouchings of the mucosa and submucosa only).
- Diverticulitis occurs when local inflammation and infection contribute to tissue necrosis with risk for mucosal micro- or macroperforation.
- Diverticulitis: Microscopy reveals inflammation with lymphocytic infiltrate, ulceration, mucin depletion, necrosis, Paneth cell metaplasia, and cryptitis.

- Alterations in intestinal microbiota contribute to chronic inflammation (1).
- Thinning of the vasa recta over the neck of the diverticula increases susceptibility to bleeding.
- Diverticular disease and irritable bowel syndrome (IBS) may represent the same disease continuum.

Genetics
- No known genetic pattern
- Asian and African populations have lower overall prevalence but develop diverticular disease with adoption of a Western lifestyle.

RISK FACTORS
- Age >40 years
- Low-fiber diet
- Sedentary lifestyle, obesity
- Previous diverticulitis. Risk rises with the number of diverticula.
- Smoking increases the risk of perforation (1).
- Risk of diverticular bleeding increases with NSAIDs, steroids, and opiate analgesics. Calcium channel blockers and statins protect against diverticular bleeding.

GENERAL PREVENTION
- High-fiber diet or nonabsorbable fiber (psyllium)
- Vigorous physical activity

COMMONLY ASSOCIATED CONDITIONS
Colon cancer, connective tissue diseases, obesity, and inflammatory bowel disease

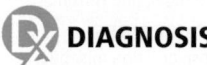

DIAGNOSIS

HISTORY
- Diverticulosis
  - 80–85% of patients are asymptomatic. Of the 15–20% with symptoms, 1–2% will require hospitalization, and 0.5% will undergo surgery.
  - The most common symptom is dull, colicky abdominal pain, typically in the LLQ. Pain can be exacerbated by eating and by passing bowel movement or flatus.
  - Diarrhea or constipation is common.
- Acute diverticulitis: uncomplicated (85%) and complicated (15%)
  - Abdominal pain: acute onset, typically in LLQ
  - Fever and/or chills
  - Anorexia, nausea (20–62%), or vomiting
  - Constipation (50%) or diarrhea (25–35%)
  - Dysuria and urinary frequency suggest bladder or ureteral irritation.
  - Pneumaturia and fecaluria with colovesical fistula
- Diverticular bleeding
  - Melena, hematochezia (0.5/1,000 person-years)
  - Painless rectal bleeding
- Immunocompromised patients may not present with fever or leukocytosis and are at higher risk for perforation and abscess formation.

PHYSICAL EXAM
- Diverticulosis
  - Exam is usually normal.
  - May have intermittent distension or tympany
  - May have heme + stools
- Acute diverticulitis
  - Abdominal tenderness (usually LLQ)
  - Abdominal distension and tympany

- Rebound tenderness, involuntary guarding, or rigidity suggests perforation and/or peritonitis.
- Palpable mass in LLQ (20%)
- Bowel sounds hypoactive (could be high-pitched and intermittent if obstruction is present)
- Rectal exam may reveal tenderness or a mass.
- Colovaginal, colovesical, and perirectal fistulae are rarely the initial presentation.

DIFFERENTIAL DIAGNOSIS
Urinary tract infection, nephrolithiasis, IBS, lactose intolerance, carcinoma, inflammatory bowel disease, fecal impaction, bowel obstruction, angiodysplasia, ischemic colitis, acute appendicitis, ectopic pregnancy

DIAGNOSTIC TESTS & INTERPRETATION
Initial Tests (lab, imaging)
- Diverticulosis: no labs or imaging needed
- Acute diverticulitis
  - WBC count is normal in up to 45% of cases. As diverticulitis worsens, WBC count becomes elevated with left shift.
  - Hemoglobin normal (unless bleeding)
  - ESR elevated
  - Urinalysis may show microscopic pyuria or hematuria
  - Urine culture: usually normal; persistent infection is suspicious for colovesical fistula.
  - Blood cultures positive in systemic cases
  - Plain films of the abdomen (acute abdominal series—supine and upright) to assess for free air under the diaphragm (bowel perforation) and signs of bowel obstruction (dilated loops of bowel)
  - CT scan with IV, oral, and/or rectal contrast (sensitivity: 98%, specificity: 99%) to stage disease and determine treatment plan (2)[A]
  - Ultrasound and MRI (sensitivity: 94%, specificity: 92%) are useful alternatives.
  - Barium enema is not recommended due to risk of peritoneal extravasation.
- Diverticular bleeding
  - Anemia with bleeding
  - Obtain coagulation panel for coagulopathy.

Diagnostic Procedures/Other
Diverticular bleeding
- Endoscopy to evaluate GI bleeding
- NG lavage to exclude upper GI bleeding
- Angiography if bleeding obscures endoscopy or when endoscopy cannot visualize a source
- 99mTc-pertechnetate–labeled RBC scan (more sensitive) with follow-up angiography to localize bleeding (not studied in a comparison trial)

TREATMENT

GENERAL MEASURES
- Diverticulosis: outpatient therapy with fiber supplementation and/or bulking agents (psyllium) (>30 g/day) (2)[A]
- Uncomplicated diverticulitis: outpatient therapy with or without oral antibiotics. 1–2% of subjects require hospitalization for toxicity, septicemia, peritonitis, or failure of symptoms to resolve. Up to 30% of patients may require surgery at first episode of diverticulitis.

- Complicated diverticulitis: hospitalization, bowel rest, and IV antibiotics. Hinchey classification (severity):
  - Stage I: diverticulitis + confined paracolic abscess
  - Stage II: diverticulitis + distant abscess
  - Stage III: diverticulitis + purulent peritonitis
  - Stage IV: diverticulitis + fecal peritonitis
- Symptomatic improvement is expected within 2 to 3 days. Antibiotics should be continued for 7 to 10 days.
- Diverticular bleeding: 80% of cases resolve spontaneously.

MEDICATION
First Line
- Symptomatic diverticulosis: cyclical rifaximin 400 mg PO BID for 7 days every month or continuous mesalamine 800 mg PO BID (2)[C]
- Acute diverticulitis
  - The routine use of antibiotics in uncomplicated diverticulitis is controversial (2,3)[C].
  - Outpatient oral antibiotics: Cover for anaerobes and gram-negatives with:
    - A fluoroquinolone (ciprofloxacin 750 mg BID or levofloxacin 750 mg QD) *plus* metronidazole 500 mg TID (may use clindamycin if metronidazole intolerant) or
    - Trimethoprim/sulfamethoxazole DS BID *plus* metronidazole 500 mg TID
    - Treat for 7 to 10 days.
  - Inpatient: Use IV antibiotics.
    - Monotherapy with a β-lactam/β-lactamase inhibitor: piperacillin/tazobactam (3,375 g IV QID) or ampicillin/sulbactam 3 g IV q6h or ertapenem (1 g IV QD)
    - Penicillin-allergic patient: quinolone (levofloxacin 750 mg IV QD plus metronidazole 500 mg IV TID)
    - Unresponsive or severe disease: imipenem or meropenem
  - Recurrences of acute diverticulitis may be decreased by using mesalamine ± rifaximin or probiotics.
- Diverticular bleeding
  - Consider vasopressin 0.2 to 0.3 U/min through selective intra-arterial catheter.
- Precautions
  - Avoid morphine and other opiates that may increase intraluminal pressure or promote ileus.
  - Increased fiber intake is not recommended in the acute management of diverticulitis.

Second Line
- Outpatient: amoxicillin/clavulanate monotherapy (875/125 mg BID) (contraindicated in patients with clearance <30 mL/min) or moxifloxacin (400 mg PO QD) *plus* metronidazole (500 mg PO TID)
- Severely ill inpatients: ampicillin (500 mg IV q6h) + metronidazole (500 mg IV TID) + a quinolone *or* ampicillin + metronidazole + an aminoglycoside

ISSUES FOR REFERRAL
- Acute diverticulitis patients should follow up with a gastroenterologist or surgeon after resolution of diverticulitis (6 to 8 weeks) for colonoscopy to exclude malignancy, fistula, strictures, or inflammatory bowel disease (2).

- Acute complicated diverticulitis should have appropriate surgical and critical care/infectious disease consultations.

SURGERY/OTHER PROCEDURES
- Acute diverticulitis
  - Indications for emergent surgery: peritonitis, uncontrolled sepsis, perforation, obstruction
  - Hinchey I and II: consultation to interventional radiology to drain large abscesses (>4 cm) (4)
  - Hinchey III or IV: may require surgery during the same hospital admission
  - Elective colon resection in recurrent diverticulitis is a case-by-case decision and is typically performed during the quiescent phase following appropriate nonoperative treatment (2).
  - Immunocompromised patients are more likely to present with acute complicated diverticulitis, fail medical management, and have complications from elective surgery.
- Diverticular bleeding
  - Endoscopy and hemostasis via epinephrine injection, electrocautery, or clipping
  - Angiography is preferred over endoscopy in unstable patients to identify the bleeding source and embolize the feeding artery.
  - Massive or recurrent bleeding requires limited or subtotal colectomy to control hemorrhage.

COMPLEMENTARY & ALTERNATIVE MEDICINE
Probiotics have been used to prevent recurrence with mixed success.

ADMISSION, INPATIENT, AND NURSING CONSIDERATIONS
- Admit for systematic toxicity, sepsis, and/or peritonitis (complicated diverticulitis).
- Admit patients who cannot tolerate oral intake or who need IV fluids, analgesics, antibiotics, and bowel rest.

 ONGOING CARE

DIET
- Bowel rest with NPO during acute diverticulitis; advance diet as tolerated as bowel function returns
- Patients with known diverticulosis or a history of diverticulitis should consume a high-fiber diet to prevent recurrence (3).
- Avoiding nuts and popcorn is not necessary (3).

PROGNOSIS
- Good with early detection and prompt treatment
- After first episode of diverticulitis, there is a 33% chance of recurrence. After a second episode, there is a 66% chance of further recurrence.
- Most complications occur during first bout of diverticulitis.
- Younger patients are more likely to have recurrence.
- Rebleeding occurs in up to 6%.

COMPLICATIONS
Hemorrhage, perforation, peritonitis, obstruction, abscess, or colovesicular/colovaginal fistula

REFERENCES
1. Strate LL, Modi R, Cohen E, et al. Diverticular disease as a chronic illness: evolving epidemiologic and clinical insights. *Am J Gastroenterol*. 2012;107(10):1486–1493.
2. Feingold D, Steele SR, Lee S, et al. Practice parameters for the treatment of sigmoid diverticulitis. *Dis Colon Rectum*. 2014;57(3):284–294.
3. Stollman N, Smalley W, Hirano I; for American Gastroenterological Association Institute Clinical Guidelines Committee. American Gastroenterological Association Institute guideline on the management of acute diverticulitis. *Gastroenterology*. 2015;149(7):1944–1949.
4. Barnert J, Messmann H. Diagnosis and management of lower gastrointestinal bleeding. *Nat Rev Gastroenterol Hepatol*. 2009;6(11):637–646.

ADDITIONAL READING
- Boynton W, Floch M. New strategies for the management of diverticular disease: insights for the clinician. *Therap Adv Gastroenterol*. 2013;6(3):205–213.
- Katz LH, Guy DD, Lahat A, et al. Diverticulitis in the young is not more aggressive than in the elderly, but it tends to recur more often: systematic review and meta-analysis. *J Gastroenterol Hepatol*. 2013;28(8):1274–1281.
- Templeton AW, Strate LL. Updates in diverticular disease. *Curr Gastroenterol Rep*. 2013;15(8):339.

 CODES

ICD10
- K57.90 Dvrtclos of intest, part unsp, w/o perf or abscess w/o bleed
- K57.30 Dvrtclos of lg int w/o perforation or abscess w/o bleeding
- K57.92 Diverticulitis of intestine, part unspecified, without perforation or abscess without bleeding

CLINICAL PEARLS
- Diverticulosis is common in elderly patients with a sedentary lifestyle who consume a Western diet.
- Patients with diverticulosis benefit from a high-fiber diet.
- Acute uncomplicated diverticulitis can be treated as an outpatient with oral antibiotics. Acute complicated diverticulitis requires hospitalization, bowel rest, and IV antibiotics.
- Surgical consultation is recommended in all cases of acute complicated diverticulitis. Surgical intervention in diverticulitis and diverticular bleeding is a case-by-case decision.
- After an episode of diverticulitis, patients should undergo colonoscopy to rule out malignancy.
- Diverticular disease is a common cause of GI bleeding.

DOMESTIC VIOLENCE

Rhonda A. Faulkner, PhD • Luis T. Garcia, MD

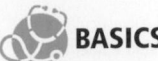 **BASICS**

DESCRIPTION

- Domestic violence (DV) is the behavior in any relationship that is used to gain or maintain power and control over an intimate partner.
- May include physical, sexual, and/or emotional abuse; economic or psychological actions; or threats of actions that influence another person
- Although women are at greater risk of experiencing DV, it occurs among patients of any race, age, sexual orientation, religion, gender, socioeconomic background, and education level.
- Synonym(s): intimate partner violence (IPV); spousal abuse; family violence

EPIDEMIOLOGY

Incidence
In the United States, lifetime estimates of DV are 22–39% of women, with 10–69% reporting physical assault by an intimate partner at some point in their lifetime. DV affects both sexes, but women are more likely to be victims than men and are more likely to report partner violence.

Prevalence
- DV occurs in 1 of 4 American families. Nearly 5.3 million incidents of DV occur each year among U.S. women aged ≥18 years and 3.2 million incidents among men.
- DV results in nearly 2 million injuries and up to 4,000 deaths annually in the United States.
- 14–35% of adult female patients in emergency departments report experiencing DV within the past year.
- Costs of DV are estimated to exceed $5.8 billion annually, of which $4.1 billion are for direct medical and mental health services.
- DV survivors have a 1.6- to 2.3-fold increase in health care use compared with the nonabused population.

Geriatric Considerations
- 4–6% of elderly are abused, with ~2 million elderly persons experiencing abuse and/or neglect each year. In 90% of cases, the perpetrator is a family member.
- Elder abuse is any form of mistreatment that results in harm or loss to an older person; may include physical, sexual, emotional, financial abuse, and/or neglect

Pediatric Considerations
- >3 million children aged 3 to 17 years are at risk of witnessing acts of DV.
- ~1 million abused children are identified in the United States each year.
- Children living in violent homes are at increased risk of physical, sexual, and/or emotional abuse; anxiety and depression; decreased self-esteem; emotional, behavioral, social, and/or physical disturbances; and lifelong poor health.

Pregnancy Considerations
DV occurs during 7–20% of pregnancies. Women with unintended pregnancy are at 3 times greater risk of DV. 25% of abused women report exacerbation of abuse during pregnancy. There is a positive correlation between DV and postpartum depression.

RISK FACTORS
- Patient/victim risk factors
  - Substance abuse
  - Poverty/financial stressors/unemployment
  - Recent loss of social support
  - Family disruption and life cycle changes
  - History of abusive relationships or witness to abuse as child

- Mental or physical disability in family
- Social isolation
- Pregnancy
- Attempting to leave the relationship
- Perpetrator risk factors
  - Substance abuse (e.g., PCP, cocaine, amphetamines, alcohol)
  - Young age
  - Unemployment
  - Low academic achievement
  - Witnessing or experiencing violence as child
  - Depression
  - Personality disorders
  - Threatening to self or others
  - Violence to children or violence outside the home
  - Owns weapons
- Relational risk factors
  - Marital conflict
  - Marital instability
  - Economic stress
  - Traditional gender role norms
  - Poor family functioning
  - Obsessive, controlling relationship

Geriatric Considerations
Factors associated with the abuse of older adults include increasing age, nonwhite race, low-income status, functional impairment, cognitive disability, substance use, poor emotional state, low self-esteem, cohabitation, and lack of social support.

Pediatric Considerations
Factors associated with child abuse or neglect include low-income status, low maternal education, nonwhite race, large family size, young maternal age, single-parent household, parental psychiatric disturbances, and presence of a stepfather.

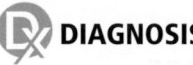 **DIAGNOSIS**

- DV is often underdiagnosed, with only 10–12% of physicians conducting routine screening.
- Although prevalence of DV in primary care settings is 7–50%, <15% are screened.
- Pregnancy increases risk.
- Barriers to screening: time constraints, discomfort with the subject, fear of offending the patient, and lack of perceived skills and resources to manage DV
- Abused patients may refuse to disclose abuse for many reasons, which include the following:
  - Not feeling emotionally ready to admit the reality of the situation
  - Shame and self-blame
  - Feelings of failure if abuse is admitted
  - Fear of rejection by the physician
  - Fear of retribution from abuser
  - Belief that abuse will not happen again
  - Belief that no alternatives or available resources exist

HISTORY
- Physicians should introduce the subject of DV in a general way (i.e., "I routinely ask all patients about domestic violence. Have you ever been in a relationship where you were afraid?").
- How to screen
  - Screen patient alone, without partner or others present.
  - Ask screening questions in patient's primary language; do not use children or other family members as interpreters.

- Partner violence screen (sensitivity 35–71%; specificity 80–94%)
  - "Have you ever been hit, kicked, punched, or otherwise, hurt by someone within the past year? If so, by whom?"
  - "Do you feel safe in your current relationship?"
  - "Is there a partner from a previous relationship who is making you feel unsafe now?"
- CDC-recommended RADAR system
  - **R**: Routinely screen every patient; make screening a part of everyday practice in prenatal, postnatal, routine gynecologic visits, and annual health screenings.
  - **A**: Ask questions directly, kindly, and be nonjudgmental.
  - **D**: Document findings in the patient's chart using the patient's own words, with details. Use body maps and photographs as necessary.
  - **A**: Assess the patient's safety and see if the patient has a safety plan.
  - **R**: Review options for dealing with DV with the patient and provide referrals.
- SAFE questions
  - **S**tress/safety: "Do you feel safe in your relationship?"
  - **A**fraid/abused: "Have you ever been in a relationship where you were threatened, hurt, or afraid?"
  - **F**riends/family: "Are your friends or family aware that you have been hurt? Could you tell them, and would they be able to give you support?"
  - **E**mergency plan: "Do you have a safe place to go and the resources you need in an emergency?"
- HITS questions: "How often does your partner:
  - **H**urt you physically?
  - **I**nsult or talk down to you?
  - **T**hreaten you with harm?
  - **S**cream or curse at you?"
- Assess pregnancy difficulties such as poor/late prenatal care, low-birth-weight babies, and perinatal deaths.
- Pelvic and abdominal pain, chronic without demonstrable pathology
- Headaches, back pain
- Gynecologic disorders
- Sexually transmitted infections (STIs), including HIV/AIDS
- Depression, suicidal ideation, anxiety, fatigue
- Substance abuse
- Eating disorders
- Overuse of health services/frequent emergency room visits
- Noncompliance

PHYSICAL EXAM
- Clinical presentation/psychological signs and symptoms
  - Delay in seeking treatment
  - Inconsistent explanation of injuries
  - Reluctance to undress
  - Signs of battered woman syndrome and/or posttraumatic stress disorder (PTSD) (flat affect/avoidance of eye contact, evasiveness, heightened startle response, sleep disturbance, traumatic flashbacks)
  - Depression, anxiety, chronic fatigue, substance abuse
  - Suspicious partner accompaniment at appointment; overly solicitous partner and/or refusal to leave exam room
- Physical signs and symptoms
  - Tympanic membrane rupture
  - Rectal or genital injury (centrally located injuries with bathing-suit pattern of distribution—concealable by clothing)

– Head and neck injuries (site of 50% of abusive injuries)
– Facial scrapes, loose or broken tooth, bruises, cuts, or fractures to face or body
– Knife wounds, cigarette burns, bite marks, welts with outline of weapon (such as belt buckle)
– Broken bones
– Defensive posture injuries
– Injuries inconsistent with the explanation given
– Injuries in various stages of healing

DIAGNOSTIC TESTS & INTERPRETATION

- The U.S. Preventive Services Task Force (USPSTF) in 2013 issued guidelines recommending that clinicians screen all women of childbearing age (14 to 46 years old) for DV and provide or refer women to intervention services when appropriate (1)[B].
- Other recommendations
  – American College of Physicians (ACP) recommends routine screening for DV for all women in primary care settings at periodic intervals and when women present for emergency care with traumatic injuries.
  – The American Medical Association (AMA) recommends that all patients be routinely screened for DV with inquiry into history of family violence.
  – The World Health Organization (WHO) recommends against DV screening or routine inquiry about exposure to DV; however, they recommend asking about exposure to DV when assessing conditions that may be caused or complicated by abuse (2)[B].
  – U.S. Surgeon General and American Academy of Family Physicians recommend that physicians consider the possibility of DV as a cause of illness and injury.
  – The Partner Violence Screen is a three-question screening tool with a high specificity.
  – There is no evidence of harm in screening for DV.

Pediatric Considerations
American Academy of Pediatrics (AAP) and AMA recommend that physicians remain alert for signs and symptoms of child physical and sexual abuse in the routine exam.

Pregnancy Considerations
American College of Obstetrics and Gynecologists (ACOG) and AMA guidelines on DV recommend that physicians routinely assess all pregnant women for DV. ACOG recommends periodic screening throughout obstetric care (at the first prenatal visit, at least once per trimester, at the postpartum checkup).

Initial Tests (lab, imaging)
Liver function tests (LFTs), amylase, lipase if abdominal trauma is suspected

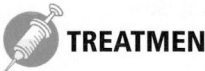 TREATMENT

- Treatment includes initial diagnosis; ongoing medical care; emotional support, counseling, and patient education regarding the DV cycle; referrals to community; and supportive services as needed.
- On diagnosis, use the SOS-DoC intervention:
  – **S**: Offer *Support* and assess *Safety*:
    ○ Support: "You are not to blame. I am sorry this is happening to you. There is no excuse for DV."
    ○ Remind patient of your commitment to confidential communication.

  ○ Safety: Listen and respond to safety issues for the patient: "Do you feel safe going home?"; "Are your children safe?"
  – **O**: Discuss *Options*, including safety planning and follow-up:
    ○ Provide information about DV and help when needed. Make referrals to local resources:
      ▪ "Do you need or want to access a safety shelter or DV service agency?"
      ▪ "Do you want police intervention and if so, would you like me to call the police so they can make a report with you?"
      ▪ Offer numbers to local resources and National DV Hotline: 1-800-799-SAFE (open 24/7; can provide physicians in every state with information on local resources).
  – **S**: Validate patient's *Strengths*:
    ○ "It took courage for you to talk with me today. You have shown great strength in very difficult circumstances."
  – **Do**: *Document* observations, assessment, and plans:
    ○ Use patient's own words regarding injury and abuse.
    ○ Legibly document injuries: Use a body map.
    ○ If possible, take instant photographs of patient's injuries if given patient consent.
    ○ Make patient safety plan. Prepare patient to get away in an emergency:
      ▪ Encourage patient to keep the following items in a safe place: keys (house and car); important papers (Social Security card, birth certificates, photo ID/driver's license, passport, green card); cash, food stamps, credit cards; medication for self and children; children's immunization records; important phone numbers/addresses (friends, family, local shelters); personal care items (e.g., extra glasses).
      ▪ Encourage patient to arrange a signal with someone to let that person know when she or he needs help.
  – **C**: Offer *Continuity*:
    ○ Offer a follow-up appointment and assess barriers to access.

GENERAL MEASURES

- Reporting child and elder abuse to protective services is mandatory in most states. Several states have laws requiring mandatory reporting of IPV.
- Contact the local DV program to find out about laws and community resources before they are needed.
- Display resource materials (National DV Hotline: 1-800-799-SAFE) in the office, all exam rooms, and restrooms.

ADDITIONAL THERAPIES

- National DV Hotline: 1-800-799-SAFE (7233)
- Post in all exam rooms posters in both English and Spanish; available at http://www.thehotline.org /resources/download-materials/

ONGOING CARE

FOLLOW-UP RECOMMENDATIONS

- Schedule prompt follow-up appointment.
- Inquire about what has happened since last visit.
- Review medical records and ask about past episodes to convey concern for the patient and a willingness to address this health issue openly.
- DV often requires multiple interventions over time before it is resolved.

PATIENT EDUCATION

- Counsel patients about nonviolent ways to resolve conflict.
- Educate patients about the cycle of violence.
- Counsel parents about developmentally appropriate ways to discipline their children.
- Educate parents about the negative consequences of arguments on children and each other.
- National Coalition Against Domestic Violence: http://www.ncadv.org/
- CDC: http://www.cdc.gov/violenceprevention/

PROGNOSIS

Most DV perpetrators do not voluntarily seek therapy unless pressured by partners or on legal mandate. Current evidence is insufficient on effectiveness of therapy for perpetrators.

REFERENCES

1. U.S. Preventive Services Task Force. *Intimate Partner Violence and Abuse of Elderly and Vulnerable Adults: Screening.* Rockville, MD: Agency for Healthcare Research and Quality; 2013.
2. Sumner SA, Mercy JA, Dahlberg LL, et al. Violence in the United States: status, challenges, and opportunities. *JAMA.* 2015;314(5):478–488.

ADDITIONAL READING

- Hamberger LK, Rhodes K, Brown J. Screening and intervention for intimate partner violence in healthcare settings: creating sustainable system-level programs. *J Womens Health (Larchmt).* 2015;24(1):86–91.
- Hegarty K, O'Doherty L, Taft A, et al. Screening and counselling in the primary care setting for women who have experienced intimate partner violence (WEAVE): a cluster randomised controlled trial. *Lancet.* 2013;382(9888):249–258.
- Lachs MS, Pillemer KA. Elder abuse. *N Engl J Med.* 2015;373(20):1947–1956.

CODES

ICD10
- T74.91XA Unspecified adult maltreatment, confirmed, initial encounter
- T74.11XA Adult physical abuse, confirmed, initial encounter
- T74.31XA Adult psychological abuse, confirmed, initial encounter

CLINICAL PEARLS

- Display resource materials in the office (e.g., posting abuse awareness posters/National DV Hotline, 1-800-799-SAFE, in both English and Spanish, in all exam rooms and restrooms).
- Given the high prevalence of DV and the lack of harm and potential benefits of screening, routine screening is recommended.
- For those who screened positive, offer resources, reassure confidentiality, and provide close follow-up.

DOWN SYNDROME

Michele Roberts, MD, PhD • Brian G. Skotko, MD, MPP

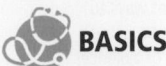

BASICS

DESCRIPTION
- Down syndrome (DS) is a congenital condition associated with intellectual disability and an increased risk of multisystem medical problems.
- System(s) affected: neurologic (100%), cardiac (40–50%), GI (8–12%)
- Synonym(s): trisomy 21

Pediatric Considerations
Murmur may not be present at birth. Delay in recognition of heart condition may lead to irreversible pulmonary hypertension.

Geriatric Considerations
- Life expectancy has increased to ~60 years.
- Age-related health issues occur at earlier age than in the general population.
- Communication difficulties may interfere with prompt recognition of some medical issues.

Pregnancy Considerations
- American College of Obstetricians and Gynecologists (ACOG) recommends all pregnant women be offered traditional prenatal screening and diagnostic testing for DS.
  - Maternal prenatal screening may be performed in the 1st or 2nd trimester.
  - Prenatal diagnostic tests include chorionic villus sampling or amniocentesis.
- ACOG and the Society for Maternal-Fetal Medicine (SMFM) acknowledge that any women may choose noninvasive prenatal screening (NIPS), although conventional screening tests might be more appropriate. American College of Medical Genetics and Genomics (ACMG) recommends all women be offered NIPS (1,2).
- Most, but not all, men with DS are believed to be infertile.
- Most women with DS are subfertile but can conceive children with and without DS.

EPIDEMIOLOGY

Incidence
In the United States, 1/792 live births, ~5,300 births per year (3)

Prevalence
~206,000 persons in the United States (4)

ETIOLOGY AND PATHOPHYSIOLOGY
- Etiology: presence of all or part of an extra chromosome 21
- Trisomy 21: 95% of DS, an extra chromosome 21 is found in all cells due to nondisjunction, usually in maternal meiosis.
- Translocation DS: 3–4% of DS, extra chromosome 21q material is translocated to another chromosome (usually 13, 14, or 21); ~25% have parental origin.
- Mosaic trisomy 21: 1–2% of DS, manifestations may be milder.

Genetics
- Online Mendelian Inheritance in Man (OMIM) 190685
- Inheritance: most commonly sporadic nondisjunction resulting in trisomy 21

- Chance of having another child with DS is
  - 1% (or age risk, whichever is greater) after conceiving a pregnancy with nondisjunction trisomy 21
  - 10–15% for mothers/sisters and 3–5% for fathers/brothers who carry balanced translocation with chromosome 21
  - 100% if the parental balanced translocation is 21;21 (45,t[21;21])
  - Unclear after child with mosaic DS but ~1%

RISK FACTORS
- DS believed to occur in all races and ethnicities with equal frequency
- Chance of having an infant with DS increases with mother's age.
- Relatively more infants with DS are born to younger mothers because younger women are more likely to become pregnant.
- Prenatal diagnosis of DS is more common in older women, and a high percentage of such pregnancies are electively terminated.

GENERAL PREVENTION
- No prevention for nondisjunction trisomy 21
- Preimplantation diagnosis with in vitro fertilization (IVF), prenatal diagnosis followed by termination, and adoption are current options for expectant parents who do not wish to raise a child with DS.

COMMONLY ASSOCIATED CONDITIONS
- Cardiac
  - Congenital heart defects (40–50%)
- GI/growth
  - Feeding problems are common in infancy.
  - Structural defects (~12%)
  - Gastroesophageal reflux
  - Constipation
  - Celiac disease (~5%)
- Pulmonary
  - Tracheal stenosis/tracheoesophageal fistula
  - Pulmonary hypertension
  - Obstructive sleep apnea (50–75%)
- Genitourinary
  - Cryptorchidism, hypospadias
- Hematologic/neoplastic
  - Transient myeloproliferative disorder (~10%): generally resolves spontaneously; can be preleukemic (acute megakaryoblastic leukemia [AMKL]) in 20–30%
  - Leukemia (AMKL or acute lymphoblastic leukemia [ALL]) in 0.5–1%
  - Decreased risk of most solid tumors; increased risk of germ cell tumors/testicular cancer
- Endocrine
  - Hypothyroidism: congenital or acquired (13–63%)
  - Diabetes
- Skeletal
  - Atlantoaxial instability (15%): ~2% symptomatic
  - Short stature is common.
  - Scoliosis (some cases have adult onset)
  - Hip problems (1–4%)
- Immune/rheumatologic
  - Abnormal immune function with increased rate of respiratory infections
  - Increased risk of autoimmune disorders, including Hashimoto thyroiditis, celiac disease, and alopecia

---

- Neurologic
  - Intellectual ability ranging from mild to severe disability. Average is moderate intellectual disability.
  - Autism spectrum disorder (<18%); autism (<6%)
  - Seizures (8%); typically occurring <1 year of age or >30 years of age
  - Alzheimer disease: At least 40% at age 40 years develop signs of dementia; percentage increases with age.
- Psychiatric
  - Attention deficit hyperactivity disorder (ADHD), obsessive-compulsive disorder (OCD), oppositional defiant disorder (ODD), and autism spectrum disorder increased frequency in children.
  - Generalized depression and anxiety with increased frequency in young adults/adults
- Sensory
  - Hearing loss (75%): mostly conductive due to high frequency of asymptomatic middle ear effusion; otitis media (50–70%)
  - Visual impairment (60%): mostly strabismus (refractive errors, 15%), nystagmus, cataracts (15%)
- Dermatologic
  - Xerosis, eczema, palmoplantar hyperkeratosis, atopic or seborrheic dermatitis, onychomycosis, syringomas, furunculosis/folliculitis

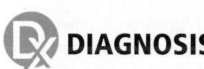

DIAGNOSIS

HISTORY
~85% of mothers of infants with DS learn of the diagnosis postnatally, although this is changing with the availability of NIPS.

PHYSICAL EXAM
- In November 2015, DS-specific growth charts were released. They describe recent growth trends in a sample of children with DS in the United States. These charts can be used as screening tools to help better assess growth and nutritional trends of children with DS, who grow differently from their typically developing peers; these charts do not represent "optimal" growth of children with DS; 50% BMI on the DS-specific growth curves corresponds to the 85% (overweight) on the standard NCHS growth curves (5).
- Infants and children
  - Brachycephaly (100%)
  - Hypotonia (80%)
  - Small ears, often low set and simplified
  - Upslanting palpebral fissure (90%)
  - Epicanthic folds (90%)
  - Brushfield spots
  - Depressed nasal bridge
  - Short neck, often with increased nuchal folds
  - Single palmar crease, single flexion crease on 5th finger
  - Increased space between toes 1 and 2, 5th finger clinodactyly, brachydactyly

DIAGNOSTIC TESTS & INTERPRETATION
Initial Tests (lab, imaging)
- Maternal prenatal screening includes the following:
  - 1st trimester: combined screen (maternal age, β-human chorionic gonadotropin [β-hCG], pregnancy-associated plasma protein A [PAPP-A], and nuchal translucency)
  - 2nd trimester: quad screen (α-fetoprotein, β-hCG, estriol, inhibin A)
  - Sequential screen (combined screen in 1st trimester, if abnormal, obtain amniocentesis or await 2nd trimester quad screening)
  - Integrated screen (combined screening in 1st trimester plus quad screen in 2nd trimester)
  - NIPS with cell-free DNA (beginning at 10 weeks' gestation) (1,2)
- Prenatal diagnosis includes the following:
  - Chorionic villus sampling: 1st trimester, ~99% accurate, ~1% miscarriage
  - Amniocentesis: 2nd trimester, ~99% accurate, ~0.25% miscarriage rate
- Postnatal diagnosis
  - Fluorescence in situ hybridization (FISH) can be performed at time of clinical suspicion, but karyotype should always be done to differentiate type of DS.
  - Parental (and adult-aged sibling) karyotype is indicated only if translocation DS found in child.
- Labs for newborns
  - Echo, with or without murmur
  - CBC with differential (to look for transient myeloproliferative disorder)
  - Thyroid-stimulating hormone (TSH)
  - Audiogram
  - Ophthalmologic exam (look for red reflex)
  - Swallowing study for those with feeding difficulties

Follow-Up Tests & Special Considerations
- After delivering a prenatal diagnosis, the physician should offer "Understanding a Down Syndrome Diagnosis" (http://understandingdownsyndrome.org).
- If the diagnosis is postnatal, the mother and her partner should be informed of the diagnosis promptly by a physician (preferably the obstetrician and pediatrician or family physician), on the basis of clinical observations and before the karyotype is available, but with consideration of extenuating circumstances (e.g., mother's medical condition). The spouse/partner and infant should be present unless this would cause undue delay. The meeting should be private. Refer to the baby by name.
- In the postnatal setting, the physician should be knowledgeable on the subject of DS and should conduct a discussion with content that is current, respectful, balanced, informative, and realistic but not overly pessimistic, concentrating on what is relevant to the 1st year of life.
- Cardiac follow-up, as indicated

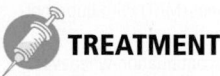 TREATMENT

GENERAL MEASURES
Genetic evaluation and counseling

ISSUES FOR REFERRAL
- Infant stimulation programs (early intervention)
- Lactation consultant
- Physical/occupational/speech therapy
- Educational inclusion supported by federal law
- Pediatric cardiologist, if indicated
- DS specialty clinics can improve medical outcomes.

SURGERY/OTHER PROCEDURES
Repair of congenital anomalies is appropriate. Plastic surgery for facial features is not recommended.

COMPLEMENTARY & ALTERNATIVE MEDICINE
- There is no evidence to support the use of antioxidant or folinic acid supplements in children with DS.
- Craniosacral manipulation is dangerous due to potential atlantoaxial instability.

ADMISSION, INPATIENT, AND NURSING CONSIDERATIONS
If the social situation indicates adoption, consider the National Down Syndrome Adoption Network (NDSAN) (http://www.ndsan.org/) national registry of families seeking to adopt a child with DS.

 ONGOING CARE

FOLLOW-UP RECOMMENDATIONS
Patient Monitoring
The American Academy of Pediatrics recommends ongoing assessment and review, at least annually, the following surveillance:
- Vision: Assess for strabismus, cataracts, and nystagmus by ophthalmologist by 6 months, annually between ages 1 and 5 years, every 2 years ages 5 to 13 years, every 3 years ages 13 to 21 years.
- Hearing: neonatal screen with auditory brainstem response (ABR) or otoacoustic emissions (OAE), then audiogram every 6 months until age 3 years, and then annually
- Thyroid: initial newborn screen. Repeat TSH at 6 months, 12 months, and then annually (5)[C].
- Screening for celiac disease (total IgA and tissue transglutaminase [tTG]-IgA) annually, if symptomatic
- Three-view cervical spine films if patient symptomatic, beginning at 3 to 5 years of age
- Hemoglobin annually to screen for iron deficiency anemia
- Repeat echocardiogram in teens if with murmur or fatigue.
- Integrating specific aspects of DS care into the electronic health record can improve adherence to guidelines that span the life of the child (6)[B].

DIET
- No special diet, but caloric needs are lower in adolescents/adults with DS than their peers.
- Obesity is prevalent at all ages.
- No scientific evidence supports megavitamin therapy or dietary supplements.

PATIENT EDUCATION
- National Down Syndrome Congress: 800-232-NDSC; https://www.ndsccenter.org/
- National Down Syndrome Society: 800-221-4602; https://www.ndss.org/
- The LuMind Down Syndrome Research Foundation provides information on the latest research for people with DS: www.lumindfoundation.org.
- Lettercase provides peer-reviewed booklet for parents who have received a prenatal diagnosis of DS and have not yet made a decision about their pregnancy: https://www.lettercase.org/.
- Down Syndrome Pregnancy provides free downloadable books and articles for expectant mothers who have decided to continue their pregnancies after a prenatal diagnosis of DS: http://downsyndromepregnancy.org/.
- Understanding a Down Syndrome Diagnosis provides an overview of DS and select resources: http://understandingdownsyndrome.org/.

PROGNOSIS
- Associated congenital anomalies are the immediate concern during the newborn period.
- 99% of young adults/adults with DS report being happy with their lives.
- Life expectancy ~60 years

REFERENCES
1. Gregg AR, Skotko BG, Benkendorf JL, et al. Non-invasive prenatal screening for fetal aneuploidy, 2016 update: a position statement of the American College of Medical Genetics and Genomics. *Genet Med*. 2016;18(10):1056–1065.
2. Committee Opinion No. 640: cell-free DNA screening for fetal aneuploidy. *Obstet Gynecol*. 2015;126(3):e31–e37.
3. de Graaf G, Buckley F, Skotko BG. Estimates of the live births, natural losses, and elective terminations with Down syndrome in the United States. *Am J Med Genet A*. 2015;167A(4):756–767.
4. de Graaf G, Buckley F, Skotko BG. Estimation of the number of people with Down syndrome in the United States. *Genet Med*. 2017;19(4):439–447.
5. Zemel BS, Pipan M, Stallings VA, et al. Growth charts for children with Down syndrome in the United States. *Pediatrics*. 2015;136(5):e1204–e1211.
6. Santoro SL, Bartman T, Cua CL, et al. Use of electronic health record integration for down syndrome guidelines. *Pediatrics*. 2018;142(3):e20174119.

ADDITIONAL READING
- Brian Skotko: http://brianskotko.com/publications/
- University of Kentucky's Human Development Institute. *National Center for Prenatal and Postnatal Down Syndrome Resources*. Lexington, KY: University of Kentucky's Human Development Institute; 2012. https://www.dsdiagnosisnetwork.org. Accessed September 21, 2018.

 SEE ALSO

Algorithm: Intellectual Disability

 CODES

ICD10
- Q90.9 Down syndrome, unspecified
- Q90.1 Trisomy 21, mosaicism (mitotic nondisjunction)
- Q90.0 Trisomy 21, nonmosaicism (meiotic nondisjunction)

CLINICAL PEARLS
- 99% of young adults/adults with DS report being happy with their lives.
- DS specialty clinics can improve medical outcomes.

DRUG ABUSE, PRESCRIPTION

Pamela R. Tsinteris, MD, MPH • Matthew A. Silva, PharmD, RPh, BCPS

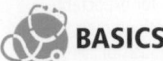

BASICS

DESCRIPTION
- Prescription drug abuse behaviors exist on a continuum and may include:
  - Use of medication for nonmedical reasons such as to get high or enhance performance
  - Use of medication for medical reasons other than what the prescriber intended
  - Use of medication for any reason by someone other than the person for whom the medication was originally prescribed
- Commonly abused prescription medications include opioid analgesics (morphine, oxycodone, hydrocodone, oxymorphone, hydromorphone, fentanyl, methadone, buprenorphine), stimulants (amphetamine, methylphenidate), benzodiazepines (alprazolam, clonazepam, lorazepam), and barbiturates (secobarbital, amobarbital).
- *Diversion* is a term used to describe the rerouting of medications from prescriptions or other legitimate supplies for recreational use or criminal activity, such as selling prescription medication for personal profit.

EPIDEMIOLOGY
- More than half of ED related visits are related to abused or misused pharmaceuticals (opioid and nonopioid).
- Almost half of opioid overdose deaths involve a prescription opioid. In 2015, there were >15,000 overdose deaths involving prescription opioids in the United States.
- Prescription opioid abuse is the strongest predictor of heroin initiation and use.

Incidence
- Predominant sex: males > females
- Predominant age: highest among adults 18 to 25 years (mean 22 years), then adolescents and teens 12 to 17 years, followed by adults ≥26 years

Prevalence
- Lifetime prevalence of prescription drug abuse is highest for opioids, benzodiazepines, and stimulants.
- 18.7 million (6.9%) of U.S. population misuse prescription drugs (opioid and nonopioids combined) and 7.5 million (2.8%) persons age 12 years or older report prescription drug misuse in the past month.
- 11.8 million (4.4%) with some form of opioid misuse
- 11.5 million used prescription opioids and analgesics.
- 6.9 million (59%) used hydrocodone.
- 3.9 million (33%) used oxycodone.
- Only 1 in 5 receives specialty treatment.

ETIOLOGY AND PATHOPHYSIOLOGY
- Opioids, benzodiazepines, stimulants, and barbiturates produce euphoria, tolerance, and dependence leading to misuse and addiction.
- Many adults perceive prescription medications to be more socially acceptable than other illicit drugs.

Genetics
Variant alleles affect the expression and function of opioid, dopamine, acetylcholine, serotonin, and GABA helping to explain susceptibility to different forms of prescription and nonprescription drugs.

RISK FACTORS
- Sociodemographic, psychiatric, pain-, and drug-related factors
- Genetics, environment, family history
- Ongoing opioid prescription (3+ months) greatly increases risk of opioid-related overdose at 1 year (4-fold) and 5 years (30-fold).

GENERAL PREVENTION
- Limit or avoid prescribing controlled medications on the first visit (until the relationship is established).
- Take a thorough history, review records, and perform periodic urine drug screens (UDSs) before deciding if controlled substance is indicated.
- Try all available nonopioid treatments for pain before prescribing opioids for chronic pain.
- Avoid prescribing benzodiazepines. Use other treatments for anxiety (CBT, mindfulness, SSRIs, PRN H1 blocker, buspirone).
- Avoid benzodiazepines and hypnotics in elderly patients.
- Patients should give good informed consent about risks of controlled medications (see "Commonly Associated Conditions" below) before starting AND at least every 3 months while continuing treatment.
- Develop/adopt standard practice agreements for prescribing and monitoring controlled substances with abuse potential.
- Wean/stop prescription analgesics for chronic pain if ineffective for improving pain and function, if aberrant behaviors suggesting opioid use present, or if patient overdoses.
- Dose reduction of chronic opioids can decrease risk while improving pain, function, and quality of life.
- Educate and reinforce safe practices for prescribing medications. Office-based, peer-to-peer education and follow-up with pharmacies help identify abuse behaviors.
- Prescription monitoring programs (PMPs) reduce doctor shopping but not ED visits for overdose and prescription drug abuse–related deaths.
- Identify and treat underlying substance abuse; involve behavioral health providers when possible.
- Prescribe intranasal naloxone to all patients prescribed chronic opioids and provide education to patient and family members on proper use in case of overdose. Intranasal naloxone programs in communities with >1 enrollment/100,000 people and 5 or more opioid-related overdose fatalities reduce new opioid-related overdose deaths.

COMMONLY ASSOCIATED CONDITIONS
- Opioids: tolerance (loss of effectiveness over time), opioid-induced hyperalgesia, dependence (uncomfortable withdrawal if loss of access), addiction (which can lead to loss of savings, job, close relationships and incarceration, HCV or HIV infection, etc.), overdose/death, depression, constipation, low testosterone, and sexual dysfunction with chronic use. Methadone is associated with QT prolongation, which increases risk for torsades de pointes.
- Benzodiazepines and barbiturates: dependence (withdrawal can cause seizures, delirium tremens, death), psychosis, anxiety, sleep driving, blackout states, cognitive impairment, impaired driving while awake; increased fall risk and mortality in elderly patients
- Stimulants: dependence, hypertension, tachyarrhythmias, myocardial ischemia, seizures, hypothermia, psychosis, hallucinations, paranoia, anxiety

DIAGNOSIS

- Initial screening: "How many times in the past year have you used an illegal drug or used a prescription medication for nonmedical reasons?"; primary care setting sensitivity of 100% and specificity of ~75% (1)[C]
- Other screening tools:
  - Drug abuse screening test (DAST) helps determine involvement with drugs over the past year. Assess alcohol use with CAGE or Alcohol Use Disorders Identification Test (AUDIT).

HISTORY
Consider aberrant behaviors when taking a history. Patient may ask for dose escalations and early refills ("spilled the bottle . . . ," "pharmacist shorted me . . . ," etc.). Patients may have a strong preference for one drug, make appointments at end of day and after hours, and/or show hostile/threatening or flattering behavior.

DIAGNOSTIC TESTS & INTERPRETATION
- Despite limited evidence of reliability and accuracy, UDSs are recommended to identify nonadherent patients (2)[C]. Random pill counts are useful for identifying patients taking more controlled substances than prescribed.
- UDS: Order an expanded panel to detect commonly used opioids (ask specifically for semisynthetics [hydrocodone, hydromorphone, oxycodone] and synthetics [methadone, fentanyl, propoxyphene, meperidine]) along with tramadol and buprenorphine.

Initial Tests (lab, imaging)
- Interpretation: Results are positive if drugs that are not prescribed are present; positive in presence of illicit drugs (i.e., marijuana, cocaine). Suspect diversion when negative for prescribed drug.
- Be suspicious if patient refuses test.
- Oxycodone (OxyContin) will be positive for oxycodone and oxymorphone.
- Hydrocodone will be positive for hydrocodone and hydromorphone.
- Codeine will be positive for codeine plus morphine.
- Heroin will be positive for morphine and 6-acetylmorphine if very recent use. Codeine can also be seen as metabolite of common impurities found in heroin.
- If the UDS is positive for morphine, it could mean ingestion of morphine, codeine, or heroin.

TREATMENT

Addiction is a treatable chronic disease. The general approach to treatment includes inpatient, residential, or outpatient detoxification as required; counseling and intensive counseling as needed; and ongoing medication-assisted treatment (MAT) with buprenorphine or injectable naltrexone.

- Begin taper to initiate discontinuation whenever there is evidence of prescription opioid abuse (2)[C]. Some situations indicate immediate discontinuation rather than taper (e.g., diversion or plan to switch to buprenorphine treatment).
- Opioid discontinuation through interdisciplinary pain care programs, buprenorphine-assisted programs, and detoxification programs have achieved opioid discontinuation rates >85% (3)[A].

- Benzodiazepines cannot be stopped abruptly for risk of seizures and death. Discontinue via slow taper or at a controlled detoxification program.
- Amphetamines can be stopped abruptly without risk of severe withdrawal or death.

GENERAL MEASURES
Alcoholics Anonymous/Narcotics Anonymous is helpful, as are Al-Anon/Alateen for family members. Nonjudgmental interactions and cognitive-behavioral therapy focused on motivational interviewing, goal setting, and brief interventions help manage anxiety, insomnia, and denial while improving willingness to change.

MEDICATION
- Short-term opioid detoxification programs use clonidine, buprenorphine/naloxone, or methadone under the direction of an addiction specialist.
- Long-term MAT with buprenorphine/naloxone, methadone, or naltrexone is more effective than short-term detoxification (4)[A].
- Buprenorphine/naloxone and methadone are similarly effective when used in long-term opioid maintenance therapy, and both are effective in the treatment of chronic pain.
- Only an addiction specialist may dispense methadone for treatment of opioid use disorder at a certified site.
- Any provider (MD, DO, NP or PA) may prescribe buprenorphine/naloxone after completing training and obtaining an X waiver. For details, see https://www.samhsa.gov/medication-assisted -treatment/buprenorphine-waiver-management.
- Buprenorphine/naloxone should be continued as long as the patient takes prescribed doses and remains engaged in care; discontinue if there is evidence of buprenorphine/naloxone diversion. The use of buprenorphine/naloxone with benzodiaz-epines, alcohol, and stimulants is risky but safer than buprenorphine/naloxone with other full-dose opioid agonists.
- Buprenorphine/naloxone doses should be titrated to the maximum of 24 mg/day for patients who continue to use other opioids. Methadone or detoxi-fication followed by naltrexone should be recom-mended for those unable to abstain from opioids on maximal buprenorphine/naloxone dosing.
- Buprenorphine/naloxone formulations discourage abuse and diversion because naloxone displaces buprenorphine binding to opioid receptors when taken parenterally (naloxone is not well absorbed sublingually).
- Buprenorphine without naloxone is prone to diver-sion and abuse because it can be crushed, snorted, or injected. Previously recommended for use in pregnant patients because of concern for possible fetal harm from naloxone, this recommendation is not evidence-based, and many clinicians prescribe the combined product in pregnancy.
- The opioid antagonist naltrexone (oral or long-acting injectable) reduces cravings for opioids and blocks opioid-euphoria when ingested and does not require special training to prescribe. Naltrexone should not be started until a full 7-day wash-out is ensured to avoid precipitating severe withdrawal (5,6)[A]. This requirement for injectable naltrexone means fewer patients will be successful starting buprenorphine/naloxone, but once started, effective-ness of injectable naltrexone is similar.
- There is neither support for using nor for converting to long half-life benzodiazepines before beginning

a slow benzodiazepine taper, although diazepam is often preferred. Carbamazepine may be useful in patients dependent on ≥20 mg diazepam equivalents daily. Antidepressants may be helpful for depression and anxiety linked to benzodiazepine withdrawal. There are no specific benefits shown using propranolol, buspirone, progesterone, or hydroxyzine to manage withdrawal symptoms.
- Atomoxetine and bupropion SR can also be helpful in managing ADHD symptoms in select patients.

ISSUES FOR REFERRAL
Enlist the help of chemical dependency groups/ addiction specialists/pain management and psychiatry/ psychology when patients have polysubstance abuse and to treat underlying mood and anxiety disorders, PTSD, and ADHD.

COMPLEMENTARY & ALTERNATIVE MEDICINE
Acupuncture, yoga, meditation, or martial arts may help with anxiety management and stress reduction.

ADMISSION, INPATIENT, AND NURSING CONSIDERATIONS
Indications for inpatient detoxification include concomitant alcohol and benzodiazepine dependence (increased risk of seizures), mental confusion/delirium, history of seizures, psychosis, active suicidal ideation, serious comorbid medical issues, or absence of social support.

 ONGOING CARE

PATIENT EDUCATION
- Controlled medication should be inaccessible to others (ideally in locked box/bag). Diverting medica-tion may result in legal charges. Patients should be aware of addiction potential when starting controlled substances and about withdrawal symp-toms if a medication is stopped abruptly. Respiratory depression and death are possible when opioids are mixed with benzodiazepines. Avoid alcohol and illicit drugs.
- Red flags include a need for higher doses, dose escalation and use to feel high or overcome stress, cravings, and preoccupation about the next dose. Create a mutual plan to stop prescription medica-tions and try something new.
- Consider and use family dynamics as an important behavioral component.

REFERENCES
1. Smith PC, Schmidt SM, Allensworth-Davies D, et al. A single-question screening test for drug use in primary care. *Arch Intern Med*. 2010;170(13): 1155–1160.
2. Manchikanti L, Abdi S, Atluri S, et al. American Society of Interventional Pain Physicians (ASIPP) guidelines for responsible opioid prescribing in chronic non-cancer pain: part I—evidence assess-ment. *Pain Physician*. 2012;15(Suppl 3):S1–S65.
3. Frank JW, Lovejoy TI, Becker WC, et al. Patient outcomes in dose reduction or discontinuation of long-term opioid therapy: a systematic review. *Ann Intern Med*. 2017;167(3):181–191.
4. Mattick RP, Breen C, Kimber J, et al. Buprenorphine maintenance versus placebo or methadone maintenance for opioid dependence. *Cochrane Database Syst Rev*. 2014;(2):CD002207.

5. Comer SD, Sullivan MA, Yu E, et al. Injectable, sustained-release naltrexone for the treatment of opioid dependence: a randomized, placebo-controlled trial. *Arch Gen Psychiatry*. 2006;63(2):210–218.
6. Lee JD, Nunes EV, Novo P, et al. Comparative effectiveness of extended-release naltrexone versus buprenorphine-naloxone for opioid relapse prevention (X:BOT): a multicentre, open-label, randomised controlled trial. *Lancet*. 2018;391(10118):309–318.

ADDITIONAL READING
- Ahrnsbrak R, Bose J, Hedden S, et al. *Key Substance Use and Mental Health Indicators in the United States: Results from the 2016 National Survey on Drug Use and Health*. Rockville, MD: Center for Behavioral Health Statistics and Quality, Substance Abuse and Mental Health Services Administration, United States Department of Health and Human Services; 2017.
- Dowell D, Haegerich TM, Chou R. CDC guideline for prescribing opioids for chronic pain—United States, 2016. *JAMA*. 2016;315(15):1624–1645. doi:10.1001/jama.2016.1464.
- Jones CM, McAninch JK. Emergency department visits and overdose deaths from combined use of opioids and benzodiazepines. *Am J Prev Med*. 2015;49(4):493–501.

 CODES

ICD10
- F19.10 Other psychoactive substance abuse, uncomplicated
- F11.10 Opioid abuse, uncomplicated
- F15.10 Other stimulant abuse, uncomplicated

CLINICAL PEARLS
- Education and PMPs help prevent prescription drug abuse.
- Standardized office practice agreements can help manage controlled substance prescriptions.
- Perform informed consent about all risks of controlled substances before starting and every 3 months while prescribing.
- Conduct frequent UDSs (weekly to every 3 months) for all patients prescribed controlled substances.
- Discontinue prescription opioid analgesics if pain or functionality does not improve or if there is evidence of abuse (i.e., positive UDSs, driving while intoxicated [DWI], overdose, early refills).
- Limit benzodiazepine use to 2 to 4 weeks.
- A single effective screening question is "How many times in the past year have you used an illegal drug or prescription medication for nonmedical reasons?"
- Buprenorphine/naloxone is an effective treatment for opioid use disorder that can be prescribed by any provider after completing training and obtaining an X waiver. Buprenorphine/naloxone can also be used to treat chronic pain in those with opioid dependence.
- Other MATs for opioid use disorder include nal-trexone (no special training required to prescribe) and methadone (although methadone can only be used to treat opioid use disorder by an addiction specialist).

DUCTAL CARCINOMA IN SITU

Bradley M. Turner, MD, MPH, MHA, FCAP, FASCP • David G. Hicks, MD

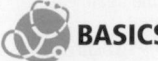 **BASICS**

DESCRIPTION
- Ductal carcinoma in situ (DCIS) is a heterogeneous group of lesions that have in common the presence of a clonal proliferation of neoplastic, *noninvasive* epithelial cells confined to ducts and lobules.
- Considered a premalignant lesion
- Classified as low, intermediate, or high grade
- Mortality from DCIS with subsequent progression to invasive breast carcinoma (IBC) is low, regardless of histologic type or type of treatment.

EPIDEMIOLOGY
Incidence
- Average annual percentage increase of 1%
- Estimated 62,117 new diagnoses of DCIS in 2018
- Estimated 62,738 new diagnoses of DCIS in 2019
- DCIS accounts for approximately 80–85% of in situ breast carcinomas (lobular carcinoma in situ [LCIS] accounts for approximately 15–20%).
- More stable incidence in women 50 to 69 years old
- Increasing incidence in women <50 and >70 years old
- Represents ~26% of all new IBC
- Incidence rate comparable in different ethnicities

ETIOLOGY AND PATHOPHYSIOLOGY
- A nonobligate precursor to IBC
- Poorly understood spectrum of polyclonal and clonal epithelial proliferative lesions—final step prior to IBC
- The changes necessary for transition to IBC are poorly understood.
- Molecular evidence suggests that low- and high-grade DCIS are genetically distinct lesions, with high-grade DCIS associated with more aggressive disease.

Genetics
- Low-grade DCIS typically expresses estrogen receptor (ER) and progesterone receptor (PR), without HER2 protein overexpression or amplification.
- High-grade DCIS not consistently ER+ or PR+; frequent HER2 protein overexpression and amplification (even more frequent compared to IBC); commonly associated with p53 gene mutations
- *BRCA1* and *BRCA2* associations observed
- Consider genetic counseling in high-risk DCIS patients.

RISK FACTORS
- Similar to IBC, although not as strongly associated
- Female gender, nulliparity, late age at first birth or menopause, first-degree relative with breast cancer, long-term use of postmenopausal combined estrogen and progestin therapy, high breast density, history of atypical ductal hyperplasia (ADH)
- Association with age, body mass index, smoking, lactation, early menarche, alcohol consumption, and oral contraceptive use is less clear.

GENERAL PREVENTION
- Controversy exists because studies have suggested that screening may result in overdiagnosis with little or no reduction in the incidence of advanced cancers.
- General screening guidelines suggested for asymptomatic women with an average risk
- Women with increased risk should have more aggressive screening (risk assessment tool available at http://www.cancer.gov/bcrisktool/Default.aspx).

- General screening guidelines—U.S. Preventive Services Task Force (USPSTF):
  – Biennial mammography for women aged 50 to 74 years (B recommendation)
  – The decision to start screening mammography in women <50 years should be an individual one.
  – If a higher value is placed on potential benefit, consider beginning biennial screening between 40 and 49 years of age (C recommendation).
  – Insufficient evidence regarding benefits and harms of screening mammography if ≥75 years old
  – Insufficient evidence to assess the benefits and harms of digital breast tomosynthesis (DBT) as a primary screening method (I statement)
  – Insufficient evidence to assess the balance of benefits and harms of adjunctive screening using breast ultrasonography, magnetic resonance imaging (MRI), DBT, or other methods in women identified to have dense breasts on an otherwise negative screening mammogram (I statement)
- General screening guidelines—National Comprehensive Cancer Network (NCCN):
  – Women should be familiar with their breasts and promptly report changes; periodic consistent BSE may facilitate breast self-awareness.
  – Age 25 to 39 years: breast awareness, CBE every 1 to 3 years
  – Age ≥40 years: breast awareness, annual CBE, annual screening mammography
- Clinical judgment when applying screening guidelines
- Mammography screening should be individualized.
- If no intervention would occur based on screening findings, patient should not undergo screening.
- Risk reduction:
  – Assess familial/genetic history.
  – Lifestyle modifications: Limit alcohol intake to <1 drink per day, exercise, maintain healthy diet, and weight control.
  – Risk reduction surgery supported for carefully selected women at high risk of breast cancer
  – Hormonal risk reduction agents (i.e., tamoxifen) recommended in certain high-risk women ≥35 years old
  – Benefits of aromatase inhibitors are less clear.
  – Recent clinical trial with anastrozole (an aromatase inhibitor) significantly decreased incidence of DCIS in postmenopausal women.

DIAGNOSIS

HISTORY
- Most DCIS is now diagnosed by screening mammography (presence of microcalcifications in approximately 72%); patients may be asymptomatic with nonpalpable mass (12%).
- More advanced lesions may present with a palpable mass, spontaneous nipple discharge, or Paget disease.

PHYSICAL EXAM
- CBE with patient in upright and supine position; evaluating for asymmetry, spontaneous discharge, skin changes (peau d'orange, erythema, scaling); nipple retraction/excoriation (Paget disease)
- Palpation of all breast quadrants, including lymph node examination (axillary, supraclavicular, and internal mammary nodes)
- Positive clinical findings: Refer for consideration of diagnostic imaging and/or surgical evaluation unless <30 years old with a low clinical suspicion (observe 1 to 2 menstrual cycles; refer if clinical findings persist).

DIFFERENTIAL DIAGNOSIS
Usual ductal hyperplasia, flat epithelial atypia, ADH, LCIS, microinvasive carcinoma

DIAGNOSTIC TESTS & INTERPRETATION
Initial Tests (lab, imaging)
- Mammography Breast Imaging Reporting and Data System (BI-RADS: categories 0 to 6) is used for uniform reporting of mammography results.
- Interpretation and screening recommendations:
  – 0: needs additional imaging: diagnostic workup with consideration for diagnostic imaging
  – 1: negative: screening recommendations
  – 2: benign findings: screening recommendations
  – 3: probably benign finding: diagnostic imaging at 6 months, every 6 to 12 months for 2 to 3 years; consider biopsy if patient anxious or follow-up uncertain.
  – 4: suspicious: diagnostic imaging with follow-up
  – 5: highly suggestive of malignancy: diagnostic imaging with follow-up
  – 6: known biopsy-proven malignancy: NCCN guidelines for breast cancer should be followed.
- Similar for diagnostic ultrasound (US)
- DCIS seen as clustered microcalcifications
- *Diagnostic* imaging will result in consideration for tissue biopsy.

Follow-Up Tests & Special Considerations
- US not recommended for *screening*
- Sensitivity of breast MRI screening > mammography with < specificity resulting in > false positives
- Screening MRI only recommended in certain women:
  – *BRCA* mutation—*commence at age 25 to 29 years*
  – First-degree relative of *BRCA* carrier—*commence at age 25 to 29 years*
  – ≥20% lifetime risk of breast cancer defined by models that are largely based on family history—*annual breast MRI to begin 10 years prior to the youngest family member but not prior to age 25 years*
  – Thoracic radiation between the ages of 10 and 30 years—*annual breast MRI to begin 10 years after radiation therapy but not prior to age 25 years*
  – Presence of Li-Fraumeni, *PTEN*, or Bannayan-Riley-Ruvalcaba syndrome in patient or first-degree relative
  – ≥20% risk of breast cancer based on gene and/or risk level: ATM, CDH1, CHEK2, PALB2, PTEN, STK11, TP53
- Insufficient evidence to recommend for or against MRI screening in the following groups: 15–20% lifetime risk of breast cancer, defined by models that are largely based on family history; heterogeneous or extremely dense breast tissue on mammography; personal history of breast cancer or DCIS
- Screening with MRI is not recommended in women with <15% lifetime risk of breast cancer.
- MRI can also complement mammography in patients with skin changes.
- Although MRI and US are complementary diagnostic methods to mammography, US is less sensitive in detecting most microcalcifications and MRI does not typically detect microcalcifications at all.
- *After a diagnosis* of DCIS, MRI has been prospectively shown to have a sensitivity of up to 98% for high-grade DCIS (1)[A].

- The NCCN Panel has included breast MRI as indicated during the initial workup of DCIS, noting that the use of MRI has not been shown to increase the likelihood of negative margins or decrease the conversion to mastectomy with DCIS.
- Pathology
  - Tissue is necessary for diagnosis: typically core needle (CN) or vacuum-assisted (VA) biopsy (mammographic/stereotactic, US, or MRI guided). Open surgical biopsy can be performed in patients not amenable to CN or VA biopsy.
  - Fine-needle aspiration (FNA) is not adequate for specific diagnosis of DCIS; however, it can suggest the presence of neoplastic cells.
  - Histologic classification
    - Classification is subjective; however, traditionally classified as either low, intermediate, or high grade based on architectural patterns (comedo, solid, cribriform, clinging, papillary, and micropapillary), nuclear grade (I, II, or III), and the absence or presence of necrosis
    - Ductal intraepithelial neoplasia (DIN) is an alternative histologic classification incorporating size as a discriminating factor.
    - Grade is more important for prognosis, risk for progression, and local recurrence.
    - Comedo-type necrosis (necrosis filling central portion of involved duct) is typically seen in high-grade DCIS, with varying degrees of necrosis in other types of DCIS.
  - Determination of ER and PR status (1)[A]
  - Studies show unclear or weak evidence of HER2 status as a prognostic indicator in DCIS.

TREATMENT

SURGERY/OTHER PROCEDURES

- Surgery is the primary treatment option. Options for surgery are based on risk of recurrence, anatomic location, extent of disease, and the ability to achieve "negative" margins (1)[A].
- Positive margins are considered "ink on tumor."
- Totality of evidence does not support the routine practice of obtaining negative margin widths wider than 2 mm (1)[C].
- Margins <1 mm considered inadequate (1)[A]
- Margins <1 mm at the breast fibroglandular boundary (chest wall or skin) do not mandate surgical excision but may be an indication for higher boost dose radiation in patients opting for breast conservation (1)[A].
- DCIS with microinvasion, defined as no invasive focus >1 mm in size, should be considered as DCIS when considering the optimal margin width (1)[C]. When there is only minimal or focal DCIS involvement near the margin, clinical judgment can be applied to determine if reexcision might be avoided in individual cases (1)[C].
- Surgical options include the following:
  - Breast conservation (lumpectomy) without lymph node procedure, without breast radiation therapy (1)[A]
  - Breast conservation (lumpectomy) without lymph node procedure, with whole breast radiation therapy, with or without boost to tumor bed (1)[A]
  - A complete axillary lymph node dissection should not be performed in the absence of evidence of invasive cancer or proven axillary metastatic disease (1)[A].

- A sentinel lymph node biopsy may be considered if the lumpectomy is in an anatomic location compromising the performance of a future sentinel lymph node procedure (1)[C].
- Radiation decreases recurrence rates by about 50% but with limited overall survival benefit.
- ~50% of recurrences are pure DCIS; ~50% are IBC (1)[A].
- Drawbacks to radiation therapy include (i) the patient's burden of daily treatment for 6 weeks and short-term side effects, such as fatigue and skin toxicity; (ii) a slightly increased risk of secondary cancers; and (iii) inability to receive radiation therapy again in the ipsilateral breast should an invasive carcinoma develop.
- Recurrence generally requires mastectomy with consideration for systemic treatment.
- Patients not amenable to margin-free lumpectomy should have total mastectomy (1)[C].
- Mastectomy with or without sentinel node biopsy plus optional breast reconstruction (1)[A]
- Mastectomy provides maximum local control.
- Rates of recurrence for DCIS and IBC are similar to lumpectomy.
- Recurrence should be treated with wide local excision, chest wall radiation, and consideration for systemic treatment (1)[A].
- Long-term cause-specific survival seems to be equivalent to lumpectomy with whole breast radiation (1)[A].
- A sentinel lymph node biopsy may also be considered in patients with seemingly pure DCIS to be treated with mastectomy (1)[C].
- Secondary chemoprevention following breast-conserving surgery for ER + DCIS:
  - Tamoxifen for premenopausal patients or tamoxifen or an aromatase inhibitor for postmenopausal patients for 5 years
  - There may be some advantage for aromatase inhibitor therapy in patients <60 years old or patients with concerns for thromboembolism (1)[C].
  - Considered in lumpectomy patients with or without whole breast radiation (1)[A]
  - Benefit of tamoxifen and trastuzumab in ER-negative/HER2-positive disease is unclear.

ONGOING CARE

FOLLOW-UP RECOMMENDATIONS

- History and physical exam every 6 to 12 months for the first 5 years and then annually
- Mammography every 12 months (first mammogram 6 to 12 months after breast conservation therapy) (1)[C]
- If treated with tamoxifen or an aromatase inhibitor, monitor per NCCN guidelines for breast cancer risk reduction (1)[C].

PROGNOSIS

- Good prognosis: 10-year breast cancer–specific survival rates of >95%; overall mortality after diagnosis of treated pure DCIS generally >98%
- Risk of local recurrence after mastectomy generally reported as 1–2% (higher in some studies)
- Higher risk of local recurrences after breast-conserving therapy in younger age (particularly before age 40 years), larger tumor size, high nuclear grade, comedo-type necrosis, and close/positive margin status (related to DCIS volume)

- ER+ tumors are associated with lower risk for recurrence.
- There is interest in identifying subsets of patients who have low rates of ipsilateral breast tumor recurrence such that they might safely forgo radiation. The Oncotype DX DCIS test may help clinicians in selecting which patients with DCIS might safely forgo radiation therapy after breast-conserving surgery (2)[C]. The test results in an Oncotype DX DCIS score, with the following risk categories: *DCIS score <39* (low risk of recurrence; radiation therapy benefits likely to be small and will not outweigh the risks of side effects); *DCIS score 39 to 54* (intermediate risk of recurrence; radiation therapy benefits unclear relative to the risks of side effects); *DCIS score 55 to 100* (high risk of recurrence; radiation therapy benefits are likely to be greater than the risks of side effects)

REFERENCES

1. National Comprehensive Cancer Network. NCCN clinical practice guidelines in oncology: breast cancer (Version 3.2018) 2018. http://www.nccn.org. Accessed November 8, 2018.
2. Wood WC, Alvarado M, Buchholz DJ, et al. The current clinical value of the DCIS Score. *Oncology (Williston Park)*. 2014;28(5 Suppl 2):C2, 1–8, C3.

ADDITIONAL READING

Siu AL; for U.S. Preventive Services Task Force. Screening for breast cancer: U.S. Preventive Services Task Force recommendation statement. *Ann Intern Med*. 2016;164(4):279–296.

 SEE ALSO

Breast Cancer

CODES

ICD10

- D05.10 Intraductal carcinoma in situ of unspecified breast
- D05.11 Intraductal carcinoma in situ of right breast
- D05.12 Intraductal carcinoma in situ of left breast

CLINICAL PEARLS

- DCIS is a heterogeneous group of *noninvasive* neoplastic breast ductal epithelial cell lesions.
- The incidence of DCIS has continued to increase in women <50 and >70 years of age, with a more stable incidence in women 50 to 69 years of age.
- The goal of DCIS treatment is to prevent recurrence and progression to IBC.
- The Oncotype DX DCIS score may help clinicians in selecting which patients with DCIS might safely forgo radiation therapy after breast-conserving surgery.
- Current standard of care is breast-conserving therapy with consideration for postoperative whole breast radiation therapy and/or postsurgical tamoxifen or aromatase inhibitor therapy, unless otherwise contraindicated.
- With appropriate therapy, the overall prognosis of pure DCIS is good.

DUPUYTREN CONTRACTURE

Rebecca M. King, MD • Karl T. Clebak, MD, FAAFP • Shawn F. Phillips, MD, MSPT

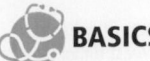 BASICS

DESCRIPTION
- Palmar fibromatosis; caused by progressive fibrous proliferation and tightening of the fascia of the palms, resulting in flexion deformities and loss of function
- Not the same as "trigger finger," which is caused by thickening of the distal flexor tendon
- Similar change rarely occurs in plantar fascia, usually appearing simultaneously.
- System(s) affected: musculoskeletal
- Dupuytren diathesis is an aggressive form that has ectopic involvement of knuckle pads, plantar fibromatosis (Ledderhose – 10%), and penile fibromatosis (Peyronie – 2%).
- Synonyms: morbus Dupuytren; Dupuytren disease; "Celtic hand;" Viking's disease; palmar fascial fibromatosis, contracture of palmar fascia

EPIDEMIOLOGY
Prevalence
- Increases with age; mean prevalence in western countries: 12%, 21%, and 29% at ages 55, 65, and 75 years, respectively. Norway: 30% of males >60 years; Spain: 19% of males >60 years
- More common in Caucasians of Scandinavian or Northern European ancestry
- Mean age of onset is 60 years.

ETIOLOGY AND PATHOPHYSIOLOGY
Unknown; possibly oxidative stress, altered wound repair, and/or abnormal immune response; occurs in three stages:
- Proliferative phase: proliferation of myofibroblasts with nodule development on palmar surface
- Involutional stage: spread along palmar fascia to fingers with cord development
- Residual phase: spread into fingers with cord tightening and contracture formation

Genetics
- Autosomal dominant with incomplete penetrance:
  – Siblings with 3-fold risk
- 68% of male relatives of affected patients develop disease at some time.
- Possible association with HLA alleles

RISK FACTORS
- Smoking (mean 16 pack-years, odds ratio: 2.8)
- Increasing age
- Male/Caucasian; male > female (range 3.5:1 to 9:1)
- Vibration exposure and manual work— risk doubles if regular (weekly) exposure

- Diabetes mellitus (DM) (increases with duration of DM, usually mild; middle and ring finger involved)
- Epilepsy
- Chronic illness (e.g., pulmonary tuberculosis, liver disease, HIV)
- Hypercholesterolemia
- Excessive alcohol consumption
- Northern European ethnicity
- Family history
- Hand trauma
- Low body weight and BMI

GENERAL PREVENTION
Avoid risk factors, especially if a strong family history.

COMMONLY ASSOCIATED CONDITIONS
- Alcoholism
- Epilepsy (inconstant data)
- DM
- Chronic lung disease
- Occupational hand trauma (vibration)
- Hypercholesterolemia
- Carpal tunnel syndrome
- Peyronie disease
- HIV
- Cancer
- Adhesive capsulitis of shoulder

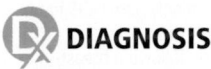 DIAGNOSIS

HISTORY
- Caucasian male aged 50 to 60 years
- Family history
- Mild pain early:
  – Begins in palm and spreads to digits
- Unilateral or bilateral (50%)
- Right hand more frequent
- Ring finger or little finger most common, but any digit can be involved
- Ulnar digits more affected than radial digits
- Flexion contracture of metacarpophalangeal (MCP) before proximal interphalangeal (PIP) joint

PHYSICAL EXAM
- Painless plaques or nodules in palmar fascia
- Cordlike band in the palmar fascia
- Skin adheres to fascia and becomes puckered.
- Palpable subcutaneous nodules
- Reduced flexibility of MCP and PIP joints
- No sign of inflammation
- Web space contractures

- Knuckle pads over PIP
  – Garrod nodes associated with severe disease
- Disease stages:
  – Early: skin pits (can also be seen in nevoid basal cell cancer and palmar keratosis)
  – Intermediate: nodules and cords. Nerves and vessels can be entwined in cords.
  – Late: contractures

DIFFERENTIAL DIAGNOSIS
- Camptodactyly: early teens; tight fascial bands on ulnar side of small finger
- Diabetic cheiroarthropathy: all four fingers
- Volkmann ischemic contracture
- Trigger finger
- Ganglion cyst

DIAGNOSTIC TESTS & INTERPRETATION
Diagnostic Procedures/Other
Diagnosis based on history and physical, testing is not routinely indicated. MRI can assess cellularity of lesions that correlate with recurrence after surgery.

Test Interpretation
- Myofibroblasts predominate.
- Nodules: Lumps fixed to skin hypercellular masses
- Cords: organized collagen type III arranged parallel and hypocellular
- First stage (proliferative): increased myofibroblasts
- Second stage (residual): dense fibroblast network
- Third stage (involutional): Myofibroblasts disappear.

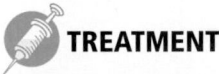 TREATMENT

GENERAL MEASURES
- Physical therapy alone is ineffective:
  – Intermittent splinting is unlikely to be effective.
  – Continuous splinting may help pre- and postop.
- Follow isolated involvement of palmar fascia conservatively.
- MCP joint involvement can be followed conservatively if flexion contracture is <30 degrees.

MEDICATION
First Line
- Clostridial collagenase injections (FDA-approved 2010):
  – Degrades collagen to allow manual rupture of diseased cord
  – Best for isolated cord of MCP joint
  – 5-year recurrence rate of 47%; comparable with surgical recurrence rates (1)[B]
  – More rapid recovery of hand function compared to limited fasciectomy with fewer serious adverse events (2)[B]

- Complications: injection site reaction, skin tear
- Can do two cords concurrently
- Can be effective for postsurgical recurrence
- Steroid injection:
  - Can treat acute nodules or painful knuckle pads
  - Serial triamcinolone injections improved long-term outcomes when combined with needle aponeurotomy (3)[B].
  - Steroid alone associated with 50% recurrence in 1 to 3 years

Second Line
Surgery for contracture >30%

ISSUES FOR REFERRAL
- Any involvement of PIP joints
- MCP joints contracted >30 degrees
- Impaired function
- Progressively worsening contracture
- Disabling deformity

ADDITIONAL THERAPIES
- Percutaneous and needle fasciotomy:
  - Best for MCP joint; improvement of 93% versus 57% for PIP joint
  - Recurrence common; 50%
  - Shown to be effective for recurrent disease
  - Better for MCP joints in patients with comorbid conditions; lower complication rate, but higher recurrence
  - At 3 months and 1 year, outcomes of needle fasciotomy and collagenase injections are the same (4)[B].

SURGERY/OTHER PROCEDURES
- Dermofasciectomy/limited fasciectomy/segmental aponeurectomy:
  - Greater initial correction over nonincisional treatment; higher complication rates
  - Percutaneous aponeurotomy and lipofilling (PALF) is a new, minimally invasive procedure that appears to have shorter convalescence, less long-term complications, similar operative contraction correction, and no significant difference at 1 year in results versus limited fasciectomy (5)[A].
- Indications:
  - Any involvement of the PIP joints
  - MCP joints contracted at least 30 degrees
  - Positive Hueston tabletop test (Patient is unable to lay palm flat on a table.)
- May require skin grafts for wound closure with severe cutaneous shrinkage
- 80% have full range of movement with early surgery.
- Amputation of 5th digit if severe and deforming
- MCP joints respond better to surgery than PIP joints, especially if contracted >45 degrees.

ONGOING CARE

FOLLOW-UP RECOMMENDATIONS
Patient Monitoring
Regular follow-up every 6 months to 1 year

PATIENT EDUCATION
- Avoid risk factors (alcohol, vibratory exposure, etc.), especially if strong family history.
- Mild disease: Passively stretch digits twice a day and avoid recurrent gripping of tools.

PROGNOSIS
- Unpredictable but usually slowly progressive
- 10% may regress spontaneously.
- Dupuytren diathesis predicts aggressive course. Features include ethnicity (Nordic), family history, bilateral lesions outside of palm, age <50 years—all factors with 71% risk of recurrence compared to baseline 23% without any risk factors.
- Prognosis better for MCP versus PIP joint after surgery and collagenase injection

COMPLICATIONS
- Complex regional pain syndrome
- Operative nerve injury
- Postoperative recurrence in 46–80%
- Postoperative hand edema and skin necrosis
- Digital infarction
- Limited hand function

REFERENCES

1. Peimer CA, Blazar P, Coleman S, et al. Dupuytren contracture recurrence following treatment with collagenase *Clostridium histolyticum* (CORDLESS [Collagenase Option for Reduction of Dupuytren Long-Term Evaluation of Safety Study]): 5-year data. *J Hand Surg Am*. 2015;40(8):1597–1605.
2. Zhou C, Hovius SE, Slijper HP, et al. Collagenase *Clostridium histolyticum* versus limited fasciectomy for Dupuytren's contracture: outcomes from a multicenter propensity score matched study. *Plast Reconstr Surg*. 2015;136(1):87–97.
3. McMillan C, Binhammer P. Steroid injection and needle aponeurotomy for Dupuytren disease: long-term follow-up of a randomized controlled trial. *J Hand Surg Am*. 2014;39(10):1942–1947.
4. Scherman P, Jenmalm P, Dahlin LB. One-year results of needle fasciotomy and collagenase injection in treatment of Dupuytren's contracture: a two-centre prospective randomized clinical trial. *J Hand Surg Eur Vol*. 2016;41(6):577–582.
5. Kan HJ, Selles RW, van Nieuwenhoven CA, et al. Percutaneous aponeurotomy and lipofilling (PALF) versus limited fasciectomy in patients with primary Dupuytren's contracture: a prospective, randomized, controlled trial. *Plast Reconstr Surg*. 2016;137(6):1800–1812.

ADDITIONAL READING

- Ball C, Pratt AL, Nanchahal J. Optimal functional outcome measures for assessing treatment for Dupuytren's disease: a systematic review and recommendations for future practice. *BMC Musculoskelet Disord*. 2013;14:131.
- Collis J, Collocott S, Hing W, et al. The effect of night extension orthoses following surgical release of Dupuytren contracture: a single-center, randomized, controlled trial. *J Hand Surg Am*. 2013;38(7): 1285.e2–1294.e2.
- Eaton C. Evidence-based medicine: Dupuytren contracture. *Plast Reconstr Surg*. 2014;133(5): 1241–1251.
- Henry M. Dupuytren's disease: current state of the art. *Hand (N Y)*. 2014;9(1):1–8.
- Lanting R, Broekstra DC, Werker PM, et al. A systematic review and meta-analysis on the prevalence of Dupuytren disease in the general population of Western countries. *Plast Reconstr Surg*. 2014;133(3):593–603.
- Michou L, Lermusiaux JL, Teyssedou JP, et al. Genetics of Dupuytren's disease. *Joint Bone Spine*. 2012;79(1):7–12.
- Sweet S, Blackmore S. Surgical and therapy update on the management of Dupuytren's disease. *J Hand Ther*. 2014;27(2):77–83.
- van Rijssen AL, Werker PM. Percutaneous needle fasciotomy for recurrent Dupuytren disease. *J Hand Surg Am*. 2012;37(9):1820–1823.

CODES

ICD10
M72.0 Palmar fascial fibromatosis [Dupuytren]

CLINICAL PEARLS
- Dupuytren contracture is a fixed flexion deformity of (most commonly) the 4th and 5th digits due to palmar fibrosis. 90% of cases are progressive; not trigger finger, which is due to thickening of the distal flexor tendon
- Refer patients with involvement of the PIP joints or MCP involvement with contractures of >30 degrees.
- Both surgical and enzymatic fasciotomy have high rate of recurrence.

D

DYSHIDROSIS

Benjamin T. Tan, DO • Tarang P. Jethwa, MD, MS • George G.A. Pujalte, MD, FACSM

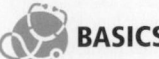

BASICS

DESCRIPTION
- A common chronic dermatitis often involving the palms and soles. The precise definition is frequently debated, with many terms being used interchangeably. Efforts are being made to more specifically define dyshidrosis, and literature supports the presence of several different classes within the family "dyshidrosis."
- Dyshidrotic eczema
  - Common, chronic, or recurrent; nonerythematous; symmetric vesicular eruption primarily of the palms, soles, and interdigital areas
  - Associated with burning, itching, and pain
- Pompholyx (from Greek "bubble")
  - Rare condition characterized by abrupt onset of large bullae
  - Often used interchangeably with dyshidrotic eczema (small vesicles); however, may be a distinct entity
- Lamellar dyshidrosis
  - Fine, spreading, exfoliation of the superficial epidermis in the same distribution as described above
- System(s) affected: dermatologic, exocrine, immunologic
- Synonym(s): cheiropompholyx, keratolysis exfoliativa, vesicular palmoplantar eczema, desquamation of interdigital spaces pompholyx, acute and recurrent vesicular hand dermatitis

EPIDEMIOLOGY
Incidence
- Mean age of onset is 40 years and younger.
- Male = female
- Comprises 5–20% of hand eczema cases

Prevalence
20 cases per 100,000 people

ETIOLOGY AND PATHOPHYSIOLOGY
- Exact mechanism unknown; thought to be multifactorial (allergies, genetics, and dermatophyte infection implicated)
- Dermatopathology: intraepidermal spongiosis without effect on eccrine sweat glands
- Vesicles remain intact due to thickness of stratum corneum of palmar/plantar skin (1).
- Immunologic reaction: theorized that rapid rise in immunoglobulin levels may precipitate vesicle formation
- Aggravating factors (debated)
  - Hyperhidrosis (in 40% of patients with the condition)
  - Detergents/solvents
  - Increased water exposure (e.g., florists, hair stylists, health care workers)
  - Climate: hot/cold weather; humidity
  - Contact sensitivity (in 30–67% of patients with the condition) (2)
  - Metals: nickel, cobalt, and chromate sensitivity (may include implanted orthopedic or orthodontic metals) (1)
  - Stress
  - Dermatophyte infection (present in 10% of patients with the condition) (2)
  - Prolonged wear of occlusive gloves
  - Cement workers
  - IV immunoglobulin therapy
  - Smoking
  - Sunlight/UVA radiation

Genetics
- Atopy: 50% of patients with dyshidrotic eczema have atopic dermatitis (1).
- Rare autosomal dominant form of pompholyx found in Chinese population maps to chromosome 18q22.1–18q22.3 (2)

RISK FACTORS
- Many risk factors are disputed in the literature, with none being consistently associated.
- Atopy
- Other dermatologic conditions
  - Atopic dermatitis (early in life)
  - Contact dermatitis (later in life)
  - Dermatophytosis
- Sensitivity to
  - Foods
  - Drugs: neomycin, quinolones, acetaminophen, and oral contraceptives
  - Contact and dietary: nickel (more common in young women), chromate (more common in men), and cobalt (1)
  - Smoking

GENERAL PREVENTION
- Control emotional stress.
- Avoid excessive sweating.
- Avoid exposure to irritants.
- Avoid diet high in metal salts (chromium, cobalt, nickel).
- Avoid smoking.

COMMONLY ASSOCIATED CONDITIONS
- Atopic dermatitis
- Allergic contact dermatitis
- Parkinson disease
- HIV (2)

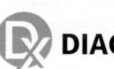

DIAGNOSIS

HISTORY
- Episodes of pruritic rash
- Recent emotional stress
- Familial or personal history of atopy
- Exposure to allergens or irritants
  - Occupational, dietary, or household
  - Cosmetic and personal hygiene products
  - Vesicular eruption typically occurs 24 hours after allergen challenge (1).
- Costume jewelry use
- IV immunoglobulin therapy
- HIV
- Smoking

PHYSICAL EXAM
- Transient, often recurrent, symmetrical vesicular eruptions located on volar and plantar surfaces and lateral fingers. Lesions may not heal completely between flares (1).
- Prodrome: Intense pruritus may occur prior to vesicular eruption.
- Early findings
  - 1 to 2 mm, clear, nonerythematous, deep-seated vesicles (lasting 2 to 3 weeks)
  - Has a "tapioca" appearance
- Late findings
  - Unroofed vesicles with inflamed bases
  - Desquamation (terminal phase)
  - Peeling, rings of scale, or lichenification common

DIFFERENTIAL DIAGNOSIS
- Vesicular tinea pedis/manuum
- Vesicular id reaction
- Contact dermatitis (allergic or irritant)
- Scabies
- Chronic vesicular hand dermatitis
- Drug reaction
- Dermatophytid
- Bullous disorders: dyshidrosiform bullous pemphigoid, pemphigus, bullous impetigo, epidermolysis bullosa (3)
- Pustular psoriasis
- Acrodermatitis continua
- Erythema multiforme
- Herpes simplex infection
- Pityriasis rubra pilaris
- Vesicular mycosis fungoides

DIAGNOSTIC TESTS & INTERPRETATION
Follow-Up Tests & Special Considerations
- Skin culture in suspected secondary infection (most commonly, *Staphylococcus aureus*) (4)
- Consider antibiotics based on culture results and severity of symptoms.

Diagnostic Procedures/Other
- Diagnosis is based on clinical exam.
- Potassium hydroxide (KOH) wet mount (if concerned about dermatophyte infection)
- Patch test (if suspecting allergic cause) (4)

Test Interpretation
- Fine, 1- to 2-mm spongiotic, intraepidermal vesicles with little to no inflammatory change
- No eccrine glandular involvement
- Thickened stratum corneum

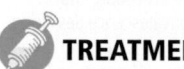

TREATMENT

GENERAL MEASURES
- Avoid possible causative factors: stress, direct skin contact with irritants, nickel, occlusive gloves, household cleaning products, smoking, sweating.
- Use moisturizers/emollients for symptomatic relief and to maintain effective skin barrier (4).
- Skin care
  - Avoid shoes with known irritants (i.e., leather, rubber soles, etc.).
  - Wear socks and gloves made of cotton and change frequently.
  - Wash infrequently in lukewarm water, carefully dry, and then apply emollient.
  - Avoid direct contact with fresh fruit (5)[C].

MEDICATION
First Line
- Mild cases: topical steroids (high potency) (2)[B]
  - Considered cornerstone of therapy but limited published evidence
  - Limited use for 2 weeks due to risk of infection (4)[B]
- Moderate to severe cases
  - Ultra high-potency topical steroids with occlusion over treated area (4)[B]
  - Prednisone 40 to 100 mg/day tapered after blister formation ceases (2)[B]
    - Limited use due to significant side effects (4)[B]
  - Psoralens plus ultraviolet (UV)-A (PUVA) therapy, either systemic/topical or immersion in psoralens (2)[B]

302

- Recurrent cases (4)[B]
  – Systemic steroids at onset of itching prodrome
  – Prednisone 60 mg PO for 3 to 4 days

Second Line
- Topical calcineurin inhibitors (mitigate the long-term risks of topical steroid use)
  – Topical tacrolimus (6)[B]
  – Topical pimecrolimus (6)[B]
  – May not be as effective on plantar surface
- Other therapies (typically with dermatology consultation)
  – Oral cyclosporine (4)[B]; monitor for hypertension and renal injury.
  – Injections of botulinum toxin type A (BTXA) (6)[B]
    ○ Newer topical forms of BTXA currently being developed show promise.
    ○ Painful, requires nerve block
  – Systemic alitretinoin (teratogenic) (5)[B]
  – Topical bexarotene (a teratogenic retinoid X receptor agonist approved for use in cutaneous T-cell lymphoma) (6)[B]
  – Methotrexate (6)[C] (significant side effects including GI intolerance and hepatotoxicity) (4)[B]
  – Azathioprine (1)[C] (6- to 8-week onset of action; must monitor for GI side effects, liver toxicity, blood dyscrasia)
  – Disulfiram or sodium cromoglycate in nickel-allergic patients (1)[C]
  – Mycophenolate mofetil (2)[C] (GI side effects; benefit: no hepatotoxicity with long-term use) (4)[B]
  – Tap water iontophoresis (2)[C]

ISSUES FOR REFERRAL
- Allergist (if allergen testing required)
- Psychologist (if stress modification needed)

ADDITIONAL THERAPIES
- Other oral agents:
  – Thalidomide (do not use in pregnancy/no available studies on efficacy)
  – Dapsone 100 to 150 mg daily (also limited literature on efficacy; may be used in combination with steroids) both significant side effects; very limited use (4)[B]
- Radiation therapy (1)[C]
- UV-free phototherapy (5)[C]
- Treat underlying dermatophytosis (1).
- BTXA in those in which excessive sweating is an exacerbating factor (4)[B]

COMPLEMENTARY & ALTERNATIVE MEDICINE
- Conservative management:
  – Antihistamines: hydroxyzine, cetirizine, loratadine
  – Soaks/cold compresses of weak solutions of potassium permanganate, Burow solution (aluminum acetate), or vinegar 15 minutes, 4 times daily (4)[C]
- Exposure to sunlight as maintenance therapy, 12 minutes every other day, 10 to 15 exposures (5)[C]
- Dandelion juice (avoid in atopic patients) (6)[C]
- Cognitive relaxation techniques (4)[B]

ONGOING CARE

FOLLOW-UP RECOMMENDATIONS
Patient Monitoring
- Dyshidrotic Eczema Area and Severity Index (DASI) (1)
- Parameters used in the DASI score
  – Number of vesicles per square centimeter
  – Erythema
  – Desquamation
  – Severity of itching
  – Surface area affected

- Grading: mild (0 to 15), moderate (16 to 30), severe (31 to 60)
- Monitor BP and glucose in patients receiving systemic corticosteroids.
- Monitor for adverse effects of medications.

DIET
- Consider diet low in metal salts if there is history of nickel sensitivity (4)[B].
- Updated recommendations for low-cobalt diet are available (1).

PATIENT EDUCATION
- Instructions on self-care, complications, and avoidance of triggers/aggravating factors
- American Academy of Dermatology: dyshidrotic eczema at: https://www.aad.org/public/diseases/eczema/dyshidrotic-eczema#overview

PROGNOSIS
- Condition is benign.
- Usually heals without scarring
- Lesions may spontaneously resolve.
- Recurrence is common.

COMPLICATIONS
- Quality of life impact: skin tightening, pain, and decreased dexterity
- Secondary bacterial infections with or without steroid use (*S. aureus* most common)
- Dystrophic nail changes
- Fissures and ulcerations
- Psychological distress
- Lymphedema

REFERENCES

1. Veien NK. Acute and recurrent vesicular hand dermatitis. *Dermatol Clin*. 2009;27(3):337–353.
2. Wollina U. Pompholyx: a review of clinical features, differential diagnosis, and management. *Am J Clin Dermatol*. 2010;11(5):305–314.
3. Basseri S, Ly TY, Hull PR. Dyshidrotic bullous pemphigoid: case report and review of literature. *J Cutan Med Surg*. 2018;22(6):614–617.
4. Lofgren SM, Warshaw EM. Dyshidrosis: epidemiology, clinical characteristics, and therapy. *Dermatitis*. 2006;17(4):165–181.
5. Letić M. Use of sunlight to treat dyshidrotic eczema. *JAMA Dermatol*. 2013;149(5):634–635.
6. Wollina U. Pompholyx: what's new? *Expert Opin Investig Drugs*. 2008;17(6):897–904.

ADDITIONAL READING

- Agner T, Aalto-Korte K, Andersen KE, et al; for European Environmental and Contact Dermatitis Research Group. Classification of hand eczema. *J Eur Acad Dermatol Venereol*. 2015;29(12):2417–2422.
- Chen JJ, Liang YH, Zhou FS, et al. The gene for a rare autosomal dominant form of pompholyx maps to chromosome 18q22.1–18q22.3. *J Invest Dermatol*. 2006;126(2):300–304.
- Gerstenblith MR, Antony AK, Junkins-Hopkins JM, et al. Pompholyx and eczematous reactions associated with intravenous immunoglobulin therapy. *J Am Acad Dermatol*. 2012;66(2):312–316.
- Guillet MH, Wierzbicka E, Guillet S, et al. A 3-year causative study of pompholyx in 120 patients. *Arch Dermatol*. 2007;143(12):1504–1508.

- Hsu CY, Wang YC, Kao CH, et al. Dyshidrosis is a risk factor for herpes zoster. *J Eur Acad Dermatol Venereol*. 2015;29(11):2177–2183.
- Kurata M, Horie C, Kano Y, et al. Pompholyx as a clinical manifestation suggesting increased serum IgG levels in a patient with drug-induced hypersensitivity syndrome/drug reaction with eosinophilia and systemic symptoms. *Br J Dermatol*. 2016;174(3):681–683.
- Molin S, Diepgen TL, Ruzicka T, et al. Diagnosing chronic hand eczema by an algorithm: a tool for classification in clinical practice. *Clin Exp Dermatol*. 2011;36(6):595–601.
- Nalluri R, Rhodes LE. Photoaggravated pompholyx. *Photodermatol Photoimmunol Photomed*. 2016;32(3):168–170.
- Nishizawa A. Dyshidrotic eczema and its relationship to metal allergy. *Curr Probl Dermatol*. 2016;51:80–85.
- Schuttelaar ML, Coenraads PJ, Huizinga J, et al. Increase in vesicular hand eczema after house dust mite inhalation provocation: a double-blind, placebo-controlled, cross-over study. *Contact Dermatitis*. 2013;68(2):76–85.
- Soler DC, Bai X, Ortega L, et al. The key role of aquaporin 3 and aquaporin 10 in the pathogenesis of pompholyx. *Med Hypotheses*. 2015;84(5):498–503.
- Stuckert J, Nedorost S. Low-cobalt diet for dyshidrotic eczema patients. *Contact Dermatitis*. 2008;59(6):361–365.
- Sumila M, Notter M, Itin P, et al. Long-term results of radiotherapy in patients with chronic palmoplantar eczema or psoriasis. *Strahlenther Onkol*. 2008;184(4):218–223.
- Tchernev G, Zanardelli M, Voicu C, et al. Impetiginized dyshidrotic eczema. *Open Access Maced J Med Sci*. 2017;5(4):539–540.
- Tzaneva S, Kittler H, Thallinger C, et al. Oral vs. bath PUVA using 8-methoxypsoralen for chronic palmoplantar eczema. *Photodermatol Photoimmunol Photomed*. 2009;25(2):101–105.

 SEE ALSO

Algorithm: Rash

 CODES

ICD10
L30.1 Dyshidrosis [pompholyx]

CLINICAL PEARLS

- Dyshidrosis is a transient, recurrent, vesicular eruption, most commonly of the palms, soles, and interdigital areas.
- Etiology and pathophysiology are unknown but are most likely related to a combination of genetic and environmental factors.
- Best prevention is effective skin care and limiting exposure to irritating agents.
- Treatments are based on disease severity; preferred treatments include topical steroids, oral steroids, and calcineurin inhibitors.
- Condition, although benign and self-healing, can be chronic and debilitating with major concern for superimposed bacterial infection that may be avoided by preventative measures, early treatment, and recognition.

DYSMENORRHEA

Maggie C. Wertz, MD

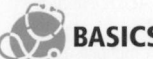

BASICS

DESCRIPTION
- Pelvic pain occurring at/around time of menses; a leading cause of absenteeism for women <30 years old
- Primary dysmenorrhea: pelvic pain without pathologic physical findings
- Secondary dysmenorrhea: often more severe, results from specific pelvic pathology; severity based on activity impairment
  - Mild: painful, rarely limits daily function, or requires analgesics
  - Moderate: daily activity affected, rare absenteeism, requires analgesics
  - Severe: daily activity affected, likelihood of absenteeism increased, limited benefit from analgesics
- System affected: reproductive
- Synonym(s): menstrual cramps

EPIDEMIOLOGY
- Predominant age
  - Primary: onset 6 to 12 months after the start of menarche, teens to early 20s
  - Secondary: 20s to 30s
- Predominant sex: women only

Prevalence
- Up to 90% of menstruating females have experienced primary dysmenorrhea (1).
- Up to 42% lose days of school/work monthly due to dysmenorrhea.
- Up to 20% reported impairment in daily activities and/or sleep.

ETIOLOGY AND PATHOPHYSIOLOGY
- Primary: Elevated prostaglandin (PGF2α) production through indirect hormonal control (decrease in progesterone at start of menses leads to increase in prostaglandins) causes nonrhythmic hypercontractility and increased uterine muscle tone with vasoconstriction and resultant uterine ischemia. Ischemia results in hypersensitization of type C pain nerve fibers; intensity of cramps directly proportional to amount of PGF2α released (1)
- Secondary
  - Endometriosis (most common cause)
  - Adenomyosis
  - Congenital abnormalities of uterine/vaginal anatomy
  - Cervical stenosis
  - Pelvic inflammatory disease
  - Ovarian cysts
  - Pelvic tumors, especially leiomyomata (fibroids) and uterine polyps

Genetics
Not well studied

RISK FACTORS
- Primary (1,2)
  - Cigarette smoking
  - Alcohol use
  - Early menarche (age <12 years)
  - Age <30 years

- Family history of dysmenorrhea
- Irregular/heavy menstrual flow
- Nonuse of oral contraceptives
- Sexual abuse/history of sexual assault
- Psychological symptoms (depression, anxiety, increased stress, etc.)
- Nulliparity
- Secondary
  - Pelvic infection
  - Use of intrauterine device (IUD) in the few months following insertion
  - Structural pelvic malformations
  - Family history of endometriosis in first-degree relative

GENERAL PREVENTION
- Primary: regular exercise; early childbirth
- Secondary: Reduce risk of sexually transmitted infections (STIs).

Pediatric Considerations
Onset with first menses raises probability of genital tract anatomic abnormality (i.e., transverse vaginal septum, imperforate or minimally perforated hymen, uterine anomalies).

COMMONLY ASSOCIATED CONDITIONS
- Irregular/heavy menstrual periods
- Longer menstrual cycle length/duration of bleeding
- Anxiety/depression
- Decreased quality of life

DIAGNOSIS

Based on characteristic history of suprapubic/low back cramping/pain occurring at or near menstrual flow onset lasting for 8 to 72 hours (2)

HISTORY
- Primary: onset once ovulatory cycles are established in adolescents; 6 to 12 months after menarche on average
- Patients may have associated nausea, vomiting, diarrhea, headache, fatigue, insomnia, pain radiating into the low back or inner thighs, and rarely syncope and fever. These are all considered to be secondary to prostaglandin release.
- Recurrence at or just before the onset of the menstrual flow
  - Pelvic pain occurring between menstrual periods is not likely to be dysmenorrhea.
  - Present with most menstrual periods (cyclic)
- Relief associated with the following:
  - Use of analgesics, especially NSAIDs
  - Local heat application
  - Orgasm
- Response to NSAIDs helps confirm diagnosis.
- Impact of symptoms on daily activities can help determine severity.
- Secondary: associated with chronic pelvic pain, midcycle pain, dyspareunia, abnormal uterine bleeding, typical onset after age 25 years, nonmidline pain, progression of severity, lack of response to NSAIDs/hormonal treatment and infertility

PHYSICAL EXAM
- Primary: Physical exam typically is normal. Examine to rule out secondary dysmenorrhea only if the history is inconsistent with primary dysmenorrhea. Pelvic exam is recommended if patient is sexually active to rule out infection.
- Secondary: Evaluate for cervical discharge, uterine enlargement, tenderness, irregularity, or fixation.

DIFFERENTIAL DIAGNOSIS
- Primary: History is characteristic.
- Secondary
  - Endometriosis (most common)
  - Pelvic/genital infection
  - Complication of pregnancy
  - Missed/incomplete abortion
  - Ectopic pregnancy
  - Uterine/ovarian neoplasm
  - UTI
  - Complication with IUD use
  - Congenital uterine or cervical anomaly
  - Adenomyosis
  - Leiomyomata (fibroids)
  - Pelvic adhesions
  - Inflammatory bowel disease
  - Irritable bowel syndrome
  - Chronic pelvic pain (idiopathic)

DIAGNOSTIC TESTS & INTERPRETATION
Initial Tests (lab, imaging)
All tests should only be performed if indicated based on history or if patient has symptoms refractory to first-line therapies; most cases of primary dysmenorrhea can be diagnosed on history alone.
- Pregnancy test
- Urine testing for infection
- Gonorrhea/chlamydia cervical testing, especially in women age <25 years and in high-prevalence areas
- Primary: Consider pelvic ultrasound to rule out secondary abnormalities.
- Secondary: ultrasound and/or laparoscopy to define anatomy for severe/refractory cases. MRI may be useful as second-line noninvasive imaging if ultrasound is nondiagnostic and fibroids, ovarian torsion, deep endometriosis, or adenomyosis is suspected.

Follow-Up Tests & Special Considerations
Counsel regarding appropriate preventive measures for STI and pregnancy.

Diagnostic Procedures/Other
Laparoscopy is rarely needed and is usually only considered in cases of suspected endometriosis or pelvic adhesions not definitively identified on transvaginal ultrasound.

Test Interpretation
- Primary: none
- Secondary: Specific anatomic abnormalities may be noted (see "Differential Diagnosis").

Pregnancy Considerations
Consider ectopic pregnancy when pelvic pain occurs with vaginal bleeding in a patient with a positive pregnancy test.

TREATMENT

- Reassure the patient that treatment success is very likely with adherence to recommendations.
- Relief may require the use of several treatment modalities at the same time.

GENERAL MEASURES

- Exercise (3)[B] and local heat (1)[A] are noninvasive general measures to relieve pain. Local heat in conjunction with the use of an NSAID is superior to an NSAID alone (1)[A].
- High-frequency transcutaneous electrical nerve stimulation (TENS) has been found to be beneficial (1,4)[A]. Low-frequency TENS is not recommended because it is not superior to placebo.
- Secondary dysmenorrhea: treatment of suspected/confirmed underlying cause of pain

MEDICATION

First Line

- NSAIDs: inhibit the peripheral production of prostaglandins. No NSAID has been found to be superior to others (5)[A]. Medication should be taken on scheduled dosing 1 to 2 days prior to onset of menses and continued for 2 to 3 days (1,2,5)[A]. If one NSAID preparation does not work, another NSAID preparation should be tried. Each preparation should be taken as prescribed for at least 3 menstrual cycles prior to determining effectiveness.
  - Ibuprofen 400 mg PO q8h
  - Naproxen sodium 500 mg PO q12h
  - Celecoxib 400 mg PO × 1 and then 200 mg PO q12h
  - Mefenamic acid 500 mg PO × 1 and then 250 mg PO q6h
- Hormonal contraceptives: recommended for primary dysmenorrhea in women desiring contraception (2)[B]. Directly suppresses ovulation and limits endometrial growth resulting in reduced prostaglandin production, intrauterine pressure, and uterine contractions. Continuous rather than cyclic dosing has been found to be superior for pain control (4)[A]. Estrogen-containing contraceptives are recommended first line for secondary dysmenorrhea due to endometriosis, although progestin-only methods have also been shown to be beneficial (2)[B].
  - Low-dose and high-dose combined oral contraceptives (COCs) along with transdermal and intravaginal combined contraceptives have all been found to be superior to placebo (1)[A].
  - Levonorgestrel IUDs are just as effective as COCs (4)[A].
  - Progestin-only contraceptions including subcutaneous and subdermal preparations appear to decrease primary dysmenorrhea but to a lesser extent than combined options and IUDs (1,2)[B].
- Potential contraindications to NSAIDs and COCs
  - Platelet disorders
  - Gastric ulceration or gastritis
  - Personal and family history of thromboembolic disorders
  - Vascular disease
  - Migraines with aura
  - Active smoking
- Precautions for all first-line options:
  - GI irritation
  - Lactation
  - Coagulation disorders
  - Impaired renal function
  - Heart failure
  - Liver dysfunction
  - Pregnancy
  - Hypertension
- Significant possible interactions
  - Coumadin-type anticoagulants
  - Aspirin with other NSAIDs

Second Line

- Acetaminophen and acetaminophen with caffeine are superior to placebo and have less side effects than NSAIDs (1)[B].
- Behavioral interventions, such as relaxation exercises including yoga, may help alleviate pain in primary dysmenorrhea.
- Nifedipine may be effective in some women and may be used in women trying to conceive (pregnancy Category C).

SURGERY/OTHER PROCEDURES

Laparoscopic uterosacral nerve ablation and presacral neurectomy have been shown to relieve pain at 6 and 12 months, respectively, but are still reserved for patients with pain resistant to all other first-line and second-line treatments (1,4)[B].

COMPLEMENTARY & ALTERNATIVE MEDICINE

- Chinese herbal medicine shows promising evidence of decreasing pain, but more evidence is needed.
- Acupuncture treatments have been shown to decrease pain in dysmenorrhea, but further randomized, well-designed studies are needed. Additionally, these treatments must be frequent and timely for effectiveness.
- Acupoint stimulation, particularly noninvasive stimulation (acupressure), has had inconclusive results for pain relief.
- Aromatherapy abdominal massage performed daily for 10 minutes, 7 days prior to onset of menses can decrease primary dysmenorrhea.
- Further research needed to determine benefit and safety for regular use of oral fennel, oral ginger, oral fenugreek, oral valerian, extracorporeal magnetic innervation, vitamin K_1 injection into the spleen-6 acupuncture point, use of high-frequency vibratory stimulation tampon, transdermal nitroglycerin, and vaginal sildenafil.

ADMISSION, INPATIENT, AND NURSING CONSIDERATIONS

Both primary and secondary dysmenorrhea are usually managed in the outpatient setting.

- Primary: outpatient care
- Secondary: usually outpatient care

 ONGOING CARE

FOLLOW-UP RECOMMENDATIONS

Normal

DIET

Insufficient evidence for any specific dietary changes

PATIENT EDUCATION

Reassure the patient that primary dysmenorrhea is treatable with the use of NSAIDs, COCs, IUD, or local heat, and that it will usually abate with age and parity.

PROGNOSIS

- Primary: reduced with age and parity
- Secondary: likely to require therapy based on underlying cause

COMPLICATIONS

- Primary: anxiety and/or depression
- Secondary: infertility from underlying pathology

REFERENCES

1. Burnett M, Lemyre M. No. 345—primary dysmenorrhea consensus guideline. *J Obstet Gynaecol Can.* 2017;39(7):585–595.
2. Osayande AS, Mehulic S. Diagnosis and initial management of dysmenorrhea. *Am Fam Physician.* 2014;89(5):341–346.
3. Brown J, Brown S. Exercise for dysmenorrhoea. *Cochrane Database Syst Rev.* 2010;(2):CD004142.
4. Oladosu FA, Tu FF, Hellman KM. Nonsteroidal anti-inflammatory drug resistance in dysmenorrhea: epidemiology, causes, and treatment. *Am J Obstet Gynecol.* 2018;218(4):390–400.
5. Lethaby A, Duckitt K, Farquhar C. Non-steroidal anti-inflammatory drugs for heavy menstrual bleeding. *Cochrane Database Syst Rev.* 2013;(1):CD000400.

ADDITIONAL READING

- Ryan SA. The treatment of dysmenorrhea. *Pediatr Clin North Am.* 2017;64(2):331–342.
- Shetty GB, Shetty B, Mooventhan A. Efficacy of acupuncture in the management of primary dysmenorrhea: a randomized controlled trial. *J Acupunct Meridian Stud.* 2018;11(4):153–158.

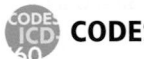 **SEE ALSO**

- Dyspareunia; Endometriosis; Menorrhagia (Heavy Menstrual Bleeding); Premenstrual Syndrome (PMS) and Premenstrual Dysphoric Disorder (PMDD)
- Algorithm: Pelvic Pain

CODES

ICD10

- N94.6 Dysmenorrhea, unspecified
- N94.4 Primary dysmenorrhea
- N94.5 Secondary dysmenorrhea

CLINICAL PEARLS

- Dysmenorrhea is a leading cause of absenteeism for women age <30 years.
- In women who desire contraception, hormonal contraceptives are the preferred treatment.
- All NSAIDs studied have been found to be equally effective in the relief of dysmenorrhea and should be initiated 1 to 2 days prior to onset of menses with scheduled dosing.

DYSPAREUNIA

Scott T. Henderson, MD

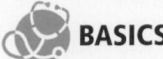 **BASICS**

DESCRIPTION

- Recurrent and persistent genital pain associated with sexual activity, which is not exclusively due to lack of lubrication or vaginismus, and is associated with distress or interpersonal difficulty
- May be the result of organic, emotional, or psychogenic causes
  - Primary: present throughout one's sexual history
    - Potential relationship exists between primary dyspareunia and vaginismus, low libido, and arousal disorders.
  - Secondary: arising from some specific event or condition (e.g., menopause, drugs)
  - Superficial: pain at, or near, the introitus or vaginal barrel associated with penetration
  - Deep: pain after penetration located at the cervix or lower abdominal area
  - Complete: present under all circumstances
  - Situational: occurring selectively with specific situations
- System(s) affected: reproductive

EPIDEMIOLOGY

- Predominant age: all ages
- Predominant sex: female > male

Incidence

>50% of all sexually active women will report dyspareunia at some time.

Geriatric Considerations

Incidence increases dramatically in postmenopausal women primarily because of vaginal atrophy.

Prevalence

Most sexually active women will experience dyspareunia at some time in their lives.

- ~15% (4–40%) of adult women will have dyspareunia on a few occasions during a year.
- ~1–2% of women will have painful intercourse on a more-than-occasional basis.
- Male prevalence is ~1%.

ETIOLOGY AND PATHOPHYSIOLOGY

- Disorders of vaginal outlet
  - Adhesions
  - Condyloma
  - Clitoral irritation
  - Episiotomy scars
  - Fissures
  - Hymenal ring abnormalities
  - Inadequate lubrication
  - Infections
  - Lichen planus
  - Lichen sclerosus
  - Postmenopausal atrophy
  - Psoriasis
  - Trauma
  - Vulvar papillomatosis
  - Vulvar vestibulitis/vulvodynia
- Disorders of vagina
  - Abnormality of vault owing to surgery or radiation
  - Congenital malformations
  - Inadequate lubrication
  - Infections
  - Inflammatory or allergic response to foreign substance
  - Masses or tumors
  - Pelvic relaxation resulting in rectocele, uterine prolapse, or cystocele
- Disorders of pelvic structures
  - Endometriosis
  - Levator ani myalgia/spasm
  - Malignant or benign tumors of the uterus
  - Ovarian pathology
  - Pelvic adhesions
  - Pelvic inflammatory disease (PID)
  - Pelvic venous congestion
  - Prior pelvic fracture
  - Uterine fibroids
- Disorders of the GI tract
  - Constipation
  - Crohn disease
  - Diverticular disease
  - Fistulas
  - Hemorrhoids
  - Inflammatory bowel disease
- Disorders of the urinary tract
  - Interstitial cystitis
  - Ureteral or vesical lesions
  - Urethritis
- Chronic disease
  - Behçet syndrome
  - Diabetes
  - Sjögren syndrome
- Male
  - Cancer of penis
  - Genital muscle spasm
  - Infection or irritation of penile skin
  - Infection of seminal vesicles
  - Lichen sclerosus
  - Musculoskeletal disorders of pelvis and lower back
  - Penile anatomy disorders
  - Phimosis
  - Prostate infections and enlargement
  - Testicular disease
  - Torsion of spermatic cord
  - Urethritis
- Psychological disorders
  - Anxiety
  - Conversion reactions
  - Depression
  - Fear
  - Hostility toward partner
  - Phobic reactions
  - Psychological trauma

RISK FACTORS

- Fatigue
- Stress
- Depression
- Diabetes
- Estrogen deficiency
  - Menopause
  - Lactation
- Previous PID
- Vaginal surgery
- Alcohol/marijuana consumption
- Medication side effects (antihistamines, tamoxifen, bromocriptine, low-estrogen oral contraceptives, SSRIs, depo-medroxyprogesterone, desipramine)

Pregnancy Considerations

- Pregnancy has a potent influence on sexuality; dyspareunia is common in late pregnancy and postpartum.
  - Breastfeeding, perineal pain, fatigue, and stress can be risk factors in postpartum period.
- Episiotomies do not have a protective effect.
  - Women who experience delivery interventions including episiotomy are at greater risk than women who deliver over an intact perineum or have an unsutured tear.

COMMONLY ASSOCIATED CONDITIONS

Vaginismus

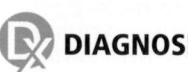 **DIAGNOSIS**

HISTORY

- Identify pain characteristics:
  - Onset
  - Duration
  - Location: entry versus deep, single versus multiple sites; positional
  - Intensity/quality: varying degrees of pelvic/genital pressure, aching, tearing, and/or burning
  - Pattern (precipitating or aggravating factors): when pain occurs (at entry, during, or after intercourse)
  - Relief measures: Avoid intercourse, change positions, and have intercourse only at certain times of the month.
- Include menstrual, obstetric, reproductive, sexual, domestic violence, and sexual assault histories with past medical, surgical, and psychosocial history.

PHYSICAL EXAM

- A complete exam, including a focused pelvic exam, to identify pathology
  - Exam must include inspection and palpation of urethra, vulva, and vaginal areas; palpation of the uterine, bladder, and adnexal structures; and a rectovaginal exam.
  - Sensory mapping with a cotton-tipped applicator to identify sensitive and painful areas
- Because examination often reproduces the pain, examiner should be cautious and sensitive to patient's anxiety.

DIFFERENTIAL DIAGNOSIS

Vaginismus (genito-pelvic pain penetration disorder)

- If pain prevents penetration, severe vaginismus may be present.

DIAGNOSTIC TESTS & INTERPRETATION

Initial Tests (lab, imaging)

Based on history and exam findings

- Wet mount
- Gonorrhea and chlamydia cultures
- Herpes culture
- Urinalysis and urine culture
- Pap smear

Follow-Up Tests & Special Considerations
- Serum estradiol if vulvodynia or atrophic vaginitis
- Voiding cystourethrogram if urinary tract involvement
- GI contrast studies if GI symptoms
- Ultrasound and CT scan are of limited value; perform if clinically indicated.

Diagnostic Procedures/Other
Based on history and exam findings
- Colposcopy and biopsy if vaginal/vulvar lesions
- Laparoscopy if complex deep-penetration pain
- Cystoscopy if urinary tract involvement
- Endoscopy if GI involvement

Test Interpretation
Depends on etiology

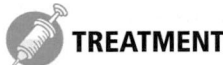 TREATMENT

GENERAL MEASURES
- Educate the patient and partner regarding the nature of the problem. Reassure both that there are solutions to the problem.
- Initiate specific treatment when initial evaluation identifies an organic cause.
- Once organic causes are ruled out, treatment is a multidimensional and multidisciplinary approach; medications alone don't resolve (1)[A].
  – Individual behavioral therapy
    ○ Indicated to help the patient deal with intrapersonal issues and assess the role of the partner
  – Couple behavioral therapy
    ○ Indicated to help resolve interpersonal problems
    ○ May involve short-term structured intervention or sexual counseling
    ○ Designed to desensitize systemically uncomfortable sexual responses and intercourse through a series of interventions over a period of weeks
    ○ Interventions range from muscle relaxation and mutual body massage to sexual fantasies and erotic massage.

MEDICATION
First Line
Depends on the etiology
- Antibiotics, antifungals, or antivirals, as indicated, for infection
- Vaginal moisturizers and lubricants for dryness
- Analgesics and topical anesthetics for pain
- Topical/vaginal estrogen for vaginal and vulvar atrophy
  – Available data support the use of estrogen over other vaginal therapies for postmenopausal vaginal symptoms (2)[A], although vaginal lubricants have an important role in management of atrophy-associated symptoms and may be tried first.
- Neuropathic pain associated with vulvar vestibulitis/vulvodynia may respond to tricyclic antidepressants (amitriptyline or nortriptyline) or gabapentin.

Second Line
- Ospemifene for moderate to severe symptoms due to menopause-related vulvovaginal atrophy (3)[C]
- TX-004HR estradiol vaginal inserts for the treatment of moderate-to-severe dyspareunia, a symptom of vulvovaginal atrophy due to menopause (4)[A]
- Intravaginal DHEA (prasterone) for moderate to severe symptoms due to menopause-related vulvovaginal atrophy

ISSUES FOR REFERRAL
Referral for long-term therapy may be necessary.

ADDITIONAL THERAPIES
Physical therapy for pelvic floor muscle pain

SURGERY/OTHER PROCEDURES
- Consideration of surgical interventions for dyspareunia due altered anatomy, uterine position, fibroids, or prior pelvic surgery
  – Laparoscopic excision of endometriotic lesions or pelvic adhesions
  – Surgical vestibulectomy can be considered if medical measures fail with vulvar vestibulitis.
  – Fractional CO_2 laser treatments demonstrate improvement in symptoms of vulvovaginal atrophy.
- FDA warns against the use of medical devices for unapproved uses including "vaginal rejuvenation" procedures.

COMPLEMENTARY & ALTERNATIVE MEDICINE
- Sitz baths may relieve painful inflammation.
- Perineal massage
- Antioxidants may improve symptoms associated with endometriosis.

ONGOING CARE

FOLLOW-UP RECOMMENDATIONS
Patient Monitoring
- Outpatient follow-up depends on therapy.
- Every 6 to 12 months once resolved

DIET
A high-fiber diet may help if constipation is a contributing cause.

PATIENT EDUCATION
- Boston Women's Health Book Collective and Judy Norsigian. Our Bodies, Ourselves. New York, NY: Touchstone; 2011.
- Kegel exercise information
- Provide couples with information about sexual arousal techniques.

PROGNOSIS
Depends on underlying cause but most patients will respond to treatment

REFERENCES

1. Weinberger JM, Houman J, Caron AT, et al. Female sexual dysfunction: a systematic review of outcomes across various treatment modalities [published online ahead of print February 3, 2018]. Sex Med Rev. doi:10.1016/j.sxmr.2017.12.004.
2. Pitsouni E, Grigoriadis T, Douskos A, et al. Efficacy of vaginal therapies alternative to vaginal estrogens on sexual function and orgasm of menopausal women: a systematic review and meta-analysis of randomized controlled trials. Eur J Obstet Gynecol Reprod Biol. 2018;229:45–56.
3. ACOG Practice Bulletin No. 141: management of menopausal symptoms. Obstet Gynecol. 2014;123(1):202–216.
4. Constantine GD, Simon JA, Pickar JH, et al; for REJOICE Study Group. The REJOICE trial: a phase 3 randomized, controlled trial evaluating the safety and efficacy of a novel vaginal estradiol soft-gel capsule for symptomatic vulvar and vaginal atrophy. Menopause. 2017;24(4):409–416.

ADDITIONAL READING
- Seehusen DA, Baird DC, Bode DV. Dyspareunia in women. Am Fam Physician. 2014;90(7):465–470.
- Sorensen J, Bautista KE, Lamvu G, et al. Evaluation and treatment of female sexual pain: a clinical review. Cureus. 2018;10(3):e2379.

SEE ALSO

- Balanitis, Phimosis, and Paraphimosis; Endometriosis; Genito-Pelvic Pain/Penetration Disorder (Vaginismus); Pelvic Inflammatory Disease; Sexual Dysfunction in Women; Vulvovaginitis, Estrogen Deficient; Vulvovaginitis, Prepubescent
- Algorithms: Discharge, Vaginal; Dyspareunia

CODES

ICD10
- N94.1 Dyspareunia
- F52.6 Dyspareunia not due to a substance or known physiol cond

CLINICAL PEARLS
- Careful history to determine if patient feels pain before, during, or after intercourse will help identify cause.
  – Pain before intercourse suggests a phobic attitude toward penetration and/or the presence of vestibulitis.
  – Pain during intercourse combined with the location of the pain is most predictive of the causes of pain.
  – Introital pain after intercourse suggests vestibulitis in women of childbearing age, hypertonic pelvic floor, or vulvovaginal dystrophia.
  – A sudden symptom onset can suggest a psychosexual etiology, whereas gradual onset of symptoms is more likely physical or anatomical.
- Potential relationship exists between primary dyspareunia and vaginismus, low libido, and arousal disorders.
- Episiotomy does not offer any benefit in the prevention of dyspareunia; an episiotomy in fact may cause more future discomfort.

DYSPEPSIA, FUNCTIONAL

Briana Lindberg, MD • Kristina Burgers, MD, FAAFP

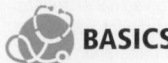 **BASICS**

DESCRIPTION
- The presence of bothersome postprandial fullness, early satiety, or epigastric pain/burning in the absence of causative structural disease (to include normal upper endoscopy) for at least 1 to 3 days per week for the preceding 3 months, with initial symptom onset at least 6 months prior to diagnosis (Rome IV criteria)
- Rome IV criteria divide patients into two subtypes:
  - Postprandial distress syndrome (PDS)
  - Epigastric pain syndrome (EPS)
- System(s) affected: GI
- Synonym(s): idiopathic dyspepsia; nonulcer dyspepsia; nonorganic dyspepsia; PDS; and EPS

EPIDEMIOLOGY
Incidence
Unknown; accounts for 70% of patients with dyspepsia and ~5% of primary care visits

Prevalence
- 10% prevalence worldwide (varies based on criteria)
- More common in Western cultures
- PDS may be more common in Eastern cultures.
- Predominant age: adults (can be seen in children)
- Predominant gender: female > male

ETIOLOGY AND PATHOPHYSIOLOGY
Unknown but proposed mechanisms or associations include gastric motility disorders, visceral pain hypersensitivity, *Helicobacter pylori* infection, alteration in upper GI microbiome, postinfectious complications, immune activation, inflammation, and gut-brain axis disorders

Genetics
Possible link to G-protein β_3 subunit 825 CC genotype, serotonin transport genes, and/or cholecystokinin-A-receptor gene polymorphisms

Geriatric Considerations
Patients age >60 years with new-onset dyspepsia should undergo endoscopy.

Pediatric Considerations
Be alert for family system dysfunction.

Pregnancy Considerations
Pregnancy may exacerbate symptoms.

RISK FACTORS
- Other functional disorders: fibromyalgia, temporomandibular joint pain, chronic fatigue syndrome
- Anxiety/depression, psychosocial stressors (e.g., divorce, unemployment)
- Smoking
- Female gender

GENERAL PREVENTION
Avoid foods and habits known to exacerbate symptoms.

COMMONLY ASSOCIATED CONDITIONS
Other functional bowel disorders

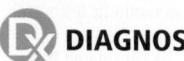 **DIAGNOSIS**

HISTORY
- Postprandial fullness (1)
- Early satiety (1)
- Epigastric pain (1)
- Epigastric burning (1)
- Symptoms for 3 months (1)
- Alarm features that may necessitate endoscopy include (2,3,4):
  - Unintended weight loss
  - Progressive dysphagia
  - Odynophagia
  - Persistent vomiting
  - GI bleeding
  - Family history of upper GI cancer
  - Age ≥60 years

PHYSICAL EXAM
- Document weight status and vital signs.
- Examine for signs of systemic illness.
  - Murphy sign for cholecystitis
  - Rebound and guarding for ulcer perforation
  - Palpate during muscle contraction to assess for abdominal wall pain.
  - Jaundice
  - Thyromegaly

DIFFERENTIAL DIAGNOSIS
- Peptic ulcer disease; gastroesophageal reflux disease
- Cholecystitis; choledocholithiasis
- Gastric or esophageal cancer; esophageal spasm
- Malabsorption syndromes; celiac disease
- Pancreatic cancer; pancreatitis
- Inflammatory bowel disease; carbohydrate malabsorption; gastroparesis
- Ischemic bowel disease
- Intestinal parasites
- Irritable bowel syndrome
- Ischemic heart disease
- Diabetes mellitus; thyroid disease
- Connective tissue disorders
- Conversion disorder
- Medication effects

DIAGNOSTIC TESTS & INTERPRETATION
Initial Tests (lab, imaging)
- Functional dyspepsia is a diagnosis of exclusion. Order labs based on clinical suspicion (2)[C].
- Test for *H. pylori* (stool antigen or urea breath test) in areas of high *H. pylori* prevalence (2,4)[A].
- CBC (if anemia or infection are suspected)
- Liver-associated enzymes/right upper quadrant ultrasound (if hepatobiliary disease is suspected)
- Pancreatic enzymes (if pancreatic disease is suspected)
- Upper endoscopy for patients age >60 years to rule out malignancy (4)[C]
- Upper endoscopy is unlikely to change outcomes or management (2,5)[C].
- Self-report questionnaires can track symptoms (3)[C].

Diagnostic Procedures/Other
- Esophageal manometry or gastric accommodation studies are rarely needed (3)[C].
- Motility studies are unnecessary, unless gastroparesis is strongly suspected (4)[C].

Test Interpretation
None (by definition, this a functional disorder)

TREATMENT

GENERAL MEASURES
- Reassurance/physician support is helpful (2,3)[C].
- Treatment is based on presumed etiologies.
- Discontinue offending medications (3)[C].
- Routine endoscopy not recommended in dyspeptic patients age <60 years even without alarm features (4)[B]

MEDICATION

First Line
- Treat *H. pylori* if confirmed on testing (3,4)[A].
- Trial of once daily proton pump inhibitor (PPI) medication (e.g., omeprazole 20 mg PO QD) or H_2 receptor antagonist (e.g., ranitidine 150 mg BID) for up to 8 weeks in patients without alarm symptoms—most effective for patients with EPS (3,4,5)[A]
- Prokinetics have been proposed as first-line agents in PDS, although efficacy data for metoclopramide, 5 to 10 mg PO TID 30 minutes before meals (only agent approved in United States) are limited (5)[C]. Prokinetics should be prescribed at the lowest effective dose to avoid potential side effects (4)[C]. Use with caution in elderly patients due to side effects of tardive dyskinesia and parkinsonian symptoms.

Second Line
- Trial of tricyclic antidepressant (TCA) medication is more helpful for EPS than PDS (e.g., amitriptyline 25 mg PO QD, can up-titrate to 50 mg PO QD), with a NNT of 6 (2,4,6)[A]. Caution in elderly. There is no benefit to SSRI/SNRI (6)[A].
- Trazodone 25 mg at bedtime is an alternative (2,5)[A]. Consider buspirone or mirtazapine if no response or if contraindications to TCA (2)[B].

ADDITIONAL THERAPIES
- Stress reduction (2,5)[C]
- Psychotherapy effective in some patients (2)[C],(3,4)[B]
- Patients should be given a positive diagnosis and reassured of benign prognosis (2)[C].

COMPLEMENTARY & ALTERNATIVE MEDICINE
Alternative medicine approaches need further study and are not currently recommended (4)[C].
- Iberogast may be helpful (2)[C].
- Probiotics have theoretical benefit but lack consistent controlled trials to support routine use (2)[C].
- Hypnotherapy may help (3)[B].
- Transcutaneous electroacupuncture may help (3)[B].

 # ONGOING CARE

FOLLOW-UP RECOMMENDATIONS
Patient Monitoring
- Provide ongoing support and reassurance.
- Upper endoscopy if persistent symptoms
- Change medications if no difference in symptoms after 4 weeks (3)[C].
- Discontinue medications once symptoms resolve (3)[C].

DIET
- Limited data to support dietary modification
- Consider limiting fatty foods (2,5)[C].
- Avoid foods that exacerbate symptoms: wheat and cow milk proteins, peppers or spices, coffee, tea, and alcohol (2,5)[C].

PATIENT EDUCATION
Reassurance and stress reduction techniques

PROGNOSIS
Long-term/chronic symptoms with symptom-free periods

COMPLICATIONS
Iatrogenic, from evaluation to rule out serious pathology

REFERENCES

1. Stanghellini V, Chan FK, Hasler WL, et al. Gastroduodenal disorders. *Gastroenterology*. 2016;150(6):1380–1392.
2. Talley NJ, Ford AC. Functional dyspepsia. *N Engl J Med*. 2015;373(19):1853–1863.
3. Miwa H, Kusano M, Arisawa T, et al; Japanese Society of Gastroenterology. Evidence-based clinical practice guidelines for functional dyspepsia. *J Gastroenterol*. 2015;50(2):125–139.
4. Moayyedi PM, Lacy BE, Andrews CN, et al. ACG and CAG clinical guideline: management of dyspepsia. *Am J Gastroenterol*. 2017;112(7): 988–1013.
5. Talley NJ, Walker MM, Holtmann G. Functional dyspepsia. *Curr Opin Gastroenterol*. 2016;32(6): 467–473.
6. Ford AC, Luthra P, Tack J, et al. Efficacy of psychotropic drugs in functional dyspepsia: systematic review and meta-analysis. *Gut*. 2017;66(3):411–420.

ADDITIONAL READING

- Du LJ, Chen BR, Kim JJ, et al. *Helicobacter pylori* eradication therapy for functional dyspepsia: systematic review and meta-analysis. *World J Gastroenterol*. 2016;22(12):3486–3495.
- Ford AC, Marwaha A, Sood R, et al. Global prevalence of, and risk factors for, uninvestigated dyspepsia: a meta-analysis. *Gut*. 2015;64(7):1049–1057.
- Koloski NA, Jones M, Talley NJ. Evidence that independent gut-to-brain and brain-to-gut pathways operate in the irritable bowel syndrome and functional dyspepsia: a 1-year population-based prospective study. *Aliment Pharmacol Ther*. 2016;44(6):592–600.
- Lu Y, Chen M, Huang Z, et al. Antidepressants in the treatment of functional dyspepsia: a systematic review and meta-analysis. *PLoS One*. 2016;11(6):e0157798.
- Mahadeva S, Ford AC. Clinical and epidemiological differences in functional dyspepsia between the East and the West. *Neurogastroenterol Motil*. 2016;28(2):167–174.

 ## SEE ALSO
- Irritable Bowel Syndrome
- Algorithm: Dyspepsia

 # CODES

ICD10
K30 Functional dyspepsia

CLINICAL PEARLS
- Dyspepsia without underlying organic disease is functional or idiopathic.
- Consider empiric acid suppression therapy as first line for functional dyspepsia.
- Extensive diagnostic testing is not recommended unless alarm symptoms are present.

D

DYSPHAGIA
Felix B. Chang Cruz, MD, FAAMA, ABIHM

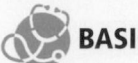 BASICS

Difficulty transmitting the alimentary bolus from the mouth to stomach

DESCRIPTION
- Oropharyngeal dysphagia: difficulty transferring food bolus from oropharynx to proximal esophagus
- Esophageal dysphagia: difficulty moving food bolus through the body of the esophagus to the pylorus

EPIDEMIOLOGY
10% of individuals >50 years of age

Prevalence
- Common primary care complaint
- Rates of impaired swallowing in nursing home residents range from 29% to 32%.

ETIOLOGY AND PATHOPHYSIOLOGY
- Oropharyngeal (transfer dysphagia):
  - Mechanical causes: pharyngeal and laryngeal cancer, acute epiglottitis, carotid body tumor, pharyngitis, tonsillitis, strep throat, lymphoid hyperplasia of lingual tonsil, lateral pharyngeal pouch, hypopharyngeal diverticulum
- Esophageal:
  - Esophageal mechanical lesions: carcinomas, esophageal diverticula, esophageal webs, Schatzki ring, structures (peptic, chemical, trauma, radiation), foreign body
  - Extrinsic mechanical lesions: peritonsillar abscess, thyroid disorders, tumors, mediastinal compression, vascular compression (enlarged left atrium, aberrant subclavius, aortic aneurysm), osteoarthritis of the cervical spine, adenopathy, esophageal duplication cyst
- Neuromuscular: achalasia, diffuse esophageal spasm, hypertonic lower esophageal sphincter, scleroderma, nutcracker esophagus, CVA, Alzheimer disease, Huntington chorea, Parkinson disease, multiple sclerosis, skeletal muscle disease (polymyositis, dermatomyositis), neuromuscular junction disease (myasthenia gravis, Lambert-Eaton syndrome, botulism), hyper- and hypothyroidism, Guillain-Barré syndrome, systemic lupus erythematosus, acute lymphoblastic leukemia, amyloidosis, diabetic neuropathy, brainstem tumors, Chagas disease
- Infection: diphtheria, chronic meningitis, tertiary syphilis, Lyme disease, rabies, poliomyelitis, CMV, esophagitis (*Candida*, herpetic)
- Globus phenomenon

RISK FACTORS
- Children: hereditary and/or congenital malformations
- Adults: age >50 years; elderly: GERD, stroke, COPD, chronic pain
- Smoking, excess alcohol intake, obesity
- Medications: quinine, potassium chloride, vitamin C, tetracycline, Bactrim, clindamycin, NSAIDs, procainamide, anticholinergics, bisphosphates
- Neurologic events or diseases: CVA, myasthenia gravis, multiple sclerosis, Parkinson disease, amyotrophic lateral sclerosis (ALS), Huntington chorea

- HIV patients with CD4 cell count <100 cells/mm³
- Trauma or irradiation of head, neck, and chest; mechanical lesions
- Extrinsic mechanical lesions: lung, thyroid tumors, lymphoma, metastasis
- Iron deficiency
- Anterior cervical spine surgery (up to 71% in the first 2 weeks postop; 12–14% at 1 year postop)
- Dysphagia lusoria (vascular abnormalities causing dysphagia): complete vascular ring, double aortic arch, right aortic arch with retroesophageal left subclavian artery and left ligamentum arteriosum, and right aortic arch with mirror-image branching and left ligamentum arteriosum

GENERAL PREVENTION
- Correct poorly fitting dentures.
- Educate patients to prolong chewing and drink adequate volumes of water at meals.
- Liquid and soft food diet as appropriate
- Avoid alcohol with meals.
- Prophylactic swallowing exercises in patients with head and neck cancer undergoing chemoradiation

COMMONLY ASSOCIATED CONDITIONS
Peptic structure, esophageal webs and rings, carcinoma; history of stroke, dementia, pneumonia

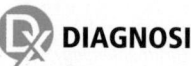 DIAGNOSIS

HISTORY
- Dysphagia to both solids and liquids from the onset of deglutition likely represents an esophageal motility disorder.
- Oropharyngeal dysphagia presents as difficulty initiating the swallowing process.
- Dysphagia for solids that progresses to involve liquids more likely reflects mechanical obstruction.
- Progressive dysphagia is usually caused by cancer or a peptic stricture. Intermittent dysphagia is most often related to a lower esophageal ring.
- Inquire about heartburn, weight loss, hematemesis, coffee ground emesis, anemia, regurgitation of undigested food particles, and respiratory symptoms.
- Inquire about regurgitation, aspiration, or drooling immediately after swallowing because this may represent oropharyngeal dysphagia.
- Does the food bolus feel stuck?
  - Upper sternum or back of throat may represent oropharyngeal dysphagia, whereas sensation over the lower sternum is typical of esophageal dysphagia.
- Is odynophagia present?
  - May represent inflammation, achalasia, diffuse esophageal spasm, esophagitis, pharyngitis, pill-induced esophagitis, cancer
- Globus sensation ("lump in the throat")?
  - Potentially indicates cricopharyngeal or laryngeal disorders
- History of sour taste in the back of the throat or chronic heartburn suggests GERD.
- Inquire about alcohol and/or tobacco use.

- Are there associated symptoms such as weight loss or chest pain?
  - Double aortic arch, right aortic arch with retroesophageal left subclavian artery and left ligamentum arteriosum
  - Anticholinergics, antihistamines, and some antihypertensives can decrease salivary production.
- Halitosis: Rule out diverticulitis.
- Prior history of a connective tissue disorder
- Changes in speech, hoarseness, weak cough, dysphonia? Rule out neuromuscular dysfunction.

PHYSICAL EXAM
- General: vital signs
- Skin: telangiectasia, sclerodactyly, calcinosis (r/o autoimmune disease); Raynaud phenomenon, sclerodactyly may be found in CREST syndrome or systemic scleroderma; stigmata of alcohol abuse (palmar erythema; telangiectasia)
- Head, eye, ear, nose, throat (HEENT):
  - Oropharyngeal: pharyngeal erythema/edema, tonsillitis, pharyngeal ulcers or thrush, odynophagia (bacterial, viral, fungal infections); tongue fasciculations (ALS)
  - Neck: masses, lymphadenopathy, neck tenderness (thyroiditis), goiter
- Neurologic:
  - Cranial nerve exam: sensory: cranial nerves V, IX, and X; motor: cranial nerves V, VII, X, XI, and XII
  - CNS, mental status exam, strength testing, Horner syndrome, ataxia, cogwheel rigidity (CVA, dementia, Parkinson disease, Alzheimer disease)
    - Eye position, extraocular motility
- Informal bedside swallowing evaluation: Observe level of consciousness, postural control-upright position, oral hygiene, mobilization of oral secretions.

DIFFERENTIAL DIAGNOSIS
See "Etiology and Pathophysiology."

DIAGNOSTIC TESTS & INTERPRETATION
Adults (1)[C]:
- Barium swallow
- Fiberoptic endoscopic examination of swallowing (FEES)
- Gastroesophageal endoscopy
- Barium cine/video esophagram
- Ambulatory 24-hour pH testing
- Esophageal manometry
- Videofluoroscopic swallowing study (VFSS): oropharyngeal dysphagia

Initial Tests (lab, imaging)
- Guided by diagnostic considerations (2)[C]
  - CBC (infection and inflammation)
  - Serum protein and albumin levels for nutritional assessment
  - Thyroid function studies to detect dysphagia associated with hypothyroidism or hyperthyroidism, cobalamin levels
  - Antiacetylcholine antibodies (myasthenia)
- Barium swallow: detects strictures or stenosis

Follow-Up Tests & Special Considerations
- CT scan of chest; MRI of brain and cervical spine
- VFSS (lips, tongue, palate, pharynx, larynx, proximal esophagus)
- Fiberoptic endoscopy and videofluoroscopy are similar in terms of diagnostic sensitivity (3)[C].

Diagnostic Procedures/Other
Endoscopy with biopsy; esophageal manometry; esophageal pH monitoring

 TREATMENT

GENERAL MEASURES
Exclude cardiac disease. Ensure airway patency and adequate pulmonary function. Assess nutritional status. Speech therapy evaluation is helpful.

MEDICATION
First Line
- For esophageal spasms: calcium channel blockers: nifedipine 10 to 30 mg TID; imipramine 50 mg at bedtime; sildenafil 50 mg/day PRN
- For esophagitis:
  - Antacids: Tums, Mylanta, Maalox
  - H_2 blockers:
    - Cimetidine: up to 1,600 mg orally per day in 2 or 4 divided doses for 12 weeks
    - Ranitidine: initial 150 mg orally 4 times daily and maintenance 150 mg orally twice daily
    - Nizatidine: 150 mg orally twice daily for 12 weeks
    - Famotidine: 20 to 40 mg orally twice daily for 12 weeks
- Proton pump inhibitors:
  - Omeprazole: 20 mg once daily for 4 to 8 weeks
  - Lansoprazole: 30 mg once daily for up to 8 weeks
  - Rabeprazole: 20 mg orally once daily for 4 to 8 weeks
  - Esomeprazole: 20 to 40 mg orally once daily for 4 to 8 weeks
  - Pantoprazole: 40 mg orally once daily for up to 8 weeks
- Prokinetic agents: rarely used
- Precautions: may need to use liquid forms of medications because patients might have difficulty swallowing pills

ISSUES FOR REFERRAL
- Gastroenterology: endoscopy, refractory symptoms
- Surgery: dilation, esophageal myotomy, biopsy

ADDITIONAL THERAPIES
Speech therapy to assess swallowing; nutritional evaluation for dietary and positioning recommendations; physical therapy for muscle-strengthening exercise; no eating at bedtime; remaining upright after eating
- Self-expanded metal stent is safe, effective, and quicker in palliating dysphagia compared to other modalities.

SURGERY/OTHER PROCEDURES
- Esophageal dilatation (pneumatic or bougie)
- Esophageal stent; laser for cancer palliation (4)[A]
- Treat underlying problem (e.g., thyroid goiter, vascular ring, esophageal atresia).
- Nd:YAG laser incision of lower esophageal rings refractory to dilation
- Photodynamic therapy (cancer) (4)[C]
- Cricopharyngeal myotomy (oropharyngeal dysphagia)
- Surgery for Zenker diverticulum, refractory strictures, or myotomy (for achalasia)
- Percutaneous endoscopic gastrostomy (PEG) decreases risk of dysphagia when compared with nasogastric tube.

COMPLEMENTARY & ALTERNATIVE MEDICINE
- Acupuncture has been used with some success for neurogenic dysphagia.
- Electroacupuncture combined with dilating granule has been used in the treatment of GERD.
- Insufficient evidence for routine use of botulinum toxin

ADMISSION, INPATIENT, AND NURSING CONSIDERATIONS
- Complete or partial esophageal obstruction associated with malnutrition or dehydration
- Need for enteral feeding
- Outpatient if patient is able to maintain nutrition and has little risk of complications
- Hospitalization with total or near-total obstruction of esophageal lumen
- Hospitalization may be needed for endoscopy and/or esophageal dilatation and is generally indicated for diagnostic or therapeutic surgical procedures.
- IV fluids for dehydrated, hypovolemic patients, and patients with impaired consciousness
- Discharge when tolerating adequate diet without nausea/pain

 ONGOING CARE

DIET
See "General Prevention."

PATIENT EDUCATION
Dietary modification; no eating at bedtime; remaining upright after eating; smoking cessation

PROGNOSIS
Vary with specific diagnosis

COMPLICATIONS
- Oropharyngeal: pneumonia, lung abscess, aspiration, airway obstruction
- Malnutrition and dehydration

REFERENCES
1. American College of Radiology. ACR appropriateness criteria for dysphagia. https://www.guidelinecentral.com/summaries/acr-appropriateness-criteria-dysphagia/. Accessed October 4, 2017.
2. Al-Hussaini A, Latif EH, Singh V. 12-minute consultation: an evidence-based approach to the management of dysphagia. *Clin Otolaryngol.* 2013;38(3):237–243.
3. Pasha SF, Acosta RD, Chandrasekhara V, et al; and ASGE Standards of Practice Committee. The role of endoscopy in the evaluation and management of dysphagia. *Gastrointest Endosc.* 2014;79(2): 191–201.
4. Dai Y, Li C, Xie Y, et al. Interventions for dysphagia in oesophageal cancer. *Cochrane Database Syst Rev.* 2014;(10):CD005048.

ADDITIONAL READING
- Jones K, Pitceathly RD, Rose MR, et al. Interventions for dysphagia in long-term, progressive muscle disease. *Cochrane Database Syst Rev.* 2016;(2):CD004303.
- Malagelada JR, Bazzoli F, Boeckxstaens G, et al. World Gastroenterology Organisation global guidelines: dysphagia—global guidelines and cascades update September 2014. *J Clin Gastroenterol.* 2015;49(5):370–378.
- Perry A, Lee S, Cotton S, et al. Therapeutic exercises for affecting post-treatment swallowing in people treated for advanced-stage head and neck cancers. *Cochrane Database Syst Rev.* 2016;(8):CD011112.

 CODES

ICD10
- R13.10 Dysphagia, unspecified
- R13.12 Dysphagia, oropharyngeal phase
- R13.14 Dysphagia, pharyngoesophageal phase

CLINICAL PEARLS
- Dysphagia is an alarm symptom that warrants prompt evaluation to define the exact cause and initiate appropriate therapy.
- Patients with oropharyngeal dysphagia usually report feeling an obstruction in the neck and point to this area when asked to identify the site of their symptoms.

ECTOPIC PREGNANCY
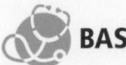
Jeremy Golding, MD, FAAFP

BASICS

DESCRIPTION
Ectopic: pregnancy implanted outside the uterine cavity. Subtypes include:
- Tubal: pregnancy implanted in any portion of the fallopian tube
- Abdominal: pregnancy implanted intra-abdominally, most commonly after tubal abortion or rupture of tubal ectopic pregnancy
- Heterotopic: pregnancy implanted intrauterine and a separate pregnancy implanted outside uterine cavity
- Ovarian: implantation of pregnancy in ovarian tissue
- Cervical: implantation of pregnancy in cervix
- Intraligamentary: implantation of pregnancy within the broad ligament

EPIDEMIOLOGY
Incidence
- The true incidence is difficult to estimate. Incidence is likely between about 6 and 20 per 1,000 pregnancies in the United States. About 1 in 10 1st trimester pregnancies presenting to the emergency with pain and/or bleeding are due to ectopic pregnancy.
- In the United States, ectopic pregnancy is the leading cause of 1st trimester maternal deaths.
- Heterotopic pregnancy, although rare (1:30,000), occurs with greater frequency in women undergoing in vitro fertilization (IVF) (1/1,000).
- Increasing incidence of nontubal, and particularly cesarean scar ectopic pregnancies, due in part to more cesarean sections and more IVF

Prevalence
~33% recurrence rate if prior ectopic pregnancy

ETIOLOGY AND PATHOPHYSIOLOGY
- 95–97% of ectopic pregnancies occur in the fallopian tube, of which, 55–80% in the ampulla, 12–25% in the isthmus, and 5–17% in the fimbria.
- One risk factor for a tubal pregnancy is impaired movement of the fertilized ovum to the uterine cavity due to dysfunction of the tubal cilia, scarring, or narrowing of the tubal lumen.
- Other locations are rare but may occur from reimplantation of an aborted tubal pregnancy or from uterine structural abnormalities (mainly cervical pregnancy).

RISK FACTORS
- History of pelvic inflammatory disease (PID), endometritis, or current gonorrhea/chlamydia infection
- Previous ectopic pregnancy
- History of tubal surgery (~33% of pregnancies after tubal ligation will be ectopic)
- Pelvic adhesive disease (infection or prior surgery)
- Use of an intrauterine device (IUD): IUD reduces absolute risk of ectopic pregnancy, but there is an increased likelihood of ectopic location if pregnancy occurs.
- Use of assisted reproductive technologies
- Maternal diethylstilbestrol (DES) exposure in utero (DES was last used in 1972)
- Tobacco use
- Patients with disorders that affect ciliary motility may be at increased risk (e.g., endometriosis, Kartagener).

GENERAL PREVENTION
- Reliable contraception or abstinence
- Screening for and treatment of STIs (i.e., gonorrhea, chlamydia) that can cause PID and tubal scarring

DIAGNOSIS

HISTORY
In >50% of presenting cases, patients have sudden-onset abdominal pain coupled with cessation of/or irregular menses and acute vaginal bleeding (the classic triad). Other common symptoms include nausea and/or vomiting, vaginal bleeding, and pain referred to the shoulder (from hemoperitoneum).

PHYSICAL EXAM
- Abdominal tenderness ± rebound tenderness
- Vaginal bleeding
- Palpable mass on pelvic exam (adnexal or cul-de-sac fullness)
- Cervical motion tenderness
- In cervical cases, an hourglass-shaped cervix might be noted.
- In cases of rupture and significant intraperitoneal bleeding, signs of shock such as pallor, tachycardia, and hypotension may be present.

DIFFERENTIAL DIAGNOSIS
- Missed, threatened, inevitable, or completed abortion (miscarriage)
- Gestational trophoblastic neoplasia ("molar pregnancy")
- Appendicitis
- Salpingitis, PID
- Ruptured corpus luteum or hemorrhagic cyst
- Ovarian tumor, benign or malignant
- Ovarian torsion
- Cervical polyp, cancer, trauma, or cervicitis

DIAGNOSTIC TESTS & INTERPRETATION
Initial Tests (lab, imaging)
- Check CBC and ABO type and antibody screen.
- Transvaginal US (TVUS) is the gold standard for diagnosis:
  - Failure to visualize a normal intrauterine gestational sac when serum human chorionic gonadotropin (hCG) is above the discriminatory level (>1,500 to 2,000 IU/L) suggests an abnormal pregnancy of unknown location (PUL).
  - An hCG level of 3,500 IU/L is associated with a 99% probability of detecting a normal intrauterine gestational sac in clinical practice (1).
  - These values are not validated for multiple gestations.
- If TVUS unavailable or inconclusive for intrauterine pregnancy (IUP), check hCG: Serial quantitative serum levels normally increase by at least 53% every 48 hours: Abnormal rise (<35%) should prompt workup for gestational abnormalities. Clinical impression of acute abdomen/intraperitoneal bleeding concurrent with a positive hCG level is indicative of ectopic pregnancy until proven otherwise.
- MRI may also be useful but costly and rarely used if TVUS is available; benefits particularly for abdominal or cesarean scar pregnancy

Follow-Up Tests & Special Considerations
- Serum progesterone level: >20 mg/mL associated with lower risk of ectopic pregnancy. In women with pain and/or bleeding who have an inconclusive US, serum progesterone level <3.2 ng/mL ruled out a viable pregnancy in 99.2% of women (2); may provide additional data for PUL but does not predict ectopic pregnancy (3)[B]
- Under investigation: evaluation of serum progesterone levels in conjunction with vascular endothelial growth factor, inhibin A, and activin A using

an algorithm. This diagnosed patients with ectopic pregnancy with 99% accuracy.

Diagnostic Procedures/Other
- In the setting of an undesired pregnancy, sampling of the uterine cavity with endometrial biopsy or D&C can identify the presence/absence of intrauterine chorionic villi. When an IUP has been evacuated by curettage, hCG levels should drop by 50% within 48 hours.
- Historically, culdocentesis was performed to confirm suspected hemoperitoneum prior to surgical management. Currently, TVUS quantification of pelvic fluid is sufficient.

Test Interpretation
Products of conception (POC; especially chorionic villi) outside the uterine cavity

TREATMENT

MEDICATION
- Methotrexate: treatment for unruptured tubal pregnancy or for remaining POCs after laparoscopic salpingostomy. Methotrexate inhibits DNA synthesis via folic acid antagonism by inactivating dihydrofolate reductase.
- If TVUS is suggestive but not diagnostic, in the hemodynamically stable patient who qualifies for medical management, confirm suspected US findings with 2 hCG levels drawn 48 hours apart. Rise <35% is consistent with nonviable pregnancy.
- Most effective when pregnancy is <3 cm diameter, hCG <5,000 mIU/mL, and no fetal heart movement is seen. Success rate is 88% if hCG <1,000 mIU/mL, 71% if hCG 1,000 to 2,000 mIU/mL, 38% if 2,000 to 5,000 mIU/mL:
  - Three main dosage regimens exist (4), but single dose regimen is preferred (X) for simplicity, safety, and comparable effectiveness to multidose regimens (4,5)[A]:
    ○ Single: IM methotrexate 50 mg/m² of body surface area (BSA); may repeat once if <15% decline in hCG between day 4 and 7. Follow hCG weekly.
    ○ Double dose: methotrexate 50 mg/m² of BSA once and then repeated on day 4; if <15% decline in hCG between day 4 and 7, may repeat third dose on day 7. Repeat hCG as needed on days 11 and 14 until decreases >15% in the interval and then weekly. If not dropping by day 14, refer for surgical management.
    ○ Multidose: methotrexate 1 mg/kg IM/IV every other day, with leucovorin 0.1 mg/kg IM in between. Maximum 4 doses until hCG drop below 15%; course may be repeated 7 days after last dose if necessary.
  - Contraindications:
    ○ Hemodynamic instability or any evidence of rupture
    ○ Moderate to severe anemia
    ○ Severe hepatic or renal dysfunction
    ○ Immunodeficiency
  - Relative contraindications
    ○ Fetal heart activity seen
    ○ Large gestational sac (>3 cm, less effective)
    ○ Noncompliance or limited access to hospital or transportation
    ○ hCG >5,000 mIU/Ml
- Precautions: immunologic, hematologic, renal, GI, hepatic, and pulmonary disease, or interacting medications
- Pretreatment testing: serum hCG, CBC, liver and renal function tests, blood type and screen

- Patient counseling: During therapy, refrain from use of alcohol, aspirin, NSAIDs, and folate supplements (decreases efficacy of methotrexate); avoid excessive sun exposure due to risk of sensitivity.
  - Adherence to scheduled follow-up appointments is critical.
  - Increased abdominal pain may occur during treatment; however, severe pain, nausea, vomiting, bleeding, dizziness, or light-headedness may indicate treatment failure and require urgent evaluation.
- Rupture of ectopic pregnancy during methotrexate treatment ranges from 7% to 14%.
- Side effects include stomatitis; conjunctivitis; abdominal cramping; and rarely neutropenia, pneumonitis, or alopecia (5).
- Systemic methotrexate may be offered in some kinds of nontubal ectopic pregnancies, but data is limited.

ISSUES FOR REFERRAL

- Consider gynecologic consultation if not experienced in medical management.
- Refer to a gynecologist for surgical care.

ADDITIONAL THERAPIES

- Physician or patient may elect for surgical treatment as primary method and then postop hCG should guide need for supplemental methotrexate.
- After evidence of medical failure or tubal rupture, surgery is necessary.
- Treatment of cervical, ovarian, abdominal, or other ectopic pregnancy is complicated and requires immediate specialist referral.
- Follow all patients treated medically to an hCG of 0 to ensure that there is no need for surgical intervention.
- Offer anti-D Rh prophylaxis at a dose of 50 μg to all Rh-negative women who have a surgical procedure to manage an ectopic pregnancy or if there has been significant bleeding or abdominal pain.
- Expectant management of ectopic (confirmed on TVUS) may be offered to women who are clinically stable and have low and decreasing hCG level initially <1,500 mIU/mL (3)[B].
- Expectant management to allow for spontaneous resolution of PUL is acceptable in asymptomatic patients with no evidence of rupture or hemodynamic instability coupled with an appropriately low hCG and no extrauterine mass suggestive of ectopic. Ruptured tubal pregnancies may occur even with extremely low hCG levels (<100 mIU/mL) (6).
- With expectant management of PUL, repeat TVUS weekly (or when hCG above discriminatory zone) until location is confirmed or clinical picture is unstable.

SURGERY/OTHER PROCEDURES

- Indications include ruptured ectopic pregnancy, inability to comply with medical follow-up, previous tubal ligation, known tubal disease, current heterotopic pregnancy, desire for permanent sterilization at time of diagnosis.
- Laparoscopy is the first-line surgical management (3)[A].
- Salpingectomy (tubal removal) is preferred and is indicated for uncontrolled bleeding, recurrent ectopic pregnancy, severely damaged tube, large gestational sac, or patient's desire for sterilization (3)[B].
- Salpingostomy (preservation of tube) is considered in patients who wish to maintain fertility particularly if contralateral tube is damaged/absent (3)[C]:
  - No difference in recurrence rate compared to salpingectomy
  - Persistent trophoblastic tissue with salpingostomy remains in the fallopian tube in 4–15% of cases; will need to follow weekly hCG

- Use of US-guided intra-amniotic injection with methotrexate and/or potassium chloride is experimental at this time.
- Surgical treatment is first line for cesarean and cornual pregnancies.

ADMISSION, INPATIENT, AND NURSING CONSIDERATIONS

- Fails criteria for methotrexate management, suspicion of rupture, orthostatic, shock, and severe abdominal pain requiring IV narcotics
- Inpatient observation in the setting of an uncertain diagnosis, particularly with an unreliable patient, may be appropriate.
- Surgical emergency
  - Two IV access lines should be placed immediately if suspicion of rupture; aggressive resuscitation as needed
  - Blood product transfusion if necessary en route to OR
  - In cases of shock, pressors and cardiac support may be necessary.
- IV fluids
  - Unnecessary for a stable ectopic pregnancy being medically treated
  - Critical for a surgical patient who is bleeding
- Strict input/output, hourly vitals, orthostatics if mobile, frequent abdominal exams, serial hematocrit, pad counts if heavy vaginal bleeding
- Discharge criteria: afebrile, abdominal pain resolving or resolved, diagnosis established, surgical treatment, and recovery is complete

 ONGOING CARE

FOLLOW-UP RECOMMENDATIONS
Patient Monitoring
- Serial serum quantitative hCG until level drops to zero:
  - After methotrexate administration, a strict monitoring protocol should be followed.
  - Following salpingostomy, weekly levels are appropriate.
  - Following salpingectomy, further follow-up may be unnecessary.
- Pelvic US for persistent or recurrent masses
- Pain control: brief course of narcotics usually necessary with medical or surgical management
- Liver and renal function tests weekly following methotrexate administration if repeat dosing is required
- Delay of subsequent pregnancy for at least 3 months after treatment with methotrexate due to teratogenicity (folate deficiency) (3)[C]

DIET
- During treatment, avoid alcohol and foods and vitamins high in folate (leafy greens, liver, edamame) due to interaction with methotrexate efficacy.
- Maintain excellent hydration.

PATIENT EDUCATION
- Signs and symptoms of ectopic pregnancy should be reviewed.
- Patients should be encouraged to plan subsequent pregnancies and seek early medical care on discovery of future pregnancies.

PROGNOSIS
- Chronic ectopic pregnancies are rare and treated with surgical removal of the fallopian tube.
- Future fertility depends on fertility prior to ectopic pregnancy and degree of tubal compromise. In women with normal fertility, treatment options have no differences in future fertility rates. In women with subfertility, expectant or medical treatments confer better future fertility (3)[C].

- ~66% of women with a history of ectopic pregnancy will have a future IUP if they are able to conceive.
- If infertility persists beyond 12 months, the fallopian tubes should be evaluated.

COMPLICATIONS
- Hemorrhage and hypovolemic shock
- Persistent trophoblastic tissue after medical or surgical management
- Infection
- Infertility
- Blood transfusions with associated infections/transfusion reaction
- Disseminated intravascular coagulation in the setting of massive hemorrhage

REFERENCES

1. Connolly A, Ryan DH, Stuebe AM, et al. Reevaluation of discriminatory and threshold levels for serum β-hCG in early pregnancy. *Obstet Gynecol*. 2013;121(1):65–70.
2. Verhaegen J, Gallos ID, van Mello NM, et al. Accuracy of single progesterone test to predict early pregnancy outcome in women with pain or bleeding: meta-analysis of cohort studies. *BMJ*. 2012;345:e6077.
3. Diagnosis and management of ectopic pregnancy: Green-top Guideline No. 21. *BJOG*. 2016;123(13):e15–e55.
4. Mergenthal MC, Senapati S, Zee J, et al. Medical management of ectopic pregnancy with single-dose and 2-dose methotrexate protocols: human chorionic gonadotropin trends and patient outcomes. *Am J Obstet Gynecol*. 2016;215(5):590.e1–590.e5.
5. Yuk JS, Lee JH, Park WI, et al. Systematic review and meta-analysis of single-dose and non-single-dose methotrexate protocols in the treatment of ectopic pregnancy. *Int J Gynaecol Obstet*. 2018;141(3):295–303.
6. ACOG Practice Bulletin No. 191 summary: tubal ectopic pregnancy. *Obstet Gynecol*. 2018;131(2):409–411.

ADDITIONAL READING

Barnhart KT. Clinical practice. Ectopic pregnancy. *N Engl J Med*. 2009;361(4):379–387.

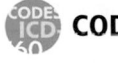 **CODES**

ICD10
- O00.9 Ectopic pregnancy, unspecified
- O00.1 Tubal pregnancy
- O00.0 Abdominal pregnancy

CLINICAL PEARLS
- Ectopic pregnancy is the leading cause of 1st trimester maternal death and accounts for 6% of U.S. pregnancy deaths.
- 97% of ectopic pregnancies occur in the fallopian tube.
- Diagnosis requires high clinical suspicion in the setting of abdominal pain and a positive pregnancy test until IUP is confirmed.

EJACULATORY DISORDERS

Payam Sazegar, MD, CCFP

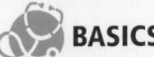 **BASICS**

DESCRIPTION
- Group of dysfunctions involving altered time and control (premature ejaculation [PE], delayed ejaculation [DE]), presence (anejaculation [AE]), direction (retrograde ejaculation [RE]), volume (perceived ejaculate volume reduction [PEVR]), or force (decreased force of ejaculation [DFE]) of ejaculation
- PE is defined (*DSM-V*, 2013) as a persistent/recurrent pattern of ejaculation occurring during partnered sexual activity within 1 minute following vaginal penetration and before the individual wishes it + present for 6 months + causing significant distress for individual.
  - Natural biologic response is to ejaculate within 2 to 5 minutes after vaginal penetration.
  - Ejaculatory control is an acquired behavior that increases with experience.
  - Comorbidities common (diabetes, hypertension, sexual desire disorder, ED)
- DE: prolonged time to ejaculate (>30 minutes) despite desire, stimulation, and erection; problematic for couples trying to conceive
- Aspermia (lack of sperm in the ejaculate):
  - AE: lack of emission or contractions of bulbospongiosus muscle
  - RE: partial or complete ejaculation of semen into the bladder
  - Obstruction: ejaculatory duct obstruction or urethral obstruction
- Also:
  - Painful ejaculation: genital or perineal pain during or after ejaculation
  - Ejaculatory anhedonia: normal ejaculation lacking orgasm or pleasure
  - Hematospermia: presence of blood in the ejaculate (often not a serious condition)

EPIDEMIOLOGY
Prevalence
- PE is common; reported prevalence in U.S. males in up to 20–30%
- DE is reported in 5–8% of men age 18 to 59 years, but <3% have the problem for >6 months.
- Predominant age: all sexually mature age groups
- Predominant sex: male only

ETIOLOGY AND PATHOPHYSIOLOGY
Male sexual response:
- Erection mediated by parasympathetic nervous system
- Normal ejaculation consists of three phases:
  - Emission phase: Semen is deposited into urethra by contraction of prostate, seminal vesicles, vas deferens; under autonomic sympathetic control
  - Ejaculation phase: semen forcibly propelled out of urethra by rhythmic contractions of the bulbospongiosus and ischiocavernosus muscles. This is mediated by the somatic nervous system on the motor branches of the pudendal nerve. Bladder neck contracture by α-adrenergic receptors ensures anterograde ejaculation.
  - Orgasm: the pleasurable sensation associated with ejaculation (cerebral cortex); smooth muscle contraction of accessory sexual organs; release of pressure in posterior urethra

- PE:
  - Hypersensitivity/hyperexcitability of glans penis
  - 5-hydroxytryptamine (5-HT) receptor sensitivity
  - Psychogenic (inexperience, anxiety/guilt, low frequency of sex, relationship problems)
  - Urologic (ED, prostatitis, urethritis)
  - Endocrine (hyperthyroid)
  - Lack of physical activity
  - Withdrawal/detox of prescription or illicit drugs
- DE:
  - Rarely due to underlying painful disorder (e.g., prostatitis, seminal vesiculitis)
  - Often has psychogenic component
  - No relation to testosterone levels
  - Sexual performance anxiety and other psychosocial factors
  - Medications may impair ejaculation (e.g., MAOIs, SSRIs, α- and β-blockers, thiazides, antipsychotics, tricyclic and quadricyclic antidepressants, NSAIDs, opiates, alcohol).
- Never any ejaculate:
  - Congenital structural disorder (müllerian duct cyst, Wolffian abnormality)
  - Acquired (radical prostatectomy, postinfectious, posttraumatic, T10–T12 neuropathy)
- AE:
  - Retroperitoneal lymph node (LN) dissection
  - Spinal cord injury or other (traumatic) sympathetic nerve injury
  - Medications (α- and β-blockers, benzodiazepines, SSRIs, MAOIs, TCAs, antipsychotics, aminocaproic acid)
  - Diabetes mellitus (DM) (neuropathy)
  - Radical prostatectomy
- RE:
  - Transurethral resection of the prostate (25%) or other prostate resection procedures
  - Surgery on the neck of the bladder
  - Extensive pelvic surgery
  - Retroperitoneal LN dissection for testicular cancer (also may produce failure of emission)
  - Neurologic disorders (MS, DM)
  - Medications (tamsulosin, other α-blockers, SSRIs, antipsychotics)
  - Urethral stricture (may be posttraumatic)
- Painful ejaculation:
  - Infection or inflammation (orchitis, epididymitis, prostatitis, urethritis)
  - Ejaculatory duct obstruction
  - Seminal vesicle calculi
  - Obstruction of the vas deferens
  - Psychological/functional
- Hematospermia (often unable to find cause):
  - Usually not a serious condition
  - Inflammation/infection
  - Calculi: bladder, seminal vesicle, prostate, urethra
  - Trauma to genital area (cycling, constipation)
  - Obstruction
  - Cyst
  - Tumor (1–3% prostate cancers present with hematospermia)
  - Arteriovenous malformations
  - Iatrogenic
  - Hypertension

COMMONLY ASSOCIATED CONDITIONS
- Neurologic disorders (e.g., multiple sclerosis)
- DM
- Prostatitis
- Ejaculatory duct obstruction
- Urethral stricture
- Psychological disorders
- Endocrinopathies
- Relationship/interpersonal difficulties

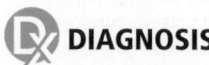 **DIAGNOSIS**

Start by asking if ejaculation occurs before individual wishes OR does not occur following normal stimulation (including masturbation).

HISTORY
Detailed sexual history, including:
- Time frame of the problem
- Quality of patient's sexual response
- Sense of ejaculatory control and sexual distress
- Overall assessment of the relationship
- Ask specific questions because patients often reluctant to discuss openly.
- Detailed history of recent and current medications
- History of past trauma or recent infections
- Past surgical history with particular attention to genitourinary (GU) surgeries
- Supplements and alternative therapies tried
- Many men do not distinguish initially between problems related to erection and ejaculation.
- Some men have unrealistic expectations of ejaculatory response and frequency.
- Include the sexual partner in the interview, especially if the patient expresses a belief that he is not meeting his partner's needs.
- In review of systems, elicit any evidence of testosterone deficiency or prolactin excess, especially if anhedonia present.

PHYSICAL EXAM
- Check vitals. Look for focal neurologic signs (MS, spinal cord injury) and psychiatric disorders.
- Thorough GU exam, including:
  - Size and texture of testes and epididymis
  - Verification of the presence of the vas deferens
  - Location and patency of urethral meatus
  - Digital rectal examination to evaluate prostate consistency, size, and possible midline lesions

DIAGNOSTIC TESTS & INTERPRETATION
- Laboratory test results may be normal.
- Fasting glucose or HgbA1c to rule out diabetes
- Postorgasmic urinalysis will confirm RE. Semen fructose level, sperm count, and viscosity can be measured. Patient may complain of cloudy urine.
- AE will have fructose negative, sperm negative, and nonviscous postorgasmic urinalysis.
- In painful ejaculation, urinalysis and urine culture needed
- If prostate cancer is considered, check prostate-specific antigen (PSA).
- In anhedonia, consider checking testosterone, prolactin, glucose, and thyroid levels.
- In hematospermia, painful ejaculation, or if ejaculatory duct obstruction is considered, transrectal ultrasound (TRUS) may be helpful.

- TRUS-guided seminal vesicle aspiration; if ejaculatory duct obstruction is present, then the aspirate will contain sperm.
- If suspicious of anatomic abnormality, can get scrotal US and/or MRI

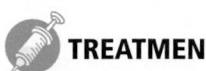

TREATMENT

GENERAL MEASURES
- Identifying any medical cause (even if not reversible) helps patient accept condition.
- Improve partner communication.
- Psychological counseling for patient and partner
- Reduce performance pressure through reassurance.
- Use of a variety of resources may be necessary (e.g., psychiatrist, psychologist, sex therapist, vascular surgeon, urologist, endocrinologist, neurologist).
- PE:
  – Use sensate focus therapy (gradual progression of nonsexual contact to sexual contact).
  – Quiet vagina: Female partner stops moving just prior to ejaculation.
  – Techniques to learn ejaculatory control (e.g., coronal squeeze technique [squeezing the glans penis until ejaculatory urge ceases] or start-and-stop technique [cessation of penile stimulation when ejaculation approaches and resumption of stimulation when ejaculatory feeling ends]) (1)[B]
- DE:
  – Change to antidepressant less likely to cause DE (citalopram, fluvoxamine, nefazodone) (2)[B]
- AE/RE:
  – Discontinue offending medications.
  – Diabetic control
  – If urethral obstruction present, refer to urology.
  – RE may be helped if intercourse occurs when bladder is full.
  – Consider penile vibratory stimulation (effective in spinal cord injuries >T10) or electroejaculation (place on monitor if lesions above T6 because autonomic dysreflexia may result) to collect sperm in AE cases.
- Painful ejaculation:
  – Counseling may be beneficial.
  – If seminal vesicle stones are possible, refer to urology.
- Hematospermia:
  – Often resolves spontaneously, without known cause. Reassure initially.
  – May try empiric antibiotic, but little evidence to support
  – If persistent or high degree of suspicion for abnormality, refer to urologist.

MEDICATION
- PE:
  – Treat underlying erectile dysfunction (if identified) with PDE5 inhibitors (3)[A].
- First line:
  – Dapoxetine, a short-acting SSRI, used "on demand" 30 to 60 mg 1 to 2 hours prior to sex has good efficacy (2,3,4)[A]; best efficacy but higher cost
  – Other "on-demand" options include clomipramine 20 to 50 mg 4 to 24 hours before intercourse, sertraline 50 mg 4 to 8 hours before intercourse, and paroxetine 20 mg 3 to 4 hours before intercourse (2,3,4)[A].

  – Daily dosing of clomipramine 20 to 50 mg, sertraline 25 to 200 mg, fluoxetine 5 to 20 mg, or paroxetine 10 to 40 mg can delay ejaculation within 1 to 3 weeks of starting (2,3)[A].
  – PDE5 inhibitor with or without SSRI (3)[A]
  – Topical anesthetic gel applied (2.5% prilocaine ± 2.5% lidocaine [EMLA]) 2.5 g under a condom for 30 minutes prior to intercourse (5)[A]
  – Tramadol 5 to 50 mg used "on demand" 2 hours before sex. Effective in many studies (6)[A]; now available in spray form
  – Second line: behavioral/sex therapy, pelvic floor muscle therapy (1,2)[B]
- DE:
  – No "approved" drugs; many options
  – Consider switching antidepressants to bupropion, nefazodone, and mirtazapine.
  – Patients who must continue SSRIs may respond to bupropion and buspirone (2,7)[B].
  – Sex therapy, self-stimulation therapies (1,2)[B]
  – Some evidence that amantadine or cyproheptadine may be helpful (2,7)[B]
- AE and RE:
  – First line: pseudoephedrine 60 mg PO daily to QID or imipramine 25 to 75 mg PO BID (8)[A]
  – α-Agonists and antihistamines can be helpful but are not approved by the FDA.
  – Second line: for RE, can try postejaculation bladder harvest of sperm (if fertility desired); for AE, can try midodrine, penile vibratory stimulation, or electroejaculation (2,8)[B]
- Painful ejaculation:
  – Treat underlying infection/inflammatory process.
  – α-Blockers may have some benefit.

ISSUES FOR REFERRAL
The following conditions, when suspected, should be referred to a urologist:
- Ejaculatory duct obstruction
- Seminal vesicle or prostatic stones
- Urethral obstruction
- Vas deferens obstruction
- Calculi
- Persistent or severe hematospermia (2)[B]

SURGERY/OTHER PROCEDURES
Surgical treatment of ejaculatory duct obstruction:
- Transurethral resection of the ejaculatory ducts

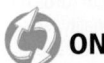

ONGOING CARE

PATIENT EDUCATION
See "General Measures."

PROGNOSIS
Often improves with therapy and counseling

COMPLICATIONS
Psychological impact on some males: signs of severe inadequacy, self-doubt, additional anxiety, and guilt

REFERENCES
1. Pastore A, Palleschi G, Fuschi A, et al. Pelvic muscle floor rehabilitation as a therapeutic option in life-long premature ejaculation: long-term outcomes. *Asian J Androl*. 2018;20(6):572–575.
2. Althof SE, McMahon CG. Contemporary management of disorders of male orgasm and ejaculation. *Urology*. 2016;93:9–21.
3. Sun Y, Yang L, Bao Y, et al. Efficacy of PDE5Is and SSRIs in men with premature ejaculation: a new systematic review and five meta-analyses. *World J Urol*. 2017;35(12):1817–1831.
4. Sridharan K, Sivaramakrishnan G, Sequeira R, et al. Pharmacological interventions for premature ejaculation: a mixed-treatment comparison network meta-analysis of randomized clinical trials. *Int J Impot Res*. 2018;30(5):215–223.
5. Wyllie MG, Powell JA. The role of local anaesthetics in premature ejaculation. *BJU Int*. 2012;110(11, Pt C):E943–E948.
6. Kirby EW, Carson CC, Coward RM. Tramadol for the management of premature ejaculation: a timely systematic review. *Int J Impot Res*. 2015;27(4):121–127.
7. Abdel-Hamid I, Ali O. Delayed ejaculation: pathophysiology, diagnosis, and treatment. *World J Mens Health*. 2018;36(1):22–40.
8. Shoshany O, Abhyankar N, Elyaguov J, et al. Efficacy of treatment with pseudoephedrine in men with retrograde ejaculation. *Andrology*. 2017;5(4):744–748.

ADDITIONAL READING
- Jiann B. The office management of ejaculatory disorders. *Transl Androl Urol*. 2016;5(4):526–540.
- Mehta A, Sigman M. Management of the dry ejaculate: a systematic review of aspermia and retrograde ejaculation. *Fertil Steril*. 2015;104(5):1074–1081.
- Sahin S, Bicer M, Yenice MG, et al. A prospective randomized controlled study to compare acupuncture and dapoxetine for the treatment of premature ejaculation. *Urol Int*. 2016;97(1):104–111.

CODES

ICD10
- F52.4 Premature ejaculation
- N53.11 Retarded ejaculation
- N53.14 Retrograde ejaculation

CLINICAL PEARLS
- If erectile dysfunction is contributing to ejaculatory difficulty, management of erectile dysfunction should precede attempted management of ejaculatory disorders.
- Medications should always be thoroughly reviewed because they may be the primary cause of ejaculatory disorders.
- PE and DE generally have both psychogenic and physical causes, whereas AE and RE are due to organic neurogenic/autonomic dysfunction.
- A multidisciplinary approach, including the primary care physician, urologists, psychologists, and other appropriate health care professionals, is essential to the proper treatment of ejaculatory disorders.

ELDER ABUSE

Nitin Budhwar, MD • Kimberly Kone, MD

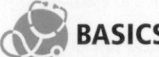 **BASICS**

DESCRIPTION
- The National Center of Elder Abuse divides abuse into three categories (age >60) (1)[A]:
  - **Domestic:** abuse from someone who has a special relationship with the elderly individual (spouse, child, friend, or in-home caregiver) that occurs in the home of the elderly or caregiver
  - **Institutional:** occurs in the setting of a facility that is responsible for caring for the elderly, such as a nursing home or long-term care facility
  - **Self-neglect:** The behavior of the elderly individual leads to harm.
- Types of abuse in estimated order of occurrence:
  - Self-neglect (estimated 50%): the most common form of abuse (2)[C]
  - Financial
  - Neglect
  - Emotional
  - Physical
  - Sexual
  - Taken advantage of: misinformation and unregulated online pharmaceutical, financial companies, and so forth, that specifically target the elderly leading to deleterious outcomes (3)[C]

EPIDEMIOLOGY
Incidence
Estimate is that as many as 1:10 have been victims of abuse, placing a conservative number at 50,000 cases per year. Majority of whom are believed to be women (4)[A].

Prevalence
A recent national survey measuring prevalence of abuse in individuals of at least 60 years and older found that 11.9% of the surveyed population suffered some form of abuse:
- 5.2% encountered financial mistreatment by family members.
- 5.1% suffered potential neglect.
- 4.6% encountered emotional mistreatment, mostly by humiliation or verbal abuse.
- 1.6% encountered physical mistreatment, mostly through battery.
- 0.6% sexually mistreated, mostly through forced intercourse.

ETIOLOGY AND PATHOPHYSIOLOGY
The etiology of elder abuse is a complex biopsychosocial combination of increased dependence on the caregiver by the victim in a suboptimal environment with poor behavioral coping methods, which is compounded by increased stress.

Genetics
Not contributory

RISK FACTORS
- The victim:
  - Advanced age
  - Exploitable resources
  - Prior history of abuse in life
  - Dementia or other cognitive impairment
  - Female gender
  - Disability in caring for him/herself
  - Depression
  - Social isolation
  - Stress: health, financial, or situational
- The abuser:
  - Mental illness
  - Financial dependency
  - Substance abuse
  - History of violence
  - Other antisocial behavior (5)[C]

GENERAL PREVENTION
- Improve patient's social contact and support.
- Identify and correct potential risk factors for elder abuse:
  - Home visit to identify for potential risks of fall hazards and barriers to ambulation that could lead to fractures and functional decline that could leave the individual vulnerable to abuse
  - Evaluate for assistive devices that help the patient independently complete his/her ADLs and prevent caregiver dependence.
  - Screen for depression using validated tools like the Geriatric Depression Scale.
  - Early identification and treatment of cognitive impairment
- Identify caregiver stress and burden; refer to community programs that aid with emotional assistance.
- Advance life directives planning, including identifying possible caregivers, choosing a medical power of attorney (MPOA), estate, and will planning, and so forth

COMMONLY ASSOCIATED CONDITIONS
Most common associated conditions with elder abuse are also identified as risk factors: social isolation, increased dependence for ADLs/IADLs, depression, cognitive impairment, and aggressive behavior (5)[C],(6)[B].

 DIAGNOSIS

A high index of suspicion when risk factors are present is important; types of abuse should be kept in mind as some types might not be obvious. It can be difficult to diagnose elder abuse in a single clinic visit, so it is important to get social services involved and to consider doing home visits, when abuse is suspected (5)[C].

HISTORY
It is important to take a detailed history with focus on the living arrangements, degree of functionality, who the caregivers are, and other risk factors listed above. Pay attention to clues such as withdrawal from normal activities or a sudden change in finances or abrupt changes to a will.

PHYSICAL EXAM
- It is important objectively to document positive and negative findings in your physical exam and to be very detailed because it can be admissible in court if abuse is suspected.
- Vital signs: Check weight and assess for progressive loss in weight; BP and pulse rate can be an indicator of dehydration that could be secondary to neglect.
- General overall appearance:
  - Wasting or cachexia
  - Poor hygiene, unkempt clothing
  - If the patient is bedbound, it is important to assess the integrity of the mattress and sheets. Look for excessive skin flakes, hair, or urine-soiled mattresses.
- Oral exam:
  - Assess for poor dentition, oral ulcers, or abscesses.
- Skin exam:
  - Most bruises from elder abuse are large (>5 cm) and located on the face, lateral arm, or back.
  - Bite or burn marks
  - It is important to check for pressure ulcers on the bony prominences of the patient: elbows, sacrum, heels, and scapula.
- Mental/psychiatric:
  - Withdrawn, anxious, fearful, blunted
- Genital/rectal exam if sexual abuse is suspected (4)[A]

DIFFERENTIAL DIAGNOSIS
- Advanced dementia can present with individuals appearing withdrawn and they are often malnourished.
- Elderly with advanced dementia of Alzheimer type or Lewy body dementia can present with delusions of persecution and aggression that can be confused for elder abuse.
- Patients with Parkinson disease often fall and may exhibit fractures and bruises on a frequent basis that may mimic recurrent physical abuse.
- Coagulopathy seen in patients in advanced malignancy with bone marrow suppression or invasion, and those on chronic antiplatelet therapy can appear with bruising that can be easily confused with elder abuse.
- Wasting from malignancy, infections, chronic disease
- Thyroid disorder can present with altered mental status (AMS), depression, or anxiety.
- Chronic lung disease can present with decreased weight.
- Delirium from acute electrolyte disturbances, infectious etiology, or cardiovascular compromise can all present similar to elder abuse.
- Impaired financial status can also be confused with self-neglect.

DIAGNOSTIC TESTS & INTERPRETATION
The following workup is recommended:
- Nutritional assessment: iron, vitamin B$_{12}$, folate, thiamine, albumin, prealbumin, CBC, LFTs, electrolytes
- Malignancy workup, as per current guidelines
- If bruising is noted, check for coagulopathies (e.g., platelets, bleeding times, PT/INR, and PTT).
- If cognitive impairment is observed, check thyroid-stimulating hormone, vitamin B$_{12}$ level; consider syphilis and HIV testing if indicated.
- Assessment of infection: may include urinalysis and culture, chest radiograph, blood count, and cultures
- Radiographic imaging of areas below soft tissue injury is indicated if there is evidence of infection (osteomyelitis) at a pressure ulcer site or bruising of a limb (fracture).
- If physical abuse is suspected and cognitive impairment present, then cranial imaging to look for hemorrhage (e.g., subdural) is indicated using CT scan or MRI.

Diagnostic Procedures/Other
- Pulse test: Check BP and pulse in presence and absence of suspected abuser. Elevation of either in the presence of the suspected abuser should raise suspicion. Useful in patients with dementia or other condition that makes history-taking difficult.
- Folstein Mini-Mental State Examination (MMSE), Montreal Cognitive Assessment (MOCA), or other validated tools to assess for cognitive impairment if suspected

- Geriatric Depression Scale if suspected
- Documentation: Practitioners may make statements of "suspected mistreatment" but should avoid making definitive diagnosis of abuse in their initial assessment, unless it is very obvious.

 TREATMENT

Most states require all health care providers to report suspected elder abuse to a local agency such as the Adult Protective Services (http://www.nccafv.org /state_elder_abuse_hotlines.htm).

MEDICATION
None

ADMISSION, INPATIENT, AND NURSING CONSIDERATIONS
- Victims of elder abuse should be admitted to the hospital if there are no safe discharge alternatives.
- Management of uncontrolled chronic conditions due to neglect (i.e., wound care from ulcers or infections)
- Cases of suspected abuse *must be reported* to the state's Adult Protective Services agency or a designated alternative (e.g., if patient resides in nursing home, then report to that state's regulatory entity). Social services may help. If physical harm has occurred, consider reporting to local law enforcement for investigation.
- Hospital security may need to be notified if restricted visitor access to a patient is required, and the patient's name may be hidden from the public hospital census.
- If the patient is a victim of elder abuse, he/she must be relocated to a safer alternative and may need admission for sequelae caused by the abuse.
- Victims should not be discharged to a potentially abusive environment. Alternatives to discharge to the unsafe environment may include:
  – Friend or family member
  – Nursing home
  – Personal care home
  – Assisted living facility
  – Local victims' rescue or sheltering program if available

 ONGOING CARE

FOLLOW-UP RECOMMENDATIONS
Victims of abuse should not be discharged without adequate follow-up, including:
- Primary care physician visit within 1 week
- Follow-up with Adult Protective Services or other agency; a home visit should be scheduled prior to discharge if the patient is going back home.

- Home Health Agency for assessment of safety (physical therapy)
- Follow-up with appropriate mental health care

Patient Monitoring
The patient should have frequent visits and be followed through the appropriate agencies to reduce continuation of abuse and to identify recurring abuse.

PATIENT EDUCATION
- For Elder Abuse Resources in your state, you can go to the National Center of Elder Abuse at https://ncea.acl.gov
- Or your local representative by calling 1-800-677-1166

PROGNOSIS
Elder abuse and self-neglect are associated with an overall increased risk in mortality (7)[B].

COMPLICATIONS
Complications of elder abuse can lead to worsening depression, increased mortality, and overall poor quality of life.

REFERENCES
1. National Center on Elder Abuse. *Elder Abuse Prevalence and Incidence*. Washington, DC: National Center on Elder Abuse; 2005.
2. Mosqueda L, Dong X. Elder abuse and self-neglect: "I don't care anything about going to the doctor, to be honest. . ." *JAMA*. 2011;306(5):532–540.
3. Liang BA, Lovett KM, Mackey TK. Elder abuse. *J Am Geriatr Soc*. 2012;60(2):398–400.
4. Committee opinion no. 568: elder abuse and women's health. *Obstet Gynecol*. 2013;122(1):187–191.
5. Halphen JM, Varas GM, Sadowsky JM. Recognizing and reporting elder abuse and neglect. *Geriatrics*. 2009;64(7):13–18.
6. Acierno R, Hernandez MA, Amstadter AB, et al. Prevalence and correlates of emotional, physical, sexual, and financial abuse and potential neglect in the United States: the National Elder Mistreatment Study. *Am J Public Health*. 2010;100(2):292–297.
7. Dong X, Simon M, Mendes de Leon C, et al. Elder self-neglect and abuse and mortality risk in a community-dwelling population. *JAMA*. 2009;302(5):517–526.

ADDITIONAL READING
- Burnett J, Dyer CB, Halphen JM, et al. Four subtypes of self-neglect in older adults: results of a latent class analysis. *J Am Geriatr Soc*. 2014;62(6): 1127–1132.
- Cooper C, Katona C, Finne-Soveri H, et al. Indicators of elder abuse: a crossnational comparison of psychiatric morbidity and other determinants

in the ad-hoc study. *Am J Geriatr Psychiatry*. 2006;14(6):489–497.
- Lachs MS, Pillemer K. Elder abuse. *Lancet*. 2004;364(9441):1263–1272.
- Lachs MS, Williams CS, O'Brien S, et al. Adult protective service use and nursing home placement. *Gerontologist*. 2002;42(6):734–739.
- Lachs MS, Williams CS, O'Brien S, et al. The mortality of elder mistreatment. *JAMA*. 1998;280(5): 428–432.
- Widera E, Steenpass V, Marson D, et al. Finances in the older patient with cognitive impairment: "He didn't want me to take over." *JAMA*. 2011;305(7):698–706.
- Wiglesworth A, Austin R, Corona M, et al. Bruising as a marker of physical elder abuse. *J Am Geriatr Soc*. 2009;57(7):1191–1196.
- Wiglesworth A, Mosqueda L, Mulnard R, et al. Screening for abuse and neglect of people with dementia. *J Am Geriatr Soc*. 2010;58(3):493–500.

 CODES

ICD10
- T74.11XA Adult physical abuse, confirmed, initial encounter
- T74.21XA Adult sexual abuse, confirmed, initial encounter
- T74.01XA Adult neglect or abandonment, confirmed, initial encounter

CLINICAL PEARLS
- Elder abuse, or elder mistreatment, is a condition in which the physical, psychological, or financial well-being of an older adult is infringed on through intentional acts or lack of action, even if harm is not intended.
- It is important to identify vulnerable individuals through proper evaluation of potential risk factors for abuse (social isolation, depression, cognitive impairment, disability requiring assistance, and financial dependence by the caregiver).
- Correction of risk factors is important to reduce the incidence of elder abuse (strengthen the patients' social support, treat depression, provide the patient with assistive devices, screen for cognitive impairment with a trial of medication if possible, and identify caregiver burn out).
- Clearly document your physical exam with only specific objective findings.
- Contact APS or your local resources if elder abuse is suspected; it is unlawful not to report suspected elder abuse.

ENCOPRESIS

Jay Fong, MD • William T. Garrison, PhD

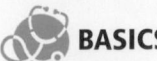 **BASICS**

DESCRIPTION
- Voluntary or involuntary fecal soilage in a (typically) previously toilet-trained child
  - Age may be chronologic or developmental.
  - No underlying organic disease
  - At least one event per month for 3 months
  - Classified into functional constipation (retentive encopresis) and functional nonretentive fecal incontinence (FNRFI); both cause fecal incontinence. There is no constipation in FNRFI. *Functional constipation is more common.*
- System(s) affected: GI; psychological
- Synonyms(s): fecal incontinence, soiling

EPIDEMIOLOGY
Incidence
Predominant sex: male > female (4 to 6:1)
Constipation accounts for 3% of general pediatric referrals; up to 84% of constipated children have fecal incontinence at some point.

Prevalence
Occurs in 1–3% of children 4 years of age

ETIOLOGY AND PATHOPHYSIOLOGY
- In 90% of cases, encopresis develops as a consequence of chronic constipation, with resulting overflow incontinence (*retentive encopresis*). The other 10% are caused by specific organic etiologies.
- Chronic constipation with irregular and incomplete evacuation results in progressive rectal distension and stretching of the internal/external anal sphincters.
- As a child habituates to chronic rectal distension, they may no longer sense the normal urge to defecate. Eventually, soft or liquid stool leaks around the retained fecal mass.
- Many children voluntarily withhold stool in response to the urge to defecate for fear of pain or a preoccupation with not interrupting social activities.
- Psychological
  - Stool withholding, fear, anxiety
  - Difficulty with toilet training, including unusual anxiety or conflict with parent
  - Resistance to using public toilet facilities, such as school bathrooms or outdoor toilets
  - Known association with sexual abuse in boys; likely similar association in girls
  - Developmental delay
- Anatomic
  - Rectal distension and desensitization
  - Anal fissure or painful defecation
  - Muscle hypotonia
  - Slow intestinal motility
  - Hirschsprung disease
  - Cystic fibrosis
  - Spinal cord defects (e.g., spina bifida)
  - Congenital anorectal malformations
  - Anal stenosis
  - Anterior displacement of the anus
  - Postoperative stricture of anus or rectum
  - Pelvic mass
  - Neurofibromatosis

- Dietary or metabolic
  - Inadequate dietary fiber
  - Excessive protein or milk intake
  - Inadequate water intake
  - Hypothyroidism
  - Hypercalcemia
  - Hypokalemia
  - Diabetes insipidus; diabetes mellitus
  - Food allergy
  - Gluten enteropathy
- Medication side effects

Genetics
None known; although incidence may be higher in children with family history of constipation

RISK FACTORS
- Male gender
- Constipation
- Very low birth weight
- Painful defecation
- Difficulty with bowel training, including social pressure related to early daycare placement
- Organic/anatomic causes
- Anxiety and depression
- Insufficient fluid or fiber intake
- Refusal to use public restrooms
- Attention deficit
- History of abuse

GENERAL PREVENTION
Family education: toilet training when ready; optimize fluid and fiber intake.

COMMONLY ASSOCIATED CONDITIONS
- Constipation, Hirschsprung disease
- Cerebral palsy, cystic fibrosis
- Developmental and behavioral diagnoses, urinary incontinence

 DIAGNOSIS

HISTORY
- Signs/symptoms of constipation:
  - Hard, large-caliber stools
  - <3 defecations per week
  - Pain or discomfort with stool passage
  - Withholding stool
  - Blood on stool or in diaper/toilet bowl
  - Decreased appetite
  - Abdominal pain that improves with stool passage
  - Hiding while defecating before child is toilet-trained; avoiding use of the toilet
  - Diet low in fiber or fluids, high in dairy products
  - No stool passage in the first 48 hours of life
  - Pasty stool on underclothes
  - Recurrent UTIs
- Abrupt onset after age 5 years more likely to be associated with psychological trauma
- Overlap with attention deficit disorder (ADD) common in children >5 years
- Medication use: opiates, phenobarbital, and tricyclic antidepressants (TCAs)
- Family history of constipation

PHYSICAL EXAM
- Neurologic exam of lower extremities and perineal area, with attention to S1–S4 distribution, perineal sensation, cremasteric reflex, and anal sphincter tone
- Genital examination and digital rectal exam: Assess for anal fissures, sphincter tone, rectal distension/impaction, occult or visible blood.
- Abdominal exam: bowel sounds, percussion note (tympany), abdominal distension; palpate for stool (most common in left lower quadrant).

DIAGNOSTIC TESTS & INTERPRETATION
Most cases diagnosed by history and physical

Initial Tests (lab, imaging)
- Only to rule out organic causes
- UA/urine culture: UTI/glucosuria
- Thyroid function tests: hypothyroidism
- Electrolyte panel, including calcium: hypokalemia, hypercalcemia, or hyperglycemia
- Abdominal plain films if impaction is suspected and not detected by abdominal or rectal exam

Follow-Up Tests & Special Considerations
- Failure to pass meconium within 48 hours of birth, failure to thrive, bloody diarrhea, or bilious vomiting in a neonate should be promptly evaluated to exclude aganglionic megacolon.
- Constipation and diarrhea, rash, failure to thrive, or recurrent pneumonia should prompt evaluation for cystic fibrosis. Patients with abdominal distension or ileus should be evaluated for possible obstruction.

Diagnostic Procedures/Other
Manometric studies may be useful in patients who have constipation that does not respond to treatment.

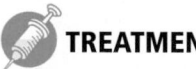 **TREATMENT**

GENERAL MEASURES
- Anticipatory toilet training advice about when children should reduce reliance on diapers or use pull-ups during the daytime hours (average age for toilet training in girls is 29 months; 31 months for boys)
- Eliminate impaction prior to maintenance therapy.
- Avoid frequent and repeated rectal exams, enemas, and suppositories, especially in infants.
- Once stools are regular in frequency, child should sit on toilet BID at the same time each day for 10 to 15 minutes and for 10 to 15 minutes after meals. Incorporate positive reinforcement for successful bowel movements.

MEDICATION
- Remove impaction and start maintenance treatment.
- No randomized, controlled studies have compared methods of disimpaction: can use oral agents, enemas, and rectal suppositories; oral agents are least traumatic. Glycerin suppositories are best option for infants.

First Line
- Disimpaction with polyethylene glycol (PEG)
  - Give 17 g (240 mL) water or juice: 1.0 to 1.5 g/kg/day for 3 days for disimpaction
  - 0.4 to 0.8 g/kg/day for maintenance
- Disimpaction with mineral oil for child >1 year; give 15 to 30 mL/year of age to max 240 mL.
  - Maintenance: 1 to 3 mL/kg/day or divided BID
  - May mix with orange juice to make palatable; avoid in infants to avoid aspiration pneumonia.
- Other maintenance regimens include the following:
  - Milk of magnesia (MOM) 400 mg (5 mL): 1 to 2 mL/kg/day BID
  - Lactulose 10 g (15 mL): 1 to 3 mL/kg/day divided BID
  - Senna syrup 8.8 g sennoside (5 mL): age 2 to 6 years: 2.5 to 7.5 mL/day divided BID; age 6 to 12 years: 5 to 15 mL/day divided BID
  - Bisacodyl suppository 10 mg: 0.5 to 1 suppository once or twice per day

ISSUES FOR REFERRAL
If symptoms do not improve after 6 months of compliance with a multifactorial treatment model, refer to pediatric gastroenterologist for further evaluation and guidance.

ADDITIONAL THERAPIES
Behavioral treatment and counseling

SURGERY/OTHER PROCEDURES
If ongoing constipation is refractory to a combination of medical and behavioral therapy, consider anorectal manometry to evaluate for internal anal sphincter achalasia (or ultrashort-segment Hirschsprung disease). If present, this condition can be treated successfully in most patients with an internal sphincter myectomy.

COMPLEMENTARY & ALTERNATIVE MEDICINE
- Children with volitional stool holding who receive behavioral treatment in addition to medications are more likely to have resolution of encopresis at 3 and 6 months than with medication alone (1)[A].
- No evidence that biofeedback training adds benefit to conventional treatment for functional fecal incontinence in children (2)[A]
- Behavioral interventions combined with laxative therapy (rather than laxative therapy alone) improve continence in children with functional fecal incontinence associated with constipation (1)[B].

ADMISSION, INPATIENT, AND NURSING CONSIDERATIONS
- Admission criteria/initial stabilization
  - Continued soiling and recurrent impaction on outpatient medical therapy, whether from lack of medication efficacy or patient nonadherence
  - Decreased intake leading to malnutrition or dehydration
  - Recalcitrant vomiting or concern for obstruction
  - Involve appropriate agencies if concern for abuse.
  - Hospital admission and abdominal films may be necessary to ensure complete removal of impaction. This may include direct gastric administration of balanced electrolyte–PEG solutions if the patient cannot tolerate by mouth. Serial abdominal films and observation of rectal effluent can help determine treatment adequacy.

- IV fluids if the patient is dehydrated and has difficulty tolerating oral intake
- Nursing to document stool output and character
- Discharge criteria
  - Stools that are looser in consistency and clearer in appearance are a successful inpatient end point.
  - Abdominal radiographs showing less fecal loading (compared with a pretreatment radiograph) with improving serial abdominal exams

 ONGOING CARE

FOLLOW-UP RECOMMENDATIONS
Patient Monitoring
- Continue maintenance treatment for 6 months to 2 years with visits every 4 to 10 weeks for support and to ensure compliance; more frequent visits with oppositional or anxious children
- Telephone or virtual visits can be used to adjust doses and to provide ongoing encouragement.
- Treat recurrences of impaction promptly.
- Emphasize compliance with medication and self-initiation of regular bathroom visits.
- Children who do not progress using a well-designed behavior plan should be referred for more in-depth mental health evaluation and counseling.

DIET
Adequate fluid and fiber intake (2)[A]. Reduce cow's milk products. Avoid excessive consumption of bananas, rice, apples, and gelatin.

PATIENT EDUCATION
- Demystify defecation.
- Carefully explain the treatment plan including medications and dietary changes.
- Avoid punishment for inadvertent soiling.
- In children >4 years of age, explain to parents how overreliance on diapers and pull-ups (while convenient) can prolong the problem.
- Always attempt to use positive reinforcement for successful toilet sits and medication compliance.
- If positive approach is unsuccessful, consider removing desired privileges (e.g., TV, video games) for noncompliance with behavioral plan. Some children respond well to a token economy (earned privileges) to promote desired behavior.

PROGNOSIS
- Many children exhibit a good response and relapse due to parental noncompliance.
- From 30% to 50% of children may still have encopresis after 5 years of treatment.
- Children with psychosocial or emotional problems preceding the encopresis are more recalcitrant to treatment.

COMPLICATIONS
- Colitis due to excessive enema/suppository
- Perianal dermatitis
- Anal fissure

REFERENCES
1. Brazzelli M, Griffiths PV, Cody JD, et al. Behavioural and cognitive interventions with or without other treatments for the management of faecal incontinence in children. *Cochrane Database Syst Rev.* 2011;(12):CD002240.
2. Tabbers MM, DiLorenzo C, Berger MY, et al; for European Society for Pediatric Gastroenterology, Hepatology, and Nutrition, North American Society for Pediatric Gastroenterology. Evaluation and treatment of functional constipation in infants and children: evidence-based recommendations from ESPGHAN and NASPGHAN. *J Pediatr Gastroenterol Nutr.* 2014;58(2):258–274.

ADDITIONAL READING
- Constipation Guideline Committee of the North American Society for Pediatric Gastroenterology, Hepatology and Nutrition. Evaluation and treatment of constipation in infants and children: recommendations of the North American Society for Pediatric Gastroenterology, Hepatology and Nutrition. *J Pediatr Gastroenterol Nutr.* 2006;43(3): e1–e13.
- Levitt M, Peña A. Update on pediatric faecal incontinence. *Eur J Pediatr Surg.* 2009;19(1):1–9.

 CODES

ICD10
- R15.9 Full incontinence of feces
- R15.1 Fecal smearing
- F98.1 Encopresis not due to a substance or known physiol condition

CLINICAL PEARLS
- 90% of encopresis results from chronic constipation.
- Address toddler constipation early by decreasing excessive milk intake, increasing fruits/vegetables intake, and ensuring adequate fluid and fiber intake.
- Eliminate fecal impaction before initiating maintenance therapy.

ENDOCARDITIS, INFECTIVE

Samantha Faryn Gottlieb, DO, MS • Theodore B. Flaum, DO, FACOFP

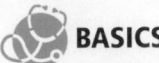

BASICS

DESCRIPTION
- An infection of the valvular (primarily) and/or mural (rarely) endocardium
- System(s) affected: cardiovascular, endocrine/metabolic, hematologic/lymphatic, immunologic, pulmonary, renal/urologic, skin/exocrine, neurologic
- Synonym(s): bacterial endocarditis; subacute bacterial endocarditis (SBE); acute bacterial endocarditis (ABE)

EPIDEMIOLOGY
Incidence
- Incidence rose in the United States from 11/100,000 in 2000 to 15/100,000 in 2011.
- 1.5–3% incidence 1 year after prosthetic valve replacement; 3–6% 5 years postreplacement
- Increasing incidence of cardiovascular device–related infections due to higher frequency of implantable devices, especially in the elderly

ETIOLOGY AND PATHOPHYSIOLOGY
- ABE: Staphylococcus aureus; Streptococcus groups A, B, C, G; Streptococcus pneumoniae; Staphylococcus lugdunensis; Enterococcus spp. (gram-positive); Haemophilus influenzae or parainfluenzae; Neisseria gonorrhoeae (gram-negative)
- SBE: α-hemolytic streptococci (viridans group strep), Streptococcus bovis, Enterococcus spp., S. aureus, Staphylococcus epidermidis (gram-positive); HACEK organisms: Haemophilus aphrophilus or paraphrophilus, Actinobacillus (Aggregatibacter) actinomycetemcomitans, Cardiobacterium hominis, Eikenella corrodens, Kingella kingae
- Endocarditis in IV drug abusers (tricuspid valve): S. aureus, Enterococcus spp. (gram-positive); Pseudomonas aeruginosa, Burkholderia cepacia, other bacilli (gram-negative); Candida spp.
- Early prosthetic valve endocarditis (<60 days after valve implantation): S. aureus, S. epidermidis (gram-positive); gram-negative bacilli; fungi: Candida spp., Aspergillus spp.
- Late prosthetic valve endocarditis (>60 days after valve implantation): α-hemolytic streptococci, Enterococcus spp., S. epidermidis (gram-positive); Candida spp., Aspergillus spp.
- Culture-negative endocarditis: 10% of cases; Bartonella quintana (homeless); Brucella spp., fungi, Coxiella burnetii (Q fever), Chlamydia trachomatis, Chlamydophila psittaci, HACEK organisms; Abiotrophia (formerly vitamin B₆–deficient streptococci); use of antibiotics prior to blood cultures
- Device-related endocarditis: coagulase-negative staphylococci or S. aureus

RISK FACTORS
- Injection drug use, IV catheterization, certain malignancies (colon cancer), poor dentition, chronic hemodialysis
- High risk with:
  - Prosthetic cardiac valve, implantable devices (pacemaker, automatic implantable-cardioverter defibrillator [AICD]), total parenteral nutrition
  - Previous infective endocarditis (IE)
  - Congenital heart disease (CHD): unrepaired cyanotic CHD, including palliative shunts and conduits; repaired CHD with prosthetic device during the first 6 months; repaired CHD with residual defects at or near prosthetic site; cardiac transplant with valvulopathy (1)[B]

GENERAL PREVENTION
- Good oral hygiene
- Antibiotic prophylaxis is only recommended for high-risk cardiac conditions (1)[B]—prosthetic heart valve, history of endocarditis, transplant with abnormal valvular function, CHD (see "Risk Factors").
- *Procedures requiring prophylaxis*
  - Oral/upper respiratory tract: any manipulation of gingival tissue or periapical region of teeth or perforation of the oral mucosa (1)[B]; invasive respiratory procedures involving incision; or biopsy of the respiratory mucosa merit prophylaxis. Amoxicillin 2 g PO (if penicillin allergic, clindamycin 600 mg PO) 30 to 60 minutes before procedure or ampicillin 2 g IV/IM are first-line prophylactic choices. For penicillin-allergic patients, use clindamycin 600 mg IV, or cephalexin 2 g PO, or azithromycin/clarithromycin 500 mg PO, or cefazolin/ceftriaxone 1 g IV/IM 30 minutes before procedure. Pediatric doses are amoxicillin 50 mg/kg PO (max 2 g), cephalexin 50 mg/kg PO (max 2 g), clindamycin 20 mg/kg PO (max 600 mg), and ampicillin or ceftriaxone 50 mg/kg (maximum 1 g) IM/IV.
  - GI/GU: Only consider coverage for Enterococcus (with penicillin, ampicillin, piperacillin, or vancomycin) for patients with an established infection undergoing procedures (1)[B].
  - Cardiac valvular surgery or placement of prosthetic intracardiac/intravascular materials: perioperative cefazolin 1 to 2 g IV 30 minutes preoperative or vancomycin 15 mg/kg (maximum 1 g) (penicillin-allergic patients) 60 minutes preoperative (1)[B]
  - Skin: incision and drainage of infected tissue; use agents active against skin pathogens (e.g., cefazolin 1 to 2 g IV q8h or vancomycin 15 mg/kg q12h; max 1 g) if penicillin-allergic or if methicillin-resistant S. aureus (MRSA) suspected.

DIAGNOSIS

- Modified Duke Criteria (1)[B] (definite: 2 major criteria, or 1 major and 3 minor criteria, or 5 minor criteria; possible: 1 major and 1 minor or 3 minor criteria)
- Major clinical criteria
  - Positive blood culture: isolation of typical microorganism for IE from two separate blood cultures or persistently positive blood culture
  - Single positive blood culture for C. burnetii or anti–phase-1 IgG antibody titer >1:800
  - Positive echocardiogram: presence of vegetation, abscess, or new partial dehiscence of prosthetic valve; must be performed rapidly if IE is suspected
  - New valvular regurgitation (change in preexisting murmur not sufficient)
- Minor criteria
  - Predisposing heart condition or IV drug use
  - Fever ≥38.0°C (100.4°F)
  - Vascular phenomena: major arterial emboli, septic pulmonary infarcts, mycotic aneurysm, intracranial hemorrhage, conjunctival hemorrhage, Janeway lesions
  - Immunologic phenomena: glomerulonephritis, Osler nodes, Roth spots, rheumatoid factor (RF)
  - Microbiologic evidence: positive blood culture not a major criterion (excluding single positive cultures for coagulase-negative staphylococci and organisms that do not cause endocarditis) or serologic evidence of infection likely to cause IE

HISTORY
- Fever (>38°C), chills, cough, dyspnea, orthopnea; especially in subacute endocarditis: night sweats, weight loss, fatigue
- Review risk factors.
- Symptoms of transient ischemic attack, cerebrovascular accident (CVA), or myocardial infarction (MI) on presentation

PHYSICAL EXAM
- Most patients with IE have new murmur or change in existing murmur; signs of heart failure (rales, edema) if valve function is compromised
- Peripheral stigmata of IE: splinter hemorrhages in fingernail beds, Osler nodes on fleshy portions of extremities, "Roth spot" retinal hemorrhages, Janeway lesions (cutaneous evidence of septic emboli), palatal or conjunctival petechiae, splenomegaly, hematuria (due to emboli or glomerulonephritis)
- Neurologic findings consistent with CVA, such as visual loss, motors weakness, and aphasia

DIFFERENTIAL DIAGNOSIS
Fever of unknown origin, infected central venous catheter, marantic endocarditis, connective tissue diseases, intra-abdominal infections, rheumatic fever, salmonellosis, brucellosis, malignancy, tuberculosis, atrial myxoma, septic thrombophlebitis

DIAGNOSTIC TESTS & INTERPRETATION
- If not critically ill; three sets of blood cultures drawn >2 hours apart from different sites *before administration of antibiotics*
- If acutely ill, draw three sets of blood cultures over 1-hour *prior to empiric therapy* (1)[A].
- Leukocytosis is common in acute endocarditis.
- Anemia; decreased C3, C4, CH50; and RF in subacute endocarditis
- ESR, C-reactive protein (CRP)
- Hematuria, microscopic or macroscopic
- Consider serologies for Chlamydia, Q fever, Legionella, and Bartonella in "culture-negative" endocarditis.
- Transthoracic (TTE) or transesophageal echocardiogram (TEE) (TEE preferred) should be performed as soon as IE is suspected (1)[A].
- CT scan may help locate embolic abscesses (e.g., spleen).
- Vegetations are composed of platelets, fibrin, and colonies of microorganisms. Destruction of valvular endocardium, perforation of valve leaflets, rupture of chordae tendineae, abscesses of myocardium, rupture of sinus of Valsalva, and pericarditis may occur.
- Emboli, abscesses, and/or infarction of any system
- Immune-complex glomerulonephritis

TREATMENT

MEDICATION

First Line

- Start empiric treatment after three sets of blood cultures have been drawn. Results guide treatment.
  - Native valves: ampicillin-sulbactam 12 g/day IV divided into 4 doses with gentamicin 3 mg/kg/day IV/IM in 2 or 3 doses. If penicillin-allergic, use vancomycin 30 mg/kg/day IV in 2 doses with gentamicin 3 mg/kg/day IV/IM in 2 or 3 doses and with ciprofloxacin 1,000 mg/day PO or 800 mg/day IV in 2 doses (2)[A].
  - Prosthetic valves: vancomycin 30 mg/kg/day IV in 2 doses with gentamicin 3 mg/kg/day IV/IM in 2 doses and rifampin 1,200 mg/day PO in 2 doses, if <12 months postsurgery. If >12 months, use native valve regimen (2)[A].
- Penicillin-susceptible viridans streptococci or *S. bovis*
  - Native valve: penicillin G 12 to 18 million U/day IV continuously or in 4 to 6 doses or ceftriaxone 2 g/day IV/IM in 1 dose, both for 4 weeks (1)[B]
  - Prosthetic valve: penicillin G 24 million U/day IV continuously or in 4 to 6 doses for 6 weeks or ceftriaxone 2 g/day IV/IM in 1 dose ± gentamicin 3 mg/kg IV/IM q24h for 2 weeks (peak gentamicin level 3 μg/mL and trough <1 μg/mL) (1)[B]
- Penicillin-resistant viridans streptococci or *S. bovis*
  - Native valve: penicillin G 24 million U/day IV, either continuously or in 4 to 6 equally divided doses + gentamicin 3 mg/kg IV/IM q24h for 2 weeks (peak gentamicin level 3 μg/mL and trough <1 μg/mL) (1)[B]
- Prosthetic valve: penicillin G 24 million U/day IV, either continuously or in 4 to 6 equally divided doses or ceftriaxone 2 g/day IV/IM in 1 dose for 6 weeks + gentamicin 3 mg/kg IV/IM q24h for 2 weeks (peak gentamicin level 3 μg/mL and trough <1 μg/mL) (1)[B] *Staphylococcus*
  - Native valve: oxacillin or nafcillin 12 g IV/day in 4 to 6 equally divided doses for 6 weeks. For oxacillin-resistant strains, use vancomycin 15 mg/kg/day IV q12h for 6 weeks for goal trough of 15 to 20 μg/mL (1)[B].
  - Prosthetic valve: oxacillin or nafcillin 12 g/day IV in 4 to 6 doses + rifampin 300 mg IV/PO q8h, for 6 weeks, + gentamicin 3 mg/kg/day IV for first 2 weeks (peak gentamicin level 3 μg/mL and trough <1 μg/mL). For oxacillin-resistant strains, use vancomycin 15 mg/kg IV q12h, + rifampin 300 mg IV/PO q8h, both for 6 weeks, + gentamicin 3 mg/kg/day IV/IM in 2 to 3 doses for the first 2 weeks (peak gentamicin level 3 μg/mL and trough <1 μg/mL) (1)[B].
- Penicillin-sensitive *Enterococcus*, native or prosthetic valve: ampicillin 2 g IV q4h or penicillin G 18 to 30 million U/day IV continuously or in 6 doses + gentamicin 3 mg/kg IV q8h for 4 to 6 weeks (peak gentamicin level 3 μg/mL and trough <1 μg/mL) (1)[B]. Consider expert consultation for penicillin-resistant enterococci.
- *HACEK* organisms: ceftriaxone 2 g IM or IV q24h for 4 weeks (1)[B] *or* ampicillin-sulbactam 12 g IV q4h for 4 weeks *or* ciprofloxacin 1 g/day PO or 800 mg/day IV in 2 equally divided doses for 4 weeks (1)[B]
  - Cardiac device–related endocarditis: device removal followed by antibiotic therapy based on organism susceptibility (3)[B]

- Precautions: Adjust dosage of penicillin G, gentamicin, cefazolin, ampicillin, ampicillin/sulbactam, ciprofloxacin, and vancomycin in patients with renal impairment. Rapid infusion of vancomycin <1 hour may cause "red-man syndrome" due to histamine release (not an allergic reaction). Treat with antihistamines and decrease infusion rate.
- Interactions: Vancomycin + gentamicin increases renal toxicity. Rifampin alters warfarin and oral hypoglycemic metabolism.

Second Line

For patients allergic to penicillin:

- Penicillin-susceptible or resistant viridans group streptococci or *S. bovis*: vancomycin 30 mg/kg/day (not to exceed 2 g/day) IV in 2 equal doses for 4 weeks (6 weeks for prosthetic valve endocarditis) for goal trough of 10 to 15 μg/mL (1)[B]
- *Enterococcus*, native or prosthetic valve: Desensitization to penicillin should be considered; vancomycin 15 mg/kg (usual dose, 1 g) IV q12h + gentamicin or streptomycin (peak gentamicin level 3 μg/mL and trough <1 μg/mL) for 4 to 6 weeks (6 weeks for prosthetic valve endocarditis) (1)[B]
- *Staphylococcus* of native valve: cefazolin 2 g IV q8h (not to be used in patients with immediate-type hypersensitivity to penicillin) for 6 weeks *or* vancomycin 30 mg/kg (usual dose, 1 g) IV q12h for a goal trough of 15 to 20 μg/mL for 6 weeks (1)[B]

SURGERY/OTHER PROCEDURES

Surgery is required in 50% of IE cases. Indications (2)[A]:

- Heart failure due to aortic or mitral valve disease
  - Prevention of embolism: aortic or mitral valve vegetations >10 mm with prior embolic episodes; isolated very large vegetation >15 mm; in patients with major ischemic stroke, surgery is delayed for at least 4 weeks, if possible (4)[C].
- Uncontrolled infection: persistent fever and positive cultures >7 to 10 days; infection caused by fungi or resistant organism; presence of abscess, fistula, false aneurysm, or enlarging vegetations
- Early prosthetic valve IE

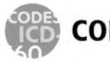

ONGOING CARE

FOLLOW-UP RECOMMENDATIONS

Patient Monitoring

- Check gentamicin peak (~3 μg/mL) and trough (<1 μg/mL) levels if used for >5 days and with renal dysfunction. Perform twice-weekly BUN and serum creatinine while on gentamicin. Consider audiometry baseline and follow-up during long-term aminoglycoside therapy.
- Check vancomycin trough (15 to 20 μg/mL) levels in all patients (typically prior to fourth dose) (2)[B].
- Baseline ECG; monitor ECG for conduction disturbances/MI in initial weeks of therapy.
- TTE at the conclusion of therapy
- Blood cultures q48h until negative

PROGNOSIS

Late complications contribute to poor prognosis. These include heart failure, reinfection, and cerebral emboli. 10-year survival is 60–90% (5)[A].

COMPLICATIONS

- Cerebral complications are the most frequent and severe, occurring in 15–20% of patients (1)[A].
- Emboli: arterial (e.g., MI, mesenteric, splenic, cerebral infarction), infectious (e.g., abscesses of heart, lung, brain, meninges, bone, pericardium)
  - Neurologic events are the most frequent complications in patients with IE requiring ICU admission. Ischemic stroke is the presenting symptom of IE in 20% of cases (5)[A].
- Inflammatory/immune disorders (e.g., arthritis, myositis, glomerulonephritis)
- Other complications: congestive heart failure (CHF), ruptured valve cusp, sinus of Valsalva aneurysm, arrhythmia, and mycotic aneurysms

REFERENCES

1. Baddour LM, Wilson WR, Bayer AS, et al; for American Heart Association Committee on Rheumatic Fever, Endocarditis, and Kawasaki Disease of the Council on Cardiovascular Disease in the Young, Council on Clinical Cardiology, Council on Cardiovascular Surgery and Anesthesia, and Stroke Council. Infective endocarditis in adults: diagnosis, antimicrobial therapy, and management of complications: a scientific statement for healthcare professionals from the American Heart Association. *Circulation*. 2015;132(15):1435–1486.
2. Hoen B, Duval X. Clinical practice. Infective endocarditis. *N Engl J Med*. 2013;368(15):1425–1433.
3. Baddour LM, Wilson WR, Bayer AS, et al. Infective endocarditis in adults: diagnosis, antimicrobial therapy, and management of complications: a scientific statement for healthcare professionals from the American Heart Association. Circulation. 2016;134(8):e113. *Circulation*. 2015;132(17):e205.
4. Byrne JG, Rezai K, Sanchez JA, et al. Surgical management of endocarditis: the society of thoracic surgeons clinical practice guideline. *Ann Thorac Surg*. 2011;91(6):2012–2019.
5. Sonneville R, Mirabel M, Hajage D, et al. Neurologic complications and outcomes of infective endocarditis in critically ill patients: the ENDOcardite en REAnimation prospective multicenter study. *Crit Care Med*. 2011;39(6):1474–1481.

CODES

ICD10

- I33.0 Acute and subacute infective endocarditis
- I39 Endocarditis and heart valve disord in dis classd elswhr
- A54.83 Gonococcal heart infection

CLINICAL PEARLS

- Antibiotic prophylaxis is recommended for patients with artificial heart valves, history of IE, CHD, and cardiac transplants with valvulopathy.
- TEE/TTE and blood cultures are the mainstays for diagnosing IE.
- The most commonly identified organisms are viridans *Streptococcus* species and *Staphylococcus*.

ENDOMETRIAL CANCER AND UTERINE SARCOMA

Michael P. Hopkins, MD, MEd

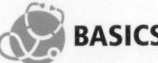 **BASICS**

DESCRIPTION

- Endometrial cancer: malignancy of the endometrial lining of the uterus
  - Two types
    - Type I: estrogen-dependent, grade 1 or grade 2, better prognosis, endometrioid histology
    - Type II: estrogen-independent, higher grade, more aggressive, includes grade 3 endometrioid and nonendometrioid: serous, clear cell, mucinous, poor prognosis (1)[A]
- Cell types: adenocarcinoma, adenosquamous (malignant squamous elements), clear cell, and papillary serous
- Sarcomas: malignancy of the uterine mesenchyme and mixed tumors
  - Mixed müllerian sarcoma (carcinosarcoma): Heterologous sarcoma elements are not native to the müllerian system (e.g., cartilage or bone); homologous sarcoma elements are native to the müllerian system (40–50% prevalence of all sarcomas).
  - Leiomyosarcoma develops in the myometrium, characterized by cellular atypic mitoses and coagulative necrosis (30% prevalence of all sarcomas).
  - Endometrial stromal sarcoma develops from the stromal component of the endometrium (15% prevalence of all sarcomas).
  - Poorer prognosis (2)[C]
- Predominant age
  - Endometrial cancer: Most patients are postmenopausal:
    - Average age of diagnosis: 63 years old
  - Sarcomas: occur in both pre- and postmenopausal:
    - Average age of diagnosis: 40 to 69 years old (2)[C]
- 70% of endometrial cancer is stage I at the time of diagnosis.
- System(s) affected: reproductive
- Synonym(s): uterine cancer; endometrial cancer; corpus cancer

Pregnancy Considerations
This malignancy is not associated with pregnancy.

EPIDEMIOLOGY

Incidence
- Endometrial cancer is the most common gynecologic malignancy, fourth most common cancer in women, and eighth leading cause of cancer-related death in women worldwide.
- In the United States, it is estimated that endometrial cancer will account for 61,380 new cases and 10,920 deaths in 2017 according to SEER database.
- Incidence higher in Caucasian than African American, but African Americans have stage matched higher mortality (3).

Prevalence
Approximately 500,000 women in the United States

ETIOLOGY AND PATHOPHYSIOLOGY
Continuous estrogen stimulation unopposed by progesterone
- Endometrial: unopposed estrogen
  - Estrogen replacement therapy without concomitant progesterone increases the risk. Addition of progesterone decreases risk to that of general population.
- Sarcomas: etiology unknown

Genetics
- Endometrial: Lynch syndrome (hereditary nonpolyposis colorectal cancer); lifetime risk up to 30% (3); Cowden syndrome (4,5)
- Sarcoma: African American, higher incidence of leiomyosarcoma, childhood retinoblastoma survivors

RISK FACTORS
- Early menarche/late menopause
- Nulliparity
- Personal or family history of colon or reproductive system cancer
- Obesity
- Diabetes mellitus
- Hypertension
- Polycystic ovarian syndrome
- Increasing age
- Estrogen-secreting tumor
- Endometrial hyperplasia
- Unopposed estrogens
- Tamoxifen use

GENERAL PREVENTION
- In young women who are obese or anovulatory, the risk of endometrial cancer can be reduced by taking oral contraceptive pills, permanently losing weight, or taking cyclic progesterone to prevent unopposed estrogen's effects on the uterus.
- Estrogen replacement therapy should always include progesterone unless the woman has had a hysterectomy.
- Cigarette smoking has been associated with a lower risk of type I endometrial cancer; however, it is not recommended secondary to its many health risks and increase risk of type II endometrial cancer.

COMMONLY ASSOCIATED CONDITIONS
- Endometrial hyperplasia: 1–25% will progress to endometrial adenocarcinoma:
  - Simple without atypia
  - Complex without atypia
  - Simple with atypia
  - Complex with atypia
    - 43% with complex hyperplasia with atypia have concurrent endometrial cancer.
- Endometrial cancer patients should be screened regularly for breast and colon cancer per routine screening guidelines.
- Patients who have breast or colon cancer are at increased risk for endometrial cancer.
- Granulosa cell tumors of the ovary produce estrogen; these patients will have an increased risk of endometrial cancer.

 DIAGNOSIS

HISTORY
- Endometrial cancer
  - Postmenopausal bleeding is the most frequent sign. Any spotting or abnormal discharge mandates evaluation.
  - Premenopausal patients with history of anovulation and heavy, irregular, or prolonged periods that fail multiple medical managements mandate evaluation.
- Sarcoma
  - Mixed müllerian sarcoma: bleeding and prolapsing tissue, pain (2)[C]
  - Leiomyosarcoma: pelvic pain, pressure, uterine mass, abnormal bleeding

PHYSICAL EXAM
Pelvic exam: enlarged uterus, fixed

DIFFERENTIAL DIAGNOSIS
- Atypical complex hyperplasia: a premalignant lesion of the endometrium
- Cervical cancer
- Ovarian cancer invading the uterus
- Endometriosis
- Adenomyosis
- Leiomyoma

DIAGNOSTIC TESTS & INTERPRETATION

Initial Tests (lab, imaging)
- Liver and renal function tests
- Transvaginal ultrasound usually shows increased endometrial thickness (>4 mm in postmenopausal patients or in patients with irregular or heavy periods if >35 years of age, 100% NPV) (1)[A].
- Levels of cancer antigen 125 (CA-125) may be elevated when intra-abdominal disease is present (1)[A].
- Chest x-ray (CXR): Most common site of metastases is the lung.
- Mammogram and colonoscopy: Endometrial cancer is associated with breast and colon cancer.
- Routine preoperative MRI, CT, or PET scan: not recommended (3)

Follow-Up Tests & Special Considerations
- Endometrial cancer is mostly localized to the uterus; therefore, preoperative evaluation for metastasis is not needed unless metastasis is already suspected (2)[A].
- CT scan, PET/CT, MRI, CA-125: not part of the routine evaluation but may be needed if metastasis is suspected, patient is a poor operative candidate, or pathology returns high grade (G3 endometrioid, papillary serous, clear cell, carcinosarcoma) (2)
- MRI has been reported to show the depth of myometrial penetration accurately but is not always cost-effective (6)[A].

Diagnostic Procedures/Other
- Office endometrial biopsy (90% accurate): If negative with high suspicion for cancer or patient continues to have bleeding, a dilation and curettage (D&C) is necessary (2)[B]. Endometrial stromal sarcoma and leiomyosarcoma rarely are diagnosed preoperatively. Any patient with history of irregular, heavy, or prolonged periods should undergo endometrial biopsy prior to endometrial ablation procedures.
- Fractional D&C is 99% accurate except in cases of sarcoma.
- If surgical approach is favored, D&C with hysteroscopic guidance is recommended over D&C alone, due to its ability to pick up discrete lesions (2)[A].
- Meta-analyses suggest hysteroscopic peritoneal dissemination of malignant cells; unknown significance of that dispersion

Test Interpretation
- International Federation of Gynecology and Obstetrics Staging System: revised 2009
  - Stage I (confined to corpus uteri)
    - A: No or <1/2 myometrial invasion
    - B: Invasion ≥1/2 the myometrium
  - Stage II: Tumor invades cervical stroma but does not extend beyond the uterus.

– Stage III: Local and/or regional spread
  ○ A: Uterine serosal and/or adnexal invasion
  ○ B: Vaginal and/or parametrial involvement
  ○ C: Metastases to pelvic and/or para-aortic lymph nodes
  ○ IIIC1: +Pelvic nodes
  ○ IIIC2: +Para-aortic lymph nodes positive pelvic lymph nodes
– Stage IV: Tumor invades bladder and/or bowel mucosa and/or distant metastases:
  ○ A: Tumor invades bladder and/or bowel mucosa.
  ○ B: Distant metastases, including intra-abdominal metastases and/or inguinal lymph nodes (1)[A]
• Uterine sarcoma criteria for diagnosis: mitotic index, cellular atypia, and areas of coagulative necrosis separated from tumor (7)[C]

 TREATMENT

GENERAL MEASURES
• Main treatment for uterine cancer is surgery.
• Radiation is used to prevent tumor recurrence at the vaginal cuff.

MEDICATION
First Line
• Endometrial
  – Chemotherapy for advanced or recurrent disease incurable with surgery and radiation
    ○ Paclitaxel + carboplatin (2)[B]
    ○ Doxorubicin + cisplatin + paclitaxel
• Hormonal therapy
  – Medroxyprogesterone acetate: for recurrence or metastases
  – Megestrol (Megace) 160 mg/day for at least 2 months for women with premalignant lesions, atypical complex hyperplasia, or well-differentiated endometrial cancer in patients desiring fertility. Follow with D&C to determine cancer resolution.
  – Levonorgestrel-containing intrauterine device: as mentioned earlier for patients who desire future fertility
• Sarcoma
  – Chemotherapy
    ○ Doxorubicin as single agent or in combination (7)[A]
• Hormonal
  – Tamoxifen or aromatase inhibitors; not fully studied, +/− progesterone
  – Progesterones

ADDITIONAL THERAPIES
Radiation therapy
• Nonoperative candidates: radiation therapy alone
• Low risk: no adjuvant radiation therapy
• Intermediate risk: Consider adjuvant vaginal brachytherapy; reduces local recurrences but has no effect on overall survival
• Vaginal brachytherapy is equivalent to whole pelvic radiation in regard to overall survival (3).
• High risk: chemotherapy and radiation therapy in some cases (6,8)[A]

SURGERY/OTHER PROCEDURES
Surgical staging
• Extrafascial hysterectomy and bilateral salpingo-oophorectomy
• Cytologic washings
• Pelvic and para-aortic lymph node dissection
• Omental sampling, as indicated, and for papillary serous (3)

• Optimal tumor debulking (1)[A], survival advantage
• LAP2 trial: minimally invasive and laparotomy similar 5-year survival (3)

Geriatric Considerations
Older (and obese) patients may be at high risk for surgery. Alternative radiation or progesterone therapy can be considered.

ADMISSION, INPATIENT, AND NURSING CONSIDERATIONS
• Admission criteria/initial stabilization
  – Excessive vaginal bleeding
  – Preoperative stabilization
• Nursing: routine; ensure postoperative pain is controlled
• Postsurgical criteria: pain controlled, tolerating diet, ambulating, and voiding

 ONGOING CARE

FOLLOW-UP RECOMMENDATIONS
Follow-up visit with speculum and rectovaginal exam every 3 to 6 months for 2 years, then every 6 months for 3 years, and then annually for life (2)[C]

Patient Monitoring
• Annual CXR is no longer recommended.
• CT scan or PET/CT scan of the chest, abdomen, and pelvis should be used only to investigate suspicion of recurrent disease, not routinely.
• Control comorbid conditions.

DIET
As tolerated and according to comorbidities

PATIENT EDUCATION
After surgery:
• No intercourse for ~6 weeks
• No lifting >10 to 15 lb
• No driving until pain free
• Do not expect resumption of full activity for 6 weeks.

PROGNOSIS
5-year survival rates
• Uterine adenocarcinoma

Stage	Survival (%)
IA	88
IB	75
II	69
IIIA	58
IIIB	50
IIIC	47
IVA	17
IVB	15

• Uterine carcinosarcoma

Stage	Survival (%)
I	70
II	45
III	30
IV	15

(6)[A]

COMPLICATIONS
• Surgical: excessive bleeding, wound infection, lymphedema, deep vein thrombosis (DVT), and damage to the urinary or intestinal systems
• Radiation: diarrhea, ileus, bowel obstruction or fistula, radiation cystitis, proctitis, vaginal stenosis, DVT
• Chemotherapy: per the drug given

REFERENCES
1. Creasman W. Revised FIGO staging for carcinoma of the endometrium. *Int J Gynaecol Obstet.* 2009;105(2):109.
2. Practice Bulletin No. 149: endometrial cancer. *Obstet Gynecol.* 2015;125(4):1006–1026.
3. Sorosky JI. Endometrial cancer. *Obstet Gynecol.* 2012;120(2, Pt 1):383–397.
4. Burke W, Orr J, Leitao M, et al; for Society of Gynecologic Oncology Clinical Practice Committee. Endometrial cancer: a review and current management strategies: part I. *Gynecol Oncol.* 2014;134(2):385–392.
5. Burke W, Orr J, Leitao M, et al; for Society of Gynecologic Oncology Clinical Practice Committee. Endometrial cancer: a review and current management strategies: part II. *Gynecol Oncol.* 2014;134(2):393–402.
6. Humber C, Tierney J, Symonds P, et al. Chemotherapy for advanced, recurrent or metastatic endometrial carcinoma. *Cochrane Database Syst Rev.* 2005;(4):CD003915.
7. Gadducci A, Cosio S, Romanini A, et al. The management of patients with uterine sarcoma: a debated clinical challenge. *Crit Rev Oncol Hematol.* 2008;65(2):129–142.
8. Einhorn N, Tropé C, Ridderheim M, et al. A systematic overview of radiation therapy effects in uterine cancer (corpus uteri). *Acta Oncol.* 2003;42(5–6):557–561.

 SEE ALSO

• Cervical Malignancy
• Algorithm: Pelvic Pain

 CODES

ICD10
• C54.1 Malignant neoplasm of endometrium
• C55 Malignant neoplasm of uterus, part unspecified
• C54.2 Malignant neoplasm of myometrium

CLINICAL PEARLS
• Most common presenting symptom is abnormal uterine bleeding.
• Any patient with history of irregular, heavy, or prolonged periods should undergo endometrial biopsy.
• Primary cause is unopposed estrogen.
• Endometrial thickness on transvaginal ultrasound of <5 mm makes endometrial cancer very unlikely.
• Primary treatment is with surgery, with possible chemotherapy ± radiation.

ENDOMETRIOSIS

Kimberly S. Tustison, MD • Maegen Dupper, MD • Kenneth A. Ballou, MD, FAAFP

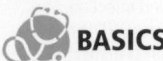 **BASICS**

DESCRIPTION
- Endometriosis is a common but potentially painful and debilitating estrogen-dependent gynecologic condition affecting women of predominately reproductive age (1)[A].
- Symptoms and signs generally consist of pelvic pain, pelvic mass, and/or decreased fertility.
- Due to estrogen-dependent implants of endometrial tissue found outside the uterus. Although endometriomas have been recorded in liver, bowel, umbilicus, lung, and other tissue, the most common pathologic sites are:
  - Peritoneum (bladder, cul-de-sac, pelvic walls, ligaments, and fallopian tubes)
  - Ovaries
  - Rectovaginal septum
- Ectopic endometrial implants proliferate and slough with the menstrual cycle.
- Stage I (minimal) to IV (severe). Staging is useful in therapeutic planning but does not correlate with pain severity.

EPIDEMIOLOGY
Prevalence
- Female only
- Affects 6–10% of fertile women (1)
- Found in 20–50% of infertile women (1)
- Found in 71–87% of women with chronic pelvic pain (1)

Pediatric Considerations
Endometriosis may begin with puberty as endometrial implants are dependent on ovarian hormones. This can lead to debilitating pelvic pain and severe dysmenorrhea associated with missed school, social, and family activities.

Pregnancy Considerations
The presence of endometriosis decreases fecundability from 15–20% per month to 2–10% per month. 25–50% of infertile women have endometriosis. However, pelvic endometriosis generally improves during pregnancy.

Geriatric Considerations
Although menopause often results in a resolution of symptoms, pelvic endometriosis may extend into menopause and may be exacerbated by hormone replacement therapy (HRT).

ETIOLOGY AND PATHOPHYSIOLOGY
- Not fully understood; several factors are believed to play a role, including immunologic changes and genetic predisposition in the presence of abnormal proliferating endometrial tissue implants causing chronic peritoneal inflammation.
- Theories include:
  - Sampson theory: Retrograde menstruation results in peritoneal implantation and disease.
  - Halban theory: Distant disease is probably caused by hematogenous/lymphatic dissemination or metaplastic transformation.
  - Coelomic metaplasia: Coelomic epithelium remains undifferentiated in the peritoneal cavity and differentiates to form functioning endometrium.

- Endometrial-associated infertility is multifactorial:
  - Pelvic inflammation
  - Anatomic disruption of pelvic structures (Involvement of the fallopian tube may cause isthmic tubal obstruction.)
  - Proliferation and activation of peritoneal macrophages (may predispose to gamete phagocytosis)
  - Alteration in eutopic endometrium

Genetics
Odds ratio of symptomatic endometriosis with a first-degree affected relative is 7.2. Those with affected first-degree relatives have a 26% chance of severe manifestations versus 12% if no first-degree affected relatives.

RISK FACTORS
- Family history
- Menstruation and ovulation
- Delayed childbirth

GENERAL PREVENTION
- Suppression of heavy menstruation and ovulation with oral contraceptives during adolescence may delay sequelae.
- Some factors are considered protective:
  - Fruits, green vegetables, n-3 long-chain fatty acids
  - Aerobic exercise may decrease pelvic pain.
- Early diagnosis and treatment might help prevent sequelae.

COMMONLY ASSOCIATED CONDITIONS
Associated with increased risks for cancer of the ovary, breast, endometrium; increased risk for cutaneous melanoma, non-Hodgkin lymphoma, autoimmune diseases, asthma, and cardiovascular disease

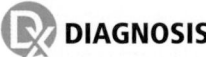 **DIAGNOSIS**

HISTORY
- Dysmenorrhea (50–90% of cases) due to deep infiltrating endometrial implants
- Dyspareunia due to lesions of the cul-de-sac, uterosacral ligaments, and posterior vaginal fornix
- Dyschezia due to involvement of the rectosigmoid colon and rectovaginal regions
- Chronic pelvic pain (≥6 months) that worsens with time and begins 1 to 2 days prior to menstrual cycles
- Hematochezia
- Cyclic nausea, abdominal distention
- Infertility (late finding)
- History of pelvic pain, infertility, and hysterectomy in first- or second-degree relative

PHYSICAL EXAM
- Focal pain/tenderness on pelvic exam is associated with endometriosis in 66% of patients.
- Pelvic mass may be present.
- Immobile pelvic organs (frozen pelvis)
- Rectovaginal exam revealing uterosacral nodules, beading, or tenderness
- An exquisitely tender "barb" stabbing pain in the region of the uterosacral ligament is found in severe cases.

DIFFERENTIAL DIAGNOSIS
Differential diagnosis of pelvic pain includes all causes of acute abdomen and
- Pelvic adhesions
- Nonspecific dysmenorrhea
- Acute salpingitis/pelvic inflammatory disease
- Ruptured ovarian cyst
- Uterine leiomyomas
- Adenomyosis
- Irritable bowel syndrome
- Inflammatory bowel disease
- Pelvic malignancy
- Complications of intrauterine/ectopic pregnancy
- Cystitis
- Depression
- History of sexual abuse
- Chronic pain syndrome

DIAGNOSTIC TESTS & INTERPRETATION
Initial Tests (lab, imaging)
- Labs are only useful to rule out other diagnoses; there are no useful labs to rule in endometriosis.
- CA-125 levels are not recommended (2)[C] due to low sensitivity.
- If history and physical exam reveal adnexal pain or tenderness with/without fullness on pelvic exam
  - Transvaginal ultrasound (US) and MRI are equally effective in detecting ovarian endometriomas: sensitivity, 80–90%; specificity, 60–98% for both
  - US is preferred (less costly).
  - Both modalities are poor in detecting peritoneal implants and adhesions.

Diagnostic Procedures/Other
Definitive diagnosis is made only by microscopic characteristics of tissue biopsied during laparoscopy or laparotomy (1).

Test Interpretation
- Laparoscopically visualized red and blue-black lesions described as "powder-burns," adhesions, and "chocolate cysts" on the ovarian and peritoneal surfaces
- Histologically described endometrial glands and stroma on analysis of biopsied lesions

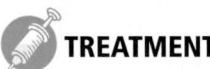 **TREATMENT**

GENERAL MEASURES
Management is dependent on multiple factors:
- Age and reproductive desires of the patient
- The certainty of the diagnosis
- The degree of degradation on quality of life due to pain and infertility
- The threat to other organ systems: GI tract, bladder

MEDICATION
Medications are used to improve the patient's quality of life through symptom relief and to prevent progression of the disease and its potential to cause organ dysfunction. Unfortunately, few studies of medical therapy report patient-relevant outcomes. Many women gain only limited or intermittent benefit from medical therapies (3)[A].

First Line

Women found to have endometriomas during incidental surgery or studies may not need any treatment. Others with minimal symptoms may find sufficient relief with NSAID medications. Increased exercise, especially aerobic, may help others.

- Cyclic combined oral contraceptive pills (OCPs) suppress ovulation.
- NSAIDs initiated at the beginning or just before menses. Evidence is inconclusive on effectiveness (4)[B].

Second Line

- Low-dose OCPs or low-dose progestins with recommendations to switch from cyclic to continuous combined contraception for 3 to 6 months if symptoms persist or if there is chronic, noncyclic pelvic pain (5)[A]. Evidence for combined hormonal contraception is of relatively low quality.
- Levonorgestrel intrauterine device (IUD) (Mirena) found to decrease recurrence of painful menstruation (although not FDA-approved for this indication)
- Medroxyprogesterone acetate 150 mg IM 3 months. Prolonged use may lead to loss of bone mineral density of uncertain clinical significance.
- Gonadotropin-releasing hormone (GnRH) agonists: inhibit pituitary gonadotropin synthesis and induce a hypoestrogenic state
- Norethindrone acetate 5 mg PO once daily plus conjugated equine estrogen 0.625 mg PO once daily

Third Line

If symptoms and signs continue, physicians should be experienced in the use and side effects of GnRH analogues prior to their use (symptoms return in as many as 70% of treated patients):

- Leuprolide acetate (Lupron Depot) 3.75 mg IM each month or 11.25 mg IM every 3 months (gluteal)
- Nafarelin (Synarel) intranasal one spray (200 μg) in one nostril each morning and the other nostril each evening (start between days 2 and 4 of menstrual cycle)
- Goserelin (Zoladex) implant 3.6 mg SC in upper abdominal wall every 28 days
- Danazol: also effective, with side effects similar to GnRH analogs
- Aromatase inhibitors (anastrozole and letrozole) prolong the remission induced by GnRH medications.

ALERT

Calcium (1,000 to 1,500 mg/day) with vitamin D 1,000 to 2,000 IU daily or low-dose estrogen with progestogen (1)[A],(6)[B] is recommended when using GnRH agonists to prevent calcium loss.

ISSUES FOR REFERRAL

- Refer early to a physician with expertise in medical and surgical treatment of endometriosis, especially if the patient desires to conceive in the future.
- Indications for referral to a specialty gynecologist include the following:
  - Need for definitive diagnosis
  - Failure to respond to a conservative or first-line therapy
  - Chronic pelvic pain
  - Delayed fertility

ADDITIONAL THERAPIES

Regular exercise and counseling for pain-management strategies. Narcotics are contraindicated for chronic pain.

SURGERY/OTHER PROCEDURES

Surgery (laparoscopy or laparotomy) is both diagnostic and therapeutic (first line or when conservative measures fail):

- Peritoneal endometriosis: laser ablation/excision/fulguration
- Ovarian endometriosis (endometriomas) >3 to 4 cm: ablation, excision, drainage
- Lysis of adhesions (LOA)
- Hysterectomy with bilateral salpingo-oophorectomy for debilitating symptoms refractory to other medical or surgical treatments:
  - Relieves pain in 80–90%, but pain recurs in 10% within 1 to 2 years after surgery
  - Postoperative HRT should include estrogen and progestogen or progesterone.
- Interruption of nerve pathways: Laparoscopic ablations and presacral neurectomy improve dysmenorrhea.
- Fertility procedures: Ablation or excision of lesions with LOA is recommended to treat infertility in stages I and II disease:
  - Spontaneous conception should be attempted for 1 year prior to assisted reproduction techniques.
  - Disease does not endanger in vitro fertilization (IVF) pregnancies.

ALERT

Surgery for endometriomas may decrease ovarian reserve in advanced disease.

COMPLEMENTARY & ALTERNATIVE MEDICINE

- Osteopathic manipulative therapy found to improve quality of life (2)[C]
- Postsurgical use of Chinese herbal medicine has been found to be effective.
- Acupuncture may be more effective than danazol to decrease pain, irregular menstruation, and perineal swelling.

 ONGOING CARE

FOLLOW-UP RECOMMENDATIONS

Routine gynecologic care

Patient Monitoring

Symptomatic and asymptomatic pelvic masses (http://www.acog.org/)

PROGNOSIS

- Excellent, especially if diagnosis and treatment plans are initiated early in disease course
- Poor for recovery of fertility if the disease has progressed to stage III/IV
- Symptoms and signs improve after bilateral oophorectomy

COMPLICATIONS

Sequelae include chronic pelvic pain, reduced quality of life, repetitive surgical intervention, depression, medication side effects and costs, and infertility.

REFERENCES

1. Practice bulletin no. 114: management of endometriosis. *Obstet Gynecol*. 2010;116(1):223–236.
2. Daraï C, Deboute O, Zacharopoulou C, et al. Impact of osteopathic manipulative therapy on quality of life of patients with deep infiltrating endometriosis with colorectal involvement: results of a pilot study. *Eur J Obstet Gynecol Reprod Biol*. 2015;188:70–73.
3. Becker CM, Gattrell WT, Gude K, et al. Reevaluating response and failure of medical treatment of endometriosis: a systematic review. *Fertil Steril*. 2017;108(1):125–136.
4. Allen C, Hopewell S, Prentice A, et al. Nonsteroidal anti-inflammatory drugs for pain in women with endometriosis. *Cochrane Database Syst Rev*. 2009;(2):CD004753.
5. Jensen JT, Schlaff W, Gordon K. Use of combined hormonal contraceptives for the treatment of endometriosis-related pain: a systematic review of the evidence. *Fertil Steril*. 2018;110(1):137–152.
6. Giudice LC. Clinical practice. Endometriosis. *N Engl J Med*. 2010;362(25):2389–2398.

ADDITIONAL READING

- Brown J, Farquhar C. Endometriosis: an overview of Cochrane Reviews. *Cochrane Database Syst Rev*. 2014;(3):CD009590.
- Davis L, Kennedy SS, Moore J, et al. Oral contraceptives for pain associated with endometriosis. *Cochrane Database Syst Rev*. 2007;(3):CD001019.
- de Ziegler D, Borghese B, Chapron C. Endometriosis and infertility: pathophysiology and management. *Lancet*. 2010;376(9742):730–738.
- Fujii S. MR imaging of endometriosis. In: Harada T, ed. *Endometriosis: Pathogenesis and Treatment*. Tottori, Japan: Springer; 2014.
- Jacobson TZ, Duffy JM, Barlow D, et al. Laparoscopic surgery for pelvic pain associated with endometriosis. *Cochrane Database Syst Rev*. 2009;(4):CD001300.
- Koga K, Yoshino O, Hirota Y, et al. Infertility treatment of endometriosis patients. In: Harada T, ed. *Endometriosis: Pathogenesis and Treatment*. Tottori, Japan: Springer; 2014.
- Practice Committee of American Society for Reproductive Medicine. Treatment of pelvic pain associated with endometriosis. *Fertil Steril*. 2008;90(Suppl 5):S260–S269.
- Schrager S, Falleroni J, Edgoose J. Evaluation and treatment of endometriosis. *Am Fam Physician*. 2013;87(2):107–113.
- Zhu X, Hamilton KD, McNicol ED. Acupuncture for pain in endometriosis. *Cochrane Database Syst Rev*. 2011;(9):CD007864.

 CODES

ICD10
- N80.9 Endometriosis, unspecified
- N80.3 Endometriosis of pelvic peritoneum
- N80.2 Endometriosis of fallopian tube

CLINICAL PEARLS

- Severe dysmenorrhea and dyspareunia are never normal. Failure to respond to NSAIDs and/or OCPs warrants further investigation.
- A rectovaginal exam can be useful in patients suspected of having endometriosis.

ENDOMETRITIS AND OTHER POSTPARTUM INFECTIONS

Justin P. Lavin Jr., MD • Ayesha Hasan, MD • Cassandra Heiselman, DO, MPH

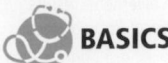 **BASICS**

DESCRIPTION
- Endometritis (infection of the endometrium) is the most common postpartum infection.
- Bacterial infection of genital tract, usually within the 1st week after delivery, can occur as late as 1 to 6 weeks postpartum.
- Postpartum infections of the myometrium and parametrial tissues are less common. Vaginal and cervical infections, perianal cellulitis, pelvic cellulitis, septic pelvic vein thrombophlebitis, and parametrial phlegmon are other postpartum infections of the pelvic region that are relatively rare.
- System(s) affected: reproductive
- Synonym(s): postpartum infection; endometritis; endoparametritis; endomyometritis; myometritis; endomyoparametritis; metritis; metritis with pelvic cellulitis

EPIDEMIOLOGY
Incidence
Occurs in women of childbearing years

Prevalence
- Occurs after 1–3% of all births
- Infection 10 times more likely after cesarean section
  - 2–15% of infections occur prior to labor.
  - 30–35% occur after labor in absence of appropriate antibiotic prophylaxis; 2–15% occur after labor with appropriate prophylaxis.
  - Fifth leading cause of maternal mortality, accounting for 11% of maternal deaths

ETIOLOGY AND PATHOPHYSIOLOGY
- Endometritis is more common in labors complicated by chorioamnionitis.
- Other infections follow trauma to the perineum, vagina, cervix, and uterus.
- Postpartum infections are typically polymicrobial, involving organisms ascending from the lower genital tract:
  - Aerobic isolates (70%): *Streptococcus faecalis, Streptococcus agalactiae, Streptococcus viridans, Staphylococcus aureus, Escherichia coli*
  - Anaerobic isolates (80%): *Peptococcus* sp., *Peptostreptococcus* sp., *Clostridium* sp., *Bacteroides bivius, Bacteroides fragilis, Fusobacterium* sp.
- Other genital *Mycoplasma*
- Consider herpes simplex virus and cytomegalovirus, particularly in immunocompromised patients failing to improve on appropriate antibiotics.
- Thrombosis of any pelvic vein, including vena cava
- Phlegmon on leaves of the broad ligament

RISK FACTORS
- Cesarean delivery is the primary risk factor.
- Chorioamnionitis
- Bacterial vaginosis
- Group B streptococcal colonization of genital tract
- HIV infection

- Prolonged labor
- Prolonged rupture of membranes
- Multiple vaginal examinations
- Internal fetal monitoring during labor
- Operative vaginal delivery; manual extraction of the placenta; care in a teaching hospital
- Low socioeconomic status
- Obesity
- Anemia

GENERAL PREVENTION
- Vaginal delivery
  - Avoid unnecessary vaginal examinations.
  - Treat chorioamnionitis during labor.
  - Avoid manual placental extraction and retained placental products.
  - Consider antibiotic prophylaxis for third- and fourth-degree laceration (1)[B].
  - Aseptic technique for operative vaginal delivery
  - Antibiotic prophylaxis not necessary for operative vaginal delivery or manual removal of the placenta
- Cesarean delivery
  - Preoperative paint and scrub with 10% povidone-iodine scrub or an alcohol-based solution decreases puerperal infection by up to 38%.
  - Prophylactic antibiotics before both emergency and scheduled cesarean deliveries prior to skin incision reduce postpartum infection (2)[A].
    - Administer antibiotics within 1 hour of the start of surgery (3)[B].
    - Appropriate administration of antibiotics results in a 40% reduction in postpartum maternal infections without any increase in neonatal infections (3)[B].
  - Extended coverage with cephalosporin and macrolide may further decrease infection risk (4)[A].
  - Vaginal preparation with povidone-iodine solution or alcohol-based solutions immediately before cesarean delivery reduces the risk of postoperative endometritis (5)[A].
  - Weight-based antibiotic dosage helps ensure appropriate tissue concentrations prior to skin incision.

COMMONLY ASSOCIATED CONDITIONS
- Chorioamnionitis
- Wound infection

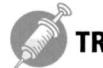 **DIAGNOSIS**

HISTORY
- History of cesarean delivery or chorioamnionitis
- Fever and chills
- Malaise
- Headache
- Anorexia
- Abdominal pain
- Heavy vaginal bleeding or foul smelling lochia

PHYSICAL EXAM
- Oral temperature >38°C (100.4°F)
- Tachycardia
- Uterine tenderness on exam
- Other localized abdominopelvic tenderness on exam
- Purulent or malodorous lochia
- Heavy vaginal bleeding
- Ileus
- Group A or B streptococcal bacteremia may have no localizing signs.

DIFFERENTIAL DIAGNOSIS
- "5 Ws": Wind (pneumonia); Water (UTI); Wound infection; Wow (mastitis); Wonder drug (medication-related fever)
- Viral syndrome; dehydration
- Thrombophlebitis
- Thyroid storm
- Appendicitis

DIAGNOSTIC TESTS & INTERPRETATION
Initial Tests (lab, imaging)
- CBC: Interpret with care. (Physiologic leukocytosis may be as high as 20,000 WBCs.)
- Two sets of blood cultures (especially with suspected sepsis)
- Diagnosis often made on clinical grounds. Potential testing includes:
  - Genital tract cultures and rapid test for group B streptococci (may be done during labor)
  - Amniotic fluid Gram stain: usually polymicrobial
  - Uterine tissue cultures: Prep the cervix with Betadine and use a shielded specimen collector or Pipelle; difficult to obtain without contamination
- If patient not responding to antibiotics in 24 to 48 hours:
  - Ultrasound for retained products of conception, pelvic abscess, or mass
  - CT or MRI looking for pelvic vein thrombophlebitis, abscess, or deep-seated wound infection

Diagnostic Procedures/Other
Paracentesis/culdocentesis with culture rarely necessary

Test Interpretation
- Superficial layer of infected necrotic tissue in microscopic sections of uterine lining
- >5 neutrophils per high-power field in superficial endometrium; ≥1 plasma cell in endometrial stroma

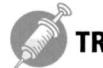 **TREATMENT**

MEDICATION
First Line
Clindamycin 900 mg IV q8h + gentamicin 5 mg/kg IV q24h (5)[A]
- Potential side effects include nephrotoxicity, ototoxicity, pseudomembranous colitis, or diarrhea (in up to 6%).

Second Line

- Ampicillin/sulbactam 3 g IV q6h
- Metronidazole 500 mg IV or PO q8–12h + penicillin 5,000,000 U IV q6h, *or*
- Ampicillin 2 g IV q6h + gentamicin 5 mg/kg IV q24h (5)[A]
- Cefoxitin 2 g IV q6h. Add ampicillin 2 g IV q6h, if clinical failure after 48 hours (5)[A].
- Cefotetan 2 g IV q12h. Add ampicillin 2 g IV q6h, if clinical failure after 48 hours (5)[A].
- Note: Base therapy on cultures, sensitivities, and clinical response.
- Contraindications
  – Drug allergy
  – Renal failure (aminoglycosides)
  – Avoid sulfa, tetracyclines, and fluoroquinolones before delivery and if breastfeeding. Metronidazole is relatively contraindicated if breastfeeding.
- Precautions:
  – Clindamycin and other antibiotics occasionally cause pseudomembranous colitis.
  – Antibiotic-associated diarrhea (*Clostridium difficile*)
- Note: Consider adding a macrolide antibiotic (for chlamydia coverage) for infections occurring after 48 hours.
- Note: Heparin typically indicated for septic pelvic vein thrombophlebitis; requires 10 days of full anticoagulation

SURGERY/OTHER PROCEDURES

- Curettage for retained products of conception
- Surgery or image-guided drainage to drain abscess
- Surgery to decompress the bowel
- Surgical drainage of a phlegmon is not advised unless it is suppurative. Surgical removal of other inflamed tissue is usually not required.

ADMISSION, INPATIENT, AND NURSING CONSIDERATIONS

- Inpatient care is recommended for postpartum infections.
- Many infections occur after hospital discharge.
- IV antibiotics and close observation for severe infections
- Open and drain infected wounds.
- Optimize fluid status.

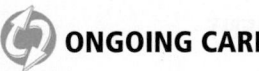 ONGOING CARE

FOLLOW-UP RECOMMENDATIONS

Patient Monitoring

- Individualize according to severity.
- IV antibiotics can be stopped when the patient is afebrile for 24 to 48 hours.
- Oral antibiotics on discharge are not necessary, unless patient was bacteremic; then continue oral antibiotics to complete a 7-day course.

DIET

As tolerated, although may be limited by ileus

PATIENT EDUCATION

- Advise patient to contact physician with fever >38°C (100.4°F) postpartum, heavy vaginal bleeding, foul-smelling lochia, or other symptoms of infection.
- Information available at http://www.healthline.com/health/pregnancy/complications-postpartum-endometritis

PROGNOSIS

With supportive therapy and appropriate antibiotics, most patients improve quickly and recover without complication.

COMPLICATIONS

- Resistant organisms; peritonitis; pelvic abscess
- Septic pelvic thrombophlebitis
- Ovarian vein thrombosis
- Sepsis; death

REFERENCES

1. Smaill FM, Grivell RM. Antibiotic prophylaxis versus no prophylaxis for preventing infection after cesarean section. *Cochrane Database Sys Rev*. 2014;(10):CD007482.
2. American College of Obstetricians and Gynecologist. ACOG Practice Bulletin No. 120: use of prophylactic antibiotics in labor and delivery. *Obstet Gynecol*. 2011;117(6):1472–1483.
3. Tita AT, Szychowski JM, Boggess K, et al; for C/SOAP Trial Consortium. Adjunctive azithromycin prophylaxis for cesarean delivery. *N Engl J Med*. 2016;375(13):1231–1241.
4. Haas DM, Morgan S, Contreras K. Vaginal preparation with antiseptic solution before cesarean section for preventing postoperative infections. *Cochrane Database Syst Rev*. 2014;(12):CD007892.
5. French LM, Smaill FM. Antibiotic regimens for endometritis after delivery. *Cochrane Database Syst Rev*. 2004;(4):CD001067.

ADDITIONAL READING

- Chibueze EC, Parsons AJ, Ota E, et al. Prophylactic antibiotics for manual removal of retained placenta during vaginal birth: a systematic review of observational studies and meta-analysis. *BMC Pregnancy Childbirth*. 2015;15:313.
- Hadiati DR, Hakimi M, Nurdiati DS, et al. Skin preparation for preventing infection following caesarean section. *Cochrane Database Sys Rev*. 2014;(9):CD007462.

- Liabsuetrakul T, Choobun T, Peeyananjarassri K, et al. Antibiotic prophylaxis for operative vaginal delivery. *Cochrane Database Syst Rev*. 2014;(10):CD004455.
- Mackeen AD, Packard RE, Ota E, et al. Antibiotic regimens for postpartum endometritis. *Cochrane Database Syst Rev*. 2015;(2):CD001067.
- Mackeen AD, Packard RE, Ota E, et al. Timing of intravenous prophylactic antibiotics for preventing postpartum infectious morbidity in women undergoing cesarean delivery. *Cochrane Database Syst Rev*. 2014;(12):CD009516.
- McKibben RA, Pitts SI, Suarez-Cuervo C, et al. Practices to reduce surgical site infections among women undergoing cesarean section: a review. *Infect Control Hosp Epidemiol*. 2015;36(8):915–921.
- Pevzner L, Swank M, Krepel C, et al. Effects of maternal obesity on tissue concentrations of prophylactic cefazolin during cesarean delivery. *Obstet Gynecol*. 2011;117(4):877–882.

 SEE ALSO

Algorithm: Pelvic Pain

 CODES

ICD10

- O86.12 Endometritis following delivery
- O86.4 Pyrexia of unknown origin following delivery
- O86.13 Vaginitis following delivery

CLINICAL PEARLS

- Postpartum endometritis follows 1–3% of all births.
- Infections are typically polymicrobial and involve organisms ascending from the lower genital tract.
- Evidence supports antibiotic prophylaxis prior to skin incision for all cesarean deliveries but not for operative vaginal deliveries.
- Clindamycin 900 mg IV q8h and gentamicin 5 mg/kg IV q24h are recommended as first-line therapy for endometritis. Treat until the patient is afebrile for 24 to 48 hours and stop antibiotics completely (unless there is documented bacteremia, which requires a 7-day course of therapy).
- If no improvement occurs on antibiotics, consider retained placental products, abscess, wound infection, hematoma, cellulitis, phlegmon, or septic pelvic vein thrombosis.

E

ENURESIS

Joseph L. Hesse, MD • Swati Avashia, MD, FAAP, FACP, ABIHM

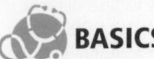

BASICS

DESCRIPTION
- Classification
  - Primary nocturnal enuresis (NE): 80% of all cases; person who has never established urinary continence on consecutive nights for a period of ≥6 months
  - Secondary NE: 20% of cases; resumption of enuresis after at least 6 months of urinary continence
- NE: intermittent nocturnal incontinence after the anticipated age of bladder control (age 5 years)
  - Primary monosymptomatic NE (PMNE): bed-wetting with no history of bladder dysfunction or other lower urinary tract (LUT) symptoms
  - Nonmonosymptomatic NE (NMNE): bed-wetting with LUT symptoms such as frequency, urgency, daytime wetting, hesitancy, straining, weak or intermittent stream, posturination dribbling, lower abdominal or genital discomfort, or sensation of incomplete emptying

ALERT
Adult-onset NE with absent daytime incontinence is a serious symptom; complete urologic evaluation and therapy are warranted.

- System(s) affected: nervous, renal/urologic
- Synonym(s): bed-wetting; sleep enuresis; nocturnal incontinence; primary NE

EPIDEMIOLOGY
Incidence
- Depends on family history
- Spontaneous resolution: 15% per year

Prevalence
- Very common; 5 to 7 million children in the United States (1)
- 10% of 7-year-olds; 3% of 11- to 12-year-olds; 0.5–1.7% at 16 to 17 years old (2)
- 1.5 to 2 times more common in males than females
- Nocturnal > day (3:1)

Geriatric Considerations
Infrequent; often associated with daytime incontinence (formerly referred to as diurnal enuresis)

ETIOLOGY AND PATHOPHYSIOLOGY
- A disorder of sleep arousal, a low nocturnal bladder capacity, and nocturnal polyuria are the three factors that interrelate to cause NE.
- Both functional and organic causes (below); many theories, none absolutely confirmed
- Detrusor instability
- Deficiency of arginine vasopressin (AVP); decreased nocturnal AVP or decreased AVP stimulation secondary to an empty bladder (Bladder distension stimulates AVP.)
- Maturational delay of CNS
- Severe NE with some evidence of interaction between bladder overactivity and brain arousability: association with children with severe NE and frequent cortical arousals in sleep
- Organic urologic causes in 1–4% of enuresis in children: urinary tract infection (UTI), occult spina bifida, ectopic ureter, lazy bladder syndrome, irritable bladder with wide bladder neck, posterior urethral valves, neurologic bladder dysfunction

- Organic nonurologic causes: epilepsy, diabetes mellitus, food allergies, obstructive sleep apnea, chronic renal failure, hyperthyroidism, pinworm infection, sickle cell disease
- NE occurs in all stages of sleep.

Genetics
Most commonly, NE is an autosomal-dominant inheritance pattern with high penetrance (90%).
- 1/3 of all cases are sporadic.
- 75% of children with enuresis have a first-degree relative with the condition.
- Higher rates in monozygotic versus dizygotic twins (68% vs. 36%)
- If both parents had NE, risk in child is 77%; 44% if one parent is affected. Parental age of resolution often predicts when child's enuresis should resolve.

RISK FACTORS
- Family history
- Stressors (emotional, environmental) common in secondary enuresis (e.g., divorce, death)
- Constipation and/or encopresis
- Organic disease: 1% of monosymptomatic NE (e.g., urologic and nonurologic causes)
- Psychological disorders
  - Comorbid disorders are highest with secondary NE: depression, anxiety, social phobias, conduct disorder, hyperkinetic syndrome, internalizing disorders.
  - Association with ADHD; more pronounced in ages 9 to 12 years
- Altered mental status or impaired mobility

GENERAL PREVENTION
No known measures

COMMONLY ASSOCIATED CONDITIONS
- Obstructive sleep apnea syndrome (10–54%) (1): Atrial natriuretic factor inhibits renin-angiotensin-aldosterone pathway leading to diuresis.
- Constipation (33–75%) (1)
- Behavioral problems (specifically ADHD in 12–17%) (1)
- Overactive bladder or dysfunctional voiding (up to 41%) (1)
- UTI (18–60%) (1)

DIAGNOSIS

HISTORY
- Age of onset, duration, severity
- LUT tract symptoms
- Daily intake patterns
- Voiding and stooling patterns (voiding diary)
- Psychosocial history
- Family history of enuresis
- Investigation and previous treatment history

PHYSICAL EXAM
- ENT: evaluation for adenotonsillar hypertrophy
- Abdomen: enlarged bladder, kidneys, fecal masses, or impaction
- Back: Look for dimpling or tufts of hair on sacrum.
- Genital urinary exam
  - Males: meatal stenosis, hypospadias, epispadias, phimosis
  - Females: vulvitis, vaginitis, labial adhesions, ureterocele at introitus; evidence of abuse
- Rectal exam: tone, fecal soiling, fecal impaction
- Neurologic exam, especially lower extremities

DIFFERENTIAL DIAGNOSIS
- Primary NE
  - Delayed physiologic urinary control
  - UTI (both)
  - Spina bifida occulta
  - Obstructive sleep apnea (both)
  - Idiopathic detrusor instability
  - Previously unrecognized myelopathy or neuropathy (e.g., multiple sclerosis, tethered cord, epilepsy)
  - Anatomic urinary tract abnormality (e.g., ectopic ureter)
- Secondary NE
  - Bladder outlet obstruction
  - Neurologic disease, neurogenic bladder (e.g., spinal cord injury)

DIAGNOSTIC TESTS & INTERPRETATION
Initial Tests (lab, imaging)
- Only obligatory test in children is urinalysis.
- Urinalysis and urine culture: UTI, pyuria, hematuria, proteinuria, glycosuria, and poor concentrating ability (low specific gravity) may suggest organic etiology, especially in adults.
- Urinary tract imaging is usually not necessary.
- If abnormal clinical findings or adult onset: renal and bladder US
- IV pyelogram, voiding cystourethrogram (VCUG), or retrograde pyelogram is rarely indicated (1).
- MRI if spinal dysraphism is suspected

Follow-Up Tests & Special Considerations
- Secondary enuresis: serum glucose, BUN, creatinine, thyroid-stimulating hormone (TSH), urine culture
- In children, imaging and urodynamic studies are helpful for significant daytime symptoms, history of UTIs, suspected structural abnormalities, and in refractory cases.

Diagnostic Procedures/Other
Urodynamic studies may be beneficial in adults and nonmonosymptomatic NE.

Test Interpretation
- Dysfunctional voiding
- Detrusor instability and/or reduced bladder capacity most common findings

TREATMENT

GENERAL MEASURES
- Use nonpharmacologic approaches as first line before prescribing medications (1)[A].
- Simple behavioral interventions (e.g., scheduled wakening, positive reinforcement, bladder training, diet changes) are effective, although less so than alarms or medications (1)[B]; found to achieve dryness in 15–20% of cases (3)
  - Explain the three pathophysiologic factors (fragmented sleep, low nocturnal bladder capacity, and increased nocturnal urine production).
  - Encourage normal drinking patterns during daytime hours and reduction of intake 2 hours prior to sleep.
  - Emphasize regular bedtime with full night's sleep.
  - Scheduled voiding before bed
  - Scheduled waking for nighttime voiding
  - Nightlights to light the way to the bathroom
  - Reward system for dry nights
  - Use pull up over regular underwear or cloth underwear with built in waterproof barrier.
  - "Cleanliness training": child helps with changing wet bedding

- Do not shame or punish bed-wetting but have the child participate in removing and laundering soiled bedding and garments.
- If behavioral interventions alone have no success, combined therapy (e.g., enuresis alarm, bladder training, motivational therapy, and pelvic floor muscle training) is more effective than each component alone or than pharmacotherapy (1)[A].
- Enuresis alarms (bells or buzzers)
  - Considered first line; most effective treatment
  - 66–70% success rate; must be used nightly for 2 to 4 months; offers cure; significant parental involvement; disruption of sleep for entire family
  - If successful, it should be used until 14 consecutive dry nights achieved (2)[B].
- See "Patient Education" for options.

MEDICATION
First Line
Desmopressin (DDAVP): synthetic analogue of vasopressin that decreases nocturnal urine output (2)[A]

- Intranasal DDAVP: adults only, 20 mg (2 sprays) intranasally at bedtime
- FDA recommends against use in children due to reports of severe hyponatremia resulting in seizures and deaths in children using intranasal formulations of desmopressin.
- Oral DDAVP: safe in children. Begin at 0.2 mg tablet taken at bedtime on empty stomach; after 14 days of inefficient treatment, can titrate to 0.4 mg (2).
  - Maximally effective in 1 hour; effect lasts 8 to 10 hours.
  - If treatment is successful, can be continued for 3 months, then stop for 2 weeks for test of dryness.
  - High relapse rate after discontinuation without a structured withdrawal program. If relapse occurs, oral desmopressin can continue to be prescribed in 3-month blocks.
  - Suspend dose in children who experience acute condition affecting fluid/electrolyte balances (fever, vomiting, diarrhea, vigorous exercise).
  - 60–70% success; 30% of children have full response and 40% have partial response.

Pediatric Considerations
FDA recommends against using intranasal formulations of desmopressin in children due to reports of severe hyponatremia resulting in seizures and deaths (3)[A].

Second Line
- Imipramine (Tofranil): tricyclic antidepressant, anticholinergic effects; increases bladder capacity, antispasmodic properties
  - Primarily in adults; use in children is reserved for resistant cases and initiated by specialists.
  - Dose: adults, 25 to 75 mg and children >6 years, 10 to 25 mg PO at bedtime; increase by 10 to 25 mg at 1- to 2-week intervals; treat for 2 to 3 months; then taper.
  - 40% success rate, but relapses after discontinuation are high (2).
  - Pretreatment ECG recommended identifying underlying rhythm disorders
- Anticholinergics: Monotherapy is not recommended in children.
  - Oxybutynin (Ditropan, Ditropan XL, Oxytrol patch): anticholinergic; smooth muscle relaxant, antispasmodic; may increase functional bladder capacity and aids in timed voiding (4)[B]
    o 30–50% success; 50% relapse after stopped
    o Ditropan: adults: 5 mg PO TID–QID; children >5 years old with overactive bladder who have failed alarm therapy and desmopressin can try 5 mg at bedtime.

    o Ditropan XL: adults: 5 mg/day PO; increase to 30 mg/day PO (5- to 10-mg tablet).
    o Oxytrol patch: 1 patch every 3 to 4 days (3.9 mg/patch) (Periodic trials of the medication, that is, weekends or weeks at a time, will help determine efficacy and resolution of primary disturbance.)
  - Tolterodine (Detrol, Detrol LA): anticholinergic; fewer side effects than Ditropan (4)[B]
    o Detrol: 1 to 2 mg PO BID in adults, 2 mg at bedtime in children >5 years old
    o Detrol LA: 2 to 4 mg/day
- Precautions
  - Oxybutynin: glaucoma, myasthenia gravis, GI or genitourinary obstruction, ulcerative colitis, constipation, megacolon; use a decreased dose in the elderly.
  - Tolterodine: urinary retention, gastric retention, constipation, uncontrolled narrow-angle glaucoma; significant drug interactions with CYP2D6, CYP3A3/4 substrates
  - Desmopressin: Avoid in patients at risk for electrolyte changes or fluid retention (congestive heart failure [CHF], renal insufficiency). Stop during gastroenteritis or other acute illness with risk of dehydration.
  - Imipramine: Do not use with monoamine oxidase inhibitors (MAOIs), hypotension, and arrhythmias; low-toxic therapeutic ratio
- Combination therapy with DDAVP and oxybutynin has better results than individual use (4)[B].

ALERT
Imipramine: cardiotoxicity and death with overdose

ISSUES FOR REFERRAL
- Primary NE: persistent enuresis despite nonpharmacologic and pharmacologic therapies
- Diurnal incontinence or nonmonosymptomatic enuresis with voiding dysfunction or underlying medical condition

ADDITIONAL THERAPIES
Individual and family psychotherapy, crisis intervention

SURGERY/OTHER PROCEDURES
Only for surgically correctable causes (e.g., tethered cord, ectopic ureter, benign prostatic hypertrophy, obstructive sleep apnea)

COMPLEMENTARY & ALTERNATIVE MEDICINE
Acupuncture has small amounts of supportive data (3)[B].

 ONGOING CARE

FOLLOW-UP RECOMMENDATIONS
Patient Monitoring
- When starting with nonpharmacologic treatment, patient should be seen in clinic every 1 to 3 months.
- If starting enuresis alarm, patient should return in 1 week to assess response.
- If starting DDAVP, patient should return in 1 to 2 weeks to assess response and then return at least every 3 months.

DIET
- Limit fluid and caffeine intake 2 hours before sleep.
- Limit dairy products 4 hours before sleep (decrease osmotic diuresis) (5).

PATIENT EDUCATION
Web resources for hypnosis scripts, alarms, and supplies
- https://www.hypnoticworld.com/hypnosis-scripts/habits-disorders/enuresis
- http://wetstop.com
- https://bedwettingstore.com
- www.dri-sleeper.com
- www.nitetrain-r.com
- Parents can search their App Store for free bed-wetting diary apps (e.g., My Dryness Tracker).

PROGNOSIS
In children, NE is usually self-limiting; 1% will persist as adult; evaluate for organic causes.

COMPLICATIONS
UTI, perineal excoriation, psychological disturbance (especially in children)

REFERENCES
1. Baird DC, Seehusen DA, Bode DV. Enuresis in children: a case based approach. *Am Fam Physician*. 2014;90(8):560–568.
2. Kuwertz-Bröking E, von Gontard A. Clinical management of nocturnal enuresis. *Pediatr Nephrol*. 2018;33(7):1145–1154.
3. Jain S, Bhatt GC. Advances in the management of primary monosymptomatic nocturnal enuresis in children. *Paediatr Int Child Health*. 2016;36(1):7–14.
4. Bayne AP, Skoog SJ. Nocturnal enuresis: an approach to assessment and treatment. *Pediatr Rev*. 2014;35(8):327–335.
5. Traisman E. Enuresis: evaluation and treatment. *Pediatr Ann*. 2015;44(4):133–137.

 SEE ALSO

- Incontinence, Urinary Adult Female; Incontinence, Urinary Adult Male
- Algorithm: Enuresis, Secondary

CODES
ICD10
- N39.44 Nocturnal enuresis
- R32 Unspecified urinary incontinence
- F98.0 Enuresis not due to a substance or known physiol condition

CLINICAL PEARLS
- Initial evaluation is history, exam, and urinalysis.
- For PMNE in children, if the condition is not distressing to child and caretakers, treatment is unnecessary.
- Behavioral and lifestyle interventions are the first-line treatment for PMNE; alarms and desmopressin are the most effective treatments.
- Dryness is possible for most children.

EPICONDYLITIS

Julie A. Creech, DO • Brooke E. Organ, DO • Sabrina L. Silver, DO, CAQSM

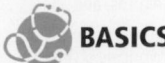 BASICS

DESCRIPTION
- Tendinopathy of the elbow characterized by pain and tenderness at the origins of the wrist flexors/extensors at the humeral epicondyles
- May be acute (traumatic) or chronic (overuse)
- Two types
  - Medial epicondylitis (ME, "golfer's elbow")
    - Involves the wrist flexors and pronators, which originate at the medial epicondyle
  - Lateral epicondylitis (LE, "tennis elbow")
    - Involves the wrist extensors and supinators, which originate at the lateral epicondyle
- May be caused by various different athletic or occupational activities
- Common in carpenters, plumbers, gardeners, and overhead athletes
- 75% of cases involve the dominant arm.

EPIDEMIOLOGY
- Predominant age: >40 years
- Predominant sex: male = female

Incidence
- Common overuse injury
- Lateral > medial
- Estimated between 1% and 3%

Prevalence
- LE: 1.3%
- ME: 0.4%

ETIOLOGY AND PATHOPHYSIOLOGY
- Acute (tendonitis)
  - Inflammatory response to injury or sudden, violent contraction
- Chronic (tendinosis)
  - Overuse injury
  - Repetitive wrist flexion or extension places strain across enthesis of flexor/extensor group.
  - Degeneration, calcium deposition, fibroblast proliferation, microvascular proliferation, hyaline cartilage destruction, absence of restorative inflammatory response
- Aggravating activities
  - Tool/racquet griping
  - Shaking hands
  - Occupational (painters, mechanics, cooks)
  - Sports (golf, tennis, archery, pitchers)

RISK FACTORS
- Repetitive wrist motions
  - Flexion/pronation: medial
  - Extension/supination: lateral
- Smoking
- Obesity
- Upper extremity forceful activities

GENERAL PREVENTION
- Limit overuse of the wrist flexors, extensors, pronators, and supinators.
- Use proper techniques when working with hand tools or playing racquet sports.
- Use lighter tools and smaller grips.

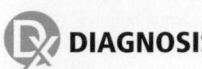 DIAGNOSIS

HISTORY
- Insidious onset
- Pain localized to lateral or medial elbow
- Aching pain, often radiates from epicondyle to forearm or wrist
- Pain with gripping
- Sensation of mild forearm weakness

PHYSICAL EXAM
- Localized pain just distal to the affected epicondyle
- ME
  - Tenderness at origin of wrist flexor tendons
  - Increased pain with resisted wrist flexion and pronation
  - Normal elbow range of motion
  - Increased pain with gripping
- LE
  - Tenderness at origin of wrist extensors
  - Increased pain with resisted wrist extension/supination
  - Normal elbow range of motion
  - Increased pain with gripping

DIFFERENTIAL DIAGNOSIS
- Elbow osteoarthritis
- Epicondylar fractures
- Posterior interosseous nerve entrapment (lateral)
- Ulnar neuropathy (medial)
- Synovitis
- Medial collateral ligament injury
- Referred pain from shoulder or neck

DIAGNOSTIC TESTS & INTERPRETATION
Initial Tests (lab, imaging)
No imaging is required for initial evaluation and treatment of a classic overuse injury.

Follow-Up Tests & Special Considerations
- Anterior-posterior/lateral radiographs if decreased range of motion, trauma, or no improvement with initial conservative therapy. Assess for fractures or signs of arthritis.
- For recalcitrant cases
  - Musculoskeletal ultrasound (US) reveals abnormal tendon appearance (e.g., hypoechoic, tendon thickening, partial tear at tendon origin, calcifications). US can also guide injections of steroid and/or anesthetic.
  - MRI can show intermediate or high T2 signal intensity within the common flexor or extensor tendon or the presence of peritendinous soft tissue edema.

Diagnostic Procedures/Other
Infiltration of local anesthetic with subsequent resolution of symptoms supports the diagnosis if clinically in doubt.

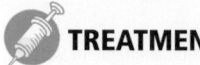 TREATMENT

GENERAL MEASURES
Initial treatment consists of activity modification, counterforce bracing, oral or topical NSAIDs, ice, and physical therapy.
- If left untreated, symptoms typically last between 6 months and 2 years. For patients with good function and minimal pain, consider conservative management using a "wait and see" approach based on patient preference.
- Modify activity, encourage relative rest, and correct faulty biomechanics.
- Bracing
  - Wrist extensor splints (WESs) inhibit contraction of extensor muscle and decreases tendon movement, thereby decreasing stress at the common extensor origin in LE (1)[B].
  - Counterforce bracing with a forearm strap is easy and inexpensive. Systematic reviews are inconclusive about overall efficacy, but initial bracing may improve the ability to perform daily activities in the first 6 weeks.
  - Consider cock-up wrist splinting for repetitive daily activities if counterforce bracing fails; can also use at nighttime to provide relative rest.
- Ice frequently after activities
- Physical therapy
  - Begin once acute pain is resolved. Infiltration of local anesthetic can reduce pain and permit better participation in physical therapy.
  - Eccentric strength training and stretching program
  - US therapy
  - Corticosteroid iontophoresis
  - Dry needling

MEDICATION

First Line

- Topical NSAIDs: Low-quality evidence suggests topical NSAIDS are significantly more effective than placebo with respect to pain and number needed to treat to benefit (NNT = 7) in the short term (up to 4 weeks) with minimal adverse effects (2)[A].
- Oral NSAIDs: unclear efficacy with respect to pain and function, but may offer short-term pain relief; associated with adverse GI effects (2)[A]

Second Line

Corticosteroid injections: short-term (≤8 weeks) reduction in pain. No benefits found for intermediate or long-term outcomes (3)[A].

ISSUES FOR REFERRAL

Failure of conservative therapy

ADDITIONAL THERAPIES

Given the mechanism of injury, many new treatments are targeted at tendon regeneration.

- Glyceryl trinitrate (GTN) transdermal patch
  - Nitric oxide (NO) is a small free radical generated by NO synthesis. NO is expressed by fibroblasts and is postulated to aid in collagen synthesis. Topical application of GTN theoretically improves healing by this mechanism. 1/4 of a 5-mg/24-hr GTN transdermal patch is applied once daily for up to 24 weeks.
  - Significant decreases in pain are seen at 3 weeks and 6 months compared to placebo patch.
- Extracorporeal shock wave therapy (ESWT) is a noninvasive, nonelectrical therapy found to be 89% effective in treating LE in some studies and is noted to be as effective as WES (1)[B].
- Prolotherapy
  - Injection of a dextrose solution into and around the tendon attachment stimulates a localized inflammatory response, leading to increased blood flow to stimulate healing.
- Platelet-rich plasma (PRP) injections
  - Injection of supraphysiologic autologous PRP leads to a local inflammatory response. Platelets degranulate, release growth factors, and stimulate the physiologic healing cascade.
  - PRP treatment of chronic LE significantly reduces pain and increases function. The benefit exceeds that of corticosteroid injection even after a follow-up of 1 year (4)[A].
- US-guided percutaneous needle tenotomy
  - Injection of a local anesthetic followed by US-guided tendon fenestration, aspiration, and abrasion of the underlying bone; thought to break apart scar tissue and stimulate inflammation and healing
  - Usually requires referral to sports medicine or orthopedic physician with specific equipment and training.

- Autologous tenocyte injection (ATI)
  - Two-step process
  - Small number of tenocytes are harvested, often from patellar tendon, and cultured.
  - Cultured tenocytes are then injected into tendon to help stimulate regeneration.
- Botulinum toxin A for chronic LE
  - Injections into the forearm extensor muscles (60 units) can be performed in the outpatient setting.

SURGERY/OTHER PROCEDURES

- Surgical intervention required in only 2.8% of patients
- Elbow surgery may be indicated in refractory cases:
  - Involves débridement and tendon release
  - Can be performed open or arthroscopically
  - Improvements in VAS, DASH scores, and grip strength seen in 5-year study (5)[B]
- Denervation of the lateral humeral epicondyle
  - Transection of the posterior cutaneous nerve of the forearm with implantation into the triceps may help with chronic symptoms and pain.

COMPLEMENTARY & ALTERNATIVE MEDICINE

Acupuncture: effective for short-term pain relief for lateral epicondyle pain

 ONGOING CARE

PROGNOSIS

Good: Majority resolve with conservative care.

REFERENCES

1. Aydın A, Atiç R. Comparison of extracorporeal shock-wave therapy and wrist-extensor splint application in the treatment of lateral epicondylitis: a prospective randomized controlled study. *J Pain Res*. 2018;11:1459–1467.
2. Pattanittum P, Turner T, Green S, et al. Non-steroidal anti-inflammatory drugs (NSAIDs) for treating lateral elbow pain in adults. *Cochrane Database Syst Rev*. 2013;(5):CD003686.
3. Krogh TP, Bartels EM, Ellingsen T, et al. Comparative effectiveness of injection therapies in lateral epicondylitis: a systematic review and network meta-analysis of randomized controlled trials. *Am J Sports Med*. 2013;41(6):1435–1446.
4. Mi B, Liu G, Zhou W, et al. Platelet rich plasma versus steroid on lateral epicondylitis: meta-analysis of randomized clinical trials. *Phys Sportsmed*. 2017;45(2):97–104.
5. Han SH, Lee JK, Kim HJ, et al. The result of surgical treatment of medial epicondylitis: analysis with more than a 5-year follow-up. *J Shoulder Elbow Surg*. 2016;25(10):1704–1709.

ADDITIONAL READING

- Cullinane FL, Boocock MG, Trevelyan FC. Is eccentric exercise an effective treatment for lateral epicondylitis? A systematic review. *Clin Rehabil*. 2014;28(1):3–19.
- Dingemanse R, Randsdorp M, Koes BW, et al. Evidence for the effectiveness of electrophysical modalities for treatment of medial and lateral epicondylitis: a systematic review. *Br J Sports Med*. 2014;48(12):957–965.
- Green S, Buchbinder R, Barnsley L, et al. Acupuncture for lateral elbow pain. *Cochrane Database Syst Rev*. 2002;(1):CD003527.
- Lin YC, Wu WT, Hsu YC, et al. Comparative effectiveness of botulinum toxin versus non-surgical treatments for treating lateral epicondylitis: a systematic review and meta-analysis. *Clin Rehabil*. 2018;32(2):131–145.
- Mattie R, Wong J, McCormick Z, et al. Percutaneous needle tenotomy for the treatment of lateral epicondylitis: a systematic review of the literature. *PM R*. 2017;9(6):603–611.
- Ozden R, Uruç V, Doğramaci Y, et al. Management of tennis elbow with topical glyceryl trinitrate. *Acta Orthop Traumatol Turc*. 2014;48(2):175–180.

 SEE ALSO

Algorithm: Pain in Upper Extremity

 CODES

ICD10

- M77.00 Medial epicondylitis, unspecified elbow
- M77.10 Lateral epicondylitis, unspecified elbow
- M77.01 Medial epicondylitis, right elbow

CLINICAL PEARLS

- ME (golfer's elbow) is characterized by pain and tenderness at the tendinous origins of the wrist flexors at the medial epicondyle.
- LE (tennis elbow) is characterized by pain and tenderness at the tendinous origins of the wrist extensors at the lateral epicondyle.
- Left untreated, symptoms typically last between 6 months and 2 years
- Most patients improve using conservative treatment with bracing, activity modification, and physical therapy.
- Newer therapies such as ATI, prolotherapy, and tenotomy are directed toward tendon regeneration.

E

EPIDIDYMITIS

David B. McCaleb, MD • Holly L. Baab, MD

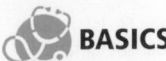

BASICS

DESCRIPTION

- Acute epididymitis: scrotal pain for <6 weeks
- Chronic epididymitis: scrotal pain for ≥3 months
- Inflammation (infectious or noninfectious) of epididymis resulting in scrotal pain and swelling, induration of the posterior epididymis, eventual scrotal wall edema, involvement of the adjacent testicle, and hydrocele formation
- Epididymitis with involvement of testis is named epididymo-orchitis.
- Classification: infectious (bacterial, viral, fungal, parasitic) versus noninfectious (chemical, traumatic, autoimmune, idiopathic, industrial, noninfectious, vasoepididymal reflux syndrome, vasal reflux syndrome); chronic versus acute
- System(s) affected: reproductive

EPIDEMIOLOGY

- Predominant age: usually younger, sexually active men or older men with UTIs; in older men, commonly secondary to bladder outlet obstruction
- Predominant sex: male only

Pediatric Considerations

In prepubertal boys: Epididymitis is found to be the most common cause of acute scrotum—more common than testicular torsion.

Incidence

- Common (600,000 cases annually in the United States) (1)
- 1 in 1,000 adult males per year
- 1.2 in 1,000 boys age 2 to 13 years per year (2,3)

Prevalence

Common

ETIOLOGY AND PATHOPHYSIOLOGY

- Infectious epididymitis
  - Retrograde passage of urinary bacteria from the prostate or urethra to the epididymis via the ejaculatory ducts and the vas deferens, rarely, hematogenous spread
  - Causative organism is identified in 80% of patients and varies according to patient age.
- Noninfectious epididymitis
  - Often no etiology is found; however, can be instigated by trauma, autoimmune disease, or vasculitis
  - Thought to likely be secondary to reflux of sterile urine causing a chemical inflammation rather than infectious
  - Can develop as a sequelae of strenuous exercise with a full bladder when urine is pushed through internal urethral sphincter (located at proximal end of prostatic urethra) or prolonged periods of sitting
  - Reflux of urine through orifice of ejaculatory ducts at verumontanum may occur with history of urethritis/prostatitis because inflammation may produce rigidity in musculature surrounding orifice to ejaculatory ducts, holding them open.
  - Exposure of epididymis to foreign fluid may produce inflammatory reaction within 24 hours.
- <14 years of age
  - Cause largely unknown although likely anatomic abnormalities resulting in urine reflux such as vesicoureteral reflux, ectopic ureter, or anorectal malformation (rectourethral fistula)
  - May also be part of postinfectious syndrome from *Mycoplasma pneumoniae*, enterovirus, or adenovirus
  - Henoch-Schönlein purpura may present as acute scrotum.

- 14 to 35 years of age
  - Usually *Chlamydia trachomatis* (serous urethral discharge) or *Neisseria gonorrhoeae* (purulent discharge) in sexually active males
  - With anal intercourse, likely *Escherichia coli* or *Haemophilus influenzae*
- >35 years
  - Commonly enteric bacteria but occasionally *Staphylococcus aureus* or *Staphylococcus epidermidis*
  - In elderly men, often with distal urinary tract obstruction, benign prostatic hyperplasia (BPH), UTI, or catheterization
  - Tuberculosis (TB), if sterile pyuria, nodularity of vas deferens (hematogenous spread), and recent infection. TB is the most common granulomatous disease affecting the epididymis (4).
  - Sterile urine reflux after transurethral prostatectomy
  - Granulomatous reaction following BCG intravesical therapy for bladder cancer
- Amiodarone may cause noninfectious epididymitis; resolves with decreasing drug dosage
- Syphilis, blastomycosis, coccidioidomycosis, and cryptococcosis are rare causes, but brucellosis can be a common cause in endemic areas.

RISK FACTORS

- UTI
- Prostatitis
- Indwelling urethral catheter
- Urethral instrumentation or transurethral surgery
- Urethral or meatal stricture
- Transrectal prostate biopsy
- Prostate brachytherapy (seeds) for prostate cancer
- Anal intercourse
- High-risk sexual activity
- Strenuous physical activity
- Prolonged sedentary periods
- Bladder obstruction (BPH, prostate cancer)
- HIV-immunosuppressed patient
- Severe Behçet disease
- Presence of foreskin
- Constipation
- Noninfectious epididymitis
  - Increased intra-abdominal pressure (due to frequent physical strain)
    - Military recruits, especially who begin physically unprepared
    - Laborers; restaurant kitchen workers
    - Full bladder during intense physical exertion

GENERAL PREVENTION

- Safer sexual practices
- Mumps vaccination
- Antibiotic prophylaxis for urethral manipulation
- Early treatment of prostatitis/BPH
- Vasectomy or vasoligation during transurethral surgery
- Avoid vigorous rectal exam with acute prostatitis.
- Emptying the bladder prior to physical exertion
- Physically conditioning the body prior to engaging in regular intense physical exertion
- Treat constipation.

COMMONLY ASSOCIATED CONDITIONS

- Prostatitis/urethritis/orchitis
- Hemospermia
- Constipation
- UTI

DIAGNOSIS

HISTORY

- Gradual onset of scrotal pain, sometimes radiating to the groin region over 1 to 2 days
- Urethral discharge or symptoms of UTI, such as frequency of urination, dysuria, cloudy urine, or hematuria
- Fever only in 11–19% (3)
- Progresses posterior-lying epididymis—body/head of epididymis
- Entire hemiscrotum becoming swollen and red; the testis becomes indistinguishable from the epididymis; the scrotal wall becomes thick and indurated; and reactive hydrocele may occur.
- Noninfectious epididymitis
  - Unilateral scrotal pain/swelling preceded by prolonged intense physical exertion with full bladder
  - No symptoms of infection

Pediatric Considerations

- Bacteremia from *H. influenzae* infection may produce acute epididymitis.
- Must rule out testicular torsion in adolescent males particularly age >13 years
- History not helpful in distinguishing epididymitis from testicular torsion

Geriatric Considerations

Diabetics with sensory neuropathy may have no pain despite severe infection/abscess.

PHYSICAL EXAM

- Epididymis is markedly tender to palpation.
- The tail of the epididymis is larger in comparison with the contralateral side.
- Elevation of the testes/epididymis reduces the discomfort (Prehn sign).
- Absence of a cremasteric reflex should raise suspicion for testicular torsion.

DIFFERENTIAL DIAGNOSIS

- Testicular/testicular appendage torsion
- Urethritis/orchitis
- Testicular trauma
- Epididymal congestion following vasectomy
- Testicular malignancy
- Epididymal cyst
- Inguinal hernia
- Spermatocele
- Hydrocele
- Hematocele
- Varicocele
- Epididymal adenomatoid tumor
- Epididymal rhabdomyosarcoma
- Vasculitis (Henoch-Schönlein purpura)

DIAGNOSTIC TESTS & INTERPRETATION

Initial Tests (lab, imaging)

- All suspected cases should be evaluated for objective evidence of inflammation by one of the following:
  - Urinalysis/urine culture preferably on first-void urine to evaluate for positive leukocyte esterase and bacteriuria
  - Urine culture/Gram stain urethral discharge; ≥2 WBC per oil immersion field; evaluate for gonococcal infection.
  - Microscopic examination of sediment from a spun first-void urine with ≥10 WBC per high power field
- Urine GC/CT testing for all suspected cases (4)[A]

- CRP >24 mg/L suggestive of epididymitis (5)[C]
- Urinalysis clear, and culture negative suggests noninfectious epididymitis
- If testicular torsion/mass cannot be excluded (especially in children), Doppler ultrasound (US) is test of choice (2,3).
- In adult men, US: sensitivity and specificity of 100% in evaluation of acute scrotum (6) compared to sensitivity of 63.6–100% and specificity of 97–100% in children (3)

Pediatric Considerations
Further radiographic imaging in children should be done to rule out anatomic abnormalities.

Diagnostic Procedures/Other
This is a clinical diagnosis.

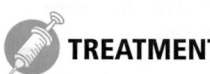 TREATMENT

GENERAL MEASURES
- Bed rest or restriction on activity
- Scrotal elevation, athletic scrotal supporter
- Ice pack wrapped in towel
- Avoid constipation.
- Spermatic cord block with local anesthesia in severe cases
- If noninfectious epididymitis
  - No strenuous physical activity and avoidance of any Valsalva maneuvers for several weeks
  - Empty bladder prior to strenuous exercises.

MEDICATION
First Line
- Sexually active adults <35 years: doxycycline 100 mg PO BID for 10 days (*C. trachomatis* coverage) PLUS ceftriaxone 250 mg IM × 1 (*N. gonorrhoeae* coverage) (2)[C],(4)[A]
- ≥35 years, not suspecting STD with enteric etiology (i.e., bacteriuria due to bladder outlet obstruction, prostate biopsy, urinary instrumentation, systemic disease, and/or immunosuppression)
  - Levofloxacin 500 mg/day PO for 10 days OR
  - Ofloxacin 300 mg PO BID for 10 days (2)[C],(4)[A]
  - Note: 2016 FDA black box warning on fluoroquinolones due to disabling and potentially permanent side effects. Consider trimethoprim-sulfamethoxazole for milder infections.
- Men who practice insertive anal intercourse: ceftriaxone 250 mg IM × 1 plus fluoroquinolone as above (2)[C],(4)[A]
- Analgesia:
  - NSAIDs (e.g., naproxen or ibuprofen) for mild to moderate pain
  - Consider steroid if patient cannot tolerate NSAID.
  - Acetaminophen with codeine or oxycodone for moderate to severe pain
- Septic or toxic patient
  - 3rd-generation cephalosporin or aminoglycoside
- For Behçet, sarcoid, Henoch-Schönlein purpura
  - Steroids, such as methylprednisolone, 40 mg/day recommended
- Chronic epididymitis: 2-week course of NSAIDs, scrotal icing/elevation; if no improvement, may add TCA or neuroleptic (2)

Second Line
- Trimethoprim-sulfamethoxazole (Bactrim, Septra) double strength PO BID for 10 to 14 days; increasing bacterial resistance may limit effectiveness.
- Add rifampin (rifampicin) or vancomycin, as required.

Pediatric Considerations
- May be postinfectious inflammatory condition; treat with anti-inflammatories and analgesics.
- Antibiotic therapy can be reserved for young infants until positive urine cultures (2).

ISSUES FOR REFERRAL
- If suspicion is high for testicular torsion, then urgent referral to urologist for possible surgery (1)[C]
- Epididymitis in ages <14 years requires a urology referral due to high incidence of associated urogenital abnormalities.
- If medical management fails, should be referred to urologist to rule out anatomic abnormality or chemical epididymitis

SURGERY/OTHER PROCEDURES
- Vasostomy to drain infected material if severe or refractory case
- Scrotal exploration if unable clinically to distinguish between epididymitis and testicular torsion
- Drainage of abscesses, epididymectomy (acute suppurative), or epididymo-orchiectomy in severe cases refractory to antibiotics
- Surgery to correct underlying anatomic abnormality or obstruction

ADMISSION, INPATIENT, AND NURSING CONSIDERATIONS
- Intractable pain
- Sepsis
- Abscess
- Persistent vomiting
- Scheduled surgery
- Purulent drainage
- Most cases can be managed with outpatient care.

 ONGOING CARE

FOLLOW-UP RECOMMENDATIONS
Patient Monitoring
- Routine follow-up in 1 week. Follow up within 72 hours if symptoms fail to improve with treatment for reevaluation of diagnosis and therapy (4)[A].
- Swelling and tenderness after antibiotic course should be evaluated for abscess, tumor, infarction, cancer, TB, and fungal epididymitis (4)[A].
- In noninfectious epididymitis, follow up in 4 weeks to assess efficacy of NSAIDs and lifestyle changes.

DIET
If constipation is contributing to pain or chemical epididymitis, then consider constipation prevention (high-fiber diet) and/or treatment.

PATIENT EDUCATION
- Stress completing course of antibiotics, even when asymptomatic.
- Early recognition and treatment of UTI or prostatitis
- Safer sexual practices. Avoid sex until antibiotic course completed and partner treated if likely STD.
- If treated for STI, refer sexual partners for evaluation of *N. gonorrhoeae* or *C. trachomatis* if sexual contact within 60 days preceding onset of symptoms or most recent sexual partner if >60 days (4)[A].
- If noninfectious epididymitis, then educate on noninfectious etiology and proper lifestyle changes.

PROGNOSIS
- Pain improves within 1 to 3 days, but induration may take several weeks/months to completely resolve.
- If bilateral involvement, sterility may result.
- In noninfectious epididymitis, symptoms usually resolve in <1 week.

COMPLICATIONS
- Recurrent epididymitis
- Infertility
- Oligospermia
- Testicular necrosis or atrophy
- Secondary abscess formation
- Fournier gangrene (necrotizing synergistic infection)

REFERENCES
1. Trojian TH, Lishnak TS, Heiman D. Epididymitis and orchitis: an overview. *Am Fam Physician*. 2009;79(7):583–587.
2. McConaghy JR, Panchal B. Epididymitis: an overview. *Am Fam Physician*. 2016;94(9):723–726.
3. Tekgul S, Dogan HS, Kocvara R, et al; for European Society for Paediatric Urology and European Association of Urology. *EAU Guidelines on Paediatric Urology*. Arnhem, Netherlands: European Association of Urology; 2016.
4. Workowski KA, Bolan GA; for Centers for Disease Control and Prevention. Sexually transmitted diseases treatment guidelines, 2015. *MMWR Recomm Rep*. 2015;64(RR-03):1–137.
5. Crawford P, Crop JA. Evaluation of scrotal masses. *Am Fam Physician*. 2014;89(9):723–727.
6. Rizvi SA, Ahmad I, Siddiqui MA, et al. Role of color Doppler ultrasonography in evaluation of scrotal swellings: pattern of disease in 120 patients with review of literature. *Urol J*. 2011;8(1):60–65.

ADDITIONAL READING
- Somekh E, Gorenstein A, Serour F. Acute epididymitis in boys: evidence of a post-infectious etiology. *J Urol*. 2004;171(1):391–394.
- Tracy CR, Steers WD, Costabile R. Diagnosis and management of epididymitis. *Urol Clin North Am*. 2008;35(1):101–108.
- Wolin LH. On the etiology of epididymitis. *J Urol*. 1971;105(4):531–533.

CODES

ICD10
- N45.1 Epididymitis
- N45.3 Epididymo-orchitis
- N45.4 Abscess of epididymis or testis

CLINICAL PEARLS

- With epididymitis, pain is gradual in onset, and the tenderness is mostly posterior to the testis. With testicular torsion, the symptoms are quite rapid in onset, the testis will be higher in the scrotum and may have a transverse lie, and the cremasteric reflex will be absent. The absence of leukocytes on urine analysis and decreased blood flow on scrotal US with Doppler will suggest torsion.
- Prostatic massage is contraindicated in epididymitis because of the risk for worsening local infection. The potential for sepsis is increased with acute prostatitis.
- Noninfectious epididymitis is a clinical diagnosis of exclusion, and infectious causes are much more common but must be considered in certain occupations, such as soldiers and laborers.

EPISCLERITIS

Sean M. Oser, MD, MPH • Daniel J. Schlegel, MD, MHA • Tamara K. Oser, MD

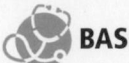

BASICS

- Episcleritis is irritation and inflammation of the episclera, a thin layer of tissue covering the sclera. It is not an infection.
- Episcleritis is the localized inflammation of the vascular connective tissue superficial to the sclera.
- Usually a self-limited condition, typically resolving within 3 weeks
- Most cases resolve without treatment.
- Topical lubricants and/or topical corticosteroid treatment may relieve symptoms while awaiting spontaneous resolution.

DESCRIPTION
- Edema and injection confined to the episcleral tissue
- Two types
  - Simple (diffuse scleral involvement—more common)
  - Nodular (focal area[s] of involvement—less common)

EPIDEMIOLOGY
Slight female predominance (~60–65%)

Incidence
- May occur at any age
- Peak incidence in 40s to 50s
- Community incidence not well-known (~20 to 50 cases per 100,000 person-years)

Prevalence
Not historically well-known; a recent community study found a prevalence of 53 cases per 100,000 persons.

ETIOLOGY AND PATHOPHYSIOLOGY
- Etiology: usually idiopathic, but other causes may be found (either nonimmune or immune)
- Pathophysiology:
  - Nonimmune (e.g., dry eye syndrome, with histology showing widespread vasodilation, edema, lymphocytic infiltration)
  - Immune (systemic vasculitis or rheumatologic disease)

COMMONLY ASSOCIATED CONDITIONS
- Usually not associated with another condition
- Less commonly associated conditions include the following:
  - Rheumatoid arthritis
  - Vasculitis
  - Inflammatory bowel disease
  - Ankylosing spondylitis
  - Systemic lupus erythematosus
  - Gout
  - Herpes zoster
  - Hypersensitivity disorders
    - Rosacea
    - Contact dermatitis
    - Penicillin sensitivity
    - Erythema multiforme

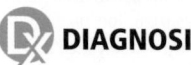

DIAGNOSIS

Episcleritis is a clinical diagnosis (1,2)[C].

HISTORY
- History should elicit potential causative factors, recurrence, or associated systemic disease (2).
- Pain is often absent; when present, it is usually mild and localized to the eye (1,2).
- Mild tearing may be present (2).

PHYSICAL EXAM
- Check visual acuity; decreased vision is very unusual with episcleritis, and its presence should raise suspicion for another condition such as scleritis (1,2).
- The white sclera will have a pink or purplish hue.
- Focal hyperemia (2,3)
- Pupils equal and reactive (2)
- Superficial episcleral vascular dilation (1,2)
- Episcleral edema (1,2)
  - Diffuse in simple episcleritis
  - Focal in nodular episcleritis
- Tenderness over involved area may be present (2) but is usually absent (3).
- Superficial episcleral vascular hyperemia blanches with topical phenylephrine (1,3).

ALERT
Recurrent episodes, difficulty confirming the diagnosis, or worsening symptoms require prompt ophthalmology referral (2)[C].

DIFFERENTIAL DIAGNOSIS
- Scleritis
- Bacterial conjunctivitis
- Viral conjunctivitis
- Herpes (ulcerative) keratitis
- Superficial keratitis
- Increased intraocular pressure (ocular hypertension)

DIAGNOSTIC TESTS & INTERPRETATION
Most patients with episcleritis do not require any further lab work or diagnostic studies (4)[C].

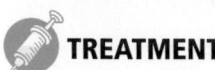

TREATMENT

MEDICATION
Treatment for episcleritis typically consists of symptomatic relief. The goal is to suppress the inflammation, which will, in turn, relieve the discomfort or pain. In most cases, treatment is not needed.

First Line
Topical lubricants such as artificial tears are typically used for initial management of symptomatic episcleritis (2)[C].

Second Line
- Topical corticosteroids are useful when discomfort is not sufficiently controlled by conservative measures (2,4,5)[C].
  - Fluorometholone 0.1% drops 4 times daily; if not effective, may increase frequency
  - Prednisolone 0.5–1% eye drops
- Refractory episcleritis may be treated with oral NSAIDs (4)[C].

ISSUES FOR REFERRAL

Recurrent episodes, uncertain diagnosis, and/or worsening symptoms should prompt ophthalmology referral. Rarely, episcleritis may progress to scleritis in which case ophthalmology referral is also recommended.

ADDITIONAL THERAPIES

- Topical NSAIDs have not been shown to have a significant benefit over artificial tears (6)[B].
- When episcleritis results from viral infection, appropriate antiviral therapy is indicated (5)[C].

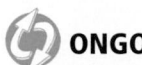 ONGOING CARE

FOLLOW-UP RECOMMENDATIONS

Episcleritis is usually self-limited (up to 21 days) and does not typically require follow-up.

PROGNOSIS

- Most patients have no ocular complications.
- Prognosis for episcleritis is excellent, with most patients making a full recovery.

COMPLICATIONS

Associated complications are rare, even at tertiary care referral centers, where referral bias likely overestimates their community incidence. When complications do occur, they tend not to be severe.

- Anterior uveitis may occur in 4–16% of cases (1,5)[C].
- Decreased vision may occur in 0–4% of cases (1,5)[C].
- Ocular hypertension has been reported in 0–3.5% of cases (1,5)[C].

REFERENCES

1. Sainz de la Maza M, Molina N, Gonzalez-Gonzalez LA, et al. Clinical characteristics of a large cohort of patients with scleritis and episcleritis. *Ophthalmology*. 2012;119(1):43–50.
2. Cronau H, Kankanala RR, Mauger T. Diagnosis and management of red eye in primary care. *Am Fam Physician*. 2010;81(2):137–144.
3. Galor A, Thorne JE. Scleritis and peripheral ulcerative keratitis. *Rheum Dis Clin North Am*. 2007;33(4):835–854.
4. Kirkwood BJ, Kirkwood RA. Episcleritis and scleritis. *Insight*. 2010;35(4):5–8.
5. Berchicci L, Miserocchi E, Di Nicola M, et al. Clinical features of patients with episcleritis and scleritis in an Italian tertiary care referral center. *Eur J Ophthalmol*. 2014;24(3):293–298.
6. Williams CP, Browning AC, Sleep TJ, et al. A randomised, double-blind trial of topical ketorolac vs artificial tears for the treatment of episcleritis. *Eye (Lond)*. 2005;19(7):739–742.

ADDITIONAL READING

- Daniel Diaz J, Sobol EK, Gritz DC. Treatment and management of scleral disorders. *Surv Ophthalmol*. 2016;61(6):702–717.
- Salama A, Elsheikh A, Alweis R. Is this a worrisome red eye? Episcleritis in the primary care setting. *J Community Hosp Intern Med Perspect*. 2018;8(1):46–48.

 CODES

ICD10

- H15.109 Unspecified episcleritis, unspecified eye
- H15.129 Nodular episcleritis, unspecified eye
- H15.102 Unspecified episcleritis, left eye

CLINICAL PEARLS

- Episcleritis typically is a benign, self-limited disorder.
- Often not painful and presents without decrease in visual acuity
- Although treatment is often not needed, when employed, the goal is symptomatic relief while awaiting spontaneous resolution.
- Topical lubricants and/or topical corticosteroid treatment may relieve symptoms.
- Associated complications are uncommon and not severe but may include anterior uveitis, decreased vision, and ocular hypertension.
- Episcleritis can be an early presentation of scleritis, which is more severe. Accurate diagnosis of episcleritis is important.

E

EPISTAXIS

Rebecca Wetzel, DO • Brian E. Neubauer, MD

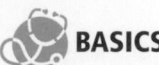 BASICS

DESCRIPTION
- Hemorrhage from the nose involving either the anterior or posterior mucosal surfaces
- Intractable or refractory epistaxis: recurrent or persistent despite appropriate packing or multiple episodes during a short period, each requiring medical attention
- Synonym(s): nosebleed

EPIDEMIOLOGY
Incidence
- Very common in the United States
- Estimated lifetime prevalence: ~60%
- Bimodal, with peaks in children up to 15 years and in adults >50 years, particularly ages 70 to 79 years
- Most common in males <49 years
- Rare in children age <2 years
- ~6% of patients require medical or surgical intervention; accounts for ~1 in 200 ER visits

ETIOLOGY AND PATHOPHYSIOLOGY
- Local versus systemic disease. Most nosebleeds are due to local causes.
- Anterior: 90–95% of all cases (Kiesselbach plexus)
- Posterior: 5–10% of cases (Woodruff plexus); usually branches of sphenopalatine arteries: may be asymptomatic or may present with other symptoms (hematemesis, hemoptysis)
- Idiopathic
- Local inflammation/irritation
  - Infection (viral URI, sinusitis, TB, syphilis)
  - Irritant inhalation (smoking, rhinitis)
  - Topical steroid or antihistamine use
  - Septal deviation (more air movement on one side)
  - Low humidity, nasal oxygen use, CPAP
  - Tumors: benign, malignant
  - Vascular malformations
- Trauma
  - Epistaxis digitorum (nose picking)
  - Foreign bodies
  - Septal perforation
  - Nasal fracture
  - Nasal surgery
- Systemic
  - Thrombocytopenia
  - Congenital or acquired coagulopathies
  - Liver or renal disease
  - Chronic alcohol abuse
  - Leukemia
  - Anticoagulant drug use
  - CHF
  - Hereditary hemorrhagic telangiectasia (HHT)
  - Collagen abnormalities
  - Mitral valve stenosis
  - Multiple myeloma
  - Polycythemia vera
  - HIV

RISK FACTORS
- Local irritation from multiple causes
- Medications/supplements including aspirin, clopidogrel, ginseng, garlic, ginkgo biloba, sildenafil, warfarin, and other anticoagulant
- Prior septoplasty/turbinate procedures, anemia, and thrombocytopenia are risk factors for recurrent epistaxis.

GENERAL PREVENTION
- Humidification at night
- Cut fingernails and minimize picking.
- For topical-nasal medication users, direct spray laterally away from septum. Use opposite hand to spray (i.e., right hand to spray in left nostril).
- Petroleum jelly to prevent anterior mucosal drying
- Control hypertension (HTN) (controversial association with increased risk for recurrent epistaxis).

COMMONLY ASSOCIATED CONDITIONS
- Vascular malformation/telangiectasia (HHT)
- Neoplasm (rare; consider if persistent and unilateral)
- Systemic
  - Coagulopathy: primary or iatrogenic
  - Thrombocytopenia
  - Cirrhosis
  - Renal failure
  - Alcoholism
- No proven association with HTN but may make control of bleeding more difficult

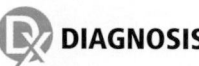 DIAGNOSIS

HISTORY
- Assess airway patency and cardiovascular stability.
- Determine on which side bleeding began, anterior or posterior, duration.
- Define trauma (including nose picking) or other precipitating events.
- Previous episodes
- Comorbid conditions (cardiovascular compromise symptoms)
- Current medications including over-the-counter and supplements
- Nausea, hematemesis, or hemoptysis may indicate a posterior and more severe bleed.

PHYSICAL EXAM
- Blood loss through one or both nostrils in most cases is due to anterior nasal septal bleeding and can often be directly visualized.
- Focus on localizing site of bleeding to anterior versus posterior nasal cavity.
- Patient is seated, head forward, to avoid blood going down the posterior pharynx.
- Use of nasal speculum improves visualization.

DIFFERENTIAL DIAGNOSIS
- Diagnosis usually apparent; the differential for the etiology is key.
- Posterior bleeding must be included in the differential for any chronic blood loss.

DIAGNOSTIC TESTS & INTERPRETATION
Lab testing is not indicated in most uncomplicated cases in which bleeding is easily controlled.

Initial Tests (lab, imaging)
- Mild cases, responsive to pressure: no labs
- For recurrent or intractable cases
  - CBC, PT/PTT, BMP
- PT/PTT if on warfarin or other medications affecting coagulation
- Crossmatch when appropriate
- Toxicology screen when nasal use of illicit drugs is suspected
- For most cases, imaging is not indicated.

Follow-Up Tests & Special Considerations
Consider neoplasm if recurrent unilateral epistaxis, especially if not responding to treatment.

Diagnostic Procedures/Other
Nasal endoscopy

Pediatric Considerations
More likely anterior, idiopathic, and recurrent

Geriatric Considerations
More likely to be posterior bleed

 TREATMENT

- Most cases are managed as outpatient (1)[B].
- Home use—Nosebleed QR: a nonprescription powder of hydrophilic polymer with potassium salt; induces scab formation
- Patient applies direct pressure by pinching the lower part of the nose (nasal ala) for 5 to 20 minutes without a break. This stops bleeding in most patients.
- Cleanse nasal cavity of blood clots by blowing nose.
- An ice pack placed over the dorsum of the nose may help with hemostasis.
- Inspect the nasal septum for the bleeding site.

GENERAL MEASURES
Resuscitation, as indicated. Use universal "airway/breathing/circulation (ABC)" approach.

MEDICATION
First Line
If general measures fail, affected naris may be sprayed with topical vasoconstrictor, such as:
- Phenylephrine: 0.5–1%
- Oxymetazoline: 0.05%
- Epinephrine: 1:1,000
- Cocaine: 4%

Second Line
- Chemical (silver nitrate) or electrical cautery
- Nasal packing: ribbon gauze, nasal tampons, nasal balloon catheter
- For intractable/refractory: Consider surgical ligation, endoscopic ligation/cautery, endovascular embolization.

ISSUES FOR REFERRAL

- Posterior bleeding frequently requires an otolaryngology consultation.
- Anterior bleeding that fails conservative measures, packing, and cauterization
- Recurrent episodes
- HHT patients should establish care with ENT.
- Concurrent anticoagulation
  - If bleeding stops with packing, may continue same dose of warfarin if INR therapeutic; decrease dose if supratherapeutic INR.
  - If bleeding persists despite packing, stop anticoagulation and administer vitamin K 10 mg IV ×1, recheck INR in 30 minutes, if still >1.5, give PCC.
  - Novel anticoagulation may be associated with lower rates of epistaxis than warfarin. When epistaxis occurs, it may be harder to control.

ADDITIONAL THERAPIES

- Nasal packing: either with ribbon gauze or preformed nasal tampons. Systemic prophylactic antibiotics are unnecessary in the majority of patients with nasal packs; topical antibiotics may be as effective and cheaper (2)[B].
- FloSeal: A biodegradable hemostatic sealant (a thrombin-type gel) in one study is more effective and better tolerated than packing (3)[B].
- Local application of tranexamic acid may reduce bleeding time as compared to anterior packing (4).
- If an actively bleeding anterior septal site is visualized, this may be treated with gentle silver nitrate cautery for ~10 seconds for definitive treatment. 75% silver nitrate is preferred. Apply in a spiral fashion, starting around the bleeding vessel, moving inward.
- Limit cautery (silver nitrate) to one side of septum, or wait 4 to 6 weeks in between treatments to reduce risk of perforation.
- Posterior: Posterior packing or tamponade with balloon devices (Foley catheter has been used). Inpatient monitoring is generally required.
- Recurrent epistaxis: Cochrane review in children shows no difference in effectiveness between antiseptic nasal cream, petroleum jelly, silver nitrate cautery, or no treatment.
  - Silver nitrate cautery followed by 4 weeks of antiseptic cream may be better than antiseptic cream alone (5).

SURGERY/OTHER PROCEDURES

- Packing
  - Layering of Vaseline ribbon gauze (1/2 inch)
    - For gauze packing, be certain that both ends of the ribbon gauze protrude from the nostril.
    - Packing is layered from the floor upward.
    - Secure packing with gauze across the outside of the nostril.
  - Nasal tampon may be used after lubricating the tip with KY Jelly or antibiotic cream or ointment.

- Additional saline may be needed to expand the tampon if the bleeding has slowed.
- Merocel and Rapid Rhino packs are easier to use than gauze packing and are usually well tolerated.
- Posterior bleed
  - In the emergent setting, this may be attempted utilizing a Foley catheter or a specific posterior packing balloon.
  - With both methods, the tubing is introduced through the nose similar to the passage of a nasogastric tube. Once it reaches the posterior oral pharynx, the balloon is inflated, and the tubing is pulled back outward to tamponade the posterior bleeding source.
    - If using a Foley catheter (10 to 14F catheter), the balloon can be inflated with 10 mL of saline.
    - Traction is maintained with an umbilical cord clamp with adequate padding between the clip and the nose to avoid injury.

ADMISSION, INPATIENT, AND NURSING CONSIDERATIONS

- Consider hospitalization for elderly or for patients with posterior bleeding or coagulopathy; may also consider if significant comorbidities
- Admission criteria/initial stabilization
  - Posterior bleed
  - Hemodynamic changes
  - Clotting dysfunction
  - Universal ABC approach. Stop blood loss.

 ONGOING CARE

FOLLOW-UP RECOMMENDATIONS

Patient Monitoring
- Hemodynamic monitoring if severe blood loss
- 24-Hour minimum for leaving packing in place; some recommend 3 to 5 days. Rebleed usually occurs between 24 and 48 hours. Longer durations of packing have increased risk of mucosal injury and toxic shock syndrome.

PATIENT EDUCATION
- Demonstrate proper pinching pressure techniques.
- Avoidance of trauma or irritants is key.
- Management of systemic illness and proper use of medication

PROGNOSIS
- Most are self-limited.
- Good results with proper treatment

COMPLICATIONS
- Septal perforation
- Pressure-induced tissue necrosis of the nasal mucosa
- Toxic shock syndrome with packing
- Arrhythmias triggered by packing (particularly posterior)

REFERENCES

1. Melia L, McGarry GW. Epistaxis: update on management. *Curr Opin Otolaryngol Head Neck Surg*. 2011;19(1):30–35.
2. Biggs TC, Nightingale K, Patel NN, et al. Should prophylactic antibiotics be used routinely in epistaxis patients with nasal packs? *Ann R Coll Surg Engl*. 2013;95(1):40–42.
3. Escabasse V, Bequignon E, Vérillaud B, et al. Guidelines of the French Society of Otorhinolaryngology (SFORL). Managing epistaxis under coagulation disorder due to antithrombotic therapy. *Eur Ann Otorhinolaryngol Head Neck Dis*. 2017;134(3):195–199.
4. Clinkard D, Barbic D. Tranexamic acid for epistaxis—a promising treatment that deserves further study. *CJEM*. 2016;18(1):72–73.
5. Calder N, Kang S, Fraser L, et al. A double-blind randomized controlled trial of management of recurrent nosebleeds in children. *Otolaryngol Head Neck Surg*. 2009;140(5):670–674.

ADDITIONAL READING

- Manes RP. Evaluating and managing the patient with nosebleeds. *Med Clin North Am*. 2010;94(5):903–912.
- Schlosser RJ. Clinical practice. Epistaxis. *N Engl J Med*. 2009;360(8):784–789.

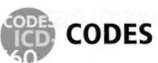 **CODES**

ICD10
R04.0 Epistaxis

CLINICAL PEARLS

- Most epistaxis is anterior and responds well to timed pressure over the anterior nares for 5 to 20 minutes.
- Most nosebleeds are idiopathic or as a result of nose picking.
- Posterior nosebleeds can be asymptomatic or present with nausea, hematemesis, or heme-positive stool.
- Consider evaluation for neoplasm in cases of recurrent unilateral epistaxis.

E

ERECTILE DYSFUNCTION

James G. Nee, MD, FAAFP

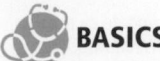 **BASICS**

DESCRIPTION

- Erectile dysfunction (ED): the consistent or recurrent inability to acquire or sustain an erection of sufficient rigidity and duration for sexual intercourse
- In the past, ED was assumed to be a symptom of the aging process in men, but it is more often the result of concurrent medical conditions of the patient or from medications that patients may be taking to treat those conditions.
- Sexual problems are frequent among older men and have a detrimental effect on their quality of life but are infrequently discussed with their physicians.
- Synonym(s): impotence

EPIDEMIOLOGY

Incidence
It is estimated that >600,000 new cases of ED will be diagnosed annually in the United States, although this may be an underestimation of the true incidence, as ED is vastly underreported.

Prevalence
Overall prevalence for some degree of ED:
- 52% in men age 40 to 70 years
- Age-related increase ranging from 12.4% in men age 40 to 49 years up to 46.6% in men age 50 to 69 years

ETIOLOGY AND PATHOPHYSIOLOGY

- ED is a neurovascular event.
  - With stimulation, there is release of nitrous oxide, which increases production of cyclic guanosine 3',5'-monophosphate (cGMP).
  - This leads to relaxation of cavernous smooth muscle, leading to increased blood flow to penis.
  - As cavernosal sinusoids distend with blood, there is passive compression of subtunical veins, which decreases venous outflow, and this leads to an erection.
- Alterations in any of these events lead to ED.
- ED may result from problems with systems required for normal penile erection.
  - Vascular: diseases that compromise blood flow
    - Peripheral vascular disease, arteriosclerosis, essential hypertension
  - Neurologic: diseases that impair nerve conduction to brain or penile vasculature
    - Spinal cord injury, stroke, diabetes
  - Endocrine: diseases associated with changes in testosterone, luteinizing hormone, prolactin levels
  - Structural: phimosis, lichen sclerosis, congenital curvature
  - Psychological: patients suffering from malaise, depression, performance anxiety
- Social habits such as smoking or excessive alcohol intake
- Medications may cause ED.
- Prostate cancer treatment
- Structural injury or trauma (bicycling accident)

Genetics
Rarely related to chromosomal disorders

RISK FACTORS
- Advancing age
- Cardiovascular disease
- Diabetes mellitus
- Metabolic syndrome
- Sedentary lifestyle
- Cigarette smoking
- Urologic surgery, radiation, trauma/injury to pelvic area or spinal cord
- Medications that induce ED
  - SSRIs, β-blockers, clonidine, digoxin, spironolactone, antiandrogens, corticosteroids, H_2 blockers, anticonvulsants
- Central neurologic and endocrinologic conditions
- Substance abuse (alcohol, cocaine, opioids, marijuana)
- Psychological conditions: stress, anxiety, or depression, sexual abuse, relationship problems

GENERAL PREVENTION
The two best ways to prevent ED are by the following:
- Making healthy lifestyle choices by exercising regularly, eating well-balanced meals, limiting alcohol, and avoiding smoking
- Treating existing health problems and working with your patients to manage diabetes, heart disease, and other chronic problems

ALERT
Aging alone is not a cause.

COMMONLY ASSOCIATED CONDITIONS
- Cardiovascular disease:
  - Men with ED have a greater likelihood of having angina, myocardial infarction, stroke, transient ischemic attack, congestive heart failure, or cardiac arrhythmia compared to men without ED (1).
- Diabetes
- Neurologic conditions
- Metabolic syndrome
- Psychiatric disorders

 DIAGNOSIS

Inability to achieve or maintain erection satisfactory for intercourse

HISTORY
- Identify concurrent medical illnesses or surgical procedures, history of trauma, and a list of current medications (e.g., antihypertensive meds).
- Psychosocial history: smoking, ethanol intake, recreational drug use, anxiety and depression, satisfaction with current relationship
- Presence or absence of morning erections
- Speed of onset and duration of symptoms
- Relationship of symptoms to libido
- Detailed sexual history important to rule out premature ejaculation, as this is frequently confused with ED
- Five-question International Index of Erectile Function (IIEF-5) is useful in rapid clinical assessment and measurement of effectiveness of ED treatments (1).

PHYSICAL EXAM
- Signs and symptoms of hypogonadism: gynecomastia, small testicles, decreased body hair
- Penile plaques (Peyronie disease)
- Detailed examination of the cardiovascular, neurologic, and genitourinary systems
  - Blood pressure, waist circumference, BMI
  - Check femoral and lower extremity pulses to assess vascular supply to genitals.
  - Check anal sphincter tone and genital reflexes, including cremasterics and bulbocavernosus.

DIFFERENTIAL DIAGNOSIS
- Premature ejaculation
- Decreased libido
- Anorgasmia
- Sudden versus chronic ED

DIAGNOSTIC TESTS & INTERPRETATION
Vascular and/or neurologic assessment and monitoring of nocturnal erections may be indicated in selected patients but not for routine workup (2)[C].

Initial Tests (lab, imaging)
- Depending on history, Hgb A1c, lipid panel, TSH, and morning total testosterone level (1)[C]
- Doppler, angiogram, and cavernosogram are available radiologic modalities but not recommended in routine practice for the diagnosis of ED (2)[C].

Follow-Up Tests & Special Considerations
Other hormonal tests, such as prolactin, should only be ordered when there is suspicion for a specific endocrinopathy.

Diagnostic Procedures/Other
Questionnaires can be offered to assess the severity of ED, including the IIEF and its validated and more easily administered abridged version, the Sexual Health Inventory for Men (SHIM) (2)[C].

 TREATMENT

- Lifestyle modifications and managing medications contributing to ED is first-line therapy for ED (3)[C]. Use least invasive therapy first; reserve more invasive therapies for nonresponders.
- Cardiovascular risk stratification and risk-factor management is recommended in all men with vasculogenic ED (4).
- Current smoking is significantly associated with ED, and smoking cessation has a beneficial effect on the restoration of erectile function (1)[A].
- Phosphodiesterase type 5 (PDE-5) inhibitors are the first-line treatment for ED (1)[A].

GENERAL MEASURES
- Psychotherapy alone or in combination with psychoactive drugs may be helpful in men whose ED is related to depression or anxiety.
- Weight loss and increased physical activity for obese men with ED. Men with metabolic syndrome should be counseled to make lifestyle modifications to reduce the risk of cardiovascular events and ED (1)[B].

MEDICATION

First Line

PDE-5 inhibitors are effective in the treatment of ED in many men, including those with diabetes mellitus and spinal cord injury and sexual dysfunction associated with antidepressants (5). Choice should be based on patient's preference (cost, ease of use, and adverse effects). There is insufficient evidence to support the superiority of one agent over the others (3)[A]:

- Sildenafil (Viagra): usual daily dose: 50 to 100 mg within at least 60 minutes of sexual intercourse
- Vardenafil (Levitra): usual daily dose 5 to 20 mg within at least 60 minutes of sexual intercourse
- Vardenafil (Staxyn): ODT: usual dose 10 mg within 60 minutes of sexual intercourse
- Tadalafil (Cialis): usual daily dose 5 to 20 mg within at least 30 minutes of sexual intercourse or 2.5 mg once daily without regard to sexual activity
- Avanafil (Stendra): usual daily dose: 50 to 200 mg within at least 15 to 30 minutes of sexual intercourse
  - Adverse effects of PDE-5 inhibitors: headache, facial flushing, dyspepsia, nasal congestion, dizziness, hypotension, increased sensitivity to light (sildenafil and vardenafil), vision changes, lower back pain (tadalafil), and priapism (with excessive doses)
  - Sildenafil and vardenafil should be taken on an empty stomach for maximum effectiveness.

Geriatric Considerations

Use doses at the lower end of the dosing range for elderly patients and evaluate exercise tolerance before prescribing.

- Sildenafil 25 mg daily
- Vardenafil 5 mg daily

Second Line

Intraurethral and intracavernosal injectables are second-line therapies shown to be effective and should be administered based on patient preference (1)[B]. Intraurethral suppositories are a less invasive treatment option than intracavernosal injections; however, they are not as effective (3)[C]. Alprostadil, also known as prostaglandin E1, causes smooth muscle relaxation of the arterial blood vessels and sinusoidal tissues in the corpora:

- Intraurethral alprostadil (Muse):
  - Urethral suppository: 125-, 250-, 500-, and 1,000-μg pellets. Administer 5 to 50 minutes before intercourse. No >2 doses in 24 hours are recommended.
- Intracavernosal alprostadil (available in 2 formulations):
  - Alprostadil (Caverject): usual dose: 10 to 20 μg, with max dose of 60 μg. Injection should be made at right angles into one of the lateral surfaces of the proximal 3rd of the penis using a 0.5-inch, 27- or 30-gauge needle. Do not use >3 times a week or more than once in 24 hours.
  - Alprostadil may also be combined with papaverine (Bimix) plus phentolamine (Tri-Mix).

ALERT

- Initial trial dose of second-line agents should be administered under supervision of a specialist or primary care physician with expertise in these therapies.
- Patient should notify physician if erection lasts >4 hours for immediate attention.

- Vacuum pump devices are a noninvasive second-line option and are available over the counter. Do not use vacuum devices in men with sickle cell anemia or blood dyscrasias.
- Testosterone supplementation in men with hypogonadism improves ED and libido (5)[B]. Available formulations include injectable depots, transdermal patches and gels, SC pellets, and oral therapy.
- Best practices in urology recommendation: Do not prescribe testosterone to men with ED who have normal testosterone levels (1).
- Contraindications:
  - Nitroglycerin (or other nitrates) and phosphodiesterase inhibitors: potential for severe, fatal hypotension
  - Precautions/side effects:
    - Testosterone: *precautions*: Exogenous testosterone reduces sperm count and thus do not use in patients wishing to keep fertility; *side effects*: acne, sodium retention
    - Intraurethral suppository: local penile pain, urethral bleeding, dizziness, and dysuria
    - Intracavernosal injection: penile pain, edema and hematoma, palpable nodules or plaques, and priapism
    - Sildenafil: hypotension (caution for patients on nitrates)
    - PDE-5 inhibitors: Use caution with congenital prolonged QT syndrome, class Ia or II antiarrhythmics, nitroglycerin, α-blockers (e.g., terazosin, tamsulosin), retinal disease, unstable cardiac disease, liver and renal failure.
    - Significant possible interactions
    - PDE-5 inhibitor concentration is affected by CYP3A4 inhibitors (e.g., erythromycin, indinavir, ketoconazole, ritonavir, amiodarone, cimetidine, clarithromycin, delavirdine, diltiazem, fluoxetine, fluvoxamine, grapefruit juice, itraconazole, nefazodone, nevirapine, saquinavir, and verapamil). Serum concentrations and/or toxicity may be increased. Lower starting doses should be used in these patients.
    - PDE-5 inhibitor concentration may be reduced by rifampin and phenytoin.

ADDITIONAL THERAPIES

Men with relationship difficulties who received therapy plus sildenafil had more successful intercourse than those who received only sildenafil (6)[A].

SURGERY/OTHER PROCEDURES

Penile prosthesis should be reserved for patients who have failed or are ineligible first- or second-line therapies.

COMPLEMENTARY & ALTERNATIVE MEDICINE

Trazodone, yohimbine, and herbal therapies are not recommended for the treatment of ED, as they have not proven to be efficacious.

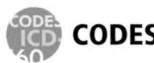 ## ONGOING CARE

FOLLOW-UP RECOMMENDATIONS

Patient Monitoring

Treatment should be assessed at baseline and after the patient has completed at least 1 to 3 weeks of a specific treatment: Monitor the quality and quantity of penile erections and monitor the level of satisfaction patient achieves.

DIET

Diet and exercise recommended to achieve a normal body mass index; limit alcohol.

PROGNOSIS

- All commercially available PDE-5 inhibitors are equally effective. In the presence of sexual stimulation, they are 55–80% effective.
  - Lower success rates with diabetes mellitus and radical prostatectomy patients who suffer from ED
- Overall effectiveness is 70–90% for intracavernosal alprostadil and 43–60% for intraurethral alprostadil (2)[B].
- Penile prostheses are associated with an 85–90% patient satisfaction rate (2)[C].

REFERENCES

1. Rew KT, Heidelbaugh JJ. Erectile dysfunction. *Am Fam Physician*. 2016;94(10):820–827.
2. McVary KT. Clinical practice. Erectile dysfunction. *N Engl J Med*. 2007;357(24):2472–2481.
3. American Urological Association. Guideline on the management of erectile dysfunction: diagnosis and treatment recommendations. http://www.auanet.org/education/guidelines/erectile-dysfunction.cfm. Accessed January 13, 2017.
4. Miner M, Nehra A, Jackson G, et al. All men with vasculogenic erectile dysfunction require a cardiovascular workup. *Am J Med*. 2014;127(3):174–182.
5. Heidelbaugh JJ. Management of erectile dysfunction. *Am Fam Physician*. 2010;81(3):305–312.
6. Melnik T, Soares BG, Nasselo AG. Psychosocial interventions for erectile dysfunction. *Cochrane Database Syst Rev*. 2007;(3):CD004825.

CODES

ICD10

- N52.9 Male erectile dysfunction, unspecified
- N52.1 Erectile dysfunction due to diseases classified elsewhere
- F52.21 Male erectile disorder

CLINICAL PEARLS

- Nitrates should be withheld for 24 hours after sildenafil or vardenafil administration and for 48 hours after use of tadalafil. PDE-5 inhibitors are contraindicated in patients taking concurrent nitrates of any form (regular or intermittent nitrate therapy), as it can lead to severe hypotension and syncope.
- Reserve surgical treatment for patients who do not respond to drug treatment.
- The use of PDE-5 inhibitors with α-adrenergic antagonists may increase the risk of hypotension. Tamsulosin is the least likely to cause orthostatic hypotension.
- Avanafil should not be used with strong CYP3A4 inhibitors and max dose should be 50 mg with moderate CYP3A4 inhibitors.
- ED may be a marker for subclinical cardiovascular disease. Thoroughly assess patients with nonpsychogenic ED for CV risks.

E

ERYSIPELAS

Fozia Akhtar Ali, MD • Barbara M. Kiersz Muller, DO • Sanna R. Bhajjan, DO

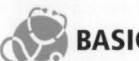 **BASICS**

DESCRIPTION
- Distinct form of cellulitis: notable for acute, well-demarcated, superficial bacterial skin infection with lymphatic involvement almost always caused by *Streptococcus pyogenes*
- Usually acute, but a chronic recurrent form can also exist (1)
- Nonpurulent
- System(s) affected: skin, exocrine

EPIDEMIOLOGY
- Predominant age: infants, children, and adults >45 years
- Greatest in elderly (>75 years)
- No gender/racial predilection

Incidence
- Erysipelas occurs in ~1/1,000 persons/year.
- Incidence on the rise since the 1980s (2)

Prevalence
Unknown

ETIOLOGY AND PATHOPHYSIOLOGY
- Group A streptococci induce inflammation and activation of the contact system, a proinflammatory pathway with antithrombotic activity, releasing proteinases and proinflammatory cytokines.
- The generation of antibacterial peptides and the release of bradykinin, a proinflammatory peptide, increase vascular permeability and induce fever and pain.
- The M proteins from the group A streptococcal cell wall interact with neutrophils, leading to the secretion of heparin-binding protein, an inflammatory mediator that also induces vascular leakage.
- This cascade of reactions leads to the symptoms seen in erysipelas: fever, pain, erythema, and edema.
- Group A β-hemolytic streptococci primarily; commonly *S. pyogenes*, occasionally, other *Streptococcus* groups C/G
- Rarely, group B streptococci/*Staphylococcus aureus* may be involved.

RISK FACTORS
- Disruption in the skin barrier (surgical incisions, insect bites, eczematous lesions, local trauma, abrasions, dermatophytic infections, intravenous drug user [IVDU])
- Chronic diseases (diabetes, malnutrition, nephrotic syndrome, heart failure)
- Immunocompromised (HIV)/debilitated
- Fissured skin (especially at the nose and ears)
- Toe-web intertrigo and lymphedema
- Leg ulcers/stasis dermatitis
- Venous/lymphatic insufficiency (saphenectomy, varicose veins of leg, phlebitis, radiotherapy, mastectomy, lymphadenectomy)
- Alcohol abuse
- Morbid obesity
- Recent streptococcal pharyngitis
- Varicella

GENERAL PREVENTION
- Good skin hygiene
- It is recommended that predisposing medical conditions, such as tinea pedis and stasis dermatitis, be appropriately managed first.

- Men who shave within 5 days of facial erysipelas are more likely to have a recurrence.
- With recurrences, search for other possible sources of streptococcal infection (e.g., tonsils, sinuses).
- Compression stockings should be encouraged for patients with lower extremity edema.
- Consider suppressive prophylactic antibiotic therapy, such as penicillin, in patients with >2 episodes in a 12-month period.

Pediatric Considerations
Group B *Streptococcus* may be a cause of erysipelas in neonates/infants.

 DIAGNOSIS

Prodromal symptoms before the skin eruption of erysipelas may include:
- Moderate- to high-grade fever
- Chills
- Headache
- Malaise
- Anorexia, usually in the first 48 hours
- Vomiting
- Arthralgias

ALERT
It is important to differentiate erysipelas from a methicillin-resistant *S. aureus* (MRSA) infection, which usually presents with an indurated center, significant pain, and later evidence of abscess formation.

PHYSICAL EXAM
- Vital signs: moderate- to high-grade fever with resultant tachycardia. Hypotension may occur.
- The presence of a fever in erysipelas can be considered a differentiating factor from other skin infections.
- Headache and vomiting may be prominent.
- Acute onset of intense erythema; well-demarcated painful plaque (3)
- Peau d'orange appearance
- Milian ear sign (Erythema involves skin of ear as well as face implies erysipelas.)
- Vesicles and bullae may form but are not uniformly present.
- Desquamation may occur later.
- Lymphangitis
- Location (most commonly unilateral; bilateral presentation should prompt consideration of alternative diagnosis)
  - Lower extremity 70–80% of cases
  - Face involvement is less common (5–20%), especially nose and ears.
  - Chronic form usually recurs at site of the previous infection and may recur years after initial episode.
- Patients on systemic steroids may be more difficult to diagnose because signs and symptoms of the infection may be masked by anti-inflammatory action of the steroids.
- Systemic toxicity resolves rapidly with treatment; skin lesions desquamate on days 5 to 10 but usually heal without scarring.
- In geriatric patients, facial involvement presents in a butterfly pattern. Pustules characteristically absent and regional lymphadenopathy with lymphangitic streaking is seen.

Pediatric Considerations
- Abdominal involvement is more common in infants, especially around umbilical stump.
- Face, scalp, and leg involvement are common in older children due to the excoriations when scratching in atopic dermatitis, allowing an easy port of entry.

Geriatric Considerations
- Fever may not be as prominent.
- 80% of cases affect the lower extremities. The rest are usually on the face.
- High-output cardiac failure may occur in debilitated patients with underlying cardiac disease.
- More susceptible to complications

DIFFERENTIAL DIAGNOSIS
- Cellulitis (Margins are less clear and do not involve ear.)
- Necrotizing fasciitis (systemic illness and more pain)
- Skin abscess (feel for area of fluctuance)
- DVT (needs to rule out if clinically suspected)
- Acute gout (Check patient history.)
- Insect bite (Check patient history.)
- Dermatophytes
- Impetigo (blistered/crusted appearance; superficial)
- Ecthyma (ulcerative impetigo)
- Herpes zoster (dermatomal distribution)
- Erythema annulare centrifugum (raised pink-red ring/bull's-eye marks)
- Contact dermatitis (no fever, pruritic, not painful)
- Giant cell urticaria (transient, wheal appearance, severe itching)
- Angioneurotic edema (no fever)
- Scarlet fever (widespread rash with indistinct borders and without edema; rash is most common early in skin folds; develops generalized "sandpaper" feeling as it progresses)
- Toxic shock syndrome (diffuse erythema with evidence of multiorgan involvement)
- Lupus (of the face; less fever, positive antinuclear antibodies)
- Polychondritis (common site is the ear)
- Other bacterial infections to consider:
  - Meat, shellfish, fish, and poultry workers: *Erysipelothrix rhusiopathiae* (known as erysipeloid)
  - Human bite: *Eikenella corrodens*
  - Cat/dog bite: *Pasteurella multocida/Capnocytophaga canimorsus*
  - Salt water exposure: *Vibrio vulnificus*
  - Fresh/brackish water exposure: *Aeromonas hydrophila*

DIAGNOSTIC TESTS & INTERPRETATION
Reserve diagnostic tests for severely ill, toxic patients, patients who failed initial antibiotic therapy, or those who are immunosuppressed.

Initial Tests (lab, imaging)
- Leukocytosis
- Blood culture (<5% positive)
- Elevated erythrocyte sedimentation rate (ESR) and C-reactive protein (CRP)
- Streptococci may be cultured from exudate/noninvolved sites.

Test Interpretation

Biopsy is not needed; however, skin findings would show

- Dermal and epidermal edema, extending into the SC tissues
- Peau d'orange appearance caused by edema in the superficial tissue surrounding the hair follicles
- Vasodilation and enlarged lymphatics
- Mixed interstitial infiltrate mainly consisting of neutrophils and mononuclear cells
- Endothelial cell swelling
- Gram-positive cocci in lymphatics and tissue with rare invasion of local blood vessels
- Fibrotic thickening of lymphatic vessel walls with possible luminal occlusion may be seen in recurrent erysipelas.

 TREATMENT

GENERAL MEASURES

- Symptomatic treatment of myalgias and fever
- Adequate fluid intake
- Local treatment with cold compresses
- Elevation of affected extremity
- Appropriate therapy for any underlying predisposing condition

MEDICATION

- Antibiotics cure 50–100% of infections, but which regimen is most successful is unclear.
- Antibiotics may be as effective when given orally versus intravenously.
- A 5-day course of antibiotics may be as effective as a 10-day course at curing (4)[A].

First Line

- Adults
  - Extremities, nondiabetic
    - Primary
      - Penicillin G: 1 to 2 million U IV q6h *or* cefazolin 1 g IV q8h
    - Alternative (if penicillin allergic)
      - Vancomycin 15 mg/kg IV q12h
      - When afebrile, penicillin VK 500 mg PO QID AC and HS
  - Total 10 days, diabetics
    - Early mild:
      - Trimethoprim-sulfamethoxazole (TMP-SMX)-DS: 1 to 2 tabs PO BID and penicillin VK 500 mg PO QID *or* cephalexin 500 mg PO QID
    - Severe disease
      - MP or MER or ERTA IV and linezolid 600 mg IV/PO BID *or* vancomycin IV or daptomycin 4 mg/kg IV q24h
  - Facial
    - Primary
      - Vancomycin: 15 mg/kg (actual weight) IV q8–12h with target trough 15 to 20
    - Alternative
      - Daptomycin 4 mg/kg IV q24h or linezolid 600 mg IV q12h
- Children
  - Penicillin G
    - 0 to 7 days, <2,000 g = 50,000 U/kg q12h
    - 8 to 28 days, <2,000 g = 75,000 U/kg q8h

  - 0 to 7 days, >2,000 g = 50,000 U/kg q8h
  - 8 to 28 days, >2,000 g = 50,000 U/kg q6h
  - >28 days = 50,000 U/kg/day
  - Cefazolin
    - 0 to 7 days, <2,000 g = 25 mg/kg q12h
    - 8 to 28 days, <2,000 g = 25 mg/kg q12h
    - 0 to 7 days, >2,000 g = 25 mg/kg q12h
    - 8 to 28 days, >2,000 g = 25 mg/kg q8h
    - >28 days = 25 mg/kg q8h
- No reported group A streptococci resistance to β-lactam antibiotics
- In chronic recurrent infections, prophylactic treatment after the acute infection resolves:
  - Penicillin G benzathine: 1.2 million U IM q4wk *or* penicillin VK 500 mg PO BID or azithromycin 250 mg PO QD
- If staphylococcal infection is suspected or if patient is acutely ill, consider a β–lactamase-stable antibiotic.
- Consider community-acquired MRSA, and depending on regional sensitivity, may treat MRSA with TMP-SMX DS 1 tab PO BID *or* vancomycin 1 g IV q12h *or* doxycycline 100 mg PO BID.

ISSUES FOR REFERRAL

Recurrent infection, treatment failure

ADDITIONAL THERAPIES

Some patients may notice a deepening of erythema after initiating antimicrobial therapy. This may be due to the destruction of pathogens that release enzymes, increasing local inflammation. In this case, treatment with corticosteroids, in addition to antimicrobials, can mildly reduce healing time and antibiotic duration in patients with erysipelas. Consider prednisolone 30 mg/day with taper over 8 days.

ADMISSION, INPATIENT, AND NURSING CONSIDERATIONS

- Admission criteria/initial stabilization
  - Patient with systemic toxicity
  - Patient with high-risk factors (e.g., elderly, lymphedema, postsplenectomy, diabetes)
  - Failed outpatient care
- IV therapy if systemic toxicity/unable to tolerate PO
- Discharge criteria: no evidence of systemic toxicity with resolution of erythema and swelling

 ONGOING CARE

FOLLOW-UP RECOMMENDATIONS

Bed rest with elevation of extremity during acute infection and then activity as tolerated

Patient Monitoring

Patients should be treated until all symptoms and skin manifestations have resolved.

PATIENT EDUCATION

Stress importance of completing prescribed medication regimen.

PROGNOSIS

- Patients should recover fully if adequately treated.
- May experience deepening of erythema after initiation of antibiotics
- Most respond to therapy after 24 to 48 hours.

- Mortality is <1% in patients receiving appropriate treatment.
- Bullae formation suggests longer disease course and often indicates a concomitant *S. aureus* infection that may require antibiotic coverage for MRSA.
- Chronic edema/scarring may result from chronic recurrent cases.
- Rarely, obstructive lymphadenitis may result from chronic recurrent cases.

COMPLICATIONS

- Recurrent infection
- Abscess (suggests staphylococcal infection)
- Necrotizing fasciitis
- Lymphedema (most prominent risk factor for recurrence) (5)
- Bacteremia, which may lead to sepsis
- Pneumonia (due to sepsis/toxin-producing organism)
- Meningitis (due to sepsis/toxin-producing organism)
- Embolism
- Gangrene
- Bursitis, septic arthritis, tendinitis, or osteitis

REFERENCES

1. Gabillot-Carré M, Roujeau JC. Acute bacterial skin infections and cellulitis. *Curr Opin Infect Dis*. 2007;20(2):118–123.
2. Celestin R, Brown J, Kihiczak G, et al. Erysipelas: a common potentially dangerous infection. *Acta Dermatovenerol Alp Pannonica Adriat*. 2007;16(3):123–127.
3. Breen JO. Skin and soft tissue infections in immunocompetent patients. *Am Fam Physician*. 2010;81(7):893–899.
4. Morris AD. Cellulitis and erysipelas. *BMJ Clin Evid*. 2008;2008:1708.
5. Inghammar M, Rasmussen M, Linder A. Recurrent erysipelas—risk factors and clinical presentation. *BMC Infect Dis*. 2014;14:270.

ADDITIONAL READING

Gilbert D, Chambers HF, Eliopoulos GM, et al, eds. *The Sanford Guide to Antimicrobial Therapy*. 44th ed. Sperryville, VA: Antimicrobial Therapy; 2014.

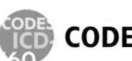 CODES

ICD10
A46 Erysipelas

CLINICAL PEARLS

- Athlete's foot is the most common portal of entry.
- Erysipelas is distinguished from cellulitis by its sharp, shiny, fiery-red, raised border.
- In recurrent cases, search for other possible source of streptococcal infection (e.g., tonsils, sinuses, intertrigo).
- Most erysipelas infections now occur on the legs, rather than the face.

E

ERYTHEMA MULTIFORME

Losika Sivaganeshan, MD, MPH • Pradeepa P. Vimalachandran, MD, MPH

BASICS

- Erythema multiforme (EM) is relatively common, acute, recurrent, self-limiting inflammatory disease.
  - Mostly (~90% of cases) triggered by infectious agents (up to 50% by herpes simplex virus [HSV]-1 or -2), or less commonly, by drugs and vaccinations (1,2)
  - Skin lesions include acrally distributed, distinct targetoid lesions with concentric color variation, sometimes accompanied by oral, genital, or ocular mucosal lesions (1,3).
  - Flat, atypical lesions and macules with or without blisters are more suggestive of Stevens-Johnson syndrome (SJS) or toxic epidermal necrolysis (TEN) (4,5).
- There are no universal diagnostic criteria, but clinical history, clinical examination, skin biopsy, laboratory studies, and special consideration of persistent EM are all included in making a diagnosis.

DESCRIPTION
- Two subtypes, erythema multiforme minor (EMm) and erythema multiforme major (EMM), with the former involving none or one mucous membrane and the latter involving at least two mucous membrane sites. EMM is now separate from SJS and TEN.
- Recurrent EM is defined as >3 attacks but has a mean number of 6 attacks (range 2 to 24) per year and a mean duration of 6 to 9.5 years (range 2 to 36) (1).

EPIDEMIOLOGY
Incidence
Annual U.S. incidence is estimated at <1% (1).

Prevalence
- Peak incidence in 20s to 40s; rare <3 years and >50 years of age
- Slight male predominance is observed.

ETIOLOGY AND PATHOPHYSIOLOGY
- The exact pathophysiology of EM is incompletely understood but appears to be the result of a TH1-mediated immune response to an inciting event such as infection or drug exposure.
- Genetic susceptibility can be a predisposing factor in some patients with EM. Different HLA alleles have been found to be consistent in patients with EM.
- HSV containing a certain *HSV pol*, a polymerase associated with the HSV-triggered EM seems to involve autoimmune activation and a cell-mediated response (1).
- With electron microscopy, there is evidence of lichenoid inflammatory infiltrate and epidermal necrosis including circulating immune complexes, deposition of C3, IgM, and fibrin around the upper dermal blood vessels.
- SJS and TEN have an increased granulysin and perforin expression within T cells than in EM (4,5).
- Previous viral infections, particularly; also Epstein-Barr, coxsackievirus, echovirus, varicella, mumps, poliovirus, hepatitis C, cytomegalovirus, HIV, molluscum contagiosum virus (1)

- Bacterial infections, particularly *Mycoplasma pneumoniae*; other reported bacterial infections include *Treponema pallidum*, *Mycobacterium tuberculosis*, and *Gardnerella vaginalis* (1).
- Medications, including NSAIDs, antibiotics, penicillin, sulfonamides, and antiepileptics (1,3)
- Vaccines: stronger association with HPV, MMR, and small pox vaccines, but also associated with hepatitis B, meningococcal, pneumococcal, varicella, influenza, diphtheria-pertussis-tetanus, and *Haemophilus influenzae* (2)
- Occupational exposures: herbicides (alachlor and butachlor), iodoacetonitrile
- Radiation therapy
- Premenstrual hormone changes (3)
- Malignancy (3)

Genetics
Strong association with HLA-DQB10301, particularly in herpes-related cases (1); possible association in recurrent cases with HLA-B35, -B62, -DR53

RISK FACTORS
Previous history of EM

GENERAL PREVENTION
- Known or suspected etiologic agents should be avoided.
- Acyclovir or valacyclovir may help prevent herpes-related recurrent EM.

COMMONLY ASSOCIATED CONDITIONS
See "Etiology and Pathophysiology" earlier.

DIAGNOSIS

Clinical

HISTORY
- Absent or mild prodromal symptoms
- Acute, self-limiting episodic course
- History of new medication
- Preceding HSV infection 10 to 15 days before the skin eruptions
- Rash involving the skin and sometimes the mucous membrane, most commonly the mouth
- Symptoms of any of the infections associated with EM, most commonly HSV and *M. pneumoniae*

PHYSICAL EXAM
- Acral extremities
- Symmetric cutaneous eruptions composed of targetoid lesions with concentric color variation
- Mucosal involvement
  - Oral involvement manifests as erythema, erosions, bullae, and ulcerations on both nonkeratinized and keratinized mucosal surfaces and on the vermilion of the lips; minimal involvement in EMm, if present, most commonly involves the mouth.
  - Can include any mucosal tissue including genital, ocular, oral, and so forth
  - At least two mucosal sites involved in EMM, including eyes (conjunctivitis, keratitis); mouth (stomatitis, cheilitis, characteristic blood-stained crusted erosions on lips); and probable trachea, bronchi, GI tract, or genital tract (balanitis and vulvitis) (5)

DIFFERENTIAL DIAGNOSIS
- SJS
  - Generalized distribution of lesions; concentrated on the trunk
  - Macular atypical targetoid lesions
  - Flat target lesions or macules with coalescence of lesions
  - Blisters and skin detachment <10% of the total body surface area (5)
  - 1–5% mortality
  - Presence of constitutional symptoms with presence of high fever (>38.5°C) more likely with SJS than EM
  - More likely to have mucosal involvement at ≥2 sites, lymphadenopathy, high C-reactive protein levels (>10 mg/dL), and hepatic dysfunction and >90% have severe mucosal involvement at least at one site (1)
- TEN
  - Similar to SJS but has full-thickness skin necrosis and skin detachment >30% of the total body surface area (5,6)
  - 34–40% mortality rate
- Urticaria
- Fixed drug eruption
- Bullous pemphigoid
- Paraneoplastic pemphigoid
- Sweet syndrome
- Rowell syndrome
- Polymorphous light eruption
- Cutaneous small-vessel vasculitis
- Mucocutaneous lymph node syndrome
- Erythema annulare centrifugum
- Acute hemorrhagic edema of infancy
- Subacute cutaneous lupus erythematosus
- Contact dermatitis
- Pityriasis rosea
- HSV
- Secondary syphilis
- Tinea corporis
- Dermatitis herpetiformis
- Herpes gestationis
- Septicemia
- Serum sickness
- Viral exanthem
- Rocky Mountain spotted fever
- Meningococcemia
- Lichen planus
- Behçet syndrome
- Recurrent aphthous ulcers
- Herpetic gingivostomatitis
- Granuloma annulare

DIAGNOSTIC TESTS & INTERPRETATION
- No lab test is indicated to make the diagnosis of EM (1).
- Skin biopsy of lesional and perilesional tissue in equivocal conditions
- Direct and indirect immunofluorescence (DIF and IIF) to differentiate EM from other vesiculobullous diseases. DIF is detected on a biopsy of perilesional skin, and IIF is detected from a blood sample (1).

- HSV tests in recurrent EM (serologic tests, swab culture, or tests using skin biopsy sample to check HSV antigens or DNA in keratinocytes by DIF or direct fluorescent antibody [DFA] or polymerase chain reaction [PCR])
- Antibody staining to IFN-γ and TNF-α to differentiate HSV from drug-associated EM
- As the second most common cause of EM, *M. pneumoniae* should be worked up with chest x-ray, swabs, and serologic test.
- In persistent EM, check complement levels (1).

Initial Tests (lab, imaging)
No imaging studies are indicated in most cases unless there is suspicion for *M. pneumoniae*.

Follow-Up Tests & Special Considerations
Chest x-ray may be necessary if an underlying pulmonary infection (*M. pneumoniae*) is suspected.

Test Interpretation
- Vacuolar interface dermatitis with CD4$^+$ T lymphocytes and histiocytes in papillary dermis and the dermal–epidermal junction
- Superficial perivascular lymphocytic inflammation
- Satellite cell necrosis
- Necrotic keratinocytes mainly in the basal layer
- Papillary dermal edema

TREATMENT

GENERAL MEASURES
- Step 1: Discontinue or treat inciting factor (1).
- Wound care for severe cases with epidermal detachment
- Oral lesions should be addressed to insure maintenance of PO intake. This can include oral anesthetic solutions and antiseptic rinses.

MEDICATION
- Acute EM
  - Discontinuation of inciting factors and treatment of underlying disease (1)[B]
  - Symptomatic treatment with oral antihistamines and topical (1)[B]
  - HSV-induced EM: Most recent sources report no proven effect on the course of EM using antivirals with acute mild EM (1)[B].
  - *M. pneumoniae*–associated EM may require antibiotics.
- Mucosal membrane EM
  - Consider high-potency topical corticosteroid gel, oral antiseptic, and oral anesthetic solutions if mild.
  - If more severe, consider prednisone 40 to 60 mg/day with dosage tapered over 2 to 4 weeks (1)[B].
  - Ophthalmology consultation is imperative for ocular involvement.

- Recurrent EM
  - First-line treatment with HSV-associated and idiopathic recurrent EM is antiviral prophylaxis; 12 to 24 months of prophylaxis is most effective (1)[B].
  - Therapy includes acyclovir 400 mg BID, valacyclovir 500 mg BID, famciclovir 250 mg BID (1)[B].
  - Second-line therapy includes dapsone (100 to 150 mg/day), azathioprine (Imuran, 100 to 150 mg/day), thalidomide (100 to 200 mg/day), tacrolimus (0.1% ointment daily), mycophenolate mofetil (CellCept, 1,000 to 1,500 mg BID), hydroxychloroquine (400 mg/day) (1)[B].

ADMISSION, INPATIENT, AND NURSING CONSIDERATIONS
- Care at home
- Hospitalization needed for fluid and electrolyte management in patient with severe mucous membrane involvement, impaired oral intake, and dehydration
- IV antibiotics if secondary infection develops

ONGOING CARE

FOLLOW-UP RECOMMENDATIONS
Patient Monitoring
- The disease is self-limiting.
- Complications are rare, with no mortality.

DIET
As tolerated, with increased fluid intake

PATIENT EDUCATION
- The disease is self-limiting. However, the recurrence risk may be 30%.
- Avoid any identified etiologic agents.

PROGNOSIS
- Rash evolves over 1 to 2 weeks and subsequently resolves within 2 to 6 weeks, generally without scarring or sequelae.
- Following resolution, there may be some postinflammatory hyper- or hypopigmentation.

COMPLICATIONS
Secondary infection

REFERENCES

1. Sokumbi O, Wetter DA. Clinical features, diagnosis, and treatment of erythema multiforme: a review for the practicing dermatologist. *Int J Dermatol*. 2012;51(8):889–902.
2. Rosenblatt AE, Stein SL. Cutaneous reactions to vaccinations. *Clin Dermatol*. 2015;33(3):327–332.
3. Levin J, Hofstra T. Recurrent erythema multiforme. *JAMA*. 2014;312(4):426–427.
4. Iwai S, Sueki H, Watanabe H, et al. Distinguishing between erythema multiforme major and Stevens-Johnson syndrome/toxic epidermal necrolysis immunopathologically. *J Dermatol*. 2012;39(9):781–786.
5. Schwartz RA, McDonough PH, Lee BW. Toxic epidermal necrolysis: part I. Introduction, history, classification, clinical features, systemic manifestations, etiology, and immunopathogenesis. *J Am Acad Dermatol*. 2013;69(2):173.e1–173.e13, quiz 185–186.
6. Schwartz RA, McDonough PH, Lee BW. Toxic epidermal necrolysis: part II. Prognosis, sequelae, diagnosis, differential diagnosis, prevention, and treatment. *J Am Acad Dermatol*. 2013;69(2):187.e1–187.e16, quiz 203–204.

ADDITIONAL READING

- Sola CA, Beute TC. Erythema multiforme. *J Spec Oper Med*. 2014;14(3):90–92.
- Wetter DA, Davis MD. Recurrent erythema multiforme: clinical characteristics, etiologic associations, and treatment in a series of 48 patients at Mayo Clinic, 2000 to 2007. *J Am Acad Dermatol*. 2010;62(1):45–53.

 SEE ALSO

Cutaneous Drug Reactions; Dermatitis Herpetiformis; Pemphigoid Gestationis; Stevens-Johnson Syndrome; Toxic Epidermal Necrolysis; Urticaria

 CODES

ICD10
- L51.9 Erythema multiforme, unspecified
- L51.8 Other erythema multiforme
- L51.0 Nonbullous erythema multiforme

CLINICAL PEARLS

- EM is diagnosed clinically by careful review of the history, thorough detailed physical exam, and by excluding other similar disorders. No lab tests are required for the diagnosis.
- Typical lesions are characteristic targetoid or "iris" lesions but can include raised targetoids.
- Lesions are symmetrically distributed on palms, soles, dorsum of the hands, and extensor surfaces of extremities and face. The oral mucosa is the most affected mucosal region in EM.
- Management of EM involves determining the etiology when possible. The first step is to treat the suspected infection or discontinue the causative drug.
- Complications are rare. Most cases are self-limited. However, the recurrence risk may be as high as 30%.
- Recurrent cases often are secondary to HSV infection. Antiviral therapy may be beneficial.

ERYTHEMA NODOSUM

Lolwa Al-Obaid, MD • Faruq Pradhan, MD • Fredric D. Gordon, MD

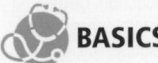 **BASICS**

DESCRIPTION

- A delayed-type hypersensitivity reaction to various antigens, or an autoimmune reaction presenting as a panniculitis (1) that affects subcutaneous fat
- Clinical pattern of multiple, bilateral, erythematous, tender nodules in a typically pretibial distribution that undergo a characteristic pattern of color changes, similar to that seen in bruises. Unlike erythema induratum, the lesions of erythema nodosum (EN) do not typically ulcerate.
- Occurs most commonly on the shins; less commonly on the thighs, forearms, trunk, head, or neck
- Often associated with nonspecific prodrome including fever, weight loss, and arthralgia
- Often idiopathic but may be associated with a number of clinical entities
- Usually remits spontaneously in weeks to months without scarring, atrophy, or ulceration
- Uncommon to have recurrences after initial presentation

Pregnancy Considerations
May have repeat outbreaks during pregnancy

Pediatric Considerations
Rare pediatric variant has lesions only on palms or soles, often unilateral; typically has a shorter duration in children than adults

EPIDEMIOLOGY

Incidence
- 1 to 5/100,000/year
- Predominant age: 20 to 30 years
- Predominant sex: female > male (6:1) in adults

Prevalence
- Varies geographically depending on the prevalence of disorders associated with EN
- Reported 1 to 5/100,000

ETIOLOGY AND PATHOPHYSIOLOGY

- Idiopathic: up to 55%
- Infectious: 44%. Streptococcal pharyngitis (most common), mycobacteria, mycoplasma, chlamydia, mycoplasma, coccidioidomycosis, rarely can be caused by *Campylobacter* spp., rickettsiae, *Salmonella* spp., psittacosis, syphilis

- Sarcoidosis: 11–25%
- Drugs: 3–10%; sulfonamides amoxicillin, oral contraceptives, bromides, azathioprine, vemurafenib
- Pregnancy: 2–5%
- Enteropathies: 1–4%; ulcerative colitis, Crohn disease, Behçet disease, celiac disease, diverticulitis
- Rare causes: <1% (2)
  - Fungal: dermatophytes, coccidioidomycosis, histoplasmosis, blastomycosis
  - Viral/chlamydial: infectious mononucleosis, lymphogranuloma venereum, paravaccinia, HIV, hepatitis B, C
  - Malignancies: lymphoma/leukemia, sarcoma, myelodysplastic syndrome
  - Sweet syndrome

RISK FACTORS
See "Etiology and Pathophysiology."

COMMONLY ASSOCIATED CONDITIONS
See "Etiology and Pathophysiology."

 **DIAGNOSIS**

HISTORY
- Often a prodrome 1 to 3 weeks prior to onset of lesions; can consist of malaise, fever, weight loss, cough, and arthralgia
- Increasingly tender nodules on the legs, usually over the shins
- Fever, malaise, chills, fatigue
- Headache
- Can precede systemic process by weeks

PHYSICAL EXAM
- Lesions initially present as warm, tender, erythematous firm nodules and become fluctuant, gradually fading to resemble a bruise over 1 to 2 months (erythema contusiformis).
- Typically pretibial, although can extend proximally to involve thighs or trunk (atypically can involve extensor surface of forearms)
- Diameter varies from 1 to 10 cm with poor demarcation.

DIFFERENTIAL DIAGNOSIS
- Nodular vasculitis or erythema induratum (warm ulcerating calf nodules)
- Superficial thrombophlebitis
- Cellulitis
- Weber-Christian disease (violaceous, scarring nodules)
- Lupus panniculitis
- Cutaneous polyarteritis nodosa
- Sarcoidal granulomas
- Cutaneous T-cell lymphoma
- EN leprosum (clinically similar to EN but shows vasculitis on histopathology)
- Subcutaneous infection (including *Staphylococcus*, *Sporothrix schenckii*, *Nocardia brasiliensis*, *Mycobacterium marinum*, *Leishmania braziliensis*)

DIAGNOSTIC TESTS & INTERPRETATION
Diagnosis is made clinically, with support of testing.

- ESR or C-reactive protein (CRP): often elevated, but can be normal in up to 40% (3)[C]
- CBC: mild leukocytosis (3)
- Urine pregnancy test (3)
- Throat culture, antistreptolysin O titer (3)
- Blood and/or stool culture, stool ova and parasites (O&P)
- Tuberculin skin testing (3)
- Seronegative rheumatoid factor

Initial Tests (lab, imaging)
CXR for hilar adenopathy or infiltrates related to sarcoidosis or tuberculosis (3)[C]

Diagnostic Procedures/Other
Deep-incisional or excisional skin biopsy including subcutaneous tissue; rarely necessary except in atypical cases with ulceration, duration >12 weeks, or absence of nodules overlying lower limbs (4)[C]

Test Interpretation
- Septal panniculitis without vasculitis
- Neutrophilic infiltrate in septa of fat tissue early in course
- Actinic radial (Miescher) granulomas, consisting of collections of histiocytes around a central stellate cleft, may be seen.
- Fibrosis, paraseptal granulation tissue, lymphocytes, and multinucleated giant cells predominate late in course (5).

TREATMENT

- Condition usually self-limited within 1 to 2 months
- All medications listed as treatment for EN are off-label uses of the medications. There are no specific FDA-approved medications.

GENERAL MEASURES
- Mild compression bandages and leg elevation may reduce pain (wet dressings, hot soaks, and topical medications are not useful).
- Discontinue potentially causative drugs.
- If specific cause is identified, treatment of the condition typically leads to resolution of EN.
- Indication for treatment is poorly defined in literature; hence, therapy specifically for EN is directed toward symptom management.

MEDICATION
First Line
- NSAIDs:
  – Ibuprofen 400 mg PO q4–6h (not to exceed 3,200 mg/day)
  – Indomethacin 25 to 50 mg PO TID
  – Naproxen 250 to 500 mg PO BID
- Precautions
  – GI upset/bleeding (avoid in Crohn or ulcerative colitis)
  – Fluid retention
  – Renal insufficiency
  – Dose reduction in elderly, especially those with renal disease, diabetes, or heart failure
  – May mask fever
  – NSAIDs can increase cardiovascular (CV) risk.
- Significant possible interactions
  – May blunt antihypertensive effects of diuretics and β-blockers
  – NSAIDs can elevate plasma lithium levels.
  – NSAIDs can cause significant elevation and prolongation of methotrexate levels.

Second Line
- Potassium iodide 400 to 900 mg/day divided BID or TID for 3 to 4 weeks (for persistent lesions); need to monitor for hyperthyroidism with prolonged use; pregnancy class D (6)[B]
- Corticosteroids for severe, refractory, or recurrent cases in which an infectious workup is negative. Prednisone 1 mg/kg/day for 1 to 2 weeks is the recommended dose/duration. Potential side effects include hyperglycemia, hypertension, weight gain, worsening gastroesophageal reflux disease, mood changes, bone loss, osteonecrosis, and proximal myopathy (2).

- For EN related to Behçet disease, one can also consider colchicine 0.6 to 1.2 mg BID. Potential side effects include GI upset and diarrhea (7)[B].

ADMISSION, INPATIENT, AND NURSING CONSIDERATIONS
Occasionally, admission may be needed for the antecedent illness (e.g., tuberculosis).

 ONGOING CARE

FOLLOW-UP RECOMMENDATIONS
- Keep legs elevated.
- Elastic wraps or support stockings may be helpful when patients are ambulating.

Patient Monitoring
Monthly follow-up or as dictated by underlying disorder

DIET
No restrictions

PATIENT EDUCATION
- Lesions will resolve over a few weeks to months.
- Scarring is unlikely.
- Joint aches and pains may persist.
- <20% recur.

PROGNOSIS
- Individual lesions resolve generally within 2 weeks.
- Total time course of 6 to 12 weeks but may vary with underlying disease
- Joint aches and pains may persist for years.
- Lesions do not scar.
- Recurrences: occurs over variable periods, averaging several years; seen most often in sarcoid, streptococcal infection, pregnancy, and oral contraceptive use. If medication induced, avoid recurrent exposure.

COMPLICATIONS
- Vary according to underlying disease
- None expected from lesions of EN

REFERENCES
1. Chowaniec M, Starba A, Wiland P. Erythema nodosum—review of the literature. *Reumatologia*. 2016;54(2):79–82.
2. Schwartz RA, Nervi SJ. Erythema nodosum: a sign of systemic disease. *Am Fam Physician*. 2007;75(5):695–700.
3. Cribier B, Caille A, Heid E, et al. Erythema nodosum and associated diseases. A study of 129 cases. *Int J Dermatol*. 1998;37(9):667–672.
4. Requena L, Yus ES. Erythema nodosum. *Dermatol Clin*. 2008;26(4):425–438.
5. Sánchez Yus E, Sanz Vico MD, de Diego V. Miescher's radial granuloma. A characteristic marker of erythema nodosum. *Am J Dermatopathol*. 1989;11(5): 434–442.
6. Horio T, Imamura S, Danno K, et al. Potassium iodide in the treatment of erythema nodosum and nodular vasculitis. *Arch Dermatol*. 1981;117(1): 29–31.
7. Yurdakul S, Mat C, Tüzün Y, et al. A double-blind trial of colchicine in Behçet's syndrome. *Arthritis Rheum*. 2001;44(11):2686–2692.

ADDITIONAL READING
- Bartyik K, Várkonyi A, Kirschner A, et al. Erythema nodosum in association with celiac disease. *Pediatr Dermatol*. 2004;21(3):227–230.
- Chong TA, Hansra NK, Ruben BS, et al. Diverticulitis: an inciting factor in erythema nodosum. *J Am Acad Dermatol*. 2012;67(1):e60–e62.
- Harris T, Henderson MC. Concurrent Sweet's syndrome and erythema nodosum. *J Gen Intern Med*. 2011;26(2):214–215.
- Jeon HC, Choi M, Paik SH, et al. A case of assisted reproductive therapy-induced erythema nodosum. *Ann Dermatol*. 2011;23(3):362–364.
- Then C, Langer A, Adam C, et al. Erythema nodosum associated with myelodysplastic syndrome: a case report. *Onkologie*. 2011;34(3):126–128.

 CODES

ICD10
- L52 Erythema nodosum
- A18.4 Tuberculosis of skin and subcutaneous tissue

CLINICAL PEARLS
- Lesions of EN appear to be erythematous patches, but when palpated, their underlying nodularity is appreciated.
- Evaluation for a concerning underlying etiology is necessary in EN, but most cases are idiopathic.
- EN in the setting of hilar adenopathy may be seen with multiple etiologies and does not exclusively indicate sarcoidosis.
- In patients with a history of Hodgkin lymphoma, EN may be an early sign of recurrence.

E

ESOPHAGEAL VARICES

Maximos Attia, MD, FAAFP • Marcelle Meseeha, MD

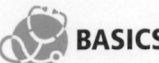 **BASICS**

DESCRIPTION
- Dilated submucosal esophageal veins connecting the portal and systemic circulations
- Most commonly results from portal hypertension (typically a result of cirrhosis)
- Variceal rupture: most common fatal complication of cirrhosis; severity of liver disease correlates with presence of varices and risk of bleeding.

EPIDEMIOLOGY
Incidence
- 30% of cirrhotic patients have varices at the time of diagnosis. This increases to 90% at 10 years.
- 1-year rate of first variceal bleeding is 5% for small varices, 15% for large varices.

Pediatric Considerations
Portal hypertension is common in chronic liver disease (CLD) in children. No clear guidelines for screening; pharmacologic or endoscopic treatment is equivalent.

Prevalence
- 50% of patients with esophageal varices experience bleeding at some point.
- Variceal bleeding: 10–20% mortality in the 6 weeks following the episode
- Gender: male > female

ETIOLOGY AND PATHOPHYSIOLOGY
- Portal hypertension causes the formation of portacaval anastomoses to decompress the portal circulation. This leads to a congested submucosal venous plexus with tortuous dilated veins, particularly in the distal esophagus. Variceal rupture results in hemorrhage.
- Pathophysiology of portal hypertension:
  - Increased resistance to portal flow at the level of hepatic sinusoids caused by
    - Intrahepatic vasoconstriction due to decreased nitric oxide production and increased release of endothelin-1 (ET-1), angiotensinogen, and eicosanoids
    - Sinusoidal remodeling causes disruption of blood flow.
  - Increased portal flow caused by hyperdynamic circulation due to splanchnic arterial vasodilation through mediators such as nitric oxide, prostacyclin, and TNF
- Causes of portal hypertension:
  - Prehepatic:
    - Extrahepatic portal vein obstruction (EHPVO)
    - Massive splenomegaly with increased splenic vein blood flow
  - Posthepatic:
    - Severe right-sided heart failure, constrictive pericarditis, and hepatic vein obstruction (Budd-Chiari syndrome)
  - Intrahepatic:
    - Cirrhosis (accounts for most cases of portal hypertension)
  - Less frequent causes are schistosomiasis, massive fatty change, diseases affecting portal microcirculation as nodular regenerative hyperplasia, and diffuse fibrosing granulomatous disease as sarcoidosis.

Genetics
Cirrhosis is rarely hereditary.

RISK FACTORS
- Cirrhosis
- In cirrhotic patients, thrombocytopenia and splenomegaly are independent predictors of esophageal varices.
- Noncirrhotic portal hypertension
- Increased bleeding risk for known varices is associated with varix size, endoscopic signs (red wale marks, cherry-red spots), vessel wall thickness, and abrupt increase in variceal pressure (i.e., Valsalva maneuver).
- MELD/Child-Pugh score; presence of portal vein thrombosis; high hepatic venous pressure gradient (HVPG)

GENERAL PREVENTION
Prevent underlying causes: Prevent alcohol abuse, administer hepatitis B vaccine, needle hygiene, IV drug use (needle exchange programs reduce risk of hepatitis); specific screening and therapy for hepatitis B and C, hemochromatosis

COMMONLY ASSOCIATED CONDITIONS
- Portal hypertensive gastropathy; varices in stomach, duodenum, colon, rectum (causes massive bleeding, unlike hemorrhoids); rarely at umbilicus (caput medusae) or ostomy sites
- Isolated gastric varices can occur due to splenic vein thrombosis/stenosis from hypercoagulability/contiguous inflammation (most commonly, chronic pancreatitis).
- Other complications of cirrhosis: hepatic encephalopathy, ascites, hepatorenal syndrome, spontaneous bacterial peritonitis, hepatocellular carcinoma

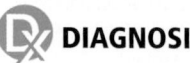 **DIAGNOSIS**

- First indication of varices is often GI bleeding: hematemesis, hematochezia, and/or melena.
- Occult bleeding (anemia): uncommon

HISTORY
- Underlying history of cirrhosis/liver disease. Variceal bleed can be initial presentation of previously undiagnosed cirrhosis.
- Alcohol abuse, exposure to blood-borne viruses through intravenous drug use or sexual practices
- Hematemesis, melena, or hematochezia
- Rapid upper GI bleed can present as rectal bleeding.

PHYSICAL EXAM
- Assess hemodynamic stability: hypotension, tachycardia (active bleeding)
- Abdominal exam—liver palpation/percussion (often small and firm with cirrhosis)
- Splenomegaly, ascites (shifting dullness; fluid shift; puddle splash—physical maneuvers have limited sensitivity)
- Visible abdominal periumbilical collateral circulation (caput medusae)
- Peripheral stigmata of alcohol abuse: spider angiomata on chest/back, palmar erythema, testicular atrophy, gynecomastia
- Rectal varices
- Hepatic encephalopathy; asterixis
- Blood on rectal exam

DIFFERENTIAL DIAGNOSIS
- Upper GI bleeding: 10–30% are due to varices.
  - In patients with known varices, as many as 50% bleed from nonvariceal sources.
  - Peptic ulcer; gastritis

- Gastric/esophageal malignancy
- Congestive gastropathy of portal hypertension
- Arteriovenous malformation
- Mallory-Weiss tears
- Aortoenteric fistula
- Hemoptysis; nosebleed
- Lower GI bleeding
  - Rectal varices; hemorrhoids
  - Colonic neoplasia
  - Diverticulosis/arteriovenous malformation
  - Rapidly bleeding upper GI site
- Continued/recurrent bleeding risk: actively bleeding/large varix, high Child-Pugh severity score, infection, renal failure

DIAGNOSTIC TESTS & INTERPRETATION
Initial Tests (lab, imaging)
- Anemia: Hemoglobin may be normal in active bleeding; may require 6 to 24 hours to equilibrate; other causes of anemia are common in patients with cirrhosis.
- Thrombocytopenia: most sensitive and specific parameter, correlates with portal hypertension, large esophageal varices
- Abnormal aspartate aminotransferase (AST), alanine aminotransferase (ALT), alkaline phosphatase, bilirubin; prolonged PT; low albumin suggests cirrhosis.
- BUN, creatinine (BUN often elevated in GI bleed)
- Sodium level; may drop in patients treated with terlipressin (1)[A]
- Esophagogastroduodenoscopy (1)[A]
  - Can identify actively bleeding varices as well as large varices and stigmata of recent bleeding
  - Can be used to treat bleeding with esophageal band ligation (preferred to sclerotherapy); prevent rebleeding; detect gastric varices, portal hypertensive gastropathy; diagnose alternative bleeding sites
  - Can identify and treat nonbleeding varices (protruding submucosal veins in the distal third of the esophagus)

Diagnostic Procedures/Other
- Transient elastography (TE) for identifying CLD patients at risk of developing clinically significant portal hypertension (CSPH) (1)[A]
- HVPG >10 mm Hg: gold standard to diagnose CSPH (normal: 1 to 5 mm Hg) (1)[A]
- HVPG response of ≥10% or to ≤12 mm Hg to intravenous propranolol identifies responders to nonselective β-blocker (NSBB) and is linked to a decreased risk of variceal bleeding (1,2)[A].
- Video capsule endoscopy screening as an alternative to traditional endoscopy
- Doppler sonography (second line): demonstrates patency, diameter, and flow in portal and splenic veins, and collaterals; sensitive for gastric varices; documents patency after ligation or transjugular intrahepatic portosystemic shunt (TIPS)
- CT- or MRI-angiography (second line, not routine): demonstrates large vascular channels in abdomen, mediastinum; demonstrates patency of intrahepatic portal and splenic vein
  - Venous-phase celiac arteriography: demonstrates portal vein and collaterals; hepatic vein occlusion
  - Portal pressure measurement using retrograde catheter in hepatic vein

TREATMENT

GENERAL MEASURES

- Treat underlying cirrhotic comorbidities.
- Variceal bleeding is often complicated by hepatic encephalopathy and infection.
- Active bleeding (3)[A]
  - IV access, hemodynamic resuscitation
  - Type and crossmatch packed RBCs. Overtransfusion increases portal pressure and increases rebleeding risk.
  - Treat coagulopathy as necessary. Fresh frozen plasma may increase blood volume and increase rebleeding risk.
  - Avoid sedation, monitor mental status, and avoid nephrotoxic drugs and β-blockers acutely.
  - IV octreotide to lower portal venous pressure as adjuvant to endoscopic management; IV bolus of 50 μg followed by drip of 50 μg/hr
  - Terlipressin (alternative): 2 mg q4h IV for 24 to 48 hours and then 1 mg q4h
  - Erythromycin 250 mg IV 30 to 120 minutes before endoscopy (1)[A]
  - Urgent upper GI endoscopy for diagnosis and treatment
    - Variceal band ligation preferred to sclerotherapy for bleeding varices; also for nonbleeding medium-to-large varices to decrease bleeding risk
    - Ligation: lower rates of rebleeding, fewer complications, more rapid cessation of bleeding, higher rate of variceal eradication
- Repeat ligation/sclerosant for rebleeding.
- If endoscopic treatment fails, consider self-expanding esophageal metal stents or per oral placement of Sengstaken-Blakemore–type tube up to 24 hours to stabilize patient for TIPS (1)[C].
- As many as 2/3 of patients with variceal bleeding develop an infection, most commonly spontaneous bacterial peritonitis, UTI, or pneumonia; antibiotic prophylaxis with oral norfloxacin 400 mg or IV ceftriaxone 1 g q24h for up to a week
- In active bleeding, avoid β-blockers, which decrease BP and blunt the physiologic increase in heart rate during acute hemorrhage.
- Prevent recurrence of acute bleeding.
  - Vasoconstrictors: terlipressin, octreotide (reduce portal pressure)
  - Endoscopic band ligation (EBL): if bleeding recurs/portal pressure measurement shows portal pressure remains >12 mm Hg
  - TIPS: second-line therapy if above methods fail; TIPS decreases portal pressure by creating communication between hepatic vein and an intrahepatic portal vein branch.

MEDICATION

Primary prevention of variceal bleeding (4)[A]
- Endoscopy: assesses variceal size, presence of red wale sign (longitudinal variceal reddish streak that suggests either a recent bleed or a pending bleed) to determine risk stratification
  - Endoscopy every 2 to 3 years if cirrhosis but no varices; every 1 to 2 years if small varices and not receiving β-blockers (2)[A]

First Line
- Not actively bleeding. NSBB reduce portal pressure and decrease risk of first bleed from 25% to 15% when used as primary prophylaxis; beneficial in cirrhosis with small varices and increased hemorrhage risk as well as cirrhosis with medium-to-large varices (2,4)[A]

- Carvedilol: 6.25 mg daily (2)[A] is more effective than NSBB in dropping HVPG (1)[A].
  - Propranolol: 20 mg BID increase until heart rate decreased by 25% from baseline
  - Nadolol 80 mg daily; increase as above
  - Contraindications: severe asthma
- Chronic prevention of rebleeding (secondary prevention): NSBBs and EBL reduce rate of rebleeding to a similar extent, but β-blockers reduce mortality, whereas ligation does not (5)[A].

Second Line
Obliterate varices with esophageal banding if not tolerant of medication prophylaxis.
- During ligation: proton pump inhibitors, such as lansoprazole 30 mg/day, until varices obliterated
- Management of Budd-Chiari syndrome: anticoagulation, angioplasty/thrombolysis, TIPS, and orthotopic liver transplantation (1)[C]
- Management of EHPVO: anticoagulation (1)[B]; mesenteric-left portal vein bypass (Meso-Rex procedure) (1)[C]

ISSUES FOR REFERRAL
Refer for endoscopy, liver transplant, and interventional radiology for TIPS.

ADDITIONAL THERAPIES
Pneumococcal and hepatitis A/B vaccine (HAV/HBV)

SURGERY/OTHER PROCEDURES
- Esophageal transection: in rare cases of uncontrollable, exsanguinating bleeding
- Liver transplantation

ADMISSION, INPATIENT, AND NURSING CONSIDERATIONS
- Inpatient to stabilize acute bleeding and hemodynamic status, therapeutic endoscopy. ICU is typically the most appropriate initial setting.
- Discharge criteria: bleeding cessation, hemodynamic stability, and appropriate plan for treating comorbidities

 ONGOING CARE

FOLLOW-UP RECOMMENDATIONS
Patient Monitoring
- Close monitoring of vital signs
- Endoscopic variceal ligation, every 1 to 4 weeks, until varices eradicated
- If TIPS, repeat endoscopy to assess rebleeding.
- Endoscopic screening in patients with known cirrhosis every 2 to 3 years; yearly in patients with decompensated cirrhosis (1)[C]
- Patients with a liver stiffness <20 kPa and with platelets >150,000 can avoid endoscopic screening (1)[A] and may follow up by annual TE and platelet count (1)[C].

PATIENT EDUCATION
National Digestive Diseases Information Clearinghouse (http://www.niddk.nih.gov/health-information/health-topics/digestive-diseases/Pages/default.aspx) or American Liver Foundation (http://www.liverfoundation.org/)

PROGNOSIS
- Depends on underlying comorbidities
- In cirrhosis, 1-year survival is 50% for those who survive at least 2 weeks following a variceal bleed.

- In-hospital mortality remains high and is related to severity of underlying cirrhosis, ranging from 0% in Child-Pugh class A disease to 32% in Child-Pugh class C disease (3).
- Prognosis in noncirrhotic portal fibrosis is better than for cirrhotic portal fibrosis.

COMPLICATIONS
- Formation of gastric varices after eradication of esophageal varices
- Esophageal varices can recur.
- Hepatic encephalopathy, renal dysfunction, hepatorenal syndrome
- Infections after banding/ligation of varices

REFERENCES
1. de Franchis R; and Baveno VI Faculty. Expanding consensus in portal hypertension: report of the Baveno VI Consensus Workshop: stratifying risk and individualizing care for portal hypertension. *J Hepatol*. 2015;63(3):743–752.
2. Tripathi D, Stanley AJ, Hayes PC, et al; for Clinical Services and Standards Committee of the British Society of Gastroenterology. U.K. guidelines on the management of variceal haemorrhage in cirrhotic patients. *Gut*. 2015;64(11):1680–1704.
3. Herrera JL. Management of acute variceal bleeding. *Clin Liver Dis*. 2014;18(2):347–357.
4. Simonetto DA, Shah VH, Kamath PS. Primary prophylaxis of variceal bleeding. *Clin Liver Dis*. 2014;18(2):335–345.
5. Albillos A, Tejedor M. Secondary prophylaxis for esophageal variceal bleeding. *Clin Liver Dis*. 2014;18(2):359–370.

ADDITIONAL READING
- Tayyem O, Bilal M, Samuel R, et al. Evaluation and management of variceal bleeding. *Dis Mon*. 2018;64(7):312–320.
- Zanetto A, Senzolo M, Ferrarese A, et al. Assessment of bleeding risk in patients with cirrhosis. *Curr Hepatol Rep*. 2015;14(1):9–18.

 SEE ALSO

Cirrhosis of the Liver; Portal Hypertension

 CODES

ICD10
- I85.00 Esophageal varices without bleeding
- I85.01 Esophageal varices with bleeding
- I85.10 Secondary esophageal varices without bleeding

CLINICAL PEARLS
- Thrombocytopenia is the most sensitive marker of increased portal pressure and large esophageal varices.
- In acute bleeding, avoid β-blockers.
- In acute bleeding, overtransfusion can elevate portal pressure and increase bleeding risk.

ESSENTIAL TREMOR SYNDROME

Jennifer E. Svarverud, DO • Pamela R. Hughes, MD

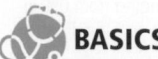 **BASICS**

DESCRIPTION
- A postural (occurring with voluntary maintenance of a position against gravity) or kinetic (occurring during voluntary movement) flexion–extension tremor that is slow and rhythmic and primarily affects the hands and forearms, head, or voice with a frequency of 4 to 12 Hz
- Older patients tend to have lower frequency tremors, whereas younger patients exhibit frequencies in the higher range.
- May be familial, sporadic, or associated with other movement disorders
- Incidence and prevalence increase with age, but symptom onset can occur at any age.
- The tremor can be intermittent and exacerbated by emotional or physical stressors, fatigue, and caffeine.
- System(s) affected include neurologic, musculoskeletal, ear/nose/throat (ENT) (voice)

EPIDEMIOLOGY
Essential tremor is the most common pathologic tremor in humans.

Incidence
- Can occur at any age but bimodal peaks exist in the 2nd and 6th decades
- Incidence rises significantly after age 49 years.

Prevalence
The overall prevalence for essential tremor has been estimated between 0.4% and 0.9% but is increased in older patients with an estimated 4.6% at age 65 years and up to 22% at age 95 years.

ETIOLOGY AND PATHOPHYSIOLOGY
- Suspected to originate from an abnormal oscillation within thalamocortical and cerebello-olivary loops, as lesions in these areas tend to reduce essential tremor
- Essential tremor is not a homogenous disorder; many patients have other motor manifestations and nonmotor features, including cognitive and psychiatric symptoms.

Genetics
- Positive family history in 50–70% of patients; autosomal dominant inheritance is demonstrated in many families with poor penetrance. Twin studies suggest that environmental factors are also involved.
- A link to genetic loci exists on chromosomes 2p22–2p25, 3q13, and 6p23. In addition, a Ser9Gly variant in the dopamine D_3 receptor gene on 3q13 has been suggested as a risk factor.

COMMONLY ASSOCIATED CONDITIONS
- Can be present in 10% of patients with Parkinson disease (PD); characteristics of PD that distinguish it from essential tremor include 3- to 5-Hz resting tremor; accompanying rigidity, bradykinesia, or postural instability; and no change with alcohol consumption.
- Patients with essential tremor have a 4% risk of developing PD.
- Resting tremor, typically of the arm, may be seen in up to 20–30% of patients with essential tremor. Although action tremor is the hallmark feature of essential tremor, it is commonly found in patients with PD as well.

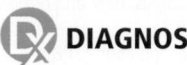 **DIAGNOSIS**

HISTORY
- Core criteria for diagnosis
  - Bilateral (less likely unilateral) action (postural or kinetic) tremor of the hands and forearms that is most commonly asymmetric
  - Absence of other neurologic signs, with the exception of cogwheel phenomenon
  - May have isolated head tremor with no signs of dystonia
- Secondary criteria include long duration (>3 years), positive family history, and beneficial response to alcohol.

PHYSICAL EXAM
- Tremor can affect upper limbs (~95% of patients).
- Less commonly, the tremor affects head (~34%), lower limbs (~30%), voice (~12%), tongue (~7%), face (~5%), and trunk (~5%).

DIFFERENTIAL DIAGNOSIS
- PD
- Wilson disease
- Hyperthyroidism
- Multiple sclerosis
- Dystonic tremor
- Cerebellar tremor
- Asterixis
- Psychogenic tremor
- Orthostatic tremor
- Drug-induced or enhanced physiologic tremor (amiodarone, cimetidine, lamotrigine, itraconazole, valproic acid, SSRIs, steroids, lithium, cyclosporine, β-adrenergic agonists, ephedrine, theophylline, tricyclic antidepressants [TCAs], antipsychotics)

DIAGNOSTIC TESTS & INTERPRETATION
Initial Tests (lab, imaging)
- No specific biologic marker or diagnostic test is available.
- Ceruloplasmin and serum copper to rule out Wilson disease
- Thyroid-stimulating hormone to rule out thyroid dysfunction
- Serum electrolytes, BUN, creatinine
- Brain MRI usually is not necessary or indicated unless Wilson disease is found or exam findings imply central lesion.

Diagnostic Procedures/Other
- Accelerometry evaluates tremor frequency and amplitude; >95% of PD cases exhibit frequencies in the 4- to 6-Hz range, and 95% of essential tremor cases exhibit frequencies in the 5- to 8-Hz range.
- Surface electromyography is less helpful in distinguishing essential tremor from PD.

Test Interpretation
Posture-related tremor seen on exam

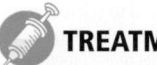 **TREATMENT**

MEDICATION
Pharmacologic treatment should be considered when tremor interferes with activities of daily living (ADLs) or causes psychological distress.

First Line
- Propranolol 60 to 320 mg/day in divided doses or in long-acting formulation reduces limb tremor magnitude by ~50%, and almost 70% of patients experience improvement in clinical rating scales. There is insufficient evidence to recommend propranolol for vocal tremor. Single doses of propranolol, taken before social situations that are likely to exacerbate tremor, are useful for some patients.
- Primidone 25 mg at bedtime, gradually titrated to 150 to 300 mg at bedtime, improves tremor amplitude by 40–50%. Maximum dose is 750 mg/day, with doses >250 mg/day typically divided to BID or TID. Low-dose therapy (<250 mg/day) is just as effective as high-dose (750 mg/day) therapy.
- Propranolol and primidone have similar efficacy when used as initial therapy for limb tremor; both carry a level A recommendation (1)[A].
- 30–50% of patients will not respond to either propranolol or primidone.

Second Line

- Topiramate at a mean dose of 292 mg/day demonstrated significantly greater reduction in Tremor Rating Scale (TRS) compared with placebo (7.70 vs. 0.08; $p < .005$; baseline TRS = 37.0) in a small study combining results of three double-blind, randomized, controlled trials following a common protocol. Use is limited by dropout rates as high as 40% due to appetite suppression, weight loss, paresthesias, and concentration difficulties (2)[B].
- Gabapentin up to 400 mg TID (3)[B]
- Sotalol, nadolol, and atenolol are alternative β-blockers; each has less evidence than propranolol to support use.
- Clonazepam and alprazolam should be used with caution because of potential abuse.
- Clozapine has shown efficacy at doses of 6 to 75 mg/day but is recommended only for refractory cases of limb tremor because of a 1% risk of agranulocytosis. The American Academy of Neurology (AAN) indicates that insufficient evidence exists to support or refute the efficacy of clozapine for chronic use (1)[A].
- Memantine, in a pilot study using doses up to 40 mg/day, showed significant benefit in a small subset of the study group. Adverse events at this dose included dizziness, somnolence, and poor energy (4)[B].
- Pramipexole, at a dose of 2.1 mg/day, demonstrated moderate efficacy in reducing severity of tremor in a pilot study of 29 patients. Immediate- and extended-release formulations were equally effective (5)[B].
- Levetiracetam and 3,4-diaminopyridine are probably ineffective at reducing limb tremor and should not be considered according to the AAN (1)[A].
- Other medications that have been evaluated for treatment of essential tremor, with limited data to support their use, include acetazolamide, clonidine, flunarizine, methazolamide, nimodipine, olanzapine, phenobarbital, pregabalin, quetiapine, sodium oxybate, and zonisamide (1)[A].
- Alcohol may provide transient improvement in symptoms, but its brief duration of action, subsequent rebound, and associated risk of developing alcohol addiction make it a less attractive option for longer term treatment. Alcohol may be an appropriate option for short-term, situation-specific improvement in symptoms.
- Botulinum toxin A injections should be offered as a treatment option for cervical dystonia (level A recommendation from AAN) and may be offered for blepharospasm, focal upper extremity dystonia, adductor laryngeal dystonia, and upper extremity essential tremor. Limited data support its use for head and vocal tremor (6)[B].

ISSUES FOR REFERRAL

Referral to a neurologist can help to differentiate those with dystonia, neuropathic tremor, PD, or drug-induced tremor.

SURGERY/OTHER PROCEDURES

- Deep brain stimulation provides a magnitude of benefit that is superior to all available medications and may be used to treat medically refractory limb tremor; it has fewer adverse effects than thalamotomy.
- Bilateral thalamic stimulation is effective in reducing tremor and functional disability; however, dysarthria is a possible complication.
- Unilateral thalamotomy may be used to treat limb tremor that is refractory to medical management.
- Bilateral thalamotomy is not recommended because of adverse side effects.

 ## ONGOING CARE

DIET
Avoid caffeine.

PATIENT EDUCATION
Although essential tremor can cause significant impairment in daily functioning, it does not decrease life expectancy.

PROGNOSIS
Tremor tends to worsen with age, increasing in amplitude.

REFERENCES

1. Zesiewicz TA, Elble RJ, Louis ED, et al. Evidence-based guideline update: treatment of essential tremor: report of the Quality Standards Subcommittee of the American Academy of Neurology. *Neurology*. 2011;77(19):1752–1755.
2. Connor GS, Edwards K, Tarsy D. Topiramate in essential tremor: findings from double-blind, placebo-controlled, crossover trials. *Clin Neuropharmacol*. 2008;31(2):97–103.
3. Gironell A, Kulisevsky J, Barbanoj M, et al. A randomized placebo-controlled comparative trial of gabapentin and propranolol in essential tremor. *Arch Neurol*. 1999;56(4):475–480.
4. Handforth A, Bordelon Y, Frucht SJ, et al. A pilot efficacy and tolerability trial of memantine for essential tremor. *Clin Neuropharmacol*. 2010;33(5):223–226.
5. Herceg M, Nagy F, Pál E, et al. Pramipexole may be an effective treatment option in essential tremor. *Clin Neuropharmacol*. 2012;35(2):73–76.
6. Simpson DM, Blitzer A, Brashear A, et al; for Therapeutics and Technology Assessment Subcommittee of the American Academy of Neurology. Assessment: botulinum neurotoxin for the treatment of movement disorders (an evidence-based review): report of the Therapeutics and Technology Assessment Subcommittee of the American Academy of Neurology. *Neurology*. 2008;70(19):1699–1706.

ADDITIONAL READING

- Bain P, Brin M, Deuschl G, et al. Criteria for the diagnosis of essential tremor. *Neurology*. 2000;54(11 Suppl 4):S7.
- Buijink AW, Contarino MF, Koelman JH, et al. How to tackle tremor—systematic review of the literature and diagnostic work-up. *Front Neurol*. 2012;3:146.
- Deuschl G, Raethjen J, Hellriegel H, et al. Treatment of patients with essential tremor. *Lancet Neurol*. 2011;10(2):148–161.
- Elias WJ, Shah BB. Tremor. *JAMA*. 2014;311(9):948–954.
- Flora ED, Perera CL, Cameron AL, et al. Deep brain stimulation for essential tremor: a systematic review. *Mov Disord*. 2010;25(11):1550–1559.
- Schuurman PR, Bosch DA, Bossuyt PM, et al. A comparison of continuous thalamic stimulation and thalamotomy for suppression of severe tremor. *N Engl J Med*. 2000;342(7):461–468.
- Sullivan KL, Hauser RA, Zesiewicz TA. Essential tremor. Epidemiology, diagnosis, and treatment. *Neurologist*. 2004;10(5):250–258.
- Thenganatt MA, Louis ED. Distinguishing essential tremor from Parkinson's disease: bedside tests and laboratory evaluations. *Expert Rev Neurother*. 2012;12(6):687–696.
- Zeuner KE, Deuschl G. An update on tremors. *Curr Opin Neurol*. 2012;25(4):475–482.

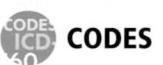 ## CODES

ICD10
G25.0 Essential tremor

CLINICAL PEARLS

- Core criteria for diagnosis of essential tremor include bilateral action or postural tremor of the hands, forearm, and/or head without a resting component.
- Beneficial response to alcohol and positive family history help to differentiate essential tremor from PD (PD is characterized by tremor at rest, bradykinesia, and rigidity, and it does not improve with alcohol use.).
- 10% of patients with PD will have both resting tremors of PD and essential tremor.
- Wilson disease, thyroid disease, and medication effect should be ruled out.
- Brain MRI is usually not necessary or indicated.
- First-line treatments include propranolol and primidone. 30–50% of patients will not benefit from these first-line treatments.

E

EUSTACHIAN TUBE DYSFUNCTION

Adam W. Kowalski, MD • Vernon Wheeler, MD, FAAFP

BASICS

DESCRIPTION

- A spectrum of disorders involving impairment of the functional valve of the eustachian tube (ET)
- ETD can be classified as *patulous dysfunction*, in which the ET is excessively open, or *dilatory dysfunction*, in which there is failure of the tubes to dilate (i.e., open) appropriately.
- Pathophysiology related to pressure dysregulation, impaired protection secondary to reflux of irritating material into the middle ear, or impaired clearance by the mucociliary system
- May occur in the setting of pressure changes (e.g., scuba diving or air travel) or acute upper airway inflammation (e.g., allergic or infectious rhinosinusitis, acute otitis media [OM])
- Chronic ETD may lead to a retracted tympanic membrane, recurrent serous effusion, recurrent OM, adhesive OM, chronic mastoiditis, or cholesteatoma.
- System(s) affected: auditory
- Synonym(s): auditory tube dysfunction; ET disorder; blocked ET; patulous ET

ALERT

- Sudden sensorineural hearing loss (SSNHL) can be misdiagnosed as ETD.
- A simple 512-Hz tuning fork test lateralizes to the opposite ear in SSNHL and to the affected ear in ETD with conductive hearing loss.
- Any SSNHL is a medical emergency and should be referred to an otolaryngologist immediately.

EPIDEMIOLOGY

- Most common in children <5 years of age, thought to be related to anatomical differences (see "Etiology and Pathophysiology" section)
- Usually decreases with age

Incidence

70% of children by age 7 years have experienced ETD.

Prevalence

- 1% of the adult population
- Males > females
- Highest prevalence among Native Americans, Inuits, Australian Aborigines, Hispanics, Africans

ETIOLOGY AND PATHOPHYSIOLOGY

- Under normal circumstances, the ET is closed, opening to release a small amount of air to equilibrate middle ear pressure with surrounding atmospheric pressure.
- ETD is failure of the ET, palate, nasal cavities, and nasopharynx to regulate middle ear and mastoid pressure.
- ET functions
  - Ventilation/regulation of middle ear pressure
  - Protection from nasopharyngeal secretions
  - Drainage of middle ear fluid
  - ET is closed at rest and opens with yawning, swallowing, and chewing.
- Cycle of dysfunction: structural or functional obstruction of the ET:
  - Negative pressure develops in middle ear.
  - Serous exudate is drawn to the middle ear by negative pressure or refluxed into the middle ear if the ET opens momentarily.
  - Infection of static fluid causes edema and release of inflammatory mediators, exacerbating the cycle of inflammation and obstruction.

- In children, a horizontal and shorter ET predisposes to difficulties with ventilation and drainage.
- Adenoid hypertrophy can block the torus tubarius (proximal opening of the ET).
- In adults, paradoxical closing of the ET with swallowing occurs in a majority of affected patients.
- Tumors that impair/occlude the ET or that invade the tensor veli palatini to impair normal swallow regulation can also lead to dysfunction.

Genetics

Twin studies show a genetic component. Specific genetic cause is undefined.

RISK FACTORS

Adult and pediatric

- Allergic rhinitis, tobacco exposure, GERD, chronic sinusitis, adenoid hypertrophy or nasopharyngeal mass, neuromuscular disease, altered immunity
- Prematurity and low birth weight, young age, daycare, crowded living conditions, low socioeconomic status, prone sleeping position, prolonged bottle use, craniofacial abnormalities (e.g., cleft palate, Down syndrome)

Pregnancy Considerations

ETD may be exacerbated by rhinitis of pregnancy; symptoms resolve postpartum.

GENERAL PREVENTION

- Control of upper airway inflammation: allergies, infectious rhinosinusitis, GERD
- Autoinsufflation of middle ear (i.e., blow gently against pinched nostril and closed mouth)
- Avoid atmospheric pressure changes (e.g., plane flight, scuba diving) in the setting of acute allergy exacerbation or URI.
- Avoid exposure to environmental irritants: tobacco smoke and pollutants.

COMMONLY ASSOCIATED CONDITIONS

- Hearing loss
- OM: acute, chronic, and serous
- Chronic mastoiditis
- Cholesteatoma
- Allergic rhinitis
- Chronic sinusitis/URI
- Adenoid hypertrophy
- GERD
- Cleft palate
- Down syndrome
- Obesity
- Nasopharyngeal carcinoma or other tumor

DIAGNOSIS

HISTORY

- Symptoms of ear pain, fullness, "plugging," hearing loss, tinnitus, popping or snapping noises, and vertigo
  - Unilateral or bilateral. Evaluate adults with persistent unilateral symptoms for nasopharyngeal tumor.
  - History of previous ear infections, surgeries, head trauma, recent flying or diving

- Voice change (hypo- or hypernasal voice, consider NP mass or palatal dysfunction)
- Differentiate patulous dysfunction, in which patient's own voice and breath sounds are amplified (autophony), from dilatory dysfunction, in which patient complains more of ear pain, "plugged" ear, hearing loss, and tinnitus.
- ETDQ-7 is a questionnaire that attempts to quantify ETD in adult patients. Based on presence and intensity of symptoms in past 1 month, severity is rated on 1 to 7 scale. A total score >14.5 categorizes patient as having ETD (1,2)[B].
  - Pressure in ears in past 1 month?
  - Pain in ears in past 1 month?
  - A feeling that ears are clogged or "under water"?
  - Ear symptoms when you have cold or sinusitis?
  - Crackling or popping sounds in the ears?
  - Ringing in ears?
  - A feeling that your hearing is muffled?

PHYSICAL EXAM

- Pneumatic otoscopy: retracted tympanic membrane, effusion, decreased drum movement
- Toynbee maneuver: View changes of the drum while patient autoinsufflates against closed lips and pinched nostrils; may show various degrees of retraction
  - Entire drum may be retracted and "lateralize" with insufflation.
  - Posterosuperior quadrant (pars flaccida) may form a retraction pocket.
- Tuning fork tests: 512-Hz fork placed on the forehead lateralizes to affected ear (Weber test); the fork will be louder behind the ear on the mastoid than in front of the ear (bone conduction > air conduction, Rinne test) in conductive hearing loss.
- Nasopharyngoscopy: adenoid hypertrophy or nasopharyngeal mass
- Anterior rhinoscopy: deviated nasal septum, polyps, mucosal hypertrophy, turbinate hypertrophy

DIFFERENTIAL DIAGNOSIS

- SSNHL (a medical emergency)
- Tympanic membrane perforation
- Barotrauma
- Temporomandibular joint disorder
- Ménière disease
- Superior semicircular canal dehiscence

DIAGNOSTIC TESTS & INTERPRETATION

Initial Tests (lab, imaging)

- No routine radiologic studies needed if clinical signs/symptoms suggest ETD
- CT scan (not necessary) may show changes related to OM or middle ear/mastoid opacification.
- Functional MRI might determine cause of ETD (in recalcitrant cases), as the ET opening can be visualized during Valsalva.

Diagnostic Procedures/Other

- Audiogram may show conductive hearing loss.
- Tympanometry: Type B or C tympanograms indicate fluid or retraction, respectively; negative middle ear peak pressures seen even with normal (type A) tympanograms

TREATMENT

- Due to limited high-quality evidence, it is difficult to recommend any one treatment option/intervention as superior (3)[C].
- Use of a "nasal balloon" shown effective for clearing OM with effusion; unclear of benefit for ETD
- General principle is to remove or fix the underlying cause (e.g., infection, tumor, perforation of TM, restore tensor palatini muscle) and reduce or eliminate the cycle of infection/inflammation.
- Although no evidence exists, some consider antibiotics for AOM; decongestants, nasal steroids, antihistamines (if allergic rhinitis is present), and surgery/procedures for recalcitrant cases
- Tympanostomy tubes ± adenoidectomy when indicated for recurrent ear infections or severe progressive retractions

MEDICATION

- Antibiotics only if infection is suspected as cause of ETD (4)[A]
- Few data support pharmacologic treatments such as decongestants, nasal steroids, or antihistamines for ETD.
- Medications treat comorbid conditions.
- Decongestants, topical, oral
  - Avoid prolonged use (>3 days); can cause rhinitis medicamentosa
  - Decongestants are most useful for acute ETD related to a resolving URI.
  - Decongestants are not typically used for relief of chronic ETD in children.
    - Phenylephrine: adults and children ≥12 years of age, 1 tablet (10 mg) q4h PRN; children 6 to 11 years of age, 5 mg q4h PRN; children 4 to 5 years of age, 2.5 mg q4h PRN
    - Pseudoephedrine: adults, 60 mg q4–6h PRN; children 6 to 12 years of age, 30 mg q4–6h PRN; children 4 to 5 years of age, 15 mg q4–6h PRN
    - Oxymetazoline: adults and children ≥6 years of age, 1 to 2 sprays each nostril q12h PRN. Limit use to ≤3 days.
    - Phenylephrine: adults, 1 to 2 sprays each nostril q4h PRN. Limit use to ≤3 days.
- Nasal steroids (may be beneficial for those with allergic rhinitis) (5)[A]
  - Beclomethasone (Beconase, Vancenase): adults and children ≥12 years of age, 1 to 2 sprays each nostril BID; children 6 to 11 years of age, 1 spray each nostril BID; not recommended for children <6 years of age
  - Budesonide (Rhinocort): adults and children ≥6 years of age, 1 spray each nostril daily
  - Ciclesonide (Omnaris) (a prodrug activated on nasal mucosa): adults and children ≥6 years of age, 2 sprays each nostril daily
  - Flunisolide (Nasarel, Nasalide): adults and children ≥6 years of age, 2 sprays each nostril BID
  - Fluticasone furoate (Veramyst): adults and children ≥12 years of age, 2 sprays each nostril daily; children 2 to 11 years of age, 1 spray each nostril daily
  - Fluticasone propionate (Flonase): adults 1 to 2 sprays each nostril daily; children ≥4 years of age, 1 spray each nostril daily
  - Mometasone (Nasonex): adults and children ≥12 years of age, 2 sprays each nostril daily; children 2 to 12 years of age, 1 spray each nostril daily
  - Triamcinolone (Nasacort): adults and children ≥6 years of age, 1 to 2 sprays each nostril daily; children 2 to 5 years of age, 1 spray each nostril daily

- 2nd-generation H₁ antihistamines (may be beneficial for those with ETD and chronic rhinitis)
  - Cetirizine (Zyrtec) (tablets, chewable tablets, liquid): adults and children ≥6 years of age, 5 to 10 mg/day PO; children 12 months to 5 years of age: 2.5 mg/day PO, may increase to BID; children 6 to <12 months of age: 2.5 mg/day PO
  - Desloratadine (Clarinex) (tablets, RediTabs, liquid): adults and children ≥12 years of age, 5 mg/day PO; children 6 to 11 years of age, 2.5 mg/day PO; children 12 months to 5 years of age, 1.25 mg/day PO; children 6 to 11 months of age, 1 mg/day PO
  - Fexofenadine (Allegra) (tablets, RediTabs, liquid): adults and children ≥12 years of age, 60 mg PO BID or 180 mg/day PO; children 2 to 11 years of age, 30 mg PO BID
  - Levocetirizine (Xyzal) (tablets, liquid): adults and children ≥12 years of age, 2.5 to 5.0 mg PO every evening; children 6 to 11 years of age, 2.5 mg PO every evening; children 6 months to 5 years of age, 1.25 mg PO every evening
- Antihistamine nasal sprays (may be beneficial for those with ETD and chronic rhinitis)
  - Azelastine (Astepro or Astelin): adults and children ≥12 years of age, 1 to 2 sprays each nostril BID; children 6 to 11 years of age, 1 spray each nostril BID
  - Olopatadine (Patanase): adults and children ≥12 years of age, 2 sprays each nostril BID; children 6 to 11 years of age, 1 spray each nostril BID

SURGERY/OTHER PROCEDURES

- Myringotomy and pressure equalization tube placement to ventilate middle ear, relieve pressure, and prevent sequelae of chronically retracted drum
- Patients with ETD during pressure changes may benefit from minimally invasive laser eustachian tuboplasty.
- Balloon tuboplasty (limited data in terms of efficacy, safety, and long-term outcomes) (6)[B]
- Adenoidectomy if hypertrophied tissue is present
  - In children, first set of tubes are typically placed alone. Adenoidectomy is performed with second set of tubes if problems recur.
  - Some advocate adenoidectomy even in absence of excess tissue; reduces frequency and number of subsequent tubes

ONGOING CARE

FOLLOW-UP RECOMMENDATIONS

- Monitor pressure equalization tubes every 6 to 8 months in children and every 6 to 12 months in adults.
- Monitor tympanic membrane retraction pocket for progression every 6 to 12 months to allow for early intervention for progression in hearing loss, obvious ossicular erosion, or cholesteatoma.

DIET

Breastfeeding is associated with lower incidence of ETD and OM.

PROGNOSIS

If symptoms of ETD persist beyond age 7 years, patient is more likely to have long-term problems and require regular monitoring.

COMPLICATIONS

Morbidity related to hearing compromise or associated sequela of chronic ear infections

REFERENCES

1. McCoul ED, Anand VK, Christos PJ. Validating the clinical assessment of eustachian tube dysfunction: the Eustachian Tube Dysfunction Questionnaire (ETDQ-7). *Laryngoscope*. 2012;122(5):1137–1141.
2. Van Roeyen S, Van de Heyning P, Van Rompaey V. Value and discriminative power of the seven-item Eustachian Tube Dysfunction Questionnaire. *Laryngoscope*. 2015;125(11):2553–2556.
3. Norman G, Llewellyn A, Harden M, et al. Systematic review of the limited evidence base for treatments of eustachian tube dysfunction: a health technology assessment. *Clin Otolaryngol*. 2014;39(1):6–21.
4. van Zon A, van der Heijden GJ, van Dongen TM, et al. Antibiotics for otitis media with effusion in children. *Cochrane Database Syst Rev*. 2012;(9):CD009163.
5. Simpson SA, Lewis R, van der Voort J, et al. Oral or topical nasal steroids for hearing loss associated with otitis media with effusion in children. *Cochrane Database Syst Rev*. 2011;(5):CD001935.
6. Gürtler N, Husner A, Flurin H. Balloon dilation of the eustachian tube: early outcome analysis. *Otol Neurotol*. 2015;36(3):437–443.

ADDITIONAL READING

- Gluth MB, McDonald DR, Weaver AL, et al. Management of eustachian tube dysfunction with nasal steroid spray: a prospective, randomized, placebo-controlled trial. *Arch Otolaryngol Head Neck Surg*. 2011;137(5):449–455.
- Williamson I, Vennik J, Harnden A, et al. Effect of nasal balloon autoinflation in children with otitis media with effusion in primary care: an open randomized controlled trial. *CMAJ*. 2015;187(13):961–969.

SEE ALSO

Algorithm: Ear Pain/Otalgia

CODES

ICD10

- H69.90 Unspecified Eustachian tube disorder, unspecified ear
- H69.00 Patulous Eustachian tube, unspecified ear
- H68.109 Unspecified obstruction of Eustachian tube, unspecified ear

CLINICAL PEARLS

- ETD can be acute or chronic. Treatment is based on the underlying etiology.
- A simple 512-Hz tuning fork test lateralizes to the opposite ear in SSNHL and to the affected ear in ETD with conductive hearing loss.
- Rule out SSNHL (medical emergency) which can be misdiagnosed as ETD, especially in patients with unilateral symptoms.

E

FACTOR V LEIDEN

Christy L. Baggett, DO • Collin R. Jones, MD • George G.A. Pujalte, MD, FACSM

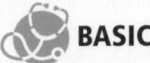 **BASICS**

DESCRIPTION
- Factor V Leiden is a genetic mutation at the activated protein C (APC) cleavage site on the factor V and Va molecule leading to the most common form of inherited thrombophilia.
- System(s) affected: cardiovascular, gastrointestinal, hemo/lymphatic/immunologic, nervous, pulmonary, reproductive
- Synonym(s): factor V Leiden thrombophilia; factor V Leiden mutation, hereditary APC resistance

Pediatric Considerations
Potential for increased thrombosis risk in patients with factor V Leiden and concomitant risks

Pregnancy Considerations
- Recurrent pregnancy loss is a possible complication.
- Increased thrombotic risk in pregnancy and postpartum (additive) especially in homozygous state
- Possible increased risk of IUGR, preeclampsia, placental abruption: evidence mixed
- Women with a history of adverse pregnancy outcomes should be tested for thrombophilia if they are planning a future pregnancy (1).

EPIDEMIOLOGY
Prevalence
Studies estimate ~5–8% occurrence of heterozygosity in Caucasians, Hispanic Americans ~2%, African American ~1%, and Asian Americans ~0.45%.

ETIOLOGY AND PATHOPHYSIOLOGY
- Factor V circulates in the plasma. When exposed to tissue factor, factor V amplifies the production of thrombin, which further promotes clotting by activating factor V into procoagulant factor Va.
- For balance, thrombin also promotes APC production, which will cleave and inactivate factor V, Va, and VIII, thereby keeping the clotting cascade in check (negative feedback loop).
- In factor V Leiden, a point mutation at the binding site of APC (Arg506Glu) renders it less able to cleave factor V or Va. This, in turn, reduces the anticoagulant role of factor V as a cofactor to APC and increases the *procoagulant* role of activated factor V because there is now 20-fold slower degradation of factor Va.

RISK FACTORS
- Risk for venous thromboembolism (VTE) is ~7-fold in heterozygous and ~80-fold in homozygous factor V Leiden individuals, compared with individuals without the mutation (2). This risk is compounded/increased by the presence of the following:
  - Having non-O blood type (A, B, or AB): 2- to 4-fold
  - Oral contraceptives: homozygotes up to 100-fold; heterozygotes, 35-fold. The increased risk is halved when the patient uses desogestrel-containing oral contraceptives.
  - Hormone replacement therapy (HRT) and selective estrogen receptor modulators (SERMs) both increase the risk of thrombosis; in patients with factor V Leiden, that risk is compounded.

- In men with an underlying thrombophilia, testosterone therapy can promote VTE (3).
- Pregnancy and *homozygous* factor V Leiden increase the risk of thrombosis 7- to 16-fold during pregnancy and the puerperium.
  - Those with combined thrombophilias and end-stage renal disease are at risk for developing calciphylaxis (4).
- Data are conflicting with regard to risk for recurrent VTE for patients with factor V Leiden but trend toward an increased risk (5,6).

GENERAL PREVENTION

ALERT
Patients with factor V Leiden without thrombosis do not require prophylactic anticoagulation.

COMMONLY ASSOCIATED CONDITIONS
Venous thrombosis

 DIAGNOSIS

HISTORY
- Previous thrombosis
- Family history of thrombosis

PHYSICAL EXAM
- Family history of factor V Leiden mutation
- Findings suggestive of VTE in any form (DVT, PE, cerebral thrombosis): 10–26% of patients with VTE are carriers of the factor V Leiden mutation.
- Thrombosis in unusual locations, such as the sagittal sinus or mesentery and portal systems, although these are less common in patients with factor V Leiden than in patients with deficiency of protein C or S
- There is a weak, however significant, association between procoagulant states (including factor V Leiden) and coronary events in younger patients (4).

DIFFERENTIAL DIAGNOSIS
- Protein C deficiency
- Protein S deficiency
- Antithrombin deficiency
- Other causes of APC resistance (e.g., antiphospholipid antibodies)
- Dysfibrinogenemia
- Dysplasminogenemia
- Homocystinemia
- Prothrombin 20210 mutation
- Elevated factor VIII levels

DIAGNOSTIC TESTS & INTERPRETATION
Initial Tests (lab, imaging)
- For evaluation of a new clot in patient at risk: CBC with peripheral smear, PT/INR, activated partial thromboplastin time (aPTT), thrombin time, lupus anticoagulant, antiphospholipid antibodies, factor VIII, anticardiolipin antibody, anti-β2 glycoprotein I antibody, APC resistance, protein S antigen and resistance, antithrombin III assay, fibrinogen, factor V Leiden, prothrombin G20210A
- Genetic test: DNA-based test for factor V mutation; will be unaffected by anticoagulation and other drugs

- Functional test: plasma-based coagulation assay using factor V–deficient plasma to which patient plasma is added along with purified APC. The relative prolongation of the aPTT is used to assay for the defect. Heparin, direct thrombin inhibitors, and factor Xa inhibitor may cause false-negative results. In the absence of exposure to anticoagulants, functional testing is preferred to genetic testing due to cost and time to diagnosis (5)[A].
- Extremity US for DVT
- V/Q scan or spiral CT for PE

Follow-Up Tests & Special Considerations
- US may not show DVT acutely; repeat in 5 to 7 days if strong suspicion.
- V/Q scan for evaluation of PE may be difficult to interpret in smokers or those with underlying lung disease.

Diagnostic Procedures/Other
Magnetic resonance angiography (MRA), venography, or arteriography to detect thrombosis

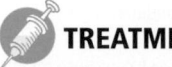 **TREATMENT**

Only indicated if with thrombotic event

GENERAL MEASURES
- Like general VTE treatment, patients with factor V Leiden and a first thrombosis should be anticoagulated initially with heparin or low-molecular-weight heparin (LMWH) and warfarin for at least 3 months.
- Factor Xa inhibitors are FDA-approved for VTE/PE prophylaxis and treatment in patients without kidney disease. These have the benefit of not requiring lab monitoring or dietary limitations. For patients with factor V Leiden and recurrence of DVT/PE, factor Xa inhibitors are indicated for prophylaxis (7).
- Treatment with LMWH is recommended over unfractionated heparin, unless the patient has severe renal failure (6)[A].
- Treat as outpatient, if possible (6)[A].
- Initiate warfarin with LMWH on the first treatment day and discontinue LMWH after minimum of 5 days and when INR >2 for 2 consecutive days (6)[A].
- Patients should be maintained on warfarin with an INR of 2 to 3 for at least 3 months (6)[A].
- For those patients with recurrence, the risks and benefits of indefinite anticoagulation need to be assessed and considered.

MEDICATION
First Line
- LMWH:
  - Enoxaparin (Lovenox): 1 mg/kg SC BID; start warfarin simultaneously; continue enoxaparin for minimum of 5 days and until INR is >2 for 2 consecutive days, at which time enoxaparin can be stopped.
  - Fondaparinux (Arixtra): 5 mg (body weight <50 kg), 7.5 mg (body weight 50 to 100 kg), or 10 mg (body weight >100 kg) SC daily

– Tinzaparin (Innohep): 175 anti-Xa IU/kg SC daily for minimum of 5 days and patient is adequately anticoagulated with warfarin (INR of at least 2 for 2 consecutive days)

– Dalteparin (Fragmin): 200 IU/kg SC daily

- Oral anticoagulant
  – Warfarin (Coumadin) PO with dose adjusted to an INR of 2 to 3 (3)[A]
  – Apixaban (Eliquis): treatment dose: 10 mg BID × 7 days and then 5 mg BID × 3 to 6 months. Nonatrial fibrillation DVT prophylaxis: 2.5 mg BID
  – Rivaroxaban (Xarelto): treatment dose: 15 mg BID × 7 days and then 20 mg daily × 3 to 6 months. Nonatrial fibrillation prophylaxis: 10 mg daily

- Contraindications
  – Active bleeding precludes anticoagulation.
  – Risk of bleeding is a relative contraindication to long-term anticoagulation.
  – Warfarin is contraindicated in patients with history of warfarin skin necrosis (6)[A].
  – Warfarin is contraindicated in pregnancy.

- Precautions
  – Observe patient for signs of embolization, further thrombosis, or bleeding.
  – Avoid IM injections. Periodically check stool and urine for occult blood; monitor CBCs, including platelets.
  – Heparin: thrombocytopenia and/or paradoxical thrombosis with thrombocytopenia
  – Warfarin: necrotic skin lesions (typically breasts, thighs, or buttocks)
  – LMWH: Adjust dosage in renal insufficiency; may also need dose adjustment in pregnancy

- Significant possible interactions
  – Agents that intensify the response to oral anticoagulants: alcohol, allopurinol, amiodarone, anabolic steroids, androgens, many antimicrobials, cimetidine, chloral hydrate, disulfiram, all NSAIDs, sulfinpyrazone, tamoxifen, thyroid hormone, vitamin E, ranitidine, salicylates, acetaminophen
  – Agents that diminish the response to anticoagulants: aminoglutethimide, antacids, barbiturates, carbamazepine, cholestyramine, diuretics, griseofulvin, rifampin, oral contraceptives

Second Line

- Heparin 80 mg/kg IV bolus followed by 18 g/kg/hr continuous infusion
- Adjust dose depending on aPTT.
- In patients requiring large daily doses of heparin, measure an anti-Xa level for dose guidance.
- Alternatively, for outpatients, weight-adjusted subcutaneous unfractionated heparin with 333 U/kg first and then 250 U/kg, without monitoring (6)[A]
- Consider deficiency of antithrombin as a comutation in patients with significant elevated heparin requirements.

ISSUES FOR REFERRAL

- Recurrent thrombosis on anticoagulation
- Difficulty anticoagulating
- Genetic counseling
- Homozygous state in pregnancy

SURGERY/OTHER PROCEDURES

- Anticoagulation must be held for surgical interventions.
- For most patients with DVT, recommendations are against routine use of inferior vena cava filter in addition to anticoagulation, except when there is contraindication for anticoagulation (6)[A].
- Thrombectomy may be necessary in some cases.

ADMISSION, INPATIENT, AND NURSING CONSIDERATIONS

- Admission criteria/initial stabilization: complicated thrombosis, such as PE
- Nursing
  – Teach LMWH and warfarin use.
  – See earlier for drug interactions.
- Discharge criteria: stable on anticoagulation

ONGOING CARE

FOLLOW-UP RECOMMENDATIONS

Patient Monitoring

Warfarin use requires periodic (~monthly after initial stabilization) INR measurements, with a goal of 2 to 3 (6)[A].

DIET

- No restrictions
- Large amounts of foods rich in vitamin K may interfere with anticoagulation with warfarin.

PATIENT EDUCATION

- Patients should be educated about the following:
  – Use of oral anticoagulant therapy
  – Avoidance of NSAIDs while on warfarin
- The role of family screening is unclear because most patients with this mutation do not have thrombosis. In a patient with a family history of factor V Leiden, consider screening during pregnancy or if considering oral contraceptive use.

PROGNOSIS

- Most patients heterozygous for factor V Leiden do not have thrombosis.
- Homozygotes have about a 50% lifetime incidence of thrombosis.
- Recurrence rates after a first thrombosis are not clear, with some investigators finding rates as high as 5% and others finding rates similar to the general population.
- Despite the increased risk for thrombosis, factor V Leiden does not increase overall mortality.

COMPLICATIONS

- Recurrent thrombosis
- Bleeding on anticoagulation

REFERENCES

1. Dłuski D, Mierzyński R, Poniedziałek-Czajkowska E, et al. Adverse pregnancy outcomes and inherited thrombophilia. *J Perinat Med.* 2018;46(4):411–417.
2. Rosendaal FR, Koster T, Vandenbroucke JP, et al. High risk of thrombosis in patients homozygous for factor V Leiden (activated protein C resistance). *Blood.* 1995;85(6):1504–1508.
3. Glueck CJ, Goldenberg N, Wang P. Thromboembolism peaking 3 months after starting testosterone therapy: testosterone-thrombophilia interactions. *J Investig Med.* 2018;66(4):733–738.
4. Dobry AS, Ko LN, St John J, et al. Association between hypercoagulable conditions and calciphylaxis in patients with renal disease: a case-control study. *JAMA Dermatol.* 2018;154(2):182–187.
5. Lijfering WM, Middeldorp S, Veeger NJ, et al. Risk of recurrent venous thrombosis in homozygous carriers and double heterozygous carriers of factor V Leiden and prothrombin G20210A. *Circulation.* 2010;121(15):1706–1712.
6. Eichinger S, Weltermann A, Mannhalter C, et al. The risk of recurrent venous thromboembolism in heterozygous carriers of factor V Leiden and a first spontaneous venous thromboembolism. *Arch Intern Med.* 2002;162(20):2357–2360.
7. Bauersachs R, Berkowitz SD, Brenner B, et al; for EINSTEIN Investigators. Oral rivaroxaban for symptomatic venous thromboembolism. *N Engl J Med.* 2010;363(26):2499–2510.

ADDITIONAL READING

Seligsohn U, Lubetsky A. Genetic susceptibility to venous thrombosis. *N Engl J Med.* 2001;344(16):1222–1231.

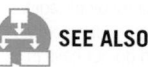 SEE ALSO

Deep Vein Thrombophlebitis

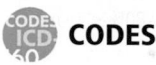 CODES

ICD10

D68.51 Activated protein C resistance

CLINICAL PEARLS

- Extremely rare in Asian and African populations
- Asymptomatic patients with factor V Leiden do not need anticoagulation.
- For pregnant women homozygous for factor V Leiden but no prior history of VTE, postpartum prophylaxis with prophylactic or intermediate-dose LMWH or vitamin K antagonists with target INR 2 to 3 for 6 weeks is recommended. Antepartum prophylaxis is added if there is positive family history of VTE.

F

FAILURE TO THRIVE
Durr-e-Shahwaar Sayed, DO

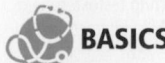 **BASICS**

DESCRIPTION
- Failure to thrive (FTT) is not a diagnosis but a sign of inadequate nutrition in young children manifested by a failure of physical growth, usually affecting weight. In severe cases, decreased length and/or head circumference may develop.
- Various parameters are used to define FTT, but in clinical practice, it is commonly defined as either weight or BMI for age that falls below the 5th percentile on more than one occasion or weight that drops two or more major percentile lines on standard growth charts OR weight-for-length falls below the 5th percentile.
- A combination of anthropometric criteria rather than one criterion should be used to identify children at risk of FTT (1)[C].

Pediatric Considerations
- Children with genetic syndromes, intrauterine growth restriction (IUGR), or prematurity follow different growth curves.
- 25% of children will decrease their weight or height crossing ≥2 major percentile lines in the first 2 years of life. These children are failing to reach their genetic potential or demonstrating constitutional growth delay (slow growth with a bone age < chronologic age). After shifting down, these infants grow at a normal rate along their new percentile and do not have FTT.

EPIDEMIOLOGY
Incidence
- Predominant age: 6 to 12 months; 80% <18 months
- Predominant sex: male = female

Prevalence
- As many as 10% of children seen in primary care have signs of growth failure.
- 1–5% of pediatric inpatient admissions are for FTT.
- Occurs more frequently in children living in poverty (1)

ETIOLOGY AND PATHOPHYSIOLOGY
- Mismatch between caloric intake and caloric expenditure
- Often grouped into four major categories:
  - Inadequate caloric intake (most frequent)
  - Inadequate caloric absorption
  - Excessive caloric expenditure
  - Defective utilization
- Traditionally, FTT was classified as organic or nonorganic, but most cases are multifactorial.
- FTT often begins with a specific event and may lead to persistent difficulties.
- Causes of FTT can be grouped by pathophysiology (including examples):
  - Inadequate intake: breastfeeding difficulty, incorrect formula preparation, poor transition to food (6 to 12 months), poor feeding habits (e.g., excessive juice, restrictive diets), mechanical problems (e.g., oromotor dysfunction, congenital anomalies, GERD, CNS, or PNS anomalies), oral aversion, poverty, neglect, poor parent–child interaction, caregiver feeding style
  - Inadequate absorption: necrotizing enterocolitis, short gut syndrome, biliary atresia, liver disease, cystic fibrosis, celiac disease, milk protein allergy, vitamin/mineral deficiency, environmental enteric dysfunction
  - Increased expenditure: hyperthyroidism, congenital/chronic cardiopulmonary disease, HIV, immunodeficiencies, malignancy, renal disease
  - Defective utilization: metabolic disorders, congenital infections (TORCH: toxoplasmosis, other agents, rubella, cytomegalovirus, herpes simplex)

Genetics
Multiple genetic disorders can cause FTT.

RISK FACTORS
- Psychosocial risks (2)
  - Poverty, parent(s) with mental health disorder or cognitive impairment, poor parenting skills or hypervigilant parents, families with unique health/nutritional beliefs, physical or emotional abuse, substance abuse, and social isolation
- Medical risks (2)
  - Intrauterine exposures, history of IUGR (symmetric or asymmetric), congenital abnormalities, oromotor dysfunction, premature or sick newborn, infant with physical deformity, acute or chronic medical conditions, developmental delay, lead poisoning, anemia

Pregnancy Considerations
FTT is linked to intrauterine exposures, IUGR, and prematurity.

GENERAL PREVENTION
- Educate parents on normal feeding and parenting skills.
- Access to supplemental feeding programs (Women, Infants, and Children [WIC])

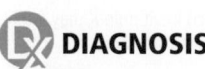 **DIAGNOSIS**

HISTORY
- Successful treatment of FTT almost always is accomplished by a careful and detailed history because most cases are due to underfeeding or inappropriate feeding.
- Prenatal and developmental history
- Past medical history: acute/chronic disease affecting caloric intake, digestion, absorption, or causing increased energy need or defective utilization
- Medication history, including complementary and alternative medications
- Family history: stature of parents and growth trajectories of siblings, chronic diseases, genetic disorders, developmental delay
- Diet history from birth: breastfeeding or formula feeding; timing and introduction of solids; who feeds the child, when, and how often; placement of child during feeds; amounts consumed/caloric intake; beverages consumed; snacking; vomiting or stooling associated with feeds; oral aversions or unusual behaviors during feeding
- Social history: family composition, socioeconomic status, hygiene practices, child-rearing beliefs, stressors, parental depression, parental substance abuse, caretaker personal history of abuse/neglect
- Review of systems: anorexia, activity level, mental status, fevers, dysphagia, vomiting, gastroesophageal reflux, stooling pattern/consistency, dysuria, urinary frequency

PHYSICAL EXAM
- A combination of anthropometric criteria, rather than one criterion, should be used, and measurements over time are required for diagnosis (1).
- Accurate measurement of height, weight, and head circumference on National Center for Health Statistics (NCHS) (https://www.cdc.gov/growthcharts/) growth charts may be more appropriate for breastfed infants (http://www.who.int/childgrowth/standards/en/).
- Growth charts exist for many other syndromes/conditions such as Down syndrome, Turner syndrome, and the premature infant.

- Exam should assess for the following:
  - Signs of dehydration or severe malnutrition are as follows:
    - Severity of malnutrition estimated via Gomez classification: Compare current weight for age with expected weight for age (50th percentile): severe, <60% of expected; moderate, 61–75%; mild, 76–90%.
  - Underlying medical disease
  - Dysmorphic features
  - Mental status (alert, responsive to stimuli)
  - Any signs of physical abuse and/or neglect
- Observe interaction with caregivers and feeding techniques, specifically bonding and social/psychological cues.

DIFFERENTIAL DIAGNOSIS
Differentiate based on growth patterns.
- FTT classically presents as low weight for age, with normal linear growth and head circumference OR low weight for age, followed by decreased linear growth OR low weight for age, leading to decreased linear growth and decreased head circumference (without neurologic signs).
  - In this situation, consider differential diagnosis as outlined in "Etiology and Pathophysiology."
- If low linear growth with normal weight for length or low linear growth and proportionately low weight and decreased head circumference:
  - Consider genetic potential (constitutional short stature or growth delay), genetic syndromes, teratogens, and endocrine disorders.
- If microcephaly with prominent neurologic signs, with poor growth secondary to presumed neurologic disorder:
  - Consider TORCH infections, genetic syndromes, teratogens, and brain injury (i.e., hypoxic/ischemic).

DIAGNOSTIC TESTS & INTERPRETATION
- Labs useful only in ~1% of cases and are generally not recommended (1,3)[C]
- A period of addressing nutritional causes is preferable prior to extensive labs and other workup.

Initial Tests (lab, imaging)
Labs should be ordered based on history and physical exam findings and the age of the patient.
- Tests often considered in initial evaluation:
  - CBC, ESR
  - Electrolytes, BUN/creatinine, liver function tests
  - Urinalysis and urine culture
  - Lead level
- Other tests as dictated by the history and exam:
  - TSH, amylase/lipase, serum zinc level, iron studies, karyotype, genetic testing, sweat chloride test, stool for ova and parasite or fat/reducing substances, guaiac, α_1-antitrypsin and elastase, radioallergosorbent test for IgE food allergies, tissue transglutaminase and total IgA (celiac sprue), p-ANCA and anti–*Saccharomyces cerevisiae* antibodies (for inflammatory bowel disease [IBD]), TB test, HIV, hepatitis A and B, other infections

Follow-Up Tests & Special Considerations
- Prospective 3-day food diary for accurate record of caloric intake should be obtained.
- Home visit by a clinician to observe infant feeding, interaction of caretakers, and home environment (3,4)[B]
- Observe breastfeeding and/or formula preparation to ensure adequacy and offer instruction.

- Additional indicated evaluations may be performed by dietitians; occupational, physical, and speech therapists; social workers; developmental specialists; psychiatrists; psychologists; visiting nurses; lactation consultants; and/or child protection services.
- Can consider
  - Skeletal survey if suspicion of physical abuse
  - Bone age if possible endocrine disorder
  - Swallowing studies, small bowel follow-through if possible oromotor dysfunction, GERD, structural abnormalities
  - Brain imaging if microcephalic and/or neurologic findings on examination
  - Echocardiogram if murmur auscultated

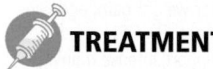 **TREATMENT**

GENERAL MEASURES
- Treat underlying conditions.
- Caregiver and infant interaction should be evaluated in infants and children with FTT.
- Age-appropriate nutritional counseling should be provided (1)[C].
  - The goal is to improve nutrition to allow catch-up growth (weight gain 2 to 3 times > average for age).
- Calculate energy needs based on recommended energy intake for age and then increase by 50%.
- Alternatively, may calculate caloric requirements for infants to achieve catch-up growth
  - kcal/kg/day required = RDA for age (kcal/kg) × ideal weight for height/actual weight, where ideal weight for height is the median weight for the patient's height
- Try various strategies to increase caloric intake, such as the following:
  - Optimize breastfeeding support; consider supplementation.
  - Higher calorie formulas
  - Addition of rice cereal or fats to current foods
  - Limit intake of milk to 24 to 32 oz/day.
  - Avoid juice and soda.
  - Vitamin and/or nutritional supplements
  - Assist with social and family problems (WIC, food stamps, and other transitional assistance).
- Rapid high-calorie intake can cause diarrhea, malabsorption, hypokalemia, and hypophosphatemia. Therefore, increasing formulas >24 kcal/oz is not recommended.
- The target energy intake should be slowly increased to goal over 5 to 7 days.
- Catch-up growth should be seen in 2 to 7 days.
- Accelerated growth should be continued for 4 to 9 months to restore weight and height.

MEDICATION
Use only for identified underlying conditions.

ISSUES FOR REFERRAL
- Refer as indicated for underlying conditions.
- Multidisciplinary care is beneficial (1)[A]. Specialized multidisciplinary clinics may be of benefit for children with complicated situations, failure to respond to initial treatment, or when the PCP does not have access to specialized services such as nutrition, psychology, PT/OT, and speech therapy.

ADDITIONAL THERAPIES
In severe cases, nasogastric tube feedings or gastrostomy may be considered.

ADMISSION, INPATIENT, AND NURSING CONSIDERATIONS
- Most cases of FTT can be managed as outpatients.
- Hospitalization should be considered if (1)[C]:
  - Outpatient management fails.
  - There is evidence of severe dehydration or malnutrition.
  - There are signs of abuse or neglect.
  - There are concerns that the psychosocial situation presents harm to child.
  - During catch-up growth, some children will develop nutritional recovery syndrome:
    - Symptoms include sweating, increased body temperature, hepatomegaly (increased glycogen deposits), widening of cranial sutures (brain growth > bone growth), increased periods of sleep, fidgetiness, and mild hyperactivity.
  - There may also be an initial period of malabsorption with resultant diarrhea.
- Catch-up growth should be seen in 2 to 7 days. If this is not seen, reevaluation of causes is needed.

 ONGOING CARE

FOLLOW-UP RECOMMENDATIONS
- If specific disease is identified, follow up as indicated.
- Close, long-term follow-up with frequent visits is important to create and maintain a healthy, supportive environment (3,4)[B].
- Children with history of FTT are at increased risk of recurrent FTT, and long-term sequelae and growth should be monitored closely (1,4)[B].
- If the family fails to comply, child protection authorities must be notified.

DIET
Nutritional requirements for a "normal" child:
- Infant
  - 120 kcal/kg/day, decreased to 95 kcal/kg/day at 6 months; if breastfed, ensure appropriate frequency and duration of feeding.
  - Between 6 and 12 months, continue breast milk and/or formula, but pureed foods should be consumed several times a day during this period.
- Toddler
  - Three meals plus two nutritional snacks, 16 to 32 oz of milk per day; avoid juice and soda and feed in a social environment.
  - Do not restrict fat and cholesterol in children <2 years.
- Rate of weight gain expected for age:
  - 0 to 3 months: 26 to 31 g/day
  - 3 to 6 months: 17 to 18 g/day
  - 6 to 9 months: 12 to 13 g/day
  - 9 to 12 months: 9 g/day
  - 1 to 3 years: 7 to 9 g/day

PATIENT EDUCATION
- Counsel parents regarding the need to avoid "food battles," which worsen the problem.
- Educate parents regarding infant social and physiologic cues, formula/food preparation, proper feeding techniques, and importance of relaxed and social mealtimes.
- When environmental deprivation is identified, educating in a nonpunitive way is essential.

- "Failure to thrive: What this means for your child," available from AAFP at: https://www.aafp.org/afp/2011/0401/p837.html
- WIC provides grants to states for supplemental foods, health care referrals, and nutrition education for low-income pregnant, breastfeeding, and nonbreastfeeding postpartum women and to infants and children up to age 5 years at nutritional risk: https://www.fns.usda.gov/wic/women-infants-and-children-wic

PROGNOSIS
- Many children with FTT show adequate improvement in dietary intake with intervention (2)[B].
- Some studies looking at children with FTT have demonstrated an association with later problems with cognitive development, behavioral issues, and growth, but there is no consensus on these long-term outcomes or their clinical significance (1,4).
- Children with FTT are at increased risk for future undernutrition, overnutrition, and eating disorders.

REFERENCES

1. Cole SZ, Lanham JS. Failure to thrive: an update. *Am Fam Physician.* 2011;83(7):829–834.
2. Black MM, Tilton N, Bento S, et al. Recovery in young children with weight faltering: child and household risk factors. *J Pediatr.* 2016;170:301–306.
3. Shields B, Wacogne I, Wright CM. Weight faltering and failure to thrive in infancy and early childhood. *BMJ.* 2012;345:e5931.
4. Black MM, Dubowitz H, Krishnakumar A, et al. Early intervention and recovery among children with failure to thrive: follow-up at age 8. *Pediatrics.* 2007;120(1):59–69.

ADDITIONAL READING

- Atalay A, McCord M. Characteristics of failure to thrive in a referral population: implications for treatment. *Clin Pediatr (Phila).* 2012;51(3):219–225.
- Homan GJ. Failure to thrive: a practical guide. *Am Fam Physician.* 2016;94(4):295–299.
- Jaffe AC. Failure to thrive: current clinical concepts. *Pediatr Rev.* 2011;32(3):100–107.
- Kerzner B, Milano K, MacLean WC Jr, et al. A practical approach to classifying and managing feeding difficulties. *Pediatrics.* 2015;135(2):344–353.
- Krugman SD, Dubowitz H. Failure to thrive. *Am Fam Physician.* 2003;68(5):879–884.

 CODES

ICD10
- R62.51 Failure to thrive (child)
- P92.6 Failure to thrive in newborn

CLINICAL PEARLS
- FTT is a sign of inadequate nutrition. It is rarely due to a medical condition.
- Underlying medical and/or social issues are generally suggested by history and physical exam, and extensive laboratory or imaging tests are rarely needed.
- A multidisciplinary team approach to diagnosis and treatment is critical to help children with FTT and their families.
- Prompt diagnosis and intervention is important to decrease the risk of adverse effects.

FEMALE ATHLETE TRIAD

Miranda Gordon-Zigel, MD • Rahul Kapur, MD, CAQSM

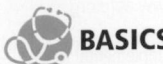 **BASICS**

Syndrome of three interrelated clinical entities: low energy availability (EA) (with or without disordered eating [DE]), menstrual dysfunction (MD), and low bone mineral density (BMD) (1). There is also emerging research to suggest an expanded syndrome referred to as Relative Energy Deficiency in Sport (RED-S), which acknowledges that male athletes maybe at risk (2).

DESCRIPTION
- Female athlete triad was first described in 1992: Patients may meet criteria for only one or two parts of the triad.
- 2014 Female Athlete Triad Coalition consensus statement and the 2007 American College of Sports Medicine (ACSM) position stand suggest (1):
  – Each component of the triad represents a spectrum ranging from health to dysfunction.
  – EA is fundamental to the propagation of the triad.
  – Full recovery is not possible without correction of low EA.
- The International Olympic Committee's updated position statement from 2014 now considers RED-S to be a more accurate representation of the psychological and physiologic stresses placed on the athlete's body.
- Metabolic rate, menstrual function, bone health, immunity, protein synthesis, and cardiovascular and psychological health are all effected (2).
- Prevention and early intervention are essential to prevent progression to serious clinical end points of eating disorders, amenorrhea, and osteoporosis.
- RED-S also takes into account the effects of relative energy deficiency on male athletes, who are often affected in weight-sensitive sports (gymnastics, wrestling, cycling, etc.) (2).
- The changes in physiology should be viewed as a spectrum, with normal EA, BMD, and regular menses at one extreme and clinical eating disorders, osteoporosis, and amenorrhea at the other (2).
- EA
  – Dietary energy intake minus exercise energy expenditure; the core element of the triad
  – Represents the amount of dietary energy remaining for bodily functions after correcting for exercise training
  – EA (kcal/kg FFM/day) = [EI (kcal/day) − EEE (kcal/day)] where EEE is effective energy expenditure and FFM is fat free mass
  – Low EA results in reduced capacity for cellular maintenance, thermoregulation, and growth.
  – Low EA serves a causal role in the induction of exercise-associated menstrual disturbances.
  – Low EA occurs either intentionally or inadvertently. Examples include increasing training disproportionately to energy intake; DE; and reducing energy intake by restricting, fasting, binging, and purging or use of diet pills, laxatives, diuretics, or enemas. Not all athletes meet diagnostic criteria from *Diagnostic and Statistical Manual of Mental Disorders*, 5th edition (*DSM-5*) for eating disorders.
- MD
  – Low EA alters the hypothalamic-pituitary axis, resulting in functional hypothalamic amenorrhea.
  – MD ranges from eumenorrhea to amenorrhea.
  – MD includes athletes who have low estrogen levels but still experience menstruation.
  – Energy deficit results in MD at ∼30 kcal/kg lean body mass per day.
  – MD includes luteal suppression (shortened luteal phase, prolonged follicular phase, and decreased

estradiol level), anovulation, oligomenorrhea (menstrual cycle >35 days), and primary and secondary hypothalamic amenorrhea.
  – Primary amenorrhea (no menarche by age 15 years), although less common, can occur in young athletes. Secondary amenorrhea is defined as the absence of menstrual cycles for >3 months after menarche has been established.
  – Although hypothalamic suppression is the most common cause of secondary amenorrhea in these athletes, other causes must be ruled out.
- BMD
  – Ranges from optimal bone health to osteoporosis
  – Peak BMD occurs at 19 years in females and 20.5 years in males.
  – Bone health encompasses bone strength as well as bone quality. The current practice standard (dual energy x-ray absorptiometry [DEXA]) measures bone density, not bone quality. This research may help providers better understand why two athletes with the same BMD may have very different bone fracture histories (3).
    ○ ACSM position stand recommends using the International Society for Clinical Densitometry (ISCD) guidelines for BMD Z-scores <−2.0 with a history of clinically significant fracture for diagnosis of osteoporosis.
    ○ Because most athletes have a higher BMD than nonathletes, ACSM recommends further workup for any athlete with a Z-score <−1, even in the absence of fracture.
  – Endothelial dysfunction
    ○ Emerging evidence suggests that the female athlete triad is associated with endothelial dysfunction. Reduced levels of estrogen alter vasodilation. Athletic amenorrhea is associated with reduced brachial artery flow-mediated dilation, which has a 95% positive predictive value for coronary endothelial dysfunction. Consequences include decreased blood flow to muscles during exercise and accelerated atherosclerosis. In the future, this clinical syndrome may be considered a tetrad (4).

EPIDEMIOLOGY
Prevalence
- Overall prevalence: 0–16% of female athletes (5). Prevalence of two criteria varies: MD + BMD 0–8% (*n* = 460), MD + LE 18% (*n* = 80), and BMD + LE 4% (*n* = 80) (3).
- DE higher than general population (3)
- MD: Prevalence of secondary amenorrhea is as high as 60% in female athletes compared to 2–5% in the general population (3).
- Bone health: Using the World Health Organization (WHO) criteria for low BMD, prevalence of osteopenia (T-score between −1 and −2) ranges from 0% to 40% in female athletes, as compared to ∼12% in the general population (3).

ETIOLOGY AND PATHOPHYSIOLOGY
- In functional hypothalamic amenorrhea, low EA disrupts the hypothalamic-pituitary-ovarian axis, decreasing pulsatile gonadotropin-releasing hormone (GnRH).
- Low GnRH levels decrease luteinizing hormone (LH) and follicle-stimulating hormone (FSH) levels, decreasing estrogen production with resultant MD.
- Estrogen deficiency negatively affects bone density. A chronic state of malnutrition reduces the rate of bone formation and increases the rate of bone resorption. Changes in bone metabolism occur within 5 days of reductions in EA.

RISK FACTORS
- History of menstrual irregularities and amenorrhea; history of stress fractures and recurrent or nonhealing injuries; history of critical comments about eating or weight from parent or coach; history of depression; history of dieting; personality factors, including perfectionism and/or obsessiveness, overtraining, and inappropriate coaching behaviors (1)
- Lean physique, sports with an aesthetic component (ballet, figure skating, gymnastics, distance running, diving, and swimming), or sports with weight classifications (martial arts and wrestling). Frequent weigh-ins, consequences for weight gain, and win-at-all-cost attitude all increase risk (2).
- A lack of family or social support; intense training hours; social isolation, or entering a new environment (boarding school or college); an athlete with comorbid psychological conditions (anxiety, depression, and/or obsessive-compulsive disorder)

GENERAL PREVENTION
- Education of athletes (middle school through college), coaches, trainers, parents, and physicians. Young athletes are extremely impressionable and may turn negative comments and unhealthy advice into maladaptive eating and exercising habits.
- General screening during preparticipation exam (PPE) and annual physicals are endorsed by AAP, AAFP, ACSM, AOSSM, and AMSSM (6).
- Female Athlete Triad Coalition has 11-question screening to use during PPE (1).
- Screen athletes presenting with "red flag" conditions such as fractures, weight changes, fatigue, amenorrhea, bradycardia, orthostatic hypotension, syncope, arrhythmias, electrolyte abnormalities, or depression.

COMMONLY ASSOCIATED CONDITIONS
- Anorexia nervosa, bulimia nervosa, avoidant or restrictive food intake disorder, and other psychological disorders, including low self-esteem, depression, and anxiety (5)
- Low BMD predisposes athletes to stress fractures and may not be fully reversible. This may lead to a higher rate of fractures after menopause.

DIAGNOSIS

- The female athlete triad is a clinical diagnosis based primarily on patient history; screening for the female athlete triad at annual sports physicals or during routine exams and acute visits if there are concerns (1,5)[A]
- EDE-17 is the gold standard for eating disorder diagnosis.

HISTORY
Assess menstrual history (including hormonal contraceptive use), fracture history, and symptoms of depression. Assess dietary practices, eating behaviors, and history of weight changes. Dietary intake logs and a nutritional assessment by a sports dietitian can help. Assess body image, fear of weight gain, fluctuations in weight, history of DE, and use of laxatives, diet pills, or enemas.

PHYSICAL EXAM
- Height, weight, body mass index (BMI) <17.5% kg/m², <85% of expected body weight in adolescents, or ≥10% weight loss in 1 month (1)
- Common findings include bradycardia, orthostatic hypotension, hypothermia, cold or cyanotic extremities, lanugo, parotid gland enlargement or tenderness, epigastric tenderness, eroded tooth enamel, and knuckle or hand calluses (Russell sign).

- Patients with amenorrhea should undergo a pelvic exam to verify the presence of a uterus and evaluate for outflow tract abnormalities. Vaginal atrophy may be present if the patient is in a low estrogen state.

DIFFERENTIAL DIAGNOSIS

Screen for anorexia nervosa, bulimia nervosa, avoidant/restrictive food intake disorder, and rumination disorder using the *DSM-5* criteria. Rule out the following in amenorrheic patients:

- Pregnancy
- Endocrine abnormalities: thyroid dysfunction, Cushing syndrome
- Hypothalamic dysfunction: psychological stress-induced amenorrhea, medication-induced amenorrhea, Kallmann syndrome
- Pituitary dysfunction: prolactinoma, Sheehan syndrome, sarcoidosis, empty sella syndrome
- Ovarian dysfunction: polycystic ovarian syndrome, premature ovarian failure, menopause, gonadal dysgenesis, Turner syndrome, ovarian neoplasm, autoimmune disease
- Uterine dysfunction: Asherman syndrome, absence of uterus

DIAGNOSTIC TESTS & INTERPRETATION

Initial Tests (lab, imaging)

- Basic metabolic panel, magnesium, phosphorus, albumin, CBC with differential, ESR, thyroid-stimulating hormone (TSH), calcium, 25-OH vitamin D, and urinalysis (1,5)
- Evaluation for secondary amenorrhea includes urine hCG and serum FSH, LH, prolactin, and TSH.
- Pelvic ultrasound in patients with hyperandrogenism to exclude polycystic ovaries or virilizing ovarian tumors
- ECG to rule out prolonged QT interval

Follow-Up Tests & Special Considerations

- BMD testing by DEXA is based on a risk stratification model (1). Risk factors include DE, eating disorders >6 months, hypoestrogenism, amenorrhea, oligomenorrhea, and/or in patients with a history of stress fractures or fractures from minimal impact.
- If components of the triad persist, ISCD 2013 guidelines suggest reevaluation by the same DEXA machine every 1 to 2 years.

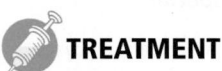 ## TREATMENT

- The goal is to optimize nutritional status and treat maladaptive behavioral disorders (1,3)[A].
- A multidisciplinary team including a physician, registered dietitian, and behavioral health provider. Build open lines of communication with coaches, trainers, and family.
- A positive EA of >30 kcal/kg of fat-free muscle mass per day is sufficient to restore menses (5)[A].
- Physically active females should strive for an EA of >45 kcal/kg of fat-free muscle mass per day (1)[A].

MEDICATION

First Line

- Increasing EA through appropriate nutrition is the best strategy for normalizing gonadotropin pulsatility and release. The use of combination oral contraceptive pills (cOCPs), hormone replacement therapy (HRT), and/or bisphosphonates has not been clearly shown to increase BMD or aid in the restoration of normal menstrual cycling. Transdermal estradiol with cyclic oral progesterone can be considered in patients with particularly low BMD Z-scores and fracture histories who do not respond to 1 year of nonpharmacologic management.

- Transdermal estradiol can also be given to minimize further bone loss in patients >16 years and <21 years who, despite adequate nutrition and body weight gain, continue to have decreasing BMD and functional hypothalamic amenorrhea.
- cOCPs do have potential to mask signs of RED-S and do not correct underlying energy deficiency. They can also suppress androgen release, potentially causing a decrease in BMD (2).
- Provide calcium (1,500 mg/day) and vitamin D supplementation to maintain serum levels within 32 to 50 mg/mL (1)[A].
- In male athletes, with RED-S, testosterone replacement therapy can be helpful in patients with hypogonadism and osteoporosis (2).

ADMISSION, INPATIENT, AND NURSING CONSIDERATIONS

Evaluate patients with eating disorders for potentially life-threatening conditions requiring hospital admission, including bradycardia, severe orthostatic hypotension, significant electrolyte imbalances, hypothermia, arrhythmias, or prolonged QT interval.

 ## ONGOING CARE

- Patients should have regular follow-up with a multidisciplinary treatment team (6)[A].
- Cognitive-behavioral therapy (CBT) is effective for exercising women with DE and may be more beneficial than nutritional counseling alone in women with DE behavior.
- "Clearance and Return to Play (RTP) Guidelines by Medical Risk Stratification" helps determine when to allow an athlete to return to competition. More research is needed to validate this model (1)[A].
- To continue training and competing, athletes with eating disorders must agree to the following stipulations as part of a behavioral contract: to comply with all treatment strategies; to be closely monitored by health care providers; to place treatment goals over training goals; and to modify the type, duration, and intensity of training or competition as necessary.
- The RED-S Risk Assessment Model can be used to aid decision to clear athletes to return to play (2).

PATIENT EDUCATION

- All young female patients should be counseled on the importance of proper nutrition, calcium and vitamin D intake, and the benefits of regular weight-bearing exercise. Patients presenting with ≥1 components of the triad should be educated about the short- and long-term effects of low BMD (1,3)[A].
- RED-S effects on performance: decrease endurance, increased injury risk, decreased training response, impaired judgment, decreased coordination, decreased concentration, irritability, depression, decreased glycogen stores, decreased muscle strength (2)

PROGNOSIS

- The short- and long-term prognosis for patients with female athlete triad depends on time to diagnosis and response to treatment.
- It is estimated that amenorrheic women will lose 2–3% of bone mass per year without intervention.
- With early diagnosis and treatment using a multidisciplinary team, the prognosis for patients with the female athlete triad is good. Patients regain normal menstrual cycling and increase BMD.
- Because the triad often occurs within the age window of optimal bone strengthening, patients with a prolonged disease course may suffer from

complications of decreased BMD throughout their adolescent and adult life.
- Patients with DE behaviors often require long-term therapy to manage their disease.

REFERENCES

1. De Souza MJ, Nattiv A, Joy E, et al. 2014 Female Athlete Triad Coalition consensus statement on treatment and return to play of the female athlete triad: 1st International Conference held in San Francisco, CA, May 2012, and 2nd International Conference held in Indianapolis, IN, May 2013. *Clin J Sport Med.* 2014;24(2):96–119.
2. Mountjoy M, Sundgot-Borgen J, Burke L, et al. The IOC consensus statement: beyond the Female Athlete Triad—Relative Energy Deficiency in Sport (RED-S). *Br J Sports Med.* 2014;48(7):491–497.
3. Barrack MT, Ackerman KE, Gibbs JC. Update on the female athlete triad. *Curr Rev Musculoskelet Med.* 2013;6(2):195–204.
4. Lanser EM, Zach KN, Hoch AZ. The female athlete triad and endothelial dysfunction. *PM R.* 2011;3(5):458–465.
5. Temme KE, Hoch AZ. Recognition and rehabilitation of the female athlete triad/tetrad: a multidisciplinary approach. *Curr Sports Med Rep.* 2013;12(3):190–199.
6. Deimel JF, Dunlap BJ. The female athlete triad. *Clin Sports Med.* 2012;31(2):247–254.

ADDITIONAL READING

Nattiv A, Loucks AB, Manore MM, et al. American College of Sports Medicine position stand. The female athlete triad. *Med Sci Sports Exerc.* 2007;39(10):1867–1882.

 ## SEE ALSO

Algorithms: Amenorrhea, Primary (Absence of Menarche by Age 16 Years); Amenorrhea, Secondary; Weight Loss, Unintentional

 ## CODES

ICD10

- F50.9 Eating disorder, unspecified
- N91.2 Amenorrhea, unspecified
- R53.83 Other fatigue

CLINICAL PEARLS

- The female athlete triad consists of low EA (with or without DE), MD, and low BMD. Athletes may exhibit varying degrees of dysfunction in any of these three areas. There is emerging research regarding an expanded syndrome called RED-S.
- Screen at-risk women and men to allow for early diagnosis and intervention.
- Early intervention by a multidisciplinary team, including physicians, registered dietitians, mental health professionals, coaches, trainers, and parents, is the most successful strategy to minimize further bone loss, recover BMD, and regain normal menstrual function.
- Current guidelines recommend screening for abnormal BMD using DEXA studies for patients with DE, eating disorders >6 months, hypoestrogenism, amenorrhea, oligomenorrhea, and/or in patients with a history of stress fractures or fractures from minimal impact.

F

FEVER OF UNKNOWN ORIGIN (FUO)

Scott T. Henderson, MD

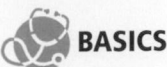 **BASICS**

DESCRIPTION

- Classic definition
  - Repeated fever >38.3°C
  - Fever duration at least 3 weeks
  - Diagnosis remains uncertain after 1 week of study in the hospital.
- The definition of fever of unknown origin (FUO) has evolved and is based on patient characteristics and presentation. The need for in-hospital evaluation has been eliminated in previously healthy people.
- Some expand the definition to include nosocomial, neutropenic (immunodeficient), and HIV-associated fevers.

EPIDEMIOLOGY

Incidence
Incidence unclear

ETIOLOGY, PATHOPHYSIOLOGY, AND DIFFERENTIAL DIAGNOSIS

- >200 causes; each with prevalence of ≤5%
- Most commonly, FUO is an atypical presentation of a common condition.
- Spectrum of causes varies widely.
  - Noninfectious inflammatory diseases are the most frequent causes in high-income countries. Common causes include temporal arteritis, polymyalgia rheumatica, or rheumatoid arthritis.
- Infection
  - Abdominal or pelvic abscesses
  - Amebic hepatitis
  - Catheter infections
  - Cytomegalovirus
  - Dental abscesses
  - Endocarditis/pericarditis
  - HIV (advanced stage)
  - Mycobacterial infection (often with advanced HIV)
  - Osteomyelitis
  - Pyelonephritis or renal abscess
  - Sinusitis
  - Wound infections
  - Other miscellaneous infections
- Neoplasms
  - Atrial myxoma
  - Colorectal cancer and other GI malignancies
  - Hepatoma
  - Lymphoma
  - Leukemia
  - Solid tumors (renal cell carcinoma)
- Noninfectious inflammatory disease
  - Connective tissue diseases
    ○ Adult Still disease
    ○ Rheumatoid arthritis
    ○ Systemic lupus erythematosus
  - Granulomatous disease
    ○ Crohn disease
    ○ Sarcoidosis
  - Vasculitis syndromes
    ○ Giant cell arteritis
    ○ Polymyalgia rheumatica

- Other causes
  - Alcoholic hepatitis
  - Cerebrovascular accident
  - Cirrhosis
  - Medications
    ○ Allopurinol, captopril, carbamazepine, cephalosporins, cimetidine, clofibrate, erythromycin, heparin, hydralazine, hydrochlorothiazide, isoniazid, meperidine, methyldopa, nifedipine, nitrofurantoin, penicillin, phenytoin, procainamide, quinidine, sulfonamides
  - Endocrine disease
  - Factitious/fraudulent fever
  - Occupational causes
  - Periodic fever
  - Pulmonary emboli/deep vein thrombosis
  - Thermoregulatory disorders
- In up to 20–30% of cases, the cause of the fever is never identified despite a thorough workup.

RISK FACTORS

- Recent travel (malaria, enteric fevers)
- Exposure to biologic or chemical agents
- HIV infection (particularly in acute infection and advanced stages)
- Elderly
- Drug abuse
- Immigrants
- Young, (typically) female health care workers (factitious fever)

Geriatric Considerations
Common causes of geriatric infections include intra-abdominal abscess, urinary tract infection, tuberculosis, (TB) and endocarditis. Other common causes of FUO in patients >65 years include malignancies (particularly hematologic cancers) and drug-induced fever.

Pediatric Considerations
- ~50% of FUO in pediatric cases are infectious. Collagen vascular disease and malignancy are common.
- Inflammatory bowel disease is a common cause of FUO in older children and adolescents.

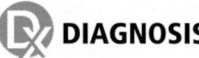 **DIAGNOSIS**

HISTORY

- Onset and pattern of fever
- Constitutional symptoms:
  - Chills, night sweats, myalgias, weight loss with an intact appetite (infectious etiology)
  - Arthralgias, myalgias, fatigue (inflammatory etiology)
  - Fatigue, night sweats, weight loss with loss of appetite (neoplastic etiology)
- Past medical history: chronic infections, abdominal diseases, transfusion history, malignancy, psychiatric illness, and recent hospitalization
- Past surgical history: type of surgery performed, postoperative complications, and any indwelling foreign material
- Comprehensive medication history, including over-the-counter and herbal products

- Family history, such as periodic fever syndromes and recent febrile illnesses in close contacts
- Social history: travel, exposures, living environment, sexual activity, recreational drug use

ALERT
Obtain a thorough travel, psychosocial, occupational, sexual, and drug use history.

PHYSICAL EXAM
Physical findings with high diagnostic yield
- Funduscopic exam for choroid tubercles or Roth spots
- Temporal artery tenderness
- Oral-mucosal lesions
- Cardiac auscultation for bruits and murmurs
- Pulmonary exam: consolidation or effusion
- Abdominal palpation for organomegaly and tenderness or peritoneal signs
- Rectal examination for blood, fluctuance, and/or tenderness
- Testicular examination
- Lymph node examination
- Skin and nail bed exam for clubbing, nodules, lesions, and erosions
- Focal neurologic signs
- Musculoskeletal exam for tenderness or effusion
- Serial exams help identify evolving physical signs (e.g., findings associated with endocarditis).

DIAGNOSTIC TESTS & INTERPRETATION

Initial Tests (lab, imaging)
- CBC, C-reactive protein, ESR
- Peripheral blood smear
- Electrolytes, BUN, and creatinine; LFT; calcium
- Lactate dehydrogenase
- HIV testing
- Blood cultures (not to exceed six sets)
- Urinalysis and urine culture
- Chest x-ray
- CT or MRI of abdomen and pelvis (with directed biopsy, if indicated) (1)[C]

Follow-Up Tests & Special Considerations
- Rheumatoid factor and antinuclear antibody test
- Serologies: Epstein-Barr, hepatitis, syphilis, Lyme disease, Q fever, cytomegalovirus, brucellosis, amebiasis, coccidioidomycosis
- Serum ferritin
- Serum procalcitonin
- Serum protein electrophoresis
- AFB smear
- Sputum and urine cultures for TB
- TB testing
  - Tuberculin skin test
    ○ May not be helpful if anergic or acute infection
    ○ If test negative, repeat in 2 weeks.
  - Interferon gamma release assay (IGRA)
    ○ Preferred in those likely to be infected with TB and/or who are BCG-vaccinated

- Thyroid function tests
- Technetium-based scan (infection tumor) (1)[B]
- FDG-PET/CT scan if infectious process, inflammatory process, or tumor suspected; PET scans have a high negative predictive value and good sensitivity (but may have false positives) (2)[A].
- Ultrasound of abdomen and pelvis (with directed biopsy, if indicated) if renal obstruction or biliary pathology suspected
- Echocardiogram if endocarditis, atrial myxomas, or pericardial effusion is suspected
- Lower extremity Doppler if deep vein thrombosis/pulmonary embolism suspected
- CT scan of chest if pulmonary embolism suspected
- Indium-labeled leukocyte scanning if inflammatory process or occult abscess suspected
- Bone scan if osteomyelitis or metastatic disease suspected

Diagnostic Procedures/Other
- Liver biopsy if granulomatous disease suspected (1)[C]
- Temporal artery biopsy, particularly in the elderly
- Lymph node, muscle, or skin biopsy, if clinically indicated
- Bone marrow aspiration biopsy with smear, culture, histologic examination, and flow cytometry
- Lumbar puncture, if clinically indicated

TREATMENT

GENERAL MEASURES
- Treatment depends on the specific etiology.
- Therapeutic trials are a last resort and should be as specific as possible based on available clinical evidence. Avoid "shotgun" approaches because they obscure the clinical picture, have untoward effects, and do not provide a diagnostic solution (1)[C].

MEDICATION

First Line
- First-line drugs depend on the diagnosis.
- Evidence does not support isolated treatment of fever (3)[C].

Second Line
Consider a therapeutic trial only if the patient has localizing symptoms associated with the fever or continues to decline. Consultation with appropriate specialists (infectious disease, rheumatology) is recommended in this case.
- Antibiotic trial based on patient's history and suspected culture negative endocarditis
- Antituberculous therapy if there is a high risk for TB pending definitive culture results
- Corticosteroid trial based on patient's history (once occult malignancy is ruled out) if temporal arteritis is suspected

ALERT
If a steroid trial is initiated, patient may have a relapse after treatment or if certain conditions (e.g., TB) have been undiagnosed.

ADDITIONAL THERAPIES
Febrile patients have increased caloric and fluid demands.

SURGERY/OTHER PROCEDURES
The need for exploratory laparotomy has been largely eliminated with the advent of more sophisticated tests and imaging modalities.

ADMISSION, INPATIENT, AND NURSING CONSIDERATIONS
- Reserved for the ill and debilitated
- Consider if factitious fever has been ruled out or an invasive procedure is indicated.

ONGOING CARE

FOLLOW-UP RECOMMENDATIONS
Patient Monitoring
If the etiology of the fever remains unknown, repeat the history, physical exam, and screening lab studies.

DIET
No specific dietary recommendations have been shown to ameliorate undiagnosed fever.

PATIENT EDUCATION
Maintain an open line of communication between physician and patient/family as the workup progresses:
- The extended time required in establishing a diagnosis can be frustrating.

PROGNOSIS
- Depends on etiology and age
  - Patients with HIV have the highest mortality.
- Prognosis worse if delay in diagnosis
- 1-year survival rates (reflecting deaths due to all causes)

Age	Survival
<35 y	91%
35–64 y	82%
>64 y	67%

COMPLICATIONS
Depends on etiology

Pregnancy Considerations
Fever increases the risk of neural tube defects in pregnancy and can also trigger preterm labor.

REFERENCES
1. Mourad O, Palda V, Detsky AS. A comprehensive evidence-based approach to fever of unknown origin. Arch Intern Med. 2003;163(5):545–551.
2. Takeuchi M, Dahabreh IJ, Nihashi T, et al. Nuclear imaging for classic fever of unknown origin: meta-analysis. J Nucl Med. 2016;57(12):1913–1919.
3. Hersch EC, Oh RC. Prolonged febrile illness and fever of unknown origin in adults. Am Fam Physician. 2014;90(2):91–96.

ADDITIONAL READING
- Cunha BA, Lortholary O, Cunha CB. Fever of unknown origin: a clinical approach. Am J Med. 2015;128(10):1138.e1–1138.e15.
- Hayakawa K, Ramasamy B, Chandrasekar PH. Fever of unknown origin: an evidence-based review. Am J Med Sci. 2012;344(4):307–316.
- Mulders-Manders C, Simon A, Bleeker-Rovers C. Fever of unknown origin. Clin Med (Lond). 2015;15(3):280–284.

 SEE ALSO

- Arteritis, Temporal; Arthritis, Juvenile Idiopathic; Colon Cancer; Cytomegalovirus (CMV) Inclusion Disease; Endocarditis, Infective; Hepatoma (Hepatocellular Carcinoma); HIV/AIDS; Lupus Erythematosus, Discoid; Osteomyelitis; Polyarteritis Nodosa; Polymyalgia Rheumatica; Pulmonary Embolism; Rectal Cancer; Rheumatic Fever; Sinusitis; Stroke, Acute (Cerebrovascular Accident [CVA])
- Algorithms: Fever in the First 3 Months of Life; Fever of Unknown Origin (FUO)

CODES

ICD10
R50.9 Fever, unspecified

CLINICAL PEARLS

- A sequential approach to FUO based on a careful history, physical examination, with targeted testing and imaging typically yields an appropriate diagnosis and avoids excessive nontargeted testing.
- Empiric therapy is indicated only for carefully defined circumstances.
- FUO cases that defy precise diagnosis after intensive investigation and prolonged observation generally have a favorable prognosis.
- FUO in older persons may represent an atypical presentation of a common disease.
- The most common causes of FUO in high-income countries are noninfectious inflammatory diseases and idiopathic causes.

F

FIBROCYSTIC CHANGES OF THE BREAST

Sharon L. Koehler, DO, FACS • Maria A. Pino, PhD, MS, Rph

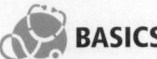 **BASICS**

DESCRIPTION
- Fibrocystic changes (FCC) is not a disease but refers to a constellation of benign histologic findings. It is the most frequent female benign clinical breast finding.
- FCC may also be described as aberrations of normal development and evolution.
- The most common symptoms are cyclic pain, tenderness, swelling, and fullness.
- The breast tissue may feel dense with areas of thicker tissue having an irregular, nodular, or ridge-like surface.
- Women may experience sensitivity to touch with a burning sensation. For some, the pain is so severe that it limits exercise or the ability to lie prone. Usually affects both breasts, most often in the upper outer quadrant where most of the milk-producing glands are located.
- Histologically, in addition to macrocysts and microcysts, FCC may contain solid elements, including adenosis, sclerosis, apocrine metaplasia, stromal fibrosis, and epithelial metaplasia and hyperplasia.
  - Depending on the presence of epithelial hyperplasia, FCC is classified as nonproliferative, proliferative without atypia, or proliferative with atypia (1).
  - Nonproliferative lesions are generally not associated with an increased risk of breast cancer.
- System(s) affected: endocrine/metabolic, reproductive
- Synonym(s): diffuse cystic mastopathy; fibrocystic disease; chronic cystic mastitis; or mammary dysplasia

EPIDEMIOLOGY
FCC occurs with great frequency in the general population. It affects women between the ages of 25 and 50 years, and it is rare at age <20 years.

Incidence
Unknown but very frequent

Prevalence
Up to 1/3 of women aged 30 to 50 years have cysts in their breasts (1). It most commonly presents in the 3rd decade, peaks in the 4th decade when hormonal function is at its peak, and sharply diminishes after menopause.
- With hormone replacement therapy, FCC may extend into menopause.
- Less common in East Asian races

ETIOLOGY AND PATHOPHYSIOLOGY
- FCC originates from an exaggerated response of breast stroma and epithelium to a variety of circulating and locally produced hormones (mainly estrogen and progesterone) and growth factors.
- Cysts may form due to dilatation of the lobular acini possibly due to imbalance of fluid secretion and resorption or due to obstruction of the duct leading to the lobule.

RISK FACTORS
- In many women, methylxanthine-containing substances (e.g., coffee, tea, cola, and chocolate) can potentiate symptoms of FCC, although a direct causality has not been established.
- Diet high in saturated fats may increase risk of FCC.

COMMONLY ASSOCIATED CONDITIONS
FCC categorized as proliferative with atypia confers a higher risk of breast cancer.

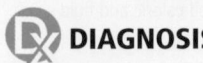 **DIAGNOSIS**

HISTORY
- Obtain personal history of breast biopsy and family history of breast disease (benign or malignant). It is important to ascertain if the patient has a known family history of *BRCA1-* or *BRCA2*-related cancer.
- Inquire regarding pertinent signs/symptoms, such as breast pain, engorgement, nipple discharge, palpable lumps, and tenderness.
  - Symptomatically, the condition is manifested as premenstrual cyclic mastalgia, with pain and tenderness to touch.

PHYSICAL EXAM
- The patient should be examined in the following positions while disrobed down to the waist:
  - With the patient standing with arms at sides, observe for elevation of the level of a nipple, dimpling, bulging, and peau d'orange.
  - With the patient's arms raised above her head, observe for dimpling and elevation/retraction of the nipple (may accentuate a mass fixed to the pectoral fascia). If so, have the patient push her hands down against her hips to flex and tense the pectoralis major muscles; move the mass to determine fixation to the underlying fascia.
  - If the patient has large and pendulous breasts, ask her to lean forward, so that her breasts hang free from the chest wall (retraction and masses may become more evident).
  - With the patient lying supine, palpate with the pads of the three middle fingers (with varying pressures from light, to medium, to deep), rotating the fingers in small circular motions and moving in vertical overlapping passes from rostral to caudal and then back caudal to rostral in the next pass. The lateral half of the breast is best palpated with the patient rolled onto the contralateral hip and the medial half with the patient supine, both with the ipsilateral hand behind the head. The entire breast from the 2nd to 6th rib and from the left sternal border to the midaxillary line must be palpated against the chest wall.
- Be certain to examine the creases under and between the breasts. If the patient has noted a lump, ask her to point it out; always palpate the opposite breast first.
- Patients with FCC have clinical breast findings that range from mild alterations in texture to dense, firm breast tissue with palpable masses.

DIFFERENTIAL DIAGNOSIS
- Pain
  - Mastitis
  - Costochondritis
  - Pectoralis muscle strain
  - Neuralgia
  - Breast cancer
  - Angina pectoris
  - Gastroesophageal reflux (GERD)
  - Superficial phlebitis of the thoracoepigastric vein (Mondor disease)
- Masses
  - Breast cancer
  - Sebaceous cyst
  - Fibroadenoma
  - Lipoma
  - Fat necrosis
  - Phyllodes tumor
- Skin changes
  - Breast cancer (peau d'orange: thickened skin similar to peel of an orange)
  - Eczema
  - Infection
  - Fungus
  - Paget disease

DIAGNOSTIC TESTS & INTERPRETATION
- Evaluation should focus on excluding breast cancer.
- Testing may be conducted based on a level of clinical suspicion.
- FCC can be evaluated with mammogram, although dense breast tissue may appear normal in women <35 years of age.
- Ultrasound (US) is the most important method in assessing a cyst.

Initial Tests (lab, imaging)
- On mammogram, FCC appears as nodular densities of breast tissue; solitary cysts can appear as round or ovoid or well-circumscribed masses, usually with low to intermediate density. FCC may also contain calcifications.
- On US, if a simple cyst is demonstrated as an anechoic structure with imperceptible wall and posterior acoustic enhancement, benign diagnosis is confirmed and no further imaging or intervention is indicated. However, if the cyst appears to be thick-walled and/or contains internal echoes, differential diagnosis should include a complicated cyst, an abscess, a galactocele, or a focal duct ectasia in the appropriate clinical contexts.
- MRI is indicated in patients with *BRCA1* or *BRCA2* mutation or in any woman with ≥25% lifetime risk for breast cancer.
- On MRI, cystic changes are well-circumscribed lesions of high-signal intensity on T2-weighted sequences and of low-signal intensity on T1-weighted images (1).

Diagnostic Procedures/Other
- Fine-needle aspiration (FNA) biopsy:
  - Allows differentiation of cystic and solid lesions
  - Aspirate may be straw-colored, dark brown, or green.
  - Cells sent for cytology can reveal cancer with high accuracy.
  - Low morbidity
- If mass disappears, no further evaluation is necessary (including cytologic evaluation of aspirated fluid).
- On the basis of the presence and degree of epithelial hyperplasia, FCC is composed of nonproliferative (approximately 65% of the total), proliferative without atypia (approximately 30% of the total), and proliferative with atypia (approximately 5–8% of the total) (2).

- Weight loss may augment the benefits of exercise.
- Strength/resistance training—mild to moderate
- Tai chi—equal or superior to aerobic exercise (4)[B]
- Aquatic exercise training
- Sleep hygiene
- Mitigate/eliminate tobacco, alcohol, and substance use.
- Pharmacologic
  - Three FDA-approved drugs: duloxetine, milnacipran, and pregabalin; others are off-label. Recent studies suggest that these agents, when used as monotherapy, only benefit a minority of responders.
  - **Caution**: Fibromyalgia patients are frequently treated with multidrug regimens; monitor closely for drug interactions, sedative, and anticholinergic effects.

MEDICATION

First Line

- Amitriptyline 10 to 50 mg PO at bedtime to treat pain, fatigue, and sleep disturbances (5)[A]. Other TCAs (imipramine, desipramine, nortriptyline) may be similarly effective.
- Duloxetine initially 30 mg/day for 1 week and then increase to 60 mg/day as tolerated. Taper if discontinued (5)[A].
- Milnacipran day 1: 12.5 mg/day; days 2 to 3, begin dividing doses: 12.5 mg BID; days 4 to 7: 25 mg BID; after day 7: 50 mg BID; max dose 100 to 200 mg BID. Taper if discontinued (5)[A].
- Pregabalin: Start with 75 mg BID, titrate over 1 week to 150 mg BID; max dose 450 mg/day (some authorities recommend up to 600 mg daily) divided BID–TID (5)[A]
- Cyclobenzaprine 5 mg qHS; titrate to 10 mg BID–TID as tolerated (3)[B].

Second Line

- Gabapentin: Start at 300 mg HS, titrate to 1,200 to 2,400 mg/day divided BID–TID; max dose 3,600 mg daily (3)[B]
- Venlafaxine XR 37.5 to 225 mg; likely to be as effective as other SNRIs (duloxetine, milnacipran)
- Tramadol 50 to 100 mg q6h; likely more effective in combination with acetaminophen (3)[C]
- Quetiapine 25 to 100 mg qHS (6)[B]
- Several agents have shown some promise of benefit, albeit with limited evidence, including pramipexole, memantine, low-dose naltrexone, cannabinoids, and hyperbaric O_2 therapy.
- Cholecalciferol may be beneficial in patients with low 25-OH vitamin D levels.

ISSUES FOR REFERRAL

In cases of unclear diagnosis or poor response to therapy, refer to rheumatology, neurology, and/or pain management.

ADDITIONAL THERAPIES

- Trigger point (<u>not</u> tender point) injections for regional myofascial dysfunction may provide relief.
- Multidisciplinary rehab (specialized clinic with physical medicine and therapy, occupational therapy, and integrated pain management)

ALERT

Ineffective or dangerous treatment modalities

- NSAIDs, full-agonist opioids (except in refractory cases), benzodiazepines, SSRIs (although may have efficacy in combination therapy with TCAs or pregabalin), magnesium, guaifenesin, thyroxine, corticosteroids, DHEA, valacyclovir, interferon, calcitonin, nabilone, and antiepileptic agents (other than those listed above) (6)[A]
- *Fibromyalgia often presents concurrently with other pain syndromes that may respond to NSAIDs, corticosteroids, opioids, and other agents.*

COMPLEMENTARY & ALTERNATIVE MEDICINE

- Acupuncture and electroacupuncture, biofeedback, hypnotherapy
- Balneotherapy (mineral-rich baths)
- Yoga, tai chi (4)[B], and qi gong
- Mindfulness-based meditation
- Myofascial massage—short- to medium-term benefit
- Limited double-blind trials have shown effectiveness of supplementation with S-adenosyl-l-methionine and acetyl-L-carnitine.
- Weak evidence for transcranial direct current and other forms of cranial electrical stimulation
- Likely to be ineffective: chiropractic treatment, multivitamin therapy, homeopathy

 ONGOING CARE

FOLLOW-UP RECOMMENDATIONS

Patient Monitoring

- For efficacy of initial therapy: at 2- to 4-week intervals, then every 1 to 6 months, tailored to patient's needs
- Advance exercise gradually to maintain tolerability.

DIET

No specific diet is recommended, but patient should make healthy choices and address negative dietary habits. Caloric or carbohydrate restriction may be helpful in obese patients.

PROGNOSIS

- 50% with partial remission after 2 to 3 years of therapy; complete remission possible but rare
- Typically has fluctuating, chronic course
- Poorer outcome tied to greater duration and severity of symptoms, depression, advanced age, lack of social support

REFERENCES

1. Wolfe F, Häuser W. Fibromyalgia diagnosis and diagnostic criteria. *Ann Med*. 2011;43(7):495–502.
2. Wolfe F, Clauw DJ, Fitzcharles MA, et al. 2016 Revisions to the 2010/2011 fibromyalgia diagnostic criteria. *Semin Arthritis Rheum*. 2016;46(3):319–329.
3. National Guideline Clearinghouse. Guideline summary NGC-7367: management of fibromyalgia syndrome in adults. http://f.i-md.com/medinfo/material/8d0/4eb2854244ae46d1d13648d0/4eb2855d44ae46d1d13648d3.pdf. Accessed September 4, 2018.
4. Wang C, Schmid CH, Fielding RA, et al. Effect of tai chi versus aerobic exercise for fibromyalgia: comparative effectiveness randomized controlled trial. *BMJ*. 2018;360:k851.
5. Welsch P, Üçeyler N, Klose P, et al. Serotonin and noradrenaline reuptake inhibitors (SNRIs) for fibromyalgia. *Cochrane Database Syst Rev*. 2018;(2):CD010292.
6. Häuser W, Walitt B, Fitzcharles MA, et al. Review of pharmacological therapies in fibromyalgia syndrome. *Arthritis Res Ther*. 2014;16(1):201.

ADDITIONAL READING

Theadom A, Cropley M, Smith HE, et al. Mind and body therapy for fibromyalgia. *Cochrane Database Syst Rev*. 2015;(4):CD001980.

 SEE ALSO

Algorithm: Fatigue

CODES

ICD10

M79.7 Fibromyalgia

CLINICAL PEARLS

- Use ACR criteria to make the formal diagnosis.
- Fibromyalgia is a disease of central sensitization; it is not a somatoform disorder and is not merely a manifestation of depression or anxiety. As with all chronic pain syndromes, fibromyalgia is frequently associated with mood and anxiety disorders.
- The best clinical outcomes occur in patients who understand their illness and actively engage in a multimodal treatment plan that includes exercise, sleep hygiene, and other lifestyle modifications, along with appropriate pharmacotherapy and CBT.

F

FOLLICULITIS

David C. Cadena Jr., MD

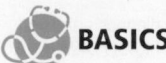 BASICS

DESCRIPTION

- Inflammation of a hair follicle (1). Subtypes include perifolliculitis and pseudofolliculitis, which occur around the follicle.
- Can occur anywhere on the body where hair is found
- Most frequent symptom is pruritus.
- Painless or tender pustules, vesicles, or pink/red papulopustules up to 5 mm in size
- Most commonly infectious in etiology:
  – *Staphylococcus aureus* bacteria
  – *Pseudomonas aeruginosa* infects areas of the body exposed to poorly chlorinated hot tubs, pools, or contaminated water.
  – *Aeromonas hydrophila* with recreational water exposure
  – Fungal (dermatophytic, *Pityrosporum, Candida*)
  – Viral (VZV, herpes simplex virus [HSV])
  – Parasitic (*Demodex* spp. mites, schistosomes)
- Noninfectious types
  – Acneiform folliculitis
  – Actinic superficial folliculitis
  – Acne vulgaris
  – Keloidal folliculitis
  – Folliculitis decalvans
  – Perioral dermatitis
  – Fox-Fordyce disease
  – Pruritus folliculitis of pregnancy
  – Eosinophilic pustular folliculitis (three variants: Ofuji disease in patients of Asian descent, HIV positive/immunocompromised, infantile)
  – Toxic erythema of the newborn
  – Eosinophilic folliculitis (seen in HIV positive/immunocompromised)
  – Follicular mucinosis
- Skin disorders that may produce a follicular eruption:
  – Pseudofolliculitis barbae: similar in appearance; occurs after shaving; affects the face, scalp, pubis, and legs; known as razor bumps, occurs frequently in black men
  – Atopic dermatitis
  – Follicular psoriasis
  – Rosacea

EPIDEMIOLOGY

Affects persons of all ages, gender, and race African ethnicities more predisposed to certain types of folliculitis

ETIOLOGY AND PATHOPHYSIOLOGY

Predisposing factors to folliculitis

- Chronic staphylococcal carrier
- Diabetes mellitus
- Malnutrition
- Pruritic skin disease (e.g., scabies, eczema)
- Exposure to poorly chlorinated swimming pools/hot tubs or water contaminated with *P. aeruginosa, A. hydrophila,* or schistosomes
- Occlusive corticosteroid use (for multiple hours)
- Bacteria
  – Most frequently due to *S. aureus* (increasing number of methicillin-resistant *S. aureus* [MRSA] cases)
  – Also due to *Streptococcus* species, *Pseudomonas* (following exposure to water contaminated with the species), or *Proteus*
  – May progress to furunculosis (painful pustular nodule with central necrosis that leaves a permanent scar after healing)

- Fungal
  – Dermatophytic (tinea capitis, tinea corporis, tinea pedis)
  – *Pityrosporum* (Pityrosporum orbiculare) commonly affecting teenagers and men, predominantly on upper chest and back
  – *Candida albicans,* although rare, has been reported with broad-spectrum antibiotic use, glucocorticoid use, immunosuppression, and in those who abuse heroin, resulting in candidemia that leads to pustules and nodules in hair-bearing areas.
- Viral
  – HSV
  – Molluscum contagiosum
- Parasitic
  – *Demodex* spp. mites (most commonly *Demodex folliculorum*), common around nasolabial area
  – Schistosomes (swimmer's itch)
- Acneiform type commonly drug induced (systemic and topical corticosteroids, lithium, isoniazid, rifampin), EGFR inhibitors
- Severe vitamin C deficiency, scurvy
- Actinic superficial type occurs within 24 to 48 hours of exposure to the sun, resulting in multiple follicular pustules on the shoulders, trunk, and arms.
- Acne vulgaris
- Keloidal folliculitis is a chronic condition affecting mostly black patients; involves the neck and occipital scalp, resulting in hypertrophic scars and hair loss; usually consequence of uncontrolled folliculitis barbae
- Folliculitis decalvans is a chronic folliculitis that leads to progressive scarring and alopecia of the scalp.
- Rosacea consists of papules, pustules, and/or telangiectasias of the face; individuals are genetically predisposed; *can be confused with folliculitis*
- Fox-Fordyce disease affects the skin containing apocrine sweat glands (i.e., axillae), resulting in chronic pruritic, annular, follicular papules.
- Eosinophilic pustular folliculitis has three variants: classic (Ofuji disease), associated with HIV infection, and infantile.
- Toxic erythema of the newborn is a self-limiting pustular eruption usually appearing during the first 3 to 4 days of life and subsequently fading in the following 2 weeks.
- *Malassezia* infections in adult males with lesions on trunk (2)

RISK FACTORS

- Hair removal (shaving, plucking, waxing, epilating agents)
- Other pruritic skin conditions: eczema, scabies
- Occlusive dressing or clothing
- Personal carrier or contact with MRSA-infected persons
- Diabetes mellitus
- Immunosuppression (medications, chemotherapy, HIV)
- Use of hot tubs or saunas
- Use of EGFR inhibitors
- Chronic antibiotic use (gram-negative folliculitis)
- Tattoo recipient

GENERAL PREVENTION

- Good hygiene practices
  – Wash hands frequently.
  – Antimicrobial soap
  – Wash towels, clothes, and linens frequently with hot water to avoid reinfection.

- Good hair removal practices
  – Exfoliate beforehand.
  – Use witch hazel, alcohol, or Tend Skin afterward.
  – Shave in direction of hair growth; use shaving gel and moisturizer.
  – Decrease frequency of shaving.
  – Use clippers primarily or single-blade razors if straight shaving is desired.

COMMONLY ASSOCIATED CONDITIONS

- Impetigo
- Scabies
- Acne
- Follicular psoriasis
- Eczema
- Xerosis
- *Staphylococcus*/MRSA colonization

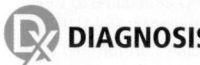 DIAGNOSIS

HISTORY

- Recent use of hot tubs, swimming pools, topical corticosteroids, certain hair styling and shaving practices, antibiotics or systemic steroids
- HIV status
- History of STDs (specifically syphilis)
- MRSA exposures/carrier status
- Home and work environment (risk/exposure potential)
- Pityrosporum folliculitis occurs more often in warm, moist climates.
- Inquire about the timeline in which the lesions have occurred, including previous similar episodes.

PHYSICAL EXAM

- Characteristic lesions are 1- to 5-mm–wide vesicles, pustules, or inflamed papules with surrounding erythema.
- Rash occurs on hair-bearing skin, especially the face (beard), proximal limbs, scalp, and pubis.
- Pseudomonal folliculitis appears as a widespread rash, mainly on the trunk and limbs.
- In pseudofolliculitis barbae, the growing hair curls around and penetrates the skin at shaved areas.

DIFFERENTIAL DIAGNOSIS

- Acne vulgaris/acneiform eruptions
- Arthropod bite
- Contact dermatitis
- Perioral dermatitis
- Cutaneous candidiasis
- Milia
- Atopic dermatitis
- Follicular psoriasis
- Hidradenitis suppurativa

DIAGNOSTIC TESTS & INTERPRETATION

Initial Tests (lab, imaging)

- Diagnosis is usually made clinically, taking risk factors, history, and locations of lesions into account.
- Culture and Gram stain may be done for larger lesions lancing or unroofing the pustule.
- KOH preparation as well as Wood lamp fluorescence to identify *Candida* or yeast
- Tzanck smear where suspicion of herpetic simplex viral folliculitis is high
- Ultrasound can be performed for questionably deeper seeding infections.

Follow-Up Tests & Special Considerations

- If risk factors or clinical suspicion exist, consider serologies for HIV or syphilis.
- If recurrent, consider HIV testing and A1C/fasting blood sugar testing to evaluate for diabetes.
- Consider punch biopsy with uncertain diagnosis.
- Treat positive bacterial culture according to sensitivities.
- Positive HIV serology: Follow up with CD4 count and punch biopsy to rule out eosinophilic folliculitis.

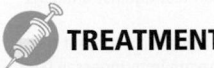 **TREATMENT**

GENERAL MEASURES

- Lesions usually resolve spontaneously.
- Avoid shaving and waxing affected areas (3)[C].
- Warm compresses may be applied TID.
- Systemic antibiotics are typically unnecessary.
- Topical mupirocin may be used in presumed *S. aureus* infection (4)[B].
- Topical antifungals for fungal folliculitis (2)[B]
- Preventive measures:
  - Antibacterial soaps (Dial soap, chlorhexidine, or benzoyl peroxide wash when showering/bathing)
  - Bleach baths (1/2 cup of 6% bleach per standard bathtub and soak for 5 to 15 minutes followed by water, rinse 1 to 2 times a week)
  - Keep skin intact; daily skin care with noncomedogenic moisturizers; avoid scratching.
  - Avoid trauma to skin: Use an electric razor as able.
  - Clean shaving instruments daily or use disposable razor, disposing after one use (5)[B].
  - Change washcloths, towels, and sheets daily.

MEDICATION

Antiseptic and supportive care is usually enough. Systemic antibiotics may be used with questionable efficacy.

First Line

- Staphylococcal folliculitis
  - Mupirocin ointment applied TID for 10 days
  - Cephalosporin (cephalexin): 250 to 500 mg PO QID for 7 to 10 days
  - Dicloxacillin: 250 to 500 mg PO QID for 7 to 10 days
- For MRSA
  - Bactrim DS: 1 to 2 tablets (160 mg/800 mg) BID PO for 5 to 10 days
  - Clindamycin: 300 mg PO TID for 10 to 14 days
  - Minocycline: 200 mg PO initially and then 100 mg BID for 5 to 10 days
  - Doxycycline: 50 to 100 mg PO BID for 5 to 10 days
- *Pseudomonas* folliculitis
  - Topical dilute acetic acid baths
  - Ciprofloxacin: 500 to 750 mg PO BID for 7 to 14 days only if patient is immunocompromised or lesions are persistent
- Eosinophilic folliculitis/eosinophilic pustular folliculitis
  - HAART treatment for HIV positive–related causes. Consider referral to appropriate treatment center.
  - High-potency topical corticosteroids for inflammation
  - Antihistamines (hydroxyzine, cetirizine) to control itching
  - Can consider: tacrolimus topically BID *or*
  - Isotretinoin 0.5 mg/kg/day PO with caution
  - Itraconazole or metronidazole

- Fungal folliculitis
  - Topical antifungals: ketoconazole 2% cream or shampoo or selenium sulfide shampoo daily *or*
  - Econazole cream applied to affected area BID for 2 to 3 weeks
    - Systemic antifungals for relapses fluconazole (100 to 200 mg/day for 3 weeks) *or* itraconazole (200 mg/day for 1 week) *or* griseofulvin (500 mg/day for 2 to 4 weeks)
    - Do not use oral ketoconazole due to risk of liver failure.
- Parasitic folliculitis
  - 5% permethrin: Apply to affected area, leave on for 8 hours, and wash off.
  - Ivermectin: 200 μg/kg PO and repeat in 1 to 2 weeks if topical application unsuccessful
- Herpetic folliculitis
  - Valacyclovir: 500 mg PO TID for 5 to 10 days or
  - Famciclovir: 500 mg PO TID for 5 to 10 days or
  - Acyclovir: 200 mg PO 5 times daily for 5 to 10 days

ISSUES FOR REFERRAL

Unusual or persistent cases should be biopsied and then referred to dermatology.

ADDITIONAL THERAPIES

- Stay informed: Testing strips can be used to test hot tubs and pools. This will help determine proper chlorine levels.
- Both hot tubs and pools should have a pH level of 7.2 to 7.8.

SURGERY/OTHER PROCEDURES

Incision and drainage is unlikely to be necessary and typically not preferred due to potential for scar formation.

 ONGOING CARE

FOLLOW-UP RECOMMENDATIONS

Patient Monitoring

- Resistant cases should be followed every 2 weeks until cleared.
- Consider prompt system therapy for worsening cases.

DIET

Caloric monitoring for obese patients; weight reduction will decrease risk of skin trauma and distension.

PATIENT EDUCATION

- Avoid shaving in involved areas.
- Monitor hot tub and pools.

PROGNOSIS

- Usually resolves with treatment; however, *S. aureus* carriers may experience recurrences.
- Mupirocin nasal treatment for carrier status and for family/household members might be helpful.
- Resistant or severe cases may warrant testing for diabetes mellitus or immunodeficiency (HIV).

COMPLICATIONS

- Primary complication is recurrent folliculitis.
- Extensive scarring with hyperpigmentation
- Progression to furunculosis or abscesses

REFERENCES

1. Laureano A, Schwartz RA, Cohen P. Facial bacterial infections: folliculitis. *Clin Dermatol*. 2014;32(6):711–714.
2. Song HS, Kim SK, Kim YC. Comparison between *Malassezia* folliculitis and non-*Malassezia* folliculitis. *Ann Dermatol*. 2014;26(5):598–602.
3. Khanna N, Chandramohan K, Khaitan BK, et al. Post waxing folliculitis: a clinicopathological evaluation. *Int J Dermatol*. 2014;53(7):849–854.
4. Lopez FA, Lartchenko S. Skin and soft tissue infections. *Infect Dis Clin North Am*. 2006;20(4):759–772.
5. Stevens DL, Bisno AL, Chambers HF, et al. Practice guidelines for the diagnosis and management of skin and soft tissue infections: 2014 update by the Infectious Diseases Society of America. *Clin Infect Dis*. 2014;59(2):147–159.

ADDITIONAL READING

- Böer A, Herder N, Winter K, et al. Herpes folliculitis: clinical, histopathological, and molecular pathologic observations. *Br J Dermatol*. 2006;154(4):743–746.
- Brooke RC, Griffiths CE. Folliculitis decalvans. *Clin Exp Dermatol*. 2001;26(1):120–122.
- Centers for Disease Control and Prevention. Rashes. https://www.cdc.gov/healthywater /swimming/swimmers/rwi/rashes.html. Accessed October 31, 2018.
- Ellis E, Scheinfeld N. Eosinophilic pustular folliculitis: a comprehensive review of treatment options. *Am J Clin Dermatol*. 2004;5(3):189–197.
- Fiorillo L, Zucker M, Sawyer D, et al. The *Pseudomonas* hot-foot syndrome. *N Engl J Med*. 2001;345(5):335–338.
- Fridkin SK, Hageman JC, Morrison M, et al; for Active Bacterial Core Surveillance Program of the Emerging Infections Program Network. Methicillin-resistant *Staphylococcus aureus* disease in three communities. *N Engl J Med*. 2005;352(14): 1436–1444.
- Luelmo-Aguilar J, Santandreu MS. Folliculitis: recognition and management. *Am J Clin Dermatol*. 2004;5(5):301–310.
- Nervi SJ, Schwartz RA, Dmochowski M. Eosinophilic pustular folliculitis: a 40 year retrospect. *J Am Acad Dermatol*. 2006;55(2):285–289.
- Parsad D, Saini R, Negi KS. Short-term treatment of pityrosporum folliculitis: a double blind placebo-controlled study. *J Eur Acad Dermatol Venereol*. 1998;11(2):188–190.

 SEE ALSO

Algorithm: Rash

 CODES

ICD10

- L73.9 Follicular disorder, unspecified
- L66.2 Folliculitis decalvans
- L73.8 Other specified follicular disorders

CLINICAL PEARLS

- Folliculitis lesions are typically 1- to 5-mm clusters of pruritic erythematous papules and pustule surrounding hair follicles.
- Most commonly due to *S. aureus*. If community has increased incidence of MRSA, consider anti-MRSA treatment.
  - It is extremely important to educate patients on proper hygiene and skin care techniques to prevent chronic or recurrent cases.

F

FOOD ALLERGY

Stanley Fineman, MD

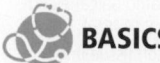 BASICS

DESCRIPTION
- Hypersensitivity reaction related to certain food exposures
- System(s) affected: gastrointestinal (GI), hemic/lymphatic/immunologic, pulmonary, skin/exocrine
- Synonym(s): allergic bowel disease; dietary protein sensitivity syndrome

EPIDEMIOLOGY
- Predominant age: all ages but more common in infants and children
- Predominant sex: male > female (2:1)

Incidence
~2.5% of infants experience hypersensitivity reactions to cow's milk in their 1st year of life (1)[B].

Prevalence
- The prevalence of IgE-mediated food allergy assessed by food challenge is 3% (1)[B].
- The self-reported prevalence of food allergy is 12% in children and 13% in adults (1)[B].
- In young children, the most common food allergies are cow's milk (2.5%), egg (1.3%), peanut (0.8%), and wheat (0.4%) (2)[B].
- Adults more commonly have allergies to shellfish (2%), peanuts (0.6%), tree nuts (0.5%), and fish (0.4%).
- Food allergy is frequently a transient phenomenon; only 3–4% of children >4 years of age have persisting food allergy (2)[B].
- 20% of children with peanut protein allergy may outgrow their sensitivity by school age.

ETIOLOGY AND PATHOPHYSIOLOGY
Allergic response triggered by immunologic mechanisms (e.g., IgE-allergic response) or non–immunologic-mediated mechanisms
- Any ingested substance can cause allergic reactions:
  - Most commonly implicated foods include cow's milk, egg whites, wheat, soy, peanuts, fish, tree nuts (walnut and pecan), and shellfish.
- Several food dyes and additives may elicit non–IgE-mediated allergic-like reactions.

Genetics
In families with a history of food hypersensitivity, the probability of food allergy in subsequent siblings may be as high as 50%.

RISK FACTORS
- Patients with allergic or atopic predisposition have increased risk of hypersensitivity reaction to food.
- Family history of food hypersensitivity

GENERAL PREVENTION
- Avoid the offending food.
- In patients at risk for anaphylaxis, epinephrine autoinjectors should be readily available.

DIAGNOSIS

HISTORY AND PHYSICAL EXAM
- Symptoms after food ingestion/exposure—usually within 30 minutes of ingestion but could be delayed 4 to 8 hours
- Document a temporal relationship between symptoms and suspected food.
- Differentiate true food allergy/hypersensitivity from food intolerance which may present with similar symptoms.
- GI
  - More common: nausea, vomiting, diarrhea, abdominal pain, occult bleeding, flatulence, and bloating
  - Less common: malabsorption, protein-losing enteropathy, eosinophilic enteritis, colitis
- Skin
  - More common: urticaria/angioedema, atopic dermatitis, pallor, or flushing
  - Less common: contact rashes
- Respiratory
  - More common: allergic rhinitis, asthma and bronchospasm, cough, serous otitis media
  - Less common: pulmonary infiltrates (Heiner syndrome), pulmonary hemosiderosis
- Neurologic
  - Less common: migraine headaches
- Other
  - Systemic anaphylaxis, vasculitis

DIFFERENTIAL DIAGNOSIS
- GI (irritable bowel syndrome, celiac sprue, dumping syndrome, inflammatory bowel diseases, etc.), dermatologic, respiratory, neurologic, psychiatric (generalized anxiety disorder, personality disorders, etc.)
- Oral allergy syndrome
  - The oral allergy syndrome is the result of cross-reacting proteins in pollens (e.g., patients sensitive to birch tree pollen frequently have cross-reactivity to fresh apples and pears).
- Galactose-α-1,3-galactose (α-gal)
  - Following a lone star tick bite, susceptible patients may develop an IgE sensitivity to α-gal which manifests as delayed anaphylaxis presenting 3 to 6 hours after ingestion of mammalian meat. Diagnosis is by history and confirmed by specific IgE to α-gal (3).

DIAGNOSTIC TESTS & INTERPRETATION
Initial Tests (lab, imaging)
- CBC with differential: Eosinophilia suggests atopy.
- Serum IgA antitissue transglutaminase (IgA-anti-tTG)
- Epicutaneous (prick or puncture) allergy skin tests document IgE-mediated immunologic hypersensitivity using commercially available extracts (variable sensitivities) or fresh food skin testing.

- Skin testing using the suspect food is helpful. If negative on skin test, an oral challenge may aid in diagnosis. The overall correlation between commercially available allergy skin testing and oral food challenge is 60%, increasing to 90% when fresh food skin testing is done (i.e., the positive skin test correlates with a positive challenge).
  - Skin testing has a high sensitivity (low false-negative rate) *but* a low specificity (high false-positive rate), so *only* skin test against antigens found on history (4)[C].
- Food-specific IgE assays (radioallergosorbent test [RAST] and fluorescent enzyme immunoassay [FEI]) detect specific IgE antibodies to offending foods and are less sensitive to skin testing.
  - Using a serum assay alone to diagnose food allergy can result in misdiagnosis of true food allergic sensitivity, particularly in children with atopic dermatitis. Do not use a panel. Test for specific IgE to foods based on patient history.
- Periodic monitoring of peanut-specific IgE levels every 2 years may be helpful. If the level of peanut-specific IgE falls to <0.5 kU/L, a supervised oral challenge can be helpful. Consider a fresh food skin test with peanut protein prior to the oral challenge (4)[B].
- Component-resolved diagnosis (CRD) is a new diagnostic tool that measures specific allergenic proteins in various foods to identify specific IgE to allergenic proteins rather than whole allergen; particularly helpful for certain nuts (e.g., peanuts) (5)[B]
- Patch testing for patients with eosinophilic esophagitis and atopic dermatitis to determine delayed-sensitivity immunologic reactions is of marginal benefit (1)[B].
- Widespread allergy skin testing or serum IgE tests are *not* recommended because of their poor predictive value without a clinical correlating history (2)[B].
- Leukocyte histamine release assays for circulating immune complexes are of limited clinical use (2)[B].
- Provocative injection and sublingual tests are of little benefit for diagnosis of food allergy.
- The leukocytotoxic assay is unproven (1)[B].
- Other unproven diagnostic procedures that are not recommended include provocative neutralization, lymphocyte stimulation, hair analysis, and applied kinesiology (2)[B].

Diagnostic Procedures/Other
Elimination and challenge testing is best for confirming food allergy:
- Eliminate the suspected food from the diet for 1 to 2 weeks.
- Monitor the patient's symptoms. If they disappear or substantially improve, perform an oral challenge with the suspected food under medical supervision.
- Optimally, this challenge should be performed in a double-blind, placebo-controlled manner.

- Patients with history of anaphylaxis should not have an oral challenge without a documented lack of IgE sensitivity.
- Most allergic reactions occur within 30 minutes to 2 hours after challenge. Late reactions have been described up to 12 to 24 hours.
- Consider referral to gastroenterology for endoscopy and continue monitoring carefully if history and testing are inconclusive.

Test Interpretation
Pathologic findings on tissue biopsy are uncommon in food allergies; inflammatory changes can sometimes be seen in the GI tract. The diagnosis of eosinophilic esophagitis is defined by >15 to 20 eosinophils per high-power field on esophageal biopsy (2)[C].

 TREATMENT

GENERAL MEASURES
- Offending food avoidance is the most effective treatment.
- Patients with severe food allergy should be meticulous about food avoidance. They should carry epinephrine for self-administration in the event that the offending food is ingested unknowingly and an immediate reaction develops.
- Immunotherapy may be effective for certain food allergies. Oral immunotherapy (OIT), sublingual immunotherapy (SLIT), and epicutaneous immunotherapy (EPIT) are still considered experimental and are not recommended for patients who are not participating in appropriately controlled and monitored clinical trials (6)[C].
- Immunotherapy or hyposensitization with food extracts are not recommended. Research studies are in progress, but immunotherapy is considered experimental at this time.

MEDICATION
- Patients with significant type 1, IgE-mediated hypersensitivity should have epinephrine available for autoinjection in case of an anaphylactic reaction.
- After receiving epinephrine for a systemic anaphylactic reaction to a food, patients should be monitored in a medical facility (15–25% of patients may require >1 dose of epinephrine).
- Symptomatic treatment for milder reactions with antihistamines is generally adequate.
- Cromolyn is not recommended for use in most patients with food allergy.

COMPLEMENTARY & ALTERNATIVE MEDICINE
Benefits of herbal medicines in food allergy are inconclusive.

 ONGOING CARE

FOLLOW-UP RECOMMENDATIONS
Patient Monitoring
As needed

DIET
- As determined by tests and clinical evaluation
- Strict avoidance of offending food

PATIENT EDUCATION
- Dietary counseling is advised to maintain a nutritionally sound diet avoiding foods to which the patient is sensitive.
- Food Allergy Research & Education, Inc.: 7925 Jones Branch Drive Suite 1100 McLean, VA 22102 Toll-Free: 800-929-4040; Web site https://www.foodallergy.org
- http://www.allergyasthmanetwork.org, https://acaai.org/ and https://www.aaaai.org

PROGNOSIS
- Most infants outgrow food hypersensitivity by 2 to 4 years:
  – It may be possible to reintroduce the offending food cautiously into the diet (especially if a particular food is difficult to avoid). Check food-specific IgE by fresh food allergy skin test to ensure negative prior to oral challenge.
  – 20% of peanut allergies resolve by age 5 years.
  – 42% of children with egg allergy and 48% of children with milk allergy develop clinical tolerance and lose their sensitivity over time (1)[C].
- Adults with food hypersensitivity (particularly to milk, fish, shellfish, or nuts) tend to maintain their allergy for many years (2)[B].

COMPLICATIONS
- Anaphylaxis
- Angioedema
- Bronchial asthma
- Enterocolitis
- Eosinophilic esophagitis
- Eczematoid lesions

REFERENCES
1. Sicherer SH, Sampson HA. Food allergy: epidemiology, pathogenesis, diagnosis, and treatment. *J Allergy Clin Immunol*. 2014;133(2):291–308.
2. Burks AW, Tang M, Sicherer S, et al. ICON: food allergy. *J Allergy Clin Immunol*. 2012;129(4):906–920.
3. Steinke JW, Platts-Mills TAE, Commins SP. The alpha gal story: lessons learned from connecting the dots. *J Allergy Clin Immunol*. 2015;135(3):589–597.
4. Sicherer SH, Wood RA. Advances in diagnosing peanut allergy. *J Allergy Clin Immunol Pract*. 2013;1(1):1–14.
5. Lieberman J, Glaumann S, Batelson S, et al. The utility of peanut components in the diagnosis of IgE-mediated peanut allergy among distinct populations. *J Allergy Clin Immunol Pract*. 2013;1(1):75–82.
6. Wood RA. Food allergen immunotherapy: current status and prospects for the future. *J Allergy Clin Immunol*. 2016;137(4):973–982.

ADDITIONAL READING
- Du Toit G, Roberts G, Sayre PH, et al; for LEAP Study Team. Randomized trial of peanut consumption in infants at risk for peanut allergy. *N Engl J Med*. 2015;372(9):803–813.
- Gernez Y, Nowak-Węgrzyn A. Immunotherapy for food allergy: are we there yet? *J Allergy Clin Immunol Pract*. 2017;5(2):250–272.
- Gupta RS, Springston EE, Warrier MR, et al. The prevalence, severity, and distribution of childhood food allergy in the United States. *Pediatrics*. 2011;128(1):e9–e17.
- Sampson HA, Aceves S, Bock SA, et al; for Joint Task Force on Practice Parameters. Food allergy: a practice parameter update—2014. *J Allergy Clin Immunol*. 2014;134(5):1016–1025.e43.

 SEE ALSO

Anaphylaxis; Celiac Disease; Irritable Bowel Syndrome

 CODES

ICD10
- T78.1XXA Oth adverse food reactions, not elsewhere classified, init
- T78.00XA Anaphylactic reaction due to unspecified food, init encntr
- L27.2 Dermatitis due to ingested food

CLINICAL PEARLS
- Up to 20% of children with peanut allergy may outgrow their sensitivity.
- Oral itching following ingestion of fresh fruit may be a warning for anaphylaxis.
- Maternal dietary restrictions during pregnancy and lactation do not appear to prevent atopic disease in infants.
- Breastfeeding is recommended for the first 6 months of life, particularly when there is a family history of atopy and food allergy.
- Delaying the introduction of solid foods beyond 6 months does not appear to have a significant protective effect on the development of allergies.
- Children 4 to 11 months of age with eczema or other food allergy may benefit from early introduction of peanut protein. Consider allergy skin testing prior to introducing peanut protein.

FOOD POISONING, BACTERIAL

Michael B. Kalinowski, DO, MS • Irfan H. Siddiqui, MD

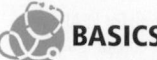 **BASICS**

DESCRIPTION
- Results from the consumption of contaminated food or water
- Symptoms commonly include vomiting, diarrhea, dehydration, abdominal discomfort, and fever (1).
- Foodborne illness may be caused by bacterial, parasitic, or viral infection (2).

EPIDEMIOLOGY
- Roughly 1 in 6 Americans (48 million) become ill, 128,000 are hospitalized, and 3,000 die of food-borne diseases annually (3).
- 80% of foodborne illness is due to unclear agents (3).
- Bacterial pathogens most commonly contributing to foodborne illness are *Salmonella* (nontyphoidal), *Campylobacter*, *Clostridium perfringens*, *Staphylococcus aureus*, *Listeria monocytogenes*, and *Escherichia coli* (1,3).
- Norovirus is the most common viral cause of foodborne illness in the United States (4).

ETIOLOGY AND PATHOPHYSIOLOGY
- Short incubation period (1 to 6 hours)
  – *Bacillus cereus* toxin
    ○ Food sources: improperly cooked rice/fried rice and red meats (2)
    ○ Symptoms: sudden onset of severe nausea and vomiting. Diarrhea may be present.
  – *S. aureus* (1)
    ○ Food sources: nonrefrigerated or improperly refrigerated meats and potato and egg salads
    ○ Symptoms: sudden onset of severe nausea and vomiting. Abdominal cramps and fever may be present.
- Medium incubation period (8 to 16 hours)
  – *B. cereus* (1)
    ○ Food sources: meat, stews, gravy, vanilla sauce
    ○ Symptoms: watery diarrhea, abdominal cramps, nausea
  – *C. perfringens* (1,2)
    ○ Food sources: dry/precooked or undercooked meats, home-canned goods
    ○ Symptoms: watery diarrhea, nausea, abdominal cramps
- Long incubation period (>16 hours)
  – Toxin-producing organisms:
    ○ *Clostridium botulinum* (1)
      ▪ Food source: commercially canned or improperly home-canned foods
      ▪ Symptoms: vomiting, diarrhea, slurred speech, diplopia, dysphagia, and descending muscle weakness/flaccid paralysis
    ○ Enterohemorrhagic *E. coli* (e.g., 0157:H7) (1,2)
      ▪ Food sources: undercooked ground beef, juice, unpasteurized milk; raw produce; and contaminated water
      ▪ Risk factors: daycare centers, nursing homes, extremes of age
      ▪ Symptoms: severe diarrhea that often becomes bloody, abdominal pain, vomiting
    ○ Enterotoxigenic *E. coli* ("traveler's diarrhea") (5)
      ▪ Food sources: food or water contaminated by human feces
      ▪ Symptoms: watery diarrhea, abdominal cramps, tenesmus, fecal urgency, and vomiting
    ○ *Vibrio cholerae* (2)
      ▪ Food sources: contaminated water, fish, and shellfish, especially food sold by street vendors
      ▪ Symptoms: profuse watery "rice water" diarrhea and vomiting, which can lead to severe dehydration and rapid death
  – Invasive organisms
    ○ *Salmonella, nontyphoidal* (1,2,4)
      ▪ Food sources: contaminated eggs, poultry; unpasteurized milk or juice; cheese; contaminated raw fruit and vegetables; and contaminated peanut butter
      ▪ Risk factors: contact with animals
      ▪ Symptoms: small volume, mucopurulent and possibly bloody diarrhea; fever; abdominal cramps; vomiting
    ○ *Campylobacter jejuni* (1,2)
      ▪ Food sources: raw and undercooked poultry, unpasteurized milk, and contaminated meats
      ▪ Symptoms: diarrhea (possibly bloody), cramps, vomiting, fever
    ○ *Shigella* (1,2)
      ▪ Food sources: contaminated water, raw produce, uncooked foods, foods handled by infected food worker
      ▪ Risk factors: MSM
      ▪ Symptoms: abdominal cramps, fever, mucopurulent and bloody diarrhea
    ○ *Vibrio parahaemolyticus* (1,2)
      ▪ Food source: undercooked or raw seafood, especially shellfish
      ▪ Risk factors: cirrhosis
      ▪ Symptoms: nausea, vomiting, diarrhea, abdominal pain
    ○ *Vibrio vulnificus* (1,2)
      ▪ Food source: undercooked or raw seafood, particularly oysters
      ▪ Symptoms: vomiting, diarrhea, abdominal pain, bacteremia, wound infections; can be fatal in patients with liver disease or those who are immunocompromised
    ○ *Yersinia enterocolitica* (2)
      ▪ Food sources: undercooked beef and pork, unpasteurized milk, tofu, contaminated water
      ▪ Risk factors: cirrhosis, hemochromatosis, blood transfusion
      ▪ Symptoms: abdominal pain, fever, diarrhea (possibly bloody), vomiting
    ○ *L. monocytogenes* (1)
      ▪ Food sources: unpasteurized/contaminated milk, soft cheese, and processed deli meats
      ▪ Risk factors: pregnancy
      ▪ Symptoms: nausea, vomiting, fever, watery diarrhea; pregnant women may have a flu-like illness leading to premature delivery or stillbirth; immunocompromised patients may develop meningitis and bacteremia.

RISK FACTORS
- Recent travel to a developing country (4)
- Food handlers, daycare attendees, nursing home residents, and recently hospitalized patients (2)
- Altered immunity due to underlying disease or use of certain medications, including antacids, H_2 blockers, and proton pump inhibitors (4)
- Cross-contamination and subsequent ingestion of improperly prepared and stored foods

GENERAL PREVENTION
- When preparing food:
  – Wash hands, cutting boards, and food preparation surfaces before and after preparing each item.
  – Wash fresh produce thoroughly before eating.
  – Keep raw meat, poultry, fish, and their juices away from other food (e.g., salad). Wear gloves when handling raw meats (6).
  – Do not put cooked protein or washed produce into containers or on surfaces where unwashed or raw food was stored.
  – Thoroughly cook meat to the following internal temperature:
    ○ Fresh beef, veal, pork, and lamb: 145°F
    ○ Ground meats and egg dishes: 160°F
    ○ Poultry: 165°F
    ○ Cook eggs thoroughly until the yolk is firm.
    ○ Seafood: 145°F
  – Refrigerate leftovers within 2 to 3 hours in clean, shallow, covered containers. If the temperature is >90°F, refrigerate within 1 hour.
- When traveling to underdeveloped countries:
  – Eat only freshly prepared foods.
  – Avoid beverages and foods prepared with nonpotable water.
  – Other risky foods include raw or undercooked meat and seafood, unpeeled raw fruits, and vegetables.
  – Bottled, carbonated, and boiled beverages are generally safe to drink.
- Improved hygiene and sanitation reduces the risk of traveler's diarrhea. The prevention strategy "Boil it, Cook it, Peel it, or Forget it" has inconsistent and limited evidence (5).
- Chemoprophylaxis for traveler's diarrhea is recommended for high-risk travelers (e.g., immunocompromised) (5).

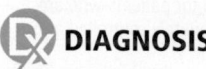 **DIAGNOSIS**

HISTORY
- Onset, duration, frequency, severity, and character (i.e., watery, bloody, mucus-filled, etc.) of diarrhea (2)
- The definition of diarrhea is >3 or more unformed stools daily or the passage of >250 g of unformed stool per day (4).
- Suspect bacterial food poisoning when multiple persons have rapid onset of symptoms after eating the same meal; high fever, blood, or mucus in stool; severe abdominal pain; signs of dehydration; or recent travel to a foreign country (2,4).
- Further evaluation and treatment with high fever (≥101.3°F), ≥6 stools per day, blood in the stools, elevated white blood cell count, signs of dehydration, or diarrheal illness that lasts >2 to 3 days (4)

PHYSICAL EXAM
- Focus on signs of dehydration: delayed capillary refill, decreased skin turgor, dry mucous membranes, and orthostatic hypotension (2).
- Fever may be suggestive of invasive or toxin-producing bacteria (2).
- Abdominal exam: Assess for pain, peritoneal signs, and bowel activity to differentiate from other acute abdominal processes (2).
- Rectal exam for blood, rectal pain, stool consistency

DIFFERENTIAL DIAGNOSIS
- Other infectious gastrointestinal illnesses (i.e., viral or parasitic)
- *Clostridium difficile* colitis
- Inflammatory bowel disease
- Appendicitis
- Acute cholecystitis
- Acute diverticulitis
- Acute hepatitis
- Malabsorption

DIAGNOSTIC TESTS & INTERPRETATION
Initial Tests (lab, imaging)
- For mild, self-limiting illness, a stool culture is not typically necessary and is unlikely to change management (1)[C].
- Testing for fecal leukocytes and fecal occult blood is not mandatory unless patients have fever or bloody diarrhea. Stool sample is preferred collection (6).
- Consider ova and parasites if dehydration, history of foreign travel, or symptoms lasting >2 weeks (4).
- CBC, BMP for severe cases with dehydration, inpatient, and nursing home exposure (4)
- Consider endoscopic evaluation for severe cases (4,6,7). Have a low threshold for endoscopy among patients with AIDS and persistent diarrhea (6).
- Abdominal CT may be helpful when intra-abdominal pathology is in the differential (4,6).

Follow-Up Tests & Special Considerations
Epidemiologic investigation may be warranted. Reporting requirements vary by state and organism (1).

 ## TREATMENT

Most cases of food poisoning are self-limited and do not require medication.

MEDICATION
First Line
- Oral rehydration is the first-line therapy for treating acute diarrheal illness (2,6).
- A balanced oral rehydration solution (ORS) is particularly recommended for elderly or pediatric patients with severe diarrhea, or for travelers with severe, cholera-like watery diarrhea (7)[B].
- Most patients with mild illness do not need formal ORS and can rehydrate with fluids and salt-rich foods (7).
- Empiric antibiotic therapy is not recommended for most cases of acute diarrhea (unless traveler's diarrhea is suspected) (7)[A].

Second Line
Consider antibiotics only for patients with severe illness requiring hospitalization and those with fever and hematochezia or when diagnostic testing confirms a bacterial source (1). Pathogen-specific therapy:
- *B. cereus* (2)
  - Supportive care only
- *C. jejuni* (2,4)
  - Mild: supportive care only—antibiotics may induce resistance
  - Severe: azithromycin 500 mg/day for 3 to 5 days. Fluoroquinolones are no longer recommended due to resistance (1).
- *C. botulinum*
  - Supportive care only. Antitoxin can be helpful early during illness.
- *C. perfringens*
  - Supportive care only
- Enterohemorrhagic *E. coli* (e.g., 0157:H7) (4)
  - Supportive care only. Closely monitor renal function, hemoglobin, and platelets. Infection associated with hemolytic uremic syndrome (HUS). Avoid antibiotics because they may increase risk.
- Enterotoxigenic *E. coli* (common cause of traveler's diarrhea) (2,4,5)
  - Generally self-limited. Antibiotics shorten course of illness (5)[A].
  - Ciprofloxacin 500 mg BID or 750 mg daily for 1 to 3 days; azithromycin 1 g × single dose or daily for 3 days; or rifaximin 200 mg TID for 3 days

- *Salmonella, nontyphoidal* (2,4,5,7)
  - No therapy in mild disease (Antibiotics may lengthen shedding.)
  - Moderate: ciprofloxacin 500 mg BID for 5 to 7 days, levofloxacin 500 mg daily for 7 to 10 days, or TMP/SMX DS 160/800 mg BID for 5 to 7 days
  - Severe diarrhea, immunocompromised, systemic signs, positive blood cultures: IV ceftriaxone 1 to 2 g daily for 7 to 10 days
- *Shigella* (2,4,7)
  - Ciprofloxacin 500 mg BID or 750 mg daily for 3 days, or 2 g single dose; alternative options: azithromycin (drug of choice secondary to quinolone resistance) 500 mg BID for 3 days, TMP/SMX DS 160/800 mg BID for 5 days, or ceftriaxone 2 to 4 g single dose
- *S. aureus* (4)
  - Supportive care only
- Noncholeraic *Vibrio* (4)
  - Ciprofloxacin 750 mg daily for 3 days or azithromycin 500 mg daily for 3 days
- *V. cholerae* (4)
  - Doxycycline 300 mg 1-time dose in most cases, or tetracycline 500 mg QID for 3 days, or erythromycin 250 mg TID for 3 days, or azithromycin 1,000 mg as single dose or 500 mg/day for 3 days
- *Yersinia* (2)
  - Usually supportive care only
  - Severe: doxycycline combine with aminoglycoside; TMP/SMX DS 160/800 mg BID for 5 days; or ciprofloxacin 500 mg BID for 7 to 10 days

ADDITIONAL THERAPIES
- For severe nausea and vomiting, promethazine is effective in adults. Ondansetron is effective in children (5).
- Loperamide 4 mg initially then 2 mg after each loose stool to a maximum of 8 mg in a 24-hour period may be used *unless* high fever, bloody diarrhea, and/or severe abdominal pain present (signs of enteroinvasion) (5).
- Bismuth subsalicylate (Pepto-Bismol) 525 mg QID is moderately effective in traveler's diarrhea (5,7).
- Evidence for the effectiveness of probiotics and prebiotics is limited and inconsistent. Use is not currently recommended outside of postantibiotic-related infectious diarrhea (6,7).
- Diligent hand washing throughout the course of illness decreases spread (2).

 ## ONGOING CARE

DIET
- Avoid food if nausea is present or vomiting prevents intake. Drink plenty of fluids in frequent sips.
- As nausea subsides, drink adequate fluids; add in bland, low-fat meals; and rest. Avoid alcohol, coffee, nicotine, and spicy foods.
- Breastfeed nursing infants on demand. Infants and older children should be offered usual food.
- For diarrhea, consider a bland diet (BRAT: Bananas, Rice, Apples, Toast-dry).
- Limiting dairy to 24 hours after last diarrhea episode may assist in symptom reduction.

PROGNOSIS
Most infections are self-limited and resolve over several days. Antibiotics for moderate to severe traveler's diarrhea shorten duration by several days (5).

COMPLICATIONS
- Dehydration (2)
- HUS following *E. coli* 0157:H7 infection (4)

- Guillain-Barré syndrome following *Campylobacter* enteritis (4)
- Reactive arthritis following salmonella, shigella, or yersinia infections (4)
- Postinfectious irritable bowel (4)

REFERENCES

1. Switaj TL, Winter KJ, Christensen SR. Diagnosis and management of foodborne illness. *Am Fam Physician*. 2015;92(5):358–365.
2. Barr W, Smith A. Acute diarrhea. *Am Fam Physician*. 2014;89(3):180–189.
3. Centers for Disease Control and Prevention. Estimates of foodborne illness in the United States. http://www.cdc.gov/foodborneburden/. Accessed November 12, 2018.
4. DuPont HL. Acute infectious diarrhea in immunocompetent adults. *N Engl J Med*. 2014;370(16):1532–1540.
5. Steffen R, Hill DR, DuPont HL. Traveler's diarrhea: a clinical review. *JAMA*. 2015;313(1):71–80.
6. Shane AL, Mody RK, Crump JA, et al. 2017 Infectious Diseases Society of America clinical practice guidelines for the diagnosis and management of infectious diarrhea. *Clin Infect Dis*. 2017;65(12):1963–1973.
7. Riddle MS, DuPont HL, Connor BA. ACG clinical guideline: diagnosis, treatment, and prevention of acute diarrheal infections in adults. *Am J Gastroenterol*. 2016;111(5):602–622.

ADDITIONAL READING
- Kalyoussef S, Feja KN. Foodborne illnesses. *Adv Pediatr*. 2014;61(1):287–312.
- U.S. Food and Drug Administration. Foodborne illness & contaminants. https://www.fda.gov/food/foodborneillnesscontaminants/default.htm. Accessed November 2, 2018.

 ## SEE ALSO

Appendicitis, Acute; Botulism; Brucellosis; Dehydration; Diarrhea, Acute; Guillain-Barré Syndrome; Hypokalemia; Intestinal Parasites; Salmonella Infection; Typhoid Fever

 ## CODES

ICD10
- A05.9 Bacterial foodborne intoxication, unspecified
- A02.0 Salmonella enteritis
- A04.5 Campylobacter enteritis

CLINICAL PEARLS
- Consider bacterial food poisoning when multiple people present after ingesting the same food with fevers and blood/mucus in stool or having recently returned from a developing nation.
- Consider culture and antibiotics if there is persistent fever with blood/mucus in stool, concern for sepsis, and/or for symptoms lasting >7 days.
- Withhold antispasmodics and antidiarrheal agents if there is concern for enteroinvasion (high prolonged fever, bloody diarrhea, severe pain, septicemia).
- Consider empiric antibiotic therapy for traveler's diarrhea in cases of moderate to severe disease.

F

FROSTBITE

Jeffrey D. Kueter, MD, FAAFP

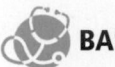

BASICS

DESCRIPTION
- A severe localized injury due to cold exposure, causing tissue to freeze, resulting in direct cellular injury and progressive dermal ischemia (most commonly of exposed hands, feet, face, and ears)
- Systems affected: integumentary, vascular, muscular, skeletal, nervous
- Synonym: dermatitis congelationis

EPIDEMIOLOGY
- Predominantly adults but can affect all ages
- Predominant sex: male = female

ETIOLOGY AND PATHOPHYSIOLOGY
- Prolonged exposure to cold
- Refreezing thawed extremities
- Ice crystals form intracellularly and extracellularly.
- Vasoconstriction reduces blood flow, and microvascular endothelial injury leads to ischemia.
- Cellular dehydration leads to abnormal electrolyte concentrations and cell death.
- In severe cases, tissue injury extends to muscle and bone leading to necrosis and mummification.
- Rewarming injured endothelium results in edema and bullae.
- Inflammatory mediators such as prostaglandins and thromboxane A2 induce vasoconstriction and platelet aggregation, worsening ischemia.

RISK FACTORS
- Prolonged exposure to below freezing temperatures, especially combined with wind and/or water exposure
- High-altitude activities, such as mountaineering
- Military operations in cold environments
- Constricting or wet clothing with inadequate insulation
- Altered mental status due to alcohol, drugs, or psychiatric illness
- Homelessness
- Previous cold-related injury
- Dehydration and/or malnutrition
- Smoking
- Raynaud phenomenon
- Peripheral vascular disease
- Diabetes

GENERAL PREVENTION
- Dress in layers with appropriate cold weather gear and avoid clothing that is too constricting.
- Cover exposed areas and extremities appropriately.
- Stay dry; avoid alcohol and minimize wind exposure.
- Ensure adequate hydration and caloric intake.
- Use supplemental oxygen at very high altitudes (>7,500 meters).
- Exercise can protect against frostbite by increasing core and peripheral temperatures.
- Appropriate use of chemical or electric hand and foot warmers can help maintain peripheral warmth.

COMMONLY ASSOCIATED CONDITIONS
- Hypothermia
- Alcohol or drug abuse

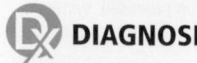

DIAGNOSIS

HISTORY
- Significant cold exposure—determine length and severity.
- Throbbing pain
- Paresthesias
- Numbness
- Loss of coordination and dexterity

PHYSICAL EXAM
- Hands, feet, face, and ears are most commonly affected.
- Before rewarming, skin may be insensate, white or grayish-yellow in color, cyanotic, or hard and waxy to touch.
- After rewarming, immediate physical exam findings can be categorized as:
  – Grade 1: no cyanosis on the extremity
  – Grade 2: cyanosis isolated to the distal phalanx
  – Grade 3: intermediate and proximal phalangeal cyanosis
  – Grade 4: cyanosis over the carpal or tarsal bones (1)[C]
- Frostbite can alternatively be categorized into four degrees (similar to burn injuries):
  – 1st degree: numbness and erythema. A white or yellow, firm, slightly raised plaque develops. No gross tissue infarction occurs; there may be slight epidermal sloughing. Mild edema is common.
  – 2nd degree: superficial skin vesiculation; a clear or milky blisters, surrounded by erythema and edema
  – 3rd degree: deeper hemorrhagic blisters
  – 4th degree: extends through the dermis to involve subcutaneous tissues, with necrosis extending into muscle and bone
  – 1st- and 2nd-degree injuries are superficial.
  – 3rd- and 4th-degree injuries are deep (2)[C].

DIFFERENTIAL DIAGNOSIS
- Frostnip: a superficial cold injury that resolves spontaneously without tissue loss
- Chilblains (pernio): a localized inflammatory reaction to cold and wet exposure without tissue freezing; typically presents as edematous, erythematous to violaceous skin lesions
- Immersion foot (trench foot): inflammatory reaction of the feet to prolonged exposure to cold and moisture

DIAGNOSTIC TESTS & INTERPRETATION
Initial Tests (lab, imaging)
- Baseline labs: CBC, CMP, UA for myoglobinuria, culture wound if suspected infection
- Technetium (Tc)-99m scintigraphy can identify tissue viability at early stage and identify candidates for thrombolytic therapy.

- MRI/MRA, duplex ultrasonography, and standard or digital subtraction angiography are occasionally used.
- Consider serial photographs at time of injury, at 24 hours and every several days until hospital discharge.

TREATMENT

GENERAL MEASURES
- Correct hypothermia.
- Assess for additional injuries.
- Remove jewelry from affected extremities.
- Initiate rewarming of affected body part only if there is no risk of refreezing.
- Warm affected parts of body in 37–39°C water for approximately 30 minutes until the involved part takes on a red or purple appearance and becomes pliable to touch.
- A whirlpool bath can help with rewarming.
- Avoid using other heat sources, such as a fire or space heater to rewarm affected parts avoided.
- Apply topical aloe vera gel before dressing.
- Selectively drain clear or cloudy blisters; leave hemorrhagic blisters intact.
- Splint and elevate affected extremity.
- Tetanus prophylaxis
- Oral hydration if patient is alert and has no GI symptoms, otherwise IV hydration with warm normal saline in small boluses
- Daily bathing in warm water with active and passive mobilization
- Dry, loose bulky dressings, including in between fingers/toes (2)[C]

ALERT
- Avoid rubbing the affected area because this can lead to further tissue damage.
- Patients should not walk on a frostbitten foot prior to definitive care.

MEDICATION
First Line
- tPA for deep injury, administered (either IV or intra-arterially) within 24 hours of injury may prevent damage from microvascular thrombosis and reduce amputation rates (3,4,5)[B].
- **Precaution**: tPA should not be used with history of recent bleeding, stroke, peptic ulcer, or recent surgery.
- Heparin is recommended as adjunctive therapy in tPA protocols. Heparin is not recommended as monotherapy (5)[C].
- Consider low-molecular-weight dextran in patients not given other systemic treatments (e.g., tPA) (2)[C].
- Aspirin 250 mg plus buflomedil 400 mg IV followed by 8 days of iloprost 0.5 to 2.0 mg/kg/min for 6 hr/day may reduce amputation rates in patients with frostbite extending to the proximal phalanx (3)[B].
- Update tetanus toxoid (2)[C].

- Ibuprofen 400 mg q12h (inhibits prostaglandins) (2)[C]
- NSAIDs for mild to moderate pain; narcotic analgesia for moderate to severe pain
- Use systemic antibiotics for proven infection. Prophylactic antibiotics are not recommended (2)[C].

Second Line
Pentoxifylline 400 mg q8 hours (6)[C]

ADDITIONAL THERAPIES
- Heated oxygen
- Warm IV fluids

SURGERY/OTHER PROCEDURES
- Urgent surgery is rarely needed.
- Fasciotomy is indicated if the patient develops elevated compartment pressures (2)[C].
- Surgical débridement, as needed, to remove necrotic tissue
- Amputation only if tissues are necrotic: may take 4 to 12 weeks for the demarcation of tissue necrosis to become definitive
- Consider imaging with 99mTc bone scan and/or MRA in severe cases to determine extent of injury; assess viability of surrounding tissue and determine need for surgery.

ADMISSION, INPATIENT, AND NURSING CONSIDERATIONS
- Hospitalization is generally recommended unless no blisters are present after rewarming (e.g., grade 1/1st-degree frostbite) (1,2)[C].
- Patients are typically best cared for in a hospital with experience treating frostbite injuries (trauma center or burn unit).
- Administer tPA in intensive care setting.
- Ensure proper hydration and nutrition.
- Treat pain (often requires narcotic analgesia).
- Wound care—clean dressings and twice daily whirlpool baths
- Apply aloe vera gel every 6 to 8 hours through resolution of blisters.
- Elevate injured extremities above heart level to minimize edema.
- Physical therapy and early mobilization
- If patient cannot tolerate oral fluids or has altered mental status, give warmed normal saline in small boluses (2)[C].

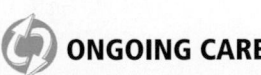 **ONGOING CARE**

FOLLOW-UP RECOMMENDATIONS
- Protect injured body parts.
- Continue physical therapy.
- Avoid smoking.
- Avoid recurrent cold exposure.
- Ensure properly fitting clothing and footwear.

Patient Monitoring
- Follow-up for physical therapy progress, infection, and other complications listed below
- Monitor growth of affected extremity in pediatric patients.

DIET
- As tolerated
- Warm oral fluids

PATIENT EDUCATION
Provide education on:
- Protection from cold injuries
- Risk factors for frostbite
- Early signs and symptoms of frostbite
- Field treatment of cold injuries
- Wound care

PROGNOSIS
- Grade 1: no amputation and no sequelae
- Grade 2: potential soft tissue amputation and nail sequelae
- Grade 3: potential bone amputation of the digit and functional sequelae
- Grade 4: potential bone amputation of the limb with functional sequelae (1)[C]

COMPLICATIONS
- Tissue loss: Distal parts of an extremity may undergo spontaneous amputation.
- Tissue necrosis requiring amputation
- Gangrene
- Hyperhidrosis due to nerve injury
- Decreased hair and nail growth
- Raynaud phenomenon
- Changes in skin color
- Joint stiffness and arthritis
- Chronic regional pain
- Neuropathy
- Localized osteoporosis
- Premature closure of epiphyses in pediatric patients

REFERENCES
1. Cauchy E, Chetaille E, Marchand V, et al. Retrospective study of 70 cases of severe frostbite lesions: a proposed new classification scheme. *Wilderness Environ Med*. 2001;12(4):248–255.
2. McIntosh SE, Hamonko M, Freer L, et al. Wilderness Medical Society practice guidelines for the prevention and treatment of frostbite. *Wilderness Environ Med*. 2011;22(2):156–166.
3. Cauchy E, Cheguillaume B, Chetaille E. A controlled trial of a prostacyclin and rt-PA in the treatment of severe frostbite. *N Engl J Med*. 2011;364(2):189–190.
4. Bruen KJ, Ballard JR, Morris SE, et al. Reduction of the incidence of amputation in frostbite injury with thrombolytic therapy. *Arch Surg*. 2007;142(6):546–553.
5. Twomey JA, Peltier GL, Zera RT. An open-label study to evaluate the safety and efficacy of tissue plasminogen activator in treatment of severe frostbite. *J Trauma*. 2005;59(6):1350–1355.
6. Hayes D Jr, Mandracchia V, Considine C, et al. Pentoxifylline. Adjunctive therapy in the treatment of pedal frostbite. *Clin Podiatr Med Surg*. 2000;17(4):715–722.

ADDITIONAL READING
- Handford C, Thomas O, Imray C. Frostbite. *Emerg Med Clin North Am*. 2017;35(2):281–299.
- Imray C, Grieve A, Dhillon S; for Caudwell Xtreme Everest Research Group. Cold damage to the extremities: frostbite and non-freezing cold injuries. *Postgrad Med J*. 2009;85(1007):481–488.
- Ingram B, Raymond T. Recognition and treatment of freezing and nonfreezing cold injuries. *Curr Sports Med Rep*. 2013;12(2):125–130.
- Jurkovich G. Environmental cold-induced injury. *Surg Clin North Am*. 2007;87(1):247–267.

 SEE ALSO

- Hypothermia
- Algorithm: Hypothermia

 CODES

ICD10
- T33.90XA Superficial frostbite of unspecified sites, init encntr
- T34.90XA Frostbite with tissue necrosis of unsp sites, init encntr
- T33.829A Superficial frostbite of unspecified foot, initial encounter

CLINICAL PEARLS
- Frostbite is a tetanus-prone injury. Provide appropriate tetanus prophylaxis.
- Avoid rewarming en route to the hospital if there is a chance of refreezing; rewarm only with water.
- Assess for additional injuries to areas which may be insensate.
- tPA can reduce amputation rates. Use within 24 hours of injury in appropriate clinical settings.
- Early assessment of the degree of tissue involvement is difficult. Delay surgery until a definite tissue demarcation of necrosis occurs (may take 4 to 12 weeks).

FURUNCULOSIS

Zoltan Trizna, MD, PhD

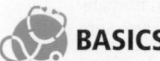

BASICS

DESCRIPTION
- Acute bacterial abscess of a hair follicle (often *Staphylococcus aureus*)
- System(s) affected: skin/exocrine
- Synonym(s): boils

EPIDEMIOLOGY

Incidence
- Predominant age
  - Adolescents and young adults
  - Clusters have been reported in teenagers living in crowded quarters, within families, or in high school athletes.
- Predominant sex: male = female

Prevalence
Exact data are not available.

ETIOLOGY AND PATHOPHYSIOLOGY
- Infection spreads away from hair follicle into surrounding dermis.
- Pathogenic strain of *S. aureus* (usually); most cases in United States are now due to community-acquired methicillin-resistant *S. aureus* (CA-MRSA), whereas methicillin-sensitive *S. aureus* (MSSA) is most common elsewhere (1).

Genetics
Unknown

RISK FACTORS
- Carriage of pathogenic strain of *Staphylococcus* sp. in nares, skin, axilla, and perineum
- Rarely, polymorphonuclear leukocyte defect or hyperimmunoglobulin E–*Staphylococcus* sp. abscess syndrome
- Diabetes mellitus, malnutrition, alcoholism, obesity, atopic dermatitis
- Primary immunodeficiency disease and AIDS (common variable immunodeficiency, chronic granulomatous disease, Chédiak–Higashi syndrome, C3 deficiency, C3 hypercatabolism, transient hypo-gammaglobulinemia of infancy, immunodeficiency with thymoma, Wiskott-Aldrich syndrome)

- Secondary immunodeficiency (e.g., leukemia, leukopenia, neutropenia, therapeutic immunosuppression)
- Medication impairing neutrophil function (e.g., omeprazole)
- The most important independent predictor of recurrence is a positive family history.

GENERAL PREVENTION
Patient education regarding self-care (see "General Measures"); treatment and prevention are interrelated.

COMMONLY ASSOCIATED CONDITIONS
- Usually normal immune system
- Diabetes mellitus
- Polymorphonuclear leukocyte defect (rare)
- Hyperimmunoglobulin E–*Staphylococcus* sp. abscess syndrome (rare)
- See "Risk Factors."

DIAGNOSIS

HISTORY
- Located on hair-bearing sites, especially areas prone to friction or repeated minor traumas (e.g., underneath belt, anterior aspects of thighs, nape, buttocks)
- No initial fever or systemic symptoms
- The folliculocentric nodule may enlarge, become painful, and develop into an abscess (frequently with spontaneous drainage).

PHYSICAL EXAM
- Painful erythematous papules/nodules (1 to 5 cm) with central pustules
- Tender, red, perifollicular swelling, terminating in discharge of pus and necrotic plug
- Lesions may be solitary or clustered.

DIFFERENTIAL DIAGNOSIS
- Folliculitis
- Pseudofolliculitis
- Carbuncles
- Ruptured epidermal cyst
- Myiasis (larva of botfly/tumbu fly)
- Hidradenitis suppurativa
- Atypical bacterial or fungal infections

DIAGNOSTIC TESTS & INTERPRETATION

Initial Tests (lab, imaging)
Obtain culture if with multiple abscesses marked by surrounding inflammation, cellulitis, systemic symptoms such as fever, or if immunocompromised.

Follow-Up Tests & Special Considerations
- Immunoglobulin levels in rare (e.g., recurrent or otherwise inexplicable) cases
- If culture grows gram-negative bacteria or fungus, consider polymorphonuclear neutrophil leukocyte functional defect.

Test Interpretation
Histopathology (although a biopsy is rarely needed)
- Perifollicular necrosis containing fibrinoid material and neutrophils
- At deep end of necrotic plug, in SC tissue, is a large abscess with a Gram stain positive for small collections of *S. aureus*.

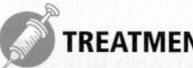

TREATMENT

GENERAL MEASURES
- Moist, warm compresses (provide comfort, encourage localization/pointing/drainage) 30 minutes QID
- If pointing or large, incise and drain: Consider packing if large or incompletely drained.
- Routine culture is not necessary for localized abscess in nondiabetic patients with normal immune system.
- Sanitary practices: Change towels, washcloths, and sheets daily; clean shaving instruments; avoid nose picking; change wound dressings frequently; do not share items of personal hygiene (2)[B].

MEDICATION

First Line
- Systemic antibiotics usually *unnecessary*, unless extensive surrounding cellulitis or fever. Other indications include a single abscess >2 cm, immunocompromise.
- If suspecting MRSA, see "Second Line."

- If multiple abscesses, lesions with marked surrounding inflammation, cellulitis, systemic symptoms such as fever, or if immunocompromised: Place on antibiotics therapy directed at *S. aureus* for 10 to 14 days.
  - Dicloxacillin (Dynapen, Pathocil) 500 mg PO QID *or* cephalexin 500 mg PO QID *or* clindamycin 300 mg TID, if penicillin-allergic

Second Line
- Resistant strains of *S. aureus* (MRSA): clindamycin 300 mg q6h or doxycycline 100 mg q12h or trimethoprim-sulfamethoxazole (TMP-SMX DS) 1 tab q8–12h or minocycline 100 mg q12h
- If known or suspected impaired neutrophil function (e.g., impaired chemotaxis, phagocytosis, superoxide generation), add vitamin C 1,000 mg/day for 4 to 6 weeks (prevents oxidation of neutrophils).
- If antibiotic regimens fail:
  - May try PO pentoxifylline 400 mg TID for 2 to 6 months
  - Contraindications: recent cerebral and/or retinal hemorrhage; intolerance to methylxanthines (e.g., caffeine, theophylline); allergy to the particular drug selected
  - Precautions: prolonged prothrombin time (PT) and/or bleeding; if on warfarin, frequent monitoring of PT

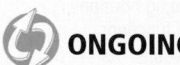 **ONGOING CARE**

FOLLOW-UP RECOMMENDATIONS
Patient Monitoring
Instruct patient to see physician if compresses are unsuccessful.

DIET
Unrestricted

PROGNOSIS
- Self-limited: usually drains pus spontaneously and will heal with or without scarring within several days
- Recurrent/chronic: may last for months or years

- If recurrent, usually related to chronic skin carriage of staphylococci (nares or on skin). Treatment goals are to decrease or eliminate pathogenic strain *or* suppress pathogenic strain.
  - Culture nares, skin, axilla, and perineum (culture nares of family members)
  - Mupirocin 2%: Apply to both nares BID for 5 days each month.
  - Culture anterior nares every 3 months; if failure, retreat with mupirocin or consider clindamycin 150 mg/day for 3 months.
- Especially in recurrent cases, wash entire body and fingernails (with nailbrush) daily for 1 to 3 weeks with povidone-iodine (Betadine), chlorhexidine (Hibiclens), or hexachlorophene (pHisoHex soap), although all can cause dry skin.

COMPLICATIONS
- Scarring
- Bacteremia
- Seeding (e.g., septal/valve defect, arthritic joint)

REFERENCES

1. Demos M, McLeod MP, Nouri K. Recurrent furunculosis: a review of the literature. *Br J Dermatol*. 2012;167(4):725–732.
2. Fritz SA, Camins BC, Eisenstein KA, et al. Effectiveness of measures to eradicate *Staphylococcus aureus* carriage in patients with community-associated skin and soft-tissue infections: a randomized trial. *Infect Control Hosp Epidemiol*. 2011;32(9):872–880.

ADDITIONAL READING

- El-Gilany AH, Fathy H. Risk factors of recurrent furunculosis. *Dermatol Online J*. 2009;15(1):16.
- Ibler KS, Kromann CB. Recurrent furunculosis–challenges and management: a review. *Clin Cosmet Investig Dermatol*. 2014;7:59–64.
- McConeghy KW, Mikolich DJ, LaPlante KL. Agents for the decolonization of methicillin-resistant *Staphylococcus aureus*. *Pharmacotherapy*. 2009;29(3):263–280.
- Rivera AM, Boucher HW. Current concepts in antimicrobial therapy against select gram-positive organisms: methicillin-resistant *Staphylococcus aureus*, penicillin-resistant pneumococci, and vancomycin-resistant enterococci. *Mayo Clin Proc*. 2011;86(12):1230–1243.

- Wahba-Yahav AV. Intractable chronic furunculosis: prevention of recurrences with pentoxifylline. *Acta Derm Venereol*. 1992;72(6):461–462.
- Winthrop KL, Abrams M, Yakrus M, et al. An outbreak of mycobacterial furunculosis associated with footbaths at a nail salon. *N Engl J Med*. 2002;346(18):1366–1371.

 SEE ALSO

Folliculitis; Hidradenitis Suppurativa

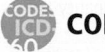 **CODES**

ICD10
- L02.92 Furuncle, unspecified
- L02.12 Furuncle of neck
- L02.429 Furuncle of limb, unspecified

CLINICAL PEARLS

- Pathogens may be different in different localities. Keep up-to-date with the locality-specific epidemiology.
- If few, furuncles/furunculosis do not need antibiotic treatment. If systemic symptoms (e.g., fever), cellulitis, or multiple lesions occur, oral antibiotic therapy is used.
- Other treatments for MRSA include linezolid PO or IV and IV vancomycin.
- Folliculitis, furunculosis, and carbuncles are parts of a spectrum of pyodermas.
- Other causative organisms include aerobic (e.g., *Escherichia coli*, *Pseudomonas aeruginosa*, and *Streptococcus faecalis*), anaerobic (e.g., *Bacteroides*, *Lactobacillus*, *Peptobacillius*, and *Peptostreptococcus*), and *Mycobacteria*.
- Decolonization (treatment of the nares with topical antibiotic) is only recommended if the colonization was confirmed by cultures because resistance is common and treatment is of uncertain efficacy.

F

GALACTORRHEA

Sarah E. Barker, DO • Chandini Rathee, MD • Kelley V. Lawrence, MD, IBCLC, FAAFP, FABM

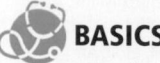 **BASICS**

DESCRIPTION

- Milky nipple discharge not associated with gestation or present >1 year after weaning. Galactorrhea does not include serous, purulent, or bloody nipple discharge.
- System(s) affected: endocrine/metabolic, nervous, reproductive

Pregnancy Considerations

- Most cases of galactorrhea during pregnancy are physiologic.
- Pregnancy stimulates lactotroph cells, so pituitary prolactin-secreting macroadenomas may increase by 21% (1)[A].

EPIDEMIOLOGY

- Predominant age: 15 to 50 years (reproductive age)
- Predominant sex: female > male (rare, e.g., in patients with multiple endocrine neoplasia type 1 [MEN1], the most common anterior pituitary tumors are prolactinomas)

Prevalence

6.8% of women referred to physicians with a breast complaint have nipple discharge.

ETIOLOGY AND PATHOPHYSIOLOGY

- Lactation is stimulated by prolactin, which is secreted in pulses by the anterior pituitary, inhibited by dopamine produced in the hypothalamus.
- Galactorrhea results either from prolactin overproduction or loss of inhibitory regulation by dopamine.
  - Afferent neural stimulation
    - Chest wall trauma
    - Chiari-Frommel, del Castillo, and Forbes-Albright syndromes
    - Herpes zoster
    - Nipple stimulation
    - Spinal cord injury
  - Organic hyperprolactinemia
    - Craniopharyngiomas
    - Irradiation
    - Meningiomas or other tumors
    - Multiple sclerosis (MS) (with hypothalamic lesion)
    - Pituitary stalk compression
    - Post-breast augmentation surgery (1%)
    - Prolactinoma
    - Sarcoid
    - Traumatic injury
    - Vascular malformations (aneurysms)
  - Functional hyperprolactinemia
    - Adrenal insufficiency
    - Breast tissue with increased sensitivity to prolactin and/or increased prolactin receptors
    - Chronic kidney disease
    - Cirrhosis
    - Hypothyroidism
    - Lung cancer
    - Renal cell cancer

- Medications/substances:
  - Cardiology
    - α-Methyldopa
    - Reserpine
    - Verapamil
  - GI
    - Domperidone
    - H$_2$ blockers
    - Metoclopramide
    - Proton pump inhibitors (2)[C]
  - Herbal
    - Anise
    - Barley
    - Blessed thistle
    - Fenugreek seed
    - Fennel
  - Illicit
    - Cocaine
    - Marijuana (3)[C]
  - Infectious disease
    - Isoniazid
    - Protease inhibitors
    - Typical and atypical antipsychotics
  - Pain
    - Opioids
  - Psych/neuro
    - Neuroleptics
    - Stimulants
    - SSRIs (prolactin not always elevated)
    - Tricyclic antidepressants
  - Reproductive
    - Estrogens
    - Copper IUD
  - Postoperative condition, especially oophorectomy
  - Idiopathic
    - Normal prolactin levels

GENERAL PREVENTION

- Frequent nipple stimulation can cause galactorrhea.
- Avoid medications that can suppress dopamine.

COMMONLY ASSOCIATED CONDITIONS

See "Etiology and Pathophysiology."

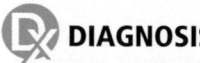 **DIAGNOSIS**

- Findings vary with causes.
- Look for signs/symptoms of associated conditions:
  - Acromegaly
  - Adrenal insufficiency
  - Chest wall conditions
  - Hypothyroidism
  - Polycystic ovarian syndrome

HISTORY

- Usually bilateral milky nipple discharge; may be spontaneous or induced by stimulation
- Determine possibility of pregnancy or recent discontinuation of lactation.
- Signs of hypogonadism from hyperprolactinemia
  - Oligomenorrhea, amenorrhea
  - Inadequate luteal phase, anovulation, infertility
  - Decreased libido (especially in affected males)

- Mass effects from pituitary enlargement
  - Headache, cranial neuropathies
  - Bitemporal hemianopsia, amaurosis, scotomata

PHYSICAL EXAM

Breast examination should be performed with attention to the presence of spontaneous or induced nipple discharge.

DIFFERENTIAL DIAGNOSIS

- Pregnancy-induced lactation or recent weaning
- Nonmilky nipple discharge
  - Intraductal papilloma
  - Fibrocystic disease
- Purulent breast discharge
  - Mastitis
  - Breast abscess
  - Impetigo
  - Eczema
- Bloody breast discharge: Consider malignancy (Paget disease, breast cancer).

DIAGNOSTIC TESTS & INTERPRETATION

Perform formal visual field testing if pituitary adenoma suspected.

Initial Tests (lab, imaging)

- Prolactin level, thyroid-stimulating hormone, pregnancy test, liver and renal functions
- Situations that may alter lab results:
  - Lab evaluation of prolactin may be falsely elevated by a recent breast examination.
  - Vigorous exercise
  - Sexual activity
  - High-carbohydrate diet
  - Consider repeating the test under different circumstances if the value is borderline (30 to 40) elevated.
- Prolactin levels may fluctuate (tend to be highest in the early morning). Elevated prolactin levels should be confirmed with at least one additional level drawn in a fasting, nonexercised state, with no breast stimulation (4)[C].
- If a breast mass is palpated in the setting of nipple discharge, evaluation of that mass is indicated with mammogram and/or ultrasound.
- Pituitary MRI with gadolinium enhancement if the serum prolactin level is significantly elevated (>200 ng/mL) or if a pituitary tumor is otherwise suspected

Follow-Up Tests & Special Considerations

- Consider evaluation of follicle-stimulating hormone and luteinizing hormone if amenorrheic.
- Consider evaluation of growth hormone levels if acromegaly suspected (1)[A].
- Measure adrenal steroids if signs of Cushing disease present.

Diagnostic Procedures/Other

If diagnosis is in question, confirm by microscopic evaluation that nipple secretions are lipoid.

TREATMENT

- Avoid excess nipple stimulation.
- Idiopathic galactorrhea (normal prolactin levels) does not require treatment.
- Discontinue causative medications, if possible.
- If SSRI is implicated, trial of mirtazapine
- Medication is preferred therapy, with surgery or radiotherapy for patients not responding to medication.
- Medical treatment is preferred except for tumors >10 mm (even if asymptomatic) which should be removed to reduce pituitary tumor size or prevent progression to avoid neurologic sequelae.
- If microadenoma, watchful waiting can be appropriate because 95% do not enlarge.

MEDICATION

- Dopamine agonists work to reduce prolactin levels and shrink tumor size. Therapy is suppressive, not curative (4)[C].
- Treatment is discontinued when tumor size has reduced or regressed completely or after pregnancy has been achieved.
- Dopamine agonists are class B in pregnancy and may be resumed if a macroadenoma grows significantly (1)[A].
- Cabergoline (Dostinex)
  – Start at 0.25 mg PO twice weekly and increase by 0.25 mg monthly until prolactin levels normalize. Usual dose ranges from 0.25 to 1.00 mg PO once or twice weekly.
  – More effective and better tolerated than bromocriptine
  – Check ESR and creatinine at baseline and then periodically.
  – ECG at baseline and every 6 to 12 months
  – DC after prolactin level normal for 6 months
- Bromocriptine
  – Start at 1.25 mg QHS PO with food and increase every 3 to 7 days by 2.5 mg/day until therapeutic response achieved (usually 2.5 to 15.0 mg/day).
  – More expensive and more frequent dosing; however, most providers have experience with this effective drug.
  – Long-term treatment can cause woody fibrosis of the pituitary gland.
  – Check creatinine, CBC, LFTs, cardiovascular evaluation; pregnancy test every 4 weeks during amenorrhea and after menses restored if period is >3 days late
- Contraindications are similar for all and include the following:
  – Uncontrolled hypertension
  – Sensitivity to ergot alkaloids
- Precautions
  – Dopamine antagonists may cause nausea, vomiting, psychosis, or dyskinesia.
- Significant possible interactions
  – H_2 blockers, CYP3A4; weak serotonin effect; hypotensive effect

– For women with microadenomas who do not wish to become pregnant, oral contraceptives may be a treatment option.

SURGERY/OTHER PROCEDURES

- Surgery
  – Macroadenomas need surgery if (i) medical management does not halt growth, (ii) neurologic symptoms persist, (iii) size >10 mm, or (iv) patient cannot tolerate medications; also considered in young patients with microadenomas to avoid long-term medical therapy
  – Transsphenoidal pituitary resection
  – 50% recurrence after surgery
- Radiotherapy
  – Radiation is an alternative tumor therapy for macroprolactinomas not responsive to other modes of treatment:
    ○ 20–30% success rate
    ○ 50% risk of panhypopituitarism after radiation
    ○ Risk of optic nerve damage, hypopituitarism, neurologic dysfunction, and increased risk for stroke and secondary brain tumors

 ONGOING CARE

FOLLOW-UP RECOMMENDATIONS

- Outpatient care unless pituitary resection required
- Bromocriptine patients need adequate hydration.
- Dopamine agonist therapy should be discontinued in pregnancy.

Patient Monitoring
- Varies with cause
- Check prolactin levels every 6 weeks until normalized and then every 6 to 12 months.
- Monitor visual fields and/or MRI at least yearly until stable for prolactinoma.

DIET
No restrictions

PATIENT EDUCATION
- Warn about symptoms of mass enlargement in pituitary.
- Discuss treatment rationale, risks of treating, and expectant management.
- Patient education material available from American Family Physician: https://www.aafp.org/afp/2012/0601/p1073-s1.html

PROGNOSIS
- Depends on underlying cause
- Symptoms can recur after discontinuation of a dopamine agonist.
- Surgery can have 50% recurrence.
- Prolactinomas <10 mm can resolve spontaneously.
- Postsurgical hyperprolactinemia is associated with better outcomes in node-negative breast cancer.

COMPLICATIONS
- If enlarging pituitary adenoma, risk of permanent visual field loss

- Panhypopituitarism can complicate radiation or surgical therapy.
- Osteoporosis if amenorrhea persists without estrogen replacement
- Hyperprolactinemia does not increase breast cancer risk.

REFERENCES

1. Molitch M. Diagnosis and treatment of pituitary adenomas: a review. *JAMA*. 2017;317(5):516–524.
2. Pipaliya N, Solanke D, Rathi C, et al. Esomeprazole induced galactorrhea: a novel side effect. *Clin J Gastroenterol*. 2016;9(1):13–16.
3. Rizvi AA. Hyperprolactinemia and galactorrhea associated with marijuana use. *Endocrinologist*. 2006;16:308–310.
4. Huang W, Molitch ME. Evaluation and management of galactorrhea. *Am Fam Physician*. 2012;85(11):1073–1080.

ADDITIONAL READING

Patel BK, Falcon S, Drukteinis J. Management of nipple discharge and the associated imaging findings. *Am J Med*. 2015;128(4):353–360.

 SEE ALSO

Hyperprolactinemia

 CODES

ICD10
- N64.3 Galactorrhea not associated with childbirth
- N64.52 Nipple discharge

CLINICAL PEARLS

- Galactorrhea is a common disorder, affecting up to 50% of reproductive-age women.
- Common causes include idiopathic, from excess nipple stimulation, **dopamine**-suppressing medications, or pituitary prolactinoma.
- Most cases may be adequately evaluated by thyroid-stimulating hormone, prolactin, and human chorionic gonadotropin measurement, with additional testing only as suggested by the presence of other symptoms or signs.
- Lab evaluation of prolactin may be falsely elevated due to recent sexual activity, breast examination, exercise, or a high-carbohydrate diet. Repeat any borderline elevation before continuing evaluation or initiating treatment.
- Evaluate prolactin >200 ng/mL (or signs of suspicion for a pituitary macroadenoma) with a gadolinium-enhanced MRI.

G

GAMING DISORDER, INTERNET

Madhavi Singh, MD • Lauren Schneekloth, MD

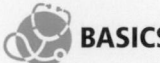 **BASICS**

DESCRIPTION

- Internet gaming disorder (IGD) is where the "gamers" play compulsively, to the exclusion of other interests resulting in clinically significant impairment or distress.
- For gaming disorder to be diagnosed, the behavior pattern must be of sufficient severity and would be evident for at least 12 months.
- IGD is identified in section III of *DSM-5* as a condition warranting more clinical research and experience before it might be considered for inclusion in the main book as a formal disorder.
- On June 18, 2018, WHO recognized gaming disorder as a mental health condition.
- Gaming disorder (digital or video) is included in ICD-11.

EPIDEMIOLOGY

Incidence
- Predominant age—adolescence
- Predominant sex—male

Prevalence
- Median prevalence of 2.0%
- Prevalence rates are highest in Eastern Asian countries and male adolescents aged 12 to 20 years (1).

ETIOLOGY AND PATHOPHYSIOLOGY

- On the molecular level, Internet addiction is characterized by an overall reward deficiency that entails decreased dopaminergic activity (2).
- On the level of neural circuitry, Internet and gaming addiction lead to neuroadaptation and structural changes that occur as a consequence of prolonged increased activity in brain areas associated with addiction (2).
- On a behavioral level, Internet and gaming addicts appear to be constricted with regards to their cognitive functioning in various domains (2).
- IGD shares multiple features with drug addictions, including elevated impulsivity, cognitive inflexibility, and attentional biases.

RISK FACTORS

The following risk factors were found to be significantly associated with IGD (3):
- Functional and dysfunctional impulsivity
- Belief self-control
- Anxiety
- Pursuit of desired appetitive goals
- Money spent on gaming
- Weekday game time
- Offline community meeting attendance
- Game community membership
- Gaming motives play a role as well.
- Gamers with psychiatric distress use it a coping strategy to improve their mood and/or attain emotional stability.
- Achievement-related motives may be related to the lack of real-life achievements that are compensated by virtual victories and successes.

COMMONLY ASSOCIATED CONDITIONS
- Anxiety disorder
- Mood disorder
- Autism spectrum disorder
- Attention deficit hyperactivity disorder
- Personality disorder
- Behavioral disorder

 DIAGNOSIS

HISTORY
- Thorough history
- *DSM-5* section III proposed symptoms of IGD include:
  - Preoccupation with gaming
  - Withdrawal symptoms when gaming is taken away or not possible (sadness, anxiety, irritability)
  - Tolerance, the need to spend more time gaming to satisfy the urge
  - Inability to reduce playing, unsuccessful attempts to quit gaming
  - Giving up other activities, loss of interest in previously enjoyed activities due to gaming
  - Continuing to game despite problems

- Deceiving family members or others about the amount of time spent on gaming
- The use of gaming to relieve negative moods, such as guilt or hopelessness
- Risk, having jeopardized or lost a job or relationship due to gaming
- Under the proposed criteria, a diagnosis of IGD would require experiencing five or more of these symptoms within a year.
- The condition can include gaming on the Internet or on any electronic device.
- Most people who develop clinically significant gaming problems play primarily on the Internet.
- 7-item Game Addiction Scale—GAS items such as relapse, conflict, withdrawal, and problems (loss of interests) were endorsed more frequently in more severe IGD stages, whereas items related to tolerance, salience (preoccupation), and mood modification (escape) were endorsed more widely among participants (including in less severe IGD stages) (4)

PHYSICAL EXAM
Mental status exam

DIFFERENTIAL DIAGNOSIS
- High-engagement Internet gaming, which is normal
- Social anxiety

 TREATMENT

GENERAL MEASURES
- Cognitive-behavioral therapy (CBT) is considered efficacious (5)[A].
- Suggested psychotherapies (6)[C]:
  - CBT is suggested to improve inhibitory control ability, recognize maladaptive cognition, and employ adaptive decision making.
  - Cognitive enhancement therapy to help improve elevated impulsivity, impaired cognitive control, and cognitive inflexibility
  - Cognitive bias modification to target attention biases
  - Mindfulness-based stress reduction to address stress-induced association of IGD

MEDICATION

Methylphenidate, bupropion, and escitalopram have been studied but showed no added benefit.

 ONGOING CARE

PATIENT EDUCATION

- American Academy of Pediatrics recommends no screen time for toddlers <18 months of age except video chatting.
- For children 2 to 5 years, limit are for 1 hr/day for high-quality content and parents should co-view.
- For children 6 years and older, should have consistent limits on screen time with designated media-free times
- For all ages, media should not be located in bedroom and video game play should not begin within half an hour before sleep.

PROGNOSIS

Fair

COMPLICATIONS

- Higher risk of mood disturbance, suicide ideation, and suicide planning in heavy gamers involved with screen times of >5 hours a day (1)
- Reduced sleep duration and disrupted sleep patterns
- Auditory hallucinations
- Enuresis
- Encopresis
- Wrist, neck, and elbow pain, tenosynovitis ("nintendinitis")
- Obesity
- Skin blisters, calluses, sore tendons
- Hand–arm vibration syndrome and peripheral neuropathy

REFERENCES

1. Paulus FW, Ohmann S, von Gontard A, et al. Internet gaming disorder in children and adolescents: a systematic review. *Dev Med Child Neurol*. 2018;60(7):645–659.
2. Griffiths MD, King DL, Demetrovics Z. *DSM-5* Internet gaming disorder needs a unified approach to assessment. *Neuropsychiatry*. 2014;4(1):1–4.
3. Rho MJ, Lee H, Lee TH, et al. Risk factors for Internet gaming disorder: psychological factors and Internet gaming characteristics. *Int J Environ Res Public Health*. 2017;15(1):40.
4. Khazaal Y, Breivik K, Billieux J, et al. Game addiction scale assessment through a nationally representative sample of young adult men: item response theory graded-response modeling. *J Med Internet Res*. 2018;20(8):e10058.
5. Torres-Rodríguez A, Griffiths MD, Carbonell X. The treatment of Internet gaming disorder: a brief overview of the PIPATIC program. *Int J Ment Health Addict*. 2018;16(4):1000–1015.
6. Dong G, Potenza MN. A cognitive-behavioral model of internet gaming disorder: theoretical underpinnings and clinical implications. *J Psychiatr Res*. 2014;58:7–11.

ADDITIONAL READING

- Gentile D. Pathological video-game use among youth ages 8 to 18: a national study. *Psychol Sci*. 2009;20(5):594–602.
- Gentile DA, Bailey K, Bavelier D, et al. Internet gaming disorder in children and adolescents. *Pediatrics*. 2017;140(Suppl 2):S81–S85.

- Higuchi S, Nakayama H, Mihara S, et al. Inclusion of gaming disorder criteria in ICD-11: a clinical perspective in favor. *J Behav Addict*. 2017;6(3):293–295.
- Király O, Griffiths MD, Demetrovics Z. Internet gaming disorder and the *DSM-5*: conceptualization, debates, and controversies. *Curr Addict Rep*. 2015;2(3):254–262.

CLINICAL PEARLS

- IGD is considered a mental health disorder where the "gamers" play compulsively, to the exclusion of other interests resulting in clinically significant impairment or distress with symptoms presence of 12 months.
- Should be differentiated from high-engagement Internet gaming, which is normal
- Most prevalent in Southeast Asian countries in young adolescent males
- Gaming disorder (digital or video) is included in ICD-11.
- CBT is considered efficacious treatment.

G

GASTRITIS
Naureen Rafiq, MBBS

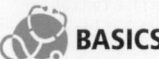 **BASICS**

DESCRIPTION
- Inflammation of the gastric mucosa
- Patchy erythema of gastric mucosa
  - Common on endoscopy; usually insignificant
- Erosive gastritis or reactive gastropathy
  - A reaction to mucosal injury by a noxious agent (especially NSAIDs or alcohol)
  - Damage to the surface epithelium caused by mucosal hypoxia or the direct action of NSAIDs
- Reflux gastritis
  - A reaction to protracted reflux exposure to biliary and pancreatic fluid
  - Typically limited to the prepyloric antrum
- Hemorrhagic gastritis (stress ulceration)
  - A reaction to hemodynamic disorder (e.g., hypovolemia or hypoxia [shock])
  - Common in ICU patients, particularly after severe burns and trauma
  - Seen rarely with certain medications (e.g., dabigatran, an oral thrombin inhibitor)
- Infectious gastritis
  - Acute and/or chronic *Helicobacter pylori* infection
  - Viral infection (reaction to systemic infection)
- Atrophic gastritis
  - Autoimmune versus environmental
  - Frequent in the elderly
  - Primarily from long-standing *H. pylori* infections
  - Prolonged proton pump inhibitor (PPI) use
  - Major risk factor for gastric cancer
  - Associated with primary (pernicious) anemia

Geriatric Considerations
Persons age >60 years often harbor *H. pylori* infection.

Pediatric Considerations
Gastritis rarely occurs in infants or children; increases in prevalence with age

EPIDEMIOLOGY
- Predominant age: all ages (more common in elderly)
- Predominant sex: male = female

ETIOLOGY AND PATHOPHYSIOLOGY
- Noxious agents cause a breakdown in the gastric mucosal barrier, exposing epithelium to injury.
- Infection: *H. pylori* (most common cause), *Staphylococcus aureus* exotoxins, and viral infections
- Alcohol
- Aspirin and other NSAIDs
- Bile reflux
- Pancreatic enzyme reflux
- Portal hypertensive gastropathy
- Emotional stress

Genetics
Unknown, but observational studies show that 10% of a given population is never colonized with *H. pylori*, regardless of exposure. Genetic variations in *TLR1* may help explain some of this observed variation in individual risk for *H. pylori* infection.

RISK FACTORS
- Age >60 years—prevalence of 50–60% by age 60 years
- Exposure to potentially noxious drugs or chemicals (e.g., alcohol or NSAIDs)
- Hypovolemia, hypoxia (shock), burns, head injury, complicated postoperative course
- Autoimmune diseases (thyroid disease and diabetes)
- Family history of *H. pylori* and/or gastric cancer
- Stress (hypovolemia or hypoxia)
- Tobacco use
- Radiation
- Ischemia
- Pernicious anemia
- Gastric mucosal atrophy

GENERAL PREVENTION
- Avoid injurious drugs or chemical agents.
- Patients with hypovolemia or hypoxia (especially ICU patients) should receive prophylaxis with H_2 receptor antagonists, prostaglandins, or sucralfate.
- Consider testing for *H. pylori* (and eradicating if present) in patients on long-term NSAID therapy.

COMMONLY ASSOCIATED CONDITIONS
- Gastric or duodenal peptic ulcer
- Primary (pernicious) anemia—atrophic gastritis
- Portal hypertension (HTN), hepatic failure
- Mucosa-associated lymphoid tissue (MALT) lymphoma

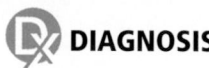 **DIAGNOSIS**

HISTORY
- Epigastric discomfort, often aggravated by eating
- Burning epigastric pain
- Anorexia
- Nausea, with or without vomiting
- Significant bleeding is unusual except in hemorrhagic gastritis.
- Rectal bleeding/melena
- Hiccups
- Bloating or abdominal fullness

PHYSICAL EXAM
- Vital signs to assess hemodynamic stability
- Abdominal exam often normal
- Mild epigastric tenderness
- May have heme-positive stool
- Examine for stigmata of chronic alcohol abuse.

DIFFERENTIAL DIAGNOSIS
- Functional abdominal pain (dyspepsia)
- Peptic ulcer disease
- Viral gastroenteritis
- Gastric cancer (elderly)
- Cholecystitis
- Pancreatic disease (inflammation vs. tumor)

DIAGNOSTIC TESTS & INTERPRETATION
Initial Tests (lab, imaging)
- Usually normal
- CBC to evaluate for blood loss/anemia
- ^{13}C-urea breath test for *H. pylori*
  - 95% specificity and sensitivity
- *H. pylori*, serology serum IgG
  - Inexpensive; 85% sensitivity, 79% specificity
  - Positive in history of colonization or prior infections; *cannot be used to assess eradication*
- Stool analysis for fecal *H. pylori* antigen
  - 95% specificity and sensitivity
- Gastric acid analysis may be abnormal but is not a reliable indicator of gastritis.
- Low serum pepsinogen I (PG I) relative to PG II is associated with fundal intestinal metaplasia.
- Drugs that may alter lab results: Antibiotics or PPIs may affect urea breath test for *H. pylori*.
  - Hold PPIs for 2 weeks, H_2 receptor antagonists for 24 hours, and antibiotics for 4 weeks prior to stool or breath tests (1)[C].

Follow-Up Tests & Special Considerations
Endoscopy for *H. pylori*
- Culture; polymerase chain reaction (PCR); histology; rapid urease testing

Diagnostic Procedures/Other
- Gastroscopy with biopsy is first-line diagnostic tool in:
  - Age >55 years with new-onset signs and symptoms
  - Weight loss, persistent vomiting, or GI bleed (1)[C]
- Gastric biopsies (multiple) in both body and antrum recommended if there is a poor response to initial treatment. *Patients must discontinue PPIs for 2 weeks prior to endoscopy to improve diagnostic accuracy.*

Test Interpretation
Acute or chronic inflammatory infiltrate in gastric mucosa, often with distortion or erosion of adjacent epithelium; presence of *H. pylori* often confirmed

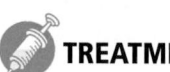 **TREATMENT**

GENERAL MEASURES
- *H. pylori* treatment is required to relieve symptoms.
- Parenteral fluid and electrolyte supplements if unable to tolerate oral intake
- Discontinue NSAID use if possible.
- Abstinence from alcohol; smoking cessation
- Endoscopy in patients not responsive to treatment

MEDICATION

First Line

- Antacids: best given in liquid form, 30 mL 1 hour after meals and at bedtime; useful mainly as an emollient
- H₂ receptor antagonists (e.g., cimetidine [Tagamet]): oral cimetidine 300 mg q6h (or ranitidine [Zantac] 150 mg BID or famotidine [Pepcid] 20 mg BID or nizatidine [Axid]); 150 mg BID not shown to be clearly superior to antacids
- Sucralfate (Carafate): 1 g q4–6h on an empty stomach; rationale uncertain but empirically helpful
- Prostaglandins (misoprostol [Cytotec]): can help allay gastric mucosal injury; dosage 100 to 200 μg QID
- PPIs if no response to antacids or H₂ receptor blockers (e.g., omeprazole 20 mg daily or BID or esomeprazole 20 mg daily or BID)
- H. pylori eradication
  - Clarithromycin triple therapy (CTT)
    - A short-course therapy (10 to 14 days) of amoxicillin 1 g BID, standard dose PPI BID (omeprazole 20 mg BID, etc.), and clarithromycin 500 mg BID (2)[A]
    - 70–85% eradication
    - Optimal treatment still undefined
    - If PCN allergic: Substitute amoxicillin with metronidazole 500 mg TID.
  - Bismuth quadruple therapy (BQT)
    - PPI (omeprazole 20 mg) BID plus bismuth (Pepto-Bismol) 30 mL liquid or 2 tablets QID plus metronidazole 250 mg QID plus tetracycline 500 mg QID for 10 to 14 days (2)[A]
    - 75–90% eradication
    - Use as initial therapy in areas of high clarithromycin resistance (>15%).
    - Consider in penicillin-allergic patients.
- Alternative H. pylori treatment: sequential antibiotic therapy with standard dose PPI (i.e., omeprazole 20 mg) and amoxicillin 1 g BID for 5 days followed by clarithromycin 500 mg and tinidazole mg BID with standard-dose PPI (omeprazole 20 mg) BID for 5 days; equivalent to triple therapy (1)[B],(2)[A]
- H. pylori treatment failure: Use a different regimen; avoid clarithromycin (unless resistance testing confirms susceptibility):
  - BQT for 7 to 14 days (1,2)[A]
  - Consider levofloxacin 250 mg BID, amoxicillin 1 g BID, and standard-dose PPI BID for 14 days in those who fail twice (1,2)[A].
- Consider probiotics in known symptomatic H. pylori. May decrease density of H. pylori in gastric antrum and body; decrease severity of gastritis, peptic ulcers; and possibly slow progression toward atrophic gastritis and gastric adenocarcinoma (3)[A],(4)[C]
  - Probiotics alone likely do not eradicate H. pylori.
  - Possible regimens as used in trials: Bifidobacterium infantis BID × 14 days (5)[C]

- Contraindications: hypersensitivity
- Precautions:
  - Bismuth may turn stool black.
- The manufacturer's profile of each drug lists precautions and potential drug interactions.

ADMISSION, INPATIENT, AND NURSING CONSIDERATIONS

- Gastritis prophylaxis in ICU patients
- Outpatient management, except for severe hemorrhagic gastritis

 ## ONGOING CARE

FOLLOW-UP RECOMMENDATIONS

Usually no restrictions

- Confirm H. pylori eradication 4+ weeks after treatment.

Patient Monitoring

- Consider repeat endoscopy after 6 weeks if gastritis was severe or if poor treatment response.
- Surveillance endoscopy every 3 to 5 years in patients with atrophic gastritis in both the antrum and body, within 1 year for patients with low-grade dysplasia (with extensive biopsy sampling), endoscopy at 6 and 12 months for patients with high-grade dysplasia

DIET

Diet restrictions (e.g., bland, light, soft foods) depend on symptom severity. In general, avoid caffeine and spicy foods and alcohol.

PATIENT EDUCATION

- Smoking cessation; limit alcohol.
- Dietary changes
- Relaxation therapy
- Avoid NSAIDs as possible.

PROGNOSIS

- Most cases clear with identification and treatment of the underlying cause.
- Recurrence of H. pylori infection requires a repeated course of treatment.

COMPLICATIONS

- Bleeding from extensive mucosal erosion or ulceration
- Clearing H. pylori before the development of chronic gastritis may prevent development of gastric cancer.

REFERENCES

1. McColl KE. Clinical practice. *Helicobacter pylori* infection. *N Engl J Med*. 2010;362(17):1597–1604.
2. Malfertheiner P, Megraud F, O'Morain CA, et al; for European Helicobacter Study Group. Management of *Helicobacter pylori* infection—the Maastricht IV/Florence consensus report. *Gut*. 2012;61(5): 646–664.
3. Patel A, Shah N, Prajapati JB. Clinical applications of probiotics in the treatment of *Helicobacter pylori* infection—a brief review. *J Microbiol Immunol Infect*. 2014;47(5):429–437.
4. Emara MH, Elhawari SA, Yousef S, et al. Emerging role of probiotics in the management of *Helicobacter pylori* infection: histopathologic perspectives. *Helicobacter*. 2016;21(1):3–10.
5. Dajani AI, Abu Hammour AM, Yang DH, et al. Do probiotics improve eradication response to *Helicobacter pylori* on standard triple or sequential therapy? *Saudi J Gastroenterol*. 2013;19(3):113–120.

ADDITIONAL READING

- Eslami L, Nasseri-Moghaddam S. Meta-analyses: does long-term PPI use increase the risk of gastric premalignant lesions? *Arch Iran Med*. 2013;16(8):449–458.
- Lopetuso LR, Napoli M, Rizzatti G, et al. Considering gut microbiota disturbance in the management of *Helicobacter pylori* infection. *Expert Rev Gastroenterol Hepatol*. 2018;12(9):899–906. doi:10.1080/17474124.2018.1503946.
- Ruggiero P. Use of probiotics in the fight against *Helicobacter pylori*. *World J Gastrointest Pathophysiol*. 2014;5(4):384–391.

 ## CODES

ICD10

- K29.70 Gastritis, unspecified, without bleeding
- K29.71 Gastritis, unspecified, with bleeding
- K29.00 Acute gastritis without bleeding

CLINICAL PEARLS

- *H. pylori* is the most common cause of gastritis.
- >50% of adult patients are colonized with *H. pylori* by age 60 years.
- *H. pylori* antibody titers rise significantly with reinfection.
- *H. pylori* antibodies decline in the year after treatment and should not be used to determine eradication.
- *H. pylori* stool antigen tests can be used before and after therapy to assess for eradication and reinfection.
- Several courses of therapy may be necessary to eradicate *H. pylori*.
- In cases of suspected gastritis, discontinue PPI 2 weeks prior to endoscopy to improve diagnostic accuracy.
- Consider probiotics as adjunct treatment in symptomatic *H. pylori* gastritis.

G

GASTROESOPHAGEAL REFLUX DISEASE

Fozia Akhtar Ali, MD • Anna Cecilia S. Tenorio, MD • Adriana S. Sanchez, MD

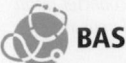 **BASICS**

DESCRIPTION
- Changes of the esophageal mucosa resulting from reflux of gastric contents into the esophagus
- Often described as "heartburn," "acid indigestion," and "acid reflux"

EPIDEMIOLOGY
Incidence
Incidence: 5/1,000 person-years
Prevalence
- 10–20% in the United States
- 40% of adults in the United States have reflux symptoms.
- 50–85% of gastroesophageal reflux disease (GERD) patients have nonerosive reflux disease.
- Chronic GERD is a risk factor for Barrett esophagus.
- 10% of patients with chronic GERD have Barrett esophagus.
- Risk of adenocarcinoma without Barrett esophagus and no dysplasia: 0.1–0.5% per patient-year
- Risk of adenocarcinoma with Barrett esophagus and high-grade dysplasia: 6–19% per patient-year
- Pediatric population: Regurgitation occurs at least once a day in 2/3 of 4-month-old infants, decreasing to 21% at age 6 to 7 months, and 5% at 10 to 12 months.

ETIOLOGY AND PATHOPHYSIOLOGY
- The pattern and mechanism of reflux varies depending on the severity of disease.
- GERD begins when acidic stomach contents contact the squamous mucosal lining of the esophagus, at the esophagogastric junction (EGJ).
- Inappropriate transient lower esophageal sphincter (LES) relaxation. Foods that are spicy; acidic; and high in fat, caffeine, alcohol, tobacco, anticholinergic medications, nitrates, smooth muscle relaxants affect LES relaxation.
- Patients with severe GERD often have evidence of a hiatal hernia, which can (1):
  - Trap acid in the hernia sac
  - Impair acid emptying
  - Increase retrograde acid flow rate
  - Reduce the EGJ sphincter pressure
  - Increase frequency of transient LES relaxations
Genetics
Genetic heterogeneity has been associated with GERD.

RISK FACTORS
- Obesity
- Hiatal hernia
- Scleroderma
- Alcohol use
- Tobacco use
- Pregnancy

GENERAL PREVENTION
- Decrease consumption of food and beverage triggers such as spicy, fatty foods, alcohol, and caffeine.
- Weight loss
- Avoid lying down after meals.
- Tobacco and alcohol cessation
- Elevate head of bed at night.
- Avoid meals close to bedtime.
- Infants: Use car seat for 2 to 3 hours after meals; thickened feedings

COMMONLY ASSOCIATED CONDITIONS
- Nonerosive esophagitis
- Erosive esophagitis
- Irritable bowel syndrome
- Peptic ulcer disease
- Extraesophageal reflux: aspiration, chronic cough, laryngitis, vocal cord granuloma, sinusitis, otitis media
- Halitosis
- Hiatal hernia: acid pocket (zone of high acidity in the proximal stomach above the diaphragm) (2)[B]
- Peptic stricture: 10% of patients with GERD
- Barrett esophagus
- Esophageal adenocarcinoma

 DIAGNOSIS

HISTORY
- Typical symptoms: acid regurgitation, heartburn, dysphagia (mostly postprandial)
- Atypical symptoms: epigastric fullness/pressure/pain, dyspepsia, nausea, bloating, belching, chest pain, lump in throat
- Extraesophageal signs and symptoms: chronic cough, bronchospasm, wheezing, hoarseness, sore throat
- Heartburn: retrosternal burning sensation
- Regurgitation; sour or acid taste in mouth ("water brash")
- Symptoms worse with bending or lying down
- Diet, alcohol and tobacco use

PHYSICAL EXAM
Often unremarkable. Make note of:
- BMI
- Epigastric tenderness or palpable epigastric mass
- Stigmata of chronic systemic disease or alcohol use
- Dental erosions

DIFFERENTIAL DIAGNOSIS
- Infectious esophagitis (*Candida*, herpes, HIV, cytomegalovirus)
- Chemical esophagitis; pill-induced esophagitis
- Eosinophilic esophagitis
- Nonulcer dyspepsia
- Biliary tract disease
- Radiation injury
- Crohn disease
- Angina/coronary artery disease
- Esophageal stricture or anatomic defect (ring, sling)
- Esophageal adenocarcinoma
- Achalasia; scleroderma
- Peptic ulcer disease

DIAGNOSTIC TESTS & INTERPRETATION
Diagnosis often based on history and clinical symptoms. Treat patients with typical symptoms of GERD and no alarm symptoms (dysphagia, odynophagia, weight loss, early satiety, anemia, new onset, male >50 years) empirically with antisecretory agents without any further diagnostic testing.

Initial Tests (lab, imaging)
- Indication for blood work depends on clinical presentation. Check for anemia (history of bleeding; or possible poor vitamin B_{12} absorption due to chronic proton pump inhibitor [PPI] use).
- Appropriately evaluate patients who present with symptoms suspicious for cardiac disease.

Diagnostic Procedures/Other
- Upper endoscopy
  - First-line diagnostic test for those with alarm signs and uncontrolled symptoms (2)[B]
  - Indications for endoscopy:
    ○ Alarm symptoms such as dysphagia, bleeding, anemia, weight loss, recurrent vomiting
    ○ Persistent typical GERD symptoms despite treatment with twice-daily PPI for 4 to 8 weeks
    ○ Men >50 years with chronic GERD (>5 years) and other risk factors: hiatal hernia, high BMI, tobacco use, high abdominal fat distribution
    ○ History of severe erosive esophagitis (Assess healing and check for UGI pathology including Barrett esophagus.)
    ○ Surveillance (history of Barrett esophagus)
  - ~50–70% of patients with heartburn have negative endoscopic findings.
  - Savary-Miller classification (endoscopic grading)
    ○ Grade I: ≥1 nonconfluent reddish spots, with or without exudate
    ○ Grade II: erosive and exudative lesions in the distal esophagus; may be confluent but not circumferential
    ○ Grade III: circumferential erosions in the distal esophagus
    ○ Grade IV: chronic complications such as deep ulcers, stenosis, or scarring with Barrett metaplasia
- Esophageal manometry
  - Not recommended for primary GERD diagnosis; a second option for those with GERD and normal endoscopy (2)[B]
  - Diagnose motility disorders: functional heartburn, achalasia, and distal esophageal spasm.
  - Used to evaluate peristaltic function preoperatively and to record LES pressure
- Ambulatory reflux (pH) monitoring
  - Evaluate excessive acid exposure in those with GERD symptoms, normal endoscopy, and no response to PPI (2)[B].
  - Used to document frequency of reflux
  - Discontinue PPI for 7 days prior to procedure.
- Barium swallow: not used for GERD diagnosis; used to evaluate complaints of dysphagia or to outline anatomic abnormalities (hiatal hernia)

Test Interpretation
- Acute inflammation (especially eosinophils)
- Epithelial basal zone hyperplasia seen in 85%
- Barrett epithelial change: Gastric columnar epithelium replaces squamous epithelium in distal esophagus (metaplasia).

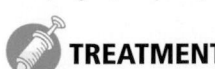 **TREATMENT**

GENERAL MEASURES
Lifestyle changes are first-line intervention:
- Elevate head of bed (2)[B].
- Avoid meals 2 to 3 hours before bedtime (2)[B].
- Avoid stooping, bending, and tight-fitting garments.

- Avoid medications that relax LES (anticholinergic drugs; calcium channel blockers).
- Promote weight loss (2)[B].
- Tobacco cessation and alcohol avoidance
- Limit consumption of patient-specific food triggers (global elimination of all reflux-causing foods is not necessary, practical, or beneficial).
- Stepped therapy
  - Phase I: lifestyle and diet modifications, antacids plus H_2 blockers or PPIs
  - Phase II: If symptoms persist, consider endoscopy.
  - Phase III: If symptoms still persist, consider surgery.

MEDICATION

First Line

- H_2 blockers in equipotent oral doses (e.g., cimetidine 800 mg BID or 400 mg QID, ranitidine 150 mg BID, famotidine 20 mg BID, or nizatidine 150 mg BID)
  - Renally dosed: Decrease dose to 50 mg and for creatinine clearance <50 mL/min.
  - Although less effective than PPIs, H_2 blockers given in divided doses provide symptomatic relief in patients with less severe symptoms (3)[A].
- PPIs: irreversibly bind proton pump (H^+/K^+ ATPase), effective onset within 4 days; omeprazole 20 to 40 mg/day, lansoprazole 15 to 30 mg/day, dexlansoprazole 30 mg/day, pantoprazole 40 mg/day, rabeprazole 20 mg/day, esomeprazole 40 mg/day
  - No major differences in efficacy among PPIs
  - Dose 30 to 60 minutes before meals with the exception of dexlansoprazole (2)[A].
  - PPIs may increase risk of hypomagnesemia, hip fracture, *Clostridium difficile* infection, vitamin B_{12} deficiency, and community-acquired pneumonia.
- PPI more effective than H_2 blocker and prokinetics for healing erosive and nonerosive esophagitis (4)[A]
- Erosive esophagitis: 8 weeks of PPI effective in 90%

Pediatric Considerations

Antacids or liquid H_2 blockers and PPIs are available. Prokinetics have a minimal role due to safety concerns and limited efficacy.

Second Line

- Antacids or barrier agents (sucralfate 1 g PO QID 1 hour before meals and at bedtime for 4 to 8 weeks) may relieve breakthrough symptoms.
- Prokinetics: metoclopramide 5 to 10 mg before meals
- Baclofen as add-on therapy with a PPI
- Precautions
  - Blood dyscrasias and anemia with PPIs and H_2 blockers
  - Metoclopramide is a dopamine blocker; risk of dystonia and tardive dyskinesia
  - Tachyphylaxis may occur with H_2 blockers.
- Significant possible interactions
  - PPIs and H_2 blockers: multiple cytochrome P450 drug interactions; warfarin, phenytoin, antifungals, digoxin

SURGERY/OTHER PROCEDURES

- Laparoscopic fundoplication (wrapping gastric fundus around distal esophagus) increases pressure gradient between stomach and esophagus.
- Bariatric surgery
  - Surgery indicated if patient desires to discontinue medical therapy, has side effects with medical therapy, has a large hiatal hernia, has esophagitis refractory to medical therapy, or has refractory symptoms (4)[A]
  - Preoperative ambulatory pH monitor mandatory in patients with no evidence of erosive esophagitis (4)[A]

- Manometry to rule out esophageal dysmotility, achalasia, or scleroderma prior to surgery (4)[A]
- Best surgical response in patients with typical symptoms who respond well to PPI therapy
- If patient is expected to require >10 years of PPI treatment, surgery may be more cost-effective.
- Consider bariatric surgery for morbidly obese patients. Gastric bypass is preferred (4)[A].

Pediatric Considerations

Surgery for severe symptoms (apnea, choking, persistent vomiting)

 ## ONGOING CARE

FOLLOW-UP RECOMMENDATIONS

Patient Monitoring

- Track symptoms over time.
- Repeat endoscopy in 4 to 8 weeks if there is a poor symptomatic response to medical therapy, especially in older patients.
- In patients with Barrett esophagus who would opt for treatment if cancer is detected, perform endoscopic surveillance every 2 to 3 years.

DIET

Avoid foods that can trigger or make symptoms worse.

PATIENT EDUCATION

Lifestyle and dietary modifications: Eat small meals; avoid lying down after meals; elevate head of bed; weight loss; smoking cessation; avoid alcohol and caffeine.

PROGNOSIS

- Symptoms and esophageal inflammation often return promptly when treatment is withdrawn. To prevent relapse of symptoms, continue antisecretory therapy (in addition to lifestyle and dietary modifications).
  - PPI maintenance therapy likely improves quality of life more than H_2 blockers.
  - Full-dose PPIs are more effective than half-dose for maintenance (4)[A].
  - In erosive esophagitis, daily maintenance therapy with PPI prevents relapse; intermittent PPI therapy not as effective (1)[A]
- Medical and surgical therapy are equally effective for symptom reduction (4)[A].
- Antireflux surgery
  - 90–94% symptom response. Patients with persistent symptoms should have repeat anatomic evaluation (endoscopy or esophagram).
  - Some surgically treated patients eventually require medical therapy due to recurrence of symptoms.
- Regression of Barrett epithelium does not routinely occur despite aggressive medical or surgical therapy.

COMPLICATIONS

- Peptic stricture: 10–15%
- Barrett esophagus: 10%
  - Adenocarcinoma cancer develops at an annual rate of 0.5%.
  - Primary treatment for Barrett esophagus with high-grade dysplasia is endoscopic radiofrequency ablation.
- Extraesophageal symptoms: hoarseness, aspiration, (including pneumonia)
- Bleeding due to mucosal injury
- Noncardiac chest pain

Geriatric Considerations

Complications more likely (e.g., aspiration pneumonia)

REFERENCES

1. Lee YY, McColl KE. Pathophysiology of gastroesophageal reflux disease. *Best Pract Res Clin Gastroenterol.* 2013;27(3):339–351.
2. Patti MG. An evidence-based approach to the treatment of gastroesophageal reflux disease. *JAMA Surg.* 2016;151(1):73–78.
3. Sigterman KE, van Pinxteren B, Bonis PA, et al. Short-term treatment with proton pump inhibitors, H2-receptor antagonists and prokinetics for gastro-oesophageal reflux disease-like symptoms and endoscopy negative reflux disease. *Cochrane Database Syst Rev.* 2013;(5):CD002095.
4. Katz PO, Gerson LB, Vela MF. Guidelines for the diagnosis and management of gastroesophageal reflux disease. *Am J Gastroenterol.* 2013;108(3):308–328.

ADDITIONAL READING

- Anderson WD III, Strayer SM, Mull SR. Common questions about the management of gastroesophageal reflux disease. *Am Fam Physician.* 2015;91(10):692–697.
- El-Serag HB, Sweet S, Winchester CC, et al. Update on the epidemiology of gastro-oesophageal reflux disease: a systematic review. *Gut.* 2014;63(6):871–880.

 ## SEE ALSO

Algorithms: Abdominal Pain, Upper; Dyspepsia

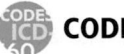 ## CODES

ICD10

- K21.9 Gastro-esophageal reflux disease without esophagitis
- K21.0 Gastro-esophageal reflux disease with esophagitis

CLINICAL PEARLS

- GERD is primarily a historical diagnosis.
- Consider GERD in nonsmokers with a chronic cough (>3 weeks).
- Antisecretory therapy is the mainstay of pharmacotherapy for GERD.
- PPIs provide the most rapid symptomatic relief and healing of esophagitis.
- Endoscopy is recommended for patients with alarm symptoms, onset age >50 years, or prolonged severe symptoms.

G

GAY HEALTH

Justin Bowen Neisler, MD • Kimberly Insel, MD, MPH

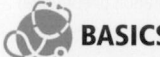 **BASICS**

DESCRIPTION

- Health disparities exist among sexual minority groups (gay or lesbian and bisexual) and between sexual minority groups and heterosexuals; disparities are far reaching and include differences in health conditions, health behaviors, health care access, and health care utilization. Sexual minority groups tend to fare worse across all realms.
- LGBT individuals may hide their orientation out of fear of stigma and discrimination, so it is important to ask all patients about sexual identity and behavior in a nonjudgmental environment.
- Structural barriers of a heterosexist and unwelcoming healthcare system and the minority stress (fear, stigma, internalized homophobia) experienced by LGBT people likely contribute to the development of health disparities. These disparities do not arise from innate characteristics of LGBT people.
- This chapter focuses on the diverse group of gay, bisexual, and other men who have sex with men (MSM). Although lesbian and transgender health are discussed separately under their respective topic headings, please note that many of the disparities and risks discussed here affect transgender women at similar or higher levels than men. Men who have sex with transgender women may need many of the same screenings and prevention strategies as MSM.
- Although this chapter reviews the important topics that disproportionally effect this population, primary care of MSM is foremost about delivering the same care delivered to all patients.

GENERAL PREVENTION

- All MSM should receive hepatitis A and B immunizations (1)[A].
- Young MSM <26 years old should be vaccinated against HPV (1)[C].
- Centers for Disease Control and Prevention (CDC) recommends at least annual screening for HIV, syphilis, gonorrhea, and chlamydia as detailed below.
- CDC recommends testing for hepatitis B (2)[A].
- Annual screening for hepatitis C is only recommended in MSM with HIV (2)[A].
- Screening for hepatitis A is not recommended.

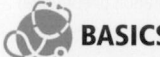 **DIAGNOSIS**

- Sexually transmitted infections (STIs)
  - STIs among MSM are increasing. In 2016, MSM accounted for approximately 58% of new cases of primary and secondary syphilis.
  - Behaviors that increase risk of non-HIV STIs also increase risk of HIV acquisition.
  - Physicians should screen for these high-risk behaviors and advocate for safer sex practices nonjudgmentally from a harm reduction perspective.

- Behavioral risk factors include the following:
  - Anonymous sexual encounters
  - Multiple active sex partners
  - Inconsistent barrier protection (condom) use
  - Substance use around and during sex
  - Receptive > insertive anal intercourse
  - Among adolescents, those who are unsure about their sexual identity report the highest rates of sexual risk-taking behavior.
  - Annual screening of all asymptomatic sexually active MSM should include:
    - Syphilis serology using both nontreponemal and treponemal testing
    - Urine testing with nucleic acid amplification test (NAAT) for *Neisseria gonorrhoeae* and *Chlamydia trachomatis* if having insertive intercourse within the last year
    - Rectal swab NAAT for *N. gonorrhoeae* and *C. trachomatis* if having anal receptive intercourse within the last year
    - Pharyngeal swab NAAT for *N. gonorrhoeae* if having oral receptive intercourse within the last year. Pharyngeal swab for *C. trachomatis* is not recommended (2)[A].
  - Screening should be increased to every 3 or 6 months in MSM at higher risk (see above) (2)[A].
  - Because of the stigma of male same-sex sexual behavior, many MSM may not volunteer STI symptoms. Providers should ask about sexual behaviors (insertive/receptive, oral/anal) and the corresponding symptoms of STIs, that is, pain with defecation seen in proctitis.

- HIV
  - 82% of new cases of HIV diagnosed in 2016 were among MSM. These disproportionately affected African American and Hispanic/Latino MSM, young MSM aged 13 to 24 years, and transgender women.
  - Up to 44% of MSM may not know their HIV status. This is more likely in men who are not open about their sexual identity and behavior (2).
  - Sexually active MSM should be screened at least annually for HIV (3)[A].
  - Educate patients having anal sex on multimodal risk reduction using condoms (63% reduction for insertive, 72% receptive), preexposure prophylaxis (PrEP, 90% reduction), and postexposure prophylaxis (PEP) in the case of an unsafe sexual encounter.
  - Indications for PrEP
    - HIV negative (confirm with RNA viral load if exposure within last 4 weeks)
    - Sexually active, but not in a monogamous relationship with an HIV-negative partner
    - *And* at least one of the following:
      - Anal sex without condoms in past 6 months (receptive or insertive)
      - Any STI diagnosed in past 6 months
      - In a sexual relationship with HIV-positive partner

  - The only FDA-approved regimen for PrEP is daily oral single-pill combination tenofovir disoproxil fumarate (TDF) 300 mg and emtricitabine(FTC) 200 mg, which has shown to be safe and effective in reducing the risk of sexual transfer of HIV (4)[A].
    - Additional medications or replacement with other antiretrovirals is not recommended (4)[A].
    - Although TDF alone is approved for other groups, it is not recommended in MSM because it has not been studied in this population (4)[A].
    - Monitor HIV status every 3 months and renal function at least every 6 months.
  - Indications for PEP
    - ≤72 hours after exposure to known HIV-positive partner
  - PEP generally involves 28-day course of highly active antiretroviral therapy (HAART) in a three-drug combination:
    - Two nucleoside reverse transcriptase inhibitors (NRTIs) and either a protease inhibitor (PI) or a nonnucleoside reverse transcriptase inhibitor (NNRTI) or integrase inhibitor
    - Selection of medications are based on side effect profiles, patient compliance, and patient convenience.
    - "Preferred" regimens include the following:
      - Efavirenz plus lamivudine or emtricitabine plus zidovudine or tenofovir
      - Lopinavir/ritonavir (Kaletra) plus lamivudine or emtricitabine plus zidovudine
    - Counsel on safer sex and risk reduction for repeated exposures, including immediate transition to PrEP after completing PEP.
- Cancer
  - Annual incidence of anal cancer is 5 times higher in HIV-negative MSM than the general population; increases to between 78 and 168 times higher in HIV-positive MSM
  - Anal carcinoma has been linked to certain high-risk subtypes of HPV, specifically types 16 and 18.
  - Screening for anal dysplasia with anal cytology may be considered for at-risk populations, especially HIV-infected MSM, but further research is needed for appropriate screening intervals (5)[A].
  - HPV vaccine is recommended for all boys age 11 to 12 years and young MSM through age 26 years to reduce the risk of anal cancer (1)[B].
- Substance and tobacco abuse
  - Tobacco use is double in LGBT populations.
    - LGBT people report not feeling mainstream tobacco cessation inventions connect with them.
  - Alcoholism has also been shown to be more prevalent among gay and bisexual men.
    - Many gay and bisexual men may find difficulty seeking aid in faith-based groups such as Alcoholics Anonymous due to the long history of religious discrimination of LGBT people.
  - Methamphetamine use is increased among MSM; some may use it during or around sexual encounters to increase pleasure and performance.
    - Substance abuse treatment programs implementing cognitive behavioral intervention from a harm reduction perspective is beneficial in reducing stimulant use and sexual risk-taking behavior.

- Mental health
  - Most LGBT people, like all people, are mentally healthy; however, risks for developing major depressive, bipolar, and anxiety disorders are 1.5 times higher in the LGBT population (6).
  - Risk of deliberate self-harm is also increased especially among youth due to stressors such as having an identity different than family and peers, isolation, bullying, family rejection, and self-nonacceptance.

Pediatric Considerations

- Normalizing nonheterosexual identities and behaviors during regular screening of sexual development during well adolescent visits could reduce stigma and decrease risk for negative mental health outcomes.
  - Rates of body image and eating disorders are increased in adolescent and young adult gay men.
  - Depression has been linked to increased sexual risk-taking behavior.
  - In addition to depression screenings recommended for all patients, regular assessments of mental health and suicide risk should include questions about family and peer support, experiences of stigma, connection to an LGBT community, and self-acceptance.
- Intimate partner violence (IPV) (domestic violence)
  - Recent study reported ~21% of sexual minority men with a history of physical abuse and ~50% with psychological abuse; highest rates reported among bisexual men
  - Despite rates of IPV among male same-sex couples being equal to heterosexual couples, there is a lack of attention to IPV among LGBT people.
  - Same-sex IPV can be complex, involving worsening of the emotional and psychological minority stress of the victim, threats to "out" partner, abuse regarding HIV status.
  - Gay and bisexual victims are less likely to have support from family or the community.
  - Providers can stigmatize male same-sex IPV as not being as serious.
  - Screen for IPV with patients alone.
  - Be prepared to respond with compassion and connection to local LGBT-welcoming resources.

ONGOING CARE

Obtaining a history

- Establish with patients that information related to sexual orientation is confidentially asked of all patients to assist in providing them the best care.
- Avoid labeling patients as gay, lesbian, bisexual, or transgender unless prompted by the patients.
- Intake forms and waiting room and marketing materials inclusive of same-sex couples and identities create a welcoming and open environment.
- Individualize regular discussions about substance and tobacco abuse, HIV/STIs, mental health, and IPV.
- Take an inclusive and complete sexual history:
  - Do you have sex with men, women, both?
  - Who are you having sex with?
  - What kind of sex do you have? Oral? Anal? Insertive/Topping? Receptive/Bottoming? Others?
  - Do you use drugs or drink alcohol before sex?
  - How do you protect yourself during sex?

- How often do you use condoms?
- Do you feel comfortable with your sexuality?
- Tell me about your support system?
- Do you have a significant other?
- Do you feel safe and supported in your relationship?
- Are you interested in PrEP?

PATIENT EDUCATION

- Educate patients on risk-reduction strategies for safer sex such as avoiding or limiting substance use around sex, condoms, PrEP, and PEP.
- Educate patients on LGBT-specific or welcoming resources in your community for substance and tobacco abuse, IPV, mental health, and suicide prevention.

REFERENCES

1. Kim DK, Riley LE, Hunter P; for Advisory Committee on Immunization Practices. Recommended immunization schedule for adults aged 19 years or older, United States, 2018. *Ann Intern Med*. 2018;168(3):210–220.
2. Workowski KA, Bolan GA; for Centers for Disease Control and Prevention. Sexually transmitted diseases treatment guidelines, 2015. *MMWR Recomm Rep*. 2015;64(RR-03):1–137.
3. DiNenno EA, Prejean J, Delaney KP, et al. Evaluating the evidence for more frequent than annual HIV screening of gay, bisexual, and other men who have sex with men in the United States: results from a systematic review and CDC expert consultation. *Public Health Rep*. 2018;133(1):3–21.
4. U.S. Public Health Service. *Preexposure Prophylaxis for the Prevention of HIV Infection in the United States—2017 Update: A Clinical Practice Guideline*. Washington, DC: U.S. Public Health Service; 2017.
5. Clarke MA, Wentzensen N. Strategies for screening and early detection of anal cancers: a narrative and systematic review and meta-analysis of cytology, HPV testing, and other biomarkers [published online ahead of print May 24, 2018]. *Cancer Cytopathol*. doi:10.1002/cncy.22018.
6. King M, Semlyen J, Tai SS, et al. A systematic review of mental disorder, suicide, and deliberate self harm in lesbian, gay and bisexual people. *BMC Psychiatry*. 2008;8:70.

ADDITIONAL READING

- Adelson S, Stroeh O, Ng Y. Development and mental health of lesbian, gay, bisexual, or transgender youth in pediatric practice. *Pediatr Clin North Am*. 2016;63(6):971–983.
- Berger I, Mooney-Somers J. Smoking cessation programs for lesbian, gay, bisexual, transgender, and intersex people: a content-based systematic review. *Nicotine Tob Res*. 2017;19(12):1408–1417.
- Blaser N, Bertisch B, Kouyos R, et al. Impact of screening and antiretroviral therapy on anal cancer incidence in HIV-positive MSM. *AIDS*. 2017;31(13):1859–1866.
- Carrico AW, Flentje A, Gruber VA, et al. Community-based harm reduction substance abuse treatment with methamphetamine-using men who have sex with men. *J Urban Health*. 2014;91(3):555–567.

- Centers for Disease Control and Prevention. Diagnoses of HIV infection in the United States and dependent areas, 2016. *HIV Surveill Rep*. 2016;28:1–125.
- Gay & Lesbian Medical Association. *Guidelines for the Care of Lesbian, Gay, Bisexual, and Transgender Patients*. San Francisco, CA: Gay & Lesbian Medical Association; 2006. http://www.glma.org. Accessed September 24, 2018.
- Institute of Medicine. *The Health of Lesbian, Gay, Bisexual, and Transgender People: Building a Foundation for Better Understanding*. Washington, DC: National Academies Press; 2011.
- Kuhar DT, Henderson DK, Struble KA, et al; and US Public Health Service Working Group. Updated US Public Health Service guidelines for the management of occupational exposures to human immunodeficiency virus and recommendations for postexposure prophylaxis. *Infect Control Hosp Epidemiol*. 2013;34(9):875–892.
- Mayer KH, Bekker LG, Stall R, et al. Comprehensive clinical care for men who have sex with men: an integrated approach. *Lancet*. 2012;380(9839): 378–387.
- Meyer IH. Prejudice, social stress, and mental health in lesbian, gay, and bisexual populations: conceptual issues and research evidence. *Psychol Bull*. 2003;129(5):674–697.
- Miranda-Mendizábal A, Castellví P, Parés-Badell O, et al. Sexual orientation and suicidal behaviour in adolescents and young adults: systematic review and meta-analysis. *Br J Psychiatry*. 2017;211(2):77–87.
- Rollè L, Giardina G, Caldarera AM, et al. When intimate partner violence meets same sex couples: a review of same sex intimate partner violence. *Front Psychol*. 2018;9:1506.

 ## CODES

ICD10

- Z11.59 Encounter for screening for other viral diseases
- Z11.4 Encounter for screening for human immunodeficiency virus
- Z72.52 High risk homosexual behavior

CLINICAL PEARLS

- Provide gay, bisexual, and MSM with the same comprehensive primary care delivered to all patients.
- Create a welcoming, open, nonjudgmental, and inclusive environment of care.
- All sexually active MSM should be offered annual screening for HIV, syphilis, rectal and urethral gonorrhea and chlamydia, and pharyngeal gonorrhea.
- Immunize all MSM for hepatitis A and B as well as all young MSM through age 26 years for HPV.
- Counsel patients on risk-reduction strategies for safer sex such as avoiding or limiting substance use around sex, condoms, PrEP, and PEP.
- Regularly screen for substance use, mental health conditions, eating disorders, suicidality, and IPV and be ready to respond with compassion and connection to LGBT-welcoming resources.

G

GENITO-PELVIC PAIN/PENETRATION DISORDER (VAGINISMUS)

Jeffrey D. Quinlan, MD, FAAFP

BASICS

Genito-pelvic pain/penetration disorder is the name of the conditions formally known as vaginismus and dyspareunia. Vaginismus results from involuntary contraction of the vaginal musculature. Primary vaginismus occurs in women who have never been able to have penetrative intercourse. Women with secondary vaginismus were previously able to have penetrative intercourse but are no longer able to do so.

DESCRIPTION
- Persistent or recurrent difficulties for 6 months or more with at least one of the following:
  - Inability to have vaginal intercourse/penetration on at least 50% of attempts
  - Marked genito-pelvic pain during at least 50% of vaginal intercourse/penetration attempts
  - Marked fear of vaginal intercourse/penetration or of genito-pelvic pain during intercourse/penetration on at least 50% of vaginal intercourse/penetration attempts
  - Marked tensing or tightening of the pelvic floor muscles during attempted vaginal intercourse/penetration on at least 50% of occasions
- The disturbance causes marked distress or interpersonal difficulty.
- Dysfunction is not as a result of:
  - Nonsexual mental disorder
  - Severe relationship stress
  - Other significant stress
  - Substance or medication effect
- Specify if with a general medical condition (e.g., lichen sclerosus, endometriosis) (1).

Pregnancy Considerations
May first present during evaluation for infertility
- Pregnancy can occur in patients with genito-pelvic pain/penetration disorder when ejaculation occurs on the perineum.
- Vaginismus may be an independent risk factor for cesarean delivery.

EPIDEMIOLOGY
Incidence
The incidence of vaginismus is thought to be about 1–17% per year worldwide. In North America, 12–21% of women have genito-pelvic pain of varying etiologies (2).

Prevalence
- True prevalence is unknown due to limited data/reporting.
- Population-based studies report prevalence rates of 0.5–30%.
- Affects women in all age groups
- Approximately 15% of women in North America report recurrent pain during intercourse.

ETIOLOGY AND PATHOPHYSIOLOGY
Most often multifactorial in both primary and secondary vaginismus
- Primary
  - Psychological and psychosocial issues
    - Negative messages about sex and sexual relations in upbringing may cause phobic reaction.
    - Poor body image and limited understanding of genital area
    - History of sexual trauma
  - Abnormalities of the hymen
  - History of difficult gynecologic examination
- Secondary
  - Often situational
  - Often associated with dyspareunia secondary to:
    - Vaginal infection
    - Inflammatory dermatitis
    - Surgical or postdelivery scarring
    - Endometriosis
    - Inadequate vaginal lubrication
    - Pelvic radiation
    - Estrogen deficiency
  - Conditioned response to pain from physical issues previously listed

RISK FACTORS
- Most often idiopathic
- Although the exact role in the condition is unclear, many women report a history of abuse or sexual trauma.
- Often associated with other sexual dysfunctions

COMMONLY ASSOCIATED CONDITIONS
- Marital stress, family dysfunction
- Anxiety
- Vulvodynia/vestibulodynia

DIAGNOSIS

DSM-5 has combined vaginismus and dyspareunia in a condition called genito-pelvic pain/penetration disorder.

HISTORY
- Complete medical history
- Full psychosocial and sexual history, including the following:
  - Onset of symptoms (primary or secondary)
  - If secondary, precipitating events, if any
  - Relationship difficulty/partner violence
  - Inability to allow vaginal entry for different purposes
    - Sexual (penis, digit, object)
    - Hygiene (tampon use)
    - Health care (pelvic examination)
  - Infertility
  - Traumatic experiences (exam, sexual, etc.)
  - Religious beliefs
  - Views on sexuality

PHYSICAL EXAM
- Pelvic examination is necessary to exclude structural abnormalities or organic pathology.
- Educating the patient about the examination and giving her control over the progression of the examination is essential because genital/pelvic examination may induce varying degrees of anxiety in patients.
- Referral to a gynecologist, family physician, or other provider specializing in the treatment of sexual disorders may be appropriate.
- Contraction of pelvic floor musculature in anticipation of examination may be seen.
- Lamont classification system aids in the assessment of severity:
  - First degree: perineal and levator spasm relieved with reassurance
  - Second degree: perineal spasm maintained throughout the pelvic exam
  - Third degree: levator spasm and elevation of buttocks
  - Fourth degree: levator and perineal spasm and elevation with adduction and retreat

DIFFERENTIAL DIAGNOSIS
- Vaginal infection
- Vulvodynia/vestibulodynia
- Vulvovaginal atrophy
- Urogenital structural abnormalities
- Interstitial cystitis
- Endometriosis

DIAGNOSTIC TESTS & INTERPRETATION
No laboratory tests indicated unless signs of vaginal infection are noted on examination. When diagnosing of this disorder has been conducted, five factors should be considered.
- Partner factors
- Relationship factors
- Individual vulnerability factors
- Cultural/religious factors
- Medical factors

Test Interpretation
Not available; may be needed to check for secondary causes

TREATMENT

- Genito-pelvic pain/penetration disorder may be successfully treated (2)[B].
- Outpatient care is appropriate.
- Treatment of physical conditions, if present, is first line (see "Secondary" under "Etiology and Pathophysiology").
- Role for pelvic floor physical therapy and myofascial release

- Some evidence suggests that cognitive-behavioral therapy may be effective, including desensitization techniques, such as gradual exposure, aimed at decreasing avoidance behavior and fear of vaginal penetration (3)[A].
- Based on a Cochrane review, a clinically relevant effect of systematic desensitization cannot be ruled out (4)[A].
- Evidence suggests that sex therapy may be effective (4)[B].
  – Involves Kegel exercises to increase control over perineal muscles
  – Stepwise vaginal desensitization exercises
    ○ With vaginal dilators that the patient inserts and controls
    ○ With woman's own finger(s) to promote sexual self-awareness
    ○ Advancement to partner's fingers with patient's control
    ○ Coitus after achieving largest vaginal dilator or three fingers; important to begin with sensate-focused exercises/sensual caressing without necessarily a demand for coitus
    ○ Female superior at first; passive (nonthrusting); female-directed
    ○ Later, thrusting may be allowed.
- Topical anesthetic or anxiolytic with desensitization exercises may be considered.
- Patient education is an essential component of treatment (see "Patient Education" section).

MEDICATION

- Antidepressants and anticonvulsants have been used with limited success. Low-dose tricyclic antidepressant (amitriptyline 10 mg) may be initiated and titrated as tolerated (3)[B].
- Topical anesthetics or anxiolytics may be used in combination with either cognitive-behavioral therapy or desensitization exercises as noted above (4)[B].
- Botulinum neurotoxin type A injections may improve vaginismus in patients who do not respond to standard cognitive behavioral and medical treatment for vaginismus.
  – Dosage: 20, 50, and 100 to 400 U of botulinum toxin type A injected in the levator ani muscle have been shown to improve vaginismus (4)[B].
- Intravaginal botulinum neurotoxin type A injection (100 to 150 U) followed by bupivacaine 0.25% with epinephrine 1:400,000 intravaginal injection (20 to 30 mL) while the patient is anesthetized may facilitate progressive placement of dilators and ultimately resolution of symptoms (5)[B].

ISSUES FOR REFERRAL

For diagnosis and treatment recommendations, the following resources may be consulted:
- Obstetrics/gynecology
- Pelvic floor physical therapy
- Psychiatry
- Sex therapy
- Hypnotherapy

SURGERY/OTHER PROCEDURES

Contraindicated

COMPLEMENTARY & ALTERNATIVE MEDICINE

- Biofeedback
- Functional electrical stimulation

 ONGOING CARE

FOLLOW-UP RECOMMENDATIONS

Desensitization techniques of gentle, progressive, patient-controlled vaginal dilation

Patient Monitoring

General preventive health care

DIET

No special diet

PATIENT EDUCATION

- Education about pelvic anatomy, nature of vaginal spasms, normal adult sexual function
- Handheld mirror can help the woman to learn visually to tighten and loosen perineal muscles.
- Important to teach the partner that spasms are not under conscious control and are not a reflection on the relationship or a woman's feelings about her partner
- Instruction in techniques for vaginal dilation
- Resources
  – American College of Obstetricians and Gynecologists (ACOG), 409 12th St., SW, Washington, DC 20024-2188; 800-762-ACOG. http://www.acog.org/
  – Valins L. *When a Woman's Body Says No to Sex: Understanding and Overcoming Vaginismus*. New York, NY: Penguin; 1992.

PROGNOSIS

Favorable, with early recognition of the condition and initiation of treatment

REFERENCES

1. American Psychiatric Association. *Diagnostic Statistical Manual of Mental Disorders*. 5th ed. Arlington, VA: American Psychiatric Association; 2013.
2. Landry T, Bergeron S. How young does vulvovaginal pain begin? Prevalence and characteristics of dyspareunia in adolescents. *J Sex Med*. 2009;6(4):927–935.
3. Crowley T, Goldmeier D, Hiller J. Diagnosing and managing vaginismus. *BMJ*. 2009;338:b2284.
4. Melnik T, Hawton K, McGuire H. Interventions for vaginismus. *Cochrane Database Syst Rev*. 2012;(12):CD001760.
5. Pacik PT. Vaginismus: review of current concepts and treatment using Botox injections, bupivacaine injections, and progressive dilation with the patient under anesthesia. *Aesthetic Plast Surg*. 2011;35(6):1160–1164.

ADDITIONAL READING

- Basson R, Wierman ME, van Lankveld J, et al. Summary of the recommendations on sexual dysfunctions in women. *J Sex Med*. 2010;7(1, Pt 2):314–326.
- Jeng CJ, Wang LR, Chou CS, et al. Management and outcome of primary vaginismus. *J Sex Marital Ther*. 2006;32(5):379–387.
- Pacik PT. Understanding and treating vaginismus: a multimodal approach. *Int Urogynecol J*. 2014;25(12):1613–1620.
- Reissing ED, Binik YM, Khalifé S, et al. Etiological correlates of vaginismus: sexual and physical abuse, sexual knowledge, sexual self-schema, and relationship adjustment. *J Sex Marital Ther*. 2003;29(1):47–59.
- Simons JS, Carey MP. Prevalence of sexual dysfunctions: results from a decade of research. *Arch Sex Behav*. 2001;30(2):177–219.
- ter Kuile MM, van Lankveld JJ, de Groot E, et al. Cognitive-behavioral therapy for women with lifelong vaginismus: process and prognostic factors. *Behav Res Ther*. 2007;45(2):359–373.

 SEE ALSO

Dyspareunia; Sexual Dysfunction in Women

 CODES

ICD10

- N94.2 Vaginismus
- N94.1 Dyspareunia

CLINICAL PEARLS

- In a patient with suspected genito-pelvic pain/penetration disorder, a complete medical history, including a comprehensive psychosocial and sexual history and a patient-centric, patient-controlled educational pelvic exam should be conducted.
- This condition can be treated effectively.
- Cognitive-behavioral therapy may be effective for the treatment of this condition.
- Botox injection therapy is in the experimental stages but looks promising for the treatment of vaginismus. Bupivacaine and dilation under general anesthesia has also been tried as a treatment for vaginismus.

G

GERIATRIC CARE: GENERAL PRINCIPLES

Erica K. Cichowski, MD • Mohammad Selim, MBBCh

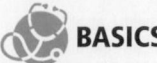 **BASICS**

DESCRIPTION
The optimal approach to caring for our elderly patient population requires an understanding of the physiology of normal aging as well as unique geriatric considerations for access to care, diagnosis, treatment, and ongoing care.

EPIDEMIOLOGY
The percentage of the U.S. population anticipated to be >65 years by the year 2050 exceeds 20%, and the percentage of those who are >85 years may reach 24%.

ETIOLOGY AND PATHOPHYSIOLOGY
Physiology of aging

- Although patients age ≥65 years are typically considered elderly, there is variability in the rate of decline in organ function associated with aging dependent on genetic, environmental, socioeconomic factors as well as disease burden.
- The aging process is not pathologic but part of the developmental continuum. However, physiologic changes associated with aging tend to diminish the body's compensatory reserve and increase susceptibility to disease.
  – Aging increases body fat and decreases total body water and lean body mass. This results in hydrophilic drugs having a smaller apparent volume of distribution. Lipophilic drugs will have an increased volume of distribution and longer half-life.
  – Aging decreases renal elimination of drugs.
  – Declines in lung capacity, oxygen uptake, cardiac output, muscle mass, glomerular filtration rate as well as blood flow to the brain, liver, and kidneys are associated with aging and must be considered in the diagnosis and treatment of elderly patients.

RISK FACTORS
Access to care

- Despite Medicare or dual health care coverage, persistent perceived barriers to health care include:
  – Lack of provider responsiveness to patient concerns
  – Mounting medical bills
  – Transportation challenges
- Barriers tend to be more prevalent in the female population and with increasing age.
- Alternatives to the traditional face-to-face visit should be considered to enhance access to care:
  – Encrypted email or home telehealth for those who are technologically equipped
  – Phone visits for those with adequate hearing

GENERAL PREVENTION
- Vaccination schedule for seniors: https://www.vaccines.gov/who_and_when/seniors/index.html
- Functional status
  – Activities of daily living (ADLs)
  – Instrumental ADLs (IADLs)
- Hearing assessment via hearing
  – Handicapped inventory
- Depression via:
  – Geriatric Depression Scale: https://consultgeri.org/try-this/general-assessment/issue-4.pdf
- Cognition via Mini Cognitive Assessment Instrument: https://www.alz.org/documents_custom/minicog.pdf

- Falls: Those with two or more falls in the past year, fall with injury requiring medical treatment, or fear of falling due to difficulty with gait or balance require a full fall risk assessment: https://www.cdc.gov/steadi/pdf/STEADI-Algorithm-a.pdf.
- Urinary incontinence: Inquire if patient has lost urine >5 times in past year.
- Polypharmacy
  – Use pill bottles, pharmacy records, patient and caregiver input to reconcile medication lists.
  – Ask about use of over-the-counter and alternative medications.
- Substance use: CAGE criteria: https://www.mdcalc.com/cage-questions-alcohol-use
- Advanced care planning
  – Completion of an advanced directive among most important interventions
  – Definition: Advanced directives are documents a person completes while still in possession of decisional capacity to ensure their values are reflected when considering how treatment decisions should be made on her or his behalf in the event she or he loses the capacity to make such decisions.
  – Instruments:
    ○ Durable power of attorney: Patient (called the principal) appoints an agent to handle specific health, legal, and financial responsibilities.
    ○ Health care proxy: a durable power of attorney specifically for health care decisions; their role is to express the patient's wishes and make health care decisions if the patient cannot speak for themselves.
    ○ Living will: a legal document that allows patients to express their wishes for end-of-life medical care, in case they become unable to communicate their decisions

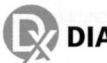 **DIAGNOSIS**

HISTORY
Optimizing communication

- Speak directly to your patient unless directed toward their surrogate.
- Use emotional intelligence to assess and manage emotionally charged interactions and overly helpful loved ones.
- Assess patient and caregiver health literacy and adjust explanations accordingly.
- Gauge the degree of social and financial support.
- Establish patient's values, preferences, and goals of care.

PHYSICAL EXAM
Geriatric-specific considerations:

- Orthostatic hypotension: contributes to poor energy, diminished functional status, increased risk of falls, and decline in renal function due to ineffective organ perfusion
- Hypothermia/hyperthermia: increased susceptibility in the elderly; less likely to mount a fever in the setting of infection; consider thyroid derangement.
- Weight loss: Assess access to food; may be presenting feature in mood disorder, thyroid derangement, dementia, malignancy
- Hearing: Check for cerumen impaction; perform Whisper Test: https://www.youtube.com/watch?v=PzRzpW6JKzQ
- Gait, balance, and proximal muscle strength: assessed via Get up and Go Test: https://www.cdc.gov/steadi/pdf/tug_test-a.pdf

DIFFERENTIAL DIAGNOSIS
Geriatric-specific presentations:

- CAD: Elderly patients with coronary heart disease often present with atypical symptoms, including exertional dyspnea. Silent myocardial ischemia is also common.
  – Constipation: In older adults, constipation may be associated with fecal impaction and overflow fecal incontinence.
  – Delirium: Nearly 30% of older patients experience delirium at some time during hospitalization.
  – Urinary tract infection (UTI): UTI is the most common infectious illness in adults age ≥65 years.
  – Depression: It is more common in elderly females.
  – Insomnia: Late-life insomnia is often persistent and may prompt self-medication with over-the-counter sleep aids or alcohol.
  – Hearing difficulties: Some studies showed increased incidence of dementia in patient with hearing difficulties (1).

DIAGNOSTIC TESTS & INTERPRETATION
Informed decision-making

- Decision-making capacity: Evaluate in four areas: ability to understand information about treatment, ability to appreciate how that information applies to their situation, ability to reason with that information, and ability to make a choice and express it: http://www.aafp.org/afp/2001/0715/p299.html.
- Surrogate decision maker
  – Patient-identified agent (durable power of attorney for health care, medical power of attorney, health care agent)
  – Court-appointed surrogate (legal guardian or conservator)

Diagnostic Procedures/Other
- Avoid unnecessary patient/caregiver burden if results will not significantly enhance the plan of care.
  – Cost
  – Time
  – Travel
  – Pain
  – Anxiety
  – Recovery time
- Avoid unnecessary risk; taking into consideration renal function, cognitive impact, cost, diagnostic yield in the geriatric population
- Factor in estimated life expectancy
- Geriatric-specific reference values (e.g., TSH, A1c)

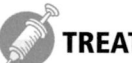 **TREATMENT**

GENERAL MEASURES
- Optimize nonpharmacologic options first.
- Align with patients' goals of care.
- Feasibility for patient and caregivers
  – Cost
  – Availability
  – Travel burden
- Compliance
- Nonpharmacologic (2)
  – OT/PT
  – Speech therapy
  – Hearing aids
  – Walking assist devices
  – Nonpharmacologic treatment of depression and insomnia

- Pharmacologic
  - Start low and go slow.
  - Dose adjustments for renal and hepatic function
  - Be respectful of pill burden, drug–drug interactions, and polypharmacy.
  - Beers criteria: assists in selecting medications with best geriatric benefit to risk ratio; http://www.americangeriatrics.org/files/documents/beers/PrintableBeersPocketCard.pdf
- Deprescribing: AGA and Choosing Wisely recommend:
  - Don't recommend percutaneous feeding tubes in patients with advanced dementia; instead, offer oral-assisted feeding.
  - Don't use antipsychotics as the first choice to treat behavioral and psychological symptoms of dementia.
  - Avoid using medications other than metformin to achieve hemoglobin A1c.
  - Don't use benzodiazepines or other sedative hypnotics in older adults as first choice for insomnia, agitation, or delirium.
  - Don't use antimicrobials to treat bacteriuria in older adults unless specific urinary tract symptoms are present.
  - Don't prescribe cholinesterase inhibitors for dementia without periodic assessment for perceived cognitive benefits and adverse gastrointestinal effects.
  - Don't recommend screening for breast, colorectal, prostate, or lung cancer without considering life expectancy and the risks of testing, overdiagnosis, and overtreatment.
  - Avoid using prescription appetite stimulants or high-calorie supplements for treatment of anorexia or cachexia in older adults; instead, optimize social supports, discontinue medications that may interfere with eating, provide appealing food and feeding assistance, and clarify patient goals and expectations.
  - Don't prescribe a medication without conducting a drug regimen review.
  - Don't use physical restraints to manage behavioral symptoms of hospitalized older adults with delirium.
- Geriatric pain management:
  - Treatment goal is to improve functionality.
  - Stepwise care
  - Nonpharmacologic:
    - Physical intervention (e.g., PT/aquatic therapy, aquapuncture, chiropractic manipulation, massage)
    - Psychoeducational interventions (such as cognitive-behavioral therapy, meditation, and patient education)
  - Pharmacologic: Consider Beers criteria.
- Assess the home environment.
  - Social work
  - Home safety evaluations
    - OT/PT
  - Diagnose and address social isolation (3):
    - Group support
    - Social activities
    - Home visitations

SURGERY/OTHER PROCEDURES
- Assess surgical risk.
- Weigh risks versus benefits.
- Explore alternatives thoroughly.
- Align with goals of care.
- Preoperative discharge planning with caregiver input

COMPLEMENTARY & ALTERNATIVE MEDICINE
- Use of CAM is on the rise in geriatric patients (4).
- Discuss potential risks and limitations.

ADMISSION, INPATIENT, AND NURSING CONSIDERATIONS
Inpatient prevention measures
- Falls
- Acute delirium
- Skin breakdown
- Pain
- Infections

 ## ONGOING CARE

FOLLOW-UP RECOMMENDATIONS
- Realistic expectations
- Consider pharmacologic débridement.

Patient Monitoring
Use team members optimally.
- Home health care
- Social work
- RN care managers

PATIENT EDUCATION
- Caregiver support (5)
  - Screening:
    - Frustrations
    - Depression
    - Social support
    - Financial burden
    - Time spent on providing care
    - Coping mechanisms
    - Need for help
  - Resources
    - Local agency on aging
    - Respite care: Taking care of an older or ill family member can be enormously rewarding, but it can be physically and emotionally draining as well. That's why it's important for caregivers to seek occasional respite from their responsibilities.
    - Support group: Alzheimer's Association 800-272-3900
    - Targeted education
    - Skills training to address caregiver concerns
  - Follow-up
    - Home and phone visits
    - Frequent touch points
- Elder mistreatment
  - Screening
    - Brief Abuse Screen for the Elderly (BASE)
    - Elder Assessment Instrument (EAI)
  - Warning signs
    - Skin findings (e.g., lacerations and bruises)
    - Fractures
    - Malnutrition
    - Dehydration
    - Pressure ulcers
    - Signs of sexual abuse
    - Change in the ability to manage and control finances
  - Forms
    - Abuse (e.g., physical, sexual)
    - Neglect
    - Financial exploitation

- Interventions:
  - Prevention by caregiver support
  - Documentation
  - Reporting
  - Social and medical interventions
- Palliative care
  - A philosophy of care for those with serious illnesses that focuses on symptom, pain and stress relief with a goal of optimizing functional status and quality of life
  - Ideal for patients with:
    - Complex or refractory symptoms, pain, or stress
    - Frequent admissions
    - Complex care needs
    - Decline in function or quality of life
- Hospice
  - A model of end-of-life care
  - Provide physical, emotional, and spiritual support to patients with <6 months life expectancy to maintain optimal quality of life and die with dignity.

REFERENCES

1. Uhlmann RF, Larson EB, Rees TS, et al. Relationship of hearing impairment to dementia and cognitive dysfunction in older adults. *JAMA*. 1989;261(13):1916–1919.
2. Abraha I, Cruz-Jentoft A, Soiza RL, et al. Evidence of and recommendations for non-pharmacological interventions for common geriatric conditions: the SENATOR-ONTOP systematic review protocol. *BMJ Open*. 2015;5(1):e007488.
3. Dickens AP, Richards SH, Greaves CJ, et al. Interventions targeting social isolation in older people: a systematic review. *BMC Public Health*. 2011;11:647.
4. Siddiqui MJ, Min CS, Verma RK, et al. Role of complementary and alternative medicine in geriatric care: a mini review. *Pharmacogn Rev*. 2014;8(16):81–87.
5. Nichols LO, Martindale-Adams J, Burns R, et al. Translation of a dementia caregiver support program in a health care system—REACH VA. *Arch Intern Med*. 2011;171(4):353–359.

ADDITIONAL READING

- Choosing Wisely. American Geriatrics Society: ten things clinicians and patients should question. http://www.choosingwisely.org/societies/american-geriatrics-society/. Accessed December 27, 2018.
- Reuben DB, Herr KA, Pacala JT, et al. *Geriatrics at Your Fingertips: 2017*. 19th ed. New York, NY: The American Geriatrics Society; 2017.

 ## CODES

ICD10
Z71.89 Other specified counseling

CLINICAL PEARLS

- Establish patient goals of care and align all clinical decisions within the context of these goals.
- Use an interdisciplinary team approach to optimize holistic care for elders and their caregivers.

GIARDIASIS

Carol H. Hungerford, DO • Pamela R. Hughes, MD

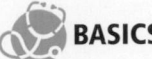 **BASICS**

DESCRIPTION
- Intestinal infection caused by the protozoan parasite *Giardia lamblia*:
  - *G. lamblia* is also called *Giardia duodenalis* and *Giardia intestinalis*.
- Infection results from ingestion of cysts, which transform into trophozoites and colonize the small intestine to cause symptoms.
  - The infectious cycle is continued when trophozoites encyst in the small intestine to be subsequently transmitted through water, food, or hands contaminated by feces of an infected person.
- Most infections result from fecal–oral transmission or ingestion of contaminated water (e.g., swimming).
- Less commonly acquired through contaminated food

EPIDEMIOLOGY
- Predominant age:
  - All ages but most common in early childhood (ages 1 to 9 years) and adults 35 to 44 years
- Predominant gender:
  - Male > female (slightly)
- Minimal seasonal variability; slight increase in summer and early fall

Pediatric Considerations
- Most common in early childhood
- Chronic infection in children can lead to intestinal malabsorption (may also be associated with growth restriction).

Prevalence
- 10% of cases of traveler's diarrhea are caused by parasites, most commonly *Giardia* (1).
- >19,000 cases per year from U.S. states where *Giardia* is reportable:
  - *Giardia* is currently not reportable in Indiana, Kentucky, Mississippi, North Carolina, and Texas.

ETIOLOGY AND PATHOPHYSIOLOGY
Giardia trophozoites colonize the surface of the proximal small intestine: The mechanism of diarrhea is unknown.

Genetics
No known genetic risk factors

RISK FACTORS
- Daycare centers
- Anal intercourse
- Wilderness camping
- Travel to developing countries
- Children adopted from developing countries
- Public swimming pools
- Pets with *Giardia* infection/diarrhea

GENERAL PREVENTION
- Hand hygiene
- Water purification when camping and when traveling to developing countries
- Properly cook all foods.

COMMONLY ASSOCIATED CONDITIONS
Hypogammaglobulinemia, IgA deficiency, and immunosuppression are associated with prolonged course of the disease and treatment failures.

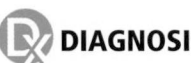 **DIAGNOSIS**

HISTORY
- 25–50% of infected persons are symptomatic.
- Symptoms usually appear 1 to 2 weeks after exposure.
- Persistent diarrhea, often >3 weeks (95%)
- Abdominal cramps (70%)
- Nausea (60%)
- Bloating (50%)
- Flatulence (50%)
- Weight loss (50%), up to 10–20% of ideal body weight
- Fever (20%), usually early on. If persistent, consider another diagnosis.

PHYSICAL EXAM
- Vital signs are typically normal.
- Nonspecific; abdominal exam; may have bloating, tenderness, or increased bowel sounds

DIFFERENTIAL DIAGNOSIS
- Cryptosporidiosis, microsporidiosis, strongyloidiasis, cyclosporiasis
- Other causes of malabsorption include celiac sprue, tropical sprue, bacterial overgrowth syndromes, and Crohn ileitis.
- Irritable bowel (diarrhea without weight loss)

DIAGNOSTIC TESTS & INTERPRETATION
Initial Tests (lab, imaging)
- Light microscopy of stool for ova and parasites:
  - Repeat 3 times on separate days.
  - Cysts in fixed or fresh stools and occasionally trophozoites are found in fresh diarrheal stools.
  - Test limitations: labor intensive; experienced operator is necessary for interpretation; intermittent shedding means that ova may not be present in stool sample.
- ELISA: sensitivity and specificity of 100% and 92% (compared to 50% and 70% with microscopy) (2)[A]
- Polymerase chain reaction (PCR) techniques are more sensitive than microscopy but have not been widely adopted due to high cost.

Follow-Up Tests & Special Considerations
String test (entero-test):
- A gelatin capsule on a string is swallowed and left in the duodenum for several hours or overnight. The string is removed and evaluated for presence of trophozoites by microscopy.

Diagnostic Procedures/Other
Esophagogastroduodenoscopy (EGD) with biopsy and sample of small intestinal fluid

Test Interpretation
Intestinal biopsy shows flattened, mild lymphocytic infiltration and trophozoites on the surface.

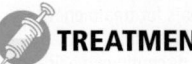 **TREATMENT**

Outpatient for mild cases; inpatient if symptoms are severe enough to cause dehydration warranting parenteral fluid replacement

GENERAL MEASURES
- No treatment required in asymptomatic patients
- Prophylactic therapy indicated for asymptomatic patients in close contact with pregnant or immunocompromised individuals
- Fluid replacement is first line for dehydration.

MEDICATION
First Line
- Metronidazole (Flagyl): 250 mg PO TID for 5 to 10 days
- Tinidazole: 2 g PO single dose (50 mg/kg up to 2 g for children)

- Albendazole: 400 mg/day PO daily for 5 days:
  - Albendazole has comparable effectiveness to metronidazole with fewer side effects (3)[A].
- Precautions:
  - Theoretical risk of carcinogenesis with metronidazole
- Significant possible interactions: occasional disulfiram reaction with metronidazole or tinidazole
- Paromomycin (Humatin): a nonaminoglycoside recommended in pregnancy due to lower risk of teratogenicity in the 1st trimester

Pregnancy Considerations
Medications to treat giardiasis are relatively contraindicated during pregnancy.

Pediatric Considerations
Limited evidence to suggest vitamin A reduces prevalence of *G. lamblia* (4)[A]

Second Line
- Nitazoxanide suspension was approved by the FDA in 2003 for treatment of giardiasis in children age 1 to 11 years; children age 1 to 4 years 100 mg BID and age 5 to 11 years 200 mg BID for 3 days
- Several other medications effective against *Giardia* are not available in the United States.
- Treat failures with a longer course of original agent or change to a different agent class.
- Multiple combination therapies have been investigated; there are no definitive guidelines for use (5)[C].

ADDITIONAL THERAPIES
Anecdotal reports of *Mentha crispa* for the treatment of *Giardia* (efficacy is unclear)

 ONGOING CARE

FOLLOW-UP RECOMMENDATIONS
Patient Monitoring
Monitor symptoms, weight, and stool exams, particularly if patients fail to improve.

DIET
Low lactose/lactose free for at least 1 month; low-fat diet generally helpful

PATIENT EDUCATION
- Hand washing is more important than water purification to prevent transmission in outdoor enthusiasts.

- Lactose intolerance may follow *Giardia* infection and cause persistent diarrhea posttreatment. Recommend patients adhere to a low-lactose/lactose-free diet to mitigate symptoms.
- CDC facts about *Giardia* and swimming pools: http://www.cdc.gov/healthywater/pdf/swimming/resources/giardia-factsheet.pdf
  - Don't swim if you have diarrhea.
  - Wash hands with soap after changing diapers before returning to the pool.
  - Do not ingest pool, lake, or river water.
  - Use chlorine to kill *Giardia* in water used for recreational activities.

PROGNOSIS
- Untreated giardiasis lasts for several weeks.
- Most (90%) patients respond to treatment within a few days:
  - Most nonresponders or relapses respond to a second course with the same or a different agent.

COMPLICATIONS
Malabsorption, weight loss, postinfectious IBS, and lactose intolerance

ALERT
Reportable disease to the CDC

REFERENCES
1. Shane A, Mody R, Crump J, et al. 2017 Infectious Diseases Society of America clinical practice guidelines for the diagnosis and management of infectious diarrhea. *Clin Infect Dis*. 2017;65(12):e45–e80.
2. Jahan N, Khatoon R, Ahmad S. A comparison of microscopy and enzyme linked immunosorbent assay for diagnosis of *Giardia lamblia* in human faecal specimens. *J Clin Diagn Res*. 2014;8(11):DC04–DC06.
3. Solaymani-Mohammadi S, Genkinger JM, Loffredo CA, et al. A meta-analysis of the effectiveness of albendazole compared with metronidazole as treatments for infections with *Giardia duodenalis*. *PLoS Negl Trop Dis*. 2010;4(5):e682.
4. Lima AA, Soares AM, Lima NL, et al. Effects of vitamin A supplementation on intestinal barrier function, growth, total parasitic, and specific *Giardia* spp infections in Brazilian children: a prospective randomized, double-blind, placebo-controlled trial. *J Pediatr Gastroenterol Nutr*. 2010;50(3):309–315.
5. Yadav P, Tak V, Mirdha B, et al. Refractory giardiasis: a molecular appraisal from a tertiary care centre in India. *Indian J Med Microbiol*. 2014;32(4):378–382.

ADDITIONAL READING
- Cañete R, Rodríguez P, Mesa L, et al. Albendazole versus metronidazole in the treatment of adult giardiasis: a randomized, double-blind, clinical trial. *Curr Med Res Opin*. 2012;28(1):149–154.
- Eissa MM, Amer EI. *Giardia lamblia*: a new target for miltefosine. *Int J Parasitol*. 2012;42(5):443–452.
- Hahn J, Seeber F, Kolodziej H, et al. High sensitivity of *Giardia duodenalis* to tetrahydrolipstatin (orlistat) in vitro. *PLoS One*. 2013;8(8):e71597.
- Mukku KK, Raju S, Yelanati R. Refractory giardiasis in renal transplantation: a case report. *Nephrology (Carlton)*. 2015;20(1):44.
- Tejman-Yarden N, Miyamoto Y, Leitsch D, et al. A reprofiled drug, auranofin, is effective against metronidazole-resistant *Giardia lamblia*. *Antimicrob Agents Chemother*. 2013;57(5):2029–2035.

 SEE ALSO

Algorithm: Diarrhea, Chronic

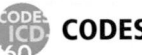 CODES

ICD10
A07.1 Giardiasis [lambliasis]

CLINICAL PEARLS
- Daycare facilities and public swimming pools are common sources of *Giardia* transmission (a history of camping or recent travel is not required for the diagnosis).
- Abdominal bloating and loose, foul-smelling stool are common presenting symptoms.
- Metronidazole is highly effective for the treatment of giardiasis (and is often poorly tolerated).
- Most treatment failures respond to a second course of antibiotics (with same or other medication).
- A single fluorescence antibody (FA) or ELISA is as sensitive as three stool samples (looking for ova and parasites) to detect *Giardia*.

G

GILBERT SYNDROME

Alethea Y. Turner, DO • Anna James, DO

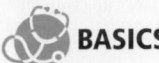 **BASICS**

DESCRIPTION
A benign, inherited syndrome, in which mild, intermittent unconjugated hyperbilirubinemia occurs in the absence of hemolysis or liver dysfunction

Pediatric Considerations
Rare for the disorder to be diagnosed before puberty

Pregnancy Considerations
The relative fasting that may occur with morning sickness can elevate bilirubin level.

EPIDEMIOLOGY
- Predominant age: present from birth but most often presents in the 2nd or 3rd decade of life
- Predominant sex: male > female (2 to 7:1)

Prevalence
Prevalence in the United States: ~8% of the population; ~1 in 3 of those affected are not aware that they have the disorder.

ETIOLOGY AND PATHOPHYSIOLOGY
Indirect hyperbilirubinemia in Gilbert syndrome (GS) results from impaired hepatic bilirubin clearance (~30% of normal) due to decreased levels of the enzyme uridine diphosphoglucuronate-glucuronosyltransferase (UDPGT). Hepatic bilirubin conjugation (glucuronidation) is thus reduced, although this may not be the only defect.

Genetics
- Inherited defects within the promoter region of the gene that encodes the enzyme UDPGT yields reduced conjugation of bilirubin with glucuronic acid.
- Once considered as an autosomal dominant condition, GS is now thought to be inherited in an autosomal recessive manner.

RISK FACTORS
- Male gender
- Family history; particularly first-degree relatives

COMMONLY ASSOCIATED CONDITIONS
GS is part of a spectrum of hereditary disorders that includes types I and II Crigler-Najjar syndrome (1). However, bilirubin levels in these cases will be >6 mg/dL.

 DIAGNOSIS

HISTORY
- A nonpruritic jaundice can occur in the setting of fasting, dehydration, infection, lack of sleep, physical exertion, or surgery. Other symptoms that may present during an episode of jaundice, including fatigue, are caused by the triggering factor and are not directly a result of GS.
- Some medications may also trigger episodes of jaundice in patients with GS due to abnormal metabolism. These include drugs that inhibit glucuronyl transferase (i.e., gemfibrozil) as well as selective protease inhibitors (i.e., atazanavir and indinavir) (2). There is some evidence that tocilizumab (3), a monoclonal antibody used to treat rheumatoid arthritis, and ribavirin, an antiviral for hepatitis C treatment, may also induce jaundice (4). Note, the aforementioned drugs have not been associated with causing liver toxicity in patients with GS.

PHYSICAL EXAM
Occasional mild jaundice precipitated by the aforementioned triggers (fasting, dehydration, infection, lack of sleep, physical exertion, surgery, and some medications). Exam should be devoid of the stigmata of chronic liver disease.

DIFFERENTIAL DIAGNOSIS
- Hemolysis
- Ineffective erythropoiesis (megaloblastic anemias, certain porphyrias, thalassemia major, sideroblastic anemia, severe lead poisoning, congenital dyserythropoietic anemias)
- Cirrhosis
- Chronic persistent hepatitis
- Pancreatitis
- Biliary tract disease

DIAGNOSTIC TESTS & INTERPRETATION
Initial Tests (lab, imaging)
- Bilirubin: elevated but <6 mg/dL (103 μmol/L) and usually <3 mg/dL (51 μmol/L) (1)[C], virtually all unconjugated (indirect), with conjugated bilirubin within the normal range and/or <20% of the total bilirubin (2)
- CBC with peripheral smear is normal.
- Reticulocyte count, haptoglobin, and lactate dehydrogenase levels are normal.
- Liver function tests (LFTs) (aspartate aminotransferase [AST], alanine transaminase [ALT], alkaline phosphatase, and γ-glutamyl transpeptidase [GGT]) are normal.
- Direct Coombs test is normal.
- Up to 60% of patients with GS have a clinically insignificant mild hemolysis that frequently can only be detected with sophisticated red cell survival studies (1).
- Drugs that may alter lab results: Bilirubin level may be raised by nicotinic acid and some other medications and lowered by phenobarbital (1).
- Disorders that may alter lab results: Bilirubin levels increase during fasting and may increase during a febrile illness.

Follow-Up Tests & Special Considerations

GS should be suspected if unconjugated hyperbilirubinemia persists in the absence of hemolysis or other liver dysfunction. A definitive diagnosis may be reported after 3 to 12 months of follow-up if the exam and diagnostic workup is otherwise normal.

Diagnostic Procedures/Other

Confirmatory testing is often unnecessary.

- A 48-hour fast is impractical and nonspecific for GS (2).
- Provocation testing with rifampin (5)[C] could be employed if there is significant diagnostic doubt:
  - After 12 hours of fasting, an increase of total bilirubin to >1.9 mg/dL 2 hours after an oral dose of rifampin 900 mg distinguishes patients with GS with a sensitivity of 100% and a specificity of 100% (5).
- Genetic testing is available in the form of polymerase chain reaction (PCR) or DNA-fragment sequencing for DNA mutations in the *UGT1A1* gene.

ALERT

A liver biopsy is not usually needed to exclude other diagnoses unless concomitant liver disease is present.

 TREATMENT

- Outpatient
- Avoid unnecessary testing and procedures.
- Specific treatment is not necessary (1)[C].

 ONGOING CARE

FOLLOW-UP RECOMMENDATIONS

Patient Monitoring

Once GS has been confidently diagnosed, no further monitoring is required.

PATIENT EDUCATION

- Reassure patients that GS is benign.
- Educate patients on common triggers for jaundice.
- Recommend patients to inform medical providers of their diagnosis.
- Instruct patients to seek medical help if severe or prolonged jaundice occurs because these may be signs of a separate disease process.

PROGNOSIS

- GS is benign with an excellent prognosis.
- Patients with GS are able to serve as donors for right lobe of liver for transplantation (6)[B].
- Preliminary evidence suggests that patients with GS may have protective properties against cardiovascular disease, type 2 diabetes mellitus, some cancers such as Hodgkin lymphoma, and all-cause mortality (7).

COMPLICATIONS

There are no known complications from GS.

ALERT

Caution before using irinotecan in patients with GS. Once metabolized, this colorectal cancer treatment affects the enzyme responsible for GS, significantly increasing risk of toxicity (7).

REFERENCES

1. Watson KJ, Gollan JL. Gilbert's syndrome. *Baillieres Clin Gastroenterol*. 1989;3(2):337–355.
2. Claridge LC, Armstrong MJ, Booth C, et al. Gilbert's syndrome. *BMJ*. 2011;342:d2293.
3. Lee JS, Wang J, Martin M, et al. Genetic variation in UGT1A1 typical of Gilbert syndrome is associated with unconjugated hyperbilirubinemia in patients receiving tocilizumab. *Pharmacogenet Genomics*. 2011;21(7):365–374.
4. Deterding K, Grüngreiff K, Lankisch TO, et al. Gilbert's syndrome and antiviral therapy of hepatitis C. *Ann Hepatol*. 2009;8(3):246–250.
5. Murthy GD, Byron D, Shoemaker D, et al. The utility of rifampin in diagnosing Gilbert's syndrome. *Am J Gastroenterol*. 2001;96(4):1150–1154.
6. Demirbas T, Piskin T, Dayangac M, et al. Right-lobe liver transplant from donors with Gilbert syndrome. *Exp Clin Transplant*. 2012;10(1):39–42.
7. Ha VH, Jupp J, Tsang RY. Oncology drug dosing in Gilbert syndrome associated with UGT1A1: a summary of the literature. *Pharmacotherapy*. 2017;37(8):956–972.

 CODES

ICD10

- E80.4 Gilbert syndrome
- E80.6 Other disorders of bilirubin metabolism

CLINICAL PEARLS

- GS is a benign, inherited syndrome, in which mild, intermittent unconjugated hyperbilirubinemia causing jaundice occurs with otherwise normal liver function.
- Reduced hepatic bilirubin conjugation (glucuronidation) occurs due to altered *UDPGT1A1* gene promotion.
- GS is diagnosed when a mild, persistent or recurrent elevation in unconjugated hyperbilirubinemia persists in the absence of hemolysis or other liver dysfunction.
- Confirmatory tests are not frequently needed, and a liver biopsy is not recommended unless there is serious concern for concomitant liver disease.
- Patient education and reassurance is essential, and unnecessary testing and procedures should be avoided.

GINGIVITIS

Karlynn Sievers, MD • Sheila O. Stille, DMD

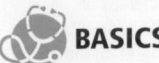

BASICS

DESCRIPTION
Gingivitis is a reversible form of inflammation of the gingiva. It is a mild form of periodontal disease. Classification includes the following:
- Plaque induced
- Not plaque induced (bacterial, viral, or fungal; e.g., necrotizing ulcerative gingivitis, Vincent disease ["trench mouth"], denture related)
- Modified by systemic factors (e.g., pregnancy, puberty, HIV, diabetes, smoking, leukemia)
- Modified by medications (calcium channel blockers, antipsychotics, antiepileptics, antirejection medications, hormones)
- Modified by malnutrition (vitamin deficiencies)
- Acute or chronic
- System(s) affected: gastrointestinal; ears, nose, throat; dental
- Synonym(s): mild periodontal disease; gum disease

Geriatric Considerations
More frequent in this age group (due more to additive effects than to increased susceptibility)

Pediatric Considerations
Cases of plaque-induced gingivitis are common in children (most common form of pediatric periodontal disease) and usually require no specific interventions other than improved oral hygiene.

Pregnancy Considerations
- Very common in pregnant women; hormonal effect
- Self-limited

EPIDEMIOLOGY
- Predominant age: children, teenagers, and young adults
- Predominant sex: slightly more males than female
- Prevalence ~50% of children
- ~90% of adolescents and adult population
- ~30–75% of pregnant women
- 42% of adults in United States have periodontal diseases (1).

ETIOLOGY AND PATHOPHYSIOLOGY
Inflammation of the marginal gingiva. This can progress to deeper, destructive inflammation; if involving supporting bone, will be classified as periodontitis, not gingivitis (2)
- Usually noncontagious
- Inadequate plaque removal
- Blood dyscrasias (pregnancy)
- Medication induced (e.g., oral contraceptives, antiepileptics)
- Allergic reactions
- Nutritional deficiencies
- Vasoconstriction (nicotine, methamphetamine)
- Endocrine/hormonal variations
  – Pregnancy, menses, menarche
- Chronic debilitating disease
- Vincent disease, necrotizing ulcerative gingivitis
  – Synergistic infection with fusiform bacillus (*Fusobacterium* spp.) and spirochete (*Borrelia vincentii*)

- Pathology
  – Acute or chronic inflammation
  – Hyperemic capillaries
  – Polymorphonuclear infiltration
  – Papillary projections in subepithelial tissue
  – Fibroblasts

Genetics
Possible genetic link (up to 30% of population); rare condition called hereditary gingival fibromatosis, where severe gingival hyperplasia covers teeth, associated with hirsutism

RISK FACTORS
- Poor dental hygiene/plaque formation
- Pregnancy
- Uncontrolled diabetes mellitus
- Malocclusion or dental crowding
- Smoking
- Mouth breathing
- Xerostomia
- Faulty dental restorations
- HIV-positive; AIDS
- Stress
- Hospitalization
- Vitamin C deficiency; coenzyme Q10 deficiency
- Dental appliances (dentures, braces)
- Eruption of primary or secondary teeth
- Necrotizing ulcerative gingivitis
  – Stress
  – Lack of sleep
  – Malnutrition
  – Viral illness
  – Typically teens and young adults
- Bronchial asthma and other respiratory diseases
- Rheumatoid arthritis
- Epilepsy

GENERAL PREVENTION
- Good oral hygiene
  – Adults
    ○ Regular twice-daily brushing with fluoride toothpaste
    ○ May be increased benefit of using circular oscillating electric brush rather than regular brush or sonic/vibration, although evidence is inconclusive (2,3)
    ○ Daily "high-quality" flossing (studies show that flossing only helps when it is done correctly) and interdental brushes (2,4)
    ○ Chlorhexidine with oral hygiene better than other oral rinse agents (2,5)
      ■ Use in acute phase (2).
  – Pediatrics
    ○ Regular twice-daily brushing with fluoride toothpaste under parental supervision until full manual dexterity (~8 years of age)
    ○ Regular flossing if no spaces between teeth
- Cleaning by a dentist or hygienist every 6 months or more frequently, as indicated (2)
- Mouth rinse with essential oils (menthol, thymol, eucalyptol; e.g., Listerine) combined with brushing (2)
  – It had been thought that long-term use of alcohol-based mouth rinse may be associated with an increased risk of oral cancer. A recent systematic review found no evidence (2).

COMMONLY ASSOCIATED CONDITIONS
- Periodontitis
- Glossitis
- Pedunculated growths (pyogenic granulomata)

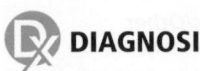

DIAGNOSIS

HISTORY
- Gingival erythema, edema, and bleeding
- Gingiva is tender to touch but otherwise painless.
- Bleeding of gingiva when brushing, flossing, or eating
- Inquire about HIV risk, pregnancy, nutritional deficiencies, diabetes, and other risk factors as indicated (see "Risk Factors").
- Smoking history
- Poor oral hygiene, infrequent dental visit history

PHYSICAL EXAM
- Normal gums should appear pink, firm, stippled, and scalloped.
- Gingivitis—marginal gingiva edematous with blunted papilla (usually painless, except to touch)
- Gingiva erythema: bright red or red-purple appearance
- Bleeding with manipulation of gingiva
- Biofilm of plaque (soft) and calculus (calcified, not easily removed)
- Edema of interdental papillae
- HIV gingivitis
  – Also called linear gingival erythema
  – Narrow band of bright red inflamed gum surrounding neck of tooth
  – Painful
  – Bleeds easily
  – Rapid destruction of gingival tissue and can progress to periodontitis with destruction of underlying support tissues (periodontal ligament, supporting alveolar bone)
- Vincent disease/necrotizing ulcerative gingivitis
  – Ulcers
  – Fever
  – Malaise
  – Regional lymphadenopathy
  – Pain
  – Mouth odor

DIFFERENTIAL DIAGNOSIS
- Periodontitis (deeper inflammation, causing destruction to connective tissue, ligaments, and alveolar bone)
- Glossitis
- Desquamative gingivitis (painful, persistent, usually middle-aged women)
- Pericoronitis (gum flap traps food and plaque over partially erupted 3rd molar), common in adolescence
- Gingival ulcers (aphthous, herpetic, malignancy, TB, syphilis)
- Specific forms of gingivitis: See "Description," including acute necrotizing ulcerative gingivitis (Vincent disease) and HIV gingivitis (linear gingival erythema), adrenal crisis, leukemia.

DIAGNOSTIC TESTS & INTERPRETATION
Initial Tests (lab, imaging)
- No tests usually needed
- Possible smear or culture to identify causative agent (HIV gingivitis includes gram-negative anaerobes, enteric strains, and yeast—*Candida*.)
- Labs for contributing conditions (HIV, pregnancy, diabetes, nutritional deficiencies)
- Increase in C-reactive protein (5)[A]

TREATMENT
GENERAL MEASURES
- Stop any contributing medications.
- Remove irritating factors (plaque, calculus, faulty dental restorations, or partial dentures).
- Good oral hygiene (see "General Prevention")
- Regular dental checkups (for scaling and polishing if plaque and/or tartar are present)
- Smoking cessation
- Warm saline rinses BID
- Special needs patients: use of tray-applied 10% carbamide peroxide gels (5)[A]

MEDICATION
First Line
- Chlorhexidine rinses or varnishes may be used. (Note: Prolonged use of chlorhexidine can lead to blackening of the tongue and taste alterations/metallic.)
- Essential oil mouthwash (EOMW) may be equally effective to chlorhexidine for reduction of gingival inflammation (although EOMW is not as effective for plaque control) (2)[A].
- Both chlorhexidine and EOMW rinses are as clinically effective as dental prophylaxis and oral hygiene instruction at 6-month recall (2)[A].
- Antibiotics indicated *only* for acute necrotizing ulcerative gingivitis (Vincent disease)
- Antibiotics for necrotizing ulcerative gingivitis:
  – Penicillin V: pediatric dose, 25 to 50 mg/kg/day divided q6h; adult dose, 250 to 500 mg q6h, *OR*
  – Metronidazole: pediatric dose, 30 mg/kg/day PO/IV divided q6h; maximum 4 g/day; adult dose, 500 mg BID or TID for 10 days *OR*
  – Amoxicillin/clavulanic acid: pediatric dose, 30 mg/kg/day PO divided q12h; information: use 125 mg/31.25 mg/5 mL suspension; adult dose, 875 mg/125 mg PO BID for 10 days
  – Erythromycin: pediatric dose, 30 to 40 mg/kg/day divided q6h; adult dose, 250 mg q6h
  – Clindamycin: penicillin allergy; pediatric dose, 8 to 20 mg/kg/day in 3 to 4 divided doses as hydrochloride; adults, 300 mg q6h (maximum 1.8 g/day)
  – Doxycycline: adult dose, 100 mg BID 1st day and then QD for 10 days
- Topical corticosteroids
  – Triamcinolone 0.1% in Orabase (spray or ointment), applied locally TID, QID
    ○ Contraindications
      ■ Allergy to specific medication
- Precautions
  – Erythromycin frequently causes GI issues.

Second Line
- Acetaminophen or ibuprofen for any pain (rare)
- Other antibiotics or antifungal rinses or systemic according to culture or smear
- Decapinol oral rinse (surfactant that acts as a physical barrier, making it harder for bacteria to stick to the polysaccharide pellicle on tooth and mucosal surfaces) to reduce bacteria (not recommended for pregnant women or children <12 years); should be used in conjunction with traditional oral hygiene practices when those practices alone are not enough

ISSUES FOR REFERRAL
- Dental referral for acute gingivitis and routine cleanings and further treatment, as needed
- If gingivitis becomes periodontitis, deep root scaling, root planing, and antibiotics may be indicated.

SURGERY/OTHER PROCEDURES
- Débridement for acute necrotizing gingivitis
- Minor surgery may be necessary to correct tissue overgrowth for gingivitis caused by medicines/hereditary gingival fibromatosis.

COMPLEMENTARY & ALTERNATIVE MEDICINE
- Bilberry: potentially helpful in reducing inflammation and stabilizing collagen tissue
- Coenzyme Q10: topically, to restore coenzyme Q10 deficiency
- Replace any other nutritional deficiencies (e.g., vitamin A, B₁₂, C).

ONGOING CARE
FOLLOW-UP RECOMMENDATIONS
- Outpatient
- No restrictions

Patient Monitoring
Until clear; dental follow-up for continued cleanings and secondary prevention

DIET
- Well-balanced diet that includes fruits, vegetables, vitamin C; avoid sugary snacks and drinks, which contribute to plaque formation.
- Soft foods during flare, if significant inflammation/bleeding

PATIENT EDUCATION
- Good oral hygiene, including twice-daily brushing with circular oscillating electric brush, fluoridated toothpaste, and daily flossing; regular dental visits
- Printable and viewable patient information available from the American Dental Association at http://www.mouthhealthy.org/en.org/en/ and the American Academy of Periodontology under "patient resources" at http://www.perio.org/ and NIDCR at http://www.nidcr.nih.gov/oralhealth/Topics/GumDiseases/PeriodontalGumDisease.htm

PROGNOSIS
- Usual course: acute, relapsing, intermittent; chronic
- Prognosis: generally favorable, responds well to appropriate treatment
- Left untreated, may progress to periodontitis (controversial), which is a major cause of tooth loss

COMPLICATIONS
Severe periodontal disease (which is associated with supporting bone loss, tooth loss, heart disease, diabetes, dementia, and preterm birth)

REFERENCES
1. Eke PI, Thornton-Evans GO, Wei L, et al. Periodontitis in US adults: National Health and Nutrition Examination Survey 2009–2014. *J Am Dent Assoc*. 2018;149(7):576–588.e6.
2. Chapple IL, Van der Weijden F, Doerfer C, et al. Primary prevention of periodontitis: managing gingivitis. *J Clin Periodontol*. 2015;42(Suppl 16):S71–S76.
3. Tilliss T, Carey CM. Insufficient evidence within a systematic review and meta-analysis of powered toothbrushes over manual toothbrushes for soft tissue health during orthodontic treatment. *J Evid Based Dent Pract*. 2018;18(2):176–177.
4. Sälzer S, Slot DE, Van der Weijden FA, et al. Efficacy of inter-dental mechanical plaque control in managing gingivitis—a meta-review. *J Clin Periodontol*. 2015;42(Suppl 16):S92–S105.
5. Prasad M, Patthi B, Singla A, et al. The clinical effectiveness of post-brushing rinsing in reducing plaque and gingivitis: a systematic review. *J Clin Diagn Res*. 2016;10(5):ZE01–ZE07.

ADDITIONAL READING
- Aarabi G, Heydecke G, Seedorf U. Roles of oral infections in the pathomechanism of atherosclerosis. *Int J Mol Sci*. 2018;19(7):E1978.
- James P, Worthington HV, Parnell C, et al. Chlorhexidine mouthrinse as an adjunctive treatment for gingival health. *Cochrane Database Syst Rev*. 2017;(3):CD008676.
- Lee YT, Lee HC, Hu CJ, et al. Periodontitis as a modifiable risk factor for dementia: a nationwide population-based cohort study. *J Am Geriatr Soc*. 2017;65(2):301–305.
- Nguyen DH, Martin JT. Common dental infections in the primary care setting. *Am Fam Physician*. 2008;77(6):797–802.

SEE ALSO
- Dental Infection; Glossitis
- Algorithm: Bleeding Gums

CODES
ICD10
- K05.10 Chronic gingivitis, plaque induced
- K05.11 Chronic gingivitis, non-plaque induced
- K05.00 Acute gingivitis, plaque induced

CLINICAL PEARLS
- Gingivitis may be prevented and treated with regular dental cleanings, good oral hygiene, and use of certain mouth rinses including chlorhexidine.
- Untreated, gingivitis may progress to periodontitis, a possible contributor to systemic inflammation and its consequences (e.g., coronary artery disease and uncontrolled diabetes)
- New-onset or difficult-to-treat gingivitis, consider differential of etiology: pregnancy, HIV, diabetes, medications, and vitamin deficiencies

G

GLAUCOMA, PRIMARY CLOSED-ANGLE

Salman S. Dar, MD • Sunil Shashikumar Bellur, MD • David A. Belyea, MD, MBA, FACS

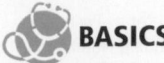 **BASICS**

DESCRIPTION

Glaucoma is a progressive decline in vision that is usually associated with elevated intraocular pressure (IOP) in the eye, which leads to damage of the optic nerve. Primary angle closure (PAC) is one reason for glaucoma and can be classified as the following:

- Primary angle-closure suspect (PACS) is >180 degrees of iridotrabecular contact (ITC), normal IOP with no optic nerve damage.
- PAC is >180 degrees ITC with peripheral anterior synechiae (PAS) or elevated IOP but with no optic neuropathy.
- Primary angle-closure glaucoma (PACG) is >180-degree ITC with PAS, elevated IOP, and optic neuropathy.

ALERT
Acute angle-closure crisis (AACC) is when the angle is occluded with symptomatic high IOP; it is a medical emergency requiring prompt treatment.

- Plateau iris configuration is any ITC persisting after a patent laser peripheral iridotomy (LPI) or a plateau iris syndrome which is any ITC persisting after a patent LPI with pressure elevation after dilation.

Geriatric Considerations
Increased risk with age and prior history of cataract, hyperopia, and/or uveitis.

Pregnancy Considerations
Medications used may cross the placenta and be excreted into breast milk. Majority of IOP-lowering medications are within class C, and the risk of adverse effects to the fetus must be balanced with risk of vision loss in the mother.

EPIDEMIOLOGY
- Older age
- Female sex
- More likely in those of Inuit and East or South Asian descent

Prevalence
In 2013, it is estimated to have a worldwide prevalence of 20.2 million people aged 40 to 80 years with majority (15.5 million) in Asia (1). PACG is not as common in the United States; accounts for 10% of all glaucoma

ETIOLOGY AND PATHOPHYSIOLOGY
- PAC happens when iris touches the trabecular meshwork at the anterior chamber angle called ITC. ITC causes obstruction of aqueous humor outflow through the trabecular meshwork, which causes elevation in IOP. Prolonged ITC can cause scarring, degradation of trabecular meshwork, and loss of vision (1).
- Most common underlying mechanism of angle closure is pupillary blockage of the aqueous flow from posterior to anterior chamber. This causes increase in pressure in the posterior chamber as compared to the anterior chamber. The buildup of pressure in the posterior chamber leads to anterior bowing of the iris and closing of the angle (1,2).
- Other mechanisms include predisposing ocular anatomy, such as plateau iris configuration (2).

Genetics
First-degree relatives have a 1–12% increased risk in whites; 6 times greater risk in Chinese patients with positive family history

RISK FACTORS
- Age >50 years
- Female gender
- Asian or Inuit descent
- Family history of angle closure
- Shallow anterior chamber
- Hyperopia
- Short axial length
- Thick crystalline lens
- Anterior positioned lens
- Plateau iris
- Drugs that can induce angle closure:
  - Adrenergic agonists (albuterol, phenylephrine), anticholinergics (oxybutynin, atropine, botulinum toxin A), topiramate, antihistamines, antidepressants including selective serotonin reuptake inhibitors (SSRIs) and tricyclic antidepressants (TCAs), sulfa-based drugs, cocaine, ecstasy

GENERAL PREVENTION
- Routine eye exam with gonioscopy for high-risk populations
- U.S. Preventive Services Task Force: insufficient evidence to recommend for or against screening adults for glaucoma without visual symptoms (3)[A]
- Prophylactic laser iridotomy may be considered in patients with PACS for preventing PACG.

COMMONLY ASSOCIATED CONDITIONS
- Cataract
- Hyperopia
- Microphthalmos
- Systemic hypertension

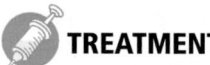 **DIAGNOSIS**

HISTORY
- Patient may be asymptomatic as in PACS or may have acute symptoms as in AACC.
- Acute symptoms commonly include unilateral:
  - Severe eye pain
  - Blurred vision
  - Eye redness
  - Halos around lights/objects
  - Frontal headache
  - Nausea and vomiting
- Patients with PACG can be asymptomatic, have subacute symptoms (intermittent subacute attacks), or compromised peripheral vision.
- Family history of acute angle-closure glaucoma
- Obtain history of prescription, over-the-counter, and herbal medications.
- Precipitating factors (dim light, medicines)
- Review of symptoms

PHYSICAL EXAM
Includes, but is not limited to, the following in the undilated eye:

- Visual acuity with refractive error (hyperopic eyes especially in older phakic patients)
- Visual field testing and ocular motility
- Pupil size and reactivity (mid-dilated, asymmetric or oval, minimally reactive, and may have relative afferent pupillary defect)
- Slit-lamp biomicroscopy—conjunctival hyperemia (in acute cases), central and peripheral anterior chamber depth narrowing, corneal swelling, iris abnormalities (diffuse and focal iris atrophy, posterior synechiae), lens changes (cataract and glaukomflecken-patchy localized anterior subcapsular lens opacities)
- IOP elevation as measured by applanation tonometry
- Gonioscopy: visualization of anatomy of the angle of both eyes and to look for ITC and PAS
- Anterior segment imaging with ultrasound (US) biomicroscopy and anterior segment optical coherence tomography (AS-OCT) to understand the angle anatomy
- Undilated fundus exam (congestion, cupping, atrophy of optic nerve)

DIFFERENTIAL DIAGNOSIS
- Acute orbital compartment syndrome
- Traumatic hyphema
- Conjunctivitis, episcleritis
- Corneal abrasion
- Glaucoma, malignant, or neovascular
- Herpes zoster ophthalmicus
- Iritis and uveitis
- Orbital/periorbital infection
- Vitreous or subconjunctival hemorrhage
- Lens-induced angle closure

DIAGNOSTIC TESTS & INTERPRETATION

Initial Tests (lab, imaging)
US biomicroscopy AS-OCT (1)[C]

Diagnostic Procedures/Other
Careful undilated ophthalmic examination including possible evaluation of fundus and optic nerve head, slit lamp biomicroscopy, gonioscopy, and tonometry (1)[C]

Test Interpretation
- Narrow or closed anterior angle
- Corneal stromal and epithelial edema
- Endothelial cell loss (guttata)
- Iris stromal necrosis
- Anterior subcapsular opacities (glaukomflecken)
- Optic nerve atrophy, pallor, or excavation

TREATMENT

ALERT
- For patients with acute symptoms (severe eye pain, blurred vision, eye redness, halos around lights/objects, frontal headache, nausea and vomiting) and asymmetric pupillary response, obtain immediate consultation with ophthalmology.

GENERAL MEASURES
- Goals of treatment (1)[C]:
  - Reverse or prevent angle-closure process
  - Control IOP
  - Prevent damage to the optic nerve
- PACS
  - Majority will not develop PAC or PACG.
  - May be either observed for development of PAC or be treated with iridotomy (1)[C]

- PAC and PACG
  - Iridotomy performed using argon or neodymium-doped yttrium aluminum garnet (Nd:YAG) laser (1)[A]
  - Complications of iridotomy: cataract; increased IOP; laser burn to the cornea, lens, vitreous, or retina; late-onset corneal edema; development of posterior synechiae; hyphema; iritis; and ocular dysphotopsia
- AACC
  - Initial treatment of AACC is to lower the IOP with medications to relieve the acute symptoms followed by iridotomy as soon as possible (1)[A]; for acute attack: ocular emergency
    - Manage nausea and pain.
    - Immediate ophthalmology consultation

MEDICATION

- During acute attack, medical therapy lowers IOP to relieve symptoms and clear corneal edema so that iridotomy can be performed as soon as possible.
- Medical therapy aims at:
  - Reduction of aqueous production:
    - Carbonic anhydrase inhibitors (CAIs): acetazolamide 10 mg/kg IV or PO. May repeat 250 mg in 4 hours to a maximum of 1 g/day. CAIs are contraindicated in sulfa allergy and hepatic insufficiency. Topical CAIs are not potent enough to break the papillary block.
    - Topical β-blockers: timolol 0.5%, levobunolol 0.5%, or carteolol 1%
    - Topical α_2-agonists: brimonidine 0.2% or apraclonidine 0.5%
  - Withdrawing aqueous from vitreous body and posterior chamber using hyperosmotic agents:
    - Glycerol 1.0 to 1.5 g/kg PO
    - Mannitol 1.0 to 1.5 g/kg IV
      - Hyperosmotic agent should be used with caution in patients with heart and kidney disease. Glycerol can increase blood sugar level and should not be given to diabetic patients.
  - Pupillary constriction to open the chamber angle: topical pilocarpine 1% or 2% or aceclidine 2%. Miotic therapy is ineffective when IOP is markedly elevated due to sphincter ischemia. They may cause forward rotation of ciliary muscle, increasing the papillary block and worsening the IOP.
- During acute attack, acetazolamide 500 mg IV is given followed by 500 mg PO. Topical therapy is initiated with 0.5% timolol maleate and 1% apraclonidine drops 1 minute apart. Reduction of inflammation is accomplished with frequent topical steroids. In addition, systemic therapy with mannitol 20% 1.5 to 2.0 g/kg infused over 30 to 60 minutes or oral glycerol (Osmoglyn) (50%) 6 oz PO may be needed. Also treat pain and nausea with analgesic and antiemetics; about an hour after initiating treatment, 2 doses of pilocarpine drops administered 15 minutes apart to cause miosis in an attempt to open the angle (2)[C]
- After corneal edema clears, a peripheral iridotomy is done.

ADDITIONAL THERAPIES

- Keep patient supine.
- Can give antiemetics if needed
- Can do retrobulbar block for nausea and pain control

SURGERY/OTHER PROCEDURES

- Definitive therapy for PAC, PACG, and AACC is Nd:YAG or argon laser iridotomy (1,2)[B].
- Surgical iridectomy may be performed if cornea is cloudy and laser iridotomy cannot be performed.
- Corneal indentation with four-mirror gonioscopic lens, cotton-tipped applicator, or muscle hook may be used to break a pupillary block in AACC (1)[C].
- Growing evidence shows cataract extraction alone can lower IOP and reduce the risk of lens-induced angle closure, thus can be considered as a treatment option in appropriate cases (1)[A]. Other procedures to reduce IOP that have been studied include argon laser peripheral iridoplasty (especially for plateau iris configuration/syndrome), anterior chamber paracentesis, goniosynechialysis, and trabeculectomy.

ADMISSION, INPATIENT, AND NURSING CONSIDERATIONS

- Patient requires metabolic $\pm$ electrolyte and volume status monitoring (with osmotic agents).
- Facilitate close ophthalmology follow-up.

 ONGOING CARE

FOLLOW-UP RECOMMENDATIONS

Schedule immediate ophthalmology follow-up.

Patient Monitoring

- Postsurgical follow-up and routine monitoring after acute attack as per ophthalmologist
- Half of the fellow eye of patients with AACC will develop AACC within 5 years. Hence, prophylactic LPI should be performed in the fellow eye as soon as possible (1)[B].

PATIENT EDUCATION

- Advise patient to seek emergency medical attention if experiencing a change in visual acuity, blurred vision, eye pain, or headache.
- Patients with PACS and no iridotomy; avoid use of decongestants, motion sickness medications, adrenergic agents, antipsychotics, antidepressants, and anticholinergic agents.
- Correct eyedrop administration technique, including the following:
  - Remove contact lenses before administration.
  - Allow at least 5 minutes between administration of multiple ophthalmic products.
- Patient education materials:
  - Glaucoma Research Foundation: http://www.glaucoma.org
  - National Eye Institute: http://www.nei.nih.gov

PROGNOSIS

- With timely treatment, most patients do not have permanent vision loss.
- Prognosis depends on ethnicity, underlying eye disease, and time to treatment.

COMPLICATIONS

- Chronic angle closure, corneal edema, corneal fibrosis, and vascularization
- Iris atrophy
- Cataract

- Optic atrophy
- Malignant glaucoma
- Central retinal artery/vein occlusion
- Permanent decrease in visual acuity
- Repeat episode
- Fellow (contralateral) eye attack

REFERENCES

1. American Academy of Ophthalmology. *Primary Angle Closure Preferred Practice Pattern*. San Francisco, CA: American Academy of Ophthalmology; 2016. http://www.aao.org. Accessed July 14, 2018.
2. European Glaucoma Society. *Terminology and Guidelines for Glaucoma*. 4th ed. Savona, Italy: PubliComm; 2014. https://www.eugs.org/eng/guidelines.asp. Accessed July 14, 2018.
3. Moyer VA; and U.S. Preventive Services Task Force. Screening for glaucoma: U.S. Preventive Services Task Force recommendation statement. *Ann Intern Med*. 2013;159(7):484–489.

ADDITIONAL READING

- Gupta D, Chen PP. Glaucoma. *Am Fam Physician*. 2016;93(8):668–674.
- Kolko M. Present and new treatment strategies in the management of glaucoma. *Open Ophthalmol J*. 2015;9:89–100.

 SEE ALSO

Glaucoma, Primary Open-Angle

 CODES

ICD10

- H40.20X0 Unsp primary angle-closure glaucoma, stage unspecified
- H40.219 Acute angle-closure glaucoma, unspecified eye
- H40.2290 Chronic angle-closure glaucoma, unsp eye, stage unspecified

CLINICAL PEARLS

- For patients with acute symptoms (severe eye pain, blurred vision, eye redness, halos around lights/objects, frontal headache, nausea and vomiting) and asymmetric pupillary response, obtain immediate consultation with ophthalmology.
- Examiner can determine if patient is hyperopic by observing the magnification of the patient's face through his or her glasses (myopic lenses minify).
- A careful history may reveal similar episodes of angle closure that resolved spontaneously. Miotics, such as pilocarpine, can be effective during mild attacks but ineffective in the setting of high IOP (due to pressure-induced iris sphincter ischemia).
- In patients with AACC, the fellow eye should undergo prophylactic laser iridotomy.

G

GLAUCOMA, PRIMARY OPEN-ANGLE

Richard W. Allinson, MD

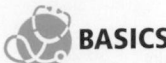

BASICS

DESCRIPTION

- Primary open-angle glaucoma (POAG) is an optic neuropathy resulting in visual field loss frequently associated with increased intraocular pressure (IOP).
- Normal IOP is 10 to 22 mm Hg. However, glaucomatous optic nerve damage also can occur with normal IOP and as a secondary manifestation of other disorders such as corticosteroid-induced glaucoma.
- System(s) affected: nervous
- Synonym(s): chronic open-angle glaucoma

Pregnancy Considerations
Prostaglandins should be avoided during pregnancy in the treatment of POAG.

EPIDEMIOLOGY

Incidence
- Predominant age: usually >40 years
- Increases with age
- Predominant gender: male = female

Prevalence
Prevalence in persons >40 years of age is ~1.8%.

Geriatric Considerations
Increasing prevalence with increasing age

ETIOLOGY AND PATHOPHYSIOLOGY

- Decreased aqueous outflow resulting in increased IOP
- Normally, aqueous is produced by the ciliary epithelium of the ciliary body and is secreted into the posterior chamber of the eye.
  - Aqueous then flows through the pupil and enters the anterior chamber to be drained by the trabecular meshwork (TM) in the iridocorneal angle of the eye. It then drains into the Schlemm canal and then into the episcleral venous system.
- 5–10% of the total aqueous outflow leaves via the uveoscleral pathway.
- Impaired aqueous outflow through the TM
  - Increased resistance within the aqueous drainage system

Genetics
- A family history of glaucoma increases the risk for developing glaucoma.
- TMCO1 genotype has been found to increase the risk of developing glaucoma among non-Hispanic whites
- The myocilin (MYOC) gene was the first gene associated with POAG.
  - MYOC cascade genetic testing for POAG allows identification of at-risk individuals (1)[C].

RISK FACTORS
- Increased IOP
- Myopia
- Diabetes mellitus (DM)
- African American
- Elderly
- Hypothyroidism
- Positive family history
- Central corneal thickness <550 μm
- Larger vertical cup-to-disc ratio (CDR)
- Larger horizontal CDR
- CDR asymmetry
- Disc hemorrhage
- Prolonged use of topical, periocular, inhaled, or systemic corticosteroids
- Obstructive sleep apnea
- Hypertension

- Corneal hysteresis (CH)
  - A measure of the viscoelastic damping of the cornea
  - Lower CH associated with faster rates of visual field loss

GENERAL PREVENTION
- Possible reduced risk of open-angle glaucoma with long-term use of oral statins among persons with hyperlipidemia
- Higher dietary nitrate and green leafy vegetable intake has been associated with a lower POAG risk.
  - Evidence suggests that nitrate, a precursor of nitric oxide, is beneficial for blood circulation.
    - The vascular endothelium regulates the microcirculation via vasoactive factors with nitric oxide being one of them.
    - Nitric oxide reduces IOP by causing relaxation of the TM and Schlemm canal, resulting in increased aqueous humor outflow.

COMMONLY ASSOCIATED CONDITIONS
DM

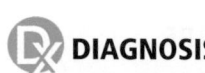

DIAGNOSIS

HISTORY
Painless, slowly progressive visual loss; patients are generally unaware of the visual loss until late in the disease. Central visual acuity remains unaffected until late in the disease.

PHYSICAL EXAM
- Visual acuity and visual field assessment
- Ophthalmoscopy to assess optic nerve for glaucomatous damage
- Increased IOP
- CDR >0.5: Normal eyes show a characteristic configuration for disc rim thickness of inferior ≥ superior ≥ nasal ≥ temporal (ISNT rule).
- Earliest visual field defects are paracentral scotomas and peripheral nasal steps.

DIFFERENTIAL DIAGNOSIS
- Normal-tension glaucoma
- Optic nerve pits
- Anterior ischemic optic neuropathy
- Compressive lesions of the optic nerve or chiasm
- Posthemorrhagic (shock optic neuropathy)

DIAGNOSTIC TESTS & INTERPRETATION

Initial Tests (lab, imaging)
Optical coherence tomography (OCT) can be useful in the detection of glaucoma.

- The retinal nerve fiber layer (RNFL) is primarily composed of the axons of the retinal ganglion cells (RGCs).
- Glaucoma involves not only the RGC axons but also the bodies and dendrites.
- RGC axonal thickness is greatest at the peripapillary retina; therefore, OCT measures the peripapillary RNFL.
- RGCs are concentrated in the macula; therefore, OCT measurements of the macular ganglion cell–inner plexiform layer (mGCIPL) can determine glaucoma progression by the thinning of the mGCIPL.
- RNFL is thinner in patients with glaucoma.
- RNFL tends to be thinner with older age, in Caucasians, greater axial length, and smaller optic disc area.
- Significant RGC loss may occur at specific location before corresponding visual field loss is detected.
  - Trend-based analysis of ganglion cell–inner plexiform layer thickness on spectral-domain OCT

may be useful for assessing glaucoma progression objectively and quantitatively (2)[C].

Diagnostic Procedures/Other
- Visual field testing: perimetry
  - A multifocal intraocular lens may reduce visual sensitivity on standard automated perimetry.
- Tonometry to measure IOP

Test Interpretation
- Atrophy and cupping of optic nerve
- Loss of RGCs and their axons produces defects and thinning in the RNFL. Assessment of RNFL thickness with OCT can detect glaucomatous damage before the appearance of visual field defects on standard automated perimetry.
- RNFL OCT utility declines in advanced glaucoma, whereas the mGCIPL OCT remains a sensitive progression detector from early to advanced glaucoma (3)[A].
- OCT angiography of the peripapillary retina and optic nerve in eyes with POAG demonstrates microvascular reduction associated with visual field defects in a region-specific manner.

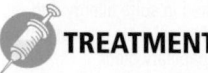

TREATMENT

GENERAL MEASURES
- Early Manifest Glaucoma Trial
  - Early treatment delays progression.
  - The magnitude of initial IOP reduction influences disease progression.
- Ocular Hypertension Treatment Study
  - Patients who only had increased IOP in the range of 24 to 32 mm Hg were treated with topical ocular hypotensive medication.
  - Treatment produced ~20% reduction in IOP.
  - At 5 years, treatment reduced the incidence of POAG by >50%: 9.5% in the observation group versus 4.4% in the medication-treated group.
- Advanced Glaucoma Intervention Study
  - Eyes were randomized to laser trabeculoplasty or filtering surgery when medical therapy failed.
  - In follow-up, if IOP was always <18 mm Hg, visual fields tended to stabilize. When IOP was >17 mm Hg, >1/2 the time, patients tended to have worsening of visual fields.
- Collaborative Initial Glaucoma Treatment Study
  - Both initial medical and surgical (trabeculectomy) treatment achieved significant IOP reduction, and both had little visual field loss over time.
  - There was a 5-year risk of endophthalmitis of 1.1% after trabeculectomy.

MEDICATION
More than one medication, with different mechanisms of action, may be needed. Ocular hypotensive agent categories include the following:

- Prostaglandin analogues: generally used as first-line treatment. Enhance uveoscleral outflow and increase aqueous outflow through the TM: latanoprost 0.005% one drop at bedtime; travoprost 0.004% one drop at bedtime; bimatoprost 0.01% one drop at bedtime.
- Latanoprostene bunod, 0.024% solution, This is a combination drug with one of the actions being the release of nitric oxide (4)[B]. Instill one drop at bedtime.
  - Contraindications/precautions
    - Prostaglandin analogues may cause increased pigmentation of the iris and periorbital tissue.

○ Increased pigmentation and growth of eyelashes
○ Should be used with caution in active intraocular inflammation (iritis/uveitis)
○ Caution is also advised in eyes with risk factors for herpes simplex, iritis, and cystoid macular edema.
○ Macular edema may be a complication associated with treatment.
○ Avoid during pregnancy.
- β-Adrenergic antagonists (nonselective and selective): decrease aqueous formation; best when used as an add-on therapy: timolol 0.25% (initial) to 0.5% one drop in affected eye q12h; gel-forming solution (0.25% or 0.5%) one drop in affected eye once daily; betaxolol 0.5% one drop affected eye BID
  − Nonselective β-adrenergic antagonists: Avoid in asthma, chronic obstructive pulmonary disease (COPD), 2nd- and 3rd-degree atrioventricular (AV) block, and decompensated heart failure. Betaxolol is a selective β-adrenergic antagonist and is safer in pulmonary disease.
  − β-Adrenergic antagonists: caution in patients taking calcium antagonists because of possible AV conduction disturbances, left ventricular failure, or hypotension
- Adrenergic agonists (selective α_2-adrenergic agonists)
  − Brimonidine tartrate 0.1%: One drop TID (α_2-adrenergic agonist) decreases aqueous formation and increases uveoscleral outflow.
    ○ Brimonidine should not be used in infants and young children because of the risk of CNS depression, apnea, bradycardia, and hypotension.
    ○ Monoamine oxidase inhibitors and tricyclic antidepressants may interfere with the metabolism of brimonidine and result in toxicity.
- Carbonic anhydrase inhibitors (oral, topical): decrease aqueous formation
  − Acetazolamide: 250 mg PO 1 to 4 times per day
  − Dorzolamide 2%: one drop TID
  − Brinzolamide 1%: one drop TID
  − Carbonic anhydrase inhibitors
    ○ Do not use with sulfa drug allergies.
    ○ Do not use with cirrhosis because of the risk of hepatic encephalopathy.
- Rho kinase (Rock) inhibitors lower IOP by increasing aqueous outflow through the trabecular outflow pathway by decreasing actomyosin-driven cellular contraction and reducing production of fibrotic extracellular matrix proteins (5)[B].
  − Netarsudil 0.02%: one drop once daily in the evening
  − Corneal verticillata, or whorl keratopathy can occur with its usage.
- Parasympathomimetics (miotic), including cholinergic (direct acting) increase aqueous outflow
  − Pilocarpine 1–4%: one drop in affected eye BID–QID (cholinergic)
  − Parasympathomimetics (miotic): cause pupillary constriction and may cause decreased vision in patients with a cataract; may cause eye pain or myopia due to increased accommodation. All miotics break down the blood–aqueous barrier and may induce chronic iridocyclitis.
- Hyperosmotic agents: increase blood osmolality, drawing water from the vitreous cavity
  − Mannitol 20% solution: administered IV at 2 g/kg of body weight
  − Glycerin 50% solution: administered PO; dosage is usually 4 to 7 oz.

- Hyperosmotic agents: caution in diabetics; dehydrated patients; and those with cardiac, renal, and hepatic disease. Contact lens wearers: Many glaucoma drops contain benzalkonium chloride; remove contact lens prior to administration and wait 15 minutes before reinsertion.
- When greater than or equal to three medications are required, compliance is difficult, and surgery may be needed.

SURGERY/OTHER PROCEDURES
- ALT
  − Can be applied up to 180 degrees of the TM
  − Improves aqueous outflow
  − The Glaucoma Laser Trial Research Group showed in newly diagnosed, previously untreated patients with POAG that ALT was as effective as topical glaucoma medication within the first 2 years of follow-up.
  − Usually reserved for patients needing better IOP control while taking topical glaucoma drops
- Selective laser trabeculoplasty (SLT)
  − 532-nm Nd:YAG laser
  − Appears to be as effective as ALT in lowering IOP
  − May be repeated if necessary
- Trabeculectomy (glaucoma filtering surgery)
  − Usually reserved for patients needing better IOP control after maximal medical therapy and who may have previously undergone an ALT/SLT
  − Mitomycin C can be applied at the time of surgery to increase the chances of a surgical success.
  − Subconjunctival bevacizumab may be a beneficial adjunctive therapy for reducing late surgical failure after trabeculectomy.
- Shunt (tube) surgery
  − For example, Molteno and Ahmed devices
  − Generally reserved for difficult glaucoma cases in which conventional filtering surgery has failed or is likely to fail
- Tube Versus Trabeculectomy (TVT) study
  − After 5 years of follow up, both procedures were associated with similar IOP reduction and the number of glaucoma medications needed.
- Ciliary body ablation: indicated to lower IOP in patients with poor visual potential or those who are poor candidates for filtering or shunt procedures
- Minimally invasive glaucoma surgery (MIGS) is frequently combined with cataract surgery; currently targeted at patients with mild to moderate glaucoma
  − Schlemm canal stents
    ○ iStent, Hydrus
  − Suprachoroidal stents
    ○ CyPass, iStent Supra
      ■ CyPass Micro-Stent demonstrated sustained reduction in IOP and glaucoma medication after a 2-year follow-up for mild to moderate POAG.
  − Subconjunctival stents
    ○ Xen, InnFocus
  − The trabectome system performs a trabeculotomy via an internal approach, removing both a strip of TM and the inner wall of the Schlemm canal.
- Cataract extraction can decrease IOP in patients with ocular hypertension.

ONGOING CARE

FOLLOW-UP RECOMMENDATIONS
Patient Monitoring
- Monitor vision and IOP every 3 to 6 months.
- Visual field testing every 6 to 18 months
- Optic nerve evaluation every 3 to 18 months, depending on POAG control

- A worsening of the mean deviation by 2 dB on the Humphrey field analyzer and confirmed by a single test after 6 months had a 72% probability of progression.
- The IOP response to ocular hypotensive agents tends to be reduced in persons with thicker corneas.

PATIENT EDUCATION
POAG is a silent robber of vision, and patients may not appreciate the significance of their disease until much of their visual field is lost.

PROGNOSIS
- With standard glaucoma therapy, the rate of visual field loss in POAG is slow.
- Patients still may lose vision and develop blindness, even when treated appropriately.
- The rate of legal blindness from POAG over a follow-up of 22 years was 19%.
- The rate of progression of visual field loss increases with older age.

COMPLICATIONS
Blindness

REFERENCES
1. Souzeau E, Tram KH, Witney M, et al. Myocilin predictive genetic testing for primary open-angle glaucoma leads to early identification of at-risk individuals. Ophthalmology. 2017;124(3):303–309.
2. Lee WJ, Kim YK, Park KH, et al. Trend-based analysis of ganglion cell-inner plexiform layer thickness changes on optical coherence tomography in glaucoma progression. Ophthalmology. 2017;124(9):1383–1391.
3. Zhang X, Dastiridou A, Francis B, et al; for Advanced Imaging for Glaucoma Study Group. Comparison of glaucoma progression detection by optical coherence tomography and visual field. Am J Ophthalmol. 2017;184:63–74.
4. Weinreb RN, Scassellati Sforzolini B, Vittitow J, et al. Latanoprostene bunod 0.024% versus timolol maleate 0.5% in subjects with open-angle glaucoma or ocular hypertension: the APOLLO study. Ophthalmology. 2016;123(5):965–973.
5. Serle JB, Katz JK, McLaurin E, et al; for the Rocket-1 and Rocket-2 Study Groups. Two phase 3 clinical trials comparing the safety and efficacy of netarsudil to timolol in patients with elevated intraocular pressure: Rho Kinase Elevated IOP Treatment Trial 1 and 2 (ROCKET-1 and ROCKET-2). Am J Ophthalmol. 2018;186:116–127.

CODES

ICD10
- H40.11X0 Primary open-angle glaucoma, stage unspecified
- H40.11X1 Primary open-angle glaucoma, mild stage
- H40.11X2 Primary open-angle glaucoma, moderate stage

CLINICAL PEARLS
- Pain is not a frequent symptom of POAG.
- Painless, slowly progressive visual loss; patients generally are unaware of the visual loss until late in the disease. Central visual acuity remains unaffected until late in the disease.
- Patients still may lose vision and develop blindness, even when treated appropriately.
- Topical or system steroids can cause the IOP to increase.

GLOMERULONEPHRITIS, ACUTE

Dayyan M. Adoor, MD • Jonathan T. Lin, MD

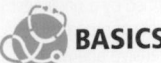

BASICS

DESCRIPTION
- Acute glomerulonephritis (GN) is an inflammatory process involving the glomerulus of the kidney, resulting in a clinical syndrome consisting of hematuria, proteinuria, and renal insufficiency, often in association with hypertension and edema.
- Acute GN may be caused by primary glomerular disease or secondary to systemic disease.
  - Infection-related GN (also postinfectious GN)
  - IgA nephropathy/Henoch-Schönlein purpura (HSP)
  - Antiglomerular basement membrane disease (anti-GBM disease)
  - Antineutrophil cytoplasmic antibody (ANCA)-associated GN
  - Membranoproliferative GN (MPGN)
  - Lupus nephritis
  - Cryoglobulin-associated GN
- Clinical severity ranges from asymptomatic microscopic or gross hematuria to a rapid loss of kidney function over days to weeks, termed rapidly progressive GN (RPGN).
  - In patients with RPGN, kidney biopsy often demonstrates crescentic GN, which usually warrants urgent and aggressive treatment.

ALERT
Urgent investigation and treatment are required to avoid irreversible loss of kidney function.

EPIDEMIOLOGY
- Infection-related GN
  - Most commonly manifests after resolution of group A β-hemolytic *Streptococcus* infection (poststreptococcal)
  - Can also occur as a result of other bacterial infections, such as infective endocarditis or shunt nephritis, or less commonly with viral or parasitic infections
  - Accounts for 80% of acute GN in children
- IgA nephropathy
  - Most common primary GN in the world
  - Most common in the 2nd and 3rd decades but can occur at any age
  - Incidence differs geographically: Asia > United States
  - Populations of East Asian ancestry are at increased risk for IgA nephropathy, and some genetic factors have been identified.
  - HSP, the form with extrarenal manifestations, can occur at any age but typically occurs in children <10 years old.
- Anti-GBM disease
  - Can cause Goodpasture disease, a notable cause of the pulmonary–renal syndrome
  - Peak distribution in 3rd and 6th decades
- ANCA-associated GN
  - Often has a relapsing and remitting course
  - Four disease presentations:
    ○ Granulomatosis with polyangiitis (GPA), formerly Wegener granulomatosis
    ○ Microscopic polyangiitis (MPA)
    ○ Isolated pauci-immune GN—when isolated to kidneys
    ○ Eosinophilic GPA, formerly Churg-Strauss disease—GN relatively common but renal involvement rarely severe
  - Older patients are more commonly affected, although this GN can affect any age group.

- MPGN
  - May be primary (idiopathic) or secondary to systemic diseases
  - Epidemiology varies depending on the mechanism of injury.
- Lupus nephritis
  - 30–70% of systemic lupus patients will have renal involvement.
  - Incidence of lupus nephritis is higher among African Americans in comparison to white Caucasian populations.
- Cryoglobulin-associated vasculitis
  - 80% of cases with hepatitis C virus infection
  - May also be associated with autoimmune disease or dysproteinemia

ETIOLOGY AND PATHOPHYSIOLOGY
- In general, systemic and/or local immune activation causes glomerular injury.
- Immune-complex mediated: from antigen–antibody formation and deposition in the kidneys
  - Postinfectious GN: host immune reaction to nephritogenic streptococci strains as a trigger
  - IgA nephropathy: abnormal glycosylation of IgA, leads to its mesangial deposition; etiology poorly understood
  - MPGN: typically secondary to systemic diseases, such as chronic infections (hepatitis C), autoimmune diseases, monoclonal gammopathies, and complement dysregulation
  - Lupus nephritis: autoimmune disease
  - Cryoglobulin-associated GN: inflammation from complexes known as cryoglobulins, named for their property of precipitating as lower temperatures
- Direct antibody-mediated injury:
  - Anti-GBM disease: caused by autoantibodies that target type IV collagen of basement membranes
- Pauci-immune GN
  - ANCA-associated GN: autoantibodies against neutrophil granules involved in pathogenesis
- Alternative complement pathway dysregulation:
  - C3 glomerulopathy: subtype of MPGN with predominant C3 without immunoglobulin staining on immunofluorescence; includes dense deposit disease (DDD) and C3GN

Genetics
Genetic factors are likely to play a role in susceptibility to many of the acute GNs, although these have not been sufficiently defined to be clinically useful in most circumstances.

RISK FACTORS
- Epidemics of nephritogenic strains of streptococci are triggers for postinfectious GN.
- Anti-GBM disease has been associated with prior pulmonary injury and inhalation exposures, such as hydrocarbon solvents.
- ANCA-associated GN may be drug induced (e.g., hydralazine, levamisole-contaminated cocaine) and is also associated with environmental exposures such as silica.
- Infection with hepatitis B or C is associated with MPGN.
- Infection with hepatitis C is a risk factor for developing cryoglobulinemic GN.
- Mutations in alternate complement pathway genes are associated with increased risk of developing complement-mediated MPGN.

GENERAL PREVENTION
Early detection is paramount.

DIAGNOSIS

HISTORY
- Patients may report cola- or tea-colored urine and decreased urine volume.
- Edema occurs in many patients, typically in face and lower extremities.
- Shortness of breath may occur with significant fluid overload.
- Generalized malaise
- Timing
  - Poststreptococcal GN typically occurs 1 to 3 weeks after pharyngitis or 2 to 6 weeks after skin infection.
- IgA nephropathy may present within several days after an acute infection.
- Patients may also present with complaints more specific to the associated disease:
  - Joint pain or rash in lupus nephritis
  - Hemoptysis in pulmonary–renal syndromes (see "Physical Exam")
  - Sinusitis, pulmonary infiltrates, arthralgias in ANCA-associated GN
  - Abdominal or joint pain and purpura in IgA–HSP
  - Purpura and skin vasculitis in cryoglobulinemia-associated GN

PHYSICAL EXAM
- A complete physical exam may discover clues to systemic disease as a potential cause.
- Majority of patients will have normal exam, but can often present with hypertension and signs of fluid overload.
- Sinus disease: often with ANCA-associated GN/GPA
- Pharyngitis or impetigo: postinfectious GN or IgA nephropathy
- Pulmonary hemorrhage (pulmonary–renal syndrome): anti-GBM disease/Goodpasture, ANCA-associated GN, or lupus nephritis
- Hepatomegaly or liver tenderness could point to cryoglobulinemia-associated GN or IgA nephropathy.
- Purpura may point to ANCA-associated GN or HSP/IgA nephropathy.

DIFFERENTIAL DIAGNOSIS
Nonglomerular hematuria: trauma, prostate diseases, urologic cancer, cystitis, nephrolithiasis, renal cysts, thrombotic microangiopathy

DIAGNOSTIC TESTS & INTERPRETATION
Initial Tests (lab, imaging)
- Urinalysis with examination of sediment
  - Dysmorphic RBCs or RBC casts on urine microscopy indicate glomerular hematuria and strongly suggest the diagnosis of an acute GN.
  - Pyuria and white blood cell casts may also be present.
- Proteinuria: 24-hour collection or random urine protein/creatinine ratio
  - Can be mild to severe proteinuria, occasionally nephrotic range
- Electrolytes, BUN, creatinine, CBC
- Serologies, depending on clinical presentation, may help clarify etiology:
  - Antistreptolysin O titer, streptozyme: often positive in poststreptococcal GN
  - Complement levels (C3, C4):
    ○ C3 low in infection-related GN
    ○ Both C3 and C4 can be low in lupus nephritis and MPGN.
    ○ C4 typically low in cryoglobulinemia
  - Antinuclear antibody (ANA) to rule out lupus nephritis

- ANCA screen: MPO and PR3 antibodies
- Anti-GBM antibody
- Hepatitis B surface antigen and antibody
- Hepatitis C antibody
- Cryoglobulins (must be sent warm)
- Rheumatoid factor
- HIV testing
- Serum free light chain to assess for monoclonal gammopathies
- A chest x-ray may be useful in the setting of hemoptysis or a suspected infiltrate on exam.

Test Interpretation
Renal biopsy
- If clinical picture is consistent with postinfectious GN in a child, a biopsy may not be required.
- If there is clinical suspicion for other causes of acute GN, renal biopsy should be done.
- Light microscopy
  - Diffuse hypercellularity suggests a proliferative disease such as IgA nephropathy, lupus nephritis, or postinfectious GN.
  - Presence of glomerular crescents correlates with RPGN and disease severity.
- Immunofluorescence
  - Pattern of IgG, IgA, IgM, C3, and C4 staining may aid in characterizing the GN.
  - Isolated mesangial IgA staining is pathognomonic for IgA nephropathy.
  - Crescentic GN in absence of immune complex staining suggests ANCA-associated GN.
  - Lupus nephritis typically positive for all immunoglobulins and complements ("full house")
- Electron microscopy: The location of immunoglobulin deposits is useful in pointing to a particular diagnosis.

TREATMENT

MEDICATION
First Line
- Hypertension
  - Diuretics are useful for management of salt retention and edema.
  - Calcium channel blockers
  - Avoid ACE inhibitors or ARBs if acute renal dysfunction is present.
- Peripheral edema: Loop diuretics are often required due to the degree of edema.
- Pulmonary edema: oxygen and diuretics

Second Line
- Each of the glomerular diseases often requires a specific treatment plan based on renal biopsy results; therefore, a nephrologist is often guiding care.
- Supportive care is adequate in postinfectious GN.
- Crescents on renal biopsy may be an indication for steroids in postinfectious GN and, in other cases, are often an indication for additional potent immunosuppressive medications (1)[C].
- Commonly used immunosuppressive medications include
  - Corticosteroids—may consider initiation in high doses even prior to kidney biopsy (1)[C]
  - Cyclophosphamide
  - Mycophenolate mofetil
  - Calcineurin inhibitors (cyclosporine, tacrolimus)
  - Rituximab
- Choice of immunosuppressive agent depends on patient characteristics and the disease process.
  - Steroids plus either cyclophosphamide, rituximab, or mycophenolate may be used to treat ANCA-associated renal disease and proliferative forms of lupus nephritis (1)[C],(2,3)[A].

- IgA nephropathy: ACE inhibitors or ARBs recommended for patients with proteinuria (1,4)[C]. Additional steroids and immunosuppression may be considered in refractory cases (1)[C].
  - MPGN: Treat underlying cause in secondary type.
  - Anti-GBM: Treatment consists of a combination of immunosuppressants and plasmapheresis (4)[C].
- Plasmapheresis may also be considered in some cases for RPGN or ANCA-associated renal disease with diffuse pulmonary hemorrhage (1)[C],(2,5)[A].
- Dialysis may be needed for uremia, hyperkalemia refractory to medical management, intractable acidosis, and diuretic-resistant pulmonary edema.

ISSUES FOR REFERRAL
- Consultation with a nephrologist is usually required to assist with renal biopsy to confirm diagnosis and assist with management.
- Consultation with a rheumatologist may also be helpful in cases with systemic manifestations.

ADMISSION, INPATIENT, AND NURSING CONSIDERATIONS
- Consider admission for patients with no urine output, rapidly deteriorating renal function, significant hypertension, and suspicion of pulmonary hemorrhage or fluid overload that is compromising heart or respiratory function.
- Hemodynamically stable patients without complications may be managed as outpatients.

 ONGOING CARE

FOLLOW-UP RECOMMENDATIONS
Patient Monitoring
- Depends on type of GN
- Regular BP checks and urinalysis to detect recurrence, assessment of renal function to detect acute or follow chronic renal disease as a result of the primary event, and regular clinical assessment to detect suspicious symptoms that may herald a recurrence (i.e., rash, joint complaint, hemoptysis)
- Periodic reassessment of serology tests to follow asymptomatic individuals

DIET
- No-added-salt diet and fluid restriction until edema and hypertension clear
- Avoid high-potassium foods if significant renal dysfunction is present.
- Avoid a high-protein diet.

PATIENT EDUCATION
National Kidney Foundation: http://www.kidney.org/atoz/content/glomerul

PROGNOSIS
- In general, the prognosis depends on the cause of the GN.
- The GN may be self-limited (as often is the case in postinfectious GN) or part of a chronic disease that makes the possibility of recurrence of acute disease likely, with the potential for progressive loss of renal function over time.
- Some forms of acute GN (including ANCA-associated and severe lupus) require long-term immunosuppression to prevent recurrence.

COMPLICATIONS
- Hypertensive retinopathy and encephalopathy
- Microscopic hematuria may persist for years.
- Chronic kidney disease
- Nephrotic syndrome (~10%)

REFERENCES

1. Beck L, Bomback AS, Choi MJ, et al. KDOQI US commentary on the 2012 KDIGO clinical practice guideline for glomerulonephritis. *Am J Kidney Dis*. 2013;62(3):403–441.
2. Walters G, Willis NS, Craig JC. Interventions for renal vasculitis in adults. *Cochrane Database Syst Rev*. 2008;(3):CD003232.
3. Stone JH, Merkel PA, Spiera R, et al; for RAVE-ITN Research Group. Rituximab versus cyclophosphamide for ANCA-associated vasculitis. *N Engl J Med*. 2010;363(3):221–232.
4. Floege J, Amann K. Primary glomerulonephritides. *Lancet*. 2016;387(10032):2036–2048.
5. Jayne DR, Gaskin G, Rasmussen N, et al; for European Vasculitis Study Group. Randomized trial of plasma exchange or high-dosage methylprednisolone as adjunctive therapy for severe renal vasculitis. *J Am Soc Nephrol*. 2007;18(7):2180–2188.

ADDITIONAL READING
- Bomback AS, Appel GB. Updates on the treatment of lupus nephritis. *J Am Soc Nephrol*. 2010;21(12):2028–2035.
- Kidney Disease: Improving Global Outcomes Glomerulonephritis Work Group. KDIGO clinical practice guideline for glomerulonephritis. *Kidney Int Suppl*. 2012;2(Suppl 2):139–274.
- Sethi S, Haas M, Markowitz GS, et al. Mayo Clinic/Renal Pathology Society consensus report on pathologic classification, diagnosis, and reporting of GN. *J Am Soc Nephrol*. 2016;27(5):1278–1287.

 SEE ALSO

- Glomerulonephritis, Postinfectious; Henoch-Schönlein Purpura; Hyperkalemia; Hypertensive Emergencies; IgA Nephropathy; Lupus Nephritis; Nephrotic Syndrome; Vasculitis
- Algorithm: Acute Kidney Injury (Acute Renal Failure); Hematuria

 CODES

ICD10
- N00.9 Acute nephritic syndrome with unsp morphologic changes
- N00.2 Acute nephritic syndrome w diffuse membranous glomrlneph
- N00.8 Acute nephritic syndrome with other morphologic changes

CLINICAL PEARLS
- Dysmorphic RBCs and RBC casts are a key component of the urinalysis in GN.
- Postinfectious GN in children is typically a self-limited disease.
- Searching for other organ involvement is useful in establishing a definitive diagnosis.
- With the discovery of a GN, monitor the initial renal function labs frequently to identify an RPGN.
- Clinical course and treatment strategies depend on the underlying disease process.

G

GLOMERULONEPHRITIS, POSTINFECTIOUS

Frances M. Rusnack, DO • Theodore B. Flaum, DO, FACOFP

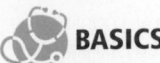 **BASICS**

DESCRIPTION
Postinfectious glomerulonephritis (PIGN) is an immune complex disease associated with nonrenal infection by certain strains of bacteria, most commonly *Streptococcus* and *Staphylococcus*. The most common form of PIGN, poststreptococcal glomerulonephritis (PSGN), is preceded by *Streptococcus* and predominantly affects children. The clinical presentation varies from asymptomatic to the acute nephritic syndrome, characterized by gross hematuria, proteinuria, edema, hypertension (HTN), and acute kidney injury.

EPIDEMIOLOGY
A global decline in incidence, especially in developed countries, is attributed to better hygiene and a decreased incidence of streptococcal skin infections. Of cases, 97% occur in developing countries. PSGN is primarily a pediatric disease, but a recent increase has been seen in nonstreptococcal GN in adults.

Incidence
- Pediatrics: 24.3 cases/100,000 persons per year in developing countries; 6 cases/100,000 persons per year in developed countries
- Adults: 2 cases/100,000 persons per year in developing countries; 0.3 cases/100,000 persons per year in developed countries
- Worldwide: 34% of cases are now seen in adults with a global burden of 68,000 cases per year.
- Male > female (2:1) (1)

ETIOLOGY AND PATHOPHYSIOLOGY
- Glomerular immune complex disease induced by specific nephritogenic strains of bacteria:
  - Group A β-hemolytic *Streptococcus* (GAS)
  - *Staphylococcus* (predominantly *Staphylococcus aureus*; more commonly methicillin-resistant *S. aureus* [MRSA], occasionally coagulase-negative *Staphylococcus*)
  - Gram-negative bacteria, including *Escherichia coli*, *Yersinia*, *Pseudomonas*, and *Haemophilus* (1)
- Proposed mechanisms for the glomerular injury (2):
  - Deposition of circulating immune complexes with streptococcal or staphylococcal antigens—these complexes can be detected in patients with streptococcal- or staphylococcal-related GN but do not correlate to disease activity (3).
  - Note: IgG is the most frequent immunoglobulin in PSGN (1).
  - In situ immune complex formation from deposition of antigens within the glomerular basement membrane (GBM) and subsequent antibody binding
  - In situ glomerular immune complex formation promoted by antibodies to streptococcal or staphylococcal antigens
  - Alteration of normal renal antigen leading to molecular mimicry that elicits an autoimmune response
- Glomerular immune complex causing complement activation and inflammation:
  - Nephritis-associated plasmin receptor (NAPlr): activates plasmin, contributes to activation of the alternative complement pathway

- Streptococcal pyrogenic exotoxin B (SPE B): binds plasmin and acts as a protease; promotes the release of inflammatory mediators
- Activation of the alternative complement pathway causes initial glomerular injury as evidenced by C3 deposition and decreased levels of serum C3. The lectin pathway of complement activation has also been recently implicated in glomerular injury (4).

RISK FACTORS
- Children 5 to 12 years of age
- Older patients (>65 years of age) (1):
  - Patients with immunocompromising comorbid conditions
  - Diabetes
  - Alcohol abuse

GENERAL PREVENTION
- Early antibiotic treatment for streptococcal and staphylococcal infections, when indicated, although efficacy in preventing GN is uncertain
- Improved hygiene
- Prophylactic penicillin treatment to be used in closed communities and household contacts of index cases in areas where PIGN is prevalent

COMMONLY ASSOCIATED CONDITIONS
Commonly streptococcal or staphylococcal infection

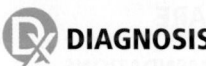 **DIAGNOSIS**

HISTORY
- Patients present with acute nephritic syndrome, characterized by sudden onset of hematuria associated with edema and HTN 1 to 2 weeks after an infection.
- A triad of edema, hematuria, and HTN is classic.
- Urine described as "tea-colored" or "cola-colored"
- PIGN in children usually follows GAS skin/throat infection.
- The latent period between GAS infection and PIGN depends on the site of infection: 1 to 3 weeks following GAS pharyngitis and 3 to 6 weeks following GAS skin infection.
- Adult PIGN most commonly follows staphylococcal infections (3 times more common than streptococcal infections) of the upper respiratory tract, skin, heart, lung, bone, or urinary tract. Studies show 7–16% of cases of adult PIGN have no preceding evidence of infection and, in 24–59%, the offending microorganism cannot be identified (5)[A].

PHYSICAL EXAM
- Edema: present in ~2 of 3 adult patients due to sodium and water retention; less common in pediatric patients
- Gross hematuria: present in 25–60% of patients
- HTN: present in 80–90% of patients and varies from mild to severe; secondary to fluid retention. Hypertensive encephalopathy is an uncommon but serious complication.
- Microscopic hematuria: subclinical cases of PIGN
- Respiratory distress: due to pulmonary edema (rare)

DIFFERENTIAL DIAGNOSIS
The diagnosis of PIGN is generally by history once the diagnosis of acute nephritis is made, with documentation of a recent infection and nephritis beginning to resolve 1 to 2 weeks after presentation. However, with progressive disease >2 weeks, persistent hematuria/HTN >4 to 6 weeks, or no adequate documentation of a GAS or other infection, the differential diagnosis of GN needs to be considered and renal biopsy ordered:
- Membranoproliferative glomerulonephritis (MPGN): The presentation of MPGN may be indistinguishable initially with hematuria, HTN, proteinuria, and hypocomplementemia after an upper respiratory infection. However, patients with MPGN continue to have persistent nephritis and hypocomplementemia beyond 4 to 6 weeks and possibly also have a further elevation in serum creatinine. Patients with PIGN tend to have resolution of their disease and a return of normal C3 and CH50 levels within 2 to 4 weeks.
- Secondary causes of GN: Lupus nephritis and Henoch-Schönlein purpura nephritis have features similar to PIGN. Extrarenal manifestations and laboratory tests for these underlying systemic diseases help differentiate them from PIGN. Hypocomplementemia is not characteristic of Henoch-Schönlein purpura, and the hypocomplementemia that occurs in lupus nephritis is with reductions in both C3 and C4, whereas C4 levels are normal in PIGN.
- IgA nephropathy often presents after an upper respiratory infection. It can be distinguished from PIGN based on a shorter time frame between the upper respiratory illness and hematuria, as well as history of gross hematuria, as PIGN recurrence is rare. IgA nephropathy is a chronic illness and will recur. Patients with IgA nephropathy have normal C3/C4 levels.
- IgA-dominant acute PIGN: a recently recognized form of PIGN occurring in poststaphylococcal GN. This differs from primary IgA nephropathy in that these patients do not have a history of renal disease. The terms IgA-dominant PIGN and poststaphylococcal GN have been debated because such cases are described in association with active staphylococcal infection. Emerging terms include IgA-dominant infection-related GN or staphylococcus-associated GN (1)[A].
- Pauci-immune crescentic GN: In elderly patients with severe renal failure and active urine sediment, this is much more common, so antineutrophil cytoplasmic antibody (ANCA) testing should be done (1)[A].

DIAGNOSTIC TESTS & INTERPRETATION
Initial Tests (lab, imaging)
Urinalysis shows hematuria; can be with/without RBC casts and pyuria. Proteinuria is present, but nephrotic range proteinuria is uncommon in children (more likely in adults).

Follow-Up Tests & Special Considerations
- Culture: PSGN usually presents weeks after a GAS infection; only ~25% of patients will have either a positive throat or skin culture.

- Complement: 90% of pediatric patients (slightly fewer adult patients) will have depressed C3 and CH50 levels in the first 2 weeks of the disease, whereas C2 and C4 levels remain normal. C3 and CH50 levels return to normal within 4 to 8 weeks after presentation.
- Creatinine: elevated to the point of renal insufficiency in 25–83% of cases, more commonly in adults (83%) (4)[A]
- Serology: Elevated titers of antibodies support evidence of a recent GAS infection. Streptozyme test measuring antistreptolysin O (ASO), antihyaluronidase (AHase), antistreptokinase (ASKase), anti–nicotinamide-adenine dinucleotidase (anti-NAD), and anti-DNAse B antibodies: positive in >95% of patients with PSGN due to pharyngitis and 80% with skin infections. In pharyngeal infection, ASO, anti-DNAse B, anti-NAD, and AHase titers are elevated. In skin infections, only the anti-DNAse and AHase titers are typically elevated.

Diagnostic Procedures/Other
Renal biopsy is rarely done in children; recommended in most adults to confirm the diagnosis and rule out other glomerulopathies with similar clinical presentations that require immunosuppressive treatment

Test Interpretation
- Light microscopy: diffuse proliferative glomerulonephritis with prominent endocapillary proliferation and numerous neutrophils within the capillary lumen. Deposits may also be found in the mesangium ("starry sky"). Severity of involvement varies and correlates with clinical findings. Crescent formation is uncommon and is associated with a poor prognosis.
- Immunofluorescence microscopy: deposits of C3 and IgG distributed in a diffuse granular pattern
- Electron microscopy: dome-shaped subepithelial electron-dense deposits that are referred to as "humps." These deposits are immune complexes, and they correspond to the deposits of IgG and C3 found on immunofluorescence. Rate of clearance of these deposits affects recovery time.
- Renal biopsy: usually not performed in most patients to confirm the diagnosis of PIGN as clinical history is highly suggestive and resolution of PIGN typically begins within 1 week of presentation. A biopsy is done when other glomerular disorders are being considered, such as in the case of persistently low C3 levels beyond 6 weeks for possible diagnosis of MPGN, recurrent episodes of hematuria suggestive of IgA nephropathy, or a progressive increase in serum creatinine not characteristic of PIGN.

 TREATMENT

MEDICATION
- No specific therapy exists for PIGN, and no randomized controlled trials indicate that aggressive immunosuppressive therapy has a beneficial effect in patients with rapidly progressive crescentic disease. Despite this, patients with >30% crescents on renal biopsy are often treated with steroids (4)[A].
- Older patients often require hospitalization to prevent and treat complications of heart failure (HF) from volume overload (1).

- Management is supportive, with focus on treating the clinical manifestations of PIGN. These include HTN and pulmonary edema:
  - General measures include salt and water restriction and loop diuretics.
  - Calcium channel blockers/angiotensin-converting enzyme (ACE) inhibitors may be used in cases of severe HTN (4)[A].
- Patients with evidence of persistent bacterial infection should be given a course of antibiotic therapy.

SURGERY/OTHER PROCEDURES
Acute dialysis is required in approximately 50% of elderly patients (1).

ADMISSION, INPATIENT, AND NURSING CONSIDERATIONS
Admission and inpatient observation may be necessary, specifically for elderly patients who are at greater risk for complications such as new-onset or exacerbation of preexisting HF (1).

 ONGOING CARE

FOLLOW-UP RECOMMENDATIONS
Patient Monitoring
- Repeat urinalysis to check for clearance of hematuria and/or proteinuria.
- Consider other diagnosis if no improvement within 2 weeks.
- Recurrence is rare.

DIET
Renal diet if requiring instances of dialysis

PROGNOSIS
- Most children with PIGN have an excellent outcome, with >90% of cases achieving full recovery of renal function.
- Elderly patients, especially adults, develop HTN, recurrent proteinuria, and renal insufficiency long after the initial illness. Adults with multiple comorbid factors have the worst prognosis and highest incidence of chronic renal injury following PIGN (1).
- Complete remission in adult PIGN is only 26–56%. This has declined since the 1990s, suggesting prognosis is worsening (5).
- The presence of diabetes, higher creatinine levels, and more severe glomerular disease (e.g., crescents) on biopsy are all risk factors for developing end-stage renal disease (1).

REFERENCES
1. Nasr SH, Radhakrishnan J, D'Agati VD. Bacterial infection-related glomerulonephritis in adults. *Kidney Int*. 2013;83(5):792–803.
2. Nadasdy T, Hebert LA. Infection-related glomerulonephritis: understanding mechanisms. *Semin Nephrol*. 2011;31(4):369–375.
3. Uchida T, Oda T, Watanabe A, et al. Clinical and histologic resolution of poststreptococcal glomerulonephritis with large subendothelial deposits and kidney failure. *Am J Kidney Dis*. 2011;58(1):113–117.
4. Ramdani B, Zamd M, Hachim K, et al. Acute postinfectious glomerulonephritis. *Nephrol Ther*. 2012;8(4):247–258.
5. Wen YK. Clinicopathological study of infection-associated glomerulonephritis in adults. *Int Urol Nephrol*. 2010;42(2):477–485.

ADDITIONAL READING
- Eison TM, Ault BH, Jones DP, et al. Post-streptococcal acute glomerulonephritis in children: clinical features and pathogenesis. *Pediatr Nephrol*. 2011;26(2):165–180.
- Glassock RJ, Alvarado A, Prosek J, et al. Staphylococcus-related glomerulonephritis and poststreptococcal glomerulonephritis: why defining "post" is important in understanding and treating infection-related glomerulonephritis. *Am J Kidney Dis*. 2015;65(6):826–832.
- Nasr SH, Fidler ME, Valeri AM, et al. Postinfectious glomerulonephritis in the elderly. *J Am Soc Nephrol*. 2011;22(1):187–195.
- Nast CC. Infection-related glomerulonephritis: changing demographics and outcomes. *Adv Chronic Kidney Dis*. 2012;19(2):68–75.
- Rodriguez-Iturbe B, Musser JM. The current state of poststreptococcal glomerulonephritis. *J Am Soc Nephrol*. 2008;19(10):1855–1864.
- Singh GR. Glomerulonephritis and managing the risks of chronic renal disease. *Pediatr Clin North Am*. 2009;56(6):1363–1382.

CODES

ICD10
- N05.9 Unsp nephritic syndrome with unspecified morphologic changes
- N00.9 Acute nephritic syndrome with unsp morphologic changes

CLINICAL PEARLS
- PIGN is an immune complex disease occurring after infection with certain strains of bacteria, most commonly group A *Streptococcus pyogenes*.
- The clinical presentation varies from asymptomatic to the acute nephritic syndrome, characterized by gross hematuria, proteinuria, edema, HTN, and acute kidney injury.
- Treatment is primarily supportive and includes treating HTN and edema, along with antibiotics for any ongoing bacterial infection.
- Persistent nephritis and low C3 levels for >2 weeks should prompt evaluation for other causes of GN, such as MPGN or systemic lupus erythematosus nephritis.

GLUCOSE INTOLERANCE

Mariya Milko, DO, MS

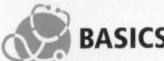 **BASICS**

DESCRIPTION
- Glucose intolerance is an intermediate stage between a normal glucose metabolism and diabetes.
- Individuals with impaired fasting glucose (IFG) and/or impaired glucose intolerance (IGT) have been referred to as having prediabetes:
  - IFG: 100 to 125 mg/dL
  - IGT: 140 to 199 mg/dL 2 hours after ingestion of 75 g oral glucose load
  - Hemoglobin A1c (HbA1c) 5.7–6.4% (1)

EPIDEMIOLOGY
- As of 2010, it is estimated that one of every three U.S. adults ≥20 years of age have prediabetes (2).
- An estimated 86 million people in the United States are living with prediabetes.
- Only 11% of people with prediabetes are aware of their condition (3).
- Prediabetes has a 37% prevalence among adults >20 years old and 51% of adults ≥65 years in the United States (4).

Incidence
- Systematic review indicates a 5-year cumulative incidence of developing diabetes of 9–25% for people with an HbA1c of 5.5–6.0% and 25–50% with an HbA1c of 6.0–6.5% (1).
- Highest incidence in American Indians/Alaska Natives, non-Hispanic blacks, and Hispanics (2)

ETIOLOGY AND PATHOPHYSIOLOGY
Progressive loss of insulin secretion on the background of insulin resistance (1)

RISK FACTORS
- Body mass index (BMI) ≥25: overweight
- Obesity and metabolic syndrome
- History of gestational diabetes mellitus (GDM)
- Sedentary lifestyle
- Medications (see "Differential Diagnosis")
- Genetic factors. Variants in 11 genes have been shown to be significantly associated with future development of type 2 diabetes and IFG. Variants in 8 of these genes have been associated with impaired β-cell function.

GENERAL PREVENTION
- Lifestyle modification with weight reduction and increased physical activity
- A decrease in excess body fat provides the greatest risk reduction.

Pregnancy Considerations
- Screening for diabetes in pregnancy is based on risk factor analysis:
  - High risk: first prenatal visit
  - Average risk: 24 to 28 weeks' gestation
- Women with GDM should be screened for diabetes 6 to 12 weeks' postpartum with 75-g OGTT and then every 1 to 3 years via any method (5).

COMMONLY ASSOCIATED CONDITIONS
- Obesity (abdominal and visceral obesity)
- Dyslipidemia with high triglycerides (TG)
- Metabolic syndrome
- PCOS
- GDM
- Low HDL
- HTN
- Congenital diseases (Down, Turner, Klinefelter, and Wolfram syndromes)

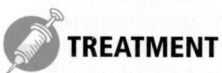 **DIAGNOSIS**

Who to screen
- BMI ≥25 or ≥23 for Asian Americans (1)[B]
- Age ≥45 years (1)[B]
- First-degree relative with diabetes
- High TG >250 mg/dL
- Low HDL <35 mg/dL
- HTN: BP >140/90 mm Hg or on treatment
- History of GDM
- Physical inactivity
- History of cardiovascular disease
- Ethnic group at increased risk (non-Hispanic black, Native American, Hispanics, Asian American, Pacific Islander)
- HbA1c ≥5.7%, IGT, or IFG on previous testing
- PCOS
- Conditions associated with insulin resistance such as severe obesity or acanthosis nigricans

HISTORY
- No clear symptoms
- Polyuria
- Polydipsia
- Weight loss
- Blurred vision
- Polyphagia

PHYSICAL EXAM
- General physical exam
- BMI assessment

DIFFERENTIAL DIAGNOSIS
- Type A insulin resistance
- Leprechaunism
- Rabson-Mendenhall syndrome
- Lipoatrophic diabetes
- Pancreatitis
- Cystic fibrosis
- Hemochromatosis
- Acromegaly
- Cushing syndrome
- Glucagonoma

- Pheochromocytoma
- Hyperthyroidism
- Somatostatinoma
- Aldosteronoma
- Drug-induced hyperglycemia
  - Thiazide diuretics (high doses)
  - β-Blockers
  - Corticosteroids (including inhaled corticosteroids)
  - Thyroid hormone
  - α-Interferon
  - Pentamidine
  - Protease inhibitors
  - Atypical antipsychotics
  - Selective serotonin reuptake inhibitors

DIAGNOSTIC TESTS & INTERPRETATION
Initial Tests (lab, imaging)
- Fasting glucose, 2-hour OGTT, or HbA1c is equally appropriate (1)[B].
- Repeat screen at 3-year intervals with normal results, sooner depending on risk status, and yearly in patients with prediabetes (1)[C].

Follow-Up Tests & Special Considerations
- Fasting lipid profile
- Creatinine and GFR
- Urinalysis
- Microalbumin-to-creatinine ratio
- Thyroid-stimulating hormone with free T_4
- Periodic measurement of vitamin B_{12} levels for patients on long-term metformin therapy especially those with anemia or peripheral neuropathy

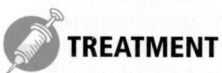 **TREATMENT**

- Therapeutic lifestyle modification to include physical activity focused on weight loss and medical nutrition therapy (preferably via a registered dietitian)
- Mediterranean diet and diets high in fiber-rich foods such as vegetables, fruits, whole grains, seeds, and nuts plus white meat sources are protective against type 2 diabetes (6).
- Patients with prediabetes should be referred to an intensive diet and physical activity behavioral counseling program adhering to the tenets of the Diabetes Prevention Program targeting a loss of 7% of body weight and should increase their moderate-intensity physical activity (such as brisk walking to at least 150 min/week) (6)[A].
- Resistance training and endurance exercise both reduce diabetes risk.
- Interrupt prolonged sitting every 30 minutes with short bouts of physical activity (6)[B].
- Follow-up counseling (6)[B]

- Diabetes prevention programs are cost-effective and should be covered by third-party payers (6)[B].
- Screening and treating for modifiable risk factors for cardiovascular disease is suggested (6)[B].
- Diabetes self-management education and support systems are appropriate venues for people with prediabetes to receive education and support to develop and maintain behaviors that can prevent or delay the onset of diabetes (6)[B].
- Technology-assisted tools including internet-based social networks, distance learning, DVD-based content, and mobile applications can be useful elements of effective lifestyle modification to prevent diabetes (6)[B].

MEDICATION

Consider metformin therapy for prevention of type 2 diabetes, especially in those with BMI >35, those aged <60 years, and women with prior GDM and/or rising HbA1c despite lifestyle intervention (6)[A].

First Line

Metformin (drug of choice): started at 500 mg BID or 500 mg XR. Observational data suggest it can be used safely down to GFR of 30 to 45 but may require dose adjustments.

Second Line

Acarbose: started at 50 mg PO once daily and titrated to 100 mg PO TID; GI upset is common.

ISSUES FOR REFERRAL

- Nutritionist
- Diabetes educator/registered dietitian upon diagnosis
- Exercise physiologist
- Lifestyle coaching

ADDITIONAL THERAPIES

Alternative/botanical therapy:

- Although studies lack large sample size and ideal design, there is some evidence that fenugreek, bitter melon, and cinnamon can reduce hyperglycemia and improve insulin sensitivity (7).

 ONGOING CARE

FOLLOW-UP RECOMMENDATIONS

Patient Monitoring

- At least annual monitoring for development of diabetes with HbA1c, 2-hour OGTT, or fasting glucose
- BP should be routinely measured.
- Annual testing for lipid abnormalities and microalbuminuria (for detection and therapy modification of incipient diabetic nephropathy)
- Monitoring of BMI

DIET

- Mediterranean diet has been shown to be beneficial. One small cohort study showed that the addition of about 10 g of extra virgin olive oil to meals improved postprandial glucose by reducing DPP4 activity and increasing insulin and GLP-1. It also showed a significant decrease in TG and apolipoprotein B-48.
- Limit high glycemic carbohydrates and sucrose-containing foods.
- Diets high in fiber, vegetables, nuts, seeds, and whole grains

PROGNOSIS

- Individuals with IFG and/or IGT have high risk for the future development of diabetes.
- Prediabetes increases the risk of developing type 2 diabetes, heart disease, and stroke.
- 20–70% of individuals with prediabetes who do not lose weight, change their dietary habits, and/or engage in moderate physical activity will progress to type 2 diabetes within 3 to 6 years.
- Lifestyle intervention reduced 3-year diabetes incidence by 58% compared to 31% with metformin.

COMPLICATIONS

- Cardiovascular disease
- Peripheral artery disease
- Stroke: 2 to 4 times higher risk
- Ketoacidosis
- Sexual dysfunction
- Gastroparesis
- Nephropathy and potential for renal failure
- Retinopathy and potential for loss of vision
- Peripheral and autonomic neuropathy

REFERENCES

1. American Diabetes Association. 2. Classification and diagnosis of diabetes. *Diabetes Care*. 2017;40(Suppl 1):S11–S24.
2. Centers for Disease Control and Prevention. *National Diabetes Statistics Report, 2014: Estimates of Diabetes and Its Burden in the United States*. Atlanta, GA: U.S. Department of Health and Human Services; 2014.
3. Centers for Disease Control and Prevention. Awareness of prediabetes—United States, 2005–2010. *MMWR Morb Mortal Wkly Rep*. 2013;62(11):209–212.
4. Centers for Disease Control and Prevention. Prediabetes. http://www.cdc.gov/diabetes/basics/prediabetes.html. Accessed January 18, 2017.
5. American Diabetes Association. 13. Management of diabetes in pregnancy. *Diabetes Care*. 2017;40(Suppl 1):S114–S119.
6. American Diabetes Association. 5. Prevention or delay of type 2 diabetes. *Diabetes Care*. 2017;40(Suppl 1):S44–S47.
7. Deng R. A review of the hypoglycemic effects of five commonly used herbal food supplements. *Recent Pat Food Nutr Agric*. 2012;4(1):50–60.

ADDITIONAL READING

- Carnevale R, Loffredo L, Del Ben M, et al. Extra virgin olive oil improves post-prandial glycemic and lipid profile in patients with impaired fasting glucose. *Clin Nutr*. 2017;36(3):782–787.
- Knowler WC, Fowler SE, Hamman RF, et al; for Diabetes Prevention Program Research Group. 10-year follow-up of diabetes incidence and weight loss in the Diabetes Prevention Program Outcomes Study. *Lancet*. 2009;374(9702):1677–1686.
- Maruthur NM, Ma Y, Delahanty LM, et al; for Diabetes Prevention Program Research Group. Early response to preventive strategies in the Diabetes Prevention Program. *J Gen Intern Med*. 2013;28(12):1629–1636.
- Stull AJ. Lifestyle approaches and glucose intolerance. *Am J Lifestyle Med*. 2016;10(6):406–416.

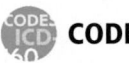 CODES

ICD10

- E74.39 Other disorders of intestinal carbohydrate absorption
- R73.09 Other abnormal glucose
- R73.01 Impaired fasting glucose

CLINICAL PEARLS

- Lifestyle optimization is essential for all patients with prediabetes.
- Research shows that you can lower your risk for type 2 diabetes by 58% by losing 7% of your body weight (or 15 lb if you weigh 200 lb).
- Recommend exercising moderately (such as brisk walking) 30 min/day, 5 days a week.
- Consider concurrent cardiovascular risks and further workup as indicated clinically.
- Patient education and lifestyle reinforcement should be emphasized in all clinical encounters.

G

GONOCOCCAL INFECTIONS

Melissa Jefferis, MD, FAAFP

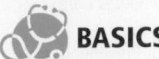 **BASICS**

DESCRIPTION

A sexually or vertically transmitted bacterial infection caused by *Neisseria gonorrhoeae*:

- *N. gonorrhoeae* is a fastidious gram-negative intracellular diplococcus (1)[A].
- Present as conjunctival, pharyngeal, urogenital, or anorectal infections. Urogenital infections are the most common (1)[A].
- Hematogenous dissemination leads to fever, cutaneous lesions, arthralgias, purulent or sterile arthritis, tenosynovitis, endocarditis, or (rarely) meningitis (1)[A].
- Asymptomatic carrier states occur in both sexes.
- In newborns, gonococcal ophthalmia neonatorum, a purulent conjunctivitis, may occur after vaginal delivery by an infected mother, potentially leading to blindness if not treated promptly (1,2)[A].
- System(s) affected: cardiovascular, musculoskeletal, nervous, reproductive, skin/exocrine
- Synonym(s): gonococcal infection; clap

EPIDEMIOLOGY

- Predominant age: 15- to 44-year-olds account for 92% of cases; highest rate among those ages 20 to 24 years
- Predominant sex: women 203/100,000; men 142/100,000

Incidence

Centers for Disease Control and Prevention (CDC) 2017: 555,608 reported cases

Prevalence

Incidence and prevalence are roughly equal. The true prevalence is higher due to asymptomatic cases (2)[A]:

- Rates peaked in mid-1970s and fell 74% over the next 20 years with national control program. Rates have been slowly increasing since 2012 (2)[A].
- Rates in men now higher than women (2)[A]

ETIOLOGY AND PATHOPHYSIOLOGY

Infection requires four steps: (i) mucosal attachment—bacterial proteins bind to receptors on host cells, (ii) local penetration/invasion, (iii) local proliferation, (iv) inflammatory response or dissemination. *N. gonorrhoeae* spreads most commonly through sexual relations.

Genetics

Deficiency of late components of complement cascade (C7–C9) makes individuals prone to develop dissemination of local gonococcal infections.

RISK FACTORS

- History of previous gonorrhea infection or other STIs
- Sexual exposure to an infected individual without appropriate use of barrier protection (condom)
- New/multiple sexual partners
- Inconsistent condom use
- Commercial sex work or drug use
- Infants: infected mother
- Children: sexual abuse by infected individual
- Autoinoculation (finger to eye)

GENERAL PREVENTION

- Condoms offer partial protection and must be used appropriately during oral, anal, and vaginal sex.
- Treat sexual contacts; consider expedited partner therapy (EPT) (2)[A].

COMMONLY ASSOCIATED CONDITIONS

Other STIs: *Chlamydia*, syphilis, HIV, hepatitis B, herpes (2,3)[A]

 DIAGNOSIS

HISTORY

- Sexual history
  - Number of partners; age of onset of sexual activity; STI history
  - New/recent change in sexual partners
  - Contact with commercial sex workers
  - Condom use
  - Menses and possibility of pregnancy
- 10% of men and 20–40% of women are asymptomatic (2)[A].
- If symptomatic, explore the onset, context, duration, timing, severity, and associated symptoms:
  - Symptoms (when present) typically appear within 1 to 14 days after exposure (1)[A].
- Ocular symptoms: discharge, itch, redness (1)[A]
- Pharyngeal symptoms: asymptomatic infection (98%), sore throat (1)[A]
- GI symptoms: acute diarrhea (1)[A]
- Urinary symptoms: frequency, urgency, dysuria (1)[A]
- Urethral symptoms: discharge (1,2)[A]
  - Males: scant to copious purulent urethral discharge (82%), dysuria (53%), asymptomatic (10%), testicular pain (1%), proctitis
  - Females: endocervical discharge (96%), asymptomatic cervical infection (20%), vaginal discharge, Bartholin gland swelling, dysmenorrhea, menometrorrhagia, abdominal pain/tenderness, dyspareunia, cervical motion tenderness, rebound, infertility, chronic pelvic pain
- Either sex, with receptive anal intercourse: rectal discharge, tenesmus, rectal burning; can also be asymptomatic
- Disseminated syndromes (1,2)[A]
  - Fever, chills, malaise, skin rash, arthralgia/arthritis
  - Endocarditis: high fevers
  - Meningitis: meningeal signs, headache, skin lesions, fever, altered mental status

PHYSICAL EXAM

- General: fever, chills (1)[A]
- Ocular: purulent discharge, conjunctivitis, chemosis, eyelid edema, corneal ulceration (1)[A]
- Pharynx: exudative pharyngitis (<1%) (1)[A]
- GI: acute diarrhea, hyperactive bowel sounds (1)[A]
- Genitourinary (GU) (1)[A]
  - Males: urethral discharge, testicular tenderness
  - Females: endocervical discharge, Bartholin gland abscess, abdominal pain/tenderness, cervical motion tenderness, rebound tenderness
- Either sex, for receptive anal intercourse: rectal discharge; rectal exam may be normal (1)[A].

- Disseminated syndromes (1)[A]:
  - Fever, chills, malaise, tenosynovitis, maculopapular–pustular rash, polyarthralgia—typically large joints (knee, wrist, ankle), purulent arthritis
  - Endocarditis: rapid cardiac valve destruction, heart murmurs, high fevers
  - Meningitis: meningeal signs, headache, skin lesions, fever, altered mental status

DIFFERENTIAL DIAGNOSIS

Chlamydia trachomatis, UTIs, other vaginitis, or urethritis (bacterial, viral, or parasitic)

DIAGNOSTIC TESTS & INTERPRETATION

Initial Tests (lab, imaging)

- Nucleic acid amplification test (NAAT) is the most sensitive and specific test for *N. gonorrhoeae* (2)[A]. Other options:
  - Genital culture
  - Add pharyngeal culture in adolescents.
  - Gram stain (recommended for urethritis)
  - Urethral smear, sensitivity in symptomatic male: ≥95%; sensitivity of endocervical smear in infected woman: 40–60%; specificity: 100%
- DNA probes and polymerase chain reaction (PCR) sensitivity: 92–99% dependent on population; specificity: >97%; can replace culture
- Blood culture is 50% sensitive in disseminated disease. Joint fluid culture is 50% sensitive in septic arthritis. Screen for additional STIs, especially chlamydia, syphilis, and HIV.
- Imaging is not generally recommended.

Follow-Up Tests & Special Considerations

- Test of cure not generally recommended (1,2)[A]
- Individuals treated for pharyngeal gonorrhea with an alternative regimen should have test of cure 14 days after treatment with NAAT or culture (2)[A].
- Consider follow-up testing in cases of recurrent infection, when oral cephalosporin treatment is used, and/or in areas with high antibiotic resistance (2)[A].
- Pelvic ultrasound or CT scan may demonstrate thick, dilated fallopian tubes or abscess formation.

Diagnostic Procedures/Other

Culdocentesis may demonstrate free purulent exudate and provide material for Gram staining and culture. Gram staining material from unroofed skin lesions may show typical organisms.

Test Interpretation

- Gram-negative intracellular diplococci
- Nonpathologic gram-negative diplococci may be found in extragenital locations. For this reason, Gram stain of pharyngeal or rectal swabs is not recommended.

 TREATMENT

GENERAL MEASURES

- STI counseling and condom use
- In children and adolescents, suspect sexual abuse.

MEDICATION

- *N. gonorrhoeae* multidrug antimicrobial resistance continues to increase. *CDC recommends dual therapy* (treat for chlamydia and drug-resistant strains) (2,3)[A].
- Quinolones are not recommended (2,4)[A].
- *If treatment fails, check culture and sensitivities and report to CDC through local health authorities* (2,3)[A].
- Treat with regimen that is also effective against uncomplicated genital chlamydial infection (2,3,4)[A].

First Line

- Uncomplicated urogenital, anorectal, and pharyngeal gonorrheal infection (2)[A]
  - Ceftriaxone 250 mg IM in a single dose *PLUS* azithromycin 1 g PO single dose; ideally administered together on the same day, preferably under direct observation
  - Azithromycin is the preferred second drug over doxycycline due to ease of administration and increased resistance to tetracycline.
  - Alternative: cefixime 400 mg PO once PLUS azithromycin 1 g PO once
- Pharyngitis: ceftriaxone 250 mg IM once PLUS treatment for chlamydia (azithromycin 1 g PO once) (1,2)[A]
- Conjunctivitis: ceftriaxone, 1 g IM single dose PLUS azithromycin 1 g PO once (1,2)[A]
- Arthritis and arthritis–dermatitis syndrome (1,2)[A]
  - Ceftriaxone 1 g IM or IV q24h until 24 to 48 hours after improvement begins to complete at least 1 week of antibiotic treatment, PLUS azithromycin 1 g PO once
  - Alternative regimens:
    - Cefotaxime 1 g IV every 8 hours until 24 to 48 hours after improvement begins to complete at least 1 week of antibiotic treatment, PLUS azithromycin 1 g PO once
    - Ceftizoxime 1 g IV every 8 hours until 24 to 48 hours after improvement begins to complete at least 1 week of antibiotic treatment, PLUS azithromycin 1 g PO once
- Meningitis and endocarditis (1,2)[A]
  - Ceftriaxone 1 to 2 g IV q12h 10 to 14 days for meningitis; 4 weeks for endocarditis PLUS azithromycin 1 g PO once
- Contraindications: Doxycycline is contraindicated in pregnancy and young children.

Pediatric Considerations

- Children >45 kg: same dosing as adults (1,2)[A]
- Children <45 kg: uncomplicated urethral, cervical, rectal, or pharyngeal gonococcal infections (1,2)[A]
  - Ceftriaxone 125 mg IM in single dose
  - Disseminated infections: ceftriaxone 50 mg/kg IV or IM daily (max dose 1 g) in single dose; bacteremia: 7 days; meningitis: 10 to 14 days; endocarditis: 4 weeks
- Ophthalmic neonatorum prophylaxis: single application of erythromycin 0.5% ophthalmic ointment to each eye immediately after delivery (1,2)[A]
- Neonatal conjunctivitis: ceftriaxone 25 to 50 mg/kg IV or IM in a single dose (not to exceed 125 mg) (1,2)[A]
- *Conjunctival exudates should be cultured for definitive diagnosis* (1,2)[A].

- Scalp abscesses (from scalp electrodes) (1,2)[A]
  - Ceftriaxone 25 to 50 mg/kg/day IV or IM in a single daily dose for 7 days. Treat for a duration of 10 to 14 days if meningitis is documented.
- Asymptomatic infants born to mothers with untreated gonorrhea (1,2)[A]
  - Ceftriaxone 25 to 50 mg/kg IV or IM, not to exceed 125 mg in a single dose

Pregnancy Considerations

- Pregnant women should be treated with dual therapy including ceftriaxone 250 mg IM once AND azithromycin 1 g PO once (2)[A].
- Alternative: gentamicin 240 mg IM once PLUS azithromycin 2 g PO once (5)[A]
- Another alternative includes treatment with spectinomycin. If spectinomycin or other regimens are not possible, consultation with an infectious disease specialist is recommended (2)[A].
- Test of cure generally not recommended if uncomplicated urogenital or rectal infections are treated with recommended/alternative regimens

Second Line

- Due to antimicrobial resistance, combination therapy using two agents with different mechanisms of action improves treatment efficacy and decreases resistance to cephalosporins (1,2)[A].
- A single 2-g oral dose of azithromycin has been used in the past, although should be avoided due to the potential to develop macrolide resistance (2)[A].
- For additional treatment options, see CDC STD treatment guidelines: http://www.cdc.gov/std/tg2015/.

ADMISSION, INPATIENT, AND NURSING CONSIDERATIONS

- Hematogenously disseminated infection
- Pneumonia or eye infection in infants

 ## ONGOING CARE

FOLLOW-UP RECOMMENDATIONS

Patient Monitoring

- U.S. Preventive Services Task Force (USPSTF) (3)[A]
  - Screen all sexually active women 24 years of age and younger and in older women at increased risk for infection for chlamydia and gonorrhea: grade B recommendation.
  - Insufficient evidence to recommend for or against screening for chlamydia and gonorrhea in men: grade I recommendation
  - Report cases of gonorrhea to public health (3,4)[A].
- CDC (6)[A]
  - Screen annually for sexually active men who have sex with men (MSM) at sites of contact (urethra, rectum, pharynx), regardless of condom use. Increase screening to every 3 to 6 months if at increased risk.

PATIENT EDUCATION

- Counseling concerning risk reduction, condom use, future fertility, and full STI testing
- Encourage patient to notify partners (from past 60 days); consider EPT.

PROGNOSIS

Complete cure with return to normal function with adequate and timely treatment

COMPLICATIONS

- Infertility
- Urethral stricture
- Corneal scarring
- Destruction of joint articular surfaces
- Cardiac valvular damage

Pediatric Considerations

Vertical transmission is a significant risk among patients with gonococcal infection at the time of delivery (1,2)[A].

REFERENCES

1. Mayor MT, Roett MA, Uduhiri KA. Diagnosis and management of gonococcal infections. *Am Fam Physician*. 2012;86(10):931–938.
2. Centers for Disease Control and Prevention. 2015 sexually transmitted diseases treatment guidelines: gonococcal infections. https://www.cdc.gov/std/tg2015/gonorrhea.htm. Accessed December 12, 2018.
3. Centers for Disease Control and Prevention. Update to CDC's sexually transmitted diseases treatment guidelines, 2010: oral cephalosporins no longer a recommended treatment for gonococcal infections. *MMWR Morb Mortal Wkly Rep*. 2012;61(31):590–594.
4. U.S. Preventive Services Task Force. Final recommendation statement: chlamydia and gonorrhea: screening. http://www.uspreventiveservicestaskforce.org/Page/Document/UpdateSummaryFinal/chlamydia-and-gonorrhea-screening?ds=1&s=Gonorrhea. Accessed December 12, 2018.
5. Committee on Gynecologic Practice. ACOG Committee Opinion No. 645: dual therapy for gonococcal infections. *Obstet Gynecol*. 2015;126(5):e95–e99.
6. Centers for Disease Control and Prevention. 2015 sexually transmitted diseases treatment guidelines: screening recommendations and considerations referenced in treatment guidelines and original sources. https://www.cdc.gov/std/tg2015/screening-recommendations.htm#modalIdString_CDCTable_5. Accessed December 12, 2018.

 ## SEE ALSO

Chlamydia Infection (Sexually Transmitted); HIV/AIDS; Pelvic Inflammatory Disease; Syphilis

CODES

ICD10

- A54.9 Gonococcal infection, unspecified
- A54.03 Gonococcal cervicitis, unspecified
- A54.31 Gonococcal conjunctivitis

CLINICAL PEARLS

- Antibiotic resistance is a significant problem because many new gonorrheal infections are resistant.
- Treatment for uncomplicated gonorrhea should include two drugs, one of which is effective against chlamydia.
- Screen patients with gonorrhea for chlamydia, syphilis, HIV, and hepatitis.

G

GOUT

David A. Ross, MD, CAQSM

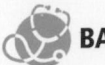

BASICS

DESCRIPTION

- Gout is an inflammatory arthritis related to a hyperuricemia (serum uric acid [SUA] level >6.8 mg/dL) (1)[C].
- Acute gouty arthritis can affect ≥1 joint; the 1st metatarsophalangeal joint is most commonly involved at presentation (podagra).
- Although hyperuricemia is necessary for the development of gout, it is not the only determining factor.
- Characterized by deposition of monosodium urate (MSU) crystals that accumulate in joints and soft tissues, resulting in acute and chronic arthritis, soft-tissue masses called tophi, urate nephropathy, and uric acid nephrolithiasis
- After an initial flare, a second flare occurs in ~60% of patients within 1 year and 78% within 2 years of the initial attack (2)[C].
- Management involves treating acute attacks and preventing recurrent disease by long-term reduction of SUA levels through pharmacology and lifestyle adjustments.

EPIDEMIOLOGY

Incidence
Annual incidence of gout (3):
- Uric acid 7.0 to 8.9 mg/dL is 0.5%.
- Uric acid >9 mg/dL is 4.5%.

Prevalence
- Increasing prevalence over the past decades (3)
- Overall prevalence of 3.9% (8.3 million) in the United States in 2008 (3):
  – Men 5.8% (6.1 million)
  – Women 2.0% (2.2 million)

ETIOLOGY AND PATHOPHYSIOLOGY

- Hyperuricemia results from urate overproduction, underexcretion, or often a combination of the two.
- Gout occurs when MSU, a product of purine metabolism, precipitates out of solution and accumulates in joints and soft tissues.
- Transient changes in urate solubility caused by local temperature decrease, trauma, or acidosis may lead to an acute gouty attack.
- Urate crystals that precipitate trigger an immune response.
- Left untreated, this crystal deposition leads to permanent joint damage and tophus formation.
- Obesity predisposes to gout by promoting insulin resistance, which in turn reduces renal urate excretion resulting in hyperuricemia (4)[A].
- Hypertension and renal disease reduce renal urate excretion due to glomerular arteriolar damage (4)[A].

Genetics
- Phosphoribosyl pyrophosphate (PRPP) deficiency and hypoxanthine guanine phosphoribosyltransferase (HGPRT) deficiency (Lesch-Nyhan syndrome) are inherited enzyme defects associated with overproduction of uric acid.
- Polymorphisms in the URAT1 and SLC2A9 (GLUT9) renal transporters are hereditary enzyme defects resulting in primary underexcretion of uric acid.

RISK FACTORS
- Age >40 years
- Male gender
- Increased purine uptake (meats and seafood)
- Alcohol intake (especially beer)
- Obesity (BMI >30)

- Heart disease and congestive heart failure
- Dyslipidemia
- Hypertension and renal disease
- Smoking
- Diabetes mellitus
- Diuretics raise SUA levels by increasing uric acid reabsorption and decreasing uric acid secretion in the kidneys (4)[A].
- Urate-elevating medications:
  – Thiazide diuretics: ethambutol
  – Loop diuretics (less of a risk vs. thiazides)
  – Niacin
  – Calcineurin inhibitors (cyclosporine and tacrolimus)

GENERAL PREVENTION
- Maintain optimal weight.
- Regular exercise
- Diet modification (purine-rich foods)
- Reduce alcohol consumption (beer and liquor).
- Smoking cessation
- Maintain fluid intake and avoid dehydration.

COMMONLY ASSOCIATED CONDITIONS
- Hypertension
- Dyslipidemia
- Nontraumatic joint disorders
- Heart disease
- Diabetes mellitus
- Metabolic syndrome
- Obesity (BMI >30)
- Renal disease

DIAGNOSIS

HISTORY
- Classic presentation of acute gouty arthritis:
  – Intense pain and tenderness in the 1st metatarsophalangeal joint (podagra)
  – Can occur in the midtarsal, ankle, or knee joints
  – Joint may be swollen, warm, and red.
  – Often awakes patients from sleep due to an intolerance to contact with clothing or bed sheets
  – There is a rapid onset of intense pain, often beginning in the early morning and progressing rapidly over 12 to 24 hours.
  – In the absence of treatment, flares can last up to 10 days.
- Fever can be present.
- Subcutaneous or intraosseous nodules, referred to as tophi, can be seen.
- Pain with urination secondary to uric acid renal stones

PHYSICAL EXAM
- Examine suspected joint(s) for tenderness, swelling, and range of motion (ROM).
- Assess for presence of firm nodules known as tophi.
- In patients with chronic gout, tophi can frequently be found in the helix of the ear, over the olecranon process, or on the Achilles tendon.
- Patients with untreated chronic gout can have evidence of joint inflammation and deformity.

DIFFERENTIAL DIAGNOSIS
Acute bursitis, tendonitis, septic arthritis, pseudogout (calcium pyrophosphate deposition disease), cellulitis, osteoarthritis

DIAGNOSTIC TESTS & INTERPRETATION
- SUA (may be normal during an acute flare)
- CBC (can see elevation of WBC during gout flare)

- Synovial fluid analysis: urate crystals (negatively birefringent under polarizing microscopy), cell count (WBC usually 2,000 to 5,000 cells/mm³); culture to rule out infection
- Screen for uric acid overproduction using 24-hour urinary uric acid in those patients with gout onset before the age of 25 years or with a history of urolithiasis (1)[C].
- Radiographs are normal early in disease but can reveal
  – Swelling in acute gout
  – Periarticular erosions with periosteum overgrowth in chronic gout
- Urate kidney stones are radiolucent and thus invisible on radiograph.
- Ultrasound evidence of urate deposition—hyperechoic enhancement over surface of hyaline cartilage
- Dual energy CT (DECT) imaging can show urate deposition at articular or periarticular sites.

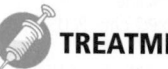

TREATMENT

GENERAL MEASURES
Topical ice as needed (5)[B]

MEDICATION
- Acute treatment
  – General principles:
    ○ Acute gouty arthritis attacks should be treated with pharmacologic therapy (5)[C].
    ○ Pharmacologic treatment should be initiated within 24 hours of acute gout attack (5)[C].
    ○ Ongoing pharmacologic urate-lowering therapy should not be interrupted during an acute gout attack (5)[C].
    ○ Choice of agent is based on severity of pain and the number of joints involved (5)[C].
  – Mild/moderate gout severity (≤6 of 10 on visual analog pain scale, particularly for an attack involving only one or a few small joints or one to two large joints)
    ○ NSAIDs:
      ▪ Naproxen (Naprosyn, Anaprox, Aleve): 750 mg followed by 250 mg q8h for 5 to 8 days (5)[C]
      ▪ Indomethacin (Indocin): 50 to 150 mg/day for 2 to 7 days (5)[C]
      ▪ Sulindac (Clinoril): 200 mg BID for 7 to 10 days (5)[C]
      ▪ Celecoxib (Celebrex)
        □ Not FDA-approved but can be considered in selected patients with contraindications or intolerance to NSAIDs (5)[C]
        □ Dose: 800 mg once, then 400 mg on day 1, and then 400 mg BID for 1 week (5)[C]
    ○ Corticosteroids
      ▪ Those with an acute flare involving one to two large joints can consider intra-articular corticosteroids; can consider using oral corticosteroids in combination
      ▪ Corticosteroids are useful in patients with acute gout flare who cannot tolerate NSAIDs or have contraindications to NSAIDs such as chronic kidney disease (CKD).
      ▪ For other acute flares, use oral corticosteroids:
        □ Prednisone (Sterapred): 0.5 mg/kg/day for 5 to 10 days followed by discontinuation or alternately 2 to 5 days at full dose followed by tapering for 7 to 10 days and then discontinuing (5)[C]
        □ Methylprednisolone (Medrol) dose pack (5)[C]

□ Triamcinolone acetonide (Trivaris): 60 mg IM single dose followed by oral corticosteroids (5)[C]
○ Colchicine (Colcrys)
- Used for gout attacks where the onset was <36 hours prior to treatment initiation (5)[C]
- Begin a loading dose of 1.2 mg followed by 0.6 mg 1 hour later, followed by 0.6 mg once or twice daily 12 hours later, until the gout attack resolves (5)[C].
- Dose reduction recommended in moderate to severe kidney disease and in those on inhibitors of cytochrome P450 3A4 and P-glycoprotein (clarithromycin, erythromycin, cyclosporine, and disulfiram) (5)[C]
- Severe gout (≥7 of 10 on visual analog pain scale, involving ≥4 joints with arthritis involving >1 region, or involving three separate large joints)
○ Initial combination therapy is an option and includes the use of full doses of the following (5)[C]:
- Colchicine and NSAIDs
- PO corticosteroids and colchicine
- Intra-articular steroids
- For patients not responding to initial pharmacologic monotherapy, add a second agent (5)[C].
• Chronic treatment
- Indications for pharmacologic urate-lowering therapy include any patient with
○ Tophus or tophi by clinical exam or imaging study (1)[C]
○ Frequent attacks of acute gouty arthritis (≥2 attacks per year) (1)[C]
○ CKD stage 2 or worse (1)[C]
○ Past urolithiasis (1)[C]
- Treat to the serum urate:
○ Minimum serum urate target is <6 mg/dL.
○ Serum urate target may need to be <5 mg/dL to improve gout signs and symptoms (1)[C].
- Urate-lowering agents can be prescribed during an acute attack provided that effective anti-inflammatory prophylaxis has been initiated prior to urate-lowering therapy (1)[C].
- Anti-inflammatory prophylaxis required when initiating urate-lowering therapy:
○ First line
- Low-dose colchicine: 0.6 mg once or twice daily (5)[C]
- Low-dose NSAIDs: naproxen 250 mg PO BID (5)[C]
○ Second line: if use of colchicine and NSAIDs both are not tolerated, contraindicated, or ineffective:
- Low-dose prednisone or prednisolone at ≤10 mg/day (5)[C]
○ Treatment duration for the greater of
- At least 6 months (5)[C] or
- 3 months after achieving serum urate appropriate for the patient with no tophi on exam (5)[C], or for 6 months after achieving serum urate appropriate for the patient with ≥1 tophi on exam (5)[C]
- Pharmacologic urate-lowering agents:
○ Allopurinol (Zyloprim): xanthine oxidase inhibitor (1)[C]
- Starting dose should be no higher than 100 mg/day (1)[C].
- Starting dose should be 50 mg/day in stage 4 CKD or worse.
- Gradually titrate the dose upward q2–5wk to appropriate maximum dose (1)[C].
- Dose can be >300 mg/day, even with renal impairment, as long as accompanied by patient education and monitoring of drug

toxicity; maximum FDA-approved dosage is 800 mg/day (1)[C].
- Regularly monitor for allopurinol hypersensitivity syndrome (AHS), pruritus, rash, elevated hepatic transaminases, and eosinophilia.
- Screening for the HLA-B*5801 allele for AHS should be performed in those of Korean descent with stage 3 CKD or worse and Chinese or Thai descent irrespective of renal function (1)[C].
○ Febuxostat: selective xanthine oxidase inhibitor (1)[C]
- No renal or hepatic adjustments needed for mild-to-moderate hepatic or renal disease
- Starting dose 40 mg/day; may be titrated to 80 mg/day
- In select instances, may dose up to 120 mg/day (not FDA-approved) (1)[C]
○ Probenecid: uricosuric agent (1)[C]
- Alternative first-line urate-lowering therapy; use if xanthine oxidase inhibitor is contraindicated or not tolerated (1)[C].
- May be used in addition to allopurinol or febuxostat if serum urate target not achieved (1)[C].
- Multiple drug interactions exist as well as risk of urolithiasis with this agent.
- Not recommended if creatinine clearance (CrCl) is <50 or with patient history of urolithiasis (1)[C]
- Starting dose is 250 mg BID; gradually titrate to 2,000 mg/day.
• Other treatment
- Losartan possesses uricosuric properties; therefore, it may be an excellent agent if patient is also hypertensive.
- Acute treatment: adrenocorticotropic hormone (ACTH): 25 to 40 IU SC (5)[C]
- Pegloticase in select severe instances

SURGERY/OTHER PROCEDURES
Large tophi that are infected or interfering with joint motion may need to be surgically removed.

 ONGOING CARE

FOLLOW-UP RECOMMENDATIONS
Patient Monitoring
• SUA q2–5wk while titrating urate-lowering treatment to goal (1)[C]
• Regularly monitor CBC, renal function, liver function test, and urinalysis.

DIET
• General lack of evidence regarding specific recommendations, although the American College of Rheumatology has outlined the following (1)[C]:
• General measures:
- Weight loss for obese patients
- Healthy overall diet and good hydration
- Smoking cessation
• Avoid
- Organ meats high in purine content (sweetbreads, liver, kidney) (1)[C]
- High-fructose corn syrup–sweetened sodas, other beverages, or foods
- Alcohol overuse (>2 servings per day for men and >1 serving per day for women) (1)[C]
- Alcohol use, especially during periods of frequent gout attacks or advanced gout under poor control
• Limit
- Beef, lamb, pork, and seafood with high purine content such as sardines and shellfish (1)[C]
- Servings of naturally sweetened fruit juices
- Sugar, sweetened beverages, and desserts

- Table salt, including in sauces and gravies
- Alcohol (particularly beer) in all patients (1)[C]
• Encourage
- Low-fat or nonfat dairy products
- Vegetables

PATIENT EDUCATION
• Dietary and lifestyle modifications (1)[C]
• Instructions on initiating treatment on signs and symptoms of an acute gout attack without the need to consult health care provider for each attack (1)[C]
• Discussion that gout is caused by excess uric acid and that effective urate-lowering therapy is essential treatment (1)[C]

PROGNOSIS
Gout can usually be successfully managed with proper treatment.

COMPLICATIONS
• Increased susceptibility to infection
• AHS
• Urate nephropathy and renal stones

REFERENCES
1. Khanna D, Fitzgerald JD, Khanna PP, et al; for American College of Rheumatology. 2012 American College of Rheumatology guidelines for management of gout. Part 1: systematic nonpharmacologic and pharmacologic therapeutic approaches to hyperuricemia. Arthritis Care Res (Hoboken). 2012;64(10):1431–1446.
2. Doghramji PP. Managing your patient with gout: a review of treatment options. Postgrad Med. 2011;123(3):56–71.
3. Zhu Y, Pandya BJ, Choi HK. Prevalence of gout and hyperuricemia in the US general population: the National Health and Nutrition Examination Survey 2007–2008. Arthritis Rheum. 2011;63(10):3136–3141.
4. Evans PL, Prior JA, Belcher J, et al. Obesity, hypertension and diuretic use as risk factors for incident gout: a systematic review and meta-analysis of cohort studies. Arthritis Res Ther. 2018;20(1):136.
5. Khanna D, Khanna PP, Fitzgerald JD, et al; for American College of Rheumatology. 2012 American College of Rheumatology guidelines for management of gout. Part 2: therapy and antiinflammatory prophylaxis of acute gouty arthritis. Arthritis Care Res (Hoboken). 2012;64(10):1447–1461.

ADDITIONAL READING
Neogi T, Jansen T, Dalbeth N, et al. 2015 Gout classification criteria: an American College of Rheumatology /European League Against Rheumatism collaborative initiative. Arthritis Rheumatol. 2015;67(10):2557–2568.

 CODES

ICD10
• M10.9 Gout, unspecified
• M10.00 Idiopathic gout, unspecified site
• M10.30 Gout due to renal impairment, unspecified site

CLINICAL PEARLS
• MSU crystals found in synovial fluid aspirate are pathognomonic for gout.
• Pharmacologic treatment should begin within 24 hours of acute gout flare.
• Asymptomatic hyperuricemia does not require treatment.

GRANULOMA ANNULARE

Stephen C. Sears, DO • Adam K. Saperstein, MD

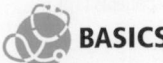 **BASICS**

DESCRIPTION
Granuloma annulare (GA) is a benign skin condition characterized by groups of skin-colored to erythematous papules that are usually in an annular (ring-like) pattern and typically located on the dorsal aspects of the hands and feet. There are five types of GA: localized, generalized, subcutaneous, patch, and perforating.

EPIDEMIOLOGY
Incidence
- GA is a relatively common, noninfectious granulomatous disease. Population-based studies to determine the incidence and/or prevalence of GA are lacking. A single study in 1980 demonstrated that 0.1–0.4% of new patients presenting to dermatologists have GA but did not report similar descriptive statistics in the primary care arena (1).
- Although most lesions resolve spontaneously within 2 years, some persist for 10 years or more.
- Predominant sex: female > male (1 to 2.5:1)
- Onset of symptoms occurs at <30 years old in 2/3 of all patients. Typical ages for onset of each subtype are:
  – Localized: <30 years old
  – Generalized: bimodal: <10 years old, 30 to 60 years old
  – Subcutaneous: 2 to 14 years old
  – Patch: >30 years old
  – Perforating: children and young adults
- Distribution of subtypes is as follows:
  – Localized: 75%
  – Generalized: 10–15%
  – Subcutaneous: <5%
  – Patch type: <5%
  – Perforating: <5%

ETIOLOGY AND PATHOPHYSIOLOGY
The etiology of GA remains unknown. It is hypothesized to be a dermatologic manifestation of a delayed-type hypersensitivity reaction to an unknown antigen in the dermis that is mediated by tumor necrosis factor alpha (TNF-α) and interleukin factors 1 and 2 (IL-1 and IL-2) (2). Characteristic histopathologic features include lymphohistiocytic infiltrates, degeneration of collagen, palisading or interstitial granulomatous inflammation, and mucin deposition.

Genetics
There is some evidence for a genetic predisposition. Two studies reported an increased frequency of HLA-Bw35 in patients with generalized GA. Of note, HLA-Bw35 has also been associated with thyroid disease (1).

RISK FACTORS
No definite risk factors have been identified. There are reported associations between GA and diabetes mellitus (DM), autoimmune thyroid disease, dyslipidemia, human immunodeficiency virus, Epstein-Barr virus, herpes simplex virus, systemic lupus erythematosus, tuberculosis, and hepatitis B and C, among others. There have also been associations with interferon-α therapy, trauma, sun exposure, insect bites, borreliosis, and malignancies (most commonly lymphoma) (2,3).

GENERAL PREVENTION
There are no known preventive measures for GA.

COMMONLY ASSOCIATED CONDITIONS
- DM: The association between GA and DM is controversial. Early studies from the 1980s showed a possible link, but recent case-controlled studies have shown no statistically significant association between GA and DM (3).
- Autoimmune thyroid disease: Multiple case reports have linked thyroid disease with both generalized and localized GA. In one case-control study, 24 women with localized GA were compared to 100 age-matched women with non-GA dermatologic disease. A statistically significant increase in the incidence of autoimmune thyroid disease among those with localized GA as compared with those with other non-GA cutaneous disease was identified (12% vs. 1%, $p = .022$) (2,3).
- Malignancy: There is no definitive relationship between GA and malignancy. A review of the literature found 14 case reports and two correlation studies in which patients who had one or more malignancies also had GA. In a majority of these cases, the malignancies were hematologic, primarily lymphoma (2,3).
- Dyslipidemia: Dyslipidemia may be associated with GA. A single case-control study ($n = 140$) demonstrated a statistically significant increase in hyperlipidemia among patients with GA compared to controls (79.3% vs. 51.9%, $p <.001$) (4).
- HIV: Among patients with GA, those who also have HIV appear more likely to have the generalized subtype. In one study of 34 patients with GA and HIV, 20 (59%) had generalized GA (2).
- Note: Conclusions regarding associations between GA and various diseases, including those listed above, are limited by both design and power. Consequently, in the absence of new research, definitive associations between GA and other diseases cannot be made.

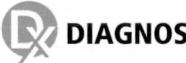 **DIAGNOSIS**

HISTORY
Cutaneous lesions of GA are generally asymptomatic. Lesions often persist for months or years, especially in patients who have generalized GA. In most cases, regardless of subtype, GA resolves spontaneously but may thereafter recur without obvious trigger.

PHYSICAL EXAM
- Localized: asymptomatic, flesh-colored or erythematous annular, or arciform plaque with a moderately firm, rope-like border and central clearing, ranging from 5 mm to 5 cm in diameter. Small 1- to 2-mm papules may be noted peripheral to the primary lesion. The most common locations are the dorsal aspects of the distal upper and lower extremities; involvement of palms is rare. It is common to have multiple lesions at the time of presentation.
- Generalized: Lesions have the same morphology as localized GA lesions but tend to be larger, greater in number (usually >10), persist for a longer period of time, and are more widespread.
- Subcutaneous: firm, nontender nodules that tend to grow rapidly; usually solitary but may occur in groups; most common location is scalp and/or anterior aspect of the lower extremities, followed by upper extremities and buttocks.
- Patch: erythematous macules and patches distributed symmetrically on the extremities and trunk. The typical annular configuration may or may not be present; often involves proximal extremities
- Perforating: Damaged collagen from dermis is extruded onto skin surface. Papules may be up to 4 mm in diameter and display yellowish umbilication, crusting, or scale. Lesions are often widely distributed on the body and cause scaring.

DIFFERENTIAL DIAGNOSIS
- Localized: tinea corporis, annular lichen planus, necrobiosis lipoidica, pityriasis rosea, erythema migrans, leprosy
- Generalized: sarcoidosis, lichen planus, cutaneous metastases, mycosis fungoides (cutaneous T-cell lymphoma)
- Patch type: erythema migrans
- Subcutaneous: rheumatoid nodules
- Perforating: molluscum contagiosum, sarcoidosis, insect bites

DIAGNOSTIC TESTS & INTERPRETATION
Initial Tests (lab, imaging)
- Diagnosis is typically established by history and physical examination; laboratory investigations are rarely needed. Microscopic evaluation of skin cells using potassium hydroxide (KOH) preparation may be useful to exclude a fungal process.
- Consider laboratory testing to evaluate comorbid dyslipidemia, DM, thyroid disease, HIV, hepatitis B/C, and malignancy as clinically indicated.

Diagnostic Procedures/Other
Punch biopsy and histologic evaluation may aid in confirming the diagnosis and identifying the subtype. Immunohistochemical streptavidin-biotin–horseradish peroxidase (HRP) analysis for CD68/KP-1 (a marker for histiocytic differentiation) may also aid in the diagnosis.

Test Interpretation

Dermal infiltrate demonstrating foci of degenerative collagen associated with palisading granulomas around an anuclear dermis with mucin deposition. Histologic variants include interstitial (histiocytic infiltrate between collagen fibers), classic (palisading dermal granulomas), and epithelioid (tuberculoid and sarcoidal granulomas).

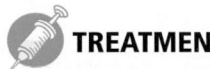 TREATMENT

GENERAL MEASURES

GA is a self-limited condition that is likely to regress spontaneously. The clinician's primary role after making the diagnosis is to educate the patient about the natural history of GA and to consider screening for conditions that may be associated with this disease.

MEDICATION

- Strength of recommendation for therapeutic interventions is B or C (3,5).
- The trauma induced by biopsy alone can cause involution of lesions through an unknown mechanism.
- Given the self-limited nature of the disease, it is incumbent on providers to assess the risk/benefit ratio of treatment. Reassurance is often all that is required for localized, asymptomatic disease.
- The following therapies have been tried with variable success (2,3,5,6). Duration of therapy is often undefined and is based on clinical response.

First Line

Corticosteroids

- High-potency topical (class I or II), with or without occlusion (3,5)[C]
- Intralesional triamcinolone: concentration of 2.5 to 5.0 mg/mL (3,5)[C]. Technique: Insert the needle into the dermis at the elevated border and slowly inject while withdrawing the needle, with enough volume to cause the lesion to begin to blanch.

Second Line

- Pimecrolimus cream: 1% BID (3)[C]
- Tacrolimus ointment: 0.1% BID (3)[C]
- Chloroquine: 250 mg/day (3)[C]
- Hydroxychloroquine: 9 mg/kg/day for 2 months, 6 mg/kg/day for month 3, 2 mg/kg/day for month 4 (3)[C]
- Doxycycline: 100 mg/day for 10 weeks (3)[C]
- Isotretinoin: 0.50 to 0.75 mg/kg/day (3)[C]
- Rifampin 600 mg, ofloxacin 400 mg, with minocycline 100 mg once daily (3)[C]
- Dapsone: 100 mg/day (3)[C]
- Cyclosporine: 3 to 4 mg/kg/day (3)[C]
- Methotrexate: 15 mg IM weekly (3)[C]
- Niacinamide: 500 mg TID (3)[C]
- Fumaric acid esters: variable dosing schemes (3)[C]

- Interferon gamma 1b: intralesional injection, 2.5 $\times$ 10^5 IU/lesion for 7 consecutive days followed by 3 times per week for 2 weeks (3)[C]
- TNF-α inhibitors, such as infliximab 5 mg/kg IV at weeks 0, 2, and 6, then variable or adalimumab 80 mg SC at week 0, and then 40 SC at week 1 and every other week, or etanercept 50 mg twice weekly (3)[C]

ADDITIONAL THERAPIES

- Cryotherapy (one 10- to 60-second freeze thaw cycle) (3)[B]
- Fractional thermolysis (e.g., YAG fractionated laser) (3)[C]
- 585- to 595-nm pulsed dye laser (3)[C]
- Narrowband ultraviolet B (NBUVB) (6)[C]
- Psoralen ultraviolet A (PUVA) (6)[C]
- Surgical excision (for subcutaneous GA) (2)[C]

 ONGOING CARE

FOLLOW-UP RECOMMENDATIONS

Routine follow-up is not required unless treatment is initiated. In such situations, follow-up is recommended to monitor for possible adverse effects of treatment. Referral to a dermatologist is prudent for patients who have generalized GA, cosmetic concerns, and for patients whose lesions persist despite conservative therapy.

PATIENT EDUCATION

Patients should be educated that GA is a benign, self-limited condition that may persist for months to years, spontaneously resolves, and spontaneously recurs. Additionally, patients may benefit from knowing that GA is not thought to be of an infectious etiology and is not transmissible to others.

PROGNOSIS

>50% of cases resolve spontaneously within 2 months to 2 years after onset, although recurrence, typically at the original site, is common (>40%). Patients <39 years tend to have a shorter duration of illness.

COMPLICATIONS

Complications of treatment are much more likely than complications from GA.

REFERENCES

1. Piette EW, Rosenbach M. Granuloma annulare: clinical and histologic variants, epidemiology, and genetics. *J Am Acad Dermatol*. 2016;75(3):457–465.
2. Piette EW, Rosenbach M. Granuloma annulare: pathogenesis, disease associations and triggers, and therapeutic options. *J Am Acad Dermatol*. 2016;75(3):467–479.
3. Keimig EL. Granuloma annulare. *Dermatol Clin*. 2015;33(3):315–329.
4. Wu W, Robinson-Bostom L, Kokkotou E, et al. Dyslipidemia in granuloma annulare: a case-control study. *Arch Dermatol*. 2012;148(10):1131–1136.
5. Cyr PR. Diagnosis and management of granuloma annulare. *Am Fam Physician*. 2006;74(10):1729–1734.
6. Cunningham L, Kirby B, Lally A, et al. The efficacy of PUVA and narrowband UVB phototherapy in the management of generalised granuloma annulare. *J Dermatolog Treat*. 2016;27(2):136–139.

ADDITIONAL READING

- De Paola MD, Batsikosta A, Feci L, et al. Granuloma annulare, autoimmune thyroiditis, and lichen sclerosus in a woman: randomness or significant association? *Case Rep Dermatol Med*. 2013;2013:289084.
- Duarte AF, Mota A, Pereira MA, et al. Generalized granuloma annulare—response to doxycycline. *J Eur Acad Dermatol Venereol*. 2009;23(1):84–85.
- Liu A, Hexsel CL, Moy RL, et al. Granuloma annulare successfully treated using fractional photothermolysis with a 1,550-nm erbium-doped yttrium aluminum garnet fractionated laser. *Dermatol Surg*. 2011;37(5):712–715.
- Plotner AN, Mutasim DF. Successful treatment of disseminated granuloma annulare with methotrexate. *Br J Dermatol*. 2010;163(5):1123–1124.
- Shanmuga SC, Rai R, Laila A, et al. Generalized granuloma annulare with tuberculoid granulomas: a rare histopathological variant. *Indian J Dermatol Venereol Leprol*. 2010;76(1):73–75.
- Werchau S, Enk A, Hartmann M. Generalized interstitial granuloma annulare—response to adalimumab. *Int J Dermatol*. 2010;49(4):457–460.

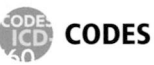 CODES

ICD10
L92.0 Granuloma annulare

CLINICAL PEARLS

- GA is benign, self-limited condition. Consider risk-to-benefit ratio when partnering with patients to determine treatment.
- When initiating therapy for localized GA, start with high-dose topical corticosteroids or intralesional corticosteroids followed by cryotherapy or other listed topical therapies. For widespread disease, consider initiating treatment with antimalarials or phototherapy (2,3)[C].
- Consider GA in the differential diagnosis of lesions that appear to be tinea, especially when these lesions lack scale and are KOH negative.
- Consider fasting lipid panel, fasting blood glucose or HbA1C, TSH, free T4, thyroid antibodies, hepatitis B and C panel, HIV screening test, and age-appropriate cancer screening, especially in those with generalized or atypical presentations of GA (3)[C].

G

GRANULOMA, PYOGENIC

Cameron S. Gilbert, MD

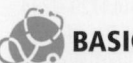 **BASICS**

DESCRIPTION

- Pyogenic granulomas (PG), also called lobular capillary hemangiomas, are benign vascular proliferations that can appear on the skin and mucus membranes. Most common sites are head and neck, the lips and oral cavity, the trunk, and the extremities (1,2).
- They are friable and tend to bleed profusely due to the vascular nature of the lesion.
- Smooth, red to purple, sessile or pedunculated, grow rapidly over several weeks
- Rarely regress completely without intervention (2)

EPIDEMIOLOGY

- The peak incidence of PG occurs in children and young adults (2).
- Commonly seen in early pregnancy

ETIOLOGY AND PATHOPHYSIOLOGY

- Definitive cause unknown
- Thought to be associated with capillary prolif-eration resulting from aberrant healing response to minor trauma
- Associated with peripheral nerve injury, inflam-matory systemic diseases, and drugs (retinoids, systemic steroids, protease inhibitors, epidermal growth factor receptor inhibitors)
- May be related to hormonal changes in pregnancy
- Not considered a hemangioma or neoplasm; no true granulomatous histology present

RISK FACTORS

- Pregnancy
- Trauma
- Intraoral trauma or surgery
- Inflammatory systemic diseases

GENERAL PREVENTION

Good oral hygiene may be helpful.

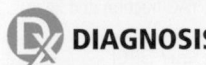 **DIAGNOSIS**

HISTORY

- Solitary lesion that develops rapidly from days to weeks after minor trauma
- Tends to bleed easily
- Grows early in pregnancy and partially regresses postpartum

PHYSICAL EXAM

- Most commonly located at the head, neck, and upper extremities, especially in children
- Among oral lesions, gingiva is the most common location.
- Usually a bright red, friable papule; can also be purple, yellow, or brown
- Moist and sometimes scaly-appearing surface
- Usually <1 cm but ranges from a few millimeters to 2 to 3 cm in diameter
- Giant lesions may occur on areas such as the foot (rare).
- Soft; pedunculated or sessile
- Solitary red papule, grows rapidly, forming a stalk, may bleed, and ulcerate

- On diascopy, red structureless areas surrounded by a white collarette intersected by white lines
- Erythematous, soft compressible papule with sero-sanguineous crusting and sharp demarcation

DIFFERENTIAL DIAGNOSIS

- Benign lesions
  - Cherry/infantile hemangioma (3)
  - Fibrous papule (1,3)
  - Bacillary angiomatosis, from by *Bartonella* (1)
- Malignant lesions
  - Basal cell carcinoma (1)
  - Squamous cell carcinoma (1)
  - Amelanotic melanoma (1)
  - Kaposi sarcoma (1)
  - Cutaneous metastases (1)

DIAGNOSTIC TESTS & INTERPRETATION

Initial Tests (lab, imaging)
No labs are necessary for the diagnosis.

Diagnostic Procedures/Other
- Excisional/shave biopsy
- Send for pathology.

Test Interpretation
Microscopic examination reveals

- Small, endothelial-lined vascular spaces
- Loose/dense connective tissue stroma
- Acute and chronic inflammatory cells
- No true granuloma formation
- Abundant mitotic activity
- Resembles granulation tissue in an edematous matrix, showing immature capillaries with interspersed tissue

TREATMENT

- Full thickness surgical excision is best to yield material for histopathologic analysis and avoid recurrence (4)[A]. Excision must be adequate to avoid recurrence. Even a small fragment of tissue left behind may lead to recurrence.
- CO_2 laser ablation results in less pain and allows for superficial dermal ablation (4)[A].
- Shave biopsy can be used for pedunculated lesions; can combine with cautery (5)[B]
- Punch biopsy acceptable for small lesions
- Electrosurgery: electrodesiccation and curettage (5)[B]

SURGERY/OTHER PROCEDURES
- Cryotherapy with liquid nitrogen (recur 2%) (5)[B]
- Pulsed dye laser or CO_2 laser (5)[B]
- Topical imiquimod (5)[B]
- Silver nitrate (5)[A]
- Topical 1.5% phenol solution may be used for periungual lesion (5)[B].
- Recurrence rate of up to 15% depending on treatment modality used

 ONGOING CARE

PATIENT EDUCATION
Patient should avoid trauma to area following excision.

PROGNOSIS
- Some lesions spontaneously resolve on their own (usually within 6 months).
- With treatment, recurrence rates are between 4% and 5% (2).

COMPLICATIONS
Recurrence: After removal or destruction of solitary lesion, multiple satellite lesions can form around original treatment site.

REFERENCES

1. Lin RL, Janniger CK. Pyogenic granuloma. *Cutis.* 2004;74(4):229–233.
2. Borden A, Harrington JW. Pyogenic granuloma: an overview of pathogenesis, diagnosis, and management. *Consultant.* 2018;58(6):e181.
3. Pagliai KA, Cohen BA. Pyogenic granuloma in children. *Pediatr Dermatol.* 2004;21(1):10–13.
4. Plachouri KM, Georgiou S. Therapeutic approaches to pyogenic granuloma: an updated review [published online ahead of print October 21, 2018]. *Int J Dermatol.* doi:10.1111/ijd.14268.
5. Lee J, Sinno H, Tahiri Y, et al. Treatment options for cutaneous pyogenic granulomas: a review. *J Plast Reconstr Aesthet Surg.* 2011;64(9):1216–1220.

ADDITIONAL READING

- Gilmore A, Kelsberg G, Safranek S. Clinical inquiries. What's the best treatment for pyogenic granuloma? *J Fam Pract.* 2010;59(1):40–42.
- Greene AK. Management of hemangiomas and other vascular tumors. *Clin Plast Surg.* 2011;38(1):45–63.
- Kroumpouzos G, Cohen LM. Dermatoses of pregnancy. *J Am Acad Dermatol.* 2001;45(1):1–19.

- Losa Iglesias ME, Becerro de Bengoa Vallejo R. Topical phenol as a conservative treatment for periungual pyogenic granuloma. *Dermatol Surg.* 2010;36(5):675–678.
- Piraccini BM, Bellavista S, Misciali C, et al. Periungual and subungual pyogenic granuloma. *Br J Dermatol.* 2010;163(5):941–953.
- Zalaudek I, Kreusch J, Giacomel J, et al. How to diagnose nonpigmented skin tumors: a review of vascular structures seen with dermoscopy: part II. Nonmelanocytic skin tumors. *J Am Acad Dermatol.* 2010;63(3):377–386.

 CODES

ICD10
- L98.0 Pyogenic granuloma
- K06.8 Oth disrd of gingiva and edentulous alveolar ridge
- K13.4 Granuloma and granuloma-like lesions of oral mucosa

CLINICAL PEARLS

- Benign, vascular tumor, usually rapidly growing, that involves exposed areas, such as distal extremities and face, as well as in the oral cavity
- Excision must be adequate to avoid recurrence.
- Excisional biopsy recommended to ensure proper diagnosis and rule out malignancy
- Excision with primary closure is superior to shave excision with cautery in terms of recurrence risk, but both are effective.

G

GRAVES DISEASE

Fozia Akhtar Ali, MD • Christina A. Majd, MD • Melida A. Juarez, MD

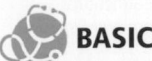

BASICS

DESCRIPTION
Autoimmune disease in which thyroid-stimulating antibodies cause increased thyroid function; most common cause of hyperthyroidism. Classic findings are goiter, ophthalmopathy (orbitopathy), and occasionally dermopathy (pretibial or localized myxedema).

EPIDEMIOLOGY
Prevalence
- Overall prevalence of hyperthyroidism in United States: ~2% for women and 0.2% for men
- More common in white and Hispanic populations in comparison to the black population
- Graves disease accounts for 60–80% of all cases of hyperthyroidism.
- Hyperthyroidism occurs in 0.2% of pregnancies, of which 95% is due to Graves disease.
- Predominant age: 30 to 40 years
- Synonym(s): Basedow disease

ETIOLOGY AND PATHOPHYSIOLOGY
- Excessive production of thyroid-stimulating hormone (TSH) receptor antibodies from B cells primarily within the thyroid, likely due to genetic clonal lack of suppressor T cells
- Binding of these antibodies to TSH receptors in the thyroid activates the receptor, stimulating thyroid hormone synthesis and secretion as well as thyroid growth (leading to goiter).
- Binding to similar antigen in retro-orbital connective tissue causes ocular symptoms.

Genetics
Higher risk with personal or family history of any autoimmune disease, especially Hashimoto thyroiditis

RISK FACTORS
- Female gender (5 to 10 times more than men)
- Postpartum period
- Family history (15% of patients with Graves disease have an affected relative)
- Medications: iodine, amiodarone, lithium, highly active antiretroviral (HAART); rarely, immune-modulating medications (e.g., interferon therapy)
- Smoking (higher risk of developing ophthalmopathy)

GENERAL PREVENTION
Screening TSH in asymptomatic patients is not recommended. No data conclusively show that treatment of subclinical thyroid dysfunction improves quality of life or clinical outcome measures.

COMMONLY ASSOCIATED CONDITIONS
- Mitral valve prolapse
- Type 1 diabetes mellitus
- Addison disease, hypokalemic periodic paralysis
- Vitiligo, alopecia areata
- Other autoimmune disorders (myasthenia gravis, celiac disease)

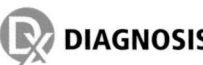

DIAGNOSIS

Hyperthyroid patients appear hypermetabolic with increased adrenergic tone.

HISTORY
- Tachycardia, palpitations
- Tremor, restlessness
- Hyperactivity, anxiety, emotional lability, insomnia
- Sweating, heat intolerance
- Pruritus, skin changes
- Weight loss with increased appetite
- Fatigue, dyspnea (due to muscle weakness)
- Oligo-/amenorrhea (women), loss of libido, erectile dysfunction (men), gynecomastia
- Loose, frequent stools
- Blurred vision or diplopia, lacrimation, photophobia, gritty sensation in eyes (ocular dryness), retro-orbital discomfort, painful eye movement, loss of color vision or visual acuity
- Worsening of chronic medical conditions (anxiety, bipolar disorder, glucose intolerance, heart failure, or angina)

Geriatric Considerations
Elderly patients may not display classic symptoms; may present with atrial fibrillation, weight loss, or shortness of breath

PHYSICAL EXAM
- Ophthalmologic (present in 50% of cases): Grittiness/discomfort in the eyes, retrobulbar pressure/pain, lid lag/retraction, proptosis, ophthalmoplegia, papilledema, and loss of color vision may signify optic neuropathy.
- Thyroid: enlarged (goiter), nontender, and without nodules; possible bruit (increased blood flow)
- Integumentary: fine hair, warm skin, onycholysis, palmar erythema, possible pretibial myxedema (orange peel appearance), possible hyperpigmented plaques (dermopathy)
- Cardiac: resting tachycardia, hyperdynamic circulation, possible atrial fibrillation
- Extremities: fine tremor, hyperreflexia, proximal myopathy; rarely, soft tissue edema of extremities and clubbing of digits (acropachy)

DIFFERENTIAL DIAGNOSIS
- Toxic multinodular goiter (multiple hormone-producing nodules)
- Toxic adenoma (single hormone-producing nodule)
- Thyroiditis (hormone leakage)
  - Subacute, usually postviral (Thyroid will be tender.)
  - Lymphocytic, including postpartum
  - Hashimoto thyroiditis (Antithyroperoxidase [TPO] antibodies may stimulate TSH receptors.)
- Iatrogenic (treatment induced)
  - Iodine induced (dietary, radiographic contrast, or medications)
  - Amiodarone
  - Thyroid hormone overreplacement (accidental or intentional)
- Tumor
  - Pituitary adenoma–producing TSH
  - Human chorionic gonadotropin (hCG)-producing tumors (stimulate TSH receptors)
  - Extraglandular thyroid hormone production (e.g., struma ovarii or metastatic thyroid cancer)

DIAGNOSTIC TESTS & INTERPRETATION
Initial Tests (lab, imaging)
- TSH is initial test: suppressed (low or undetectable)
- TSH <0.1 mU/L has >98% sensitivity and >92% specificity in confirming suspected thyroid disease.
- Elevated free T_4 with low TSH confirms hyperthyroidism.
- Thyroid peroxidase antibodies (present in 70–80% of patients with Graves disease) and TSH receptor antibodies (thyroid binding inhibitory immunoglobulin) may be useful in differentiating between Graves disease and toxic multinodular goiter.
- After confirming suppressed TSH and high T_4, perform radioactive iodine uptake (RAIU) and scan. Patients with Graves disease will have diffuse, elevated RAIU (vs. localized/nodular elevated uptake in adenoma and multinodular goiter and decreased uptake in thyroiditis or exogenous thyroid hormone).
- Thyroid ultrasound is not always required but may be used to distinguish nodular forms of Graves disease from nodular nonautoimmune causes of hyperthyroidism.

Pregnancy Considerations
- Increase in serum T_4-binding globulin concentration and initial stimulation of TSH by hCG results in a total T_4 and T3 rise during first half of pregnancy. The TSH level is decreased throughout pregnancy and should be compared to the trimester-specific ranges for pregnancy. Measurement of thyrotropin receptor autoantibody (TRAb) is positive in 95% of patients with Graves and should be used if diagnosis is unclear in pregnancy (1)[A].
- Ultrasonography is the primary modality of imaging during pregnancy.

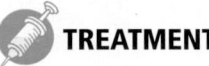

TREATMENT

MEDICATION
Goal is to correct hypermetabolic state with the fewest side effects and lowest incidence of posttreatment hypothyroidism.

First Line
- β-Blockers provide prompt control of adrenergic symptoms; start while workup is in progress (2)[A]. Long-acting propranolol is used most commonly and titrated to symptom control (40 to 160 mg/day).
- RAI
  - Concentrates in the thyroid gland and destroys thyroid tissue
  - Radioiodine plus prednisone therapy might have the least probability of leading to an exacerbation or new appearance of ophthalmopathy, and radioiodine therapy might have the least probability of causing a recurrence (3)[A].
  - Treatment of choice for definitive therapy of hyperthyroidism, in the absence of moderate or severe orbitopathy (1)[A]
  - High cure rate with single treatment, especially with high-dose regimen

– Risks: side effects (neck soreness, flushing, decreased taste); worsening ophthalmopathy (15% incidence, higher in smokers); posttreatment hypothyroidism (80% incidence, not dosage dependent); radiation thyroiditis (1% incidence); need to adhere to safety precautions until radiation is eliminated from the body

– Pretreatment with antithyroid medication should be considered in patients with severe disease and the elderly, to reduce risk of posttreatment transient hyperthyroidism and posttreatment radiation thyroiditis as well as quicker return to normal thyroid function.

– May be repeated in as soon as 3 months if minimal response or after 6 months if not euthyroid (2)[A]

Pregnancy Considerations
RAI is contraindicated in pregnancy and during breastfeeding.

• Antithyroid drugs: methimazole (MMI) and propylthiouracil (PTU)

– Compete with the thyroid for iodine, thereby decreasing the synthesis of thyroid hormone; propylthiouracil blocks peripheral conversion of T_4 to T_3.

– Treatment of choice for children and for adults who refuse RAI

– May use as pretreatment for older or cardiac patients before RAI or surgery

– Methimazole is now almost exclusively used except during the 1st trimester of pregnancy. It has longer duration of action, allowing for once daily dosing, more rapid efficacy, and lower incidence of side effects (2)[A].

– No improvement in remission rates were noted with higher dose methimazole; lowest effective dose should be used (1)[B].

– Minor side effects (<5% incidence): controlled by switching from one agent to another: skin rash (3–5%), fever, arthralgias, GI side effects

– Major side effects necessitating change in treatment: polyarthritis (1–2%), idiopathic granulocytopenia (0.5%), and cholestasis/jaundice (rare)

– Evidence suggests that the optimal duration of antithyroid drugs is 12 to 18 months; no increased benefit to treatment beyond 18 months (3)[A]

– Relapse rates up to 50% in patients who respond initially; higher rates if smoker, large goiter, or positive thyroid-stimulating antibodies at end of treatment

Pregnancy Considerations
Propylthiouracil is preferred in 1st trimester of pregnancy due to teratogenic effects of methimazole. Switch to methimazole in 2nd and 3rd trimesters due to risk of PTU-induced hepatotoxicity (4)[A].

ISSUES FOR REFERRAL
• Endocrinologist for RAI therapy; if patient is pregnant or breastfeeding
• Graves ophthalmopathy
• Surgery if failed drug therapy or refusing RAI; obstruction or cosmesis

ADDITIONAL THERAPIES
• Symptom control may be achieved with iodides, which block conversion of T_4 to T_3 and inhibit TSH release. Use for pregnant patients who do not tolerate antithyroid medication or in conjunction with antithyroid medications; should not be used long term (may cause paradoxical increase in TSH release) or in combination with RAI
• For corneal protection: tinted glasses when outdoors, artificial tears, patching/taping the lids at night
• For orbitopathy: Mild cases can be treated with lubricants, nocturnal ointments, botulinum toxin injection for upper lid retraction, and smoking cessation. Moderate to severe cases should be treated with pulse-dose IV glucocorticoid if no contraindications. Alternative is PO steroid (prednisone 60 to 80 mg/day for 2 to 4 weeks and then taper off).
• For dermopathy, use medium- to high-potency topical corticosteroids.

SURGERY/OTHER PROCEDURES
With regard to ophthalmopathy progression, postoperative bleeding, permanent hypoparathyroidism, temporary and permanent recurrent laryngeal nerve palsy—total thyroidectomy (TT) is consistent with subtotal thyroidectomy (ST) in patients with Graves disease. However, TT is associated with a reduced incidence of recurrent hyperthyroidism and results in an increase in temporary hypoparathyroidism (5)[A].

ADMISSION, INPATIENT, AND NURSING CONSIDERATIONS
Indications for hospital admission:
• Severe thyrotoxicosis with hemodynamic compromise (thyroid storm). ICU management is indicated.
• Severe ophthalmopathy with visual compromise

 ONGOING CARE

FOLLOW-UP RECOMMENDATIONS
Patient Monitoring
• Monitoring is for the resolution of hyperthyroidism and for the development of hypothyroidism.
• Check TSH and T_4 levels every 1 to 2 months for the first 6 months after treatment, then every 3 months for a year, and then every 6 to 12 months thereafter. For patients on treatment with propylthiouracil and methimazole, check CBC yearly. Also, check anti-TSH receptor antibodies at 12 months of treatment to determine possibility of discontinuing medication.

Pregnancy Considerations
Postpartum exacerbation of hyperthyroidism is common for women not currently under treatment, so TSH and symptoms should be monitored.

PATIENT EDUCATION
Adherence to both follow-up surveillance and medication regimens is the most important way to achieve a good outcome.

PROGNOSIS
• Generally good with treatment
• May have irreversible ocular, cardiac, and psychiatric consequences
• Increased morbidity and mortality due to osteoporosis, atherosclerotic disease, insulin resistance and obesity, and endothelial cell dysfunction (thromboembolic risk)

COMPLICATIONS
Hypothyroidism is the most common consequence of treatment. The percentage of patients with Graves disease who become hypothyroid within the 1st year after treatment varies with treatment modality.

REFERENCES
1. Ren Z, Qin L, Wang JQ, et al. Comparative efficacy of four treatments in patients with Graves' disease: a network meta-analysis. *Exp Clin Endocrinol Diabetes*. 2015;123(5):317–322.
2. Bahn Chair RS, Burch HB, Cooper DS, et al; for American Thyroid Association and American Association of Clinical Endocrinologists. Hyperthyroidism and other causes of thyrotoxicosis: management guidelines of the American Thyroid Association and American Association of Clinical Endocrinologists. *Thyroid*. 2011;21(6):593–646.
3. Abraham P, Avenell A, McGeoch SC, et al. Antithyroid drug regimen for treating Graves' hyperthyroidism. *Cochrane Database Syst Rev*. 2010;(1):CD003420.
4. Stagnaro-Green A, Abalovich M, Alexander E, et al; and American Thyroid Association Taskforce on Thyroid Disease During Pregnancy and Postpartum. Guidelines of the American Thyroid Association for the diagnosis and management of thyroid disease during pregnancy and postpartum. *Thyroid*. 2011;21(10):1081–1125.
5. Guo Z, Yu P, Liu Z, et al. Total thyroidectomy vs bilateral subtotal thyroidectomy in patients with Graves' diseases: a meta-analysis of randomized clinical trials. *Clin Endocrinol (Oxf)*. 2013;79(5):739–746.

 SEE ALSO

Algorithms: Anxiety; Cardiac Arrhythmias; Weight Loss, Unintentional

CODES

ICD10
• E05.00 Thyrotoxicosis w diffuse goiter w/o thyrotoxic crisis
• E05.01 Thyrotoxicosis w diffuse goiter w thyrotoxic crisis or storm
• E05.20 Thyrotoxicosis w toxic multinod goiter w/o thyrotoxic crisis

CLINICAL PEARLS
• Graves disease accounts for 60–80% of all cases of hyperthyroidism.
• Potential morbidities of hyperthyroidism include ophthalmopathy, atrial fibrillation, congestive heart failure (CHF), stroke, seizure, and osteopenia/osteoporosis.

G

Grant M. Reed, DO • Simon B. Griesbach, MD

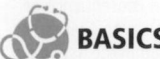

BASICS

DESCRIPTION

- A group of acquired autoimmune disorders causing acute peripheral neuropathy and ascending paralysis that progressively worsens for up to 4 weeks followed by a slow spontaneous recovery of function
- Subtypes classified by pattern of neural injury:
  - *Acute inflammatory demyelinating polyradiculoneuropathy* (AIDP): progressive limb weakness with areflexia (~95% of GBS cases in Europe and North America)
  - Axonal subtypes:
    - *Acute motor axonal neuropathy* (AMAN): pure motor neuropathy strongly associated with *Campylobacter jejuni* and a higher rate of respiratory failure (~5% of cases in Europe and North America but 30–47% of cases in China, Japan, and Central and South America)
    - *Acute motor-sensory axonal neuropathy* (AMSAN): combined motor–sensory neuropathy; poor prognosis with prolonged course
  - Regional subtypes:
    - *Miller Fisher syndrome* (MFS): triad with ophthalmoplegia, ataxia, and areflexia; antibodies to GQ1b present in 90% of patients with MFS
    - *Bickerstaff encephalitis*: possible variant of MFS with encephalopathy, ophthalmoplegia, ataxia, and hyperreflexia
    - *Pharyngeal-cervical-brachial GBS*: Parasympathetic and cholinergic dysfunction leads to neck, arm, and oropharyngeal weakness along with upper extremity areflexia
  - Sensory subtypes:
    - *Acute pandysautonomia*: orthostatic hypotension, gastroparesis, ileus, constipation/diarrhea, sudomotor/pupillary abnormalities, and neuropathic pain
    - *Acute sensory ataxic neuropathy* (ASAN): controversial variant with sensory loss and ataxia
- *Polyneuritis cranialis*: bilateral cranial nerve involvement and severe peripheral sensory loss associated with cytomegalovirus (CMV) infections
- Synonym(s): GBS, AIDP; Landry-Guillain-Barré-Strohl syndrome, acute inflammatory idiopathic polyneuritis; acute autoimmune neuropathy; Landry ascending paralysis

ALERT
Rapidly progressing paralysis and respiratory failure occur in 20–30% of patients. Some require mechanical ventilation within 48 hours.

ALERT
Areflexia is a red flag for GBS in patients with rapidly progressive limb weakness.

ALERT
A history of weakness preceded by respiratory or GI infection suggests GBS.

EPIDEMIOLOGY

Incidence
- Most common acute paralytic disease in Western countries
- 0.6 to 2.0/100,000 worldwide
- U.S. incidence: 0.9 to 1.8/100,000

- Increases with age: 0.8/100,000 in children <18 years of age; 3/100,000 in adults >60 years
- 1.5 times higher incidence in males

ETIOLOGY AND PATHOPHYSIOLOGY
- Autoimmune process targets Schwann cell surface membrane, myelin, and/or gangliosides causing peripheral nerve destruction and demyelination.
- Pathogenesis thought to involve molecular mimicry (i.e., an immune response to antigenic targets that are coincidentally shared by infectious organisms and host peripheral nerve tissue)

Genetics
Host factors appear to play a role in GBS, but no clear genetic risk has been identified.

RISK FACTORS
Influenza vaccinations
- Inactivated seasonal flu vaccines associated with an increase in GBS risk equivalent to one case/million vaccines above background incidence (far less than the 17 cases of GBS per million people *infected* with influenza virus)
- Incidence of GBS associated with influenza vaccine has steadily decreased over time.
- *Of historical note*: Increased incidence during 1976 U.S. National H1N1 Immunization Program had vaccine-attributable risk of 8.8 per million recipients compared to 1.6 per million recipients in the 2009 H1N1 vaccination campaign.

COMMONLY ASSOCIATED CONDITIONS
Infection of the respiratory (22–53%) or GI tract (6–26%) in preceding 6 weeks
- *C. jejuni*: most common precipitant of GBS, (21–40% of cases):
  - Associated with axonal degeneration, slower recovery, more severe residual disability
- CMV: Primary CMV infection precedes 10–22% of cases.
- Rarely associated with *Mycoplasma pneumoniae*, influenza infection, Epstein-Barr virus, varicella-zoster virus, HIV infection, and some arboviral infections

DIAGNOSIS

HISTORY
- AIDP presents with onset of progressive limb weakness that reaches its worst within 4 weeks (73% reach a functional nadir in 1 week).
- Preceding respiratory or gastrointestinal infection
- Earliest symptoms include pain, numbness, paresthesias, or limb weakness typically affecting distal extremities and spread proximally.
- Neuropathic pain, sometimes severe, occurs in 30–50%, most commonly in the back and lower extremities.
- Purely sensory symptoms exclude GBS.

PHYSICAL EXAM
Diagnostic criteria for typical GBS:
- Required for diagnosis:
  - Progressive weakness reaching nadir between 12 hours and 28 days
  - Affects >1 limb
  - Areflexia/hyporeflexia
- Strongly supportive:
  - Paresthesias with only mild changes in objective sensory function (e.g., pinprick, light touch)

  - Relative symmetry
  - Cranial nerve involvement, especially bilateral/symmetric weakness of facial muscles
  - Recovery beginning within 4 weeks after progression ceases
  - Autonomic dysfunction
  - Absence of fever at onset

DIFFERENTIAL DIAGNOSIS
Differential diagnosis of acute flaccid paralysis:
- Brain: basilar artery stroke, brainstem encephalitis
- Spinal cord: transverse myelitis, cord compression
- Motor neuron: poliomyelitis
- Peripheral neuropathy other than GBS: vasculitis, critical illness polyneuropathy, infectious disease (e.g., diphtheria, Lyme disease), chronic inflammatory demyelinating polyradiculoneuropathy (CIDP), acute intermittent porphyria
- Neuromuscular junction: myasthenia gravis, Eaton-Lambert syndrome, botulism, toxins (e.g., heavy metals, inhalant abuse, organophosphates)
- Muscle: electrolyte disturbance (hypokalemia, hypophosphatemia), inflammatory myopathy, critical illness myopathy, acute rhabdomyolysis, trichonosis, periodic paralysis
- Psychological causes of weakness

DIAGNOSTIC TESTS & INTERPRETATION

Initial Tests (lab, imaging)
- Studies to establish the diagnosis:
  - Lumbar puncture (LP): Increased CSF protein without pleocytosis is present in ~80% of cases (CSF protein is often normal within the first 48 hours of symptom onset).
  - Nerve conduction study (NCS): *most useful confirmatory test*; conduction velocities abnormal in 85% of patients with demyelination, even early in the disease. If nondiagnostic, repeat after 1 to 2 weeks.
- Imaging generally not required. MRI demonstrates spinal nerve root and/or cauda equina enhancement.
- Studies to find underlying cause:
  - Stool culture and serology for *C. jejuni*
  - Acute and convalescent serology for CMV, EBV, HIV, and *M. pneumoniae*
  - Anti-GQ1b antibodies in MFS variant

Follow-Up Tests & Special Considerations
- Analyze CSF prior to treatment with intravenous immunoglobulin (IVIG), which can cause aseptic meningitis.
- A repeat NCS 3 to 8 weeks after onset can classify the subtype of GBS.

Diagnostic Procedures/Other
Sural nerve biopsy not indicated except to rule out vasculitis or amyloidosis

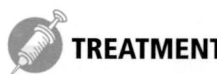

TREATMENT

GENERAL MEASURES
- Pain treatment: NSAIDs helpful but often insufficient. Gabapentin and carbamazepine decrease opioid requirements in patients with GBS. One is not superior to others (1)[A].
- DVT prophylaxis recommended in nonambulatory patients (2)[C]
- Neostigmine or erythromycin may be effective for ileus, if present (2)[C].

MEDICATION

First Line

- IVIG 0.4 g/kg/day for 5 days or (less commonly) 1 g/kg/day for 2 days
  - In severe disease, IVIG started within 2 weeks of onset hastens recovery as much as plasma exchange (PE) (3)[A].
  - In children, IVIG hastens recovery compared with supportive care alone (3)[A].
  - Combined treatment with IVIG and PE confers no clinically significant benefit (3)[A].
- PE:
  - Compared with supportive treatment alone, those treated with PE are quicker to recover walking (NNT 7), have less requirement and shorter duration for mechanical ventilation (NNT 8), recover full muscle strength more quickly (NNT 8), and have fewer severe sequelae at 1 year (NNT 17) (4)[A].
  - Higher risks of relapse found with PE versus supportive care with no difference in severe infection or mortality (4)[A]
  - In mild GBS, two sessions of PE are superior to none. In moderate GBS, four sessions are superior to two. In severe GBS, six sessions are not significantly better than four (4)[A].
  - PE is most beneficial if started within 7 days of disease onset. PE still helpful up to 30 days (4)[A].
  - Value of PE in children <12 is unknown.

Second Line

- Corticosteroids: not beneficial as monotherapy or as combined treatment. Low-quality evidence suggests steroids delay recovery (5)[A].
- CSF filtration is no different than PE (6)[B].
- Interferon β and brain-derived neurotrophic factor no different than placebo (6)[B]

ADDITIONAL THERAPIES

- Physical and occupational therapy improves fatigue and functional abilities (2)[C].
- Speech and language therapy improves swallowing function, if affected (2)[C].

COMPLEMENTARY & ALTERNATIVE MEDICINE

Tripterygium polyglycoside hastened recovery significantly more than corticosteroids (NNT 4), in one small trial (6)[A].

ADMISSION, INPATIENT, AND NURSING CONSIDERATIONS

- Admit patients with suspected GBS.
- Closely monitor respiratory status with serial measurement of vital capacity (VC) and static inspiratory and expiratory pressures (PI_{max} and PE_{max}).
- Predictors of respiratory failure:
  - Rapid progression: ≥3 days between onset of weakness and hospital admission
  - Facial and/or bulbar weakness
  - VC decrease >30%
  - Medical Research Council (MRC) sum score indicating muscle weakness: 0 to 5/5 muscle strength grading for bilateral upper arm abductors, elbow flexors, wrist extensors, hip flexors, knee extensors, and foot dorsal flexors totaling 60 points

- Indications for intubation:
  - VC <20 mL/kg
  - PI_{max} <30 cm H_2O
  - PE_{max} <40 cm H_2O
- Prevent complications of immobilization with DVT prophylaxis and frequent turning.
- Respiratory care, aspiration precautions, pulmonary toilet
- Monitor bowel and bladder function for ileus and urinary retention.
- Begin immediate physical therapy to preserve passive range of motion.
- Mildly affected patients who can walk unaided and are stable for >2 weeks are unlikely to experience disease progression and may be managed as outpatients. Monitor bowel and bladder function for ileus and urinary retention.

 ONGOING CARE

FOLLOW-UP RECOMMENDATIONS

Patient Monitoring

- Patients require close monitoring of respiratory, cardiac, and hemodynamic function, typically in the ICU setting.
- Pulmonary function testing (VC, respiratory frequency) q2–6h in the progressive phase and q6–12h in the plateau phase
- Monitor bulbar weakness and ability to handle airway secretions.
- Telemetry in patients with severe disease

PATIENT EDUCATION

Emphasize expectation for significant recovery and explain phases of illness.

PROGNOSIS

- If untreated, three phases of illness:
  - Initial progressive phase up to 4 weeks with highest risk of death and complication
  - Variable plateau phase
  - Recovery phase (weeks to months): return of proximal then distal strength
- Most recovery occurs within the 1st year.
- 80% recover within 6 to 12 months with maximum 18 months past onset.
- 20% with residual disability after 1 year:
  - Bilateral foot drop, intrinsic hand muscle wasting, sensory ataxia, dysesthesia
  - Half with severe disability
- Factors associated with poor functional outcome:
  - Age >60 years, rapid progression, severe disease indicated by GBS disability score or MRC sum score, preceding diarrhea, positive *C. jejuni* or CMV serology, axonal degeneration, need for mechanical ventilation

COMPLICATIONS

- 3–7% mortality in Europe and North America. Older patients, those with severe disease, have highest risk.
- 20–30% require mechanical ventilation.
- 70% develop autonomic dysfunction with hemodynamic instability, urinary retention, ileus, and anhidrosis.
- 10% have relapse.
- ~2% develop relapsing CIDP.

REFERENCES

1. Liu J, Wang LN, McNicol ED. Pharmacological treatment for pain in Guillain-Barré syndrome. *Cochrane Database Syst Rev.* 2015;(4):CD009950.
2. Hughes RA, Wijdicks EF, Benson E, et al; for Multidisciplinary Consensus Group. Supportive care for patients with Guillain-Barré syndrome. *Arch Neurol.* 2005;62(8):1194–1198.
3. Hughes RA, Swan AV, van Doorn PA. Intravenous immunoglobulin for Guillain-Barré syndrome. *Cochrane Database Syst Rev.* 2014;(9):CD002063.
4. Chevret S, Hughes RA, Annane D, et al. Plasma exchange for Guillain-Barré syndrome. *Cochrane Database Syst Rev.* 2017;(2):CD001798.
5. Hughes RA, Brassington R, Gunn A, et al. Corticosteroids for Guillain-Barré syndrome. *Cochrane Database Syst Rev.* 2016;(10):CD001446.
6. Pritchard J, Hughes RA, Hadden RD, et al. Pharmacological treatment other than corticosteroids, intravenous immunoglobulin and plasma exchange for Guillain-Barré syndrome. *Cochrane Database Syst Rev.* 2016;(11):CD008630.

ADDITIONAL READING

- Rinaldi S. Update on Guillain-Barré syndrome. *J Peripher Nerv Syst.* 2013;18(2):99–112.
- Sejvar JJ, Baughman AL, Wise M, et al. Population incidence of Guillain-Barré syndrome: a systematic review and meta-analysis. *Neuroepidemiology.* 2011;36(2):123–133.
- Vellozzi C, Iqbal S, Broder K. Guillain-Barre syndrome, influenza, and influenza vaccination: the epidemiologic evidence. *Clin Infect Dis.* 2014;58(8):1149–1155.

CODES

ICD10
G61.0 Guillain-Barre syndrome

CLINICAL PEARLS

- Suspect GBS in cases of ascending flaccid paralysis with areflexia and an antecedent history of viral respiratory illness or gastroenteritis.
- When GBS is suspected, evaluate VC and inspiratory force for signs of respiratory compromise.
- Uncomplicated GBS has a slow spontaneous recovery. Treatment with IVIG or PE speeds rate of recovery and reduces disability.
- The most useful diagnostic tests for GBS are NCS and LP.
- GBS risk following native influenza virus infection is 40 to 70 times greater than after seasonal influenza vaccination.

G

GYNECOMASTIA

Franklyn C. Babb, MD, FAAFP

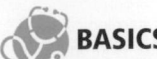 BASICS

DESCRIPTION
- Benign glandular proliferation of male breast tissue
- Increase in estrogens relative to androgens leads to the development of gynecomastia.
- Gynecomastia can be transient and may represent the normal physiologic changes that occur in utero or in adolescence. However, gynecomastia presenting or persisting in adulthood is typically pathologic in nature.
- Pseudogynecomastia which is lipomastia (subareolar fat)

EPIDEMIOLOGY
- 60–90% of infants have transient gynecomastia (1).
- 50–60% of pubertal males have mild transient gynecomastia (onset at 10 to 12 years of age and resolution by age 18 years in most individuals) (1).
- Up to 70% of men between 50 and 69 years of age report gynecomastia (1).

ETIOLOGY AND PATHOPHYSIOLOGY
Increase in estrogen activity relative to androgen activity leads to the development of gynecomastia (2). Estrogen stimulates ductal cell hyperplasia, facilitates ductal branching and lengthening, increases vascularity, and results in the proliferation of periductal fibroblasts. These changes occur within 12 months and are followed by fibrosis in the later stages of gynecomastia. Multiple factors can alter the estrogen to androgen ratio and precipitate gynecomastia:
- Decrease in androgen production
- Increase in estrogen production
- Increase in peripheral conversion to estrogen
- Inhibition of the androgen receptor
- Increase in the level of sex hormone–binding globulin (SHBG) or the affinity of androgens to SHBG (decreases free or bioavailable testosterone)
- Displacement of estrogen relative to testosterone from SHBG due to medications

RISK FACTORS
Gynecomastia can be physiologic or pathologic in nature.
- Physiologic gynecomastia presents in infants and adolescent boys and resolves spontaneously.
  - Neonatal gynecomastia: The placenta converts dehydroepiandrosterone (DHEA) and dehydro-epiandrosterone sulfate (DHEA-S) to estrone and estradiol resulting in transient gynecomastia.
  - Adolescent gynecomastia: Transient increases in estradiol levels at the onset of puberty lead to gynecomastia.
- Pathologic gynecomastia refers to persistent or adult-onset gynecomastia. 25% of cases are idiopathic in nature most likely secondary to age-associated decline in free testosterone and adipose tissue–mediated aromatase activity.
- Multiple medications have been implicated (1).

ALERT
- Illicit drugs: marijuana, heroin, methadone, alcohol, amphetamines, and over-the-counter body building supplements
- Hormones: androgens, anabolic steroids, estrogens, estrogen agonist, and human chorionic gonadotropin (hCG)
- Antiandrogens or inhibitors of androgen synthesis: bicalutamide, flutamide, nilutamide, cyproterone, and GnRH agonists (leuprolide and goserelin)
- Anti-infectives: metronidazole, ketoconazole, minocycline, isoniazid

- Antiulcer medications: cimetidine, ranitidine, meto-clopramide, and proton pump inhibitors
- Cytotoxic agents: methotrexate, alkylating agents, and vinca alkaloids
- Cardiovascular drugs: Digoxin, spironolactone, calcium channel blockers, ACEIs, amiodarone, methyldopa, reserpine, minoxidil, and recently statins can be added to this list (3).
- Psychoactive drugs: antidepressants, benzodiazepines, phenothiazines, antipsychotics (typical and atypical) (i.e., haloperidol and risperidone)
- Medications: HIV medications like efavirenz, phenytoin, penicillamine, sulindac, or theophylline
- Causes to rule out:
  - Primary hypogonadism: androgen insensitivity syndromes (defect in the androgen receptor), Klinefelter syndrome
  - Testicular tumor: germ cell (secretes hCG), Leydig cell (secretes estrogen), Sertoli cell (excessive aromatization to estrogens)
  - Adrenal tumors (secrete DHEA-S and estrogens)
  - Ectopic hCG tumors (hepatoblastoma, gastric tumors, renal cell carcinomas)
  - Cirrhosis
  - Secondary hypogonadism: Kallmann syndrome or prolactinemia, which can also stimulate milk production in breast tissue
  - Hyperthyroidism
  - Renal disease or dialysis
  - Malnutrition/starvation
  - Rare (true hermaphroditism [both testicular and ovarian tissue present])

Pediatric Considerations
Transient gynecomastia is seen in neonates or pubertal boys; typically resolves within 6 to 24 months

Geriatric Considerations
Age-associated decline in testosterone production and increase in SHBG production leads to low free testosterone levels in the elderly population. Furthermore, the increased ratio of fat mass to lean mass noted with aging leads to adipose tissue–mediated peripheral conversion of androgens to estrogen. Medications also play a significant role in the development of gynecomastia in this population.

COMMONLY ASSOCIATED CONDITIONS
- Prostate carcinoma—treatment with estrogen and antiandrogen leads to gynecomastia in 50–75% of patients.
- Cirrhosis
- Primary hypogonadism; especially Klinefelter syndrome—congenital abnormality leads to primary hypogonadism and gynecomastia. These patients are at risk for breast cancer and need regular breast exams.
- Testicular tumors; Leydig or Sertoli cell tumors especially when associated with Peutz-Jeghers syndrome or Carney complex

Dx DIAGNOSIS

HISTORY
- Inquire about duration of breast growth, increase in breast tissue size, and associated breast pain and discharge.
- If suspicious of hypogonadism, ask about erectile dysfunction, muscle mass, and decreased shaving frequency and libido.

- Obtain a complete medical history including headache, loss of vision, loss of appetite, weight loss, malignancy, thyroid disorders, liver disease, renal disease, and genetic abnormalities.
- Obtain a family history including Carney complex and Peutz-Jeghers syndrome.
- Review medication list extensively and inquire about the use of illicit substances.
- Question about herbal supplements, marijuana use, and OTC cimetidine (Tagamet) use.

PHYSICAL EXAM
- Careful breast exam to evaluate characteristics:
  - Firm, concentric glandular tissue beneath the nipple and areola palpable by pinching the thumb and forefinger together from either side of the breast toward the nipple
  - May involve one or both breasts
  - Usually asymptomatic but may be painful or tender if it is of recent onset
  - Off center, hard, fixed mass is concerning for malignancy, although palpation of subareolar fat is more consistent with pseudogynecomastia.
  - Breast discharge should raise concern for malignancy or prolactinemia. In the latter, the discharge is typically clear or milky.
- Thyroid exam (Evaluate for diffuse enlargement and palpable nodules and check extremities for tremor and brisk reflexes.)
- Abdominal exam (Evaluate for masses and liver size.)
- Genitourinary exam (Evaluate for testicular size, hair pattern, and presence of ovary or uterus.)
- Visual field exam (Evaluate for peripheral field defect.)

DIFFERENTIAL DIAGNOSIS
- Pseudogynecomastia—fat deposition without glandular proliferation often seen in obesity
- Breast cancer—on exam, the lesion is typically unilateral; firm; eccentric to the nipple; and associated with skin dimpling, nipple retraction/discharge, and lymphadenopathy.
- Lipomas
- Sebaceous cyst
- Dermoid cyst
- Mastitis
- Hematoma
- Hamartoma

DIAGNOSTIC TESTS & INTERPRETATION
- Laboratory and radiologic investigations should be tailored to fit history and physical exam findings.
- Idiopathic gynecomastia is a diagnosis of exclusion, and therefore, laboratory tests to rule out medical conditions associated with gynecomastia is recommended.

Initial Tests (lab, imaging)
- Luteinizing hormone (LH)—elevated in primary hypogonadism and decreased in secondary hypogonadism (4)[C]
- Morning total and free testosterone—decreased testosterone level in hypogonadism (4)[C]
- hCG—elevated in germ cell tumors and ectopic hCG tumors (4)[C]
- Estradiol—elevated in Leydig cell tumors, Sertoli cell tumors, adrenal tumors, and with increased aromatase activity (4)[C]
- DHEA-S levels, which can be increased in adrenal tumors
- Urine for drugs of abuse (UDA)
- Other tests to consider include creatinine, liver function test, thyroid function tests, and prolactin.

Follow-Up Tests & Special Considerations

Consider imaging studies based on laboratory findings.

- Testicular ultrasound (testicular tumor)
- Chest x-ray (CXR) and abdominal CT/MRI (extragonadal germ cell tumor, ectopic hCG tumor, and adrenal tumor)
- MRI of pituitary (pituitary tumor)

Diagnostic Procedures/Other

Based on physical exam findings, consider biopsy of breast mass to rule out malignancy (i.e., off center, hard, fixed, discharge).

Test Interpretation

- Elevated hCG: Check testicular ultrasound. If positive for a mass, likely a testicular germ cell tumor. If the ultrasound is negative, consider extragonadal germ cell tumor or hCG-secreting neoplasm and order a CXR and CT abdomen (4)[C].
- Elevated LH: if in relation to low testosterone, likely primary hypogonadism. If elevated in relation to high testosterone, check thyroid-stimulating hormone (TSH) and free thyroxine (FT_4). If FT_4 is elevated and TSH is suppressed, likely hyperthyroidism; if TSH and FT_4 are normal, likely androgen resistance (4)[C]
- Normal or decreased LH in relation to low testosterone: Check prolactin level. If prolactin is elevated, likely due to a prolactin-secreting pituitary tumor; if normal, likely due to secondary hypogonadism (4)[C]
- Normal or decreased LH in relation to increased estradiol: Check testicular ultrasound. If positive for a mass, likely Leydig or Sertoli cell tumor. If negative for mass, check CT abdomen to evaluate the adrenals. If mass is present, possible adrenal neoplasm versus adenoma; if no mass is detected, then likely due to increased aromatase activity in extraglandular tissue (4)[C]
- hCG, LH, testosterone, and estradiol are normal: likely idiopathic or medication/drug-induced gynecomastia (4)[C]

TREATMENT

GENERAL MEASURES

- Gynecomastia usually regresses spontaneously within 6 months of onset. This is true even for adult males. Therefore, patients can be monitored for the first 6 months and treatment considered if gynecomastia persists.
- The histologic changes early in the disease process can be reversed with medical therapy. However, with the development of fibrotic tissue, surgery is typically required. Typically, 1 to 2 years after the onset of gynecomastia, fibrotic changes can be seen and medical intervention is less effective (5)[C].
- Neonatal and pubertal gynecomastia spontaneously resolves within 6 to 24 months. Persistent pubertal gynecomastia (>24 months) occurs in 8% of pubertal boys. In adult males, 75% of gynecomastia is secondary to persistent pubertal gynecomastia, medications, and idiopathic conditions. Only 25% is related to an underlying medical condition.
- All illicit drug use and offending medications should be stopped if appropriate and patients monitored for clinical improvement.
- Underlying medical conditions need to be treated (i.e., testosterone replacement for hypogonadal men, dopamine agonist for prolactinoma, appropriate treatment for thyrotoxicosis, and tumor resection).
- Medical and surgical therapy to reduce gynecomastia should be considered in patients with significant physical or psychological discomfort.

MEDICATION

There are no FDA-approved medications for the treatment of gynecomastia, but clinical trials involving selective estrogen receptor modulators (SERMs) and aromatase inhibitors demonstrate partial regression and symptom relief (i.e., breast tenderness).

- SERMs: Clinical trials of both tamoxifen (10 to 20 mg/day) and raloxifene (60 mg/day) showed partial reduction in pubertal gynecomastia in 90% of study participants after 3 to 9 months, but 40% of patients in both treatment groups were not satisfied with the final results and underwent surgical removal (5)[B]. Tamoxifen has also been shown to reduce breast tenderness and prevent the development of gynecomastia in prostate cancer patients on androgen deprivation therapy. Therefore, SERMs (particularly tamoxifen) can be considered in men with 6 to 12 months of severe, painful gynecomastia symptoms (6)[B].
- Aromatase inhibitors block peripheral conversion of androgens to estrogens. In prostate cancer patients, anastrozole prevented the development of gynecomastia in patients undergoing androgen deprivation therapy (2)[B].

ISSUES FOR REFERRAL

- Refer patients to an endocrinologist if abnormally elevated hormone levels are confirmed.
- If patients have refractory gynecomastia despite medical therapy and have prolonged gynecomastia characterized by the late fibrotic stage or symptoms concerning for breast cancer, referral to a surgeon would be appropriate.

ADDITIONAL THERAPIES

In clinical trials, prophylactic radiotherapy (10 to 15 Gy in one fraction over 3 days) prevented the development of gynecomastia in prostate cancer patients on androgen deprivation therapy. Higher doses (20 Gy in five fractions) improved pain symptoms in the same population (6)[B].

SURGERY/OTHER PROCEDURES

Surgery to remove breast tissue is recommended if:

- Gynecomastia does not regress within 12 months either spontaneously or after medical therapy.
- Significant discomfort (i.e., pain, tenderness)
- Causes embarrassment or anxiety
- Biopsy suspicious for malignancy

ONGOING CARE

FOLLOW-UP RECOMMENDATIONS

Patient Monitoring

- Every 3 to 6 months for 24 months; consider medical therapy (i.e., tamoxifen) if severe, painful symptoms persist after 6 to 12 months and surgery after 12 to 24 months. In individuals with asymptomatic or mild disease, routine yearly breast and physical exam is recommended.
- Patients with Klinefelter syndrome are at increased risk of breast cancer and should have routine breast exams done.

PATIENT EDUCATION

Patients should be encouraged to do periodic breast examination and to alert their clinical provider if a nodule is palpated in the breast or axilla, skin discoloration occurs, or nipple discharge develops.

PROGNOSIS

- Good in physiologic cases because they often regress spontaneously within 3 to 6 months (4)

- Majority of patients experience regression once underlying disorder is treated or offending agents are eliminated (4).
- The majority of patients, who undergo surgery, are satisfied with the postoperative cosmetic appearance (7).

REFERENCES

1. Johnson RE, Murad MH. Gynecomastia: pathophysiology, evaluation, and management. *Mayo Clin Proc.* 2009;84(11):1010–1015.
2. Boccardo F, Rubagotti A, Battaglia M, et al. Evaluation of tamoxifen and anastrozole in the prevention of gynecomastia and breast pain induced by bicalutamide monotherapy of prostate cancer. *J Clin Oncol.* 2005;23(4):808–815.
3. Skeldon SC, Carleton B, Brophy JM, et al. Statin medications and the risk of gynecomastia. *Clin Endocrinol (Oxf).* 2018;89(4):470–473.
4. Braunstein GD. Clinical practice. Gynecomastia. *N Engl J Med.* 2007;357(12):1229–1237.
5. Lawrence SE, Faught KA, Vethamuthu J, et al. Beneficial effects of raloxifene and tamoxifen in the treatment of pubertal gynecomastia. *J Pediatr.* 2004;145(1):71–76.
6. Fagerlund A, Cormio L, Palangi L, et al. Gynecomastia in patients with prostate cancer: a systematic review. *PLoS One.* 2015;10(8):e0136094.
7. Lemaine V, Cayci C, Simmons PS, et al. Gynecomastia in adolescent males. *Semin Plast Surg.* 2013;27(1):56–61.

ADDITIONAL READING

- Dickson G. Gynecomastia. *Am Fam Physician.* 2012;85(7):716–722.
- Nuttall FQ, Warrier RS, Gannon MC. Gynecomastia and drugs: a critical evaluation of the literature. *Eur J Clin Pharmacol.* 2015;71(5):569–578.

 SEE ALSO

Algorithm: Gynecomastia

CODES

ICD10

N62 Hypertrophy of breast

CLINICAL PEARLS

- Gynecomastia can be transient and may represent the normal physiologic changes in neonates or adolescents. However, gynecomastia presenting or persisting in adulthood is typically pathologic in nature.
- Thorough history and physical exam should be performed on all patients and offending medications eliminated.
- Lab and radiologic studies should be conducted to rule out medical conditions associated with gynecomastia including thyrotoxicosis, prolactinemia, hypogonadism, testicular tumors, adrenal tumors, and ectopic hCG tumors. Treatment should be tailored to exam findings.
- ~25% of gynecomastia is idiopathic in nature, and treatment should focus on symptom control.
- Clinical trials of SERMs, aromatase inhibitors, and radiation therapy seem promising. Surgery is the treatment of choice for refractory gynecomastia.

HAMMER TOES
Neil Feldman, DPM

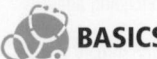 **BASICS**

Contraction deformities of the toes

DESCRIPTION
- Hammer toes include three distinct types of deformity.
  - Hammer toe (as defined) involves a plantar flexion deformity of the proximal interphalangeal (PIP) joint with varying degrees of hyperextension of the metatarsophalangeal (MTP) and distal interphalangeal (DIP) joint; primarily in sagittal plane (1)
  - Claw toe involves a plantar flexion deformity of the PIP and DIP joint with varying degrees of hyperextension of the MTP.
  - Mallet toe involves a plantar flexion deformity of the DIP joint only.
- Each can be flexible, semirigid, or fixed.
  - Flexible: passively correctable to neutral position
  - Semirigid: partially correctable to neutral position
  - Fixed: not correctable to neutral position without intervention

EPIDEMIOLOGY
Most common deformity of lesser digits, typically affecting only one or two toes:
- 2nd toe is the most commonly involved.
- Hallux malleus is term used when the great toe (hallux) is involved.

Incidence
- Undefined
- Increases with age, duration of deformity (from flexible to rigid)

Prevalence
- Predominant sex: female > male (2)
  - Female predominance from 2.5:1 to 9:1, depending on age group
- Can range from 1% to 20% of population studied
- Blacks are more often affected than whites (2).

ETIOLOGY AND PATHOPHYSIOLOGY
- Can be congenital or acquired
- Three categories of acquired hammer toes
  - Extensor substitution (most common with pes cavus). Occurs during the swing phase of gait. The extensor digitorum longus (EDL) muscle remains overactive, substituting for dysfunctional hip and ankle extensors.
  - Flexor substitution. Least common cause and seen commonly with pes cavus. The flexor digitorum longus (FDL) muscle remains overactive with relative weakness/dysfunction to the Achilles and flexor hallucis longus (FHL), which are the main foot flexors.
  - Flexor stabilization (most common cause and occurs in pronated foot/foot with pes planus). The FDL muscle remains overactive, overutilizing the toes to assist in relative foot instability.
- Biomechanical dysfunction results in muscle/tendon imbalance between the EDL tendon at the PIP joint and the FDL tendon at the MTP joint; the imbalance at the MTP joint level leads to the altering of the stabilizing force of the intrinsic muscles inserting into the extensor sling and wing apparatus of the MTP joint. In the case of classic hammer toes, the toe(s) sublux dorsally as the MTP hyperextends. This results in plantar flexion of the PIP joint and hyperextension of the MTP joint (2).

- Specific pathomechanics vary by etiology:
  - Toe length discrepancy or narrow footwear toe box induces PIP joint flexion by forcing digit to accommodate shoe.
    - May also lead to MTP joint synovitis secondary to overuse, with elongation of plantar plate and MTP joint hyperextension
    - 4th and 5th toes commonly assume an adductovarus attitude, which can make the toes appear to sit on their side.
  - Rheumatoid arthritis (RA) causes MTP joint destruction and resultant subluxation.
  - Any condition that compromises intra-articular and periarticular tissues, such as second ray longer than first, inflammatory joint disease, neuromuscular conditions, improper-fitting shoes, and trauma (3)
  - Damage to joint capsule, collateral ligaments, or synovia leads to unstable PIP joint or MTP joint.

Genetics
- Significant heritability rates of 49–90% (4)
- Specific genetic markers are not identified.

RISK FACTORS
- Pes cavus, pes planus
- Hallux valgus
- Metatarsus adductus
- Ankle equinus
- Neuromuscular disease (rare)
- Trauma; improperly fitted shoes (narrow toe box) and/or tight hosiery
- Abnormal metatarsal and/or digit length
- Inflammatory joint disease (e.g., RA)
- Connective tissue disease
- Diabetes mellitus

GENERAL PREVENTION
- Proper fitting of shoes. Use of pressure-dispersive footwear helps reduce pain.
- Foot orthoses modulate biomechanical dysfunction and muscular imbalance, preventing progression (2).
- Limiting use of shoes in the growing foot. Use of zero drop shoes when necessary. Traditional shoes have an elevated heel relative to the ball of the foot (MTP joints). Therefore, at rest, the toes are positioned in dorsal subluxation at the MTP joints and forced to be contracted (termed toe spring).
- Control of predisposing factors (e.g., inflammatory joint disease) may also slow progression.

COMMONLY ASSOCIATED CONDITIONS
- Hallux valgus
- Cavus foot (pes cavus)
- Flat foot (pes planus)
- Metatarsus adductus
- Dorsal callus

 DIAGNOSIS

History and physical exam are typically sufficient for diagnosis of hammer toes. Additional tests are available to exclude other conditions.

HISTORY
- Location, duration, severity, and rate of progression of foot deformity
- Type, location, duration of pain
  - Patients often relate sensation of lump on plantar aspect of MTP joint.

- Degree of functional impairment
- Improving/exacerbating factors
- Type of footwear and hosiery worn
- Peripheral neurologic symptoms
- Any prior treatment rendered

PHYSICAL EXAM
- Note MTP joint hyperextension, PIP joint flexion, and DIP joint extension or flexion.
- Observe any adjacent toe deformities (e.g., hallux valgus, flexion contractures).
- Assess degree of flexibility and reducibility of deformity in both weight-bearing and non–weight-bearing positions (2).
- Note any hyperkeratosis over the joint, ulcers, clavi (dorsal PIP joint, metatarsal head), adventitious bursa, erythema, or skin breakdown or ulceration (2).
- Palpate for pain over dorsal aspect of PIP joint or MTP joint.
- Drawer test of MTP joint
- Palpate web spaces to exclude interdigital neuroma.
- Neurovascular evaluation (e.g., pulses, sensation, muscle bulk)

DIFFERENTIAL DIAGNOSIS
- Hammer toe: hyperextension of the MTP and DIP joints and plantar flexion of the PIP joint
- Claw toe: dorsiflexion of MTP joint and plantar flexion of the DIP joint
- Mallet toe: fixed or flexible deformity of the DIP joint of the toe
- Overlapping 5th toe
- Interdigital neuroma
- Plantar plate rupture
- Nonspecific synovitis of MTP joint
- Fracture; exostosis
- Arthritis (e.g., rheumatoid, psoriatic)

DIAGNOSTIC TESTS & INTERPRETATION
Initial Tests (lab, imaging)
- Not required unless clinically indicated to rule out suspected metabolic or inflammatory arthropathies (2)[C]: rheumatoid factor, antinuclear antibodies (ANA), HLA-B27 serologies for inflammatory disease
- Weight-bearing x-rays of affected foot in anteroposterior (AP), lateral, and oblique views (2)[C]:
  - AP view superior for assessing transverse plane MTP subluxation or dislocation
  - Lateral view is best for the evaluation of hammer toe.

Follow-Up Tests & Special Considerations
MRI or bone scan if osteomyelitis is suspected

Diagnostic Procedures/Other
- Nerve conduction studies or EMG if neurologic disorder is suspected
- Doppler or plethysmography if impaired circulation and surgery is considered
- Computerized weight-bearing pressure testing is indicated only in setting of neuromuscular deficiencies.

Test Interpretation
Histologic evaluation is not necessary before treatment.

TREATMENT

- Goal of treatment is to relieve symptoms and help patients return to their normal activity level.
- Surgical and nonsurgical interventions are available.
- Mild and asymptomatic cases may not require treatment.

GENERAL MEASURES

Nonsurgical (conservative) treatments include

- Shoe modifications (wider and/or deeper toe box) to accommodate the deformity and decrease the pressure over osseous prominences. Avoid high-heeled shoes (2)[C].
- Toe sleeve or orthodigital padding of the hammer toe prominence (5)[C]
- Metatarsal pads in reducible deformities and crest pads in nonreducible deformities
- Dynamic toe splints for MTP joint subluxations or dislocations with (semi)reducible deformity
- Hammer toe—straightening orthotics or taping to reduce flexible deformities
- Débridement of hyperkeratotic lesions can reduce symptoms. Topical keratolytics may be helpful (2)[C].
- Shoe orthotics mitigates abnormal biomechanics.
- Physical therapy for stretching and strengthening of the toes helps preserve flexibility, which include intrinsic muscle strengthening (short foot exercises).

MEDICATION

For pain relief

First Line

NSAIDs may be helpful in managing symptoms of pain as well as soft tissue and joint inflammation.

ISSUES FOR REFERRAL

If nonsurgical (conservative) treatment is unsuccessful and/or impractical or patient has combined deformity of MTP joint, PIP joint, and/or DIP joint, then patient may be referred to a podiatric physician/surgeon or orthopedic surgeon.

SURGERY/OTHER PROCEDURES

- Surgical procedures for the correction of hammer toes depend on the degree and flexibility of the contracture(s) and related abnormalities.
- Surgical interventions for *flexible* hammer toes include (1,3,5,6,7)[C]
  – PIP joint arthroplasty or arthrodesis (most common)
  – Flexor tenotomy for reducible or mallet toe deformities with distal ulceration
  – Extensor tendon lengthening/tenotomy/MTP joint capsulotomy
  – Flexor tendon transfer with digital arthrodesis
  – Exostosectomy
  – Implant arthroplasty
- Surgical interventions for semirigid/rigid hammer toes include (1,3,5,7)[C]
  – PIP joint resection arthroplasty or arthrodesis
  – Girdlestone-Taylor flexor-to-extensor transfer
  – Metatarsal shortening (Weil osteotomy)
  – Exostosectomy
  – Middle phalangectomy (more common in 5th toe)
  – Soft tissue releases/lengthening
  – Diaphysectomy of the proximal phalanx (less common)
  – Phalangeal base resection as part of Hoffman-Clayton procedure for RA mutilans
- Procedures may be performed as isolated operations or in conjunction with other procedures.
- Contraindications for surgery: active infection, inadequate vascular supply, and desire for cosmesis alone

 ONGOING CARE

FOLLOW-UP RECOMMENDATIONS

- Obtain radiographs immediately following surgery or at the first postoperative visit; subsequent x-rays as needed
- Full weight-bearing in a postoperative (surgical) shoe or other device based on the procedure(s) performed and the individual patient
- Pinning often used across the MTP joint, which requires limited to non–weight-bearing to the forefoot for 3 to 5 weeks
- Elevate the foot to minimize swelling.
- Return to regular shoe wear after pain is controlled, swelling has subsided, and wounds have healed.
- Role and efficacy of postoperative physical therapy unclear

Patient Monitoring

In the absence of complications, the patient should be seen initially within the 1st week following the procedure(s). Frequency of subsequent visits is determined based on the procedure(s) performed and the postoperative course.

PATIENT EDUCATION

- Patients should be aware of mild to moderate swelling and plantar foot discomfort that may persist for many (1 to 6) months after surgery and may limit footwear options until resolved.
- MTP joint and PIP joint may remain stiff for extended periods of time.
- "Molding" of the operative toe (assuming the contours of adjacent toes) is common.
- Encourage patients to wear shoes of adequate size with "roomy" (rounded or squared) toe box.

PROGNOSIS

- Nonoperative (conservative) treatment in mild deformities usually alleviates pain; however, the deformity may progress.
- Surgical treatment of flexible hammer toe deformity reliably corrects the deformity and alleviates pain. Recurrence and progression are common, especially if the patient continues to wear ill-fitting shoes.
- Surgical treatment of fixed hammer toe deformity provides reliable deformity correction and pain relief. Recurrence is uncommon.

COMPLICATIONS

- Common complications specific to digital surgery include but are not limited to
  – Persistent edema
  – Recurrence of deformity
  – Residual pain
  – Excessive stiffness
  – Metatarsalgia
- Less common complications include
  – Numbness (e.g., digital nerve palsy)
  – Flail toe
  – Symptomatic osseous regrowth
  – Malposition of toe
  – Malunion/nonunion
  – Infection
  – Sausage toe
  – Vascular impairment (e.g., toe ischemia, gangrene)

REFERENCES

1. Shirzad K, Kiesau CD, DeOrio JK, et al. Lesser toe deformities. *J Am Acad Orthop Surg.* 2011;19(8):505–514.
2. Thomas JL, Blitch EL IV, Chaney DM, et al; and Clinical Practice Guideline Forefoot Disorders Panel. Diagnosis and treatment of forefoot disorders. Section 1: digital deformities. *J Foot Ankle Surg.* 2009;48(3):418.e1–418.e9.
3. Zelen CM, Young NJ. Digital arthrodesis. *Clin Podiatr Med Surg.* 2013;30(3):271–282.
4. Hannan MT, Menz HB, Jordan JM, et al. High heritability of hallux valgus and lesser toe deformities in adult men and women. *Arthritis Care Res (Hoboken).* 2013;65(9):1515–1521.
5. Smith BW, Coughlin MJ. Disorders of the lesser toes. *Sports Med Arthrosc Rev.* 2009;17(3):167–174.
6. Kwon JY, De Asla RJ. The use of flexor to extensor transfers for the correction of the flexible hammer toe deformity. *Foot Ankle Clin.* 2011;16(4):573–582.
7. Sung W, Weil L Jr, Weil LS Sr. Retrospective comparative study of operative repair of hammertoe deformity. *Foot Ankle Spec.* 2014;7(3):185–192.

ADDITIONAL READING

- Marx RC, Mizel MS. What's new in foot and ankle surgery. *J Bone Joint Surg Am.* 2013;95(10):951–957.
- Miller JM, Blacklidge DK, Ferdowsian V, et al. Chevron arthrodesis of the interphalangeal joint for hammertoe correction. *J Foot Ankle Surg.* 2010;49(2):194–196.
- Schuberth JM. Hammer toe syndrome. American College of Foot and Ankle Surgeons. *J Foot Ankle Surg.* 1999;38(2):166–178.

 SEE ALSO

Algorithm: Foot Pain

 CODES

ICD10
- M20.40 Other hammer toe(s) (acquired), unspecified foot
- M20.41 Other hammer toe(s) (acquired), right foot
- M20.42 Other hammer toe(s) (acquired), left foot

CLINICAL PEARLS

- Hammer toe is a plantar flexion deformity of the PIP joint. Claw toe and mallet toe are additional types of hammer toes.
- Initial management of hammer toe deformity is conservative. Consider surgery if pain persists or the deformity worsens.
- Properly fitting footwear helps minimize recurrence. Patients should be aware of mild to moderate swelling and plantar foot discomfort that may persist for months after surgery and may limit footwear options until resolved.

H

HAND-FOOT-AND-MOUTH DISEASE

M. Tyler Melson, DO • John M. Doan, DO

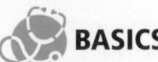 **BASICS**

DESCRIPTION
- Common clinical syndrome caused by enterovirus serotypes
- Prevalent cause of viral exanthem often easily recognized
- Classic appearance of oral enanthem along with rash of hands and feet (classically) and potentially located elsewhere
- Rash may be macular, maculopapular, and/or vesicular.
- Synonym(s): herpangina (when affecting oral mucosa and posterior pharynx)

EPIDEMIOLOGY
- Self-limiting illness resolves in 7 to 10 days.
- Moderately contagious
- Infection is spread by direct contact with nasal secretions, saliva, blister fluid, or stool.
- Infected individuals are most contagious during the 1st week of the illness but may continue to spread illness for days to weeks after. Some exposed individuals (especially adults) may be asymptomatic but still contagious.
- The viruses that cause hand-foot-and-mouth disease (HFMD) can persist for weeks after symptoms have resolved, most commonly in stool, allowing transmission following resolution of symptoms.
- The incubation period is 3 to 7 days (1).

Incidence
- Children <5 years of age are most commonly affected, especially in daycare facilities (1,2).
- Can occur as isolated cases, outbreaks, or epidemics
- Occurs worldwide

- Vertical transmission is possible.
- Most large outbreaks occur in Southeast Asia.

ETIOLOGY AND PATHOPHYSIOLOGY
- HFMD is not the same as foot (hoof) and mouth found in cattle, and there is no cross species infectious concern (3).
- Transmission by the fecal–oral route or contact with skin lesions or oral secretions; caused by viruses that belong to the *Enterovirus* genus and replicated in the GI tract (3)
- Most commonly coxsackievirus A16
- Also coxsackieviruses A5, A7, A9, A10, B2, B5, and enterovirus 71

GENERAL PREVENTION
- Hand washing, especially around food handling or diaper changes
- Exclusion of children from group settings during the first few days of the illness in the presence of open lesions in the mouth or on the skin may reduce the spread of infection.
- Hand hygiene measures are effective in reducing transmission.
- Pregnant woman should avoid contact with infected individuals.

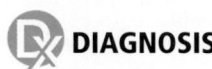 **DIAGNOSIS**

HISTORY
- 1- to 2-day prodrome of fever, anorexia, malaise, abdominal pain, upper respiratory symptoms
- Fever may last 3 to 4 days.
- Maculopapular rash on hands, feet, and mouth. Oral lesions may precede skin.

- Sore throat (follows fever)
- Often history of sick contacts

PHYSICAL EXAM
- Oral enanthem along with tender vesicles becoming ulcers on buccal mucosa, sides of tongue, and palate
- May persist for up to 1 week
- Cutaneous vesicles 3 to 5 mm in diameter start as painful maculopapular eruptions, occur typically on dorsal aspect of fingers and toes.
- May also occur on the palms, soles, buttocks, and groin
- Adults are less likely to have cutaneous findings.
- Nail dystrophies are not uncommon and may persist weeks after.
- Be mindful of CNS symptoms. Although rare, CNS involvement is possible.

DIFFERENTIAL DIAGNOSIS
- Herpetic gingivostomatitis
- Aphthous stomatitis
- Scabies
- Chickenpox
- Measles
- Rubella
- Scarlet fever
- Roseola infantum
- Fifth disease
- Other enteroviral infections
- Kawasaki disease
- Viral pharyngitis
- Varicella
- Rickettsial infection (RFSF)

DIAGNOSTIC TESTS & INTERPRETATION
Clinical diagnosis is typically adequate.

Initial Tests (lab, imaging)
Culture for responsible virus (virus isolation) can be obtained from oral lesions, cutaneous vesicles, naso-pharyngeal swabs, stool, and CSF, although not typically performed. PCR of throat swabs and vesicle fluid is the most efficient test if enterovirus 71 is suspected (3).

 TREATMENT

- Symptomatic
- Avoid spicy or acidic foods to limit oral pain.
- IV fluids may be required in more severe cases of dehydration.

MEDICATION
- Symptomatic care using ibuprofen or acetaminophen for pain from oral ulcers or fever
- Soothing mouthwashes ("magic mouthwash") containing lidocaine do not appear to be superior to placebo and have risk of side effects when absorbed systemically (4)[B].

Pediatric Considerations
Avoid aspirin use in treating febrile illness in children due to concern of Reye syndrome—an encephalopathy associated with aspirin use in viral illness in children.

ADMISSION, INPATIENT, AND NURSING CONSIDERATIONS
- Patients with CNS manifestations or autonomic dysregulation should require hospitalization.
- Admit those with dehydration unable to maintain adequate oral hydration.

 ONGOING CARE

DIET
- Encourage cold liquids (e.g., ice cream, popsicles) to prevent dehydration.
- Avoid acidic, salty, and spicy foods because they will increase pain.

COMPLICATIONS
- Dehydration most common due to painful oral ulcerations
- CNS involvement (i.e., aseptic meningitis) is a rare complication
- Fever >3 days and lethargy are associated with CSF pleocytosis.
- Enterovirus 71 has caused outbreaks and has been implicated in more severe disease associated with CNS infection (5).
- Cardiopulmonary complications include myocarditis, pneumonitis, and pulmonary edema.
- Nail dystrophies (loss of nails, Beau lines) are common.

REFERENCES

1. Centers for Disease Control and Prevention. Hand, foot, and mouth disease (HFMD). http://www.cdc.gov/hand-foot-mouth/. Accessed January 5, 2018.
2. Centers for Disease Control and Prevention. Notes from the field: severe hand, foot, and mouth disease associated with coxsackievirus A6—Alabama, Connecticut, California, and Nevada, November 2011-February 2012. MMWR Morb Mortal Wkly Rep. 2012;61(12):213–214.
3. World Health Organization: Western Pacific Region. A guide to clinical management and public health response for hand, foot and mouth disease (HFMD). http://www.wpro.who.int/publications/docs/GuidancefortheclinicalmanagementofHFMD.pdf. Accessed January 5, 2015.
4. Hopper SM, McCarthy M, Tancharoen C, et al. Topical lidocaine to improve oral intake in children with painful infectious mouth ulcers: a blinded, randomized, placebo-controlled trial. Ann Emerg Med. 2014;63(3):292–299.
5. Hamaguchi T, Fujisawa H, Sakai K, et al. Acute encephalitis caused by intrafamilial transmission of enterovirus 71 in adult. Emerg Infect Dis. 2008;14(5):828–830.

 CODES

ICD10
- B08.4 Enteroviral vesicular stomatitis with exanthem
- B34.1 Enterovirus infection, unspecified
- B08.5 Enteroviral vesicular pharyngitis

CLINICAL PEARLS
- Most common: May to October
- Children <5 years of age tend to have worse symptoms than older children.
- HFMD is the most common cause of mouth sores in pediatric patients.
- Dehydration is a common problem secondary to swallowing aversions.
- Usually self-limiting, resolving in 7 to 10 days
- Careful hand washing to limit dissemination

H

HEADACHE, CLUSTER
Samuel C. Wang, MD, FAAFP • Sumana Basu, MD

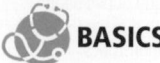

BASICS

DESCRIPTION
- Primary headache disorder
- Multiple attacks of unilateral, excruciating, sharp, searing, or piercing pain; typically localized in the periorbital area and temple accompanied by signs of ipsilateral parasympathetic autonomic features, along with restlessness and agitation
- Autonomic symptoms: parasympathetic hyperactivity signs (ipsilateral lacrimation, eye redness, nasal congestion) and sympathetic hypoactivity (ipsilateral ptosis and miosis)
- Patients often pace the floor during an acute attack because lying down seems to exacerbate the pain.
- Symptoms usually remain on the same side during a single cluster attack.
- Individual attacks last 15 to 180 minutes if untreated and occur from once every other day to 8 times per day.
- Attacks usually occur in series (cluster periods) that are often seasonal, lasting for weeks or months; separated by remission periods usually lasting months or years
- About 10–15% of patients have chronic symptoms without remissions (i.e., chronic cluster headache [cH]).

EPIDEMIOLOGY
Incidence
1-year incidence: 2 to 10/100,000
Prevalence
- Lifetime prevalence: 124/100,000
- Predominant sex: male > female; 2.1:1 overall
- Women often develop earlier in life (20s).
- Mean age of onset: 30 years
- Episodic/chronic ratio: 6:1

ETIOLOGY AND PATHOPHYSIOLOGY
- Complex and incompletely understood
- Proposed mechanism include the following:
  - Posterior hypothalamus activation may trigger an attack by activating trigeminal nociceptive pathways through perivascular activation and increased parasympathetic outflow, causing unilateral pain.

Genetics
- Usually sporadic: autosomal dominant in 5% of cases; autosomal recessive or multifactorial in other families
- Evidence varies: First-degree relatives carry 5- to 8-fold and second degree 1- to 3-fold increased relative risk of disease.
- >50% with migraine and 18% with CH in family history

RISK FACTORS
- Male gender
- Age (70% onset before age 30 years)
- Cigarette smoking or childhood exposure to cigarette smoke
- Family history of CH
- Head trauma

COMMONLY ASSOCIATED CONDITIONS
- Depression (24%)
- Increased risk of suicide secondary to the extreme nature of the pain
- Medication-overuse headache
- Asthma (9%)

- History of migraine, frequently in female patients
- Sleep apnea (30–80%)
- Increased prevalence of cardiac right-to-left shunt and patent foramen ovale (relationship unclear)

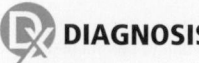

DIAGNOSIS

- Diagnosis is clinical.
- *International Classification of Headache Disorders* (3rd edition) criteria
- At least five attacks of severe or very severe unilateral orbital, supraorbital, and/or temporal pain lasting 15 to 180 minutes if untreated
- At least one of the following:
  - Ipsilateral
    - Conjunctival injection and/or lacrimation
    - Nasal congestion and/or rhinorrhea
    - Eyelid edema
    - Forehead and facial sweating/flushing
    - Sensation of fullness in the ear
    - Miosis and/or ptosis
- Restlessness or agitation during acute attack
- Attack frequency: one every other day to eight per day for more than half of the time during cluster periods
- Episodic CH (eCH): at least two cluster periods lasting 7 days to 1 year, separated by a pain-free interval of >1 month (80–90% of cases)
- Chronic CH (cCH): cluster-free interval of <1 month, for at least a year

HISTORY
- Episodic periods of headache described as excruciating, unilateral, sharp, searing, or piercing pain, typically localized in the periorbital area
- Eye redness, tearing, nasal congestion, clear rhinorrhea, sweating
- Timing of headaches often circadian in nature, usually early morning (12 AM to 3 AM) and early evening, often occurring at the same time each day
- Presence of triggers, including vasodilators (e.g., alcohol, nitroglycerin, sildenafil), histamine, or strong odors
- Seasonal pattern of cluster periods, often recurring around the same time of the year

PHYSICAL EXAM
- Patients are usually seen between attacks, so physical exam is often unremarkable.
- Acute distress, crying, screaming, restlessness, and/or agitation during acute attack
- Ipsilateral lacrimation, injected conjunctivae, ptosis, and miosis during acute attack
- Edematous nasal mucosa or rhinorrhea during acute attack

DIFFERENTIAL DIAGNOSIS
- Other trigeminal autonomic cephalgias (e.g., paroxysmal hemicrania, short-lasting unilateral neuralgiform headache attacks with conjunctival injection and tearing [SUNCT], hemicrania continua, hypnic headaches, trigeminal and other facial neuralgias, migraine, temporal arteritis, herpes zoster)
- Secondary CH:
  - Vertebral or carotid artery dissection, brain arteriovenous malformations, intracranial artery aneurysms
  - Pituitary tumors
  - Nasopharyngeal carcinoma
  - Maxillary sinus with foreign body/sinusitis
  - Cavernous hemangioma
  - Meningiomas/carcinomas/metastases

DIAGNOSTIC TESTS & INTERPRETATION
- Diagnosis is primarily clinical.
- Diagnosis is often delayed (>40% report 5-year delay in diagnosis).
- Consider neuroimaging (MRI/CT head and vascular imaging of brain) if:
  - Abnormal neurologic exam
  - Suspect secondary CH
  - "Red flag" headache symptoms are present.

TREATMENT

Many of the medications discussed in the following section are used off-label in the treatment of CH.

GENERAL MEASURES
- Avoid major changes in sleep habits.
- Stop smoking.
- Avoid use of alcohol during cluster period.
- Avoid extreme changes in altitude due to changes in oxygen levels.
- Avoid exposure to chemical agents/solvents or other known triggers for the patient.

MEDICATION
- Avoid pain medications, especially narcotic analgesics, for acute attacks.
- Goal is abortion of acute attack and transitional prophylaxis for expected duration of the cluster period; long-term prophylaxis used for cCH
- Assess cardiovascular risk before instituting a vasoactive drug, such as triptans or ergot derivatives.

First Line
- For acute attacks:
  - Oxygen
    - 100% at 7 to 12 L/min for 15 minutes via nonrebreather mask or demand valve oxygen mask while sitting or standing provides relief within 15 minutes. High flow used if resistant to low-flow oxygen; excellent side-effect profile (1,2)[A]

ALERT
Avoid high-flow oxygen in severe chronic obstructive pulmonary disease (COPD) because it might reduce respiratory drive.

  - Sumatriptan
    - 6 mg SC, max 2 times per day with at least 1 hour between injections is most effective medication for acute attacks; NNT = 2.4 and 3.3 for headache relief and pain free in 15 minutes, respectively
    - Nasal spray: 20 mg; may repeat in 2 hours, max dose 40 mg/24 hr; NNT = 3.2 for headache relief at 30 minutes (1,3)[A]
  - Zolmitriptan
    - Nasal spray: 5- and 10-mg dosage both effective; may repeat in 2 hours, max 2 times per day; NNT = 12 and 4.9 for headache relief in 15 minutes for 5 and 10 mg, respectively
    - Tablet: 5- and 10-mg dosage both effective; may repeat in 2 hours, max dose 10 mg/24 hr; NNT = 6.7 and 4.5 for headache relief in 30 minutes for 5 and 10 mg, respectively (1,3)[A]

ALERT
Triptans are contraindicated in ischemic cardiac disease, stroke, uncontrolled hypertension, Prinzmetal angina, basilar migraine, hemiplegic migraine, ischemic bowel disease, and peripheral vascular disease.

- For prophylaxis:
  - Used at start of cluster period to prevent and shorten further attacks. Start as soon as possible:
    - Verapamil
      - Start at 80 mg TID and increase by 80 mg/week to 480 mg and then 80 mg every 2 weeks if needed. Short- or long-acting equivalent. Most patients respond to daily dose of 200 to 480 mg, but up to 960 mg/day may be needed; NNT = 1.2 (4)[C]

ALERT
ECG monitoring is required for verapamil dose >400 mg/day because of risk of bradycardia, prolonged PR interval, RBBB, or complete heart block. Avoid grapefruit juice due to CYP3A4 inhibition (4)[C].

Second Line
- For acute attacks:
  - Lidocaine/cocaine: 10 mg (1 mL) of lidocaine or 40 to 50 mg of 10% cocaine intranasal. No well-controlled randomized controlled trials (RCTs) done. Most common side effects are nasal congestion and unpleasant taste.
  - Octreotide: SC 100 μg. Can be considered in patients when triptans are contraindicated. Main side effect is GI upset.
- For prophylaxis:
  - Melatonin: 10-mg regular-release tablet in late evening showed reduction in headache frequency versus placebo in small RCT. No side effects were reported.
  - Lithium: Start 300 mg BID; titrate to therapeutic range of 0.4 to 0.8 mEq/L. Can increase to 300 mg TID in 1 week and then as tolerated. Two RCTs done; one was positive, one was negative. Must monitor drug levels, liver, renal, and thyroid function. Caution with nephrotoxic drugs, diuretics. Monitor for CNS side effects.
  - Civamide: 100 μL of 0.025% into each nostril daily. Only studied in eCH in one trial of 28 patients. Most common side effects were nasal burning, lacrimation, pharyngitis, and rhinorrhea (not available in the United States).
  - Capsaicin: 0.025% ipsilateral nostril for 7 days showed benefit in one small RCT.
  - Warfarin: for refractory cCH. One crossover RCT showed reduction in attack frequency during treatment period compared to placebo period. Patients were treated to an INR goal of 1.5 to 1.9. NNT = 2.6 (1)[B]. Weigh risk of bleeding complications against benefit.

ADDITIONAL THERAPIES
Transitional prophylaxis:
- Used to reduce attack frequency until longer term preventive treatment becomes effective. Longer term maintenance agents are started concurrently.
- Steroids: Several open studies suggested benefit but no rigorous trials to prove efficacy. Studies support 60 to 80 mg/day (initial dose) prednisone with a taper no longer than 18 days to avoid side effects; adverse effects for short-term use: insomnia, psychosis, hyponatremia, edema, hyperglycemia, peptic ulcer (4)[C]
- Suboccipital steroid injection: 3.75 mg of cortivazol injected into the suboccipital area on the ipsilateral side of the headache; single injection or series of three injections, given 48 to 72 hours apart, reduces attack frequency during cluster period when used as add-on therapy to verapamil; NNT = 2.5 (5)[B]
- Dihydroergotamine (DHE): 1 mg injected SC/IM BID–TID for up to a week. Controlled studies are lacking (4)[C].

ALERT
Ergotamines are contraindicated in patients with CV disease and cannot be used with triptans; black box warning against using concomitantly with 3A4 inhibitors, such as protease inhibitors and macrolide antibiotics

Pregnancy Considerations
- Collaboration between headache specialist, obstetrician, pediatrician, and lactation specialist is recommended.
- Patient should be informed of limited data on treatment efficacy versus safety.
- For acute treatment, oxygen is most appropriate first-line therapy. Intranasal lidocaine (pregnancy Category B) can be used as second-line therapy and has no adverse effects with breastfeeding (6)[C].
- For transitional prophylaxis, steroids (pregnancy Category C/D) can be used, but systemic use should be avoided in 1st trimester (6)[C].
- As preventive therapy, verapamil (pregnancy Category C) remains the preferred option. Use of SC or intranasal sumatriptan and zolmitriptan (pregnancy Category C) should be limited as much as possible. Avoid ergotamines (pregnancy Category X) (6)[C].

ISSUES FOR REFERRAL
Consider a neurology or headache center referral for refractory or complicated patients.

SURGERY/OTHER PROCEDURES
- No evidence for Botox or hyperbaric oxygen treatment
- Surgery may be considered only for patients who are refractory to, or have contraindications to, medical therapy.
- Various techniques focus on stimulation or ablation of segments of trigeminal nerve root and sphenopalatine ganglion. Techniques are often invasive and/or involve implantation of devices. Other techniques are aimed at decreasing pain and inflammation surrounding the greater occipital nerve.
- Neurostimulation
  - Multicenter RCT showed efficacy of sphenopalatine ganglion stimulation (SPG) compared to sham treatment; CINTHA Trial ongoing
  - Bilateral occipital nerve stimulation (ONS) has been shown to reduce severity and attack frequency in cCH patients.
  - Deep brain stimulation (DBS) of the hypothalamus has shown a positive response rate but carries risks of stroke, hemorrhage, and death.
  - One open-label, sham-controlled study of noninvasive vagal nerve stimulation (nVNS) used in acute eCH and acute cCH did not show any significant overall difference between groups (nVNS vs. sham), although nVNS was superior to sham in eCH only. Another RCT noted sustained reductions in cCH when used in conjunction with standard therapy.

ADMISSION, INPATIENT, AND NURSING CONSIDERATIONS
- Intractable, severe pain
- Suicidal ideation

ONGOING CARE

FOLLOW-UP RECOMMENDATIONS
Patient Monitoring
- Anticipate cluster bouts and initiate early prophylaxis.
- Monitor for depression and suicidal ideation, especially in those with cCH.
- Watch for adverse medication responses and side effects, such as unmasking of underlying cardiovascular disorder, when using medications to treat CH.

PROGNOSIS
- Unpredictable but often chronic course
- With increasing age, attack frequency often decreases.
- Possibility of transformation of eCH to cCH

COMPLICATIONS
- Depression and suicide
- Side effects of medication, including unmasking of coronary artery disease

REFERENCES
1. Robbins M, Starling A, Pringsheim T, et al. Treatment of cluster headache: the American Headache Society evidence-based guidelines. *Headache*. 2016;56(7):1093–1106.
2. Petersen A, Barloese M, Jensen R. Oxygen treatment of cluster headache: a review. *Cephalalgia*. 2014;34(13):1079–1087.
3. Law S, Derry S, Moore RA. Triptans for acute cluster headache. *Cochrane Database Syst Rev*. 2013;(7):CD008042.
4. Becker WJ. Cluster headache: conventional pharmacological management. *Headache*. 2013;53(7):1191–1196.
5. Leroux E, Valade D, Taifas I, et al. Suboccipital steroid injections for transitional treatment of patients with more than two cluster headache attacks per day: a randomised, double-blind, placebo-controlled trial. *Lancet Neurol*. 2011;10(10):891–897.
6. VanderPluym J. Cluster headache: special considerations for treatment of female patients of reproductive age and pediatric patients. *Curr Neurol Neurosci Rep*. 2016;16(1):5.

ADDITIONAL READING
- Gaul C, Diener HC, Silver N, et al. Non-invasive vagus nerve stimulation for PREVention and Acute treatment of chronic cluster headache (PREVA): a randomised controlled study. *Cephalalgia*. 2016;36(6):534–546.
- International Headache Society: http://www.ihs-headache.org
- Láinez MJ, Guillamón E. Cluster headache and other TACs: pathophysiology and neurostimulation options. *Headache*. 2017;57(2):327–335.

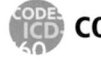 ## CODES

ICD10
- G44.009 Cluster headache syndrome, unspecified, not intractable
- G44.019 Episodic cluster headache, not intractable
- G44.029 Chronic cluster headache, not intractable

CLINICAL PEARLS
- CHs are uncommon but very disabling.
- Patients are often agitated and restless during the acute attack.
- High-flow oxygen and triptans, not narcotics, are first-line therapy for acute attacks.
- Among triptans, injected forms are more effective than nasal sprays, which are more effective than oral tablets.
- Abortive, transitional, and prophylactic treatment must all be considered.

HEADACHE, MIGRAINE

Benjamin N. Schneider, MD

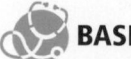 **BASICS**

DESCRIPTION

Recurrent headache disorder manifesting in attacks lasting 4 to 72 hours. Typical characteristics are unilateral location, pulsating quality, moderate or severe intensity, aggravation by physical activity, and association with nausea and/or photophobia and phonophobia (1).

- Most frequent subtypes of migraine (1):
  – Without aura (common migraine): defining >80% of attacks, often associated with nausea, vomiting, photophobia, and/or phonophobia
  – With aura (classic migraine): visual or other types of fully reversible neurologic phenomenon lasting 5 to 60 minutes
  – Chronic (transformed) migraine: chronic headache pattern evolving from episodic migraine. Migraine-like attacks are superimposed on a daily or near-daily headache pattern (e.g., tension headaches) >15 headache days/month for at least 3 months.
  – Menstrual-related (molimina) migraine: associated with onset of menstrual period
- Rare but important subtypes (1):
  – Status migrainosus: debilitating migraine lasting >72 hours
  – With brainstem aura (basilar migraine): brainstem symptoms—dysarthria, vertigo, tinnitus, or ataxia, which are fully reversible, lasting 5 to 60 minutes
  – Hemiplegic migraine: aura consisting of fully reversible hemiplegia and/or hemiparesis
  – Recurrent painful ophthalmoplegic neuropathy (ophthalmoplegic migraine): neuralgia accompanied by paresis of an ocular cranial nerve with ipsilateral headache
  – Retinal: repeated attacks of monocular visual disturbance, including scintillations, scotomata, or blindness, associated with migraine headache

EPIDEMIOLOGY

Female > male (3:1)

Prevalence

- Affects >28 million Americans
- Adults: women 18%; men 6%

ETIOLOGY AND PATHOPHYSIOLOGY

Trigeminovascular hypothesis: Hyperexcitable trigeminal sensory neurons in brainstem are stimulated and release neuropeptides, such as substance P and calcitonin gene-related peptide (CGRP), leading to vasodilation and neurogenic inflammation.

Genetics

- >80% of patients have a positive family history.
- Familial hemiplegic migraine has been shown to be linked to chromosomes 1, 2, and 19 (1).

RISK FACTORS

- Family history of migraine
- Female gender
- Stress
- Menstrual cycle, hormones
- Sleep pattern disruption
- Diet: skipped meals (48%), alcohol (32%), chocolate (20%), cheese (13%), caffeine overuse (14%), monosodium glutamate (MSG) (12%), and artificial sweeteners (e.g., aspartame, sucralose)
- Medications: estrogens, vasodilators

GENERAL PREVENTION

- Avoid precipitants of attacks.
- Lifestyle modifications are the cornerstone of prevention: sleep hygiene, stress management, healthy diet, and regular exercise.
- Biofeedback, education, and psychological intervention
- Prophylactic medication if attacks are frequent, severely debilitating, or not controlled by acute interventions

COMMONLY ASSOCIATED CONDITIONS

- Depression, psychiatric disorders
- Sleep disturbance (e.g., sleep apnea)
- Cerebral vascular disease
- Peripheral vascular disease
- Seizure disorders
- Irritable bowel syndrome
- Obesity
- Medication overuse headache (MOH)

 DIAGNOSIS

Migraine is a clinical diagnosis; thorough history and neuro examination are usually all that are necessary.

HISTORY

- Screening mnemonic "POUND": **P**ulsating, duration of 4 to 72 h**O**urs, **U**nilateral, **N**ausea, **D**isabling
  – + Likelihood ratio (LR) = 24 for migraine diagnosis if 4 of 5 criteria present
  – + LR = 0.41 for migraine diagnosis if ≤2 criteria present (2)
- Headache usually begins with mild pain escalating into unilateral (30–40% bilateral) throbbing (40% nonthrobbing) pain lasting 4 to 72 hours.
- Intensified by movement and associated with systemic manifestations: nausea (87%), vomiting (56%), diarrhea (16%), photophobia (82%), phonophobia (78%), muscle tenderness (65%), light-headedness (72%), and vertigo (33%)
- May be preceded by aura
  – Visual disruptions are most common—scotoma, hemianopsia, fortification spectra, geometric visual patterns, and occasionally hallucinations.
  – Somatosensory disruption in face or arms
  – Speech difficulties
- Obtain headache profile: episodes per month, HA days per month, frequency, and amount and effect of medications used.
- Migraine disability assessment (MiDAS) is a useful tool to assess level of disability and correlates well with headache diaries.
- Identify possible triggers (e.g., stress, sleep disturbance, food, caffeine, alcohol).

PHYSICAL EXAM

Neurologic exam should be performed including funduscopy; abnormalities consistent with other causes for severe headaches may include:

- Gait abnormalities or other cerebellar findings
- Loss of gross and/or fine motor function
- Altered mental status including possible hallucinations (visual, auditory, olfactory)
- Short-term memory loss
- Papilledema

DIFFERENTIAL DIAGNOSIS

- Other primary headache syndromes
- Secondary headaches: tumor, infection, vascular pathology, prescription, or illicit drug use (MOH)
- If focal neurologic signs/symptoms are present, consider transient ischemic attack (TIA) or stroke.
- Psychiatric disease
- Rarely, atypical forms of epilepsy

DIAGNOSTIC TESTS & INTERPRETATION

Neuroimaging is appropriate ONLY with suspicious symptomatology and/or an abnormality on physical examination (3). Other red flags include the following:

- New onset in patient >50 years of age
- Change in established headache pattern
- Atypical pattern or unremitting/progressive neurologic symptoms
- Prolonged or bizarre aura
- Data are insufficient to make evidence-based recommendations regarding use of MRI versus CT in the evaluation of migraine or other nonacute headache.
- EEG is NOT indicated unless evaluating loss of consciousness or altered mental status.

Pediatric Considerations

NSAIDs and triptans are effective for the acute treatment of children and adolescents with migraine. Triptans may have better efficacy than NSAIDs but also have higher rates of side effects. Not all triptans are approved for use in children (4).

Pregnancy Considerations

- Frequency may decrease in 2nd and 3rd trimesters.
- Nonpharmacologic methods are preferred.
- No treatment drug has FDA approval in pregnancy.
  – Acetaminophen (category C) triptans, antiemetics, and short-acting opioids can be considered for acute headaches during pregnancy.
  – Ergotamines are contraindicated (category X).
  – Avoid herbal remedies.
  – Sumatriptan, naratriptan, and opiates are pregnancy Category C—risk cannot be ruled out, but early data suggest no increase in birth defects.
  – Sumatriptan by injection is ideal for breastfeeding women with disabling migraines.
  – Propranolol (category C) is effective for prophylaxis during pregnancy and lactation.

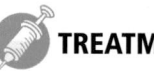 **TREATMENT**

GENERAL MEASURES

- Most patients manage attacks with self-care.
- Cold compresses to area of pain
- Withdrawal from stressful surroundings
- Sleep is desirable.
- See also "General Prevention."

MEDICATION

- First-line abortive treatments
  – Mild to moderate attacks:
    ○ Acetaminophen is effective and when combined with metoclopramide has relief rates similar to triptans (5)[A].
    ○ NSAIDs are inexpensive and effective in up to 60% of cases (5)[B].
    ○ Aspirin-acetaminophen–caffeine (Excedrin Migraine) is an inexpensive, OTC treatment with efficacy higher than its components (5)[B].

- Moderate to severe attacks:
  - Triptans when OTC agents fail for moderate attacks OR first line for severe attacks (6)[B]
  - All triptans have similar efficacy/tolerability, but patients often respond better to one triptan over another (5)[C]. Suggested initial doses:
    - Sumatriptan 100 mg PO; 6 mg subcut; 20 mg intranasal. subcut is most rapid.
    - Eletriptan 40 mg PO
    - Rizatriptan 10 mg PO
    - Zolmitriptan 2.5 mg PO; 5 mg intranasal
    - Naratriptan 2.5 mg PO
    - Frovatriptan 2.5 mg PO
      - 44–77% of patients taking triptans report complete pain relief within 2 hours.
      - Frovatriptan and naratriptan have slow onset but long half-lives—best for people with long migraine duration/recurrence.
  - Combination triptan and NSAID: Sumatriptan 85 mg/naproxen 500 mg PO at onset of headache show improved efficacy over either alone.
  - Monoclonal antibodies: Erenumab (Aimovig), FDA-approved in 2018, is one of four novel medications in late-stage trials targeting CGRP.
  - Antiemetics: Dopamine antagonists are excellent adjunctive medications (5)[B].
- Contraindications to treatments
  - Avoid triptans and ergots in coronary artery or peripheral vascular disease, uncontrolled hypertension, and complicated migraine (e.g., brainstem or hemiplegic migraine).
  - Do not combine triptans or use with ergots or MAOIs.
  - Avoid opioids or butalbital in patients with frequent migraines.
- Precautions
  - Frequent use of acute-treatment drugs can result in MOH.
  - Triptan's adverse reactions are common and include chest pressure, flushing, weakness, dizziness, feeling of warmth, and paresthesias.
- Second-line abortive treatment
  - Dihydroergotamine: drug of choice in status migrainosus and triptan resistance
  - Opiate use can contribute to MOH with use as few as 8 days per month.
- First-line preventative treatment
  - Should not be limited to pharmacologic agents; trigger reduction, biofeedback, relaxation techniques, and CBT have evidence of efficacy.
  - Lifestyle modifications should be recommended for all migraine sufferers.
  - ~38% of migraineurs need preventive therapy, but only 3–13% use it. Trial and error is needed to determine optimal therapy.
- The American Migraine Prevalence and Prevention Study suggests prophylactic treatment when:
  - Quality of life is severely impaired.
  - ≥6 headache days per month, ≥4 headache days per month of moderate severity, or ≥2 headache days per month of severe impairment
  - Migraines do not respond to abortive treatment.
  - Frequent, very long, or uncomfortable auras occur.
- Prevention of *episodic migraine*: Divalproex, valproate, topiramate, metoprolol, and timolol are effective in reducing frequency/severity.
  - NSAIDs appear effective for prevention in people with predictable triggers (menses, etc.) but pose a risk for MOH.
  - For treatment/prevention of *chronic migraine*, botulinum toxin A (Botox) significantly reduces frequency of headache days by 2 days relative to placebo (6)[B].

ISSUES FOR REFERRAL
- Obscure diagnosis, concomitant medical conditions, significant psychopathology
- Unresponsive to usual treatment
- Analgesic-dependent headache patterns

COMPLEMENTARY & ALTERNATIVE MEDICINE
- Riboflavin (vitamin B_2): 400 mg/day (7)[B]
- Magnesium: 400 mg/day (7)[B]
- MIG-99 (Feverfew): 6.25 mg TID (7)[B]
- Histamine subcut: 1 to 10 ng twice weekly (7)[B]
- Melatonin: 3 mg nightly
- Acupuncture is as effective as prophylactic drug treatment and has fewer adverse effects.
- Butterbur use is controversial. Although effective, recent safety concerns in Europe limit its use.

ADMISSION, INPATIENT, AND NURSING CONSIDERATIONS
- Admission is rarely necessary, unless diagnosis is not clear or in the case of status migrainosus.
- Hydration and antiemetics are central to management. Various IV dihydroergotamine protocols can be found.
- Discharge criteria judgment based on patient's overall clinical status and patient's ability to tolerate PO medications

 ONGOING CARE

FOLLOW-UP RECOMMENDATIONS
- Early intervention is key at the onset of an attack.
- Preventive treatment to decrease frequency and severity of attacks, make acute treatments more efficacious, and minimize adverse drug reactions
- Prophylactic medications can be recommended to any patient but should be offered if attacks are frequent, severely debilitating, or not controlled by acute interventions.

Patient Monitoring
- Like many chronic conditions, patients suffering from migraine headaches tend to benefit from regular office visits. Quarterly or even more frequent appointments may be necessary when headaches are suboptimally controlled.
- Monitor frequency of attacks, pain behaviors, and medication usage via headache diary.
- Encourage lifestyle modifications. Counsel patients and manage expectations.
- Regular lab monitoring is not recommended, but given that migraine (especially with aura) is a risk factor for stroke, lipid assessment and other harm reduction such as tobacco cessation are reasonable.

PATIENT EDUCATION
Patient education is central to the treatment of migraines.
- Trigger identification and modification can significantly improve headache frequency.
- Setting expectations is also critical, especially with regard to prophylactic medications where success is often defined as a reduction of 50% in severity or frequency of headaches.

PROGNOSIS
- With increasing age, there may be a reduction in severity, frequency, and disability of attacks.
- Most attacks subside within 72 hours.

COMPLICATIONS
- Status migrainosus (>72 hours)
- MOH: headache 10 or more days per month for >3 months due to regular overuse of an acute or symptomatic headache medication; likelihood with butalbital > opiates > triptans > NSAIDs
- Cerebral ischemic events (rare)

REFERENCES
1. Headache Classification Committee of the International Headache Society. The International Classification of Headache Disorders, 3rd edition (beta version). *Cephalalgia*. 2013;33(9):629–808.
2. Detsky ME, McDonald DR, Baerlocher MO, et al. Does this patient with headache have a migraine or need neuroimaging? *JAMA*. 2006;296(10):1274–1283.
3. Loder E, Weizenbaum E, Frishberg B, et al; for American Headache Society Choosing Wisely Task Force. Choosing wisely in headache medicine: the American Headache Society's list of five things physicians and patients should question. *Headache*. 2013;53(10):1651–1659.
4. Richer L, Billinghurst L, Linsdell MA, et al. Drugs for the acute treatment of migraine in children and adolescents. *Cochrane Database Syst Rev*. 2016;(4):CD005220.
5. Becker WJ. Acute migraine treatment in adults. *Headache*. 2015;55(6):778–793.
6. Herd CP, Tomlinson CL, Rick C, et al. Botulinum toxins for the prevention of migraine in adults. *Cochrane Database Syst Rev*. 2018;(6):CD011616.
7. Holland S, Silberstein SD, Freitag F, et al. Evidence-based guideline update: NSAIDs and other complementary treatments for episodic migraine prevention in adults: report of the Quality Standards Subcommittee of the American Academy of Neurology and the American Headache Society. *Neurology*. 2012;78(17):1346–1353.

 SEE ALSO

Algorithm: Headache, Chronic

 CODES

ICD10
- G43.909 Migraine, unsp, not intractable, without status migrainosus
- G43.109 Migraine with aura, not intractable, w/o status migrainosus
- G43.409 Hemiplegic migraine, not intractable, w/o status migrainosus

CLINICAL PEARLS
- Migraine is a chronic headache disorder of unclear etiology often characterized by unilateral, throbbing headaches that may be associated with additional neurologic symptoms.
- Accurate diagnosis of migraine is crucial.
- Consider nonspecific analgesics and antiemetics for mild attacks; migraine-specific treatments for more severe attacks
- Avoid opiates and barbiturates as well as frequent (>8 per month) use of triptans or NSAIDs to avoid creating a MOH.
- All patients should be counseled on lifestyle modifications and trigger identification.
- In those with frequent or highly debilitating migraines, prophylactic treatment should be encouraged.

H

HEADACHE, TENSION
Assim AlAbdulKader, MD, MPH • Jason Chao, MD, MS

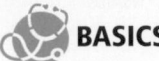

BASICS

DESCRIPTION
- Typically characterized by bilateral mild to moderate pain or pressure without other associated symptoms
- Three types of tension-type headache (TTH):
  – Infrequent episodic TTH: <1 day per month
  – Frequent episodic TTH: ≥1 but <15 days per month
  – Chronic TTH: ≥15 days per month for >3 months
- TTHs replaced older terms: muscle contraction headache, stress or tension headache, and psychogenic headache

EPIDEMIOLOGY
The most common type of primary headache

Prevalence
- Peak age of prevalence in the United States: the 4th decade
- Lifetime prevalence: men (69%); women (88%)
- Prevalence of episodic TTH decreases with age, whereas the prevalence of chronic TTH increases with age.

ETIOLOGY AND PATHOPHYSIOLOGY
- Debatable: peripheral and/or central mechanisms
- Activation of peripheral nociceptors leads to myofascial pain in episodic TTH.
- Prolonged stimulation of nociceptors sensitizes the central pain pathways leading to chronic TTH.
- Nitric oxide may play an important role in TTH.

Genetics
An increased genetic risk has been suggested by studies, particularly for chronic TTH.

RISK FACTORS
Associated with triggers/precipitating factors:
- Stress (mental or physical): the most common
- Change in sleep regimen
- Skipping meals
- Certain foods (caffeine, alcohol, chocolate)
- Dehydration
- Physical exertion
- Environmental factors (sun glare, odors, smoke, noise, lighting)
- Poor or sustained posture
- Female hormonal changes
- Medications (e.g., nitrates, SSRIs, antihypertensives)
- Overuse of abortive headache medication

GENERAL PREVENTION
- Identify and avoid triggers/precipitating factors.
- Minimize physical and emotional stress.
- Encourage relaxation techniques: biofeedback, relaxation therapy, and physical therapy.
- Consider counseling/psychotherapy.

COMMONLY ASSOCIATED CONDITIONS
- 83% of patients with migraine headaches also suffer from TTHs.
- Debatable: increased prevalence of comorbid anxiety and depression

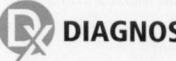

DIAGNOSIS

HISTORY
Obtain a thorough pain history to rule out other headache disorders, including onset, location, radiation, quality of pain, severity, associated symptoms; concurrent medical conditions and medications; and recent trauma or other procedures.

- Diagnosis is based on clinical symptoms.
  – Diagnostic criteria provided by the International Headache Society (1):
    ○ Headache lasting 30 minutes to 7 days
    ○ At least two of the following:
      ▪ Bilateral location
      ▪ Pressing/tightening (nonpulsating) quality
      ▪ Mild or moderate intensity
      ▪ Not aggravated by routine physical activity
    ○ Not associated with nausea or vomiting (chronic type may be associated with nausea)
    ○ No more than one of the following: photophobia or phonophobia
  – Headache not due to another disorder
  – Fronto-occipital or generalized pain (dull, pressing, or bandlike)
  – Associated symptoms:
    ○ Fatigue
    ○ Irritability
    ○ Difficulty concentrating
    ○ Muscular tightness, tenderness, or stiffness in neck, occipital, and frontal regions

PHYSICAL EXAM
- General physical exam: vital signs, funduscopic and cardiovascular assessment, palpation of the head and neck
- Neurologic exam: mental status, pupillary responses, motor-strength testing, deep tendon reflexes, sensation, cerebellar function, gait testing, signs of meningeal irritation

DIFFERENTIAL DIAGNOSIS
- Migraine headache
- Cluster headache
- Head trauma
- Subarachnoid hemorrhage (SAH)
- Subdural hematoma
- Unruptured vascular malformation
- Ischemic cerebrovascular disease
- Temporal arteritis
- Arterial hypertension (HTN)
- Cerebral venous thrombosis
- Benign intracranial HTN
- Intracranial neoplasm, infection, or meningitis
- Low CSF pressure
- Medication (nonprescription analgesic dependency, nitrates)
- Caffeine dependency
- Metabolic disorders (hypoxia, hypercapnia, hypoglycemia)
- Toxic effects from drugs or fumes
- Temporomandibular joint syndrome

- Eyes: glaucoma, refractive errors
- Sinusitis or middle ear infection
- Cervical spondylosis
- Severe anemia or polycythemia
- Uremia and hepatic disorders
- Paget disease of bone

DIAGNOSTIC TESTS & INTERPRETATION
- Most primary headaches with typical features do not require lab testing or diagnostic imaging.
- Labs and neuroimaging (CT or MRI) are only necessary when a secondary cause is suspected:
  – Atypical pattern of headache (does not fit specific category such as migraine, cluster, or tension)
  – Rapid increase in frequency
  – Unexplained focal neurologic findings
  – New onset after age 40 years
  – Sudden onset or worsening with exertion
- MRI with and without contrast is the test of choice. However, head CT is preferred in emergency settings.
- If acute SAH is suspected, head CT should be performed before lumbar puncture (1)[C].

TREATMENT

- Nonsteroidal anti-inflammatory drugs (NSAIDs), acetaminophen, and aspirin are effective for short-term relief of episodic TTH (2,3)[B].
- Amitriptyline should be considered first line for prophylaxis of chronic TTH (2,3)[B].

GENERAL MEASURES
Relief measures: relaxation routines; rest in quiet, dark room; hot bath or shower; massage of back of neck and temples

MEDICATION
Choice of simple analgesic is based on patient-specific parameters:
- NSAIDs may be more effective than acetaminophen for episodic TTH (2)[C]: Ibuprofen and naproxen may be preferred due to better GI tolerability.
- Acetaminophen should be considered for patients taking warfarin, unable to tolerate NSAIDs, or allergic to aspirin or NSAIDs.

First Line
- For acute treatment in episodic TTH:
  – NSAIDs:
    ○ Ibuprofen (Motrin, Advil): 200 to 400 mg; may repeat q8h PRN (max 3.2 g/day)
    ○ Naproxen sodium (Naprosyn): 220 to 550 mg BID PRN (max 1,250 mg base per day)
    ○ Contraindications: aspirin or NSAID allergy or bronchospasm, renal disease, bleeding disorders, increased risk of cardiovascular events (myocardial infarction [MI], stroke, new onset or worsening of HTN)
    ○ Drug interactions: antihypertensives, anticoagulants, antiplatelet drugs, aspirin, lithium, methotrexate
    ○ Adverse effects: epigastric distress, peptic ulcer

– Aspirin: 650 to 1,000 mg; may repeat q6h PRN (max 4 g/day):
  ○ Contraindication: aspirin or NSAID allergy or bronchospasm, bleeding disorders, peptic ulcer
  ○ Drug interactions: anticoagulants, antiplatelet drugs, ACE inhibitors, β-blockers, corticosteroids, NSAIDs, sulfonylureas
  ○ Adverse effects: GI irritation/bleeding, thrombocytopenia
– Acetaminophen (Tylenol): 1,000 mg; may repeat q6h PRN (max 3 to 4 g/day):
  ○ Adverse effects (rare): rash, pancytopenia, liver damage
  ○ Precaution: hepatic impairment, consumption of ≥3 per day alcoholic beverages
- For prophylaxis in frequent episodic and chronic TTH:
  – Tricyclic antidepressants (TCAs): Amitriptyline [Elavil]: Start at 10 mg, may slowly up-titrate to 100 mg QHS.
    ○ Not FDA-approved for chronic TTH
    ○ Consider if patient has depression, anxiety, or insomnia.
    ○ Contraindications: acute recovery phase of MI, use of monoamine oxidase inhibitors (MAOIs) within 14 days
    ○ Drug interactions: clonidine, MAOIs, quinolone antibiotics, SSRIs, sympathomimetics, azole antifungals, valproic acid
    ○ Adverse effects: drowsiness, dry mouth, tachycardia, heart block, blurred vision, urinary retention, seizure

Second Line
- For acute treatment in episodic TTH:
  – Caffeine combinations: 130-mg caffeine with 500-mg acetaminophen and/or 500-mg aspirin q6h PRN (2)[C]
  – Ketorolac: 60 mg IM once, for severe episodes
  – Opioids (e.g., codeine), butalbital, or their combination: not recommended. Consider secondary causes of headache or secondary gain such as drug-seeking behavior for personal use or diversion/sale.
- For prophylaxis in frequent episodic and chronic TTH:
  – Mirtazapine: 15 to 30 mg/day (not FDA-approved for chronic TTH) (2,3)[B]
  – Venlafaxine XR (Effexor XR): 37.5 mg, may be slowly up-titrated to goal dose of 75 to 150 mg/day (not FDA-approved for chronic TTH) (2,3)[B]

ALERT
Use of abortive agents >2 days/week may lead to *medication-overuse headaches*; must withdraw acute treatment to diagnose

Pediatric Considerations
Aspirin and antidepressants are contraindicated.

ADDITIONAL THERAPIES
- The combination of stress management therapy and a TCA (amitriptyline) may be most effective for chronic TTH.
- Topiramate: 100 mg/day (limited clinical evidence for prevention of chronic TTH; not FDA-approved for chronic TTH)

- Alternative TCAs: limited evidence of benefit (4)[B]
  – Desipramine (Norpramin): 50 to 100 mg/day
  – Imipramine (Tofranil): 50 to 100 mg/day
  – Nortriptyline (Pamelor): 25 to 50 mg/day
  – Protriptyline (Vivactil): 25 mg/day
- Drugs with conflicting clinical evidence for chronic TTH (not FDA-approved for chronic TTH):
  – Tizanidine: 2 to 6 mg TID
  – Memantine: 20 to 40 mg/day
- Botulinum toxin type A is not likely to be effective for episodic TTH or chronic TTH.

COMPLEMENTARY & ALTERNATIVE MEDICINE
- Tiger Balm or peppermint oil (not FDA-approved for TTH) applied topically to the forehead may be effective for episodic TTH (5)[B].
- Cognitive-behavioral therapy may be helpful (2,5)[C].
- Electromyography (EMG) biofeedback may be effective and is enhanced when combined with relaxation therapy (2,5)[C].
- Physical therapy, including positioning, ergonomic instruction, massage, transcutaneous electrical nerve simulation, and application of heat/cold may help.
- Chiropractic spinal manipulation has equivocal evidence in the management of episodic and chronic TTH (5)[B].
- Acupuncture may decrease symptoms frequency; NNT = 3 to have at least 50% reduction in headache frequency, compared to routine care (6)[B]

ADMISSION, INPATIENT, AND NURSING CONSIDERATIONS
Typical symptoms usually managed in the outpatient setting. However, red flag symptoms may prompt emergent evaluation (thunderclap onset, fever and meningismus, papilledema with focal signs); or urgent management (temporal arteritis, relevant systemic illness, papilledema without focal signs, elderly patient with new headache and cognitive changes).

ONGOING CARE

FOLLOW-UP RECOMMENDATIONS
- Keep headache diary to identify triggers, monitor progress, and prevent medication-overuse headache.
- Regulate sleep schedule.
- Regular exercise

DIET
- Identify and avoid dietary triggers.
- Regulate meal schedule.

PATIENT EDUCATION
- National Headache Foundation: http://www.headaches.org/resources
- Family Doctor by AAFP: https://familydoctor.org/condition/headaches

PROGNOSIS
- Usually follows a chronic course when life stressors are not changed
- Most cases are intermittent and decreases with age.

COMPLICATIONS
- Lost days of work and productivity (more with CTTH)
- Cost to health system
- Medication-overuse headache
- Dependence/addiction to narcotic analgesics
- GI bleeding from NSAID use

REFERENCES
1. Headache Classification Committee of the International Headache Society (IHS) The International Classification of Headache Disorders, 3rd edition. *Cephalalgia.* 2018;38(1):1–211.
2. Bendtsen L, Jensen R. Treating tension-type headache—an expert opinion. *Expert Opin Pharmacother.* 2011;12(7):1099–1109.
3. Becker WJ, Findlay T, Moga C, et al. Guideline for primary care management of headache in adults. *Can Fam Physician.* 2015;61(8):670–679.
4. Verhagen AP, Damen L, Berger MY, et al. Lack of benefit for prophylactic drugs of tension-type headache in adults: a systematic review. *Fam Pract.* 2010;27(2):151–165.
5. Sun-Edelstein C, Mauskop A. Complementary and alternative approaches to the treatment of tension-type headache. *Curr Pain Headache Rep.* 2012;16(6):539–544.
6. Linde K, Allais G, Brinkhaus B, et al. Acupuncture for the prevention of tension-type headache. *Cochrane Database Syst Rev.* 2016;(4):CD007587.

SEE ALSO

Algorithm: Headache, Chronic

CODES

ICD10
- G44.209 Tension-type headache, unspecified, not intractable
- G44.219 Episodic tension-type headache, not intractable
- G44.229 Chronic tension-type headache, not intractable

CLINICAL PEARLS
- Don't perform neuroimaging studies in patients with stable headache.
- Don't recommend frequent or prolonged use of over-the-counter (OTC) pain medications for headache.
- Medication-overuse headaches must be avoided by limiting use of abortive agents to no more than 2 days/week.
- Chronic TTH is difficult to treat, and these patients are more likely to develop medication-overuse headache.
- Don't prescribe opioids or butalbital-containing medications as first-line treatment for recurrent headaches.
- Consider secondary causes of headaches if there are unexplained focal signs, atypical presentation, late onset (>50 years of age), or when usual treatment fails.

H

HEARING LOSS
Susan L. Steffans, DO

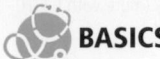 **BASICS**

DESCRIPTION
- Decrease in the ability to perceive and comprehend sound. It can be partial, complete, unilateral, or bilateral.
- Types of hearing loss include conductive hearing loss (CHL or air–bone gap), sensorineural hearing loss (SNHL), or mixed hearing loss.
- System(s) affected: auditory; outer and middle ear (CHL) or inner ear, auditory nerve, and/or brainstem (SNHL)

EPIDEMIOLOGY
- All ages affected; common in children (CHL) and elderly (SNHL)
- Usually more severe at an earlier age in men

Incidence
- Increases with age
- Sudden sensorineural hearing loss (SSHL) occurs in 5 to 20 per 100,000 persons per year.

Prevalence
WHO estimates that 538 million people affected worldwide

Geriatric Considerations
- 24.7% of 60 to 69 year olds in United States have bilateral speech-frequency hearing loss.
- ~80% of people aged >85 years have hearing loss.
- Hearing aids are underused.
- Loss of communication is a source of emotional stress and a physical risk for the elderly.

Pediatric Considerations
- Congenital hearing loss
  - 1 to 6/1,000 infants have hearing loss.
  - Mandatory screening in >97% of newborns with otoacoustic emission (OAE) and auditory brainstem response (ABR) testing
- Audiologic testing after major intracranial infection (meningitis)
- Significant hearing loss at birth and infancy can lead to speech, language, and cognitive delays. Early diagnosis and treatment improves outcome.

Pregnancy Considerations
- Otosclerosis can worsen during pregnancy.
- Maternal infections cause permanent pediatric hearing loss.

ETIOLOGY AND PATHOPHYSIOLOGY
- CHL: Hearing loss can result from middle ear effusion, obstruction of canal (cerumen/foreign body, osteomas/exostoses, cholesteatoma, tumor), loss of continuity (ossicular discontinuity), stiffening of the components (myringosclerosis, tympanosclerosis, and otosclerosis), and loss of the pressure differential across the tympanic membrane (TM) (perforation).
- SNHL: damage along the pathway from oval window, cochlea, auditory nerve, and brainstem. Examples include vascular/metabolic insult, mass effect, infection and inflammation, and acoustic trauma.
  - Noise-induced hearing loss is caused by acoustic insult that affects outer hair cells in the organ of Corti, causing them to be less stiff. Over time, severe damage occurs with fusion and loss of stereocilia; eventually may progress to inner hair cells and auditory nerve as well

- Large vestibular aqueduct or superior canal dehiscence: Third mobile window shunts acoustic energy away from cochlea.

Genetics
- Connexin 26 (13q11–13q12): most common cause of nonsyndromic genetic hearing loss
- Mitochondrial disorders (may predispose to aminoglycoside ototoxicity)
- Otosclerosis: familial
- Most common congenital syndromes
  - Alport syndrome
  - Stickler syndrome
  - Congenital cytomegalovirus
  - Usher syndrome
  - Branchio-oto-renal syndrome
  - Pendred syndrome
  - CHARGE association
  - Neurofibromatosis type 2
  - Waardenburg syndrome

RISK FACTORS
- Conductive
  - Eustachian tube dysfunction
    - Chronic sinusitis; allergy
    - Adenoid hypertrophy; nasopharyngeal mass
    - Cigarette smoking
  - Sleep apnea with continuous positive airway pressure (CPAP) use
  - Neuromuscular disease
  - Family history/heredity
  - Prematurity and low birth weight
  - Craniofacial abnormalities (e.g., cleft palate, Down syndrome)
  - Third mobile window (superior canal dehiscence or large vestibular aqueduct)
- Sensorineural
  - Aging/older age
  - Loud noise/acoustic trauma
  - Dizziness/vertigo: especially Ménière disease or history of labyrinthitis
  - Medications (aminoglycosides, loop diuretics, aspirin, quinine, chemotherapeutic agents, especially cisplatin)
  - Bacterial meningitis
  - Head trauma
  - Atherosclerosis
  - Vestibular schwannoma/skull base neoplasm
  - Previous ear surgery
- Sensorineural, pediatric specific
  - Perinatal asphyxia
  - Mechanical ventilation lasting ≥5 days
  - Congenital infections (toxoplasmosis, other agents, rubella, cytomegalovirus, herpes simplex [TORCH] syndrome)
  - Toxemia of pregnancy
  - Maternal diabetes
  - Rh incompatibility
  - Prematurity or birth weight <1,500 g
  - Severe hyperbilirubinemia; exchange transfusions
  - Anomalous temporal bone (Mondini or large vestibular aqueduct)
  - Infectious diseases: chickenpox, measles, encephalitis, influenza, mumps, bacterial meningitis

GENERAL PREVENTION
- Limit noise exposure; use hearing protection.
- Avoid ear canal instrumentation (e.g., cotton swabs).
- Limit ototoxic medications.

 DIAGNOSIS

HISTORY
- The U.S. Preventive Services Task Force concludes that the current evidence is insufficient to assess the balance of benefits and harms of screening for hearing loss in asymptomatic adults aged 50 years or older.
- Social problems and comments from friends and family members are often the first presentation of presbycusis (age-related hearing loss) because patients are often not aware of the degree of hearing loss they experience and how it affects their life; insidious onset and progression
- Difficulty hearing
  - Rapid versus gradual decline: Rapid loss (<3 days) is a medical emergency. Urgent ENT referral and steroid therapy are recommended.
  - Difficulty with discrimination of sounds, hearing in crowds, or turning up the volume of television sets
  - Frequently having to ask speakers to repeat
  - Friends/family complain of hearing loss.
- Tinnitus, bilateral or unilateral
- Otalgia
- Otorrhea, clear or purulent
- Dizziness or vertigo
- Aural fullness
- Autophony (hearing own voice louder or echoing)
- History of ear infections or ear surgeries
- History of trauma or noise exposure
- Family history of hearing loss
- History of recent viral infection

PHYSICAL EXAM
- Whispered voice test: A whisper heard from ~2 feet away is a good screen for intact hearing. Patients with SNHL have difficulty with this because their hearing loss is usually in the high frequency range.
- A simple 512-Hz tuning fork test lateralizes to unaffected ear in sudden SNHL (emergency) and lateralizes to the affected ear in CHL (not an emergency).
- 512-Hz tuning fork tests:
  - Sensorineural loss
    - Placed on the forehead: lateralizes to unaffected ear (Weber test)
    - Base of tuning fork placed on the mastoid and then fork end placed next to ear; heard louder next to ear-Air > Bone (+Rinne test)
  - Conductive loss
    - Placed on the forehead or teeth lateralizes to affected or symptomatic ear
    - Placed on the mastoid and then next to ear; heard louder behind the ear on the side of conductive deficit Bone > Air (−Rinne Test)
- Otoscopy: Assess for deformity, canal patency, and otorrhea; TM integrity/retraction/mobility with insufflation, canal, or middle ear mass
- Facial symmetry
- Cranial nerve exam
- Nasopharyngoscopy: adenoid hypertrophy or nasopharyngeal mass (mandatory in adult patient with new unilateral serous effusion)
- Pediatric: Survey for syndromic anomalies.

DIFFERENTIAL DIAGNOSIS
- Conductive
  - Cerumen impaction/foreign body
  - Perforation of TM
  - Middle ear fluid (serous otitis media)
  - Acute otitis media/adhesive otitis media

– Ossicular erosion (infection, cholesteatoma)
– Myringosclerosis/tympanosclerosis
– Temporal bone fracture
– Otosclerosis
– Glomus tumor
• Sensorineural
– Presbycusis (age-related hearing loss)
– Noise induced (recreational, occupational)
– Ménière disease
– Ototoxicity (aspirin, aminoglycosides)
– Viral labyrinthitis
– Cerebellopontine angle (CPA) tumor
– Large vestibular aqueduct syndrome
– Syndromic hearing loss
– Congenital cochlear malformation
– Syphilis
– Cytomegalovirus; rubella
– Temporal bone fracture
– Metabolic (hyper-/hypothyroidism)
– Paget disease
– Perilymphatic (inner ear) fistula

DIAGNOSTIC TESTS & INTERPRETATION
Often, labs are not needed. If indicated

• MRI of the brain and brainstem with gadolinium to evaluate SNHL in congenital, early onset, and asymmetric hearing loss
• Fine-cut CT temporal bones without contrast may help in the evaluation of CHL.
• Newborn screening with OAE and/or ABR
• Any pediatric patient with SNHL: Consider genetic testing for connexin 26, mitochondrial studies.
• TORCH screening (congenital infection)
• Rapid plasma reagin (RPR) or venereal disease research laboratory (VDRL) confirmed by fluorescent treponemal antibody absorption (FTA-ABS)
• Lyme titer in endemic areas
• Antinuclear antibodies and sedimentation rate as a screen for autoimmune disease
• Pendred syndrome (goiter, mental retardation + SNHL): perchlorate test, thyroid function tests
• Alport syndrome (nephritis + SNHL): urinalysis, renal function tests
• Jervell and Lange-Nielsen syndrome (syncope, family history of sudden death + profound SNHL): ECG

Diagnostic Procedures/Other
• Audiometry: pure tone (air and bone), speech testing, and impedance (middle ear pressure) testing
• Tympanometry: Type B or C tympanograms indicate fluid or retraction, respectively. Negative middle ear peak pressures were seen even with normal (type A) tympanograms.
• Other tests
– ABR
– OAEs: "echo" of the cochlea
– Behavioral (visual reinforcement) audiometry; used in children 6 months to 5 years old
• Myringotomy and tubes can be considered for persistent fluid with hearing loss.

Test Interpretation
Varies depending on etiology

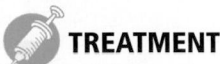

TREATMENT

MEDICATION
• Depends on cause
• Clinical practical guidelines for sudden hearing loss include the following (1)[C]:
– Distinguishing SNHL from CHL; testing for bilateral sudden hearing loss in patients with unilateral sudden hearing loss; obtaining an MRI, ABR, or audiometric follow-up to evaluate for retrocochlear pathology; offer intratympanic steroid perfusion for refractory cases after initial management fails to treat idiopathic sudden SNHL (ISSNHL) and follow-up within 6 months of diagnosis.
– May offer corticosteroids as initial therapy to patients with ISSNHL and hyperbaric oxygen within 3 months of ISSNHL diagnosis
– Recommend against prescribing antivirals, thrombolytics, vasodilators, vasoactive substances, or antioxidants to patients with ISSNHL.
– Recommend against routine laboratory tests in patients with ISSNHL.
• Treatment should begin ASAP, ideally within 1 to 2 weeks of onset with high-dose oral steroids: 1 mg/kg or 60 to 100 mg/day prednisone or 12 to 16 mg/day dexamethasone for 7 to 14 days, followed by a taper.
• Intratympanic steroids show similar efficacy to oral steroids and reduce systemic side effects (2)[A].
• Newer studies are suggesting benefit of combined therapy (oral systemic steroid and intratympanic steroid injections) for first-line treatment of sudden SNHL (3)[A].

ISSUES FOR REFERRAL
• Required for failure of newborn screen, but 32% lost to follow-up
– Collaborating with Women, Infants, and Children (WIC) program to provide targeted follow-up improved loss to follow-up rates, decreased age at hearing confirmation by 1 month, and addressed reported care barriers (4)[B].
• Audiology: If hearing loss is suspected, refer to audiology for formal evaluation. Audiologists also provide hearing aid options and maintenance.
• Genetics: if congenital syndrome or familial hearing loss is suspected
• Speech therapist: if speech delay or speech impediment is present
• Endocrinology: Pendred syndrome, other associated endocrine disorder (hypo-/hyperthyroidism)
• Cardiology: Jervell and Lange-Nielsen syndrome
• Ophthalmology: Usher syndrome
• Neurology and neurosurgery: CPA lesion, intracranial complication of middle ear disease

ADDITIONAL THERAPIES
Aural rehabilitation: interdisciplinary approach involving audiologists, speech language pathologists, otologist, family physician, and other members of health care team as needed

SURGERY/OTHER PROCEDURES
• CHL often has surgical options for repair.
– Tympanostomy and tube placement
– Tympanoplasty
– Mastoidectomy
– Ossicular chain reconstruction
– Stapedectomy/stapedotomy
– Canaloplasty
• Those with profound bilateral SNHL may qualify for cochlear implantation.

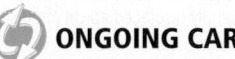

ONGOING CARE

FOLLOW-UP RECOMMENDATIONS
Patient Monitoring
Audiogram and clinical exam are the primary means of monitoring patient. Patients with hearing assistive devices benefit from audiology involvement.

DIET
Salt restriction to 2 g/day is helpful for patients with Ménière disease.

PATIENT EDUCATION
• To prevent damage that leads to noise-induced hearing loss, practice noise exposure moderation.
– Avoid excessive noise.
– Avoid prolonged noise exposure.
– Use protective devices.
• National Institute on Deafness and Other Communication Disorders (NIDCD): http://www.nidcd.nih.gov/health/hearing/Pages/Default.aspx

PROGNOSIS
• SNHL is usually permanent and may be progressive. However, amplification devices (e.g., hearing aids) may help improve functionality.
• ISSNHL may recover spontaneously in 32–70% of cases, but urgent referral and treatment is recommended to maximize recovery. No factors have been proven to predict recovery (5).

COMPLICATIONS
Acute middle ear problems may become chronic (perforations, cholesteatoma).

REFERENCES
1. Stachler RJ, Chandrasekhar SS, Archer SM, et al. Clinical practice guideline: sudden hearing loss. *Otolaryngol Head Neck Surg*. 2012;146(Suppl 3): S1–S35.
2. Lai D, Zhao F, Jalal N, et al. Intratympanic glucocorticoid therapy for idiopathic sudden hearing loss: meta-analysis of randomized controlled trials. *Medicine (Baltimore)*. 2017;96(50):e8955.
3. Han X, Yin X, Du X, et al. Combined intratympanic and systemic use of steroids as a first-line treatment for sudden sensorineural hearing loss: a meta-analysis of randomized, controlled trials. *Otol Neurotol*. 2017;38(4):487–495.
4. Hunter LL, Meinzen-Derr J, Wiley S, et al. Influence of the WIC program on loss to follow-up for newborn hearing screening. *Pediatrics*. 2016;138(1):e20154301.
5. Walling AD, Dickson GM. Hearing loss in older adults. *Am Fam Physician*. 2012;85(12): 1150–1156.

 CODES

ICD10
• H91.90 Unspecified hearing loss, unspecified ear
• H90.2 Conductive hearing loss, unspecified
• H90.5 Unspecified sensorineural hearing loss

CLINICAL PEARLS
• In sudden hearing loss, if a 512-Hz tuning fork test (Weber test) lateralizes to the *unaffected ear*, suspect sensorineural causes (emergent evaluation needed), but if it lateralizes to the *affected* ear, the diagnosis is CHL (not an emergency).
• ~80% of people aged >85 years have hearing loss; encourage screening and treatment, especially in patients with early dementia.
• Best way to prevent noise-induced hearing loss is to protect against noise exposure.

HEART FAILURE, ACUTELY DECOMPENSATED
Muhammad Durrani, DO, MS • Eric P. Blazar, MD

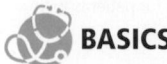 **BASICS**

DESCRIPTION
Acute decompensated heart failure (ADHF) is a rapid-onset cardiac pump function impairment, structurally or functionally, resulting in inefficient perfusion, yielding symptoms due to excessive fluid accumulation and due to reduction in cardiac output. ADHF can be a new diagnosis or worsening of preexisting chronic heart failure (HF).

EPIDEMIOLOGY
Incidence
- HF hospitalization places a major strain on health care resources, and Medicare spends more to diagnose and treat HF than any other medical condition. HF is the most common cause of admission and readmission in the United States. In 2012, the total cost of HF was $30.7 billion. By 2030, total cost will increase 127% to $69.7 billion. In the United States, there are 915,000 new cases annually. HF is the primary cause of >55,000 deaths each year and a contributing factor in >280,000 deaths.
- >1 million hospital discharges per year, unchanged from 2000 to 2010, and about half of people who have HF die within 5 years of diagnosis. One in nine deaths has HF mentioned on the death certificate.

Prevalence
- ~6.5 million people age >20 in the United States carry an HF diagnosis; prevalence is expected to increase 46% from 2012 to 2030, resulting in >8 million cases in patients >18 years of age.
- HF is primarily a disease of the elderly; 75% of hospital admissions for HF are in persons >65 years of age.
- African Americans have the highest risk of developing HF, followed by Hispanics, whites, and Chinese Americans, which reflects differences in prevalence of hypertension (HTN), diabetes mellitus, and socioeconomic status.

ETIOLOGY AND PATHOPHYSIOLOGY
- Two potential pathophysiologic conditions lead to the clinical findings of HF, namely systolic and/or diastolic heart dysfunction.
  - Systolic dysfunction: an *inotropic* abnormality, due to myocardial infarction (MI) or dilated or ischemic cardiomyopathy (CM), resulting in diminished systolic emptying (ejection fraction <45%)
  - Diastolic dysfunction: a *compliance* abnormality, due to hypertensive CM, in which ventricular relaxation is impaired (ejection fraction >45%), resulting in decreased filling
  - In attempt to adopt a more pragmatic classification system, one that has been accepted by both the European and American HF guidelines, the terms HF with reduced, midrange, or preserved LVEF (HFrEF, FHmrEF, and HFpEF, respectively) have been adopted recently.
- ADHF can result from the following conditions:
  - Myocardial disease:
    - Exacerbation of preexisting chronic HF heralded by noncompliance or infection
    - Any of the following as cause of new HF or exacerbation of preexisting chronic HF: coronary artery disease (CAD), MI, toxic damage, immune-mediated and inflammatory damage, infiltrative diseases, metabolic derangements, and genetic abnormalities
  - Abnormal loading conditions:
    - HTN, valvular and myocardial structural defects, pericardial and endomyocardial pathologies, high-output states, volume overload

- Arrhythmias:
  - Atrial fibrillation, tachyarrhythmias, high-grade heart block, bradyarrhythmias

Genetics
Familial CM is a predisposition to development of HF (rare).

RISK FACTORS
- CAD and MI: RR 8.1
- Diabetes mellitus: RR 1.9
- Cigarette smoking: RR 1.6
- Valvular heart disease: RR: 1.5
- HTN, systemic or pulmonary: RR 1.4
- Dietary sodium intake: RR 1.4
- Obesity: RR 1.3

GENERAL PREVENTION
Mortality reduction has been attributed to treating HF risk factors (see above), with implementation of ACE inhibitors, β-blockers, coronary revascularization, implantable cardioverter-defibrillators, and cardiac resynchronization strategies in patients.

- Some recommend B-type natriuretic peptide (BNP) screening in conjunction with guideline-directed management/therapies for at-risk populations to aid in prevention of new-onset HF and to delay development of left ventricular (LV) dysfunction in existing HF.

COMMONLY ASSOCIATED CONDITIONS
- Dysrhythmia followed by pump failure is the leading cause of death in ADHF. Most patients have >5 comorbidities (especially CAD, chronic kidney disease, and diabetes) and take >5 medications.
- Cardiogenic shock

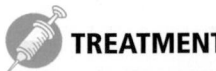 DIAGNOSIS

Requires a multifaceted clinical approach with no gold standard diagnostic test: No single historical, physical exam (PE), ECG, or radiographic finding can rule out HF.

HISTORY
- Patients typically have a history of HF, MI, uncontrolled HTN, and other risk factors.
- Dyspnea on exertion and orthopnea are the only symptoms with high sensitivity but suffer from low specificity.
- Other symptoms include deteriorating exercise capacity, fatigue, general weakness, chest pain/discomfort if acute coronary syndrome (ACS) is present, paroxysmal nocturnal dyspnea, nocturnal nonproductive cough, wheezing (especially nocturnal) in absence of history of asthma, or infection (cardiac asthma).
- Edema, abdominal bloating (ascites), anasarca, cyanosis, weight gain (>2 kg/week)

PHYSICAL EXAM
- S_3 has highest likelihood ratio (LR) in respects to PE with positive LR ranging from 1.6 to 13.0. No PE finding has sensitivity >70%.
- Peripheral pitting edema, cool extremities, cyanosis, hepatomegaly, hepatojugular reflux, cardiac murmur, hypotension, laterally displaced apical impulse
- Lung exam: rales (crackles) and sometimes wheezing, Cheyne-Stokes respirations

DIFFERENTIAL DIAGNOSIS
Rule out life-threatening diagnoses first: pulmonary embolism, MI, tamponade, pneumothorax, ARDS, sepsis, COPD, pneumonia, constrictive pericarditis, high-output states (anemia, hyperthyroidism).

DIAGNOSTIC TESTS & INTERPRETATION
Laboratory data are adjunctive and help with prognostication and clinical course.

Initial Tests (lab, imaging)
- First, assess BP and other vital signs and rule out hemodynamic instability and cardiogenic shock state.
- Cardiac troponins, ECG to evaluate for ACS. Note that elevated troponins are detected in the majority of HF patients, often without obvious myocardial ischemia (1)[C].
- BUN, creatinine, electrolytes, liver function tests, TSH (new onset), glucose, and CBC (1)[C].
- Routine ABG is not indicated (1)[C].
- Transthoracic echocardiogram: recommended immediately in hemodynamically unstable ADHF patients and within 48 hours when cardiac structure and function are either not known or may have changed since previous studies (1)[C]
- BNP and/or N-type pro-BNP (BT-BNP): Measurement of BNP or NT-proBNP is recommended in all patients with acute dyspnea and suspected ADHF to help in the differentiation of ADHF from noncardiac causes (1)[A].
  - BNP <100 essentially will rule out HF with negative LR of 0.2 and sensitivity of 93.5% (2)[A]. BNP >500 have specificity of 89.8% (2)[A]. BNP 100 to 400 may indicate HF or may be due to a variety of cardiac and noncardiac conditions (1)[A].
  - BNP has a relative increase in women, is lower with obesity, and higher with renal dysfunction (1)[A].
- NT-proBNP values >450 pg/mL for people age <50 years, >900 pg/mL ages 50 to 75 years, and >1,800 pg/mL for people >75 years are highly suggestive of HF (sensitivity 90%, specificity of 84%) (3)[B].
- Chest x-ray: to assess for pulmonary congestion and to detect other cardiac or noncardiac diseases that may cause or contribute to the patient's symptoms: cardiomegaly, vascular redistribution (cephalization) with "butterfly" pattern of pulmonary edema, interstitial and alveolar edema, Kerley B lines, pleural effusions (1)[C]
- Lung ultrasound (LUS): emerging as a diagnostic tool for ADHF with a positive LUS defined by presence of >3 B lines in two bilateral lung zones yielding a specificity of 92.7% and LR of 7.4 (2)[A]

Follow-Up Tests & Special Considerations
Please see "Heart Failure, Chronic" topic.

Diagnostic Procedures/Other
Cardiac catheterization may be considered when CAD is suspected. Pulmonary artery catheterization may be performed to guide therapy in severe cases with cardiogenic shock.

Test Interpretation
Cardiac pathology depends on the etiology of HF. Please refer to "Heart Failure, Chronic" topic.

TREATMENT

Goal of treatment is to improve hemodynamics and organ perfusion, alleviate symptoms, limit cardiac and renal damage, restore oxygenation, and minimize hospital length of stay as well as identify the etiology or precipitating factors. See "Heart Failure, Chronic" chapter as well.

MEDICATION

ALERT

Contemporary therapies for ADHF remain suboptimal, and many therapies do not favorably impact morbidity or mortality. Diuretics are used initially in fluid overload ADHF, with nitrates added as needed. Once ADHF is stabilized, guideline suggests an ACE inhibitor, ARB, or ARNI and β-blocker be started in patients with reduced systolic function. Use of new agent ivabradine has also been touted in select patients. Avoid NSAIDs and COX-2 inhibitors. There are no class IA drug recommendations for ADHF.

First Line

- IV loop diuretics recommended for all patients with ADHF and symptoms of fluid overload in hemodynamically stable patients (contraindicated if systolic blood pressure [SBP] <90 mm Hg, severe hyponatremia, acidosis) (1)[C]; be cautious of electrolyte abnormalities if kidney disease is present. Diuresis should be instituted early in ADHF, continuous infusion is no better than bolus, and high dose is not significantly better than low dose (1)[B].
  - Furosemide (Lasix): New-onset ADHF patients should get boluses of 20 to 40 mg IV (1)[B].
  - If on furosemide (Lasix) chronically, initial IV dose should be equal or exceed chronic oral daily dose (1.0-2.5 times home dose) (1)[B]. Monitor for appropriate urine output.
- Thiazides in combination with loop diuretics may be useful if ineffective diuresis hydrochlorothiazide [HCTZ] 25 mg PO). Thiazides and spironolactone or eplerenone (25 to 50 mg PO) may be used in combination with loop diuretics if excessive volume overload (1)[C].
- Metolazone (Zaroxolyn): 2.5 to 20.0 mg/day PO, can be added as second diuretic to loop diuretic in cases of ineffective diuresis
- Vasodilators: Consider in ADHF with SBP >90 mm Hg, and patients with hypertensive ADHF should get IV vasodilators as initial therapy to reduce congestion (1)[B]. Use in chronic HF is not effective (3)[B].
  - IV nitroglycerin may be of short-term benefit to decrease preload, afterload, and systemic resistance (IV 10 to 20 μg/min, increase up to 200 μg/min) (1)[B].
  - IV nitroprusside: Administer with caution, start with 0.3 μg/kg/min, and increase up to 5.0 μg/kg/min (1)[B].
- Bilevel positive airway pressure (BIPAP)/NPPV: NPPV decreases early mortality in ADHF. See "Additional Therapies" section.

Second Line

- Tolvaptan (an oral vasopressin antagonist) for severe hypervolemic hyponatremia refractory to water restriction and medical therapy
- Inotropes: reserved for patients with severe systolic dysfunction occurring most often in hypotensive ADHF. Withdraw as hemodynamics improve due to increased short- and medium-term mortality. ECG monitoring is required because they can induce ischemia and arrhythmias.
  - Phosphodiesterase inhibitors (milrinone, enoximone) decrease pulmonary resistance; may be used for patients on β-blockers but may increase medium-term mortality in CAD patients
  - Dobutamine infusion 2 to 20 μg/kg/min requires close BP monitoring; avoid in cardiogenic shock or with tachyarrhythmias.
  - Low-dose dopamine infusion may be considered (3 to 5 μg/kg/min).

- Levosimendan (calcium sensitizer) improves hemodynamic parameters but not survival compared to placebo while improving hemodynamic parameters and survival compared to dobutamine.
- Vasopressors: Consider in patients with cardiogenic shock despite treatment with another inotrope (1)[B].
  - Norepinephrine 0.2 to 1.0 μg/kg/min compared with dopamine has fewer side effects and lower mortality (1)[C].
  - Epinephrine restricted to patients with persistent hypotension despite other agents (1)[C]
- Nesiritide, a BNP analog, is not recommended secondary to higher rates of hypotension, no benefit on death, or rehospitalization rates.
- Ultrafiltration renal replacement therapy: Routine use of ultrafiltration is not recommended and should be used only in patients with refractory volume overload (1)[C].

ADDITIONAL THERAPIES

- Oxygen: Begin treatment early; ideally, arterial oxygen saturation >92% (90% if COPD)
- Cochrane review shows that one death can be avoided for every 14 ADHF patient treated with NPPV and one death for every 9 ADHF patients treated with CPAP. Avoid mechanical ventilation for patients with right HF if possible.
- Treat anemia with transfusion: conservative trigger Hgb <8; target Hgb 10. IV iron replacement may help with New York Heart Association (NYHA) II and III patients. Avoid erythropoietin-stimulating agents.
- For patients with new-onset arrhythmias, consider pacing and/or antiarrhythmics.
- Please refer to "Heart Failure, Chronic" for maintenance treatments.

SURGERY/OTHER PROCEDURES

- Heart valve surgery if valvular disease is responsible
- PCI/CABG for patients with CAD/MI if applicable

ADMISSION, INPATIENT, AND NURSING CONSIDERATIONS

- Admission criteria considerations:
  - Evidence of severely decompensated HF, including hypotension, worsening renal function, altered mental status, dyspnea at rest, decreased oxygenation, arrhythmias, electrolyte disturbances, associated comorbid conditions, newly diagnosed HF
  - Consider observation unit stay for stable patients with preexisting HF and the following:
    ○ No acute interventions needed for comorbid condition, SBP >120 mm Hg, RR <32 bpm, BUN <40 mg/dL, creatinine <3.0 mg/dL, no evidence of ischemia or elevated troponins, and BNP <1,000, N-type pro-BNP <5,000 (2)[B]
    ○ Clinical impression that patient could be discharged in the next 24 hours
- Inpatient: continuous pulse oxygen; daily weights; monitor input and output; fluid restriction; 2-g sodium diet; echocardiogram if necessary; monitor for worsening HF; assess treatment response.
- 1.5 to 2.0 L/day fluid restriction may be useful to reduce congestive symptoms.
- Discharge criteria: improved symptoms, SBP normalized at 100 to 120 mm Hg, good urine output, serum sodium >135 mEq/L, HF outpatient education

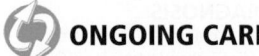 **ONGOING CARE**

FOLLOW-UP RECOMMENDATIONS
Patient Monitoring
Rapid follow-up and a multidisciplinary care to reduce hospitalization and mortality (1)[A]

DIET
Reduce sodium (2 g); maintain cardiac or diabetic diet if these comorbidities are present.

PATIENT EDUCATION
- Monitoring and self-care; record daily weight; know how/when to use health care systems to increase diuretic dose with weight gain or dyspnea.
- Medications: Understand indications, dose, effects, and side effects of drugs.
- Adherence: Value treatment plan maintenance.
- Alcohol, smoking, and drugs: abstinence recommended in alcohol-induced CM; smoking and illicit drug cessation
- Exercise: Understand the benefits of exercise.

PROGNOSIS
- The ADHERE risk tree stratifies ADHF patients for inpatient mortality using SBP, BUN, and creatinine.
- S_3 on PE correlates with poor prognosis.
- After diagnosis, 1-year survival ~75%, 5-year survival <50%, 10-year survival <25%
- Consider predischarge BNP to establish postdischarge prognosis in hospitalized patients (3)[C].

COMPLICATIONS
Arrhythmia, pulmonary edema, hyponatremia, death

REFERENCES

1. Ponikowski P, Voors AA, Anker SD, et al; for ESC Scientific Document Group. 2016 ESC guidelines for the diagnosis and treatment of acute and chronic heart failure: the task force for the diagnosis and treatment of acute and chronic heart failure of the European Society of Cardiology (ESC). Developed with the special contribution of the Heart Failure Association (HFA) of the ESC. *Eur Heart J.* 2016;37(27):2129–2200.
2. Martindale JL, Wakai A, Collins SP, et al. Diagnosing acute heart failure in the emergency department: a systematic review and meta-analysis. *Acad Emerg Med.* 2016;23(3):223–242.
3. Yancy CW, Jessup M, Bozkurt B, et al. 2017 ACC/AHA/HFSA focused update of the 2013 ACCF/AHA guideline for the management of heart failure: a report of the American College of Cardiology/American Heart Association Task Force on Clinical Practice Guidelines and the Heart Failure Society of America. *Circulation.* 2017;136(6):e137–e161.

 CODES

ICD10
- I50.9 Heart failure, unspecified
- I50.21 Acute systolic (congestive) heart failure
- I50.31 Acute diastolic (congestive) heart failure

CLINICAL PEARLS

- BNP in ADHF is best reserved for situations in which diagnosis of ADHF is unclear.
- Look for underlying cause of each episode of ADHF.
- IV diuretics are used initially in fluid-overload acute HF, with nitrates added if needed, especially if patient is hypertensive.
- Using early noninvasive ventilation for the treatment of pulmonary edema can bridge care while awaiting the effects of diuretics and can decrease morbidity and mortality associated with intubation.

H

Jeffrey A. Shih, MD

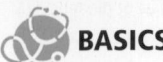

BASICS

DESCRIPTION

- Heart failure (HF) is the condition resulting from inability of the heart to fill and/or pump blood sufficiently to meet tissue metabolic needs. Alternatively, HF may occur when adequate cardiac output can be achieved only at the expense of elevated filling pressures. It is the principal complication of heart disease.
- HF is the preferred term over congestive HF because patients are not always congested (fluid overloaded).
- HF may involve the left heart, the right heart, or be biventricular. The New York Heart Association (NYHA) classification is a subjective grading scale used for classifying patients with HF: NYHA I: asymptomatic; NYHA II: symptomatic with moderate exertion; NYHA III: symptomatic with mild exertion and may limit activities of daily living; NYHA IV: symptomatic at rest. For acute HF, see "Heart Failure, Acutely Decompensated."

EPIDEMIOLOGY

The annual direct and indirect cost of HF in the United States is ~$34.4 billion.

Incidence

In the United States, 550,000 new cases diagnosed annually with >250,000 deaths per year

Prevalence

- ~6.5 million people in the United States have HF; <1% in those age <50 years, increasing to 10% of those age >80 years
- Primarily a disease of the elderly; 75% of hospital admissions for HF are for persons >65 years of age.

ETIOLOGY AND PATHOPHYSIOLOGY

Two physiologic components explain most of the clinical findings of HF and result in classifications of patients in four general categories:

- HF with reduced ejection fraction (HFrEF) or systolic HF: an *inotropic* abnormality, often due to myocardial infarction (MI) or dilated cardiomyopathy (CM), resulting in diminished systolic emptying (ejection fraction [EF] ≤40%)
- HF with preserved ejection fraction (HFpEF) or diastolic HF: a *compliance* abnormality, often due to hypertensive CM, in which the ventricular relaxation is impaired (EF ≥50%)
- Borderline HFpEF (EF 41–49%): mild systolic dysfunction but clinically behaves like HFpEF
- Improved HFpEF (EF >40%): previously HFrEF but with improvement in systolic function
- Patients with systolic dysfunction may also have diastolic dysfunction.
- Most common etiologies: coronary artery disease (CAD)/MI and hypertension (HTN)
- Myocarditis and CM: alcoholic, viral, long-standing HTN, drugs (e.g., chemotherapeutic agents), muscular dystrophy, infiltrative (e.g., amyloidosis, sarcoidosis), postpartum state, infectious (e.g., Chagas disease, HIV), hypertrophic CM (HCM), inherited familial dilated CM, left ventricular (LV) noncompaction
- Valvular and vascular abnormalities: any valvular stenosis or regurgitation, rheumatic heart; renal artery stenosis, usually bilateral, may cause recurrent "flash" pulmonary edema, especially in setting of severe chronic HTN.
- Chronic lung disease and pulmonary HTN (cor pulmonale)

- Iatrogenic volume overload (requires extreme overload in patients with normal hearts and kidneys)
- Arrhythmias (atrial fibrillation and other tachyarrhythmias, high-grade heart block)
- Miscellaneous: high-output states: hyperthyroidism, anemia; cardiac depressants (β-blocker overdose), stress induced
- Idiopathic: 20–50% of idiopathic dilated cardiomyopathies are familial.
- HF is progressive—manifested by the remodeling (altered heart geometry) process.

Genetics

Multiple genetic abnormalities responsible for a variety of phenotypes have been identified (HCM, arrhythmogenic right ventricular [RV] dysplasia, LV noncompaction, dilated CM). Consider genetic screening for first-degree relatives of HCM and arrhythmogenic RV dysplasia.

RISK FACTORS

For development of HF: CAD/MI, HTN (80% of cases of HF in the United States caused by either CAD or HTN), valvular heart disease, diabetes mellitus, cardiotoxic medications (e.g., anthracyclines, tyrosine-kinase inhibitors, TNF-α inhibitors), obesity, older age

GENERAL PREVENTION

Control HTN and other risk factors. Thiazide diuretics and angiotensin-converting enzyme inhibitors (ACE-I) are superior to other agents in preventing development of HF.

COMMONLY ASSOCIATED CONDITIONS

Sudden cardiac death and progressive pump failure are the leading causes of death. Most patients have >5 comorbid medical conditions and take >5 medications.

DIAGNOSIS

HISTORY

- Dyspnea on exertion: *cardinal sign of left-sided HF*. Deteriorating exercise capacity: easy fatigued, general weakness
- Nocturnal nonproductive cough, orthopnea, and paroxysmal nocturnal dyspnea; sometimes frothy or pink sputum. Wheezing, especially nocturnal, in absence of history of asthma or infection (cardiac asthma); Cheyne-Stokes respirations
- Anorexia and/or fullness or dull pain in right upper quadrant (hepatic congestion). Nausea and poor appetite may indicate advanced HF.

PHYSICAL EXAM

- Increased filling pressures: rales and sometimes wheezing, peripheral edema, S_3 gallop, hepatomegaly, jugular venous distention, hepatojugular reflux, ascites
- Remodeling: enlarged or displaced point of maximal impulse
- Poor cardiac output: hypotension, pulsus alternans, tachycardia, narrow pulse pressure, cool extremities, cyanosis

DIFFERENTIAL DIAGNOSIS

Simple dependent edema, pulmonary embolism, exertional asthma, cardiac ischemia, asthma/COPD, constrictive pericarditis, nephrotic syndrome, cirrhosis, venous occlusive disease with subsequent peripheral edema, high-output states: anemia, sepsis, hyperthyroidism, lymphedema, tamponade

DIAGNOSTIC TESTS & INTERPRETATION

Diagnosis should be primarily clinical, with laboratory data as adjunctive and indicative of complications.

Initial Tests (lab, imaging)

- β-Type natriuretic peptide (BNP) and N-terminal pro-BNP (NT-BNP) are helpful in the acute setting to differentiate the cause of dyspnea (BNP <100 essentially rules out HF) (1)[A]. A BNP level in those with risk factors for developing HF or with structural heart disease but no symptoms of HF can help predict the development of symptomatic HF (2)[A]. Other, non-HF conditions, such as pulmonary embolism, renal failure, and acute coronary syndromes, may cause elevated BNP. Obesity may lower BNP levels. The use of BNP-guided therapy in chronic HF and acutely decompensated HF is not well established, although a predischarge BNP can predict risk of readmission and survival (2)[A].
- Lab findings include respiratory alkalosis, mild azotemia, decreased ESR, proteinuria (usually <1 g/day), elevated creatinine (cardiorenal syndrome), dilutional hyponatremia (poor prognosis), hyperuricemia, and hyperbilirubinemia.
- Chest x-ray (changes lag clinical symptoms by up to 6 hours): increased heart size, vascular redistribution (cephalization) with "butterfly" pattern of pulmonary edema, interstitial and alveolar edema, Kerley B lines, and pleural effusions. Findings of pulmonary edema may be absent in long-standing HF.

Diagnostic Procedures/Other

Determination of left ventricular ejection fraction (LVEF) is critical to proper diagnosis and management:

- Echocardiogram is the most useful test to determine LVEF, RV function, diastolic dysfunction, ventricular size, wall thickness, and valvular abnormalities; may be repeated if change suspected in underlying cardiac status
- Nuclear imaging to estimate ventricular sizes; assess for ischemia or infarction, ATTR-wild type amyloidosis, and systolic function.
- Cardiac MRI can be considered in select circumstances: suspicion of cardiac sarcoidosis, arrhythmogenic RV CM, acute myocarditis, amyloidosis, and hemochromatosis.
- Cardiac catheterization is important for excluding CAD as an etiology in the setting of risk factors.
- Endomyocardial biopsy should not be performed routinely, only in special circumstances (e.g., suspected giant cell myocarditis) that may change therapy (1)[C].

Test Interpretation

Cardiac pathology depends on underlying etiology.

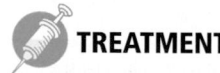

TREATMENT

GENERAL MEASURES

Correct and treat risk factors for HF. The treatment of chronic HF is focused on improving hemodynamics, relieving symptoms, and blocking the neurohormonal response to improve survival.

MEDICATION

Diuretics are used initially in fluid overload acute HF. The addition of ACE-I and aldosterone antagonists can be added at any time. Once acute HF is stabilized, a β-blocker should be started. Avoid nonsteroidal anti-inflammatory drugs (NSAIDs), which markedly worsen HF. Avoid the use of diltiazem and verapamil in patients with systolic dysfunction because they may increase mortality and have negative inotropic effects.

First Line

- ACE-I: used to decrease afterload. Shown to increase survival, improve symptoms, and overall exercise capacity in patients in all NYHA classifications; benefit greatest for patients with systolic dysfunction and post-MI. Number needed to treat (NNT) ~25 per year for mortality. All ACE-Is considered equally effective. Initiate at low doses and titrate as tolerated to target doses.
- Angiotensin receptor blockers (ARBs) are indicated for those who are intolerant to ACE-Is. Avoid combination of ACE-I and ARB.
- β-Blockers: used in systolic or diastolic HF (Note: Initiate in hemodynamically stable/compensated patients at low dose and titrate upward slowly.); NNT = 25 for mortality. Mortality decreased in systolic HF; evidence for titration to heart rate (HR) rather than specific dose (1)[A]
  - Carvedilol: 3.125 mg PO BID to a target of 25 mg PO BID; metoprolol succinate extended release: 12.5 mg/day PO to a target of 200 mg/day PO; or bisoprolol: 1.25 to 10.00 mg once daily (currently not FDA-approved for the treatment of HF)
- Sacubitril/valsartan (Entresto) is an angiotensin receptor blocker and neprilysin inhibitor (ARNI) shown to reduce the risk of CV death and HF hospitalizations in patients with HFrEF. In patients with HFrEF and NYHA class II and III symptoms who tolerate an ACE-I or ARB, and CrCl >30, replacement by an ARNI is recommended to further reduce morbidity and mortality (NNT to prevent one CV death >3.5 years: 31). ACE-Is should be discontinued at least 36 hours prior to starting ARNIs. The most common adverse effects include hypotension, angioedema, and renal insufficiency (3)[A]. Cost is >$500/month. Diuretics are helpful to manage volume overload/reduce preload.
  - Furosemide (Lasix): 20 to 320 mg/day IV/IM/PO divided dose; bumetanide (Bumex): 0.5 mg to 10.0 mg/day IV/PO divided dose; torsemide (Demadex): 10 to 200 mg/day PO divided dose (1)[C]
  - Metolazone (Zaroxolyn): 2.5 to 20.0 mg/day PO divided dose; hydrochlorothiazide: 12.5 to 100.0 mg/day PO divided dose; chlorothiazide (Diuril): 250 to 2,000 mg/day IV/PO divided dose
  - Spironolactone, eplerenone (improve mortality when added to standard therapy in NYHA class II to IV + EF <35%): spironolactone 12.5 to 25.0 mg/day PO; maximum 50 mg/day PO; eplerenone 25 to 50 mg/day; caution regarding hyperkalemia and chronic kidney disease (CKD) (1)[A]
- Digoxin reduces symptoms but has not clearly shown any positive effect on mortality: In patients with preserved renal function (CrCl >50 mL/min), the recommended dose is 0.125 mg/day. Levels lower than used for atrial fibrillation are effective and safer (1)[B].
- The combination of hydralazine (75 mg/day divided BID or TID) and isosorbide dinitrate (40 mg QID) is effective for improving survival and reducing hospitalizations in patients with HfrEF. In patients who are at least 40 days post-MI; LVEF ≤35%, NYHA class II or III HF (1)[A], or LVEF ≤30%, NYHA I HF (1)[B]; and on optimal medical therapy and >1 year estimated survival; generally not indicated in American Heart Association (AHA) stage D (end-stage) HF
- Ivabradine (Corlanor) can be considered in patients with NYHA II and III HF, EF ≤35%, on maximally tolerated β-blockers with HRs >70 to reduce hospitalization from worsening HF (2)[B]. Ivabradine is contraindicated in ADHF, hypotension (<90/50 mm Hg), severe hepatic impairment, pacemaker-dependence, bradyarrhythmias, or strong CYP3A4 inhibitors. It should not be administered to patients that are currently in atrial fibrillation and should be discontinued if atrial fibrillation develops (3)[A].

- Intravenous iron replacement might improve functional status and quality of life in patients with NYHA II and III HF and iron deficiency (ferritin <100 ng/mL or 100 to 300 ng/mL if transferrin saturation <20%) (1)[B].
- In diastolic HF, no medical therapy has improved survival (1)[A]. ARBs and spironolactone can be used to potentially reduce hospitalizations (1,2)[A].

ADDITIONAL THERAPIES

Device therapy including implantable cardioverter-defibrillators (ICDs) and cardiac resynchronization therapy (CRT) shown to improve outcomes.

- CRT is recommended for patients in sinus rhythm with a QRS width ≥150 ms due to left bundle branch block (LBBB) and LVEF ≤35% and persistent mild to moderate HF (NYHA II and III) despite optimal medical therapy. CRT may be considered for ambulatory NYHA class IV patients in sinus rhythm with a QRS width ≥150 ms, LBBB, and LVEF ≤35% (1)[A].
- CRT may be considered for patients with LVEF ≤35%, sinus rhythm, QRS width ≥150 ms, non-LBBB pattern, and NYHA III or ambulatory NYHA IV symptoms (1)[A].
- CRT may also be considered for patients with a QRS width between 120 and 150 ms, LBBB, LVEF ≤35%, and persistent mild to severe HF (NYHA II to IV) despite optimal medical therapy (1)[B].
- ICDs are recommended for primary prevention in patients with *nonischemic* CM and *ischemic* CM who are at least 40 days post-MI; LVEF ≤35%, NYHA class II or III HF (1)[A], or LVEF ≤30%, NYHA I HF (1)[B]; and on optimal medical therapy and >1 year estimated survival; generally not indicated in American Heart Association (AHA) stage D (end-stage) HF
- CRT is recommended in patients with reduced LVEF and chronic RV pacing or with bradyarrhythmias and an anticipated need for a pacemaker (4)[A].

SURGERY/OTHER PROCEDURES

- Heart valve surgery if defective heart valve is responsible; mitral valve repair especially helpful if mitral regurgitation is the primary issue and not functional
- Advanced therapies such as cardiac transplantation and LV assist device (LVAD) implantation can be considered in patients with HF refractory to conventional medical/device therapies without other disqualifying medical and psychosocial conditions. Cardiac transplantation is generally considered for patients ≤70 years old with a predicted 1-year survival worse than that afforded by transplantation. Consideration can be made for patients >70 years with few comorbid conditions. Indications for LVAD implantation are generally similar to cardiac transplantation but are evolving.

ADMISSION, INPATIENT, AND NURSING CONSIDERATIONS

- See "Heart Failure, Acutely Decompensated."
- Admit patients with hemodynamic/respiratory compromise, hypoxia/hypoxemia, change in mental status, acute renal insufficiency, significant volume overload, and significant electrolyte abnormalities (e.g., hyponatremia).
- Discharge criteria: subjective improvement, euvolemia on clinical assessment, resting HR <100 bpm, systolic BP >80 mm Hg, HF outpatient education performed

ONGOING CARE

FOLLOW-UP RECOMMENDATIONS

- Critical patient education performed at all outpatient and inpatient physician visits
- Rapid office follow-up (7 days) after hospitalization

Patient Monitoring

Home health monitoring by specially trained nurses have both been shown to decrease frequency of hospitalizations. Readmissions remain problematic.

DIET

Reduce sodium load (<1.5 to 2.0 g/day). Optimal level is unknown.

PATIENT EDUCATION

AHA: www.americanheart.org

PROGNOSIS

After diagnosis: 1-year survival ~75%, 5-year survival <50%, and 10-year survival <25%

COMPLICATIONS

Sudden death (arrhythmic), acute pulmonary edema, death, progressive pump failure

REFERENCES

1. Yancy CW, Jessup M, Bozkurt B, et al. 2013 ACCF/AHA guideline for the management of heart failure: a report of the American College of Cardiology Foundation/American Heart Association Task Force on Practice Guidelines. *J Am Coll Cardiol.* 2013;62(16):e147–e239.
2. Yancy CW, Jessup M, Bozkurt B, et al. 2017 ACC/AHA/HFSA focused update of the 2013 ACCF/AHA guideline for the management of heart failure: a report of the American College of Cardiology/American Heart Association Task Force on Clinical Practice Guidelines and the Heart Failure Society of America. *Circulation.* 2017;136(6): e137–e161.
3. Yancy CW, Jessup M, Bozkurt B, et al. 2016 ACC/AHA/HFSA focused update on new pharmacological therapy for heart failure: an update of the 2013 ACCF/AHA guideline for the management of heart failure: a report of the American College of Cardiology/American Heart Association Task Force on Clinical Practice Guidelines and the Heart Failure Society of America. *J Am Coll Cardiol.* 2016;68(13):1476–1488.
4. Curtis AB, Worley SJ, Adamson PB, et al. Biventricular pacing for atrioventricular block and systolic dysfunction. *N Engl J Med.* 2013;368(17):1585–1593.

 SEE ALSO

Algorithm: Congestive Heart Failure: Differential Diagnosis

 CODES

ICD10
- I50.9 Heart failure, unspecified
- I50.1 Left ventricular failure
- I50.22 Chronic systolic (congestive) heart failure

CLINICAL PEARLS

- Have patients weigh themselves daily and report weight gains of >2 lb in a day or 5 lb above dry weight.
- β-Blockers, ACE-I, and aldosterone antagonists are the core medications for management of chronic HF.
- Consider referral for biventricular pacing in patients with LBBB and ICD in those with low EF.

H

HEAT ILLNESS: HEAT EXHAUSTION AND HEAT STROKE
Sean C. Robinson, MD, CAQSM • Matthew G. Chan, MD

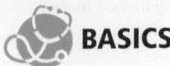

BASICS

DESCRIPTION
- A continuum of increasingly severe heat illnesses caused by dehydration, electrolyte losses, and failure of the body's thermoregulatory mechanisms when exposed to elevated environmental temperatures
  - Heat exhaustion is a mild to moderate form of heat illness displaying dehydration type symptoms with a normal to elevated temperature <104°F (1).
  - Heat stroke is characterized by an elevated core temperature >104°F with central nervous system abnormalities and is a true medical emergency (1,2).
- System(s) affected: endocrine/metabolic, nervous, hepatic, hematologic
- Synonym(s): heat illness; heat injury; hyperthermia; heat collapse; heat prostration

Geriatric Considerations
Elderly persons are more susceptible.

Pediatric Considerations
Children are more susceptible.

Pregnancy Considerations
Pregnant women may be more susceptible to volume depletion with heat stress.

EPIDEMIOLOGY
- Predominant age: more likely in children or elderly
- Predominant sex: male = female

Incidence
- Depends on intensity of heat; estimate of 20/100,000 persons per season (3)
- Concern for increasing incidence because ambient environmental temperatures continue to rise

Prevalence
- Depends on predisposing conditions in combination with environmental factors
- Roughly 600 deaths per year in the United States

ETIOLOGY AND PATHOPHYSIOLOGY
- Excess heat has direct cellular toxicity. Excess heat also leads to an imbalance between inflammatory and anti-inflammatory cytokines as well as vascular endothelial damage causing end-organ dysfunction.
- Interplay between failure of heat-dissipating mechanisms, an overwhelming heat stress, and an exaggerated acute-phase inflammatory response

RISK FACTORS
- Poor acclimatization to heat
- Poor physical conditioning
- Salt or water depletion
- Obesity
- Acute febrile or GI illnesses
- Chronic illnesses: uncontrolled diabetes mellitus, hypertension, cardiac disease
- Alcohol and other substance abuse
- High heat and humidity, poor environmental air circulation
- Heavy, restrictive clothing
- Nutritional supplements (e.g., ephedra) (2)
- Medications (α-adrenergics, anticholinergics, antihistamines, antipsychotics, benzodiazepines, β-blockers, calcium channel blockers, clopidogrel, diuretics, laxatives, neuroleptics, phenothiazines, thyroid agonists, tricyclic antidepressants) (1)

GENERAL PREVENTION
- The most important factor in preventing heat illness is activity modification and adequate fluid replacement.
- Allow acclimatization to hot weather through proper conditioning and activity modification.
- Dress appropriately with loose-fitting, open-weaved, light-colored clothing.
- Consume a proper volume of fluids, particularly during physical activity in hot environments.
- Never leave children (or pets) unattended in cars during hot weather.
- Try to gain access to air-conditioned environments during hot weather.

PROGNOSIS
- If mental function is not altered and serum chemistries are normal, the prognosis is good and recovery within 24 to 48 hours is typical.
- The mortality rate for heat stroke (10–80%) is directly related to the duration and intensity of hyperthermia as well as to the speed and effectiveness of diagnosis and treatment (3).

COMPLICATIONS
- May involve failure of any major organ system
- Cardiac arrhythmias or infarction
- Pulmonary edema, acute respiratory distress syndrome
- Coma, seizures
- Acute renal failure
- Rhabdomyolysis
- Disseminated intravascular coagulation (DIC)
- Hepatocellular necrosis

DIAGNOSIS

- Heat exhaustion: Symptoms are milder than in heat stroke, and there are no CNS derangements:
  - Fatigue, lethargy, weakness, dizziness, nausea, vomiting, myalgias, headache, profuse sweating, tachycardia, hypotension, thirst, hyperventilation
  - Core temperature usually elevated but can be normal; if elevated, usually <104°F (40°C)
- Heat stroke: marked by mental status changes and elevated core temperature
  - *Classic*: caused by environmental exposure, primarily in elderly or chronically ill patients, and may develop gradually over days
    - Delirium
    - Confusion
    - Coma
    - Core temperature >104°F (>40°C)
    - Hot, flushed, dry skin
  - *Exertional*: typically younger, very active patients; rapid onset
    - Exhaustion
    - Confusion, disorientation
    - Delirium
    - Coma
    - Hot, flushed skin, typically with sweating
    - Core temperature >104°F (>40°C) (1,2)

DIFFERENTIAL DIAGNOSIS
- Febrile illnesses, sepsis
- Drug-induced fluid loss
- Cardiac arrhythmia or infarction
- Acute cocaine intoxication
- Neuroleptic malignant syndrome
- Malignant hyperthermia (an autosomally inherited disorder of skeletal and cardiac muscle in which patients have abnormal muscle metabolism on exposure to halothane or skeletal muscle reactants)

DIAGNOSTIC TESTS & INTERPRETATION
Detect end-organ damage

Initial Tests (lab, imaging)
- Creatinine, BUN, electrolytes (sodium in particular)
- Liver enzymes, muscle enzymes (creatine phosphokinase)

- CBC—hemoconcentration
- Urinalysis: increased urine specific gravity
- Drugs that may alter lab results: diuretics

Diagnostic Procedures/Other
Rectal temperature (*Don't rely on oral temperature.*) (1,2)

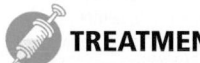 ## TREATMENT

GENERAL MEASURES
- For heat stroke: immediate body immersion in ice water to cool core temperature. Monitor hemodynamics and airway status (1,3)[C].
- Careful fluid and electrolyte replacement with normal saline; avoid hypotonic fluids. Follow sodium (1,2)[C].
- Consider CVP monitoring.
- For heat exhaustion, consider:
  – Evaporative cooling: spraying water over the patient and using fans to facilitate evaporative and convective heat loss (1,3)[C]
  – Immerse hands and forearms in cold water (3)[C].
  – Ice or cold packs on the neck, groin, and axillae (1,2)[C]
- No clear superiority of any one method for heat exhaustion (1)

MEDICATION
First Line
- No medications are required in the initial management. Use isotonic saline solution to rehydrate (1,3)[C].
- Do not use antipyretics to lower core temperature in heat illness.

Second Line
- For severely ill, consider immunomodulators such as corticosteroids (patients in ICU setting).
- Iced gastric, bladder, or peritoneal lavage (3)[C]
- If DIC, consider appropriate replacement therapy.

ADMISSION, INPATIENT, AND NURSING CONSIDERATIONS
- *Cool patient immediately* (prior to transport even) if heat stroke is suspected.
- Rapid cooling: Remove clothing, wet patient down, and apply ice packs.
- Emergency treatment; best in a hospital setting

 ## ONGOING CARE

FOLLOW-UP RECOMMENDATIONS
Rest with legs elevated (3)[C].

Patient Monitoring
- Rectal temperature monitoring: Cooling may be discontinued when the core temperature drops to 102°F (38.9°C) and stabilizes.
- Heat stroke patients may require airway management, hemodynamic monitoring, and careful fluid and electrolyte administration and monitoring.
- Consider CVP monitoring.

DIET
- Cool or cold clear liquids only (noncarbonated)
- Avoid caffeine.
- Unrestricted sodium

PATIENT EDUCATION
- Proper hydration is the key to prevention.
- Proper conditioning and acclimatization
- Recognize signs and symptoms of heat stress—fatigue and headache.
- Skin exposure facilitates heat loss in hot, humid conditions (use proper sun protection).

REFERENCES
1. Lipman GS, Eifling KP, Ellis MA, et al. Wilderness Medical Society practice guidelines for the prevention and treatment of heat-related illness: 2014 update. *Wilderness Environ Med*. 2014;25(Suppl 4):S55–S65.
2. Becker JA, Stewart LK. Heat-related illness. *Am Fam Physician*. 2011;83(11):1325–1330.
3. Yeo TP. Heat stroke: a comprehensive review. *AACN Clin Issues*. 2004;15(2):280–293.

ADDITIONAL READING
- Armstrong LE, Casa DJ, Millard-Stafford M, et al. American College of Sports Medicine position stand. Exertional heat illness during training and competition. *Med Sci Sports Exerc*. 2007;39(3):556–572.
- Atha WF. Heat-related illness. *Emerg Med Clin North Am*. 2013;31(4):1097–1108.

CODES

ICD10
- T67.5XXA Heat exhaustion, unspecified, initial encounter
- T67.0XXA Heatstroke and sunstroke, initial encounter
- T67.3XXA Heat exhaustion, anhydrotic, initial encounter

CLINICAL PEARLS
- Exertional heat stroke is a life-threating medical emergency that requires immediate whole body cooling (cold/ice water immersion preferred).
- The diagnosis of heat stroke includes an elevated core temperature and signs of CNS dysfunction (e.g., irritability, ataxia, confusion, seizures, or coma).
- Start the cooling process immediately when heat exhaustion is recognized, beginning with wetting the skin with a cool mist and giving oral rehydration solutions if the patient is alert and oriented.
- If in the field (e.g., sporting events, wilderness), cooling should be priority prior to transport.
- Do not rely on oral temperature—a rectal temperature is always preferred.

H

HEMATURIA

Tracy O. Middleton, DO, FACOFP

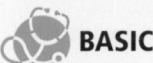 **BASICS**

DESCRIPTION
Gross (visible) or microscopic (nonvisible) blood in the urine, either symptomatic or asymptomatic

EPIDEMIOLOGY
Prevalence
- Children: gross: 0.13%; asymptomatic microscopic hematuria (AMH): 0.4–4.1%
- Adults: AMH: 0.9–17%, depending on population

ETIOLOGY AND PATHOPHYSIOLOGY
- Trauma
  - Exercise induced (resolves within 24 hours of ceasing activity)
  - Abdominal trauma or pelvic fracture with renal, bladder, or ureteral injury
  - Iatrogenic from abdominal or pelvic surgery, indwelling catheters, or foreign body
  - Physical/sexual abuse
- Neoplasms
  - Urologic malignancies or benign tumors
  - Endometriosis of the urinary tract (suspect in females with cyclic hematuria)
- Inflammatory/infectious causes
  - UTI: most common cause of hematuria in adults
  - Renal diseases: radiation nephritis and cystitis, acute/chronic tubulointerstitial nephritis (due to drugs, infections, systemic disease)
  - Glomerular disease
    ○ Goodpasture syndrome (antiglomerular basement membrane disease; autoimmune; associated pulmonary hemorrhage)
    ○ IgA nephropathy
    ○ Lupus nephritis
    ○ Henoch-Schönlein purpura
    ○ Membranoproliferative, poststreptococcal, or rapidly progressive glomerulonephritis (GN)
    ○ Wegener granulomatosis
  - Endocarditis/visceral abscesses
  - Other infections: schistosomiasis, TB, syphilis
- Metabolic causes
  - Stones (85% have hematuria)
    ○ Hypercalciuria: common cause of both gross and microscopic hematuria in children
    ○ Hyperuricosuria
- Congenital/familial causes
  - Cystic disease: polycystic, solitary renal cyst
  - Benign familial hematuria or thin basement membrane nephropathy (autosomal dominant)
  - Alport syndrome (X-linked in 85%; hematuria, proteinuria, hearing loss, corneal abnormalities)
  - Fabry disease (X-linked recessive inborn error of metabolism; vascular kidney disease)
  - Nail–patella syndrome (autosomal dominant; nail and patella hypoplasia; hematuria in 33%)
  - Renal tubular acidosis type 1 (autosomal dominant or autoimmune)
- Hematologic causes
  - Bleeding dyscrasias (e.g., hemophilia)
  - Sickle cell anemia/trait (renal papillary necrosis)
- Vascular causes
  - Hemangioma
  - Arteriovenous malformations (rare)
  - Nutcracker syndrome: compression of left renal vein with renal parenchymal congestion
  - Renal artery/vein thrombosis
  - Arterial emboli to kidney

- Chemical causes
  - Aminoglycosides, cyclosporine, analgesics, oral contraceptives, Chinese herbs
- Obstruction
  - Strictures or posterior urethral valves
  - Hydronephrosis from any cause
  - Benign prostatic hyperplasia: Rule out other causes of hematuria.
- Other causes: loin pain hematuria (most often in young women on oral contraceptives)

RISK FACTORS
- Smoking
- Occupational exposures (dyes, rubber, or tire manufacturing)
- Medications (e.g., cyclophosphamide, pioglitazone therapy >1 year)
- Pelvic radiation
- Chronic infection, especially with calculi
- Recent upper respiratory tract infection
- Positive family history of stones, GN, or cancer
- Chronic indwelling foreign body

 DIAGNOSIS

HISTORY
Considerations
- Burning, urgency, frequency: UTI
- Dark cola-colored urine: glomerular origin
- Clots: extraglomerular bleeding
- Arthritis/arthralgias/rash: lupus, vasculitis, Henoch-Schönlein purpura
- Flank pain: stones, infarction, pyelonephritis
- Recent upper respiratory infection (URI): poststreptococcal GN, membranoproliferative GN
- Concurrent URI: IgA nephropathy
- Excessive vitamin use: stones
- Marathon runner: traumatic, rhabdomyolysis
- Travel: schistosomiasis, TB
- Painless hematuria and/or weight loss: malignancy
- Family history: Alport disease (hereditary nephritis), sickle cell, polycystic, IgA nephropathy, thin basement membrane disease, von Willebrand
- In patients with microscopic hematuria, any episode of visible hematuria (VH) in the urine, even if transient, is associated with an OR of 7.2 for the prevalence of urologic cancers.

PHYSICAL EXAM
Considerations
- Elevated BP, edema, and weight gain: glomerular disease
- Fever: infection
- Palpable kidney: neoplasm, polycystic
- Genitalia: Look for meatal erosion, lesions.

DIAGNOSTIC TESTS & INTERPRETATION
A hematuria risk index may assist in stratifying patients at risk for urothelial malignancies who require more intensive testing. High-risk indicators are VH, age >50 years, male gender, and smoking.

Initial Tests (lab, imaging)
- If acute cystitis/UTI is ruled out, guidelines recommend evaluating AMH with upper urinary tract imaging and cystoscopy; none recommend cytology or urine markers for initial AMH evaluation (1)[C].

- Urine dipstick (sensitivity 91–100%; specificity 65–99%)
  - False negatives are rare but can be caused by high-dose vitamin C.
  - False positives: oxidizers used to cleanse the perineum, alkaline urine (>9), semen; free hemoglobin (hemolysis) and myoglobin (rhabdomyolysis)
  - Heme-negative red urine: food dyes, beets, rhubarb, porphyria, rifampin, phenytoin; phenazopyridine may discolor the dipstick, making interpretation difficult.
  - Any proteinuria >2+ raises concern for glomerular disease
- Microscopic urinalysis should always be done to confirm dipstick findings and quantify RBCs (1)[C].
  - American Urological Association (AUA) defines clinically significant microscopic hematuria as ≥3 RBCs/HPF on a properly collected urinary specimen when there is not an obvious benign cause (1,2)[C].
  - Positive dipstick, but a negative microscopic exam should be followed by three repeat tests. If anyone is positive, proceed with a workup (1,2)[C].
  - Exclude factitious or nonurinary causes, such as menstruation, mild trauma, exercise, poor collection technique, or chemical/drug causes, through cessation of activity/cause and a repeat urinalysis (1)[C].
  - RBC casts are pathognomonic for glomerular origin; dysmorphic cells are also suggestive.
- Renal function tests (eGFR, BUN, creatinine), albumin, and electrolytes to differentiate intrinsic renal disease and to evaluate for risks for imaging with contrast (1)[C]
  - Indicators of renal disease are significant (>500 mg/day) proteinuria, red cell casts, dysmorphic RBCs, increased creatinine, and albumin:creatinine ratio ≥30 mg/mmol (1,2)[C].
- Urine culture if suspected infection/pyuria
- Multidetector CT urography (MDCTU); sensitivity 95%, specificity 92% (3)[C]
  - The initial imaging of choice in nonpregnant adults without contraindications to contrast or radiation with unexplained hematuria per the AUA and the American College of Radiology (ACR) (1,3)[C]
  - Highly specific and relatively sensitive for the diagnosis of upper urinary tract neoplasms, especially when >1 cm (3)[C]
  - Higher radiation dose; weigh risk of disease versus risk of radiation exposure.
  - Does not obviate the need for cystoscopy, particularly in high-risk patients (3)[C]
  - Presence of calculi on noncontrast does not exclude another diagnosis or need for contrast phase.
  - Visualization of ureters is discontinuous.
  - Less cost-efficient
- CT
  - Noncontrast CT is preferred first line in adult patients with acute flank pain suspicious of stones.
  - Perform unenhanced helical CT for suspected stone disease in children if US is negative (4)[C].
  - Perform CT abdomen and pelvis with contrast in children with traumatic hematuria (4)[C].
- Renal and bladder US (RBUS)
  - Best for differentiating cystic from solid masses
  - Sensitive for hydronephrosis; point of care US in the emergency room may help avoid CT in patients with suspected stones.

- No radiation or iodinated contrast exposure
- Cost-efficient
- US can be used first line in patients with contraindications to CTU or at low risk of malignancy (3)[C].
- Sensitivity and NPV: for renal cancer = 85.7% and 99.9% and for upper tract urothelial cancer = 14.3% and 99.7%
- Poor sensitivity for renal masses <3 cm
- Main disadvantage is inability to fully evaluate the urothelium for transitional cell cancer.
- Magnetic resonance urography (MRU)
  - High sensitivity/specificity for renal parenchyma; less useful for collecting system or stones
  - Can be used in patients with contraindications to MDCTU (2,3)[C]
- MRI
  - Similar to CT in sensitivity for renal masses
  - No radiation exposure
  - Least cost-efficient
  - Limited ability to reliably detect urinary tract calcifications (3)[C]
  - Can be combined with retrograde pyelogram (RPG) for patients who cannot tolerate MDCTU or MRU (2)[C]

Follow-Up Tests & Special Considerations
- Other tests depend on suspected etiology: STD testing, antineutrophil cytoplasmic antibody (ANCA), C3, C4, antistreptolysin O (ASO) titer, hemoglobin electrophoresis, PT/INR for patients on warfarin.
- Consider genetic testing in patients suspected of having familial hematuria.
- Voided urine cytology (sensitivity 0–100%; specificity 62.5–100%)
  - Not recommended for routine evaluation of AMH; may be considered in those with significant risk factors for urinary malignancy (1,2)[C]
- Insufficient evidence to recommend routine use of urinary tumor markers (5)[C]
- Malignancies are detected in up to 6.5% of patients with AMH and up to 40% of patients with VH.
- Summary positive predictive value of VH for bladder/renal cancer in age >15 years is 5.1%; risk increases with age and male gender.

Diagnostic Procedures/Other
- Flexible cystoscopy (sensitivity 62%; specificity 43–98%)
  - Best for evaluation of bladder, especially small urothelial lesions; NPV for bladder tumors is 99%.
  - AUA recommends all patients with hematuria who are ≥35 years of age and all patients with risk factors for bladder cancer regardless of age to receive cystoscopy in addition to imaging (1,2)[C].
- Renal biopsy
  - Not routine but may be necessary to diagnose GN or in the face of increasing renal insufficiency
- RPG
  - Reserved for patients in which findings on MDCTU are equivocal or in addition to US or noncontrast studies in patients who are contraindicated for contrast or MRI (2,3)[C]
  - Sensitive for small lesions of supravesicular collecting system
  - Requires cystoscopy
- Ureteroscopy/pyeloscopy
  - For visualization of suspected supravesical collecting system lesions
  - Biopsy, excision, fulguration, or extraction of lesions/stones possible

- Requires anesthesia and cystoscopy
- Risk of injury to collecting system

Pregnancy Considerations
US is initial imaging choice for pregnant patients (3)[C]. MRU or RPG combined with either MRI or US are alternatives (2)[C].

Pediatric Considerations
- Consider GN, Wilms tumor, child abuse, and hypercalciuria.
- Isolated ASM may not need full workup; these patients rarely need cystoscopy; observe for development of hypertension, gross hematuria, or proteinuria (6)[C].
- In patients with ASM, most common diagnoses on renal biopsy are hypercalciuria (30–35%), hyperuricemia (5–20%), and glomerulonephritides, such as IgAN and thin basement membrane disease.
- Gross or symptomatic hematuria needs a full workup.
  - If eumorphic RBCs, consider US and urinary Ca:Cr ratio. Urine Ca:Cr ratio >0.2 is suggestive of hypercalciuria in children >6 years of age (6)[C].
- If dysmorphic RBCs, consider renal consult.
- Renal US identifies most congenital and malignant conditions; CT is reserved for cases of suspected trauma (with contrast) or stones (without contrast) (4,6)[C].

 ## TREATMENT

MEDICATION
None indicated for undiagnosed hematuria

ISSUES FOR REFERRAL
- Nephrology referral for proteinuria, red cell casts, elevated serum creatinine, and albumin:creatinine ratio ≥30 mg/mmol (2)[C]
- Urology referral for stones, vascular/anatomic anomalies, or nutcracker syndrome

SURGERY/OTHER PROCEDURES
Clots may require continuous bladder irrigation with a large-bore Foley catheter to prevent clot retention.

 ## ONGOING CARE

FOLLOW-UP RECOMMENDATIONS
Patient Monitoring
Some experts still recommend periodic urinalysis; recent literature suggests that, after thorough initial negative investigations (imaging, cystoscopy), no follow-up is indicated for the patient with AMH unless symptoms or frank hematuria develop. AUA recommends annual urinalyses in these patients, until two consecutive are negative and the consideration for a repeat workup at 3 to 5 years if hematuria is persistent (1,2)[C].

DIET
Increased fluids for stones or clots

PROGNOSIS
- Generally excellent for common causes of hematuria
- Poorer for malignant tumors and certain types of nephritis
- Persistent AMH is associated with an increased risk of end-stage renal disease in patients aged 16 to 25 years.

REFERENCES

1. Linder BJ, Bass EJ, Mostafid H, et al. Guideline of guidelines: asymptomatic microscopic haematuria. *BJU Int*. 2018;121(2):176–183.
2. Davis R, Jones JS, Barocas DA, et al; for American Urological Association. Diagnosis, evaluation and follow-up of asymptomatic microhematuria (AMH) in adults: AUA guideline. *J Urol*. 2012;188(Suppl 6): 2473–2481.
3. Shen L, Raman SS, Beland MD, et al; for Expert Panel on Urologic Imaging. *ACR Appropriateness Criteria® Hematuria*. Reston, VA: American College of Radiology; 2014.
4. Dillman JR, Rigsby CK, Iyer RS, et al; for Expert Panel on Pediatric Imaging. *ACR Appropriateness Criteria® Hematuria—Child*. Reston, VA: American College of Radiology; 2018.
5. Nielsen M, Qaseem A; for High Value Care Task Force of the American College of Physicians. Hematuria as a marker of occult urinary tract cancer: advice for high-value care from the American College of Physicians. *Ann Intern Med*. 2016;164(7):488–497.
6. Massengill SF. Hematuria. *Pediatr Rev*. 2008;29(10):342–348.

ADDITIONAL READING
- DeGeorge KC, Holt HR, Hodges SC. Bladder cancer: diagnosis and treatment. *Am Fam Physician*. 2017;96(8):507–514.
- Tan WS, Sarpong R, Khetrapal P, et al; for DETECT I Trial Collaborators. Can renal and bladder ultrasound replace computerized tomography urogram in patients investigated for microscopic hematuria? *J Urol*. 2018;200(5):973–980.

 ## SEE ALSO

Algorithm: Hematuria

 ## CODES

ICD10
- R31.9 Hematuria, unspecified
- R31.1 Benign essential microscopic hematuria
- R31.0 Gross hematuria

CLINICAL PEARLS
- Screening asymptomatic patients for microscopic hematuria is an "I" recommendation from the USPSTF.
- AMH and hematuria persisting after treatment of UTIs must be evaluated.
- Patients with bladder cancer can have intermittent microscopic hematuria; a thorough evaluation in high-risk patients is needed after just one episode.
- In patients with AMH, a history of anticoagulant use does not preclude the need for an evaluation (1)[C].
- Signs of underlying renal disease indicate the need for a nephrologic workup, but a urologic evaluation is still needed in the presence of persistent hematuria (2)[C].

H

HEMOCHROMATOSIS

Alethea Y. Turner, DO • Farrah J. Parker, DO

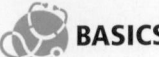 **BASICS**

DESCRIPTION

Hereditary hemochromatosis (HHC) is a hereditary multisystem disorder that results in iron overload and subsequent deposition into various tissues.

- HHC includes at least four types of iron overload conditions, which involve gene mutations that alter iron metabolism.
- There is no mechanism to excrete excess iron, so the surplus is stored in tissue, including the liver, pancreas, and heart, eventually resulting in severe damage to the affected organ(s).
- Patients are often asymptomatic, but early clinical features can include fatigue, malaise, arthralgia, and decreased libido.
- Late effects may include diabetes, liver cirrhosis, hypermelanotic pigmentation of the skin, porphyria cutanea tarda, cardiomyopathy, and cardiac arrhythmias.
- Cirrhosis may ultimately result in hepatocellular carcinoma.
- Synonym(s): bronze diabetes; Troisier-Hanot-Chauffard syndrome

EPIDEMIOLOGY

Incidence
- Predominant age: Metabolic abnormality is congenital, but symptoms typically present between the 3rd and 5th decades for HHC types 1, 3, and 4; type 2 juvenile hemochromatosis typically presents between the 1st and 3rd decades of life, and neonatal presentation is exceedingly rare.
- Predominant sex: Gene frequency is equal between male and female, although clinical signs are more frequent in men.

Prevalence
- Prevalence in the United States for carrying an *HFE* gene mutation (type 1 HHC) is 5.4% for the *C282Y* gene and 13.5% for the *H63D* gene; prevalence for homozygosity is 0.3% for *C282Y* and 1.9% for *H63D* (1).
- Type 1 accounts for >90% of HHC cases in the United States and primarily occurs in people of northern European descent; ~1 in 200 white adults in the United States are *C282Y* homozygous (1,2).

Pediatric Considerations
Juvenile (type 2) HHC is rare but can present in young patients (between 1st and 3rd decades of life) with hypogonadism and cardiomyopathy.

ETIOLOGY AND PATHOPHYSIOLOGY
- HHC type 1 is caused by mutations in the *HFE* gene (most commonly *C282Y* and/or *H63D*), type 2 by mutations in either the *HJV* or *HAMP* gene, type 3 by mutations in the *TFR2* gene, and type 4 by mutations in the *SLC11A3* gene.
- Types 1 to 3 involve a deficiency in an iron-regulating hormone named hepcidin, which causes increased intestinal absorption of iron through excessive expression of ferroportin (a transmembrane protein that transports iron out of the cell and into the bloodstream).
- Type 4 is caused by an insensitivity of ferroportin to hepcidin (4a) or an inactivity of ferroportin itself (4b); the latter leads to iron accumulation within mesenchymal tissue.

- Other rare types of HHC exist as a result of different gene mutations.
- Increased plasma iron and transferrin saturation leads to elevated levels of unbound iron, which are then absorbed into various tissue, eventually causing organ dysfunction.

Genetics
- Genetically heterogeneous disorder of iron overload; types 1, 2, and 3 are autosomal recessive; type 4 is autosomal dominant.
- Penetrance is incomplete; expressivity is variable; ~13.5% disease penetrance of *C282Y* homozygosity (CI 13.5%) (3)
- Factors contributing to variable expressivity include different mutations in the same gene, mitigating or exacerbating genes, and environmental factors.

RISK FACTORS
- Family history
- White men between the ages of 30 and 50 years (particularly for HFE-related HHC)
- Loss of blood, such as that which occurs during menstruation and pregnancy, delays the onset of symptoms in women; alcohol consumption because it increases the absorption of iron and synergistically damages the liver along with the oxidative effects of iron

GENERAL PREVENTION
First-degree relatives of those with HHC should be screened; typically, with fasting transferrin saturation and ferritin levels

> **ALERT**
> Screening of the general population is *not* recommended because only a small subset of patients with HHC will develop symptoms or advanced disease (2,4)[B].

COMMONLY ASSOCIATED CONDITIONS
See "Complications."

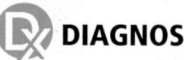 **DIAGNOSIS**

HISTORY
- Fatigue
- Weakness
- Arthralgias
- Abdominal pain
- Loss of libido or impotency
- Symptoms of diabetes
- Skin pigmentation or blistering
- Dyspnea on exertion

PHYSICAL EXAM
- Hepatomegaly and/or splenomegaly
- Increased skin pigmentation
- Hepatic tenderness
- Peripheral edema
- Jaundice
- Gynecomastia
- Ascites
- Testicular atrophy
- Hepatic tenderness

DIFFERENTIAL DIAGNOSIS
- Inflammatory syndromes
- Various causes of hepatitis
- Biliary or alcoholic cirrhosis
- Repeated transfusions
- Sideroblastic anemia
- β-Thalassemia major

DIAGNOSTIC TESTS & INTERPRETATION
Initial Tests (lab, imaging)
There is currently no evidence to support a concrete relationship between symptoms and the degree of iron overload (1).

- Serum ferritin (SF): ≥300 μg/L for men and postmenopausal women and 200 μg/L for premenopausal women; may be elevated for a number of other reasons including but not limited to inflammation (consider checking inflammatory markers); if elevated with suspicion of hemochromatosis, obtain fasting transferrin saturation.
- Fasting transferrin saturation (serum iron concentration ÷ total iron-binding capacity × 100) is the earliest biochemical marker to be increased in HHC: ≥45% is suspicious for HHC but warrants further evaluation because it can be elevated in other disease processes including chronic anemias.
- Confirmatory testing should be done through HFE gene mutation analysis (2).

Follow-Up Tests & Special Considerations
- After the diagnosis is established, check the following to determine need for phlebotomy:
  – ALT and AST
- Assess for complications of HHC and order testing as deemed appropriate; for instance:
  – HbA1c to rule out diabetes
  – ECG to evaluate an arrhythmia
  – Echocardiogram if concerned for cardiomyopathy
  – Total testosterone if symptoms of hypogonadism are present
- Consider screening for osteoporosis in patients >50 years with additional risk factors (i.e., alcohol or tobacco use) (2).
- Test for viral hepatitis if transaminitis exists to rule out concomitant disease.
- Monitor for liver lesions with an abdominal ultrasound every 6 months if severe liver fibrosis or cirrhosis is present (2).

Diagnostic Procedures/Other
- Liver biopsy or hepatic MRI should be done to measure liver iron content if hepatomegaly is present, SF is >1,000 μg/L, and/or ALT/AST are elevated.
- Consider liver biopsy in these cases to determine the degree of liver damage and prognosis (2,4)[C]; SF <1,000 μg/L, normal AST, and the absence of hepatomegaly have a negative predictive value of 95% for severe fibrosis or cirrhosis (3).

Test Interpretation
- MRI signal intensity of liver to muscle should be <0.88 in the setting of high iron content (~87% sensitive, 90% specific) (3).
- Liver biopsy will reveal increased hepatic parenchymal iron stores and evidence of any fibrosis or cirrhosis.

TREATMENT

GENERAL MEASURES

Due to a lack in evidence-based data, there is debate regarding when treatment should be initiated (particularly in asymptomatic patients), what the target serum indices, and frequency of phlebotomy should be. American and European liver associations recommend initiating treatment when SF is above the normal limit (see "Initial Tests (lab, imaging)"). If HCC diagnosis is confirmed, there is no liver involvement, SF remains normal, and the patient is asymptomatic, it is reasonable to monitor SF at least annually (2)[C].

- Phlebotomy (~500 mL per session) is the mainstay of therapy and is performed once or twice weekly in the initial treatment phase and may take up to 2 to 3 years to deplete iron stores (1,4)[C].
- When the patient finally becomes iron deficient, a lifelong maintenance program of ~2 to 6 phlebotomies a year is required to keep iron storage normal or below normal (3,4)[C].
- Erythrocytapheresis is an alternative to phlebotomy because it involves removing only red cells from the blood; however, it is expensive, not widely available, and there is no evidence to support a benefit over phlebotomy (1,3).

MEDICATION

- If phlebotomy is not feasible or if it is contraindicated (anemia or severe heart disease), a 2nd tier option is chelation therapy with parenteral deferoxamine (contraindicated in severe renal disease) or oral deferasirox (contraindicated in severe hepatic impairment) (2); monitor patients for auditory or visual changes annually if on chelation therapy.
- The daily use of pantoprazole 40 mg has been shown to reduce the number of phlebotomies needed to keep the ferritin level <100 μg/L in HHC patients homozygous for p.C282Y (5)[B].
- Testosterone replacement in men with HHC can improve symptoms of erectile dysfunction and decreased libido (6)[B].
- Hepatitis A and hepatitis B immunizations should be provided if there is no evidence of previous exposure (2)[C].
- Pneumococcal vaccination (PPSV23) should be given if cirrhosis is present (2).

ALERT

Caution is advised for prescribing androgens in the setting of hypogonadism secondary to risk of hepatotoxicity (2).

ISSUES FOR REFERRAL

- Refer to a gastroenterologist if liver biopsy is indicated and for the management of concomitant liver disease.
- Refer to a cardiologist if cardiac involvement is suspected.
- Refer to endocrinology if male infertility is present.

ADMISSION, INPATIENT, AND NURSING CONSIDERATIONS

Need for hospitalization is typically rare and necessary only for the management of severe complications including need for organ transplant.

ONGOING CARE

FOLLOW-UP RECOMMENDATIONS

Patient Monitoring

- Measure hematocrit before each phlebotomy; skip phlebotomy if hemoglobin is <11 g/dL (2).
- In the initial phases of treatment, check SF every 3 months (3,4).
- Once iron stores are depleted, phlebotomy every 1 to 6 months (adjusted based on patient's need) should be performed to maintain SF between 50 and 100 μg/L; consider targeting SF to <50 μg/L (3).
- During maintenance therapy, measure transferrin saturation and SF yearly.

DIET

- Avoid consumption of iron-fortified foods, oysters, uncooked shellfish, vitamin C, and iron-containing supplements (2)[C].
  - Natural sources of vitamin C and iron are considered safe (2,4).
- Black tea chelates iron and may be drank with meals (2)[C].

PATIENT EDUCATION

- Adequate hydration prior to phlebotomy is recommended (2).
- Blood collected through phlebotomy may be donated (3,4).
- http://www.hemochromatosis.org/

PROGNOSIS

- Patients diagnosed and treated before the development of cirrhosis or diabetes have a normal life expectancy (2).
- Life expectancy is reduced in patients with cirrhosis and/or diabetes (4).
- Cirrhosis is associated with an increased risk of hepatocellular carcinoma (annual incidence of 3–4%) and mortality (4).
- Cirrhosis is irreversible; arthralgias and symptoms of hypogonadism may not improve with phlebotomies, but other symptoms and complications may be averted with successful management (2,4).

COMPLICATIONS

Complications develop as a result of untreated HHC.

- Arthritis, chondrocalcinosis
- Diabetes mellitus
- Hypogonadism
- Arrhythmia
- Congestive heart failure
- Cirrhosis (prevalence of 20–45% in *C282Y* homozygotes with SF >1,000 μg/L) (4)
- Hepatocellular carcinoma
- Osteoporosis
- Infection from *Listeria monocytogenes*, *Yersinia enterocolitica*, or *Vibrio vulnificus* is rare, but those with iron overload are at increased risk (4).

REFERENCES

1. Buzzetti E, Kalafateli M, Thorburn D, et al. Interventions for hereditary haemochromatosis: an attempted network meta-analysis. *Cochrane Database Syst Rev*. 2017;(3):CD011647.
2. Powell LW, Seckington RC, Deugnier Y. Haemochromatosis. *Lancet*. 2016;388(10045):706–716.
3. European Association for the Study of the Liver. EASL clinical practice guidelines for HFE hemochromatosis. *J Hepatol*. 2010;53(1):3–22.
4. Bacon BR, Adams PC, Kowdley KV, et al. Diagnosis and management of hemochromatosis: 2011 practice guideline by the American Association for the Study of Liver Diseases. *Hepatology*. 2011;54(1):328–343.
5. Vanclooster A, Van Deursen C, Jaspers R, et al. Proton pump inhibitors decrease phlebotomy need in HFE hemochromatosis: double-blind randomized placebo-controlled trial. *Gastroenterology*. 2017;153(3):678–680.
6. Kley HK, Stremmel W, Kley JB, et al. Testosterone treatment of men with idiopathic hemochromatosis. *Clin Investig*. 1992;70(7):566–572.

ADDITIONAL READING

U.S. Preventive Services Task Force. Screening for hemochromatosis: recommendation statement. *Ann Intern Med*. 2006;145(3):204–208.

CODES

ICD10

- E83.110 Hereditary hemochromatosis
- E83.118 Other hemochromatosis
- E83.111 Hemochromatosis due to repeated red blood cell transfusions

CLINICAL PEARLS

- Screening of the general population for hemochromatosis is not recommended, but testing is recommended if there is clinical suspicion or family history. An elevated transferrin saturation is the earliest abnormality in hemochromatosis. Ferritin is a sensitive measure of iron overload but can be elevated in a variety of infectious and inflammatory conditions without iron overload being present.
- Genetic testing is recommended to confirm type 1 hemochromatosis, which is the most common type.
- Patients with hemochromatosis who have hepatomegaly, transaminitis, and/or serum transferrin >1,000 μg/L should be evaluated for liver iron content via MRI or liver biopsy; liver biopsy is necessary to determine degree of liver damage and clarify prognosis.
- Initiate once or twice weekly phlebotomy when SF levels are elevated, particularly when symptoms or clinical findings are present.
- Goal is to achieve and then maintain SF levels 50 to 100 μg/L and possibly even <50 μg/L; maintenance phlebotomy is less frequent and patient specific.
- Consider adding a daily proton pump inhibitor because it may reduce the overall number of phlebotomies.

H

HEMOPHILIA

Toussaint L. Mears-Clarke, MD

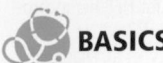

BASICS

DESCRIPTION
- Deficiency of factor VIII (hemophilia A) or factor IX (hemophilia B) coagulation proteins leading to bleeding tendencies in affected individuals. The majority of cases are due to inherited genetic mutations in factor VIII or factor IX coagulation proteins. However, an estimated 30% of all hemophilia cases result from spontaneous mutations.
- Hemophilia A and B are clinically indistinguishable but can be differentiated by assays that detect levels of factors VIII and IX, respectively.
- Disease severity correlates with the relative levels of coagulation factors present in serum analysis:
  - Severe: frequent spontaneous bleeding (factor activity <1%)
  - Moderate: bleeding with mild to moderate trauma (factor activity 1–5%)
  - Mild: bleeding with major trauma, tooth extraction, or surgery (factor activity 5–40%)
- Bleeding frequency is similar in hemophilia A and B with similar levels of factor deficiency.

EPIDEMIOLOGY
- Worldwide, an estimated 400,000 people are affected with hemophilia; estimated frequency of 1 in 10,000 births (1)[A]
- Hemophilia A represents 80–85% of the total hemophilia population; hemophilia B comprises the remaining 15–20%.

ETIOLOGY AND PATHOPHYSIOLOGY
- Damage to vascular endothelium leads to exposure of subendothelial tissue factors, which interact with platelets, plasma proteins, and coagulation factors to produce a localized platelet plug contributing to hemostasis. Complexes involving factors VIII and IX participate in the intrinsic coagulation pathway to activate factor X, FXa. Downstream interactions involving FXa culminate in the conversion of prothrombin to thrombin, mediating platelet activation and fibrin deposition necessary for stabilization of the platelet plug.
- Deficiencies of factor VIII or factor IX result in decreased production of FXa, leading to an unstable platelet plug and impaired hemostasis.

Genetics
- Exhibits an X-chromosome linked inheritance pattern. Males are almost exclusively affected; females are asymptomatic carriers, unless their factor activity is <40% of normal.
- Carriers with symptomatically low clotting factor levels are treated similarly to patients with the trait:
  - May bleed at the time of surgery
- Males within the same family share similar deficiencies and level of severity owing to the same genetic defect.

GENERAL PREVENTION
- Patients should carry medical ID tags listing their bleeding disorder or factor deficiency, inhibitor status, type of treatment products used, and initial treatment doses for mild, moderate, or severe bleeding.
- Immediate family members of affected patients should have factor VIII and IX levels checked prior to invasive procedures, childbirth, and if bleeding tendencies occur.
- Genetic testing should be offered to at-risk female family members to facilitate genetic counseling.
- Regular dental care and good oral hygiene are recommended to prevent gum bleeding.

DIAGNOSIS

- History and initial presentation
  - 2/3 of presenting hemophilic patients have a positive family history. All male infants born to known carriers should have factor level testing.
  - Prolonged bleeding with circumcision, dental work, surgery, or injury
  - Excessive or easy bruising in early childhood
  - Spontaneous bleeding, especially in joints, muscle, or soft tissue
  - Typical age of presentation: mild (36 months), moderate (8 months), severe (1 month)
  - *Pregnancy considerations*: Treat all males born to a carrier as if they have hemophilia; recommend planned caesarean delivery if male infant is potentially affected. Avoid fetal scalp electrode placement, vacuum/forceps deliveries.
  - Test infant at birth (2)[B]. Cord blood can be used for testing (3)[A].
- Life-threatening bleeds
  - Intracranial hemorrhage: generally resulting from trauma; incidence of 1:10; fatal in 30% of cases
  - Hematomas of bowel wall can cause obstruction or intussusception and pain mimicking appendicitis.
  - Neck or throat bleeds: can lead to airway obstruction
- Serious bleeds
  - Hemarthrosis, most commonly of ankles, elbows, and knees
    - Infants may present with irritability or decreased use of limb.
    - Adults may have prodromal stiffness, acute pain, and swelling of joint.
    - Arthropathy results from repeated bleeding into joints, damaging cartilage, and subchondral bone:
      - Can result in fixed joints, muscle wasting, and significantly impaired mobility
  - Muscular hematomas most commonly occur in quadriceps, iliopsoas, and forearm:
    - May result in compartment syndrome and ischemic nerve damage, such as femoral nerve neuropathy due to undetected retroperitoneal hemorrhage
  - Mucous membrane bleeding, such as in the genitourinary tract, leading to hematuria
  - Pseudotumor syndrome: untreated hemorrhage causing a hematoma, which calcifies (named because it can be mistaken for cancer)

DIFFERENTIAL DIAGNOSIS
- von Willebrand disease
- Vitamin K deficiency, anticoagulant (i.e., warfarin, rivaroxaban, heparin) therapy (factor IX is vitamin K dependent)
- Other factor deficiencies (i.e., hemophilia C, acquired hemophilia A), afibrinogenemia, dysfibrinogenemia, fibrinolytic defects, platelet disorders
- Child abuse

DIAGNOSTIC TESTS & INTERPRETATION
Initial Tests (lab, imaging)
- Screening tests: CBC with platelet count, PT, aPTT, platelet function (preferred), or bleed time
  - aPTT usually prolonged. aPTT may be normal in patients with mild hemophilia.
  - PT, platelet count, and function are normal.
- Follow-up tests: mixing study, vWF, factor activity levels (factor VIII:C and factor IX)
  - Mixing study: Patient's plasma is mixed with pooled normal plasma. Prolonged aPTT corrects in

absence of inhibitors, that is, lupus anticoagulant and acquired factor inhibitors.
  - vWF is normal.
- Diagnosis based on factor VIII:C or IX activity
  - Normal factor levels: 50 to 150 IU/dL
  - Mild: 5 to 40 IU/dL
  - Moderate: 1 to 5 IU/dL
  - Severe: <1 IU/dL

Follow-Up Tests & Special Considerations
- Genetic counseling, and participation in genotyping project for affected individuals and family, is recommended; the information may help predict inhibitor risk, bleeding severity, and individualize treatment (4)[A].
- Inhibitors to factor VIII and IX (see "Complications"):
  - Should be periodically measured using the Nijmegen or Bethesda assay, which quantifies the alloantibody titer
  - Screen before invasive procedures and at regular intervals.

Diagnostic Procedures/Other
Prenatal diagnosis via genetic testing of a sample of chorionic villus or fluid obtained at amniocentesis is not recommended (2)[B].

Test Interpretation
Pathology of affected joints: synovial hemosiderosis, articular cartilage degeneration, thickening of periarticular tissues, bony hypertrophy

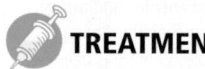

TREATMENT

GENERAL MEASURES
- Integrated, multidisciplinary, comprehensive care model, including hematologist, physical therapist, and social worker, is recommended (1,5)[A].
- Avoid aspirin or other NSAIDs.
- Treat early; acute bleeds should be treated as quickly as possible, preferable within 2 hours (1)[A].
- For surgical prophylaxis
  - If major surgery is undertaken, factor levels should be maintained at >50% for at least 2 to 3 weeks after the procedure:
    - Fibrin glue products may be beneficial for oozing.
  - Dental extractions: Antifibrinolytics (Amicar, tranexamic acid) may be used.
  - Minor procedures: may use desmopressin (DDAVP) in hemophilia A
- Hepatitis A and B vaccinations are recommended.
- Encourage physical activity: Patients should avoid high-impact contact sports. Organized sports should be encouraged (1)[A].

MEDICATION
First Line
- Principles of therapy
  - Primary prophylaxis: administration of specific factor replacement therapy in the absence of bleeding to maintain adequate baseline plasma levels sufficient for hemostasis in all categories of severity (1)[A]
    - Lower frequency of acute bleeds and episodes of life-threatening hemorrhage compared to on-demand therapy
    - Standard of care for children with severe hemophilia A or B to prevent joint bleeds and joint degeneration

- Additionally, bispecific monoclonal antibody for FIXa and FX (emicizumab-kxwh) is available for prophylaxis for hemophilia A with/without inhibitors (6)[B].
  - Dosing, frequency, duration of therapeutic regimens tailored to individual patient needs in clinical practice
  - Gene therapy is currently under development to reduce the risk of bleeding (7)[B].
- On-demand therapy: treatment administered in response to occurrence of bleeding (1)[A]
  - Amount and duration of factor replacement depends on location and severity of bleeding:
    - Mild bleeds correct to a factor level of >30% major hemorrhages, and large muscle bleeds require correction to levels between 50% and 100%.
    - Life-threatening bleeds require levels between 80% and 100%, sustained with bolus dosing or continuous infusion.
- Specific agents:
  - Hemophilia A: Replacement with factor VIII concentrates is the treatment of choice: two sources for the factor available (1)[A]:
    - Purified plasma-derived factor VIII: Donor pool is screened, and the plasma-derived factor is treated to inactivate viruses (HIV, hepatitis B, and hepatitis C). Theoretical risks still exist.
    - Recombinant factor VIII
      - Dosing: 1 IU of factor VIII (the amount in 1 mL of plasma)/kg body weight administered will raise the plasma level of the recipient by 2%.
  - Hemophilia B: Replacement with factor IX concentrates is the treatment of choice:
    - Plasma-derived factor IX and recombinant factor IX (preferred) are commercially available.
      - Dosing: 1 IU/kg body weight administered will raise plasma factor IX levels 1%.
- Hemophilia patients with inhibitors (neutralizing alloantibodies to factors VIII or IX) (1)[A]
  - Inhibitor formation should be suspected when replacement with the deficient factor fails to correct coagulopathy.
  - Low-titer (<5 BU/mL) patients: Replace with high doses of the deficient factor to overcome the circulating inhibitor concentration.
  - High-titer patients: Treat using products that *bypass* the factor neutralized by the alloantibody or emergently with high doses of the specific deficient factor:
    - Two bypassing agents are available; both are efficacious at providing 80% of bleeding episodes:
      - Activated prothrombin complex concentrate
      - Recombinant activated factor VII
- Immune tolerance induction (ITI): protocols to promote immune tolerance through repeated exposure to high-dose factor VIII therapy over 12 to 18 months, with or without immunosuppressive therapy (corticosteroids, cyclophosphamide, rituximab). Success rates are 60–80%.
  - Home therapy allows immediate access to clotting factor, resulting in decreased pain, dysfunction, and long-term disability (2)[B].

Second Line
- Cryoprecipitate and fresh frozen plasma (FFP) can be used in instances where the specific factor concentrate is unavailable for *emergent hemostasis*.
  - FFP: contains all coagulation factors but generally difficult to attain high levels of factors VIII or IX
    - Starting dose: 15 to 20 mL/kg

- Cryoprecipitate: derived from precipitates of cooled FFP; contains significant levels of factor VIII (up to 100 IU/bag) but *not* factor IX:
  - Dosing: 1 mL cryoprecipitate has ~3 to 5 IU factor VIII.
- Desmopressin (DDAVP): synthetic vasopressin; stimulates endogenous release of factor VIII (and *vWF*) from endothelial stores; used in mild hemophilia A
  - IV or SC: 0.3 μg/kg infused 30 minutes prior to procedure; may repeat if needed
  - Intranasal (150 μg/spray): adult dose, 1 spray to each nostril (300 μg total). Alternate dose if <50 kg: 150 μg once.
  - Adverse effect: hyponatremic seizures, especially in children; restrict fluids and watch sodium levels and urine output.
- Antifibrinolytic agents: inhibit plasminogen activation, thereby stabilizing the clot
  - Effective in controlling mucosal bleeding, such as bleeding in oral cavity, epistaxis, and menorrhagia; can also be used prophylactically (e.g., prior to tooth extractions)
    - Tranexamic acid (25 mg/kg PO q6–8h or 10 mg/kg IV q6–8h)
    - Aminocaproic acid (Amicar) is less frequently used.

 ## ONGOING CARE

FOLLOW-UP RECOMMENDATIONS
Patient Monitoring
Regular evaluations every 6 to 12 months, including a musculoskeletal evaluation, an inhibitor screen, liver tests, and tests for antibodies to hepatitis viruses and HIV

PATIENT EDUCATION
- National Hemophilia Foundation: http://www.hemophilia.org/
- World Federation of Hemophilia: http://www.wfh.org/
- Center for Disease Control and Prevention: https://www.cdc.gov/ncbddd/hemophilia/index.html

PROGNOSIS
- Survival is normal for those with mild disease; mortality is increased 2- to 6-fold in those with moderate to severe disease.
- Intracranial hemorrhage is a leading cause of death in hemophilia.
- Hemophilic arthropathy is the main cause of morbidity in patients with severe hemophilia.

COMPLICATIONS
- Hemophilic arthropathy: Symptoms include pain, limitation of motion, and contractures.
- Theoretical transmission of blood-borne infections, such as hepatitis A, B, C, and D and HIV; this risk has been greatly reduced with current testing of blood products.
- Development of inhibitor autoantibodies
  - More common in hemophilia A (20–30% of patients with severe hemophilia compared to 5% in hemophilia B) and in patients with severe disease requiring multiple transfusions
  - In severe hemophilia A, inhibitors develop by median age of 3 years; in mild/moderate hemophilia, inhibitors develop by median age 30 years.
  - Risk of inhibitor development in hemophilia B associated with family history and/or specific genetic defects
  - High incidence (up to 50%) of severe allergic reactions, including anaphylaxis, with factor IX administration in hemophilia B patients with inhibitors
  - No increased risk of bleeding, but when bleeding occurs, it is more difficult to achieve hemostasis due to decreased response to factor replacement.

REFERENCES
1. Srivastava A, Brewer AK, Mauser-Bunschoten EP, et al; for Treatment Guidelines Working Group on Behalf of the World Federation of Hemophilia. Guidelines for the management of hemophilia. *Haemophilia*. 2013;19(1):e1–e47.
2. Tsui NB, Kadir RA, Chan KC, et al. Noninvasive prenatal diagnosis of hemophilia by microfluidics digital PCR analysis of maternal plasma DNA. *Blood*. 2011;117(13):3684–3691.
3. National Hemophilia Foundation. MASAC guidelines for perinatal management of women with bleeding disorders and carriers of hemophilia A and B. http://www.hemophilia.org/Researchers-Healthcare-Providers/Medical-and-Scientific-Advisory-Council-MASAC/MASAC-Recommendations/MASAC-Guidelines-for-Perinatal-Management-of-Women-with-Bleeding-Disorders-and-Carriers-of-Hemophilia-A-and-B. Accessed September 20, 2018.
4. National Hemophilia Foundation. MASAC recommendations on the NHF genotyping project for persons with hemophilia. https://www.hemophilia.org/Researchers-Healthcare-Providers/Medical-and-Scientific-Advisory-Council-MASAC/MASAC-Recommendations/MASAC-Recommendations-on-the-NHF-Genotyping-Project-for-Persons-with-Hemophilia. Accessed September 15, 2018.
5. Pai M, Key NS, Skinner M, et al. NHF-McMaster guideline on care models for haemophilia management. *Haemophilia*. 2016;22(Suppl 3):6–16.
6. Oldenburg J, Mahlangu J, Kim B, et al. Emicizumab prophylaxis in hemophilia A with inhibitors. *N Engl J Med*. 2017;377(9):809–818.
7. Rangarajan S, Walsh L, Lester W, et al. AAV5-Factor VIII gene transfer in severe hemophilia A. *N Engl J Med*. 2017;377(26):2519–2530.

ADDITIONAL READING
Hartmann J, Croteau S. 2017 clinical trials update: innovations in hemophilia therapy. *Am J Hematol*. 2016;91(12):1252–1260.

 ## CODES

ICD10
- D66 Hereditary factor VIII deficiency
- D67 Hereditary factor IX deficiency
- Z14.01 Asymptomatic hemophilia A carrier

CLINICAL PEARLS
- Deficiency of factor VIII (hemophilia A) or factor IX (hemophilia B) coagulation proteins leading to bleeding tendencies in affected individuals
- The majority of hemophilia cases are due to inherited genetic mutations in factor VIII or factor IX.
- An estimated 30% of all hemophilia cases result from spontaneous mutations.
- Exhibits an X-chromosome linked inheritance pattern. Males are almost exclusively affected.
- Diagnosis based on decreased factor VIII:C or IX activity
- Initial site of bleeding and bleeding severity dependent on coagulation factor levels
- Survival is normal for those with mild disease; mortality is increased 2- to 6-fold in those with moderate to severe disease.

H

HEMORRHOIDS

Donna I. Meltzer, MD

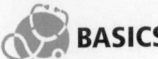 **BASICS**

DESCRIPTION
- Varicosities of the hemorrhoidal venous plexus
- External hemorrhoids
  - Located below the dentate line; visceral innervation (painful)
  - Covered by squamous epithelium
- Internal hemorrhoids
  - Located above the dentate line; somatic innervation (painless)
  - Covered by columnar epithelium
  - Classification of internal hemorrhoids (1):
    - Grade I: Hemorrhoid vessel bulges without prolapse.
    - Grade II: Hemorrhoid prolapses with straining but reduces spontaneously.
    - Grade III: Hemorrhoid prolapses with straining and requires manual reduction.
    - Grade IV: chronically prolapsed—can't be reduced
- Internal and external hemorrhoids often coexist.
- Although often asymptomatic, hemorrhoids can present with itching, bleeding, soilage, prolapse, or pain.
- Pain and Thrombosis more common with external than internal hemorrhoids.

Geriatric Considerations
Hemorrhoids and rectal prolapse are more common in elderly.

Pediatric Considerations
- Uncommon in infants and children; most common cause is chronic liver failure; other findings (rectal polyps, skin tags, condyloma) often misdiagnosed as hemorrhoids
- In adolescents, chronic constipation and prolonged toilet time can result in hemorrhoids.

Pregnancy Considerations
- Common in pregnancy
- Usually resolves after delivery
- No treatment required, unless extremely painful

EPIDEMIOLOGY
- Predominant age: adults; peak from 45 to 65 years (2)
- Predominant sex: male = female

Incidence
Common

Prevalence
- ~4–5% in general population in the United States
- 39% prevalence on routine screening colonoscopy (2)

ETIOLOGY AND PATHOPHYSIOLOGY
- Exact pathophysiology is unknown.
- There are three primary hemorrhoidal cushions—typically located in left lateral, right anterior, and right posterior positions. Hemorrhoidal cushions augment anal closing pressure and protect the anal sphincter during stool passage. During Valsalva, increased intra-abdominal pressure raises pressure within the hemorrhoidal cushions. Mechanisms implicated in symptomatic hemorrhoidal disease include:
  - Dilated veins of hemorrhoidal plexus
  - Tight internal anal sphincter

- Abnormal distention of the arteriovenous anastomosis
- Prolapse of the cushions and the surrounding connective tissues

Genetics
No known genetic pattern

RISK FACTORS
- Pregnancy
- Pelvic space-occupying lesions
- Liver disease; portal HTN
- Constipation
- Occupations that require prolonged sitting
- Loss of perianal muscle tone due to old age, rectal surgery, birth trauma/episiotomy, anal intercourse
- Obesity
- Chronic diarrhea

GENERAL PREVENTION
- Avoid constipation by consuming high-fiber diet (>30 g/day) and ensuring proper hydration.
- Maintain appropriate weight.
- Avoid prolonged sitting or straining on the toilet.

COMMONLY ASSOCIATED CONDITIONS
- Liver disease; cirrhosis, ascites
- Pregnancy
- Constipation

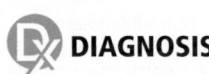 **DIAGNOSIS**

Diagnosis is typically straightforward through history and inspection of the perineum, rectal exam, and anoscopy.

HISTORY
- Symptoms (1)
  - Bleeding (~60%)
  - Classically, bright red blood per rectum, may range from scant blood on toilet paper to copious blood in the toilet bowl
  - Pruritus (~55%)
  - Perianal discomfort (~20%)
  - Soiling (~10%)
  - Constipation or diarrhea
  - Straining with defecation
- External hemorrhoids
  - Episodic bleeding on stool or toilet paper, pruritus, and irritation from compromised hygiene and pain
- More extensive internal hemorrhoids
  - Feeling of incomplete evacuation
- Thrombosed hemorrhoids present as acute painful mass.
- Ask about diet (fiber, fluid intake), bowel patterns (frequency, consistency), bowel habits (prolonged sitting), change in stools, systemic symptoms (weight loss, pain, fever).
- Ask about past medical history and family history (gastrointestinal disease, colorectal cancer).

PHYSICAL EXAM
- Visual anorectal inspection with Valsalva
- Digital exam with anoscopy
  - Internal hemorrhoid appears as purple mass on lumen wall.
  - Look for other anorectal pathology (mass, abscess, fissure, fistula).

- Attempt to reduce prolapsed hemorrhoids.
- Abdominal exam to exclude mass
- Peripheral stigmata of cirrhosis and portal HTN (caput, telangiectasias, palmar erythema)

DIFFERENTIAL DIAGNOSIS
- Rectal or anal neoplasia
- Condyloma
- Skin tag
- Inflammatory bowel disease
- Anal fistula, fissure, or abscess
- Rectal polyp
- Rectal prolapse

DIAGNOSTIC TESTS & INTERPRETATION
Initial Tests (lab, imaging)
Not indicated unless anemia is suspected

Diagnostic Procedures/Other
Sigmoidoscopy or colonoscopy depending on risk factors for malignancy in patients with rectal bleeding

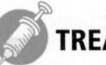 **TREATMENT**

Prevention
- Fiber supplements
- Stool softeners
- Anal hygiene

GENERAL MEASURES
- Hemorrhoids are a recurrent disease, even after surgical excision. Preventive measures should be continued indefinitely.
- For mild symptoms or prevention
  - Avoid prolonged sitting during bowel movements.
  - Avoid straining.
  - Avoid constipation by eating a high-fiber diet or by taking fiber supplements; if necessary, take regular stool softeners.
  - Regular exercise, weight loss if indicated
- Pruritus or mild discomfort after stooling might respond to topical corticosteroid ointment, anesthetic ointments or sprays, and warm sitz baths.
- Constipation relief, anal hygiene, local ointments, and sitz baths are effective through the stage of easy reduction (grade II). More severe stages often require ligation or surgery.

MEDICATION
First Line
- Dietary modification with adequate fluid (generally ≥2 L water per day) and high fiber (25 to 35 g/day) is first-line, nonoperative therapy for symptomatic hemorrhoids (1).
- Fiber helps relieve overall symptoms and bleeding (3)[A].
- Stool softener or bulk-forming laxative to soften stool
- Sitz bath with warm water for pain relief
- Witch hazel (Tucks) as a wipe after stooling may be useful for astringent properties.
- Topic anesthetics (benzocaine, lidocaine, pramoxine), steroids, emollients to alleviate symptoms; these over-the-counter (OTC) products have been traditionally used but lack strong evidence for long-term use.
  - Local anesthetics for relief of pain and itch; applied to perianal area (not inserted into rectum)

- Dibucaine 1% ointment (Nupercainal), pramoxine 1% foam, ointment, wipe (Proctofoam); benzocaine 20% spray, ointment (Americaine). Use sprays with caution as alcohol in product may cause burning sensation.
  - Anti-inflammatory agents (corticosteroids) to decrease swelling and for discomfort and itch
    - Hydrocortisone ointment, cream (0.25–2.5%) (Anusol HC, Cortifoam). Rectal suppositories are for short-term use only.
  - Astringents to help dry skin
    - Witch hazel solution, pads (Preparation H, Tucks)
  - Vasoconstrictors to shrink hemorrhoids and ameliorate swelling, pain, itch
    - 0.25% phenylephrine ointment, suppository (Preparation H, Rectacaine)

Second Line
Treatment for special cases
- Thrombosed external hemorrhoids: if present within 72 hours after pain onset, recommend incision and clot evacuation or excision of hemorrhoid complex. Early surgical excision may resolve symptoms faster and lower incidence of recurrence (3)[C].
- Strangulated hemorrhoid: untreated irreducible hemorrhoid can progress to ulceration and thrombosis. Treatment requires urgent or emergent hemorrhoidectomy (4)[A].
- Acute hemorrhoidal bleeding associated with portal HTN can be life-threatening. Treatment should involve medical management and correction of coagulopathy; sclerotherapy, suture ligation, and surgical shunts (if necessary)

SURGERY/OTHER PROCEDURES
- Indications: failure of medical and nonoperative therapy, symptomatic grade III or IV hemorrhoids in presence of a concomitant anorectal condition requiring surgery, or patient preference
- Office-based procedures for patients with grade I or II (or III) internal hemorrhoids who have failed conservative management
  - Rubber band ligation (RBL) most common and most effective office-based procedure for symptomatic internal hemorrhoids. Avoid if on anticoagulants (3)[A],(5).
  - Infrared photocoagulation: Infrared light waves cause necrosis within hemorrhoid; similar or slightly higher recurrence rates compared to RBL; less postoperative pain and fewer complications (1,3)[B],(2)[A]
  - Sclerotherapy: submucosal injections causing local thrombosis; might be best for patients at increased bleeding risk (anticoagulated, advanced liver disease); care must be taken to inject proper site; not for advanced disease or if evidence of infection, inflammation, and ulceration is present
  - Cryotherapy is no longer recommended due to high rate of complications.
- Surgery for patients with symptomatic grade III or IV disease who have failed nonoperative treatments (3)[A]
  - Conventional hemorrhoidectomy
  - Closed hemorrhoidectomy—closure of mucosal defect
  - Open hemorrhoidectomy—tissue removed and mucosal defect left open
  - Different technologies are now used to excise hemorrhoidal tissue: diathermy, lasers, ultrasonic dissectors; associated with less pain.

- Newer techniques reduce surgical time, early postoperative pain, urinary retention, and time to return to normal activity.
  - Doppler-guided/assisted hemorrhoidal artery ligation (HAL): Anoscope or proctoscope with Doppler probe identifies hemorrhoidal artery which is then ligated; favorable in terms of outcome and postoperative pain in advanced hemorrhoidal disease (6)[B]
  - Stapled hemorrhoidopexy—for advanced internal hemorrhoidal disease. Excises submucosa; shorter recovery but more recurrent disease than conventional hemorrhoidectomy (2,5)[A],(6)[B]
  - LigaSure hemorrhoidectomy: reduces operating time, is superior in terms of patient tolerance, and is equal to conventional hemorrhoidectomy in long-term symptom control (2)[A]

COMPLEMENTARY & ALTERNATIVE MEDICINE
- Oral bioflavonoids have shown beneficial effect on bleeding, pruritus, and recurrence (3)[A].
- Topical nifedipine (compounded by pharmacist) can relieve pain of thrombosed hemorrhoids.
- Topical nitroglycerin (0.4%) has been used to decrease anal sphincter spasm in thrombosed hemorrhoids; headache is primary side effect.
- Botulinum toxin injection into anal sphincter to relieve spasm and pain of thrombosed hemorrhoid
- Aloe vera cream on the surgical site after hemorrhoidectomy reduces postoperative pain and decreases healing time and analgesic requirements.

 ONGOING CARE

FOLLOW-UP RECOMMENDATIONS
- Encourage physical fitness, weight management, and dietary compliance.
- Avoid prolonged sitting and straining on the toilet.

Patient Monitoring
As needed, depending on treatment

DIET
High-fiber with a target of 30 g of insoluble fiber per day through sources such as wheat bran cereals, oatmeal, peanuts, artichokes, beans, corn, peas, spinach, potatoes, apples, apricots, blackberries, raspberries, prunes, pears, bananas; adequate fluids (6 to 8 glasses of water per day); avoid excessive caffeine.

PATIENT EDUCATION
Top fiber-rich foods list: http://www.todaysdietitian.com/newarchives/063008p28.shtml

PROGNOSIS
- Spontaneous resolution
- Recurrence

COMPLICATIONS
- Thrombosis
- Ulceration
- Anemia (rare)
- Incontinence
- Pelvic sepsis following hemorrhoidectomy

REFERENCES
1. Jacobs D. Clinical practice. Hemorrhoids. *N Engl J Med*. 2014;371(10):944–951.
2. Mott T, Latimer K, Edwards C. Hemorrhoids: diagnosis and treatment options. *Am Fam Physician*. 2018;97(3):172–179.
3. Davis BR, Lee-Kong SA, Migaly J, et al. The American Society of Colon and Rectal Surgeons clinical practice guidelines for the management of hemorrhoids. *Dis Colon Rectum*. 2018;61(3):284–292.
4. Song S, Kim S. Optimal treatment of symptomatic hemorrhoids. *J Korean Soc Coloproctol*. 2011;27(6):277–281.
5. Lohsiriwat V. Treatment of hemorrhoids: a coloproctologist's view. *World J Gastroenterol*. 2015;21(31):9245–9252.
6. Brown SR. Haemorrhoids: an update on management. *Ther Adv Chronic Dis*. 2017;8(10):141–147.

ADDITIONAL READING
- Brown SR, Watson A. Comments to "rubber band ligation versus excisional haemorrhoidectomy for haemorrhoids." *Tech Coloproctol*. 2016;20(9):659–661.
- Hall JF. Modern management of hemorrhoidal disease. *Gastroenterol Clin North Am*. 2013;42(4):759–772.
- Jacobs DO. Hemorrhoids: what are the options in 2018? *Curr Opin Gastroenterol*. 2018;34(1):46–49.
- Klein JW. Common anal problems. *Med Clin North Am*. 2014;98(3):609–623.
- Wald A, Bharucha AE, Cosman BC, et al. ACG clinical guideline: management of benign anorectal disorders. *Am J Gastroenterol*. 2014;109(8):1141–1157.
- Yeo D, Tan KY. Hemorrhoidectomy—making sense of the surgical options. *World J Gastroenterol*. 2014;20(45):16976–16983.

 SEE ALSO

Colon Cancer; Portal Hypertension; Rectal Cancer

 CODES

ICD10
- K64.9 Unspecified hemorrhoids
- K64.0 First degree hemorrhoids
- K64.1 Second degree hemorrhoids

CLINICAL PEARLS
- Hemorrhoids are very common. Internal hemorrhoids are typically painless. External hemorrhoids are typically painful.
- All patients should be encouraged to consume 25 to 35 g of fiber per day.
- More advanced hemorrhoidal disease requires intervention with ligation or surgery.

H

HENOCH-SCHÖNLEIN PURPURA

Shani I. Muhammad, MD

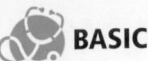

BASICS

DESCRIPTION
- Henoch-Schönlein purpura (HSP) is a nonthrombo-cytopenic, predominantly IgA-mediated, small vessel vasculitis that affects multiple organ systems and occurs in both children and adults.
- HSP is often self-limited, with the greatest morbidity and mortality attributable to long-term renal damage.
- Characterized by a tetrad of purpuric skin lesions, arthralgia, abdominal pain, and nephropathies

EPIDEMIOLOGY

Incidence
- Annual incidence: 135/1 million children and 3.4 to 14.3/1 million adults
- Mean age of patients affected is 6 years; 90% <10 years of age but has been reported in patients age 6 months to 75 years old
- Gender: Male-to-female ratio is 1.2:1.
- Race/ethnicity: most common in Caucasians and Asians, less common among African Americans

Prevalence
- Annual prevalence: 10 to 22/100,000 persons
- Year-round occurrence; more common in late fall to early spring

ETIOLOGY AND PATHOPHYSIOLOGY
- Autoimmune disorder in which IgA production is increased in response to trigger(s), IgA1 immune complexes then activate the complement pathway, leading to production of inflammatory cytokines and chemokines.
- Immune complex deposition results in small vessel inflammation; fibrosis; and necrosis within skin, intestinal mucosa, joints, and kidneys.
- No single etiologic agent has been identified.
- Known triggers include infection, drugs, vaccinations, and insect bites.
- Infectious antigens include (but are not limited to) group A *Streptococcus* (may be present in up to 30% of HSP-associated nephritis), parvovirus B19, *Bartonella henselae*, *Helicobacter pylori*, *Haemophilus parainfluenzae*, coxsackievirus, adenovirus, hepatitis A and B viruses, *Mycoplasma*, Epstein-Barr virus, varicella, *Campylobacter*, methicillin-resistant *Staphylococcus aureus*.
- Drugs: acetaminophen, quinolones, etanercept, codeine, clarithromycin
- Vaccinations: MMR (mumps, measles, rubella), pneumococcal, meningococcal, influenza, hepatitis B

Genetics
Associated with α_1-antitrypsin deficiency, familial Mediterranean fever, *HLA-DRB1*01*, *HLA-B35*

COMMONLY ASSOCIATED CONDITIONS
- Malignancy (rare): Greatest association is not only with solid tumors, including lymphoma, prostate cancer, and non–small cell lung cancer but also associated with multiple myeloma.
- Studies suggest a possible relationship with *H. pylori* infection (1)[A].

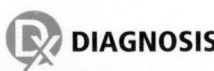

DIAGNOSIS

Palpable purpura and *at least one* of the following:
- Diffuse abdominal pain
- Biopsy with predominant IgA deposition
- Arthralgia or arthritis
- Renal involvement (hematuria or proteinuria)
- Direct immunofluorescense showing IgA deposition (2)[A]

HISTORY
- History of exposure to known trigger, including recent infection (particularly upper respiratory infection), vaccination, foods, or offending drug (3)
- Rash (most common presenting symptom): purpuric, palpable; distribution often symmetric on lower extremities and buttocks; may present on upper extremities, trunk, and face; typical duration 3 to 10 days; no definitive temporal association with other symptoms
- Fatigue
- Low-grade fever
- Nausea/vomiting
- Abdominal pain (diffuse, colicky, may be transient or constant)
- Hematochezia/melena
- Polyarthritis (often symmetric involvement of knees and ankles)
- Gross hematuria
- Rare symptoms: periorbital or scrotal swelling, headache, neuropathy, hemoptysis

PHYSICAL EXAM
- Rash (96% of cases, 74% primary presenting symptom):
  - May start as urticaria, develops into nonblanching purpura, with or without petechiae and ecchymoses, may also be bullous
  - Distribution usually symmetric, most commonly involving the lower extremities but may involve the face and trunk
- Abdominal tenderness (66% of cases, 12% primary presenting symptom):
  - Evidence of GI hemorrhage (28% of cases)
- Joint tenderness (64% of cases, 15% primary presenting symptom):
  - Mainly affects knees or ankles; may have associated warmth and limited range of motion, less commonly effusion; erythema is absent.
  - Mostly nonmigratory, transient, and nondeforming
- Orchitis (5%):
  - Presents as scrotal swelling and tenderness, may have associated torsion
- Renal disease (<1% primary presenting symptom):
  - Hypertension (HTN) may be present.
- Rarely, patients present with CNS or pulmonary involvement, which may manifest as signs of cerebral hemorrhage or diffuse interstitial pneumonia, respectively.

DIFFERENTIAL DIAGNOSIS
- Infection:
  - Meningococcemia
  - Rocky Mountain spotted fever
  - Bacterial endocarditis
  - Rheumatic fever
- Immune-mediated:
  - Polyarteritis nodosa
  - Wegener granulomatosis
  - Systemic lupus erythematosus
  - Kawasaki disease
- Other:
  - Inflammatory bowel disease
  - Idiopathic thrombocytopenic purpura
  - Juvenile rheumatoid arthritis
  - Leukemia
  - Acute surgical abdomen
  - Child abuse

DIAGNOSTIC TESTS & INTERPRETATION
- No single lab test confirms the diagnosis of HSP.
- Labs directed toward excluding other illnesses and assessing degree of renal involvement

Initial Tests (lab, imaging)
The following are generally accepted as initial labs for HSP:
- CBC:
  - Leukocytosis and thrombocytosis may occur. Thrombocytopenia indicates an alternative cause of purpura.
  - Hemoglobin is variable, depending on whether GI hemorrhage occurs.
- Basic serum chemistry panel (electrolytes, BUN, creatinine):
  - Electrolyte imbalances or elevated creatinine indicate renal dysfunction.
- Urinalysis:
  - Gross or microscopic hematuria, proteinuria, and red cell casts indicate renal dysfunction.
- PT and PTT:
  - Normal in HSP
- Imaging is not part of the routine workup for HSP but may be performed to rule out alternative etiologies or for evaluation of suspected complications, particularly in cases of GI and renal involvement. Initial imaging modalities to consider include the following:
  - Abdominal radiographs, with or without barium enema: Evaluate for free abdominal air suggestive of bowel perforation.
  - Abdominal ultrasound: sensitive for the detection of intramural bleeding in HSP and may also show thickened bowel wall, reduced peristalsis, intussusception
- Renal ultrasound: evaluates for hydronephrosis in cases of renal failure

Follow-Up Tests & Special Considerations
The following labs are also useful in diagnosing HSP:
- Blood culture:
  - To rule out sepsis/bacteremia when diagnosis is unclear
- Acute phase reactants:
  - Expect mild elevation.
- IgA level:
  - Often elevated, although nonspecific, nonsensitive
- Visfatin levels (4)
- Degree of elevation correlates with disease severity and likelihood of renal involvement (4).
- Complement levels:
  - Normal; sometimes decreased
- Antinuclear antibody/antineutrophil cytoplasmic antibody:
  - Negative
- Antistreptolysin-O titer:
  - Evaluates for preceding streptococcal infection
- Stool guaiac if suspected GI hemorrhage
- CT arteriography may be necessary to identify the location of bleeding in patients with GI hemorrhage.

Diagnostic Procedures/Other
- Renal biopsy: Obtain if diagnosis is uncertain or if nephrotic range proteinuria shows mesangial IgA deposition, mesangial proliferation, or, in severe cases, crescentic glomerulonephritis.
- Skin biopsy of purpura: IgA deposition in the dermis on immunofluorescence (2)[A]

- Endoscopy may be considered in cases of GI hemorrhage given symptomatic overlap of HSP with inflammatory bowel disease.
- Barium enema may be therapeutic in some instances of intussusception, although surgical correction is commonly needed.

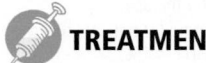

TREATMENT

GENERAL MEASURES
Rest and elevation of affected areas may limit purpura.

MEDICATION
- In the absence of renal dysfunction or complication, HSP is usually self-limited and best managed with supportive care.
- NSAIDs effective for symptomatic joint pain. Caution is advised in cases of GI hemorrhage; avoid use in cases of renal involvement and consider acetaminophen as an alternative.
- Steroids given early in disease course using oral prednisone 1 to 2 mg/kg/day for 1 to 2 weeks decrease both duration of abdominal pain and severity of joint pain and may have benefit in preventing GI bleeding and causes of surgical abdomen, including intussusception.
- Steroids have benefit in treatment of severe and/or bullous purpura.
- Steroids given early in disease are effective for the acute treatment of crescentic nephritis and may prevent chronic renal disease in such patients.
- Early steroids have no effect on prevention or development of renal involvement after 1 year.
- High-dose IV pulse steroids (0.5 g to 1.0 g) may be considered in cases of mesenteric vasculitis and severe renal impairment. Evidence is very limited to support use of cyclophosphamide, plasmapheresis, and intravenous immunoglobulin (IVIG) for severe renal and GI involvement, as well as colchicine for severe skin lesions.
- Mycophenolate mofetil (MMF) could be valuable in the treatment of complicated HSP (4,5)[A].

ISSUES FOR REFERRAL
- Consider nephrology referral for renal biopsy if nephrotic range proteinuria at any time or proteinuria >100 mg/mmol for 3 months after diagnosis.
- Dermatology referral for skin biopsy

ADMISSION, INPATIENT, AND NURSING CONSIDERATIONS
- Admission criteria/initial stabilization
  – Insufficient oral intake
  – Renal insufficiency
  – Severe abdominal pain
  – Severe GI bleeding
  – Altered mental status
  – Mobility restriction due to arthritis
  – HTN
  – Nephrotic syndrome
- IV fluids: Hydration should be maintained.

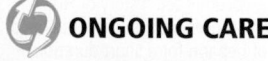

FOLLOW-UP RECOMMENDATIONS
Patient Monitoring
- Patients should be seen weekly during the acute illness. Visits should include history and physical exam to include BP measurement and urinalysis.
- Because ~100% of patients who develop renal involvement will do so within 6 months of HSP diagnosis, all patients should be followed at least monthly with BP and urinalysis for a duration of no <6 months.

- Women with a history of HSP should be monitored for proteinuria and HTN during pregnancy.
- Consider workup for occult malignancy in patients with adult-onset HSP.

PATIENT EDUCATION
- American Family Physician handout on HSP available at: http://www.aafp.org/afp/1998/0801/p411.html
- National Kidney and Urologic Diseases Information Clearinghouse (NKUDIC): http://www.niddk.nih.gov/health-information/health-topics/kidney-disease/henoch-sch%C3%B6nlein-purpura-hsp/Pages/facts.aspx

PROGNOSIS
- Long-term prognosis heavily dependent on presence and severity of nephritis
- HSP is self-limited in 94% of children and 89% of adults.
- Most cases of HSP resolve within 4 weeks of diagnosis. Recurrence rate within 6 months of diagnosis is 33%.
- Factors associated with poorer prognosis include age >8 years, fever at presentation, purpura above the waist, elevated ESR or IgA concentration, and increasing severity of renal histology grade.
- Chronic renal disease occurs in up to 20% of children with nephritic and nephrotic syndrome compared with 50% of adults who had any renal involvement. Risk of long-term renal failure is ≤5%.
- Risk factors that may result in renal failure include old age, HTN, elevated serum creatinine, and nephrotic and mixed nephritic–nephrotic syndrome at the onset of disease (4)[A].

COMPLICATIONS
- Nephrotic/nephritic syndrome and renal failure
- HTN
- Hemorrhagic cystitis
- Ureteral obstruction
- Intestinal infarction, perforation, obstruction, stricture
- GI hemorrhage
- Intussusception
- Alveolar hemorrhage
- CNS complications, including cerebral hemorrhage and seizure
- Anterior uveitis
- Myocarditis
- Orchitis
- Testicular torsion

REFERENCES
1. Kutlubay Z, Zara T, Engin B, et al. Helicobacter pylori infection and skin disorders. *Hong Kong Med J*. 2014;20(4):317–324.
2. Mysorekar VV, Sumathy TK, Shyam Prasad AL. Role of direct immunofluorescence in dermatological disorders. *Indian Dermatol Online J*. 2015;6(3):172–180.
3. Karakayali B, Yilmaz S, Çakir D, et al. Henoch-Schonlein purpura associated with primary active Epstein-Barr virus infection: a case report. *Pan Afr Med J*. 2017;27:29.
4. Nikibakhsh AA, Mahmoodzadeh H, Karamyyar M, et al. Treatment of severe Henoch-Schonlein purpura nephritis with mycophenolate mofetil. *Saudi J Kidney Dis Transpl*. 2014;25(4):858–863.
5. Antoon JW, Keane MW. Migratory polyarthritis in a child. *Clin Pediatr (Phila)*. 2012;51(4):401–403.

ADDITIONAL READING
- Batu ED, Ozen S. Pediatric vasculitis. *Curr Rheumatol Rep*. 2012;14(2):121–129.
- Boulis E, Majithia V, McMurray R. Adult-onset Henoch-Schonlein purpura with positive c-ANCA (anti-proteinase 3): case report and review of literature. *Rheumatol Int*. 2013;33(2):493–496.
- Cao N, Chen T, Guo ZP, et al. Elevated serum levels of visfatin in patients with Henoch-Schönlein purpura. *Ann Dermatol*. 2014;26(3):303–307.
- Dillon MJ, Ozen S. A new international classification of childhood vasculitis. *Pediatr Nephrol*. 2006;21(9):1219–1222.
- González LM, Janniger CK, Schwartz RA. Pediatric Henoch-Schönlein purpura. *Int J Dermatol*. 2009;48(11):1157–1165.
- Hoyer PF. Prevention of renal disease in Henoch-Schonlein purpura: clear evidence against steroids. *Arch Dis Child*. 2013;98(10):750–751.
- Jithpratuck W, Elshenawy Y, Saleh H, et al. The clinical implications of adult-onset Henoch-Schonelin purpura. *Clin Mol Allergy*. 2011;9(1):9.
- Kawasaki Y. The pathogenesis and treatment of pediatric Henoch-Schönlein purpura nephritis. *Clin Exp Nephrol*. 2011;15(5):648–657.
- McCarthy HJ, Tizard EJ. Clinical practice: diagnosis and management of Henoch-Schönlein purpura. *Eur J Pediatr*. 2010;169(6):643–650.
- Ozen S, Pistorio A, Iusan SM, et al. EULAR/PRINTO/PRES criteria for Henoch-Schönlein purpura, childhood polyarteritis nodosa, childhood Wegener granulomatosis and childhood Takayasu arteritis: Ankara 2008. Part II: final classification criteria. *Ann Rheum Dis*. 2010;69(5):798–806.
- Reamy BV, Williams PM, Lindsay TJ. Henoch-Schönlein purpura. *Am Fam Physician*. 2009;80(7):697–704.
- Sohagia AB, Gunturu SG, Tong TR, et al. Henoch-Schonlein purpura—a case report and review of the literature. *Gastroenterol Res Pract*. 2010;2010:597648.
- Trnka P. Henoch-Schönlein purpura in children. *J Paediatr Child Health*. 2013;49(12):995–1003.
- Weiss PF, Klink AJ, Localio R, et al. Corticosteroids may improve clinical outcomes during hospitalization for Henoch-Schönlein purpura. *Pediatrics*. 2010;126(4):674–681.

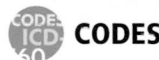 CODES

ICD10
D69.0 Allergic purpura

CLINICAL PEARLS
- HSP is a systemic small vessel vasculitis characterized by clinical tetrad of palpable purpura, abdominal pain, arthralgia, and renal dysfunction.
- The main form of treatment is supportive care, but oral corticosteroids are beneficial in certain circumstances.
- In all patients with HSP, regardless of renal involvement at presentation, it is reasonable to check BP and urinalysis at weekly to monthly intervals for no <6 months after diagnosis to monitor for developing renal dysfunction.

H

HEPARIN-INDUCED THROMBOCYTOPENIA

Tipsuda Junsanto-Bahri, MD • Maria A. Pino, PhD, MS, RpH

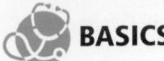

BASICS

DESCRIPTION

- A life-threatening complication of heparin use
  - Minimum platelet count falls between 30% and 50% from baseline.
- Antibody-mediated prothrombotic disorder initiated by heparin administration
- Unlike other thrombocytopenias, heparin-induced thrombocytopenia (HIT) is an idiosyncratic reaction that results in thrombosis rather than bleeding.
- Two types: nonimmune heparin-associated thrombocytopenia (previously called HIT type I) and heparin-induced thrombocytopenia/thrombosis (HITT) (immune induced; previously called HIT type II)
  - Nonimmune heparin-associated thrombocytopenia (HIT): more common, onset 1 to 4 days after starting heparin, mild thrombocytopenia ($>$100,000/mm³), few complications
  - Immune HITT: less common, onset 5 to 14 days after primary exposure to heparin, thrombocytopenia often $<$100,000/mm³ but usually $>$20,000/mm³; high risk of thrombosis and mortality

EPIDEMIOLOGY

Incidence

- 0.1–5% of heparin-treated patients will experience thrombocytopenia, regardless of dose, schedule, or route of administration.
- 25–50% of these patients will develop HITT (1).

ETIOLOGY AND PATHOPHYSIOLOGY

- Nonimmune heparin-associated thrombocytopenia: potentially a result of direct platelet membrane binding with heparin
- HITT: Heparin can cause an increase in the blood concentration of platelet factor 4 (PF4), a chemokine. PF4 will form a complex with heparin.
- Heparin/PF4 complex can, in turn, stimulate the production of specific antiheparin/PF4 complex antibodies. These antibodies cause platelet activation and a prothrombotic state. Ultimately, this hypercoagulable state leads to thromboembolic complications in many patients.
- Sources of heparin
- Heparin flushes (e.g., for arterial lines or heparin locks)
- Heparin-bonded catheters
- Unfractionated heparin (UFH)
- Low-molecular-weight heparin (LMWH) (enoxaparin, dalteparin)

RISK FACTORS

- Postsurgical $>$ medical $>$ obstetric
  - Post-cardiopulmonary bypass (CPB) is the most significant risk factor.
- Bovine UFH $>$ porcine UFH $>$ LMWH
- Female $>$ male
- Heparin duration $>$5 days
- Rare in pregnant females

GENERAL PREVENTION

- Inquire about recent heparin exposure and any history of HIT.
- Use of LMWH (vs. unfractionated), for a shorter duration, can reduce the risk of developing HIT.
- Properly document past HIT reactions in patient's medical record. Develop a HIT recognition and treatment protocol.
- No form of heparin should be administered once the diagnosis of HIT is confirmed.

COMMONLY ASSOCIATED CONDITIONS

- Venous thrombosis: deep venous thrombosis (DVT), pulmonary embolism (PE), adrenal vein thrombosis with hemorrhagic infarction; seen more frequently among medical and postoperative orthopedic surgery patients
- Arterial thrombosis: myocardial infarction, stroke, mesenteric infarction, limb ischemia; seen more frequently among vascular and cardiac surgery patients
- Skin lesions (skin necrosis at site of injection)
- Acute systemic reactions

DIAGNOSIS

- Nonimmune heparin-associated thrombocytopenia (HIT): asymptomatic drop in platelet count
- HITT: thrombocytopenia or thrombosis with the presence of heparin-dependent antibodies
  - The foundation for diagnosis is based on both clinical and serologic findings.

HISTORY

- Duration of current heparin therapy
- Previous exposure to heparin, including heparin flushes and heparin-coated catheters
- In patients being treated with heparin for thrombosis, in which thrombosis recurs during therapy, consider HITT as a potential cause.
- Clinical scoring systems:
  - Pretest probability for HIT can be calculated using the commonly used "4 Ts" methodology:
    ○ Thrombocytopenia of new onset
    ○ Timing of thrombocytopenia (5 to 10 days after exposure)
    ○ Thrombosis of new onset
    ○ Thrombocytopenia by other causes is ruled out.
  - The HIT Expert Probability score is an effective pretest probability tool (2).
  - The post-CPB scoring system

PHYSICAL EXAM

- Signs of venous or arterial thrombosis
- Skin necrosis (begins with erythema, progresses to ecchymosis and necrosis)
- Ischemic changes (signs of limb, renal, splenic, mesenteric ischemia)
- Bleeding (less common)
- Acute systemic reactions after IV bolus of heparin (e.g., signs of anaphylaxis)

DIFFERENTIAL DIAGNOSIS

Other potential causes of thrombocytopenia include (list is not all inclusive)
- Sepsis and other infections
- Drug reactions
- Autoimmune
- Transfusion reactions
- Physical destruction (e.g., during CPB)

DIAGNOSTIC TESTS & INTERPRETATION

- Serial platelet counts in patients receiving heparin who have a possible risk of HITT $>$1%: Check platelets at baseline and then every 2 to 3 days from days 4 to 14 of heparin therapy:
  - Withhold platelet monitoring for patients receiving heparin with risk of HITT $<$1%.
- Confirmatory lab tests needed for a clinical diagnosis can be divided into two major categories:
  - Antigen assay to detect presence of anti-PF4 antibodies:
    ○ ELISA: up to 99% sensitive, poor specificity; has a high negative predictive value for HIT
  - Functional assay to detect evidence of platelet activation in the presence of heparin:
    ○ Serotonin release assay (SRA), gold standard for diagnosis: high specificity and high sensitivity
    ○ Heparin-induced platelet activation (HIPA): high specificity and low sensitivity
- Antigenic assay should be the initial test.
  - Either a functional assay or an antigenic assay alone may not be adequate for clinical diagnosis; their use in combination is usually recommended.
- The diagnostic interpretation of these laboratory tests must be made in the context of the clinical estimation of the pretest probability because HIT is a clinico-pathologic syndrome. Patients may form heparin-dependent antibodies and still not develop HIT.

TREATMENT

Treatment is by prompt withdrawal of heparin and replacement with a suitable alternative anticoagulant.

GENERAL MEASURES

- Discontinue all heparin products, including flushes and heparin-coated catheters.
- All patients with a diagnosis of HIT should receive alternative anticoagulation because they are of high thrombotic risk.
- Nonimmune heparin-associated thrombocytopenia generally resolves when heparin is stopped.

ALERT

- Platelet transfusions can increase thrombosis. Give platelet transfusions only if bleeding or during an invasive procedure with a high risk of bleeding.
- Warfarin should not be administered until platelet recovery. If warfarin has been administered, vitamin K should be given due to depletion of proteins S and C and increased risk for venous limb gangrene.
  - Among patients with HIT, 7.1% received platelet transfusion. Of these patients, 20.6% experienced thrombotic complications (3)[A].
- Adverse reaction to heparin should be clearly documented in the patient's medical record with instruction to avoid all heparin products.
- For patients with a documented history of HIT, under special circumstances only (such as the need for CPB), the use of heparin for a short duration may be acceptable if the absence of heparin/PF4 complex antibodies can be documented. Patients who develop antibodies to the heparin/PF4 complex have a significantly higher rate of postoperative thrombotic events than patients who lack these antibodies (1,4)[A].

MEDICATION

- Most patients require anticoagulation because of
  - Preexisting thrombosis *or*
  - Risk of thrombosis during 30 days after HIT diagnosis (consider anticoagulation for 30 days)
- Dosing of anticoagulant depends on indication (prophylaxis vs. treatment):
  - In cases with a clinically low suspicion/pretest probability of HIT and laboratory confirmation is pending, it may be appropriate to continue antithrombotic prophylaxis using nonheparin anticoagulants.
  - In cases with high suspicion/pretest probability of HITT and laboratory confirmation is pending, it is appropriate to begin anticoagulation treatment with a nonheparin product (1,4)[A].
- Direct thrombin inhibitors (DTIs) (argatroban and bivalirudin)
  - Reduce relative risk of thrombosis by 30% and are associated with a 5–10% risk of bleeding.
  - Can produce misleading elevation in international normalized ratio (INR) (most likely an in vitro reaction)
    - Argatroban > bivalirudin (4)[A]
  - Argatroban
    - Currently approved for treatment of HITT or in patients undergoing percutaneous coronary intervention when heparin is contraindicated
    - Initial dose, 2 μg/kg/min by continuous IV infusion; decrease dose (0.5 to 1.2 μg/kg/min) for patients with reduced hepatic function or with critical illness.
    - Dose adjustments based to achieve activated partial thromboplastin time (aPTT) 1.5 to 3 times the baseline
    - Dose adjustment required for patients with hepatic dysfunction
  - Bivalirudin
    - Off-label use for HIT, complicated by thrombosis
    - Reduced risk of bleeding in patients undergoing percutaneous artery interventions (PCIs) and other cardiac procedures
    - Initial dose of 0.15 to 0.20 mg/kg/hr; adjust aPTT 1.5 to 2.5 times the baseline.
- Factor Xa inhibitors
  - Reports of factor Xa treatment are theorized to be useful; however, minimal data support its efficacy for HIT, and an ideal dose has yet to be determined.
  - Rivaroxaban has been frequently studied and provides evidence for HIT management (5)[B],(6)[A].
  - Fondaparinux has not been recommended due to lack of evidence.
- Warfarin transition
  - Must anticoagulate with an immediate-acting agent before starting warfarin
  - Begin warfarin after platelet count is >150,000/mm³.
  - Discontinue other anticoagulant and continue only warfarin after INR is therapeutic (2 to 3) for at least 5 days. This management differs from the normal heparin-to-warfarin transition in other conditions requiring anticoagulation (1,4)[A].
- LMWH
  - Although LMWH has a lower risk of initiating a HIT reaction, it should not be used when antibodies are already present, which cross-react with LMWH and induce thrombosis and thrombocytopenia.

ADMISSION, INPATIENT, AND NURSING CONSIDERATIONS

- Avoid heparin flushes.
- Avoid platelet transfusion.
- Clearly document reaction in all medical records to control the future use of heparin.
- HIT in pregnancy is rare. Safety of therapeutic agents has not been established but may be effective in the prevention of thrombotic complications (6)[A].

ONGOING CARE

FOLLOW-UP RECOMMENDATIONS

- The transition period of anticoagulation with a DTI and warfarin in patients with HIT can be problematic.
- The INR while administering both a DTI and warfarin should be therapeutic (2 to 3) for at least 5 days before discontinuing the DTI.
- Warfarin therapy should not be commenced until the platelet count has stabilized within a normal range.
- Warfarin therapy should continue for a minimum of 3 months.
- DTIs can prolong INR; therefore, if INR is <4 while on both warfarin and a DTI, temporarily hold the DTI for 4 to 6 hours and recheck INR; this second INR will represent only the anticoagulant effect of warfarin.
- Monitor use of concurrent drugs with warfarin.

Patient Monitoring

- Serial platelet counts
- Monitor PTT or INR as determined by the anticoagulation agent.

PATIENT EDUCATION

- Patient should inform all health care providers of any previous adverse reaction to heparin.
- HIT information available at http://medlibrary.org /medwiki/Heparin-induced_thrombocytopenia

PROGNOSIS

- Thrombosis in HIT has 20–30% mortality, with additional morbidity from stroke and limb ischemia.
- Platelet counts normalize within weeks after stopping heparin.
- Risk of delayed thrombosis, especially in the first 30 days

REFERENCES

1. Salter BS, Weiner MM, Trinh MA, et al. Heparin-induced thrombocytopenia: a comprehensive clinical review. *J Am Coll Cardiol*. 2016;67(21):2519–2522.
2. Cuker A, Arepally G, Crowther MA, et al. The HIT Expert Probability (HEP) Score: a novel pre-test probability model for heparin-induced thrombocytopenia based on broad expert opinion. *J Thromb Haemost*. 2010;8(12):2642–2650.
3. Goel R, Ness PM, Takemoto CM, et al. Platelet transfusions in platelet consumptive disorders are associated with arterial thrombosis and in-hospital mortality. *Blood*. 2015;125(9):1470–1476.
4. Linkins LA, Dans AL, Moores LK, et al. Treatment and prevention of heparin-induced thrombocytopenia: Antithrombotic Therapy and Prevention of Thrombosis, 9th ed: American College of Chest Physicians Evidence-Based Clinical Practice Guidelines. *Chest*. 2012;141(Suppl 2):e495S–e530S.
5. Tran PN, Tran MH. Emerging role of direct oral anticoagulants in the management of heparin-induced thrombocytopenia. *Clin Appl Thromb Hemost*. 2018;24(2):201–209
6. Chaudhary RK, Nepal C, Khanal N, et al. Management and outcome of heparin-induced thrombocytopenia in pregnancy: a systematic review. *Cardiovasc Hematol Agents Med Chem*. 2015;13(2): 92–97.

ADDITIONAL READING

- Onwuemene O, Arepally G. Heparin-induced thrombocytopenia: research and clinical updates. *Hematology Am Soc Hematol Educ Program*. 2016;2016(1):262–268.
- Smythe MA, Mehta TP, Koerber JM, et al. Development and implementation of a comprehensive heparin-induced thrombocytopenia recognition and management protocol. *Am J Health Syst Pharm*. 2012;69(3):241–248.
- Walenga JM, Prechel M, Jeske WP, et al. Rivaroxaban—an oral, direct Factor Xa inhibitor—has potential for the management of patients with heparin-induced thrombocytopenia. *Br J Haematol*. 2008;143(1):92–99.
- Warkentin TE, Maurer BT, Aster RH. Heparin-induced thrombocytopenia associated with fondaparinux. *N Engl J Med*. 2007;356(25):2653–2655.

CODES

ICD10

D75.82 Heparin induced thrombocytopenia (HIT)

CLINICAL PEARLS

- Heparin exposure through virtually any preparation (including LMWH), any dose, or any route can cause HITT, a life-threatening condition which is associated with severe and extensive thromboembolism.
- LMWH, warfarin, and platelet transfusion are contraindicated in HIT, although LMWH is less likely to cause HIT. Once HIT is present, the antibodies will cross-react and continue to cause a HIT reaction.
- If a patient is suspected of HIT (with or without confirmatory testing), immediately discontinue all forms of heparin.
- Patients will require anticoagulation either because of preexisting thrombosis or the risk of thrombosis in first 30 days after HIT.
- A DTI should be used until a patient's INR is therapeutic (2 to 3) on warfarin for at least 5 days.
- The key to avoiding sequelae from HIT is awareness, vigilance, and a high degree of suspicion.

H

HEPATIC ENCEPHALOPATHY

Walter M. Kim, MD, PhD • Jyoti Ramakrishna, MD, MPH

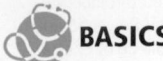 **BASICS**

DESCRIPTION

- Reversible altered mental and neuromotor functioning occurring in association with acute or chronic liver disease and/or portal systemic shunting
- The prominent features are confusion, impaired arousability, and a "flapping tremor" (asterixis).
- System(s) affected: gastrointestinal (GI); nervous
- Synonym(s): portosystemic encephalopathy (PSE); hepatic coma; liver coma

EPIDEMIOLOGY

Predominant sex: male = female (reflects prevalence of underlying liver disease)

Prevalence

- Overt hepatic encephalopathy (HE) occurs in 30–45% of cirrhotic patients.
- Occurs in all cases of fulminant hepatic failure
- Present in ~50% of patients requiring liver transplantation
- Parallels the age predominance of fulminant liver disease: peaks in the 40s; cirrhosis peaks in the late 50s; may occur at any age

ETIOLOGY AND PATHOPHYSIOLOGY

- There is no defined pathophysiology for the development of HE. Three classifications have been proposed (1):
  - Type A: resulting from acute liver failure
  - Type B: resulting from portosystemic bypass or shunting
  - Type C: resulting from cirrhosis
- Several metabolic factors implicated in HE based on the failure of the liver to detoxify noxious CNS agents (e.g., ammonia, mercaptan, fatty acids)
- Increased aromatic and reduced branched chain amino acids in blood may act as false neurotransmitters, possibly interacting with the γ-aminobutyric acid (GABA) receptor and causing clinical symptoms.
- HE presents most commonly in long-standing cirrhosis with spontaneous shunting of intestinal blood through collateral vessels or surgical portacaval shunts.
- Asterixis is the inability to maintain a particular posture due to metabolic encephalopathy. Abnormal diencephalic function leads to the characteristic liver flap noted when the arms and wrists are held in extension. Asterixis is also present in patients with uremia, barbiturate toxicity, and some cases of pulmonary disease. As such, asterixis is not pathognomonic for HE.

Genetics

- Unknown
- Conditions that predispose an individual to developing chronic liver disease such as cystic fibrosis, α_1-antitrypsin deficiency, hemochromatosis, and Wilson disease can contribute to the development of HE.

RISK FACTORS

In patients with underlying liver disease, precipitating factors include:

- Infection (overt or occult, including spontaneous bacterial peritonitis [SBP])
- GI hemorrhage
- Use of sedative or opiate drugs
- Fluid or electrolyte disturbance (Na^+, K^+, Mg^{2+} most common)
- Transjugular intrahepatic portosystemic shunt (TIPS—a radiologically inserted shunt to lower portal pressure)—elderly patients and those with worse liver function are at increased risk of HE following TIPS

GENERAL PREVENTION

- Recognize early signs and seek prompt treatment.
- Avoid nonessential medications, particularly opiates, benzodiazepines, and sedatives.
- Consider lactulose therapy as secondary prophylaxis for recurrence of HE (2)[B].

COMMONLY ASSOCIATED CONDITIONS

- May occur as a complication of acute fatty liver of pregnancy
- Occurs rarely in patients with a portacaval shunt but normal liver function

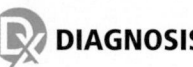 **DIAGNOSIS**

HISTORY

- Preexisting liver disease
- Confusion; altered mental status
- Impaired arousability
- Constipation

PHYSICAL EXAM

- Age 10 to 60 years
  - Five grades of confusion and degree of obtundation (West Haven classification) (1):
    ○ Minimal: psychometric or neuropsychological alterations without mental status changes
    ○ Grade I: lack of awareness, anxiety, shortened attention span, impaired arithmetic, altered sleep rhythm
    ○ Grade II: asterixis, lethargy, disorientation to time, personality change, inappropriate behavior
    ○ Grade III: somnolence to stupor, confusion, gross disorientation, bizarre behavior
    ○ Grade IV: coma
  - Prominent signs of underlying liver disease (50%); jaundice is most common, ascites is second most common.
  - GI bleeding with hematemesis or melena (20%)
  - Systemic infection, urinary tract infection, or pulmonary infection (20%)
- Age >60 years
  - Signs of underlying liver disease diminish (25%).
  - Confusion more prominent
  - Precipitating GI hemorrhage or infection is less often identified.
  - Progression is slower.

- Age <10 years
  - Signs of underlying liver disease are prominent; fulminant hepatic failure or advanced cirrhosis
  - Progression is very rapid, often over hours.
  - Wilson disease can imitate HE.
- Vital signs:
  - Bradycardia
  - Increased blood pressure suggestive of increased intracranial pressure
- Jaundice, ascites, other correlates of liver disease
- CNS exam: Assess short-term memory and presence of asterixis ("liver flap"—a flapping of the wrist when arms and wrists are extended).
- Pupillary reaction regresses from normal to sluggish and then absent with worsening HE.

DIFFERENTIAL DIAGNOSIS

- Metabolic encephalopathy related to anoxia, hypoglycemia, hypokalemia, hypo- or hypercalcemia, or uremia
- Head trauma, concussion, subdural hematoma
- Transient ischemic attack (TIA), ischemic stroke
- Alcohol intoxication
- Alcohol withdrawal syndrome
- Confusion due to medications or illicit drugs
- Meningitis, encephalitis
- Wilson disease
- Reye syndrome
- Wernicke-Korsakoff syndrome

DIAGNOSTIC TESTS & INTERPRETATION

- Clinical findings diagnostic in 80% of cases
- Response to treatment often confirms the diagnosis.
- EEG (limited utility): symmetric slowing of basic (α) rhythm (also common with other metabolic encephalopathies)
- Visual evoked potential: specific in grades II to IV
- Number connection test (NCT), line drawing test, critical flicker frequency (CFF) test, digit symbol test (DST), continuous reaction time (CRT) test, inhibitory control test (ICT), repeatable battery for the assessment of neuropsychological status (RBANS) and other psychometric tests may be used to assess minimal HE.

Initial Tests (lab, imaging)

- Liver function tests, including aspartate aminotransferase (AST), alanine aminotransferase (ALT), and serum albumin
- Prothrombin time (PT) and international normalized ratio (INR) often elevated
- Serum ammonia level is elevated in 90% of patients with HE; levels affected by infusion of amino acid solutions, opiate administration (constipation), uremia, tissue breakdown, burns, trauma, or infection
- CBC: anemia and leukocytosis
- Complete metabolic profile to identify hypokalemia, hyperbilirubinemia, altered calcium concentration, hypomagnesemia, and hypoglycemia
- BUN: Creatinine >20 mg/dL suggests dehydration or GI bleeding.
- Diagnostic paracentesis to rule out SBP
- Blood, urine, sputum, and ascitic fluid cultures to identify infection, as clinically indicated
- Consider arterial blood gas measurement.

- Toxicology screen
- Head CT to identify frontal cortical atrophy and/or edema
- MRI may demonstrate increased T1 signal within the globus pallidus.

Test Interpretation
- Brain edema is seen in 100% of fatal cases.
- Glial hypertrophy in chronic encephalopathy

 # TREATMENT

GENERAL MEASURES
- Identify and treat precipitating causes: GI bleeding, infection, electrolyte imbalance.
- Eliminate offending medications.
- Grade I or higher: Ensure adequate fluid and caloric ≥1,000 kcal (4.19 MJ) intake; avoid hypoglycemia.
- Consider enema for patients without diarrhea.
- If clumsiness and poor judgment are prominent, institute fall precautions.
- Avoid sedatives, benzodiazepines, opiates, diphenoxylate, and atropine.

MEDICATION
First Line
- Lactulose syrup (nonabsorbable disaccharide with laxative action that decreases colonic transit time and bacterial digestion that acidifies the colon to promote ammonia excretion): 30 to 45 mL PO up to every hour for goal of 3 to 6 bowel movements per day. Decrease to 15 to 30 mL BID when ≥3 bowel movements per day (3)[A].
- Lactulose enema (for patients who cannot tolerate oral lactulose or have suspected ileus): 300 mL lactulose plus 700 mL tap water, retained for 1 hour
- If worsening occurs acutely or there is no improvement in 2 days, add antibiotics:
  – Rifaximin: 400 mg PO TID or 550 mg PO BID (nonabsorbable antibiotic); highly effective in reversing minimal HE (4)[B]
- Contraindications:
  – Total ileus
  – Hypersensitivity reaction
- Precautions:
  – Hypokalemia
  – Electrolyte imbalance
  – Dehydration and renal failure

Second Line
- Neomycin: 1 to 2 g/day PO divided q6–8h, if renal function is within normal limits
- Polyethylene glycol may be effective as an alternative to lactulose in management of acute HE (5)[B].
- Metronidazole is an alternative antibiotic.
- Flumazenil may be of benefit in select patients.

ISSUES FOR REFERRAL
Refer early to experienced transplant center.

SURGERY/OTHER PROCEDURES
- Artificial liver perfusion devices are useful in fulminant hepatic failure as a bridge to transplantation.
- Consider liver transplant in grade II to IV HE.

COMPLEMENTARY & ALTERNATIVE MEDICINE
Probiotics and prebiotics have been associated with improvement of HE through modulation of gut flora (1)[C].

ADMISSION, INPATIENT, AND NURSING CONSIDERATIONS
- Monitor clinical status closely in grades I and II when diagnosis is clear and watch for progression.
- Evaluate patients with grades II to IV HE in fulminant hepatic failure for liver transplantation.

 # ONGOING CARE

FOLLOW-UP RECOMMENDATIONS
Activity as tolerated once resolved

Patient Monitoring
- Trail-making test (a pencil/paper connect-the-dots according to numbers) and assessment of asterixis help to monitor HE patients. Periodic evaluation helps determine maintenance treatment and diet. Test daily at first and then at each visit when changes in drugs and diet are made.
- See patients biweekly if there are changes on the trail-making test.
- Stable patients should be seen monthly.
- NCT or line drawing test at each office visit can also help with patient monitoring.
- In cirrhosis, evaluate for transplantation and periodically monitor Model for End-Stage Liver Disease (MELD) score.

DIET
- Regular protein diet (1.2 to 1.5 g/kg/day); vegetable protein diets are better tolerated than animal protein diets in patients with advanced cirrhosis; special IV/enteral formulations with increased branched chain amino acids are available.
- Grades III to IV patients need parenteral nutrition or jejunal feeds.

PATIENT EDUCATION
American Association for the Study of Liver Diseases, 1729 King Street, Suite 200, Alexandria, VA 22314; 703-299-9766; www.aasld.org

PROGNOSIS
- With appropriate treatment, acute HE often resolves.
- Chronic liver disease
  – HE recurs.
  – With each recurrence, HE is more difficult to treat—the degree of improvement with treatment is reduced and the mortality rate approaches 80%.

COMPLICATIONS
- Recurrence
- With many recurrences, permanent basal ganglion injury (non-Wilsonian hepatolenticular degeneration)
- Hepatorenal syndrome

REFERENCES
1. Vilstrup H, Amodio P, Bajaj J, et al. Hepatic encephalopathy in chronic liver disease: 2014 practice guideline by the American Association for the Study of Liver Diseases and the European Association for the Study of the Liver. *Hepatology*. 2014;60(2):715–735.
2. Agrawal A, Sharma BC, Sharma P, et al. Secondary prophylaxis of hepatic encephalopathy in cirrhosis: an open-label, randomized controlled trial of lactulose, probiotics, and no therapy. *Am J Gastroenterol*. 2012;107(7):1043–1050.
3. Gluud LL, Vilstrup H, Morgan MY. Non-absorbable disaccharides versus placebo/no intervention and lactulose versus lactitol for the prevention and treatment of hepatic encephalopathy in people with cirrhosis. *Cochrane Database Syst Rev*. 2016;(5):CD003044.
4. Bass NM, Mullen KD, Sanyal A, et al. Rifaximin treatment in hepatic encephalopathy. *N Engl J Med*. 2010;362(12):1071–1081.
5. Rahimi RS, Singal AG, Cuthbert JA, et al. Lactulose vs polyethylene glycol 3350—electrolyte solution for treatment of overt hepatic encephalopathy: the HELP randomized clinical trial. *JAMA Intern Med*. 2014;174(11):1727–1733.

ADDITIONAL READING
- McGee RG, Bakens A, Wiley K, et al. Probiotics for patients with hepatic encephalopathy. *Cochrane Database Syst Rev*. 2011;(11):CD008716.
- Sturgeon JP, Shawcross DL. Recent insights into the pathogenesis of hepatic encephalopathy and treatments. *Expert Rev Gastroenterol Hepatol*. 2014;8(1):83–100.
- Wijdicks EFM. Hepatic encephalopathy. *N Engl J Med*. 2016;375(17):1660–1670.

 ## SEE ALSO

Algorithm: Delirium

 ## CODES

ICD10
- K72.90 Hepatic failure, unspecified without coma
- K72.91 Hepatic failure, unspecified with coma

CLINICAL PEARLS
- HE includes a spectrum of neuropsychiatric findings that occur in patients with significant alterations in hepatic function.
- Lactulose is a cornerstone of therapy for HE.
- Asterixis ("liver flap") is the classic physical finding associated with HE.

H

HEPATITIS A

Uthman A. Alamoudi, MBBS • Adam B. Greenfest, MD • Marie L. Borum, MD, EdD, MPH, MACP, FACG, AGAF

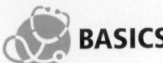 BASICS

DESCRIPTION
One of the world's most common infections, the hepatitis A virus (HAV) primarily involves the liver.

EPIDEMIOLOGY
Incidence
- 1.4 million cases globally each year
- Since routine use of hepatitis A vaccine (1995), the incidence of HAV has decreased by 95%.
- Approximately 2,000 HAV infections in 2016
- Incidence in the United States: 0.4/100,000
- No difference based on sex
- As many as 1/2 of current HAV infections in the United States are acquired during travel to endemic countries.
- Incubation period averages 28 days but can be as long as 50 days (range 15 to 50 days).

Prevalence
Serologic evidence of prior HAV infection is present in ~1/3 of U.S. population. Anti-HAV prevalence relates to age, ranging from 9% in children ages 6 to 11 years to 75% of those >70 years; relates inversely to income

Pediatric Considerations
- Often, milder or asymptomatic in children; severity increases with age.
- Infections asymptomatic in 70% of children <6 years
- <50% of 13- to 17-year-olds in the United States are vaccinated.

Pregnancy Considerations
- Increased risk of complications including preterm labor and premature rupture of membranes
- Vertical transmission has been reported; fecal–oral transmission during birth is possible.
- Breastfeeding is not contraindicated.

ETIOLOGY AND PATHOPHYSIOLOGY
- HAV is a single-stranded linear RNA enterovirus of the *Picornaviridae* family.
- Infection is limited to hepatocytes and macrophages.
- HAV is excreted into the bile and then stool, providing major route of spread.
- Primary transmission is fecal–oral.
- Humans are the only natural host.
- Incubation is 2 to 6 weeks (mean 4 weeks).
- Greatest infectivity is the 2 weeks before and 1 week after onset of clinical illness.
- Infection occurs primarily after consuming food or water contaminated with HAV or via direct contact.
- Outbreaks occur through exposure to a common food or water source.
- Virus is stable in water and on surfaces but is easily killed with high heat or cleaning agents.
- Shellfish (clams and oysters) may be contaminated if harvested from waters contaminated with HAV.
- Blood-borne transmission is rare.
- HAV is not a chronic disease but can last for months.

Genetics
Autoimmune hepatitis is rarely associated with human leukocyte antigen class II; DR3 and DR4 after active infection with HAV

RISK FACTORS
- Travel to developing countries accounts for >50% of cases in North America and Europe.
- Employment in health care
- Household exposure
- Intimate exposure, especially men who have sex with other men
- Injection of illicit drugs
- Child care centers, schools
- Institutionalized individuals
- Clotting factor disorders, such as hemophilia
- Blood exposure/transfusion (rare)
- No identifiable risk factor in 50%

GENERAL PREVENTION
- Proper sanitation and personal hygiene (hand washing), especially for food handlers, health care, and daycare workers
- Active immunization: HAV vaccines: Havrix and Vaqta; Twinrix—combination HAV and HBV
- Vaccine lasts ~25 years or more.
- Vaccine is recommended for (1)[C],(2)[A]:
  - All children aged 12 to 23 months, with catch-up administration until 18 years old
  - All travelers to countries with high endemic rate of hepatitis A
  - Men who have sex with men
  - Illicit IV drug users
  - Anyone with chronic liver disease (including pre– and post–liver transplant)
  - Individuals with a clotting factor disorder
  - Household members and close contacts of children adopted from countries with a high HAV prevalence (prior to arrival)
  - Anyone exposed during an outbreak
- Routine vaccination is no longer routinely recommended for food service, child care, or health care workers (1)[C].
- HIV-infected patients who are negative for HAV IgG should receive HAV vaccine series, preferably early in course of HIV infection.
  - If CD4 count is <200 cells/mm³ or the patient has symptomatic HIV disease, defer vaccination until several months after initiation of antiretroviral (ARV) therapy to maximize antibody response.
  - Hepatitis A vaccine can be given to immunocompromised patients with CD4 count >200.
  - Hepatitis A vaccine is recommended for pregnant women with additional medical conditions (higher risk for HAV infection).
- HAV is *not* killed by freezing.
- HAV is killed by
  - Heating to 185°F for 60 seconds
  - Chlorine
  - Iodine

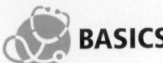 DIAGNOSIS

HISTORY
- Onset is often abrupt. Common symptoms include nausea, emesis and diarrhea, and headache.
- Symptom severity increases with age.
- Pediatric cases (<6 years) frequently asymptomatic
- Other symptoms:
  - Fever, malaise, fatigue, myalgias, anorexia, joint pain
  - Dark urine (bilirubinuria)
  - Right upper abdominal pain
  - Pruritus (can suggest cholestasis)

PHYSICAL EXAM
- Fever (variable)
- Jaundice and icterus present in >70% of adults and older children
- Hepatomegaly is common; splenomegaly is less common.
- Right upper quadrant abdominal tenderness
- Rare: lymphadenopathy (cervical), arthritis, or rash
- Asterixis suggests acute hepatic failure.

DIFFERENTIAL DIAGNOSIS
- Hepatitis B, C, D, E. Not clinically distinguishable from other forms of viral hepatitis; diagnosis may be suspected with typical symptoms during an outbreak.
- Drug-induced hepatitis; toxin-induced hepatitis
- Alcoholic hepatitis; autoimmune hepatitis
- Hemochromatosis (adults) or Wilson disease
- Malaria
- Epstein-Barr virus (EBV), cytomegalovirus (CMV), herpes simplex virus, yellow fever
- Primary or secondary hepatic malignancy
- Ischemic hepatitis or Budd-Chiari syndrome
- Nonhepatobiliary disease (elevated AST/ALT): celiac disease, congestive heart failure, thyroid disease
- Bacterial infections (Q fever, leptospirosis, syphilis, Rocky Mountain spotted fever)
- Parasites (liver flukes or toxocariasis)

DIAGNOSTIC TESTS & INTERPRETATION
Initial Tests (lab, imaging)
- Anti-HAV IgM: positive at time of onset of symptoms sensitivity and specificity >95%; primary test used to diagnose acute infection
- Anti-HAV IgG: appears soon after IgM and generally persists from years to lifetime
- AST/ALT elevated ~500 to 5,000: ALT usually > AST
- Alkaline phosphatase: mildly elevated
- Bilirubin: Conjugated and unconjugated fractions usually increased. Bilirubin rises typically following rise in ALT/AST, consistent with hepatocellular injury pattern.
- Prothrombin time and partial thromboplastin time usually remain normal or near normal.
  - Significant rises should raise concern for acute hepatic failure or coexisting chronic liver disease.
- CBC: mild leukocytosis; aplasia and pancytopenia
  - Thrombocytopenia may predict illness severity.
  - Autoimmune hemolytic anemia (rare)
- Albumin, electrolytes, and glucose to evaluate for hepatic and renal function (rare renal failure)
- Urinalysis (not clinically necessary): bilirubinuria
- Consider ultrasound (US) to rule out biliary obstruction only if lab pattern is cholestatic.

Follow-Up Tests & Special Considerations

Illness usually resolves within 4 weeks of symptom onset. Repeat labs are not indicated unless symptoms persist or new symptoms develop.

Diagnostic Procedures/Other

Liver biopsy is usually not necessary. US can evaluate other causes (e.g., thrombosis or concurrent cirrhosis).

Test Interpretation

- Positive serum markers in hepatitis A
  - Acute disease: anti-HAV IgM only
  - Recent disease (last 6 months): anti-HAV IgM and IgG positive
  - Previous disease or prior vaccination: anti-HAV IgM negative and IgG positive
- If liver biopsy obtained, shows portal inflammation; immunofluorescent stains for HAV antigen positive

 TREATMENT

GENERAL MEASURES

- Maintain appropriate nutrition/hydration.
- Avoid alcohol.
- Universal precautions to prevent spread
- Monitor coagulation defects, fluid, electrolytes, acid–base imbalance, hypoglycemia, and renal function.
- Report cases to local public health department.
- Laboratory evaluation including coagulation factors to rule out hepatic failure
- Referral to liver transplant center for fulminant failure (rare)

MEDICATION

- Preexposure vaccination per recommended guidelines. Both hepatitis A vaccines in the United States (Havrix, Vaqta) require 2 doses.
- The ACIP recommends administering the first dose as soon as possible in travelers to endemic areas (1)[C].
  - For healthy individuals <40 years, vaccinate up to the day or departure (1)[C].
  - Give immunoglobulin (0.02 mL/kg) to those >40 years or with chronic medical conditions if <2 weeks from planned departure (1)[C].
- Give postexposure prophylaxis to persons who have not previously received HAV vaccine within 2 weeks of exposure to HAV (3)[A],(4)[C].
  - Administer hepatitis A vaccine to healthy persons between the ages of 1 and 40 years (5)[A].
  - Administer immunoglobulin (0.02 mL/kg) to persons <1 or >40 years of age or to patients with significant comorbidities (immunosuppression, liver disease) who are at risk for poor immune response (3)[A],(4)[C].
- Use immunoglobulin for passive preexposure prophylaxis if not eligible for the vaccine (3)[A],(4)[C].
  - 0.02 mL/kg provides 1 to 2 months of coverage; 0.06 mL/kg provides 3 to 5 months of coverage.
  - Long-term prophylaxis should be with 0.06 mL/kg every 5 months for sustained risk (e.g., travelers).
  - Use immunoglobulin alone in children <1 year and unvaccinated pregnant women who will be traveling.
  - Do not give immunoglobulin with the MMR or varicella vaccines.

First Line

- No antiviral medications indicated; spontaneous resolution occurs in almost all patients.
- Caution with acetaminophen. If used, limit to 2 g/day or less.
- Avoid hepatotoxic agents.

Second Line

- Antiemetics (e.g., ondansetron)
- IV fluids
- Pruritus: diphenhydramine 50 mg PO IM q6h; consider cholestyramine 4 g BID if cholestasis.

ISSUES FOR REFERRAL

- Dictated by severity of illness
- Hepatic failure, refer to a high-volume liver transplant program.

SURGERY/OTHER PROCEDURES

Liver transplant in fulminant hepatic failure—rare

COMPLEMENTARY & ALTERNATIVE MEDICINE

Avoid potentially hepatotoxic botanicals including barberry, comfrey, golden ragwort, groundsel, huang qin, kava kava, pennyroyal, sassafras, senna, valerian, wall germander, and wood sage.

ADMISSION, INPATIENT, AND NURSING CONSIDERATIONS

- Treatment is usually outpatient unless signs of liver failure; dictated by severity of illness
- Treat dehydration and electrolyte imbalances.
- Enteric isolation. Private rooms, gowns, and masks are not necessary. Frequent hand washing. Use gloves when handling potentially contaminated material.
- 1:100 bleach dilution can be used to clean surfaces.

 ONGOING CARE

FOLLOW-UP RECOMMENDATIONS

Return to work/school 10 to 14 days after onset of symptoms with diligence to hygiene (patients remain infectious for up to 4 weeks from symptom onset).

Patient Monitoring

Monitor coagulation defects, fluid and electrolytes, acid–base imbalance, hypoglycemia, and renal function.

DIET

- Adequate balanced nutrition
- Avoid alcohol.

PATIENT EDUCATION

- Segregate food handlers with HAV.
- HAV immunity persists after infection.
- CDC hepatitis A FAQs link: http://www.cdc.gov/hepatitis/hav/afaq.htm

PROGNOSIS

- Excellent; mortality is 0.3%.
- Risk increased with underlying chronic liver disease and in the elderly (1.8% mortality age >50 years)

COMPLICATIONS

- Coagulopathy, encephalopathy, and renal failure
- Relapsing HAV: usually milder than the initial case
- Positive anti-HAV IgM; total duration typically <9 months

- Prolonged cholestasis: characterized by protracted periods of jaundice and pruritus (>3 months); resolves without intervention (supportive care only)
- Autoimmune hepatitis: can be seen after HAV infection; good response to steroids
- Hepatic failure: rare (1–2%)
- Postviral encephalitis, Guillain-Barré syndrome, pancreatitis, aplastic or hemolytic anemia, agranulocytosis, thrombocytopenic purpura, pancytopenia, arthritis, vasculitis, and cryoglobulinemia (all rare)

REFERENCES

1. Centers for Disease Control and Prevention. Hepatitis A questions and answers for health professionals. https://www.cdc.gov/hepatitis/hav/havfaq.htm. Accessed November 3, 2018.
2. Irving GJ, Holden J, Yang R, et al. Hepatitis A immunisation in persons not previously exposed to hepatitis A. *Cochrane Database Syst Rev*. 2012;(7):CD009051.
3. Liu JP, Nikolova D, Fei Y. Immunoglobulins for preventing hepatitis A. *Cochrane Database Syst Rev*. 2009;(2):CD004181.
4. Fiore AE, Wasley A, Bell BP; and Advisory Committee on Immunization Practices. Prevention of hepatitis A through active or passive immunization: recommendations of the Advisory Committee on Immunization Practices (ACIP). *MMWR Recomm Rep*. 2006;55(RR-7):1–23.
5. Victor JC, Monto AS, Surdina TY, et al. Hepatitis A vaccine versus immune globulin for postexposure prophylaxis. *N Engl J Med*. 2007;357(17):1685–1694.

ADDITIONAL READING

Chaudhry SA, Koren G. Hepatitis A infection during pregnancy. *Can Fam Physician*. 2015;61(11):963–964.

 SEE ALSO

- Hepatitis B; Hepatitis C
- Algorithms: Cirrhosis; Hyperbilirubinemia and Jaundice

CODES

ICD10

B15.9 Hepatitis A without hepatic coma

CLINICAL PEARLS

- HAV vaccine is indicated for all children, travelers (particularly to endemic areas), those at elevated risk of disease, and patients with liver impairment.
- Check HAV IgG in all HIV-positive patients; provide HAV vaccine if results are negative.
- HAV disease severity directly correlates with age; children are often asymptomatic.
- Treatment of acute HAV is supportive.
- Eligible patients should receive postexposure prophylaxis within 14 days of exposure.

HEPATITIS B

Navpreet K. Singh, MD • Jason Chao, MD, MS

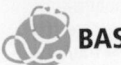

BASICS

DESCRIPTION
Systemic viral infection associated with acute and chronic liver disease and hepatocellular carcinoma (HCC)

EPIDEMIOLOGY

Incidence
- Predominant age: can infect patients of all ages
- Predominant sex: fulminant hepatitis B virus (HBV): male > female (2:1)
- In the United States, ~3,200 cases of acute HBV in 2016
- African Americans have the highest rate of acute HBV infection in the United States.
- Overall rate of new infections is down 82% since 1991 (due to national immunization strategy). There has been a slight increase in new infections since 2014 (associated with increased IV drug use).
- Vaccine coverage for the birth dose ~72% in United States

Prevalence
- In the United States, 800,000 to 1.4 million with chronic HBV
- Asia and the Pacific Islands have the largest populations at risk for HBV.
- Chronic HBV worldwide: 350 to 400 million persons
  - 1 million deaths annually
    - Second most important carcinogen (behind tobacco)
    - Of chronic carriers with active disease, 25% die due to complications of cirrhosis or HCC.
    - Of chronic carriers, 75% are Asian.

ETIOLOGY AND PATHOPHYSIOLOGY
HBV is a DNA virus of the Hepadnaviridae family; highly infectious via blood and secretions

Genetics
Family history of HBV and/or HCC

RISK FACTORS
- Screen the following high-risk groups for HBV with HBsAg/sAb. Vaccinate if seronegative (1)[A]:
  - Persons born in endemic areas (45% of world)
  - Hemodialysis patients
  - IV drug users (IVDUs), past or present
  - Men who have sex with men (MSM)
  - HIV- and HCV-positive patients
  - Household members of HBsAg carriers
  - Sexual contacts of HBsAg carriers
  - Inmates of correctional facilities
  - Patients with chronically elevated AST/ALT levels
- Additional risk factors:
  - Needle stick/occupational exposure
  - Recipients of blood/products; organ transplant recipients
  - Intranasal drug use
  - Body piercing/tattoos
  - Survivors of sexual assault

Pediatric Considerations
- Shorter acute course; fewer complications
- 90% of vertical/perinatal infections become chronic.

Pregnancy Considerations
- Screen all prenatal patients for HBsAg (1)[A].
- If HBsAG (+), obtain HBV DNA.

- Consider treating patients with high viral load at 28 weeks or history of previous HBV (+) infant with oral nucleos(t)ide medication beginning at 32 weeks to reduce perinatal transmission (2)[C].
- Infants born to HBV-infected mothers require hepatitis B immune globulin (HBIg) (0.5 mL) and HBV vaccine within 12 hours of birth.
- Breastfeeding is safe if HBIg and HBV vaccines are administered and the areolar complex is without fissures or open sores. Oral nucleos(t)ide medications are not recommended during lactation.
- HIV coinfection increases risk of vertical transmission.
- Continue medications if pregnancy occurs while on an oral antiviral therapy to prevent acute flare.

GENERAL PREVENTION
Most effective: HBV vaccination series (3 doses)
- Vaccinate
  - All infants at birth and during well-child care visits
  - All at-risk patients (see "Risk Factors")
  - Health care and public safety workers
  - Sexual contacts of HBsAg carriers
  - Household contacts of HBsAg carriers
- Proper hygiene/sanitation by health care workers, IVDUs, and tattoo/piercing artists
  - Barrier precautions, needle disposal, sterilize equipment, cover open cuts
- Do not share personal items exposed to blood (e.g., nail clipper, razor, toothbrush).
- Safe sexual practices (condoms)
- HBsAg carriers cannot donate blood or tissue.
- Postexposure (e.g., needle stick): HBIg 0.06 mL/kg in <24 hours in addition to vaccination

COMMONLY ASSOCIATED CONDITIONS
HIV, hepatitis C coinfection

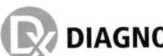

DIAGNOSIS

HISTORY
- Exposure: detailed family and social history
- Acute HBV
  - Fever, malaise, fatigue, arthralgias, myalgias
  - Anorexia, nausea, vomiting
  - Jaundice, scleral icterus
  - Dark urine, pale stools
  - Right upper quadrant (RUQ) abdominal pain
- Chronic HBV: typically asymptomatic

PHYSICAL EXAM
Acute disease: ill; jaundice/scleral icterus; RUQ tenderness; hepatomegaly

DIFFERENTIAL DIAGNOSIS
- Epstein-Barr virus (EBV); cytomegalovirus (CMV); hepatitis A, C, or E
- Drug-induced, alcoholic, or autoimmune hepatitis
- Wilson disease or rheumatologic/immunologic disorders

DIAGNOSTIC TESTS & INTERPRETATION

Initial Tests (lab, imaging)
- AST/ALT: markedly elevated in acute HBV (particularly ALT-hundreds to several thousand IU/mL). Transaminases may be normal or mildly elevated in chronic HBV:
  - Transaminases elevate before bilirubin.

- Bilirubin (conjugated/unconjugated): normal to markedly elevated in acute HBV
  - Last test to normalize as acute infection resolves
- Alkaline phosphatase: mild elevation
- HBcAb IgM may be the only early finding ("window period," before HBsAg turns positive).
- For acute hepatitis:
  - PT, albumin, electrolytes, glucose, and CBC
  - If severe acute HBV, check for superinfection with hepatitis D (HDV Ag and HDV Ab).
  - Hepatitis B serologic markers
- Hepatitis B e-antigen (HBeAg+) indicates high replication/infectivity; confirmed with high HBV DNA ($\geq 10^5$ copies/mL); benefit from medical therapy
- HBV precore mutants have undetectable HBeAg despite active viral replication (confirm with HBV DNA level) as well as antibody to e-antigen (HBeAb+).
- Screen for HDV, HIV, HCV, and immunity to hepatitis A virus (HAV Ab total/IgG).
- Ultrasound to document ascites, organomegaly, signs of portal hypertension, hepatic or portal obstruction, and to screen for HCC
- Contrast CT or MRI if ultrasound is abnormal or if α-fetoprotein (AFP) is elevated

Follow-Up Tests & Special Considerations
HBsAg+ persistence >6 months defines chronic HBV:
- Measure HBV DNA level and ALT every 3 to 6 months.
- If age >40 years and ALT borderline or mildly elevated, consider liver biopsy.
- Measure baseline AFP.
- Follow HBeAg for elimination (every 6 to 12 months).
- Lifetime monitoring for progression, need for treatment, and screening for HCC

Diagnostic Procedures/Other
- Liver biopsy
- Noninvasive tests (Hepascore, FibroTest) or measurement of elastography (FibroScan) to assess for hepatic fibrosis

Test Interpretation
Liver biopsy in chronic HBV may show interface hepatitis and inflammation, necrosis, cholestasis, fibrosis, cirrhosis, or chronic active hepatitis.

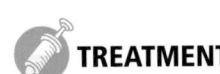

TREATMENT

GENERAL MEASURES
- Vaccinate for HAV if seronegative.
- Monitor CBC, coagulation, electrolytes, glucose, renal function, and phosphate.
- Monitor ALT and HBV DNA; increased ALT and reduced DNA implies response to therapy.
- Screen for HCC if HBsAg+.

MEDICATION

First Line
- Acute HBV
  - Supportive care; spontaneously resolves in 95% of immunocompetent adults
  - Antiviral therapy not indicated except for fulminant liver failure or immunosuppressed

Marker	Acute Infection	Chronic Infection	Inactive Carrier	Resolved Infection	Susceptible to Infection	Vaccinated
HBsAg	+	+	+	−	−	−
HBsAb	−	−	−	+	−	+
HBcAb	+IgM	−IgM; +total/IgG	+	+	−	−
HBeAg	+	±	−	−	−	−
HBeAb	−	±	+	±	−	−
HBV DNA	Present	Present	Low negative	−	−	−
ALT	Marked elevation	Normal to mildly elevated	Normal	Normal	Normal	Normal

- Chronic HBV: Treatment is based on HBeAg status:
  - FDA-approved drugs: lamivudine 100 mg, adefovir 10 mg, entecavir 0.5 to 1.0 mg, telbivudine 600 mg, or tenofovir 300 mg, all given PO every day (dose based on renal function); pegylated interferon (peg-IFN) α2a, α2b SC weekly (3)[A]
- Entecavir, tenofovir, and peg-IFN are preferred first-line agents (3)[A].
- Extended oral regimens are indicated (3)[A]:
  - If HBeAg+, treat 6 to 12 months post disappearance of HBeAg and gain of HBeAb, and monitor after cessation.
  - If HBeAg−, treat indefinitely or until HBsAg clearance and HBsAb development.
- Change/add drug based on resistance:
  - Confirm medication adherence prior to assuming drug resistance.
  - Adherence to therapy lowers rate of resistance.
- Adjust dosing for renal function.
- Peg-IFN preferred to standard interferon:
  - Weekly peg-IFN (Pegasys) injections for 48 weeks
  - Most efficacious for genotype A
  - Contraindicated if decompensated cirrhosis
- Goals of therapy: undetectable HBV DNA, normal ALT, loss of HBeAg, gain of HBeAb; loss of HBsAg and gain of HBsAb
- Precautions:
  - Oral drugs: renal insufficiency
  - Peg-IFN: coagulopathy, myelosuppression, depression/suicidal ideation

ISSUES FOR REFERRAL
- Refer all persistent HBsAg+ patients for potential antiviral therapy.

- Immediate referral for liver transplant if fulminant acute hepatitis, end-stage liver disease, or HCC

SURGERY/OTHER PROCEDURES
Liver transplantation, operative resection, radiofrequency ablation for HCC

ADMISSION, INPATIENT, AND NURSING CONSIDERATIONS
- Worsening course (marked increase in bilirubin, transaminases, or symptoms)
- Hepatic failure (high PT, encephalopathy)

 ONGOING CARE

FOLLOW-UP RECOMMENDATIONS
Patient Monitoring
- Serial ALT and HBV DNA:
  - High ALT + low HBV DNA associated with favorable response to therapy
- CBC for WBC and platelets if on interferon therapy
- Monitor HBV DNA q3–6mo during therapy:
  - Undetectable DNA at week 24 of oral drug therapy associated with low resistance at year 2
- Monitor for complications (ascites, encephalopathy, variceal bleed) in cirrhosis
- Vaccinate household contacts and sexual partners.
- Ultrasound q6–12mo to screen for HCC starting at age 40 years in men and age 50 years in women (3)[B]

DIET
Avoid alcohol.

PATIENT EDUCATION
- Acute HBV
  - Review transmission precautions.
- Chronic HBV
  - Alcohol and tobacco use accelerate progression.
  - Emphasize medication compliance to prevent flare.
- Patient education materials: http://www.cdc.gov /hepatitis/Resources/PatientEdMaterials.htm

COMPLICATIONS
- Hepatic necrosis; cirrhosis; hepatic failure
- HCC (all chronic HBV patients are at risk)
- Severe flare of chronic HBV with corticosteroids and other immunosuppressants: Avoid if possible.
- Reactivation of infection if immunosuppressed. Premedicate prophylactically if HBsAg+ or if HBcAb+ and receiving systemic chemotherapy (1)[A].

REFERENCES
1. Weinbaum CM, Williams I, Mast EE, et al. Recommendations for identification and public health management of persons with chronic hepatitis B virus infection. *MMWR Recomm Rep.* 2008;57(RR-8):1–20.
2. Borgia G, Carleo MA, Gaeta GB, et al. Hepatitis B in pregnancy. *World J Gastroenterol.* 2012;18(34):4677–4683.
3. McMahon BJ. Chronic hepatitis B virus infection. *Med Clin North Am.* 2014;98(1):39–54.

ADDITIONAL READING
- Schillie S, Vellozzi C, Reingold A, et al. Prevention of hepatitis B virus infection in the United States: recommendations of the Advisory Committee on Immunization Practices. *MMWR Recomm Rep.* 2018;67(1):1–31.
- Terrault NA, Bzowej NH, Chang KM, et al. AASLD guidelines for treatment of chronic hepatitis B. *Hepatology.* 2016;63(1):261–283.

 SEE ALSO

Cirrhosis of the Liver; Hepatitis A; Hepatitis C

 CODES

ICD10
- B19.10 Unspecified viral hepatitis B without hepatic coma
- B16.9 Acute hepatitis B w/o delta-agent and without hepatic coma
- B18.1 Chronic viral hepatitis B without delta-agent

CLINICAL PEARLS
- Screen all patients born in countries with endemic disease for HBV infection using HBsAg.
- Patients with chronic HBV need lifetime monitoring for disease progression and HCC.
- HBV is the second most common worldwide carcinogen (behind tobacco).

H

Chronic Hepatitis B Therapy

HBeAg	HBV DNA Viral Load	ALT*	Recommend
+	≥20,000 IU/mL	Elevated	Treat with antiviral or interferon.
−	≥2,000 IU/mL	Elevated	Consider biopsy or serum fibrosis marker and treatment.
+	≤20,000 IU/mL	Any	Monitor q6–12mo.
−	≥2,000 IU/mL	Normal	Biopsy; treat if disease.
+	≥20,000 IU/mL	Normal	Observe, consider treatment if ALT elevated. Biopsy if age >40 years or ALT is high normal to mild elevation.
−	≤2,000 IU/mL	Any	Monitor q6–12mo.
Cirrhosis	Any	Any	Treat with mono or combination treatment.
Liver failure	Any	Any	Treat and refer for transplant.

*ALT elevated if >2 × ULN; ULN for male = 30 IU/mL and for female = 19 IU/mL

HEPATITIS C
Jennifer L. Bauer, MD • Christopher Lin-Brande, MD

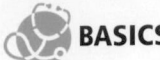

BASICS

DESCRIPTION
Hepatitis C virus (HCV) is a systemic viral infection (acute and chronic) primarily involving liver.

EPIDEMIOLOGY
- Highest incidence between ages 20 and 39 years; highest prevalence between 40 and 59 years of age
- Males and non-Hispanic blacks (1)
- IV drug use accounts for 70% of new HCV infections.

Geriatric Considerations
Patients >60 years are less responsive to therapy; important to initiate treatment early

Pregnancy Considerations
- Routine HCV testing is not indicated.
- Vertical transmission 6/100 births; risk doubles with HIV coinfection.
- Breastfeeding is safe if no cracks or fissures.

Pediatric Considerations
- Prevalence: 0.3%
- Test children born to HCV-positive mothers with HCV Ab at 18 months or HCV RNA at 1 to 2 months.
- More likely to clear spontaneously; slower rate of progression

Incidence
Incidence of acute HCV infection increased nearly 3-fold from 2010 to 2015. In 2015, there were 2,436 cases of acute HCV reported to the CDC, with an estimated 33,900 total new cases in the United States.

Prevalence
- Approximately 3.5 million persons in the United States have chronic HCV (Ab+).
- Prevalence highest if born 1945 to 1965 (2.6%) (1)
- HCV-related deaths are more common than HIV-related deaths.
- HCV is the most common cause of chronic liver disease and transplantation in the United States.
- Six known genotypes (GT) with 50 subtypes. GT 1 is predominant form in the United States (75%). GT predicts response to treatment.

ETIOLOGY AND PATHOPHYSIOLOGY
Single-stranded RNA virus of *Flaviviridae* family

RISK FACTORS
- Exposure risks
  - Chronic hemodialysis
  - Blood/blood product transfusion or organ transplantation before July 1992
  - Hemophilia treatment before 1987
  - Household or health care–related exposure to HCV-infected body fluids (1.8% risk)
  - Children born to HCV-positive mothers
- Risk behaviors and/or medical conditions
  - Prior history of injection drug use
  - Intranasal illicit drug use
  - History of incarceration
  - Tattooing in unregulated settings
  - High-risk sexual behaviors
  - HIV and hepatitis B infection

GENERAL PREVENTION
- *Primary prevention*
  - Do not share razors/toothbrushes/nail clippers.
  - Use and dispose needles properly through harm reduction programs.
  - Practice safe sex.
  - Cover cuts and sores.
- *Secondary prevention*
  - No vaccine or postexposure prophylaxis available
  - Substance abuse treatment
  - Reinforce use of barrier contraception for HIV-seropositive coinfected with HCV.
  - Assess for degree of liver fibrosis/cirrhosis.

COMMONLY ASSOCIATED CONDITIONS
Diabetes, metabolic syndrome, iron overload, depression, substance abuse/recovery, autoimmune and hematologic disease; cutaneous manifestations (necrotizing vasculitis, mixed cryoglobulinemia, porphyria cutanea tarda, lichen planus, erythema multiforme, erythema nodosum), HIV, and hepatitis B coinfection

DIAGNOSIS

HISTORY
- Determine exposure risk: *detailed* social history, including alcohol and IV drug use, psychiatric and medical comorbidities, and coinfections.
- Chronic HCV: Most cases are mildly symptomatic (nonspecific fatigue) or asymptomatic (elevated alanine/aspartate aminotransferase [ALT, AST]).
- Acute HCV: *if* symptoms develop (rare)
  - Onset typically 4 to 12 weeks postexposure
  - Jaundice, dark urine, steatorrhea, nausea, abdominal pain (right upper quadrant [RUQ]), fatigue, low-grade fevers, myalgias, arthralgias

PHYSICAL EXAM
- Typically normal unless advanced fibrosis/cirrhosis
- May have RUQ tenderness/hepatomegaly
- Spider angioma, caput medusa, palmar erythema, jaundice, gynecomastia, Terry nails
- Arthralgias/myalgias, neuropathy, glomerulonephritis, livedo reticularis, lichen planus, pruritus, sicca syndrome, cold agglutinin disease

DIFFERENTIAL DIAGNOSIS
Hepatitis A or B; Epstein-Barr virus (EBV), cytomegalovirus (CMV); alcoholic hepatitis; nonalcoholic steatohepatitis (NASH); hemochromatosis; Wilson disease, α_1-antitrypsin deficiency; ischemic, drug-induced, or autoimmune hepatitis

DIAGNOSTIC TESTS & INTERPRETATION
Initial Tests (lab, imaging)
- Screen adults born between 1945 and 1965, those with exposure risks, current and former IV drug users, HIV-positive individuals, people who engage in high-risk sexual behaviors (partner either HCV positive or IV drug user, multiple partners, or unprotected sex), and patients with persistently elevated ALT.
- CDC algorithm
  - HCV Ab
    - If nonreactive, no further action unless exposure within last 6 months is suspected (test with HCV RNA).
    - If reactive, test HCV RNA.
  - HCV RNA
    - If not detected, no current HCV infection; no further action (2)[A]
- HCV Ab detected 3 to 12 weeks after infection
- HCV RNA detected 1 to 2 weeks after infection
- RNA detectability precedes ALT elevation.
- AST/ALT: often normal, but elevations may persist in chronic HCV; ALT usually is 1 to 2 times upper limit of normal; AST may be normal/elevated.
  - Acute hepatitis C can elevate transaminases and bilirubin (direct and indirect).
- AST/ALT ratio ≥1 associated with cirrhosis
  - If AST/ALT ratio >2, rule out alcohol abuse.
- Persistent HCV RNA >6 months = chronic HCV

Follow-Up Tests & Special Considerations
- Once diagnosed, test for HCV GT and resistance.
- CBC, metabolic panel, TSH (if using PEG), hepatic function panel, coagulation factors
- IL28B testing: (CC homozygote more likely to clear)
- HBV and HIV coinfection
- Vaccinate if seronegative for hepatitis A/B.
- Pneumococcal polysaccharide vaccine (PPSV23)

Diagnostic Procedures/Other
Evaluate for hepatic fibrosis:
- Indirect markers include multiple clinical prediction models that are based on factors such as age, gender, AST, ALT, platelets, bilirubin. No one model has emerged as the standard. Models include AST to Platelet Ratio Index (APRI), Fibrosis-4 score, FibroIndex, Forns index, HepaScore, and FibroSure.
- Liver imaging: ultrasound (US), CT scan, MRI, transient US elastography, MR elastography
- Liver biopsy (gold standard)
  - Indications: discordant indirect marker results, concurrent non-HCV liver disease, elastography not available
  - Not necessary if diagnosis of hepatocellular carcinoma (HCC) is definitive based on imaging

Test Interpretation
- Biopsy measures grade (degree of inflammation) and stage (amount of existing fibrosis).
- Scoring systems: Batts and Ludwig, Metavir, International Association for the Study of the Liver (IASL)
  - Metavir: F0—no fibrosis; F1—portal fibrosis; F2—portal fibrosis with few septa; F3—septal fibrosis; F4—cirrhosis; A (necroinflammation): A0—absent; A1—mild; A2—moderate; A3—severe

TREATMENT

GENERAL MEASURES
- Report acute HCV to health department.
- Treat patients with virologic evidence of HCV (except patients with a short life expectancy whose prognosis would not be changed by treatment).
- Pretreatment counseling includes a thorough behavioral health and substance abuse history.
- Treat comorbidities prior to initiating antiviral therapy.
- Discuss treatment plan and likelihood of success based on individual factors such as BMI, GT, race, stage of fibrosis, and viral load.
- Sustained virologic response (SVR): undetectable HCV RNA after 12 to 24 weeks of treatment. This is considered a virologic cure of HCV infection.
- HCV cascade: Only 50% of patients with chronic HCV are diagnosed; 25% are HCV RNA confirmed, 15% are prescribed treatment, and 10% achieve SVR (3).

Medications*	Standard Dose	Common Side Effects; Contraindications
A: Elbasvir-grazoprevir (Zepatier)	50 mg/100 mg daily	Fatigue, headaches, nausea; avoid with OATPIB1/3 inhibitors or CYP3A inducers.
B: Glecaprevir-pibrentasvir (Mavyret)	300 mg/120 mg daily	Fatigue, headaches, nausea, diarrhea; avoid with atazanavir or rifampin.
C: Ledipasvir-sofosbuvir (Harvoni)	90 mg/400 mg daily	Fatigue, headaches, weakness, irritability, insomnia, dizziness, depression, nausea, diarrhea, myalgia, cough, dyspnea
D: Sofosbuvir-velpatasvir (Epclusa)	400 mg/100 mg daily	Fatigue, headaches, irritability, insomnia, depression, rash, nausea, weakness

Genotype, Regimen,† Duration, Evidence (4)

1A—without cirrhosis: A for 12 weeks [A], B for 8 weeks [A], C for 12 weeks [A], C for 8 weeks‡ [B]

1A—with compensated cirrhosis: A for 12 weeks [A], B for 12 weeks [A], C for 12 weeks [A], D for 12 weeks [A]

1B—without cirrhosis: A for 12 weeks [A], B for 8 weeks [A], C for 12 weeks [A], C for 8 weeks†‡ [B], D for 12 weeks [A]

1B—with compensated cirrhosis: A for 12 weeks [A], B for 12 weeks [A], C for 12 weeks [A], D for 12 weeks [A]

2—without cirrhosis: B for 8 weeks [A], D for 12 weeks [A]

2—with compensated cirrhosis: D for 12 weeks [A], B for 12 weeks [B]

3—without cirrhosis: B for 8 weeks [A], D for 12 weeks [A]

3—with compensated cirrhosis: B for 12 weeks [A], D for 12 weeks [A]

4—without cirrhosis: B for 8 weeks [A], D for 12 weeks [A], A for 12 weeks [B], C for 12 weeks [B]

4—with compensated cirrhosis: D for 12 weeks [A], B for 12 weeks [B], A for 12 weeks [B], C for 12 weeks [B]

5 or 6—without cirrhosis: B for 8 weeks [A], D for 12 weeks [B], C for 12 weeks [B]

5 or 6—with compensated cirrhosis: B for 12 weeks [A], D for 12 weeks [B], C for 12 weeks [B]

*Other medications still in use, although recommended for specific circumstances include ombitasvir, paritaprevir, ritonavir, and dasabuvir, ribavirin, simeprevir, daclatasvir, and voxilaprevir.

†Alternative regimens may be available but may have limitations for use in certain patient populations or lower quality of supporting evidence.

‡If non-black, HIV non-infected, HCV RNA <6 m IU/mL.

MEDICATION
First Line
- Acute HCV: OK to delay treatment for 12 to 16 weeks after suspected inoculation to allow for spontaneous clearance. Regimen is the same as for chronic HCV.
- Chronic HCV treatment with traditional agents, pegylated interferon (PEG-IFN) and ribavirin, is often poorly tolerated and no longer preferred.

ISSUES FOR REFERRAL
- Consult a specialist experienced in HCV care.
- Refer to liver transplant program if fulminant acute hepatitis, complication of end-stage disease, or HCC.

COMPLEMENTARY & ALTERNATIVE MEDICINE
No evidence for effective complementary therapy in HCV/cirrhosis/HCC

 ## ONGOING CARE

FOLLOW-UP RECOMMENDATIONS
- Treat early to prevent fibrosis. If cirrhosis is present, treatment may not prevent decompensation.
- Monitor serial viral load only if on antiviral therapy.
- Some experts recommend abdominal US every 6 months to monitor for HCC.
- Screen for varices with endoscopy if cirrhosis present.

Patient Monitoring
- Serial ALT/AST, renal function, and CBCs
- For 12-week course, follow up 4 weeks after starting therapy and 12 weeks after completing therapy.
  - 4-week HCV RNA: If detectable, recheck at week 6. If RNA has increased >10 times, stop therapy.
  - SVR12: Undetectable HCV RNA 12 weeks after completing therapy generally translates to long-term cure (goal of therapy).
- SVR decreases risk of portal hypertension, hepatic decompensation, and HCC. Monitor for decompensation (low albumin, ascites, encephalopathy, GI bleed).

DIET
- Low-fat, high-fiber diet and exercise to treat obesity/fatty liver
- Extra protein and fluids while on IFN therapy

PATIENT EDUCATION
- Avoid alcohol, tobacco, and illicit drugs (including marijuana); refer to rehabilitation/12-step program and monitor for relapse as appropriate.
- Caution with nutritional supplements and herbal medications (may contain hepatotoxins)
- http://www.cdc.gov/knowmorehepatitis/

PROGNOSIS
- For every 100 persons infected with HCV
  - 75 to 85 will develop chronic infection.

- 60 to 70 will develop chronic liver disease.
- 10 to 20 will develop cirrhosis over 20 to 30 years (more rapid if older age at infection, male gender, alcohol/substance abuse, HIV/HBV coinfection, or diabetes/insulin resistance)
  - 1–5% annual risk of HCC
  - 3–6% annual risk of hepatic decompensation
- Chronic HCV is *curable* in ~70% of cases; in noncirrhotic GT 2 or 3, cure rate is ~90%.

COMPLICATIONS
- Fibrosis and cirrhosis typically develop within the first 5 to 10 years of infection.
- Acute/subacute hepatic necrosis, liver failure, HCC, transplant and complications, death
- Risk factors for cirrhosis: age, white race, hypertension, alcohol use, anemia; risk for decompensation: diabetes, hypertension, anemia

REFERENCES
1. Denniston MM, Jiles RB, Drobeniuc J, et al. Chronic hepatitis C virus infection in the United States, National Health and Nutrition Examination Survey 2003 to 2010. *Ann Intern Med.* 2014;160(5):293–300.
2. Centers for Disease Control and Prevention. Testing for HCV Infection: an update of guidance for clinicians and laboratorians. *MMWR Morb Mortal Wkly Rep.* 2013;62(18):362–365.
3. Yehia BR, Schranz AJ, Umscheid CA, et al. The treatment cascade for chronic hepatitis C virus infection in the United States: a systematic review and meta-analysis. *PLoS One.* 2014;9(7):e101554.
4. American Association for the Study of Liver Diseases and the Infectious Diseases Society of America. Initial testing for HCV infection. http://www.hcvguidelines.org/treatment-naive. Accessed September 9, 2018.

ADDITIONAL READING
Leoni MC, Ustianowski A, Farooq H, et al. HIV, HCV and HBV: a review of parallels and differences [published online ahead of print September 4, 2018]. *Infect Dis Ther.* doi:10.1007/s40121-018-0210-5.

 ## SEE ALSO

- Cirrhosis of the Liver; Hepatitis A; Hepatitis B; HIV/AIDS
- Algorithm: Hyperbilirubinemia and Jaundice
- http://www.hepatitisc.uw.edu/

 ## CODES

ICD10
- B19.20 Unspecified viral hepatitis C without hepatic coma
- B17.10 Acute hepatitis C without hepatic coma
- B18.2 Chronic viral hepatitis C

CLINICAL PEARLS
- 1 of every 10 patients with hepatitis C has no identifiable risk factors.
- 15–25% of HCV-infected persons spontaneously resolve the infection without specific treatment.
- Assess for coinfections (HBV/HIV) and comorbid substance abuse in patients infected with HCV.

H

HERNIA

Yuhamy Curbelo-Peña, MD • Yulibeth Curbelo Peña, MD • Nolberto Adrián Medina-Gallardo, MD, PhD

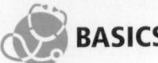 **BASICS**

DESCRIPTION

Areas of weakness or disruption of the abdominal wall through which structures can pass

- Types
  - Inguinal
    - Direct: acquired; herniation through defect in transversalis fascia of abdominal wall medial to inferior epigastric vessels; increased frequency with age as fascia weakens
    - Indirect: congenital; herniation lateral to the inferior epigastric vessels through internal inguinal ring into inguinal canal. A "complete hernia" descends into the scrotum, an "incomplete hernia" remains in the inguinal canal.
  - Pantaloon: combination of direct and indirect inguinal hernia with protrusion of abdominal wall on both sides of the epigastric vessels
  - Femoral: herniation descending through the femoral canal deep to the inguinal ligament; has a narrow neck and is especially prone to incarceration and strangulation
  - Incisional or ventral: herniation through a defect in the anterior abdominal wall at the site of a prior surgical incision
  - Congenital: herniation through defect in abdominal wall fascia due to collagen deficiency disease
  - Umbilical: defect at umbilical ring
  - Epigastric: protrusion through the middle line above the level of the umbilicus
  - Spigelian hernia: herniation through Spigelian line (lateral border of the rectus abdominis) for a lateral ventral hernia result
  - Sports hernia (not a true hernia): strain or tear of soft tissue of groin or lower abdomen
  - Others: obturator, sciatic, perineal
- Definitions
  - Reducible: Extruded sac and its contents can be returned to intra-abdominal position spontaneously or with gentle manipulation.
  - Irreducible/incarcerated: Extruded sac and its contents cannot be returned to original intra-abdominal position.
  - Strangulated: Blood supply to hernia sac contents is compromised.
  - Richter: Partial circumference of the bowel is incarcerated or strangulated. Partial wall damage may occur, increasing potential for bowel rupture and peritonitis.
  - Sliding: Wall of a viscus forms part of the wall of the inguinal hernia sac (i.e., right side—cecum, left side—sigmoid colon).

Geriatric Considerations

Abdominal wall hernias increase with advancing age, with significant increase in risk during surgical repair.

Pregnancy Considerations

- Increased intra-abdominal pressure and hormone imbalances with pregnancy may contribute to increased risk of abdominal wall hernias.
- Umbilical hernias are associated with multiple, prolonged deliveries.

EPIDEMIOLOGY

Incidence

- 75–80% groin hernias: inguinal and femoral
- 2–20% incisional/ventral, depends if prior surgery was associated with infection or contamination
- 3–10% umbilical, considered congenital
- Groin
  - 6–27% lifetime risk in adult men
  - Two peaks: most inguinal hernias present before 1 year of age or after 55 years of age
  - ~50% of children <2 years of age have a patent processus vaginalis, decreasing to 40% after age 2 years. Only between 25% and 50% are clinically significant.
  - Inguinal hernia in <5% of newborns male-to-female ratio 10:1
  - Increased incidence in premature infants
  - Increased incidence in patients with abdominal aortic aneurysms
  - Femoral <10% of all groin hernias, 40% present as a surgical emergency
- Incisional/ventral: ~10–23% of abdominal surgeries complicated by an incisional hernia, most common in upper midline incisions
- Incidence ratio: male = female
- Umbilical: 10–20% of newborns; most close by age 5 years

Prevalence

- Groin and inguinal hernias are more prevalent in men; femoral and umbilical more prevalent in women
- Most inguinal hernias are indirect in men and women.
- Incisional/ventral hernias (IVH) are more prevalent in smokers and obese individuals.

ETIOLOGY AND PATHOPHYSIOLOGY

Loss of tissue strength and elasticity (especially with aging or congenital defect in abdominal fascia) results in a fascial defect of the abdominal wall. Most pediatric hernias are congenital (e.g., patent processus vaginalis). Most adult hernias are a result of acquired weakness in the tissues of the anterior abdominal wall.

Genetics

No known genetic pattern

RISK FACTORS

- Increased abdominal pressure, coughing, heavy lifting, constipation, pregnancy, ascites, prostatism, obesity, advancing age (loss of tissue turgor), smoking, steroid use, low birth weight, prematurity
- Age: Femoral and scrotal hernias, along with recurrent groin hernias, are associated with increased risk for acute hernia surgery.

COMMONLY ASSOCIATED CONDITIONS

Obesity, chronic obstructive pulmonary disease, multiple abdominal surgeries, pregnancy, advanced age, Ehlers-Danlos syndrome, Marfan syndrome, polycystic kidney disease (PKD), osteogenesis imperfecta, Down syndrome, abdominal aortic aneurysm

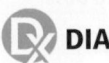 **DIAGNOSIS**

HISTORY

- May observe protrusion through abdominal wall during increased intra-abdominal pressure (Valsalva maneuver or cough)
- Pain, nausea, vomiting, bloating; relieved with reclining; may signal complication (e.g., strangulation)

PHYSICAL EXAM

- Examine initially with patient standing. During palpation, the patient should cough, strain, or perform Valsalva maneuver to determine the extent of intracavitary content movement. Repeat exam with patient in supine position.
- Inguinal (superior to inguinal ligament)
  - Direct inguinal hernia: Finger in inguinal canal finds defect of the transversalis fascia as a deep (posterior to anterior) bulge palpated with increased intra-abdominal pressure.
  - Indirect inguinal hernia: Finger in inguinal canal finds a persistent process vaginalis as a bulge (lateral to medial) that may extend into scrotum.
- Femoral (inferior to inguinal ligament): bulge in upper middle thigh; neck of the sac protrudes lateral to and below a finger placed on the pubic tubercle.
- Umbilical: palpable protrusion at umbilicus
- Incisional/ventral: palpable protrusion at site of prior abdominal incision or midline superior to the umbilicus
- Epigastric: palpable protrusion off midline above umbilicus

DIFFERENTIAL DIAGNOSIS

Lymphadenopathy, hydrocele, lipoma, varices, cryptorchidism, abscess, tumor, sports hernia (athletic pubalgia), pelvic fractures, adductor tears, omphalomesenteric duct, urachal cyst

DIAGNOSTIC TESTS & INTERPRETATION

Imaging rarely required; reserve for suspected abdominal hernia or unclear diagnosis; plain radiographs to rule out obstruction

- Ultrasound (US) can assess inguinal hernias.
- CT or tangential radiography for incisional and abdominal wall hernias and postsurgical patients with complaints of abdominal pain
- Herniography is no longer recommended.

Follow-Up Tests & Special Considerations

Diagnostic laparoscopy may be beneficial for occult hernias poorly appreciated on exam or with imaging.

 TREATMENT

- Elective
  - Elective surgical repair is associated with significantly lower morbidity and mortality.
- Acute setting
  - Pain management for symptomatic hernias
  - Strangulated hernias should be surgically repaired early to prevent complications such as necrosis and viscus perforation.

– Manual reduction of incarcerated hernias improves outcomes by allowing for elective repair after swelling and inflammation subside.
– Complication rate is greater with emergent pediatric inguinal hernia repairs compared to elective procedures.
– Acute hernia repair carries a higher morbidity and lower survival rate.
– Laparoscopic repair of IVH is safe, has fewer complications, shorter hospital stays, and possibly a shorter surgical time. Postoperative pain and recurrence rates are similar to open repair.
– For patients undergoing repair, operative times are shorter for extraperitoneal laparoscopic repair compared to open mesh repair with no difference in complication rates (1)[B].
– Mesh is generally preferred for hernia repairs; there have been numerous FDA product recalls in the past—primarily related to complications of bowel perforation and obstruction (https://www.fda.gov/medicaldevices/productsandmedicalprocedures/implant).

MEDICATION
- Antibiotics: Prophylaxis does not reduce wound infections after groin hernia repairs.
- Pain: Local anesthetic during surgical repair results in significant reduction of postoperative pain. Tension-free procedures (e.g., Lichtenstein) may be performed under local anesthesia.

ISSUES FOR REFERRAL
Warn patients of symptoms or signs of incarceration or strangulation (acute abdominal pain, fever, bloody bowel movements), which mandate immediate evaluation.

ADDITIONAL THERAPIES
Geriatric Considerations
Use of a truss (external supportive device) for direct inguinal hernias is common; no data regarding efficacy

SURGERY/OTHER PROCEDURES
All inguinal hernias should be surgically repaired. Watchful waiting in asymptomatic patients is safe if the patient has significant comorbidities that may compromise urgent repair.
- Incarceration and strangulation are absolute indications for hernia repair.
- Contraindications: patients who are not surgical candidates based on risk factors
  – Avoid elective repair in pregnant patients or patients with active infections.
- Special considerations
  – Umbilical hernias <0.5 cm can usually be followed clinically.
  – Umbilical hernias in children age 2 to 4 years typically close spontaneously.
  – Operative times and complication rates are similar when comparing single-incision laparoscopic inguinal hernia repair versus traditional multiport laparoscopic repair (2)[B].
  – "Watchful waiting" is recommended in pregnancy. Elective postpartum repair has similar outcomes and no increased risk of incarceration or strangulation before or during delivery.

– Women have lower recurrence rates using laparoscopic compared with open method.
– Ascites is not a strict contraindication for repair.
- Gold standard
  – Inguinal hernia
    ○ Open: Lichtenstein with mesh (37%): decreased recurrence rates
    ○ Laparoscopic (14%) with mesh: decreased hospital stay and postoperative pain
      ▪ Requires general anesthesia
      ▪ Transabdominal preperitoneal (TAPP) versus total extraperitoneal (TEP)
    ○ Pediatric: Laparoscopic percutaneous repair is an efficient, safe, and effective alternative to open repair. It is associated with reduced operative times and no increase in complication or recurrence rates. Avoid mesh in pediatric patients (3)[B].
  – Incisional/ventral
    ○ Laparoscopic repair is effective for most patients with primary or recurrent ventral hernias; there is <10% recurrence rate.
  – Umbilical
    ○ Pediatric: open excision with suture closure
    ○ Adult: Open repair with mesh may reduce hernia recurrence.
- Complications
  – Recurrence
  – Seromas
  – Postoperative pain, temporary or chronic: less with laparoscopic versus open technique
  – Wound infection
  – Injury to cord structures in inguinal herniorrhaphy; with nerve injury, most symptoms will resolve.

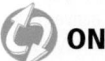 **ONGOING CARE**

PATIENT EDUCATION
Cleveland clinic: http://my.clevelandclinic.org/disorders/hernia/hic_hernia.aspx

PROGNOSIS
- Groin (pediatric): low recurrence rates (<3%) with surgery; may spontaneously resolve in infants
- Groin (adult): ≥1% per year risk of bowel strangulation without surgical treatment; 0–10% postoperative recurrence rates, depending on surgeon experience and procedure type
- Incisional/ventral: 3–5% postoperative occurrence; 2–17% postrepair recurrence, increased to 20–46% in larger hernias
- Umbilical (pediatric)
  – High rate of spontaneous resolution
  – Hernia less likely to close further in older children and in children with larger defects
- Umbilical (adult): up to 11% postoperative recurrence
- Epigastric: most ultimately become incarcerated and/or strangulated without surgical treatment. Recurrence is high due to frequency of missed defects during repair.

REFERENCES
1. Lockhart K, Dunn D, Teo S, et al. Mesh versus non-mesh for inguinal and femoral hernia repair. *Cochrane Database Syst Rev.* 2018;(9):CD011517.
2. Buckley FP III, Vassaur H, Monsivais S, et al. Comparison of outcomes for single-incision laparoscopic inguinal herniorrhaphy and traditional three-port laparoscopic herniorrhaphy at a single institution. *Surg Endosc.* 2014;28(1):30–35.
3. Timberlake MD, Sukhu TA, Herbst KW, et al. Laparoscopic percutaneous inguinal hernia repair in children: review of technique and comparison with open surgery. *J Pediatr Urol.* 2015;11(5):262.e1–262.e6.

ADDITIONAL READING
- Pereira JA, López-Cano M, Hernández-Granados P, et al. Initial results of the National Registry of Incisional Hernia. *Cir Esp.* 2016;94(10):595–602.
- Schmidt L, Öberg S, Andresen K, et al. Recurrence rates after repair of inguinal hernia in women: a systematic review [published online ahead of print October 31, 2018]. *JAMA Surg.* doi:10.1001/jamasurg.2018.3102.

 SEE ALSO

Algorithms: Abdominal Pain, Lower; Intestinal Obstruction; Pelvic Pain

 CODES

ICD10
- K46.9 Unspecified abdominal hernia without obstruction or gangrene
- K40.90 Unil inguinal hernia, w/o obst or gangr, not spcf as recur
- K41.90 Unil femoral hernia, w/o obst or gangrene, not spcf as recur

CLINICAL PEARLS
- Inguinal hernias are either direct or indirect:
  – Direct: acquired herniation through defect in transversalis fascia of abdominal wall medial to inferior epigastric vessels
  – Indirect: congenital herniation lateral to the inferior epigastric vessels; a "complete hernia" descends into the scrotum; an "incomplete hernia" remains within the inguinal canal.
- Pantaloon: combined direct and indirect inguinal hernia
- Femoral: descends through the femoral canal deep to the inguinal ligament
- Incisional or ventral: iatrogenic, herniation through a defect at site of a prior surgical incision
- Umbilical: Defect occurs at umbilical ring tissue. Most pediatric umbilical hernias close spontaneously within the first few years of life.
- Incarceration and strangulation are the primary complications associated with hernias.

H

HERPES EYE INFECTIONS

Stephanie L. Conway, PharmD • Gerald Gleich, MD

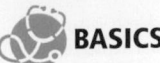

BASICS

DESCRIPTION
- Eye infection (blepharitis, conjunctivitis, keratitis, stromal keratitis, uveitis, retinitis, glaucoma, or optic neuritis) caused by herpes simplex virus (HSV) types 1 or 2 or varicella-zoster virus (VZV, also known as human herpes virus type 3 [HHV3])
- Categories
  - HSV: can affect many parts of the eye but most often affects the cornea (herpes keratoconjunctivitis); HSV1 > HSV2; can be further divided into primary and recurrent
  - VZV: When VZV is reactivated and affects the ophthalmic division of the 5th cranial nerve, this is known as herpes zoster ophthalmicus (HZO), a type of shingles.
- System(s) affected: eye, skin, central nervous system (CNS) (neonatal)

EPIDEMIOLOGY
- Predominant age: HSV—mean age of onset 37.4 years but can occur at any age, including primary infection in newborns; VZV usually advancing age (>50 years)
- Predominant sex: HSV—male = female; HZO—female > male

Incidence
- HSV keratitis: In the United States, approximated at 18.2 per 100,000 person-years. Incidence is 1.5 million per year worldwide (1).
- VZV: 1 million new cases of shingles per year in the United States; 25–40% develop ophthalmic complications. Temporary keratitis is most common.

Prevalence
- Ocular HSV prevalence estimated at 500,000 in the United States (1)
- VZV: Prevalence of herpes zoster infection is 20–30%. Ocular involvement in 50% if not treated with antivirals (2); overall lifetime prevalence of HZO: 1%.

ETIOLOGY AND PATHOPHYSIOLOGY
- HSV and VZV are Herpesviridae dsDNA viruses.
- HSV: primary infection from direct contact with infected person via saliva, genital contact, or birth canal exposure (neonates)
  - Primary infection may lead to severe disease in neonates, including eye, skin, CNS, and disseminated disease.
  - Recurrent infection is more common overall cause of herpetic eye infections.
- VZV: Primary infection from direct contact with infected person may cause varicella ("chickenpox") and/or lead to a latent state within trigeminal ganglia.
  - Reactivation of the virus may affect any dermatome (resulting in herpes zoster or "shingles"), including the ophthalmic branch (HZO).

RISK FACTORS
- HSV: personal history of HSV or close contact with HSV-infected person
  - General risk factors for reactivation: stress, trauma, fever, UV light exposure, other viral infections
  - Risk factors for HSV keratitis: UV laser eye treatment, some topical ocular medications such as prostaglandin analogues and primary/secondary immunosuppression

- HZO
  - History of varicella infection, advancing age (>50 years), sex (female > male), acute/painful prodrome, trauma, stress, immunosuppression (1,3)

ALERT
Consider primary/secondary immunodeficiency disorders in all zoster patients <40 years of age (e.g., AIDS, malignancy).

GENERAL PREVENTION
- Contact precautions with active lesions (HSV and VZV)
- VZV can be spread to those who have not had chickenpox and are not immunized.
- Varicella recombinant zoster vaccine (Shingrix) (VZV only): 2 doses 2 to 6 months apart recommended by the CDC for all persons age 50 years and older; preferred over older vaccine (Zostavax), which can still be used for persons age >60 years unable to take Shingrix (4)
  - Do not give varicella vaccine during an acute infection.
- Acyclovir can be used prophylactically to prevent recurrence of ocular HSV.
- HSV immunization currently being researched (1)

ALERT
Zoster vaccination is contraindicated if HIV-positive or other immunocompromised state, pregnancy, or in active untreated tuberculosis (TB).

Pregnancy Considerations
- Pregnant women without history of chickenpox should avoid contact with persons with active zoster.
- Pregnancy increases risk of recurrence of HSV/VZV.
- Shingrix and Zostavax vaccinations are both contraindicated during pregnancy.

COMMONLY ASSOCIATED CONDITIONS
Primary and secondary immunocompromised states

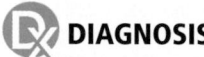

DIAGNOSIS

HISTORY
- Varies according to the virus and the ocular structures involved
- History of varicella or herpes simplex infection
- Acute onset, eye pain, headache, photophobia, tearing, ocular redness, decreased or blurry vision (3)
- May present with a prodromal period of fever, malaise, headache, and eye pain before skin eruptions and eye lesions (HZO) (3)

PHYSICAL EXAM
- Varies according to the virus and ocular structures involved
  - HSV most commonly affects the corneal epithelium (1).
  - VZV most commonly affects corneal stroma and uvea (3).
- Typically unilateral in presentation
  - HZO presents as early as 1 to 2 days after unilateral vesicular eruption in a dermatomal pattern (3).
- Decreased visual acuity
- Conjunctival injection near the limbus
- Decreased corneal sensation
- Slit-lamp exam

ALERT
Unilateral dermatomal vesicular rash most commonly in ophthalmic branch (V_1) of trigeminal nerve (VZV):
- Hutchinson sign: Vesicular lesion on nose from VZV indicates an increased risk of HZO due to involvement of nasociliary branch of trigeminal nerve, which also innervates the eye (3)[A].

DIFFERENTIAL DIAGNOSIS
- Any other cause of red, painful eye
  - Bacterial, fungal, allergic, or other viral conjunctivitis
  - Acute angle-closure glaucoma
- Corneal abrasion, recurrent corneal erosion, toxic conjunctivitis
- Temporal arteritis
- Trigeminal neuralgia

DIAGNOSTIC TESTS & INTERPRETATION
Initial Tests (lab, imaging)
- Typically none needed, as diagnosis is primarily based on history and physical exam (3)[A]
- Other
  - Corneal swab for HSV DNA by polymerase chain reaction (PCR) (PPV = 96%)
  - If vesicle present, can perform a Tzanck smear for VZV or HSV (multinucleated giant cells)
  - Antibody titers to assess exposure only; direct fluorescent antibody (DFA); tissue culture

ALERT
Urgent ophthalmology referral necessary for slit-lamp exam, dilated fundus exam, and intraocular pressure measurement

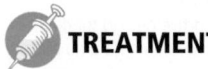

TREATMENT

GENERAL MEASURES
- Avoid contact with nonimmune people.
- No contact lenses should be worn during treatment period.
- Cool compresses
- Artificial tears
- Oral pain medications

MEDICATION
First Line
- HSV corneal epithelial disease
  - Trifluridine 1%: Apply 1 drop q2h while awake to a max of 9 drops daily until reepithelialization occurs and then 1 drop q4h for another 7 days.
  - Acyclovir: 400 mg PO 5 times per day for 10 days
  - Ganciclovir: 0.15% gel: Apply 1 drop in eye q3h while awake, ~5× daily, until reepithelialization occurs, and then 1 drop q8h for 7 days.
  - Trifluridine and acyclovir cure about 90% of treated eyes within 2 weeks with no significant differences in effectiveness (5)[A].
  - Evidence conflicting as to whether ganciclovir is as good as or better than acyclovir (5)[A]
  - Epithelial débridement by an ophthalmologist: may accelerate healing in combination with treatment as above (5)[A]
  - Avoid topical steroids.

- Utility of PO antivirals unclear HSV stromal keratitis or uveitis (without epithelial disease): combination of antiviral and steroid treatment; requires ophthalmology evaluation
  - Prednisolone acetate: 1% drops QID with slow taper (6)[A]
  - Consider systemic steroids in severe uveitis (6)[A].
  - Trifluorothymidine: 1% drops QID for prophylaxis while on topical steroids
- HZO
  - Valacyclovir (Valtrex) 1 g PO TID for 7 to 10 days or famciclovir (Famvir) 500 mg PO TID for 7 to 10 days or acyclovir 800 mg PO 5 times a day for 7 to 10 days
  - Valacyclovir and famciclovir result in significant reduction in PHN compared to acyclovir (number needed to treat [NNT] = 3) with equivalent efficacy (7)[A].
  - Topical antibiotic ophthalmic ointment to protect ocular surfaces (e.g., bacitracin, polymyxin B): 0.5-inch ribbon BID to TID for 7 to 10 days (8)[C]
  - If immunocompromised: acyclovir 10 to 15 mg/kg IV q8h for 10 days
  - Prednisolone acetate: 1% drops QID with slow taper with an ophthalmologist (8)[C]
- Cycloplegic agent if anterior uveitis present; intraocular pressure-lowering agent if necessary

Second Line
- HSV: acyclovir 2 g/day PO in divided doses over 10 days in patients intolerant of topical antivirals
- Topical idoxuridine, acyclovir, brivudine, although approved internationally, are not approved for use in the United States.
- Concomitant treatment with interferon may also improve outcomes but is not currently available.

ALERT
HZO: Antiviral therapy is most effective within the first 72 hours of rash onset but should still be initiated >72 hours after onset because of the possible complications of HZO (2)[C].

- Topical antiviral agents
  - Toxic to corneal epithelium, especially after 10 to 14 days of continuous use
- Acyclovir: Reduce dosage in renal insufficiency.
- Topical steroids
  - Should only be prescribed by an ophthalmologist
  - Contraindicated with active corneal epithelial disease, which is best monitored with a slit lamp
  - Can increase intraocular pressure; cause corneal thinning; and, with long-term use, cause cataracts
- Prednisone: caution in immunocompromised patients

ISSUES FOR REFERRAL
Emergent or urgent ophthalmology referral, depending on severity of disease

ADDITIONAL THERAPIES
- Recurrent HSV requires suppressive therapy.
- HZO leading to PHN is very common and can be treated with gabapentin or pregabalin, TCAs, opioids, and/or lidocaine gel.

SURGERY/OTHER PROCEDURES
Corneal transplantation for severe scarring or perforation

ADMISSION, INPATIENT, AND NURSING CONSIDERATIONS
- Admission criteria/initial stabilization
  - Severe systemic VZV disease
  - Systemic HSV in neonates—see "Herpes Simplex Virus, Pediatric."
- Discharge criteria: resolution of systemic disease

 ## ONGOING CARE

FOLLOW-UP RECOMMENDATIONS
Patient Monitoring
- Monitor with slit-lamp exam q1–2d until improvement and then q3–4d until epithelial defect resolves.
- Weekly after epithelial disease resolves until off topical antivirals

PATIENT EDUCATION
Educate patients about the importance of early recognition of recurrent symptoms and need for prompt evaluation and treatment.

PROGNOSIS
- Many cases are self-limited but, depending on the ocular structure involved, can lead to permanent blindness, especially in the setting of recurrent disease.
- Ocular HSV is the number one cause of infectious blindness worldwide (1).
- Recurrent ocular HSV
  - HSV epithelial disease without treatment
  - Without sequelae, 40% resolve.
  - With treatment, 90–95% resolve without complication.

Pediatric Considerations
- Neonatal primary HSV often disseminated, with high mortality rate; 37% develop vision worse than 20/200.
- Pediatric cases more likely to be bilateral (26%), recurrent (48% in 15 months), and may cause amblyopia

COMPLICATIONS
- Recurrence
- Corneal neovascularization and scarring resulting in poor vision
- Neurotrophic ulcer with perforation
- Secondary bacterial or fungal infection
- Secondary glaucoma in 10%
- PHN in 20–40% with VZV, typically longer lasting in older patients
- Vision loss from optic neuritis or chorioretinitis

REFERENCES
1. Faroog AV, Shukla D. Herpes simplex epithelial and stromal keratitis: an epidemiologic update. *Surv Opththalmol.* 2012;57(5):448–462.
2. Carter WP III, Germann CA, Baumann MR. Ophthalmic diagnoses in the ED: herpes zoster ophthalmicus. *Am J Emerg Med.* 2008;26(5): 612–617.
3. Liesegang TJ. Herpes zoster ophthalmicus natural history, risk factors, clinical presentation, and morbidity. *Ophthalmology.* 2008;115(Suppl 2):S3–S12.
4. Dooling KL, Guo A, Patel M, et al. Recommendations of the Advisory Committee on Immunization Practices for use of herpes zoster vaccines. *MMWR Morb Mortal Wkly Rep.* 2018;67(3):103–108. doi:10.15585/mmwr.mm6703a5.
5. Wilhelmus KR. Antiviral treatment and other therapeutic interventions for herpes simplex virus epithelial keratitis. *Cochrane Database Syst Rev.* 2015;(1):CD002898.
6. Knickelbein JE, Hendricks RL, Charukamnoetkanok P. Management of herpes simplex virus stromal keratitis: an evidence-based review. *Surv Ophthalmol.* 2009;54(2):226–234.
7. McDonald EM, de Kock J, Ram FS. Antivirals for management of herpes zoster including ophthalmicus: a systematic review of high-quality randomized controlled trials. *Antivir Ther.* 2012;17(2):255–264.
8. Dworkin RH, Johnson RW, Breuer J, et al. Recommendations for the management of herpes zoster. *Clin Infect Dis.* 2007;44(Suppl 1):S1–S26.

ADDITIONAL READING
Rowe AM, St Leger AJ, Jeon S, et al. Herpes keratitis. *Prog Retin Eye Res.* 2013;32:88–101.

 ## SEE ALSO

- Herpes Simplex; Herpes Simplex Virus, Pediatric; Herpes Zoster (Shingles)
- Algorithm: Eye Pain

 ## CODES

ICD10
- B00.50 Herpesviral ocular disease, unspecified
- B02.30 Zoster ocular disease, unspecified
- B00.52 Herpesviral keratitis

CLINICAL PEARLS
- HSV and VZV can lead to a wide array of ocular manifestations, ranging from self-limited disease to potentially vision-threatening disease and complications.
- An exam with fluorescein stain should be performed on all patients with possible HSV keratitis or HZO.
- Topical antiviral treatment is appropriate for HSV, but systemic PO antiviral treatment is necessary for HZO.
- An ophthalmologist should be consulted before prescribing topical steroids. All HZO patients should be referred to an ophthalmologist.
- Hutchinson sign (vesicular lesion on nose from VZV) is a strong indicator of HZO.
- Shingrix and Zostavax are both effective at preventing zoster and HZO as well as decreasing the duration of PHN.

H

HERPES SIMPLEX

Sonia Rivera-Martinez, DO • Sharon L. Koehler, DO, FACS

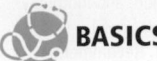

BASICS

DESCRIPTION

- Characteristic vesicular rash primarily located in oral and genital regions as the result of infection with:
  - Herpes simplex virus (HSV)-1 blisters mostly on lips, in mouth, face, eyes
  - HSV-2 primarily genital herpes, although cross-reactivity is common (HSV-1 can cause genital sores through oral–genital contact)
- Associated with a wide range of sequelae. Complexity and variation of presentation depends on the age and immune status of host, whether the infection is primary or recurrent and the degree of dissemination.
- Viral shedding is typically greatest in the first (primary) infection and lessens with recurrences.
- Meningitis/encephalitis and pneumonia are serious systemic manifestations associated with HSV infection.

EPIDEMIOLOGY

- Predominant age: affects all ages; however, most HSV-1 is acquired in childhood, and most HSV-2 is acquired in young–middle adulthood.
- Predominant sex: male = female

Incidence

- >1 million new cases of HSV per year
- HSV can reactivate, causing recurrent disease.

Prevalence

- Widespread; 1–25% of adults may shed HSV-1 or HSV-2 at any given time. Many are unaware of their infection status.
- Prevalence of antibodies to HSV-1 is 90% by adulthood in the general population. 30% of adults have antibodies to HSV-2.

ETIOLOGY AND PATHOPHYSIOLOGY

HSV-1 and HSV-2 are double-stranded DNA viruses from the family *Herpesviridae*. HSV-1 and HSV-2 are transmitted by contact with infected skin during periods of viral shedding. Transmission also occurs vertically during childbirth. Most often, HSV-1 is associated with oral lesions and HSV-2 with genital lesions.

RISK FACTORS

- Immunocompromised state
  - Chemotherapy, malignancy/chronic disease states such as diabetes or AIDS, old age
- Atopic eczema, especially in children
- Prior HSV infection
- Sexual intercourse with infected person (Condoms help minimize HSV transmission, but lesions outside condom-protected areas can spread virus.)
- Occupational exposure
  - Dental professionals at higher risk for HSV-1 and resulting herpetic whitlow
  - Neonatal herpes simplex: Primary infection is life-threatening and usually acquired by vaginal birth to an infected mother; risk is greatest in mothers with primary genital herpes infection; incubation is usually from 5 to 7 days (rarely 4 weeks); cutaneous, mucous membrane, or ocular signs seen in only 70%

GENERAL PREVENTION

- If active lesions are present, avoid direct contact with immunocompromised people, elderly, and newborns.
- Hand hygiene
- Kissing, sharing beverages, and sharing utensils/toothbrushes can transmit HSV.
- Genital herpes: Avoid sexual contact if active lesions (herpes simplex is also transmitted when disease appears to be inactive); discuss condom benefits and limits; consider antiviral therapy to reduce viral shedding; encourage safe sex.

COMMONLY ASSOCIATED CONDITIONS

- Erythema multiforme: 50% of cases associated with HSV-1 or HSV-2
- Screen all severe, treatment-resistant, or unusual HSV for concurrent HIV infection.

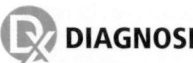

DIAGNOSIS

HISTORY

- Many patients are unaware of a known exposure.
- Prodrome of fatigue, low-grade fever, itching, tingling, or hot skin for several days immediately prior to outbreak of characteristic vesicular rash
- Herpes labialis is precipitated by sunlight, fever, trauma, menses, and stress; prodrome of pain, burning, and itching commonly occurs 6 to 48 hours before vesicles appear.

PHYSICAL EXAM

- Vesicles are often clustered and become painful ulcerated lesions, often with erythematous base.
- Primary genital herpes: See "Herpes, Genital."
- Primary herpetic gingivostomatitis and pharyngitis: usually in early childhood; incubation from 2 to 12 days, followed by fever, sore throat, pharyngeal edema, and erythema
  - Small vesicles develop on pharyngeal and oral mucosa, rapidly ulcerate, and increase in number to involve soft palate, buccal mucosa, tongue, floor of mouth, lips, and cheeks; tender, bleeding gums; cervical adenopathy; fever, general toxicity, poor oral intake, and excess salivation contribute to dehydration; autoinoculation of other sites may occur; resolves in 10 to 14 days
- Primary herpes keratoconjunctivitis: unilateral conjunctivitis with regional adenopathy, blepharitis with vesicles on lid marginal keratitis with dendritic lesions or with punctate opacities; lasts 2 to 3 weeks; systemic involvement prolongs process.
- Eczema herpeticum: diffuse pox-like eruption complicating atopic dermatitis; sudden appearance of lesions in typical atopic areas (upper trunk, neck, head); high fever, localized edema, adenopathy
- Herpetic whitlow: localized infection of affected finger with intense itching and pain, followed by vesicles that may coalesce with swelling and erythema. Mimics pyogenic paronychia; neuralgia and axillary adenopathy are possible; heals in 2 to 3 weeks
- Congenital infection through transplacental transfer may present with jaundice, hepatosplenomegaly, disseminated intravascular coagulation (DIC), encephalitis, seizures, temperature instability, chorioretinitis, and conjunctivitis with/without vesicles.
- Recurrent diseases from endogenous reactivation
  - Herpes labialis: recurrent lesions with HSV-1; usually <1 recurrence per 6 months, but 5–25% may have >1 attack per month; vesicles often at vermilion border, ulcerate and crust within 48 hours; heal within 8 to 10 days; may have local adenopathy
  - Ocular herpes: may recur as keratitis, blepharitis, or keratoconjunctivitis; dendritic ulcers, decreased corneal sensation, decreased visual acuity; uveitis may cause permanent visual loss.

DIFFERENTIAL DIAGNOSIS

- Impetigo: honey-crusted vesicles
- Aphthous stomatitis: grayish, shallow erosions with ring of hyperemia of anterior in mouth and lips
- Herpes zoster: unilateral dermatome distribution
- Syphilitic chancre: painless ulcer
- Folliculitis: may mimic "shave bumps" in genital area
- Herpangina: Vesicles predominate on anterior tonsillar pillars, soft palate, uvula, and oropharynx but not more anteriorly on lips/gums (usually caused by group A coxsackievirus).
- Stevens-Johnson syndrome

DIAGNOSTIC TESTS & INTERPRETATION

- Screen for other sexually transmitted infections (STIs) in patients with primary genital herpes.
- Viral: HIV, hepatitis B and C, and human papillomavirus (HPV) have crossover.
- Bacterial: Screen for concurrent gonorrhea, chlamydia in new primary genital outbreaks.

Initial Tests (lab, imaging)

- Tzanck smear shows multinucleated giant cells often with eosinophilic intranuclear inclusions (scrape material from lesion to slide, fix with ethanol/methanol, stain with Giemsa or Wright stain); varicella (herpes zoster) has identical findings.
- HSV culture: Swab and plate on viral-specific media. Sample may need to be refrigerated; can take up to 6 days to be positive; highly specific, hence, reliable if positive but has 20% false-negative rate
- HSV type–specific antibody tests distinguish between HSV-1 and HSV-2.
  - Polymerase chain reaction (PCR), direct fluorescent antibody (DFA), ELISA, and Western blot
  - 3 weeks after infection, 50% of those infected test positive; 70%, 6 weeks after infection; by 16 weeks, nearly all infected test positive

Diagnostic Procedures/Other

Biopsy is occasionally needed to confirm diagnosis.

Test Interpretation

- Intraepithelial edema (ballooning degeneration) and intracellular edema
- Brain biopsy (in encephalitis) shows hemorrhagic necrosis of gray and white matter with acute and chronic inflammation, thrombosis, and fibrinoid necrosis of parenchymal vessels; intranuclear inclusions in astrocytes, oligodendroglia, and neurons

TREATMENT

GENERAL MEASURES
- Cool dressings moistened with aluminum acetate solution
- Pouring a cup of warm water over genitals while urinating or by sitting in a warm bath while urinating (sitz baths) if lesions are causing urinary difficulty
- Children with gingivostomatitis who resist oral intake due to pain or extensive skin disease (eczema herpeticum) may require IV hydration.

MEDICATION
First Line
- Begin promptly, preferably in prodromal phase.
- Acyclovir (generic)
  - Mucocutaneous (or genital) HSV
    o Primary/first infection: 400 mg TID or 200 mg 5 times per day for 7 to 10 days
    o If severe, start with IV q8h dosing for the first few days, then complete 10-day course PO route.
    o Recurrence: 400 mg PO TID for 5 days *or* 800 mg BID for 5 days *or* 800 mg TID for 2 days
    o Suppression: 400 mg BID daily (1)[B]
  - Keratitis HSV: 400 mg PO 5 times per day; topical treatment is preferred as first line.
  - Pediatric dosing: neonatal herpes simplex or encephalitis: 60 mg/kg/day IV divided q8h for 14 to 21 days (2)[B]
    o Older (>3 months of age) immunocompetent is weight-based dosing (40 to 80 mg/kg/day [max 1,000 mg/day] divided q8h for 5 to 7 days).
  - Safe in pregnancy and lactation—Category B
  - Recurrent herpes labialis: 800 to 1,600 mg/day for prevention (3,4)[B]
- Penciclovir (Denavir): 1% cream. Apply to oral lesions q2h during waking hours for 4 days (5)[B].
- Valacyclovir (Valtrex)
  - Primary genital herpes: 1 g PO BID for 7 to 10 days. Recurrent genital herpes: 500 mg PO BID for 3 days; suppression: 500 to 1,000 mg PO daily (depending on frequency of outbreaks); labialis HSV (cold sores/oral lesions): 2,000 mg PO q12h for 1 day (3,4,6)[B]
  - 500-mg daily dose if suppression is needed/desired
  - Recurrent herpes labialis: 500 mg/day for 4 months for prevention (3)[B]
- Famciclovir (Famvir)
  - Primary genital herpes: 250 mg PO TID for 7 to 10 days
  - Recurrence: 125 mg PO BID for 5 days or 1,000 mg PO BID for 1 day
  - Suppression: 250 mg PO BID
- Precautions
  - Renal dosing for all oral antivirals
  - Significant possible interactions: Probenecid with IV acyclovir and possibly probenecid with valacyclovir may reduce renal clearance and elevate antiviral drug levels.

Second Line
- Foscarnet
  - Drug of choice for acyclovir resistance in immunocompromised persons with systemic HSV
  - 40 mg/kg IV q8h (Assume valacyclovir and famciclovir resistance also if acyclovir resistance occurs.)

- Other topicals
  - Ophthalmic preparations for herpes keratoconjunctivitis; acyclovir, vidarabine (Vira-A), ganciclovir, trifluridine
  - Topical acyclovir and penciclovir improve recurrent herpes labialis healing times by ~10% (3)[B].
  - Topical analgesics: Lidocaine 2% or 5% helps reduce pain associated with vulvar and penile outbreaks.
- Over-the-counter topical antivirals: docosanol

ISSUES FOR REFERRAL
Refer recurrent cases of herpes keratoconjunctivitis to an ophthalmologist.

ADMISSION, INPATIENT, AND NURSING CONSIDERATIONS
- Pregnancy considerations
  - Cesarean section and/or acyclovir are indicated if any active genital lesions (or prodrome) present at time of delivery; consider cesarean delivery if primary genital herpes is suspected within previous 4 weeks (5,6)[B].
  - Daily oral antivirals after 36 weeks of pregnancy in women with history of genital herpes help to prevent outbreak around the time of delivery.
  - Avoid fetal scalp electrodes, forceps, vacuum extractor, and artificial rupture of membranes if mother has history of genital HSV.
  - Risk of viral shedding at delivery from asymptomatic recurrent genital HSV is low (~1.6%).
- Pediatric considerations
  - Neonates with likely exposure (high index of suspicion) at birth or those who exhibit signs of HSV infection should have body fluids cultured and immediately start treatment (IV acyclovir).

ONGOING CARE

FOLLOW-UP RECOMMENDATIONS
- For most routine cases, follow-up is not necessary. Lesions and symptoms resolve rapidly within 10 days. Extensive cases should be rechecked in 1 week; monitor for secondary bacterial infections.
- Consider long-term suppression.

DIET
If oral lesions are present, avoid salty, acidic, or sharp foods (e.g., snack chips, orange juice).

PATIENT EDUCATION
- Explain the natural history that timing of exposure is difficult to determine and that the virus will remain in the body indefinitely. Acknowledging and discussing psychological impact of the diagnosis helps to reduce stigmatization.
- Emphasize personal hygiene to avoid self-spreading to other body areas (autoinoculation) or exposing others. Frequent hand washing; avoid scratching; cover active, moist lesions.
- Reinforce safe sexual practices.

PROGNOSIS
- Usual duration of primary disease is 5 days to 2 weeks.
- Antiviral treatment shortens duration, reduces complications, and mitigates recurrences (if used for suppression).
- Viral shedding during recurrence is briefer than with primary disease; frequency of recurrence is variable and depends on individual host factors.

- Newborns/immunocompromised individuals are at highest risk for major morbidity/mortality.
- HSV is never eliminated from the body but stays dormant in dorsal root ganglia and can reactivate, causing recurrent symptoms and lesions.

COMPLICATIONS
- Herpes encephalitis: Brain biopsy may be needed for diagnosis.
- Herpes pneumonia

REFERENCES
1. Sauerbrei A. Optimal management of genital herpes: current perspectives. *Infect Drug Resist.* 2016;9:129–141.
2. Pinninti SG, Kimberlin DW. Neonatal herpes simplex virus infections. *Pediatr Clin North Am.* 2013;60(2):351–365.
3. Rahimi H, Mara T, Costella J, et al. Effectiveness of antiviral agents for the prevention of recurrent herpes labialis: a systematic review and meta-analysis. *Oral Surg Oral Med Oral Pathol Oral Radiol.* 2012;113(5):618–627.
4. Sawleshwarkar S, Dwyer DE. Antivirals for herpes simplex viruses. *BMJ.* 2015;351:h3350.
5. Lee R, Nair M. Diagnosis and treatment of herpes simplex 1 virus infection in pregnancy. *Obstet Med.* 2017;10(2):58–60.
6. Obiero J, Mwethera PG, Wiysonge CS. Topical microbicides for prevention of sexually transmitted infections. *Cochrane Database Syst Rev.* 2012;(6):CD007961.

ADDITIONAL READING
Harmenberg J, Oberg B, Spruance S. Prevention of ulcerative lesions by episodic treatment of recurrent herpes labialis: a literature review. *Acta Derm Venereol.* 2010;90(2):122–130.

SEE ALSO
- Herpes, Genital
- Algorithm: Genital Ulcers

CODES
ICD10
- B00.9 Herpesviral infection, unspecified
- A60.00 Herpesviral infection of urogenital system, unspecified
- B00.1 Herpesviral vesicular dermatitis

CLINICAL PEARLS
- Up to 25–30% of the U.S. population has serologic evidence of genital herpes (HSV-2), and >80% is seropositive for HSV-1.
- Most individuals are unaware they are infected, allowing for asymptomatic viral transmission.
- Viral suppression for patients with frequent recurrences reduces transmission and decreases outbreak frequency.

HERPES ZOSTER (SHINGLES)

Edwin Y. Choi, MD • Lea S. Choi, DO • Shane L. Larson, MD

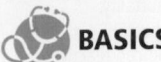 **BASICS**

DESCRIPTION
- Results from reactivation of latent varicella-zoster virus (VZV) (human herpesvirus type 3) infection
- Postherpetic neuralgia (PHN) is defined as pain persisting at least 1 month after rash has healed. The term *zoster-associated pain* is more clinically useful.
- Usually presents as a painful unilateral vesicular eruption with a dermatomal distribution
- System(s) affected: nervous; integumentary; exocrine
- Synonym(s): shingles

EPIDEMIOLOGY
Incidence
- Incidence increases with age—2/3 of cases occur in adults age ≥50 years. Incidence is increasing overall as the U.S. population ages.
- Herpes zoster: 4/1,000 person-years
- PHN: 18% in adult patients with herpes zoster; 33% in patients ≥79 years of age
- Individual lifetime risk of 30% in the United States

Prevalence
~1 million new cases of herpes zoster annually in the United States

Pregnancy Considerations
May occur during pregnancy

Geriatric Considerations
- Increased incidence of zoster outbreaks
- Increased incidence of PHN

Pediatric Considerations
- Occurs less frequently in children
- Has been reported in newborns infected in utero

ETIOLOGY AND PATHOPHYSIOLOGY
Reactivation of VZV from dorsal root/cranial nerve ganglia. Upon reactivation, the virus replicates within neuronal cell bodies, and virions are carried along axons to dermatomal skin zones, causing local inflammation and vesicle formation.

RISK FACTORS
- Increasing age
- Immunosuppression (malignancy or chemotherapy)
- Physical trauma
- Female
- HIV infection
- Spinal surgery

GENERAL PREVENTION
- Herpes zoster vaccination (Shingrix) is approved and recommended by the CDC for adults 50 years and older (1).
- Shingrix is recommended for adults who previously received Zostavax and is the preferred vaccine.

- Live VZV vaccine (Zostavax) (recommended for >60 years) is contraindicated in immunosuppressed persons, patients with HIV and CD4 counts <200, patients undergoing cancer treatment, and patients with hematologic or lymphatic (1,2).
- Patients with active zoster may transmit disease-causing varicella virus—typically through direct contact.

COMMONLY ASSOCIATED CONDITIONS
Immunocompromised states, HIV infection, posttransplantation, immunosuppressive drugs, and malignancy

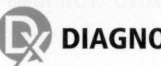 **DIAGNOSIS**

HISTORY
- Prodromal phase (sensory changes over involved dermatome prior to rash)
  - Tingling, paresthesias
  - Itching
  - Boring "knife-like" pain
  - Allodynia and hyperalgesia
- Acute phase
  - Constitutional symptoms (e.g., fatigue, malaise, headache, low-grade fever) are variable.
  - Dermatomal rash

PHYSICAL EXAM
- Acute phase
  - Rash: initially erythematous and maculopapular; evolves to characteristic grouped vesicles usually in one dermatome but may affect two to three adjacent dermatomes
  - Thoracic and lumbar dermatomes are most commonly involved sites (2).
  - Vesicles become pustular and/or hemorrhagic in 3 to 4 days.
  - Weakness in distribution of rash (1%)
  - Rash crusts and resolves by 14 to 21 days.
- Possible sine herpete (zoster without rash) and other chronic disorders associated with VZV without the typical rash
  - Herpes zoster ophthalmicus (HZO). Vesicles on tip of the nose (Hutchinson sign) indicate involvement of the external branch of cranial nerve V; associated with increased incidence of HZO
- Chronic phase
  - PHN is the most common complication (15% overall; increases with age).
  - 1–5% of cases may affect the motor nerves, causing weakness (*zoster motorius*), facial nerve (e.g., Ramsay Hunt syndrome), spinal motor radiculopathies
  - Lesions usually heal 2 to 4 weeks after onset, but scarring and pigmentation changes are common (2).

DIFFERENTIAL DIAGNOSIS
Rash
- Herpes simplex virus
- Coxsackievirus
- Contact dermatitis
- Superficial pyoderma

DIAGNOSTIC TESTS & INTERPRETATION
Initial Tests (lab, imaging)
Rarely necessary. Clinical appearance is distinct.

Follow-Up Tests & Special Considerations
- Viral culture
- Tzanck smear (does not distinguish from herpes simplex, and false-negative results occur)
- Polymerase chain reaction
- Immunofluorescent antigen staining
- Varicella-zoster–specific IgM

Test Interpretation
- Multinucleated giant cells with intralesional inclusion
- Lymphatic infiltration of sensory ganglia with focal hemorrhage and nerve cell destruction

 TREATMENT

GENERAL MEASURES
- Treat to control symptoms and prevent complications.
- Antiviral therapy decreases viral replication; lessens inflammation, nerve damage; and reduces the severity and duration of long-term pain.
- Prompt analgesia may shorten the duration of zoster-associated pain.
- Calamine and colloidal oatmeal may help reduce itching and burning.

MEDICATION
First Line
- Acute treatment
  - Antiviral agents initiated within 72 hours of skin lesions help relieve symptoms, speed resolution, and prevent or mitigate PHN (3)[A].
  - Antivirals do not significantly reduce the incidence of PHN (4)[A].
  - Valacyclovir: 1,000 mg PO TID for 7 days
  - Famciclovir: 500 mg PO TID for 7 days
  - Acyclovir: 800 mg q4h (5 doses daily) for 7 days
  - In children, oral acyclovir is the drug of choice.
- Analgesics (acetaminophen, NSAIDs)

- Corticosteroids do not prevent PHN but may accelerate resolution of acute neuritis.
  - Tricyclic antidepressants (TCAs); amitriptyline 10 to 25 mg at bedtime and other low-dose TCAs relieve pain acutely and may reduce pain duration; dose may be titrated up to 75 to 150 mg/day as tolerated.
  - Lidocaine patch 5% (Lidoderm) applied over painful areas (limit three patches simultaneously or trim a single patch) for up to 12 hours may be effective.
  - Gabapentin: 300 to 600 mg TID for pain; limited by adverse effects
  - Capsaicin cream and other analgesics may be useful adjuncts. Use opioids sparingly.
  - Capsaicin 8% patch or plaster provides pain relief for patients with PHN (5)[C]; better tolerated when initially applied with topical anesthetic
  - Pregabalin: 150 to 300 mg/day divided BID or TID reduces pain; use is limited by side effects.
- Prevention of PHN and zoster-associated pain: Nothing prevents PHN entirely, but treatment may shorten duration and/or reduce severity.
  - Antiviral therapy with valacyclovir, famciclovir, or acyclovir given during acute skin eruption may decrease the duration of pain.
  - Low-dose amitriptyline (25 mg at bedtime) started within 72 hours of rash onset and continued for 90 days may reduce PHN incidence/duration.
  - Paravertebral blockade: Nerve blocks during the acute phase shorten the duration of pain; somatic blocks, paravertebral blocks, and repeated/continuous epidural blocks can be used to prevent PHN (6)[A].
  - Insufficient evidence to suggest that corticosteroids reduce incidence, severity, or duration of PHN
- Precautions
  - Assess renal function prior to using valacyclovir, famciclovir, acyclovir, gabapentin, and pregabalin.
  - Valacyclovir, famciclovir, and acyclovir are pregnancy Category B.

Second Line
Numerous therapies have been advocated, but supporting evidence to routinely recommend is lacking.

COMPLEMENTARY & ALTERNATIVE MEDICINE
Cupping therapy (traditional Chinese medicine) shows potential benefit, but evidence is conflicting.

ADMISSION, INPATIENT, AND NURSING CONSIDERATIONS
- Outpatient treatment, unless disseminated or occurring as complication of serious underlying disease requiring hospitalization
- Consultation with ophthalmology for ophthalmic involvement (VZO).

 ## ONGOING CARE

FOLLOW-UP RECOMMENDATIONS
Refer to ophthalmology if concern that ophthalmic branch of the trigeminal nerve is involved.

Patient Monitoring
Follow duration of symptoms—particularly PHN. Consider hospitalization if symptoms are severe; patients are immunocompromised; >2 dermatomes are involved; serious bacterial superinfection, disseminated zoster, or meningoencephalitis develops.

DIET
No special diet

PATIENT EDUCATION
- The rash typically lasts 2 to 3 weeks.
- Encourage good hygiene and proper skin care.
- Warn of potential for dissemination (dissemination must be suspected with constitutional illness signs and/or spreading rash).
- Warn of potential PHN.
- Warn of potential risk of transmitting illness (chickenpox) to susceptible persons.
- Seek medical attention if any eye involvement.

PROGNOSIS
- Immunocompetent individuals should experience spontaneous and complete recovery within a few weeks.
- Acute rash typically resolves within 14 to 21 days.
- PHN may occur in patients despite antiviral treatment.

COMPLICATIONS
- PHN
- HZO: 10–20%
- Superinfection of skin lesions
- Meningoencephalitis
- Disseminated zoster
- Hepatitis; pneumonitis; myelitis
- Cranial and peripheral nerve palsies
- Acute retinal necrosis

REFERENCES
1. Centers for Disease Control and Prevention. Shingles (herpes zoster). https://www.cdc.gov/shingles/vaccination.html. Accessed October 18, 2018.
2. Saguil A, Kane S, Mercado M, et al. Herpes zoster and postherpetic neuralgia: prevention and management. *Am Fam Physician*. 2017;96(10):656–663.
3. McDonald EM, de Kock J, Ram FS. Antivirals for management of herpes zoster including ophthalmicus: a systematic review of high-quality randomized controlled trials. *Antivir Ther*. 2012;17(2):255–264.
4. Chen N, Li Q, Zhang Y, et al. Vaccination for preventing postherpetic neuralgia. *Cochrane Database Syst Rev*. 2011;(3):CD007795.
5. Massengill JS, Kittredge JL. Practical considerations in the pharmacological treatment of postherpetic neuralgia for the primary care provider. *J Pain Res*. 2014;7:125–132.
6. Kim HJ, Ahn HS, Lee JY, et al. Effects of applying nerve blocks to prevent postherpetic neuralgia in patients with acute herpes zoster: a systematic review and meta-analysis. *Korean J Pain*. 2017;30(1):3–17.

ADDITIONAL READING
Langan SM, Smeeth L, Margolis DJ, et al. Herpes zoster vaccine effectiveness against incident herpes zoster and post-herpetic neuralgia in an older US population: a cohort study. *PLoS Med*. 2013;10(4):e1001420.

 ## SEE ALSO

- Bell Palsy; Chickenpox (Varicella Zoster); Herpes Eye Infections; Herpes Simplex
- Algorithm: Genital Ulcers

 ## CODES

ICD10
- B02.9 Zoster without complications
- B02.29 Other postherpetic nervous system involvement

CLINICAL PEARLS
- Antiviral therapy within 72 hours of the onset of rash is most effective.
- Patients with active herpes zoster can transmit clinically active disease (chickenpox) to susceptible individuals.
- Shingrix is the recommended vaccine for healthy adults 50 years and older, including those who previously received Zostavax, to prevent shingles and related complications.

H

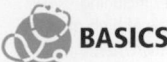

BASICS

DESCRIPTION

- Chronic, recurrent herpes simplex virus (HSV) type 1 or 2 infection of any area innervated by the sacral ganglia
- HSV-1 causes anogenital and orolabial lesions.
- HSV-2 causes anogenital lesions.
- Primary episode: occurs in the absence of preexisting antibodies to HSV-1 or HSV-2 (may be asymptomatic)
- First episode nonprimary: initial genital eruption; preexisting antibodies are present.
- Reactivation: recurrent episodes
- Synonym(s): herpes genitalis

EPIDEMIOLOGY

- Most commonly infected from age 15 to 30 years; prevalence increases with age due to cumulative likelihood of exposure.
- Predominant sex: female > male
- Predominant race: non-Hispanic blacks

Incidence

>700,000 new cases per year in the United States

Prevalence

- Overall prevalence of HSV-2 is 10–40% in the general population and up to 60–95% in the HIV-positive population (1).
- Between the ages of 14 and 49 years, the prevalence of HSV-1 in the United States is ~48%. The prevalence of HSV-2 ~12%. The prevalence of HSV-1 was highest (72%) in Mexican Americans and HSV-2 was highest (35%) in non-Hispanic blacks.
- Up to 90% of those who are seropositive lack formal diagnosis.
- Globally, it is estimated that 3.7 billion people are infected with HSV-1 and 140 million with HSV-2.

ETIOLOGY AND PATHOPHYSIOLOGY

- HSV is a double-stranded DNA virus of the *Herpeto-viridae* family (1).
- Spread via genital-to-genital contact, oral-to-genital contact, and via maternal–fetal transmission (2)
- Incubation is 4 to 7 days after exposure.
- Risk of transmission highest when lesions are present
- Viral shedding is possible in the absence of lesions, increasing the risk of transmission (precautions—abstinence, condom use—may not be followed). Viral shedding occurs intermittently and unpredictably.
- HSV infection increases the risk for HIV.

RISK FACTORS

- Risk increases with age, number of lifetime partners, history of sexually transmitted infections (STIs), history of HIV, sexual encounters before the age of 17 years, and partner with HSV-1 or HSV-2.
- Infection with HSV-1 confers 3-fold risk of infection with HSV-2.
- Immunosuppression, fever, stress, and trauma increase risk of reactivation.

COMMONLY ASSOCIATED CONDITIONS

Syphilis, HIV, chlamydia, gonorrhea, and other STIs

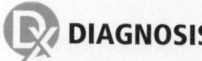

DIAGNOSIS

HISTORY

- Many patients are asymptomatic (74% of HSV-1 and 63% of HSV-2) or do not recognize clinical manifestations of disease (2).
- If symptoms are present during primary episode, they are often more severe, longer in duration, and associated with constitutional symptoms.
- Common presenting symptoms (primary episode): multiple genital ulcers, dysuria, pruritus, fever, tender inguinal lymphadenopathy, headache, malaise, myalgias, cervicitis/dyspareunia, urethritis (watery discharge)
- First episode, nonprimary: In general, symptoms are less severe than primary episode.
- Common presenting symptoms for recurrent episodes: prodrome of tingling, burning, or shooting pain (2 to 24 hours before lesion appears); single ulcer; lesion can be atypical in appearance; dysuria; pruritus (lasting 4 to 6 days on average)
- Recurrent episodes are more frequent with HSV-2 than with HSV-1, especially the 1st year after infection. Recurrences are less frequent over time.
- Less common presentations: constipation (from anal involvement causing tenesmus), proctitis, stomatitis, pharyngitis, sacral paresthesias

PHYSICAL EXAM

- Lesions around groin/perineum and within anus, vagina, and on cervix
- Lesion may appear as papular, vesicular, pustular, ulcerated, or crusted; can be in various stages
- Inguinal lymphadenopathy
- Extragenital manifestations include meningitis, recurrent meningitis (Mollaret syndrome), sacral radiculitis/paresthesias, encephalitis, transverse myelitis, and hepatitis.

Pediatric Considerations

- Neonatal infection occurs in 20 to 50/100,000 live births; 80% of infections result from asymptomatic maternal viral shedding during an undiagnosed primary infection in the 3rd trimester.
- Transmission ranges from 30% to 50% if the primary episode is near time of delivery. This risk is higher with HSV-1 than with HSV-2. Neonatal disease is associated with high morbidity and mortality.
- Suspect sexual abuse with genital lesions in children.

DIFFERENTIAL DIAGNOSIS

- HIV; syphilis; chancroid
- Herpes zoster
- Ulcerative balanitis
- Granuloma inguinale; lymphogranuloma venereum
- Cytomegalovirus; Epstein-Barr virus
- Drug eruption; trauma
- Behçet syndrome
- Neoplasia

DIAGNOSTIC TESTS & INTERPRETATION

Initial Tests (lab, imaging)

- Confirm clinical diagnosis with laboratory testing.
- Viral isolation (swab or scraping) for culture or PCR
  - Use Dacron or polyester-tipped swabs with plastic shafts (cotton tips/wood shafts inhibit viral growth and/or replication) (1).
  - Culture by unroofing vesicle to obtain fluid sample. Specificity >99%; sensitivity depends on sample: 52–93% for vesicle, 41–72% for ulcer, 19–30% for crusted lesion (1,3).
  - Culture requires timely transport of live virus to the laboratory in appropriate medium at 4°C.
  - PCR has the greatest sensitivity (98%) and specificity (>99%) but is also expensive and not readily available. It can increase detection rates by up to 70% (4); used primarily for CSF (1)
- Type-specific serologic assays
  - Seroconversion occurs 10 days to 4 months after infection (3). *Antibody testing is not necessary if a positive culture or PCR has been obtained.*
  - *IgM antibody testing is not useful because HSV IgM is often present with recurrent disease and does not distinguish new from old infection.*
  - Western blot (gold standard) and type-specific IgG antibody (glycoprotein G) enzyme-linked immunosorbent assay (ELISA) are used to discriminate between HSV-1 and HSV-2 (3)[B].
  - Western blot is >97–99% sensitive and specific but labor intensive and not readily available (1,3).
  - ELISA 81–100% sensitive; 93–100% specific (1) for HSV-2 but lower for HSV-1 detection. False positives are possible.
  - Screening with type-specific antibody is not generally recommended for (3):
    ○ Asymptomatic patients with HIV infection
    ○ Discordant couples (one partner with known HSV, the other without)
    ○ Recurrent symptoms but no active lesions

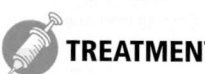

TREATMENT

GENERAL MEASURES

- Ice packs to perineum, sitz baths, topical anesthetics
- Analgesics, NSAIDs

MEDICATION

Start antiviral medications within 72 hours of onset of symptoms (including prodrome). After 3 days, antivirals may help if new lesions form or for significant pain.

First Line

- Acyclovir (4)[A]: the most studied antiviral in genital herpes; decreases pain, duration of viral shedding, and time to full resolution
  - Primary episode
    - 400 mg PO TID for 7 to 10 days
    - 200 mg PO 5 times a day for 7 to 10 days
    - Longer if needed for incomplete healing
  - Episodic therapy
    - 200 mg 5 times per day for 5 days
    - 400 mg TID for 5 days
    - 800 mg BID for 5 days
    - 800 mg TID for 2 days
  - Daily suppression
    - 400 mg BID
  - Severe, complicated infections (IV therapy)
    - 5 to 10 mg/kg/dose q8h until clinical improvement; switch to PO therapy to complete a 10-day course.
  - HIV infection: 400 mg PO 3 to 5 times per day until clinical resolution is attained
  - Precautions
    - Modify dose in renal insufficiency.
- Valacyclovir (Valtrex) (4)[A]: prodrug of acyclovir, improved bioavailability, less frequent dosing
  - Primary episode
    - 1 g PO BID for 7 to 10 days
  - Episodic therapy
    - 500 mg PO BID for 3 to 5 days
    - 1 g PO daily for 5 days
  - Daily suppression
    - 500 mg PO daily
    - 1 g PO daily
- Famciclovir (Famvir) (4)[A]
  - Primary episode
    - 250 mg PO TID for 7 to 10 days
  - Episodic therapy
    - 125 mg PO BID for 5 days
    - 1 g PO BID for 1 day
  - Daily suppression: 250 mg PO BID

ISSUES FOR REFERRAL

For acyclovir-resistant HSV, in consultation with infectious disease specialist (4)[A]:

- Foscarnet: 40 mg/kg/dose IV q8h until clinical resolution
  - Associated with significant toxicity
- Cidofovir: 5 mg/kg IV once weekly

Pregnancy Considerations

ACOG clinical management guidelines (4)[A],(5)[C]:

- Screening: Pregnant women negative for HSV-1 and HSV-2 antibodies should avoid sexual contact in the 3rd trimester if their partner is antibody positive.
- Suppressive therapy: Pregnant women with a history of genital herpes should be offered suppression treatment starting at 36 gestational weeks until delivery to decrease reactivation rate and reduce the risk of neonatal infection:
  - Acyclovir 400 mg PO TID
  - Valacyclovir 500 mg PO BID
- Monitor for outbreaks during pregnancy and examine for any lesions at the onset of labor. C-section is recommended if prodromal symptoms or lesions are present at onset of labor.

Pediatric Considerations

- High-risk infants include those with active symptoms or lesions, those delivered vaginally with maternal lesions present, and those born during a primary maternal episode. Monitor closely; obtain diagnostic laboratory specimens (HSV PCR and ocular, nasal, anal, and oral cultures). If symptomatic, require prolonged treatment:
  - Acyclovir 20 mg/kg IV q8h for 14 days if skin or mucosal lesions present, 21 days if disseminated or CNS disease (4)[A]
- Low-risk infants who are asymptomatic can be observed while obtaining serum HSV PCR and ocular, nasal, anal, and oral cultures.
- Infants with possible HSV infection should be isolated from other neonates; maternal separation is not necessary, and breastfeeding is not contraindicated.

 ONGOING CARE

GENERAL PREVENTION

- Use barrier contraception and avoid sexual contact when symptoms/lesions are present.
- Abstinence is the only means of complete protection.

Patient Monitoring

Test for HIV and other STIs.

PATIENT EDUCATION

- Patient education helps in treatment of subsequent outbreaks and to reduce risk of transmission:
  - Options include daily suppressive therapy and episodic therapy.
  - Alert partners of history prior to sexual activity.
  - Avoid sexual contact when symptoms or lesions are present.
  - Viral shedding and transmission can occur when symptoms/lesions are NOT present.
    - Shedding increased with HSV-2 and HIV.
  - 100% condom use reduces HSV-2 transmission risk by 30%.
  - Sexual activity between concordant couples (i.e., both partners with the same type of herpes [HSV-1 or HSV-2]) does not increase risk of outbreaks.
  - Ensure maternity care team knows HSV status.
- Herpes Resource Center: http://www.ashasexualhealth.org/stdsstis/herpes/
- Centers for Disease Control and Prevention: http://www.cdc.gov/

PROGNOSIS

- Resolution of signs/symptoms: 3 to 21 days
- Average recurrence rate is one to four episodes per year (2).
- Antivirals do not eliminate virus from body but can reduce transmission, shedding, and outbreaks.

Pediatric Considerations

Neonatal infection survival rates: localized >95%, CNS 85%, systemic 30%

COMPLICATIONS

Behavioral issues include lowered self-esteem, guilt, anger, depression, fear of rejection, and fear of transmission to partner.

REFERENCES

1. LeGoff J, Péré H, Bélec L. Diagnosis of genital herpes simplex virus infection in the clinical laboratory. *Virol J*. 2014;11:83.
2. Hofstetter AM, Rosenthal SL, Stanberry LR. Current thinking on genital herpes. *Curr Opin Infect Dis*. 2014;27(1):75–83.
3. Groves MJ. Genital herpes: a review. *Am Fam Physician*. 2016;93(11):928–934.
4. Centers for Disease Control and Prevention. 2015 Sexually transmitted diseases treatment guidelines. http://www.cdc.gov/std/tg2015. Accessed September 9, 2018.
5. ACOG Committee on Practice Bulletins. ACOG practice bulletin. Clinical management guidelines for obstetrician-gynecologists. No. 82 June 2007. Management of herpes in pregnancy. *Obstet Gynecol*. 2007;109(6):1489–1498.

ADDITIONAL READING

- Dhankani V, Kutz JN, Schiffer JT. Herpes simplex virus-2 genital tract shedding is not predictable over months or years in infected persons. *PLoS Comput Biol*. 2014;10(11):e1003922.
- Gnann JW Jr, Whitley RJ. Clinical practice. Genital herpes. *N Engl J Med*. 2016;375(7):666–674.
- Kimberlin DW, Baley J; and Committee on Infectious Diseases, Committee on Fetus and Newborn. Guidance on management of asymptomatic neonates born to women with active genital herpes lesions. *Pediatrics*. 2013;131(2):e635–e646.
- McQuillan G, Kruszon-Moran D, Flagg EW, et al. Prevalence of herpes simplex virus type 1 and type 2 in persons aged 14–49: United States, 2015–2016. *NCHS Data Brief*. 2018;(304):1–8.

 SEE ALSO

Algorithm: Genital Ulcers

 CODES

ICD10

- A60.00 Herpesviral infection of urogenital system, unspecified
- A60.04 Herpesviral vulvovaginitis
- A60.09 Herpesviral infection of other urogenital tract

CLINICAL PEARLS

- Genital herpes is caused by HSV-1 and/or HSV-2.
- Many seropositive individuals are unaware that they are infected.
- Most primary episodes are asymptomatic.
- Viral shedding occurs in the absence of lesions.
- Meticulous (100%) condom use decreases transmission of HSV.

H

HICCUPS

Maria Montanez Villacampa, MD • Renee F. del Carmen, MD • Nida Hussain, MD

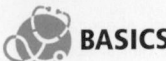 **BASICS**

DESCRIPTION

- Hiccups are caused by a repetitive sudden involuntary contraction of the inspiratory muscles (predominantly the diaphragm) and terminated by the abrupt closure of the glottis, which stops the inflow of air and produces a characteristic sound.
- Hiccups are classified based on their duration: Hiccup bouts last up to 48 hours; persistent hiccups last >48 hours but <1 month; intractable hiccups last for >1 month.
- System(s) affected: nervous, pulmonary
- Synonym(s): hiccoughs; singultus

Geriatric Considerations
Can be a serious problem, particularly among the elderly

Pregnancy Considerations
- Fetal hiccups are rhythmic fetal movements (confirmed sonographically) that can be confused with contractions.
- Fetal hiccups are a sign of normal neurologic development (1).

EPIDEMIOLOGY
- Predominant age: all ages (including fetus)
- Predominant sex: male > female (4:1)

Prevalence
Self-limited hiccups are extremely common, as are intra- and postoperative hiccups.

ETIOLOGY AND PATHOPHYSIOLOGY
- Results from stimulation of ≥1 limbs of the hiccup reflux arc (vagus and phrenic nerves) with a "hiccup center" located in the upper spinal cord and brain (2)
- In men, >90% have an organic basis; whereas in women, a psychogenic cause is more common.
- Specific underlying causes include:
  - CNS disorders: vascular lesions (AV malformation), infectious causes (meningitis, encephalitis), structural lesions (intracranial /brainstem mass lesions, multiple sclerosis, hydrocephalus, syringomyelia)
  - Seizure disorder
  - Diaphragmatic irritation (tumors, pericarditis, eventration, splenomegaly, hepatomegaly, peritonitis)
  - Irritation of the tympanic membrane
  - Nerve irritation: pharyngitis, laryngitis, neck tumors
  - Mediastinal and other thoracic lesions (pneumonia, aortic aneurysm, tuberculosis [TB], myocardial infarction [MI], lung cancer, rib exostoses)
  - Esophageal lesions (reflux esophagitis, achalasia, *Candida* esophagitis, carcinoma, obstruction)
  - Gastrointestinal disorders (gastritis, GERD, PUD, distention, cancer)
  - Hepatic lesions (hepatitis, hepatoma)
  - Pancreatic lesions (pancreatitis, pseudocysts, cancer)
  - Inflammatory bowel disease
  - Cholelithiasis, cholecystitis
  - Prostatic disorders
  - Appendicitis
  - Postoperative, particularly with abdominal procedures
  - Metabolic causes (uremia, hyponatremia, gout, diabetes)
  - Drug-induced (dexamethasone, methylprednisolone, anabolic steroids, benzodiazepines, α-methyldopa, propofol)
  - Psychogenic causes (hysterical neurosis, grief, malingering)
  - Idiopathic

RISK FACTORS
- Overeating
- Consuming carbonated beverages
- Excessive alcohol consumption
- Excitement or emotional stress
- Changes in ambient or gastrointestinal temperature

GENERAL PREVENTION
- Identify and correct relevant underlying cause(s).
- Avoid gastric distention.
- Acupuncture shows promise compared to chronic drug therapy for controlling hiccups (3).

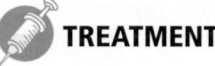 **DIAGNOSIS**

- Hiccup attacks usually occur at brief intervals and last seconds or minutes. Persistent bouts lasting >48 hours often imply an underlying physical or metabolic disorder.
- Intractable hiccups may occur continuously for months or years (4).
- Hiccups usually have a frequency of 4 to 60 per minute (4).
- Persistent and intractable hiccups warrant further evaluation.

HISTORY
- Severity and duration of hiccup bouts
- Associated medical conditions that could be causative—gastrointestinal, cardiac, neurologic, or pulmonary disorders
- Recent surgery (especially genitourinary)
- Behavioral health history
- Review of medications
- Alcohol and illicit drug use

PHYSICAL EXAM
- Correlate exam with potential etiologies (e.g., rales with pneumonia; organomegaly with splenic or hepatic disease).
- Examine the ear canal for foreign bodies.
- Head and neck masses and lymphadenopathy
- Complete neurologic exam

DIFFERENTIAL DIAGNOSIS
Hiccups are rarely be confused with burping (eructation).

DIAGNOSTIC TESTS & INTERPRETATION
- In hiccups lasting >48 hours, if an underlying etiology is suspected, consider condition-specific testing as appropriate (e.g., CBC, electrolytes, BUN, creatinine, LFTs, amylase/lipase, metabolic panel, chest x-ray).
- Fluoroscopy can evaluate hemidiaphragm movement.

Diagnostic Procedures/Other
- Upper endoscopy; CT scan (or other imaging) of brain, thorax, abdomen, and pelvis to look for underlying causes
- Head MRI with contrast, lumbar puncture
- The extent of the workup is often in proportion to the duration and severity of the hiccups (2).

TREATMENT

- Outpatient (usually)
- Inpatient (if elderly, debilitated, or intractable hiccups)
- Many hiccup treatments are purely anecdotal.

GENERAL MEASURES
- Evaluate frequent bouts or persistent hiccups.
- Treat underlying cause when identified (2,4)[C].
  - Dilate esophageal stricture or obstruction.
  - Treat ulcers or reflux disease.
  - Remove hair or foreign body from ear canal.
  - Angostura bitters for alcohol-induced hiccups
  - Catheter stimulation of pharynx for operative and postoperative hiccups
  - Antifungal treatment for *Candida* esophagitis
  - Correct electrolyte imbalance.
- Medical measures
  - Relieve gastric distention (gastric lavage, nasogastric aspiration, induced vomiting).
  - Cautious counterirritation of the vagus nerve (supraorbital pressure, carotid sinus massage, digital rectal massage)
  - Respiratory center stimulants (breathing 5% CO_2)
  - Behavioral health modification (hypnosis, meditation, paced respirations)
  - Phrenic nerve block or electrical stimulation (or pacing) of the dominant hemidiaphragm
  - Acupuncture
  - Miscellaneous (cardioversion)

MEDICATION

First Line

- Physical maneuvers: breath holding, Valsalva maneuver, breathing into a bag, fright, ice water gargles
- Others: swallowing granulated sugar, hard bread, or peanut butter; biting on a lemon, pulling knees to chest or leaning forward to compress chest
- Drug therapy if physical maneuvers have failed or treatment is directed toward a specific cause of hiccups
- Pharmacologic therapy (5)[B]
  - Chlorpromazine (FDA-approved for hiccups): 25 to 50 mg PO/IV TID
  - Metoclopramide: 5 to 10 mg PO QID
  - Baclofen: 5 to 10 mg PO TID (2,4,6)[B]
  - Haloperidol: 2 to 5 mg PO/IM followed by 1 to 2 mg PO TID
  - Phenytoin: 200 to 300 mg PO HS
  - Nifedipine: 10 to 20 mg PO daily to TID
  - Amitriptyline: 10 mg PO TID
  - Viscous lidocaine 2%: 5 mL PO daily to TID
  - Gabapentin (Neurontin): 300 mg PO HS; may increase up to 1,800 mg/day PO in divided doses (4)[B]; 1,200 mg/day PO for 3 days and then 400 mg/day PO for 3 days in patients undergoing stroke rehabilitation or in the palliative care setting where chlorpromazine adverse effects are undesirable (4)[B]
  - Combination of lansoprazole 15 mg PO daily, clonazepam 0.5 mg PO BID, and dimenhydrate 25 mg PO BID (5)[B]
  - Contraindications: Refer to manufacturer's literature.
    - Chlorpromazine is not recommended in elderly patient with dementia.
  - Baclofen is not recommended in patients with stroke or other cerebral lesions or in severe renal impairment. Avoid abrupt withdrawal of baclofen.
- Other possible drug therapies (2,5,6)[C]
  - Amantadine, carbidopa and levodopa in Parkinson disease
  - Steroid replacement in Addison disease
  - Antifungal agent in *Candida* esophagitis
  - Ondansetron in carcinomatosis with vomiting
  - Nefopam (a nonopioid analgesic with antishivering properties related to antihistamines and antiparkinsonian drugs) is available outside the United States in both IV and oral formulations.
  - Olanzapine 10 mg QHS
  - Pregabalin 375 mg/day

ISSUES FOR REFERRAL

For acupuncture or phrenic nerve crush, block, or electrostimulation; cardioversion

SURGERY/OTHER PROCEDURES

- Phrenic nerve crush or transaction or electrostimulation of the dominant diaphragmatic leaflet
- Resection of rib exostoses

COMPLEMENTARY & ALTERNATIVE MEDICINE

- Acupuncture is increasingly used to manage persistent or intractable hiccups, especially in cancer patients (3,4)[A].
- Home remedies (2)[C]
  - Swallowing a spoonful of sugar
  - Sucking on hard candy or swallowing peanut butter
  - Holding breath and increasing pressure on diaphragm (Valsalva maneuver)
  - Tongue traction
  - Lifting the uvula with a cold spoon
  - Inducing fright
  - Smelling salts
  - Rebreathing into a paper (not plastic) bag
  - Sipping ice water
  - Rubbing a wet cotton-tipped applicator between hard and soft palate for 1 minute

ADMISSION, INPATIENT, AND NURSING CONSIDERATIONS

Most patients can be managed as outpatients; those with severe intractable hiccups may require rehydration, pain control, IV medications, or surgery.

 ONGOING CARE

FOLLOW-UP RECOMMENDATIONS

Patient Monitoring

Until hiccups cease

DIET

Avoid gastric distension from overeating, carbonated beverages, and aerophagia.

PATIENT EDUCATION

See "General Measures."

PROGNOSIS

- Hiccups often cease during sleep.
- Most acute benign hiccup bouts resolve spontaneously or with home remedies.
- Intractable hiccups may last for years or decades.
- Hiccups have persisted despite bilateral phrenic nerve transection.

COMPLICATIONS

- Inability to eat
- Weight loss
- Exhaustion, debility
- Insomnia
- Cardiac arrhythmias
- Wound dehiscence
- Death (rare)

REFERENCES

1. Witter F, Dipietro J, Costigan K, et al. The relationship between hiccups and heart rate in the fetus. *J Matern Fetal Neonatal Med*. 2007;20(4):289–292.
2. Calsina-Berna A, García-Gómez G, González-Barboteo J, et al. Treatment of chronic hiccups in cancer patients: a systematic review. *J Palliat Med*. 2012;15(10):1142–1150.
3. Ge AX, Ryan ME, Giaccone G, et al. Acupuncture treatment for persistent hiccups in patients with cancer. *J Altern Complement Med*. 2010;16(7):811–816.
4. Thompson DF, Brooks KG. Gabapentin therapy of hiccups. *Ann Pharmacother*. 2013;47(6):897–903.
5. Maximov G, Kamnasaran D. The adjuvant use of lansoprazole, clonazepam and dimenhydrinate for treating intractable hiccups in a patient with gastritis and reflux esophagitis complicated with myocardial infarction: a case report. *BMC Res Notes*. 2013;6:327.
6. Moretto EN, Wee B, Wiffen PJ, et al. Interventions for treating persistent and intractable hiccups in adults. *Cochrane Database Syst Rev*. 2013;(1):CD008768.

ADDITIONAL READING

- Berger TJ. A rash case of hiccups. *J Emerg Med*. 2013;44(1):e107–e108.
- Chang FY, Lu CL. Hiccup: mystery, nature and treatment. *J Neurogastroenterol Motil*. 2012;18(2):123–130.
- Choi TY, Lee MS, Ernst E. Acupuncture for cancer patients suffering from hiccups: a systematic review and meta-analysis. *Complement Ther Med*. 2012;20(6):447–455.
- Hurst DF, Purdom CL, Hogan MJ. Use of paced respiration to alleviate intractable hiccups (singultus): a case report. *Appl Psychophysiol Biofeedback*. 2013;38(2):157–160.
- Rizzo C, Vitale C, Montagnini M. Management of intractable hiccups: an illustrative case and review. *Am J Hosp Palliat Care*. 2014;31(2):220–224.

 CODES

ICD10

- R06.6 Hiccough
- F45.8 Other somatoform disorders

CLINICAL PEARLS

- Most hiccups resolve spontaneously.
- An organic cause is more likely in men and individuals with intractable hiccups.
- Rule out foreign body in the ear canal as a trigger.
- Baclofen and gabapentin are the only pharmacologic agents proven to be clinically effective.
- Acupuncture may be effective for persistent hiccups.

H

HIDRADENITIS SUPPURATIVA

Rachel L. Storey, DO • Cody E. Homistek, DO • Christopher A. Zagar, MD, FAAFP

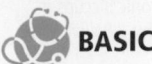 **BASICS**

DESCRIPTION
- Chronic inflammatory skin disease manifested as recurrent inflammatory nodules, abscesses, sinus tracts, and complex scar formation
- Areas affected are tender, malodorous, often with exudative drainage.
- Common in intertriginous skin regions: axillae, groin, perianal, perineal, inframammary skin
- System affected: skin, psychosocial
- Synonym(s): acne inversa; Verneuil disease; apocrinitis; hidradenitis axillaris

Geriatric Considerations
Rare after menopause

Pediatric Considerations
Rarely occurs before puberty; occurrence in children is associated with premature adrenarche.

Pregnancy Considerations
No Accutane (isotretinoin) or tetracycline treatment during pregnancy. Disease may ease during pregnancy and rebound after parturition.

EPIDEMIOLOGY
- Predominant sex: female > male (3:1)
- African Americans

Incidence
Peak onset during 2nd and 3rd decades of life

Prevalence
0.05–4.10% (1)

ETIOLOGY AND PATHOPHYSIOLOGY
- Not fully understood; previously considered a disorder of apocrine glands but more recently thought to be due to a follicular epithelium defect. Deregulation of the local immune system may also play a role.
- Inflammatory disorder of the hair follicle triggered by follicular plugging within apocrine gland–bearing skin
- Hormonally induced ductal keratinocyte proliferation leads to a failure of follicular epithelial shedding, causing follicular occlusion.
- Mechanical stress on skin (intertriginous regions) precipitates follicular rupture and immune response.
- Bacterial involvement is a secondary event.
- Rupture and reepithelialization cause sinus tracts to form.

Genetics
- Familial occurrences suggest single gene transmission (autosomal dominant), but the condition may also be polygenic.
- Estimated 40% of patients have an affected family member.

RISK FACTORS
- Obesity
- Smoking
- Hyperandrogenism
- Lithium may trigger onset of or exacerbate this condition.

GENERAL PREVENTION
- Lose weight if overweight or obese.
- Smoking cessation
- Avoid constrictive clothing/synthetic fabrics, frictional trauma, heat exposure, excessive sweating, shaving, depilation, and deodorants.
- Use of antiseptic soaps

COMMONLY ASSOCIATED CONDITIONS
- Acne vulgaris, acne conglobate
- Perifolliculitis capitis abscedens et suffodiens (dissecting cellulitis of scalp)
- Pilonidal disease
- Metabolic syndrome/obesity
- Polycystic ovary syndrome (PCOS) and androgen dysfunction
- Thyroid disease
- Arthritis and spondyloarthritis (seronegative)
- Irritable bowel disease (Crohn disease)
- Squamous cell carcinoma
- PAPASH syndrome (pyogenic arthritis, pyoderma gangrenosum, acne, and suppurative hydradenitis)

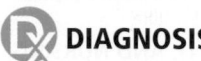 **DIAGNOSIS**

HISTORY
- Diagnostic criteria adopted by the 2nd International Conference on Hidradenitis Suppurativa, 2009 (2)
- All three criteria (morphology, location, progression) must be present for diagnosis:
  - Typical lesions: painful nodules, abscesses, draining sinus, bridged scars, and "tombstone" double-ended pseudocomedones in secondary lesions
  - Typical topography: axillae, groins, perineal and perianal region, buttocks, infra- and intermammary folds
  - Chronicity and recurrences, commonly refractory to initial treatments

PHYSICAL EXAM
- Tender dome-shaped nodules 0.5 to 3.0 cm in size are present.
  - Location corresponds with the distribution of apocrine-related mammary tissue and terminal hair follicles dependent on low androgen concentrations.
  - Sites ordered by frequency of occurrence: axillary, inguinal, perianal and perineal, mammary and inframammary, buttock, pubic region, chest, scalp, retroauricular, eyelid
  - Large lesions are often fluctuant; comedones may be present.
- Possible malodorous discharge
- Hurley clinical staging system
  - **Stage I**: nodule/abscess formation without sinus tracts or scarring
  - **Stage II**: more than one lesion widely spaced with tract and scar formation
  - **Stage III**: diffuse, multiple interconnected tracts and abscesses with scarring
- Sartorius clinical staging system (points attributed)
  - Anatomic region involved
  - Quantity and quality of lesions
  - Distance between lesions
  - Presence or absence of normal skin between lesions

DIFFERENTIAL DIAGNOSIS
- Acne vulgaris, conglobate
- Furunculosis/carbuncles
- Infected Bartholin or sebaceous cysts
- Lymphadenopathy/lymphadenitis
- Cutaneous Langerhans cell histiocytosis
- Actinomycosis
- Granuloma inguinale
- Lymphogranuloma venereum
- Apocrine nevus

- Crohn disease with anogenital fistula(s) (may coexist with hidradenitis suppurativa)
- Fox-Fordyce disease

DIAGNOSTIC TESTS & INTERPRETATION
Initial Tests (lab, imaging)
- Cultures of skin or aspirates of boils are most commonly negative. When positive, cultures are often polymicrobial and commonly grow *Staphylococcus aureus* and *Staphylococcus epidermidis*.
- Lesion biopsy usually unnecessary; useful to rule out other disorders such as squamous cell carcinoma
- May note increased erythrocyte sedimentation rate (ESR), leukocytosis, decreased serum iron, normocytic anemia, or changes in serum electrophoresis pattern

Follow-Up Tests & Special Considerations
- Consider biopsy of concerning lesions due to increased risk of squamous cell carcinoma.
- If the patient is female, overweight, and/or hirsute, consider evaluating the following:
  - Dehydroepiandrosterone sulfate
  - Testosterone: total and free
  - Sex hormone–binding globulin
  - Progesterone

Diagnostic Procedures/Other
- Incision and drainage, culture and biopsy
- Ultrasound may be useful in planning an excision to identify the full extent of sinus tracts.

Test Interpretation
- Dermis shows granulomatous inflammation and inflammatory cells, giant cells, sinus tracts, subcutaneous abscesses, and extensive fibrosis.
- Hair follicular dilatation and occlusion by keratinized stratified squamous epithelium

 TREATMENT

Despite the prevalence of this condition, most trials have been small and underpowered. Evidence is therefore generally of poor quality (3)[A]. Treatment goals: Reduce extent of disease, prevent new lesions, remove chronic disease, and limit scar formation.

- Conservative treatment includes all items under "General Prevention," plus use of warm compresses, sitz baths, topical antiseptics for inflamed lesions, and nonopioid analgesics.
- Weight loss and smoking cessation result in marked improvement (1).
- Corticosteroids, isotretinoin, and zinc gluconate
- For stages I and II, attempt medical treatment.
- Short medical trial may be appropriate in stage III prior to moving on to surgical therapies.
- Only FDA-approved medication for this condition is adalimumab. Other biologics may be effective. No medications are curative; relapse is almost inevitable, but the disease may be controlled. Usually must fail other treatments before starting biologics. They can be a costly option.

GENERAL MEASURES
- Education and psychosocial support
- Appropriate hygiene including avoidance of shearing stress to skin (light clothing), daily cleansing with antibacterial soap
- Diet: Avoid dairy, high glycemic loads.
- Symptomatic treatment for acute lesions

- Improve environmental factors that cause follicular blockage (see "General Prevention").
- Smoking cessation and weight loss

MEDICATION

First Line

- Stage I disease: Consider either systemic or topical antibiotics.
  - Topical antibiotics (clindamycin was studied in clinical trials) (1)[B]
    ○ Clindamycin 0.1% solution BID for 12 weeks with or without benzoyl peroxide 5–10% solution
    ○ Chlorhexidine 4% solution
  - Systemic antibiotics (initial 7- to 10-day course)
    ○ Tetracycline 500 mg BID
    ○ Doxycycline 100 mg q12h
    ○ Augmentin 875 mg q8–12h
    ○ Clindamycin 300 mg BID (4)[B]
  - Intralesion corticosteroids: limited evidence; possible reduction in pain, erythema, edema, and lesion size (1). (triamcinolone acetonide 10 mg/mL usually 0.2 to 2.0 mL injection)
- Stages II and III disease
  - Address overlying bacterial infection with broad-spectrum coverage. Base antibiotic selection on disease location and characteristics; best evidence for antibiotic treatment with combinations of clindamycin and rifampicin, or ertapenem followed by combination rifampicin, moxifloxacin, and metronidazole for 6 months (1)[A]
  - Minor surgical procedures (punch débridement, local unroofing) to treat individual lesions or sinus tracts
- Other modalities (rarely used)
  - Hormonal therapy: antiandrogenic therapy such as cyproterone acetate (may not be available in the United States), estrogen/norgestrel oral contraceptive, finasteride (5 mg daily)

Second Line

- Dapsone 50 to 150 mg daily
- Metformin: significant reduction in Sartorius score
- Oral retinoids (isotretinoin): poor efficacy, limited therapeutic effect
- TNF-α inhibitors:
  - Adalimumab 40 mg weekly (a high dose) produces statistically significant differences versus placebo in treated patients, but clinical effect size is small (Cochrane) (1)[A], and long-term safety is unknown (5)[A].
  - Infliximab: A majority of patients in the treatment group had a 50% or greater decrease in disease, improving quality of life (5)[A].
  - Etanercept: no difference versus placebo

ISSUES FOR REFERRAL

- Lack of response to treatment, stages II and III disease, or concern for malignancy (squamous cell carcinoma) is a reason to refer for surgical excision or radiation/laser treatment (stage II).
- If significant psychosocial stress exists secondary to disease, refer for stress management or psychiatric evaluation.
- Suspicion of hyperandrogenic states (e.g., PCOS) should prompt investigation or referral.
- Severe perianal/perivulvar disease or otherwise very extensive disease may prompt referral to plastic surgeon or reconstructive urologist.

SURGERY/OTHER PROCEDURES

- Important mode of treatment; necessary if wanting to permanently remove tunnels and scarring
- Could be used in conjunction with antibiotics or if first-line therapy fails

- Various surgical approaches have been used for stages II and III disease.
  - Incision and drainage: necessary to treat acute flare-ups when abscess is present
  - Deroofing of sinus tracts and skin tissue–sparing excision with electrosurgical peeling (STEEP) allow for healing by secondary intention. Recurrences remain common but usually are smaller than original lesions.
  - Wide full-thickness excision with healing by granulation or flap placement is the most definitive treatment and rarely has local recurrence if all sinus tracts are excised with a clear 1- to 2-cm margin. Rates of local recurrence (within 3 to 72 months): axillary (3%), perianal (0%), inguino-perineal (37%), submammary (50%)
- Laser therapy for Hurley stages I and II disease (rarely used); no consensus on the benefit
  - Monthly treatments with neodymium-doped yttrium aluminum garnet (Nd:YAG) laser for 3 to 4 months
  - CO_2 laser ablation with healing by secondary intention
- Cryotherapy and photodynamic therapy have shown variable results; they are not routinely recommended.
- Potential role for combined therapy consisting of radical resection plus biologic in advanced cases

 ## ONGOING CARE

FOLLOW-UP RECOMMENDATIONS

Follow up monthly or sooner to evaluate progress and to assist with symptom management.

DIET

- Avoid dairy and high glycemic loads.
- Healthy diet that promotes weight loss
- May benefit from zinc supplementation

PATIENT EDUCATION

- Severity can range from only two to three papules per year to extensive draining sinus tracts.
- Medications are temporizing measures, rarely curative. Attempts at local surgical "cures" do not affect recurrence at other sites.
- Smoking cessation and weight loss can improve symptoms significantly.
- Hidradenitis Suppurativa Foundation: www.hs-foundation.org

PROGNOSIS

- Individual lesions heal slowly in 10 to 30 days.
- Recurrences may last for several years.
- Relentlessly progressive scarring and sinus tracts are likely with severe disease.
- Radical wide-area excision, with removal of all hair-bearing skin in the affected area, shows the greatest chance for cure.
- Increased all-cause mortality

COMPLICATIONS

- Contracture and stricturing of the skin after extensive abscess rupture, scarring, and healing; or at sites of surgical excisions
- Lymphatic obstruction, lymphedema
- Psychosocial: anxiety, malaise, depression, self-injury
- Anemia, amyloidosis, and hypoproteinemia (due to chronic suppuration)
- Lumbosacral epidural abscess, sacral bacterial osteomyelitis

- Squamous cell carcinoma may develop in indolent sinus tracts.
- Disseminated infection or septicemia (rare)
- Urethral, rectal, or bladder fistula (rare)

REFERENCES

1. Saunte D, Jemec G. Hidradenitis suppurativa: advances in diagnosis and treatment. *JAMA.* 2017;318(20):2019–2032.
2. Rambhatla PV, Lim HW, Hamzavi I. A systematic review of treatments for hidradenitis suppurativa. *Arch Dermatol.* 2012;148(4):439–446.
3. van der Zee HH, Boer J, Prens EP, et al. The effect of combined treatment with oral clindamycin and oral rifampicin in patients with hidradenitis suppurativa. *Dermatology.* 2009;219(2):143–147.
4. Wang S, Wang S, Sibbald R. Hidradenitis suppurativa: a frequently missed diagnosis, part 1: a review of pathogenesis, associations, and clinical features. *Adv Skin Wound Care.* 2015;28(7):325–332.
5. Falola R, DeFazio M, Anghel E, et al. What heals hidradenitis suppurativa: surgery, immunosuppression, or both? *Plast Reconstr Surg.* 2016;138 (Suppl 3):219S–229S.

ADDITIONAL READING

- Alikhan A, Lynch PJ, Eisen DB. Hidradenitis suppurativa: a comprehensive review. *J Am Acad Dermatol.* 2009;60(4):539–563.
- Blok JL, van Hattem S, Jonkman MF, et al. Systemic therapy with immunosuppressive agents and retinoids in hidradenitis suppurativa: a systematic review. *Br J Dermatol.* 2013;168(2):243–252.
- Grant A, Gonzalez T, Montgomery MO, et al. Infliximab therapy for patients with moderate to severe hidradenitis suppurativa: a randomized, double-blind, placebo-controlled crossover trial. *J Am Acad Dermatol.* 2010;62(2):205–217.
- Jemec GB. Clinical practice. Hidradenitis suppurativa. *N Engl J Med.* 2012;366(2):158–164.
- van der Zee HH, Prens EP, Boer J. Deroofing: a tissue-saving surgical technique for the treatment of mild to moderate hidradenitis suppurativa lesions. *J Am Acad Dermatol.* 2010;63(3):475–480.
- Verdolini R, Clayton N, Smith A, et al. Metformin for the treatment of hidradenitis suppurativa: a little help along the way. *J Eur Acad Dermatol Venereol.* 2013;27(9):1101–1108.

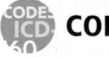 ## CODES

ICD10
L73.2 Hidradenitis suppurativa

CLINICAL PEARLS

- Chronic inflammatory disease of the skin, often difficult to control with behavior changes and medication alone
- First-line treatment for mild disease is topical and/or systemic antibiotics.
- For patients with refractory or severe disease, wide local excision provides the only chance at a cure. Success rates depend on the location and extent of excision.
- This is a difficult to treat disease that can greatly affect the patient's quality of life.

H

HIRSUTISM

Natasha S. Kadakia, DO • Ruchita Patel, DO

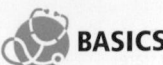

BASICS

DESCRIPTION
- Presence of excessive terminal (coarse, pigmented) hair of body and face, in a male pattern
- May be present in normal adults as an ethnic characteristic or may develop as a result of androgen excess
- Often seen in polycystic ovary syndrome (PCOS) which is characterized by hirsutism, acne, menstrual irregularities, and obesity
- System(s) affected: dermatologic, endocrine, metabolic, reproductive

EPIDEMIOLOGY
Prevalence
5–10% of reproductive age women

ETIOLOGY AND PATHOPHYSIOLOGY
- Hirsutism is due to increased androgenic (male) hormones, either from increased peripheral binding (idiopathic) or increased production from the ovaries, adrenals, or body fat.
- Exogenous medications can also cause hirsutism.

Genetics
Multifactorial

RISK FACTORS
- Family history
- Ethnicity—increased in Ashkenazi Jews and Mediterranean backgrounds
- Anovulation
- Obesity

GENERAL PREVENTION
Women with late-onset congenital adrenal hyperplasia (CAH) should be counseled that they may be carriers for the severe early-onset childhood disease.

COMMONLY ASSOCIATED CONDITIONS
- PCOS: the most common cause of premenopausal hirsutism (1)
- Insulin resistance, common
- Prolonged amenorrhea and anovulation, common
- Emotional distress and depression, common
- Acne, common
- Central obesity
- Hypothyroidism/hyperthyroidism, rare
- Hyperprolactinemia, rare
- Risk for endometrial hyperplasia or carcinoma, rare
- Virilization (rapid onset, clitoromegaly, balding, deepening voice) (2)
- Cushing syndrome: characterized by moon facies, striae, hypertension, rare
- Acromegaly, rare
- Vitamin D deficiency

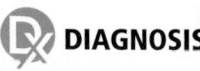

DIAGNOSIS

HISTORY
- Severity, time course, and age of onset of hirsutism
- Weight
- Psychosocial impact on patient
- Menstrual and fertility history, anovulation (defined as ovulatory cycle >35 days)

- Severe acne, especially if treatment resistant
- Presence of virilization
- Medication history: Look for use of valproic acid, testosterone, danazol, glucocorticoids, topical androgen use by partner, and athletic performance drugs.
- The presence of galactorrhea

PHYSICAL EXAM
- Increased hair growth in premenopausal women, particularly over the chin, neck, sideburns, lower back, sternum, abdomen, shoulders, buttocks, perineal area, and inner thighs
- Check skin for acne, striae, acanthosis nigricans (velvety black skin in the axillae or neck).
- Virilization: Deep voice, male pattern balding, increased muscle mass, and clitoromegaly indicate risk of tumor.
- The Ferriman-Gallwey scale (an instrument that rates hair growth in nine areas on a scale of 0 to 4, with >8 being positive) may be used for diagnosis but underrates patient's perception of hirsutism and altered by previous cosmetic treatment. Scores between 8 and 15 are considered to be mild hirsutism, 16 to 25 moderate, and >25 severe (1,2).

DIFFERENTIAL DIAGNOSIS
- PCOS (72–82%)—irregular menses, elevated androgens, polycystic ovaries on US, infertility, insulin resistance
- Idiopathic hyperandrogenemia (6–15%)—hirsutism with normal ovaries on US, elevated androgen levels, no other explainable cause
- Idiopathic hirsutism (4–7%)—hirsutism with normal menses, androgen levels, and ovaries on ultrasonography, no other explainable cause
- Late-onset CAH (2–4%), a genetic enzyme deficiency associated with more severe and earlier onset hirsutism in amenorrheic patients presents in adolescence with severe hirsutism and irregular menses.
- Androgen-secreting tumor (0.2%)—ovaries (benign or malignant) or adrenals (commonly malignant); have rapid onset, virilization, resistance to treatment
- Ovarian hyperthecosis—increase in testosterone by theca cells. Gradual onset of hirsutism, frank virilization; mostly affects postmenopausal women
- Thyroid dysfunction
- Hyperprolactinemia if accompanied by galactorrhea or amenorrhea
- Rare endocrine disorders—Cushing, acromegaly

DIAGNOSTIC TESTS & INTERPRETATION
- Testing for elevated androgen levels in all women with an abnormal hirsutism score. Guidelines recommend screening hyperandrogenemic women for NCCAH due to 21-hydroxylase deficiency by measuring early morning 17-hydroxyprogesterone levels (2).
- PCOS is diagnosed by having two out of three signs: menstrual dysfunction, clinical or biochemical hyperandrogenemia, polycystic ovaries on US (2)[C].
- Lab testing is performed to rule out underlying tumor and pituitary diseases, which are rare.

Initial Tests (lab, imaging)
- Basic workup of moderate hirsutism is a total testosterone level +/− thyroid screen (TSH) (1)[C].
- Testosterone: Random total testosterone level is usually sufficient.
- Normal upper limit for serum total testosterone in adult women is approximately 40 to 60 ng/dL (1.4 to 2.1 nmol/L). Patients who have clinical features consistent with PCOS but have normal total testosterone should have repeat testing, preferably an early morning serum free testosterone level calculated from sex hormone-binding globulin (SHBG). A morning free testosterone is 50% more sensitive (1,3).
- If testosterone is >150 (some use 200) ng/dL, consider ovarian or adrenal tumor (2,4). Testosterone is made by both the ovaries and adrenals, so both areas should be imaged. US is best for the ovaries, and CT is best for the adrenals.
- The workup for PCOS recommended by the American College of Obstetricians and Gynecologists (ACOG) includes the above plus:
  – Screening for metabolic syndrome with a fasting and 2-hour glucose after 75-g glucose load, lipid panel, waist circumference, and blood pressure (4)[C]
- Ovarian US to look for polycystic ovaries
- If the patient is amenorrheic, check prolactin, FSH, LH, TSH, and a pregnancy test (5)[C]. An LH/FSH ratio >2 indicates PCOS.

Follow-Up Tests & Special Considerations
- 17α-Hydroxyprogesterone (17α-OHP)
  – Elevations of 17α-OHP (>300) can indicate late-onset CAH.
  – Consider in patients with onset in early adolescence or high-risk group (Ashkenazi Jews) (2)[C].
  – If elevated, order corticotropin stimulation test.
- If prolactin level is high, MRI the pituitary
- If PCOS is diagnosed, ACOG recommends screening for dyslipidemia and DM type 2 (4)[C].
- New studies show an inverse correlation between vitamin D levels and insulin resistance in women with PCOS. Screening women who are at risk of vitamin D deficiency and supplementation with vitamin D could be considered.
- Dehydroepiandrosterone sulfate (DHEA-S) is no longer recommended routinely but should be checked in virilization (5)[C].
  – Levels >700 may indicate adrenal tumor.

TREATMENT

GENERAL MEASURES
- Treatment in mild hirsutism depends on patient preference and psychosocial effect.
- If patient desires pregnancy, induction of ovulation may be necessary.
- Provide contraception, as needed.
- Encourage patient to maintain ideal weight with lifestyle modification. A calorie-restricted diet is recommended in all overweight patients with PCOS. Weight loss has positive effects on fertility, metabolic profile, and may improve hirsutism (5).
- Treat accompanying acne.

MEDICATION

First Line

- Treatment goal is to decrease new hair growth and improve metabolic disorders.
- Direct hair removal or pharmacologic therapy is recommended for mild hirsutism (2)[B].
- Oral contraceptives are first line to manage menstrual abnormalities and hirsutism/acne (3)[A]; they will suppress ovarian androgen production and increase SHBG, improve metabolic syndrome, and slow but not reverse hair growth.
  - Doses of 20 to 35 μg ethinyl estradiol effectively decrease ovarian androgen production. Those containing the progestins, norgestimate, desogestrel, or drospirenone have more androgen-blocking effects, but desogestrel and drospirenone are associated with more DVTs especially in severely obese patients (3,4)[C].
  - They take 6 months to show effect and are continued for years.
  - Oral preparations, compared to vaginal or transdermal, are better at controlling hirsutism and acne; by passing through the liver, they induce SHBG production (1).
- Progesterone (depot or intermittent oral) can be used if estrogens are contraindicated (4).
- Eflornithine (Vaniqa) HCl cream: Apply BID at least 8 hours apart; reduces facial hair in 40% of women (must be used indefinitely to prevent regrowth); only FDA-approved hirsutism treatment
- Combination oral contraceptives and antiandrogen is contraindicated first line unless those with severe hirsutism and significant emotional distress or no success with oral contraceptives alone (2)[B].

Second Line

- Antiandrogenic drugs will further reduce hirsutism to 15–25%. Usually begun 6 months after first-line therapy if results are suboptimal. Must be used in combination with oral contraceptives to prevent menorrhagia and potential fetal toxicity. All should be avoided in pregnancy (2,5)[C].
  - Spironolactone, 50 to 200 mg/day: Onset of action is slow; use with oral contraceptives to prevent menorrhagia. Watch for hyperkalemia, especially with drospirenone-containing OCP (Yasmin); avoid use in pregnancy.
  - Finasteride: 5 mg/day decreases androgen binding; not approved by FDA. Use with contraception (pregnancy Category X).
  - Cyproterone, not available in the United States: 12.5 to 100.0 mg/day for days 5 to 15 of cycle combined with ethinyl estradiol 20 to 50 μg for days 5 to 25 of cycle
  - Flutamide is not recommended due to potential hepatotoxicity (2).
  - Topical antiandrogen therapy is not recommended.
- It is suggested against using insulin-lowering drugs as the sole indication of treating hirsutism (2).
- Steroids: used in late-onset CAH
  - Dexamethasone: 2 mg/day
- Cosmetic treatment: includes many methods of hair removal
  - Temporary: shaving, chemical depilation, plucking, waxing

- Permanent: Laser epilation and photoepilation are preferred to electrolysis (4)[C].
- If hair removal therapy is chosen, pharmacologic therapy is suggested to minimize hair regrowth (2).

Pregnancy Considerations

- May have related infertility. Offer intervention, if desired.
- As hormone balance improves, fertility may increase; provide contraception, as needed.
- Several medications used for treatment are contraindicated in pregnancy.

COMPLEMENTARY & ALTERNATIVE MEDICINE

Several herbals including spearmint tea, saw palmetto, licorice, fennel, and soy have been shown in small (<50 people) and short (<12 weeks) studies to decrease hair size or lower androgen levels (5)[C].

 ONGOING CARE

FOLLOW-UP RECOMMENDATIONS

No special activity

Patient Monitoring

Monitor for known side effects of medications.

DIET

Diet consisting of low-calorie, low-glycemic index foods improve fertility in obese PCOS patients with anovulatory infertility.

PATIENT EDUCATION

- Hormonal treatment stops further hair growth and will improve but not reverse present hair.
  - Treatment takes 6 months to take effect and may need to be lifelong.
- Cosmetic measures may be needed for the already present hair (see above).

PROGNOSIS

- Good (with long-term therapy) for halting further hair growth
- Moderate to poor for reversing current hair growth

COMPLICATIONS

- If PCOS is present, dysfunctional uterine bleeding may lead to anemia.
- If PCOS is present, anovulation may increase endometrial hyperplasia and uterine cancer risk.
- Androgenic excess may adversely affect lipid status, cardiac risk, and bone density.
- Poor self-image

REFERENCES

1. Azziz R, Carmina E, Dewailly D, et al; for Task Force on the Phenotype of the Polycystic Ovary Syndrome of the Androgen Excess and PCOS Society. The Androgen Excess and PCOS Society criteria for the polycystic ovary syndrome: the complete task force report. *Fertil Steril*. 2009;91(2):456–488.
2. Martin KA, Anderson RR, Chang RJ, et al. Evaluation and treatment of hirsutism in premenopausal women: an endocrine society clinical practice guideline. *J Clin Endocrinol Metab*. 2018;103(4):1233–1257.
3. Goodman NF, Cobin RH, Futterweit W, et al; for American Association of Clinical Endocrinologists, American College of Endocrinology, Androgen Excess and PCOS Society. American Association of Clinical Endocrinologists, American College of Endocrinology, and Androgen Excess and PCOS Society disease state clinical review: guide to the best practices in the evaluation and treatment of polycystic ovary syndrome—part 1. *Endocr Pract*. 2015;21(11):1291–1300.
4. Rosenfield RL. Clinical practice. Hirsutism. *N Engl J Med*. 2005;353(24):2578–2588.
5. Williams T, Mortada R, Porter S. Diagnosis and treatment of polycystic ovary syndrome. *Am Fam Physician*. 2016;94(2):106–113.

ADDITIONAL READING

- Bode D, Seehusen DA, Baird D. Hirsutism in women. *Am Fam Physician*. 2012;85(4):373–380.
- Brown J, Farquhar C, Lee O, et al. Spironolactone versus placebo or in combination with steroids for hirsutism and/or acne. *Cochrane Database Syst Rev*. 2009;(2):CD000194.
- Krul-Poel YHM, Snackey C, Louwers Y, et al. The role of vitamin D in metabolic disturbances in polycystic ovary syndrome: a systematic review. *Eur J Endocrinol*. 2013;169(6):853–865.
- National Institute of Health. Evidence-based methodology workshop on PCOS. https://prevention.nih.gov/docs/programs/pcos/FinalReport.pdf. Accessed September 22, 2016.

 SEE ALSO

Acne Vulgaris; Infertility; Polycystic Ovarian Syndrome (PCOS)

 CODES

ICD10

- L68.0 Hirsutism
- E28.2 Polycystic ovarian syndrome

CLINICAL PEARLS

- PCOS is the most common cause of hirsutism (diagnosed with two out of three: menstrual dysfunction, clinical or biochemical hyperandrogenemia, polycystic ovaries on US).
- Diagnosis is based on androgen level in all women with abnormal hirsutism score; total testosterone and TSH for initial testing
- Patients suspected of PCOS should also get prolactin, lipid panel, blood pressure, and pregnancy test.
- Treatment is long term and often lifelong.
- Virilization (clitoromegaly, balding, deepening voice): Suspect if testosterone >150 ng/dL; look for adrenal and ovarian tumor.
- Lifestyle modification and OCPs are first-line therapy for hirsutism, menstrual irregularities, and acne.

H

HIV/AIDS

Carol H. Hungerford, DO • Pamela R. Hughes, MD

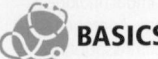 **BASICS**

DESCRIPTION
- HIV is a retrovirus (subgroup lentivirus) that integrates into CD4 T lymphocytes, altering cell-mediated immunity and causing cell death, severe immunodeficiency, opportunistic infections, and malignancies if not treated.
- The natural history of untreated HIV infection includes viral transmission, acute retroviral syndrome, recovery and seroconversion, asymptomatic chronic HIV infection, and symptomatic HIV infection or AIDS.
- Without treatment, the average patient progresses to AIDS ~10 years after acquiring the virus.
- HIV-infected persons with CD4 <200 cells/mm³ or with AIDS-defining illnesses are categorized as persons living with AIDS.

EPIDEMIOLOGY
Incidence
In the United States, HIV incidence has decreased 5% since 2011. There were approximately 39,000 new cases in 2016 (1). There were approximately 1.8 million new cases of HIV worldwide in 2016 (1).

Prevalence
- 1.1 million persons in the United States are living with HIV, ~15% are not aware they are infected (1).
- Worldwide, >35 million people are living with HIV. >75% are in sub-Saharan Africa.
- In 2016, ~1 million people died from AIDS (1).

ETIOLOGY AND PATHOPHYSIOLOGY
- HIV primarily infects CD4+ cells. HIV is a single-stranded, positive-sense, enveloped RNA virus. After entering target cells, viral RNA is transcribed to DNA (through reverse transcription), imported to the host cell nucleus and incorporated into host DNA. The virus can become latent or produce new viral RNA with proteins that are released to infect other CD4+ cells. Host CD8+ cells are activated as part of the seroconversion response.
- There are two types of HIV. HIV-1 was first described and is more virulent, causing the majority of HIV infections worldwide. HIV-2 is less infective and seen primarily in West Africa.

RISK FACTORS
- Sexual activity (>90% of transmission): Ulcerative urogenital lesions promote transmission (1).
- Injection drug use
- Children of HIV-infected women
  - Maternal HIV-1 RNA level predicts transmission.
  - HIV can also be transmitted in breast milk. HIV+ women should not breastfeed their infants unless there is no other alternative. In this case, consider antiretroviral therapy (ART) (2).
- Recipients of blood products prior to 1985
- Occupational exposure (health care workers)

GENERAL PREVENTION
- Avoid unprotected, high-risk sex and intravenous drug use, particularly with shared needles.
- Preexposure prophylaxis (PrEP) is recommended by WHO for persons at high risk of acquiring HIV.

- General guidelines for PrEP: (i) exclude acute or chronic HIV infection before initiating therapy, (ii) repeat HIV testing every 3 months during therapy, (iii) renal function testing at baseline and every 6 months
- Postexposure prophylaxis (PEP) should be started within 72 hours of exposure and continued for 28 days with a three-drug regimen (1).

COMMONLY ASSOCIATED CONDITIONS
- Syphilis is more aggressive in HIV-infected persons.
- Tuberculosis (TB) is coepidemic with HIV; test all patients for TB. Dually infected patients (TB and HIV) have 100 times greater risk of developing active TB.
- Patients coinfected with hepatitis B or hepatitis C have a more rapid progression to cirrhosis.
- Increased risk for cervical cancer, lymphoma, and skin malignancies

 DIAGNOSIS

- Acute retroviral syndrome: CD4 lymphocyte count declines with increase in viral load 1 to 4 weeks after transmission; confirmed by high-HIV RNA in the absence of HIV antibody
- Acute retroviral syndrome presents as a mononucleosis-like syndrome:
  - Fever, adenopathy, pharyngitis, rash, myalgias/ arthralgias
  - Seroconversion: positive HIV antibody 4 weeks to 6 months after exposure
- Clinical latency (asymptomatic): variable duration (average is 8 to 10 years) accompanied by a gradual decline in CD4 cell counts and relatively stable HIV RNA levels (the viral "set point"). Patients often develop persistent generalized lymphadenopathy (>1 cm in size, at ≥2 extrainguinal sites) and may develop fever, weight loss, myalgias, and gastrointestinal problems if unrecognized.
- Associated conditions:
  - Fever or diarrhea >1 month, bacillary angiomatosis, thrush, persistent candidal vulvovaginitis, cervical dysplasia or carcinoma in situ, oral hairy leukoplakia, herpes zoster, idiopathic thrombocytopenic purpura, pelvic inflammatory disease, peripheral neuropathy or myelopathy.
- AIDS: defined by a CD4 cell count <200, a CD4 cell percentage of total lymphocytes <14%, or an AIDS-related opportunistic infections: *Pneumocystis jiroveci* (*carinii*) pneumonia, cryptococcal meningitis, recurrent bacterial pneumonia, candida esophagitis, CNS toxoplasmosis, TB, non-Hodgkin lymphoma (NHL), progressive multifocal encephalopathy, HIV nephropathy, Kaposi sarcoma, Hodgkin lymphoma, invasive cervical cancer
- Advanced HIV disease: CD4 cell count <50. Most AIDS-related deaths occur at this time. Common late opportunistic infections: cytomegalovirus (CMV) disease (retinitis, colitis) or disseminated *Mycobacterium avium* complex

HISTORY
- Complete medical history, including risk exposures, and social/occupational history
- Review of systems: fever, chills, night sweats, weight loss, fatigue, adenopathy, diarrhea, oral sores, odynophagia (esophageal candidiasis), cough, shortness of breath and dyspnea on exertion (early *P. jiroveci* pneumonia), sinusitis, visual changes (CMV retinitis), neurologic symptoms (CNS infection, malignancy, or dementia), skin rash
- Review immunization record.

PHYSICAL EXAM
Focus on weight, skin, retinal exam, oropharynx, lymph nodes, liver, spleen, mental status, neurologic, genital, and rectal examinations.

DIFFERENTIAL DIAGNOSIS
Burkitt lymphoma, candidiasis, CMV, coccidioldomycosis, cryptococcus, EBV, herpes simplex, influenza, lymphoma, mononucleosis, TB, toxoplasmosis

DIAGNOSTIC TESTS & INTERPRETATION
Initial Tests (lab, imaging)
- Screening: Rapid oral test is FDA-approved. Two FDA-approved home testing kits are available.
- Fourth-generation HIV testing combines antibody/ antigen immunoassay for HIV-1/HIV-2 (3)[A].
  - Can be positive within 2 to 3 weeks of exposure
  - Is considered a confirmatory test
- Obtain HIV RNA if acute HIV infection is suspected using quantitative PCR; detects infection within 12 days of exposure
- CD4 cell count and percentage (3)[A]
- HIV RNA viral load (3)[A]
- CBC with differential; lipid levels
- Western blot confirmation is no longer recommended.
- Serologies: hepatitis A/B/C, syphilis
- Screen for STI (chlamydia, gonorrhea, herpes).
- Cervical cytology
- Purified protein derivative (PPD) or interferon-γ release assay (IGRA) to screen for latent TB infection; chest x-ray (CXR) if pulmonary symptoms or positive PPD
- HLAB*5701 testing if abacavir planned for treatment (3)[A]
- Genotypic tests for resistance to antiretrovirals for patients with pretreatment HIV RNA >1,000 copies/mL; transmitted resistance to at least one drug seen in 6–16% of patients (3)[A]
- Tropism assay if considering CCR5 antagonist

 TREATMENT

- Initiate ART in patients meeting eligibility requirements. Select/change regimens based on resistance testing.
- Consider dosing frequency, pill burden, adverse toxic effect profiles, comorbidities, and drug interactions.
- Pregnancy, AIDS-defining conditions, acute opportunistic infections, CD4 <200, HIV-associated nephropathy, acute/early infection, HIV/HBV coinfection, HIV/HCV coinfection, rapidly declining CD4 counts (>100 cells/mm³ per year), and high viral loads (>100,000 copies/mL) increase urgency for immediate therapy (3)[A].

- In women of childbearing age, use ART regimen that decreases viral load with minimal teratogenicity (2)[A].
- Genotypic testing is recommended to guide therapy in patients who are naive to ART.
- Tenofovir/emtricitabine (Truvada) 300 mg/200 mg PO daily is FDA-approved for PrEP in adults at high risk (4)[A].

GENERAL MEASURES
- The goal of ART is to reduce viral load (below limits of detection) and delay immune suppression. Viral load is the most important indicator of response to ART.
- Assess drug resistance before starting ART (3).
- Assess substance abuse, economic factors (unstable housing, food insecurity), social support, mental illness, comorbidities, high-risk behaviors, and factors known to impair adherence and promote transmission.
- Prophylactic antimicrobial agents and vaccines:
  - *P. jiroveci* prophylaxis: trimethoprim/sulfamethoxazole (TMP-SMX) if CD4 <200 cells/mm^3, prior *P. jiroveci*, thrush, or unexplained fever for >2 weeks
  - *Mycobacterium tuberculosis*: Treat for latent TB if positive PPD or positive IGRA without prior prophylaxis or treatment, with negative CXR, recent TB contact, or history of inadequately treated TB that healed.
  - *Toxoplasma gondii* prophylaxis: 33% per year risk of infection in untreated patients with CD4 <100 cells/mm^3; prophylaxis: TMP-SMX 1 DS tab daily
  - *M. avium* complex prophylaxis: 20–40% risk with CD4 <50 and no ART. Azithromycin 1,200 mg PO weekly is preferred prophylaxis.
  - *Streptococcus pneumoniae*: 50 to 100 times increased risk of invasive infection compared with general population; Prevnar and Pneumovax at least 8 weeks apart, every 5 years
  - Influenza vaccine annually (no live vaccine)
  - Hepatitis A and B vaccines
  - Tdap vaccination every 10 years. Substitute one-time dose of Tdap vaccine at time of next booster.

MEDICATION
- Recommended regimens for ART-naive (3)[A]
  - Integrase strand transfer inhibitor-based regimens:
    ○ Dolutegravir/abacavir/lamivudine (50 mg/600 mg/300 mg PO daily)—only for patients who are HLA-B*5701 negative
    ○ Bictegravir/tenofovir/emtricitabine (50 mg/25 mg/200 mg PO daily)
    ○ Dolutegravir (50 mg PO daily) plus tenofovir disoproxil fumarate/emtricitabine (300 mg/200 mg PO daily)
    ○ Elvitegravir/cobicistat/tenofovir/emtricitabine (150 mg/150 mg/300 mg/200 mg PO daily)—only for patients with pre-ART CrCl >70 mL/min
    ○ Raltegravir (400 mg PO BID) plus tenofovir/emtricitabine (300 mg/200 mg PO daily)
  - Protease inhibitor-based regimen:
    ○ Darunavir and ritonavir (800 mg PO daily and 100 mg PO daily) plus tenofovir/emtricitabine (300 mg/200 mg PO daily)
- Drug failure: Before selecting regimen, review clinical symptoms, history of ART, and adherence. Perform resistance testing.
- ART, especially the protease inhibitors, have interactions with other medications, such as antacids, steroids, contraceptives.

ONGOING CARE

FOLLOW-UP RECOMMENDATIONS
Patient Monitoring
- HIV RNA (viral load) 2 to 8 weeks after starting therapy and repeated every 3 to 6 months until suppressed (3)
- Monitor HIV RNA, CD4, and CBC every 3 to 4 months for first 2 years of ART or if the CD4 count is <300 cells/mm^3 (3).
- Space CD4 monitoring to 12 months if suppressed viral load and CD4 >300 cells/mm^3
- Monitor HIV RNA and CBC every 6 months (3).
- Annual HIV RNA and CD4 count once viral load undetectable and stable
- Once viral load has been suppressed consistently for >2 years and CD4 cell counts are consistently >500/μL, monitoring CD4 cell counts is optional unless virologic failure occurs (or there are intercurrent immunosuppressive treatments or conditions).
- Confirm HIV-1 RNA level is >50 copies/mL within 4 weeks of medication management decisions.
- Annual fasting lipids and fasting glucose; basic metabolic panel, AST/ALT, total/direct bilirubin every 6 to 12 months (3)
- Annual cervical cytology annually (regardless of age) until three negative screens and then every 3 years
- Pregnancy test in women of childbearing age (3)
- Urinalysis every 6 to 12 months or as clinically indicated (3)
- Hepatitis C as clinically indicated (3)

DIET
- Encourage good nutrition; avoid raw eggs and unpasteurized dairy products.
- Discuss unknown and potentially harmful effects of supplement use including drug–drug interactions.

PATIENT EDUCATION
Provide nonjudgmental, sex-positive prevention counseling, reviewing high-risk behaviors and viral transmission. American Foundation for AIDS Research: 212-719-0033 (new treatments and research) https://aidsinfo.nih.gov/

PROGNOSIS
- Untreated HIV infection leading to the diagnosis of AIDS has an associated life expectancy of about 3 years, and if the patient has an opportunistic infection, the life expectancy is about 1 year.
- AIDS-defining opportunistic infections usually do not develop until CD4 <200.
- Adherence failure—not drug resistance—is the most common cause of treatment failure.

COMPLICATIONS
- Immunodeficiency
- Opportunistic infections
- Neurologic complications:
  - AIDS dementia complex (ADC), cryptococcal meningitis, CMV encephalitis, progressive multifocal leukoencephalopathy (PML), neurosyphilis, herpes encephalitis, toxoplasma encephalitis, vacuolar myelopathy, and psychological and neuropsychiatric disorders (5)
- Respiratory complications such as acute bronchitis, bacterial pneumonia, *P. carinii* pneumonia with CD4 <200 cells/mm^3 and *M. avium*
- Malignancy, including cervical or anal cancer

REFERENCES
1. Centers for Disease Control and Prevention. HIV/AIDS basic statistics. https://www.cdc.gov/hiv/basics/statistics.html. Updated June 26, 2018. Accessed September 8, 2018.
2. U.S. Department of Health and Human Services. Recommendations for the use of antiretroviral drugs in pregnant women with HIV infection and interventions to reduce perinatal HIV transmission in the United States. https://aidsinfo.nih.gov/contentfiles/lvguidelines/perinatalgl.pdf. Updated May 2018. Accessed September 8, 2018.
3. U.S. Department of Health and Human Services. Guidelines for the use of antiretroviral agents in adults and adolescents living with HIV. http://aidsinfo.nih.gov/contentfiles/lvguidelines/adultandadolescentgl.pdf. Updated May 2018. Accessed September 8, 2018.
4. Centers for Disease Control and Prevention. Updated guidelines for antiretroviral postexposure prophylaxis after sexual, injection drug use, or other nonoccupational exposure to HIV—United States, 2016. http://www.cdc.gov/hiv/guidelines/index.html. Accessed September 8, 2018.
5. National Institute of Neurological Disorders and Stroke. Neurological complications of AIDS Fact Sheet. https://www.ninds.nih.gov/Disorders/Patient-Caregiver-Education/Fact-Sheets/Neurological-Complications-AIDS-Fact-Sheet. Accessed September 8, 2018.

ADDITIONAL READING
- Centers for Disease Control and Prevention. Statistics overview: HIV surveillance report. http://www.cdc.gov/hiv/statistics/overview/index.html. Accessed September 8, 2018.
- Lucas S, Nelson AM. HIV and the spectrum of human disease. *J Pathol*. 2015;235(2):229–241.

 CODES

ICD10
- Z21 Asymptomatic human immunodeficiency virus infection status
- B20 Human immunodeficiency virus [HIV] disease
- R75 Inconclusive laboratory evidence of human immunodef virus

CLINICAL PEARLS
- Acute HIV seroconversion illness mimics mononucleosis and is characterized by fever, sore throat, adenopathy, myalgias, and rash.
- Transmitted drug resistance is increasing. Evaluate for resistance prior to initiating ART.
- Provide necessary vaccinations and prophylactic antibiotics to HIV+ patients based on clinical history and CD4 count.
- Discuss prevention strategies, including PrEP, with individuals who are at high risk of HIV infection.
- Consider HIV testing in at-risk patients reporting unintended weight loss, fatigue, night sweats, or rash.

H

HODGKIN LYMPHOMA

Rory M. Shallis, MD • John L. Reagan, MD

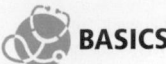

BASICS

DESCRIPTION
Historical background:
- Described in 1832 by Thomas Hodgkin in "On some morbid appearance of the absorbent glands and spleen"
- First neoplasm to be (i) defined by cytologic grounds based on presence of Reed-Sternberg (RS) cells, (ii) clinically staged neoplastic disease, and (iii) treated with chemotherapy and/or radiotherapy
- Neoplastic RS cells of monoclonal lymphoid B-cell origin within inflammatory background of lymphocytes (T-helper type 2 and regulatory T cells), eosinophils, histiocytes, and plasma cells
- Two subtypes: classic Hodgkin lymphoma (CHL, 95% of cases) and nodular lymphocyte predominant Hodgkin lymphoma (NLPHL, 3–8% of cases)
  - NLPHL: B cells, neoplastic luteinizing hormone (LH) cells with multilobulated nuclei, small nucleoli, and popcorn-like appearance
  - CHL histologic subdivisions: nodular sclerosing (60%), mixed cellularity (30%), lymphocyte depleted (<10%), lymphocyte rich (<10%)
  - Frequency of lymph node involvement: cervical > mediastinal > axillary > paraaortic

EPIDEMIOLOGY
- Incidence: 2.6/100,000/year
- Predominance: 8% of lymphoid malignancies
- Typically diagnosed at age 20 to 34 years with median age 39 years at diagnosis given decreasing bimodal age distribution
- 1.3:1 male-to-female ratio

Geriatric Considerations
Poorer prognosis if present at ≥60 years:
- Less likely to tolerate intensive chemotherapy
- Less likely to be included in clinical trial

Pediatric Considerations
Young females (<30 years of age) treated with thoracic radiation are at high risk for breast cancer, and early breast cancer screening is recommended.

Pregnancy Considerations
- Abdominal ultrasonography to detect subdiaphragmatic disease
- Treatment:
  - Delay until after delivery if asymptomatic and early stage.
  - ABVD safely used in 2nd and 3rd trimesters
  - Vinblastine monotherapy to control symptoms
  - 1st trimester: ABVD may or may not cause fetal malformations.

Incidence
Approximately 8,500 new cases in the United States annually

Prevalence
Approximately 220,000 living with Hodgkin lymphoma in the United States as of 2015

ETIOLOGY AND PATHOPHYSIOLOGY
- RS cells likely derived from germinal center B cells with mutations in immunoglobulin variable chain
- Seasonal features and higher frequencies with Epstein-Barr virus (EBV) suggest environmental factors.
- T-lymphocyte defects persist even after successful treatment.

- Human leukocyte antigen (HLA) is strongly associated with increased risk.
- EBV positivity associated with increased risk
- Genome-wide association studies identified 19p13.3 at intron 2 of *TCF3*.

Genetics
- First-degree relative: 3 to 9 times risk
- Siblings of younger patients: 7 times risk
- Weak correlation between familial HL and HLA class I regions containing HLA-A1, HLA-B5, HLA-B8, HLA-B18 alleles

RISK FACTORS
- Immunodeficiency (inherited or acquired)
- Autoimmune disorders
- EBV
- Seasonal factors

COMMONLY ASSOCIATED CONDITIONS
In HIV:
- AIDS-defining illness
- Predominantly mixed-cellularity or lymphocyte-depleted histologic subtypes
- At diagnosis: widespread disease, extranodal involvement, systemic symptoms

DIAGNOSIS

HISTORY
- Asymptomatic lymphadenopathy (cervical/supraclavicular)
- Pel-Ebstein (cyclic) fever
- Constitutional symptoms: night sweats, weight loss, fatigue, anorexia
- Alcohol-induced pain
- Pruritus

PHYSICAL EXAM
- Lymphadenopathy 70% (cervical > supraclavicular > axillary)
- Splenomegaly
- Hepatomegaly

DIFFERENTIAL DIAGNOSIS
Non-Hodgkin lymphoma, infectious lymphadenopathy, solid tumor metastases, sarcoidosis, autoimmune disease, AIDS/HIV, drug reaction

DIAGNOSTIC TESTS & INTERPRETATION
Initial Tests (lab, imaging)
- CBC with differential
- Comprehensive metabolic panel
- LFT, LDH
- ESR
- HIV, EBV, HCV
- Pregnancy test for women of childbearing age
- Echocardiogram (in anticipation of treatment with anthracycline)
- Pulmonary function tests (diffusion capacity of the lung for CO in anticipation of treatment with bleomycin)
- Chest x-ray
- Computed tomography (CT) with contrast of chest, abdomen, and pelvis
- Positron emission tomography (PET): for initial staging, midtreatment decision making, and end-of-treatment evaluation

Follow-Up Tests & Special Considerations
- Fertility considerations:
  - Semen cryopreservation if chemotherapy or pelvic radiation therapy (RT)
  - In vitro fertilization or ovarian tissue/oocyte cryopreservation
- RT considerations:
  - Splenic RT: pneumococcal, *Haemophilus influenzae*, meningococcal vaccine

Diagnostic Procedures/Other
- Excisional lymph node biopsy
- Immunohistochemistry
- Bone marrow biopsy if cytopenia with negative PET

Test Interpretation
RS cell characteristics include the following:
- Diameter: 20 to 50 μm
- Abundant acidophilic cytoplasm
- Bi- or polylobulated nucleus
- Acidophilic nucleoli
- CD30+, CD15+, CD45−, CD3−, CD20+ in 40% of cases
- RS cells necessary but not sufficient for diagnosis (needs inflammatory background)

TREATMENT

- Ann Arbor staging with Cotswold modification
  - Stage I: single lymph node or of a single extralymphatic organ or site
  - Stage II: ≥2 lymph node regions on the same side of diaphragm alone or with involvement of extralymphatic organ or tissue
  - Stage III: node groups on both sides of the diaphragm
  - Stage IV: dissemination involving extranodal organs (except the spleen, which is considered lymphoid tissue)
  - Subclasses: A = no systemic symptoms; B = systemic symptoms (fever, night sweats, weight loss >10% body weight); X = bulky disease (>1/3 intrathoracic, diameter, or >10-cm nodal mass)
  - Classified into three groups: early stage (I or II) favorable, early stage unfavorable (I or II with presence of either B symptoms, large mediastinal adenopathy, three or more nodal sites of disease, extranodal involvement, or an ESR ≥50), or advanced stage (III or IV)
- Goal: Aim for cure.
- All subsequent treatment and follow-up care recommendations based on National Comprehensive Cancer Network (NCCN) consensus. Please refer to NCCN Practice Guidelines in Oncology for Hodgkin lymphoma.

MEDICATION
Hodgkin lymphoma

First Line
- Early stage disease: combined modality treatment *or* chemotherapy
- Advanced stage disease: chemotherapy
- PET/CT used after cycle 2 (PET-2) to guide either escalation or de-escalation of therapy (1)
- ABVD (doxorubicin, bleomycin, vinblastine, dacarbazine):
  - Highly emetic, severe phlebitis
  - Doxorubicin: risk of cardiotoxicity; monitor LVEF.

- Bleomycin: risk of pulmonary toxicity, death; test dose may be administered prior to first cycle.
- Dacarbazine cannot be omitted without loss of efficacy.
- Stage I/II favorable: ABVD × 2 then 20 Gy involved site radiation therapy (ISRT); can also use Stanford V × 8 weeks +/− 30 Gy ISRT pending PET/CT response
- Stage I/II unfavorable: ABVD × 2 then PET-2. If PET-2 negative, then ABVD × 2 + ISRT or AVD [dropped bleomycin (2)] × 4. If PET-2 positive, then ABVD × 2 + ISRT or escalated BEACOPP + ISRT; can also use Stanford V × 12 weeks + 30 to 36 Gy
- Stage III/IV: ABVD × 2 is preferred then AVD [dropped bleomycin (2)] × 4 if PET-2 negative. If PET-2 positive, then ABVD × 2 + ISRT or escalated BEACOPP × 4 +/− ISRT; can also use Stanford V × 12 + ISRT unless refractory or BEACOPP × 6 +/− ISRT pending PET/CT response; also can consider brentuximab vedotin (anti-CD30 chimeric antibody conjugated to synthetic antimicrotubule agent monomethyl auristatin E) FDA-approved for use in combination with AVD based on results of ECHELON-1 phase 3 trial which showed reduced "modified" PFS compared to ABVD (HR 0.77; 95% CI, 0.60–0.98; $p = .04$), although "modified" PFS criteria controversial and no difference between groups >65 years

Second Line
- Reserved for patients with relapsed/refractory (R/R) disease
- Standard is for chemotherapy agents not used for initial treatment and then high-dose therapy with autologous stem cell transplant (HDT/ASCT) +/− ISRT.
  - HDT/ASCT shows improved EFS/PFS compared with conventional chemotherapy but not overall survival; can achieve disease-free survival in 30–40% of patients after auto SCT
  - Allogeneic SCT to be considered if failed autologous SCT (used in trials only)
- Brentuximab vedotin FDA-approved for use as maintenance therapy × 1 year in relapsed HL after HDT/ASCT or failed two prior lines of multiagent chemotherapy. Strongly encouraged if Deauville of 4 on restaging PET after HDT/ASCT or in patients at high risk for relapse. Improves PFS in those at risk for relapse or progression after transplantation (3). Initial phase II study data showed 73% response rate and 34% CR. 3-year follow-up confirmed responses with OS and PFS rates of 75% and 58%, respectively (4).
  - Side effects include peripheral neuropathy, nausea, fatigue, neutropenia, diarrhea.
  - May also be used prior to HDT/ASCT to avoid toxicity with HDT
- Pembrolizumab (anti-PD1) FDA-approved for patients with R/R CHL who have failed three lines of therapy. Phase 2 study (KEYNOTE-087) showed ORR and CR rate of 68% and 29%, respectively.
- Nivolumab (another anti-PD1) in a phase 2 study of R/R CHL showed ORR 69% with durable response and favorable safety profile (5).
- Third-line novel agents undergoing studies: NF-κB inhibitors (bortezomib), mammalian target of rapamycin (mTOR) inhibitors (everolimus), immunomodulators (lenalidomide), cell signaling targets histone deacetylase (HDAC) inhibitors (vorinostat, panobinostat, mocetinostat)

- Median survival <3 years if fail second-line therapy, including HDT/ASCT
- NLPHL
  - Treated with rituximab + CHOP (CD20 positive)

 ## ONGOING CARE

FOLLOW-UP RECOMMENDATIONS
Patient Monitoring
- During therapy: CBC, nutrition, and hydration
- Restage with PET after 2 to 4 cycles of chemotherapy: sensitive prognostic indicator
- Posttreatment monitoring:
  - History and physical: q3–6mo for first 2 years, then q6–12mo for next 3 to 5 years, and then annually
  - Laboratory studies
    - CBC, platelets, BMP, ESR (if elevated at time of diagnosis), as indicated clinically
    - Thyroid-stimulating hormone (TSH) annually if radiation to neck
  - Imaging:
    - CT is appropriate 6, 12, and 24 months posttreatment as well as when clinically indicated.
    - Annual breast mammogram beginning 8 to 10 years after therapy or at age 40 years (whichever first) if chest or axillary irradiation (annual breast MRI as well if initially radiated between ages 10 and 30 years) according to the American Cancer Society
    - Surveillance PET should not be done routinely due to risk of false-positive findings.
- Annual influenza vaccine

PATIENT EDUCATION
- Reproductive impact
- Risks of secondary malignancy
- Oral and dental care during therapy
- Leukemia & Lymphoma Society (http://www.lls.org/)

PROGNOSIS
- Cure rate for CHL: 80%
- Relapse or progression of disease rate: 5–20%
- Overall survival rates:
  - 1-year survival: 92%
  - 5-year survival: 87% (93% if localized)
  - 10-year survival: 80%
- International prognostic score for advanced disease:
  - Age >45 years
  - Male gender
  - Albumin <4 g/dL
  - Hemoglobin <10.5 g/dL
  - Lymphocytopenia: <600 lymphocyte cells/dL or lymphocytes <8% of WBC
  - WBC ≥15,000 cells/dL
  - Stage IV disease
- Main cause of death
  - Initial 5 years: Hodgkin lymphoma
  - After 5 to 10 years: leukemia, myelodysplastic syndrome
  - After 20 years: second primary malignancy, cardiovascular disease

REFERENCES

1. Barrington SF, Kirkwood AA, Franceschetto A, et al. PET-CT for staging and early response: results from the Response-Adapted Therapy in Advanced Hodgkin Lymphoma study. *Blood*. 2016;127(12):1531–1538.
2. Johnson P, Federico M, Kirkwood A, et al. Adapted treatment guided by interim PET-CT scan in advanced Hodgkin's lymphoma. *N Engl J Med*. 2016;374(25):2419–2429.
3. Moskowitz CH, Nademanee A, Masszi T, et al. Brentuximab vedotin as consolidation therapy after autologous stem-cell transplantation in patients with Hodgkin's lymphoma at risk of relapse or progression (AETHERA): a randomised, double-blind, placebo-controlled, phase 3 trial. *Lancet*. 2015;385(9980):1853–1862.
4. Gopal AK, Chen R, Smith SE, et al. Durable remissions in a pivotal phase 2 study of brentuximab vedotin in relapsed or refractory Hodgkin lymphoma. *Blood*. 2015;125(8):1236–1243.
5. Armand P, Engert A, Younes A, et al. Nivolumab for relapsed/refractory classic Hodgkin lymphoma after failure of autologous hematopoietic cell transplantation: extended follow-up of the multicohort single-arm phase II CheckMate 205 trial. *J Clin Oncol*. 2018;36(14):1428–1439.

ADDITIONAL READING

- American Cancer Society. *American Cancer Society Recommendations for Early Breast Cancer Detection in Women without Breast Symptoms*. Atlanta, GA: American Cancer Society; 2013.
- Centers for Disease Control and Prevention. *Vaccines that Might Be Indicated for Adults Aged 19 Years or Older Based on Medical and Other Indications*. Atlanta, GA: Centers for Disease Control and Prevention; 2016. https://www.cdc.gov/vaccines/schedules/downloads/adult/adult-combined-schedule.pdf. Accessed October 9, 2017.
- National Cancer Institute, Surveillance, Epidemiology, and End Results Program. Cancer Stat Facts: Hodgkin lymphoma. http://seer.cancer.gov/statfacts/html/hodg.html. Accessed July 7, 2017.
- National Comprehensive Cancer Network. NCCN clinical practice guidelines in oncology. Hodgkin lymphoma. http://www.nccn.org/. Accessed July 8, 2017.

 ## CODES

ICD10
- C81.90 Hodgkin lymphoma, unspecified, unspecified site
- C81.91 Hodgkin lymphoma, unsp, lymph nodes of head, face, and neck
- C81.92 Hodgkin lymphoma, unspecified, intrathoracic lymph nodes

CLINICAL PEARLS

- Neoplastic disease of lymphatics
- RS cells of monoclonal lymphoid B-cell origin within inflammatory background of lymphocytes
- Two subtypes: CHL 95% of cases and NLPHL 5% of cases
- CHL cure rate: 80%; 5-year survival: 87%; relapse or progression of disease rate: 5–20%
- Incorporation of anti-CD30 therapy into frontline therapy and immunotherapy with PD1 blockade currently underway and promising

H

HOMELESSNESS

Dana Sprute, MD, MPH, FAAFP • Feba Thomas, MD, MS

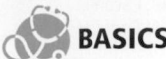 **BASICS**

DESCRIPTION

Defined as the condition in which (i) an individual lacks a fixed, regular, and adequate nighttime residence; or (ii) an individual who has a primary nighttime residence that is (a) a supervised publicly or privately operated shelter designed to provide temporary living accommodations (including welfare hotels, congregate shelters, and transitional housing for the mentally ill); (b) an institution that provides a temporary residence for individuals intended to be institutionalized; and (c) a public or private place not designed for, or ordinarily used as, a regular sleeping accommodation for human beings

EPIDEMIOLOGY

Prevalence

As of January 2017, there are 553,742 homeless individuals in the United States on any given night: 33% are homeless families, 7.2% were veterans, 7.4% were unaccompanied children and young adults (1).

- From 2016 to 2017, homelessness increased for the first time in 7 years, reflective of a 9% increase in number of people experiencing homelessness in unsheltered locations and specific changes happening within cities. Risk for becoming homeless remains high in certain populations (see "Risk Factors") (1).
- Although many people experiencing homelessness reside in temporary housing or shelters, 35% live unsheltered (1).
- There was a 12% increase in individuals with chronic patterns of homelessness in 2017 when compared to 2016, both in sheltered and unsheltered populations. However, the number of individuals experiencing chronic homelessness has declined by 18% between 2010 and 2017 (1,2).

RISK FACTORS

- Economic factors
  - Poverty
    - 2018 federal poverty definition: $25,100 annual income for four-person household in the lower 48 states and District of Columbia, slightly higher in Alaska and Hawaii (3)
    - In 2016, 12.7% of the U.S. population fell below federal poverty definition (U.S. Census Bureau).
  - Unemployment: U.S. rate 4.4% in June 2017 (U.S. Bureau of Labor Statistics)
  - Lack of affordable health care: In 2016, 8.8% of people in the United States were uninsured for the entire calendar year, a 0.3% decrease since 2015 (4).
    - Young adults (ages 19 to 34 years) are disproportionately uninsured (12.1%) compared with the average for all ages (9.1%); the uninsured rate for ages 19 to 25 years decreased by 12% between 2009 and 2016, following Affordable Care Act provision allowing individuals in this age group to stay on parental insurance plans (4).
    - The number of uninsured nonelderly Americans has dropped 43% since October 2013 (4).
  - Lack of affordable housing: Housing is considered affordable if ≤30% of household income is devoted to housing costs.
    - An estimated 12 million households are "severely housing cost burdened" (≥50% of income is spent on housing).

- Additional at-risk populations: intimate partner violence (IPV), victims of violence; youth (particularly those aging out of foster care); veterans; rural; addiction; psychiatric illness; disabled due to chronic medical disease, psychiatric illness, or substance use disorder; reentry after incarceration/prison
  - IPV: 12% of overall homeless population, and as many as 1 in 5 families, will have reported experiencing IPV; IPV leads directly to homelessness in many cases (2).
  - Youth: In 2017, Department of Housing and Urban Development (HUD) estimates 40,799 unaccompanied individual homeless youths (up to age 24 years) and another 9,800 persons in families where the parent is a youth (1). Approximately 550,000 youths in a year will experience homelessness lasting longer than a week (2).
  - Veterans: 7.4% of homeless adults; homelessness rate decreased by about half between 2010 and 2017 (1).
  - Transgender individuals: In 2017, fewer than 1% of all persons experiencing homelessness were either transgender or did not identify as male, female, or transgender, but there was an increase in this group from 2016.
  - Addiction disorders: 46% of homeless individuals report alcohol and/or drug use as a major factor contributing to homelessness (2).
  - Psychiatric illness: 45% of homeless report indicators of a mental health issue in the past year; 25% of homeless adults suffer from chronic mental illness (2).
  - Reentry after incarceration: Up to 50,000 people each year enter homeless shelters from jails or prisons (2).
- Fundamental issues in homelessness and health care that require ongoing consideration:
  - Unstable housing, limited access to nutritious food and water, lack of transportation
  - Higher risk for abuse and violence
  - Physical/cognitive impairments, behavioral health problems
  - Developmental discrepancies for children: speech delay, chronic ear infection, insufficient opportunity to practice gross and fine motor skills
  - Higher risk for communicable disease
  - Lack of health insurance/resources, discontinuous/inaccessible health care, lack of a medical home, barriers to disability assistance
  - Cultural/linguistic barriers: racial and ethnic groups overrepresented in homeless population
  - Limited education/literacy
  - Lack of social supports: Alienation from family and friends precipitate homelessness.
  - Criminalization of homelessness: frequent arrests for loitering, sleeping in public places

GENERAL PREVENTION

- Policy and funding for community programs to provide emergency/rapid housing, housing stabilization, and case management services
- Increased Medicaid eligibility for homeless and expanded home and community-based services and case management to the homeless population (5)
- HUD: increasing permanent supportive housing units, increasing services for veterans and those with disabilities (5)

- Social justice policy recommendations: permanent affordable housing, foreclosure and homelessness prevention, increased funds for HUD McKinney-Vento programs (emergency, transitional, and permanent housing) and National Housing Trust Fund, rural homeless assistance, universal health care, universal livable income, employment/workforce services, prevention of hate crimes against the homeless, decriminalization of homelessness

COMMONLY ASSOCIATED CONDITIONS

- Hunger
- Worsening of chronic medical conditions: lack of healthy food, places to store medications, or medical equipment; lack of restful sleep; decreased health literacy; limited transportation to appointments
  - Infectious diseases
    - Tuberculosis (TB), HIV/AIDS, STI
    - Skin/nail infections and infestation (lice, bedbugs, and scabies)
    - Liver disease (e.g., hepatitis B or C, or alcohol related)
  - Cognitive impairment: traumatic brain injury (TBI), cerebrovascular accident (CVA), substance use
  - Dental problems
  - Exposure-related conditions (frostbite, heatstroke)
  - Psychiatric illness
  - Trauma: increased risk of assault, victims of hate crimes

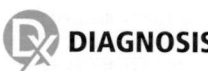 **DIAGNOSIS**

HISTORY

- Living conditions: location, access to food, restrooms, place to store medicines, safety
- Prior homelessness: causes and circumstances
- Individual/family history of reactive airway disease (RAD), chronic otitis media, anemia, diabetes, cardiovascular disease (CVD), TB, HIV/STIs, hospitalizations
- Family members, especially dependent children
- Medications: include OTC medication, dietary supplements, medication "borrowed" from others
- Prior providers: oral health, primary and specialty care, current medical home
- Mental health: stress, anxiety, appetite, sleep, concentration, mood, speech, memory, thought process and content, auditory/visual hallucinations, suicidal/homicidal ideation, insight, judgment, impulse control, social interactions; symptoms of brain injury (headaches, seizures, memory loss, irritability, dizziness, insomnia, poor organizational/decision-making skills), trauma history
- Alcohol/nicotine/drug use: amount, frequency, duration
- Gender identity/orientation, behaviors, rape, pregnancies, hepatitis, HIV, other STIs
- History of or current abuse: emotional, physical, sexual; patient safety
- Legal problems/violence: history of incarceration
- Activities: routines (treatment feasibility); level of strenuous activity
- Work: previous types of jobs, length held, veteran status, occupational injuries/toxic exposures; vocational skills, interest
- Education: highest level; ever in special education; assess ability to read/language skills/English fluency.
- Nutrition/hydration: diet, food resources, preparation skills, liquid intake

- Cultural heritage/affiliations: family, friends, faith community, other sources of support
- Strengths: coping skills, job skills, resourcefulness, abilities, interests

PHYSICAL EXAM

- Comprehensive exam: height/weight, BMI, especially abdominal, cardiopulmonary, dermatologic, oral, feet, neurologic, mental status
- Focused exams: for patients uncomfortable with full-body, unclothed exam at first visit
- Dental assessment: age-appropriate teeth, obvious caries, dental/referred pain, diabetes, CVD

DIAGNOSTIC TESTS & INTERPRETATION
Initial Tests (lab, imaging)

- Mental health: Patient Health Questionnaire (PHQ-9, PHQ-2), MHS-III, MDQ, GAD-7
- Cognitive assessment: Mini-Mental State Examination (MMSE), Traumatic Brain Injury Questionnaire (TBIQ), Repeatable Battery for the Assessment of Neuropsychological Status (RBANS)
- Developmental assessment: Ages & Stages Questionnaires, Parents' Evaluation of Developmental Status (PEDS), Denver II, or other screening tool
- Interpersonal violence: IPV, sexual assault, TBI
- Forensic evaluation: if indicated by history
- Baseline labs: as needed to address suspected medical concerns
- TB screening: PPD or T-SPOT/QuantiFERON-TB Gold if available
- STI screening: HIV, chlamydia, gonorrhea, syphilis, hepatitis B, hepatitis C, trichomonas
- Substance abuse: Simple Screening Instrument for Alcohol and Other Drugs (SSI-AOD), urine drug screen

Follow-Up Tests & Special Considerations

- Reproductive health care and STIs: Obtain detailed sexual history (sexual identity, orientation, behaviors/sexual practices, number of partners). Consider patient exploitation, especially if mental illness/developmental disability suspected. Communicate willingness to initiate contraception first visit without exam. Genital exam recommended, but be sensitive to patient needs, if possible sexual abuse history. If pelvic exam is refused, consider empiric treatment for STI (and possibility of multiple orifice infection). Dispense medications on site; facilitate partner treatment.
- Pediatric care: complete exam every visit; use each visit to identify/address problems and provide vaccinations because homeless families may not see a medical provider unless child is sick. Vision and hearing screening at every visit. Facilitate referrals as able.

 TREATMENT

- Establish rapport: Many patients will have had negative health care experiences.
- Enlist community resources: mental health and substance abuse programs, free clinics, case management.
- Health care maintenance: vaccinations (hepatitis A and B, Pneumovax, Tdap, influenza), cancer and chronic disease screening for adults; Early and Periodic Screening, Diagnosis, and Treatment (EPSDT) program screening and vaccinations for children
- Care plan
  – Basic needs: Food, clothing, and housing may be higher priorities than health care.
  – Patient goals and priorities: immediate/long-term health needs. Address patient concerns first.

– Action plan: simple language, pocket card
– After hours: extended clinic hours and access
– Safety plan: violence and abuse; mandatory reporting requirements
– Emergency plan: location of nearest emergency department (ED), preparation for evacuation
– Adherence plan: use of interpreter; identification of potential barriers

MEDICATION

- Simple regimen: low pill count, once-daily dosing
- Dispensing: small amounts on site to promote follow-up, decrease loss/theft/misuse. Determine resources for written prescriptions.
- Storage of medications: If no access, avoid medications requiring refrigeration.
- Patient assistance: free/low-cost drugs depending on available local options
- Aids to adherence: harm reduction, outreach/case management, directly observed therapy
- Side effects: Primary reason for medication nonadherence are drugs causing diarrhea, polyuria, nausea, and/or disorientation.
- Analgesia/symptomatic treatment: Consider pain contract, single provider for pain medication refills.
- Dietary supplements: multivitamins with minerals, nutritional supplements
- Managed care: generics, if possible; assistance getting prescription filled
- Lab monitoring: Monitor patients on antipsychotic medications for metabolic disorders using available laboratory resources.

ADDITIONAL THERAPIES

- Associated problems/complications
  – Fragmented care: multiple providers. Use electronic medical record (EMR) as possible; list prescribed medication on wallet-sized card.
  – Masked symptoms/misdiagnosis: for example, weight loss, dementia, edema, lactic acidosis
  – Focus on immediate concerns, not possible future consequences.
  – Integrated treatment for concurrent mental illness/substance use disorders
  – Support for parent of child abused by others and for abused parent
  – Large appointment burdens: For those individuals who suffer from multiple chronic illnesses, specialty care may be difficult to obtain due to the many barriers to care listed above.
- Follow-up
  – Reliable phone/e-mail contact for patient/friend/family/case manager
  – Frequent follow-up, incentives, nonjudgmental care regardless of adherence
  – Anticipate/accommodate unscheduled clinic visits.
  – Provide car fare, tokens, and help with transportation services.
  – Monitor school attendance and address health/developmental problems with family/school.

ADMISSION, INPATIENT, AND NURSING CONSIDERATIONS

- Homeless likely to benefit from admission if living conditions are suboptimal to treat medical, psychiatric, and substance use disorders.
- Discharge criteria
  – Bed rest, extended periods of elevation, rest, or icing are not feasible in most instances.
  – Plans requiring multiple return visits likely to fail if no transportation.
  – Admission to inpatient rehabilitation if appropriate and possible

 ONGOING CARE

FOLLOW-UP RECOMMENDATIONS

- Patients with a history of nonadherence need additional support (e.g., case manager, outreach) to succeed in ongoing care after hospital discharge.
- Limited telephone access to schedule appointments; may be unable to receive telephone messages with test results or rescheduled appointment times. Some social service agencies will provide phone, mail, e-mail, Internet, and laundry services.
- Arrange appointments prior to discharge.
- Document the best way to contact the individual.
- Work with experienced health care agency designed to address physical/mental health services and substance use treatment.

PATIENT EDUCATION

- https://www.nhchc.org/
- http://www.endhomelessness.org/pages/mentalphysical_health

PROGNOSIS

Mortality rates for homeless adults are 3 to 4 times higher compared with general U.S. population (6)[C].

REFERENCES

1. U.S. Department of Housing and Urban Development, Office of Community Planning and Development. The 2017 annual homeless assessment report (AHAR) to congress. https://www.hudexchange.info/resources/documents/2017-AHAR-Part-1.pdf. Accessed July 17, 2018.
2. National Alliance to End Homelessness: https://www.endhomelessness.org.
3. U.S. Department of Health and Human Services. Annual update of the HHS poverty guidelines. http://www.gpo.gov/fdsys/pkg/FR-2017-01-31/pdf/2017-02076.pdf. Accessed July 17, 2018.
4. Barnett JC, Berchick ER. Health Insurance Coverage in the United States: 2016. https://www.census.gov/content/dam/Census/library/publications/2017/demo/p60-260.pdf. Accessed July 17, 2018.
5. United States Interagency Council on Homelessness. Opening doors: federal strategic plan to prevent and end homelessness, update 2015. http://usich.gov/opening_doors/. Accessed July 17, 2018.
6. Maness DL, Khan M. Care of the homeless: an overview. *Am Fam Physician.* 2014;89(8):634–640.

CODES

ICD10
- Z59.0 Homelessness
- Z59.1 Inadequate housing
- Z59.8 Other problems related to housing and economic circumstances

CLINICAL PEARLS

- Permanent supportive housing is an important step toward ending homelessness, in accordance with a Housing First approach.
- Assistance in gaining access to benefits or providing help to support basic needs decreases stress, improves therapeutic relationship, and allows individuals to focus on physical and mental health.

H

HORDEOLUM (STYE)

Konstantinos E. Deligiannidis, MD, MPH, FAAFP

BASICS

DESCRIPTION
- An acute inflammation or infection of the eyelid margin involving the sebaceous gland of an eyelash (external hordeolum) or a meibomian gland (internal hordeolum)
- System(s) affected: skin/exocrine
- Synonym(s): internal hordeolum; external hordeolum; zeisian sty; meibomian stye; stye

EPIDEMIOLOGY
- Predominant age: none
- Predominant sex: male = female

Incidence
Unknown: Although external hordeolum is common, internal hordeolum is rare.

ETIOLOGY AND PATHOPHYSIOLOGY
- Bacterial infection of sweat or sebaceous glands, causing an acute inflammatory reaction
- In an internal hordeolum, the meibomian gland may become obstructed, leading to a pustule on the conjunctival surface as opposed to the margin of the eyelid.
- Most commonly caused by *Staphylococcus aureus* (~90–95% of all cases) or by *Staphylococcus epidermidis*
- Seborrhea can predispose to infections of the eyelid.

Genetics
No known genetic pattern

RISK FACTORS
- Poor eyelid hygiene
- Previous hordeolum
- Contact lens wearers
- Application of makeup
- Seborrheic dermatitis
- Predisposing blepharitis (low-grade infections of the eyelid margin)
- Ocular rosacea

GENERAL PREVENTION
Eyelid hygiene

COMMONLY ASSOCIATED CONDITIONS
- Acne
- Seborrhea
- An association may exist between hordeolum during childhood and developing rosacea in adulthood.

DIAGNOSIS

HISTORY
- Localized inflammation (vs. involvement of the entire eyelid or surrounding skin)
- Foreign body sensation in the eye
- Prior episodes are common.

PHYSICAL EXAM
- Localized inflammation of the eyelashes or a small pustule at the margin of the eyelid
- Localized swelling and tenderness on the internal or external aspect of the eyelid with an opening to either side
- To determine if an internal hordeolum is obstructed, the eyelid should be gently everted to examine for a pustule on the tarsal conjunctiva.
- Itching or scaling of the eyelids; collection of discharge, redness, and irritation leading to localized tenderness and pain
- The size of the swelling usually correlates to the severity of the hordeolum.

DIFFERENTIAL DIAGNOSIS
- Chalazion
- Blepharitis
- Eyelid neoplasms
- Periorbital cellulitis
- Dacryocystitis
- Squamous cell carcinoma

DIAGNOSTIC TESTS & INTERPRETATION
Culture of the eyelid margins usually is not necessary.

Diagnostic Procedures/Other
History and eye exam

Test Interpretation
Bacterial contamination and white cells in eyelid discharge

TREATMENT

GENERAL MEASURES
- The hordeolum should not be expressed.
- Warm compresses to the area of inflammation can help increase blood supply and encourage spontaneous drainage.
- Good personal hygiene with attention to cleansing the eyelids on a daily basis helps to prevent recurrent infections.

MEDICATION
First Line
- A Cochrane review found no evidence for or against nonsurgical treatment of internal hordeolum. External hordeola were not considered (1)[A].
- Usually, a hordeolum spontaneously drains, aided by warm compresses to the area.
- Also, lid scrubs, digital massage, and alternative medicine have been used to reduce healing time and relieving symptoms.
- Application of an antibiotic ointment (e.g., erythromycin) to the margin of the eyelid after proper cleansing (except in children age <12 years, in whom there is a risk of blurred vision and amblyopia) helps reduce bacterial proliferation. There is little evidence that any topical therapy is effective. Erythromycin ophthalmic ointment may be applied up to 6 times per day for 7 to 10 days or an antibiotic ointment containing bacitracin (2,3)[C].
- Treat underlying dry eye with artificial tears.

Second Line

- Occasionally, the use of an aminoglycoside ophthalmic ointment, such as gentamicin or tobramycin, may be necessary if condition is refractory to simpler treatment (case reports).
- Oral dicloxacillin or cephalexin for 2 weeks if refractory to topical antibiotics

ISSUES FOR REFERRAL

Consider referral if unresponsive to oral antibiotics.

SURGERY/OTHER PROCEDURES

- If the infection becomes localized to a single gland, incision, drainage, or curettage sometimes is necessary. This is an in-office procedure with a local anesthetic: Exercise caution because ocular perforation has been reported with the injection of an anesthetic to an infected lid.
- Use of combined antibiotic ointment (neomycin sulfate, polymyxin B sulfate, and gramicidin) after surgery was not shown to have any statistically significant benefit compared with artificial tears.

COMPLEMENTARY & ALTERNATIVE MEDICINE

- Broncasma berna is a polyvalent antigen vaccine that may be useful in the treatment of recurrent hordeolum.
- A Cochrane review found low-quality evidence that acupuncture (with or without antibiotics and/or warm compresses) may increase the chance of improvement of hordeolum compared to antibiotics and/or warm compresses (4)[A].

ADMISSION, INPATIENT, AND NURSING CONSIDERATIONS

Outpatient

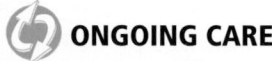 ## ONGOING CARE

FOLLOW-UP RECOMMENDATIONS

No restrictions

Patient Monitoring

The patient should be seen within several weeks to assess the effectiveness of therapy or should at least call the physician's office with a progress report.

DIET

No special diet

PATIENT EDUCATION

- The patient should be instructed in proper cleansing of the eyelids using a solution of tap water and baby shampoo or a commercially prepared hypoallergenic cleanser.
- The stye should not be squeezed or incised.

PROGNOSIS

- Usually responds well to good hygiene and warm compresses
- Inflammation usually improves within a week.
- Hordeolum tends to recur in some patients, usually due to incomplete elimination of bacteria.

COMPLICATIONS

An internal hordeolum, if untreated, may lead to chalazion, infections of adjacent glands, or generalized cellulitis of the lid.

REFERENCES

1. Lindsley K, Nichols JJ, Dickersin K. Non-surgical interventions for acute internal hordeolum. *Cochrane Database Syst Rev.* 2017;(1):CD007742.
2. Wald ER. Periorbital and orbital infections. *Pediatr Rev.* 2004;25(9):312–320.
3. Mueller JB, McStay CM. Ocular infection and inflammation. *Emerg Med Clin North Am.* 2008;26(1):57–72.
4. Cheng K, Law A, Guo M, et al. Acupuncture for acute hordeolum. *Cochrane Database Syst Rev.* 2017;(2):CD011075.

ADDITIONAL READING

- Bamford JT, Gessert CE, Renier CM, et al. Childhood stye and adult rosacea. *J Am Acad Dermatol.* 2006;55(6):951–955.
- Hirunwiwatkul P, Wachirasereechai K. Effectiveness of combined antibiotic ophthalmic solution in the treatment of hordeolum after incision and curettage: a randomized, placebo-controlled trial: a pilot study. *J Med Assoc Thai.* 2005;88(5):647–650.
- Kim JH, Yang SM, Kim HM, et al. Inadvertent ocular perforation during lid anesthesia for hordeolum removal. *Korean J Ophthalmol.* 2006;20(3):199–200.
- Nakatani M. Treatment of recurrent hordeolum with broncasma berna. *Eye (Lond).* 1999;13(Pt 5):692.
- Wald ER. Periorbital and orbital infections. *Infect Dis Clin North Am.* 2007;21(2):393–408, vi.

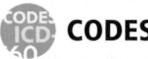 ## CODES

ICD10

- H00.019 Hordeolum externum unspecified eye, unspecified eyelid
- H00.029 Hordeolum internum unspecified eye, unspecified eyelid
- H00.039 Abscess of eyelid unspecified eye, unspecified eyelid

CLINICAL PEARLS

- A hordeolum should not be expressed.
- Warm compresses to the area of inflammation can encourage spontaneous drainage.
- Application of an antibiotic ointment (e.g., erythromycin) to the margin of the eyelid after proper cleansing helps reduce bacterial proliferation but may have no effect on the healing of the stye.
- Good personal hygiene with attention to cleansing the eyelids on a daily basis can prevent recurrent infections.

H

HORNER SYNDROME

Jairo J. Tejada-Tejada, MD • Jose L. Perez-Lara, MD • Manjeet Dhallu, MD

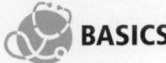

BASICS

DESCRIPTION

- Horner syndrome is a constellation of neurologic signs and symptoms manifested as a classic triad of ipsilateral miosis, eyelid ptosis, and anhidrosis of the ipsilateral midface and/or neck (with iris heterochromia in children).
- It is caused by the interruption or lesion along the sympathetic nerve supply to the head, neck, and eye.
- Oculosympathetic pathway anatomy:
  - First-order neuron: Sympathetic nerve fibers originate in the hypothalamus, descend through the brainstem, and synapse at the ciliospinal center (of Budge) located at approximately the C8–T2 levels of the spinal cord.
  - Second-order neuron: exits the spinal column at the T1 level primarily, arches over the apex of the lung and under the subclavian artery, ascending to the superior cervical ganglion at the level of the carotid bifurcation and angle of the jaw
  - Third-order neuron: ascends along the adventitia of the internal carotid artery, through the cavernous sinus in proximity to cranial nerve (CN) VI, and joins CN VI to innervate the iris dilator muscle and Müller muscle in the eye
- System(s) affected: nervous, skin/exocrine
- Synonym(s): Bernard-Horner syndrome; Bernard syndrome; Horner syndrome; cervical sympathetic syndrome; oculosympathetic syndrome; oculosympathetic paralysis; oculosympathetic deficiency; oculosympathetic paresis

EPIDEMIOLOGY

- Predominant age: none
- Predominant sex: male = female

Incidence
Unknown

Prevalence
Unknown

ETIOLOGY AND PATHOPHYSIOLOGY

- The constellation of signs and symptoms will be produced when sympathetic innervation is lesioned anywhere along the track producing ipsilateral Horner syndrome.
- Syndrome characteristics based on lesion locations:
  - Central or preganglionic lesion (complete syndrome):
    - First-order Horner syndrome (central): lesion located in the sympathetic tracts in the brainstem or cervicothoracic spinal cord; most common cause (MCC) lateral medullary infarction which present Horner syndrome as part of Wallenberg syndrome
    - Second-order Horner syndrome (preganglionic): due to trauma or surgery involving spinal cord, thoracic outlet or lung apex
  - Peripheral postganglionic lesion (incomplete syndrome, given by anhidrosis): third-order Horner syndrome; lesions usually located in internal carotid artery (e.g., dissection, thrombosis, cavernous sinus aneurysm, surgical endarterectomy, or stenting)
- Sympathetic fibers innervating sweat glands and vasodilatory muscles branch off before the cervical sympathetic ganglion traveling along the external carotid artery, so distal lesions will not result in anhidrosis; idiopathic (40%), congenital, or acquired

- Best classified by which order neuron is affected as mentioned above and by age (pediatric vs. adult)
- Etiology adult:
  - First-order neuron (13%)—central mostly located in hypothalamus/brainstem (lateral medulla)/spinal cord (cervical thoracic):
    - Arnold-Chiari malformation
    - Basal meningitis (e.g., syphilis)
    - Tumors
    - Cerebral vascular accident: lateral medullary (Wallenberg) syndrome
    - Cervical cord trauma
    - Demyelinating disease (multiple sclerosis)
    - Intrapontine hemorrhage
    - Neck trauma
    - Pituitary tumor
    - Syringomyelia
    - Unintended subdural placement of lumbar epidural catheter
  - Second-order neuron (44%)—preganglionic: pulmonary or thoracic upper lesions
    - Aneurysm/dissection of aorta
    - Central venous catheterization
    - Chest tubes
    - 1st rib fracture
    - Lymphadenopathy (Hodgkin, leukemia, tuberculosis, mediastinal tumors, sarcoid)
    - Mandibular tooth abscess
    - Neurofibromatosis types I and II
    - Pancoast tumor or infection of lung apex
    - Proximal common carotid artery dissection
    - Trauma/surgical injury
  - Third-order neuron lesions (43%)—postganglionic lesions located in superior cervical ganglion, internal carotid artery, skull base lesions, cavernous sinus lesions
    - Carotid cavernous fistula or other pathology
    - Carotid endarterectomy or carotid artery stenting
    - Cluster headaches
    - Internal carotid artery dissection
    - Herpes zoster
    - Lesions of the middle ear (acute otitis media)
    - Lyme disease
    - Nasopharyngeal cancer
    - Tonsillectomy
    - Raeder paratrigeminal syndrome
- Etiology children: Common causes are birth-related injuries (in neck and shoulder), neuroblastoma (paraspinal), vascular anomalies, and chest surgical interventions.
- MCC birth-related: associated injury to lower brachial plexus presenting ipsilateral forearm and hand weakness (Klumpke paralysis)
- Drugs: acetophenazine, alseroxylon, bupivacaine, butaperazine, carphenazine, chloroprocaine, deserpidine, diacetylmorphine, diethazine, ethopropazine, etidocaine, guanethidine, influenza virus vaccine, levodopa, lidocaine, mepivacaine, mesoridazine, methdilazine, methotrimeprazine, oral contraceptives, perazine, prilocaine, procaine, prochlorperazine, promazine, propoxycaine, reserpine, thioproperazine, thioridazine, trifluoperazine

Genetics
Rare autosomal dominant inheritance

RISK FACTORS

- Most common: apical bronchogenic carcinoma (Pancoast tumor) in smokers
- Aneurysm of the carotid or subclavian artery

- Injuries to the carotid artery high in the neck
- Dissection of the carotid arteries
- Carotid artery occlusion
  - 15% of patients with carotid artery occlusion develop ipsilateral Horner syndrome.
  - May occur without evidence of cerebral ischemia, neck injuries, or operative procedures
- Cluster headaches
  - 20% have an ipsilateral Horner syndrome.

COMMONLY ASSOCIATED CONDITIONS

- Wallenberg syndrome
- Pancoast tumor
- C8 radiculopathy

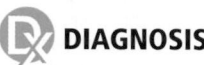

DIAGNOSIS

HISTORY

- Symptoms presented from birth? Presentation is acute or progressive?
- Is there any associated headaches or double vision?
- Does the degree of ptosis vary over the course of the day or with fatigue?
- Ask questions regarding anhidrosis or hypohidrosis (difficult to appreciate by patients or clinicians):
  - Ipsilateral side of the body: suggests central lesion
  - Ipsilateral face: suggests preganglionic lesion
  - Medial portion of forehead and side of nose: suggests postganglionic lesion

Pediatric Considerations
In infants and children, loss of facial flushing is appreciated more than anhidrosis (harlequin sign).

ALERT
Horner syndrome in the presence of pain merits urgent evaluation and referral to the emergency room:

- Axial, shoulder, scapula, arm, or hand pain may be related to Pancoast tumor.
- Acute-onset, ipsilateral facial or neck pain: Consider carotid artery dissection until proven otherwise.
- Paratrigeminal syndromes:
  - Raeder paratrigeminal syndrome type I: orbital pain, miosis, ptosis, with associated ipsilateral lesions of CN III to VI; suspect middle cranial fossa mass lesion.
  - Raeder paratrigeminal syndrome type II: episodic retrobulbar or orbital pain, miosis, ptosis with no CN lesions; suspect migraine variant, syphilis, herpes zoster, hypertension.

PHYSICAL EXAM

- Measure pupillary diameter in dim and bright light and reactivity to light and accommodative response (1):
  - Anisocoria is greatest in dark, with affected pupil failing to dilate.
  - Redilation (after light is removed) may lag 15 to 20 seconds on the affected side.
- Examine the upper lids for ptosis (<2 mm).
- Miosis examine if associated with dilated lag
- Examination of the lower lids for "upside-down ptosis": elevation of lower lid due to Müller muscle weakness
  - Illusion of enophthalmos secondary to narrowing of palpebral fissure
- Ipsilateral impaired flushing may be found.

- Loss of ciliospinal reflex. Pinching the skin on back of the neck normally produces ipsilateral pupil dilation (unreliable).
- Biomicroscopic exam of the papillary margin and iris structure and color
  - In congenital Horner syndrome, long-standing Horner syndrome, or Horner syndrome that occurs in children <2 years: Iris shows reduced pigmentation, blue-gray, and mottling of the affected eye (heterochromia iridis) because formation of iris pigment early in life is under sympathetic control.
- Observe for the presence of nystagmus, facial swelling, lymphadenopathy, or vesicular eruptions.
- Ophthalmoparesis, specifically CN VI palsy with Horner syndrome, is suggestive of cavernous sinus lesion.
- Neurologic and chest exams for associated physical findings

DIFFERENTIAL DIAGNOSIS

- Physiologic anisocoria (15–30% population)
- Neurologic diseases versus neuromuscular junctional disease (myasthenia gravis, botulinum toxin)
- Myogenic disease (mitochondrial myopathy, myotonic dystrophy, pseudoptosis)
- 3rd nerve palsy
- Blepharoptosis
- Unilateral use of miotics
- Unilateral use of mydriatics
- Adie tonic pupil
- Iris sphincter muscle damage
- Pharmacologic causes

DIAGNOSTIC TESTS & INTERPRETATION

Initial Tests (lab, imaging)

CBC, fluorescent treponemal antibody absorption test, venereal disease research laboratory, purified protein derivative; vanillylmandelic acid, homovanillic acid to rule out neuroblastoma in pediatric patients

- Chest x-ray if patient is a smoker (apical bronchogenic carcinoma)
- Computed tomography (CT)/magnetic resonance imaging (MRI), and/or angiography (MRA) of the brain, chest, and spinal cord
  - If painful, order MRI/MRA to evaluate for carotid artery dissection emergently.
- Ultrasound/duplex may be considered for evaluation of internal carotid artery.

Pediatric Considerations

In a child of any age without contributory history, MRI brain, neck, and chest to exclude a mass lesion (2)[B]

Diagnostic Procedures/Other

- When in doubt of Horner syndrome, confirmation test is required:
  - Topical 0.5% apraclonidine drops (3)[A],(4,5)[B]
  - 4–10% topical cocaine drops:
    ○ Used to confirm diagnosis of Horner syndrome when subtle symptoms but will not identify location of lesion
    ○ If the diagnosis is clear clinically, then confirmatory test is not required as it may interrupt with other test to localize lesions.
  - Test interpretation:
    ○ A normal pupil will dilate. The miotic pupil in Horner syndrome (regardless of location of lesion) will not dilate or will dilate poorly after 45 minutes because of the absence of norepinephrine at the nerve endings of the third-order neuron (3)[A].
    ○ Positive test is anisocoria of ≥1 mm.

- Mechanism of action:
  ○ Cocaine blocks the reuptake of norepinephrine at the level of sympathetic neuron. It has no effect in impaired sympathetic innervation regardless of site of lesion.
  ○ Apraclonidine is a direct α-adrenergic agonist, weak α-1 (mediates pupil dilation in Horner pupils) with strong α-2 receptor agonist (mediates pupil constriction in normal pupil).
- Test to localize level of the lesion:
  - Topical 1% hydroxyamphetamine drops (3)[A]
    ○ If there is a first- or second-order neuron lesion, dilation will take place.
    ○ Failure of the pupil to dilate, or poor dilation, indicates a third-order neuron lesion (positive when anisocoria increases by ≥1 mm).
    ○ No pharmacologic test exists to differentiate between a first- and second-order neuron lesion.
    ○ Hydroxyamphetamine causes release of endogenous norepinephrine stored in the postganglionic neuron.
    ○ Alternative test: 1% topical pholedrine drops
- Must wait 24 to 72 hours between the cocaine and hydroxyamphetamine tests

Pediatric Considerations

Due to transsynaptic degeneration in children, the hydroxyamphetamine test is not reliable.

Test Interpretation

- Brainstem lesion
- Massive hemisphere lesion
- Cervical cord lesion
- Root lesion
- Sympathetic chain lesion

 TREATMENT

GENERAL MEASURES

- Horner syndrome itself does not produce any disability or necessarily require treatment.
- Treat the underlying etiology.
- Search for a tumor or other compressive lesion.

MEDICATION

Carotid artery dissection: Pharmacologic treatment options include thrombolysis, antithrombotic therapy with anticoagulation, or antiplatelet therapy. No randomized control trials have compared these treatment options (6)[C].

ISSUES FOR REFERRAL

- Neurologic, neuro-ophthalmic, oculoplastic
- Neurologic or vascular surgery: interventional in cases of suspected carotid artery dissection or aneurysm
- Neurosurgery, surgical oncology, oncology, or radiotherapy consultation depends on the particular etiology.

SURGERY/OTHER PROCEDURES

- Surgical care depends on etiology.
- Consider ptosis repair surgery (oculoplastics).

 ONGOING CARE

PROGNOSIS

- Postganglionic: usually benign
- Central and preganglionic: poorer prognosis

COMPLICATIONS

- Chronic pupillary constriction
- Cosmesis

REFERENCES

1. Gross J, McClelland C, Lee M. An approach to anisocoria. *Curr Opin Ophthalmol*. 2016;27(6): 486–492.
2. Knyazer B, Smolar J, Lazar I, et al. Iatrogenic Horner syndrome: etiology, diagnosis and outcomes. *Isr Med Assoc J*. 2017;19(1):34–38.
3. Antonio-Santos AA, Santo RN, Eggenberger ER. Pharmacological testing of anisocoria. *Expert Opin Pharmacother*. 2005;6(12):2007–2013.
4. Koc F, Kavuncu S, Kansu T, et al. The sensitivity and specificity of 0.5% apraclonidine in the diagnosis of oculosympathetic paresis. *Br J Ophthalmol*. 2005;89(11):1442–1444.
5. Chen PL, Chen JT, Lu DW, et al. Comparing efficacies of 0.5% apraclonidine with 4% cocaine in the diagnosis of Horner syndrome in pediatric patients. *J Ocul Pharmacol Ther*. 2006;22(3):182–187.
6. Sadaka A, Schockman SL, Golnik KC. Evaluation of Horner syndrome in the MRI era. *J Neuroophthalmol*. 2017;37(3):268–272.

ADDITIONAL READING

- Ahmadi O, Saxena P, Wilson BK, et al. First rib fracture and Horner's syndrome: a rare clinical entity. *Ann Thorac Surg*. 2013;95(1):355.
- Almog Y, Gepstein R, Kesler A. Diagnostic value of imaging in Horner syndrome in adults. *J Neuroophthalmol*. 2010;30(1):7–11.
- Bazari F, Hind M, Ong YE. Horner's syndrome—not to be sneezed at. *Lancet*. 2010;375(9716):776.
- Davagnanam I, Fraser CL, Miszkiel K, et al. Adult Horner's syndrome: a combined clinical, pharmacological, and imaging algorithm. *Eye (Lond)*. 2013;27(3):291–298.
- Lyrer PA, Brandt T, Metso TM, et al; for Cervical Artery Dissection and Ischemic Stroke Patients Study Group. Clinical import of Horner syndrome in internal carotid and vertebral artery dissection. *Neurology*. 2014;82(18): 1653–1659.
- Reede DL, Garcon E, Smoker WR, et al. Horner's syndrome: clinical and radiographic evaluation. *Neuroimaging Clin N Am*. 2008;18(2):369–385.

 CODES

ICD10
- G90.2 Horner's syndrome
- S14.5XXA Injury of cervical sympathetic nerves, initial encounter

CLINICAL PEARLS

- Horner syndrome triad: ipsilateral miosis, eyelid ptosis, and anhidrosis caused by a lesion of the oculosympathetic pathway
- Horner syndrome in the presence of acute-onset, ipsilateral facial or neck pain: Consider carotid artery dissection until proven otherwise.
- Ptosis is mild, usually <2 mm.
- Red flags: If associated with pain, suspect central or preganglionic lesion.
- Confirm the diagnosis clinically with topical cocaine to the affected eye.
- Use hydroxyamphetamine to differentiate which order neuron is affected.
- Order imaging studies based on history and physical and hydroxyamphetamine testing.

H

HYDROCELE

Jared M. Patton, MD, MS • John E. Laird, MD, FAAFP, FAAMA

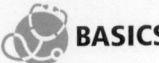 **BASICS**

DESCRIPTION

A collection of fluid between the parietal and visceral layers of the tunica vaginalis within the scrotum

- Communicating hydrocele (patent processus vaginalis)
  - Direct communication with the peritoneal cavity
  - Contains peritoneal fluid
  - Almost always with associated indirect inguinal hernia
  - Decreases in size with recumbent position
- Noncommunicating hydrocele (The processus vaginalis is not patent.)
  - No direct connection to the peritoneal cavity
  - Fluid contained is from the mesothelial lining.
  - Can be isolated to the cord with the distal and proximal portions of the processus vaginalis closed
- Acute hydrocele: fluid collection resulting from an acute process within the tunica vaginalis, typically involving only the scrotum
- System(s) affected: urogenital

Pediatric Considerations

In a communicating hydrocele, consider contralateral inguinal exploration to rule out an occult indirect hernia.

EPIDEMIOLOGY

Predominant age: childhood

Incidence

Estimated at 0.7–4.7% of male infants

Prevalence

- 1,000/100,000
- Estimated at 1% of adult men

ETIOLOGY AND PATHOPHYSIOLOGY

- Incomplete closure of the processus vaginalis trapping peritoneal fluid anywhere along the length of the tunica vaginalis
- Failure of closure of the processus vaginalis maintaining a communication to the peritoneal cavity

- Imbalance of the secretion and reabsorption of fluid from the lining of the tunica vaginalis
- Infection
- Tumors
- Trauma
- Ipsilateral renal transplantation

RISK FACTORS

- Ventriculoperitoneal shunt
- Exstrophy of the bladder
- Cloacal exstrophy
- Ehlers-Danlos syndrome
- Peritoneal dialysis

COMMONLY ASSOCIATED CONDITIONS

- Testicular tumors
- Scrotal trauma
- Ventriculoperitoneal shunt
- Nephrotic syndrome
- Renal failure with peritoneal dialysis

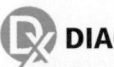 **DIAGNOSIS**

HISTORY

- Acute, subacute, or chronic swelling of the scrotum or inguinal canal
- Frequent changes in size of the hydrocele with position change or activity (indicative of communicating)
- Usually painless unless acute onset
- Sensation of heaviness or pressure in the scrotum
- Pain radiating to the flank/back

PHYSICAL EXAM

- Swelling in the scrotum or inguinal canal
- Scrotal mass, usually fluctuant
- Fluctuation in size with change of position (communicating hydrocele)
- Scrotal mass that transilluminates

DIFFERENTIAL DIAGNOSIS

- Indirect inguinal hernia
- Orchitis

- Epididymitis
- Varicocele
- Traumatic testicular injury
- Testicular torsion or torsion of appendix testes
- Testicular neoplasm

DIAGNOSTIC TESTS & INTERPRETATION

Initial Tests (lab, imaging)

- Inguinoscrotal ultrasound (US): can demonstrate the presence of bowel (e.g., distinguish incarcerated hernia from a hydrocele of the cord) as well as the presence of testicular torsion
- Testicular MRI when US is unable to distinguish etiology
- Doppler US or testicular nuclear scan can distinguish testicular torsion.

> **ALERT**
> Aspiration of a hydrocele for diagnosis is not indicated and may lead to severe complications if herniated bowel is present.

Test Interpretation

Patent processus vaginalis on imaging in communicating hydroceles

 TREATMENT

ISSUES FOR REFERRAL

- Urology referral for symptomatic adults or if underlying diagnosis is unclear
- Pediatric urology/surgery referral for children with symptomatic noncommunicating hydrocele
- Children with communicating hydroceles can be expectantly managed until at least 2 years of age to allow time for spontaneous resolution, unless there is a concern for inguinal hernia (1)[C].
- New onset hydrocele in late childhood and pre-adolescent patients typically resembles the adult type hydrocele pathology (2)[B].

SURGERY/OTHER PROCEDURES

- Children: Surgical treatment is generally deferred until 2 years of age because many hydroceles will spontaneously resolve. Some evidence shows that delaying longer than 2 years may be appropriate and decreases unnecessary surgery (1)[C].
  - When surgery is indicated, children with communicating hydroceles may undergo either open or laparoscopic approach.
    - Open inguinal approach involves ligation of the processus vaginalis and excision, distal splitting, or drainage of hydrocele sac (in a hydrocele of cord, the sac can be completely removed).
    - Open scrotal approach involves ligation and removal of the processus vaginalis. The benefit of this approach is improved cosmesis and decreased operative time (3)[B].
    - Laparoscopic repair offers the benefit of contralateral exploration.
- Adults: No therapy is needed unless the hydrocele causes discomfort or unless there is a significant underlying cause such as a tumor.
  - Aspiration of the hydrocele with instillation of a sclerosing agent has been successfully used in adults (4)[A].
  - If resection is indicated, a scrotal approach with resection of hydrocele sac has the lowest recurrence rate.
    - Postoperative complications as well as cost and time to work resumption were less in treatment by aspiration and sclerotherapy versus resection, but the recurrence rate was higher (5)[A].
    - The recurrence rate and low patient satisfaction may relegate aspiration and sclerotherapy as an alternative option only when resources for surgery are limited (6)[A].

ADMISSION, INPATIENT, AND NURSING CONSIDERATIONS

- Open inguinal or scrotal approach is typically performed as an outpatient.
- Laparoscopic approach in pediatric patients may require 24-hour admission for postoperative monitoring.
- Sclerotherapy is a same-day office procedure.

 ## ONGOING CARE

FOLLOW-UP RECOMMENDATIONS
Patient Monitoring
- Depending on method of treatment, initial follow-up is generally in the first 4 to 6 weeks.
- With sclerotherapy, follow-up is for confirmation of resolution or to proceed with retreatment.
- Postoperative follow-up at 2 to 4 weeks and subsequent 2- to 3-month intervals until resolution of any postoperative complications

PROGNOSIS
Low risk of long-term sequelae with either treatment method

COMPLICATIONS
- Complication rate for a scrotal approach may reach 30%.
- Postoperative traumatic hydrocele is common and usually resolves spontaneously.
- Injury to vas deferens or spermatic vessels
- Suture granuloma
- Hematoma
- Wound infection
- Recurrence

REFERENCES

1. Hall NJ, Ron O, Eaton S, et al. Surgery for hydrocele in children—an avoidable excess? *J Pediatr Surg*. 2011;46(12):2401–2405.
2. Koutsoumis G, Patoulias I, Kaselas C. Primary new-onset hydroceles presenting in late childhood and pre-adolescent patients resemble the adult type hydrocele pathology. *J Pediatr Surg*. 2014;49(11):1656–1658.
3. Alp BF, Irkilata HC, Kibar Y, et al. Comparison of the inguinal and scrotal approaches for the treatment of communicating hydrocele in children. *Kaohsiung J Med Sci*. 2014;30(4):200–205.

4. Lund L, Kloster A, Cao T. The long-term efficacy of hydrocele treatment with aspiration and sclerotherapy with polidocanol compared to placebo: a prospective, double-blind, randomized study. *J Urol*. 2014;191(5):1347–1350.
5. Shakiba B, Heidari K, Jamali A, et al. Aspiration and sclerotherapy versus hydrocoelectomy for treating hydrocoeles. *Cochrane Database Syst Rev*. 2014;(11):CD009735. doi:10.1002/14651858. CD009735.pub2.
6. Khaniya S, Agrawal C, Koirala R, et al. Comparison of aspiration-sclerotherapy with hydrocelectomy in the management of hydrocele: a prospective randomized study. *Int J Surg*. 2009;7(4):392–395.

CODES

ICD10
- N43.3 Hydrocele, unspecified
- N43.2 Other hydrocele
- P83.5 Congenital hydrocele

CLINICAL PEARLS

- A hydrocele can usually be diagnosed by physical exam and transillumination. If there is any concern for other underlying process, a formal US is recommended.
- Aspiration alone is not indicated as the primary treatment of a hydrocele due to high recurrence rate.
- Attempted aspiration of an unconfirmed hydrocele could lead to bowel injury in an undiagnosed inguinal hernia and should not be attempted.
- Expectant management of children with hydrocele until >2 years of age is acceptable to allow sufficient time for spontaneous resolution, decreasing the likelihood of an unnecessary procedure.
- In adults, surgical resection costs more and has more complications but has a much lower recurrence rate and a much higher patient satisfaction rate.

H

HYDROCEPHALUS, NORMAL PRESSURE

Dennis E. Hughes, DO, FAAFP, FACEP

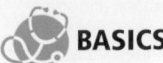 **BASICS**

DESCRIPTION
- Normal pressure hydrocephalus (NPH) is a clinical triad of gait instability, incontinence, and dementia (mnemonic: *wet, wobbly, wacky*); originally described by Hakim in 1957
- Two forms of the disorder: idiopathic and obstructive (the latter usually due to physical insult—posttrauma, meningitis, or subarachnoid hemorrhage)
- Absence of papilledema on clinical exam and normal CSF pressures at lumbar puncture

ALERT
Idiopathic NPH (iNPH) primarily affects persons >60 years; extremely rare before 40 years

EPIDEMIOLOGY
Incidence
- Varies from 1.1% to 5.5% in various surrogate analysis of shunt data. Arriving at accurate data is hampered by uncertain diagnosis.
- iNPH form primarily affects elderly, at least >40 years of age.
- Secondary form can occur at any age.
- Male = female

Prevalence
- Ranges from 0.2% in the 70- to 79-year age group and increases to 5.9% in those 80 years and older. It is estimated that approximately 700,000 are affected in the United States (compared with 400,000 with MS) (1).
- Estimated to be a contributing factor in 6% of all cases of dementia

ETIOLOGY AND PATHOPHYSIOLOGY
- Idiopathic form is a communicating hydrocephalus, a disorder of decreased CSF absorption (not overproduction). In iNPH, the leading theory suggests that poor venous compliance impairs the subarachnoid granulations' ability to maintain baseline removal of CSF. In secondary NPH, scarring is likely.
- The result is a pressure gradient between the subarachnoid space and ventricular system.
- CSF production decreases in the face of an increased pressure set point (but still in excess of the amount of CSF absorbed).
- Elevated pressure distends ventricles and compresses the brain parenchyma.

- As a result of compression, ischemic changes occur in the parenchymal vasculature with subsequent tissue damage and loss.
- Some believe that the idiopathic form is a result of persistently insufficient removal of CSF by immature subarachnoid granulations from childhood.
- Secondary NPH may result from the following:
  - Head trauma (most common)
  - Subarachnoid hemorrhage
  - Resolved acute meningitis
  - Chronic meningitis (tuberculosis, syphilis)
  - Paget disease of the skull

RISK FACTORS
- Idiopathic risk is unknown (case reports suggest a possible genetic link but unsubstantiated).
- Secondary form is due to head trauma, subarachnoid hemorrhage, meningitis, or encephalitis.

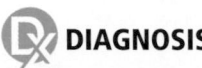 **DIAGNOSIS**

Detailed history and careful examination is the key to early diagnosis.

HISTORY
- Insidious and usually progressive; gait instability usually manifests initially, followed by changes in mentation, and eventually, urinary incontinence.
- Behavioral changes noted in many cases: Depression, mania, and psychotic features in many cases precede the physical findings and respond poorly to usual treatment (1).
- Difficulty with initiation of movement: Feet appear "glued to the floor." Gait is wide-based, shuffling, and turning appears "en bloc."
- Inattention, forgetfulness, and lack of spontaneity often are seen with the subcortical dementia of NPH.
- Urinary urgency initially, followed by lack of inhibition and then frank incontinence
- A minimum duration of at least 3 to 6 months of symptoms and progression over time
- A remote trauma or infection suggests secondary versus the idiopathic form.
- A lack of psychiatric, neurologic, or other medical conditions to explain the symptoms (including structural reasons for CSF flow restriction) (2)
- Because memory impairment may be present, it is important to include a knowledgeable informant who is familiar with the patient's premorbid state.
- Frontal lobe function is affected disproportionately to the memory impairment (objective testing may lead to an early diagnosis).

PHYSICAL EXAM
- Decreased step height and length
- Reduced speed of walking (cadence)
- Widened standing base
- Swaying of trunk during walking
- Decreased fine motor speed and accuracy
- Recall impaired for recent events
- Impaired ability to do multistep tasks or interpret abstractions

DIFFERENTIAL DIAGNOSIS
- Alzheimer disease (may be a comorbid condition in as many as 75%)
- Parkinson disease
- Chronic alcoholism
- Intracranial infection
- Multi-infarct dementia
- Subdural hematoma
- Carcinomatous meningitis
- Collagen vascular disorders
- Depression
- Syphilis
- B_{12} deficiency
- Urologic disorders
- Other hydrocephalus disorders

DIAGNOSTIC TESTS & INTERPRETATION
Initial Tests (lab, imaging)
- Thyroid-stimulating hormone (TSH)
- Syphilis serology
- CBC
- Serum B_{12}, folate
- Metabolic profile
- Blood alcohol, analysis for drugs of abuse
- Urinalysis
- CSF analysis, including an opening pressure <245 mm H_2O (a value greater than this rules out iNPH by definition)
- Imaging is essential.
  - Either CT or MRI (preferred imaging study) shows the ventriculomegaly (particularly lateral and 3rd ventricles) with preservation of the cerebral parenchyma (as opposed to ventricular enlargement seen in other forms of dementia where brain atrophy is present). A narrow subarachnoid space ("tight convexity") was recently shown to correlate to probable or definite iNPH (3)[A].
  - MRI can allow detection of other features, such as signs of altered brain water content and callosal angles. However, these supportive findings are not independently diagnostic of NPH.

Diagnostic Procedures/Other

CSF removal aids in the definitive diagnosis as well as predicting response to surgical treatment.

- High-volume (30 to 70 mL) CSF removal via spinal tap ("tap test")
- Comparison of gait analysis before and after CSF removal should be performed within 24 hours (a ≥20% improvement indicates a positive test), especially when combined with coexisting executive function improvement. Testing should be done with a quantifiable gait scale (Berg Balance Scale, Timed Get UP and Go Test, etc.) (4)[B].

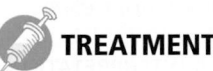

TREATMENT

MEDICATION

- No medication is significantly helpful.
- Use of carbonic anhydrase inhibitors (acetazolamide) with repeat lumbar punctures has provided mild and transient relief but is only supported by anecdotal evidence.
- Use of levodopa to rule out Parkinson disease may be helpful (NPH will display little, if any, significant improvement to dopamine agonist).

ISSUES FOR REFERRAL

- Neurology or neurosurgical consultation is helpful in suspected cases when other reversible medical conditions are ruled out.
- Recent cohort studies have demonstrated clinical improvement after surgical shunts. Perimeters of urinary continence, gait stability, and cognitive scores all improved at 1 year postshunt.

ADDITIONAL THERAPIES

Gait training and use of ambulation assist devices, as indicated, but limited efficacy

SURGERY/OTHER PROCEDURES

- Current therapy is limited to placement of ventricle-peritoneal or ventricle-atrial shunt from a lateral ventricle tunneled SC and drained into the peritoneal cavity (or right atrium). Recent work demonstrated that use of a lumbar-peritoneal shunt to be noninferior is technically easier and associated with less complications.
- Patients whose symptoms have been present for a shorter period (<2 years) have a greater chance of improvement with shunting. Age has not been shown to negatively affect response to shunting. Improvement has been seen in patients with symptoms present for many years and previously undiagnosed (5)[B].

ADMISSION, INPATIENT, AND NURSING CONSIDERATIONS

Usually only for planned surgical treatment

 ## ONGOING CARE

FOLLOW-UP RECOMMENDATIONS

- Assessment and modification of environment for fall risks
- Evaluation for ability to operate a motor vehicle safely (if driving)

Patient Monitoring

- Repeat neuropsychological testing to evaluate the status of the dementia after treatment.
- Improvement in the incontinence and walking speed can also be objectively measured.

PATIENT EDUCATION

Information at: http://www.ninds.nih.gov/disorders /normal_pressure_hydrocephalus/normal _pressure_hydrocephalus.htm

PROGNOSIS

Natural history is progressive deterioration. Patient's axial skeletal stability worsens with inability to walk, stand, sit, or turn over in bed.

COMPLICATIONS

- In patients treated surgically, cerebral infarcts, hemorrhage, infection, and seizures (in addition to the usual surgical risks): all usual age-related illnesses (as NPH is a condition affecting those age >65 years)
- Shunt malfunction (especially when symptoms recur after successful shunt placement)
- Falls due to gait instability
- UTIs
- Skin breakdown, pressure ulcers, infections as movement dysfunction progresses

REFERENCES

1. Nassar BR, Lippa CF. Idiopathic normal pressure hydrocephalus: a review for general practitioners. *Gerontol Geriatr Med*. 2016;2:2333721416643702.
2. Williams MA, Relkin NR. Diagnosis and management of idiopathic normal-pressure hydrocephalus. *Neurol Clin Pract*. 2013;3(5):375–385.
3. Hashimoto M, Ishikawa M, Mori E, et al; for Study of INPH on neurological improvement (SINPHONI). Diagnosis of idiopathic normal pressure hydrocephalus is supported by MRI-based scheme: a prospective cohort study. *Cerebrospinal Fluid Res*. 2010;7:18.

4. Allali G, Laidet M, Beauchet O, et al. Dual-task related gait changes after CSF tapping: a new way to identify idiopathic normal pressure hydrocephalus. *J Neuroeng Rehabil*. 2013;10:117.
5. Williams MA, Malm J. Diagnosis and treatment of idiopathic normal pressure hydrocephalus. *Continuum (Minneap Minn)*. 2016;22(2 Dementia):579–599.

ADDITIONAL READING

- Andrén K, Wikkelsø C, Tisell M, et al. Natural course of idiopathic normal pressure hydrocephalus. *J Neurol Neurosurg Psychiatry*. 2014;85(7):806–810.
- Halperin JJ, Kurlan R, Schwalb JM, et al. Practice guideline: idiopathic normal pressure hydrocephalus: response to shunting and predictors of response: report of the Guideline Development, Dissemination, and Implementation Subcommittee of the American Academy of Neurology. *Neurology*. 2015;85(23):2063–2071.
- Jaraj D, Rabiei K, Marlow T, et al. Prevalence of idiopathic normal-pressure hydrocephalus. *Neurology*. 2014;82(16):1449–1454.

 ## SEE ALSO

Algorithm: Ataxia

 ## CODES

ICD10

- G91.2 (Idiopathic) normal pressure hydrocephalus
- G91.0 Communicating hydrocephalus

CLINICAL PEARLS

- NPH is a clinical triad of gait instability, incontinence, and dementia (mnemonic: wet, wobbly, wacky).
- NPH is insidious and usually progressive; gait instability usually manifests initially, followed by changes in mentation, and eventually, urinary incontinence.
- Consider in unexplained dementia or behavioral change.
- Poor prognosis without therapy

H

HYDRONEPHROSIS

Monzurul H. Chowdhury, MD • Pang-Yen Fan, MD

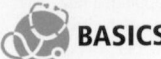

BASICS

DESCRIPTION
- Hydronephrosis refers to a structural finding—dilatation of the renal calyces and pelvis.
  - May occur with urinary tract infection (UTI), vesicoureteral reflux (VUR), high urine output, or physiologic changes in pregnancy
  - Can be accompanied with hydroureter
  - Presentation varies from incidental finding to discovery during workup for UTI or for flank or abdominal pain, or for acute kidney injury.
- Hydronephrosis should not be used interchangeably with obstructive uropathy, which refers to the damage to renal parenchyma resulting from urinary tract obstruction (UTO).

EPIDEMIOLOGY
- The incidence is more common in men than women and in children than adults (congenital anomalies).
- Acute unilateral hydronephrosis is more common than bilateral.

ETIOLOGY AND PATHOPHYSIOLOGY
- Hydronephrosis develops with increased pressure in the urinary collecting system.
- Increased pressure can cause calyceal fornix rupture and urinary extravasation.
- Over time, pressures return to normal, but kidney function declines from intense renal vasoconstriction.
- With concomitant urinary infection, bacteria can enter the renal vasculature, resulting in sepsis.
- Hydronephrosis may be acute/chronic, partial/complete, and uni-/bilateral.
  - Intraluminal obstruction: calculi, sloughed renal papillae, blood clot, fungal ball
  - Intrinsic abnormality of the urinary collecting system: transitional cell carcinomas, benign prostatic hypertrophy, prostate cancer, congenital ureteropelvic junction (UPJ) obstruction, uretero-cele, neurogenic bladder (functional obstruction), urethral stricture or tuberculosis (TB) (can cause ureteral narrowing)
  - Extrinsic compression of the urinary collecting system: extraurinary malignancy (lymphoma, colon, cervix), aortic/iliac aneurysm, retroperitoneal fibrosis, uterine prolapse (15% affected), endometriosis, ovarian vein syndrome, IgG4-related disease
  - Transplant hydronephrosis: Consider BK virus infection.
- Hydronephrosis in transplanted kidney is more common than native kidneys, specifically in immediate posttransplant period. It is due to ureteral strictures and lymphoceles (ureteral compression and bladder dysfunction).
- VUR resulting in varying degrees of hydroureteronephrosis
- Hydronephrosis due to high urine output (e.g., diabetes insipidus, psychogenic polydipsia)
- Hydronephrosis of infection: due to bacterial toxins inhibiting smooth muscle contraction of the renal pelvis and ureter

Pediatric Considerations
- Antenatal hydronephrosis is diagnosed in 1–5% of pregnancies, usually by US, as early as the 12th to 14th week of gestation.
- Children with antenatal hydronephrosis are at greater risk of postnatal pathology.
- Postnatal evaluation begins with US exam; further studies, such as voiding cystourethrogram (VCUG), based on the severity of postnatal hydronephrosis
- In neonates, it is the most common cause of abdominal mass.
- Common etiologies in children are VUR, congenital UPJ obstruction, neurogenic bladder, and posterior urethral valves.
- Pediatric diagnostic algorithm differs from adult due to different differential diagnosis necessitating age-appropriate testing.

Pregnancy Considerations
- Physiologic hydronephrosis in pregnancy is more prominent on the right than left and can be seen in up to 80% of pregnant women.
- Dilatation is caused by hormonal effects, external compression from expanding uterus, and intrinsic changes in the ureteral wall.
- Despite high incidence, most cases are asymptomatic.
- If symptomatic and refractory to medical management, ureteric calculus should be considered and urinary infection must be excluded.

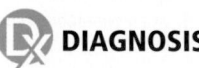

DIAGNOSIS

HISTORY
- Symptoms vary according to cause, chronicity, location, and degree of obstruction.
- Although often asymptomatic, hydronephrosis can be associated with pain ranging from vague, intermittent discomfort to severe renal colic.
- Nausea and vomiting may be associated with pain or infection.
- Fever, chills with coexisting infection
- Anuria, if complete obstruction of bilateral or a solitary kidney
- Polyuria may occur due to impaired urinary concentration in partial obstruction or postobstructive diuresis.
- Symptoms of chronic kidney disease (CKD): anorexia, malaise, weight gain, edema, shortness of breath, mental state changes, tremors from long-standing obstruction
- Dietl crisis: sudden attack of flank pain due to distension of renal pelvis caused by rapid ingestion of large amount of liquid or kinking of a ureter, producing temporary occlusion of urine flow
- Symptoms of bladder outlet obstruction: weak urine stream, nocturia, straining to void, overflow incontinence, urgency, and frequency
- General medical and surgical history: malignancy (extrinsic compression), radiotherapy (ureteric stricture/fibrosis), surgery (iatrogenic obstruction), trauma (hematoma or fibrosis), gynecologic disease (endometriosis, ovarian masses, uterine prolapse), smoking (urothelial cancer), drugs (methysergide-induced retroperitoneal fibrosis)

PHYSICAL EXAM
- General signs
  - Volume overload (edema, rales, hypertension [HTN]) from renal failure
  - Diaphoresis, tachycardia, tachypnea with pain
  - High-grade fever, if infection
- Abdominal exam: CVA tenderness, palpable bladder, rarely palpable abdominal mass (may be visible, particularly in thin children)
- Pelvic exam: pelvic mass, uterine prolapse, palpable enlarged prostate (cancer or benign), urethral meatal stenosis, phimosis

DIAGNOSTIC TESTS & INTERPRETATION
- Urinalysis with microscopy: hematuria, proteinuria, crystalluria, pyuria
- Midstream urine culture and sensitivity: Exclude UTI.
- Basic metabolic panel: Elevated urea and creatinine may indicate obstructive uropathy. Hyperkalemic nonanion gap metabolic acidosis may indicate type 4 distal RTA due to obstruction.
- CBC: anemia of CKD, leukocytosis; if infection, check platelet count prior to considering ureteral instrumentation.
- Prostate-specific antigen (PSA): adult males age >50 years or with abnormal digital rectal exam or bladder outlet obstruction signs or symptoms
- Urine cytology: for malignant cells in urothelial malignancies
- US and noncontrast CT scanning are effective in diagnosing presence and cause of obstruction in most cases.
- US: screening test of choice for hydronephrosis
  - Sensitivity 90%, specificity 84.5% compared with IVU. Does not assess function and rarely detects cause and level of obstruction. Degree of hydronephrosis does not correlate with duration or severity of the obstruction.
  - Advantages: detects renal parenchymal disease (decreased renal size, increased cortical echogenicity, cortical thinning, cysts); no exposure to radiation or contrast; safe in pregnancy, contrast allergy, and renal dysfunction
  - False-positive findings 15.5%: normal extrarenal pelvis, parapelvic cysts, VUR, excessive diuresis
  - False-negative findings 10%: dehydration, acute obstruction, calyceal dilatation misinterpreted as renal cortical cysts, and retroperitoneal fibrosis
- Noncontrast helical CT (NHCT): test of choice for suspected nephrolithiasis
  - Reported sensitivity 94–96%, specificity 94–100%. Stone is most commonly found at levels of ureteric luminal narrowing: UPJ, pelvic brim, and the vesicoureteric junction.
  - Typical findings in acute obstruction are hydronephrosis with hydroureter proximal to the level of obstruction, perinephric stranding, and renal swelling. If chronic, renal atrophy may be noted.
  - Advantages: no contrast exposure, time-saving, cost-effective, identifies extraurinary pathology (1)
  - Disadvantages: does not assess function or degree of obstruction; higher radiation exposure, although low radiation dose protocols have shown comparable accuracy

- DTPA or MAG-3 radionuclide renal scan (diuretic renal scintigraphy)
  - Indicated only for evaluation of hydronephrosis without apparent obstruction
  - Determines presence of true obstruction as well as total and split (right vs. left) renal function
  - Furosemide is given 20 minutes after the tracer and the T1/2 for the tracer's washout is measured. T1/2; <10 minutes is unobstructed, >20 minutes is obstructed, and 10 to 20 minutes is equivocal; some experts consider <15 minutes normal.
  - Advantages: no contrast exposure, safe in contrast allergy and renal dysfunction
  - False-positive findings: delayed excretion due to renal failure, massive dilatation causing a water-reservoir effect of delayed excretion without obstruction
  - False-negative findings: dehydration or inadequate diuretic challenge
- Multiphase contrast-enhanced CT
  - Nonenhanced phase detects stones and swelling.
  - Parenchymal phase demonstrates decreased enhancement of renal parenchyma with acute obstruction; can identify extraurinary causes of obstruction and determine the relative glomerular filtration rate (GFR) of each kidney with accuracy equal to radionuclide renal scan
  - Delayed phase allows visualization of the collecting system and soft tissue filling defects (e.g., urothelial cancer).
- Magnetic resonance urography (MRU): indicated when US and NHCT are nondiagnostic
  - Provides anatomic, functional, and prognostic information; sensitivity not superior to US or NHCT for nephrolithiasis (70%) but superior for soft tissue causes including strictures
  - Advantages: no radiation exposure, safe in pregnancy
  - Disadvantages: more expensive and time-consuming (35 minutes vs. 5 minutes) and less available compared with CT. Gadolinium is contraindicated in renal failure especially when GFR is <30 mL/min due to risk of nephrogenic systemic fibrosis.

Diagnostic Procedures/Other
Cystoscopy, retrograde pyelogram ± ureteroscopy, and biopsy are occasionally used to determine the cause of obstruction (e.g., small urothelial cancer missed on imaging) or to confirm a normal distal ureter prior to pyeloplasty. In addition, such procedures are often needed to establish a definitive pathologic diagnosis for mass lesions.

TREATMENT

GENERAL MEASURES
- Medical treatment: correction of fluid and electrolyte abnormalities, pain control, antibiotics as an adjunct to drainage if infection present
- Relief of obstruction: prompt drainage indicated in the presence of UTI, compromised renal function, or uncontrollable/persistent pain
  - Bladder outlet obstruction: urethral or suprapubic catheter
  - Ureteric obstruction: retrograde (cystoscopic) or antegrade (percutaneous) stenting (2)

- VUR is often managed conservatively with antibiotics; surgical management required in severe cases in children or women of childbearing age
- Medical expulsive therapy (MET) with α-blockers or calcium channel blockers indicated for urethral stones <10 mm in patients with controlled pain, no signs of sepsis, with good renal function (3)[C]

SURGERY/OTHER PROCEDURES
- Hydronephrosis due to obstruction
  - Congenital UPJ obstruction: Pyeloplasty (open or laparoscopic) and minimally invasive stricture incision (endopyelotomy) are used with comparable results.
  - Nephrolithiasis: Extracorporeal shock wave lithotripsy (ESWL) is the initial treatment of choice for management of impacted upper urethral stones ≤2 cm. Ureteroscopy with or without intracorporeal lithotripsy has lower retreatment but higher complication rates and longer hospital stay; ureteral stenting pre-ESWL or postureteroscopy associated with no additional benefit and more discomfort and morbidity (4)[A]
  - Transitional cell cancer: nephroureterectomy
  - Idiopathic retroperitoneal fibrosis: ureterolysis (frees ureters from inflammatory mass)
  - Prostate disorders: various treatment modalities, including transurethral resection of the prostate (TURP) and radical prostatectomy
- Nonobstructed hydronephrosis
  - VUR: ureteric reimplantation, endoscopic suburethral injection

ADMISSION, INPATIENT, AND NURSING CONSIDERATIONS
Obstruction coexisting with infection (pyonephrosis) is a true urologic emergency requiring urgent drainage. Typically, this requires placement of percutaneous nephrostomy tube(s) because retrograde (cystoscopic) stenting is often difficult, but both are equally effective.

 ## ONGOING CARE

FOLLOW-UP RECOMMENDATIONS
- Serial monitoring of kidney function (electrolytes, BUN, and creatinine) and BP until renal function stabilizes. Frequency of monitoring depends on severity of renal dysfunction.
- Follow-up US after stabilization of renal function to assess for resolution of hydronephrosis. If hydronephrosis persists, consider diuretic radionuclide study to rule out persistent obstruction.

PROGNOSIS
- Recovery of renal function depends on etiology, presence or absence of UTI, and degree and duration of obstruction.
- Significant recovery can occur despite days of complete obstruction, although some irreversible injury may develop within 24 hours. Delays in therapy can lead to irreversible renal damage (5).
- Diagnostic testing is of poor predictive value. Course of incomplete obstruction is highly unpredictable.

COMPLICATIONS
- Urine stasis: increased risk of infection and stones formation
- Obstruction causes progressive atrophy of kidney with irreversible loss of function.
- Spontaneous rupture of a calyx may occur with urine extravasation in the perinephric space.
- Postobstructive diuresis: marked polyuria after relief of obstruction:
  - Caused mostly by fluid and solute overload but may be exacerbated by impaired renal tubular concentrating ability. Urine output may be >500 mL/hr.
  - Replace urine losses with hypotonic fluid (usually with 0.45% NaCl) and only enough to avoid volume depletion. Replacement of urine output with equal amounts of saline will perpetuate the diuresis.

REFERENCES

1. Worster A, Preyra I, Weaver B, et al. The accuracy of noncontrast helical computed tomography versus intravenous pyelography in the diagnosis of suspected acute urolithiasis: a meta-analysis. *Ann Emerg Med*. 2002;40(3):280–286.
2. Ramsey S, Robertson A, Ablett MJ, et al. Evidence-based drainage of infected hydronephrosis secondary to ureteric calculi. *J Endourol*. 2010;24(2):185–189.
3. Seitz C, Liatsikos E, Porpiglia F, et al. Medical therapy to facilitate the passage of stones: what is the evidence? *Eur Urol*. 2009;56(3):455–471.
4. Aboumarzouk OM, Kata SG, Keeley FX, et al. Extracorporeal shock wave lithotripsy (ESWL) versus ureteroscopic management for ureteric calculi. *Cochrane Database Syst Rev*. 2011;(12):CD006029.
5. Cohen EP, Sobrero M, Roxe DM, et al. Reversibility of long-standing urinary tract obstruction requiring long-term dialysis. *Arch Intern Med*. 1992;152(1):177–179.

ADDITIONAL READING

Shen P, Jiang M, Yang J, et al. Use of ureteral stent in extracorporeal shock wave lithotripsy for upper urinary calculi: a systematic review and meta-analysis. *J Urol*. 2011;186(4):1328–1335.

 ## CODES

ICD10
- N13.30 Unspecified hydronephrosis
- N13.39 Other hydronephrosis
- Q62.0 Congenital hydronephrosis

CLINICAL PEARLS
- US and noncontrast CT identify most causes of hydronephrosis.
- Relief of obstruction, when present, is the primary treatment.

H

HYPERCHOLESTEROLEMIA
Cameron D. Blegen, MD • James E. Hougas III, MD, FAAFP

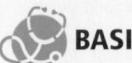

BASICS

DESCRIPTION
- Elevated cholesterol is a significant risk factor for atherosclerotic cardiovascular disease (ASCVD).
- Lipoprotein subtypes:
  - Low-density lipoproteins (LDL): atherogenic; primary target of therapy
  - High-density lipoproteins (HDL): atheroprotective
  - Triglycerides (TG)
- System(s) affected: cardiovascular (CV)

EPIDEMIOLOGY
- Nearly 37% of U.S. adults have LDL cholesterol levels above treatment thresholds (1).
- Only 55% of U.S. adults who warrant cholesterol medication are currently taking it (1).
- 7% of U.S. children and adolescents ages 6 to 19 years have high total cholesterol (1).

Prevalence
Disease incidence and prevalence increases with age.

ETIOLOGY AND PATHOPHYSIOLOGY
- Pathophysiology
  - Deposition of cholesterol in vascular walls creates fatty streaks which become fibrous plaques.
  - Inflammation causes plaque instability, leading to plaque rupture.
- Etiology
  - Primary: genetic causes (familial dyslipidemia)
  - Secondary: obesity, diet, excessive alcohol intake, hypothyroidism, diabetes, nephrotic syndrome, liver disease, chronic renal failure, medications (thiazide diuretics, carbamazepine, cyclosporine, progestins, anabolic steroids, corticosteroids, protease inhibitors)

Genetics
- Familial hypercholesterolemia (FH)
  - Elevated LDL levels from birth
  - Prevalence is 1:500 in the United States.
  - Predisposition to atherosclerotic disease in early adulthood and high coronary heart disease risk at younger ages (40s and 50s)
  - Tendon xanthomas on Achilles and extensor tendons of the hands are common.
  - Early lipid-lowering drug therapy has been shown to reduce ASCVD risk.
- Early cholesterol testing of first-degree relatives is recommended and beneficial.

RISK FACTORS
Obesity (BMI >30 kg/m²), physical inactivity, heredity, cigarette smoking, excessive alcohol use. Unclear relationship between diet rich in saturated fat and hypercholesterolemia. The relationship of diet to disease is very complex and is not explained by how much cholesterol is present in an individual's diet. Eggs and whole fat dairy sources are likely *not* significant contributors to atherosclerosis.

GENERAL PREVENTION
- Regular physical activity
- Weight control (see "Ongoing Care")

COMMONLY ASSOCIATED CONDITIONS
Hypertension (HTN), diabetes mellitus (DM), obesity

DIAGNOSIS

Screening recommendations:
- U.S. Preventive Services Task Force (USPSTF) (2)[A]: TC and HDL cholesterol (HDL-C) every 5 years
  - Men and women ≥40 years
  - No recommendation for or against screening in adults aged 21 to 39 years
  - No recommendation for or against screening in children and adolescents
- American Diabetes Association: yearly dyslipidemia screening for patients with diabetes

Pediatric Considerations
- National Heart, Lung, and Blood Institute (NHLBI): Recommend lipid screening on all children between 9 and 11 years. This remains controversial because of the absence of data showing improved outcomes and concern about potential harms. Selective screening of children with FH is not controversial.
- USPSTF: insufficient evidence to recommend for or against screening children and adolescents

HISTORY
- Review possible secondary etiologies (see "Etiology and Pathophysiology").
- Review medications which may alter lipid levels.
- Assess other ASCVD risk factors.

PHYSICAL EXAM
Nonspecific findings; may calculate BMI and examine for xanthomas

DIAGNOSTIC TESTS & INTERPRETATION
Initial Tests (lab, imaging)
- Lipid panel (fasting labs do not significantly affect lab values): TC, LDL, HDL, TG: LDL is usually a calculated value and is accurate if TG <350 mg/dL.
- Consider genetic etiology in very high LDL (>190 mg/dL) or TG (>500 mg/dL).

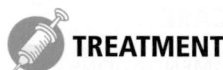

TREATMENT

ALERT
The 2013 American College of Cardiology/American Heart Association (ACC/AHA) cholesterol guidelines no longer recommend treatment to an LDL goal. ACC/AHA and USPSTF guidelines recommend statin therapy based on patients' risk of an ASCVD event. Efficacy of statin medication for reduction in myocardial infarction (MI) and death is likely due to mechanisms other than cholesterol lowering alone. Risk stratifying patients should be reserved for primary prevention as patients with established CV disease should be considered high risk (secondary prevention).

- United States: ACC/AHA cholesterol guidelines (3)[C]
  - Four groups benefit from statin therapy:
    - Clinical ASCVD
      - <75 years old: high-intensity statin
      - >75 years old or not candidate for high-intensity statin: moderate-intensity statin
    - Primary elevation of LDL-C >190 mg/dL: high-intensity statin
    - Diabetics (type 1 or 2) ages 40 to 75 years with LDL-C 70 to 189 mg/dL:
      - 10-year ASCVD risk <7.5%: moderate-intensity statin
      - 10-year ASCVD risk >7.5%: high-intensity statin

- Without above but estimated 10-year ASCVD risk >7.5% based on Pooled Cohort Equations http://tools.acc.org/ASCVD-Risk-Estimator: moderate- to high-intensity statin depending on risk
  - Definition of clinical ASCVD:
    - Acute coronary syndrome or history of MI
    - Stable or unstable angina
    - Coronary or other arterial revascularization
    - Stroke or TIA
    - Peripheral arterial disease
  - Significant controversy over threshold calculated risk with which to treat patients:
    - Concern that Pooled Cohort Equations significantly *overestimates* ASCVD risk
  - Concern for significant overtreatment: One study shows 96% of men and 66% of women >55 years of age on statins based on recommendations.
- United States: USPSTF statin recommendations (2)[A]
  - Adults aged 40 to 75 years with no history of CVD, one or more CVD risk factors, and a calculated 10-year CVD event risk of 10% or greater: low to moderate dose statin
  - Adults aged 40 to 75 years with no history of CVD, one or more CVD risk factors, and a calculated 10-year CVD event risk of 7.5–10%: low to moderate dose statin
  - Adults 76 years and older with no history of CVD: insufficient evidence to make recommendation
- Many patients treated and medications used in the United States than elsewhere in the world without substantial evidence for improved outcomes
- United Kingdom: National Institute for Health and Care Excellence (NICE) cholesterol guidelines (4)[C]
  - 10-year risk to be calculated using QRISK2: http://www.qrisk.org/
  - If 10-year risk of CVD >10% and no history of CVD, start atorvastatin 20 mg.
  - If 10-year risk of CVD >10% in presence of known CVD, start atorvastatin 80 mg.
  - If eGFR <60 or type I diabetes, start atorvastatin 20 mg regardless of risk.
  - Check nonfasting lipid panel before treatment initiation and at 3 months of treatment: goal reduction of 40% in non–HDL-C
- U.S. Veterans Affairs 2014 Guideline (5)[A] advises moderate-dose statin for 10-year CVD risk >12%, or LDL-C ≥190, or DM with HTN or smoking.

ALERT
Elevated serum TG
- If >500 mg/dL, TG lowering becomes primary target until TG <500 to prevent acute pancreatitis. Statin therapy is usually recommended as treatment unless TGs remain >500 after statin added. Fibrates may be used cautiously with statins (increased risk of rhabdomyolysis).

MEDICATION
- Therapeutic lifestyle changes are cornerstone therapies to be attempted before drug therapy (diet and regular exercise; see "Ongoing Care").
- Available data do not support initiation of statin therapy for primary prevention in most adults age >75 years (ALLHAT-LLT and other trials).
- Check lipid panel 4 to 12 weeks after starting medication to evaluate response/compliance.
  - High-intensity statin: should lower LDL-C >50%
  - Moderate-intensity statin: should lower LDL-C 30–50%
  - Subsequent monitoring not generally indicated unless question of patient adherence

First Line
HMG-CoA reductase inhibitors (statins)
- Categorized based on intensity
  - High intensity
    - Atorvastatin 40 to 80 mg/day
    - Rosuvastatin 20 to 40 mg/day
  - Moderate intensity
    - Atorvastatin 10 to 20 mg/day
    - Rosuvastatin 5 to 10 mg/day
    - Simvastatin 20 to 40 mg/day
    - Pravastatin 40 to 80 mg/day
    - Lovastatin 40 mg/day
    - Fluvastatin XL 80 mg/day
    - Fluvastatin 40 mg BID
    - Pitavastatin 2 to 4 mg/day
  - Low intensity
    - Simvastatin 10 mg/day
    - Pravastatin 10 to 20 mg/day
    - Lovastatin 20 mg/day
    - Fluvastatin 20 to 40 mg/day
    - Pitavastatin 1 mg/day
- To be taken in the evening or at bedtime for best effect because majority of cholesterol synthesis appears to occur at night
- Effect is greatest in lowering LDL-C; shown to decrease coronary heart disease incidence and all-cause mortality (2), although number needed to treat may be high in primary prevention, depending on risk
- Contraindications: pregnancy, lactation, or active liver disease
- Drug interactions: cyclosporine, macrolide antibiotics, various antifungal agents, HIV protease inhibitors, fibrates/nicotinic acid (to be used with caution)
- Adverse reactions:
  - Mild myalgia is common.
  - Liver transaminase elevations: ALT before therapy to establish baseline; if ALT >3 times upper limit of normal, do not start statin; routine monitoring is not recommended.
  - Association with increased cases of diabetes: 0.1 excess cases of diabetes per 100 persons on moderate-intensity statin and 0.3 excess cases per 100 persons on high-intensity statin
  - Myopathies (considered rare but not well studied):
    - Creatine kinase (CK) baseline reasonable for those at increased risk for adverse muscle events; routine monitoring not recommended
    - Instruct patients to report new onset of myalgias or weakness.
    - If myopathy or rhabdomyolysis is suspected, discontinue statin and draw serum CK, creatinine, and urine analysis.
    - Can rechallenge statin at lower dose or different type after resolution of symptoms
  - Statin intolerance
    - Consider use of a different statin.
    - Dose reduction
    - Alternate day therapy.
    - A majority of patients who had previously discontinued statins due to side effects are able to restart the same or another statin and tolerate them (6).

ALERT
FDA-alert: Simvastatin should no longer be prescribed at 80 mg/day doses due to increased risk of myopathy. Patients who have been at this drug dosage for >1 year can continue if no signs of myopathy. Dose restrictions to reduce myopathy risk include the following:
- Do not exceed simvastatin 10 mg/day with amiodarone, verapamil, and diltiazem.
- Do not exceed simvastatin 20 mg/day with amlodipine and ranolazine.

ALERT
Avoid grapefruit juice with statins, it increases the risk of statin myopathy.

Pregnancy Considerations
- Statins contraindicated during pregnancy: class X
- Lactation: possibly unsafe

Second Line
- Second-line drugs are no longer recommended for primary prevention due to lack of evidence of improved patient outcomes, especially in patients already on statin therapy (3)[C]. However, for secondary prevention in high-risk patients, adjunctive therapy may be indicated to lower LDL even more.
- Ezetimibe
  - Can be taken by itself or in combination with a statin: monotherapy (10 mg/day) or ezetimibe/simvastatin (10/10, 10/20, 10/40)
  - Effect: lowers LDL-C; one RCT shows combination therapy with statin has small benefit in reducing CV events and CV-related mortality after acute coronary syndromes.
  - Adverse reactions: generally well tolerated
- Fibrates
  - Types: gemfibrozil 600 mg BID, fenofibrate
  - Effect: most effective in lowering TG with moderate effect in lowering LDL and raising HDL. More recent studies fail to show benefit in most patients.
  - Contraindications: severe hepatic or renal insufficiency
  - Possible interactions: potentiates effects of warfarin and oral hypoglycemic agents
  - Adverse reactions: GI complaints; increased likelihood of gallstones
- Niacin raises HDL but no evidence for improved outcomes in recent trials and significant potential harms; should no longer be used in routine practice
- Bile acid sequestrant (e.g., cholestyramine) causes significant GI side effects, no evidence for improved outcomes, rarely used.
- Proprotein convertase subtilisin/kexin type 9 (PCSK9) inhibitors (e.g., alirociumab, evolocumab)
  - Monoclonal antibody requiring SC injections every 2 to 4 weeks
  - Current evidence shows decreased incidence of CVD in secondary prevention without affecting incidence of all-cause mortality; active research ongoing
  - Very expensive and unclear role in therapy at this time

COMPLEMENTARY & ALTERNATIVE MEDICINE
- Omega-3 fatty acids and fish oil intake:
  - Sources—fish oil (salmon), plants (flaxseed, canola oil, soybean oil, nuts)
  - Effect—mainly lowers TG level (dose dependent) but has some benefit in lowering LDL and raising HDL, although overall CV benefit and mortality reduction is uncertain
- β-Sitosterols and red yeast rice (contains small amount of natural lovastatin analogue) can reduce TC and LDL. However, there is significant variability across commercial preparations.

 ## ONGOING CARE

FOLLOW-UP RECOMMENDATIONS
Exercise: sustained exercise for 30 minutes, 3 to 4 times per week: increases HDL, lowers TC, and helps control weight

Patient Monitoring
- Routine monitoring of LDL levels in patients on statin is not necessary.
- Routine monitoring of LFTs is no longer recommended if initial ALT is within normal range.

REFERENCES
1. Centers for Disease Control and Prevention. High cholesterol facts. https://www.cdc.gov/cholesterol/facts.htm. Accessed September 28, 2018.
2. U.S. Preventive Services Task Force. Final recommendation statement: statin use for the primary prevention of cardiovascular disease in adults: preventive medication. https://www.uspreventiveservicestaskforce.org/Page/Document/RecommendationStatementFinal/statin-use-in-adults-preventive-medication1. Accessed September 28, 2018.
3. Stone NJ, Robinson JG, Lichtenstein AH, et al. 2013 ACC/AHA guideline on the treatment of blood cholesterol to reduce atherosclerotic cardiovascular risk in adults: a report of the American College of Cardiology/American Heart Association Task Force on Practice Guidelines. Circulation. 2014;129(25 Suppl 2):S1–S45.
4. National Institute for Health and Care Excellence. Cardiovascular disease: risk assessment and reduction, including lipid modification. https://www.nice.org.uk/guidance/cg181. Accessed September 28, 2018.
5. U.S. Veterans Affairs/Department of Defense. Clinical practice guideline: the management of dyslipidemia for cardiovascular risk reduction (lipids) 2014. https://www.healthquality.va.gov/guidelines/cd/lipids/index.asp. Accessed September 28, 2018.
6. Zhang H, Plutzky J, Skentzos S, et al. Discontinuation of statins in routine care settings: a cohort study. Ann Intern Med. 2013;158(7):526–534.

ADDITIONAL READING
Last AR, Ference JD, Menzel ER. Hyperlipidemia: drugs for cardiovascular risk reduction in adults. Am Fam Physician. 2017;95(2):78–87.

 ## SEE ALSO
Diabetes Mellitus, Type 2; Hypertension, Essential; Obesity

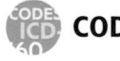 ## CODES
ICD10
E78.0 Pure hypercholesterolemia

CLINICAL PEARLS
- Hypercholesterolemia is a significant risk factor for ASCVD, but ASCVD is a multifactorial disease with many different risk factors.
- Diet and exercise should be tried before pharmaceutical interventions.
- Statins are considered first-line medications for hypercholesterolemia. Other medications show little evidence of benefit.

HYPEREMESIS GRAVIDARUM

Emma Brooks, MD

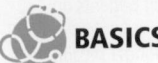

BASICS

DESCRIPTION
- Hyperemesis gravidarum is persistent vomiting in a pregnant woman that interferes with fluid and electrolyte balance as well as nutrition:
  - Usually associated with the first 8 to 20 weeks of pregnancy
  - Believed to have biomedical and behavioral aspects
  - Associated with high estrogen and human chorionic gonadotropin (hCG) levels
  - Symptoms usually begin ~2 weeks after first missed period.
- System(s) affected: endocrine/metabolic; gastrointestinal; reproductive
- Synonym(s): morning sickness

Pregnancy Considerations
Common condition during pregnancy, typically in the 1st and 2nd trimesters but may persist into the 3rd trimester

EPIDEMIOLOGY
Incidence
Hyperemesis gravidarum occurs in 1–2% of pregnancies.

Prevalence
Hyperemesis gravidarum is the most common cause of hospitalization in the first half of pregnancy and the second most common cause of hospitalization of pregnant women.

ETIOLOGY AND PATHOPHYSIOLOGY
- Unknown
- Possible psychological factors
- Hyperthyroidism
- Hyperparathyroidism
- Gestational hormones
- Liver dysfunction
- Autonomic nervous system dysfunction
- CNS neoplasm
- Addison disease

RISK FACTORS
- Obesity
- Nulliparity
- Multiple gestations
- Gestational trophoblastic disease
- Gonadotropin production stimulated
- Altered GI function
- Hyperthyroidism
- Hyperparathyroidism
- Liver dysfunction
- Female fetus
- *Helicobacter pylori* infection

GENERAL PREVENTION
Anticipatory guidance in 1st and 2nd trimesters regarding dietary habits in hopes of avoiding dehydration and nutritional depletion

Pregnancy Considerations
- 2% of pregnancies have electrolyte disturbances.
- 50% of pregnancies have at least some GI disturbance.

COMMONLY ASSOCIATED CONDITIONS
Hyperthyroidism

DIAGNOSIS

HISTORY
- Hypersensitivity to smell
- Alteration in taste
- Excessive salivation
- Poor appetite
- Nausea
- Vomiting with retching
- Decreased urine output
- Fatigue
- Dizziness with standing

DIAGNOSTIC TESTS & INTERPRETATION
Initial Tests (lab, imaging)
- Urinalysis: may see glucosuria, albuminuria, granular casts, and hematuria (rare); ketosis more common
- Thyroid-stimulating hormone (TSH), T_4
- Electrolytes, BUN, creatinine:
  - Electrolyte abnormalities due to nausea and vomiting and subsequent dehydration
  - Acidosis
- Calcium
- Uric acid
- Albumin
- No imaging is indicated for the diagnosis of hyperemesis gravidarum unless there is concern for hydatidiform mole or multiple gestation, in which case ultrasound may be obtained.

Follow-Up Tests & Special Considerations
- If hypercalcemia, consider checking parathyroid hormone (PTH) for hyperparathyroidism.
- Drugs are unlikely to alter lab results.

Diagnostic Procedures/Other
Indicated only if it is necessary to rule out other diagnoses, as listed in the following section

DIFFERENTIAL DIAGNOSIS
Other common causes of vomiting must be considered:
- Gastroenteritis
- Gastritis
- Reflux esophagitis
- Peptic ulcer disease
- Cholelithiasis
- Cholecystitis
- Pyelonephritis
- Anxiety
- Hyperparathyroidism
- *H. pylori* infection

TREATMENT

Pyridoxine and doxylamine (pregnancy Category A) are first-line treatments for hyperemesis gravidarum (1)[C]. This is followed by metoclopramide or ondansetron (pregnancy Category B) and then prochlorperazine (pregnancy Category C), methylprednisolone (pregnancy Category C), or promethazine (pregnancy Category C).

GENERAL MEASURES
- Patient reassurance
- Bed rest
- If dehydrated, IV fluids, either normal saline or 5% dextrose normal saline (with consideration for potential thiamine deficiency). Repeat if there is a recurrence of symptoms following initial improvement.
- For severe cases, consider PO thiamine 25 to 50 mg TID or IV 100 mg in 100 mL of normal saline over 30 minutes once weekly and potential parental nutrition if needed.
- Ondansetron carries an FDA warning regarding concerns for QT prolongation, but this is in the setting of high-dose IV administration and in patients with heart disease. It has unclear risk in the setting of pregnancy. The majority of the current studies appear to show no increased risk of fetal malformation with the use of ondansetron, but this is still an area of controversy.

MEDICATION
- Pyridoxine (vitamin B_6) 25 mg PO or IV every 8 hours
- Antihistamines (e.g., diphenhydramine [25 to 50 mg q4–6h] or doxylamine [12.5 mg PO BID]) (2)[C]
- Combination product Diclegis (sustained-release pyridoxine 10 mg and doxylamine 10 mg) dosed (start 2 tabs PO QHS; if symptoms persist, increase to 1 tab in AM and 2 QHS; if symptoms still persist, take 1 tab q AM, 1 midday, and 2 QHS; max 4 tablets/day)
- Phenothiazines (e.g., promethazine or prochlorperazine):
  - Precautions: Phenothiazines are associated with prolonged jaundice, extrapyramidal effects, and hyper- or hyporeflexia in newborns.
- Meclizine 25 mg PO q6h
- Metoclopramide 10 mg PO q6–8h

- Methylprednisolone 16 mg PO/IV q8h for 2 to 3 days and then taper over 2 weeks if initial 3-day treatment is effective; reserved for severe cases with unclear benefit
- Ondansetron 4 to 8 mg PO q8h

Pregnancy Considerations
All medications taken during pregnancy should balance the risks and benefits both to the mother and the fetus.

COMPLEMENTARY & ALTERNATIVE MEDICINE
- Ginger 350 mg PO TID may help (3)[A].
- Evidence is mixed regarding the impact of acupressure and acupuncture in treating hyperemesis gravidarum. Acupressure bands at the Neiguan point are effective adjuvant treatment in severe hyperemesis (4)[A].
- Medical hypnosis may be a helpful adjunct to the typical medical treatment regimen, but further study is needed.

ADMISSION, INPATIENT, AND NURSING CONSIDERATIONS
- Typically outpatient therapy
- In some severe cases, parenteral therapy in the hospital or at home may be required.
- Enteral volume and nutrition repletion may be indicated, but early enteral tube feeding does not improve maternal or perinatal outcomes (5)[A].

 ONGOING CARE

FOLLOW-UP RECOMMENDATIONS
- Activity as tolerated after improvement
- Overall quality of life and future fertility plans can be impacted by severity of nausea and vomiting (6)[B].

Patient Monitoring
- In severe cases, follow-up on a daily basis for weight monitoring
- Special attention should be given to monitor for ketosis, hypokalemia, or acid–base disturbances due to hyperemesis.

DIET
- NPO for first 24 hours if patient is ill enough to require hospitalization
- For outpatient: a diet rich in carbohydrates and protein, such as fruit, cheese, cottage cheese, eggs, beef, poultry, vegetables, toast, crackers, rice. Limit intake of butter. Patients should avoid spicy meals and high-fat foods. Consider cold foods. Encourage small amounts at a time every 1 to 2 hours.

PATIENT EDUCATION
- Attention should be given to psychosocial issues, such as possible ambivalence about the pregnancy.
- Patients should be instructed to take small amounts of fluid frequently to avoid volume depletion.

- Avoid individual foods known to be irritating to the patient.
- Wet-to-dry nutrients (sherbet, broth, gelatin to dry crackers, toast)

PROGNOSIS
- Self-limited illness with good prognosis if patient's weight is maintained at >95% of prepregnancy weight
- With complication of hemorrhagic retinitis, mortality rate of pregnant patient is 50%.

COMPLICATIONS
- Patients with >5% weight loss are associated with intrauterine growth retardation and fetal anomalies.
- Poor weight gain is associated with slightly increased risk for small for gestational age infant <2,500 g and premature birth <37 weeks (7)[A].
- Hemorrhagic retinitis
- Liver damage
- CNS deterioration, Wernicke encephalopathy secondary to thiamine deficiency, coma

REFERENCES
1. Maltepe C, Koren G. The management of nausea and vomiting of pregnancy and hyperemesis gravidarum—a 2013 update. *J Popul Ther Clin Pharmacol*. 2013;20(2):e184–e192.
2. Boelig RC, Barton SJ, Saccone G, et al. Interventions for treating hyperemesis gravidarum. *Cochrane Database Syst Rev*. 2016;(5):CD010607.
3. Viljoen E, Visser J, Koen N, et al. A systematic review and meta-analysis of the effect and safety of ginger in the treatment of pregnancy-associated nausea and vomiting. *Nutr J*. 2014;13:20.
4. Adlan A, Chooi K, Mat Adenan N. Acupressure as adjuvant treatment for the inpatient management of nausea and vomiting in early pregnancy: a double-blind randomized controlled trial. *J Obstet Gynaecol Res*. 2017;43(4):662–668.
5. Grooten I, Koot M, van der Post J, et al. Early enteral tube feeding in optimizing treatment of hyperemesis gravidarum: the Maternal and Offspring outcomes after Treatment of HyperEmesis by Refeeding (MOTHER) randomized controlled trial. *Am J Clin Nutr*. 2017;106(3):812–820.
6. Heitmann K, Nordeng H, Havnen GC, et al. The burden of nausea and vomiting during pregnancy: severe impacts on quality of life, daily life functioning and willingness to become pregnant again—results from a cross-sectional study. *BMC Pregnancy Childbirth*. 2017;17(1):75.
7. Veenendaal MV, van Abeelen AF, Painter RC, et al. Consequences of hyperemesis gravidarum for offspring: a systematic review and meta-analysis. *BJOG*. 2011;118(11):1302–1313.

ADDITIONAL READING
- Abas MN, Tan PC, Azmi N, et al. Ondansetron compared with metoclopramide for hyperemesis gravidarum: a randomized controlled trial. *Obstet Gynecol*. 2014;123(6):1272–1279.
- Anderka M, Mitchell AA, Louik C, et al. Medications used to treat nausea and vomiting of pregnancy and the risk of selected birth defects. *Birth Defects Res A Clin Mol Teratol*. 2012;94(1):22–30.
- Boelig R, Barton S, Saccone G, et al. Interventions for treating hyperemesis gravidarum: a Cochrane systematic review and meta-analysis. *J Matern Fetal Neonatal Med*. 2018;31(18):2492–2505.
- Jarvis S, Nelson-Piercy C. Management of nausea and vomiting in pregnancy. *BMJ*. 2011;342:d3606.
- Matthews A, Haas DM, O'Mathúna DP, et al. Interventions for nausea and vomiting in early pregnancy. *Cochrane Database Syst Rev*. 2015;(9):CD007575.
- McCarthy FP, Lutomski JE, Greene RA. Hyperemesis gravidarum: current perspectives. *Int J Womens Health*. 2014;6:719–725.
- McCormack D. Hypnosis for hyperemesis gravidarum. *J Obstet Gynaecol*. 2010;30(7):647–653.
- McParlin C, O'Donnell A, Robson S, et al. Treatments for hyperemesis gravidarum and nausea and vomiting in pregnancy: a systematic review. *JAMA*. 2016;316(13):1392–1401.
- Pasternak B, Svanström H, Hviid A. Ondansetron in pregnancy and risk of adverse fetal outcomes. *N Engl J Med*. 2013;368(9):814–823.
- Tan PC, Omar SZ. Contemporary approaches to hyperemesis during pregnancy. *Curr Opin Obstet Gynecol*. 2011;23(2):87–93.

 CODES

ICD10
- O21.9 Vomiting of pregnancy, unspecified
- O21.0 Mild hyperemesis gravidarum
- O21.1 Hyperemesis gravidarum with metabolic disturbance

CLINICAL PEARLS
- Do not allow patients to become volume depleted. Once this occurs, it is more difficult to interrupt the process.
- Do not be hesitant to use medications to assist the patient because this may help avoid volume depletion.
- Consider secondary causes of hyperemesis if it develops after 12 weeks of gestation.

H

HYPERKALEMIA

Merima Bucaj, DO, FAAFP • Roselyn Jan W. Clemente-Fuentes, MD, FAAFP • Ian J. McDowell, DO

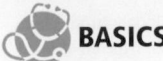

BASICS

DESCRIPTION
- Hyperkalemia is a common electrolyte disorder that may be defined as a plasma potassium (K) concentration >5.5 mEq/L (>5 mmol/L).
- Hyperkalemia depresses cardiac conduction and can lead to fatal arrhythmias.
- Normal K regulation
  - Ingested K enters portal circulation; pancreas releases insulin in response. Insulin facilitates K entry into cells.
  - K in renal circulation causes renin release from juxtaglomerular cells, leading to activation of angiotensin I, which is converted to angiotensin II in lungs. Angiotensin II acts in adrenal zona glomerulosa to stimulate aldosterone secretion. Aldosterone, at the renal collecting ducts, causes K to be excreted and sodium to be retained.
- Four major causes
  - Increased load: either endogenous from tissue release or exogenous from a high intake, usually in association with decreased excretion
  - Decreased excretion: due to decreased glomerular filtration rate or impaired aldosterone secretion
  - Cellular redistribution: shifts from intracellular space (majority of K is intracellular) to extracellular space
  - Pseudohyperkalemia: related to red cell lysis during collection or transport of blood sample, thrombocytosis, or leukocytosis

Geriatric Considerations
Increased risk for hyperkalemia because of decreases in renin and aldosterone as well as comorbid conditions

EPIDEMIOLOGY
Prevalence
- 1–10% of hospitalized patients
- 2–3% in general population but as high as 50% in patients with chronic kidney disease (1)
- Predominant sex: male = female
- No age-related predilection

ETIOLOGY AND PATHOPHYSIOLOGY
- Pseudohyperkalemia
  - Hemolysis of red cells in phlebotomy tube (spurious result is most common)
  - Thrombolysis
  - Leukocytosis
  - Thrombocytosis
  - Hereditary spherocytosis
  - Infectious mononucleosis
  - Traumatic venipuncture or fist clenching during phlebotomy (spurious result)
  - Familial pseudohyperkalemia
- Transcellular shift (redistribution)
  - Metabolic acidosis
  - Insulin deficiency
  - Hyperglycemia (diabetic ketoacidosis or hyperosmolar hyperglycemic state)
  - Tissue damage (rhabdomyolysis, burns, trauma)
  - Tumor lysis syndrome

- Cocaine abuse
- Exercise with heavy sweating
- Mannitol
- Impaired K excretion
  - Renal insufficiency/failure
  - Addison disease
  - Mineralocorticoid deficiency
  - Primary hyporeninemia, primary hypoaldosteronism
  - Type IV renal tubular acidosis (hyporeninemic hypoaldosteronism)
  - Obstructive uropathy
  - Cirrhosis
  - Congestive heart failure
  - Sickle cell disease
  - Amyloidosis
  - Systemic lupus erythematosus
- Medication-induced
  - Excess K supplementation
  - Statins
  - ACE inhibitors
  - Angiotensin receptor blockers
  - β-Blockers
  - Cyclosporine
  - Digoxin toxicity
  - Ethinyl estradiol/drospirenone
  - Heparin
  - Lithium
  - NSAIDs
  - Penicillin G potassium
  - Pentamidine
  - Spironolactone
  - Succinylcholine
  - Tacrolimus
  - Trimethoprim, particularly with other medications associated with hyperkalemia (2)

Genetics
Associated with some inherited diseases and conditions
- Familial hyperkalemic periodic paralysis
- Congenital adrenal hyperplasia

RISK FACTORS
- Impaired renal excretion of K
- Acidemia
- Massive cell breakdown (rhabdomyolysis, burns, trauma)
- Use of K-sparing diuretics
- Excess K supplementation
- Comorbid conditions: chronic kidney disease, diabetes, heart failure, liver disease

GENERAL PREVENTION
Low K diet and oral supplement compliance in those at risk

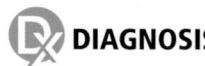

DIAGNOSIS

HISTORY
- Neuromuscular cramps
- Abdominal pain
- Palpitations

- Myalgias
- Numbness
- Muscle weakness or paralysis

PHYSICAL EXAM
- Decreased deep tendon reflexes
- Flaccid paralysis of extremities

DIAGNOSTIC TESTS & INTERPRETATION
- Serum electrolytes
- Renal function: BUN, creatinine
- Urinalysis: K, creatinine, osmoles (to calculate fractional excretion of K and transtubular K gradient; both assess renal handling of K)
- Disorders that may alter lab results
  - Acidemia: K shifts from the intracellular to extracellular space.
  - Insulin deficiency
  - Hemolysis of sample
- Cortisol, aldosterone, and renin levels to check for mineralocorticoid deficiency when other causes are ruled out

Diagnostic Procedures/Other
ECG abnormalities usually occur when K ≥7 mEq/L.
- Peaked T wave with shortened QT interval in precordial leads (most common, usually earliest ECG change; however, neither sensitive nor specific) (3)
- Lengthening of PR interval
- Loss of P wave
- Widened QRS
- Sine wave at very high K
- Can eventually lead to arrhythmias including bradycardia, ventricular fibrillation, and asystole

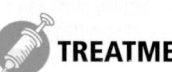

TREATMENT

MEDICATION
- Stabilize myocardial membranes; initial treatment with calcium gluconate IV 1,000 mg (10 mL of 10% solution) over 2 to 3 minutes (2)[A]
  - With constant cardiac monitoring
  - Can repeat after 5 minutes if needed
  - Effect begins within minutes but only lasts 30 to 60 minutes and should be used in conjunction with definitive therapies.
  - Can also use calcium chloride (3 times as concentrated; however, central or deep vein administration is necessary to avoid tissue necrosis).
- Drive extracellular K into cells
  - Nebulized albuterol (at 10 to 20 mg/4 mL saline >10 minutes—4 to 8 times bronchodilation dose) and other β-agonists have an additive effect with insulin and glucose (2)[B].
  - Dextrose 50% 1 amp (if plasma glucose <250 mg/dL) and insulin 10 U IV may drive K intracellularly but does not decrease total body K and may result in hypoglycemia (close monitoring advised, especially 1 to 2 hours postinjection) (2)[B].
  - Sodium bicarbonate not routinely recommended but some possible benefits in severe metabolic acidosis (4)[C]

- Remove excess K from body.
  - Cation exchange resins definitive treatment but require several doses and best used with rapidly acting transient therapies above and when dialysis not readily available (5)[A]
  - Gastrointestinal cation exchangers, patiromer calcium (Veltassa), sodium polystyrene sulfonate (Kayexalate), and zirconium cyclosilicate bind K in the intestinal tract. Patiromer in particular is favored for improved tolerance and decreased side effects in both acute and chronic settings (6)[C].
  - Patiromer calcium (Veltassa): 8.4 g PO daily (dose may vary 4.2 to 16.8 g BID in studies)
    - This requires ~7 to 24 hours to lower K. This may be repeated q12h, if necessary (7)[C].
  - Sodium polystyrene sulfonate (Kayexalate): 15 g PO or 30 g rectally
    - This requires 1 to 4 hours to lower K. This may be repeated q6h, if necessary.
    - Enema has faster effect than PO (2)[C].
  - Hemodialysis is the definitive therapy when other measures are not effective. This may be required particularly when conditions, such as digitalis toxicity, rhabdomyolysis, end-stage renal disease, severe chronic kidney disease, or acute kidney injury, are present; should watch for postdialysis rebound (2)[A]
  - Little clinical evidence for the use of diuretics (loop and thiazides), however, can consider for control of chronic hyperkalemia (2)[B]

ALERT

- Sodium polystyrene sulfonate provides a sodium load that may exacerbate fluid overload in patients with cardiac or renal failure.
- Avoid sodium polystyrene sulfonate use in patients who are postoperative or with a bowel obstruction or ileus due to high risk of intestinal necrosis.
- Rapid administration of calcium in patients with suspected digitalis toxicity may result in a fatal dysrhythmia. Calcium should be administered slowly over 20 to 30 minutes in 5% dextrose with extreme caution. Preferred therapy is digoxin-specific antibody fragments.

ADMISSION, INPATIENT, AND NURSING CONSIDERATIONS

- If hyperkalemia is severe, treat first and then do diagnostic investigations.
- Consider early consultation of nephrologist.
- IV calcium to stabilize myocardium (caution in setting of digoxin toxicity because definitive treatment may cause hypokalemia)
- Insulin (usually 10 U IV, given with 50 mL of 50% glucose [if serum glucose <250 mg/dL] to avoid hypoglycemia); consider repeating if elevation persists.
- Inhaled β_2-agonist (nebulized albuterol)
- Discontinue any medications that may increase K (e.g., K-sparing diuretics, exogenous K).
- Admit for cardiac monitoring if ECG changes are present or if K is >6 mEq/L (6 mmol/L).

 ## ONGOING CARE

FOLLOW-UP RECOMMENDATIONS
Patient Monitoring
- Reduction of plasma K should begin within the first hour of treatment initiation.
- Serum K levels should be rechecked every 2 to 4 hours until the patient has stabilized, and recurrent hyperkalemia is no longer a threat.
- Identification and elimination of possible causes and risk factors for hyperkalemia are essential.

DIET
Recommend ≤80 mEq (≤80 mmol) of K per 24 hours. Many foods contain K. Those that are particularly high in K (>6.4 mEq/serving) include bananas, orange juice, other citrus fruits and their juices, figs, molasses, seaweed, dried fruits, nuts, avocados, lima beans, bran, tomatoes, tomato juice, cantaloupe, honeydew melon, peaches, potatoes, and salt substitutes. Multiple herbal medications can also increase K levels, including alfalfa, dandelion, horsetail nettle, milkweed, hawthorn berries, toad skin, oleander, foxglove, and ginseng.

PATIENT EDUCATION
Consult with a dietitian about a low-K diet.

PROGNOSIS
- Associated with poor prognosis in patients with heart failure and chronic kidney disease
- Associated with poor prognosis in disaster medicine, with trauma, tissue necrosis, K^+ supplementation, metabolic acidosis, if calcium gluconate administered for treatment of hyperkalemia, if AKI, or if prolonged duration of hyperkalemia (4)

COMPLICATIONS
- Life-threatening cardiac arrhythmias
- Hypokalemia
- Potential complications of the use of ion-exchange resins for the treatment of hyperkalemia include volume overload and intestinal necrosis (6)[C].

REFERENCES

1. Palmer BF, Clegg DJ. Hyperkalemia. *JAMA*. 2015;314(22):2405–2406.
2. Viera AJ, Wouk N. Potassium disorders: hypokalemia and hyperkalemia. *Am Fam Physician*. 2015;92(6):487–495.
3. Wong R, Banker R, Aronowitz P. Electrocardiographic changes of severe hyperkalemia. *J Hosp Med*. 2011;6(4):240.
4. Khanagavi J, Gupta T, Aronow WS, et al. Hyperkalemia among hospitalized patients and association between duration of hyperkalemia and outcomes. *Arch Med Sci*. 2014;10(2):251–257.
5. Sterns RH, Rojas M, Bernstein P, et al. Ion-exchange resins for the treatment of hyperkalemia: are they safe and effective? *J Am Soc Nephrol*. 2010;21(5):733–735.
6. Ingelfinger JR. A new era for the treatment of hyperkalemia? *N Engl J Med*. 2015;372(3):275–277.
7. Bushinsky DA, Williams GH, Pitt B, et al. Patiromer induces rapid and sustain potassium lowering in patients with chronic kidney disease and hyperkalemia. *Kidney Int*. 2015;88(6):1427–1433.

ADDITIONAL READING

- Harel Z, Harel S, Shah PS, et al. Gastrointestinal adverse events with sodium polystyrene sulfonate (Kayexalate) use: a systematic review. *Am J Med*. 2013;126(3):264.e9–264.e24.
- Jain N, Kotla S, Little BB, et al. Predictors of hyperkalemia and death in patients with cardiac and renal disease. *Am J Cardiol*. 2012;109(10):1510–1513.
- Mahoney BA, Smith WA, Lo DS, et al. Emergency interventions for hyperkalaemia. *Cochrane Database Syst Rev*. 2005;(2):CD003235.
- Noori N, Kalantar-Zadeh K, Kovesdy CP, et al. Dietary potassium intake and mortality in long-term hemodialysis patients. *Am J Kidney Dis*. 2010;56(2):338–347.
- Pepin J, Shields C. Advances in diagnosis and management of hypokalemic and hyperkalemic emergencies. *Emerg Med Pract*. 2012;14(2):1–18.
- Riccardi A, Tasso F, Corti L, et al. The emergency physician and the prompt management of severe hyperkalemia. *Intern Emerg Med*. 2012;7(Suppl 2):S131–S133.
- Weisberg LS. Management of severe hyperkalemia. *Crit Care Med*. 2008;36(12):3246–3251.

 ### SEE ALSO

- Addison Disease; Hypokalemia
- Algorithm: Hyperkalemia

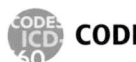 ## CODES

ICD10
E87.5 Hyperkalemia

CLINICAL PEARLS

- Emergency and urgent management of hyperkalemia takes precedent to a thorough diagnostic workup. Urgent treatment includes stabilization of the myocardium with calcium gluconate to protect against arrhythmias and pharmacologic strategies to move K from the extracellular (vascular) space into cells.
- Calcium and dextrose/insulin are only temporizing measures and do not actually lower total body K levels; definitive treatment with either dialysis or cation exchange resin (sodium polystyrene sulfonate) necessary
- To lower a patient's risk of developing hyperkalemia, have the patient follow a low-K diet, use selective β_1-blockers, such as metoprolol or atenolol, instead of nonselective β-blockers such as carvedilol. Avoid NSAIDs. Concomitant use of kaliuretic loop diuretics may be useful.

H

HYPERNATREMIA

Sasmit Roy, MD, MBBS • Pang-Yen Fan, MD

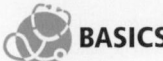 **BASICS**

DESCRIPTION
- Serum sodium (Na) concentration >145 mEq/L (1)
- Usually represents a state of hypertonicity (1,2)
- Na concentration reflects balance between total body water (TBW) and total body Na. Hypernatremia occurs from deficit of water relative to Na.
- Hypernatremia results from net water loss or, more rarely, from primary Na gain (1).
- May exist with hypo-, hyper-, or euvolemia, although hypovolemia is by far most common type
  - Hypovolemic: occurs with a decrease in TBW and a proportionately smaller decrease in total body Na
  - Euvolemic: no change in TBW with a proportionate increase in total body Na
  - Hypervolemic: increase in TBW and a proportionately greater increase in total body Na
- It has been shown to be an indicator for higher mortality in critically ill patients and patients with chronic kidney disease (CKD) (3)[B].
- Hypernatremia will not develop if thirst mechanism is intact and water is available.

EPIDEMIOLOGY
Incidence
- More common in elderly and young
- Occurs in 1% of hospitalized elderly patients (4)
- Seen in about 9% of ICU patients (4). Gastroenteritis with diarrhea is the most common cause of hypernatremia in infants.
- Women are at an increased risk due to decreased TBW, as compared with men.

ETIOLOGY AND PATHOPHYSIOLOGY
- Water loss (total body Na normal). Hypernatremia due to water loss occurs only in patients who can't access water such as infants, elderly, patients with altered mental status and hypodipsia (5).This is called dehydration and differs from hypovolemia where both salt and water are lost. The following conditions lead to water loss:
  - Insensible loss
    - Burns
    - Hyperventilation
    - Excessive sweating, such as with fever, infants under radiant heaters, and exercise
  - Renal loss
    - Nephrogenic diabetes insipidus (DI) (congenital or due to renal dysfunction, hypercalcemia, hypokalemia, medication-related, e.g., lithium)
    - Central DI (due to head trauma, stroke, meningitis) (4)
    - Osmotic diuresis: glucose, urea, and mannitol
    - Post-ATN diuresis
  - Gastrointestinal loss
    - Osmotic diarrhea: lactulose, malabsorption, and some types of infectious diarrhea
    - Enterocutaneous fistula
    - Vomiting, NG suction
  - Hypothalamic disorders leading to impaired thirst or osmoreceptor function
    - Primary hypodipsia

- Reset osmostat due to volume expansion in mineralocorticoid excess.
- Essential hypernatremia with loss of osmoreceptor function
- Excess Na (increase in total body Na) resulting from the following:
  - IV NaCl or NaHCO₃ during cardiopulmonary resuscitation, metabolic acidosis, or hyperkalemia (4)
  - Sea water ingestion
  - Excessive use of NaHCO₃ antacid
  - Incorrect infant formula preparation
  - Intrauterine NaCl for abortion
  - Excessive Na in dialysate solutions
  - Disorders of the adrenal axis (Cushing syndrome, Conn syndrome, congenital adrenal hyperplasia)
  - Tube feeding
- With acute hypernatremia, the rapid decrease in brain volume can cause rupture of the cerebral veins, leading to focal intracerebral and subarachnoid hemorrhages and possibly irreversible neurologic damage (2).

Genetics
Some forms of DI may be hereditary.

RISK FACTORS
- Patients at increased risk include those with an impaired thirst mechanism or restricted access to water as well as those with increased water loss
- Infants/children
- Elderly patients (may also have a diminished thirst response to osmotic stimulation via an unknown mechanism)
- Patients who are intubated/have altered mental status
- Diabetes mellitus
- Prior brain injury
- Surgery
- Diuretic therapy, especially loop diuretics
- Lithium treatment

GENERAL PREVENTION
- Treatment/prevention of underlying cause
- Properly prepare infant formula and never add salt to any commercial infant formula.
- Keep patients well hydrated.

COMMONLY ASSOCIATED CONDITIONS
- Gastroenteritis
- Altered mental status
- Burns
- Hypermetabolic conditions
- Head injury
- Renal dysfunction

 **DIAGNOSIS**

HISTORY
- Excessive thirst, nausea, vomiting, diarrhea, oliguria, polyuria
- Fever, myalgia, muscle weakness
- Neurologic symptoms common: altered mental status, seizure (especially if rapid development of hypernatremia), twitching, lethargy, irritability, coma, anophthalmos

- Severe symptoms are likely to occur with acute increases in plasma Na levels or at concentrations >160 mEq/L.
- Obtain list of current and recent medications.
- Review recent illnesses and activities.

PHYSICAL EXAM
- Sinus tachycardia, hypotension, orthostatic hypotension, poor O₂ saturation
- Dry mucous membranes, cool/gray skin
- Neurologic abnormalities: lethargy, weakness, focal deficits (in cases of intracerebral bleeding/lesion), confusion, coma, seizures

DIFFERENTIAL DIAGNOSIS
- DI
- Hyperosmotic coma
- Salt ingestion
- Hypertonic dehydration
- Hypothyroidism
- Cushing syndrome

DIAGNOSTIC TESTS & INTERPRETATION
Initial Tests (lab, imaging)
- Serum Na, potassium, BUN, creatinine, calcium, and osmolality (serum lithium if appropriate)
- Urine Na and osmolality
  - DI: urine osmolality (usually <300 mOsmol/kg) < serum osmolality, and urine Na usually low normal/slightly low (due to dilution) (5)
  - Partial DI and central DI with volume depletion can give a urine osmolarity of 300 to 800 mOsm/kg.
  - Osmotic diuresis: urine osmolality intermediate, urine Na low/low-normal, total daily osmole excretion high
  - Salt ingestion: increased urine osmolality (>600 mOsmol/kg) and high urine Na
  - Hypertonic dehydration: increased urine osmolality and decreased urine Na
- Serum glucose
- Special tests for DI
  - Water deprivation test: In DI, urine osmolality does not increase because it normally should when hypernatremic.
  - Antidiuretic hormone (ADH) stimulation: distinguishes central versus nephrogenic DI
    - Urine osmolality does not increase after ADH or desmopressin in nephrogenic DI.
- Head CT/MRI in DI to rule out craniopharyngioma, other brain tumor or masses, or median cleft syndrome

Diagnostic Procedures/Other
History, physical, laboratory studies, family history for central DI

 **TREATMENT**

GENERAL MEASURES
- The treatment of hypernatremia involves treating the underlying cause and correcting the water deficit.
- Goal for corrected Na is 145 mEq/L (1).

- Speed of correction depends on symptom severity and rate of development of hypernatremia. Avoid rapid correction to prevent development of cerebral edema if chronic hypernatremia (>24 hours):
  – Maximum of 0.5 mEq/L/hr or 10 mEq/L/day
  – May correct at up to 1 mEq/L/hr if acute hypernatremia (<24 hours) (1)
- Treat volume depletion first and then hypernatremia:
  – Restore intravascular volume with IV fluids to normalize serum Na levels.
- Replace water orally if patient is conscious.
- Important formulas in determining rate of fluid administration
  – TBW = coefficient × wt (kg), where coefficient = 0.6 for men and children, 0.5 for women and elderly men, 0.45 for elderly women
  – Calculated free water deficit (liters) = TBW × (PNa / 140 − 1), where PNa = plasma Na+, TBW = total body water
  – Change in serum Na per 1 L infusate = [(infusate Na + infusate K) − serum Na] / (TBW + 1)
  – Example: A 45-year-old male weighing 70 kg is admitted with head injury. Labs show a serum Na of 160.
    ◦ Free water deficit = 70 × 0.6 × (160 / 140 − 1) = 6 L
    ◦ Remember the 6 L should be given over a 48-hour period to avoid over correction.
- Account for ongoing fluid losses during calculation of rate of fluid administration (i.e., insensible water loss through skin and water lost through urine, stool).
- Dialysis can be considered if acute kidney injury is present concomitantly and if conventional treatment has failed (6)[B].

MEDICATION

First Line
- See "General Measures" for overall approach.
- Volume depletion: Use isotonic fluids initially if signs of hemodynamic compromise and then change to hypotonic fluids when stable:
  – Hypotonic fluids (0.45% NaCl or dextrose 5% in water)
    ◦ Important not to decrease serum Na by >10 mEq/L/day to prevent cerebral edema (5)[C]
- Hypervolemia: Give furosemide along with hypotonic fluids. Dose varies depending on desired urine output. Loop diuretics with fluid restriction worsen hypernatremia (5)[C].
- Central DI
  – Desmopressin acetate (DDAVP): Use parenteral form for acute symptomatic patients, and use intranasal or oral form for chronic therapy (5).
  – Free water replacement: may use 2.5% dextrose in water if giving large volumes of water in DI to avoid glycosuria
  – May consider sulfonylureas/thiazide diuretics for chronic but not acute treatment
- Nephrogenic DI
  – Treat with diuretics and NSAIDs.
  – Lithium-induced nephrogenic DI: hydrochlorothiazide 25 mg PO BID or indomethacin 50 mg PO TID, or amiloride hydrochloride 5 to 10 mg PO BID

- Precautions
  – Rapid correction of hypernatremia can cause cerebral edema, central pontine myelinolysis, seizures, or death.
  – Hypocalcemia and more rarely acidosis can occur during correction.
  – DI: High rates of dextrose 5% in water can cause hyperglycemia and glucose-induced diuresis.

Second Line
- Consider NSAIDs in nephrogenic DI.
- Modalities requiring further investigations
- Continuous renal replacement therapy (CRRT): Multiple case reports and case series have shown success and safety in using CRRT to treat hypernatremia in critically ill patients with CHF and severe burns (6).

ISSUES FOR REFERRAL
Underlying renal involvement associated with hypernatremia would benefit from a nephrology referral.

ADMISSION, INPATIENT, AND NURSING CONSIDERATIONS
- Symptomatic patient with serum Na >155 mEq/L requires IV fluid therapy.
- IV fluids: Refer to "Medication" section.
- Bed rest until stable or underlying condition resolved/controlled
- Discharge criteria: Stabilization of serum Na level and symptoms are minimal.

 ONGOING CARE

FOLLOW-UP RECOMMENDATIONS
Patient Monitoring
- Frequent reexams in an acute setting
- Frequent electrolytes and blood glucose: initially q4–6h
- Urine osmolality and urine output in DI
- Ensure adequate ingestion of calories because patients may ingest so much water that they feel full and do not eat.
- Measure ongoing losses of water and solute and replace as needed.
- Daily weights

DIET
- Ensure proper nutrition during acute phase.
- After resolution of acute phase, may want to consider Na-restricted diet for patient
- Low-salt, low-protein diet in nephrogenic DI

PATIENT EDUCATION
Patients with nephrogenic DI must avoid salt and drink large amounts of water.

PROGNOSIS
Most recover but neurologic impairment can occur.

COMPLICATIONS
- CNS thrombosis/hemorrhage
- Seizures
- Mental retardation
- Hyperactivity
- Chronic hypernatremia: >2 days duration has higher mortality.
- Serum Na >180 mEq/L (>180 mmol/L): often results in residual CNS damage
- More common if rapid development of hypernatremia

REFERENCES
1. Adrogué HJ, Madias NE. Hypernatremia. *N Engl J Med*. 2000;342(20):1493–1499.
2. Sterns RH. Disorders of plasma sodium—causes, consequences, and correction. *N Engl J Med*. 2015;372(1):55–65.
3. Kovesdy CP, Lott EH, Lu JL, et al. Hyponatremia, hypernatremia, and mortality in patients with chronic kidney disease with and without congestive heart failure. *Circulation*. 2012;125(5):677–684.
4. Bagshaw SM, Townsend DR, McDermid RC. Disorders of sodium and water balance in hospitalized patients. *Can J Anaesth*. 2009;56(2):151–167.
5. Hannon MJ, Finucane FM, Sherlock M, et al. Clinical review: disorders of water homeostasis in neurosurgical patients. *J Clin Endocrinol Metab*. 2012;97(5):1423–1433.
6. Huang C, Zhang P, Du R, et al. Treatment of acute hypernatremia in severely burned patients using continuous veno-venous hemofiltration with gradient sodium replacement fluid: a report of nine cases. *Intensive Care Med*. 2013;39(8):1495–1496.

ADDITIONAL READING
Waite MD, Fuhrman SA, Badawi O, et al. Intensive care unit–acquired hypernatremia is an independent predictor of increased mortality and length of stay. *J Crit Care*. 2013;28(4):405–412.

 SEE ALSO

- Diabetes Insipidus
- Algorithm: Hypernatremia

CODES

ICD10
E87.0 Hyperosmolality and hypernatremia

CLINICAL PEARLS

- Occurs from water deficit in comparison to total body Na stores
- Common causes include dehydration, DI, impaired access to fluids.
- Determine if the patient has hypervolemic, euvolemic, or hypovolemic hypernatremia in the differential diagnosis of etiology; most commonly hypovolemic; other entities rare
- Avoid rapid correction of hypernatremia to prevent development of cerebral edema when hypernatremia is chronic (goal rate is 10 mEq/L in 24 hours).
- Use hypotonic fluids unless patient has hemodynamic compromise, which necessitates use of isotonic fluids.
- Use oral replacement in conscious patients if possible.
- Use the estimated water deficit, desired rate of correction, and estimation of ongoing free water losses to calculate a fluid repletion regimen.

H

HYPERPARATHYROIDISM

Michael Morkos, MD, MS • Sandy Botros, MD

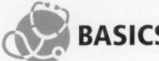

BASICS

DESCRIPTION

A dysfunction of the body's normal regulatory feedback mechanisms resulting in excess production of parathyroid hormone (PTH)

- Primary hyperparathyroidism (HPT): intrinsic parathyroid gland dysfunction resulting in excessive secretion of PTH with a lack of response to feedback inhibition by elevated calcium
- Secondary HPT: excessive secretion of PTH in response to potential hypocalcemia and/or hyperphosphatemia. This is commonly caused by vitamin D deficiency or renal failure.
- Tertiary HPT: autonomous hyperfunction of the parathyroid gland in the setting of long-standing secondary HPT

EPIDEMIOLOGY

Incidence
- Predominantly postmenopausal females
- Female > male (3:1)

Prevalence
Primary HPT is 1 in 500 to 1 in 1,000 in the United States.

ETIOLOGY AND PATHOPHYSIOLOGY

- PTH is synthesized by the four parathyroid glands, which are located behind the four poles of the thyroid gland (locations can vary).
- Ectopic (abnormal locations and most common is the thymus) or supernumerary glands (more than four glands)
- PTH releases calcium from bone by osteoclastic stimulation (increasing bone resorption).
- PTH increases reabsorption of calcium in the distal tubules of the kidneys.
- PTH stimulates conversion of 25-hydroxycholecalciferol (25[OH]D) to 1,25-dihydroxycholecalciferol (1,25[OH]$_2$D or active vitamin D) in the kidneys. 1,25(OH)$_2$D increases calcium and phosphate absorption from the GI tract and kidneys, and stimulates osteoclastic activity and bone resorption.
- Primary HPT: unregulated PTH production and release due to the loss of normal feedback control by extracellular calcium, causing increase in serum calcium
  - Solitary adenoma (80–85%)
  - Diffuse hyperplasia (10–15%) of the four parathyroid glands, either sporadically or in association with multiple endocrine neoplasia (MEN) types I or II
  - Parathyroid carcinoma (<1%), a very rare and severe form
- Secondary HPT: adaptive parathyroid gland hyperplasia and hyperfunction
  - Dietary: vitamin D or calcium deficiency
  - Chronic renal disease resulting in the following:
    ○ Renal parenchymal loss causing hyperphosphatemia
    ○ Impaired calcitriol production causing hypocalcemia
    ○ General skeletal and renal resistance to PTH
- Tertiary HPT: autonomous oversecretion of PTH following prolonged parathyroid stimulation

Genetics
- MEN types I and II: Patients with multiple gland hyperplasia in the absence of renal disease should be screened for MEN-I gene mutation.
- Neonatal severe primary HPT
- HPT—jaw tumor syndrome
- Familial hypocalciuric hypercalcemia (FHH)
- Familial isolated HPT

RISK FACTORS
Chronic kidney disease, increasing age, poor nutrition, radiation, and/or family history

GENERAL PREVENTION
Adequate intake of calcium and vitamin D may help prevent secondary HPT.

COMMONLY ASSOCIATED CONDITIONS
- Vitamin D deficiency
- Chronic renal failure
- MEN syndromes types I and II

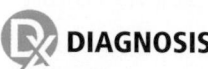

DIAGNOSIS

HISTORY
- History of present illness
  - Almost 80% of patients are asymptomatic.
  - Kidney stones (15–20%)
  - Osteitis fibrosa cystica (<5%) characterized by subperiosteal resorption of phalanges, tapering of distal clavicles, bone cysts, brown tumors of long bones, and "salt and pepper" appearance of the skull
  - Symptoms due to hypercalcemia like polyuria, polydipsia, constipation, bone pain, decreased concentration, fatigue, and muscle weakness
- Past medical history
  - The following conditions may be associated with HPT:
    ○ MEN syndrome (MEN-associated conditions include pancreatic cancer, pituitary adenomas, medullary thyroid cancer, and pheochromocytoma), nephrolithiasis (in 20–30%), nephrocalcinosis, pancreatitis, gastroduodenal ulcer, hypertension, short QT interval, left ventricular hypertrophy, osteitis fibrosa cystica, cystic bone lesions, spontaneous fracture, vertebral collapse, osteoporosis, gout, pseudogout, anxiety, depression, psychosis, coma, conjunctivitis, band keratopathy, conjunctival calcium deposits, radiation to the neck
- Medications: hydrochlorothiazide or lithium (decreases parathyroid sensitivity to calcium in small subset of patients)

PHYSICAL EXAM
- Limited usefulness; 70–80% of patients have no obvious symptoms or signs of disease.
- Physical findings related to the underlying cause of HPT may be found.

DIFFERENTIAL DIAGNOSIS
- Increased PTH: Ectopic PTH production is rare. In most of the cases, it establishes the diagnosis of primary HPT, but first rule out:
  - FHH
  - Thiazide diuretics and lithium
- Nonparathyroid causes
  - Malignancy: lung (squamous cell) carcinoma, breast carcinoma, multiple myeloma, lymphoma, leukemia, prostate cancer, Paget disease
  - Granulomatous diseases: sarcoidosis, tuberculosis, berylliosis, histoplasmosis, coccidioidomycosis
  - Drugs: vitamin D intoxication, milk-alkali syndrome
  - Endocrine: hyperthyroidism, acute adrenal insufficiency

DIAGNOSTIC TESTS & INTERPRETATION

Initial Tests (lab, imaging)
- The disease is often detected by an incidental finding of hypercalcemia on routine labs. The best modality is to check ionized calcium, but it is not done routinely.
- The best next step is to calculate the corrected calcium: [serum calcium in mg/dL + 0.8 × (4 − patient's albumin in g/dL)]. Some patients will have mild hypercalcemia for years, and it won't be detected as the uncorrected calcium is normal.
- If hypercalcemia is confirmed, follow with intact PTH level (1)[B].
  - PTH-dependent: High or (abnormally) normal PTH suggests primary HPT.
  - PTH-independent: Undetectable or low PTH suggests PTH-independent hypercalcemia.
- Other findings may include low serum phosphate and high 24-hour urine calcium excretion.
- In secondary HPT, an elevated phosphorus suggests chronic renal failure; a low phosphorus suggests another cause, commonly 25(OH)D deficiency. Both are common causes of elevated PTH levels while having normal corrected calcium levels.

Follow-Up Tests & Special Considerations
- A 24-hour urine calcium concentration to creatinine clearance ratio >0.02 suggests primary HPT; a ratio <0.01 may be normal or indicate FHH; an important finding because FHH does not require surgery (1)[C].
- Routine measurement of 25(OH)D levels is recommended in all patients with primary HPT. In case of vitamin D deficiency (<20 ng/mL or <50 nmol/L), defer management decisions until levels are maintained >20 ng/mL (50 nmol/L) (1)[C].

Diagnostic Procedures/Other
- Imaging is not required for diagnosis. It is required for surgical planning, especially for minimally invasive parathyroidectomy (MIP) (2)[C].
  - Imaging is also indicated to localize hyperplasia or an ectopic parathyroid gland in repeat surgery.

- Imaging options for presurgical localization
  - Technetium-99m sestamibi with or without single-photon emission computed tomography (SPECT): it has the greatest reported success in localizing single parathyroid adenomas but often inaccurate in multigland disease (3)[B].
  - Neck ultrasound (US): painless, noninvasive, and does not expose the patient to radiation; however, its accuracy is operator-dependent (4)[C].
  - Four-dimensional CT (4D-CT) may be more effective for primary localization than both US and sestamibi-SPECT (4)[B].
  - Positron emission tomography (PET) using C-methionine (MET-PET) is comparable to US and technetium-99m sestamibi with SPECT in terms of diagnostic use (2)[B].
  - CT and MRI are mostly used to localize ectopic mediastinal glands.

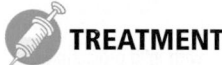 ## TREATMENT

MEDICATION

- Primary HPT: Operative management is curative; indications for surgical intervention are mentioned below. For those awaiting or unable to have surgery:
  - Bisphosphonates (alendronate): reduce bone turnover and help to maintain bone density; avoid in kidney disease (GFR ≤35).
  - Calcimimetics (cinacalcet) (1)[B]: activates calcium-sensing receptor in parathyroid gland thereby inhibiting PTH secretion. FDA-approved for symptomatic patients who are unfit for surgery; no long-term data on its effect on constitutional, neuropsychological symptoms or fractures
  - Selective estrogen receptor modulator therapy (raloxifene): antagonizes PTH-mediated bone resorption
  - Hormone replacement therapy with estrogens is not recommended as first-line treatment; must weigh benefit with risks of known systemic effects
    - Can be used in postmenopausal women who do not undergo or refuse surgery
- Secondary HPT
  - Calcium replacement
  - Vitamin D analogues (paricalcitol and calcitriol)
  - Phosphorus-binding agents (sevelamer)
  - Calcimimetic (cinacalcet)
- Tertiary HPT
  - Medical treatment is not curative and generally not indicated.

SURGERY/OTHER PROCEDURES

- Operative management is curative for patients with primary HPT in 95–98% of patients.
- Indications for parathyroidectomy
  - Symptomatic primary HPT
    - Nephrolithiasis
    - Fragility fractures
    - Osteitis fibrosa cystica
  - Asymptomatic primary HPT (1)[C]
    - Serum Ca$^+$ level >1 mg/dL above normal
    - Age <50 years
    - Creatinine clearance <60 mL/min
    - 24-hour urine for calcium >400 mg/day (>10 mmol/day) and increased stone risk by biochemical stone risk analysis
    - Presence of nephrolithiasis or nephrocalcinosis by x-ray, US, or CT
    - Bone density loss with a T-score <−2.5 at the lumbar spine, femoral neck, total hip, or distal 1/3 radius

- Tertiary HPT
- Surgical removal of diseased gland or tissue is only proven curative therapy for HPT.
- Surgical options include the following:
  - Bilateral open neck exploratory surgery
  - MIP using preoperative sestamibi scan with SPECT/US/4D-CT and intraoperative PTH levels (high sensitivity 79–95% to predict location of single parathyroid adenoma) (5), which result in decreased pain, smaller incisions, improved cosmetic results, lower morbidity, and decreased length of hospital stay when compared with open neck exploratory surgery
- Follow postoperative serum calcium, magnesium, and phosphorus levels; monitor closely for hypocalcemia "hungry bone" syndrome.
- Patients may need IV calcium infusion postoperatively with oral calcitriol and calcium supplementation initially. Hungry pain syndrome can be severe, although less common now.
- Patients also at risk for bleeding and airway compromise
- Monitor renal function closely.

ADMISSION, INPATIENT, AND NURSING CONSIDERATIONS

Critical hypercalcemia requires IV fluid rehydration, IV bisphosphonate therapy, and SC calcitonin (4 U/kg q12h) for severe symptoms.

 ## ONGOING CARE

FOLLOW-UP RECOMMENDATIONS

Asymptomatic patients with primary HPT require serial monitoring of calcium and PTH.

Patient Monitoring

In patients with primary HPT who are asymptomatic, measurement of serum calcium and creatinine annually and bone density scan every 1 to 2 years is sufficient (1)[C].

DIET

- In the presence of hypercalciuria or elevated 1,25(OH)$_2$D levels, dietary calcium restriction is recommended. Otherwise, daily calcium intake should be maintained at up to 1,000 mg.
- Restrict dietary phosphate in secondary HPT.

PATIENT EDUCATION

- Importance of periodic lab testing
- Signs of severe hypercalcemia

PROGNOSIS

Prognosis after surgery is excellent in primary HPT, with resolution of many of the preoperative symptoms.

COMPLICATIONS

Related to high levels of PTH and/or elevated calcium

REFERENCES

1. Bilezikian JP, Brandi ML, Eastell R, et al. Guidelines for the management of asymptomatic primary hyperparathyroidism: summary statement from the Fourth International Workshop. *J Clin Endocrinol Metab*. 2014;99(10):3561–3569.
2. Caldarella C, Treglia G, Isgrò MA, et al. Diagnostic performance of positron emission tomography using ^{11}C-methionine in patients with suspected parathyroid adenoma: a meta-analysis. *Endocrine*. 2013;43(1):78–83.
3. Caldarella C, Treglia G, Pontecorvi A, et al. Diagnostic performance of planar scintigraphy using ^{99}mTc-MIBI in patients with secondary hyperparathyroidism: a meta-analysis. *Ann Nucl Med*. 2012;26(10):794–803.
4. Cheung K, Wang TS, Farrokhyar F, et al. A meta-analysis of preoperative localization techniques for patients with primary hyperparathyroidism. *Ann Surg Oncol*. 2012;19(2):577–583.
5. Kunstman JW, Kirsch JD, Mahajan A, et al. Clinical review: parathyroid localization and implications for clinical management. *J Clin Endocrinol Metab*. 2013;98(3):902–912.

 ## CODES

ICD10

- E21.3 Hyperparathyroidism, unspecified
- E21.0 Primary hyperparathyroidism
- E21.1 Secondary hyperparathyroidism, not elsewhere classified

CLINICAL PEARLS

- 80% of patients with primary HPT are asymptomatic.
- HPT is often detected by an incidental finding of hypercalcemia on a routine serum chemistry analysis.
- Classic symptoms of HPT include painful bones, renal stones, abdominal pain, and behavioral changes (stones, bones, moans, and groans).
- Repeat calcium (elevated), correct for serum albumin, and obtain intact PTH levels to make an initial diagnosis.
- Secondary HPT is due to excessive secretion of PTH in response to hypocalcemia, which can be caused by vitamin D deficiency or renal failure.
- The most commonly used imaging modalities in HPT are technetium-99m sestamibi scan, US, and 4D-CT.
- Surgery is curative for most cases of primary HPT.
- Recommend normal daily calcium intake (1,000 mg) in asymptomatic patients with primary HPT who don't qualify for surgery.
- In patients with primary HPT who are asymptomatic, measurement of serum calcium and creatinine annually and bone density scan every 1 to 2 years is sufficient.

H

HYPERPROLACTINEMIA

D'Ann Somerall, DNP, MAEd, CRNP, FNP-BC • William E. Somerall Jr., MD, MEd

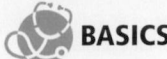 **BASICS**

DESCRIPTION

Hyperprolactinemia is an abnormal elevation in the serum prolactin level with multiple possible etiologies.

EPIDEMIOLOGY

Prevalence

- Predominant age: reproductive age
- Predominant sex: female > male
- More readily detected in females because a slight elevation in prolactin causes changes in menstruation and galactorrhea

ETIOLOGY AND PATHOPHYSIOLOGY

- Prolactin, which is produced by lactotrophs in the anterior pituitary, is regulated by:
  - Inhibitory factors, primarily dopamine, produced in the hypothalamus and delivered via the hypothalamic-pituitary vessels in the pituitary stalk
  - Stimulatory factors, primarily thyrotropin-releasing hormone (TRH)
- Causes of hyperprolactinemia include the following:
  - Physiologic
  - Pregnancy due to increased estrogen
  - Breastfeeding
  - Nipple stimulation
  - Stress, including postoperative state
  - Medications
    - Dopamine (D_2) blockers: prochlorperazine, metoclopramide
    - Dopamine depleters: α-methyldopa, reserpine
    - Antidepressants: selective serotonin reuptake inhibitors (SSRIs), tricyclic antidepressants (SSRIs do not appear to cause clinically significant hyperprolactinemia.)
    - Verapamil (but no other calcium channel blockers; thought to decrease hypothalamic synthesis of dopamine)
    - Antipsychotics: haloperidol, fluphenazine, risperidone
  - Hypothyroidism (due to elevated TRH)
  - Chest wall conditions:
    - Herpes zoster
    - After thoracotomy
    - Trauma
  - Prolactin-secreting adenoma (anterior pituitary), categorized:
    - Microadenoma: <1 cm
    - Macroadenoma: >1 cm
  - Pituitary stalk compression/disruption:
    - Craniopharyngioma
    - Rathke cleft cyst
    - Meningioma
    - Astrocytoma
    - Metastases
    - Head trauma
    - Infiltrative/inflammatory disorders
  - Diminished prolactin clearance:
    - Chronic renal failure
    - Cirrhosis
- Cocaine

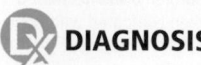 **DIAGNOSIS**

HISTORY

- Galactorrhea
- Amenorrhea
- Oligomenorrhea
- Infertility
- Osteoporosis/osteopenia
- Decreased libido, impotence
- Weight gain
- Also may have signs and symptoms of pituitary enlargement:
  - Headache
  - Visual field impairment (bitemporal hemianopia)
  - Hypopituitarism (secondary to tumor pressure on surrounding structures)
- Also may have signs and symptoms of associated conditions:
  - Hypothyroidism
  - Cushing disease
  - Acromegaly
  - Multiple endocrine neoplasia (MEN)-1 syndrome

PHYSICAL EXAM

- Visual field testing
- Cranial nerve exam

DIFFERENTIAL DIAGNOSIS

Macroprolactinemia: Macroprolactin, a polymer of several units of prolactin, is detected by immunologically based lab tests but is not biologically active. If patient is asymptomatic but found to have elevated prolactin, consider this diagnosis and notify the lab. No treatment is required.

DIAGNOSTIC TESTS & INTERPRETATION

- Serum prolactin (most accurate results if checked fasting, in morning) <25 μg/L normal; >25 μg/L abnormal; >250 μg/L often indicates a prolactinoma (1)[A].
- Pregnancy test
- Thyroid-stimulating hormone (TSH)
- Luteinizing hormone (LH)/follicle-stimulating hormone (FSH) if amenorrheic
- Chemistry, renal function
- LFTs

Initial Tests (lab, imaging)

A single measurement of serum prolactin; a level above the upper limit of normal confirms the diagnosis.

- Pituitary MRI: single best imaging
- CT scan if MRI is contraindicated
- Levels should be drawn prior to breast exam.

Follow-Up Tests & Special Considerations

Formal visual field testing if pituitary adenoma is suspected

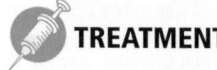 **TREATMENT**

GENERAL MEASURES

- Discontinue offending medications, if any (1)[A].
- Treat underlying causes (1)[A].
- For asymptomatic patients with mild prolactin elevations, observation alone may be considered (1,2)[A].
- Medications indicated for (1)[A]:
  - Symptoms of hypogonadism, such as decreased libido
  - Galactorrhea (if bothersome to patient)
  - Restoration of fertility
  - Pituitary adenoma
  - Prevention of osteoporosis

MEDICATION

Dopamine agonists: decrease serum prolactin concentrations and decrease the size of most lactotroph adenomas

- Cabergoline (Dostinex): This is now a first-line choice due to efficacy and favorable side effect profile (1,3)[A]: dosed twice weekly. Cabergoline was more effective than bromocriptine in reducing persistent hyperprolactinemia, galactorrhea, and amenorrhea/oligomenorrhea (2)[A]. Has recently been reported to be associated with significant improvements in the body mass index, total HDL and LDL cholesterol levels, and insulin sensitivity; decrease in proinflammatory markers; and carotid intima-media thickness, indicated with bromocriptine failure or resistance; has been shown to reduce erectile dysfunction in hyperprolactinemic men (1)[A].
  - Adverse effects (better tolerated if start with low dose, slow titration, given at night with food):
    - Nausea/vomiting
    - Headache
    - Dizziness
    - Fatigue
    - Light-headedness

○ Postural hypotension (2)[A]
○ Contraindications
  ▪ Uncontrolled hypertension
  ▪ Cardiac valvular disorders
  ▪ Pulmonary, pericardial, or retroperitoneal fibrotic disorders
• Bromocriptine (Parlodel): This has the longest clinical history: dosed BID; preferred by some clinicians when infertility is an indication for treatment (2,4)[A]
• Both are effective for reducing tumor size and improving symptoms (2)[A].
• SE less with cabergoline than bromocriptine (2)[A]. Pergolide (Permax) is no longer used in the United States. If patient is still on med, do not withdraw abruptly.

ADDITIONAL THERAPIES
Patients with medically and surgically refractory prolactinomas; radiotherapy produced a reduction in prolactin levels in nearly all patients and normalization in over a quarter of patients with low complication rates (2)[A].

SURGERY/OTHER PROCEDURES
• For adenomas, medical treatment will be successful in 80–90% of patients. In some cases, surgery is indicated (1).
• Indications
  – Intolerance or resistance to medical treatment
  – Headache
  – Visual field loss
  – CSF leak due to tumor apoplexy or shrinkage
  – Cranial nerve deficit
• Risks
  – High recurrence rate (up to 40%)
  – CSF leakage
  – Meningitis
  – Transient diabetes insipidus (5)
• Pituitary insufficiency

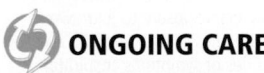

ONGOING CARE

FOLLOW-UP RECOMMENDATIONS
Patient Monitoring
• Depends on etiology
• After at least 2 years of treatment, no tumor and prolactin levels normal may consider decreasing and stopping medication; must be followed closely because tumor may grow back (1)
• Consider:
  – Formal visual field testing yearly (4)[A]
  – Serial MRIs if clinically indicated (4)[A]

Pregnancy Considerations
• If pregnancy is desired in a woman with hyperprolactinemia, dopamine agonists are not approved during pregnancy and should be discontinued once pregnancy is confirmed, but their use is recommended if neurologic findings are present (1)[A].
• With microprolactinoma: Treat with bromocriptine if symptomatic; monthly pregnancy tests; discontinue bromocriptine when pregnancy is confirmed.
• With macroprolactinomas: a definitive, individualized plan is made. Options include discontinuation of bromocriptine at conception and careful monitoring of prolactin levels and VS, with or without MRI scan evidence of tumor enlargement; prepregnancy transsphenoidal surgery with debulking of tumor; continuation of bromocriptine throughout gestation, with a risk to the fetus.
• Careful monitoring of visual fields in each trimester; no need to monitor prolactin levels because they are normally high due to pregnancy (1)[A]

PATIENT EDUCATION
• Discuss risks of untreated hyperprolactinemia:
  – Headache
  – Visual field loss
  – Decreased bone density
  – Infertility
• Patient guide to hyperprolactinemia diagnosis and treatment

PROGNOSIS
• Tends to recur after discontinuation of medical therapy (1)
• >10 years, 7% chance of progression of prolactin-secreting microadenoma (4)

COMPLICATIONS
• Depends on underlying cause
• If pituitary adenoma, risk of permanent visual field loss

REFERENCES
1. Hoffman AR, Melmed S, Schlechte J. Patient guide to hyperprolactinemia diagnosis and treatment. *J Clin Endocrinol Metab*. 2011;96(2):35A–36A.
2. Wang AT, Mullan RJ, Lane MA, et al. Treatment of hyperprolactinemia: a systematic review and meta-analysis. *Syst Rev*. 2012;1:33.
3. Wong A, Eloy JA, Couldwell WT, et al. Update on prolactinomas. Part 2: treatment and management strategies. *J Clin Neurosci*. 2015;22(10):1568–1574.
4. Casanueva FF, Molitch ME, Schlechte JA, et al. Guidelines of the Pituitary Society for the diagnosis and management of prolactinomas. *Clin Endocrinol (Oxf)*. 2006;65(2):265–273.
5. Bloomgarden E, Molitch ME. Surgical treatment of prolactinomas: cons. *Endocrine*. 2014;47(3):730–733.

ADDITIONAL READING
• Inancli SS, Usluogullari A, Ustu Y, et al. Effect of cabergoline on insulin sensitivity, inflammation, and carotid intima media thickness in patients with prolactinoma. *Endocrine*. 2013;44(1):193–199.
• Inder WJ, Castle D. Antipsychotic-induced hyperprolactinaemia. *Aust N Z J Psychiatry*. 2011;45(10):830–837.
• Klibanski A. Clinical practice. Prolactinomas. *N Engl J Med*. 2010;362(13):1219–1226.
• Melmed S, Casanueva FF, Hoffman AR, et al. Diagnosis and treatment of hyperprolactinemia: an Endocrine Society clinical practice guideline. *J Clin Endocrinol Metab*. 2011;96(2):273–288.
• Molitch ME. Pituitary gland: can prolactinomas be cured medically? *Nat Rev Endocrinol*. 2010;6(4):186–188.

CODES

ICD10
E22.1 Hyperprolactinemia

CLINICAL PEARLS
• If a cause for hyperprolactinemia cannot be found by history, examination, and routine laboratory testing, an intracranial lesion might be the cause and brain MRI with specific pituitary cuts and intravenous contrast media should be performed.
• Treatment of hyperprolactinemia should be targeted at correcting the cause (hypothyroidism, discontinuation of offending medications, etc.).
• There is a difference among antipsychotics in influencing prolactin levels. In general, those with the highest potency D_2 antagonism are most likely to elevate prolactin levels. Among the newer atypical antipsychotics, risperidone has been identified as more likely to elevate prolactin.
• High prolactin levels decrease testosterone by inhibiting gonadotropin-releasing hormone (GnRH), LH, and FSH secretion and by decreasing central dopamine activity, both of which are important in mediating sexual arousal.

H

HYPERSENSITIVITY PNEUMONITIS

Han Q. Bui, MD

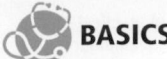

BASICS

DESCRIPTION
- Hypersensitivity pneumonitis (HP) is also called extrinsic allergic alveolitis (EAA).
- HP is a diffuse inflammatory disease of the lung parenchyma caused by an immunologic reaction to aerosolized antigenic particles found in a variety of environments. Classification depends on time frame involved:
  - Acute: fever, chills, diaphoresis, myalgias, nausea; cough and dyspnea common but not necessarily present. Occurs 4 to 12 hours after heavy exposure to an inciting agent. Symptoms subside within 12 hours to several days after removal from exposure. Complete resolution occurs within weeks.
  - Subacute: mainly caused by continual low-level antigen exposure, could have a low-grade fever in 1st week; cough, dyspnea, fatigue, anorexia, weight loss—develops over days to weeks
  - Chronic: from recurrent exposure either acute or subacute cases; prolonged and progressive cough, dyspnea, fatigue, weight loss; could lead to fibrosis and respiratory failure
- Farmer's lung is an old term of this disease, a type of HP, particular to the farmer population; causative agent is a bacterium found in moldy hay or straw. Farmer's lung now has new and different etiologies due to modernization of farming practices (1,2).

EPIDEMIOLOGY
- Not well defined; tends to occur in adults as a result of occupation-related exposure, but some home environmental exposures are also seen
- HP is increasingly recognized as an important cause of fibrotic interstitial lung disease (3).

Incidence
0.9/100,000

Prevalence
- Farmers: 1–19% exposed farmers
- Bird fanciers: 6–20% exposed individuals
- Others: 1–8% exposed

ETIOLOGY AND PATHOPHYSIOLOGY
- Hypersensitivity reaction involving immune complexes: Inhaled antigens bind to IgG, triggering complement cascade (types III and IV immunologic reactions) (3).
- Cellular-mediated reaction: T cell–mediated immune inflammatory response
- Farming, vegetable, or dairy cattle workers (1,2)
  - Moldy hay, grain, silage: thermophilic actinomycetes, such as *Faenia rectivirgula*
  - Mold on pressed sugar cane: *Thermoactinomyces sacchari*, *Thymus vulgaris*
  - Tobacco plants: *Aspergillus* sp., *Scopulariopsis brevicaulis*
  - Mushroom worker's lung: *Saccharopolyspora rectivirgula*, *T. vulgaris*, *Aspergillus* spp.
  - Potato riddler's lung: thermophilic actinomycetes, *T. vulgaris*, *F. rectivirgula*, *Aspergillus* sp.
  - Wine maker's lung: *Mucor stolonifer*
  - Cheese washer's lung: *Penicillium caseifulvum*, *Aspergillus clavatus*
  - Coffee worker's lung: coffee bean dust
  - Tea grower's lung: tea plants

- Ventilation and water-related contamination (1,2)
  - Contaminated humidifiers and air conditioners: amoebae, nematodes, yeasts, bacteria
  - Unventilated shower: *Epicoccum nigrum*
  - Hot-tub lung: *Cladosporium* sp., *Mycobacterium avium* complex
  - Sauna taker's lung: *Aureobasidium* sp.
  - Summer-type pneumonitis: *Trichosporon cutaneum*
  - Swimming pool lifeguard's lung: aerosolized endotoxin and *M. avium* complex
  - Contaminated basement pneumonitis: *Cephalosporium* and *Penicillium* spp.
- Bird and poultry handling (1)
  - Bird fancier's lung: droppings, feathers, serum proteins
  - Poultry worker's lung: serum proteins
  - Turkey-handling disease: serum proteins
  - Canary fancier's lung: serum proteins
  - Duck fever: feathers, serum proteins
- Veterinary work and animal handling (1,2)
  - Laboratory worker's lung: urine, serum, pelts, proteins
  - Pituitary snuff taker's disease: dried, powdered neurohypophysis
  - Furrier's lung: animal pelts
  - Bat lung: bat serum protein
  - Fish meal worker's lung: fish meal
  - Coptic lung: cloth wrapping of mummies
  - Mollusc shell HP: sea-snail shell
  - Pearl oyster shell pneumonitis: oyster shells
- Grain and flour (1,2)
  - Grain measurer's lung: cereal grain, grain dust
  - Miller's lung: *Sitophilus granarius*
  - Malt worker's disease: *Aspergillus fumigatus*, *A. clavatus*
- Lumber milling, construction, wood stripping, paper, wallboard manufacture (1,2)
  - Wood dust pneumonitis: *Alternaria* sp., *Bacillus subtilis*
  - Sequoiosis: *Graphium*, *Pullularia*, *Trichoderma* sp., *Aureobasidium pullulans*
  - Maple bark disease: *Cryptostroma corticale*
  - Wood trimmer's disease: *Rhizopus* sp., *Mucor* sp.
  - Wood pulp worker's disease: *Penicillium* sp.
  - Suberosis: *Trogon viridis*, *Penicillium glabrum*
- Plastic manufacturing, painting, electronics, chemicals (1)
  - Chemical HP: diphenyl diisocyanate, toluene diisocyanate
  - Detergent worker's lung: *B. subtilis* enzymes
  - Pauli reagent alveolitis: sodium diazobenzene sulfate
  - Vineyard sprayer's lung: copper sulfate
  - Pyrethrum: *Pyrethrum*
  - Epoxy resin lung: phthalic anhydride
  - Bible printer's lung: moldy typesetting water
  - Machine operator's lung: *Pseudomonas fluorescens*, aerosolized metal working fluid
- Textile workers
  - Byssinosis: cotton mill dust
  - Velvet worker's lung: nylon, tannic acid, potato starch
  - Upholstery fabric: aflatoxin-producing fungus, *Fusarium* sp.
  - Lycoperdonosis: puffball spores

Genetics
No evidence of clear genetic susceptibility; possible genetic predisposition involving tumor necrosis factor alpha (TNF-α) and major histocompatibility complex (MHC) class II genes (1,3)[B]

RISK FACTORS
- Contact with organic antigens increases the risk of developing HP. Viral infection at time of exposure could also increase risk.
- Nonsmokers have an increased incidence of HP compared with smokers. The mechanisms that account for the "protective" effect of smoking are poorly understood, but nicotine is thought to inhibit macrophage activation and lymphocyte proliferation and function (3).
  - Smokers have a diminished antibody response to inhaled antigens.
  - However, smokers who develop disease tend to have the chronic form, and mortality is higher.

GENERAL PREVENTION
Avoidance of offending antigen and/or use of protective equipment

COMMONLY ASSOCIATED CONDITIONS
Constrictive bronchiolitis

DIAGNOSIS

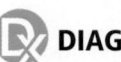

- Diagnosis criteria most widely used but not validated: (i) history and physical and pulmonary function tests (PFTs) indicating restriction or diffusion disease, (ii) radiologic imaging consent with interstitial lung disease, (iii) exposure to a recognized cause, (iv) proof of sensitization in bronchoalveolar lavage (BAL) fluids (serum precipitins and/or lymphocytosis) (2)
- Six significant predictors: exposure to a known antigen, positive antibodies precipitating, (if identified) recurrent episodes of symptoms, inspiratory crackles, symptoms 4 to 8 hours after exposure, weight loss (3)
- Acute form: develops 4 to 12 hours following exposure. Cough, dyspnea without wheezing, fever, chills, diaphoresis, headache, nausea, malaise, chest tightness. Symptoms last hours to days.
- Sequela (prior subacute, chronic): gradual or progressive productive cough, dyspnea, fatigue, anorexia, weight loss can lead to respiratory failure; develops over days, weeks to months
- Symptomatic improvement when away from work or home

PHYSICAL EXAM
- Acute: fever, tachypnea, diffuse fine rales
- Sequela or chronic: inspiratory crackles, progressive hypoxia, weight loss, diffuse rales, clubbing, rarely wheezing

DIFFERENTIAL DIAGNOSIS
- Acute: acute infectious pneumonia: influenza (or other viral pneumonia), mycoplasma, *Pneumocystis jiroveci* pneumonia, asthma, aspiration
- Chronic: sarcoidosis, chronic bronchitis, chronic obstructive pulmonary disease, tuberculosis, collagen vascular disease, idiopathic pulmonary fibrosis, lymphoma, fungal infections, *P. jiroveci* pneumonia

DIAGNOSTIC TESTS & INTERPRETATION

- Testing for positive precipitating antibodies is NOT diagnostic because up to 40% may have positive antibody without disease; antigens that cover most cases: pigeon and parakeet sera, dove feather, *Aspergillus* sp., *Penicillium*, *S. rectivirgula*, and *Thalassomonas viridans*
- PFTs: Typical profile is a restrictive pattern with low diffusing capacity; could also have an obstructive pattern (4)
- BAL with serum precipitins and lymphocytosis: usually with low CD4-to-CD8 ratio; findings not unique to HP (1,4)
- Positive antigen–specific inhalation challenge testing: reexposure to the environment, inhalation challenge to the suspected antigen in a hospital setting, but it lacks standardization (3)
- Chest x-ray (CXR): used to rule out other diseases
  - Acute: ground-glass infiltrates, nodular or striated patchy opacities, interstitial pattern in a variety of distributions in lung field. Up to 20% could be normal.
  - Sequela/chronic: upper lobe fibrosis, nodular or ground-glass opacities, volume loss, emphysematous changes
- CT scan of chest; patterns not specific to HP:
  - Acute: ground-glass opacities, poorly defined centrilobular nodules, and ground-glass opacities and air trapping on expiratory images (3,5)
  - Chronic: fibrosis, ground-glass attenuation, irregular opacities, bronchiectasis, loss of lung volume, honeycombing, emphysematous changes (3,5)
- High-resolution CT (HRCT) mid-to-upper zone predominance of centrilobular ground glass or nodular opacities with signs of air trapping (3)
- Usually start with CXR; may progress to HRCT based on findings (3)

Diagnostic Procedures/Other

Lung biopsy:

- Transbronchial: reveals small, poorly formed non-caseating granulomas near respiratory or terminal bronchioles, large foam cells, peribronchial fibrosis
- Open lung biopsy: highest yield in advanced disease; reveals varying patterns of organizing pneumonia, centrilobular and perilobular fibrosis, multinucleated giant cells with clefts

ALERT

HP in farmers must be distinguished from febrile, toxic reactions to inhaled dusts (organic dust toxic syndrome [ODTS]). Nonimmunologic reactions occur 30–50% more commonly than HP in farmers. ODTS is associated with intense exposure occurring on a single day.

 ## TREATMENT

GENERAL MEASURES

Outpatient, except for acute pneumonitis cases and admission for workup (BAL, lung biopsy)

MEDICATION

First Line

- Avoidance of offending antigen is primary therapy and results in disease regression (3).
- Corticosteroids: help control the symptoms of exacerbations but do not improve long-term outcomes
  - Prednisone: 20 to 50 mg daily (3,4)
  - For severe symptomatic patients, initial course of 1 to 2 weeks with taper (3,4)[C]

Second Line

- Bronchodilators and inhaled corticosteroids may symptomatically improve patients with wheeze and chest tightness (4)[C].
- Oxygen may be needed in advanced cases.
- Lung transplantation may be the last resort in severe cases unresponsive to therapy.

ISSUES FOR REFERRAL

Referral to pulmonologist/immunologist

ADMISSION, INPATIENT, AND NURSING CONSIDERATIONS

Supportive management, as needed, to maintain oxygenation and ventilation:

- Unstable ventilation, oxygen requirement, mental status changes
- Need for invasive evaluation (lung biopsy)

 ## ONGOING CARE

FOLLOW-UP RECOMMENDATIONS

Patient Monitoring

- Initial follow-up should be weekly to monthly, depending on severity and course.
- Follow treatments with serial CXR, PFTs, and circulating antibody levels.

DIET

No dietary restrictions

PATIENT EDUCATION

Note that chronic exposure may lead to a loss of acute symptoms with exposure (i.e., the patient may lose awareness of exposure–symptom relationship).

PROGNOSIS

- Presence of fibrosis is a poor prognosis factor (3).
- Acute: good prognosis with reversal of pathologic findings if elimination of offending antigen early in disease (2)
- Sequela/chronic: Corticosteroids have been found to improve lung function acutely but offer no significant difference in long-term outcome (3)[C].

COMPLICATIONS

- Progressive interstitial fibrosis with eventual respiratory failure
- Cor pulmonale and right-sided heart failure

REFERENCES

1. Girard M, Cormier Y. Hypersensitivity pneumonitis. *Curr Opin Allergy Clin Immunol*. 2010;10(2): 99–103.
2. Costabel U, Bonella F, Guzman J. Chronic hypersensitivity pneumonitis. *Clin Chest Med*. 2012;33(1):151–163.
3. Spagnolo P, Rossi G, Cavazza A, et al. Hypersensitivity pneumonitis: a comprehensive review. *J Investig Allergol Clin Immunol*. 2015;25(4):237–250.
4. Lacasse Y, Girard M, Cormier Y. Recent advances in hypersensitivity pneumonitis. *Chest*. 2012;142(1):208–217.
5. D'souza RS, Donato A. Hypersensitivity pneumonitis: an overlooked cause of cough and dyspnea. *J Community Hosp Intern Med Perspect*. 2017;7(2):95–99.

CODES

ICD10

- J67.9 Hypersensitivity pneumonitis due to unspecified organic dust
- J67.0 Farmer's lung
- J67.2 Bird fancier's lung

CLINICAL PEARLS

- Skin testing is not useful for the diagnosis of HP.
- Diagnosis should be suspected in every patient with unexplained cough and dyspnea on exertion, functional impairment (restriction or diffusion defect), and unclear fever, especially if exposure to potential antigens is known (workplace, domestic bird keeping, moldy walls in the home) (2).
- HP may mimic viral upper respiratory illness or asthma exacerbation. Misdiagnosis has critical therapeutic and prognostic implications because it may delay proper treatment, result in significant morbidity, unnecessary hospitalizations, and irreversible fibrosis to the lungs (3).
- Once the disease is established, smoking does not appear to attenuate its severity, and it may predispose to more chronic and severe course.
- Use of protective gear on individual with high-risk exposure occupations can prevent HP.
- Chronic HP is increasingly recognized as an important mimic of other fibrotic lung diseases (3).

H

HYPERSPLENISM

Shadi Hamdeh, MD • Adil Abdalla, MD

 BASICS

DESCRIPTION

- Hypersplenism is defined as overactivity of the spleen and presents as the following:
  - Splenomegaly (commonly but not always)
  - Cytopenias with respective bone marrow hyperplasia of precursors
  - Resolution of cytopenias with splenectomy
- Splenomegaly is not synonymous with hypersplenism. Overactivity of the spleen can occur without enlargement, as is seen in immune thrombocytopenic purpura (ITP) and autoimmune hemolytic anemia. Similarly, splenomegaly is not always associated with hypersplenism.

EPIDEMIOLOGY

May be as common as 30–70% in patients with cirrhosis and portal hypertension (HTN)

ETIOLOGY AND PATHOPHYSIOLOGY

- Enlargement of the spleen results in sequestration of formed blood elements, leading to peripheral cytopenias and concomitant bone marrow precursor hyperplasia.
- Many of the common etiologies are listed below. Almost any process involving the spleen or the hematologic system can result in hypersplenism:
  - Infectious
    - Tuberculosis
    - Brucellosis
    - Malaria
    - Leishmaniasis
    - Ehrlichiosis
    - Schistosomiasis
    - Histoplasmosis
    - Candidiasis
    - Viral
    - Syphilis
    - Infective endocarditis
  - Hematologic
    - Myeloproliferative disorders
    - Polycythemia vera
    - Primary hypersplenism
    - ITP
    - Hemolytic anemias
  - Neoplastic
    - Hematologic malignancies
    - Melanoma
    - Various carcinomas
    - Metastatic cancers
  - Storage diseases
    - Gaucher disease
    - Niemann-Pick disease
    - Amyloidosis
    - Glycogen storage disease
  - Inflammatory
    - Sarcoidosis
    - Systemic lupus erythematosus
    - Felty syndrome
  - Congestive
    - Cirrhosis
    - Heart failure
    - Portal or splenic vein thrombosis
    - Congenital malformations of the portal vein

 DIAGNOSIS

HISTORY

- Patients may complain of abdominal fullness or protrusion of the spleen through the abdominal wall; may complain of early satiety if the spleen is compressing stomach
- Patients may complain of tenderness in the left upper quadrant, especially with viral infections. In lymphoproliferative disorders, spleen may be enlarged but asymptomatic unless there is splenic infarction. Given location of the spleen next to the diaphragm, a sense of fullness may be referred through the phrenic nerve to the C3–C5 dermatomes in the left shoulder.
- Symptoms related to the underlying cause of hypersplenism may be present.

PHYSICAL EXAM

Splenomegaly

- The normal spleen is not palpable. A palpable spleen always indicates underlying abnormality such as splenomegaly and, in turn, hypersplenism in the appropriate clinical context or may indicate a wandering spleen. Also, spleen can be palpated in chronic obstructive pulmonary disease and acute asthma exacerbation, without coexisting splenomegaly.
- Begin by percussing Traube semilunar space, demarcated laterally by left anterior axillary line, inferiorly by the left costal margin, and superiorly by the left 6th rib. This space is usually hollow. Splenic enlargement may cause dullness to percussion in this area. Other processes that may cause dullness include pleural or pericardial effusions. Additionally, if the patient recently ate a large meal, this area may be dull to percussion.
- With patient supine, rest hand gently on the abdomen to prevent sudden tensing of the abdominal musculature, which may obscure palpation. Better abdominal relaxation can be obtained by flexing the knees toward the abdomen. As the spleen enlarges, it moves caudally and medially. Start by palpating in the right lower quadrant and moving toward the umbilicus, toward the left upper quadrant. If there is doubt about whether the spleen has moved beyond the costal margin, ask patient to take a large breath, which will push the diaphragm, and, in turn, the spleen toward the examiner's hands.
- Jaundice: if hemolytic anemia is present or in advanced cirrhosis
- Petechiae, purpura, or ecchymosis: if thrombocytopenia is present
- Lymphadenopathy: in hematologic or solid organ malignancies. It also can be seen in infectious etiologies.

DIAGNOSTIC TESTS & INTERPRETATION

On CBC, any and all cell lines may be decreased, resulting in the following:

- Anemia
- Leukopenia
- Thrombocytopenia

Initial Tests (lab, imaging)

- CBC
- Reticulocyte count if anemia
- If there is hemolysis, there should be an elevated reticulocyte count, elevated LDH, decreased haptoglobin, along with evidence of hyperbilirubinemia (unconjugated).
- US
- CT
- Tc-99m sulfur colloid scintigraphy
- PET
- MRI

Follow-Up Tests & Special Considerations

Based on other historical and exam findings, testing for specific infectious etiologies may be warranted:

- Blood parasite smear for malaria and other parasitic infections
- EBV serologies
- HIV ELISA with Western blot
- JAK2 mutation in polycythemia vera
- PPD for tuberculosis
- Hgb electrophoresis in hereditary hemoglobinopathies

Diagnostic Procedures/Other

- Bone marrow biopsy
- Liver biopsy for cirrhosis and storage diseases

Test Interpretation

Hyperplasia of bone marrow precursors, especially those correlating with the patient's individual cytopenias

TREATMENT

MEDICATION

- No specific medication can be recommended for patients with hypersplenism. The most important intervention is to treat the underlying disorder.
- If ITP is the cause, the patient may benefit from the following:
  - Prednisone or methylprednisolone
  - IVIG
  - Rituximab
- If an infectious cause is discovered, treatment with appropriate antibiotic therapy may help to improve the cytopenias.

SURGERY/OTHER PROCEDURES

- Many patients with severe uncontrolled cytopenias undergo splenectomy.
- Laparoscopic splenectomy is preferred over open splenectomy (1)[A].

ALERT

Splenectomized patients should receive immunization to pneumococcus, meningococcus, *Haemophilus influenzae*, and influenza at least 14 days prior to splenectomy (2)[A].

- If this cannot be done (i.e., in cases of emergent splenectomy), wait at least 14 days postsplenectomy to immunize.
  - Pneumococcal vaccine
    - Pneumococcal polyvalent-23 vaccine (PPSV23) for use in adults and fully immunized children ≥2 years of age

- ○ Pneumococcal polyvalent-13 vaccine (PCV13) for infants and young children ≥2 months of age as part of routine immunization schedule (3)[A]
- ○ PCV13 for children >2 years of age, adolescents and adults in addition to PPSV23; refer to CDC for timing of administration.
- ○ Current guidelines recommend single revaccination of PPSV23 5 years after the initial dose and again at age of ≥65 years, at least 5 years after the previous dose.
- – *H. influenzae* vaccine
  - ○ All unvaccinated individuals ≥5 years of age should be given 1 dose of *H. influenzae* type B (Hib) conjugate vaccine.
  - ○ Children <5 years old should also be vaccinated. Refer to CDC for timing.
  - ○ Vaccinated individuals can also be given additional dose of vaccine (4)[A].
- – Meningococcal vaccine (5)[A]
  - ○ Meningococcal conjugate vaccine (MCV4) for use in patients between 2 and 55 years
  - ○ Meningococcal polysaccharide vaccine (MPSV4) for use in patients >55 years of age
  - ○ Revaccination is recommended every 5 years.
- – Influenza vaccine should be administered yearly based on prevalent circulating strains. Although patients are not at higher risk from influenza itself, infection with influenza may place patients at higher risk for secondary bacterial infections.
- Radiofrequency ablation (RFA) is becoming more available and can be successful at preventing recurrence of hypersplenism. It is not currently known whether there are differences between RFA and splenectomy in terms of postprocedure infectious risks. Other alternatives to splenectomy include total and partial splenic embolization and shunting, although these techniques are evolving and additional studies are needed to evaluate efficacy and morbidity as compared to splenectomy.

ADMISSION, INPATIENT, AND NURSING CONSIDERATIONS

- Hypersplenism alone generally does not warrant admission. However, all patients should be monitored closely for complications of the resulting cytopenias, including bleeding and infection, as well as complications of splenomegaly, including increased risk of splenic rupture. In some patients, the large spleen compresses the stomach and prevents adequate oral intake.
- Splenectomized patients are at increased risk of infection and postsplenectomy sepsis, especially with *Streptococcus pneumoniae*. Fevers, chills, or pain concerning for underlying infection warrant immediate attention because clinical decompensation can occur within hours. Empiric broad-spectrum antibiotics should not be delayed while evaluation is ongoing. Common empiric regimens include the following:
  - – Ceftriaxone: 2 g IV q24h and vancomycin 1 g IV q12h
  - – Levofloxacin: 750 mg IV q24h and vancomycin 1 g IV q12h in β-lactam–allergic patients

 ONGOING CARE

- Adult patients who are splenectomized should be advised to monitor closely for fever or rigors at home, which may be an early sign of bacteremia. They should be instructed to begin antibiotics immediately prior to proceeding to a medical facility for evaluation. Early antibiotics have been shown to reduce the mortality from overwhelming postsplenectomy sepsis.
- Controlled trials have not been performed, but some regimens include the following:
  - – Amoxicillin-clavulanate: 875 mg PO BID
  - – Cefuroxime axetil: 500 mg PO BID
- Patients allergic to β-lactam antibiotics can be given an extended-spectrum fluoroquinolone such as levofloxacin 750 mg PO *or* moxifloxacin 400 mg PO daily.
- In children with splenectomy, daily antibiotic prophylaxis for overwhelming postsplenectomy sepsis with penicillin VK or amoxicillin is recommended until age 5 years or at least 3 years after splenectomy:
  - – Age 2 months to 5 years: 125 mg PO BID
  - – >5 years old: 250 mg PO BID

PATIENT EDUCATION

Patients who are splenectomized should be counseled extensively about the risk of overwhelming postsplenectomy sepsis and the need to obtain prompt medical evaluation in the event of fevers, chills, or any other concerning symptoms.

REFERENCES

1. Bai YN, Jiang H, Prasoon P. A meta-analysis of perioperative outcomes of laparoscopic splenectomy for hematological disorders. *World J Surg*. 2012;36(10):2349–2358.
2. Advisory Committee on Immunization Practices. Recommended adult immunization schedule: United States, 2012. *Ann Intern Med*. 2012;156(3):211–217.
3. American Academy of Pediatrics. Children with asplenia or functional asplenia. In: Pickering LK, Baker CJ, Kimberlin DW, et al, eds. *Red Book: 2009 Report of the Committee on Infectious Diseases*. 28th ed. Elk Grove Village, IL: American Academy of Pediatrics; 2009:72.
4. American Academy of Pediatrics Committee on Infectious Diseases: *Haemophilus influenzae* type b conjugate vaccines: recommendations for immunization with recently and previously licensed vaccines. *Pediatrics*. 1993;92(3):480–488.
5. Centers for Disease Control and Prevention. Updated recommendations for use of meningococcal conjugate vaccines—Advisory Committee on Immunization Practices (ACIP), 2010. *MMWR Morb Mortal Wkly Rep*. 2011;60(3):72–76.

ADDITIONAL READING

- Abdella HM, Abd-El-Moez AT, Abu El-Maaty ME, et al. Role of partial splenic arterial embolization for hypersplenism in patients with liver cirrhosis and thrombocytopenia. *Indian J Gastroenterol*. 2010;29(2):59–61.
- Di Sabatino A, Carsetti R, Corazza GR. Postsplenectomy and hyposplenic states. *Lancet*. 2011;378(9785):86–97.
- Feng K, Ma K, Liu Q, et al. Randomized clinical trial of splenic radiofrequency ablation versus splenectomy for severe hypersplenism. *Br J Surg*. 2011;98(3):354–361.
- Iriyama N, Horikoshi A, Hatta Y, et al. Localized, splenic, diffuse large B-cell lymphoma presenting with hypersplenism: risk and benefit of splenectomy. *Intern Med*. 2010;49(11):1027–1030.
- Jandl JH, Aster RH, Forkner CE, et al. Splenic pooling and the pathophysiology of hypersplenism. *Trans Am Clin Climatol Assoc*. 1967;78:9–27.
- Kapoor P, Singh E, Radhakrishnan P, et al. Splenectomy in plasma cell dyscrasias: a review of the clinical practice. *Am J Hematol*. 2006;81(12):946–954.
- Mourtzoukou EG, Pappas G, Peppas G, et al. Vaccination of asplenic or hyposplenic adults. *Br J Surg*. 2008;95(3):273–280.
- Shatz DV, Schinsky MF, Pais LB, et al. Immune responses of splenectomized trauma patients to the 23-valent pneumococcal polysaccharide vaccine at 1 versus 7 versus 14 days after splenectomy. *J Trauma*. 1998;44(5):760–766.

 SEE ALSO

Anemia, Autoimmune Hemolytic; Malaria; Polycythemia Vera; Tuberculosis

 CODES

ICD10
D73.1 Hypersplenism

CLINICAL PEARLS

- Splenectomy is not necessary to make the diagnosis.
- Avoid splenectomy in patients unless absolutely necessary. Splenectomized patients are at lifelong risk for overwhelming postsplenectomy infection and sepsis.
- If splenectomy is to be performed, give immunization for pneumococcus, meningococcus, *H. influenzae*, and influenza at least 14 days prior to surgery. Otherwise, wait until the 14th postoperative day to immunize.

H

HYPERTENSION, ESSENTIAL

Ronald N. Adler, MD, FAAFP • Jeremy Golding, MD, FAAFP

BASICS

DESCRIPTION

- Essential hypertension (HTN) is HTN without an identifiable cause; it is also known as primary HTN and benign HTN. Although its importance as a risk factor for cardiovascular and other morbidity and mortality is well-established, there is significant and increasing controversy regarding recommended thresholds for diagnosis and treatment.
- HTN is defined (Joint National Committee [JNC] 8) as ≥2 elevated BPs (1).
  – Age <60 years: systolic BP (SBP) ≥140 mm Hg and/or diastolic BP (DBP) ≥90 mm Hg at ≥2 visits
  – Age ≥60 years: SBP ≥150 mm Hg and/or DBP ≥90 mm Hg at ≥2 visits
  – With diabetes or chronic kidney disease (CKD): SBP ≥140 and/or DBP ≥90 mm Hg
- Synonym(s): benign, chronic, idiopathic, familial, or genetic HTN; high BP

Geriatric Considerations

- Isolated systolic HTN is common.
- Therapy has been shown to be effective and beneficial at preventing stroke, although target SBP is higher than in younger patients (~150 mm Hg systolic), and adverse reactions to medications are more frequent (2)[A]. The benefit of therapy has been conclusively demonstrated in older patients for SBP ≥160 mm Hg. More aggressive targets may be appropriate for higher risk individuals (2)[A].

Pediatric Considerations

- Measure BP during routine exams for >3 years of age.
- Defined as SBP or DBP ≥95th percentile on repeated measurements
- Pre-HTN: SBP or DBP between 90th and 95th percentile

Pregnancy Considerations

- Elevated BP during pregnancy may represent chronic HTN, pregnancy-induced HTN, or preeclampsia. ACE inhibitors and angiotensin II receptor blockers (ARBs) are contraindicated.
- Maternal and fetal mortality are reduced with treatment of severe HTN. Evidence is not clear for treatment of mild HTN (see topic "Preeclampsia and Eclampsia (Toxemia of Pregnancy)").
- Preferred agents: methyldopa, labetalol, hydralazine, or nifedipine

EPIDEMIOLOGY

Incidence

Incidence and prevalence is higher among men. Depending on the definition used, 32–46% of adults in the United States have HTN.

ETIOLOGY AND PATHOPHYSIOLOGY

- >90% of cases of HTN have no identified cause.
- For differential diagnosis and causes of secondary HTN, see "Hypertension, Secondary and Resistant."

Genetics

BP levels are strongly familial, but no clear genetic pattern exists. Familial risk for cardiovascular diseases (CVDs) should be considered.

RISK FACTORS

Family history, obesity, alcohol use, excess dietary sodium, stress, physical inactivity, tobacco use, insulin resistance

DIAGNOSIS

Despite more aggressive guidelines issued by the ACC/AHA in 2017 (3)[C], many experts consider recommendations from JNC 8 to retain primacy. Critics of the ACC/AHA guidelines note multiple methodologic concerns, especially the fact the guidelines were heavily influenced by the findings of SPRINT, which was conducted in a relatively high-risk population and therefore less applicable to many patients seen in primary care. Embracing the low diagnostic threshold (<130/80) endorsed by AHA/ACC compared to JNC 8 would result in the diagnosis of and treatment for HTN of millions more people, with unclear benefits and likely harm. Therefore, this chapter uses JNC 8 as its basis but focuses on recommendations that are relevant regardless of the specific guideline which is being applied. These include the approach to diagnosis and using assessment of overall CV risk to guide decisions regarding treatment.

HISTORY

- HTN is asymptomatic except in extreme cases or after related cardiovascular complications develop.
- Headache can be seen with higher BP, often present on awakening and occipital in location.

PHYSICAL EXAM

- Body mass index (BMI), waist circumference
- BP in both arms (see below for correct technique—essential to accurate diagnosis and treatment)
- Complete cardiac and peripheral pulse exam: Compare radial and femoral pulse for differences in volume and timing, auscultation for carotid and femoral bruits.
- Evaluate for signs of end-organ damage.
- Funduscopic exam for arteriolar narrowing, AV compression, hemorrhages, exudates, and papilledema

DIFFERENTIAL DIAGNOSIS

- Secondary HTN: Because of the low incidence of reversible secondary HTN, special tests should be considered only if the history, physical exam, or basic laboratory evaluation suggest a higher likelihood. Also consider for patients who prove nonresponsive to treatment (see "Hypertension, Secondary and Resistant").
- White coat HTN: elevation of BP in office setting and normal BP outside office
- Masked HTN: elevated BP at home and normal BP in office

DIAGNOSTIC TESTS & INTERPRETATION

Incorrect BP determination a common cause of overdiagnosis

ALERT

- Measuring BP:
  – Caffeine, exercise, and smoking avoided >30 minutes before measurement
  – Patient seated quietly for 5 minutes with feet on floor
  – Patient's arm supported at heart level
  – Correct cuff size
  – Deflate cuff slowly or use an automated device.
  – Average of two or more measurements
  – Avoid "rounding" results.
- A diagnosis of HTN should be made under the following circumstances:
  – Age <60 years: SBP ≥140 mm Hg and/or DBP ≥90 mm Hg at ≥2 visits
  – Age ≥60 years: SBP ≥150 mm Hg and/or DBP ≥90 mm Hg at ≥2 visits
  – Age ≥60 years with CKD or diabetes: SBP ≥140 mm Hg and/or DBP ≥90 mm Hg at ≥2 visits

Initial Tests (lab, imaging)

- Hemoglobin or hematocrit or CBC
- Complete urinalysis (may reveal proteinuria, hematuria/nephritis)
- Potassium, calcium, creatinine, and uric acid
- Lipid panel (total, HDL, LDL, triglyceride)
- Fasting blood glucose or hemoglobin A1c
- ECG to evaluate possible presence of left ventricular hypertrophy (LVH) or rhythm abnormalities

Follow-Up Tests & Special Considerations

- Special tests only if suggested by history, physical, or labs. Consider possibility of sleep apnea with high BMI.
- Ambulatory (24-hour) BP monitoring if "white coat" HTN is suspected, episodic HTN, or autonomic dysfunction
- Home BP monitoring is effective; elevated home BPs correlate with adverse outcomes, possibly more so than office BPs, and normal readings are reassuring.
- Cardiovascular risk assessment should be performed. The AHA/ACC risk tool based on Framingham data likely significantly overestimates risk (50–75%). Others have used a definition of "low risk" that excludes patients with a history of CVD, DM, CKD, or FH of premature CAD (4).

TREATMENT

GENERAL MEASURES

- The treatment discussed follows JNC 8 guidelines. More intensive therapy may be warranted for certain high-risk individuals (5)[B].
- Individual treatment goals should be jointly established with patients after discussion of the anticipated potential benefits and harms (shared decision making) (1)[A],(2)[C].
- Recommend lifestyle improvements, including diet, exercise, and reducing or eliminating tobacco/alcohol.
- Benefit of pharmacologic treatment of low-risk patients with class I HTN (SBP 140 to 150 mm Hg, DBP 90 to 99 mm Hg) remains uncertain (4,6)[A], with harms including syncope, kidney injury, and electrolyte abnormalities.
- Treating patients age <60 years or with CKD or diabetes to lower-than-standard BP targets, <140/90 mm Hg, does not further reduce mortality or morbidity. Individualize goal BP based on risk factors.
- A target SBP at or just below 150 mm Hg in patients >60 years of age is acceptable in the general population (1).
- The majority of treatment benefit is attained with initial 2 to 3 medications. Striving for small additional drops in BP to achieve a "target" is less clinically beneficial and more likely to cause adverse effects.
- Lower than standard DBP targets are not associated with decreased morbidity/mortality.
- More aggressive treatment should be considered in patients meeting enrollment criteria for SPRINT because aggressive treatment does show improvement in outcomes, but 61 nondiabetic patients would need to be treated (NNT) for 3 years to a goal of SBP <120 to prevent a major cardiovascular outcome and 90 to prevent one death (5)[B].

MEDICATION

- Multiple drugs at submaximal dose may achieve target BP with fewer side effects. In patients on >1 medication, divide between morning and night time for better 24-hour antihypertensive effect.
- Sequential monotherapy attempts should be tried with different classes because individual responses vary.
- Many patients will require multiple medications.
- For initial monotherapy, choose from 1 of 4 classes of medications: ACE inhibitors, ARBs, calcium channel blockers (CCBs), or diuretics (1)[A].
- Thiazide diuretics or CCB preferred as first line in the general black population
- Chlorthalidone has a longer half-life than HCTZ and is the preferred diuretic based on established trial evidence of benefit.
- If concomitant conditions, choose first-line agent based on comorbidity.
- β-Blockers had been strongly recommended until recent meta-analyses. Atenolol may be particularly *ineffective* in reducing adverse outcomes of HTN (except in patients with left ventricle hypertrophy undergoing dialysis).
- β-Blockers might benefit patients with ischemic heart disease, CHF, migraine, and patients with history of ST-segment elevation myocardial infarction (STEMI).
- ACE inhibitors should be used in patients with diabetes, proteinuria, atrial fibrillation, or heart failure with reduced ejection fraction (HFrEF) but *not in pregnancy.*
- α-Adrenergic blockers are not a first choice for monotherapy but remain as second line after combination therapy of first-line agents; might benefit males with benign prostatic hypertrophy (BPH)
- CCB could be considered in patients with isolated systolic HTN, atherosclerosis, angina, migraine, or asthma; well documented to reduce risk of stroke

First Line

- Thiazide diuretics (5)[A] may not be effective with creatinine clearance <30.
  - Chlorthalidone: 12.5 to 25.0 mg/day (more potent than hydrochlorothiazide but causes more hyponatremia and hypokalemia)
  - Hydrochlorothiazide: 12.5 to 50.0 mg/day
  - Indapamide: 1.25 to 2.50 mg/day
  - Metolazone: 2.5 to 5.0 mg daily is more effective in patients with impaired renal function.
- ACE inhibitors
  - Lisinopril: 5 to 40 mg/day
  - Enalapril: 5 to 40 mg/day
  - Ramipril: 2.5 to 20.0 mg/day
  - Benazepril: 10 to 40 mg/day
- CCB
  - Diltiazem CD: 180 to 360 mg/day
  - Nifedipine (sustained release): 30 to 90 mg/day
  - Verapamil (sustained release): 120 to 480 mg/day
  - Amlodipine: 2.5 to 10.0 mg/day
- ARBs
  - Losartan: 25 to 100 mg in 1 or 2 doses; has unique but modest uricosuric effect
  - Valsartan: 80 to 320 mg daily
  - Irbesartan: 75 to 300 mg daily
  - Candesartan: 4 to 32 mg daily
  - Renin inhibitor: aliskiren 150 to 300 mg daily
- Contraindications
  - Thiazide diuretics may worsen gout.
  - β-Blockers (relative) in reactive airway disease, heart block, diabetes, and peripheral vascular disease; probably should be avoided in patients with metabolic syndrome or insulin-requiring diabetes

- Diltiazem or verapamil: Do not use with systolic dysfunction or heart block. Amlodipine may cause peripheral edema.

Second Line

- Before escalating therapy, ensure that patient is adherent to prescribed regimen.
- Many may be combined. Choose additional medications with complementary effects (i.e., ACE inhibitors/ARBs with diuretic or a vasodilator with a diuretic or β-blocker). Don't combine ACE inhibitor and ARB.
- Medication-refractory HTN: Spironolactone 25 to 100 mg/day or eplerenone 50 mg once to twice daily are especially effective.
- Centrally acting α-2 agonists: clonidine 0.1 to 1.2 mg BID or weekly patch 0.1 to 0.3 mg/day, guanfacine 1 to 3 mg daily, or methyldopa 250 to 2,000 mg BID
- α-Adrenergic antagonists: prazosin 1 to 10 mg BID, terazosin 1 to 20 mg/day, or doxazosin 1 to 16 mg/day
- Vasodilators
  - Hydralazine: 10 to 25 mg QID; risk of tachycardia, so generally combined with β-blocker; also drug-induced systemic lupus erythematosus (SLE)
  - Minoxidil: rarely used due to adverse effects; may be more effective than other medications in renal failure and refractory HTN
- Metolazone and loop diuretics may be used with more severe renal impairment, but outcomes data are absent; loop diuretics (for volume overload): furosemide 20 to 320 mg/day or bumetanide 0.5 to 2.0 mg/day
- K+-sparing diuretics in patients with hypokalemia while taking thiazides: amiloride 5 to 10 mg/day or triamterene 50 to 150 mg/day

COMPLEMENTARY & ALTERNATIVE MEDICINE

- Biofeedback and relaxation exercise
- Dietary supplements such as garlic have been suggested for lowering BP, but evidence is lacking.

 ONGOING CARE

FOLLOW-UP RECOMMENDATIONS

Patient Monitoring

- Reevaluate patients q3–6mo until stable and then q6–12mo. Consider use of home self-BP monitoring; quality-of-life issues including sexual function should be considered.
- Poor medication adherence is a leading cause of apparent medication failure.
- At least annual creatinine and potassium for patients on diuretics, ACE inhibitors, and ARBs

DIET

- ~20% of patients will respond to reduced-salt diet (<100 mmol/day; <6 g NaCl or <2.4 g Na).
- Consider Dietary Approaches to Stop HTN (DASH) diet: http://www.nhlbi.nih.gov/files/docs/public/heart/hbp_low.pdf.
- Limit alcohol consumption to <1 oz/day.

PATIENT EDUCATION

- Emphasize the asymptomatic nature of HTN.
- Printed aids for high BP education available: http://www.nhlbi.nih.gov/health/public/heart

COMPLICATIONS

Heart failure, renal failure, LVH, myocardial infarction, retinal hemorrhage, stroke, hypertensive heart disease, drug side effects, erectile dysfunction

REFERENCES

1. James PA, Oparil S, Carter BL, et al. 2014 Evidence-based guideline for the management of high blood pressure in adults: report from the panel members appointed to the Eighth Joint National Committee (JNC 8). *JAMA.* 2014;311(5):507–520.
2. Qaseem A, Wilt TJ, Rich R, et al. Pharmacologic treatment of hypertension in adults aged 60 years or older to higher versus lower blood pressure targets: a clinical practice guideline from the American College of Physicians and the American Academy of Family Physicians. *Ann Intern Med.* 2017;166(6):430–437.
3. Whelton PK, Carey RM, Aronow WS, et al. 2017 ACC/AHA/AAPA/ABC/ACPM/AGS/APhA/ASH/ASPC/NMA/PCNA guideline for the prevention, detection, evaluation, and management of high blood pressure in adults: executive summary: a report of the American College of Cardiology/American Heart Association Task Force on Clinical Practice Guidelines. *Hypertension.* 2018;71(6):1269–1324.
4. Sheppard JP, Stevens S, Stevens R, et al. Benefits and harms of antihypertensive treatment in low-risk patients with mild hypertension. *JAMA Intern Med.* 2018;178(12):1626–1634.
5. Wright JT Jr, Williamson JD, Whelton PK, et al; for SPRINT Research Group. A randomized trial of intensive versus standard blood-pressure control. *N Engl J Med.* 2015;373(22):2103–2116.
6. Diao D, Wright JM, Cundiff DK, et al. Pharmacotherapy for mild hypertension. *Cochrane Database Syst Rev.* 2012;(8):CD006742.

 SEE ALSO

Hypertension, Secondary and Resistant; Hypertensive Emergencies; Polycystic Kidney Disease

 CODES

ICD10

I10 Essential (primary) hypertension

CLINICAL PEARLS

- Treatment of HTN reduces risk of many serious medical conditions with NNT to prevent one serious MACE ranging from ~20 patients per year for severe HTN to more than several hundred per year for milder HTN.
- Multiple submaximal doses are likely to have fewer side effects and more effectiveness than fewer maximum-dosed drugs.
- Treatment decisions should be informed by BP measured by proper technique; accurate measures obtained outside the clinical office may be more predictive of CV risk.
- Appropriate lifestyle changes should be recommended before and during pharmacologic treatment.
- Overly aggressive treatment may cause significant harms, including syncope and electrolyte abnormalities; effects are more likely and often more significant in the elderly.
- Treatment goals should be informed by risk assessment and periodically revisited and jointly established through shared decision making, informed by anticipated potential benefits and harms.

H

HYPERTENSION, SECONDARY AND RESISTANT

George Maxted, MD

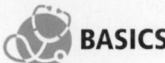 BASICS

DESCRIPTION

Uncontrolled hypertension (HTN) comprises the following entities (see "Alert" below):

- Resistant HTN: defined as blood pressure (BP) that remains above goal in spite of the concurrent use of three antihypertensive agents of different classes. Ideally, one of the three agents should be a diuretic, and all agents should be prescribed at optimal dose amounts (1)[C].
- Secondary HTN: elevated BP that results from an identifiable underlying mechanism (1)
- The 2017 revised ACC/AHA guideline recommends a change in the classification of HTN. For the purposes of this chapter, we will be considering stage 2 HTN: systolic blood pressure (SBP) ≥140 mm Hg or diastolic blood pressure (DBP) ≥90 mm Hg. The guideline is controversial (2). Many experts still adhere to the JNC 8 guideline, which allows for a goal of <150/90 mm Hg for patients age >60 years (3)[C].

Geriatric Considerations

- Onset of HTN in adults >60 years of age is a strong indicator of secondary HTN.
- In patients >80 years of age, consider a higher target SBP of ≥150 mm Hg. Be cautious to avoid excessive diastolic lowering.
- Elderly are particularly responsive to diuretics and dihydropyridine calcium channel blockers.
- Systolic HTN is particularly problematic in the elderly.
- Secondary causes more common in the elderly include sleep apnea, renal disease, renal artery stenosis, and primary aldosteronism (PA).
- Noncompressible arteries (Osler phenomenon)—mostly in elderly with arteriosclerosis: Brachial and radial artery pulsations are present at high cuff pressures.

ALERT
Pseudoresistance

- Inaccurate measurement of BP
  - Cuff too small
  - Patient not at rest; sitting quietly for 5 minutes
- Poor adherence: In primary care settings, this has been estimated to occur in 40–60% of patients with HTN.
- White coat effect: prevalence 20–40%. Do not make clinical decisions about HTN based solely on measurement in the clinic setting. Home BP monitoring and/or ambulatory BP monitoring is more reliable. See USPSTF recommendations.
- Inadequate treatment

EPIDEMIOLOGY

- Predominant age: In general, HTN has its onset between ages 30 and 50 years. Patients with resistant HTN are more likely to experience the combined outcomes of death, myocardial infarction, congestive heart failure (CHF), stroke, or chronic kidney disease.
- Depending on etiology, age of onset can vary. Age of onset <20 or >50 years increases likelihood of a secondary cause for HTN.

- The strongest predictors for resistant HTN are age (>75 years), presence of left ventricular hypertrophy (LVH), obesity (body mass index [BMI] >30), and high baseline SBP. Other predictors include chronic kidney disease, diabetes, living in the southeastern United States, African American race (especially women), and excessive salt intake.

Prevalence

- Prevalence of resistant HTN is unknown. NHANES analysis indicates only 53% of adults are controlled to a BP of <140/90 mm Hg.
- Secondary HTN occurs in about 5–10% of adults with chronic HTN.

ETIOLOGY AND PATHOPHYSIOLOGY

- Obstructive sleep apnea (OSA): One study diagnosed OSA in 83% of treatment-resistant hypertensives.
- Primary hyperaldosteronism (17–22% of resistant HTN cases)
- Chronic renal disease (2–5% of hypertensives)
- Renovascular disease (0.2–0.7%, up to 35% of elderly, 20% of patients undergoing cardiac catheterization)
- Cushing syndrome (0.1–0.6%)
- Pheochromocytoma (0.04–0.1% of hypertensives)
- Other rare causes: hyperthyroidism, hyperparathyroidism, aortic coarctation, intracranial tumor
- Drug-related causes
  - Medications, especially NSAIDs (may also blunt effectiveness of ACE inhibitors), decongestants, stimulants (e.g., amphetamines, attention deficient hyperactivity disorder [ADHD] medications), anorectic agents (e.g., modafinil, ephedra, guarana, ma huang, bitter orange), erythropoietin, natural licorice (in some chewing tobacco), yohimbine, glucocorticoids
  - Oral contraceptives: unclear association; mainly epidemiologic and with higher estrogen pills
  - Cocaine, amphetamines, other illicit drugs; drug and alcohol withdrawal syndromes
- Lifestyle factors: Obesity and dietary salt may negate the beneficial effect of diuretics. Excessive alcohol may cause or exacerbate HTN. Physical inactivity also contributes.

RISK FACTORS

A recent large cohort study revealed that those with resistant HTN (16.2%) were more likely to be male, Caucasian, older, and diabetic. They were also more likely to be taking β-blockers, calcium channel blockers, and α-adrenergic blockers compared with other drug classes. Factors predictive of resistant or secondary HTN: female sex, African American race, obesity, diabetes, worsening of control in previously stable hypertensive patient, onset in patients age <20 years or >50 years, lack of family history of HTN, significant target end-organ damage, stage 2 HTN (SBP >160 mm Hg or DBP >100 mm Hg), renal disease, and alcohol or drug use

GENERAL PREVENTION

The prevention of resistant and secondary HTN is thought to be the same as for primary or essential HTN: Adopting a Dietary Approaches to Stop Hypertension (DASH) diet, a low-sodium diet, weight loss in obese patients, exercise, limitation of alcohol intake, and smoking cessation may all be of benefit. Relaxation techniques may be of help, but data are limited.

 DIAGNOSIS

HISTORY

- Ask or review at every visit: SANS mnemonic: (i) Salt intake, (ii) Alcohol intake, (iii) NSAID use, (iv) Sleep (author's suggestion, based on reference listed) (2)
- Review home BP readings; consider ambulatory BP monitoring.
- History will vary with etiology of HTN.
- Pheochromocytoma: episodes of headache, palpitations, sweating
- Cushing syndrome: weight gain, fatigue, weakness, easy bruising, amenorrhea
- OSA: loud snoring while asleep, daytime somnolence
- Increased intravascular volume: swelling

PHYSICAL EXAM

- Ensure that the BP is measured correctly. The patient should be sitting quietly with back supported for at least 5 minutes before measurement. Proper cuff size: bladder encircling at least 80% of the arm. Support arm at heart level. Minimum of two readings at least 1 minute apart. Check BP in both arms. Also check standing BP for orthostasis.
- The USPSTF recommends "obtaining measurements outside of the clinical setting for diagnostic confirmation." Attention to findings related to possible etiologies: renovascular HTN: systolic/diastolic abdominal bruit; pheochromocytoma: diaphoresis, tachycardia; Cushing syndrome: hirsutism, moon facies, dorsal hump, purple striae, truncal obesity; thyroid disease: enlarged thyroid, tremor, exophthalmos, tachycardia; coarctation of the aorta: upper limb HTN with decreased or delayed femoral pulses
- Funduscopic exam

DIAGNOSTIC TESTS & INTERPRETATION

- ECG performed as part of the initial workup; LVH is an important marker of resistant HTN.
- Sleep study if history and physical indicate. The Epworth Sleepiness Scale is recommended.
- Home-based polysomnography has been shown to be accurate in screening for OSA. Overnight oximetry is not helpful.

Initial Tests (lab, imaging)

Initial limited diagnostic testing should include urinalysis, CBC, potassium, sodium, glucose, creatinine, lipids, thyroid-stimulating hormone (TSH), and calcium. 50% of patients with hyperaldosteronism may have normal potassium levels.

- Imaging tests listed are necessary only if history, physical, or lab data indicate.
- Abdominal US: if renal disease is suspected
- Duplex ultrasonography may be the preferred test for renovascular disease. MR angiography (MRA) of renal vasculature is sensitive but has low specificity and potentially more harmful. Conventional catheter angiography or CT angiography may be required to confirm the diagnosis.
- Adrenal "incidentaloma" frequently arises in this era of multiple CT studies. If present in the setting of resistant HTN, consider hyperaldosteronism or hyperadrenal corticoid states.

Follow-Up Tests & Special Considerations

Further testing for PA may be considered.

- Empiric treatment with an aldosterone inhibitor may be preferable and more clinically relevant: spironolactone or eplerenone. Amiloride may be more effective in African Americans.
- Plasma aldosterone-to-renin ratio (ARR) is the preferred lab test, but the test is difficult to perform and interpret properly. Consult your reference lab and interpret results with caution.
  - Further testing for pheochromocytoma: plasma metanephrines
  - Other tests to consider for resistant or secondary HTN: 24-hour urine for free cortisol, calcium, parathyroid hormone (PTH), overnight 1-mg dexamethasone suppression test, urine toxicology screen

Diagnostic Procedures/Other

Consider 24-hour ambulatory BP monitoring, especially if white coat effect is suspected. Home BP monitor results predict mortality, stroke, and other target organ damage better than office BP. Optimal protocol involves two paired measurements: morning and evening (four measurements) over 4 to 7 days.

- Oscillometric, electronic, upper arm, fully automatic device with memory: average multiple readings over several days
- See http://www.dableducational.org/ for validated monitors.

 TREATMENT

- Treatment modality depends on etiology of HTN. Please see each etiology listed for information on proper treatment.
- Emphasize adherence to JNC 8 and/or AHA/ACC guidelines, with emphasis on lifestyle modification (2,3)[C].
  - Obese patients, African Americans, and elderly may be particularly responsive to diuretics.
  - Tolerance to diuretics may occur: long-term adaptation to thiazides or the "braking effect." Consider increasing the dose of thiazide or adding an aldosterone inhibitor.
- Treatment specific to certain secondary etiologies
  - PA: aldosterone receptor antagonist: spironolactone or eplerenone
  - Cushing syndrome: aldosterone receptor antagonist
  - OSA: continuous positive airway pressure (CPAP) ± oxygen, surgery, weight loss
    - Mandibular advancement devices may be equally effective in some patients.
  - Nocturnal hypoxia: oxygen supplementation
  - Renal sympathetic denervation has been largely disproven as an effective strategy. New techniques/approaches are under study.
- The treatment of atherosclerotic renal artery stenosis (ARAS) is controversial. A recent meta-analysis again questions the value of percutaneous stenting (4)[B].

MEDICATION

- Follow treatment guidelines and algorithms by JNC 8 and AHA/ACC/CDC, understanding the differences between them (2,3)[C].

- Adding a medication to the regimen may have greater efficacy than increasing the dose of medications (see JNC 8 management algorithm option B) (3).
- Aldosterone antagonists may offer significant benefit (5)[B].
- Central-acting agents (e.g., clonidine) are effective at reducing BP, but outcome data are lacking.

ALERT

- Agents specific for treatment of HTN emergencies should be initiated in those situations, in which immediate BP reduction will prevent or limit end-organ damage (see "Hypertensive Emergencies").
- Renovascular HTN: Angioplasty is the treatment of choice for fibromuscular dysplasia of a renal artery.
- The recent CORAL study concluded that in patients with atherosclerotic renovascular disease and HTN, renal artery stenting did not improve outcomes over medical therapy alone.
- Referral to an HTN specialist or clinic: Retrospective studies indicate improved control rates for patients with resistant HTN referred to special HTN clinics.

First Line

- For non-black patients: thiazide diuretics, ACEi or ARB (not both), CCB
- For black patients: thiazide diuretics, CCBs

Second Line

Combine thiazide diuretic with ACEi, ARB, or CCB or add a K^+-sparing diuretic.

Third Line

Add agent not used in second line; if this does not adequately lower BP, initiate workup for secondary causes (chronic NSAID use, alcohol abuse, RAS, etc.).

ADMISSION, INPATIENT, AND NURSING CONSIDERATIONS

Hospitalization may be necessary for hypertensive urgency or emergency general measures.

 ONGOING CARE

FOLLOW-UP RECOMMENDATIONS

Encourage aerobic activity of 30 min/day, depending on patient's condition.

DIET

- Reduced salt may lower BP in some patients.
- Recommend the Mediterranean diet or DASH.

PATIENT EDUCATION

Home BP monitoring is recommended.

REFERENCES

1. Calhoun DA, Jones D, Textor S, et al. Resistant hypertension: diagnosis, evaluation, and treatment. A scientific statement from the American Heart Association Professional Education Committee of the Council for High Blood Pressure Research. *Hypertension.* 2008;51(6):1403–1419.
2. Whelton PK, Carey RM, Aronow WS, et al. 2017 ACC/AHA/AAPA/ABC/ACPM/AGS/APhA/ASH/ASPC/NMA/PCNA guideline for the prevention, detection, evaluation, and management of high blood pressure in adults: executive summary: a report of the American College of Cardiology/American Heart Association Task Force on Clinical Practice Guidelines. *Hypertension.* 2018;71(6):1269–1324.
3. James PA, Oparil S, Carter BL, et al. 2014 Evidence-based guideline for the management of high blood pressure in adults: report from the panel members appointed to the Eighth Joint National Committee (JNC 8). *JAMA.* 2014;311(5):507–520.
4. Balk EM, Raman G, Adam GP, et al. *Renal Artery Stenosis Management Strategies: An Updated Comparative Effectiveness Review.* Rockville, MD: Agency for Healthcare Research and Quality; 2016. https://effectivehealthcare.ahrq.gov/topics/renal-update/research/. Accessed October 17, 2016.
5. Calhoun DA. Low-dose aldosterone blockade as a new treatment paradigm for controlling resistant hypertension. *J Clin Hypertens (Greenwich).* 2007;9(1 Suppl 1):19–24.

ADDITIONAL READING

- Agarwal R, Bills JE, Hecht TJ, et al. Role of home blood pressure monitoring in overcoming therapeutic inertia and improving hypertension control: a systematic review and meta-analysis. *Hypertension.* 2011;57(1):29–38.
- Bell KJL, Doust J, Glasziou P. Incremental benefits and harms of the 2017 American College of Cardiology/American Heart Association high blood pressure guideline. *JAMA Intern Med.* 2018;178(6):755–757.
- Rimoldi SF, Scherrer U, Messerli FH. Secondary arterial hypertension: when, who, and how to screen? *Eur Heart J.* 2014;35(19):1245–1254.

 SEE ALSO

Aldosteronism, Primary; Coarctation of the Aorta; Cushing Disease and Cushing Syndrome; Hyperparathyroidism; Hypertension, Essential; Hyperthyroidism; Pheochromocytoma

CODES

ICD10

- I15.9 Secondary hypertension, unspecified
- I15.8 Other secondary hypertension
- I15.0 Renovascular hypertension

CLINICAL PEARLS

- Onset of HTN in adults >60 years of age is a strong indicator of secondary HTN.
- Common causes of resistant HTN: OSA, excessive salt intake, medication nonadherence, alcohol, NSAIDs
- Common secondary causes include sleep apnea, renal disease, renal artery stenosis, and PA.
- Aldosterone inhibitors should be considered in all cases of resistant HTN.
- Home BP monitoring predicts outcomes better than office monitoring of BP.

H

HYPERTHYROIDISM

Anup Sabharwal, MD, MBA, FACE • Atil Y. Kargi, MD

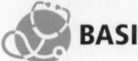 **BASICS**

- Hyperthyroidism or thyrotoxicosis is composed of a spectrum of clinical findings consistent with thyroid hormone excess. The former describes excess from the thyroid gland, whereas the latter can be produced from another source.
- In general, patients with thyrotoxicosis have hyperthyroidism. However, this is not always the case. Patients could suffer from thyrotoxicosis not due to a prolonged elevation in thyroid hormone synthesis. Examples include subacute thyroiditis, exogenous thyrotoxicosis, and radiation-induced thyroiditis.
- Also, medications (such as amiodarone and interferon-α) have cytotoxic effects on thyroid cells resulting in thyrotoxicosis from preformed thyroid hormones.

DESCRIPTION

- Graves disease (GD): the most common form; diffuse goiter and thyrotoxicosis are common characteristics. Infiltrative orbitopathy is seen in up to 50% of patients. Infiltrative dermopathy is rare. Autoantibodies are directed at the thyroid-stimulating hormone (TSH) receptors.
- Toxic multinodular goiter (TMNG): second most common; most common cause of hyperthyroidism in patients age >65 years; patients >40 years, insidious onset, frequent in iodine-deficient areas
- Toxic adenoma (Plummer disease): younger patients, autonomously functioning nodules
- Iodine-induced hyperthyroidism
- Thyroiditis: transient autoimmune process:
  - Subacute thyroiditis/de Quervain: granulomatous giant cell thyroiditis, benign course; viral infections have been involved.
  - Postpartum thyroiditis
  - Drug-induced thyroiditis: amiodarone, interferon-α, interleukin-2, lithium
  - Miscellaneous: thyrotoxicosis factitia, TSH-secreting pituitary tumors, and functioning trophoblastic tumors (1)[B]
- Subclinical hyperthyroidism: suppressed TSH with normal thyroxine (T_4); may be associated with osteoporosis and atrial fibrillation
- Thyroid storm: rare hyperthyroidism; fever, tachycardia, gastrointestinal (GI) symptoms, CNS dysfunction (e.g., coma); up to 50% mortality

Geriatric Considerations
- Characteristic symptoms and signs may be absent.
- Atrial fibrillation is common when TSH <0.1 mIU/L (2)[A].

Pediatric Considerations
- Neonates and children are treated with antithyroids for 12 to 24 months.
- Radioactive iodine treatment is controversial in patients <15 to 18 years.

Pregnancy Considerations
Propylthiouracil is currently the drug of choice during 1st trimester of pregnancy, and methimazole is preferred in the 2nd and 3rd trimester (3)[A]. Treat with lowest effective dose. Avoid treatment-induced hypothyroidism. Radioiodine therapy is contraindicated.

EPIDEMIOLOGY
- 1.3% of population
- Predominant sex: female > male (7 to 10:1)
- Predominant age: autoimmune thyroid disease (GD) in 2nd and 3rd decades; TMNG more common in patients >40 years

Incidence
- Female: 1/1,000
- Male: 1/3,000

ETIOLOGY AND PATHOPHYSIOLOGY
- GD: autoimmune disease
- TMNG: 60% TSH receptor gene abnormality; 40% unknown
- Toxic adenoma: point mutation in TSH receptor gene with increased hormone production
- Thyroiditis:
  - Hashitoxicosis: autoimmune destruction of the thyroid; antimicrosomal antibodies present
  - Subacute/de Quervain thyroiditis: granulomatous reaction; genetic predisposition in specific human leukocyte antigens; viruses, such as coxsackievirus, adenovirus, echovirus, and influenza virus, have been implicated; self-limited course, 6 to 12 months
  - Suppurative: infectious
  - Drug-induced thyroiditis: Amiodarone produces an autoimmune reaction and a destructive process. Lithium, interferon-α, and interleukin-2 cause an autoimmune thyroiditis.
  - Postpartum thyroiditis: autoimmune thyroiditis that lasts up to 8 weeks, and in 60% of patients, hypothyroidism manifests in the future

Genetics
Concordance rate for GD among monozygotic twins is 35%.

RISK FACTORS
- Positive family history, especially in maternal relatives
- Female
- Other autoimmune disorders
- Iodide repletion after iodide deprivation, especially in TMNG

COMMONLY ASSOCIATED CONDITIONS
- Autoimmune diseases
- Down syndrome
- Iodine deficiency

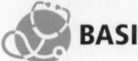 **DIAGNOSIS**

HISTORY
- Thyrotoxicosis is a hypermetabolic state in which energy production exceeds needs, causing increased heat production, diaphoresis, and even fever.
- Thyrotoxicosis affects several different systems:
  - Constitutional: fatigue, weakness, increased appetite, weight loss
  - Neuropsychiatric: agitation, anxiety, emotional lability, psychosis, coma, and poor concentration and memory
  - GI: increased appetite, hyperdefecation
  - Gynecologic: oligomenorrhea, amenorrhea
  - Cardiovascular: tachycardia (most common) and chest discomfort that mimics angina

Geriatric Considerations
Apathetic hyperthyroidism in the elderly

PHYSICAL EXAM
- Adults:
  - Skin: warm, moist, pretibial myxedema (GD only)
  - Head, eye, ear, nose, throat (HEENT): exophthalmos, lid lag
  - Endocrine: hyperhidrosis, heat intolerance, goiter, gynecomastia, low libido, and spider angiomata (males)
  - Cardiovascular: tachycardia, atrial fibrillation, cardiomegaly
  - Musculoskeletal: skeletal demineralization, osteopenia, osteoporosis, fractures
  - Neurologic: tremor, proximal muscle weakness, anxiety and lability, brisk deep tendon reflexes
  - Rarely: thyroid acropathy (clubbing), localized dermopathy
- Children:
  - Linear growth acceleration
  - Ophthalmic abnormalities more common

DIFFERENTIAL DIAGNOSIS
- Anxiety
- Malignancy
- Diabetes mellitus
- Pregnancy
- Menopause
- Pheochromocytoma
- Depression
- Carcinoid syndrome

DIAGNOSTIC TESTS & INTERPRETATION
- 95% have suppressed TSH and elevated free T_4. Total T_4 and triiodothyronine (T_3) represent the bound hormone and can be affected by pregnancy and hepatitis (1)[A].
- T_3: elevated, especially in T_3 toxicosis or amiodarone-induced thyrotoxicosis (AIT): Presence of TSH receptor antibody or thyroid-stimulating immunoglobulin is diagnostic of GD.
- Free thyroxine index (FTI): calculated from T_4 and thyroid hormone—binding ratio; corrects for misleading results caused by pregnancy and estrogens
- Inappropriately normal or elevated TSH with high T_4 suspicious for pituitary tumor or thyroid hormone resistance
- Drugs may alter lab results: estrogens, heparin, iodine-containing compounds (including amiodarone and contrast agents), phenytoin, salicylates, and steroids (e.g., androgens, corticosteroids).
- Exogenous biotin supplements can interfere with immunoassays for thyroid hormones, TSH, thyroglobulin, and TSH receptor binding inhibiting antibody (4)[B].
- Drug precautions: Amiodarone and lithium may induce hyperthyroidism; methimazole may cause warfarin resistance.
- Other findings that can occur: anemia, granulocytosis, lymphocytosis, hypercalcemia, transaminase, and alkaline phosphate elevations

Initial Tests (lab, imaging)
- TSH, free T_4, total T_4, and T_3 will establish the hyperthyroid diagnosis (5)[A].
- Thyrotropin receptor antibody (TRAb) (6)[A]
- TSH receptor antibodies (TSH-R Abs): The routine assay is the TSH-binding inhibitor immunoglobulin assay (TBII). TSH-R Abs are useful in the prediction of postpartum Graves thyrotoxicosis and neonatal thyrotoxicosis (5)[A].
- Thyroxine/triiodothyronine ratio: The T_4-to-T_3 ratio may be a useful tool when the iodine uptake testing is not available/contraindicated. ~2% of thyrotoxic patients have "T_3 toxicosis."
- Nuclear medicine uptake and scanning (^{123}I or ^{131}I): The reference-range value for 24-hour radioiodine uptake is between 5% and 25%.
- Increased thyroid iodine uptake is seen with TMNG, toxic solitary nodule, and GD.

- GD shows a diffuse uptake and can have a paradoxical finding of high uptake at 4 to 6 hours but normal uptake at 24 hours because of the rapid clearance.
- TMNG will show a heterogeneous uptake, whereas solitary toxic nodule will show a warm or "hot" nodule.
- In iodine-deficient areas, an increased uptake is associated with low urine iodine levels.
- Causes of thyrotoxicosis with low iodine uptake:
  - Acute thyroiditis, thyrotoxicosis factitia, and iodine intoxication with amiodarone or contrast material can cause low-uptake transient thyrotoxicosis. After thyroiditis resolves, the patient can become euthyroid or hypothyroid.
  - Iodine loading can cause iodine trapping and decreased iodine uptake (Wolff-Chaikoff effect).
  - Thyrotoxicosis factitia: Thyroglobulin levels are low in exogenous intake and high in endogenous production.
  - Other extrathyroidal causes include struma ovarii and metastatic thyroid carcinoma.
  - Technetium-99m scintigraphy: controversial because it has a 33% discordance rate with radioactive iodine scanning

Follow-Up Tests & Special Considerations
In severe cases, such as thyroid storm, hospitalize until stable, especially if >60 years of age, because of the risk of atrial fibrillation.

Diagnostic Procedures/Other
Neck ultrasound will show increased diffuse vascularity in GD.

Test Interpretation
- GD: hyperplasia
- Toxic nodule: nodule formation

 ## TREATMENT

- Decision of which patients to treat and how to treat should be individualized.
- Observation may be appropriate for patients with mild hyperthyroidism (TSH >0.1 or with no symptoms) especially those who are young and with low risk of complications (atrial fibrillation, osteoporosis).
- Antithyroid medication is contraindicated in patients with thyroiditis. Treatment for subacute thyroiditis is supportive with NSAIDs and β-blockers. Steroids can be used for 2 to 3 weeks (3). GD or TMNG can be managed by either antithyroid medication, radioactive iodine therapy (RAIT), or thyroidectomy.
- RAIT: most common definitive treatment used in United States for GD and TMNG
- Pretreatment with antithyroid drugs is preferred to avoid worsening thyrotoxicosis after RAIT. Methimazole is preferred over propylthiouracil as pretreatment because of decreased relapse, but it is held 3 to 5 days before therapy (3)[A].
- Usually, patients become hypothyroid 2 to 3 months after RAIT; therefore, antithyroid medications are continued after ablation.
- Glucocorticoids: reduce the conversion of active T_4 to the more active T_3. In Graves ophthalmopathy, the use of prednisone before and after RAIT prevents worsening ophthalmopathy (3)[B].
- Smoking in GD patients is a risk factor for ophthalmopathy, especially after RAIT.
- For GD, due to the chance of remission, 12- to 18-month trial of antithyroid medications may be considered prior to offering RAIT.

- For TMNG, the treatment of choice is RAIT. Medical therapy with antithyroid medications has shown a high recurrence rate. Surgery is considered only in special cases (3)[B].
- For AIT type I, the treatment is antithyroid drugs and β-blockers. Thyroidectomy is the last option. AIT type II is self-limited but may use glucocorticoids.

MEDICATION
First Line
- Antithyroid drugs: Methimazole and propylthiouracil are thioamides that inhibit iodine oxidation, organification, and iodotyrosine coupling. Propylthiouracil can block peripheral conversion of T_4 to active T_3. Both can be used as primary treatment for GD and prior to RAIT or surgery (1)[A].
- Duration of treatment: 12 to 18 months; 50–60% relapse after stopping; treatment beyond 18 months did not show any further benefit on remission rate. The most serious side effects are hepatitis (0.1–0.2%), vasculitis, and agranulocytosis; baseline CBC recommended:
  - Methimazole (preferred): adults: 10 to 15 mg q12–24h; children aged 6 to 10 years: 0.4 mg/kg/day PO once daily
  - Propylthiouracil: adults (preferred in thyroid storm and 1st trimester of pregnancy): 100 to 150 mg PO q8h, not to exceed 200 mg/day during pregnancy
- β-Adrenergic blocker: Propranolol in high doses (>160 mg/day) inhibits T_3 activation by up to 30%. Atenolol, metoprolol, and nadolol can be used and are also useful in relieving palpitations and in slowing the heart rate in patients with sinus tachycardia (7)[A].
- Glucocorticoids: reduce the conversion of active T_4 to the more active T_3
- Cholestyramine: anion exchange resin that decreases thyroid hormone reabsorption in the enterohepatic circulation; dose: 4 g QID (1)[B]
- Other agents:
  - Lithium: inhibits thyroid hormone secretion and iodotyrosine coupling; use is limited by toxicity.
  - Lugol solution or saturated solution of potassium iodide (SSKI); blocks release of hormone from the gland but should be administered at least 1 hour after thioamide was given; otherwise, acts as a substrate for hormone production (Jod-Basedow effect)
  - RAIT: See "Treatment" section.

ISSUES FOR REFERRAL
Patients with Graves ophthalmopathy should be referred to an experienced ophthalmologist.

SURGERY/OTHER PROCEDURES
Thyroidectomy for compressive symptoms, masses, and thyroid malignancy may be performed in the 2nd trimester of pregnancy only.

 ## ONGOING CARE

FOLLOW-UP RECOMMENDATIONS
Patient Monitoring
- Repeat thyroid tests q3mo, CBC, and liver function tests (LFTs) on thioamide therapy; continue therapy with thioamides for 12 to 18 months.
- After RAIT, thyroid function tests at 6 weeks, 12 weeks, 6 months, and annually thereafter if euthyroid; TSH may remain undetectable for months even after patient is euthyroid; follow T_3 and T_4.

DIET
Sufficient calories to prevent weight loss

PROGNOSIS
Good (with early diagnosis and treatment)

COMPLICATIONS
- Surgery: hypoparathyroidism, recurrent laryngeal nerve damage, and hypothyroidism
- RAIT: postablation hypothyroidism
- GD: high relapse rate with antithyroid drug as primary therapy
- Graves ophthalmopathy, worsening heart failure if cardiac condition, atrial fibrillation, muscle wasting, proximal muscle weakness, increased risk of cerebrovascular accident (CVA), and cardiovascular mortality

REFERENCES
1. Bahn Chair RS, Burch HB, Cooper DS, et al. Hyperthyroidism and other causes of thyrotoxicosis: management guidelines of the American Thyroid Association and American Association of Clinical Endocrinologists. *Thyroid*. 2011;21(6):593–646.
2. Cappola AR, Fried LP, Arnold AM, et al. Thyroid status, cardiovascular risk, and mortality in older adults. *JAMA*. 2006;295(9):1033–1041.
3. Bahn RS, Burch HB, Cooper DS, et al. Hyperthyroidism and other causes of thyrotoxicosis: management guidelines of the American Thyroid Association and American Association of Clinical Endocrinologists. *Endocr Pract*. 2011;17(3):456–520.
4. Barbesino G. Misdiagnosis of Graves' disease with apparent severe hyperthyroidism in a patient taking biotin megadoses. *Thyroid*. 2016;26(6):860–863.
5. Abraham P, Avenell A, Park CM, et al. A systematic review of drug therapy for Graves' hyperthyroidism. *Eur J Endocrinol*. 2005;153(4):489–498.
6. Abraham-Nordling M, Törring O, Hamberger B, et al. Graves' disease: a long-term quality-of-life follow up of patients randomized to treatment with antithyroid drugs, radioiodine, or surgery. *Thyroid*. 2005;15(11):1279–1286.
7. Ross DS, Burch HB, Cooper DS, et al. 2016 American Thyroid Association guidelines for diagnosis and management of hyperthyroidism and other causes of thyrotoxicosis. *Thyroid*. 2016;26(10):1343–1421.

CODES

ICD10
- E05.90 Thyrotoxicosis, unspecified without thyrotoxic crisis or storm
- E05.20 Thyrotoxicosis w toxic multinod goiter w/o thyrotoxic crisis
- E06.1 Subacute thyroiditis

CLINICAL PEARLS
- Not all thyrotoxicoses are secondary to hyperthyroidism.
- GD presents with hyperthyroidism, ophthalmopathy, and goiter.
- Medical treatment for GD has a high relapse rate after stopping medications.
- Thyroid storm is a medical emergency that needs hospitalization and aggressive treatment.
- Serum TSH level may be misleading and remain low in the early period after initiating treatment, even when T_4 and T_3 levels have decreased.

H

HYPERTRIGLYCERIDEMIA
S. Lindsey Clarke, MD, FAAFP

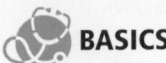

BASICS

DESCRIPTION
- Hypertriglyceridemia (HTG) is a common form of dyslipidemia characterized by an excess fasting plasma concentration of triglycerides (TGs).
  - TGs are fatty molecules that occur naturally in vegetable oils and animal fats and are major sources of dietary energy.
  - TGs are packaged into chylomicrons and very low-density lipoproteins (VLDL).
- HTG is a risk factor for acute pancreatitis at levels ≥1,000 mg/dL.
  - Risk is 10–20% at these TG levels.
  - Third leading cause of acute pancreatitis
- HTG also is independently associated with cardio-vascular disease at levels ≥200 mg/dL.
  - A large Danish population study in 2018 showed that TG ≥264 mg/dL conferred a 10-year risk of major adverse cardiovascular events comparable to that of statin eligible individuals.
  - The degree to which excess TGs cause atherosclerosis is uncertain and debatable. Evidence for a causal relationship comes mainly from Mendelian randomization studies.
  - Lowering TG has not been proven to reduce cardiovascular risk.
- The American Association of Clinical Endocrinologists classifies HTG as follows based on fasting TG levels:
  - Normal: <150 mg/dL
  - Borderline high: 150 to 199 mg/dL
  - High: 200 to 499 mg/dL
  - Very high: ≥500 mg/dL
  - Divide by 88.5 to convert to mmol/L.
- TGs are considered high in children when TGs exceed the 95th percentiles for age:
  - ≥100 mg/dL for ages 0 to 9 years
  - ≥130 mg/dL for ages 10 to 19 years

EPIDEMIOLOGY
- Predominant gender: male > female
- Predominant race: Hispanic, white > black

Prevalence
- 33% of U.S. population has TG levels ≥150 mg/dL.
- 1.7% has TG levels ≥500 mg/dL.
- Highest prevalence at age 50 to 70 years
- The most common genetic syndromes with HTG, familial combined hyperlipidemia and familial HTG, each affect ≤1% of general population.

ETIOLOGY AND PATHOPHYSIOLOGY
- Primary
  - Familial
  - Acquired (sporadic)
- Secondary
  - Obesity and overweight
  - Physical inactivity
  - Cigarette smoking
  - Excess alcohol intake
  - Very high carbohydrate diets (>60% of total caloric intake)

- Certain medications
  - Atypical antipsychotics (e.g., quetiapine)
  - β-Blockers other than carvedilol
  - Cyclosporine
  - Glucocorticoids
  - Interferon-α
  - Isotretinoin
  - Oral estrogens
  - Protease inhibitors (e.g., ritonavir, darunavir)
  - Tamoxifen
- Medical conditions
  - Type 2 diabetes mellitus
  - Hypothyroidism
  - Chronic renal failure, nephrotic syndrome
  - Autoimmune disorders (e.g., systemic lupus erythematosus)
  - Paraproteinemias (e.g., macroglobulinemia, myeloma, lymphoma, lymphocytic leukemia)
  - Pregnancy (usually physiologic and transient)

Genetics
- Familial chylomicronemia (type 1 dyslipidemia): autosomal recessive inheritance of lipoprotein lipase deficiency; 0.0001% prevalence
- Familial combined hyperlipidemia (type IIb): usually autosomal dominant, caused by overproduction of apolipoprotein (APO) B-100; approximately 1% prevalence
- Familial dysbetalipoproteinemia (type III): usually autosomal recessive, caused by lipoprotein overproduction due to inheritance of two APOE2 variants; 0.01% prevalence
- Familial HTG (type IV): autosomal dominant, caused by an inactivating mutation of the lipoprotein lipase gene; 1% prevalence
- Primary mixed HTG (type V)

RISK FACTORS
- Genetic susceptibility
- Obesity, overweight
- Lack of exercise
- Diabetes
- Alcoholism
- Certain medications (see "Etiology and Pathophysiology")
- Medical conditions (see "Etiology and Pathophysiology")

GENERAL PREVENTION
- Weight reduction
- Moderation of dietary fat and carbohydrates
- Regular aerobic exercise

COMMONLY ASSOCIATED CONDITIONS
- Coronary artery disease
- Diabetes mellitus type 2 and insulin resistance
- Dyslipidemias
  - Decreased high-density lipoprotein (HDL) cholesterol
  - Increased LDL, non-HDL, and total cholesterol
  - Small, dense LDL particles
- Metabolic syndrome (three of the following):
  - Abdominal obesity (waist circumference >40 inches in men, >35 inches in women)

- TG ≥150 mg/dL
- Low levels of HDL cholesterol (<40 mg/dL in men, <50 mg/dL in women)
- BP ≥130/85 mm Hg
- Fasting glucose ≥100 mg/dL
- Nonalcoholic steatohepatitis
- Pancreatitis
- Polycystic ovary syndrome

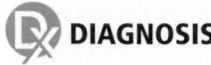

DIAGNOSIS

HISTORY
- Usually asymptomatic
- Patients with chylomicronemia syndrome can have memory loss, headache, vertigo, dyspnea, and paresthesias.
- Pancreatitis: epigastric pain, nausea, and vomiting
- Assess for other cardiac risk factors.
- Family history of coronary artery disease

PHYSICAL EXAM
- Obesity, overweight (body mass index ≥25 kg/m²)
- Eruptive cutaneous, tuberous, and striate palmar xanthomas
- Lipemia retinalis
- Epigastric tenderness in pancreatitis
- Hepatomegaly in NASH and chylomicronemia

DIFFERENTIAL DIAGNOSIS
Primary and secondary HTG

DIAGNOSTIC TESTS & INTERPRETATION
Initial Tests (lab, imaging)
- Serum: turbid with milky supernatant
- Fasting lipid profile (12-hour fast)
  - Routine screening every 5 years beginning at age 35 years for men and age 45 years for women
  - Begin screening earlier in those at higher risk for coronary heart disease.
  - For interpretation, see "Description."
- Secondary causes
  - Glycosylated hemoglobin, fasting or postprandial glucose for type 2 diabetes mellitus
  - Creatinine, urinary protein measurement for nephrotic syndrome, renal failure
  - Thyroid-stimulating hormone for hypothyroidism
  - Human chorionic gonadotropin for pregnancy
- Atherosclerosis: cardiac stress imaging, coronary angiography, CT arteriography
- Pancreatitis: serum lipase; CT scan, US of pancreas

Follow-Up Tests & Special Considerations
- Repeat lipid panel after 2 months of therapy.
- High levels of APO B (≥90 mg/dL) are a strong predictor of coronary death in patients whose LDL cannot be calculated because of very high TGs. However, evidence for routine clinical use is lacking.

Test Interpretation
- Chylomicronemia syndrome: lipid-laden macrophage (foam cell) infiltration of visceral organs, bone marrow, and skin
- Atherosclerosis
- Pancreatitis

TREATMENT

GENERAL MEASURES

- Cardiovascular risk reduction through LDL lowering should be prioritized over TG lowering unless patient is at risk for pancreatitis because of very high TG (≥500 mg/dL) (1)[C].
- Therapeutic lifestyle changes are first-line interventions for all patients and can reduce TG by as much as 50% (1)[C]:
  - Dietary modification (by decreasing carbohydrate intake to <50% of calories and limiting alcohol intake)
  - Moderate-intensity physical activity can reduce TG by 20–30%.
  - Weight loss of 5–10% can reduce TG by 20%.
  - Persons with very high TG should abstain from alcohol.
- Search for correctable secondary causes, treat underlying illness, or remove offending drug.
- Improve glycemic control if diabetic.
- Control other cardiac risk factors, such as hypertension, diabetes mellitus, and smoking.
- Primary HTG: Screen other family members.

MEDICATION

First Line

- Fibrates: the most effective agents for reducing TG up to 50%; used primarily to reduce risk of pancreatitis when TGs are severe or very severe; have been shown to decrease nonfatal myocardial infarction but not all-cause mortality (1)[C],(2)[A]:
  - Fenofibrate: 30 to 200 mg daily
  - Gemfibrozil: 600 mg BID
  - Adverse reactions: GI upset, hepatotoxicity, cholelithiasis, myalgias, rhabdomyolysis (when combined with a statin), gemfibrozil-warfarin interaction (enhanced anticoagulation)
  - Gemfibrozil should be avoided in combination with statins due to high risk of muscle injury. If combination therapy is needed, use fenofibrate.
- Statins: the most effective agents for reducing cardiovascular risk; primarily affect LDL but also may lower TG 15–30% (3)[A]; dosing depends on intensity of statin desired based on 10-year cardiovascular risk; 2013 ACC/AHA guidelines recommend initiating therapy for 7.5% 10-year risk and other clinical factors (4)[C]:
  - Rosuvastatin: 5 to 40 mg/day
  - Atorvastatin: 10 to 80 mg/day
  - Adverse reactions: myalgias, myopathy, rhabdomyolysis (especially if combined with fibrates); contraindicated in pregnancy and lactation

Second Line

Omega-3 fatty acids

- Lovaza, others: 4 g daily or 2 g BID (5)[C]
- May lower TG 30–50%
- Limited tolerability due to adverse GI effects (diarrhea in up to 15%; also nausea, abdominal pain, dysgeusia, eructation, dyspepsia)
- Limited outcomes data

ISSUES FOR REFERRAL

- HTG refractory to treatment
- Familial HTG syndromes

ADMISSION, INPATIENT, AND NURSING CONSIDERATIONS

- Acute pancreatitis
- Acute coronary syndrome
- In acute hypertriglyceridemic pancreatitis with TG >1,000 mg/dL, the following interventions can be used to lower TG rapidly and safely to <500 mg/dL:
  - Apheresis (therapeutic plasma exchange) for 1 to 3 days
  - Insulin infusion
    - Regular insulin 0.1 to 0.3 U/hr IV for 3.5 to 4 days
    - Administer separate infusion of dextrose 5% if blood glucose <200 mg/dL.
- Discharge criteria: stabilization of acute complicating illness

 ONGOING CARE

FOLLOW-UP RECOMMENDATIONS

2 months after initiation or modification of therapy (repeat fasting lipid profile)

Patient Monitoring

- Fasting lipid profile q6–12mo
- Maintain TG <1,000 mg/dL to reduce risk of acute pancreatitis.
- Hepatic transaminases
- Creatine phosphokinase if patient has myalgias

DIET

- Restrict dietary fat to 30% of total caloric intake; restrict further to 15% of caloric intake if TG ≥1,000 mg/dL (1)[C].
- Limit carbohydrates (especially simple carbohydrates and sugars) to 60% of total caloric intake.
- Mediterranean-style diet reduces TG 10–15% more than a low-fat diet.
- Increase marine-derived omega-3 polyunsaturated fatty acids (4 g/day reduces TG by 25–30%, dose–response relationship).
- Eliminate trans fatty acids.
- Increase dietary fiber.
- Avoid concentrated sugars such as fructose.
- Moderate alcohol intake (<1 oz/day or complete abstinence if TGs are very high)

PATIENT EDUCATION

Smoking cessation for cardiovascular risk reduction

PROGNOSIS

- Good with correction of TG levels
- Patients with primary HTG usually require lifelong treatment.

COMPLICATIONS

- Atherosclerosis
- Chylomicronemia syndrome
- Pancreatitis

REFERENCES

1. Miller M, Stone NJ, Ballantyne C, et al. Triglycerides and cardiovascular disease: a scientific statement from the American Heart Association. *Circulation.* 2011;123(20):2292–2333.
2. Wang D, Liu B, Tao W, et al. Fibrates for secondary prevention of cardiovascular disease and stroke. *Cochrane Database Syst Rev.* 2015;(10):CD009580.
3. Karlson BW, Palmer MK, Nicholls SJ, et al. A VOYAGER meta-analysis of the impact of statin therapy on low-density lipoprotein cholesterol and triglyceride levels in patients with hypertriglyceridemia. *Am J Cardiol.* 2016;117(9):1444–1448.
4. Stone NJ, Robinson JG, Lichtenstein AH, et al. 2013 ACC/AHA guideline on the treatment of blood cholesterol to reduce atherosclerotic cardiovascular risk in adults: a report of the American College of Cardiology/American Heart Association Task Force on Practice Guidelines. *Circulation.* 2014;129(25 Suppl 2):S1–S45.
5. Kastelein JJ, Maki KC, Susekov A, et al. Omega-3 free fatty acids for the treatment of severe hypertriglyceridemia: the EpanoVa fOr Lowering Very high triglyceridEs (EVOLVE) trial. *J Clin Lipidol.* 2014;8(1):94–106.

ADDITIONAL READING

- Jellinger PS, Handelsman Y, Rosenblit PD, et al. American Association of Clinical Endocrinologists and American College of Endocrinology guidelines for management of dyslipidemia and prevention of cardiovascular disease. *Endocr Pract.* 2017;23(Suppl 2): 1–87.
- Madsen CM, Varbo A, Nordestgaard BG. Unmet need for primary prevention in individuals with hypertriglyceridaemia not eligible for statin therapy according to European Society of Cardiology/European Atherosclerosis Society guidelines: a contemporary population-based study. *Eur Heart J.* 2018;39(7):610–619.

 SEE ALSO

- Hypercholesterolemia; Pancreatitis, Acute
- Algorithm: Hypertriglyceridemia

CODES

ICD10

E78.1 Pure hyperglyceridemia

CLINICAL PEARLS

- HTG is a risk factor for pancreatitis at levels ≥1,000 mg/dL and for coronary artery disease at levels ≥200 mg/dL.
- Diet and exercise are first-line interventions for all patients who have HTG.
- For patients with TG levels ≥500 mg/dL, the greatest amount of TG lowering is achieved with fibrates; however, the magnitude of clinical benefit is uncertain.
- In patients with TG levels <500 mg/dL, the primary pharmacologic strategy for cardiovascular risk management is statins.

H

HYPOGLYCEMIA, DIABETIC

Joseph A. Florence, MD • Emily K. Flores, PharmD, BCPS

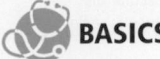

BASICS

DESCRIPTION

- Abnormally low concentration of glucose in circulating blood of a patient with diabetes mellitus (DM); often referred to as an *insulin reaction*
- Classification of hypoglycemia (1,2)[A]:
  - Level 1: hypoglycemia alert value. <70 mg/dL (3.9 mmol/L): may or may not be accompanied by symptoms; asymptomatic hypoglycemia if symptoms not present
  - Level 2: clinically significant hypoglycemia. <54 mg/dL (3.0 mmol/L)
  - Level 3: severe hypoglycemia. No specific glucose threshold: hypoglycemia associated with severe cognitive impairment requiring external assistance for recovery
- Probable symptomatic hypoglycemia: event with symptoms but glucose not tested
- Pseudohypoglycemia: an event with typical symptoms but glucose ≥70 mg/dL (3.9 mmol/L)
- Hypoglycemia is the leading limiting factor in the glycemic management of type 1 DM (T1DM) and type 2 DM (T2DM). Severe or frequent hypoglycemia requires modification of treatment regimens, including higher treatment goals.

ALERT
Severe hypoglycemia associated with increased mortality

- Hypoglycemia unawareness
  - Major risk factor for severe hypoglycemic reactions
  - Most commonly found in patients with long-standing T1DM and children age <7 years

EPIDEMIOLOGY

Incidence
- From the ACCORD study, the annual incidence of hypoglycemia was the following:
  - 3.14% in the intensive treatment group
  - 1.03% in the standard group
  - Increased risk among women, African Americans, those with less than high school education, aged participants, and those who used insulin at trial entry
- From the RECAP-DM study: Hypoglycemia was reported in 35.8% of patients with T2DM who added a sulfonylurea or thiazolidinedione to metformin therapy during the past year.

ETIOLOGY AND PATHOPHYSIOLOGY
- Loss of hormonal counterregulatory mechanism in glucose metabolism
- Too little food (skipping or delaying meals), decreased CHO intake
- Too much insulin or oral hypoglycemic agent (improper dose, timing, or erratic absorption)
- Unplanned or excessive exercise/physical activity
- Alcohol consumption
- Vomiting or diarrhea

RISK FACTORS
- Nearly 3/4 of severe hypoglycemic episodes occur during sleep.
- Severe hypoglycemia is associated with comorbid conditions in patients aged ≥65 years and in users of a long-acting sulfonylurea.
- Intensive insulin therapy (further lowering HgbA1C from 7% to 6%) is associated with higher rate of hypoglycemia.

- Comorbidities: renal/liver disease, congestive heart failure (CHF), hypothyroidism, hypoadrenalism, gastroenteritis, gastroparesis (unpredictable CHO delivery), autonomic neuropathy, pregnancy, anxiety, depression, disordered eating behavior, illness/stress, and unplanned life events
- Duration of DM >5 years
- Young children with type 1 diabetes
- Advanced age
- Reduced cognitive function, dementia
- Starvation, prolonged fasting, weight loss, or food insecurity
- Current smokers with T1DM
- Alcoholism: Alcohol consumption may increase risk of delayed hypoglycemia, especially if on insulin or insulin secretagogues. Evening consumption of alcohol is associated with an increased risk of nocturnal and fasting hypoglycemia, especially in patients with T1DM.
- Insulin secretagogues: Sulfonylureas (glyburide, glimepiride, glipizide, etc.) and glinide derivatives (repaglinide, nateglinide) stimulate insulin secretion.
- Hypoglycemia is rare in diabetics not treated with insulin or insulin secretagogues.
- Other antidiabetes medications such as dipeptidyl peptidase 4 (DPP-4) inhibitors, glucagon-like peptide-1 (GLP-1) agonists, and sodium-glucose contransporter-2 (SGLT-2) agents carry a lower but present risk of hypoglycemia, which may increase when combining agents from different categories.

Geriatric Considerations
- American Geriatric Society Beers Criteria recommend avoiding glyburide and chlorpropamide due to their prolonged half-life in older adults and risk for prolonged hypoglycemic episodes. Medications should be dosed for age and renal function.
- Individualize pharmacologic therapy in older adults to reduce the risk of hypoglycemia, avoid overtreatment, and simplify complex regimens if possible while maintaining the HgbA1C target (1)[A].

Pediatric Considerations
Children may not realize when they have hypoglycemia, needing increased supervision during times of higher activity. Children may have higher glycemic goals for this reason. Caregivers should be instructed in use of glucagon (1,2)[A].

Pregnancy Considerations
Hypoglycemia management and avoidance education should be reemphasized and blood glucose monitoring increased due to more stringent glycemic goals and increased risk in early pregnancy (1)[A].

GENERAL PREVENTION
- Maintain routine schedule of diet (consistent CHO intake), medication, and exercise (1)[A].
- Regular self-monitoring of blood glucose (SMBG) or continuous glucose monitoring (CGM)
  - Particularly helpful for asymptomatic hypoglycemia
  - Use if taking insulin or secretagogue.
  - Utilize ≥3 times daily testing if multiple injections of insulin, insulin pump therapy, or pregnant diabetic; frequency and timing dictated by needs and treatment goals
- Diabetes treatment and teaching programs (DTTPs) especially for high-risk type 1 patients, which teach flexible insulin therapy to enable dietary freedom
- Hypoglycemia may be decreased with use of insulin analogs, continuous SC insulin infusion (CSII) pumps, and CGM systems (1)[A].

COMMONLY ASSOCIATED CONDITIONS
- Autonomic neuropathy
- Neuropathies
- Cardiomyopathies

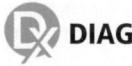

DIAGNOSIS

HISTORY
- Discuss timing of episodes, awareness, frequency, and causes (1).
- Symptoms vary considerably between individuals.
- Adrenergic symptoms
  - Hunger, trembling, pallor, sweating, shaking, pounding heart, anxiety, urinary incontinence
- Neurologic symptoms
  - Dizziness, poor concentration, drowsiness, weakness, confusion, light-headedness, slurred speech, blurred vision, double vision, unsteadiness, poor coordination
  - Hypoglycemia causes a significant deterioration in reading span and subject-verb agreement, demonstrating that language processing is impaired during moderate hypoglycemia (3).
- Behavioral symptoms
  - Tearfulness, confusion, fatigue, irritability, aggressiveness
- If altered cognition, consider hypoglycemia.

PHYSICAL EXAM
- General: confusion, lethargy
- HEENT: diplopia
- Coronary: tachycardia
- Neurologic: tremulousness, weakness, paresthesia, stupor, seizure, or coma
- Mental status: irritability, anxiety, inability to concentrate, or short-term memory loss
- Skin: pale, diaphoresis
- End-organ damage: microvascular, macrovascular, ophthalmologic, neurologic, renal

DIFFERENTIAL DIAGNOSIS
Hypoglycemia not associated with DM may be seen in:
- Chronic alcoholics and binge drinkers
- GI dysfunction causing postprandial hypoglycemia or alimentary reactive hypoglycemia
- Hormonal deficiency states (hormonal reactive hypoglycemia)
- Hypoglycemia of sepsis
- Islet cell tumors
- Factitious hypoglycemia from surreptitious injection of insulin

DIAGNOSTIC TESTS & INTERPRETATION
- Plasma, serum, or whole-blood glucose
- SMBG and CGM are especially useful for asymptomatic hypoglycemia (2)[A].
- A hypoglycemic reading from a CGM sensor should be verified by SMBG fingerstick glucose testing prior to treatment, unless specific device is approved otherwise (1)[A].
- Low HgbA1c level may be due to chronic hypoglycemia.
- Disorders that may alter lab results
  - Conditions that affect erythrocyte turnover, such as hemolysis or blood loss, and hemoglobin variants may alter HgbA1c (1)[A].

TREATMENT

GENERAL MEASURES

- Glucose: pure glucose preferred; any form of CHO that contains glucose should be effective (see "Medication" section below) (1)[A].
- Glucagon should be prescribed proactively to patients at significant risk of clinically significant hypoglycemia. People in close contact with these individuals should be instructed in using an emergency glucagon kit (1)[A].
- Insulin-treated patients with hypoglycemia unawareness or an episode of clinically significant hypoglycemia should have glycemic targets raised to strictly avoid hypoglycemia (1)[A].
- α-Glucosidase inhibitors (acarbose) prevent digestion of complex CHOs; therefore, hypoglycemia must be treated with monosaccharides, such as glucose tablets.
- Patients with T1DM should use insulin analogs to reduce hypoglycemia risk (1)[A].
- Address medications (i.e., insulin, sulfonylureas, GLP-1 agonists, thiazolidinediones) that may induce hypoglycemia.
- CGM-augmented CSII with automated insulin suspension when blood glucose falls below a threshold value reduces the combined rate of severe and moderate hypoglycemia in T1DM and reduces nocturnal hypoglycemia without increasing HgbA1c levels in patients >16 years old (1,4)[A].

MEDICATION

- Conscious patients (1)[A]:
  - Glucose (15 to 20 g) is preferred, although any form of CHO may be used.
    - Any sugar-containing food or beverage that can be rapidly absorbed: juice or nondiet soda (4 to 5 oz), candy (5 to 6 pieces of hard candy), or OTC glucose tablets (4 tablets = 16 g CHO)
    - Takes ~15 minutes for CHOs to be digested and enter bloodstream as glucose
    - Blood glucose value may correct prior to symptoms resolving.
    - "Rule of 15": 15 to 20 g CHO (~60 to 80 calories simple CHO) repeated q15min until blood sugar is ≥70 mg/dL
  - Once sugar has normalized, a meal or snack may need to be consumed to prevent recurrence of hypoglycemia.
- Loss of consciousness at home (4)[A]:
  - Administer glucagon.
  - IM or SC in the deltoid or anterior thigh
    - Age <6 years and/or weight <20 to 25 kg: 0.50 mg
    - Age ≥6 years and/or weight >20 to 25 kg: 1 mg
    - May repeat dose in 15 minutes if needed
- In unconscious, with emergency medical personnel present or patient hospitalized (4)[A]:
  - Give 25 g IV 50% dextrose every 5 to 10 minutes until patient awakens.
  - Then, feed orally and/or administer 5% dextrose IV at level that will maintain blood glucose >100 mg/dL.
  - Patients with hypoglycemia secondary to oral hypoglycemics should be monitored for 24 to 48 hours because hypoglycemia may recur after apparent clinical recovery.
- Significant possible interactions:
  - Overtreatment may cause hyperglycemia. Clearance of certain oral hypoglycemics may be prolonged in persons with renal or liver disease.

ISSUES FOR REFERRAL

Frequent or recurring episodes that do not readily respond to treatment. If anxiety and fear of hypoglycemia are uncontrolled, refer to mental health provider.

ADMISSION, INPATIENT, AND NURSING CONSIDERATIONS

- A hypoglycemia prevention and management protocol should be adopted and implemented by each hospital or hospital system (1)[A].
- Admission criteria/initial stabilization
  - Any doubt of cause
  - Expectation of prolonged hypoglycemia (e.g., caused by sulfonylurea drug)
  - Inability to drink
  - Treatment has not resulted in prompt sensory recovery.
  - Seizures, coma, or altered behavior (e.g., ataxia, disorientation, unstable motor coordination, dysphasia) secondary to documented or suspected hypoglycemia
- Discharge criteria: Normoglycemia and risk of severe hypoglycemia are negligible.

 ONGOING CARE

FOLLOW-UP RECOMMENDATIONS

Rest until glucose is normal. Individuals with poor cognitive function or severe hypoglycemia should have their glycemic therapy tailored to avoid significant hypoglycemia (1)[A]. Patients with hypoglycemia unawareness or unexplained severe hypoglycemia should raise their glycemic targets to avoid further hypoglycemia for several weeks to partially reverse hypoglycemia unawareness and reduce risk of additional episodes (1)[A]. Less stringent HgbA1c goals should be used in patients with history of severe hypoglycemia or frequent hypoglycemia (1)[A].

Patient Monitoring
SMBG

DIET

- Alcohol consumption may place patients with diabetes at increased risk for delayed hypoglycemia (1)[A].
- CHO sources high in protein should not be used to treat or prevent hypoglycemia (1)[A].
- Fats may slow absorption of CHOs and may retard and then prolong the acute glycemic response (1)[A].
- Food insecurity increases risk of hypoglycemia due to inadequate or erratic carbohydrate consumptions following administration of sulfonylureas or insulin (1)[A].

PATIENT EDUCATION

- Always have access to quick-acting CHO.
- For exercise, consider ingestion of added CHO if preexercise blood sugar <100 mg/dL or a reduced insulin dose.
- Educate patients and their relatives, close friends, teachers, and supervisors to be aware of DM diagnosis and signs/symptoms of hypoglycemia and treatment.
- Teach SMBG and self-adjustment for insulin therapy, diet control, and exercise regimen.
- Wear medical alert identification bracelet or necklace.

PROGNOSIS

Full recovery usually depends on rapidity of diagnosis and treatment.

COMPLICATIONS

- Coma, seizure, myocardial infarction, stroke (especially in elderly)
- Prolonged or severe hypoglycemia may cause permanent neurologic damage and/or cognitive impairment.
- Children with T1DM have a greater vulnerability to neurologic manifestations of hypoglycemia.

ALERT

The ACCORD trial (adults with T2DM) demonstrated that intensively lowering blood glucose below current recommendations increased the risk of death versus standard treatment strategy.

REFERENCES

1. American Diabetes Association. 6. Glycemic targets: *standards of medical care in diabetes—2018*. *Diabetes Care*. 2018;41(Suppl 1):S55–S64.
2. Seaquist ER, Anderson J, Childs B, et al; for American Diabetes Association, Endocrine Society. Hypoglycemia and diabetes: a report of a workgroup of the American Diabetes Association and the Endocrine Society. *J Clin Endocrinol Metab*. 2013;98(5):1845–1859.
3. Allen KV, Pickering MJ, Zammitt NN, et al. Effects of acute hypoglycemia on working memory and language processing in adults with and without type 1 diabetes. *Diabetes Care*. 2015;38(6):1108–1115.
4. Cryer PE, Axelrod L, Grossman AB, et al; for Endocrine Society. Evaluation and management of adult hypoglycemic disorders: an Endocrine Society clinical practice guideline. *J Clin Endocrinol Metab*. 2009;94(3):709–728.

ADDITIONAL READING

Thompson AE. JAMA patient page. Hypoglycemia. *JAMA*. 2015;313(12):1284.

 SEE ALSO

- Diabetes Mellitus, Type 1
- Algorithm: Hypoglycemia

 CODES

ICD10
- E11.649 Type 2 diabetes mellitus with hypoglycemia without coma
- E10.649 Type 1 diabetes mellitus with hypoglycemia without coma
- E13.649 Oth diabetes mellitus with hypoglycemia without coma

CLINICAL PEARLS

- Address hypoglycemia in every visit with patients at risk.
- Best treatment includes:
  - Patient education and empowerment
  - Frequent SMBG or CGM
  - Flexible insulin (or other drug) regimens
  - Regular professional guidance and support
  - Individualized glycemic goals based in part on the risk of hypoglycemia
- Hypoglycemia unawareness should be recognized and addressed by less aggressive glycemic goals.
- Any form of CHO that contains glucose should be effective, such as sugar-containing food or beverage that can be rapidly absorbed:
  - Using the "rule of 15" is an easy way to teach patients to manage hypoglycemia at home. "Rule of 15": 15 to 20 g CHO (~60 to 80 calories simple CHO) SMBG and repeated q15min until blood sugar is ≥70 mg/dL

H

HYPOGLYCEMIA, NONDIABETIC

Matthew A. Silva, PharmD, RPh, BCPS • Pablo Hernandez Itriago, MD, MHCM, FAAFP

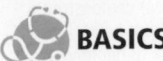 BASICS

DESCRIPTION
- Hypoglycemia defined by the Whipple triad
  - Low plasma glucose level (≤60 mg/dL) with hypoglycemic symptoms that are relieved when glucose is corrected
  - Occurs commonly in patients with diabetes receiving sulfonylurea or insulins; less commonly in patients without diabetes
- Reactive hypoglycemia occurs in response to a meal, drugs, herbal substances, or nutrients and may occur 2 to 3 hours postprandially or later (1).
  - Symptoms are generally observed with serum glucose ≤60 mg/dL, lower in patients with hypoglycemic unawareness.
  - Also seen after GI surgery (in association with dumping syndrome in some patients)
- Spontaneous (fasting) hypoglycemia may be associated with primary conditions including hypopituitarism, Addison disease, myxedema, or disorders related to hepatic dysfunction or renal failure (1,2).
  - If hypoglycemia presents as a primary disorder, consider hyperinsulinism and extrapancreatic tumors.

EPIDEMIOLOGY
Incidence
- True incidence is unknown.
- 0.5–8.6% of hospitalized patients ≥65 years (3,4,5)
  - Asymptomatic in 25% of cases

Prevalence
True prevalence is unknown:
- Predominant age: older adult
- Predominant sex: female > male

ETIOLOGY AND PATHOPHYSIOLOGY
- Reactive, postprandial
  - Alimentary hyperinsulinism
  - Meals high in refined carbohydrate
  - Certain nutrients, including fructose, galactose, leucine
  - Glucose intolerance (prediabetes)
  - GI surgery, especially gastric bypass
  - Idiopathic (unknown cause)
- Spontaneous
  - Fasting
  - Alcohol or prescription medication–associated (6) (insulin, sulfonylureas, thiazolidinediones, incretin mimetics, DPP-IV inhibitors, β-blockers, salicylates, quinine, hydroxychloroquine, fluoroquinolones, doxycycline, sertraline, disopyramide, pentamidine, gabapentin, tramadol)
  - Nonprescription over-the-counter (OTC) agents, including performance-enhancing agents. Adulterated versions of phosphodiesterase inhibitors and performance-enhancing agents are routinely imported and may contain sulfonylureas and other hypoglycemic agents.
  - Consider medication errors as a source of unexplained hypoglycemia even in patients without diabetes.
  - Surreptitious drug use (self-injection of insulin or ingestion of oral hypoglycemic medications in patients with diabetes)
  - Natural medicines or herbs (bitter melon, caffeine, cassia cinnamon, chromium, fenugreek, ginseng, guarana, mate, stevia, vanadium)
  - Postsurgical (e.g., bariatric surgery, gastrectomy, Roux-en-Y) hypoglycemia/dumping syndrome
  - Islet cell hyperplasia or tumor (insulinoma)
  - Extrapancreatic insulin-secreting tumor
  - Autoimmune hypoglycemia (Hirata disease)
  - Hepatic disease
  - Glucagon deficiency
  - Adrenal insufficiency
  - Catecholamine deficiency
  - Hypopituitarism
  - Hypothyroidism
  - Eating disorders
  - Exercise
  - Fever
  - Pregnancy
  - Renal glycosuria
  - Large tumors
  - Ketotic hypoglycemia of childhood
  - Enzyme deficiencies or defects
  - Severe malnutrition
  - Sepsis
  - Total parenteral nutrition therapy
  - Hemodialysis

Genetics
Some aspects may involve genetics (e.g., hereditary fructose intolerance).

RISK FACTORS
Refer to "Etiology and Pathophysiology."

GENERAL PREVENTION
- Follow dietary and exercise guidelines.
- Patient recognition of early symptoms and knowledge of corrective action

Pediatric Considerations
- Usually divided into two syndromes
  - Transient neonatal hypoglycemia
  - Hypoglycemia of infancy and childhood
- Screening infants for hypoglycemia is appropriate when pregnancy was complicated by maternal diabetes.
- Cases of hypoglycemia observed in children taking propranolol for infantile hemangioma
- Associated with indomethacin when treating patent ductus arteriosus

Geriatric Considerations
- More likely to have underlying disorders or be caused by medications
- Iatrogenic hypoglycemia is common in the hospitalized elderly with renal insufficiency.

COMMONLY ASSOCIATED CONDITIONS
- Severe liver disease; alcoholism
- Addison disease; adrenocortical insufficiency
- Myxedema
- Malnutrition (patients with renal failure)
- GI surgery
- Panhypopituitarism
- Insulinoma

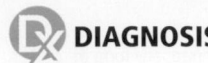 DIAGNOSIS

HISTORY
- CNS (neuroglycopenic) symptoms predominate with gradual glucose reduction:
  - Headache
  - Confusion
  - Light-headedness
  - Fatigue and weakness
  - Visual disturbances
  - Changes in personality
- Adrenergic symptoms: more prominent in acute drop in glucose
  - Anxiety
  - Tremulousness
  - Dizziness
  - Diaphoresis
  - Warmth/flushing
  - Heart palpitations
- GI symptoms
  - Hunger
  - Nausea
  - Belching

PHYSICAL EXAM
- CNS (neuroglycopenic) symptoms predominate with gradual glucose reduction:
  - Convulsions
  - Coma
  - Hypotension
- Adrenergic symptoms: more prominent in acute drop in glucose
  - Tremulousness
  - Diaphoresis
  - Warmth/flushing
  - Heart palpitations

DIFFERENTIAL DIAGNOSIS
CNS disorders
- Psychogenic
- Pseudohypoglycemia: symptoms of hypoglycemia or self-diagnosis in patients in whom low blood glucose may not be detectable and may be impossible to convince that they do not suffer from hypoglycemia after all tests are found to be normal

DIAGNOSTIC TESTS & INTERPRETATION
Initial Tests (lab, imaging)
- Blood glucose ≤45 mg/dL (≤2.5 mmol/L) when symptomatic followed by symptom resolution with feeding (2)[C]
- Plasma glucose overnight fasting: ≤60 mg/dL (≤3.33 mmol/L); confirm on ≥2 occasions (2)[C].
- Plasma glucose 72-hour fasting: ≤45 mg/dL (≤2.5 mmol/L) for females; ≤55 mg/dL (≤3.05 mmol/L) for males; fasting may be ended when Whipple triad is achieved or hypoglycemia is demonstrated (2)[C].
- Abdominal CT to rule out abdominal tumor

Follow-Up Tests & Special Considerations

- Misinterpretation of glucose tolerance tests may lead to misdiagnosis of hypoglycemia; ≥1/3 of normal patients have hypoglycemia, with or without symptoms, during the 4-hour glucose tolerance test. These patients may be at future risk for type 2 diabetes.
- C-peptide measurement (2)[C]
- Check liver studies, serum insulin, adrenocorticotropic hormone (ACTH), and cortisol. Serum insulin should be suppressed when glucose is <60 mg/dL.
- Serum β-hydroxybutyrate (2)[C]
- Insulin radioimmunoassay: Elevated insulin levels suggest islet cell hyperplasia or tumor.
- Drugs that may alter lab results: Many drugs can affect glucose levels; refer to drug or laboratory reference.

Diagnostic Procedures/Other

- For definitive diagnosis, patient should have
  - Documented low glucose levels
  - Symptoms when glucose levels are low
  - Evidence that symptoms are relieved specifically by ingestion of sugar or other food
  - Identification of the specific type of hypoglycemia
- Serum β-hydroxybutyrate <2.7 mg/dL in the presence of high-serum insulin, C-peptide, and low-serum glucose suggests excessive insulin production (2)[C].

TREATMENT

GENERAL MEASURES

- Outpatient except for severe cases; may also be inpatient for testing
- Oral carbohydrate for alert patient without drug overdose (2 to 3 tbsp of sugar in glass of water or fruit juice, 1 to 2 cups of milk, piece of fruit, or several soda crackers)
- If unable to swallow: Use glucagon IM or SC.
- If caused by medication or nutrients: Avoid or control causative agents.
- If triggered by meals: Try high-protein diet with carbohydrate restriction.
- Nonhypoglycemic hypoglycemia or pseudohypoglycemia
  - Many patients (often women aged 20 to 45 years) present with diagnosis of reactive hypoglycemia (self-diagnosed or misinterpretation of tests).
  - Symptoms may pertain to chronic fatigue and somatic complaints (stress often plays a role in these symptoms).
  - Management difficult; listening is important. Try 120-g carbohydrate diet.
  - Counseling may be useful for stress and other problems.

MEDICATION

- Once diagnosis is established, begin therapy appropriate for underlying disorder.
- If unable to swallow: glucagon 1 mg (1 unit) IM or SC. If no response, give IV bolus of 25 to 50 g of 50% glucose solution followed by continuous infusion until patient able to take by mouth.
- Postsurgical gastrectomy patients unresponsive to dietary changes may benefit from propantheline, psyllium, fiber, or oat bran to delay gastric emptying.
- Insulinoma

SURGERY/OTHER PROCEDURES

If islet cell tumor (insulinoma) or other insulin-secreting tumor, surgery is treatment of choice; if inoperable, diazoxide may relieve symptoms (1)[C].

ADMISSION, INPATIENT, AND NURSING CONSIDERATIONS

Hypoglycemia unresponsive to oral intake

 ONGOING CARE

FOLLOW-UP RECOMMENDATIONS

- Exercise routine or daily activity may need to be reevaluated.
- Patients with recurrent hypoglycemia should have glucose source at hand for immediate ingestion during symptoms.

Patient Monitoring

- Depends on type and severity of symptoms and treatment of underlying cause
- Hypoglycemia from sulfonylureas can last for hours to days depending on half-life and renal function.

DIET

- High protein, high fiber, complex carbohydrates from multigrain, and whole foods in moderation
- Frequent small feedings (six daily)
- Avoid fasting.

PATIENT EDUCATION

- Dietary instruction
- Counseling for stress, if appropriate
- Recognition of early symptoms of hypoglycemia and how to take corrective action

PROGNOSIS

Favorable, with appropriate treatment

COMPLICATIONS

- Insulinoma: If tumor identified and removed, some surgical risk is involved.
- Organic brain syndrome: may occur with extensive, prolonged hypoglycemia

REFERENCES

1. Guettier JM, Gorden P. Hypoglycemia. *Endocrinol Metab Clin North Am*. 2006;35(4):753–766.
2. Cryer PE, Axelrod L, Grossman AB, et al. Evaluation and management of adult hypoglycemic disorders: an Endocrine Society clinical practice guideline. *J Clin Endocrinol Metab*. 2009;94(3):709–728.
3. Kagansky N, Levy S, Rimon E, et al. Hypoglycemia as a predictor of mortality in hospitalized elderly patients. *Arch Intern Med*. 2003;163(15): 1825–1829.
4. Mannucci E, Monami M, Mannucci M, et al. Incidence and prognostic significance of hypoglycemia in hospitalized non-diabetic elderly patients. *Aging Clin Exp Res*. 2006;18(5):446–451.
5. Nirantharakumar K, Marshall T, Hodson J, et al. Hypoglycemia in non-diabetic in-patients: clinical or criminal? *PLoS One*. 2012;7(7):e40384.
6. Ben Salem C, Fathallah N, Hmouda H, et al. Drug-induced hypoglycaemia: an update. *Drug Saf*. 2011;34(1):21–45.

ADDITIONAL READING

- Cansu DU, Korkmaz C. Hypoglycaemia induced by hydroxychloroquine in a non-diabetic patient treated for RA. *Rheumatology (Oxford)*. 2008;47(3):378–379.
- Singh M, Jacob JJ, Kapoor R, et al. Fatal hypoglycemia with levofloxacin use in an elderly patient in the post-operative period. *Langenbecks Arch Surg*. 2008;393(2):235–238.
- Vaurs C, Brun JF, Bertrand M, et al. Post-prandial hypoglycemia results from a non-glucose-dependent inappropriate insulin secretion in Roux-en-Y gastric bypassed patients. *Metabolism*. 2016;65(3):18–26.

 SEE ALSO

- Hypoglycemia, Diabetic; Insulinoma
- Algorithm: Hypoglycemia

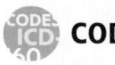 **CODES**

ICD10
- E16.2 Hypoglycemia, unspecified
- E16.1 Other hypoglycemia
- P70.4 Other neonatal hypoglycemia

CLINICAL PEARLS

- Symptoms coincide with low blood glucose levels and resolve with PO/IV glucose or glucagon.
- Avoid known agents/nutrients that trigger hypoglycemia.
- Treat underlying cause.

H

HYPOKALEMIA

James Auteri Ferguson, MD, MPH, CPH • Jason Chao, MD, MS

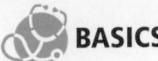 **BASICS**

DESCRIPTION

Hypokalemia is defined as a serum potassium concentration <3.5 mEq/L (normal range, 3.5 to 5.0 mEq/L).

- Mild hypokalemia (serum potassium 3.0 to 3.5 mEq/L)
- Moderate hypokalemia (serum potassium 2.5 to 3.0 mEq/L)
- Severe hypokalemia (serum potassium <2.5 mEq/L)

EPIDEMIOLOGY

Predominant sex: male = female

Incidence

- Electrolyte abnormality is commonly encountered in clinical practice and in the elderly.
- Found in >20% of hospitalized patients (when defined as potassium <3.6 mEq/L)
- Higher incidence (5–20%) in individuals with eating disorders
- >10% of inpatients with alcoholism
- Higher incidence in patients with AIDS
- Higher incidence in patients receiving diuretics
- 12–18% in patients with CKD
- Associated risk after bariatric surgery

ETIOLOGY AND PATHOPHYSIOLOGY

Most common causes:

- Decreased intake: deficient diet in alcoholics and elderly; anorexia nervosa
- GI loss: vomiting, diarrhea, nasogastric tubes, laxative abuse, villous adenoma, uretero-sigmoidostomy, malabsorption, chemotherapy, radiation enteropathy, bulimia
- Intracellular shift of potassium: metabolic alkalosis, insulin excess, β-adrenergic catecholamine excess (acute stress, β_2-agonists), hypokalemic periodic paralysis, intoxications (theophylline, caffeine, barium, toluene), refeeding syndrome (1)[C]
- Renal potassium loss
  - Drugs: diuretics (especially loop and thiazides), amphotericin B, aminoglycosides
  - Mineralocorticoid excess states: primary hyperaldosteronism; secondary hyperaldosteronism (congestive heart failure [CHF], cirrhosis, nephrotic syndrome, malignant hypertension, renin-producing tumors); renovascular hypertension; Bartter syndrome; Gitelman syndrome; congenital adrenogenital syndromes; exogenous mineralocorticoids (glycyrrhizic acid in licorice, carbenoxolone, steroids in nasal sprays); Liddle syndrome; vasculitis
  - Osmotic diuresis (e.g., poorly controlled diabetes)
  - Renal tubular acidosis (type I and II)
  - Magnesium depletion

- Glucocorticoid excess states: Cushing syndrome, exogenous steroids, ectopic adrenocorticotrophic hormone production, 11-β-hydroxysteroid dehydrogenase deficiency, refeeding syndrome

Genetics

Some rare, familial disorders can cause hypokalemia.

- Familial hypokalemic periodic paralysis: hypokalemia after a high-carbohydrate or high-sodium meal or after exercise
- Congenital adrenogenital syndromes
- Liddle syndrome: increases K+ secretion
- Familial interstitial nephritis

GENERAL PREVENTION

When initiating a diuretic, especially loop and thiazide diuretics, advise patients to increase their dietary potassium intake (see "Diet").

COMMONLY ASSOCIATED CONDITIONS

- Acute GI illnesses with severe vomiting or diarrhea
- Increased risk of cardiac arrhythmias; atrial fibrillation
- Hypokalemia is a predictor of development of severe alcohol withdrawal syndrome.

 DIAGNOSIS

- Patients with hypokalemia often have no symptoms, especially if the hypokalemia is mild (serum potassium 3.0 to 3.5 mEq/L).
- Neuromuscular (most prominent manifestations)
  - Easy fatigability, cramping, myalgias
  - Skeletal muscle weakness (proximal > distal muscles, lower limbs > upper limbs) may range from mild weakness to total paralysis, including respiratory muscles; it may lead to rhabdomyolysis and/or respiratory acidosis/arrest in severe cases.
  - Smooth muscle involvement may lead to GI hypomotility, producing ileus and constipation.
- Cardiovascular
  - Ventricular arrhythmias; higher risk if underlying CHF, left ventricular failure (LVF), cardiac ischemia
  - Increased risk of atrial fibrillation
  - Hypotension
  - Cardiac arrest
- Renal: polyuria, polydipsia, nocturia owing to impaired ability to concentrate, myoglobinuria
- Metabolic: hyperglycemia, alkalosis

HISTORY

Muscle weakness, hypotension, vomiting, diarrhea, polyuria, polydipsia

PHYSICAL EXAM

Decreased skin turgor in dehydration, hypotension, orthostasis, pulmonary congestion/rales, peripheral edema in heart failure

DIFFERENTIAL DIAGNOSIS

- Spurious hypokalemia occurs when blood with high WBC count (>100,000/mm³) is allowed to stand at room temperature (WBCs extract potassium from plasma).
- Thyrotoxicosis

DIAGNOSTIC TESTS & INTERPRETATION

- Serum potassium <3.5 mEq/L (<3.5 mmol/L)
- Disorders that may alter lab results: leukemia and other conditions with high WBCs

Initial Tests (lab, imaging)

- ECG
- If source of potassium loss not likely to be medications or GI tract: serum electrolytes, urinary potassium
- Calculate plasma anion gap (anion gap = Na − [Cl + HCO_3]); normal values, 12 ± 4 mEq/L. Must correct calculated anion gap for hypoalbuminemia. Increase calculated anion gap by 2.5 mEq/L for each 1 g/dL decrease in albumin <4 g/dL.
- CT scan of adrenal glands if there is evidence of mineralocorticoid excess

Follow-Up Tests & Special Considerations

- If excessive renal potassium loss (>20 mEq/day) and hypertension, plasma renin and aldosterone levels should be determined to differentiate adrenal from nonadrenal causes of hyperaldosteronism. If hypertension is absent and the patient is acidotic, renal tubular acidosis should be considered.
- In severe hypokalemia, rhabdomyolosis may result.
- Hypokalemia increases the myocyte resting potential, which increases the refractory period; this can lead to cardiac arrhythmias.

Test Interpretation

- If hypertension is absent and serum pH is normal to alkalotic
  - High urine chloride (>10 mEq/day [>10 mmol/day])—diuretics or Bartter and Gitelman syndromes
  - Low urine chloride (<10 mEq/day [<10 mmol/day])—GI losses likely
- ECG
  - Flattening or inversion of T waves
  - Increased prominence of U waves (small, positive deflection after T wave, best seen in V_2 and V_3)
  - Depression of ST segment
  - Ventricular ectopia

TREATMENT

GENERAL MEASURES
- Underlying cause of hypokalemia should be identified.
- For asymptomatic patients treated with oral replacement, outpatient follow-up is sufficient.
- Patients with cardiac manifestations require IV replacement with cardiac monitoring in an intensive care setting.

MEDICATION
- Nonemergent conditions (serum potassium >2.5 mEq/L [>2.5 mmol/L], no cardiac manifestations)
  - Oral therapy preferred: 40 to 120 mEq/day (40 to 120 mmol/day) in divided doses usually is adequate.
  - IV potassium should be given only when oral administration is not feasible (e.g., vomiting, postoperative state). Rate should not exceed 10 mEq/hr, and concentration should not exceed 40 mEq/L. Up to 40 mEq in 100 mL over 1 hour can be given safely through a central venous line. The patient's cardiac rhythm should be closely monitored.
  - Potassium chloride is suitable for all forms of hypokalemia.
  - Other potassium salts may be indicated if a coexisting disorder is present: potassium bicarbonate or bicarbonate precursor (gluconate, acetate, or citrate) in metabolic acidosis or phosphate in phosphate deficiency (2)[C].
- Emergent situations (serum potassium <2.5 mEq/L [<2.5 mmol/L], arrhythmias), IV replacement: Rate of administration should not exceed 20 mEq/hr (20 mmol/hr); maximum recommended concentration, 60 mEq/L (60 mmol/L) of saline for peripheral administration; administration through central venous lines preferred for rates >20 mEq/hr
- Check serum magnesium and replace, if needed; cannot adequately replace potassium in a setting of low magnesium
- Precautions
  - Any form of potassium replacement carries the risk of hyperkalemia.
  - Serum potassium should be checked more frequently in groups at higher risk: the elderly, diabetic patients, and patients with renal insufficiency.
  - Patients receiving digitalis and patients with diabetic ketoacidosis in whom intracellular shift in potassium is expected after insulin therapy is initiated must have more aggressive replacement.
- Significant possible interactions: Concomitant administration of potassium-sparing diuretics (spironolactone, triamterene, amiloride, ACE inhibitors) magnifies risk of hyperkalemia.

Geriatric Considerations
May need to correct magnesium depletion

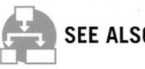 ONGOING CARE

FOLLOW-UP RECOMMENDATIONS
Patient Monitoring
- Patients receiving IV therapy should have cardiac monitoring and serum potassium level checked frequently (q4–6h).
- Patients requiring potassium supplements should have serum potassium studied at intervals and magnesium level dictated by clinical judgment and patient compliance (3)[C].

DIET
In patients with mild hypokalemia (potassium, 3.0 to 3.5 mEq/L [3.0 to 3.5 mmol/L]) not caused by GI losses, dietary supplementation may be sufficient; potassium-rich foods include oranges, bananas, cantaloupes, prunes, raisins, dried beans, dried apricots, and squash.

PATIENT EDUCATION
- Instructions for appropriate diet
- If potassium supplementation is necessary, stress the need for compliance.

PROGNOSIS
- Associated with higher morbidity and mortality because of cardiac arrhythmias
- Ease of correction of hypokalemia and need for prolonged treatment rest on the primary cause; if it can be eliminated (e.g., resolution of diarrhea, discontinuation of diuretics, removal of adrenal tumor), hypokalemia can be expected to resolve, and no further treatment is indicated.

COMPLICATIONS
- Hyperkalemia can occur during the course of treatment.
- Increased risk of digoxin toxicity
- Increased risk of atrial fibrillation (4)[B]

REFERENCES

1. Palmer BF. A physiologic-based approach to the evaluation of a patient with hypokalemia. *Am J Kidney Dis*. 2010;56(6):1184–1190.
2. Asmar A, Mohandas R, Wingo CS. A physiologic-based approach to the treatment of a patient with hypokalemia. *Am J Kidney Dis*. 2012;60(3):492–497.
3. Unwin RJ, Luft FC, Shirley DG. Pathophysiology and management of hypokalemia: a clinical perspective. *Nat Rev Nephrol*. 2011;7(2):75–84.
4. Krijthe BP, Heeringa J, Kors JA, et al. Serum potassium levels and the risk of atrial fibrillation: the Rotterdam Study. *Int J Cardiol*. 2013;168(6):5411–5415.

ADDITIONAL READING

- Ben Salem C, Hmouda H, Bouraoui K. Drug-induced hypokalaemia. *Curr Drug Saf*. 2009;4(1):55–61.
- Ernst ME, Moser M. Use of diuretics in patients with hypertension. *N Engl J Med*. 2009;361(22):2153–2164.
- Osadchii OE. Mechanisms of hypokalemia-induced ventricular arrhythmogenicity. *Fundam Clin Pharmacol*. 2010;24(5):547–559.
- Viera A, Wouk N. Potassium disorders: hypokalemia and hyperkalemia. *Am Fam Physician*. 2015;92(6):487–495.

 SEE ALSO

- Hyperkalemia
- Algorithm: Hypokalemia

CODES

ICD10
E87.6 Hypokalemia

CLINICAL PEARLS

- In patients without heart disease, a mildly low potassium level will rarely cause cardiac disturbances. In an otherwise healthy patient, gentle repletion using oral potassium or an increase in potassium-rich foods should be adequate.
- In patients with cardiac ischemia, heart failure, or left ventricular hypertrophy, even mild to moderate hypokalemia can cause arrhythmias. These patients should receive potassium repletion as well as cardiac monitoring.
- To safely prevent hypokalemia in diabetic and renal insufficiency patients, ensure adequate dietary potassium intake with foods rich in potassium, including spinach, tomatoes, broccoli, squash, potatoes, bananas, cantaloupe, and oranges. Avoid potassium-wasting diuretics, if possible.
- Uncorrected hypomagnesemia can hinder the correction of hypokalemia. Check magnesium levels and replete as necessary.
- Hypokalemia in an otherwise healthy young woman should prompt evaluation for bulimia nervosa.

H

HYPONATREMIA

Caitlin E. Jones, MD • Patricia Martinez Quinones, MD • Cassandra Q. White, MD, FACS

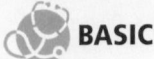 BASICS

DESCRIPTION
- Hyponatremia is a plasma sodium (Na^+) concentration of ≤135 mEq/L.
- Hyponatremia itself does not provide information about the "total body water (TBW)" state of the patient. Patients with hyponatremia may be hypervolemic, hypovolemic, or euvolemic.
- System(s) affected: endocrine/metabolic, renal, cardiovascular, central nervous system (CNS)

EPIDEMIOLOGY
Incidence
- Most common electrolyte disorder seen in the general hospital population
- Predominant age: all ages
- Predominant sex: male = female

Prevalence
- 2.5% of hospitalized patients
- 20–30% in hospitalized patients (1)
- 7.7% outpatients (1)

Geriatric Considerations
The elderly have lower TBW, a decreased thirst mechanism, and decreased urinary concentrating ability; their kidneys are less responsive to antidiuretic hormone (ADH), and they show decreased renal mass, renal blood flow, and glomerular filtration rate, putting them at higher risk for hyponatremia. Presenting symptoms may be frequent falls and gait disturbances.

Pediatric Considerations
Children <16 years of age have less intracranial space and are at increased risk of brain herniation from cerebral edema.

ETIOLOGY AND PATHOPHYSIOLOGY
- Assess serum osmolality and volume status to determine etiology. The etiology directs the management.
- Hypertonic hyponatremia: serum osmolarity (Osm) >295 mOsm
- Shift of water from intracellular fluid (ICF) to extracellular fluid (ECF), resulting in dilution
  – Unchanged TBW and Na^+
  – Causes: hyperglycemia, mannitol, sorbitol, radiologic contrast
- Isotonic hyponatremia ("pseudohyponatremia"): serum Osm 275 to 295 mOsm
  – Excessive osmoles leading to dilution
  – Unchanged TBW and Na^+
  – Causes: hyperlipidemia, hyperproteinemia (e.g., multiple myeloma), laboratory artifact, irrigant solutions
- Hypotonic hyponatremia: serum Osm <275 mOsm
  – Subdivided by volume status into hypovolemic, euvolemic, or hypervolemic
    ○ Hypovolemic hyponatremia: subtype of hypotonic hyponatremia with decreased TBW and Na^+
  – Signs include orthostatic hypotension, decreased skin turgor, dry mucous membranes.
  – Urine Na^+ <20 mmol/L; indicates extrarenal loss
    ○ Causes include GI loss (vomiting, diarrhea), third spacing (pancreatitis, peritonitis, burns, rhabdomyolysis), skin loss (burns, cystic fibrosis, sweating), and heat-related illnesses.
  – Urine Na^+ >20 mmol/L; indicates renal loss
    ○ Causes include cerebral salt-wasting syndrome, adrenal insufficiency, diuretics, and osmotic diuresis.

- Euvolemic hyponatremia: most common subtype of hypotonic hyponatremia with increased TBW and normal Na^+
  – Signs include a nonedematous state.
  – Urine Osm >100 mOsm/kg
    ○ Causes include syndrome of inappropriate antidiuretic hormone (SIADH), hypothyroidism, adrenal insufficiency, medications (e.g., thiazide diuretics, loop diuretics, carbamazepine, clofibrate, cyclosporine, levetiracetam, oxcarbazepine, SSRIs, TCAs, vincristine).
  – Urine Osm <100 mOsm/kg
    ○ Causes include primary polydipsia, beer potomania (massive consumption of beer, which is poor in solutes and electrolytes), and exercise-induced.
- Hypervolemic hyponatremia: subtype of hypotonic hyponatremia with increased TBW and Na^+
  – Signs include edematous state.
  – Urine Na^+ <20 mmol/L
    ○ Causes include congestive heart failure (CHF), cirrhosis, nephrotic syndrome, hypoalbuminemia, psychogenic polydipsia.
  – Urine Na^+ >20 mmol/L
    ○ Causes include CHF, liver cirrhosis, nephrotic syndrome, and chronic renal failure.

Genetics
- Polymorphisms have been demonstrated.
- Mutations have been associated with nephrogenic syndrome of inappropriate antidiuresis (NSIAD; SIADH).

GENERAL PREVENTION
Depends on underlying etiology

COMMONLY ASSOCIATED CONDITIONS
- Hypothyroidism
- Hypopituitarism
- Cirrhosis
- CHF
- Nephrotic syndrome
- Adrenocortical hormone deficiency
- HIV patients
- SIADH is associated with cancers, pneumonia, tuberculosis, encephalitis, meningitis, head trauma, cerebrovascular accident, HIV infection.
- Traumatic brain injury
- Marathon runners in hot environments
- Beer potomania
- Tea-and-toast diet
- Ecstasy use

 DIAGNOSIS

- Symptoms related to the rate of fall in serum Na^+, onset and degree of hyponatremia (2)
- Acute (≤48 hours): no time for full adaptation, more likely to present with moderate or severe symptoms
- Chronic: develops gradually, organ systems adapt to Na^+ concentration, associated with minimal symptoms
- Mild (serum Na^+ 130 to 135 mEq/L): usually asymptomatic, fatigue, loss of appetite
- Moderate (serum Na^+ 120 to 130 mEq/L): nausea, vomiting, lethargy
- Severe (serum Na^+ 115 to 120 mEq/L): headache, lethargy, restlessness, disorientation
- Severe/rapid decrease in serum Na^+ can cause seizures, coma, brain herniation, respiratory arrest, and may be fatal.

- Other signs and symptoms: weakness, muscle cramps, anorexia, hiccups, depressed deep tendon reflexes, hypothermia, positive Babinski responses, cranial nerve palsies, orthostatic hypotension

ALERT
Low Na^+ creates an osmotic gradient between plasma and cells, resulting in fluid shift into cells. This causes cerebral edema and increased intracranial pressure; eventually, this can lead to hyponatremic encephalopathy and brain herniation.

HISTORY
- Symptoms include headache, nausea, vomiting, muscle cramps.
- Can progress to lethargy or restlessness and disorientation

PHYSICAL EXAM
- Volume status: skin turgor, jugular venous pressure, heart rate, orthostatic blood pressure measurement
- Evaluate for underlying illness: signs of CHF, cirrhosis, hypothyroidism.
- Decreased reflexes may be seen.

DIFFERENTIAL DIAGNOSIS
See "Etiology and Pathophysiology."

DIAGNOSTIC TESTS & INTERPRETATION
Initial Tests (lab, imaging)
- Comprehensive metabolic profile (BUN, creatinine, glucose, electrolytes, liver function studies, etc.)
- Thyroid-stimulating hormone (TSH)
- Lipid panel
- Serum osmolality
- Urine Na^+ and osmolality
- Chest x-ray to rule out pulmonary pathology if SIADH is diagnosed

Follow-Up Tests & Special Considerations
CT scan of head if pituitary problem is suspected or if SIADH from CNS problem is suspected

 TREATMENT

GENERAL MEASURES
- Assess all medications patient is taking.
- Institute seizure precautions.
- Institute fluid restriction.
- Indications for 3% hypertonic saline versus normal saline solution: acute hyponatremia, symptomatic hyponatremia, association with intracranial pathology already at risk for cerebral edema

MEDICATION
ALERT
Rapid correction of severe symptomatic hyponatremia has been associated with central pontine myelinolysis, a neurologic disorder of loss of myelin and supportive structures in pons and occasionally in other areas of the brain (3). This results in irreversible injury. Symptoms are apparent 2 to 6 days after injury and include seizure, coma, spastic paraparesis, dysarthria, and dysphagia. Patients at increased risk are those with Na^+ <105, alcoholism, hypokalemia, malnutrition, and advanced liver disease liver transplant recipients. MRI is not required for diagnosis because it may not be positive until 4 weeks after symptom onset.

- Treatment is tailored to etiology, degree of hyponatremia, onset, and symptomatology.
- Some general principles apply:
  - Expected change in serum Na^+ with selected infusate: $\Delta Na = [(\text{infusate } Na^+ + \text{infusate } K^+ - \text{serum } Na^+) / (TBW + 1)]$
  - TBW = a coefficient × weight (kg) as in the following table:

Total Body Water

Children	0.6 × weight
Women	0.5 × weight
Men	0.6 × weight
Elderly women	0.45 × weight
Elderly men	0.5 × weight

  - Formula to determine correction available at http://www.medcalc.com/sodium.html
- Asymptomatic, euvolemic patients can be treated with fluid restriction; etiology must be addressed.
- For severely hyponatremic/symptomatic patients, administer 3% hypertonic saline, 2 mL/kg up to 100 mL, over a 20-minute period. Check serum Na^+ levels after infusion. Repeat as necessary until a 5 mmol/L increase in serum Na^+ is seen. Admit to ICU and check Na^+ every 2 hours.
  - If symptoms improve after a 5 mmol/L increase, discontinue the hypertonic saline and switch to 0.9% isotonic saline solution. Increase serum Na^+ with a limit of 10 mmol/L during the first 24 hours and then 8 mmol/L every day afterward until serum Na^+ is 130 mmol/L.
  - If symptoms do not improve after a 5 mmol/L increase, continue the hypertonic saline infusion until 1 mmol/L/hr increase in serum Na^+ is achieved. Discontinue infusion if symptoms improve, serum Na^+ increases by 10 mmol/L, or serum Na^+ is 130 mmol/L.
- For mild to moderate hyponatremia, use isotonic saline solution (0.9%). For moderate to severe hyponatremia, consider specialist consultation for use of hypertonic saline (3%) via central venous access at a rate of 1 to 2 mL/kg/hr; increasing serum Na^+ levels by 0.5 mmol/L/hr and monitoring frequently the plasma Na^+ level (approximately every 2 hours)
- In patients with severe hyponatremia (euvolemic and hypervolemic state) who do not respond to the aforementioned approach, consider the use of vasopressin V2-receptor antagonists, such as tolvaptan or conivaptan (4)[A].
- Treat underlying etiology.
- Chronic hyponatremia resulting from SIADH (5): demeclocycline (inhibits ADH action at the collecting duct) if fluid restriction alone is not effective
  - Contraindications: drug allergy, pregnancy, children <8 years old; caution in renal and hepatic disease
  - In doses of 600 to 1,200 mg/day, the drug produces nephrogenic diabetes insipidus.
  - Significant possible interactions: oral anticoagulants, oral contraceptives, penicillin
  - In case of overcorrection, relower Na^+ concentration. Begin with infusion of 3 mL/kg of 5% dextrose in water over 1 hour. Repeat Na^+ measurement. Be cautious; dextrose infusion rates >250 to 300 mL/hr can cause significant hyperglycemia in both diabetic and nondiabetic patients and may lead to osmotic diuresis and subsequent free water loss with increased serum Na^+ concentration. Consider 2 to 4 μg IV desmopressin every 8 hours to prevent overcorrection.

ALERT

Caution: If severe, consider hypertonic saline (3% Na^+ chloride) with central line access, exercise extreme caution, and monitor serum Na^+ as frequently as every 1 to 2 hours.

ADMISSION, INPATIENT, AND NURSING CONSIDERATIONS

- Admission is mandatory if the patient has acute hyponatremia or is symptomatic; acute hyponatremia (developing over <48 hours) increases the risk of cerebral edema.
- Admission is advised if patient is asymptomatic and has a serum Na^+ <125 mEq/dL.

 ## ONGOING CARE

DIET

- Euvolemic hyponatremia: Restrict water to 1 L/day.
- Hypervolemic hyponatremia: water and Na^+ restriction

PROGNOSIS

- In hospitalized patients, hyponatremia is associated with an elevated risk of adverse clinical outcomes and higher mortality (1)[B].
- Recently, in community-dwelling, middle-aged, and elderly adults, mild hyponatremia has been shown to be an independent predictor of death.
- Associated with poor prognosis in patients with acute pulmonary embolism
- Associated with poor prognosis in patients with liver cirrhosis and those waiting for liver transplant; it is associated with significant postoperative risk and short-term graft loss.

COMPLICATIONS

- Occult tumor may be present if SIADH is identified.
- Hypervolemia if isotonic saline solution is used
- Osmotic demyelination (central pontine and extrapontine irreversible myelinolysis) (1)
- Hyponatremia is the cause of 30% new-onset seizures in intensive care settings.
- Can cause hyponatremic encephalopathy and brain herniation if severe and untreated, especially in young women and children (2)
- Chronic hyponatremia is associated with increased risk of osteoporosis, attention deficit, gait disturbances, falls, and fractures.

REFERENCES

1. Rondon-Berrios H, Agaba EI, Tzamaloukas AH. Hyponatremia: pathophysiology, classification, manifestations and management. *Int Urol Nephrol*. 2014;46(11):2153–2165.
2. Williams DM, Gallagher M, Handley J, et al. The clinical management of hyponatraemia. *Postgrad Med J*. 2016;92(1089):407–411.
3. Singh TD, Fugate JE, Rabinstein AA. Central pontine and extrapontine myelinolysis: a systematic review. *Eur J Neurol*. 2014;21(12):1443–1450.

4. Rozen-Zvi B, Yahav D, Gheorghiade M, et al. Vasopressin receptor antagonists for the treatment of hyponatremia: systematic review and meta-analysis. *Am J Kidney Dis*. 2010;56(2):325–337.
5. Basu A, Ryder RE. The syndrome of inappropriate antidiuresis is associated with excess long-term mortality: a retrospective cohort analyses. *J Clin Pathol*. 2014;67(9):802–806.

ADDITIONAL READING

- Abraham WT, Hensen J, Gross PA, et al; for LIBRA Study Group. Lixivaptan safely and effectively corrects serum sodium concentrations in hospitalized patients with euvolemic hyponatremia. *Kidney Int*. 2012;82(11):1223–1230.
- De Picker L, Van Den Eede F, Dumont G, et al. Antidepressants and the risk of hyponatremia: a class-by-class review of literature. *Psychosomatics*. 2014;55(6):536–547.
- Friedman B, Cirulli J. Hyponatremia in critical care patients: frequency, outcome, characteristics, and treatment with the vasopressin V2-receptor antagonist tolvaptan. *J Crit Care*. 2013;28(2): 219.e1–219.e12.
- Sahay M, Sahay R. Hyponatremia: a practical approach. *Indian J Endocrinol Metab*. 2014;18(6):760–771.
- Sood L, Sterns RH, Hix JK, et al. Hypertonic saline and desmopressin: a simple strategy for safe correction of severe hyponatremia. *Am J Kidney Dis*. 2013;61(4):571–578.
- Zieg J. Pathophysiology of hyponatremia in children. *Front Pediatr*. 2017;5:213.

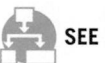 ## SEE ALSO

Algorithm: Hyponatremia

 ## CODES

ICD10

E87.1 Hypo-osmolality and hyponatremia

CLINICAL PEARLS

- Assess all medications patient is taking because many are associated with hyponatremia.
- Alcohol-dependent individuals with vitamin deficiencies, elderly women taking thiazide diuretics, and people with hypokalemia or burns are at increased risk of central pontine myelinolysis from too rapid correction of hyponatremia. Chronic hyponatremia is also a risk factor.
- Bronchogenic carcinoma and pancreatic, duodenal, and prostate cancer, as well as thymoma, lymphoma, and mesothelioma, are neoplastic diseases associated with SIADH.
- Formulas have been developed (Adrogue and Madias) for safe correction of hyponatremia and are available online (see http://www.medcalc.com/sodium.html).

H

HYPOPARATHYROIDISM

Cherry Onaiwu, MD, MS • Luay Sarsam, MD • Carrie Valenta, MD, FACP, FHM

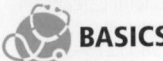 **BASICS**

DESCRIPTION

- Deficient or absent secretion of parathyroid hormone (PTH), a major hormone regulator of serum calcium and phosphorus levels in the body (1)
- Acute hypoparathyroidism: tetany that is mild (muscle cramps, perioral numbness, paresthesias of hands and feet) or severe (carpopedal spasm, laryngospasm, heart failure, seizures, stridor)
- Chronic: often asymptomatic; lethargy, anxiety/depression, urolithiasis and renal impairment, dementia, blurry vision from cataracts or kerato-conjunctivitis, parkinsonism or other movement disorders, mental retardation, dental abnormalities, and dry, puffy, coarse skin
- System(s) affected: endocrine/metabolic, musculoskeletal, nervous, ophthalmologic, renal

Pediatric Considerations
- May occur in premature infants
- Neonates born to hypercalcemic mothers may experience suppression of developing parathyroid glands.
- Congenital absence of parathyroids
- May appear later in childhood as autoimmune

Geriatric Considerations
Hypocalcemia is fairly common in elderly, however, rarely secondary to hypoparathyroidism.

Pregnancy Considerations
- Use of magnesium as a tocolytic may induce functional hypoparathyroidism.
- For women with hypoparathyroidism, calcitriol requirements decrease during lactation.

EPIDEMIOLOGY
More common in women; affects all ages

Incidence
Most common after surgical procedure of the anterior neck (75% of all cases). Transient hyperparathyroidism is seen after 6.9–46% of thyroidectomies, whereas permanent hypoparathyroidism, 0.9–1.6% at experienced centers.

Prevalence
- Affects 24 to 37/100,000 persons per year (1)
- Autosomal dominant hypocalcemia with hypercalciuria (ADHH): 1/70,000 typically in infancy with hypocalcemic seizures

ETIOLOGY AND PATHOPHYSIOLOGY
- PTH aids in regulating calcium homeostasis:
  - Mobilizes calcium and phosphorus from bone stores
  - Increases calcium absorption from the intestine by stimulating formation of 1,25-dihydroxy vitamin D
  - Stimulates reabsorption of calcium in the distal convoluted tubule and phosphate excretion in proximal tubule
- Reduced or absent PTH action results in hypocalcemia, hyperphosphatemia, and hypercalciuria.
- Acquired hypoparathyroidism
  - Surgical: removal or damage to parathyroid glands or their blood supply; thyroid, parathyroid, or neck surgery for head and neck cancers (2)
  - Autoimmune: isolated or combined with other endocrine deficiencies in polyglandular autoimmune (PGA) syndrome

- Deposition of heavy metals in gland: copper (Wilson disease) or iron (hemochromatosis, thalassemias), radiation-induced destruction, and metastatic infiltration
- Functional hypoparathyroidism: may result from hypomagnesemia or hypermagnesemia because magnesium is crucial for PTH secretion and activation of the PTH receptor
- Congenital
  - Calcium-sensing receptor (CaSR) abnormalities: hypocalcemia with hypercalciuria
  - HDR or Barakat syndrome: deafness, renal dysplasia
  - Familial: mutations of the *TBCE* gene; abnormal PTH secretions
  - 22q11.2 deletion syndrome
- Autoimmune: genetic gain-of-function mutation in CaSR
- Infiltrative: metastatic carcinoma, hemochromatosis, Wilson disease, granulomas
- Hypo- (alcoholics) or hypermagnesemia: chronic iron overloads

Genetics
- X-linked or in autosomal recessive mutations in the transcription factor glial cell missing B (GCMB)
- Mutations in transcription factors or regulators of parathyroid gland development
  - Component of a larger genetic syndrome (APS-1 or DiGeorge syndrome) or in isolation (X-linked hypoparathyroidism) (3)
  - May be autosomal dominant (DiGeorge), autosomal recessive (APS-1), or X-linked recessive (X-linked hypoparathyroidism) (3)
  - Congenital syndromes
    - 22q11.2 deletion syndrome, familial hypomagnesemia, hypoparathyroidism with lymphedema (3)
    - Hypoparathyroidism with sensorineural deafness
    - ADHH: mutations gain-of-function of the CaSR gene suppressing the parathyroid gland, without elevation of PTH
  - PGA syndrome type I: mucocutaneous candidiasis, hypoparathyroidism, and Addison disease

RISK FACTORS
Neck surgery and neck trauma, neck malignancies, family history of hypocalcemia, PGA syndrome

GENERAL PREVENTION
Intraoperative identification and preservation of parathyroid tissue

COMMONLY ASSOCIATED CONDITIONS
- DiGeorge syndrome
- Bartter syndrome
- PGA syndrome type I
- Multiple endocrine deficiency autoimmune candidiasis (MEDAC) syndrome
- Juvenile familial endocrinopathy
- Addison disease
- Moniliasis (HAM) syndrome: a polyglandular deficiency syndrome, possibly genetic, characterized by hypoparathyroidism

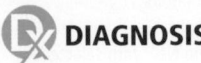 **DIAGNOSIS**

HISTORY
Often asymptomatic; ask about previous neck trauma or surgery, head or neck irradiation, family history of hypocalcemia, or presence of other autoimmune endocrinopathies.
- Cardinal clinical feature: neuromuscular hyperexcitability
- Also includes: fatigue, circumoral or distal extremity paresthesias, muscle spasm, seizures, neuropsychiatric symptoms

PHYSICAL EXAM
- Surgical scar on neck
- Chvostek sign: ipsilateral twitching of the upper lip on tapping the facial nerve on the cheek. 15% of normocalcemic people have positive sign (1).
- Trousseau sign: painful carpal spasm after 3-minute occlusion of brachial artery with BP cuff. BP cuff inflation to above systolic BP for 3 minutes leads to carpal spasm (flexion of metacarpophalangeal [MCP] joints, extension of interphalangeal [IP] joints, adduction of fingers and thumb).
- Tetany, laryngo- or bronchospasm, cardiac arrhythmias, refractory heart failure, dyspnea, edema
- Dry, coarse, puffy hair; brittle nails
- Loss of deep tendon reflexes
- Dysrhythmias (secondary hypocalcemia)
- Cataracts or ectopic calcifications
- Tooth enamel defects
- Vitiligo

DIFFERENTIAL DIAGNOSIS
- Vitamin D deficiency/resistance
- Pseudohypoparathyroidism, which presents in childhood; kidney and bone unresponsiveness to PTH; characterized by hypocalcemia, hyperphosphatemia, and, in contrast to hypoparathyroidism, elevated rather than reduced PTH concentrations
- Hypoalbuminemia, renal failure, malabsorption, familial hypocalcemia, hypomagnesemia

DIAGNOSTIC TESTS & INTERPRETATION

Initial Tests (lab, imaging)
- Calcium: ionized (low) and total (low) (correct serum calcium level for albumin)
  - Corrected serum calcium = total serum calcium + 0.8 (4 — serum albumin)
- Phosphorus (high)
- Intact or "whole" PTH (low); how to distinguish from pseudohypoparathyroidism or secondary causes
- Magnesium (low may be cause of hypoparathyroidism; may also be normal)
- BUN, creatinine, 25-OH vitamin D level (especially in elderly)
- Urinary calcium (normal or high)
- Calcium should be monitored after thyroid or parathyroid surgery.
- Radiographs may show absent tooth roots, calcification of cerebellum, choroid plexus, or cerebral basal ganglia.

Follow-Up Tests & Special Considerations

- ECG: prolongation of ST and QTc intervals, nonspecific repolarization changes, dysrhythmias
- Urine calcium: Creatinine ratio (normal 0.1 to 0.2) may be low before treatment but should be monitored to prevent stones due to hypercalciuria.
- Gene sequencing: Evaluation of other hormone levels may be required to diagnose APS-1.
- Hungry bone syndrome (transient hypoparathyroidism after parathyroid surgery)
  - Hypocalcemia due to hungry bone syndrome may persist despite recovery of PTH secretion from the remaining normal glands. Thus, serum PTH concentrations may be low, normal, or even elevated.
- Infiltrative: osteoblastic metastasis of prostate, breast, or lung cancer
- Metabolic/nutritional: renal failure, neonatal hypocalcemia, hypoalbuminemia, malabsorption, calcium (Ca^{++}) chelators, and hypomagnesemia
- Familial hypocalcemia, acute hyperphosphatemia (rare), vitamin D deficiency
- Autoantibodies against NACHT leucine-rich-repeat protein 5 (NALPS) found in 49% of 73 patients with APS-1 and hypoparathyroidisms

TREATMENT

GENERAL MEASURES

- Monitor ECG during calcium repletion.
- Maintenance therapy: may require lifelong treatment with calcium and calcitriol
  - Maintain serum calcium in low normal range: 8 to 8.5 mg/dL (2.00 to 2.12 mmol/L).
- If hypercalcemia occurs, hold therapy until calcium returns to normal. Treat magnesium deficiency if present.
- Phosphate binders are required if high calcium-phosphate product.
- Thiazide diuretics combined with a low-salt diet may be used to prevent hypercalciuria, nephrocalcinosis, and nephrolithiasis.
- Oral calcium administration and vitamin D supplementation after thyroidectomy may reduce the risk for symptomatic hypocalcemia after surgery.

MEDICATION

- Acute hypoparathyroidism
  - Hypoparathyroid with severe symptoms (tetany, seizures, cardiac failure, laryngospasm, bronchospasm)
    - IV calcium gluconate: 1 or 2 g, each infused over a period of 10 minutes. Central venous catheter is preferred because calcium-containing solutions can irritate surrounding tissues. Follow with infusion of 10 g calcium gluconate in 1 L 5% dextrose water at a rate of 1 to 3 mg calcium gluconate per kg body weight per hour (2)[B].
  - Hypomagnesemia: acutely: 1 to 2 g IV q6h; long-term magnesium oxide tablets (600 mg) once or twice per day
  - Maintenance: See "First Line" treatment for chronic hypoparathyroidism.
- Chronic hypoparathyroidism

First Line

- Adults
  - Oral calcium carbonate: calcium salts: Start with 1 to 3 g/day PO but dose varies. For geriatric patients, those on a PPI or those who have constipation on the carbonate form, consider using calcium citrate instead (4)[B].

- Calcitriol (vitamin D 1, 25-dihydroxycholecalciferol): 0.25 μg/day. Doses 0.5 to 2.0 μg/day are usually required (3)[A].
  - Either parental form of vitamin D (D_2 ergocalciferol or D_3 cholecalciferol) for tissues to generate their own 1,25 form
  - For hypercalciuria, consider a thiazide diuretic.
  - For phosphate level well above normal (>6.5 mg/dL), use low phosphate diet or phosate binder.
- Children
  - Oral elemental calcium: 25 to 50 mg/kg daily
  - Calcitriol: 0.25 μg daily for age >1 year

ISSUES FOR REFERRAL

Endocrinologist, nephrologist, ophthalmologist

ADDITIONAL THERAPIES

PTH peptides 1-34 and 1-84 SC

- rhPTH 1-84—FDA-approved, 50 μg SC daily
- For patients with frequent episodes of hyper- and hypocalcemia, nephrolithiasis, nephrocalcinosis, GFR <60 mL/min, persistently high phosphate (4)[B]
- Treatment goal: Eliminate use of active vitamin D_3, reduce supplemental calcium to 500 mg daily; maintain consistent Ca level in low normal range.
- Improved well-being and increased bone mineral density have been shown for these patients.

SURGERY/OTHER PROCEDURES

Autotransplantation of cryopreserved parathyroid tissue: restores normocalcemia in 23% of cases

ADMISSION, INPATIENT, AND NURSING CONSIDERATIONS

- Admission criteria/initial stabilization: laryngospasm, seizures, tetany, QT prolongation
- Discharge criteria: resolution of hypocalcemic symptoms, patient educated on hypoparathyroidism and treatment

ONGOING CARE

FOLLOW-UP RECOMMENDATIONS

Patient Monitoring

- Goal is a total corrected serum calcium level in low normal range (8.0 to 8.5 mg/dL or 2.00 to 2.12 mmol/L), 24-hour urine calcium <300 mg, and calcium-phosphate product <55. If Ca <2.0 mmol/L or <8.0 mg/dL, then treat even if asymptomatic (4)[B].
- Outpatient measurement of serum calcium, phosphate, magnesium, and creatinine weekly to monthly during initial management; for changes in medication, check weekly or every other week; when stable, measure every 6 months (4)[B].
- 24-hour urine for calcium and Cr secretion yearly
- If symptoms of renal stone disease or increasing Cr, get renal imaging every 5 years (4)[B].
- Annual slit-lamp and ophthalmologic evaluations are recommended.
- DEXA scan: standard monitoring recommended (4)[B]

DIET

Low-phosphate diet in patients with hyperphosphatemia

PATIENT EDUCATION

https://www.hypopara.org/

PROGNOSIS

Hypoparathyroidism following neck surgery is often transient. Length of required treatment may vary depending on origin.

COMPLICATIONS

- Reversible: due to low calcium levels, most likely to improve with adequate treatment
  - Neuromuscular symptoms: Paresthesias (circumoral, fingers, toes), tetany, seizures, parkinsonian symptoms; pseudotumor cerebri has been described.
  - Renal: hypercalciuria, nephrocalcinosis, nephrolithiasis
  - Cardiovascular: heart failure, arrhythmias
- Irreversible: when condition starts early in childhood and will not improve with calcium and vitamin D treatment
  - Stunting of growth
  - Enamel defects and hypoplasia of teeth
  - Atrophy, brittleness, and ridging of nails
  - Cataracts and basal ganglia calcifications

REFERENCES

1. Abate E, Clarke B. Review of hypoparathyroidism. *Front Endocrinol (Lausanne).* 2017;7:172.
2. Al-Azem H, Khan A. Hypoparathyroidism. *Best Pract Res Clin Endocrinol Metab.* 2012;26(4): 517–522.
3. Bilezikian JP, Khan A, Potts JT Jr, et al. Hypoparathyroidism in the adult: epidemiology, diagnosis, pathophysiology, target-organ involvement, treatment, and challenges for future research. *J Bone Miner Res.* 2011;26(10):2317–2337.
4. Brandi M, Bilezikian D, Shoback D, et al. Management of hypoparathyroidism: summary statement and guidelines. *J Clin Endocrinol Metab.* 2016;101(6):2273–2283.

ADDITIONAL READING

- Bollerslev J, Rejnmark L, Marcocci C, et al. European Society of Endocrinology clinical guideline: treatment of chronic hypoparathyroidism in adults. *Eur J Endocrinol.* 2015;173(2):G1–G20.
- Michels TC, Kelly KM. Parathyroid disorders. *Am Fam Physician.* 2013;88(4):249–257.
- Stack BC Jr, Bimston DN, Bodenner DL, et al. American Association of Clinical Endocrinologists and American College of Endocrinology disease state clinical review: postoperative hypoparathyroidism—definitions and management. *Fndocr Pract.* 2015;21(6):674–685.

 ## CODES

ICD10

- E20.9 Hypoparathyroidism, unspecified
- P71.4 Transitory neonatal hypoparathyroidism
- E89.2 Postprocedural hypoparathyroidism

CLINICAL PEARLS

Often asymptomatic; consider if hypocalcemic with fatigue and circumoral or distal extremity paresthesias.

- Correct the serum calcium level for albumin level.
- Monitor calcium after thyroid or parathyroid surgery.
- Distinguish hypoparathyroidism from pseudohypoparathyroidism and secondary causes by PTH level.
- Not much clinical difference between 2nd- and 3rd-generation PTH assays
- Serum levels of magnesium and 25-OH should be measured to rule out deficiency that could contribute to reduced serum calcium levels.

H

HYPOTHERMIA

Scott T. Henderson, MD

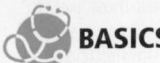

BASICS

DESCRIPTION
- A core temperature of <35°C (95°F)
- May take several hours to days to develop
- Patients with cold-water immersion may appear dead but can sometimes still be resuscitated.
- System(s) affected: all body systems
- Synonym(s): accidental hypothermia

EPIDEMIOLOGY
- Predominant age: very young and the elderly
- Predominant sex: male > female

Geriatric Considerations
More common in elderly due to lower metabolic rate, impaired ability to maintain normal body temperature, and impaired ability to detect temperature changes

Prevalence
Estimates vary widely; typically a secondary issue

ETIOLOGY AND PATHOPHYSIOLOGY
- Overwhelming environmental cold stress
- Decreased heat production
- Increased heat loss
- Impaired thermoregulation

RISK FACTORS
- Alcohol consumption
- Bronchopneumonia
- Cardiovascular disease
- Cold-water immersion
- Dermal dysfunction (burns, erythrodermas)
- Drug intoxication
- Endocrinopathies (myxedema, severe hypoglycemia)
- Excessive fluid loss
- Hepatic failure
- Hypothalamic and central nervous system (CNS) dysfunction
- Malnutrition
- Mental illness; Alzheimer disease
- Prolonged cardiac arrest
- Prolonged environmental exposure
- Renal failure
- Sepsis
- Trauma (especially head)
- Uremia

GENERAL PREVENTION
- Appropriate clothing, with particular attention to head, feet, and hands
- For outdoor activities, carry survival bags with rescue foil blanket for use if stranded or injured.
- Avoid alcohol.
- Alertness to early symptoms and initiating preventive steps (e.g., drinking warm fluids)
- Identify medications that may predispose to hypothermia (e.g., neuroleptics, sedatives, hypnotics, tranquilizers).

COMMONLY ASSOCIATED CONDITIONS
- Addison disease
- CNS dysfunction
- Congestive heart failure
- Diabetes
- Hypopituitarism
- Hypothyroidism
- Ketoacidosis
- Pulmonary infection
- Sepsis
- Uremia

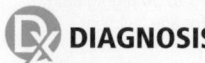

DIAGNOSIS

HISTORY
Presentation varies with the temperature of the patient at the time of presentation.

ALERT
History of prolonged exposure to cold may make the diagnosis obvious, but hypothermia may be overlooked in other situations, especially in comatose patients. Always obtain a core temperature if hypothermia is suspected.

PHYSICAL EXAM
- Esophageal temperature is most accurate, minimally invasive method of assessing core temperature (1)[C].
  - Must have secure airway
  - Probe inserted into lower 3rd of esophagus
  - Peripheral thermometers (tympanic membrane, temporal artery, axillary, or oral) associated with reduced accuracy
- Exam findings vary with the temperature of the patient at the time of presentation.
  - Mild (32–35°C)
    - Lethargy and mild confusion
    - Shivering
    - Tachypnea
    - Tachycardia
    - Loss of fine motor coordination
    - Increased BP
    - Peripheral vasoconstriction
    - Hyperactive reflexes
  - Moderate (28–32°C)
    - Delirium
    - Bradycardia
    - Hypotension
    - Hypoventilation
    - Cyanosis
    - Arrhythmias (prolonged PR interval, AV junctional rhythm, accelerated idioventricular rhythm, prolonged QT interval, altered T waves)
    - Semicoma and coma
    - Muscular rigidity
    - Generalized edema
    - Slowed reflexes
  - Severe (<28°C)
    - Very cold skin
    - Rigidity
    - Apnea
    - Bradycardia
    - No pulse: ventricular fibrillation or asystole
    - Areflexia
    - Unresponsive
    - Pupils (dilated <27°C; fixed and dilated <27°C)

ALERT
Use specially designed thermometers that can record low temperatures and measure core temperatures.

Pediatric Considerations
- Infants may present with bright red, cold skin and very low energy.
- A child's body temperature drops faster than an adult does when immersed in cold water.

DIFFERENTIAL DIAGNOSIS
- Cerebrovascular accidents
- Intoxication
- Drug overdose
- Complications of diabetes, hypothyroidism, hypopituitarism

DIAGNOSTIC TESTS & INTERPRETATION
Initial Tests (lab, imaging)
- Arterial blood gases (corrected for temperature)
- CBC and platelet counts
- Serum electrolytes; BUN/creatinine; glucose; calcium; magnesium
- Urinalysis
- Coagulation studies; fibrinogen level
- Blood culture
- Liver function studies; amylase
- Cardiac enzymes
- Alcohol level and toxicology screen
- Cervical spine, chest, and abdomen x-rays, if appropriate
- Bedside ultrasound to assess hemodynamics
- CT of the head for any concern regarding mental status

Follow-Up Tests & Special Considerations
Serum cortisol and TSH if underlying endocrine dysfunction (hypothalamus stimulates release of hormones in response to hypothermia)

Diagnostic Procedures/Other
ECG

Test Interpretation
Serum potassium >12 mmol/L associated with nonsurvival

TREATMENT

GENERAL MEASURES
- Prehospital (1)[C]
  - Factors to guide treatment
    - Level of consciousness
    - Shivering intensity
    - Cardiovascular stability based on blood pressure and cardiac rhythm
    - ABCs of basic life support
    - Remove wet garments.
      - Dry patient.
    - Protect against heat loss and wind chill.
    - If far from definitive care, begin active rewarming but do not delay transport.
      - Mild hypothermic patients with shivering ability will have improved comfort and might have a reduced cold-stress response with active rewarming (2)[B].
    - Give warm humidified oxygen if available.
- See "Admission, Inpatient, and Nursing Considerations."

MEDICATION

- For sepsis or bacterial infections: antibiotics based on site and etiology
- For hypoglycemia: D50W at a dose of 1 mg/kg
- Thiamine: 100 mg, if alcoholic or cachectic
- Naloxone: 2 mg
- Levothyroxine: 150 to 500 μg for myxedema
- For severe acidosis: sodium bicarbonate
- Precautions
  - Medications including epinephrine, lidocaine, and procainamide can accumulate to toxic levels if used repeatedly; should be avoided until core temperature is >30°C:
    - When temperature reaches >30°C, IV medications are indicated. Administer slowly.
  - Consider vasopressors according to standard ACLS algorithm with concurrent rewarming in setting of cardiac arrest.
- Significant possible interactions:
  - Use all drugs cautiously due to impaired metabolism and renal elimination.
- Once rewarming has occurred, there is mobilization of depot stores.
- Routine use of steroids or antibiotics does not increase survival or decrease postresuscitative damage.

ADMISSION, INPATIENT, AND NURSING CONSIDERATIONS

- Rewarming depends on severity of hypothermia and presence of cardiac arrest.
- If no cardiac arrest, consider active external rewarming (3)[B].
- If cardiac arrest is present, consider active internal rewarming (3)[B].
- Warm center of body first (4)[C].
- The rate of rewarming is determined by whether a perfusing cardiac output is present.
  - If a perfusing cardiac output is present, 1–2°C/hr is appropriate.
  - If not, then a faster rate of >2°C/hr should be used.
- Monitor core temperature; use a consistent method.
- Monitor BP and cardiac rhythm.
- Correct metabolic acidosis.
- Evaluate for frostbite and other trauma.
- Mild hypothermia
  - Passive rewarming
  - Administration of heated IV solutions
  - Provide warm fluids by mouth if fully alert.
- Moderate hypothermia
  - Active external rewarming
- Severe hypothermia (active internal [core] rewarming)
  - Minimally invasive
  - Heated IV fluids
  - Heated humidified oxygen
  - Body cavity lavage
    - Thoracic cavity lavage (40–45°C)
    - Peritoneal lavage (40–45°C)
  - Extracorporeal blood rewarming
    - Cardiopulmonary bypass
    - Extracorporeal membrane oxygenation
    - Continuous arteriovenous rewarming
    - Hemodialysis and hemofiltration
- Cardiac arrhythmias
  - Atrial fibrillation and sinus bradycardia are common—patients usually convert to normal sinus rhythm with rewarming.
  - If ventricular fibrillation is present, treat with one shock. If patient does not respond, consider deferring further attempts until rewarm has occurred.
  - Do not treat transient ventricular arrhythmias.
  - If cardiac pacing required, preferable to use external noninvasive pacemaker.
- Admit patients, preferably to the ICU, with underlying disease, physiologic abnormalities, or core temperature <32°C.
- Normal saline is preferred as fluid of choice (1)[C].
- Heat IVs from 40°C to 45°C if possible—should at least be no colder than patient core temperature.

ALERT
- Avoid fluid overload.
- Avoid overheating dextrose solutions; dextrose caramelizes at 60°C.
- Avoid lactated Ringer solution because of decreased lactate metabolism.
- Heart is irritable and susceptible to arrhythmias; take care transporting.
- Electrolytes may fluctuate with rewarming, check electrolytes (particularly potassium) frequently.
- Discharge from emergency department once normothermic, if mild hypothermia and no predisposing conditions or complications and has suitable place to go. All others require admission.

 ONGOING CARE

FOLLOW-UP RECOMMENDATIONS
Patient Monitoring
- During acute episode
  - Monitor cardiac rhythm.
  - Monitor electrolytes and glucose frequently.
  - Monitor urinary output.
  - Follow blood gases.
- Following acute episode
  - Continued therapy for any underlying disorder

DIET
Warm fluids only if alert and able to swallow
- Alcohol intake increases risk of becoming hypothermic in cold conditions.
- Encourage persons with cardiovascular disease to avoid outdoor exercise in cold weather.
- Refer to social service agency for help with adequate housing, heat, and/or clothing, if appropriate.

PROGNOSIS
- Mortality rates are decreasing due to increased recognition and advanced therapy.
- Mortality usually depends on age and the severity of underlying cause and comorbidities.
  - Mortality rate in healthy patients is <5%.
  - Mortality rate with coexisting illness is >50%.
  - Alcohol or drug poisoning seen in 10% of deaths

Geriatric Considerations
Mortality rates increase with increasing age. Over half of deaths are seen in patients >65 years.

COMPLICATIONS
- Core temperature after drop
- Cardiac arrhythmias
- Hypotension
- Hyperkalemia, hypoglycemia
- Rhabdomyolysis
- Sepsis
- Pneumonia (aspiration and bronchopneumonia), pulmonary edema
- Acute respiratory distress syndrome
- Pancreatitis, peritonitis, GI bleeding, ileus
- Acute tubular necrosis, bladder atony
- Intravascular thromboses/disseminated intravascular coagulation
- Metabolic acidosis
- Gangrene of extremities
- Compartment syndromes
- Seizures, cerebral ischemia, delirium

REFERENCES

1. Zafren K, Giesbrecht GG, Danzl DF, et al. Wilderness Medical Society practice guidelines for the out-of-hospital evaluation and treatment of accidental hypothermia: 2014 update. *Wilderness Environ Med*. 2014;25(Suppl 4):S66–S85.
2. Lundgren P, Henriksson O, Naredi P, et al. The effect of active warming in prehospital trauma care during road and air ambulance transportation—a clinical randomized trial. *Scand J Trauma Resusc Emerg Med*. 2011;19:59.
3. Kempainen RR, Brunette DD. The evaluation and management of accidental hypothermia. *Respir Care*. 2004;49(2):192–205.
4. van der Ploeg GJ, Goslings JC, Walpoth BH, et al. Accidental hypothermia: rewarming treatments, complications and outcomes from one university medical centre. *Resuscitation*. 2010;81(11):1550–1555.

ADDITIONAL READING

- Petrone P, Asensio JA, Marini CP. Management of accidental hypothermia and cold injury. *Curr Probl Surg*. 2014;51(10):417–431.
- Rischall ML, Rowland-Fisher A. Evidence-based management of accidental hypothermia in the emergency department. *Emerg Med Pract*. 2016;18(1):1–24.

 SEE ALSO

- Frostbite; Nonfatal Drowning
- Algorithm: Hypothermia

 CODES

ICD10
- T68.XXXA Hypothermia, initial encounter
- T68.XXXD Hypothermia, subsequent encounter
- T68.XXXS Hypothermia, sequela

CLINICAL PEARLS

- The most common cause of hypothermia in the United States is cold exposure due to alcohol intoxication.
- With a severely decreased core temperature, begin resuscitation (if possible) unless there are obvious lethal injuries. Continue resuscitation and rewarm to 33–35°C ("not dead until warm and dead").
- ECG changes associated with hypothermia: slowing of sinus rate with T-wave inversion; QT, QRS, and PR interval prolongation; atrial and ventricular arrhythmias; J waves (Osborn waves)

H

HYPOTHYROIDISM, ADULT

Adithi Naidu, MD, ABFM, CCFP • Faraz Ahmad, MD, MPH • Hiba Ahmad, PharmD

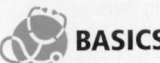 **BASICS**

DESCRIPTION
- Clinical and metabolic state resulting from decreased levels of free thyroid hormone or from resistance to hormone action
- Primary (intrinsic thyroid disease) or central (secondary or tertiary resulting from hypothalamic-pituitary disease)
- Subclinical: serum TSH above the upper reference limit with a normal free thyroxine (T₄) and normal hypothalamic-pituitary-thyroid axis (1)
- Overt: elevated TSH, usually >10 mIU/L with a subnormal free T₄

EPIDEMIOLOGY
Incidence
- Women: 3.5/1,000 persons per year
- Men: 0.6/1,000 persons per year

Prevalence
- The National Health and Nutrition Examination Survey III (NHANES III), subclinical hypothyroidism 9.3%, overt 0.3–3.7% in an unselected U.S. population age >12 years, with upper limit TSH 4.5
- Framingham study, 5.9% of women and 2.3% of men age >60 years had a serum TSH >10 mIU/L.

ETIOLOGY AND PATHOPHYSIOLOGY
- Primary: abnormality at the thyroid gland (>95% of cases)
- Most common cause worldwide: environmental iodine deficiency (1)[A]
- Most common cause in the United States: Hashimoto thyroiditis (chronic autoimmune thyroiditis)
  - Hashimoto is characterized pathologically by infiltration of the thyroid with sensitized T lymphocytes and serologically by circulating antithyroid antibodies.
  - Autoimmunity to the thyroid gland is an inherited defect in immune surveillance, leading to abnormal regulation of immune responsiveness or alteration of presenting antigen in the thyroid (1).
- Postablative/posttherapeutic: follows radioactive iodine therapy or hemithyroidectomy for hyperthyroidism; radiotherapy or surgery for thyroid cancer, benign nodular thyroid disease, or neck malignancies
- Transient hypothyroidism: de Quervain syndrome (viral), postpartum, silent thyroiditis (2)
- Drug use: propylthiouracil, methimazole, lithium, amiodarone, antiepileptic drugs, and newer chemotherapeutic agents such as tyrosine kinase inhibitors (sunitinib), interleukin-2, or interferon-α
- Central: hypothyroidism due to insufficient stimulation by TSH of an otherwise normal thyroid gland
- Can be secondary (level of the pituitary) or tertiary (level of the hypothalamus)
- Etiology involves genetic defects, tumors, vascular, empty sella syndrome, inflammatory, infiltrative, iatrogenic, posttrauma, or drug related.

RISK FACTORS
- Women >60 years of age
- Personal or family history of autoimmune diseases
- Pregnant women or those with previous postpartum thyroiditis
- Previous head or neck irradiation
- Past history of thyroid dysfunction or thyroid surgery
- Abnormal thyroid examination, presence of goiter and/or TPOAb positivity

- Treatment with amiodarone, lithium, interferon-α, sunitinib, or sorafenib
- Down syndrome or Turner syndrome

COMMONLY ASSOCIATED CONDITIONS
- Diabetes mellitus type 1 and 2
- Pernicious anemia
- Primary adrenal failure (Addison disease)
- Myasthenia gravis
- Celiac disease
- Rheumatoid arthritis
- Systemic lupus erythematosus
- Vitiligo
- Depression
- Genetic syndromes that have multiple autoimmune endocrinopathies (MAE) such as type 1 MAE and type 2 MAE

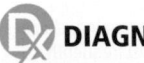 **DIAGNOSIS**

HISTORY
- Lethargy
- Fatigue
- Cold intolerance
- Slowed thinking
- Hearing impairment
- Constipation
- Dry skin
- Muscle cramps, arthralgias, paresthesias
- Modest weight gain (10 lb [4.5 kg])
- Menstrual disturbances
- Depression
- Change in voice (hoarseness)
- Carpal tunnel syndrome
- Symptoms can vary and can be nonspecific.

PHYSICAL EXAM
- Dry, coarse, thickened skin
- Hair loss/brittle hair
- Coarsening of voice
- Periorbital puffiness
- Swelling of hands and feet (nonpitting)
- Bradycardia
- Reduced systolic BP; increased diastolic BP
- Delayed relaxation of deep tendon reflexes
- Macroglossia
- Goiter (particularly in patients with Hashimoto thyroiditis)

Geriatric Considerations
- Characteristic signs and symptoms frequently nonspecific, changed, or absent
- Normal serum thyrotropin ranges are higher (in those >65 years of age).

DIFFERENTIAL DIAGNOSIS
- Chronic fatigue syndrome
- Depression
- Euthyroid sick syndrome
- Congestive heart failure
- Primary amyloidosis
- Dementia from other causes
- Primary adrenal insufficiency
- Thyrotropin-secreting pituitary adenoma

DIAGNOSTIC TESTS & INTERPRETATION
Initial Tests (lab, imaging)
- Primary hypothyroidism
  - Elevated TSH (>4.5 mIU/L)
  - Decreased serum free T₄ (2)[A]
- Central (secondary or tertiary) hypothyroidism
  - Assess only free T₄ or free T₄ index, not TSH (1)[A].
  - Decreased serum free T₄
  - Antithyroid antibodies absent
  - TRH stimulation test, especially if free T₄ and/or TSH is low-normal and patient has hypothalamo-pituitary pathology
  - Imaging of the hypothalamus and pituitary gland
- Subclinical hypothyroidism
  - Elevated serum TSH (>4.5 mIU/L)
  - Normal serum free T₄ (3)[A]
  - Note: Serum free triiodothyronine (T₃) or total T₃ should not be done to diagnose hypothyroidism (1)[A].

Follow-Up Tests & Special Considerations
- Antithyroid antibodies may define the cause of primary hypothyroidism but are not necessary in all settings.
- Drugs that may alter lab results:
  - Drugs that decrease TSH:
    - Thyroid supplement, cortisone, dopamine, octreotide
  - Drugs that increase TSH:
    - Phenytoin, amiodarone, dopamine antagonist (metoclopramide/domperidone, salicylates, oral cholecystographic dyes [sodium ipodate]), or estrogen or androgen in excess
  - Drugs that increase free T₄:
    - Heparin, high intake of biotin
- Disorders that may alter lab results
  - Any severe illness, pregnancy, chronic protein malnutrition, hepatic failure, or nephrotic syndrome

Test Interpretation
Screening
- Patient with risks factors as described above (1)[A]
- Patient with laboratory or imaging abnormalities
  - Substantial hyperlipidemia or change in lipid pattern
  - Hyponatremia, often resulting from inappropriate production of antidiuretic hormone
  - High serum muscle enzyme concentrations
  - Macrocytic anemia
  - Pericardial or pleural effusion
  - Pituitary or hypothalamic disorder
- Pregnant women
  - Personal or family history of thyroid disease
  - Diabetes mellitus type 1
  - H/o recurrent miscarriage, morbid obesity, or infertility; TPOAb should be considered (1)[A].
  - Universal screening not recommended for patients pregnant or planning pregnancy
- U.S. Preventive Services Task Force found insufficient evidence for or against screening nonpregnant, asymptomatic children or adults (2)[A].
- Recommendations by expert groups:
  - ATA recommends screening in all adults at age 35 years and every 5 years thereafter (1)[A].
  - AACE recommends screening older patients (age not specified), especially women.
  - AAFP recommends against routine screening in asymptomatic patients <60 years.
  - ACOG recommends women with h/o autoimmune disease or strong family h/o thyroid disease should be screened at age 19 years.

TREATMENT

MEDICATION

First Line

- Levothyroxine (Synthroid, Levothroid)
  - 1.5 to 1.8 μg/kg/day (use ideal body weight) (2)[A]; titrate by 12.5 to 25.0 μg/day every 4 to 8 weeks until TSH in normal range.
  - Dosage requirements may vary with age, gender, residual secretory capacity of thyroid gland, other drugs being taken by patient, and intestinal function (1)[A].
  - Use caution when changing between capsule, tablet, and injection because dose conversions are not a 1:1 ratio.
  - Elderly patients may require 2/3 of dose used in young adults because clearance is decreased.
  - Levothyroxine should be taken on an empty stomach, ideally an hour before breakfast. Administering at bedtime may result in higher levels than administering in the morning (4)[A].
  - Medications that interfere with its absorption should be taken 4 hours after the T_4 dose: ferrous sulfate, proton pump inhibitors, calcium carbonate, bile acid resins.
- Contraindications
  - Thyrotoxic heart disease
  - Uncorrected adrenocorticoid insufficiency
  - MI, acute
  - TSH suppression, preexisting
- Precautions
  - If elderly or known coronary artery disease, start with lower doses, such as 12.5 to 25.0 μg.
  - Diabetic patients may need readjustment of hypoglycemic agents with institution of T_4.
  - Dosage of oral anticoagulants may need adjustment; monitor prothrombin time while initiating treatment.
  - Patients on digoxin may need close monitoring.
  - Elderly patients more susceptible to AFib and osteoporotic fracture with thyroid hormone excess
  - Patients requiring doses that are higher than expected should be evaluated for GI disorders (*Helicobacter pylori*, celiac disease).
- Possible interactions with the following medications:
  - Oral anticoagulants, insulin, oral hypoglycemic, estrogen, OCP, PPI, cholestyramine
  - Ferrous sulfate, calcium carbonate, antacids, laxatives, colestipol, sucralfate, ciprofloxacin, and cholestyramine may decrease absorption.
- Controversy exists whether subclinical hypothyroidism should be treated. Cochrane Review found no improvement in survival, cardiovascular morbidity, or health-related quality of life. Some evidence indicates improvement in lipid profiles and left ventricular function. Subclinical hypothyroidism should be treated in patients with iron deficiency anemia and in patients with TSH >10 (3,5)[B],(6).
- If surgery is elective, render patient euthyroid prior to procedure.
- If surgery is urgent, proceed with individualized replacement therapy preoperatively and postoperatively.
- Brand and generic T_4 formulations available. Questionable equivalent efficacy of preparation when switching between manufactures; can measure serum TSH 6 weeks after changing manufactures

Pregnancy Considerations

- Replacement therapy may need adjustment; average dose increases from 25% to 50% (6)[A].
- TSH levels should be monitored monthly during 1st trimester; goal TSH of 2.0 to 2.5 mIU/L for 1st trimester, <3.0 mIU/L for 2nd trimester, and <3.5 mIU/L for 3rd trimester (6)[A]

- Postpartum: Check TSH levels at 6 weeks (6)[A].
- Painless subacute thyroiditis may occur in postpartum period, leading to transient hypothyroidism lasting 3 months. Treatment with replacement therapy may be warranted. Up to 30% of these individuals develop permanent hypothyroidism.

Second Line

- No benefit to adding T_3 to T_4 (6)[A]
- Desiccated thyroid hormone is not recommended for the treatment of hypothyroidism (1).
- Liothyronine (T_3) or desiccated thyroid hormone (T_3 and T_4) may be an alternative for patients who do not feel balanced on T_4 alone.

ISSUES FOR REFERRAL

- Children and infants
- Pregnancy or women planning conception
- Patient in whom it is difficult to maintain a euthyroid state
- Cardiac disease
- Presence of goiter, nodule, or other structural changes in the thyroid gland
- Presence of adrenal or pituitary disorders (1)[C]

ADMISSION, INPATIENT, AND NURSING CONSIDERATIONS

- Myxedema coma (decompensated severe untreated hypothyroidism)
- True clinical emergency (requires ICU care)
- Profound hypothermia and unconsciousness
- Increased risk of shock and potentially fatal arrhythmias
- Postponing surgery for initiating therapy for hypothyroidism is not indicated.

ONGOING CARE

FOLLOW-UP RECOMMENDATIONS

Patient Monitoring

- Monitor TSH and free T_4 every 4 to 8 weeks after initiating treatment or after change in dose. Once stabilized, periodic TSH level should be done after 6 months and then at 12-month intervals or more frequently if the clinical situation dictates otherwise (1)[B].
- Monitor cardiac function closely in older patients.
- Check TSH more frequently during pregnancy, initiation of estrogen supplementation, or after large changes in body weight.
- In central hypothyroidism, TSH is unreliable; must monitor free T_4 and T_3
- Thyroid hormones should not be used to treat obesity in euthyroid patients (1)[A].

PATIENT EDUCATION

- Stress importance of compliance with thyroid replacement therapy.
- Explain need for lifelong treatment.
- Further education required for patients taking multiple medications that may interact
- Instruct to report to physician any signs of infection or heart problems.
- Describe signs of thyrotoxicity.
- High-bulk diet may help avoid constipation.

PROGNOSIS

- Return to normal state is the rule.
- Relapses will occur if treatment is interrupted.
- If untreated, may progress to myxedema coma

COMPLICATIONS

- Mortality and complication rates from surgery are similar between hypothyroid and euthyroid patients.
- Myxedema coma: mortality 30–60%
- Increased susceptibility to infection
- Megacolon
- Sexual dysfunction
- Organic psychosis with paranoia
- Infertility
- Hypersensivity to opiates
- Treatment over long periods can lead to bone demineralization.
- Iatrogenic thyrotoxicosis can lead to AFib and osteoporosis.
- Can lead to adrenal crisis with vigorous treatment, especially in patients with undiagnosed polyendocrine syndromes
- Treatment-induced congestive heart failure in people with coronary artery disease

REFERENCES

1. Garber JR, Cobin RH, Gharib H, et al. Clinical practice guidelines for hypothyroidism in adults: cosponsored by the American Association of Clinical Endocrinologists and the American Thyroid Association. *Endocr Pract*. 2012;18(6):988–1028.
2. Chaker L, Bianco AC, Jonklaas J, et al. Hypothyroidism. *Lancet*. 2017;390(10101):1550–1562.
3. Cooper DS, Biondi B. Subclinical thyroid disease. *Lancet*. 2012;379(9821):1142–1154.
4. Khandelwal D, Tandon N. Overt and subclinical hypothyroidism: who to treat and how. *Drugs*. 2012;72(1):17–33.
5. Jonklaas J, Bianco AC, Bauer AJ, et al. Guidelines for the treatment of hypothyroidism: prepared by the American Thyroid Association Task Force on Thyroid Hormone Replacement. *Thyroid*. 2014;24(12):1670–1751.
6. Alexander EK, Marqusee E, Lawrence J, et al. Timing and magnitude of increases in levothyroxine requirements during pregnancy in women with hypothyroidism. *N Engl J Med*. 2004;351(3):241–249.

CODES

ICD10

- E03.9 Hypothyroidism, unspecified
- E06.3 Autoimmune thyroiditis
- E89.0 Postprocedural hypothyroidism

CLINICAL PEARLS

- Monitor TSH and free T_4 every 4 to 8 weeks after initiating treatment or after change in dose. Once stabilized, periodic TSH level should be done after 6 months and then at 12-month intervals or more frequently if the clinical situation dictates otherwise (1)[B].
- Screening test: TSH levels (1)[A]
- Serum free T_3 or total T_3 should not be done to diagnose hypothyroidism (1)[A].
- Dosage requirements may vary with age, gender, residual secretory capacity of thyroid gland, other drugs being taken by patient, and intestinal function (1)[A].

H

ID REACTION

Sahil Mullick, MD

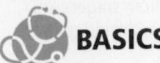

BASICS

DESCRIPTION
A generalized skin reaction associated with various infectious (fungal, bacterial, viral, or parasitic) or inflammatory cutaneous conditions distant from the primary disease site (1)

- "Id" is often combined with a root to reflect the causative factor (i.e., bacterid, syphilid, and tuberculid). Dermatophytid is the most frequently referenced id reaction. A dermatophytid is an autosensitization reaction in which a secondary cutaneous reaction occurs at a site distant to a primary fungal infection. The eruption typically begins within 1 to 2 weeks of the onset of the main lesion or following exacerbation of the main lesion.
- Most commonly localized vesicular lesions, erythema nodosum, and erythema multiforme
- System(s) affected: skin/exocrine
- Synonym(s): dermatophytid, trichophytid, autoeczematization

EPIDEMIOLOGY
- Predominant age: all ages
- Predominant sex: male = female
- Predominant race: all races

Incidence
Unknown

Prevalence
Common

ETIOLOGY AND PATHOPHYSIOLOGY
Precise pathophysiology is uncertain. Circulating antigens may react with antibodies at sensitized areas of the skin. An abnormal immune recognition of autologous skin antigens may also occur. Inflammation may lower the irritation threshold of the skin, and hematogenous spread of cytokines from the primary site of inflammation may also play a role (1).

- Etiology
  - Infectious
    - Fungal infections: *Trichophyton mentagrophytes*, *Trichophyton rubrum*, *Epidermophyton floccosum*, and *Candida* spp.
    - Bacterial infections: *Streptococcus pyogenes*, *Staphylococcus aureus*, and *Mycobacterium tuberculosis*
    - Viral infections: HSV, *Molluscum contagiosum*, orf, and milker's nodules
    - Parasitic infections: *Sarcoptes scabiei* and *Leishmania* spp.
  - Allergic
    - Id reactions occur in patients with nickel and aluminum allergy.
  - Miscellaneous
    - Id reaction rarely develops due to retained postoperative sutures, ionizing radiation, and blunt trauma.
    - Rarely, id reaction has been documented in patients receiving intravesical BCG live therapy for transitional cell carcinoma.

RISK FACTORS
- Fungal infection of the skin, especially tinea pedis
- Stasis dermatitis

GENERAL PREVENTION
- Good skin hygiene (particularly in intertriginous areas) to minimize risk of developing fungal infections
- Promptly treat any developing fungal infection.

COMMONLY ASSOCIATED CONDITIONS
- Primary fungal infection
- Stasis dermatitis

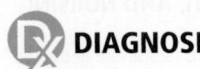

DIAGNOSIS

HISTORY
Itchy rash: Inquire about presence of lesions (typically fungal or bacterial) that could have incited the id reaction in the preceding days to weeks.

PHYSICAL EXAM
- Common
  - Symmetric, pruritic vesicles on the palms and, most commonly, on lateral aspects of fingers
  - Tinea infection on the feet; contact or other eczematous dermatitis; bacterial, fungal, or viral infection of the skin
- Less common
  - Papules
  - Lichenoid eruption
- Eczematoid eruption

DIFFERENTIAL DIAGNOSIS
- Pompholyx (dyshidrotic eczema)
- Contact dermatitis
- Drug eruptions
- Pustular psoriasis
- Folliculitis
- Scabies

DIAGNOSTIC TESTS & INTERPRETATION
- Potassium hydroxide (KOH) or fungal culture of primary lesion
- No fungal elements are present at the site of the id reaction.
- Special tests: Skin shows a positive trichophyton reaction. A wheal >10 mm at 20 minutes and induration >5 mm at 72 hours is a positive response.

Follow-Up Tests & Special Considerations
- The id reaction resolves with successful eradication of the primary skin condition.
- It is important to distinguish dermatophytids from drug-induced allergic reactions because continued treatment is essential to clear the underlying infection.

Test Interpretation
Histology
- Vesicles in the upper dermis
- Superficial perivascular lymphohistiocytic infiltrate with small numbers of eosinophils and increased granular cell layer
- No infectious agents present in biopsy specimen.

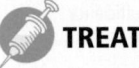

TREATMENT

GENERAL MEASURES
- Outpatient treatment of the underlying infection or eczematous dermatitis
- Symptomatic treatment of pruritus with antihistamines and/or topical steroids if needed (may require class 1 or 2 steroid)
- Treatment for secondary bacterial infection

MEDICATION
First Line
- PO antihistamines for pruritus (2)
  - Chlorpheniramine: 4 mg PO q4–6h PRN; max 24 mg/24 hr (pediatric: 6 to 11 years 2 mg PO q4–6h PRN; max 12 mg/24 hr; ≥12 years, refer to adult dosing)
  - Diphenhydramine: 25 to 50 mg PO q4–6h PRN; max 400 mg/24 hr (pediatric: 5 mg/kg/24 hr divided q6h PRN; 2 to 5 years max 37.5 mg/24 hr; 6 to 11 years max 150 mg/24 hr; ≥12 years, refer to adult dosing)
  - Hydroxyzine: 25 to 100 mg PO q6–8h PRN; max 600 mg/24 hr (pediatric: 2 mg/kg/24 hr divided q6h PRN)

- Topical treatments for pruritus
  - Triamcinolone 0.1% ointment TID
  - Hydrocortisone 0.5%, 1%, 2.5%: up to QID
  - Capsaicin 0.025%, 0.075% cream: Apply TID–QID; EMLA (2.5% lidocaine + 2.5% prilocaine) applied 30 to 60 minutes prior to capsaicin may minimize burning.
  - Doxepin 5% cream: Apply QID for up to 8 days (to max of 10% of the body).
  - Permethrin 5% cream (for scabies)
    - Apply from neck down after bath.
    - Wash off thoroughly with water in 8 to 12 hours.
    - May repeat in 7 days
  - Permethrin 1% cream rinse (for lice)
    - Shampoo, rinse, towel dry, saturate hair and scalp (or other affected area), leave on 10 minutes and then rinse.
    - May repeat in 7 days
  - White petroleum emollients: Apply after short bath/shower in warm (not hot) water.
- Systemic steroids only if reaction is severe or generalized (e.g., prednisone 20 mg)

Second Line
- Topical and/or systemic antifungals for identified associated fungal infection (common)
  - Tinea cruris/corporis
    - Topical azole antifungal compounds econazole (Spectazole) and ketoconazole (Nizoral): usually applied BID for 2 to 4 weeks
    - Terbinafine (Lamisil): over-the-counter (OTC) compound; can be applied daily or BID for 1 to 2 weeks
    - Butenafine (Mentax): applied once daily for 2 weeks; also very effective
  - Tinea capitis
    - PO griseofulvin for *Trichophyton* and *Microsporum* sp.; microsized preparation available; dosage 20 to 25 mg/kg/day divided BID or as a single dose daily for 6 to 12 weeks
    - PO terbinafine can be used for *Trichophyton* sp. at 62.5 mg/day in patients weighing 10 to 20 kg, 125 mg/day if weight 20 to 40 kg, 250 mg/day if weight >40 kg, and use for 4 to 6 weeks.

- Topical or systemic antibiotics for any secondary bacterial infection
- Treatment with antiviral agents for erythema multiforme associated with HSV is required.

 ONGOING CARE

PATIENT EDUCATION
Avoid hot, humid conditions that promote fungal growth. Aerate susceptible body areas (e.g., wear sandals or open footwear). If possible, wear loose-fitting clothing and undergarments, dry wet skin after bathing, and use powders and antiperspirants to discourage fungal growth. Treat primary dermatitis promptly.

PROGNOSIS
After appropriate treatment, complete resolution in days to weeks

COMPLICATIONS
- Secondary bacterial infection (cellulitis)
- After resolution of dermatophytid, postinflammatory hyperpigmentation is common and disappears without treatment in 1 month.

REFERENCES
1. Ilkit M, Durdu M, Karakaş M. Cutaneous id reactions: a comprehensive review of clinical manifestations, epidemiology, etiology, and management. *Crit Rev Microbiol.* 2012;38(3):191–202.
2. Cotes ME, Swerlick RA. Practical guidelines for the use of steroid-sparing agents in the treatment of chronic pruritus. *Dermatol Ther.* 2013;26(2):120–134.

ADDITIONAL READING
- Elmariah SB, Lerner EA. Topical therapies for pruritus. *Semin Cutan Med Surg.* 2011;30(2):118–126.
- Paulsen LL, Geller DD, Guggenbiller M. Symmetrical vesicular eruption on the palms. *Am Fam Physician.* 2012;85(8):811–812.
- Stachler RJ, Al-khudari S. Differential diagnosis in allergy. *Otolaryngol Clin North Am.* 2011;44(3):561–590, vii–viii.
- Veien NK. Acute and recurrent vesicular hand dermatitis. *Dermatol Clin.* 2009;27(3):337–353, vii.
- Yosipovitch G, Bernhard JD. Clinical practice. Chronic pruritus. *N Engl J Med.* 2013;368(17):1625–1634.

 CODES

ICD10
- L30.2 Cutaneous autosensitization
- B35.9 Dermatophytosis, unspecified

CLINICAL PEARLS
- When one skin eruption follows another closely in time, consider an id reaction.
- When assessing an itchy rash, inquire about potential fungal or bacterial lesions in the preceding days to weeks as a potential prelude to the id reaction.

IMMUNE THROMBOCYTOPENIA (ITP)

Pedro Emilio Alcedo, MD • Gabriela Sanchez Petitto, MD • Cristhiam Rojas-Hernandez, MD

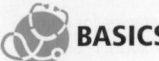 BASICS

DESCRIPTION

- Immune thrombocytopenia (ITP) is a condition characterized by the immunologic destruction of normal platelets and/or impaired thrombopoiesis in response to an unknown stimulus.
- It is defined as a platelet count $<100 \times 10^9$/L, once other causes of thrombocytopenia have been ruled out (1).
- ITP nomenclature:
  - Newly diagnosed (<3 months), persistent (3 to 12 months), and chronic (>12 months)
  - Primary when it presents in isolation; secondary when associated with other disorders
- ITP is a relatively common disease of childhood that typically follows a viral infection. Onset is within 1 week, and spontaneous resolution occurs within 2 months in $>80\%$ of patients.
- In adults, ITP is usually a chronic disease and spontaneous remission is rare.
- Synonym(s): idiopathic thrombocytopenic purpura; immune thrombocytopenic purpura; and Werlhof disease

EPIDEMIOLOGY

- Peak age
  - Pediatric ITP: 2 to 4 years
  - Chronic ITP: >50 years with incidence 2 times higher in persons 60 years than those <60 years of age
- Predominant gender
  - Pediatric ITP: male = female
  - Chronic ITP: female $>$ male (1.2 to 1.7:1)

Incidence

- Pediatric acute ITP: 1.9 to 6.4/100,000 children per year (2)
- Adult ITP: 1.6/100,000 per year (1)

Prevalence

Limited data; in one population (in Oklahoma) (3):

- Overall prevalence of 11.2/100,000 persons
- In children (<16 years): 8.1/100,000 with average age of 6 years
- In adults (>16 years): 12.1/100,000 persons with average age of 55 years

ETIOLOGY AND PATHOPHYSIOLOGY

- Accelerated platelet uptake and destruction by reticuloendothelial phagocytes results from action of IgG autoantibodies against platelet membrane glycoproteins IIb/IIIa. There is also cell-mediated platelet destruction by CD8$^+$ T cells.
- Autoantibodies interfere with megakaryocyte maturation, resulting in decreased production.
- Fc-independent desialylated platelet clearance has been proposed as the mechanism of refractoriness to therapies that target the classic FC-dependent pathway.

RISK FACTORS

- Autoimmune thrombocytopenia (e.g., Evans syndrome)
- Common variable immunodeficiency (CVID)
- Drug side effect (e.g., quinidine, vancomycin, penicillin, sulfonamides)
- Infections: *Helicobacter pylori*, hepatitis C, HIV, CMV, varicella zoster, measles, rubella, influenza, EBV, Whipple disease

- Vaccination side effect. Live virus vaccinations carry a lower risk than natural viral infection: 2.6/100,000 cases MMR vaccine doses versus 6 to 1,200/100,000 cases of natural rubella or measles infections.
- Bone marrow transplantation side effect
- Connective tissue disease, such as systemic lupus erythematosus, antiphospholipid antibody syndrome
- Lymphoproliferative disorders

 DIAGNOSIS

A careful history, physical exam, and review of CBC and peripheral blood smear remain the key components of the diagnosis of ITP.

HISTORY

- Often asymptomatic; found incidentally on routine CBC
- Posttraumatic bleeding occurs at counts of 40 to 60×10^9/L.
- With counts $<30 \times 10^9$/L, bruising tendency, epistaxis, menorrhagia, and gingival bleeding are common.
- Spontaneous bleeding may occur with platelet count $<20 \times 10^9$/L.
- Intracerebral bleeding is rare and may occur with counts $<20 \times 10^9$/L and associated trauma or vascular lesions, resulting in neurologic symptoms.
- Female sex and exposure to NSAIDs have been associated with bleeding.

PHYSICAL EXAM

- Ecchymoses, petechiae, epistaxis, and gingivorrhagia are common.
- Abnormal uterine bleeding may be present.
- Hemorrhagic bullae on buccal mucosa reflect acute, severe thrombocytopenia.
- Absence of splenomegaly, hepatomegaly, lymphadenopathy, stigmata of congenital disease

DIFFERENTIAL DIAGNOSIS

- Acute leukemia
- Thrombotic thrombocytopenic purpura
- Hemolytic uremic syndrome
- Factitious: platelet clumping on peripheral smear
- Thrombocytopenia secondary to sepsis
- Myelodysplastic syndrome, particularly in older patients
- Decreased marrow production: malignancy, drugs, viruses, megaloblastic anemia
- Posttransfusion
- Gestational thrombocytopenia
- Isoimmune neonatal purpura
- Congenital thrombocytopenias
- Disseminated intravascular coagulation
- Alcohol-induced thrombocytopenic purpura

DIAGNOSTIC TESTS & INTERPRETATION

Initial Tests (lab, imaging)

- CBC with differential and peripheral smear:
  - Isolated decreased platelet count $<100 \times 10^9$/L
  - Giant platelets are usually present.
  - Normal red and white blood cell morphology
- For patients with history, exam, CBC, and peripheral smear typical of ITP, consider the following:
  - PT/PTT is normal.
  - In adults, serologies for hepatitis B, hepatitis C, and HIV infections are recommended (1)[B].

- In pediatric ITP, immunoglobulin levels to exclude CVID are commonly obtained (1)[B].
- Other tests are not necessary for patients with typical ITP presentation: antiplatelet, antinuclear, antiphospholipid antibodies; *H. pylori* testing; thrombopoietin; platelet parameters; direct antiglobulin test; reticulocyte count; urinalysis; and thyroid function tests (1)[C].
- Further studies should be considered if the patient with thrombocytopenia also presents with:
  - Fever
  - Arthralgia
  - Lymphadenopathy
  - Family history of bleeding disorder
  - Risk factors for HIV
  - Abnormalities in other cell lines

Diagnostic Procedures/Other

- Imaging is not necessary.
- Bone marrow aspiration/biopsy
  - Not necessary for diagnosis in children (1)[B] and adults (1,2)[C]
  - Can be considered for a patient with atypical symptoms, such as fever and weight loss and multiple abnormalities in blood count

Test Interpretation

- Peripheral smear: normal red and white cells with large or giant platelets but diminished in number
- Marrow reveals normal to abundant megakaryocytes with normal erythroid and myeloid precursors.

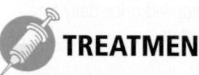 TREATMENT

GENERAL MEASURES

- Management is based on both platelet count and hemorrhagic manifestations.
- Current evidence-based guidelines recommend treatment should be administered for newly diagnosed patients with a platelet count $<30 \times 10^9$/L (1,2)[C].
- The main goal is to achieve a platelet count associated with adequate hemostasis, rather than a normal count (1).
- Outpatient management unless patient has platelet count $<20 \times 10^9$/L and is at risk for bleeding
- Admit patients with active bleeding.

MEDICATION

First Line

- Pediatric
  - First-line treatment:
    - For children with no or mild bleeding (bruising and petechiae only with no mucosal bleeding), observation alone regardless of platelet count (1)[B]
    - For children with significant bleeding
      - Single-dose intravenous immunoglobulin (IVIG) 0.8 to 1.0 g/kg, especially when a more rapid increase in platelet count is desired (1)[B]. Do not administer in patients with IgA deficiencies because of anaphylaxis risk.
      - A short course of corticosteroids (e.g., PO prednisone 2 mg/kg/day for 2 weeks with 3 weeks taper) (1)[B]
      - Single dose of anti-Rho(D) immunoglobulin (anti-D), 50 to 75 g/kg for nonsplenectomized children who are Rh-positive, with negative direct antiglobulin test (1),(2)[B]. Do not use in children with low hemoglobin or evidence of hemolysis (1)[C].

- Second and other treatments for pediatric and adolescent with ITP
  - Splenectomy for chronic or persistent ITP (1)[B]
  - Rituximab (Rituxan) 375 mg/m² weekly for 4 weeks (1,2)[C]
  - High-dose dexamethasone 0.6 mg/kg/day for 4 days every 4 weeks (1,2)[C]
  - Others without adequate data: azathioprine, cyclosporin A, danazol, mycophenolate mofetil, anti-CD52 monoclonal antibody, and interferon
  - Phase 3 clinical trials have shown that thrombopoietin receptor agonists induce good response in children with chronic ITP (4).
- Adult
  - First line, adult ITP
    - Treatment is recommended for newly diagnosed patients with platelet count <30 × 10⁹/L (1,2)[C].
    - Longer courses of steroids are preferred over shorter courses of steroids or IVIG (5).
    - If corticosteroids are contraindicated:
      - IVIG: 1 to 2 g/kg once, repeating as necessary (1,2)[C] OR
      - Anti-D: 50 to 75 μg/kg once, repeating as necessary for Rh⁺, nonsplenectomized patients. Do not use anti-D in patients with low hemoglobin or evidence of hemolysis (1,2)[C].
  - Second line, adult ITP
    - Splenectomy for patients who failed corticosteroid therapy (1)[B]
    - For patients for whom splenectomy is contraindicated and have risk of bleeding, thrombopoietin receptor agonists (1)[B]: eltrombopag (Promacta), 50 mg/day PO OR romiplostim (Nplate), 1 μg/kg SC weekly
    - Rituximab, 375 mg/m² IV weekly for 4 weeks, for patients at high risk of bleeding who have failed one line of therapy or postsplenectomy (1,2)[C]
    - Others to consider: azathioprine, cyclosporine A, cyclophosphamide, danazol, dapsone, mycophenolate mofetil, and vincristine
    - Asymptomatic patients after splenectomy, with platelet counts >30 × 10⁹/L, do not require treatment (1)[C].
    - FDA has approved avatrombopag and fostamatinib recently.
- ITP in pregnancy
  - Preeclampsia or gestational thrombocytopenia may cause thrombocytopenia unrelated to ITP.
  - Corticosteroids or IVIG are considered safe and are considered first line (1)[C].
  - Do not use danazol or cyclophosphamide.
  - ITP management at time of delivery is based on maternal bleeding risks, and mode of delivery should be based on obstetric indications (1,2)[C]. Platelet autoantibodies can cross the placenta and cause neonatal thrombocytopenia.
  - Cesarean section can be considered if platelet count >50 × 10⁹/L.
  - Prednisone and/or IVIG may be considered 2 to 3 weeks prior to delivery.
- ITP secondary to HIV
  - Antivirals should be considered before other treatment (1)[A].
  - If treatment required, corticosteroids, IVIG, or anti-D are first-line options, and splenectomy is a second-line option (1,2)[C].
- ITP secondary to HCV
  - Antivirals should be considered before other treatment (1,2)[C].
  - If treatment required, IVIG is initial treatment (1,2)[C].
  - Based on recent studies, TPO mimetics are approved for HCV-related ITP because they increase platelets to a level required to initiate antiviral therapy (6).

- ITP and *H. pylori*
  - Screen for *H. pylori* in patients in whom eradication therapy would be considered if result is positive (1,2)[C].
- Emergency treatment
  - Patients with intracranial or GI bleeding, massive hematuria, internal hematoma, or who need emergent surgery
  - IV corticosteroids (e.g., IV methylprednisolone, 1 g/day for 3 doses) (1)[B] with caution in patients with GI bleeding and/or IVIG 1 g/kg; repeat following day for count <50 × 10⁹/L (1)[B].
  - Platelet transfusions with IVIG may also be considered for significant bleeding (1)[C].
  - Other agents that may be considered: Recombinant factor VIIa (1)[C] not only promotes hemostasis but also increases risk of thrombosis. Efficacy of antifibrinolytic agents, aminocaproic acid and tranexamic acid, is unproved in randomized trials; they may be used as adjunctive treatments only. Emergent splenectomy has been reported.

ISSUES FOR REFERRAL
Hematology consultation is recommended for acute bleeding or for those who fail to respond to first-line therapies.

SURGERY/OTHER PROCEDURES
Splenectomy

- Mortality rate is very low (<1%) even in patients with severe thrombocytopenia.
- Necessary vaccinations prior to splenectomy: polyvalent pneumococcal vaccine and quadrivalent meningococcal vaccine every 3 to 5 years and one-time *Haemophilus influenzae B* (Hib)
- Consider lifelong prophylactic antibiotics with penicillin or erythromycin.
- Should raise the platelet count to at least 20 × 10⁹/L prior to surgery
- Reported 5- to 10-year efficacy is ~65% for all patients.
- Laparoscopic splenectomy has similar long-term outcomes compared to open splenectomy and has better short-term outcomes in medically suitable patients (1)[C].

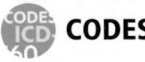 ONGOING CARE

FOLLOW-UP RECOMMENDATIONS
Patient Monitoring
Platelet counts weekly for patients on prednisone and monthly for stable patients are reasonable.

DIET
- Evidence demonstrating benefit of an anti-inflammatory diet in ITP is lacking.
- The following foods and supplements can cause significant bleeding: garlic, ginger, *Ginkgo biloba*, and saw palmetto.
- Some foods and supplements that may inhibit platelets: evening primrose oil, fish oil, feverfew, ginseng, licorice, soy, vitamin C, vitamin E, and wintergreen
- Partial list of foods and supplements with coumarin or salicylate components: alfalfa, angelica, anise, asafetida, aspen bark, birch, black cohosh, celery, chamomile, cinnamon, dandelion, fenugreek, heartsease, horse chestnut, meadowsweet, poplar, prickly ash, *Quassia*, sarsaparilla, sweet birch, sweet clover, and willow bark

PATIENT EDUCATION
- Modified activity to prevent injury or bruising; avoid contact sports.
- Avoid anticoagulants, aspirin and other platelet-inhibiting drugs, and NSAIDs.

PROGNOSIS
- Acute ITP
  - ~80–85% of patients completely recover within 2 months.
  - 15% proceed to chronic ITP.
- Chronic ITP
  - ~10–20% of the patients recover spontaneously.
  - Remainder with diminished platelets for months to years
  - May see spontaneous remissions (5%) and relapses
- ~10% are refractory (fail medical therapy and splenectomy).

COMPLICATIONS
- Related to thrombocytopenia: 1% mortality due to intracranial hemorrhage and severe blood loss
- Related to treatment: for example, corticosteroid adverse effects, anaphylaxis and renal failure with IVIG, hepatotoxicity with eltrombopag, reports of progressive multifocal leukoencephalopathy with rituximab, hemolysis with anti-D, and septicemia for splenectomized patients

REFERENCES
1. Neunert C, Lim W, Crowther M, et al; for American Society of Hematology. The American Society of Hematology 2011 evidence-based practice guideline for immune thrombocytopenia. *Blood*. 2011;117(16):4190–4207.
2. Terrell DR, Beebe LA, Vesely SK, et al. The incidence of immune thrombocytopenic purpura in children and adults: a critical review of published reports. *Am J Hematol*. 2010;85(3):174–180.
3. Terrell DR, Beebe LA, Neas BR, et al. Prevalence of primary immune thrombocytopenia in Oklahoma. *Am J Hematol*. 2012;87(9):848–852.
4. Tarantino MD, Bussel JB, Blanchette VS, et al. Romiplostim in children with immune thrombocytopenia: a phase 3, randomised, double-blind, placebo-controlled study. *Lancet*. 2016;388(10039):45–54.
5. Wei Y, Ji XB, Wang YW, et al. High-dose dexamethasone vs prednisone for treatment of adult immune thrombocytopenia: a prospective multicenter randomized trial. *Blood*. 2016;127(3):296–370.
6. Afdhal NH, Dusheiko GM, Giannini EG, et al. Eltrombopag increases platelet numbers in thrombocytopenic patients with HCV infection and cirrhosis, allowing for effective antiviral therapy. *Gastroenterology*. 2014;146(2):442–452.e1.

CODES

ICD10
D69.3 Immune thrombocytopenic purpura

CLINICAL PEARLS
- ITP: platelet counts of <100 × 10⁹/L caused by accelerated destruction and/or impaired thrombopoiesis by antiplatelet antibodies
- Pediatric ITP: relatively common, with spontaneous remission in 2 months
- Adult ITP: usually persistent; requires treatment, with rare spontaneous remission
- Goal of treatment is to achieve adequate hemostasis.

IMPETIGO

Elisabeth L. Backer, MD

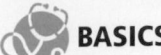 BASICS

DESCRIPTION
- A contagious, superficial, intraepidermal infection occurring prominently on exposed areas of the face and extremities, most often seen in children
- Primary impetigo (pyoderma): invasion of previously normal skin
- Secondary impetigo (impetiginization): invasion at sites of minor trauma (abrasions, insect bites, underlying eczema)
- Infected patients usually have multiple lesions.
- Cultures are positive in >80% cases for *Staphylococcus aureus* either alone or combined with group A β-hemolytic streptococci; *S. aureus* is the more common pathogen since the 1990s.
- Nonbullous impetigo: most common form of impetigo. Formation of vesiculopustules that rupture, leading to crusting with a characteristic golden appearance; local lymphadenopathy may occur.
- Bullous impetigo: staphylococcal impetigo that progresses from small to large flaccid bullae (newborns/young children) caused by epidermolytic toxin release; ruptured bullae leaving brown crust; less lymphadenopathy; trunk more often affected; <30% of patients
- Folliculitis: considered by some to be *S. aureus* impetigo of hair follicles
- Ecthyma: a deeper, ulcerated impetigo infection often with lymphadenitis
- System(s) affected: skin/exocrine
- Synonym(s): pyoderma; impetigo contagiosa; impetigo vulgaris

EPIDEMIOLOGY
Incidence
- Predominant sex: male = female
- Predominant age: children ages 2 to 5 years

Prevalence
In the United States: not reported but common

Pediatric Considerations
- Poststreptococcal glomerulonephritis may follow impetigo (in young children).
- Impetigo neonatorum may occur due to nursery contamination.

ETIOLOGY AND PATHOPHYSIOLOGY
- Coagulase-positive staphylococci: pure culture ~50–90%; more contagious via contact
- β-Hemolytic streptococci: pure culture only ~10% of the time (primarily group A)

- Mixed infections of streptococci and staphylococci are common; data suggest increasing importance of staphylococci over the past decades.
- Methicillin-resistant *S. aureus* (MRSA) detected in some cases
- Direct contact or insect vector
- Can result from contamination at trauma site
- Regional lymphadenopathy

RISK FACTORS
- Warm, humid environment
- Tropical or subtropical climate
- Summer or fall season
- Minor trauma, insect bites, breaches in skin
- Poor hygiene, poverty, crowding, epidemics, wartime
- Familial spread
- Poor health with anemia and malnutrition
- Complication of pediculosis, scabies, chickenpox, eczema/atopic dermatitis
- Contact dermatitis (*Rhus* spp.)
- Burns
- Contact sports
- Children in daycare
- Carriage of group A *Streptococcus* and *Staphylococcus aureus*

GENERAL PREVENTION
- Close attention to family hygiene, particularly hand washing among children
- Covering of wounds
- Avoidance of crowding and sharing of personal items
- Treatment of atopic dermatitis

COMMONLY ASSOCIATED CONDITIONS
- Malnutrition and anemia
- Crowded living conditions
- Poor hygiene
- Neglected minor trauma
- Any chronic/underlying dermatitis
- Can occur as coinfection with scabies

DIAGNOSIS

HISTORY
- Lesions are often described as painful.
- May be slow and indolent or rapidly spreading
- Most frequent on face around mouth and nose or at site of trauma

PHYSICAL EXAM
- Tender red macules or papules as early lesions (contact dermatitis presents with pruritic lesions)
- Thin-roofed vesicles to bullae: usually nontender
- Pustules
- Weeping, shallow, red ulcers
- Honey-colored crusts
- Satellite lesions
- Often multiple sites
- Bullae on buttocks, trunk, face

DIFFERENTIAL DIAGNOSIS
- Nonbullous
  - Contact dermatitis
  - Chickenpox
  - Herpes
  - Folliculitis
  - Erysipelas
  - Insect bites
  - Severe eczematous dermatitis
  - Scabies
  - Tinea corporis
- Bullous
  - Burns
  - Pemphigus vulgaris
  - Bullous pemphigoid
- Stevens-Johnson syndrome

DIAGNOSTIC TESTS & INTERPRETATION
Initial Tests (lab, imaging)
- None usually necessary in typical presentations; cultures of pus/bullae fluid may be helpful if no response to empiric therapy.
  - Culture: taken from the base of lesion after removal of crust; will grow both staphylococci and group A streptococci
  - Antistreptolysin-O (ASO) titer: can be weak positive for streptococci but overall not useful
  - Antideoxyribonuclease B (anti-DNase B) and antihyaluronidase (AHT) response more reliable than ASO response
  - Streptozyme: positive for streptococci
- Disorders that may alter lab results: Streptococcal pharyngitis will alter streptococcal enzyme tests.

Follow-Up Tests & Special Considerations
- Monitor for spread of disease and systemic manifestations.
- Serologic testing is helpful in context of impetigo with subsequent poststreptococcal glomerulonephritis.

TREATMENT

GENERAL MEASURES
- Treatment speeds healing, improves cosmetic appearance, and avoids spread of disease.
- Prevent with mupirocin ointment TID to sites of minor skin trauma.
- Remove crusts; clean with gentle washing 2 to 3 times daily; and clean with antibacterial soap, chlorhexidine, or Betadine.
- Washing of entire body may prevent recurrence at distant sites.

MEDICATION
- In 2014, the Infectious Diseases Society of America (IDSA) recommended topical treatment for limited lesions and oral medication when the disease is more severe/extensive (1)[A]. A 2017 Canadian systematic review found that topical mupirocin is equally, or more effective than oral treatments for nonextensive impetigo (2)[A]. Penicillin and macrolide therapy is no longer recommended. Fluoroquinolones are not indicated due to resistance patterns.
- Consult the local hospital or health department for microbial resistance information.
- Nonbullous (minor spread, treat 7 days; widespread, treat 10 days); bullous (treat 10 days)
  - Mupirocin (Bactroban) 2% topical ointment applied TID for 5 to 7 days (nonbullous only); not as effective on scalp as around mouth
  - Retapamulin 1% ointment to be applied BID for 5 days (very expensive)
  - Dicloxacillin: adult 250 mg PO QID; pediatric <40 kg: 12 to 25 mg/kg/day divided q6h; >40 kg: 125 to 250 q6h
- Dicloxacillin, cephalexin, topical mupirocin, and fusidic acid are effective, unless local staphylococcal strains are resistant. For MRSA infections, treatment options include clindamycin, tetracyclines, or trimethoprim-sulfamethoxazole. Oral doses given for 7 days are usually sufficient (3)[C].
- 1st-generation cephalosporins
  - Children
    - Cephalexin 25 to 50 mg/kg/day divided, q6–12h
    - Cefaclor 20 to 40 mg/kg/day divided q8h
    - Cephradine 25 to 50 mg/kg/day divided q6–12h
    - Cefadroxil 30 mg/kg/day divided BID
  - Adults
    - Cephalexin 250 mg up to QID
    - Cefaclor 250 mg TID
    - Cephradine 500 mg BID
    - Cefadroxil 1 g/day in divided doses

- Clindamycin 300 mg q6–8h
- Severe bullous disease may require IV therapy such as nafcillin or cefazolin.

ISSUES FOR REFERRAL
If resistant or extensive infections occur, especially in immunocompromised patients

ADDITIONAL THERAPIES
Monitor for microbial resistance patterns.

ONGOING CARE

FOLLOW-UP RECOMMENDATIONS
- Athletes are restricted from contact sports.
- School and daycare contagious restrictions
- Children can return to school 24 hours after initiation of antimicrobial treatment.

Patient Monitoring
If not clear within 7 to 10 days, culture the lesions.

PATIENT EDUCATION
Avoidance of infection spread is the key; hand washing is vital, especially for reducing spread in children.

PROGNOSIS
- Complete resolution in 7 to 10 days with treatment
- Antibiotic treatment will not prevent or halt glomerulonephritis, as it will in rheumatic fever.
- If not clear within 7 to 10 days, culture is necessary to find resistant organism.
- Recurrent impetigo: Evaluate for carriage of *S. aureus* in nares (also perineum, axillae, toe web). Apply mupirocin ointment to nares BID for 5 days for decolonization.

COMPLICATIONS
- Ecthyma
- Erysipelas
- Poststreptococcal acute glomerulonephritis
- Cellulitis
- Bacteremia
- Osteomyelitis
- Septic arthritis
- Pneumonia
- Lymphadenitis

REFERENCES
1. Stevens DL, Bisno AL, Chambers HF, et al. Practice guidelines for the diagnosis and management of skin and soft tissue infections: 2014 update by the Infectious Diseases Society of America. *Clin Infect Dis*. 2014;59(2):147–159.
2. Edge R, Argáez C. *Topical Antibiotics for Impetigo: A Review of the Clinical Effectiveness and Guidelines*. Ottawa, Ontario, Canada: Canadian Agency for Drugs and Technologies in Health; 2017.
3. Del Giudice P, Hubiche P. Community-associated methicillin-resistant *Staphylococcus aureus* and impetigo. *Br J Dermatol*. 2010;162(4): 905–906.

ADDITIONAL READING
- Bowen AC, Mahé A, Hay RJ, et al. The global epidemiology of impetigo: a systematic review of the population prevalence of impetigo and pyoderma. *PLoS One*. 2015;10(8):e0136789.
- George A, Rubin G. A systematic review and meta-analysis of treatments for impetigo. *Br J Gen Pract*. 2003;53(491):480–487.
- Koning S, van der Sande R, Verhagen AP, et al. Interventions for impetigo. *Cochrane Database Syst Rev*. 2012;(1):CD003261.
- Parish LC, Jorizzo JL, Breton JJ, et al; for SB275833/032 Study Team. Topical retapamulin ointment (1%, wt/wt) twice daily for 5 days versus oral cephalexin twice daily for 10 days in the treatment of secondarily infected dermatitis: results of a randomized controlled trial. *J Am Acad Dermatol*. 2006;55(6):1003–1013.
- Stanley JR, Amagai M. Pemphigus, bullous impetigo, and the staphylococcal scalded-skin syndrome. *N Engl J Med*. 2006;355(17):1800–1810.

SEE ALSO

Algorithm: Rash

CODES

ICD10
- L01.00 Impetigo, unspecified
- L01.01 Non-bullous impetigo
- L01.03 Bullous impetigo

CLINICAL PEARLS
- Superficial, intraepidermal infection
- Predominantly staphylococcal in origin
- Microbial resistance patterns need to be monitored.
- Topical treatment is recommended for limited lesions and oral medication only when the disease is more severe/extensive.

INCONTINENCE, FECAL
Kalyanakrishnan Ramakrishnan, MD

BASICS

Defined as continuous or recurrent involuntary passage of fecal material through the anal canal for >1 month in an individual at least 4 years of age
- Involves recurrent, involuntary loss of solid/liquid stool
- Requires careful rectal exam to assess rectal tone, voluntary squeeze, and rule out overflow incontinence from fecal impaction
- Endorectal ultrasound (EUS) is the simplest, most reliable, and least invasive method to detect anatomic anal sphincter defects.
- The goal of treatment is to restore continence and/or improve quality of life.

DESCRIPTION
Major incontinence is the involuntary evacuation of feces. Minor incontinence (fecal soilage) includes incontinence to flatus and occasional seepage of liquid stool.

Geriatric Considerations
- The prevalence of fecal incontinence increases with age. It is an important cause for nursing home placement among the elderly.
- Idiopathic fecal incontinence is more common in older women.

EPIDEMIOLOGY
Incidence
Patients often do not report fecal incontinence unless specifically queried ("silent affliction"). The number of affected patients is likely significantly underestimated.

Prevalence
- Women > men
- 7% of adults; 15% of adults age >90 years
- 56–66% of hospitalized older patients and >50% of nursing home residents
- 50–70% of patients who have urinary incontinence also suffer from fecal incontinence.

Pregnancy Considerations
Obstetric injury to the pelvic floor may result in either temporary or persistent incontinence.

Geriatric Considerations
- Fecal impaction and overflow diarrhea leading to fecal incontinence is common in older patients.
- Surgical history—particularly anal surgery, including hemorrhoidectomy, anal fissure repair (sphincterotomy), anal dilatation, or prior pelvic floor surgeries

ETIOLOGY AND PATHOPHYSIOLOGY
- Continence requires the complex orchestration of pelvic musculature, nerves, and reflex arcs.
- Stool volume and consistency, colonic transit time, anorectal sensation, rectal compliance, anorectal reflexes, external and internal sphincter muscle tone, puborectalis muscle function, and mental capacity each plays a role in maintaining fecal continence.
- Disease processes or structural defects impacting any of these factors may contribute to incontinence.
- Diabetes is the most common metabolic disorder leading to fecal incontinence through pudendal nerve neuropathy.
- Congenital: spina bifida and myelomeningocele with spinal cord damage
- Trauma: anal sphincter damage from vaginal delivery or surgical procedures
- Medical: diabetes mellitus, stroke, spinal cord trauma, degenerative disorders of the nervous system, inflammatory bowel disorders, rectal neoplasia

RISK FACTORS
- Poor functional status—older age, female sex, obesity, limited physical activity contributory
- Neuropsychiatric conditions (dementia, depression)
- Multiple sclerosis, spinal cord injury, stroke, diabetic neuropathy
- Prostatectomy, radiation
- Trauma: Risk factors for perineal trauma at the time of vaginal delivery include occipitoposterior presentation, prolonged second stage of labor, assisted vaginal delivery (forceps or vacuum-assist), and episiotomy.
- Diarrhea, inflammatory bowel disease (IBD), irritable bowel syndrome (IBS), menopause, smoking, constipation
- Potential association with child abuse and sexual abuse
- Congenital abnormalities, such as imperforate anus/rectal prolapse
- Fecal impaction

GENERAL PREVENTION
- Behavioral and lifestyle changes: Obesity, limited physical activity/exercise, poor diet, and smoking are modifiable risk factors.
- Postmeal bowel regimen—defecate regularly after meals to maximize effect of gastrocolic reflex.
- Pelvic floor muscle training during and after pregnancy and pelvic surgery
- Increase fiber intake (>30 g/day)

COMMONLY ASSOCIATED CONDITIONS
- Increasing age (>65 years)
- Urinary incontinence/pelvic organ prolapse
- Chronic medical conditions—diabetes mellitus, dementia, stroke, spinal cord compression, depression, immobility, chronic obstructive pulmonary disease, IBS, and IBD
- Perineal trauma (obstetric)
- Anorectal surgery
- History of pelvic/rectal irradiation

DIAGNOSIS

Diagnosis is based on history and physical findings.

HISTORY
- Patients seldom volunteer information about fecal incontinence. Direct questioning is important.
- Problem-specific history includes (1)[C]:
  - Severity of soiling by liquid stool or gross incontinence of solid stool
  - Onset and duration (recent onset vs. chronic)
  - Frequency, presence of constipation/diarrhea
- Medication review
- Review diet, medical and obstetric history, lifestyle, and mobility.
- Evaluate for social withdrawal and depression.

PHYSICAL EXAM
- Inspect the perineum for chemical dermatitis, hemorrhoids, fistula, surgical scars, skin tags, rectal prolapse, soiling, and ballooning of the perineum (sarcopenia of pelvic musculature).
- A patulous anal orifice may indicate myopathy or a neurologic disorder.
- Evaluate the external sphincter response to perineal skin stimulation (anal wink). Absence suggests neuropathy.
- Ask the patient to bear down, preferably in standing position, to assess for rectal prolapse.

- Digital rectal exam to assess anal canal pressure sphincter tone, rectal bleeding, hemorrhoids, neoplasm, fecal consistency, and diarrhea/distal fecal impaction
- General neurologic examination, including perianal sensation (1)[C]
- Evaluate mental status.

DIFFERENTIAL DIAGNOSIS
- Anorectal disorders
  - Inflammatory/infectious gastrointestinal disorders
  - Bowel neoplasms, radiation proctitis, ischemic colitis, fistulas
  - Prolapsed internal hemorrhoids; rectal prolapse
  - Trauma: obstetric, surgical, radiation, accidental, sexual
- Neurologic disorders
  - Stroke, dementia, neoplasms, spinal cord injury, and/or diseases causing altered level of consciousness
  - Pudendal neuropathy, neurosyphilis, multiple sclerosis, diabetes mellitus
- Miscellaneous causes
  - Infectious diarrhea, fecal impaction and overflow, IBS, laxative abuse, IBD, short bowel syndrome, myopathies, senescence and frailty, collagen vascular disease, psychological and behavioral problems

DIAGNOSTIC TESTS & INTERPRETATION
The approach to fecal incontinence in older patients should be individualized, minimally invasive, and practically feasible. History and physical examination are generally sufficient for diagnosis. If uncertainty remains, consider the following:
- EUS is the most reliable and least invasive test for defining anatomic defects in the external and internal anal sphincters, rectal wall, and the puborectalis muscle (1)[B]. EUS can reliably predict therapeutic response to sphincteroplasty.
- Plain abdominal x-ray (fecal impaction, constipation)
- Sigmoidoscopy/anoscopy/colonoscopy (hemorrhoids, colitis, neoplasm)

Initial Tests (lab, imaging)
- If history of travel, antibiotics, tube feedings, or signs and symptoms of sepsis, consider stool studies:
  - Culture
  - Ova and parasites
  - *Clostridium difficile* toxin assay
- Thyroid-stimulating hormone (TSH), electrolytes, and BUN in elderly patients
- EUS may demonstrate structural abnormalities of the anal sphincters, rectal wall, or puborectalis muscle.
- EUS may detect a sphincter injury in over 1/3 of primiparous vaginal deliveries and nearly half of multiparous vaginal deliveries.

Follow-Up Tests & Special Considerations
- Defecography can measure the anorectal angle, evaluate pelvic descent, and detect occult/overt rectal prolapse.
- MRI defecography (dynamic MRI) can further define pelvic floor anatomy.
- Anorectal manometry measures parameters such as maximal resting anal pressure, amplitude and duration of squeeze pressure, the rectoanal inhibitory reflex, threshold of conscious rectal sensation, rectal compliance, and anorectal pressures during straining.

- Pudendal nerve terminal motor latency (PNTML) measures neuromuscular integrity between the pudendal nerve and the anal sphincter; is operator-dependent and has poor correlation with clinical and histologic findings
- Electromyography can assess neurogenic/myopathic damage.

TREATMENT

GENERAL MEASURES
- In ambulatory patients, scheduled (or prompted) defecation is effective, particularly in those with overflow incontinence.
- Kegel exercises to strengthen pelvic floor
- If bed-bound, scheduled osmotic or stimulant laxatives for constipation
- Enemas, laxatives, and suppositories may help promote more complete bowel emptying in impacted patients and minimize postdefecation leakage.
- Use of stool deodorants (Peri-Wash, Derifil, Devrom)

MEDICATION
Limited evidence that antidiarrheals (loperamide, codeine) and drugs enhancing sphincter tone (phenylephrine gel, sodium valproate) are of benefit (2)[B]. Cholestyramine, colestipol useful in diarrhea following malabsorption or cholecystectomy; alosetron in diarrhea due to IBS, amitriptyline in idiopathic fecal incontinence

First Line
Specific treatment of underlying disorder (e.g., infectious diarrhea/IBD) may improve fecal continence.

Second Line
- Increasing dietary fiber in milder forms of fecal incontinence reduces symptoms (1)[B]. Stool-bulking agents include high-fiber diet, psyllium products, or methylcellulose.
- Antidiarrheal agents, such as adsorbents or opium derivatives, may reduce diarrhea-associated incontinence (1)[C].
- Disimpacting patients with fecal impaction and overflow incontinence and treating with a bowel regimen to prevent recurrence

ADDITIONAL THERAPIES
- Biofeedback: initial treatment modality in motivated patients with some voluntary sphincter control (1)[C]; teaches patients to recognize rectal distension and contract the external anal sphincter while keeping intra-abdominal pressure low
- Biofeedback plus electrical stimulation of the anal sphincters is more effective than either alone.
- Patients with systemic neurologic disorders, anal deformities, or frequent episodes of incontinence respond poorly.

SURGERY/OTHER PROCEDURES
- Surgery should be considered only when nonsurgical approaches have failed.
- Sphincter repair should be offered for highly symptomatic patients with well-defined defect of external anal sphincter (1)[A].
- Injectable therapy (tissue-bulking agent injected into the anorectal submucosa or the intersphincteric space) appears safe and effective (40% efficacy) for patients with internal anal sphincter dysfunction (3)[A].

- Artificial anal sphincter implantation/dynamic graciloplasty (where gracilis muscle transposed into anus as modified sphincter) considered in patients with severe fecal incontinence and irreparable sphincter damage (4)[B]
- Stoma (colostomy/ileostomy) creation may be appropriate in patients with disabling fecal incontinence when other available therapeutic options have failed or if preferred by patient (1)[B]. A continent stoma created using the appendix or the cecum as the point of entry is a less radical option and enables using antegrade continence enema to flush the colon in these patients.
- Anal plugs minimize fecal leakage in patients who do not benefit from other treatment modalities, especially immobilized, institutionalized, or neurologically disabled patients; plugs often poorly tolerated (1)[C]
- Sacral nerve stimulation (neuromodulation) via implantation of SC electrodes delivering low-amplitude electrical stimulation to sphincter muscles improves overall rectal tone, especially in patients with a coexistent sphincter defect (5)[B].
- SECCA procedure (radiofrequency anal sphincter remodeling)—temperature-controlled radiofrequency energy delivered to the anorectal junction distal to the dentate line causing tissue damage, scarring, and anal canal narrowing; minimally invasive, ambulatory procedure useful in mild-to-moderate fecal incontinence (1)[C]
- Magnetic anal sphincter (MAS) devices—series of interlinked titanium beads (14 to 20) with internal magnetic cores placed to form a flexible ring that encircles the external anal sphincter 3 to 5 cm from the anal verge. During expulsion of feces, the beads separate allowing evacuation. After evacuation, the beads approximate closing the canal (5)[C]; useful in moderate and severe incontinence
- A vaginally placed bowel control device that the patient inflates to control leakage and deflates to defecate is well tolerated and effective in 86% (5)[B].
- Percutaneous posterior tibial nerve stimulation at the ankle for 30 minutes weekly for 12 weeks (50% efficacy) and the TOPAS pelvic floor repair system (self-fixating polypropylene mesh placed behind the anorectum to support the puborectalis) (55% efficacy) are other recent advances in controlling fecal incontinence (5)[B].

ADMISSION, INPATIENT, AND NURSING CONSIDERATIONS
- If secondary to fecal impaction, manual evacuation of fecal mass (after lubrication with lidocaine jelly)
- Avoid catharsis.
- No hot water, soap, or hydrogen peroxide enemas
- Outpatient care

ONGOING CARE

FOLLOW-UP RECOMMENDATIONS
Periodic rectal exam

Patient Monitoring
Consider impaction if there is <1 bowel movement every other day in patients with fecal incontinence.

DIET
- High fiber (20 to 30 g/day) and at least 1.5 L fluid daily
- Avoid precipitants (caffeine).

PATIENT EDUCATION
Kegel/sphincter training exercises are helpful but not sufficient for treating fecal incontinence.

PROGNOSIS
- Reimpaction likely if bowel regimen discontinued
- 50% failure rate over 5 years following overlapping sphincteroplasty

COMPLICATIONS
- Depression and social isolation
- Skin ulcerations
- Artificial bowel sphincter: infection, erosion, mechanical failure

REFERENCES

1. Tjandra JJ, Dykes SL, Kumar RR, et al. Practice parameters for the treatment of fecal incontinence. *Dis Colon Rectum.* 2007;50(10):1497–1507.
2. Omar MI, Alexander CE. Drug treatment for faecal incontinence in adults. *Cochrane Database Syst Rev.* 2013;(6):CD002116.
3. Hong KD, Kim JS, Ji WB, et al. Midterm outcomes of injectable bulking agents for fecal incontinence: a systematic review and meta-analysis. *Tech Coloproctol.* 2017;21(3):203–210.
4. Rao SSC. Current and emerging treatment options for fecal incontinence. *J Clin Gastroenterol.* 2014;48(9):752–764.
5. Rosenblatt P. New developments in therapies for fecal incontinence. *Curr Opin Obstet Gynecol.* 2015;27(5):353–358.

ADDITIONAL READING

Rao SSC. Fecal incontinence. In: Feldman M, Friedman LS, Brandt LJ, eds. *Sleisenger and Fordtran's Gastrointestinal and Liver Disease: Pathophysiology/Diagnosis/Management.* 10th ed. Philadelphia, PA: Saunders/Elsevier; 2015:251–269.

CODES

ICD10
- R15.9 Full incontinence of feces
- R15.2 Fecal urgency
- R15.0 Incomplete defecation

CLINICAL PEARLS

- Scheduled defecation after meals, bulking agents, and scheduled enemas minimize impaction and are helpful in mild/moderate fecal incontinence.
- Differentiate true incontinence from pseudoincontinence (overflow or functional incontinence).
- New onset fecal incontinence may indicate spinal cord compression if accompanied by other neurologic signs or symptoms.

INCONTINENCE, URINARY ADULT FEMALE

Cara Marshall, MD • Chelsea Harris, MD • Julia Tse, MD

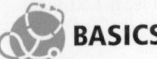

BASICS

DESCRIPTION
- Urinary incontinence: involuntary loss of urine
- Stress incontinence: associated with increased intra-abdominal pressure, such as coughing, laughing, sneezing, or exertion
- Urge incontinence: sudden uncontrollable loss of urine, preceded or accompanied by urgency, or a sudden compelling desire to urinate that is difficult to delay. Urge incontinence may be associated with overactive bladder or detrusor overactivity.
- Mixed incontinence: loss of urine from a combination of stress and urge incontinence
- Overflow incontinence: high residual or chronic urinary retention leading to urinary spillage from an overdistended bladder
- Functional incontinence: loss of urine due to deficits of cognition and/or mobility
- Total incontinence: continuous leakage of urine; leakage without awareness

EPIDEMIOLOGY
- Overall prevalence—38% of women age >60 years. A 2012 survey showed stress incontinence affected 37.5% of women age 30 to 50 years (1).
- Prevalence in women >75 years is 75%, and 6% of nursing home admissions are directly attributable to incontinence (2).

ETIOLOGY AND PATHOPHYSIOLOGY
- Stress incontinence: occurs with increased intra-abdominal pressure. Two types:
  - Anatomic: due to urethral hypermobility from lack of pelvic support
  - Intrinsic sphincter deficiency (ISD): impaired closure of urethra. Urethral mucosal seal and inherent closure from collagen, fibroelastic tissue, and smooth and striated muscles may be lost secondary to surgical scarring, radiation, or hormonal and age-related changes.
- Urge incontinence: may be due to detrusor overactivity or may be idiopathic
- Overflow incontinence: urinary retention (usually from neurogenic bladder)
- Total incontinence: constant loss of urine. Ectopic ureters in females usually open in the urethra distal to the sphincter or in the vagina, causing continuous leakage; may also occur with fistulous connections between bladder, ureters, or urethra and vagina or uterus
- Women with urge urinary incontinence report poorer quality of life than those with stress incontinence (2).

RISK FACTORS
Advanced age, impaired functional status, obesity (BMI >30), history of gestational diabetes, pregnancy, vaginal childbirth, pelvic surgery or radiation, urethral diverticula, genital prolapse, smoking, chronic obstructive pulmonary disease (COPD), cognitive impairment, constipation, caffeine, and pelvic floor dysfunction

GENERAL PREVENTION
Obesity and caffeine avoidance, smoking cessation, high-fiber diet to reduce constipation

COMMONLY ASSOCIATED CONDITIONS
Pelvic organ prolapse, UTI, COPD, diabetes mellitus, neurologic disease, obesity, chronic constipation, depression, low libido, dyspareunia, and any disease that results in chronic cough

DIAGNOSIS

HISTORY
- Important to screen for symptoms because only 45% of women who reported at least twice weekly urine leakage on a U.S. survey sought care for their symptoms (2)
- Age: Stress incontinence is more common in women aged 19 to 64 years, whereas mixed incontinence is more common in women >65 years. Onset from childhood indicates congenital causes (e.g., ectopic ureter).
- Amount and frequency of leakage; pad usage
- Stress incontinence: occurs in small spurts; patients typically remain dry at night in bed.
- Urge incontinence: sudden urge followed by leakage of large amounts, usually associated with frequency and nocturia. Sensory stimuli may trigger (e.g., cold).
- Continuous slow leakage in between regular voiding indicates ectopic ureter or urinary fistula.
- Pain: Suprapubic pain with dysuria implies urinary infection or interstitial cystitis.
- Medical history
  - Neurologic conditions or suggestive symptomatology: cerebrovascular accident, parkinsonism, multiple sclerosis, myelodysplasia, diabetes, spinal cord injury
  - Radiation to pelvic and vaginal areas: causes ISD, overactive bladder, fibrotic changes of pelvic floor musculature, and low bladder compliance
  - Obstetric history: Weakness of the pelvic floor is more likely in multiparous women.
  - History of smoking and COPD with a chronic cough can aggravate incontinence.
  - Constipation can aggravate incontinence.
  - Surgical history: Pelvic surgery, including gynecologic and bowel surgery, can injure the pelvic floor musculature and affect neurologic function.
- Medications
  - Sympatholytic α-blockers (terazosin, prazosin, doxazosin, tamsulosin, alfuzosin, silodosin) can cause or worsen incontinence.
  - Sympathomimetic agents, tricyclic antidepressants, anticholinergics, and opioids can cause retention with overflow incontinence.
- International Consultation on Incontinence Questionnaire (ICIQ) is highly recommended for assessment of patient's perspective of symptoms of incontinence and his or her impact on quality of life.
- Can use 3-day voiding diary to evaluate fluid intake, caffeine intake, timing of leakage, and patient habits

PHYSICAL EXAM
- General status
  - Obesity (BMI)
- General neurologic examination
  - Mental status, speech, intellectual performance
  - Motor status: gait, generalized or focal weakness, rigidity, tremor
  - Sensory status: impairment of perineal–sacral area sensation
- Urologic examination
  - Abdomen: masses, incisional scars of previous surgeries
  - Suprapubic tenderness: may indicate cystitis
  - Palpable, distended bladder: chronic urinary retention
- Pelvic examination
  - Examination of the perineum and external genitalia, including tissue quality and sensation
  - Vaginal (half-speculum) examination for prolapse
  - Bimanual pelvic and anorectal examination for pelvic masses, fecal impaction, pelvic floor function, and so forth
    - Assessment of pelvic floor resting tone and function (ability to isolate and contract pelvic floor musculature) (3); can use Oxford scale to grade strength
  - Urethral mobility (cotton swab test): displacement angle of urethra-bladder neck at least 30 degrees from horizontal with Valsalva (2)
  - Stress test: positive with involuntary loss of urine from urethral meatus with cough or Valsalva maneuver. If test is negative in supine position, can try in standing position. Ensure that patient has a comfortably full bladder (4). Test has 98% positive predictive value for SUI (3).
  - Cystocele: if evident, should stage (grade 0 to 4)
  - Rectocele: if evident, should stage (stage 0 to 4)

DIFFERENTIAL DIAGNOSIS
- Nocturnal enuresis: idiopathic, detrusor overactivity, neurogenic, cardiogenic, or sleep apnea
- Continuous leakage: ectopic ureter, urinary fistulas
- Postvoid dribbling: urethral diverticulum, idiopathic, iatrogenic, surgical
- Pelvic pain/dyspareunia: interstitial cystitis, STI
- Pelvic organ prolapse
- Hematuria/recurrent UTI/pelvic mass: malignancy

DIAGNOSTIC TESTS & INTERPRETATION
Initial Tests (lab, imaging)
- Urinalysis and urine culture
- Renal function assessment: recommended if renal impairment is suspected
- Imaging is unnecessary in uncomplicated patients.
- Bladder scan to evaluate postvoid residual (PVR) if overflow suspected (>100 mL) (5)
- TSH if constipation is present
- Upper tract imaging if upper tract involvement is suspected: renal ultrasound

Follow-Up Tests & Special Considerations
With a positive urine culture, initial treatment is reasonable. However, treatment of asymptomatic bacteriuria will not improve UI in the elderly (5)[B].

Diagnostic Procedures/Other
- Urodynamic studies and cystoscopy are not indicated in initial workup and should only be performed after failing conservative treatment; this includes cystometric study of detrusor function and pressure flow studies looking at bladder emptying (1,5)[B].
- Cystoscopy should be performed in women with microscopic hematuria and may be helpful in evaluating recurrent UTIs (3).
- Results of urodynamic testing are not predictive of treatment success (2)[A] and are not necessary prior to surgery for uncomplicated patients with known SUI (3)[C].

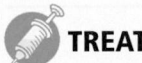 **TREATMENT**

GENERAL MEASURES
- Treat correctable causes (e.g., UTI).
- Encourage weight loss in obese patients.
- Aggressively correct constipation.
- Treat mixed for primary symptom type (5)[C].

MEDICATION
First Line
- Lifestyle changes:
  – Reduce BMI to <25; can reduce weekly incontinence episodes by 28–47% (2)[A]. Even moderate weight loss (5–10%) can help (6)[A].
  – Bladder diaries (fluid intake, voids, leakage)
  – Decrease fluid intake before bedtime.
  – Reduce caffeine to <1 cup coffee per day (2)[B].
  – Aggressive treatment of constipation: Limit medications that may induce constipation. Treat constipation with polyethylene glycol 3350 (PEG 3350), increased fluid intake, and nutrition (5)[C].
- Pelvic floor muscle training with Kegel exercises may be used alone or in combination with bladder training, biofeedback, or electrical stimulation (2).
  – Proper technique should be confirmed on exam by trained physical therapists. Recommend 3 sets of 10 contractions held for 10 seconds each (1)[C].
  – Women who undergo pelvic floor muscle training are 8 times more likely to report cure than with no treatment (6)[A].
- Bladder training:
  – Scheduled voiding, urge suppression between voids
- No differences in treatment efficacy by type of incontinence so reasonable to start with lifestyle changes in all types (2)[A]

Second Line
- Stress incontinence
  – Surgical management for stress incontinence
    ○ Mesh midurethral sling (most common, most studied surgical intervention) (2)[C],(4)[A]
    ○ Women with moderate to severe stress incontinence have better outcomes at 1 year with midurethral slings than pelvic floor muscle training (2)[A].
    ○ Main approaches with similar effectiveness: retropubic (more perioperative complications) versus transobturator (more groin pain) (2,4)[A]
    ○ Autologous fascial bladder neck slings should be considered in severe incontinence and fixed urethra, urethral diverticula or fistula, or with complications from previously placed mesh (2)[C].
    ○ Pelvic organ prolapse may unmask incontinence in up to 40% of women; consider repair of both during same surgery (2)[A].
    ○ Periurethral bulking agents (silicone polymers, collagen) can increase periurethral resistance in women who have recurrent symptoms after surgery or who cannot tolerate surgery. However, they are 2 to 5 times less effective than surgery and often require repeat injections (2)[A].
    ○ Occlusive and supportive devices (e.g., cones, pessaries) are a low risk alternative to surgery (4,5,6)[C].
- Urge incontinence: anticholinergic agents (inhibit involuntary detrusor contractions) (1)[A]
  – Tolterodine (Detrol LA): 2 to 4 mg/day PO
  – Oxybutynin (Ditropan XL): 5 to 15 mg/day PO
  – Solifenacin (VESIcare): 5 to 10 mg/day PO
  – Darifenacin (Enablex): 7.5 to 15.0 mg/day PO
  – Trospium chloride (Sanctura XR): 20 to 60 mg/day PO—does not cross blood–brain barrier (3)

  – Transdermal oxybutynin gel (Gelnique): 10%, 1 g applied daily
  – Transdermal oxybutynin patch (Oxytrol): twice weekly—available over the counter (OTC)
  – Fesoterodine (Toviaz): 4 to 8 mg/day PO
  – Fesoterodine may be more effective than tolterodine, at the expense of greater adverse effects (1)[B].
  – No single agent has been shown to be overall superior (5).
  – Extended-release and transdermal medications cause fewer side effects (1)[C].
  – Dry mouth, dry eyes, constipation, impaired cognitive function, and other anticholinergic side effects can limit use.
  – Higher doses are more effective but have higher risk of side effects (4)[B].
  – Avoid with narrow-angle glaucoma, urinary retention (PVR >250 mL), impaired gastric emptying, frail elders (3); may worsen existing cardiac arrhythmias (1)

Third Line
- Stress incontinence
  – Duloxetine (Cymbalta) 40 mg is effective but causes GI and CNS side effects; no differences between SUI and MUI (5)[A]
  – Estrogen may be beneficial in topical form for symptoms of urgency and frequency in postmenopausal women with vaginal atrophy, but transdermal or PO estrogen may worsen symptoms (1)[B],(2)[C].
  – Acupuncture (1)[B]
- Urge incontinence
  – Intradetrusor onabotulinumtoxinA 100 to 200 U (urinary retention common, temporary self-catheterization may be needed) (5)[A]
  – Sacral nerve stimulation: 61% of patients found this treatment effective and efficacy maintained at mean 30 months; invasive with frequent complications (3)[B]
  – Posterior tibial nerve stimulation: office-based therapy, requires frequent visits (3)[B]
  – Bladder augmentation: At average 6-year follow-up, only 53% were continent (5)[B].

Geriatric Considerations
Anticholinergics (oxybutynin, in particular) can worsen cognition and delirium; the effects are cumulative and increase with length of exposure (5).

- β_3 Agonist (leads to detrusor muscle relaxation and increased bladder capacity): mirabegron (Myrbetriq ER): 25 to 50 mg/day PO (1)[B]; onset of action delayed ~8 weeks; increases BP (avoid use in those with uncontrolled HTN, end-stage renal disease, or significant liver impairment); safe in geriatric patients (5); recommend BP check 2 weeks after starting (3)[C].
- Can consider dual therapy with mirabegron and low-dose anticholinergics (3,5)

 ONGOING CARE

FOLLOW-UP RECOMMENDATIONS
Patient Monitoring
Periodic long-term follow-up with outcome-based questionnaire surveys

PATIENT EDUCATION
Instructions on self-care and warning signs are available at PubMed Health: Urinary incontinence: https://medlineplus.gov/urinaryincontinence.html.

PROGNOSIS
Significant improvements are usually obtained with most patients.

COMPLICATIONS
- Prolonged exposure to urine causes skin breakdown and dermatitis, which may lead to ulceration and secondary infection.
- Inability to self-care (including toileting) is the precipitating factor for many nursing home admissions.
- Increased risk for falls
- Social isolation/depression
- Weight gain (due to self-limiting exercise from fear of leakage)
- Impaired sexual function
- Impaired quality of life

REFERENCES
1. Lukacz ES, Santiago-Lastra Y, Albo ME, et al. Urinary incontinence in women: a review. *JAMA*. 2017;318(16):1592–1604.
2. Committee on Practice Bulletins—Gynecology and the American Urogynecologic Society. ACOG Practice Bulletin No. 155: urinary incontinence in women. *Obstet Gynecol*. 2015;126(5):e66–e81.
3. Elser DM. Recognizing and managing common urogynecologic disorders. *Obstet Gynecol Clin North Am*. 2017;44(2):271–284.
4. Kobashi KC, Albo ME, Dmochowski RR, et al. Surgical treatment of female stress urinary incontinence: AUA/SUFU guideline. *J Urol*. 2017;198(4):875–883.
5. Burkhard F, Bosch J, Cruz F, et al. *Guidelines on Urinary Incontinence*. Arnhem, Netherlands: European Association of Urology; 2017.
6. Lavelle ES, Zyczynski HM. Stress urinary incontinence: comparative efficacy trials. *Obstet Gynecol Clin North Am*. 2016;43(1):45–57.

ADDITIONAL READING
- Gormley EA, Lightner DJ, Burgio KL, et al. Diagnosis and treatment of overactive bladder (non-neurogenic) in adults: AUA/SUFU guideline. *J Urol*. 2012;188(Suppl 6):2455–2563.
- Riemsma R, Hagen S, Kirschner-Hermanns R, et al. Can incontinence be cured? A systematic review of cure rates. *BMC Med*. 2017;15(1):63.
- Smith A, Bevan D, Douglas HR, et al. Management of urinary incontinence in women: summary of updated NICE guidance. *BMJ*. 2013;347:f5170.

CODES

ICD10
- R32 Unspecified urinary incontinence
- N39.3 Stress incontinence (female) (male)
- N39.41 Urge incontinence

CLINICAL PEARLS
- Rule out infection (UTI or STI) and hematuria.
- Aggressively treat constipation.
- Try lifestyle changes first for all types of urinary incontinence.
- If lifestyle changes do not work for stress incontinence, mesh midurethral sling surgery has high success rates.
- If lifestyles changes do not work for urge incontinence, anticholinergic medications and/or mirabegron should be trialed.

INCONTINENCE, URINARY ADULT MALE

William Dabbs, MD • Justin Jenkins, DO, MBA • Taylor Wright, MD

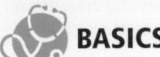

BASICS

DESCRIPTION

- Urinary incontinence (UI) is a pathologic condition of an acute or chronic nature that refers to the involuntary loss of urine leading to medical, financial, social, or hygienic problems. Five main types of UI have been described: stress, urge, mixed, overflow (urinary retention), and functional UI (1).
- Stress incontinence: involuntary urine leaks secondary to increased intra-abdominal pressure being greater than the sphincter can control; may be precipitated by sneezing, laughing, coughing, exertion
- Urge incontinence: Involuntary leakage of urine associated with urgency is believed to be secondary to uncontrolled contraction of the urinary bladder. It is also called detrusor overactivity.
- Mixed incontinence: involuntary leakage of urine with urgency and with stress, such as sneezing, laughing, coughing, exertion
- Overflow incontinence: also known as urinary retention; this occurs with bladder overdistention due to impaired detrusor contraction or bladder outlet obstruction (due to benign prostatic hyperplasia [BPH], bladder stones, bladder tumors, pelvic tumors, urethral strictures, or spasms).
- Functional UI: urine leakage variable, often due to environmental or physical barriers to toileting (i.e., reduced mobility)
- Polyuria is defined by excessive amounts of urine (≥2.5 to 3.0 L) >24 hours.
- Nocturnal polyuria is where >33% of total daily urine output occurs during sleeping hours.

EPIDEMIOLOGY

- Stress incontinence in men is rare and is often attributable to prostate surgery, neurologic disease, or trauma.
- Involuntary detrusor overactivity may be spontaneous or provoked and may be neurogenic or idiopathic in cause.
- Reported rates of incontinence range from 1% after transurethral resection to 2–66% after radical prostatectomy and 1–15% following transvesical prostatectomy, although rates decline with time (1).

Prevalence

- 12.4% prevalence of UI in community-dwelling adult men in the United States as based on the National Health and Nutrition Examination Survey (NHANES) as of 2008
- 4.5% reported moderate to severe UI, of which 48.6% experienced urge, 23.5% experienced other UI, 15.4% experienced mixed, and 12.5% experienced stress incontinence as per the NHANES report in 2010.
- UI is common in nursing home patients, with a prevalence of about 70% in the Southeastern United States from 1999 to 2002.
- Incontinence in men of all ages is approximately half as prevalent as it is in women; however, after 80 years of age, both sexes are affected equally (1).

ETIOLOGY AND PATHOPHYSIOLOGY

- Incontinence secondary to bladder abnormalities
  - Detrusor overactivity results in urge incontinence.
  - Detrusor overactivity commonly is associated with bladder outlet obstruction from BPH.
- Incontinence secondary to outlet abnormalities
  - Sphincteric damage secondary to pelvic surgery or radiation

- Sphincteric dysfunction secondary to neurologic disease
  - Commonly associated with BPH due to compression of the urethra, affecting urinary flow
- Mixed incontinence is caused by abnormalities of both the bladder and the outlet overflow or by enlarged prostate/bladder neck contracture from prostate surgery.
- Stress incontinence is caused by weakened urethral sphincter and/or pelvic floor weakness.

RISK FACTORS

- Age
- Diabetes
- Hypertension (HTN)
- History of urinary tract infections
- Major depression
- Neurologic disease
- Pelvic trauma
- Polypharmacy
- Prostate surgery

GENERAL PREVENTION

Proper management of conditions, such as symptomatic bladder outlet obstruction caused by BPH early in the course, may prevent continence problems later in life; no evidence for screening in men unless patient is experiencing symptoms using the 3 Incontinence Questions tool to evaluate the type of UI (2).

COMMONLY ASSOCIATED CONDITIONS

- Benign prostatic hypertrophy
- Neurologic disease (cerebrovascular accident, parkinsonism, multiple sclerosis, myelodysplasia, spinal cord injury, normal pressure hydrocephalus, and cognitive impairment)
- Major depression
- Pelvic surgery, radiation, or trauma

DIAGNOSIS

HISTORY

- Voiding symptoms
  - Duration and characteristics of incontinence
  - Precipitants, severity, timing, and associated symptoms (BPH, fluid intake, etc.)
  - Use of pads, briefs, diapers
  - Alteration in bowel habits
  - Previous treatments and effect on incontinence
- Associated conditions, such as diabetes mellitus, neurologic disease, cardiopulmonary disorders, renal disorders, sleep disturbance, mental health or cognitive impairment, erectile dysfunction
- Transient causes: UTI, delirium, medications, constipation, immobility
- Geriatric patients: Assess cognitive levels (dementia/delirium), psychological disorders, mobility problems.
- Medication use: diuretics, drugs for BPH, opioids, muscle relaxants, anticholinergics, antidepressants
- Alcohol and drug use, including caffeine
- Surgery
  - Pelvic surgery or radiation
  - Bowel, back, genitourinary procedures
  - Abdominoperineal resection
  - Prostatectomy: radical for cancer, open/transurethral for benign disease

- Red flag symptoms requiring rapid referral to specialist management
  - Pain, hematuria, recurrent UTI, history of prostate irradiation, history of radical pelvic surgery (i.e., prostate surgery), constant leakage suggesting fistula, voiding difficulty, suspected neurologic disease

PHYSICAL EXAM

- Cardiovascular
  - Look for signs of volume overload.
- Abdominal examination
  - Suprapubic mass suggests retention.
  - Suprapubic tenderness suggests UTI.
  - Surgical scars suggesting prior pelvic surgery
  - Skin lesions associated with neurologic disease (e.g., neurofibromatosis and café au lait spots)
- Genitourinary examination
  - External genitalia
  - DRE (prostate)
- Musculoskeletal (look for neurogenic or functional causes)
  - Extremities and spine
  - Skeletal deformities
  - Scars from previous spinal surgery
  - Sacral abnormalities may be associated with neurogenic bladder dysfunction.
- Neurologic
  - Motor, sensory, reflexes

DIFFERENTIAL DIAGNOSIS

- Transient (infections, meds, constipation, etc.)
- Chronic
  - Urge incontinence
  - Stress incontinence
  - Mixed incontinence
  - Overflow incontinence
  - Functional UI

DIAGNOSTIC TESTS & INTERPRETATION

Initial Tests (lab, imaging)

- Urinalysis and urine culture to check for glucosuria, pyuria, proteinuria, and/or blood
  - If UTI is present, treat and then reassess need for further workup as this frequently causes UI (3)[C]
- Voiding diary, the 3 Incontinence Questions (1)[C]
- Pad test if quantity of leakage or objective outcome measure is desired (low sensitivity) (3)
- Do not routinely perform urodynamics before conservative treatment for UI (4)[B].
- Postvoid residual (PVR) volume if difficulty voiding or other lower urinary tract symptoms using ultrasound (US) to measure PVR: PVR persistently ≥100 mL indicates voiding dysfunction (1)[C].
- Uroflowmetry
- PSA only if diagnosis of prostate cancer will influence treatment or if levels can help decision making for patients at risk for BPH
- Renal function if renal impairment or hydronephrosis is suspected or if considering surgical treatment for lower urinary tract symptoms
- Voiding cystogram in select cases

Diagnostic Procedures/Other

- Urodynamics is useful for confirming bladder outlet obstruction as a possible cause of detrusor overactivity (4)[B].
- Prostate US and biopsy if indicated by physical exam or PSA level

- Urethrocystoscopy to exclude suspected bladder or urethral pathology or before invasive therapies if findings might influence treatment
- Imaging of upper and lower urinary tract is not routinely indicated as part of UI assessment.
- Consider US (preferred) or MRI of lower urinary tract if indicated.
  - US is rarely required to diagnose or rule out BPH in patients with UI because DRE can diagnose and guide treatment in most patients.
  - Consider US of prostate if it assists with choice of drug therapy for lower urinary tract symptoms.
  - Consider US of prostate to assess for intravesical prostatic protrusion (IPP) if considering surgical treatment.
  - Consider US of upper urinary tract in patients with large PVR, hematuria, or history of urolithiasis.

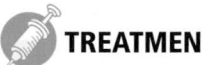 **TREATMENT**

Conservative, nonmedication interventions, such as behavioral modification, timed voiding, bladder training, and pelvic floor muscle training, should be considered *first-line therapies*, prior to initiating any pharmacologic therapy.

GENERAL MEASURES
- Bladder diaries are invaluable in helping patients understand patterns of incontinence (2)[A].
- Bladder training and timed voiding are effective (4)[A].
- Pelvic floor muscle training speeds recovery of continence following radical prostatectomy (4)[B], and preoperative PFMT seems to confer benefit in men undergoing radical prostatectomy (3)[B].
- Obesity increases the risk of UI, and weight loss may improve UI symptoms (3)[C].
- Patients with underlying or associated disease states should have appropriate medical therapy for those diseases (5)[A].
- Constipation is associated with UI, but treatment for constipation has not been shown to improve UI (4)—patients with constipation should receive standard care for their constipation (3)[C].
- Reduction in caffeine intake does not improve UI but may improve urgency and frequency (2)[B].
- Stopping smoking has not been shown to reduce UI, but patients should all be counseled to quit (4)[A].
- Pads may be used for urine containment in UI as well as external sheaths (1)[B]—external sheaths may have similar rates of UTIs with indwelling catheters but result in better QoL (1)[B]. Penile clamps may also be used, and hinge type clamps are more effective than circular clamps (3)[B].

MEDICATION
First Line
- Urge incontinence: There is no consistent evidence that drug therapy is better than behavioral therapy in UUI (1)[B], and behavioral therapy results in higher patient satisfaction (1)[B].
- Antimuscarinic agents are first-line drug therapy in UUI (1)[B], and there is no evidence that any one agent is superior for UUI (1)[A].
- Oxybutynin (Ditropan XL) 5 to 15 mg PO every day
- Tolterodine (Detrol LA) 2 to 4 mg PO every day
- Darifenacin (Enablex) 7.5 to 15.0 mg PO every day
- Solifenacin (VESIcare) 5 to 10 mg PO every day
- Trospium chloride (Sanctura XR) 60 mg PO every day
- Transdermal oxybutynin (Gelnique) 10% apply daily (EAU Grade B)—no dry mouth
- Fesoterodine (Toviaz) 4 to 8 mg PO every day

- Mirabegron, a β_3-agonist, has been shown in some trials and systematic reviews to be as efficacious as antimuscarinics (3)[B].
- Mirabegron (Myrbetriq): 25 to 50 mg PO daily. *Caution*: HTN
- Review efficacy and side effects 4 to 6 weeks after treatment initiation.
- Most patients will stop antimuscarinic therapy within 3 months due to adverse effects, nonefficacy, or cost (2).
- Caution in those with bladder outlet obstruction and PVR >250 to 300 mL: In men with urgency associated with BPH, consider α-blockers (i.e., tamsulosin, alfuzosin, silodosin) as monotherapy or in combination with antimuscarinic for residual overactive bladder (5).
- Stress incontinence
  - No generally accepted drug therapy
  - Mixed stress and urge incontinence; ER formulations are preferred due to reduced side effects.

Second Line
- Urge incontinence
- Tricyclic antidepressants
  - Imipramine 10 to 25 mg PO BID/TID
- Desmopressin (DDAVP) for occasional short-term relief of UI
  - 25 to 50 μg PO or intranasal at bedtime
- Intradetrusor botulinum toxin injections 100 U intravesical injections (not FDA-approved)
- Duloxetine for temporary improvements of incontinence with dose titration (mixed stress/urge)

Geriatric Considerations
- Anticholinergics and tricyclics may result in significant cognitive impairment in elderly patients.
- DDAVP should be avoided in patients with known/potential cardiac disease.

ADDITIONAL THERAPIES
- Pelvic floor rehabilitation (Kegel exercises) may significantly reduce both stress and urge incontinence in male patients and should be considered a part of initial management for stress UI.
- Overflow incontinence is usually caused by poor bladder contractility with urinary retention.
  - Indwelling or intermittent catheterization
  - Evaluate for outlet obstruction.

SURGERY/OTHER PROCEDURES
- Urge incontinence
  - Sacral nerve stimulation with behavioral therapy
  - Augmentation cystoplasty and urinary diversion
  - Botulinum toxin injection via cystoscopy
- Stress incontinence (4)[B]
  - Urethral bulking agents: modest success rates with low cure rates
  - Male sling procedures: promising short-term and intermediate results but no long-term studies
  - Artificial urinary sphincter implant has excellent long-term continence rates and is considered gold standard (6).

COMPLEMENTARY & ALTERNATIVE MEDICINE
Alternative modalities such as acupuncture, chiropractic, are not effective.

 ONGOING CARE

FOLLOW-UP RECOMMENDATIONS
Patient Monitoring
Must monitor residual volume after voiding in patients taking anticholinergic medications; monitor side effects.

PROGNOSIS
Continence can be improved in almost all patients.

COMPLICATIONS
- Dermatitis
- Candidiasis
- Skin breakdown
- Social isolation
- Avoidance of sex
- Weight gain

REFERENCES
1. Khandelwal C, Kistler C. Diagnosis of urinary incontinence. *Am Fam Physician*. 2013;87(8):543–550.
2. Gravas A, Bachmann A, Descazeaud A, et al. *EAU Guidelines on the Management of Non-neurogenic Male Lower Urinary Tract Symptoms (LUTS), Including Benign Prostatic Obstruction (BPO)*. Arnhem, Netherlands: European Association of Urology; 2014.
3. Nambiar AK, Bosch R, Cruz F, et al. EAU guidelines on assessment and nonsurgical management of urinary incontinence. *Eur Urol*. 2018;73(4):596–609.
4. Lucas MG, Bedretdinova D, Bosch JL, et al. *EAU Guidelines on Urinary Incontinence*. Arnhem, Netherlands: European Association of Urology; 2014.
5. Gormley EA, Lightner DJ, Burgio KL, et al; for American Urological Association, Society of Urodynamics, Female Pelvic Medicine & Urogenital Reconstruction. Diagnosis and treatment of overactive bladder (non-neurogenic) in adults: AUA/SUFU guideline. *J Urol*. 2012;188(Suppl 6):2455–2463.
6. Herschorn S, Bruschini H, Comiter C, et al; for Committee of the International Consultation on Incontinence. Surgical treatment of stress incontinence in men. *Neurourol Urodyn*. 2010;29(1):179–190.

ADDITIONAL READING
- Bauer RM, Bastian PJ, Gozzi C, et al. Postprostatectomy incontinence: all about diagnosis and management. *Eur Urol*. 2009;55(2):322–333.
- Markland AD, Goode PS, Redden DT, et al. Prevalence of urinary incontinence in men: results from the National Health and Nutrition Examination Survey. *J Urol*. 2010;184(3):1022–1027.

 CODES

ICD10
- R32 Unspecified urinary incontinence
- N39.3 Stress incontinence (female) (male)
- N39.41 Urge incontinence

CLINICAL PEARLS
- Think "outside" the lower urinary tract: Comorbid medical illness and impairments are independently associated with UI; treat contributing comorbidities and rule out secondary causes.
- Always check PVR to rule out overflow incontinence.
- Have patient complete the International Prostate Symptom Score and do uroflow, PSA if indicated.
- Pelvic floor rehabilitation handouts may be a good alternative for male patients, rather than physical therapy–mediated pelvic floor rehabilitation.

Dennis E. Hughes, DO, FAAFP, FACEP

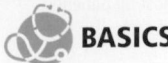

BASICS

DESCRIPTION
- Epstein-Barr virus (EBV) is a member of the herpes virus family; human herpes virus 4 (1)
  - Two subtypes: ST1 predominates in Western Hemisphere, Southeast Asia; ST1 and ST2 equally prevalent in Africa
- Primary infection typically occurs in childhood; responsible for infectious mononucleosis (IM) (most common); also linked to numerous cancers
- WHO classified EBV as "tumor virus" (group I carcinogen) due to cancer association (1).

EPIDEMIOLOGY

Prevalence
Worldwide, infects >90% of people (antibody positive)

Incidence
- Military recruits, college students, and others living in cloistered and crowded populations have highest infection rate. Overall rate in United States is 500/100,000 (2).
- Predominant age of primary infection is 15 to 24 years; 200 to 800/100,000 affected (2)
  - Primary clinical manifestation is IM.
  - Early childhood infections are usually asymptomatic.
- Seroconversion occurs later in childhood in developed countries; there is suggestion of race/ethnicity disparity in the United States with higher seroprevalence in non-Hispanic black, Asian, and Hispanic populations (2).

ETIOLOGY AND PATHOPHYSIOLOGY
- After inoculation, the virus replicates in the nasopharyngeal epithelium with resulting cell lysis, virion spread, and viremia. The reticuloendothelial system is affected, resulting in a host response and the appearance of atypical lymphocytes in the peripheral blood. Viral genome can be detected in the oral cavity 1 week prior to symptoms.
- A polyclonal B-cell proliferative response follows. Relatively few (<0.1%) of the circulating lymphocytes are infected by EBV in the acute illness.
- A persistent (asymptomatic) state ensues with the EBV genome invisible to the immune system.
- During this period, coinfection increases risk for an EBV-associated condition (e.g., malignancy).
- Either through B-cell stimulation or diminished EBV-specific immune modulation, the previously latent EBV-infected B cells replicate, allowing clinical expression of the EBV genome. The proteins produced may either modify host response to or contribute directly to subsequent malignancy (1,3).
- Immunosuppression (organ transplant/acquired immune deficiency) can result in transformation and lymphoproliferative disorders.

RISK FACTORS
- Age (highest incidence in adolescent, young adults)
- Socio-hygienic level ("crowded conditions")
- Geographic location
- Close, intimate contact; especially "deep kissing" in adolescents and young adults (4)
- Immunosuppression

GENERAL PREVENTION
- Avoid close physical contact with symptomatic EBV/IM patients.
- Meticulous hand washing and hygiene
- General precautions with potential blood exposure (EBV can be transmitted via blood contamination as well as hematopoietic cell and solid organ transplant.)
- EBV vaccines under investigation—limited efficacy

COMMONLY ASSOCIATED CONDITIONS
- IM: Symptomatic primary EBV infection is common in otherwise healthy adolescents and young adults.
  - Clinical features vary in severity and duration: In children age <10 years, generally mild; in adolescents and adults, symptoms can be more severe and protracted.
  - Incubation period is 30 to 50 days.
- X-linked lymphoproliferative syndrome (XLP—rare, inherited extreme vulnerability to EBV infection)
- Lymphoproliferative syndromes due to EBV infections in transplant recipients
- Lymphomas (B-cell lymphoblastic, T cell)
- Lymphocytic interstitial pneumonitis
- Hairy leukoplakia of the tongue, leiomyosarcoma, and CNS lymphomas in patients with AIDS
- Burkitt lymphoma (most common childhood tumor in Africa and Papua New Guinea where malaria is also endemic and may be a cofactor)
- Nasopharyngeal carcinoma (particularly in SE China)
- Parotid carcinoma
- Hodgkin lymphoma (most common EBV-associated malignancy in United States, European Union)
- Postulated to be associated with multiple sclerosis (2 to 3 times incidence in EBV-positive individuals)
- Chronic active Epstein-Barr virus (CAEBV) due to loss of host control of viral replication

DIAGNOSIS

HISTORY
- May be either abrupt or insidious in onset
- Syndrome of fatigue, malaise, and sore throat
- In adults, temperature may rise to 103°F (39.4°C) and gradually fall over a variable period of 7 to 10 days; in severe cases, temperature elevations of 104–105°F (40.0–40.6°C) may persist for 2 weeks.
- Children typically have low-grade fever or are afebrile.
- Rash
- Chest pain (myocarditis and pericarditis)

PHYSICAL EXAM
- Fever, lymphadenopathy, pharyngitis in >50%, with palatal petechiae and hepatosplenomegaly in ~10%
- Diffuse hyperemia and hyperplasia of oropharyngeal lymphoid tissue
- Gelatinous, grayish-white exudative tonsillitis persists for 7 to 10 days in 50%.
- Petechiae at border of hard and soft palates in 60%.
- Axillary, epitrochlear, popliteal, inguinal, mediastinal, and mesenteric lymphadenopathy (95% of patients)
- Lymph node enlargement subsides over days/weeks.
- Tender lymphadenopathy (Cervical nodes are most commonly enlarged.)
- Splenomegaly in 50%
- Skin manifestations in 3–16%
  - Erythematous macular/maculopapular rash
  - Petechial and purpuric exanthems reported
  - Rash typically on trunk and upper arms; occasionally, the face and forearms are involved.

DIFFERENTIAL DIAGNOSIS
- Streptococcal pharyngitis and tonsillitis
- Diphtheria
- Blood dyscrasias
- Rubella
- Measles
- Viral hepatitis
- Cytomegalovirus
- Toxoplasmosis

DIAGNOSTIC TESTS & INTERPRETATION

Initial Tests (lab, imaging)
- CBC with differential
- Lymphocytes and atypical lymphocytes
  - Increased numbers of lymphocytes (especially atypical lymphocytes; may be up to 70% of leukocytes) in peripheral blood
  - In 1st week after onset, WBC count is normal/moderately decreased. Due to EB-related neutrophil fragility, automated processing can result in pseudoneutropenia (5).
    - By week 2, atypical lymphocytosis develops.
  - During early illness, atypical lymphocytes are B cells transformed by the EBV; later, atypical cells are activated CD8 T lymphocytes (4).
- Antibodies
  - Heterophile antibodies in 80–90% of adults
  - Heterophile antibody is an IgM response, which appears during the first 2 weeks of illness; disappears in 4 to 6 weeks
  - In general, agglutinin titer is higher in IM than other disorders; an unabsorbed heterophile titer >1:128 and ≥1:40 is significant.
- Specific antibodies to EBV-associated antigens
  - Develop regularly in IM
  - Viral capsid-specific IgM and IgG are present early in illness.
  - Viral capsid-IgM disappears after several weeks; viral capsid-IgG persists for life.
- Liver tests: Transaminitis, hyperbilirubinemia are common; jaundice is rare.

- Atypical lymphocytes are not specific for EBV infections and may be present in other clinical conditions, including rubella, infectious hepatitis, allergic rhinitis, asthma, and atypical pneumonia.
- Routine abdominal ultrasound to monitor for splenic enlargement is not necessary.
- Consider ultrasound for those wishing to return to strenuous activity/contact sports at day 21 of illness to exclude splenomegaly.

Follow-Up Tests & Special Considerations
- Abnormal hepatic enzymes persist in 80% of patients for several weeks; hepatomegaly in 15–20%
- In transplant recipients, quantitative polymerase chain reaction (PCR) used to monitor EBV loads

Diagnostic Procedures/Other
Chest x-ray
- Hilar adenopathy may be observed in IM with extensive lymphoid hyperplasia.

Test Interpretation
- Mononuclear infiltrations of lymph nodes, tonsils, spleen, lungs, liver, heart, kidneys, adrenal glands, skin, and CNS
- Bone marrow hyperplasia with small granulomas formation may be present; these findings are non-specific and have no prognostic significance.

TREATMENT
- Treatment is mostly supportive.
- NSAIDs or acetaminophen
- During acute stage, limit activity for 4 weeks to reduce potential complications (e.g., splenic rupture).
- Transplant recipients who develop EBV infection may require reduction in immunosuppression and administration of monoclonal anti-CD20 (rituximab).

MEDICATION
- In primary infections:
  – Antimicrobial agents (usually penicillin) only if throat culture is positive for group A β-hemolytic streptococci. Previously, ampicillin rash in presumed group B Streptococcus (GBS) was thought to be highly suggestive of IM. Incidence of rash is much lower than historically thought (4)[B].
  – Warm saline gargles for oropharyngeal pain
  – Corticosteroids
    o May provide some symptomatic relief but no improvement in resolution of illness
    o Consider in severe pharyngotonsillitis with oropharyngeal edema and airway encroachment. Dexamethasone 0.3 mg/kg/day may be used for 1 to 3 days.
    o Also for patients with marked toxicity/major complications (e.g., hemolytic anemia, thrombocytopenic purpura, neurologic sequelae, myocarditis, pericarditis) (6)[B]
- Antiviral medications (acyclovir) have been found to shorten recovery time and improve subjective symptoms in acute EBV infection in small studies.

ISSUES FOR REFERRAL
Most cases can be managed as an outpatient without the need for specialty referral. Consider referral for complications such as oropharyngeal edema with airway compromise.

SURGERY/OTHER PROCEDURES
- Splenectomy may be necessary with profound thrombocytopenia that is refractory to corticosteroids.
- Only current effective treatment for XLP is hematopoietic stem cell transplantation.
- Splenic rupture

 ## ONGOING CARE

FOLLOW-UP RECOMMENDATIONS

ALERT
Rupture of the spleen may be fatal if not recognized; it requires blood transfusions, treatment for shock, and splenectomy. Occurrence is estimated at 0.1%.

Patient Monitoring
- Avoid contact sports, heavy lifting, and excess exertion until spleen and liver have returned to normal size (ultrasound can verify). Current consensus is that if after 3 weeks and normal exam, no fever, and no constitutional symptoms, patients may return to contact sport activities.
- Eliminate alcohol/exposure to other hepatotoxic drugs until LFTs return to normal.
- Rates of complications are highest during the first 3 weeks of illness.
- Symptoms (malaise, fatigue, intermittent sore throat, lymphadenopathy) may persist for months.

DIET
No restrictions. Hydration is important.

PROGNOSIS
- Most recover in ~4 weeks.
- Fatigue may persist for months.

COMPLICATIONS
- Neurologic (rare)
  – Aseptic meningitis, meningoencephalitis
  – Bell palsy, Guillain-Barré syndrome
  – Transverse myelitis
  – Cerebellar ataxia
  – Acute psychosis
- Hematologic (rare)
  – Thrombocytopenia, early in illness
  – Hemolytic anemia with neutropenia (early)
  – Hemophagocytic syndrome (splenomegaly, fever, cytopenia)
  – Agammaglobulinemia
- Pneumonitis
- Airway obstruction
- Splenic rupture
  – Rare, but most often occurs in first 21 days of illness

REFERENCES
1. Stanfield BA, Luftig MA. Recent advances in understanding Epstein-Barr virus. F1000Res. 2017;6:386. doi:10.12688/f1000research.10591.1.
2. Williams-Harmon YJ, Jason LA, Katz BZ. Incidence of infectious mononucleosis in universities and U.S. military settings. J Diagn Tech Biomed Anal. 2016;5(1). doi:10.4172/2469-5653.1000113.
3. Thorley-Lawson DA, Hawkins JB, Tracy SI, et al. The pathogenesis of Epstein-Barr virus persistent infection. Curr Opin Virol. 2013;3(3):227–232.
4. Dunmire SK, Hogquist KA, Balfour HH. Infectious mononucleosis. Curr Top Microbiol Immunol. 2015;390(Pt 1):211–240.
5. Loudin M, Deloughery T, Shatzel J. Mononucleosis-induced pseudo neutropenia. Am J Hematology. 2017;92(2):219.
6. Odumade O, Hogquist K, Balfour H Jr. Progress and problems in understanding and managing primary Epstein-Barr virus infections. Clin Microbiol Rev. 2011;24(1):193–209.

ADDITIONAL READING
- Grimm JM, Schmeling DO, Dunmire SK, et al. Prospective studies of infectious mononucleosis in university students. Clin Transl Immunology. 2016;5(8):e94.
- Womack J, Jimenez M. Common questions about infectious mononucleosis. Am Fam Physician. 2015;91(6):372–376.

 ## CODES

ICD10
- B27.00 Gammaherpesviral mononucleosis without complication
- B27.09 Gammaherpesviral mononucleosis with other complications
- B27.01 Gammaherpesviral mononucleosis with polyneuropathy

CLINICAL PEARLS
- 98% of patients with acute IM present with some combination of fever, sore throat, cervical node enlargement, and tonsillar hypertrophy.
- False-negative monospot (heterophile antibody) is common in the first 10 to 14 days of illness. 90% will have heterophile antibodies by week 3 of illness.
- Lymphocytosis (not monocytosis) is common in IM.
- Treatment of IM is primarily supportive.

I

INFERTILITY
LuDane Simmons, MD • Sahil Mullick, MD

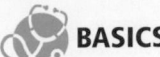 **BASICS**

DESCRIPTION
Definition: failure of a couple to conceive after 1 year of normal sexual activity without contraceptives. Primary: Couple has never been pregnant. Secondary: Couple has been pregnant. Fecundability: the probability of achieving pregnancy in one menstrual cycle

EPIDEMIOLOGY
Incidence
Incidence is the probability of achieving a pregnancy within 1 year. The incidence of infertility increases with age, with a decline in fertility in the early 30s, accelerating in the late 30s. ~85% of couples will conceive within 12 months of unprotected intercourse.

Prevalence
- About 25% of couples experience infertility at some point in their reproductive lives.
- ~11.5% couples between ages 15 and 34 years and 42% between ages 35 and 44 years meet the criteria for being infertile.
- May increase as more women delay childbearing; 20% of women in the United States have their first child >35 years.
- CDC National Survey of Family Growth noted 12% of U.S. women >15 to 44 years old have impaired fecundity.

ETIOLOGY AND PATHOPHYSIOLOGY
- Most cases multifactorial: approximately 50% of cases due to female factors (of which 20% are due to ovulatory dysfunction and 30% due to tubal and pelvic pathology); ~40% due to male factors; 20% unknown etiology
- Acquired: Most common cause of infertility in the United States is pelvic inflammatory disease (PID) secondary to chlamydia (1), endometriosis, polycystic ovary syndrome (PCOS), premature ovarian failure, and increased maternal age.
- Diminished ovarian reserve (DOR): low fertility due to low quantity or functional quality of oocytes
- Congenital: anatomic and genetic abnormalities

Genetics
- Higher incidence of genetic abnormalities among infertile population, including Klinefelter syndrome (47,XXY), Turner syndrome (45X or mosaic), and fragile X syndrome
- Y chromosomal microdeletions are associated with isolated defects of spermatogenesis → found in 16% of men with azoo-/severe oligospermia.
- Cystic fibrosis transmembrane conductance regulator (CFTR) gene mutation causing congenital bilateral absence of vas deferens (CBAVD)

RISK FACTORS
- Female
  - Gynecologic history: irregular/abnormal menses, sexually transmitted infections (STIs), dysmenorrhea, fibroids, prior pregnancy
  - Medical history: endocrinopathy, autoimmune disease, undiagnosed celiac disease, collagen vascular diseases, thrombophilia, obesity, and cancer
  - Surgical history: appendicitis, pelvic surgery, intrauterine surgery, tubal ligation
  - Social history: smoking, alcohol/substance abuse, eating disorders, exercise, advanced maternal age
- Male
  - Medical history: STI, prostatitis, medication use (i.e., β-blockers, calcium channel blocker, antiulcer medication), endocrinopathy, cancer

- Surgical history: orchiopexy, hernia repair, vasectomy with/without reversal
- Social: smoking, alcohol/substance abuse, anabolic steroids, environmental exposures, occupations leading to increased scrotal temperature (frequent use of saunas, hot tubs, or tight underwear), prescription drugs that impair male potency

GENERAL PREVENTION
Normal diet and exercise, avoid smoking and other substance abuse, prevention of STIs

COMMONLY ASSOCIATED CONDITIONS
- Sexual behavior increasing risk for STIs
- Pelvic pathology: endometriosis, ovarian cysts, endometrial polyps, and uterine fibroids
- Endocrine dysfunction (thyroid, glucose metabolism, menstrual cycle abnormalities, prolactin)
- Anovulation is commonly associated with hyperandrogenism and PCOS.

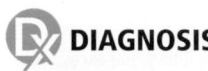 **DIAGNOSIS**

HISTORY
- Complete reproductive history:
  - Age at menarche, regularity of menstrual cycle, physical development, previous methods of contraception, history of abnormal Pap smears and treatment
  - History of abortion, D&Cs, bilateral tubal ligation, vasectomy, or other pelvic/abdominal surgery
- Frequency of intercourse and sexual dysfunction
- Abdominal pain or other abdominal symptoms
- History of STI
- History of endocrine abnormalities
- History of malignancy or chronic illness
- Family history: close relatives with congenital abnormalities or mental retardation; infertility or early menopause in close relatives of female partner
- Medications: drug abuse, allergies, occupation, and exposure to environmental hazards

PHYSICAL EXAM
- BMI, distribution of body fat, and waist circumference
- Female
  - Pubertal development with Tanner staging
  - Signs of PCOS: androgen excess, obesity, signs of insulin resistance
  - Breast exam: galactorrhea
  - Vaginal exam: Describe rugation, discharge, anatomic variation.
  - Uterine size/shape, mobility, tenderness
  - Adnexal tenderness infection or mass
- Male
  - Abnormalities of the penis or urethral meatus
  - Testes: volume, symmetry, masses (varicocele, hydrocele), presence/absence of vas deferens

DIAGNOSTIC TESTS & INTERPRETATION
Initial Tests (lab, imaging)
Evaluation is directed by history:
- Assessment of ovulation
  - Irregular or infrequent menses, not accompanied by consistent premenstrual or moliminal characteristics, which are inconsistent in flow and duration, are indicative of ovulatory dysfunction.
  - Elevated FSH and luteinizing hormone (LH) but low estradiol indicate ovarian insufficiency. High LH alone suggests PCOS. Luteal-phase progesterone ≥3 ng/mL confirms ovulation has recently occurred but does not indicate when it occurred.

- Assessment of ovarian reserve
  - Women >35 years old need to have ovarian reserve assessed. On day 3 of menses, an FSH >15 to 20 IU/L is suggestive.
  - Anti-müllerian hormone (AMH) and antral follicle counts (AFCs): The number of antral follicles measured by transvaginal ultrasound (US) is termed the "antral follicle count." AMH is secreted by the granulosa cells of the antral follicles and decreases as a woman approaches menopause. AMH can be measured any time during the cycle and not affected by hormones. AMH <0.7 μ/dL and total AFC <10 during the follicular phase indicates decreased reserve.
  - Clomiphene challenge test: After administration of clomiphene from day 5 to 9, measure FSH of ≥10 mIU/mL on day 10 to help confirm the diagnosis of DOR.
- Semen analysis
  - Warranted in all infertile couples. Semen analysis alone is not used to predict male fertility potential.
  - Semen collection: collected after 2 to 5 days of abstinence. Repeat test 2 to 3 times due to inherent variability within the same individual.
  - Parameters for male subfertility: sperm concentration <13.5 million/mL, sperm motility <32%, sperm morphology <9% normal
- Additional labs
  - Prolactin, thyroid-stimulating hormone, 17-hydroxyprogesterone, androgen levels
  - HIV, HSV 1 and 2, chlamydia, gonorrhea, RPR, hepatitis B and C, CMV
  - Genetic testing based on family history
- Transvaginal US for anatomic abnormality
- Hysterosalpingogram (HSG) to evaluate patency of tubes and contour of the cavity; may be both diagnostic and therapeutic
- Sonohysterography (SHG) may provide a more detailed evaluation of the uterine cavity, if indicated.

Follow-Up Tests & Special Considerations
- Abnormal lab values warrant reevaluation/referral.
- Abnormal imaging may require surgical evaluation.

Diagnostic Procedures/Other
- Hysteroscopy: gold standard, used to directly visualize the endometrial cavity; may be indicated to evaluate filling defects on HSG or SHG
- Laparoscopy: used to directly visualize the peritoneal cavity and may be indicated to evaluate abnormal findings on HSG. Laparoscopy is the only way to definitively diagnose endometriosis.

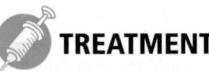 **TREATMENT**

GENERAL MEASURES
- Couples may wish to begin with simpler methods for determining ovulation and timing intercourse, depending on duration of infertility and resources available. Basal body temperature (BBT) tracking and/or detection of LH surge may be helpful for some. BBT: ~1 degree increase in BBT taken upon wakening indicates ovulation has occurred: Greatest fertility spans 7 days PRIOR to rise in BBT; LH testing kit: identifies midcycle LH surge, which occurs approximately 14 to 26 hours prior to ovulation. Greatest fertility on day of LH surge until 2 days after; predicts time of ovulation in advance so couples can time intercourse

- Be aware of insurance coverage for each patient. Be mindful of the couple's emotional state: Depression, anger, anxiety, and marital discord are common. Many patients benefit from counseling and support measures.
- All female fertility patients should be given folate supplementation 1 mg/day by mouth.
- Additionally, dietary carotenoids in males may improve sperm quality (2,3).
- IVF is the most effective infertility treatment available:
  - Eggs are removed from the female and fertilized outside the body. The embryo is monitored for 3 to 5 days and then implanted into the uterus on day 3 or day 5.
  - Anatomic causes should be referred immediately for IVF, although surgical consult may be required.
  - Fewer complications have been reported for individuals undergoing IVF for anatomic causes rather than ovulatory dysfunction (low APGAR scores, DM) (4)[A].
  - Donor eggs may be obtained.
- Male factor
  - Consider lifestyle changes.
  - Intrauterine insemination (IUI): Sperm is placed via a catheter directly in the uterus. IUI effectively increases the sperm count.
  - Intracytoplasmic sperm injection (ICSI) is performed in conjunction with IVF for males with severe abnormalities (i.e., <5 million sperm) or those who have failed to conceive with IUI. A single sperm is injected directly into the cytoplasm of the egg. Fertilization occurs ~70% of the time.
  - Donor sperm may be obtained.

MEDICATION
First Line
- Treatment of infertility depends on the etiology.
- Anovulation: must determine if HYPOgonadotropic or NORMOgonadotropic
  - Hypogonadotropic patients: Standard treatment to induce ovulation consists of daily injections of both FSH and LH, which need to be carefully monitored to avoid overstimulation, resulting in ovarian hyperstimulation syndrome (OHSS).
  - Normogonadotropic patients: most commonly due to PCOS. Ovulation induction with letrozole (aromatase inhibitor) is possibly superior to clomiphene for patients with PCOS. Clomiphene citrate (Clomid). Regimen: 50 mg/day for 5 days beginning typically on CD 5 after spontaneous or progestin-induced withdrawal bleed. If no ovulation, increase dose to 100 mg/day in subsequent cycles; maximum 150 mg/day. Some will increase dose with ovulation but no pregnancy; most effective with ~10% body weight loss if obese
- Unexplained infertility: The first-line therapy might be controlled ovarian hyperstimulation, as with clomiphene citrate and IUI. IVF may be recommended as second line.
- Coital or cervical problems: IUI
- Endometriosis: either IVF or surgery; medical therapy does not increase pregnancy rates.

Second Line
If clomiphene and letrozole fail to induce ovulation:
- Metformin beneficial in anovulatory women with PCOS, especially those with glucose intolerance; initiate with 500 mg daily and increase to ~1,500 mg/day; monitor renal function; might take up to 3 months to be effective

- Consider also oral contraceptive pills (OCPs) for ≥2 cycles and then retry the clomiphene immediately after stopping the OCPs.
- Cabergoline or bromocriptine used if prolactin is elevated or if no withdrawal bleed after progesterone administration. Once pregnancy has occurred, the medication can be stopped.
- Human menopausal gonadotropins (hMGs) or recombinant FSH is indicated if there is resistance to clomiphene or if there is hypogonadotropism.

ISSUES FOR REFERRAL
Reproductive endocrinology and/or urology: Specialized lab prep is needed for IUI. FSH + LH therapies and IVF warrant referral in most cases.

ADDITIONAL THERAPIES
Consider using surrogate pregnancy if female cannot conceive.

SURGERY/OTHER PROCEDURES
Reproductive surgery may be necessary in those with anatomic causes of infertility. Polypectomy could be beneficial for large polyps obstructing the lumen of the uterus. Myomectomy may increase pregnancy success rates for intramural fibroids that obstruct or distort the uterine cavity. Salpingectomy is recommended and increases fertility in those with hydrosalpinx. In males with a varicocele, surgical treatment may improve sperm characteristics. Aspiration of sperm using transepidermal or microsurgical techniques may be useful.

COMPLEMENTARY & ALTERNATIVE MEDICINE
Acupuncture may increase live birth rates with IVF.

ADMISSION, INPATIENT, AND NURSING CONSIDERATIONS
Rarely needed; however, may be needed occasionally for problems in early pregnancy and OHSS

 ## ONGOING CARE

FOLLOW-UP RECOMMENDATIONS
Patients should be referred to a specialist and consider more aggressive options if not successful after 3 to 6 cycles of oral ovulation induction.

Patient Monitoring
Cycle monitoring may decrease risks. US can show the number of developing follicles per cycle, which may help to predict OHSS and risk of multiple gestations.

DIET
A diet with sufficient calories to maintain a BMI permissive for ovulation. If obese, weight loss is recommended.

PATIENT EDUCATION
- Many reproductive-age women lack knowledge regarding the adverse effects of STI, irregular menses, and obesity on reproduction. Infertility treatment should focus on patient education (5)[A].
- American Society for Reproductive Medicine (http://www.asrm.org)
- Resolve: patient advocacy group (http://www.resolve.org)

PROGNOSIS
Most couples will achieve a pregnancy if minor (even multiple) disorders can be identified and treated. For those without identified cause following evaluation, 60% will achieve pregnancy within 3 years.

COMPLICATIONS
Anxiety (stress levels are high during treatment), multiple pregnancy (rates increase with all medical ovulation induction therapies and IVF), OHSS (very rare with oral medications but more common with FSH treatments). Couples with infertility may have a slightly increased risk of congenital abnormalities in offspring.

REFERENCES
1. Tsevat DG, Wiesenfeld HC, Parks C, et al. Sexually transmitted diseases and infertility. *Am J Obstet Gynecol*. 2017;216(1):1–9.
2. Ruder EH, Hartman TJ, Reindollar RH, et al. Female dietary antioxidant intake and time to pregnancy among couples treated for unexplained infertility. *Fertil Steril*. 2014;101(3):759–766.
3. Zareba P, Colaci DS, Afeiche M, et al. Semen quality in relation to antioxidant intake in a healthy male population. *Fertil Steril*. 2013;100(6):1572–1579.
4. Grigorescu V, Zhang Y, Kissin DM, et al. Maternal characteristics and pregnancy outcomes after assisted reproductive technology by infertility diagnosis: ovulatory dysfunction versus tubal obstruction. *Fertil Steril*. 2014;101(4):1019–1025.
5. Lundsberg LS, Pal L, Gariepy AM, et al. Knowledge, attitudes, and practices regarding conception and fertility: a population-based survey among reproductive-age United States women. *Fertil Steril*. 2014;101(3):767–774.

ADDITIONAL READING
- Humphries L, Chang O, Humm K, et al. Influence of race and ethnicity on in vitro fertilization outcomes: systematic review. *Am J Obstet Gynecol*. 2016;214(2):212.e1–212.e17.
- Practice Committee of American Society for Reproductive Medicine. Diagnostic evaluation of the infertile female: a committee opinion. *Fertil Steril*. 2012;98(2):302–307.
- Practice Committee of American Society for Reproductive Medicine. Diagnostic evaluation of the infertile male: a committee opinion. *Fertil Steril*. 2012;98(2):294–301.

 ## SEE ALSO
- Amenorrhea; Endometriosis; Metabolic Syndrome; Polycystic Ovarian Syndrome (PCOS)
- Algorithm: Infertility

 ## CODES

ICD10
- N97.9 Female infertility, unspecified
- N46.9 Male infertility, unspecified
- N97.1 Female infertility of tubal origin

CLINICAL PEARLS
- Women <35 years of age should be evaluated for infertility after failing to conceive after 1 year of unprotected intercourse, those ≥35 years should receive evaluation after 6 months, and those ≥40 years should receive assistance immediately.
- Medical therapy for endometriosis does not increase pregnancy rates, but surgical treatment does.

INFLUENZA
Kai-Soon "David" Yang, MD • Bassem M. Mostafa Elsawy, MD, FAAFP, CMD

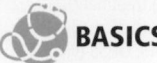 BASICS

DESCRIPTION
- Acute, typically self-limited, febrile infection caused by orthomyxovirus influenza types A and B
- Marked by inflammation of nasal mucosa, pharynx, conjunctiva, and respiratory tract
- Outbreaks have varying degrees of severity and generally peak in winter.
- Influenza virus can undergo antigenic shift (abrupt change) leading to viral strains with little immunologic resistance in a population. This can result in pandemic outbreaks. Minor seasonal variations are called *antigenic drift*.
- System(s) affected: typical cases: head/eyes/ears /nose/throat, pulmonary; complicated cases: cardiac and CNS involvement
- Synonym(s): flu; grippe; acute catarrhal fever

EPIDEMIOLOGY
- Predominant age: children (3 months to 16 years) and young adults
  - Morbidity: seasonal morbidity and rates of hospitalization highest in very young (preschool), elderly (>75 years of age), and individuals with comorbid illness (lung disease, malignancy)
- Predominant sex: male = female

Incidence
- Seasonal influenza in preuniversal vaccination: 95 million cases per year, typically fall/winter
- Attack rates in healthy children: 10–40% each year, prior to routine influenza vaccination
- Weekly reports: https://www.cdc.gov/flu/weekly

ETIOLOGY AND PATHOPHYSIOLOGY
Orthomyxovirus (influenza types A [majority] and B); influenza A virus subtypes HxNx based on hemagglutinin and neuraminidase
- Incubation is 1 to 4 days; infected persons are most contagious during peak symptoms.
- Spread by aerosolized droplets or contact with respiratory secretions
- Hemagglutinin binds to columnar respiratory epithelium where replication occurs, and neuraminidase protein facilitates spread along respiratory epithelium.

RISK FACTORS
- For contracting disease
  - Crowded environments such as nursing homes, barracks, schools, and correctional facilities
- For complications
  - Neonates, infants, elderly
  - Pregnancy, especially in 3rd trimester
  - Chronic pulmonary diseases
  - Cardiovascular diseases, including valvular pathology and congestive heart failure (CHF)
  - Metabolic disease, morbid obesity
  - Hemoglobinopathies
  - Malignancy; immunosuppression
  - Neuromuscular diseases that limit respiratory function and ability to handle secretions

GENERAL PREVENTION
- Vaccination: All persons >6 months should be vaccinated annually unless contraindication present.
  - Inactivated influenza vaccine (IIV) is available with either 3 (IIV3) or 4 (IIV4) strains of influenza. IIV also is available as high-dose, intradermal, cell culture–based (ccIIV3), MF59-adjuvanted (aIIV3), and recombinant hemagglutinin vaccine (RIV3).
  - Live attenuated influenza vaccine (LAIV) is an intranasal quadrivalent vaccine.
- IIV recommended annually for the following:
  - All persons aged ≥6 months
  - Vaccine should be administered annually as soon as the vaccine is available.
  - Protection occurs 1 to 2 weeks after immunization.
  - Typically, mild side effects include low-grade fever and local reaction at vaccination site.
  - Inactivated IM dose: ≥3 years of age: 0.5 mL; children 6 to 35 months of age: 0.25 mL
  - Intradermal formulation for 18- to 64-year-olds uses a short 30-gauge needle in a single-use prefilled syringe with 0.1 mL vaccine; somewhat higher local reactions when given intradermal
  - Single annual dose except for children <9 years of age, who should receive 2 doses (4 weeks apart) the 1st year they receive influenza vaccine
  - Vaccine contraindication: Severe allergy such as anaphylaxis to IIV components, allergies from eggs are not considered a contraindication; observe all patients for 15 minutes after vaccination; no skin testing with influenza vaccine is needed in egg-allergic patients. RIV is safe in patients with an egg allergy.
  - Precaution: Guillain-Barré syndrome within 6 weeks after a previous dose of influenza vaccine
- LAIV is recommended for 2018 to 2019 influenza season.
- IIV-HD: high-dose quadrivalent IIV
  - Contains 4 times the antigen concentration of IIV
  - Licensed for persons ≥65 years of age
  - Results in higher antibody levels but somewhat higher rates of local reactions
  - Advisory Committee on Immunization Practices does not express a preference for/against IIV-HD.
- Antiviral prophylaxis depends on current resistance patterns each year; see https://www.cdc.gov/flu/ for patterns or check with local health department.
  - In high-risk groups that have not been vaccinated or need additional control measures during epidemics; *not* a substitute for vaccination unless vaccine is contraindicated (1)[A]
  - During influenza season, for those with contraindications to vaccine who have been exposed to the virus (1)[A]
  - For staff and residents in nursing home outbreaks
  - For immune-deficient persons who are expected not to respond to vaccination after viral exposure

Pediatric Considerations
- Vaccinate children 6 months and older annually.
- Recommend all household members with children <6 months be vaccinated (2)[A].
- For children who need 2 doses, administer first dose as soon as available for second dose to be given before the end of October (2)[A].

- For prophylaxis, oseltamivir dosage varies by weight and is recommended by the CDC for prophylaxis for children ≥3 months; zanamivir is approved for prophylaxis for children ≥5 years of age at a dosage of 2 inhalations per day. Prophylaxis treatment duration is 7 days. For prophylaxis, the dosage of amantadine and of rimantadine is 5 mg/kg/day up to 150 mg in 2 divided doses. Currently, amantadine and rimantadine are not recommended due to resistance.

Pregnancy Considerations
- The CDC recommends vaccinating all women who will be pregnant during influenza season.
- If unvaccinated at the time of flu season, pregnant women should receive IIV or RIV.
- Oseltamivir, zanamivir, peramivir, rimantadine, and amantadine are pregnancy Category C.

COMMONLY ASSOCIATED CONDITIONS
Bacterial pneumonia

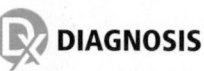 DIAGNOSIS

Look for:
- Systemic symptoms
- Cough
- Not being able to cope with daily activities
- Being confined to bed

HISTORY
Sudden onset of:
- Fever (37.7–40.0°C), especially within 3 days of illness onset
- Anorexia
- Chills, sweats, malaise, myalgia, arthralgia
- Headache
- Sore throat/pharyngitis
- Nonproductive cough
- Rhinorrhea, nasal congestion

PHYSICAL EXAM
- Physical exam is not specific for influenza.
- Physical examination should exclude complications such as otitis media, pneumonia, sinusitis, and tracheobronchitis.

DIFFERENTIAL DIAGNOSIS
- Respiratory viral infections including respiratory syncytial virus, parainfluenza, adenovirus, enterovirus ("influenza-like illness")
- Infectious mononucleosis
- Coxsackievirus infections
- Viral or streptococcal tonsillitis
- Atypical mycoplasmal pneumonia
- *Chlamydia pneumoniae*
- Q fever
- Less likely possibilities include severe acute respiratory syndrome, primary HIV infection, acute myeloid leukemia, tuberculosis, anthrax, and malaria.

DIAGNOSTIC TESTS & INTERPRETATION
Initial Tests (lab, imaging)
- During influenza season, diagnosis is based solely on clinical findings. If additional testing is needed:
  - Viral culture is gold standard for diagnosis but is of limited practical value due to the time it takes for results to become available.
  - Reverse transcription polymerase chain reaction (RT-PCR) from nasopharyngeal swab or aspirate is the test of choice for diagnostic confirmation.
  - CBC: typically shows normal WBC count or mild leukopenia. Leukocytosis may indicate bacterial complications.
  - Direct fluorescent antibody or indirect fluorescent antibody staining for influenza antigen; results available in hours (dependent on lab expertise)
  - Commercial rapid enzyme-linked immunosorbent assay antigen tests are available. Some rapid tests diagnose influenza A, others diagnose A and B. Sensitivity and specificity vary by manufacturer, strain of influenza, and age of patient. False-negative results are common, particularly during peak influenza activity.
  - Viral isolation is not useful except during periods of low influenza activity (if making the correct diagnosis is critical).
- Imaging
  - Chest x-ray if pneumonia is suspected

TREATMENT

- Symptomatic treatment (saline nasal spray, analgesic gargle, antipyretics, analgesics)
- Cool-mist or ultrasonic humidifier to increase moisture of inspired air
- Droplet precautions: See https://www.cdc.gov/HAI/settings/outpatient/basic-infection-control-prevention-plan-2011/transmission-based-precautions.html#c.
- 5 days is the average period of viral shedding in immunocompetent hosts.
- Hospitalized patients may require oxygen or ventilatory support.
- Tobacco cessation

MEDICATION
- Antiviral treatment depends on yearly resistance patterns; check https://www.cdc.gov/flu/ or with local health department. Antivirals are most effective if administered within first 48 hours in laboratory-confirmed (or highly suspected based on clinical findings) influenza cases.
- Antivirals within 48 hours of symptom onset are recommended for patients at risk of complications (i.e., diabetes, CHD, COPD, asthma, etc.) (1)[A].
- Antivirals are recommended if hospitalized (3)[A].
- Antivirals include baloxavir, oseltamivir, zanamivir, and peramivir. Amantadine and rimantadine *currently are not recommended due to resistance*.
- Consider antivirals for patients whose onset of symptoms is within the past 48 hours and who wish to shorten the duration of illness and further reduce their relatively low risk of complications (1)[A].
- Symptomatic treatment is preferred for those patients *without risk factors* and *without* signs of lower respiratory tract infection (3)[A].

- Effect is 24-hour reduction of symptoms and a reduction in complication rates.
  - Baloxavir dose: oral, 1-time dose
    - 40 to <80 kg, 40 mg
    - >80 kg, 80 mg
    - For children >12 years, use adult dosing.
  - Zanamivir dose: 2 inhalations BID for 5 days (age ≥7 years)
  - Oseltamivir dose: 75 mg PO BID for 5 days (age ≥13 years)
  - If severe renal impairment, 75 mg/day PO
  - Oseltamivir for children ≥1 year of age
    - <15 kg, 30 mg BID
    - >15 to 23 kg, 45 mg BID
    - >23 to 40 kg, 60 mg BID
    - >40 kg, 75 mg BID
  - Oseltamivir for children <1 year of age: 3 mg/kg/dose BID
  - Peramivir dose: 600 mg IV infusion over 15 to 30 minutes for adults ≥18 years of age
- Antipyretics
  - Acetaminophen: in children
- Precautions
  - Zanamivir may cause bronchospasm if the patient has COPD or asthma; the patient should have a bronchodilator available.
  - Amantadine has anticholinergic properties and should be used with caution in those with psychiatric, addiction, or neurologic disorders because it may increase risk for suicide attempts or increase neurologic symptoms.
  - Rimantadine may increase the risk of seizures in those with an underlying seizure disorder.
  - Oseltamivir may cause nausea and vomiting; may be less severe if taken with food
  - Peramivir may cause serious skin reactions.
- Decrease dose of certain antivirals if creatinine clearance <60 mL/min.
- Ibuprofen or other NSAIDs for symptomatic relief
- Aspirin: should not be used in children <16 years due to risk of Reye syndrome
- Outpatient treatment is sufficient except for cases with severe complications or in high-risk groups.

ONGOING CARE

FOLLOW-UP RECOMMENDATIONS
- Mild cases: Usually, no follow-up is required.
- Moderate or severe cases: Follow up until symptoms and any secondary sequelae resolve.

DIET
Increase fluid intake.

PATIENT EDUCATION
CDC: https://www.cdc.gov/flu/

PROGNOSIS
Good

COMPLICATIONS
- Otitis media; acute sinusitis
- Croup; bronchitis
- Pneumonia (primary viral or secondary bacterial)

- Apnea in neonates
- Reye syndrome
- Rhabdomyolysis/myositis
- Postinfluenza asthenia
- COPD or CHF exacerbation
- Encephalopathy, death

Geriatric Considerations
Complications requiring hospitalization are more likely in elderly patients.

REFERENCES
1. Centers for Disease Control and Prevention. Influenza antiviral medications: summary for clinicians. https://www.cdc.gov/flu/professionals/antivirals/summary-clinicians.htm. Accessed November 30, 2018.
2. Grohskopf LA, Sokolow LZ, Broder KR, et al. Prevention and control of seasonal influenza with vaccines: recommendations of the advisory committee on immunization practices—United States, 2018–19 influenza season. *MMWR Recomm Rep.* 2018;67(3):1–20.
3. Harper SA, Bradley JS, Englund JA, et al. Seasonal influenza in adults and children—diagnosis, treatment, chemoprophylaxis, and institutional outbreak management: clinical practice guidelines of the Infectious Diseases Society of America. *Clin Infect Dis.* 2009;48(8):1003–1032.

ADDITIONAL READING
Centers for Disease Control and Prevention. Influenza (flu). https://www.cdc.gov/flu/index.htm. Accessed November 30, 2018.

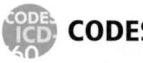

CODES

ICD10
- J11.1 Influenza due to unidentified influenza virus with other respiratory manifestations
- J10.1 Flu due to oth ident influenza virus w oth resp manifest
- J11.00 Flu due to unidentified flu virus w unsp type of pneumonia

CLINICAL PEARLS
- Influenza is an acute, (typically) self-limited, febrile infection caused by influenza virus types A and B.
- With rare exceptions, all persons >6 months should be vaccinated against influenza on an annual basis.
- Complications from influenza are most common in the very young, very old, and individuals with comorbid disease.
- Hand hygiene either with soap and water (slightly superior) or with alcohol-based hand rubs and covering coughs are simple ways to reduce the spread of influenza.

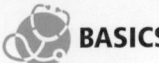

INGROWN TOENAIL

Sally-Ann L. Pantin, MD, FAAFP • Thomas A. Waller, MD

BASICS

DESCRIPTION
- In an ingrown toenail, the distal margin of the nail plate grows into the lateral nail fold, causing irritation, inflammation, and sometimes bacterial or fungal infection:
  - Stage 1 (inflammation): erythema, edema, tenderness to palpation of lateral nail fold
  - Stage 2 (abscess): increased pain, erythema, and edema as well as drainage (purulent or serous)
  - Stage 3 (granulation): Chronic inflammation leads to further erythema, edema, and pain, often with granulation tissue growing over the nail plate and significant nail fold hypertrophy.
- Can reoccur
- Synonym(s): onychocryptosis, unguis incarnatus

EPIDEMIOLOGY
- Great toenail is most often affected.
- Lateral edge of nail is more commonly affected than the medial edge.
- Most common in males aged 14 to 25 years
- Infrequent, but more often in elderly females than in elderly males
- More common in those with lower incomes

Prevalence
- 24.5/1,000 overall
- 50/1,000 ≥65 years

ETIOLOGY AND PATHOPHYSIOLOGY
- Nail plate penetrates the nail fold, causing a foreign body reaction (inflammation).
- Bacteria or fungi may enter through the opening in the nail fold, causing infection and abscess formation.
- The inflamed and infected area leads to granulation tissue and hypertrophy of the nail fold.

RISK FACTORS
- Genetic factors
  - Increased nail fold width
  - Decreased nail thickness
  - Medial rotation of the toe
- Many others proposed; none proven, including the following:
  - Distorted, thickened nail (onychogryphosis)
  - Fungal infection (onychomycosis)
  - Hyperhidrosis
  - Improper trimming of the lateral nail plate
  - Poorly fitting shoes
  - Trauma to nail or nail fold
  - Conditions that predispose to pedal edema (i.e., thyroid dysfunction, diabetes, obesity, heart failure, renal disease)

GENERAL PREVENTION
- Properly fitting shoes
- Proper nail trimming (see "Patient Education")

DIAGNOSIS

HISTORY
- Patients most often present with pain, redness, and swelling in the toe along one or both sides of the nail.
- Drainage can occur as inflammation and/or infection develop.

PHYSICAL EXAM
- Nail fold tenderness
- Erythema and edema
- Drainage (serous or purulent)
- Granulation tissue
- Lateral nail fold hypertrophy

DIFFERENTIAL DIAGNOSIS
- Cellulitis
- Felon (pulp abscess on plantar aspect of toe)
- Onychogryphosis (gross thickening and hardening of the nail)
- Onycholysis (separation of nail from nail bed)
- Onychomycosis (fungal infection of the nail)
- Osteomyelitis
- Paronychia (infection or inflammation around the nail fold)
- Subungual exostosis (bony projection from distal phalanx)
- Subungual osteochondroma (benign bone tumor)

DIAGNOSTIC TESTS & INTERPRETATION
Initial Tests (lab, imaging)
None usually needed
- Consider MRI, x-ray, or bone scan if osteomyelitis is suspected.
- Consider x-ray if subungual exostosis or osteochondroma is suspected.

TREATMENT

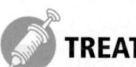

GENERAL MEASURES
- Majority of cases respond to conservative therapy.
- Warm, soapy water or Epsom salt soaks for 10 to 20 minutes 3 times per day until symptoms resolve (1)
- Bluntly insert a cotton wisp or dental floss underneath the ingrown portion of the nail. The patient can continue to replace the insert until the nail grows beyond the fold.

- Use tape to pull the lateral nail fold away from the nail plate until the nail grows beyond the fold.
- Stage 2 ingrown nails often respond to conservative treatment, as above, especially cotton wool, or a trial of cryotherapy.

MEDICATION
- NSAIDs are usually adequate for analgesia.
- Topical antibiotic can be applied after soaking (1).
- Neither oral nor topical antibiotics are useful as an adjunct to surgical treatment.

SURGERY/OTHER PROCEDURES
- Surgical interventions are more effective than nonsurgical interventions in preventing recurrence (2,3)[A].
- Nail avulsion techniques are more effective than nail fold debulking techniques (not described in this topic) (3)[A].
  - Partial avulsion of the nail with phenol nail matrix ablation
    - Obtain surgical consent after explaining the risks, benefits, and alternatives.
    - Achieve local anesthesia with a digital wing or ring block.
    - May consider placing a tourniquet around the base of the toe to assist with hemostasis (caution in patients with diabetes or peripheral vascular disease)
    - Elevate the ingrown part of the nail from the nail bed with a periosteal (Freer) elevator or hemostat.
    - Incise the nail longitudinally with scissors or a nail splitter a few millimeters from the ingrown border, starting at the distal edge and proceeding to the matrix.
    - Grasp, down to the cuticle, the avulsed fragment with a hemostat and pull this portion gently out with a hemostat, utilizing longitudinal traction, as well as rotation to the lateral nail fold if needed.
    - Remove the tourniquet once hemostasis is attained.
    - Dip a urethral swab in 80–88% phenol solution (phenol use is contraindicated in pregnancy).
    - Apply the phenol 3 times for 30 seconds to the nail matrix under the proximal nail fold. Wash the area with 70% isopropyl (rubbing) alcohol to neutralize phenol.
- Nonsurgical interventions, such as a flexible gutter splint, are another option for treatment of stage 2 or 3 ingrown nails (4,5)[B].
  - J Flexible gutter splint
    - Cut a 1- to 2-cm long piece of sterilized plastic tube, such as IV tubing, 2 to 3 mm in diameter (alternatively, you may use a cap from a 29-gauge needle).

- ○ Make a slit in the tubing lengthwise and cut the end off at an angle.
- ○ Apply local anesthesia with a digital wing or ring block.
- ○ Release the ingrown edge of the nail from the nail fold with a hemostat.
- ○ Slide the tube, angled end first, along the ingrown edge of the nail.
- ○ Consider fixing the tube in place with self-curing formable acrylic resin (used for dentures and sculptured nails), tape, or a single suture through the nail plate.
- ○ Leave the tube in place until nail has grown beyond the nail fold.
- Bilateral partial matricectomy should be considered in patients with severe ingrown toenail or recurrence.
- Permanent destruction of the germinal matrix can be used to prevent recurrence. The use of phenol for nail bed ablation is probably more effective than nail avulsion alone in preventing recurrence (2,3)[A].
  - Other options for nail bed ablation:
    - ○ Sodium hydroxide (NaOH)
    - ○ Cryotherapy
    - ○ Electrocautery with a special flattened tip coated with Teflon on one side to protect the proximal nail fold
    - ○ Carbon dioxide laser
    - ○ Surgical excision of the nail matrix

ONGOING CARE

FOLLOW-UP RECOMMENDATIONS

- Dress with antibiotic ointment or sterile petroleum jelly; cover with sterile gauze and tube gauze.
- Postop instructions should include the following:
  - Rest and elevate the foot for 12 to 24 hours.
  - Take NSAIDs for discomfort.
  - Change dressing and wash with soap and water at least daily for 1 to 2 weeks following procedure.
  - Expect a sterile exudate for 2 to 6 weeks.
  - Avulsed nails may take 6 to 12 months to grow completely out (if no matrix ablation).
  - Call for increasing pain, redness, or swelling.
  - Average time to return to normal activities is 2 weeks.
- Patients treated conservatively should be followed up in the office every 7 to 10 days until marked improvement is noted.

PATIENT EDUCATION

- Trim nails straight across perpendicular to long axis of the nail (do not round corners) and not too short.
- Wear properly fitting, comfortable shoes.

COMPLICATIONS

- Cellulitis after surgical procedure (uncommon)
- Damage to fascia or periosteum from overly aggressive matrix ablation
- Damage to nail bed
- Distal toe ischemia due to prolonged use of a tourniquet during surgery (rare)
- Nail plate deformity (due to nail matrix damage)
- Osteomyelitis (rare)
- Permanent narrowing of nail (if partial matrix ablation is performed)
- Persistent postoperative wound drainage particularly with excessive phenolization of adjacent tissues
- Recurrence (40–80% with avulsion alone, 0.6–14% with matrix ablation, 6–13% with gutter splint)

REFERENCES

1. Heidelbaugh J, Lee H. Management of the ingrown toenail. *Am Fam Physician*. 2009;79(4):303–308.
2. Eekhof JA, Van Wijk B, Knuistingh Neven A, et al. Interventions for ingrowing toenails. *Cochrane Database Syst Rev*. 2012;(4):CD001541.
3. Park DH, Singh D. The management of ingrowing toenails. *BMJ*. 2012;344:e2089.
4. Arai H, Arai T, Nakajima H, et al. Formable acrylic treatment for ingrowing nail with gutter splint and sculptured nail. *Int J Dermatol*. 2004;43(10):759–765.
5. Nazari S. A simple and practical method in treatment of ingrown nails: splinting by flexible tube. *J Eur Acad Dermatol Venereol*. 2006;20(10):1302–1306.

ADDITIONAL READING

- Bos AM, van Tilburg MW, van Sorge AA, et al. Randomized clinical trial of surgical technique and local antibiotics for ingrowing toenail. *Br J Surg*. 2007;94(3):292–296.
- Bryant A, Knox A. Ingrown toenails: the role of the GP. *Aust Fam Physician*. 2015;44(3):102–105.

- Chapeskie H. Ingrown toenail or overgrown toe skin? Alternative treatment for onychocryptosis. *Can Fam Physician*. 2008;54(11):1561–1562.
- Reyzelman AM, Trombello KA, Vayser DJ, et al. Are antibiotics necessary in the treatment of locally infected ingrown toenails? *Arch Fam Med*. 2000;9(9):930–932.
- Richert B. Basic nail surgery. *Dermatol Clin*. 2006;24(3):313–322.
- Woo SH, Kim IH. Surgical pearl: nail edge separation with dental floss for ingrown toenails. *J Am Acad Dermatol*. 2004;50(6):939–940.

 SEE ALSO

For a video of this Nail Avulsion and Matrixectomy procedure, go to http://5minuteconsult.com/procedure/1508006.

 CODES

ICD10
L60.0 Ingrowing nail

CLINICAL PEARLS

- The best treatment for a stage 1 ingrown toenail is to insert a wisp of cotton or dental floss between the nail plate and lateral nail fold.
- The best treatment for a stage 3 ingrown toenail is partial nail avulsion with phenol matrix ablation.
- Patients can prevent ingrown toenails by trimming nails properly and wearing properly fitting shoes.
- Oral and topical antibiotics are not useful in the treatment of ingrown nails in conjunction with surgical treatment.

INJURY AND VIOLENCE

Jonathan R. Ballard, MD, MPH, MPhil • Tisha K. Johnson, MD, MPH

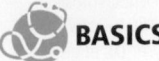 **BASICS**

DESCRIPTION

- Injury, intentional or not, is often predictable and preventable.
- Unintentional injuries are no longer considered "accidents" given that most injuries are preventable.
- As of 2016, unintentional injury is the 4th leading cause of death, and intentional self-harm is the 10th leading cause of death in the United States.
- Injury is the leading cause of death of people aged 1 to 44 years and a leading cause of disability for people of all ages, regardless of sex, race/ethnicity, or socioeconomic status.
- Violence-related deaths accounted for 55,693 deaths in the United States in 2016 (74% suicide, 26% homicide).

EPIDEMIOLOGY

Incidence

Leading Cause of Death by Age Group, United States, 2016

Age	Most Common	Number of Deaths
<1 y	Congenital anomalies	4,816
1–44 y	Unintentional injury	61,749
45–64 y	Malignant neoplasm	157,655
≥65 y	Heart disease	507,118

Source: Centers for Disease Control and Prevention (CDC) Web-based Injury Statistics Query and Reporting System (WISQARS)

- Children mostly die of unintentional injuries: motor vehicle accidents (MVAs), drowning, fire/burn, and suffocation.
- MVAs are the most common type of unintentional injury deaths in adolescents, followed by poisoning deaths.

ALERT

Poisoning, which includes drug overdose, has been the leading cause of injury deaths in the United States overall since 2011 and is particularly deadly for persons ages 15 to 64 years, as the leading cause of injury deaths among 25 to 64 years and the second leading cause of unintentional injury deaths for 15 to 24 years.

- Approximately 5.8 million people worldwide die yearly secondary to injuries, of which all forms of violence combine to cause nearly 1/3 of these deaths (World Health Organization [WHO]).
- Unintentional motor vehicle traffic deaths rank second in the United States for overall injury deaths, first in those aged 5 to 24 years and second in those aged 1 to 4 years and 25 to >65 years.
- Among leading causes of injury deaths in the United States, firearms (related suicide and homicide deaths combined) rank third overall.
- Homicide is the third leading cause of death in 2016 for persons 15 to 34 years in the United States.

ALERT

Consider homicide as cause of unexplained death in young children.

ETIOLOGY AND PATHOPHYSIOLOGY

Multifactorial

RISK FACTORS

- MVAs:
  – MVAs accounted for 40,528 deaths in 2016 with an age-adjusted rate of 12.2 deaths per 100,000 persons.
  – >2.5 million adult drivers and passengers were treated in emergency departments (EDs) in 2015.
  – Young adults (20 to 24 years old) have the highest crash-related injury rates.
  – In the United States, 1 in 3 deaths involved drunk driving and almost 1 in 3 deaths involved implicated speeding.
  – Motorcyclists are more likely to die in a motor vehicle crash than car occupants. The risk of death is reduced by 37% with helmets.
  – Risk factors for involvement in an MVA include high speed, teenage drivers, consumption of alcohol or drugs affecting the central nervous system, fatigue, and distracted driving (handheld mobile phones and inadequate visibility).
  – Increased risk of death by MVA: male driver, inexperience, nighttime driving, speeding, tailgating, driving with other teenagers, cell phone use, unrestrained occupants, use of older cars, nonuse of crash helmets, alcohol, and drug use. In elderly, poor vision, medical conditions, and comorbidities increase risk of death by an MVA (CDC, National Center for Injury Prevention and Control [NCIPC], and WHO).
- Pedestrians:
  – 5,376 pedestrians were killed by motor vehicles and nearly 129,000 were treated in EDs for nonfatal injuries (2015; CDC, NCIPC).
- Bicycles (WHO):
  – Risk of death from crash with motor vehicle increases if speed >30 km/hr (~18 mph) and if there is impact with front of vehicle.
  – Risk factors for cyclist injury include alcohol consumption, shared use motorways, poor visibility, lack of understanding of road safety, and design/type of impacting vehicle.
- Sports- and recreation-related injury (CDC):
  – >2.6 million children (0 to 19 years) treated in EDs each year; males, deconditioned adults, and athletes playing collision or contact sports are at also increased risk.
- Drowning: a leading cause of unintentional injury death among all children, particularly 1 to 4 years of age; children at increased risk include African Americans and those unattended in bathtubs, swimming pools, and recreational water activities (CDC, NCIPC).
- Suffocation: increased risk for children <1 year, unsafe sleeping environments (CDC)
- Falls (CDC, NCIPC):
  – The leading cause of nonfatal injuries and most common cause of traumatic brain injuries (TBIs)
  – Poor vision, psychotropic medications and diuretics, arthritis, impaired mobility, inappropriate footwear and walking aids, cognitive impairment, gait imbalance, environmental risk factors (1)
- **Violence**: risk factors: adverse childhood exposures (ACEs); lack of access to social capital, community organization, and economic resources; familial instability; community and family violence; access to firearms; mental health; personal or household member alcohol and drug use; exposure to suicidal behavior; history of aggressive behavior; cognitive deficits; poor supervision; poor peer-to-peer interaction; academic failure; poverty; lower socioeconomic class (CDC)
- Homicide: third leading cause of death for persons aged 15 to 34 years in the United States (CDC). Most common victims are young males. Firearms are used in more than half of U.S. homicides.
- Suicide: Females are more likely to have suicidal thoughts, but males are 4 times more likely to complete suicide. Most common methods are firearms for males and poisoning for females (CDC, NCIPC).
- Adolescent violence (CDC):
  – In 2015, nearly 8% of students participated in ≥1 fights at school in the last year.
  – >5% of high schoolers reported not going to school on ≥1 day(s) in the last 30 days because they felt unsafe at school or on their way to school.
  – 4% of students have carried a weapon to school; 6% of students have been threatened or injured by a weapon at school.
- Bullying (CDC):
  – 20% of 9th- to 12th-grade students bullied on school property in the last year
  – 15% of students report cyberbullying.
  – Bullying is associated with social, emotional, and academic difficulties.
- Interpersonal and intimate partner violence (IPV):
  – WHO reports about 38% of female homicides were killed by partners, similar to CDC reports of 40% of female homicide victims.
  – In their lifetime, approximately 8.5 million women and >4 million men report physical violence, rape, or stalking from an intimate partner many before the age of 18 years (CDC).
  – Dating violence: Of high school students who dated in the previous 12 months, 12% of girls and 7% of boys experienced physical violence, and 16% of girls and 5% of boys experienced sexual violence (CDC).
  – Increased risk for female, history of IPV or sexual assault or child abuse, alcohol or drugs, marital difficulties, unemployment, emotional or mental health problems, income or educational disparity, poverty

ALERT

Poisonings (CDC):

- The United States' epidemic of drug overdoses (poisonings) includes more than half a million deaths from 2000 to 2015, mainly from opioids (>6 out of 10, ~91 deaths per day).
- Since 1999, prescription opioids sold in the United States have almost quadrupled, and deaths from prescription opioids have more than quadrupled.
- >33,000 people died from opioid overdoses in 2015; a 15% increase in opioid-death rates from 2014 to 2015 is likely due to illicit opioids, including synthetic opioids (72%) such as fentanyl and fentanyl analogs and heroin (20%).
- Overlapping prescriptions of pain relievers or other sedating drugs; high doses, history of mental illness or substance abuse, uninsured or Medicaid, low income increase risk for overdose deaths.
- Consider opioid-induced poisonings in unexplained altered mental status.

DIAGNOSIS

HISTORY

- Mechanism, timing, and location of injury:
  - Blunt versus penetrating; intentional versus unintentional; others injured versus isolated injury; circumstances (weather, substance use, restrained vs. unrestrained)
  - Does history correlates with level of injury (i.e., level of suspicion for abuse [elderly, child, or partner])?
  - Is further evaluation required (blood and/or urine testing, response to opioid receptor antagonists, imaging)?
- IPV: neurologic deficits, seizures, chronic pain, GI, STI, pregnancy, psychiatric presentations
  - Screen women of childbearing age for IPV and intervene if screening results are positive.

 TREATMENT

- Prevention: The primary focus for reducing injury and violence is individually tailored prevention based on risk factors combined with population-level prevention (2). The "three Es": education, engineering strategies, and enforcement of laws (2). The "Haddon Matrix" describes injury events in terms of three influencing factors (host, agent/vector, environment) and three phases (preevent, event, postevent) (1,2).
- Primary (i.e., prevent crash), secondary (i.e., prevent injury from crash), and tertiary (i.e., prevent poor outcomes from injury) prevention (1,2)[C]
- Acute setting: Follow basic life support (BLS), advanced trauma life support (ATLS), advanced cardiovascular life support (ACLS), and pediatric advanced life support (PALS) guidelines (2,3)[A].
- Motor vehicle injuries (CDC):
  - Infants, toddlers, and children: age-appropriate child safety seats and passenger restraints with distribution programs, education programs for parents and caregivers, safety seat checkpoints, penalties for drivers transporting children under the influence of drugs and/or alcohol, legislation regarding restraint of motor vehicle occupants (1)[A]
  - Adolescents and adults: seat belts, air bags, graduated driver licensing programs, blood alcohol concentration laws, minimum drinking age laws, sobriety checkpoints, ignition interlocks, programs for alcohol servers, zero-alcohol tolerance laws for young drivers, school-based education programs on drinking and driving. Emergency medical services (EMS) response times, engineering cars for rapid extraction, organized trauma systems; collapsible automobile steering columns have been shown to decrease injury mortality and morbidity; texting and driving penalties (1)[B]
  - Older adults: alternative transportation programs, screening for high-risk drivers, gradual curtailment of driving privileges, more frequent license renewal process (1)[B]
  - Bicycle helmets can reduce risk of head injury by 63–88%. Canadian helmet legislation decreased mortality by 52% (1)[B].
  - Pedestrian injury: pedestrian safety education, reflective clothing, use of crosswalks, limit mobile phone use while crossing roads (1)[B], street lighting for pedestrians (1)[A], fluorescent clothing for pedestrians and cyclists (1)[A]
  - Cyclists injury: flashing lights and reflectors at night (2)[B], helmet use and laws (1)[A], cyclists separation for motor vehicles (1)[B]

- Sports-related injuries:
  - Proper equipment: Helmets can prevent bicyclist head injuries and mortality (1)[A].
  - Plan of action for dealing with concussion and head injury in young athletes, with guidelines regarding if or when it is safe to return to play (CDC)[A]
- Drowning:
  - Improved supervision of young children, especially for those with epilepsy; swimming lessons; trained lifeguard supervision; fencing; locked gates and pool alarms; no use of alcohol in recreation aquatic activities; personal flotation devices and boating safety awareness; parental and caregiver certification in CPR (1)[B]
- Falls:
  - Home safety assessments, installation of handrails and grab bars, removal of tripping hazards, nonslip mats, exercise programs such as tai chi to improve strength and balance, night lights, cataract surgery, gradual withdrawal of psychotropic medication (1)[B]
  - In April 2018, USPSTF recommends exercise interventions to prevent falls in community-dwelling adults aged 65 years or older who are at increased risk for falls (4)[B].
- Violence (homicide, suicide, assaults) (CDC):
  - Primary prevention: Most effective strategies focus on younger age groups to change individual attitudes and behaviors (1)[C].
  - Secondary prevention: Detect and identify violence in early stages (1)[B]. The USPSTF recommends that clinicians screen women of childbearing age for IPV, such as domestic violence, and provide or refer women who screen positive to intervention services (4)[B].
  - Tertiary prevention: IPV reduced by alcoholism treatment for partner; intense advocacy interventions of >12 hours (1)[A]
  - Suicide: access to mental health services, improved family and community support, development of healthy coping and problem-solving skills (CDC)[B]
  - USPSTF recommends screening adults for depression when depression care supports are in place to assure accurate diagnosis, effective treatment, and follow-up (4)[B].
  - Dating violence: self-reported dating violence reduced by school- and community-based programs for prevention of dating violence (1)[A]

ALERT

Poisonings (CDC): In response to the opioid epidemic, the *CDC Guideline for Prescribing Opioids for Chronic Pain—United States, March 2016* was released to **improve prescribing practices**, to aid in early identification of those at high risk for addiction, and to prevent opiate and heroin addiction and deaths.

- Prevent and treat opioid abuse: prescription drug monitoring programs; state prescription drug laws; insurance strategies (prior authorization, quantity limits, drug utilization review); prescribing practice quality improvement programs; substance abuse counseling and medication-assisted treatment.
- In April 2018, the U.S. Surgeon General issued an advisory emphasizing the importance of the overdose-reversing drug naloxone.
- *Consider use of* naloxone *to counter the effects of opioid overdose.*
- *Multiple doses of* naloxone *may be required because the duration of many opioids is greater than that of* naloxone.
- Follow acute care guidelines and call 911; may contact Poison Control Center hotline after discovered ingestion of toxin for recommendations (5)[A]

 ONGOING CARE

COMPLICATIONS

Social burden of injury: loss of productivity, emotional loss, nonmedical expenditures, reduced quality of life, litigation, rehabilitation, mental health costs, altered family and peer relationships, chronic pain, substance use and abuse, changes in lifestyle (1,CDC)

REFERENCES

1. Curry P, Ramaiah R, Vavilala MS. Current trends and update on injury prevention. *Int J Crit Illn Inj Sci*. 2011;1(1):57–65.
2. Sleet DA, Dahlberg LL, Basavaraju SV, et al; for Centers for Disease Control and Prevention. Injury prevention, violence prevention, and trauma care: building the scientific base. *MMWR Suppl*. 2011;60(4):78–85.
3. Neumar RW, Shuster M, Callaway CW, et al. Part 1: executive summary: 2015 American Heart Association guidelines update for cardiopulmonary resuscitation and emergency cardiovascular care. *Circulation*. 2015;132(18 Suppl 2): S315–S367.
4. U.S. Preventive Services Task Force. Recommendations for primary care practice. https://www.uspreventiveservicestaskforce.org /Page/Name/recommendations. Accessed July 20, 2018.
5. Mowry JB, Spyker DA, Brooks DE, et al. 2015 Annual report of the American Association of Poison Control Centers' National Poison Data System (NPDS): 33rd annual report. *Clin Toxicol (Phila)*. 2016;54(10):924–1109.

ADDITIONAL READING

- CDC WISQARS (Web-based Injury Statistics Query and Reporting System): https://www.cdc.gov/injury /wisqars
- National Center for Injury Prevention and Control: https://www.cdc.gov/injury
- The Surgeon General's Report on Alcohol, Drugs, and Health: https://addiction.surgeongeneral.gov/
- WHO Violence and Injury Prevention: http://www .who.int/violence_injury_prevention

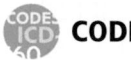 CODES

ICD10

- T14.90 Injury, unspecified
- T14.8 Other injury of unspecified body region
- R29.6 Repeated falls

CLINICAL PEARLS

- Injury and violence are predictable and preventable.
- Unintentional injury is a leading cause of death in the United States.
- Injury is the primary source of lost years of productive life for individuals age <44 years.
- MVAs cause most deaths in children and adolescents.
- Opioid overdose is increasing as a serious cause of unintentional injury and death.

INSOMNIA

Susanne Wild, MD

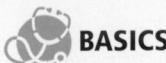 BASICS

DESCRIPTION
- Difficulty initiating or maintaining sleep or nonrestorative sleep despite adequate opportunity and circumstances for sleep
- Causes at least one of the following forms of daytime impairment related to nighttime sleep difficulty:
  - Fatigue or malaise
  - Attention, concentration, or memory impairment
  - Social or vocational dysfunction or poor school performance
  - Mood disturbance or irritability
  - Daytime sleepiness
  - Motivation, energy, or initiative reduction
  - Proneness for errors or accidents at work or while driving
  - Tension, headaches, or GI symptoms in response to sleep loss
  - Concerns or worries about sleep

EPIDEMIOLOGY
- Predominant age: increases with age
- Predominant sex: female > male (5:1)

Prevalence
- Insomnia (transient and chronic): 5–35% of the population; 10–15% associated with daytime impairment
- Chronic insomnia: 10% middle-aged adults; 1/3 of people >65 years

ETIOLOGY AND PATHOPHYSIOLOGY
- Transient/intermittent (<30 days)
  - Stress/excitement/bereavement
  - Shift work
  - Medical illness
  - High altitude
- Chronic (>30 days)
  - Medical: gastroesophageal reflux disease, sleep apnea, chronic pain, congestive heart failure, Alzheimer disease, Parkinson disease, chronic fatigue syndrome, irritable bowel syndrome
  - Psychiatric: mood, anxiety, psychotic disorders
  - Primary sleep disorder: idiopathic, psychophysiologic (heightened arousal and learned sleep-preventing associations), paradoxical (sleep state misperception)
  - Circadian rhythm disorder: irregular pattern, jet lag, delayed/advanced sleep phase, shift work
  - Environmental: light (liquid crystal display [LCD] clocks), noise (snoring, household, traffic), movements (partner/young children/pets)
  - Behavioral: poor sleep hygiene, adjustment sleep disorder
  - Substance induced
  - Medications: antihypertensives, antidepressants, corticosteroids, levodopa-carbidopa, phenytoin, quinidine, theophylline, thyroid hormones

Pregnancy Considerations
Transient insomnia occurs secondary to change of sleep position, nocturia, gastritis, back pain, and anxiety.

RISK FACTORS
- Age
- Female gender
- Medical comorbidities
- Unemployment
- Psychiatric illness
- Impaired social relationships
- Lower socioeconomic status
- Shift work
- Separation from spouse or partner
- Drug and substance abuse

GENERAL PREVENTION
- Practice consistent sleep hygiene:
  - Fixed wake-up times and bedtimes regardless of amount of sleep obtained (weekdays and weekends)
  - Go to bed only when sleepy.
  - Avoid naps.
  - Sleep in a cool, dark, quiet environment.
  - No activities or stimuli in bedroom associated with anything but sleep or sex
  - 30-minute wind-down time before sleep
  - If unable to sleep within 20 minutes, move to another environment and engage in quiet activity until sleepy.
- Limit caffeine intake to mornings.
- No alcohol after 4 PM
- Fixed eating times
- Avoid medications that interfere with sleep.
- Regular moderate exercise

COMMONLY ASSOCIATED CONDITIONS
- Psychiatric disorders
- Painful musculoskeletal conditions
- Obstructive sleep apnea
- Restless leg syndrome
- Drug or alcohol addiction/dependence

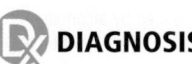 DIAGNOSIS

HISTORY
- Daytime sleepiness and napping
- Unintended sleep episodes (driving, working)
- Insomnia history
  - Duration, time of problem
  - Sleep latency, difficulty in maintaining sleep (repeated awakening), early morning awakening, nonrestorative sleep, or patterns (weekday vs. weekend, with or without bed partner, home vs. away)
- Sleep hygiene
  - Bedtime/wakening time
  - Physical environment of sleep area: LED clocks, TV, room lighting, ambient noise
  - Activity: nighttime eating, exercise, sexual activity
  - Intake: caffeine, alcohol, herbal supplements, diet pills, illicit drugs, prescriptions, over-the-counter (OTC) sleep aids
- Symptoms or history of depression, anxiety, obsessive-compulsive disorder, or other major psychological symptomatology
- Symptoms of restless leg syndrome and periodic limb movement disorder
- Symptoms of heightened arousal
- Snoring and other symptoms of sleep apnea
- Symptoms or history of drug or alcohol abuse
- Current medication use
- Chronic medical conditions
- Acute change or stressors such as travel or shift work
- Sleep diary: sleep log for 7 consecutive days

DIFFERENTIAL DIAGNOSIS
- Sleep-disordered breathing such as obstructive sleep apnea
- CNS hypersomnias (e.g., narcolepsy)
- Circadian rhythm sleep disturbances
- Sleep-related movement disorders (e.g., restless leg syndrome)
- Substance abuse
- Insomnia due to medical or neurologic disorder
- Mood and anxiety disorders such as depression or anxiety

DIAGNOSTIC TESTS & INTERPRETATION
- Diagnostic testing usually not required; consider polysomnography if sleep apnea or periodic limb movement disorder is suspected (1)[C].
- Primary insomnia
  - Symptoms for at least 1 month: difficulty in initiating/maintaining sleep or nonrestorative sleep
  - Impairment in social, occupational, or other important areas of functioning
  - Does not occur exclusively during narcolepsy, breathing-related sleep disorder, circadian rhythm sleep disorder, or parasomnia
  - Does not occur exclusively during major depressive disorder, generalized anxiety disorder, delirium
  - Is not secondary to physiologic effects of substance or general medical condition
  - Sleep disturbance (or resultant daytime fatigue) causes clinically significant distress.
- Secondary insomnia
  - Due to substance abuse, medication induced (diuretics, stimulants, etc.), primary depressive disorder, generalized anxiety disorder or phobias, acute situational stress, posttraumatic stress disorder, pain

Initial Tests (lab, imaging)
Testing to consider based on history and physical exam:
- Thyroid-stimulating hormone
- Urine toxicology

Diagnostic Procedures/Other
Polysomnography or multiple sleep latency test not routinely indicated but may be considered if
- Initial diagnosis is uncertain.
- Treatment interventions have proven unsuccessful.

TREATMENT

- Transient insomnia
  - May use medications for short-term use only; hypnotic sedatives favored
  - Self-medicating with alcohol can increase awakenings and sleep-stage changes.
- Chronic insomnia
  - Treatment of underlying condition (major depressive disorder, generalized anxiety disorder, medications, pain, substance abuse)
  - Advise good sleep hygiene.
  - Cognitive-behavioral therapy is first-line treatment for chronic insomnia, especially in >60 years population, especially when sedatives are not advantageous (2)[A].
  - Behavioral therapy is an effective treatment for insomnia and a potentially more effective long-term treatment than pharmacotherapy (3)[B].
  - Ramelteon is the only agent without abuse potential (4)[B].

MEDICATION

- Reserved for transient insomnia such as with jet lag, stress reactions, transient medical condition
- Nonbenzodiazepine hypnotics
  - Act on benzodiazepine receptor, so have abuse potential
    - Zaleplon (Sonata) 5 to 20 mg; half-life 1 hour
    - Zolpidem (Ambien) 5 to 10 mg (males); 5 mg (females); half-life 2.5 to 3.0 hours
    - Zolpidem (Ambien CR) 6.25 to 12.50 mg (males); 6.25 mg (females); half-life 2.5 to 3.0 hours
    - Eszopiclone (Lunesta) 1 to 3 mg; half-life 6 hours
- Benzodiazepine hypnotics
  - Short acting
    - Triazolam (Halcion) 0.25 mg; half-life 1.5 to 5.5 hours
  - Intermediate acting
    - Temazepam (Restoril) 7.5 to 30.0 mg; half-life 8.8 hours
    - Estazolam (Prosom) 1 to 2 mg; half-life 10 to 24 hours
  - Long acting
    - Flurazepam (Dalmane) 15 to 30 mg; half-life 40 to 100 hours
    - Quazepam (Doral) 7.5 to 15.0 mg; half-life 39 hours (parent drug), 73 hours (active metabolite)
- Contraindications/precautions are as follows:
  - Not indicated for long-term treatment due to risks of tolerance, dependency, daytime attention and concentration compromise, incoordination, rebound insomnia
  - Long-acting benzodiazepines associated with higher incidence of daytime sedation and motor impairment
  - Avoid in elderly, pregnant, breastfeeding, substance abusers, and patients with suicidal or parasuicidal behaviors.
  - Avoid in patients with untreated obstructive apnea and chronic pulmonary disease.
  - No good evidence for benzodiazepines for patients undergoing palliative care (4)[A]
  - Nonbenzodiazepine receptor agonists may occasionally induce parasomnias (sleepwalking, sleep eating, sleep driving)
- Melatonin receptor agonist
  - Ramelteon (Rozerem) 8 mg; half-life 1.0 to 2.6 hours
    - Recommended as first-line pharmacologic treatment option per AASM consensus
    - Effective to reduce sleep time onset for short- and long-term use in adults, without abuse potential; no comparative studies with older agents have been completed. Onset of effect may take up to 3 weeks.
- Sedating antidepressants
  - Doxepin (Silenor) 10 to 50 mg; half-life 15 hours
    - Only antidepressant with FDA approval for insomnia
    - New formulation of medication is available at dosage 3 to 6 mg QHS.
  - Trazodone (Oleptro) 25 to 200 mg; half-life 3 to 9 hours
  - Mirtazapine (Remeron) 7.5 to 15.0 mg; half-life 20 to 40 hours
  - Amitriptyline (Elavil) 25 to 100 mg; half-life 10 to 26 hours
- Orexin receptor agonists
  - Suvorexant (Belsomra) 10 to 20 mg; half-life 12 hours

- Sedating antihistamines are not recommended and should be used conservatively for insomnia due to insufficient evidence of efficacy and significant concerns about risks of these medications.
- Evidence for use of antipsychotics is weak. They should only be prescribed if the patient has a concurrent psychiatric diagnosis warranting their use.

Geriatric Considerations

Caution (risk of falls and confusion) when prescribing benzodiazepines or other sedative hypnotics; if absolutely necessary, use short-acting nonbenzodiazepine agonists at half the dosage or melatonin agonists for short-term treatment.

ADDITIONAL THERAPIES

Associated with hypertension, congestive heart failure, anxiety and depression, and obesity; management of these chronic conditions will help with incidence and symptoms of insomnia.

COMPLEMENTARY & ALTERNATIVE MEDICINE

- Melatonin: decreases sleep latency when taken 30 to 120 minutes prior to bedtime, but there is no good evidence for efficacy in insomnia, and long-term effects are unknown (5)[B]
- Valerian: Inconsistent evidence supporting efficacy and its slow onset of action (2 to 3 weeks) makes it unsuitable for the acute treatment of insomnia.
- Acupuncture: insufficient evidence on effect of needle acupuncture and its variants
- Antihistamines: insufficient evidence; should not be recommended for use
- Cognitive-behavioral therapy (including relaxation therapy): effective and considered more useful than medications; recommended initial treatment for patients with chronic insomnia; no improvement of efficacy when combined with medication
- Mindfulness awareness practices: improved sleep quality and sleep-related daytime impairment for older adults per small randomized trial

 ONGOING CARE

FOLLOW-UP RECOMMENDATIONS

- Daily exercise improves quality of sleep and may be more effective than medication.
- Avoid exercise within 4 hours of bedtime.

Patient Monitoring

- Reassess need for medications periodically; avoid standing prescriptions.
- Caution patients that nonbenzodiazepine agonists (zolpidem, zaleplon, eszopiclone), as well as benzodiazepines, can be habit forming.
- Studies suggest an association between receiving a hypnotic prescription and a >3-fold increase in hazards of death, even when prescribed <18 pills per year (6)[B].

DIET

- Avoid caffeine or reserve for morning only.
- Avoid heavy late-night snacks (light snack at bedtime may help).
- Avoid alcohol within 6 hours of bedtime.

PROGNOSIS

- Situational insomnia should resolve with time.
- Treatment of underlying etiology and consistent sleep hygiene are the mainstays of treatment.

COMPLICATIONS

- Transient insomnia can become chronic.
- Daytime sleepiness, cognitive dysfunction
- Pulmonary hypertension if chronic sleep apnea left untreated
- Sleep apnea may lead to hypertension, stroke, or cardiac ischemia.

REFERENCES

1. Kushida CA, Littner MR, Morgenthaler T, et al. Practice parameters for the indications for polysomnography and related procedures: an update for 2005. *Sleep*. 2005;28(4):499–521.
2. Montgomery P, Dennis J. Cognitive behavioural interventions for sleep problems in adults aged 60+. *Cochrane Database Syst Rev*. 2003;(1):CD003161.
3. Ebben MR, Spielman AJ. Non-pharmacological treatments for insomnia. *J Behav Med*. 2009;32(3):244–254.
4. Hirst A, Sloan R. Benzodiazepines and related drugs for insomnia in palliative care. *Cochrane Database Syst Rev*. 2002;(4):CD003346.
5. Verster GC. Melatonin and its agonists, circadian rhythms and psychiatry. *Afr J Psychiatry (Johannesbg)*. 2009;12(1):42–46.
6. Kripke DF, Langer RD, Kline LE. Hypnotics' association with mortality or cancer: a matched cohort study. *BMJ Open*. 2012;2(1):e000850.

ADDITIONAL READING

Glass J, Lanctôt KL, Herrmann N, et al. Sedative hypnotics in older people with insomnia: meta-analysis of risks and benefits. *BMJ*. 2005;331(7526):1169.

 SEE ALSO

- Anxiety (Generalized Anxiety Disorder); Depression; Fibromyalgia; Sleep Apnea, Obstructive
- Algorithms: Anxiety; Insomnia, Chronic; Restless Legs Syndrome

CODES

ICD10

- G47.00 Insomnia, unspecified
- F51.02 Adjustment insomnia
- F51.01 Primary insomnia

CLINICAL PEARLS

- Treatment of underlying etiology of the insomnia and consistent sleep hygiene are key.
- Most medications are indicated for short-term use only.
- Sedative hypnotics are not recommended in the elderly because risks may outweigh benefits.
- Patients with chronic insomnia benefit from sleep hygiene education and cognitive-behavioral therapy.

INTELLECTUAL DISABILITY (INTELLECTUAL DEVELOPMENTAL DISORDER)

Jennifer L. Ayres, PhD

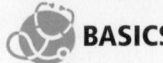 BASICS

- A global deficit in cognitive functioning evidenced by a significant difference in mental and chronologic ages (IQ) and significantly impaired adaptive functioning (1)
- The term "*mental retardation*" was deleted from the *DSM-5* and replaced with "intellectual disability" (ID) or "intellectual developmental disorder." The term "mental retardation" is pejorative and insensitive and should be avoided.
- Although cognitive issues typically have a pervasive impact, patients with ID display highly variable levels of functioning and subsequent service needs.
- Tailor evaluation and treatment to individual needs.

DESCRIPTION
- ID is defined as an IQ ≤70 + 5 and a significant impairment in intellectual functioning. This include verbal and nonverbal reasoning, planning, academic learning, problem solving, and experiential learning. Intellectual function is confirmed by IQ testing and clinical assessment (1).
- A diagnosis of ID also requires deficits in adaptive functioning, such as communication, socialization, and independent living (1).
- By definition, ID is a neurodevelopmental disorder that is typically present from birth or recognized during early childhood because developmental milestones are delayed (1).
- ID is currently subgrouped according to adaptive function and level of needed support: *mild* (typical development in some domains, mild impairment in others), *moderate* (skills are markedly behind typically developing, same-age peers), *severe* (skills quite limited compared to peers), *profound* (limited awareness of concepts, language; dependent on others for adaptive functioning) (1).
- The three most common causes of ID are Down syndrome, fragile X syndrome, and fetal alcohol syndrome (FAS).
- If ID reflects a loss of previously acquired intellectual skills, consider a comorbid neurocognitive disorder.
- Stereotypes of people with ID (e.g., always happy, poor prognosis, unable to function independently) have been categorically refuted. People with ID show levels of functional variability that parallels the non-ID population.
- Under the Individuals with Disabilities Education Act (IDEA), caregivers should familiarize themselves with their child's legal rights to facilitate coordination of services with the school district.
- Under the Americans with Disabilities Act (1990), people with ID cannot be discriminated against based on their disability, and employers are legally required to ensure that appropriate accommodations are in place.

ALERT
For some causes of ID, prenatal testing is available.

EPIDEMIOLOGY
Incidence
- 1 of 6 children (2)
- Predominant sex: male > female: 1.6:1 for mild ID, 1.2:1 for severe ID (1)

Prevalence
In the United States, 1% of the general population. The prevalence of severe ID is 6/1,000 (1).

ETIOLOGY AND PATHOPHYSIOLOGY
- Causes:
  - Maternal substance abuse (e.g., alcohol); FAS is a leading environmental cause of ID.
  - Maternal infections: TORCH viruses (toxoplasma, other infections, rubella, cytomegalovirus, and herpes simplex virus)
  - Down syndrome
  - Sex chromosome abnormalities: fragile X, Turner syndrome, Klinefelter syndrome
  - Autosomal dominant conditions: neurocutaneous syndromes (e.g., neurofibromatosis, tuberous sclerosis)
  - Autosomal recessive conditions:
    ○ Amino acid metabolism (e.g., phenylketonuria, maple syrup urine disease)
    ○ Carbohydrate metabolism (e.g., galactosemia, fructosuria)
    ○ Lipid metabolism
    ○ Tay-Sachs disease
    ○ Gaucher disease
    ○ Niemann-Pick disease; mucopolysaccharidosis
    ○ Purine metabolism (e.g., Lesch-Nyhan disease)
    ○ Other (e.g., Wilson disease)
- Maternal medications (e.g., isotretinoin, Dilantin)
- Perinatal factors:
  - Prematurity
  - Birth injuries
  - Perinatal anoxia
- Postnatal factors:
  - Childhood diseases (e.g., meningitis, encephalitis, hypothyroidism, seizure disorders)
  - Trauma (e.g., accidents, physical abuse, hypoxia)
  - Severe deprivation
  - Poisoning (e.g., lead, carbon monoxide, household products)

Genetics
A number of genetic and epigenetic causes are known, and more are under investigation.

RISK FACTORS
- Maternal substance abuse during pregnancy
- Maternal infection during pregnancy
- For some causes, family history

GENERAL PREVENTION
- Reduce alcohol and drug use by pregnant women.
- Prenatal folic acid supplementation

COMMONLY ASSOCIATED CONDITIONS
- Seizures
- Mood disorders
- Behavioral disorders
- Constipation

 DIAGNOSIS

The diagnosis of ID requires a thorough assessment conducted by an appropriately credentialed mental health professional who is formally trained and licensed to conduct appropriate psychodiagnostic testing.

HISTORY
- Children with profound/severe ID are typically diagnosed at birth or during the newborn period. They may have pathognomonic dysmorphic features.
- Children with ID are often identified because they fail to meet motor/language milestones.

PHYSICAL EXAM
Certain morphologic features suggest a specific etiology for ID (e.g., microcephaly).

DIFFERENTIAL DIAGNOSIS
- Auditory, visual, and/or speech/language impairment
- Autism spectrum disorder (language and social skills are more affected than other cognitive abilities); however, 75% of individuals with an autistic disorder may meet criteria for a comorbid diagnosis of ID.
- Expressive/receptive language disorders
- Cerebral palsy
- Brain tumors
- Emotional/behavioral disturbance
- Learning disorders (reading, math, written expression)
- Auditory/sensory processing difficulties
- Lack of environmental opportunities for appropriate development

DIAGNOSTIC TESTS & INTERPRETATION
- Visual and hearing tests to rule these out as the cause of impairment and to provide an assessment of visual and auditory functioning (often impaired in children and adults with ID)
- Formal testing of intellectual and adaptive functioning:
  - A child's communication skills must be considered in test selection. For example, a patient with auditory processing issues/limited expressive/receptive language skills may need to be assessed using a nonverbal IQ test, such as the Leiter-R, *Test of Nonverbal Intelligence*, or other nonverbal measures.
  - Commonly used intelligence tests (e.g., Bayley Scales of Infant Development, Stanford-Binet Intelligence Scale, Wechsler Intelligence Scales) are determined by age/developmental level.
  - Common tests of adaptive functioning include the *Vineland Adaptive Behavior Scales, 2nd ed.* and *Adaptive Behavior Assessment System, 2nd ed.* These tests assess areas of functioning such as age-appropriate communication, social skills, activities of daily living, and motor skills.
- Metabolic screening as indicated by history and physical exam or if no newborn screening was previously performed (3).

Initial Tests (lab, imaging)

- Lead levels (3)[B]
- Thyroid-stimulating hormone if systemic features are present or no newborn screening was done (3)[B]
- Routine cytogenetic testing (karyotype) (3)[B]:
  - Fragile X screening (FMR1 gene), particularly with a family history of ID
  - Rett syndrome (MECP2 gene) in women with unexplained moderate to severe ID (3)
- Molecular screening (e.g., array comparative genomic hybridization) is increasing in use.
- Neuroimaging (MRI more sensitive than CT) is routinely recommended. The presence of physical findings (microcephaly, focal motor deficit) increase yield (3)[B].
- MRI may show mild cerebral abnormalities but is unlikely to establish etiology of ID.

Follow-Up Tests & Special Considerations

Electroencephalography is not routinely used unless a specific epileptiform diagnosis is present (3)[C].

 ## TREATMENT

- Tailor early intervention services to individual needs.
- Caregiver support, including:
  - Train caregiver(s) to address behavioral issues, discipline, and social development.
  - Encourage caregivers to create a structured home environment based on the child's developmental level and specific needs rather than routine age-appropriate expectations.
  - Offer caregiver(s) an opportunity to address their reactions to the diagnosis and their child's special needs.
  - Inform caregivers about advocacy groups and available resources (4).
  - Encourage caregiver(s) to seek social support to increase their own overall sense of well-being.
  - Encourage caregivers to intermittently seek respite care to promote self-care.
- Individualized education plans, social skills, and behavioral plans/training
- Refer to job training programs and independent living opportunities, if appropriate.
- Note changes in behavior, which may be indicative of pain/illness, particularly in individuals with limited communication skills.
- Assess for abuse and neglect.

MEDICATION

Medication may be appropriate for comorbid conditions (e.g., anxiety, ADHD, depression).

 ## ONGOING CARE

Match provider communication of procedures, results, and treatment recommendations to patient level of cognitive functioning and receptive language skills.

- Most patients with mild ID are fully capable of understanding information when provided at the appropriate level.
- Provide oral and written explanations directly to the patient instead of solely to caregivers. Respect patient dignity at all times. Provide honest information, respond to patient's questions with respect, and do not infantilize the patient due to the ID.

FOLLOW-UP RECOMMENDATIONS

Link to community-based resources for job training, independent living, caregiver support, school-based services

Patient Monitoring

- A quality of life assessment provides information about a patient's general sense of well-being and life satisfaction. Quality of life may be difficult to assess when significant behavioral issues confound an individual's self-report and socialization.
- Vision testing at least once before age 40 years (age 30 years in Down syndrome) and every 2 years thereafter
- Hearing evaluations every 5 years after age 45 years (every 3 years throughout life in Down syndrome)
- Screen for sexual activity and offer contraception and testing for STIs as appropriate.
- Screen annually for abuse and neglect, more frequently if behavior change is noted. Report abuse/neglect to appropriate protective agencies.
- Dysphagia and aspiration are common; consider speech pathology evaluation and swallowing study.

DIET

No restrictions, except in cases of metabolic and storage disorders (e.g., phenylketonuria)

PATIENT EDUCATION

- The Arc: www.thearc.org
- American Association on Intellectual and Developmental Disabilities: www.aaidd.org
- Family support groups (Parent to Parent, Local Down Syndrome, or Autism Association)
- Special Olympics: www.specialolympics.org

PROGNOSIS

- Although ID is a lifelong diagnosis, most individuals with ID are capable of fulfilling, purposeful lives that include career, independent living, participating in a committed relationship, and becoming a parent.
- The level of severity and support needed may vary over the course of the individual's life.

COMPLICATIONS

- Constipation is a commonly overlooked problem and can lead to significant morbidity.
- Polypharmacy, often associated with psychotropic medication use to control behaviors, should be addressed to minimize adverse side effects.

REFERENCES

1. American Psychiatric Association. *Diagnostic and Statistical Manual of Mental Disorders*. 5th ed. Arlington, VA: American Psychiatric Association; 2013.
2. Centers for Disease Control and Prevention. Developmental disabilities. http://www.cdc.gov/ncbddd/developmentaldisabilities/index.html. Accessed November 11, 2018.
3. Shevell M, Ashwal S, Donley D, et al. Practice parameter: evaluation of the child with global developmental delay: report of the Quality Standards Subcommittee of the American Academy of Neurology and the Practice Committee of the Child Neurology Society. *Neurology*. 2003;60(3):367–380.
4. Shogren KA, Bradley VJ, Gomez SC, et al. Public policy and the enhancement of desired outcomes for persons with intellectual disability. *Intellect Dev Disabil*. 2009;47(4):307–319.

ADDITIONAL READING

- Kripke C. Adults with developmental disabilities: a comprehensive approach to medical care. *Am Fam Physician*. 2018;97(10): 649–656.
- Ratti V, Hassiotis A, Crabtree J, et al. The effectiveness of person-centred planning for people with intellectual disabilities: a systematic review. *Res Dev Disabil*. 2016;57:63–84.

 ## CODES

ICD10

- F79 Unspecified intellectual disabilities
- F70 Mild intellectual disabilities
- F71 Moderate intellectual disabilities

CLINICAL PEARLS

- "Mental retardation" is an insensitive and disrespectful term that should not be used. ID or intellectual developmental disorder is preferred.
- Multiple factors (including appropriateness of school placement/special education services, exposure to early intervention, behavioral therapy, parent training, self-esteem, and social skills) influence overall functional ability for individuals with ID.
- Children with developmental disabilities are at higher risk of abuse.
- The diagnosis of ID should be confirmed through psychodiagnostic testing by an appropriately licensed professional.

I

INTERSTITIAL CYSTITIS

Sarah R. Hollis, MD • Montiel T. Rosenthal, MD

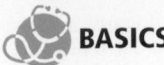

BASICS

DESCRIPTION
- A condition of pain or discomfort in the bladder associated with a need to urinate frequently and urgently
- A disease of unknown cause, probably representing a final common pathway from several etiologies
- Likely, pathogenesis is disruption of urothelium, impaired lower urinary tract defenses, and loss of bladder muscular wall elasticity. The symptoms in many patients are insidious, and the disease progresses for years before diagnosis is established.
- Newer research implicates urine and serum inflammatory proteins antiproliferative factor, epidermal growth factor, heparin-binding epidermal growth factor, glycosaminoglycans, and bladder nitric oxide as contributing factors.
- Mild: normal bladder capacity under anesthesia; ulceration, cracking, or glomerulation of mucosa (or not) with bladder distention under anesthesia; no incontinence symptoms wax and wane and may not progress. Interstitial cystitis is a bladder sensory problem.
- Severe: progressive bladder fibrosis; small true bladder capacity under anesthesia; poor bladder wall compliance. In 5–10% of cases, Hunner ulcers present at cystoscopy; may have overflow incontinence and/or chronic bacteriuria unresponsive to antibiotics
- When examined under scanning electron microscope, patients with painful bladder syndrome/interstitial cystitis were found to have defects of umbrella cell integrity of which the severity of damage coincided with severity of symptoms.
- System(s) affected: renal/urologic
- Synonym(s): urgency frequency syndrome; IC/bladder pain syndrome

Pregnancy Considerations
Unpredictable symptom improvement or exacerbation during pregnancy; no known fetal effects from interstitial cystitis; usual problems of unknown effect on fetus with medications taken during pregnancy

EPIDEMIOLOGY
- Occurs predominantly among whites
- Predominant sex: female > male (10:1)
- Patients <30 years have predominant symptoms: dysuria, frequency, urinary urgency, pain in external genitals, and dyspareunia, and those >60 years more commonly have nocturia, urinary incontinence, or Hunner ulcer disease.
- Predominant age
  - Mild: 20 to 40 years
  - Severe: 20 to 70 years

Pediatric Considerations
- <10 years old and again at 13 to 17 years
- Daytime enuresis, dysuria without infection

Prevalence
In the United States:
- Up to 1 million affected, but many cases likely are unreported
- 0.052% but may be higher up to 10%

ETIOLOGY AND PATHOPHYSIOLOGY
- Unknown but is not primarily psychosomatic
- Possible causes
  - Subclinical urinary infection
  - Damage to glycosaminoglycan mucus layer increasing bladder wall permeability to irritants such as urea
  - Autoimmune
  - Mast cell histamine release
- Neurologic upregulation/stimulation

RISK FACTORS
Unknown

COMMONLY ASSOCIATED CONDITIONS
- Fibromyalgia
- Allergies
- Chronic fatigue syndrome
- Depression
- Vulvodynia
- Sexual dysfunction
- Sleep disturbance
- Migraines
- Syncope
- Dyspepsia
- Chronic prostatitis
- Chronic pelvic pain
- Irritable bowel syndrome
- Anal/rectal disease

DIAGNOSIS

- Frequent, urgent, relentless urination day and night; >8 voids in 24 hours
- Pain with full bladder that resolves with bladder emptying (except if bacteriuria is present)
- Urge urinary incontinence if bladder capacity is small
- Sleep disturbance
- Dyspareunia, especially with full bladder
- Secondary symptoms from chronic pain and sleeplessness, especially depression

HISTORY
- Pelvic Pain and Urgency/Frequency patient symptom scale: self-reporting questionnaire for screening potential interstitial cystitis patients (http://www.wgcaobgyn.com/files/urgency_frequency_pt_symptom_scale.pdf)
- Frequent UTIs, vaginitis, or symptoms during the week before menses
- O'Leary/Sant Voiding and Pain Indices (http://www.ichelp.org/wp-content/uploads/2015/06/OLeary_Sant.pdf)

PHYSICAL EXAM
- Perineal/prostatic pain in men
- Anterior vaginal wall pain in women

DIFFERENTIAL DIAGNOSIS
- Uninhibited bladder (urgency, frequency, urge incontinence, less pain, symptoms usually decrease when asleep)
- Urinary infection: cystitis, prostatitis

- Bladder neoplasm
- Bladder stone
- Neurologic bladder disease
- Nonurinary pelvic disease (STIs, endometriosis, pelvic relaxation)

DIAGNOSTIC TESTS & INTERPRETATION
Initial Tests (lab, imaging)
- Urinalysis: normal except with chronic bacteriuria (rare)
- Urine culture from catheterized specimen: normal except with chronic bacteriuria (rare) or partial antibiotic treatment
- Urine cytology
  - Normal: reserve for men >40 years old and women with hematuria

Diagnostic Procedures/Other
- Cystoscopy (especially in men >40 years old or women with hematuria)
  - Bladder wall visualization
  - *Hydraulic distention: no improved diagnostic certainty over history and physical alone*
  - No role for urodynamic testing
- Intravesical lidocaine can help to pinpoint the bladder as the source of pain in patients with pelvic pain; this can be both diagnostic and therapeutic.
- Potassium sensitivity test
  - *Insert catheter, empty bladder, instill 40 mL H_2O over 2 to 3 minutes, rank urgency on scale of 0 to 5 in intensity, rank pain on scale of 0 to 5 in intensity, drain bladder, instill 40 mL potassium chloride (KCl) 0.4 mol/L solution.*
  - *If immediate pain, flush bladder with 60 mL H_2O and treat with bladder instillations.*
    - *If no immediate pain, wait for 5 minutes and rate the urgency and pain.*
- If urgency or pain >2, treat as above.
- Pain or urgency >2 is considered a positive test and strongly correlates with interstitial cystitis if no radiation cystitis or acute bacterial cystitis is present.

Test Interpretation
- Nonspecific chronic inflammation on bladder biopsies
- Urine cytology negative for dysplasia and neoplasia
- Possible mast cell proliferation in mucosa

TREATMENT

GENERAL MEASURES
- Appropriate health care: outpatient
- Self-care (Eliminate foods and liquids that exacerbate symptoms on individual basis, fluid management.) (1)[C]
- Biofeedback bladder retraining (1)[C]

MEDICATION
- Randomized controlled trials of most medications for interstitial cystitis demonstrate limited benefit over placebo; there are no clear predictors of what will benefit an individual. Prepare the patient that treatment may involve trial and error.

- Behavioral therapy combined with oral agents found improved outcomes compared to medications alone.
- Intravesical injections of botulinum toxin are not effective in the treatment of ulcer-type interstitial cystitis.

First Line
- Note: AUA consensus states medicines should be considered second-line therapy after patient education, pain management, general relaxation, stress reduction, behavior modification, and self-care (1)[C].
- Pentosan polysulfate (Elmiron) 100 mg TID on empty stomach; may take several months (3 to 6) to become effective; rated as modestly beneficial in systematic drug review (only FDA-approved treatment for interstitial cystitis)
- Amitriptyline: most effective at higher doses (≥50 mg/day); however, initiate with lower doses to minimize side effects (2)[B].
- Hydroxyzine 25 to 50 mg HS
- Sildenafil 25 mg/day (3)[B]
- Cimetidine 400 mg BID (3)[C]
- Triple-drug therapy: 6 months of pentosan, hydroxyzine, doxepin
- Antibacterials for bacteriuria
- Oxybutynin, hyoscyamine, tolterodine, and other anticholinergic medications decrease frequency.
- Prednisone (only for ulcerative lesions)
- Montelukast has shown some benefit.
- NSAIDs for pain and any inflammatory component
- Bladder instillations
  - Lidocaine, sodium bicarbonate, *and* heparin *or* pentosan polysulfate sodium
  - *Dimethyl sulfoxide (DMSO) every 1 to 2 weeks for 3 to 6 weeks and then PRN*
  - Heparin *sometimes added to DMSO*
  - *Intravesical liposomes*
  - *Other agents: steroids,* silver nitrate, *oxychlorosene (Clorpactin)*
  - Contraindication
  - *No anticholinergics for patients with close-angle glaucoma*
  - Significant possible interaction
  - *Refer to manufacturer's profile of each drug.*

Second Line
- Cystoscopy under anesthesia with hydrodistention (3)[B]
- Treatment of Hunner lesions if found

Third Line
- Phenazopyridine, a local bladder mucosal anesthetic, usually is not very effective.
- Intravesicular injection of botulinum type A for nonulcer interstitial cystitis

Fourth Line
- Cyclosporin A (1)[C]
- Hyaluronic acid instillations (4)[C]
- Chondroitin sulfate instillations (single or in combination with hyaluronic acid) have shown mixed results (4)[C].

ISSUES FOR REFERRAL
- Need for clarity with respect to diagnosis
- Surgical intervention

ADDITIONAL THERAPIES
Myofascial physical therapy (targeted pelvic, hip girdle, abdominal trigger point massage) (5)[B]

SURGERY/OTHER PROCEDURES
- Hydraulic distention of bladder under anesthesia: symptomatic but transient relief
- Cauterization of bladder ulcer
- Augmentation cystoplasty to increase bladder capacity and decrease pressure with or without partial cystectomy. Expected results in severe cases: much improved, 75%; with residual discomfort, 20%; unchanged, 5%
- Urinary diversion with total cystectomy only if disease is completely refractory to medical therapy
- Sacral neuromodulation
- Transurethral electro- or laser fulguration (effective for Hunner lesions). Pain relief may persist from several months to 2 years (4)[C].

COMPLEMENTARY & ALTERNATIVE MEDICINE
Guided imagery

 ## ONGOING CARE

FOLLOW-UP RECOMMENDATIONS
Patient Monitoring
Not specifically needed unless symptoms are unresponsive to treatment

DIET
- Variable effects from person to person
- Common irritants include caffeine, chocolate, citrus, tomatoes, carbonated beverages, potassium-rich foods, spicy foods, acidic foods, and alcohol.

PATIENT EDUCATION
Interstitial Cystitis Association, 110 Washington St. Suite 340, Rockville, MD 20850; 1-800-HELPICA: http://www.ichelp.org/

PROGNOSIS
- Mild: exacerbations and remissions of symptoms; may not be progressive; does not predispose to other diseases
- Severe: progressive problems that usually require surgery to control symptoms

COMPLICATIONS
Severe, with long-term, continuous high bladder pressure could be associated with renal damage.

REFERENCES

1. Hanno PM, Erickson D, Moldwin R, et al; for American Urological Association. Diagnosis and treatment of interstitial cystitis/bladder pain syndrome: AUA guideline amendment. *J Urol*. 2015;193(5):1545–1553.
2. Foster HE Jr, Hanno PM, Nickel JC, et al; and Interstitial Cystitis Collaborative Research Network. Effect of amitriptyline on symptoms in treatment naïve patients with interstitial cystitis/painful bladder syndrome. *J Urol*. 2010;183(5):1853–1858.
3. Chen H, Wang F, Chen W, et al. Efficacy of daily low-dose sildenafil for treating interstitial cystitis: results of a randomized, double-blind, placebo-controlled trial—treatment of interstitial cystitis/painful bladder syndrome with low-dose sildenafil. *Urology*. 2014;84(1):51–56.
4. Homma Y, Ueda T, Tomoe H, et al. Clinical guidelines for interstitial cystitis and hypersensitive bladder updated in 2015. *Int J Urol*. 2016;23(7):542–549.
5. FitzGerald MP, Payne CK, Lukacz ES, et al; for Interstitial Cystitis Collaborative Research Network. Randomized multicenter clinical trial of myofascial physical therapy in women with interstitial cystitis/painful bladder syndrome and pelvic floor tenderness. *J Urol*. 2012;187(6):2113–2118.

ADDITIONAL READING

Rais-Bahrami S, Friedlander JI, Herati AS, et al. Symptom profile variability of interstitial cystitis/painful bladder syndrome by age. *BJU Int*. 2012;109(9):1356–1359.

 ## SEE ALSO

- Urinary Tract Infection (UTI) in Females
- Algorithm: Pelvic Girdle Pain (Pregnancy or Postpartum Pelvic Pain)

 ## CODES

ICD10
- N30.10 Interstitial cystitis (chronic) without hematuria
- N30.11 Interstitial cystitis (chronic) with hematuria

CLINICAL PEARLS

- The potassium sensitivity test has been the most useful in confirming an initial diagnosis of interstitial cystitis.
- Potassium sensitivity test
  - *Insert catheter, empty bladder, instill 40 mL H_2O over 2 to 3 minutes, rank urgency on scale of 0 to 5 in intensity, rank pain on scale of 0 to 5 in intensity, drain bladder, and instill 40 mL KCl 0.4 mol/L solution.*
  - *Submucosal petechial hemorrhages and/or ulceration at the time of bladder distention and cystoscopy further support the diagnosis.*
- At present, there is no definitive treatment for interstitial cystitis.
- Most patients with severe disease receive multiple treatment approaches. Regular multidisciplinary follow-up, pharmacologic therapy, avoidance of symptom triggers, and psychological and supportive therapy are all important because this disease tends to wax and wane. Monitor patients for comorbid depression.
- Empowering patients to manage their symptoms, communicate regularly with their physicians, and learn as much as they can about this disease, which may help them to optimize their outcome

I

INTERSTITIAL NEPHRITIS

Narothama Reddy Aeddula, MD, FACP, FASN • Samata Pathireddy, MD • Subhasish Bose, MD, FASN

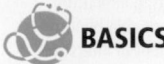

BASICS

DESCRIPTION
- Acute and chronic tubulointerstitial diseases result from the interplay of renal cells and inflammatory cells. Lethal or sublethal injury to renal cells leads to new local antigen expression, inflammatory cell infiltration, and proinflammatory activation and cytokines. Cytokines are produced by macrophages, lymphocytes, and renal cells (i.e., proximal tubule, vascular endothelial cells, interstitial cells, fibroblasts). The outcome is acute interstitial nephritis (AIN) or chronic interstitial nephritis (CIN).
- Central component in AIN is altered tubular function, which precedes decrements in filtration rate.
- AIN presents as acute kidney injury (AKI) after the use of offending drugs or agents (OFA) and is associated with typical findings of proteinuria, hematuria, and white cell casts. Less frequently, AIN is secondary to infections, systemic diseases, and mixed connective tissue disease (MCTD).
- System(s) affected: renal/urologic, endocrine/metabolic, immunologic
- Synonym(s): acute interstitial allergic nephritis

EPIDEMIOLOGY
Pediatric Considerations
- Children with history of lead poisoning are more likely to develop CIN as young adults.
- Tubulointerstitial nephritis with uveitis (TINU) presents in adolescent females with mean age of 15 years.

Incidence
- AIN account for 15–20% of AKI.
- Peak incidence in women 60 to 70 years of age

Geriatric Considerations
Elderly (≥65 years) have severe disease and increased risk of permanent damage given polypharmacy, specifically drug-induced AIN (87% vs. 64%), proton pump inhibitor–induced AIN (18% vs. 6%), but less AIN from autoimmune or systemic causes (7% vs. 27%) than younger adults (1)[B].

ETIOLOGY AND PATHOPHYSIOLOGY
- AIN
  - Delayed drug hypersensitivity reactions
  - Causes AKI
  - Renal dysfunction generally is partially or completely reversible, possibly reflecting the regenerative capacity of tubules with a preserved basement membrane.
  - Hypersensitivity to drugs (75%): not dose dependent. The top three drug causes were omeprazole (12%), amoxicillin (8%), and ciprofloxacin (8%) (2)[C].
    ○ Antibiotics (e.g., penicillins, cephalosporins, sulfonamides, tetracycline, vancomycin, fluoroquinolones, macrolides, TB meds)
    ○ Proton pump inhibitors
    ○ Antivirals (indinavir)
    ○ NSAIDs (all, including Cox-2 inhibitors)
    ○ Diuretics (thiazide, loop, and triamterene)
    ○ Miscellaneous (allopurinol, H₂ blockers, diphenylhydantoin, and 5-aminosalicylates such as sulfasalazine [Azulfidine] and mesalamine)
  - Infections: *Legionella*, *Leptospira*, streptococci, CMV, *Mycobacterium tuberculosis* (5–10%)
  - Autoimmune disorders (e.g., SLE, Sjögren syndrome, sarcoidosis, Wegener granulomatosis, cryoglobulinemia) (10–15%)
  - Toxins (e.g., snake bite venom)

- CIN
  - Follows long-term exposure to OFA (e.g., heavy metals, especially lead)
  - Often found on routine labs or evaluation for hypertension (HTN)
  - Characterized by interstitial scarring, fibrosis, and tubular atrophy, resulting in progressive chronic kidney disease (CKD)

GENERAL PREVENTION
- Early recognition and prompt discontinuation of OFA
- Avoid further nephrotoxic substances.

COMMONLY ASSOCIATED CONDITIONS
CIN
- Chronic pyelonephritis
- Abuse of analgesics
- Lithium use
- Gout and gout therapy
- Immune disorders
- Malignancy (lymphoma, multiple myeloma)
- Amyloidosis
- Exposure to heavy metals (e.g., lead, cadmium)
- Renal papillary necrosis

DIAGNOSIS

- AIN: suspected in a patient with nonspecific signs and symptoms of AKI (e.g., malaise, fever, nausea, vomiting) with an elevated serum creatinine and an abnormal urinalysis
  - AKI
    ○ Elevated creatinine, BUN, and electrolyte abnormalities (e.g., hyperkalemia, low serum bicarbonate)
    ○ Decreased urine output (oliguria in 51%)
    ○ Signs of fluid overload or depletion
  - Signs of systemic allergy (e.g., fever [27%], maculopapular rash [15%], peripheral eosinophilia [23%], arthralgias [45%] but less commonly found when NSAIDs are the OFA)
  - Eosinophilia and eosinophiluria
  - Urine—WBC, RBC, and white cell casts
- CIN
  - HTN
  - Decreased urine output or polyuria
  - Inability to concentrate urine
  - Polydipsia
  - Metabolic acidosis
  - Anemia
  - Fanconi syndrome

HISTORY
- Medications: Onset of AIN following drug exposure ranges from 3 to 5 days (as occurs with a second exposure to an OFA) to as long as several weeks to many months (the latter with NSAIDs, especially) (2).
- Infections: symptoms related to an associated infection or systemic condition
- TINU patients present with interstitial nephritis and uveitis and occasionally systemic findings.
- Exposure to heavy metals
- Postorgan transplant

PHYSICAL EXAM
- Increased BP
- Fluid retention/extremity swelling/weight gain
- Rash accompanying renal findings in acute AIN
- Lung crackles/rales
- Pericardial rub if uremic pericarditis

DIFFERENTIAL DIAGNOSIS
- AKI secondary to other causes:
  - Prerenal (e.g., hypovolemia, shock, sepsis, renal artery emboli)
  - Intrarenal (e.g., acute tubular necrosis, hypertensive nephropathy, DM nephropathy)
  - Postrenal (e.g., obstructive uropathy)
  - Some OFA that cause AIN can produce other forms of AKI as well:
    ○ NSAIDs can exacerbate prerenal disease.
    ○ Aminoglycosides can cause acute tubular necrosis.
- CKD secondary to long-standing HTN, diabetes, and chronic pyelonephritis

DIAGNOSTIC TESTS & INTERPRETATION
Initial Tests (lab, imaging)
- Chemistry
  - Elevated creatinine: seen in all patients, with 40% requiring dialysis
  - Hyperkalemia and acidosis
- CBC
  - Eosinophilia (80%): NSAID-induced AIN is only associated with eosinophilia in ~15% of cases.
  - Anemia
- Urinalysis with urine electrolytes
  - Hematuria (95%)
  - Mild and variable proteinuria: usually <1 g/24 hr, except in AIN associated with NSAIDs where it is higher
  - Urine sediment: WBC, RBC, white cell casts. Red blood cell casts are rare.
  - Eosinophiluria but has no clinical utility specific for AIN (3)[C]
  - Fractional excretion of sodium (FE$_{Na}$ >1%) indicative of tubular damage
  - Normal urinalysis does not rule out AIN.
- CXR to evaluate for pulmonary tuberculosis, sarcoidosis, and infections
- Serologies for immunologic disease (e.g., sarcoidosis, Sjögren syndrome, Wegener granulomatosis, Behçet syndrome) or infectious causes (e.g., histoplasmosis, coccidioidomycosis, toxoplasmosis, EBV)
  - Serum levels of angiotensin-converting enzyme and serum Ca^{++} for sarcoidosis
  - Antinuclear antibody (ANA) and dsDNA to exclude SLE
  - ANCA
  - Urinary *Legionella* antigen
  - C3 and C4 to evaluate for SLE and IgG4-related disease
  - Serum protein electrophoresis
  - Anti-Ro/SSA, anti-La/SSB antibodies, CRP, and rheumatoid factor to exclude Sjögren syndrome
- Liver function tests: elevated serum transaminase levels in patients with associated drug-induced liver injury
- Renal US may demonstrate kidneys that are normal to enlarged in size with increased cortical echogenicity, but no reliable confirmatory US findings for AIN.
- IV pyelography (IVP) and CT scans with contrast are relatively contraindicated given nephrotoxicity and limited diagnostic yield.

Follow-Up Tests & Special Considerations
Patients who do not recover and with CIN should receive follow-up care to protect from further nephrotoxic therapies.

Diagnostic Procedures/Other

- Renal biopsy is the definitive method of establishing the diagnosis of AIN. Should be considered:
  - Patients on an OFA known to cause AIN but have normal urinalysis
  - Patients considered for steroid therapy
  - Patients not on glucocorticoid therapy and do not have recovery following cessation of the OFA
  - Patients with advanced renal failure of recent onset (<3 months)
  - Patients with any features (e.g., high-grade proteinuria) that makes AIN diagnosis uncertain
- Contraindications: Biopsy is contraindicated in bleeding diathesis, solitary kidney, end-stage renal disease (ESRD) with small kidneys, uncontrolled HTN and sepsis, or renal parenchymal infection.

Test Interpretation

- Acute
  - Biopsy shows marked interstitial infiltrate consisting of T lymphocytes and monocytes. Eosinophils, plasma cells, and neutrophils may be found.
  - Tubulitis is found when inflammatory cells invade the tubular basement membrane.
  - Generally, the urinary findings will distinguish AIN from other causes (e.g., acute tubular necrosis, glomerulonephritis).
- Chronic: CIN is characterized by tubular atrophy, fibrosis, and cellular infiltration with mononuclear cells.

TREATMENT

For AIN, data on corticosteroids' efficacy have been limited (4)[B].

GENERAL MEASURES

- Discontinue offending agent including topical NSAIDs.
- Reduce exposure to nephrotoxic agents (e.g., furosemide, aminoglycosides).
- Supportive measures:
  - Maintain adequate hydration.
  - Symptomatic relief for fever and rash
  - Control of BP and anemia
  - Correct acidosis and electrolyte imbalances.
  - Short-term dialysis until renal recovery

MEDICATION

- Mainstay is supportive therapy.
- If patient is on multiple OFA, a reasonable approach is substitution of the suspected drug with another medication.
- If AKI persists after removing OFA, attempt medication therapy.

First Line

- Unknown optimal therapy because no randomized controlled trials (RCTs) or large observational studies
- Immunosuppression if no improvement within 3 to 7 days after OFA discontinuation
- Renal biopsy to confirm AIN and to exclude others or CIN, where immunosuppressive prescription not indicated
- Prednisone 1 mg/kg/day PO or equivalent IV dose to a max of 40 to 60 mg/day for 1 to 2 weeks, beginning a gradual taper after serum creatinine has returned to near baseline for a duration of 2 to 3 months, followed by a gradual taper over 3 to 4 weeks (4)[B]. Complete recovery is noted in 49% and partial in 39% (1)[C].
  - Steroids started within 7 days of withdrawal of OFA more likely to recover than those who started later (odds ratio [OR] 6.6).

Second Line

- Limited experience with treating AIN in patients who are steroid dependent (i.e., relapse during prednisone taper), steroid resistant (as with NSAID-induced disease), or cannot tolerate steroids
- Mycophenolate mofetil may be considered in biopsy-proven AIN patients. Prescription may need to be continued for 1 to 3 years (5).
- Lead toxicity: Chelation may improve function.
  - Succimer 10 mg/kg (max 500 mg) PO q8h for 5 days, then q12h for 14 days, or
  - EDTA 2 g IV/IM; if IM, use with 2% lidocaine.
- SLE nephritis: steroids + cyclophosphamide or azathioprine
- Urate nephropathy: urate-lowering agents
  - Allopurinol starting at 100 mg/day, increasing to 300 mg/day to achieve serum urate level <6 mg/dL
  - Dose need to be adjusted depending on level of renal impairment.
  - Allopurinol itself can be a cause of AIN.
  - Discontinue thiazide.
- Lithium-induced nephritis: Use amiloride as adjunct.
- Indinavir-induced nephritis: Use probenecid as adjunct.

ISSUES FOR REFERRAL

Patients presenting with AKI, proteinuria, and acid-base and/or electrolyte disorders require consultation with a nephrologist.

ADMISSION, INPATIENT, AND NURSING CONSIDERATIONS

Patients with AKI and/or with serious electrolyte or acid-base disorders require hospitalization.

- Admission criteria/initial stabilization
  - Persistent oliguria or anuria
  - Severe acidosis and/or electrolyte abnormalities
  - ECG changes
- Discharge criteria
  - Stable vitals; correction of all electrolyte imbalances and improved eGFR
  - Normal urine production

 # ONGOING CARE

FOLLOW-UP RECOMMENDATIONS

Patient Monitoring

If patients must remain on nephrotoxic agents, measure renal function, electrolytes, and phosphorus frequently.

DIET

- Low potassium (<2 g/day)
- Low sodium
- Low protein

PATIENT EDUCATION

Printed materials for patients are available at the National Kidney Disease Education Program, (866) 4-KIDNEY, http://www.niddk.nih.gov/health-information/health-communication-programs/nkdep/Pages/default.aspx.

PROGNOSIS

- If AIN is detected early (within 1 week of the rise in serum creatinine) and the OFA is discontinued promptly, the long-term outcome is favorable; however, it is often incomplete with persistent serum creatinine noted in up to 40% of patients, especially in NSAID-induced AIN.
- Renal biopsy reveals extent of damage.

- AIN
  - Recovery within weeks to months
  - Acute dialysis is needed for 1/3 of patients before resolution.
  - Progresses to ESRD in 10% patients
- CIN: can progress to ESRD
  - Renal disease may remit in 1 year if untreated.
  - TINU has relapsing course, requiring systemic corticosteroids.
- Untreated severe AKI has 45–70% mortality.
- AIN prognosis in sarcoidosis or infection is not well described.

COMPLICATIONS

- Chronic tubulointerstitial disease may progress to ESRD, requiring dialysis or transplantation.
- Analgesics increase the risk of transitional cell cancers of the uroepithelium.

REFERENCES

1. Muriithi AK, Leung N, Valeri AM, et al. Clinical characteristics, causes and outcomes of acute interstitial nephritis in the elderly. *Kidney Int*. 2015;87(2):458–464.
2. Muriithi AK, Leung N, Valeri AM, et al. Biopsy-proven acute interstitial nephritis, 1993–2011: a case series. *Am J Kidney Dis*. 2014;64(4):558–566.
3. Muriithi AK, Nasr SH, Leung N. Utility of urine eosinophils in the diagnosis of acute interstitial nephritis. *Clin J Am Soc Nephrol*. 2013;8(11):1857–1862.
4. Clarkson MR, Giblin L, O'Connell FP, et al. Acute interstitial nephritis: clinical features and response to corticosteroid therapy. *Nephrol Dial Transplant*. 2004;19(11):2778–2783.
5. Preddie DC, Markowitz GS, Radhakrishnan J, et al. Mycophenolate mofetil for the treatment of interstitial nephritis. *Clin J Am Soc Nephrol*. 2006;1(4):718–722.

ADDITIONAL READING

- Fouque D, Laville M. Low protein diets for chronic kidney disease in non diabetic adults. *Cochrane Database Syst Rev*. 2009;(3):CD001892.
- Raghavan R, Eknoyan G. Acute interstitial nephritis—a reappraisal and update. *Clin Nephrol*. 2014;82(3):149–162.

CODES

ICD10

- N12 Tubulo-interstitial nephritis, not spcf as acute or chronic
- N10 Acute tubulo-interstitial nephritis
- N11.9 Chronic tubulo-interstitial nephritis, unspecified

CLINICAL PEARLS

- First step in treatment is to remove OFA.
- Most common OFA in elderly is proton pump inhibitors and antibiotics.
- A renal biopsy is preferred to confirm AIN.
- Immunosuppressive therapy is employed if no subsequent improvement within 3 to 7 days after discontinuation of OFA.

IRRITABLE BOWEL SYNDROME

Naureen Rafiq, MBBS

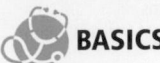 **BASICS**

DESCRIPTION
- A gastrointestinal disorder characterized by
  - Chronic and/or recurrent abdominal pain or discomfort and alteration in bowel habits
- May be characterized as diarrhea-predominant or constipation-predominant; may alternate between
- Synonym(s): spastic colon; irritable colon

EPIDEMIOLOGY
Irritable bowel syndrome (IBS) accounts for up to 50% of visits to gastroenterologists:
- Second only to upper respiratory infection as cause of lost workdays

Prevalence
Pooled estimate of 11% IBS prevalence internationally; ranges from South Asia (7%) to South America (21%) (1)
- Predominant age: 20 to 39 years
- If age >50 years, consider other diagnoses.
- Predominant sex: in the United States, female > male (2:1)
- More common in low socioeconomic communities

ETIOLOGY AND PATHOPHYSIOLOGY
- The etiology is unknown; associated with abnormalities of intestinal motility and enhanced sensitivity to visceral stimuli
- The trigger may be luminal or environmental.
- Evidence for the role of small intestinal bacterial overgrowth (SIBO) in IBS and association with antibiotic therapy is controversial; older age and female gender are predictors of SIBO in IBS patients.

Genetics
Unknown but more common in families of IBS patients

RISK FACTORS
- Other family members with similar GI disorder
- History of childhood sexual abuse
- Sexual/domestic abuse (primarily in women)
- Depression
- Gastrointestinal infection

Pregnancy Considerations
No risk to mother or fetus

GENERAL PREVENTION
See "Diet."

COMMONLY ASSOCIATED CONDITIONS
- Chronic migraine
- Fibromyalgia
- Chronic fatigue syndrome
- Sleep disorders
- Psychiatric disorders: major depression, anxiety, somatoform disorders, and posttraumatic stress
- Chronic pelvic pain
- Temporomandibular joint dysfunction

 DIAGNOSIS

HISTORY
- Rome IV criteria: recurrent abdominal pain >1 day/week, on average, in the previous 3 months with an onset >6 months before diagnosis
- Abdominal pain and at least two of the following:
  - Pain related to defecation
  - Change in frequency of stools
  - Change in form (appearance) of stools
- Patient has no warning signs:
  - Age >50 years, no previous colon cancer screening and presence of symptoms
  - Recent change in bowel habit
  - Evidence of overt GI bleeding (melena or hematochezia)
  - Nocturnal pain or passage of stools
  - Unintentional weight loss
  - Family history of colorectal cancer or inflammatory bowel disease
  - Palpable abdominal mass or lymphadenopathy
  - Evidence of iron deficiency anemia on blood testing
  - Positive fecal occult blood

PHYSICAL EXAM
- Complete exam to exclude other causes
- Vital signs and general exam are typically normal.
- There is typically an absence of jaundice and organomegaly, but there may be tenderness to palpation.

DIFFERENTIAL DIAGNOSIS
- Inflammatory bowel disease
- Lactose intolerance; fructose malabsorption
- Infections (*Giardia lamblia, Entamoeba histolytica, Salmonella, Campylobacter, Yersinia, Clostridium difficile*)
- Celiac sprue; microscopic colitis
- Laxative abuse; magnesium-containing antacids
- Hypo-/hyperthyroidism
- Pancreatic insufficiency
- Small bowel bacterial overgrowth
- Somatization; depression
- Villous adenoma
- Endocrine tumors
- Diabetes mellitus
- Radiation damage to colon or small bowel

DIAGNOSTIC TESTS & INTERPRETATION
- With a typical history and no warning signs (anemia or weight loss), obtain baseline labs to rule out other causes and begin treatment.
- In patients who do not respond to treatment, further evaluation with imaging and/or endoscopy is warranted to exclude organic pathology.

Initial Tests (lab, imaging)
Rule out pathology specific to the patient's symptoms:
- Diarrhea-predominant: ESR, CBC, tissue transglutaminase, thyroid-stimulating hormone (TSH), and stool for ova and parasites
- Constipation-predominant: CBC, TSH, electrolytes, calcium (2)
- Abdominal pain: LFTs and amylase
- When obtained, abdominal CT scan and ultrasound are generally normal.
- Consider small bowel series or video capsule endoscopy to rule out Crohn disease (typically normal).
- Sitz marker study may be used to evaluate colonic transit in patients with constipation.

Follow-Up Tests & Special Considerations
Consider lactulose breath test to assess for small bowel bacterial overgrowth associated with IBS.

Diagnostic Procedures/Other
Sigmoidoscopy/colonoscopy may be used to rule out inflammatory bowel disease or microscopic colitis.

ALERT
Screen all persons >50 years of age (or those with warning signs/red flags) for colorectal cancer.

Test Interpretation
None

 TREATMENT

- Goals: Relieve symptoms, improve quality of life (2).
  - Determine if diarrhea-predominant, constipation-predominant, or mixed type.
- Lifestyle modification
  - Exercise 3 to 5 times per week decreases severity (2).
  - Food diary to determine triggers (2)

- Medications
  - Fiber supplementation (psyllium) increases stool bulk; does not typically relieve abdominal pain; may be used for all types (2)[B]
- Medications that improve abdominal pain, global symptoms, and symptom severity in all types:
  - Antispasmodics such as hyoscyamine 0.125 to 0.250 mg PO/SL q4h PRN and dicyclomine 20 to 40 mg PO BID can be used for all types but have adverse effects such as dry mouth, dizziness, and blurred vision (2).
  - Probiotics such as *Lactobacillus*, *Bifidobacterium*, and *Streptococcus* (3)[C]
- Diarrhea-predominant
  - Antidiarrheal such as loperamide 4 to 8 mg/day orally divided 1 to 3 times per day as needed to decrease stool frequency and increase stool consistency; does not help with abdominal pain; may also use diphenoxylate and atropine (2)
  - Antibiotics such as 2-week course of rifaximin improve bloating, pain, and stool consistency (4).
  - Alosetron (Lotronex; 0.5 mg PO BID), for women with severe symptoms; associated with ischemic colitis, constipation, and death in a small number of patients
  - Ondansetron was found to reduce symptoms severity other than pain (5).
- Constipation-predominant
  - Laxatives such as polyethylene glycol (MiraLAX) may improve stool frequency but not pain.
  - Antibiotics such as neomycin and selective chloride channel activators such as lubiprostone (Amitiza) 8 mg BID can improve global symptoms and severity (2)[B].
  - Linaclotide (guanylate cyclase 2C agonist) has been shown to improve bowel function and reduces abdominal pain and overall severity in adults only (6).
- Mixed
  - Use medications to match symptoms (2).
- Treat underlying behavioral issues:
  - Tricyclic antidepressants can help control IBS symptoms in moderate to severe cases.
  - Behavioral therapy helps reduce symptoms (4).

ISSUES FOR REFERRAL
- Behavioral health referral may help with management of affective or personality disorders.
- Gastroenterology referral for difficult to control cases

ADDITIONAL THERAPIES
Probiotics use may result in reducing IBS symptoms and decreasing pain and flatulence. There is no difference among *Lactobacillus*, *Streptococcus*, *Bifidobacterium*, and combinations of probiotics.

 ONGOING CARE

FOLLOW-UP RECOMMENDATIONS
Patient Monitoring
The IBS Severity Scoring System is a validated measure to assess the severity of IBS symptoms and can help monitor response to treatment.
- IBS Severity Scoring System:
  - How severe has your abdominal pain been over the last 10 days?
  - On how many of the last 10 days did you get pain?
  - How severe has your abdominal distension (bloating, swollen, or tight) been over the last 10 days?
  - How satisfied have you been with your bowel habit (frequency, ease, etc.) over the last 10 days?
  - How much has your IBS been affecting/interfering with your life in general over the last 10 days?

DIET
- Low FODMAPs diet: This diet contains fermentable oligosaccharides, disaccharides, and monosaccharides, and polyols that are carbohydrates (sugars) found in foods. FODMAPs are osmotic, so they may not be digested or absorbed well and could be fermented upon by bacteria in the intestinal tract when *eaten in excess*.
- A low FODMAP diet may help reduce symptoms.
  - Increase fiber slowly to avoid excess intestinal gas production.
  - Initially, consider 2 weeks of lactose-free diet to rule out lactose intolerance.
  - Avoid large meals, fatty foods, and caffeine, which can exacerbate symptoms.
  - A gluten-free diet resolves symptoms for some patients (especially diarrhea-predominant IBS) despite negative testing for celiac disease.

PATIENT EDUCATION
IBS is not a psychiatric illness.

PROGNOSIS
- IBS is a disorder that reduces quality of life. Many patients have behavioral health issues. IBS does not increase mortality (1).
- Expect recurrences, especially when under stress.
- Evidence suggests that "symptom shifting" occurs in some patients, whereby resolution of functional bowel symptoms is followed by the development of functional symptoms in another system (1).

REFERENCES
1. Canavan C, West J, Card T. The epidemiology of irritable bowel syndrome. *Clin Epidemiol*. 2014;6: 71–80.
2. Chey WD, Kurlander J, Eswaran S. Irritable bowel syndrome: a clinical review. *JAMA*. 2015;313(9): 949–958.
3. Ciorba MA. A gastroenterologist's guide to probiotics. *Clin Gastroenterol Hepatol*. 2012;10(9):960–968.
4. Schey R, Rao SS. The role of rifaximin therapy in patients with irritable bowel syndrome without constipation. *Expert Rev Gastroenterol Hepatol*. 2011;5(4):461–464.
5. Garsed K, Chernova J, Hastings M, et al. A randomised trial of ondansetron for the treatment of irritable bowel syndrome with diarrhoea. *Gut*. 2014;63(10):1617–1625.
6. Videlock EJ, Cheng V, Cremonini F. Effects of linaclotide in patients with irritable bowel syndrome with constipation or chronic constipation: a meta-analysis. *Clin Gastroenterol Hepatol*. 2013;11(9): 1084.e3–1092.e3.

 SEE ALSO

Algorithm: Diarrhea, Chronic

 CODES

ICD10
- K58.9 Irritable bowel syndrome without diarrhea
- K58.0 Irritable bowel syndrome with diarrhea

CLINICAL PEARLS
- Use Rome III criteria to establish the diagnosis of IBS.
- Goals of treatment are to relieve symptoms and improve quality of life.
- If patients do not respond to initial treatment, consider further evaluation (including imaging and/or referral for endoscopy) to exclude organic pathology.

KAWASAKI SYNDROME
Scott P. Grogan, DO, MBA, FAAFP

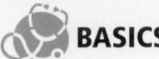 **BASICS**

DESCRIPTION
- Kawasaki syndrome (KS) is a self-limited acute, febrile, systemic vasculitis of small- and medium-sized arteries that predominantly affects patients age 6 months to 5 years and is the most prominent cause of acquired coronary artery disease in pediatric populations.
  - Vasculitis of coronary arteries resulting in aneurysms/ectasia, further leading to myocardial infarction (MI)/ischemia or sudden death
- System(s) affected: cardiovascular, gastrointestinal, hematologic/lymphatic/immunologic, musculoskeletal, nervous, pulmonary, renal/urologic, skin/exocrine
- Synonym(s): mucocutaneous lymph node syndrome (MCLS), infantile polyarteritis, Kawasaki disease

ALERT
KS should be considered in any child with extended high fever unresponsive to antibiotics or antipyretics, rash, and nonexudative conjunctivitis.

EPIDEMIOLOGY
Incidence
- Worldwide: affects all races but most prevalent in Asia; Japan annual incidence rate 265/100,000 in children <5 years of age
- In the United States, the annual incidence in children <5 years is 19/100,000. In comparison to Caucasians, African Americans have a 1.5 times risk, and Asian Americans have a 2.5 times increased risk. Highest state incidence is in Hawaii.
- Leading cause of acquired heart disease in children in developed countries
  - Predominant age: 1 to 5 years
  - 85% of cases are children <5 years of age and 50% <2 years of age.
  - Male-to-female ratio = 1.5:1

Prevalence
- Highest to lowest prevalence: Asians > African Americans > Hispanics > Caucasians
- Seasonal variation: increased in winter and early spring in temperate places, summer in Asia, and outbreaks at 2- to 3-year intervals

ETIOLOGY AND PATHOPHYSIOLOGY
- Acute KS causes a necrotizing arteritis in the smooth muscle layer of medium extraparenchymal arteries that destroys arterial walls into the adventitia, especially in coronary arteries.
- Inflammatory cells in the media secrete cytokines (TNF-α), interleukins 1 and 6, and matrix metalloproteases that cause fragmentation of the internal elastic lamina.
- A prominence of IgA plasma cells and IgA deposits are characteristic features and may be found in the lungs.
- As the acute process resolves, active neutrophilic inflammatory cells are succeeded by a subacute/chronic, lymphocytic vasculitis; fibroblasts and monocytes cause tissue repair/remodeling that may cause vascular fibrosis and stenosis.
- Unknown; believed to be an exaggerated immune response to infectious agent due to the acute, self-limited nature; community-wide outbreaks; age distribution; seasonality; and laboratory features indicating respiratory route of entry

Genetics
- Siblings of patients in Japan have a 10- to 30-fold increased risk, and >50% develop KS within 10 days of first case; increased occurrence of KS in children whose parents also had illness in childhood

- Populations at higher risk and family link suggest a genetic predisposition.
- Single-nucleotide polymorphisms in six different genes have been implicated in KS (Fcγ receptor 2A, CASP3, HLA class II, B-cell lymphoid kinase, IPTKC, CD40).
- Coronary aneurisms are associated with variants in TGF-β signaling pathways.

GENERAL PREVENTION
No preventive measures available

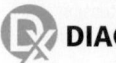 **DIAGNOSIS**

≥5 days of fever and ≥4 of the following 5 principal clinical features; or <4 features and presence of coronary artery disease on 2D echocardiography:
- Bilateral conjunctival injection with limbic sparing
- Erythematous mouth and pharynx, tongue, and lips
- A polymorphous, generalized, erythematous rash
- Changes in the skin of the peripheral extremities
- Cervical lymphadenopathy

Pediatric Considerations
- Prolonged fever without rash and treated with antibiotics may cause clinicians to believe that later rash development is due to a drug reaction.
- Can be diagnosed on day 4 of illness if ≥4 principal features are present
- Incomplete KS
  - ≥5 days of fever, 2 to 3 principal clinical features, labs indicating systemic inflammation, and exclusion of other diseases
  - Incomplete cases that exhibit <4 clinical criteria often occur in infants ≤6 months of age or older children/adolescents. The frequency of coronary artery aneurysms (CAAs) is often higher in patients with missed diagnosis/delayed treatment. Therefore, in infants with prolonged fever and few or no clinical features, consider echocardiography and inflammatory labs.

HISTORY
- Fever is the first sign during the acute phase.
- Symptoms may not occur all at once but usually occur in close proximity.

PHYSICAL EXAM
- High-spiking and remittent fever for ≥5 days
  - Fever is high (102–105°F [39.4–40.5°C]) and unresponsive to antibiotics.
  - May be prolonged up to 3 to 4 weeks
  - Extreme irritability is a very common feature.
- Bilateral, painless, nonpurulent, conjunctival injection without corneal ulceration or edema. Limbic sparing is usually seen.
- Changes in lips and oral cavity
  - Redness and swelling of lips in the acute stage; cracking, fissuring, bleeding in subacute phase
  - Strawberry/erythematous tongue
- Extensive erythematous polymorphous rash: within 5 days of fever
  - Morbilliform is most common. May be maculopapular, scarlatiniform; can resemble erythema multiforme, erythroderma, urticarial exanthem; rarely micropustular
  - Perineal desquamation, especially in skin folds
- Extremity changes
  - Reddened palms and soles on days 3 to 5
  - Edema of hands and feet on days 4 to 7; painful induration
  - Desquamation of fingers and toes that begins in periungual area at 2 to 3 weeks

- Acute, unilateral cervical lymphadenopathy (least common symptom)
  - ≥1 lymph nodes >1.5 cm, firm, nonfluctuant, and usually with no to slight tenderness
- Cardiac exam: tachycardia, gallop rhythms, hyperdynamic precordium, innocent flow murmurs, depressed contractility
- Other organ system involvement
  - Cardiovascular: myocarditis; pericarditis (often subclinical), CAAs, and other medium-sized arterial aneurysms
  - Gastrointestinal: anorexia, abdominal pain, vomiting/diarrhea, acute gallbladder hydrops, hepatic enlargement, jaundice
  - Renal: proteinuria, sterile pyuria
  - Joints: polyarthritis of small joints in acute phase; weight-bearing joints affected after 10th day from onset of fever
  - Neurologic: irritability, aseptic meningitis, peripheral neuropathy (unilateral facial palsy), transient high-frequency hearing loss

DIFFERENTIAL DIAGNOSIS
- Bacterial: staphylococcal scalded-skin syndrome, toxic shock syndrome, scarlet fever, bacterial cervical lymphadenitis, *Mycoplasma* infection, leptospirosis, Lyme disease, Rocky Mountain spotted fever
- Viral: measles, adenovirus, Epstein-Barr virus
- Toxoplasmosis
- Reiter syndrome
- Hypersensitivity drug reactions (erythema multiforme minor, Stevens-Johnson syndrome)
- Juvenile rheumatoid arthritis
- Acrodynia (mercury poisoning)

DIAGNOSTIC TESTS & INTERPRETATION
- Initial workup: CBC with differential, urinalysis (UA)/culture, blood culture; lumbar puncture if signs of meningitis or if <90 days old
  - Leukocytosis (12,000 to 40,000 cells/mm^3) with immature and mature granulocytes
  - Anemia: normochromic, normocytic
  - Thrombocytosis (500,000 to >1,000,000/mm^3) in 2nd and 3rd week. Thrombocytopenia during acute phase is associated with CAA and MI.
- Elevated C-reactive protein (CRP) (>35 mg/L in 80% cases), erythrocyte sedimentation rate (ESR) (>60 mm/hr in 60% cases), and α_1-antitrypsin
- Normal ESR, CRP, and PLTs after day 7 suggest diagnosis other than KS.

ALERT
ESR can be artificially high after intravenous immunoglobulin (IVIG) therapy.

- Hyponatremia
- Moderately elevated AST, ALT, GGT, and bilirubin
- Decreased albumin and protein
- CSF pleocytosis may be seen (lymphocytic with normal protein and glucose).
- N-terminal brain natriuretic peptide might be elevated in acute phase, but definitive cut-off values have not been established.
- Sterile pyuria but not seen in suprapubic collection
- Nasal swab to rule out adenovirus

Initial Tests (lab, imaging)
- If KS is suspected, obtain ECG and echocardiogram.
  - ECG may show arrhythmias, prolonged PR interval, and ST/T wave changes.

- Echocardiography has a high sensitivity and specificity for detection of abnormalities of proximal left main coronary artery, and right coronary artery may show perivascular brightening, ectasia, decreased left ventricular contractility, pericardial effusion, or aneurysms.
- Repeat echocardiography frequency determined by degree of abnormal more significant findings should be followed twice weekly until aneurismal progression halts.
- Cardiac stress test if CAA seen on echocardiogram
- Baseline chest x-ray (CXR): may show pleural effusion, atelectasis, and congestive heart failure (CHF)
- Hydrops of the gallbladder may be associated with abdominal pain or may be asymptomatic.

Diagnostic Procedures/Other
- No laboratory study is diagnostic; diagnosis rests on constellation of clinical features and exclusion of other illnesses.
- Magnetic resonance coronary angiography is non-invasive modality to visualize coronary arteries for stenosis, thrombi, and intimal thickening (1).
- Patients with complex coronary artery lesions may benefit from coronary angiography after the acute inflammatory process has resolved; generally recommended in 6 to 12 months

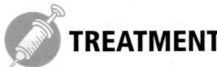 TREATMENT

GENERAL MEASURES
Use antibiotics until bacterial etiologies are excluded (e.g., sepsis or meningitis).

MEDICATION
- Optimal therapy is IVIG 2 g/kg IV over 10 to 12 hours with high-dose aspirin preferably within 7 to 10 days of fever, followed by low-dose aspirin until follow-up echocardiograms indicate a lack of coronary abnormalities.
  - IVIG lowers the risk of CAA and may shorten fever duration.
  - The extreme irritability often resolves very quickly after IVIG is given.
- Retreatment with IVIG if clinical response is incomplete or fever persists/returns >36 hours after start of IVIG treatment
  - ≥10% of patients do not respond to initial IVIG treatment. 2/3 of nonresponders respond to the second dose of IVIG.
  - Nonresponders tend to have ↑ bands, ↓ albumin, and an abnormal echo.
- Aspirin 80 to 100 mg/kg/day in 4 doses beginning with IVIG administration. Switch to low-dose aspirin (3 to 5 mg/kg/day) when afebrile for 48 to 72 hours, or continue until day 14 of illness. Maintain low dose for 6 to 8 weeks until follow-up echocardiogram is normal and CRP and/or ESR are normal. Continue salicylate regimen in children with coronary abnormalities, long term or until documented regression of aneurysm (2)[C].
- Aspirin does not appear to reduce CAA (3)[B].
- Corticosteroids have conflicting evidence for use and:
  - Should not be used as first-line agent in all KS patients (1)[B]
  - Should be used in conjunction with IVIG and ASA as initial treatment to decrease risk of CAAs in those at highest risk of IVIG failure (4)[A]
- Contraindications
  - IVIG: documented hypersensitivity, IgA deficiency, anti-IgE/IgG antibodies, severe thrombocytopenia, coagulation disorders

- Aspirin: vitamin K deficiency, bleeding disorders, liver damage, documented hypersensitivity, hypoprothrombinemia
- Precautions
  - No statistically significant difference is noted between different preparations of IVIG.
  - High-dose aspirin therapy can result in tinnitus, decreased of renal function, and increased transaminases.
  - Do not use ibuprofen in children with CAAs who are taking aspirin for antiplatelet effects.
  - Significant possible interactions: Aspirin therapy has been associated with Reye syndrome in children who develop viral infections, especially influenza B and varicella. Yearly influenza vaccination thus is recommended for children requiring long-term treatment with aspirin. Delay any live vaccines for 11 months after IVIG treatment.

Second Line
- In patients refractory to IVIG and steroids, consider infliximab or cyclosporine (5)[B].
- Plasma exchange may decrease likelihood of CAA in IVIG nonresponders (6)[B].

ISSUES FOR REFERRAL
Pediatric cardiologist if abnormalities on echo or if extensive stenosis

ADDITIONAL THERAPIES
- Treatment and prevention of thrombosis are crucial.
- Antiplatelet agents (clopidogrel, dipyridamole), heparin, low-molecular-weight heparin, or warfarin are sometimes added to the low-dose aspirin regimen, depending on severity of CAAs.
- Clarithromycin given with IVIG may reduce relapse rates and length of hospital stay.

SURGERY/OTHER PROCEDURES
- Rarely needed; coronary artery bypass grafting for severe obstruction/recurrent MI. Younger patients have a higher mortality rate.
- Coronary revascularization via percutaneous coronary intervention for patients with evidence of ischemia on stress testing

ADMISSION, INPATIENT, AND NURSING CONSIDERATIONS
- Normal saline (NS) for rehydration and 1/2 NS for maintenance
- Discharge if afebrile after IVIG treatment for 24 hours.

ONGOING CARE

FOLLOW-UP RECOMMENDATIONS
With aneurysms, contact and high-risk sports should be avoided.

Patient Monitoring
- Repeat ECG and echocardiogram at 6 to 8 weeks. If abnormal, repeat at 6 to 12 months.
- Patients with complex coronary artery lesions may benefit from coronary angiography at 6 to 12 months.

PROGNOSIS
- Usually self-limited
- Moderate-sized aneurysms usually regress in 1 to 2 years, resolving in 50–66% of cases.
- Recurrence (3% in Japan, <1% in the United States)
- Sudden death in early adulthood (rare)

COMPLICATIONS
- 15–25% of untreated patients develop CAAs in convalescent phase.
- 2–7% of treated patients develop aneurysms. 1% develop giant aneurysms.

- Risk factors for aneurysm
  - Male, <1 year of age, ↑ ESR >4 weeks, fever >2 weeks, fever >48 hours after IVIG treatment
- Mortality of 0.08–0.17% is due to cardiac disease.

REFERENCES
1. McCrindle BW, Rowley AH, Newburger JW, et al; for American Heart Association Rheumatic Fever, Endocarditis, and Kawasaki Disease Committee of the Council on Cardiovascular Disease in the Young, Council on Cardiovascular and Stroke Nursing, Council on Cardiovascular Surgery and Anesthesia, Council on Epidemiology and Prevention. Diagnosis, treatment, and long-term management of Kawasaki disease: a scientific statement for health professionals from the American Heart Association. *Circulation*. 2017;135(17):e927–e999.
2. Baumer JH, Love SJ, Gupta A, et al. Salicylate for the treatment of Kawasaki disease in children. *Cochrane Database Syst Rev*. 2006;(4):CD004175.
3. Lee G, Lee SE, Hong YM, et al. Is high-dose aspirin necessary in the acute phase of Kawasaki disease? *Korean Circ J*. 2013;43(3):182–186.
4. Chen S, Dong Y, Kiuchi MG, et al. Coronary artery complication in Kawasaki disease and the importance of early intervention: a systematic review and meta-analysis. *JAMA Pediatr*. 2016;170(12):1156–1163.
5. Patel RM, Shulman ST. Kawasaki disease: a comprehensive review of treatment options. *J Clin Pharm Ther*. 2015;40(6):620–625.
6. Hokosaki T, Mori M, Nishizawa T, et al. Long-term efficacy of plasma exchange treatment for refractory Kawasaki disease. *Pediatr Int*. 2012;54(1):99–103.

ADDITIONAL READING
- Huang SK, Lin MT, Chen HC, et al. Epidemiology of Kawasaki disease: prevalence from national database and future trends projection by system dynamics modeling. *J Pediatr*. 2013;163(1):126.e1–131.e1.
- Nanishi E, Nishio H, Takada H, et al. Clarithromycin plus intravenous immunoglobulin therapy can reduce the relapse rate of Kawasaki disease: a phase 2, open-label, randomized control study. *J Am Heart Assoc*. 2017;6(7):e005370.
- Oates-Whitehead RM, Baumer JH, Haines L, et al. Intravenous immunoglobulin for the treatment of Kawasaki disease in children. *Cochrane Database Syst Rev*. 2003;(4):CD004000.
- Singh S, Vignesh P, Burgner D. The epidemiology of Kawasaki disease: a global update. *Arch Dis Child*. 2015;100(11):1084–1088.
- Takahashi K, Oharaseki T, Yokouchi Y. Update on etio and immunopathogenesis of Kawasaki disease. *Curr Opin Rheumatol*. 2014;26(1):31–36.

CODES

ICD10
M30.3 Mucocutaneous lymph node syndrome [Kawasaki]

CLINICAL PEARLS
- The diagnosis of KS rests on a constellation of clinical features.
- Once KS is suspected, all patients need an inpatient cardiac evaluation, including ECG and echocardiogram.
- Expert recommendation for optimal therapy is IVIG 2 g/kg IV over 10 hours, with high-dose aspirin 80 to 100 mg/kg/day in 4 doses.

K

KERATOACANTHOMA

Patrick M. Zito, DO • Kenneth Beer, MD

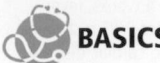 **BASICS**

DESCRIPTION

- Most common is a solitary, rapidly proliferating, dome-shaped, erythematous or flesh-colored papule or nodule with a central keratinous plug, typically reaching 1 to 2 cm in diameter.
- Clinically and microscopically resemble squamous cell carcinoma (SCC)
- Other presentations include grouped, multiple, keratoacanthoma (KA) centrifugum marginatum, intraoral, subungual, regressing, nonregressing, generally eruptive (1).
- Majority are benign and resolve spontaneously, but lesions do have the potential for invasion and metastasis, therefore require treatment.
- Three clinical stages of KAs (1):
  - Proliferative: rapid growth of the lesion over weeks to several months
  - Maturation/stabilization: Lesion stabilizes and growth subsides.
  - Involution: spontaneous resolution of the lesion, leaving a hypopigmented, depressed scar; most but not all lesions will enter this stage.
- System(s) affected: integumentary

EPIDEMIOLOGY

- Greatest incidence age >50 years but may occur at any age
- Presentation increased during summer and early fall seasons
- Most frequently on sun-exposed, hair-bearing skin but may occur anywhere
- Predominant sex: male > female (2:1)
- Most commonly in fair-skinned individuals; highest rates in Fitzpatrick I to III
- 104 cases per 100,000 individuals

ETIOLOGY AND PATHOPHYSIOLOGY

- Derived from an abnormality causing hyperkeratosis within the follicular infundibulum
- Squamous epithelial cells proliferate to extend upward around the keratin plug and proceed downward into the dermis; followed by invasion of elastic and collagen fibers
- Cellular mechanism responsible for the hyperkeratosis is currently unknown; role of human papillomavirus (HPV) has been discussed but has no established causality (2).
- Regression may be due to immune cytotoxicity or terminal differentiation of keratinocytes.
- Multiple etiologies have been suggested:
  - UV radiation
  - May be provoked by surgery, cryotherapy, chemical peels, or laser therapy
  - Viral infections: HPV or Merkel cell polyomavirus
  - Genetic predisposition: Muir-Torre syndrome, xeroderma pigmentosum, Ferguson-Smith syndrome
  - Immunosuppression
  - BRAF inhibitors (1)
  - Chemical carcinogen exposure

Genetics

- Mutation of *p53* or H-*ras*
- Ferguson-Smith (AD)
- Witten-Zak (AD)
- Muir-Torre (AD)
- Xeroderma pigmentosum (AR)
- Grzybowski (periodic)
- Incontinentia pigmenti (XLD)

RISK FACTORS

- UV exposure/damage: outdoor and/or indoor tanning
- Fitzpatrick skin types I to III
- Trauma (typically appears within 1 month of injury): laser resurfacing, surgery, cryotherapy, tattoos
- Chemical carcinogens: tar, pitch, and smoking
- Immunocompromised state
- Discoid lupus erythematosus
- HPV infection

GENERAL PREVENTION

Sun protection

COMMONLY ASSOCIATED CONDITIONS

- Frequently, the patient has concurrent sun-damaged skin: solar elastosis, solar lentigines, actinic keratosis, nonmelanoma skin cancers (basal cell carcinoma, SCC).
- In Muir-Torre syndrome, KAs are found with coexisting sebaceous neoplasms and malignancy of the GI and GU tracts; may have sebaceous differentiation known as a seboacanthoma

DIAGNOSIS

HISTORY

- Lesion begins as a small, solitary, pink macule that undergoes a rapid growth phase; classically reaching a diameter of 1 to 2 cm; size may vary.
- Once the proliferative stage has subsided, lesion size remains stable.
- May decrease in size, indicating regression
- Asymptomatic, occasionally tender
- If multiple lesions present, important to elicit a family history and recent therapies or treatments
- If sebaceous neoplasms present, must review history for signs/symptoms of GI or GU malignancies

PHYSICAL EXAM

- Firm, solitary, erythematous or flesh-colored, dome-shaped papule or nodule with a central keratin plug, giving a crateriform appearance
- Surrounding skin and borders of lesion may show telangiectasia, atrophy, or dyspigmentation.
- Usually solitary; multiple lesions can occur.
- Most commonly seen on sun-exposed areas: face, neck, scalp, dorsum of upper extremities, and posterior legs
- May also be seen on areas without sun exposure: buttocks, anus, subungual, mucosal surfaces
- Subungual KAs are very painful and seen on the first 3 digits of the hands.
- Examine for regional lymphadenopathy due to chance of lesion invasion and metastasis.
- Dermoscopy (3)
  - Central keratin highest sensitivity to distinguish from SCC (4)
  - White circles, blood spots; white circles highest specificity (4)
  - Cannot reliably distinguish between KA and SCC

DIFFERENTIAL DIAGNOSIS

- SCC
- Nodular or ulcerative basal cell carcinoma
- Cutaneous horn
- Hypertrophic actinic keratosis
- Amelanotic melanoma
- Merkel cell carcinoma
- Metastasis to the skin
- Molluscum contagiosum
- Prurigo nodularis
- Verruca vulgaris
- Verrucous carcinoma
- Sebaceous adenoma
- Hypertrophic lichen planus
- Hypertrophic lupus erythematosus
- Deep fungal infection
- Atypical mycobacterial infection
- Nodular Kaposi sarcoma

DIAGNOSTIC TESTS & INTERPRETATION

- Excisional biopsy, including the center of the lesion as well as the margin, is the best diagnostic test (2)[C].
- A shave biopsy may be insufficiently deep to distinguish KA from an SCC.
- If unable to perform an excisional biopsy, a deep shave (saucerization) of the entire lesion, extending into the subcutaneous fat, can be done.
- Punch biopsies should be avoided because they give an insufficient amount of tissue to represent the entire lesion.

Initial Tests (lab, imaging)

- Subungual KA: radiograph of the digit to monitor for osteolysis (cup-shaped radiolucent defect)
- Aggressive tumors may need CT with contrast for evaluation of lymph nodes and MRI if there is concern of perineural invasion.
- Most lesions do not need any form of imaging.

Test Interpretation

- Pathology of biopsy: a well-demarcated central core of keratin surrounded by well-differentiated, mildly pleomorphic, atypical squamous epithelial cells with a characteristic glassy eosinophilic cytoplasm
- Histopathology: keratin-filled crater encompassed with epithelial lips
- May see elastic and collagen fibers invading into the squamous epithelium
- Histologic differentiation of a KA from an SCC may be difficult and unreliable, although immunochemical staining for cellular protein Ki-67 may help do this (4).
- KAs have a greater tendency than SCC to display fibrosis and intraepidermal abscesses of neutrophils and eosinophils.
- Regressing KA shows flattening and fibrosis at base of lesion.

TREATMENT

- Treatment of choice is an excisional procedure plus electrodessication and curettage (ED&C); however, there are many treatment options available (2)[C].
- Aggressive tumors (>2 cm) or lesions in cosmetically sensitive areas (face, digits, genitalia) that require tissue sparing, consider Mohs micrographic surgery
  - Mohs is the treatment of choice in cases with perineural or perivascular invasion.
- Small lesions (<2 cm) of the extremities may undergo ED&C.
- Immunocompromised patients should receive immediate surgical treatment.

MEDICATION

- Nonsurgical management is a viable and relatively cost-effective option in these select cases not amenable to surgery due to lesion number, size, or location; also for patients with multiple comorbidities who are unwilling or unable to withstand surgery
- Evidence for the following treatments based on case reports and retrospective reviews:
  - Intralesional methotrexate 12.5 to 25.0 mg in 0.5 mL normal saline every 2 to 3 weeks for 1 to 4 treatment sessions (5)[B]
    - Monitor for pancytopenia with complete blood count (5)[C].
  - 5% imiquimod cream 3 times per week for 11 to 13 weeks (5)[B]
  - Topical 5% 5-fluorouracil cream daily, 61–92% cure rate (5)[B]
  - Intralesional 5-fluorouracil of 50 mg/mL on a weekly basis for 3 to 8 treatment sessions—98% cure rate (5)[B]
  - Intralesional IFN α-2a or α-2b (83%, 100% cure rate, respectively) (5)[B]
  - Intralesional bleomycin—100% cure rate (5)[B]
  - Isotretinoin oral 0.5 to 1.0 mg/kg/day

ISSUES FOR REFERRAL

Dermatology referral if lesions are >2 cm, numerous, mucosal, or subungual

ADDITIONAL THERAPIES

- Photodynamic therapy with methyl aminolevulinic acid and red light, successful case reports (1)[B] but also reported aggravation following treatment
- Cryotherapy (1)
- Argon or YAG lasers
- Radiotherapy, primary or adjuvant: KAs may regress with low doses of radiation but may require doses up to 25 to 50 Gy in low-dose (5 to 10 Gy) fractions for possible SCC (1)[B].
- Erlotinib (EGFR inhibitor) 150 mg daily for 21 days, single case report (1)[B]

SURGERY/OTHER PROCEDURES

Excisional and office-based procedures as discussed above

 ONGOING CARE

FOLLOW-UP RECOMMENDATIONS

After the surgical site has healed or lesion has resolved, patient should be seen every 6 months due to increased risk of developing new lesions or skin cancers, annually at minimum (3)[C].

Patient Monitoring

- Skin self-exams should be routinely performed with detailed instructions (see "Additional Reading").
- If multiple KAs are present in patient or family members, evaluate for Muir-Torre syndrome and obtain a colonoscopy beginning at age 25 years as well as testing for genitourinary cancer (3)[C].

PATIENT EDUCATION

- Sun protection measures: sun block with SPF >30, wide-brimmed hats, long sleeves, dark clothing, avoiding indoor tanning
- Arc welding may produce harmful UV radiation and skin should not be exposed.
- Tar, pitch, and smoking should be avoided.

PROGNOSIS

- Atrophic scarring and hypopigmentation can occur with self-resolution but may be significantly reduced by intervention.
- 52 of 445 cases (12%) spontaneously regressed without treatment and none of these recurred (2).
- 393 (88%) regressed following medical or excisional treatment (2).
- 445 cases reported with no metastases or deaths attributable to the KA (2)
- 4–8% recurrence
- Mucosal and subungual lesions do not regress; must undergo treatment

REFERENCES

1. Kwiek B, Schwartz RA. Keratoacanthoma (KA): an update and review. *J Am Acad Dermatol.* 2016;74(6):1220–1233.
2. Savage JA, Maize JC Sr. Keratoacanthoma clinical behavior: a systematic review. *Am J Dermatopathol.* 2014;36(5):422–429.
3. Cavicchini S, Tourlaki A, Lunardon L, et al. Amelanotic melanoma mimicking keratoacanthoma: the diagnostic role of dermoscopy. *Int J Dermatol.* 2013;52(8):1023–1024.
4. Scola N, Segert HM, Stücker M, et al. Ki-67 may be useful in differentiating between keratoacanthoma and cutaneous squamous cell carcinoma. *Clin Exp Dermatol.* 2014;39(2):216–218.
5. Chitwood KL, Etzkorn J, Cohen G. Topical and intralesional treatment of nonmelanoma skin cancer: efficacy and cost comparisons. *Dermatol Surg.* 2013;39(9):1306–1316.

ADDITIONAL READING

- The American Academy of Dermatology: https://www.aad.org/spot-skin-cancer/learn-about-skincancer/types-of-skin-cancer
- The Skin Cancer Foundation: http://www.skincancer.org/

 SEE ALSO

Squamous Cell Carcinoma, Cutaneous

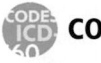 CODES

ICD10

- D23.9 Other benign neoplasm of skin, unspecified
- D48.5 Neoplasm of uncertain behavior of skin
- L85.8 Other specified epidermal thickening

CLINICAL PEARLS

- Suspect KA with a solitary, dome-shaped, erythematous or flesh-colored papule or nodule with a central keratinous plug.
- If KA is in the differential diagnosis, elicit time frame of onset during patient encounter; rapid onset supports diagnosis.
- Due to the broad differential diagnosis of a suspected KA and unreliable clinical differentiation between these, strongly consider surgical excision as first-line diagnostic test and therapy.
- Medical and radiation therapies are reasonable and effective options available for patients who are not surgical candidates or for lesions that are not amenable for surgery.

K

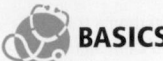

BASICS

DESCRIPTION

- Common, usually multiple, premalignant lesions of sun-exposed areas of the skin. Many resolve spontaneously, and a small proportion progresses to squamous cell carcinoma (SCC).
- Common consequence of excessive cumulative ultraviolet (UV) light exposure
- Synonym(s): solar keratosis

Geriatric Considerations
Frequent problem

Pediatric Considerations
Rare (if child, look for freckling and other stigmata of xeroderma pigmentosum)

EPIDEMIOLOGY

Incidence
- Rates vary with age group and exposure to sun.
- Predominant age: ≥40 years; progressively increases with age
- Predominant sex: male > female
- Common in those with blonde and red hair; rare in darker skin types

Prevalence
- Age-adjusted prevalence rate for actinic keratoses (AKs) in U.S. Caucasians is 6.5%.
- For 65- to 74-year-old males with high sun exposure: ~55%; low sun exposure: ~18%

ETIOLOGY AND PATHOPHYSIOLOGY

- The epidermal lesions are characterized by atypical keratinocytes at the basal layer with occasional extension upward. Mitoses are present. The histopathologic features resemble those of SCC in situ or SCC, and the distinction depends on the extent of epidermal involvement.
- Cumulative UV exposure

Genetics
The *p53* chromosomal mutation has been shown consistently in both AKs and SCCs. Many new genes have been shown recently to have similar expression profiles in AKs and SCCs.

RISK FACTORS

- Exposure to UV light (especially long-term and/or repeated exposure due to outdoor occupation or recreational activities, indoor or outdoor tanning)
- Skin type: burns easily, does not tan
- Immunosuppression, especially organ transplantation

GENERAL PREVENTION

Sun avoidance and protective techniques are helpful.

COMMONLY ASSOCIATED CONDITIONS

- SCC
- Other features of chronic solar damage: lentigines, elastosis, and telangiectasias

DIAGNOSIS

HISTORY

- The lesions are frequently asymptomatic; symptoms may include pruritus, burning, and mild hyperesthesia.
- Lesions may enlarge, thicken, or become more scaly. They also may regress or remain unchanged.
- Most lesions occur on the sun-exposed areas (head and neck, hands, forearms).

PHYSICAL EXAM

- Usually small (<1 cm), often multiple red, pink, or brown macules, papules, or plaques that are rough to palpation
- Yellow or brown adherent scale is often present on top of the lesion.
- Several clinical variants exist.
  - Atrophic: dry, scaly macules with indistinct borders and an erythematous base
  - Hypertrophic: Overlying hyperkeratosis (in an extreme form, cutaneous horn) may be impossible to differentiate from SCC clinically.
  - Pigmented: smooth tan/brown plaque, spreading centrifugally
  - Bowenoid: red scaly plaques with distinct borders
  - Actinic cheilitis: inflammatory lesion involving usually the lower lip

DIFFERENTIAL DIAGNOSIS

- SCC (hypertrophic type)
- Keratoacanthoma
- Bowen disease
- Basal cell carcinoma
- Verruca vulgaris
- Less likely: verrucous nevi, warty dyskeratoma, lichenoid keratoses, seborrheic keratoses, porokeratoses, seborrheic dermatitis or psoriasis (near hairline), lentigo maligna, solar lentigo, discoid lupus erythematosus

DIAGNOSTIC TESTS & INTERPRETATION

Diagnostic Procedures/Other
- The diagnosis is usually made clinically, except where there is a suspicion of carcinoma.
- Skin biopsy is especially recommended if large, ulcerated, indurated, or bleeding, or if the lesions are nonresponsive to treatment.

Test Interpretation
- Dysplastic keratinocytes in lower levels of epidermis with a dermal lymphocytic infiltrate
- Neoplastic cells, mostly found in the lower epidermal layers, are cytologically identical to those of SCCs.
- If neoplastic cells extend throughout entire epidermis or into the dermis, the lesions will qualify as an SCC in situ or invasive SCC, respectively.
- Malignant cells are sparse except of the bowenoid variety.
- Hypertrophic, atrophic, bowenoid, acantholytic, and pigmented varieties show the corresponding epidermal findings.

TREATMENT

- First-line treatment is cryotherapy (technically, this is considered surgery, especially by insurance companies) (1,2)[A]. Medical therapy is usually reserved for extensive AKs ("field therapy").
- Cryotherapy combined with a topical approach resulted in significantly higher complete clearance rates than monotherapy (3)[A].

GENERAL MEASURES
- Sun-protective techniques
- Sunscreens and physical sun protection recommended

MEDICATION
First Line
- Topical treatments target both visible and subclinical lesions.
- With the exception of generic 5-fluorouracil, medication cost is high ($600 to $1,200 per course).
- Topical fluorouracil (Efudex, Carac, Fluoroplex cream, Fluoroplex solution)
  - Every day—BID for 3 to 6 weeks, depending on the brand, concentration, and formulation
  - Can be very irritating
  - May be most effective of the topical treatments listed in this section (3)[A]
- Topical imiquimod (Aldara) 5% cream
  - Apply 2 days per week at HS for up to 16 weeks to an area not larger than the forehead or one cheek.
  - Can be irritating
- Topical imiquimod (Zyclara) 3.75% cream
  - Apply once a day for 2 weeks, followed by no treatment for the next 2 weeks, and then apply once a day for another 2 weeks.
  - Can be irritating
- Topical ingenol mebutate (Picato) 0.015% and 0.05% gel
  - Apply to the face and scalp once a day for 3 consecutive days.
  - Apply to the trunk and extremities once a day for 2 consecutive days.
    - It should only be used on one contiguous skin area of not >25 cm^2.
    - Cases of severe allergic reactions (including anaphylaxis) and herpes zoster reactivation unrelated to application errors have been reported.
- Diclofenac (Solaraze) 3% gel
  - Apply BID for 60 to 90 days.

Second Line
- Topical tretinoin (Retin-A) or tazarotene (Tazorac): may be used to enhance the efficacy of topical fluorouracil
- Systemic retinoids: used infrequently

ADDITIONAL THERAPIES
Close monitoring with no treatment is an appropriate option for mild lesions.

SURGERY/OTHER PROCEDURES
- Cryosurgery ("freezing," liquid nitrogen)
  - Most common method for treating AK
  - Cure rate: 75–98.8%
  - May cause atrophy and hypopigmentation
  - May be superior to photodynamic therapy for thicker lesions
- Photodynamic therapy with a photosensitizer (e.g., aminolevulinic acid) and "blue light"
  - May clear >90% of AKs
  - Less scarring than cryotherapy
  - May be superior to cryotherapy, especially in the case of more extensive skin involvement
- Curettage and electrocautery (electrodesiccation and curettage [ED&C]; "scraping and burning")
- Medium-depth peels, especially for the treatment of extensive areas
- CO$_2$ laser therapy
- Dermabrasion
- Surgical excision (excisional biopsy)

  ## ONGOING CARE

FOLLOW-UP RECOMMENDATIONS
Patient Monitoring
Depends on associated malignancy and frequency with which new AKs appear

PATIENT EDUCATION
- Teach sun-protective techniques.
  - Limit outdoor activities between 10 AM and 4 PM.
  - Wear protective clothing and wide-brimmed hat.
  - Proper use (including reapplication) of sunscreens with SPF >30, preferably a preparation with broad-spectrum (UV-A and UV-B) protection
- Teach self-examination of skin (melanoma, squamous cell, basal cell).
- Patient education materials
  - http://dermnetnz.org/lesions/solar-keratoses.html

PROGNOSIS
Very good. A significant proportion of the lesions may resolve spontaneously (4), with regression rates of 20–30% per lesion per year.

COMPLICATIONS
- AKs are premalignant lesions that may progress to SCCs. The rate of malignant transformation is unclear; the reported percentages vary but range from 0.1% to a few percent per year per lesion.
- Patients with AKs are at increased risk for other cutaneous malignancies.
- Approximately 60% of SCCs arise from an AK precursor.

REFERENCES
1. Helfand M, Gorman AK, Mahon S, et al. *Actinic Keratoses: Final Report*. Rockville, MD: Agency for Healthcare Research and Quality; 2001.
2. de Berker D, McGregor JM, Hughes BR; for British Association of Dermatologists Therapy Guidelines and Audit Subcommittee. Guidelines for the management of actinic keratoses. *Br J Dermatol*. 2007;156(2):222–230.
3. Heppt MV, Steeb T, Ruzicka T, et al. Cryosurgery combined with topical interventions for actinic keratosis: a systematic review and meta-analysis [published online ahead of print November 17, 2018]. *Br J Dermatol*. doi:10.1111/bjd.17435.
4. Criscione VD, Weinstock MA, Naylor MF, et al; for Department of Veterans Affairs Topical Tretinoin Chemoprevention Trial Group. Actinic keratoses: natural history and risk of malignant transformation in the Veterans Affairs Topical Tretinoin Chemoprevention Trial. *Cancer*. 2009;115(11):2523–2530.

ADDITIONAL READING
Feldman SR, Fleischer AB Jr. Progression of actinic keratosis to squamous cell carcinoma revisited: clinical and treatment implications. *Cutis*. 2011;87(4):201–207.

CODES

ICD10
L57.0 Actinic keratosis

CLINICAL PEARLS
- AKs are premalignant lesions, although most will not progress to squamous cell cancer and many will regress with time.
- Often more easily felt than seen
- Therapy-resistant lesions should be biopsied, especially on the face.

K

KERATOSIS, SEBORRHEIC

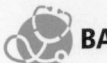

Christopher J. Weber, MD • Cesar R. Mojica Vazquez, MD

BASICS

DESCRIPTION
- Common benign tumor of the epidermis
- Formed from keratinocytes
- Frequently appears in multiples on the head, neck, and trunk of older individuals but may occur on any hair-bearing area of the body. Lesions spare the palms and soles.
- Typically can present as multiple, well circumscribed, yellow to brown raised lesions that feel greasy, velvety, or warty usually described as having "stuck-on" appearance
- Clinical variants include the following:
  - Common seborrheic keratosis
  - Dermatosis papulosa nigra
  - Stucco keratosis
  - Flat seborrheic keratosis
  - Pedunculated seborrheic keratosis
- System(s) affected: integumentary
- Synonym(s): SK, verruca seborrhoica; seborrheic wart; senile wart; basal cell papilloma; verruca senilis; basal cell acanthoma; benign acanthokeratoma; barnacles of aging

EPIDEMIOLOGY
Incidence
- Predominant age
  - Rarely seen before 30 years
- Predominant sex: slightly more common and more extensive involvement in males
- Most common among Caucasians, except for the dermatosis papulosa nigra variant, which usually presents in darker skinned individuals

Prevalence
- 69–100% in patients >50 years of age (1)
- The prevalence rate increases with advancing age.

ETIOLOGY AND PATHOPHYSIOLOGY
- Seborrheic keratoses are monoclonal tumors.
- Etiology still is largely unclear.
- Ultraviolet (UV) light and genetics are thought to be involved.
- The role of human papillomavirus is uncertain.

Genetics
An autosomal dominant inheritance pattern is suggested.

RISK FACTORS
- Advanced age
- Exposure to UV light and genetic predisposition are possible factors (1).

GENERAL PREVENTION
Sun protection methods may help prevent seborrheic keratoses from developing.

COMMONLY ASSOCIATED CONDITIONS
- Sign of Leser-Trélat: a paraneoplastic syndrome characterized by a sudden outbreak of multiple seborrheic keratoses in association with an internal malignancy, most commonly adenocarcinoma of the stomach (2). Seborrheic keratosis may resolve with treatment of the malignancy and reappear with neoplasm recurrence (1).
- Documentation of other cutaneous lesions, such as basal cell carcinoma, malignant melanoma, Bowen disease, or squamous cell carcinoma, growing adjacent to or within a seborrheic keratosis, has been reported. The exact relationship between lesions is unclear.

DIAGNOSIS

HISTORY
- Usually asymptomatic
- Trauma or irritation of the lesion may result in pruritus, erythema, bleeding, pain, and/or crusting.

PHYSICAL EXAM
- Typically begin as oval- or round-shaped, flat, dull, sharply demarcated patches
- As they mature, may develop into thicker, elevated, uneven, verrucous-like papules, plaques, or peduncles with a waxy or velvety surface, and appear "stuck on" to the skin (1)
- Commonly appear on sun-exposed areas of the body, predominately the head, neck, or trunk but may appear on any hair-bearing skin
- Vary in color from black, brown, tan, gray to white, or skin-colored; and range in size from several millimeters to several centimeters, but the average diameter is 0.5 to 1.0 cm (1)
- Usually occur as multiples; patients having >100 is not uncommon.
- If irritated, may be bleeding, inflamed, painful, pruritic, or crusted
- Common clinical variants include the following (3):
  - Common seborrheic keratoses: on hair-bearing skin, usually on the face, neck, and trunk; verrucous-like, waxy, or velvety lesions that appear "stuck on" to the skin
  - Dermatosis papulosa nigra: Small black papules that usually appear on the face, neck, chest, and upper back; most common in darker skinned individuals, more common in females; most have a positive family history.
  - Stucco keratoses: small gray-white, rough, verrucous papules; usually occur in large numbers on the lower extremities or forearms; more common in men
  - Flat seborrheic keratoses: oval-shaped, brown patches or macules on face, chest, and upper extremities; increases with age
  - Pedunculated seborrheic keratoses: Hyperpigmented peduncles appear on areas of friction (neck, axilla).

DIFFERENTIAL DIAGNOSIS
Consider the following diagnoses if the seborrheic keratosis is:
- Pigmented
  - Malignant melanoma
  - Melanocytic nevus
  - Angiokeratoma
  - Pigmented basal cell carcinoma
- Lightly pigmented
  - Basal cell carcinoma
  - Bowen disease
  - Condyloma acuminatum
  - Fibroma
  - Verruca vulgaris
  - Eccrine poroma
  - Invasive squamous cell carcinoma
  - Acrochordon
  - Acrokeratosis verruciformis of Hopf
  - Follicular infundibulum tumor
- Flat
  - Solar lentigo
  - Verrucae planae juveniles
- Hyperkeratotic
  - Actinic keratosis

DIAGNOSTIC TESTS & INTERPRETATION
Initial Tests (lab, imaging)
Not needed unless internal malignancy is suspected

Diagnostic Procedures/Other
- Diagnosis is made clinically.
- Dermoscopy
  - If uncertain, can aid in diagnosis
  - Common findings are comedo-like openings, fissures, ridges, sharply demarcated borders, milia-like cysts, pseudofollicular openings, hairpin vessels, and horn pseudocysts (4,5).
- Biopsy and histologic exam should be performed if the seborrheic keratosis
  - Is atypical
  - Has inflammation
  - Recently changed in appearance
  - Diagnosis remains unclear.

Test Interpretation
- Histologic findings include the following:
  - Acanthosis and papillomatosis due to basaloid cell proliferation
  - "Squamous eddies" or squamous epithelial cell clusters
  - Hyperpigmentation
  - Hyperkeratosis
  - Horn cysts
  - Pseudocysts
- Several histologic variants exist.

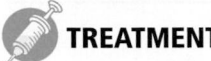 **TREATMENT**

- Treatment is not usually necessary due to the benign nature of the lesions.
- Removal of seborrheic keratoses may be indicated if
  – Symptomatic (e.g., easily irritated, gets caught on clothing or jewelry)
  – Aesthetically displeasing or undesirable (common)
  – There is a question of malignancy.

MEDICATION
Current topical treatments of seborrheic keratoses are less effective than a surgical approach.

ISSUES FOR REFERRAL
- New seborrheic keratoses appear abruptly.
- A seborrheic keratosis becomes inflamed or changes in appearance.

SURGERY/OTHER PROCEDURES
- A surgical approach to treatment is preferred.
- Choice depends on physician preference and availability of the treatment.
- The following procedures are used:
  – Cryotherapy (liquid nitrogen)
    ○ Spray flat lesions for 5 to 10 seconds; may require more time or additional treatments if the seborrheic keratosis is thicker
    ○ Possible complications include scarring, hypopigmentation, recurrence.
  – Curettage
    ○ Requires local anesthesia
    ○ Metal hand tool with small scoop at the tip (curette) used to scrape off the lesion
  – Electrodessication
    ○ Requires local anesthesia
    ○ Requires tool with needle-like metal tip that uses electric current to destroy affected tissue
  – Shave excision
    ○ Requires local anesthesia
    ○ Requires scalpel to remove lesion
  – Laser
    ○ Requires local anesthesia
    ○ Uses intense beam of light that burns and vaporizes the lesion
  – Chemical peel
    ○ Involves application of chemical solution (e.g., Trichloroacetic acid) to remove top layer of skin
- No statistically significant differences were found in patient's ratings of cosmetic appearance between cryotherapy and curettage. The majority of patients preferred cryotherapy over curettage due to decreased postoperative wound care, despite the increased discomfort experienced and increased frequency of seborrheic keratosis remaining after cryotherapy when compared to curettage (6).

 ONGOING CARE

FOLLOW-UP RECOMMENDATIONS
Patient Monitoring
After initial diagnosis, follow-up is not usually required unless

- Inflammation or irritation develops.
- There is a change in appearance.
- New seborrheic keratoses suddenly appear.

PATIENT EDUCATION
- Sun-protective methods may help reduce seborrheic keratosis development.
- Patient education materials
  – http://www.aad.org/public/diseases/bumps-and-growths/seborrheic-keratoses
  – www.cdc.gov/cancer/skin/basic_info/prevention.htm

PROGNOSIS
- Seborrheic keratoses generally do not become malignant.
- Sign of Leser-Trélat usually represents a poor prognosis.

COMPLICATIONS
- Irritation and inflammation due to mechanical irritation (i.e., from clothing, jewelry)
- Possible complications of surgical treatment include hypopigmentation, hyperpigmentation, scarring, incomplete removal, and recurrence.
- Misdiagnosis (rare)

REFERENCES

1. Hafner C, Vogt T. Seborrheic keratosis. *J Dtsch Dermatol Ges*. 2008;6(8):664–677.
2. Husain Z, Ho JK, Hantash BM. Sign and pseudo-sign of Leser-Trélat: case reports and a review of the literature. *J Drugs Dermatol*. 2013;12(5):e79–e87.
3. Noiles K, Vender R. Are all seborrheic keratoses benign? Review of the typical lesion and its variants. *J Cutan Med Surg*. 2008;12(5):203–210.
4. Marghoob AA, Usatine RP, Jaimes N. Dermoscopy for the family physician. *Am Fam Physician*. 2013;88(7):441–450.
5. Takenouchi T. Key points in dermoscopic diagnosis of basal cell carcinoma and seborrheic keratosis in Japanese. *J Dermatol*. 2011;38(1):59–65.
6. Wood LD, Stucki JK, Hollenbeak CS, et al. Effectiveness of cryosurgery vs curettage in the treatment of seborrheic keratoses. *JAMA Dermatol*. 2013;149(1):108–109.

ADDITIONAL READING

- Culbertson GR. 532-nm diode laser treatment of seborrheic keratoses with color enhancement. *Dermatol Surg*. 2008;34(4):525–528.
- Draelos ZD, Rizer RL, Trookman NS. A comparison of postprocedural wound care treatments: do antibiotic-based ointments improve outcomes? *J Am Acad Dermatol*. 2011;64(Suppl 3):S23–S29.
- Garcia MS, Azari R, Eisen DB. Treatment of dermatosis papulosa nigra in 10 patients: a comparison trial of electrodesiccation, pulsed dye laser, and curettage. *Dermatol Surg*. 2010;36(12):1968–1972.
- Georgieva IA, Mauerer A, Groesser L, et al. Low incidence of oncogenic EGFR, HRAS, and KRAS mutations in seborrheic keratosis. *Am J Dermatopathol*. 2014;36(8):635–642.
- Herron MD, Bowen AR, Krueger GG. Seborrheic keratoses: a study comparing the standard cryosurgery with topical calcipotriene, topical tazarotene, and topical imiquimod. *Int J Dermatol*. 2004;43(4):300–302.
- Higgins JC, Maher MH, Douglas MS. Diagnosing common benign tumors. *Am Fam Physician*. 2015;92(7):601–607.
- Krupashankar DS; and IADVL Dermatosurgery Task Force. Standard guidelines of care: CO₂ laser for removal of benign skin lesions and resurfacing. *Indian J Dermatol Venereol Leprol*. 2008;74(Suppl 7):S61–S67.
- Luba MC, Bangs SA, Mohler AM, et al. Common benign skin tumors. *Am Fam Physician*. 2003;67(4):729–738.
- Rajesh G, Thappa DM, Jaisankar TJ, et al. Spectrum of seborrheic keratoses in South Indians: a clinical and dermoscopic study. *Indian J Dermatol Venereol Leprol*. 2011;77(4):483–488.
- Saeed AK, Salmo N. Epidermal growth factor receptor expression in mice skin upon ultraviolet B exposure—seborrheic keratosis as a coincidental and unique finding. *Adv Biomed Res*. 2012;1:59.
- Taylor SC, Averyhart AN, Heath CR. Postprocedural wound-healing efficacy following removal of dermatosis papulosa nigra lesions in an African American population: a comparison of a skin protectant ointment and a topical antibiotic. *J Am Acad Dermatol*. 2011;64(Suppl 3):S30–S35.

 CODES

ICD10
- L82.1 Other seborrheic keratosis
- L82.0 Inflamed seborrheic keratosis

CLINICAL PEARLS

- Seborrheic keratoses are one of the most common benign tumors of the epidermis.
- Prevalence increases with age.
- Underlying internal malignancy should be considered if large numbers of seborrheic keratoses appear suddenly.

K

KNEE PAIN

Scott M. Goldberg, MD • J. Herbert Stevenson, MD

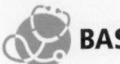 BASICS

DESCRIPTION

A common outpatient complaint with a broad differential
- Knee pain may be acute, chronic, or an acute exacerbation of a chronic condition.
- Trauma, overuse, and degenerative change are frequent causes.
- A detailed history, including patient's age, pain onset and location, mechanism of injury, and associated symptoms can help narrow the differential diagnosis.
- A thorough and focused examination of the knee (as well as the back, hips, and ankles) helps to establish the correct diagnosis and appropriate treatment.

EPIDEMIOLOGY

Incidence
- Knee complaints account for 12.5 million primary care visits annually.
- The incidence of knee osteoarthritis (OA) is 240 cases per 100,000 person-years.

Prevalence
- The knee is a common site of lower extremity injury.
  - Patellar tendinopathy and patellofemoral syndrome are the most common causes of knee pain in runners.
- OA of the hip/knee is 11th cause of global disability and 38th most common cause of disability-adjusted life years (DALYs).

ETIOLOGY AND PATHOPHYSIOLOGY
- Trauma (ligament or meniscal injury, fracture, dislocation)
- Overuse (tendinopathy, patellofemoral syndrome, bursitis, apophysitis)
- Age (arthritis, degenerative conditions in older patients; apophysitis in younger patients)
- Rheumatologic (rheumatoid arthritis [RA], systemic lupus erythematosus [SLE])
- Crystal arthropathies (gout, pseudogout)
- Infectious (bacterial, postviral, Lyme disease)
- Referred pain (hip, back)
- Vascular: popliteal artery aneurysm, deep vein thrombosis
- Others: tumor, cyst, plica

RISK FACTORS
- Obesity
- Malalignment
- Poor flexibility, muscle imbalance, or weakness
- Rapid increases in training frequency and intensity
- Improper footwear, training surfaces, technique
- Activities that involve cutting, jumping, pivoting, deceleration, kneeling
- Previous injuries

GENERAL PREVENTION
- Maintain normal body mass index.
- Proper exercise technique, volume, and equipment; avoid overtraining.
- Correct postural strength and flexibility imbalances.

COMMONLY ASSOCIATED CONDITIONS
- Fracture, contusion
- Effusion, hemarthrosis
- Patellar dislocation/subluxation
- Meniscal or ligamentous injury
- Tendinopathy, bursitis
- Osteochondral injury
- OA, septic arthritis
- Muscle strain

DIAGNOSIS

HISTORY
- Pain location, quality, and mechanism of injury guide diagnostic reasoning (also see "Differential Diagnosis"):
  - Diffuse pain: OA, patellofemoral pain syndrome, chondromalacia
  - Pain ascending/descending stairs: meniscal injury, patellofemoral pain syndrome
  - Pain with prolonged sitting, standing from sitting: patellofemoral pain syndrome
  - Mechanical symptoms (locking): meniscal injury
- Mechanism of injury:
  - Hyperextension, deceleration, cutting: anterior cruciate ligament (ACL) injury
  - Hyperflexion, fall on flexed knee, "dashboard injury": posterior cruciate ligament (PCL) injury
  - Lateral force (valgus load): medial collateral injury
  - Twisting on planted foot: meniscal injury
- Effusion:
  - Rapid onset (2 hours): ACL tear, patellar subluxation, tibial plateau fracture. Hemarthrosis is common.
  - Slower onset (24 to 36 hours), smaller: meniscal injury, ligament sprain, arthritis
  - Swelling behind the knee: popliteal (Baker) cyst

PHYSICAL EXAM
- Observe gait (antalgia); patellar tracking
- Inspect for malalignment, atrophy, swelling, ecchymosis, or erythema.
- Palpate for effusion, warmth, and tenderness.
- Evaluate active and passive range of motion (ROM) and flexibility of quadriceps and hamstrings.
- Evaluate strength and muscle tone.
- Note joint instability, locking, and catching.
- Evaluate hip ROM, strength, and stability.
- Special tests:
  - Patellar apprehension test: patellar instability; patellar grind test: patellofemoral pain or OA (1)
  - Lachman test (more sensitive and specific), pivot shift, anterior drawer: ACL integrity
  - Posterior drawer, posterior sag sign: PCL integrity
  - Valgus/varus stress test: medial/lateral collateral ligament (MCL/LCL) integrity
  - McMurray test, Apley grind test, Thessaly test: meniscal injury
  - Ober test: iliotibial band (ITB) tightness

  - Dial test: positive with posterolateral corner laxity
  - Patellar tilt test and squatting may help suggest patellofemoral pain syndrome.
  - Patella facet tenderness suggests OA or patellofemoral pain syndrome (1).

DIFFERENTIAL DIAGNOSIS
- Acute onset: fracture, contusion, cruciate or collateral ligament tear, meniscal tear, patellar dislocation/subluxation; if systemic symptoms: septic arthritis, gout, pseudogout, Lyme disease, osteomyelitis
- Insidious onset: patellofemoral pain syndrome/chondromalacia, ITB syndrome, OA, RA, bursitis, tumor, tendinopathy, loose body, bipartite patella, degenerative meniscal tear
- Anterior pain: patellofemoral pain syndrome, patellar injury, patellar tendinopathy, pre- or suprapatellar bursitis, tibial apophysitis, fat pad impingement, quadriceps tendinopathy, OA (1)
- Posterior pain: PCL injury, posterior horn meniscal injury, popliteal cyst or aneurysm, hamstring or gastrocnemius injury, deep venous thrombosis (DVT)
- Medial pain: MCL injury, medial meniscal injury, pes anserine bursitis, medial plica syndrome, OA
- Lateral pain: LCL injury, lateral meniscal injury, ITB syndrome, OA

DIAGNOSTIC TESTS & INTERPRETATION

Initial Tests (lab, imaging)
- Suspected septic joint, gout, pseudogout:
  - Arthrocentesis with cell count, Gram stain, culture, protein/glucose, synovial fluid analysis
- Suspected RA:
  - CBC, erythrocyte sedimentation rate (ESR), rheumatoid factor
- Consider Lyme titer.
- Radiographs to rule out fracture in patients with acute knee trauma (Ottawa Rules):
  - Age >55 years *or*
  - Tenderness at the patella or fibular head *or*
  - Inability to bear weight four steps *or*
  - Inability to flex knee to 90 degrees
- Radiographs help diagnose OA, osteochondral lesions, patellofemoral pain syndrome:
  - Weight-bearing, upright anteroposterior, lateral, merchant/sunrise, notch/tunnel views

Follow-Up Tests & Special Considerations
- MRI is "gold standard" for soft tissue imaging.
- Ultrasound may help diagnose tendinopathy (2)[B].
- CT can further elucidate fracture.

Diagnostic Procedures/Other
Arthroscopy may be beneficial in the diagnosis of certain conditions, including meniscus and ligament injuries.

Geriatric Considerations
OA, degenerative meniscal tears, and gout are more common in middle-aged and elderly populations.

Pediatric Considerations
- 3 million pediatric sports injuries occur annually.
- Look for physeal/apophyseal and joint surface injuries in skeletally immature:
  - Acute: patellar subluxation, avulsion fractures, ACL tear
  - Overuse: patellofemoral pain syndrome, apophysitis, osteochondritis dissecans, patellar tendinitis, stress fracture
  - Others: neoplasm, juvenile RA, infection, referred pain from slipped capital femoral epiphysis

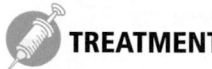 TREATMENT

GENERAL MEASURES
Acute injury: PRICEMM therapy (**p**rotection, **r**elative rest, **i**ce, **c**ompression, **e**levation, **m**edications, **m**odalities)

MEDICATION
First Line
- Oral medications:
  - Acetaminophen: up to 3 g/day; safe and effective in OA
  - Nonsteroidal anti-inflammatory drugs (NSAIDs):
    - Ibuprofen: 200 to 800 mg TID
    - Naproxen: 250 to 500 mg BID:
      - Useful for acute sprains, strains
      - Useful for short-term pain reduction in OA. Long-term use is not recommended due to side effects.
      - Not recommended for fracture, stress fracture, chronic muscle injury; may be associated with delayed healing; low dose and brief course only if necessary
  - Tramadol/opioids: not recommended as first-line treatment; can be used with acute injuries for severe pain
  - Celecoxib: 200 mg QD may be effective in OA with less GI side effects than NSAIDs (3)[A].
- Topical medications:
  - Topical NSAIDs provide pain relief in OA and may be more tolerable than oral medications (4)[A].
  - Topical capsaicin may be an adjuvant for pain management in OA.
- Injections:
  - Intra-articular corticosteroid injection may provide short-term benefit in knee OA stage 2 or 3 (2)[A].
  - Viscosupplementation may reduce pain and improve function in patients with OA (2)[A]. Peak effectiveness is 5 to 13 weeks.
  - Equivocal evidence for platelet-rich plasma (PRP) compared to viscosupplementation
  - Stem cell therapy with insufficient data

ISSUES FOR REFERRAL
- Acute trauma, young athletic patient
- Joint instability
- Lack of improvement with conservative measures
- Salter-Harris physeal fractures (pediatrics)

ADDITIONAL THERAPIES
- Physical therapy is recommended as initial treatment for patellofemoral pain (5) and tendinopathies (2)[A].
- Muscle strengthening improves outcome in OA.
- Foot orthoses, taping, acupuncture
- May need bracing for stability (5)[B]

SURGERY/OTHER PROCEDURES
- Surgery may be indicated for certain injuries (e.g., ACL tear in competitive athletes or grade IV OA).
- Chronic conditions refractory to conservative therapy may require surgical intervention.

COMPLEMENTARY & ALTERNATIVE MEDICINE
May reduce pain and improve function in early OA:
- Glucosamine sulfate (500 mg TID)
- Chondroitin (400 mg TID)
- Turmeric or curcumin 1,000 mg/day (6)
- Collagen hydrolysates 10 g daily
- S-adenosyl-l-methionine (SAMe), ginger extract, methylsulfonylmethane: less reliable improvement with inconsistent supporting evidence
- Acupuncture: need to do 4 weeks or 10 sessions

 ONGOING CARE

FOLLOW-UP RECOMMENDATIONS
- Activity modification in overuse conditions
- Rehabilitative exercise in OA:
  - Low-impact exercise: walking, swimming, cycling
  - Strength, ROM, and proprioception training

Patient Monitoring
- Rehabilitation after initial treatment of acute injury
- In chronic and overuse conditions, assess functional status, rehabilitation adherence, and pain control at follow-up visit.

DIET
Weight reduction by 10% improved function by 28%.

PATIENT EDUCATION
- Review activity modifications.
- Encourage active role in the rehabilitation process.
- Review medication risks and benefits.

PROGNOSIS
Varies with diagnosis, injury severity, chronicity of condition, patient motivation to participate in rehabilitation, and whether surgery is required

COMPLICATIONS
- Disability
- Arthritis
- Chronic joint instability
- Deconditioning

REFERENCES

1. Hong E, Kraft MC. Evaluating anterior knee pain. *Med Clin North Am*. 2014;98(4):697–717.
2. Ayhan E, Kesmezacar H, Akgun I. Intraarticular injections (corticosteroid, hyaluronic acid, platelet rich plasma) for the knee osteoarthritis. *World J Orthop*. 2014;5(3):351–361.
3. Bijlsma JW, Berenbaum F, Lafeber FP. Osteoarthritis: an update with relevance for clinical practice. *Lancet*. 2011;377(9783):2115–2126.
4. Zeng C, Wei J, Persson MSM, et al. Relative efficacy and safety of topical non-steroidal anti-inflammatory drugs for osteoarthritis: a systematic review and network meta-analysis of randomised controlled trials and observational studies. *Br J Sports Med*. 2018;52(10):642–650.
5. Rothermich MA, Glaviano NR, Li J, et al. Patellofemoral pain: epidemiology, pathophysiology, and treatment options. *Clin Sports Med*. 2015;34(2):313–327.
6. Cross M, Smith E, Hoy D, et al. The global burden of hip and knee osteoarthritis: estimates from the global burden of disease 2010 study. *Ann Rheum Dis*. 2014;73(7):1323–1330.

ADDITIONAL READING
- Collins NJ, Bisset LM, Crossley KM, et al. Efficacy of nonsurgical interventions for anterior knee pain: systematic review and meta-analysis of randomized trials. *Sports Med*. 2012;42(1):31–49.
- Lopes AD, Hespanhol LC Jr, Yeung SS, et al. What are the main running-related musculoskeletal injuries? A systematic review. *Sports Med*. 2012;42(10): 891–905.
- Nunes GS, Stapait EL, Kirsten MH, et al. Clinical test for diagnosis of patellofemoral pain syndrome: systematic review with meta-analysis. *Phys Ther Sport*. 2013;14(1):54–59.
- Patel S, Dhillon MS, Aggarwal S, et al. Treatment with platelet-rich plasma is more effective than placebo for knee osteoarthritis: a prospective, double-blind, randomized trial. *Am J Sports Med*. 2013;41(2):356–364.
- Ziltener JL, Leal S, Fournier PE. Non-steroidal anti-inflammatory drugs for athletes: an update. *Ann Phys Rehabil Med*. 2010;53(4):278–288.

 SEE ALSO

Algorithms: Knee Pain; Popliteal Mass

 CODES

ICD10
- M25.569 Pain in unspecified knee
- M17.9 Osteoarthritis of knee, unspecified
- M76.50 Patellar tendinitis, unspecified knee

CLINICAL PEARLS
- A careful history (location/quality of pain and mechanism of injury) targets diagnosis for most causes of knee pain.
- Consider ligamentous injury, meniscal tear, and fracture for patients presenting with acute knee pain.
- Consider OA, patellofemoral pain syndrome, tendinopathy, bursitis, and stress fracture in patients presenting with more chronic symptoms.
- Consider physeal, apophyseal, or articular cartilage injury in young patients presenting with knee pain.
- The presence of an effusion in a patient <30 years of age indicates a significant injury.
- Referred pain from the hip (slipped capital femoral epiphysis, Legg-Calvé-Perthes disease) can present as knee pain.

K

LABYRINTHITIS

John Kerr, DO • Wayne K. Robbins, DO

 BASICS

DESCRIPTION
- The sudden onset of vertigo, accompanied by sensorineural hearing loss and tinnitus, lasting hours to days, and caused by acute inflammation or infection of the labyrinth
- Can be categorized as suppurative or serous/toxic labyrinthitis (1)
- Labyrinthitis is a clinical diagnosis in absence of neurologic deficits.
- Typically presents with a subjective sense of motion or room-spinning vertigo lasting for hours or days and often sudden unilateral sensorineural hearing loss
- Often associated with vestibular hypofunction of the involved ear. Peripheral vertigo improves over time with central compensation. Hearing loss generally improves in the case of serous labyrinthitis but is permanent in the case of suppurative labyrinthitis.
- System(s) affected: nervous, special sensory (auditory and vestibular)

ALERT
- "Vertigo" and "dizziness" are commonly used terms. Clarify symptoms by giving options of alternative descriptions such as light-headedness, disequilibrium, room-spinning vertigo, or imbalance.
- Hearing loss and duration of symptoms can help narrow the differential diagnosis in patients with vertigo.
- Vestibular neuritis/neuronitis occurs due to inflammation of the vestibular nerve causing vertigo lasting hours to days without the auditory symptoms of labyrinthitis (2).
- Benign paroxysmal positional vertigo (BPPV) is the most common cause of vertigo. Unlike labyrinthitis, BPPV is episodic, with severe symptoms lasting <1 minute. BPPV is diagnosed using the Dix-Hallpike maneuver. Unlike labyrinthitis, it is not associated with hearing loss.
- Vestibular migraine is the second most common cause of recurrent vertigo, lasting hours and usually with a history of migraine. Up to 10% of cases can occur without headaches (2).

EPIDEMIOLOGY
- Data is lacking for labyrinthitis alone.
- Most common in 30 to 50 years of age (3)
- 10% of all patients seen for dizziness, if vestibular neuritis is included (4)
- Predominant sex: female = male

Incidence
- Estimated incidence of 3.5 per 100,000 if including vestibular neuritis (3)
- Viral labyrinthitis is the most common etiology.
- Suppurative labyrinthitis secondary to otitis media or meningitis is increasingly rare.

Prevalence
20–30% of adults see a health care provider for vertigo in their lifetimes (3). True labyrinthitis is rare.

ETIOLOGY AND PATHOPHYSIOLOGY
- Acute inflammation and damage to the labyrinth, involving both the vestibular apparatus and cochlea.
- Viral or bacterial toxins may pass into the labyrinth directly from the middle ear to labyrinth via the round or oval window, in the case of serous labyrinthitis.

- Bacterial invasion of the inner ear, either from a middle ear infection or meningitis, occurs in suppurative labyrinthitis (1).
- Infections
  - Common viral: cytomegalovirus, mumps, varicella zoster, rubeola, influenza, parainfluenza, herpes simplex, adenovirus, coxsackievirus, respiratory syncytial virus, HIV
  - Common bacterial: *Streptococcus pneumoniae, Haemophilus influenzae, Moraxella catarrhalis, Neisseria meningitidis, Streptococcus* spp., *Staphylococcus* spp., *Borrelia burgdorferi*
  - Treponemal: *Treponema pallidum*

Genetics
No known genetic link

RISK FACTORS
- Viral upper respiratory infection
- Otitis media
- Cholesteatoma
- Head trauma
- Meningitis

GENERAL PREVENTION
- Early treatment of acute otitis media to prevent complications
- Scheduled immunizations (to prevent common viral pathogens)
- Prevent maternal transmission of pathogens, including syphilis and HIV.

COMMONLY ASSOCIATED CONDITIONS
- Viral upper respiratory infection
- Otitis media
- Cholesteatoma
- Head injury

 DIAGNOSIS

HISTORY
- Vertigo *AND* sensorineural hearing loss in one ear
- Vertigo is acute in onset and lasts hours to days.
- Nausea and vomiting are common.
- Fullness of affected ear
- Tinnitus of affected ear (roaring, ringing)
- Upper respiratory tract infection symptoms
- Otorrhea or otalgia (not common with viral causes)
- Severe headache, fever, and nuchal rigidity in the setting of meningitis
- Recurrent symptoms should raise suspicion for autoimmune causes.
- Profound imbalance or associated focal neurologic signs are not typical and should prompt imaging.

PHYSICAL EXAM
- Nystagmus
  - Fast-beating nystagmus toward affected ear during the acute phase
  - Fast-beating nystagmus away from affected ear during the convalescent phase, 48 to 72 hours later
- Symptoms abate with eyes open and visual fixation.
- Otologic exam may be unremarkable in the setting of viral labyrinthitis.
- Serous/purulent effusion may be present in the middle ear.
- Retraction of the tympanic membrane and keratinaceous debris may be present with cholesteatoma.

DIFFERENTIAL DIAGNOSIS
- Vestibular neuritis/neuronitis (vertigo without hearing loss)
- BPPV: episodic, vertigo lasting seconds/minutes, worse when lying down or looking up
- Ménière disease: episodic vertigo lasting minutes to hours, associated with the triad of episodic vertigo, tinnitus, and hearing loss
- Vestibular migraine
- Autoimmune inner ear disease
- Postconcussive syndrome
- Acute otitis media
- Ototoxicity
- Cardiovascular accident (CVA)/brainstem infarct
- Cerebellopontine-angle tumors (e.g., vestibular schwannoma)
- Less common etiologies: parainfectious encephalomyelitis or cranial polyneuritis, Ramsay Hunt syndrome, HIV infection, syphilis, temporal lobe epilepsy, perilymphatic fistula, superior canal dehiscence, idiopathic sudden single-sided deafness, multiple sclerosis, vasculitis (cerebral or systemic)

DIAGNOSTIC TESTS & INTERPRETATION
- Routine lab studies are not helpful in making the diagnosis unless an autoimmune cause is highly suspected.
- Consider culture of otorrhea or middle ear fluid to direct antibiotic choice.
- CT of the temporal bone may be indicated in the setting of complicated otitis media or cholesteatoma.
- Consider lumbar puncture only if meningitis is suspected.
- Consider screening for syphilis or HIV when clinically indicated by risk factors or clinical history.
- Imaging is not required for the diagnosis of acute labyrinthitis.
- With acute sensorineural hearing loss or other associated neurologic symptoms, an MRI of the IACs and/or MRA of the brain and brainstem are recommended.

Follow-Up Tests & Special Considerations
Labyrinthitis ossificans is fibrosis of the internal auditory canal following bacterial meningitis and is thought to occur due to a suppurative labyrinthitis. This can occur rapidly, especially after *S. pneumoniae* meningitis.

Diagnostic Procedures/Other
- Audiogram should be obtained.
- Vestibular tests are not typically indicated in the acute setting. If vertigo and dizziness persist after expected resolution of symptoms, videonystagmography should be used.

Test Interpretation
- Audiogram may show varying degrees of both sensorineural hearing loss and discrimination loss.
- Caloric testing may show relative weakness of the horizontal semicircular canal of the affected side. Sensitivity and specificity of this test are variable within literature.

TREATMENT

- Symptom management and reassurance in the acute phase
- Vestibular suppressants as needed (see "Medication") for severe acute attacks of vertigo only. Patients should be advised *NOT* to use these medications as scheduled medications or for prophylaxis without symptoms because this can delay central compensation (2)[B].
- Sudden single-sided sensorineural hearing loss should be managed with high-dose steroids (oral and/or intratympanic) as soon as possible, ideally within 2 weeks. Steroids have not been found to definitively improve vestibular symptoms (5)[B].
- Vestibular rehabilitation is the mainstay of treatment for persistent vertigo and dizziness and has been shown to be safe and effective management for unilateral peripheral vestibular dysfunction (6)[A].
- Patients should begin exercises as soon as the acute phase resolves and movement is tolerable, generally within 2 to 3 days of onset (4).
- For suppurative labyrinthitis, appropriate antibiotics to eradicate infection. Surgical intervention may also be required with tympanostomy tubes or mastoidectomy, depending on the extent of middle ear involvement.

GENERAL MEASURES
Vestibular exercises for prolonged symptoms and unilateral vestibular loss have been shown to alleviate postural control.

MEDICATION
Use of the following drugs should be on a PRN basis. Benzodiazepines can also assist with the anxiety associated with vertigo. No patient should take vestibular suppressants as a chronic medication because they can block central compensation.

- Vestibular suppressants
  - Lorazepam (Ativan): 0.5 to 2.0 mg SL/PO BID PRN or diazepam (Valium) 2 to 5 mg QID PO PRN
  - Meclizine (Antivert, Bonine, Zentrip [dissolvable]) 12.5 to 25.0 mg PO BID–TID PRN
  - Dimenhydrinate (Dramamine) 25 to 50 mg PO q4–6h PRN
- Antiemetics
  - Ondansetron (Zofran) 4 to 8 mg PO TID PRN or granisetron (Kytril) 1 mg PO TID PRN
  - Meclizine (Antivert, Bonine) 12.5 to 25.0 mg PO q4h PRN
  - Promethazine (Phenergan) 12.5 to 25.0 mg PO/PR QID PRN or prochlorperazine (Compazine) 25 mg PR BID PRN
  - Metoclopramide (Reglan) 10 mg PO TID PRN
- Antivirals
  - Acyclovir 800 mg PO 5 times per day for 7 days can be used in cases associated with herpes.
- Steroids
  - Prednisone 1 mg/kg/day up to maximum 60 mg daily for 1 week, followed by 1 week taper
  - Methylprednisolone initially 100 mg PO daily and then tapered to 10 mg PO daily over 3 weeks
  - Dexamethasone 0.4 to 0.8 mL of 24 mg/mL strength given via transtympanic injection for three to four sessions; can be used for salvage therapy
  - Given early in the setting of bacterial meningitis, may decrease the otologic sequelae, specifically labyrinthitis ossificans
  - Used in treatment of labyrinthitis for associated sudden sensorineural hearing loss, ideally within the first 2 weeks

Geriatric Considerations
- Elderly are less likely to compensate fully and may report symptoms of disequilibrium lasting weeks to months after resolution of the acute vertigo.
- Avoid excessive use of scopolamine, meclizine, and other vestibular suppressants following the initial event because this will delay central compensation.
- Benzodiazepines are the preferred vestibular suppressant treatment but do increase the risk of falls in older persons.

Pregnancy Considerations
Dimenhydrinate, diphenhydramine, ondansetron, granisetron, and metoclopramide are pregnancy Category B.

First Line
- Benzodiazepines, which are better vestibular suppressants, are preferred over antihistamine/anticholinergics such as meclizine. Sublingual benzodiazepines are very effective for vertigo and should be considered first-line therapy.
- Urgent steroid treatment in acute setting

ISSUES FOR REFERRAL
- Consider neurology referral for suspected central causes of vertigo or dizziness.
- Consider otolaryngology/neurotology referral for progressive hearing loss and vertigo, or in cases of suppurative labyrinthitis requiring surgical intervention.

ADMISSION, INPATIENT, AND NURSING CONSIDERATIONS
- Patients with systemic infection, young age, or intractable vertigo with nausea and vomiting may need to be hospitalized for intravenous fluids and medications.
- Usually outpatient management

ONGOING CARE

FOLLOW-UP RECOMMENDATIONS
Patient Monitoring
Follow hearing loss weekly with audiograms until hearing stabilizes. Acute vertiginous symptoms may last up to 6 weeks. Residual symptoms have been documented to last months or years.

DIET
Avoid alcohol because this may exacerbate symptoms.

PATIENT EDUCATION
Opening eyes with visual fixation should improve symptoms, whereas closing eyes may make symptoms worse. Otherwise, encourage activity as tolerated. Minimize rapid head movement until symptoms resolve. Avoid vestibular suppressants long term because this can inhibit central compensation.

PROGNOSIS
Prognosis depends on cause of labyrinthitis.

COMPLICATIONS
Permanent hearing loss, more common with bacterial causes, and chronic impairment of balance

REFERENCES
1. Kaya S, Schachern PA, Tsuprun V, et al. Deterioration of vestibular cells in labyrinthitis. *Ann Otol Rhinol Laryngol*. 2017;126(2):89–95.
2. Sandhu J, Rea PA. Clinical examination and management of the dizzy patient. *Br J Hosp Med (Lond)*. 2016;77(12):692–698.
3. Neuhauser HK, Lempert T. Vertigo: epidemiologic aspects. *Semin Neurol*. 2009;29(5):473–481.
4. Wipperman J. Dizziness and vertigo. *Prim Care*. 2014;41(1):115–131.
5. Yoo MH, Yang CJ, Kim SA, et al. Efficacy of steroid therapy based on symptomatic and functional improvement in patients with vestibular neuritis: a prospective randomized controlled trial. *Eur Arch Otorhinolaryngol*. 2017;274(6):2443–2451.
6. McDonnell M, Hillier SL. Vestibular rehabilitation for unilateral peripheral vestibular dysfunction. *Cochrane Database Syst Rev*. 2015;(1):CD005397.

ADDITIONAL READING
- Lee HK, Ahn SK, Jeon SY, et al. Clinical characteristics and natural course of recurrent vestibulopathy: a long-term follow-up study. *Laryngoscope*. 2012;122(4):883–886.
- Romoli M, Allais G, Airola G, et al. Ear acupuncture and fMRI: a pilot study for assessing the specificity of auricular points. *Neurol Sci*. 2014;35(Suppl 1):189–193.
- Sokolova L, Hoerr R, Mishchenko T. Treatment of vertigo: a randomized, double-blind trial comparing efficacy and safety of *Ginkgo biloba* extract EGb 761 and betahistine. *Int J Otolaryngol*. 2014;2014:682439.
- Wei BP, Mubiru S, O'Leary S. Steroids for idiopathic sudden sensorineural hearing loss. *Cochrane Database Syst Rev*. 2006;(1):CD003998.

SEE ALSO

Ménière Disease; Postconcussion Syndrome (Mild Traumatic Brain Injury); Tinnitus

CODES

ICD10
- H83.09 Labyrinthitis, unspecified ear
- H83.01 Labyrinthitis, right ear
- H83.02 Labyrinthitis, left ear

CLINICAL PEARLS
- Ask patients to describe symptoms in their own words; alternative symptoms include light-headedness, vertigo, disequilibrium, or imbalance.
- Benzodiazepines are better vestibular suppressants and are preferred over antihistamine/anticholinergics such as meclizine. Vestibular suppressants should be used for short duration only because these will delay central compensation.
- Episodic vertigo tends to be caused by BPPV or Ménière disease, whereas persistent vertigo with sensorineural hearing loss and tinnitus is more consistent with labyrinthitis. Vestibular neuritis would be considered if there was no hearing involvement.

L

LACTOSE INTOLERANCE

Nihal K. Patel, MD

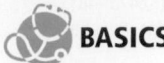 **BASICS**

DESCRIPTION
- Lactose intolerance is a syndrome of abdominal pain, bloating, and flatulence after the ingestion of lactose.
- Lactose malabsorption results from a reduction in lactase activity in the brush border of the small intestinal mucosa.
- Lactase activity peaks at birth then decreases after the first few months of life, declining continuously throughout life. 75% of adults worldwide exhibit a decline in lactase activity after birth. *Only 50% of lactase activity is needed to digest lactose without causing symptoms of lactose intolerance.*
  - Congenital lactose intolerance: very rare
  - Primary lactose intolerance: common in adults who develop low lactase levels after childhood
  - Secondary lactose intolerance: inability to digest lactose caused by any condition injuring the intestinal mucosa (e.g., infectious enteritis, celiac disease, eosinophilic gastroenteritis, or inflammatory bowel disease) or a reduction of available mucosal surface (e.g., resection)
- Lactose malabsorption may be asymptomatic and is equally common in healthy patients and in those with functional bowel disorders.
- System(s) affected: endocrine/metabolic, gastrointestinal

Pediatric Considerations
- Primary lactose intolerance begins in late childhood.
- No consensus on whether young children (<5 years of age) should avoid lactose following diarrheal illness
- Lactose-free formulas are available.
- Exclude milk protein allergy.

EPIDEMIOLOGY
Incidence
- ≥50% of infants with acute or chronic diarrheal disease have lactose intolerance; particularly common with rotavirus infection
- Lactose intolerance is common with giardiasis, ascariasis, irritable bowel syndrome (IBS), tropical and nontropical sprue, and AIDS malabsorptive syndrome.

Prevalence
- In South America, Africa, and Asia, rates of lactose intolerance are >50%.
- In the United States, the prevalence is 15% among whites, 53% among Hispanics, and 80% among African Americans.
- In Europe, lactose intolerance varies from 15% in Scandinavian countries to 70% in Italy.
- Predominant age:
  - Primary: teenage and adult
  - Secondary: depends on underlying condition
- Predominant sex: male = female

ETIOLOGY AND PATHOPHYSIOLOGY
- Primary lactose intolerance: The normal decline in lactase activity in the intestinal mucosa is genetically determined and permanent after weaning from breast milk.
- Secondary lactose intolerance: associated with gastroenteritis in children; also associated with any gastrointestinal infection or inflammation of the small intestine with resultant lactose malabsorption in both adults and children

Genetics
- In whites, lactase deficiency is associated with a single nucleotide polymorphism (SNP) consisting of a nucleotide switch of T for C 13910 bp on chromosome 2. This results in variants of CC-13910 (lactase nonpersistence) OR CT-13910/TT-13910 (lactase persistence) (1).
- SNP (C/T-13910) is associated with lactase persistence in northern Europeans.
- Other SNPs (G/C-14010, T/G-13915, and C/G-13907) have been linked to lactase persistence in some patients of African descent.

RISK FACTORS
- Adult-onset lactase deficiency has wide geographic variation.
- Age:
  - Signs and symptoms usually do not become apparent until after age 6 to 7 years.
  - Symptoms may not be apparent until adulthood, depending on dietary lactose intake and rate of decline of intestinal lactase activity.
  - Lactase activity correlates with age, regardless of symptoms.

GENERAL PREVENTION
Lactose avoidance relieves symptoms. Patients can learn what level of lactose is tolerable in their diet.

COMMONLY ASSOCIATED CONDITIONS
- Tropical or nontropical sprue
- Giardiasis
- IBS or other functional bowel disorders
- Small intestinal bacterial overgrowth (SIBO)
- Celiac disease

DIAGNOSIS

- Lactose intolerance can be presumed in patients manifesting mild symptoms after ingestion of significant amounts of lactose (such as >2 servings of dairy per day), with resolution of symptoms after avoidance of lactose-containing foods for 1 week.
- A positive lactose hydrogen breath test is confirmatory.
- Lactose intolerance can mimic symptoms of functional gastrointestinal disorders. Lactose intolerance can also be a coexisting condition.

HISTORY
- Assess daily lactose consumption.
- A single dose of lactose (12 g, equivalent to 1 cup of milk) consumed alone produces no or minor symptoms in persons with lactose intolerance.
- Lactose doses of 15 to 18 g are well tolerated with other nutrients. Doses >18 g cause progressively more symptoms, and quantities >50 g elicit symptoms in most individuals.
- Symptoms arise 30 minutes to 2 hours after consumption of lactose-containing products.
- Symptoms include bloating, flatulence, cramping abdominal discomfort, and diarrhea or loose stools. Vomiting may be noted in adolescents.
- Abdominal pain may be crampy in nature and often is localized to the periumbilical area or lower quadrant.
- Stools usually are bulky, frothy, and watery, although diarrhea may be rare in adults.
- Only 20–30% of individuals with lactose malabsorption develop symptoms.

PHYSICAL EXAM
- Vital signs and general appearance are typically normal.
- Audible bowel sounds (borborygmi) on physical examination (may be particularly bothersome to the patient). The exam is otherwise typically normal or nonspecific.

DIFFERENTIAL DIAGNOSIS
- Functional GI disorder (e.g., IBS)
- SIBO
- Celiac disease
- Inflammatory bowel disease
- Infectious enteritis such as giardiasis
- Drug or radiation induced enteritis
- Sucrase deficiency
- Cow's milk protein allergy

DIAGNOSTIC TESTS & INTERPRETATION
Initial Tests (lab, imaging)
- The lactose breath test (LBT) is a confirmatory for lactose intolerance. It is noninvasive, easy to perform (sensitivity 78%; specificity 98%) (2).
- Intestinal bacteria digest carbohydrates and produce measurable hydrogen and methane in expired breath:
  - Administer lactose when fasting (2 g/kg; max dose 25 g in children; 50 g in adults). Note any symptoms; sample breath hydrogen at baseline and at 30-minute intervals for 3 hours. Compare postlactose and baseline values. A rise in hydrogen concentration value of 20 ppm over baseline is diagnostic for lactose malabsorption. An early peak (15 to 30 minutes) suggests SIBO.
- Small bowel biopsy for histology and direct measurement of lactase activity (rarely needed).
- A positive LBT confirms lactose malabsorption but does not determine etiology.

Diagnostic Procedures/Other
- Lactose tolerance test is an alternative to LBT in adults and measures lactose absorption through serum glucose measurements. Following oral administration of a 50-g test dose in adults (2 g/kg in children), blood glucose levels are monitored at 0, 60, and 120 minutes. An increase in blood glucose of <20 mg/dL (1.1 mmol/L) with the concurrent development of symptoms is diagnostic. False-negative results may occur in patients with diabetes or bacterial overgrowth.
- Stool electrolyte testing, if done, may indicate a stool osmotic gap >125 mOsm/kg, although this is not specific to lactose intolerance.

Test Interpretation
Low lactase enzyme activity in intestinal mucosa, tested by small bowel biopsy, may be patchy or focal.

TREATMENT

There is insufficient evidence to recommend any particular treatment (including probiotics, colonic adaptation, and other supplements) as definitive first line.

- In the absence of a correctable underlying disease, treatment includes four general principles (3)[B].
  - Avoid milk/dairy products to improve symptoms.
  - Up to 12 to 15 g of lactose can be tolerated in without significant symptoms (1 cup of milk).
  - Gradually reintroduce lactose as symptoms allow. Spreading lactose servings throughout the day improves tolerance.
  - If symptoms persist, substitute fermented and matured milk products for lactose.
- Certain strains, concentrations, and preparations of probiotics may alleviate symptoms.
- Incrementally increasing doses of lactose to induce adaptation have limited success.
- Insufficient evidence to routinely recommend lactose-reduced or hydrolyzed milk, lactase supplements taken with milk or probiotics.
- Maintain calcium and vitamin D intake.

MEDICATION
First Line
Lactase (Lactaid, Lactrase):
- Commercially available "lactase" preparations are bacterial or yeast β-galactosidases.
- Take 1 to 2 capsules or tablets prior to ingesting dairy products.
- Effectiveness at preventing symptoms varies.
- Can add tablets or contents of capsules to milk (1 to 2 caps/tabs per quart of milk) before drinking; also commercially available in milk in some areas
- Not effective for all people with lactose intolerance

COMPLEMENTARY & ALTERNATIVE MEDICINE
Certain probiotic formulations taken with meals may alleviate some symptoms of lactose intolerance (4)[B].

ONGOING CARE

DIET
- Reduce or restrict dietary lactose to control symptoms—patient-specific "trial and error."
- Yogurt and fermented products such as hard cheese are often better tolerated than milk.
- Supplement calcium (e.g., calcium carbonate).
- Prehydrolyzed milk (Lactaid) is available.

PATIENT EDUCATION
- Read labels on commercial products—milk sugar is used in many products and may cause symptoms.
- Patients may tolerate whole milk or chocolate milk better than skim milk (slower rate of gastric emptying)
- Lactose consumed with other food products is better tolerated than when consumed with milk alone.
- Primary lactase deficiency is permanent; secondary lactose intolerance usually is temporary, although it may persist for months after the inciting event.
- 20% of prescription drugs and 6% of over-the-counter (OTC) medicines may contain lactose as a base.
- Most patients with lactose intolerance or malabsorption can tolerate 12 to 15 g of lactose per day.

PROGNOSIS
- Normal life expectancy
- Symptoms can be controlled through diet alone if lactase tablets are ineffective.

COMPLICATIONS
Calcium deficiency: Avoidance of milk and other dairy products can lead to reduced calcium intake, which may increase the risk for osteoporosis and fracture.

REFERENCES

1. Mattar R, de Campos Mazo DF, Carrilho FJ. Lactose intolerance: diagnosis, genetic, and clinical factors. *Clin Exp Gastroenterol*. 2012;5:113–121.
2. Gasbarrini A, Corazza GR, Gasbarrini G, et al; and 1st Rome H2-Breath Testing Consensus Conference Working Group. Methodology and indications of H2-breath testing in gastrointestinal diseases: the Rome Consensus Conference. *Aliment Pharmacol Ther*. 2009;29(Suppl 1):1–49.
3. Shaukat A, Levitt MD, Taylor BC, et al. Systematic review: effective management strategies for lactose intolerance. *Ann Intern Med*. 2010;152(12):797–803.
4. Deng Y, Misselwitz B, Dai N, et al. Lactose intolerance in adults: biological mechanism and dietary management. *Nutrients*. 2015;7(9):8020–8035.

ADDITIONAL READING

- Almeida CC, Lorena SL, Pavan CR, et al. Beneficial effects of long-term consumption of a probiotic combination of *Lactobacillus casei* Shirota and *Bifidobacterium breve* Yakult may persist after suspension of therapy in lactose-intolerant patients. *Nutr Clin Pract*. 2012;27(2):247–251.
- Fernández-Bañares F. Reliability of symptom analysis during carbohydrate hydrogen-breath tests. *Curr Opin Clin Nutr Metab Care*. 2012;15(5):494–498.
- Tan-Dy CR, Ohlsson A. Lactase treated feeds to promote growth and feeding tolerance in preterm infants. *Cochrane Database Syst Rev*. 2013;(3):CD004591.

CODES

ICD10
- E73.9 Lactose intolerance, unspecified
- E73.8 Other lactose intolerance
- E73.1 Secondary lactase deficiency

CLINICAL PEARLS

- The diagnosis of lactose intolerance is based on clinical history and confirmed by hydrogen breath testing.
- Most lactose-intolerant patients can tolerate up to 12 to 15 g of lactose per day (equivalent to 1 cup of milk).
- Lactose-intolerant patients may tolerate yogurt and fermented products better than milk and cheese.
- A diary helps identify problematic foods.
- Patients should read ingredient labels to look for milk, lactose, whey, and curd.
- Lactose-intolerant patients may tolerate whole milk or chocolate milk better than skim milk due to a slower rate of gastric emptying.
- Many patients with lactose intolerance unnecessarily avoid all dairy products, potentially causing an inadequate intake of calcium and vitamin D.

LARYNGITIS

Sheila O. Stille, DMD • Karlynn Sievers, MD

BASICS

DESCRIPTION
- Laryngitis is inflammation, erythema, and edema of the mucosa of the larynx and/or vocal cords characterized by hoarseness, loss of voice, throat pain, coughing, and often a negative impact on a person's quality of life and daily activities.
- There is a range of severity, but most cases are acute and are associated with viral upper respiratory infection, irritation, or acute vocal strain.
- System(s) affected: pulmonary; ears, nose, throat (ENT)
- Synonym(s): acute laryngitis; chronic laryngitis; croup or laryngotracheitis (in children)

EPIDEMIOLOGY
- Predominant age: affects all ages
- Children more susceptible than adults due to increased risk of symptomatic inflammation from smaller airways
- Predominant sex: male = female

Incidence
Common

Prevalence
Common; approximately 1.7% of population have dysphonia with 50% of this being caused by acute laryngitis. Prevalence rates are increasing but difficult to calculate because many patients do not seek medical attention.

ETIOLOGY AND PATHOPHYSIOLOGY
- Misuse or abuse of voice
- Infectious
  - Viral: influenza A, B; parainfluenza; adenovirus; coronavirus; rhinovirus; human papillomavirus; cytomegalovirus; varicella-zoster virus; herpes simplex virus; respiratory syncytial virus; coxsackievirus
  - Fungal: uncommon but thought to be underdiagnosed, potentially accounting for up to 10% of presentations in both immunocompromised and immunocompetent patients; risk factors include recent antibiotic or inhaled corticosteroid use (1): histoplasmosis, blastomycosis, *Coccidioides*, *Cryptococcus*, and *Candida*.
  - Bacterial (uncommon): β-hemolytic streptococcus, *Streptococcus pneumoniae*, *Haemophilus influenzae*, tuberculosis (TB), leprosy, *Moraxella catarrhalis*, *Mycoplasma pneumoniae*, *Chlamydophila pneumoniae*
  - Secondary syphilis if left untreated
  - Leprosy (in 30–55% of those with leprosy, larynx is affected; in tropical and warm countries)
- Irritants
  - Inhalation of irritating substances (e.g., air pollution, cigarette smoke)
  - Aspiration of caustic chemicals

- Gastroesophageal reflux disease (GERD)/laryngopharyngeal reflux disease (LPRD)
  - Excessively dry environment
  - Allergy exposures (including pollens)
- Anatomic
  - Aging changes: muscle atrophy, loss of moisture in larynx, and bowing of vocal cords
  - Vocal cord nodules/polyps ("singer's nodes")
  - Local cancer
- Iatrogenic: inhaled steroids such as those used to treat asthma, surgical injury, endotracheal intubation injury
- Idiopathic
- Neuromuscular disorder (e.g., myasthenia gravis); stroke
- Rheumatoid arthritis
- Trauma (e.g., blunt or penetrating trauma to neck)

RISK FACTORS
- Acute:
  - Infection or trauma
  - Upper respiratory tract viral infection (e.g., influenza, rhinovirus, adenovirus, parainfluenza)
  - Voice overuse—excess talking, singing, or shouting
  - Pneumonia—viral or bacterial
  - Coughing
  - Lack of immunization for pertussis or diphtheria
  - Immunocompromised
  - Recent endotracheal intubation or local surgery
- Chronic (persists beyond 3 weeks):
  - Allergic laryngitis (2)
  - Chronic rhinitis/sinusitis
  - Voice abuse
  - GERD/LPRD (1)
  - Smoking: primary or secondhand
  - Excessive alcohol use
  - Autoimmune disorders (e.g., rheumatoid arthritis) (1,3)
  - Granulomatous diseases (e.g., sarcoidosis) (1)
  - Stroke
  - Environmental pollution; constant exposure to dust or other irritants such as chemicals at workplace
  - Medications: inhaled steroids, anticholinergics, antihistamines, anabolic steroids

Geriatric Considerations
May be more ill, slower to heal; need to consider neoplasm

Pediatric Considerations
- Common in this age group
- Consider congenital/anatomic causes.

GENERAL PREVENTION
- Avoid overuse of voice (speech therapy/voice training is helpful for vocal musicians/public speakers).
- Influenza virus vaccine is recommended.
- Quit smoking and avoid secondhand smoke.

- Limit or avoid alcohol/caffeine/acidic foods.
- Control GERD/LPRD.
- Maintain proper hydration status.
- Avoid allergens.
- Wear mask around chemical/environmental irritants.
- Good hand washing (infection prevention)

COMMONLY ASSOCIATED CONDITIONS
- Viral pharyngitis
- Diphtheria (rare): Membrane can descend into the larynx.
- Pertussis: larynx involved as part of the respiratory system
- Bronchitis
- Pneumonitis
- Croup, epiglottitis, in children

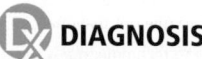

DIAGNOSIS

HISTORY
- Hoarseness, throat "tickle," dry cough, and rawness (4)
- Dysphonia (abnormal-sounding voice)
- Constant urge to clear the throat
- Possible fever
- Malaise
- Dysphagia/odynophagia
- Regional cervical lymphadenopathy
- Stridor or possible airway obstruction in children (1)
- Cough may be worse at night in children.
- Hemoptysis
- Laryngospasm or sense of choking
- Allergic rhinitis/rhinorrhea/postnasal drip (PND) (4)
- Occupation or other reasons for voice overuse
- Smoking history
- Blunt or penetrating trauma to neck
- GERD/LPRD

PHYSICAL EXAM
- Head and neck exam, including airway patency, cervical nodes; cranial nerve exam
- Visualization of the larynx: preferably with a flexible or rigid endoscope or with an indirect mirror examination as a screening technique to dictate further appropriate testing (4)
- Note quality of voice (i.e., hoarse, breathy, wet, "hot potato like," asthenic [weak], strained) (2).

DIFFERENTIAL DIAGNOSIS
- Diphtheria
- Vocal nodules or polyps
- Laryngeal malignancy
- Thyroid malignancy
- Upper airway malignancy (2,4)[A]
- Epiglottitis
- Pertussis

- Laryngeal nerve trauma/injury
- Foreign body (in children)
- Autoimmune (rheumatoid arthritis) (3)[A]

DIAGNOSTIC TESTS & INTERPRETATION
- Rarely needed
- WBCs elevated in bacterial laryngitis
- Viral culture (seldom necessary)

Follow-Up Tests & Special Considerations
- Barium swallow, only if needed for differential diagnosis
- CT scan if foreign body suspected

Diagnostic Procedures/Other
- Fiber-optic or indirect laryngoscopy: looking for red, inflamed, and occasionally hemorrhagic vocal cords; rounded edges and exudate (Reinke edema)
- Consider otolaryngologic evaluation and biopsy: laryngitis lasting >2 weeks in adults with history of smoking or alcohol abuse, to rule out malignancy.
- pH probe (24-hour): no difference in incidence of pharyngeal reflux as measured by pH probe between patients with chronic reflux laryngitis and healthy adults (2)[A]
- Strobovideo laryngoscopy for diagnosis of subtle lesions (e.g., vocal cord nodules or polyps) (4)[A]

TREATMENT
- Limited but good evidence that treatment beyond supportive care is ineffective (4)[A]
- Supportive care consists of hydration, voice rest, humidification, and limitation of caffeine (1)[A].
- Antibiotics appear to have no benefit because etiologies are predominantly viral (1,5)[A].
- Corticosteroids in severe cases of laryngitis to reduce inflammation such as croup
- May need voice training, if voice overuse
- Nebulized epinephrine reduces croup symptoms 30 minutes posttreatment; evidence does not favor racemic epinephrine or L-epinephrine or IPPB over simple nebulization. Racemic epinephrine reduces croup symptoms at 30 minutes, but effect lasts only 2 hours (5)[A].

GENERAL MEASURES
- Acute:
  – Usually a self-limited illness lasting <3 weeks and not severe
  – Antibiotics of no value (5)[A]
  – Avoid excessive voice use, including whispering.
  – Steam inhalations or cool-mist humidifier
  – Increase fluid intake, especially in cases associated with excessive dryness.
  – Avoid smoking (or secondhand exposure).
  – Warm saltwater gargles
- Chronic:
  – Symptomatic treatment as above
  – Voice therapy (for patients with intermittent dysphagia and vocal abuse)
  – Smoking cessation

– Reduction or cessation of alcohol intake
– Occupational change or modification, if exposure driven
– Allergen avoidance
– Consider discontinuing offending medication (e.g., inhaled steroids) (5)[A].
- Reflux laryngitis: elevate head of bed, diet changes, other antireflux lifestyle change management; proton pump inhibitors (1)[A]

MEDICATION
Usually none

First Line
- Analgesics
- Antipyretics (rare)
- Cough suppressants
- Throat lozenges
- Plenty of fluids

Second Line
- Inhaled corticosteroids (consider only if allergy induced) (2)
- Oral corticosteroids: only if urgent need in adults (presenter, singer, actor)
- Oral corticosteroids: Evidence of benefit has been studied with single-dose dexamethasone in children ages 6 months to 5 years for moderate-severity croup; reduces symptoms within 6 hours; reduces hospitalizations, hospital length of stay, and revisits to office (5)[A]
- Standard of care is to prescribe proton pump inhibitors for chronic laryngitis if GERD or LPRD is suspected; however, evidence suggests only a modest benefit, if any (1)[A].
- Treat nonviral infectious underlying causes.
- Candidal laryngitis:
  – Mild cases: oral antifungal (fluconazole)
  – Amphotericin B or echinocandin can be given in life-threatening cases (1)[A].

ISSUES FOR REFERRAL
- Immediate emergency ENT referral for patients with stridor or respiratory distress (1)[A]
- ENT referral for persistent symptoms (>2 to 3 weeks) or concern for foreign body
- Consider otolaryngologic evaluation and biopsy for laryngitis lasting >3 weeks in adults, especially in those with history of smoking or alcohol abuse to rule out malignancy.
- Consider GI consult to rule out GERD/LPRD.

SURGERY/OTHER PROCEDURES
- Vocal cord biopsy of hyperplastic mucosa and areas of leukoplakia if cancer or TB is suspected
- Removal of nodules or polyps if voice therapy fails

COMPLEMENTARY & ALTERNATIVE MEDICINE
Some experts, although not well studied, have recommended the following:
- Barberry, black currant, *Echinacea*, *Eucalyptus*, German chamomile, goldenrod, goldenseal, warmed lemon and honey, licorice, marshmallow, peppermint, saw palmetto, slippery elm, vitamin C, zinc

 ONGOING CARE

PATIENT EDUCATION
- Educate on the importance of voice rest, including whispering.
- Provide assistance with smoking cessation.
- Help the patient with modification of other predisposing habits or occupational hazards.

PROGNOSIS
Complete clearing of the inflammation without sequelae

COMPLICATIONS
Chronic hoarseness

REFERENCES
1. Wood JM, Athanasiadis T, Allen J. Laryngitis. *BMJ*. 2014;349:g5827.
2. Platt MP, Brook CD, Kuperstock J, et al. What role does allergy play in chronic ear disease and laryngitis? *Curr Allergy Asthma Rep*. 2016;16(10):76.
3. Hamdan AL, Sarieddine D. Laryngeal manifestations of rheumatoid arthritis. *Autoimmune Dis*. 2013;2013:103081.
4. Reiter R, Hoffmann TK, Pickhard A, et al. Hoarseness—causes and treatments. *Dtsch Arztebl Int*. 2015;112(19):329–337.
5. Reveiz L, Cardona AF. Antibiotics for acute laryngitis in adults. *Cochrane Database Syst Rev*. 2015;(5):CD004783.

ADDITIONAL READING
- Benninger MS, Holy CE, Bryson PC, et al. Prevalence and occupation of patients presenting with dysphonia in the United States. *J Voice*. 2017;31(5): 594–600.
- Russell KF, Liang Y, O'Gorman K, et al. Glucocorticoids for croup. *Cochrane Database Syst Rev*. 2011;(1):CD001955.

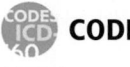 **CODES**

ICD10
- J04.0 Acute laryngitis
- J37.0 Chronic laryngitis
- J04.2 Acute laryngotracheitis

CLINICAL PEARLS
- Laryngitis is usually self-limited and needs only comfort care. Standard treatment is voice rest, hydration, humidification, and limit caffeine intake.
- Refer to ENT for direct visualization of vocal cords for prolonged laryngitis.
- Corticosteroids have some benefits for children with moderately severe croup.
- Voice training useful for chronic laryngitis

L

LEAD POISONING

Jason Chao, MD, MS

 BASICS

DESCRIPTION
- Disease resulting from a high body burden of lead (Pb)—an element with no known physiologic value
- Synonym(s): lead poisoning, inorganic

EPIDEMIOLOGY
- Predominant age: 1 to 5 years, adult workers
- Predominant sex: male > female (1:1 in childhood)

Prevalence
- Centers for Disease Control and Prevention (CDC) estimates half a million U.S. children aged 1 to 5 years have blood Pb levels >5 μg/dL. Levels vary among communities and populations.
- In 2016, 12,574 children in the United States were noted with a blood Pb level ≥10 μg/dL, down from 17,246 in 2012.

ETIOLOGY AND PATHOPHYSIOLOGY
- Inhalation of Pb dust or fumes, or ingestion of Pb
- Pb replaces calcium in bones. Pb interferes with heme synthesis, causes interstitial nephritis, and interferes with neurotransmitters, especially glutamine; high levels affect blood–brain barrier and lead to encephalopathy, seizures, and coma.
- Early life Pb exposure causes methylation changes leading to epigenetic alterations that may predispose to brain dysfunction.

RISK FACTORS
- Children with pica or with iron-deficiency anemia
- Residence in or frequent visitor to deteriorating pre-1960 housing with Pb-painted surfaces or recent renovation
- Soil/dust exposure near older homes, Pb industries, or urban roads
- Sibling or playmate with current or past Pb poisoning
- Dust from clothing of Pb worker or hobbyist
- Pb dissolved in water from Pb or Pb-soldered plumbing (e.g., Flint, Michigan 2014 to 2015)
- Pb-glazed ceramics leach (especially with acidic food or drink)
- Folk remedies and cosmetics
  - Mexico: Azarcon, Greta
  - Dominican Republic: litargirio, a topical agent
  - Asia and Middle East: chuifong tokuwan, payloo-ah, ghasard, bali goli, kandu, ayurvedic herbal medicine from South Asia, kohl (alkohl, ceruse), surma, saoott, cebagin
- Hobbies: target shooting, glazed pottery making, Pb soldering, preparing Pb shot or fishing sinkers, stained-glass making, car/boat repair, home remodeling
- Occupational exposure: plumbers, pipe fitters, Pb miners, auto repairers, glass manufacturers, ship builders, printer operators, plastic manufacturers, Pb smelters and refiners, steel welders or cutters, construction workers, rubber product manufacturers, battery manufacturers, bridge reconstruction workers, firing range workers, military and law enforcement

- Dietary: zinc or calcium deficiency
- Imported toys with Pb
- Retained bullet fragments

Pediatric Considerations
- Children are at increased risk because of incomplete development of the blood–brain barrier prior to 3 years of age (allowing more Pb into the CNS).
- Ingested Pb has 40% bioavailability in children (10% in adults).
- Common childhood behaviors such as frequent hand-to-mouth activity and pica (repeated ingestion of nonfood products) increase the risk of Pb ingestion.

Pregnancy Considerations
Cross-sectional studies suggest an association between elevated blood Pb and preeclampsia.

GENERAL PREVENTION
- Counsel families on sources of Pb and how to decrease exposure. Screen high-risk children (1)[C].
- Warn parents about unsafe home renovations.
- Wet mopping and dusting with a high-phosphate solution (e.g., powdered automatic dishwasher detergent with 1/4 cup per gallon of water) helps control Pb-bearing dust. High-phosphate detergent is no longer available in some states.
- If tap water is potentially Pb contaminated, use cold water instead of hot water and run for 30 to 60 seconds to flush pipes. Use Pb-free water source if possible (bottled or distilled water).
- Screen at-risk pregnant women (2)[C].

COMMONLY ASSOCIATED CONDITIONS
Iron-deficiency anemia

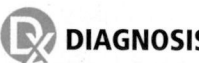 **DIAGNOSIS**

HISTORY
- Often asymptomatic
- Mild-to-moderate toxicity:
  - Myalgias, paresthesias, fatigue, irritability, lethargy
  - Abdominal discomfort, arthralgia, difficulty concentrating, headache, tremor, vomiting, weight loss, muscular exhaustibility
- Severe toxicity: three major clinical syndromes:
  - Alimentary type: anorexia, metallic taste, constipation, severe abdominal cramps due to intestinal spasm and sometimes associated with abdominal wall rigidity
  - Neuromuscular type (characteristic of adult plumbism): peripheral neuritis, usually painless and limited to extensor muscles
  - Cerebral type or Pb encephalopathy (more common in children): seizure, coma, and long-term sequelae, including neurologic defects, delayed mental development, and chronic hyperactivity
- Chronic exposure may cause renal failure.

PHYSICAL EXAM
Often normal, but abdominal tenderness may be severe. Neurologic exam may reveal neuropathy or encephalopathy. Historical feature is "crackpot skull"—resonant cranium secondary to hydrocephalus.

DIFFERENTIAL DIAGNOSIS
- Alimentary type may present as acute abdomen.
- Neuromuscular type presents similar to other polyneuropathies.
- May be confused with ADD, intellectual disability, autism, dementia, and other causes of seizures
- Elevated erythrocyte protoporphyrin may be caused by iron-deficiency anemia or (less commonly) hemolytic anemia.
- Erythropoietic protoporphyria produces a very high erythrocyte protoporphyrin level.

DIAGNOSTIC TESTS & INTERPRETATION
- Venous blood Pb >5 μg/dL (0.24 μmol/L)
- Confirm screening capillary Pb levels >5 μg/dL (0.24 μmol/L) with a venous sample.
- Hemoglobin and hematocrit slightly low; eosinophilia; basophilic stippling on peripheral smear (not diagnostic of Pb toxicity)
- Renal function is decreased in late stages.
- Abdominal radiograph for Pb particles in gut if recent ingestion is suspected
- Radiograph of long bones may show metaphyseal changes (resulting from growth arrest). Films are not routinely recommended.

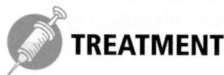 **TREATMENT**

Blood Level (μg/dL)	Time to Confirmation Testing
≥ref value–9	1–3 mo
10–44	1 wk–1 mo
45–59	48 hr
60–69	24 hr
≥70	Urgently as emergency test

ALERT
- For blood Pb levels persistently >15 μg/dL, contact local public health department for home inspection.
- For Pb levels between 5 and 45 μg/dL, higher levels require urgent confirmation.
- For any elevated level, educate on sources of Pb exposure.
- 5 Pb level-45: complete history and physical exam, follow-up Pb monitoring; complete inspection of home or workplace to determine source of Pb and Pb-hazard reduction; neurodevelopmental monitoring: iron status, hemoglobin, or hematocrit (3)[C]
- Pb level 45 to 69 μg/dL: treatment to lower level plus free erythrocyte protoporphyrin, oral chelation therapy, or hospitalization if Pb-safe environment cannot be ensured (3)[C]
- Pb >70 μg/dL: Hospitalize for chelation therapy (4)[C].

MEDICATION

- Consider oral chelation for asymptomatic and Pb >45 and <70; chelation (preferably parenteral) for Pb >70 or symptomatic Pb <70 (4)[C]
- Do not begin chelation until Pb particles present in gut are cleared (5)[C].

First Line

- Oral chelation: succimer (Chemet), dimercaptosuccinic acid (DMSA) 350 mg/m^2 or 10 mg/kg q8h for 5 days and then q12h for 2 weeks. This may be repeated after 2 weeks off if Pb levels are not stabilized at <15 μg/dL (<0.72 μmol/L) (4)[C].
- Parenteral chelation (begin after establishment of adequate urine output):
  - Dimercaprol (British anti-Lewisite [BAL]) 75 mg/m^2 given deep IM, then BAL 450 mg/m^2/day divided q4h for 5 days plus Ca edetate calcium disodium (EDTA) 1,500 mg/m^2/day continuous IV infusion for 5 days. If rebound Pb level ≥45 μg/dL (≥2.17 μmol/L), chelation may be repeated after 2-day interval if symptomatic or after 5-day interval if asymptomatic.
  - Ca EDTA 1,000 mg/m^2/day for 5 days; may be repeated after 5 to 7 days
- Diazepam for initial control of seizures; further control maintained with paraldehyde
- Contraindications: Do not give BAL to patients with a peanut allergy (the drug solution contains peanut oil).
- Precautions
  - Succimer: GI upset, rash, nasal congestion, muscle pains, elevated liver function tests
  - BAL: nausea, vomiting, fever, headache, transient hypertension, hepatocellular damage
  - Ca EDTA: renal failure; increased excretion of zinc, copper, and iron
- Significant possible interactions
  - Do not give vitamins with oral chelation.
  - BAL may precipitate hemolytic crisis in a patient with glucose-6-phosphate dehydrogenase deficiency.

Second Line

Oral chelation with penicillamine (D-penicillamine, Depen, Cuprimine) (5)[C]

- Penicillin-allergic patient should not receive penicillamine (cross-sensitivity is common).
- 10 to 15 mg/kg/day given BID mixed in apple juice/sauce on empty stomach (not FDA-approved)
- Penicillamine may cause GI upset, renal failure, granulocytopenia, liver dysfunction, iron deficiency, and drug-induced lupus-like syndrome.

ISSUES FOR REFERRAL

Consider consultation if parenteral chelation is required.

ADDITIONAL THERAPIES

Remove patient from potential source of Pb if Pb level >45 until complete home inspection is performed.

COMPLEMENTARY & ALTERNATIVE MEDICINE

Garlic has been used to treat mild to moderate Pb poisoning in adults.

ADMISSION, INPATIENT, AND NURSING CONSIDERATIONS

- Blood Pb level >70 μg/dL
- If symptomatic, blood Pb level >35 μg/dL

- Outpatient care unless parenteral chelation or immediate removal from contaminated environment is required
- If Pb source is in the home, the patient must reside elsewhere until the abatement process is completed.
- Avoid visit to any site of potential contamination.

 ONGOING CARE

FOLLOW-UP RECOMMENDATIONS

Patient Monitoring

- Check for rebound Pb level 7 to 10 days after chelation therapy. Monitor biweekly or monthly thereafter.
- Correct iron or other detected nutritional deficiencies.
- Once Pb <35 μg/dL, repeat testing every 1 to 3 months until level <25 μg/dL is achieved. Then, monitor every 3 to 6 months until level <10 μg/dL. Once <9 μg/dL, test every 6 to 9 months (3)[C].

DIET

- If symptomatic, avoid excessive fluids.
- Avoid pica.
- Adequate calcium, iron, zinc, and vitamin C to reduce absorption and retention of Pb (5)[B]

PATIENT EDUCATION

- National Lead Information Center, 422 South Clinton Avenue, Rochester, NY 14620; 800-424-5323; https://www.epa.gov/lead
- National Safety Council, 1121 Spring Lake Drive, Itasca, IL 60143-3201; 800-621-7615; http://www.nsc.org/learn/safety-knowledge/Pages/Lead-Poisoning-Prevention.aspx

PROGNOSIS

- Symptomatic Pb poisoning without encephalopathy generally improves with chelation, but subtle CNS toxicity may be long-lasting or permanent.
- Children with high Pb levels at age 11 years have lower IQ score and socioeconomic status in adulthood.
- With Pb encephalopathy, permanent sequelae (e.g., mental retardation, seizure disorder, blindness, and hemiparesis) occurs in 25–50%.

COMPLICATIONS

- CNS toxicity may be long-lasting or permanent.
- Long-term Pb exposure may cause chronic renal failure (Fanconi-like syndrome), gout, or Pb line (blue–black) on gingival tissue.
- Pb exposure in pregnancy is associated with reduced birth weight and premature birth.
- Pb is an animal teratogen.

REFERENCES

1. Council on Environmental Health. Prevention of childhood lead toxicity. Pediatrics. 2016;138(1):e20161493.
2. Centers for Disease Control and Prevention. Guidelines for the Identification and Management of Lead Exposure in Pregnant and Lactating Women. Atlanta, GA: Centers for Disease Control and Prevention; 2010.
3. Centers for Disease Control and Prevention. Low Level Lead Exposure Harms Children: A Renewed Call for Primary Prevention. Atlanta, GA: Centers for Disease Control and Prevention; 2012.
4. American Academy of Pediatrics Committee on Environmental Health. Lead exposure in children: prevention, detection, and management. Pediatrics. 2005;116(4):1036–1046.
5. Woolf AD, Goldman R, Bellinger DC. Update on the clinical management of childhood lead poisoning. Pediatr Clin North Am. 2007;54(2):271–294.

ADDITIONAL READING

- Centers for Disease Control and Prevention. CBLS national table. https://www.cdc.gov/nceh/lead/data/CBLS-National-Table-508.pdf. Accessed September 8, 2018.
- Neuwirth LS. Resurgent lead poisoning and renewed public attention towards environmental social justice issues: a review of current efforts and call to revitalize primary and secondary lead poisoning prevention for pregnant women, lactating mothers, and children within the U.S. Int J Occup Environ Health. 2018;24(3-4):86–100.
- Reuben A, Caspi A, Belsky DW, et al. Association of childhood blood lead levels with cognitive function and socioeconomic status at age 38 years and with IQ change and socioeconomic mobility between childhood and adulthood. JAMA. 2017;317(12):1244–1251.
- Zahran S, McElmurry SP, Sadler RC. Four phases of the Flint water crisis: evidence from blood lead levels in children. Environ Res. 2017;157:160–172.

 SEE ALSO

Anemia, Iron Deficiency

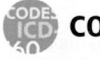 CODES

ICD10

- T56.0X4A Toxic effect of lead and its compounds, undetermined, init
- T56.0X1A Toxic effect of lead and its compounds, accidental, init

CLINICAL PEARLS

- Screen the following children:
  - 6 to 11 months of age with ≥1 risk factors:
    - Living in or visit a house built before 1960 with peeling paint or recent renovation
    - Sibling/playmate with elevated Pb
    - Living with adult with job or hobby involving Pb
    - Living near industry likely to release Pb
  - Children living in high-risk communities (>12% elevated Pb) should be tested annually from 1 to 5 years of age.
  - Newly arrived refugees
- There is no clear safe Pb level. Many experts consider Pb levels >4 μg/dL as elevated.
- There are no studies that show benefit of chelation for asymptomatic children with Pb <45. Removal of sources of Pb within the environment is critical.

L

LEGIONNAIRES' DISEASE

Andrew G. Alexander, MD • Kenneth A. Ballou, MD, FAAFP • Maegen Dupper, MD

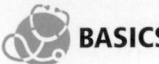 **BASICS**

DESCRIPTION
- *Legionnaires' disease* was named for an epidemic of lower respiratory tract disease at an American Legion convention in Philadelphia in 1976. The previously unrecognized causative bacterium was isolated, identified, and named *Legionella pneumophila*. The organism primarily causes pneumonia and flulike illness. *Legionella* preferentially colonizes commercial water systems (e.g., hotels, hospitals, air conditioning cooling towers).
  - It is one of the three most common causes of pneumonias and the most common atypical pneumonia.
- System(s) affected: pulmonary, gastrointestinal (GI)
- Synonym(s): *Legionella* pneumonia; legionellosis

EPIDEMIOLOGY
- Predominant age: 15 months to 84 years; 74–91% of patients are >50 years old.
- Predominant gender: male > female

Incidence
- U.S. cases of Legionnaires' disease have increased 4-fold since 2000; >6,000 cases reported in 2015 (1)
- Outbreaks most common in late summer/early fall
- ~2–9% of all cases of pneumonia in the United States

ETIOLOGY AND PATHOPHYSIOLOGY
- *L. pneumophila* is a weak gram-negative aerobic saprophytic freshwater bacterium. It is widely distributed in soil and water. Bipolar flagella provide motility; grow optimally at 40–45°C
- Exists in nature as protozoan parasite and within fresh water biofilms
- Serogroups 1 to 6 account for clinical disease.
- Serogroup 1 represents 70–92% of all clinical cases of *Legionella* in the United States.
- In the lung, *Legionella* infects alveolar macrophages.
- The organism is transmitted by breathing in contaminated water droplets or by aspiration of contaminated water (e.g., contaminated shower water responsible for the inaugural Philadelphia outbreak).
- Recently, community outbreaks associated with whirlpools, spas, fountains, and aboard cruise ships

RISK FACTORS
- Impaired cellular immunity (*Legionella* are intracellular pathogens.)
- Male gender
- Smoking; alcohol abuse
- Immunosuppression; HIV; diabetes; organ transplant recipients; corticosteroid use
- Chronic cardiopulmonary disease
- Advanced age
- Use of antimicrobials within the past 3 months

GENERAL PREVENTION
- *Not transmitted person to person* (Respiratory isolation is unnecessary.)
- Superheat and flush water systems: Heat water to 70°C and flush for 30 minutes (2)[C].
- Ultraviolet light and copper–silver ionization are bactericidal.
- Monochloramine disinfection of municipal water supplies decreases risk for *Legionella* infection.
- 0.2 micron water filters—change regularly
- Keep water heaters >60°C, cold water <20°C.

COMMONLY ASSOCIATED CONDITIONS
Pontiac fever: self-limited flulike illness without pneumonia caused by *Legionella* species

 DIAGNOSIS

- Illness ranges from asymptomatic seroconversion and mild febrile illness to severe pneumonia.
- Wound infections with *Legionella* also reported
- Incubation period is 2 to 14 days.

HISTORY
- Signs and symptoms (with associated percentage):
  - Cough: 92% (typically dry; rarely productive)
  - Fever/chills: 90%
  - Dyspnea: 62%
  - Pleuritic chest pain: 35%
  - Headache: 48%
  - Myalgia/arthralgia: 40%
  - Watery diarrhea: 50%
  - Nausea and vomiting: 49%
  - Neuropsychiatric symptoms include encephalopathy, confusion, disorientation, obtundation, depression, hallucinations, insomnia, and seizure: 53%.
- History of immunosuppression increases risk.

PHYSICAL EXAM
- Fever
- Relative bradycardia (key sign)
  - Temperature ≥102°F with an inappropriately low pulse pressure <100 beats/min (Normal compensatory reaction to fever is >110 beats/min.)
- Rales and signs of consolidation (pectoriloquy; egophony; tactile fremitus)

DIFFERENTIAL DIAGNOSIS
- Other bacterial pneumonias, especially atypical pneumonias: *Mycoplasma pneumoniae*, Q fever (*Coxiella burnetii*), *Chlamydophila pneumoniae*, *Chlamydophila psittaci*, *Francisella tularensis*
- Viral pneumonias, such as adenovirus, influenza (human, avian, swine), cytomegalovirus (CMV)

DIAGNOSTIC TESTS & INTERPRETATION
Indications for *Legionella* testing:
- Failed outpatient antibiotic treatment for community-acquired pneumonia (CAP)
- Severe pneumonia, particularly those requiring intensive care
- Immunocompromised patients with pneumonia

- Patients with a history of traveling away from their home within 10 days of illness onset
- Pneumonia in the setting of a known Legionnaires' disease outbreak
- Pneumonia beginning ≥48 hours after hospital admission

Initial Tests (lab, imaging)
Diagnosis:
- *Legionella* PCR detects ~100% of all *Legionella* species from lower respiratory secretions (3)[C].
- Urinary antigen test (UAT) detects serogroup 1 (which causes 80% of disease). UATs are highly specific (95–100%) but variably sensitive. *Legionella* culture (gold standard) requires an adequate sputum sample and special media (buffered charcoal yeast extract [BCYE] agar). Culture has variable sensitivity (10–80%) and time delays of up to 7 days for results.
- Other lab abnormalities:
  - Hyponatremia
  - Hypophosphatemia (transient)
  - Lymphopenia
  - Mildly elevated serum transaminases; elevated LDH; elevated creatine kinase
  - Microscopic hematuria
  - Highly elevated C-reactive protein (CRP) (>30)
  - Highly elevated ferritin (≥2 times normal)
- Chest radiograph
  - Not specific for *Legionella*
  - Commonly shows unilateral lower lobe patchy alveolar infiltrate with consolidation
  - Cavitation and abscess formation are more common in immunocompromised patients.
  - Pleural effusion occurs in up to 50%.
  - May take 1 to 4 months for radiographic findings to resolve. Progression of infiltrate on x-ray can be seen despite antibiotic therapy.

Diagnostic Procedures/Other
Transtracheal aspiration/bronchoscopy occasionally necessary to obtain sputum/lung samples

Test Interpretation
- Multifocal pneumonia with alveolitis and bronchiolitis and fibrinous pleuritis; may have serous or serosanguineous pleural effusion
- Abscess formation occurs in up to 20% of patients.
- Progression of infiltrates on x-ray (despite appropriate therapy) suggests Legionnaires'. Radiographic improvement may not correlate with clinical findings (longer lag times).

 TREATMENT

GENERAL MEASURES
- Supportive care:
  - Oxygenation, hydration, and electrolyte balance with antibiotic therapy
- Extrapulmonary complications and higher mortality in patients with AIDS
- In severe pneumonia, obtain UAT and start empiric antibiotics to include coverage for *Legionella* (4)[C].

MEDICATION

First Line

- Antibiotics that achieve high intracellular concentrations (e.g., macrolides, tetracyclines, fluoroquinolones) are most effective; first-line treatment is levofloxacin; no prospective randomized controlled trials have compared fluoroquinolones to macrolides for the treatment of *Legionella*; levofloxacin associated with more rapid defervescence, fewer complications, decreased hospital stay by 3 days, and decreased mortality (4% vs. 10.9%) compared with macrolide antibiotics (4)[A]
- Start antibiotics parenterally if sufficiently ill due to the GI symptoms associated with *Legionella*:
  - Levofloxacin is the preferred agent:
    - Levofloxacin 750 mg/day IV (switch to PO when patient is afebrile/tolerating PO) for 5 days or 750 mg/day for 7 to 10 days
  - Azithromycin may also be used first line. It requires a shorter duration of treatment than levofloxacin due to a longer half-life:
    - Azithromycin 500 mg/day IV (switch to PO when afebrile/tolerating PO) for 7 to 10 days
- Contraindications: hypersensitivity reactions
- Precautions: liver disease
- Significant drug interactions:
  - Can increase theophylline, carbamazepine, and digoxin levels; can increase activity of oral anticoagulants
  - May decrease the effectiveness of digoxin, quinidine, oral contraceptives, and hypoglycemic agents
- Longer courses of treatment (up to 21 days) may be needed in immunocompromised patients or valvular heart disease.

Second Line

- Doxycycline 100 mg IV/PO q12h for 14 days; for severe infections, initial dose is 200 mg IV/PO q12h.
- Doxycycline should not be used in pregnant patients and is not approved for children <8 years.

ADMISSION, INPATIENT, AND NURSING CONSIDERATIONS

- Inability to tolerate oral antibiotics
- Hypoxemia
- Criteria for direct admission to the ICU:
  - Any major criteria for severe CAP:
    - Septic shock requiring vasopressor support
    - Acute respiratory failure requiring intubation and/or mechanical ventilation
  - Three or more minor criteria for severe CAP:
    - $RR \geq 30$ breaths/min, $PaO_2:FiO_2$ ratio ≤ 250, multilobular infiltrates, confusion/disorientation, uremia (BUN ≥ 20 mg/dL), leukopenia (WBC <4,000 cells/mm^3), thrombocytopenia (PLT <100,000 cells/mm^3), hypothermia (temperature <36°C), hypotension requiring aggressive fluid resuscitation
- Discharge criteria
  - Afebrile
  - Able to tolerate oral antibiotics
  - Normal room air oxygen saturation

 ONGOING CARE

FOLLOW-UP RECOMMENDATIONS

Patient Monitoring

- Monitor respiratory status, hydration, and electrolyte status closely.
- Chest radiography lags behind the clinical status and may not help with monitoring clinical response.

PATIENT EDUCATION

- Disease prevention: Eliminate pathogens from water supplies, low-emission cleaning of cooling towers with control measurements of water and air samples.
- *Legionella* is not spread person to person.

PROGNOSIS

- Improved prognosis when appropriate antibiotics are started early in the disease course
- Recovery is variable:
  - Patients may clinically worsen despite appropriate initial treatment (first 1 to 2 days of therapy).
  - Improvement with defervescence in 3 to 5 days and complete recovery in 6 to 10 days is typical. Some have a more protracted course.
- Mortality in nosocomial infections as high as 15–34%

COMPLICATIONS

- Dehydration
- Hyponatremia
- Respiratory insufficiency requiring ventilator support
- Bacteremia/lung abscess formation in up to 20%
- Extrapulmonary diseases:
  - Endocarditis (most common extrapulmonary site)
  - Cellulitis
  - Sinusitis
  - Pancreatitis
  - Pyelonephritis
  - Encephalitis
  - Pericarditis
  - Perirectal abscess
- Renal failure
- Disseminated intravascular coagulation
- Multiple organ dysfunction syndrome (MODS)
- Coma
- Death occurs in 8–12% of treated immunocompetent patients and in up to 80% of untreated immunocompromised patients.

REFERENCES

1. Adams DA, Thomas KR, Jajosky RA, et al; for Nationally Notifiable Infectious Conditions Group. Summary of notifiable infectious diseases and conditions—United States, 2015. *MMWR Morb Mortal Wkly Rep*. 2017;64(53):1–143.
2. Walser SM, Gerstner DG, Brenner B, et al. Assessing the environmental health relevance of cooling towers—a systematic review of legionellosis outbreaks. *Int J Hyg Environ Health*. 2014;217(2–3):145–154.
3. Botelho-Nevers E, Grattard F, Viallon A, et al. Prospective evaluation of RT-PCR on sputum versus culture, urinary antigens and serology for Legionnaire's disease diagnosis. *J Infect*. 2016;73(2):123–128.
4. Burdet C, Lepeule R, Duval X, et al. Quinolones versus macrolides in the treatment of legionellosis: a systematic review and meta-analysis. *J Antimicrob Chemother*. 2014;69(9):2354–2360.

ADDITIONAL READING

- Mandell LA, Wunderink RG, Anzueto A, et al; for Infectious Diseases Society of America, American Thoracic Society. Infectious Diseases Society of America/American Thoracic Society consensus guidelines on the management of community-acquired pneumonia in adults. *Clin Infect Dis*. 2007;44(Suppl 2):S27–S72.
- Mercante JW, Winchell JM. Current and emerging *Legionella* diagnostics for laboratory and outbreak investigations. *Clin Microbiol Rev*. 2015;28(1):95–133.
- Phin N, Parry-Ford F, Harrison T, et al. Epidemiology and clinical management of Legionnaires' disease. *Lancet Infect Dis*. 2014;14(10):1011–1021.

 SEE ALSO

Pneumonia, Bacterial

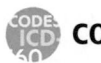 CODES

ICD10

- A48.1 Legionnaires' disease
- A48.2 Nonpneumonic Legionnaires' disease [Pontiac fever]

CLINICAL PEARLS

- *Legionella* is an intracellular organism that can only be grown on BCYE agar.
- Serology is not useful in early stages of the disease (an increase in *Legionella* antibody titers cannot be detected until 3 to 4 weeks after symptom onset).
- UAT and *Legionella* sputum PCR are the most sensitive and practical initial tests. Sputum culture is definitive but can take up to 7 days.
- Consider Legionnaires' disease in cases of nosocomial pneumonia.
- Consider Legionnaires' disease in patients with pneumonia who have GI and other extrapulmonary findings (atypical CAP) and a relative bradycardia. Relative lymphopenia, mildly elevated serum transaminases (aspartate aminotransferase/alanine aminotransferase), highly increased ferritin levels, or hypophosphatemia are other laboratory clues to *Legionella* infection.

L

LESBIAN HEALTH

Tina D'Amato, DO

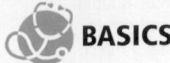 **BASICS**

DESCRIPTION

- A lesbian is a woman who has her primary emotional and sexual relationships with women.
- Other sexual minorities include bisexual, transgender, and transsexual women.
- Sexual behaviors
  - May be celibate, sexually active only with women or with both men and women
  - ~75% of self-reported lesbians have reported prior or ongoing sexual contact with men.
- Sexual orientation and gender nonconformity are complex concepts, and defining them can be challenging.

EPIDEMIOLOGY

Prevalence
- Estimated to be between 1% and 5%
- Approximately 1.4 million women living in the United States identify as lesbians. Another 2.6 million women identify as bisexual.
- 2016 American Community Survey from United States Census Bureau estimates 451,594 households are headed by female same-sex couples.

RISK FACTORS

Higher incidence for the following risk factors compared to heterosexual women:

- Elevated BMI
  - Lesbian women have a higher prevalence of overweight/obesity than all other female sexual orientation groups.
- Alcohol use
  - More common use than reported in heterosexual women
  - Age 20 to 34 years is at highest risk for daily use and heavy use of alcohol. Those numbers decline in older age groups.
- Tobacco use
  - 2 times more likely to smoke than heterosexual women
- Sexual minority stress (1)
  - Increased risk for health issues secondary to greater exposure to social stresses related to prejudice and stigma
- The above factors can increase risks for
  - Cardiovascular disease (CVD)
  - Type 2 diabetes
  - Hepatic disease
  - Cancers

COMMONLY ASSOCIATED CONDITIONS

- Cervical cancer
  - Lesbians are equally at risk for developing cervical cancer compared to heterosexual women.
  - HPV can be transmitted genitally skin to skin, oral to genitals, and digital to genitals.
  - Risk of cervical cancer is highest in lesbians:
    ○ With prior HPV infection/abnormal Pap smear
    ○ Who have had a history of heterosexual intercourse
  - Lesbian and bisexual women are 10 times less likely to have adequate cervical cancer screening compared to heterosexual women.
  - Tobacco use influences cervical cell atypia.

- Breast cancer
  - Risk factors same as heterosexual women
    ○ Moderate or heavy alcohol consumption
    ○ Obesity
    ○ Nulliparity or first child born after age 30 years
  - Mammogram screening rates lower among lesbians
  - Data suggest lesbians have increased mortality rate compared to heterosexual women (2).
- Ovarian cancer
  - Elevated BMI and tobacco use increases risks.
  - Lesbians less likely to have been on hormonal contraception for 5 years or longer
  - Lesbians less likely to have been pregnant or breastfed an infant before age 30 years
  - Lesbians at increased risk for ovarian cancer may want to explore potential benefits of long-term progestin-containing contraception to reduce risk.
- CVD
  - Lesbians have higher rates of obesity, smoking, and stress, which increase risks for CVD.
- Mental health diagnoses
  - 2 times more likely to see general physician for mental/emotional complaint
    ○ Depression
      ▪ Double the rate compared to heterosexual women
      ▪ Discrimination stress proposed factor
    ○ Anxiety disorders
      ▪ 2- to 4-fold higher rate of generalized anxiety disorder
      ▪ Higher rates of PTSD, panic, phobia
      ▪ Multiple diagnoses
      ▪ 3 times risk
    ○ Alcohol abuse
      ▪ Greatest in lesbians ages 20 to 34 years
      ▪ Bar culture
      ▪ May not feel comfortable in traditional Alcoholics Anonymous environment
      ▪ Sexual minority females more likely than heterosexual counterparts to be current alcohol users, binge drinkers, and heavy drinkers (3)
- Sexually transmitted infections (STI)
  - Many lesbians underestimate their STI risks.
  - Difficult to ascertain accurate statistics because of lack of research and the confounding factors of relying on identifiers of sexual orientation versus sexual behaviors
  - Lesbian sexual practices include the following:
    ○ High risk: oral–vaginal contact, genital–genital contact, oral–anal contact, digital stimulation/penetration, and sharing of sex toys
  - Lower risk: kissing, rubbing genitals against partner's body
- Bacterial vaginosis
  - Higher rate than heterosexual women
    ○ Estimated 25–52% prevalence
  - Increased incidence with smoking, receptive oral sex, symptomatic partner, and new partner
  - Often found in monogamous lesbian couples suggesting it can be sexually transmitted
- Chlamydia
  - Can be transmitted woman to woman (WTW)
- Gonorrhea
  - Can be transmitted WTW

- Hepatitis B
  - Can be transmitted WTW
- Herpes
  - Can be transmitted WTW
- HPV
  - Can be transmitted WTW
  - Up to 30% of women who have sex with women (WSW) have genital HPV (4).
  - 12% of WSW report genital warts.
  - 25% of WSW report cervical abnormalities.
  - WSW may not get HPV vaccine due to perceived decreased risk.
- HIV
  - Transmission between women rare but possible
  - WSW more likely to have sexual contact with men having sex with men (MSM) than heterosexual women
- Syphilis
  - Can be transmitted WTW
- Trichomonas
  - Can be transmitted WTW
- STI screening and prevention
  - Screen based on woman's history.
  - Encourage safer sex practices:
    ○ Avoid menstrual blood/open sores.
    ○ Dental dams for oral sex
    ○ Condoms on sex toys and cleaning immediately after use
    ○ Vinyl/latex gloves for manual sex
- Psychosocial considerations
  - Sexual abuse
    ○ 3 times more likely than heterosexual women to report having been sexually assaulted
    ○ 43% of lesbians reported at least one sexual assault in their lifetime.
    ○ History of childhood sexual abuse can be associated with more complicated and difficult "coming out."
  - Intimate partner violence
    ○ 17–45% of lesbians report at least one act of physical violence at the hands of a lesbian partner.
  - Parenthood
    ○ A reported 41% of lesbians desire to have a child.
      ▪ Perinatal depression is common and may be more common than in heterosexual women.
    ○ >30% have biologic children.
      ▪ Often from previous heterosexual relationship
      ▪ Adoption
      ▪ Assisted reproductive technology/donor insemination
      ▪ Some will engage in high-risk sexual behaviors (MSM, "one-night stand") in an attempt to get pregnant.
      ▪ Providers should discuss parenting with their lesbian patients.
      ▪ Encourage both partners or nonbiologic parent to adopt child to ensure permanent legal relationship to child.
      ▪ Discuss durable power of attorney for health care and finances in the event of death or separation.
      ▪ Adolescents who have been reared in lesbian mother families since birth demonstrate healthy psychological adjustment.

- Adolescent lesbians
  - Increased risk for eating disorders
  - Higher rates of substance use particularly polysubstance abuse
  - If also having sexual contact with males, higher rates of pregnancy compared to heterosexual counterparts due to (5)
    - High rates of early sexual initiation
    - Greater number of partners
    - Less contraceptive use
  - Higher rates of physical and/or sexual abuse
    - Childhood sexual abuse does not cause children to become LGBTQ.
- Aging lesbians
  - Elders aging "back into the closet"
    - Discrimination by religious and other groups that own nursing homes
    - Fear of discrimination by caregivers/health care workers
    - Few elder care programs specifically directed at LGBT persons

 TREATMENT

GENERAL MEASURES

- Create a safe practice environment for lesbian patients.
  - Have nondiscrimination policy posted where it is visible to patients.
  - Educate staff to be comfortable dealing with the needs of lesbian patients and their families.
  - Brochures/photos should feature both same-sex and heterosexual couples.
  - Intake forms should include options for patient to indicate sexual preference and include options for partnered status.
  - Use "gender-neutral" language.
    - "Do you have a significant other?"
  - Avoid heterosexist assumptions ("What do you use for birth control?" asking instead "Do you plan to become pregnant or have a child? Do you need birth control?").
- Ask about sexual orientation.
  - Many physicians do not ask.
  - Intake/annual physical forms should include questions about orientation/activity.
  - Twice as likely to identify as a sexual minority if questions ask in an indirect way
- Take a detailed sexual history.
  - Sexual identity and sexual behaviors not always strongly correlated
  - Ask about behaviors ("Do you have sex with women, men, or both?"); do not just assume current/past sexual activity with women.
  - STI screening based on reported history/activity
  - Address contraception when appropriate.
  - Some physicians may create barriers by believing a patient's sexual self-identity and behaviors are not pertinent to competent care (6).
- Respect the partners.
  - Treat her as you would any other spouse/partner.
  - Assure access if partner hospitalized.
  - Recommend durable power of attorney if couple is not legally married.
- Follow same preventive screening guidelines and lifestyle recommendations as for heterosexual women (Pap smear, mammography, colonoscopy screening, safer sex, exercise, diet, alcohol moderation, and tobacco avoidance).

- Legal/U.S. government
  - Healthy People 2010 identified lesbian/gay Americans as 1 of 6 population groups affected by health care disparities.
  - Healthy People 2020 goals to increase routine data collection efforts on LGBT populations via health care surveys
  - Access to health insurance was increased with supreme court decisions on *United States v. Windsor* in 2013 and *Obergefell v. Hodges* in 2015.
    - Some states still recognize same-sex civil union, but access to health insurance varies by state.
  - Affordable Care Act (ACA)
    - Prohibits discrimination based on sexual orientation in any program receiving federal funds (Medicare/Medicaid)
    - Increased emphasis on research and data collections in LGBT population
    - National Health Interview Survey (NHIS)
      - 2013 survey added a question about sexual orientation.
      - This was the first time nationally representative U.S. data on sexual orientation and health was made available.

REFERENCES

1. Frost DM, Lehavot K, Meyer IH. Minority stress and physical health among sexual minority individuals. *J Behav Med*. 2015;38(1):1–8.
2. Boehmer U, Ozonoff A, Miao X. Breast cancer mortality's association with sexual orientation. *Sex Res Soc Policy*. 2013;10(4):279–284.
3. Medley G, Lipari RN, Bose J, et al. Sexual orientation and estimates of adult substance use and mental health: results from the 2015 National Survey on Drug Use and Health. NSDUH data review. https://www.samhsa.gov/data/sites/default/files/NSDUH-SexualOrientation-2015/NSDUH-SexualOrientation-2015-NSDUH-SexualOrientation-2015.htm.
4. McRee AL, Katz ML, Paskett ED, et al. HPV vaccination among lesbian and bisexual women: findings from a national survey of young adults. *Vaccine*. 2014;32(37):4736–4742.
5. Committee on Adolescence. Office-based care for lesbian, gay, bisexual, transgender, and questioning youth. *Pediatrics*. 2013;132(1):198–203.
6. Knight DA, Jarrett D. Preventive health care for women who have sex with women. *Am Fam Physician*. 2017;95(5):314–321.

ADDITIONAL READING

- Ard KL, Makadon H. Addressing intimate partner violence in lesbian, gay, bisexual, and transgender patients. *J Gen Intern Med*. 2011;26(8):930–933.
- Boehmer U, Bowen DJ, Bauer GR. Overweight and obesity in sexual-minority women: evidence from population-based data. *Am J Public Health*. 2007;97(6):1134–1140.
- Buchmueller T, Carpenter CS. Disparities in health insurance coverage, access, and outcomes for individuals in same-sex versus different-sex relationships, 2000–2007. *Am J Public Health*. 2010;100(3):489–495.
- Everett B. Sexual orientation disparities in sexually transmitted infections: examining the intersection between sexual identity and sexual behavior. *Arch Sex Behav*. 2013;42(2):225–236.

- Gartrell N, Bos H. US National Longitudinal Lesbian Family Study: psychological adjustment of 17-year-old adolescents. *Pediatrics*. 2010;126(1):28–36.
- Gates GJ. *How Many People Are Lesbian, Gay, Bisexual, and Transgender?* Los Angeles, CA: The Williams Institute, UCLA School of Law; 2011.
- Gay and Lesbian Medical Association and LGBT Health Experts. *Healthy People 2010 Companion Document for Lesbian, Gay, Bisexual, and Transgender (LGBT) Health*. San Francisco, CA: Gay and Lesbian Medical Association; 2010. http://www.glma.org. Accessed July 28, 2018.
- Institute of Medicine Committee on Lesbian, Gay, Bisexual, and Transgender Health Issues and Research Gaps and Opportunities. *The Health of Lesbian, Gay, Bisexual, and Transgender People: Building a Foundation for Better Understanding*. Washington, DC: National Academies Press; 2011.
- Kates J, Ranji U, Beamesderfer A, et al. Health and access to care and coverage for lesbian, gay, bisexual, and transgender individuals in the U.S. http://files.kff.org/attachment/Issue-Brief-Health-and-Access-to-Care-and-Coverage-for-LGBT-Individuals-in-the-US. Accessed July 30, 2018.
- Kelly-Barton C. Creating a welcoming environment for LGBT seniors in assisted living. National Resource Center on LGBT Aging. https://www.lgbtagingcenter.org. Accessed July 29, 2018.
- Makadon HJ, Mayer KH, Potter J, et al, eds. *The Fenway Guide to Lesbian, Gay, Bisexual, and Transgender Health*. Philadelphia, PA: American College of Physicians; 2008.
- Marrazzo JM, Gorgos LM. Emerging sexual health issues among women who have sex with women. *Curr Infect Dis Rep*. 2012;14(2):204–211.
- Ross LE, Steele L, Goldfinger C, et al. Perinatal depressive symptomatology among lesbian and bisexual women. *Arch Womens Ment Health*. 2007;10(2):53–59.
- The Joint Commission. *Advancing Effective Communication, Cultural Competence, and Patient- and Family-Centered Care for the Lesbian, Gay, Bisexual, and Transgender Community: A Field Guide*. Oak Brook, IL: The Joint Commission; 2011. http://www.jointcommission.org/assets/1/18/LGBTField Guide.pdf. Accessed July 29, 2018.

 CODES

ICD10

- E66.3 Overweight
- Z72.0 Tobacco use
- F10.10 Alcohol abuse, uncomplicated

CLINICAL PEARLS

- Create a safe health care environment for all patients.
- Use gender-neutral language.
- Do not assume heterosexuality or sexual practices.
- Take a detailed history and avoid assumptions.
- Be aware that some patients may openly identify as lesbian, but others may only identify when asked directly. Some may be engaging in a same-sex relationship and not identify as a lesbian.
- Follow same preventive screening guidelines and lifestyle recommendations as for heterosexual women.
- Discuss durable power of attorney for health care needs to ensure partner's involvement in care.

L

LEUKEMIA, ACUTE LYMPHOBLASTIC (ALL) IN ADULTS

Katyayini Aribindi, MD • Adrian DaSilva-DeAbreu, MD • Mark A. Farnie, MD

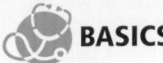 **BASICS**

DESCRIPTION
- Acute lymphoblastic leukemia (ALL) in adults is the result of a clonal proliferation, survival, and impaired differentiation of immature lymphocytes. The World Health Organization (WHO) defines ALL as the presence of ≥25% lymphoblasts in the bone marrow (1), whereas the National Comprehensive Cancer Network (NCCN) uses a ≥20% as cutoff (2).
- ALL and lymphoblastic lymphoma (LBL) can arise from the same precursor cell line, and therefore can be considered diseases along the same spectrum:
  – LBL presents as a mass, possibly, but not limited to, the mediastinum, with <25% blasts in the bone marrow.
  – ALL may present with a mass lesion but contains ≥25% bone marrow involvement.
- Any organ can be affected.

Pregnancy Considerations
Many chemotherapy (CTX) drugs are teratogenic.

Pediatric Considerations
ALL is the most common malignancy in children—it accounts for 30% of all pediatric malignancies and 80% of pediatric leukemias (see "Acute Lymphoblastic Leukemia, Pediatric").

Geriatric Considerations
Patients >60 years with ALL have a 42% mortality during induction CTX. The cause of death is usually CTX-related complications or relapse. Survival is often reduced due to poor tolerance of CTX, thus leading to dose reductions and ineffective medication delivery.

EPIDEMIOLOGY
- Incidence of ALL is 1.7/100,000 per year.
- Higher incidence in males, whites, those with history of radiation, CTX, or certain genetic disorders
- Bimodal distribution: early peak at 4 to 5 years of age, second peak at ~50 years
- 80% of cases occur in children, 20% in adults.

ETIOLOGY AND PATHOPHYSIOLOGY
Unknown in most patients

Genetics
- Higher rates in monozygotic and dizygotic twins
- Increased risk of ALL with diseases related to chromosomal instability: Bloom syndrome, Fanconi anemia, ataxia-telangiectasia, neurofibromatosis
- Increased risk with inherited chromosomal abnormalities: Down syndrome, Klinefelter syndrome, etc.
- See "Follow-Up Tests & Special Considerations."

RISK FACTORS
- Age >70 years, radiation exposure, and infection with HIV are risk factors for developing ALL.
- Human T-cell lymphotropic virus type 1 is associated with adult T-cell ALL.
- Epstein-Barr virus is associated with mature B-cell ALL.

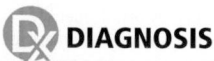 **DIAGNOSIS**

HISTORY
- Symptoms arise from sequelae of bone marrow suppression and/or from leukemic cell organ infiltration.
- B symptoms: fever, weight loss, night sweats
- Anemia: fatigue, shortness of breath, light-headedness, angina, headache

- Thrombocytopenia: easy bruising
- Neutropenia: fever, infection
- Lymphocytosis: bone pain
- CNS: confusion
- Organ infiltration: organ-specific symptoms and signs

PHYSICAL EXAM
- Thrombocytopenia: petechiae, ecchymoses, epistaxis, retinal hemorrhages
- Anemia: pallor
- Neutropenia: fever, infections
- Lymphocytosis: lymphadenopathy; splenomegaly; less often, hepatomegaly
- CNS: cranial nerve palsies, meningeal signs
- Testicular invasion: abnormal testicular exam

DIFFERENTIAL DIAGNOSIS
- Malignant disorders: other leukemias, especially AML, chronic myeloid leukemia in lymphoid blast phase, prolymphocytic leukemia, malignant lymphomas; multiple myeloma, bone marrow metastases from solid tumors (breast, prostate, lung, renal), and myelodysplastic syndromes
- Nonmalignant disorders: aplastic anemia, myelofibrosis, autoimmune diseases (Felty syndrome, lupus), infectious mononucleosis, pertussis, autoimmune thrombocytopenic purpura, leukemoid reaction to infection

DIAGNOSTIC TESTS & INTERPRETATION
Initial Tests (lab, imaging)
- CBC with differential:
  – Anemia: normocytic, normochromic
  – Thrombocytopenia
  – Peripheral blood lymphoblasts (B cell or T cell)
- Hepatitis B/C, HIV, CMV Ab testing, LDH
- Pregnancy test if indicated
- Tumor lysis panel: uric acid, potassium, calcium, phosphorus
- CT of the neck, chest, abdomen, and pelvis with contrast and PET/CT if suspicion of lymphomatous involvement
- CT/MRI of head with contrast if neurologic symptoms are present
- Scrotal US if abnormal testicular exam

Follow-Up Tests & Special Considerations
- Immunophenotyping of marrow/blood lymphoblasts: B lineage (CD19, CD20, CD22, CD24), T lineage (CD2, CD3, CD5, CD7), common ALL antigen (CD10); human leukocyte antigen (HLA)-DR, terminal deoxynucleotidyl transferase (TdT), aberrant myeloid antigens (CD13, CD33), and stem cell antigen (CD34)
- Cytochemical stains: myeloperoxidase negative; Sudan black B usually negative; TdT positive; periodic acid–Schiff ± is variable, depending on subtype.
- Cytogenetics: Specific recurring chromosomal abnormalities have independent diagnostic and prognostic significance (hyperdiploidy >50 chromosomes or t[14q11q13] are favorable; the Philadelphia [Ph] chromosome, t[9;22], t[4;11], −7, and +8 are unfavorable). A translocation t(8;14) or t(2;8) or t(8;22) identifies Burkitt-type mature B-cell leukemia that requires specific therapy.
- Reverse transcription polymerase chain reaction for rapid diagnosis of BCR/ABL1+ ALL

- Genomic analysis by next-generation sequencing: detection of mutations associated with Ph-like ALL
- HLA typing of patient and siblings for hematopoietic stem cell transplantation

Diagnostic Procedures/Other
- Bone marrow aspiration/biopsy with immunohisto-chemistry, immunophenotyping, cytogenetics, and molecular diagnostics
- Lymph node biopsy if available
- Lumbar puncture is mandatory and typically done both for diagnosis of CNS involvement and for intrathecal (IT) CTX. It should be done at diagnosis and immediately if neurologic symptoms or signs are present. Repeat lumbar puncture after bone marrow remission is achieved to evaluate occult CNS involvement and continue prophylactic CNS treatment.

Test Interpretation
Diagnosis of ALL is generally based on the presence of ≥20% (NCCN definition) (2) or ≥25% (WHO definition) (1) lymphoblasts in the bone marrow. In some cases, the diagnosis of ALL can be made based on the presence of certain mutations (1), even if the percentage of blasts is lower than these numbers. The bone marrow biopsy typically shows diffuse replacement of marrow and lymph node architecture by sheets of malignant lymphoblasts, T-cell or B-cell lineage determined by CD expression.

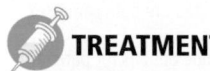 **TREATMENT**

GENERAL MEASURES
- Three phases to treatment:
  – Induction + CNS prophylaxis
  – Consolidation
  – Prolonged maintenance
- Treatment for initial induction and relapse is changing based on Ph receptor status and should be managed by a specialist.
- Hyperleukocytosis with WBC >50,000 or 100,000 can lead to leukostasis, a medical emergency with microvascular white cell plugs. Patients may present with neurologic deficits or respiratory distress and should be treated with fluids, and cytoreductive therapy (hydroxyurea, plasmapheresis, or remission induction CTX).

MEDICATION
- Induction
  – The mainstay of treatment is a regimen called hyper-CVAD (3)[A]: hyperfractionated cyclophosphamide, vincristine, anthracyclines, and dexamethasone. Hyper-CVAD is the most widely used regimen for ALL in adolescents and young adults.
  – Hyper-CVAD consists of eight alternating treatment cycles of parts A and B:
    ○ Part A: Hyper-CVAD
    ○ Part B: high-dose methotrexate and cytarabine
    ○ Granulocyte colony-stimulating factors are given after each cycle to prevent delay in treatment and hasten bone marrow recovery (4)[A].
    ○ CNS prophylaxis: IT CTX consistent of IT-methotrexate or cytarabine or 6-mercaptopurine (6-MP) throughout all three phases (2)[A]
    ○ Those with CNS leukemia at diagnosis will need twice a week IT therapy until CSF is cleared on three subsequent lumbar punctures (2)[A].

- <40 years of age with complete remission after the first induction, the next step is either consolidation CTX or allogeneic stem cell transplant based on risk donor availability.
  - Minimal residual disease (MRD), measured by flow cytometry in the US, signifies CTX refractory disease, usually in 8 months from start of treatment with continued CTX. These patients should be evaluated for an allogeneic bone marrow transplant (2)[A].
- Consolidation
  - Purpose is to eliminate residual leukemic cells after induction therapy.
  - Induction phase drugs are used.
  - Peg-asparaginase is used in children but has poorer outcomes and toxicities in adults (5)[A].
- Prolonged maintenance
  - Purpose is to prevent relapse and prolong remission.
  - Consist of POMP: daily 6-MP, weekly methotrexate, monthly vincristine, with pulses of prednisone for 2 to 3 years. Little benefit has been shown for >3 years of prolonged maintenance (3,6)[A].
  - Dexamethasone can be substituted for prednisone, a.k.a DOMP.
- Special considerations
  - Besides hyper-CVAD, some pediatric ALL regimens have shown superior complete remission outcomes for adults from 15 to 39 years. These usually contain vincristine and peg-asparaginase, nonmyelosuppressive agents.
  - Allogeneic stem cell transplantation is also recommended with relapsed ALL during the first remission or if there are high-risk genetic features.
  - Burkitt leukemia requires only 18 weeks of treatment and has better outcomes with methotrexate and alkylating agents in the initial therapy. Rituximab (anti-CD20 monoclonal antibody) also improves outcomes.
  - Rituximab improves outcomes if CD20 expression is >20% of blast cells in ALL.
  - Immunotherapy:
    - Bispecific anti-CD19/anti-CD3 antibody blinatumomab is approved for relapsed/refractory ALL.
  - Ofatumumab is a 2nd-generation anti-CD20 monoclonal antibody undergoing trials with concomitant hyper-CVAD in pre–B-cell ALL with CD20 expression >1%.
  - Ph-positive ALL have improved prognosis with tyrosine kinase inhibitors (TKIs) targeting BCR-ABL1 translocation. Consolidation/maintenance with a TKI may be used instead of allogeneic stem cell transplant in these patients.
  - Adult T-cell ALL is much less common than B-cell ALL and unfortunately has a relapse rate up to 50% with traditional hyper-CVAD therapy. Nelarabine is a T cell–specific purine nucleoside and currently is approved for relapsed T-cell ALL, with additional clinical trials studying a combination of hyper-CVAD and nelarabine as part of induction therapy.
  - Patients with unfavorable cytogenetic subtypes should undergo allogeneic stem cell transplantation on first remission if an HLA-identical donor is available.
  - A novel agent, inotuzumab-ozogamicin combination, has shown higher rates of complete remission and longer progression free and overall survival in patients with relapsed or refractory ALL when compared to standard therapy (7)[A].

ISSUES FOR REFERRAL
ALL can quickly become a fatal disorder, and thus, when the diagnosis is suspected, patients should be referred to and treated by an oncologist immediately, preferably at a comprehensive cancer center where medication regimen can be tailored as appropriate with a combination of multiple modalities.

SURGERY/OTHER PROCEDURES
In some centers, patients may undergo surgical placement of a port for CTX. Nevertheless, PICC lines are preferred because they can be easily removed after CTX cycles to decrease the risk of infections. This is very important because these patients can get neutropenic.

COMPLEMENTARY & ALTERNATIVE MEDICINE
Unproven; may result in adverse drug interactions with CTX

 ONGOING CARE

FOLLOW-UP RECOMMENDATIONS
Ambulatory as tolerated

Patient Monitoring
- Requires inpatient admission during induction CTX for continuous infusion and monitoring of metabolic and infectious complications
- Weekly clinic visits with remission consolidation CTX
- Monthly clinic visits during maintenance therapy
- Outpatient follow-up every 3 months thereafter

DIET
- Nutritional support; enteral nutrition is preferred over IV hyperalimentation.
- Avoid alcohol.
- Calcium and vitamin D for steroid-induced osteoporosis

PATIENT EDUCATION
- Neutropenic precautions with avoidance of fresh fruit and vegetables
- Early physical rehabilitation is always recommended due to high risk of deconditioning.
- All patients should be counseled to stop smoking, regardless of ALL diagnosis.

PROGNOSIS
~80–90% of adults <60 years will achieve a complete remission; however, only 40–50% will remain cured due to relapses. Only 30–40% of adults have a 5-year overall survival as opposed to 90% in children.

COMPLICATIONS
- Tumor lysis syndrome (elevated uric acid, potassium, and phosphate with decreased calcium, leading to renal failure, disseminated intravascular coagulation, and cardiac arrhythmias) may be prevented by administering allopurinol prior to CTX. Allopurinol doses should be reduced if used with mercaptopurine or azathioprine. Increased fluids should be given; IV urate oxidase (rasburicase) can be used to treat hyperuricemia rapidly (if not G6PD deficient).
- Neutropenia from myelosuppression
- High-dose cyclophosphamide causes severe nausea and vomiting. Use appropriate antiemetic regimen.
- Vincristine can cause neurotoxicity and ileus.
- AVN or osteonecrosis may occur with alkylating agents and corticosteroids.
- Steroid-induced hyperglycemia may require starting patients on insulin/oral antihyperglycemics.

- Anthracyclines can cause cardiotoxicity and require assessment of left ventricular ejection fraction by transthoracic echocardiography before hyper-CVAD initiation begins and monitoring during treatment.
- Asparaginase therapy increases the risks for deep vein thromboses and veno-occlusive disease.
- Infections (*Pneumocystis carinii* pneumonia, bacterial pneumonia or sepsis, fungal pneumonia)
- Adverse reactions from blood product transfusions for pancytopenia
- CTX can cause sterility.
- Arachnoiditis and CNS effects from IT CTX, high-dose methotrexate, and irradiation
- Pancreatitis and liver dysfunction from CTX
- Relapse of ALL in marrow or extramedullary sites (CNS, testis)

REFERENCES
1. Vardiman JW, Thiele J, Arber DA, et al. The 2008 revision of the World Health Organization (WHO) classification of myeloid neoplasms and acute leukemia: rationale and important changes. *Blood*. 2009;114(5):937–951.
2. National Comprehensive Cancer Network. Acute lymphoblastic leukemia. Version 1.2018. https://www.nccn.org/professionals/physician_gls/pdf/all.pdf. Updated March 12, 2018. Accessed July 21, 2018.
3. Kantarjian HM, O'Brien S, Smith TL, et al. Results of treatment with hyper-CVAD, a dose-intensive regimen, in adult acute lymphocytic leukemia. *J Clin Oncol*. 2000;18(3):547–561.
4. Larson RA, Dodge RK, Linker CA, et al. A randomized controlled trial of filgrastim during remission induction and consolidation chemotherapy for adults with acute lymphoblastic leukemia: CALGB study 9111. *Blood*. 1998;92(5):1556–1564.
5. Patel B, Kirkwood A, Dey A, et al. Feasibility of pegylated-asparaginase (PEG-ASP) during induction in adults with acute lymphoblastic leukaemia (ALL): results from UK phase 3 multicentre trial UKALL14. *Blood*. 2013;122:3900.
6. Jabbour E, O'Brien S, Konopleva M, et al. New insights into the pathophysiology and therapy of adult acute lymphoblastic leukemia. *Cancer*. 2015;121(15):2517–2528.
7. Kantarjian HM, DeAngelo DJ, Stelljes MS, et al. Inotuzumab ozogamicin versus standard therapy for acute lymphoblastic leukemia. *N Engl J Med*. 2016;375(8):740–753.

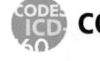 **CODES**

ICD10
- C91.00 Acute lymphoblastic leukemia not having achieved remission
- C91.01 Acute lymphoblastic leukemia, in remission
- C91.02 Acute lymphoblastic leukemia, in relapse

CLINICAL PEARLS
- The diagnosis of ALL is based on the presence of ≥20% (NCCN) or 25% (WHO) lymphoblasts or characteristic mutations in the bone marrow.
- Hyper-CVAD is still the main therapy; however, newer immunotherapeutic agents targeting specific mutations in ALL are currently being investigated.
- Treatment at an appropriate cancer center allows for tailored therapy based on mutations in ALL cells.
- Patients need to be monitored closely for CTX toxicities and progression of disease.

LEUKEMIA, ACUTE MYELOID

Jan Cerny, MD, PhD

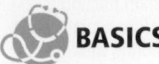 **BASICS**

DESCRIPTION
- Acute myeloid leukemia (AML) is characterized by proliferation and accumulation of abnormal immature myeloid progenitors (blasts) with reduced capacity to differentiate into more mature cellular elements. This leads to bone marrow failure and results in a variety of systemic symptoms.
- Previously, the French–American–British (FAB) classification system divided AML based on the cell morphology with the addition of cytogenetics (subtypes M0 to M7).
- The World Health Organization (WHO) classification attempts to provide more meaningful prognostic information.
  - AML with characteristic genetic abnormalities: translocation t(8;21), t(15;17), and inversion in chromosome 16 inv(16)
  - AML with multilineage dysplasia: presence of a prior myelodysplastic syndrome (MDS) or myelo-proliferative neoplasm (MPN) that transformed into AML
  - AML and MDS, therapy related
  - AML not otherwise categorized
  - Acute leukemias of ambiguous lineage (*biphenotypic acute leukemia*)

EPIDEMIOLOGY
- ~19,950 cases estimated in 2016 making it the most common type of leukemia in adults
- Predominant sex: male ≥ female

Incidence
The incidence of AML increases with age, and median age is 67 years.

ETIOLOGY AND PATHOPHYSIOLOGY
Precise causes unknown, but some risk factors have been identified (see "Risk Factors")

Genetics
- Unknown; some are familial.
- Cytogenetics and genetics play an important role in diagnosis and prognosis of AML and have implications for therapy.
- Three risk groups
  - Good risk: inv(16), t(8;21), t(15;17)
  - Standard risk: normal karyotype
  - Poor risk: monosomy 5 and 7 (typically secondary AML), deletion 5q, abnormalities of 11q23 or complex karyotype
- *FLT3* gene mutations, especially internal tandem duplications (FLT3-ITD), have been associated with poor survival in AML. These and growing list of (onco)gene (e.g., *NPM1*, *DNMT3A*, and *P53*) mutations have been studied to further risk-stratify patients (1,2)[A].

RISK FACTORS
- Genetic predisposition (e.g., Down syndrome); other familial disorders are Bloom syndrome (~25% develop AML), Fanconi anemia (52%), neurofibromatosis, Li-Fraumeni syndrome, Wiskott-Aldrich syndrome, Kostmann syndrome, and Diamond-Blackfan anemia.
- Radiation exposure
- Immunodeficiency states

- Chemical and drug exposure (nitrogen mustard and alkylating agents; benzene)
- MDS
- Cigarette smoking

GENERAL PREVENTION
None currently identified, but treatment of high-risk MDS with demethylating agents (5-azacitidine [Vidaza]) has been shown to prolong time to transformation from MDS into AML (3)[A]

COMMONLY ASSOCIATED CONDITIONS
The following are oncologic emergencies:
- Disseminated intravascular coagulopathy (DIC) especially in acute promyelocytic leukemia (APL) but may be seen in any AML
- Leukostasis (high blast number and increased adhesive ability of blasts)
- Tumor lysis syndrome (TLS): spontaneous or in response to chemotherapy

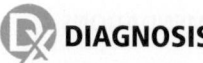 **DIAGNOSIS**

HISTORY
Fatigue (anemia or tumor burden); bleeding (low platelets or DIC); difficulty clearing infections (neutropenia or immune dysregulation)

PHYSICAL EXAM
- Mostly nonspecific and related to marrow or tissue infiltration
  - Fever
  - Bleeding
  - Pallor
  - Splenomegaly
  - Hepatosplenomegaly
  - Lymphadenopathy (usually reactive)
- If CNS is involved, symptoms of increased intracranial pressure can be present.
- Occasionally, patients will present with prominent extramedullary sites of leukemia (e.g., skin infiltration or ultimately as a myeloid sarcoma).

DIFFERENTIAL DIAGNOSIS
- Virus-induced cytopenia, lymphadenopathy, and organomegaly
- Immune cytopenias (including systemic lupus erythematosus [SLE])
- Drug-induced cytopenias
- Other marrow failure and infiltrative diseases (e.g., aplastic anemia, paroxysmal nocturnal hemoglobinuria, MDS, Gaucher disease)

DIAGNOSTIC TESTS & INTERPRETATION
- CBC shows subnormal RBCs, neutrophils, and platelets.
- Bone marrow for histology, flow cytometry, and cytogenetics to establish diagnosis and prognosis
- ESR
- Lactate dehydrogenase (LDH) and uric acid can be elevated (e.g., TLS).
- Coagulation profile can be normal or prolonged (e.g., DIC).
- Drugs that may alter lab results: chemotherapy agents, corticosteroids

- Other special tests: Spinal tap may reveal fluid with leukemic cells.
- Ultrasonography or CT scan of the abdomen may discover organomegaly.

Diagnostic Procedures/Other
Bone marrow studies are usually necessary to make the diagnosis.
- Aspirates: for cell morphology, cytochemistries, immunophenotyping (can confirm differentiation stage of AML); cytogenetics: chromosomal aberration (prognostic value; see "Genetics")
- Biopsies provide valuable information for cellularity, architecture, and so forth.

Test Interpretation
- Marrow is usually hypercellular and the normal architecture effaced; leukemic blast count is 20% or more.
- Liver and spleen may be infiltrated with leukemic cells.

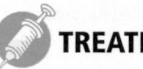 **TREATMENT**

- Chemotherapy is the backbone of AML therapy; it consists of induction and consolidation phase ± maintenance (APL).
- Bone marrow transplantation (BMT) for high-risk AML
- Only modest improvements have been made in AML induction chemotherapy. Supportive care had improved significantly.

GENERAL MEASURES
- Ongoing assessment of bone marrow, liver, heart, and kidney functions during therapy
- Close monitoring of coagulation parameters (risk for DIC)
- Supportive therapy with
  - Good hydration
  - Transfusions of packed RBCs and platelets based on patient's needs (threshold as for platelets as low as 5,000); use leukoreduced, irradiated blood products because all patients can be considered for BMT.
  - Avoid antiplatelet agents (e.g., aspirin products).
  - Follow febrile neutropenic guidelines in neutropenic patient who becomes febrile (even low-grade fever).

Geriatric Considerations
- Older patients (>60 to 65 years of age) remain a therapeutic challenge. These patients are offered so-called reduced-intensity or nonmyeloablative BMT.
- Adding growth factors (granulocyte colony-stimulating factor [G-CSF]) may reduce toxicity in older patients (but is not broadly accepted).
- Hypomethylating agent, such as 5-azacitidine, significantly prolongs survival in older adults with low marrow blast count (<30%).

Pediatric Considerations
Tolerate intense treatments better.

Pregnancy Considerations
Chemotherapy is a viable option in the 2nd and 3rd trimesters.

MEDICATION

First Line

- APL (APL, AML with t[15;17])
  - All-trans retinoic acid (ATRA) and arsenic trioxide both promote maturation to granulocytes.
  - Idarubicin is often added to induction therapy.
- Treatment of AML in younger adults: AML (other than APL)
  - Induction (daunorubicin or idarubicin [anthracycline and cytarabine]): The generally accepted combination is 3 + 7 (anthracycline is given for 3 days and cytarabine for 7 days) or more intensive regimens with high-dose cytarabine (HiDAC) or high dose of anthracycline.
  - Liposomal preparation of daunorubicin and cytarabine is now available for AML with MDS changes or therapy-related AML.
- Remission is typically consolidated in younger patients by the following:
  - In good-risk AML, 3 to 4 cycles of HiDAC and BMT is reserved for time of recurrence.
  - In poor-risk patients, 1 to 2 cycles of HiDAC (until donor is identified) are followed by allogeneic BMT.
  - Intermediate-risk AML should be treated based on individual patient's features, donor availability, and access to clinical trials. A meta-analysis showed that even intermediate-risk patients benefit from allogeneic BMT (4)[A].
- Treatment of AML in older adults (>65 years of age) remains a challenge. These patients have poor performance status, more likely secondary AML, higher incidence of unfavorable cytogenetics, comorbidities, shorter remissions, and shorter overall survival.
  - Intensive chemotherapy may be feasible for patients with good performance status; alternative regimens with mitoxantrone, fludarabine, and clofarabine. New drugs (hypomethylating agents as above, FLT3 inhibitors, monoclonal antibodies, etc.) are being studied in clinical trials (5)[A].
- Contraindications: comorbidities; therapy has to be individualized.
- Precautions
  - If organ failure, some drugs may be avoided or dose reduced (e.g., no anthracyclines in patients with preexisting cardiac problems).
  - Patients will be immunosuppressed during treatment. Avoid live vaccines. Administer varicella-zoster or measles immunoglobulin as soon as exposure of patient occurs.
- Significant possible interactions: Allopurinol accentuates the toxicity of 6-mercaptopurine.
- Novel targeted therapies: midostaurin for AML with FLT3 mutations (both ITD and TKD). Ivosidenib (IDH1 inhibitor) and enasidenib (IDH2 inhibitor) for relapsed/refractory AML with respective IDH mutations; gemtuzumab ozogamicin (anti-CD33 monoclonal antibody) for relapsed/refractory AML with CD33 expression

Second Line

Healthy, younger patients usually are offered reinduction chemotherapy and allogeneic BMT.

ISSUES FOR REFERRAL

- AML should be managed by specialized team led by a hematologist/oncologist.
- Refer patient to a transplant center early because a search for a donor may be necessary.

SURGERY/OTHER PROCEDURES

- BMT: Decision between myeloablative and nonmyeloablative approach should be based on patient's performance status, comorbidities, and AML risk factors.
  - Allogeneic BMT is usually indicated in first remission in intermediate- or high-risk AML or in second remission in all other AML patients. Matched related donor used to be preferred over matched unrelated donor (lower risk of graft versus host disease); recent data suggest equal outcomes because allogeneic transplant regimens and posttransplant care have improved significantly.
- Haploidentical transplants and cord blood have emerged as alternative sources of hematopoietic stem cells for adults that show comparable outcomes as well.
- Autologous BMT may be acceptable in specific situations (e.g., no donor is available).

ADMISSION, INPATIENT, AND NURSING CONSIDERATIONS

- Induction treatment for AML requires inpatient care, usually on a specialized ward. Episodes of febrile neutropenia typically require admission and IV antibiotics.
- Appropriate hydration to prevent TLS
- IV may lead to chemical burns in the event of extravasation.

 ONGOING CARE

FOLLOW-UP RECOMMENDATIONS

Ambulatory, as tolerated; no intense or contact sports; no aspirin due to risk of bleeding

Patient Monitoring

- Repeat bone marrow studies to document remission and also if a relapse is suspected.
- Follow CBC with differential, coagulation studies, uric acid level, and other chemistries related to TLS (creatinine, potassium, phosphate, calcium); monitor urinary function at least daily during induction phase and less frequently later.
- Physical evaluation, including weight and BP, should be done frequently during treatment.

DIET

Ensure adequately balanced calorie/vitamin intake; total parenteral nutrition (TPN) in case of severe mucositis

PATIENT EDUCATION

- Leukemia Society of America, 600 Third Avenue, New York, NY 10016, 212-573-8484
- National Cancer Institute, Bethesda, MD, has pamphlets and telephone education.
- Baker LS. *You and Leukemia: A Day at a Time.* Philadelphia, PA: Saunders; 1978.

PROGNOSIS

AML remission rate is 60–80%, with only 20–40% long-term survival. The wide variable prognosis is due to prognostic group (age, cytogenetics, and genetics).

COMPLICATIONS

- Acute side effects of chemotherapy, including febrile neutropenia
- TLS
- DIC
- Late-onset cardiomyopathy in patients treated with anthracyclines
- Chronic side effects of chemotherapy (secondary malignancies)
- Graft versus host disease in patients who have received allogeneic BMT

REFERENCES

1. Döhner H, Estey EH, Amadori S, et al; for European LeukemiaNet. Diagnosis and management of acute myeloid leukemia in adults: recommendations from an international expert panel, on behalf of the European LeukemiaNet. *Blood.* 2010;115(3):453–474.
2. Patel JP, Gönen M, Figueroa ME, et al. Prognostic relevance of integrated genetic profiling in acute myeloid leukemia. *N Engl J Med.* 2012;366(12):1079–1089.
3. Fenaux P, Mufti GJ, Hellstrom-Lindberg E, et al; for International Vidaza High-Risk MDS Survival Study Group. Efficacy of azacitidine compared with that of conventional care regimens in the treatment of higher-risk myelodysplastic syndromes: a randomised, open-label, phase III study. *Lancet Oncol.* 2009;10(3):223–232.
4. Koreth J, Schlenk R, Kopecky KJ, et al. Allogeneic stem cell transplantation for acute myeloid leukemia in first complete remission: systematic review and meta-analysis of prospective clinical trials. *JAMA.* 2009;301(22):2349–2361.
5. Fenaux P, Mufti GJ, Hellström-Lindberg E, et al. Azacitidine prolongs overall survival compared with conventional care regimens in elderly patients with low bone marrow blast count acute myeloid leukemia. *J Clin Oncol.* 2010;28(4):562–569.

ADDITIONAL READING

O'Donnell MR, Appelbaum FR, Coutre SE, et al. Acute myeloid leukemia. *J Natl Compr Canc Netw.* 2008;6(10):962–993.

 SEE ALSO

Disseminated Intravascular Coagulation; Leukemia, Acute Lymphoblastic (ALL) in Adults; Leukemia, Chronic Myelogenous; Myelodysplastic Syndromes (MDS); Myeloproliferative Neoplasms

 CODES

ICD10

- C92.00 Acute myeloblastic leukemia, not having achieved remission
- C92.01 Acute myeloblastic leukemia, in remission
- C92.02 Acute myeloblastic leukemia, in relapse

CLINICAL PEARLS

- Prognosis of leukemia depends on the cytogenetic and molecular profile of the disease.
- Allogeneic transplant remains the only therapy with curative potential for patients with intermediate- and high-risk AML.

L

LEUKEMIA, CHRONIC LYMPHOCYTIC

Jan Cerny, MD, PhD • Amy E. Pratt, DO

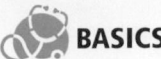 **BASICS**

DESCRIPTION
- Chronic lymphocytic leukemia (CLL) is a monoclonal disorder characterized by a progressive accumulation of mature but functionally incompetent lymphocytes.
- CLL should be distinguished from prolymphocytic leukemia (PLL); based on percentage of prolymphocytes, the disease may be regarded as CLL (<10% prolymphocytes), PLL (>55% prolymphocytes), or CLL/PLL (>10% and <55% prolymphocytes).
- Small lymphocytic lymphoma is a lymphoma variant of CLL.
- System(s) affected: hematologic, lymphatic, immunologic

EPIDEMIOLOGY
Incidence
- CLL represents the most common form of leukemia in adults in the United States with an estimated 18,960 new cases diagnosed in 2016 (1)[A].
- In 2016, an estimated 4,660 adults in the United States died from CLL, which makes it the second leading cause of death among adults with leukemia in the United States after acute myeloid leukemia (1)[A].
- Predominant age: CLL primarily affects elderly individuals, median age of diagnosis being 70 years. Incidence continues to rise in those age >55 years.
- Predominant sex: male > female (1.7:1)
- The incidence is higher among Caucasians than among African Americans.

ETIOLOGY AND PATHOPHYSIOLOGY
- The cell of origin in CLL is a clonal B cell arrested in the B-cell differentiation pathway, intermediate between pre–B cells and mature B cells. In the peripheral blood, these cells resemble mature lymphocytes and typically show B-cell surface antigens: CD19, CD20, CD21, and CD23. In addition, they express CD5 (usually found on T cells).
- The Bcl2 proto-oncogene is overexpressed in B-CLL. Bcl2 is a known suppressor of apoptosis (programmed cell death), resulting in extremely long life of the affected lymphocytes.
  - Genetic mutations leading to disrupted function and prolonged survival of affected lymphocytes are suspected but unknown.

Genetics
CLL is an acquired disorder, and reports of truly familial cases are exceedingly rare. CLL has been shown, however, to occur at higher frequency among first-degree relatives of patients with the disease, and several somatic gene mutations have been identified at significantly higher rates among CLL patients.

RISK FACTORS
- As in the case of most malignancies, the exact cause of CLL is uncertain.
- Possible chronic immune stimulation is suspected but is still being evaluated.
- Monoclonal B-cell lymphocytosis: 1% risk progression to CLL

GENERAL PREVENTION
Unknown

COMMONLY ASSOCIATED CONDITIONS
- Immune system dysregulation is common.
- Conditions that may accompany CLL:
  - Autoimmune hemolytic anemia (AIHA)
  - Immune thrombocytopenia purpura (ITP)
  - Pure red cell aplasia (PRCA)

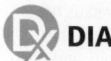 **DIAGNOSIS**

HISTORY
- Insidious onset. It is not unusual for CLL to be discovered incidentally (up to 40% of patients are asymptomatic at the time of diagnosis).
- Others may have the following symptoms:
  - B symptoms: fevers, night sweats, >10% weight loss
  - Fatigue and/or other symptoms of anemia
  - Enlarged lymph nodes (lymphadenopathy = LAD)
  - Mucocutaneous bleeding and/or petechiae
  - Early satiety and/or abdominal discomfort related to an enlarged spleen
  - Recurrent infection(s)

PHYSICAL EXAM
- Lymphadenopathy (localized or generalized)
- Organomegaly (splenomegaly, hepatomegaly)
- Mucocutaneous bleeding (thrombocytopenia)
- Skin: petechiae (thrombocytopenia), pallor (anemia), rash (leukemia cutis)

DIFFERENTIAL DIAGNOSIS
- Infectious:
  - Bacterial (tuberculosis, pertussis)
  - Viral (mononucleosis)
- Neoplastic:
  - Leukemic phase of non-Hodgkin lymphomas
  - Hairy cell leukemia
  - PLL
  - Large granular lymphocytic leukemia
  - Waldenstrom macroglobulinemia

DIAGNOSTIC TESTS & INTERPRETATION
Initial Tests (lab, imaging)
- CBC with differential: B cell absolute lymphocytosis with >5,000 B lymphocytes per μL; often also shows anemia and/or thrombocytopenia
- Blood smear: ruptured lymphocytes ("smudge" cells) and morphologically small mature-appearing lymphocytes
- Confirm diagnosis with immunophenotyping: CLL cells are positive for CD19, CD20, CD23, and CD5; low levels of surface membrane immunoglobulin (Ig)—either IgM or IgM&D; only a single Ig light chain is expressed (κ or λ) confirming monoclonality.
- Additional labs:
  - Hemolysis labs (in cases associated with high disease activity or AIHA): high LDH and indirect bilirubin, low haptoglobin, +/– elevated reticulocyte count (bone marrow infiltration)
  - High plasma β_2-microglobulin (poor prognosis)
  - Hypogammaglobulinemia
- Liver/spleen ultrasound: may demonstrate organomegaly and enlarged abdominal lymph nodes
- CT scan of chest/abdomen/pelvis: not necessary for staging but may identify compression of organs or internal structures from enlarged lymph nodes
- Positron emission tomography (PET) scan: not recommended unless Richter transformation suspected and biopsy necessary (see "Prognosis")

Follow-Up Tests & Special Considerations
Frequency and type of follow-up depend on severity of symptoms as well as risk factors (see "Prognosis").

Diagnostic Procedures/Other
- Bone marrow biopsy: has prognostic value (diffuse infiltration is a risk factor) but not performed routinely
- Lymph node biopsy: Consider if lymph node(s) begins to rapidly enlarge in a patient with known CLL to assess the possibility of transformation to a high-grade lymphoma (Richter syndrome), especially when accompanied by fever, weight loss, and painful lymphadenopathy.

Test Interpretation
- Bone marrow biopsy aspirate usually shows >30% lymphocytes.
- Cytogenetics (fluorescence in situ hybridization) may show chromosomal changes, which are prognostic:
  - Unfavorable: del(17p), del(11q)
  - Neutral: normal, trisomy 12
  - Favorable: del(13q), del(6q)

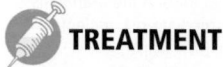 **TREATMENT**

GENERAL MEASURES
Patients with CLL with frequent infections associated with hypogammaglobulinemia are likely to benefit from infusions of intravenous immunoglobulin (IVIG).

MEDICATION
First Line
- Standard of care for new diagnosis with no symptoms or early stage disease: observation
- Standard of care for new diagnosis with symptoms (B symptoms, symptomatic anemia and/or thrombocytopenia, AIHA and/or thrombocytopenia poorly responsive to corticosteroids, progressive organomegaly) or progressive lymphocytosis (increase >50% in 2 months or a doubling time of <6 months): Initiate treatment.
- Low-risk disease, Rai stage 0, and Binet stage A: observation with periodic follow-up
- Intermediate-risk group, Rai stages I and II, and Binet stage B: Observe until evidence of disease progression or development of symptoms.
- High-risk patients, Rai stage III and IV, and Binet stage C: Initiate treatment.
- Selection of first-line therapy depends on patient factors: age, performance status, and medical comorbidities.
- Three main groups of chemotherapeutic drugs:
  - Alkylators: cyclophosphamide (C), chlorambucil, and bendamustine
  - Purine analogs: fludarabine (F) and pentostatin
  - Monoclonal antibodies: rituximab (R) (chimeric anti-CD20) and alemtuzumab (anti-CD52)
- Commonly used single-agent regimens: bendamustine, cyclophosphamide (historically, the standard of care in older patients with comorbidities), and fludarabine

- Commonly used fludarabine- and rituximab-based combination regimens: FC, FR (lower toxicity), FCR (preferred first-line regimen if tolerable to patient), and PCR
- Steroids, high dose: useful in autoimmune manifestations of CLL (AIHA, ITP)

Second Line
- Second-line therapy consists of combinations of chemotherapeutic agents that patient did not fail yet or, occasionally, retreatment with a drug used previously.
- Novel agents (listed below) have also shown promising activity in CLL:
  - Ibrutinib (Bruton tyrosine kinase inhibitor): showed favorable findings in older patients with comorbidities and previously untreated CLL (2)[A]
  - Idelalisib (PI3Kδ kinase inhibitor): Combination of this drug with rituximab compared to placebo with rituximab significantly improved the rate of progression-free survival in patients with comorbidities and relapsed CLL unable to undergo standard chemotherapy (3)[A].
  - Venetoclax (βCL-2 inhibitor): ongoing studies for use in relapsed/refractory CLL and in patients with 17p deletion
  - Obinutuzumab (humanized anti-CD20 monoclonal antibody): Combination of this drug with chlorambucil improved response rates and prolonged progression-free survival in patients with comorbidities and previously untreated CLL (4)[A].
  - Ofatumumab (anti-CD20 monoclonal antibody distinct from rituximab)
- Lenalidomide, a thalidomide derivative, is sometimes first line for elderly patients or second line when combined with rituximab for relapsed/refractory disease.
- Alemtuzumab (anti-CD52) is second line when used for relapsed/refractory disease.
- Allogenic (nonmyeloablative conditioning) and autologous hematopoietic stem cell transplant (hSCT) may be considered in high-risk and younger patients, particularly those with refractory disease (limited data available as still considered experimental therapy).

ISSUES FOR REFERRAL
- Surgical consultation for splenectomy in patients with progressive splenomegaly +/− refractory cytopenias
- Radiation oncology consultation for large or bulky lymphadenopathy, particularly those causing compressive symptoms

ADDITIONAL THERAPIES
- Patients requiring therapy who are high risk for tumor lysis syndrome should be given allopurinol to prevent uric acid nephropathy.
- Vaccinations (avoid live vaccines):
  - Annual influenza vaccine
  - Pneumococcal vaccine every 5 years

SURGERY/OTHER PROCEDURES
See "Issues for Referral" above.

ADMISSION, INPATIENT, AND NURSING CONSIDERATIONS
No specific criteria but may require inpatient admission for complications of disease (AIHA) or of therapy (febrile neutropenia, tumor lysis syndrome)

 ONGOING CARE

FOLLOW-UP RECOMMENDATIONS
Patient Monitoring
Patients with low-risk CLL and/or patients in remission:
- CBC with differential (lymphocytosis), LDH, and β_2-microglobulin every 3 to 6 months
- Physical exam (lymphadenopathy, organomegaly)

DIET
- Ensure adequately balanced calorie/vitamin intake.
- Follow weights.

PATIENT EDUCATION
Leukemia and Lymphoma Society has educational pamphlets: https://www.lls.org/resource-center/download-or-order-free-publications?language=English&category=Leukemia&sortby=alpha

PROGNOSIS
- Two staging systems are used, but neither is completely satisfactory: Rai system in the United States and Binet system in Europe
- Rai staging system:
  - Stage 0: lymphocytosis only; low risk status
  - Stage I: lymphocytosis and adenopathy; intermediate risk status
  - Stage II: lymphocytosis +/− adenopathy and splenomegaly and/or hepatomegaly; intermediate risk status
  - Stage III: lymphocytosis and anemia (hemoglobin <11 g/dL); high risk status
  - Stage IV: lymphocytosis and thrombocytopenia (platelets <100 × 10⁹/L); high risk status
- Binet staging system:
  - Stage A: hemoglobin ≥10 g/dL, platelets ≥100 × 10⁹, and <3 lymph node areas involved (Rai stages 0, I, and II); survival >120 months
  - Stage B: hemoglobin and platelet levels as in stage A and ≥3 lymph node areas involved (Rai stages I and II); survival 61 months
  - Stage C: hemoglobin <10 g/dL, platelets <100 × 10⁹, and any number of lymph nodes involved (Rai stages III and IV); survival 32 months
- Adverse risk factors:
  - Advanced Rai or Binet stage
  - Peripheral lymphocyte doubling time <12 months
  - Diffuse marrow infiltration
  - Increased number of prolymphocytes or cleaved cells
  - Poor response to chemotherapy
  - High β_2-microglobulin and thymidine kinase levels and low micro RNAs (miRNAs)
  - Abnormal karyotyping: del(17p) and del(11q)
  - Mutated immunoglobulin heavy chain variable (IgHV) genes (Expression of ZAP-70 >20% or CD38 >30% evaluated by immunophenotyping are surrogate markers.)
  - NOTCH1 mutation (associated with unmutated IgVH)

COMPLICATIONS
- Acute or long-term effects of chemotherapy
- Richter syndrome
- AIHA (Some cases may be related to the use of fludarabine.)

- Slightly increased risk of solid tumors (especially Kaposi sarcoma, malignant melanoma, laryngeal cancer, lung cancer, colon cancer)
- Infection
- Membranoproliferative glomerulonephritis (MPGN) or other glomerular pathology

REFERENCES
1. Siegel RL, Miller KD, Jemal A. Cancer statistics, 2016. *CA Cancer J Clin*. 2016;66(1):7–30.
2. Burger JA, Tedeschi A, Barr PM, et al; and RESONATE-2 Investigators. Ibrutinib as initial therapy for patients with chronic lymphocytic leukemia. *N Engl J Med*. 2015;373(25):2425–2437.
3. Furman RR, Sharman JP, Coutre SE, et al. Idelalisib and rituximab in relapsed chronic lymphocytic leukemia. *N Engl J Med*. 2014;370(11):997–1007.
4. Goede V, Fischer K, Busch R, et al. Obinutuzumab plus chlorambucil in patients with CLL and coexisting conditions. *N Engl J Med*. 2014;370(12):1101–1110.

ADDITIONAL READING
- Chiorazzi N, Rai KR, Ferrarini M. Chronic lymphocytic leukemia. *N Engl J Med*. 2005;352(8):804–815.
- National Comprehensive Cancer Network guidelines: http://www.nccn.org/.
- Shanafelt TD, Kay NE. Comprehensive management of the CLL patient: a holistic approach. *Hematology Am Soc Hematol Educ Program*. 2007;2007(1):324–331.

 CODES

ICD10
- C91.10 Chronic lymphocytic leukemia of B-cell type not achieve remission
- C91.11 Chronic lymphocytic leukemia of B-cell type in remission
- C91.12 Chronic lymphocytic leukemia of B-cell type in relapse

CLINICAL PEARLS
- CLL is the most common form of leukemia in adults in the United States.
- CLL primarily affects elderly individuals, median age of diagnosis being 70 years. Incidence continues to rise in those age >55 years.
- Clinical monitoring of asymptomatic and low-risk patients is a reasonable approach ("watch and wait").
- High-risk patients, patients with bulky disease, and patients who fail fludarabine- and rituximab-based therapies typically have poor prognoses and may require intensive therapies, including allogeneic hematopoietic stem cell transplantation.
- Several novel agents are being developed to improve therapeutic approaches to CLL.

L

LEUKEMIA, CHRONIC MYELOGENOUS

Jan Cerny, MD, PhD

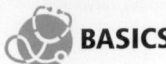

BASICS

DESCRIPTION
- Chronic myelogenous leukemia (CML) is a myeloproliferative neoplasm characterized by clonal proliferation of myeloid precursors in the bone marrow with continuing differentiation into mature granulocytes.
- Hallmark of CML is Philadelphia chromosome (translocation t[9;22]).
- Natural history of the disease evolves in three clinical phases: a chronic phase, an accelerated phase, and a blast phase or crisis (transformation to acute leukemia).

EPIDEMIOLOGY
Incidence
- Per year, 1.6 cases/100,000 persons
- Predominant age: 50 to 60 years
- Predominant sex: male > female (1.3:1)

Prevalence
Accounts for 15–20% of adult leukemias

ETIOLOGY AND PATHOPHYSIOLOGY
Philadelphia chromosome is a balanced translocation between *BCR* (on chromosome 22) and *ABL* (on chromosome 9) genes t(9;22)(q34;q11). This fusion gene, *BCR-ABL*, codes for an abnormal, constitutively active tyrosine kinase that affects numerous signal transduction pathways, resulting in uncontrolled cell proliferation and reduced apoptosis.

Genetics
Acquired genomic changes

RISK FACTORS
Ionizing radiation exposure (uncommon)

GENERAL PREVENTION
None currently identified

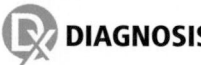

DIAGNOSIS

85–90% of patients present in the chronic phase, and the disease can be found accidentally during routine screening.

HISTORY
- Chronic phase: fatigue, weight loss, night sweats, abdominal fullness owing to enlarged spleen, early satiety, dyspnea, and bleeding. Rare: bruising, left upper quadrant abdominal pain, sternal pain (owing to expanding bone marrow), and gouty arthritis; up to 30% of patients are asymptomatic.

- Accelerated phase progressive splenomegaly and left upper quadrant abdominal pain occasionally referred to the left shoulder (owing to splenic infarction or rupture), progressive weight loss and sweats, unexplained fever or bone pain, chloromas (extramedullary tumors)
- Blast phase: bleeding, bruising, infections, prominent constitutional symptoms

PHYSICAL EXAM
- Splenomegaly (50–90%), hepatomegaly (up to 50%)
- Less common: splenic friction rub, lymphadenopathy

DIFFERENTIAL DIAGNOSIS
- Chronic myelomonocytic leukemia, chronic neutrophilic leukemia, chronic eosinophilic leukemia, juvenile myelomonocytic leukemia, infectious mononucleosis, leukemoid reaction, polycythemia vera, and treatment with granulocyte-stimulating factors
- Acute myelogenous leukemia resembles blast crisis with myeloid blasts, and acute lymphoblastic leukemia resembles blast crisis with lymphoid blasts.
- Atypical CML is a chronic myeloproliferative disorder with a clinical hematologic picture similar to CML, but it lacks Philadelphia chromosome and *BCR-ABL* rearrangement.

DIAGNOSTIC TESTS & INTERPRETATION
- CBC
  - Hematocrit: may be normal, slightly increased, or decreased
  - WBC count: markedly increased (50,000 to 100,000/μL), with granulocytes in all stages of development, including occasional blasts <10% in chronic phase, basophilia, eosinophilia
  - Platelets: normal, elevated (34%), or occasionally low
  - In accelerated phase: anemia, 10–19% blood or marrow blasts, basophils plus eosinophils >20%, thrombocytopenia
  - Blast phase: blood or marrow blasts >20%
- Genetics
  - Demonstration of the Philadelphia chromosome, t(9;22), by cytogenetic techniques, fluorescence in situ hybridization (FISH), or reverse transcription-polymerase chain reaction (RT-PCR)
  - Additional cytogenetic abnormalities occur in the accelerated and blast phases (monosomy 7; t[3,21]; trisomies 8 and 19; Philadelphia chromosome duplication; abnormalities of chromosome 17 such as monosomy, trisomy, and isochromosome mutations). These may contribute to resistance to tyrosine kinase inhibitors (TKIs; e.g., imatinib). Further molecular testing (mutations within *BCR-ABL*) is suggested in case of loss of response to therapy.

- Others:
  - Low or absent leukocyte alkaline phosphatase in neutrophils
  - High lactate dehydrogenase (LDH)
  - Elevated uric acid

Initial Tests (lab, imaging)
- CBC, LDH, uric acid, bone marrow biopsy and aspiration, cytogenetics on bone marrow, and FISH for *BCR-ABL*, RT-PCR, LFTs
- Abdominal ultrasound or CT scan shows splenomegaly; not mandatory

Follow-Up Tests & Special Considerations
- Mutation analysis of tyrosine kinase domain of *ABL* kinase because they may cause resistance to therapy with TKIs
- HLA-A*02 positive is associated with CML, and a protective effect is seen with the HLA-B*35 allele (pooled odds ratio 0.64, 95% CI 0.48–0.86).

Diagnostic Procedures/Other
Bone marrow aspiration and biopsy

Test Interpretation
Myeloid hyperplasia with elevated myeloid: erythroid ratio, normal maturation, marrow basophilia, and increased reticulin fibrosis

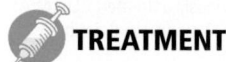

TREATMENT

MEDICATION
- TKIs (e.g., imatinib) provide durable, long-term control of disease.
- The response to TKIs is assessed at specific time points from the beginning of treatment and is categorized as follows:
  - Complete hematologic response (CHR): normalization of peripheral counts, no disease symptoms, no immature cells
  - Minor/partial/complete cytogenetic response (CCR): 1–34%, 35–90%, no Philadelphia-positive metaphases
  - Major molecular response (MMR): decreased level of *BCR-ABL* transcript by PCR 3-log
  - Complete molecular response (CMR): *BCR-ABL* transcript is undetectable by PCR.

First Line
- Imatinib mesylate (Gleevec), an oral TKI, 400 mg/day
- Side effects: thrombocytopenia, anemia, elevated liver enzymes, edema, GI disturbances, rash
- International Randomized Study of Interferon versus STI571 (IRIS) established imatinib as first-line therapy (1)[A].

- Imatinib dose can be increased to 600 and 800 mg/day if only suboptimal response is achieved with standard dose.
- 2nd-generation TKIs have shown higher efficacy and fewer side effects and are approved for first-line therapy of chronic phase CML: nilotinib (Tasigna) and dasatinib (Sprycel) (2,3)[A]. Bosutinib is now approved for front-line setting as well.

Second Line
- Dasatinib, 2nd-generation TKI; active against most of *BCR-ABL* mutants; not active in *T315I* mutation
  - 100 mg/day in patients resistant or intolerant to imatinib and 70 mg BID or 140 mg/day for patients in accelerated or blastic phase
  - Side effects: pleural effusions, cytopenias
- Nilotinib, also 2nd-generation TKI; highly selective and more potent *BCR-ABL* TKI; active against most *BCR-ABL* mutants; not active in *T315I* mutation
  - 400 mg PO BID in patients resistant or intolerant to imatinib in chronic or accelerated phase
  - Side effects: cytopenias, QTc prolongation, pancreatitis
- Bosutinib and omacetaxine are now approved for patient who failed or did not tolerate two TKIs previously. Ponatinib has now more restricted approval, but together with omacetaxine, in addition, they are the only effective agents in patients with *T315I* mutation. Agents targeting leukemic stem cells are being developed for clinical use.

ISSUES FOR REFERRAL
All patients with CML should be referred to a hematologist. Patients with inadequate response to TKIs or with *T315I* mutation should consult with a bone marrow transplant (BMT) physician.

SURGERY/OTHER PROCEDURES
Allogeneic BMT
- It is the only known cure; however, 71% of patients who achieve CCR with imatinib maintain that response beyond 7 years, and no patient progressed on the trial between years 5 and 6 of treatment.
- Most effective in patients <50 years of age who are in the chronic phase
- Initial mortality is higher (related to the use of myeloablative regimens) than medical management but provided higher rates of survival in pre-TKI era.
- Significant improvement in transplant techniques leading to better outcomes, such as alternative sources of stem cells; nonmyeloablative regimens have shown improvements in transplant-related mortality.
- Transplant option should be thoroughly discussed with young patients in chronic phase and considered an alternative to TKIs, especially if the patient does not tolerate TKIs or disease is not responding.
- Can be considered in patients who fail to achieve CHR by 3 months, have no cytogenetic response or cytogenetic relapse, or have *T315I* mutation

ADMISSION, INPATIENT, AND NURSING CONSIDERATIONS
- Acute abdominal symptoms (infarcted or ruptured spleen); tumor lysis syndrome owing to initial therapy; complications of BMT
  - Hydroxyurea might be given, with the goal of reduction of the WBC count, but it has minimal impact on patient response to TKIs.
  - Induction chemotherapy (for acute leukemia) in setting of blastic phase
  - Allopurinol to prevent tumor lysis syndrome in patients with very high counts; however, probably not necessary when TKIs are used
- Discharge criteria: abatement of acute symptoms

 ONGOING CARE

FOLLOW-UP RECOMMENDATIONS
- Frequency depends on stage at presentation and response to first-line therapy.
- Although splenomegaly persists, avoid contact sports or trauma to abdomen.

Patient Monitoring
- CBC with differential: weekly until blood counts stable and then every 2 to 4 weeks during CHR; once in CCR and stable, patient can be followed less frequently (3-month intervals).
- Bone marrow cytogenetics (evaluation for clonal evolution) every 6 months while in CHR, every 12 to 18 months while in CCR, MMR, CMR
- Quantitative RT-PCR every 3 months (peripheral blood)
- ECGs (concern for QT prolongation), LFTs while on TKIs. Nilotinib, bosutinib, and ponatinib can cause pancreatitis.
- Blood pressure monitoring because several TKIs have been associated with elevated blood pressure and related cardiovascular complications

PROGNOSIS
- With treatment and good response, the survival is similar to the normal population.
- Without treatment: CML invariably will progress to accelerated phase within 2 to 5 years and blast phase within several months of the accelerated phase.
- Poor prognosis: patients presenting in accelerated or blastic phase or presenting with very large spleen size, platelets >700,000/μL, and patients resistant to TKIs (*T315I* mutation)

COMPLICATIONS
- Splenic infarct or rupture
- Progression to accelerated or blastic phase
- Thrombotic events owing to elevated platelets
- Bleeding owing to low or dysfunctional platelets
- Sequelae of anemia

REFERENCES
1. O'Brien SG, Guilhot F, Goldman JM, et al. International Randomized Study of Interferon versus STI571 (IRIS) 7-year follow-up: sustained survival, low rate of transformation and increased rate of major molecular response (MMR) in patients (pts) with newly diagnosed chronic myeloid leukemia in chronic phase (CMLCP) treated with imatinib (IM). *Blood*. 2008;112(11):76.
2. Saglio G, Kim DW, Issaragrisil S, et al; for ENESTnd Investigators. Nilotinib versus imatinib for newly diagnosed chronic myeloid leukemia. *N Engl J Med*. 2010;362(24):2251–2259.
3. Kantarjian H, Shah NP, Hochhaus A, et al. Dasatinib versus imatinib in newly diagnosed chronic-phase chronic myeloid leukemia. *N Engl J Med*. 2010;362(24):2260–2270.

ADDITIONAL READING
- Kantarjian HM, Baccarani M, Jabbour E, et al. Second-generation tyrosine kinase inhibitors: the future of frontline CML therapy. *Clin Cancer Res*. 2011;17(7):1674–1683.
- Kantarjian H, Pasquini R, Hamerschlak N, et al. Dasatinib or high-dose imatinib for chronic-phase chronic myeloid leukemia after failure of first-line imatinib: a randomized phase 2 trial. *Blood*. 2007;109(12):5143–5150.
- Naugler C, Liwski R. Human leukocyte antigen class I alleles and the risk of chronic myelogenous leukemia: a meta-analysis. *Leuk Lymphoma*. 2010;51(7):1288–1292.

 CODES

ICD10
- C92.10 Chronic myeloid leukemia, BCR/ABL-positive, not having achieved remission
- C92.11 Chronic myeloid leukemia, BCR/ABL-positive, in remission
- C92.12 Chronic myeloid leukemia, BCR/ABL-positive, in relapse

CLINICAL PEARLS
- CML belongs to the myeloproliferative disorders group.
- The gold standard for diagnosis of CML is detection of the Philadelphia chromosome or its products, *BCR-ABL* mRNA, and fusion protein.
- TKIs provide durable, long-term control of the disease and have dramatically altered treatment.
- Atypical CML is a form of clinically typical CML but without the presence of the typical *BCR-ABL* translocation.
- Blast crisis is a form of acute leukemia that is a possible complication of CML.

L

LEUKOPLAKIA, ORAL

Kathya M. Chartre, MD • Robert C.M. Ander, MD • Rajitha Kota, MD, MPH

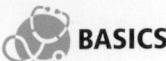 BASICS

DESCRIPTION
- Oral leukoplakia is a white plaque or patches on the oral mucosa, generally precancerous.
- System(s) affected: gastrointestinal
- Hyperplasia of squamous epithelium

EPIDEMIOLOGY
- Develops in middle age, increases with age
- Most common in India, where more people smoke and chew tobacco and areca nuts

Prevalence
- 1–3% of the worldwide population is affected (1).
- Age of onset is >40 years old with peak in the 60s (1).
- Males 3 times more likely to be affected as females (1)
- Smokers 6 times more likely to be affected than nonsmokers (1)

Geriatric Considerations
Malignant transformation to carcinoma is more common in older patients.

ETIOLOGY AND PATHOPHYSIOLOGY
Hyperkeratosis or dyskeratosis of the oral squamous epithelium
- Tobacco use in any form
- Alcohol consumption/alcoholism
- Periodontitis
- *Candida albicans* infection may induce dysplasia and increase malignant transformation.
- Human papillomavirus, types 16 and 18
- Sunlight
- Vitamin deficiency
- Syphilis
- Dental restorations/prosthetic appliances
- Estrogen therapy
- Chronic trauma or irritation
- Epstein-Barr virus (oral hairy leukoplakia)
- Areca nut/betel (Asian populations)
- Mouthwash preparations and toothpaste containing the herbal root extract sanguinaria

Genetics
- Dyskeratosis congenital and epidermolysis bullosa increase the likelihood of oral malignancy.
- P53 overexpression, PTEN allelic loss correlates with leukoplakia and particularly squamous cell carcinoma.

RISK FACTORS
- 70–90% of oral leukoplakia is related to tobacco, particularly smokeless tobacco or areca/betel nut use.
- Similar to risk factors for squamous cell carcinoma
- Alcohol increases risk 1.5-fold.
- Repeated or chronic mechanical trauma from dental appliances or cheek biting
- Chemical irritation to oral regions
- Diabetes
- Age
- Socioeconomic status

- Risk factors for malignant transformation of leukoplakia
  - Female
  - Long duration of leukoplakia
  - Nonsmoker (idiopathic leukoplakia)
  - Located on tongue or floor of mouth
  - Size >200 mm^2
  - Nonhomogenous type
  - Presence of epithelial dysplasia

GENERAL PREVENTION
- Avoid tobacco of any kind, alcohol, habitual cheek biting, tongue chewing.
- Use well-fitting dental prosthesis.
- Regular dental check-ups to avoid bad restorations
- Diet rich in fresh fruits and vegetables may help to prevent cancer.
- HPV vaccination may be preventive.

COMMONLY ASSOCIATED CONDITIONS
- HIV infection is closely associated with hairy leukoplakia.
- Erythroplakia in association with leukoplakia, "speckled leukoplakia," or erythroleukoplakia is a marker for underlying dysplasia.
- 1–20% of lesions will progress to carcinoma within 10 years.

 DIAGNOSIS

Leukoplakia is an asymptomatic white patch on the oral mucosa.

HISTORY
- Usually asymptomatic
- History of tobacco or alcohol use or oral exposure to irritants

PHYSICAL EXAM
- Location
  - 50% on tongue, mandibular alveolar ridge, and buccal mucosa
  - Also seen on maxillary alveolar ridge, palate, and lower lip
  - Infrequently seen on floor of the mouth and retromolar areas
  - Floor of mouth, ventrolateral tongue, and soft palate complex are more likely to have dysplastic lesions.
- Appearance
  - Varies from homogeneous, nonpalpable, faintly translucent white areas to thick, fissured, papillomatous, indurated plaques
  - May feel rough or leathery
  - Lesions can become exophytic or verruciform.
  - Color may be white, gray, yellowish white, or brownish gray.
  - Cannot be wiped or scraped off
- World Health Organization classification
  - Homogeneous refers to color.
    - Flat, corrugated, wrinkled, or pumice
  - Nonhomogeneous refers to color and texture (more likely to be dysplastic or malignant).
    - Erythroleukoplakia (mixture of red and white)
    - Proliferative verrucous leukoplakia (PVL) (multifocal, mostly women)

DIFFERENTIAL DIAGNOSIS
- White oral lesions that can be rubbed off: acute pseudomembranous candidiasis
- White oral lesions that cannot be rubbed off (2):
  - Developmental/genetic (rare):
    - Cannon white sponge nevus (diffuse bilateral white plaques of buccal mucosa, tongue)
    - Hereditary benign intraepithelial dyskeratosis
    - Pachyonychia congenita
  - Reactive/frictional:
    - Leukoedema (delicate gray-white lines, disappear with stretching)
    - Contact desquamation
    - Morsicatio mucosae oris (cheek/gum biting)
    - Benign alveolar ridge keratosis (ill-fitting dentures)
    - Hairy tongue (elongated filiform papillae, may become pigmented from food/bacteria)
    - Nicotinic stomatitis and smokeless tobacco keratosis (South Asian "paan" or "gutka"; American/Swedish snuff; Ethiopian "toombak")
  - Infectious:
    - Candidiasis
    - Hairy leukoplakia (associated with EBV and HIV-infected individuals)
  - Immune-mediated:
    - Lichen planus (typically symmetric, bilateral, reticular white lesions)
    - Lichenoid lesions
    - Benign migratory glossitis
  - Autoimmune:
    - SLE
    - Chronic graft versus host disease

DIAGNOSTIC TESTS & INTERPRETATION
Biopsy with histopathologic examination is the gold standard.

Initial Tests (lab, imaging)
- Laboratory tests generally are not indicated.
  - Consider saliva culture if *C. albicans* infection is suspected.
- No imaging is indicated.

Follow-Up Tests & Special Considerations
- Biopsy is necessary to rule out carcinoma if lesion is persistent, changing, or unexplained.
- Consider CBC, rapid plasma reagin (RPR).

Diagnostic Procedures/Other
- Oral cytology is superior to conventional oral examination (3)[A].
- Computer-assisted cytology or liquid-based cytology is not superior to oral cytology (3)[A].
- Noninvasive brush biopsy and analysis of cells with DNA–image cytometry constitute a sensitive and specific screening method.
- Patients with dysplastic or malignant cells on brush biopsy should undergo more formal excisional biopsy.
- Excisional biopsy is definitive procedure.

Test Interpretation

- Biopsy specimens range from hyperkeratosis to keratosis of unknown significance (KUS) to dysplasia to invasive carcinoma.
- At initial biopsy, 6% are invasive carcinoma.
- 0.13–6% subsequently undergo malignant transformation.
- Location is important: 60% on floor of mouth or lateral border of tongue are cancerous; buccal mucosal lesions are generally not malignant but require biopsy if not resolving.

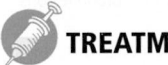 **TREATMENT**

- All oral leukoplakias should be treated because they are potentially malignant.
- Treatment may include the following:
  - For 2 to 3 circumscribed lesions, surgical excision is treatment of choice (4)[C].
  - For multiple or large lesions where surgery would cause unacceptable deformity, consider cryosurgery or laser surgery (4)[C].
  - Abstinence from predisposing habits (alcohol and tobacco)
- Complete excision is standard treatment for dysplasia or malignancy.
- After treatment, up to 30% of leukoplakia recurs, and some leukoplakia still transforms to squamous cell carcinoma (4)[B].
- Oral hairy leukoplakia may be treated with podophyllin with acyclovir cream.

GENERAL MEASURES

- Eliminate habitual lip biting.
- Correct ill-fitting dental appliances, bad restorations, or sharp teeth.
- Stop smoking and using alcohol.
- Some small lesions may respond to cryosurgery.
- β-Carotene, lycopene, retinoids, and cyclooxygenase 2 (COX-2) inhibitors may cause partial regression.
- For hairy tongue: tongue brushing

MEDICATION

Carotenoids; vitamins A, C, and K; bleomycin; and photodynamic therapy ineffective to prevent malignant transformation and recurrence

ISSUES FOR REFERRAL

Consider otolaryngologist or oral surgery referral for extensive disease.

SURGERY/OTHER PROCEDURES

- Scalpel excision, laser ablation, electrocautery, or cryoablation
- Cryotherapy slightly less effective than photodynamic therapy response (73% vs. 90%) and recurrence (27% vs. 24%) (5)[A]
- CO_2 laser had 20% recurrence and 10% malignant transformation within 5 years (6)[B].
- Biopsy/excision algorithm (2)[C]:
  - KUS that is poorly demarcated and likely frictional: Rebiopsy and follow up.
  - KUS that is well demarcated and >3 cm: Follow up every 3 months; rebiopsy every 12 months.
  - KUS that is <3 cm: Excise/ablate with narrow margins; follow up every 3 months; if recurs, excise with wider margins.
  - PVL: Follow up every 3 months; excise verrucous or nodular areas.
  - Dysplastic/SCC: Excise.

ADMISSION, INPATIENT, AND NURSING CONSIDERATIONS

- Eliminate etiologic factors.
- Reevaluate in 7 to 14 days.
- Biopsy if lesion is persistent

 ONGOING CARE

FOLLOW-UP RECOMMENDATIONS

Patient Monitoring

- Regular, close follow-up, even after successful treatment
- Biopsy as needed

DIET

Regular

PATIENT EDUCATION

- If biopsy is negative, stress importance of periodic and careful follow-up.
- Initiate a dental referral to eliminate dental factors.
- Stress importance of stopping tobacco and alcohol use.
- Encourage participation in smoking cessation program.

PROGNOSIS

- Most leukoplakia is benign.
- Leukoplakia may regress, remain stable, or progress.
- 0.13–6% of initially benign lesions subsequently develop into cancer.
- Size >4 cm increases risk of malignant transformation.
- 5-year survival rate of oral cancer is 50%.

COMPLICATIONS

- New lesions may develop after treatment.
- Risk of malignant transformation to squamous cell carcinoma is approximately 5–17%.
- Larger lesions and nonhomogeneous leukoplakia are associated with higher rates of malignant transformation.

REFERENCES

1. Nadeau C, Kerr A. Evaluation and management of oral potentially malignant disorders. *Dent Clin North Am.* 2018;62(1):1–27.
2. Villa A, Woo S. Leukoplakia—a diagnostic and management algorithm. *J Oral Maxillofac Surg.* 2017;75(4):723–734.
3. Fuller C, Camilon R, Nguyen S, et al. Adjunctive diagnostic techniques for oral lesions of unknown malignant potential: systematic review with meta-analysis. *Head Neck.* 2015;37(5):755–762.
4. Feller L, Lemmer J. Oral leukoplakia as it relates to HPV infection: a review. *Int J Dent.* 2012;2012:540561.
5. Kawczyk-Krupka A, Waśkowska J, Raczkowska-Siostrzonek A, et al. Comparison of cryotherapy and photodynamic therapy in treatment of oral leukoplakia. *Photodiagnosis Photodyn Ther.* 2012;9(2):148–155.
6. Jerjes W, Upile T, Hamdoon Z, et al. CO2 laser of oral dysplasia: clinicopathological features of recurrence and malignant transformation. *Lasers Med Sci.* 2012;27(1):169–179.

ADDITIONAL READING

- Messadi DV. Diagnostic aids for detection of oral precancerous conditions. *Int J Oral Sci.* 2013;5(2):59–65.
- Nair DR, Pruthy R, Pawar U, et al. Oral cancer: premalignant conditions and screening—an update. *J Cancer Res Ther.* 2012;8(Suppl 1):S57–S66.
- Reamy BV, Derby R, Bunt CW. Common tongue conditions in primary care. *Am Fam Physician.* 2010;81(5):627–634.

 SEE ALSO

HIV/AIDS; Infectious Mononucleosis, Epstein-Barr Virus Infections

 CODES

ICD10

- K13.21 Leukoplakia of oral mucosa, including tongue
- K13.3 Hairy leukoplakia

CLINICAL PEARLS

- Excisional biopsy is indicated for any undiagnosed leukoplakia.
- After treatment, up to 30% of leukoplakia recurs, and some leukoplakia still transforms to squamous cell carcinoma; thus, long-term surveillance is essential.
- To lessen risk of malignant transformation, encourage tobacco and alcohol cessation and consider *C. albicans* eradication.

L

LICHEN PLANUS

Mercedes E. Gonzalez, MD • Herbert P. Goodheart, MD

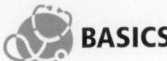 **BASICS**

Lichen planus (LP) is an idiopathic eruption with characteristic shiny, flat-topped (Latin: *planus*, "flat") purple (violaceous) papules and plaques on the skin, often accompanied by characteristic mucous membrane lesions. Itching may be severe.

DESCRIPTION
- Classic (typical) LP is a relatively uncommon inflammatory disorder of the skin and mucous membranes; hair and nails may also be affected.
  - Skin lesions are small, flat, angular, red-to-violaceous, shiny, pruritic papules and/or plaques with overlying fine, white lines (called Wickham striae), or gray-white puncta; most commonly seen on the flexor surfaces of the upper extremities, extensor surfaces of the lower extremities, the genitalia, and on the mucous membranes
  - On the oral mucosa, lesions typically appear as raised white lines in a lacelike pattern seen most often on the buccal mucosa.
  - Onset is abrupt or gradual. Course is unpredictable; may resolve spontaneously, recur intermittently, or persist for many years
- Drug-induced LP
  - Clinical and histopathologic findings may mimic those of classic LP. Lesions usually lack Wickham striae (see in the following text) and oral involvement is rare.
  - There is generally a latent period of months from drug introduction until lesions appear.
  - Lesions resolve when the inciting agent is discontinued, often after a prolonged period.
- LP variants
  - Follicular: also called lichen planopilaris; typically seen on the scalp, can lead to scarring alopecia
  - Annular: Papules spread centrifugally as central area resolves; occur on glans penis, axillae, and oral mucosa
  - Linear: may be an isolated finding
  - Hypertrophic: itchy, hyperkeratotic, thick plaques on dorsal legs and feet
  - Atrophic: rare, most often the result of resolved lesions
  - Bullous LP: Intense inflammation in the dermis leads to blistering of epidermis.
  - LP pemphigoides: a combination of LP and bullous pemphigoid (IgG autoantibodies to collagen 17)
  - Nail LP: affects the nail matrix, lateral thinning, longitudinal ridging, and fissuring
- System(s) affected: skin/exocrine
- Synonym(s): lichenoid eruptions

EPIDEMIOLOGY
- Predominant age: 30 to 60 years old; rare in children and the geriatric population
- Predominant sex: female > male

Prevalence
In the United States, 450/100,000

ETIOLOGY AND PATHOPHYSIOLOGY
LP is considered to be a T cell–mediated autoimmune response to self-antigens on damaged keratinocytes.

RISK FACTORS
Exposure to certain drugs or chemicals
- Thiazides, furosemide, β-blockers, sulfonylureas, antimalarials, penicillamine, gold salts, and angiotensin-converting enzyme inhibitors
- Rarely: photo-developing chemicals, dental materials, tattoo pigments

COMMONLY ASSOCIATED CONDITIONS
- An association has been noted between LP and hepatitis C virus infection, particularly in certain geographic regions (Asia, South America, the Middle East, Europe) (1). Hepatitis should be considered in patients with widespread presentations of LP and those with primarily oral disease.
- In addition, chronic active hepatitis, lichen nitidus, and primary biliary cirrhosis have been noted to coexist with LP.
- Association with dyslipidemia has been reported (2)[B].
- LP has also been reported in association with other diseases of altered immunity, more often than would be expected by chance.
  - Bullous pemphigoid
  - Alopecia areata
  - Myasthenia gravis
  - Vitiligo
  - Ulcerative colitis
  - Graft versus host reaction
  - Lupus erythematosus (lupus erythematosus–LP overlap syndrome)
  - Morphea and lichen sclerosus et atrophicus

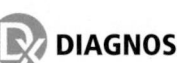 **DIAGNOSIS**

LP is most commonly diagnosed by its appearance despite its range of clinical presentations. A skin biopsy should be performed if the diagnosis is in doubt.

HISTORY
A minority of patients have a family history of LP. Affected families have an increased frequency of human leukocyte antigen B7 (HLA-B7). A thorough drug history should be performed.

PHYSICAL EXAM
- Skin (often severe pruritus)
  - Papules: 1 to 10 mm, shiny, flat-topped (planar) lesions that occur in crops; lesions may have a fine scale.
  - Evidence of scratching (i.e., crusts and excoriations) is usually absent.
  - Color: violaceous, with white lacelike pattern (Wickham striae) on surface of papules. Wickham striae are best seen after topical application of mineral oil and, if present, are virtually pathognomonic for LP.
  - Shape: polygonal or oval. Annular lesions may appear on trunk and mucous membranes. Various shapes and sizes may be noted (polymorphic).
  - Arrangement: may be grouped, linear, or scattered individual lesions
  - Koebner phenomenon (isomorphic response): New lesions may be noted at sites of minor injuries, such as scratches or burns.

- Distribution: ventral surface of wrists and forearms, dorsa hands, glans penis, dorsa feet, groin, sacrum, shins, and scalp. Hypertrophic (verrucous) lesions may occur on lower legs and may be generalized.
- Postinflammatory hyperpigmentation: Lesions typically heal, leaving darkly pigmented macules in their wake.
- Mucous membranes (40–60% of patients with skin lesions; 20% have mucous membrane lesions without skin involvement.)
  - Most commonly asymptomatic, nonerosive, milky-white lines with an elegant, lacy, netlike streaked pattern
  - Usually seen on buccal mucosa but may appear on tongue, gingiva, palate, or lips
  - Less commonly, LP may be erosive; rarely bullous
  - Painful, especially if ulcers present
  - Lesions may develop into squamous cell carcinoma (1–3%).
  - Glans penis, labia minora, vaginal vault, and perianal areas may be involved.
- Hair/scalp
  - LP of the hair follicle (lichen planopilaris) presents with keratotic plugs at the follicle orifice with a violaceous rim; may result in atrophy and permanent destruction of hair follicles (scarring alopecia)
- Nails (10%)
  - Involvement of nail matrix may cause proximal-to-distal linear grooves and partial or complete destruction of nail bed with pterygium formation.

DIFFERENTIAL DIAGNOSIS
- Skin
  - Lichen simplex chronicus
  - Eczematous dermatitis
  - Psoriasis
  - Discoid lupus erythematosus
  - Other lichenoid eruptions (those that resemble LP)
  - Pityriasis rosea
  - Lichen nitidus
- Oral mucous membranes
  - Leukoplakia
  - Oral hairy leukoplakia
  - Candidiasis
  - Squamous cell carcinoma (particularly in ulcerative lesions)
  - Aphthous ulcers
  - Herpetic stomatitis
  - Secondary syphilis
- Genital mucous membranes
  - Psoriasis (penis and labia)
  - Nonspecific balanitis, Zoon balanitis
  - Fixed drug eruption (penis)
  - Candidiasis (penis and labia)
  - Pemphigus vulgaris, bullous pemphigoid, and Behçet disease (all rare)
- Hair and scalp
  - Scarring alopecia (central centrifugal cicatricial alopecia)

DIAGNOSTIC TESTS & INTERPRETATION
If suggested by history
- Serology for hepatitis
- Liver function tests

Diagnostic Procedures/Other
- Skin biopsy
- Direct immunofluorescence helps to distinguish LP from discoid lupus erythematosus.

Test Interpretation
- Dense, bandlike (lichenoid) lymphocytic infiltrate of the upper dermis
- Vacuolar degeneration of the basal layer
- Hyperkeratosis and irregular acanthosis, increased granular layer
- Basement membrane thinning with "saw-toothing"
- Degenerative keratinocytes, known as colloid or Civatte bodies, are found in the lower epidermis.
- Melanin pigment in macrophages

 TREATMENT

Although LP can resolve spontaneously, treatment is usually requested by patients who may be severely symptomatic or troubled by its cosmetic appearance.

GENERAL MEASURES
- Goal is to relieve itching and resolve lesions.
- Asymptomatic oral lesions require no treatment.

MEDICATION
First Line
- Skin
- Superpotent topical steroids (e.g., 0.05% clobetasol propionate) twice daily
  - Potent topical steroids such as triamcinolone acetonide 0.1% or fluocinonide 0.05% under occlusion
  - Intralesional corticosteroids (e.g., triamcinolone [Kenalog] 5 to 10 mg/mL) for recalcitrant and hypertrophic lesions
  - Antihistamines (e.g., hydroxyzine 25 mg PO q6h) have limited benefit for itching but may be helpful for sedation at bedtime.
  - "Soak and smear" technique: can lead to a rapid improvement of symptoms in even 1 to 2 days and may obviate the need for systemic steroids. Soaking allows water to hydrate the stratum corneum and allows the anti-inflammatory steroid in the ointment to penetrate more deeply into the skin. Smearing of the ointment traps the water in the skin because water cannot move out through greasy materials.
    - Soaking is done in a bathtub using lukewarm plain water for 20 minutes and then, without drying the skin, the affected area is immediately smeared with a thin film of the steroid ointment containing clobetasol or another superpotent topical steroid.
    - Soak and smear may be done for 4 to 5 days or longer, if necessary. The treatments are best done at night because the greasy ointment applied to the skin gets on pajamas (instead of on daytime clothes) and the ointment is on the skin during sleep. A topical steroid cream is applied thereafter during the daytime hours, if necessary.
- Mucous membranes
  - For oral, erosive, painful LP, a Cochrane review found at best weak evidence for the effectiveness of any intervention (3)[A].
    - Topical corticosteroids (0.1% triamcinolone [Kenalog] in Orabase) or 0.05% clobetasol propionate ointment BID
    - Intralesional corticosteroids

- Topical 0.1% tacrolimus (Protopic ointment) BID or 1% pimecrolimus (Elidel) cream BID. A Cochrane review found no evidence that calcineurin inhibitors are better than placebo (4)[A].
- Topical retinoids (e.g., 0.05% tretinoin [retinoic acid] in Orabase)

Pediatric Considerations
Children may absorb a proportionally larger amount of topical steroid because of larger skin surface-to-weight ratio.

Second Line
Skin and mucous membranes
- Intralesional corticosteroids
- Topical 0.1% tacrolimus (Protopic ointment) BID or topical 1% pimecrolimus (Elidel) cream BID
- Oral prednisone: used only for a short course (e.g., 30 to 60 mg/day for 2 to 4 weeks) or IM triamcinolone (Kenalog) 40 to 80 mg every 6 to 8 weeks
  - Precautions with systemic steroids
    - Systemic absorption of steroids may result in hypothalamic-pituitary-adrenal axis suppression, Cushing syndrome, hyperglycemia, or glucosuria.
    - Increased risk with high-potency topical steroids (i.e., use over large surface area, prolonged use, occlusive dressings)
    - In pregnancy: usually safe, but benefits must outweigh the risks
- Oral retinoids: Isotretinoin in doses of 10 mg PO daily for 2 months, acitretin 30 mg, or alitretinoin 30 mg PO daily have resulted in improvement in some refractory cases. Observe carefully for resultant dyslipidemia.
- Oral metronidazole 500 mg BID for 20 to 60 days can be given as a safer alternative to systemic corticosteroids.
- Cyclosporine may be used in severe cases, but cost and potential toxicity limit its use; topical use for severe oral involvement refractory to other treatments
- Thalidomide
- Psoralen ultraviolet-A (PUVA), broad- or narrow-band ultraviolet B (UVB) (5)[A]
- Low-level laser therapy and photodynamic therapy
- Griseofulvin (5)[A]
- Azathioprine
- Mycophenolate mofetil
- Metronidazole

ALERT
Avoid oral and topical retinoids during pregnancy.

ADMISSION, INPATIENT, AND NURSING CONSIDERATIONS
Outpatient care

 ONGOING CARE

FOLLOW-UP RECOMMENDATIONS
Patient Monitoring
Serial oral examinations for erosive/ulcerative lesions

PATIENT EDUCATION
- Oral, erosive, or ulcerative LP: annual follow-up to screen for malignancy (6)[A]
- Avoid spicy foods, cigarettes, and excessive alcohol.
- Avoid dry, crispy foods such as corn chips, pretzels, and toast.

PROGNOSIS
- Spontaneous resolution in weeks is possible, but disease may persist for years, especially oral lesions and hypertrophic lesions on the shins.
- There is a tendency toward relapse.
- Recurrence in 12–20%, especially in those with generalized involvement

COMPLICATIONS
- Alopecia
- Nail destruction
- Squamous cell carcinoma of the mouth or genitals

REFERENCES
1. Shengyuan L, Songpo Y, Wen W, et al. Hepatitis C virus and lichen planus: a reciprocal association determined by a meta-analysis. *Arch Dermatol*. 2009;145(9):1040–1047.
2. Arias-Santiago S, Buendía-Eisman A, Aneiros-Fernández J, et al. Cardiovascular risk factors in patients with lichen planus. *Am J Med*. 2011;124(6):543–548.
3. Cheng S, Kirtschig G, Cooper S, et al. Interventions for erosive lichen planus affecting mucosal sites. *Cochrane Database Syst Rev*. 2012;(2):CD008092.
4. Thongprasom K, Carrozzo M, Furness S, et al. Interventions for treating oral lichen planus. *Cochrane Database Syst Rev*. 2011;(7):CD001168.
5. Atzmony L, Reiter O, Hodak E, et al. Treatments for cutaneous lichen planus: a systematic review and meta-analysis. *Am J Clin Dermatol*. 2016;17(1): 11–22.
6. Fitzpatrick SG, Hirsch SA, Gordon SC. The malignant transformation of oral lichen planus and oral lichenoid lesions: a systematic review. *J Am Dent Assoc*. 2014;145(1):45–56.

ADDITIONAL READING
- Fazel N. Cutaneous lichen planus: a systematic review of treatments. *J Dermatolog Treat*. 2015;26(3):280–283.
- Kolios AG, Marques Maggio E, Gubler C, et al. Oral, esophageal and cutaneous lichen ruber planus controlled with alitretinoin: case report and review of the literature. *Dermatology*. 2013;226(4):302–310.

 CODES

ICD10
- L43.9 Lichen planus, unspecified
- L43.0 Hypertrophic lichen planus
- L43.1 Bullous lichen planus

CLINICAL PEARLS
- Remember the 7 P's of LP: **p**urple, **p**lanar, **p**olygonal, **p**olymorphic, **p**ruritic (not always), **p**apules that heal with **p**ostinflammatory hyperpigmentation.
- Serial oral or genital exams are indicated for erosive/ulcerative LP lesions to monitor for the development of squamous cell carcinoma.
- An association has been noted between LP and hepatitis C virus infection, chronic active hepatitis, and primary biliary cirrhosis.
- The "soak and smear" technique can lead to a rapid improvement of symptoms in 1 to 2 days and may obviate the need for systemic steroids.

L

LICHEN SIMPLEX CHRONICUS

Jeremy Golding, MD, FAAFP

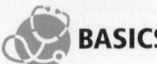 **BASICS**

DESCRIPTION
- Lichen simplex chronicus (LSC) is a chronic derma-titis resulting from chronic, repeated rubbing or scratching of the skin. Skin becomes thickened with accentuated lines ("lichenification").
- System(s) affected: skin
- Synonym(s): LSC; lichen simplex; localized neurodermatitis; neurodermatitis circumscripta

EPIDEMIOLOGY
Geriatric Considerations
Most common in middle aged and elderly

Pediatric Considerations
Rare in preadolescents

Incidence
- Common
- Peak incidence 35 to 50 years
- Predominant sex: females > males (2:1)

Prevalence
Common

ETIOLOGY AND PATHOPHYSIOLOGY
- Itch–scratch cycle leads to a chronic dermatosis. Repeated scratching or rubbing causes inflammation and pruritus, which leads to continued scratching.
- Primary LSC: scratching secondary to nonorganic pruritus, habit or a conditioned response to stress/anxiety
- Common triggers are excess dryness of skin, heat, sweat, and psychological stress.
- Secondary LSC: begins as a pruritic skin disease that evolves into neurodermatitis, which persists after resolution of the primary condition. Precursor dermatoses include atopic dermatitis, contact dermatitis, lichen planus, stasis dermatitis, psoriasis, tinea, and insect bites.
- There is a possible relation between disease development and underlying neuropathy, particularly radiculopathy or nerve root compression.
- Pruritus-specific C neurons are temperature sensitive, which may explain itching that occurs in warm environments.

RISK FACTORS
- Anxiety disorders
- Dry skin
- Insect bites
- Pruritic dermatosis

GENERAL PREVENTION
Avoid common triggers such as psychological distress, environmental factors such as heat and excessive dryness, skin irritation, and the development of pruritic dermatoses.

COMMONLY ASSOCIATED CONDITIONS
- Prurigo nodularis is a nodular variety of the same disease process.
- Atopic dermatitis
- Anxiety, depression, and obsessive-compulsive disorders

 DIAGNOSIS

HISTORY
- Gradual onset
- Begins as a localized area of pruritus
- Most patients acknowledge that they respond with vigorous rubbing, itching, or scratching, which brings temporary satisfaction.
- Pruritus is typically paroxysmal, worse at night, and may lead to scratching during sleep.
- Can be asymptomatic with patient scratching at night while asleep

PHYSICAL EXAM
- Well-circumscribed lichenified plaques with varying amounts of overlying excoriation or scaling
- Lichenification: accentuation of normal skin lines
- Hyperpigmentation or hypopigmentation can be seen.
- Scarring is uncommon with typical LSC; can be seen following ulcer formation or secondary infection
- Most commonly involves easily accessible areas
  - Lateral portions of lower legs/ankles
  - Nape of neck (lichen simplex nuchae)
  - Vulva/scrotum/anus
  - Extensor surfaces of forearms
  - Palmar wrist
  - Scalp

DIFFERENTIAL DIAGNOSIS
- Lichen sclerosis
- Psoriasis
- Atopic dermatitis
- Contact, irritant, or stasis dermatitis
- Extramammary Paget disease
- Lichen planus
- Mycosis fungoides
- Lichen amyloidosis
- Tinea
- Nummular eczema

DIAGNOSTIC TESTS & INTERPRETATION
Initial Tests (lab, imaging)
- No specific diagnostic test
- Microscopy (i.e., KOH prep) and culture preparation may be helpful in identifying possible bacterial or fungal infection.

Diagnostic Procedures/Other
- Skin biopsy if diagnosis is in question
- Patch testing may be used to rule out a contact dermatitis.

Test Interpretation
- Hyperkeratosis
- Acanthosis
- Lengthening of rete ridges
- Hyperplasia of all components of epidermis
- Mild to moderate lymphohistiocytic inflammatory infiltrate with prominent lichenification

 TREATMENT

GENERAL MEASURES
- Patient education is critical.
- Low likelihood of resolution if patient unable to avoid scratching
- Treatment aimed at reducing inflammation and pruritus

MEDICATION
First Line
- Reducing inflammation
  - Topical steroids are first-line agents (1)[C].
  - High-potency steroids alone, such as 0.05% beta-methasone dipropionate cream or 0.05% clobetasol propionate cream, can be used initially but should be avoided on the face, anogenital region, or intertriginous areas. They should be used on small areas only, for no longer than 2 weeks except under the close supervision of a physician.
  - Switch to intermediate- or low-potency steroids as response allows.
  - An intermediate-potency steroid, such as 0.1% triamcinolone cream, may be used for initial, brief treatment of the face and intertriginous areas, and for maintenance treatment of other areas.
  - A low-potency steroid, such as 1% hydrocortisone cream, should be used for maintenance treatment of the face and intertriginous areas.
  - Steroid tape, flurandrenolide, has optimized penetration and provides a barrier to continued scratching. Change tape once daily.
  - Intralesional steroids, such as triamcinolone acetate, are also safe and effective for severe cases.
- Preventing scratching
  - Topical antipruritic agents
  - 1st-generation oral antihistamines such as diphenhydramine and hydroxyzine for antipruritic and sedative effects
  - Sedating tricyclics, such as doxepin and amitriptyline, for nighttime itching
  - Itching may occur at night while the patient is asleep; occlusive dressings may be helpful in these cases.

> **ALERT**
> High-dose and prolonged treatment with topical steroids can cause dermal/epidermal atrophy as well as pigmentary changes and should not be used on the face, intertriginous areas, or anogenital region. Duration of treatment on other parts of the body should not exceed 3 weeks without close physician supervision.

Second Line
All recommendations
- Topical aspirin has been shown to be helpful in treating neurodermatitis (2)[C].
- Topical 5% doxepin cream has significant antipruritic activity (2)[C].
- Topical capsaicin cream can be helpful for treatment of early disease manifestations (2)[C].

- 0.1% tacrolimus applied twice daily over 6 weeks as an effective alternative treatment (3)[C]
- Gabapentin was found to decrease symptoms in patients who are nonresponsive to steroids.
- Topical lidocaine can be effective in decreasing neuropathic pruritus (2)[C].
- Intradermal botulinum toxin injections have been reported to improve symptoms in patients with recalcitrant pruritus.
- Transcutaneous electrical nerve stimulation may relieve pruritus in patients for whom topical steroids were not effective (4)[C].
- A case report showed NB-UVB as a possible off-label treatment of refractory LSC (5)[C].
- SSRIs may be effective in controlling compulsive scratching secondary to psychiatric diagnosis.

ISSUES FOR REFERRAL
- No response to treatment
- Presence of signs and symptoms suggestive of a systemic cause of pruritus
- Consultation with a psychiatrist for patients with severe stress, anxiety, or compulsive scratching
- Consultation with an allergist for patients with multisystem atopic symptoms

ADDITIONAL THERAPIES
- Cooling of the skin with ice or cold compresses
- Soaks and lubricants to improve barrier layer function
- Occlusion of lesion with bandages or Unna boots
- Nail trimming
- Silk underwear to decrease friction in genital LSC

COMPLEMENTARY & ALTERNATIVE MEDICINE
- Acupuncture has been shown as an effective treatment for pruritus (6)[C].
- Cognitive-behavioral therapy may improve awareness and help to identify coping strategies.
- Hypnosis may be beneficial in decreasing pruritus and preventing scratching.
- Homeopathic remedies (i.e., thuja and graphite) have been used.

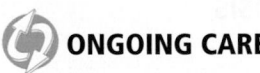 ## ONGOING CARE

FOLLOW-UP RECOMMENDATIONS
Patient Monitoring
Patients should be followed for response to therapy, complications from therapy (especially topical steroids), and secondary infections.

DIET
Regular balanced diet

PATIENT EDUCATION
- Patients should understand the cause of this disease and the critical role they play in its resolution:
  – Emphasize that scratching and rubbing must stop for lesions to heal; medications ineffective if scratching continues
- Stress reduction techniques can be useful for patients for whom stress plays a role.
- Avoid exposure to known triggers.

PROGNOSIS
- Often chronic and recurrent
- Good prognosis if the itch–scratch cycle can be broken
- After healing, the skin should return to normal appearance but may also retain accentuated skin markings or post inflammatory pigmentary changes that may be slow to resolve.

COMPLICATIONS
- Secondary infection
- Scarring is rare without ulceration or secondary infection.
- Complications related to therapy, as mentioned in medication precautions
- Squamous cell carcinoma within affected regions is rare.

REFERENCES
1. Lynch PJ. Lichen simplex chronicus (atopic/neurodermatitis) of the anogenital region. *Dermatol Ther*. 2004;17(1):8–19.
2. Patel T, Yosipovitch G. Therapy of pruritus. *Expert Opin Pharmacother*. 2010;11(10):1673–1682.
3. Tan ES, Tan AS, Tey HL. Effective treatment of scrotal lichen simplex chronicus with 0.1% tacrolimus ointment: an observational study. *J Eur Acad Dermatol Venereol*. 2015;29(7):1448–1449.
4. Mohammad Ali BM, Hegab DS, El Saadany HM. Use of transcutaneous electrical nerve stimulation for chronic pruritus. *Dermatol Ther*. 2015;28(4):210–215.
5. Virgili A, Minghetti S, Borghi A, et al. Phototherapy for vulvar lichen simplex chronicus: an "off-label use" of a comb light device. *Photodermatol Photoimmunol Photomed*. 2014;30(6):332–334.
6. Ma C, Sivamani RK. Acupuncture as a treatment modality in dermatology: a systematic review. *J Altern Complement Med*. 2015;21(9):520–529.

ADDITIONAL READING
- Aschoff R, Wozel G. Topical tacrolimus for the treatment of lichen simplex chronicus. *J Dermatolog Treat*. 2007;18(2):115–117.
- Engin B, Tufekci O, Yazici A, et al. The effect of transcutaneous electrical nerve stimulation in the treatment of lichen simplex: a prospective study. *Clin Exp Dermatol*. 2009;34(3):324–328.
- Gencoglan G, Inanir I, Gunduz K. Therapeutic hotline: treatment of prurigo nodularis and lichen simplex chronicus with gabapentin. *Dermatol Ther*. 2010;23(2):194–198.
- Goldstein AT, Parneix-Spake A, McCormick CL, et al. Pimecrolimus cream 1% for treatment of vulvar lichen simplex chronicus: an open-label, preliminary trial. *Gynecol Obstet Invest*. 2007;64(4):180–186.
- Heckmann M, Heyer G, Brunner B, et al. Botulinum toxin type A injection in the treatment of lichen simplex: an open pilot study. *J Am Acad Dermatol*. 2002;46(4):617–619.
- Hercogová J. Topical anti-itch therapy. *Dermatol Ther*. 2005;18(4):341–343.
- Kirtak N, Inaloz HS, Akçali C, et al. Association of serotonin transporter gene-linked polymorphic region and variable number of tandem repeat polymorphism of the serotonin transporter gene in lichen simplex chronicus patients with psychiatric status. *Int J Dermatol*. 2008;47(10):1069–1072.
- Konuk N, Koca R, Atik L, et al. Psychopathology, depression and dissociative experiences in patients with lichen simplex chronicus. *Gen Hosp Psychiatry*. 2007;29(3):232–235.
- Lotti T, Buggiani G, Prignano F. Prurigo nodularis and lichen simplex chronicus. *Dermatol Ther*. 2008;21(1):42–46.
- Shenefelt PD. Biofeedback, cognitive-behavioral methods, and hypnosis in dermatology: is it all in your mind? *Dermatol Ther*. 2003;16(2):114–122.
- Solak O, Kulac M, Yaman M, et al. Lichen simplex chronicus as a symptom of neuropathy. *Clin Exp Dermatol*. 2009;34(4):476–480.
- Wu M, Wang Y, Bu W, et al. Squamous cell carcinoma arising in lichen simplex chronicus. *Eur J Dermatol*. 2010;20(6):858–859.
- Yosipovitch G, Sugeng MW, Chan YH, et al. The effect of topically applied aspirin on localized circumscribed neurodermatitis. *J Am Acad Dermatol*. 2001;45(6):910–913.
- Yüksek J, Sezer E, Aksu M, et al. Transcutaneous electrical nerve stimulation for reduction of pruritus in macular amyloidosis and lichen simplex. *J Dermatol*. 2011;38(6):546–552.

 ## CODES

ICD10
L28.0 Lichen simplex chronicus

CLINICAL PEARLS
- LSC is a chronic inflammatory condition that results from repeated scratching and rubbing.
- Primary LSC originates de novo, whereas secondary LSC occurs in the setting of a preexisting pruritic dermatologic condition.
- LSC is a clinical diagnosis based on history and skin examination with biopsy only indicated in difficult or unclear cases.
- Stopping the itch–scratch cycle through patient education, skin lubrication, and topical medications is key.
- Treatment aimed at decreasing both inflammation and pruritus utilizing topical steroids and antipruritics

L

LONG QT INTERVAL

Henry DeYoung, MD • Yousef Ahmed, MD • Derek Lodico, DO

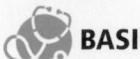

BASICS

DESCRIPTION

- QT interval: the measurement interval from the beginning of the QRS complex to the end of the T wave on the surface electrocardiogram (ECG). This represents the period from the onset of depolarization to completion of repolarization of the ventricular myocardium.
- Corrected QT interval (QTc): The QT interval has an inverse relationship with heart rate. The QTc is the QT interval corrected for heart rate. See formulas.
- Prolonged QTc is generally defined as >450 ms for adult males and >470 ms for adult females (1):
  – 430 to 450 ms considered borderline in men
  – 450 to 470 ms considered borderline in women (1,2,3)
  – 440 to 460 ms considered borderline in children aged 1 to 15 years old (4)
- Most cases of prolonged QT are acquired, but several genetic mutations cause inherited long QT syndrome (LQTS) (3).
- Prolonged QTc from any cause can precipitate polymorphic ventricular tachycardia (VT) called torsade de pointes (TdP), leading to dizziness, syncope, and sudden cardiac death from ventricular fibrillation (VF).

EPIDEMIOLOGY

Incidence

Incidence of medication-induced QTc prolongation and TdP varies with medication and a host of other factors. Exact incidences are difficult to estimate but may be 1:2,000 to 1:2,500 (2).

Prevalence

- Hereditary LQTS is estimated to occur in 1/2,500 to 1/7,000 births.
- Five thousand people across the United States may die yearly due to LQTS-related cardiac arrhythmia.

ETIOLOGY AND PATHOPHYSIOLOGY

- Acquired
  – Demographics: increasing age, female sex
  – Electrolyte abnormalities: hypokalemia, hypocalcemia, and hypomagnesemia
  – Noncardiac disease: hypothyroidism renal impairment, and hepatic impairment
  – Cardiac disease: heart failure, LVH, and myocardial ischemia (2)
  – Scenarios: rapid increase in the QT interval >60 ms, conversion from atrial fibrillation/bradycardia (5)
  – Medications (3)
    ○ Antiarrhythmic medications (quinidine, procainamide, dronedarone, dofetilide, sotalol, disopyramide, and amiodarone)
    ○ Antipsychotic medications: especially if given IV (haloperidol*, chlorpromazine*, thioridazine*, pimozide*)
    ○ Antidepressants: most commonly used drugs responsible (SSRIs, SNRIs, trazodone, TCAs)
    ○ Antibiotics/antivirals/antifungals/antiprotozoals/antimalarials: macrolides (clarithromycin*, erythromycin* also CYP3A4 inhibitors), fluoroquinolones, quinine, and chloroquine
    ○ Antiemetics: metoclopramide, ondansetron, promethazine
    ○ Opioids: methadone*, buprenorphine

○ Antihistamines: cetirizine, hydroxyzine, diphenhydramine
○ Decongestants: pseudoephedrine, phenylephrine
○ Stimulants: albuterol, phentermine
○ Misc: chloroquine*, pentamidine*, various antimuscarinics, and anticonvulsants
○ *Denote "high-risk" medication for TdP (2,5)
- Congenital
  – Loss of function mutations in several potassium ion membrane channels or gain of function mutations in the sodium or calcium ion membrane channels in cardiac myocytes (6)
- Pathophysiology
  – Depolarization (phase 0) of the myocardium results from the rapid influx of sodium through sodium channels (I_{Na}) causing myocyte contraction during systole; seen on ECG as the QRS complex
  – Repolarization occurs through the efflux of potassium from the cell (phases 2 and 3) by rapid (I_{Kr}) and slow (I_{Ks}) components of the delayed rectifier; represented by the T wave on an ECG
  – Drug-induced QT prolongation most often due to blockade of the I_{Kr} channel leading to delay in phase 3 rapid repolarization (2)
  – In both cases, deviation from normal ion channel function leads to transmural dispersion of repolarization currents across the myocardium triggering early after depolarizations which may devolve into TdP (3,6).
  – Prolonged QT interval alone does not denote imminent risk for TdP; TdP is often self-limited, but TdP can cause syncope or degrade to VF (2).

Genetics

- 13+ distinct genotypes are linked to LQTS (1,6).
- Penetrance is highly variable making both diagnosis and management challenging (3).
- LQT1 (40–55%) is the most common cause of LQTS. Loss of function in the KCNQ1 gene coding for the I_{Ks} transport protein; arrhythmias triggered by sympathetic activation (stress/exercise—especially swimming), leading to shorter ventricular repolarization
- LQT2 (30–45%) results from a mutation in the KCNH2 gene causing a defect in the I_{Kr} transport protein; at risk for cardiac events due to abrupt catecholamine surges like auditory stimuli/emotional arousal (postpartum)
- LQT3 (5–10%) is caused by a mutation in the SCN5A gene leading to a gain of function in the alpha subunit of the I_{Na} transport protein. Excessive sodium accumulates in the cell, increasing repolarization time; prominent during sleep due to amplified inward flow of sodium at low heart rates (1,3,6)
- LQT4 to LQT13—<1% of the total frequency
- Jervell and Lange-Nielsen syndrome (JLNS): autosomal recessive inheritance through homozygous or compound heterozygous mutations of the KCNQ1 or KCNE1 genes. Reduced function in the I_{Ks} transport protein; associated with sensorineural hearing loss
- Romano-Ward syndrome (RWS): most common. Results from any of the 13 identified gene mutations; autosomal dominant with variable penetrance and normal hearing
- Others: Andersen-Tawil syndrome (LQT7), Timothy syndrome (LQT8). Both are very rare (3,6).

RISK FACTORS

For the feared complication, TdP, risk factors include the following (2,5):
- Female (~2 times increased risk)
- QTc >500 ms (2 to 3 times increased risk)
- QTc >60 ms over previous baseline
- For every 10 ms increase in the QTc, there is a 5–7% increased risk for developing TdP.
- History of syncope or presyncope
- History of TdP
- Bradycardia
- Liver or kidney disease (by increasing blood levels of QT-prolonging medications)
- Medications that cause QTc prolongation
  – High doses
  – Fast infusions
  – Combination of medications
- Medications that inhibit CYP3A4
- Electrolyte abnormalities
  – Hypokalemia
  – Hypomagnesemia
  – Hypocalcemia
- For hereditary LQTS
  – Catecholamine surges from exercise, emotional stress, loud noises, postpartum

GENERAL PREVENTION

- Avoid (or use with caution) causative medications, including combinations with potentially additive effects (1,2,5)[C].
- Replete electrolytes (goal Mg >2, K 4.5 to 5.0) (2)[C].
- Treat underlying diseases.
- Avoid strenuous sports in LQTS.
- Avoid sudden loud noises in LQTS (alarm clocks, doorbells, telephones).
- 36th Bethesda Conference recommends restriction of athletes from participation to class 1A activities (e.g., bowling, golf, riflery), although evidence of safe participation is emerging (3)[C].

DIAGNOSIS

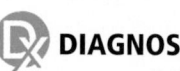

HISTORY

- Incidental finding on ECG in asymptomatic patients
- Evaluate for syncope, presyncopal episodes, palpitations, and associated precipitating events (emotional triggers, swimming, diving).
- Family history of syncope or sudden cardiac death
- History of seizures in patient or family members (tonic–clonic movement may due to cerebral hypoperfusion during episodes of ventricular arrhythmia or syncope)
- Detailed medication history
- Congenital deafness

PHYSICAL EXAM

- The physical exam is typically unremarkable.
- Signs of underlying cardiac disease
- Signs of hypothyroidism, liver, or renal impairment
- Congenital deafness present in many forms of LQTS

DIAGNOSTIC TESTS & INTERPRETATION

Initial Tests (lab, imaging)

- ECG
- Metabolic panel: especially calcium, magnesium, and potassium
- TSH

Follow-Up Tests & Special Considerations

- Echocardiogram to evaluate for cardiomyopathy
- Outpatient cardiac rhythm monitoring
- Consider provocative testing (epinephrine infusion, exercise stress testing) to evaluate for QTc interval changes and/or for coronary artery disease (2)[C].
- Genetic testing for LQTS mutations

Test Interpretation

- The QT interval is best measured from the onset of the QRS to the completion of the T wave; most commonly measured in lead II or V_2
- QTc calculation can be performed in several ways using RR interval immediately preceding the QT interval for calculation. The Bazett formula is most commonly used method (1,2).
  - Framingham formula: $QT + 0.154 (1 - RR)$
  - Bazett formula: $QTc = QT / \sqrt{RR}$ (all measurements in seconds, and RR obtained by direct measurement or 60/heart rate)
  - Fridericia formula is similar to Bazett but uses the cube root RR interval. $QTc = QT / (RR)^{1/3}$

TREATMENT

GENERAL MEASURES

- Treat VT, TdP, and VF emergently per ACLS guidelines.
- Withdraw offending agents and correct electrolytes. (2)[C].
- Transvenous cardiac pacing or isoproterenol may be used for drug-induced TdP to prevent bradycardia. Maintain heart rate 90 to 110 beats/min.

MEDICATION

First Line

- For TdP: magnesium sulfate 2 g infused over 2 to 5 minutes, followed by continuous infusion of 2 to 4 mg/min if needed. Flushing is a normal side effect of bolus injections. Monitor for magnesium toxicity in those with renal insufficiency (1,2)[C].
- For hereditary LQTS, to prevent life-threatening arrhythmias: propranolol or nadolol generally regarded as the best β-blockers for management of LQTS, although rigorous studies are lacking (7)[B].
- β-Blockers are effective in decreasing but not eliminating the risk of fatal arrhythmias.
- For high-risk patients who remain symptomatic on a β-blocker, implantable cardiac defibrillators (ICDs) with or without pacemaker may be indicated (2,6)[B].

Second Line

Atenolol or metoprolol may be used, although switching β-blockers may precipitate lethal or near-lethal events (7)[B].

ISSUES FOR REFERRAL

- Refer to cardiologist to establish diagnosis, especially for hereditary LQTS.
- Symptomatic prolonged QT

SURGERY/OTHER PROCEDURES

- ICD for those with a history of major cardiac events
- Left cervical-thoracic sympathetic denervation was used for symptomatic LQTS prior to the advent of β-blockers. It is still an option for those patients with LQTS who are refractory to β-blocker therapy (3)[B].

ADMISSION, INPATIENT, AND NURSING CONSIDERATIONS

- Treat TdP, VT, and VF promptly as per ACLS guidelines. Correct electrolytes on an emergent basis. Evaluate for acquired QT prolongation. If no cause is found, consider hereditary LQTS.

- Patients with prolonged QTc and syncope/near syncope should be monitored on telemetry.
- Obtain a baseline ECG if initiating or combining medications with QT-prolonging medications, then when the drug reaches steady state, at 30 days, and annually thereafter.
- Avoid QT-prolonging medications in patients with congenital LQTS.
- Patients at risk of LQTS should be educated on symptoms arrhythmia.
- Monitor electrolytes, urgently treat hypomagnesemia and hypokalemia, and discontinue/change offending medications (1,2)[C].
- Avoid sudden loud noises or emotional stress for those who have LQTS.
- Review adherence to β-blocker therapy.
- Clinical decision support systems may be useful to assess the risk of drug-induced risk of QT prolongation while considering clinical scenario (5).
- Notify others if telemetry monitoring reveals prolonged QT interval.

ONGOING CARE

FOLLOW-UP RECOMMENDATIONS

On routine visits, ask about syncope, presyncope, and palpitations in those who have QTc prolongation.

- Consider ECG and/or outpatient cardiac rhythm monitoring with medication additions or dosage changes.
- Prompt evaluation is warranted for symptomatic QTc prolongation of any cause.
- Check and correct for electrolyte imbalances.

PATIENT EDUCATION

- Educate patients with QTc prolongation about medication side effects and medication interactions.
- Patients with congenital forms of LQTS should be aware of and avoid triggers (depending on their specific gene mutation).
- Consider the emotional and psychological impacts. Additional reading by Fortescue shares personal impact of LQTS.
- Information and support from groups listed may be helpful (see "Additional Reading").

PROGNOSIS

Acquired LQTS will resolve after withdrawal of offending agents and normalization of metabolic abnormalities. Patients with underlying cardiovascular disease may be at increased risk of mortality and require further intervention. Prognosis for congenital LQTS if untreated is quite poor. Perhaps 20% of untreated patients presenting with syncope die within 1 year, 50% within 10 years (4,6).

REFERENCES

1. Kramer DB, Zimetbaum PJ. Long-QT syndrome. *Cardiol Rev*. 2011;19(5):217–225.
2. Kallergis EM, Goudis CA, Simantirakis EN, et al. Mechanisms, risk factors, and management of acquired long QT syndrome: a comprehensive review. *ScientificWorldJournal*. 2012;2012:212178.
3. Abrams DJ, Macrae CA. Long QT syndrome. *Circulation*. 2014;129(14):1524–1529.
4. Clarke CJ, McDaniel GM. The risk of long QT syndrome in the pediatric population. *Curr Opin Pediatr*. 2009;21(5):573–578.
5. Schwartz PJ, Woosley RL. Predicting the unpredictable: drug-induced QT prolongation and torsades de pointes. *J Am Coll Cardiol*. 2016;67(13):1639–1650.

---

6. Schwartz PJ, Crotti L, Insolia R. Long-QT syndrome: from genetics to management. *Circ Arrhythm Electrophysiol*. 2012;5(4):868–877.
7. Wilde AA, Ackerman MJ. Beta-blockers in the treatment of congenital long QT syndrome: is one beta-blocker superior to another? *J Am Coll Cardiol*. 2014;64(13):1359–1361.

ADDITIONAL READING

- Cardiac Arrhythmias Research and Education Foundation: http://www.longqt.org
- CredibleMeds: http://www.crediblemeds.org
- Drug and Therapeutics Bulletin. QT interval and drug therapy. *BMJ*. 2016;353:i2732.
- Fortescue EB. A piece of my mind. Keeping the pace. *JAMA*. 2014;311(23):2383–2384.
- Morita H, Wu J, Zipes DP. The QT syndromes: long and short. *Lancet*. 2008;372(9640):750–763.
- Priori SG, Blomström-Lundqvist C, Mazzanti A, et al. 2015 ESC guidelines for the management of patients with ventricular arrhythmias and the prevention of sudden cardiac death. *Rev Esp Cardiol (Engl Ed)*. 2016;69(2):176.
- Sudden Arrhythmia Death Syndromes Foundation: http://www.sads.org
- van Noord C, Eijgelsheim M, Stricker BH. Drug- and non-drug-associated QT interval prolongation. *Br J Clin Pharmacol*. 2010;70(1):16–23.
- Yap YG, Camm AJ. Drug induced QT prolongation and torsades de pointes. *Heart*. 2003;89(11):1363–1372.
- Zipes DP, Camm AJ, Borggrefe M, et al. ACC/AHA/ESC 2006 guidelines for management of patients with ventricular arrhythmias and the prevention of sudden cardiac death: a report of the American College of Cardiology/American Heart Association Task Force and the European Society of Cardiology Committee for Practice Guidelines (writing committee to develop guidelines for management of patients with ventricular arrhythmias and the prevention of sudden cardiac death): developed in collaboration with the European Heart Rhythm Association and the Heart Rhythm Society. *Circulation*. 2006;114(10):e385–e484.

SEE ALSO

Algorithms: Cardiac Arrhythmias; Torsade de Pointes (TdP): Variant Form of Polymorphic Ventricular Tachycardia (VT)

CODES

ICD10
I45.81 Long QT syndrome

CLINICAL PEARLS

- Evaluate for acquired causes before making a diagnosis of hereditary LQTS.
- For accurate diagnosis, calculate QTc manually.
- The ideal management of TdP is prevention; avoid multiple "stacking" risk factors and seek alternates to high-risk medications, correct electrolytes, and monitor treatment with serial ECGs if no alternatives exist.
- Magnesium sulfate is the treatment of choice during ACLS for TdP.
- β-Blockers are initial treatment of choice for hereditary LQTS.

LUNG, PRIMARY MALIGNANCIES

Zeeshan Mirza, MD • Mohammad Razaq, MD

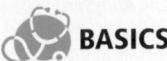

BASICS

DESCRIPTION

- Primary lung cancers are the leading cause of cancer-related deaths in the United States (estimated 154,050 deaths in 2018, 25.3% of all cancer-related deaths).
- Divided into two broad categories
  - Non–small cell lung cancer (NSCLC) (>85% of all lung cancers); normally originate in periphery
    ○ Adenocarcinoma (~40% of NSCLC): most common type in the United States and also nonsmokers; metastasizes earlier than squamous cell; lepidic growth, a subtype of adenocarcinoma has better prognosis.
    ○ Squamous cell carcinoma (SCC) (also known as epidermoid carcinoma) (~25% of NSCLC): dose-related effect with smoking; slower growing than adenocarcinoma
    ○ Large cell (~10% of NSCLC): prognosis similar to adenocarcinoma
  - Small cell lung cancer (SCLC) (16% of all lung cancers): centrally located, early metastases, aggressive
- Others: mesothelioma and carcinoid tumor
- Staging
  - Both NSCLC and SCLC: staged from I to IV based on: primary tumor (T), lymph node status (N), and presence of metastasis (M)
  - SCLC further staged by:
    ○ Limited disease: confined to ipsilateral hemithorax
    ○ Extensive disease: beyond ipsilateral hemithorax (stages IIIB and IV), which may include malignant pleural or pericardial effusion or hematogenous metastases (stage IV)
    ○ Tumor locations: upper: 60%; lower: 30%; middle: 5%; overlapping and main stem: 5%
    ○ May spread by local extension to chest wall, diaphragm, pulmonary vessels, vena cava, phrenic nerve, esophagus, or pericardium
    ○ Most commonly metastasize to lymph nodes (pulmonary, mediastinal), then liver, adrenal glands, bones, brain

EPIDEMIOLOGY

Incidence

- Estimated 234,030 new cases in the United States in 2018
- Usual age of diagnosis: between 65 and 74 years; peak at 70 years
- Predominant sex: male > female

Prevalence

- Most common cancer worldwide
- Lifetime probability: men: 1 in 15; women: 1 in 17

ETIOLOGY AND PATHOPHYSIOLOGY

Multifactorial; see "Risk Factors."

Genetics

NSCLC
- Oncogenes: Ras family (H-ras, K-ras, N-ras)
- Tumor suppressor genes: retinoblastoma, *p53*

RISK FACTORS

- Smoking
- Secondhand smoke exposure
- Radon
- Environmental and occupational exposures
  - Asbestos exposure (synergistic increase in risk for smokers)
  - Air pollution

- Ionizing radiation
- Mutagenic gases (halogen ethers, mustard gas, aromatic hydrocarbons)
- Metals (inorganic arsenic, chromium, nickel)
- Lung scarring from tuberculosis
- Radiation therapy to the breast or chest

GENERAL PREVENTION

- Smoking cessation and prevention programs
- Screening recommended by NCCN and shown to reduce mortality in National Lung Screening Trial (NLST) (1)[A]
- Annual screening recommended with low-dose computed tomography (CT) in adults aged 55 to 74 years who have a 30 pack-year smoking history and currently smoke or have quit within the past 15 years
- Screening should be discontinued once a person has not smoked for 15 years or develops a health problem that substantially limits life expectancy or the ability or willingness to have curative lung surgery.
- Prevention via aggressive smoking cessation counseling and therapy; a 20–30% risk reduction occurs within 5 years of cessation.
- Avoid hormone replacement therapy in postmenopausal smokers or former smokers (increased risk of death from NSCLC).

COMMONLY ASSOCIATED CONDITIONS

- Paraneoplastic syndromes: hypertrophic pulmonary osteoarthropathy, Lambert-Eaton syndrome, Cushing syndrome, hypercalcemia from ectopic parathyroid-releasing hormone, syndrome of inappropriate antidiuretic hormone (SIADH)
- Hypercoagulable state
- Pancoast syndrome
- Superior vena cava syndrome
- Pleural effusion
- Chronic obstructive pulmonary disease (COPD), other sequelae of cigarette smoking

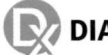

DIAGNOSIS

HISTORY

- May be asymptomatic for most of course
- Respiratory
  - Cough (new or change in chronic cough)
  - Wheezing and stridor
  - Dyspnea
  - Hemoptysis
  - Pneumonitis (fever and productive cough)
- Constitutional
  - Malaise
  - Bone pain (metastatic disease)
  - Fatigue
  - Weight loss, anorexia
  - Fever
  - Anemia
- Other presentations
  - Chest pain (dull, pleuritic)
  - Shoulder/arm pain (Pancoast tumors)
  - Dysphagia
  - Plethora (redness of face or neck)
  - Hoarseness (involvement of recurrent laryngeal nerve)
  - Horner syndrome
  - Neurologic abnormalities (e.g., headaches, syncope, weakness, cognitive impairment)
  - Pericardial tamponade (pericardial invasion)

PHYSICAL EXAM

- General: fever, chills, night sweats, weight loss
- Head, eye, ear, nose, throat (HEENT): Horner syndrome, dysphonia, stridor, scleral icterus, dysphagia
- Neck: supraclavicular/cervical lymph nodes, mass
- Lungs: effusion, wheezing, airway obstruction, dyspnea
- Abdomen/groin: hepatomegaly or lymphadenopathy
- Extremities: signs of hypertrophic pulmonary osteoarthropathy, deep venous thrombosis (DVT), fingernail clubbing
- Neurologic: headache, syncope, weakness, cognitive impairment

DIFFERENTIAL DIAGNOSIS

- COPD (may coexist)
- Granulomatous (tuberculosis, sarcoidosis)
- Cardiomyopathy
- Congestive heart failure (CHF)

DIAGNOSTIC TESTS & INTERPRETATION

Initial Tests (lab, imaging)

- Serum
  - CBC
  - Comprehensive metabolic panel (CMP)
  - Hypercalcemia (paraneoplastic syndrome)
  - Hyponatremia (SIADH)
  - Lactate dehydrogenase (LDH)
- Sputum cytology
- Chest x-ray (CXR) (compare with prior XRs)
  - Nodule or mass, especially if calcified
  - Persistent infiltrate
  - Atelectasis
  - Mediastinal widening
  - Hilar enlargement
  - Pleural effusion
- CT scan of chest (with IV contrast)
  - Nodule or mass (central or peripheral)
  - Lymphadenopathy
- Evaluation for metastatic disease
  - Positron emission tomography (PET) scan to evaluate metastasis mediastinal lymphadenopathy (replacing CT abdomen/pelvis and bone scan)
  - Brain MRI: Lesions may be necrotic, bleeding.

Follow-Up Tests & Special Considerations

CBC, BUN, serum creatinine, LFTs prior to each cycle of chemotherapy

Diagnostic Procedures/Other

- Biopsy with pathology review using
  - Bronchoscopy with transbronchial biopsy (WANG needle)
  - CT-guided biopsy of lung mass or metastatic site
  - Endobronchial ultrasound (EBUS)-guided fine-needle aspiration
  - Enlarged mediastinal lymph nodes necessitate staging by mediastinoscopy, video-assisted thoracoscopy, EBUS-guided fine-needle aspiration.
- Video-assisted thoracoscopy (associated pleural disease and suspected mediastinal nodal spread)
- Pulmonary function tests
- In patients with advanced NSCLC, determination of epidermal growth factor receptor (EGFR)-activating mutations, BRAF mutation, *KRAS/NRAS* mutations, *ALK* gene rearrangements, and ROS1 fusions in patients with non-SCC (NSCC) or mixed squamous histology
- PD-L1 testing
- Bone marrow aspirate (small cell)

Test Interpretation

Pathologic changes from smoking are progressive: basal cell proliferation, development of atypical nuclei, stratification, metaplasia of squamous cells, carcinoma in situ, and then invasive disease.

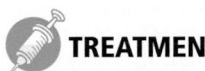

TREATMENT

GENERAL MEASURES

- NSCLC
  - Stage I, stage II, and selected stage III tumors are surgically resectable. Neoadjuvant or adjuvant therapy is recommended for many patients with high risk IB, II, and IIIA NSCLC. Patients with resectable disease who are not surgical candidates may receive radiation therapy.
  - Patients with unresectable or N2, N3 disease are treated with concurrent chemoradiation. Selected patients with T3 or N2 disease can be treated effectively with surgical resection and either pre- or postoperative chemotherapy or chemoradiation therapy.
  - Patients with distant metastases (M1B) can be treated with chemotherapy, targeted therapy, immunotherapy, or radiation therapy for palliation or best supportive care alone.
- SCLC
  - Limited stage: concurrent chemoradiation
  - Extensive stage: combination chemotherapy
  - Consider prophylactic cranial irradiation (PCI) in patients achieving a complete or partial response (2)[A].
- Quality-of-life assessments: Karnofsky Performance Status (KPS) scale (http://www.hospicepatients.org/karnofsky.html); Eastern Cooperative Oncology Group (ECOG)
- Discussions with patient and family about end-of-life care

MEDICATION

- Chemotherapies, targeted therapies, and immunotherapies are the mainstay of treatment.
- Adjuvant chemotherapy following surgery improves survival in patients with fully resected stages II and III NSCLC.
- Palliative measures: analgesics
- Dyspnea: oxygen, morphine

First Line

- NSCLC
  - Stages II and III: neoadjuvant or adjuvant chemotherapy
    - Cisplatin-based doublets (combination with paclitaxel, etoposide, vinorelbine, docetaxel, gemcitabine)
    - Carboplatin alternative for patients unlikely to tolerate cisplatin
    - Cisplatin plus pemetrexed (NSCC)
  - Unresectable stages IIA, IIIB
    - Concurrent chemoradiation
      - Cisplatin plus etoposide, vinblastine, or pemetrexed (NSCC) plus concurrent radiation
      - Carboplatin plus paclitaxel plus concurrent radiation
      - Carboplatin plus pemetrexed (NSCC) plus concurrent radiation
- Stage IV
  - No chemotherapy regimen can be recommended for routine use.
  - Cisplatin- or carboplatin-based doublets
  - +/− Bevacizumab (NSCC)
  - Erlotinib, afatinib, gefitinib, or osimertinib for patients with EGFR mutations

- Dabrafenib with trametinib for untreated patients with BRAF V600E mutations
- Pembrolizumab with pemetrexed and carboplatin for NSCC regardless of PD-L1 expression
- Pembrolizumab monotherapy for NSCLC with PD-L1 expression ≥50% of tumor cells
- Alectinib, dacomitinib for untreated ALK-positive NSCLC
- Crizotinib for patients with EML4-ALK translocations or ROS1-positive NSCLC
  - Ceritinib, brigatinib for patients who fail or are intolerant to crizotinib
- Maintenance therapy after 4 to 6 cycles in patients achieving a response or stable disease
  - Continuation of bevacizumab, pemetrexed (NSCC), gemcitabine or pembrolizumab or switch to pemetrexed (NSCC), erlotinib (EGFR mutations), docetaxel or observation
- SCLC
  - Cisplatin or carboplatin plus etoposide

Second Line

- NSCLC
  - Cisplatin-based doublets +/− bevacizumab (NSCC) if not previously used
  - Docetaxel, pemetrexed (NSCC), erlotinib, gemcitabine, ramucirumab plus docetaxel, or nivolumab (squamous cell)
  - Atezolizumab if progressed during or after first-line platinum-based drug
  - Brigatinib or alectinib, ceritinib for ALK-positive patients who failed crizotinib
- SCLC
  - Topotecan or CAV (cyclophosphamide, doxorubicin, vincristine), gemcitabine, docetaxel, paclitaxel, nivolumab

ADDITIONAL THERAPIES

- Smoking cessation counseling
- Consider IV bisphosphonates or denosumab in patients with bone metastases to reduce skeletal-related events.

SURGERY/OTHER PROCEDURES

- Resection for NSCLC, for stages I, II, and IIIA, if medically fit to undergo surgery
- Resection of isolated, distant metastases has been achieved and may improve survival.
- Resection involves lobectomy in 71%, wedge in 16%, and complete pneumonectomy in 18%.
- Resection should be accompanied by lymph node dissection for pathologic staging.

 ONGOING CARE

FOLLOW-UP RECOMMENDATIONS

Patient Monitoring

- Depends on clinical history; in general, postoperative visits every 3 to 6 months in the first 2 years after surgery with physical exam and CT scan
- Follow-up usually lifelong with CT scans, following NCCN criteria

PATIENT EDUCATION

- National Cancer Institute: https://www.cancer.gov/
- Smokefree.gov: https://smokefree.gov/

PROGNOSIS

- For combined, all types and stages, 5-year survival rate is 18.6%.
- NSCLC 5-year survival
  - Localized disease: for stages IA1, IA2, and IA3 is 92%, 83%, and 77%, respectively; stages IB and IIA is 68% and 60%, respectively

- Regional disease: for stages IIIA, IIIB, and IIIC is 36%, 26%, and 13%, respectively
- Distant metastatic disease: for stages IVA and IVB is 10% and <1%, respectively
- SCLC
  - Without treatment: median survival from diagnosis of only 2 to 4 months
  - 5-year survival rate: ranges from 2% (stage IV) to 31% (stage I)
  - Extensive-stage disease: median survival of 6 to 12 months; long-term disease-free survival is rare.

COMPLICATIONS

- Development of metastatic disease
- Local recurrence of disease
- Postoperative complications
- Side effects of chemotherapy or radiation

REFERENCES

1. Aberle DR, Adams AM, Berg CD, et al; and National Lung Screening Trial Research Team. Reduced lung-cancer mortality with low-dose computed tomographic screening. *N Engl J Med*. 2011;365(5):395–409.
2. Slotman B, Faivre-Finn C, Kramer G, et al; for EORTC Radiation Oncology Group and Lung Cancer Group. Prophylactic cranial irradiation in extensive small-cell lung cancer. *N Engl J Med*. 2007;357(7):664–672.

ADDITIONAL READING

National Cancer Institute. Lung cancer—health professional version. https://www.cancer.gov/types/lung/hp. Accessed September 29, 2018.

CODES

ICD10

- C34.90 Malignant neoplasm of unsp part of unsp bronchus or lung
- C34.10 Malignant neoplasm of upper lobe, unsp bronchus or lung
- C34.30 Malignant neoplasm of lower lobe, unsp bronchus or lung

CLINICAL PEARLS

- Two types: NSCLC and SCLC
  - NSCLC (>85% of all lung cancers); normally originate in periphery
    - Adenocarcinoma (~40% of NSCLC)
    - SCC (~25% of NSCLC)
    - Large cell (~10% of NSCLC)
  - SCLC centrally located, early metastases, aggressive
- Prognosis and treatment of lung cancer differ greatly between small cell and non–small cell histologies.
- Adjuvant cisplatin-based chemotherapy improves survival in patients with completely resected stages II and III NSCLC.
- Chemotherapy, with or without radiation, can be offered to patients with advanced NSCLC or SCLC.
- There is little role for surgery in the treatment of SCLC.

L

LUPUS ERYTHEMATOSUS, SYSTEMIC (SLE)

Katherine M. Tromp, PharmD • Hershey S. Bell, MD, MS, FAAFP

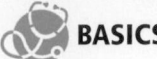

BASICS

DESCRIPTION

- Systemic lupus erythematosus (SLE) is a multisystem autoimmune inflammatory disease characterized by a chronic relapsing/remitting course; can be mild to severe and may be life-threatening (CNS and renal forms)
- System(s) affected: mucocutaneous; musculoskeletal; renal; nervous; pulmonary; cardiac; hematologic; vascular; gastrointestinal (GI)
- Synonym(s): SLE; lupus

ALERT
Women with SLE have a 7- to 50-fold increased risk of coronary artery disease and may present with atypical/nonspecific symptoms.

EPIDEMIOLOGY
Predominant age: 15 to 45 years

Incidence
- Per year, 1.6 to 7.6/100,000 and increasing due to better diagnosis
- Most common: African American women (8.1 to 11.4/100,000/year)
- Least common: Caucasian men (0.3 to 0.9/ 100,000/year)

Prevalence
Occurs in 30 to 50/100,000 and increasing due to increased survival

ETIOLOGY AND PATHOPHYSIOLOGY
- Skin: photosensitivity; scaly erythematous, plaques with follicular plugging, dermal atrophy, and scarring; nonscarring erythematous psoriasiform/annular rash; alopecia; mucosal ulcers
- Musculoskeletal: nonerosive arthritis; ligament and tendon laxity, ulnar deviation, and swan neck deformities; avascular necrosis
- Renal: glomerulonephritis
- Pulmonary: pleuritis, pleural effusion, alveolar hemorrhage, pneumonitis, interstitial fibrosis, pulmonary hypertension, pulmonary embolism (PE)
- Cardiac: nonbacterial verrucous endocarditis, pericarditis, myocarditis, atherosclerosis
- CNS: thrombosis of small intracranial vessels ± perivascular inflammation resulting in micro- or macroinfarcts ± hemorrhage
- Peripheral nervous system: mononeuritis multiplex, peripheral neuropathy
- GI: pancreatitis, peritonitis, colitis
- Hematologic: hemolytic anemia, thrombocytopenia, leukopenia, lymphopenia
- Vascular: vasculitis, thromboembolism
- Most cases are idiopathic with possible environmental factors.
- Drug-induced lupus: hydralazine, D penicillamine, quinidine, procainamide, minocycline, isoniazid, etc.

Genetics
- Identical twins: 24–58% concordance
- Fraternal twins and siblings: 2–5% concordance
- 8-fold risk if first-degree relative with SLE
- Major histocompatibility complex associations: HLA-DR2, HLA-DR3
- Deficiency of early complement components, especially C1q, C1r/s, C2, and C4

- Immunoglobulin receptor polymorphisms: *FCγR2A, FCγR3A, and others*
- Polymorphism in genes associated with regulation of programmed cell death, protein tyrosine kinases, and interferon production

RISK FACTORS
- Race: African Americans, Hispanics, Asians, and Native Americans
- Predominant sex: females > males (10:1)
- Environmental: UV light, infectious agents, stress, diet, drugs, hormones, vitamin D deficiency, and tobacco

COMMONLY ASSOCIATED CONDITIONS
- Overlap syndromes: rheumatoid arthritis (RA), Sjögren syndrome, scleroderma
- Antiphospholipid syndrome; coronary artery disease; nephritis; depression

DIAGNOSIS

Consider SLE in multisystem disease including fever, fatigue, and signs of inflammation.

HISTORY
- Fever, fatigue, malaise, weight loss, headache
- Rash (discoid [LR+] = 18, malar [LR+] = 14), photosensitivity (LR+) = 11, alopecia
- Oral/nasal ulcers (usually painless)
- Arthritis, arthralgia, myalgia, weakness
- Pleuritic chest pain, cough, dyspnea, hemoptysis
- Early stroke (age <50 years), unexplained seizure/psychosis (LR+) = 13, cognitive deficits
- Proteinuria, cellular casts
- Hemolytic anemia, leukopenia, lymphopenia, thrombocytopenia
- Abdominal pain, anorexia, nausea, vomiting
- Raynaud phenomenon

PHYSICAL EXAM
- Vital signs: fever, hypertension
- Malar, discoid, psoriasiform, or annular rash, alopecia
- Oral/nasal ulcers (*often minimally symptomatic*)
- Lymphadenopathy, splenomegaly
- Acrocyanosis
- Inflammatory arthritis, tenosynovitis
- Pleural/pericardial rub, heart murmur
- Bibasilar rales
- Cranial/peripheral neuropathies

DIFFERENTIAL DIAGNOSIS
Undifferentiated connective tissue disease, Sjögren syndrome, fibromyalgia, RA, vasculitis, idiopathic thrombocytopenia purpura, antiphospholipid antibody syndrome, drug-induced lupus

DIAGNOSTIC TESTS & INTERPRETATION
Initial Tests (lab, imaging)
American College of Rheumatology (ACR) and Systemic Lupus International Collaborating Clinics (SLICC) criteria

- ACR and the SLICC have established diagnostic criteria for SLE.
- ACR requires at least 4 of 11 criteria be met (95% specificity; 85% sensitivity).

- SLICC requires at least 4 of 13 criteria including at least 1 abnormal clinical criterion and 1 abnormal immunologic criterion or patient must have biopsy—confirmed lupus nephritis and elevated ANA or anti-dsDNA levels (97% specificity; 84% sensitivity).
- ACR remains the gold standard; SLICC not yet endorsed by ACR
  - Cardiac/pulmonary: ACR: pleuritic or pericarditis; SLICC: serositis
  - Hematologic: ACR: hemolytic anemia or leukopenia or lymphopenia or thrombocytopenia; SLICC: hemolytic anemia, leukopenia or lymphopenia more than once, thrombocytopenia
  - Immunologic: ACR: positive antinuclear antibody (ANA), elevated anti double-stranded DNA (anti-dsDNA), anti-Smith (anti-Sm) or antiphospholipid antibodies; SLICC: positive ANA, elevated anti-dsDNA, anti-Sm, or phospholipid antibodies, low complement (C3, C4, CH50) or direct Coombs test (in absence of hemolytic anemia), chronic cutaneous lupus, nonscarring alopecia, oral or nasal ulcers
  - Musculoskeletal: ACR: nonerosive arthritis involving two or more joints; SLICC: synovitis involving two or more joints, or tenderness at two or more joints and at least 30 minutes of morning stiffness
  - Neuropsychiatric: ACR: seizure or psychosis; SLICC: seizures, psychosis, mononeuritis complex, myelitis, or peripheral or cranial neuropathy
  - Renal: ACR: persistent proteinuria >0.5 g per day or >3+ on urine dipstick, or cellular casts; SLICC: urinary creatinine (or 24-hour urinary protein) >500 mg or red blood cell casts
  - Skin/mucosal: ACR: malar rash; SLICC: acute or subacute cutaneous lupus
- Initial imaging is dependent on presenting symptoms.
- Radiograph of involved joints
- Chest x-ray: infiltrates, pleural effusion, low lung volumes
- Chest CT scan, ventilation/perfusion (V/Q) scan, duplex ultrasound for PE or deep vein thrombosis
- Head CT scan: ischemia, infarct, hemorrhage
- Brain MRI: focal areas of increased signal intensity
- Echocardiogram: pericardial effusion, valvular vegetations, pulmonary hypertension
- Contrast angiography for medium-size artery vasculitis: mesenteric/limb ischemia, CNS symptom

Follow-Up Tests & Special Considerations
- Hemolytic anemia: elevated reticulocyte count and indirect bilirubin, low haptoglobin, positive direct Coombs test
- Confirm positive phospholipid antibodies results in 12 weeks.
- If phospholipid antibodies are initially negative, but symptoms arise, repeat because they may become positive over time.
- 24-hour urine collection/spot protein/creatinine to quantify proteinuria
- Histone antibodies present in >95% of drug-induced lupus (vs. 80% of idiopathic SLE)
- Fasting lipid panel and glucose
- Follow vitamin D(25[OH]) levels and replenish PRN.

Diagnostic Procedures/Other
- Renal biopsy to diagnose lupus nephritis (if UA abnormal)
- Skin biopsy with immunofluorescence on involved and uninvolved non–sun-exposed skin (*lupus band test*) may help differentiate SLE rash from others.

- Lumbar puncture in patients with fever and CNS/meningeal symptoms
- EEG for seizures/global CNS dysfunction
- Neuropsychiatric testing for cognitive impairment
- EMG/nerve conduction study (NCS) for peripheral neuropathy and myositis
- Nerve and/or muscle biopsy
- ECG, cardiac enzymes, stress tests

Test Interpretation
- Skin: vascular/perivascular inflammation, immune-complex deposition at dermal–epidermal junction, mucinosis, basal layer vacuolar changes
  - Similar findings seen in other connective tissue disorders such as dermatomyositis
- Renal: mesangial hypercellularity/matrix expansion, subendothelial/subepithelial immune deposits, glomerular sclerosis, fibrous crescents
  - Vary depending on degree of involvement
- Vascular: immune-complex deposition in vessel walls with fibrinoid necrosis and perivascular mononuclear cell infiltrates, intraluminal fibrin thrombi

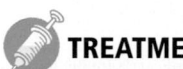

TREATMENT

GENERAL MEASURES
- Education, counseling, and support
- Influenza/pneumococcal vaccines are safe; weigh risk versus benefit for live vaccines in immunocompromised patients.
- Low-estrogen oral contraceptives safe in mild SLE

MEDICATION
First Line
- Antimalarial agents and NSAIDs are first-line therapy for patients with mild SLE (1)[A].
  - Hydroxychloroquine for constitutional and musculoskeletal symptoms, rash, mild serositis; may reduce flares and increase long-term survival (1)[A],(2)[C]; recommended maximum dose is 5 mg/kg based on actual body weight (3)[C].
  - NSAIDs for musculoskeletal manifestations, mild serositis, headache, and fever (1)[A]
- Systemic glucocorticoids (prednisone or equivalent)
  - Low dose (<0.5 mg/kg) for minor disease activity not responsive to NSAIDs or when NSAIDs are contraindicated (1)[A]
  - High dose (1 to 2 mg/kg/day) (1)[A] or IV pulse methylprednisolone for organ-threatening disease, particularly CNS and renal; often combined with immunosuppressive agent (1)[A]
- Topical corticosteroids for skin manifestations

Second Line
- Methotrexate (4)[C], azathioprine (4)[C], mycophenolate mofetil (4)[C], or leflunomide as steroid-sparing agent for persistent active disease or to maintain remission
  - Requires laboratory monitoring for toxicity
- Belimumab as adjunct for preventing flares in patients with active lupus despite first-line therapy (5)[B]
  - 10 mg/kg IV q2wk × 3 doses and then monthly
- Treatments under investigation: rituximab, epratuzumab, abatacept, interferon-α inhibitors
- Immunosuppressive agents for severe disease
  - Cyclophosphamide (1)[A]: adequate hydration to reduce risk of hemorrhagic cystitis
  - Mycophenolate mofetil (1)[A]: more efficacious for lupus nephritis (4)[A]

SURGERY/OTHER PROCEDURES
Renal transplant for end-stage renal disease

COMPLEMENTARY & ALTERNATIVE MEDICINE
Biofeedback, visual imagery, cognitive therapy

ADMISSION, INPATIENT, AND NURSING CONSIDERATIONS
- Difficult to differentiate SLE flare from infection; may need to treat both pending full evaluation
- IV pulse Solu-Medrol 1 g/day for 3 to 5 days for life- or organ-threatening disease (1)[A]

 ## ONGOING CARE

FOLLOW-UP RECOMMENDATIONS
Patient Monitoring
- Clinical evaluation for signs and symptoms
  - Weekly to monthly for active disease
  - Every 3 to 6 months for mild/inactive disease
- Measures of disease activity and damage: Systemic Lupus Erythematosus Disease Activity Index, British Isles Lupus Assessment Group Index, European Consensus Lupus Activity Measure
- Laboratory studies
  - CBC with differential
  - Serum creatinine, UA
  - Vitamin D
  - Declining C3/C4 and rising dsDNA and ESR may correlate with disease activity
- Monitor for adverse effects of treatment.
  - NSAIDs: GI bleeding and/or ulceration
  - Glucocorticoids: glucose, lipids, bone density
  - Hydroxychloroquine: ophthalmologic exam every 6 to 12 months
  - Methotrexate: CBC, creatinine, albumin, aspartate aminotransferase (AST), alanine aminotransferase (ALT) every 2 months
  - Azathioprine and mycophenolate mofetil: CBC every 1 to 3 months
  - Cyclophosphamide
    ○ CBC, creatinine, UA every 2 weeks, and liver function tests monthly during treatment
    ○ UA every 6 to 12 months for life

DIET
- No special diet unless for complications such as renal failure, diabetes, hyperlipidemia (1)[A]
- Adequate calcium/vitamin D intake in patients on corticosteroids (1)[A]
- Low glycemic index or calorie-restricted diet in patients on corticosteroids

PATIENT EDUCATION
- Avoid UV light exposure: sunscreens (SPF ≥30), protective clothing (1)[A].
- Weight control, smoking cessation, exercise (1)[A]
- Stress avoidance/management

PROGNOSIS
- Permanent treatment-free remission is uncommon.
- 5-year survival after diagnosis is 95%.
- Poor prognostic factor: major organ involvement
- Drug-induced lupus resolves within weeks to months after discontinuation of the offending drug.

COMPLICATIONS
Infections, neoplasms, cardiac disease, nephritis, neuropsychiatric lupus; depression

Pregnancy Considerations
- Exacerbations during pregnancy are less common when in remission for 6 months prior to conception.
- Fetal loss is increased, especially in those with active lupus/antiphospholipid antibodies.

- A 2% risk of congenital heart block if anti–SS-A (Ro) or anti–SS-B (La) antibodies are present
- See "Antiphospholipid Antibody Syndrome" for recommendations regarding use of aspirin and heparin to prevent pregnancy complications.

REFERENCES

1. Bertsias G, Ioannidis JP, Boletis J, et al. EULAR recommendations for the management of systemic lupus erythematosus. Report of a Task Force of the EULAR Standing Committee for International Clinical Studies Including Therapeutics. *Ann Rheum Dis*. 2008;67(2):195–205.
2. Ruiz-Irastorza G, Ramos-Casals M, Brito-Zeron P, et al. Clinical efficacy and side effects of antimalarials in systemic lupus erythematosus: a systematic review. *Ann Rheum Dis*. 2010;69(1):20–28.
3. Marmor MF, Kellner U, Lai TYY, et al; for American Academy of Ophthalmology. Recommendations on screening for chloroquine and hydroxychloroquine retinopathy (2016 revision). *Ophthalmology*. 2016;123(6):1386–1394.
4. Yildirim-Toruner C, Diamond B. Current and novel therapeutics in the treatment of systemic lupus erythematosus. *J Allergy Clin Immunol*. 2011;127(2):303–314.
5. Navarra SV, Guzmán RM, Gallacher AE, et al; for BLISS-52 Study Group. Efficacy and safety of belimumab in patients with active systemic lupus erythematosus: a randomised, placebo-controlled, phase 3 trial. *Lancet*. 2011;377(9767):721–731.

ADDITIONAL READING
- Lam NC, Ghetu MV, Bieniek ML. Systemic lupus erythematosus: primary care approach to diagnosis and management. *Am Fam Physician*. 2016;94(4):284–294.
- Lisnevskaia L, Murphy G, Isenberg D. Systemic lupus erythematosus. *Lancet*. 2014;384(9957):1878–1888.
- van Assen S, Agmon-Levin N, Elkayam O, et al. EULAR recommendations for vaccination in adult patients with autoimmune inflammatory rheumatic diseases. *Ann Rheum Dis*. 2011;70(3):414–422.

 ### SEE ALSO

Antiphospholipid Antibody Syndrome

 ## CODES

ICD10
- M32.9 Systemic lupus erythematosus, unspecified
- M32.10 Systemic lupus erythematosus, organ or system involv unsp
- M32.14 Glomerular disease in systemic lupus erythematosus

CLINICAL PEARLS
- Aggressiveness of therapy should reflect intensity of disease.
- Most important diagnostic test is the UA: if abnormal, order kidney biopsy; serum and urine lab values often do not reveal extent of kidney disease.
- Atherosclerotic and atheroembolic complications are the major cause of death; address modifiable cardiovascular risk factors.

LUPUS NEPHRITIS

Neena R. Gupta, MD

BASICS

DESCRIPTION
- The renal manifestation of systemic lupus erythematosus (SLE)
- American College of Rheumatology (ACR) criteria: persistent proteinuria >500 mg/day or ≥3 on dipstick and/or presence of cellular casts; alternatively, spot urine protein-to-creatinine ratio >0.5 and "active urinary sediment" (>5 RBC/HPF, >5 WBC/HPF in absence of infection, or cellular casts—RBC or WBC casts) (1)
- Clinical manifestations primarily due to immune complex–mediated glomerular disease. Tubulointerstitial and vascular involvement often coexist. Diagnosis is based on clinical findings, urine abnormalities, autoantibodies, and renal biopsy.
- Treatment and prognosis depend on International Society of Nephrology/Renal Pathology Society (ISN/RPS) histologic class—risk of end-stage renal disease (ESRD) highest in class IV.
- Delay in diagnosis/treatment increases risk of ESRD.

EPIDEMIOLOGY
- Peak incidence of SLE is 15 to 45 years of age.
- Predominant sex: female > male (10:1)
- Once SLE develops, lupus nephritis (LN) affects both genders equally; it is more severe in children and men and less severe in older adults.

Incidence
- SLE: 1.4 to 22/100,000
- Up to 60% of SLE patients develop LN over time; 25–50% of SLE patients have nephritis as the initial presentation.

Pediatric Considerations
LN is more common and more severe in children: 60–80% of children have LN at or soon after SLE onset.

Prevalence
SLE: 7.4 to 159.4/100,000

ETIOLOGY AND PATHOPHYSIOLOGY
- Immune complex–mediated inflammation injures glomeruli, tubules, interstitium, and vasculature.
- Glomeruli: Varying degrees of mesangial proliferation, crescent formation, and fibrinoid necrosis cause reduced glomerular filtration rate (GFR).
- Persistent inflammation (chronicity) leads to sclerosis and glomerular loss.
- Tubulointerstitial injury (edema, inflammatory cell infiltrate acutely; tubular atrophy in chronic phase) with or without tubular basement membrane immune complex deposition leads to reduced renal function.
- Vascular lesions: immune complex deposition and noninflammatory necrosis in arterioles
- SLE is a multifactorial disease, with multigenic inheritance; exact etiology remains unclear.
- Defective T-cell autoregulation and polyclonal B-cell hyperactivity contribute to dysregulated apoptosis. Impaired clearance of apoptotic cells inhibits self-tolerance to nuclear antigen.
- Anti-DNA, anti-C1q, anti–α-actin, and other nuclear component autoantibodies develop.

- Deposition of circulating immune complexes or autoantibodies attaching to local nuclear antigens leads to complement activation, inflammation, and tissue injury.
- Interaction of genetic, hormonal, and environmental factors leads to great variability in LN severity.

Genetics
Multigenic inheritance; clustering in families, ~25% concordance in identical twins

RISK FACTORS
Younger age, African American or Hispanic race, more ACR criteria for SLE, longer disease duration, hypertension, lower socioeconomic status, family history of SLE, anti-dsDNA antibodies

COMMONLY ASSOCIATED CONDITIONS
Skin, hematologic, cerebral, pulmonary, GI, and cardiopulmonary systems are often involved in SLE.

DIAGNOSIS

HISTORY
Assess for risk factors and other signs/symptoms of SLE: rash, photosensitivity, arthritis, neurologic complaints, fever, weight loss, alopecia.

PHYSICAL EXAM
- Hypertension, fever
- Pleural/pericardial rub
- Skin rash
- Edema
- Arthritis
- Alopecia
- Oral ulcers

DIFFERENTIAL DIAGNOSIS
- Primary glomerular disease
- Secondary renal involvement in other systemic disorders such as antineutrophil cytoplasmic antibody (ANCA)-associated vasculitis, Henoch-Schönlein purpura (HSP), antiglomerular basement membrane disease, and viral infections
- Mixed connective tissue disorder may have glomerulonephritis indistinguishable from LN.

DIAGNOSTIC TESTS & INTERPRETATION
- Renal biopsy is the gold standard for diagnosing and classifying LN.
- Combine clinical data with serologic and renal biopsy patterns to differentiate LN from other conditions.
- Active urine sediment suggests nephritis.
- Autoantibodies, low C3, C4, and CH50 complement levels support LN diagnosis.

Initial Tests (lab, imaging)
- Urinalysis may show hematuria, proteinuria, and active urine sediment (2)[C].
- Serum electrolytes, BUN, creatinine, albumin, routine serologic markers of SLE such as antinuclear antibody (ANA), anti-dsDNA, anti-Ro, anti-La, anti-RNP, anti-Sm, antiphospholipid antibody, C3, C4, CH50, CBC with differential, and C-reactive protein (CRP) (2)[C]
- CBC may show anemia, thrombocytopenia, and leukopenia.
- Renal ultrasound (2)[C]

Follow-Up Tests & Special Considerations
- Monitor disease activity q3mo (2)[C]: urinalysis for hematuria and proteinuria; blood for C3, C4, anti-dsDNA, serum albumin, and creatinine.
- Patients with estimated glomerular filtration rate (eGFR) of <60 mL should be managed according to the National Kidney Foundation guidelines for chronic kidney disease (CKD): http://www.kdigo.org/clinical_practice_guidelines/pdf/CKD/KDIGO_2012_CKD_GL.pdf.

Pregnancy Considerations
- Pregnancy leads to worsening of renal function in LN. Risk factors include renal impairment at baseline, active disease, hypertension, and proteinuria.
- Risk factors for fetal loss include elevated serum creatinine, heavy proteinuria, hypertension, and anticardiolipin antibodies.
- Mycophenolate mofetil (MMF) is contraindicated in pregnancy; azathioprine can be safely used.

Test Interpretation
- Adequate renal biopsy (at least 10 glomeruli for light microscopy or total 20 to 25 glomeruli) is essential. Light, immunofluorescence, and electron microscopy are needed for accurate classification.
- On immunofluorescence microscopy: Immune complex deposits consisting of IgG, IgA, IgM, C1q, and C3 ("full house") are highly suggestive of LN.
- Revised ISN/RPS histologic classification guides therapeutic decisions: http://jasn.asnjournals.org/content/15/2/241.full.pdf.
- LN is classified as purely mesangial (classes I and II), focal proliferative: <50% glomeruli (class III), diffuse proliferative: ≥50% (class IV), membranous (class V), and advanced sclerosis (class VI); subdivisions for activity (A) and chronicity (C) in class III/IV and for segmental (S) or global (G) glomerular involvement in class IV (class III A, C, A/C and class IV S[A], G[A], S[A/C], S[C], G[C])
- LN may change class over time or with therapy.
- Focal and diffuse proliferative LN (classes III and IV) are common and most likely to progress to ESRD.

TREATMENT

GENERAL MEASURES
- Monitor bone density; optimize vitamin D and calcium intake in patients on glucocorticoid therapy.
- Low-salt diet for hypertension and edema. For eGFR <60 mL: Follow National Kidney Foundation guidelines for CKD.
- Avoid sun or ultraviolet light exposure.

MEDICATION
Note: Other than methylprednisolone and prednisone, no other medications listed below are FDA-approved for LN.

First Line
- Class I + II LN: No specific therapy is needed because long-term renal prognosis is good; renin-angiotensin system blockade (ACE inhibitors or angiotensin receptor blockers) to manage BP and proteinuria (e.g., lisinopril 5 to 40 mg/day PO, losartan 25 to 100 mg/day PO)
- Proliferative LN (class III, IV, V + III/IV): Induce remission by steroids + IV cyclophosphamide or MMF and maintenance of remission by low-dose steroids and azathioprine or MMF (1).

- Principles of treatment:
  - Avoid delay; induce remission quickly (3 to 6 months).
  - Maintain response and avoid iatrogenic morbidity.
- INDUCTION: steroids + immunosuppressive agent (for mild class III, high-dose steroids may be sufficient):
  - Glucocorticoids: methylprednisolone pulse 0.5 to 1.0 g/day for 3 days followed by oral prednisone 0.5 to 1.0 mg/kg/day PO (max 60 mg/day, taper after 4 to 8 weeks) (3)[A] AND
  - Cyclophosphamide: IV cyclophosphamide (high dose = 0.5 to 1.0 g/m² monthly for 6 doses—NIH regimen; low dose = 0.5 g q2wk for 6 doses—Euro-Lupus regimen) OR
  - MMF: 1 to 3 g/day PO divided BID (target 3 g/day as tolerated) for 6 months. MMF is as effective as cyclophosphamide in achieving remission with fewer side effects (3)[A].
  - Combination of tacrolimus and MMF has been found to have higher complete remission and total response rate than cyclophosphamide in some studies (4)[C].
- MAINTENANCE:
  - Glucocorticoids: oral prednisone tapered to low doses (generally <10 mg/day by 6 months) AND
  - MMF 1 to 2 g/day divided BID PO OR azathioprine: 1.0 to 2.5 mg/kg/day PO (3)[A]
  - MMF shown to be equal to azathioprine for maintenance therapy in mostly Caucasian population (5)[A].
  - Cyclophosphamide IV quarterly for 1 to 2 years after renal remission; not used now due to availability of less toxic regimen
  - Optimum duration of maintenance therapy is unclear, but periods ranging from 3 to 10 years have been studied in clinical trials (5,6).
- Class V LN: good prognosis, no standardized treatment
  - For subnephrotic patients, no specific treatment except renin-angiotensin system blockade
  - Options for nephrotic patients include steroids with either calcineurin inhibitors, IV cyclophosphamide, azathioprine, or MMF (3)[B].
  - Class V LN with presence of class III or class IV biopsy findings needs aggressive combination regimen as for class III/IV.

Second Line
Other treatments in selected patients: rituximab, plasma exchange, IVIG, calcineurin inhibitors. Belimumab was approved by FDA in 2011, but trials excluded patients with severe active LN (3)[C].

ISSUES FOR REFERRAL
Nephrology consults for initial management and relapses

ADDITIONAL THERAPIES
- KDIGO guidelines for LN state that all patients with LN of any class be treated with hydroxychloroquine (maximum daily dose of 6.0 to 6.5 mg/kg ideal body weight), unless they have a specific contraindication.
- BP control; treat dyslipidemia and other modifiable cardiovascular risk factors.
- Anticoagulation for symptomatic antiphospholipid antibody syndrome

SURGERY/OTHER PROCEDURES
- Renal transplant for ESRD when indicated
- Patient and graft survival rates similar to non-SLE patients
- Risk of recurrent LN in renal transplant recipients ranges between 0% and 30%; graft loss due to recurrence is rare.

ADMISSION, INPATIENT, AND NURSING CONSIDERATIONS
- Admission criteria/initial stabilization
  - Uncontrolled hypertension, acute kidney injury
  - Severe extrarenal manifestation
  - Control hypertension and proteinuria, if present.
  - Labs to help confirm SLE/LN, renal ultrasound
  - Nephrology to manage input and renal biopsy
- Patients who have nephrotic syndrome or acute kidney injury should be fluid restricted.
- Once the patient is stabilized and renal biopsy is performed, manage safely as an outpatient.

 ONGOING CARE

FOLLOW-UP RECOMMENDATIONS
Patient Monitoring
- Monitor urine protein-to-creatinine ratio, urine microscopy, serum albumin and creatinine, antibody titers (especially anti-dsDNA), C3, C4, BP at least every 3 months for first 2 to 3 years (2)[C].
- Once stable on maintenance therapy with no active disease, follow up every 6 to 12 months (2)[C].
- Cyclophosphamide: CBC; ensure adequate hydration.
- MMF: CBC, LFT, SrCr
- Azathioprine: CBC

DIET
Low-salt diet. For eGFR <60 mL: Follow National Kidney Foundation guidelines for CKD.

PATIENT EDUCATION
Medication adherence and self-monitoring for relapse

PROGNOSIS
- 10-year survival of 88% and 94% in SLE patients with and without renal involvement (1)
- Relapse rate is ~35%. 10–20% of patients progress to ESRD within 10 years.
- 5-year renal survival of class IV LN <30% before 1970 has improved to >80% in last 2 decades.
- Early and complete remission of proteinuria with treatment is the best prognostic factor. Other predictors of remission include low baseline proteinuria, normal creatinine, Caucasian race, and treatment initiated within 3 months of diagnosis.
- Indicators of poor prognosis: diffuse proliferative LN (especially crescentic), higher activity/chronicity index, African American race, lower socioeconomic status, poor response to treatment, high creatinine at baseline, uncontrolled hypertension, and relapse

COMPLICATIONS
- Risks of immunosuppressive therapy: infections, malignancy
- Treatment side effects: Cyclophosphamide causes primary amenorrhea.

- MMF may cause GI upset and nausea and is a teratogen (azathioprine recommended for women who desire pregnancy).
- Risk of vascular thromboses (hypercoagulable state from antiphospholipid antibodies)
- About 10–20% of patients develop ESRD from progressive disease refractory to treatment requiring dialysis/kidney transplantation.

REFERENCES

1. Hahn BH, McMahon MA, Wilkinson A, et al. American College of Rheumatology guidelines for screening, treatment, and management of lupus nephritis. *Arthritis Care Res (Hoboken)*. 2012;64(6):797–808.
2. Mosca M, Tani C, Aringer M, et al. European League Against Rheumatism recommendations for monitoring patients with systemic lupus erythematosus in clinical practice and in observational studies. *Ann Rheum Dis*. 2010;69(7):1269–1274.
3. Parikh SV, Rovin BH. Current and emerging therapies for lupus nephritis. *J Am Soc Nephrol*. 2016;27(10):2929–2939.
4. Chen Y, Sun J, Zou K, et al. Treatment for lupus nephritis: an overview of systematic reviews and meta-analyses. *Rheumatol Int*. 2017;37(7): 1089–1099.
5. Tamirou F, D'Cruz D, Sangle S, et al; and MAINTAIN Nephritis Trial Group. Long-term follow-up of the MAINTAIN nephritis trial, comparing azathioprine and mycophenolate mofetil as maintenance therapy of lupus nephritis. *Ann Rheum Dis*. 2016;75(3):526–531.
6. Dooley MA, Jayne D, Ginzler EM, et al; for ALMS Group. Mycophenolate versus azathioprine as maintenance therapy for lupus nephritis. *N Engl J Med*. 2011;365(20):1886–1895.

ADDITIONAL READING

- Almaani S, Meara A, Rovin BH. Update on lupus nephritis. *Clin J Am Soc Nephrol*. 2017;12(5): 825–835.
- Kidney Disease: Improving Global Outcomes (KDIGO) Glomerulonephritis Work Group. KDIGO clinical practice guideline for glomerulonephritis. *Kidney Int Suppl*. 2012;2(2):139–274.

 CODES

ICD10
M32.14 Glomerular disease in systemic lupus erythematosus

CLINICAL PEARLS
- Early diagnosis, correct classification (requires renal biopsy), and rapid treatment improve renal survival in patients with LN.
- Treat proliferative/progressive LN with a short induction course followed by maintenance therapy using glucocorticoids and immunosuppressants.
- Survival rates for patients with LN have improved dramatically over the past several decades.

L

LYME DISEASE

Felix B. Chang Cruz, MD, FAAMA, ABIHM • Roberto S. Amado, MD

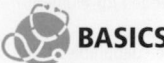 **BASICS**

DESCRIPTION
- A multisystem infection caused by *Borrelia* spirochetes, transmitted primarily by ixodid ticks
  - *Ixodes scapularis* (deer ticks) in the Northeast and Great Lakes areas
  - *Ixodes pacificus* in the West (black-legged ticks and Western black-legged ticks)
  - *Ixodes ricinus* in Europe
  - *Ixodes persulcatus* in Asia and Russia
- Early localized Lyme disease includes a characteristic expanding skin rash (erythema migrans [EM]) (80%) and constitutional flulike symptoms (1).
- Early neurologic manifestations 15%: cranial nerve palsy, meningitis, acute radiculopathy, or mononeuropathy
- Disseminated Lyme disease presents with involvement of ≥1 organ systems; most commonly neurologic, cardiac, and pauciarticular arthritis
- Lyme carditis: AV block, myopericarditis 1%
- Post–Lyme disease syndrome includes arthritis (50%) and chronic neurologic syndromes.
- System(s) affected: hemic/lymphatic/immunologic; musculoskeletal; skin/exocrine; cardiac; neurologic
- Synonym(s): Lyme arthritis; Lyme borreliosis

EPIDEMIOLOGY
Incidence
- 95% of U.S. cases (2015) reported from 14 states—primarily Connecticut, Delaware, Maine, Massachusetts, Minnesota, New Hampshire, New Jersey, New York, Pennsylvania, Rhode Island, Vermont, Virginia, Wisconsin (1)
- During 2016 >26,000 confirmed U.S. cases (1)
- In endemic states, the incidence is 0.5 per 1,000 but can be substantially higher in certain areas.
- Cases have been reported from all 50 states.

Prevalence
- The most reported vector-borne illness in the United States
- Estimated 106 cases per 100,000 persons
- Predominant age: most common in children ages 5 to 14 years and in adults aged 55 to 70 years of age
- Predominant sex: male > female in the United States

ETIOLOGY AND PATHOPHYSIOLOGY
- Infection with spirochete *Borrelia burgdorferi* in the United States, or *Borrelia afzelii* or *Borrelia garinii* in Europe, transmitted by the bite of ixodid ticks
- Approximately 90% of cases are transmitted during the nymph stage of the tick life cycle.
- Average incubation period 7 to 10 days
- Most transmissions occur in late May to September when nymphal tick activity is highest.
- If a tick is infected, the chance of transmission increases with time attached: 12% at 48 hours, 79% at 72 hours, and 94% at 96 hours of attachment.
- Primary animal reservoir is the white-footed mouse.
- Spirochetes multiply and spread within dermis. Host response results in characteristic (EM) rash. Hematogenous dissemination results in disease within CNS, cardiovascular, or other organ systems.
- Star ticks (*Amblyomma americanum*), the American dog tick (*Dermacentor variabilis*), the Rocky Mountain wood tick (*Dermacentor andersoni*), and the brown dog tick (*Rhipicephalus sanguineus*) are not known to transmit Lyme disease.

Genetics
Human leukocyte antigen: Patients with haplotype DR4 or DR2 may be more susceptible to prolonged arthritis.

RISK FACTORS
- Exposure in tick-infested area, particularly from April to November
- Those who reside or are employed in endemic areas where ixodid ticks are found are at increased risk.
- Ixodid ticks are common on deer; hunters at increased risk

GENERAL PREVENTION
- "Tick checks": Examine skin after outdoor activities.
- Remove ticks within 36 hours to limit transmission.
- Wear clothing covering the ankles in endemic areas.
- Use insect repellents containing N,N-diethyl-meta-toluamide (DEET).
- Apply permethrin to clothes, shoes, and tents.
- Antibiotic prophylaxis is recommended for the prevention of Lyme disease in endemic areas following an *Ixodes* tick bite.
- Prophylactic treatment with 1 dose of 200 mg of doxycycline within 72 hours of a tick bite in highly endemic areas is 87% effective. Contraindicated in pregnancy and in children; no prophylactic agent is approved for these groups (1)[A].

COMMONLY ASSOCIATED CONDITIONS
- Coinfection (e.g., babesiosis) increasingly reported
- Southern tick–associated rash illness may be mistaken for Lyme disease. It is seen in the Southeastern and South Central United States and is associated with the bite of the lone star tick, *A. americanum*.
- Comorbid human granulocytic anaplasmosis and/or babesiosis in patients living in endemic regions

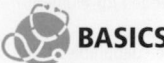 **DIAGNOSIS**

HISTORY
- History of a tick bite followed by EM and/or illness. About 1/3 of patients recall tick bite.
- Round, flat or raised, erythematous lesion that expands in diameter over days to weeks may have area of central clearing.
- Common EM sites: axilla, back, abdomen, groin, or popliteal fossa
- 75–80% presenting with EM having a single lesion
- Early Lyme disease: incubation period 3 to 30 days
  - Some patients may be asymptomatic (2).
  - Fever; headache; myalgias; arthralgias, regional lymphadenopathy
- Disseminated Lyme disease
  - Carditis (pleuritic chest pain; palpitations)
  - Facial palsies or other cranial neuropathies
  - Joint pain (polyarthritis/polyarthralgia; late disease: monoarthritis-like knee)
  - Iritis, conjunctivitis
  - Migratory musculoskeletal pain
- Late Lyme disease arises months after exposure.
  - Recurrent synovitis
  - Recurrent tendonitis and bursitis
  - Encephalopathic symptoms
    - Severe headaches and neck stiffness
    - *Cognitive slowing*
    - Confusion
    - Profound fatigue
    - Facial palsy
    - Nerve pain

- Symptoms mimicking other CNS diseases
  - Multiple sclerosis–like symptoms
  - Stroke-like symptoms
  - Transverse myelitis
- Peripheral neuropathic symptoms: motor, sensory, or autonomic neuropathies
- Meningitis
- Acrodermatitis chronic atrophicans: fibrosing skin process often involving extremities

PHYSICAL EXAM
- Early Lyme disease
  - EM 70–80%
- Disseminated Lyme disease
  - Multiple EM
  - Facial palsies or other cranial neuropathies
  - Heart block—irregular pulse
  - Pericarditis—friction rub
  - Arthritis
  - Other focal neurologic findings

DIFFERENTIAL DIAGNOSIS
- Other rickettsial disease (Rocky Mountain spotted fever [RMSF])
- Juvenile rheumatoid arthritis (RA); systemic lupus erythematosus (SLE); RA
- Viral syndromes
- Coinfection: ehrlichiosis; babesiosis
- Contact dermatitis; cellulitis; granuloma annulare (mimic EM)
- Syphilis
- AV block
- Malignant neoplastic diseases

DIAGNOSTIC TESTS & INTERPRETATION
Initial Tests (lab, imaging)
- Testing and treatment not indicated if tick attached for <48 hours
- Diagnosis is based mainly on clinical findings in endemic areas (2).
- Serology: enzyme-linked immunosorbent assay (ELISA) for IgM and IgG *B. burgdorferi* antibodies, followed by a Western blot test if positive or equivocal, or an indirect immunofluorescence assay
- Culture of CSF for *B. burgdorferi*
- Plasma polymerase chain reaction (PCR) testing is of little value (only exception is synovial fluid analysis).
- No imaging routinely indicated
- For non-EM presentations: Two-tier serologic testing is recommended, synovial fluid when arthritis is suspected, and CSF analysis when neurologic involvement suspected.
- Tests yet to be validated:
  - Urine antigen capture assays
  - Culture, immunofluorescence staining, or cell sorting of cell wall-deficient or cystic forms of *B. burgdorferi*
  - Lymphocyte transformation tests
  - Quantitative CD57 lymphocyte assays
  - "Reverse Western blots"
  - In-house criteria for interpretation of immunoblots
  - Measurements of antibodies in joint fluid (synovial fluid)
  - IgM or IgG tests without a previous ELISA/EIA/IFA

Follow-Up Tests & Special Considerations
Disorders that may alter lab results: false-positive response with RMSF, syphilis, SLE, and RA
- Arthritis: Serology + PCR of synovial fluid is both sensitive and specific.
- Neuroborreliosis: serology + CSF pleocytosis (PCR of CSF has a very low sensitivity.)

- Late-stage disease with negative serology may be seen in patients receiving early antibiotic treatment.
- After an infection, antibodies may persist for months to years. *Serologic tests do not distinguish active from past infection* (3).
- Antibodies are not protective.

Diagnostic Procedures/Other
Lumbar puncture when neurologic findings are present, with ELISA or CSF for *B. burgdorferi* antibodies (2)

Test Interpretation
Culture of *B. burgdorferi* from blood or skin has low yield.

TREATMENT

GENERAL MEASURES
Early and disseminated Lyme disease can usually be treated as an outpatient except when complicated by carditis or meningitis (requires parenteral antibiotics).

MEDICATION
First Line
- EM (4,5)[A]
  - Doxycycline 100 mg PO BID for 10 to 21 days (do not use in children <8 years old or in pregnant women) (3)[A]; *or*
  - Amoxicillin 500 mg PO TID for 14 to 21 days (pediatric dose 50 mg/kg/day); *or*
  - Cefuroxime axetil 500 mg PO BID for 14 to 21 days
    - Doxycycline has the advantage of covering other tick-borne infections such as ehrlichiosis, anaplasmosis, and RMSF.
    - Alternative: azithromycin 500 mg QD for 7 to 10 days or clarithromycin 500 mg BID for 14 to 21 days
- Neurologic disease
  - Normal CSF, treat for 14 to 21 days.
  - Doxycycline 100 mg PO BID or amoxicillin 500 mg PO TID
  - Abnormal CSF, treat for 4 weeks: ceftriaxone 2 g QD IV, cefotaxime 2 g q8h, *or* penicillin G 5 mIU q6h
  - Cardiac disease
    - Mild (first-degree AV block, PR <300 ms): doxycycline 100 mg PO BID or amoxicillin 500 mg PO TID for 14 to 21 days
    - More serious: ceftriaxone 2 g QD IV for 30 days
- Arthritis without neurologic disease
  - Oral treatment for 28 days with doxycycline 100 mg BID or amoxicillin 500 mg TID
  - If oral treatment fails, repeat oral regimen for 28 days or begin IV treatment with ceftriaxone 2 g QD for 2 to 4 weeks.
- Contraindications
  - Allergy to specific medication
  - Doxycycline is contraindicated in children and in women who are pregnant or breastfeeding.
- Precautions
  - In ~15% of patients treated with IV therapy, a Jarisch-Herxheimer–type reaction develops within 24 hours of initiation of therapy.
- Significant possible interactions:
  - Oral anticoagulants may require dose adjustments.
  - Oral contraceptives may be less effective.

Pediatric Considerations
- Amoxicillin is the drug of choice in children; 50 mg/kg/day PO divided in 3 doses
- Tetracyclines are contraindicated.

Pregnancy Considerations
- Because *B. burgdorferi* can cross the placenta, pregnant patients with active disease should be treated with parenteral antibiotics.
- Doxycycline should not be used in pregnancy.

Second Line
- Azithromycin, 500 mg PO daily for 7 days, can be used for those allergic to β-lactams and unable to take tetracyclines but is less effective (4,5)[A].
- There is no evidence for meaningful clinical benefit from prolonged treatment or retreatment of patients with persistent unexplained symptoms despite previous antibiotic treatment of Lyme disease.

ADMISSION, INPATIENT, AND NURSING CONSIDERATIONS
- Admission is recommended for patients with Lyme carditis and symptoms of chest pain, syncope, or dyspnea and for those with second- or third-degree heart block or first-degree heart block of ≥300 ms.
- Admission is also recommended for patients with symptoms of meningitis.

ONGOING CARE

FOLLOW-UP RECOMMENDATIONS
Patient Monitoring
Based on the severity of symptoms, patients with Lyme carditis, neurologic syndromes, or arthritis may require prolonged follow-up.

DIET
No restrictions

PATIENT EDUCATION
- In endemic areas, patients should be advised to protect themselves against tick exposure.
- Avoid "painting" the tick with nail polish or petroleum jelly, or using heat to make the tick detach from the skin. Remove the tick as quickly as possible.
- Prevention
  - Use repellents that contain 20–30% DEET on exposed skin and clothing for protection lasting several hours.
  - Use 0.5% permethrin on clothing.
  - Bathe or shower as soon as possible after coming indoors (preferably within 2 hours) and perform regular tick checks after outdoor activities.

PROGNOSIS
- Early treatment with antibiotics can shorten the duration of symptoms and prevent later disease.
- Response of late-stage disease to treatment is variable. Symptoms may take weeks to resolve after beginning treatment.
- Untreated rash usually resolves in 3 to 4 weeks.
- Excellent long-term prognosis with early antibiotic treatment
- Neurologic symptoms arise in about 15% of untreated Lyme disease patients.

COMPLICATIONS
- Recurrent synovitis, tendonitis, bursitis
- Chronic neurologic symptoms
- Peripheral neuropathies
- Posttreatment Lyme disease syndrome: 10–20% lingering symptoms of fatigue, pain, or joint and muscle aches; can last for 6 months
- Lyme carditis >40% syncopal presentation

REFERENCES

1. Schwartz AM, Hinckley AF, Mead PS, et al. MMWR surveillance for Lyme disease—United States, 2008–2015. *MMWR Surveill Summ*. 2017;66(22):1–12.
2. Marques A, Telford SR III, Turk SP, et al. Xenodiagnosis to detect *Borrelia burgdorferi* infection: a first-in-human study. *Clin Infect Dis*. 2014;58(7):937–945.
3. Nadelman RB, Hanincová K, Mukherjee P, et al. Differentiation of reinfection from relapse in recurrent Lyme disease. *N Engl J Med*. 2012;367(20):1883–1890.
4. Wormser GP, Dattwyler RJ, Shapiro ED, et al. The clinical assessment, treatment, and prevention of Lyme disease, human granulocytic anaplasmosis, and babesiosis: clinical practice guidelines by the Infectious Diseases Society of America. *Clin Infect Dis*. 2006;43(9):1089–1134.
5. Sanchez E, Vannier E, Wormser GP, et al. Diagnosis, treatment, and prevention of Lyme disease, human granulocytic anaplasmosis, and babesiosis: a review. *JAMA*. 2016;315(16):1767–1777.

ADDITIONAL READING

- Borchers AT, Keen CL, Huntley AC, et al. Lyme disease: a rigorous review of diagnostic criteria and treatment. *J Autoimmun*. 2015;57:82–115.
- Centers for Disease Control and Prevention. *Tickborne Diseases of the United States: A Reference Manual for Health Care Providers*. 4th ed. Atlanta, GA: U.S. Department of Health and Human Services, Centers for Disease Control and Prevention; 2017. https://www.cdc.gov/lyme/resources/tickbornediseases.pdf. Accessed August 25, 2018.
- Centers for Disease Control and Prevention. Tick removal and testing. https://www.cdc.gov/lyme/removal/index.html. Updated May 21, 2018. Accessed September 13, 2018.
- Centers for Disease Control and Prevention. Treatment. https://www.cdc.gov/lyme/treatment/index.html. Accessed August 27, 2018.
- Centers for Disease Control and Prevention. Two-step laboratory testing process. https://www.cdc.gov/lyme/diagnosistesting/labtest/twostep/index.html. Accessed August 26, 2018.

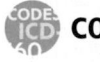

CODES

ICD10
- A69.20 Lyme disease, unspecified
- A69.23 Arthritis due to Lyme disease

CLINICAL PEARLS

- The presence of EM following a tick bite in an endemic area is an indication for empiric antibiotic treatment for presumptive Lyme disease.
- Lyme disease during pregnancy may lead to infection of the placenta and possible stillbirth.
- Ticks must be attached for at least 36 to 48 hours to transmit Lyme disease.
- The Lyme disease vaccine is no longer available.
- Never crush a tick with your fingers. Dispose of a live tick by putting it in alcohol, placing it in a sealed bag/container, wrapping it tightly in tape, or flushing down the toilet.
- Sometimes, EM clears as it enlarges, resulting in a target or "bull's eye" appearance.
- Perform routine tick checks after outdoors activities in endemic areas and remove any attached ticks as quickly as possible.

L

LYMPHANGITIS
Amar Kapur, DO

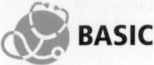 **BASICS**

DESCRIPTION
Acute or chronic inflammation of lymphatic channels; presents as red, tender streaks extending to regional lymph nodes
- May result from compromised lymphatic drainage following surgical procedures
- May be infectious or noninfectious

ETIOLOGY AND PATHOPHYSIOLOGY
- Acute infection
  - Usually caused by group A β-hemolytic *Streptococcus*
  - Less commonly caused by:
    - *Staphylococcus aureus*
    - *Pasteurella multocida*
    - *Erysipelothrix*
    - *Spirillum minus* (rat bite disease)
    - *Pseudomonas*
    - Other *Streptococcus* sp.
    - Immunocompromised patients can be infected with gram-negative rods, gram-negative bacilli, or fungi.
    - In fresh water exposures, *Aeromonas hydrophila*
- Nodular lymphangitis
  - Also known as sporotrichoid lymphangitis
  - Painful or painless nodular subcutaneous swellings along lymphatic vessels
  - Lesions may ulcerate with accompanying regional lymphadenopathy.
  - Typical of infections from: *Sporothrix schenckii*, *Nocardia brasiliensis*, *Mycobacterium marinum*, leishmaniasis, tularemia, and systemic mycoses
  - Pathology may show granulomas.
- Noninfectious granulomatous lymphangitis
  - Rare-acquired lymphedema of the genitalia in children
  - May be due to atypical Crohn disease or sarcoidosis (1)[C]
- Filarial lymphangitis
  - Mosquito bites transmit parasites causing lymphatic inflammation and dilatation; can predispose to secondary bacterial infection
  - Usually caused by nematodes *Wuchereria bancrofti*. Other causes include *Brugia malayi* and *Brugia timori*.
- Lymphangitis can occur after surgical procedures and lymph node dissection.
- Cutaneous lymphangitis carcinomatosa is rare. Represents ~5% of all skin metastases; caused by neoplastic occlusion of dermal lymphatic vessels (2)
- Sclerosing lymphangitis of the penis
  - Swelling around coronal sulcus of penis as a result of vigorous sexual activity or masturbation

RISK FACTORS
- Impaired lymphatic drainage due to surgery, nodal dissection, or irradiation
- Diabetes mellitus
- Chronic steroid use
- Peripheral venous catheter
- Varicella infection
- Immunocompromising condition
- Human, animal, or insect bites; skin trauma
- Fungal, bacterial, or mycobacterial skin infections
- IV drug abuse
- Residence in endemic areas of filariasis

GENERAL PREVENTION
- Reduce chronic lymphedema with compression devices or by treating underlying process.
- Insect repellant; arthropod bite precautions
- Proper wound and skin care

COMMONLY ASSOCIATED CONDITIONS
- Lymphedema
- Prior lymph node dissection
- Tinea pedis (athlete's foot)
- Sporotrichosis
- Cellulitis, erysipelas
- Filarial infection (*W. bancrofti*)

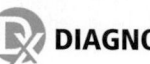 **DIAGNOSIS**

HISTORY
- Trauma to skin, cut, abrasion, or fungal infection
- Systemic symptoms:
  - Malaise
  - Fever and chills
  - Loss of appetite
  - Headache
  - Muscle aches
- Travel to a tropical zone or region with filariasis

PHYSICAL EXAM
Local signs:
- Erythematous, macular linear streaks from site of infection toward regional lymph nodes
- Tenderness and warmth over affected skin or lymph nodes
- Blistering of affected skin
- Fluctuance, swelling, or purulent drainage
- Nodular lymphangitis can present with subcutaneous swellings along the lymphatic channels.
- Sporotrichosis may present with papulonodular lesions that may ulcerate.
- Sites may be painless.

DIFFERENTIAL DIAGNOSIS
- Superficial thrombophlebitis
  - Thrombus or infection within the thrombosis (septic thrombophlebitis)
- Contact dermatitis
- Allergic reaction: less likely to be allergic if >24 hours after exposure (e.g., insect bite)
- Lymphangitis carcinomatosa
- Malignancy-related inflammation

DIAGNOSTIC TESTS & INTERPRETATION
- CBC may show leukocytosis; blood smear may show filarial infection.
- Blood or wound cultures
- Biopsy cultures
- FNAC for filariasis of testiculoscrotal swelling but not for other superficial locations (3)

Initial Tests (lab, imaging)
Plain films are unnecessary; consider lymphangiography for lymphedema (4)[C].

Diagnostic Procedures/Other
- Swab, aspirate, and/or biopsy primary site; purulent discharge; nodule or distal ulcer for culture; acid fast staining; histology; and microscopy
- Blood cultures if systemically ill
- Serology (e.g., *Francisella tularensis*, histoplasma)
- Blood film/smear (e.g., filaria)
- Lymphangiography to determine lymphedema or lymphatic obstruction

 TREATMENT

GENERAL MEASURES
- Hot, moist compresses to affected area
- Compression garments and weight loss may help lymphedema.
- Abstinence from sexual activity (for sclerosing lymphangitis)

MEDICATION
- Treat common organisms empirically. Use culture and susceptibility to guide antibiotic treatment.
- If mild disease, outpatient oral antibiotics
- If no improvement after 48 hours of oral antibiotics, reassess and consider IV antibiotics and/or hospitalization.
- IV antibiotics if systemically ill
- If necrotizing fasciitis is suspected, treat aggressively with antibiotics and surgical intervention.

First Line
Antibiotics for group A streptococcal infection
- Amoxicillin (if known group A *Streptococcus*)
  - Dosing
    - Adults
      - Mild to moderate: 500 mg PO q12h
      - Severe: 875 mg PO q12h or 500 mg PO q8h

- Children <3 months: 30 mg/kg/day PO divided q12h
- Children ≥3 months, ≤40 kg
  - Mild to moderate: 25 mg/kg/day PO divided q12h or 20 mg/kg/day divided q8h
  - Severe: 45 mg/kg/day PO divided q12h or 40 mg/kg/day divided q8h
- Children ≥40 kg same as adult dosing
  - Common adverse effects
    - Diarrhea
  - Serious adverse effects
    - Anaphylaxis, Stevens-Johnson syndrome (SJS), toxic epidermal necrolysis (TEN)
  - Drug interactions
    - Methotrexate, venlafaxine, warfarin, hormonal contraceptives
  - Contraindications
    - Hypersensitivity to penicillin
- Ampicillin/sulbactam
  - Dosing
    - Adults and children ≥40 kg: 1.5 to 3.0 g IV/IM q6h
    - Children <40 kg: 200 mg/kg/day IV infusion, in divided doses q6h; maximum 8 g ampicillin per day
  - Common adverse effects
    - Diarrhea, injection site reactions
  - Serious adverse effects
    - *Clostridium difficile* diarrhea, pseudomembranous enterocolitis
  - Drug interactions
    - Hormonal contraceptives
  - Contraindications
    - Hypersensitivity reactions
- Ceftriaxone
  - Dosing
    - Adults: 1 to 2 g IV/IM q24h
    - Children: 50 to 75 mg/kg/day IV/IM once daily or in divided doses q12h; maximum 2 g/day
  - Common adverse effects
    - Injection site reactions, diarrhea
  - Serious adverse effects
    - Same as amoxicillin or ampicillin
  - Drug interactions
    - Do not administer calcium-containing solutions in the same IV line.
  - Contraindications
    - Hypersensitivity to cephalosporins
    - Concurrent calcium-containing IV fluids
    - Increased risk of kernicterus, salt precipitation in lungs and kidneys in neonates <28 days (use cefotaxime instead)
- Cephalexin
  - Dosing
    - Adults: 500 mg PO q12h
    - Children: 25 to 50 mg/kg/day divided q12h
  - Common adverse effects
    - Diarrhea
  - Serious adverse effects
    - SJS, TEN, interstitial nephritis, renal failure, pseudomembranous enterocolitis, anaphylaxis
  - Contraindications
    - Hypersensitivity to cephalosporins

- Azithromycin (if penicillin or cephalosporin allergy)
  - Dosing
    - Adults: 500 mg PO on day 1 followed by 250 mg/day PO on days 2 to 5
    - Children ≥2 years: 12 mg/kg/day PO (maximum dose: 500 mg/day) once daily for 5 days (FDA off-label use for skin infections in children)
  - Common adverse effects
    - Abdominal pain, nausea, vomiting, diarrhea, headache
  - Serious adverse effects
    - Prolonged QT interval, torsades de pointes, liver failure, Lambert-Eaton syndrome, myasthenia gravis, corneal erosion, anaphylaxis
  - Drug interactions
    - Nelfinavir, warfarin, other medications with potential to prolong QT interval
  - Contraindications
    - Hepatic dysfunction or cholestatic jaundice with prior treatment
    - Hypersensitivity to macrolide (azithromycin, erythromycin, clarithromycin)
- Diethylcarbamazine, ivermectin, albendazole, and doxycycline are used to treat filarial infection.
- Acetaminophen or ibuprofen (NSAIDs) for pain and fever

SURGERY/OTHER PROCEDURES
- Incision and drainage of abscess if present
- Necrotizing fasciitis requires surgical evaluation and likely débridement.
- Nodular lymphangitis may benefit from I&D.

ADMISSION, INPATIENT, AND NURSING CONSIDERATIONS
- Admit for signs of serious illness: fluids if in hypotensive shock.
- Fever, chills, systemic toxicity
- IV antibiotics, ICU, or surgery as indicated
- Discharge on oral antibiotics after systemic symptoms resolve. Home IV antibiotics are an option depending on clinical setting.

 ONGOING CARE

FOLLOW-UP RECOMMENDATIONS
- Elevate affected area.
- 48-hour follow-up to ensure improvement
- Work up recurrent lymphangitis to ascertain underlying cause (other infectious organism, anatomic abnormality, etc.).

Patient Monitoring
Close follow-up to ensure decreasing inflammation

PATIENT EDUCATION
Instruct patients on proper wound and skin care.

PROGNOSIS
- Good prognosis for uncomplicated cases
- Antimicrobial therapy is effective in 90% of patients.
- Untreated, can spread rapidly, especially group A *Streptococcus*

COMPLICATIONS
Sepsis, cellulitis, necrotizing fasciitis, myositis

REFERENCES
1. Taylor MJ, Hoerauf A, Bockarie M. Lymphatic filariasis and onchocerciasis. *Lancet*. 2010;376(9747):1175–1185.
2. Prat L, Chouaid C, Kettaneh A, et al. Cutaneous lymphangitis carcinomatosa in a patient with lung adenocarcinoma: case report and literature review. *Lung Cancer*. 2013;79(1):91–93.
3. Khare P, Kala P, Jha A, et al. Incidental diagnosis of filariasis in superficial location by FNAC: a retrospective study of 10 years. *J Clin Diagn Res*. 2014;8(12):FC05–FC08.
4. Falagas ME, Bliziotis IA, Kapaskelis AM. Red streaks on the leg. Lymphangitis. *Am Fam Physician*. 2006;73(6):1061–1062.

ADDITIONAL READING
- Babu AK, Krishnan P, Andezuth DD. Sclerosing lymphangitis of penis—literature review and report of 2 cases. *Dermatol Online J*. 2014;20(7):13030/qt7gq9h1v9.
- Cohen BE, Nagler AR, Pomeranz MK. Nonbacterial causes of lymphangitis with streaking. *J Am Board Fam Med*. 2016;29(6):808–812.
- Raja A, Seshadri RA, Sundersingh S. Lymphangitis carcinomatosa: report of a case and review of literature. *Indian J Surg Oncol*. 2010;1(3):274–276.

 CODES

ICD10
- I89.1 Lymphangitis
- L03.91 Acute lymphangitis, unspecified
- N48.29 Other inflammatory disorders of penis

CLINICAL PEARLS
- Lymphangitis classically presents with erythematous linear streaks of the skin from site of entry (e.g., bite, cut, abrasion) to regional lymph nodes.
- Patients with prior surgical lymph node dissection are predisposed to lymphangitis.
- Patients with severe systemic symptoms should be admitted for treatment with IV antibiotics.
- Parasitic or fungal infections can cause acute or chronic lymphangitis.
- Treatment of underlying skin infection (such as tinea pedis) may prevent recurrence.

L

LYMPHEDEMA

Khalid Bashir, MD • Jon S. Parham, DO, MPH, FAAFP

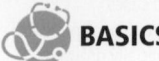 BASICS

DESCRIPTION
- Accumulation of lymphatic fluid in the interstitial tissue causing swelling
- Lymphedema can develop when lymphatic vessels are missing or impaired (primary) or when lymph vessels are damaged or lymph nodes are removed (secondary).
- Most common in the lower limb(s) (80%) but also can occur in the arm(s), face, trunk, and external genitalia

EPIDEMIOLOGY

Incidence
- Predominant sex: female > male
- Predominant age: any age
- 13% of patients with breast cancer treated with surgery; 42% of those treated with surgery and radiation therapy; 25% after GYN cancer surgery
- Milroy disease presents at birth; estimated to be between 1/6,000 and 1/300 live births
- Meige disease develops during puberty.

Prevalence
- 120 million people worldwide are affected with lymphatic filariasis in 73 countries but no primary infections in United States.
- 10 million people are affected by nonfilarial secondary lymphedema in the United States.

ETIOLOGY AND PATHOPHYSIOLOGY
Secondary lymphedema:
- Postoperative: gradual failure of distal lymphatics, which have to "pump" lymph at a greater pressure through damaged proximal ducts
- Risk is higher with postoperative radiation because radiation reduces regrowth of ducts due to fibrous scarring.
- Trauma; recurrent infection; malignancy, including metastatic disease, and marked obesity
- Lymphangiogenesis inhibition and tissue fibrosis promotion by T cells appear to promote lymphedema.
- Developing countries: Most common cause is filariasis (*Wuchereria bancrofti*).

Genetics
- Milroy disease: autosomal dominant; diagnosed either at birth or the 1st year of life
- Lymphedema praecox has onset between the ages of 1 and 35 years.
- Lymphedema tarda occurs in those >35 years of age.
- Genetics referral: primary and lymphedema tarda

RISK FACTORS
- Filariasis: most common cause worldwide
- Mastectomy, melanoma surgery
- Prior trauma, serious burns, infection of affected limb
- Lymphadenectomy or radiation therapy for malignancy

- Obesity (>50 body mass index)
- Inflammatory disorders: arthritis, sarcoidosis, dermatitis

GENERAL PREVENTION
Healthy body weight maintenance; treatment of congestive heart failure (CHF), early recognition of infection and cancer, and venous insufficiency

COMMONLY ASSOCIATED CONDITIONS
Venous disease, morbid obesity, regional cancer, filarial disease (Africa and Asia)

DIAGNOSIS

HISTORY
Recent surgery: Vein stripping can significantly exacerbate mild lymphedema:
- First symptom: painless swelling
- Feeling of heaviness in the limb, especially at the end of the day and in hot weather

> **ALERT**
> After 1st year, edema becomes nonpitting.

PHYSICAL EXAM
- Initial: pitting edema, can spread proximally or distally
- Later: nonpitting; after 1st year, does not spread proximally/distally, but spreads radially
- Hyperkeratosis (thicker skin)
- Papillomatosis (rough skin)
- Increase in skin turgor
- Positive Stemmer sign (inability to pinch the skin of the dorsum of the second toe between the thumb and forefinger), false positives are rare.

DIFFERENTIAL DIAGNOSIS
- CHF, renal failure, lipedema
- Hypoalbuminemia, protein-losing nephropathy
- DVT, chronic venous disease
- Postoperative complications following ipsilateral surgery
- Cellulitis, Baker cyst, idiopathic edema

DIAGNOSTIC TESTS & INTERPRETATION
- Lack of response to elevation or diuretic therapy may indicate a lymphatic insufficiency.
- Diuretics increase excretion of salt and water, thereby decreasing plasma volume, venous capillary pressure, and filtration. Diuretics improve filtration edema but do not improve lymph drainage over the long term.
- Some relevant protein biomarkers for lymphedema have been identified and show promise for early- and latent-stage diagnosis.

Initial Tests (lab, imaging)
- Comprehensive chemistry panel: hepatic or renal impairment
- TSH: hypothyroidism
- Urinalysis: protein-losing nephropathy

- Ultrasound: evaluates for acute/chronic DVT; gives information about soft tissue changes but does not inform about truncal anatomy of the lymphatics
- Duplex ultrasound: Lymphedema causes gradual impedance of venous return that aggravates the edema; 82% of patients with unexplained limb edema were diagnosed using a combination of duplex ultrasound and lymphoscintigram.

Follow-Up Tests & Special Considerations
- Lymphangiogram: direct cannulation of lymphatics through the skin; risk for infection, local inflammation; rarely used now
- Fluorescence microlymphography may be highly sensitive (91.4%) and specific (85.7%), atraumatic, and is without radiation in diagnosis of leg lymphedema.
- Lymphoscintigram: radiolabeled protein technetium-99m–labeled colloid
  - Measures lymphatic function, lymph movement, lymph drainage, and response to treatment
  - Sensitivity, 73–97%; specificity, 100%
  - Best to use 1 hour and delayed images together
- Indocyanine green lymphography: reported
  - Superior to lymphoscintigraphy in early diagnosis of arm
  - Accurately screens postsurgically for subclinical lymphedema (1)[B]
- CT scan: calf skin thickening, thickening of the SC compartment, increased fat density, thickened perimuscular aponeurosis; typical honeycomb appearance
- MRI: circumferential edema, increased volume of SC tissue, honeycomb pattern above the fascia between the muscle and subcutis; cannot differentiate primary from secondary lymphedema

TREATMENT

GENERAL MEASURES
- Seek optimal weight; early treatment of cellulitis; avoid trauma to affected area (direct injury, venipunctures, inept nail care, extreme heat/cold).
- Achieve mechanical reduction and maintenance of limb size: compression garments via professionals.
- Elevate affected limb/area, but avoid stasis.
- Avoid BP cuffs and other focal constriction in affected limbs.
- Prevent skin infection with daily cleansing, inspection, and skin care (with emollients).
- Nonsurgical treatment of varicose veins in some
- Doubtful that air travel is associated with increased limb volumes

MEDICATION

> **ALERT**
> No medications, including diuretics, are useful.

ISSUES FOR REFERRAL

- Refer to physical therapist with lymphedema training for manual decongestive therapy.
  – In patients with recurrent or metastatic disease, discuss with oncologist prior to initiation of complete decongestive therapy in order not to promote the spread of cancer.
- Provide education for patient/family for self-administration of therapy in future.
- Education for family about bandaging
- Fitting for compression garments (2)[A]

ADDITIONAL THERAPIES

- Exercise: Lymph flow occurs as a result of inspiratory reduction in the intrathoracic pressure associated with inspiration. Best results are achieved with combination of flexibility, strength, and aerobic training.
- Compression with custom-made elastic stocking (minimum pressure is 40 mm Hg)
  – Protection against external incidental trauma
  – Decreases the intrinsic trauma on the skin due to chronically increased interstitial pressures, which cause stretch of the skin and SC tissues
  – No data on preference of custom made versus prefabricated
  – Replace every 3 to 6 months or when starting to lose elasticity.
- Multilayer bandaging: inner layer of tubular stockinette followed by foam and padding to protect the joint flexures and to even out the contours of the limb so that pressure is distributed evenly; outer layer of at least two short-stretch extensible bandages; more effective than hosiery alone
- Pneumatic pumps develop high pressures like systolic BP and can reduce limb girth significantly; wear a compression sock afterward (2)[A].
- Advanced pneumatic compression devices (APCDs) are programmable, offer a more individualized fit, reduced rates of cellulitis by at least 75%, and reduce early treatment costs by 37–54% depending on health care setting (3)[B].

SURGERY/OTHER PROCEDURES

- Bypass procedures: Creation of lymphatic–venous anastomosis or lymph node transplantation (most effective) via microsurgery showed a reduction in use of conservative compression therapy (4)[C]: reserved for refractory cases only
- Low-level laser therapy in smaller studies was shown to be noninferior to manual lymphatic drainage or in combination in arm volume reduction among breast cancer patients in half the treatment time (4)[C].
- Axillary reverse mapping during axillary node dissection in selected preclinical breast cancer can significantly reduce lymphedema incidence (5)[A].
- Thoracic sympathetic ganglion block for breast cancer–related lymphedema, a new treatment showed better life quality and arm size reduction >50%, especially in patients with high-grade lymphedema.
- Debulking procedures (Charles procedure): radical excision of SC tissue with primary or staged skin grafting
  – Men had less improvement than women.
  – Main risk is infection and necrosis of the skin graft.
  – Liposuction is cosmetically preferred to debulking (4)[C].

COMPLEMENTARY & ALTERNATIVE MEDICINE

- Heat therapy: Microwave and electromagnetic irradiation may be helpful.
- Selenium ingestion has been reported to reduce lymphedema volume (not approved indication in United States).
- Benzopyrene oral medicine (flavonoids and coumarin; neither are approved in the United States)
  – Flavonoids: Micronized purified flavonoid fraction (Daflon 500 mg) reported to decrease venous stasis and idiopathic cyclic edema, chronic venous insufficiency, and postmastectomy lymphedema.
  – Coumarin reduces edema fluid by increasing the number of macrophages and enhancing proteolysis, resulting in the removal of protein, some reports of bleeding, and hepatotoxicity (4)[C].

ADMISSION, INPATIENT, AND NURSING CONSIDERATIONS

- Systemic signs of infection
  – May admit to specialized rehabilitation unit for combination treatment in patients with heart failure or severe pulmonary disease
  – IV antibiotics for infection; cellulitis is most common.
- Affected extremity positioning with some distal elevation
- Encourage patient mobilization/exercise.
- Patient education for bandaging/wound care
- Discharge criteria
  – Improved signs/symptoms of infection (e.g., elevated WBC count, fever, abnormal vital signs)
  – Clinical improvement in wound appearance

 ## ONGOING CARE

FOLLOW-UP RECOMMENDATIONS

Lymphedema will return in several days if patient stops wearing compression garments during the day and bandaging at night.

Patient Monitoring
- Daily visit to therapist for acute treatment
- Monthly visits for maintenance care

DIET
Lower sodium, healthy protein, and weight loss-oriented (if needed)

PATIENT EDUCATION
- Use compression garments, especially when exercising.
- Avoid affected limb(s) being dependent for long period of time: Patient should perform daily skin examination.
- http://www.nlm.nih.gov/medlineplus/lymphedema.html

PROGNOSIS
No cure, but treatment can produce good results with daily care.

COMPLICATIONS
- Infection (local vs. systemic): common
- Risk of wound formation (punctures/abrasions) that are difficult to heal: common
- Lymphangiosarcoma: found in lymphedematous arms of patients following radical mastectomy, also in patients with Milroy disease. Treatment is radiotherapy with surgery; reserved for patients with discrete nonmetastatic disease.

REFERENCES

1. Keo HH, Husmann M, Groechenig E, et al. Diagnostic accuracy of fluorescence microlymphography for detecting limb lymphedema. *Eur J Vasc Endovasc Surg*. 2015;49(4):474–479.
2. Rogan S, Taeymans J, Luginbuehl H, et al. Therapy modalities to reduce lymphoedema in female breast cancer patients: a systematic review and meta-analysis. *Breast Cancer Res Treat*. 2016;159(1):1–14.
3. Karaca-Mandic P, Hirsch AT, Rockson SG, et al. The cutaneous, net clinical, and health economic benefits of advanced pneumatic compression devices in patients with lymphedema. *JAMA Dermatol*. 2015;151(11):1187–1193.
4. Merchant SJ, Chen SL. Prevention and management of lymphedema after breast cancer treatment. *Breast J*. 2015;21(3):276–284.
5. Han C, Yang B, Zuo W-S, et al. The feasibility and oncological safety of axillary reverse mapping in patients with breast cancer: a systematic review and meta-analysis of prospective studies. *PLoS One*. 2016;11(2):e0150285.

ADDITIONAL READING

- Choi E, Nahm FS, Lee PB. Sympathetic block as a new treatment for lymphedema. *Pain Physician*. 2015;18(4):365–372.
- Gardenier JC, Kataru RP, Hespe GE, et al. Topical tacrolimus for the treatment of secondary lymphedema. *Nat Commun*. 2017;8:14345.
- Yen TWF, Laud PW, Sparapani RA, et al. An algorithm to identify the development of lymphedema after breast cancer treatment. *J Cancer Surviv*. 2015;9(2):161–171.

 ## CODES

ICD10
- I89.0 Lymphedema, not elsewhere classified
- Q82.0 Hereditary lymphedema
- I97.89 Oth postproc comp and disorders of the circ sys, NEC

CLINICAL PEARLS

- Refer primary lymphedema and lymphedema tarda to genetics.
- Affected skin with heavy feeling, painless swelling initially, later nonpitting swelling
- Rule out DVT if unilateral limb or CHF if bilateral.
- Early referral to lymphedema therapist for manual therapy, compression devices/wrappings
- Aggressive weight loss and health promotion as needed
- High risk for cutaneous-sourced infections, so promote therapeutic skin care.
- Lymphoscintigram is standard diagnostic if clinically diagnosis is uncertain.

L

MACULAR DEGENERATION, AGE-RELATED

Richard W. Allinson, MD

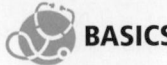 **BASICS**

DESCRIPTION
- Age-related macular degeneration (ARMD) is the leading cause of irreversible, severe visual loss in persons age >65 years.
- ARMD results in pigmentary changes in the macula or typical drusen associated with visual loss to the 20/30 level or worse, not caused by cataract or other eye disease, in individuals >50 years of age, although some definitions exclude age or visual acuity criteria.
- Stages
  - Atrophic/nonexudative
  - Neovascular/exudative
- System(s) affected: nervous
- Synonym(s): senile macular degeneration; subretinal neovascularization (SRN)

EPIDEMIOLOGY
- Neovascular/exudative form is rare in blacks and more common in whites.
- Predominant sex: female

Incidence
- In the Framingham Eye Study (FES), drusen were noted in 25% of all participants who were ≥52 years of age. ARMD-associated visual loss was noted in 5.7%.
- Atrophic/nonexudative stage accounts for 20% of cases of severe visual loss.
- Neovascular/exudative stage accounts for 80% of cases of severe visual loss.

Prevalence
Per FES study:
- People 65 to 74 years old: 11%
- People ≥75 years old: 27.9%

ETIOLOGY AND PATHOPHYSIOLOGY
- Breaks in the Bruch membrane allow choroidal neovascular membranes (CNVMs) to invade the retinal pigment epithelium (RPE) and grow into the subretinal space.
- Atrophic/nonexudative: drusen and/or pigmentary changes in the macula
- Neovascular/exudative: growth of blood vessels underneath the retina
  - Polypoidal choroidal vasculopathy is a subtype of exudative ARMD.
- Visible light can result in the formation and accumulation of metabolic by-products in the RPE, a pigment layer underneath the retina that normally helps remove metabolic by-products from the retina. Excess accumulation of these metabolic by-products interferes with the normal metabolic activity of the RPE and can lead to the formation of drusen.
- Neovascular stage generally arises from the atrophic stage.
- Most do not progress beyond the atrophic/nonexudative stage; however, those who do are at a greater risk of severe visual loss.

Genetics
- Genetic susceptibility may be a factor in ARMD: ~25% genetically determined
- Complement factor H is an important susceptibility gene for ARMD.
- Although the development of ARMD may be predicted by specific alleles, the clinical response to antivascular endothelial growth factor (VEGF) is not.

RISK FACTORS
- Obesity
- Ethnicity: non-Hispanic whites
- Cigarette smoking
- *Chlamydia pneumoniae* infection
- Family history
- Excess sunlight exposure
- Blue or light iris color
- Hyperopia
- History of cardiovascular disease
- Short stature
- High plasma high-density lipoprotein cholesterol levels are associated with an increased risk for ARMD.
- Physical activity is associated with lower risk of early and late ARMD in white populations.
- Aspirin use
- Female sex

GENERAL PREVENTION
- Ultraviolet (UV) protection for eyes
- Routine ophthalmologic visits
  - Every 2 to 4 years for patients age 40 to 64 years
  - Every 1 to 2 years after age 65 years
- Patients who take statins, which modify lipid profiles, may have a reduced risk.

COMMONLY ASSOCIATED CONDITIONS
- Presumed ocular histoplasmosis syndrome
- Exudative retinal detachment
- Vitreous hemorrhage
- Other causes of CNVMs

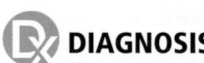 **DIAGNOSIS**

HISTORY
- Patients frequently notice distortion of central vision.
- Patients may notice straight lines appear crooked (e.g., telephone poles).

PHYSICAL EXAM
- Atrophic/nonexudative stage retinal exam
  - Drusen (small yellowish white lesions)
    - Subtypes: hard drusen and soft drusen
  - Atrophy of the RPE
    - When the area of absent or attenuated RPE is contiguous, the condition is termed geographic atrophy (GA) of the RPE.
- Neovascular/exudative stage retinal exam
  - Blood vessels growing underneath the retina from the choroid are called *CNVMs* or SRN. The choroid is the vascular layer underneath the RPE.
  - Subretinal fluid or hemorrhage
  - Exudates
  - On Amsler grid testing, the horizontal or vertical lines may become broken, distorted, or missing.
- Disciform scar: an advanced stage resulting in a fibrovascular scar

DIFFERENTIAL DIAGNOSIS
- Idiopathic SRN
- Presumed ocular histoplasmosis syndrome
- Diabetic retinopathy
- Hypertensive retinopathy
- Central serous chorioretinopathy
- Topiramate can cause a macular neurosensory retinal detachment.

DIAGNOSTIC TESTS & INTERPRETATION
Diagnostic Procedures/Other
- Amsler grid testing
- Fluorescein angiography
  - Detection of CNVMs
  - Differentiates between atrophic and neovascular ARMD
- Indocyanine green video angiography: may identify occult or hidden CNVMs
- Optical coherence tomography (OCT) is useful in determining the presence of subretinal fluid, the degree of retinal thickening, and the presence of a pigment epithelial detachment (PED).
  - Newer generation OCT modalities, including spectral domain OCT (SD-OCT) and OCT angiography (OCTA) are preferred for evaluating ARMD.
  - OCT visualized anatomic subtypes of neovascularization include type 1 (sub-RPE), type 2 (subretinal), and type 3 (intraretinal vascular proliferation).

Test Interpretation
Drusen: deposits of hyaline material between the RPE and Bruch membrane (the limiting membrane between the RPE and the choroid)

 **TREATMENT**

GENERAL MEASURES
Low-vision aids may be helpful.

MEDICATION
First Line
- Ranibizumab (Lucentis)
  - Antibody fragment that inhibits all active forms of VEGF
  - Approved for neovascular (wet) ARMD
  - Injected intravitreally, at a dose of 0.5 mg, every 4 weeks
  - 1 year after treatment, up to 40% of patients treated with ranibizumab gained at least three lines of vision, and ~95% maintained vision.
  - Ranibizumab is superior to verteporfin in the treatment of predominately classic CNVMs.
  - The PrONTO study demonstrated OCT-guided, variable-dosing regimen with ranibizumab resulted in similar results to the MARINA (minimally classic/occult CNVM trial) and ANCHOR (predominantly classic CNVM trial) studies with monthly injections of ranibizumab.
  - When comparing ranibizumab and bevacizumab in a multicenter study, both treatments were effective in stabilizing visual loss, and no difference was found in the visual outcome between the two treatment groups. A slightly higher rate of serious systemic adverse events was noted in the bevacizumab group.
    - In this study, treatment as needed resulted in less gain in visual acuity, whether instituted at enrollment or after 1 year of monthly treatment.
    - Visual gains during the first 2 years were not maintained at 5 years. At the 5-year visit, 50% of eyes had vision of 20/40 or better and 20% had vision of 20/200 or worse (1)[A].
    - Cystoid macular edema is a marker for poorer visual outcomes in patients with CNVMs.
  - Eyes with ≥50% of the lesion composed of blood had a similar visual prognosis compared to other treated eyes in the Comparison of Age-related Macular Degeneration Treatments Trials (CATT). Neovascular ARMD lesions composed of >50% blood can be managed similarly to those with less or no blood.

– The treat and extend regimen (TER) is commonly used to decrease the treatment burden. Once no signs of CNVM activity are detected, patient follow-ups and treatments are then extended by intervals of 2 weeks as long as no signs of CNVM activity are present, up to a maximum interval of 12 weeks. If examination shows any sign of recurrence, the interval is shortened by 2 weeks at a time, until the disease is considered to be inactive. Interval extension is then restarted, with the maximum final interval being 2 weeks less than the period when the previous recurrence was observed.

– Ranibizumab and bevacizumab had equivalent effects on visual acuity at 1 year using the TER. The visual acuity results at 1 year were comparable to those of other clinical trials with monthly treatment.

- VEGF Trap-Eye/aflibercept (Eylea)

– A decoy VEGF receptor that inhibits all isoforms of VEGF-A and placental growth factor (PGF), the members of the VEGF family in mammals primarily involved in ocular neovascularization

– Approved for neovascular (wet) ARMD

– Injected intravitreally, at a dose of 2 mg, every 4 weeks for 12 weeks and then every 8 weeks

– Dosed as needed after the 12-week fixed dosing schedule resulted in a 5.3-letter gain in best corrected visual acuity at 52 weeks.

– Routine use of prophylactic antibiotics after intravitreal injections (IVIs) may be unnecessary.

– May be beneficial in patients who are not responding to ranibizumab or bevacizumab

– Anti-VEGF treatment with either ranibizumab or aflibercept showed limited efficacy for the complete resolution of PED.

  o Patients with a PED tend to have worse outcomes when switched from a fixed regimen to a PRN strategy.

  o Patients with PEDs and intraretinal cysts have a worse visual prognosis.

  o PEDs treated with aflibercept showed a better anatomical response than eyes treated with ranibizumab, but the visual outcomes were the same.

Second Line

- Bevacizumab (Avastin) is a full-length antibody to VEGF, administered intravitreally at a dose of 1.25 mg; widely used off-label because of its lower cost

- Brolucizumab is being investigated. It is a humanized single-chain antibody fragment that inhibits all isoforms of VEGF-A. It is the smallest of the anti-VEGF antibodies. A 12-week treatment cycle may be a viable option, which would help reduce the frequency of IVIs (2)[B].

- Fovista, a platelet-derived growth factor (PDGF) antagonist, when administered in combination with ranibizumab demonstrated more favorable outcomes compared with ranibizumab monotherapy. This drug is not U.S. Food and Drug Administration (FDA)-approved (3)[B].

- No FDA-approved stem cell therapies for retinal disease exist.

SURGERY/OTHER PROCEDURES

- Laser treatment for CNVMs located ≥200 microns from the center of the macula has been evaluated in the Macular Photocoagulation Study (MPS).

– Anti-VEGF treatment is first-line therapy for subfoveal CNVMs.

- Vitrectomy has been used to remove CNVMs, but this is generally not recommended.

- CNVMs can bleed spontaneously, leaving blood underneath the retina. Vitrectomy to remove subretinal blood may be of benefit and should be performed within 7 days of the bleed. Tissue plasminogen activator (tPA) instilled into the eye may help remove a subretinal hemorrhage. In some cases, intravitreal gas with or without tPA may displace submacular blood:

– Intravitreal anti-VEGF monotherapy may be helpful in the treatment of neovascular ARMD associated with a submacular hemorrhage.

- Photodynamic therapy (PDT) with verteporfin is not frequently used anymore.

– Patients should be informed of a <4% risk of acute, severe vision loss after PDT.

– Ranibizumab has greater clinical efficacy than PDT.

– Combination treatment with intravitreal ranibizumab and PDT appears to offer similar gain in visual acuity when compared with ranibizumab monotherapy.

– Combination treatment with ranibizumab and PDT may reduce the number of ranibizumab retreatments.

COMPLEMENTARY & ALTERNATIVE MEDICINE

Free radical formation in the retina, induced by visible light, may play a role in cellular damage that results in atrophic/nonexudative macular degeneration. The Age-Related Eye Disease Study (AREDS) found that a high-dose regimen of antioxidant vitamins and mineral supplements reduced progression of ARMD in some cases.

- Recommended daily doses: vitamin C 500 mg, vitamin E 400 IU, β-carotene 15 mg, zinc oxide 80 mg, and cupric oxide 2 mg

– Exercise caution with β-carotene use in smokers due to potential link to lung cancer.

- The AREDS2 found the addition of lutein with zeaxanthin alone or in combination with omega-3 fatty acids had no overall effect in further reducing the risk of progression to advanced ARMD.

ONGOING CARE

FOLLOW-UP RECOMMENDATIONS
Patient Monitoring

- Amsler grid can aid in discovering visual disturbances.

- Patients with soft drusen or pigmentary changes in the macula are at an increased risk of visual loss. They should monitor their vision, such as by daily Amsler grid testing, and subjective measures of visual acuity, such as reading ability; if no new symptoms, follow-up examination in 6 to 12 months

DIET

- Eating dark green, leafy vegetables (spinach/collard greens), which are rich in carotenoids, may decrease the risk of developing the neovascular/exudative stage.

- Fish consumption with omega-3 fatty acid intake reduces the risk of ARMD.

- A Western-type diet characterized by higher intake of red meat, processed meat, high-fat dairy products, French fries, refined grains, and eggs increases the risk of ARMD as compared to an Oriental-type diet characterized by higher intake of vegetables, legumes, fruit, whole grains, tomatoes, and seafood which decreases the risk of ARMD.

– A Mediterranean diet may reduce the risk of developing ARMD.

PATIENT EDUCATION

Instruct visually impaired patients to check with the local low-vision center for aids.

PROGNOSIS

- Patients with bilateral soft drusen and pigmentary changes in the macula, but no evidence of exudation, have an increased likelihood of developing CNVMs and subsequent visual loss.

- Patients with bilateral drusen carry a cumulative risk of 14.7% over 5 years of suffering significant visual loss in one eye from the neovascular stage of ARMD.

- Patients with neovascular stage in one eye and drusen in the opposite eye are at an annual risk of 5–14% of developing the neovascular stage in the opposite eye with drusen.

- Macular atrophy progression and severity were the primary anatomic determinants of visual outcomes 7 years after treatment with ranibizumab.

- High incidence of recurrence after thermal laser treatment for CNVMs

COMPLICATIONS

- Blindness

- The intraocular pressure should be monitored in eyes receiving intravitreal anti-VEGF injections.

– Seven or more IVI of bevacizumab annually is associated with a higher risk of glaucoma surgery compared to less frequent administration (4)[B].

REFERENCES

1. Maguire MG, Martin DF, Ying GS, et al; for Comparison of Age-related Macular Degeneration Treatments Trials (CATT) Research Group. Five-year outcomes with anti-vascular endothelial growth factor treatment of neovascular age-related macular degeneration: the comparison of age-related macular degeneration treatments trials. *Ophthalmology.* 2016;123(8):1751–1761.

2. Dugel PU, Jaffe GJ, Sallstig P, et al. Brolucizumab versus aflibercept in participants with neovascular age-related macular degeneration: a randomized trial. *Ophthalmology.* 2017;124(9):1296–1304.

3. Jaffe GJ, Ciulla TA, Ciardella AP, et al. Dual antagonism of PDGF and VEGF in neovascular age-related macular degeneration: a phase IIb, multicenter, randomized controlled trial. *Ophthalmology.* 2017;124(2):224–234.

4. Eadie BD, Etminan M, Carleton BC, et al. Association of repeated intravitreous bevacizumab injections with risk for glaucoma surgery. *JAMA Ophthalmol.* 2017;135(4):363–368.

CODES

ICD10

- H35.30 Unspecified macular degeneration
- H35.32 Exudative age-related macular degeneration
- H35.31 Nonexudative age-related macular degeneration

CLINICAL PEARLS

- Patients frequently notice distortion of central vision.

- Patients may notice straight lines appear crooked (e.g., telephone poles).

- Hyperopia is a risk factor for ARMD.

- The AREDS found that a high-dose regimen of antioxidant vitamins and mineral supplements reduces progression of ARMD in some cases.

- Tobacco cessation should be strongly encouraged.

M

MALARIA

Kathrine R. Tan, MD, MPH

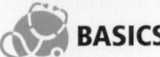 **BASICS**

DESCRIPTION

- Acute or chronic infection transmitted to humans by *Anopheles* spp. mosquitoes
- Most morbidity and mortality is caused by *Plasmodium falciparum*. An estimated 216 million cases occur annually, including 445,000 deaths, most of which occur in children <5 years in sub-Saharan Africa (1).
- Nonimmune individuals are most susceptible to rapid progression to severe disease.
- System(s) affected: cardiovascular, hematologic, renal, respiratory, cerebral, lymphatic, immunologic

EPIDEMIOLOGY

- Cases imported to the United States: 67% *P. falciparum*; 12% *Plasmodium vivax*; 3% *Plasmodium malariae*; 4% *Plasmodium ovale*; 1% mixed; 13% unknown
- Occurs worldwide in tropical latitudes: *P. falciparum*, *P. malariae*, *P. vivax*, and *P. ovale*; *Plasmodium knowlesi* in parts of Southeast Asia

Incidence

- Most U.S. cases (>99%) are imported.
- ~1,700 cases and 5 deaths per year in the United States (2)

Prevalence

- Predominant age: all ages
- Predominant sex: male = female

ETIOLOGY AND PATHOPHYSIOLOGY

- Malarial parasites digest red blood cell (RBC) proteins and alter the RBC membrane, causing hemolysis, increased splenic clearance, and anemia.
- RBC lysis stimulates release of cytokines and tumor necrosis factor (TNF-α) causing fever and systemic symptoms.
- *P. falciparum* alters RBC viscosity, causing obstruction and end-organ ischemia.

Genetics

Unknown genetic predilection, but inherited conditions may affect disease severity and susceptibility (glucose-6-phosphate dehydrogenase deficiency, sickle cell disease or trait, and hereditary elliptocytosis).

RISK FACTORS

- Travel to or migration from endemic areas (primarily sub-Saharan Africa)
- Rarely, blood transfusion, mother-to-fetus transmission, and local autochthonous transmission

GENERAL PREVENTION

- Mosquito avoidance: Use insect repellent, wear clothing to cover exposed skin, use mosquito nets treated with permethrin, and avoid outdoor activity from dusk to dawn.
- *Malarial chemoprophylaxis when in endemic area*
  - Mefloquine: Begin at least 2 weeks before arrival and continue for 4 weeks after leaving area. Adults, 250 mg (1 tablet) weekly; children ≤9 kg, 5 mg/kg; children >9 to 19 kg, 1/4 tablet weekly; children >19 to 30 kg, 1/2 tablet weekly; children >30 to 45 kg, 3/4 tablet weekly; children >45 kg as adult dosing
    - Caution: mefloquine-resistant areas; don't use if history of psychiatric disorders.

- Atovaquone/proguanil: Begin 1 to 2 days before arrival and continue for 1 week after leaving area. Adults, 1 adult tablet daily; children 5 to 8 kg, 1/2 pediatric tablet daily; children 9 to 10 kg, 3/4 pediatric tablet daily; children 11 to 20 kg, 1 pediatric tablet daily; children 21 to 30 kg, 2 pediatric tablets daily; children 31 to 40 kg, 3 pediatric tablets daily; children >40 kg, 1 adult tablet daily
- Doxycycline: Begin 1 to 2 days before arrival and continue for 4 weeks after leaving area. Adults, 100 mg daily; children, 2 mg/kg up to 100 mg daily (not for children <8 years old)
- Chloroquine: Begin 1 to 2 weeks before arrival and continue for 4 weeks after leaving area. Adults, 500 mg (300-mg base) weekly; children, 8.3 mg/kg (5-mg base/kg) weekly up to 300 mg
  - Caution: chloroquine-resistant areas
- Primaquine: Begin 1 to 2 days before arrival and continue for 1 week after leaving area; adults, 30 mg/day; children, 0.5 mg/kg/day up to adult dose
  - For use only in areas predominantly endemic for *P. vivax*
  - Caution: Glucose-6-phosphate dehydrogenase deficiency must be excluded prior to first use.
- Tafenoquine: Take daily 3 days before arrival, weekly during travel, and 1 week after leaving area; adults 200 mg per dose
  - Caution: Glucose-6-phosphate dehydrogenase deficiency must be excluded prior to first use, don't use if history of psychotic disorders.

COMMONLY ASSOCIATED CONDITIONS

Bacterial coinfections sometimes occur.

 DIAGNOSIS

HISTORY

- Initial malaria symptoms are nonspecific. Suspect malaria in ill patients returning from endemic area with:
  - Fever, malaise, myalgias, chills, headache, nausea, splenomegaly (with chronic infection), hypotension, anemia (with chronic or severe disease), thrombocytopenia, jaundice, vomiting, and/or diarrhea (resembling gastroenteritis)
- *P. falciparum*
  - Incubation usually 12 to 14 days, symptoms within 1 month of infection in most individuals (Partially immune individuals such as immigrants may become ill up to 1 year after last exposure.)
  - Severe disease and complications: vascular collapse, CNS impairment, renal failure, and acute respiratory distress syndrome
- *P. vivax* and *P. ovale*
  - Incubation period 12 to 18 days for primary infection and up to 12 months (and longer) for relapses; generally presents with fevers
  - Dormant parasites may remain in liver and reactivate years after initial infection.
  - Can be severe
- *P. malariae*
  - Incubation period ~35 days
  - May become chronic; untreated can persist asymptomatically in human host for years
- *P. knowlesi*
  - Incubation period ~12 days
  - Possibly severe

PHYSICAL EXAM

- Often not specific
- General: elevated temperature, fatigue, tachycardia, tachypnea, jaundice

- Neurologic: mental status and motor–sensory exam (cerebral malaria)
- Cardiopulmonary exam: hemodynamic stability and signs of vascular leak (effusion)
- Skin exam: pallor, rash
- Abdominal exam: organomegaly

DIFFERENTIAL DIAGNOSIS

- Infections (disseminated or localized): abscess, viral, gastroenteritis, typhoid/paratyphoid, other bacteremias, rickettsial disease, mycobacteria
- Collagen vascular disease (systemic lupus erythematosus [SLE], vasculitides)
- Neoplasms (lymphoma, leukemia, other blood dyscrasias, other tropical causes of splenomegaly)
- Severe malaria infection may mimic hepatitis, pneumonia, meningitis, stroke, or sepsis.

DIAGNOSTIC TESTS & INTERPRETATION

- Malaria microscopy, thick and thin blood smears (3)[A]
  - Blood is spread on a slide in both a thick and thin preparation, stained with Giemsa smear, and examined under 100× oil immersion.
  - Thick smear used to evaluate for presence of parasite forms (rings, trophozoites, schizonts)
  - Thin smear used to determine species and quantify the percentage of RBCs that are infected (gametocytes are not counted)
  - Perform test on site—results immediately available.
- Rapid antigen testing: can detect the presence of malaria parasites within minutes. Cannot determine species or quantify parasitemia. Positive and negative results must always be confirmed by microscopy.
- Other tests: species-specific PCR; species confirmation by PCR is encouraged.
- General laboratory findings (nonspecific)
  - In uncomplicated infection
    - Elevated liver function tests and lactate dehydrogenase
    - Thrombocytopenia, anemia, and leukopenia
- Note: A low to low-normal platelet count or a slightly high bilirubin should alert the clinician to the diagnosis after exposure in an endemic setting.
- Note: Incomplete antimalarial prophylaxis may reduce parasitemia.

Initial Tests (lab, imaging)

- CBC with differential and platelets
- Basic chemistry panel, including bilirubin
- Malaria thick and thin blood films (If negative, repeat q12–24h for at least three sets.)
- Imaging necessary only for respiratory disease (chest x-ray) or cerebral malaria (CT scan prior to lumbar puncture)

Follow-Up Tests & Special Considerations

Submit specimens from suspected or confirmed malaria cases to the CDC for diagnostic confirmation, speciation, and drug resistance surveillance.

Test Interpretation

- Microscopy: Results should include both species of malaria and percent of red cells infected to determine the most appropriate treatment regimen.
- Rapid diagnostic test: use as a preliminary determination of presence of malaria infection, not to determine species of malaria. Perform smears to confirm results, determine species, and quantify percentage of red cells infected.

TREATMENT

MEDICATION

First Line

- For uncomplicated chloroquine-resistant *P. falciparum* (most *P. falciparum*), chloroquine-resistant *P. vivax* (New Guinea has highest rates of chloroquine-resistant *P. vivax*), or when species is unknown, the following regimens are recommended:
  - Atovaquone-proguanil (Malarone): adult tablet: 250 mg atovaquone and 100 mg proguanil. Pediatric tablet: 62.5 mg atovaquone and 25 mg proguanil. Adults: 4 adult tablets QD for 3 days. Children 5 to 8 kg: 2 pediatric tablets QD for 3 days; children 9 to 10 kg: 3 pediatric tablets QD for 3 days; children 11 to 20 kg: 1 adult tablet QD for 3 days; children 21 to 30 kg: 2 adult tablets QD for 3 days; children 31 to 40 kg: 3 adult tablets QD for 3 days; children >40 kg: 4 adult tablets QD for 3 days
  - Artemether-lumefantrine (Coartem): Tablet contains 20 mg artemether and 120 mg lumefantrine. Treatment schedule is a total of 6 doses over 3 days. On day 1, the initial dose is given and then second dose is 8 hours later. On days 2 and 3, doses are given BID. Persons 5 to <15 kg: 1 tablet per dose; persons 15 to <25 kg: 2 tablets per dose; persons 25 to <35 kg: 3 tablets per dose; persons ≥35 kg: 4 tablets per dose. (Call 1-855-COARTEM to locate pharmacy with stock.)
  - Quinine sulfate plus doxycycline or clindamycin: adults: quinine sulfate 650 mg (salt) TID for 3 days (should be extended to 7 days for infections acquired in Southeast Asia). Doxycycline 100 mg BID for 7 days. Clindamycin 20 mg (base)/kg/day divided TID for 7 days; children: quinine sulfate 10 mg (salt)/kg TID for 3 days (should be extended to 7 days for infections acquired in Southeast Asia) plus clindamycin dosed as above
  - Mefloquine: adults: 750 mg followed by 500 mg 8 hours later; children: 15 mg/kg followed by 10 mg/kg 8 hours later (max total dose: 1,250 mg)
- PO therapy for *P. ovale*, *P. malariae*, chloroquine-sensitive *P. falciparum* (rare), and chloroquine-sensitive *P. vivax*; in addition to the treatment regimens listed above, other options include:
  - Chloroquine: adults: 1 g (600-mg base) followed by 500 mg (300-mg base) at 6, 24, and 48 hours after first dose; children: 16.6 mg/kg (10-mg base/kg) on day 1 (max 1,000 mg [600-mg base]) and then 8.3 mg/kg (5-mg/kg base) at 6, 24, and 48 hours after first dose
  - Primaquine (add to acute treatment regimen for cure of dormant forms of *P. vivax* and *P. ovale*): adults: 30-mg base (52.6 mg) daily for 2 weeks; children: 0.6-mg base/kg/day for 2 weeks
    - Caution: Glucose-6-phosphate dehydrogenase deficiency must be excluded prior to first use.
  - Tafenoquine (add to the acute treatment regimen to cure dormant forms of *P. vivax* and *P. ovale*): patients age >16; 300 mg single dose
    - Caution: Exclude glucose-6-phosphate dehydrogenase deficiency prior to first use.
- Therapy for severe malaria
  - Clinical features defining severe malaria:
    - Impaired level of consciousness (LOC)
    - Respiratory distress, jaundice
    - Repeated convulsions, shock
    - Renal failure
  - Laboratory features:
    - Parasitemia >5%
    - Hypoglycemia
    - Acidosis (usually lactic acidosis)

- Parenteral therapy
  - Quinidine gluconate 10 mg/kg in normal saline over 1 to 2 hours followed by 0.02 mg/kg/min continuous infusion
  - Intensive care monitoring is necessary, especially when initiating quinidine therapy.
- In severe malaria, contact the CDC for assistance; CDC Malaria Branch: 770-488-7100; http://www.cdc.gov/Malaria/
- Artesunate available in the United States for severe malaria in special circumstances under investigational protocol. Contact the CDC for assistance.

ISSUES FOR REFERRAL

Infectious disease or tropical medicine consultation. Malaria is reportable https://www.cdc.gov/malaria/report.html.

ADDITIONAL THERAPIES

None

Pediatric Considerations

- Children are particularly susceptible to severe disease.
- All children, even infants, should receive chemoprophylaxis if traveling to an endemic area.
- Malaria can resemble acute gastroenteritis in children.
- Children with severe disease are prone to hypoglycemia. Use IV fluids with glucose for maintenance and monitor blood glucose frequently.

Pregnancy Considerations

- Chloroquine is safe in the doses recommended for prevention and treatment of malaria. Mefloquine is safe in the doses recommended for prevention and treatment of malaria.
- Artemether-lumefantrine (Coartem) is safe in the 2nd and 3rd trimesters in the doses recommended for the treatment of malaria (4)[A]. There is some evidence for its safety in the 1st trimester.
- Atovaquone-proguanil (Malarone) has not been studied in pregnant women; it has not been shown to cause birth defects or other problems in animal studies.
- No primaquine, tafenoquine, or tetracyclines should be used in pregnancy or lactation.
- Quinine/quinidine should be used during pregnancy because benefit outweighs risk.

SURGERY/OTHER PROCEDURES

Rarely, splenectomy must be performed in patients with splenic rupture.

COMPLEMENTARY & ALTERNATIVE MEDICINE

None. Deaths have resulted from using unapproved alternatives to recommended medications.

ADMISSION, INPATIENT, AND NURSING CONSIDERATIONS

- Inpatient care for all cases of *P. falciparum* malaria. Hospitalize patients with signs of severe illness, regardless of species; outpatient care for others
- Nonimmune patients with *P. falciparum* may progress from mild symptoms to death within 12 hours.
- Follow up all patients treated as an outpatient within 24 hours.
- Add glucose to maintenance IV fluids because of risk of hypoglycemia if unable to tolerate fluids by mouth. Excess fluids may promote pulmonary edema.
- Observe for fluid excess, renal insufficiency (reduced urine output), and hypoglycemia.
- Discharge criteria: clinical improvement and ability to tolerate oral medications and fluids, with documented decreasing parasitemia levels

ONGOING CARE

PATIENT EDUCATION

- Malaria chemoprophylaxis prior to travel
- Travel information may be obtained at the CDC travel Web site: http://www.cdc.gov/travel.

PROGNOSIS

Malaria infection (particularly *P. falciparum*) can carry a high mortality if untreated. If diagnosed early and treated appropriately, the prognosis is excellent.

COMPLICATIONS

- If not treated early: cerebral malaria, acute renal failure, acute gastroenteritis, respiratory distress syndrome, and massive hemolysis
- Other complications: seizures, anuria, delirium, coma, dysentery, algid malaria, blackwater fever, hyperpyrexia
- *P. malariae*: Nephrotic syndrome may develop in patients with chronic infection.

REFERENCES

1. World Health Organization. *World Malaria Report 2017*. Geneva, Switzerland: WHO Press; 2017.
2. Mace KE, Arguin PM, Tan KR. Malaria surveillance—United States, 2015. *MMWR Surveill Summ*. 2018;67(7):1–28.
3. Centers for Disease Control and Prevention. Guidance for malaria diagnosis in patients suspected of Ebola infection in the United States. http://www.cdc.gov/malaria/new_info/2014/malaria_ebola.htm. Accessed June 27, 2018.
4. Ballard SB, Salinger AS, Arguin PM, et al. Updated CDC recommendations for using artemether-lumefantrine for the treatment of uncomplicated malaria in pregnant women in the United States. *MMWR Morb Mortal Wkly Rep*. 2018;67(14):424–431.

ADDITIONAL READING

Centers for Disease Control and Prevention. Infectious diseases related to travel. https://wwwnc.cdc.gov/travel/yellowbook/2018/infectious-diseases-related-to-travel/malaria#1939. Accessed September 9, 2018.

CODES

ICD10

- B54 Unspecified malaria
- B50.9 Plasmodium falciparum malaria, unspecified
- B51.9 Plasmodium vivax malaria without complication

CLINICAL PEARLS

- Consider malaria in travelers returning from endemic areas presenting with fever or flulike illness.
- Early identification and aggressive treatment of persons with suspected or confirmed *P. falciparum* malaria is essential.
- Treat patients with clinical malaria with a different medication than what was used for chemoprophylaxis.
- *P. falciparum* malaria can be rapidly fatal; inpatient treatment is recommended.

M

MARIJUANA (CANNABIS) USE DISORDER

J.E. Lambrecht, MD, PharmD, FACP, FSHM • Paul G. Millner, MD

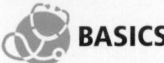 BASICS

DESCRIPTION
- Marijuana use leading to clinically significant impairment or distress, manifested by two or more of the following symptoms within a 12-month period:
  - Taken in larger amounts and over a longer period of time than intended
  - Persistent desire or unsuccessful efforts to cut down or control amount used
  - Inordinate amount of time spent in activities is necessary to obtain, use, or recover from use.
  - Presence of craving for the substance
  - Recurrent use resulting in failure to fulfill major role obligations at work, school, or home
  - Continued use despite having persistent or recurrent social or interpersonal problems due to cannabis use
  - Important social, occupational, or recreational activities are given up or reduced.
  - Recurrent use in physically hazardous situations
  - Use is continued despite knowledge of having a persistent physical or psychological problem caused or exacerbated by cannabis.
  - Tolerance defined by using increased amounts of cannabis to achieve the desired effect or intoxication or diminished effect with continued use of the same amount
  - Withdrawal
- According to *DSM-5*, marijuana or cannabis use disorder is classified into different categories (mild, moderate, or severe) depending on how many symptoms are present. Mild: 2 to 3; moderate: 4 to 5; severe: 6+ (1)

EPIDEMIOLOGY
- The United States is ranked first among 17 European and North American countries by the World Health Organization for prevalence of marijuana use.
- Cannabis is the most widely used illicit psychoactive substance in the United States (2).
- In 2014, an estimated 22 million Americans, age >12 years, self-identified as current marijuana users
- Prevalence of marijuana use disorder rose from 1.5% to 2.9% over the last decade.
- 45% of 12th graders have tried marijuana.
- Approximately 30% of students have used marijuana at the time of college entry (3).
- In the United States, 10% of marijuana users become daily users, 20–30% become weekly users.
- Younger users have a higher rate of addiction; 1 in 6 adolescents become addicted with repeated use.
- Marijuana use is increasing in pregnant women. In 2002, 2% reported using in the last month. In 2014, 7% of pregnant women aged 18 to 25 years reported use.

- In the United States, the legal landscape is changing rapidly. 30 states and the District of Columbia have legalized marijuana in some form, whereas eight states and the District of Colombia have legalized recreational marijuana.
- Popular opinion has changed over time. In 1969, only 12% of people approved of legalizing marijuana. In 2015, 58% approved of legalization.

ETIOLOGY AND PATHOPHYSIOLOGY
- Currently, there are two well-known therapeutically active cannabinoids in marijuana, δ9-tetrahydrocannabinol (THC) and cannabidiol.
- THC is responsible for marijuana's analgesic, antiemetic, and intoxicating properties.
- Cannabidiol is the nonpsychoactive component responsible for marijuana's antianxiety, antidepressant, antipsychotic, antispastic, anticonvulsant, and antineoplastic properties.
- In terms of bioavailability, smoking marijuana results in 25–50% absorption of THC, which rapidly passes into the circulation. When ingested, the oral bioavailability of THC is much less (3–10%).
- Effects of smoked marijuana occur within minutes and last several hours.
- Effects from marijuana consumed in foods or beverages appear after 30 minutes to 1 hour and can last up to 4 hours.
- Cannabinoid receptors (CBRs) are associated with memory, thinking, concentration, sensory/time perception, pleasure, movement, and coordination.
- THC artificially stimulates the CBRs, disrupting the function of endogenous cannabinoids. A marijuana "high" results from overstimulation of these receptors.
- With time, overstimulation alters the function of CBRs, leading to addiction and withdrawal.

RISK FACTORS
- Family history of chemical dependence including THC
- Comorbid psychiatric disorders (i.e., antisocial personality disorder)
- Other substance use (i.e., alcohol, tobacco)
- Lower educational achievement (rates of dependence are lowest among college graduates)
- Low socioeconomic status
- Ease of acquisition of marijuana

 DIAGNOSIS

- Significant impairment or distress results from use (1)[A].
- Screen for marijuana (similar to tobacco and alcohol).
- Ask for frequency and amount used (e.g., "How often do you use marijuana? Daily? Weekly?"; "How long does a typical 'eighth' [1/8 oz] last?").
- Usage is defined by: occasional = 1/8 oz/week, moderate = 1/4 oz/week, heavy = 1/2 oz/week.

- Unexplained deterioration in school or work performance is a red flag for abuse.
- Problems with, or changes in, social relationships (e.g., spending more time alone or with persons suspected of using drugs) and recreational activities (e.g., giving up activities that were once pleasurable) may also indicate abuse.
- If possible, obtain information from concerned parents or significant others.

HISTORY
- Clinical presentation of acute intoxication:
  - Euphoria, elation, laughter, heightened sensory perception, altered perception of time, increased appetite
  - Poor short-term memory, concentration
  - Fatigue, depression
  - Occasionally, distrust, fear, anxiety, panic
  - With large doses, acute psychosis: delusions, hallucinations, loss of sense of identity (4)
- Withdrawal symptoms include:
  - Nausea
  - Weight loss
  - Decreased appetite
  - Insomnia
  - Depressed mood

PHYSICAL EXAM
- Evaluate for:
  - Conjunctival injection
  - Xerostomia
  - Nystagmus
  - Increased heart rate
  - Decreased coordination
  - Altered mental status
- Withdrawal findings (nonspecific) include:
  - Restlessness/agitation
  - Irritability
  - Tremor
  - Diaphoresis
  - Increased body temperature

DIAGNOSTIC TESTS & INTERPRETATION
Positive urine drug screen: Cannabinoids can be detected in urine weeks to months after marijuana use. Blood testing is preferred for interpreting acute effects and levels. In the United States, there is no consensus for acceptable legal limits for marijuana levels while driving. Hair testing can be unreliable and may reflect second-hand exposure. In general, testing identifies cannabis use (not necessarily cannabis use disorder).

TREATMENT

- *DSM-5* does not specify treatment options for cannabis use disorder. No intervention has proved consistently effective for marijuana abuse. Users often have a hard time quitting (1)[A].
- Several methods of behavioral-based interventions:
  - Cognitive-behavioral therapy
  - Motivational interviewing
  - Contingency management
  - Social network behavior therapy

- 12-step approach
- Family-oriented therapy
- Brief intervention
- Relapse prevention
- Community reinforcement approach
- Trials on cognitive-behavioral therapy and contingency management show better outcomes for reducing use and maintaining abstinence (5).
- The addition of a comprehensive parenting training curriculum does not further enhance efficacy (5).
- Among patients suffering from comorbid psychiatric disorders, treating the mental health disorder may help reduce use, particularly among heavy users.
- Advice to help manage withdrawal:
  - Reduce amount used before quitting entirely.
  - Delay first use of marijuana until later in the day.
  - Consider nicotine replacement therapy if concomitant tobacco use is present.
  - Relaxation, distraction
  - Avoid cues and triggers associated with use.
- Prescribe short-term analgesia and sedation for withdrawal symptoms, if required.
- With marked irritability and restlessness, consider very low-dose diazepam for 3 to 4 days.
- Provide user and family members with information regarding abuse and withdrawal to increase understanding of abuse and reduce likelihood of relapse.
- Withdrawal symptoms peak on day 2 or 3; generally subside by day 7. Vivid dreams can continue for 2 to 3 weeks.

MEDICATION
- No effective medication currently exists to treat marijuana abuse.
- Oral THC may help abate marijuana withdrawal in individuals who are trying to quit.
- Medications used to treat other drug use disorders, such as buspirone, lithium, and fluoxetine, may have therapeutic benefit.

 ONGOING CARE

FOLLOW-UP RECOMMENDATIONS
- Monitor cessation by testing urine over several weeks for the inactive cannabis metabolites (carboxy-THC).
- Drug screening of heavy smokers may remain positive for marijuana up to 6 weeks after last use.

PATIENT EDUCATION
National Institute on Drug Abuse (NIDA):
- http://www.drugabuse.gov
- https://drugpubs.drugabuse.gov/promotions/back-to-school
- http://www.drugabuse.gov/drugs-abuse/marijuana
- https://teens.drugabuse.gov/

COMPLICATIONS
Acute adverse effects
- Acute panic or paranoid reactions can occur, especially in drug-naive individuals or those with a history of psychosis or other behavioral health conditions.
- Psychotic symptoms can present with high doses.

- Driving while intoxicated on marijuana likely increases the risk of motor vehicle accidents.
- Chronic adverse effects: abnormal brain development; diminished lifetime achievement
- Chronic bronchitis and impaired respiratory function in regular smokers
- Smoking marijuana is likely harmful in transplant patients and other immunosuppressed individuals with an increased risk of inhaled aspergillosis or and other infections.
- Marijuana use has been associated with an increased risk of fibrosis in hepatitis C patients.
- Psychotic symptoms in heavy users, especially those with a personal or family history of schizophrenia
- Addiction to other substances
- An increased risk of overall mortality has been suggested in heavy cannabis users.
- Higher mortality rates due to hypertension have been shown in marijuana users. There also appears to be increased risk of ischemic stroke.
- Cannabinoid hyperemesis syndrome is characterized by episodes of cyclic nausea and vomiting in association with chronic cannabis use.

REFERENCES

1. American Psychiatric Association. Substance-related and addictive disorders. In: *Diagnostic and Statistical Manual of Mental Disorders*. 5th ed. Arlington, VA: American Psychiatric Association; 2013.
2. Suerken CK, Reboussin BA, Sutfin EL, et al. Prevalence of marijuana use at college entry and risk factors for initiation during freshman year. *Addict Behav*. 2014;39(1):302–307.
3. Hall W, Degenhardt L. Adverse health effects of non-medical cannabis use. *Lancet*. 2009;374(9698):1383–1391.
4. Abayomi O, Adelufosi AO. Psychosocial interventions for cannabis abuse and/or dependence among persons with co-occurring cannabis use and psychotic disorders. *Cochrane Database Syst Rev*. 2015;(1):CD011488.
5. Stanger C, Ryan SR, Scherer EA, et al. Clinic- and home-based contingency management plus parent training for adolescent cannabis use disorders. *J Am Acad Child Adolesc Psychiatry*. 2015;54(6):445–453.e2.

ADDITIONAL READING

- Center for Behavioral Health Statistics and Quality. *2015 National Survey on Drug Use and Health*. Rockville, MA: Substance Abuse and Mental Health Services Administration; 2016.
- Freeman MJ, Rose DZ, Myers MA, et al. Ischemic stroke after use of the synthetic marijuana "spice." *Neurology*. 2013;81(24):2090–2093.

- Hooper SR, Woolley D, De Bellis MD. Intellectual, neurocognitive, and academic achievement in abstinent adolescents with cannabis use disorder. *Psychopharmacology (Berl)*. 2014;231(8):1467–1477.
- Manrique-Garcia E, Ponce de Leon A, Dalman C, et al. Cannabis, psychosis, and mortality: a cohort study of 50,373 Swedish men. *Am J Psychiatry*. 2016;173(8):790–798.
- National Institute of Drug Abuse. Marijuana. https://www.drugabuse.gov/drugs-abuse/marijuana. Accessed November 13, 2017.
- Yankey BA, Rothenberg R, Strasser S, et al. Effect of marijuana use on cardiovascular and cerebrovascular mortality: a study using the National Health and Nutrition Examination Survey linked mortality file. *Eur J Prev Cardiol*. 2017;24(17):1833–1840.

 CODES

ICD10
- F12.10 Cannabis abuse, uncomplicated
- F12.20 Cannabis dependence, uncomplicated
- F12.288 Cannabis dependence with other cannabis-induced disorder

CLINICAL PEARLS
- Marijuana abuse may result in poor performance in school or work, legal problems, and family dysfunction.
- Effects of smoked marijuana have an almost immediate onset and can last 1 to 3 hours. Effects from foods or beverages containing marijuana appear later, usually in 30 minutes to 1 hour but can last up to 4 hours. Smoking marijuana delivers significantly more THC into the bloodstream than eating or drinking the drug.
- Acute marijuana intoxication is manifested by conjunctival injection, increased heart rate, euphoria, heightened sensory perception, altered perception of time, increased appetite, poor short-term memory and concentration, and fatigue. Large doses may result in acute psychosis, panic or paranoid reactions, delusions, or hallucinations.
- Withdrawal symptoms include weight loss, decreased appetite, insomnia, and depressed mood. These symptoms peak on day 2 or 3 and resolve by day 7.
- Cognitive-behavioral therapy, motivational interviewing, motivational enhancement therapy, and contingency management are four methods of behavioral-based interventions used to treat marijuana abuse.

M

MASTITIS

Anne C. Adams, MD • Montiel T. Rosenthal, MD

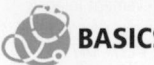

BASICS

DESCRIPTION
- Mastitis is an inflammation of the breast parenchyma and possibly associated tissues (areola, nipple, subcutaneous [SC] fat).
- Usually associated with bacterial infection (and milk stasis in the postpartum mother)
- Usually an acute condition but can become chronic cystic mastitis

EPIDEMIOLOGY
- Predominantly affects females
- Mostly in the puerperium; epidemic form rare in the age of reduced hospital stays for mothers and newborns
- Neonatal form
- Posttraumatic: ornamental nipple piercing increases risk of transmission of bacteria to deeper breast structures: *Staphylococcus aureus* is the predominant organism.

Incidence
- 3–20% of breastfeeding mothers develop nonepidemic mastitis.
- Greatest incidence among breastfeeding mothers 2 to 6 weeks postpartum
- Neonatal form occurs at 1 to 5 weeks of age, with equal gender risk and unilateral presentation.
- Pediatric form
- Around or after puberty
- 82% of cases in girls

ETIOLOGY AND PATHOPHYSIOLOGY
- Microabscesses along milk ducts and surrounding tissues
- Inflammatory cell infiltration of breast parenchyma and surrounding tissues
- Nonpuerperal (infectious)
  - *S. aureus*, *Bacteroides* sp., *Peptostreptococcus*, *Staphylococcus* (coagulase neg.), *Enterococcus faecalis*
  - *Histoplasma capsulatum*
  - *Salmonella enterica*
  - Rare case of *Actinomyces europaeus*
- Puerperal (infectious)
  - *Staphylococcus aureus*, *Streptococcus pyogenes* (group A or B), *Corynebacterium* sp., *Bacteroides* sp., *Staphylococcus* (coagulase neg.), *Escherichia coli*, *Salmonella* sp.
  - Methicillin-resistant *S. aureus* (MRSA)
- Rare secondary site for tuberculosis in endemic areas (1% of mastitis cases in these areas): single breast nodule with mastalgia
- *Corynebacterium* sp. associated with greater risk for development of chronic cystic mastitis
- Granulomatous mastitis
  - Idiopathic
    - Predilection for Asian and Hispanic women
    - Association with α_1-antitrypsin deficiency, hyperprolactinemia with galactorrhea, oral contraceptive use, *Corynebacterium* sp. infection, and breast trauma
    - Most women have a history of lactation in previous 5 years.
  - Lupus; autoimmune

- Puerperal
  - Retrograde migration of surface bacteria up milk ducts
  - Bacterial migration from nipple fissures to breast lymphatics
  - Secondary monilial infection in the face of recurrent mastitis or diabetes
  - Seeding from mother to neonate in cyclical fashion
- Nonpuerperal
  - Ductal ectasia
  - Breast carcinoma
  - Inflammatory cysts
  - Chronic recurring SC or subareolar infections
  - Parasitic infections: *Echinococcus*; filariasis; Guinea worm in endemic areas
  - Herpes simplex
  - Cat-scratch disease
- Lupus

RISK FACTORS
- Breastfeeding
- Milk stasis
  - Inadequate emptying of breast
    - Scarring of breast due to prior mastitis
    - Scarring due to previous breast surgery (breast reduction, biopsy, or partial mastectomy)
  - Breast engorgement: interruption of breastfeeding
- Nipple trauma increases risk of transmission of bacteria to deeper breast structures: *S. aureus* predominant organism
- Neonatal colonization with epidemic *Staphylococcus*
- Neonatal
  - Bottle-fed babies
  - Manual expression of "witch's milk"
  - Can predispose to lethal necrotizing fasciitis
- Maternal diabetes
- Maternal HIV
- Maternal vitamin A deficiency (in animal models)

GENERAL PREVENTION
Regular emptying of both breasts and nipple care to prevent fissures when breastfeeding; also good hygiene, including hand washing and washing breast pumps after each use (1)[A]

COMMONLY ASSOCIATED CONDITIONS
Breast abscess

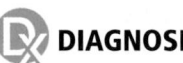

DIAGNOSIS

- Fever >38.5°C and malaise
- Nausea ± vomiting
- Localized breast tenderness, heat, swelling, and redness
- Possible breast mass

HISTORY
- Breast pain
- "Hot cords burning in chest wall"
- Consider yeast infection if nipple pain and burning and/or infant with thrush.

PHYSICAL EXAM
- Breast tenderness
- Localized breast induration, redness, and warmth
- Peau d'orange appearance to overlying skin

DIFFERENTIAL DIAGNOSIS
- Abscess (bacterial, idiopathic granulomatous mastitis, fungal, tuberculosis)
- Tumor
  - Idiopathic granulomatous mastitis
  - Inflammatory breast cancer
  - Wegener granulomatosis
  - Sarcoidosis
  - Foreign body granuloma
  - Vasospasm (may be presentation for Raynaud) (2)[B]
- Ductal cyst (ductal ectasia)
- Consider monilial infection in lactating mother, especially if mastitis is recurrent.

DIAGNOSTIC TESTS & INTERPRETATION
Initial Tests (lab, imaging)
Mastitis is typically a clinical diagnosis. Labs rarely needed. In those ill enough to need hospitalization, consider the following:
- CBC
- Blood culture
- In epidemic puerperal mastitis
  - Milk leukocyte count
  - Milk culture
  - Neonatal nasal culture
- No imaging required for postpartum mastitis in a breastfeeding mother who responds to antibiotic therapy
- Mammography for women with nonpuerperal mastitis
- Breast ultrasound (US) to rule out abscess formation in women
  - Special consideration for this in women with breast implants who have mastitis

Follow-Up Tests & Special Considerations
Lactating mothers produce salty milk from affected side (higher Na and Cl concentrations) as compared with unaffected side. Consider breast milk culture if suspect MRSA. Also consider testing for tuberculosis as may be initial presentation.

Diagnostic Procedures/Other
Options if further progression to abscess formation
- Needle aspiration
- Incision and drainage
- Excisional biopsy
- US-guided core needle biopsy is diagnostic method of choice for idiopathic granulomatous mastitis.

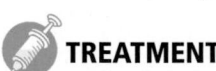

TREATMENT

A Cochrane review found that insufficient evidence exists to confirm or refute the effectiveness of antibiotic therapy for the treatment of lactational mastitis (3)[A]. If present <24 hours and symptoms are mild, conservative management with milk removal and supportive measures is recommended.

MEDICATION

- Prioritized on the basis of likelihood of MRSA as etiologic factor and clinical severity of condition.
- Treat for 10 to 14 days.
- For idiopathic granulomatous mastitis and localized infection, usually resolves with antibiotics and drainage

First Line

- Outpatient
  - Effective milk removal is most important management step (4)[A].
  - Dicloxacillin 500 mg QID
  - Cephalexin 500 mg QID
  - Trimethoprim/sulfamethoxazole (TMP/SMX); DS BID (If mastitis not improving within 48 hours after starting first-line treatment, consider MRSA.)
  - *Lactobacillus fermentum* or *Lactobacillus salivarius* 9 log 10 CFU/day
- Inpatient
  - Nafcillin 2 g q4h
  - Oxacillin 2 g q4h
  - Vancomycin 1 g q12h (MRSA possible)
- Breastfeeding beyond 1 month
  - Penicillin, ampicillin, or erythromycin
- If idiopathic granulomatous mastitis, consider corticosteroids ± methotrexate (5)[B]; surgical excision reserved for refractory cases (6)[C]

Pediatric Considerations

TMP/SMX given to breastfeeding mothers with mastitis can potentiate jaundice for neonates.

Second Line

- If mastitis is odoriferous and localized under areola, add metronidazole 500 mg TID IV or PO.
- If yeast is suspected in recurrent mastitis, add topical and oral nystatin.

ISSUES FOR REFERRAL

- Abscess formation
- Need for breast biopsy

ADDITIONAL THERAPIES

- Warm packs to improve blood flow and milk letdown and/or ice packs to reduce inflammation to affected breast for comfort
- The use of a breast pump may aid in breast emptying, especially if the infant is unable to assist in doing this.
- Wear supporting bra that is not too tight.

SURGERY/OTHER PROCEDURES

In cases of biopsy-proven idiopathic granulomatous mastitis, surgical removal can result in a 5–50% chance of recurrence, fistula formation, and poor wound healing.

ADMISSION, INPATIENT, AND NURSING CONSIDERATIONS

- If a new mother is admitted to the hospital for treatment of her mastitis, rooming-in of the infant with the mother is mandatory so that breastfeeding can continue (4)[C]. In some hospitals, rooming-in may require hospital admission of the infant.

- Admission criteria/initial stabilization
  - Failure of outpatient/oral therapy
    - Patient unable to tolerate oral therapy
    - Patient noncompliant with oral therapy
    - Severe illness without adequate supportive care at home
  - Neonatal mastitis
  - Antibiotics
  - Frequent emptying of breasts, if breastfeeding
  - Analgesics for pain
    - Ibuprofen
    - Acetaminophen
- Breastfeeding/pumping of breasts encouraged
- Start infant with feedings on affected side.
- Abscess drainage is not a contraindication for breastfeeding.
- Massage in direction from blocked area toward nipple.
- Positioning infant at breast with chin or nose pointing to blockage will help drain affected area.
- Discharge criteria
  - Afebrile
  - Tolerating oral antibiotics well

 ## ONGOING CARE

FOLLOW-UP RECOMMENDATIONS

Rest for lactating mothers, up to bathroom

DIET

- Encourage oral fluids.
- Multivitamin, including vitamin A

PATIENT EDUCATION

- Encourage oral fluids.
- Rest is essential.
- Regular emptying of both breasts with breastfeeding
- Nipple care to prevent fissures

PROGNOSIS

- Puerperal
  - Good with prompt (within 24 hours of symptom onset) antibiotic treatment and breast emptying; 96% success rate
  - 11% risk of abscess if left untreated with antibiotics
  - Antibodies develop in breast glands within first few days of infection, which may provide protection against infection or reinfection.
  - Rare risk of abscess formation beyond 6 weeks postpartum if no recurrent mastitis
- Idiopathic granulomatous mastitis recurrence rates high, encourage close follow-up (6)[C]

COMPLICATIONS

- Breast abscess 3% of women with puerperal mastitis
- Recurrent mastitis with resumption of breastfeeding or with breastfeeding after next pregnancy
- Bacteremia
- Sepsis

REFERENCES

1. Crepinsek MA, Crowe L, Michener K, et al. Interventions for preventing mastitis after childbirth. *Cochrane Database Syst Rev.* 2012;(10):CD007239.
2. Buck ML, Amir LH, Cullinane M, et al. Nipple pain, damage, and vasospasm in the first 8 weeks postpartum. *Breastfeed Med.* 2014;9(2):56–62.
3. Jahanfar S, Ng CJ, Teng CL, et al. Antibiotics for mastitis in breastfeeding women. *Cochrane Database Syst Rev.* 2013;(2):CD005458.
4. Amir LH; for Academy of Breastfeeding Medicine Protocol Committee. ABM clinical protocol #4: mastitis, revised March 2014. *Breastfeed Med.* 2014;9(5):239–243.
5. Sheybani F, Sarvghad MR, Naderi HR, et al. Treatment for and clinical characteristics of granulomatous mastitis. *Obstet Gynecol.* 2015;125(4):801–807.
6. Mathew M, Siwawa P, Misra S. Idiopathic granulomatous mastitis: an inflammatory breast condition with review of the literature. *BMJ Case Rep.* 2015;2015. doi:10.1136/bcr-2014-208086.

ADDITIONAL READING

Spencer JP. Management of mastitis in breastfeeding women. *Am Fam Physician.* 2008;78(6):727–731.

 ## SEE ALSO

Algorithms: Breast Discharge; Breast Pain

 ## CODES

ICD10

- N61 Inflammatory disorders of breast
- O91.22 Nonpurulent mastitis associated with the puerperium
- O91.23 Nonpurulent mastitis associated with lactation

CLINICAL PEARLS

- Complete emptying of the breasts on a regular schedule, avoiding constrictive clothing or bras that might obstruct breast ducts, meticulous attention to nipple care, "adequate rest," and a liberal intake of oral fluids for the mother can all reduce the risk of a breastfeeding mother's developing mastitis.
- First-line treatment for puerperal mastitis is dicloxacillin 500 mg PO QID for 10 to 14 days. Most mastitis can be treated with oral therapy.
- Among breastfeeding mothers, if the symptoms of mastitis fail to resolve within several days of appropriate management, including antibiotics, further investigations may be required to confirm resistant bacteria, abscess formation, an underlying mass, or inflammatory or ductal carcinoma.
- More than two recurrences of mastitis in the same location or with associated axillary lymphadenopathy warrant evaluation with US or mammography to rule out an underlying mass.

M

MASTOIDITIS

Renata Scalabrin Reis, MD • Cristian P. Fernandez Falcon, MD, DABFM, CAQGM, CAQHPM, CMD

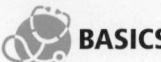

BASICS

An inflammatory process of the mastoid air cells and/or posterior process of the temporal bone, most commonly a suppurative complication of acute otitis media (AOM)

DESCRIPTION

- Clinical manifestations of mastoiditis typically appear 3 weeks after the first middle ear symptoms.
- Stiffness and thickening of the tympanic membrane (TM) is common.
- Acute mastoiditis: symptoms <1 month in duration; subdivided according to the pathologic stages:
  - Acute mastoiditis with periostitis (incipient mastoiditis): purulent material in the mastoid cavities
  - Coalescent mastoiditis (acute mastoid osteitis): destruction of the thin bony septae between air cells; followed by the formation of abscess cavities pus dissecting into adjacent areas
- Masked mastoiditis (subacute mastoiditis): low grade, persistent infection with destruction of the bony septae between air cells; occurs in patients with persistent middle ear effusion or recurrent episodes of inadequately treated AOM
- Chronic mastoiditis: associated with failed treatment of chronic otitis media. Often associated with cholesteatoma; symptoms last months to years.

EPIDEMIOLOGY

Highest incidence in children <2 years

- Routine prescription of antibiotics and routine childhood immunizations have reduced the number of cases of AOM and mastoiditis.

Incidence

1 to 4 cases per 100,000 children per year (1)

ETIOLOGY AND PATHOPHYSIOLOGY

- Subclinical stage begins with AOM and inflammation of mastoid air cells.
- Obstruction of the aditus ad antrum (connecting the tympanic cavity and mastoid)
  - Blocks outflow tract of mastoid air cells
  - Edema and accumulation of purulent material with penetration of periosteum (acute mastoiditis with periosteitis)
- Increased pressure from fluid within the air cells leads to destruction of bony septae (acute mastoid osteitis/acute coalescent mastoiditis).
- Acute mastoid osteitis can spread to adjacent areas in head and neck with abscess formation:
  - Subperiosteal abscess (most common complication), Bezold abscess, suppurative labyrinthitis, suppurative CNS complications
- AOM: *Haemophilus influenzae, Streptococcus pneumoniae*
- Acute mastoiditis: *S. pneumoniae* (most common), *Streptococcus pyogenes, H. influenzae, Staphylococcus aureus* (including methicillin-resistant *S. aureus* [MRSA])
- Chronic mastoiditis: *Pseudomonas aeruginosa, S. aureus*, Enterobacteriaceae, anaerobic bacteria, polymicrobials (2)

Genetics

No known genetic pattern

RISK FACTORS

- Cholesteatoma
- Recurrent AOM or chronic suppurative otitis media
- Immunocompromised state

GENERAL PREVENTION

- Ensure appropriate vaccinations (particularly pneumococcal vaccine).
- Referral to ENT for chronic otitis media
- Appropriate diagnosis and treatment of AOM
- Prevent recurrent AOM.
- Treat chronic eustachian tube dysfunction (pressure equalization tubes).
- Early diagnosis of cholesteatoma

DIAGNOSIS

HISTORY

- Most common symptoms in infancy (1)[A]
  - Lethargy/malaise/irritability
  - Fever
  - Poor feeding/decreased appetite
- Otalgia/possible otorrhea
- Hearing loss
- Headache
- Pain/redness/swelling noted over mastoid
- At time of admission (1)[A]
  - 42% of children have history of otologic disease.
  - 54% on antibiotic therapy
  - Average duration of symptoms: 10 days
- Suspicion for mastoiditis increases when symptoms of AOM persist >2 weeks.

PHYSICAL EXAM

- Postauricular changes: erythema, tenderness, edema, and/or fluctuance (81–85%) (1)[A]
- Bulging, erythematous, or dull TM (60–71%)
- Protrusion of auricle (79%)
- Fever (76%)
- Otorrhea if TM is perforated
- Edema of external auditory canal
- TM normal in 10%

DIFFERENTIAL DIAGNOSIS

- Postauricular cellulitis or inflammatory adenopathy
- Severe otitis externa
- Benign neoplasm: aneurysmal bone cyst, fibrous dysplasia
- Malignant neoplasm: rhabdomyosarcoma, neuroblastoma
- Deep neck space infections
- Parotitis

DIAGNOSTIC TESTS & INTERPRETATION

Initial Tests (lab, imaging)

- CBC with differential: elevated WBC count (3)[C]
- Elevated erythrocyte sedimentation rate (ESR) and C-reactive protein (CRP) (2,3)
- Blood cultures
- Myringotomy/tympanocentesis: Send for cultures, Gram stain, acid-fast stain (1)[B].
- Plain mastoid radiographs have low diagnostic yield. They may show distortion of mastoid outline or clouding of mastoid air cells. These changes are not diagnostic and can also be seen in AOM.
- Preferred: CT of the temporal bone (97% sensitivity; 94% positive predictive value) (4). Findings:
  - Clouding/opacification of air cells (also in AOM)
  - Mastoid air cell coalescence
  - Cortical bone erosion
  - Rim-enhancing fluid collections
  - Absence of mastoid opacification excludes the diagnosis.
- Use CT with contrast if complications are suspected (suppurative extension) (5)[C].
- Indications for CT scan in children (4)[C]:
  - Neurologic signs
  - Vomiting/lethargy
  - Suspected cholesteatoma
  - Fever after 48 to 72 hours of therapy
  - Concern for local disease progression
- Technetium-99m bone scan is more sensitive to osteolytic changes than CT.
- MRI: partial-to-complete opacification of the mastoid air cells +/− middle ear cleft

Follow-Up Tests & Special Considerations

Interpret normal WBC with caution in symptomatic, immunocompromised patients.

Diagnostic Procedures/Other

- Tympanocentesis to obtain middle ear fluid for culture and sensitivity (1)[B]
- Myringotomy with culture (also therapeutic)
- Audiography if suspected hearing loss
- Obtain CSF if intracranial extension suspected.
- Biopsy tissue protruding through TM or tympanostomy tube

TREATMENT

- IV antibiotics and myringotomy (± tympanostomy tubes) is the preferred treatment for uncomplicated acute mastoiditis (reflecting a shift away from more invasive surgical treatment).
- To avoid intracranial complications, simple mastoidectomy is recommended if patients do not respond to treatment after 3 to 5 days (6)[C].

GENERAL MEASURES
- Inpatient care during acute phase for IV antibiotics
- Keep the affected ear dry.

MEDICATION
First Line
- Empiric antibiotics against most common organisms: *S. pneumoniae* (including multiple resistant strains), *S. pyogenes*, *S. aureus* (including MRSA), *P. aeruginosa*
- Use combination therapy with 3rd-generation cephalosporin (ceftriaxone or cefotaxime) plus clindamycin with coverage for resistant strains (5,6)[C].
- Ceftriaxone 2 g IV q24h
  - Pediatric dosing: 50 to 75 mg/kg/day IV divided q12–24h
  - Precaution: Adjust dose with renal impairment.
  - Consider levofloxacin 750 mg IV q24h if severe β-lactam allergy.
- Clindamycin for coverage of ceftriaxone-resistant *S. pneumoniae* in pediatric patients (5)[C]:
  - Clindamycin pediatric dosing: 20 to 40 mg/kg/day IV divided q6–8h
- Cefotaxime 1 to 2 g IV q4–8h, depending on severity
  - Pediatric dosing: 100 to 200 mg/kg/day q6–8h
- Add vancomycin 30 to 60 mg/kg/day divided q8–12h if concerned for MRSA or acute on chronic exacerbation:
  - Pediatric dosing: 15 mg/kg/dose q6–8h
  - Precaution: Adjust dose with renal impairment.
- For patients with a history of recurrent AOM or recent antibiotic administration, treat with piperacillin and tazobactam 3.375 g IV q6h:
  - Pediatric dosing: 300 mg/kg/day based on piperacillin component divided q6–8h
- For other significant contraindications, precautions, or interactions, refer to the manufacturer's literature.

Second Line
- Oral antibiotics after 7 to 10 days of IV antibiotics and once myringotomy/blood cultures identify pathogen and sensitivities. Common oral antibiotics:
  - Amoxicillin-clavulanate (Augmentin) or clindamycin + 3rd-generation cephalosporin for 3 weeks or total treatment duration of 4 weeks
- For chronic mastoiditis: Use topical drops, ofloxacin otic solution (0.3%) or neomycin, polymyxin B, hydrocortisone 3 drops, 3 to 4 times per day.

ISSUES FOR REFERRAL
Consult ENT for mastoiditis in adults and children.

SURGERY/OTHER PROCEDURES
- Perform tympanocentesis to obtain cultures and guide antibiotic choice (1)[B].
- Myringotomy and tympanostomy tubes allow for middle ear drainage (6)[C].
- Mastoidectomy is the definitive treatment for patients who fail to improve within 24 to 48 hours despite IV antibiotics and myringotomy and for those with meningeal or intracranial complications (4,6)[C].
- Simple mastoidectomy is most effective for management of subperiosteal abscesses, if a trial of conservative therapy with drainage, myringotomy, and IV antibiotics fails (7)[C].

- Clean ear canal under microscopic guidance to ensure pressure-equalization tube patency and adequate drainage of middle ear.
- Topical antibiotic drops after insertion of pressure-equalization tubes

ADMISSION, INPATIENT, AND NURSING CONSIDERATIONS
- Admission criteria/initial stabilization
  - Clinical or imaging evidence of acute mastoiditis
  - Hospitalize patients with acute mastoiditis and start IV antibiotics immediately.
- Avoid getting affected ear wet.
- Discharge criteria
  - Afebrile for 48 hours before IV antibiotics are discontinued
  - Clinical improvement
  - Able to tolerate oral antibiotics

 ONGOING CARE

FOLLOW-UP RECOMMENDATIONS
- Oral antibiotics for 3 weeks following course of IV antibiotics (total duration of antibiotics is 4 weeks)
- For chronic mastoiditis, consider several months of antimicrobial prophylaxis with amoxicillin.

Patient Monitoring
- Assess for hearing loss postoperatively (audiogram) after acute condition has subsided.
- Follow-up with ENT, particularly patients with intracranial complications or hearing loss

PATIENT EDUCATION
Avoid getting the affected ear wet.

PROGNOSIS
- Depends on severity and stage of disease
- Conductive hearing loss may require reconstructive surgery.
- Most cases of mastoiditis recover fully if the diagnosis is made early and treated appropriately.

COMPLICATIONS
Complication rate is ~18% (2).
- Extracranial
  - Subperiosteal abscess (most common)
  - Bezold abscess (abscess of sternocleidomastoid muscle, insidious, risk of mediastinitis)
  - Citelli abscess (osteomyelitis of the calvaria)
  - Osteomyelitis of the temporal bone
  - Suppurative labyrinthitis (resulting in deafness)
  - Facial nerve paralysis
- Intracranial
  - Intracranial abscess: epidural/subdural/cerebral
  - Meningitis/cerebritis/periosteitis
  - Gradenigo syndrome (palsy of the 6th cranial nerve, draining ear, and retro-orbital pain)
  - Sigmoid sinus thrombophlebitis
  - Central venous sinus thrombosis

REFERENCES
1. van den Aardweg MT, Rovers MM, de Ru JA, et al. A systematic review of diagnostic criteria for acute mastoiditis in children. *Otol Neurotol*. 2008;29(6):751–757.
2. Chien JH, Chen YS, Hung IF, et al. Mastoiditis diagnosed by clinical symptoms and imaging studies in children: disease spectrum and evolving diagnostic challenges. *J Microbiol Immunol Infect*. 2012;45(5):377–381.
3. Bilavsky E, Yarden-Bilavsky H, Samra Z, et al. Clinical, laboratory, and microbiological differences between children with simple or complicated mastoiditis. *Int J Pediatr Otorhinolaryngol*. 2009;73(9):1270–1273.
4. Bakhos D, Trijolet JP, Morinière S, et al. Conservative management of acute mastoiditis in children. *Arch Otolaryngol Head Neck Surg*. 2011;137(4):346–350.
5. Lin HW, Shargorodsky J, Gopen Q. Clinical strategies for the management of acute mastoiditis in the pediatric population. *Clin Pediatr (Phila)*. 2010;49(2):110–115.
6. Psarommatis IM, Voudouris C, Douros K, et al. Algorithmic management of pediatric acute mastoiditis. *Int J Pediatr Otorhinolaryngol*. 2012;76(6):791–796.
7. Psarommatis I, Giannakopoulos P, Theodorou E, et al. Mastoid subperiosteal abscess in children: drainage or mastoidectomy? *J Laryngol Otol*. 2012;126(12):1204–1208.

ADDITIONAL READING
- Minks DP, Porte M, Jenkins N. Acute mastoiditis—the role of radiology. *Clin Radiol*. 2013;68(4):397–405.
- Pritchett CV, Thorne MC. Incidence of pediatric acute mastoiditis: 1997–2006. *Arch Otolaryngol Head Neck Surg*. 2012;138(5):451–455.

 CODES

ICD10
- H70.90 Unspecified mastoiditis, unspecified ear
- H70.009 Acute mastoiditis without complications, unspecified ear
- H70.099 Acute mastoiditis with other complications, unspecified ear

CLINICAL PEARLS
- Suspect mastoiditis if symptoms of AOM persist >2 weeks despite a normal-appearing TM.
- Hospitalize patients with acute mastoiditis for IV antibiotics. Consult ENT for drainage procedure.
- Treat with broad-spectrum IV antibiotics; collect middle ear fluid cultures to guide-specific therapy. Total duration of antibiotics is 4 weeks.
- If conservative treatment fails after 3 to 5 days, perform mastoidectomy to avoid intracranial complications.

M

MEASLES (RUBEOLA)
Nicholas E. Seeliger, MD

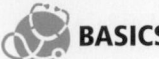

BASICS

DESCRIPTION
- A highly communicable, acute viral illness characterized by an exanthematous maculopapular rash that begins at the head and spreads inferiorly to the trunk and extremities
- Rash is preceded by fever and the classic triad of cough, coryza, and conjunctivitis (3 Cs). Koplik spots are pathognomonic lesions of the oral mucosa.
- Public health problem in the developing world, with significant morbidity and mortality; rising incidence in developed nations with declining vaccination rates
- System(s) affected: hematologic; lymphatic; immunologic; pulmonary; skin
- Synonym(s): rubeola

EPIDEMIOLOGY
- Transmission: direct contact with infectious droplets; highly contagious; 90% of nonimmune close contacts likely to become infected on exposure
  - Droplets can remain in the air for hours.
- Infectivity is greatest during the prodromal phase.
  - Patients are considered contagious from 4 days before symptoms until 4 days after rash appears.
  - Immunocompromised patients are considered contagious for the entire duration of disease.
- Incubation period: averages 12.5 days from exposure to onset of prodromal symptoms
- Predominant age: varies based on local vaccine practices and disease incidence. In developing countries, most cases occur in children <2 years.

Incidence
- No longer considered an endemic disease in the United States; isolated outbreaks still occur.
- In 2018, 22 cases of measles were reported to CDC. Between January and June 2017, 108 cases occurred including an outbreak in Minnesota with at least 65 cases related to a decline in measles, mumps, and rubella (MMR) vaccination.
- Worldwide: An estimated 20 million measles cases occur each year, with 122,000 measles deaths in 2012. >95% of measles deaths occur in poor countries with limited health infrastructure (1).

ETIOLOGY AND PATHOPHYSIOLOGY
Measles virus enters through the respiratory mucosa and replicates locally. It spreads to regional lymphatic tissues and other reticuloendothelial sites via the bloodstream.
- Measles virus is a spherical, enveloped, nonsegmented, single-stranded, negative-sense RNA virus of genus *Morbillivirus*, family *Paramyxoviridae*.
- Humans are the only natural host.

RISK FACTORS
- For developing measles:
  - Lack of adequate vaccination (2 doses)
  - Travel to countries where measles is endemic
  - Contact with exposed individuals
- For severe measles or measles complications:
  - Immunodeficiency
  - Malnutrition
  - Pregnancy
  - Vitamin A deficiency
  - Age <5 years or >20 years

GENERAL PREVENTION
- 100% preventable with proper vaccination
- Measles vaccine (active immunization)
  - Vaccine is usually given in combination with MMR or with added varicella (MMRV; ProQuad).
  - Primary vaccination requires 2 doses.
    - First dose at 12 to 15 months of age; 95% develop immunity.
    - Second dose at time of school entry (4 to 6 years of age) or any time >4 weeks after first measles vaccine; the 5% of initial nonresponders almost always develop immunity after the second dose.
    - Health care workers should have immunity verified and, if not immune, should receive the vaccine if not contraindicated.
  - Common adverse reactions to vaccine
    - Fever
    - Febrile seizures are rare (<5%) and occur 6 to 12 days after vaccination. Risk of febrile seizures increases if initial immunization is delayed past age 15 months (2).
    - Transient, mild, measles-like rash 7 to 10 days after vaccination (2%, with decreasing incidence during second vaccination)
    - If hypersensitivity reaction occurs, test for immunity; if immune, second dose not needed
    - *There is no substantiated link between MMR vaccine and autism.*
  - Contraindications
    - Live viral vaccines are contraindicated in immunosuppressed patients. For MMR, vaccinate asymptomatic HIV-infected children with adequate CD4 count.
    - Live vaccine is contraindicated in pregnancy (risk of fetal infection).
    - Anaphylactic reaction to gelatin or neomycin; consult allergist before vaccination.
    - Egg anaphylaxis is not a contraindication.

COMMONLY ASSOCIATED CONDITIONS
- Immunosuppression
- Malnutrition

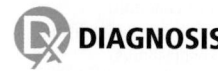

DIAGNOSIS

HISTORY
- Prodromal period: usually 2 to 3 days before rash (may be up to 8 days)
  - Fever
    - May begin 8 to 12 days after exposure; can persist until 2 to 3 days after rash onset
    - Temperature often >102°F (39–40.5°C); can precipitate febrile seizures
    - Fever onset >3 days after rash suggests complicated course.
  - "3 Cs" triad: cough, coryza, and conjunctivitis
  - Cough may persist for 2 weeks.
  - Prodromal symptoms typically intensify over 2 to 4 days, peaking on 1st day of rash before subsiding.
- Other symptoms: loose stools, malaise, irritability, photophobia (from iridocyclitis), sore throat, headache, and abdominal pain

PHYSICAL EXAM
- Koplik spots
  - Pathognomonic of prodromal measles
  - 2- to 3-mm, gray-white, raised lesions on erythematous base on buccal mucosa
  - Occur ~48 hours before measles exanthem
- Exanthematous rash (characteristic but not pathognomonic)
  - Maculopapular blanching rash
  - Begins at ears and hairline and spreads head to toe, reaching hips by day 2
  - Discrete erythematous patches become confluent over time, particularly on the upper body.
  - Clinical improvement usually occurs within 48 hours after rash appears.
  - Rash fades in 3 to 4 days changing to a brownish color, followed by fine desquamation.
- Lymphadenopathy and pharyngitis may be seen during exanthematous period.

DIFFERENTIAL DIAGNOSIS
- Drug eruptions
- Rubella
- *Mycoplasma pneumoniae* infection
- Infectious mononucleosis
- Parvovirus B19 infection, roseola
- Enteroviruses
- Rocky Mountain spotted fever, dengue
- Toxic shock syndrome
- Meningococcemia
- Kawasaki disease

DIAGNOSTIC TESTS & INTERPRETATION
Initial Tests (lab, imaging)
- Obtain serum sample and throat (or nasopharyngeal) swab. Molecular testing of serum and respiratory specimens is the most accurate method to confirm measles infection; IgM assay and measles RNA by real-time polymerase chain reaction (RT-PCR)
- Measles virus–specific IgM assay from serum and saliva. Antibodies may be undetectable on 1st day of exanthem but are usually detectable by day 3.
  - Sensitivity: 77% within 72 hours of rash onset; 100% within 4 to 11 days after rash onset. If negative but rash lasts >72 hours, repeat.
  - IgM falls to undetectable levels 4 to 8 weeks after rash onset.
- Measles virus–specific IgG may be undetectable up to 7 days after exanthem; levels peak 14 days after exanthem.
  - A 4-fold increase in IgG titers 14 days after an initial titer that was measured at least 7 days after rash onset is confirmatory.
- Viral cultures for measles are not usually performed.
- Mild neutropenia is common.
- Liver transaminases and pancreatic amylase may be elevated, particularly in adults.
- Chest x-ray if concern for secondary pneumonia

ALERT
Report suspected measles cases to public health authorities.

TREATMENT

GENERAL MEASURES

- Place all patients with measles in respiratory isolation until 4 days after onset of rash; immunocompromised patients should be isolated for duration of illness.
- Supportive therapy (i.e., antipyretics, antitussives, humidification, increased oral fluid consumption)

MEDICATION

- No approved antiviral therapy is available. Immunosuppressed children with severe measles have been treated with IV or aerosolized ribavirin. No controlled trial data exist; use is not FDA-approved.
- Vitamin A: WHO recommends daily dosages for 2 consecutive days:
  - Children <6 months of age 50,000 IU
  - Children 6 to 12 months of age 100,000 IU
  - Children >12 months of age 200,000 IU
- Ribavirin
  - Measles virus is susceptible to ribavirin in vitro; data is limited.
  - In one randomized trial including 100 children with measles treated with ribavirin or supportive care, ribavirin group had a shorter duration of fever, constitutional symptoms, and length of hospitalization.
- Antibiotics
  - Reserve for patients with clinical signs of bacterial superinfection (pneumonia, purulent otitis, pharyngitis/tonsillitis) (3)
  - A small trial resulted in an 80% (number needed to treat [NNT] = 7) decrease in measles-associated pneumonia with prophylactic antibiotics; consider in patients with a high risk of complications (4).
- Outbreak control
  - A single case of measles constitutes an outbreak.
  - Immunize contacts (individuals exposed or at risk of having been exposed) within 72 hours.
    - Monovalent vaccine may be given to infants 6 months to 1 year of age, but 2 further doses of vaccine after 12 months must be given for adequate immunization.
    - Monovalent or combination vaccine may be given to all measles-exposed susceptible individuals age >1 year if not contraindicated.
    - Individuals not immunized within 72 hours of exposure should be excluded from school, child care, and health care settings (social quarantine) until 2 weeks after onset of rash in last case of measles.
  - Immunoglobulin therapy (passive immunity) for high-risk individuals exposed to measles for whom vaccine is inappropriate:
    - Children age <1 year (infants 6 to 12 months of age may receive MMR vaccine in place of immunoglobulin if given within 72 hours of exposure)
    - Pregnant women
    - Severe immunosuppression
    - Give IM immunoglobulin within 6 days of measles exposure; CDC recommends 0.25 mL/kg to maximum of 15 mL for infants and pregnant women; dose for immunocompromised is 0.5 mL/kg to a maximum of 15 mL.

ADMISSION, INPATIENT, AND NURSING CONSIDERATIONS

- Inpatient setting: airborne transmission precautions for 4 days after the onset of rash in otherwise healthy patients and for the duration of illness in immunocompromised patients
- Outpatient care is appropriate, except where complications develop (e.g., encephalitis, pneumonia).

ONGOING CARE

FOLLOW-UP RECOMMENDATIONS

Signs of complications needing close follow-up:
- Difficulty breathing or noisy breathing
- Changes in vision
- Changes in behavior, confusion
- Chest or abdominal pain

PATIENT EDUCATION

- Adhere to recommended immunization schedules.
- Avoid exposure, particularly to unimmunized children and adults, pregnant women, and immunocompromised persons, until 4 days after rash onset.
- Avoid contact with potential pathogens until respiratory symptoms resolve.
- Centers for Disease Control and Prevention: measles: www.cdc.gov/measles/about/index.html

PROGNOSIS

- Typically self-limited; prognosis good
- High fatality rates may be seen among malnourished or immunocompromised children, particularly in developing countries.

COMPLICATIONS

- Otitis media (5–15%)
- The immune response to measles infection paradoxically depresses response to non–measles-virus antigens, rendering individuals more susceptible to pneumonia and diarrhea.
- Respiratory complications:
  - Bronchopneumonia (5–10%)
    - Accounts for most measles-related deaths
    - May be viral or bacterial
  - Interstitial pneumonitis (immunocompromised patients)
  - Laryngotracheobronchitis ("measles croup"): occurs in younger age group (<2 years)
- GI complications: diarrhea (may lead to dehydration)
- Neurologic complications
  - Febrile seizures
  - Acute disseminated encephalomyelitis with seizures and neurologic abnormalities (occurs in 1/1,000 cases): presents within 2 weeks of rash, probably an autoimmune response
  - Inclusion body encephalitis is rare but fatal in those with defective cellular immunity.
  - Subacute sclerosing panencephalitis
    - Rare degenerative CNS disease resulting from persistent measles infection following natural disease; usually fatal
    - Presents 5 to 15 years after infection
    - Most often in persons infected before age 2 years
- Ocular complications
  - Keratitis
    - Can lead to permanent scarring, blindness
    - Vitamin A deficiency predisposes to more severe keratitis and its complications.

- Other secondary bacterial infections
- Death: results from complications, mainly pneumonia, rather than the virus itself. CDC statistics show that for every 1,000 children who get measles, 1 or 2 will die.

REFERENCES

1. Orenstein W, Seib K. Mounting a good offense against measles. *N Engl J Med.* 2014;371(18):1661–1663.
2. Rowhani-Rahbar A, Fireman B, Lewis E, et al. Effect of age on the risk of fever and seizures following immunization with measles-containing vaccines in children. *JAMA Pediatr.* 2013;167(12):1111–1117.
3. Kabra SK, Lodha R. Antibiotics for preventing complications in children with measles. *Cochrane Database Syst Rev.* 2013;(8):CD001477.
4. Garly ML, Balé C, Martins CL, et al. Prophylactic antibiotics to prevent pneumonia and other complications after measles: community based randomised double blind placebo controlled trial in Guinea-Bissau. *BMJ.* 2006;333(7581):1245.

ADDITIONAL READING

- Drutz J. Measles. *Pediatr Rev.* 2016;37(5):220–221.
- Pal G. Effects of ribavirin on measles. *J Indian Med Assoc.* 2011;109(9):666–667.
- Papania MJ, Wallace GS, Rota PA, et al. Elimination of endemic measles, rubella, and congenital rubella syndrome from the Western hemisphere: the US experience. *JAMA Pediatr.* 2014;168(2):148–155.

CODES

ICD10

- B05.9 Measles without complication
- B05.2 Measles complicated by pneumonia
- B05.89 Other measles complications

CLINICAL PEARLS

- There is no substantiated link between MMR vaccine and autism.
- Measles is a highly communicable viral disease whose natural transmission has been halted in the United States by mass immunization.
- A single case of measles constitutes an outbreak.
- Report suspected measles cases to state or local health departments immediately.
- Immunization requires 2 doses: one at 12 to 15 months of age and one at school age (4 to 6 years of age).
- The clinical presentation of measles includes a prodrome of fever, cough, coryza, and conjunctivitis, followed by a descending maculopapular rash beginning on the face and progressing to the chest and lower body (centrifugal).
- Consider measles in the differential diagnosis of a febrile rash illness (especially in unvaccinated individuals with recent international travel).
- Measles-associated pneumonia is the most common cause of mortality.

M

MEASLES, GERMAN (RUBELLA)

Cody D. Mead, DO, FAAFP • Jeffrey M. Milch, DO

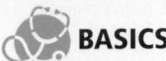 **BASICS**

DESCRIPTION

- A generally self-limited viral infection of children and adults, characterized by a mild, maculopapular rash, lymphadenopathy, and slight fever. Complications in normal populations are rare. Nonimmune women infected with rubella while pregnant may have devastating fetal effects.
- 25–50% of all rubella infections are asymptomatic (1,2)[A].
- System(s) affected: hematologic; nervous; pulmonary; exocrine; ophthalmologic; skeletal
- Synonym(s): German measles; 3-day measles

Pregnancy Considerations

- Pregnancy-associated rubella infection may lead to congenital rubella syndrome (CRS) with potentially devastating fetal outcomes.
- CRS is present in up to 90% of fetuses exposed during the 1st trimester (2)[A].
- Screening pregnant women for rubella immunity and vaccinating nonimmune women is the most effective strategy to prevent CRS (2)[A].
- Although no case of vaccine-associated CRS has been reported, women should not become pregnant for at least 28 days after vaccination because vaccine-type virus can cross the placenta (2)[A].
- Polymerase chain reaction (PCR) determination of viral RNA in amniotic fluid and fetal blood sampling allow for rapid diagnosis of fetal infection after 15 weeks' gestation (3)[B].

EPIDEMIOLOGY

- 50- to 70-nm RNA togavirus of genus *Rubivirus* (1)
- 13 genotypes have been identified (4).
- A live attenuated vaccine has been available in the United States since 1969. Primary use is to prevent CRS.
- Since 2004, all U.S. cases of rubella have been imported, most are inadequately immune travelers (1).
- Average incubation: 14 days; ranges 12 to 23 days
- Infectious period between 7 days before and 5 to 7 days after rash onset
- Transmitted primarily via respiratory droplets
- Most common in late winter and early spring
- Humans are only natural hosts (1).

Incidence

- U.S. incidence: <10/100,000 since 2001
- Declared eliminated (no endemic transmission for 12+ months) from the United States in 2004. However, primarily due to disease in international travelers, vaccine avoidance, and lack of routine pediatric care in migrant populations, cases are still reported annually.
- 667 cases from 27 states (a record number) reported to the CDC in 2015
- Still occurs in developing countries with 100,000 cases of CRS reported annually worldwide

ETIOLOGY AND PATHOPHYSIOLOGY

- Virus invades the respiratory epithelium, replicates in nasopharynx and regional lymph nodes, and spreads hematogenously. Infected patients shed virus from the nasopharynx 3 to 8 days after inoculation. Shedding lasts 7 or more days after onset of rash.

- Disease typically progresses from a prodromal stage (1 to 5 days) to lymphadenopathy (5 to 10 days) to an exanthematous, pruritic, maculopapular rash. Petechiae on the soft palate (Forchheimer spots) may precede or accompany the rash. Rash starts on the face and spreads outward to the trunk and extremities, sparing the palms and soles (14 to 17 days after onset of prodromal symptoms). The rash typically lasts an average of 3 days.
- Rubella first described by German scientists in the early 1800s as a variant of measles or scarlet fever
- 1962 to 1965: global pandemic resulting in an estimated 12.5 million cases in the United States, with 2,000 cases of encephalitis; 11,250 cases of therapeutic or spontaneous abortions; 2,100 neonatal deaths; and 20,000 infants born with CRS (1)[A]

Genetics

Children with CRS and children with type 1 diabetes share a high frequency of HLA-DR3 histocompatibility Ag and a high prevalence of islet cell Ab.

RISK FACTORS

Inadequate immunization, inadequate immunity after prior vaccination, immunodeficiency states, immunosuppressive therapy, crowded living/working conditions, international travel (1)[A]

GENERAL PREVENTION

- Vaccination is the most effective preventive strategy.
- Available combined with mumps, measles, rubella (MMR) or with varicella (MMR-V). Isolated rubella vaccine is not available in the United States.
  - Adults: 1- or 2-dose MMR vaccine schedule is recommended for those born after 1957. When 2 doses are used, each must be ≥28 days apart.
  - Pediatric: A 2-dose MMR vaccine schedule is recommended with the first dose given at ages 12 to 15 months; second dose recommended either at 4 to 6 years or at 11 to 12 years of age
  - Special pediatric cases: In special circumstances (e.g., upcoming international travel), the second dose may be given prior to 4 years of age but no sooner than 28 days since the initial dose.
  - Children 6 to 11 months of age may also receive a single dose prior to international travel but should be revaccinated with full 2-dose schedule starting at 12 months of age.
  - Children with HIV should receive MMR vaccine at 12 months of age if no contraindications exist. In the event of an outbreak, immediate vaccination of infants 6 to 11 months old is recommended (2)[A].
  - Vaccination is recommended for nonimmune people in the following groups: prepubertal boys and girls, all women of reproductive age, college students, daycare personnel, health care workers, and military personnel.
- Contraindications to vaccine: pregnancy, immunodeficiency (except HIV infection), within 3 months of IVIG or blood administration, severe febrile illness, or hypersensitivity to vaccine components. Patients who receive rubella vaccine do not transmit rubella to others, although the virus can be isolated from the pharynx. Breastfeeding is not a contraindication to vaccination (1)[A].
- During outbreaks, serologic screening before vaccination is *not* recommended because rapid mass vaccination is needed to stop disease spread (2)[A].

- MMR vaccine *is not associated with autism* (4)[A],(5)[B].
- Children who receive the MMR-V vaccine have a 2-fold increase in risk of febrile seizures compared with those who receive MMR and varicella vaccines separately (5)[B].
- Routine rubella antibody (IgG) screening is recommended during pregnancy (4)[A].

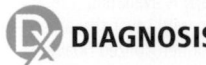 **DIAGNOSIS**

Council of State and Territorial Epidemiologists (CSTE) case definition classifications of rubella (1)[A]

- Clinical case definition
  - Acute onset of pink, coalescent macules on the face spreading to the trunk and extremities, becoming discrete macules that become confluent over (on average) 3 days
  - Temperature >99°F (37.2°C; if measured)
  - Arthralgia or arthritis, lymphadenopathy, or conjunctivitis
- Laboratory criteria for diagnosis
  - Isolation of virus from throat or nasopharynx, serum, CSF, urine, or cataracts (postmortem)
  - 4-fold rise in acute- and convalescent-phase titers of serum IgG Ab
  - Positive serologic test for IgM Ab
  - PCR positive for virus

HISTORY

- Most cases of postnatal rubella are inadequately immunized travelers returning from endemic areas.
- Rubella spreads quickly if living in close quarters.
- Postnatal rubella: low-grade fever, lymphadenopathy (postcervical, occipital, and postauricular), sore throat, nausea, anorexia, arthritis, arthralgia, malaise. 25–50% are asymptomatic.
- CRS: parental concerns about hearing or vision impairment, jaundice, or developmental delay
- Deafness could be the only manifestation and may not be noticed until 2nd year of life (2).

PHYSICAL EXAM

- Postnatal rubella: low-grade fever, lymphadenopathy (posterior auricular, occipital, posterior cervical), exanthem (mild, pink, discrete 1- to 4-mm maculopapular rash), soft palate petechiae (Forchheimer sign) (20%) (1)
- CRS: microcephaly, large anterior fontanelle, sensorineural hearing loss (58%), cataracts, glaucoma, microphthalmia, pigmentary retinopathy, purpuric ("blueberry muffin") skin lesions, murmur (50%) consistent with patent ductus arteriosus (PDA), hepatosplenomegaly, jaundice, cryptorchidism, inguinal hernia, radiolucent bone disease (2)

DIFFERENTIAL DIAGNOSIS

- Postnatal rubella
  - Measles virus (rubeola)
  - Scarlet fever (strep A)
  - Infectious mononucleosis
  - Erythema infectiosum (parvovirus B19)
  - Roseola infantum (i.e., exanthem subitum)
  - Toxoplasmosis
  - Drug eruptions
  - Other exanthematous enteroviral infections
- Congenital rubella
  - Measles
  - Parvovirus B19
  - Human herpesvirus 6
  - Other exanthematous entero- or arboviruses

DIAGNOSTIC TESTS & INTERPRETATION

Initial Tests (lab, imaging)

- Because 50% of cases are subclinical, laboratory testing to confirm the diagnosis is preferred (1,2)[A].
- Detection of wild-type virus is gold standard (1)[A].
- Enzyme immunoassay (EIA): preferred testing for IgM antibodies, which may not be detectable until 5 days after the onset of rash (1)[A]
- Hemagglutination inhibition (HAI) test: A 4-fold increase of IgG Ab levels from acute to convalescent phase is diagnostic for recent infection (1)[A].
- Latex agglutination (LA) test: sensitive and specific but dependent on experience of lab personnel (1)[A]
- Immunofluorescent antibody (IFA) assay: used for detection of viral IgG and IgM Ab (1)[A]
- Avidity test: not routinely used; use only in reference labs; distinguishes recent versus past infections (1)[A]
- Most rubella cases are virus positive on the day of the rash onset and remain positive for the next 7 to 10 days. Perform serum collection during this period. When testing for IgM, repeat collection may be necessary if sample taken before day 5. When testing for seroconversion, collect a second IgG sample 2 to 3 weeks after the first (acute to convalescent phase); IgG usually detectable 8 days after rash onset (1)[A]
- Virus may also be isolated from 1 week prior to 2 weeks after the onset of rash. Maximal viral shedding occurs up to day 4 after rash onset. Best results are from throat swab samples (1)[A].
- Epidemiologically, viral genotyping by reverse transcription (RT)-PCR helps determine the country of origin. Collect throat swabs 4 days after the rash onset and send to CDC (1)[A].
- Reserve viral cultures of CSF for suspected cases of CRS or rubella encephalitis (1)[A].
- If a pregnant female is exposed, amniotic fluid PCR or fetal blood sampling may be done at 15 weeks' gestation for viral detection. Placental biopsy (less common) may be done at 12 weeks' gestation. If positive, offer genetic counseling (1)[A].
- As the incidence of rubella decreases, the positive predictive value (PPV) of IgM results decreases. False-positive findings occur in patients with parvovirus B19, mononucleosis, and positive rheumatoid factor (1)[A].
- After reexposure, individuals with a low level of Ab (from past infection or prior vaccination) may acutely show a small rise in Ab levels. This is not associated with a high risk of contagion to others or fetal complications (1)[A].

Follow-Up Tests & Special Considerations

- Reporting is state dependent. Send samples to the CDC for genotyping. Report cases of CRS to the National Congenital Rubella Syndrome Registry (1,2)[A].
- Infants with CRS may shed virus up to 1 year; contact isolation precautions during all hospitalizations until child turns 1 year old (unless child has two negative throat cultures and urine specimens a month apart after 3 months of age) (2)[A]

 TREATMENT

- Supportive for mild cases
- Isolate patients for 5 to 7 days after rash onset.
- Postnatal rubella: mild and self-limited; treat symptomatically. Hospitalize for complications: idiopathic thrombocytopenic purpura (ITP) or encephalitis (1)[A].
- CRS: supportive care unless neurologic or hemorrhagic complications develop; phototherapy may be indicated for jaundice; multidisciplinary management of long-term complications (2)[A]

MEDICATION

No specific therapy available for mild cases

First Line

- Age- and dose-appropriate antipyretics
- NSAIDs can be used for arthritis and arthralgias in adults and infants age >6 months.
- IVIG can be given for severe thrombocytopenia; most cases, however, are self-limited.

 ONGOING CARE

FOLLOW-UP RECOMMENDATIONS

Patient Monitoring

- Individuals immune to rubella through natural infection or vaccine may be reinfected when reexposed; such infection is usually asymptomatic and detectable only by serology. Those who have received the vaccine have lower measurable IgG levels than those who had the natural disease.
- In CRS, it is important to detect auditory and visual impairment early (2)[A].
- 2/3 of internationally adopted children have no written record of immunizations (4)[A].

PATIENT EDUCATION

http://www.cdc.gov/rubella/

PROGNOSIS

- Postnatal rubella: Complete recovery is typical.
- CRS
  – Varied and unpredictable spectrum, ranging from stillbirth to normal infancy/childhood (1,2)[A]
  – Detectable levels of IgG persist for years and then may decline (does not drop at the expected 2-fold dilution per month). By age 5 years, 20% have no detectable antibody (2)[A].
  – IgM may not be detectable until 1 month after birth and may persist for 6 to 12 months (2)[A].
  – Overall mortality (up to 10%) is greatest during first 6 months.
  – 70% of encephalitis cases develop residual neurologic defects, including autistic syndrome.
  – Prognosis is excellent if only minor congenital defects are present.

COMPLICATIONS

- Leads to arthralgia/arthritis in up to 70% of women (6)
- Postinfectious encephalitis (1/5,000 cases)
- Thrombocytopenic purpura (1/3,000 cases)
- CRS: incidence dependent on trimester exposed
- Rubella vaccine may rarely cause encephalitis or ITP.
  – ITP is self-limited and is not a contraindication to vaccination.

REFERENCES

1. Lanzieri T, Redd S, Abernathy E, et al. Chapter 14: rubella. In: Roush SW, Baldy LM, Hall MAK, eds. *Manual for the Surveillance of Vaccine-Preventable Diseases*. 5th ed. Atlanta, GA: Centers for Disease Control and Prevention; 2014:1–11. http://www.cdc.gov/vaccines/pubs/surv-manual/chpt14-rubella.html. Accessed September 9, 2018.
2. Lanzieri T, Redd S, Abernathy E, et al. Chapter 15: congenital rubella syndrome. In: Roush SW, Baldy LM, Hall MAK, eds. *Manual for the Surveillance of Vaccine-Preventable Diseases*. 5th ed. Atlanta, GA: Centers for Disease Control and Prevention; 2014:1–7. http://www.cdc.gov/vaccines/pubs/surv-manual/chpt15-crs.html. Accessed September 9, 2018.
3. Abernathy ES, Hübschen JM, Muller CP, et al. Status of global virologic surveillance for rubella viruses. *J Infect Dis*. 2011;204(Suppl 1):S524–S532.
4. McLean HQ, Fiebelkorn AP, Temte JL, et al; and Centers for Disease Control and Prevention. Prevention of measles, rubella, congenital rubella syndrome, and mumps, 2013: summary recommendations of the Advisory Committee on Immunization Practices (ACIP). *MMWR Recomm Rep*. 2013;62(RR-04):1–34.
5. Lai J, Fay KE, Bocchini JA. Update on childhood and adolescent immunizations: selected review of US recommendations and literature: part 2. *Curr Opin Pediatr*. 2011;23(4):470–481.
6. White SJ, Boldt KL, Holditch SJ, et al. Measles, mumps, and rubella. *Clin Obstet Gynecol*. 2012;55(2):550–559.

ADDITIONAL READING

- Centers for Disease Control and Prevention. Measles cases and outbreaks. https://www.cdc.gov/measles/cases-outbreaks.html. Accessed September 9, 2018.
- Centers for Disease Control and Prevention. Rubella. In: Hamborsky J, Kroger A, Wolfe C, eds. *Epidemiology and Prevention of Vaccine-Preventable Diseases*. 13th ed. Atlanta, GA: Centers for Disease Control and Prevention; 2012:325–340. https://www.cdc.gov/vaccines/pubs/pinkbook/rubella.html. Accessed September 9, 2018.
- Papania MJ, Wallace GS, Rota PA, et al. Elimination of endemic measles, rubella, and congenital rubella syndrome from the Western hemisphere: the US experience. *JAMA Pediatr*. 2014;168(2):148–155.

 CODES

ICD10

- B06.9 Rubella without complication
- B06.00 Rubella with neurological complication, unspecified
- P35.0 Congenital rubella syndrome

CLINICAL PEARLS

- Rubella is typically a self-limited viral exanthematous infection of children and adults.
- Nonimmune women who are infected with rubella while pregnant may have devastating fetal effects due to CRS.
- Immunization is the key prevention strategy.

M

MEDIAL TIBIAL STRESS SYNDROME (MTSS)/SHIN SPLINTS

Vasilios Chrisostomidis, DO • Frank J. Domino, MD

BASICS

DESCRIPTION
- The term medial tibial stress syndrome (MTSS) is currently preferred to "shin splints." MTSS is aching pain along the inner edge of the tibial shaft that develops when the musculature and/or periosteum in the (lower) leg become irritated by repetitive activity. The condition is part of a continuum of stress-related injuries to the lower leg. MTSS does not encompass pain from ischemia (compartment syndrome) or stress fractures.
- Tendonitis/periostitis of the medial soleus muscles, anterior tibialis, and posterior tibialis muscles
- Synonyms: tibial stress reaction, anterior muscle syndrome, tibial periostitis, perimyositis, soleus syndrome, shin splints

EPIDEMIOLOGY
Incidence
Common, can account for between 5% and 35% of novice-running injuries; frequently occurs bilaterally (1)

Pediatric Considerations
MTSS may account for up to 31% of all overuse injuries in high school athletes.

ETIOLOGY AND PATHOPHYSIOLOGY
- Multifactorial anatomic and biomechanical factors
  - Overuse injuries causing or limited by
    - Microtrauma from repetitive motion leading to periosteal inflammation
    - Overpronation of the subtalar joint and tight gastrocnemius/soleus complex with increased eccentric loading of musculature inserting along the medial shin
    - Interosseous membrane pain
    - Periostitis
    - Tears of collagen fibers
    - Enthesopathy
  - Anatomic structures affected include:
    - Flexor hallucis longus
    - Tibialis anterior
    - Tibialis posterior
    - Soleus
    - Crural fascia
- Pathogenesis: theorized to be due to (i) calf muscle traction on periosteum and (ii) persistent repetitive loading on tibia, which leads to inadequate bone remodeling with subsequent tibial cortex changes and possible microfissures causing pain without evidence of fracture or ischemia

RISK FACTORS
- Intrinsic (personal) risk factors:
  - Greater ranges of internal and external (>65 degrees) hip rotation
  - Significant overpronation at the ankle
  - Imbalance of musculature of the ankle and foot (inversion/eversion misbalance)
  - Female gender
  - Lean calf girth
  - Femoral neck anteversion
  - Navicular drop
  - Genu varum
  - History of previous MTSS
- External (environmental) risk factors
  - Lack of physical fitness
  - Inexperienced runners—particularly those with rapid increases in mileage and inadequate prior conditioning
  - Excessive overuse or distance running, particularly on hard or inclined (crowned) surfaces
  - Prior injury
  - Equipment (shoe) failure
- Other risk factors
  - Elevated BMI
  - Lower bone mineral density
  - Tobacco use
- Those typically affected by MTSS include:
  - Runners
  - Military personnel—common in recruit/boot camp
  - Gymnasts, soccer, and basketball players
  - Ballet dancers

GENERAL PREVENTION
- Proper technique for guided calf stretching and lower extremity strength training, although supplementary gastrocnemius and soleus stretching has no statistical significance in reducing risk of shin splints
- Rehabilitate prior injuries adequately.
- Other recommendations
  - Gait analysis and retraining, particularly for overpronation
  - Orthotic footwear inserts

COMMONLY ASSOCIATED CONDITIONS
- Rule out stress fracture and compartment syndrome.
- Pes planus (flat feet)

DIAGNOSIS

HISTORY
- Patients typically describe dull, sharp, or deep pain along the lower leg that is resolved with rest.
- Patients are often able to run through the pain in early stages.
- Pain is commonly associated with exercise (also true with compartment syndrome), but in severe cases, pain may persist with rest.

PHYSICAL EXAM
- Tenderness to palpation is typically elicited along the posteromedial border of the middle-to-distal 3rd of the tibia.
- Pain with plantar flexion
- Preservation of neurovascular integrity via palpable distal pulses, intact sensation, reflexes, and muscular strength

DIFFERENTIAL DIAGNOSIS
- Bone
  - Tibial stress fractures
    - Typically, pain persists at rest or with weight-bearing activities.
    - Focal tenderness over the anterior tibia
- Muscle/soft tissue injury
  - Strain, tear, tendinopathy
  - Muscle hernia
- Fascial
  - Chronic exertional compartment syndrome (2)[C]
    - Pain without direct tenderness on exam
    - Pain increases with exertion and resolves at rest.
    - Pain is described as cramping or squeezing.
    - Pain with possible weakness or paresthesias on exam
  - Interosseous membrane tear
- Nerve
  - Spinal stenosis
  - Lumbar radiculopathy
  - Common peroneal nerve entrapment
- Vascular
  - DVT
  - Popliteal arterial entrapment
    - Rare but limb-threatening disease
    - History of intermittent unilateral claudication
    - MRI reveals compression of the artery by the medial head of the gastrocnemius muscle.
- Infection
  - Osteomyelitis
- Malignancy
  - Bone tumors

DIAGNOSTIC TESTS & INTERPRETATION

- Plain radiographs help rule out stress fractures if >2 weeks of symptoms (3).
- Bone scintigraphy
  - Diffuse linear vertical uptake in the posterior tibial cortex on the lateral view
  - Stress fractures demonstrate a focal ovoid uptake.
- High-resolution MRI reveals abnormal periosteal and bone marrow signals, which are useful for early discrimination of tibial stress fractures.
- Increased pain and localized tenderness warrant further imaging with MRI due to concern for tibial stress fracture.
- Exclude compartment syndrome using intracompartmental pressure testing.

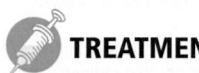

TREATMENT

GENERAL MEASURES

- Activity modification with a gradual return to training based on improvement of symptoms
- Running on flat and firm surfaces can help minimize pain.
- Patients should maintain fitness with low-impact activities such as swimming and cycling.
- Continue activity modification until pain free on ambulation.

MEDICATION

- Analgesia with acetaminophen or other oral nonsteroidal anti-inflammatory agent
- Cryotherapy (ice massage) is also advised to relieve acute-phase symptoms (4)[C].

ADDITIONAL THERAPIES

- Calf stretch, peroneal stretch, TheraBand exercises, and eccentric calf raises may improve endurance and strength (5)[A].
- Compression stockings have been used to treat MTSS with mixed results.
- Structured running programs with warm-up exercises have not been demonstrated to reduce pain in young athletes (6)[B].
- CAM boot for people with significant pain with weight-bearing

SURGERY/OTHER PROCEDURES

- Surgical intervention includes a posterior medial fascial release in individuals with both
  - Severe limitation of physical activity and
  - Failure of 6 months of conservative treatment
  - Counsel patients that complete return of activity to sport may not be always achieved postoperatively. Surgical risks include infection and hematoma formation.
- Extracorporeal shock wave therapy (ESWT) may decrease recovery time when added to a running program (5)[A].

COMPLEMENTARY & ALTERNATIVE MEDICINE

- Individualized polyurethane orthoses may help chronic running injuries.
- Special insoles, low-energy laser treatment, pulsed electromagnetic field, and knee braces have not been shown to improve outcomes (5)[A].
- Ultrasound, acupuncture, aquatic therapy, electrical stimulation, whirlpool baths, cast immobilization, taping, and steroid injection may help improve pain.
- Physical therapy approaches including Kinesio tape and fascial distortion massage may yield quicker return to activity.

 ONGOING CARE

FOLLOW-UP RECOMMENDATIONS
Patient Monitoring
- Avoid premature return to preinjury running pace.
- Maintain stretching and strengthening exercises.
- Identify and correct preinjury training errors.
- Good supportive footwear is recommended as is replacing running shoes every 350 to 450 miles.
- Allow a gradual return to activity dictated by symptoms (pain).

PROGNOSIS
The condition is usually self-limiting, and most patients respond well with rest and nonsurgical intervention.

COMPLICATIONS
- Stress fractures and compartment syndrome
- Undiagnosed MTSS or chronic exertional compartment syndrome can lead to a complete fracture or tissue necrosis, respectively.

REFERENCES

1. Fullem BW. Overuse lower extremity injuries in sports. *Clin Podiatr Med Surg*. 2015;32(2): 239–251.
2. Hutchinson M. Chronic exertional compartment syndrome. *Br J Sports Med*. 2011;45(12): 952–953.
3. Chang GH, Paz DA, Dwek JR, et al. Lower extremity overuse injuries in pediatric athletes: clinical presentation, imaging findings, and treatment. *Clin Imaging*. 2013;37(5):836–846.
4. Fields KB, Sykes JC, Walker KM, et al. Prevention of running injuries. *Curr Sports Med Rep*. 2010;9(3):176–182.

5. Winters M, Eskes M, Weir A, et al. Treatment of medial tibial stress syndrome: a systematic review. *Sports Med*. 2013;43(12):1315–1333.
6. Moen MH, Holtslag L, Bakker E, et al. The treatment of medial tibial stress syndrome in athletes; a randomized clinical trial. *Sports Med Arthrosc Rehabil Ther Technol*. 2012;4:12.

ADDITIONAL READING

- Abelson B. The tibialis anterior stretch–kinetic health. https://www.youtube.com/watch?v=6Z6XM63x2TM. Accessed June 19, 2014.
- Hamstra-Wright KL, Bliven KC, Bay C. Risk factors for medial tibial stress syndrome in physically active individuals such as runners and military personnel: a systematic review and meta-analysis. *Br J Sports Med*. 2015;49(6):362–369.
- Reshef N, Guelich DR. Medial tibial stress syndrome. *Clin Sports Med*. 2012;31(2):273–290.
- Yeung SS, Yeung EW, Gillespie LD. Interventions for preventing lower limb soft-tissue running injuries. *Cochrane Database Syst Rev*. 2011;(7):CD001256.

 CODES

ICD10
- S86.899A Other injury of other muscle(s) and tendon(s) at lower leg level, unspecified leg, initial encounter
- S86.891A Other injury of other muscle(s) and tendon(s) at lower leg level, right leg, initial encounter
- S86.892A Other injury of other muscle(s) and tendon(s) at lower leg level, left leg, initial encounter

CLINICAL PEARLS

- MTSS is the preferred term for "shin splints."
- Diagnosis is based on a reliable history of repetitive overuse accompanied by characteristic shin pain; imaging only if strong suspicion for stress fracture
- MTSS pain is typically along the middle and distal 3rd of the posteromedial tibial surface, worsened with activity and relieved with rest.
- Treatment includes ice, activity modification, analgesics, eccentric stretching, gait retraining, and a gradual return to activity.
- Symptoms recur if return to activity is "too much too fast."

M

MEDICAL MARIJUANA

Krishna M. Baradhi, MD • Narothama Reddy Aeddula, MD, FACP, FASN • Yugandhar Manda, MD

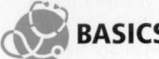 BASICS

Medical marijuana refers to the use of cannabis or cannabinoids as medical therapy to treat disease or alleviate symptoms.

DESCRIPTION
- Marijuana contains >100 pharmacologically active compounds ("cannabinoids").
- The most commonly isolated active ingredients include Δ-9-tetrahydrocannabinol (THC) and cannabidiol (CBD). Most of the psychoactive properties come from THC.
- Routes of administration include inhaled, intranasal, oral (extract, mixed into food, or made into tea), sublingual, and topical.
- Cannabinoids can be taken in herbal form, extracted naturally from the plant, gained by isomerization of CBD, or manufactured synthetically.

EPIDEMIOLOGY
- Cannabis is the most widely consumed illicit substance worldwide.
- An estimated 192 million people aged 15 to 64 years used cannabis in 2016.
- In the United States in 2016, 8.9% of individuals 12 years old had smoked cannabis in the previous month and 13.9% in the past year, and 46% of 12- to 17-year-olds have used marijuana in 2016.
- Use among high school seniors now exceeds tobacco use and is commonly seen in lower socio-economic groups.
- More than half of the states in United States have legalized marijuana, although it remains illegal under federal law (schedule 1 substance).

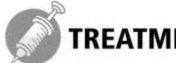 TREATMENT

In order to qualify for medical marijuana in states where it is legal, patients have to fail first- and second-line therapies, including an FDA-approved cannabinoid, and cannot have a substance-use disorder, psychotic disorder, or unstable mood disorder.

MEDICATION
FDA-approved cannabinoids and indications
- Dronabinol (Marinol): capsule with synthetically derived THC dissolved in oil
  - Refractory chemotherapy-induced nausea and vomiting
  - Anorexia resulting in weight loss in patients with AIDS

- Nabilone (Cesamet): capsule with synthetic cannabinoid that mimics THC
  - Indications above as dronabinol, additionally
  - Spasticity due to spinal cord injury
- Nabiximols (Sativex): an oromucosal spray containing THC and CBD in 1:1 ratio
- Used for treating spasticity in multiple sclerosis (MS), cancer-related pain, and neuropathic pain
- Conditions
  - Chronic pain (1)[B]
    ○ May benefit in refractory pain, neuropathic pain, and pain associated with cancer. In a recent meta-analysis of 27 randomized trials, there is low-strength evidence that cannabis alleviates neuropathic pain but insufficient evidence in other pains.
    ○ Head-to-head studies have failed to show superiority to codeine or amitriptyline.
    ○ Dronabinol has been shown to have longer lasting pain reduction and fewer side effects than non–FDA-approved cannabinoids.
  - MS (2)[B]
    ○ Spasticity: In a meta-analysis of 11 studies, cannabinoids improved spasticity, but effect did not reach statistical significance.
    ○ Pain: Oral cannabinoid extracts reduced pain in a small number of studies, but these results were limited by significant placebo effect and were also lacking statistical power.
    ○ Bladder dysfunction: no consistent evidence showing benefit
    ○ Tremor: Available data shows probably ineffective
    ○ Smoked marijuana has unclear efficacy and has been shown to negatively affect posture and balance.
    ○ Several studies showed an increase in cognitive impairment among MS patients who use cannabis. This occurred even in patients who used as infrequently as once per month.
    ○ Side effects of increased weakness, mood changes including suicidal ideation, dizziness, and fatigue were noted, which MS patients are already at risk of experiencing.
  - HIV/AIDS
    ○ Low-quality evidence showed some weight gain on dronabinol, although the effect was similar to megestrol (1)[A].
    ○ Concern for exacerbation of HIV-associated cognitive deficits (3)[C]
    ○ Evidence of any long-term benefit and/or change in morbidity and mortality is lacking.

  - PTSD (4)[B]
    ○ Conflicting data exist for the use of marijuana for PTSD. Most of these studies showed negative outcomes and worsening of PTSD symptoms.
  - Seizures (5)[B]
    ○ Insufficient evidence per American Academy of Neurology
    ○ Best available meta-analysis includes only 48 patients in four studies. Included studies have multiple major flaws including no information on randomization, data reported only on side effects but not primary outcome. One study is an abstract only with no statistical analysis performed.
    ○ One study showed totally seizure freedom compared to placebo group (two patients); all other studies showed no improvement.
    ○ Overall well tolerated, mild drowsiness noted in one study
  - Chemotherapy-induced nausea and vomiting
    ○ Low-quality evidence suggests that cannabinoids are associated with improvements in nausea and vomiting due to chemotherapy (dronabinol and nabiximols) (3)[C].
    ○ Improvement was more noticeable for nausea than vomiting due to limitations of oral route of administration and length of time to peak plasma level.
    ○ Repeated use has been linked with increased nausea and vomiting in some patients.
  - Inflammation
    ○ Cannabinoids induce apoptosis, inhibit cell proliferation, and suppress cytokine production.
    ○ Initial studies in animal models suggest possible benefit in rheumatoid arthritis and inflammatory bowel disease, but this research is in very preliminary stages.
    ○ A recent study in patients with MS failed to show any effect on disease progression.
  - Probably not effective
    ○ Acute pain
    ○ Glaucoma
    ○ Other neurologic conditions: tremor, Tourette syndrome, Huntington disease, and Parkinson disease

ONGOING CARE

- Side effects
  - Dizziness, dry mouth, nausea, vomiting, fatigue, somnolence, disorientation, drowsiness, confusion, loss of balance, and hallucination
  - Acute psychological effects include euphoria, dysphoria, sedation, and altered perception.
  - Acute intoxication can cause tachycardia, hypertension, ataxia, paranoia, and psychosis.
  - Withdrawal syndrome can include symptoms of irritability, sleeping difficulties, dysphoria, craving marijuana, and anxiety.

ALERT

Overdose by children can cause respiratory depression. Several states with legalized marijuana have noted an increase in hospitalizations after accidental ingestion by children.

- Long-term complications
  - Respiratory (3)[C]:
    - Chronic bronchitis
    - Increased rates of respiratory infections and pneumonia
  - Cardiovascular risk:
    - Associated with hypertension, dyslipidemia, and increased caloric intake
    - 4.8-fold increase in incidence of myocardial infarction (MI) in 1st hour after use but became nonsignificant after 2nd hour
    - 4.2-fold increase in MI mortality rate for marijuana users versus nonusers
    - Several case reports of cerebrovascular events related to marijuana in patients with no other risk factors (17% increased risk among users)
    - Possible mechanisms include increased platelet coagulability, detrimental effects on microcirculation, and artery spasm.
  - Cancer risk:
    - Associated with increased incidence of lung cancer and upper airway/esophageal cancer; however, association disappeared when adjusted for cigarette smoking
    - Recent review of six studies showed no association.

- Psychological (3)[C]:
  - Increased anxiety, psychosis, and depression (noncausal association)
  - Increased risk of schizophrenia in early chronic users
  - Addiction occurs in 9% of all users, with higher rates among adolescents (17%) and daily users (20–25%).
  - Interference with cognitive function and short-term memory results in difficulty learning.
  - Increased motor vehicle accidents, relative risk (RR) = 2, compared to RR = 5 for blood alcohol level >.08
  - "Gateway drug" phenomenon persists even in states where marijuana use is legal.
    - Marijuana reduces dopamine activity in reward centers, increasing susceptibility to drug abuse.
    - Concurrent use primes brain for enhanced response to other drugs.

Pediatric Considerations

Adolescents have increased vulnerability to adverse long-term outcomes (3)[C].
- Brain endocannabinoid system actively develops during adolescence.
- Initial use during adolescence is associated with long-term brain changes:
  - Increased school drop out
  - Lower IQ
  - Diminished life satisfaction

Pregnancy Considerations

- Marijuana use is associated with decreased sperm count and reduced sperm motility.
- Also thought to interfere with ovulation
- Chemicals produced by marijuana use are known to cross the placenta and into breast milk.
- Current evidence suggests that cannabis use during pregnancy and lactation may adversely affect neurodevelopment of fetal brain, with effects on neuropsychiatric, behavioral, and executive functioning.
- Use is strongly discouraged because of concern for impact on fetal and infant neurocognitive development.
- Areas of future consideration
  - The risk of secondhand marijuana smoke exposure is unstudied.
  - Increasing legal status contributes to public misconception of safety. The frequency of use and population health effects of recent changes in law should be carefully monitored.

REFERENCES

1. Whiting PF, Wolff RF, Deshpande S, et al. Cannabinoids for medical use: a systematic review and meta-analysis. *JAMA.* 2015;313(24):2456–2473.
2. Koppel BS, Brust JC, Fife T, et al. Systematic review: efficacy and safety of medical marijuana in selected neurologic disorders: report of the Guideline Development Subcommittee of the American Academy of Neurology. *Neurology.* 2014;82(17):1556–1563.
3. Volkow ND, Baler RD, Compton WM, et al. Adverse health effects of marijuana use. *N Engl J Med.* 2014;370(23):2219–2227.
4. Shishko I, Oliveira R, Moore TA, et al. A review of medical marijuana for the treatment of posttraumatic stress disorder: real symptom re-leaf or just high hopes? *Ment Health Clin.* 2018;8(2):86–94.
5. Gloss D, Vickrey B. Cannabinoids for epilepsy. *Cochrane Database Syst Rev.* 2014;(3):CD009270.

ADDITIONAL READING

- Donnelly J, Young M. The legalization of medical/recreational marijuana: implications for school health drug education programs. *J Sch Health.* 2018;88(9):693–698.
- Hasin DS. US epidemiology of cannabis use and associated problems. *Neuropsychopharmacology.* 2018;43(1):195–212.
- Keehbauch J, Rensberry M. Effectiveness, adverse effects, and safety of medical marijuana. *Am Fam Physician.* 2015;92(10):856–863.
- Kramer JL. Medical marijuana for cancer. *CA Cancer J Clin.* 2015;65(2):109–122.
- Rezkalla S, Kloner R. Recreational marijuana use: is it safe for your patient? *J Am Heart Assoc.* 2014;3(2):e000904.

CODES

ICD10

F12.90 Cannabis use, unspecified, uncomplicated

CLINICAL PEARLS

- There is scant robust clinical evidence supporting benefits of medical marijuana, and little to no evidence that alternate formulations have increased benefits compared to FDA-approved formulations.
- Medical marijuana has a narrow therapeutic index, with significant patient-to-patient variability in benefits and adverse effects.
- Chronic use in adolescents must be avoided due to increased risk of long-term negative outcomes.

M

MELANOMA

Katherine E. Haga, DO • Lloyd A. Runser, MD, MPH, FAAFP

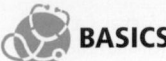 **BASICS**

DESCRIPTION

- Melanoma is a tumor arising from malignant transformation of pigment-containing cells called melanocytes, which are found in the stratum basale of the epidermis.
  - Most arise in the skin but may also present as a primary lesion in any tissue: ocular (uvea), GI, GU, lymph node, paranasal sinuses, nasal cavity, anorectal mucosa, and leptomeninges.
  - Extracutaneous sites have an adverse prognosis.
  - Metastatic spread to any site in the body
- Types of invasive cutaneous melanomas include:
  - Superficial-spreading melanoma: approximately 70% of cases; occurs in sun-exposed areas (trunk, back, and extremities); most <1 mm thick at diagnosis; when seen in younger patients, presents as a flat, slow growing, irregularly bordered lesion
  - Nodular: 15–30% of cases; present in older patients; tendency to ulcerate and hemorrhage; most commonly thick and pigmented; most common melanoma >2 mm
  - Lentigo maligna (subtype of melanoma in situ): slowest growing; older population; occurs in sun-exposed areas (head, neck, forearms). Lentigo maligna melanoma (LMM) is its invasive counterpart seen in 10–15% of cases; it is most commonly seen in elderly patients most often in the head and neck regions.
  - Acral lentiginous: <5% of all melanomas; however, most common melanoma in black or Asian patients; found in palmar, plantar, and subungual areas; can mimic other skin abnormalities, including warts, calluses, tinea pedis, or ingrown toenails
    - An important subtype of acral lentiginous melanoma is subungual melanoma. From the nail matrix, presents as dark stripe under the nail plate; Hutchinson nail sign when brown or black pigment extends from the nail to the cuticle and proximal or lateral nail folds
  - Amelanotic melanoma (<5%): can be missed and diagnosed at a later stage because it can mimic benign skin conditions, and thus is referred to as a "great pretender"
  - Desmoplastic melanoma (~1%): "neurotropic melanoma" or "spindled melanoma" with an abundance of fibrous tissue; demonstrates sarcoma-like tendencies with increased hematogenous spread; presents as a slow-growing lesion that is scar-like (no history of injury at the site is noted); often seen in the head and neck
- System(s) affected: skin/exocrine

Geriatric Considerations
Lentigo maligna is most common in elderly patients. This type is usually found on the face, beginning as a circumscribed macular patch of mottled pigmentation showing shades of dark brown, tan, or black.

Pediatric Considerations
Large congenital nevi (>5 cm) are risk factors and have a >2% lifetime risk of malignant conversion. Blistering sunburns in childhood significantly increase risk.

Pregnancy Considerations
No increased risk of melanoma in pregnancy. In the case of recent melanoma treatment, it is recommended to wait 1 to 2 years prior to becoming pregnant because melanoma can spread to the placenta.

EPIDEMIOLOGY

Incidence
- In 2018, an estimated 91,270 Americans were diagnosed with melanoma, with approximately 9,320 expected deaths (1).
- Predominant age: median age at diagnosis 64 years (https://www.cancer.gov/); >50% of all individuals with melanoma are between 20 and 40 years of age.
- Predominant sex: male > female (1.5 times)
- Melanoma is >20 times more common in whites than in African Americans (1).
- Minority groups demonstrate increased rates of metastasis, advanced stages at diagnosis, thicker initial lesions, earlier age at diagnosis, and overall poorer outcomes.
- Low socioeconomic status associated with higher incidence of melanoma

Prevalence
- Lifetime risk: men: 1/27; female: 1/42
- Lifetime risk in whites is ~2.6% (1/38), 0.1% (1/1,000) in blacks, and 0.58% (1/172) in Hispanics (1).
- 1.5% of all cancer deaths

ETIOLOGY AND PATHOPHYSIOLOGY
- DNA damage by UVA/UVB exposure
- Tumor progression: initially may be confined to epidermis with lateral growth, may then grow into dermis with vertical growth

Genetics
- Dysplastic nevus syndrome is a risk factor for development of melanoma. Close surveillance is warranted.
- 8–12% of patients with melanoma have a family history of disease.
- Mutations in *BRAF (V600E)* implicated in 50–60% of cutaneous melanomas
- Familial atypical mole malignant melanoma (FAMMM) syndrome characterized by >50 atypical moles, +FH of melanoma, clinical diagnosis (2)

RISK FACTORS
- Genetic predisposition, personal/family history of melanoma
- UVA and UVB exposure
- History of >5 sunburns during lifetime, blistering sunburns in childhood
- Previous pigmented lesions (especially dysplastic melanocytic nevi)
- Fair complexion, freckling, blue eyes, blond/red hair
- Highest predictor of risk is increased number of nevi (>50).
- 70% of melanomas are de novo, not existing from previous nevi (2).
- Tanning bed use: 75% increased risk if first exposure before age 35 years
- Changing nevus (see ABCDE criteria)
- Large (>5 cm) congenital nevi
- Chronic immunosuppression (chronic lymphocytic leukemia, non-Hodgkin lymphoma, AIDS, or posttransplant)
- Living at high altitude (>700 meters or 2,300 feet above sea level)
- Occupational exposure to ionizing radiation

GENERAL PREVENTION
- Avoidance of sunburns, especially in childhood. Seek shade and avoid midday sun.
- Use of broad-spectrum sunscreen with at least SPF 30 to all skin exposed to sunlight reapplying regularly and after toweling or swimming
- Avoid tanning beds; class 1 carcinogen by World Health Organization (WHO)
- Screening of high-risk individuals, especially males >50 years
- Education for proper diagnosis plays a large factor in prevention.
- Any suspicious lesions should be biopsied with a narrow excision encompassing the entire breadth plus sufficient depth of the lesion. Options include elliptical excisions, punch, or shave biopsies.

COMMONLY ASSOCIATED CONDITIONS
- Dysplastic nevus syndrome
- >50 nevi. These individuals have higher lifetime risk of melanoma than the general population because 30% of all melanoma arise in preexisting nevi (3).
- Giant congenital nevus: 6% lifetime incidence of melanoma
- Xeroderma pigmentosum is a rare condition associated with an extremely high risk of skin cancers, including melanoma.
- Psoriasis after psoralen-UV-A (PUVA) therapy

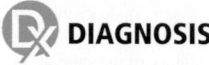 **DIAGNOSIS**

HISTORY
- Change in a pigmented lesion: either hypo- or hyperpigmentation, bleeding, scaling, ulceration, or changes in size or texture
- Obtain family and personal history of melanoma or nonmelanoma skin cancer.
- Obtain social history including occupation, sunbathing, tanning, and other sun exposure.

PHYSICAL EXAM
- ABCDE: Asymmetry, Border irregularity, Color variegation (especially red, white, black, blue), Diameter >6 mm, Evolution over time
- Any new and/or changing nevus, bleeding/ulcerated
- Location on Caucasians is primarily back and lower leg; on African Americans, it is the hands, feet, and nails.
- May include mucosal surfaces (nasopharynx, conjunctiva)
- Individuals at high risk for melanoma should have careful ocular exam to assess for presence of melanoma in the iris and retina.

DIFFERENTIAL DIAGNOSIS
- Dysplastic and blue nevi
- Vascular skin tumor
- Pigmented actinic keratosis
- Traumatic hematoma
- Pigmented basal cell carcinomas, seborrheic keratoses, other changing nevi
- Common or atypical melanocytic nevi
- Lentigo
- Pyogenic granuloma

DIAGNOSTIC TESTS & INTERPRETATION
- Lactate dehydrogenase (LDH), chest/abdomen/pelvic CT with or without PET/CT at baseline and in monitoring progression in metastatic disease (stage IV); brain MRI if any CNS symptoms or physical findings (4)
- Imaging studies only helpful in detecting and evaluating for progression of metastatic disease

Diagnostic Procedures/Other

- Dermoscopy allows for magnification of lesions; evidence limited on utility (2)[C]
- Full-thickness excisional biopsy remains the gold standard for diagnosis. Any suspicious nevus should be excised, either by elliptical excision, punch biopsy, or a scoop shave (saucerization) biopsy may be appropriate. Avoid superficial shave of suspicious lesion. Goal for full-thickness excision with 1 to 3 mm margins. Orient excisional biopsy to optimize future treatment (4)[C].
- Sentinel lymph node biopsy, a staging procedure, remains an important factor for prognosis (4)[A].

Test Interpretation

- Nodular melanoma is primarily vertical growth, whereas the other three types are horizontal.
- Estimated that 1/10,000 dysplastic nevi become melanoma annually.
- Immunohistochemical testing increases sensitivity of lymph node biopsies.
- Staging is based on the tumor-node-metastasis (TNM) criteria by current American Joint Committee on Cancer (AJCC) criteria, including:
  - (T) thickness (mm) and ulceration
  - (N) number of regional lymph nodes involved
  - (M) distant metastases and serum LDH
  - See https://www.cancer.org/cancer/melanoma -skin-cancer/detection-diagnosis-staging /melanoma-skin-cancer-stages.html for more information.

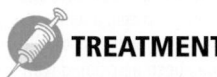

TREATMENT

GENERAL MEASURES

Full surgical excision of melanoma is the standard of care. See below for recommended surgical margins.

MEDICATION

- For stages I to III, surgical excision is curative in most cases; in patients with stage IV disease, systemic treatment with chemotherapy is recommended.
- Preferred regimens (4)[A] include the following:
  - Anti PD-4 monotherapy
  - Pembrolizumab
  - Nivolumab
  - Nivolumab with ipilimumab
  - Combo therapy demonstrated 61% response versus ipilimumab alone (5)[B].
  - If BRAF V600 activating mutation is present, can opt for target therapy with combinations of:
    ○ Dabrafenib/trametinib
    ○ Vemurafenib/cobimetinib
    ○ Encorafenib/binimetinib
- Additional active regimens (e.g., dacarbazine [DTIC], temozolomide, paclitaxel, carmustine [BCNU], cisplatin, carboplatin, vinblastine) often limited to those who are not candidates to preferred regimens
- Imatinib (Gleevec) in tumors with c-KIT mutation
- Interferon-α as adjuvant therapy received FDA approval in 1995 (high dose) and 2011 (pegylated) to treat stage IIB to III melanoma; shown to improve 4-year relapse rate but no overall effect on survival; 1/3 of patients will discontinue due to toxicity (granulocytopenia, hepatotoxicity) (4)[B].

ISSUES FOR REFERRAL

- Consultation with oncologist for consideration of chemotherapeutic options
- Surgical specialties may be required based on the extent of nodal and/or metastatic disease, if present.

SURGERY/OTHER PROCEDURES

- Standard of care for melanoma includes early surgical excision with the following recommended margins (4)[A]:
  - In situ tumors: 0.5 to 1.0 cm
  - Thickness of 1.01 to 2.00 mm: 1 to 2 cm margins
  - Thickness of >2.00 mm: 2 cm margins
- Sentinel lymph node biopsy is indicated in patients with T1b, T2-, T3-, and T4-staged melanomas.
  - Not recommended in melanoma in situ or T1a
- Mohs micrographic surgery is being increasingly used for melanoma in situ, but in general, it is not considered a treatment modality for melanoma because it relies on frozen section technique.
- Radiotherapy can be used to treat lentigo maligna in addition to certain head and neck lesions.
- Palliative radiation therapy can be used with metastatic melanoma.

COMPLEMENTARY & ALTERNATIVE MEDICINE

Molecular and mouse tumor model studies support role of topical silymarin (milk thistle derivative) in decreasing UV radiation–induced inflammation, oxidative stress, and carcinogenesis.

ADMISSION, INPATIENT, AND NURSING CONSIDERATIONS

Most monitoring and treatment completed in the outpatient setting.

 ONGOING CARE

FOLLOW-UP RECOMMENDATIONS

After diagnosis and treatment, close follow-up and skin protection (i.e., sunblock, UV protective clothing) are highly advised.

Patient Monitoring

- Routine screening clinical skin examination annually for all persons >40 years is controversial and without proven benefit.
- Total body photography and dermoscopy should be used for surveillance of skin lesions, most commonly used for patients with >5 atypical nevi.
- For patients with a history of cutaneous melanoma, NCCN guidelines recommend screening every 3 to 12 months depending on recurrence risk (4)[C], with annual examinations if there is no disease progression for 5 years.
- Lab and imaging tests after diagnosis and treatment of stage I to II melanoma are low yield, have high false-positive rates, and are not recommended (4)[B].

PATIENT EDUCATION

- Teach all patients to perform regular full-body skin examinations looking for ABCDEs, especially those at high risk, or who have had melanoma.
- High-risk patients should perform monthly skin self-examinations and be taught to examine inaccessible areas.
- Patients with a history of melanoma or dysplastic nevus syndrome should have regular total body examinations by a dermatologist.

PROGNOSIS

- Breslow depth (thickness) in millimeters remains among strongest predictors of prognosis.
- Median age at death is 68 years.
- Highest survival seen in women <45 years of age at diagnosis

- Metastatic melanoma has an average survival of 6 to 9 months; 15–20% 5-year survival with current treatment
- Stages I and II, appropriately treated, have 20-year survival rates of 90% and 80%, respectively.

COMPLICATIONS

- Metastatic spread and subsequent death
- Often referred to as the "great imitator," given that metastatic disease may present in a variety of ways
- Unsatisfactory cosmetic results

REFERENCES

1. Siegel R, Miller K, Jemal A. Cancer statistics, 2018. *CA Cancer J Clin*. 2018;68(1):7–30.
2. Bichakjian CK, Halpern AC, Johnson TM, et al; for American Academy of Dermatology. Guidelines of care for the management of primary cutaneous melanoma. American Academy of Dermatology. *J Am Acad Dermatol*. 2011;65(5):1032–1047.
3. Pampena R, Kyrgidis A, Lallas A, et al. A meta-analysis of nevus-associated melanoma: prevalence and practical implications. *J Am Acad Dermatol*. 2017;77(5):938.e4–945.e4.
4. Coit DG, Thompson JA, Algazi A, et al. NCCN guidelines insights: melanoma, version 3.2016. *J Natl Compr Canc Netw*. 2016;14(8):945–958.
5. Schachter J, Ribas A, Long GV, et al. Pembrolizumab versus ipilimumab for advanced melanoma: final overall survival results of a multicentre, randomised, open-label phase 3 study (KEYNOTE-006). *Lancet*. 2017;390(10105):1853–1862.

ADDITIONAL READING

- American Cancer Society. Survival rates for melanoma skin cancer, by stage. https://www.cancer.org /cancer/melanoma-skin-cancer/detection-diagnosis -staging/survival-rates-for-melanoma-skin-cancer-by -stage.html. Accessed December 13, 2018.
- Melanoma Prediction Tools: http://www.melanomaprognosis.net/
- Perkins A, Duffy RL. Atypical moles: diagnosis and management. *Am Fam Physician*. 2015;91(11):762–767.
- Shenenberger D. Cutaneous malignant melanoma: a primary care perspective. *Am Fam Physician*. 2012;85(2):161–168.

 SEE ALSO

Atypical Mole (Dysplastic Nevus) Syndrome

 CODES

ICD10

- C43.9 Malignant melanoma of skin, unspecified
- C43.30 Malignant melanoma of unspecified part of face
- C43.4 Malignant melanoma of scalp and neck

CLINICAL PEARLS

- Remember that amelanotic melanomas exist; pigmentation is not required.
- 70% of melanomas are de novo, not from preexisting nevi. Still, any changing nevi should be biopsied, preferably utilizing an excisional method to ensure that complete margins are taken (2).
- The prognosis is excellent with early detection and treatment.

M

MÉNIÈRE DISEASE

Jason E. Cohn, DO • Nadir Ahmad, MD, FACS • Thomas C. Spalla, MD

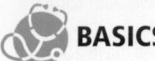 **BASICS**

DESCRIPTION
- An inner ear (labyrinthine) disorder characterized by recurrent attacks of hearing loss, tinnitus, vertigo, and sensations of aural fullness due to an increase in the volume and pressure of the inner ear endolymph fluid (endolymphatic hydrops)
- Often unilateral initially; nearly half become bilateral over time.
- Severity and frequency of vertigo may diminish with time, but hearing loss is often progressive and/or fluctuating.
- Usually idiopathic (Ménière disease) but may be secondary to another condition causing endolymphatic hydrops (Ménière syndrome)
- System(s) affected: nervous
- Synonym(s): Ménière syndrome; endolymphatic hydrops

EPIDEMIOLOGY
- Predominant age of onset: 40 to 60 years
- Predominant gender: female > male (1.3:1)
- Race/ethnicity: white, Northern European > blacks

Incidence
Estimates 1 to 150/100,000 per year

Prevalence
Varies from 7.5 to >200/100,000

ETIOLOGY AND PATHOPHYSIOLOGY
- Not fully understood; theories include increased pressure of the endolymph fluid due to increased fluid production or decreased resorption. This may be caused by endolymphatic sac pathology, abnormal development of the vestibular aqueduct, or inflammation caused by circulating immune complexes. Increased endolymph pressure may cause rupture of membranes and changes in endolymphatic ionic gradient.
- Ménière syndrome may be secondary to injury or other disorders (e.g., reduced middle ear pressure, allergy, endocrine disease, lipid disorders, vascular, viral, syphilis, autoimmune). Any disorder that could cause endolymphatic hydrops could be implicated in Ménière syndrome.

Genetics
Some families show increased incidence, but genetic and environmental influences are incompletely understood.

RISK FACTORS
May include
- Stress
- Allergy
- Increased salt intake
- Caffeine, alcohol, or nicotine
- Chronic exposure to loud noise
- Family history of Ménière
- Certain vascular abnormalities (including migraines)
- Certain viral exposures (especially herpes simplex virus [HSV])

GENERAL PREVENTION
Reduce known risk factors: stress; salt, alcohol, and caffeine intake; smoking; noise exposure; ototoxic drugs (e.g., aspirin, quinine, aminoglycosides).

COMMONLY ASSOCIATED CONDITIONS
- Anxiety (secondary to the disabling symptoms)
- Migraines
- Hyperprolactinemia
- Hypothyroidism

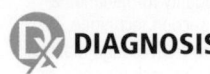 **DIAGNOSIS**

Diagnosis is clinical.

HISTORY
- Symptomatic episodes are typically spontaneous but may be preceded by an aura of increasing fullness in the ear and tinnitus. These may occur in clusters, with long periods of symptom-free remissions.
- Formal criteria for diagnosis from American Academy of Otolaryngology–Head and Neck Surgery:
  – At least two episodes of rotational-horizontal vertigo >20 minutes in duration
  – Tinnitus or aural fullness
  – Hearing loss: Low frequency (sensorineural) is confirmed by audiometric testing.
  – Other causes (e.g., acoustic neuroma) excluded
  – During severe attacks: pallor, sweating, nausea, vomiting, falling, prostration
  – Symptoms are exacerbated by motion.

PHYSICAL EXAM
- Physical exam rules out other conditions; no finding is unique to Ménière disease.
- Horizontal nystagmus may be seen during attacks.
- Otoscopy is typically normal.
- Triggering of attacks in the office with Dix-Hallpike maneuver suggests diagnosis of benign paroxysmal positional vertigo, not Ménière disease.

DIFFERENTIAL DIAGNOSIS
- Acoustic neuroma or other CNS tumor
- Syphilis
- Third window syndromes
- Endolymphatic sac tumor
- Viral labyrinthitis
- Transient ischemic attack (TIA), migraine
- Vertebrobasilar disease
- Other labyrinthine disorders (e.g., Cogan syndrome, benign positional vertigo, temporal bone trauma)
- Diabetes or thyroid dysfunction
- Vestibular neuronitis
- Medication side effects
- Otitis media
- Autoimmune inner ear disease
- Autosomal dominant sensorineural hearing loss

DIAGNOSTIC TESTS & INTERPRETATION
Testing is done to rule out other conditions but does not necessarily confirm or exclude Ménière disease.

Initial Tests (lab, imaging)
- Consider serologic tests specific for *Treponema pallidum* in at-risk populations.
- Thyroid, fasting blood sugar, and lipid studies
- Consider MRI to rule out acoustic neuroma or other CNS pathology, including tumor, aneurysm, and multiple sclerosis (MS).

Diagnostic Procedures/Other
- Auditory
  – Audiometry using pure tone and speech to show low-frequency sensorineural (nerve) loss and impaired speech discrimination; usually shows low-frequency sensorineural hearing loss
  – Tuning fork tests (i.e., Weber and Rinne), ABR, or MRI to rule out acoustic neuroma
  – Electrocochleography may be useful to confirm etiology.
- Vestibular
  – Caloric testing: Reduced activity on either side is consistent with Ménière diagnosis but is not itself diagnostic.
  – Head-impulse testing (1)[C]

Test Interpretation
- Histologic temporal bone analysis (at autopsy); dilation of inner ear fluid system, neuroepithelial damage with hair cell loss, basement membrane thickening, and perivascular microvascular damage
- Cytochemical analysis can reveal altered AQP4 and AQP6 expression in the supporting cell, altered cochlin, and mitochondrial protein expression (2)[B].
- Familial Ménière disease has been associated with DTNA and FAM136A genes (3)[B].

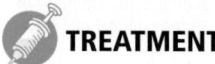 **TREATMENT**

- Usually managed in outpatient setting
- A paucity of evidence-based guidelines exists; therefore, there is no gold standard treatment.
- Medications are primarily for symptomatic relief of vertigo and nausea.
- During attacks, bed rest with eyes closed prevents falls. Attacks rarely last >4 hours.

MEDICATION
First Line
- Acute attack: Initial goal is stabilization and symptom relief; for severe episodes
  – Benzodiazepines (such as diazepam): decrease vertigo and anxiety
  – Antihistamines (meclizine/dimenhydrate): decrease vertigo and nausea
  – Anticholinergics (transdermal scopolamine): reduce nausea and emesis associated with motion sickness
  – Antidopaminergic agents (metoclopramide, promethazine): decrease nausea, anxiety
  – Rehydration therapy and electrolyte replacement
  – Steroid taper for acute hearing loss

- Maintenance (goal is to prevent/reduce attacks)
  - Lifestyle changes (e.g., low-salt diet) are needed.
  - Diuretics may help reduce attacks by decreasing endolymphatic pressure and volume; there is insufficient evidence to recommend routine use:
    - Hydrochlorothiazide; hydrochlorothiazide/triamterene (Dyazide, Maxzide)
    - Acetazolamide (Diamox)
- Contraindications/warnings:
  - Atropine: cardiac disease, especially supraventricular tachycardia and other arrhythmias, prostatic enlargement
  - Scopolamine: children and elderly, prostatic enlargement
  - Diuretics: electrolyte abnormalities, renal disease
- Precautions:
  - Sedating drugs should be used with caution, particularly in the elderly. Patients are cautioned not to operate motor vehicles or machinery. Atropine and scopolamine should be used with particular caution.
  - Diuretics: Monitor electrolytes.
- Significant possible interactions: transdermal scopolamine: anticholinergics, antihistamines, tricyclic antidepressants, other

Second Line
- Steroids, both intratympanic and systemic (PO or IV), have been used for longer treatment of hearing loss:
  - Addition of prednisone 30 mg/day to diuretic treatment reduced severity and frequency of tinnitus and vertigo in one pilot study.
- In Europe, betahistine, a histamine agonist, is routinely used (unavailable in the United States). Other vasodilators, such as isosorbide dinitrate, niacin, and histamine, have also been used; evidence of their effectiveness is incomplete.
- Evidence is lacking for routine use of Famvir; may improve hearing more than balance
- Intratympanic gentamicin has shown to improve vertigo (4)[B].

ISSUES FOR REFERRAL
- Consider ear, nose, throat/neurology referral.
- Patients should have formal audiometry to confirm hearing loss.

ADDITIONAL THERAPIES
- Application of intermittent pressures via a myringotomy using a Meniett device has been shown to relieve vertigo (5)[B]:
  - Safe; requires a long-term tympanostomy tube
- Vestibular rehabilitation may be beneficial for patients with persistent vestibular symptoms:
  - Safe and effective for unilateral vestibular dysfunction

SURGERY/OTHER PROCEDURES
- Interventions that preserve hearing:
  - Endolymphatic sac surgery, either decompression or drainage of endolymph into mastoid or subarachnoid space
    - Less invasive; may decrease vertigo; may influence hearing/tinnitus

---

  - Endolymphatic sac surgery is effective in controlling vertigo in short- and long-term follow-up in at least 75% of patients with Ménière disease who failed medical therapy (6)[A].
  - Vestibular nerve section (intracranial procedure)
    - More invasive
    - Decreases vertigo and preserves hearing
  - Tympanostomy tube: may decrease symptoms by decreasing the middle ear pressure
- Interventions for patients with no serviceable hearing:
  - Labyrinthectomy: very effective at controlling vertigo but causes deafness
  - Vestibular neurectomy
  - Endoscopic vestibular nerve section (7)[B]
  - Cochlear implantation

COMPLEMENTARY & ALTERNATIVE MEDICINE
Insufficient evidence to support effectiveness, but many integrative techniques have been tried, including the following:

- Acupuncture, acupressure, tai chi
- Niacin, bioflavonoids, Lipo-flavonoid, ginger, *Ginkgo biloba*, and other herbal supplements

 ONGOING CARE

FOLLOW-UP RECOMMENDATIONS
Patient Monitoring
Due to the possibility of progressive hearing loss despite decrease in vertiginous attacks, it is important to monitor changes in hearing and to monitor for more serious underlying causes (e.g., acoustic neuroma).

DIET
- Diet is usually not a factor, unless attacks are brought on by certain foods.
- A low salt is often recommended but not proven effective in randomized controlled trials.

PROGNOSIS
- Alert patients about the nature of alternating attacks and remission.
- Between attacks, patient may be fully active but is often limited due to fear or lingering symptoms. This can be severely disabling.
- 50% resolve spontaneously within 2 to 3 years.
- Some cases last >20 years.
- Severity and frequency of attacks diminish, but hearing loss is often progressive.
- 90% can be treated successfully with medication; 5–10% of patients require surgery for incapacitating vertigo.

COMPLICATIONS
Loss of hearing; injury during attack; inability to work

REFERENCES

1. Lee SU, Kim HJ, Koo JW, et al. Comparison of caloric and head-impulse tests during the attacks of Meniere's disease. *Laryngoscope.* 2017;127(3):702–708.
2. Ishiyama G, Lopez IA, Sepahdari AR, et al. Meniere's disease: histopathology, cytochemistry, and imaging. *Ann N Y Acad Sci.* 2015;1343:49–57.
3. Frejo L, Giegling I, Teggi R, et al. Genetics of vestibular disorders: pathophysiological insights. *J Neurol.* 2016;263(Suppl 1):S45–S53.
4. Casani AP, Cerchiai N, Navari E, et al. Intratympanic gentamicin for Meniere's disease: short- and long-term follow-up of two regimens of treatment. *Otolaryngol Head Neck Surg.* 2014;150(5):847–852.
5. Ahsan SF, Standring R, Wang Y. Systematic review and meta-analysis of Meniett therapy for Meniere's disease. *Laryngoscope.* 2015;125(1):203–208.
6. Setty P, Babu S, LaRouere MJ, et al. Fully endoscopic retrosigmoid vestibular nerve section for refractory Meniere disease. *J Neurol Surg B Skull Base.* 2016;77(4):341–349.
7. Sood AJ, Lambert PR, Nguyen SA, et al. Endolymphatic sac surgery for Ménière's disease: a systematic review and meta-analysis. *Otol Neurotol.* 2014;35(6):1033–1045.

 SEE ALSO

- Hearing Loss; Labyrinthitis; Tinnitus
- Algorithm: Dizziness

CODES

ICD10
- H81.09 Meniere's disease, unspecified ear
- H81.01 Meniere's disease, right ear
- H81.02 Meniere's disease, left ear

CLINICAL PEARLS

- Ménière disease is characterized by vertigo, hearing loss, and tinnitus +/– aural fullness.
- There is a wide differential diagnosis for Ménière disease; therefore, one must fully investigate symptoms.
- Multiple medical, surgical, and rehabilitative treatments are available to decrease the severity and frequency of attacks.

M

MENINGITIS, BACTERIAL

Felix B. Chang Cruz, MD, FAAMA, ABIHM

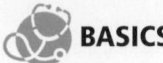 **BASICS**

DESCRIPTION
- Life-threatening bacterial infection of the meninges
- System affected: nervous

EPIDEMIOLOGY
- Predominant age: neonates, infants, and elderly
- Predominant sex: male = female

Incidence
Varies by age and pathogen
- In 2016 year 0.12
- 0 to 4 years 0.78/100,000
- 5 to 9 years 0.13/100,000
- 10 to 14 years 0.09/100,000
- 15 to 19 years 0.31/100,000
- 20 to 24 years 0.3/100,000
- 25 to 29 years 0.18/100,000
- 30 to 34 years 0.14/100,000
- 35 to 39 years 0.13/100,000
- 40 to 44 years 0.13/100,000
- 45 to 49 years 0.14/100,000
- 50 to 54 years 0.17/100,000
- 55 to 59 years 0.16/100,000
- 60 to 64 years 0.17/100,000
- 65 to 69 years 0.20/100,000
- >70 years 0.24 to 0.55/100,000
- *Streptococcus pneumoniae*: 0.81/100,000
- Group B *Streptococcus*: 0.25/100,000
- *Neisseria meningitidis*: 0.19/100,000
- *Haemophilus influenzae*: 0.08/100,000
- *Listeria monocytogenes*: 0.05/100,000

ETIOLOGY AND PATHOPHYSIOLOGY
Bacterial infection causes inflammation of the pia mater, arachnoid, and ventricular fluid. Age and likely pathogens guide empiric antibiotic choice. Tailor therapy to culture results whenever possible (1):

- Community-acquired bacterial meningitis is most commonly due to *S. pneumoniae* (50%) and *N. meningitidis* (30%).
- Nosocomial or postsurgical meningitis occurs after manipulation of the CNS space allowing for entry of pathogens.
- Newborns (<2 months)
  - Group B *Streptococcus*
  - *Escherichia coli*
  - *L. monocytogenes*
- Infants and children
  - *S. pneumoniae*
  - *N. meningitidis*
  - *H. influenzae*
- Adolescents and young adults
  - *N. meningitidis*
  - *S. pneumoniae*
- Immunocompromised adults
  - *S. pneumoniae*, *L. monocytogenes*, gram-negative bacilli such as *Pseudomonas aeruginosa*
  - Mixed bacterial infection in <1% of cases
- Older adults
  - *S. pneumoniae* 50%
  - *N. meningitidis* 30%
  - *L. monocytogenes* 5%
  - 10% gram-negatives bacilli: *E. coli*, *Klebsiella*, *Enterobacter*, *P. aeruginosa*

Genetics
Some Native American populations appear to have genetic or acquired susceptibility to invasive disease.

RISK FACTORS
- Immunocompromised
- Alcoholism, diabetes, chronic disease
- Neurosurgical procedure/head injury
- Close living quarters
- Neonates: prematurity, low birth weight, premature rupture of membranes, maternal peripartum infection, and urinary tract abnormalities
- Abnormal communication between nasopharynx and subarachnoid space (congenital, trauma), dural fistula
- Parameningeal source: otitis, sinusitis, mastoiditis
- Trauma: skull fracture
- Adults age >65 years, immunocompromised patients, and pregnant women are at risk for listeriosis.
- Complement component deficiencies C3, C5 to C9, properdin, factor H, and factor D
- Functional or anatomic asplenia

GENERAL PREVENTION
- Consider CSF fistula in cases of recurrent meningitis.
- Aseptic techniques for head wounds or skull fractures
- Meningitis caused by *H. influenzae* type B has decreased 55% with routine vaccination.
- Conjugate vaccines against *S. pneumoniae* may reduce the burden of disease in childhood.
- Chemoprophylaxis for close contacts of meningococcal meningitis patients (2)[A]

COMMONLY ASSOCIATED CONDITIONS
Factors associated with a worse prognosis:
- Alcoholism, old age, infancy, diabetes mellitus, multiple myeloma, head trauma, seizures
- Coma, sepsis, sinusitis

 **DIAGNOSIS**

HISTORY
- Antecedent upper respiratory infection
- Fever, headache, vomiting, photophobia
- Seizures, confusion
- Nausea, rigors; sweats, weakness
- Elderly: subtle findings including confusion
- Infants: irritability, lethargy, poor feeding
- Altered mental status
- Food exposures (e.g., *L. monocytogenes*)

PHYSICAL EXAM
The triad of fever, neck stiffness, and altered mental status has low sensitivity (44%) (3). 95% of patients present with at least two of the following: headache, fever, neck stiffness, and altered mental status.
- Meningismus
- Focal neurologic deficits
- Meningococcal rash: macular and erythematous at first, then petechial or purpuric
- Purpura fulminans: more common with meningococcus
- Papilledema
- Brudzinski sign: Passive flexion of neck elicits involuntary flexing of knees in supine position.
- Kernig sign: resistance or pain with passive knee extension following 90-degree hip flexion in supine position
- Late signs and symptoms: hemiparesis, stroke, cognitive impairment, coma, epilepsy, hearing loss, permanent visual impairment

DIFFERENTIAL DIAGNOSIS
- Bacteremia, sepsis, brain abscess
- Seizures, other nonbacterial meningitides

- Aseptic meningitis
- Inflammatory noninfectious: Behçet disease, systemic lupus erythematosus (SLE), sarcoidosis
- Stroke

DIAGNOSTIC TESTS & INTERPRETATION
Initial Tests (lab, imaging)
- Prompt lumbar puncture (1)[A]
  - Head CT first if focal neurologic findings, papilledema, or altered mentation
  - Typical CSF analysis: turbid
  - Adults
    - >500 cells/mL WBCs
    - Glucose <40 mg/dL
    - <2/3 blood-to-glucose ratio
    - CSF protein >200 mg/dL
    - CSF opening pressure >30 cm
    - Suspect ruptured brain abscess when WBC count is unusually high (>100,000).
- CSF Gram stain and cultures
- Polymerase chain reaction (PCR) of CSF (particularly in suspected viral meningitis)
- Reserve bacterial antigen tests for cases where initial CSF Gram stain is negative and CSF culture is negative at 48 hours.
- Serum blood cultures, serum electrolytes
- Evaluate clotting function if petechiae or purpura is present.
- Chest radiograph may reveal pneumonitis or abscess.
- C-reactive protein (CRP): Normal CRP has high negative predictive value (3)[A].
- Later in course, head CT if hydrocephalus, brain abscess, subdural effusions, and subdural empyema are suspected or if no clinical response after 48 hours of appropriate antibiotics
- Lactate concentration not recommended for suspected community-acquired bacterial meningitis

Diagnostic Procedures/Other
Lumbar puncture

- CT recommended prior to lumbar puncture if: immunocompromised, history of central nervous system disease (stroke, mass lesion, focal infection), papilledema, focal neurologic defect including fixed dilated pupil, gaze palsy, weakness of extremity, visual field cut, new-onset seizure <12 weeks prior to presentation, abnormal level of consciousness (3)[A]
- Lumbar puncture contraindications: signs of increased intracranial pressure (decerebrate posturing, papilledema), skin infection at site of lumbar puncture, CT or MRI evidence of obstructive hydrocephalus, cerebral edema, herniation

 TREATMENT

GENERAL MEASURES
- Initiate empiric antibiotic therapy immediately after lumbar puncture (lumbar puncture > Abx). If head CT scan is needed, initiate antibiotic therapy immediately after blood cultures (Abx > CT > lumbar puncture).
- Watch for seizures and aspiration precautions.

MEDICATION
Empiric antibiotic IV therapy (with dexamethasone for known or suspected *S. pneumoniae* meningitis) until culture results are available
- Consider local bacterial sensitivity patterns.

First Line
- Neonates
- Ampicillin: 150 mg/kg/day divided q8h *AND*
- Cefotaxime: 150 mg/kg/day divided q8h
- Infants >4 weeks of age (3,4)[A]
  - Ceftriaxone: 100 mg/kg/day divided q12–24h or cefotaxime 225 to 300 mg/kg/day divided q6–8h *AND*
  - Vancomycin: 60 mg/kg/day divided q6h
- Adults (3,4)[A]
  - Vancomycin: loading dose 25 to 30 mg/kg IV and then 15 to 20 mg/kg q8–12h with goal trough of 15 to 20 *AND*
  - Ceftriaxone: 2 g IV q12h *OR*
  - Cefotaxime: 2 g IV q4–6h
  - >50 years, add ampicillin: 2 g IV q4h for *Listeria*
  - Immunocompromised: Use vancomycin, ampicillin, ceftazidime, and acyclovir.
- Precaution: aminoglycoside ototoxicity
- Penicillin-allergic patients (3,4)[A]
  - Chloramphenicol: 1 g IV q6h *AND*
  - Vancomycin: loading dose 25 to 30 mg/kg IV and then 15 to 20 mg/kg q8–12h (goal trough of 15 to 20)
- Treatment duration
  - *S. pneumoniae*: 10 to 14 days
  - *N. meningitidis, H. influenzae*: 7 to 10 days
  - Group B *Streptococcus* organisms, *E. coli, L. monocytogenes*: 14 to 21 days
  - Neonates: 12 to 21 days or at least 14 days after a repeated culture is sterile
  - No reliable evidence to support the use preadmission antibiotics for suspected cases of nonsevere meningococcal disease (5)[A]
- Corticosteroids (5)[A]
  - Pediatrics
    - Early treatment with dexamethasone (0.15 mg/kg IV q6h for 2 to 4 days) decreases mortality and morbidity for patients >1 month of age with acute bacterial meningitis with no increased risk of GI bleeding.
    - Corticosteroids are associated with lower rates of hearing loss and neurologic sequelae.
- Adults (5)[A]
  - Initiate in adults and continue only if CSF Gram stain shows gram-positive diplococcus or if blood or CSF positive for *S. pneumoniae*.
  - Nonsignificant reduction in mortality (RR) 0.90, 95% CI 0.53–1.05; *p* value = .009
  - Lower rates of severe hearing loss (RR 0.67, 95% CI 0.51–0.88), any hearing loss (RR 0.74, 95% CI 0.63–0.87), and neurologic sequelae (RR 0.83, 95% CI 0.69–1.00)
  - Decreased mortality in *S. pneumoniae* (RR 0.8, 95% CI 0.20–0.59) but not in *H. influenzae* or *N. meningitidis*
  - Associated with increased recurrence of fever (RR 1.27, 95% CI 1.09–1.47)
- Dexamethasone: 0.15 mg/kg IV q6h (start 15 to 20 minutes before or with antibiotic) for 4 days
- Dexamethasone should only be continued if the CSF Gram stain and/or CSF or blood culture reveal *S. pneumoniae*.

Second Line
Antipseudomonal penicillins should be given in combination with other appropriate agents.
- Aztreonam 2 g IV q6–8h
- Fluoroquinolones (e.g., ciprofloxacin) IV 400 mg q8–12h
- Meropenem IV 2 g q8h

ISSUES FOR REFERRAL
Consultation from infectious disease and/or critical care specialist

ADMISSION, INPATIENT, AND NURSING CONSIDERATIONS
- Bacterial meningitis requires hospitalization.
  - ICU monitoring may be needed.
  - Patients with suspected meningococcal infection require respiratory isolation for 24 hours.
- Consider home therapy to complete IV antibiotics once clinically stable and culture/sensitivity results are known.

ONGOING CARE

FOLLOW-UP RECOMMENDATIONS
Patient Monitoring
- Brainstem auditory—evoked response hearing test for infants before hospital discharge
- Vaccinations
  - 4 doses *Hib* conjugate vaccine recommended during infancy
  - Meningococcal conjugate vaccine quadrivalent (MCV4) is given to children aged 11 to 12 years with a booster at 16 years.
  - Immunizing infants <3 months old with MCV4 does not reduce morbidity or mortality, and vaccinating pregnant women does not reduce infant infections.
  - Administer 2 doses MCV4 at least 2 months apart to adults with the following:
    - HIV, functional asplenia
    - Persistent complement deficiencies
  - Administer 1 dose of meningococcal vaccine to:
    - Military recruits
    - Microbiologists routinely exposed to isolates of *N. meningitidis*
    - Those who travel to or live in countries where meningitis is hyperendemic or epidemic
    - 1st-year college students up through age 21 years who live in residence halls if they have not received a dose on or after their 16th birthday
  - MCV4 is preferred for adults ≤55 years of age; meningococcal polysaccharide vaccine (MPSV4) is preferred for adults aged ≥56 years.
  - Revaccination with MCV4 every 5 years is recommended for adults previously vaccinated with MCV4 or MPSV4 who are at increased risk.
  - For patient with complement deficiencies, CDC recommends meningococcal conjugate vaccine and serogroup B meningococcal vaccine.
  - Patients taking eculizumab are at increased risk for meningococcal disease.
- Prophylaxis (2)[A]
  - Only for close contacts of patients, effective up to 2 weeks after treatment without leading to resistance
  - Rifampin is effective in eradicating *N. meningitidis* up to 4 weeks after treatment but may lead to resistance.
  - Rifampin: 600 mg PO BID for 2 days
  - Ciprofloxacin: 500 mg PO for 1 dose
  - Ceftriaxone: 250 mg IM for 1 dose

DIET
Regular, as tolerated, except with syndrome of inappropriate secretion of antidiuretic hormone

PROGNOSIS
- Overall case fatality: 10–14%
- Bacterial meningitis is fatal in 5–40% of children and 20–50% of adults despite treatment.
- Mortality rate of untreated disease approaches 100%.

COMPLICATIONS
- Seizures: 20–30% focal neurologic deficit
- Cranial nerve palsies (III, VI, VII, VIII) in 10–20% of cases; usually transient
- Sensorineural hearing loss: 10% in children
- Neurodevelopmental sequelae: 30% with subtle learning deficits
- Obstructive hydrocephalus, subdural effusion
- Inappropriate antidiuretic hormone secretion
- Elevated intracranial pressure: herniation, brain swelling

REFERENCES
1. Centers for Disease Control and Prevention. Meningitis. https://www.cdc.gov/meningitis/bacterial.html. Accessed December 6, 2018.
2. Zalmanovici Trestioreanu A, Fraser A, Gafter-Gvili A, et al. Antibiotics for preventing meningococcal infections. *Cochrane Database Syst Rev*. 2013;(10): CD004785.
3. Heckenberg SG, Brouwer MC, van de Beek D. Bacterial meningitis. *Handb Clin Neurol*. 2014;121:1361–1375.
4. Liu C, Bayer A, Cosgrove SE, et al; for Infectious Diseases Society of America. Clinical practice guidelines by the Infectious Diseases Society of America for the treatment of methicillin-resistant *Staphylococcus aureus* infections in adults and children. *Clin Infect Dis*. 2011;52(3):e18–e55.
5. Brouwer MC, McIntyre P, Prasad K, et al. Corticosteroids for acute bacterial meningitis. *Cochrane Database Syst Rev*. 2015;(9):CD004405.

ADDITIONAL READING
- McGill F, Heyderman RS, Panagiotou S, et al. Acute bacterial meningitis in adults. *Lancet*. 2016;388(10063):3036–3047.
- Tunkel A, Hasbun R, Bhimraj A, et al. 2017 Infectious Diseases Society of America's clinical practice guidelines for healthcare-associated ventriculitis and meningitis. *Clin Infect Dis*. 2017;64(6):e34–e65.

 CODES

ICD10
- G00.9 Bacterial meningitis, unspecified
- G00.2 Streptococcal meningitis
- G00.8 Other bacterial meningitis

CLINICAL PEARLS
- Consider meningococcal infection in the differential diagnosis of any patient presenting with the sudden onset of febrile illness, especially when petechiae and/or meningeal signs are present.
- Use droplet precautions for 24 hours after institution of antibiotic therapy in patient with suspected or confirmed *N. meningitidis* infection.
- Prophylaxis for close contacts of confirmed cases of *N. meningitidis*

M

MENINGITIS, VIRAL

Christine M. Broszko, MD • James E. Hougas III, MD, FAAFP

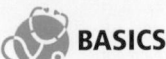

BASICS

DESCRIPTION
- A clinical syndrome characterized by signs/symptoms of acute meningeal inflammation from a viral etiology
- Viral meningitis (VM) is the most common cause of aseptic meningitis (no identifiable bacterial pathogen in CSF).
- System(s) affected: nervous

EPIDEMIOLOGY
Incidence
- Estimated 30,000 to 75,000 VM cases and 26,000 to 42,000 VM hospitalizations annually in United States
- Most common form of infectious meningitis
  - The annual incidence of VM is higher than all other causes of meningitis combined.
- Peaks June 1 to October 31
  - Nonpolio enteroviruses and arthropod-borne viruses predominate in warm months (70% of cases July to October).
  - Mumps usually occurs in the winter and spring, often in epidemics; rare due to MMR vaccination

ETIOLOGY AND PATHOPHYSIOLOGY
- In immunocompetent hosts, VM is generally caused by virus with neurotropic predilection.
- Less commonly, direct neural transmission occurs from an acute flare of a chronic viral illness (such as HSV) already present in an immunocompetent host.
- 85–95% of VM cases are caused by enterovirus family (often transmitted by the fecal–oral route), including coxsackievirus A and B, echovirus, and nonpolio E variants: E9 and E30.
- Less common: HSV-1, HSV-2, varicella-zoster virus (VZV), adenovirus, lymphocytic choriomeningitis virus (LCMV), cytomegalovirus (CMV), Epstein-Barr virus (EBV), HIV, parvovirus B19, mumps, Toscana virus
- Parechovirus 3 is the most common cause of VM in infants <90 days old.
- Arthropod-borne viruses: West Nile virus, St. Louis encephalitis virus, California encephalitis virus
- Recurrent benign lymphocytic (Mollaret) meningitis is 80% associated with HSV-2.

Genetics
None identified

RISK FACTORS
- Close contact with known cases of VM
- Age (common in children <5 years)
- Immunocompromised host (more susceptible to CMV, HSV, and adenovirus)

Geriatric Considerations
Cases of VM in the elderly are rare (most common cause is VZV, HSV); consider alternative diagnoses (e.g., carcinomatous meningitis, medication-induced aseptic meningitis).

GENERAL PREVENTION
Limit exposure to known hosts; hand washing and general hygiene procedures

COMMONLY ASSOCIATED CONDITIONS
Encephalitis; neurologic deficits; myopericarditis; neonatal enteroviral sepsis

DIAGNOSIS

HISTORY
Predominant adult symptoms include acute onset (hours to days) of:
- Fever (in 76–100% of patients)
- Headache (prominent early symptom)
- Photophobia
- Myalgias
- Nausea, vomiting
- Malaise
  - In infants, nonspecific symptoms are more common including poor feeding, fever, and irritability.
- Nuchal rigidity (>50%)
  - Note: If altered mental status (AMS), consider encephalitis. Encephalitis is associated with neurologic dysfunction, such as behavioral change, focal neurologic deficits, etc. There is a continuum between meningitis and encephalitis: "meningoencephalitis."
- Also document:
  - Travel and exposure history
  - Sexual activity (e.g., HSV, HIV)
  - Outdoor activities (Lyme disease)
  - Exposure to rodent feces and/or urine (LCMV)
  - Solid-organ transplant (LCMV, CMV)
  - Immunocompromised host (CMV, HSV, adenovirus)
  - History of VZV infection
  - Immunization status (mumps virus, VZV)

PHYSICAL EXAM
- AMS (consider encephalitis)
- Fever (>100.4°F/38°C)
- Full neurologic exam
- Meningeal signs (should not be used exclusively to diagnose or rule out meningitis):
  - Nuchal rigidity: new neck stiffness
  - Brudzinski sign: Neck flexion elicits involuntary hip and knee flexion in supine patient.
  - Kernig sign: resistance to knee extension following flexion of hips to 90 degrees by physician
  - Jolt accentuation test: Rapid horizontal rotation of the head accentuates the headache.
- Genital lesions (85% of HSV-2 cases have active lesions; can precede meningeal symptoms by up to a week)
- Parotitis (mumps)
- Asymmetric flaccid paralysis (West Nile virus)
- Infants: bulging fontanelle possible
- Mucocutaneous findings
  - Vesicular rash in hand, foot, and mouth disease (coxsackievirus)
  - Herpangina (coxsackievirus A)
  - Herpes zoster rash or recent VZV vaccination
  - Erythema migrans or cranial neuropathy (Lyme disease [Borrelia burgdorferi])
  - Generalized maculopapular rash (echovirus 9, syphilis, HIV, Rocky Mountain spotted fever)
  - Oropharyngeal thrush (HIV)
  - Petechial rash (Neisseria meningitidis)

DIFFERENTIAL DIAGNOSIS
- Bacterial meningitis (BM)
- Encephalitis
- Other infectious agents:
  - Tuberculosis; syphilis; leptospirosis; Lyme disease; Rocky Mountain spotted fever; ehrlichiosis; Coccidioides; Cryptococcus neoformans; amebiasis; Rickettsial infection

- Parameningeal infections (e.g., subdural empyema)
- Postinfectious encephalomyelitis
- Viral syndrome (e.g., influenza)
- Leukemia, lymphoma, or carcinomatous meningitis
- Migraine/tension headache
- Acute metabolic encephalopathy
- Chemical meningitis
- Postoperative aseptic meningitis
- Drug-induced meningitis (NSAIDs, IVIG, TMP/SMX, amoxicillin, cetuximab, natalizumab, lamotrigine)
- Brain/epidural abscess
- Inflammatory disorders (e.g., Behçet, sarcoidosis, SLE)

DIAGNOSTIC TESTS & INTERPRETATION
Initial Tests (lab, imaging)
- Rule out BM:
  - There is debate over whether patients with low suspicion of BM need a lumbar puncture (LP). Currently, LP remains the standard of care for suspected VM or BM.
  - Bacterial Meningitis Score (BMS): a validated clinical decision rule to identify children (≥29 days of age) at very low risk of BM. Sensitivity of 99%. Not all institutions support use of clinical decision tools to rule in/out BM.
    - Gram stain of CSF positive (2 points)
    - CSF protein >80 mg/dL (1 point)
    - Blood ANC ≥10,000/mm^3 (1 point)
    - Seizures with illness (1 point)
    - CSF neutrophils >1,000/mm^3 (1 point)
      - 0 points: VM likely
      - 1 point: VM less likely
      - 2 to 6 points: BM more likely
  - CSF bacterial culture is positive in 80–90% of BM patients who did not receive antibiotics for 2 to 4 hours prior to LP.
  - Risk factors for cerebral herniation with LP: signs of increased intracranial pressure (e.g., focal neurologic findings, papilledema, AMS, vomiting), known ventricular obstruction, new-onset seizure, immunocompromised state, hypertension with bradycardia, spinal cord trauma. Consider head CT before LP.
  - Contraindications for LP: local infection over potential LP site, suspected epidural abscess, use of anticoagulation or coagulopathy, and possibility of cardiorespiratory compromise due to patient positioning during procedure
  - Post-LP headache: occurs in 37% of patients within 48 hours. Consider the use of an atraumatic LP needle to decrease the risk of post-LP headache.
  - CSF analysis: glucose, protein, WBC count with differential, RBC count, Gram stain, culture; consider CSF lactate.
    - CSF lactate elevation helps differentiate BM from VM (decreased sensitivity if pretreated with antibiotics) (1,2)[A].
- Typical CSF findings in VM
  - Elevated WBC count: 10 to 500/mm^3 (can be up to 1,000), classically lymphocyte predominance (>50% lymphocytes—less consistent in younger patients). Note: more cases without lymphocytic pleocytosis noted in enterovirus VM; may show neutrophilic predominance in first 48 hours, especially in pediatric population
  - Decreased or normal glucose (relative to serum)
  - Protein normal to slightly elevated (<150 mg/dL)
  - Negative Gram stain and bacterial culture

- Elevated opening pressure
- RBCs in CSF (Consider HSV meningitis/encephalitis.)
- Pathogen identification:
  ○ Current practice: polymerase chain reaction (PCR), with sensitivity of 95–100% for HSV-1 and 2, EBV, enterovirus. Sensitivity for enterovirus may decrease if CSF collected >48 hours after onset of symptoms.
  ○ RT PCR test is approved for enteroviral meningitis; results in 2 to 3 hours
  ○ Serology can be performed for many arthropod-borne viruses.
- Other labs: CBC, blood culture, blood glucose; consider serum CRP and procalcitonin (PCT).
  - CBC: normal or mildly elevated WBC
  - Serum PCT elevation has been correlated with BM. PCT levels of >0.25 to 0.28 are 96% sensitive and 99% specific for BM. Elevated serum CRP was 82% sensitive and 81% specific (1)[B],(3)[A].
  - PCT has also been validated in children (sensitivity 87.5–100%, specificity 66–100%); however, cutoff ranges vary from 0.2 to 3.3 ng/mL between studies and are assay dependent (4)[A]. There may be a role for CSF PCT to help differentiate BM from VM.
- EEG if concern for encephalitis
- Fungal, mycobacterial cultures, VDRL if clinically indicated
- Indication for imaging depends on clinical scenario. Consider CT versus MRI if abnormal hospital course of VM (e.g., prolonged course or increased symptoms).
- Historic gold standard: CSF viral culture for enteroviruses, HSV, and mumps. This has low sensitivity (<6–20%); viral culture may yield no additional information over nucleic acid amplification.

Follow-Up Tests & Special Considerations
Disorders that may alter lab results:
- Diabetes: Consider current blood sugar level to correlate with CSF glucose level.
- Preexisting neurologic diseases (e.g., intracranial neoplasm, demyelinating disease)

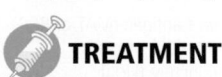

TREATMENT

GENERAL MEASURES
Management includes supportive care (e.g., pain control, IV fluids) and low threshold for empiric antibiotics for BM.

MEDICATION

First Line
- Analgesics (adult doses; titrate doses to pain relief)
  - Morphine 2.5 to 5.0 mg IV q3–4h
  - Hydromorphone (Dilaudid) 0.2 to 2.0 mg IV q2–3h
  - Hydrocodone (Norco) 5/325 mg 1 to 2 tablets PO q6h OR oxycodone (Percocet) 5/325 mg 1 to 2 tablets PO q4–6h
- Antiemetics
  - Ondansetron (Zofran) 4 to 8 mg IV q8h
  - Metoclopramide (Reglan) 10 to 20 mg IV/IM q4–6h
- Antipyretics: acetaminophen (Tylenol) 650 mg PO or rectal suppository q4h
- Antiviral agents (adult dose): Initiate empiric acyclovir at 10 mg/kg IV q8h for patients with CSF pleocytosis, negative Gram stain, and suspicion for HSV while awaiting results of definitive (e.g., HSV PCR) testing.

- Antibiotics (targeted to most likely pathogen)
  - Not indicated for treatment of VM; however, low threshold for empiric treatment if BM is suspected. Consider especially in elderly, those pretreated with antibiotics, and immunocompromised patients. In pediatrics, treat with antibiotics in suspected VM if ill-appearing, <3 months old, or immunocompromised.
  - If unclear etiology but very low risk for BM, treat symptomatically and observe in the inpatient setting pending laboratory results.
- IVIG
  - Research currently underway investigating possible benefit
- Corticosteroids
  - Not indicated for treatment in VM
  - Consider if concerned for BM.

ADMISSION, INPATIENT, AND NURSING CONSIDERATIONS
- Generally VM is treated as outpatient once BM is excluded. Hospitalize for VM with complications (e.g., encephalitis), empiric antibiotic therapy, pain/fluid control, immunocompromised patient, or <1 year old.
  - Most children with VM are hospitalized (91%).
- IV fluids: crystalloid bolus or continuous infusion, based on hydration status and clinical presentation
- Neurologic monitoring for changes in mental status, fever, neck stiffness, HA, etc., to assess disease progression
- Contact precautions; private room until BM ruled out
- Encourage hand washing.
- Discharge depends on likelihood of BM, WBC count, and clinical parameters (dehydration, functional level, social circumstances, and ability to follow up).

 ## ONGOING CARE

FOLLOW-UP RECOMMENDATIONS
Primary care follow-up to ensure resolution

Patient Monitoring
- Monitor for relapse or exacerbation of symptoms.
- Monitor for neurologic/neuroendocrine complications:
  - Seizures, cerebral edema, syndrome of inappropriate antidiuretic hormone (SIADH)
  - Assess ability to have companion monitor change in mental/neurologic status if patient discharged.

DIET
Consider NPO if nausea or vomiting. Advance to clear fluids/regular diet as tolerated.

PATIENT EDUCATION
- Discuss low probability of transmission to contacts.
- Expected duration of illness is 5 to 10 days.
- Recurrence of headache, myalgia, weakness is possible over 2 to 3 weeks.

PROGNOSIS
- Complete recovery generally within 7 to 10 days
- Headaches and other neurologic symptoms may intermittently persist for weeks to months.
- Only 0.6% of hospitalizations for VM result in death.
- European studies suggest potential residual postmeningeal cognitive impairment.
- In neonatal population, enteroviral meningitis has been associated with normal growth and development at 1 year in most patients.

COMPLICATIONS
- Common: fatigue, irritability, muscle weakness
- Rare: seizures, abscess, mastoiditis

REFERENCES

1. Viallon A, Desseigne N, Marjollet O, et al. Meningitis in adult patients with a negative direct cerebrospinal fluid examination: value of cytochemical markers for differential diagnosis. *Crit Care*. 2011;15(3):R136.
2. McGill F, Griffiths MJ, Solomon T. Viral meningitis: current issues in diagnosis and treatment. *Curr Opin Infect Dis*. 2017;30(2):248–256.
3. Vikse J, Henry BM, Roy J, et al. The role of serum procalcitonin in the diagnosis of bacterial meningitis in adults: a systematic review and meta-analysis. *Int J Infect Dis*. 2015;38:68–76.
4. Henry BM, Roy J, Ramakrishnan PK, et al. Procalcitonin as a serum biomarker for differentiation of bacterial meningitis from viral meningitis in children: evidence from a meta-analysis. *Clin Pediatr (Phila)*. 2016;55(8):749–764.

ADDITIONAL READING
- Drysdale SB, Kelly DF. Fifteen-minute consultation: enterovirus meningitis and encephalitis—when can we stop the antibiotics? *Arch Dis Child Educ Pract Ed*. 2017;102(2):66–71.
- Mohseni MM, Wilde JA. Viral meningitis: which patients can be discharged from the emergency department? *J Emerg Med*. 2012;43(6):1181–1187.
- Talan DA. Bacterial cause of suspected meningitis cannot be safely excluded without cerebrospinal fluid analysis. *Ann Emerg Med*. 2012;59(3):227–228.

 ### SEE ALSO

- Meningitis, Bacterial
- Algorithm: Delirium

CODES

ICD10
- A87.9 Viral meningitis, unspecified
- A87.1 Adenoviral meningitis
- A87.0 Enteroviral meningitis

CLINICAL PEARLS
- VM cannot be reliably distinguished from BM based on clinical findings alone.
- Potential cases of BM should be hospitalized for evaluation and treatment with broad-spectrum antibiotics until BM has been ruled out.
- VM is more common than BM, especially if vaccine rates are high.
- Antibiotic administration in the hours prior to LP and CSF analysis may result in "partially treated" BM lab results, mimicking VM.
- Morbidity with VM is low but increases if there is associated encephalitis.

M

MENINGOCOCCAL DISEASE

Han Q. Bui, MD

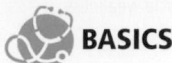

BASICS

DESCRIPTION
- Meningococcemia is a blood-borne infection caused by *Neisseria meningitidis*.
- Bacteremia without meningitis: Patient is acutely ill and may have skin manifestations (rashes, petechiae, and ecchymosis) and hypotension.
- Bacteremia with meningitis: sudden onset of fever, nausea, vomiting, headache, decreased ability to concentrate, and myalgias
- Disease progresses rapidly (within hours).
- Skin findings and hypotension may be present.
  - A petechial rash appears as discrete lesions 1 to 2 mm in diameter; most frequently on the trunk and lower portions of the body; seen in >50% of patients on presentation
  - Purpura fulminans is a severe complication of meningococcal disease and occurs in up to 25% of cases. It is characterized by acute onset of cutaneous hemorrhage and necrosis due to vascular thrombosis and disseminated intravascular coagulopathy.

EPIDEMIOLOGY
Incidence
- The mortality rate is ~13%.
  - 11–19% of survivors suffer serious sequelae, including deafness, neurologic deficits, or limb loss due to peripheral ischemia.
- Disease is seasonal, peaks in December/January.
- In 2016, there were 375 cases of reported meningococcal disease (incidence rate of 0.18 cases per 100,000 persons) (1).
  - Most common in adolescents and young adults, followed by infants <1 year

ETIOLOGY AND PATHOPHYSIOLOGY
- *N. meningitidis* is a gram-negative diplococcus with at least 13 serotypes.
- *N. meningitidis* has an outer coat that produces disease-causing endotoxin.
- Major serogroups in the United States are B, C, Y, and W-135.
  - Serogroup B is the predominant cause of meningococcemia in children <1 year.
  - Serogroup C is the most common cause of meningococcal disease in the United States.
  - Serogroup Y is the predominant cause of meningococcemia in the elderly (2).
- Major serogroups worldwide are A, B, C, Y, and W-135.
  - W-135 is the major cause of disease in the "meningitis belt" of sub-Saharan Africa.

Genetics
Late complement component deficiency has an autosomal recessive inheritance.

RISK FACTORS
- Age: 3 months to 1 year
- Late complement component deficiency (C5, C6, C7, C8, or C9)
- Asplenia (1)
- Living in close quarters (e.g., household contacts, nursery/daycare, dormitories, military barracks)
- Exposure to active (and/or) passive tobacco smoke (1)

GENERAL PREVENTION
- Two vaccines are currently licensed for use in the United States. Each contains antigens to serogroups A, C, Y, and W-135. Neither provides immunity against serotype B, which is responsible for 1/3 of U.S. cases (3).
  - Meningococcal polysaccharide vaccine (MPSV-4): recommended for patients ≥55 years at elevated risk (1)
    ○ Short duration of protection: 1 to 3 years for patients age <5 years; 3 to 5 years for adolescents and adults (3)
    ○ Often used for patients requiring short duration of protection—traveling to endemic areas, college freshmen, community outbreaks (3)
  - Meningococcal conjugate vaccine (MCV-4): recommended for patients 2 to 55 years of age (1)
- The FDA has licensed two serogroup B meningococcal (MenB) vaccines. The first (MenB-FHbp) is a 3-dose series. The second (MenB-4C) is a 2-dose series. Both vaccines were approved for use in persons aged 10 to 25 years. Individuals aged ≥10 years who are at increased risk for meningococcal disease due to persistent complement component deficiencies, anatomic or functional asplenia, should receive MenB vaccine (3).
- Protective levels of antibody are achieved ~7 to 10 days after primary immunization (2).
- Vaccine is recommended for everyone aged 11 to 18 years and individuals 19 to 55 years who are at increased risk for meningococcal disease.
  - Guillain-Barré syndrome has been associated with the MCV-4 vaccine; therefore, a personal history of Guillain-Barré is a relative contraindication for this vaccine.
- CDC international travel advisory
  - Vaccine is required by the government of Saudi Arabia for Hajj pilgrims >2 years of age.
  - The vaccine should be given to travelers to sub-Saharan Africa ("meningitis belt").

DIAGNOSIS

HISTORY
Symptoms
- Sudden onset of fever, nausea, vomiting, headache, myalgias, chills, rigor, and/or sore throat (nonsuppurative)
  - Pharyngitis may be mistaken for streptococcal disease (strep throat).
  - Myalgia may be mistaken for severe "flu," which also has a peak incidence in winter.
- Changes in mental status, decreased ability to concentrate, stiff neck, convulsions
- Assess possible exposures.

PHYSICAL EXAM
- Fever, hypotension, tachycardia
- Neurologic: nuchal rigidity, focal neurologic findings, coma, seizure
  - Focal neurologic findings and seizures are more commonly seen with *Haemophilus influenzae* or *Streptococcus pneumoniae*.
- Cardiopulmonary: signs of heart failure with pulmonary edema—gallop, rales
- Dermatologic: maculopapular rash, petechiae, ecchymosis, purpura
- Onset of specific meningitis symptoms (e.g., neck stiffness, photophobia, bulging fontanelle) can occur within 12 to 15 hours (4).

- Late signs of meningitis (e.g., unconsciousness, delirium, or seizures) occur after ~15 hours in infants <1 year and after ~24 hours in older children.

DIFFERENTIAL DIAGNOSIS
- Sepsis; bacterial meningitis (other organisms)
- Gonococcemia
- Acute bacterial endocarditis
- Rocky Mountain spotted fever
- Hemolytic uremic syndrome
- Gonococcal arthritis dermatitis syndrome
- Influenza

DIAGNOSTIC TESTS & INTERPRETATION

ALERT
- Isolation of *N. meningitidis* from a sterile site (blood or CSF) is the gold standard for diagnosing systemic meningococcal infection.
- Antibiotic administration may render blood and/or CSF culture negative within 2 hours.

Initial Tests (lab, imaging)
- CBC with differential
  - Leukocytosis (left shift; toxic granulation) or leukopenia, thrombocytopenia
- Lactic acidosis
- Procalcitonin; often elevated in bacterial meningitis (5)
- Coagulation studies
  - Prolonged prothrombin time/partial thromboplastin time
  - Low fibrinogen
  - Elevated fibrin degradation products
- Blood culture
  - Blood culture positive for *N. meningitidis*
  - Cultures positive in 50–60% of cases
- CSF
  - Grossly cloudy
  - Increased WBCs with polymorphonuclear predominance
  - Gram stain showing gram-negative diplococci
  - Glucose-to-blood glucose ratio <0.4
  - Protein >45 mg/dL
  - Positive for *N. meningitidis* antigen (MAT or PCR)
  - CSF culture positive in 80–90% of cases
- Head CT prior to lumbar puncture (LP) if concern for space-occupying lesions or if focal findings on neurologic examination

Test Interpretation
- Disseminated intravascular coagulation (DIC)
- Meningeal exudates
- Polymorphonuclear infiltration of meninges
- Hemorrhage of adrenal glands

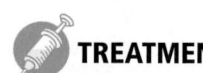

TREATMENT

MEDICATION
First Line
- Antibiotics (5)[A]
  - Begin treatment as soon as meningococcal meningitis is suspected.
  - Age guides empiric treatment.
    ○ Preterm to <1 month: ampicillin plus cefotaxime or ampicillin plus gentamicin
      ■ Cefotaxime
        □ 0 to 7 days: 50 mg/kg q12h
        □ 8 to 28 days: 50 mg/kg q8h

- Ampicillin
  - \>2,000 g
    - 0 to 7 days: 50 mg/kg q8h
    - 8 to 28 days: 50 mg/kg q6h
  - <2,000 g
    - 0 to 7 days: 50 mg/kg q12h
    - 8 to 28 days: 50 mg/kg q8h
  - 1 month to 50 years: cefotaxime or ceftriaxone plus vancomycin
    - If severe penicillin allergy: chloramphenicol plus trimethoprim-sulfamethoxazole (TMP-SMX) plus vancomycin
  - \>50 years of age or patients with significant comorbidity, alcohol abuse, or impaired immunity: ampicillin plus ceftriaxone plus vancomycin
    - Ampicillin: 2 g IV q4h
    - Ceftriaxone: 2 g IV q12h
    - Vancomycin: 30 to 45 mg/kg/day IV divided q6h
    - If severe penicillin allergy: TMP-SMX plus vancomycin
- Penicillin G
  - Effective if the isolate is penicillin-sensitive
  - Penicillin can be used if the isolate has a penicillin minimum inhibitory concentration (MIC) of <0.1 μg/mL.
  - For isolates with a penicillin MIC of 0.1 to 1.0 μg/mL, a 3rd-generation cephalosporin is preferred.
  - Penicillin G: 4 million units IV q4h (pediatric dose: 0.25 mU/kg/day IV divided q4–6h) OR ampicillin: 2 g IV q4h (pediatric dose: 200 to 300 mg/kg/day IV divided q6h)
- Duration of treatment: 7 days (4)
- Dexamethasone
  - Indications
    - Known or suspected pneumococcal meningitis in selected adults
    - Children with *H. influenzae* type B meningitis
- Dexamethasone is often given initially in adults and children with suspected bacterial meningitis while awaiting microbiologic study results.
- Dexamethasone has not been shown to be of benefit in meningococcal meningitis and should be discontinued once the diagnosis is established.
- Dosage
  - Infants and children >6 weeks: IV 0.15 mg/kg/dose q6h for the first 2 to 4 days of antibiotic treatment
  - Start 10 to 20 minutes before or with the first dose of antibiotic.
- Chemoprophylaxis
  - Indications
    - Close contacts: those with prolonged (>8 hours) close contact (<3 feet) to the patient or those directly exposed to the patient's oral secretions between 1 week before the onset of the patient's symptoms and until 24 hours after initiation of appropriate antibiotic therapy (2)
      - Examples: household members; close contacts in nursery, daycare centers, nursing homes, dormitories, military barracks, correctional facilities, and other closed institutional settings
    - No chemoprophylaxis is indicated for casual contacts, including most health care workers, unless exposed to respiratory secretions.

- Timing
  - Ideally <24 hours after case identification
  - Chemoprophylaxis should not be administered if >14 days since exposure.
- Prophylactic regimens
  - Rifampin, ciprofloxacin, and ceftriaxone
    - Ceftriaxone
      - Recommended for pregnant women
      - Adults: 250 mg IM as a single dose
    - Rifampin (meningococcal prophylaxis)
      - Adult: 600 mg IV or PO q12h for 2 days
      - Pediatric
        - <1 month: 10 mg/kg/day in divided doses q12h for 2 days
        - Infants and children: 20 mg/kg/day in divided doses q12h for 2 days (max 600 mg/dose)
      - Ciprofloxacin
      - Adults: 500 mg PO as a single dose
- Vaccination
  - For household contacts (if the case is from a vaccine-preventable serogroup)
- Precautions
  - Adjust the dosage of medications in patients with severe renal dysfunction.

Second Line
- For meningitis
  - Chloramphenicol: 1 g IV q6h (pediatric dose: 75 to 100 mg/kg/day divided q6h) or ceftriaxone 2 g IV q12h (pediatric dose: 80 to 100 mg/kg/day divided q12–24h)
  - In large outbreaks, a single dose of long-acting chloramphenicol has been used. Single-dose ceftriaxone shows equal efficacy in one randomized controlled trial.
- Precautions
  - Ceftriaxone should not be used in patients with a history of anaphylactic reactions to penicillin (e.g., hypotension, laryngeal edema, wheezing, hives).
  - Chloramphenicol may cause aplastic anemia.

ISSUES FOR REFERRAL
Potential complications
- Seizure activity
- DIC
- Acute respiratory distress syndrome
- Renal failure
- Adrenal failure
- Multisystem organ failure

ADMISSION, INPATIENT, AND NURSING CONSIDERATIONS
- Begin antibiotics (± corticosteroids) and obtain LP immediately if meningitis is suspected.
- Droplet isolation for 24 hours after starting antibiotics
- IV fluids: Replace volume as needed; with septic shock, large volumes of crystalloid may be required.

 ONGOING CARE

PATIENT EDUCATION
Educate family and close contacts regarding the risk of contracting meningococcal infection.

PROGNOSIS
Overall mortality is 13%.

COMPLICATIONS
- DIC
- Acute tubular necrosis
- Neurologic: sensorineural hearing loss, cranial nerve palsy, seizures
- Obstructive hydrocephalus
- Subdural effusions
- Acute adrenal hemorrhage
- Waterhouse-Friderichsen syndrome

REFERENCES

1. Centers for Disease Control and Prevention. Meningococcal disease: technical and clinical information. https://www.cdc.gov/meningococcal/clinical-info.html. Accessed November 5, 2018.
2. Gardner P. Clinical practice. Prevention of meningococcal disease. *N Engl J Med*. 2006;355(14):1466–1473.
3. Folaranmi T, Rubin L, Martin SW, et al. Use of serogroup B meningococcal vaccines in persons aged ≥10 years at increased risk for serogroup B meningococcal disease: recommendations of the Advisory Committee on Immunization Practices, 2015. *MMWR Morb Mortal Wkly Rep*. 2015;64(22):608–612.
4. Wei TT, Hu ZD, Qin BD, et al. Diagnostic accuracy of procalcitonin in bacterial meningitis versus nonbacterial meningitis: a systematic review and meta-analysis. *Medicine (Baltimore)*. 2016;95(11):e3079.
5. Tunkel AR, Hartman BJ, Kaplan SL, et al. Practice guidelines for the management of bacterial meningitis. *Clin Infect Dis*. 2004;39(9):1267–1284.

ADDITIONAL READING

- Visintin C, Mugglestone MA, Fields EJ, et al; for Guideline Development Group, National Institute for Health and Clinical Excellence. Management of bacterial meningitis and meningococcal septicaemia in children and young people: summary of NICE guidance. *BMJ*. 2010;340:c3209.
- Wright C, Wordsworth R, Glennie L. Counting the cost of meningococcal disease: scenarios of severe meningitis and septicemia. *Paediatr Drugs*. 2013;15(1):49–58.

 CODES

ICD10
- A39.4 Meningococcemia, unspecified
- A39.0 Meningococcal meningitis
- A39.2 Acute meningococcemia

CLINICAL PEARLS
- Invasive meningococcal disease can be rapidly fatal. Rapid identification and early treatment is essential to promote good clinical outcomes. Treat then test in suspected cases.
- Provide chemoprophylaxis to close contacts.
- Vaccinate at-risk populations to prevent disease.

M

MENISCAL INJURY

Jennifer B. Schwartz, MD

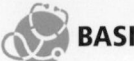

BASICS

DESCRIPTION
- The menisci are fibrocartilaginous structures between the femoral condyles and tibial plateaus.
- The menisci help stabilize the knee and distribute forces across the joint.
- There are acute/traumatic and chronic/degenerative meniscal tears.

Geriatric Considerations
Meniscal tears in older patients are typically due to chronic degeneration.

Pediatric Considerations
- Meniscal injuries are rare in children <10 years old and are often due to a discoid meniscus (anatomic variant that is thicker and wider).
- MRI is less sensitive and specific for diagnosing meniscal tears in children <12 years of age.

EPIDEMIOLOGY
Bimodal age distribution—young athletes (traumatic) and older patients >40 years (degenerative)

Incidence
Medial meniscus more commonly injured

Prevalence
One of the most common musculoskeletal injuries

ETIOLOGY AND PATHOPHYSIOLOGY
- Acute/traumatic tears occur due to a twisting motion of the knee with foot planted.
- Chronic/degenerative tears occur with minimal trauma, overuse.
- More common >40 years old

Genetics
Presence of a discoid meniscus increases the risk for a meniscal tear. No specific gene locus has been identified.

RISK FACTORS
- Acute/traumatic
  - High degree of physical activity (especially cutting sports)
  - Anterior cruciate ligament (ACL) insufficiency
- Chronic/degenerative:
  - Increased age (>60 years)
  - Obesity
  - Work related kneeling/squatting/climbing stairs

GENERAL PREVENTION
- Treatment and rehabilitation of previous knee injuries, particularly ACL injuries
- Strengthening and increased flexibility of quadriceps and hamstring muscles

COMMONLY ASSOCIATED CONDITIONS
- Acute/traumatic:
  - ACL is concomitantly torn in 1/3 of cases.
- Degenerative
  - Baker cyst—association with medial meniscal tears
  - Osteoarthritis (OA)—degenerative tears can be considered as an early stage of OA.

DIAGNOSIS

HISTORY
- Pain with descending stairs
- Noncontact twisting mechanism
  - Knee pain (increased with knee flexion)
- ± Locking, catching
  - Limited association between self-reported mechanical symptoms and presence of meniscal tear on arthroscopy (1)

PHYSICAL EXAM
- Effusion—typically >24 hour postinjury
- Joint line tenderness
- Decreased range of motion, locking
- Pain with full flexion (posterior horn tear) or extension (anterior horn tear)
- Accuracy of special tests varies.
  - McMurrays and Apley grind tests are neither sensitive nor specific (1).

DIFFERENTIAL DIAGNOSIS
- ACL or collateral ligament tear
- Pathologic plica
- Osteochondritis dissecans
- Loose body or fracture
- OA
- Patellofemoral syndrome
- Gout, pseudogout, rheumatoid arthritis

DIAGNOSTIC TESTS & INTERPRETATION
- Laboratory evaluation not indicated unless signs of septic arthritis
- Plain radiographs can detect fractures, loose bodies, or arthritic changes.
- Ultrasound may help identify meniscal tears.
- MRI is the primary imaging study for meniscal tears.

Follow-Up Tests & Special Considerations
- Meniscal tears are often found incidentally on MRI and may not be the cause of patient's symptoms.
- Asymptomatic tears increase with age and OA.
- Meniscal tears are present on MRI in ~20% of people without knee symptoms.

Diagnostic Procedures/Other
Arthroscopy may be needed if the MRI is indeterminate.

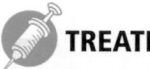

TREATMENT

GENERAL MEASURES
- Conservative treatments: rest, ice, activity modification, OTC medications, physical therapy, intra-articular corticosteroid injections
  - Effective first-line options for many patients, especially those with degenerative tears
- Surgical intervention: Consider if:
  - Concurrent injuries (i.e., ACL tear)
  - Persistent symptoms following 3 to 6 months of conservative treatment
  - Young patients (<30 years) or active patients with an acute tear
  - Mechanical symptoms—may or may not be justification for arthroscopy with degenerative meniscal tears
- For degenerative tears:
  - Recommend physical therapy/conservative treatment first—no increased benefit from surgery versus PT with degenerative meniscal tears age >40 years (2)[B]
  - Meniscal surgery should not be recommended as a first-choice treatment age >40 years; should be considered only when no response to conservative management (3)[C]
  - Partial meniscectomy did not improve function or reduce pain compared to conservative treatment (4)[B].

- For traumatic tears:
  - Consider surgery—no evidence for best treatment (surgical vs. nonsurgical) in patients <40 years with traumatic tear. These patients generally improve more after surgery compared with patients with degenerative tears (5)[C].
  - Good clinical outcomes for meniscal repairs in younger/pediatric patients (6)[B]

MEDICATION

First Line
NSAIDs, opioid analgesics if severe pain

ISSUES FOR REFERRAL
Surgical consult for patients meeting operative criteria or wishing surgical repair

ADDITIONAL THERAPIES
- Rehabilitation is required for both surgical and nonsurgical patients.
- Weight control: Weight gain is associated with increased cartilage loss and pain.
- Platelet-rich plasma (PRP) may or may not improve symptoms of meniscal tears.

SURGERY/OTHER PROCEDURES
- Meniscectomy removes the injured portion of the meniscus.
  - Both partial and total meniscectomy can lead to articular cartilage degeneration and OA.
  - Higher risk if >40 years of age, high BMI, valgus malalignment
- Meniscal repair or replacement is preferred over meniscectomy when possible and may have better outcomes.

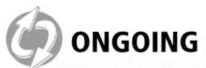 **ONGOING CARE**

FOLLOW-UP RECOMMENDATIONS
- Return to play requires that the patient be pain free, have full range of motion, and full strength.
- Following meniscal repair, patients can generally return to activities in 3 to 6 months.

PATIENT EDUCATION
Patients should be aware of the risks and benefits of surgery compared with conservative treatment.

PROGNOSIS
Prognosis better if surgery is done within 8 weeks (acute tear), patient is <30 years of age, or tear is peripheral/lateral <2.5 cm

COMPLICATIONS
- Meniscectomies may eventually lead to OA.
- Risk of developing OA increases 6-fold 20 years after a meniscectomy.

REFERENCES

1. Pihl K, Turkiewicz A, Englund M, et al. Association of specific meniscal pathologies and other structural pathologies with self-reported mechanical symptoms: a cross-sectional study of 566 patients undergoing meniscal surgery [published online ahead of print July 31, 2018]. *J Sci Med Sport*. doi:10.1016/j.jsams.2018.07.018.
2. Hohmann E, Glatt V, Tetsworth K, et al. Arthroscopic partial meniscectomy versus physical therapy for degenerative meniscus lesions: how robust is the current evidence? A critical systematic review and qualitative synthesis. *Arthroscopy*. 2018;34(9):2699–2708.
3. Lee DY, Park YJ, Kim HJ, et al. Arthroscopic meniscal surgery versus conservative management in patients aged 40 years and older: a meta-analysis. *Arch Orthop Trauma Surg*. 2018;138(12):1731–1739.
4. Lee SH, Lee OS, Kim ST, et al. Revisiting arthroscopic partial meniscectomy for degenerative tears in knees with mild or no osteoarthritis: a systematic review and meta-analysis of randomized controlled trials [published online ahead of print June 29, 2018]. *Clin J Sport Med*. doi:10.1097/JSM.0000000000000585.
5. Thorlund JB, Rodriguez Palomino J, Juhl CB, et al. Infographic. Exercise therapy for meniscal tears: evidence and recommendations [published online ahead of print June 23, 2018]. *Br J Sports Med*. doi:10.1136/bjsports-2018-099492.
6. Ferrari MB, Murphy CP, Gomes JLE. Meniscus repair in children and adolescents: a systematic review of treatment approaches, meniscal healing, and outcomes [published online ahead of print May 23, 2018]. *J Knee Surg*. doi:10.1055/s-0038-1653943.

ADDITIONAL READING

- Beaufils P, Becker R, Kopf S, et al. The knee meniscus: management of traumatic tears and degenerative lesions. *EFORT Open Rev*. 2017;2(5):195–203.
- Monk P, Garfjeld Roberts P, Palmer AJ, et al. The urgent need for evidence in arthroscopic meniscal surgery. *Am J Sports Med*. 2017;45(4):965–973.
- Siemieniuk RAC, Harris IA, Agoritsas T, et al. Arthroscopic surgery for degenerative knee arthritis and meniscal tears: a clinical practice guideline. *Br J Sports Med*. 2018;52(5):313.
- Smith BE, Thacker D, Crewesmith A, et al. Special tests for assessing meniscal tears within the knee: a systematic review and meta-analysis. *Evid Based Med*. 2015;20(3):88–97.

 SEE ALSO

Algorithm: Knee Pain

 CODES

ICD10
- S83.209A Unsp tear of unsp meniscus, current injury, unsp knee, init
- S83.249A Oth tear of medial meniscus, current injury, unsp knee, init
- S83.289A Oth tear of lat mensc, current injury, unsp knee, init

CLINICAL PEARLS

- Chronic/degenerative meniscal tears are common in patients >40 years old and are generally managed conservatively.
- Acute/traumatic meniscal tears are more common in young athletes and may require surgery.
- MRI is imaging modality of choice to identify meniscal tears.
- In patients opting for surgery, meniscal repairs have a better functional outcome and decreased risk of OA compared with meniscectomy.

M

MENOPAUSE

Jill Patton, DO • Christiana Shoushtari, MD

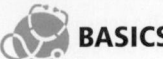 **BASICS**

DESCRIPTION

- Natural menopause: defined retrospectively after 12 consecutive months of amenorrhea in a nonpregnant woman ≥40 years of age; mean age of 51 years
  - Results from loss of ovarian activity
  - Not associated with a pathologic etiology
- Perimenopause/menopausal transition (MT): the period from the onset of irregular menses to the final menstrual cycle. Begins on average 4 years before menopause; starts at mean age of 47 years
- Postmenopause: usually >1/3 of a woman's life
- Primary ovarian insufficiency: irregular or cessation of menses before age 40 years
- Surgical menopause: removal of functioning ovaries leading to immediate menopause

EPIDEMIOLOGY

- The median age of menopause is 51 years.
- 5% of women undergo menopause after age 55 years; another 5% between ages 40 and 45 years
- Occurs earlier in Hispanic women and later in Japanese American women as compared with Caucasians

Incidence

In the United States, 1.3 million women reach menopause annually.

ETIOLOGY AND PATHOPHYSIOLOGY

- As women age, the number of ovarian follicles decreases: Ovarian production of estrogen varies and then decreases. Follicle-stimulating hormone (FSH) production varies and then increases.
- Inadequate estradiol production leads to absence of the luteinizing hormone (LH) surge and failure to ovulate. These cycles result in anovulation and lack of progesterone production.
- Eventual failure to produce estradiol leads to thinning of endometrial lining and eventual menses cessation.
- Estrone (produced by adipose tissue) becomes the dominant form of estrogen during menopause.

RISK FACTORS

- Aging
- Oophorectomy/hysterectomy
- Sex chromosome abnormalities (e.g., Turner syndrome and fragile X syndrome)
- Family history of early menopause
- Smoking (earlier age of onset by 2 years)
- Chemotherapy and/or pelvic radiation

GENERAL PREVENTION

Menopause is a physiologic event and associated with increased risk of long-term medical issues, including cardiovascular disease (CVD) and osteoporotic fractures.

- Decrease risk of CVD by:
  - Increasing exercise
  - Maintaining healthy diet and losing weight
  - Avoiding tobacco use
  - Treating hypertension, hyperlipidemia, and diabetes mellitus
  - Taking daily low-dose aspirin
- Decrease risk of osteoporotic fractures with:
  - Weight-bearing exercise and fall prevention
  - Avoidance of smoking and excessive alcohol intake
  - Dietary calcium of 1,200 mg/day
  - Adequate vitamin D intake (800 to 1,200 IU daily)
  - Fall prevention

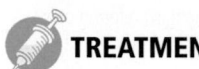 **DIAGNOSIS**

HISTORY

- Cessation of menses:
  - Generally preceded by a period of irregular cycles with heavy vaginal bleeding followed by diminished vaginal bleeding
- Vasomotor symptoms reported by 80%:
  - Sudden feeling of warmth, most commonly over face, neck, and chest, typically lasting 1 to 5 minutes; intervals unpredictable
  - Generally begin 2 years before the final menstrual period, peak during 1 year after the final menstrual period, and then diminish
  - Frequency and duration varies: 87% of women who report flushes experience them daily; ~33% have >10 per day. Mean duration of symptoms lasts 4 to 10.2 years and may begin during MT and extend well past menopause.
  - Varies with ethnicity: greatest in African and Hispanic women and least in Asian women
  - More common in obese women
- Urogenital atrophy in 50%:
  - Vaginal/vulvar dryness, discharge, itching, dyspareunia, and possible sexual dysfunction
  - Alkaline vaginal pH and atrophy increases risk of vaginal infections and UTIs.
  - Persists or worsens with aging
- Urologic symptoms (urgency, frequency, dysuria, incontinence) not clearly correlated with MT
- Anxiety/depression: Some studies show a new diagnosis of depression is 2.5 times more likely to occur during the MT as compared to premenopause.
- Sleep disturbance: Arousal from sleep and chronic insomnia may be linked with vasomotor symptoms.
- Joint pain: unclear link to loss of estrogen
- Change in intensity and severity of migraines
- Skin thinning, mild hirsutism, brittle nails

Geriatric Considerations

Vaginal bleeding in postmenopausal women is abnormal; thus, endometrial cancer/endometrioid adenocarcinoma (EAC) must be ruled out.

PHYSICAL EXAM

- Decrease in breast size and change in breast texture
- External, speculum, and bimanual pelvic exams:
  - Atrophic vulva and vaginal mucosa
  - Increased risk for uterine prolapse

DIFFERENTIAL DIAGNOSIS

Pregnancy, hyperthyroidism and other thyroid diseases, pituitary adenoma, Sheehan syndrome, hypothalamic dysfunction, anorexia nervosa, Asherman syndrome, and obstruction of uterine outflow tract

DIAGNOSTIC TESTS & INTERPRETATION

Initial Tests (lab, imaging)

- Lab testing for menopause is not required; the patient's age and symptoms establish the diagnosis.
- If laboratory confirmation is desired:
  - Elevated serum FSH level >30 mIU/mL indicates ovarian failure.
  - Symptoms may precede lab changes.
- Infertility evaluation: may use elevated day 3 FSH, decreased anti-müllerian hormone levels, and decreased antral follicle count to predict decreased ovarian reserve
- Estrogens, androgens, and oral contraceptive pills (OCPs) may alter lab results.

Follow-Up Tests & Special Considerations

- Pregnancy test
- TSH and prolactin level if pituitary disease is suspected
- Vaginal bleeding in a postmenopausal patient should be evaluated by TVUS and/or EMB. If endometrial stripe is <5 mm on TVUS, EAC is unlikely.
- U.S. Preventive Services Task Force (USPSTF) recommends mammogram every 2 years from ages 50 to 74 years.
- USPSTF recommends bone mineral density (BMD) screening with dual energy x-ray absorptiometry (DEXA) scan in postmenopausal women >65 years or <65 years if the risk for fracture is equivalent to that of a 65-year-old woman (using the FRAX tool to assess, https://www.sheffield.ac.uk/FRAX/). Risk factors include a previous history of fractures, low body weight, cigarette smoking, and family history of osteoporotic fracture.

Test Interpretation

- Abnormal BMD and DEXA scan results:
  - T-score on DEXA of −1 to −2.5 = osteopenia
  - T-score <−2.5 = osteoporosis
  - Defer to femoral neck T-score over spine T-score.
- Z-score measures age-matched mean bone density (not clinically useful).

TREATMENT

MEDICATION

First Line

Hormone therapy (HT): Developing an individual risk–benefit profile is essential. Treatment goal is to minimize menopausal symptoms to improve quality of life (1).

- The primary indication for HT is the treatment of moderate to severe vasomotor symptoms.
  - Oral estrogen or estrogen-progestin mix can reduce weekly hot flush frequency ~75% (2).
- HT also helpful with sleep disorders, urogenital atrophy, and lowers risk of osteoporotic fractures; may help with mood symptoms (3)
- In women with an intact uterus, give estrogen with progestin because unopposed estrogen carries an increased risk of EAC.
- Treatment regimens include but are not limited to:
  - Standard dose: conjugated equine estrogen (CEE) 0.625 mg/day OR micronized estradiol 17β 1.0 mg/day OR transdermal estradiol 17β 0.0375 to 0.050 mg/day
  - Low dose: CEE 0.30 to 0.45 mg/day OR micronized estradiol 17β 0.5 mg/day OR transdermal estradiol 17β 0.025 mg/day
  - Ultra-low dose: micronized estradiol 17β 0.025 mg/day OR transdermal estradiol 17β 0.014 mg/day
  - Micronized progesterone 100 mg/day can be used as progestin. Alternative: medroxyprogesterone acetate (MPA) 2.5 mg/day. Combination estradiol/progestin transdermal treatments have either levonorgestrel or norethindrone as progestin source. Although NOT approved for postmenopausal women, the levonorgestrel intrauterine system (IUS) has been used.
  - Bazedoxifene + conjugated estrogens for relief of vasomotor symptoms and bone loss prevention

- MenoPro app is free for iPhones and iPad from The North American Menopause Society (NAMS). It has two modes: one for clinicians and one for patients to aid in shared decision-making. It allows users to progress through questions to evaluate cardiovascular and reproductive organ cancer risk (4).
- American College of Obstetricians and Gynecologists (ACOG) recommends HT should be individualized with lowest effect dose given for the shortest duration of time needed to relieve vasomotor symptoms. Lower doses have similar symptom reduction profiles for many patients. Results of ultra-low-dose regimens are mixed.
- Although generally well tolerated, side effects of HT include breast tenderness, vaginal bleeding, bloating, and headaches.
- Precautions:
  - Women's Health Initiative (WHI) study demonstrate women who take CEE with MPA versus placebo had increased CHD events, invasive breast cancer, stroke, pulmonary embolism, dementia, gallbladder disease, urinary incontinence; benefits included decreased hip fractures, diabetes, and vasomotor symptoms.
  - Breast cancer risk not seen until 5 years of use
  - Cardiovascular risks not seen until after age 60 years or 10 years from menopause
  - Women on estrogen alone had no increased risk of breast cancer in the 8 years of the study and showed later cardiovascular risk compared to estrogen + progestin.
  - HT should NOT be used for cardioprotective benefit as risk outweighs benefit (5).
  - Higher doses of estrogen can cause hypercoagulability, breast tenderness, gallbladder disease, and hypertension.
  - Contraindications to HT:
    - Estrogen-dependent malignancies
    - Unexplained uterine bleeding
    - History of thromboembolism or stroke
    - CAD
    - Active liver disease
- For osteoporosis: Women with a history of hip or vertebral fracture or personal history of osteoporosis should be treated with one of the following:
  - Bisphosphonates to inhibit osteoclast action and resorption of bone:
    - Alendronate: 70 mg/week or 10 mg/day
    - Risedronate: 35 mg once a week or 5 mg/day
    - Zoledronic acid: 5 mg IV annually
    - Ibandronate: 150 mg/month PO or 3 mg IV q3mo
  - Selective estrogen receptor modulators (SERMs) selectively inhibit or stimulate estrogen-like action with stimulation of osteoblasts:
    - Raloxifene: 60 mg/day
      - Decreases the risk of vertebral fracture
    - Bazedoxifene + conjugated estrogens (0.45 mg/20 mg)
      - FDA-approved for moderate to severe vasomotor symptoms and osteoporosis
  - Denosumab (60 mg SC every 6 months) is a monoclonal antibody that prevents RANKL (receptor activator of nuclear factor kappa-B ligand) from accelerating osteoclast generation; reduces incidence of vertebral and hip fractures in postmenopausal women
  - Parathyroid hormone—rarely used due to the adverse effect on bone but shown to reduce fracture risk in menopausal women with osteoporosis
- For vulvar/vaginal atrophy:
  - Topical estrogen therapy (ET) reverses vaginal atrophy, enhances blood flow, and reduces UTI.

Continue for as long as distressing symptoms remain. Initiate treatment daily for 1 to 2 weeks and then decrease to 2 times weekly. Comes as estradiol cream, tablet, or ring. No evidence of difference in efficacy between various intravaginal estrogenic preparations. Apply vaginally:
  - Estradiol cream 0.01% (1 g), conjugated estrogen 0.625 mg/g (0.5 g), vaginal tablet (10 μg) used twice weekly, or vaginal ring (7.5 μg daily lasting for 3 months)
  - Ospemifene: 60 mg PO daily; SERM for moderate to severe dyspareunia associated with vaginal atrophy
  - Vaginal lubricant may be as effective as topical estrogen for some.
- Although there is no increased risk of endometrial hyperplasia or EAC, women with bleeding on these treatments should be evaluated with TVUS or EMB. Patients with h/o hormone-dependent cancer should meet with a gynecologist before using medication.

Second Line

Nonhormonal treatments may be helpful to treat vasomotor symptoms in women who wish to or need to avoid HT (e.g., breast cancer):

- Paroxetine (7.5 mg/day) is approved for treatment of vasomotor symptoms. This SSRI demonstrated modest decrease in hot flushes.
- Other SSRI/SRNIs: Venlafaxine (37.5 to 75.0 mg/day) or fluoxetine (20 mg/day) and citalopram (20 mg/day) shown to reduce hot flushes as compared to placebo.
- Gabapentin (300 to 900 mg/day) shown to have an effect on lowering hot flushes compared to placebo.
- Clonidine (0.05 mg BID) may be used to treat mild hot flashes, less effective than SSRI/SRNIs.
- Note that most trials of second-line therapies have been brief (i.e., a few months).

COMPLEMENTARY & ALTERNATIVE MEDICINE

Trials of nonprescribed therapies are difficult to interpret due to variability of components and doses:

- Soy isoflavone in placebo-controlled trials showed a mixed effect in reducing hot flashes.
- Red clover, black cohosh, reflexology, aerobics, and magnet therapy showed no impact on hot flashes when compared with placebo.
- Small clinical trials of evening primrose, dong quai, ginseng, and wild yam do not support use for relief of hot flashes.

 ## ONGOING CARE

FOLLOW-UP RECOMMENDATIONS
Patient Monitoring
A DEXA scan is indicated at age 65 years for all women and for younger women with risk equivalent to age 65 years.

DIET
Calcium-rich diet and vitamin D supplementation (800 to 1,200 IU/day). Calcium supplements may have adverse effects including increased risk of kidney stone and increased risk of cardiac events.

PATIENT EDUCATION
Encourage lifestyle modifications:

- Smoking cessation, reducing alcohol intake
- Weight-bearing exercise >30 minutes, 3 times weekly
- Healthy diet to maintain appropriate weight
- Address cardiovascular risk factor modification.

PROGNOSIS
If untreated:

- Ultimate disappearance of vasomotor symptoms
- Worsening of vaginal/vulvar atrophy
- Osteoporosis: possible fractures of the hip, vertebrae, and wrists

COMPLICATIONS

- Osteoporosis: At menopause, women have accelerated bone loss up to 3–5% per year for 5 to 7 years.
- Increased risk of CVD following menopause

REFERENCES

1. North American Menopause Society. The 2012 hormone therapy position statement of the North American Menopause Society. *Menopause*. 2012;19(3):257–271.
2. Maclennan AH, Broadbent JL, Lester S, et al. Oral oestrogen and combined oestrogen/progestogen therapy versus placebo for hot flushes. *Cochrane Database Syst Rev*. 2004;(4):CD002978.
3. Grant MD, Marbella A, Wang AT, et al. *Menopausal Symptoms: Comparative Effectiveness of Therapies*. Rockville, MD: Agency for Healthcare Research and Quality; 2015. Report No. 15-EHC005-EF.
4. Manson JE, Ames JM, Gass MLS, et al. MenoPro: a mobile app for women bothered by menopause symptoms. http://www.menopause.org/for-women/-i-menopro-i-mobile-app. Accessed December 2, 2018.
5. Marjoribanks J, Farquhar C, Roberts H, et al. Long-term hormone therapy for perimenopausal and postmenopausal women. *Cochrane Database Syst Rev*. 2017;(1):CD004143.

ADDITIONAL READING

- ACOG Practice Bulletin No. 141: management of menopausal symptoms. *Obstet Gynecol*. 2014;123(1):202–216.
- Mørch LS, Løkkegaard E, Andreasen AH, et al. Hormone therapy and ovarian cancer. *JAMA*. 2009;302(3):298–305.
- Takahashi TA, Johnson KM. Menopause. *Med Clin North Am*. 2015;99(3):521–534. doi:10.1016/j.mcna.2015.01.006.
- U.S. Preventive Services Task Force. Breast cancer: screening. https://www.uspreventiveservicestaskforce.org/Page/Document/UpdateSummaryFinal/breast-cancer-screening. Accessed December 2, 2018.

CODES

ICD10

- E28.310 Symptomatic premature menopause
- N95.1 Menopausal and female climacteric states
- Z78.0 Asymptomatic menopausal state

CLINICAL PEARLS

- Menopause is usually diagnosed by history alone.
- HT can be used short term for relief of moderate to severe vasomotor symptoms but should not be used for long-term prevention of CVD.

M

MENORRHAGIA (HEAVY MENSTRUAL BLEEDING)

Miguel A. Palacios, MD • Maizal Cuauhtemoc Rivera, FNP

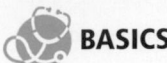 **BASICS**

DESCRIPTION
- The current preferred terminology for menorrhagia is "heavy menstrual bleeding" (HMB).
- HMB is an excessive amount (≥80 mL/cycle, compared with normal average of 30 to 60 mL/cycle) or periods lasting longer than 7 days.
- Clinically, HMB is an excessive menstrual blood loss which interferes with the woman's physical, emotional, social, and material quality of life.
- Other patterns of abnormal uterine bleeding (AUB) which may overlap with HMB include:
  - Intermenstrual bleeding (IMB; previously metrorrhagia): bleeding between regular menses
  - Polymenorrhea: menstrual cycle length <21 days
- HMB applies only to ovulatory menses and is a subcategory of "abnormal uterine bleeding."
- A classification system called the PALM-COEIN was developed to describe AUB in women of reproductive age.
- It includes the structural causes (polyp, adenomyosis, leiomyoma [submucosal or other myoma], and malignancy and hyperplasia) and nonstructural causes (coagulopathy, ovulatory dysfunction, endometrial, iatrogenic, and not yet classified).
- System affected: reproductive

EPIDEMIOLOGY
Prevalence
- HMB affects >10 million American women each year or about one out of every five women (1).
- Puberty and the perimenopause typically are associated with AUB and are considered to be physiologic in these circumstances (2).

Pediatric Considerations
- Genital bleeding before puberty is not menstrual bleeding by definition and requires further evaluation.
- Due to immaturity of the hypothalamic-pituitary-ovarian axis, adolescents are at risk of irregular bleeding and HMB.
- Adolescents with HMB should be evaluated for possible bleeding disorders, especially von Willebrand disease (3)[C].

Pregnancy Considerations
Bleeding in pregnancy is not menstrual bleeding by definition and requires further evaluation. Pregnancy test should be obtained as part of the evaluation of AUB.

Geriatric Considerations
Menopause is diagnosed after 12 months of amenorrhea in the absence of other causes and is typically preceded by irregular bleeding. All postmenopausal bleeding requires additional workup for malignancy.

ETIOLOGY AND PATHOPHYSIOLOGY
- No cause is identified in about 1/2 of patients.
- Bleeding disorders
  - Von Willebrand disease
  - ITP and other platelet disorders
  - Factor deficiencies

- Medication side effect most commonly related to anticoagulants including warfarin
  - Renal failure leading to uremic platelet dysfunction
  - Cirrhosis leading to coagulopathy
- Uterine fibroids, typically submucosal
- Endometrial polyps
- Hypothyroidism
- Iatrogenic causes including copper intrauterine device (IUD)
- Endometriosis
- Adenomyosis
- Pelvic inflammatory disease
- Some causes more typically presenting as irregular menstrual bleeding include:
  - Polycystic ovarian syndrome (PCOS)
  - Hypothalamic-pituitary dysfunction, often postmenarchal or during menopausal transition
  - Endometrial or ovarian neoplasia
  - Some forms of hormonal birth control
  - Hyperthyroidism
  - Hyperprolactinemia
- HMB has been associated with increased production and sensitivity to prostaglandins.

GENERAL PREVENTION
- Combined oral contraceptives may prevent HMB, particularly when progesterone is dominant. Lower estrogen doses result in less menstrual bleeding.
- NSAIDs including ibuprofen inhibit prostaglandin production and result in decreased blood loss and pain during menses.
- Progesterone-only contraceptives may reduce overall blood loss but often result in irregular bleeding.

COMMONLY ASSOCIATED CONDITIONS
Iron deficiency anemia

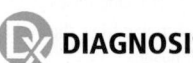 **DIAGNOSIS**

HISTORY
- Suggestive historical features for HMB:
  - Bleeding substantially heavier than patient's usual flow
  - Changing sanitary products every 1 to 2 hours or the need to change protection overnight
  - Menses lasting >7 days
  - Passage of clots larger than a quarter in diameter
- Symptoms that suggest bleeding is ovulatory:
  - Regular menstrual interval
  - Midcycle pain (mittelschmerz)
  - Premenstrual symptoms: breast soreness, mood changes
- Abdominal pain or cramps at other times of the cycle may be associated with structural causes:
  - Polyps
  - Adenomyosis
  - Leiomyoma
  - Ovarian tumors

- Symptoms that suggest an underlying bleeding disorder include:
  - Epistaxis
  - Mucosal bleeding (e.g., gums)
  - Easy bruising
  - Family history of bleeding disorder
- Review of medications, with particular attention to contraceptive and anticoagulant medication
- Other medical conditions that may relate to HMB:
  - Renal or hepatic disease
  - Thyroid disease
- Evaluate for symptoms of anemia including fatigue and dyspnea.

PHYSICAL EXAM
- Prompt assessment for signs of hemodynamic instability, including orthostatic vital signs (4)
- Thyroid nodule or goiter suggests thyroid disease.
- Signs of a bleeding disorder include petechiae and ecchymoses.
- Pelvic examination, including speculum and bimanual examination, may reveal the following:
  - Cervical or vaginal source of bleeding
  - Pelvic or adnexal mass
  - Evidence of reproductive tract infection such as cervical motion tenderness
  - Uterine enlargement
- Hirsutism, acne, and obesity are suggestive of PCOS.

DIFFERENTIAL DIAGNOSIS
- Normal menses
- Anovulatory bleeding
- IMB
- Complications of pregnancy
  - Spontaneous abortion
- Other sources of bleeding:
  - Cervical
  - Vaginal
  - Gastrointestinal

DIAGNOSTIC TESTS & INTERPRETATION
Initial Tests (lab, imaging)
- Pregnancy test
- CBC to assess for:
  - Anemia
  - Thrombocytopenia
  - Leukocytosis may suggest infection.
- Thyroid-stimulating hormone (TSH) test (2)[B]
- Labs to consider in select cases:
  - Coagulation panel for evaluation for bleeding disorder in adolescent or adult with history suggestive of bleeding disorder (2)[A]
  - Workup of anovulatory bleeding may also include prolactin, androgens, FSH, LH, and estrogen.
  - Appropriate cervical cancer screening
  - Evaluation for infection including gonorrhea and chlamydia (2)[B]
- Imaging should be obtained based on clinician judgment and should begin with transvaginal ultrasonography.
- Transabdominal ultrasonography should be performed if transvaginal approach does not provide full assessment of anatomy.

- Some experts recommend transvaginal ultrasonography as the initial screening test for AUB and MRI as a second-line test to be used when the diagnosis is inconclusive, when further delineation would affect patient management, or when coexisting uterine myomas are suspected (2)[C].
- Endometrial biopsy should be performed in patients with AUB who are >45 years as a first-line test (2)[C].

Follow-Up Tests & Special Considerations
- Saline infusion sonohysterography is recommended if ultrasound suggests intracavitary pathology and is more sensitive and specific than transvaginal ultrasound (2)[C].
  - Sonohysterography is superior to transvaginal ultrasonography in the detection of intracavitary lesions, such as polyps and submucosal leiomyomas (2)[A].
- Hysteroscopy can be performed if direct visualization is desired.

Diagnostic Procedures/Other
Endometrial biopsy to assess for malignancy and hyperplasia is recommended in some situations including (2,4)[C]:
- Any AUB, including HMB, after age 45 years in an ovulatory (premenopausal) woman
- Woman <45 years with persistent or refractory AUB, risk factors such as unopposed estrogen exposure, or concerning endometrial imaging

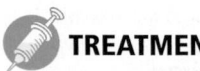

TREATMENT

GENERAL MEASURES
Treat underlying conditions (e.g., hypothyroidism) when possible.

MEDICATION
First Line
- For acute control of severe bleeding (5):
  - Obtain IV access and consider blood transfusion or clotting factor administration.
  - Estrogen, conjugated equine: 25 mg IV every 4 to 6 hours for 24 hours
  - Monophasic combined oral contraceptive that contains 35 μg ethinyl estradiol: 3 times per day for 7 days
  - Medroxyprogesterone acetate: 20 mg orally 3 times per day for 7 days
  - Tranexamic acid: 1.3 g orally or 10 mg/kg IV 3 times per day for 5 days, antifibrinolytic agent
- For less severe bleeding (typical case) or after control of acute bleeding has been achieved (5):
  - Levonorgestrel IUD (Mirena IUD): typically results in light bleeding or amenorrhea with patient satisfaction similar to hysterectomy and endometrial ablation (6)[A]
  - Combination estrogen-progestin oral contraceptive: may be prescribed in cyclic, extended, or continuous dosing and typically results in regular, lighter, and less painful menses
  - Depot medroxyprogesterone acetate: 150 mg/1 mL IM every 3 months, typically results in amenorrhea or light irregular bleeding

---

- Tranexamic acid: 1.3 g orally for 5 days during menses; antifibrinolytic agent that is option for women who desire nonhormonal treatment
- NSAIDs (e.g., naproxen, mefenamic acid, ibuprofen) can reduce blood loss and dysmenorrhea. Those with bleeding disorders or platelet function abnormalities should avoid NSAIDs (5).

Second Line
- Noncontraception estrogen-progestin oral contraceptives (ultra-low-dose estrogen): may be considered when a relative contraindication to estrogen is present
- Oral progestins: multiple formulations and dosing; typically used in women who have contraindications to estrogen or are trying to conceive

SURGERY/OTHER PROCEDURES
- Dilation and curettage can be considered in the setting of acute severe bleeding.
- For women who desire fertility, myomectomy may be considered for treatment of uterine leiomyomas (fibroids).
- For women who do not desire fertility, consider endometrial ablation, uterine artery embolization, or hysterectomy.
- Conservative surgery (i.e., myomectomy, endometrial ablation, or uterine artery embolization) is more effective for controlling bleeding symptoms at 1 and 2 years than oral medications or the levonorgestrel-releasing IUD, but by 5 years, there is no difference in long-term results or patient satisfaction (1)[B].
  - Patients who undergo endometrial ablation still require contraception.
  - Uterine artery embolization is used to treat uterine leiomyomas.
- In women of reproductive age with chronic HMB, hysterectomy is the most effective treatment for controlling symptoms (1).
  - Hysterectomy is curative but with more severe adverse effects and is typically reserved for failure of medical management or presence of another indication such as malignancy (1).

ONGOING CARE

DIET
Iron supplementation may help correct for increased blood loss.

PATIENT EDUCATION
Patient and provider should engage in informed decision making with understanding of treatment risks and benefits.

PROGNOSIS
Most patients respond well to medical management, and surgical interventions are curative options in appropriate cases. Surgical interventions (hysterectomy or conservative surgeries) are initially more effective and satisfactory than medical treatments, but that the levonorgestrel-releasing intrauterine system yields similar long-term results and patient satisfaction compared with conservative surgical interventions (1).

COMPLICATIONS
- Iron deficiency anemia
- Acute severe blood loss

REFERENCES
1. Marjoribanks J, Lethaby A, Farquhar C. Surgery versus medical therapy for heavy menstrual bleeding. *Cochrane Database Syst Rev*. 2016;(1): CD003855.
2. Committee on Practice Bulletins—Gynecology. Practice bulletin no. 128: diagnosis of abnormal uterine bleeding in reproductive-aged women. *Obstet Gynecol*. 2012;120(1):197–206.
3. Mullins T, Miller R, Mullins E. Evaluation and management of adolescents with abnormal uterine bleeding. *Pediatr Ann*. 2015;44(9):e218–e222.
4. Matthews ML. Abnormal uterine bleeding in reproductive-aged women. *Obstet Gynecol Clin North Am*. 2015;42(1):103–115.
5. American College of Obstetricians and Gynecologists. ACOG committee opinion no. 557: management of acute abnormal uterine bleeding in nonpregnant reproductive-aged women. *Obstet Gynecol*. 2013;121(4):891–896.
6. Lethaby A, Hussain M, Rishworth JR, et al. Progesterone or progestogen-releasing intrauterine systems for heavy menstrual bleeding. *Cochrane Database Syst Rev*. 2015;(4):CD002126.

CODES

ICD10
- N92.0 Excessive and frequent menstruation with regular cycle
- N92.3 Ovulation bleeding
- N92.2 Excessive menstruation at puberty

CLINICAL PEARLS
- Women with HMB are at high risk for iron deficiency anemia.
- A thorough menstrual history is critical to differentiate HMB from similar conditions including anovulatory bleeding.
- Teenagers presenting with HMB should be evaluated for an underlying bleeding disorder.
- All postmenopausal bleeding and bleeding during pregnancy requires additional workup.
- The levonorgestrel (Mirena, Kyleena, generics) IUD may be used for HMB and is associated with high patient satisfaction rates.

M

MESOTHELIOMA

Khalid Bashir, MD

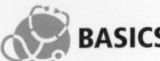 **BASICS**

DESCRIPTION
- Mesothelioma is a rare, aggressive malignancy of the mesothelial or serous tissues primarily found in the pleura (65–70%) or peritoneum (20–33%), tunica vaginalis (1–2%) or pericardium (1–2%) (1).
- Inhalation of asbestos is the predominant cause of mesothelioma, most often from occupational exposure.

EPIDEMIOLOGY
Incidence
- The incidence in the United States is decreasing, but it is increasing in other countries, particularly Great Britain and Australia.
- It is expected that rates of mesothelioma will start to drop after 2015 to 2025 related to reduced exposure and better understanding of the process of development of mesothelioma after exposure to asbestos (2).
- The incidence increases with age, peaking in the 6th decade, with 70% of pleural disease occurring in males. Peritoneal involvement is slightly higher in women.
- Main risk factor is asbestos exposure, but tumors have arisen after prior radiation or exposure to talc, erionite, or mica or in patients with familial Mediterranean fever and diffuse lymphocytic leukemia.

Prevalence
There are 3,300 cases of mesothelioma diagnosed in the United States annually (3).

ETIOLOGY AND PATHOPHYSIOLOGY
- The predominant cause of mesothelioma is exposure to asbestos (hydrated magnesium silicate fibrous minerals).
- There is a long latent period of up to 44 years between exposure and development of mesothelioma (2).
- Inhaled or ingested asbestos fibers become trapped in pleural or peritoneal membranes, causing changes of irritation and inflammation.

Genetics
Loss of nuclear deubiquitinase BAP1 is associated with incidence of mesothelioma in some families as well as with other cancers such as melanoma.

RISK FACTORS
- The predominant risk factor is exposure to asbestos.
- Occupational exposures involve mining or milling of fibers, work with textiles, cement, friction materials, insulation, or shipbuilding.
- Nonoccupational exposures include renovation or destruction of asbestos-containing buildings, exposure to industrial sources in the community or natural geologic sources, or exposure to soiled clothing of asbestos workers (1,3,4).
- Radiation exposure, smoking, proximity to naturally occurring asbestos deposits, or inhalation of other fibrous silicates can contribute to malignant mesothelioma.

GENERAL PREVENTION
- Avoidance of asbestos exposure
- Strict adherence to protective protocols for workers in buildings where asbestos is found
- Continued aggressive remediation of asbestos-affected buildings and homes

DIAGNOSIS

HISTORY
- Symptoms are usually nonspecific and occur when disease is advanced. General fatigue, night sweats, and weight loss may be present.
- Pleural mesothelioma presents with gradual onset of pulmonary symptoms, chest pain, dyspnea, and cough.
- Peritoneal disease presents with vague abdominal pain, increased abdominal girth, nausea, anorexia, and weight loss.

PHYSICAL EXAM
- Pulmonary findings consistent with pleural effusion, including decreased breath sounds, dullness to percussion, and asymmetric chest wall expansion, are found.
- Abdominal findings consistent with ascites, including abdominal distension, fluid wave, and tenderness, are found.

DIFFERENTIAL DIAGNOSIS
- Pleural mesothelioma's differential diagnosis includes inflammatory reactions (empyema, pleural effusion), metastatic tumor from other sites, fibrosarcoma, malignant fibrous histiocytoma, sarcomatoid carcinoma, and synovial sarcoma.
- Peritoneal mesothelioma's differential diagnosis includes peritoneal carcinomatosis, serous peritoneal carcinoma, ovarian carcinoma in women, lymphomatosis, and tuberculous peritonitis.

DIAGNOSTIC TESTS & INTERPRETATION
Initial Tests (lab, imaging)
- At present, there is no tumor marker or serum chemistry that is of value in establishing the diagnosis of mesothelioma.
- Biomarkers that may be elevated in mesothelioma include fibulin-3, mesothelin, and osteopontin. However, they do not have an established role in diagnosis or monitoring response to therapy (2)[A].
- Pleural mesothelioma diagnosis requires tissue. Thoracentesis for cytology and closed pleural biopsy may be adequate, but often, more invasive procedures such as video-assisted thoracoscopic surgery (VATS) is needed to obtain an adequate specimen (1,2)[A].

Follow-Up Tests & Special Considerations
Seeding of biopsy sites and tracks may occur in mesothelioma, which can be prevented with prophylactic radiation therapy to the scar or biopsy site (5)[A].

Diagnostic Procedures/Other
- CT, MRI, PET, or integrated PET-CT helps with clinical staging in pleural and peritoneal disease (1,2,3,4),(5)[A].
- Mediastinoscopy, bronchoscopy, and laparoscopy can assist in full surgical staging of pleural disease (2)[A].
- Endobronchial ultrasound for staging is under investigation for pleural disease.

Test Interpretation

- The tumor, node, metastasis (TNM) staging system is most commonly used, although some centers use other staging systems.
- Butchart staging system is the oldest and still used in some parts of the world.
- Brigham staging system attempts to define resectability and lymph node involvement.

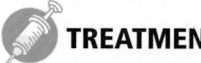

TREATMENT

GENERAL MEASURES

- A multidisciplinary team is important in management and should include thoracic surgery, oncology, pathology, pulmonary, and radiology for patient-specific planning of management.
- Pain assessment and control should follow principles of cancer pain management (5).

MEDICATION

First Line

- In pleural disease, combined therapy with cisplatin + gemcitabine or cisplatin + pemetrexed are associated with longer median survival than cisplatin alone (2),(4)[A].
- Vinflunine is showing some potential for first-line treatment in pleural disease (2)[A].
- Hyperthermic intraoperative or early postoperative intraperitoneal chemotherapy can increase drug concentration in the peritoneum and decrease systemic side effects. Use cisplatin, mitomycin C, fluorouracil, doxorubicin, and/or paclitaxel (1,2),(3)[A].

Second Line

- Palliative benefit in pleural disease with mitomycin C, vinblastine, cisplatin, and pemetrexed alone or in combination with carboplatin (2,3),(4)[A].
- Systemic therapy for peritoneal disease may include pemetrexed + cisplatin; vinorelbine or gemcitabine alone or in combination (1),(5)[A]

ISSUES FOR REFERRAL

- Pulmonary, oncology, and surgical follow-up after discharge as indicated
- Anger and depression may require psychological or psychiatric services (5).

ADDITIONAL THERAPIES

Immunotherapy in pleural disease uses humanized anti-CB3 AB (OKT3), cytotoxic T lymph (CTL), interferon α-2a, and autovaccine in advanced disease (1,2,3,4,5).

- Gene therapy
- Photodynamic therapy
- Radiotherapy in some cases of pleural disease
- Vascular endothelial growth factor (anti-VEGF-2) in combination with chemotherapy (2)
  - Vaccines are under study (5).

SURGERY/OTHER PROCEDURES

- For pleural mesothelioma, the role of surgery is not as clear cut. Pleurectomy with tumor decortication and extrapleural pneumonectomy reduces the tumor load, but there remains no clear effect on mortality (2,4,5).
- Radical resection of the peritoneum and cytoreductive surgery is associated with a better prognosis (1).

ADMISSION, INPATIENT, AND NURSING CONSIDERATIONS

- Based on overall condition
- IV fluids as indicated by general condition
- Nursing as indicated by condition
- Discharge criteria as indicated by general condition

 ONGOING CARE

FOLLOW-UP RECOMMENDATIONS

- Smoking cessation
- Immunization for pneumococcal pneumonia and influenza

Patient Monitoring

Monitor for paraneoplastic phenomenon, including fever, thrombocytosis, malignancy-related thrombosis, hypoglycemia, and rare Coombs-positive hemolytic anemia.

DIET

No specific restrictions

PROGNOSIS

- Prognosis is based on gender, stage, and level of completeness of cytoreduction.
- Poorly differentiated tumor grade, failure to undertake surgical resection, advanced age, and male gender are all independent predictors of poorer prognosis (2,3).
- Average survival is 17 to 92 months, with 5-year survival rate at 63%.

COMPLICATIONS

Relapses and progression, infection and dysphagia

Geriatric Considerations

Age >65 years is associated with significantly increased morbidity and mortality.

Pediatric Considerations

Rarely a pediatric issue because most disease occurs after the 5th decade of life

Pregnancy Considerations

Rarely an issue with pregnancy because most disease occurs after the 5th decade of life

REFERENCES

1. Bridda A, Padoan I, Mencarelli R, et al. Peritoneal mesothelioma: a review. *MedGenMed*. 2007;9(2):32.
2. Weder W. Mesothelioma. *Ann Oncol*. 2010;21(Suppl 7):vii326–vii333.
3. Mott FE. Mesothelioma: a review. *Ochsner J*. 2012;12(1):70–79.
4. Fuhrer G, Lazarus AA. Mesothelioma. *Dis Mon*. 2011;57(1):40–54.
5. van Meerbeeck JP, Scherpereel A, Surmont VF, et al. Malignant pleural mesothelioma: the standard of care and challenges for future management. *Crit Rev Oncol Hematol*. 2011;78(2):92–111.

CODES

ICD10

- C45.9 Mesothelioma, unspecified
- C45.0 Mesothelioma of pleura
- C45.1 Mesothelioma of peritoneum

CLINICAL PEARLS

- Mesothelioma remains a rare but universally fatal disease in part due to long latency.
- Multimodal treatment has decreased recurrence rates and has extended survival time.
- Main risk factor is asbestos exposure, but tumors have arisen after prior radiation or exposure to talc, erionite, or mica or in patients with familial Mediterranean fever and diffuse lymphocytic leukemia.

M

METABOLIC SYNDROME
Naomi Parrella, MD, FAAFP, Dipl. ABOM

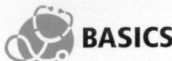 **BASICS**

DESCRIPTION
- Progressive metabolic abnormalities, including insulin resistance, a proinflammatory and prothrombotic state that manifest with at least three of (1):
  - Increased waist circumference (WC)
  - Elevated blood pressure (BP)
  - Elevated triglycerides (TG) ≥150 mg/dL or treatment
  - Decreased high-density lipoprotein (HDL-C) in men <40 mg/dL, women <50 mg/dL or treatment
  - Elevated fasting glucose ≥100 mg/dL or treatment
- Metabolic syndrome (MetS) predicts increased risk for type 2 diabetes mellitus (T2DM), cardiovascular disease, stroke, nonalcoholic fatty liver disease (NAFLD), certain cancers, and all-cause mortality.

EPIDEMIOLOGY
Prevalence
- Affects 34.2% of U.S. adults aged ≥18 years; increasing with the aging population and the prevalence of obesity (2)
- MetS is a rapidly growing epidemic worldwide. From 1988 to 2012, prevalence of MetS in the United States had the largest increase in non-Hispanic black men, non-Hispanic white women, non-Hispanic black women, and persons of low socioeconomic status (2).
- Predominant sex: female (34.9%) > male (33.4%) (2)
- Prevalence increases with age with >50% of person >70 years old with MetS (2).
- Predominant ethnicity: non-Hispanic white men and women and non-Hispanic black women (2)

Pediatric Considerations
- Obese children and adolescents are at high risk of MetS (prevalence of 29.2% in the United States). Risk factors in children and adolescents include ethnicity; heredity; maternal gestational diabetes; low birth weight; childhood excess weight gain and obesity; endocrine abnormalities, including polycystic ovarian syndrome (PCOS); and poor health habits (eating refined carbohydrates, drinking daily fruit juice or sugar sweetened beverages, sedentariness, inadequate sleep) (2).
- International Diabetes Federation (IDF) consensus report defined criteria in three age groups (6 to ≤10 years; 10 to ≤16 years; 16+ years, adult criteria applicable). Obesity defined by WC ≥90th percentile; rest of the diagnostic criteria (TG, HDL-C, hypertension [HTN], and fasting blood sugar/T2DM) are largely the same as in adults for children ≥10 years, with some exceptions, and warrant treatment to optimize diet and physical activity.
- Clinical significance of MetS in pediatric population is not well established using these criteria. WC alone is better than using IDF criteria to predict development of MetS, abnormal BP, dyslipidemia, and insulin resistance (3). Focus on healthy weight management and promoting healthy lifestyle habits for the whole family rather than diagnosis.

ETIOLOGY AND PATHOPHYSIOLOGY
- Increase in intra-abdominal and visceral adipose tissue
- Adipose tissue dysfunction, insulin resistance, and leptin resistance
- Decreased levels of adiponectin, an adipocytokine, known to protect against T2DM, HTN, atherosclerosis, and inflammation

- Abnormal fatty acid metabolism, endothelial dysfunction, systemic inflammation (increased IL-6, tumor necrosis factor-α [TNF-α], resistin, CRP), oxidative stress, elevated renin-angiotensin system activation, and a prothrombotic state (increased tissue plasminogen activator inhibitor-1) are also associated.
- The main etiologic factors are the following:
  - Central obesity (particularly abdominal)/excess visceral adipose tissue
  - Insulin resistance
  - Other contributing factors:
    - Advancing age
    - Proinflammatory state
    - Genetics
    - Sedentary lifestyle
- Endocrine (e.g., postmenopausal state)
- Prescription medications (e.g., corticosteroids, antipsychotics, β-blockers)

Genetics
Genetic factors contribute to causation. Most identified genes are transcription factors or regulators of transcription and translation. It is a multifactorial disease with evidence of complex interactions between genetics and environment.

RISK FACTORS
- Obesity/intra-abdominal obesity, insulin resistance
- Childhood obesity
- Older age, postmenopausal status
- Ethnicity
- Family history
- Physical inactivity
- High-carbohydrate diet
- Sugar-sweetened beverages daily
- Smoking
- Low socioeconomic status
- Alteration of gut flora

GENERAL PREVENTION
- Effective weight loss and maintenance of the body weight long term
- Built environment to promote healthy lifestyle choices
- Regular and sustained physical activity
- Diet low in processed carbohydrates and simple sugars; avoidance of sugar-sweetened beverages

COMMONLY ASSOCIATED CONDITIONS
- PCOS
- Acanthosis nigricans
- NAFLD
- Obstructive sleep apnea (OSA)
- Depression
- Cognitive impairment
- Gallstones (cholesterol)
- Chronic renal disease
- Erectile dysfunction
- Hyperuricemia and gout
- Vitamin D deficiency
- Subclinical hypothyroidism

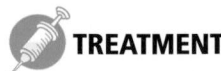 **DIAGNOSIS**

HISTORY
Not necessary for diagnosis of MetS; useful in identifying risk factors and beneficial preventive strategies
- Family history of MetS, T2DM, and cardiovascular disease
- Symptoms indicating cardiovascular disease or diabetes or PCOS

- Comprehensive lifestyle history:
  - Diet, including timing (night eating) and intake of carbohydrates especially added sugars and caloric beverages
  - Weight history, including onset of obesity and previous weight loss attempts
  - Exercise regimen, daily activity level
  - Alcohol intake
  - Sleep patterns, duration, and quality
- Cigarette smoking
- Assess cardiovascular risk with cardiovascular risk assessment tool.

PHYSICAL EXAM
- Abdominal obesity: men >102 cm, women >88 cm (lower threshold in populations susceptible to insulin resistance, especially Asian Americans)
- BP ≥130/85 mm Hg or treatment
- Additional exam findings suggestive of insulin resistance such as acanthosis nigricans, hirsutism

DIFFERENTIAL DIAGNOSIS
- T2DM
- OSA, PCOS, thyroid abnormalities, Cushing syndrome, medication effect (especially psychotropic, chronic steroids, β-blockers, and thiazide diuretic medications) may also be considered in the differential.

DIAGNOSTIC TESTS & INTERPRETATION
Initial Tests (lab, imaging)
- Fasting TGs ≥150 mg/dL or treatment
- HDL: men <40 mg/dL, women <50 mg/dL or treatment
- Fasting glucose ≥100 mg/dL or treatment

Follow-Up Tests & Special Considerations
- Formal 75-mg oral glucose tolerance test or hemoglobin A1C for diagnosis of impaired glucose tolerance (IGT) or chronically elevated blood glucose
- Liver function tests (Assess for NAFLD.)
- Measurement of fasting insulin levels is controversial.
- Consider evaluation for vitamin D deficiency.
- Consider evaluation for hyperuricemia and microalbuminuria.
- May consider further risk factor evaluation for cardiovascular disease such as advanced lipid profile analysis, hs-CRP, or homocysteine
- Consider evaluation of OSA.

Diagnostic Procedures/Other
- Home BP monitoring or 24-hour BP monitoring may be used to rule out white coat HTN.
- ECG, stress test, coronary calcium test, and coronary angiography may be used for further cardiovascular risk assessment.
- Ultrasound of liver may be considered to evaluate for fatty liver.

TREATMENT

Primary therapeutic goal is to prevent or reduce obesity and risk factors. Aggressive lifestyle modification (diet and exercise) is considered first-line therapy and most clinically effective (4).

GENERAL MEASURES
- Aggressive treatment of individual risk factors
- Increase daily physical activity
- Stop smoking.
- Avoid excess alcohol intake.
- Avoid sugar-sweetened beverages.

- Avoid high glycemic load meals and snacks that cause rapid insulin release.
- Increase leafy green vegetables.
- Maintain healthy sleep patterns and stress management.

MEDICATION

- Consider daily aspirin for patients with cardiovascular disease or those at high risk.
- Consult clinical guidelines for treatment of dyslipidemia, HTN, IGT, prediabetes, and diabetes.
- Multiple medications may be required to achieve adequate BP control.
- Diagnosis and treatment of insulin resistance is controversial.

First Line

Lifestyle modification alone because initial strategy is applicable to individuals with low 10-year risk for coronary artery disease (CAD). In individuals with higher 10-year risk, more aggressive risk factor–based approach is recommended in addition to lifestyle modifications:

- Obesity: Lifestyle changes are the cornerstone of treatment. Aim for a ~5–10% weight reduction. Any amount of weight loss is associated with significant benefits. See section on "Obesity."
- Physical activity: Exercise improves MetS (5)[A]. 30 to 60 minutes of moderate-intensity aerobic activities such as brisk walking 5 to 7 days/week; increase in daily lifestyle activities and resistance training 1 to 2 days/week. In patients with established CAD, assess detailed history of physical activity and exercise tolerance to guide activity prescription. Advise medically supervised programs for high-risk population (recent acute coronary syndrome [ACS], congestive heart failure, recent revascularization). Cumulative exercise time over the day contributes to health benefit.
- Tobacco use: See section on "Smoking Cessation."
- OSA: See section on "Obstructive Sleep Apnea."
- Dyslipidemia: See section on "Dyslipidemia."
- HTN: Aim for similar targets to patients with diabetes. See section on "Hypertension." β-Blockers may lead to weight gain and worsen MetS.
- IGT and/or prediabetes: intensive lifestyle interventions (ILI) to decrease the development of diabetes. Metformin (875 mg twice daily), although less efficacious than ILI, has also been demonstrated to decrease the incidence of diabetes in patients with MetS (6)[A]. If CAD or T2DM is already evident, treat as per guidelines. Use ASA 81 mg for primary prevention as indicated per USPSTF if benefits outweigh bleeding risk.

ISSUES FOR REFERRAL

- Obesity management
- Nutrition therapy
- Exercise planning
- Smoking cessation
- Cardiovascular disease management
- Worsening glycemic control
- Liver function tests suggesting liver disease
- Suspected OSA
- Weight-related mental health concerns (e.g., binge eating disorder)

SURGERY/OTHER PROCEDURES

- Bariatric surgery can treat MetS in severely obese patients who have failed trials of lifestyle modification and pharmacotherapy; surgery is recommended in appropriate individual if body mass index (BMI) >40 or BMI >35 with obesity-related comorbidities.
- Liposuction of abdominal adipose tissue does not reduce insulin resistance or cardiovascular risk factors.

COMPLEMENTARY & ALTERNATIVE MEDICINE

Chromium picolinate 500 to 1,000 μg/day and selenium 200 mg/day may improve insulin resistance, and plant sterol esters may be used for cardioprotective effects; insufficient evidence on the use of cinnamon or fish oil for improved insulin sensitivity (4)[A]

ADMISSION, INPATIENT, AND NURSING CONSIDERATIONS

- Management usually does not require admission.
- Admission criteria/initial stabilization
  – Serious complications (e.g., ACS, hypertensive crisis, diabetic coma)

 ONGOING CARE

FOLLOW-UP RECOMMENDATIONS

- Regular exercise will improve all components of the MetS. Cumulative small periods of exercise over the day provide significant health benefits. Encourage small increases in physical activity over time.
- Encourage replacing sedentary activity choices (e.g., sitting at desk, driving car, taking elevator, and the like) to more active ones (e.g., standing desk, walking, cycling, stationary walking during commercials).
- Weight reduction to improve abdominal obesity is a primary goal achieved by dietary modification and increased physical activity.
- Regular monitoring of weight, WC, and BP. Fasting TG, HDL, and sugar levels may be routinely monitored to assess progress and to focus treatment efforts.

DIET

- Dietary recommendations may include limiting sugars and simple carbohydrates in diet; intermittent fasting or time-restricted feeding; eating a low carbohydrate, Mediterranean, New Nordic (4,7)[A], or DASH (Dietary Approaches to Stop Hypertension) diet (7)[A].
- To reduce risk of developing T2DM, encourage increasing intake of vegetables and fiber and keep fruit and alcohol in moderation (4,7)[A].
- Avoid processed red meats, refined grains, fruit juice, and sugar-sweetened beverages (4,7)[A].

PROGNOSIS

Increased risk of T2DM (~5-fold), CAD (~1.5- to 3-fold), acute myocardial infarction (~2.5-fold), and all-cause mortality (~1.5-fold)

COMPLICATIONS

Long-term complications are primarily CAD and T2DM. Recent evidence demonstrates an increased risk of NAFLD, stroke, chronic kidney disease, cognitive decline, and an increased risk of developing certain cancers, especially breast cancer in postmenopausal women. Finally, individuals with infertility may find fertility is restored, and unexpected pregnancy may occur when MetS is appropriately treated.

REFERENCES

1. Alberti KG, Eckel RH, Grundy SM, et al. Harmonizing the metabolic syndrome: a joint interim statement of the International Diabetes Federation Task Force on Epidemiology and Prevention; National Heart, Lung, and Blood Institute; American Heart Association; World Heart Federation; International Atherosclerosis Society; and International Association for the Study of Obesity. *Circulation*. 2009;120(16):1640–1645.
2. Moore JX, Chaudhary N, Akinyemiju T. Metabolic syndrome prevalence by race/ethnicity and sex in the United States, National Health and Nutrition Examination Survey, 1988–2012. *Prev Chronic Dis*. 2017;14:E24.
3. Al-Hamad D, Raman V. Metabolic syndrome in children and adolescents. *Transl Pediatr*. 2017;6(4):397–407.
4. Via MA, Mechanick JI. Nutrition in type 2 diabetes and the metabolic syndrome. *Med Clin North Am*. 2016;100(6):1285–1302.
5. Paley CA, Johnson MI. Abdominal obesity and metabolic syndrome: exercise as medicine? *BMC Sports Sci Med Rehabil*. 2018;10:7.
6. Diabetes Prevention Program Research Group. Long-term effects of lifestyle intervention or metformin on diabetes development and microvascular complications over 15-year follow-up: the Diabetes Prevention Program Outcomes Study. *Lancet Diabetes Endocrinol*. 2015;3(11):866–875.
7. Forouhi NG, Misra A, Mohan V, et al. Dietary and nutritional approaches for prevention and management of type 2 diabetes. *BMJ*. 2018;361:k2234.

ADDITIONAL READING

- Diet Doctor: https://www.dietdoctor.com
- Intensive Dietary Management: https://idmprogram.com/tag/metabolic-syndrome/

 CODES

ICD10

E88.81 Metabolic syndrome

CLINICAL PEARLS

- Routine WC should be measured as part of a cardiovascular risk assessment.
- Consider further evaluation for MetS when history and/or physical exam demonstrates findings consistent with sedentary lifestyle, sleep apnea, increasing WC, elevation of BP or treatment, increased TG:HDL ratio, evidence of insulin resistance, or abnormal screening labs or treatment for lipids or blood glucose.
- Prevention or reduction of obesity and cardiovascular risk factors is the cornerstone of management of MetS.
- Consider alternatives for medications known to increase risk of MetS such as atypical antipsychotic medications and chronic steroids.
- Risks associated with MetS may be reduced or resolved by following a diet limiting daily sugars and carbohydrates.
- In addition to regular 30- to 60-minute exercise regimen, there is significant benefit to decreasing sedentariness and increasing cumulative physical activity over the day.
- Consider evaluation and treatment of sleep disorders that may affect metabolic risk factors.
- Unexpected pregnancy may occur with the treatment of MetS.
- Aggressive lifelong lifestyle modification is the first line and most potent treatment for all patients.

M

METATARSALGIA

Ammar Shahid, MD • Marc W. McKenna, MD

 BASICS

DESCRIPTION
- Metatarsalgia is defined as pain in the forefoot under one or more metatarsal heads.
- There are three groups:
  - Primary: due to anatomical issues
  - Secondary: due to conditions that increase metatarsal loading via indirect mechanisms, such as chronic synovitis
  - Iatrogenic

EPIDEMIOLOGY
Incidence
Especially common in athletes engaging in high-impact sports (running, jumping, dancing), in rock climbers (12.5%), and in older active adults

Prevalence
Common

ETIOLOGY AND PATHOPHYSIOLOGY
- The 1st metatarsal head bears significant weight when walking or running. A normal metatarsal arch ensures this balance. The 1st metatarsal head normally has adequate padding to accommodate increased forces.
- Reactive tissue can build a callus around the metatarsal head, compounding the pain.
  - Excessive or repetitive stress. Forces are transmitted to the forefoot during several stages (midstance and push off) of walking and running. These forces are translated across the metatarsal heads at nearly 3 times the body weight (1)[C].
  - A pronated splayfoot disturbs this balance, causing equal weight-bearing on all metatarsal heads.
  - Any foot deformity changes distribution of weight, impacting areas of the foot that do not have sufficient padding.
  - Soft tissue dysfunction: intrinsic muscle weakness, laxity in the Lisfranc ligament
  - Abnormal foot posture: forefoot varus or valgus, cavus or equinus deformities, loss of the metatarsal arch, splayfoot, pronated foot, inappropriate footwear
  - Dermatologic: warts, calluses (2)[C]
- Great toe
  - Hallux valgus (bunion), either varus or rigidus
- Lesser metatarsals
  - Freiberg infraction (i.e., aseptic necrosis of the metatarsal head usually due to trauma in adolescents who jump or sprint)
  - Hammer toe or claw toe
  - Morton syndrome (i.e., long 2nd metatarsal)

RISK FACTORS
- Obesity
- High heels, narrow shoes, or overly tight-fitting shoes (rock climbers typically wear small shoes)
- Competitive athletes in weight-bearing sports (e.g., ballet, basketball, running, soccer, baseball, football)
- Foot deformities or changes in ROM (e.g., pes planus, pes cavus, tight Achilles tendon, tarsal tunnel syndrome, hallux valgus, prominent metatarsal heads, excessive pronation, hammer toe deformity, tight toe extensors) (2)[C]

Geriatric Considerations
- Concomitant arthritis
- Metatarsalgia is common in older athletes.
- Age-related atrophy of the metatarsal fat pad may increase the risk for metatarsalgia.

Pediatric Considerations
- Muscle imbalance disorders (e.g., Duchenne muscular dystrophy) cause foot deformities in children.
- In adolescent girls, consider Freiberg infraction.
- Salter I injuries may affect subsequent growth and healing of the epiphysis.

Pregnancy Considerations
- Forefoot pain during pregnancy usually results from change in gait, center of mass, and joint laxity.
- Wear properly fitted low-heeled shoes.

GENERAL PREVENTION
- Wear properly fitted shoes with good padding.
- Start weight-bearing exercise programs gradually.
- Adequate stretching, particularly of the calf muscles
- Weight loss if overweight

COMMONLY ASSOCIATED CONDITIONS
- Arthritis
- Morton neuroma
- Sesamoiditis
- Plantar keratosis—callous formation

DIAGNOSIS

HISTORY
- Pain gradually develops and persists over the heads of one or more metatarsals. Pain is usually on the plantar surface and worse during midstance gait phase.
- Pain is often chronic.
- Predisposition with pes cavus and hyperpronation
- Pain often described as walking with a pebble in the shoe; aggravated during midstance or propulsion phases of walking or running

PHYSICAL EXAM
- Point tenderness over plantar metatarsal heads
- Pain in the interdigital space or a positive metatarsal squeeze test suggests Morton neuroma.
- Plantar keratosis
- Tenderness of the metatarsal head(s) with pressure applied by the examiner's finger and thumb
- Erythema and swelling (occasionally)

DIFFERENTIAL DIAGNOSIS
- Stress fracture (most commonly 2nd metatarsal)
- Morton neuroma (i.e., interdigital neuroma)
- Tarsal tunnel syndrome
- Sesamoiditis or sesamoid fracture
- Salter I fracture in children
- Arthritis (e.g., gouty, rheumatoid, inflammatory, osteoarthritis, septic, calcium pyrophosphate dihydrate crystal deposit disease [CPPD])
- Lisfranc injury
- Avascular necrosis of the metatarsal head
- Ganglion cyst
- Foreign body
- Vasculitis (diabetes)
- Bony tumors

DIAGNOSTIC TESTS & INTERPRETATION
Initial Tests (lab, imaging)
- Weight-bearing radiographs: anteroposterior, lateral, and oblique views:
  - Occasionally, metatarsal or sesamoid axial films (to rule out sesamoid fracture) or skyline view of the metatarsal heads to assess the plantar declination of the metatarsal heads: obtained with the metatarsophalangeal (MTP) joints in dorsiflexion (to evaluate alignment)
- Ultrasound and MRI in recalcitrant cases especially if concern for stress fracture (3)[C]
- MR arthrography of the MTP joint can delineate capsular tears, typically of the distal lateral border of the plantar plate (an often underrecognized cause of metatarsalgia).
- Only if diagnosis is in question
  - Erythrocyte sedimentation rate or C-reactive protein
  - Rheumatoid factor
  - Uric acid
  - Glucose
  - CBC with differential

Diagnostic Procedures/Other
Plantar pressure distribution analysis may help distinguish pressure distribution patterns due to malalignment.

TREATMENT

Treatment for metatarsalgia is typically conservative.
- Relieve pain.
- Ice initially
- Rest: temporary alteration of weight-bearing activity; use of cane or crutch. For more physically active patients, suggest an alternative exercise or cross-training:
  – Moist heat later
  – Taping or gel cast
  – Stiff-soled shoes will act as a splint.
  – Gastrocnemius stretching exercises
- Relieve the pressure beneath the area of maximal pain by redistributing the pressure load of the foot, which can be achieved by weight loss.

MEDICATION
Nonsteroidal anti-inflammatory medications for 7 to 14 days if no contraindications toward use

ISSUES FOR REFERRAL
High-level athletes may benefit from early podiatric or orthopedic evaluation.

ADDITIONAL THERAPIES
- Physical therapy to restore normal foot biomechanics
- Low-heeled (<2 cm height) wide-toe-box shoes
- Metatarsal bars, pads, and arch supports. Metatarsal bars are often more effective than pads.
- Orthotics/rocker bar (Prescriptive orthotics have been shown to be effective treatment.)
- Thick-soled shoes
- Shaving the callus may provide temporary relief. Callus excision is not recommended.
- Corticosteroid injection may benefit interdigital neuritis but should be used with caution because it may cause MTP instability and fat pad atrophy.
- Improve flexibility and strength of the intrinsic muscles of the foot with:
  – Exercises (e.g., towel grasps, pencil curls)
  – Physical therapy to maintain range of motion and restore normal biomechanics

SURGERY/OTHER PROCEDURES
- If no improvement with conservative therapy for 3 months, refer to foot/ankle orthopedic surgeon or podiatrist.
- Surgery may help correct anatomic abnormality: bunionectomy, partial osteotomy, or surgical fusion. Success rates vary depending on procedure.
- Direct plantar plate repair (grade II tear) combined with Weil osteotomy can restore normal alignment of the MTP joint, leading to diminished pain with improved functional scores.

- Callus removal is generally not recommended.
- Morton neurectomy and ultrasound-guided alcohol ablation of Morton neuroma are options (4)[C].
- Surgery only as a last resort if no anatomic abnormality is present.

COMPLEMENTARY & ALTERNATIVE MEDICINE
Magnetic insoles are not effective for chronic nonspecific foot pain.

ADMISSION, INPATIENT, AND NURSING CONSIDERATIONS
Patients generally admitted only for surgery

 ONGOING CARE

FOLLOW-UP RECOMMENDATIONS
Patient Monitoring
If stress fracture has been ruled out and patient's condition has not improved >3 months of conservative treatment, consider surgical evaluation.

PATIENT EDUCATION
- Instruct about wearing proper shoes and gradual return to activity.
- Cross-training until symptoms subside. Goal is to restore normal foot biomechanics, relieve abnormal pressure on the plantar metatarsal heads, and relieve pain (5)[C].

PROGNOSIS
Outcome depends on the severity of the problem and whether surgery is required to correct it.

COMPLICATIONS
- Back, knee, and hip pain due to change in gait
- Transfer metatarsalgia following surgical intervention, which subsequently transfers stress to other areas.

REFERENCES
1. Hockenbury RT. Forefoot problems in athletes. *Med Sci Sports Exerc*. 1999;31(Suppl 7):S448–S458.
2. DiPreta JA. Metatarsalgia, lesser toe deformities, and associated disorders of the forefoot. *Med Clin North Am*. 2014;98(2):233–251.
3. Besse, JL. Metatarsalgia. *Orthop Traumatol Surg Res*. 2017;103(Suppl 1):S29–S39.
4. Musson RE, Sawhney JS, Lamb L, et al. Ultrasound guided alcohol ablation of Morton's neuroma. *Foot Ankle Int*. 2012;33(3):196–201.
5. Espinosa N, Brodsky JW, Maceira E. Metatarsalgia. *J Am Acad Orthop Surg*. 2010;18(8):474–485.

ADDITIONAL READING
- Birbilis T, Theodoropoulou E, Koulalis D. Forefoot complaints—the Morton's metatarsalgia. The role of MR imaging. *Acta Medica (Hradec Kralove)*. 2007;50(3):221–222.
- Burns J, Landorf KB, Ryan MM, et al. Interventions for the prevention and treatment of pes cavus. *Cochrane Database Syst Rev*. 2007;(4):CD006154.
- Deshaies A, Roy P, Symeonidis PD, et al. Metatarsal bars more effective than metatarsal pads in reducing impulse on the second metatarsal head. *Foot (Edinb)*. 2011;21(4):172–175.
- Pace A, Scammell B, Dhar S. The outcome of Morton's neurectomy in the treatment of metatarsalgia. *Int Orthop*. 2010;34(4):511–515.
- Thomas JL, Blitch EL IV, Chaney DM, et al; and Clinical Practice Guideline Forefoot Disorders Panel. Diagnosis and treatment of forefoot disorders. Section 2. Central metatarsalgia. *J Foot Ankle Surg*. 2009;48(2):239–250.

 SEE ALSO

Morton Neuroma (Interdigital Neuroma)

 CODES

ICD10
- M77.40 Metatarsalgia, unspecified foot
- G57.60 Lesion of plantar nerve, unspecified lower limb
- M77.42 Metatarsalgia, left foot

CLINICAL PEARLS
- Metatarsalgia refers to pain of the plantar surface of the forefoot in the region of the metatarsal heads.
- Metatarsalgia is common in athletes who participate in high-impact sports involving the lower extremities.
- Patients describe as "walking with a pebble in the shoe." Pain is worse during midstance or propulsion phases of walking or running. The most common physical finding is point tenderness over the plantar metatarsal heads.
- Typical treatment is conservative, including rest and ice, activity modification, and ensuring proper padding under the foot.
- Pregnant patients should wear properly fitted, low-heeled shoes to reduce incidence of metatarsalgia.

M

METHICILLIN-RESISTANT *STAPHYLOCOCCUS AUREUS* (MRSA) SKIN INFECTIONS

Stephen A. Martin, MD, EdM • Paul P. Belliveau, PharmD

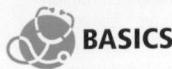

BASICS

DESCRIPTION

- Community-acquired methicillin-resistant *Staphylococcus aureus* (CA-MRSA) has unique properties that allow the organism to cause skin and soft tissue infections (SSTIs) in healthy hosts:
  - CA-MRSA has a different virulence and disease pattern than hospital-acquired MRSA (HA-MRSA).
- CA-MRSA infections impact patients who have not been recently (<1 year) hospitalized or had a medical procedure (e.g., dialysis, surgery, catheters).
- Incidence of CA-MRSA increased in the United States before plateauing between 2005 and 2010.
- CA-MRSA typically causes mild to moderate SSTIs (abscesses, furuncles, and carbuncles):
  - Severe or invasive CA-MRSA disease is less frequent but can include:
    o Necrotizing pneumonia with abscesses
    o Necrotizing fasciitis
    o Septic thrombophlebitis
    o Sepsis
    o Osteomyelitis
- Although less frequent, HA-MRSA can still cause SSTIs in the community.
- System(s) affected: skin, soft tissue

EPIDEMIOLOGY
- Predominant age: all ages, generally younger
- Predominant sex: female > male

Incidence
- 316/100,000/year (2004 to 2005)
- 46/100,000 per year pediatric MRSA SSTI hospitalizations
- The incidence of MRSA-related hospitalizations decreased from 2010 to 2014.
- The incidence of MRSA-related skin abscesses among people who inject drugs is increasing.

Prevalence
- Local epidemiology patterns vary.
- 25–30% of U.S. population colonized with *S. aureus*; up to 7% are colonized with MRSA.
- CA-MRSA isolated in ~60% of SSTIs presenting to emergency departments (range 15–74%)
- CA-MRSA accounts for up to 75% of all community staphylococcal infections in children.

ETIOLOGY AND PATHOPHYSIOLOGY
- First noted in 1980. Current epidemic began in 1999. The USA300 clone is predominant.
- CA-MRSA is distinguished from HA-MRSA by
  - Lack of a multidrug-resistant phenotype
  - Presence of exotoxin virulence factors
  - Type IV *Staphylococcus* cassette cartridge (contains the methicillin-resistant gene *mecA*)

RISK FACTORS
- ~50% of patients have no obvious risk factor.
- Antibiotic use in the past month
- Abscess
- Reported "spider bite"
- Intravenous (IV) drug use
- History of MRSA infection
- Close contact with a similar infection
- Children, particularly in daycare centers
- Competitive athlete
- Incarceration
- Hospitalization in the past 12 months

GENERAL PREVENTION
- Colonization (particularly of the anterior nares) is a risk factor for subsequent *S. aureus* infection. Not certain if similar for CA-MRSA. Oropharyngeal and inguinal colonization are equally prevalent.
- CA-MRSA transmitted easily through environmental and household contact
- Health care workers are a primary MRSA vector for hospitalized patients, reinforcing the need for meticulous cleaning of hands and medical equipment.
- Vaccine under development
- CDC guidance for prevention of MRSA in athletes: http://www.cdc.gov/mrsa/community/team-hc-providers/advice-for-athletes.html

COMMONLY ASSOCIATED CONDITIONS
Many patients are otherwise healthy.

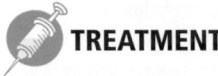

DIAGNOSIS

HISTORY
- Review risk factors.
- "Spider bite" is commonly confused with MRSA—patients often report an unclear history of spider bite.
- Prior MRSA skin infection
- Risk factors alone cannot rule in or rule out a CA-MRSA infection.

PHYSICAL EXAM
- Furuncles and/or carbuncles, sometimes with surrounding cellulitis. Nonsuppurative cellulitis is a less common presentation of CA-MRSA.
- Erythema, warmth, tenderness, swelling
- Fluctuance
- Folliculitis, pustular lesions
- Appearance like an insect or spider bite
- Tissue necrosis

DIFFERENTIAL DIAGNOSIS
SSTIs due to other organisms

DIAGNOSTIC TESTS & INTERPRETATION
Initial Tests (lab, imaging)
- Wound cultures establish definitive diagnosis. Guidelines recommend culture of a purulent lesion with systemic signs of illness or if the patient is immunocompromised (1)[B].
- Susceptibility testing; many labs use oxacillin instead of methicillin.

- "D-zone disk-diffusion test" evaluates for inducible clindamycin resistance if CA-MRSA is resistant to erythromycin.
- Ultrasound may help identify abscesses (2,3)[A].
- Look for fascial plane edema on CT or MRI if necrotizing fasciitis is suspected. DO NOT DELAY surgical intervention to obtain imaging in such cases.

Diagnostic Procedures/Other
Incision and drainage (I&D) purulent lesions; needle aspiration not recommended (1)

TREATMENT

- Use antibiotics that are active against MRSA for patients with carbuncles or abscesses if patients do not respond to initial antibiotic treatment, have markedly impaired host defenses, or present with systemic inflammatory response (SIRS) and hypotension (1).
- Extended antibiotic coverage for CA-MRSA not warranted for nonsuppurative cellulitis (4)[A]
- Routine elimination of MRSA colonization is not recommended in patients with active infection or their close contacts.
- Most CA-MRSA infections are localized SSTIs and do not require hospitalization or vancomycin.
- Base initial antibiotic coverage on local CA-MRSA prevalence and individual risk factors.
- http://www.cdc.gov/mrsa/pdf/Flowchart_pstr.pdf

GENERAL MEASURES
- Modify therapy based on culture and susceptibility.
- Determine if household/close contacts have SSTI.
- Treat underlying conditions (e.g., tinea pedis).
- Restrict contact (e.g., sports competition) if wound cannot be covered.
- Elevate affected area.

MEDICATION

ALERT
Consider surgical drainage, wound culture, and narrow-spectrum antimicrobials for purulent infections:

- I&D may have more impact than antibiotics in mild cases for both adults and children.
- Patients with an abscess are frequently cured by I&D alone. The addition of clindamycin or trimethoprim/sulfamethoxazole (TMP/SMX) for abscesses <5 cm results in modestly improved cure rates at 7 to 14 days (number needed to treat is 7 to 14) (5).
- Packing may not improve outcomes (3)[A].
- Moist heat may work for small furuncles.

First Line
Antibiotics for CA-MRSA SSTIs: 7- to 14-day course (depends on severity and clinical response):
- TMP/SMX: DS (160 mg TMP and 800 mg of SMX) 1 to 2 tablet(s) PO q12h; children, 8 to 12 mg/kg/day PO of trimethoprim component in 2 divided doses
- Doxycycline or minocycline: 100 mg PO q12h. Children, >8 years and <45 kg, 2 to 5 mg/kg/day PO in 1 to 2 divided doses, not to exceed 200 mg/day; >8 years and >45 kg, use adult dosing; taken with a full glass of water

- Clindamycin: 300 to 450 mg PO q6h. Children, 30 to 40 mg/kg/day PO in 3 divided doses. Taken with full glass of water. Check D-zone test in erythromycin-resistant, clindamycin-susceptible *S. aureus* isolates (a positive test indicates induced resistance—choose a different antibiotic).
- CA-MRSA is resistant to β-lactams (including oral cephalosporins and antistaphylococcal penicillins) and often macrolides, azalides, and quinolones.
- Although most CA-MRSA isolates are susceptible to rifampin, this drug should *never* be used as a single agent because of concerns regarding resistance. The role of combination therapy with rifampin in CA-MRSA SSTIs is not clearly defined.
- There has been increasing resistance to clindamycin, both initial (~33%) and induced.
- Although CA-MRSA isolates are susceptible to vancomycin, oral vancomycin cannot be used for CA-MRSA SSTIs due to limited absorption.

Second Line
Treat severe CA-MRSA SSTIs requiring hospitalization and HA-MRSA SSTIs using

- Vancomycin: Generally, 1 g IV q12h (30 mg/kg/day IV in 2 divided doses). Children: 40 mg/kg/day IV in 4 divided doses. Vancomycin-like antibiotics that require only 1 or 2 doses are also available (6)[A].
- Linezolid: 600 mg IV/PO q12h. Children, uncomplicated: <5 years of age, 30 mg/kg/day IV/PO in 3 divided doses; 5 to 11 years of age, 20 mg/kg/day IV/PO in 2 divided doses; >11 years, use adult dosing. Children, complicated: birth to 11 years, 30 mg/kg/day IV/PO in 3 divided doses; older, use adult dosing.
  - Linezolid seems to be more effective than vancomycin for treating people with SSTIs, but current studies have high risk of bias.
- Clindamycin: 600 mg IV q8h; children, 10 to 13 mg/kg/dose IV q6–8h up to 40 mg/kg/day
- Daptomycin: 4 mg/kg/day IV; children, 1 to <2 years, 10 mg/kg IV once daily; 2 to 6 years, 9 mg/kg IV once daily; 7 to 11 years, 7 mg/kg IV once daily; 12 to 17 years, 5 mg/kg IV once daily; ≥18 years, adult dosing
  - Do not use if pulmonary involvement.
- Ceftaroline: 600 mg IV q12h; children, 2 months to <2 years, 8 mg/kg IV q8h; ≥2 years to <18 years and ≤33 kg, 12 mg/kg IV q8h; ≥2 years to <18 years and >33 kg, 400 mg IV q8h OR 600 mg IV q12h; ≥18 years, adult dosing

Pediatric Considerations
- Tetracyclines not recommended for patients age <8 years for CA-MRSA (in contrast with their position as treatment of choice in tickborne rickettsial diseases)
- TMP/SMX not recommended for patients <2 months
- Daptomycin is not recommended in pediatric patients <1 year of age (risk of potential muscular, neuromuscular, and/or nervous system side effects).
- Daptomycin dosage adjustment for pediatric patients with renal impairment has not been established.
- Ceftaroline dosage adjustment for pediatric patients with CrCl <50 mL/min/1.73 m² has not been established.

Pregnancy Considerations
- Tetracyclines are contraindicated.
- TMP/SMX not recommended in 1st or 3rd trimester

Geriatric Considerations
A recent review notes no prospective trials in this age group and recommends use of general adult guidelines.

ISSUES FOR REFERRAL
Consider consultation with infectious disease if
- Refractory CA-MRSA infection
- Plan to attempt decolonization

SURGERY/OTHER PROCEDURES
Concern for serious SSTIs (including necrotizing fasciitis) mandates prompt surgical evaluation.

ADMISSION, INPATIENT, AND NURSING CONSIDERATIONS
- Consider admission if
  - Systemically ill
  - Comorbidities that may delay or complicate resolution of SSTI
  - Presence of SSTI complications (sepsis, necrotizing fasciitis) and comorbidities
  - Alternatives to inpatient admission include observation units and outpatient parenteral antimicrobial therapy (OPAT) in carefully selected cases.
- Nursing: contact precautions
- If admitted for IV therapy, assess the following before discharge:
  - Afebrile for 24 hours
  - Clinically improved
  - Able to take oral medication
  - Has adequate social support and is available for outpatient follow-up

 ## ONGOING CARE

FOLLOW-UP RECOMMENDATIONS
Patient Monitoring
For outpatients:
- Promptly return for care with systemic symptoms, worsening local symptoms, or failure to improve within 48 hours. Consider a follow-up within 48 hours of initial visit to assess response and review culture.

PATIENT EDUCATION
- Cover draining wounds with clean, dry bandages.
- Clean hands regularly with soap and water or alcohol-based gel; hot soapy shower daily
- Do not share items that may be contaminated (including razors or towels).
- Clean clothes, towels, and bed linens.
- National MRSA Education Initiative: https://www.cdc.gov/mrsa/
- A mixture of 1/4 cup household bleach diluted in 1 gallon of water can be used to clean potentially contaminated surfaces.

PROGNOSIS
In outpatients, improvement should occur within 48 hours.

COMPLICATIONS
- Necrotizing pneumonia or empyema (after an influenza-like illness)
- Necrotizing fasciitis
- Sepsis syndrome
- Pyomyositis and osteomyelitis
- Purpura fulminans
- Disseminated septic emboli
- Endocarditis

REFERENCES
1. Stevens DL, Bisno AL, Chambers HF, et al; for Infectious Diseases Society of America. Practice guidelines for the diagnosis and management of skin and soft tissue infections: 2014 update by the Infectious Diseases Society of America. *Clin Infect Dis*. 2014;59(2):e10–e52.
2. Mistry RD. Skin and soft tissue infections. *Pediatr Clin North Am*. 2013;60(5):1063–1082.
3. Singer AJ, Talan DA. Management of skin abscesses in the era of methicillin-resistant *Staphylococcus aureus*. *N Engl J Med*. 2014;370(11):1039–1047.
4. Shuman EK, Malani PN. Empirical MRSA coverage for nonpurulent cellulitis: swinging the pendulum away from routine use. *JAMA*. 2017;317(20):2070–2071.
5. Daum RS, Miller LG, Immergluck L, et al; for DMID 07-0051 Team. A placebo-controlled trial of antibiotics for smaller skin abscesses. *N Engl J Med*. 2017;376(26):2545–2555.
6. Chambers HF. Pharmacology and the treatment of complicated skin and skin-structure infections. *N Engl J Med*. 2014;370(23):2238–2239.

ADDITIONAL READING
- Bystritsky R, Chambers H. Cellulitis and soft tissue infections. *Ann Intern Med*. 2018;168(3): ITC17–ITC32.
- Fenster DB, Renny MH, Ng C, et al. Scratching the surface: a review of skin and soft tissue infections in children. *Curr Opin Pediatr*. 2015;27(3):303–307.
- Lee AS, de Lencastre H, Garau J, et al. Methicillin-resistant *Staphylococcus aureus*. *Nat Rev Dis Primers*. 2018;4:18033.
- Loewen K, Schreiber Y, Kirlew M, et al. Community-associated methicillin-resistant *Staphylococcus aureus* infection: literature review and clinical update. *Can Fam Physician*. 2017;63(7):512–520.
- Ramakrishnan K, Salinas RC, Agudelo Higuita NI. Skin and soft tissue infections. *Am Fam Physician*. 2015;92(6):474–483.

 ## CODES

ICD10
- A49.02 Methicillin resis staph infection, unsp site
- A41.02 Sepsis due to Methicillin resistant Staphylococcus aureus
- J15.212 Pneumonia due to Methicillin resistant Staphylococcus aureus

CLINICAL PEARLS
- Incise and drain abscesses and send purulent material for culture and sensitivity.
- Local susceptibility patterns of CA-MRSA dictate antibiotic treatment (http://www.cdc.gov/mrsa/pdf/Flowchart_pstr.pdf).
- CA-MRSA skin lesions are commonly misidentified as "spider bites."

M

MILD COGNITIVE IMPAIRMENT

Birju B. Patel, MD, FACP, AGSF • N. Wilson Holland, MD, FACP

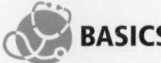

BASICS

DESCRIPTION
- Mild cognitive impairment (MCI) is defined as significant cognitive impairment in the absence of dementia, as measured by standard memory tests:
  – Concern regarding change in cognition
  – Preservation of independence in functional activities (ADLs)
  – Impairment in ≥1 cognitive domains (attention, executive dysfunction, memory, visuospatial, language)
  – Other terms used in the literature relating to MCI: isolated memory impairment; cognitive impairment not dementia (CIND); predementia; mild cognitive disorder; age-associated memory impairment; age-related cognitive decline; benign senescent forgetfulness. Some of these conditions do not progress to dementia (i.e., benign senescent forgetfulness, age-associated memory impairment, age-related cognitive decline). *DSM-5* mentions "mild neurocognitive disorder" (mNCD), which may be a precursor to Alzheimer disease and has many of the same features as MCI.
- Older adults with MCI are 3 times more likely to progress to dementia in 2 to 5 years than age matched cohorts (1)[A].

EPIDEMIOLOGY

Incidence
- Predominant sex: male > female
- Predominant age:
  – Higher in older persons and in those with less education
  – 12 to 15/1,000 person-years in those age ≥65 years
  – 54/1,000 person-years in those age ≥75 years

Prevalence
- MCI is more prevalent than dementia in the United States.
- 12–18% for those age ≥60 years (2)

ETIOLOGY AND PATHOPHYSIOLOGY
- Subtypes of MCI:
  – Single-domain amnestic
  – Multiple-domain amnestic
  – Nonamnestic single-domain
  – Nonamnestic multiple-domain
- The amnestic subtype is higher risk for progression to Alzheimer disease.
- Vascular, degenerative, traumatic, metabolic, psychiatric, or a combination

Genetics
Apolipoprotein (APO) E4 genotype: Various pathways exist leading to amyloid accumulation and deposition thought to be associated with dementia.

RISK FACTORS
- Age
- Diabetes
- Hypertension
- Hyperlipidemia
- Cerebrovascular disease
- Smoking
- Sleep apnea
- APO E4 genotype

COMMONLY ASSOCIATED CONDITIONS
See "Risk Factors."

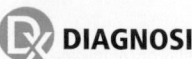

DIAGNOSIS

HISTORY
- Focus on cognitive deficits and impairment. MCI is meant to reflect a change in cognition and not lifelong impaired cognition.
- Review all medications that may affect cognition; give emphasis to anticholinergic medications (patients on these may mistakenly be classified as having MCI).
- Rule out depression. The prevalence of depression in patients with MCI is higher than age-matched cohorts.
- Assess function (ADLs, instrumental ADLs) and subtle changes in daily function (e.g., in the workplace).
- Impact on interpersonal relationships and caregiver stress
- Assess vascular risk factors (hypertension, diabetes, hyperlipidemia, and cerebrovascular disease).
- Assess behavioral changes.
- Olfactory dysfunction may be associated with amnestic MCI and progression to Alzheimer dementia. This can be easily evaluated in patients with memory impairment (3).

PHYSICAL EXAM
- A general exam focusing on clinical clues to identifying vascular disease (e.g., bruits, abnormal BP)
- Neurologic exam to rule out reversible CNS causes cognitive impairment or other causes of cognitive impairment (e.g., Parkinson disease).
- Office measures of cognitive function, depression, and functional status

DIFFERENTIAL DIAGNOSIS
- Delirium
- Dementia
- Depression
- "Reversible" cognitive impairment
  – Medications (anticholinergics and medications with anticholinergic properties)
  – Hypothyroidism
  – Vitamin B$_{12}$ deficiency

- Reversible CNS conditions
- Give consideration to sleep conditions, especially sleep apnea, that can contribute to cognitive deficits.

DIAGNOSTIC TESTS & INTERPRETATION

Initial Tests (lab, imaging)
- CBC
- Comprehensive metabolic profile
- Thyroid-stimulating hormone
- Vitamin B$_{12}$
- Lipids
- Consider HIV testing in the appropriate risk setting.
- Imaging tests are helpful when there are focal neurologic deficits or rapid or atypical presentations:
  – CT scan can detect structural CNS conditions leading to cognitive impairment:
    ○ Subdural hematoma
    ○ Normal pressure hydrocephalus
    ○ Metastatic disease
  – MRI further evaluates vascular, infectious, neoplastic, and inflammatory conditions.
- Cognitive testing is important (e.g., Montreal Cognitive Assessment [MoCA] and Saint Louis University Mental Status [SLUMS]); MoCA may be more sensitive for detecting and following MCI.
- Neuropsychological testing is recommended for all patients with MCI.
- Vascular risk factor reduction and treatment

Follow-Up Tests & Special Considerations
- Document progression of functional impairment, cognitive decline, concurrent depression, and comorbid conditions.
- Advanced planning while patient is competent
- Early education of caregivers on safety, maintaining structure, managing stress, and future planning
- Neuropsychological testing should be done at 1- to 2-year intervals depending on subjective concerns and ongoing diagnosis of MCI.

Test Interpretation
- Little is known about MCI pathology due to a lack of longitudinal studies.
- Alzheimer dementia pathophysiology:
  – Neurofibrillary tangles in hippocampus
  – Senile plaques (amyloid deposition)
  – Neuronal degeneration
- Those with MCI have intermediate amounts of pathologic findings of Alzheimer disease with amyloid deposition and neurofibrillary tangles in the mesial temporal lobes compared with those with dementia.
- Amnestic MCI is associated with white matter hyperintensity volume on MRI, whereas nonamnestic MCI is associated with infarcts.

TREATMENT

GENERAL MEASURES

Atherosclerotic risk factors should be treated aggressively.

MEDICATION

The use of cholinesterase inhibitors (ChEIs) in MCI is not associated with any delay in the onset of Alzheimer disease or dementia. Moreover, the safety profile showed that the risks associated with ChEIs are significant. Therefore, ChEIs are not routinely recommended (1)[B].

ISSUES FOR REFERRAL

Consider referral to a memory specialist (i.e., geriatrician, neurologist, geropsychiatrist, neuropsychologist) to evaluate and differentiate subtypes of MCI and specific cognitive deficits.

ADDITIONAL THERAPIES

There may be benefit in terms of improvement in performance on tests for global cognitive functioning with cognitive training and physical exercise.

COMPLEMENTARY & ALTERNATIVE MEDICINE

No evidence suggests the efficacy of vitamin E in the prevention or treatment of people with MCI. More research is needed to identify the role of vitamin E, if any, in the management of cognitive impairment.

- Long-term use of Ginkgo biloba extract has shown to have no benefit in the treatment of MCI and in terms of progression to dementia. In addition, Ginkgo biloba can be associated with increase in bleeding risk including CNS bleeds (4)[B].

ADMISSION, INPATIENT, AND NURSING CONSIDERATIONS

Delirium is more common in patients hospitalized with all forms of cognitive impairment.

- Avoid medications that may worsen or pre-cipitate cognitive decline (e.g., anticholinergics, antihistamines).
- Patients may be extremely sensitive to the hospital environment:
  - Moderate level of stimulation is best.
  - Avoid sensory deprivation. Make sure that patients have access to hearing aids and eyeglasses.
  - Use frequent cueing and have caregivers or family in the room whenever possible with patient.
  - Frequently orient patients to date and time.

ONGOING CARE

FOLLOW-UP RECOMMENDATIONS

Patients should be reevaluated every 6 to 12 months to determine if symptoms are progressing.

Patient Monitoring

Appropriate cognitive and functional testing should be used to evaluate progression, along with clinical history and exam. If a medication is started, patients need to be followed more frequently to evaluate for efficacy, side effects, dose titration, and so forth. Declining executive function may be an early marker to progression of MCI to dementia, and clinicians should monitor and advise patients and families pro-actively to look for this. Impairments in ADL function is a good clue to progression to dementia from MCI.

DIET

Diets that are promoted by the American Heart Association to minimize atherosclerotic risk factors should be emphasized.

PATIENT EDUCATION

- Encourage lifestyle changes:
  - Physical activity, such as walking 30 minutes daily on most days of the week
  - Mental activity that stimulates language skills and psychomotor coordination should be encour-aged. Computer activities, reading books, crafts, crossword puzzles, and games may be linked to decreased risk of development of MCI (5)[C].
- Cognitive rehabilitation strategies may be beneficial in helping with daily activities relating to memory tasks in MCI.
- Participation in exercise programs modestly improved some measures of cognition in some studies.
- Treatment of vascular risk factors (hypertension, diabetes, cerebrovascular disease, and hyperlipid-emia) is important in lowering risk of progression to dementia.

PROGNOSIS

- Older adults with MCI have 3 times higher risks of progression to dementia in 2 to 5 years.
- Amnestic subtypes of MCI are most likely to prog-ress to dementia.
- Neuropsychological testing measures, cerebrospinal fluid (CSF) biomarkers, and neuroimaging studies are being used in specialty settings to predict con-version to dementia. These are not widely available or cost-effective and are not used in general use.

REFERENCES

1. Petersen RC, Lopez O, Armstrong MJ, et al. Practice guideline update summary: mild cognitive impairment: report of the Guideline Development, Dissemination, and Implementation Subcommittee of the American Academy of Neurology. *Neurology*. 2018;90(3):126–135.
2. Petersen RC. Mild cognitive impairment. *Continuum (Minneap Minn)*. 2016;22(2 Dementia):404–418.
3. Roberts RO, Christianson TJ, Kremers WK, et al. Association between olfactory dysfunc-tion and amnestic mild cognitive impairment and Alzheimer disease dementia. *JAMA Neurol*. 2016;73(1):93–101.
4. Vellas B, Coley N, Ousset PJ, et al; for GuidAge Study Group. Long-term use of standardised Ginkgo biloba extract for the prevention of Alzheimer's disease (GuidAge): a randomised placebo-controlled trial. *Lancet Neurol*. 2012;11(10):851–859.
5. Marshall GA, Rentz DM, Frey MT, et al. Executive function and instrumental activities of daily living in mild cognitive impairment and Alzheimer's disease. *Alzheimers Dement*. 2011;7(3):300–308.

ADDITIONAL READING

Sanford AM. Mild cognitive impairment. *Clin Geriatr Med*. 2017;33(3):325–337.

CODES

ICD10

G31.84 Mild cognitive impairment, so stated

CLINICAL PEARLS

- Amnestic MCI affects primarily memory and is more likely to progress to Alzheimer dementia.
- Screen for reversible factors, particularly anticholin-ergic medications, depression, and sleep disorders.
- Look closely at vascular risk factors and modify them as best as possible.
- ChEIs should not be used routinely unless memory complaints are affecting quality of life in patients. Potential side effects of these medications should be thoroughly discussed with patients and their families. A baseline ECG should be done prior to initiation of ChEIs due to risk of bradycardia and syncope.
- Neuropsychological testing is recommended in indi-viduals suspected of having MCI. Patients with MCI and with prominent subjective complaints should have follow-up testing to evaluate for progression between 1 and 2 years after the initial assessment.
- Brain MRI should be performed in those with MCI to exclude structural disease and assess the extent of atrophy and vascular disease.

M

MISCARRIAGE (EARLY PREGNANCY LOSS)

Clara M. Keegan, MD

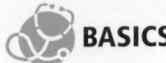 **BASICS**

DESCRIPTION
- Miscarriage, also known as spontaneous abortion (SAb), is the failure or loss of a pregnancy before 13 weeks' gestational age (WGA).
- Related terms
  - Anembryonic gestation: gestational sac on ultrasound (US) without visible embryo after 6 WGA
  - Complete abortion: entire contents of uterus expelled
  - Ectopic pregnancy: pregnancy outside the uterus
  - Embryonic or fetal demise: cervix closed; embryo or fetus present in the uterus without cardiac activity
  - Incomplete abortion: abortion with retained products of conception, generally placental tissue
  - Induced or therapeutic abortion: evacuation of uterine contents or products of conception medically or surgically
  - Inevitable abortion: cervical dilatation or rupture of membranes in the presence of vaginal bleeding
  - Recurrent abortion: ≥3 consecutive pregnancy losses at <15 WGA
  - Threatened abortion: vaginal bleeding in the 1st trimester of pregnancy
  - Septic abortion: a spontaneous or therapeutic abortion complicated by pelvic infection; common complication of illegally performed induced abortions
- Synonym(s): miscarriage; early pregnancy loss
  - Missed abortion and blighted ovum are used less frequently in favor of terms representing the sonographic diagnosis.

EPIDEMIOLOGY
Predominant age: increases with advancing age, especially >35 years; at age 40 years, the loss rate is twice that of age 20 years.

Incidence
- Threatened abortion (1st-trimester bleeding) occurs in 20–25% of clinical pregnancies.
- Between 10% and 15% of all clinically recognized pregnancies end in SAb, with 80% of these occurring within 12 weeks after last menstrual period (LMP) (1).
- When both clinical and biochemical (β-hCG detected) pregnancies are considered, about 30% of pregnancies end in SAb.
- One in four women will have a SAb during her lifetime (1).

ETIOLOGY AND PATHOPHYSIOLOGY
- Chromosomal anomalies (50% of cases)
- Congenital anomalies
- Trauma
- Maternal factors: uterine abnormalities, infection (toxoplasma, other viruses, rubella, cytomegalovirus, herpesvirus), maternal endocrine disorders, hypercoagulable state

Genetics
Approximately 50% of 1st-trimester SAbs have significant chromosomal anomalies, with 50% of these being autosomal trisomies and the remainder being triploidy, tetraploidy, or 45X monosomies.

RISK FACTORS
Most cases of SAb occur in patients without identifiable risk factors; however, risk factors include the following:
- Chromosomal abnormalities
- Advancing maternal age

652

- Uterine abnormalities
- Maternal chronic disease (antiphospholipid antibodies, uncontrolled diabetes mellitus, polycystic ovarian syndrome, obesity, hypertension, thyroid disease, renal disease)
- Other possible contributing factors include smoking, alcohol, cocaine use, infection, and luteal phase defect.

GENERAL PREVENTION
- Insufficient evidence supports the use of aspirin and/or other anticoagulants, bed rest, hCG, immunotherapy, progestogens, uterine muscle relaxants, or vitamins for general prevention of SAb before or after threatened abortion is diagnosed.
- By the time hemorrhage begins, half of pregnancies complicated by threatened abortion already have no fetal cardiac activity.
- Recurrent miscarriage: Women with a history of ≥3 prior SAbs may benefit from progestogens (OR 0.39, 95% CI 0.21–0.72) (2)[A].
- Antiphospholipid syndrome: The combination of unfractionated heparin and aspirin reduces risk of SAb in women with antiphospholipid antibodies and a history of recurrent abortion (RRR 46%, 95% CI 0.29–0.71).

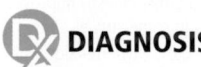 **DIAGNOSIS**

HISTORY
- The possibility of pregnancy should be considered in a reproductive-age woman who presents with nonmenstrual vaginal bleeding.
- Vaginal bleeding
  - Characteristics (amount, color, consistency, associated symptoms), onset (abrupt or gradual), duration, intensity/quantity, and exacerbating/precipitating factors
  - Document LMP if known: allows calculation of estimated gestational age
- Abdominal pain/uterine cramping as well as associated nausea/vomiting/syncope
- Rupture of membranes
- Passage of products of conception
- Prenatal course: toxic or infectious exposures, family or personal history of genetic abnormalities, past history of ectopic pregnancy or SAb, endocrine disease, autoimmune disorder, bleeding/clotting disorder

PHYSICAL EXAM
- Orthostatic vital signs to estimate hemodynamic stability
- Abdominal exam for tenderness, guarding, rebound, bowel sounds (peritoneal signs more likely with ectopic pregnancy)
- Speculum exam for visual assessment of cervical dilation, blood, and products of conception (confirms diagnosis of SAb)
- Bimanual exam to assess for uterine size–dates discrepancy and adnexal tenderness or mass

DIFFERENTIAL DIAGNOSIS
- Ectopic pregnancy: potentially life-threatening; must be considered in any woman of childbearing age with abdominal pain and vaginal bleeding
- Physiologic bleeding in normal pregnancy (implantation bleeding)
- Subchorionic bleeding
- Cervical polyps, neoplasia, and/or inflammatory conditions

- Hydatidiform mole pregnancy
- hCG-secreting ovarian tumor

DIAGNOSTIC TESTS & INTERPRETATION
Initial Tests (lab, imaging)
- Quantitative hCG
  - Particularly useful if intrauterine pregnancy (IUP) has not been documented by US
  - Serial quantitative serum hCG measurements can assess viability of the pregnancy. Serum hCG should rise at least 53% every 48 hours through 7 weeks after LMP. An inappropriate rise, plateau, or decrease of hCG suggests abnormal IUP or possible ectopic pregnancy.
- Complete blood count (CBC) with differential
- Rh type
- Cultures: gonorrhea/chlamydia
- US exam to evaluate fetal viability and to rule out ectopic pregnancy (3)[A]
  - hCG >2,000 mIU/mL necessary to detect IUP via transvaginal US (TVUS), >5,500 mIU/mL for abdominal US
  - TVUS criteria for nonviable intrauterine gestation: 7-mm fetal pole without cardiac activity or 25-mm gestational sac without a fetal pole, IUP with no growth over 1 week, or previously seen IUP no longer visible
  - Structures and timing: with TVUS, gestational sac of 2 to 3 mm generally seen around 5 WGA; yolk sac by 5.5 WGA; fetal pole with cardiac activity by 6 WGA

Follow-Up Tests & Special Considerations
- In the case of vaginal bleeding with no documented IUP and hCG <2,000 mIU/mL, follow serum hCG levels weekly to zero.
- If levels plateau, consider ectopic pregnancy or retained products of conception. If levels are very high, consider gestational trophoblastic disease.
- If initial hCG level does not permit documentation of IUP by TVUS, follow serum hCG in 48 hours to document appropriate rise.
- Repeat US once hCG is at a level commensurate with visualization on US (see above).
- Provide patient with ectopic precautions in interim: worsening abdominal pain, dizziness/syncope, nausea/vomiting.
- In a pregnancy of unknown location with hCG rise <53% in 48 hours, offer methotrexate for treatment of presumed ectopic pregnancy.

Diagnostic Procedures/Other
- Fetal heart tones can be auscultated with Doppler starting between 10 and 12 WGA in a viable pregnancy.
- In threatened abortion, fetal cardiac activity at 7 to 11 WGA is 90–96% predictive of continued pregnancy (1).

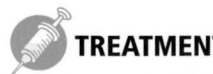 **TREATMENT**

GENERAL MEASURES
- Discuss contraception plan at the time of diagnosis of SAb, as ovulation can occur prior to resumption of normal menses.
- Expectant management ("watchful waiting") is 90% effective for incomplete abortion, although it may take several weeks for the process to be complete (1)[A]. This approach is only recommended in the 1st trimester and is more effective in women with symptoms of impending pregnancy loss (4)[C].

MEDICATION

- Rates of complete miscarriage and of need for surgical evacuation are equivalent with expectant management and medication (5)[A].
- Long-term conception rate and pregnancy outcomes are similar for women who undergo expectant management, medical treatment, or surgical evacuation.
- Infection rates are lower with medical versus surgical management.

First Line

- Misoprostol: most common agent for inducing passage of tissue in incomplete abortion or embryonic demise
  - Off-label use; has not been submitted to the FDA for consideration for use in treatment of early pregnancy failure; recognized by the World Health Organization (WHO) as a life-saving medication for this indication
  - Efficacy: complete expulsion of products of conception in 71% by day 3, 84% by day 8
  - Efficacy depends on route of administration, gestational age of pregnancy, and dose.
  - Recommended dose is 800 μg vaginally; alternate regimens include the WHO regimen of 600 μg sublingually q3h for up to 3 doses; multidose regimens and oral dosing (including buccal and sublingual) may result in increased side effects.
- Common adverse effects include abdominal pain/cramping, nausea, and diarrhea. Pain increases at higher doses but is manageable with oral analgesia.
- Recommended for stable patients who decline surgery but do not want to wait for spontaneous passage of products of conception

Second Line

- Rh-negative patients should be given Rh immunoglobulin (RhoGAM) 50 μg IM following a SAb.
- Women with evidence of anemia should receive iron supplementation.

ISSUES FOR REFERRAL

Patients should be monitored for up to 1 year for the development of pathologic grief. There is insufficient evidence to support counseling to prevent development of anxiety or depression related to grief following SAb.

SURGERY/OTHER PROCEDURES

- Uterine aspiration (suction dilation and curettage [D&C] or manual uterine aspiration [MUA]), also known as manual vacuum aspiration (MVA), is the conventional treatment.
- Indications: septic abortion, heavy bleeding, hypotension, persistent IUP after medical or expectant management, patient choice
- Risks (all rare): anesthesia (usually local), uterine perforation, intrauterine adhesions, cervical trauma, infection that may lead to infertility or increased risk of ectopic pregnancy
- When compared with expectant management, surgical intervention leads to fewer days of vaginal bleeding, with a lower risk of incomplete abortion and heavy bleeding and a similar risk of infection (6)[A].
- Vacuum aspiration (manual or electric) is considered preferable to sharp curettage because aspiration is less painful, takes less time, involves less blood loss, and does not require general anesthesia. The WHO supports use of suction curettage over rigid metal curettage.
- Although data from induced abortions suggest that antibiotic prophylaxis with doxycycline 100 mg BID reduces the already rare risk of postprocedure infection, data are insufficient to support use of antibiotics after aspiration for SAb.

COMPLEMENTARY & ALTERNATIVE MEDICINE

A systematic review of Chinese herbal medicine alone and in conjunction with Western medicine showed benefit over Western medicine alone in achieving continued viability at 28 weeks (number needed to treat [NNT] = 4.8 pregnancies with combined therapy). However, the available studies did not meet international standards for reporting quality.

ADMISSION, INPATIENT, AND NURSING CONSIDERATIONS

- If the patient has orthostatic vital signs, initiate resuscitation with IV fluids and/or blood products, if needed.
- Hemodynamically unstable patients may require IV fluids and/or blood products to maintain BP.

 ONGOING CARE

FOLLOW-UP RECOMMENDATIONS

All patients should be offered follow-up in 2 to 6 weeks to monitor for resolution of bleeding, return of menses, and symptoms related to grief as well as to review the contraception plan.

Patient Monitoring

- If SAb occurs in setting of previously documented IUP and abortion is completed with resumption of normal menses, it is not necessary to check or follow serum hCG to 0.
- After medical management, confirm complete expulsion with US or serial serum β-hCG (4)[C].
- If pregnancy is not immediately desired, offer effective contraception. Immediate insertion of an intrauterine device is both acceptable and safe.
- If pregnancy is desired, provide preconception counseling. There is no evidence that it is necessary to wait a certain number of cycles before attempting conception again.

DIET

NPO if patient is to undergo D&C under general anesthesia

PATIENT EDUCATION

- Pelvic rest for 1 week after D&C or MVA
- Advise patients to call with excessive bleeding (soaking two pads per hour for 2 hours), fever, pelvic pain, or malaise, which could indicate retained products of conception or endometritis.
- A patient fact sheet on miscarriage is available through the American Academy of Family Physicians at http://www.aafp.org/afp/2011/0701/p85.html.

PROGNOSIS

- Prognosis is excellent once bleeding is controlled.
- Recurrent miscarriage: Prognosis depends on etiology; up to 70% rate of success with subsequent pregnancy

COMPLICATIONS

- D&C or MVA: uterine perforation, bleeding, adhesions, cervical trauma, and infection that may lead to infertility or increased risk of ectopic pregnancy. Bleeding and adhesions more common with D&C than with MUA; all complications rare
- Retained products of conception

REFERENCES

1. Prine LW, MacNaughton H. Office management of early pregnancy loss. *Am Fam Physician*. 2011;84(1):75–82.
2. Haas DM, Ramsey PS. Progestogen for preventing miscarriage. *Cochrane Database Syst Rev*. 2013;(10):CD003511.
3. Doubilet PM, Benson CB, Bourne T, et al; for Society of Radiologists in Ultrasound Multispecialty Panel on Early First Trimester Diagnosis of Miscarriage and Exclusion of a Viable Intrauterine Pregnancy. Diagnostic criteria for nonviable pregnancy early in the first trimester. *N Engl J Med*. 2013;369(15):1443–1451.
4. Committee on Practice Bulletins—Gynecology. The American College of Obstetricians and Gynecologists Practice Bulletin No. 150. Early pregnancy loss. *Obstet Gynecol*. 2015;125(5):1258–1267.
5. Kim C, Barnard S, Neilson JP, et al. Medical treatments for incomplete miscarriage. *Cochrane Database Syst Rev*. 2017;(1):CD007223.
6. Nanda K, Lopez LM, Grimes DA, et al. Expectant care versus surgical treatment for miscarriage. *Cochrane Database Syst Rev*. 2012;(3):CD003518.

ADDITIONAL READING

- Empson M, Lassere M, Craig J, et al. Prevention of recurrent miscarriage for women with antiphospholipid antibody or lupus anticoagulant. *Cochrane Database Syst Rev*. 2005;(2):CD002859.
- Li L, Dou L, Leung PC, et al. Chinese herbal medicines for threatened miscarriage. *Cochrane Database Syst Rev*. 2012;(5):CD008510.
- May W, Gülmezoglu AM, Ba-Thike K. Antibiotics for incomplete abortion. *Cochrane Database Syst Rev*. 2007;(4):CD001779.

 SEE ALSO

- Ectopic Pregnancy
- Algorithm: Recurrent Pregnancy Loss

 CODES

ICD10

- O03.9 Complete or unspecified spontaneous abortion without complication
- O03.4 Incomplete spontaneous abortion without complication
- O02.1 Missed abortion

CLINICAL PEARLS

- Any pregnant woman with abdominal pain and/or vaginal bleeding must be evaluated to rule out ectopic pregnancy, which is potentially life threatening.
- As all options have similar long-term outcomes, patient preference should determine whether management is expectant, medical, or surgical.

M

MITRAL REGURGITATION

Yongkasem Vorasettakarnkij, MD, MSc

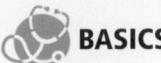 **BASICS**

DESCRIPTION

- Disorder of mitral valve (MV) closure, either primary or secondary (functional), resulting in a backflow of the left ventricular (LV) stroke volume into the left atrium (LA); uncompensated, this leads to LV and LA enlargement, elevated pulmonary pressures, atrial fibrillation, heart failure (HF), and sudden cardiac death.
- Types of mitral regurgitation (MR):
  - Acute versus chronic
  - Primary versus secondary (functional)
    - Primary: abnormalities at any level of the MV structures (annulus, leaflets, chordae tendineae, and papillary muscles)
    - Secondary: No valvular abnormalities are found. The abnormal and dilated LV causes papillary muscle displacement, resulting in leaflet tethering with annular dilatation that prevents coaptation.
- System(s) affected: cardiac; pulmonary

EPIDEMIOLOGY
Moderate to severe MR affects 2.5 million people in the United States (2000 data). It is the most common valvular disease and is expected to double by 2030 (1).

Prevalence
- By severity on echocardiography:
  - Mild MR: 19% (up to 40% if trivial jets included)
  - Moderate MR: 1.9%
  - Severe MR: 0.2%
- By category (1)
  - Degenerative (myxomatous disease, annular calcification): 60–70%
  - Ischemic: 20%
  - Endocarditis: 2–5%
  - Rheumatic: 2–5%

ETIOLOGY AND PATHOPHYSIOLOGY
- Acute MR
  - Leaflet perforation: infective endocarditis, trauma
  - Chordae tendineae rupture: trauma, spontaneous rupture, infective endocarditis, or rheumatic fever
  - Papillary muscle rupture or dysfunction: acute myocardial infarction (MI), severe myocardial ischemia, or trauma
- Chronic MR
  - Primary
    - Degenerative: mitral annular calcification, MV prolapse (MVP)
    - Infective endocarditis
    - Rheumatic heart disease (RHD)
    - Inflammatory diseases: lupus, eosinophilic endocardial disease
    - Anorectic drugs
    - Congenital (cleft leaflet)
  - Secondary (functional)
    - Ischemic: coronary artery disease (CAD)/MI
    - Nonischemic: cardiomyopathy from any cause, annular dilatation from chronic atrial fibrillation, dyssynchrony from right ventricular pacing
- Acute MR: Acute MV damage leads to sudden LA and LV volume overload. Sudden rise in LV volume load without LV remodeling results in impaired forward cardiac output and possible cardiogenic shock.
- Chronic MR: LV eccentric hypertrophy compensates for increased regurgitant volume to maintain forward cardiac output and alleviate pulmonary congestion. However, LV remodeling can result in LV dysfunction. LA compensatory dilatation for the larger regurgitant volume predisposes patients to develop AF.

- Ischemic MR: papillary muscle rupture, ischemia during acute MI, and incomplete coaptation of leaflets or restricted valve movement from chronic ischemia

RISK FACTORS
Age, hypertension, RHD, endocarditis, anorectic drugs

GENERAL PREVENTION
- Risk factor modification for CAD
- Antibiotic prophylaxis for poststreptococcal RHD
- Endocarditis prophylaxis is no longer recommended.

COMMONLY ASSOCIATED CONDITIONS
MVP with MR common in Marfan syndrome

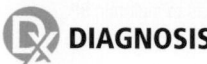 **DIAGNOSIS**

HISTORY
- Associated conditions: RHD, prior MI, connective tissue disorder
- Acute MR
  - Sudden onset of dyspnea
  - Orthopnea, paroxysmal nocturnal dyspnea
- Chronic MR
  - Exertional dyspnea, fatigue
  - Palpitation: paroxysmal/persistent AF

PHYSICAL EXAM
- Acute MR
  - Rapid and thready pulses
  - Signs of poor tissue perfusion with peripheral vasoconstriction
  - Hyperdynamic precordium without apical shift
  - S_3 and S_4 (if in sinus rhythm)
  - Systolic murmur at left sternal border and base
    - Early, middle, or holosystolic murmur
    - Often soft, low-pitched decrescendo murmur
  - Rales
- Chronic MR
  - Brisk upstroke of arterial pulse
  - Leftward displaced LV apical impulse
  - Systolic thrill at the apex (suggests severe MR)
  - Soft S_1 and widely split S_2, S_3 gallop
  - Loud P_2 (if pulmonary hypertension)
  - Holosystolic murmur at apex that radiates to axilla or to left parasternal boarder
  - Ankle edema, jugular venous distension, and ascites, if development of right-sided HF

DIFFERENTIAL DIAGNOSIS
- Aortic stenosis (AS): usually midsystolic but can be long; difficult to distinguish from holosystolic, at apical area, and radiating to the carotid arteries (unlike MR)
- Tricuspid regurgitation: holosystolic but at left lower sternal border, does not radiate to axilla, and may increase in intensity with inspiration (unlike MR)
- Ventricular septal defect (VSD): harsh holosystolic murmur at lower left sternal border but radiates to right sternal border (not axilla)

DIAGNOSTIC TESTS & INTERPRETATION
- Chest x-ray (CXR)
  - Acute MR: pulmonary edema, normal heart size
  - Chronic MR: LA and LV enlargement
- ECG
  - Acute MR: varies depending on etiologies (e.g., AMI)
  - Chronic MR
    - P mitrale from LA enlargement, AF
    - LV hypertrophy
    - Q waves from prior MI

Initial Tests (lab, imaging)
- Cardiac enzymes brain natriuretic peptide, if appropriate
- Transthoracic echocardiogram (TTE)
  - Indications for TTE (2)
    - Baseline evaluation of LV size and function, right ventricular function and LA size, pulmonary artery pressure, and severity of MR
    - Delineation of mechanism of MR
    - Surveillance of asymptomatic moderate to severe LV dysfunction (ejection fraction [EF] and end-systolic dimension [ESD])
    - Evaluate MV apparatus and LV size and function after a change in sign/symptom in MR patient.
    - Evaluate after MV repair or replacement.
  - Findings in acute MR
    - Evidence of etiology: flail leaflet or vegetations
    - Normal LA and LV size
  - Findings in chronic MR
    - Evidence of degenerative, rheumatic, ischemic, congenital, and other causes
    - Enlarged LA and LV

Follow-Up Tests & Special Considerations
- Intervals for follow-up TTE: See "Follow-Up Recommendations."
- Cardiovascular magnetic resonance (CMR):
  - TTE results are not satisfactory to assess LV and RV volumes, function, or MR severity (2)[B].
- Transesophageal echocardiogram (TEE)
  - Intraoperatively to define the anatomic basis of MR and to guide repair (2)[B]
  - Nondiagnostic information about severity, mechanism of MR, and/or status of LV function from noninvasive imaging (2)[C]
- Exercise hemodynamics with either Doppler echocardiography or cardiac catheterization (2)[B].
  - Discrepancy between symptoms and the severity of MR from resting TTE in symptomatic patients with chronic primary MR
- Exercise treadmill testing (2)[C]
  - To establish symptom status and exercise tolerance in asymptomatic patients with chronic primary MR
- Noninvasive imaging (stress nuclear/position emission tomography, CMR, stress echocardiography, cardiac CT angiography)
  - To establish etiology of chronic secondary MR and/or to assess myocardial viability (2)[C]

Diagnostic Procedures/Other
Cardiac catheterization (2)[C]

- Left ventriculography and hemodynamic measurement
  - Noninvasive tests are inconclusive regarding severity of MR, LV function, and the need for surgery.
- Coronary angiography: prior to MV surgery in patients at risk for CAD

Test Interpretation
Quantification of severe MR requires integration of the following structural parameters:

- LA size: dilated, unless acute
- LV size: dilated, unless acute
- Leaflets: abnormal
- Doppler parameters
- Quantitative parameter

TREATMENT

MEDICATION

- Acute, severe MR
  - Medical therapy has a limited role and is aimed to stabilize hemodynamics preoperatively.
  - Vasodilators (nitroprusside, nicardipine): to improve hemodynamic compensation but is often limited by systemic hypotension (2,3)[C]
- Chronic MR
  - Primary
    - Asymptomatic: no proven long-term medical therapy
    - Symptomatic: diuretics, β-blockers, angiotensin-converting enzyme inhibitors (ACE-I) or angiotensin receptor blockers (ARBs), and possibly aldosterone antagonists as indicated in standard therapy for HF (2)[B],(3)[C]
  - Secondary: LV dysfunction or symptomatic (stages B to D)
    - ACE-I or ARBs, β-blockers, and/or aldosterone antagonists as indicated in standard therapy for HF (2)[B],(3)[C]

SURGERY/OTHER PROCEDURES

- Isolated MV surgery is not indicated for patients with mild to moderate MR.
- Acute, severe MR secondary to acute MI
  - Acute rupture of papillary muscle: emergency MV repair/replacement
  - Papillary muscle displacement
    - Aggressive medical stabilization and intra-aortic balloon pump
    - Valve surgery usually required in addition to revascularization
- Chronic severe MR
  - Severe primary MR (2,3,4)
    - MV surgery
      - Symptomatic patients (stage D)
        □ Absence of severe LV dysfunction (EF >30%) (2,3)[B]
        □ May be considered if presence of severe LV dysfunction (EF ≤30%) (2,3)[C]
      - Asymptomatic patients
        □ Mild/moderate LV dysfunction (EF 30–60% and/or ESD ≥40 mm, stage C2) (2)[B]
        □ MV repair is reasonable for asymptomatic patients (stage C1) with preserved LV function (EF >60% and ESD <40 mm):
          • The likelihood of a successful and durable repair without residual MR is >95% and expected mortality <1% when performed at a heart valve center of excellence (2)[B].
      - Progressive increase in LV size or decrease in EF on serial imaging studies (4)[B]
      - Nonrheumatic MR with new onset of AF or resting pulmonary hypertension (pulmonary artery systolic pressure >50 mm Hg) and the likelihood of a successful and durable repair is high (2,3)[B].
    - MV repair is recommended over MV replacement in patients with
      - MR limited to the posterior leaflet (2)[B]
      - MR involving the anterior leaflet or both leaflets when a successful and durable repair can be accomplished (2)[B]
    - Transcatheter MV repair:
      - May be considered for severely symptomatic patients (NYHA class III/IV) despite optimal GDMT for HF, who have a favorable anatomy for the repair, and a reasonable life expectancy but a prohibitive surgical risk from severe comorbidities (2)[B].

  - Severe secondary MR (2,3,4)
    - MV surgery
      - Undergoing coronary artery bypass graft (CABG) (2,3)[C]
      - Undergoing aortic valve replacement (2)[C]
      - May be considered for severely symptomatic patients (NYHA classes III and IV) despite optimal GDMT for HF (2)[B],(3)[C]
      - Chordal-sparing MVR is preferred over downsized annuloplasty repair in ischemic MR patients (4)[B].
    - Cardiac resynchronization therapy is recommended for symptomatic patients (stages B to D) who meet the indications for device therapy (2)[C].

Geriatric Considerations

- Medical therapy alone for patients >75 years of age with MR is preferred, owing to increased operative mortality and decreased survival (compared with those with AS), especially with preexisting CAD or need for MV replacement.
- MV repair is preferable than MV replacement.

ADMISSION, INPATIENT, AND NURSING CONSIDERATIONS

Acute MR: Stabilize airway, breathing, circulation (ABCs). Initiate IV, O₂, and monitoring. Nitroprusside (plus dobutamine and/or aortic balloon counterpulsation if hypotensive). Treat underlying causes (e.g., MI). Treat acute pulmonary edema with furosemide and morphine. Obtain urgent surgical consultation.

 ONGOING CARE

FOLLOW-UP RECOMMENDATIONS

Chronic MR: asymptomatic

- Mild MR with normal LV size and function and no pulmonary hypertension: annual clinical evaluation and TTE every 3 to 5 years
- Moderate MR: annual clinical evaluation and TTE every 1 to 2 years
- Severe MR: clinical evaluation, TTE every 6 to 12 months
- Consider serial CXRs and ECGs, and consider stress test if exercise capacity is doubtful.

PATIENT EDUCATION

- Exercise after MV repair: Avoid sports with risk for bodily contact or trauma. Low-intensity competitive sports are allowed.
- Competitive athletes with MR
  - Asymptomatic with normal LV size and function, normal pulmonary artery pressures, and sinus rhythm: no restrictions
  - Mildly symptomatic and those with LV dilatation: activities with low to moderate dynamic and static cardiac demand allowed
- AF and anticoagulation: no contact sports

PROGNOSIS

- Acute, severe MR: Mortality risk with surgery is 50%; mortality risk with medical therapy alone is 75% in first 24 hours and 95% at 2 weeks.
- Chronic MR: asymptomatic severe MR with normal LVEF: 10% yearly rate of progression to symptoms and subnormal resting LVEF. Symptomatic severe MR: 8-year survival rate, 33% without surgery; mortality rate, 5% yearly

Pregnancy Considerations

MR with NYHA functional classes III and IV at high risk for maternal and/or fetal risk

COMPLICATIONS

Acute pulmonary edema, CHF, AF, bleeding risk with anticoagulation, endocarditis, sudden cardiac death

REFERENCES

1. Enriquez-Sarano M, Akins CW, Vahanian A. Mitral regurgitation. *Lancet*. 2009;373(9672):1382–1394.
2. Nishimura RA, Otto CM, Bonow RO, et al. 2014 AHA/ACC guideline for the management of patients with valvular heart disease: a report of the American College of Cardiology/American Heart Association Task Force on Practice Guidelines. *Circulation*. 2014;129(23):e521–e643.
3. Baumgartner H, Falk V, Bax JJ, et al; for European Society of Cardiology Scientific Document Group. 2017 ESC/EACTS Guidelines for the management of valvular heart disease. *Eur Heart J*. 2017;38(36):2739–2791.
4. Nishimura RA, Otto CM, Bonow RO, et al. 2017 AHA/ACC focused update of the 2014 AHA/ACC guideline for the management of patients with valvular heart disease: a report of the American College of Cardiology/American Heart Association Task Force on clinical practice guidelines. *Circulation*. 2017;135(25):e1159–e1195.

ADDITIONAL READING

- Acker MA, Parides MK, Perrault LP, et al; for Cardiothoracic Surgical Trials Network. Mitral-valve repair versus replacement for severe ischemic mitral regurgitation. *N Engl J Med*. 2014;370(1):23–32.
- El Sabbagh A, Reddy YNV, Nishimura RA. Mitral valve regurgitation in the contemporary era: insights into diagnosis, management, and future directions. *JACC Cardiovasc Imaging*. 2018;11(4):628–643.
- Michler RE, Smith PK, Parides MK, et al; for Cardiothoracic Surgical Trials Network. Two-year outcomes of surgical treatment of moderate ischemic mitral regurgitation. *N Engl J Med*. 2016;374(20):1932–1941.
- Yancy CW, Jessup M, Bozkurt B, et al. 2017 ACC/AHA/HFSA focused update of the 2013 ACCF/AHA guideline for the management of heart failure: a report of the American College of Cardiology/American Heart Association Task Force on Clinical Practice Guidelines and the Heart Failure Society of America. *Circulation*. 2017;136(6):e137–e161.

 CODES

ICD10

- I34.0 Nonrheumatic mitral (valve) insufficiency
- I05.1 Rheumatic mitral insufficiency
- Q23.3 Congenital mitral insufficiency

CLINICAL PEARLS

- Follow-up for mild to moderate MR: serial exam and/or echo (mild, every 3 to 5 years, moderate 1 to 2 years) unless LV structural changes
- Severe MR is usually managed with MV repair.
- Endocarditis prophylaxis is not recommended.

M

MITRAL STENOSIS

Gene Pershwitz, MD • Harish C. Devineni, MD

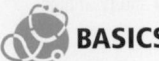 **BASICS**

DESCRIPTION
- The mitral apparatus is made up of the apparatus, anterior and posterior leaflets which are attached to the anterolateral and posteromedial papillary muscles via the chordae.
- Mitral stenosis (MS) is the narrowing of the valve area causing obstruction of the left ventricular inflow, resulting in increased left atrial pressures and consequent elevation of pulmonary venous and atrial pressures.
- Normal valve orifice 4 to 5 cm^2; symptoms typically seen when orifice is <2.5 cm^2 (1)
- Staging of the disease is used to guide appropriate treatment regimen. Stages vary from A (with risk factors), B (hemodynamically obstruction), C (severe but no symptoms), to D (symptomatic) (1).
- The most common etiology for MS is rheumatic heart disease (RHD), and MS is the most common valvular disease secondary to RHD.
- Other etiologies will be discussed below.

EPIDEMIOLOGY
- Globally, the prevalence of RHD is 30 million. Approximately 470,000 new cases are reported and 233,000 deaths are attributed to RHD yearly (2).
- Predominant age: Symptoms primarily occur in 3rd to 4th decades. Predominant sex: female > male (3:1)

Incidence
Incidence of rheumatic disease in the continental United States remains low. Annual incidence of acute rheumatic fever in the continental United States is unknown, because it is no longer nationally reportable, but is higher in Hawaii and American Samoa. Global burden remains significant (3).

ETIOLOGY AND PATHOPHYSIOLOGY
- Narrowing of the valve orifice leads to obstruction of blood flow between LA and LV. This impairs LV filling during diastole and causes increased LA pressure.
- Increased LA pressure is transmitted passively ("back pressure") to the pulmonary circulation causing pulmonary hypertension (HTN) and pulmonary congestion over time.
- Chronic LA pressure overload results in atrial dilation and fibrosis, resulting in atrial fibrillation.
- Rheumatic fever: most common (see "Risk Factors")
- Pathognomonic commissural fusion, leaflet thickening, and "fish mouth appearance" seen with RHD
- Aging (extension of mitral annular calcification)
- Rare causes: congenital (associated with mucopolysaccharidoses), autoimmune: systemic lupus erythematosus (SLE), rheumatoid arthritis, malignant carcinoid, Whipple disease, methysergide therapy, and other acquired: LA myxoma, LA thrombus, endomyocardial fibrosis

RISK FACTORS
- Rheumatic fever is the greatest risk factor.
  - 30–40% of rheumatic fever patients eventually develop MS, presenting 20 years after diagnosis of rheumatic fever.
  - Acute rheumatic fever occurs 2 to 3 weeks after an episode of untreated pharyngitis caused by rheumatogenic group A streptococci (GAS) organism in a genetically susceptible host.
  - Recurrent infections can accelerate the progression of the disease.
  - Low socioeconomic status (i.e., crowded conditions) favors the spread of streptococcal infection.
- Aging (increasing valvular calcification)
- Chest irradiation (increasing tissue fibrosis)

GENERAL PREVENTION
- Prompt recognition and treatment of GAS infection in at-risk populations; recognition of cardinal signs and symptoms of acute rheumatic fever via Jones criteria
- Ultrasound-based screening has been shown to increase diagnosis of RHD in asymptomatic patients residing in areas of high prevalence.

COMMONLY ASSOCIATED CONDITIONS
- Atrial fibrillation (30–40% of symptomatic patients)
- Associated valve lesions due to chronic inflammation (aortic stenosis, aortic insufficiency)
- Pulmonary HTN and right heart failure
- Systemic embolism, stroke, pulmonary embolism (10%)
- Infection, including infectious endocarditis (1–5%)
- Chronic rheumatic myocarditis

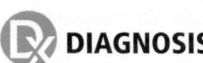 **DIAGNOSIS**

HISTORY
- History of rheumatic fever
- Severity depends on valve area; most early cases will be asymptomatic.
- Mean age of symptom onset in rheumatic valvular disease is in the late 30s to 40s. Latent period 20 to 40 years after infection. Rapid progression can be seen in some high prevalence areas.
- Presenting features usually include dyspnea on exertion, decrease exercise tolerance, chest pain, embolic events, palpitations, hoarseness, hemoptysis, fatigue, paroxysmal nocturnal dyspnea, atrial fibrillation, and embolic events.
- In advanced disease, symptoms of pulmonary HTN and right heart failure predominate: jugular venous distention, hepatomegaly, ascites, and peripheral edema.
- Other presentations: hemoptysis (due to pulmonary vein rupture and bronchial circulation causing intra-parenchymal hemorrhage), hoarseness (compression of recurrent laryngeal nerve by enlarged pulmonary artery or LA, Ortner syndrome), dysphagia (compression of bronchi), chronic cough (due to LA compressing the bronchi), and infective endocarditis
- Not infrequently, symptoms are first noted in pregnancy: mitral faces, plethoric cheeks, and bluish patches.

PHYSICAL EXAM
- Elevated jugular venous pressure, left parasternal heave; apical impulse may be displaced, diastolic thrill in the left lateral decubitus position.
- Auscultation
  - Classic murmur: accentuated S$_1$, opening snap, apical early decrescendo diastolic rumble with presystolic accentuation (presystolic accentuation of murmur is lost with atrial fibrillation). Murmur is low pitch and best heard at the apex in the left lateral decubitus position.
  - Murmur is accentuated with exercise and decreased with rest and Valsalva.
    - With mobile, noncalcified valve, murmur persists throughout diastole and S$_1$, and the opening snap remains loud.
    - With increasing severity of MS, murmur often is difficult to hear. Duration of murmur reflective of severity. S$_1$ and the opening snap may be soft to absent.
    - A shorter S$_2$ to O$_2$ interval indicates more severe MS.
    - Further evaluation is required while looking for concomitant murmurs.

- If pulmonary HTN is present: Increased P$_2$, high-pitched decrescendo diastolic murmur of pulmonic insufficiency is heard (Graham Steell murmur); may have signs of right heart failure. RV lift can also be seen.
- May also find associated aortic or tricuspid murmurs due to involvement from RHD

DIAGNOSTIC TESTS & INTERPRETATION
Initial Tests (lab, imaging)
- ECG (4,5)[C]
  - LA enlargement (manifested by broad, notched P waves in lead II [P mitrale], with P wave duration >0.12 seconds with a negative terminal deflection of the P wave in lead V$_1$)
  - Atrial fibrillation is a common finding.
  - Right ventricular hypertrophy (RVH), right axis deviation, and an R to S ratio >1 in V$_1$ are possible.
- Chest radiograph (4,5)[C]
  - LA enlargement, straightening of the left heart border, a "double density," in the cardiac silhouette, and elevation of the left main stem bronchus
  - Prominent pulmonary arteries at the hilum with rapid tapering, RVH, and edema pattern with Kerley A and B lines (late presentation)
- Transthoracic echo (TTE) recommended in all patients with signs of symptoms of MS (1)[B],(5)[C]
  - Used for diagnosis of MS
    - Assess doming of the valve, mitral orifice size, and commissural fusion.
    - Extent of involvement based on degree of commissural fusion, calcification, and subvalvular fibrosis
    - Hockey stick, fish mouth appearance, which is due to narrowing of the valve orifice
  - Assess for concomitant valvulopathies.
- TEE should be performed if TTE images are nondiagnostic or if being considered for a percutaneous mitral balloon commissurotomy (PMBC) to exclude thrombus in LA and evaluate severity of MR (1)[B].
- Exercise stress testing can also be considered in patients with MS who have a discrepancy in their symptoms and signs and resting echo findings (1)[C].
- Cardiac catheterization indications (1,5)[C]
- Using Gorlin formula; pressures obtained via transseptal puncture
  - Class I recommendations
    - When echo is inconclusive
    - Discrepancy between echo, symptoms, and severity
  - Class II recommendations
    - Assess cause of severe pulmonary HTN that out of proportion to echo results.
  - Class III recommendations: satisfactory result of echo
  - CT ordered prior to surgery as many at risk for CAD

Follow-Up Tests & Special Considerations
- If valve area >1.5 cm^2 and mean pressure gradient <5 mm Hg, clinical follow-up in 3 to 5 years is recommended.
- Otherwise, follow-up is usually symptom based. Symptomatic patients with severe MS need further evaluation for interventional/surgical treatment.
- Holter monitor placement in order to rule out paroxysmal atrial fibrillation

Diagnostic Procedures/Other

- Exercise testing is recommended for those with clinical discrepancy.
- Wilkins score evaluates valvular anatomy from a TTE in order to see if patient is a candidate for surgery.

Test Interpretation

- Rheumatic fever–induced pathologic changes: leaflet thickening, leaflet calcification, commissural fusion, chordal shortening
- MV area defined (1)
  - Normal: 4 to 6 cm^2, progressive MS: >1.5 cm^2, severe MS: <1.5 cm^2, very severe: <1.0 cm^2

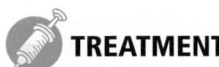

TREATMENT

GENERAL MEASURES

- Treatment is dependent on severity of stenosis and symptoms.
- Patients who have a valvular area >1.5 cm^2 and no symptoms can be managed medically
- MS is generally progressive, and medical therapy only delays the need for definitive therapy. It entails (i) treatment to prevent recurrence of rheumatic fever, (ii) treatments aimed at improving dyspnea and exercise tolerance, (iii) controlling the ventricular rate whether in sinus rhythm or atrial fibrillation, and (iv) anticoagulation for prevention of thromboembolic events.

MEDICATION

First Line

- Antibiotic prophylaxis against rheumatic fever and/or carditis is recommended for patients with history of rheumatic fever (1)[C]. Secondary prophylaxis is dependent on many factors: number of previous attacks, time since previous infection, risk for getting GAS, age of patient, and absence or presence of cardiac involvement.
- Antibiotic prophylaxis against infective endocarditis is not routinely recommended, unless there are other indications (1)[B].
- Diuretics for congestive symptoms (1)[A]
- β-Blockers or nondihydropyridine calcium channel blockers used for controlling heart rate both in sinus rhythm and atrial fibrillation to allow adequate diastolic filling and decrease LA diastolic pressure tachycardia or exertional symptoms (class IIa) (1)
- Ivabradine *helpful because it doesn't affect myocardial contraction*
- Consider cardioversion, especially in patients with mild MS and recent diagnosis of atrial fibrillation (<6 months).
- Use of anticoagulation (1)[B]
  - Class I recommendations
    - MS and atrial fibrillation or history of atrial fibrillation, MS, and prior embolic event or MS and LA thrombus
  - Class IIB recommendations
    - Patients with enlarged LA and spontaneous contrast on echo
- Warfarin is the only accepted modality for anticoagulation in patients with rheumatic mitral valve disease (international normalized ratio range 2 to 3).
- Heparin in the acute atrial fibrillation setting
- The new oral anticoagulants (factor Xa inhibitor and direct thrombin inhibitor) are not approved for use in atrial fibrillation that is secondary to MS.

Second Line

One can also consider amiodarone or digitalis if β-blockers and CCBs are not proven beneficial (2)[C].

SURGERY/OTHER PROCEDURES

- Surgical techniques include balloon valvotomy, open mitral commissurotomy, or closed mitral commissurotomy and mitral valve replacement.
- Patients with severe MS and symptoms consistent with NYHA classes III and IV are candidates for surgery.
- Any patient with a valve area >1.5 cm^2, LA thrombus, moderate MR, severe bicommissural calcifications, severe aortic valve disease, moderate TR or TS, and concomitant coronary artery disease are not candidates for PMBC.
- PMBC is recommended for those with severe MS symptoms and favorable valve morphology (1)[A], in asymptomatic patient with very severe MS and favorable valve anatomy in the absence of symptoms(1)[C], and in patients with suboptimal valvular anatomy, with a high risk for surgery (1)[C].
- Balloon valvotomy: symptomatic patients with NYHA class II, III, or IV symptoms with valves that look favorable and with favorable comorbidities (1)[A]
- MV surgery: when MS is severe with severe symptoms (NYHA classes III and IV), who are not high-risk surgical candidates, and balloon valvotomy is contraindicated or failed PMBC (1)[B]; patients with MS requiring left atrial appendage excision
- Patient's age, bleeding risk, and other comorbidities prior to deciding if patient should have a prosthetic versus mechanical valve

Pregnancy Considerations

- Volume expansion during pregnancy can exacerbate heart failure symptoms. Patients with known severe MS, prepregnancy discussions should be pursued with a cardiologist.
- Pregnant patients can safely use β-blockers. Despite some concerns of teratogenic affects with diuretics, furosemide has been used in symptomatic MS patients during pregnancy with minimal adverse effects.
- Coumadin is considered relatively safe in the 2nd and 3rd trimesters if anticoagulation is required. However, unfractionated heparin is preferred prior to labor and delivery.

ONGOING CARE

FOLLOW-UP RECOMMENDATIONS

- Counsel patients that MS usually is slowly progressive but can have sudden onset of atrial fibrillation, which could become rapidly fatal. Call 911 for marked worsening of symptoms.
- Echocardiographic surveillance in asymptomatic patients in any degree of MS: very severe (<1.0 cm^2) MS: yearly, severe (≤ 1.5 cm^2) MS: every 1 to 2 years, mild or moderate MS: every 3 to 5 years
- Follow-up will depend on the severity of the MS and the patient's symptoms.
  - Asymptomatic patients: annual history and examination
  - Symptomatic patients are followed closely based on clinical response to adjust therapy and plan definitive treatment (1)[C].

DIET

Salt restriction for pulmonary congestion

PROGNOSIS

Natural history

- Asymptomatic latent period after rheumatic fever for 10 to 30 years. 10-year survival for asymptomatic or minimally symptomatic patients is 80%.
- 10-year survival after onset of debilitating symptoms is only 0–15%.
- Mean survival with significant pulmonary HTN is <3 years.
- Commissurotomy is an effective means of reducing stenosis but is not curative. Restenosis sometimes occurs and can be early (<5 years) or late (>20 years).

COMPLICATIONS

- Left and right heart failure, atrial fibrillation and systemic embolization, pulmonary HTN, pulmonary vasoconstriction hepatic congestion, and bacterial endocarditis
- Pulmonary pressures >50 mm Hg increase surgical risk.

REFERENCES

1. Nishimura RA, Otto CM, Bonow RO, et al. 2014 AHA/ACC guideline for the management of patients with valvular heart disease: a report of the American College of Cardiology/American Heart Association Task Force on Practice Guidelines. *J Thorac Cardiovasc Surg.* 2014;148(1):e1–e132.
2. Carapetis JR, Steer AC, Mulholland EK, et al. The global burden of group A streptococcal diseases. *Lancet Infect Dis.* 2005;5(11):685–694.
3. Centers for Disease Control and Prevention. Group A streptococcal (GAS) disease. https://www .cdc.gov/groupastrep/diseases-hcp/acute-rheumatic -fever.html. Accessed October 22, 2018.
4. Anderson JL, Halperin JL, Albert NM, et al. Management of patients with atrial fibrillation (compilation of 2006 ACCF/AHA/ESC and 2011 ACCF/AHA/HRS recommendations): a report of the American College of Cardiology/American Heart Association Task Force on Practice Guidelines. *J Am Coll Cardiol.* 2013;61(18):1935–1944.
5. Manyemba J, Mayosi BM. Penicillin for secondary prevention of rheumatic fever. *Cochrane Database Syst Rev.* 2002;(3):CD002227.

CODES

ICD10

- I05.0 Rheumatic mitral stenosis
- I05.8 Other rheumatic mitral valve diseases
- I34.2 Nonrheumatic mitral (valve) stenosis

CLINICAL PEARLS

- Asymptomatic patients may be followed clinically with yearly exams for development of symptoms with periodic echo to evaluate valve area.
- Once symptoms of MS develop, initiate appropriate medical therapy, but advise patient that, for most, surgical therapy will be needed to prolong survival. Almost all cases of MV stenosis progress in severity over time.
- MS often presents during the intrapartum period. For patients with known severe MS, intervention should be pursued prior to pregnancy. Pregnancy in a patient with severe MS has a high rate of both maternal and fetal complications, including death.

M

MITRAL VALVE PROLAPSE

Praneeth Katrapati, MD • Brandon D. Coons, MD • Prashanth S. Katrapati, MD, FACC

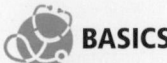

BASICS

DESCRIPTION

- Mitral valve prolapse (MVP) is a systolic billowing of one or both mitral leaflets into the left atrium (LA) during systole ± mitral regurgitation (MR).
- More specifically, MVP is a single or bileaflet prolapse of at least 2 mm superior displacement into the LA during systole on the parasternal long-axis annular plane of the valve on echocardiogram ± leaflet thickening.
  - Classic: prolapse with >5 mm of leaflet thickening
  - Nonclassic: prolapse with <5 mm of leaflet thickening
- Synonym(s): systolic click-murmur syndrome; billowing mitral cusp syndrome; myxomatous mitral valve; floppy valve syndrome; redundant cusp syndrome; Barlow syndrome

EPIDEMIOLOGY

Incidence

- Predominant age: MVP has been described in all age groups.
- Initial descriptions based on clinical examinations suggested a 2:1 female predominance. Using modern echocardiogram criteria, men and women are affected equally (1).
- The most serious consequences of hemodynamically significant MR occur in patients age >50 years (1).

Prevalence

MVP is the most common valvular abnormality, affecting 2–3% of the general population (1).

ETIOLOGY AND PATHOPHYSIOLOGY

- The pathology causing MVP is multifactorial and includes the following:
  - Abnormal valve tissue
    - Myxomatous degeneration: redundant layers of leaflet "hooding" the cords, chordal elongation, and annular dilatation
    - Myxoid leaflets are more elastic and less stiff than normal valves.
    - Chordal rupture is more common.
  - Disparity in size between the mitral valve and the left ventricle (LV)
  - Connective tissue disorders
- MVP is often associated with variable degrees of MR, which occurs in 9% of patients.
- The degree of MR depends on the degree of leaflet thickening and amount of flail or partially flail segments (2). When this occurs, 10-year mortality is 37% (2).
- Frequently, there is enlargement of the LA and LV.
- Mitral annulus is often dilated.
- Involvement of other valves may occur (tricuspid valve prolapse 40%, pulmonic prolapse and aortic prolapse 2–10%).
- Possible increased vagal tone
- Possible increased urine epinephrine and norepinephrine
- MVP patients often have orthostatic hypotension and tachycardia.
- Genetics causes proliferation of the spongiosa layer of the leaflets and fibrosis on the surface of them (1).

- Thinning and elongation of chordae tendineae
- The mitral valve differentiates during days 35 to 42 of fetal development, the same time as differentiation of the vertebrae and ribs.

Genetics

- Familial MVP is inherited as an autosomal dominant trait but with variable expressivity and incomplete penetrance.
- Two genetic loci identified
  - *MMVP1* on chromosome 16p11.2–p12.1
  - *MMVP2* on chromosome 11p15.4

RISK FACTORS

- MVP is a primary cardiovascular disorder.
- MVP is more likely to occur in patients with connective tissue disorders (see "Commonly Associated Conditions").
- Physical characteristics associated with MVP
  - Straight thoracic spine
  - Pectus excavatum
  - Asthenic body habitus
  - Low body mass index (BMI)
  - Scoliosis or kyphosis
  - Hypermobility of the joints
  - Arm span > height
  - Narrow anteroposterior (AP) diameter of the chest

COMMONLY ASSOCIATED CONDITIONS

- Marfan syndrome (91% of Marfan syndrome patients have MVP, although large majority of MVP patients do not meet criteria for Marfan.)
- Ehlers-Danlos syndrome
- Hypertrophic cardiomyopathy
- Pseudoxanthoma elasticum
- Osteogenesis imperfecta
- von Willebrand disease
- Primary hypomastia
- Graves disease
- Rheumatic heart disease

DIAGNOSIS

Physical exam and echocardiography

HISTORY

- Most patients are asymptomatic.
- The most frequent symptom is palpitations.
- Symptoms related to autonomic dysfunction
  - Anxiety and panic attacks
  - Arrhythmias
  - Exercise intolerance
  - Palpitations and chest pains that are atypical for coronary artery disease (CAD)
  - Fatigue
  - Orthostasis, syncope, or presyncope
  - Neuropsychiatric symptoms
- Symptoms related to progression of MR
  - Fatigue
  - Dyspnea
  - Exercise intolerance
  - Orthopnea
  - Paroxysmal nocturnal dyspnea
  - Congestive heart failure (CHF)
- Symptoms occur as a result of an associated complication (stroke, arrhythmia).

PHYSICAL EXAM

- Auscultatory examination
  - Mid to late systolic click
    - May vary in timing and intensity based on ventricular beat-to-beat volume variations
    - At low ventricular volumes, the valve may prolapse earlier during systole and further into the LA than during volume overload.
    - It may or may not be followed by a high-pitched, mid to late systolic murmur at the cardiac apex.
  - Murmur: a mid to late crescendo systolic murmur best heard at apex, middle to high pitched, occasionally musical or honking in quality
  - Occasionally, only the ejection click is present.
  - The duration of the murmur corresponds with the severity of MR.
- Dynamic auscultation
  - Maneuvers that move the click and murmur toward S_1
    - Arterial vasodilation
    - Amyl nitrite
    - Valsalva
    - Augmented contractility
    - Decreased venous return (which can be induced by standing up)
  - Maneuvers that move the click and murmur toward S_2
    - Squatting
    - Leg raise
    - Isometric exercise
  - Valsalva maneuver may help differentiate hypertrophic obstructive cardiomyopathy (HOCM) from MVP because it increases the intensity of the murmur in HOCM, whereas it makes it longer but not louder in MVP.

DIFFERENTIAL DIAGNOSIS

- MR
- Tricuspid regurgitation
- Tricuspid valve prolapse
- Papillary muscle dysfunction
- Hypertrophic cardiomyopathy
- Ejection clicks (do not change timing with systole)

DIAGNOSTIC TESTS & INTERPRETATION

Initial Tests (lab, imaging)

- Echocardiogram (test of choice) (3)[B]
  - In asymptomatic individuals with physical signs of MVP, an echocardiogram is indicated for diagnosis (3)[B].
  - Parasternal long-axis view is most specific for diagnosis (3).
  - Findings that may be seen with MVP
    - Anterior leaflet billowing
    - Leaflet thickening of ≥5 mm
    - Leaflet redundancy
    - MR
    - Posterior leaflet displacement
  - Nondiagnostic transthoracic echocardiogram: ≤10%
  - Transesophageal echocardiography particularly with 3D imaging may be considered to further visualize the anatomy if an intervention is being planned (2)[B].
  - Stress echocardiograms may reveal exercise-induced MR or latent LV dysfunction (3)[B].

- Angiography
  - Rarely used for diagnostic purposes
  - Recommended for hemodynamic assessment when noninvasive options or inconclusive (3)[C]
- ECG is usually normal.
  - May be nonspecific ST to T wave changes
  - T-wave inversions, prominent Q waves, or prolonged QT may also occur.
- A chest x-ray (CXR) is not necessary for diagnosis.
  - Typically, the CXR is normal.
  - Other findings
    - Possible pulmonary edema: Pulmonary edema may be asymmetric with acute chordal rupture and flail leaflet.
    - Possible calcification of the mitral annulus
- Holter monitoring is optional if patient has palpitations. Order Holter monitoring as usual for syncope or dizziness.
- Tilt table testing may be of value in patients with MVP who presents with syncope of unknown etiology (3)[C].

Follow-Up Tests & Special Considerations
- Periodic monitoring with TTE is recommended in asymptomatic patients with known VHD at intervals depending on valve lesion, severity, ventricular size, and ventricular function (3)[C].
- Patients with a family history of MVP should be screened with echocardiography (3)[B].

Test Interpretation
- Myxomatous proliferation of the middle layer (spongiosa) of the valve, resulting in increased mucopolysaccharide deposition and myxomatous degeneration
- By electron microscopy, the collagen fibers in the valve leaflets are disorganized and fragmented.
- With increased stroma deposition, the valve leaflets enlarge and become redundant.
- The endothelium is usually noncontiguous and a frequent site for thrombus or infective vegetation.

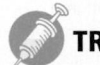 TREATMENT

GENERAL MEASURES
Treat MVP with orthostatic symptoms by liberalizing fluid and salt intake. If severe, mineralocorticoids may rarely be used. Support stockings may also be beneficial; in the absence of MR, no definitive treatment for MVP (2)

MEDICATION
- Asymptomatic MVP is treated with reassurance; normal lifestyle and regular exercise is encouraged.
- MVP with palpitations is treated with β-blockers and/or recommendation to discontinue alcohol, cigarettes, and caffeine.
- MVP and transient ischemic attacks are treated with aspirin 75 to 325 mg daily (3)[C].
- MVP with history of cryptogenic stroke or atrial fibrillation with CHADS$_2$ (acronym for **C**ongestive heart failure, **H**ypertension, **A**ge >75 years, **D**iabetes mellitus, and prior **S**troke or transient ischemic attack) score <2 is generally treated with aspirin 75 to 325 mg daily (3)[C].
- MVP with atrial fibrillation with CHADS$_2$ score ≥2 is treated with warfarin (3)[C].

- MVP with high-risk echocardiographic features (thickening >5 mm or valve redundancy) and a history of stroke; warfarin therapy may be considered (3)[C].

ADDITIONAL THERAPIES
- Endocarditis prophylaxis is no longer recommended for patients with MVP.
- Patients with prior endocarditis undergoing dental, respiratory tract, infected skin, or musculoskeletal procedures should receive prophylaxis for endocarditis with amoxicillin 30 to 60 minutes prior to procedure. Ampicillin, cefazolin, or ceftriaxone IM or IV may be used if unable to tolerate oral medications (3)[B].

SURGERY/OTHER PROCEDURES
- Referral for surgery is recommended based on severity of symptoms for patients with severe MR or impaired LV systolic function or flail leaflet owing to ruptured chordae tendineae (3)[B].
- One recent meta-analysis of observational studies suggests a benefit for an early surgical approach to MVP with severe MR (4)[A] even for asymptomatic patients; prospective studies are lacking.
- Minimally invasive mitral valve repair currently being used for high-risk patients; did not reduce MR as much as surgery but similar clinical outcomes (2)[C]
- Surgical repair of MR due to isolated posterior leaflet prolapse is associated with a low reoperation rate (5)[A].
- Asymptomatic patients with atrial fibrillation or pulmonary hypertension should be considered for intervention as well (3)[C].

 ONGOING CARE

FOLLOW-UP RECOMMENDATIONS
- Asymptomatic MVP patients with no significant MR can be followed clinically every 3 to 5 years (3)[C].
- Patients who are symptomatic or have high-risk features on initial echocardiogram, including moderate to severe MR, may need serial echocardiograms and should be followed clinically once per year (3)[C].
- Patients with MVP and severe MR may require coronary angiography and transesophageal echocardiography if cardiac surgical referral is planned (3)[C].

PATIENT EDUCATION
- No contraindication to pregnancy
- Restriction from competitive sports if patient has MVP with one of the following features:
  - A history of syncope associated with documented arrhythmia
  - A family history of MVP-related sudden cardiac death
  - Sustained or repetitive and nonsustained supraventricular tachycardia or frequent and/or complex ventricular tachyarrhythmias on ambulatory Holter monitoring
  - Severe MR
  - A prior embolic event
  - LV systolic dysfunction
- Explain the hereditary nature of familial MVP.

PROGNOSIS
- Excellent prognosis for asymptomatic patients
- For patients with severe MR or reduced ejection fraction, the prognosis is similar to that for nonischemic MR.

COMPLICATIONS
- Sudden cardiac death: not clearly established; may be secondary to ventricular arrhythmias especially if significant MR is present
- Chordae rupture with acute mitral insufficiency (higher risk of cardiac death; up to 2% per year)
- Infectious endocarditis (risk increased if murmur present)
- Cerebrovascular ischemic event
- Fibrin emboli
- Heart failure with progressive MR
- Arrhythmias such as atrial and ventricular premature beats, paroxysmal supraventricular tachycardias may all be seen. Risk increases with coexistent MR.
- Pulmonary hypertension

REFERENCES
1. Delling FN, Vasan RS. Epidemiology and pathophysiology of mitral valve prolapse: new insights into disease progression, genetics, and molecular basis. *Circulation*. 2014;129(21):2158–2170.
2. Guy TS, Hill A. Mitral valve prolapse. *Annu Rev Med*. 2012;63:277–292.
3. Nishimura RA, Otto CM, Bonow RO, et al. 2017 AHA/ACC focused update of the 2014 AHA/ACC guideline for the management of patients with valvular heart disease: a report of the American College of Cardiology/American Heart Association Task Force on Clinical Practice Guidelines. *Circulation*. 2017;135(25):e1159–e1195.
4. Goldstone AB, Patrick WL, Cohen JE, et al. Early surgical intervention or watchful waiting for the management of asymptomatic mitral regurgitation: a systematic review and meta-analysis. *Ann Cardiothorac Surg*. 2015;4(3):220–229.
5. Johnston DR, Gillinov AM, Blackstone EH, et al. Surgical repair of posterior mitral valve prolapse: implications for guidelines and percutaneous repair. *Ann Thorac Surg*. 2010;89(5):1385–1394.

ADDITIONAL READING
Otto CM, Bonow RO, eds. *Valvular Heart Disease: A Companion to Braunwald's Heart Disease*. 4th ed. Philadelphia, PA: Elsevier; 2014.

 CODES

ICD10
I34.1 Nonrheumatic mitral (valve) prolapse

CLINICAL PEARLS
- MVP patients may have orthostatic hypotension and tachycardia.
- Asymptomatic MVP patients with no significant MR can be followed clinically every 3 to 5 years. Patients who are symptomatic or have high-risk features on initial echocardiogram, including moderate to severe MR, may need serial echocardiograms and should be followed clinically once per year.
- Consider an early surgical approach for MVP with severe MR.
- Endocarditis prophylaxis is no longer recommended for MVP.

M

MOLLUSCUM CONTAGIOSUM

Erica F. Crannage, PharmD, BCPS, BCACP • Dawn M. Davis, MD, MPH

BASICS

DESCRIPTION

Molluscum contagiosum is a common, benign, viral (poxvirus) skin infection, characterized by small (2 to 5 mm), waxy white or flesh-colored, dome-shaped papules often with central umbilication. Lesions contain a cheesy grayish white material. Molluscum contagiosum is highly contagious and spreads by autoinoculation, skin-to-skin contact, sexual contact, and shared clothing/towels. Molluscum contagiosum is a self-limited infection in immunocompetent patients but can be difficult to treat and disfiguring in immunocompromised patients.

EPIDEMIOLOGY

Prevalence
- 1% in the United States, occurring mainly in children 2 to 15 years and sexually active young adults
- 5–18% HIV population

ETIOLOGY AND PATHOPHYSIOLOGY
- DNA virus; Poxviridae family
- Four genetic virus types, clinically indistinguishable
- Virions invade and replicate in cytoplasm of epithelial cells causing abnormal cell proliferation.
- Genome encodes proteins to evade host immune system.
- Incubation period: 2 to 6 weeks
- Time to resolution: 6 to 24 months
- Not associated with malignancy
- No cross-hybridization or reactivation by other poxviruses

RISK FACTORS
- Skin-to-skin contact with infected person
- Contact sports
- Swimming
- Eczema, atopic dermatitis
- Sexual activity with infected partner
- Immunocompromised: HIV, chemotherapy, corticosteroid therapy, transplant patients

GENERAL PREVENTION
- Avoid skin-to-skin contact with host (e.g., contact sports, sexual activity).
- Avoid sharing clothing and towels.

COMMONLY ASSOCIATED CONDITIONS
- Atopic dermatitis
- Immunosuppression medications: corticosteroids, biologics, chemotherapy, etc.
- HIV/AIDS

DIAGNOSIS

HISTORY
- Contact with known infected person
- Participation in contact sports
- Sexual activity

PHYSICAL EXAM
- Perform thorough skin exam including conjunctiva and anogenital area.
- Discrete, firm papules with a central umbilication
- White curdlike core under umbilicated center
- Lesions are flesh, pearl, or red in color and frequently located in intertriginous areas.
- May have surrounding erythema or dermatitis
- Immunocompetent hosts: average of 11 to 20 lesions, 2 to 5 mm diameter (range: 1 to 10 mm)
- Hosts with HIV/AIDS: hundreds of widespread lesions
- Sexually active: inner thighs, anogenital area

Pediatric Considerations
- Infants <3 months: Consider vertical transmission.
- Children: fever, >50 lesions, limited response to therapy; consider immunodeficiency.
- Children: anogenital lesions; consider autoinoculation/possible sexual abuse.

DIFFERENTIAL DIAGNOSIS
- Verruca vulgaris
- AIDS patients: cryptococcus, penicilliosis, histoplasmosis, coccidioidomycosis
- Basal cell carcinoma
- Benign appendageal tumors: syringomas, hidrocystomas, ectopic sebaceous glands
- Condyloma acuminatum
- Dermatofibroma
- Eyelid: abscess, chalazion, foreign-body granuloma
- Folliculitis/furunculosis
- Keratoacanthoma
- Oral squamous cell carcinoma
- Trichoepithelioma
- Warty dyskeratoma
- Amelanotic melanoma

DIAGNOSTIC TESTS & INTERPRETATION

Initial Tests (lab, imaging)
- Virus cannot be cultured.
- Culture lesion if concern is secondary infection.
- Sexual transmission: Test for other sexually transmitted infections, including HIV.
- Microscopy: scrape lesion
  - Core material has characteristic Henderson-Paterson intracytoplasmic viral inclusion bodies.
  - Crush prep with 10% potassium hydroxide will show characteristic inclusion bodies as well.
  - Alternatively, hematoxylin-eosin-stained formalin-fixed tissue shows same confirmatory features.

Diagnostic Procedures/Other
Clinical; using magnifying lens

Test Interpretation
Molluscum cytoplasmic inclusion bodies within keratinocytes

TREATMENT

GENERAL MEASURES
- In healthy patients, molluscum contagiosum is generally self-limited and resolves spontaneously; therefore, treatment is optional (1)[A].
- No single intervention is shown to be convincingly more effective than any other in treating molluscum contagiosum (1)[A].
- There are no FDA-approved treatments for molluscum contagiosum.
- Three categories of treatment: destructive, immune-enhancing, and antiviral
- Imiquimod is no longer recommended as treatment.

MEDICATION

First Line
Cantharidin 0.7–0.9% solution: In office application to lesions, cover with dressing; wash off in 2 to 6 hours or sooner if blistering. Repeat treatment every 2 to 4 weeks until lesions resolve (1)[B].

- Not commercially available in the United States but may be prepared in United States by compounding pharmacy from powder; might be available as solution from Canada
- Adverse effects: blistering, erythema, pain, pruritus
- Precautions: Do not use on face or on genital mucosa.

Second Line

- Benzoyl peroxide 10% cream: Apply to each lesion twice daily for 4 weeks (1)[B].
  - Inexpensive
  - Adverse effects: mild dermatitis
- For immunocompromised patients with refractory lesions, consider
  - Starting or maximizing HAART in patients with HIV/AIDS (2)[C]
  - Cidofovir
    - 3% cream applied to lesions once daily, 5 days/week for 8 weeks or 1% cream applied to lesions once daily, 5 days/week for 2 weeks; repeat in 1 month, if necessary (2)[C].
    - Adverse effects with topical use: erythema, pain, pruritus, erosions
    - 3 to 5 mg/kg IV weekly for 1 to 2 weeks, followed by IV infusions every other week, until clinical clearance or up to 9 infusions (3)[C]
    - Adverse effects with IV use: nephrotoxicity, neutropenia
    - Monitoring with IV use: renal function and complete blood counts prior to and 24 to 48 hours after infusions
    - Precaution: must coadminister oral probenecid and provide IV hydration with each IV infusion; refer to cidofovir manufacturer's recommendations on probenecid dosing.

SURGERY/OTHER PROCEDURES

Considered first-line treatment, if treatment is pursed

- Cryotherapy: 5 to 10 seconds with 1- to 2-mm margins; repeat every 3 to 4 weeks as needed until lesions disappear (4)[B].
  - Adverse effects: erythema, edema, pain, blistering
  - Contraindications: cryoglobulinemia, Raynaud disease
- Curettage under local or topical anesthesia (1)[A]
  - Adverse effects: pain, scarring

COMPLEMENTARY & ALTERNATIVE MEDICINE

- Australian lemon myrtle oil: Apply 10% solution once daily for 21 days (1)[B].
- Potassium hydroxide 5–10% solution: Apply 1 to 2 times a day until the lesions disappeared completely (1)[B].

Pediatric Considerations

- Due to the self-limiting nature of the disease, for immunocompetent children, treatment is optional.
- Surgical interventions: second line in small children due to associated pain
- Pain control: Pretreat with topical lidocaine or EMLA before surgical treatment.
- Note: adverse effect:
  - Lidocaine or EMLA over large body surface area: Methemoglobinemia and CNS toxicity. Refer to manufacturer's recommendations on dosing and use in children.

Pregnancy Considerations

Treatments safe in pregnancy: curettage, cryotherapy, incision, and expression

 ## ONGOING CARE

FOLLOW-UP RECOMMENDATIONS

Patient Monitoring

Depends on type of treatment

PATIENT EDUCATION

- Cover lesions to prevent spread.
- Avoid scratching to prevent autoinoculation.
- Avoid sharing towels and clothing.
- Avoid sexual activity when lesions present.

PROGNOSIS

- Immunocompetent: self-limited, resolves in 3 to 12 months (range: 2 months to 4 years)
- Immunocompromised: lesions difficult to treat; may persist for years

COMPLICATIONS

- Secondary infection
- Scarring, hyper-/hypopigmentation—(generally only occurs as a result of treatment, not when lesions resolve spontaneously)

REFERENCES

1. van der Wouden JC, van der Sande R, Kruithof EJ, et al. Interventions for cutaneous molluscum contagiosum. *Cochrane Database Syst Rev.* 2017;(5):CD004767.
2. Chen X, Anstey AV, Bugert JJ. Molluscum contagiosum virus infection. *Lancet Infect Dis.* 2013;13(10):877–888.
3. Erikson C, Driscoll M, Gaspari A. Efficacy of intravenous cidofovir in the treatment of giant molluscum contagiosum in a patient with human immunodeficiency virus. *Arch Dermatol.* 2011;147(6):652–654.
4. Al-Mutairi N, Al-Doukhi A, Al-Farag S, et al. Comparative study on the efficacy, safety, and acceptability of imiquimod 5% cream versus cryotherapy for molluscum contagiosum in children. *Pediatr Dermatol.* 2010;27(4):388–394.

ADDITIONAL READING

- Basdag H, Rainer BM, Cohen BA. Molluscum contagiosum: to treat or not to treat? Experience with 170 children in an outpatient clinic setting in the northeastern United States. *Pediatr Dermatol.* 2015;32(3):353–357.
- Olsen JR, Gallacher J, Piguet V, et al. Epidemiology of molluscum contagiosum in children: a systematic review. *Fam Pract.* 2014;31(2):130–136.
- Ting PT, Dytoc MT. Therapy of external anogenital warts and molluscum contagiosum: a literature review. *Dermatol Ther.* 2004;17(1):68–101.

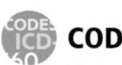 ## CODES

ICD10

B08.1 Molluscum contagiosum

CLINICAL PEARLS

- Observation is preferred treatment in healthy patients as lesions will spontaneously resolve.
- Reassure parents that lesions will heal naturally and generally resolve without scarring.
- No specific treatment has been identified as superior to any other.
- Consider topical corticosteroids for pruritus or associated dermatitis.

M

MORTON NEUROMA (INTERDIGITAL NEUROMA)

Scott M. Goldberg, MD • J. Herbert Stevenson, MD

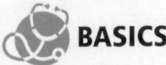 **BASICS**

DESCRIPTION

- Painful condition of the webbed spaces of the toes
- Features perineural fibrosis of the common digital nerve as it passes between metatarsals
  - The interspace between the 3rd and 4th metatarsals is most commonly affected.
  - The interspace between the 2nd and 3rd metatarsals is the next most common site.
- Systems affected: musculoskeletal, nervous
- Synonyms: plantar digital neuritis; Morton metatarsalgia; intermetatarsal neuroma

EPIDEMIOLOGY

Prevalence
- Unknown
- Mean age: 45 to 50 years
- Predominant sex: female > male (8:1)

ETIOLOGY AND PATHOPHYSIOLOGY
- Lateral plantar nerve joins a portion of medial plantar nerve, creating a nerve with a larger diameter than those going to other digits.
- Etiology not fully understood. Four main theories:
  - Chronic traction damage
  - Inflammatory environment due to intermetatarsal bursitis
  - Compression by the deep transverse intermetatarsal ligament
  - Ischemia of vasa nervorum
- Nerve lies in SC tissue, deep to the fat pad of foot, just superficial to the digital artery and vein.
- Overlying, the nerve is the strong, deep transverse metatarsal ligament that holds the metatarsal bones together.
- With each step the patient takes, the inflamed nerve becomes compressed between the ground and the deep transverse metatarsal ligament. This can generate perineural fibrotic reaction with subsequent neuroma formation.

RISK FACTORS
- High-heeled shoes
  - Transfer more weight to the forefoot.
- Shoes with tight toe boxes
  - Cause lateral compression
- Pes planus (flat feet)
  - Pulls nerve medially, increasing irritation
- Obesity
- Female gender

- Ballet dancing, particularly associated with the demi-pointe position
- Basketball, aerobics, tennis, running, and similar activities
- Hyperpronation

GENERAL PREVENTION
- Wear properly fitting shoes.
- Avoid high heels and shoes with narrow toe boxes.

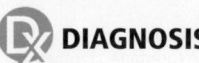 **DIAGNOSIS**

HISTORY
- Most common complaint is pain localized to interspace between 3rd and 4th toes.
- Pain is less severe when not bearing weight.
- Pain, cramping, or numbness of the forefoot during weight-bearing or immediately after strenuous foot exertion
- Radiation of pain to the toes
- Pain is relieved by removing shoes and massaging the foot.
- Patients often complain of "walking on a marble."
- Burning pain in the ball of the foot radiating to the toes
- Tingling or numbness in the toes
- Aggravated by wearing tight or narrow shoes

PHYSICAL EXAM
- Intense pain when pressure applied between metatarsal heads, sometimes with a palpable nodule
- Assess midfoot motion and digital motion to determine if arthritis or synovitis.
- Palpate along metatarsal shafts to assess for metatarsalgia or stress fractures.
- Special testing (see "Diagnostic Procedures/Other")

DIFFERENTIAL DIAGNOSIS
- Stress fracture
- Hammer toe
- Metatarsophalangeal synovitis
- Metatarsalgia
- Arthritis
- Traumatic neuroma
- Osteomyelitis
- Bursitis
- Foreign body
- Freiberg infraction (avascular necrosis of the metatarsal head, most commonly in adolescent females at the 2nd metatarsal)

- Neoplasm (malignancy, osteochondroma, neurofibroma)
- Gout

DIAGNOSTIC TESTS & INTERPRETATION
Initial Tests (lab, imaging)
- Predominantly a clinical diagnosis; imaging should be reserved for when the diagnosis is unclear (1)[A].
- Imaging may be helpful if more than one web space is involved.
- Radiographs may help to rule out osseous pathology if diagnosis is in question, but plain films usually are normal in patients with a Morton neuroma (1)[A].
- Ultrasound (US) has 79% specificity and 99% sensitivity for Morton neuromas but is poor at assessing the size of the lesion. Specificity declines to 50% for lesions <6 mm (1)[A].
- MRI can rule out an osseous tumor and help with surgical planning; MRI has a sensitivity of 83% and a specificity of 99% for diagnosis of Morton neuroma (1)[A].

Diagnostic Procedures/Other
- Five special tests have been described: thumb index finger squeeze test, Mulder sign, foot squeeze test, plantar percussion test, and toe tip sensation deficit.
  - Thumb index finger squeeze test is the most sensitive and specific (96% and 96%, respectively); positive when pain elicited by squeezing the symptomatic intermetatarsal space between the index finger and thumb (2)[B]
  - Mulder sign is a painful "click" produced by squeezing the metatarsal heads together while compressing the neuroma between the thumb and index finger of the other hand; sensitivity 40–84% (1)[A]
  - Foot squeeze test is positive when pain is induced in the symptomatic web space when the metatarsal heads are compressed by grasping the foot; sensitivity 40% (2)[B]
  - Plantar and dorsal percussion tests are positive when percussion of the affected webspace elicits pain.
  - Toe tip sensation deficit exists when the sensation of the toe distal to the affected web space is decreased relative to the other toes.
- More than one of the above tests being positive increases the diagnostic accuracy (3)[B].

Test Interpretation

Pathologic examination shows chronic fibrosis and thickening within and around the digital nerve. Arterial thickening and thrombosis of the common digital artery is sometimes present.

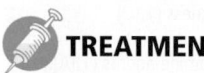

TREATMENT

GENERAL MEASURES

- Stepwise treatment, with typical progression from conservative measures followed by infiltrative treatment, and ultimately surgical treatment
- Surgical treatments are the most successful (89%) followed by infiltrative (84%) then conservative (48%) as assessed by patient satisfaction with pain reduction at 6 months or greater (4)[A].
- Conservative treatments include
  - Flat shoes with a roomy toe box
  - Plantar pads may help with alignment of metatarsal heads to provide relief.
- NSAIDs for temporary symptom relief. There is no evidence for the use of supinatory insoles (5)[A].

MEDICATION

First Line

Injectable steroids (e.g., betamethasone phosphate/acetate or methylprednisolone): number needed to treat (NNT) for significant benefit over conservative measures at 6 months = 2.3 (4,6)[A]

Second Line

US-guided alcohol ablation therapy to sclerose the nerve is effective and has a lower complication rate than surgery (4)[A].

ISSUES FOR REFERRAL

- Continued pain despite conservative treatments and injections
- Large interdigital neuromas (>5 mm diameter) or young patients, who may benefit from earlier operative intervention

SURGERY/OTHER PROCEDURES

- Surgical removal of the neuroma or shortening of the metatarsals, with or without release of the transverse metatarsal ligament, have an 89% success rate at 6 months defined by satisfaction scores (4)[A].
- Small trials have been conducted using other invasive, nonsurgical techniques including injection with botulinum toxin, cryoablation, radiofrequency ablation, and platelet-rich plasma, but evidence is limited at this time.

ONGOING CARE

FOLLOW-UP RECOMMENDATIONS

At diagnosis, or if no improvement after 3 months of conservative treatment, consider corticosteroid injection.

- May repeat injection if no improvement after 2 to 4 weeks, or consider referring for surgical management
- 21–51% of patients receiving a single corticosteroid injection require surgical intervention within 2 to 4 years (7)[B].
- Size >5 mm and younger patients are more likely to undergo invasive treatment (7)[B].

PATIENT EDUCATION

Wear properly fitting comfortable shoes.

PROGNOSIS

- 48% satisfaction rate with conservative treatment
- 85% satisfaction rate with infiltrative treatment
- 89% satisfaction rate with operative treatment (4)[A]

COMPLICATIONS

- Hip and knee pain can develop secondary to gait changes.
- Complications vary by treatment type.
- Failure rate is 47% with conservative treatment; 9–23% with invasive, nonsurgical treatment; 4% with surgical treatment (4)[A].
- Surgical complications vary by specific procedure and include keloid, CRPS, and stiffness. There was a global complication rate of 21% with operative treatment (4)[A].

REFERENCES

1. Sharp RJ, Wade CM, Hennessy MS, et al. The role of MRI and ultrasound imaging in Morton's neuroma and the effect of size of lesion on symptoms. *J Bone Joint Surg Br*. 2003;85(7):999–1005.
2. Mahadevan D, Venkatesan M, Bhatt R, et al. Diagnostic accuracy of clinical tests for Morton's neuroma compared with ultrasonography. *J Foot Ankle Surg*. 2015;54(4):549–553.
3. Owens R, Gougoulias N, Guthrie H, et al. Morton's neuroma: clinical testing and imaging in 76 feet, compared to a control group. *Foot Ankle Surg*. 2011;17(3):197–200.
4. Valisena S, Petri GJ, Ferrero A. Treatment of Morton's neuroma: a systematic review. *Foot Ankle Surg*. 2018;24(4):271–281.
5. Thomson CE, Gibson JN, Martin D. Interventions for the treatment of Morton's neuroma. *Cochrane Database Syst Rev*. 2004;(3):CD003118.
6. Saygi B, Yildirim Y, Saygi EK, et al. Morton neuroma: comparative results of two conservative methods. *Foot Ankle Int*. 2005;26(7):556–559.
7. Mahadevan D, Salmasi M, Whybra N, et al. What factors predict the need for further intervention following corticosteroid injection of Morton's neuroma? *Foot Ankle Surg*. 2016;22(1):9–11.

ADDITIONAL READING

- Jain S, Mannan K. The diagnosis and management of Morton's neuroma: a literature review. *Foot Ankle Spec*. 2013;6(4):307–317.
- Schreiber K, Khodaee M, Poddar S, et al. Clinical inquiry. What is the best way to treat Morton's neuroma? *J Fam Pract*. 2011;60(3):157–168.

CODES

ICD10

- G57.60 Lesion of plantar nerve, unspecified lower limb
- G57.61 Lesion of plantar nerve, right lower limb
- G57.62 Lesion of plantar nerve, left lower limb

CLINICAL PEARLS

- Morton neuroma is usually a clinical diagnosis but can be further evaluated with US or MRI.
- Typical treatment is stepwise with conservative, then infiltrative, and then operative treatment.
- Morton neuromas with >5 mm diameter are more likely to require operative treatment.
- Younger patients are more likely to require operative treatment.
- Neurectomy is the definitive treatment. Patients should be aware of surgical complications.

M

MOTION SICKNESS

Gina Henry, MD • Alexandra Jubran, DO, MPH • Cory N. Mitchell, MD

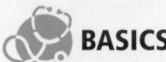 **BASICS**

DESCRIPTION
- Motion sickness is a physiologic response in affected individuals to a situation in which sensory conflict about body motion exists among visual receptors, vestibular receptors, and body proprioceptors.
- Also can be induced when patterns of motion differ from those previously experienced
- System affected: nervous, gastrointestinal
- Synonym(s): car sickness; sea sickness; air sickness; space sickness; physiologic vertigo

EPIDEMIOLOGY
Incidence
Predominant sex: female > male

Prevalence
Estimation is complex; syndrome occurs in ~25% due to travel by air, ~29% by sea, and ~41% by road. Estimates for vomiting are 0.5% by air, 7% by sea, and 2% by road.

ETIOLOGY AND PATHOPHYSIOLOGY
- Precise etiology unknown; thought to be due to a mismatch of vestibular and visual sensations
- Rotary, vertical, and low-frequency motions produce more symptoms than linear, horizontal, and high-frequency motions.
- Nausea and vomiting occur as a result of increased levels of dopamine and acetylcholine, which stimulate chemoreceptor trigger zone and vomiting center in CNS.

Genetics
Heritability estimates range from 55% to 75%.

RISK FACTORS
- Motion (auto, plane, boat, amusement rides)
- Visual stimuli (e.g., moving horizon)
- Poor ventilation (fumes, smoke, carbon monoxide)
- Emotions (fear, anxiety)
- Zero gravity
- Pregnancy, menstruation, oral contraceptive use
- History of migraine headaches, especially vestibular migraine

GENERAL PREVENTION
See "General Measures."

Pediatric Considerations
- Rare in children <2 years of age
- Incidence peaks between 3 and 12 years of age.
- Antihistamines may cause excitation in children.

Geriatric Considerations
- Age confers some resistance to motion sickness.
- Elderly are at increased risk for anticholinergic side effects from treatment.

Pregnancy Considerations
- Pregnant patients are more likely to experience motion sickness.
- Treatment with medications is thought to be safe during morning sickness (e.g., meclizine, dimenhydrinate).
- Scopolamine, meclizine, diphenhydramine, and promethazine generally considered safe during breastfeeding

COMMONLY ASSOCIATED CONDITIONS
- Migraine headache
- Vestibular syndromes

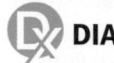 **DIAGNOSIS**

HISTORY
Presence of the following signs and symptoms in the context of a typical stimulus (1):
- Nausea
- Vomiting
- Stomach awareness (feeling of fullness in epigastrium)
- Diaphoresis
- Facial and perioral pallor
- Hypersalivation
- Yawning
- Hyperventilation
- Anxiety
- Panic
- Malaise
- Fatigue
- Weakness
- Confusion
- Dizziness

PHYSICAL EXAM
No specific findings

DIFFERENTIAL DIAGNOSIS
- Mountain sickness
- Vestibular disease, central and peripheral
- Gastroenteritis
- Metabolic disorders
- Toxin exposure

DIAGNOSTIC TESTS & INTERPRETATION
None usually indicated, can consider pregnancy test

 TREATMENT

- Follow guidelines under "General Measures" section to prevent motion sickness (1)[C].
- Premedicate before travel with antidopaminergic, anticholinergic, or antihistamine agents (1)[A]:
  - For extended travel, consider treatment with scopolamine transdermal patch (2)[A].
- Conflicting data exist on the efficacy of acupressure for nausea and vomiting associated with motion sickness (3)[B].
- Benzodiazepines suppress vestibular nuclei but would not be considered first line due to sedation and addiction potential (4)[C].
- Serotonin receptor agonist (rizatriptan) may be effective for migraineurs with motion sickness (5)[C].

GENERAL MEASURES
- Avoid noxious types of motions. Travelling in inclement weather may exacerbate symptoms.
- Improve ventilation; avoid noxious stimuli.
- Eat before travel (light, soft, bland, low-fat, and low-acid foods); avoid alcohol; avoid empty stomach.
- Increase airflow around face.
- Use semirecumbent seating or lay supine.
- Fix vision on horizon; avoid fixation on moving objects; keep eyes fixed on still, distant objects.
- Avoid reading while actively traveling.
- Frequent and graded exposure to stimulus that triggers nausea (habituation)
- Counsel patient on minimizing motion (airplanes: over the wing; automobiles: driver's or front passenger seat, facing forward; boat: facing toward the waves, away from rocking bow, near surface of the water; buses: near the front, at lowest level, facing forward; trains: at lowest level, facing forward).
- Acupressure on point PC6 (*Neiguan* on pericardium meridian) has been shown to reduce feelings of nausea and vomiting during pregnancy, after surgery, and in cancer chemotherapy. However, limited evidence of efficacy has been found for motion sickness; point PC6: 2 cm proximal of transverse crease of palmar side of wrist between tendons of the palmaris longus and the flexor carpi radialis (3)[B].

MEDICATION
First Line

- Scopolamine transdermal patch (Transderm Scop; $25.56 each): Apply 2.5-cm^2 (4 mg) patch behind ear over the mastoid at least 4 hours (preferably 6 to 12 hours) before travel and replace every 3 days (2)[A].
- Promethazine (Phenergan; $0.49 each 12.5 mg): Take 30 to 60 minutes before travel.
  - Adults: 25 mg q12h; 25 to 50 mg IM if already developed severe motion sickness
  - Children and adolescents: 0.5 mg/kg q12h, maximum 25 mg BID; *caution*: increased risk of dystonic reaction in this age group
- Dimenhydrinate (Dramamine; $0.30 each 50 mg): Take 30 to 60 minutes before travel.
  - Adults and adolescents: 50 to 100 mg q4–6h, maximum 400 mg/day
  - Children 6 to 12 years of age: 25 to 50 mg q6–8h, maximum 150 mg/day
  - Children 2 to 5 years of age: 12.5 to 25.0 mg q6–8h, maximum 75 mg/day
- Meclizine (Travel Ease; $0.03 each 25 mg): Take 60 minutes before travel.
  - Adults and adolescents >12 years of age: 25 to 50 mg q24h
  - Children <12 years of age: not recommended
- Diphenhydramine (Benadryl; $0.02 to 0.06 per 25 mg): Take 30 minutes before travel.
  - Adults and adolescents: 25 to 50 mg q6–8h, maximum 300 mg/day
  - Children 6 to 12 years of age: 5 mg/kg or 12.5 to 25.0 mg q4–6h, maximum 150 mg/day
- Contraindications: patients at risk for acute angle-closure glaucoma.
- Precautions:
  - Young children
  - Elderly
  - Pregnancy
  - Urinary obstruction
  - Pyloric duodenal obstruction
- Adverse reactions:
  - Drowsiness
  - Dry mouth
  - Blurred vision
  - Confusion
  - Headache
  - Urinary retention
- Significant possible interactions:
  - Sedatives (antihistamines, alcohol, antidepressants)
  - Anticholinergics (belladonna alkaloids)

Second Line

- Benzodiazepines: Take 1 to 2 hours before travel.
  - Diazepam 2 to 10 mg PO q6–12h
  - Lorazepam 1 to 2 mg PO q8h
- Contraindications:
  - Severe respiratory dysfunction
  - Severe liver dysfunction
- Precautions:
  - Alcohol/drug abuse
  - Elderly
  - Sedation
  - Addiction is possible.

COMPLEMENTARY & ALTERNATIVE MEDICINE

Ginger: 1.0 to 1.5 g per 24 hours (250 mg 4 times a day); take 4 hours before travel; studies have shown ginger to be an effective treatment for nausea and vomiting (6)[B].

 ONGOING CARE

DIET

- Eat before travel, avoid empty stomach; eat light, soft, bland, low-fat, and low-acid foods.
- Avoid alcohol.

PROGNOSIS

- Symptoms should resolve when motion exposure ends.
- Resistance to motion sickness seems to increase with age.

COMPLICATIONS

- Hypotension
- Dehydration
- Depression
- Panic
- Syncope

REFERENCES

1. Brainard A, Gresham C. Prevention and treatment of motion sickness. *Am Fam Physician.* 2014;90(1):41–46.
2. Spinks AB, Wasiak J. Scopolamine (hyoscine) for preventing and treating motion sickness. *Cochrane Database Syst Rev.* 2011;(6):CD002851.
3. Lee EJ, Frazier SK. The efficacy of acupressure for symptom management: a systematic review. *J Pain Symptom Manage.* 2011;42(4):589–603.
4. Soto E, Vega R. Neuropharmacology of vestibular system disorders. *Curr Neuropharmacol.* 2010;8(1):26–40.
5. Furman JM, Marcus DA, Balaban CD. Rizatriptan reduces vestibular-induced motion sickness in migraineurs. *J Headache Pain.* 2011;12(1):81–88.
6. Marx W, Kiss N, Isenring L. Is ginger beneficial for nausea and vomiting? An update of the literature. *Curr Opin Support Palliat Care.* 2015;9(2):189–195.

ADDITIONAL READING

- Bertolini G, Straumann D. Moving in a moving world: a review on vestibular motion sickness. *Front Neurol.* 2016;7:14.
- Murdin L, Golding J, Bronstein A. Managing motion sickness. *BMJ.* 2011;343:d7430.

 SEE ALSO

Algorithm: Dizziness

 CODES

ICD10

T75.3XXA Motion sickness, initial encounter

CLINICAL PEARLS

- The scopolamine transdermal patch is first line for prevention of motion sickness. It should be applied at least 4 hours before travel, although it is most effective if placed 12 hours before departure.
- First-generation antihistamines are also effective, although sedating. They should be administered 30 to 60 minutes before departure.
- Nonsedating antihistamines, ondansetron, and ginger root are not effective in the prevention or treatment of motion sickness.
- Although acupressure wristbands have been found to be effective by systematic reviews in postoperative and chemotherapy-induced nausea and vomiting, as well as hyperemesis gravidarum, conflicting data exist for use with motion sickness.

M

MULTIPLE MYELOMA
Nida (Joy) Emko, MD, FAAFP

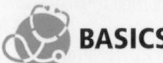

BASICS

DESCRIPTION
- Multiple myeloma (MM) is a clonal proliferation of malignant plasma cells.
- This clonal proliferation in the bone marrow (BM) can cause extensive skeletal destruction with osteolytic lesions and pathologic fractures.
- The malignant plasma cells produce monoclonal protein in the blood and urine.
- MM is also characterized by hypercalcemia, increased susceptibility to infections, renal impairment, and end-organ damage.
- Monoclonal gammopathy of undetermined significance (MGUS) is a common disorder with limited monoclonal plasma cell proliferation that can progress to MM at rate of ~1% per year.
- MGUS can progress to smoldering or asymptomatic MM and eventually to symptomatic MM.
- Synonym(s): plasma cell myeloma; plasma cell leukemia

EPIDEMIOLOGY
- Accounts for 1.8% of all cancers and slightly >10% of hematologic malignancies in the United States
- Median age of diagnosis is 66 years.
- Slight male predominance. Blacks about 2 to 3 times more commonly affected than whites; less common in Asians

Incidence
6 to 7 new cases per 100,000 annually in the United States

Prevalence
In 2015, there were ~124,733 cases in the United States.

ETIOLOGY AND PATHOPHYSIOLOGY
- Clonal proliferation of plasma cells derived from postgerminal center B cells
- Plasma cells undergo multiple chromosomal mutations to progress to MM.
- Genetic damage in developing B lymphocytes at time of isotype switching, transforming normal plasma cells into malignant cells, arising from single clone
- Earliest chromosomal translocations involve immunoglobulin (Ig) heavy chains on chromosome 14q32, with the translocation at t(4;14), t(14;16), t(14;20), and deletion, del(17p) having a poorer prognosis.
- Malignant cells multiply in BM, suppressing normal BM cells and producing large quantities of monoclonal Ig (M) protein.
- Malignant cells stimulate osteoclasts that cause bone resorption and inhibit osteoblasts that form new bone, causing lytic bone lesions.

Genetics
Rare family clusters; the hyperphosphorylated form of paratarg-7, a protein of unknown significance, is inherited as an autosomal dominant trait in familial cases of MM and MGUS, suggesting a potential pathogenic role.

RISK FACTORS
- Most cases have no known risks associated.
- Older age; immunosuppression; and chemicals like dioxin, herbicides, insecticides, petroleum, heavy metals, plastics, and ionizing radiation increase the risk of MM.
- MGUS stage consistently precedes MM.

COMMONLY ASSOCIATED CONDITIONS
Secondary amyloidosis commonly due to MM

DIAGNOSIS

HISTORY
- 34% of patients are asymptomatic at the time of presentation.
- Hypercalcemia (28%): anorexia, abdominal pain, somnolence, polydipsia, polyuria, dehydration
- Elevated creatinine (48%)
- Anemia (73%)
- Bony lesions (80%): lytic lesions causing bone pain (58%) (1), osteoporosis, or pathologic fracture (26–34%)
- Other symptoms: fatigue (32%), peripheral neuropathy (PN), weight loss (24%), recurrent infections, hyperviscosity syndrome, and cord compression

PHYSICAL EXAM
- Dehydration
- Skin findings of amyloidosis: waxy papules, nodules, or plaques that may be evident in the eyelids, retroauricular region, neck, or inguinal and anogenital regions; petechiae and ecchymosis; "pinch purpura"
- Extramedullary plasmacytomas can present as large, purplish, subcutaneous masses.
- Hyperviscosity syndrome in 7%: retinal hemorrhages, prolonged bleeding, neurologic changes
- Tender bones and masses

DIFFERENTIAL DIAGNOSIS
- MGUS
- Smoldering MM (SMM)
- Metastatic carcinoma (kidney, breast, non–small cell lung cancer)
- Waldenström macroglobulinemia
- AL amyloidosis
- Solitary plasmacytoma
- Polyneuropathy, organomegaly, endocrinopathy, M protein, skin changes (POEMS) syndrome

DIAGNOSTIC TESTS & INTERPRETATION
Criteria for diagnosis: The diagnosis of MM requires the following (2)[A]:
- BM involvement with ≥10% of plasma cells or the presence of a plasmacytoma and any one or more of the following myeloma-defining events:
  - Evidence of end-organ damage that can be attributed to the underlying plasma cell proliferative disorder, specifically:
    - Hypercalcemia: serum calcium >0.25 mmol/L (>1 mg/dL) higher than the upper limit of normal or >2.75 mmol/L (>11 mg/dL)
    - Renal insufficiency: creatinine clearance <40 mL/min or serum creatinine >177 μmol/L (>2 mg/dL)
    - Anemia: hemoglobin value of >20 g/L below the lower limit of normal or a hemoglobin value <100 g/L
    - Bone lesions: one or more osteolytic lesions on skeletal radiography, CT, or PET-CT
  - Any one or more of the following biomarkers of malignancy:
    - Clonal BM plasma cell percentage ≥60%
    - Involved:uninvolved serum free light chain (FLC) ratio ≥100
    - >1 focal lesion on MRI studies

Initial Tests (lab, imaging)
- CBC with differential to evaluate anemia and other cytopenias with evaluation of peripheral blood smear
- BUN, creatinine (elevated creatinine due to myeloma cast nephropathy)
- Serum electrolytes, serum albumin, serum calcium
- Serum lactate dehydrogenase (LDH), β_2-microglobulin
- Serum protein electrophoresis (SPEP), serum immunofixation electrophoresis (SIFE): M protein level elevated
- Quantitative serum Ig levels: IgG, IgA, and IgM
- Quantitative serum FLC levels: κ and λ chains
- ESR, C-reactive protein: elevated
- Urine analysis: 24-hour urine for protein, urine protein electrophoresis (UPEP), urine immunofixation electrophoresis (UIFE); 20% positive urine protein (3)[A]:
  - Urinalysis dip is often negative for protein because this test identifies albumin, and the protein in MM is Bence Jones (BJ) monoclonal protein.
- CRAB: hypercalcemia, renal insufficiency, anemia, and bone lesions
- Cross sectional imaging is preferred over plain radiographs for the detection of bone involvement (4)[A].
- Recommend whole body low-dose CT as a baseline assessment of bone involvement because it is quick, convenient, relatively sensitive, and cost effective.
- Skeletal surveys are reserved for patients who are unable to undergo low-dose whole body CT, MRI, and PET.

Follow-Up Tests & Special Considerations
- For patients with suspected SMM (no bone lesions on CT), a whole body MRI or MRI of the spine and pelvis is recommended to evaluate for cord compression.
- For patients with suspected extramedullary disease outside of the spine, a whole body PET/CT is recommended.
- Baseline bone densitometry may be indicated (3)[A].
- BM aspiration and biopsy for histology, immunohistochemistry, flow cytometry, cytogenetics, and fluorescence in situ hybridization (FISH) as well as to monitor response to treatment
- SPEP with SIFE: M protein helps to track progression of myeloma and response to treatment.
- Serum Igs and FLCs can be used to monitor response or relapse.
- Plasma cell labeling index may be helpful to identify the fraction of the myeloma cell population that is proliferating (3)[A].

Diagnostic Procedures/Other
Staging to determine disease burden:
- Durie-Salmon stage
  - Stage I: low tumor cell mass: <0.6 × 10^{12} cells/m^2 plus all of the following: hemoglobin >10 g/dL, M protein <5 g/dL if IgG or <3 g/dL if IgA, normal serum calcium, urine BJ protein <4 g/24 hr, no generalized lytic bone lesions
  - Stage II: neither stage I nor stage III
  - Stage III: high tumor cell mass: >1.2 × 10^{12} cells/m^2 plus one or more of the following: hemoglobin <8.5 g/L, serum calcium >12 mg/dL, bone lesions, M protein >7 g/dL if IgG and >5 g/dL if IgA, urine BJ protein >12 g/24 hr, advanced lytic bone lesions
- International Staging System (ISS)
  - Stage I: albumin ≥3.5 g/dL and β_2-microglobulin <3.5 μg/mL
  - Stage II: neither stage I nor stage III
  - Stage III: β_2-microglobulin ≥5.5 μg/mL
  - Revised ISS (R-ISS) combines ISS information with chromosomal abnormalities and LDH to provide better prognostic information for MM (5)[A].

- Mayo Stratification of Myeloma and Risk-Adapted Therapy (mSMART)
  - Standard risk: >t(11;14), t(6;14), and hyperdiploidy
  - Intermediate risk: t(4;14), del(13q) by cytogenetics, hypodiploidy
  - High risk: t(14;16), t(14;20), del(17 p), and plasma cell labeling index >3%

Test Interpretation
BM involvement with plasma cells ≥10%; Russell bodies

TREATMENT

- Treatment varies depending on level of disease activity and stage of MM.
- Key determinant factor in choosing chemotherapy regimen is to establish if the patient is an autologous stem cell transplant (ASCT) candidate or not.
- Treatment protocols vary by institution and patient.
- ASCT following induction chemotherapy is standard of care for patients with symptomatic disease.

GENERAL MEASURES
Maintain adequate hydration to prevent renal insufficiency. All patients receiving primary melanoma therapy should be given bisphosphonates initially (3)[A].

MEDICATION
- Induction chemotherapy for ASCT-eligible patients (6)[C]:
  - Preferred treatments for transplant candidates: bortezomib/lenalidomide/dexamethasone or bortezomib/cyclophosphamide/dexamethasone (preferred in acute renal insufficiency)
  - Other recommended regimens: bortezomib/doxorubicin/dexamethasone, carfilzomib/lenalidomide/dexamethasone or ixazomib/lenalidomide/dexamethasone
  - Three-drug regimens preferred; two-drug regimens can be used for elderly or frail patients.
  - Lenalidomide is recommended for maintenance therapy after ASCT; lower rates of progressive disease but higher rates of second primary cancers
  - Bortezomib an option for maintenance therapy after ASCT
- Induction chemotherapy for ASCT-ineligible patients:
  - Same regimens as ASCT-eligible patients as well as lenalidomide/low-dose dexamethasone or daratumumab/bortezomib/melphalan/prednisone
  - Other recommended regimens: carfilzomib/lenalidomide/dexamethasone, carfilzomib/cyclophosphamide/dexamethasone, or ixazomib/lenalidomide/dexamethasone
  - Lenalidomide or bortezomib are options for maintenance therapy for non-ASCT patients after primary treatment.

First Line
- Proteasome inhibitors
  - Blocks ubiquitin-proteasome catalytic pathway in cells by binding to the 20S proteasome complex
  - Consider herpes simplex virus (HSV) prophylaxis.
  - Bortezomib: IV or SC; SC has lower risk of PN. Toxicity: PN, cytopenia, nausea, anorexia, leukopenia, thrombocytopenia, rash
  - Carfilzomib: IV, 2nd-generation proteasome inhibitor. Better progression free survival and overall survival than bortezomib. Toxicity: fever, diarrhea, anemia, thrombocytopenia, fatigue; can have hypersensitivity reaction after infusion
  - Ixazomib—PO. Toxicity: PN, diarrhea, thrombocytopenia, neutropenia, back pain, edema

- Cyclophosphamide
  - Nitrogen mustard–derivative alkylating agent
  - Often used in combination with prednisone or thalidomide in cases of relapsed disease
  - Toxicity: cytopenia, anaphylaxis, interstitial pulmonary fibrosis, secondary malignancy, impaired fertility
- Immunomodulators
  - Thalidomide and lenalidomide
    - Works by antiangiogenesis inhibition, immunomodulation, and inhibition of tumor necrosis factor
    - Toxicity: birth defects, deep vein thrombosis (DVT), neuropathy, rash, nausea, bradycardia
    - DVT prophylaxis, usually with aspirin
- Dexamethasone
  - Low doses (40 mg/wk) superior to higher doses
  - Increases risk of DVT
- Bisphosphonates (3)[A]
  - No effect on mortality but decrease pain, pathologic vertebral fractures, and fractures of other bones
  - No evidence of superior outcomes for any particular aminobisphosphonate or non-aminobisphosphonate; zoledronate was shown to be better than placebo and etidronate for improving certain outcomes.
  - Dose-adjust/monitor renal function.
  - Monitor for osteonecrosis of jaw.

Second Line
- Multiple regimens can be used as salvage therapy to treat relapsed or refractory M (7)[A].
- If relapse occurs >6 months after completing initial primary treatment, can use same regimen for retreatment
- Daratumumab: IgGκ1 monoclonal Ab against CD38. Toxicity: fatigue, back pain, lymphocytopenia, neutropenia, anemia, thrombocytopenia, cough, infusion-related reaction
- Elotuzumab: IgG1 immunostimulatory monoclonal antibody directed against CS1 (SLAMF7). Toxicity: fatigue, PN, hyperglycemia, hypocalcemia, infection, cough

ISSUES FOR REFERRAL
For spinal or other bone pathology, refer to orthopedics for support.

ADDITIONAL THERAPIES
- Local radiation therapy for bone pain
- Effective pain management; avoid NSAIDs due to nephrotoxicity.
- Aspirin 81 to 325 mg is recommended for patients treated with immunomodulators.
- Kyphoplasty/vertebroplasty: Consider for symptomatic vertebral compressions.
- Plasmapheresis for hyperviscosity syndrome
- Erythropoietin for selected patients with anemia
- Patients should receive vaccines for pneumococcus and influenza.
- Do not administer live-virus vaccines.

ADMISSION, INPATIENT, AND NURSING CONSIDERATIONS
Indications: pain, infections, cytopenia, renal failure, bone complications, spinal cord compression
- Avoid IV radiographic contrast materials due to risk for contrast-induced nephropathy.
- Adequate hydration
- Manage hypercalcemia and control hyperuricemia.

 ONGOING CARE

PATIENT EDUCATION
- http://myeloma.org/Main.action
- http://www.nccn.org/patients/guidelines/myeloma/

PROGNOSIS
- The 5-year survival rate is around 50%.
- Median survival by R-ISS stage:
  - Stage I: has not been reached
  - Stage II: 83 months
  - Stage III: 43 months
- Median survival in patients with high-risk MM (see staging for definition) is <2 to 3 years, even after ASCT; standard risk has median overall survival of 6 to 7 years.

COMPLICATIONS
Many, including infection, pain, lytic bone lesions, hypercalcemia, hyperuricemia, spinal cord compression, anemia, hyperviscosity syndrome, amyloidosis, renal insufficiency

REFERENCES
1. Palumbo A, Anderson K. Multiple myeloma. *N Engl J Med*. 2011;364(11):1046–1060.
2. Rajkumar SV, Dimopoulos MA, Palumbo A, et al. International Myeloma Working Group updated criteria for the diagnosis of multiple myeloma. *Lancet Oncol*. 2014;15(12):e538–e548.
3. Mhaskar R, Kumar A, Miladinovic B, et al. Bisphosphonates in multiple myeloma: an updated network meta-analysis. *Cochrane Database Syst Rev*. 2017;(12):CD003188.
4. Hillengass J, Moulopoulos LA, Delorme S, et al. Whole-body computed tomography versus conventional skeletal survey in patients with multiple myeloma: a study of the International Myeloma Working Group. *Blood Cancer J*. 2017;7(8):e599.
5. Palumbo A, Avet-Loiseau H, Oliva S, et al. Revised international staging system for multiple myeloma: a report from International Myeloma Working Group. *J Clin Oncol*. 2015;33(26):2863–2869.
6. National Comprehensive Cancer Network. NCCN clinical practice guidelines in oncology: multiple myeloma. https://www.nccn.org/professionals/physician_gls/default.aspx#myeloma. Accessed October 30, 2018.
7. Rajkumar SV. Multiple myeloma: 2018 update on diagnosis, risk-stratification, and management. *Am J Hematol*. 2018;93:1091–1110.

CODES

ICD10
- C90.00 Multiple myeloma not having achieved remission
- C90.01 Multiple myeloma in remission
- C90.02 Multiple myeloma in relapse

CLINICAL PEARLS
- MM is a plasma cell malignancy that causes end-organ damage.
- Look for presence of "CRAB."
- Suspect MM if high total protein-to-albumin ratio is present.
- Maintain high index of suspicion for spinal cord compression.
- Avoid nephrotoxins (radiographic contrast material, NSAIDs, dehydration).
- Patients with MM are immunocompromised.

M

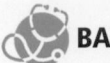

MULTIPLE SCLEROSIS

Jack R. Stacey, MD • Andrew J. McDermott, MD, FAAFP

BASICS

DESCRIPTION

- An autoimmune disease directed against components of the myelin sheath causing demyelination often leading to progressive axonal loss and eventual CNS atrophy affecting primarily white matter but may also damage grey matter and overlying meninges
- Four clinical subtypes of multiple sclerosis (MS):
  - Clinically isolated syndrome (CIS): a patient's initial symptom characteristic of CNS demyelination that may be due to MS but does not fulfill the criteria of dissemination in time. Approximately 60% of individuals diagnosed with CIS will later relapse and be diagnosed with MS.
  - Relapsing-remitting multiple sclerosis (RRMS): episodic flare-ups occurring over days to weeks between periods of neurologic stability. During attacks, new symptoms may present, whereas previous symptoms may worsen. Complete recovery of residual deficits may ensue following each bout (~90% of patients).
  - Secondary progressive multiple sclerosis (SPMS): a gradual decline in disease status after an initial relapsing-remitting disease course. Progressive phase may be associated with acute exacerbations. SPMS is often diagnosed retrospectively.
  - Primary progressive multiple sclerosis (PPMS): a progressive decline in disease status and accumulation of disability from onset of disease without an initial relapsing-remitting disease course (~10% of patients) (1)

Pregnancy Considerations

- Pregnancy is not precluded in MS; however, multidisciplinary pregnancy planning is essential.
- In most cases, MS treatment should be discontinued during pregnancy.
- A majority of patients experience reduced disease exacerbations during pregnancy, but frequency of relapse typically increases in the postpartum period.
- MS therapy should be promptly resumed after delivery, particularly for individuals with very active disease prior to conception.
- All drugs licensed for MS treatment are contraindicated during breastfeeding. Patients desiring to breastfeed should carefully consider risk of delaying MS treatment (2).

EPIDEMIOLOGY

MS is a complex condition that is multifactorial, and although advances in genomics and immunology have increased our understanding of the disease process, much is yet to be discovered. It most often affects Caucasian women in their 2nd and 3rd generations of life and is more common in those with first-degree relatives with the disease.

Incidence

- Women (worldwide): 3.6 cases per 100,000 person-years
- Men (worldwide): 2.0 cases per 100,000 person-years

Prevalence

- United States: ~400,000 MS patients
- Worldwide: ~2,500,000 MS patients

ETIOLOGY AND PATHOPHYSIOLOGY

- Predominately an autoimmune process driven by T cells and B cells against the myelin sheath. Dysregulation and mistaken antigen identity lead CD4 T cells to cross the blood–brain barrier and recognize proteins on the surface of the myelin sheath. Cytokines, interferon-γ, and tumor necrosis factor-α are subsequently released, and activation of macrophages and B cells leads to oligodendrocyte and myelin destruction.
- Following demyelination, faster salutatory nerve conduction velocities (impulses jumping between nodes of Ranvier) are replaced with considerably slower continuous nerve velocities. These changes in the acute setting lead to the focal neurologic deficits associated with MS.
- Oligodendrocytes, which have survived, or ones formed from precursor cells, are able to partially remyelinate stripped axons, producing scars which overtime can lead to irreversible axonal loss and brain atrophy.
- The majority of axons are typically lost from the lateral corticospinal (motor) tracts of the spinal cord. MS was once thought to be a disease of strictly affecting white matter tracts; however, there is increasing evidence of inflammatory damage within the cortical grey matter and overlying meninges (1).

Genetics

- MS is polygenic and does not follow a mendelian inheritance pattern. Those with affected first-degree relatives are 5 to 7 times more likely to be diagnosed.
- Over 100 genetic loci have been associated with MS suggesting that it is ultimately an antigen-specific autoimmune process. Most commonly, these are mapped to the class II region of the HLA gene cluster. The most common being the HLA-DRB1 locus on chromosome 6. These produce major histocompatibility complexes with high-binding affinity for myelin basic proteins.
- Although not fully understood, variations of natural killer cells and their polymorphic killer-immunoglobulin-like receptors are thought to play a major role in the MS disease process (1).

RISK FACTORS

- Age: peak incidence ages 15 to 45 years, mean age 28 to 31 years (slightly earlier in women than men)
- Race: Caucasian > Afro-Caribbean > East-Asian
- Gender: 2 to 3 times more common in women
- Infectious: prior infections with Epstein-Barr virus and history of infectious mononucleosis
- Substance: tobacco smoking
- Geographic: Historically, proximity to the equator and its correlation with increased vitamin D exposure were inversely proportional to MS incidence. However, recently this association has been less obvious and may be due to lifestyle changes that have led to decreased sun exposure in these locations (1).

GENERAL PREVENTION

No known prevention strategies

COMMONLY ASSOCIATED CONDITIONS

- Internuclear ophthalmoplegia: Injury to the medial longitudinal fasciculus causes impaired adduction of the affected eye.
- Optic neuritis: inflammation of optic nerve resulting in loss of vision
- Associated with numerous other autoimmune processes

DIAGNOSIS

A person with MS can present with a number of neurologic signs and symptoms depending on the locations of the lesion. The essential means of diagnoses is to demonstrate evidence of CNS lesions that are separated by both time and space that are not more likely due to a separate disease process.

HISTORY

Symptoms can vary widely but may include fatigue, epilepsy, dizziness, visual disturbances, facial palsy, dysphagia, muscle weakness or spasms, hyperesthesia or paresthesia, pain, bowel or bladder incontinence, urinary frequency or retention, or impotence (1).

PHYSICAL EXAM

- Weakness
- Internuclear ophthalmoplegia
- Gait disturbance
- Foot drop
- Hyperesthesia or paresthesia
- Cerebellar dysarthria (scanning speech)
- Spasticity (especially in lower extremities)
- Uhthoff phenomenon: Symptoms worsen with exposure to higher than usual temperature.
- Lhermitte sign: electric-like shocks extending down the spine caused by neck movement, especially flexion

DIFFERENTIAL DIAGNOSIS

- Lyme disease
- Systemic lupus erythematosus
- Antiphospholipid antibody syndrome
- Neuromyelitis optica
- Epilepsy
- Progressive multifocal leukoencephalopathy
- CNS neoplasms
- Guillain-Barré syndrome
- Metachromatic leukodystrophy
- Neurosarcoidosis
- Stroke
- Primary cerebral angiitis
- Neurosyphilis
- Cobalamin (vitamin B_{12}) deficiency
- Acute disseminated encephalomyelitis
- Behçet disease
- Normal pressure hydrocephalus

DIAGNOSTIC TESTS & INTERPRETATION

- MRI of head/spine: Periventricular and callosal lesions are relatively specific for MS. The additions of gadolinium can help identify active lesions.
- Lumbar puncture: Cerebrospinal fluid can reveal elevated or normal total protein levels. Oligoclonal immunoglobulin G bands are seen in approximately 90% of MS but may be absent early in the disease process. Positive findings are not diagnostic for MS but may be beneficial if other diagnostic criteria are equivocal.
- Blood tests: Antinuclear antibody, antineutrophil cytoplasmic antibody, anti–double-stranded DNA antibody, extractable nuclear antigen, antiphospholipid antibody, compliment, erythrocyte sedimentation rate, immunoglobulin G, immunoglobulin M, rheumatoid factor, and Lyme disease antibody can be used to rule out alternative diagnosis (1)[B].

- McDonald criteria for diagnosing MS: must demonstrate dissemination in space and time of CNS lesions (3)[C]
  - Dissemination in space: ≥1 T_2 lesion on MRI in at least 2 of 4 CNS regions typically affected by MS: periventricular, juxtacortical, infratentorial, or spinal cord or by waiting for another clinical event implying a different CNS location
  - Dissemination in time: simultaneous presentation of asymptomatic gadolinium-enhanced and nonenhancing lesions at any moment or a new T_2 and/or gadolinium-enhanced lesion on an MRI when compared baseline scans

Diagnostic Procedures/Other
Evoked potentials: Assess function of visual, auditory, and somatosensory motor CNS pathways by measuring CNS electric potentials evoked by neural stimulation. A marked delay, without a clinical manifestation, is suggestive of a demyelinating disorder. Visual evoked potentials are delayed in 80–90% of individuals with MS (1).

TREATMENT

GENERAL MEASURES
- Holistic multidisciplinary team approach is paramount.
- Three main categories currently exist for MS treatment: treatment for acute relapses, treatment for reducing MS-related activity using disease-modifying agents, and symptomatic therapy.
- The use of disease-modifying treatments early in the disease process is likely to slow overall disease progression and should be managed by a MS specialist (1)[C].

MEDICATION
- Acute relapse treatment (1,4)[A]
  - Methylprednisolone 0.5 g PO daily for 5 days or 1 g IV daily for 3 to 5 days; without subsequent oral tapering; a second course may be given.
    - Side effects: increased infection risk, adrenal insufficiency, Cushing syndrome, fluid retention, hypokalemia, GI disturbances, headache, emotional lability
  - ACTH gel 80 U IM or SC daily for 5 to 15 days
    - Side effects: similar to methylprednisolone
  - Plasmapheresis
- Disease-modifying treatment (1,5)[B]
  - IFN-β_{1a} (Avonex) 30 μg IM weekly
  - IFN-β_{1a} (Rebif) 22 or 44 μg SC 3 times per week
  - IFN-β_{1b} (Betaseron/Betaferon/Extavia) 250 μg SC every other day
    - Monitoring: CBC, LFTs, TSH
    - Side effects: flu-like symptoms, depression, skin site reactions, thyroid dysfunction, liver enzyme abnormalities
  - Glatiramer acetate (Copaxone) 20 mg SC daily
    - Monitoring: none
    - Side effects: skin site reactions, immediate postinjection reaction, lipoatrophy
  - Dimethyl fumarate (Tecfidera) 120 to 240 mg PO twice daily
    - Monitoring: CBC, LFTs
    - Side effects: diarrhea, cramps, LFT elevation, nausea, flushing
  - Teriflunomide (Aubagio) 7 to 14 mg PO daily
    - Monitoring: CBC, LFTs, UA
    - Side effects: nasopharyngitis, headache, diarrhea, fatigue, back pain, influenza, hair thinning, LFT elevation, nausea, UTI

- Natalizumab (Tysabri) 300 mg IV every 28 days
  - Monitoring: CBC, LFTs
  - Side effects: headache, fatigue, UTI, hypersensitivity reaction
- Alemtuzumab (Lemtrada) 12 to 24 mg IV for 5 days then 3 days 12 months after initial treatment
  - Monitoring: CBC, LFTs, TSH
  - Side effects: immune thrombocytopenic purpura, autoimmune thyroid-related problems, headaches, flushing
- Fingolimod (Gilenya) 0.5 mg PO daily
  - Monitoring: ECG, CBC, LFTs, eye exam
  - Side effects: 1st degree AV block, bradycardia, macular edema, shingles, worsening pulmonary function, skin cancer, back pain
- Symptomatic therapies (1)[B]
  - Spasticity: baclofen, dantrolene, diazepam, tizanidine, cannabis extract (nabiximols), botulinum toxin, physiotherapy
  - Pain: amitriptyline, pregabalin, gabapentin, cannabis extract (nabiximols)
  - Bladder dysfunction: oxybutynin, tolterodine, cannabis extract (nabiximols), catheterization, intravesical botulinum toxin
  - Constipation: natural or other laxatives, stool softeners, bulk-producing agents
  - Erectile dysfunction: sildenafil
  - Fatigue: amantadine, modafinil
  - Tremors: clonazepam, primidone, β-blockers
  - Depression: SSRI (citalopram), SSNRI (venlafaxine), TCA (amitriptyline)
  - Walking: fampridine

ADDITIONAL THERAPIES
- Cognitive behavioral therapy
- Physical, occupational, and speech therapy
- Yoga and water-based exercise
- Massage therapy

ONGOING CARE

FOLLOW-UP RECOMMENDATIONS
Patient Monitoring
Assessing the severity of neurologic impairment from MS can be done using the Kurtzke Expanded Disability Status Scale (EDSS): The EDSS quantifies severity of disability using eight functional systems (FS): pyramidal, cerebellar, brainstem, sensory, bowel and bladder, visual, and cerebral. EDSS scoring system (6)[C]:
- 1.0—no disability, minimal signs in 1 FS
- 2.0—minimal disability in 1 FS
- 3.0—moderate disability in 1 FS or mild disability in 3 to 4 FS, but fully ambulatory
- 4.0—ambulatory without aid or rest for ~500 m
- 5.0—ambulatory without aid or rest for ~200 m
- 6.0—intermittent/constant unilateral assistance (cane, crutch, or brace); must be able to walk 100 m
- 7.0—unable to walk beyond 5 m even with aid; essentially restricted to wheelchair, wheels self and transfers alone; active in wheelchair for ~12 hr/day
- 8.0—essentially restricted to bed, chair, or wheelchair; may be out of bed most of the day; retains self-care functions, generally effective use of arms
- 9.0—helpless, bedbound; but patient can communicate, eat
- 10.0—death due to MS

DIET
High fiber and fluids to prevent constipation

PATIENT EDUCATION
National Multiple Sclerosis Society: 1-800-344-4867 or www.nationalmssociety.org/

PROGNOSIS
- Differs in each individual based on numerous factors
- Approximately half of all patients will be unable to maintain a career 10 years after MS onset.
- Almost a third of patients will ultimately be wheelchair bound.
- Average life expectancy is 5 to 10 years less than the unaffected population (1).

COMPLICATIONS
Mortality secondary to MS relapse is unusual; death more commonly associated with a complication of MS such as infection in a person with more disability

REFERENCES
1. Raffel J, Wakerley B, Nicholas R. Multiple sclerosis. *Medicine*. 2016;44(9):537–541.
2. Amato MP, Bertolotto A, Brunelli R, et al. Management of pregnancy-related issues in multiple sclerosis patients: the need for an interdisciplinary approach. *Neurol Sci*. 2017;38(10):1849–1858.
3. Polman CH, Reingold SC, Banwell B, et al. Diagnostic criteria for multiple sclerosis: 2010 revisions to the McDonald criteria. *Ann Neurol*. 2011;69(2):292–302.
4. Berkovich R. Treatment of acute relapses in multiple sclerosis. *Neurotherapeutics*. 2013;10(1):97–105.
5. Castro-Borrero W, Graves D, Frohman TC, et al. Current and emerging therapies in multiple sclerosis: a systematic review. *Ther Adv Neurol Disord*. 2012;5(4):205–220.
6. Kurtzke JF. Rating neurologic impairment in multiple sclerosis: an expanded disability status scale (EDSS). *Neurology*. 1983;33(11):1444–1452.

ADDITIONAL READING
Dendrou CA, Fugger L, Friese MA. Immunopathology of multiple sclerosis. *Nat Rev Immunol*. 2015;15(9):545–558.

CODES

ICD10
G35 Multiple sclerosis

CLINICAL PEARLS
- MS is an immune-mediated inflammatory disease causing demyelination, neuronal loss, and scarring within the CNS.
- Diagnosis is made with the McDonald criteria and must demonstrate damage to the CNS disseminated in space and time.
- Disease treatments consist of acute relapse, disease-modifying agents, and symptomatic therapies.
- MS treatment modalities are complex and rapidly changing. A patient's treatment should be guided by a MS specialist, but multiprofessional therapy is necessary.
- New approaches to manipulate inflammation, neurodegeneration, and remyelination such as hematopoietic stem cell transplants are being testing in clinical trials and may dramatically alter treatment and prevention of MS in the future (1).

M

MUMPS

Frances Y. Wu, MD, FAAFP

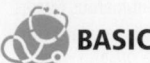 **BASICS**

An acute, generalized paramyxovirus infection typically presenting with unilateral or bilateral parotitis

DESCRIPTION
- Can be asymptomatic in 1/3 of nonimmune individuals and 60% of previously vaccinated cases
- Painful parotitis in 95% of symptomatic mumps cases
- Epidemics in late winter and spring; transmission by respiratory secretions
- Incubation period is 14 to 24 days.
- System(s) affected: hematologic/lymphatic/immunologic, reproductive, skin, exocrine
- Synonym(s): epidemic parotitis; infectious parotitis

EPIDEMIOLOGY
- 85% of mumps cases occur prior to 15 years of age.
- Adult cases are typically more severe.
- Predominant sex: male = female
- Geriatric population: Most adults are immune.
- Acute epidemic mumps
  - Most cases occur in unvaccinated children 5 to 15 years of age.
  - Multiple recent outbreaks in U.S. college students
- Mumps is unusual in children <2 years of age.
- Period of maximal communicability is 24 hours before to 72 hours after onset of parotitis.

Incidence
- From January 1 to August 11, 2018, 1,665 cases reported in United States from 47 states and District of Columbia
- Since 1967 (national vaccination program), case rate has dropped from 100/100,000 to 1.8/100,000.
- Occasional regional epidemic outbreaks

Prevalence
- 0.0064/100,000 persons in United States
- 90% of adults are seropositive.

ETIOLOGY AND PATHOPHYSIOLOGY
Mumps virus replicates in glandular epithelium of parotid gland, pancreas, and testes, leading to interstitial edema and inflammation.
- Interstitial glandular hemorrhage may occur.
- Pressure caused by testicular edema against the tunica albuginea can lead to necrosis and loss of function.

RISK FACTORS
- Foreign travel: Most of Africa, southern Asia, and Japan do *not* vaccinate for mumps.
- Crowded environments such as dormitories, barracks, or detention facilities increase risk of transmission.
- Immunity wanes after single-dose vaccination. With 2 dose schedule, immunity drops from 95% to 86% after 9 years.

GENERAL PREVENTION
- Vaccination
  - 2 doses of live mumps vaccine or mumps, measles, rubella (MMR) vaccine recommended, first at 12 to 15 months and second at 4 to 6 years. Start at 6 months if foreign travel is planned.
  - 95% effective in clinical studies; field trials show 68–95% efficacy, which may be insufficient for herd immunity to prevent spread.
  - Prevention may require 95% first dose and >80% second-dose adherence.
  - Adverse effects: fever 8/100,000; seizure 25/100,000; thrombocytopenic purpura 3/100,000
  - *No relationship between MMR vaccine and autism celiac disease or multiple sclerosis*
- Immunoglobulin (Ig) does not prevent mumps.
- Postexposure vaccination does not protect from recent exposure (1)[B].
- Isolate hospitalized patients for 5 days after onset.
- Isolate nonimmune individuals for 26 days after last case onset (social quarantine).
- In an epidemic situation, a third dose of MMR is indicated to decrease the attack rate (2)[A].
- Vaccine neutralizing antibodies are still effective against variant strains of mumps virus.
- Live vaccines are contraindicated in immunocompromised such as HIV with CD4 <200, although no reports of disseminated mumps from MMR vaccine in HIV patients.

Pregnancy Considerations
- Live viral vaccines are typically contraindicated in pregnancy; however, vaccination of children should not be delayed due to a pregnant family member.
- Immunization of contacts protects against future (but not current) exposures.

DIAGNOSIS

HISTORY
- Parotid swelling peaks in 1 to 3 days; lasts 3 to 7 days
- Clinical diagnosis (swelling of one or both parotid glands):
  - Lasting ≥2 days
  - No other apparent cause
  - Meningitis without parotitis (rare; 1–10%)
- 1/3 of individuals with mumps may be asymptomatic.
- Rare prodrome of fever, neck ache, and malaise
- Sour foods cause pain in parotid gland region.
- Moderate fever, usually not >104°F (40°C):
  - High fever frequently is associated with complications.

PHYSICAL EXAM
- Painful parotid swelling (unilateral or bilateral) obscures angle of mandible and elevates earlobe.
- Meningeal signs (15%); encephalitis (<1%)
- 2–6% orchitis, polyarthritis, thyroiditis, mastitis, pancreatitis, oophoritis, myocarditis, profound hearing loss. Complications may occur after days to weeks.
- Rare maculopapular, erythematous rash
- Up to 50% of cases are mild.
- Redness at opening of Stensen duct without pus
- Sternal swelling (rare and pathognomonic for mumps)

DIFFERENTIAL DIAGNOSIS
- If not epidemic, other viruses are more common: parainfluenza parotitis, Epstein-Barr virus, coxsackievirus, adenovirus, parvovirus B19, influenza parotitis—several hundred reported in 2016.
- Suppurative parotitis: often associated with *Staphylococcus aureus* (Presence of pus within Wharton duct with parotid massage essentially excludes diagnosis of mumps.)
- Recurrent allergic parotitis
- Salivary calculus with intermittent swelling
- Lymphadenitis from any cause, including HIV infection
- Cytomegalovirus parotitis (immunocompromised)
- Mikulicz syndrome: chronic, painless parotid and lacrimal gland swelling of unknown cause that occurs in tuberculosis, sarcoidosis, lupus, leukemia, lymphosarcoma, and salivary gland tumors
- Sjögren syndrome, diabetes mellitus, uremia, malnutrition
- Drug-related parotid enlargement (iodides, guanethidine, phenothiazine)
- Complications of mumps: 1–10% meningo/encephalitis, orchitis, oophoritis, pancreatitis, polyarthritis, nephritis, myocarditis, prostatitis
- Mumps orchitis must be differentiated from testicular torsion and from chlamydial or bacterial orchitis.

DIAGNOSTIC TESTS & INTERPRETATION
- Buccal swab and serum tests recommended https://www.cdc.gov/mumps/lab/specimen-collect.html
  - IgM titer (positive by day 5 in 100% of nonimmunized patients), rapid EIA for IgM
  - Swab of parotid duct or other affected salivary ducts for rRT-PCR plus viral culture—send to state lab or CDC; most sensitive before day 3 of parotitis
  - Rise in IgG titer samples; order if patient previously immunized: first, sample within 5 days of onset and second, 2 weeks later

- Other potential findings: elevated serum amylase; CSF leukocytosis, or leukopenia
- Testicular ultrasound may help differentiate mumps orchitis from testicular torsion.

Diagnostic Procedures/Other
If meningitis symptoms present, lumbar puncture to exclude bacterial process; CSF pleocytosis, usually lymphocytic, in 65% of patients with parotitis

Test Interpretation
Periductal edema and lymphocytic infiltration of affected glands on biopsy

 ## TREATMENT

- No specific antiviral therapy; supportive care (2)[A]
- Analgesics to relieve pain
- Avoid corticosteroids for mumps orchitis because they can reduce testosterone and increase testicular atrophy.
- IVIG can reduce certain autoimmune-based sequelae:
  – Postinfectious encephalitis; Guillain-Barré syndrome; ITP
- Interferon-α2b improves bilateral orchitis but not testicular atrophy (3)[B].

GENERAL MEASURES
- Hospitalize patients with high fever, pancreatitis, or CNS symptoms for supportive care, steroids, or interferon. Use isolation precautions.
- Orchitis
  – Ice packs to scrotum can help to relieve pain.
  – Scrotal support with adhesive bridge while recumbent and/or athletic supporter while ambulatory

MEDICATION
First Line
- Analgesics and anti-inflammatory medications (acetaminophen, nonsteroidal anti-inflammatory drugs [NSAIDs]) may diminish pain and swelling in acute orchitis and arthritis of mumps.
- May use acetaminophen for fever and/or pain
- Precautions: Avoid aspirin for pain in children as previously associated with Reye syndrome.

Second Line
- Interferon-α2b (3)[B]
- Medicinal herbs and acupuncture have not shown benefit in randomized controlled trials.

ADMISSION, INPATIENT, AND NURSING CONSIDERATIONS
- Hospitalize only if CNS symptoms occur.
- Outpatient supportive care if no complications
- IV fluids if severe nausea or vomiting accompanies pancreatitis

 ## ONGOING CARE

FOLLOW-UP RECOMMENDATIONS
Mumps orchitis:
- Bed rest and local supportive clothing (e.g., two pairs of briefs) or adhesive-tape bridge
- Withhold from school until no longer contagious (9 days after onset of pain).

Patient Monitoring
Most cases will be mild. Monitor hydration status.

DIET
Liquid diet if unable to chew

PATIENT EDUCATION
Orchitis is common in older children but rarely results in sterility, even if bilateral.

PROGNOSIS
- Complete recovery is typical; immunity is lifelong.
- Transient sensorineural hearing loss in 4% of adults
- Recurrence after 2 weeks may be nonepidemic other viral parotitis, but mumps RNA has been found in some recurrent parotitis swabs.

COMPLICATIONS
- May precede, accompany, or follow salivary gland involvement and may occur (rarely) without primary involvement of the parotid gland
- Orchitis more common (6–30%) in postpubertal boys:
  – Starts within 8 days of onset of parotitis
  – Impaired fertility in 13%; absolute sterility is rare.
- Meningitis may present 5 to 10 days after first symptoms. Aseptic meningitis is typically mild, but meningoencephalitis may lead to seizures, paralysis, hydrocephalus, or (in 2% of encephalitis cases) death.
- Acute cerebellar ataxia has been reported after mumps infections; self-resolving in 2 to 3 weeks
- Oophoritis in 7% of postpubertal females; no decreased fertility
- Pancreatitis, usually mild
- Nephritis, thyroiditis, and arthralgias are rare.
- Myocarditis: usually mild but may depress ST segment; may be linked to endocardial fibroelastosis
- Deafness: 1/15,000 unilateral nerve deafness; may not be permanent
- Inflammation about the eye (keratouveitis) is rare.
- Dacryoadenitis, optic neuritis

Pediatric Considerations
- Orchitis is more common in adolescents.
- Young children are less likely to develop complications.
- Most complications occur in postpubertal group.
- Avoid aspirin use in children with viral symptoms.

Pregnancy Considerations
May increase risk of spontaneous pregnancy loss in first trimester. Perinatal mumps often has a benign course.

REFERENCES
1. Fiebelkorn AP, Lawler J, Curns AT, et al. Mumps postexposure prophylaxis with a third dose of measles-mumps-rubella vaccine, Orange County, New York, USA. *Emerg Infect Dis*. 2013;19(9):1411–1417.
2. Albertson JP, Clegg WJ, Reid HD, et al. Mumps outbreak at a university and recommendation for a third dose of measles-mumps-rubella vaccine—Illinois, 2015–2016. *MMWR Morb Mortal Wkly Rep*. 2016;65(29):731–734.
3. Rubin S, Eckhaus M, Rennick LJ, et al. Molecular biology, pathogenesis and pathology of mumps virus. *J Pathol*. 2015;235(2):242–252.

ADDITIONAL READING
- Morita S, Fujiwara K, Fukuda A, et al. The clinical features and prognosis of mumps-associated hearing loss: a retrospective, multi-institutional investigation in Japan. *Acta Otolaryngol*. 2017;137 (Suppl 565):S44–S47.
- Tiffany A, Shannon D, Mamtcheung W, et al. Notes from the field: mumps outbreak—Alaska, May 2017–July 2018. *MMWR Morb Mortal Wkly Rep*. 2018;67(33):940–941.

 ## CODES

ICD10
- B26.9 Mumps without complication
- B26.1 Mumps meningitis
- B26.2 Mumps encephalitis

CLINICAL PEARLS
- Mumps is a clinical diagnosis based on swelling of ≥1 parotid glands for ≥2 days without other obvious cause. Confirm with buccal swab PCR, viral culture, and IgM and IgG serology to identify early in epidemic setting.
- Report positive results to public health authorities.
- Ultrasound helps distinguish testicular torsion from testicular pain related to mumps orchitis.
- A history of vaccination with MMR does not exclude mumps.
- The MMR vaccine is 68–95% effective after two immunizations. Immunity wanes over time.

MUSCULAR DYSTROPHY

Nimmy Thakolkaran, MD • George G.A. Pujalte, MD, FACSM

BASICS

- Primary inherited myopathies caused by dysfunctional proteins of muscle fibers and extracellular matrix
- Distribution of weakness, other associated symptoms, and disease prognosis depend on the specific gene affected and severity of the mutation.

DESCRIPTION

- Duchenne muscular dystrophy (DMD)
  - Highest incidence muscular dystrophy, X-linked inheritance, early onset, progressive
  - Patients are wheelchair-dependent by age 13 years.
- Becker muscular dystrophy (BMD)
  - Less severe phenotype compared to DMD; also caused by mutation in *DMD* gene; later onset and milder clinical course
  - Distinction from DMD is clinical: Patients are usually wheelchair-dependent at age 16 years.
  - Collectively referred to as dystrophinopathies
- Myotonic muscular dystrophy (MMD)
  - Myotonia (slow relaxation after muscle contraction), distal and facial weakness
  - Second most common inherited muscle disease
- Facioscapulohumeral muscular dystrophy (FSHMD)
  - Facial and shoulder muscles most affected
  - Third most common inherited muscle disease
- Limb-girdle muscular dystrophy (LGMD)
  - Proximal weakness and atrophy, variable prognosis with many different identified mutations
- Oculopharyngeal muscular dystrophy (OPMD)
  - Usually adult-onset, affects extraocular and pharyngeal muscles; presents with ptosis and dysphagia
- Emery-Dreifuss muscular dystrophy (EDMD)
  - Triad of early development of joint contractures, slowly progressive muscle wasting, and cardiomyopathy; can present as sudden death in apparently healthy, young adults
- Congenital muscular dystrophies (CMD)
  - Heterogeneous group of autosomal recessive myopathic diseases presenting in infancy, with generally poor prognosis
  - Include Fukuyama CMD, Ullrich CMD, Walker-Warburg syndrome, muscle-eye-brain disease

EPIDEMIOLOGY

Incidence

- Duchenne: 1/3,600 male births (1)
- Myotonic dystrophy: 1/10,000 births
- CMD: 0.99 per 100,000
- Other muscular dystrophies vary widely by population but are generally rare.

ETIOLOGY AND PATHOPHYSIOLOGY

Mutations affect proteins connecting cytoskeleton to cell membrane and extracellular matrix, causing muscle fibers to become fragile and easily damaged; muscle weakness and atrophy result.

- DMD/BMD
  - Defective protein is dystrophin, product of the largest human gene, *DMD*; Duchenne phenotype results from mutations that cause profound loss of dystrophin, the protein involved in calcium transport in muscle cells and stabilizing fibers during contraction.
  - Becker phenotype results from less severe mutations in *DMD* gene; patients have low but detectable levels of functional dystrophin.

- MMD: Trinucleotide repeat expansion in the untranslated region of the gene *DMPK* on chromosome 19; encodes myotonin–protein kinase
- LGMD: mutations in genes encoding proteins associated with dystrophin: Calpain-, dysferlin-, and fukutin-related proteins are affected most commonly.
- EDMD: Dysfunctional proteins are associated with the nuclear membrane in muscle fibers; emerin in X-linked form, lamin A/C in autosomal forms
- OPMD: Trinucleotide repeat expansion in *PABPN1* results in nuclear inclusions in muscle cells by hampering normal transport of mRNA from the nucleus.
- FSHMD: deletion in untranslated region of chromosome 4; function of deleted genes is unclear, although the most accepted concept is that they likely affect the expression of multiple genes by epigenetic effects.

Genetics

- X-linked
  - Duchenne and Becker muscular dystrophies
  - Gene located at Xp21
    - 30% of affected males have a de novo mutation (mother is not a carrier).
    - 20% of female carriers have some manifestation of the mutation (usually mild muscle weakness or cardiomyopathy).
- Autosomal dominant
  - Generally later onset and less severe than diseases with recessive or X-linked inheritance
  - FSHMD, OPMD, some forms of LGMD and EDMD
  - Myotonic dystrophy
    - Trinucleotide repeat expansion with more severe phenotype in subsequent generations due to accumulation of repeats
- Autosomal recessive
  - Most types of CMD

GENERAL PREVENTION

Genetic counseling for carriers and prenatal diagnosis

COMMONLY ASSOCIATED CONDITIONS

- Decreased IQ: on average, 1 *SD* below the mean in DMD; speech and language delay
- Dilated cardiomyopathy and conduction abnormalities
  - Can be severe in EDMD
  - Can affect otherwise asymptomatic female carriers of DMD
  - Progressive scoliosis

DIAGNOSIS

HISTORY

- DMD: normal attainment of early motor milestones with subsequent abnormal gait and slowing gross motor development: clumsiness, waddling gait, frequent falls, difficulty running, or climbing stairs
- BMD: progressive difficulty with ambulation and frequent falls in later childhood
- MMD: slurred speech, muscle wasting, difficulty with ambulation; often with family history
- LGMD: back pain, lordosis/inability to rise from a chair, climb stairs, and use arms overhead
- FSHMD: facial weakness, inability to close eyes completely
- EDMD: contractures of elbows and ankles, difficulty with ambulation in teenage years
- OPMD: ptosis and dysphagia; often with family history

PHYSICAL EXAM

- DMD/BMD
  - Proximal muscle weakness; Gower sign: use of arms to push upper body into standing posture from lying prone
  - Trendelenburg gait (hip waddling)
  - Hyporeflexia/areflexia
  - Winged scapulae and lordosis
  - Pseudohypertrophy of the calf (caused by replacement of muscle with fibroadipose tissue)
  - Contractures of lower extremity joints and elbows
- MMD
  - Characteristic facial appearance: narrow face, open triangular mouth, high-arched palate, concave temples, drooping eyelids, frontal balding in males
  - Myotonia: inability to relax muscles after contraction
  - Distal muscle weakness and wasting
- CMD
  - Arthrogryposis (multiple joint contractures); diffuse hypotonia and muscle wasting in an infant

DIFFERENTIAL DIAGNOSIS

- Glycogen storage diseases and other metabolic myopathies
- Mitochondrial myopathies: MELAS (**M**itochondrial **E**ncephalopathy, **L**actic **A**cidosis, and **S**troke-like episodes), MERRF (**M**yoclonus with **E**pilepsy and **R**agged-**R**ed **F**ibers)
- Inflammatory myopathies: polymyositis, dermatomyositis, inclusion-body myositis
- Neuromuscular junction diseases: myasthenia gravis, Lambert-Eaton syndrome
- Motor neuron diseases: amyotrophic lateral sclerosis, spinal muscular atrophy
- Charcot-Marie-Tooth disease
- Friedreich ataxia

DIAGNOSTIC TESTS & INTERPRETATION

Initial Tests (lab, imaging)

- Creatine kinase (CK): initial screening test if MD is suspected (2)[A]
- Elevated in DMD (10 to 100 times); elevated at birth, peaks at time of presentation, and falls during illness
- Initial detected lab abnormality may be elevated aspartate transaminase/alanine transaminase (AST/ALT) originating from muscle.
- Genetic testing/molecular diagnosis
  - For definitive diagnosis in patient with characteristic presentation and elevated CK
  - Deletion and duplication analysis (MLPA or CGH) will identify most patients; followed by genomic sequencing of *DMD* gene for point mutations (3)[A]
  - Genetic testing is available clinically for most other muscular dystrophies.

Diagnostic Procedures/Other

- Muscle biopsy: rarely performed in DMD (dystrophin protein absent); may be helpful in other cases (4)[A]
- Electromyography and nerve conduction studies are not necessary unless considering alternative diagnoses.
- ECG: abnormalities found in >90% of males and up to 10% of female carriers of DMD; Q waves in anterolateral leads, tall R waves in V1, shortened PR interval, arrhythmias, resting sinus tachycardia

Test Interpretation

- Heterogenic muscle fibers: atrophy and hypertrophy of fibers with proliferation of connective tissue in muscle
- Immunohistochemical staining for dystrophin protein
  - DMD: no detectable dystrophin in most fibers; occasional revertant fibers with normal dystrophin
  - BMD: highly variable staining for dystrophin throughout muscle

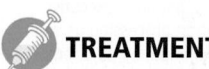 **TREATMENT**

Trials of agents that affect gene expression, such as antisense oligonucleotides, and small molecules that cause skipping of premature stop codons (ataluren) are ongoing; however, steroid treatment is the only clinically available therapy that affects disease progression.

GENERAL MEASURES

- Ambulation prolonged by knee-ankle-foot orthoses
- Serial casting to treat contractures
- Diagnose sleep apnea with polysomnography; treat with noninvasive ventilation.
- Adaptive devices to improve function
- Avoid overexertion and strenuous exercise.

MEDICATION

- Prednisone 0.75 mg/kg/day (4)[A]
  - Slows the decline in muscle function, progression to scoliosis, and degradation of pulmonary function; prolongs functional ambulation; prolongs lifespan; improved cardiac outcomes
  - Therapy should be initiated when there is no longer progress in motor skills, but prior to decline (2).
  - Monitor adverse effects.
    - Bisphosphonates should be considered for preventing loss of bone density; annual exam for cataracts; hypertension should be monitored; no NSAIDs due to risk of peptic ulcer disease (PUD); stress-dose steroids during surgeries and illnesses due to adrenal suppression
    - Patients should be aware of immune suppression and notify emergency providers.
- Deflazacort (0.9 mg/kg) is a recently approved oral corticosteroid in DMD; it acts on muscle regeneration and differentiation (5).
- ACE inhibitors
  - Treatment of cardiomyopathy; may be used in conjunction with β-blockers

ISSUES FOR REFERRAL

- Refer to neuromuscular diseases center for definitive diagnosis and coordinated multidisciplinary care (4).
- Cardiology for management of cardiomyopathy
- Pulmonology for monitoring of pulmonary function and clearance regimen
- Physical medicine and rehabilitation for management of adaptive devices
- Nutrition/swallowing: for normal weight gain, attention for dysphagia
- Psychosocial: learning/behavior and coping assessment, social development (2)

ADDITIONAL THERAPIES

Novel medication: Ataluren interferes with premature stop codons, allowing expression of dystrophin protein. In the 15% of DMD patients with nonsense mutation; FDA approved orphan drug designation (3), completed ACT DMD trial

SURGERY/OTHER PROCEDURES

- Spinal surgery for scoliosis diminishes rate of deformity progression (5)[A].
- Scapular fixation for scapular winging may be beneficial; however, also lacking clinical trials.
- Consider surgical treatment of ankle/knee contractures.
- Surgical procedures should be performed at a center experienced in DMD; total IV anesthesia should be used.

COMPLEMENTARY & ALTERNATIVE MEDICINE

Whole body vibration exercises

ADMISSION, INPATIENT, AND NURSING CONSIDERATIONS

Recognize and mitigate adrenal suppression resulting from corticosteroid dependence (5).

 ONGOING CARE

- Individualized education plan and developmental evaluation for school accommodations
- Maintenance of current influenza and pneumococcal vaccination status

FOLLOW-UP RECOMMENDATIONS
Patient Monitoring

- Electrocardiogram (ECG), echocardiogram, and consultation with a cardiologist at diagnosis and annually after age 10 years
  - Female carriers of DMD mutation should be monitored every 5 years.
- Annual spinal radiography for scoliosis
- Dual energy x-ray absorptiometry (DEXA) scanning and serum marker testing for osteoporosis
- Pulmonary function testing twice yearly if no longer ambulatory
- Psychosocial: coping, emotional adjustment, depression

DIET

- Obesity is common due to steroid treatment and wheelchair confinement: Weight control can improve quality of life.
- Diet may be limited by dysphagia; swallow evaluation can determine appropriate foods; may require gastrostomy
- Calcium and vitamin D supplementation for patients on steroids; monitor vitamin D levels.

PATIENT EDUCATION

- Muscular Dystrophy Association: http://www.mda.org
- Parent Project Muscular Dystrophy: http://www.parentprojectmd.org.

PROGNOSIS

- DMD/BMD
  - Progressive weakness, contractures, inability to walk
  - Kyphoscoliosis and progressive decline in respiratory vital capacity with recurrent pulmonary infections
  - Significantly shortened lifespan (DMD: 16 ± 4 years; BMD: 42 ± 16 years). Respiratory failure cause of death in 90%; remaining due to myocardial disease (heart failure and dysrhythmia) (6)
- Other types: slow progression and near-normal lifespan with functional limitations

COMPLICATIONS

- Cardiac arrhythmia, cardiomyopathy
- Dysphagia, gastroesophageal reflux disease (GERD), constipation
- Scoliosis, joint contractures

- Obstructive sleep apnea
- Malignant hyperthermia–like reaction to anesthesia
- Respiratory failure and early death

REFERENCES

1. Chung J, Smith AL, Hughes SC, et al. Twenty-year follow-up of newborn screening for patients with muscular dystrophy. *Muscle Nerve*. 2016;53(4):570–578.
2. Bushby K, Finkel R, Birnkrant DJ, et al; for DMD Care Considerations Working Group. Diagnosis and management of Duchenne muscular dystrophy, part 1: diagnosis, and pharmacological and psychosocial management. *Lancet Neurol*. 2010;9(1):77–93.
3. Falzarano MS, Scotton C, Passarelli C, et al. Duchenne muscular dystrophy: from diagnosis to therapy. *Molecules*. 2015;20(10):18168–18184.
4. Bushby K, Finkel R, Birnkrant DJ, et al; for DMD Care Considerations Working Group. Diagnosis and management of Duchenne muscular dystrophy, part 2: implementation of multidisciplinary care. *Lancet Neurol*. 2010;9(2):177–189.
5. Kinnett K, Noritz G. The PJ Nicholoff steroid protocol for Duchenne and Becker muscular dystrophy and adrenal suppression. *PLoS Curr*. 2017;9.
6. Roberto R, Fritz A, Hagar Y, et al. The natural history of cardiac and pulmonary function decline in patients with Duchenne muscular dystrophy. *Spine (Phila Pa 1976)*. 2011;36(15):E1009–E1017.

ADDITIONAL READING

- Manzur AY, Kuntzer T, Pike M, et al. Glucocorticoid corticosteroids for Duchenne muscular dystrophy. *Cochrane Database Syst Rev*. 2008;(1):CD003725.
- McDonald CM, Campbell C, Torricelli RE, et al; for Clinical Evaluator Training Group and the ACT DMD Study Group. Ataluren in patients with nonsense mutation Duchenne muscular dystrophy (ACT DMD): a multicenter, randomised, double-blind, placebo-controlled, phase 3 trial. *Lancet*. 2017;390(10101):1489–1498. doi:10.1016/S0140-6736(17)31611-2.
- van der Kooi EL, Lindeman E, Riphagen I. Strength training and aerobic exercise training for muscle disease. *Cochrane Database Syst Rev*. 2005;(1):CD003907.

 CODES

ICD10

- G71.0 Muscular dystrophy
- G71.11 Myotonic muscular dystrophy
- G71.2 Congenital myopathies

CLINICAL PEARLS

- Primary care providers should have a low threshold to obtain serum CK as a screening test in the face of gross motor delay/muscular weakness, especially in boys.
- Steroids should be initiated in patients with DMD when gross motor function ceases to progress.
- High-quality care of patients requires a medical home; a multidisciplinary team of physicians, therapists, and other providers; and extensive patient and family support.

M

MYALGIC ENCEPHALOMYELITIS/CHRONIC FATIGUE SYNDROME (CFS)

Naureen Rafiq, MBBS

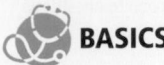 **BASICS**

DESCRIPTION
- A complex physical illness characterized by a new or definitive onset of debilitating fatigue that persists for >6 months and significantly reduces a person's ability to perform usual activities. Key features include:
  - Impaired memory or concentration
  - Joint and muscle pain
  - Unrefreshing sleep
  - Postexertional malaise
  - Orthostatic intolerance (i.e., dizziness and light-headedness when standing up)
- Synonyms: myalgic encephalomyelitis, chronic Epstein-Barr virus syndrome, postviral fatigue syndrome, chronic fatigue immune dysfunction, and systemic exertion intolerance disease (1)
- Fatigue is not relieved by rest and results in >50% reduction in previous activities (occupational, educational, social, and personal).
- Other potential medical causes must be ruled out (2).

EPIDEMIOLOGY
- Usually sporadic or isolated cases, although cluster outbreaks have occurred in different parts of the world—Iceland (1948); London, England (1955); New Zealand (1984); and the United States (1984 and 1985)
- Onset usually from age 30 to 50 years; can affect all ages (1)[B]
- Females affected 3 to 4 times more than male
- Estimated annual cost from loss of productivity and medical bills ranges from $17 to 24 billion in the United States.

Prevalence
- Affects all racial and ethnic groups; more prevalent in minority and low socioeconomic groups
- An estimated 836,000 to 2.5 million Americans suffer from chronic fatigue syndrome (CFS) (1)[B].

ETIOLOGY AND PATHOPHYSIOLOGY
- Unknown and likely multifactorial
  - Possible interaction between genetic predisposition, environmental factors, an initiating stressor, and perpetuating factors
- A recent theory attributes possible neuroendocrine immunologic and biochemical effects in CFS to dysbiosis of the gut microbiome.
- Physiologic or environmental stressors are potential precipitants.
- Many patients with chronic fatigue recall significant stressors (e.g., major medical procedure, loss of a loved one, loss of employment) in months before symptom onset.
- History of childhood trauma is common.
- Systems hypothesized to contribute include:
  - Neuroendocrine (e.g., diminished cortisol response to increased corticotropin concentrations)
  - Immune (e.g., increased C-reactive protein and β_2-microglobulin)
  - Neuromuscular (e.g., dysfunction of oxidative metabolism)
  - Autonomic (orthostatic hypotension)
  - Serotonergic (e.g., hyperserotonergic mechanisms or upregulation of serotonin receptors)

Genetics
Higher concordance among monozygotic twins compared with dizygotic twins

RISK FACTORS
Possible predisposing factors:
- Personality characteristics (neuroticism and introversion)
- Lifestyle
  - Childhood inactivity or overactivity
  - Inactivity in adulthood after infectious mononucleosis
  - Familial predisposition
  - Comorbid depression or anxiety
- Long-standing medical conditions in childhood
- Childhood trauma (emotional, physical, sexual abuse)
- Prolonged idiopathic chronic fatigue
- Postinfectious fatigue and CFS have been noted to follow mononucleosis, Ross River virus, *Coxiella burnetii*, herpes zoster, Q fever, and *Giardia lamblia*.
- Due to concern for possible infectious etiology, CFS patients excluded from donating blood by the American Red Cross in 2010

COMMONLY ASSOCIATED CONDITIONS
Common comorbidities include:
- Fibromyalgia (more common in women)
- Irritable bowel syndrome
- Gynecologic conditions (pelvic pain, endometriosis) and GYN surgeries (hysterectomy, oophorectomy) (2)
- Anxiety disorders
- Major depression
- Posttraumatic stress disorder (including physical and/or past sexual abuse)
- Domestic violence
- Attention deficit hyperactivity disorder (ADHD)
- Postural orthostatic tachycardia syndrome (POTS)
- Sleep disorders, including OSA
- Reduced left ventricular size and mass

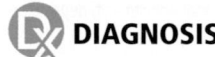 **DIAGNOSIS**

HISTORY
A thorough medical history and psychosocial history is required for accurate diagnosis. Box 1 shows updated diagnostic criteria proposed by the Institute of Medicine (IOM).

ALERT
Box 1. 2015 IOM Criteria for Diagnosis of Myalgic Encephalomyelitis/Chronic Fatigue Syndrome (1)

- Three symptoms and at least one of two additional manifestations are required for diagnosis. The three required symptoms are:
  - A substantial reduction or impairment in the ability to engage in preillness levels of activity (occupational, educational, social, or personal life) that:
    ○ Lasts for >6 months
    ○ Is accompanied by fatigue that is:
      ■ Often profound
      ■ Of new onset (not lifelong)
      ■ Not the result of ongoing or unusual excessive exertion
      ■ Not substantially alleviated by rest
  - Postexertional malaise*—worsening of symptoms after physical, mental, or emotional exertion that would not have caused a problem before the illness. PEM often puts the patient in relapse that may last days, weeks, or even longer.

  - Unrefreshing sleep*—patients with ME/CFS may not feel better or less tired even after a full night of sleep despite the absence of specific objective sleep alterations
- At least one of the following two additional manifestations must be present:
  - Cognitive impairment*—patients have problems with thinking, memory, executive function, and information processing as well as attention deficit and impaired psychomotor functions. All can be exacerbated by exertion, effort, prolonged upright posture, stress, or time pressure and may have serious consequences on a patient's ability to maintain a job or attend school full time.
  - Orthostatic intolerance—patients develop a worsening of symptoms upon assuming and maintaining upright posture as measured by objective heart rate and blood pressure abnormalities during standing, bedside orthostatic vital signs, or head-up tilt testing. Orthostatic symptoms including lightheadedness, fainting, increased fatigue, cognitive worsening, headaches, or nausea are worsened with quiet upright posture (either standing or sitting) during day-to-day life and are improved (although not necessarily fully resolved) with lying down. Orthostatic intolerance is often the most bothersome manifestation of ME/CFS among adolescents.

*The frequency and severity of these symptoms need to be evaluated.

- Common illnesses to exclude (2):
  - Anemias
  - Autoimmune diseases (rheumatoid arthritis, lupus)
  - Significant cardiac or pulmonary disease
  - Endocrine disorders (diabetes, Addison disease, thyroid disorder)
  - Infectious disease (tuberculosis, HIV/AIDS, chronic hepatitis, Lyme disease)
  - Intestinal diseases (celiac or Crohn)
  - Neurologic disorders (such as multiple sclerosis, Parkinson disease, myasthenia gravis)
  - Primary psychiatric disorders and substance abuse (clinical depression not included)
  - Primary sleep disorders such as sleep apnea
  - Malignancies

PHYSICAL EXAM
Complete physical exam to rule out other medical causes for symptoms. A complete mental status examination should be performed as well.

DIFFERENTIAL DIAGNOSIS
- Idiopathic chronic fatigue (i.e., fatigue of unknown cause for >6 months without meeting criteria for CFS)
- Psychiatric disorders
  - Major depression
  - Somatization disorder
- Physiologic fatigue (sleep disturbance, menopause)
- Pregnancy until 3 months postpartum
- Insomnia: primary (no clear etiology) versus secondary (e.g., due to anxiety, depression, environmental factors, poor sleep hygiene)
- Other known or defined systemic disease
- Endocrine disorder (hypothyroidism, Addison disease, Cushing syndrome, diabetes mellitus)
- Localized infection (e.g., occult abscess)
- Chronic or subacute bacterial disease (e.g., endocarditis)

- Lyme disease
- Fungal disease (e.g., histoplasmosis, coccidioidomycosis)
- Parasitic disease (e.g., amebiasis, giardiasis, helminth infestation)
- HIV or related disease
- Iatrogenic (e.g., medication side effects)
- Toxic agent exposure
- Obesity
- Malignancy
- Autoimmune disease
- Chronic inflammatory disease (sarcoidosis, Wegener)
- Neuromuscular disease (MS, myasthenia gravis)

DIAGNOSTIC TESTS & INTERPRETATION
No validated diagnostic test available and finding an abnormal result is not always the same as discovering the cause of fatigue. Renew the search if the suspected problem is treated and the patient remains fatigued.

Initial Tests (lab, imaging)
- Standard laboratory tests are recommended to rule out other causes for symptoms:
  – CBC; complete metabolic panel
  – Urinalysis
  – Thyroid-stimulating hormone (TSH) and free T_4
  – ESR or C-reactive protein
  – Magnesium and phosphorus level
  – Screen for drugs of abuse.
  – Age-/gender-appropriate cancer screening
- Additional studies, based on clinical findings:
  – Creatine kinase
  – Antinuclear antibodies and rheumatoid factor
  – Tuberculin skin test
  – Serum cortisol
  – HIV; RPR; VDRL
  – Lyme serology
  – IgA tissue transglutaminase
- Screen for domestic violence:
  – "Have you ever been hit, kicked, punched, or otherwise, hurt by someone within the past year? If so, by whom?"
  – "Do you feel safe in your current relationship?"
  – "Is there a partner from a previous relationship who is making you feel unsafe now?"
- No definitive imaging tests. EEG and/or MRI may help if patient has CNS symptoms; polysomnography, if patient has increased somnolence

Follow-Up Tests & Special Considerations
- Assess for comorbid psychiatric disorders.
- Assess for personality and psychosocial factors and maladaptive coping styles.
- In patients with sleep disturbance, polysomnography may reveal a treatable comorbid disease.

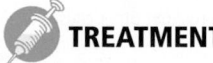

TREATMENT
- No treatment yet proven effective by large randomized trials; recommendations based on expert opinion and standard symptom management (1,2)
- Focus on changes in lifestyle and insight, with a goal to avoid complicating treatments (e.g., addictive medications, invasive testing) or interventions that support secondary gain.
- A multidisciplinary approach is recommended.

GENERAL MEASURES

ALERT
No definitive cure. Treatment involves symptom management and guided self-management. The aim is to reduce symptoms and improve quality of life

by establishing a good therapeutic relationship. It is helpful to identify troublesome symptoms (pain and insomnia) and address those first. Both cognitive-behavioral therapy (CBT) and graded exercise therapy (GET) are effective. Medication is often of little value.

- Individual CBT: Challenge fatigue-related cognition; plan social and occupational rehabilitation.
- GET: Track amount of exercise patient can do without exacerbating symptoms and gradually increase intensity and duration. Both involve a careful balance between activity and rest. Fear of movement and avoidance of physical activity are common in CFS.
- Patients learn how to gradually increase activity in a way that will not exacerbate their illness. Vigorous exercise can trigger relapse, perhaps related to immune dysregulation.
- Improves functional capacity and diminishes fatigue
- GET is more effective with educational interventions using telephone reminders.
- Duration of illness does not predict treatment outcome; aggressive combined care indicated for all

MEDICATION
- No established pharmacologic treatments
- If medications are needed, use the lowest effective dose and increase cautiously.
- Studies have been conducted with antivirals, antidepressants, immunoglobulins, hydrocortisone, and modafinil. None show clear benefit.
- Agomelatine, an antidepressant with agonist activity at melatonin receptors, is promising in early studies.
- If insomnia is present, use of nonaddicting sleep aids (hydroxyzine, trazodone, doxepin, etc.) may improve outcomes.

ISSUES FOR REFERRAL
- Psychiatrist to manage comorbid behavioral disorders
- Rehabilitative medicine
- Sleep or pain management specialist

COMPLEMENTARY & ALTERNATIVE MEDICINE
- Acupuncture, massage, and chiropractic have been shown to be benefit pain for some patients (2)[B].
- Other helpful nonpharmacologic interventions may include physical therapy, stretches, hydrotherapy, yoga, tai chi, and meditations. Hot or cold packs, warm baths as well as electrical massagers, transcutaneous electrical nerve stimulations can also be considered.
- Equivocal evidence for homeopathy and biofeedback

 ## ONGOING CARE

FOLLOW-UP RECOMMENDATIONS
Patient Monitoring
Although no consensus exists, periodic reevaluation is appropriate for support, relief of symptoms, and assessment for other possible causes of symptoms.

DIET
- Well-balanced diet, including recommended daily allowance of vitamins and minerals
- No particular diet program has been shown to be effective for treatment of CFS.
- Whether weight loss improves symptoms in obese CFS patients is unknown

PATIENT EDUCATION
- Gradual increase in physical exercise
- Avoid extended periods of rest, but ensure adequate rest between sessions.
- Patient education is important—promote the benefits of cognitive therapies, lifestyle changes,

and pharmacologic therapy; job modification as needed
- Chronic Fatigue and Immune Dysfunction Syndrome Association of America: http://solvecfs.org/
- CDC, Chronic Fatigue Syndrome: http://www.cdc.gov/cfs/

PROGNOSIS
- Fluctuating course is common.
- Generally, improvement is slow over months to years.
- An estimated 15% full recovery rate
- Patients with poor social adjustment, a strong belief in an organic etiology, financial secondary gain, or age >50 years are less likely to improve.

COMPLICATIONS
- CFS patients may reduce physical activity out of fear that it may worsen symptoms.
- Depression
- Unemployment: Although studies document improvement with treatment, <1/3 of patients in trials return to work.
- The Social Security Administration considers CFS to be a disability.
- Receipt of third-party disability pay (secondary gain) has been associated with treatment nonresponse.
- Polypharmacy
- Chronic immune activation or an associated infection may play a role in an increased risk for non-Hodgkin lymphoma in elderly (>80 years) CFS patients.

REFERENCES
1. Unger ER, Lin JS, Brimmer DJ, et al. CDC grand rounds: chronic fatigue syndrome—advancing research and clinical education. *MMWR Morb Mortal Wkly Rep.* 2016;65(50–51):1434–1438.
2. Friedberg F, Bateman L, Bested AC, et al. *ME/CFS: A Primer for Clinical Practitioners*. Chicago, IL: International Association for Chronic Fatigue Syndrome/ Myalgic Encephalomyelitis; 2014.

ADDITIONAL READING
Yancey JR, Thomas SM. Chronic fatigue syndrome: diagnosis and treatment. *Am Fam Physician*. 2012;86(8):741–746.

 SEE ALSO

Algorithm: Fatigue

CODES

ICD10
R53.82 Chronic fatigue, unspecified

CLINICAL PEARLS
- No pharmacologic agents (e.g., antidepressants, immune modulators) have been shown to be consistently effective in treating CFS.
- ~70% of patients show improvement with CBT; 55% with GET; in many cases, the combination of these two treatments is helpful.
- There are many more patients with idiopathic chronic fatigue than true CFS. To diagnose CFS, use the IOM diagnostic criteria.
- Standardized instruments (SF-36, symptom index, and Multidimensional Fatigue Inventory [MFI]) help to diagnose CFS and to follow patient progress.

M

MYASTHENIA GRAVIS

Melody A. Jordahl-Iafrato, MD, FAAFP

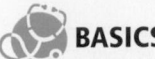

BASICS

DESCRIPTION
Primary disorder of neuromuscular transmission characterized by fluctuating muscle weakness:
- Ocular myasthenia gravis (MG) (15%): weakness limited to eyelids and extraocular muscles
- Generalized MG (85%): commonly affects ocular as well as a variable combination of bulbar, proximal limb, and respiratory muscles
- 50% of patients who present with ocular symptoms develop generalized MG within 2 years.
- Onset may be sudden and severe, but it is typically mild and intermittent over many years, maximum severity reached within 3 years for 85%.
- System(s) affected: neurologic, hematologic, lymphatic, immunologic, musculoskeletal

EPIDEMIOLOGY
Occurs at any age but a bimodal distribution to the age of onset:
- Female predominance: 20 to 40 years
- Male predominance: 60 to 80 years

Incidence
Estimated annual incidence 2 to 21/1 million

Prevalence
In the United States, 200/1 million; increasing over the past 5 decades

Pediatric Considerations
A transient form of neonatal MG seen in 10–20% of infants born to mothers with MG. It occurs as a result of the transplacental passage of maternal antibodies that interfere with function of the neuromuscular junction; resolves in weeks to months. Autoimmune juvenile MG makes up 10–15% of cases of MG in North America.

ETIOLOGY AND PATHOPHYSIOLOGY
- Reduction in the function of acetylcholine receptors (AChRs) at muscle end plates, resulting in insufficient neuromuscular transmission
- Antibody-mediated autoimmune disorder
- Antibodies are present in most cases of MG.
  - Seropositive/antiacetylcholine receptor (anti-AChR): a humoral, antibody-mediated, T-cell–dependent attack of the AChRs or receptor-associated proteins at the postsynaptic membrane of the neuromuscular junction. Found in 85% of generalized MG and 50% of ocular MG; thymic abnormalities common (1)
  - Muscle-specific kinase (MuSKs): 5% of generalized MG patients. Typically females. Is a severe form, respiratory and bulbar muscles involved. Thymic abnormalities are rare (1).
  - In remainder of seronegative, 12–50% with anti-LRP4, a molecule that forms a complex with MuSK, mild generalized weakness most common (1)
  - Seronegative MG (SNMG): 5%; may have anti-AChR detectable by cell-based assay. Clinically similar to anti-AChR; thymic hyperplasia may be present (1).
- Also documented immediately after viral infections (measles, Epstein-Barr virus [EBV], HIV, and human T-lymphotropic virus [HTLV])

Genetics
- Congenital MG syndrome describes a collection of rare hereditary disorders. This condition is not immune-mediated but instead results from the mutation of a component of the neuromuscular junction (autosomal recessive).
- Familial predisposition is seen in 5% of cases.

RISK FACTORS
- Familial MG
- D-penicillamine (drug-induced MG)
- Other autoimmune diseases

COMMONLY ASSOCIATED CONDITIONS
- Thymic hyperplasia (60–70%)
- Thymoma (10–15%)
- Autoimmune thyroid disease (3–8%)

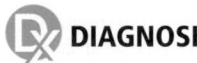

DIAGNOSIS

Myasthenia Gravis Foundation of America Clinical Classification (2)[C]:
- Class I: any eye muscle weakness, possible ptosis, no other evidence of muscle weakness elsewhere
- Class II: eye muscle weakness of any severity; mild weakness of other muscles:
  - Class IIa: predominantly limb or axial muscles
  - Class IIb: predominantly bulbar and/or respiratory muscles
- Class III: eye muscle weakness of any severity; moderate weakness of other muscles:
  - Class IIIa: predominantly limb or axial muscles
  - Class IIIb: predominantly bulbar and/or respiratory muscles
- Class IV: eye muscle weakness of any severity; severe weakness of other muscles:
  - Class IVa: predominantly limb or axial muscles
  - Class IVb: predominantly bulbar and/or respiratory muscles (can also include feeding tube without intubation)
- Class V: intubation needed to maintain airway

HISTORY
The hallmark of MG is fatigability.
- Fluctuating weakness, often subtle, that worsens during the day and after prolonged use of affected muscles, may improve with rest
- Early symptoms are transient with asymptomatic periods lasting days or weeks.
- With progression, asymptomatic periods shorten, and symptoms fluctuate from mild to severe.
- >50% of patients present with ocular symptoms (ptosis and/or diplopia). Eventually, 90% of patients with MG develop ocular symptoms.
- Ptosis might be unilateral, bilateral, or shifting from eye to eye.
- 15% present with bulbar symptoms.
- <5% present with proximal limb weakness alone.

ALERT
Myasthenic crisis: respiratory muscle weakness producing respiratory insufficiency and pending respiratory failure

PHYSICAL EXAM
- Ptosis may worsen with propping of opposite eyelid (curtain sign) or sustained upward gaze.
- "Myasthenic sneer," in which the midlip rises but corners of mouth do not move
- Muscle weakness is usually proximal and symmetric.
- Test for muscle fatigability by repetitive or prolonged use of individual muscles.
- Important to test and monitor respiratory function

DIFFERENTIAL DIAGNOSIS
- Thyroid ophthalmopathy
- Oculopharyngeal muscular dystrophy
- Myotonic dystrophy
- Kearns-Sayre syndrome
- Chronic progressive external ophthalmoplegia
- Brainstem and motor cranial nerve lesions
- Botulism
- Motor neuron disease (e.g., amyotrophic lateral sclerosis [ALS])
- Lambert-Eaton myasthenic syndrome
- Drug-induced myasthenia
- Congenital myasthenic syndrome
- Dermatomyositis/polymyositis
- Neurosarcoidosis
- Tolosa-Hunt syndrome

DIAGNOSTIC TESTS & INTERPRETATION
Initial Tests (lab, imaging)
- Anti-AChR antibody (74–85% are seropositive):
  - Generalized myasthenia: 75–85%
  - Ocular myasthenia: 50%
  - MG and thymoma: 98–100%
  - Poor correlation between antibody titer and disease severity (1)[C]
  - False-positive results in thymoma without MG, Lambert-Eaton myasthenic syndrome, small cell lung cancer, and rheumatoid arthritis treated with penicillamine
- Anti-MuSK antibody:
  - Used if MG is suspected, patient seronegative
  - Strong correlation between titer and disease severity (1)[C]
- LRP4 and clustered anti-AChR:
  - Used if MG suspected, patient seronegative
- Thyroid and other autoimmune testing antistriated muscle (anti-SM) antibody:
  - Present in 84% of patients with thymoma who are <40 years of age
  - Can be present without thymoma in patients >40 years of age
- Chest radiographs or CT scans may identify a thymoma.
- MRI of brain and orbits to rule out other causes of cranial nerve deficit

Diagnostic Procedures/Other
- Tensilon (edrophonium) test:
  - Initial 2-mg IV dose, followed by another 2 mg every 60 seconds up to a maximum dose of 10 mg
  - A positive test shows improvement of strength within 30 seconds of administration.
  - Sensitivity 80–90% (3)[C]

– Cardiac disease and bronchial asthma are relative contraindications, especially in elderly.
– Atropine: 0.4 to 0.6 mg IV may rarely be required as antidote; must be available
– Can also do trial of other cholinesterase inhibitors (neostigmine or oral) and monitor response
- Ice pack test:
  – Ice pack applied to closed eyelid for 60 seconds, then removed; extent of ptosis immediately assessed
  – Ice will decrease the ptosis induced by MG.
  – Sensitivity 80% in patients with prominent ptosis
- Electrophysiology testing:
  – Repetitive nerve stimulation (RNS):
    ○ Widely available, most frequently used
    ○ Moderately sensitive for both generalized MG (75%) and ocular MG (50%) (3)[C]
  – Single-fiber electromyogram (SFEMG):
    ○ Assesses temporal variability between two muscle fibers within same motor unit (jitter)
    ○ Sensitive (90–95%) but less specific
    ○ Technically difficult to perform; limited availability, use if suspected and negative RNS (3)[C]

Test Interpretation
- Lymphofollicular hyperplasia of thymic medulla occurs in 65% of patients with MG, thymoma in 15%.
- Immunofluorescence: IgG antibodies and complement on receptor membranes in seropositive patients

TREATMENT

GENERAL MEASURES
- Treatment based on age, gender, and disease severity and progression
- Three basic approaches: symptomatic, immunosuppressive, and supportive. Few should receive a single therapeutic modality.

MEDICATION
First Line
Symptomatic treatments (anticholinesterase agents)
- Pyridostigmine bromide (Mestinon):
  – *Most commonly prescribed because available in oral tablet*
  – Starting dose of 30 mg PO TID with food
  – Maximum dose: 120 mg q3–4h
  – Long acting available but effect not consistent
- Neostigmine methylsulfate (Prostigmin):
  – Starting dose of 0.5 mg SC or IM q3h
  – Titrate dosage to clinical need.
- Patients with anti-MuSK may not respond well to these medications.

Second Line
- Immunosuppressants: Oral corticosteroids are the first choice of drugs when immunosuppression is necessary.
  – Prednisone: Start as inpatient with a 60 mg/day PO; taper the dosage every 3 days; switch to alternate-day regimen within 2 weeks. Taper very slowly to establish the minimum dosage necessary to maintain remission (4)[B].
  – Cyclophosphamide: adults: 1 to 5 mg/kg/day PO; children: 2 to 8 mg/kg/day PO (4)[B]

– Cyclosporine: adults: 5 mg/kg/day PO (nephrotoxicity and drug interactions) (4)[B]
– Mycophenolate: 1 g PO or IV BID
– Azathioprine: 100 to 200 mg/day PO (4)[B]
  ○ *Most frequently used for long-term immunomodulation*, similar efficacy to steroids and IVIG
  ○ Benefit may not be apparent for up to 18 months after initiation of therapy.
  ○ Prednisolone + azathioprine may be effective when used as a corticosteroid-sparing agent.
- Acute immunomodulating treatments:
  – Plasmapheresis: bulk removal of 2 to 3 L of plasma 3 times per week, repeated until rate of improvement plateaus (5)[B]
    ○ Improves weakness in nearly all and can last up to 3 months
  – Immunoglobulin: 2 g/kg IV over 2 to 5 days (4)[B]
  – *Plasmapheresis and immunoglobulin have comparable efficacy in treating moderate to severe MG* (5)[C].
  – Rapid onset of effect but short duration of action
  – Used for acute worsening of MG to improve strength prior to surgery, prevent acute exacerbations induced by corticosteroids, and as a chronic intermittent treatment to provide relief in refractory MG
- Other immunosuppressant therapies:
  – Tacrolimus
  – Rituximab:
    ○ Seronegative MuSK-antibody positive MG patients may have better response to rituximab than conventional therapies.

> **ALERT**
> Use caution with drugs that can precipitate weakness: aminoglycosides, fluoroquinolones, β-blockers, calcium channel blockers, neuromuscular blockers, statins, diuretics, oral contraceptives, gabapentin, phenytoin, lithium, among others.

SURGERY/OTHER PROCEDURES
- Thymectomy recommended for patients with thymic abnormalities
- May be beneficial for patients without thymic abnormalities in those <60 years of age especially in patients with elevated anti-AChR

Pediatric Considerations
Infants with severe weakness from transient neonatal myasthenia may be treated with oral pyridostigmine; general support is necessary until the condition clears.
- Corticosteroids limited only to severe disease
- Side effects of many medications must be closely monitored in juvenile patients especially because some may affect long-term fertility or are consider carcinogenic.

ADMISSION, INPATIENT, AND NURSING CONSIDERATIONS
- Management of pulmonary infections
- Myasthenic/cholinergic crises
- Plasmapheresis
- IV γ-globulin

ONGOING CARE

PATIENT EDUCATION
Myasthenia Gravis Foundation of America (MGFA): http://www.myasthenia.org/

PROGNOSIS
- Overall good but highly variable
- Myasthenic crisis associated with substantial morbidity and 4% mortality
- Seronegative patients are more likely to have purely ocular disease, and those with generalized SNMG have a better outcome after treatment.

COMPLICATIONS
Acute respiratory arrest; chronic respiratory insufficiency

REFERENCES

1. Berrih-Aknin S, Frenkian-Cuvelier M, Eymard B. Diagnostic and clinical classification of autoimmune myasthenia gravis. *J Autoimmun*. 2014; 48–49:143–148.
2. Jaretzki A III, Barohn RJ, Ernstoff RM, et al. Myasthenia gravis: recommendations for clinical research standards. Task Force of the Medical Scientific Advisory Board of the Myasthenia Gravis Foundation of America. *Neurology*. 2000;55(1):16–23.
3. Pasnoor M, Dimachkie MM, Farmakidis C, et al. Diagnosis of myasthenia gravis. *Neurol Clin*. 2018;36(2):261–274.
4. Gotterer L, Li Y. Maintenance immunosuppression in myasthenia gravis. *J Neurol Sci*. 2016;369:294–302.
5. Barth D, Nabavi Nouri M, Ng E, et al. Comparison of IVIg and PLEX in patients with myasthenia gravis. *Neurology*. 2011;76(23):2017–2023.

ADDITIONAL READING

- Angelini C. Diagnosis and management of autoimmune myasthenia gravis. *Clin Drug Investig*. 2011;31(1):1–14.
- Meriggioli MN. Myasthenia gravis: immunopathogenesis, diagnosis, and management. *Continuum Lifelong Learn Neurol*. 2009;15(1):35–62.

CODES

ICD10
- G70.00 Myasthenia gravis without (acute) exacerbation
- G70.01 Myasthenia gravis with (acute) exacerbation
- P94.0 Transient neonatal myasthenia gravis

CLINICAL PEARLS
- An autoimmune disease, marked by abnormal fatigability and weakness of selected muscles, which is relieved by rest
- Anticholinesterase medication and a thymectomy lessen symptom severity.
- Steroid therapy, plasma exchange, or immunoglobulin can be used in severely affected patients.

M

MYELODYSPLASTIC SYNDROMES (MDS)

Gabriela Sanchez Petitto, MD • Pedro Emilio Alcedo, MD • Guillermo Garcia-Manero, MD

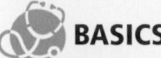 **BASICS**

DESCRIPTION

- Myelodysplastic syndromes (MDS) are a heterogeneous group of clonal stem cell disorders characterized by peripheral blood cytopenias: anemia, thrombocytopenia, and/or neutropenia.
- Dysplasia refers to an abnormality of development or differentiation in specific cell lines. In MDS, these changes take place in the bone marrow and confer a tendency for leukemic transformation.

EPIDEMIOLOGY

Incidence
The incidence in the United States is approximately 3 to 4 cases per 100,000 population per year, expanding to 30 cases per 100,000 population per year, for patients age >70 years.

Prevalence
In 2012, >60,000 people with MDS resided in the country.

ETIOLOGY AND PATHOPHYSIOLOGY

- MDS is clinically characterized by peripheral cytopenias, consequence of ineffective marrow hematopoiesis (premature cell death).
- Nongenetic mechanisms encompass apoptosis, pyroptosis, deregulated immunity, and inflammatory cytokine amplification (see "Genetics" for genetic mechanisms) (1,2).
- Low-risk MDS (LR-MDS) are characterized by deregulated immunity and apoptosis, whereas high-risk MDS (HR-MDS) are characterized by clonal expansion and transformation to acute myelogenous leukemia (AML).
- A changing interplay of proapoptotic versus antiapoptotic signals is central in the progression of the disease.
- In LR-MDS, stem cell programmed death occurs by different mechanisms: apoptosis, pyroptosis, and potentially autophagy.
  - *Apoptosis:* Tumor necrosis factor (TNF)-α, TNF-related apoptosis-inducing ligand (TRAIL), Fas ligand, and proapoptotic cytokines (TNF-α and IL-6) play a major role in stem cell apoptosis in LR-MDS.
  - *Pyroptosis:* It is an inflammatory cell death different from apoptosis that is considered sterile in nature.
    - Activation of nod-like receptors leads to formation of the inflammasome complex and caspase 1 activation that leads to pore formation in the plasma membrane of the cells; creates ionic gradients, water influx, cell swelling, and cell death (3)
    - This potentially also explains the morphologic changes seen in MDS (macrocytosis, enlarged cells).

- Evolution to AML has been associated with upregulation of NFκB, enhanced activity of the Bcl2 and the inhibitors of apoptosis protein (IAP) families.
  - This is thought to be a mechanism of bypassing the apoptotic phenomenon in the bone marrow microenvironment.

Genetics
- Recurrent somatic mutations are observed in >90% of MDS patients.
- Mutated genes are involved in:
  - Epigenetic regulation: TET2, EZH2, IDH1, IDH2, DNMT3A, ASXL1
  - DNA repair: TP53
  - Transcriptional regulation: BCOR, ETV6, RUNX1
  - RNA splicing: U2AF35, ZRSR2, SF3B1, SRSF2
  - Cohesin complex: STAG2
  - Signal transduction: JAK2, CBL, NRAS
- Mutations in the epigenetic modifiers: The concept is that any gain of function mutations in the DNA methyltransferases (DNMT3A and DNMT3B) leads to hypermethylation (a gene silencing mechanism that contributes to clonal evolution).
- It is unclear how these different molecular and genetic mechanisms translate into the same phenotypic manifestation of myelodysplasia and cytopenias.

RISK FACTORS
- Age: increased risk in patients >60 years old
- Tobacco use
- Chronic exposure to chemicals: benzene, pesticides, insecticides, and petroleum
- Prior chemotherapy or radiation therapy
- Inherited disorders: Fanconi anemia, Shwachman-Diamond syndromes, severe congenital neutropenia, and familial platelet disorder

GENERAL PREVENTION
Avoiding known cancer-causing industrial chemicals, such as benzene, and also tobacco, might lower the risk of developing MDS.

COMMONLY ASSOCIATED CONDITIONS
Myeloproliferative disorders and paroxysmal nocturnal hemoglobinuria

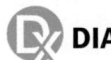 **DIAGNOSIS**

HISTORY
- The clinical course of MDS patients is driven by the type and degree of cytopenias.
- Recurrent infections, bleeding issues, fatigue, weight loss and exertional dyspnea, are common symptoms reported.

PHYSICAL EXAM
- Generalized pallor and ecchymosis as result of the anemia and thrombocytopenia respectively
- Rarely hepatosplenomegaly as consequence of extramedullary hemopoiesis is present, especially in MDS/MPN overlapping syndromes. Lymphadenopathies are infrequent.

DIFFERENTIAL DIAGNOSIS
- Acute leukemia: AML
- Vitamin B_{12} and folate deficiencies can manifest as a hypoproliferative anemia.
- Infections of the bone marrow: human immunodeficiency virus, tuberculosis, atypical mycobacterium and Epstein-Barr virus
- Indolent myeloid hematopoietic disorders that do not fulfill diagnostic criteria for MDS: idiopathic cytopenia of unknown significance, idiopathic dysplasia of unknown significance, clonal hematopoiesis of indeterminate potential (CHIP), and clonal cytopenia of unknown significance

DIAGNOSTIC TESTS & INTERPRETATION

Initial Tests (lab, imaging)
- A complete blood count, chemistry, viral studies (HIV and hepatitis panel), and vitamin levels (B_{12} and folate) should be evaluated.
- The International Working Group (IWG) recommended minimal diagnostic prerequisites:
  - Stable cytopenia for ≥6 months or for 2 months with karyotype or bilineage dysplasia
  - Exclusion of other potential reasons for dysplasia/cytopenia
- In addition, the diagnosis of MDS requires ≥1 of 3 decisive criteria:
  - Dysplasia (≥10% in ≥1 of the 3 major bone marrow lineages)
  - Blast cell count of 5–19%
  - Specific MDS-associated karyotypes: del(5q), del(20q), +8, or −7/del(7q)

Diagnostic Procedures/Other
- *Histopathology.* A bone marrow is essential to distinguish MDS from AML and to perform karyotype studies, fluorescent in situ hybridization (FISH), and mutational studies.
  - Blast %: <20% is consistent with MDS; ≥20% is diagnostic of AML.
- *Cytogenetics.* Clonal chromosome abnormalities are observed in 30–80% of MDS patients. In the rest of the patients (20–70%), submicroscopic alterations (microdeletions, point mutations) provide diagnostic evidence.
- In cases of uncertainty, analysis of somatic mutations and flow cytometry of bone marrow can evidence clonal disease.

Initial Tests (lab, imaging)

If clinical suspicion of MPN, obtain a CBC and peripheral blood smear; if suggestive, obtain bone marrow biopsy.

- PMF: radiographic osteosclerosis in 25–66%

Diagnostic Procedures/Other

- CML: diagnosis with identification of Philadelphia chromosome: Fluorescence in situ hybridization is more sensitive than karyotyping and is routinely used. Polymerase chain reaction (P210) is done at baseline to help monitor response to tyrosine kinase inhibitors (TKIs).
  – Bone marrow biopsy: increased cellularity and increased myeloid to erythroid ratio
- PMF, ET, and PV: genotypic analysis and bone marrow biopsy as described in earlier WHO criteria; "dry tap" is common in PMF.
- Risk stratification
  – CML: three phases
    ○ (i) Chronic phase (85% patients at diagnosis; <5% blast counts)
    ○ (ii) Accelerated phase (poorly controlled splenomegaly regardless of treatment, 10–19% blast counts, worsening anemia, basophil ≥20%)
    ○ (iii) Blast crisis (resembles acute myeloid or lymphoid leukemia, >20% blast counts)
    ○ PMF: International Prognostic Scoring System (IPSS) at diagnosis and Dynamic IPSS (DIPSS-plus) throughout disease
      ■ IPSS: age >65 years, constitutional symptoms, hemoglobin <10 g/dL, leukocyte count >25 × 10⁹/L, circulating blasts >1%
        □ Low risk = 0 of above, intermediate-1 risk = 1 of above, intermediate-2 risk = 2 of above, high risk = ≥3 of above
      ■ DIPSS-plus: same five risk factors in the IPSS + need for red cell transfusion, platelets <100 × 10⁹/L, and unfavorable karyotype
        □ Low risk = 0 of above, intermediate-1 risk = 1 of above, intermediate-2 risk = 2 to 3 of above, high risk = ≥4 of above
  – ET: low risk = age <40 years, no prior thromboembolic events, no cardiovascular risk factors, platelet count <1,500 × 10⁹/L; intermediate risk = age 40 to 59 years, presence of cardiovascular risk factors, platelet count <1,500 × 10⁹/L; high risk = age ≥60 years and/or prior thromboembolic or hemorrhagic episode and/or platelet count >1,500 × 10⁹/L
  – IPSET score includes presence of JAK-2 mutation to these conventional risk factors.
  – PV: low risk = age <60 years, no history of thrombosis/cardiovascular risk factors; intermediate risk = platelets >1,000 × 10⁹/L and cardiovascular risk factors; high risk = age >60 years or a history of thrombosis

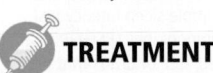

TREATMENT

GENERAL MEASURES

Low-dose aspirin for ET and PV

MEDICATION

First Line

- CML: TKIs are mainstay of treatment.
  – Chronic phase: imatinib mesylate (Gleevec): 400 mg/day is the safest choice.
- Other options: dasatinib (avoid in GI bleed), nilotinib (avoid in CHF and prolonged QT interval), or bosutinib. Accelerated or blast phase: Increase imatinib to 800 mg/day or switch to nilotinib or dasatinib.
  – While awaiting confirmation of diagnosis, hydroxyurea can be used to lower the WBC count.

- Numerous studies show 40–50% patients have durable molecular response, and TKI can be discontinued at that point.
- PMF: Main goal is symptomatic relief:
  – Low risk: symptom-directed therapy
  – Intermediate and high risk: Consider allogeneic SCT (aSCT).
  – JAK2 inhibitor ruxolitinib is approved for intermediate or high-risk myelofibrosis. It is also approved for post-PV and post-ET myelofibrosis (2).
  – Supportive treatment
    ○ Anemia: transfusions, erythropoiesis-stimulating agents, androgens, danazol, thalidomide, lenalidomide, or splenectomy
    ○ Splenomegaly: ruxolitinib, hydroxyurea, splenectomy, splenic radiation, or IV cladribine for refractory cases
    ○ Thrombosis: hydroxyurea and low-dose aspirin
    ○ Blast phase PMF: cytoreduction and transplant if eligible
- ET: in low and intermediate risk: "Watch and wait" + low-dose aspirin if microvascular disturbances are present and no contraindications. In high risk: hydroxyurea 15 mg/kg/day in divided doses to reduce platelet count to <450 × 10⁹/L (2). Anagrelide is an additional cytoreductive option.
- PV
  – Low and intermediate risk: phlebotomy with goal hematocrit <45% and low-dose aspirin
  – High risk (or those who do not tolerate phlebotomy): hydroxyurea 500 to 1,000 mg/day (2); ruxolitinib if poor response to or intolerance of hydroxyurea

Second Line

- CML: Only curable treatment is aSCT; reserved for accelerated/blast phase due to high rates of morbidity and mortality with aSCT
  – 2nd-generation TKIs: dasatinib, nilotinib, and bosutinib; increasing evidence for improved, deeper responses with these medications resulting in use of 2nd-generation TKIs for first-line therapy. Ponatinib is a 3rd-generation TKI that has activity in cases of TKI resistance due to a T315I mutation for which all the other available TKIs are ineffective. Sokal score can be used to predict achievement of molecular response and survival outcomes; patients with higher Sokal score may perform better with 2nd-generation TKIs.
- PMF: Only curable treatment is aSCT; reserved for intermediate- or high-risk patients
  – If unresponsive to hydroxyurea, use pegylated interferon-α; tolerance may be an issue.
- ET: If resistant/intolerant to hydroxyurea, use anagrelide.
  – If resistant/intolerant to hydroxyurea or anagrelide, pregnant, or age <40 years, use interferon-α.
- PV: if resistant or intolerant to hydroxyurea, can use ruxolitinib

ISSUES FOR REFERRAL

Patients with MPNs are usually referred to hematology/oncology.

SURGERY/OTHER PROCEDURES

- May require splenectomy/palliative radiation for foci of extramedullary hematopoiesis
- Hematopoietic stem cell transplant if eligible

ADMISSION, INPATIENT, AND NURSING CONSIDERATIONS

- Severe cachexia; renal failure and hepatomegaly secondary to extramedullary hematopoiesis; massive splenomegaly requiring treatment; severe thrombotic/hemorrhagic episodes; anemia; tumor lysis syndrome
- Optimal hydration to prevent tumor lysis syndrome

 ## ONGOING CARE

PROGNOSIS

- CML: 10-year survival rate ~80% from time of diagnosis; 85% will die in blast crisis; 12- to 18-month median survival for accelerated phase; 3- to 6-month median survival for blast phase
- PMF: worst prognosis of the MPNs; drug therapy does not modify disease course but treats the symptoms; median survival for IPSS low risk = 135 months, intermediate-1 risk = 95 months, intermediate-2 risk = 48 months, high risk = 27 months
- PV: median survival often >10 years
- ET: near-normal life expectancy

COMPLICATIONS

- CML: blast crisis, transformation to acute leukemia, gout, or nephropathy due to hyperuricemia
- PMF: 10% develop acute myeloid leukemia; anemia, massive hepatosplenomegaly, thrombohemorrhagic events, osteosclerosis, secondary gout, splenic infarcts, paraspinal/epidural extramedullary hematopoiesis
- ET: <10% develop post-ET myelofibrosis, 2% develop acute myeloid leukemia; thrombohemorrhagic events
- PV: 15–20% develop post-PV myelofibrosis, 5% develop leukemia; erythromelalgia, pruritus, secondary gout, headaches, vascular occlusive events

REFERENCES

1. Fava C, Rege-Cambrin G, Saglio G. The choice of first-line chronic myelogenous leukemia treatment. *Ann Hematol*. 2015;94(Suppl 2):S123–S131.
2. Geyer HL, Mesa RA. Therapy for myeloproliferative neoplasms: when, which agent, and how? *Blood*. 2014;124(24):3529–3537.

ADDITIONAL READING

Patel AB, Vellore NA, Deininger MW. New strategies in myeloproliferative neoplasms: the evolving genetic and therapeutic landscape. *Clin Cancer Res*. 2016;22(5):1037–1047.

 ## SEE ALSO

Leukemia, Chronic Myelogenous; Polycythemia Vera

 ## CODES

ICD10

- D47.1 Chronic myeloproliferative disease
- C92.10 Chronic myeloid leukemia, BCR/ABL-positive, not having achieved remission
- D45 Polycythemia vera

CLINICAL PEARLS

- MPNs are a group of clonal disorders that share a common cell of origin in the pluripotent hematopoietic stem cell.
- MPNs are characterized by proliferation of cells of myeloid lineage—granulocytic, erythroid, megakaryocytic, or mast cell. They share common clinical features including risk of thrombosis, spleen and/or liver enlargement, and constitutional symptoms related to a hypermetabolic state.
- Splenectomy as an option for symptom and cytopenia control is associated with high risk of postsplenectomy mortality and complications including thrombosis.

M

NARCOLEPSY

Waiz Wasey, MD • Brynn Dredla, MD

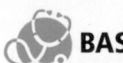

BASICS

DESCRIPTION
- Narcolepsy is a chronic incurable neurologic sleep disorder mainly characterized by excessive daytime sleepiness (EDS) and may be associated with cataplexy (sudden loss of muscle control), hypnagogic hallucinations (vivid perceptual experiences while falling asleep), or sleep paralysis (temporary inability to move or speak that happens during transition from sleeping to awake state).
- Mainly two types identified by American Academy of Sleep Medicine:
  - Type 1 (60–70%) (formerly narcolepsy with cataplexy) and type 2 (formerly narcolepsy without cataplexy) (1)
- Usually diagnosed late—5 to 15 years after the onset of symptoms (2)
- No cure, symptomatic management

EPIDEMIOLOGY
Incidence
- Affects 0.03 to 0.16% general population with incidence 1/2,000 worldwide (3)
- Bimodal distribution, age of onset peak at 15 years and again at 35 years of age
- Predominant sex: male > female (1.6:1)
- 5% familial cases (1)

Prevalence
- Narcolepsy type 1 (with cataplexy): 25 to 50/100,000 people
- Narcolepsy type 2 (without cataplexy): 20 to 34/100,000 people (1)
- Highest in Japan, lowest in Israel

ETIOLOGY AND PATHOPHYSIOLOGY
- Primarily caused by degeneration of hypothalamic neurons that produce orexin (hypocretin). Postmortem studies show 85% loss of these neurons in type 1 and about 33% loss in type 2 (1).
- Orexin is crucial to promote wakefulness, it stimulates the RAS (reticular activating system) and inhibits REM.
- Neurodegeneration may be caused by autoimmune process, probably stimulated by infections (such as influenza or *Streptococcus*) or environmental factors (occurs commonly in late spring) (2).
- Alterations in the L-PGDS (lipocalin-type prostaglandin D synthase) level also seem to be involved in causing EDS in narcolepsy (1).
- Rarely by insult to hypothalamus due to sarcoidosis, stroke, tumor, or paraneoplastic disorder (2)
- International Classification of Sleep Disorders 3rd edition (ICSD-3) classification:
  - Narcolepsy
  - Narcolepsy type 1 (with hypocretin deficiency)
  - Narcolepsy type 2 (without hypocretin deficiency)
  - Narcolepsy due to medical conditions

Genetics
- Usually sporadic but increased incidence in families with positive history: 1–2% in first-degree relative of index case (10 to 40 times the general population) (2)
- Twin concordance is 25–31% (suggests environmental contribution).
- 98% of patients with narcolepsy type 1 have human leukocyte antigen (HLA) DQB1*0602; 40–50% of patients with narcolepsy type 2 express this antigen. HLA DQB1*0602 is present in 12–30% of the general population (2).

- Heterozygous subjects have 7- to 25-fold increased risk, whereas homozygous have 2- to 4-fold increased risk (1).
- Presence of DQB1*0602 gene increased risk of narcolepsy by a factor of 200 (2).
- Autosomal recessive inheritance pattern
- Affects 12% of Asians, 25% of whites, and 38% of African Americans are gene carriers

RISK FACTORS
- Age (peaks at 15 and 35 years)
- Obesity
- Head trauma
- CNS infectious disease
- Anesthesia
- Psychological stress
- Positive family history
- Recent influenza A, streptococcal infection, or H1N1 vaccine

COMMONLY ASSOCIATED CONDITIONS
Obstructive sleep apnea (OSA) (up to 25%), obesity, anxiety

DIAGNOSIS

HISTORY
- Classic tetrad of EDS, cataplexy, sleep paralysis, and hypnagogic hallucinations (four most common symptoms): Only 10–20% of patients have all four symptoms.
- EDS and sleep attacks (cardinal symptom):
  - EDS is present in 100% of patients, usually the first initial symptom.
  - ICDS-3 classification for both type 1 and 2 requires EDS occurring almost daily for at least 3 months (1).
  - Patients may report refreshing daytime naps, with possible return of EDS in 1 to 2 hours (2).
  - Sudden sleep attacks (5 to 20 minutes) during stimulating situations such as driving and walking (4)
  - Sleep attacks are longer in children (up to 2 hours).
  - Patients may report nocturnal insomnia.
- Cataplexy (60–70% patients)
  - Mainly associated with type 1 narcolepsy (1)
  - Sudden transient (seconds to minutes) episode of total or partial loss of motor tone, triggered by strong emotions (such as laughing, anger, or fright) (4)
  - Consciousness and memory are not impaired.
  - May affect all or segmental muscles (sparing diaphragm and extraocular)
  - If seen in type 2, suggests progression of disease (1)
  - *Status cataplecticus* is a rare, prolonged episode of cataplexy (lasting hours) that is more likely in children or those withdrawing off drugs.
- Sleep paralysis
  - Transient (seconds to minute) inability to move or speak either while falling asleep or upon awakening (4)
  - Patients are aware of their surroundings.
  - Seen in 50% of patients with type 1 narcolepsy
- Hypnagogic or hypnopompic hallucinations:
  - Vivid dreamlike experience in 30–60% patients with type 1 narcolepsy that occur during awakening (hypnopompic hallucinations) or at sleep onset (hypnagogic) (4)
  - Hallucination may either be visual, tactile, or auditory.
  - Characteristic hallucinations include being attacked by animals or feeling that someone else is in the room (2).
  - 15% of type 2 patients may experience these as well.

- Other reported history
  - Nocturnal insomnia and sleep fragmentation
  - Increased N1 stage of sleep
  - Retrograde amnesia
  - Increased periodic limb movements
  - Depression
  - Dream enactment behaviors
  - Weight gain

PHYSICAL EXAM
- Unremarkable exam, but complete physical may help rule out other causes of EDS
- Deep tendon reflexes are either diminished or absent during an episode of cataplexy.

DIFFERENTIAL DIAGNOSIS
EDS is present in 4% of the general population, although most individuals are not narcoleptic. Possible etiologies include the following:
- Sleep apnea syndromes
- Epileptic seizures and syncope
- Idiopathic hypersomnia (5–10% with EDS)
- Psychiatric (depression, substance abuse/withdrawal)
- Sleep-related movement disorders (restless leg syndrome, periodic limb movements of sleep)
- Iatrogenic/secondary to medication (benzodiazepines; opioids; antihistamines; β-blockers; and some antipsychotics, antidepressants, and anticonvulsants)
- Poor sleep hygiene and habits leading to sleep deficit and chronic sleep deprivation (1)
- Circadian rhythm disorders (jet lag, shift work, delayed or advanced sleep phase disorders)
- Cataplexy disorders (Niemann-Pick type C, Prader-Willi syndrome, Norrie disease) (1)
- Hypersomnia in Parkinson disease
- Kleine-Levin syndrome (recurrent hypersomnia that lasts days to weeks and recurs months later)
- Menstrual-associated hypersomnia
- Stroke (slurred speech and facial sagging seen in partial cataplexy) (2)

Pediatric Considerations
Narcolepsy is rare before the age of 5 years. EDS is more often attributable to OSA, poor sleep hygiene, and the increased sleep requirements early in life. Recommended amount of sleep decreases with age: newborns 16 to 18 hr/day; preschool-aged children 11 to 12 hr/day; school-aged children and teens 10 hr/day; adults 7 to 8 hr/day. Children can gain excessive weight, from 20 to 40 lb (2). Symptoms of EDS, sleep paralysis, and cataplexy might last longer than compared to adult population.

DIAGNOSTIC TESTS & INTERPRETATION
- Sleep log/actigraphy: First, ensure patient is getting 6 hours of sleep at night for at least 7 to 14 days.
- Prerequisites for valid multiple sleep latency test (MSLT) → normal polysomnography (PSG) with at least 360 minutes of sleep, free of drugs that may alter sleep for at least 2 weeks, standardized sleep schedule for 7 days
- Primary diagnostic tool
  - PSG: Once patient reports symptoms and narcolepsy is suspected, an overnight PSG is performed (for ages ≥6 years), mainly to rule out other causes of EDS.
  - MSLT: performed the day after PSG if at least 6 hours of sleep and no sleep disorder explained by PSG (2)
    - Four to five 20-minute naps at 2-hour intervals
    - Positive if rapid onset of REM (<15 minutes) in at least 2 of 5 sleeps (including baseline PSG) and shortened mean sleep latency (<8 minutes)

- If MSLT negative, but strong clinical suspicion, repeat the test.
- Antidepressants and stimulants should be discontinued prior to the test for at least 2 weeks (2).
- Scoring tools
  - Epworth Sleepiness Scale: Score ranges from 0 to 24, and >10 is suggestive of a sleep disorder rather than generalized fatigue; helpful for detecting response to medications (2)
  - Stanford Sleepiness Scale: Patients select 1 of 7 statements that best describe energy level, concentration, and sleepiness. Statements 4 to 7 may indicate excessive sleepiness.
  - Narcolepsy Severity Scale: a 15-item scale to assess the frequency, severity, and consequences of symptoms of narcolepsy type 1

Follow-Up Tests & Special Considerations

- Orexin: obtained via lumbar puncture, a level of 110 pg/mL or less in the CSF is indicative of narcolepsy; rarely performed
- HLA typing: particularly in children. It is supportive of diagnosis, lacks specificity.

Diagnostic Procedures/Other

- Narcolepsy type 1 (2)[C]
  - EDS daily for ≥3 months
  - One of the following:
    - Cataplexy with positive MSLT
    - Low CSF orexin level <110 pg/mL or <1/3 of mean values in normal subjects
- Narcolepsy type 2 (2)[C]
  - All of the above without the cataplexy and normal orexin
- It is a diagnosis of exclusion.

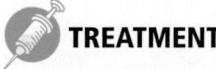# TREATMENT

GENERAL MEASURES

- Medications do not cure, but the goal is to minimize EDS and cataleptic episodes.
- First step is proper sleep hygiene and regular sleep schedule.
- Well-timed 15- to 20-minute naps may be helpful.
- Drug therapy, if used, should be supplemented by various behavioral strategies.
- Avoid stimulus (alcohol, heavy meals, caffeine, nicotine).
- Maneuvers such as altering thoughts, placing tension on muscles, or pressing against a firm support might rapidly terminate cataplectic episodes.
- Maintaining warmer body temperature and consuming warm meals/drinks may improve wakefulness (5).
- Use safety precautions, particularly when driving. Untreated patients are at 10-fold at risk of accidents.
- Adequate control can be obtained in 60–80% of patients.

MEDICATION

First Line

- EDS
  - Modafinil (Provigil) (5)[A]:
    - First-line treatment for mild to moderate EDS
    - Works on dopaminergic, adrenergic, and histaminergic receptors of hypothalamus
    - Dose: 200 mg/day, maybe divided BID. Start with 100 mg; max dose 400 mg/day
    - Half-life of 14 hours
    - Fewer adverse effects (headache, GI upset, increased metabolism of oral contraceptives) with less rebound hypersomnia and does not affect BP; tolerance limited
    - Caution in patients with cardiac diseases, may cause tachycardia

- Armodafinil (Nuvigil):
  - Enantiomeric form of modafinil with slightly longer half-life of 15 hours
  - Dose: 150 to 250 mg every morning
- Pitolisant (Wakix): new promising drug for narcolepsy and cataplexy approved for treatment in the EU (5)[A]
- Other emerging prescription: hypocretin agonists administered via intranasal route, atomoxetine and clarithromycin (1)
- Cataplexy:
  - Sodium oxybate (Xyrem):
    - Only medication proven effective and FDA-approved for both EDS and cataplexy (5)
    - Used for moderate to severe cases
    - Best option for improving nighttime sleep and FDA-approved for the same (5)
    - Dose: 6 to 9 g/day divided BID; start with 2.25 g and increase by 1.5 g/day qwk; max dose: 9 g/day
    - May take 8 to 12 weeks for full response
    - Is a date rape drug; abuse potential
    - May worsen sleep-disordered breathing in patients with OSA
    - Overdose may lead to coma.
  - Tricyclic antidepressants
    - Protriptyline: dose: 5 to 60 mg/day. Taper dose gradually.
    - Clomipramine: dose: 25 to 75 mg/day
    - High side effect profile (anticholinergic): dry mouth, sedation, urinary retention, impotence
  - Serotonin-norepinephrine reuptake inhibitors
    - Venlafaxine: dose: 75 to 300 mg/day. Start at 37.5 mg, max dose 375 mg/day. Taper dose to discontinue.
    - Fluoxetine: dose: 20 to 80 mg/day
    - Work by suppressing REM sleep
    - Not FDA-approved
  - The patient may develop a tolerance to the anti-cataplectic drugs and can have rebound cataplexy when a drug is withdrawn. Most require tapered dosing to discontinue.
- Auxiliary symptoms (e.g., hypnagogic hallucination, sleep paralysis) require treatment less often than EDS and cataplexy, but anticataplectics are useful when symptoms are problematic.

Second Line

- EDS
  - Amphetamines: used if first line fail or patient unable to tolerate
    - Methylphenidate (Ritalin): dose: initial dose 5 to 10 mg/day divided BID or TID; max dose 60 mg/day (5)[B], short acting, most potent amphetamine available; can be used in combination with modafinil and armodafinil
    - Dextroamphetamine: dose: initial dose 10 mg/day; can increase by 10 mg qwk to a max dose 60 mg/day divided BID or TID (5)[B]
    - Contraindicated in patients with hypertension (HTN)
    - Adverse reactions: headaches, irritability, HTN, psychosis, anorexia, habituation, rebound hypersomnia
    - If the patient develops a tolerance to stimulants, switch drug or drug holidays rather than increasing dose.
    - Highly addictive; high doses have been associated with frequent hospitalizations, arrhythmias, and psychiatric disturbances (5).
- Cataplexy
  - Selegiline: selective MAO-B inhibitor
    - Anticataplectic effective for EDS; 20 to 40 mg/day divided morning and noon
    - Doses >20 mg require a low-tyramine diet because the drug begins to lose selectivity

ISSUES FOR REFERRAL

- Unresponsive to primary medications
- Patient support groups can be very beneficial.
- Severe case of cataplexy may need neurology referral.

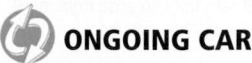# ONGOING CARE

FOLLOW-UP RECOMMENDATIONS

Patient Monitoring

- Monitoring using scoring tools to gauge treatment effectiveness and symptom control
- Frequent BP checks and regular follow-ups (approximately every 6 months) are recommended for those on medication.

DIET

Selegiline: Doses >20 mg require a low-tyramine diet because the drug begins to lose selectivity.

PATIENT EDUCATION

- Narcolepsy information from the National Institute of Neurological Disorders and Stroke at https://www.ninds.nih.gov/Disorders/Patient-Caregiver-Education/Fact-Sheets/Narcolepsy-Fact-Sheet
- Narcolepsy Network, Inc., North Kingstown, RI 02852; www.narcolepsynetwork.org

PROGNOSIS

Narcolepsy is a lifelong disease. Symptoms can worsen with aging. In women, symptoms can improve after menopause.

REFERENCES

1. Zhang J, Han F. Sleepiness in narcolepsy. *Sleep Med Clin*. 2017;12(3):323–330.
2. Scammell T. Narcolepsy. *N Engl J Med*. 2015;373(27):2654–2662.
3. Calik MW. Update on the treatment of narcolepsy: clinical efficacy of pitolisant. *Nat Sci Sleep*. 2017;9:127–133.
4. Iranzo A. Current diagnostic criteria for adult narcolepsy. In: Baumann CR, Bassetti CL, Scammell TE, eds. *Narcolepsy Pathophysiology, Diagnosis, and Treatment*. New York, NY: Springer; 2011:369–381.
5. Bhattarai J, Sumerall S. Current and future treatment options for narcolepsy: a review. *Sleep Sci*. 2017;10(1):19–27.

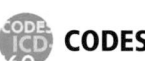# CODES

ICD10

- G47.429 Narcolepsy in conditions classified elsewhere w/o cataplexy
- G47.411 Narcolepsy with cataplexy
- G47.419 Narcolepsy without cataplexy

CLINICAL PEARLS

- Narcolepsy is an incurable, REM disorder, with an average of 15 years of symptoms before a definitive diagnosis is made.
- The classic tetrad of symptoms includes EDS, cataplexy, sleep paralysis, and hypnagogic hallucinations, but only cataplexy is pathognomonic for the disorder.
- The ICSD has specific diagnostic criteria for narcolepsy.
- Medications help minimize symptoms but not curative.

N

NASAL POLYPS

Andrew Dinh, DO • Tharani Ravi, MD

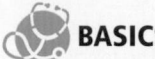 BASICS

- Chronic inflammatory lesion of nasal mucosa
- Arise from ethmoidal cells but can arise from maxillary sinus mucosa although less common

DESCRIPTION

- Appearance of edematous pedunculated mass in the nasal cavity or within the paranasal sinus
- Often causes symptoms of blockage, discharge, or loss of smell
- Most commonly bilateral; if unilateral, malignancy should be on differential.

EPIDEMIOLOGY

Prevalence

- ~4% in general population
- Much rarer in children: ~0.1% and associated with cystic fibrosis
- Increases with age
- Female > male (2:1)
- Asthma is present in 65% of patients.

ETIOLOGY AND PATHOPHYSIOLOGY

Genetics

- No clearly delineated pathway; research has demonstrated separate TH1- and TH2-driven pathways (1)[B].
- Development of condition remains unclear; multiple inflammatory and infectious pathways resulting from chronic rhinosinusitis is most common.

GENERAL PREVENTION

Use of intranasal corticosteroids after polyp removal surgery has shown effectiveness against recurrence.

COMMONLY ASSOCIATED CONDITIONS

- Asthma
- Bronchiectasis
- Aspirin hypersensitivity
- Allergic rhinitis
- Chronic sinusitis
- Allergic fungal sinusitis
- Cystic fibrosis
- Primary ciliary dyskinesia (Kartagener syndrome)
- Laryngopharyngeal reflux

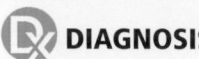 DIAGNOSIS

- Symptoms
  - Rhinorrhea
  - Nasal congestion
  - Postnasal drainage
  - Hyposmia
  - Inability to breathe through nose
  - Dull headaches
  - Facial pain/pressure over the middle third of the face
  - In some cases, there may be no symptoms.
- Pale, translucent mass on anterior rhinoscopy
  - Most commonly on lateral wall of middle meatus
- Flexible/rigid endoscopy is required to assess the nasal cavity fully.
  - Gold standard for diagnosis
- If large posterior nasal polyps, examine tympanic membrane for Eustachian tube dysfunction.
- If unilateral polyp, consider histologic exam to exclude malignancy.
- Benign versus malignant tumor:
  - Papilloma
  - Fibroma
  - Hemangioma
  - Neurilemmoma
  - Osteoma
  - Adenoma
  - Chondroma
  - Mycetoma
  - Encephalocele
  - Squamous cell carcinoma
  - Malignant melanoma
- Test for cystic fibrosis in children with multiple benign polyps.
- CT scanning (2):
  - May be helpful to corroborate history and endoscopic findings
  - Unable to differentiate polyp from other soft tissue masses
  - Reveals extent of disease and is necessary to formulate a plan for surgical intervention if indicated
- MRI (2):
  - May aid in diagnosis if concern for neoplasia, mycetoma, or encephalocele

TREATMENT

- Goal is to reduce the size or eliminate nasal polyps because they can obstruct the nasal cavity and impair sense of smell, restrict breathing ability through nose, and obstruct drainage of sinuses.
- Daily intranasal corticosteroid use with saline irrigation is first-line therapy.
  - Treat for a minimum of 12 weeks; minimal systemic absorption, side effects rare—minor nose bleeding is most common (1)
    - Budesonide 256 μg/day
    - Beclomethasone dipropionate 320 μg/day
    - Fluticasone propionate 400 μg/day
    - Mometasone furoate 200 μg BID
    - For children, mometasone furoate is preferred.

- Consider short course of oral corticosteroids (14 to 21 days) and/or doxycycline (21 days) in symptomatic patients despite initial therapy (3).
  - Prednisone 30 to 50 mg daily (taper when indicated)
  - Prednisolone 20 to 60 mg daily (taper when indicated)
  - Doxycycline 200 mg once, followed by 100 mg daily (3)[A]
- Patients with persistent symptoms and have concurrent allergic rhinitis, consider:
  - Systemic antihistamine
  - Leukotriene pathway antagonist
  - Allergy immunotherapy

ISSUES FOR REFERRAL

Consider referral to otorhinolaryngologist for endoscopic sinus surgery if severe obstruction symptoms or conservative management ineffective.

SURGERY/OTHER PROCEDURES

Recurrence ~5–10% (4)

- Most surgeries are approached endonasally.
  - The external (Caldwell-Luc) approach is used for more difficult cases but carries higher risk of complications.
- Functional endonasal sinus surgery has slightly lower revision rate than intranasal polypectomy. Both modalities provide effective symptom relief.
- Postoperative use of nasal corticosteroids delay the recurrence of nasal polyps and hence the timing of revision surgery (1).
- Postoperative use of steroid-releasing stents to prevent polyp recurrence by decreasing mucosal inflammation (1)

COMPLEMENTARY & ALTERNATIVE MEDICINE

Based on one randomized clinical trial, the addition of subcutaneous dupilumab to topical corticosteroids reduced endoscopic nasal polyp burden after 16 weeks, but further studies are needed to determine efficacy (3).

 ## ONGOING CARE

- Acute/chronic sinus infection
- Use of intranasal corticosteroids after polyp removal surgery has shown effectiveness against recurrence.
- Recurrence twice as likely in those with asthma
- Heterotrophic bone formation within the sinus cavity may occur.

REFERENCES

1. Poetker DM, Jakubowski LA, Lal D, et al. Oral corticosteroids in the management of adult chronic rhinosinusitis with and without nasal polyps: an evidence-based review with recommendations. *Int Forum Allergy Rhinol*. 2013;3(2):104–120.
2. DeMarcantonio MA, Han JK. Nasal polyps: pathogenesis and treatment implications. *Otolaryngol Clin North Am*. 2011;44(3):685–695.
3. Bachert C, Mannent L, Naclerio R, et al. Effect of subcutaneous dupilumab on nasal polyp burden in patients with chronic sinusitis and nasal polyposis: a randomized clinical trial. *JAMA*. 2016;315(5):469–479.
4. Fokkens WJ, Lund VJ, Mullol J, et al. EPOS 2012: European position paper on rhinosinusitis and nasal polyps 2012. A summary for otorhinolaryngologists. *Rhinology*. 2012;50(1):1–12.

ADDITIONAL READING

- Bachert C. Evidence-based management of nasal polyposis by intranasal corticosteroids: from the cause to the clinic. *Int Arch Allergy Immunol*. 2011;155(4):309–321.
- Håkansson K, Thomsen SF, Konge L, et al. A comparative and descriptive study of asthma in chronic rhinosinusitis with nasal polyps. *Am J Rhinol Allergy*. 2014;28(5):383–387.

- Rimmer J, Fokkens W, Chong LY, et al. Surgical versus medical interventions for chronic rhinosinusitis with nasal polyps. *Cochrane Database Syst Rev*. 2014;(12):CD006991.
- Rudmik L, Soler ZM. Medical therapies for adult chronic sinusitis: a systematic review. *JAMA*. 2015;314(9):926–939.
- Sharma R, Lakhani R, Rimmer J, et al. Surgical interventions for chronic rhinosinusitis with nasal polyps. *Cochrane Database Syst Rev*. 2014;(11):CD006990.

 ## CODES

ICD10
- J33.9 Nasal polyp, unspecified
- J33.0 Polyp of nasal cavity
- J33.8 Other polyp of sinus

CLINICAL PEARLS

- Intranasal corticosteroid use has been demonstrated to reduce polyp size and recurrence as well as to improve nasal congestion.
- Short-course oral corticosteroids and/or doxycycline may be considered in those with persistent symptoms.
- Asthma is a common concomitant diagnosis and is often previously undiagnosed.
- Aggressive medical and surgical treatment improves asthma outcomes.
- Allergy testing can be helpful.
- Patients with severe obstruction should be referred for surgery.
- Unilateral nasal polyp needs malignancy workup (MRI).

N

NEPHROTIC SYNDROME

Hanadi Abou Dargham, MD • Nandhini Veeraraghavan, MD, CAQSM, FAAFP

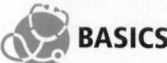 **BASICS**

DESCRIPTION

- A clinical syndrome of massive proteinuria (>3.5 g/1.73 m²/24 hr), hypoalbuminemia (<3 g/dL), severe hyperlipidemia (total cholesterol often >10 mmol/L) (380 mg/dL), clinical evidence of peripheral edema, with risk for thrombotic disease
- Includes both primary (idiopathic) and secondary forms
- Associated with many types of kidney disease

EPIDEMIOLOGY

Based on definitive diagnosis

- Diabetic nephropathy: most common cause of secondary nephrotic syndrome (1)
- Minimal change disease (MCD)
  - Most common cause of nephrotic syndrome in children <10 years (90%)
  - Peaks at 2 to 8 years of age
  - Associated with drugs (mainly NSAIDs) or lymphoma in adults
- Amyloidosis: 7–14% of idiopathic nephrotic syndrome—two renal types primary (AL) and secondary (AA)
- Lupus nephropathy (LN): Adult women are affected about 10 times more often than men.
- Focal segmental glomerulosclerosis (FSGS)
  - 35% of nephrotic syndrome in adults
  - Most common primary nephrotic syndrome in African Americans
  - Has both primary (idiopathic) and secondary forms (associated with HIV, morbid obesity, reflux nephropathy, previous glomerular injury)
- Membranous nephropathy
  - Most common cause of primary nephrotic syndrome in adults (40%)
  - May be primary or secondary associated with malignancy, Hep B, autoimmune diseases, thyroiditis, and certain drugs
- Membranoproliferative glomerulonephritis (MGN)
  - May be primary or secondary
  - May present in the setting of a systemic viral or rheumatic illness

ETIOLOGY AND PATHOPHYSIOLOGY

- Increased glomerular permeability to protein macromolecules, especially albumin
- Podocytes injury is the most common finding in diseases that cause primary nephrotic syndrome.
- Mutations in number of genes regulating podocyte proteins were identified in families with inherited nephrotic syndrome.
- Edema results primarily from renal salt retention, with arterial underfilling from decreased plasma oncotic pressure playing an additional role.
- Hyperlipidemia is thought to be a consequence of increased hepatic synthesis resulting from low oncotic pressure and urinary loss of regulatory proteins.
- The hypercoagulable state that can occur in some nephrotic states is likely due to loss of antithrombin III in urine.
- Primary renal disease:
  - MCD
  - FSGS
  - MGN
  - IgA nephropathy

- Secondary renal disease (associated primary renal disease shown in parentheses):
  - Diabetic nephropathy
  - Amyloidosis
  - LN
  - FSGS
  - Infections (MGN)
  - Cancer (MCD or MGN)
  - Drugs (MCD or MGN)

Genetics
Genetic factors are likely to play a role in the susceptibility and clinical unresponsiveness to glucose steroids, but the exact mechanism remains largely unknown.

RISK FACTORS
- Drug addiction (e.g., heroin [FSGS])
- Hepatitis B and C, HIV, other infections
- Immunosuppression
- Nephrotoxic drugs
- Vesicoureteral reflux (FSGS)
- Cancer (usually MGN, may be MCD)
- Chronic analgesic use/abuse (NSAIDs)
- Preeclampsia
- Diabetes mellitus

GENERAL PREVENTION
In general, there are few preventive measures, including avoidance of known causative medications including NSAIDs, gold, penicillamine, and captopril; avoidance of heroin abuse and tight glycemic control

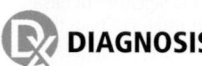 **DIAGNOSIS**

HISTORY
The history is key in pinpointing the cause of nephrotic syndrome.

- Inquire about signs or symptoms of systemic disease: joint complaint, rash, edema, infectious complaint, fevers, anorexia, oliguria, foamy urine, acute flank pain, and hematuria.
- Obtain a recent drug history for medications that may be causative, especially NSAIDs.
- Assess for risk factors.

PHYSICAL EXAM
A complete physical exam may discover clues to systemic disease as a potential cause and/or may suggest the severity of disease.

- Fluid retention: abdominal distention, abdominal fluid shift, extremity edema, puffy eyelids, scrotal swelling, weight gain, shortness of breath. Pericardial rub and decreased breath sounds with pleural effusions may develop.
- Arterial hypertension is found in 25% of the cases.
- Orthostatic hypotension
- Macroscopic hematuria is rare, but microscopic hematuria is present in 20% of the cases.

ALERT
The potential for thromboembolic disease leading to pulmonary embolism is one of the most life-threatening aspects of a patient who is actively nephrotic.

DIFFERENTIAL DIAGNOSIS
- Edema and proteinuria: See "Etiology and Pathophysiology."
- Edema alone: Other diseases to rule out in patients who have edema without proteinuria include congestive heart failure, cirrhosis, hypothyroidism, nutritional hypoalbuminemia, protein-losing enteropathy.

DIAGNOSTIC TESTS & INTERPRETATION
No guidelines are available for the investigation of nephrotic syndrome. Blood workup should be based on the clinical presentation.

Initial Tests (lab, imaging)
- Confirm proteinuria if present: by urine dipstick initially (3+ or 4+ readings) and then quantitate by 24-hour urine or spot urine protein-to-creatinine ratio.
- Rule out urine infection with urine culture.
- Full blood count and coagulation screen
- Renal function tests: BUN, creatinine with estimated glomerular filtration rate (GFR)
- Glucose to rule out overt diabetes
- Serum albumin that is often <2.5 g/dL in NS.
- Consider blood cultures to rule out a postinfectious process.
- Lipid panel
- Liver function tests to exclude liver disease or infection
- Look for autoimmune disease.
  - Antinuclear antibody and/or antidouble-stranded DNA positivity suggest lupus.
  - Complement levels (C3/C4 and total hemolytic complement): A low C3 may suggest a postinfectious or membranoproliferative process, whereas both low C3 and C4 point to lupus.
- Serum protein electrophoresis/urine immune electrophoresis to rule in a paraproteinemia
- Hepatitis B and C screen
- Measurement of cryoglobulins
- HIV and syphilis serology
- Urinalysis to evaluate for the presence of cellular casts
- Renal US to verify the presence of two kidneys of normal shape and size
- Chest x-ray to detect presence of pleural effusion or infection
- If thrombosis is suspected:
  - Doppler US of the legs
  - MRI or venography for renal vein thrombosis
  - Ventilation/perfusion nuclear medicine lung scan and/or CT angiography may be required to rule out pulmonary embolism.

Diagnostic Procedures/Other
Renal biopsy is standard in determining the underlying cause of nephrotic syndrome.

- Rarely done in children with first episode of nephrotic syndrome because MCD is common and empiric steroid therapy is the standard of care
- Required to confirm the clinical diagnosis in adults and assist with making a treatment plan (1)
- Contraindications to renal biopsy include small kidneys, renal tumor or bilateral renal cysts, active infection, severe malignant hypertension, hydronephrosis, bleeding diathesis, uncooperative patient.

Test Interpretation
- Light microscopy
  - May see nothing (e.g., MCD)
  - Sclerosis (e.g., FSGS or diabetic nodules in diabetes)
  - Diffuse hypercellularity suggests a proliferative disease such as IgA nephropathy, LN, or postinfectious GN.
- Immunofluorescence: Mesangial IgA suggests IgA nephropathy, Henoch-Schönlein purpura; other staining patterns are specific for other disease processes.
- Electron microscopy: The location of immunoglobulin deposits is useful in pointing to a particular diagnosis.

TREATMENT

MEDICATION

First Line
- Edema: salt restriction and salt-wasting diuretics (loop and thiazide diuretics) (2)[A]:
  – Salt restriction to <2 to 3 g sodium per day
  – Restrict fluid intake to <1.5 L/day if hyponatremic.
  – Target weight loss of 0.5 to 1.0 kg/day (1 to 2 lb/day)
- Edema should be corrected slowly to avoid acute hypovolemia, electrolyte disturbances, acute renal failure, and thromboembolism as a result of hemoconcentration, and diuretic dose should be increased in comparison to the general population.
- Hyperlipidemia:
  – Is reversed with resolution of the disease
  – The role of dietary modification is unproven yet.
- Statins have been shown to improve endothelial function (2)[A] and may decrease proteinuria (3)[A], but effect on GFR and preservation of renal function is small. The major role for statin use is in cardiovascular risk reduction.
- ACE inhibitors or angiotensin II receptor blockers are thought to reduce proteinuria, hyperlipidemia, thrombotic tendencies, progression of renal failure, and to control hypertension, if present (4)[A].
- For steroid-responsive disease (MCD and FSGS), steroids dosed in consultation with nephrologist

Second Line
- Many of the nephrotic diseases will require escalation in therapy above steroids. These include rapidly relapsing forms as well as MGN, LN, and IgA nephropathy. Bolus steroids and other immunosuppressives are required in this circumstance (cyclophosphamide, mycophenolate mofetil, chlorambucil, cyclosporine) (5)[A].
- Rituximab, anti-CD20 and abatacept, anti–B7-1, combined with steroids or other immunosuppressive agents, has demonstrated early promise in the treatment of refractory nephrotic syndrome (6)[B].
- Randomized controlled data have been insufficient to determine which patients require prophylactic anticoagulation (7)[A] and for how long. Common practice is to anticoagulate with heparin and then warfarin in patients who have persistent nephrotic-range proteinuria. This decision is made based on the patient's history of edema, hypoalbuminemia, thromboembolism, or immobility.
- Hypocalcemia from vitamin D loss should be treated with oral vitamin D.

ISSUES FOR REFERRAL
Consultation with a nephrologist is often required to assist with renal biopsy to confirm diagnosis and to assist with management of edema. Cytotoxic medications may be called for, depending on the disease process, and this may best be handled by a nephrologist.

ADDITIONAL THERAPIES
Ambulation or range of motion exercises to lower risk of deep vein thrombosis (DVT)

ADMISSION, INPATIENT, AND NURSING CONSIDERATIONS
- Admission criteria/initial stabilization: respiratory distress, sepsis/severe infection, thrombosis, renal failure, hypertensive urgency/emergency, or other complications

- Discharge criteria: Hemodynamically stable patients without complications may be managed as outpatients.

 ONGOING CARE

FOLLOW-UP RECOMMENDATIONS
Patient Monitoring
- Frequent monitoring is required for relapse, disease progression, and for detecting signs of toxicity of medical management.
- Reevaluate for azotemia, urine protein, hypertension, edema, loss of renal function, cholesterol, and weight.

DIET
Muscle wasting and malnutrition are major problems in severe nephrotic syndrome. Optimal diet includes:
- Normal protein (1 g/kg/day)
- Low fat (cholesterol)
- Reduced sodium (<2 g/day)
- Supplemental multivitamins and minerals, especially vitamin D and iron
- Fluid restriction if hyponatremic

PATIENT EDUCATION
- Printed material for patients: National Kidney Foundation, 30 E. 33rd Street, Suite 1100, New York, NY 10016; 800-622-9010
  – Childhood nephrotic syndrome
  – Diabetes and kidney disease
  – Focal glomerulosclerosis
- Web site: National Institutes of Health: nephrotic syndrome

PROGNOSIS
- Nephrotic syndrome in children (MCD) is typically self-limited and carries a good prognosis. In the adult, the prognosis is variable. Proteinuria is the most important adverse prognostic factor that leads to rapid progression to end-stage renal failure.
- Complete remission is expected if the basic disease is treatable (infection, malignancy, drug induced); otherwise, a relapsing and remitting course is possible, with progression to dialysis seen in more aggressive forms (diabetic glomerulosclerosis and FSGS).

COMPLICATIONS
- Thromboembolism:
  – Deep vein, renal vein, or central venous thrombosis may occur. Arterial thrombosis is very rare.
  – The risk appears to be greater the lower the serum albumin.
  – Pulmonary embolism is a known complication.
- Pleural effusion
- Symptomatic hypovolemia
- Ascites
- Hyperlipidemia, cardiovascular disease
- Acute renal failure, progressive renal failure
- Protein malnutrition/muscle wasting
- Infection secondary to low serum IgG concentrations, reduced complement activity, and depressed T-cell function: peritonitis, pneumonia, or cellulitis
- Loss of vitamin D (vitamin D–binding protein loss in urine) leading to bone disease
- Proximal tubular dysfunction resulting in glucosuria, aminoaciduria, phosphaturia, bicarbonaturia, and vitamin D deficiency

REFERENCES
1. Kodner C. Diagnosis and management of nephrotic syndrome in adults. *Am Fam Physician*. 2016;93(6):479–485.
2. Crew RJ, Radhakrishnan J, Appel G. Complications of the nephrotic syndrome and their treatment. *Clin Nephrol*. 2004;62(4):245–259.
3. Fried LF, Orchard TJ, Kasiske BL. Effect of lipid reduction on the progression of renal disease: a meta-analysis. *Kidney Int*. 2001;59(1):260–269.
4. Kunz R, Friedrich C, Wolbers M, et al. Meta-analysis: effect of monotherapy and combination therapy with inhibitors of the renin angiotensin system on proteinuria in renal disease. *Ann Intern Med*. 2008;148(1):30–48.
5. Hodson EM, Willis NS, Craig JC. Interventions for idiopathic steroid-resistant nephrotic syndrome in children. *Cochrane Database Syst Rev*. 2010;(11):CD003594.
6. Kamei K, Okada M, Sato M, et al. Rituximab treatment combined with methylprednisolone pulse therapy and immunosuppressants for childhood steroid-resistant nephrotic syndrome. *Pediatr Nephrol*. 2014;29(7):1181–1187.
7. Kulshrestha S, Grieff M, Navaneethan SD. Interventions for preventing thrombosis in adults and children with nephrotic syndrome (protocol). *Cochrane Database Syst Rev*. 2006;(2):CD006024.

ADDITIONAL READING
- Bierzynska A, Saleem M. Recent advances in understanding and treating nephrotic syndrome. *F1000Res*. 2017;6:121.
- Boyer O, Baudouin V, Bérard E, et al. Idiopathic nephrotic syndrome [in French]. *Arch Pediatr*. 2017;24(12):1338–1343.

 SEE ALSO

Acute Kidney Injury; Amyloidosis; Diabetes Mellitus, Type 1; Diabetes Mellitus, Type 2; Glomerulonephritis, Acute; HIV/AIDS; Lupus Erythematosus, Discoid; Multiple Myeloma

 CODES

ICD10
- N04.9 Nephrotic syndrome with unspecified morphologic changes
- N04.1 Nephrotic syndrome w focal and segmental glomerular lesions
- N04.2 Nephrotic syndrome w diffuse membranous glomerulonephritis

CLINICAL PEARLS
- Nephrotic syndrome is a clinical syndrome of >3.5 g/day proteinuria, hypoalbuminemia, hyperlipidemia, and edema often associated with diabetes and NSAIDs use.
- Pediatric nephrotic syndrome typically carries a good prognosis and is more easily treated with steroids, although recurrences are common.
- Nondiabetic adults with nephrotic syndrome will require a renal biopsy to determine cause.
- Have a high index of suspicion for symptoms that may represent an embolic event in patients with nephrotic syndrome.

NEUROFIBROMATOSIS TYPE 1

Michele Roberts, MD, PhD

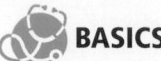 **BASICS**

DESCRIPTION

- Neurofibromatosis types 1 (NF1) and 2 (NF2) are neurocutaneous syndromes (phakomatoses). Although they share a name, they are unrelated.
  - NF1, the most common of the phakomatoses, is a multisystem disorder that may affect any organ: It is characterized by café au lait spots, axillary and inguinal freckling, neurofibromas, Lisch nodules, choroidal freckling.
  - NF2 is a rare condition that causes bilateral vestibular schwannomas.
- System(s) affected: musculoskeletal; nervous; skin/exocrine; cardiovascular; neuro-ophthalmologic
- Synonym(s): von Recklinghausen disease, formerly peripheral NF

EPIDEMIOLOGY

Incidence
- Predominant sex for NF1: male = female
- Birth incidence NF1: 1:2,500 to 3,000

Prevalence
1:3,000 to 1:4,000

ETIOLOGY AND PATHOPHYSIOLOGY

- Neurofibromin is a guanosine triphosphatase–activating protein that acts as a tumor suppressor by downregulating a cellular proto-oncogene, *p21-ras*, which enhances cell growth and proliferation.
- Neurofibromata are benign tumors composed of Schwann cells, fibroblasts, mast cells, and vascular components that develop along nerves.
- The two-hit hypothesis has been invoked to explain malignant transformation in *NF1*.

Genetics
- Online Mendelian Inheritance in Man 162200
- Caused by a mutation in the *NF1* gene on chromosome 17q11.2; autosomal dominant inheritance; protein product is called *neurofibromin*.
- 50% of cases are due to de novo mutations, mostly paternal; likelihood increases with paternal age.
- Prenatal diagnosis is possible if mutation is known.
- Penetrance is nearly 100%; expressivity is highly variable, even within a family.
- Gene is large, with a variety of mutations causing NF1. Molecular technology can detect 95% of clinically important *NF1* mutations, but clinical diagnosis frequently can be made in childhood.
- ~5% of individuals with NF1 have a large deletion of the *NF1* gene; usually a more severe phenotype
- *Segmental NF* is limited to a single body region and is caused by mosaicism for the *NF1* mutation.

RISK FACTORS

- Having an affected first-degree relative is a diagnostic criterion for NF1, although relatives may be unaware that they have NF1.
- Affected individuals with a positive family history (or a new mutation) have a 50% risk of transmitting NF1 to each offspring; 1 in 12 will be severely affected.
- Segmental NF1: may have gonadal mosaicism and may be at risk for transmission of the mutated gene

COMMONLY ASSOCIATED CONDITIONS

- Congenital heart disease, pulmonary stenosis, hypertension, renal artery stenosis
- Learning disabilities (50–75%)

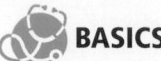 **DIAGNOSIS**

- NF1 can be diagnosed by routine exam by age 4 years, with attention to skin stigmata; diagnostic criteria include ≥2 of the following (1):
  - ≥6 café au lait (light brown) macules, ≥5 mm in prepubertal individuals, or ≥15 mm in adults
  - ≥2 neurofibromata of any type or 1 plexiform (uncircumscribed) neurofibroma
  - Axillary or inguinal freckling
  - ≥2 Lisch nodules (benign iris hamartomas)
  - Optic glioma by MRI
  - Characteristic osseous lesions: sphenoid dysplasia, long-bone cortical thinning, ribbon ribs, angular scoliosis
  - First-degree relative with NF1 by above criteria
- Prenatal diagnosis is possible with known mutation or by linkage testing (with positive family history), although not predictive of clinical course.
- With increasingly precise molecular analysis and newly recognized clinical signs, including nevus anemicus, unidentified bright objects, choroidal hamartomas, and a characteristic neuropsychological phenotype, 1988 clinical criteria may be due for revision (2).

HISTORY

- Family history of a first-degree relative with NF1
- Manifestations generally are not visible at birth, although plexiform neurofibromata are usually congenital, and tibial bowing is congenital.
- In addition to cutaneous lesions, NF1 may present with painful neurofibromata, pathologic fractures, or headaches secondary to hypertension caused by pheochromocytomas.
- Optic gliomata may present as involuntary eye movement, squinting, loss of vision, or as diencephalic syndrome.

PHYSICAL EXAM

- Skin
  - Café au lait macules, usually the presenting feature of NF1, develop before age 3 years. Evenly pigmented, irregularly shaped (coast of California), light brown macules seen in 97% of patients with NF1; many unaffected individuals have 1 to 3 such macules.
  - Neurofibromata: can be soft or firm, cutaneous, subcutaneous, or plexiform; buttonhole invagination is pathognomonic. Cutaneous neurofibromata usually appear during late childhood or adolescence.
  - Plexiform neurofibromata present in up to 50%
    - Usually congenital; may be subtle in infancy
    - Freckling or hypertrichosis may be present over plexiform neurofibromata; may affect underlying structures or focal hyperplasia
    - Many are internal, not obvious on exam.
    - Most grow slowly, but can have rapid growth, especially in early childhood.
  - Evaluate for new or progressive lesions. Rapidly growing cutaneous lesions should be evaluated.
  - Axillary freckling (Crowe sign) or inguinal freckling (91%)
- Ophthalmologic
  - Lisch nodules in 30%: well-defined, dome-shaped, gelatinous hamartomatous lesions projecting from the iris, varying from clear yellow to brown
  - Essentially unique to NF, Lisch nodules are asymptomatic; significant only for diagnosis
  - Pallor or atrophy of optic disc, bulging of orbit, and loss of vision may be signs of optic glioma
  - Choroidal freckling (3)

- Skeletal
  - Scoliosis and vertebral angulation
  - Localized bone hypertrophy, especially of the face
  - Limb abnormalities:
    - Pseudoarthrosis of the tibia
    - Tibial dysplasia (anterolateral bowing of the tibia) is congenital.
    - Nonossifying fibromas of the long bones in adolescents and adults are uncommon but can increase risk of fracture.
- Pay particular attention to neurologic examination (asymmetry) or new focal pain.
- Measure blood pressure (BP) yearly. Hypertension is more common in patients with NF1 and could be secondary to renal artery stenosis, aortic stenosis, and pheochromocytoma.
- Evaluate neurodevelopmental progress in children. Learning disabilities occur in 50–75%.

DIFFERENTIAL DIAGNOSIS

Familial café au lait spots (autosomal dominant, no other NF1 features), Legius syndrome, constitutional mismatch repair deficiency syndrome (CMMRD), NF2, Watson syndrome, LEOPARD syndrome, McCune-Albright syndrome, neurocutaneous melanosis, proteus syndrome, lipomatosis, Jaffe–Campanacci syndrome

Geriatric Considerations
In NF1, cutaneous lesions and tumors increase in size and number with age.

Pediatric Considerations
- Children who have inherited the *NF1* gene of an affected parent usually are identified by age 1 year, but external stigmata may be subtle.
- If no stigmata noted by age 2 years, NF is unlikely, but the child should be reexamined. Diagnosis usually can be made by age 4 years using NIH criteria (1), although young children may have multiple café au lait spots but no other stigmata.
- Molecular confirmation may be appropriate, especially with atypical presentation (4).

DIAGNOSTIC TESTS & INTERPRETATION

- Molecular genetic testing often not necessary for diagnosis: https://www.genetests.org/
- Confirmatory genetic testing is appropriate in those suspected of having NF1 but do not fulfill diagnostic criteria or for prenatal diagnosis or preimplantation genetic diagnosis (PGD) (5).
- Molecular genetic testing of the *NF1* gene can identify mutations in ~95% of those with a clinical diagnosis.
- Multistep pathogenic variant detection with cDNA and gDNA sequence analysis recommended if molecular genetic testing is indicated (6). NF1 is caused by a wide variety of mutations in the NF1 gene.

Initial Tests (lab, imaging)
- Characteristic radiographic findings: sphenoid dysplasia, long bone cortical thinning, ribbon ribs, angular scoliosis. Screening radiographs of the knees in adolescents is controversial. CT can demonstrate bony changes.
- MRI findings of the orbits, brain, or spine (86%). Routine head MRI scanning in asymptomatic individuals is controversial. Optic gliomata (on MRI, 11–15%) may lead to blindness. Although areas of increased T_2 signal intensity (unidentified bright objects) are common on brain MRI, they are not diagnostic of NF1 and likely of no clinical significance.

- The NIH Consensus Development Conference does not recommend routine neuroimaging as a means of establishing a diagnosis, although modification of diagnostic criteria is discussed (1)[C].

Diagnostic Procedures/Other

- Ophthalmologic evaluation, including slit-lamp exam of the irides; visual field testing to evaluate optic gliomata
- Neuropsychological testing: intelligence usually normal but may have significant deficits in language, visuospatial skills, and neuromotor skills

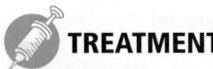

TREATMENT

MEDICATION

First Line

No specific therapeutic agents; symptoms are treated as they arise (e.g., anticonvulsants for seizures, medications for ADHD, management of BP).

Second Line

- In treating plexiform neurofibromas, tipifarnib, sirolimus, and pirfenidone have shown insufficient benefit. Small trials of imatinib have shown some tumor shrinkage. Selumetinib has shown promising results in a small study.
- Multiple clinical trials for NF1 are recruiting patients (see https://www.clinicaltrials.gov/).

ISSUES FOR REFERRAL

- Patients with more than minimal manifestations of NF1: Refer to a multidisciplinary NF clinic.
- Referral for psychosocial issues
- Educational intervention for children with learning disabilities or ADHD (40%)
- Early referral to orthopedics for congenital tibial bowing

ADDITIONAL THERAPIES

- Occupational therapy for children with NF1 who present with fine motor difficulties
- Laser therapy not recommended for café au lait spots
- The Children's Tumor Foundation (CTF) has established the NF Clinical Trials Consortium and the CTF NF Clinic Network to facilitate clinical trials.

SURGERY/OTHER PROCEDURES

- Surgical treatment for dystrophic scoliosis or malignancy (especially malignant peripheral nerve sheath tumors [MPNST]). Surgery for plexiform neurofibromata is often unsatisfactory.
- Treatment of optic gliomata unnecessary unless symptomatic

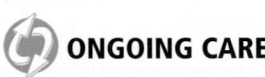

ONGOING CARE

FOLLOW-UP RECOMMENDATIONS

NF1 health supervision 2008 guidelines:

- Infancy to 1 year (7)[C]
  - Growth and development: mild short stature, macrocephaly (increased brain volume); aqueductal stenosis/obstructive hydrocephalus
  - Check for focal neurologic signs or asymmetric neurologic exam.
  - Skeletal abnormalities, especially spine and legs
  - Neurodevelopmental progress
- 1 to 5 years (7)[C]
  - Café au lait spots and axillary freckling have no clinical significance.
  - Annual ophthalmologic exam
  - Brain MRI for visual changes, persistent headaches, seizures, marked increase in head size, plexiform neurofibroma of the head

- Assess speech and language: hypernasal speech due to velopharyngeal insufficiency and delayed expressive language development.
- Developmental evaluation of learning and motor abilities; may benefit from speech/language and/or motor therapy, and special education
- Monitor BP annually.
- 5 to 13 years (7)[C]
  - Evaluate for skin tumors causing disfigurement, and obtain consultation if surgery is desired to improve appearance or function.
  - Evaluate for premature or delayed puberty. If sexual precocity is noted, evaluate for an optic glioma or hypothalamic lesion. Review the effects of puberty on NF.
  - Evaluate for learning disabilities and ADHD.
  - Evaluate social adjustment, development, and school placement.
  - Monitor ophthalmologic status yearly until age 8 years; complete eye exam every 2 years
  - Monitor BP annually.
  - Refer patient to a clinical psychologist or child psychiatrist for problems with self-esteem.
  - Discuss growth of neurofibromata during adolescence and pregnancy.
  - Counsel parents about discussing diagnosis with child.
- 13 to 21 years (7)[C]
  - Examine the adolescent for abnormal pubertal development.
  - Skin examination for plexiform neurofibromata and neurologic exam for findings suggestive of deep plexiform neurofibromata; surgical consultation for signs of pressure on deep structures
  - Continue to monitor BP yearly.
  - Ophthalmologic exam every 2 years until age 18 years
  - Discuss genetics of NF1 or refer for genetic counseling.
  - Discuss sexuality, contraception, and reproductive options.
  - Discuss effects of pregnancy on NF1, if appropriate. Neurofibromata may enlarge, and new tumors may develop during pregnancy.
  - Review prenatal diagnosis or refer to a geneticist.

PATIENT EDUCATION

- Genetic counseling and patient education regarding future complications about family planning
- Support groups are important: http://www.ctf.org/.

PROGNOSIS

Variable; most patients have a mild expression of NF1 and lead normal lives.

COMPLICATIONS

- Disfigurement: Skin neurofibromata develop primarily on exposed areas. The number tends to increase with puberty or pregnancy.
- Scoliosis: 10–30% (most cases mild); bowing of long bones, 2%; osteopenia and osteoporosis
- A large head is common but rarely associated with hydrocephalus.
- Increased risk of malignancy: MPNST (5–10%) usually in adults (1), especially within the field of previous radiotherapy for plexiform neurofibroma
- CNS tumors (5–15%), optic pathway glioma most common, most often asymptomatic but usually presents before age 6 years if symptomatic; symptomatic lesions usually stable or slowly progressive
- High relative risk (RR) for uncommon malignancies
- Increased risk for pheochromocytoma, rhabdomyosarcoma, leukemia, Wilms tumor

- RR for cancer of the esophagus (3.3), stomach (2.8), colon (2.0), liver (3.8), lung (3.0), bone (19.6), thyroid (4.9), malignant melanoma (3.6), non-Hodgkin lymphoma (3.3), chronic myeloid leukemia (6.7), female breast (2.3), and ovary (3.7)
- Learning disability: ~50%; may be associated with ADHD; cognitive impairment in 4–8%
- Neuropsychological phenotype
- GI neurofibromata may cause GI disturbances.
- Seizures: 6–7%
- Hypertension frequent in adults, may occur in childhood
- Disorders of puberty

Pregnancy Considerations

Increased risk of perinatal complications, stillbirth, intrauterine growth constriction; risk of cord compression and outlet obstruction by pelvic neurofibromata

REFERENCES

1. DeBella K, Szudek J, Friedman JM. Use of the National Institutes of Health Criteria for diagnosis of neurofibromatosis 1 in children. *Pediatrics*. 2000;105(3, Pt 1):608–614.
2. Tadini G, Milani D, Menni F, et al. Is it time to change the neurofibromatosis 1 diagnostic criteria? *Eur J Intern Med*. 2014;25(6):506–510.
3. Parrozzani R, Clementi M, Frizziero L, et al. In vivo detection of choroidal abnormalities related to NF1: feasibility and comparison with standard NIH diagnostic criteria in pediatric patients. *Invest Ophthalmol Vis Sci*. 2015;56(10):6036–6042.
4. Burkitt Wright EM, Sach E, Sharif S, et al. Can the diagnosis of NF1 be excluded clinically? A lack of pigmentary findings in families with spinal neurofibromatosis demonstrates a limitation of clinical diagnosis. *J Med Genet*. 2013;50(9):606–613.
5. National Institutes of Health Consensus Development Conference statement: neurofibromatosis. Bethesda, Md., USA, July 13–15, 1987. *Neurofibromatosis*. 1988;1(3):172–178.
6. Sabbagh A, Pasmant E, Imbard A, et al. NF1 molecular characterization and neurofibromatosis type I genotype-phenotype correlation: the French experience. *Hum Mutat*. 2013;34(11):1510–1518.
7. Hersh JH; for American Academy of Pediatrics Committee on Genetics. Health supervision for children with neurofibromatosis. *Pediatrics*. 2008;121(3):633–642.

 SEE ALSO

Tuberous Sclerosis Complex; Von Hippel-Lindau Syndrome

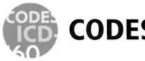 CODES

ICD10

Q85.01 Neurofibromatosis, type 1

CLINICAL PEARLS

- Marked clinical variability. External stigmata may be subtle or absent in young children. Minimally affected children may become severely affected adults.
- A single café au lait spot is of no concern in a child, but having ≥6 is a diagnostic criterion for NF1.

N

NEUROPATHIC PAIN

Michael J. Arnold, MD

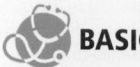 **BASICS**

DESCRIPTION
- Defined as pain caused by direct nerve injury
- An injury to either the peripheral or central nervous system (CNS) can lead to neuropathic pain.
- Can exist without ongoing disease
- Can arise from damage to nerve pathways at any point from terminals of the peripheral nociceptors to cortical neurons in the brain
- Causes include traumatic nerve injury, infection, metabolic injury, autoimmune disease, neoplasm, drugs, radiation, and neurovascular disorders.

EPIDEMIOLOGY
Prevalence
Includes chronic conditions that affect up to 10% of the population (1)
- Cancer—up to 20% have neuropathic pain from either cancer or treatment
- Herpes zoster—lifetime incidence is ~25%. Up to 10% develop chronic postherpetic neuralgia (1).
- HIV—33 million people infected across the world; ~35% have neuropathic pain.
- Diabetic neuropathy—affects 0.8% of population (1)

ETIOLOGY AND PATHOPHYSIOLOGY
- Positive symptoms due to changes in peripheral nerves, loss of inhibitory mechanisms in CNS, and central sensitization
- Negative symptoms (sensory deficits) reflect neural damage.
- Associated with numerous conditions, including:
  - Demyelinating disorders (multiple sclerosis, Guillain-Barré syndrome)
  - Neoplasm (primary/metastatic)
  - Neurovascular (central poststroke syndrome, diabetes, trigeminal neuralgia)
  - Autoimmune disease (Sjögren syndrome, polyarteritis nodosa)
  - Structural disease (herniated disc disease) (2)

RISK FACTORS
- General risk factors include older age, female gender, physical inactivity, and manual occupation.
- There is growing evidence of genetic factors.
- Includes conditions that cause nerve damage or potentiate symptoms from damaged nerves:
  - Diabetes
  - Herpes zoster
  - Trigeminal neuralgia
  - HIV
  - Lyme disease
  - Cancer and chemotherapy
  - Stroke
  - Multiple sclerosis
  - Trauma
  - Surgery
  - Limb amputation
  - Nutritional deficiencies
  - Medications

COMMONLY ASSOCIATED CONDITIONS
- Depression/anxiety
- Insomnia
- Substance abuse

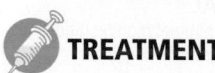 **DIAGNOSIS**

Diagnosis is based primarily on history (e.g., underlying disorder and distinct pain qualities) and the findings on physical examination (e.g., pattern of sensory disturbance) (2,3)[C].

HISTORY
- History should include:
  - Onset and duration of symptoms: location, intensity, character, temporal profile, exacerbating factors, concomitant symptoms, and effect on symptoms. Past medical and surgical history, psychosocial history, substance use (especially alcohol) can highlight possible etiologies.
  - Sensory descriptors: numbness, weakness, reduced sensation to touch, pinprick, temperature, or vibration; decreased proprioception
- Pain often described as burning, shock-like, or tingling (2,3)
- No single feature is diagnostic (3).

PHYSICAL EXAM
- Positive symptoms and signs (3)
  - Hyperalgesia: (abnormally increased pain response to stimulus) including sharp or blunt pressure, heat or cold
  - Allodynia: (pain from nonpainful stimulus) evoked by light touch, clothing, or bed sheets
- Negative symptoms—can be present in the same area as positive (3)
  - Hypoesthesia (abnormally reduced sensation of a tactile stimulus) to touch or temperature
- Motor (3)
  - Symptoms may include weakness, fatigability, decreased range of motion, joint stiffness, and spontaneous muscle spasm.
  - Signs may include hypotonia, tremor, dystonia, ataxia, hypo-/hyperreflexia, motor neglect.
- Sensory examination (2,3)
  - Light touch, pinprick, vibration sense, and proprioception may be diminished or amplified in the involved nerve territory.
  - Sensory disturbance may extend beyond a discrete nerve territory.
- Skin examination
  - Alterations in temperature, color, sweating, and hair growth suggestive of sympathetic nervous system involvement, such as in complex regional pain syndrome (CRPS) (3)
  - Residual dermatomal scars can indicate previous herpes or herpes zoster (shingles) infection.
  - Acanthosis nigricans can indicate diabetes.

DIFFERENTIAL DIAGNOSIS
- Nociceptive pain: induced by transmission impulses along peripheral nociceptors due to tissue damage
- Differentiate by clinical signs and symptoms, mechanisms, and therapeutic management.

DIAGNOSTIC TESTS & INTERPRETATION
Lab tests may suggest etiology of pain. Neurologic testing establishes distribution but does not yet provide benefit in determining treatment (4).

Initial Tests (lab, imaging)
None specifically for neuropathic pain but can rule in or out a cause of symptoms
- Serum vitamin B_{12}
- Thyroid-stimulating hormone (TSH)
- Rapid plasma reagin (RPR) or venereal disease research laboratory (VDRL) test
- Fasting glucose/hemoglobin A1c, creatinine, Lyme serology

Follow-Up Tests & Special Considerations
- Neuroimaging of affected area—only useful for verifying pathology for procedure or surgery
- Nerve conduction study (NCS): Focus on large nerves limits utility for most neuropathic pain; exceptions include compression neuropathies such as carpal tunnel syndrome (2).
- Electromyography: also large nerve focus, results do not apply to Aδ and C pain fibers (2).
- Quantitative sensory testing: measures patient perceptual response to quantified pain stimulus; being studied to find sensory types of neuropathic pain in hopes of improving therapy (2)
- Skin biopsy: used for population studies, decreased nerve fiber density seen in some neuropathic conditions (fibromyalgia, HIV neuropathy) (2)

TREATMENT

GENERAL MEASURES
- Due to multiple neuropathic pain pathways, all medications have limited efficacy and minority of patients have significant benefit at tolerable doses.
- Physical and occupational therapy can help with functional goals.
- Cognitive-behavioral therapy has proven benefit (4)[B].

MEDICATION
- The efficacy of systemic drug treatments is generally not dependent on the etiology of the underlying disorder (3).
- Combined therapy (polypharmacy) likely more effective
- Treatment needs to be individualized.
- Thought to be resistant to acetaminophen or NSAIDs but often used with some benefit (3)[C]

First Line
- Calcium channel α2δ ligands
  - Gabapentin: number needed to treat (NNT) = 7.2 for significant pain improvement (5)[A]
    - Dosing: up to 3,600 mg in 3 divided doses
    - Precautions: requires renal dosing
    - Common side effects: sedation, dizziness, peripheral edema, weight gain
  - Pregabalin NNT = 7.7 (6)[A]
    - Dosing: up to 600 mg in 2 doses
    - Precautions: requires renal dosing
    - Common side effects: sedation, dizziness, peripheral edema, weight gain

- Tricyclic antidepressants: NNT = 3.6 (6)[A]
  - Nortriptyline, desipramine, amitriptyline clomipramine, imipramine
    - Dosing: Start 10 to 25 mg at bedtime and then increase by 10 to 25 mg every 4 to 7 days up to 150 mg/day to efficacy and side effects.
    - Precautions: cardiac disease, glaucoma, prostatic adenoma, seizure, tramadol use
    - Geriatric: falls; limit dose to <75 mg.
    - Common side effects: somnolence, weight gain, anticholinergic effects
- Serotonin norepinephrine reuptake inhibitors (SNRIs): NNT = 6.4 (6)[A]
  - Duloxetine
    - Dosing: 20 mg once daily to 60 mg twice daily; effective doses 60 to 120 mg daily
    - Precautions: hepatic disorder, tramadol use, hypertension
    - Common side effect: nausea
  - Venlafaxine
    - Dosing: 37.5 mg to 225.0 mg daily
    - Effective doses: 150 to 225 mg daily
    - Precautions: cardiac disease, tramadol use, hypertension
    - Common side effects: nausea, hypertension at higher doses
- Lidocaine, 5% patches (6)[B]
  - As effective as pregabalin for localized neuropathic pain from diabetes or herpes
  - Dosage: 1 to 3 patches for 12 hours daily to cover the painful area
  - Precautions: none
  - Common side effects: local erythema, itch, rash

Second Line
Capsaicin high-concentration patches (8%): NNT = 10.6 (6)[A]
- Dosing: 1 to 4 patches to cover the painful area; 30 minutes application to feet, 60 minutes application to remainder of body; avoid use on face; benefits for up to 3 months
- Precautions: caution in progressive neuropathy
- Common side effects: pain (initial increase), erythema, itching, rare hypertension
- No benefit from low concentration capsaicin cream

Third Line
- Opioids (including tramadol): no proven long-term benefit; utility for neuropathic pain questioned
  - Chronic opioids decrease number and sensitivity of μ-opioid receptors, increasing hyperalgesia.
  - Tests show chronic pain patients on chronic opioids have higher pain sensitivity.
- Botulinum toxin type A (6)[B]
  - Limited evidence for peripheral syndromes
    - Dosage: 50 to 200 units subcutaneously to the painful area; repeat every 3 months.
    - Precautions: local infection
    - Common side effects: pain at injection site, weakness
- Cannabinoids (dronabinol and nabilone): low quality evidence (5)[A]
  - NNT = 20 for 50% improvement in pain
  - Number needed to harm (NNH) = 3 for adverse events
    - NNH = 10 for psychiatric adverse events
    - NNH = 25 for withdrawal due to adverse events

ISSUES FOR REFERRAL
- Physical or occupational therapy and psychology referrals part of standard multidisciplinary care
- Refer to pain clinic if refractory to initial treatment for trial of additional therapies.

ADDITIONAL THERAPIES
- Acupuncture: limited evidence for improvement in pain and quality of life, especially when combined with medication
- Interventional pain management (epidural or peripheral nerve injections) will provide partial, lasting relief in 40–60% of patients (4)[A].
- Spinal cord stimulation (SCS): Pain that is continuous and unchanging responds best. Best evidence for failed back surgery syndrome with leg pain. Less common indications are peripheral nerve injury, CRPS, and painful peripheral neuropathy (4)[B].
- Peripheral nerve stimulation (PNS): Indications include pain in the distribution of an accessible peripheral nerve.
- Intrathecal drug delivery: reserved for refractory pain; ziconotide has demonstrated efficacy (4)[B].
- Transcutaneous electrical nerve stimulation is widely used; evidence of efficacy is poor (4).

SURGERY/OTHER PROCEDURES
Nerve destructive procedures haven't shown effectiveness and may cause additional insult/injury (an exception is treatment of terminal cancer) (4)[B].
- Sympathectomy dorsal root entry zone lesion (dorsal rhizotomy)
- Lateral cordotomy
- Trigeminal nerve ganglion ablation

 ONGOING CARE

FOLLOW-UP RECOMMENDATIONS
- Multidisciplinary team
- Periodic evaluation to rule out other treatable conditions

Patient Monitoring
- Pain management requires ongoing evaluation, patient education, and reassurance.
- Patient compliance and adequacy of analgesic drug titrations should be continually evaluated and documented, especially opioids.

PROGNOSIS
Chronic course of pain symptoms often requires management with numerous medications and adjunctive therapies. Complete pain relief is rare.

COMPLICATIONS
Long-term disability and drug addiction are possible.

REFERENCES
1. van Hecke O, Austin SK, Khan RA, et al. Neuropathic pain in the general population: a systematic review of epidemiological studies. *Pain*. 2014;155(4):654–662.
2. Fillingim RB, Loeser JD, Baron R, et al. Assessment of chronic pain: domains, methods, and mechanisms. *J Pain*. 2016;17(Suppl 9):T10–T20.
3. Gilron I, Baron R, Jensen T. Neuropathic pain: principles of diagnosis and treatment. *Mayo Clin Proc*. 2015;90(4):532–545.
4. Jones RC III, Lawson E, Backonja M. Managing neuropathic pain. *Med Clin North Am*. 2016;100(1):151–167.
5. Mücke M, Phillips T, Radbruch L, et al. Cannabis-based medicines for chronic neuropathic pain in adults. *Cochrane Database Syst Rev*. 2018;(3):CD012182.
6. Finnerup NB, Attal N, Haroutounian S, et al. Pharmacotherapy for neuropathic pain in adults: a systematic review and meta-analysis. *Lancet Neurol*. 2015;14(2):162–173.

ADDITIONAL READING
- Attal N, Bouhassira D. Pharmacotherapy of neuropathic pain: which drugs, which treatment algorithms? *Pain*. 2015;156(Suppl 1):S104–S114.
- Baron R, Allegri M, Correa-Illanes G, et al. The 5% lidocaine-medicated plaster: its inclusion in international treatment guidelines for treating localized neuropathic pain, and clinical evidence supporting its use. *Pain Ther*. 2016;5(2):149–169.
- Hill KP. Medical marijuana for treatment of chronic pain and other medical and psychiatric problems: a clinical review. *JAMA*. 2015;313(24):2474–2483.
- Ju ZY, Wang K, Cui HS, et al. Acupuncture for neuropathic pain in adults. *Cochrane Database Syst Rev*. 2017;(12):CD012057.
- Kerstman E, Ahn S, Battu S, et al. Neuropathic pain. *Handb Clin Neurol*. 2013;110:175–187.
- Straube S, Derry S, Moore RA, et al. Cervico-thoracic or lumbar sympathectomy for neuropathic pain and complex regional pain syndrome. *Cochrane Database Syst Rev*. 2013;(9):CD002918.
- Zhang Y, Ahmed S, Vo T, et al. Increased pain sensitivity in chronic pain subjects on opioid therapy: a cross-sectional study using quantitative sensory testing. *Pain Med*. 2015;16(5):911–922.

CODES

ICD10
- M79.2 Neuralgia and neuritis, unspecified
- E10.40 Type 1 diabetes mellitus with diabetic neuropathy, unsp
- E11.40 Type 2 diabetes mellitus with diabetic neuropathy, unsp

CLINICAL PEARLS
- Neuropathic pain is a common syndrome, affecting up to 10% of the population with major impacts on quality of life.
- Due to numerous mechanisms in neuropathy, potential benefit from any single treatment is limited.
- Narcotics likely to have more harm than benefit, and chronic narcotics likely increase pain.
- Functional goals and realistic pain targets are essential.
- Physical therapy, occupational therapy, and psychological treatment should be standard elements of multidisciplinary care.

N

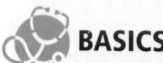

NEUROPATHY, PERIPHERAL
Aruna S. Khan, MD • Sally-Ann L. Pantin, MD, FAAFP

BASICS

DESCRIPTION
- Peripheral neuropathy (PN) is a functional or structural disorder of the peripheral nervous system (PNS).
- PN affects any combination of motor, sensory, or autonomic nerves.
- The motor PNS comprises spinal cord motor neurons, their nerve roots that combine to form plexus, and branches that form individual nerves innervating skeletal muscles. Peripheral motor involvement causes muscle atrophy, weakness, cramps, and fasciculations.
- The sensory PNS consists of sensory organs, which transmit touch, vibration, and position sensation in large-diameter myelinated fibers; pain and temperature in small-diameter, lightly myelinated and unmyelinated C fibers to the dorsal root ganglia. Sensory signals are relayed to the central nervous system (CNS) for integration. Disorders of sensory nerves produce negative phenomena (loss of sensibility, lack of balance) or heightened phenomena (tingling or pain). Large sensory fiber dysfunction impairs touch and vibration sensation, whereas small fiber sensory neuropathy (SFSN) affects pin and thermal sensation and causes neuropathic pain.
- The autonomic nervous system (ANS) includes the sympathetic and parasympathetic systems. ANS dysfunction causes cardiovascular, gastrointestinal, and sudomotor symptoms.
- The PNS can be affected from the cell body (sensory ganglionopathy or motor neuronopathy), root (radiculopathy), or plexus (plexopathy) to the nerve (demyelinating or axonal neuropathy).

EPIDEMIOLOGY
Prevalence
Approximately 2.4% of general population, to an estimated 8% of people >55 years old, are affected by distal symmetric PN, the most common form of PN.

ETIOLOGY AND PATHOPHYSIOLOGY
- PN can be acquired or hereditary.
- The most common cause of acquired PN is diabetes mellitus.
- Other categories of acquired PN with illustrative examples are the following:
  – Vascular: ischemia, vasculitis
  – Infectious: HIV, hepatitis C, cryoglobulinemia, Lyme disease
  – Traumatic: compression, crush, or transection
  – Autoimmune: rheumatoid arthritis, Sjögren, postinfectious Guillain-Barré syndrome (GBS), chronic inflammatory demyelinating polyneuropathy (CIDP), sarcoidosis
  – Metabolic: diabetes, renal failure, hypothyroidism, vitamin B_{12} deficiency, celiac disease
  – Iatrogenic/toxic: chemotherapy, platinum, taxanes, metronidazole, colchicine, infliximab, alcoholism
  – Idiopathic: 30% of PN
  – Neoplastic/paraneoplastic: paraproteinemia, Waldenström macroglobulinemia, multiple myeloma, amyloidosis, neurofibromatosis
- PN occurs due to demyelination or axonal degeneration.
- Demyelination results from Schwann cell dysfunction, mutations in myelin protein genes, or direct damage to myelin sheaths.
- Axonal degeneration occurs when injury/dysfunction occurs at the cell body or axon.

Genetics
- Approximately 50% of undiagnosed PN is hereditary.
- Currently, there are >70 known genetic causes of hereditary PN.
- Charcot-Marie-Tooth (CMT) neuropathies: the most common hereditary PN
  – CMT1A (duplication of the *PMP22* gene) is the most common CMT.
  – A *PMP22* deletion causes hereditary neuropathy with liability to pressure palsy (HNPP).

RISK FACTORS
Systemic disorders predispose to PN.

GENERAL PREVENTION
- Healthy nutrition and avoidance of alcoholism and of pressure at nerve entrapment sites
- Surveillance for glucose dysmetabolism and tight glycemic control may prevent diabetic PN.

DIAGNOSIS

HISTORY
- A detailed inquiry for symptoms of sensory, motor, or autonomic dysfunction:
  – Numbness, tingling, prickling, burning pain, a "tightly wrapped" sensation, and an "unsteady gait"
  – Distal weakness manifests as foot drop (tripping, foot slapping) or difficulty with grip; proximal weakness (e.g., difficulty arising from a chair) is less common.
  – Orthostatic dizziness, abnormal sweating, constipation, or voiding difficulties
- Symptom onset:
  – Acute: Consider infection (e.g., Lyme disease), postinfectious dysimmune process (e.g., GBS), ischemia (e.g., vasculitis), toxin, or trauma.
  – Subacute: Consider metabolic, neoplastic, paraneoplastic, or dysimmune processes.
  – Chronic: Consider dysimmune process (CIDP), idiopathic, or hereditary.
- Progression: stable or indolent; slowly or rapidly progressive; monophasic or relapsing or remitting
- Anatomic pattern: focal, multifocal, diffuse

PHYSICAL EXAM
- Based on exam, a functional (*sensory*: small fiber vs. large fiber vs. mixed, *sensorimotor*, *motor*, *autonomic*) and anatomic pattern of PN (*distal symmetric*, *multifocal*, or *focal*) should be established.
- Cognition preserved in isolated PN
- Cranial nerves may be involved with focal or multifocal PN (e.g., bifacial weakness may occur with GBS, Lyme disease, sarcoidosis, among other causes).
- Stocking/glove sensory loss is typical of distal symmetric sensory PN (e.g., diabetes).
- Isolated reduced pin or thermal sensation or allodynia suggests a pure SFN.
- Reduced vibration and proprioception suggests large-fiber sensory neuropathy; when severe, a Romberg sign is present, and gait is wide based or ataxic.
- Distal muscle atrophy and weaknesses of toe extension and finger abduction are often present with distal symmetric axonal PN.
- In acquired demyelinating PN (e.g., GBS or CIDP), weakness is commonly both proximal and distal.

- Deep tendon reflexes may be reduced or absent, distally at the ankles in large-fiber axonal PN, or diffusely in demyelinating PN.
- High arched or flat feet or hammer toes suggest hereditary PN.

ALERT
- Hemibody deficits or sensory loss below a spinal cord level suggests a CNS process.
- Hyperreflexia and spasticity are upper motor neuron signs not seen with isolated PN.

DIFFERENTIAL DIAGNOSIS
The following categories of PN can be identified (differential diagnosis [DDx] listed when applicable):
- Pure sensory neuropathy
  – DDx: SFN, sensory ganglionopathy, polyradiculopathy
- Distal symmetric sensorimotor axonal PN
  – Most common type of PN
  – DDx: distal acquired demyelinating symmetric (DADS) PN
- Motor predominant PN
  – DDx: motor neuron disease, polyradiculopathy, immune-mediated multifocal motor neuropathy (MMN)
- Mononeuropathy
  – Most likely due to compression, entrapment, or trauma
  – DDx: monoradiculopathy
- Mononeuropathy multiplex
  – DDx: plexopathy, polyradiculopathy

DIAGNOSTIC TESTS & INTERPRETATION
Initial Tests (lab, imaging)
- Blood tests
  – CBC, BUN, Cr, FBG, HbA1C, vitamin B_{12} with methylmalonic acid, LFTs, serum protein immunofixation electrophoresis (SPIEP), TSH
- Nerve conduction studies and electromyography (NCS/EMG)
  – Delineate axonal versus demyelinating, anatomic pattern, chronicity, and severity of PN
- Test of small nerve fiber function
  – Autonomic reflex screen, testing of sweat function, quantitative sensory testing, epidermal skin biopsy
- Specialized epidermal skin biopsy
  – In clinically suspected SFN if NCS/EMG is normal
  – Analysis of lower limb epidermal nerve fiber density (ENFD) (1)[A]
- Neuroimaging
  – Generally not indicated in evaluation of PN but useful in evaluation of brachial plexopathies, radiculopathies, or where findings are attributable to the CNS

Follow-Up Tests & Special Considerations
- Additional blood tests are done based on the medical history, the PN type, and NCS/EMG findings.
- For example: vitamin A, vitamin D, vitamin E, zinc, copper, ESR, CRP, ANA, Hep B/C, antitissue transglutaminase
- Genetic testing for diagnosis of hereditary PN should be ordered by neurologists with expertise in PN.
- Screen patients with distal symmetric PN for unhealthy alcohol use with CAGE-AID or AUDIT-C.

Diagnostic Procedures/Other
- Nerve biopsy (sural or superficial peroneal nerve): useful if vasculitis, amyloidosis, granulomatous disorders, or neoplastic infiltration is suspected; rarely helpful in late-onset chronic, slowly progressive distal symmetric PN
- Lumbar puncture
  - Cytoalbuminologic dissociation in GBS or CIDP
  - Infection, inflammation, or neoplasia in polyradiculopathies

Test Interpretation
- Demyelinating PN: disproportionate slowing of conduction velocities or prolonged distal latencies on NCS
- Axonal PN: reduced amplitude in sensory or motor responses, with relatively preserved conduction velocities on NCS
- Reduced ENFD on distal leg skin biopsies is supportive of SFN.

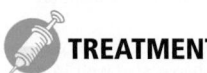 **TREATMENT**

GENERAL MEASURES
- Counsel on foot care and properly fitted footwear.
- Monitor feet for early signs of ulcer and injury.
- Targeted treatment for underlying systemic conditions:
  - Glycemic control, thyroid hormone supplementation, vitamin supplementation, antimicrobial therapy (e.g., Lyme disease, HIV), glucocorticoids for sarcoidosis, and cytotoxic therapy for vasculitis

MEDICATION
First Line
- Treatment of neuropathic pain: evidence of efficacy derived from clinical trials in diabetic painful neuropathy (DPN), postherpetic neuralgia (PHN), or trigeminal neuralgia:
  - Anticonvulsants: gabapentin, for PHN; gabapentin (off-label), for DPN; or pregabalin, for DPN and PHN
  - SNRI: duloxetine for DPN
  - Tricyclic antidepressants (TCA): amitriptyline or nortriptyline; carbamazepine, for trigeminal neuralgia
  - Patches: lidocaine 5%, capsaicin 8%
  - Supplements: α-lipoic acid, acetyl-L-carnitine

Second Line
- Venlafaxine: for DPN
- Tramadol: off-label for DPN

Third Line
Tapentadol: for DPN

ISSUES FOR REFERRAL
- Rapidly progressive symptoms, suspected demyelinating PN, or hereditary PN should be referred to a neurologist with expertise in neuromuscular disorders.
- Patients with vasculitic PN should be referred to rheumatology.
- Patients with progressive painful PN, dysautonomia, and/or cardiomyopathy should be evaluated for transthyretin (TTR)-related familial amyloidosis.
- Patients with paraproteinemia should have a skeletal bone survey and be referred to hematology.
- Patients with imbalance, ataxia, or falls should be referred to physical therapy for gait and balance training.

ADDITIONAL THERAPIES
- Combination therapy (e.g., gabapentin with TCA or venlafaxine or tramadol) can be more effective than monotherapy for neuropathic pain.
- Long-acting opiates can be considered for refractory neuropathic pain.
- Additional immunosuppressant agents (e.g., cyclophosphamide) may be used in refractory chronic dysimmune PN.
- Immunotherapy for dysimmune PN
  - Intravenous immunoglobulin (IVIG): within the first 2 weeks of GBS to hasten recovery (2)[A]; as a first-line alternative to corticosteroids for treatment of CIDP (3)[A]; and for prevention of secondary axonal loss in MMN (4)[A]
    ○ Loading dose 2 g/kg body weight divided into 2 to 5 days; maintenance regimen variable for CIDP and MMN
    ○ Adverse effects (AE): headache, fever, hypertension, and rarely pulmonary embolism
  - Plasma exchange: first agent shown to improve functional outcome for patients with GBS (5)[A]; short-term benefit in CIDP (5)[A]
    ○ AE: catheter complication, hypotension, and others
  - Corticosteroids: a first-line option in treatment of CIDP (5)[C]; oral or pulsed IV regimen can induce remission.
- Treatment of autonomic symptoms
  - Compression stockings, hydration, midodrine, and fludrocortisone for orthostatic hypotension
  - Pyridostigmine for immune-mediated dysautonomia (off-label)

SURGERY/OTHER PROCEDURES
- Decompressive surgery for entrapment neuropathy (e.g., carpal tunnel syndrome)
- Foot and ankle surgery to improve symptoms or function in hereditary PN
- Radiation, surgery, or bone marrow transplantation for plasmacytoma or osteosclerotic myeloma or POEMS syndrome
- Liver transplantation for amyloidotic PN

COMPLEMENTARY & ALTERNATIVE MEDICINE
Low-intensity transcutaneous electrical nerve stimulation (TENS), acupuncture, meditation, supplements (G-agmatine, methylcobalamin, inositol)

ADMISSION, INPATIENT, AND NURSING CONSIDERATIONS
- Patients with suspected GBS should be admitted for diagnosis, monitoring (30–60% may develop cardiovascular or respiratory failure), and for acute treatment.
- Elective intubation may be required in GBS when forced vital capacity is <15 mL/kg body weight.
- Other rapidly progressive undiagnosed PNs that impair independent ambulation may require admission.

 ONGOING CARE

FOLLOW-UP RECOMMENDATIONS
- Physical therapy and gait assistive devices as needed
- Flu vaccination should be avoided in the 1st year following GBS.

PROGNOSIS
- Late-onset idiopathic distal symmetric axonal PNs are indolent.
- 80% of GBS have a near complete or good recovery. 80% of CIDP have moderate or good response with treatment but can be relapsing.

REFERENCES
1. Lauria G, Hsieh ST, Johansson O, et al. European Federation of Neurological Societies/Peripheral Nerve Society Guideline on the use of skin biopsy in the diagnosis of small fiber neuropathy. Report of a joint task force of the European Federation of Neurological Societies and the Peripheral Nerve Society. Eur J Neurol. 2010;17(7):903–912, e44–e49.
2. Hughes RA, Swan AV, van Doorn PA. Intravenous immunoglobulin for Guillain-Barré syndrome. Cochrane Database Syst Rev. 2014;(9):CD002063.
3. Nobile-Orazio E, Cocito D, Jann S, et al; for IMC Trial Group. Intravenous immunoglobulin versus intravenous methylprednisolone for chronic inflammatory demyelinating polyradiculoneuropathy: a randomised controlled trial. Lancet Neurol. 2012;11(6):493–502.
4. Cats EA, van der Pol WL, Piepers S, et al. Correlates of outcome and response to IVIg in 88 patients with multifocal motor neuropathy. Neurology. 2010;75(9):818–825.
5. Nobile-Orazio E, Gallia F. Update on the treatment of chronic inflammatory demyelinating polyradiculoneuropathy. Curr Opin Neurol. 2015;28(5):480–485.

ADDITIONAL READING
- Callaghan BC, Price RS, Chen KS, et al. The importance of rare subtypes in diagnosis and treatment of peripheral neuropathy: a review. JAMA Neurol. 2015;75(12):1510–1518.
- Watson JC, Dyck PJ. Peripheral neuropathy: a practical approach to diagnosis and symptom management. Mayo Clin Proc. 2015;90(7):940–951.

 CODES

ICD10
- G62.9 Polyneuropathy, unspecified
- G60.9 Hereditary and idiopathic neuropathy, unspecified
- G60.8 Other hereditary and idiopathic neuropathies

CLINICAL PEARLS
- There are many causes of PN. Diagnosis is made by history and physical exam, targeted laboratory testing, NCS/EMG, skin biopsy, or ANS testing.
- Consider hereditary neuropathy if patient has an early age of PN symptom onset, family history of PN, or foot deformity.
- GBS is monophasic and progresses for up to 4 weeks; CIDP progresses beyond 8 weeks, and if untreated, usually has a progressive course.

N

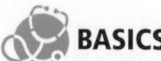

NICOTINE ADDICTION
Kamala M. Nyamathi, MD • Benjamin N. Schneider, MD

BASICS

DESCRIPTION
The compulsive use of nicotine products coupled with a lack of control over using, withdrawal symptoms, and/or continued use despite knowledge of or experiencing adverse consequences

EPIDEMIOLOGY
Prevalence
Approximately 38 million people in the United States ≥18 years of age are current tobacco users. In the past year, 58.7 million individuals smoked cigarettes, 13.3 million smoked cigars, 2.1 million smoked pipes, and 8.6 million used smokeless tobacco. An estimated 3 million middle and high school students use at least one tobacco product, and about 80% of these individuals will continue smoking into adulthood. E-cigarette use among youth has increased 10-fold for high school and middle school students from 2011 to 2015 and has been associated with nicotine addiction in adulthood.

Cost and Impact
Nearly 500,000 Americans die prematurely each year from smoking, including 41,000 deaths from second-hand smoke exposure. The estimated economic costs attributable to smoking approach $300 billion annually, with direct medical costs of at least $130 billion. Life expectancy of smokers is, on average, 10 to 12 years shorter than nonsmokers.

ETIOLOGY AND PATHOPHYSIOLOGY
- Similar to other addictive drugs, nicotine affects neural pathways that control reward and pleasure.
- Nicotine exerts its biologic effects through nicotinic acetylcholine receptors (nAChRs), which modulate neurotransmission with acetylcholine and other chemical messengers including glutamate, GABA, dopamine, serotonin, acetylcholine, and norepinephrine. In this way, it induces euphoria, assists in information processing, reduces anxiety, and mitigates fatigue.
- Upregulation of these receptors occurs over time, leading to tolerance and dependence.
- Polymorphisms in neuronal nAChR genes are associated with increased susceptibility to dependence.
- Nicotine is metabolized by cytochrome P450 2A6 (CYP2A6). Individuals who are fast metabolizers tend to smoke more cigarettes, are more likely to suffer intense withdrawal symptoms, and have a lower probability of quitting than slow metabolizers.
- Nicotine withdrawal involves the release of corticotropin-releasing factor in the amygdala, which induces the perception of anxiety and stress.

Pregnancy Considerations
- Smoking is a risk factor associated with placenta previa, abruptio placentae, decreased maternal thyroid function, preterm premature rupture of membranes, and ectopic pregnancy.
- Carbon monoxide and nicotine interfere with fetal oxygen supply, resulting in decreased birth weights and intrauterine growth restriction.
- Maternal smoking adversely affects fetal lung development, with lifelong decreases in pulmonary function and increased risk of asthma.
- Maternal smoking is associated with increased risk for sudden infant death syndrome, learning and behavioral problems, and obesity.

RISK FACTORS
- Mental illness (depression, posttraumatic stress disorder, bipolar disorder, and schizophrenia)
- Low socioeconomic status
- Low educational status
- Early firsthand nicotine experience
- Concurrent substance abuse
- Home and peer influence

GENERAL PREVENTION
- The U.S. Preventive Services Task Force (USPSTF) strongly recommends (1)[A]:
  - Screening all adults for tobacco use, providing cessation interventions for those who screen positive
  - Screening all pregnant women for tobacco use and providing pregnancy-tailored counseling to those who screen positive (1)
- The USPSTF recommends that clinicians provide interventions, including education or brief counseling to prevent initiation of tobacco use among school-age children and adolescents (1)[B].

DIAGNOSIS

HISTORY
- Identify types, amount, and duration of nicotine products used.
- Review previous attempts to quit (methods used and duration of cessation).

PHYSICAL EXAM
- Pulmonary exam: wheezing, decreased breath sounds, prolonged expiration
- Cardiovascular exam: tachycardia, hypertension
- HEENT exam: epithelial dysplasia, squamous cell carcinoma, leukoplakia, stained teeth, hoarseness

DIAGNOSTIC TESTS & INTERPRETATION
- Lung cancer screening with low-dose CT is recommended annually by USPSTF for patients between 55 and 80 years old with a history of 30+ pack years of tobacco use who are currently smoking or have quit within the past 15 years (except those with life-limiting comorbidities).
- Neither spirometry nor regular chest x-rays are recommended for routine screening.

TREATMENT

Counseling (2)[A]
- Counseling interventions (individual, telephone, or group) improve quit rates compared to minimal support (relative risk [RR] of 1.76 [95% CI 1.58–1.96]) (1).
- Combined behavioral and pharmaceutical interventions increased cessation (RR, 1.82 [95% CI 1.66–2.00]) (1).
- More intensive interactions (i.e., motivational interviewing, close follow-up) may result in higher rates of quitting.
- Brief strategies to help the patient willing to quit tobacco use—the "5 As" (2)[A]
  - Ask patient if he or she uses nicotine.
  - Advise him or her to quit.
  - Assess willingness to make a quit attempt.
  - Assist those willing to make a quit attempt.
  - Arrange follow-up contact to prevent relapse.
- Enhancing motivation to quit: the "5 Rs" (2)[A]
  - Relevance: Encourage patient to indicate why quitting is personally relevant.
  - Risks: Ask patient to identify potential negative consequences of use.
  - Rewards: Ask patient to identify potential benefits of cessation.
  - Roadblocks: Ask patient to identify barriers to quitting and provide treatment (e.g., problem-solving counseling or medication) that could address barriers.
  - Repetition: Repeat motivational intervention each visit.
- Users should be given a choice of methods to quit.
- Quit rates appear to be higher with abrupt quitting rather than gradual reduction prior to the quit date (49% vs. 39% at 4 weeks and 22% vs. 15% at 6 months). Over 4 weeks, there was no significant difference between groups in withdrawal symptoms or urge intensity, both of which declined over time (3)[B].

MEDICATION
- There are currently seven FDA-approved medications: nicotine replacement therapy (NRT), both long-acting (i.e., patch) and short-acting (i.e., gum, inhaler, lozenge, nasal spray) types, and non-NRT meds, bupropion SR and varenicline.
- With few exceptions, the choice of a first-line medication depends on patient preference.
- NRT (RR, 1.60 [95% CI 1.53–1.68]) (1)[A] (Gum: pregnancy Category C. All other formulations are Category D.)
  - Patch: For <10 cigarettes per day or <2 cans per pouches of smokeless tobacco, start with 14 mg/day for 6 weeks and then 7 mg/day for 2 weeks; for 10 to 29 cigarettes per day or 2 to 3 cans per pouches of tobacco, start 21 mg/day for 6 weeks, then 14 mg/day for 2 weeks, and then 7 mg/day for 2 weeks; for 30 to 39 cigarettes per day or 3+ pouches per cans of tobacco, start 35 mg (21 mg/day + 14 mg/day patch) for 4 weeks and then 21 mg/day for 2 weeks, 14 mg/day for 2 weeks, 7 mg/day for 2 weeks; for 40+ cigarettes per day, start 42 mg (21 mg/day patch for 2 weeks) for 4 weeks and then 21 mg/day for 2 weeks, 14 mg/day for 2 weeks, 7 mg/day for 2 weeks. Extending use of the patch beyond 8 to 10 weeks may improve abstinence rates.
  - Gum: For >25 cigarettes per day, start 4 mg gum q1–2h for 6 weeks; for <25 cigarettes per day, start 2 mg gum q1–2h for 6 weeks; then double dosing interval every 3 weeks (i.e., q2–4h and then q4–8h). Chew then tuck between cheek and gingiva once nicotine flavor is released, repeat for up to 30 minutes and then discard. Avoid using with acidic foods (i.e., coffee, soda), which decrease nicotine absorption.
  - Lozenges: For patients who smoke their first cigarette within 30 minutes of waking, start 4 mg lozenge PO q1–2h for 6 weeks; if first cigarette >30 minutes after waking, start 2 mg lozenge PO q1–2h for 6 weeks; then double dosing interval every 3 weeks (i.e., q2–4h and then q4–8h).
  - Nasal spray: Start 1 to 2 sprays (0.5 mg per spray) each nostril q1h for 8 weeks and then taper; max 10 sprays per hour and 80 sprays per day
  - Inhaler: 6 to 16 cartridges inhaled (4 mg per cartridge) per day for 6 to 12 weeks and then taper; incorporates the behavioral and sensory aspects of smoking
- Combination NRT: All forms of NRT increase quit rate 50–70% (4)[A]. Combining long-acting maintenance with short-acting breakthrough NRTs is more effective than using any single method alone. If combining patch with lozenge or gum, limit to 1–3 two mg. Avoid combined NRT use for patients with serious arrhythmias, unstable angina, MI within the prior 2 weeks, or those age <18 years old.

- Bupropion SR (RR, 1.62 [95% CI 1.49–1.76]) (1)[A] is an atypical antidepressant and norepinephrine-dopamine reuptake inhibitor (pregnancy Category C). Contraindications: history of seizure, stroke, brain injury, brain tumors, anorexia/bulimia, recent use of MAOI (within 14 days)
  - Start 1 week before target quit date due to time needed to reach steady state.
  - Use 150 mg/day for 3 days and then 150 mg BID for 7 to 12 weeks.
- Varenicline (RR, 2.27 [95% CI 2.02–2.55]) is a nicotinic acetylcholine partial agonist (pregnancy Category C) (1)[A]. Contraindications: known history of skin reactions or hypersensitivity. Associated neuropsychiatric symptoms may include vivid dreams, sleepwalking, depression, suicidal ideation/attempts in patients with and without preexisting psychiatric conditions—close monitoring recommended.
  - Starter pack: 0.5 mg/day for 3 days, 0.5 mg BID for 4 days, 1 mg/day starting day 7
  - Maintenance pack of 1 mg BID for 12 weeks; if successful, may continue for another 12 weeks
- Varenicline + bupropion is not more effective than either alone and confers increased side effects.
- Varenicline + NRT is more effective at 6 months than varenicline alone (NNT 6).
- Nortriptyline (off-label use) is a tricyclic antidepressant (pregnancy Category D). Contraindications: narrow-angle glaucoma, heart disease (CAD, heart block, long QT)
  - Start 25 mg/day, gradually increase to 75 to 100 mg/day and continue for 12 weeks.
  - Set quit date 2 to 4 weeks after initiation.
- E-cigarette is an electronic device that delivers aerosolized liquid with or without nicotine and includes various flavorings and other chemicals. Insufficient evidence exists regarding this product's safety and efficacy. Low-quality evidence suggests that e-cigarettes can help patients cut down on the number of cigarettes smoked but not nicotine consumption. Other research demonstrates poor efficacy of abstinence with long-term follow-up. Long-term safety has not been established (5).

Pregnancy Considerations
- Tobacco cessation prior to 15 weeks' gestation provides the greatest benefit for both the woman and fetus, but quitting any time is beneficial.
- ACOG recommends that pregnant and breastfeeding women be offered behavioral therapy and education as first-line treatment. NRT and medications should be reserved for patients in need of additional assistance given limited safety data.
- NRT is metabolized faster in pregnant women, which may lead to higher dose requirements.

Pediatric Considerations
- Behavioral therapy (including CBT) is recommended as first-line treatment. There is evidence that group counseling is superior to individual counseling and group messaging for tobacco cessation in youth (RR, 1.35 [95% CI 1.03–1.77]) (6)[A].
- There are currently no FDA-approved pharmacologic treatments for youth.
- AAP recommends using NRT only for youth with moderate to severe substance use disorder.
- Risk of long-term addiction is much higher when smoking is initiated in adolescence than later in life, likely reflecting changes induced by nicotine in the developing brain. The biology of addiction, including withdrawal, occurs with fewer daily cigarettes in teens than in adults. Explanation of these biologic factors may help adolescents to stop or defer smoking.

COMPLEMENTARY & ALTERNATIVE MEDICINE
- Acupuncture: no consistent evidence of efficacy
- Hypnotherapy: no consistent evidence of efficacy

ADMISSION, INPATIENT, AND NURSING CONSIDERATIONS
- Consider NRT for inpatients who use nicotine to decrease withdrawal symptoms (use with caution in patients with unstable angina, serious arrhythmias, or MI within the previous 2 weeks).
- Bupropion may not adequately control acute withdrawal symptoms.

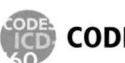 ONGOING CARE

FOLLOW-UP RECOMMENDATIONS
- Patients who have initiated therapy should follow up after 1 to 2 weeks to monitor response and side effects.
- Monitor for signs of nicotine withdrawal syndrome and start medication-assisted treatment or adjust dosage:
  - Increased appetite/weight gain (4 to 5 kg over 10 years)
  - Dysphoric, depressed mood, or anhedonia
  - Insomnia
  - Irritability, frustration, or anger
  - Anxiety
  - Difficulty concentrating
  - Restlessness
- Follow-up should continue periodically in person or via telephone, especially during the first 3 months.
- Pharmacotherapy is generally recommended for 2 to 3 months duration.

PATIENT EDUCATION
- http://smokefree.gov
- http://women.smokefree.gov/
- http://teen.smokefree.gov
- http://www.nicotine-anonymous.org
- http://quitnet.meyouhealth.com
- 1-800-QUIT-NOW (1-800-784-8669)

PROGNOSIS
- Roughly 50% of all smokers will die from a tobacco-related illness.
- Former smokers have a 50% reduction in risk of CAD 1 year after quitting, a 50% reduction in head and neck cancers by 2 to 5 years, and a 50% reduction in lung cancer mortality by 10 years. The risk of stroke is reduced to that of nonsmokers 2 to 5 years after quitting.
- 22% of smokers relapse within 3 months of quitting. Multiple attempts are often required.
- Approximately 50% of women who quit smoking in pregnancy resume smoking by 6 months postpartum.
- Individuals receiving support from significant others are more likely to quit.

COMPLICATIONS
- Chronic obstructive pulmonary disease (COPD) (emphysema and chronic bronchitis)
- Cancers (i.e., lung, oral/pharyngeal, kidney, bladder, cervical, anal, squamous cell)
- Atherosclerotic disease
- Insulin resistance
- Periodontal disease
- Osteoporosis and hip fracture (in women)
- Peptic ulcer disease
- Delayed wound healing
- Pregnancy and neonatal complications (discussed elsewhere)

REFERENCES
1. U.S. Preventive Services Task Force. Final recommendation statement: tobacco smoking cessation in adults, including pregnant women: behavioral and pharmacotherapy interventions. https://www.uspreventiveservicestaskforce.org/Page/Document/RecommendationStatementFinal/tobacco-use-in-adults-and-pregnant-women-counseling-and-interventions1. Accessed July 2, 2018.
2. Stead LF, Buitrago D, Preciado N, et al. Physician advice for smoking cessation. Cochrane Database Syst Rev. 2013;(5):CD000165.
3. Lindson-Hawley N, Banting M, West R, et al. Gradual versus abrupt smoking cessation: a randomized, controlled noninferiority trial. Ann Intern Med. 2016;164(9):585–592.
4. Hartmann-Boyce J, Chepkin S, Ye W, et al. Nicotine replacement therapy versus control for smoking cessation. Cochrane Database Syst Rev. 2018;(5):CD000146.
5. Malas M, van der Tempel J, Schwartz R, et al. Electronic cigarettes for smoking cessation: a systematic review. Nicotine Tob Res. 2016;18(10):1926–1936.
6. Fanshawe T, Halliwell W, Lindson N, et al. Tobacco cessation interventions for young people. Cochrane Database Syst Rev. 2017;(11):CD003289.

ADDITIONAL READING
- Centers for Disease Control and Prevention. Smoking & tobacco use. http://www.cdc.gov/tobacco/index.htm. Accessed October 13, 2018.
- Cochrane Tobacco Addiction: http://tobacco.cochrane.org/evidence
- DiFranza JR. Who are you going to believe? Adolescents and nicotine addiction. J Adolesc Health. 2011;48(1):1–2.
- National Tobacco Cessation Collaborative: http://www.tobacco-cessation.org/resources/tools.html#clinicians

CODES

ICD10
- F17.200 Nicotine dependence, unspecified, uncomplicated
- F17.201 Nicotine dependence, unspecified, in remission
- F17.203 Nicotine dependence unspecified, with withdrawal

CLINICAL PEARLS
- Nicotine dependence is a chronic disease and will often require repeated interventions and multiple cessation attempts.
- Follow-up is key to continuing engagement and providing additional support as needed.
- Treatments, including but not limited to medications, can significantly increase rates of long-term abstinence.
- No single type of medication is best; thus, the choice should be based on patient preference and risk factors for side effects.
- Provide anticipatory guidance in adolescence.

N

NONALCOHOLIC FATTY LIVER DISEASE (NAFLD)

Jill T. Wei Doherty, MD • Daniel T. Lee, MD, MA

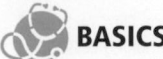

BASICS

- A spectrum of fatty liver diseases not due to excess alcohol consumption ranging from nonalcoholic fatty liver (NAFL), to nonalcoholic steatohepatitis (NASH), to cirrhosis with hepatocyte injury with/without fibrosis
- Leading cause of chronic liver disease; implicated in up to 90% of patients with asymptomatic, mild aminotransferase elevation not caused by alcohol, viral hepatitis, or medications

DESCRIPTION
- NAFL (1)
  - Reversible condition in which large vacuoles of triglyceride fat accumulate in hepatocytes
  - Liver biopsy: fatty deposits in >30% of cells, no hepatocyte necrosis, no fibrosis
  - Alanine aminotransferase/aspartate aminotransferase (ALT/AST) enzymes usually normal but may be elevated, rarely >3 to 4 times ULN
  - Minimal risk of progressing to cirrhosis or liver failure
  - Synonym: steatosis
- NASH: progressive form of NAFL (1)
  - Liver biopsy: fatty deposits in >50% of cells with ballooning, acute/chronic inflammation, ± fibrosis
  - ALT and AST elevated, generally <3 to 4 times ULN
  - 30% with NASH may progress to fibrosis over 5 years, may progress to cirrhosis, liver failure, and rarely hepatocellular cancer
- NASH cirrhosis (1)
  - Presence of cirrhosis with current or previous histologic evidence of steatosis or steatohepatitis

EPIDEMIOLOGY
- Nonalcoholic fatty liver disease (NAFLD): most common chronic liver disease globally; usually benign, asymptomatic
- Predicted to become the most frequent indication for liver transplantation by 2030 (2)
- NASH may be symptomatic with progressive inflammation and fibrosis.
  - Predominant age: 40s to 50s; can occur in children
  - Predominant sex: male > female (slight)

Incidence
Estimates vary widely from 31 to 86 cases of NAFLD per 10,000 person-years to 29/100,000 person-years (1).

Prevalence
- United States estimate: 30–40%
- Worldwide: 6–33%, median 20–25% (1)
- Present in 58–74% of obese persons (BMI >30) and 90% of morbidly obese persons (BMI >39) (1)
- Among individuals with type 2 diabetes mellitus, rate of 69–87%; in patients with dyslipidemia, rate of 50% (1)

ETIOLOGY AND PATHOPHYSIOLOGY
Primary mechanism is thought to be *insulin resistance*, leading to increased lipolysis, triglyceride synthesis, and increased hepatic uptake of fatty acids.
- NAFLD: excessive triglyceride accumulation in the liver and impaired ability to remove fatty acids
- NASH: multiple hit theory that inflammation precedes steatosis in environmentally and genetically predisposed people. Multiple insults, including insulin resistance, hormones from adipose tissue, nutritional factors, endotoxins released by the gut microbiota, oxidative stress damage, and genetic factors. These "hits" act on liver parenchymal cells via toll-like receptors to lead to the progression of NASH (3).

Genetics
Largely unknown: Some familial clustering and increased heritability. NAFL: more first-degree relatives with cirrhosis than matched controls; NASH: 18% with affected first-degree relative. Carriers of hemochromatosis gene are more likely to be affected. Patatin-like phospholipase (PNPLA3) polymorphism implicated in NAFLD, hypertriglyceridemia, and insulin resistance (1,2).

RISK FACTORS
- Obesity (BMI >30), visceral obesity (waist circumference >102 cm for men or >88 cm for women), hypertension, dyslipidemia, high serum triglycerides and low serum high-density lipoprotein (HDL) levels, metabolic syndrome
- Type 2 diabetes mellitus, cardiovascular disease, and chronic kidney disease (2)
- Possible associations with hypothyroidism, hypopituitarism, hypogonadism, obstructive sleep apnea, pancreaticoduodenal resection, osteoporosis, psoriasis, and polycystic ovary syndrome (2)
- Increasing age associated with increased prevalence, severity, advanced fibrosis, and mortality
- High fructose intake linked to intestinal dysbiosis and metabolic stress (4)
- Protein–calorie malnutrition; total parenteral nutrition (TPN) >6 weeks
- Severe weight loss (starvation, bariatric surgery)
- Organic solvent exposure (e.g., chlorinated hydrocarbons, toluene); vinyl chloride; hypoglycin A
- Gene for hemochromatosis/other conditions with increased iron stores
- Smoking
- Drugs: tetracycline, glucocorticoids, tamoxifen, methotrexate, amiodarone, antiretroviral agents for HIV, valproic acid, fialuridine, many chemotherapy regimens, and nucleoside analogues

Pregnancy Considerations
Acute fatty liver of pregnancy: rare but serious complication in 3rd trimester. 50% of cases are associated with preeclampsia.
- Symptoms: nausea, vomiting, headache, fatigue, right upper quadrant or epigastric pain, jaundice
- Elevated ALT and AST >300 IU/L but usually <1,000 IU/L; elevated bilirubin
- Liver biopsy confirms diagnosis (do not delay treatment for biopsy).
- Early recognition and prompt delivery is key.
- Recurrence is rare.

Pediatric Considerations
- Increasing prevalence of NAFLD among children parallels rise in pediatric obesity.
- Reports of NAFLD as early as age 2 years and NASH-related cirrhosis as early as age 8 years
- Treat with intensive lifestyle modification.
- Vitamin E of possible benefit.

- Reye syndrome: fatty liver syndrome with encephalopathy usually following viral illness
  - Vomiting with dehydration
  - Confusion, progressive CNS damage
  - Hepatomegaly with extensive fatty vacuolization
  - Hypoglycemia
- Etiology unknown; viral URIs and drugs (especially salicylates) have been implicated; mortality rate: 50%
- Treat with mannitol, IV glucose, and FFP.

GENERAL PREVENTION
- Avoid excess alcohol: ≤2 standard drinks per day (men); ≤1 standard drink per day (women)
- Maintain appropriate BMI.
- Prevention and optimal management of diabetes
- Avoid hepatotoxic medications.
- HAV and HBV vaccination if not immune
- Pneumococcal and annual influenza vaccinations

COMMONLY ASSOCIATED CONDITIONS
Central obesity; hypertension; type 2 diabetes; insulin resistance; hyperlipidemia; preeclampsia in pregnancy; CVD and arrhythmias; hypothyroidism; hypogonadism; OSA (2)

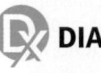

DIAGNOSIS

- Routine screening not recommended
- Consider NAFLD in patients with asymptomatic aminotransferase elevations (1)[A].
- Can occur with normal AST/ALT levels (1)[A]
- NAFLD has no distinguishing historical/lab features to distinguish from other chronic liver disorders.
- Index of suspicion is higher with risk factors, such as metabolic syndrome, insulin resistance, or obesity.
- May present as cryptogenic cirrhosis
- Noninvasive biomarkers of steatosis/fibrosis are not sufficiently reliable; no validated test yet available
- Liver biopsy is the definitive diagnostic test but should only be considered if results will change management.

HISTORY
- Typically asymptomatic
- Possible fatigue and/or abdominal fullness
- Vague right upper quadrant pain
- History of medications, alcohol use, family history

PHYSICAL EXAM
Most common signs (all are infrequent)
- Liver tenderness
- Mild to marked hepatomegaly
- Splenomegaly
- In advanced cases: cutaneous stigmata of chronic liver disease or portal hypertension (e.g., palmar erythema, spider angiomata, ascites)

DIFFERENTIAL DIAGNOSIS
- Viral hepatitis
- Alcoholic fatty liver
- Drug- or toxin-induced hepatitis
- Metabolic liver disease
- Autoimmune hepatitis
- Celiac disease
- Muscle disease, if nonhepatic cause of elevated enzymes is possible

DIAGNOSTIC TESTS & INTERPRETATION

Initial Tests (lab, imaging)

- ALT and AST may be elevated.
  - Nonalcoholic, usually AST/ALT >1
  - If alcohol induced, usually AST/ALT ≥2
  - Nonspecific enzyme abnormalities may exist or may be normal with advanced cirrhosis (1,3).
- Level of enzyme elevation does NOT correlate with degree of fibrosis (1).
- Serum ferritin (1.5 times normal), alkaline phosphatase (2 to 3 times normal), and total/direct bilirubin may be elevated (1).
- Severity and chronicity are characterized by defects in ability to produce plasma proteins (serum albumin, PT) and thrombocytopenia—marker for cirrhosis (1).
- Lipids abnormalities are common and include elevated cholesterol, low-density lipoprotein (LDL), and triglyceride and decreased HDL (1).
- Biomarkers of inflammation, increased oxidative stress, or hepatocyte apoptosis such as leptin, adiponectin, CRP, serum caspase, and cytokeratin 18 may help differentiate NASH from NAFLD (1)[B].
- Serologic studies to exclude other causes of liver disease (celiac, α_1-antitrypsin, iron, copper, HepA IgG, HepB SAg, HepB SAb, HepB cAb, HepC Ab, anti–smooth muscle antibody, ANA, serum gammaglobulin) (1)[B]
- Ultrasound (US) is first-line imaging modality for assessing liver chemistry abnormalities: Fatty liver is hyperechoic on US. MRI/CT may also be used (1)[B].
- Liver-derived microparticles released in response to free-fatty acid–induced lipotoxicity and volatile organic compounds (VOCs) in exhaled breath (5)[C].

Follow-Up Tests & Special Considerations

- Imaging modalities help noninvasively quantify fibrosis by estimating liver stiffness (5)[B]: (i) vibration-controlled transient elastography (VCTE) or FibroScan, (ii) acoustic radiation force impulse (ARFI), (iii) magnetic resonance elastography (MRE).
- No imaging modality has been found to accurately distinguish and diagnose simple steatosis from steatohepatitis (6)[B].

Diagnostic Procedures/Other

Liver biopsy is the gold standard for diagnosis and prognosis—must have likelihood of changing management prior to biopsy (1)[B].

Test Interpretation

- The NAFLD activity score (NAS) is used to grade diagnosis, based on three histologic features: steatosis (0 to 3), inflammation (0 to 3), and hepatocyte ballooning (0 to 2), for score between 0 and 8. NASH is very likely with scores ≥5 (3).
- Staging scale (0 to 4) is based on fibrosis (1,3).

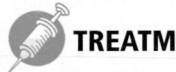

TREATMENT

- Sustained weight loss (3–5% body weight) through lifestyle modification is most successful treatment (1,7)[A]. Weight loss for those who are overweight or obese is the only therapy that has good evidence of benefits and safety.
- Bariatric surgery not proven to improve NASH (1)[B]
- Aerobic exercise 3 to 5 times per week for 20 to 45 minutes with reduced calorie intake/diet modifications (1)[B]

- Tight diabetes control (1,7)[B]
- Treatment of metabolic syndrome—hypertension, dyslipidemia, and obesity (1,7)[B]
- Avoid or limit alcohol consumption (7)[A].
- Avoid hepatotoxic medications (1)[B].

MEDICATION

- Currently no effective medication treatment (1,7)[A]
- Some promising agents include the following:
  - Peroxisome proliferator-activator receptor agonists, most notably thiazolidinediones (pioglitazone) (1)[B]
  - Vitamin E 400 to 800 IU daily, although long-term safety concerns at high doses (1)[C]
    - Statins
    - Probiotics
    - Obeticholic acid (bile acid derivative)
    - GLP-1 receptor agonists, exenatide and liraglutide
    - Pentoxifylline
    - Agents targeting apoptosis, fibrosis, and the gut microbiome are in early trials.

ISSUES FOR REFERRAL

Patients with persistent AST/ALT elevations 2 to 3 times ULN or fibrosis on biopsy benefit from hepatology consult (1)[A].

SURGERY/OTHER PROCEDURES

Bariatric procedures: NAFLD is not a contraindication in otherwise eligible obese patients. There is a lack of data to definitively assess benefits and harms of surgery in treating patients with NASH (1)[B].

 ONGOING CARE

FOLLOW-UP RECOMMENDATIONS

- Annual monitoring of LFTs (1,7)[B]
- Consider surveillance with US or CT scan to evaluate for disease progression (7)[B]. Improvements provide motivation for lifestyle changes.
- Routine liver biopsy is not recommended but may be repeated 5 years after baseline biopsy if progression of fibrosis is suspected (1,7)[B].
- Hepatic fibrosis staging is the strongest predictor for all-cause and disease-specific mortality in patients with histologically confirmed NAFLD (2)[B].

DIET

Low in saturated and trans fat; low in simple carbohydrates; avoid excessive alcohol (protective or worsening effect of light/moderate consumption inconclusive).

PATIENT EDUCATION

Extensive counseling on sustained lifestyle changes in nutrition, exercise, and alcohol use

PROGNOSIS

Within the spectrum of NAFLD, only NASH has been shown to be progressive, potentially leading to cirrhosis, hepatocellular carcinoma, cholangiocarcinoma, and/or liver failure:

- Cirrhosis develops in up to 20% of patients but may not always be present. Up to 41.7% of patients develop HCC without showing cirrhosis (3).
- Transplantation is effective, but NASH may recur after transplantation due to ongoing risk factors.

COMPLICATIONS

Progressive disease may lead to decompensated cirrhosis and portal hypertension with complications such as ascites, encephalopathy, bleeding varices, and hepatorenal or hepatopulmonary syndromes.

REFERENCES

1. Chalasani N, Younossi Z, Lavine JE, et al. The diagnosis and management of non-alcoholic fatty liver disease: practice guideline by the American Gastroenterological Association, American Association for the Study of Liver Diseases, and American College of Gastroenterology. *Gastroenterology*. 2012;142(7):1592–1609.
2. Byrne CD, Targher G. NAFLD: a multisystem disease. *J Hepatol*. 2015;62(Suppl 1):S47–S64.
3. Borrelli A, Bonelli P, Tuccillo FM, et al. Role of gut microbiota and oxidative stress in the progression of non-alcoholic fatty liver disease to hepatocarcinoma: current and innovative therapeutic approaches. *Redox Biology*. 2018;15:467–479.
4. Sharma M, Mitnala S, Vishnubhotla RK, et al. The riddle of nonalcoholic fatty liver disease: progression from nonalcoholic fatty liver to nonalcoholic steatohepatitis. *J Clin Exp Hepatol*. 2015;5(2):147–158.
5. Alkhouri N, Feldstein AE. Noninvasive diagnosis of nonalcoholic fatty liver disease: are we there yet? *Metabolism*. 2016;65(8):1087–1095.
6. Lee SS, Park SH. Radiologic evaluation of nonalcoholic fatty liver disease. *World J Gastroenterol*. 2014;20(23):7392–7402.
7. Nascimbeni F, Pais R, Bellentani S, et al. From NAFLD in clinical practice to answers from guidelines. *J Hepatol*. 2013;59(4):859–871.

ADDITIONAL READING

- Oseini AM, Sanyal AJ. Therapies in non-alcoholic steatohepatitis (NASH). *Liver Int*. 2017;37(Suppl 1): 97–103.
- Spengler EK, Loomba R. Recommendations for diagnosis, referral for liver biopsy, and treatment of nonalcoholic fatty liver disease and nonalcoholic steatohepatitis. *Mayo Clin Proc*. 2015;90(9):1233–1246.

 SEE ALSO

Alcohol Use Disorder (AUD); Cirrhosis of the Liver; Diabetes Mellitus, Type 2; Metabolic Syndrome

 CODES

ICD10

K76.0 Fatty (change of) liver, not elsewhere classified

CLINICAL PEARLS

- NAFLD is a major cause of liver disease. Spectrum ranges from NAFL to NASH, advanced fibrosis, and cirrhosis.
- NAFLD is the most common chronic liver disease in children; there has been a parallel rise in childhood obesity and NAFLD.
- Lifestyle changes with targeted weight loss are the cornerstones of therapy for NAFLD.
- NAFLD is a common cause of asymptomatic mild serum aminotransferase elevation.

N

NONFATAL DROWNING

Joseph L. Steele, MPAS, APA-C • Natasha J. Pyzocha, DO, FAWM, FAAFP

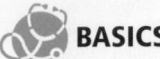

BASICS

DESCRIPTION
- Respiratory impairment from submersion in liquid (1)
- System(s) affected: cardiovascular, nervous, pulmonary, renal
- Synonym(s): submersion injury; terms such as "near-drowning," "secondary drowning," and "wet drowning" should be avoided.

EPIDEMIOLOGY
Incidence
- From 2005 to 2014, an average of 3,536 fatal unintentional drownings in the United States (2)
- Three age-related peaks: toddlers and young children (1 to 5 years), adolescents and young adults (15 to 25 years), and the elderly
- 80% of people who die from drowning are male (2).
- Greater incidence in minorities; African Americans age 5 to 19 years old are affected 5.5 times more frequently than Caucasians (2).

Prevalence
- Most common injury-related cause of death for children 1 to 4 years in the United States (3)
- For every child age <15 years who dies from drowning, five more children are seen in the emergency room for nonfatal submersion injuries.

ALERT
Proper water supervision and safety techniques are critical in avoiding morbidity and mortality from drowning.

ETIOLOGY AND PATHOPHYSIOLOGY
Hypoxemia via aspiration and/or reflex laryngospasm causing cerebral hypoxia and multisystem organ dysfunction
- 10–20% of victims drown without aspiration; likely due to prolonged laryngospasm
- Bathtub and bucket drowning in children <1 year
- Swimming pool drowning in children and young adults
- Motor vehicle accidents (vehicle submerged in water)
- Head trauma while swimming or diving
- Suicide
- Pulmonary: morbidity primarily caused by hypoxia. Aspiration causes dilution of surfactant with decreased gas transfer across alveoli, atelectasis, development of intrapulmonary right-to-left shunting; acute respiratory distress syndrome (ARDS); obstruction due to laryngospasm and bronchospasm
- Cardiac: hypoxic-ischemic injury and arrhythmia (primary or secondary)
- Renal: acute tubular necrosis from hypoxemia, shock, hemoglobinuria, myoglobinuria

- Neurologic: hypoxic-ischemic brain injury with damage especially to the hippocampus, insular cortex, and basal ganglia; cerebral edema
- Coagulation: hemolysis and coagulopathy

RISK FACTORS
- Inadequate physical barriers surrounding pools
- Alcohol ingestion; male sex
- Low socioeconomic status
- Use of illicit drugs
- Seizure disorder
- Inability to swim
- Hyperventilation prior to underwater swimming
- Boating mishaps and trauma during water sports, particularly when not wearing a life jacket
- Scuba diving
- Inadequate adult supervision of children; lack of appropriate instruction on how to swim
- Concomitant stroke or myocardial infarction (MI)
- Hypothermia
- Cardiac arrhythmias: familial long QT and polymorphic ventricular tachycardia (VT)

GENERAL PREVENTION
- Periodic education regarding proper supervision and drowning prevention for caretakers of young children
- Proper adult supervision of children, particularly around water
- Pool alarms, buddy system
- Knowledge of water safety guidelines
- Mandatory physical barriers surrounding pools; four-sided fencing, self-closing gate at least 48 inches above the ground (2)
- Avoid alcohol or recreational drugs around water.
- Swimming instruction at an early age
- Cardiopulmonary resuscitation (CPR) instruction for pool owners and parents
- Boating safety knowledge
- Personal flotation device and rescue equipment (e.g., preserver, if necessary)

Pediatric Considerations
Children should never be left alone near water. Young children can drown in very small amounts of water (bathtubs, buckets, and toilets).

COMMONLY ASSOCIATED CONDITIONS
- Trauma
- Seizure disorder
- Alcohol or illicit drug use
- Hypothermia
- Concomitant stroke or MI
- Cardiac arrhythmias: familial long QT and familial polymorphic VT
- Hyperventilation

DIAGNOSIS

HISTORY
The Utstein approach to the evaluation of drowning victims standardizes reporting data and provides guidance for the history, physical exam, and appropriate management:
- Gender, age, birthdate, event date
- Time call received and emergency medical services (EMS) start resuscitation
- Precipitating event
- Location of drowning
- Duration of submersion
- Loss of consciousness
- Period of apnea
- Artificial ventilation/CPR performed
- History of associated trauma
- Approximate water temperature (hypothermia)
- Recent use of alcohol or drugs
- Known seizure disorder, cardiac disease, syncopal event

PHYSICAL EXAM
- Airway status and degree of respiratory distress
- Pulse: absent, weak, or normal
- Vital signs, including pulse oximetry
- Glasgow Coma Scale (GCS)
- Pulmonary: rales, wheezing
- Cardiac: rate, rhythm
- Neurologic examination

DIFFERENTIAL DIAGNOSIS
Syncopal event, head trauma, arrhythmia, seizure, MI, stroke, alcohol or other substance overdose, nonaccidental trauma

DIAGNOSTIC TESTS & INTERPRETATION
Initial Tests (lab, imaging)
Unnecessary if initial GCS and pulse oximetry are normal (and remain so for 6 to 8 hours)
- CBC with differential
- Arterial blood gas (ABG): hypoxia, hypercarbia, acidosis
- Electrolytes: hypokalemia, hyponatremia, hypernatremia
- Blood glucose: Increased levels may impair neurologic recovery after ischemic brain injury.
- BUN, creatinine: acute tubular necrosis
- ECG, cardiac monitoring, and serial troponin: MI
- Creatine kinase (CK) and urine myoglobin: rhabdomyolysis
- Coagulation studies: coagulopathy
- Toxicology screen
- Blood alcohol level
- Chest x-ray (CXR) unnecessary if all of the following:
  - Normal initial GCS and pulse oximetry
  - No evidence of respiratory distress
  - No change after 6 to 8 hours of observation
- CXR may show evidence of aspiration, atelectasis, pneumothorax, or ARDS in more severe cases.
- Head CT and/or C-spine imaging for trauma

Follow-Up Tests & Special Considerations

- Observe patients with an initial GCS of 15 and pulse oximetry >95% for 6 to 8 hours in the emergency department (ED).
- CXR findings may be minimal or absent early on.

Diagnostic Procedures/Other

- Continuous cardiac monitoring and pulse oximetry
- Continuous core temperature monitoring if hypothermic
- 12-lead ECG
- Central venous pressure (CVP) monitoring for critically ill with hypotension refractory to IV fluids
- Electroencephalogram (EEG) if seizure suspected

 TREATMENT

Early resuscitation and reversal of hypoxemia are key.

GENERAL MEASURES

- Prehospital
  - Never approach a struggling victim alone.
  - Initiate basic life support (BLS) and advanced cardiovascular life support (ACLS) evaluation (4).
  - Rescue breathing may be helpful if the victim is in the water and cannot be removed; chest compressions not as effective while in the water and may harm the rescuer and the victim (4)[C]
  - Remove the victim from the water and begin effective resuscitation as quickly as possible (5).
  - Immediate CPR (airway, breathing, and circulation [ABC] sequence) (4)[A]
  - Start CPR if pulse is not definitely felt within 10 seconds, even in the hypothermic victim whose heart rate may be severely bradycardic (4)[C].
  - Routine cervical collar use and spinal precautions are not needed unless trauma suspected (5)[C].
  - Supplemental oxygen and early intubation with mechanical ventilation, if needed (1)[A]
  - Rapid crystalloid infusion if hypotension not corrected by oxygenation (1)[A]
  - If patient is breathing on his or her own and does not need spinal precautions, consider placing in the right lateral decubitus position to prevent aspiration of vomit or gastric contents (1).
- ED
  - Oxygen, as needed, to maintain saturation between 92% and 96% (1)
  - Continuous positive airway pressure (CPAP), bilevel positive airway pressure (BiPAP), or intubation if supplemental oxygen alone is inadequate.
  - If intubation is indicated, employ lung-protective ventilator settings (lower end-inspiratory airway pressures, lower tidal volumes of 6 mL/kg, higher positive end-expiratory pressures of 6 to 12 cm H_2O) to avoid barotrauma (4)[A].
  - Indications for intubation
    - Neurologic deterioration
    - Inability to protect the airway
    - Inability to maintain oxygen saturation >90% or PaO_2 >60 mm Hg on high-flow supplemental oxygen
    - $PaCO_2$ >50 mm Hg
  - Remove wet clothing and initiate rewarming.
  - Obtain core temperature to rule out hypothermia.
  - If hypothermic, rewarm with minimally invasive core techniques such as warm IV fluids, warm/humidified oxygen, and external blanketing.
  - Active core rewarming only for refractory cases

MEDICATION

First Line

- High-flow oxygen, as needed (1)[A]
- For bronchospasm: aerosolized bronchodilator (3)[C]: albuterol (Proventil, Ventolin), 3 mL of 0.083% solution or 0.5 mL of 0.5% solution diluted in 3 mL of saline
- Vasopressors, as needed, for hypotension refractory to IV fluid resuscitation
- Prophylactic antibiotics are not recommended (1)[B].

Second Line

For pneumonia: antibiotics based on sputum or endotracheal lavage culture (1)[A]

ADMISSION, INPATIENT, AND NURSING CONSIDERATIONS

- Admit all symptomatic patients or patients with abnormal vital signs, mental status, oxygenation, CXR, or laboratory analysis.
- Monitor vital signs and reassess neurologic status, continuous cardiac, and pulse oximetry monitoring.
- After initial resuscitation, induce hypothermia with core temp maintained between 32°C and 34°C for 24 hours; may be neuroprotective for patients that remain comatose or have neurologic deterioration (1)
- Patients can be discharged from the ED after 6 to 8 hours of observation if the following criteria are met:
  - GCS = 15
  - Normal CXR, if indicated
  - Lack of clinical evidence of respiratory difficulty
  - Normal lung exam
  - Normal vital signs
  - Oxygen saturation ≥95% on room air (5)

 ONGOING CARE

FOLLOW-UP RECOMMENDATIONS

Appropriate follow-up with primary care provider, orthopedic, neurologic, cardiac, pulmonary, and additional specialists as indicated

Patient Monitoring

- ABG monitoring, as indicated
- A pulmonary artery catheter may be needed for hemodynamic monitoring in unstable patients (3)[C].
- Intracranial pressure monitoring in selected patients (3)[C]
- Serum electrolyte determinations

DIET

NPO until mental status normalizes

PATIENT EDUCATION

Reemphasize preventive measures on discharge from hospital and educate parents regarding supervision and preventive practices.

PROGNOSIS

- 75% of drowning victims survive; 6% will have residual neurologic deficits (1).
- Patients with an initial GCS ≥13 and an oxygen saturation ≥95% have a low risk of complications and an excellent chance for a full recovery (1).
- Patients who are comatose or receiving CPR at the time of presentation and those who have dilated and fixed pupils and no spontaneous respiratory activity have a poor prognosis.
- Neurogenic pulmonary edema may occur within 48 hours of initial presentation.

COMPLICATIONS

- Early
  - Bronchospasm, vomiting, aspiration
  - Hypoglycemia, hypothermia, seizures
  - Hypovolemia, electrolyte abnormalities
  - Arrhythmia from hypoxia or hypothermia (rarely from electrolyte imbalance)
  - Hypotension
- Late
  - ARDS, pneumonia, lung abscess, empyema
  - Anoxic encephalopathy, barotrauma, seizure
  - Renal failure, coagulopathy, sepsis

REFERENCES

1. Szpilman D, Bierens J, Handley AJ, et al. Drowning. *N Engl J Med*. 2012;366(22):2102–2110.
2. Centers for Disease Control and Prevention. Unintentional drowning: get the facts. http://www.cdc.gov/HomeandRecreationalSafety/Water-Safety/waterinjuries-factsheet.html/. Accessed June 22, 2018.
3. Mott T, Latimer K. Prevention and treatment of drowning. *Am Fam Physician*. 2016;93(7):576–582.
4. Vanden Hoek TL, Morrison LJ, Shuster M, et al. Part 12: cardiac arrest in special situations: 2010 American Heart Association guidelines for cardiopulmonary resuscitation and emergency cardiovascular care. *Circulation*. 2010;122(18 Suppl 3): S829–S861.
5. Salomez F, Vincent JL. Drowning: a review of epidemiology, pathophysiology, treatment and prevention. *Resuscitation*. 2004;63(3):261–268.

CODES

ICD10

- T75.1XXA Unsp effects of drowning and nonfatal submersion, init
- T75.1XXD Unsp effects of drowning and nonfatal submersion, subs
- T75.1XXS Unsp effects of drowning and nonfatal submersion, sequel

CLINICAL PEARLS

- The most important treatment for near-drowning victims is prompt reversal of any hypoxia.
- Water safety education (combining physical and behavioral techniques) has the greatest impact on drowning prevention.
- Encourage pool owners and parents with young children to become CPR certified.
- Patients remain at risk for ARDS for hours after submersion. All resuscitated patients require careful monitoring.
- Use lung-protective ventilator settings for intubated patients to prevent barotrauma.
- Patients with an initial GCS ≥13 and an oxygen saturation ≥95% have a low risk of complications and an excellent chance for a full recovery.

N

OBESITY
Kimberly Bombaci, MD

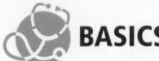 **BASICS**

DESCRIPTION
- Excess adipose tissue, typically quantified in adults by body mass index (BMI) ([kg] / [m²]), ≥30 kg/m²
- Obesity categorized into three classes:
  - Class 1 obesity is BMI 30 to 34.9 kg/m².
  - Class 2 obesity is BMI 35 to 39.9 kg/m².
  - Class 3 obesity (also called severe obesity) is BMI >40 kg/m².
- Obesity is associated with negative health outcomes. Abdominal obesity increases the risk of morbidity and mortality.
- System(s) affected: endocrine/metabolic, cardiac, respiratory, gastrointestinal (GI), musculoskeletal, dermatologic, mental health
- Synonym(s): overweight; adiposity

Geriatric Considerations
Underweight BMI (≤18) is also associated with an increased risk of mortality.

EPIDEMIOLOGY
- Predominant age: Incidence rises in the early 20s.
- Predominant sex: female > male

Prevalence
- 35% of U.S. adults are obese (1,2).
- 40% of men and 25% of women are overweight.

Pediatric Considerations
- The USPSTF recommends that clinicians screen for obesity in children and adolescents ≥6 years and refer them to comprehensive, intensive behavioral interventions to promote improvements in weight status (grade B recommendation).
- Pediatric obesity is defined as a BMI ≥95th percentile, by age- and sex-specific WHO or CDC growth curves.
- Obesity during adolescence and young adulthood is strongly associated with obesity in adulthood.

ETIOLOGY AND PATHOPHYSIOLOGY
- Obesity is caused by an imbalance between food intake, absorption, and energy expenditure.
- Underlying organic causes include psychiatric disturbances, hypothyroidism, hypothalamic disorders, insulinoma, and Cushing syndrome. It is likely that an individual's gut microbiome may cause obesity and/or make it difficult to lose weight.
- Medications that contribute to obesity include corticosteroids, neuroleptics (particularly atypical antipsychotics), and antidepressants.

Genetics
- Genetic syndromes such as Prader-Willi and Bardet-Biedl are found in a minority of people with obesity.
- Multiple genes are implicated in obesity.

RISK FACTORS
- Parental obesity
- Sedentary lifestyle
- Consumption of calorie-dense food
- Low socioeconomic status
- Stress and mental illness
- Medications

GENERAL PREVENTION
- Encourage at least 1 hour of daily exercise, limited television viewing, and moderation in portion size.
- Avoid calorie-dense and nutrient-poor foods such as sugar-sweetened beverages and processed foods.

DIAGNOSIS

HISTORY
- Diet and exercise habits
- Prior attempts at weight loss
- Reported readiness to change lifestyle
- Social support and resources
- Comorbidities: diabetes mellitus type 2, hypertension (HTN), hyperlipidemia, sleep apnea
- Psychiatric history
- Symptoms suggesting hypothyroidism, Cushing syndrome, and genetic syndromes

PHYSICAL EXAM
- Elevated BMI:
  - Overweight: BMI = 25 to 29.9 kg/m²
  - Obese: BMI 30 to 39.9 kg/m²
  - Morbid obesity: BMI ≥40 kg/m²
- Abdominal circumference:
  - Measure at the level of the umbilicus. Elevated:
    - Male: >40 inches (102 cm)
    - Female: >35 inches (88 cm)

DIAGNOSTIC TESTS & INTERPRETATION
- Screen for underlying physiologic causes as well as associated comorbid conditions.
- Glucose, total insulin, hemoglobin A1C, lipids
- Thyroid function tests
- LFTs (fatty liver)

TREATMENT

GENERAL MEASURES
- Assess:
  - Motivation to lose weight
  - Patient-specific goals of therapy
  - Need for intensive counseling to enhance adherence with diet, exercise, and behavior modification recommendations
- Goal is to achieve and sustain loss of at least 10% of body weight.

- Track nutritional intake and physical activity habits.
- Use of commercial weight loss programs (e.g., Weight Watchers) can be more effective than "standard of care" counseling (3)[B].
- Behavior therapy and cognitive behavioral methods result in modest weight loss and are most effective when combined with dietary and exercise treatments.
- Diet
  - Long-term studies suggest net calorie reduction (500 to 1,000 kcal/day) and ease of use are more important than the composition of the particular diet for long-term results:
    - A reduction of 500 kcal/day can result in ~1 lb (0.45 kg) weight loss per week.
    - Portion-control is essential.
  - Very low calorie diet (400 to 800 kcal/day)
    - Can result in more rapid weight loss than higher calorie diets but is less effective in the long term
    - Complications include dehydration, orthostatic hypotension, fatigue, muscle cramps, constipation, headache, and cold intolerance.
    - Relapse common if diet discontinued
    - Contraindications: recent myocardial infarction or cerebrovascular accident, renal disease, cancer, pregnancy, insulin-dependent diabetes mellitus, and some psychiatric disturbances

MEDICATION
- Include diet, exercise, and behavior therapy for all patients without comorbid conditions who are considering pharmacologic treatment.
- NIH guidelines suggest at least 6 months nonpharmacologic treatment.
- Consider medication for unsatisfactory weight loss in those with:
  - BMI ≥30
  - BMI ≥27 combined with associated risk factors (e.g., coronary artery disease, diabetes, sleep apnea, HTN, hyperlipidemia)
- Relapse is common after medications are discontinued.
- Treat comorbidities (such as diabetes and hyperlipidemia).

First Line
- When compared to placebo, medications have been associated with at least 5% weight loss at 52 weeks (4)[A]. Orlistat (Xenical) is a lipase inhibitor that decreases the absorption of dietary fat. Dose: 120 mg PO TID with meals containing fat; omit dose if meal is skipped or does not contain fat. Patients must avoid taking fat-soluble vitamin supplements within 2 hours of taking orlistat. The FDA has approved orlistat (Alli) 60 mg PO TID to be sold over the counter as a weight loss aid; adverse effects mainly GI (cramps, flatus, fecal incontinence)
- Contraindications
  - Orlistat: chronic malabsorption syndromes, cholestasis, pregnancy

Second Line
- Appetite suppressants recommended for short-term treatment (≤6 months) (5)[A]
- Only beneficial in patients who exercise and eat reduced calorie diet
  - Naltrexone/bupropion (Contrave): 8 mg naltrexone/90 mg bupropion per tablet; slow titration up to 2 tablets PO BID by week 4; contraindicated if uncontrolled HTN, seizure disorder, chronic opioid use, pregnancy
  - Liraglutide (Saxenda): 1.203 mg SC once daily; GLP-1 agonist recently approved for obesity; discontinue if weight loss is <4% after 16 weeks.
  - Topiramate: Initiate with 25 mg BID and increase by 50 mg/week up to 100 mg PO BID; not FDA-approved for the treatment of obesity; tolerance is a concern (paresthesias, somnolence, difficulty concentrating).
- Schedule IV drugs:
  - Lorcaserin (Belviq) 10 mg PO BID (D/C if weight loss is <5% after 12 weeks); works as serotonin agonist; avoid in those with CrCl <30 mL/min; contraindicated in pregnancy; avoid use with other serotonergic drugs.
  - Phentermine: 15, 30, 37.5 mg PO every morning; discontinue if tolerance or no response after 4 weeks; contraindicated if history of CV disease, hyperthyroidism, history of substance abuse, pregnancy
  - Phentermine/topiramate (Qsymia, 3.75 to 23.00 mg, 7.5 to 46.0 mg, 11.25 to 69.00 mg, 15 to 92 mg); initiate 3.75 to 23.00 mg PO once daily; requires enrollment into Risk Evaluation and Mitigation Strategy (REMS); women of childbearing age require negative pregnancy test prior to initiation and monthly thereafter.
  - Diethylpropion: 25 mg PO before meals TID; discontinue if no response after 4 weeks; contraindicated if severe HTN, hyperthyroidism, history of substance abuse

SURGERY/OTHER PROCEDURES
- Bariatric (weight loss) surgery for obesity is considered when other treatments have failed.
- Surgical treatment is the most effective long-term weight-loss treatment available for morbidly obese patients, but there is insufficient evidence on long-term outcomes (6)[A].
- Requires complex presurgical evaluation, surgery, and follow-up in a skilled treatment center
- Surgical procedures include biliopancreatic diversion, Roux-en-Y gastric bypass, sleeve gastrectomy, adjustable gastric banding, vagal blocking therapy (Maestro Rechargeable System), and gastric aspiration (AspireAssist).

 ONGOING CARE

FOLLOW-UP RECOMMENDATIONS
- Physical activity is an integral part of any weight loss program, yet physical activity alone rarely results in significant weight loss.
- Combination of weight training and aerobic activity is preferred over aerobic activity alone.

Patient Monitoring
Long-term routine follow-up may prevent relapse after weight loss or further weight gain.

PATIENT EDUCATION
- Healthy diet and physical activity patterns
- Focus on behaviors (not numbers).
- Recommended Web site:
  - https://www.nal.usda.gov/fnic/foodcomp/search for the FDA nutritional content in common foods

PROGNOSIS
- Lowest mortality associated with a BMI of 22
- Long-term maintenance of weight loss is difficult.
- Patient motivation is associated with successful weight loss (7).

COMPLICATIONS
- Cardiovascular disease
- Stroke (in men)
- Thromboembolism
- Heart failure
- HTN
- Hypoventilation and sleep apnea syndromes
- Higher death rates from cancer: colon, breast, prostate, endometrial, gallbladder, liver, kidney
- Diabetes mellitus
- Skin changes
- Hyperlipidemia
- Gallbladder disease
- Osteoarthritis
- Gout
- Poor self-esteem
- Discrimination
- Increased sick leave

REFERENCES

1. Ogden CL, Carroll MD, Flegal KM. Prevalence of obesity in the United States. *JAMA.* 2014;312(2):189–190.
2. Ogden CL, Carroll MD, Fryar CD, et al. Prevalence of obesity among adults and youth: United States, 2011–2014. *NCHS Data Brief.* 2015;(219):1–8.
3. Jebb SA, Ahern AL, Olson AD, et al. Primary care referral to a commercial provider for weight loss treatment versus standard care: a randomised controlled trial. *Lancet.* 2011;378(9801):1485–1492.
4. Khera R, Murad MH, Chandar A, et al. Association of pharmacological treatments for obesity with weight loss and adverse events: a systematic review and meta-analysis. *JAMA.* 2016;315(22):2424–2434.
5. Dombrowski SU, Knittle K, Avenell A, et al. Long term maintenance of weight loss with non-surgical interventions in obese adults: systematic review and meta-analyses of randomised controlled trials. *BMJ.* 2014;348:g2646.
6. Puzziferri N, Roshek TB III, Mayo HG, et al. Long-term follow-up after bariatric surgery: a systematic review. *JAMA.* 2014;312(9):934–942.
7. Ogden LG, Stroebele N, Wyatt HR, et al. Cluster analysis of the national weight control registry to identify distinct subgroups maintaining successful weight loss. *Obesity (Silver Spring).* 2012;20(10):2039–2047.

 CODES

ICD10
- E66.9 Obesity, unspecified
- E66.3 Overweight
- R63.5 Abnormal weight gain

CLINICAL PEARLS
- A majority of American adults are overweight or obese.
- Modification in dietary and physical activity patterns remains the cornerstone of therapy for obesity. Consider bariatric surgery in patients with a BMI >40 who have failed more conservative treatment, particularly if there are associated risk factors.
- Medication may be indicated when nonpharmacologic treatment for 6 months has been ineffective and the patient has a BMI >30 or a BMI >27 with associated risk factors.

OBSESSIVE-COMPULSIVE DISORDER (OCD)

Amar Kapur, DO • Nanako Negome-Kapur, PsyD

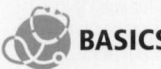

BASICS

DESCRIPTION
- An anxiety disorder characterized by pathologic obsessions (recurrent intrusive thoughts, ideas, or images) and compulsions (repetitive, ritualistic behaviors or mental acts) causing significant distress
- Not to be confused with obsessive-compulsive personality disorder

EPIDEMIOLOGY

Incidence
- Predominant age: mean age of onset 22 to 36 years
  - Male = female (males present at younger age)
  - Child/adolescent onset in 33% of cases 1/3 of cases present by age 15 years
  - 85% of cases present at <35 years of age
  - Diagnosis rarely made at >50 years of age
- Predominant gender: female > males but males more commonly affected in childhood

Pediatric Considerations
Insidious onset; consider brain insult in acute presentation of childhood obsessive-compulsive disorder (OCD).

Geriatric Considerations
Consider neurologic disorders in new-onset OCD.

Prevalence
- 2.3% lifetime in adults
- 1–2.3% prevalence in children/adolescents (1)

ETIOLOGY AND PATHOPHYSIOLOGY
- Exact pathophysiology/etiology unknown
- Dysregulation of serotonergic pathways
- Dysregulation of corticostriatal-thalamic-cortico (CSTC) path
- Genetic and environmental factors
- Pediatric autoimmune disorder associated with streptococcal infections (controversial)

Genetics
- Greater concordance in monozygotic twins
- Positive family history: prevalence rates of 7–15% in first-degree relatives of children/adolescents with OCD

RISK FACTORS
- Exact cause of OCD is not fully elucidated.
- Combination of biologic and environmental factors likely involved the following:
  - Link between low serotonin levels and development of OCD
  - Link between brain insult and development of OCD (i.e., encephalitis, pediatric streptococcal infection, or head injury)

GENERAL PREVENTION
- OCD cannot be prevented.
- Early diagnosis and treatment can decrease patient's distress and impairment.

COMMONLY ASSOCIATED CONDITIONS
- Major depressive disorder
- Panic disorder
- Phobia/social phobia
- Tourette syndrome/tic syndromes
- Substance abuse
- Eating disorder/body dysmorphic disorder

DIAGNOSIS

HISTORY
- Patient presents with either obsessions or compulsions, which cause marked distress, are time-consuming (>1 hr/day) and cause significant occupational/social impairment.
- Four criteria support diagnosis of obsessions:
  - Patients are aware that they are thinking the obsessive thoughts; thoughts are not imposed from outside (as in thought insertion).
  - Thoughts are not just excessive worrying about real-life problems.
  - Recurrent thoughts are persistent, intrusive, and inappropriate, causing significant anxiety and distress.
  - Attempts to suppress intrusive thoughts are made with some other thought/activity.
- Two criteria support a diagnosis of compulsions:
  - The response to an obsession is to perform repetitive behaviors (e.g., hand washing) or mental acts (e.g., counting silently) rigidly.
  - Although done to reduce stress, the responses are either not realistically connected with the obsession or they are excessive.
  - In children, check for precedent streptococcal infection.

PHYSICAL EXAM
- Dermatologic problems caused by excessive hand washing may be observed.
- Hair loss caused by compulsive pulling/twisting of the hair (trichotillomania) may be observed.

DIFFERENTIAL DIAGNOSIS
- Obsessive-compulsive personality disorder
  - In personality disorder, traits are ego-syntonic and include perfectionism and preoccupation with detail, trivia, or procedure and regulation. Patients tend to be rigid, moralistic, and stingy. These traits are often rewarded in the patient's job as desirable.
- Impulse-control disorders: compulsive gambling, sex, or substance abuse: The compulsive behavior is not in response to obsessive thoughts, and the patient derives pleasure from the activity.
- Major depressive disorder
- Eating disorder
- Tics (in tic disorder) and stereotyped movements
- Schizophrenia: Patient perceives thought to be true and coming from an external source.
- Generalized anxiety disorder, phobic disorders, separation anxiety: similar response on heightened anxiety, but presence of obsessions and rituals signifies OCD diagnosis
- Anxiety disorder due to a general medical condition: Obsessions/compulsions are assessed to be a direct physiologic consequence of a general medical condition.

DIAGNOSTIC TESTS & INTERPRETATION
According to *DSM-5*, diagnostic criteria for OCD are the following (2)[C]:
- Presence of obsessions, compulsions, or both
- Obsessions are defined by:
  - Recurrent or persistent thoughts, urges, or images that are experienced as intrusive and unwanted, and that cause marked anxiety or distress
  - The individual attempts to ignore or suppress such thoughts, urges, or images or to neutralize them with some other thought or actions (i.e., by performing compulsion).
- Compulsions are defined by the following:
  - Repetitive behavior (e.g., hand washing, ordering, checking) or mental acts (e.g., praying, counting, repeating words silently) that the individual feels driven to perform in response to an obsession or according to rules that must be applied rigidly
  - The behavior or mental acts are aimed at preventing or reducing anxiety or distress or preventing some dreaded event or situation. However, these behavior or mental acts are not connected in a realistic way with what they are designed to neutralize or prevent or are clearly excessive.
- The obsessions or compulsions are time-consuming (e.g., take >1 hr/day) or cause clinically significant distress or impairment in social, occupational, or other important areas of functioning.
- The obsessive-compulsive symptoms are not attributable to the physiologic effects of a substance (e.g., a drug of abuse, a medication, or other medical condition).
- The disturbance is not better explained by the symptoms of another mental disorder (e.g., excessive worries, as in generalized anxiety disorder, preoccupation with appearance, as in body dysmorphic disorder or skin picking).
- Specify if:
  - With good or fair insight: The individual recognizes the OCD beliefs are definitely or probably not true or that they may or may not be true.
  - With poor insight: The individual thinks that OCD beliefs are probably true.
  - With absent insight/delusional beliefs: The individual is completely convinced that OCD beliefs are true.
- Specify if:
  - Tic related: The individual has a current or past history of tic disorder.

Diagnostic Procedures/Other
- Yale-Brown Obsessive-Compulsive Scale (Y-BOCS) or CY-BOCS for children (1)[C]
- Maudsley Obsessive-Compulsive Inventory (MOCI) (3)[C]

Test Interpretation
- Compulsions are designed to relieve the anxiety of obsessions; they are not inherently enjoyable (ego-dystonic) and do not result in completion of a task.
- Common obsessive themes
  - Harm (i.e., being responsible for an accident)
  - Doubt (i.e., whether doors/windows are locked or the iron is turned off)
  - Blasphemous thoughts (i.e., in a devoutly religious person)
  - Contamination, dirt, or disease
  - Symmetry/orderliness
- Common rituals or compulsions
  - Hand washing, cleaning
  - Checking
  - Counting
  - Hoarding
  - Ordering, arranging
  - Repeating
- Neither obsessions nor compulsions are related to another mental disorder (i.e., thoughts of food and presence of eating disorder).
- 80–90% of patients with OCD have obsessions and compulsions.
- 10–19% of patients with OCD are pure obsessional.

TREATMENT

GENERAL MEASURES

- Cognitive-behavioral therapy (CBT) composed of exposure with response prevention and cognitive therapy is recommended as first-line treatment (1)[A].
- Five phases of treatment for CBT:
  – Family and individual psychoeducation
  – Cognitive training
  – Mapping OCD
  – Graded exposure and response training
  – Relapse prevention and generalization training
- Combined medications and CBT is most effective (1,2)[A].
- Brain modulation available for severe OCD includes electroconvulsive therapy and transcranial magnetic stimulation in small groups of patients.

MEDICATION

First Line

- Adequate trial at least 10 to 12 weeks
- Doses may exceed typical doses for depression.
- Optimal duration for pediatrics unknown but recommended minimum of maintenance treatment: 6 months
- Varying degrees of efficacy between agents (1)
- SSRIs recommended first-line agents (1,4,5)[A]
  – Fluoxetine (Prozac)
    ○ Adults: 20 mg/day; increase by 10 to 20 mg every 4 to 6 weeks until response; range: 20 to 80 mg/day
    ○ Children (7 to 17 years of age): 10 mg/day; increase 4 to 6 weeks until response; range: 20 to 60 mg/day
  – Sertraline (Zoloft)
    – Adults: 50 mg/day; increase by 50 mg every 4 to 7 days until response; range: 50 to 200 mg/day; may divide if >100 mg/day
    – Children (6 to 17 years of age): 25 mg/day; increase by 25 mg every 7 days until response; range: 50 to 200 mg/day
  – Paroxetine (Paxil)
    – Adults: 20 mg/day; increase by 10 mg every 4 to 7 days until response; range: 40 to 60 mg/day
    – Children: Safety and effectiveness in patients <18 years have not been established.
  – Citalopram (Celexa)
    – Not approved by the FDA for use in OCD but used frequently due to good tolerability
    – Black box warning of no more than 40 mg/day due to arrhythmia risk
  – Absolute SSRI contraindications
    – Hypersensitivity to SSRIs
    – Concomitant use within 14 days of monoamine oxidase inhibitor (MAOI)
  – Relative SSRI contraindications
    – Severe liver impairment
    – Seizure disorders (lower seizure threshold)
  – Precautions
    – Watch for suicidal behavior/worsening depression during first few months of therapy/after dosage changes with antidepressants, particularly in children, adolescents, and young adults.
    – Long half-life of fluoxetine (>7 days) may be troublesome if patient has an adverse reaction.
    – May cause drowsiness and dizziness when therapy was initiated; warn patients about driving and heavy equipment hazards.

Pregnancy Considerations

All SSRIs are pregnancy Category C, except paroxetine, which is Category D.

Second Line

- Try switching to another SSRI.
- 40–60% of patients will remain refractory to SSRI.
- Tricyclic acid (TCA), clomipramine (Anafranil)
  – Adults: 25 mg/day; increase gradually over 2 weeks to 100 mg/day and then to 250 mg/day (max dose) over next several weeks, as tolerated.
  – Children (10 to 17 years of age): 25 mg/day; titrate as needed and tolerated up to 3 mg/kg/day or 200 mg/day (whichever is less).
  – Absolute clomipramine contraindications
    ○ Within 6 months of a myocardial infarction (MI)
    ○ Hypersensitivity to clomipramine or other TCA
    ○ Concomitant use within 14 days of a MAOI
    ○ 3rd-degree atrioventricular (AV) block
  – Relative clomipramine contraindications
    ○ Narrow-angle glaucoma (increased intraocular pressure)
    ○ Prostatic hypertrophy (urinary retention)
    ○ 1st- or 2nd-degree AV block, bundle-branch block, and congestive heart failure (proarrhythmic effect)
    ○ Pregnancy Category C
  – Precautions
    ○ Dangerous in overdose
    ○ Pretreatment ECG for patients >40 years of age; potential arrhythmia (4)
    ○ Watch for suicidal behavior/worsening depression during first few months of therapy or after dosage changes with antidepressants, particularly in children, adolescents, and young adults.
    ○ May cause drowsiness and dizziness when therapy is initiated; warn patients about driving and heavy equipment hazards (4).
    ○ Side effect profile worse than SSRIs as a whole (4)

ISSUES FOR REFERRAL

- Psychiatric referral for CBT (in vivo exposure and prevention of compulsions)
- Psychiatric evaluation if obsessions and compulsions significantly interfere with patient's functioning in social, occupational, or educational situations

ADDITIONAL THERAPIES

Dopamine receptor antagonists (antipsychotic agents) alone are not effective in treatment of OCD. They can be used as augmentation to SSRI therapy for treatment-resistant OCD; they also can worsen OCD symptoms (4) [C]. Some evidence show that addition of quetiapine or risperidone to antidepressants will increase efficacy; data with olanzapine too limited to draw conclusions (4)[A]

- Risperidone (Risperdal): initial dose: 0.5 mg/day; target dose: 0.5 to 2.0 mg/day
- Quetiapine (Seroquel): initial dose: 25 mg/day; target dose: 600 mg/day

 ONGOING CARE

FOLLOW-UP RECOMMENDATIONS

Y-BCOS or MOCI surveys to track progress

Patient Monitoring

Monitor for decrease in obsessions and time spent performing compulsions.

DIET

No dietary modifications/restrictions recommended

PATIENT EDUCATION

- Importance of medication adherence
- Importance of psychotherapy (CBT)
- International OCD Foundation: https://iocdf.org/
- Obsessive Compulsive Anonymous: http://obsessive compulsiveanonymous.org

PROGNOSIS

- Chronic waxing and waning course in most patients:
  – 24–33% fluctuating course
  – 11–14% phasic periods of remission
  – 54–61% chronic progressive course
- Early onset a poor predictor
- Few studies address how long to continue therapy; poor results for those that do with high elapse rate (53% on placebo compared to 23% on stable escitalopram) (4)
- Patients who are classified as "responders" will continue to have symptoms, often significantly impacting their lives.

COMPLICATIONS

- Depression in 1/3 patients with OCD
- Avoidant behavior (phobic avoidance)
  – Children may drop out of education.
  – Adults may become homebound.
- Anxiety and panic-like episodes associated with obsessions

REFERENCES

1. Skarphedinsson G, Weidle B, Thomsen PH, et al. Continued cognitive-behavior therapy versus sertraline for children and adolescents with obsessive-compulsive disorder that were non-responders to cognitive-behavior therapy: a randomized controlled trial. *Eur Child Adolesc Psychiatry*. 2015;24(5):591–602.
2. American Psychiatric Association. *Diagnostic and Statistical Manual of Mental Disorders*. 5th ed. Arlington, VA: American Psychiatric Association; 2013.
3. McKay D, Sookman D, Neziroglu F, et al. Efficacy of cognitive-behavioral therapy for obsessive-compulsive disorder. *Psychiatry Res*. 2015;225(3):236–246.
4. Pittenger C, Bloch M. Pharmacological treatment of obsessive-compulsive disorder. *Psychiatr Clin North Am*. 2014;37(3):375–391.
5. Komossa K, Depping AM, Meyer M, et al. Second-generation antipsychotics for obsessive compulsive disorder. *Cochrane Database Sys Rev*. 2010;(12):CD008141.

ADDITIONAL READING

Kakhi S, Soomro GM. Obsessive compulsive disorder in children and adolescents: duration of maintenance drug treatment. *BMJ Clin Evid*. 2015;2015:1019.

 CODES

ICD10

- F42 Obsessive-compulsive disorder
- F63.9 Impulse disorder, unspecified
- F63.3 Trichotillomania

CLINICAL PEARLS

- CBT is the initial treatment of choice for mild OCD.
- CBT plus an SSRI or an SSRI alone is the treatment choice for more severe OCD.
- The majority of patients with OCD respond to first SSRI treatment.
- Improvement in symptoms, however, is often incomplete, ranging from 25% to 60%.

OCULAR CHEMICAL BURNS

Ian J. McDowell, DO

BASICS

DESCRIPTION
- Chemical exposure to the eye can result in rapid, devastating, and permanent damage and is one of the true emergencies in ophthalmology.
- Types of chemical exposure:
  - Alkali burns: more severe. Alkaline compounds are lipophilic, penetrating rapidly into eye tissue; saponification of cells leads to necrosis and may produce injury to lids, conjunctiva, cornea, sclera, iris, and lens (cataracts).
  - Acid burns: Acid usually does not damage internal structures because its associated anion causes protein denaturation, creating a barrier to further acid penetration (hydrofluoric acid is an exception to this rule; see below). Injury is often limited to lids, conjunctiva, and cornea.
- System(s) affected: nervous, skin/exocrine
- Synonym(s): chemical ocular injuries

EPIDEMIOLOGY
- Predominant age: can occur at any age, peak from 20 to 40 years of age
- Predominant sex: male > female

Incidence
- Estimated 300/100,000 per year
- Chemical burns account for 11.5–22.1% of all ocular injuries.
- Alkali burns are twice as common as acid burns.

ETIOLOGY AND PATHOPHYSIOLOGY
- Alkaline compounds
  - Lipophilic compounds that penetrate into deep structures on disassociation into cations and hydroxide
  - Hydroxide causes saponification of fatty acids in cell membranes, leading to cell death.
  - Cation causes hydration of glycosaminoglycans, leading to corneal opacification and hydration of collagen, resulting in rapid shortening and thickening of collagen fibrils that leads to an acute elevation in intraocular pressure (IOP) secondary to shrinking and contraction of the cornea and sclera.
  - Long-term elevation in IOP may occur from accumulation of inflammatory debris within the trabecular meshwork.
  - Penetration into deep structures may also affect perfusing vessels, leading to ischemia of affected area.
- Acidic compounds
  - Anion leads to protein denaturing and protective barrier formation by coagulation necrosis forming an eschar. This more superficial mechanism of injury tends to have prominent scarring that may lead to vision loss:
    - Hydrofluoric acid is an exception. In its nonionized form, it behaves like an alkaline substance, capable of penetrating the corneal stroma and leading to extensive anterior segment lesions. When ionized, it may combine with intracellular calcium and magnesium to form insoluble complexes, leading to potassium ion movements and cell death. Once systemically absorbed, severe hypocalcemia can occur.

Sources of Alkaline and Acidic Compounds

Alkaline Compounds	Typical Sources
Calcium hydroxide (lime)	Cement, plaster, mortar, whitewash
Sodium/potassium hydroxide (lye)	Drain cleaner, airbags
Ammonia	Cleaning agents
Ammonium hydroxide	Fertilizers
Acidic Compounds	**Typical Sources**
Sulfuric acid	Car batteries
Sulfurous acid	Bleach, refrigerant
Hydrochloric acid	Chem labs, swimming pools
Acetic acid	Vinegar
Hydrofluoric acid	Glass polish

RISK FACTORS
- Construction work (plaster, cement, whitewash)
- Use of cleaning agents (drain cleaners, ammonia)
- Automobile battery explosions (sulfuric acid)
- Industrial work, including work in industrial chemical laboratories
- Alcoholism
- Any risk factor for assault (~10% of injuries due to deliberate assault)

GENERAL PREVENTION
Safety glasses/goggles to safeguard eyes

COMMONLY ASSOCIATED CONDITIONS
Facial (including eyelids) cutaneous chemical or thermal burns

DIAGNOSIS

HISTORY
- Most often, complaints of pain, photophobia, blurred vision, and a foreign body sensation
- Important to assess chemical involved, duration of exposure, velocity of impact, and involved area
- In alkali burns, can have initial pain that later diminishes
- Mild burns: pain and blurred vision
- Moderate to severe burns: severe pain and markedly reduced vision

PHYSICAL EXAM
- Alkaline compounds may present with corneal opacification secondary to glycosaminoglycan hydration; however, severe acid burns may also present with this finding.
- Acidic compound may present with a ground-glass appearance secondary to superficial scar formation.
- Mild burns
  - Blurry vision
  - Eyelid skin erythema and edema
  - Corneal epithelial defects or superficial punctate keratitis
  - Conjunctival chemosis, hyperemia, and hemorrhages without perilimbal ischemia
  - Mild anterior chamber reaction

- Moderate to severe burns
  - Decreased visual acuity
  - 2nd- and 3rd-degree burns of eyelid skin
  - Corneal edema and opacification
  - Corneal epithelial defects
  - Marked conjunctival chemosis and perilimbal blanching
  - Moderate anterior chamber reaction
  - Increased IOP
  - Local necrotic retinopathy

DIFFERENTIAL DIAGNOSIS
- Thermal burns
- Ocular cicatricial pemphigoid
- Other causes of corneal opacification
- Ultraviolet radiation keratitis
- Foreign body
- Acute angle glaucoma
- Conjunctivitis

DIAGNOSTIC TESTS & INTERPRETATION
Not necessary unless suspicion of intraocular or orbital foreign body is present. In this case, CT should be used and MRI is contraindicated.

Diagnostic Procedures/Other
- Measure pH of tear film with litmus paper or electronic probe:
  - Irrigating fluid with nonneutral pH (e.g., normal saline has pH of 4.5) may alter results.
- Careful slit-lamp exam, fundus ophthalmoscopy, tonometry, and measurement of visual acuity
- Full extent of damage from alkali burns may not be apparent until 48 to 72 hours after exposure.

Test Interpretation
- Corneal epithelial defects or superficial punctate keratitis, edema, opacification
- Conjunctival chemosis, hyperemia, and hemorrhages
- Perilimbal ischemia
- Anterior chamber reaction
- Increased IOP

TREATMENT

Copious irrigation and removal of corneal or conjunctival foreign bodies are always the initial treatment and paramount to minimize long-term sequelae (1,2,3,4)[A]:
- Passively open patient's eyelid and have patient look in all directions while irrigating.
- Be sure to remove all reservoirs of chemical from the eyes via lid eversion.
- Continue irrigation until the tear film and superior/inferior cul-de-sac is of neutral pH (7 ± 0.1) and pH is stable, testing every 15 minutes (1,3)[A]:
  - Severe burns should be irrigated for at least 15 to 30 minutes to as much as 2 to 4 hours; this irrigation should not be interrupted during transportation to hospital (1,3)[B].
  - Irrigation via Morgan lens (polymethylmethacrylate scleral lens) is a good way to achieve continuous irrigation over a prolonged period of time.
  - It is impossible to overirrigate.
- Initial pH testing should be done on both eyes even if the patient claims to only have unilateral ocular pain/irritation so that a contralateral injury is not neglected.

- Use whatever nontoxic fluid is available for irrigation on scene. In hospital, sterile water, normal saline, normal saline with bicarbonate, balanced salt solution (BSS), lactated Ringer solution, Diphoterine or Cederroth eye wash may be used.
  - Diphoterine or Cederroth eye wash has shown better patient comfort and healing but should not prevent prompt irritation if not readily available (2)[B].
- A topical anesthetic can be used to provide patient comfort (e.g., proparacaine, tetracaine).
- Sweep the conjunctival fornices every 12 to 24 hours to prevent adhesions (3)[C].

MEDICATION

First Line

- Further treatment aims to decrease inflammation and collagen degradation and aid in collagen synthesis and recovery of corneal epithelium. Selection depends on severity and associated conditions.
  - Topical prophylactic antibiotics: any broad-spectrum agent (e.g., bacitracin–polymyxin B ointment q2–4h, ciprofloxacin drops q2–4h)
    - Some experts suggest adding systemic tetracycline 250 mg PO q6h and especially derivatives such as doxycycline 100 mg PO BID may be beneficial to encourage healing and prevent corneal ulceration (1,2)[C].
  - Tear substitutes: carboxymethylcellulose (Refresh Plus) drops q4h
    - Promotes re-epithelialization, reduces recurrent erosion risk, and increases visual rehab (1,2)[A]
  - Cycloplegics for photophobia and/or uveitis: cyclopentolate 1% TID or scopolamine 1/4% BID (3,4)[C]
  - Corticosteroids for intraocular inflammation: prednisolone 1% or equivalent q2h for 7 to 10 days; if severe, prednisone 20 to 60 mg PO daily for 5 to 7 days. Taper rapidly if epithelium is intact, by day 10 to 14 (1,3)[C]:
    - Using vitamin C in conjunction with steroids reduces incidence of corneal thinning, ulceration, and perforation (1,2,3)[A].
  - Vitamin C (ascorbic acid) 500 mg PO QID and topical 10% q2h ascorbate solution in artificial tears
  - Acetylcysteine (Mucomyst) 10–20% topically q4h may promote wound healing (1,3)[B].
  - Antiglaucoma for increased IOP >30 to reduce risk of optic nerve damage: latanoprost 0.005% q24h, timolol 0.5% BID, or levobunolol 0.5% BID, and/or acetazolamide 125 to 250 mg PO q6h, or methazolamide 25 to 50 mg PO BID (2,3)[B]
  - Bandage contact lens: Lenses with high oxygen permeability and hydrophilic properties aid in epithelial migration/adhesion and basement membrane regeneration (3,4)[B].
- Precautions
  - Timolol and levobunolol: history of cardiac/pulmonary disease or bradycardia
  - Acetazolamide and methazolamide: history of nephrolithiasis or metabolic acidosis
  - Mannitol: history of HF or renal failure
  - Scopolamine: history of urinary retention
  - Ascorbic acid: history of renal impairment
  - Tetracycline/doxycycline: Avoid systemic use in children <8 years old and pregnant patients.

- Topical corticosteroids must be used with caution in the presence of damaged corneal epithelium because iatrogenic infection can occur. Use of corticosteroids >6 days may inhibit repair and cause corneoscleral melt (1)[B]. Daily follow-up or consultation with an ophthalmologist is recommended.
- Consider adjunctive treatments.
  - Biologic fluids with consultation to ophthalmology: umbilical cord serum 20% q2–3h, autologous serum 20% q2–3h, platelet-rich plasma q2–3h, or amniotic membrane suspension 30–50% q1h. These consist of growth factors, vitamins, cytokines, and anti-inflammatory factors to improve dry eyes, reduce pain, persistent epithelial defects, recurrent erosion syndrome, and neurotrophic ulcers (1,2)[B].

SURGERY/OTHER PROCEDURES

- Goal of subacute treatment is restoration of the normal ocular surface anatomy, control of glaucoma, and restoration of corneal clarity.
- Surgical options include the following:
  - Débridement of necrotic tissue, removing inflammatory debris (1,4)[A]
  - Conjunctival/tenon advancement (tenoplasty) to restore vascularity in severe burns
  - Tissue adhesive (e.g., isobutyl cyanoacrylate) for impending or actual corneal perforation
    - Tectonic keratoplasty for acute perforation >1 mm
  - Limbal autograft transplantation for epithelial stem cell restoration
  - Amniotic membrane transplantation or umbilical cord serum drops to promote faster epithelial regeneration and improvement in visual acuity (1)[B]
  - Conjunctival or mucosal membrane transplant to restore ocular surface in severe injury

ADMISSION, INPATIENT, AND NURSING CONSIDERATIONS

Based on ophthalmologic consultation and concomitant burn injuries

 ONGOING CARE

FOLLOW-UP RECOMMENDATIONS

Patient Monitoring

- Depending on severity of ocular injury
  - From daily to weekly visits initially
- May be inpatient
- If on mannitol or prednisone, consider frequent serum electrolytes.

PATIENT EDUCATION

- Safety glasses
- Need for immediate ocular irrigation with any available water following chemical exposure to the eyes

PROGNOSIS

- Depends on severity of initial injury: Increased limbal involvement in clock hours and greater percentage of conjunctival involvement correlate with poorer prognosis (Dua classification system).
- For mildly injured eyes, complete recovery is common.
- For severely injured eyes, permanent loss of vision is not uncommon.

COMPLICATIONS

- Orbital compartment syndrome
- Persistent epitheliopathy

- Keratoconjunctivitis sicca (dry eye)
- Fibrovascular pannus
- Corneal ulcer/perforation
- Corneal scarring
- Progressive symblepharon
- Neurotrophic keratitis
- Lid malposition due to cicatricial ectropion/entropion
- Glaucoma
- Cataract
- Hypotony
- Phthisis bulbi
- Blindness

REFERENCES

1. Sharma N, Kaur M, Agarwal T, et al. Treatment of acute ocular chemical burns. *Surv Ophthalmol*. 2018;63(2):214–235.
2. Baradaran-Rafii A, Eslani M, Haq Z, et al. Current and upcoming therapies for ocular surface chemical injuries. *Ocul Surf*. 2017;15(1):48–64.
3. Singh P, Tyagi M, Kumar Y, et al. Ocular chemical injuries and their management. *Oman J Ophthalmol*. 2013;6(2):83–86.
4. Eslani M, Baradaran-Rafii A, Movahedan A, et al. The ocular surface chemical burns. *J Ophthalmol*. 2014;2014:196827.

ADDITIONAL READING

- Chau JP, Lee DT, Lo SH. A systematic review of methods of eye irrigation for adults and children with ocular chemical burns. *Worldviews Evid Based Nurs*. 2012;9(3):129–138.
- Sharma N, Lathi SS, Sehra SV, et al. Comparison of umbilical cord serum and amniotic membrane transplantation in acute ocular chemical burns. *Br J Ophthalmol*. 2015;99(5):669–673.

 SEE ALSO

Burns

 CODES

ICD10

- T26.50XA Corrosion of unsp eyelid and periocular area, init encntr
- T26.60XA Corrosion of cornea and conjunctival sac, unsp eye, init
- S05.00XA Inj conjunctiva and corneal abrasion w/o fb, unsp eye, init

CLINICAL PEARLS

- Prompt irrigation of all chemical burns, even prior to arrival to the emergency department, is essential to ensure the best outcomes. It is impossible to overirrigate.
- All patients with chemical injuries to their eyes should have urgent ophthalmology consultation and/or referral.

ONYCHOMYCOSIS
Lauren M. Simon, MD, MPH

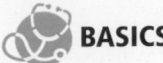

BASICS

DESCRIPTION
- Fungal infection of fingernails/toenails
- Caused mostly by dermatophytes but also yeasts and nondermatophyte molds
- Toenails are more commonly affected than fingernails.
- System(s) affected: skin, exocrine
- Synonym(s): tinea unguium; ringworm of the nail

EPIDEMIOLOGY
Prevalence
- Occurs in 2–10% of general population
- Predominant age: 20% in adults >60 years of age
- Rare before puberty
- Prevalence 15–40% in persons with human immunodeficiency infection (1)

ETIOLOGY AND PATHOPHYSIOLOGY
- Dermatophytes: *Trichophyton* (*Trichophyton rubrum* most common), *Epidermophyton*, *Microsporum*
- Yeasts: *Candida albicans* (most common), *Candida parapsilosis*, *Candida tropicalis*, *Candida krusei*
- Molds: *Scopulariopsis brevicaulis*, *Hendersonula toruloidea*, *Aspergillus* sp., *Alternaria tenuis*, *Cephalosporium*, *Scytalidium hyalinum*
- Dermatophytes cause 90% of toenail and most of fingernail onychomycoses.
- Fingernail onychomycosis is more often caused by yeasts, especially *Candida*.
- Dermatophytes can invade normal keratin, whereas nondermatophyte molds invade altered keratin (dystrophic/injured nails).

RISK FACTORS
- Older age
- Tinea pedis
- Occlusive footwear
- Cancer/diabetes/psoriasis
- Peripheral vascular disease
- Cohabitation with others with onychomycosis
- Immunodeficiency
- Communal swimming pools
- Smoking
- Peripheral vascular disease
- History of nail trauma
- Autosomal dominant genetic predisposition

COMMONLY ASSOCIATED CONDITIONS
- Immunodeficiency/chronic metabolic disease (e.g., diabetes)
- Tinea pedis/manuum

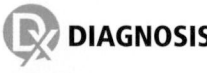

DIAGNOSIS

PHYSICAL EXAM
- Dermatophytes: commonly preceded by dermatophyte infection at another site; 80% involve toenails, especially hallux; simultaneous infection of fingernails and toenails is rare. Five clinical forms occur.
  - Distal/lateral subungual onychomycosis (most common): mainly due to *T. rubrum*. Spreads from distal/lateral margins to nail bed to nail plate; subungual hyperkeratosis; onycholysis; nail dystrophy; discoloration—yellow-white or brown-black, yellow streaking laterally; can progress proximally, *bois vermoulu* ("worm-eaten wood"); onychomadesis

- Proximal subungual onychomycosis (rare <1% of cases): hands/feet; leukonychia—begins at proximal part of nail plate, appearing to occur from the proximal underside of the nail (or direct invasion of the nail plate from above); spreads to nail plate and lunula; seen with immunosuppressive conditions
- Superficial (formerly known as superficial white onychomycosis) about 10% of cases: hallux is preferentially affected; infection of outer surface of nail plate; opaque white spots on nail plate eventually merge to involve entire surface of the nail; most commonly due to *Trichophyton mentagrophytes*
- Endonyx onychomycosis involves interior of nail plate, sparing nail bed. Nail develops milky white appearance with indentations. Subungual hyperkeratosis is absent.
- Totally dystrophic onychomycosis causes complete destruction of nail plate by fungus, resulting in thickened and ridged nail bed covered with keratotic debris.
- Candidal
  - Hands, 70%, especially for the dominant hand
  - Middle finger is most common.
  - Pain is mild, unless secondarily infected.
  - Increases on prolonged contact with water
  - Primarily affects tissue surrounding nail
  - Begins with cuticle detachment
  - White or white-yellow nail discoloration
  - Secondary ungual changes: convex, irregular, striated nail plate with dull, rough surface
  - Onycholysis, especially on hands
  - Distal subungual onychomycosis may occur.
  - Primary involvement of the nail plate is uncommon (thin, crumbly, opaque, brownish nail plate deformed by transverse grooves).
  - Periungual edema/erythema may occur (club-shaped, bulbous fingertips).
- Molds (nondermatophyte)
  - More common in those >60 years of age
  - More common in nails of hallux
  - Resembles distal and lateral onychomycosis

Pediatric Considerations
- Candidal infection presents more commonly as superficial onychomycosis.
- The U.S. Food and Drug Administration (FDA) has not approved any systemic antifungal agents for treatment of onychomycosis in children. Efficacy and safety profiles in children for some systemic antifungals are similar to those previously reported in adults (2).

DIFFERENTIAL DIAGNOSIS
- Psoriasis (most common alternate diagnosis)
- Traumatic dystrophy
- Lichen planus
- Onychogryphosis ("ram's horn nails")
- Eczematous conditions
- Hypothyroidism
- Drugs and chemicals
- Yellow nail syndrome
- Neoplasms (0.7–3.5%) of all melanoma cases are subungual. In a brownish yellow nail, if dark pigment extends into periungual skin fold, consider subungual melanoma.

DIAGNOSTIC TESTS & INTERPRETATION
- Accurate diagnosis requires both laboratory and clinical evidence.
- About 50% of nail dystrophy seen on visual inspection is not fungal in origin, so laboratory assessment improves diagnostic accuracy.

- If onychomycosis is suspected clinically and initial diagnostic laboratory tests are negative, the tests should be repeated.
- A nail plate biopsy or partial/full removal of nail with culture is needed to diagnose proximal subungual onychomycosis.

Initial Tests (lab, imaging)
- Direct microscopy with potassium hydroxide (KOH) preparation (1)[C]
  - Clean nail with 70% isopropyl alcohol.
  - Using sterile clippers, remove diseased, discolored nail plate.
  - Collect debris from stratum corneum of most proximal area (beneath nail or crumbling nail itself) with 1-mm curette/scalpel.
  - Place sample on microscope slide with drop of 5–10% KOH. View after 5 minutes.
  - Gentle heat applied to slide can enhance keratin breakdown.
  - High sensitivity if >2 preparations were examined
  - Look for hyphae, pseudohyphae, or spores.
- Cultures: False-negative finding in 30% (secondary to loss of dermatophyte viability; improved by immediate culture on Sabouraud cell culture medium); results may take 3 to 6 weeks.
- In office dermatophyte test, medium culture indicates dermatophyte growth with yellow-to-red color change of the medium; results in 3 to 7 days; limited studies
- Histologic examination of nail clippings/nail plate punch biopsy: proximal lesions; stain both with periodic acid–Schiff (PAS) stain (1)[C].
- KOH-treated nail clipping stained with PAS: significantly higher rates of detection of onychomycosis as compared with standard methods of KOH preparation and fungal culture (3)[C]
- Polymerase chain reaction (PCR) increases sensitivity of detection of dermatophytes in nail specimen; results available within 3 days can be used as complementary to direct microscope exam and fungal culture; not widely available
- Fluorescence microscopy can be used as a rapid screening tool for identification of fungi in nail specimens.
- Commercial laboratories may use KOH with calcofluor white stain to improve view of fungal elements in fluorescent microscopy.
- Discontinue all topical medication for at least 1 week before obtaining a sample.

Test Interpretation
Pathogens within the nail keratin

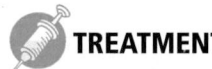

TREATMENT

GENERAL MEASURES
- Avoid factors that promote fungal growth (i.e., heat, moisture, occlusion, tight-fitting shoes).
- Treat underlying disease risk factors.
- Treat secondary infections.

MEDICATION
Pregnancy Considerations
Oral antifungals and ciclopirox are pregnancy Category B (terbinafine, ciclopirox) or C (itraconazole, fluconazole, and griseofulvin). Griseofulvin is not advised in pregnancy due to risks of teratogenicity and conjoined twins. Ideally postpone treatment of onychomycosis until after pregnancy.

First Line

- Oral antifungals are preferred due to higher rates of cure but have systemic adverse effects and many drug–drug interactions.
- Terbinafine: 250 mg/day PO for 6 weeks for fingernails and 12 weeks for toenails; most effective in cure and prevention of relapse compared with other antifungals and with itraconazole pulse in meta-analysis for toenail onychomycosis (4)[A]
- Itraconazole pulse: 200 mg PO BID for 1 week and then 3 weeks off, repeat for two cycles for fingernails and three to four cycles for toenails; does not need to monitor liver function tests (LFTs) with pulse dosing
- Itraconazole continuous: 200 mg/day PO for 6 weeks for fingernails and 12 weeks for toenails (less effective than itraconazole pulse for dermatophytes, more effective than terbinafine for *Candida* and molds)

Second Line

- Fluconazole pulse: 150 to 300 mg PO weekly for 6 months (lower cure rate); not FDA-approved for onychomycosis
- Griseofulvin: 500 to 1,000 mg/day PO for up to 18 months (lower cure rate, continue until the diseased nail is replaced)
- Posaconazole: 100, 200, or 400 mg once daily for 24 weeks; 400 mg once daily for 12 weeks; higher cost
- Topical agents: Use limited to disease not involving the lunula (proximal nail plate). Topical therapy does not cause systemic toxicity but is less effective than oral therapy. Head-to-head comparison of efficacy of available agents is generally not available.
- Efinaconazole solution 10%, apply directly to affected nails once daily for 48 weeks; complete or almost-complete cure after 48 weeks in range of 15–18% (NNT compared to vehicle 7 to 10)
- Ciclopirox: 8% nail lacquer (available generically): Apply once daily to affected nails (if without lunula involvement) for up to 48 weeks; remove lacquer with alcohol every 7 days, and then file away loose nail material and trim nails (low-cure rate, avoids systemic adverse effects, less cost-effective). Application after PO treatment may reduce recurrences; systematic review >60% failure rate after 48 weeks of use (5)[A]
- Tavaborole 5% solution, a topical oxaborole antifungal, is indicated for onychomycosis of the toenails due to *T. rubrum* or *T. mentagrophytes*; complete or almost-complete cure 15–18% after 48 weeks (NNT compared to vehicle approximately 7)
- Contraindications for oral antifungals
  - Hepatic disease
  - Pregnancy (see "Pregnancy Considerations")
  - Current/history of congestive heart failure (CHF) (itraconazole)
  - Ventricular dysfunction (itraconazole)
  - Porphyria (griseofulvin)
- Precautions/adverse effects
  - Oral antifungals
    ○ Hepatotoxicity/neutropenia
    ○ Hypersensitivity
    ○ Photosensitivity, lupus-like symptoms, proteinuria (griseofulvin)
    ○ Chronic kidney disease (Avoid terbinafine for patients with creatinine clearance [CrCl] <50 mL/min, decrease fluconazole dose.)
    ○ CHF, peripheral edema, pulmonary edema (itraconazole)
    ○ Rhinitis (itraconazole)

- Ciclopirox topical: side effects: rash, nail disorders; avoid contact with skin except along nail edge; caution with broken skin or vascular compromise
- Oral agents: numerous significant drug–drug interactions; need to check each medication:
  - Terbinafine (inhibits cytochrome P450 2D6 [CYP2D6] isoenzyme): for example, β-blockers, monoamine oxidase inhibitors (MAOIs), SSRIs, tricyclic antidepressants (TCAs), warfarin, oxycodone
  - Itraconazole (inhibit CYP3A4): for example, antiarrhythmics, benzodiazepines, ergot alkaloids, 3-hydroxy-3-methylglutaryl coenzyme A (HMG-CoA) reductase inhibitors, calcium channel blockers, corticosteroids, hydrochlorothiazide, hypoglycemics, oral contraceptives (OCPs), warfarin, zolpidem
  - Griseofulvin: for example, OCPs, salicylates, warfarin

SURGERY/OTHER PROCEDURES

- Nail débridement to remove infected keratin (efficacy not well studied): Use for few nails involved or if not, for candidate of systemic therapy.
  - Mechanical: Soften with occlusive dressing with 40% urea gel; detach from nail bed with tweezers, file with abrasive stone or curette.
  - Chemical: Protect peripheral tissue with adhesive strips; apply ointment of 30% salicylic acid, 40% urea, or 50% potassium iodide under occlusive dressing.
  - Débridement may be combined with topical antifungal therapy.
  - Surgical avulsion if few nails are involved; for pain control
- Laser treatment has shown some positive results but poor statistical power and limited efficacy or safety data (6)[A].
- Photodynamic therapy using topical photosensitizing agents and irradiation with appropriate light source some success for treatment of superficial nail infections; limited data

COMPLEMENTARY & ALTERNATIVE MEDICINE

- *Melaleuca alternifolia* (tea tree oil) Cochrane review found no evidence of benefit (5)[A].
- Vicks VapoRub application to nails daily for 48 weeks has been found safe, but efficacy is uncertain.

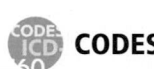

ONGOING CARE

FOLLOW-UP RECOMMENDATIONS

- Formation of a new fingernail takes 4 to 6 months, and a new toenail takes 12 to 18 months.
- Cure defined as:
  - Clinical cure, 100% absence of clinical signs, and/or
  - Mycotic cure, negative mycology with ≥1 of the following clinical signs:
    ○ Distal subungual hyperkeratosis/onycholysis leaving <10% of the nail plate affected
    ○ Nail plate thickening that does not improve with treatment because of comorbid condition

Patient Monitoring

- Topical agents: Slow response is expected; visits every 6 to 12 weeks
- Terbinafine, griseofulvin: baseline, and as needed, LFTs and CBC
- Itraconazole continuous: baseline, and as needed, LFTs

PATIENT EDUCATION

- Advise patient to:
  - Keep affected area clean and dry.
  - Avoid rubber/other occlusive, tight-fitting footwear.
  - Wear absorbent cotton socks.
  - Launder clothing and towels frequently in hot water.
  - Avoid sharing nail implements or use on both normal and abnormal nails.
- Cure of all toenails may not be attainable.
- Nails may not appear normal after cure.

PROGNOSIS

- Complete clinical cure in 25–50% (higher mycologic cure rates) with oral therapy
- Recurrence is 10–50% (relapse/reinfection).
- Poor prognostic factors
  - Areas of nail involvement >50%
  - Significant proximal/lateral disease
  - Subungual hyperkeratosis >2 mm
  - White/yellow or orange/brown streaks in the nail (includes dermatophytoma)
  - Total dystrophic onychomycosis (with matrix involvement)
  - Nonresponsive organisms (e.g., *Scytalidium* mold)
  - Patients with immunosuppression
  - Diminished peripheral circulation

COMPLICATIONS

- Secondary infections with progression to soft tissue infection/osteomyelitis
- Toenail discomfort/pain that can limit physical mobility or activity
- Anxiety, negative self-image

REFERENCES

1. Westerberg DP, Voyack MJ. Onychomycosis: current trends in diagnosis and treatment. *Am Fam Physician*. 2013;88(11):762–770.
2. Gupta AK, Paquet M. Systemic antifungals to treat onychomycosis in children: a systematic review. *Pediatr Dermatol*. 2013;30(3):294–302.
3. Eisman S, Sinclair R. Fungal nail infection: diagnosis and management. *BMJ*. 2014;348:g1800.
4. Gupta AK, Ryder JE, Johnson AM. Cumulative meta-analysis of systemic antifungal agents for the treatment of onychomycosis. *Br J Dermatol*. 2004;150(3):537–544.
5. Crawford F, Hollis S. Topical treatments for fungal infections of the skin and nails of the foot. *Cochrane Database Syst Rev*. 2007;(3):CD001434.
6. Ameen M, Lear J, Madan V, et al. British Association of Dermatologists' guidelines for the management of onychomycosis 2014. *Br J Dermatol*. 2014;171(5):937–958.

CODES

ICD10

- B35.1 Tinea unguium
- B37.2 Candidiasis of skin and nail

CLINICAL PEARLS

- Psoriasis and chronic nail trauma are commonly mistaken for fungal infection.
- Diagnosis should be based on both clinical and mycologic laboratory evidence.

OPTIC NEURITIS

Olga Cerón, MD • Pablo Hernandez Itriago, MD, MHCM, FAAFP

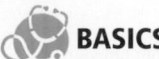 **BASICS**

DESCRIPTION
- Inflammation of the optic nerve (cranial nerve II)
- Most common form is acute demyelinating optic neuritis (ON), but other causes include infectious disease and systemic autoimmune disorders.
- Optic disc may be normal in appearance at onset (retrobulbar ON, 67%) or swollen (papillitis, 33%).
- Key features:
  – Abrupt visual loss (typically monocular)
  – Periorbital pain with eye movement (90%)
  – Pain in the distribution of the first division of the trigeminal nerve
  – Dyschromatopsia: color vision deficits
  – Relative afferent pupillary defect (RAPD)
- Usually unilateral in adults; bilateral disease more common in children
- Presenting complaint in 25% of patients with multiple sclerosis (MS)
- In children, headaches are common.
- System(s) affected: nervous
- Synonym(s): papillitis, demyelinating optic neuropathy; retrobulbar ON

EPIDEMIOLOGY
Incidence
- 5/100,000 cases per year
- More common in northern latitudes
- More common in spring season
- More common in whites than in other races
- Predominant age: 18 to 45 years; mean age 30 years
- Predominant sex: female > male (3:1)

ETIOLOGY AND PATHOPHYSIOLOGY
- In both MS-associated and isolated monosymptomatic ON, the cause is presumed to be a demyelinating autoimmune reaction.
- Possible mechanisms of inflammation in immune-mediated ON are the cross-reaction of viral epitopes and host epitopes and the persistence of a virus in CNS glial cells.
- Neuromyelitis optica (NMO) IgG autoantibody, which targets the water channel aquaporin-4
- Primarily idiopathic
- MS
- Viral infections: measles, mumps, varicella-zoster, coxsackievirus, adenovirus, hepatitis A and B, HIV, herpes simplex virus, cytomegalovirus
- Nonviral infections: syphilis, tuberculosis, meningococcus, cryptococcosis, cysticercosis, bacterial sinusitis, *Streptococcus* B, *Bartonella*, typhoid fever, Lyme disease, fungus
- Systemic inflammatory disease: sarcoidosis, systemic lupus erythematosus, vasculitis
- Local inflammatory disease: intraocular or contiguous with the orbit, sinus, or meninges
- Toxic: lead, methanol, arsenic, radiation
- Vascular lesions affecting the optic nerve
- Posterior uveitis (i.e., birdshot retinochoroidopathy, toxoplasmosis, toxocariasis)
- Tumors
- Medications: ethambutol, chloroquine, isoniazid, chronic high-dose chloramphenicol, tumor necrosis factor α-antagonist, infliximab (Remicade), adalimumab (Humira), etanercept (Enbrel)

COMMONLY ASSOCIATED CONDITIONS
- MS (common): ON is associated with an increased risk of MS.
- Other demyelinating diseases: Guillain-Barré syndrome, Devic NMO, multifocal demyelinating neuropathy, acute disseminated encephalomyelitis

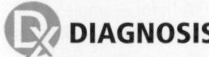 **DIAGNOSIS**

HISTORY
- *Decreased visual acuity*, deteriorating in hours to days, usually reaching lowest level after 1 week
- Usually unilateral but can also be bilateral
- Brow ache, globe tenderness, deep orbital *pain* exacerbated by *eye movement* (92%)
- Retro-orbital pain may precede visual loss.
- Desaturation of color vision (dull or faded colors), especially red tones
- Apparent dimness of light intensities
- Impairment of depth perception (80%); worse with moving objects (*Pulfrich phenomenon*)
- Transient increase in visual symptoms with increased body temperature and exercise (*Uhthoff phenomenon*)
- *Phosphenes*: fleeting colors and flashes of light (30%)
- May present with a recent flulike viral syndrome
- Detailed history and review of systems, looking for a history of demyelinating, infectious, or systemic inflammatory disease

PHYSICAL EXAM
Complete general exam, full neurologic exam, and ophthalmologic exam looking for the following:
- Decreased visual acuity and color perception
- Central, cecocentral, arcuate, or altitudinal visual field deficits
- Papillitis: (1/3) swollen disc ± peripapillary flame-shape hemorrhage or often (2/3) normal disc exam
- Temporal disc pallor seen later *at 4 to 6 weeks* (1)[A]
- *RAPD*: The pupil of the affected eye dilates with a swinging light test unless disease is bilateral.

DIFFERENTIAL DIAGNOSIS
- Demyelinating disease, especially MS
- Infectious/systemic inflammatory disease
- Neuroretinitis: virus, toxoplasmosis, *Bartonella*
- Toxic or nutritional optic neuropathy
- Acute papilledema (bilateral disc edema)
- Compression:
  – Orbital tumor/abscess compressing the optic nerve
  – Intracranial tumor/abscess compressing the afferent visual pathway
  – Orbital pseudotumor
  – Carotid–ophthalmic artery aneurysm
- Temporal arteritis or other vasculitides
- Trauma or radiation
- NMO (Devic disease)
- Anterior ischemic optic neuropathy
- Leber hereditary optic neuropathy

- Kjer-type autosomal dominant optic atrophy
- Severe systemic hypertension
- Diabetic papillopathy

DIAGNOSTIC TESTS & INTERPRETATION
Initial Tests (lab, imaging)
- In typical presentations, erythrocyte sedimentation rate (ESR) is standard, but other labs are unnecessary. Antinuclear antibodies (ANAs), angiotensin-converting enzyme (ACE) level, fluorescent treponemal antibody absorption (FTA-ABS), and chest x-ray (CXR) have been shown to have no value in typical cases (1)[A].
- In atypical presentations, including absence of pain, a very swollen optic nerve, >30 days without recovery, or retinal exudates, labs may be indicated to rule out underlying disorders:
  – CBC
  – ANA test
  – Rapid plasma reagin test
  – FTA-ABS test
- MRI of brain and orbits to evaluate risk of etiology of ON from MS: thin cuts (2 to 3 mm) gadolinium-enhanced and fat-suppression images to look for Dawson fingers of MS (periventricular white matter lesions oriented perpendicular to the ventricles) and also to look for enhancement of the optic nerve; baseline MRI provides prognostic information for MS and assists in stratifying risk of development of MS depending on absence or presence of white matter lesions in brain.
- CT scan of chest to rule out sarcoidosis if clinical suspicion is high
- Optical coherence tomography (OCT) of the retinal nerve fiber layer (RNFL); a noninvasive imaging technique of the optic nerve; may serve as a diagnostic tool to quantify thickness of the nerve fiber layer objectively and thus, monitor structural change (axonal loss) of the optic nerve in the course of the disease

Follow-Up Tests & Special Considerations
- Visual field test (Humphrey 30–2) to evaluate for visual field loss: diffuse and central visual loss more predominant in the affected eye at baseline (2)[A]
- OCT of the optic nerve RNFL to detect and monitor axonal loss in the anterior visual pathways
- Low-contrast visual acuity (as a measure of disease progression)
- A blood test serum marker: *NMO-IgG* checks for antibodies for NMO

Diagnostic Procedures/Other
- In atypical cases, including bilateral deficits, young age, or suspicion of infectious etiology, lumbar puncture (LP) with neurology consultation is indicated.
- LP for suspected MS is a physician-dependent decision. Some studies indicate that it may not add value to MRI for MS detection (1)[A], but no consensus on the subject exists.

TREATMENT

Most persons with ON recover spontaneously.

MEDICATION
First Line
- IV methylprednisolone has been shown to speed up the rate of visual recovery but without significant long-term benefit; consider for patients who require fast recovery (i.e., monocular patients or those whose occupation requires high-level visual acuity). For significant vision loss, parenteral corticosteroids may be considered on an individualized basis: Optic Neuritis Treatment Trial (ONTT):
  - Observation and corticosteroid treatment are both acceptable courses of action.
  - High-dose IV methylprednisolone (250 mg q6h for 3 days) followed by oral corticosteroids (1 mg/kg/day PO for 11 days, taper over 1 to 2 weeks) (3)[A]
- Others use IV Solu-Medrol infusion (1 g in 250 mL D_5 1/2 normal saline infused over 1 hour daily for 3 to 5 days):
  - No evidence of long-term benefit (1)[A]
  - May decrease recovery time (3)[A]
  - May decrease risk of MS at 2 years but not 5 years (3)[A]
- Give antiulcer medications with steroids.
- Discuss benefits and potential side effects of corticosteroids with patient (i.e., weight gain, osteoporosis, mood changes, gastrointestinal disturbances, hyperglycemia, insomnia).

Second Line
- Disease-modifying agents, such as interferon-β1a (IFN-β1a; Avonex, Rebif) and IFN-β1b (Betaseron), are used to prevent or delay the development of MS in people with ON who have ≥2 brain lesions evident on MRI.
  - These medications have been proposed for use in patients with one episode of ON (clinically isolated syndrome) at high risk of developing MS (1+ lesion on brain MRI).
- Decisions should be made individually with neurology consultation.

ALERT
NEVER use oral prednisone alone as the *primary* treatment because this *may increase the risk for recurrent ON* (3)[A].

Pediatric Considerations
- No systematic study defining high-dose corticosteroids in children with ON have been conducted.
  - Consensus recommends: 3 to 5 days of IV methylprednisolone (4 to 30 mg/kg/day), followed by a 2- to 4-week taper of oral steroids (4)[C]
- Optic disc swelling and bilateral disease are more common in children as is severe loss of visual acuity (20/200 or worse).
- Consider infectious and postinfectious causes of optic nerve impairment.

ISSUES FOR REFERRAL
Referral to a neurologist and/or ophthalmologist

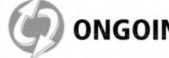 **ONGOING CARE**

FOLLOW-UP RECOMMENDATIONS
Patient Monitoring
Monthly follow-up to monitor visual changes and steroid side effects

PATIENT EDUCATION
- Provide reassurance about recovery of vision.
- If the disease is believed to be secondary to demyelinating disease, patient should be informed of the risk of developing MS.
- For patient education materials favorably reviewed on this topic, contact:
  - North American Neuro-Ophthalmology Society (NANOS), 5841 Cedar Lake Road, Suite 204, Minneapolis, MN 55416, 952-646-2037, Fax: 952-545-6073; http://www.nanosweb.org (click on section for patients); http://www.nanosweb.org/files/Patient%20Brochures/English/OpticNeuritis_English.pdf (available in other languages)

PROGNOSIS
- Orbital pain usually resolves within 1 week.
- Visual acuity
  - Rapid spontaneous improvement at 2 to 3 weeks and continues for several months (may be faster with IV corticosteroids)
  - Often returns to normal or near-normal levels (20/40 or better) within 1 year (90–95%), even after near blindness
- Other visual disturbances (e.g., contrast sensitivity, stereopsis) often persist after acuity returns to normal.
- Recurrence risk of 35% within 10 years: 14% affected eye, 12% contralateral, 9% bilateral; recurrence is higher in MS patients (48%).
- ON is associated with an increased risk of developing MS: 35% risk at 7 years, 58% at 15 years (5)[A].
  - Brain MRI helps to predict risk (by number of lesions):
    - 0 lesions: 16%
    - 1 to 2 lesions: 37%
    - 3+ lesions: 51%
- The presence of brain MRI abnormalities at the time of ON episode is a strong predictor of the 15-year risk of MS.
- Poor prognostic factors:
  - Absence of pain
  - Low initial visual acuity
  - Involvement of intracanalicular optic nerve
- Children with bilateral visual loss have a better prognosis than adults.

Monosymptomatic or clinically isolated syndrome cases of ON MRI provides prognostic information for MS development	Low MS Risk	High MS Risk
Risks of Developing MS	**Normal MRI**	**+ MRI Hyperintensities**
5 yr	15%	50%
10 yr	20%	60%
15 yr	25%	70%

Optic Neuritis—2012 American Academy of Ophthalmology NANOS and AAO Quality of Care Secretariat, Hoskins Center for Quality Eye Care
Comprehensive Ophthalmology, Neuro-Ophthalmology/Orbit
Based on results form 15-year ONTT follow-up study.

COMPLICATIONS
Permanent loss of vision

REFERENCES
1. Vedula SS, Brodney-Folse S, Gal RL, et al. Corticosteroids for treating optic neuritis. *Cochrane Database Syst Rev*. 2007;(1):CD001430.
2. Keltner JL, Johnson CA, Cello KE, et al; for Optic Neuritis Study Group. Visual field profile of optic neuritis: a final follow-up report from the Optic Neuritis Treatment Trial from baseline through 15 years. *Arch Ophthalmol*. 2010;128(3):330–337.
3. Simsek I, Erdem H, Pay S, et al. Optic neuritis occurring with anti-tumour necrosis factor alpha therapy. *Ann Rheum Dis*. 2007;66(9):1255–1258.
4. Bonhomme GR, Mitchell EB. Treatment of pediatric optic neuritis. *Curr Treat Options Neurol*. 2012;14(1):93–102.
5. Optic Neuritis Study Group. Visual function 15 years after optic neuritis: a final follow-up report from the Optic Neuritis Treatment Trial. *Ophthalmology*. 2008;115(6):1079.e5–1082.e5.
6. Arnold AC. Evolving management of optic neuritis and multiple sclerosis. *Am J Ophthalmol*. 2005;139(6):1101–1108.
7. Balcer LJ. Clinical practice. Optic neuritis. *N Engl J Med*. 2006;354(12):1273–1280.

ADDITIONAL READING
- Balk LJ, Cruz-Herranz A, Albrecht P, et al. Timing of retinal neuronal and axonal loss in MS: a longitudinal OCT study. *J Neurol*. 2016;263(7):1323–1331.
- Syc SB, Saidha S, Newsome SD, et al. Optical coherence tomography segmentation reveals ganglion cell layer pathology after optic neuritis. *Brain*. 2012;135(Pt 2):521–533.

 SEE ALSO

Multiple Sclerosis

 CODES

ICD10
- H46.9 Unspecified optic neuritis
- H46.00 Optic papillitis, unspecified eye
- H46.10 Retrobulbar neuritis, unspecified eye

CLINICAL PEARLS
- MRI is the procedure of choice for determining relative risk and possible therapy for MS prevention.
- The ONTT showed that high-dose IV methylprednisolone followed by oral prednisone accelerated visual recovery but did not improve the 6-month or 1-year visual outcome compared with placebo, whereas treatment with oral prednisone alone did not improve the outcome and was associated with an increased rate of recurrence of ON (1,2)[A],(6)[B],(7)[C].

OSGOOD-SCHLATTER DISEASE (TIBIAL APOPHYSITIS)

David P. Sealy, MD • Robert J. Tiller, MD, FAAFP

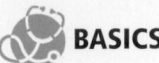
BASICS

DESCRIPTION
- Osgood-Schlatter disease (OSD) is a syndrome associated with traction apophysitis and patellar tendinosis that is most common in adolescent boys and girls.
  - Patients present with pain and swelling of the anterior tibial tubercle.
- System(s) affected: musculoskeletal
- Synonym: tibial tubercle apophysitis

EPIDEMIOLOGY
Incidence
Incidence in girls increasing with increased participation in organized youth sports; still more common in boys

Prevalence
- A common apophysitis in childhood and adolescence affecting athletes (21%) and nonathletes (4.5%) (1)
- Approximately 10% remain symptomatic as adults (2).
- 10% of all adolescent knee pain is due to OSD.

ETIOLOGY AND PATHOPHYSIOLOGY
Traction apophysitis of the tibial tubercle due to repetitive strain on the secondary ossification center of the tibial tuberosity, concurrent patellar tendinosis, and disruption of the proximal tibial apophysis
- Basic etiology unknown, exacerbated by exercise
  - Jumping and pivoting sports place highest strain on the tibial tubercle. Repetitive trauma is the most likely inciting factor.
- Possible association with tight hip flexors and tight quadriceps; increased quadriceps strength in adolescence relative to hamstring strength
- Early sports specialization increases the risk for OSD 4-fold (3)[B].

RISK FACTORS
- Affects children and adolescents most commonly from the ages of 8 to 18 years
  - Girls 8 to 14 years
  - Boys 10 to 18 years
- OSD is slightly more common in boys.
- Rapid skeletal growth
- Increased weight
- Quadriceps tightness
- Participation in repetitive-jumping sports and sports with heavy quadriceps activity (football, volleyball, basketball, hockey, soccer, skating, gymnastics)
- Ballet (2-fold risk compared with nonathletes)

GENERAL PREVENTION
- Avoid sports with heavy quadriceps loading (especially deceleration activities—eccentric loading).
- Patients may compete if pain is minimal.
- Increase hamstring and quadriceps flexibility.
- Possibly reduce sports specialization

COMMONLY ASSOCIATED CONDITIONS
- Shortened (tight) rectus femoris found in 75% with OSD
- Possible association with ADD/ADHD; adolescents with ADD/ADHD are at risk for other musculoskeletal injuries.
- Sinding-Larsen-Johansson apophysitis

DIAGNOSIS

HISTORY
- Unilateral or bilateral (30%) pain of the tibial tuberosity
- Pain exacerbated by exercise, especially jumping and landing after jumping
- Pain upon kneeling on the affected side(s)
- Antalgic or straight-legged gait

PHYSICAL EXAM
- Knee pain with squatting or crouching
- Absence of effusion or condyle tenderness
- Tibial tuberosity swelling and tenderness
- Pain increased with resisted knee extension or kneeling
- Erythema over tibial tuberosity
- Functional testing: Single-leg squat (SLS) and standing broad jump reproduce pain (3).

DIFFERENTIAL DIAGNOSIS
- Stress fracture of the proximal tibia
- Pes anserinus bursitis
- Quadriceps tendon avulsion
- Patellofemoral stress syndrome
- Chondromalacia patellae (retropatellar pain)
- Proximal tibial neoplasm
- Osteomyelitis of the proximal tibia
- Tibial plateau fracture
- Sinding-Larsen-Johansson syndrome (patellar apophysitis)—pain over inferior patellar tendon
- Patellar fracture or stress fracture
- Infrapatellar bursitis
- Patellar tendinitis—pain over inferior patellar tendon and inferior pole of patella
- Osteochondroma of the tibial tubercle
- Tibial tuberosity fracture
- Patellar tendon lipoma
- Osteosynchondroses
- Osteochondritis dissecans
- Iliotibial band syndrome
- Hoffa disease (infrapatellar fat pad syndrome)
- Saphenous neuritis

DIAGNOSTIC TESTS & INTERPRETATION
Initial Tests (lab, imaging)
- Generally a clinical diagnosis. No tests are indicated unless other diagnoses are under consideration.
- Radiographic imaging of the proximal tibia and knee may show heterotopic calcification in the patellar tendon:
  - X-rays are rarely diagnostic, but appearance of a separate fragment at the tibial tuberosity identifies candidates for potential surgical intervention.
  - Calcified thickening of the tibial tuberosity with irregular ossification at tendon insertion on the tibial tubercle (4)[B]

Diagnostic Procedures/Other
- Bone scan may show increased uptake in the area of the tibial tuberosity:
  - Increased uptake in apophysitis is normal in children, but with OSD, there *may be more uptake on the opposite side*.
- Ultrasound is an excellent alternative, showing thickening of the distal patellar tendon and infrapatellar bursa effusion.
- MRI shows fragmentation of the tibial tubercle and hyperintense T2 signal of the apophysis and patellar tendon insertion.

Test Interpretation
Biopsy is not necessary but would show osteolysis and fragmentation of the tibial tubercle.

TREATMENT

GENERAL MEASURES
- Frequent ice applications 2 to 3 times per day for 15 to 20 minutes
- Rest and activity modification—avoid activities that increase pain and/or swelling.
- Physical therapy helps with hamstring and quadriceps strengthening and stretching.
- Open- and closed-chain eccentric quadriceps strengthening
- Avoid aggressive stretching if pain is significant to avoid risk of tibial tubercle avulsion (1)[B].
- Consult orthopedic surgery for tibial tuberosity fracture or complete avulsion.
- Electrical stimulation and iontophoresis may be beneficial (1)[B].
- Patients with marked pronation may benefit from orthotics.
- A single study showed benefit from an infrapatellar strap, and many experts recommend the use of a knee brace with an H- or U-shaped buttress (1)[C].

MEDICATION

First Line
- Any analgesic may be considered.
- NSAIDs may help control pain.
- Opioids are not recommended as first line.

Second Line
- More potent analgesics, such as opioids, may ONLY be considered for short-term use in extreme situations.
- Corticosteroid injections are not recommended.
- Hypertonic glucose and/or Xylocaine injections have shown recent benefit (5)[C].
- Autologous platelet injections (PRP) have shown benefit in one study (6)[C].
- Acupuncture

ISSUES FOR REFERRAL
When conservative therapy is unsuccessful and symptoms persist into adulthood, consider surgical referral.

SURGERY/OTHER PROCEDURES
- Débridement of a thickened, cosmetically unsatisfactory tibial tubercle (rare) or removal of mobile heterotopic bone
- Surgical excision of a painful tibial tubercle is rarely needed (<5%) and may be successfully done with bursoscopy instead of an open procedure (4)[C].
- Recent report of successful pain elimination in OSD with percutaneous screw fixation of the tibial tuberosity (2)[C]
- Reduction wedge osteotomy has been recently reported as 100% successful in a small case series (6)[C].

ONGOING CARE

FOLLOW-UP RECOMMENDATIONS
- Athletes may return to play if pain is controlled.
- Presence of pain does not preclude competition.

Patient Monitoring
With worsening of symptoms only

PATIENT EDUCATION
- Avoid jumping sports or reduce activities that increase pain and swelling.
- Assure family that symptoms and findings will diminish with time and rest.
- Patients can safely play sports with mild pain.
- Quadriceps stretching and strengthening are important.
- Surgical options are rarely needed, but good results can be expected.

PROGNOSIS
- Except in rare cases, this is a self-limiting illness that resolves within 2 years of full skeletal maturation.
- 10% of patients with OSD as adolescents will have symptoms in adulthood. Up to 60% of adults with prior OSD report occasional symptoms and pain with kneeling.
- Most patients with OSD have residual "knots" of tibial tubercles that never completely resolve.

COMPLICATIONS
- Rarely, a heavily fragmented and inflamed tibial ossicle will avulse and require surgery.
- Rare complications in adulthood include pseudarthrosis of the tibial tubercle, genu recurvatum, patella alta, and ossicle fragmentation possibly leading to osteoarthritis of the knee.

REFERENCES

1. Kabiri L, Tapley H, Tapley S. Evaluation and conservative treatment for Osgood-Schlatter disease: a critical review of the literature. *Intl J Ther Rehab*. 2014;21(2):91–96.
2. Hall R, Barber Foss K, Hewett TE, et al. Sports specialization's association with an increased risk of developing anterior knee pain in adolescent female athletes. *J Sport Rehabil*. 2015;24(1):31–35.
3. Eun SS, Lee SA, Kumar R, et al. Direct bursoscopic ossicle resection in young and active patients with unresolved Osgood-Schlatter disease. *Arthroscopy*. 2015;31(3):416–421.
4. Topol GA, Podesta LA, Reeves KD, et al. Hyperosmolar dextrose injection for recalcitrant Osgood-Schlatter disease. *Pediatrics*. 2011;128(5):e1121–e1128.
5. Pagenstert G, Wurm M, Gehmert S, et al. Reduction osteotomy of the prominent tibial tubercle after Osgood-Schlatter disease. *Arthroscopy*. 2017;33(8):1551–1557.
6. Danneberg D. Successful treatment of Osgood-Schlatter disease with autologous-conditioned plasma in two patients. *Joints*. 2017;5(3):191–194.

ADDITIONAL READING

- Kaya DO, Toprak U, Baltaci G, et al. Long-term functional and sonographic outcomes in Osgood-Schlatter disease. *Knee Surg Sports Traumatol Arthrosc*. 2013;21(5):1131–1139.

- Morris E. Acupuncture in Osgood-Schlatter disease. *BMJ Case Rep*. 2016;2016:bcr2015214129.
- Narayan N, Mitchell PD, Latimer MD. Complete resolution of the symptoms of refractory Osgood-Schlatter disease following percutaneous fixation of the tibial tuberosity. *BMJ Case Rep*. 2015;2015:bcr2014206734.
- Nierenberg G, Falah M, Keren Y, et al. Surgical treatment of residual Osgood-Schlatter disease in young adults: role of the mobile osseous fragment. *Orthopedics*. 2011;34(3):176.
- Sailly M, Whiteley R, Johnson A. Doppler ultrasound and tibial tuberosity maturation status predicts pain in adolescent male athletes with Osgood-Schlatter's disease: a case series with comparison group and clinical interpretation. *Br J Sports Med*. 2013;47(2):93–97.

 ## CODES

ICD10
- M92.50 Juvenile osteochondrosis of tibia and fibula, unsp leg
- M92.51 Juvenile osteochondrosis of tibia and fibula, right leg
- M92.52 Juvenile osteochondrosis of tibia and fibula, left leg

CLINICAL PEARLS
- Infrapatellar pain in an adolescent athlete undergoing a rapid growth spurt is OSD, patellar tendinosis, or Sinding-Larsen-Johansson syndrome.
- Always consider lumbar disc disease, osteogenic sarcoma, or hip pathology in the differential diagnosis of OSD.
- OSD is generally self-limited. Athletes should modify activity based on pain. Mild pain is not a contraindication to athletic participation.
- Treatment focuses on strengthening and stretching of the hamstrings and quadriceps.
- 10% of adolescents with OSD will be symptomatic as adults.
- Persistent employment hampering symptoms in adults often require surgery.

OSTEOARTHRITIS
Patrick Wakefield Joyner, MD, MS

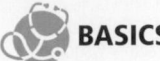 **BASICS**

DESCRIPTION
- Progressive loss of articular cartilage with reactive changes at joint margins and in subchondral bone
- Primary osteoarthritis (OA)
  - Idiopathic: categorized by clinical features (localized, generalized, erosive)
- Secondary OA
  - Posttraumatic
  - Childhood anatomic abnormalities (e.g., congenital hip dysplasia, slipped capital femoral epiphysis [SCFE], Legg-Calvé-Perthes disease)
  - Inheritable metabolic disorders (e.g., Wilson disease, alkaptonuria, hemochromatosis)
  - Neuropathic arthropathy (Charcot joints)
  - Hemophilic arthropathy
  - Endocrinopathies: acromegalic arthropathy, hyperparathyroidism, hypothyroidism
  - Paget disease
  - Noninfectious inflammatory arthritis (e.g., rheumatoid arthritis [RA], spondyloarthropathies)
  - Gout, calcium pyrophosphate deposition disease (pseudogout)
  - Septic or tuberculous arthritis
  - Femoral acetabular impingement (FAI)
- System(s) affected: musculoskeletal
- Synonym(s): osteoarthrosis; degenerative joint disease (DJD)

EPIDEMIOLOGY
- Symptomatic OA most common in patients >40 years
- Leading cause of disability in patients >65 years
- Predominant sex: male = female
- 90% of hip OA is primary.
- Hip OA is more common in whites.

Prevalence
- ~60 million patients
- Increases with age; radiographic evidence of OA is present in many patients >65 years old.
- Moderate to severe hip OA in 3–6% of whites; <1% in East Indians, blacks, Chinese, and Native Americans

ETIOLOGY AND PATHOPHYSIOLOGY
- Failure of chondrocytes to maintain the balance between degradation and synthesis of extracellular collagen matrix. Collagen loss results in alteration of proteoglycan matrix and increased susceptibility to degenerative change.
- Biomechanical, biochemical, inflammatory, and immunologic factors contribute to cartilage loss. Attempts at repair most commonly manifest as osteophyte formation.

Genetics
- Up to 65% of OA may have a genetic component.
- The heritability of end-stage hip OA is up to 27%.
- Twin studies in women show 50% (hip, knee) to 65% (hip) heritability rates of OA.

RISK FACTORS
- Increasing age: >50 years
- Age as a risk factor is greatest for hip and knee OA.
- Hand OA is most common in postmenopausal women.
- Obesity (weight-bearing joints); BMI >35
- Small critical shoulder angle (<30 degrees) can predispose to shoulder OA.
- Trauma, infection, or inflammatory arthritis
- Female gender (knee and hand)

 DIAGNOSIS

HISTORY
- Distinguish OA from other types of arthritis by:
  - Absence of systemic findings
  - Minimal articular inflammation
  - Distribution of involved joints (e.g., distal and proximal interphalangeal joints)
- OA characterized by slowly developing joint pain. Pain often described as aching or burning in nature. Anecdotally, many patients describe pain changes with alterations in weather conditions.
- Transient stiffness (especially after awakening in morning and after sitting) that tends to lessen 10 to 15 minutes after joint movement
- OA more commonly affects hands, spine, and large weight-bearing joints (hip, knee).

PHYSICAL EXAM
- Joint bony enlargement (Heberden nodes of distal interphalangeal joints; Bouchard nodes of proximal interphalangeal joints)
- Decreased range of motion of affected joints
- Mechanical symptoms (clicking, locking) may be present, especially in knees with degenerative meniscal injury.
- Crepitation is a late sign.
- Local pain and stiffness with OA of spine; radicular pain (if compression of nerve roots)
- Changes in joint alignment (genu varum [bowlegs] and genu valgum [knock-knees])

DIFFERENTIAL DIAGNOSIS
- Crystalline arthropathies (gout; pseudogout): inflammatory arthritides (RA), spondyloarthropathies (reactive arthritis; psoriatic arthritis), septic arthritis
- Fibromyalgia; avascular necrosis; Lyme disease

DIAGNOSTIC TESTS & INTERPRETATION
Initial Tests (lab, imaging)
- Routine chemistries are not helpful in diagnosis.
- X-rays are usually normal early in disease process.
- As OA progresses, plain films show:
  - Narrowed, asymmetric joint space
  - Osteophyte formation
  - Subchondral bony sclerosis
  - Subchondral cyst formation
- Erosions may occur on surface of distal and proximal interphalangeal joints (erosive OA).
- MRI may particularly demonstrate chondral degeneration and associated meniscal tears. 5–10% weight loss is associated with slowing of arthritic changes and decreased chondral loss on follow-up studies (1).

Follow-Up Tests & Special Considerations
- May be useful in monitoring treatment with NSAIDs (renal insufficiency and GI bleeding)
- In secondary OA, abnormal lab results associated with underlying disorder (e.g., hemochromatosis [abnormal iron studies])

Diagnostic Procedures/Other
Joint aspiration (not usually necessary for diagnosis)
- Can help distinguish OA from other arthritides
- OA: cell count usually <500 cells/mm^3, predominantly mononuclear
- Inflammatory: cell count usually >2,000 cells/mm^3, predominantly neutrophils
- Birefringent crystals in gout (−) and pseudogout (+)

Test Interpretation
- Macroscopic patchy cartilage damage and bony hypertrophy
- Histologic phases:
  - Extracellular matrix edema and cartilage microfissures
  - Subchondral fissuring and pitting
  - Erosion and formation of osteocartilaginous loose bodies
- Subchondral bone trabecular microfractures and sclerosis with osteophyte formation
- Degradation secondary to release of proteolytic and collagenolytic enzymes, prostaglandins, and associated immune response

TREATMENT

GENERAL MEASURES
- Weight management combined with exercise/physical therapy demonstrates most improvement in patients with OA.
- Physical therapy to maintain or regain joint motion and muscle strength
  - Quadriceps-strengthening exercises relieve knee pain and disability.
- Transition to non–weight-bearing exercises (i.e., elliptical, stationary bike, swimming)
- Exercise must be maintained; benefits are lost 6 months after exercise cessation.
- Protect joints from overuse; ambulatory aides are beneficial as is proper-fitting footwear.
- Bracing, joint supports, or insoles in patients with biomechanical instability:
  - Bracing is more beneficial in patients with unicompartmental disease of the knee.
- For knee OA in particular, several nonpharmacologic modalities are strongly recommended: aerobic, aquatic, and/or resistance exercise and weight loss.
- Nonpharmacologic modalities that are conditionally recommended for knee OA include medial wedge insoles for valgus knee OA, subtalar strapped lateral insoles for varus knee OA, medially directed patellar taping, manual therapy, walking aids, thermal agents, tai chi, self-management programs, and psychosocial intervention.

MEDICATION
First Line
- Manage pain and inflammation:
  - Acetaminophen up to 1,000 mg TID–QID: effective for pain relief in OA of knee and hip
  - Topical NSAID gels, creams have short-term (<4 weeks) benefits. Topical NSAIDs are a core treatment for hand and joints with minimal soft tissue–coverage (i.e., hand) OA. Diclofenac gel 1% can be applied as needed up to QID.
  - If acetaminophen or topical NSAIDs are insufficient, consider an oral NSAID/COX-2 inhibitor. Use the lowest effective dose for the shortest time possible.
  - May use nonacetylated salicylates (e.g., salsalate, choline-magnesium salicylate) or low-dose ibuprofen ≤1,600 mg/day
  - Topical NSAIDs and capsaicin as alternatives to oral analgesic/anti-inflammatory medications in knee OA
- NSAID contraindications:
  - All PO NSAIDs/COX-2 inhibitors have analgesic effects of a similar magnitude but vary in their potential GI and cardiorenal toxicity.

– NSAIDs should be avoided in patients with renal disease, CHF, HTN, active peptic ulcer disease, and previous hypersensitivity to an NSAID or aspirin (asthma, nasal polyps, hypotension, urticaria/angioedema).
– Combination of NSAIDs and full-strength aspirin (325 mg) is contraindicated.
– In patients at high cardiovascular risk: Combination of a nonselective NSAID and low-dose aspirin (81 mg) is recommended.
– Oral or parenteral corticosteroids are contraindicated.

ALERT
http://www.health.harvard.edu/blog/fda-strengthens-warning-that-nsaids-increase-heart-attack-and-stroke-risk-201507138138

- Precautions:
  – If PO NSAID/COX-2 inhibitor use is necessary for a patient aged >65 years or a patient <65 years with increased GI-bleeding risk factors, proton pump inhibitors are recommended.
  – Significant possible interactions:
    ○ NSAIDs reduce effectiveness of ACE inhibitors and diuretics.
    ○ Aspirin and NSAIDs (except COX-2 inhibitors) may increase effects of anticoagulants.
    ○ Salicylates reduce effectiveness of spironolactone (Aldactone) and uricosurics.
    ○ Corticosteroids and some antacids increase salicylate excretion, whereas ascorbic acid and ammonium chloride reduce salicylate excretion and may cause toxicity.

Pregnancy Considerations
- ASA and NSAIDs have reported fetal risk during 1st and 3rd trimesters of pregnancy.
- Compatible with breastfeeding

Second Line
- Topical capsaicin is an adjunct therapy for knee and hand OA.
- Topical NSAIDs (e.g., diclofenac gel) can lower gastric and renal risks associated with oral NSAIDs.
- Rubefacients (e.g., oil of wintergreen) are not recommended.
- Physical therapy: Core strengthening for hip OA and knee muscle strengthening for knee OA decrease joint reactive forces and can relieve pain.
- Physical therapy demonstrates minimal benefit compared to sham treatment in randomized trial in patients with severe hip OA (2)[A].
- Bracing; medial and lateral unloader braces are effective; long leg alignment x-rays can help determine the appropriate brace.
- TENS modalities for pain may be more beneficial than hyaluronic acid (HA) injection (3)[A].

Third Line
- Intra-articular corticosteroid injections can be used for acute flares and for patients failing first- and second-line treatments. Minimize injections (<2 per joint per year).
- Long-lasting corticosteroid injections are increasingly available; outcomes have not yet been definitively compared to traditional corticosteroid injections.
- The use of viscosupplementation injections for OA remains controversial. There is no clear evidence for benefit from HA injections.
- Platelet-rich plasma (PRP) is more effective than HA injections for early-stage knee OA (4)[B].
- Bone marrow aspirate concentrate (BMAC) demonstrates good outcomes for patients with mild to moderate knee OA; not recommended for patients with severe knee OA (5,6)[C]

- HA combined with PRP demonstrated better outcomes in patients with knee OA than either in isolation (7)[A].
- TENS is effective for pain relief in large-joint OA.
- Ultrasound improves injection accuracy.

ADDITIONAL THERAPIES
Address psychosocial factors (i.e., self-efficacy, coping skills). Screen for and appropriately treat anxiety and depression. Improve social support.

SURGERY/OTHER PROCEDURES
- Total knee arthroplasty (TKA) may be necessary if conservative management fails.
- Knee arthroscopy is not routinely recommended for the treatment of OA in the absence of clear mechanical symptoms (i.e., locking, clicking, etc.).

COMPLEMENTARY & ALTERNATIVE MEDICINE
- Nutritional supplements (glucosamine and chondroitin sulfate) may benefit some patients and have low toxicity. There is lack of standardized outcome assessments. Trial results using glucosamine and chondroitin have been mixed. If no response is apparent within 6 months, discontinue use.
- TENS, yoga, and acupuncture have shown benefit.

 ## ONGOING CARE

FOLLOW-UP RECOMMENDATIONS
Patient Monitoring
- Regularly assess range of motion and functional status.
- Monitor for GI blood loss and cardiac, renal, and mental status in older patients on NSAIDs or aspirin.
- Periodic CBC, renal function tests, stool for occult blood in patients on chronic NSAID therapy

PATIENT EDUCATION
- American College of Rheumatology: http://www.rheumatology.org/public/factsheets/index.asp?aud=pat
- Arthritis Foundation: http://www.arthritis.org

PROGNOSIS
- Progressive disease: early in course, pain relieved by rest; later, pain may persist at rest and at night.
- Joint effusions and enlargement may occur (especially in knees) as disease progresses.
- Osteophyte (spur) formation, especially at joint margins
- Advanced stage with full-thickness loss of cartilage at which point joint replacement is a consideration

COMPLICATIONS
- Leading cause of musculoskeletal pain and disability
- Decompensated CHF, GI bleeding, decreased renal function on chronic NSAID or aspirin therapy

REFERENCES
1. Gersing AS, Schwaiger BJ, Nevitt MC, et al. Is weight loss associated with less progression of changes in knee articular cartilage among obese and overweight patients as assessed with MR imaging over 48 months? Data from the Osteoarthritis Initiative. *Radiology.* 2017;284(2):508–520.
2. Bennell KL, Egerton T, Martin J, et al. Effect of physical therapy on pain and function in patients with hip osteoarthritis: a randomized clinical trial. *JAMA.* 2014;311(19):1987–1997.

3. Chen WL, Hsu WC, Lin YJ, et al. Comparison of intra-articular hyaluronic acid injections with transcutaneous electric nerve stimulation for the management of knee osteoarthritis: a randomized controlled trial. *Arch Phys Med Rehabil.* 2013;94(8):1482–1489.
4. Guler O, Mutlu S, Isyar M, et al. Comparison of short-term results of intraarticular platelet-rich plasma (PRP) and hyaluronic acid treatments in early-stage gonarthrosis patients. *Eur J Orthop Surg Traumatol.* 2015;25(3):509–513.
5. Chahla J, Dean CS, Moatshe G, et al. Concentrated bone marrow aspirate for the treatment of chondral injuries and osteoarthritis of the knee: a systematic review of outcomes. *Orthop J Sports Med.* 2016;4(1):2325967115625481.
6. Kim JD, Lee GW, Jung GH, et al. Clinical outcome of autologous bone marrow aspirates concentrate (BMAC) injection in degenerative arthritis of the knee. *Eur J Orthop Surg Traumatol.* 2014;24(8):1505–1511.
7. Yu W, Xu P, Huang G, et al. Clinical therapy of hyaluronic acid combined with platelet-rich plasma for the treatment of knee osteoarthritis. *Exp Ther Med.* 2018;16(3):2119–2125.

ADDITIONAL READING
- Hall M, Castelein B, Wittoek R, et al. Diet-induced weight loss alone or combined with exercise in overweight or obese people with knee osteoarthritis: a systematic review and meta-analysis [published online ahead of print June 21, 2018]. *Semin Arthritis Rheum.* doi:10.1016/j.semarthrit.2018.06.005.
- Jiang L, Tian W, Wang Y, et al. Body mass index and susceptibility to knee osteoarthritis: a systematic review and meta-analysis. *Joint Bone Spine.* 2012;79(3):291–297.

 ## CODES

ICD10
- M19.90 Unspecified osteoarthritis, unspecified site
- M19.91 Primary osteoarthritis, unspecified site
- M19.93 Secondary osteoarthritis, unspecified site

CLINICAL PEARLS
- Patients with OA typically have morning stiffness lasting for <15 minutes.
- OA most commonly affects the hips, knees, and hands (PIP and DIP joints).
- If used, intra-articular steroid injections should be limited to no more than 2 per joint per year.
- PRP and/or BMAC are (higher-cost) options for early-stage knee OA.
- Some professional organizations recommend against the use of HA injections for OA.
- Base long-term therapy on patient pain management and activity goals.

OSTEOMYELITIS

Matthew Mandell, DO • Adam N. Treitman, MD

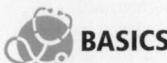 **BASICS**

DESCRIPTION

- An acute or chronic bone infection with associated inflammation; can occur as a result of hematogenous seeding, contiguous spread of infection, or direct inoculation into intact bone (trauma or surgery)
- Two major classification systems:
  - Lew and Waldvogel
    ○ Classified according to duration (acute or chronic) and mechanism of infection (hematogenous, contiguous)
  - Cierny-Mader classification
    ○ Based on the portion of bone affected, physiologic status of the host, and risk factors
- Special situations
  - Vertebral osteomyelitis
    ○ Also results from hematogenous seeding (most common), direct inoculation, or contiguous spread
    ○ Back pain is most common initial symptom.
    ○ Lumbar spine is most commonly involved, followed by thoracic spine.
    ○ Neurologic symptoms in 1/3 of patients (1)[C]
    ○ Surgery is required if neurologic symptoms or infected spinal implant. Uncomplicated acute hematogenous vertebral osteomyelitis can be treated with 6 weeks of antibiotics alone (1)[C].
  - Infections of prosthetic joints
    ○ X-ray and three-phase bone scan. MRI/CT is of limited use with prostheses.
    ○ Treat with pathogen-directed antibiotic therapy; may include rifampin (4 to 6 weeks) for higher success rate—penetrates biofilm
  - Posttraumatic infections depend on type and severity of fracture; level of contamination
    ○ Tibia is the most commonly involved.

EPIDEMIOLOGY

- Predominant age: more common in older adults
- Predominant sex: male > female
- Hematogenous osteomyelitis
  - Adults (most >50 years of age): vertebral
  - Children: long bones
- Contiguous osteomyelitis: related to diabetic foot infections (DFIs), decubitus ulcers, and infected total joint arthroplasties in older adults; trauma and surgery in younger adults
- *Mycobacterium tuberculosis* (MTB) is the most common cause of vertebral osteomyelitis worldwide. It is more likely to involve multiple vertebral bodies—especially of the thoracic spine—and is associated with paraspinal abscess formation.

Incidence

Generally low; normal bone is resistant to infection.

Prevalence

Up to 66% of diabetics with foot ulcerations

ETIOLOGY AND PATHOPHYSIOLOGY

- Acute: suppurative infection of bone with edema and vascular compromise leading to sequestrum (segments of necrotic bone, may contain pus)
- Chronic: presence of necrotic bone or sequestrum or recurrence of previous infection
- Hematogenous osteomyelitis (typically monomicrobial)
  - *Staphylococcus aureus* (most common)
  - Coagulase-negative staphylococci and aerobic gram-negative bacteria

- *Pseudomonas aeruginosa* (intravenous [IV] drug user)
- *Salmonella* sp. (sickle cell disease)
- MTB and fungi (rare) in endemic areas or in immunocompromised hosts
- Contiguous focus osteomyelitis (polymicrobial)
  - Diabetes or vascular insufficiency
    ○ Coagulase-positive and coagulase-negative staphylococci
    ○ Streptococci, gram-negative bacilli, anaerobes (*Peptostreptococcus* sp.)
  - Sacral decubitus ulcer
    ○ Pressure-related skin ulceration and necrosis
    ○ May require débridement to healthy bone and/or soft tissue coverage/surgical flap procedure (2)[C]
  - Nail puncture through a shoe
    ○ *P. aeruginosa*
- Prosthetic device
  - Coagulase-negative staph and *S. aureus*

RISK FACTORS

- Diabetes mellitus (particularly, diabetic foot ulcer)
- Recent trauma/surgery
- Foreign body (e.g., prosthetic implant)
- Neuropathy and vascular insufficiency
- Immunosuppression
- Sickle cell disease
- Injection drug use
- Previous osteomyelitis
- Bacteremia

GENERAL PREVENTION

- Comprehensive annual foot exam for diabetic patients
- Screen for peripheral artery disease.
- Optimize glycemic control in diabetes.
- Antibiotic prophylaxis for posttraumatic infection
  - Clean bone surgery.
    ○ Administer IV antibiotics within an hour of skin incision; continue ≤24 hours postprocedure.
  - Closed fractures
    ○ Cefazolin, cefuroxime, clindamycin (β-lactam allergy), or vancomycin (β-lactam allergy or MRSA infection)
  - Open fractures
    ○ In patients who can receive antibiotics within 3 hours of injury with prompt operative treatment, 1st-generation cephalosporins are preferred (clindamycin or vancomycin if allergic). Ceftriaxone for type III fractures. Add metronidazole if associated with soil or fecal matter contamination.

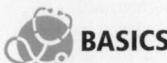 **DIAGNOSIS**

HISTORY

- Fever, chills, pain, swelling, and erythema, particularly in acute osteomyelitis. These features may be absent in chronic osteomyelitis.
- Hematogenous osteomyelitis
  - Elicit a history of conditions predisposing to bacteremia (diabetes, hemodialysis, invasive procedures, IV drug use, immunosuppression).
- Contiguous osteomyelitis and vascular insufficiency
  - Recent trauma/surgery within 1 to 2 months
  - Presence of prosthetic device
  - History of diabetes/DFI
- Chronic osteomyelitis
  - History of acute osteomyelitis
  - Draining sinus tract

PHYSICAL EXAM

- Fever, restricted range of motion, tenderness, signs of localized inflammation
- Motor and sensory deficits (vertebral infection)
- Probe to bone test in DFI has high pooled sensitivity and specificity for osteomyelitis of 0.87 (95% CI 0.75–0.93) and 0.83 (95% CI 0.65–0.93), respectively (3)[A].
- Exposed bone in the setting of DFI (4)[A]
- Ulcer >2-cm wide and >2-cm deep increases likelihood for osteomyelitis in DFI (positive LR, 7.2; 95% CI 1.1–49; negative LR, 0.48; 95% CI 0.31–0.76) (5)[A].
- Positive probe to bone test and ulcer area >2 cm² are physical exam findings that best support osteomyelitis in the setting of DFI (5)[A].
- Classic signs and symptoms of infection may be masked in diabetics due to vascular disease and neuropathy.

DIFFERENTIAL DIAGNOSIS

- Systemic infection from other source
- Aseptic bone infarction
- Localized inflammation or infection of overlying skin and soft tissues (e.g., gout)
- Brodie abscess (subacute osteomyelitis)
- Neuropathic joint disease (Charcot foot)
- Fractures/trauma
- Tumor

DIAGNOSTIC TESTS & INTERPRETATION

Initial Tests (lab, imaging)

Labs
- WBC is not reliable (can be normal) (1)[A],(5)[C].
- CRP is usually elevated (nonspecific).
- ESR is high in most cases:
  - ESR >70 mm/hr increases likelihood (LR, 11; 95% CI 1.6–79) (5)[A].
- Procalcitonin may also be elevated.
- Antibiotics given prior to culture may alter results.
- Other disorders that may alter lab results: immunosuppression (including diabetes), chronic inflammatory disease, other sites of infection
- Routine radiography is first-line imaging: Classic triad for osteomyelitis is demineralization, periosteal reaction, and bone destruction:
  - Bone destruction is not apparent on plain films until after 10 to 21 days of infection.
  - Bone scan is first test after plain x-ray for evaluation of prosthesis-related infection.
- Radionuclide scanning (e.g., technetium, indium, or gallium) helps if diagnosis is ambiguous or unsure of extent of disease; limited by low sensitivity/specificity
- MRI
  - Best for visualization of septic arthritis, spinal infection, and DFI (1)[C],(4)[A]
  - T1-weighted image: low signal intensity
  - T2-weighted image: high signal intensity
  - MRI: sensitivity 90% and specificity 83% for osteomyelitis in diabetic foot ulcers (5)[A]
  - For diabetic foot ulcer, a positive MRI increases the likelihood of osteomyelitis (positive LR, 3.8; 95% CI 2.5–5.8) (5)[A].
  - A normal MRI makes osteomyelitis less likely (negative LR, 0.14; 95% CI 0.08–0.20) (5)[A].
  - MRI does not help assess the response to therapy due to persistence of bony edema.
- CT
  - Better than standard radiography to evaluate bony fragments and sequestration; inferior to MRI for soft tissue and bone marrow assessment

Follow-Up Tests & Special Considerations

- A persistently elevated CRP (4 to 6 weeks) can be associated with osteomyelitis but is nonspecific.
- Monitor patients receiving prolonged antimicrobial therapy with weekly labs.

Diagnostic Procedures/Other

Blood cultures and bone biopsy

- For vertebral/hematogenous osteomyelitis, definitive diagnosis is made by vertebral disc aspiration or blood culture.
- Patients with positive blood cultures (with a pathogen likely to cause vertebral/hematogenous osteomyelitis) and with radiographic evidence of osteomyelitis do not need bone biopsy.
- For contiguous osteomyelitis, definitive diagnosis is made by bone biopsy for culture and histology.
- Avoid wound swabs or needle aspiration in DFI and decubitus ulcers because these do not correlate well with bone biopsy culture (2)[A],(4)[C].
- Can obtain bone biopsy at same time as surgical débridement

Test Interpretation

Pathology of bone revealing inflammatory process with pyogenic bacteria and necrosis

TREATMENT

GENERAL MEASURES

Adequate nutrition, smoking cessation, glycemic control

MEDICATION

- In clinically stable patients, delay initiation of empiric antibiotics until biopsy and/or blood cultures have been obtained.
- Direct empiric therapy toward probable organism and tailor according to culture results.
- Optimal antimicrobial concentration at infected site is essential (consider vascular perfusion).
- Adjust antibiotic dosing according to renal function.
- 4 to 6 weeks of therapy is appropriate for most cases of acute osteomyelitis. In the setting of amputation or complete removal of infected bone, a 2-week course of pathogen-directed antibiotics may be adequate (2)[C].
- If a prosthetic joint or other orthopedic hardware cannot be removed or completely débrided, a prolonged 6-week course of parenteral antibiotics is indicated. Some patients may subsequently require long-term oral antimicrobial suppression.
- Consider longer treatment courses for chronic osteomyelitis or MRSA infection (minimum 8 weeks).
- Empiric therapy:
  - For vertebral/hematogenous osteomyelitis, include coverage for MRSA and gram-negative organisms.
  - IV vancomycin plus 3rd- or 4th-generation IV cephalosporin +/- metronidazole for DFI/contiguous osteomyelitis

First Line

- *S. aureus* or coagulase-negative staphylococci
  - MSSA: β-lactam at high dose (nafcillin or oxacillin 2 g IV q4h) *or* cefazolin 1 to 2 g IV q8h (use 2 g for patients >80 kg)
  - MRSA: vancomycin 15 to 20 mg/kg IV q8–12h (use q8h interval if CrCl >70 mL/min) with target trough of 15 to 20 μg/mL, not to exceed 2 g/dose

- *Streptococcus* sp.
  - Ceftriaxone 2 g IV q24h or cefazolin 2 g IV q8h
- *Enterobacter* sp.
  - Ciprofloxacin 750 mg PO q12h (or 400 mg IV q12h) or cefepime 2 g IV q12h
- *P. aeruginosa*
  - Cefepime 2 g IV q8h or ciprofloxacin 750 mg PO q12h (or 400 mg IV q8h)

Second Line

- *S. aureus*
  - MSSA: ceftriaxone 2 g IV q24h
  - MRSA: linezolid 600 mg PO/IV q12h *or* daptomycin 6 mg/kg IV q24h
- *Streptococcus* sp.
  - Penicillin G 4 million U q4–6h
- *Enterobacter* sp. (quinolone-resistant, including extended-spectrum β-lactamase–producing *Escherichia coli*)
  - Carbapenem (imipenem/cilastatin) 500 mg IV q6h
- *P. aeruginosa*
  - Piperacillin-tazobactam 3.375 q IV q6h

ALERT

The combination of vancomycin plus piperacillin-tazobactam can increase risk of acute kidney injury (number needed to harm 11) (6)[A].

ADDITIONAL THERAPIES

Evidence does not support the use of hyperbaric oxygen therapy, growth factors, maggots, or topical negative pressure for diabetic foot osteomyelitis (4)[A].

SURGERY/OTHER PROCEDURES

- Surgical drainage, minimizing dead space, adequate soft tissue coverage, restoration of blood supply, and removal of necrotic tissues improve cure rates.
- Débridement of necrotic bone was once thought to be the cornerstone to management; however, recent evidence suggests antibiotics alone may be sufficient for DFI (4)[A].

ADMISSION, INPATIENT, AND NURSING CONSIDERATIONS

- Off-load pressure
- Discharge criteria: clinical and laboratory evidence of resolving infection and appropriate outpatient therapy

ONGOING CARE

FOLLOW-UP RECOMMENDATIONS

Patient Monitoring

Blood levels of antimicrobial agents, ESR, CRP, and repeat plain radiography as clinical course dictates. CRP correlates more closely with clinical response to therapy than ESR.

PATIENT EDUCATION

Diabetic glycemic control and foot care

PROGNOSIS

- Superficial and medullary osteomyelitis treated with antimicrobial and surgical therapy have a response rate of 90–100%.
- Up to 36% recurrence rate in diabetics
- Increased mortality after amputation

COMPLICATIONS

- Abscess formation
- Bacteremia
- Fracture/nonunion
- Loosening of prosthetic implant

- Postoperative infection
- Sinus tract formation can be associated with neoplasms, especially in presence of long-standing infection.

REFERENCES

1. Zimmerli W. Clinical practice. Vertebral osteomyelitis. *N Engl J Med*. 2010;362(11):1022–1029.
2. Schmitt SK. Osteomyelitis. *Infect Dis Clin North Am*. 2017;31(2):325–338.
3. Lam K, van Asten SA, Nguyen T, et al. Diagnostic accuracy of probe to bone to detect osteomyelitis in the diabetic foot: a systematic review. *Clin Infect Dis*. 2016;63(7):944–948.
4. Berendt AR, Peters EJ, Bakker K, et al. Diabetic foot osteomyelitis: a progress report on diagnosis and a systematic review of treatment. *Diabetes Metab Res Rev*. 2008;24(Suppl 1):S145–S161.
5. Butalia S, Palda VA, Sargeant RJ, et al. Does this patient with diabetes have osteomyelitis of the lower extremity? *JAMA*. 2008;299(7):806–813.
6. Luther MK, Timbrook TT, Caffrey AR, et al. Vancomycin plus piperacillin-tazobactam and acute kidney injury in adults: a systematic review and meta-analysis. *Crit Care Med*. 2018;46(1):12–20.

ADDITIONAL READING

- Malhotra R, Chan CS, Nather A. Osteomyelitis in the diabetic foot. *Diabet Foot Ankle*. 2014;5. doi:10.3402/dfa.v5.24445.
- Nickerson EK, Sinha R. Vertebral osteomyelitis in adults: an update. *Br Med Bull*. 2016;117(1):121–138.
- Wong D, Holtom P, Spellberg B. Osteomyelitis complicating sacral pressure ulcers: whether or not to treat with antibiotic therapy. *Clin Infect Dis*. 2019;68(2):338–342.

 ## CODES

ICD10

- M86.9 Osteomyelitis, unspecified
- M86.00 Acute hematogenous osteomyelitis, unspecified site
- M86.10 Other acute osteomyelitis, unspecified site

CLINICAL PEARLS

- Hematogenous osteomyelitis is usually monomicrobial. Osteomyelitis due to contiguous spread or direct inoculation is usually polymicrobial.
- Pain associated with acute osteomyelitis typically is gradual in onset.
- Treatment of chronic osteomyelitis often requires both surgical débridement and at least 6 weeks of antimicrobial therapy.
- Unlike diabetic foot ulcers, a positive probe-to-bone test (or frankly exposed bone) and abnormal MRI findings are not diagnostic of osteomyelitis in stage IV sacral pressure ulcers.
- Definitive treatment of osteomyelitis in stage IV sacral pressure ulcers often requires surgical débridement to healthy bone.
- Follow-up MRI is not needed for patients who are clinically improving with appropriate treatment.
- In diabetic foot wounds, if there are no signs or symptoms of soft tissue or bone infection, antibiotic therapy is unnecessary.

OSTEOPOROSIS AND OSTEOPENIA
Caitlin Nicholson, MD • Rahul Kapur, MD, CAQSM

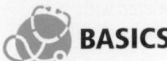 **BASICS**

DESCRIPTION
A skeletal disease characterized by low bone mass, deterioration of bone tissue, and disruption of bone architecture that leads to compromised bone strength and an increased risk of fracture

EPIDEMIOLOGY
- Most common bone disease in humans
- Predominant age: elderly >60 years of age
- Predominant sex: female > male (80%/20%)

Incidence
There is poor data on the incidence of osteoporosis and osteopenia; however, there are an estimated 9 million fractures annually attributed to osteoporosis worldwide.

Prevalence
- >10.2 million Americans have osteoporosis.
- >43.4 million Americans have osteopenia.
- Women >50 years of age: osteoporosis 15.4% and osteopenia 51.4%
- Men >50 years of age: osteoporosis 4.3% and osteopenia 35.2%
- One in three women and one in five men will experience an osteoporotic fracture.

ETIOLOGY AND PATHOPHYSIOLOGY
- Imbalance between bone resorption and bone formation
- Aging
- Hypoestrogenemia

Genetics
- Familial predisposition
- More common in Caucasians and Asians than in African Americans and Hispanics

RISK FACTORS
- Nonmodifiable
  - Advanced age (>65 years)
  - Female gender and menopause
  - Caucasian or Asian
  - Family history of osteoporosis
  - History of atraumatic fracture
- Modifiable
  - Low body weight (58 kg or body mass index [BMI] <21)
  - Calcium/vitamin D deficiency
  - Inadequate physical activity
  - Cigarette smoking
  - Excessive alcohol intake (>3 drinks per day)
  - Medications: See "Commonly Associated Conditions."

GENERAL PREVENTION
The aim in the prevention and treatment of osteoporosis is to prevent fracture:
- Regularly perform weight-bearing exercise.
- Consume a diet that includes adequate calcium (1,000 mg/day for men aged 50 to 70 years, 1,200 mg/day for women aged 51+ years and men 70+ years), and vitamin D (800 to 1,000 IU/day).
- The USPSTF recommends against vitamin D supplementation to prevent falls in community-dwelling adults aged 65 years or older who are not known to have osteoporosis or vitamin D deficiency (1)[A].
- Evidence is insufficient to assess the balance of the benefits and harms of daily supplementation with >400 IU of vitamin D_3 and >1,000 mg of calcium for the primary prevention of fractures in community-dwelling postmenopausal women (2)[B].

- USPSTF recommends against daily supplementation with 400 IU or less of vitamin D_3 and 1,000 mg or less of calcium for the primary prevention of fractures in noninstitutionalized postmenopausal women (2)[B].
- Avoid smoking.
- Limit alcohol consumption (<3 drinks per day).
- Fall prevention (home safety assessment, correction of visual impairment)
- Screen (USPSTF recommendations):
  - All women ≥65 years of age (2)[B]
  - Women >50 years of age with ≤10-year fracture risk (using the WHO's Fracture Risk Assessment [FRAX] Tool) >9.3%
  - The current evidence is insufficient to recommend screening for osteoporosis in men; however, the National Osteoporosis Foundation recommends screening men age >70 years, especially if at increased risk.

COMMONLY ASSOCIATED CONDITIONS
- Malabsorption syndromes: gastrectomy, inflammatory bowel disease, celiac disease
- Hypoestrogenism: menopause, hypogonadism, eating disorders, female athlete triad
- Endocrinopathies: hyperparathyroidism, hyperthyroidism, hypercortisolism, diabetes mellitus
- Hematologic disorders: hemophilia, sickle cell disease, multiple myeloma, thalassemia, hemochromatosis
- Other disorders: multiple sclerosis, end-stage renal disease, rheumatoid arthritis, lupus, chronic obstructive pulmonary disease (COPD), HIV/AIDS
- Medications: antiepileptics, aromatase inhibitors (raloxifene), chronic corticosteroids (>5 mg prednisone or equivalent for >3 months), medroxyprogesterone acetate, heparin, SSRI, thyroid hormone (in supraphysiologic doses), PPI

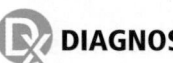 **DIAGNOSIS**

HISTORY
- Review modifiable and nonmodifiable risk factors.
- Online risk factor assessment tools are available:
  - FRAX: http://www.shef.ac.uk/FRAX/
- Assess for any commonly associated conditions.

PHYSICAL EXAM
- Thoracic kyphosis, poor balance, deconditioning
- Historical height loss >1.5 cm (difference between current height and peak height at age 20 years)
- Prospective height loss >2 cm (difference between current height and previously documented height)

DIFFERENTIAL DIAGNOSIS
- Multiple myeloma/other neoplasms
- Osteomalacia
- Type I collagen mutations
- Osteogenesis imperfecta

DIAGNOSTIC TESTS & INTERPRETATION
Dual energy x-ray absorptiometry (DEXA) of the lumbar spine/hip is considered the gold standard for the diagnosis of osteoporosis.

Initial Tests (lab, imaging)
Consider screening for secondary osteoporosis:
- Serum 25-hydroxyvitamin D and parathyroid hormone
- Complete blood count
- Serum chemistry including calcium, phosphorus, magnesium, total protein, albumin, liver enzymes, creatinine, alkaline phosphatase, and TSH

- Urinalysis (24-hour collection) for calcium, sodium, and creatinine to identify calcium malabsorption or hypercalciuria
- DEXA of the lumbar spine/hip is the gold standard for measuring bone mineral density (BMD).
- A BMD at the hip or lumbar spine that is ≤2.5 standard deviations (SDs) below the mean BMD of a young-adult reference population is diagnostic of osteoporosis.
- A minimum of 2 years may be needed to reliably measure a change in BMD.
- BMD is expressed in terms of T-scores and Z-scores:
  - T-score is the number of SDs a patient's BMD deviates from the mean for young, normal (age 25 to 40 years) control individuals of the same sex.
  - WHO defines normal BMD as a T-score ≥−1, osteopenia as a T-score between −1 and −2.5, and osteoporosis as a T-score ≤−2.5.
  - WHO thresholds can be used for postmenopausal women and men >50 years of age.
  - The Z-score is a comparison of the patient's BMD with an age-matched population.
  - A Z-score <−2 should prompt evaluation for causes of secondary osteoporosis.
- Plain radiographs lack sensitivity to diagnose osteoporosis, but an abnormality (e.g., widened intervertebral spaces, rib fractures, vertebral compression fractures) should prompt evaluation.

Follow-Up Tests & Special Considerations
Further labs depending on initial evaluation, Z-score −2.5 or lower, or young age
- Iron and ferritin (hemochromatosis)
- Testosterone levels (hypogonadism in men)
- Serum protein electrophoresis and free κ and λ light chains (multiple myeloma)
- Urinary-free cortisol (Cushing disease)
- Tissue transglutaminase antibodies (celiac disease)

Diagnostic Procedures/Other
Bone biopsy may be recommended for patients with bone disease and renal failure to establish the correct diagnosis because it can assess the degree of mineralization and microarchitecture and specific bone loss mechanisms.

Test Interpretation
- In osteoporosis, can see reduced skeletal mass; trabecular bone thinned or lost more than cortical bone
- Can assess osteoclast and osteoblast relative activity
- Can rule out other metabolic bone diseases
- Can assess if bone marrow is normal or atrophic

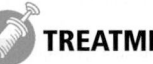 **TREATMENT**

- Criteria for patients who benefit from treatment for their osteoporosis includes:
  - All patients with a T-score ≤−2.5 with no risk factors
  - All postmenopausal women and men >50 years old who have had an osteoporotic vertebral/hip fracture
  - All postmenopausal women who have BMD values consistent with osteoporosis (T-score ≤2.5) at the lumbar spine, femoral neck, or total hip region
  - Postmenopausal women and men >50 years old with T-scores from −1.0 to −2.5 and a 10-year risk, based on FRAX calculator of an osteoporotic fracture (spine, hip, shoulder, and wrist) of at least 20% or risk of hip fracture of at least 3%

- All men >50 years of age who present with a hip or vertebral fracture or a T-score <−2.5 after appropriate evaluation; however, evidence for the effectiveness of treatment of osteoporosis in men is limited.
  - For osteopenia, treatment should only focus on risk modification: weight-bearing exercise, vitamin D supplementation (2,000 to 4,000 IU/day), limiting alcohol, and smoking cessation.

MEDICATION
Vitamin D 2,000 to 4,000 IU/day

First Line
- Bisphosphonates: Mechanism is inhibition of bone resorption by osteoclasts in skeletal tissue, reducing the incidence of vertebral and nonvertebral fractures.
  - Alendronate 10 mg PO daily or 70 mg PO weekly
  - Risedronate 5 mg PO daily, 35 mg PO weekly, or 150 mg PO monthly
  - Zoledronic acid 5 mg IV yearly
- Zoledronic acid appeared to be the most effective in preventing vertebral and nonvertebral fractures (3)[A].
- The side effects are similar for all bisphosphonates and include gastrointestinal problems such as difficulty swallowing and inflammation of the esophagus and stomach.
- Osteonecrosis of the jaw is a risk, particularly in patients with cancer who receive high doses and those who receive IV treatment (4).
- There is a possible risk of midfemur fractures in patients receiving bisphosphonates for >5 years (3).
- Avoid oral bisphosphonates in patients with
  - Delayed esophageal emptying
  - Inability to stand/sit upright for at least 30 to 60 minutes after taking the bisphosphonates
  - Hypocalcemia (Correct prior to initiating therapy.)
  - Severe renal impairment (creatinine clearance [CrCl] ≤30 for risedronate and ≤35 mL/min for alendronate and zoledronic acid)

Second Line
- Denosumab: 60 mg SQ every 6 months
  - Human monoclonal antibody receptor activator of nuclear factor kappa-B ligand (RANKL) receptor
  - Inhibits osteoclast formation
- Teriparatide 20 mg SQ daily
  - Recombinant formulation of PTH
  - Works anabolically to stimulate the growth of bone through osteoblastic activation
  - Studies have shown a reduction in the incidence of vertebral fractures by 65% and nonvertebral fractures by 53%.
  - No data exist on its safety and efficacy after >2 years of use.
- Estrogen 0.625 mg PO daily (with progesterone if patient has a uterus): effective in prevention and treatment of osteoporosis (34% reduction in hip and vertebral fractures after 5 years of use), but the risks (e.g., increased rates of myocardial infarction, stroke, breast cancer, pulmonary embolus, and deep vein thrombosis) must be weighed against the benefits
- Raloxifene 60 mg PO daily is a selective estrogen receptor modulator with positive effects on BMD and vertebral fracture risk but no stimulatory actions on breasts/uterus. It can be considered in the treatment and prevention of osteoporosis in postmenopausal women with high risk for invasive breast cancer; however, this must be weighed against the risks of DVT, PE, or stroke (especially in postmenopausal women at risk for coronary heart disease) (3).
- Strontium 2 g PO daily
  - Appears to inhibit bone resorption and increase bone formation
  - Available for use in Europe

- Calcitonin
  - PTH antagonist that reduces osteoclastic activity therefore decreasing bone turnover
  - FDA-approved for treatment of osteoporosis in women who are at least 5 years postmenopausal when alternative treatments are not suitable
  - Reduces vertebral fracture occurrence in those with prior vertebral fracture
  - Associated with an increased risk for malignancy

ISSUES FOR REFERRAL
Endocrinology for recurrent bone loss/fracture

ADDITIONAL THERAPIES
- Weight-bearing exercise 30 minutes 3 times per week
- Counseling on fall prevention
- Smoking cessation
- Physical therapy to help with muscle strengthening

SURGERY/OTHER PROCEDURES
Options for patients with painful vertebral compression fractures failing medical treatment:
- Vertebroplasty: Orthopedic cement is injected into the compressed vertebral body.
- Kyphoplasty: A balloon is expanded within the compressed vertebral body to reconstruct volume of vertebrae. Cement is injected into the space.

COMPLEMENTARY & ALTERNATIVE MEDICINE
- Isoflavones not better than placebo for fracture risk
- Beneficial effect of Chinese herbal medicines in improving BMD is still uncertain.

ADMISSION, INPATIENT, AND NURSING CONSIDERATIONS
- Inpatient care for pain control of acute back pain secondary to new vertebral fractures and for acute treatment of femoral and pelvic fractures
- Rehabilitation, nursing home, or home care may be needed following hospitalization for fractures.

 ## ONGOING CARE

FOLLOW-UP RECOMMENDATIONS
Patient Monitoring
- Weight-bearing exercises such as walking, jogging, stair climbing, and tai chi have been shown to decrease falls and fracture risk.
- Yearly height measurement is essential to determination of osteoporosis treatment efficacy. Patients who lose >2 cm in height should have repeat vertebral imaging to determine if any new vertebral fractures have occurred (5).
- Although there is no consensus, most recommendations suggest repeating a DEXA scan to assess BMD 2 years after starting bisphosphonate therapy.
- A comprehensive risk assessment should be performed after 3 to 5 years of treatment. If BMD at the hip is >−2.5 (T-score) and the patient has not had a hip or vertebral fracture, consider discontinuing treatment. If BMD remains low or if the patient is at high risk for fractures, the patient may benefit from continuing treatment beyond 5 years (6).
- Physicians prescribing bisphosphonates should advise patients of the small risk of osteonecrosis of the jaw and encourage dental examinations (6).

DIET
- Diet to maintain normal body weight.
- Calcium and vitamin D (see "General Prevention")

PATIENT EDUCATION
National Osteoporosis Foundation: http://nof.org/

PROGNOSIS
- With treatment, 80% of patients stabilize skeletal manifestations, increase bone mass and mobility, and have reduced pain.
- 15% of vertebral and 20–40% of hip fractures may lead to chronic care and/or premature death.

COMPLICATIONS
Severe, disabling pain and recurrent fractures

REFERENCES
1. US Preventive Services Task Force. Interventions to prevent falls in community-dwelling older adults: US Preventive Services Task Force recommendation statement. *JAMA*. 2018;319(16):1696–1704.
2. Christenson ES, Jiang X, Kagan R, et al. Osteoporosis management in post-menopausal women. *Minerva Ginecol*. 2012;64(3):181–194.
3. Zhou J, Ma X, Wang T, et al. Comparative efficacy of bisphosphonates in short-term fracture prevention for primary osteoporosis: a systematic review with network meta-analyses. *Osteoporos Int*. 2016;27(11):3289–3300.
4. Cosman F, de Beur SJ, LeBoff MS, et al; for National Osteoporosis Foundation. Clinician's guide to prevention and treatment of osteoporosis. *Osteoporos Int*. 2014;25(10):2359–2381.
5. Qaseem A, Forciea MA, McLean RM, et al; for Clinical Guidelines Committee of the American College of Physicians. Treatment of low bone density or osteoporosis to prevent fractures in men and women: a clinical practice guideline update from the American College of Physicians. *Ann Intern Med*. 2017;166(11):818–839.
6. McClung M, Harris ST, Miller PD, et al. Bisphosphonate therapy for osteoporosis: benefits, risks, and drug holiday. *Am J Med*. 2013;126(1):13–20.

CODES

ICD10
- M85.80 Other specified disorders of bone density and structure, unspecified site
- M81.0 Age-related osteoporosis w/o current pathological fracture
- M80.00XA Age-rel osteopor w current path fracture, unsp site, init

CLINICAL PEARLS
- Regular weight-bearing exercise from adolescence onward is recommended for prevention.
- Screen all women ≥65 years of age with DEXA scans.
- Premenopausal women with osteoporosis should be screened for secondary causes such as malabsorption syndromes, hyperparathyroidism, hyperthyroidism, and medication sensitivity.
- Evaluate and treat all patients presenting with fractures from minimal trauma.
- Bisphosphonates are first line for treatment of osteoporosis in most patients.
- For osteopenia, treat with counseling on fall prevention, weight-bearing exercise, diet high in calcium, vitamin D, limiting alcohol, and smoking cessation.
- If the patient is not responding to treatment, consider screening for a secondary, treatable cause of osteoporosis.

OTITIS EXTERNA
Douglas S. Parks, MD

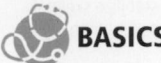 **BASICS**

DESCRIPTION
Inflammation of the external auditory canal:
- Acute diffuse otitis externa: the most common form; an infectious process; usually bacterial; occasionally fungal (10%)
- Acute circumscribed otitis externa: synonymous with furuncle; associated with infection of the hair follicle, a superficial cellulitic form of otitis externa
- Chronic otitis externa: same as acute diffuse but of longer duration (>6 weeks)
- Eczematous otitis externa: may accompany typical atopic eczema or other primary skin conditions
- Necrotizing malignant otitis externa: an infection that extends into the deeper tissues adjacent to the canal; may include osteomyelitis and cellulitis; rare in children
- System(s) affected: skin/exocrine
- Synonym(s): swimmer's ear

EPIDEMIOLOGY
Incidence
- Unknown; higher in the summer months and in warm, wet climates
- Predominant age: all ages
- Predominant sex: male = female
Prevalence
- Acute, chronic, and eczematous: common
- Necrotizing: uncommon

ETIOLOGY AND PATHOPHYSIOLOGY
- Acute diffuse otitis externa
  - Traumatized external canal (e.g., from use of cotton swab)
  - Bacterial infection (90%): *Pseudomonas* (67%), *Staphylococcus*, *Streptococcus*, gram-negative rods
  - Fungal infection (10%): *Aspergillus* (90%), *Candida, Phycomycetes, Rhizopus, Actinomyces, Penicillium*
- Chronic otitis externa: bacterial infection: *Pseudomonas*
- Eczematous otitis externa (associated with primary skin disorder)
  - Eczema
  - Seborrhea
  - Psoriasis
  - Neurodermatitis
  - Contact dermatitis
  - Purulent otitis media
  - Sensitivity to topical medications
- Necrotizing otitis externa
  - Invasive bacterial infection: *Pseudomonas*, increasing incidence of methicillin-resistant *Staphylococcus aureus* (MRSA)
  - Associated with immunosuppression

RISK FACTORS
- Acute and chronic otitis externa
  - Traumatization of external canal
  - Swimming
  - Hot, humid weather
  - Hearing aid use
- Eczematous: primary skin disorder
- Necrotizing otitis externa in adults
  - Advanced age
  - Diabetes mellitus (DM)
  - Debilitating disease
  - AIDS
  - Immunosuppression
- Necrotizing otitis externa in children (rare)
  - Leukopenia
  - Malnutrition
  - DM
  - Diabetes insipidus

GENERAL PREVENTION
- Avoid prolonged exposure to moisture.
- Use preventive antiseptics (acidifying solutions with 2% acetic acid [white vinegar] diluted 50/50 with water or isopropyl alcohol or 2% acetic acid with aluminum acetate [less irritating]) after swimming and bathing.
- Treat predisposing skin conditions.
- Eliminate self-inflicted trauma to canal with cotton swabs and other foreign objects.
- Diagnose and treat underlying systemic conditions.
- Use ear plugs when swimming.

 DIAGNOSIS

HISTORY
Variable length history of itching, plugging of ear, ear pain, and discharge from ear

PHYSICAL EXAM
- Ear canal: red, containing purulent discharge and debris
- Pain on manipulation of the pinnae
- Possible periauricular adenitis
- Possible eczema of pinna
- Cranial nerve (VII, IX to XII) involvement (extremely rare)

DIFFERENTIAL DIAGNOSIS
- Idiopathic ear pain
- Otitis media with perforation
- Hearing loss
- Cranial nerve (VII, IX to XII) palsy with necrotizing otitis externa
- Wisdom tooth eruption
- Basal cell or squamous cell carcinoma

DIAGNOSTIC TESTS & INTERPRETATION
- Gram stain and culture of canal discharge (occasionally helpful)
- Antibiotic pretreatment may affect results.
- Radiologic evaluation of deep tissues in necrotizing otitis externa with high-resolution CT scan, MRI, gallium scan, and bone scan

Test Interpretation
- Acute and chronic otitis externa: desquamation of superficial epithelium of external canal with infection
- Eczematous otitis externa: pathologic findings consistent with primary skin disorder; secondary infection on occasion
- Necrotizing otitis externa: vasculitis, thrombosis, and necrosis of involved tissues; osteomyelitis

 TREATMENT

Outpatient treatment, except for resistant cases and necrotizing otitis externa

GENERAL MEASURES
- Cleaning the external canal may facilitate recovery.
- Analgesics as appropriate for pain
- Antipruritic and antihistamines (eczematous form)
- Ear wick (Pope) for nearly occluded ear canal

MEDICATION
- Trial data is of generally poor quality and may not be fully relevant to primary care settings (1)[A].
- Resistance is an increasing problem. *Pseudomonas* is the most common bacteria, and it is more susceptible to fluoroquinolones such as ciprofloxacin or ofloxacin, whereas *Staphylococcus* is equally susceptible to both fluoroquinolones and polymyxin B combinations (2)[B]. If a patient has recurring episodes or is not improved in 2 weeks, change the class of antibacterial and consider cultures and sensitivities.
- There is evidence that using of a topical antibiotic with a corticosteroid shortens time to symptom resolution, although there is no evidence that it increases overall cure rate. There is not enough evidence to demonstrate that any antibiotic regimen is clearly superior to any other (3)[B],(4)[A].
- Oral antibiotics are indicated only if there is associated otitis media. Oral antibiotics alone are not effective and markedly increase the risk of progressing to chronic otitis externa.
- Analgesics as needed; narcotics may be necessary. Recurrent otitis externa may be prevented by applying equal parts white vinegar and isopropyl alcohol (over-the-counter [OTC] rubbing alcohol) to external auditory canals after bathing and swimming.

First Line
- Acute bacterial and chronic otitis externa
  - Ciprofloxacin 0.3% and dexamethasone 0.1% suspension (expensive as brand): 4 drops BID for 7 days or ofloxacin 0.3% solution (inexpensive generic): 10 drops once a day for 7 days (1)[A]; less ototoxicity and reported antibiotic resistance (5)[A]
  - Neomycin/polymyxin B/hydrocortisone (Cortisporin, generics): 5 drops QID. If the tympanic membrane is ruptured, use the suspension; otherwise, the solution may be used; may be ototoxic and resistance-developing in *Staphylococcus* and *Streptococcus* sp.; not expensive
  - Acetic acid 2% with hydrocortisone 1%: 3 to 5 drops q4–6h for 7 days; may cause minor local stinging. An inexpensive generic. This is as effective as neomycin–polymyxin B. It may take up to 2 days longer to achieve resolution of symptoms (3)[A]. A wick may be helpful in severe cases by keeping the canal open and keeping antibiotic solution in contact with infected skin.
- Fungal otitis externa
  - Topical therapy, antiyeast for *Candida* or yeast: 2% acetic acid 3 to 4 drops QID; clotrimazole 1% solution; itraconazole oral
  - Parenteral antifungal therapy: amphotericin B
  - Patients with Ramsay Hunt syndrome: acyclovir IV
- Eczematous otitis externa: topical therapy
  - Acetic acid 2% in aluminum acetate
  - Aluminum acetate (5%; Burow solution)
  - Steroid cream, lotion, ointment (e.g., triamcinolone 0.1% solution)
  - Antibacterial, if superinfected
- Necrotizing otitis externa
  - Parenteral antibiotics: antistaphylococcal and antipseudomonal
  - 4 to 6 weeks of therapy
  - Fluoroquinolones PO for 2 to 4 weeks

Second Line
- Acute bacterial and chronic otitis externa
  - Betamethasone 0.05% solution may be as effective as a polymyxin B combination without the risk of ototoxicity or antibiotic resistance. However, the data are not very robust, and more study is needed (3)[A].
- Azole antifungals for fungal otitis externa

ISSUES FOR REFERRAL
Resistant cases or those requiring surgical intervention

SURGERY/OTHER PROCEDURES
For necrotizing otitis externa or furuncle

COMPLEMENTARY & ALTERNATIVE MEDICINE
- OTC white vinegar; 3 drops in affected ear for minor case
- Tea tree oil in various concentrations has been used as an antiseptic. Ototoxicity has been reported in animal studies at very high doses.
- Grapefruit seed extract in various concentrations has been described as useful in the lay literature.

ADMISSION, INPATIENT, AND NURSING CONSIDERATIONS
- Admission criteria/initial stabilization: necrotizing otitis media requiring parenteral antipseudomonal antibiotics
- Discharge criteria: resolution of infection

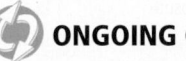 ONGOING CARE

FOLLOW-UP RECOMMENDATIONS
No restrictions

Patient Monitoring
- Acute otitis externa
  - 48 hours after therapy instituted to assess improvement
  - At the end of treatment
- Chronic otitis externa
  - Every 2 to 3 weeks for repeated cleansing of canal
  - May require alterations in topical medication, including antibiotics and steroids
- Necrotizing otitis externa
  - Daily monitoring in hospital for extension of infection
  - Baseline auditory and vestibular testing at beginning and end of therapy

DIET
No restrictions

PROGNOSIS
- Acute otitis externa: rapid response to therapy with total resolution
- Chronic otitis externa: With repeated cleansing and antibiotic therapy, most cases will resolve. Occasionally, surgical intervention is required for resistant cases.
- Eczematous otitis externa: Resolution will occur with control of the primary skin condition.
- Necrotizing otitis externa: usually can be managed with débridement and antipseudomonal antibiotics; recurrence rate is 100% when treatment is inadequate. Surgical intervention may be necessary in resistant cases or if there is cranial nerve involvement. Mortality rate is significant, probably secondary to the underlying disease (6)[C].

COMPLICATIONS
- Mainly a problem with necrotizing otitis externa; may spread to infect contiguous bone and CNS structures
- Acute otitis externa may spread to pinna, causing chondritis.

REFERENCES

1. Kaushik V, Malik T, Saeed SR. Interventions for acute otitis externa. *Cochrane Database Syst Rev*. 2010;(1):CD004740.
2. Dohar JE, Roland P, Wall GM, et al. Differences in bacteriologic treatment failures in acute otitis externa between ciprofloxacin/dexamethasone and neomycin/polymyxin B/hydrocortisone: results of a combined analysis. *Curr Med Res Opin*. 2009;25(2):287–291.
3. Rosenfeld RM, Schwartz SR, Cannon CR, et al. Clinical practice guideline: acute otitis externa. *Otolaryngol Head Neck Surg*. 2014;150(Suppl 1):S1–S24.
4. Lorente J, Sabater F, Rivas MP, et al. Ciprofloxacin plus fluocinolone acetonide versus ciprofloxacin alone in the treatment of diffuse otitis externa. *J Laryngol Otol*. 2014;128(7):591–598.
5. Mösges R, Nematian-Samani M, Hellmich M, et al. A meta-analysis of the efficacy of quinolone containing otics in comparison to antibiotic-steroid combination drugs in the local treatment of otitis externa. *Curr Med Res Opin*. 2011;27(10):2053–2060.
6. Sylvester MJ, Sanghvi S, Patel VM, et al. Malignant otitis externa hospitalizations: analysis of patient characteristics. *Laryngoscope*. 2017;127(10):2328–2336.

ADDITIONAL READING

Block SL. Otitis externa: providing relief while avoiding complications. *J Fam Pract*. 2005;54(8):669–676.

 SEE ALSO

Algorithm: Ear Pain/Otalgia

 CODES

ICD10
- H60.90 Unspecified otitis externa, unspecified ear
- H60.339 Swimmer's ear, unspecified ear
- H60.509 Unsp acute noninfective otitis externa, unspecified ear

CLINICAL PEARLS
- Acute diffuse otitis externa is the most common form: bacterial (90%), occasionally fungal (10%).
- Acute circumscribed otitis externa is associated with infection of a hair follicle.
- Chronic otitis externa is the same as acute diffuse but of longer duration (>6 weeks).
- Eczematous otitis externa may accompany typical atopic eczema or other primary skin conditions.
- Necrotizing malignant otitis externa is an infection that extends into the deeper tissues adjacent to the canal. It may include osteomyelitis and cellulitis; it is rare in children.

OTITIS MEDIA

Sarah Renna, MD • Sahil Mullick, MD

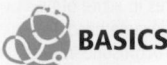

BASICS

DESCRIPTION
- Inflammation of the middle ear; usually accompanied by fluid collection
- Acute otitis media (AOM): inflammation of the middle ear. Rapid onset; cause may be infectious, either viral (AOM-v) or bacterial (AOM-b), but there is also a sterile etiology (AOM-s).
- Recurrent AOM: ≥3 episodes in 6 months or ≥4 episodes in 1 year with ≥1 in the past 6 months
- Otitis media with effusion (OME): fluid in the middle ear without signs or symptoms of infection
- Chronic otitis media with or without cholesteatoma
- System(s) affected: nervous
- Synonym(s): secretory or serous otitis media

EPIDEMIOLOGY
Incidence
- AOM
  - Predominant age: 6 to 24 months; declines >7 years; rare in adults
  - Predominant gender: male > female
  - By age 3 year, ~60% of children have had ≥1 episodes of AOM; 24% have had ≥3.
  - Placement of tympanostomy tubes is second only to circumcision as the most frequent surgical procedure in infants.
  - Increased incidence in the fall and winter
- OME
  - By age 4 years, 90% of children have had at least one episode.

Prevalence
- Most common infection for which antibacterial agents are prescribed in the United States
- >5 million cases diagnosed per year in the United States

ETIOLOGY AND PATHOPHYSIOLOGY
- AOM-b (bacterial): Usually, a preceding viral upper respiratory infection (URI) produces eustachian tube dysfunction, leading to reduced clearance.
  - *Streptococcus pneumoniae, Haemophilus influenzae, Moraxella catarrhalis* are most frequent pathogens. Less frequent: *Streptococcus pyogenes, Mycoplasma spp.*
- AOM-v (viral): 15–44% of AOM infections are caused primarily by viruses (e.g., rhinovirus, respiratory syncytial virus, parainfluenza, influenza, enteroviruses, adenovirus, human metapneumovirus, and bocavirus).
- AOM-s (sterile/nonpathogens): 25–30%
- OME: middle ear inflammation and eustachian tube dysfunction; allergic causes are rarely substantiated.

Genetics
- Strong genetic component in twin studies for recurrent and prolonged AOM
- May be influenced by skull configuration or immunologic defects

RISK FACTORS
- Age—AOM before age 1 year is a risk for recurrent AOM
- Male gender

- Bottlefeeding while supine
- Routine daycare attendance
- Family history of AOM
- Frequent pacifier use after 6 months of age
- Environmental smoke exposure
- Absence of breastfeeding
- Low socioeconomic status
- Atopy
- Underlying ENT disease (e.g., cleft palate, allergic rhinitis)

GENERAL PREVENTION
- Pneumococcal vaccine (PCV)-7 immunization reduces the number of cases of AOM by about 29% (1)[B] (however, evidence shows that this is offset by an increase in AOM caused by other bacteria).
- Influenza vaccine (2)[B]
- Breastfeeding for ≥6 months is protective (2)[B].
- Avoiding supine bottlefeeding, passive smoke, and pacifiers >6 months may be helpful.
- Secondary prevention: Adenoidectomy and adenotonsillectomy for recurrent AOM have limited short-term efficacy and are associated with their own adverse risks.
- Vitamin D supplementation (1,000 IU/day to maintain vitamin D levels >30) may be helpful in reducing recurrent AOM, but further trials are needed.

COMMONLY ASSOCIATED CONDITIONS
URI

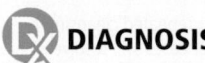

DIAGNOSIS

HISTORY
- AOM: acute history, signs, and symptoms of middle ear inflammation and effusion
  - Otalgia
  - Preceding or accompanying URI symptoms
  - Decreased hearing
- In adults, otalgia without fever or hearing loss may be the only presenting feature.

ALERT
- AOM in infants and toddlers:
  - May cause few symptoms in the first few months of life
  - Irritability may be the only symptom.
- OME: usually asymptomatic
  - Decreased hearing

PHYSICAL EXAM
- Infectious AOM:
  - Fever (not required for diagnosis)
  - Decreased eardrum mobility (with pneumatic otoscopy)
  - Moderate to severe bulging of tympanic membrane
  - Red, yellow, or cloudy tympanic membrane
  - Otorrhea
- OME:
  - Eardrum often dull but not bulging
  - Decreased eardrum mobility (pneumatic otoscopy)
  - Presence of air-fluid level
  - Weber test is positive to affected ear for an ear with effusion.

DIFFERENTIAL DIAGNOSIS
- Tympanosclerosis
- Trauma
- Referred pain from the jaw, teeth, or throat
- TMJ in adults
- Otitis externa
- Otitis-conjunctivitis syndrome
- Temporal arteritis in adults

DIAGNOSTIC TESTS & INTERPRETATION
Initial Tests (lab, imaging)
WBC count may be higher in bacterial AOM than in sterile AOM, but this is almost never useful.

Diagnostic Procedures/Other
- To document the presence of middle ear fluid, pneumatic otoscopy can be supplemented with tympanometry and acoustic reflex measurement.
- Hearing testing is recommended when hearing loss persists for ≥3 months or at any time suspecting language delay, significant hearing loss, or learning problems.
- Language testing should be performed for children with hearing loss.
- Tympanocentesis for microbiologic diagnosis is recommended for treatment failures; may be followed by myringotomy

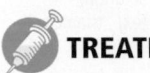

TREATMENT

- Significant disagreement exists about the usefulness of antibiotic treatment for this often self-resolving condition. Studies suggest number needed to treat for an additional beneficial outcome (NNTB) is 20 when looking at relief of pain at 2 to 3 days after start of antibiotics; the number needed to harm (primarily diarrhea and vomiting) is 9.
- 2/3 children will recover without antibiotic treatment.
- American Academy of Pediatrics/American Academy of Family Physicians (AAP/AAFP) guidelines recommend the following for observation versus antibacterial therapy, although these guidelines are not rigorously evidence based:
  - <6 months of age: Treat with amoxicillin if >2 weeks old.
  - >6 months: Antibacterial therapy is recommended with severe otitis media (i.e., moderate to severe otalgia, otalgia >48 hours or fever ≥39°C) (3)[B] or otorrhea or bilateral otitis media between 6 months and 2 years of age.
  - Observation is an option with nonsevere otitis media at >6 months of age.
- OME: Watchful waiting for 3 months per AAP/AAPP guidelines for those not at risk (see "Complications"). Of these cases, 25–90% will recover spontaneously over this period; no benefit of antihistamines or decongestants or systemic steroids (3), nor significant net benefit for antibiotics (3)

GENERAL MEASURES
- Assess pain.
- Although unusual in adults, the treatment is the same.
- Acetaminophen, ibuprofen, benzocaine drops (additional but brief benefit over acetaminophen)

MEDICATION

First Line

- AOM: AAP/AAFP consensus guideline recommends amoxicillin, 80 to 90 mg/kg/day in 2 divided doses (2)[B] *or*
- Amoxicillin-clavulanate 90 mg/kg/day of amoxicillin, with 6.4 mg/kg/day of clavulanate in 2 divided doses; recommended in children who have taken amoxicillin in the previous 30 days and those with concurrent conjunctivitis or history of AOM unresponsive to amoxicillin
- Treatment duration: 10-day course for children <2 years; 5- to 7-day course for children ≥2 years (4)
- If penicillin allergic:
  - Cefdinir, 14 mg/kg/day in 1 to 2 doses; cefpodoxime, 10 mg/kg/day in 2 divided doses; cefuroxime 30 mg/kg/day in 2 divided doses; or ceftriaxone 50 mg/kg IM/IV per day for 1 to 3 days (3)
- A single dose of azithromycin has been approved by the FDA, but studies did not include otitis-prone children or have criteria for AOM diagnosis.
- OME: See "General Measures"; no benefit to treatment. Medications promote transitory resolution in 10–15%, but the effect is short-lived.

Second Line

- Alternative antibiotics are indicated for the following AOM patients:
  - Persistent symptoms after 48 to 72 hours of amoxicillin
  - AOM within 1 month of amoxicillin therapy
  - Severe earache
  - Age <6 months with high fever
  - Immunocompromised
    - Amoxicillin-clavulanate, 90 mg/kg to 6.4 mg/kg/day, divided BID
    - Ceftriaxone, 50 mg/kg IM or IV q24h for 3 consecutive days can be reserved for those who are too sick to take oral medications or who unsuccessfully took amoxicillin-clavulanate. Neither erythromycin nor trimethoprim-sulfamethoxazole should be used as a second-line agent in treatment failures.
- Recurrent AOM: Antibiotic prophylaxis for recurrent AOM (>3 distinct, well-documented episodes in 6 months) is not recommended (2)[B].

SURGERY/OTHER PROCEDURES

- Recurrent AOM: Consider referral for surgery if ≥3 episodes of well-documented AOM within 6 months, ≥4 episodes within 12 months with ≥1 episode in previous 6 months, or AOM episodes occur while on chemoprophylaxis.
- Tympanostomy tubes may be effective in selective patients, particularly children age <2 years with recurrent AOM (5)[A].
- Adenoidectomy has limited or no effect.
- Adenotonsillectomy reduced the rate of AOM by 0.7 episode per child only in the 1st year after surgery and had a 15% complications rate.
- OME: Referral for surgery for tympanostomy should be individualized. It can be considered if >4 to 6 months of bilateral OME and/or >6 months of unilateral OME and/or hearing loss >25 dB or for high-risk individuals at any time.

- Tympanostomy tubes may reduce recurrence of AOM minimally, but it does not lower the risk of hearing loss (3).
- Adenoidectomy is indicated in specific cases; tonsillectomy or myringotomy is never indicated.

COMPLEMENTARY & ALTERNATIVE MEDICINE

- It is unclear whether alternative and homeopathic therapies are effective for AOM, including mixed evidence about the effectiveness of zinc supplementation of reducing AOM.
- Xylitol, probiotics, herbal ear drops, and homeopathic interventions may be beneficial in reducing pain duration, antibiotic use, and bacterial resistance.

ADMISSION, INPATIENT, AND NURSING CONSIDERATIONS

Outpatient management is appropriate, except if surgery is indicated or for AOM in febrile infants age <2 months or children requiring ceftriaxone who also require monitoring for 24 hours.

 ONGOING CARE

FOLLOW-UP RECOMMENDATIONS

Patients with otitis media who do not respond within 48 to 72 hours should be reevaluated:

- If therapy was delayed and diagnosis is confirmed, start therapy with high-dose amoxicillin.
- If therapy was initiated, consider changing the antibiotic; options are limited because macrolides have limited benefit against *H. influenzae* over amoxicillin, and most oral cephalosporins have no improved outcomes.

Patient Monitoring

- AOM: Up to 40% may have persistent middle ear effusion at 1 month, with 10–25% at 3 months.
- OME: Repeat otoscopic or tympanometric exams at 3 months, as indicated, as long as OME persists or sooner if there are red flags (see earlier discussion).

PROGNOSIS

- See "General Measures."
- Recurrent AOM and OME: usually subsides in school-aged children; few have complications.

COMPLICATIONS

- AOM: Serious complications are rare: tympanic membrane perforation/otorrhea, acute mastoiditis, facial nerve paralysis, otitic hydrocephalus, meningitis, hearing impairment (6).
- OME: Speech and language disabilities may occur. Hearing loss is not caused by OME, but in children who are at risk for speech, language, or learning problems (e.g., autism spectrum, syndromes, craniofacial disorders, developmental delay, and children already with speech/language delay), it could lead to further problems because they are less tolerant of a hearing impairment.
- Recurrent AOM and OME: atrophy and scarring of eardrum, chronic perforation and otorrhea, cholesteatoma, permanent hearing loss, chronic mastoiditis, other intracranial suppurative complications

REFERENCES

1. Kaur R, Morris M, Pichichero ME. Epidemiology of acute otitis media in the postpneumococcal conjugate vaccine era. *Pediatrics*. 2017;140(3):e20170181.
2. Lieberthal A, Carroll A, Chonmaitree T, et al. The diagnosis and management of acute otitis media. *Pediatrics*. 2013;131(3):e964–e999.
3. Harmes K, Blackwood A, Burrows HL, et al. Otitis media: diagnosis and treatment. *Am Fam Physician*. 2013;88(7):435–440.
4. Hoberman A, Paradise J, Rockette H, et al. Shortened antimicrobial treatment for acute otitis media in young children. *N Engl J Med*. 2016;375(25):2446–2456.
5. Kujala T, Alho OP, Luotonen J, et al. Tympanostomy with and without adenoidectomy for the prevention of recurrences of acute otitis media: a randomized controlled trial. *Pediatr Infect Dis J*. 2012;31(6):565–569.
6. Venekamp RP, Sanders SL, Glasziou PP, et al. Antibiotics for acute otitis media in children. *Cochrane Database Syst Rev*. 2015;(6):CD000219.

ADDITIONAL READING

- Marchisio P, Consonni D, Baggi E, et al. Vitamin D supplementation reduces the risk of acute otitis media in otitis-prone children. *Pediatr Infect Dis J*. 2013;32(10):1055–1060.
- Rettig E, Tunkel DE. Contemporary concepts in management of acute otitis media in children. *Otolaryngol Clin North Am*. 2014;47(5):651–672.
- Venekamp RP, Burton MJ, van Dongen TM, et al. Antibiotics for otitis media with effusion in children. *Cochrane Database Syst Rev*. 2016;(6):CD009163.

 SEE ALSO

Algorithm: Ear Pain/Otalgia

 CODES

ICD10

- H66.90 Otitis media, unspecified, unspecified ear
- H66.40 Suppurative otitis media, unspecified, unspecified ear
- H65.199 Other acute nonsuppurative otitis media, unspecified ear

CLINICAL PEARLS

- Pneumatic otoscopy is the single most specific and clinically useful test for diagnosis.
- Consider a delay of antibiotics for 24 to 48 hours in uncomplicated presentations (>6 months of age) who do not have severe illness or otorrhea.
- First-line treatment is amoxicillin, 80 to 90 mg/kg/day for 10 days for children age <2 years; consider a 5- to 7-day course in >2 years of age.
- Erythema and effusion can persist for weeks.
- Antibiotics, antihistamines, and steroids are not indicated for OME.
- OME rarely develops in adults. Persistent unilateral effusion should be investigated to rule out neoplasm, particularly if there is a cranial nerve palsy.

OTITIS MEDIA WITH EFFUSION

Hobart Lee, MD, FAAFP

 BASICS

DESCRIPTION
- Also called serous otitis media, secretory otitis media, nonsuppurative otitis media, "ear fluid," or "glue ear"
- Otitis media with effusion (OME) is defined as the presence of fluid in the middle ear in the absence of acute signs or symptoms of infection.
- More commonly, a pediatric disease
- May occur spontaneously from poor eustachian tube function or as an inflammatory response after acute otitis media (AOM)

EPIDEMIOLOGY
Incidence
Approximately 90% of children have OME before school age, mostly between the ages of 6 months and 4 years.

Prevalence
- Approximately 2.2 million new cases annually in the United States
- Less prevalent in adults and is usually associated with an underlying disorder

ETIOLOGY AND PATHOPHYSIOLOGY
- Chronic inflammatory condition where an underlying stimulus causes an inflammatory reaction with increased mucin production creating a functional blockage of the eustachian tube and thick accumulation of mucin-rich middle ear effusion
- Young children are more prone to OME due to shorter and more horizontal eustachian tubes, which become more vertical around 7 years of age.
- Biofilms, anatomic variations, and AOM caused by viruses or bacteria have been implicated as stimuli causing OME. The common pathogens causing AOM include nontypeable *Haemophilus influenzae*, *Streptococcus pneumoniae*, and *Moraxella catarrhalis*.
- In adults, OME is often associated with paranasal sinus disease (66%), smoking-induced nasopharyngeal lymphoid hyperplasia and adult onset adenoidal hypertrophy (19%), or head and neck tumors (4.8%).

RISK FACTORS
- Risk factors include a family history of OME, early daycare, exposure to cigarette smoke, bottlefeeding, and low socioeconomic status (1).
- Eustachian tube dysfunction may be a predisposing factor, although the evidence is unclear (2).
- Gastroesophageal reflux is associated with OME (2).

GENERAL PREVENTION
OME is generally not preventable, although lowering smoke exposure, breastfeeding, and avoiding daycare centers at an early age may decrease the risk.

 DIAGNOSIS

HISTORY
- OME is transient and asymptomatic in many pediatric patients.
- Most common reported symptom is hearing loss (2). There may be mild discomfort present in the ear, fullness, or "popping."
- Infants may have ear rubbing, excessive irritability, sleep problems, or failure to respond appropriately to voices or sounds.
- Clinical features may include "a history of hearing difficulties, poor attention, behavioral problems, delayed speech and language development, clumsiness, and poor balance" (2).
- There may be a history of recent or recurrent episodes of AOM or a recent upper respiratory tract infection (2).

PHYSICAL EXAM
- Cloudy tympanic membrane (TM) with distinctly impaired mobility. Air-fluid level or bubble may be visible in the middle ear (1,2).
- Color may be abnormal (yellow, amber, or blue), and the TM may be retracted or concave (2).
- Distinct redness of the TM may be present in approximately 5% of OME cases (1).
- Clinical signs and symptoms of acute illness should be absent in patients with OME (1).

DIFFERENTIAL DIAGNOSIS
- AOM
- Bullous myringitis
- Tympanosclerosis (may cause decreased/absent motion of the TM)
- Sensorineural hearing loss

DIAGNOSTIC TESTS & INTERPRETATION
Diagnostic Procedures/Other
- The primary standard to make the diagnosis is pneumatic otoscopy, which demonstrates reduced/absent mobility of the TM secondary to fluid in the middle ear. Pneumatic otoscopy has 94% sensitivity and 80% specificity for diagnosing OME. Accuracy of diagnosis with an experienced examiner is between 70% and 79% (1)[C].
- Myringotomy is the gold standard but is not practical for clinical use (2)[C].
- Tympanometry may also be used to support or exclude the diagnosis in infants >4 months old, especially when the presence of middle ear effusion is difficult to determine (1)[C].

- Acoustic reflectometry (64% specificity and 80% sensitivity) may be considered instead of tympanometry (3)[B].
- Audiogram may show mild conductive hearing loss (2)[C].
- Hearing tests are recommended for OME lasting >3 months (1)[C].
- Language testing is recommended for children with abnormal hearing tests (1)[C].

 TREATMENT

- OME improves or resolves without medical intervention in most patients within 3 months, especially if secondary to AOM (1)[C].
- Current guidelines support a 3-month period of observation with optional serial exams, tympanometry, and language assessment during that wait time (1,2)[C].
- Adults found to have OME should be screened for an underlying disorder and treated accordingly (2)[C].

MEDICATION
- The 2016 AAOHNS guideline recommends against routine use of antibiotics in treatment of OME. A 2016 Cochrane review, however, found that children treated with oral antibiotics were more likely to have tympanogram confirmed OME resolution in 2 to 3 months (number needed to treat = 5). Adverse events included diarrhea, vomiting, skin rash, and allergic reactions (number needed to harm = 20). Importantly, there were no reported patient-oriented outcomes (e.g., cognitive development, language, quality of life, or speech). Outcomes regarding short-term hearing, reduction of AOM infections, or need for ventilation tubes are unknown (1)[C],(4)[A].
- The 2016 AAOHNS and a 2006 Cochrane review found that antihistamines and decongestants have no benefit over placebo in the treatment of OME with possible adverse side effects such as insomnia, hyperactivity, and drowsiness (5)[A].
- The 2016 AAOHNS guideline recommends against administering oral or intranasal corticosteroids. No long-term benefit was shown, and adverse side effects such as weight gain and behavioral changes are possible (1)[C].
- In adults, eustachian tube dysfunction secondary to allergic rhinitis or recent upper respiratory infection can be the cause of OME. It is unknown whether decongestants, antihistamines, or nasal steroids improve outcomes in adults.

ISSUES FOR REFERRAL

The following are indications for referral to a surgeon for evaluation of tympanostomy tube placement (6)[C]:

- Chronic bilateral OME (≥3 months) with hearing difficulty
- Chronic OME with symptoms (e.g., vestibular problems, poor school performance, behavioral issues, ear discomfort, or reduced quality of life)
- At-risk children (speech, language, or learning problems due to baseline sensory, physical, cognitive, or behavioral factors) with chronic OME or type B (flat) tympanogram

ADDITIONAL THERAPIES

- Hearing aids may be an acceptable alternative to surgery (2)[C].
- Autoinflation, which refers to the process of opening the eustachian tube by raising intranasal pressure (e.g., by forced exhalation with closed mouth and nose), may be beneficial in improving patients' tympanogram or audiometry and quality of life scores (6)[A].

SURGERY/OTHER PROCEDURES

- Tympanostomy tubes are recommended as initial surgery. Risks include purulent otorrhea, myringosclerosis, retraction pockets, and persistent TM perforations (1)[C].
- Adenoidectomy with myringotomy has similar efficacy to tympanostomy tubes in children >4 years of age but with added surgical and anesthetic risks (1)[C].
- Adenoidectomy should not be performed in children with persistent OME alone unless there is a distinct indication for the procedure for another problem (e.g., adenoiditis/chronic sinusitis/nasal obstruction) (1)[C],(6)[A].
- Adenoidectomy (and concurrent tube placement) may be considered when repeat surgery for OME is necessary (e.g., when effusion recurs after tubes have fallen out or are removed). In these cases, adenoidectomy has been shown to decrease the need for future procedures for OME (1,2)[C].
- Tonsillectomy or myringotomy alone is not recommended for treatment (1)[C].

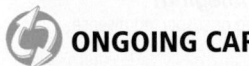 ONGOING CARE

FOLLOW-UP RECOMMENDATIONS

Patient Monitoring

- Children who are at risk for developmental difficulties should be evaluated for OME at the time of diagnosis and at 12 to 18 months (if initial diagnosis occurred <12 months). At-risk conditions include permanent hearing loss independent of OME, suspected or confirmed speech and language delay, autism spectrum disorder or other pervasive developmental disorder, Down syndrome or other craniofacial disorder, blindness or other uncorrectable visual impairment, cleft palate, and unspecified developmental delay (1)[C].

- For patients diagnosed with OME, reevaluation and repeat hearing tests should be performed every 3 to 6 months until the effusion has resolved or until the child develops an indication for surgical referral (1)[C].

PROGNOSIS

Approximately 50% of children >3 years of age have OME resolution within 3 months.

COMPLICATIONS

- The most significant complication of OME is permanent hearing loss, leading to possible language, speech, and developmental delays.
- Underventilation of the middle ear can cause a cholesteatoma (1)[C].

REFERENCES

1. Rosenfeld RM, Shin JJ, Schwartz SR, et al. Clinical practice guideline: otitis media with effusion executive summary (update). *Otolaryngol Head Neck Surg*. 2016;154(2):201–214.
2. Qureishi A, Lee Y, Belfield K, et al. Update on otitis media—prevention and treatment. *Infect Drug Resist*. 2014;7:15–24.
3. Shekelle P, Takata G, Chan LS, et al. Diagnosis, natural history, and late effects of otitis media with effusion. *Evid Rep Technol Assess (Summ)*. 2002;(55):1–5.
4. Venekamp RP, Burton MJ, van Dongen TM, et al. Antibiotics for otitis media with effusion in children. *Cochrane Database Syst Rev*. 2016;(6):CD009163.
5. Griffin G, Flynn CA. Antihistamines and/or decongestants for otitis media with effusion (OME) in children. *Cochrane Database Syst Rev*. 2011;(9):CD003423.
6. Perera R, Haynes J, Glasziou P, et al. Autoinflation for hearing loss associated with otitis media with effusion. *Cochrane Database Syst Rev*. 2006;(4):CD006285.

ADDITIONAL READING

- Browning GG, Rovers MM, Williamson I, et al. Grommets (ventilation tubes) for hearing loss associated with otitis media with effusion in children. *Cochrane Database Syst Rev*. 2010;(10):CD001801.
- Casselbrant ML, Mandel EM, Rockette HE, et al. Adenoidectomy for otitis media with effusion in 2-3-year-old children. *Int J Pediatr Otorhinolaryngol*. 2009;73(12):1718–1724.

- Cheng X, Sheng H, Ma R, et al. Allergic rhinitis and allergy are risk factors for otitis media with effusion: a meta-analysis. *Allergol Immunopathol (Madr)*. 2017;45(1):25–32.
- Rosenfeld RM, Schwartz SR, Pynnonen MA, et al. Clinical practice guideline: tympanostomy tubes in children. *Otolaryngol Head Neck Surg*. 2013;149(Suppl 1):S1–S35.
- Simpson SA, Lewis R, van der Voort J, et al. Oral or topical nasal steroids for hearing loss associated with otitis media with effusion in children. *Cochrane Database Syst Rev*. 2011;(5):CD001935.
- van Zon A, van der Heijden GJ, van Dongen TM, et al. Antibiotics for otitis media with effusion in children. *Cochrane Database Syst Rev*. 2012;(9):CD009163.
- Williamson I, Vennik J, Harnden A, et al. Effect of nasal balloon autoinflation in children with otitis media with effusion in primary care: an open randomized controlled trial. *CMAJ*. 2015;187(13): 961–969.

 CODES

ICD10

- H65.90 Unspecified nonsuppurative otitis media, unspecified ear
- H65.00 Acute serous otitis media, unspecified ear
- H65.20 Chronic serous otitis media, unspecified ear

CLINICAL PEARLS

- OME is defined as the presence of a middle ear effusion in the absence of acute signs of infection.
- In children, OME most often arises following an AOM. In adults, it often occurs in association with eustachian tube dysfunction.
- The primary standard for diagnosis is pneumatic otoscopy.
- There may be a small benefit of oral antibiotics in tympanogram testing resolution of OME in children. Clinically significant outcomes (e.g., hearing loss, language delay, etc.) are unknown. There is no benefit in antihistamines, decongestants, or corticosteroids for the treatment of OME in children.
- Management usually includes watchful waiting and surgery (when indicated); which strategy is chosen depends on many factors, including the risk/presence of any associated speech, language, or learning delays, and on the severity of any associated hearing loss.

OVARIAN CANCER

Nidha Mattappally, MD • Susan L. Zweizig, MD

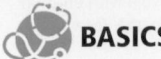 BASICS

There are >22,000 new cases of ovarian cancer annually in the United States, and approximately 14,000 women will die of their disease, making this the most lethal of gynecologic cancers. This accounts for 2.3% of all cancer deaths nationally.

DESCRIPTION

Malignancy that arises from the epithelium (90–95%), sex cord stromal, or germ cells of the ovary as well as tumors metastatic to the ovary. Histologic types include the following:

- Epithelial
  - High grade serous (most common, 70–80%)
  - Low grade serous
  - Mucinous
  - Endometrioid
  - Clear cell
  - Malignant Brenner tumor (transitional cell epithelium)
  - Carcinosarcoma (malignant mixed müllerian tumor)
- Sex cord stromal
  - Granulosa cell tumor
  - Sertoli-Leydig cell tumors
  - Lipid (steroid) cell tumor
  - Fibrosarcoma
- Germ cell
  - Teratoma (immature)
  - Dysgerminoma
  - Embryonal carcinoma
  - Endodermal sinus tumor (yolk sac tumor)
  - Choriocarcinoma
- Metastatic disease from the following:
  - GI tract (Krukenberg tumor)
  - Breast
  - Endometrium
  - Lymphoma
- System(s) affected: GI, genitourinary, endocrine

EPIDEMIOLOGY

Incidence

- 22,440 new cases per year in the United States; 14,070 deaths per year
- Leading cause of gynecologic cancer death in women
- Majority of ovarian cancer is diagnosed at an advanced stage.
- Average age of diagnosis
  - Epithelial: 63 years
  - Sex cord stromal: 50 years
  - Germ cell: 10 to 30 years

Prevalence

Lifetime risk for general population: 1 in 78 American women develop ovarian cancer.

ETIOLOGY AND PATHOPHYSIOLOGY

- Malignant transformation of the ovarian epithelium may result from repeated trauma and inflammation during ovulation.
- Ovarian, fallopian tube, and primary peritoneal carcinomas have identical histologic and morphologic features. A higher percentage of ovarian cancers are now known to originate in the fallopian tube and other components of the secondary müllerian system, including primary peritoneal cancers.

Genetics

- Hereditary breast/ovarian cancer syndrome: early-onset breast or ovarian cancer, autosomal dominant transmission with variable penetrance, usually associated with *BRCA-1* or *BRCA-2* (tumor suppressor gene) mutation

- Lynch syndrome: autosomal dominant inheritance; increased risk for colorectal, endometrial, stomach, small bowel, breast, pancreas, and ovarian cancers; defect in DNA mismatch repair genes

RISK FACTORS

- 90% of ovarian cancer is sporadic and not inherited, but family history is the most significant risk factor. Multiple relatives with breast or ovarian cancer increase risk: Refer these patients for genetic counseling. Individuals in families with familial cancer syndromes have 20–60% risk of developing ovarian cancer.
- Risk factors: older age, white race, infertility, nulligravidity, early menarche or late menopause, endometriosis, postmenopausal estrogen replacement therapy, residence in an industrialized Western country (i.e., North America, Northern Europe)
- Association between fertility medications and risk of ovarian cancer is controversial, but women with infertility who have a successful live birth do not have an increased risk of ovarian cancer.

GENERAL PREVENTION

- Use of oral contraceptives: 5 years of use decreases risk by 20%; 15 years of use decreases risk by 50% (1)[A]
- Multiparity
- Breastfeeding
- Tubal ligation or hysterectomy
- Risk-reducing salpingo-oophorectomy
- Protective effect of aspirin and NSAIDs in ovarian cancer is controversial.
- Recommendations for high-risk (family history of a hereditary ovarian cancer syndrome) population (2)[A]
  - Women should undergo pelvic examinations, CA-125 level measurement, and transvaginal US every 6 to 12 months beginning at age 30 or 10 years prior to the earliest age of diagnosis of ovarian cancer in the family.
  - Women with family histories of ovarian cancer or premenopausal breast cancer should be referred for genetic counseling.
  - Prophylactic oophorectomy is advised for mutation carriers after childbearing is completed or by age 35 years.
    - Risk of primary peritoneal carcinoma remains 1–2% after prophylactic oophorectomy.
- Screening: No effective screening exists for ovarian cancer in the general population (2)[A].
  - Routine use of CA-125 and transvaginal US for screening in women of average risk is NOT recommended. Annual pelvic examinations may be performed, particularly in postmenopausal women. An adnexal mass in a premenarchal female or a palpable adnexa in a postmenopausal female warrants further evaluation.

COMMONLY ASSOCIATED CONDITIONS

- Ascites
- Pleural effusion
- Carcinomatosis
- Bowel obstruction
- Breast cancer
- Endometrial cancer

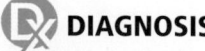 DIAGNOSIS

HISTORY

- Acute presentation:
  - Shortness of breath (pleural effusion)
  - Nausea, vomiting, decreased oral intake (bowel obstruction)

- Calf pain, shortness of breath (venous thromboembolism)
- Severe abdominal or pelvic pain (ovarian torsion or rupture)
- Subacute presentation:
  - Bloating, sense of abdominal fullness, increased abdominal size
  - Early satiety, anorexia, dyspepsia
  - Abdominal or pelvic pain/cramping
  - Dyspareunia
  - Urinary frequency or urgency in absence of infection
  - Fatigue, weight loss
  - Precocious puberty (sex cord stromal or germ cell tumors)

PHYSICAL EXAM

- Pelvic mass
- Cul-de-sac and/or pelvic nodularity (rectovaginal exam)
- Fluid wave (ascites)
- Decreased or absent breath sounds (pleural effusion)
- Abdominal mass (omental caking)
- Cachexia
- Lymphadenopathy
- Hirsutism in androgen-secreting tumors

DIFFERENTIAL DIAGNOSIS

- GI or endometrial malignancies
- Benign or borderline neoplasms
- Tubo-ovarian abscess or hydrosalpinx
- Uterine fibroids
- Endometriomas
- Physiologic cysts
- Irritable bowel syndrome
- Colitis
- Hepatic failure with ascites
- Diverticulitis
- Pelvic kidney

DIAGNOSTIC TESTS & INTERPRETATION

Initial Tests (lab, imaging)

- Obtain with confirmed or suspected disease.
- CBC
- Liver function tests (LFTs) to rule out hepatic disease
- Urinalysis
- Serum albumin
- Tumor markers:
  - Epithelial tumors: CA-125, CA 19-9, CEA
    - CA-125: Levels are elevated in 90% of women with malignant nonmucinous tumors, but 50% of stage I ovarian cancers will have a falsely negative CA-125 and common benign gynecologic conditions (PID, endometriosis, fibroids, pregnancy, menstruation) can cause elevations. Additionally, CA-125 levels can be elevated with ascites, pleural effusion, congestive heart failure, pancreatitis, systemic lupus erythematosus, and liver disease.
    - CA 19-9 and CEA: better indicators of disease in mucinous tumors, helpful if GI primary suspected
  - Nonepithelial tumors: inhibin A/B (granulosa cell tumor), HCG (dysgerminoma, choriocarcinoma, embryonal carcinoma), AFP (endodermal sinus tumor, embryonal carcinoma), LDH (dysgerminoma)
- Pelvic US
- CT abdomen and pelvis with contrast
- CXR or CT chest to evaluate for pleural effusions or lung nodules

Follow-Up Tests & Special Considerations

- Patients with ovarian cancer should be up-to-date with screening recommendations—mammograms, Pap smear, and colonoscopy.
- Colonoscopy (or other test to evaluate the colon—barium enema, CT colonography) is needed if a colonic primary is suspected.

Diagnostic Procedures/Other

- Endometrial biopsy if abnormal uterine bleeding present to evaluate for dual primary
- Consider paracentesis or thoracentesis (or IR biopsy of pelvic mass) if patient not an operative candidate.
  - IR biopsy: Epithelial ovarian cancer commonly involves the peritoneal surfaces of the abdomen and pelvis.

Test Interpretation

Pathologic diagnosis (with surgery, IR biopsy, or cytology) is necessary for definitive diagnosis.

 TREATMENT

GENERAL MEASURES

- Surgical exploration with staging and debulking is critical. Optimal cytoreduction of tumor burden enhances effectiveness of adjuvant therapy and is associated with longer survival.
- In patients with bulky advanced disease in epithelial ovarian cancer where optimal cytoreduction with primary surgery is unlikely, it is reasonable to consider neoadjuvant chemotherapy (NACT), preoperative chemotherapy, after consultation with a gynecologic oncologist (3)[A].

MEDICATION

First Line

- After surgery, most patients will require chemotherapy or adjuvant therapy. Those with stage IA, grade 1, and most stage IB, grade 1 tumors who are optimally staged do not require adjuvant therapy (4)[A]. Patients with clear cell histology, grade 3 tumors or tumors stage IC or worse, do require adjuvant therapy. Patients should be encouraged to participate in clinical trials whenever possible.
- Adjuvant chemotherapy in early stage epithelial ovarian cancer: carboplatin IV and paclitaxel (Taxol) IV every 3 weeks for 6 cycles
- Adjuvant chemotherapy in advanced stage epithelial cancer for patients with optimal cytoreduction: paclitaxel (Taxol) IV on day 1, cisplatin intraperitoneal (IP) on day 2, and paclitaxel (Taxol) IP on day 8 to repeat every 21 days for 6 cycles
- Women with suboptimal cytoreduction are not candidates for IP chemotherapy. Instead, recommend carboplatin IV every 3 weeks with paclitaxel (Taxol) weekly (or every 3 weeks) for 6 cycles.
- IP chemotherapy in combination with IV chemotherapy improves survival in advanced ovarian cancer. IP chemotherapy is associated with more toxicity (5)[A].
- Germ cell or sex cord–stromal cancers: bleomycin, etoposide, and cisplatin IV
- Contraindications to chemotherapy: poor functional status, excessive toxicity, hypersensitivity
- Precautions: All regimens cause bone marrow suppression. Cisplatin is associated with ototoxicity, renal toxicity, and peripheral neuropathy. Paclitaxel (Taxol) can cause neuropathy and alopecia.
- Antiemetics: ondansetron (Zofran), aprepitant (Emend), metoclopramide (Reglan), prochlorperazine (Compazine), promethazine (Phenergan)

Second Line

- Liposomal doxorubicin (Doxil)
- Carboplatin/gemcitabine
- Topotecan
- Etoposide
- Bevacizumab
- Cyclophosphamide
- Tamoxifen

ADDITIONAL THERAPIES

Patients receiving NACT typically receive subsequent interval surgery for debulking of disease if there is a good response to treatment followed by additional cycles of chemotherapy after surgery.

SURGERY/OTHER PROCEDURES

- For epithelial malignancies, staging and tumor excision/debulking include the following:
  - Cytologic evaluation of peritoneal fluid (pelvic washings)
  - Bilateral salpingo-oophorectomy with total hysterectomy and tumor reductive surgery
  - Excision of omentum
  - Inspection and palpation of peritoneal surfaces
  - Cytologic smear of right hemidiaphragmatic surface
  - Biopsy of adhesions or any suspicious areas
  - Biopsies of paracolic recesses, pelvic sidewalls, posterior cul-de-sac, and bladder peritoneum
  - Bilateral pelvic and paraaortic lymph node biopsies
  - Appendectomy for mucinous tumors or if appendix appears abnormal
- Goal of surgery is optimal cytoreduction (<1 cm of maximum tumor diameter remaining).
- Germ cell or sex cord–stromal cancers (less likely to be bilateral): salpingo-oophorectomy (unilateral if only one ovary involved) in young patient for fertility sparing management

 ONGOING CARE

FOLLOW-UP RECOMMENDATIONS

Patient Monitoring

- Physical exam every 3 months for the first 2 years after diagnosis, every 6 months until 5 years, and then annually thereafter
- If CA-125 elevated at diagnosis, follow levels after treatment to detect recurrence.
- Germ cell/sex cord–stromal cancer: physical exam and tumor markers every 3 months for the first 2 years after diagnosis and then annually
  - Tumor markers for sex cord–stromal cancers should be checked every 6 months for 10 years because recurrences can occur remote from initial diagnosis.
- CT scan of chest, abdomen, and pelvis and/or PET scan when recurrence suspected
- Routine screening with imaging not recommended

PROGNOSIS

- Recurrence rates for epithelial cancer
  - Early-stage disease: 20%
  - Advanced disease: >80%
- 5-year survival rates for ovarian cancer based on International Federation of Gynecology and Obstetrics (FIGO) data

Stage I	A 90%	B 86%	C 83%
Stage II	A 78%	B 73%	—
Stage III	A 47%	B 42%	C 33%
Stage IV	19%	—	—

COMPLICATIONS

- Pleural effusion
- Pseudomyxoma peritonei
- Ascites
- Toxicity of chemotherapy
- Bowel obstruction
- Malnutrition
- Electrolyte disturbances
- Fistula formation

REFERENCES

1. Beral V, Doll R, Hermon C, et al; and Collaborative Group on Epidemiological Studies of Ovarian Cancer. Ovarian cancer and oral contraceptives: collaborative reanalysis of data from 45 epidemiological studies including 23,257 women with ovarian cancer and 87,303 controls. *Lancet.* 2008;371(9609):303–314.
2. Schorge JO, Modesitt SC, Coleman RL, et al. SGO white paper on ovarian cancer: etiology, screening and surveillance. *Gynecol Oncol.* 2010;119(1):7–17.
3. Morrison J, Haldar K, Kehoe S, et al. Chemotherapy versus surgery for initial treatment in advanced ovarian epithelial cancer. *Cochrane Database Syst Rev.* 2012;(8):CD005343.
4. Trimbos JB, Vergote I, Bolis G, et al. Impact of adjuvant chemotherapy and surgical staging in early-stage ovarian carcinoma: European Organisation for Research and Treatment of Cancer-Adjuvant Chemotherapy in Ovarian Neoplasm trial. *J Natl Cancer Inst.* 2003;95(2):113–125.
5. Armstrong DK, Bundy B, Wenzel L, et al; for Gynecologic Oncology Group. Intraperitoneal cisplatin and paclitaxel in ovarian cancer. *N Engl J Med.* 2006;354(1):34–43.

ADDITIONAL READING

- Prat J; for FIGO Committee on Gynecologic Oncology. Staging classification for the cancer of the ovary, fallopian tube, and peritoneum. *Int J Gynaecol Obstet.* 2014;124(1):1–5.
- Salani R, Backes F, Fung M, et al. Posttreatment surveillance and diagnosis of recurrence in women with gynecologic malignancies: Society of Gynecologic Oncologists recommendations. *Am J Obstet Gynecol.* 2011;204(6):466–478.

 CODES

ICD10

- C56.9 Malignant neoplasm of unspecified ovary
- C56.1 Malignant neoplasm of right ovary
- C56.2 Malignant neoplasm of left ovary

CLINICAL PEARLS

- Family history of ovarian cancer or early-onset breast cancer is the most significant risk factor for the development of ovarian cancer, yet the vast majority of cases remain sporadic.
- The diagnosis of ovarian cancer should be suspected in women with persistent bloating, upper abdominal discomfort, or GI symptoms of unknown etiology.
- Surgery is the mainstay of diagnosis and treatment for ovarian cancer. Many patients benefit from adjuvant chemotherapy.
- The prognosis of advanced ovarian cancer is poor and requires close follow-up by physical exam, tumor markers, and imaging when indicated.

OVARIAN CYST, RUPTURED

Glency Sue Marie S. Corominas, MD • Adriana Arocha, MD • Marcy Wiemers, MD

BASICS

- Ovarian cysts are frequent in reproductive-aged women.
- Most ovarian cysts are benign physiologic follicles created by the ovary at the time of ovulation.
- Ovarian cysts can cause symptoms when they become enlarged and exert a mass effect on surrounding structures, or when they rupture and the cyst contents cause irritation of the peritoneum or nearby pelvic organs.
- Patients with a symptomatic ruptured cyst will usually complain of acute onset unilateral lower abdominal pain.
- Rupture can be caused by sexual intercourse, luteal phase, exercise, trauma, or pregnancy.
- Evaluation of the patient should include exclusion of other emergent causes: ectopic pregnancy, ovarian torsion, and nongynecologic sources of acute unilateral lower abdominal pain.
- Once the diagnosis of a ruptured cyst is confirmed, most patients can be managed conservatively as outpatients with adequate pain control. Surgical intervention is rarely indicated.
- OCPs are not an effective treatment for existing ovarian cysts.

DESCRIPTION
A suspected ruptured ovarian cyst should be treated as an unknown adnexal mass (mass of the ovary, fallopian tube, and surrounding tissue) until proven otherwise.

EPIDEMIOLOGY
- The actual incidence of ovarian cysts is difficult to calculate because many ruptured cysts are asymptomatic or found incidentally.
- Ovarian cysts can be seen on transvaginal ultrasounds in nearly all premenopausal women and in up to 18% of postmenopausal women. The vast majority of these cysts are benign or functional.
- Most ruptured ovarian cysts are physiologic events and self-limited; expectant management with pain control is usually sufficient.
- About 13% of ovarian masses in reproductive-aged women are malignant, as opposed to 45% in postmenopausal women. About 70% of ovarian malignancies are diagnosed at a late stage.
- Ruptured ovarian cysts most commonly affect the right ovary, 63%.

RISK FACTORS
Medications or conditions associated with increased ovulation and/or increased risk of cyst rupture
- Ovulation induction agents (i.e., Clomid, aromatase inhibitors, GnRH agonists)
- Tamoxifen increases the risk of ovarian cysts in reproductive-aged women.
- Polycystic ovarian syndrome (common)
- Fibrous dysplasia/McCune-Albright syndrome (rare)

GENERAL PREVENTION
Ovulation suppression with combined oral contraceptives is the mainstay therapy for prevention of recurrent ovarian cysts.

DIAGNOSIS

- When a ruptured ovarian cyst is suspected, a pregnancy test should be performed to rule out an ectopic pregnancy (1)[C].
- Sonographic imaging along with CT and MRI can aid in diagnosis of gynecologic emergencies (2)[C].
- CT is useful to confirm a hemoperitoneum, and MRI can assist when the diagnosis remains unclear after CT and ultrasound (2)[C].
- Ultrasound and CT imaging for diagnosis has decreased the need for diagnostic surgical intervention (3)[B].
- Additionally, ultrasound is useful in confirming normal Doppler flow to the affected ovary and adnexa (1)[C].

HISTORY
- A general past medical and surgical history should be reviewed.
- Specific questions that should be addressed if you suspect a ruptured cyst include:
  - Onset and characteristics of pain
  - Pain associated with timing of sexual intercourse, strenuous activity, or trauma
  - Date of last menstrual period
  - Vaginal bleeding
  - Nausea or vomiting
  - Shoulder or upper abdominal pain due to subphrenic extravasation
- Symptoms of circulatory collapse, including palpitations, shortness of breath, sensation of being hot or clammy, dizziness
- Additional information that will guide diagnosis should include patient age, known or previous ovarian cysts, and reproductive history.

ALERT
Patients with bleeding diathesis or undergoing anticoagulation therapy may experience significant bleeding from hemorrhagic cysts.

PHYSICAL EXAM
- Vital signs are usually normal unless significant blood loss has occurred.
- Rupture characterized by significant blood loss may be present in the form of pallor, pale mucosal membranes, and tachycardia.
- Patients will have significant tenderness to palpation or an acute abdomen if the peritoneum is irritated or inflamed.
- On some occasions, a palpable adnexal mass can be felt on bimanual exam. Care should be taken not to cause further injury with a forceful exam.

DIFFERENTIAL DIAGNOSIS
Includes all causes of acute abdominal pain, both gynecologic and nongynecologic

ALERT
- Ectopic pregnancy should always be excluded with a negative pregnancy test (1)[C].
- Benign gynecologic etiologies include:
  - Functional ovarian cysts
  - Ovarian torsion

- Tubo-ovarian abscess
- Teratomas
- Fibroids
- Endometrioma
- Cystadenoma (mucinous or serous)
- Hydrosalpinx
- Malignant gynecologic etiologies can usually be attributed to the various gynecologic cancers of the reproductive tract.
- Benign nongynecologic causes of acute lower abdominal pain include:
  - Appendicitis
  - Diverticulitis
  - Infections of the urinary tract
  - Renal colic
- Malignant nongynecologic causes of acute lower abdominal pain can be attributed to neoplastic processes of the lower GI tract.

DIAGNOSTIC TESTS & INTERPRETATION
- In all premenopausal women, pregnancy must be ruled out by a urine test. Serial quantitative β-hCG tests are helpful in evaluating an ectopic pregnancy (1)[C].
- Complete blood count will evaluate baseline levels to determine a significant drop in hematocrit if there is ongoing hemorrhage (3)[B]. Leukocytosis should raise the suspicion of an infectious process (1)[C].
- Urinalysis and STD testing should be obtained to evaluate for infectious causes, PID, or symptomatic renal stones (1)[A].
- A type and screen is indicated if surgical intervention is planned or blood products are being considered.
- Ultrasonography is the first-line imaging modality (1)[C].
- CA-125 may assist in evaluation but can be elevated in a number of conditions (1)[C].

TREATMENT

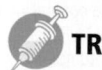

GENERAL MEASURES
- For many patients, pain associated with a ruptured cyst will be transient and self-limiting.
- Cyst rupture in a stable healthy patient can be managed conservatively in 80% of cases due to advances in imaging (3)[B].
- Patient with anticoagulation can also be managed conservatively with cyst rupture using a multidisciplinary team (4)[C].
- Scheduled NSAIDs or oral narcotics can be prescribed depending on pain severity.
- For patients with multiple episodes or a single severe occurrence, OCPs can be considered for ovulation suppression and prevention. They are not effective for treatment of ovarian cysts which are already present (5)[A].
- Unstable patients with hemodynamic compromise or patients with significant hemoperitoneum should be resuscitated, and laparoscopy or a laparotomy should be considered. Surgical exploration should also be considered if there is a concern for malignancy.

ISSUES FOR REFERRAL

- OB/GYN
  - Consider referral to an obstetrician if an adnexal mass is diagnosed during pregnancy. Such masses have a low risk of malignancy or acute complication for the pregnancy.
  - Most cysts resolve without intervention within 2 to 3 weeks; those that do not resolve in 12 weeks require prompt referral for surgical intervention (5)[A].
- Gynecologic oncology
  - Referral to a gynecologic oncologist should be considered for complex adnexal masses with an elevated CA-125 and associated symptoms concerning for malignancy such as ascites, early satiety, pleural effusion, enlarging abdominal mass, or bowel obstruction.
- General surgery
  - Acute lower abdominal pain that is nongynecologic and suspicious for bowel involvement should be referred to general surgery or a gastroenterologist.

SURGERY/OTHER PROCEDURES

- Although the need for surgical intervention is rare, it is usually of an emergent nature.
- Patients with a low diastolic blood pressure and a large amount of hemoperitoneum have an increased rate of surgical intervention (3)[B].
- In most cases, laparoscopy is diagnostic and therapeutic. The decision to proceed with cystectomy or oophorectomy should be made intraoperatively after a thorough evaluation of the intra-abdominal environment has been completed.
- The advantages of a laparoscopic approach include a shorter length of stay, faster recovery, small scar, and few adhesions. Postoperative recovery time as well as patient satisfaction is significantly improved with a minimally invasive approach.
- Laparotomy should be performed in cases of critical hemodynamic instability or lack of laparoscopically trained surgeons. If there is concern for malignancy or metastases, laparotomy may be the preferred method of surgery.

ADMISSION, INPATIENT, AND NURSING CONSIDERATIONS

Patients who require inpatient management should be managed with serial abdominal exams, analgesia, and intravenous resuscitation as indicated by their initial presentation.

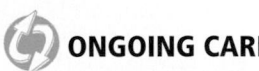 **ONGOING CARE**

FOLLOW-UP RECOMMENDATIONS

- Follow-up for patients managed conservatively should be scheduled in 72 hours from the initial onset of symptoms. Patients should present sooner for new or worsening symptoms.
- Patients with complete resolution of symptoms within a few days can follow up as needed. However, these patients should be counseled on risk of reoccurrence and options for prevention.

- Patient in whom surgical intervention was indicated, postop follow-up should be scheduled 2 weeks from the date of surgery.
- Patients in whom an ovarian cyst was diagnosed incidentally should follow up based on the size of their cyst.

Pregnancy Considerations

Most adnexal masses in pregnancy can be managed expectantly because the risk of malignancy is low (1)[C]. There is a risk for ruptured endometriotic cyst, and early surgical intervention can reduce the effects of endometriotic cyst fluid, and thus prevent adhesions and preserve fertility. MRI can help further characterize a mass safely in pregnancy (1)[C].

PATIENT EDUCATION

Reassurance of the benign nature of most ovarian cysts is an important cornerstone of patient education.

REFERENCES

1. Biggs W, Marks S. Diagnosis and management of adnexal masses. *Am Fam Physician*. 2016;93(8):676–681.
2. Iraha Y, Okada M, Iraha R, et al. CT and MR imaging of gynecologic emergencies. *Radiographics*. 2017;37(5):1569–1586.
3. Kim JH, Lee SM, Lee JH, et al. Successful conservative management of ruptured ovarian cysts with hemoperitoneum in healthy women. *PLoS One*. 2014;9(3):e91171.
4. Gupta A, Gupta S, Manaktala U, et al. Conservative management of corpus luteum haemorrhage in patients on anticoagulation: a report of three cases and review of the literature. *Arch Gynecol Obstet*. 2105;291(2):427–431.
5. Seehusen D, Earwood J. Oral contraceptive are not an effective treatment for ovarian cyst. *Am Fam Physician*. 2014;90(9):623.

ADDITIONAL READING

- Abduljabbar H, Bukhari Y, Al Hachim EG, et al. Review of 244 cases of ovarian cysts. *Saudi Med J*. 2015;36(7):834–838.
- American College of Obstetricians and Gynecologists Committee on Practice Bulletins—Gynecology. Practice Bulletin No. 174: evaluation and management of adnexal masses. *Obstet Gynecol*. 2016;128(5):e210–e226.
- Bottomley C, Bourne T. Diagnosis and management of ovarian cyst accidents. *Best Pract Res Clin Obstet Gynaecol*. 2009;23(5):711–724.
- Collins MT, Singer FR, Eugster E. McCune-Albright syndrome and the extraskeletal manifestations of fibrous dysplasia. *Orphanet J Rare Dis*. 2012;7(Suppl 1):S4.

- Farghaly SA. Current diagnosis and management of ovarian cysts. *Clin Exp Obstet Gynecol*. 2014;41(6):609–612.
- Glanc P, Salem S, Farine D. Adnexal masses in the pregnant patient: a diagnostic and management challenge. *Ultrasound Q*. 2008;24(4):225–240.
- Huang YH, Hsieh CL, Shiau CS, et al. Suitable timing of surgical intervention for ruptured ovarian endometrioma. *Taiwan J Obstet Gynecol*. 2014; 53(2):220–223.
- Kaunitz AM. Oral contraceptive health benefits: perception versus reality. *Contraception*. 1999;59(Suppl 1):29S–33S.
- Legendre G, Catala L, Morinière C, et al. Relationship between ovarian cysts and fertility: what surgery and when? *Fertil Steril*. 2014;101(3):608–614.
- Miller RW, Ueland FR. Risk of malignancy in sonographically confirmed ovarian tumors. *Clin Obstet Gynecol*. 2012;55(1):52–64.
- Mimoun C, Fritel X, Fauconnier A, et al. Epidemiology of presumed benign ovarian tumors [in French]. *J Gynecol Obstet Biol Reprod (Paris)*. 2013;42(8):722–729.
- Raziel A, Ron-El R, Pansky M, et al. Current management of ruptured corpus luteum. *Eur J Obstet Gynecol Reprod Biol*. 1993;50(1):77–81.
- Saunders BA, Podzielinski I, Ware RA, et al. Risk of malignancy in sonographically confirmed septated cystic ovarian tumors. *Gynecol Oncol*. 2010;118(3):278–282.
- Stany MP, Hamilton CA. Benign disorders of the ovary. *Obstet Gynecol Clin North Am*. 2008;35(2):271–284.
- Suzuki S, Yasumoto M, Matsumoto R, et al. MR findings of ruptured endometrial cyst: comparison with tubo-ovarian abscess. *Eur J Radiol*. 2012;81(11):3631–3637.

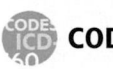 **CODES**

ICD10

- N83.20 Unspecified ovarian cysts
- N83.0 Follicular cyst of ovary
- N83.1 Corpus luteum cyst

CLINICAL PEARLS

- Functional ovarian cysts are very common in reproductive-age women and are usually self-limiting.
- Always exclude ectopic pregnancy.
- Management of symptomatic ruptured cysts is usually accomplished with outpatient pain control and follow-up.
- In cases where the patient with a ruptured cyst is unstable or presents with signs of an acute abdomen, surgical intervention is indicated.

PALLIATIVE CARE

Erika Zimmons, DO, MS

BASICS

Palliative care is a specialty that focuses on preventing and alleviating suffering of patients (and their families) living with life-limiting illness at any stage.

DESCRIPTION
- The principal goal of palliative care is to prevent and alleviate suffering—whether physical (pain, breathlessness, nausea, etc.), emotional, social, or spiritual regardless of underlying diagnosis.
- Palliative care is an interdisciplinary approach to caring for patients and families.
- Palliative care aims to improve or maintain quality of life for patients and families despite serious illness.
- Palliative care is available for patients with serious, life-limiting illness, at any stage of their disease, with or without concurrent curative care.
- Patients and their families may access palliative care services in the hospital, rehabilitation or skilled nursing facility, and ambulatory setting.
- Hospice: In the United Sates, hospice is available for patients whose average life expectancy is 6 months or less and whose principal goal is to stay home (including long-term care or assisted living facility), avoid hospitalizations, and forego disease-directed care with a curative intent. Unlike regular home nursing services, hospice does not require a patient to be homebound and offers backup support for patients 24 hours a day and 7 days per week.

COMMONLY ASSOCIATED CONDITIONS
Common symptoms/syndromes in palliative care:
- Pain
  - Chronic pain
  - Headache
  - Neuropathic pain
  - Pain from bone metastases

- GI symptoms (~60% incidence)
  - Ascites
  - Anorexia/cachexia
  - Nausea (and vomiting)
    ○ Consider underlying etiology and treat accordingly.
    ■ GI causes: constipation, bowel (full or partial) obstruction, ileus, heart burn, reflux, inflammation
    ■ Intrathoracic causes: cardiac, effusions (cardiac, pulmonary), mediastinal causes, esophageal disease
    ■ Autonomic dysfunction
    ■ Centrally mediated: intracranial pressure change, inflammation, cerebellar, vestibular, medication or metabolic cause stimulating vomiting center, and/or chemoreceptor trigger zone
  - Bowel obstruction
  - Constipation and impaction of stool
  - Diarrhea
  - Dysphagia
  - Mucositis/stomatitis
  - Sialorrhea
- General medical
  - Delirium (40–85%)
- Pulmonary symptoms
  - Cough, chronic
  - Breathlessness or dyspnea (60%): which may be due to heart failure, COPD, lung cancer, etc.
- Psychological symptoms
  - Anxiety
  - Depression
  - Insomnia
- Skin
  - Decubitus ulcer
  - Pruritus
  - Complex wounds (fungating tumors, etc.)

DIAGNOSIS

The PEACE tool evaluates (1):
- **P**hysical symptoms
- **E**motive and cognitive symptoms
- **A**utonomy and related issues
- **C**ommunication: contribution to others and closure of life affairs–related issues
- **E**conomic burden and other practical issues, including transcendent and existential concerns

HISTORY
A comprehensive palliative care assessment includes:
- Underlying medical conditions and associated physical symptoms
- Communication with empathic inquiry and open-ended questions
- Comprehensive pain assessment and review of systems (e.g., Edmonton Symptom Assessment Scale)
- Psychological symptom assessment
- Cultural, social, financial, and practical concerns
- Spiritual and existential issues
  - FICA assessment (**F**aith, **I**mportance and influence, **C**ommunity, **A**ddress—how does the patient wish these items to be addressed?) (2)
  - HOPE (sources of **H**ope/strength/comfort, **O**rganized religion's role, **P**ersonal spirituality and practices, **E**ffects on medical care and end-of-life care) (3)
- Presence and sources of suffering (personhood concerns)
- Goals of care: posthospital care, practical needs, hopes, and fears
- Prognosis: functional status and interest in knowing prognosis

PHYSICAL EXAM
Comprehensive physician examination directed by underlying diagnosis, symptoms, and functional decline

DIAGNOSTIC TESTS & INTERPRETATION
Initial Tests (lab, imaging)
Dependent on underlying diagnosis and associated symptoms. Avoid unnecessary testing.

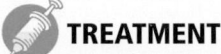

TREATMENT

GENERAL MEASURES

- Targeted interventions to maximize quality of life and minimize symptom burden considering patient values, goals, fears, and social setting
- Treatment should involve an interdisciplinary team to address potential and realized suffering (physical, emotional, social, and/or spiritual).

MEDICATION

- Minimize polypharmacy; discontinue medications that offer little improvement in the quality of life if possible.
- Medications should focus on symptom management.
- Continue use of disease-modifying medications especially if they lessen symptom burden and enhance immediate quality of life.
- Improve compliance by addressing:
  - *Pain* (4)[A]
    - Use immediate-release opioids—titrate to adequate control.
    - Once pain is controlled, convert to long-acting opioids with short-acting agents made available because tolerance develops and/or patient develops breakthrough pain.
  - Bone pain: NSAIDs added to narcotics are more effective than narcotics alone.
  - Neuropathic pain: may use adjuvant treatment, such as gabapentin or other anticonvulsants. Glucocorticoids may also help.

ALERT
Avoid morphine in patients with renal failure; can induce delirium, hyperalgesia, agitation, and seizures

- *Vomiting* associated with a particular opioid may be relieved by substitution with an equianalgesic dose of another opioid or a sustained-release formulation (5).
  - Dopamine receptor antagonists (metoclopramide, prochlorperazine) may improve nausea symptoms.
  - Droperidol: insufficient evidence on the use for the management of nausea and vomiting
- *Constipation*: Consider prophylactic stool softeners (docusate), stimulants (bisacodyl or senna), or osmotic laxatives.

ALERT
Consider laxatives with opioid treatment to avoid constipation.

- SC methylnaltrexone may be used for inducing bowel movements without inducing withdrawal in opioid-induced constipation.
- Dyspnea: Consider oxygen. Consider benzodiazepines if increased anxiety.
  - Treat the underlying cause of breathlessness. In addition, as the disease advances, low-dose opioids may be beneficial to patients (4,6)[C]. Immediate-release opioids PO/IV treat dyspnea effectively and typically at doses lower than necessary for the relief of moderate pain.
- *Delirium*: lowest doses necessary of benzodiazepines or antipsychotics (haloperidol or risperidone, etc.)
  - Monitor patient safety and use nonpharmacologic strategies to assist orientation (clocks, calendars, environment, and redirection).
- Pruritus: no optimal therapy
- Anxiety: insufficient data for recommendations of specific medication
- Megestrol acetate improves appetite and slight weight gain in patients with anorexia-cachexia syndrome.

ISSUES FOR REFERRAL
- Referral to palliative care
  - Any patient with a serious, life-limiting illness who could use help with burdensome symptoms or suffering and/or complex goals of care discussion
  - Early referral to palliative care may improve quality of life and longevity for patients with advanced cancer.
- Referral to hospice care
  - Any patient with an average life expectancy of 6 months or less
  - Consider the question, "Would you be surprised if the patient died within the next 6 months?" If the answer is no, they likely meet criteria for hospice.
    - Consider patients who have multiple hospitalizations and/or emergency department visits in the prior 6 months.
    - Refer to local hospice guidelines for additional disease-specific criteria.

REFERENCES

1. Okon TR, Evans JM, Gomez CF, et al. Palliative educational outcome with implementation of PEACE tool integrated clinical pathway. *J Palliat Med*. 2004;7(2):279–295.
2. Borneman T, Ferrell B, Puchalski CM. Evaluation of the FICA Tool for Spiritual Assessment. *J Pain Symptom Manage*. 2010;40(2):163–173.
3. Anandarajah G, Hight E. Spirituality and medical practice: using the HOPE questions as a practical tool for spiritual assessment. *Am Fam Physician*. 2001;63(1):81–89.
4. Lorenz KA, Lynn J, Dy SM, et al. Evidence for improving palliative care at the end of life: a systematic review. *Ann Intern Med*. 2008;148(2):147–159.
5. Smith HS, Smith JM, Smith AR. An overview of nausea/vomiting in palliative medicine. *Ann Palliat Med*. 2012;1(2):103–114.
6. Ben-Aharon I, Gafter-Gvili A, Paul M, et al. Interventions for alleviating cancer-related dyspnea: a systematic review. *J Clin Oncol*. 2008;26(14):2396–2404.

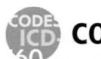 CODES

ICD10
Z51.5 Encounter for palliative care

CLINICAL PEARLS

- Early referral to palliative care helps enhance the quality of life of patients living with serious illness.
- The addition of adjuvant treatments may be more effective than narcotics alone.
- Laxatives should be started with opioid treatment to avoid constipation.

PANCREATIC CANCER

Marcelle Meseeha, MD • Maximos Attia, MD, FAAFP

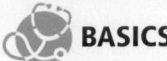 **BASICS**

DESCRIPTION
- Adenocarcinoma of the exocrine pancreas (90% of pancreatic cancers) is the fourth most common cause of cancer death in the United States and the ninth most common cancer in women.
- Rarely curable: overall 5-year relative survival rate of 7.7%
- 60% occur in the head, 20% in the body and tail, and 20% diffusely involve the gland.
- As few as 9% are localized at diagnosis. For localized, small cancers (<2 cm) with no lymph node metastases and no extension beyond the capsule, surgical resection has 5-year survival of about 29%.
- Majority of tumors have metastasized at diagnosis and are thus, largely incurable and have a 5-year survival rate of 2–3%.
- In apparently resectable disease, 20–40% have unresectable lesions at surgery.
- Ampullary, duodenal, or distal bile duct tumors may mimic pancreatic carcinoma and are more likely to be resectable and curable.
- For advanced or unresectable cancers, survival is <1% at 5 years; most patients die within 1 year.

EPIDEMIOLOGY
During 2003 to 2007, median age at diagnosis was 70 years; rare <40 years; after 45 years of age, occurrence rises.

Incidence
- According to the American Cancer Society, an estimated 55,440 diagnoses and 44,330 deaths in the United States in 2018
- About 3% of all cancers and about 7% of cancer deaths
- Lifetime risk is about 1 in 65 (1.5%).
- More common in black and white races, 16.7 and 10.3 in 100,000 men and 14.4 and 10.3 in 100,000 women, respectively. Among Hispanic and Asian/Pacific Islanders, there is an incidence of 10.9 and 8.3 in 100,000 men and 10.1 and 8.3 in 100,000 women, respectively.

Prevalence
In 2008 in the United States, ~34,600 men and women (16,811 men and 17,846 women) were alive who had a history of pancreatic cancer.

RISK FACTORS
- Smoking: relative risk (RR) 2 to 3; correlates with amount smoked
- Diabetes: RR 2.1 (95% CI 1.6–2.8); 1 in 6 become diabetic within 6 months before diagnosis.
- Prior partial gastrectomy or cholecystectomy: 2- to 5-fold increased risk 15 to 20 years after gastrectomy
- Familial aggregation/genetic factors: 5–10% of patients have a first-degree relative with the disease, which confers a 9-fold increase in risk versus the general population; subgroup may carry germline mutations of DNA repair genes (*BRCA2*).
- Hereditary chronic pancreatitis (autosomal dominant, highly penetrant): Cumulative risk by ages 50 and 75 years is 10% and 54%, respectively.
- Peutz-Jeghers syndrome: RR 30 to 40
- Familial atypical multiple mole and melanoma syndrome (p16): RR 10 to 20
- Hereditary nonpolyposis colon cancer (Lynch syndrome): RR 4
- Sporadic chronic pancreatitis

- Non–O blood type: RR 1 to 2
- High dietary fat, red meat, obesity, *Helicobacter pylori*
- Alcohol: Recent data indicate a modest increase in risk confined to heavy alcohol consumers.
- Coffee intake and NSAID use *NOT* regarded as risk factors

GENERAL PREVENTION
No effective screening modality exists to detect early cancer. Even with a strong family history or predisposition syndromes, use and cost-effectiveness of screening are unclear.

COMMONLY ASSOCIATED CONDITIONS
- Chronic pancreatitis, diabetes mellitus, cystic fibrosis
- KRAS mutations are present in >90% of pancreatic ductal adenocarcinomas.
- Mutation inactivation of tumor suppressors (SMAD4, p53, *CDKN2A*) allows for tumor progression.
- Subsets of familial pancreatic cancer involve germline cationic trypsinogen or *PRSS1* mutations (hereditary pancreatitis), *BRCA2* mutations (usually with hereditary breast–ovarian cancer syndrome), *CDKN2* mutations (familial atypical mole, multiple melanoma), or DNA repair gene mutations (e.g., *ATM* and *PALB2*, apart from *BRCA2*).
- Majority of familial pancreatic cancers have no genetic underpinnings.
- Precursor lesions are potentially curable—pancreatic intraepithelial neoplasia, intraductal papillary mucinous neoplasm, and mucinous cystic neoplasms.

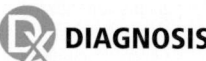 **DIAGNOSIS**

HISTORY
- Depends on tumor location; majority become symptomatic late in disease. About 60–70% of pancreatic cancers develop in the pancreatic head and block the periampullary bile duct, causing obstructive jaundice.
- Weight loss 90%; pain 75% (progressive midepigastric dull ache that often radiates to the back); malnutrition 75%; jaundice 70%; anorexia 60%; pruritus 40%; diabetes mellitus 50%; weakness, fatigue, malaise 30–40%; alcoholic stools, dark urine, steatorrhea; depression is common.
- Pancreatic cancer is a consideration in acute pancreatitis in the elderly and with new-onset diabetes, but most new-onset diabetes are not associated with cancer; thus, evaluation for cancer is warranted only in selected cases.
- Uncommon: unexplained thrombophlebitis; acute pancreatitis from tumor obstruction of pancreatic duct; duodenal obstruction or GI bleeding

PHYSICAL EXAM
- Muscle wasting and malnutrition are common; skin lesions are indicative of pruritus. Exam can be normal.
- Palpable abdominal mass or ascites in 20%
- Jaundice: 70% if tumor obstructs bile duct; 10% with body or tail carcinoma
- Courvoisier sign (painless jaundice with a palpable gallbladder): uncommon; usually associated with pancreatic head tumors, periampullary or primary bile duct tumors; hepatomegaly in advanced disease
- Virchow node (left supraclavicular) and Sister Mary Joseph node (umbilical) in metastatic disease; palpable rectal shelf (nonspecific sign of carcinomatosis)
- Migratory thrombophlebitis (Trousseau sign) (uncommon) due to hypercoagulability in mucin-producing pancreatic cancer

- GI bleeding from tumor erosion into adjacent viscera (colon); portal hypertension-related bleeding (uncommon)
- Pancreatic panniculitis: subcutaneous areas of nodular fat necrosis

DIFFERENTIAL DIAGNOSIS
- Chronic pancreatitis, duodenal cancer, cholangiocarcinoma, lymphoma, islet cell tumor, sarcoma, cystic neoplasms, tumor metastatic to pancreas (rare)
- Nonmalignant conditions: choledocholithiasis, acute or chronic pancreatitis, biliary tract stricture, adenoma; chronic mesenteric ischemia
- Tuberculosis or fungal abscess in AIDS
- Patients may present with back pain mimicking musculoskeletal disease.

DIAGNOSTIC TESTS & INTERPRETATION
- Cross-sectional imaging (usually CT scan as first-line choice) to evaluate symptoms or abnormal lab results (1)[B]
- Endoscopic ultrasound (EUS)-guided biopsy: best modality for tissue diagnosis; sensitivity 75–90%; specificity ~100% for diagnosis of a mass (1)[A]
- Routine laboratory tests may reveal elevated serum bilirubin and alkaline phosphatase (cholestasis), anemia, or decreased serum albumin (malnutrition).

Initial Tests (lab, imaging)
- Most patients do not require measurement of serum tumor markers (CA19-9) for diagnosis or management. Some evidence suggests use in predicting outcome and response to adjuvant chemotherapy.
- CEA and CA19-9 are not recommended as screening tests; useful in following patients with known disease (2)[A]
- Elevated CA19-9 antigen: 80% sensitivity; 90% specificity; individuals with Lewis-negative blood group antigen phenotype (5–10%) are unable to synthesize CA19-9; elevations can occur in benign pancreatic or biliary diseases and in nonpancreatic malignancy.
- *MUC5AC* helps in differentiation.

Follow-Up Tests & Special Considerations
- During therapy, increase in CA19-9 may identify progressive tumor growth. Normal CA19-9 does not exclude recurrence.
- CT scan (pancreatic protocol) using thin section, multiphase multidetector helical CT with a pancreatic protocol is the choice for diagnosis and staging: 85–90% sensitivity; 90–95% specificity; useful for evaluation of distant metastasis and prediction of resectability.
- Abdominal ultrasound (US): common initial test to assess jaundice and duct dilatation; less sensitive than CT for pancreatic masses
- EUS is accurate for tissue biopsy, local tumor and node staging, predicting vascular invasion (90% specificity; 73% sensitivity), and when no mass is identified on CT.
- Endoscopic retrograde cholangiopancreatography (ERCP): 90% sensitivity; 95% specificity for ductal cancer; useful if endoscopic stent is indicated for biliary obstruction; generally confined to high probability for therapeutic intervention on biliary or pancreatic ductal systems
- MRI: no advantage over contrast-enhanced CT
- MR cholangiopancreatography: 90% sensitivity; 95% specificity. Preferred in specific settings: gastric outlet or duodenal stenosis or after surgical

rearrangement (Billroth II) or ductal disruption; to detect bile duct obstruction, after attempted ERCP is unsuccessful or provides incomplete information
- Cystic pancreatic lesions may be benign or malignant; must be differentiated from pancreatic pseudocysts. Cystadenocarcinomas have better prognoses than typical pancreatic cancers.

Diagnostic Procedures/Other
- Percutaneous fine-needle biopsy with US or CT guidance: 80–90% sensitivity; 98–100% specificity
- EUS-guided biopsy: 85–90% sensitivity; virtually 100% specificity for pancreatic mass
- Staging laparoscopy and US: 92% sensitivity; 88% specificity; 89% accuracy
- Positive peritoneal cytology has a positive predictive value of 94%, specificity of 98%, and sensitivity of 25% for determining unresectability.
- PET scan: 90% sensitivity but 70% specificity; limited anatomic information
- Tumor staging
  - Stage Ia: T1 N0 M0 (tumor ≤2 cm)
  - Stage Ib: T2 N0 M0 (tumor >2 cm and ≤4 cm)
  - Stage IIa: T3 N0 M0 (tumor >4 cm)
  - Stage IIb: T1–T3 N1 M0 (N1 is metastasis in 1 to 3 regional lymph nodes.)
  - Stage III: T1–T3 N2 M0 (N2 is metastasis in ≥4 regional lymph nodes), T4 any N M0 (Tumor involves celiac axis, superior mesenteric artery, and/or common hepatic artery, regardless of size.)
  - Stage IV: any T any N M1 (distant metastases)

Test Interpretation
- Duct cell carcinoma: 90%
- Other less common tumors: acinar, papillary mucinous, signet ring, adenosquamous, mucinous, giant or small cell, cystadenocarcinoma, undifferentiated, unclassified carcinoma

ALERT
Chronic pancreatitis can present with similar pain, weight loss, jaundice, and an inflammatory mass on imaging.

 # TREATMENT

- Surgical resection: only chance of cure; no role for pancreatic resection in metastatic disease. As few as 15–20% are candidates for resection.
- Criteria for unresectability: extrapancreatic spread, encasement or occlusion of major vessels, distant metastases
- New combination chemotherapy regimens may offer advantages over gemcitabine. Standard therapies remain unsatisfactory; thus, patients should be considered for clinical trials (2)[B].

MEDICATION
- Analgesics
- Stages I and II
  - Radical pancreatic resection plus chemotherapy
  - ESPAC-3 trial after resection: Compared with 5-fluorouracil (5-FU) and folinic acid, gemcitabine did not improve overall survival.
  - Currently, postoperative gemcitabine alone or in combination with 5-FU–based chemoradiation is the current standard of care; preoperative neoadjuvant treatment trials are in progress (1)[A].
- Stage III
  - Standard: 6 months of chemotherapy with gemcitabine-based regimens (1)[A]; added chemoradiation (capecitabine and radiotherapy) is controversial (1)[B].

- FOLFIRINOX (leucovorin, fluorouracil, irinotecan, and oxaliplatin) and gemcitabine plus nab-paclitaxel were recently shown to have a benefit in patients with metastatic disease; may be tried in patients with locally advanced disease. These regimens are used for patients with no or minimal performance restrictions (1,3)[A].
  - Palliation of biliary obstruction by endoscopic, surgical, or radiologic methods
  - Intraoperative radiation therapy and/or implantation of radioactive substances
- Stage IV
  - Chemotherapy: Gemcitabine ± erlotinib or capecitabine may modestly prolong survival compared with gemcitabine alone. This regimen is used for patients with significant performance restrictions (1,3)[A].
  - Oxaliplatin- and irinotecan-containing regimens (including fluoropyrimidines) have similar efficacy when used after first-line gemcitabine-based therapy in stage IV patients (4)[A].
  - In gemcitabine-refractory pancreatic cancer, S-1 (a fluoropyrimidine not available in the United States) combination regimens have a higher response rate and longer progression-free survival (PFS) than oral S-1 monotherapy (5)[A].
  - Pain-relieving procedures (celiac or intrapleural block); supportive care; palliative decompression
  - Duodenal obstruction: endoscopic expandable metal stent placement rather than surgery (1)[C]
  - Biliary obstruction: Endoscopic biliary stenting is safer than percutaneous insertion and is as successful as surgical hepaticojejunostomy (1)[A].

ADDITIONAL THERAPIES
- For resected tumors: postoperative radiation therapy with other chemotherapeutic agents
- Intraoperative radiation therapy and/or implantation of radioactive substances (ongoing trials)
- Biliary decompression with endoprothesis or transhepatic drainage for bile duct obstruction
- Celiac axis and intrapleural nerve blocks can provide effective pain relief for some patients.
- Opiates may be needed for pain control.

SURGERY/OTHER PROCEDURES
- Standard treatment options
  - Pancreaticoduodenectomy, Whipple procedure, en bloc resection of the head of the pancreas, distal common bile duct, duodenum, jejunum, and gastric antrum
  - Total pancreatectomy
  - Distal pancreatectomy for body and tail tumors
- Nonstandard surgeries
  - Pylorus-preserving pancreaticoduodenectomy, regional pancreatectomy
  - Palliative bypass
    - Biliary decompression; gastrojejunostomy for gastric outlet obstruction; duodenal endoprosthesis for obstruction

 # ONGOING CARE

DIET
- Anorexia, asthenia, pain, and depression may contribute to cachexia.
- Fat malabsorption due to exocrine pancreatic insufficiency may contribute to malnutrition; pancreatic enzyme replacement may help to alleviate symptoms.
- Fat-soluble vitamin deficiency may require replacement therapy.

PROGNOSIS
- 90% diagnosed with pancreatic cancer die from the disease, predominantly from metastatic disease (2).
- 5-year survival: ~30% if node-negative; 10% if node-positive. Median survival: 10 to 20 months
- Metastatic cancer: 1–2% 5-year survival
- For localized disease and small cancers (<2 cm) with no lymph node involvement and no extension beyond the capsule, complete surgical resection can yield a 5-year survival of 18–24%.
- Detection of curable precursor lesions is a focus of current efforts to improve diagnosis and prognosis.

COMPLICATIONS
- Diabetes mellitus, malabsorption, thrombophlebitis
- Duodenal or distal bile duct obstruction
- Surgical complications: intra-abdominal abscess, postgastrectomy syndromes, pancreaticojejunostomy, gastric and biliary anastomotic leaks; operative mortality varies.

REFERENCES
1. Ducreux M, Cuhna AS, Caramella C, et al; for ESMO Guidelines Committee. Cancer of the pancreas: ESMO clinical practice guidelines for diagnosis, treatment and follow-up. *Ann Oncol*. 2015;26(Suppl 5):v56–v68.
2. Ryan DR, Hong TS, Bardeesy N. Pancreatic adenocarcinoma. *N Engl J Med*. 2014;371(11):1039–1049.
3. Sohal DP, Mangu PB, Khorana AA, et al. Metastatic pancreatic cancer: American Society of Clinical Oncology clinical practice guideline. *J Clin Oncol*. 2016;34(23):2784–2796.
4. Petrelli F, Inno A, Ghidini A, et al; and GISCAD (Gruppo Italiano per lo Studio dei Carcinomi dell'Apparato Digerente) and Cremona Hospital. Second line with oxaliplatin- or irinotecan-based chemotherapy for gemcitabine-pretreated pancreatic cancer: a systematic review. *Eur J Cancer*. 2017;81:174–182.
5. Zhong S, Qie S, Yang L, et al. S-1 monotherapy versus S-1 combination therapy in gemcitabine-refractory advanced pancreatic cancer: a meta-analysis (PRISMA) of randomized control trials. *Medicine (Baltimore)*. 2017;96(30):e7611.

ADDITIONAL READING
- Gurusamy KS, Kumar S, Davidson BR, et al. Resection versus other treatments for locally advanced pancreatic cancer. *Cochrane Database Syst Rev*. 2014;(2):CD010244.
- Siegel RL, Miller KD, Jemal A. Cancer statistics, 2018. *Ca Cancer J Clin*. 2018;68(1):7–30.

CODES

ICD10
- C25.9 Malignant neoplasm of pancreas, unspecified
- C25.0 Malignant neoplasm of head of pancreas
- C25.1 Malignant neoplasm of body of pancreas

CLINICAL PEARLS
- Sudden onset of diabetes mellitus in nonobese adults aged >40 years may warrant consideration of pancreatic cancer in selected cases.
- Presence of occult peritoneal tumor cells denotes a worse survival in resectable pancreatic cancer patients.
- Diagnostic laparoscopy may decrease the rate of unnecessary laparotomy in pancreatic cancer found to be resectable on CT.

PANCREATITIS, ACUTE
Robert L. Frachtman, MD • Marni L. Martinez, APRN

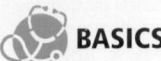 **BASICS**

DESCRIPTION
Acute inflammation of the pancreas with variable involvement of regional tissue or remote organ systems
- Inflammatory episode with symptoms related to intrapancreatic activation of enzymes with pain, nausea and vomiting, and associated intestinal ileus
- Varies widely in severity, complications, and prognosis, accounting for ~280,000 hospital admissions per year in the United States
- Complete structural and functional recovery if there is no necrosis or pancreatic ductal disruption

EPIDEMIOLOGY
Incidence
- 1 to 5/10,000
- Predominant age: none
- Predominant sex: male = female

Prevalence
- Acute: 19/10,000
- Acute pancreatitis is the most common gastrointestinal diagnosis for inpatient hospitalization.

ETIOLOGY AND PATHOPHYSIOLOGY
- Alcohol
- Gallstones (including microlithiasis)
- Trauma/surgery
- Acute discontinuation of medications for diabetes or hyperlipidemia
- Following endoscopic retrograde cholangiopancreatography (ERCP)
- Medications (most common, not an exhaustive list)
  – ACE inhibitors; angiotensin receptor blockers (ARBs); thiazide diuretics and furosemide
  – Antimetabolites (mercaptopurine and azathioprine)
  – Corticosteroids; glyburide; exenatide
  – Mesalamine; pentamidine
  – Sulfamethoxazole/trimethoprim
  – Valproic acid
  – HMG-CoA reductase inhibitors
  – Review all medications and continue only if benefit outweighs risk.
- Metabolic causes
  – Hypertriglyceridemia (classically >1,000 mg/dL); even nonfasting levels as low as ~≥177 mg/dL have been associated with acute pancreatitis.
  – Hypercalcemia; acute renal failure
  – Diet with high glycemic load
  – Systemic lupus erythematosus/polyarteritis
  – Autoimmune; with/without elevated IgG4
  – Infections
    ○ Mumps, coxsackie, CMV, EBV, cryptosporidiosis, ascaris, clonorchis
- Penetrating peptic ulcer (rare)
- Cystic fibrosis and CFTR gene mutations
- Tumors (e.g., pancreatic, ampullary)
- Miscellaneous obstruction
  – Celiac disease
  – Crohn disease
  – Pancreas divisum
  – Sphincter of Oddi dysfunction
- Scorpion venom; vascular disease
- Acute fatty liver of pregnancy
- Idiopathic
- Associated coexisting risk factors
  – Obesity
  – Type II diabetes
  – Smoking

- Pathophysiology—enzymatic "autodigestion" of the pancreas, interstitial edema with severe interstitial acute fluid accumulation ("third spacing"), hemorrhage, necrosis, release of vasoactive peptides (within 6 weeks), pseudocyst or acute necrotic collection (>6 weeks), pancreatic ductal disruption, injury to surrounding vascular structures-splenic vein (thrombosis) and splenic artery (pseudoaneurysm)
- The severity of the first episode of acute pancreatitis, alcohol abuse, and smoking all increase the risk of acute recurrent pancreatitis, which, in turn, increases the risk of progression to chronic pancreatitis.
- Clinical features associated with an increasing severity of acute pancreatitis: age ≥60 years; obesity; long-term, heavy alcohol use

Genetics
- Hereditary pancreatitis is rare; autosomal dominant
- Polymorphisms and mutations in multiple genes

GENERAL PREVENTION
- Avoid excess alcohol consumption.
- Tobacco cessation
- Correct underlying metabolic processes (hypertriglyceridemia or hypercalcemia).
- Discontinue offending medications.
- Cholecystectomy (symptomatic cholelithiasis)
- Diet: There is an increased risk of gallstone pancreatitis with diets high in saturated fats, cholesterol, red meat, and eggs. Decreased risk of gallstone pancreatitis with diet high in fiber and vitamin D. There is a decreased risk of nongallstone pancreatitis with diets high in fiber, coffee, and caffeine.

COMMONLY ASSOCIATED CONDITIONS
- Alcohol withdrawal, alcoholic hepatitis, diabetic ketoacidosis, and ascending cholangitis
- Morbid obesity, a pro-inflammatory state, increases severity and adverse outcomes (organ failure, mortality).

DIAGNOSIS
Symptoms don't always correlate with objective findings.

HISTORY
- Acute onset of "boring" epigastric pain, which may radiate toward the back
- Nausea/vomiting
- Alcohol use
- Personal or family history of gallstones
- Medication use
- Abdominal trauma
- Recent significant rapid weight loss

PHYSICAL EXAM
- Vital signs—assess hemodynamic stability; fever
- Abdominal findings: epigastric tenderness, loss of bowel sounds, peritoneal signs
- Other findings, jaundice, rales/percussive dullness
- Rare (with hemorrhagic pancreatitis)
  – Flank discoloration (Grey Turner sign) or umbilical discoloration (Cullen sign)

DIAGNOSTIC TESTS & INTERPRETATION
- Interpret laboratory and radiographic findings in the context of the clinical history—false-positive and false-negative findings are common.
- Bedside Index in Severity in Acute Pancreatitis (BISAP) score
  – Patients receive 1 point for each element in the first 24 hours: BUN >25 mg/dL, impaired mental status,

systemic inflammatory response syndrome (SIRS)—a score of 0 predicts mortality of <1%, and a score of 5 correlates with a mortality rate of 22%.
- Ranson criteria is an older model of predicting severity of pancreatitis. It includes 11 criteria, 5 of which are measured at admission, and 6 are measured in the following 48 hours. A score of 3 or less represents mild pancreatitis, and as the score increases, the mortality rises sharply.
- American College of Gastroenterology requires at least two of the three following elements to make a diagnosis of acute pancreatitis: characteristic abdominal pain, specific radiographic findings, and lipase level 3 times the upper limits of normal (ULN).
- Elevated serum amylase >3 times ULN (Severity is not related to degree of elevation.)
- Elevated serum lipase >3 times ULN (may stay elevated longer than amylase in mild cases)
- Elevated total bilirubin. If >3 mg/dL, consider common bile duct obstruction.
- A 3-fold elevation in the alanine aminotransferase (ALT) in the setting of acute pancreatitis has a 95% positive predictive value for gallstone pancreatitis. Triglyceride levels >1,000 mg/dL suggest hypertriglyceridemia as the cause.
- Glucose and calcium increased in severe disease.
- WBC elevation to 10,000 to 25,000/μL possible and not indicative of active infection
- Elevated baseline hematocrit >44 or rising hematocrit is poor prognostic sign (severe third spacing with associated hemoconcentration).
- Rising BUN and creatinine imply volume depletion or acute renal failure.

DIFFERENTIAL DIAGNOSIS
- Penetrating peptic ulcer
- Acute cholecystitis or cholangitis
- Macroamylasemia, macrolipasemia
- Mesenteric vascular occlusion and/or infarction
- Intestinal obstruction; perforated viscus
- Aortic aneurysm (dissecting or rupturing)
- Inferior wall myocardial infarction
- Lymphoma

Initial Tests (lab, imaging)
- Use follow-up labs to assess renal function, hydration, sepsis, biliary obstruction, and tissue oxygenation.
- Chest x-ray (CXR) to evaluate for early acute respiratory distress syndrome (ARDS) and pleural effusion; can also rule out subdiaphragmatic air (perforated viscus)
- Ultrasound to look for gallbladder/biliary stones
- CT scan
  – Confirms the diagnosis, assesses severity, establishes a baseline, and rules out most other pathologies (excluding noncalcified cholelithiasis)
  – IV contrast is not essential for the initial CT scan; avoid contrast in volume-depleted patients.
  – If not contraindicated, a CT scan with IV contrast on day 3 can assess the degree of necrosis if necrotizing pancreatitis is suspected.
- Magnetic resonance cholangiopancreatography (MRCP) helps assess choledocholithiasis, pancreas divisum, dilated pancreatic duct, and ductal changes.
- Esophagogastroduodenoscopy (EGD) may be necessary to rule out a penetrating duodenal ulcer or an obstructing ampullary neoplasm.
- ERCP may be necessary to decompress common bile duct due to an impacted stone.

- Endoscopic ultrasonography (EUS) is useful if patients present with "idiopathic pancreatitis."
- EUS-guided fine needle aspiration if autoimmune pancreatitis is suspected

Follow-Up Tests & Special Considerations

If renal function is stable, a contrast-enhanced CT scan at day 3 to assess for necrosis. CT guidance assists aspiration and drainage of abscess—mainly recommended if a fungal or drug-resistant infection is suspected.

TREATMENT

MEDICATION

First Line

- Analgesia: no consensus; guidelines vary: hydromorphone (Dilaudid) 0.5 to 1.0 mg IV q1–2h PRN
  - AVOID meperidine (Demerol) due to the potential of accumulation of a toxic metabolite.
- Antibiotics
  - In the clear absence of infection, the use of prophylactic antibiotics is no longer recommended (even with necrotizing pancreatitis).
  - In patients with ascending cholangitis or necrotizing pancreatitis, if there is a strong suspicion of active infection, consider empiric β-lactam/β-lactamase inhibitor (e.g., piperacillin/tazobactam 4.5 g IV q8h) for initial treatment before cultures (especially aspirates) return.
  - Levofloxacin 500 mg QD IV if cholangitis and there is an allergy to penicillin
  - Be vigilant for fungal superinfections when giving prophylactic antibiotics.

GENERAL MEASURES

Most cases of acute pancreatitis require hospitalization; ICU if multiorgan dysfunction or hypotension/respiratory failure; 15–20% of cases of acute pancreatitis progress from mild to severe (including persistent organ failure).

- Fluid resuscitation
  - Significant volume deficit due to third spacing
  - Infuse bolus of 1,000 to 2,000 mL (lactated Ringer may be better than normal saline, unless hypercalcemic), followed by 250 to 300 mL/hr, adjusted on the basis of age, weight, hemodynamic response, and comorbid conditions.
  - Target urine output should be 0.5 to 1.0 mL/kg/hr. Lower the infusion rate when this goal is achieved or once BUN decreases; 4 L should be the maximum total fluid on day 1.
  - Fluid resuscitation is of limited value after 24 hours, and fluid overload results in significant complications (1)[A].
- Eliminate unnecessary medications, especially those implicated as causes of pancreatitis.
- Nasogastric (NG) tube for intractable emesis
- Follow renal function, volume status, calcium, and oxygenation. Organ failure is more important prognostic indicator than pancreatic necrosis.
- DVT prophylaxis
- Begin oral alimentation after pain, tenderness, and ileus have resolved; small amounts of high-carbohydrate, low-fat, and low-protein foods; advance as tolerated; NPO or NG tube if vomiting persists. In cases of mild pancreatitis, a soft low-fat diet may be started even before enzymes elevation and pain have completely resolved (1)[A].
- Enteral nutrition at level of ligament of Treitz if oral feeding not possible within 5 to 7 days (preferable

to total parenteral nutrition [TPN] due to decreased infection rate and decreased mortality). Discontinue with increases in pain, increases in amylase/lipase levels, or fluid retention.
- TPN (without lipids if triglycerides are elevated) if oral or nasoenteric feedings are not tolerated (2)[A]

ISSUES FOR REFERRAL

Refer to a tertiary center if pancreatitis is severe or actively evolving and when advanced imaging or endoscopic therapy is being considered.

SURGERY/OTHER PROCEDURES

- Consider cholecystectomy before discharge in patients with cholelithiasis and nonnecrotizing pancreatitis to reduce risk of recurrence.
- Necrosectomy should be performed nonsurgically for either infected or noninfected necrosis. Walled-off necrosis should be observed for 4 weeks (treated with antibiotics if infected), followed by percutaneous or dual-modality drainage if available (3)[B]. Drainage may not be required if there are no signs of infection. Aspiration and culture are not required if infection is suspected and if patient is responding to appropriate antibiotic therapy (1)[A].
- ERCP early if evidence of acute cholangitis or at 72 hours if evidence of ongoing biliary obstruction; ERCP with pancreatic ductal stent placement, if ductal disruption persists longer than 1 to 2 weeks
- Resection or embolization for bleeding pseudoaneurysms
- Plasma exchange with insulin within 24 hours of presentation if severe necrotizing pancreatitis secondary to hypertriglyceridemia (4)[C]

ADMISSION, INPATIENT, AND NURSING CONSIDERATIONS

Discharge criteria
- Pain controlled
- Tolerating oral diet
- Alcohol rehabilitation and tobacco cessation
- Low-grade fever and mild leukocytosis do not necessarily indicate infection and may take weeks to resolve. Infections may occur even after 10 days (33% of patients with necrotizing pancreatitis) due to secondary infection of necrotic material, requiring surgical débridement.

ONGOING CARE

FOLLOW-UP RECOMMENDATIONS

- Follow-up imaging in several weeks if the original CT scan showed a fluid collection or necrosis or if the amylase/lipase continues to be elevated. Follow-up findings may include:
  - Pseudocyst (occurs in 10%) or abscess (sudden onset of fever): Conservative management is an option for asymptomatic pseudocysts up to 6 cm in diameter.
  - Splenic vein thrombosis (Gastric variceal hemorrhage rarely occurs.)
  - Pseudoaneurysm (splenic, gastroduodenal, intrapancreatic) hemorrhage can be life-threatening.
- Mild exocrine and endocrine dysfunction is usually subclinical. Patients with necrotizing pancreatitis, steatorrhea, or ductal obstruction, however, should receive enzyme supplementation.
- After the first episode of acute pancreatitis, the risk of lifetime diabetes doubles.
- After the first episode of acute pancreatitis, the risk of developing acute recurrent pancreatitis is ~17%. The risk for developing chronic pancreatitis is ~8%.

DIET

Advance diet as tolerated; reduce fat, alcohol, and added sugars.

PROGNOSIS

85–90% of cases of acute pancreatitis resolve spontaneously; 3–5% mortality (17% in necrotizing pancreatitis)

REFERENCES

1. Forsmark CE, Vege SS, Wilcox CM. Acute pancreatitis. *N Engl J Med.* 2016;375(20):1972–1981.
2. Gravante G, Garcea G, Ong SL, et al. Prediction of mortality in acute pancreatitis: a systematic review of the published evidence. *Pancreatology.* 2009;9(5):601–614.
3. Trikudanathan G, Attam R, Arain MA, et al. Endoscopic interventions for necrotizing pancreatitis. *Am J Gastroenterol.* 2014;109(7):969–982.
4. Gulati A, Papachristou GI. Update on the management of acute pancreatitis and its complications. *The New Gastroenterologist.* 2017;2017:12–17.

ADDITIONAL READING

- Crockett SD, Wani S, Gardner TB, et al; for American Gastroenterological Association Institute Clinical Guidelines Committee. American Gastroenterological Association Institute guideline on initial management of acute pancreatitis. *Gastroenterology.* 2018;154(4):1096–1101.
- Lu X, Aoun E. Complications of acute pancreatitis. *Pract Gastroenterol.* 2012;36:11–22.
- Nitsche CJ, Jamieson N, Lerch MM, et al. Drug induced pancreatitis. *Best Pract Res Clin Gastroenterol.* 2010;24(2):143–155.
- Setiawan VW, Pandol SJ, Porcel J, et al. Dietary factors reduce risk of acute pancreatitis in a large multiethnic cohort. *Clin Gastroenterol Hepatol.* 2017;15(2):257–265.e3.
- Wu BU, Banks PA. Clinical management of patients with acute pancreatitis. *Gastroenterology.* 2013;144(6):1272–1281.

CODES

ICD10
- K85.9 Acute pancreatitis, unspecified
- K85.8 Other acute pancreatitis
- K85.2 Alcohol induced acute pancreatitis

CLINICAL PEARLS

- Pancreatitis is a common cause of hospitalization.
- Gallstones and alcohol misuse are the leading causes of pancreatitis.
- The BISAP score is easier to apply than Ranson criteria and just as accurate for predicting mortality in patients with acute pancreatitis.
- Review all medications and discontinue any that may cause (or contribute to) pancreatitis.
- Start oral feeding as soon as possible in the absence of severe pain, vomiting, or ileus.
- Patients with mild pancreatitis can progress to severe pancreatitis over the initial 48 hours, often due to inadequate fluid replacement.
- Refer to tertiary center if acute pancreatitis is severe or evolving/worsening.

PANIC DISORDER
Jay Winner, MD, FAAFP

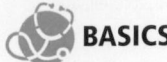 **BASICS**

DESCRIPTION
- A classic panic attack that is characterized by rapid onset of a brief period of sympathetic nervous system hyperarousal accompanied by intense fear
- In panic disorder, multiple panic attacks occur (including at least two without a recognizable trigger). Patients experience at least 1 month of worried anticipation of additional attacks and/or maladaptive (e.g., avoidance) behaviors.

EPIDEMIOLOGY
Incidence
- Predominant age: all ages; in school-aged children, panic disorder can be confused with conduct disorder and school avoidance.
- Median age of onset 24 years. Prevalence significantly decreases after 60 years.
- Predominant sex: female > male (2:1)

Prevalence
- Lifetime prevalence: 4.7%
- 4–8% of patients in a primary care practice population have panic disorder.
- Of patients presenting with chest pain in the emergency room, 25% have panic disorder.
- Chest pain is more likely due to panic if atypical, younger age, female, and known problems with anxiety.

ETIOLOGY AND PATHOPHYSIOLOGY
Remain unproven
- Biologic theories focus on limbic system malfunction in dealing with anxiety-evoking stimuli.
- Psychological theories posit deficits in managing strong emotions such as fear and anger.
- Patients resist the initial surge of adrenaline which exacerbates the symptoms—in essence, they get anxious about being anxious. Concerns about a dangerous cause of symptoms and worries about going crazy or losing control also exacerbate symptoms.
- Noradrenergic neurotransmission from the locus coeruleus causes increased sympathetic stimulation throughout the body.
- Current neurobiologic research focuses on abnormal responses to anxiety-producing stimuli in the hippocampus, amygdala, and prefrontal cortex; for example, there appears to be limbic kindling in which an original frightening experience dominates future responses even when subsequent exposures are not objectively threatening.
- Brain pH disturbances (e.g., excess lactic acid) from normal mentation in genetically vulnerable patients may activate the amygdala and generate unexpected fear responses.
- Twin studies have suggested a heritability of approximately 40% with contributions of 10% from common familial environment and >50% from individual-specific environmental effects. Some monoamine-related genes, such as serotonin transporter and monoamine oxidase A genes, have been proven to play a role in panic disorder.

RISK FACTORS
- Life stressors of any kind can precipitate attacks.
- History of sexual or physical abuse; anxious, overprotective parents
- Substance abuse, bipolar disorder, major depression, obsessive-compulsive disorder (OCD), and simple phobia

COMMONLY ASSOCIATED CONDITIONS
- Of patients with panic disorder, >70% also have ≥1 other psychiatric diagnoses: PTSD (recalled trauma precedes panic attack), social phobia (fear of scrutiny precedes panic attack), simple phobia (fear of something specific precedes panic), major depression, bipolar disorder, substance abuse, OCD, separation anxiety disorder.
- Panic disorder is more common in patients with asthma, migraine headaches, hypertension, mitral valve prolapse, reflux esophagitis, interstitial cystitis, irritable bowel syndrome, fibromyalgia, nicotine dependence.
- Panic disorder increases the risk of suicide attempts and ideation.

℞ DIAGNOSIS

- Panic attack: an abrupt surge of intense fear, reaching a peak within minutes in which ≥4 of the following symptoms develop abruptly: (i) palpitations, pounding heart, or accelerated heart rate; (ii) sweating; (iii) trembling or shaking; (iv) sensation of shortness of breath or smothering; (v) a choking sensation; (vi) chest pain or discomfort; (vii) nausea or abdominal distress; (viii) feeling dizzy, unsteady, light-headed, or faint; (ix) derealization (feelings of unreality) or depersonalization (feeling detached from oneself); (x) fear of losing control or going crazy; (xi) fear of dying; (xii) paresthesias; (xiii) chills or hot flashes (1)[C]
- Panic disorder: recurrent unexpected panic attacks not better accounted for by another psychiatric condition (e.g., PTSD, OCD, separation anxiety disorder, social anxiety disorder, or specific phobia) *and* not induced by drugs of abuse, medical conditions, or prescribed drugs *and* with >1 month of at least one of the following: (i) worry about additional attacks or worry about the implications of the attack (e.g., losing control, having a heart attack, "going crazy"), (ii) a significant maladaptive change in behavior related to the attacks (1)[C]
- Panic attack specifier can be diagnosed for patients with panic attacks who do not meet the criteria for panic disorder (1)[C].
- Unlike *DSM IV*, *DSM-5* defines agoraphobia as separate from panic disorder (1)[C].

HISTORY
- The best way to get a good history is through tactful, nonjudgmental questioning. Information should be elicited about physical and emotional symptoms, current life stress, separations, recent deaths, patient's concerns and fears, interpersonal problems.
- A thorough medication and substance abuse history is important.
- Patients must have a month of fear of out-of-the-blue panic attacks to diagnose panic disorder. Ask for avoidance patterns that have developed since the onset of panic attacks.

PHYSICAL EXAM
- During an attack, there can be tachycardia, hyperventilation, and diaphoresis.
- Check the thyroid for fullness or nodules. Look for exophthalmos or lid lag.
- Cardiac exam to check for a murmur or arrhythmias
- Lung exam to rule out asthma (limited airflow, wheezing)

DIFFERENTIAL DIAGNOSIS
- Medication use may mimic panic disorder and create anxiety: Paradoxically, antidepressants used to treat panic may, initially, worsen panic; antidepressants in bipolar patients can cause anxiety/mania/panic; short-acting benzodiazepines (alprazolam), β-blockers (propranolol), and short-acting opioids can cause interdose rebound anxiety; benzodiazepine treatment causes panic when patients take too much and run out of these medicines early; bupropion, levodopa, amphetamines, steroids, albuterol, sympathomimetics, fluoroquinolones, and interferon can cause panic.
- Substances withdrawal or abuse: alcohol withdrawal, benzodiazepine withdrawal, opioid withdrawal, caffeine, marijuana (panic with paranoia), amphetamine abuse, MDMA, hallucinogens (PCP, LSD), dextromethorphan abuse, synthetic cathinones (bath salts) abuse
- Medical conditions: cardiovascular (tachyarrhythmias, myocardial infarction (MI), mitral valve prolapse), pulmonary (asthma, COPD, reflux esophagitis with hyperventilation, hypoxia, pulmonary embolism), endocrine (hypo-/hyperthyroidism, premenstrual dysphoric disorder, menopause, pregnancy, hypoglycemia [in diabetes], carcinoid syndrome, pheochromocytoma, Cushing syndrome, hyperaldosteronism, Wilson disease, hyperparathyroidism), neurologic (transient ischemic attacks [TIAs], pre- and postictal states, e.g., in TLE), miscellaneous (autoimmune disease, e.g., SLE; inner ear disturbances, e.g., labyrinthitis, anaphylaxis, heavy metal poisoning, heavy metal poisoning), sleep apnea (when nocturnal panic attacks)
- Psychiatric conditions that have overlapping symptomatology include mood, anxiety, and personality disorders such as major depression, bipolar disorder, PTSD, borderline personality disorder, social phobia, OCD, and generalized anxiety disorder. In PTSD, there is always a recollection or visual image that precedes the panic attack. In social phobia, fear of scrutiny precedes the panic attack. In bipolar disorder, major depression, borderline personality disorder, and particularly substance abuse, the patient often complains first of panic symptoms and anxiety and minimizes other potentially relevant symptoms and behaviors.
- Somatic symptom disorder is also an illness of multiple unexplained medical symptoms, but the presenting picture is usually one of chronic symptoms rather than the acute, dramatic onset of a panic attack. Somatic symptom disorder and panic disorder can be (and often are) diagnosed together.

DIAGNOSTIC TESTS & INTERPRETATION
Consider electrocardiogram (ECG) and pulse oximetry to rule out certain serious causes of panic; consider Holter monitoring. No specific lab tests are indicated except to rule out conditions in the differential diagnosis.
- Fingerstick blood sugar in acute setting in a diabetic patient
- Thyroid-stimulating hormone (TSH), complete metabolic panel, CBC
- Consider ordering echocardiogram if you suspect mitral valve prolapse.
- If chest discomfort, do appropriate workup which could include stress test, chest CT with contrast, etc.
- If nocturnal panic attacks, consider sleep study.

Diagnostic Procedures/Other
- If a medical cause of anxiety is strongly suspected, do the workup appropriate for that condition.
- Panic Disorder Severity Scale (PDSS) is a physician or self-administered instrument for monitoring changes in severity of symptoms and response to treatment.
  – https://www.outcometracker.org/library/PDSS.pdf

TREATMENT

The two options psychotherapy and medical therapy. Studies have shown that both have comparable results and neither has advantage over the other. Combined antidepressant therapy and psychotherapy is superior to either alone during initial treatment for panic disorder (2)[A]. Most effective therapy includes cognitive-behavioral therapy (CBT), mindfulness-based therapy, and exposure therapy. Psychotherapy provides long-lasting treatment, often without subsequent need for medications.

GENERAL MEASURES
Patient education is a vital part of treatment. This can be supplemented by video and written material. Instruct how symptoms can be caused by panic and the associated hyperventilation. Teach how resisting and pushing away the anxiety makes symptoms worse. Instead, rename the panic as an energy burst and see if they can use or at least feel the energy. Also teach patients mindful diaphragmatic breathing and to mindfully notice thoughts without believing or resisting all their thoughts. If appropriate, exposure to anxiety-provoking conditions can coupled with relaxation exercises.

MEDICATION
- Medication management is indicated if psychotherapy is not successful (or not available) and may be combined with psychotherapy. It is also indicated if the patient lacks the motivation or ability to participate in psychotherapy.
- Antidepressants like selective serotonin reuptake inhibitor (SSRI), serotonin-norepinephrine reuptake inhibitor (SNRI), tricyclic antidepressant (TCA), monoamine oxidase inhibitor (MAOI), and benzodiazepines have shown efficacy in treating panic disorder.
- If medications are started, they should be maintained for at least 1 year after symptom control to reduce risk of relapse.

First Line
- SSRIs and SNRIs are first line given efficacy, benign side effect profile, and lack of abuse potential.
- Start a low-dose SSRI, for example, fluoxetine 5 mg, paroxetine 10 mg, sertraline 25 mg, citalopram 10 mg, and escitalopram 5 mg once daily in the morning. Titrate up slowly every 1 to 2 weeks to therapeutic doses over a period of 6 weeks. Side effects include irritability, diarrhea, and sexual dysfunction. Suicidality can be seen in young patients. When stopping SSRI, taper over few months (3)[A]. This is more important for medications with a shorter half-life like paroxetine compared with medications such as fluoxetine.
- Among SNRIs, venlafaxine extended release (ER) is effective. Start at 37.5 mg/day and titrate up to 75 mg/day after 7 days (maximum dose of 225 mg/day). Taper slowly over weeks to discontinue; risk of hypertension at higher doses (4)[A]
- Patients with associated mental disorders may benefit from a combination of SSRI and psychotherapy.

Second Line
- TCAs, particularly imipramine (start 25 mg/day in the evening and increase up to 25 mg every 3 days to a maximum of 200 mg/day); slower titration and lower doses are often as effective. Imipramine is as efficacious as SSRIs in the treatment of panic disorder. TCAs are considered second line because of difficulty in dosing, more side effects, and greater risk associated with overdose compared with SSRIs (5)[A]. Screen for cardiac conduction system in patients >40 years of age with an ECG.
- Mirtazapine can be used started at 15 mg QHS and potentially increasing to 30 mg QHS. Side effects of sedation and weight gain may limit use, but for people suffering from weight loss and insomnia, this medication could be helpful.
- MAOIs like phenelzine and tranylcypromine are also efficacious compared to placebo. Avoid with serotonergic agents given risk for serotonin syndrome. There are also dietary restrictions and multiple other drug interactions that limit use of these medications.
- Benzodiazepines like alprazolam (start 0.25 mg TID PRN) and clonazepam (start at 0.5 mg BID PRN) are FDA-approved for panic disorder. Clonazepam has a longer half-life, less interdose anxiety, and lower abuse potential than alprazolam. Benzodiazepines are associated with sedation, dependence, increased falls, increased car accidents, and increased mortality. Therefore, in general, benzodiazepines should be used just for crisis and short-term relief of severe symptoms. Prescribing benzodiazepines to patients on opiates increases risk of overdose.
- There is limited data supporting the use of supplements for the treatment of anxiety disorders. Kava kava should be avoided because of the risks of liver failure. A 2018 meta-analysis did show potential reduction in anxiety from omega-3 fatty acids 2 g daily with EPA <60% (would start at 1 g daily).

ISSUES FOR REFERRAL
- Refer to a counselor who specializes in anxiety treatment which usually consists of CBT, mindfulness-based therapy, and/or exposure therapy.
- Consider referral to a psychiatrist for panic disorder that is comorbid with bipolar disorder, borderline personality disorder, schizophrenia, suicidality, alcohol, or substance abuse.

ADDITIONAL THERAPIES
- Aerobic exercise may reduce symptoms.
- Stress reduction classes can be helpful such as Mindfulness-Based Stress Reduction (MBSR).

ADMISSION, INPATIENT, AND NURSING CONSIDERATIONS
- If certain life-threatening mimics of panic disorder have not been ruled out, such as an MI or PE, hospitalize patient to complete the evaluation.
- If a panic disorder patient has concrete suicidal ideation, a psychiatric admission is indicated.

ONGOING CARE

PATIENT EDUCATION
- Video on "Dealing with Panic and Anxiety" at StressRemedy.com/videos
- www.nlm.nih.gov/medlineplus/panicdisorder.html
- Patient information handouts in *American Family Physician.* 2005;71:740 and 2006;74:1393
- http://www.nimh.nih.gov/health/publications/panic -disorder-when-fear-overwhelms/index.shtml
- *Relaxation on the Run: Simple Methods to Reduce Stress in Seconds Plus Practical Lifestyle Tips for a Happier and Healthier Life* by Jay Winner

- *The Anxiety and Phobia Workbook* by Edmund Bourne
- *Hope and Help for Your Nerves* by Claire Weekes
- *Don't Panic: Taking Control of Anxiety Attacks* by Reid Wilson

PROGNOSIS
Panic disorder is a chronic or intermittent disease. Remission occurs in 64.5% of patients with a mean time to remission of about 5.7 months. Recurrence does occur in 21.4% in those who achieved remission. Predictors of remission are female gender, absence of ongoing stressors, and a low initial frequency of attacks.

COMPLICATIONS
- Iatrogenic benzodiazepine dependence
- Iatrogenic mania in bipolar patients treated for panic with unopposed antidepressants
- Misdiagnosis of panic in patients with difficult-to-treat psychiatric conditions

REFERENCES
1. American Psychiatric Association. *Diagnostic and Statistical Manual of Mental Disorders.* 5th ed. Arlington, VA: American Psychiatric Association; 2013.
2. Furukawa TA, Watanabe N, Churchill R. Combined psychotherapy plus antidepressants for panic disorder with or without agoraphobia. *Cochrane Database Syst Rev.* 2007;(1):CD004364.
3. Pollack MH, Lepola U, Koponen H, et al. A double-blind study of the efficacy of venlafaxine extended-release, paroxetine, and placebo in the treatment of panic disorder. *Depress Anxiety.* 2007;24(1):1–14.
4. Batelaan NM, de Graaf R, Penninx BW, et al. The 2-year prognosis of panic episodes in the general population. *Psychol Med.* 2010;40(1):147–157.
5. Su KP, Tseng PT, Lin PY, et al. Association of use of omega-3 polyunsaturated fatty acids with change in severe anxiety symptoms: a systematic review and meta-analysis. *JAMA Netw Open.* 2018;1(5):e182327.

ADDITIONAL READING
- Chen MH, Tsai SJ. Treatment-resistant panic disorder: clinical significance, concept and management. *Prog Neuropsychopharmacol Biol Psychiatry.* 2016;70: 219–226.
- Winston S, Martin S. *What Every Therapist Needs to Know About Anxiety Disorders: Key Concepts, Insights, and Interventions.* Abingdon, United Kingdom: Routledge; 2014.

 SEE ALSO

Algorithm: Anxiety

 CODES

ICD10
- F41.0 Panic disorder without agoraphobia
- F40.01 Agoraphobia with panic disorder
- F43.0 Acute stress reaction

CLINICAL PEARLS
- For medically stable patients, 10 minutes of vigorous aerobic exercise at onset of a panic attack often helps patient to feel safe during an attack.
- Always evaluate a patient with panic for suicidality because patients with panic disorder are at increased risk for suicide, particularly if depressed.

PARKINSON DISEASE

Sireesha Teegala, MD • Arlene Reyes, MD • Fozia Akhtar Ali, MD

 BASICS

DESCRIPTION
- Parkinson disease (PD) is a progressive neurodegenerative disorder caused by loss of dopaminergic neurons in the substantia nigra pars compacta as well as other dopaminergic regions of the brain.
- Cardinal symptoms include resting tremor, rigidity, bradykinesia, and postural instability.
- Diagnosis is primarily clinical.

EPIDEMIOLOGY
Incidence
- 8 to 18.6 per 100,000 person-years
- Average age of onset: ~60 years
- Slightly more common in men than women

Prevalence
- Second most common neurodegenerative disease after Alzheimer disease
- 3.3/1,000 persons
- 0.3% of general population and 1–2% of those ≥60 years of age and up to 4% of those ≥80 years of age
- Affects approximately 1 million people in the United States and 5 million worldwide

ETIOLOGY AND PATHOPHYSIOLOGY
Dopamine depletion in the substantia nigra and the nigrostriatal pathways results in the major motor complications of PD.
- Pathologic hallmark: selective loss of dopamine-containing neurons in the pars compacta of the substantia nigra
- Loss of neurons accompanied by presence of Lewy bodies (hyaline inclusion bodies) and Lewy neuritis

Genetics
Mutations in multiple autosomal dominant and autosomal recessive genes are linked to PD/parkinsonian syndrome particularly when the age at symptom onset is <50 years. Genes investigated in PD include *SNCA*, Parkin, PINK1, DJ-1, and *LRRK2*.

RISK FACTORS
- Age and family history of PD or tremor. Weak association with exposure to toxins (herbicides and insecticides); relationship is not clear.
- Repeated head trauma and living in rural areas, drinking well water, working in a wood pulp mill
- History of smoking as well as coffee and caffeine intake may reduce risk.

COMMONLY ASSOCIATED CONDITIONS
Cognitive abnormalities, autonomic dysfunction (e.g., constipation, urinary urgency), sleep disturbances, mental status changes (depression, psychosis, hallucinations, dementia), orthostatic hypotension, and pain

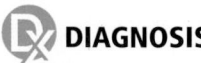 DIAGNOSIS

- Diagnosis is based on clinical features and response to dopaminergic therapy.
- Gold standard for diagnosis is neuropathologic exam.
- Generally, bradykinesia plus either tremor or rigidity must be present in order to make the diagnosis of idiopathic PD.

HISTORY
Symptoms often subtle or attributed to aging
- Decreased emotion displayed in facial features
- General motor slowing and stiffness (One or both arms do not swing with walk.)
- Resting tremor (often initially one hand)
- Speech soft/mumbling
- Falls/difficulty with balance; seen with disease progression

PHYSICAL EXAM
- Tremor
  - Resting tremor (4 to 6 Hz) that is often asymmetric
  - Disappears with voluntary movement
  - Frequently emerges in a hand while walking and may present as pill rolling
  - May also present in jaw, chin, lips, tongue
- Bradykinesia
- Rigidity: cogwheel (catching and releasing) or lead pipe (continuously rigid)
- Postural instability

DIFFERENTIAL DIAGNOSIS
- Essential tremor: Bradykinesia is not present; often symmetric and occurs mostly during action or when holding hands outstretched, nonresponsive to L-DOPA
- SWEDD: scans without evidence of dopaminergic deficit; isolated upper extremity resting and postural tremor resembling PD but failing to progress to generalized PD; no akinesia
- Dementia with Lewy bodies: characterized clinically by visual hallucinations, fluctuating cognition, and parkinsonism; dementia occurs concomitantly with or before the development of parkinsonism.
- Corticobasal degeneration: asymmetric parkinsonism, absence of tremor, no response to levodopa
- Multiple system atrophy: presets with parkinsonism and varying degrees of dysautonomia, cerebellar involvement, and pyramidal signs
- Progressive supranuclear palsy: impairment in vertical eye movements (particularly down gaze), hyperextension of neck, and early falling; pseudobulbar palsy
- Idiopathic basal ganglia calcification
- Associated neurodegenerative disorders: late stages of Alzheimer disease, Huntington disease, frontotemporal dementia, spinocerebellar ataxias
- Secondary parkinsonism:
  - Drug induced: reversible; may take weeks/months after offending medication is stopped; often bilateral symptoms
  - Neuroleptics (most common cause)
  - Antiemetics (e.g., prochlorperazine and promethazine), metoclopramide
  - SSRIs
  - Calcium channel blockers (e.g., flunarizine and cinnarizine)
  - Amiodarone
  - Lithium/valproic acid
  - Cholinergics
  - Chemotherapeutics
  - Amphotericin B
  - Estrogens

DIAGNOSTIC TESTS & INTERPRETATION
Initial Tests (lab, imaging)
- Diagnosis is mainly clinical, and there are no confirmatory physiologic or blood tests.
- Clear benefit from dopaminergic therapy is indicative of PD.
- Reduction in α-synuclein and DJ-1 protein can act as a qualitative feature in PD diagnosis.

- MRI of brain is nondiagnostic but can be used to rule out structural abnormalities.
- DaTscan: Striatal dopamine transporter imaging can distinguish PD and other parkinsonian syndromes but cannot differentiate between them.
- PET and single-photon emission CT may be helpful with diagnosis but are not required.

 TREATMENT

GENERAL MEASURES
- Multidisciplinary rehabilitation with standard physical and occupational therapy components to improve functional outcomes
- Physiotherapy to help with gait reeducation, enhancement of aerobic capacity, improvement in movement initiation, improvement in functional independence, and help with home safety

MEDICATION
- PD goal: Improve motor and nonmotor deficits.
- Agents are chosen based on patient age and symptoms present.

First Line
- First-line agents in early PD: levodopa, dopamine agonists, monoamine oxidase B (MAO-B) inhibitors (1)[A]
  - Levodopa combined with carbidopa is still the most effective treatment for symptoms of PD, particularly bradykinesia.
  - Levodopa versus dopamine agonist is controversial (2)[B]:
    ○ Most patients eventually will develop involuntary motor fluctuations or dyskinesias with levodopa. Younger patients are more likely to develop dyskinesias. Some recommend delaying initiation of levodopa to decrease drug-induced dyskinesias early in the disease.
    ○ Older patients often are less able to tolerate the adverse events of dopamine agonists.
    ○ All patients eventually will require levodopa.
  - MAO-B inhibitors (rasagiline) should be considered as initial monotherapy; currently being investigated for potential neuroprotective effects (2)[B]
- Carbidopa + levodopa (Carbidopa inhibits peripheral conversion of levodopa.)
  - Immediate release (Sinemet)
  - Tablets (mg): 10/100, 25/100, 25/250
  - Usual initial maintenance dose: 25/100 mg PO TID. Watch for nausea/vomiting, orthostatic hypotension, sedation, and vivid dreams.
  - Orally disintegrating (Parcopa)
  - Tablets (mg): 10/100, 25/100, 25/25
  - Sustained release (Sinemet CR):
  - Tablets (mg): 25/100, 50/200
  - Dose agents initially BID
- Carbidopa + levodopa + entacapone (Stalevo)
  - Tablets (mg): 12.5/50/200, 18.75/75/200, 25/100/200, 31.25/125/200, 37.5/150/200, 50/200/200
  - Addition of entacapone as a single agent should be initiated prior to use of this combination:
    ○ Once daily dose of carbidopa/levodopa has been identified, may convert to Stalevo
    ○ Dose of levodopa may need to be decreased with the addition of entacapone.
  - Side effects are the same, plus diarrhea and brownish orange urine.
- Dopamine-receptor agonists (nonergot): side effects: nausea, vomiting, hypotension, sedation, edema,

vivid dreaming, compulsive behavior, confusion, light-headedness, and hallucinations:
- Pramipexole (Mirapex): tablets (mg): 0.125, 0.25, 0.5, 1, 1.5
- Start with 0.125 mg TID; gradually increase every 5 to 7 days; usual maintenance of 0.5 to 1.5 mg TID
- CrCl 30 to 59 mL/min 0.125 mg PO BID
- CrCl 15 to 29 mL/min 0.125 mg PO daily
- Pramipexole ER (Mirapex ER): tablets (mg): 0.375, 0.75, 1.5, 3, 4.5; start with 0.375 PO daily.
- Ropinirole (Requip): tablets (mg): 0.25, 0.5, 1, 2, 3, 4, 5; start with 0.25 mg TID; increase gradually to 3 to 8 mg TID.
- Requip XL: tablets (mg): 2, 4, 6, 8, 12; start at a 2-mg dose once daily; increase in 1 to 2 weeks.
- Selective MAO-B inhibitors: side effects: insomnia, jitteriness, hallucinations; mostly found with selegiline; rasagiline similar adverse events as placebo in clinical trials. Rasagiline is metabolized via *CYP1A2*; caution with other medications using this enzyme system (e.g., ciprofloxacin):
  - Both agents contraindicated with meperidine and numerous other agents metabolized via *CYP1A2*
  - At therapeutic doses, unlikely to induce a "cheese reaction" (tyramine storm)
- Selegiline (Eldepryl)
  - Tablets: 5 mg; initiate 5 mg PO BID.
  - Orally disintegrating tablet (Zelapar): 1.25 mg; 1.25 mg PO daily for 6 weeks; increase as needed to max of 2.5 mg daily.
- Rasagiline (Azilect): tablets: 0.5 mg, 1.0 mg; initiate 0.5 to 1.0 mg daily.

Second Line
- Second-line agents in early PD: β-adrenergic antagonists (postural tremor), amantadine, anticholinergics (young patients with tremor); lack of good evidence for symptom control (1)[A]
- Dopamine agonists (ergot): Increased adverse event profile makes these agents nonpreferred to nonergot dopamine agonists; bromocriptine (Parlodel)
- Treatment of levodopa-induced motor complications
  - End of dose wearing off
  - Entacapone (with each levodopa dose) or rasagiline preferred (3)[B]
  - May also consider dopamine agonist, apomorphine, selegiline (4)[B]
  - Dyskinesias: typically occur at peak dopamine level
  - Amantadine may be considered; however, its efficacy is questionable (1)[B].
- Anticholinergic agents: avoided due to lack of efficacy (only useful for tremor) and increased adverse event profile, including blurred vision, confusion, constipation, dry mouth, memory difficulty, sedation, and urinary retention
  - Trihexyphenidyl
    - Tablets: 2 mg, 5 mg
    - Start with 1 to 2 mg daily; increase by 2 mg every 3 to 5 days until usual dose is 6 to 10 mg in 3 to 4 divided doses.
  - Benztropine (Cogentin)
    - Tablets: 0.5 mg, 1 mg, 2 mg
    - Start with 0.5 to 1.0 mg in 1 to 2 divided doses; increase by 0.5 mg every 5 to 6 days; usual dose is 1 to 2 mg/day in divided doses.
- *N*-methyl-D-aspartic acid antagonist: exact mechanism unknown, efficacy is questionable; may be useful for dyskinesias. Side effects: confusion, dizziness, dry mouth, livedo reticularis, and hallucinations
  - Amantadine (Symmetrel)
    - Tablets: 100 mg
    - Start with 100 mg BID; increase to 300 mg daily in divided doses; renally adjusted

- Catechol O-methyltransferase (COMT) inhibitors: entacapone preferred due to hepatotoxicity associated with tolcapone. Adverse events include nausea and orthostatic hypotension:
  - Entacapone (Comtan)
    - Tablets: 200 mg
    - 200 mg with each dose of carbidopa/levodopa; max dose 1,600 mg/day
  - Tolcapone (Tasmar)
    - Tablets: 100 mg, 200 mg
    - Start 100 mg TID; max dose 600 mg/day; must be taken with carbidopa/levodopa
    - Requires LFT monitoring
- Apomorphine (Apokyn): nonergot-derived dopamine agonist given SC for off episodes in advanced disease; adverse events: nausea, vomiting, dizziness, hallucinations, orthostatic hypotension, somnolence
  - Only for "off" episodes with levodopa therapy
  - Requires initial "test" dose (2 mg); monitor for orthostatic hypotension after initial dose; initiate an antiemetic (e.g., trimethobenzamide) 3 days prior to start and continue for 2 months. Avoid ondansetron (combination contraindicated due to profound hypotension) and dopamine antagonists, such as prochlorperazine and metoclopramide.
  - Effective dose ranges from 2 to 6 mg per injection.

ISSUES FOR REFERRAL
Early specialty referral (neurology) for patients with suspected PD to receive a more thorough clinical assessment and for treatment recommendations

ADDITIONAL THERAPIES
- Emotional and psychological support of patient family
- Physical therapy and endurance exercise has been shown to improve balance, muscle strength, walking speed.
- Speech therapy: may be helpful in improving speech volume and maintaining voice quality
- Nutrition should be high-fiber diet with adequate hydration and regular exercise.
- Treatment of nonmotor symptoms
  - Sildenafil to treat erectile dysfunction (5)[C]
    - Tablets: 25 mg, 50 mg, 100 mg
    - Take once daily 1 hour prior to sexual activity.
    - Caution with orthostatic hypotension; avoid with nitrates.
  - Polyethylene glycol to treat constipation (5)[C]
    - Mix 17 g in 8 oz of water once daily.
    - May titrate to one soft bowel movement per day
  - Carbidopa + levodopa to treat periodic limb movements (5)[B]

SURGERY/OTHER PROCEDURES
Deep brain stimulation is an effective therapeutic option for patients with motor complications refractory to best medical treatment who are healthy, have no significant comorbidities, are responsive to levodopa, and do not have depression or dementia.

 ## ONGOING CARE

DIET
- Increase dietary fluids and fiber for constipation.
- For dysphagia, consider soft food, swallowing evaluation, and increased time for meals.
- Avoid large, high-fat meals that slow digestion and interfere with medication absorption.

PATIENT EDUCATION
- www.apdaparkinson.org
- www.parkinson.org

PROGNOSIS
- PD is a chronic progressive disease; prognosis varies based on patient-specific symptoms.
- Increased mortality in PD; on average, survival is reduced by 5% every year of follow-up (4).

COMPLICATIONS
Most commonly, the result of adverse effects of medications used to treat PD

REFERENCES
1. Diaz NL, Waters CH. Current strategies in the treatment of Parkinson's disease and a personalized approach to management. *Expert Rev Neurother.* 2009;9(12):1781–1789.
2. Gazewood JD, Richards DR, Clebak K. Parkinson disease: an update. *Am Fam Physician.* 2013;87(4):267–273.
3. Nalls MA, Plagnol V, Hernandez DG, et al; and International Parkinson Disease Genomics Consortium. Imputation of sequence variants for identification of genetic risks for Parkinson's disease: a meta-analysis of genome-wide association studies. *Lancet.* 2011;377(9766):641–649.
4. Olanow CW, Stern MB, Sethi K. The scientific and clinical basis for the treatment of Parkinson disease (2009). *Neurology.* 2009;72(21 Suppl 4):S1–S136.
5. Zesiewicz TA, Sullivan KL, Arnulf I, et al; for Quality Standards Subcommittee of the American Academy of Neurology. Practice parameter: treatment of nonmotor symptoms of Parkinson disease: report of the Quality Standards Subcommittee of the American Academy of Neurology. *Neurology.* 2010;74(11):924–931.

ADDITIONAL READING
Macleod AD, Taylor KS, Counsell CE. Mortality in Parkinson's disease: a systematic review and meta-analysis. *Mov Disord.* 2014;29(13):1615–1622.

 ## CODES

ICD10
- G20 Parkinson's disease
- G21.9 Secondary parkinsonism, unspecified
- G31.83 Dementia with Lewy bodies

CLINICAL PEARLS
- The classic description for PD is shaky (pill-rolling tremor at rest), stiff (cogwheel rigidity), slow (bradykinesia), and stumbling (shuffling gait).
- No cure—goals are to delay disease progression and relieve symptoms.
- Emphasize the importance of exercise and movement to help preserve function.
- Pharmacotherapeutic regimens need to be individualized based on age/specific symptoms.

PARONYCHIA

Nancy V. Nguyen, DO

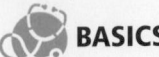

BASICS

DESCRIPTION
- Superficial inflammation of the lateral and posterior folds of skin surrounding the fingernail or toenail
  - Acute: characterized by pain, erythema, and swelling; usually a bacterial infection appears after trauma. It can progress to abscess formation.
  - Chronic: characterized by swelling, tenderness, cuticle elevation, and nail dystrophy and separation lasting at least 6 weeks, or recurrent episodes of acute eponychial inflammation and drainage
  - May be considered work-related among bartenders, waitresses, nurses, and others who often wash their hands
- System(s) affected: skin and nail bed
- Synonym(s): eponychia, perionychia

Pediatric Considerations
Less common in pediatric age groups. Thumb/finger-sucking is a risk factor (anaerobes and *Escherichia coli* may be present).

EPIDEMIOLOGY
Incidence
- Common in the United States
- Predominant age: all ages
- Predominant sex: female > male

ETIOLOGY AND PATHOPHYSIOLOGY
- Acute: *Staphylococcus aureus* (1) most common and *Streptococcus pyogenes* (1); less frequently, *Pseudomonas pyocyanea* and *Proteus vulgaris*. In digits exposed to oral flora especially in pediatric age group, consider *Eikenella corrodens*, *Fusobacterium*, and *Peptostreptococcus*.
- Chronic: eczematous reaction with secondary *Candida albicans* (~95%)
- A paronychial infection commonly starts in the lateral nail fold.
- Recurrent inflammation, persistent edema, and fibrosis of nail folds cause nail folds to round up and retract, exposing nail grooves to irritants, allergens, and pathogens.
- Inflammation compromises ability of proximal nail fold to regenerate cuticle leading to decreased vascular supply. This can cause decrease efficacy of topical medications.
- Early in the course, cellulitis alone may be present. An abscess can form if the infection does not resolve quickly.

RISK FACTORS
- Acute: direct or indirect trauma to cuticle or nail fold, manicure/sculptured nails, nail biting, and thumb sucking and predisposing conditions such as diabetes mellitus (DM)
- Chronic: frequent immersion of hands in water with excoriation of the lateral nail fold (e.g., chefs, bartenders, housekeepers, swimmers, dishwashers, nurses), DM, immunosuppression (reported association with antiretroviral therapy for HIV and with use of epidermal growth factor inhibitors)

GENERAL PREVENTION
- Acute: Avoid trauma such as nail biting; prevent thumb sucking.
- Chronic: Avoid allergens; keep fingers/hands dry; wear rubber gloves with a cotton liner. Prevent excoriation of the skin.
- Keep nails short. Avoid manicures. Apply moisturizer after washing hands.
- Good glycemic control in diabetic patients

COMMONLY ASSOCIATED CONDITIONS
- DM
- Eczema or atopic dermatitis
- Certain medications: antiretroviral therapy (2) (especially protease inhibitors, indinavir, and lamivudine, in which toes more commonly involved) (2)
- Immunosuppression (3)

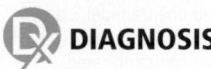

DIAGNOSIS

HISTORY
- Localized pain or tenderness, swelling, and erythema of posterior or lateral nail folds
  - Acute: fairly rapid onset
  - Chronic: at least 6 weeks' duration
- Previous trauma (bitten nails, ingrown nails, manicured nails)
- Contact with herpes infections
- Contact with allergens or irritants (frequent water immersion, latex) (3)

PHYSICAL EXAM
- Acute: red, warm, tender, tense posterior or lateral nail fold ± abscess
- Chronic: swollen, tender, boggy nail fold ± abscess
- Occasional elevation of nail bed
- Separation of nail fold from nail plate
- Red, painful swelling of skin around nail plate
- Fluctuance, purulence at the nail margin, or purulent drainage
- Secondary changes of nail platelike discoloration
- Suspect *Pseudomonas* if with green changes in nail (chloronychia).
- Positive fluctuation when mild pressure over the area causes blanching and demarcation of the abscess.
- Chronic: retraction of nail fold and absence of adjacent healthy cuticle, thickening of nail plate with prominent transverse ridges known as Beau lines and discoloration; multiple digits typically involved

DIFFERENTIAL DIAGNOSIS
- Felon (abscess of fingertip pulp; urgent diagnosis required)
- Eczema
- Herpetic whitlow (similar in appearance, very painful, often associated with vesicles)
- Allergic contact dermatitis (latex, acrylic)

- Psoriasis especially acute flare
- Proximal/lateral onychomycosis (nail folds not predominantly involved)
- Pemphigus vulgaris
- Acute osteomyelitis of the distal phalanx
- Reiter disease
- Pustular psoriasis
- Dermatomyositis
- Malignancy: squamous cell carcinoma of the nail, malignant melanoma, metastatic disease

DIAGNOSTIC TESTS & INTERPRETATION
None required unless condition is severe; resistant to treatment or if recurrence or methicillin-resistant *S. aureus* (MRSA) is suspected, then
- Gram stain
- Culture and sensitivity
- Potassium hydroxide wet mount plus fungal culture especially in chronic
- Drugs that may alter lab results: use of over-the-counter antimicrobials or antifungals

Diagnostic Procedures/Other
- Incision and drainage recommended for suppurative cases or cases not responding to conservative management or empiric antibiotics
- Tzanck testing or viral culture in suspected viral cases
- Biopsy in cases not responding to conservative management or when malignancy suspected

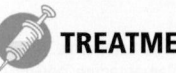

TREATMENT

GENERAL MEASURES
- Acute: warm compresses/soaks, elevation, splint protection if pain severe
- Abscesses should be opened to promote drainage.
- Insert nail elevator or hypodermic needle at junction of the affected nail fold and nail to facilitate drainage. If no drainage occurs, use a needle or scalpel to open skin directly above abscess.
- Chronic: Keep fingers dry; apply moisturizing lotion after hand washing; avoid exposure to irritants; improved diabetic control

MEDICATION
First Line
- Tetanus booster when indicated
  - Acute (mild cases, no abscess formation) Burow solution (aluminum acetate solution) and vinegar (acetic acid) combined with warm soaks
  - Topical antibiotic cream alone or in combination with a topical steroid
  - Antibiotic cream applied TID–QID after warm soak (e.g., mupirocin or gentamicin or a topical fluoroquinolone) for 5 to 10 days
  - If eczematous, low potent topical steroid applied BID (e.g., betamethasone 0.05% cream) for 7 to 14 days

- Acute (no exposure to oral flora). Treat for 7 days.
  - Dicloxacillin 250 mg QID
  - Cephalexin 500 mg TID–QID
- Acute (exposure to oral flora). Treat for 7 days. Cover for *Eikenella*.
  - Amoxicillin clavulanate: 875 mg/125 mg BID; pediatric, 45 mg/kg q12h (for <40 kg) doxycycline 100 mg BID or trimethoprim/sulfamethoxazole BID or ciprofloxacin 500 to 750 mg BID; *plus* clindamycin 300 to 450 mg TID–QID; pediatric, 10 mg/kg q8h or metronidazole 500 mg TID
- Acute (suspected MRSA). Treat for 7 days.
  - Trimethoprim/sulfamethoxazole 160 mg/800 mg BID
  - Doxycycline 100 mg BID
  - Clindamycin 300 to 450 mg TID–QID
- Chronic
  - Topical steroids: betamethasone 0.05%; applied BID for 7 to 14 days (4)[B]
  - Topical antifungal: clotrimazole or nystatin; applied topically TID for up to 30 days
  - Other topical: Tacrolimus 0.1% ointment BID for up to 21 days has been shown to be effective but is more expensive.
  - Doxycycline 100 mg BID for paronychia caused by antiepidermal growth factor receptor antibodies

Second Line
- Systemic antifungals (rarely needed, use if topical fails)
  - Itraconazole 200 mg for 90 days (may have longer action because it is incorporated into nail plate); pulse therapy may be useful (i.e., 200 mg BID for 7 days, repeated monthly for 2 months) (1)[C].
  - Terbinafine 250 mg/day for 6 weeks (fingernails) or 12 weeks (toenails)
  - Fluconazole 100 mg daily for 7 to 14 days
  - Ciclopirox 0.77% topical suspension BID for 2 to 4 weeks along with strict irritant avoidance (5)[B]
- Antipseudomonal drugs (e.g., ceftazidime, aminoglycosides) when pseudomonas is suspected

ISSUES FOR REFERRAL
Chronic: In treatment failure, consider biopsy and/or, in cases of chronic paronychia, referral for possible partial excision of the nail fold or eponychial marsupialization with or without complete nail removal or Swiss roll technique.

SURGERY/OTHER PROCEDURES
- Incision and drainage of abscess, if present
- A subungual abscess or ingrown nail requires partial or complete removal of nail with phenolization of germinal matrix.
- Swiss roll technique for chronic and severe acute paronychia with runaround abscess involving both nail folds (4)[A]
- Recalcitrant cases may also need nail removal.

 ## ONGOING CARE

FOLLOW-UP RECOMMENDATIONS
- Acute: Postdrainage care consists of warm soaks or soaking with Burow solution or acetic acid BID–TID for 2 to 3 days unless Swiss roll technique used (1)[C].
- Chronic: Avoid frequent immersion, triggers, allergens, or nail biting and finger sucking.

DIET
If patient is diabetic, consider appropriate dietary and medication changes for better control.

PATIENT EDUCATION
- Avoid trimming cuticles, avoid nail trauma, and stress importance of good diabetic control and diabetic education.
- Avoid contact irritants; use rubber gloves with cotton liners to avoid exposure to excess moisture.
- Use moisturizing lotion after washing hands; do not bite nails/suck on fingers.

PROGNOSIS
- With adequate treatment and prevention, healing can be expected in 1 to 2 weeks.
- Chronic paronychia may respond slowly to treatment, taking weeks to months.
- If no response in chronic lesions, rarely benign or malignant neoplasm may be present and referral should be considered.

COMPLICATIONS
- Acute: subungual abscess
- Chronic: nail thickening, discoloration of nail, and nail loss

REFERENCES

1. Leggit JC. Acute and chronic paronychia. *Am Fam Physician*. 2017;96(1):44–51.
2. Wollina U. Acute paronychia: comparative treatment with topical antibiotic alone or in combination with corticosteroid. *J Eur Acad Dermatol Venereol*. 2001;15(1):82–84.
3. Tosti A, Piraccini BM, D'Antuono A, et al. Paronychia associated with antiretroviral therapy. *Br J Dermatol*. 1999;140(6):1165–1168.
4. Relhan V, Goel K, Bansal S, et al. Management of chronic paronychia. *Indian J Dermatol*. 2014;59(1):15–20.
5. Daniel CR III, Daniel MP, Daniel J, et al. Managing simple chronic paronychia and onycholysis with ciclopirox 0.77% and an irritant-avoidance regimen. *Cutis*. 2004;73(1):81–85.

ADDITIONAL READING

- Chiriac A, Brzezinski P, Foia L, et al. Chloronychia: green nail syndrome caused by *Pseudomonas aeruginosa* in elderly persons. *Clin Interv Aging*. 2015;10:265–267.
- Hengge UR, Bardeli V. Images in clinical medicine. Green nails. *N Engl J Med*. 2009;360(11):1125.
- Iorizzo M. Tips to treat the 5 most common nail disorders: brittle nails, onycholysis, paronychia, psoriasis, onychomycosis. *Dermatol Clin*. 2015;33(2):175–183.
- Rigopoulos D, Gregoriou S, Belyayeva E, et al. Efficacy and safety of tacrolimus ointment 0.1% vs. betamethasone 17-valerate 0.1% in the treatment of chronic paronychia: an unblinded randomized study. *Br J Dermatol*. 2009;160(4):858–860.
- Rockwell PG. Acute and chronic paronychia. *Am Fam Physician*. 2001;63(6):1113–1116.
- Shroff PS, Parikh DA, Fernandez RJ, et al. Clinical and mycological spectrum of cutaneous candidiasis in Bombay. *J Postgrad Med*. 1990;36(2):83–86.
- Tosti A, Piraccini BM, Ghetti E, et al. Topical steroids versus systemic antifungals in the treatment of chronic paronychia: an open, randomized double-blind and double dummy study. *J Am Acad Dermatol*. 2002;47(1):73–76.

 ## SEE ALSO

Onychomycosis

 ## CODES

ICD10
- L03.019 Cellulitis of unspecified finger
- L03.039 Cellulitis of unspecified toe
- L03.011 Cellulitis of right finger

CLINICAL PEARLS
- Consider tetanus booster when indicated.
- Consider incision and drainage when appropriate. Send culture.
- For chronic paronychia, topical steroid is first-line treatment. Consider other differentials in nonresponders (e.g., rare causes: Raynaud, metastatic cancer, psoriasis, drug toxicity).
- For suspected pseudomonal infections, use a topical fluoroquinolone and acetic acid.
- For chronic nonhealing lesion, consider dermatology referral.
- Consider possibility of cancer if chronic inflammatory process is unresponsive to treatment.
- Consider presence of more than one nail disease at the same time (e.g., paronychia and onychomycosis).

PAROTITIS, ACUTE AND CHRONIC

Jeanne R. Delgado, MD • Kathy Ferrer, MD, AAHIVS

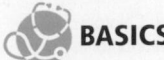 BASICS

DESCRIPTION
- Parotitis is inflammation of the parotid gland caused by infection, noninfectious systemic illnesses, mechanical obstruction, or medications.
- Can be unilateral or bilateral, acute or chronic
- The parotid gland is the largest of the salivary glands, located lateral to the masseter muscle anteriorly and extending posteriorly over the sternocleidomastoid muscle behind the angle of the mandible.
- It produces exclusively serous secretions, which lack the bacteriostatic properties of mucinous secretions, making the parotid gland more susceptible to infection than other salivary glands.
- The parotid duct, also called the Stensen duct, pierces the buccinator muscle to enter the buccal mucosa just opposite the 2nd maxillary molar.
- The branches of the 7th cranial nerve or "facial nerve" bisect the gland into lobes.
- The parotid gland contains 3 to 24 lymph nodes.

EPIDEMIOLOGY
- Viral parotitis is the most common cause of parotitis in children; exact incidence is unknown and has decreased since the advent of the mumps vaccine.
- Acute bacterial parotitis occurs more frequently in elderly patients, neonates (especially preterm infants), and postoperative patients.
- Juvenile recurrent parotitis (JRP) is the second most common inflammatory cause of parotitis in children in the United States; first episode usually occurs between the ages of 3 and 6 years.
- Chronic parotitis mainly affects adults, more often females. The average age of presentation is between 40 and 60 years.
- Chronic bilateral parotid enlargement is a common manifestation of HIV infection; for perinatally HIV-infected children, the average age of onset for parotid enlargement is 5 years.

ETIOLOGY AND PATHOPHYSIOLOGY
- Acute viral parotitis begins as a systemic infection that localizes to the parotid gland, resulting in inflammation and swelling of the gland.
  - Mumps, or paramyxovirus, has a predilection for the parotid gland and classically has been linked to parotitis. The virus replicates in the upper respiratory tract and spreads by direct contact or airborne transmission.
  - Symptoms usually begin 16 to 18 days after infection.
- Acute bacterial parotitis results from stasis of salivary flow that allows retrograde introduction of bacterial pathogens into the gland, resulting in localized infection.
- Acute parotitis pathogens
  - Viral
    - Paramyxovirus (mumps), parainfluenza virus types 1 and 3, influenza A, coxsackievirus, Epstein-Barr virus (EBV)
    - Cytomegalovirus (CMV) and adenovirus have been seen in patients with HIV.
  - Bacterial
    - *Staphylococcus aureus* and anaerobes (oral flora) most commonly
    - *Streptococcus pneumoniae*, viridans streptococci, *Escherichia coli*, and *Haemophilus influenzae* (less common)

- Other gram-negative rods, such as *Klebsiella*, *Enterobacter*, and *Pseudomonas*, can be seen in chronically ill or hospitalized patients.
  - *Bartonella henselae* in patients with cat exposure (rare)
  - Fungal
    - *Candida* has been isolated in chronically ill or hospitalized patients.
    - *Actinomyces* in patients with a history of trauma or dental caries
- Acute, recurrent parotitis
  - JRP may be secondary to chronic inflammation; etiology is unknown, but a genetic predisposition may exist.
  - Mechanical: Repeated sialolith formation leads to ductal wall damage, fibrosis, and stricture formation.
  - Pneumoparotitis may occur when air is trapped in the ducts of the parotid gland; seen in wind instrument players, glass blowers, scuba divers, and with dental cleaning
  - Certain medications and chronic diseases (see "Risk Factors") predispose to chronic parotitis.
  - "Anesthesia mumps": Possible mechanisms include transient mechanical compression of the Stensen duct by airway devices, loss of muscle tone around the Stensen orifice after neuromuscular relaxants, increased salivary secretion, and increased flexion or rotation of the head during general anesthesia.
- Chronic parotitis in HIV-infected patients can be due to presence of benign lymphoepithelial cysts, follicular hyperplasia of parotid lymph nodes, or diffuse infiltrative lymphocytosis syndrome (DILS), causing infiltration of the parotid gland by CD8 cells.
  - Parotitis may be secondary to immune reconstitution after initiation of antiretroviral therapy.
- Pediatric considerations include case reports of acute parotitis as a symptom of Kawasaki disease.

RISK FACTORS
- Acute viral parotitis: lack of mumps, measles, rubella (MMR) vaccination
- Acute bacterial parotitis
  - Conditions that predispose to salivary stasis, such as dehydration, debilitation, poor oral hygiene, Sjögren syndrome, cystic fibrosis, bulimia/anorexia, sialolithiasis (stones), ductal stenosis, trauma
  - Immunosuppression, HIV, chemotherapy, radiation, malnutrition, alcoholism
- Neonatal parotitis: prematurity, dehydration, low birth weight, ductal obstruction, oral trauma, structural abnormalities, immunosuppression
- JRP: dental malocclusion, congenital duct malformation, genetic factors, immunologic anomalies
- Drug-induced parotitis: medications such as anticholinergics, ACE inhibitors (captopril), antihistamines, tricyclic antidepressants, antipsychotics (phenylbutazone, thioridazine, clozapine), iodine (contrast media), and L-asparaginase
- Chronic parotitis: ductal stenosis, HIV, tuberculosis, Sjögren syndrome, sarcoidosis, uremia, diabetes, gout, and atopy

GENERAL PREVENTION
- MMR vaccination with the first dose between 12 and 15 months and second dose between 4 and 6 years of age; childhood mumps vaccination does not guarantee prevention, due to possibility of waning immunity with time.
  - Students in post–high school education without documented mumps immunity should receive 2 doses of the MMR vaccine, 28 days apart.

- Pregnant women should not receive the mumps vaccine, and pregnancy should be avoided for 4 weeks after vaccination.
- Maintain adequate hydration and good dental hygiene; smoking cessation, abstinence from alcohol, and avoidance of chronic purging

COMMONLY ASSOCIATED CONDITIONS
Mumps, HIV, Sjögren syndrome, sarcoidosis, sialolithiasis

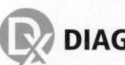 DIAGNOSIS

HISTORY
- Acute parotitis presents with sudden-onset pain and swelling of the cheek typically extending to and obscuring the angle of the mandible.
  - Viral parotitis is usually bilateral and accompanied by a prodrome of malaise, anorexia, headaches, myalgias, arthralgias, and fever; typically, overlying skin is not warm or erythematous, and no pus is reported at the opening of Stensen duct.
  - Bacterial parotitis is typically unilateral with induration, warmth, and erythema over the affected cheek; fever is often present.
  - JRP is usually unilateral; pain and swelling resolve within 2 weeks, and exacerbations occur until puberty; purulent exudate not typical unless superinfection occurs
  - Sialolithiasis is characterized by recurrent acute swelling and pain, exacerbated by eating; sialolithiasis affects the submandibular gland more frequently.
  - Other reported symptoms include trismus (inability to open mouth), pain exacerbated by chewing or worsened by foods that stimulate production of saliva, dry mouth with abnormal taste, difficulty with drinking/eating, anorexia, or dehydration.
- Chronic parotitis presents with recurrent or chronic nontender swelling of one or both parotid glands; can have periods of remission lasting weeks to years
  - Sjögren syndrome, sarcoidosis, HIV, tuberculosis
  - May predispose to superinfection, which would present similarly to acute parotitis

PHYSICAL EXAM
- Parotitis is characterized by swelling or enlargement of the parotid gland(s) overlying the masseter muscle; may obscure the angle of the mandible or cause the ear to protrude upward and outward
- Palpation of the parotid gland is best done by using one hand to start at the attachment of the earlobe and palpating anteriorly and inferiorly along the mandibular ramus while the other hand simultaneously palpates the Stensen duct orifice inside the oral cavity.
  - Tender and bilateral suggest viral etiology, whereas tender, erythematous, warm, and unilateral suggest bacterial etiology.
  - Nontender in chronic parotitis (HIV, tuberculosis, Sjögren syndrome, sarcoidosis)
- Trismus, halitosis, and dental decay may be noted.
- Pus from the Stensen duct is suggestive of bacterial parotitis or superinfection; opening of duct may appear edematous and erythematous in both bacterial and viral parotitis.
- In JRP, the Stensen duct is often enlarged, dilated, erythematous, and swollen.
- Facial nerve palsy can be seen in severe cases.

DIFFERENTIAL DIAGNOSIS
- Lymphoma, neoplasm, lymphangitis, cervical adenitis, otitis externa, dental abscess, odontogenic infections, Ludwig angina, and cellulitis

- Parotid swelling or enlargement typically obscures the angle of the mandible (unlike cervical adenitis).
- Involvement of the Stensen duct is unique to parotitis.

DIAGNOSTIC TESTS & INTERPRETATION

- History and physical exam are usually sufficient for diagnosis.
- Performing aerobic culture and Gram stain of purulent drainage from Stensen duct or aerobic and anaerobic culture from needle aspiration of gland or abscess can be helpful to identify causative organism.
  - Anaerobic culture from Stensen duct will likely contain oropharyngeal contamination; it is recommended to perform anaerobic cultures only from needle aspirate fluid.
- Acute bacterial parotitis often demonstrates an elevated white blood cell count and amylase.
- For suspected mumps, the CDC recommends collecting a buccal/oral swab for mumps RT-PCR and a blood specimen for IgM and IgG serologies. Mumps RT-PCR is best obtained from a buccal swab within 1 to 3 days of parotitis onset by massaging the parotid gland area for 30 seconds prior to collection. In areas of high vaccination rates, IgM may be falsely negative necessitating correlation with clinical symptoms. A 4-fold increase of mumps IgG antibody from acute to convalescent phase indicates infection; normal <1:20
- Consider sending EBV titers and respiratory virus PCR panel if suspected viral parotitis; CMV titers should be sent in immunocompromised patients.
- For chronic, recurrent, or nontender parotitis, obtain HIV test, PPD, SS-A/SS-B antibodies, rheumatoid factor, and antinuclear antibodies to evaluate for underlying etiology.
- Consider obtaining ultrasound or CT scan of parotid area to assess for abscess, cystic masses, tumors, ductal stenosis, or sialolithiasis if no response to initial treatment. JRP patients have diffuse microcalcifications on US.
- Consider sialography for chronic parotitis to assess the anatomy and functional integrity of the gland; can be diagnostic and therapeutic

Diagnostic Procedures/Other

Consider performing a biopsy or fine-needle aspiration of gland if there is suspicion for tuberculosis, Sjögren syndrome, or sarcoidosis.

Test Interpretation

- Findings characteristic of HIV are described in the "Etiology and Pathophysiology" section.
- Noncaseating granulomas may be seen in sarcoidosis, and caseating granulomas may be found in tuberculosis and *B. henselae* infections.

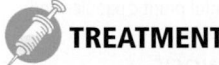 ## TREATMENT

GENERAL MEASURES

- Usually a self-limiting course that requires supportive treatment with rest, adequate hydration, analgesia, and antipyretics
  - Can stimulate glands to produce saliva by sucking on hard candies or glycerin swabs
  - Local heat and gentle massage of gland
  - For chronic presentations, encourage good dental hygiene and treat underlying etiology of parotitis.
- Patients diagnosed with mumps should be isolated with standard and droplet precautions for 5 days after onset of parotid swelling. Mumps is a nationally reportable disease.
- During a mumps outbreak, the CDC supports administration of MMR vaccine even in fully vaccinated individuals.

- A third vaccine dose has been shown to decrease risk of mumps and improve outbreak control, especially in individuals whose second MMR was >13 years prior (1)[A].
- Underimmunized individuals should get 2 doses of the MMR vaccine separated by at least 28 days. This will not change the disease course if the person is already infected but will help prevent future infection.

MEDICATION

- Viral parotitis: There is no evidence for the role of immunoglobulin for PEP or treatment; may initiate the below antibiotics if patient is toxic appearing or has an unclear diagnosis
- Acute bacterial parotitis
  - Outpatient management: amoxicillin/clavulanate or ciprofloxacin and clindamycin
  - Chronically ill or hospitalized: ampicillin/sulbactam or clindamycin and nafcillin; if MRSA is probable, consider vancomycin or linezolid.
- Sjögren syndrome recurrent parotitis: Pilocarpine and cevimeline can stimulate saliva production and inhibit ascending infection as well as provide symptomatic relief. Alternatively, botulism toxin injection may be a consideration in these patients because it limits production of saliva and sialectasis (2)[B].

SURGERY/OTHER PROCEDURES

- Consider needle aspiration for bacterial parotitis with abscess formation or clinical deterioration with increasing pain, erythema, and swelling not responding to medication.
- For sialolithiasis, ductal stenosis, chronic obstruction related to Sjögren syndrome, or for patients with >1 recurrences per year, consult otolaryngologist for possible sialendoscopy, duct ligation, ductoplasty, or parotidectomy (3)[B].
- Consider superficial parotidectomy for severe recurrent parotid infections in patients with underlying predisposing etiology.
- Pediatric considerations: Sialendoscopy with steroid irrigation is effective and safe for the treatment of JRP; irrigation alone may be just as effective; performing parotid ultrasound is recommended first to differentiate JRP from ductal stones (4)[A].
- Sclerotherapy with methyl violet or tetracycline has been shown to be effective in the treatment of cysts in HIV parotitis and is also considered definitive treatment for chronic parotitis (5)[C].

ADMISSION, INPATIENT, AND NURSING CONSIDERATIONS

- Admission is recommended for patients with comorbidities, systemic involvement, and inability to tolerate PO as well as neonates and patients for whom close outpatient follow-up is not feasible.
- Referral to otolaryngology is needed if salivary gland mass is seen, malignancy is suspected, or no improvement with antibiotic therapy.

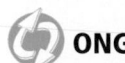 ## ONGOING CARE

FOLLOW-UP RECOMMENDATIONS

Antibiotic therapy for bacterial parotitis combined with adequate hydration should result in improvement within 48 hours; if not, patient should be reevaluated.

DIET

- Ensure adequate fluid intake.
- Hard or sour candies to promote salivary flow

PROGNOSIS

- Viral infection in immunocompetent individuals often resolves with excellent prognosis.

- Parotid cysts found in HIV-infected patients are usually benign lymphoepithelial lesions with infrequent malignant transformation.
- Increased incidence of malignant lymphoma or lymphoepithelial carcinoma may be seen in patients with Sjögren syndrome.

COMPLICATIONS

- For mumps, potential complications include orchitis, oophoritis, mastitis, aseptic meningitis, encephalitis, pancreatitis, myocarditis, sensorineural hearing loss, and nephritis.
- Untreated bacterial parotitis can lead to local extension, abscess formation, and facial paralysis.

REFERENCES

1. Cardemil CV, Dahl RM, James L, et al. Effectiveness of a third dose of MMR vaccine for mumps outbreak control. *N Engl J Med*. 2017;377(10):947–956.
2. O'Neil LM, Palme CE, Riffat F, et al. Botulinum toxin for the management of Sjögren syndrome-associated recurrent parotitis. *J Oral Maxillofac Surg*. 2016;74(12):2428–2430.
3. Guo YF, Sun NN, Wu CB, et al. Sialendoscopy-assisted treatment for chronic obstructive parotitis related to Sjogren syndrome. *Oral Surg Oral Med Oral Pathol Oral Radiol*. 2017;123(3):305–309.
4. Berlucchi M, Rampinelli V, Ferrari M, et al. Sialoendoscopy for treatment of juvenile recurrent parotitis: the Brescia experience. *Int J Pediatr Otorhinolaryngol*. 2018;105:163–166.
5. Berg EE, Moore CE. Office-based sclerotherapy for benign parotid lymphoepithelial cysts in the HIV-positive patient. *Laryngoscope*. 2009;119(5):868–870.

ADDITIONAL READING

- Armstrong MA, Turturro MA. Salivary gland emergencies. *Emerg Med Clin North Am*. 2013;31(2):481–499.
- Brook I. The bacteriology of salivary gland infections. *Oral Maxillofac Surg Clin North Am*. 2009;21(3):269–274.
- Hamborsky J, Kroger A, Wolfe S. *Epidemiology and Prevention of Vaccine-Preventable Diseases*. 13th ed. Washington, DC: Public Health Foundation; 2015.
- Hernandez S, Busso C, Walvekar RR. Parotitis and sialendoscopy of the parotid gland. *Otolaryngol Clin North Am*. 2016;49(2):381–393.

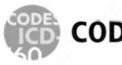 ## CODES

ICD10

- K11.20 Sialoadenitis, unspecified
- K11.21 Acute sialoadenitis
- K11.23 Chronic sialoadenitis

CLINICAL PEARLS

- History and physical exam are usually sufficient for diagnosis (parotid swelling and tenderness with or without purulent drainage from the Stensen duct).
- In recurrent or chronic cases, consider other underlying etiologies, such as HIV.
- *S. aureus* and anaerobes are the most common organisms isolated in acute bacterial parotitis.
- Encouraging good oral hygiene and adequate hydration in chronically ill, debilitated, and hospitalized patients can reduce occurrence.

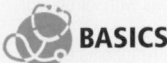

PARVOVIRUS B19 INFECTION

David L. Anderson, MD

BASICS

DESCRIPTION
- Human parvovirus B19 is the primary cause of acute erythema infectiosum (EI, or fifth disease).
- Individuals with increased RBC turnover (e.g., sickle cell anemia [SS]) are more susceptible to transient aplastic crisis (TAC). In immunocompromised individuals, pure red cell aplasia (PRCA) and chronic anemia are significant complications. In normal hosts, arthritis and arthralgias are common complications.
- System(s) affected: hematologic/lymphatic/immunologic, musculoskeletal, skin/exocrine, possibly central nervous system (CNS), cardiac, renal

Pregnancy Considerations
A documented acute infection during pregnancy should prompt referral to a maternal–fetal medicine specialist. Maternal parvovirus B19 infection between 9 and 20 weeks' gestation has the highest fetal risk.

EPIDEMIOLOGY
- Parvovirus infection is common in childhood.
- EI has an extremely low mortality rate.
- Peak age for EI is 4 to 12 years.
- Males and females are equally affected.
- Women more likely to develop postinfectious arthritis
- No known racial predilection
- In temperate climates, infections often occur from late winter to early summer.
- Local outbreaks may occur every 2 to 4 years.

Prevalence
Extremely common in the United States. Based on IgG serology:
- 1 to 5 years of age: 2–15% seropositive
- 6 to 15 years of age: 20–40% seropositive
- 16 to 40 years of age: 50–60% seropositive
- >40 years of age: 70–85% seropositive

ETIOLOGY AND PATHOPHYSIOLOGY
- Small (20 to 25 mm), nonenveloped, single-stranded DNA virus in *Parvoviridae* family
  - Only known parvovirus to infect humans
- Natural host of B19 is human erythroid progenitor.
- Respiratory, hematogenous, and vertical transmission are sources of human spread.
- 4- to 14-day incubation. Rash and joint symptoms occur 2 to 3 weeks after initial infection.
- Most contagious 5 to 10 days after exposure
- EI rash thought to be autoimmune due to IgM complexes concurrent with viral clearance
- Cytotoxic infection of proerythroblasts reduces RBC production.

Genetics
Erythrocyte P antigen–negative individuals are resistant to infection.

RISK FACTORS
- School-related epidemic and nonimmune household contacts have a secondary attack rate of 20–50%.
- Highest secondary attack rates are for daycare providers and school personnel in contact with affected children.
- Increased cell turnover (e.g., hemoglobinopathy, SS, thalassemia) increases risk for TAC.
- Immunodeficiency (e.g., HIV, congenital) increases risk of PRAC and chronic anemia.
- As many as 40% of pregnant women are not immune; 1.5% seroconversion rate per year

GENERAL PREVENTION
- Respiratory spread; hand washing and barrier precautions
- Droplet precautions are recommended around patients with TAC, chronic infection, or anemia.
- Difficult to eliminate exposure because the period of maximal contagion occurs prior to the onset of clinical symptoms (rash)
- Pregnant health care workers should not care for patients with TAC.
- No significant risk of infection based on occupational exposure. Exclusion from the workplace is neither necessary nor recommended.
- No preventive vaccine is available.

COMMONLY ASSOCIATED CONDITIONS
- Nondegenerative arthritis
  - In adults, 80% of patients may manifest polyarthritis and/or arthralgia (female > male).
  - In children, joint symptoms are less common.
  - Knees, hands, wrists, and ankles (frequently symmetric) are most commonly involved.
  - Joint symptoms usually subside within 3 weeks but may persist for months. Routine radiography is not necessary.
- TAC
  - Involves patients with increased RBC turnover (SS, spherocytosis, thalassemia) or decreased RBC production (iron deficiency anemia)
  - Presents with fatigue, weakness, lethargy, and pallor (anemia)
  - Aplastic event may be life-threatening but is typically self-limited. Reticulocytes typically reappear in 7 to 10 days with full recovery in 2 to 3 weeks.
  - In children with sickle cell hemoglobinopathies and heredity spherocytosis, fever is the most common symptom (73%); rash uncommon in these patients
- Chronic anemia
  - Seen in immunocompromised individuals (HIV, cancer, transplant) with poor IgM response
  - Usually no clinical manifestations (fever, rash, or joint symptoms)

- Fetal/neonatal infection (1)
  - Risk of transplacental spread of virus is ~33% in infected mothers.
  - Test pregnant women with a rash or arthralgias consistent with parvovirus B19.
  - Clinical manifestations vary. Many patients seroconvert without symptoms and have a normal pregnancy. Other patients develop variable degrees of fetal hydrops. 2nd- and 3rd-trimester pregnancy loss can occur without hydrops.
  - Suspect B19 infection in cases of nonimmune fetal hydrops.
  - Fetal bone marrow is primarily impacted. RBC survival is shortened resulting in anemia and (potentially) high-output cardiac failure.
  - >95% of fetal complications (fetal hydrops and death) occur within 12 weeks of acute maternal parvovirus B19 infection.
  - Risk of fetal loss is highest (2–5%) in the 1st trimester.
  - Infants requiring intrauterine transfusions due to parvovirus B19 infection are at risk for long-term neurodevelopmental impairment.
- Papular purpuric gloves and socks syndrome (PPGSS) is an uncommon dermatosis associated with parvovirus B19 infection. It results in a petechial and ecchymotic rash of the hands and feet associated with febrile tonsillopharyngitis and oral ulcerations (2).

 DIAGNOSIS

HISTORY
- Rash
- Headache
- Pharyngitis
- Coryza and rhinorrhea
- Arthralgias and arthritis
- Nausea and GI disturbances are more frequent and severe in adults (nonspecific flulike illness).
- Pruritus (especially soles of feet)
- Fever, myalgia, and malaise

PHYSICAL EXAM
- "Slapped cheek" appearance is a well-known facial rash that spares the nasolabial folds.
- A lacy, reticular rash on the trunk, buttocks, and limbs often follows 1 to 4 days later lasting 1 to 6 weeks.
- The rash may be pruritic and recurrent, exacerbated by bathing, exercise, sun exposure, heat, or emotional stress.
- B19 may manifest as painful pruritic papules and purpura on the hands and feet.

DIFFERENTIAL DIAGNOSIS
- Rubella
- Enteroviral disease
- Systemic lupus erythematosus
- Drug reaction
- Lyme disease
- Rheumatoid arthritis

DIAGNOSTIC TESTS & INTERPRETATION

Initial Tests (lab, imaging)

- No need for routine lab studies in typical cases. Diagnosis is clinical; illness is mild and self-limiting.
- IgG and IgM serology in immunocompetent patients
- B19-specific DNA polymerase chain reaction (PCR) testing for fetal infection (via cord blood or amniotic fluid) as well as for patients with chronic infection or those who are immunocompromised
- PCR increases diagnostic sensitivity and specificity to confirm infections in IgM-negative patients.
- For patients with TAC, anemia and reticulocytopenia are noted. IgM antibodies are present by day 3, and IgG antibodies are detectable at time of clinical recovery. PCR shows high levels of viremia.
- Pregnant women exposed to B19 require serial IgG and IgM serology to assess fetal risk.

Follow-Up Tests & Special Considerations

Fetal/neonatal infection (3)[C]

- To exclude congenital B19 in infants with negative B19 IgM, follow IgG serology over the 1st year of life.
- Maternal serum α-fetoprotein may be increased with hydrops fetalis.
- Serial fetal ultrasound (US) to assess for hydrops in cases of documented acute maternal infection in the 1st trimester, looking for ascites, pericardial effusion, oligohydramnios, cardiomegaly, and placental thickening
- Weekly peak systolic velocity measurements of the middle cerebral artery by Doppler US is recommended to evaluate for heart failure, fetal anemia, and the potential need for intrauterine transfusion (>1.5 MoM).
- Cerebral MRI to assess for CNS damage in infected neonates with prolonged hydrops fetalis or hematocrit <15%

Diagnostic Procedures/Other

- Skin biopsy is usually normal but may show mild inflammation consisting of perivascular infiltrates of mononuclear cells.
- In stillbirths related to maternal B19 infection, virus can be detected in all tissues.
- In hydrops fetalis, nucleated RBCs may have intranuclear inclusion bodies.

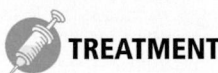

TREATMENT

GENERAL MEASURES

- No therapy is usually needed (4)[C].
- Cessation of immunosuppressive therapy allows some patients to clear chronic infections.
- B19-associated anemia in HIV-positive patients may resolve with highly active antiretroviral therapy.

MEDICATION

First Line

- Anti-inflammatory agents for arthritic symptoms
- Antipyretics for fever. Avoid aspirin in children.

Second Line

- RBC transfusions for aplastic crisis
- Intravenous immunoglobulin (IVIG) for B19-related refractory anemia or PRAC, especially in immunodeficient states (5)[C]
- Intrauterine RBC transfusions reduce mortality in cases of fetal hydrops.

ISSUES FOR REFERRAL

- Acute infection during pregnancy should prompt referral to a maternal–fetal medicine specialist.
- TAC patients require treatment by a hematologist.
- Patients with chronic or abnormal B19 infections may benefit from consultation with immunology or infectious disease specialists.

ADMISSION, INPATIENT, AND NURSING CONSIDERATIONS

- Outpatient management is typical for EI.
- Inpatient management for aplastic crisis, which may require RBC transfusions

 ## ONGOING CARE

FOLLOW-UP RECOMMENDATIONS

Patient Monitoring

Periodic blood counts for anemic patients

PATIENT EDUCATION

- Parvovirus B19 (fifth disease): http://www.cdc.gov/parvovirusB19/fifth-disease.html
- Parvovirus B19: What You Should Know: http://www.aafp.org/afp/2007/0201/p377.html
- Parvovirus B19 infection and pregnancy: http://www.cdc.gov/parvovirusB19/pregnancy.html
- March of Dimes Fifth Disease and Pregnancy: http://www.marchofdimes.org/complications/fifth-disease-and-pregnancy.aspx
- Pregnant women should avoid exposure to patients with active/chronic infections. Exclusion of pregnant women from the workplace where EI is occurring is not recommended because of likelihood of prior exposure.
- Children with typical rash are no longer infectious and may attend childcare or school.

PROGNOSIS

- Usually self-limited
- Joint symptoms subside in weeks (often by 2 weeks but may last months).
- ~20% of infections result in delayed virus elimination and viremia persisting for several months to years.
- Full recovery from aplastic crisis in 2 to 3 weeks

COMPLICATIONS

Conditions associated with B19 but where causality is unconfirmed

- Chronic fatigue syndrome
- Glomerulonephritis, nephrotic syndrome, and other renal diseases
- Hepatitis
- Neurologic manifestations/stroke/meningoencephalitis
- Henoch-Schönlein purpura, idiopathic thrombocytopenic purpura, and vasculitis
- Myocarditis and pericarditis
- Hemophagocytic syndrome

REFERENCES

1. de Jong EP, de Haan TR, Kroes AC, et al. Parvovirus B19 infection in pregnancy. *J Clin Virol*. 2006;36(1):1–7.
2. Santonja C, Nieto-González G, Santos-Briz Á, et al. Immunohistochemical detection of parvovirus B19 in "gloves and socks" papular purpuric syndrome: direct evidence for viral endothelial involvement. Report of three cases and review of literature. *Am J Dermatopathol*. 2011;33(8):790–795.
3. de Jong EP, Walther FJ, Kroes AC, et al. Parvovirus B19 infection in pregnancy: new insights and management. *Prenat Diagn*. 2011;31(5):419–425.
4. Servey JT, Reamy BV, Hodge J. Clinical presentations of parvovirus B19 infection. *Am Fam Physician*. 2007;75(3):373–376.
5. Orange JS, Hossny EM, Weiler CR, et al. Use of intravenous immunoglobulin in human disease: a review of evidence by members of the Primary Immunodeficiency Committee of the American Academy of Allergy, Asthma and Immunology. *J Allergy Clin Immunol*. 2006;117(Suppl 4):S525–S553.

ADDITIONAL READING

- Azevedo KM, Setúbal S, Camacho LA, et al. Parvovirus B19 seroconversion in a cohort of human immunodeficiency virus-infected patients. *Mem Inst Oswaldo Cruz*. 2012;107(3):356–361.
- Beigi RH, Wiesenfeld HC, Landers DV, et al. High rate of severe fetal outcomes associated with maternal parvovirus B19 infection in pregnancy. *Infect Dis Obstet Gynecol*. 2008;2008:524601.
- De Jong EP, Lindenburg IT, van Klink JM, et al. Intrauterine transfusion for parvovirus B19 infection: long-term neurodevelopmental outcome. *Am J Obstet Gynecol*. 2012;206(3):204.e1–204.e5.
- Lamont RF, Sobel JD, Vaisbuch E, et al. Parvovirus B19 infection in human pregnancy. *BJOG*. 2011;118(2):175–186.
- Snyder M, Wallace R. Clinical inquiry: what should you tell pregnant women about exposure to parvovirus? *J Fam Pract*. 2011;60(12):765–766.

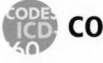 ## CODES

ICD10

- B34.3 Parvovirus infection, unspecified
- B08.3 Erythema infectiosum [fifth disease]

CLINICAL PEARLS

- Parvovirus B19 infection is usually a benign, self-limited illness with no long-term effects.
- The rash of EI, a "slapped cheek" appearance, signifies that the patient is no longer infectious.
- Patients with increased RBC turnover (SS, thalassemia) are at risk for TAC.
- Immunocompromised patients are at risk for chronic anemia.
- Documentation of acute infection in pregnant women <20 weeks' gestation merits maternal–fetal consultation.

PATELLOFEMORAL PAIN SYNDROME (PFPS)

David L. Lee, MD • Munima Nasir, MD

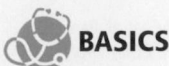

BASICS

DESCRIPTION
- Pain in or around the patella that increases after prolonged sitting, squatting, kneeling, or ascending/descending stairs
- Synonyms: anterior knee or retropatellar pain syndrome, chondromalacia patella, runner's knee
- System(s) affected: musculoskeletal

EPIDEMIOLOGY
Prevalence
- Annual prevalence of 29% in adolescents and 23% in adults (1)
- In a military population, prevalence of 12% in males and 15% in females (2)

ETIOLOGY AND PATHOPHYSIOLOGY
Multifactorial etiology, including:
- Weakness and incorrect firing of knee extensors (3)
- Impaired gluteal muscle function resulting in increased hip joint adduction and internal rotation (3)
- Decreased strength and altered recruitment patterns of core muscles during movement (3)
- Decreased muscle length, particularly of the quadriceps, may also contribute (3).

Genetics
Unknown

RISK FACTORS
- Recent research has found that age, height, weight, body mass index, body fat, Q angle, and hip weakness are no longer considered risk factors for patellofemoral pain syndrome (PFPS) (4).
- In a military population: quadriceps weakness (4)
- In adolescents: increased hip adduction strength, although this may represent increased activity level (4)

GENERAL PREVENTION
Strengthening and stretching exercises, particularly hip abductors and terminal extension of the quadriceps

COMMONLY ASSOCIATED CONDITIONS
- Overuse
- Knee ligament injury/surgery

- Patellar tendinopathy
- Prolonged synovitis
- IT band friction syndrome

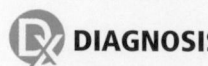

DIAGNOSIS

HISTORY
- An accurate history to differentiate between pain and instability (pain quality, location, swelling, giving way, locking, grinding, inciting events, overuse, and history of trauma)
- Most common symptom: diffuse anterior knee pain exacerbated during or after physical activity
- Pain with squatting, descending or ascending stairs, ambulating over uneven surfaces, or running (2)

PHYSICAL EXAM
- Single leg squat: 80% of patients with PFPS will demonstrate pain with this maneuver (2)[A].
- Palpation: In patients with pain on palpation of the patellar edges, 75% are found to have PFPS (2)[A].
- Evaluate knee range of motion (ROM) and for effusion.
- Compression/patellar grind test: With patient supine, place one hand superior to the patella and push the patella inferiorly. Ask the patient to contract the quadriceps; pain upon contraction is consistent with PFPS; grinding may indicate chondromalacia of the patellofemoral joint. These maneuvers have low sensitivity and limited diagnostic accuracy for diagnosing PFPS (2)[A]

DIFFERENTIAL DIAGNOSIS
- Prepatellar bursitis
- Patellar and quadriceps tendinitis/tendinopathy
- Chondromalacia patella
- Patellofemoral arthrosis
- Patellar subluxation and dislocation
- Knee ligamentous and meniscal pathology
- IT band syndrome
- Plica syndrome
- Osteochondral defect
- Osteochondritis dissecans

- Sinding-Larsen-Johansson syndrome
- Osgood-Schlatter disease
- Knee infection
- Neuroma or nerve entrapment
- Benign or malignant tumors
- Referred pain from hip or spine

DIAGNOSTIC TESTS & INTERPRETATION
- None indicated. In general, imaging is unnecessary and not helpful in the diagnosis of PFPS. If imaging is indicated because of severity, atypical symptoms, or persistence of symptoms despite treatment, plain films with four views of the knee are recommended to view patellar tilt and to rule out other etiologies of anterior knee pain:
  - Lateral
  - Merchant (also called sunrise)
  - Standing anteroposterior
  - Posteroanterior tunnel views
- CT can be used to grade patellar malalignment.
- Radiographic findings may not correlate with symptoms.

Follow-Up Tests & Special Considerations
Radiographic images may be normal until late stages, when the posterior patellar surface becomes irregular and cartilage erosion is radiographically detectable.

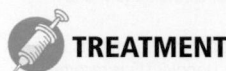

TREATMENT

GENERAL MEASURES
- Conservative therapy is the gold standard (3,5)[A].
- Initial goal of therapy is to increase strength, flexibility, and ROM to enable practice of correct motion (3)[A].
- Supervised therapy should focus on hip abductors and external rotators, knee extensors, and core muscles (3,5)[A].
- Stretching of the muscles surrounding the hip and knee, particularly proprioceptive neuromuscular facilitation stretches (5)[A]

MEDICATION

- Acetaminophen or NSAIDs for pain management
- The evidence for oral glucosamine and chondroitin sulfate and hyaluronic acid injections is lacking and is not routinely recommended for treatment of patellofemoral pain.

ISSUES FOR REFERRAL

- Referral for surgery after all conservative measures fails. Surgery is rarely needed.
- Recalcitrant cases can be associated with psychosocial issues including depression and abuse. Referral to a mental health care professional is critical in these cases.

ADDITIONAL THERAPIES

- Ice packs after activity have been found to improve clinical symptoms.
- Combination therapy in addition to an exercise program with other modalities such as patellar taping or manual therapy may be beneficial (1)[A].
- Ankle and foot orthoses may offer some relief in the short term, but there is lack of strong evidence to support its use, particularly in the long term (1,5)[B].

SURGERY/OTHER PROCEDURES

- Exercise therapy is first line.
- For patients with a tight lateral retinaculum and lateral patellar tilt: operative realignment of the patella
- For patients with a defect in the cartilage of the patellofemoral joint, cartilage resurfacing/restoration

 ## ONGOING CARE

PATIENT EDUCATION

- Educate patient on importance of participation and compliance in a specialized exercise program with a physical therapist.
- Provide a list of physical therapy locations for the patient.

PROGNOSIS

- PFPS is not self-limiting and can become chronic (6).
- Patellofemoral pain for longer than 12 months duration is associated with long-term pain (6).
- Long-term PFPS is not associated with structural patellofemoral joint OA (6).

REFERENCES

1. Collins NJ, Barton CJ, van Middelkoop M, et al. 2018 Consensus statement on exercise therapy and physical interventions (orthoses, taping and manual therapy) to treat patellofemoral pain: recommendations from the 5th International Patellofemoral Pain Research Retreat, Gold Coast, Australia, 2017. *Br J Sports Med*. 2018;52(18):1170–1178.
2. Crossley KM, Stefanik JJ, Selfe J, et al. 2016 Patellofemoral pain consensus statement from the 4th International Patellofemoral Pain Research Retreat, Manchester. Part 1: terminology, definitions, clinical examination, natural history, patellofemoral osteoarthritis and patient-reported outcome measures. *Br J Sports Med*. 2016;50(14):839–843.
3. Hiemstra LA, Kerslake S, Arendt EA. Clinical rehabilitation of anterior knee pain: current concepts. *Am J Orthop (Belle Mead NJ)*. 2017;46(2):82–86.
4. Neal BS, Lack SD, Lankhorst NE, et al. Risk factors for patellofemoral pain: a systematic review and meta-analysis. *Br J Sports Med*. pii:bjspors-2017-098890.
5. van der Heijden RA, Lankhorst NE, van Linschoten R, et al. Exercise for treating patellofemoral pain syndrome. *Cochrane Database Syst Rev*. 2015;(1):CD010387.
6. Lankhorst NE, van Middelkoop M, Crossley KM, et al. Factors that predict a poor outcome 5–8 years after the diagnosis of patellofemoral pain: a multicentre observational analysis. *Br J Sports Med*. 2016;50(14):881–886.

ADDITIONAL READING

- Callaghan MJ, Selfe J. Patellar taping for patellofemoral pain syndrome in adults. *Cochrane Database Syst Rev*. 2012;(4):CD006717.
- Fredericson M, Yoon K. Physical examination and patellofemoral pain syndrome. *Am J Phys Med Rehabil*. 2006;85(3):234–243.
- Heintjes E, Berger MY, Bierma-Zeinstra SM, et al. Pharmacotherapy for patellofemoral pain syndrome. *Cochrane Database Syst Rev*. 2004;(3):CD003470.

- Matthews M, Rathleff MS, Claus A, et al. Can we predict the outcome for people with patellofemoral pain? A systematic review on prognostic factors and treatment effect modifiers. *Br J Sports Med*. 2017;51(23):1650–1660.
- Saltychev M, Dutton RA, Laimi K, et al. Effectiveness of conservative treatment for patellofemoral pain syndrome: a systematic review and meta-analysis. *J Rehabil Med*. 2018;50(5):393–401.
- Smith BE, Selfe J, Thacker D, et al. Incidence and prevalence of patellofemoral pain: a systematic review and meta-analysis. *PLoS One*. 2018;13(1):e0190892.
- Rothermich MA, Glaviano NR, Li J, et al. Patellofemoral pain: epidemiology, pathophysiology, and treatment options. *Clin Sports Med*. 2015;34(2):313–327.

 ## SEE ALSO

Algorithm: Knee Pain

 ## CODES

ICD10

- M25.569 Pain in unspecified knee
- M25.561 Pain in right knee
- M25.562 Pain in left knee

CLINICAL PEARLS

- PFPS is the most common cause of anterior knee pain in active adults.
- The clinical diagnosis is made by an accurate history and physical exam.
- Well-designed exercises geared at core, hip, and lower extremity flexibility and strength are the most effective evidence-based treatments.
- PFPS is not self-limiting and needs to be treated.

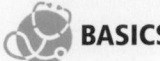

PEDICULOSIS (LICE)
Muhammad M. Hossain, DO • Sangili Chandran, MD, MS(ortho)

BASICS

DESCRIPTION
- A contagious parasitic infection caused by ectoparasitic blood-feeding insects (lice)
- Two species of lice infest humans:
  - *Pediculus humanus* has two subspecies: the head louse (var. *capitis*) and the body louse (var. *corporis*). Both species are 1 to 3 mm long, flat, and wingless and have three pairs of legs that attach closely behind the head.
  - *Pthirus pubis* (pubic or crab louse): resembles a sea crab and has widespread claws on the 2nd and 3rd legs
- System(s) affected: skin/exocrine
- Synonym(s): lice; crabs

EPIDEMIOLOGY
Incidence
- In the United States: 6 to 12 million new cases per year
- Predominant age
  - Head lice: most common in children 3 to 12 years of age; more common in girls than boys
  - Pubic lice: most common in adults

Prevalence
Head lice: 1–3% in industrialized countries

ETIOLOGY AND PATHOPHYSIOLOGY
- Characteristics of lice:
  - Adult louse is dark grayish and moves quickly but does not jump or fly.
  - Eggs (nits) camouflage with the individuals' hair color and are cemented to the base of the hair shaft (within 4 mm of the scalp).
  - Nits (empty egg casings) appear white (opalescent) and remain cemented to the hair shaft.
  - Lice feed solely on human blood by piercing the skin, injecting saliva (anticoagulant properties to allow for blood meal), and then ingesting blood.
  - Itching is a hypersensitivity reaction to the saliva of the feeding louse.
- Transmission: direct human-to-human contact
  - Head lice: direct head-to-head contact or contact with infested fomite (less likely)
  - Body lice: contact with contaminated clothing or bedding
  - Pubic lice: typically transmitted sexually (fomite transmission much less likely)

RISK FACTORS
- General: overcrowding and close personal contact
- Head lice
  - School-aged children, gender (girls; longer hair)
  - Sharing combs, hats (including helmets), clothing, and bed linens
  - African Americans rarely have head lice; theories include twisted hair shaft and increased use of pomades
- Body lice: poor hygiene, homelessness
- Pubic lice: promiscuity (very high transmission rate)

GENERAL PREVENTION
- Environmental measures: Wash, dry-clean, or vacuum items that may have contacted infected individuals.
- Screen and treat affected household contacts.
- Head lice: Follow-up by school nurses may help to prevent recurrence and spread.

- Pubic lice: Limit the number of sexual partners (condoms do not prevent transmission nor does shaving pubic hair).
- Body lice: proper body hygiene

COMMONLY ASSOCIATED CONDITIONS
Up to 1/3 of patients with pubic lice have at least one concomitant STI.

DIAGNOSIS

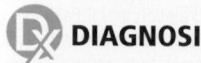

HISTORY
- Pruritus is common, often worse at night.
- Often associated with "outbreak" in school settings
- Investigate contacts of infected individuals.

PHYSICAL EXAM
- Diagnosis is confirmed by visualization of live lice.
- *P. capitis* (head lice)
  - Found most often on the back of the head and neck and behind the ears (warmer areas)
  - Eyelashes may be involved.
  - Eggs, found cemented on the base of a hair shaft, are difficult to remove.
  - Pruritus may be accompanied by local erythema and small papules.
  - May see excoriations around hairline
  - Scratching can cause inflammation and secondary bacterial infection.
  - Pyoderma and lymphadenopathy may occur in severe infestation.
- *P. corporis* (body lice)
  - Poor general hygiene
  - Adult lice and nits in the seams of clothing
  - Intense pruritus involving area covered by clothing (trunk, axillae, and groin)
  - Uninfected bites present as erythematous macules, papules, and wheals.
  - Pyoderma and excoriation may be seen.
- *P. pubis* (pubic lice)
  - Pubic hair is the most common site, but lice may spread to hair around anus, abdomen, axillae, chest, beard, eyebrows, and eyelashes.
  - Eggs are present at the base of hair shafts.
  - Anogenital pruritus
  - Blue macules may be seen in surrounding skin.
  - Delay in treatment may lead to development of groin infection and regional adenopathy.

DIFFERENTIAL DIAGNOSIS
- Scabies and other mite species that can cause cutaneous reactions in humans
- Dandruff and other hair debris sometimes look like head lice eggs and nits but are less adherent.

DIAGNOSTIC TESTS & INTERPRETATION
- Diagnosis is based on visualization of live louse.
- Head lice: Comb hair thoroughly with a fine-toothed louse comb (0.2 to 0.3 mm between teeth) to identify live lice (1)[C]. Wet the hair to limit static electricity, which repels lice. Simple visual inspection has same sensitivity as wet combing but is only ~25% as effective as dry combing with a metal comb (2).
- Body lice: Examine the seams of clothing to locate lice and eggs (3).
- Lice and eggs are more easily visualized with a microscope.
- In contrast to dandruff, eggs and nits cannot be removed easily from a hair shaft.

Follow-Up Tests & Special Considerations
- Empty nits remain on hair shafts for months after eradication of the live infestation. Wood lamp exam: Live nits fluoresce white and empty nits fluoresce gray.
- Pubic lice: Evaluate for concurrent STIs.

TREATMENT

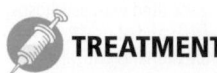

GENERAL MEASURES
- Head lice: Clean items that have been in contact with the head of the infected individual within 48 hours.
- Wash all bedding, towels, clothes, headgear, combs, brushes, and hair accessories in hot water (60°C).
- Vacuum furniture and carpets.
- Seal any personal articles that cannot be washed in hot water, dry-cleaned, or vacuumed in a plastic bag and store for at least 2 weeks.
- Examine and treat household members and close contacts concurrently.
- Insecticide sprays are not necessary.
- Pubic lice: Avoid sexual activity until all partners are successfully treated.
- Nit and egg removal
  - Remove eggs within 1 cm of the scalp to prevent reinfestation.
  - After treatment with shampoo or lotion, eggs and nits remain in the scalp or pubic hair until mechanically removed. Hair conditioner facilitates nit removal.
  - Eggs and nits best removed with a fine nit comb

MEDICATION
Permethrin (over the counter [OTC]), synergized pyrethrin (OTC), spinosad (Rx), benzyl alcohol (Rx), malathion (Rx), and topical ivermectin (Rx) are all effective for head lice (1)[A],(2)[C]. Permethrin, synergized pyrethrin, and malathion are effective for pubic lice (2)[C]:
- Permethrin generally preferred because it may have residual activity for up to 3 weeks. However, use of newer shampoos and conditioners may reduce the residual effect (1)[C].
- Malathion and spinosad are considered second line for head lice but may not require a second application due to ovicidal activity (1)[B],(2)[C].
- Ivermectin 0.5% lotion and benzyl alcohol 5% lotion are also effective for head lice (1,2)[C].

First Line
- Head and pubic lice:
  - Pyrethrum insecticides: Permethrin 1% cream rinse (Nix) or pyrethrins 0.33% with piperonyl butoxide 4% (synergized pyrethrin, Rid, Pronto) are first line unless there is proven resistance in the community.
    - Apply for 10 minutes and then wash.
    - Reapply synergized pyrethrin in 7 to 10 days (day 9 is optimal); also be necessary with permethrin, if live lice are observed
    - Side effects: application-site erythema, ocular erythema, and application-site irritation
- Body lice: best treated with synergized pyrethrin lotion applied once and left on for several hours
- Eyelash infestation: Apply petroleum jelly BID for 10 days.

- Precautions:
  - Pyrethrin: Avoid in patients with ragweed allergy (may cause respiratory symptoms).
  - Pediculicides should never be used to treat eyelash infections.

Second Line

- Head lice and pubic lice
  - Malathion 0.5% lotion (Ovide)
    - Apply for 8 to 12 hours and then wash off.
    - Excipients isopropyl alcohol (78%) and terpineol (12%) may contribute to its efficacy:
      - Flammable and has a bad odor
      - Despite ovicidal activity, a second application may be necessary after 7 to 10 days (day 9 is optimal) if live lice are observed.
  - Lindane 1% shampoo, no longer recommended
    - Apply for 4 minutes and then wash (do not repeat).
    - Side effects: neurotoxicity (seizures, muscle spasms), aplastic anemia
    - Contraindications: uncontrolled seizure disorder, premature infants
    - Precautions: Do not use on excoriated skin, in immunocompromised patients, conditions that increase seizure risk, or with medications that decrease seizure threshold.
    - Possible interactions: concomitant use with medications that lower the seizure threshold
- Head lice
  - Spinosad 0.9% lotion (Natroba)
    - Apply to dry hair and scalp for 10 minutes and then rinse with warm water. Repeat in 7 days if live lice are observed.
    - Side effects: application-site erythema, ocular erythema, and application-site irritation
  - Benzyl alcohol 5% lotion (Ulesfia)
    - Apply to dry hair using enough to saturate scalp and hair (amount depends on hair length), rinse after 10 minutes; repeat in 1 week.
    - Side effects: pruritus, erythema, pyoderma, ocular irritation, application-site irritation
  - Ivermectin 0.5% lotion (Sklice)
    - Apply to dry hair by using enough to saturate the scalp and hair (max. 4 oz) and then rinse after 10 minutes.
    - Side effects: burning sensation at application site, dandruff, dry skin, eye irritation
- Mechanical removal of lice and nits by wetting hair and then systematically combing with a fine-toothed comb every 3 to 4 days for 2 weeks to remove all lice as they hatch

ALERT

Lindane: FDA black box warning of severe neurologic toxicity (use only when first-line agents have failed). The National Pediculosis Association strongly advises against using lindane at all.

Pediatric Considerations

- Avoid synergized pyrethrin and permethrin in infants <2 months of age. Avoid benzyl alcohol, topical ivermectin, and spinosad in children <6 months of age and avoid malathion in children <2 years of age.
- Lindane: not recommended

Pregnancy Considerations

Permethrin, synergized pyrethrin, malathion, spinosad, and benzyl alcohol are pregnancy Category B. Lindane and topical ivermectin are pregnancy Category C.

ADDITIONAL THERAPIES

- For "difficult to treat" cases of head lice, oral ivermectin 400 μg/kg (not approved by the FDA for lice), given twice at a 7-day interval, is superior to topical 0.5% malathion lotion (4,5)[B].
- Ivermectin: 200 μg/kg PO repeated after 10 days or 300 μg/kg PO repeated after 7 days
  - Should not be used in children <15 kg; pregnancy Category C
  - Not approved by the FDA for lice
- Dual therapy with permethrin 1% and oral trimethoprim/sulfamethoxazole (TMP/SMX) only for cases of multiple treatment failures or suspected cases of lice-related resistance to therapy (TMP/SMX is not approved by the FDA for lice)
- Permethrin 5% cream (Rx) is not FDA-approved for lice and is unlikely to be effective for lice that are resistant to 1% cream rinse (1)[B].

COMPLEMENTARY & ALTERNATIVE MEDICINE

- Cetaphil lotion: dry-on, suffocation-based pediculicide (not approved by the FDA for lice)
  - Apply thoroughly to hair, comb, and then dry with hair dryer; shampoo after 8 hours.
  - Repeat once a week until cured, up to a maximum of three applications.
- Dimethicone 4% lotion: Apply to hair for 8 hours; repeat in 1 week (not approved by the FDA for lice).
- No home remedies (e.g., vinegar, isopropyl alcohol, olive oil, ylang ylang oil, mayonnaise, melted butter, and petroleum jelly) are proven as effective.
- Herbal shampoos and pomades have not been evaluated in clinical trials.
- Lavender oil and tea tree oil have been implicated in triggering prepubertal gynecomastia in boys and should not be used to treat lice.
- Electronic louse combs have not proven effective and are not approved by the FDA.

 ## ONGOING CARE

FOLLOW-UP RECOMMENDATIONS

Children may return to school after completing topical treatment, even if nits remain in place. No-nit policies are unnecessary.

Patient Monitoring

Drug resistance should be suspected if no dead lice are observed 8 to 12 hours after treatment.

PATIENT EDUCATION

- National Pediculosis Association: http://www.headlice.org/
- CDC: https://www.cdc.gov/parasites/lice/
- http://www.guideline.gov/content.aspx?id=46429&search=lice

PROGNOSIS

- With appropriate treatment, >90% cure rate
- Recurrence is common, mainly from reinfection or treatment nonadherence. Resistance to synthetic pyrethroids is increasing.

COMPLICATIONS

- Poor sleep due to pruritus
- Persistent itching may be caused by too frequent use of the pediculicide.
- Missed school; social stigma
- Secondary bacterial infections
- Body lice can transmit typhus and trench fever.

REFERENCES

1. Devore CD, Schutze GE; for Council on School Health and Committee on Infectious Diseases, American Academy of Pediatrics. Head lice. *Pediatrics*. 2015;135(5):e1355–e1365.
2. Burgess IF. Current treatments for pediculosis capitis. *Curr Opin Infect Dis*. 2009;22(2):131–136.
3. Gunning K, Pippitt K, Kiraly B, et al. Pediculosis and scabies: treatment update. *Am Fam Physician*. 2012;86(6):535–541.
4. Chosidow O, Giraudeau B, Cottrell J, et al. Oral ivermectin versus malathion lotion for difficult-to-treat head lice. *N Engl J Med*. 2010;362(10):896–905.
5. Feldmeier H. Treatment of pediculosis capitis: a critical appraisal of the current literature. *Am J Clin Dermatol*. 2014;15(5):401–412.

ADDITIONAL READING

- Cole SW, Lundquist LM. Spinosad for treatment of head lice infestation. *Ann Pharmacother*. 2011;45(7–8):954–959.
- Sanchezruiz WL, Nuzum DS, Kouzi SA. Oral ivermectin for the treatment of head lice infestation. *Am J Health Syst Pharm*. 2018;75(13):937–943.
- Webber E, McConnell S. Lice update: management and treatment in the home. *Home Healthc Now*. 2018;36(5):289–294.

 ## SEE ALSO

Arthropod Bites and Stings; Scabies

CODES

ICD10

- B85.0 Pediculosis due to Pediculus humanus capitis
- B85.1 Pediculosis due to Pediculus humanus corporis
- B85.3 Phthiriasis

CLINICAL PEARLS

- School-based no-nit policies are not necessary because empty nits may remain on hair shafts for months after successful eradication.
- Improper product application is a common cause of treatment failure.
- Prevalence of resistant infestations is increasing; if no dead lice are observed 8 to 12 hours after treatment, suspect resistance and use an alternative agent.
- Routine retreatment on day 9 is recommended for nonovicidal products (permethrin and synergized pyrethrin).
- With all treatment options, reinspect hair after 7 to 9 days, and if live lice are detected, repeat treatment on day 9.

PELVIC INFLAMMATORY DISEASE

Juliana Zamora Cubillos, MD • Miguel A. Palacios, MD

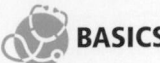

BASICS

DESCRIPTION
- Pelvic inflammatory disease (PID) is an infectious and inflammatory disorder of the upper female genital tract, including the uterus, fallopian tubes, ovaries, and adjacent pelvic structures. It is community acquired from sexually transmitted organisms (1).
- Salpingitis is the most important component due to its impact on future fertility.
- Mild to moderate PID is defined as the absence of a tubo-ovarian abscess (TOA). Severe disease is defined as severe systemic symptoms OR the presence of a TOA (2).
- Diagnosis may be challenging due to variation in signs and symptoms because many patients with PID have subtle or nonspecific symptoms (3).

EPIDEMIOLOGY
- Predominant age: 15 to 25 years; this number has remained constant since early 1900s.
- Predominant sex: female only

Incidence
PID is the most common gynecologic reason for admission in the United States accounting for 18 per 10,000 recorded hospital discharges (2). The estimated prevalence of self-reported lifetime PID was 4.4% in sexually experienced women ages 18 to 44 years (4).
- Lifetime prevalence has decreased steadily since 1995 across all races (4).
- Among those with no history of prior STI, lifetime PID prevalence was higher in black versus white women (6% vs. 2.7%). Among women with a prior STI, lifetime prevalence of PID was similar by race (10% vs. 10.3%) (4).

ETIOLOGY AND PATHOPHYSIOLOGY
Multiple organisms may be etiologic agents in PID. Most cases are polymicrobial. The proportion of PID cases due to *Chlamydia trachomatis* and *Neisseria gonorrhoeae* appears to be declining. Fewer than 50% of women diagnosed with acute PID have a test positive for either of these organisms.
- *C. trachomatis*, *N. gonorrhoeae*, genital tract mycoplasmas (particularly *Mycoplasma genitalium*), aerobic and anaerobic (*Bacteroides fragilis*), and vaginal flora (e.g., *Prevotella*, peptostreptococci, *Gardnerella vaginalis*, *Escherichia coli*, *Haemophilus influenzae*) are recognized as etiologic agents. Mixed infections are common (1,5,6).
- Many nongonococcal, nonchlamydial microorganisms recovered from upper genital tract in acute PID are associated with bacterial vaginosis.
- The precise mechanism by which microorganisms ascend from the lower genital tract is unclear. Possible mechanisms include the following: (i) travel from cervix to endometrium to salpinx to peritoneal cavity; (ii) lymphatic spread via infection of the parametrium (from an IUD); and (iii) hematogenous route, although this is rare.
- Of cases, 75% occur within 7 days of menses, when cervical mucus favors ascent of organisms.

RISK FACTORS
- Sexually active and age <25 years
- First sexual activity at young age (<15 years)
- New/multiple sexual partners
- Nonbarrier contraceptive methods (i.e., oral contraceptive pills)

- Previous history of PID; 20–25% will have a recurrence.
- Cervical ectopy
- History of *C. trachomatis*; 10–40% will develop PID.
- History of gonococcal cervicitis; 10–20% will develop PID.
- Gynecologic procedures that break the cervical barrier such as endometrial biopsy, curettage, hysterosalpingography, hysteroscopy, in vitro fertilization, and insertion of IUD in the last 6 weeks

GENERAL PREVENTION
- Educational programs about safer sex practices such as barrier contraceptives, especially condoms and spermicidal creams or sponges, provide some protection.
- The U.S. Preventive Services Task Force recommends screening for chlamydia in all sexually active women <25 years and in those 25 years and older at increased risk (new sex partner/multiple sex partners). Moderate-quality evidence suggests that chlamydia screening reduces cases of PID (3)[A].
- Routine STI screening in pregnancy
- Early medical care with occurrence of genital lesions or abnormal discharge

COMMONLY ASSOCIATED CONDITIONS
- If PID is suspected in a patient with an IUD and a pelvic abscess is present, an *Actinomyces* infection requiring penicillin treatment may be present.
- Rupture of an adnexal abscess is rare but life threatening. Early surgical exploration is mandatory (5).
- Chlamydial or gonococcal perihepatitis may occur with PID. This combination is called Fitz-Hugh–Curtis (FHC) syndrome and is characterized by severe pleuritic right upper quadrant pain. FHC syndrome complicates 10% of PID cases.
- Plasma cell endometritis has also been seen in the majority of females with PID; the density of plasma cell infiltration has been related to severity of symptoms (5).

DIAGNOSIS

- The diagnosis of PID is based primarily on clinical evaluation.
- The positive predictive value of clinical diagnosis is 65–90% compared with laparoscopy (2).
- The CDC recommends empiric treatment for PID in sexually active female or other female at risk with pelvic or lower abdominal pain with no other cause identified and if one or more of the following is present:
  – Cervical motion tenderness
  – Uterine tenderness
  – Adnexal tenderness
- Additional criteria used to enhance specificity: fever >101°F, new/abnormal cervical mucopurulent discharge or cervical friability, presence of abundant numbers of WBCs on wet prep, elevated C-reactive protein (CRP), elevated ESR, and laboratory documentation of cervical infection with *N. gonorrhoeae* or *C. trachomatis* (1,7)
- Most specific criteria for diagnosing PID: Endometrial biopsy reveals endometritis, transvaginal ultrasound showing thickened, fluid-filled salpinges, and laparoscopic abnormalities consistent with PID (1,3).

HISTORY
- Lower abdominal or pelvic pain: typically described as dull, aching or crampy, bilateral, and constant; accentuated by motion, exercise, or coitus
- New/abnormal vaginal discharge (~75% of cases)
- Fever, chills, cramping, dyspareunia
- Low back pain
- Urinary discomfort
- Unanticipated vaginal bleeding, often postcoital, is reported in about 40% of cases.
- Recent hysterosalpingogram (HSG)
- IUD insertion within the past 21 days (1)

PHYSICAL EXAM
- Fever
- Lower abdominal pain and particularly cervical motion tenderness
- Findings of cervicitis with/without vaginal discharge (1)

DIFFERENTIAL DIAGNOSIS
- Appendicitis
- Constipation
- Gastroenteritis
- Ectopic pregnancy
- Ovarian tumor/torsion
- Hemorrhagic/ruptured ovarian cyst
- Endometriosis/dysmenorrhea
- Functional pelvic pain
- Inflammatory bowel disease
- Diverticulitis
- UTI/pyelonephritis
- Nephrolithiasis (1)

DIAGNOSTIC TESTS & INTERPRETATION
Initial Tests (lab, imaging)
- Pregnancy test must be performed to rule out ectopic pregnancy and complications of an intrauterine pregnancy.
- Specific testing for chlamydia and gonorrhea (usually nucleic acid amplification test [NAAT] and/or ligase chain reaction), negative results does not exclude PID
- Urinalysis
- Saline microscopy of vaginal fluid (for WBC)
- Consider CBC: WBC count $\geq 10,500/mm^3$, although $\leq 50\%$ of PID cases present with leukocytosis.
- CRP (optional) is nonspecific and often normal in mild/moderate PID.
- Consider transvaginal ultrasound: not necessary for diagnosis; may show thickened, fluid-filled tubes (hydrosalpinges) ± free fluid, or TOA.

Pediatric Considerations
- ESR >15 mm/hr or elevated CRP used in some diagnostic criteria
- Consider HIV testing in patients with PID.
- Follow-up ultrasound as outpatient for resolution of adnexal abscess

Diagnostic Procedures/Other
- Culdocentesis with culture is rarely necessary.
- Laparoscopy is best used for confirming, as opposed to making, the diagnosis of PID and should be reserved for the following situations:
  – Ill patient with competing diagnosis (e.g., appendicitis)
  – Ill patient who has failed outpatient treatment
  – Any patient not improving after 72 hours of inpatient treatment
- Endometrial biopsy (rarely indicated): reveals endometritis/plasma cells (5)

TREATMENT

- Patient education: Avoid unprotected intercourse until patient and partner(s) have been treated and emphasis on the long-term implications for their/partner(s) health.
- Outpatient treatment, if appropriate
- Criteria for hospitalization and parenteral treatment are described below.

GENERAL MEASURES
- IUD removal is NOT required for mild PID.
- Treatment should cover principal pathogens, regardless of the test results.

MEDICATION
First Line
- Several antibiotic regimens are highly effective, with no single regimen of choice (5)[A].
- Outpatient treatment regimen
  - Ceftriaxone 250 mg IM single dose *plus* doxycycline 100 mg PO BID for 14 days
- The addition of metronidazole 500 mg PO BID for 14 days should be considered where risk of infection with anaerobic organisms is considered high like in pelvic abscess, trichomonas vaginalis infection, bacterial vaginosis, or recent gynecologic instrumentation. Also, clindamycin 450 mg PO every 6 hours can be considered as an alternative to metronidazole.
- On the basis of the recent emergence of fluoroquinolone-resistant gonococci, the CDC no longer recommends the use of fluoroquinolones for the treatment of gonococcal infections and associated conditions such as PID.

Second Line
- Because of emerging resistance in gonococci, resistance testing and confirmation of treatment success is advisable (5).
- Outpatient treatment regimen
  - Cefoxitin 2 g IM single dose and probenecid 1 g PO, or cefotaxime (1 g IM) or ceftizoxime (1 g IM) administered concurrently in single dose *plus* doxycycline 100 mg PO BID for 14 days ± metronidazole 500 mg PO BID for 14 days
- In persons with documented severe allergic reactions to penicillin or cephalosporins:
  - Azithromycin PO 2 g once or spectinomycin might be an option for therapy of uncomplicated gonococcal infections.
- Special consideration
  - Refer sex partners for appropriate evaluation and treatment if they had sexual contact with patient during preceding 60 days or most recent sexual contact. Partners should be treated with regimens effective against chlamydia and gonorrhea (5).
  - HIV-infected women with acute PID should be treated similar to non–HIV-infected women (6).

SURGERY/OTHER PROCEDURES
Reserved for failures of medical treatment and for suspected ruptured adnexal abscess with resulting acute surgical abdomen

ADMISSION, INPATIENT, AND NURSING CONSIDERATIONS
- Criteria for hospitalization if any of following (5)[C]:
  - Surgical emergencies (e.g., appendicitis) cannot be excluded.
  - Patient is pregnant.
  - Patient does not respond clinically within 72 hours of initiation with oral antimicrobial therapy.

- Failure to either tolerate or respond to outpatient therapy; the patient has severe illness, nausea and vomiting, or high fever, or the patient has a TOA.
- For inpatient treatment of PID, the CDC recommends following treatment regimens (7):
  - Parenteral regimen A
    - Cefotetan 2 g IV every 12 hours or cefoxitin 2 g IV q6h + doxycycline 100 mg PO or IV every 12 hours
    - Parenteral therapy for 24 hours after clinical improvement. Doxycycline should be preferred orally when possible as oral and IV provides similar bioavailability. Continue doxycycline for a total of 14 days (3).
  - Parenteral regimen B
    - Clindamycin 900 mg IV every 8 hours plus gentamicin loading dose IV or IM (2 mg/kg of body weight) followed by a maintenance dose (1.5 mg/kg) q8h or single daily dosing at 3 to 5 mg/kg can be substituted (3).
    - Parenteral therapy may be discontinued 24 hours after clinical improvement, and oral therapy with doxycycline as aforementioned or clindamycin 450 mg PO QID for a total of 14 days should be continued.
  - Parenteral regimen C
    - Ampicillin/sulbactam 3 g IV every 6 hours plus doxycycline 100 mg PO or IV every 12 hours
- PID is rare in pregnant patients, however, may appear prior to 12 weeks' gestation before mucous plug appears. Change doxycycline to azithromycin + 2nd-generation cephalosporin (7).

 ONGOING CARE

FOLLOW-UP RECOMMENDATIONS
Patient Monitoring
- Follow up in 72 hours after initiation of treatment is recommended particularly for patients with moderate or severe clinical presentation (3).
- Observe for clinical signs and symptoms particularly for fever, leukocytosis, abdominal, and cervical motion tenderness.
- Retest for gonorrhea and chlamydia in 3 to 6 months. The likelihood of reinfection is high.
- Follow adnexal abscess size and position with serial ultrasounds.

PATIENT EDUCATION
- Abstinence from any type of sexual contact until treatment of patient/partner (if necessary) is complete
- Consistent and correct condom use should be enforced.
- Hepatitis B and human papilloma virus (HPV) vaccines should be given to patients who meet criteria.
- Advise comprehensive STI screening (7).

PROGNOSIS
- PID has a high morbidity; about 20% of affected women become infertile, 40% develop chronic pelvic pain, and 1% of those who conceive have an ectopic pregnancy (1).
- Wide variation with good prognosis if early effective therapy is instituted and further infection is avoided
- Poor prognosis related to late therapy and continued high-risk sexual behavior
- Nongonococcal, nonchlamydial PID is more often associated with severe PID and with worse prognosis for future fertility.

COMPLICATIONS
- TOA will develop in ~7–16% of patients with PID.
- Recurrent infection occurs in 20–25% of patients.
- Risk of ectopic pregnancy is increased 7- to 10-fold among women with a history of PID.
- Tubal infertility occurs in 8%, 19.5%, and 40% of women after 1, 2, and 3 episodes of PID, respectively.
- Chronic pelvic pain occurs in 20% of cases and is related to adhesion formation, chronic salpingitis, or recurrent infection (1,4).
- Hydrosalpinx: After PID resolves, fallopian tube may fill with sterile fluid and become blocked; it may be associated with pain and infertility related to negative outcomes with IVF.

REFERENCES
1. Brunham R, Gottlieb S, Paavonen J. Pelvic inflammatory disease. *N Engl J Med*. 2015;372(21):2039–2048.
2. Ross J. Pelvic inflammatory disease. *Am Fam Physician*. 2014;90(10):725–726.
3. Low N, Redmond S, Uusküla A, et al. Screening for genital chlamydia infection. *Cochrane Database Syst Rev*. 2016;(9):CD010866.
4. Kreisel K, Torrone E, Bernstein K, et al. Prevalence of pelvic inflammatory disease in sexually experienced women of reproductive age—United States, 2013–2014. *MMWR Morb Mortal Wkly Rep*. 2017;66(3):80–83.
5. Judlin P. Current concepts in managing pelvic inflammatory disease. *Curr Opin Infect Dis*. 2010;23(1):83–87.
6. Ross J, Guaschino S, Cusini M, et al. 2017 European guideline for the management of pelvic inflammatory disease. *Int J STD AIDS*. 2018;29(2):108–114.
7. Workowski KA, Bolan GA; for Centers for Disease Control and Prevention. Sexually transmitted diseases treatment guidelines, 2015. *MMWR Recomm Rep*. 2015;64(RR-03):1–137.

 CODES

ICD10
- N73.9 Female pelvic inflammatory disease, unspecified
- N73.0 Acute parametritis and pelvic cellulitis
- N70.93 Salpingitis and oophoritis, unspecified

CLINICAL PEARLS
- Most often, PID starts with gonorrhea or chlamydia infection, but it is often polymicrobial.
- Physicians should treat on the basis of clinical judgment (pelvic pain with cervical motion tenderness or adnexal tenderness or uterine tenderness in a patient at risk) without waiting for confirmation from laboratory or imaging tests. PID is a common cause of infertility.
- Complications include hydrosalpinx, adhesions, pelvic pain, and 10-fold increased risk of ectopic pregnancy.
- Three major predictors of preserved post-PID fertility: (i) short duration of symptoms (<72 hours) prior to initiation of treatment, (ii) first episode of PID, and (iii) nongonococcal PID

PEPTIC ULCER DISEASE

Fozia Akhtar Ali, MD • Anh V. Dinh, MD • Paula A. Shelton, MD

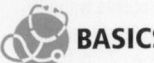 **BASICS**

Peptic ulcer disease is characterized by defects in the stomach and/or duodenal mucosa through the muscularis mucosa, leading to inflammation of the underlying tissue by gastric acid and pepsin.

DESCRIPTION
- Duodenal ulcer
  - Most common form of peptic ulcer
  - Usually located in the proximal duodenum
  - Multiple ulcers or ulcers distal to the second portion of duodenum raise possibility of gastrinoma (Zollinger-Ellison syndrome).
- Gastric ulcer
  - Less common than duodenal ulcer in absence of NSAID use
  - Commonly located along lesser curvature of the antrum
- Esophageal ulcers
  - Located in the distal esophagus; usually secondary to gastroesophageal reflux disease (GERD); also seen with gastrinoma
- Ectopic gastric mucosal ulceration
  - May develop with Meckel diverticulum

EPIDEMIOLOGY
Incidence
- Predominant sex: male = female
- Predominant age
  - 70% of ulcers occur between ages 25 and 64 years.
  - Duodenal/gastric ulcer incidence increases with age.
- Peptic ulcer: 500,000 new cases per year
- Recurrence: 4 million per year
- Global incidence rate: 0.1–0.19%

Prevalence
- Peptic ulcer: 2% in the United States
- The lifetime prevalence is higher (10–20%) in *Helicobacter pylori*–positive patients, compared to the general population (5–10%).

ETIOLOGY AND PATHOPHYSIOLOGY
Genetics
Increased incidence of PUD in families is likely due to familial clustering of *H. pylori* infection and inherited genetic factors reflecting response to the organism.

RISK FACTORS
- *H. pylori* infection (95% of duodenal and 70% of gastric ulcers)
- Chronic use of NSAIDs, including aspirin and COX-2 inhibitors
- Tobacco use
- Stress (after acute illness, ventilator support, extensive burns, head injury)
- Hypersecretion syndromes: gastrinoma (Zollinger-Ellison), systemic mastocytosis, carcinoid syndrome; alcohol use
- Medications: corticosteroids (high-dose and/or prolonged therapy), bisphosphonates, potassium chloride, clopidogrel, sirolimus chemotherapeutic agents
- Radiation therapy

GENERAL PREVENTION
- NSAID ulcers: Use acetaminophen (instead of NSAIDs) when appropriate, and discontinue NSAID use (or add a proton pump inhibitor [PPI]) in patients with previous NSAID-related ulcer.
  - If NSAIDs are absolutely necessary, use lowest possible dose to decrease risk of ulcerogenesis and use in combination with a PPI or misoprostol.
  - To reduce ulcer risk, consider testing for and eradicating *H. pylori*, particularly before starting therapy with NSAIDs.
- Maintenance therapy with PPIs or H₂ blockers is indicated for patients with a history of ulcer complications, recurrences, refractory ulcers, or persistent *H. pylori* infection.
- Consider maintenance PPI treatment in patients with *H. pylori*–negative, non–NSAID-induced ulcer.
  - *H. pylori* infection: present in 95% of duodenal and 70% of gastric ulcers; annual risk of duodenal ulcer in those with *H. pylori* infection: ≤1%

COMMONLY ASSOCIATED CONDITIONS
- Gastrinoma (Zollinger-Ellison syndrome)
- Multiple endocrine neoplasia type 1
- Carcinoid syndrome
- Chronic illness: Crohn disease, chronic obstructive pulmonary disease (COPD), chronic renal failure, hepatic cirrhosis, cystic fibrosis
- Hematopoietic disorders (rare): systemic mastocytosis, myeloproliferative disease, hyperparathyroidism, polycythemia rubra vera

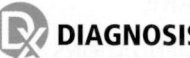 **DIAGNOSIS**

HISTORY
- Signs and symptoms:
  - Duodenal ulcer
    - Midepigastric pain
    - Gnawing or burning, nonradiating, recurring pain that is often is episodic and relieved by food or antacids.
  - Gastric ulcer
    - Midepigastric pain
    - Aggravated by food, relieved by antacids
- Nonspecific dyspeptic symptoms: indigestion, nausea, vomiting, loss of appetite, heartburn, and epigastric fullness
- Red flag or alarm symptoms
  - Onset of symptoms after age 55 years
  - Progressive dysphagia
  - Recurrent vomiting
  - Blood in stool, melena, hematemesis, anemia
  - Progressive dysphagia
  - Persistent or recurrent vomiting
  - Severe abdominal pain
  - Weight loss, anorexia, or family history of gastric malignancy
- NSAID-induced ulcers are often silent; perforation or bleeding may be the initial presentation.

PHYSICAL EXAM
Physical exam for uncomplicated peptic ulcer may be nonspecific: Check vital signs for hemodynamic stability, conjunctival pallor (anemia); epigastric tenderness (absent in at least 30% of older patients); guaiac-positive stool from occult blood loss

DIFFERENTIAL DIAGNOSIS
Functional dyspepsia, gastritis, GERD, biliary colic, gastroenteritis, pancreatitis, cholecystitis, Crohn disease, intestinal ischemia, cardiac ischemia, GI malignancy

DIAGNOSTIC TESTS & INTERPRETATION
Initial Tests (lab, imaging)
- Lab tests to consider:
  - CBC: Rule out anemia.
  - Fecal occult blood test
  - If multiple/refractory ulcers: Consider fasting serum gastrin to rule out gastrinoma.
- Indications for *H. pylori* testing: new-onset PUD, prior history of PUD, persistent symptoms after empiric antisecretory therapy, gastric mucosa–associated lymphoid tissue (MALT) lymphoma, noninvestigated dyspepsia in patients <50 years of age without alarm symptoms *H. pylori* diagnostic tests:
  - False-negative results may occur if patient was recently treated with antibiotics, bismuth, or PPIs, or in patients with active bleeding.
  - Diagnostic yield improved with two different tests:
    ○ Noninvasive tests:
      ■ Serology: *H. pylori* serologic testing is a cost-effective approach in untreated patients with dyspepsia but cannot be used to document successful eradication (sensitivity, 85%; specificity, 79%).
      ■ Urea breath test: identifies active *H. pylori* infection; also used for posttreatment testing (sensitivity, >95%; specificity, >90%).
      ■ Stool antigen: easy to obtain and accurate but can be effected by antibiotics, bismuth, and PPIs; can be used for screening and posttreatment testing (sensitivity, 91%; specificity, 94%)
      ■ To prove eradication, use urea breath test or stool antigen. Stop antibiotics and bismuth for at least 4 weeks and PPIs for 1 week prior to testing because of high false-negative rates.
    ○ Invasive tests:
      ■ Diagnostic upper endoscopy (sensitivity, >95%; specificity, >95%) is most accurate for diagnosing PUD and active *H. pylori* infection. Endoscopy is costly and invasive and recommended only for patients with "red flag" symptoms (1)[B].
      ■ Rapid urease test: conducted on gastric biopsies (sensitivity, 93–97%; specificity, 95%)
- Barium or Gastrografin contrast radiography (double-contrast hypotonic duodenography): indicated when endoscopy is unsuitable or not feasible

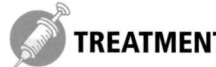 **TREATMENT**

MEDICATION
First Line
- Acid suppression: PPIs. PPIs have higher efficacy than H₂ blockers. 95% of duodenal ulcers heal on PPI therapy within 4 weeks.
  - Omeprazole 20 mg/day PO; lansoprazole 30 mg/day PO; rabeprazole 20 mg/day PO; esomeprazole 40 mg/day PO; pantoprazole 40 mg/day PO; dexlansoprazole 30 mg/day PO
  - Administer PPIs on an empty stomach and before breakfast.
  - Administer PPI for 4 weeks to treat duodenal ulcer and 8 weeks to treat gastric ulcer.
- H₂ blockers: ranitidine or nizatidine 150 mg PO BID or 300 mg PO at bedtime; cimetidine 400 mg PO BID or 800 mg PO at bedtime; famotidine 20 mg PO BID or 40 mg PO at bedtime

- Treat ulcers for 8 to 12 weeks or until healing is confirmed in patients with complicated ulcers.
- PPIs help heal peptic ulcers more rapidly.
- Precautions:
  - Renal insufficiency: Decrease H_2 blocker dosage by 50% if CrCl <50 mL/min cimetidine: Use caution with theophylline, warfarin, phenytoin, and lidocaine.
  - PPIs may decrease bone density. Obtain interval bone densitometry with long-term PPI use (2).
  - PPIs may cause hypomagnesemia. Consider baseline and interval levels in patients, especially for long-term use and in patients taking diuretics.
  - PPIs may be associated with increased risk of *Clostridium difficile* infection (2). Short-term use associated with development of community-acquired pneumonia; long-term use does not appear to have an increased risk.
  - Despite earlier concerns, PPIs do not appear to decrease the efficacy of clopidogrel (2).
- NSAID-induced ulcers
  - Discontinue NSAID use.
  - Treat with PPIs for 8 to 12 weeks; may use as maintenance for patients with recurrent, complicated, or idiopathic ulcers; or in patients who require long-term aspirin or NSAID use.
- *H. pylori*–induced ulcers
  - *H. pylori* eradication regimens: Preferred duration of therapy is 14 days.
  - Triple therapy: standard dose PPI given BID plus clarithromycin 500 mg PO BID plus amoxicillin 1 g PO BID or metronidazole 500 mg PO BID in patients with allergy to amoxicillin; bacterial resistance: clarithromycin 10%; amoxicillin 1.4%; metronidazole 37%: Culture-guided choice of triple therapy is preferred (3).

Second Line

- For *H. pylori* eradication: Use second-line therapy if first-line fails (3):
  - Bismuth quadruple therapy for 14 days
    - Bismuth subsalicylate 525 mg PO QID plus
    - Metronidazole 250 mg PO QID plus
    - Tetracycline 500 mg PO QID plus
    - Standard dose PPI PO BID
- Sequential therapy
  - Standard-dose PPI PO BID plus amoxicillin 1,000 mg PO QID for 5 days followed by
  - Standard-dose PPI PO BID plus clarithromycin 500 mg PO BID plus tinidazole (or metronidazole) 500 mg PO BID for 5 days
    - Levofloxacin 250 mg PO BID may be substituted in those with PCN allergy or in areas of high clarithromycin resistance rates.
  - Another alternative salvage therapy:
    - Rifabutin 300 mg PO daily plus
    - Amoxicillin 1,000 mg PO BID plus
    - PPI orally BID
  - Alternative ulcer-healing drugs:
    - Sucralfate and antacids are additional options; however, antisecretory options are preferred.
- Significant possible interactions:
  - Cimetidine inhibits cytochrome P450 isozymes (avoid with theophylline, warfarin, phenytoin, and lidocaine).
  - Omeprazole may prolong elimination of diazepam, warfarin, and phenytoin.
  - Sucralfate reduces absorption of tetracycline, norfloxacin, ciprofloxacin, and theophylline; it leads to subtherapeutic levels.

Pregnancy Considerations

PPIs are *not* associated with an increased risk for major birth defects, spontaneous abortions, or preterm delivery.

- Breastfeeding
  - Both ranitidine and esomeprazole are secreted in breast milk; at considerably lower doses than used for treatment in infants with reflux disease. Use in breastfeeding women is generally safe.

SURGERY/OTHER PROCEDURES

- Endoscopy is indicated for patients age >55 years with new onset of dyspeptic symptoms, those who do not respond to treatment, and patients of any age with alarm/red flag symptoms (4)[B].
- During endoscopy:
  - Biopsy stomach for *H. pylori* testing (CLO test)
  - Biopsy ulcer margin to exclude malignancy
  - Interventions to stop active bleeding or prevent rebleeding in those with certain stigmata include injection with epinephrine, heater probe treatment, or placement of endoscopic clips (2).
- Indications for surgery: ulcers that are refractory to treatment and patients at high risk for complications (e.g., transplant recipients, patients dependent on steroids/NSAIDs); surgery also may be needed acutely to treat perforation and bleeding refractory to endoscopic therapy (5).
- Surgical options:
  - Duodenal ulcers: truncal vagotomy and drainage (pyloroplasty/gastrojejunostomy), selective vagotomy (preserving the hepatic and/or celiac branches of the vagus) and drainage, or highly selective vagotomy (1)
  - Gastric ulcers: partial gastrectomy, Billroth I or II
  - Perforated ulcers: laparoscopy/open patching (1)
- Emerging options: Vonoprazan is a novel acid blocker that blocks the hydrogen-potassium ATPase.

ADMISSION, INPATIENT, AND NURSING CONSIDERATIONS

- Discontinue ulcerogenic agents (e.g., NSAIDs).
- Bleeding peptic ulcers
  - Stable: Give PPI to reduce transfusion requirements, need for surgery, and duration of hospitalization (6).
  - Unstable: fluid/packed RBC resuscitation followed by emergent esophagogastroduodenoscopy (EGD); use IV PPI.
  - Insufficient evidence for high-dose PPI treatment over lower doses in peptic ulcer bleeding (2)[A]
- Oral PPI equivalent to IV after endoscopic treatment (6)
- Perforated peptic ulcers are a surgical emergency (1).

ONGOING CARE

FOLLOW-UP RECOMMENDATIONS

Patient Monitoring

- *H. pylori* eradication: expected in >90% (with double antibiotic regimen): Confirm eradication with urea breath test.
- Acute duodenal ulcer: Monitor clinically.
- Acute gastric ulcer: Confirm healing via endoscopy after 12 weeks; biopsies (if not done initially) to confirm benign mucosa
- Tobacco cessation

PROGNOSIS

After *H. pylori* eradication (4):

- Low ulcer relapse rate; if relapse, consider surreptitious use of NSAIDs.
- Reinfection rates <1% per year
- Low risk of rebleeding
- Decreased NSAID ulcer recurrence (4)

COMPLICATIONS

- Hemorrhage: up to 25% of patients (initial presentation in 10%)
- Perforation: <5% of patients
- Gastric outlet obstruction: up to 5% of duodenal or pyloric channel ulcers; male predilection found
- Risk of gastric adenocarcinoma is increased in *H. pylori*–infected patients.
- Refractory peptic ulcer disease (5–10% after eradication of *H. pylori* or completion of 12 weeks of PPI)

REFERENCES

1. Lanas A, Chan FKL. Peptic ulcer disease. *Lancet*. 2017;390(10094):613–624.
2. Neumann I, Letelier LM, Rada G, et al. Comparison of different regimens of proton pump inhibitors for acute peptic ulcer bleeding. *Cochrane Database Syst Rev*. 2013;(6):CD007999.
3. Luther J, Higgins PD, Schoenfeld PS, et al. Empiric quadruple vs. triple therapy for primary treatment of *Helicobacter pylori* infection: systematic review and meta-analysis of efficacy and tolerability. *Am J Gastroenterol*. 2010;105(1):65–73.
4. Gisbert JP, Calvet X, Cosme A, et al; and *H. pylori* Study Group of the Asociación Española de Gastroenterología (Spanish Gastroenterology Association). Long-term follow-up of 1,000 patients cured of *Helicobacter pylori* infection following an episode of peptic ulcer bleeding. *Am J Gastroenterol*. 2012;107(8):1197–1204.
5. Laine L, Jensen DM. Management of patients with ulcer bleeding. *Am J Gastroenterol*. 2012;107(3):345–361.
6. Yen HH, Yang CW, Su WW, et al. Oral versus intravenous proton pump inhibitors in preventing re-bleeding for patients with peptic ulcer bleeding after successful endoscopic therapy. *BMC Gastroenterol*. 2012;12:66.

ADDITIONAL READING

Echizen H. The first-in-class potassium-competitive acid blocker, vonoprazan fumarate: pharmacokinetic and pharmacodynamic considerations. *Clin Pharmacokinet*. 2016;55(4):409–418.

CODES

ICD10

- K27.9 Peptic ulc, site unsp, unsp as ac or chr, w/o hemor or perf
- K26.9 Duodenal ulcer, unspecified as acute or chronic, without hemorrhage or perforation
- K25.9 Gastric ulcer, unspecified as acute or chronic, without hemorrhage or perforation

CLINICAL PEARLS

- PPIs have higher efficacy than H_2 blockers for healing duodenal ulcers.
- In patients with PUD, eradicate *H. pylori* to assist healing and reduce the risk of recurrence.
- Upper endoscopy is indicated for patients with suspected peptic ulcers and red flag symptoms and for those who do not respond to treatment.

PERICARDITIS

Veronica J. Ruston, DO

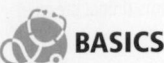 **BASICS**

DESCRIPTION

Inflammation of the pericardium, with or without associated pericardial effusion. Myopericarditis or perimyocarditis refers to cases that have myocardial involvement in addition to involvement of the pericardium.

EPIDEMIOLOGY

Incidence

Epidemiologic studies are lacking. Exact incidence is unknown but occurs in up to 5% of patients evaluated in the ER for chest pain without myocardial infarction (MI); appears to be a slightly increased prevalence in men

ETIOLOGY AND PATHOPHYSIOLOGY

- Inflammation of the pericardial sac can be *acute* or *chronic* (recurrent). Chronic/recurrent inflammation may result in constrictive pericarditis.
- Can produce serous/purulent fluid/dense fibrinous material (depending on etiology), which may or may not lead to hemodynamic compromise
- Idiopathic: 85–90% of cases; likely related to viral infection, which may trigger immune-related process
- Infectious
  - Viral: coxsackievirus, echovirus, adenovirus, Epstein-Barr virus, cytomegalovirus, hepatitis viruses, influenza virus, HIV, measles, mumps, varicella
  - Bacterial: gram-positive and gram-negative organisms
  - Fungal (more common in immunocompromised populations): *Blastomyces dermatitidis*, *Candida* sp., *Histoplasma capsulatum*
  - Mycobacterial: *Mycobacterium tuberculosis*
  - Parasites: *Echinococcus*
- Noninfectious causes
  - Acute MI (2 to 4 days after MI), Dressler syndrome (weeks to months after MI)
  - Aortic dissection
  - Renal failure, uremia, dialysis-associated
  - Malignancy (e.g., breast cancer, lung cancer, Hodgkin disease, leukemia, lymphoma)
  - Radiation therapy
  - Trauma
  - Postpericardiotomy
  - After cardiac procedures (e.g., catheterization, pacemaker placement, ablation)
  - Autoimmune disorders: connective tissue disorders, systemic lupus erythematosus (SLE), rheumatoid arthritis, scleroderma, hypothyroidism, inflammatory bowel disease, Wegener granulomatosis, spondyloarthropathies
  - Sarcoidosis
- Medication-induced: dantrolene, doxorubicin, hydralazine, isoniazid, mesalamine, methysergide, penicillin, phenytoin, procainamide, rifampin

Genetics

No known factors

COMMONLY ASSOCIATED CONDITIONS

Depends on etiology

 DIAGNOSIS

HISTORY

- Prodrome of fever, malaise, myalgias, viral upper respiratory
- Acute, sharp, stabbing chest pain

- Duration typically hours to days
- Pleuritic pain
- Pain reduced by leaning forward, worsened by lying supine
- Shortness of breath

PHYSICAL EXAM

- Heart rate is usually regular and may be rapid.
- Pericardial friction rub: coarse, high-pitched sound best heard during end expiration at left lower sternal border with patient leaning forward. Highly specific for diagnosis (but not sensitive); may be transient and mono-, bi-, or triphasic
- New S_3 may suggest myopericarditis.
- Cardiac tamponade
- Diagnostic clinical criteria
  - Acute pericarditis (at least two of four criteria)
    ○ Typical (pleuritic) chest pain
    ○ Pericardial friction rub
    ○ ECG changes with widespread ST elevation
    ○ New/increasing pericardial effusion
  - Myopericarditis
    ○ Definite pericarditis *plus*
    ○ Symptoms (dyspnea, chest pain, or palpitations) *and* ECG changes not previously documented (ST/T wave abnormalities, supraventricular/ventricular tachycardia) *or* focal/diffuse depressed left ventricular (LV) function documented on imaging study
    ○ Absence of evidence of other cause
    ○ One of the following: elevated cardiac enzymes (creatine kinase [CK]-MB, troponin I or T) *or* new focal/diffuse depressed LV function *or* abnormal imaging consistent with myocarditis (MRI with gadolinium, gallium-67 scanning, antimyosin antibody scanning)
  - Case definitions
    ○ *Suspected myopericarditis*: criteria 1, 2, and 3
    ○ *Probable myopericarditis*: criteria 1, 2, 3, and 4
    ○ *Confirmed myopericarditis*: histopathologic evidence of myocarditis by endomyocardial biopsy (EMB) or autopsy (Note: In the clinical setting, for self-limited cases with predominantly pericarditis, EMB is rarely indicated.)

DIAGNOSTIC TESTS & INTERPRETATION

Initial Tests (lab, imaging)

- It is not necessary to order tests for uncomplicated cases or when the diagnosis is clear. Following labs may be helpful (1)[C]:
  - CBC: typically shows leukocytosis
  - Inflammatory markers: elevated erythrocyte sedimentation rate (ESR), C-reactive protein (CRP), and lactate dehydrogenase (LDH)
  - Cardiac biomarkers: typically elevated CK, troponins
    ○ Elevated troponins associated with younger age, male sex, pericardial effusion at presentation, and ST segment elevation on ECG
    ○ Adverse outcomes are not predicted by elevated troponin.
- ECG: Findings include widespread upward concave ST segment elevation (in all or most leads, a diffuse, nonregional process) and PR segment depression that may evolve through four stages. ECG may be normal/show nonspecific abnormalities:
  - Stage 1: diffuse ST segment elevation and PR segment depression
  - Stage 2: Normalization of the ST and PR segments and T waves begin to flatten and invert.

- Stage 3: widespread T wave inversions
- Stage 4: normalization of T waves; may have persistent inversions if chronic pericarditis
- ECG may demonstrate low voltage and electrical alternans with tamponade.
- Transthoracic echocardiogram is recommended to evaluate for the presence of pericardial effusion, tamponade, or myocardial disease (presence of effusion helps to confirm diagnosis of pericarditis) (1)[C].
- Chest x-ray (CXR) is performed to rule out pulmonary/mediastinal pathology. Enlarged cardiac silhouette suggests large pericardial effusion (at least 200 mL).
- CT and MRI allow visualization of pericardium to assess for complications or if initial workup is inconclusive (1)[C].
- Additional testing (if clinically appropriate based on history or atypical presentation or course) may include tuberculin skin test, sputum cultures, rheumatoid factor, antinuclear antibody, and HIV serology (1)[C].
- Viral cultures and antibody titers rarely clinically useful (1)[C]

Diagnostic Procedures/Other

- Pericardiocentesis indicated for cardiac tamponade; for suspected purulent, tuberculous, or neoplastic pericarditis; and for effusions >20 mm on echocardiography (2)[C]
- Surgical drainage with pericardial biopsy recommended if recurrent tamponade, ineffective pericardiocentesis, or hemodynamic instability (2)[C]

Test Interpretation

- Microscopic examination may reveal hyperemia, leukocyte accumulation, or fibrin deposition.
- Purulent fluid with neutrophilic predominance if bacterial etiology
- Lymphocytic predominance in viral, tuberculous, and neoplastic pericarditis

TREATMENT

- Goal of treatment is to relieve pain and reduce complications (e.g., recurrence, tamponade, chronic restrictive pericarditis).
- Outpatient therapy is reported to be successful in 85% patients with low-risk features.

GENERAL MEASURES

Specific therapy directed toward underlying disorder for patients with identified cause other than viral/idiopathic disease. Restrictions of physical activity are important part of treatment for recurrences.

MEDICATION

First Line

- NSAIDs are considered the mainstay of therapy for acute pericarditis:
  - Ibuprofen 400 to 800 mg TID for 1 to 2 weeks (2 to 4 weeks for recurrence) then taper (3)[C]
  - Aspirin 650 to 975 mg TID–QID for 1 to 2 weeks (2 to 4 weeks for recurrence) then taper; preferable for patients with recent MI because other NSAIDs impair scar formation in animal studies (4)[C]
  - Indomethacin 50 mg TID for 1 to 2 weeks (2 to 4 weeks for recurrence) then taper; should avoid in elderly due to flow restrictions to coronaries (3)[C]

- Ketorolac 15 to 30 mg IV/IM q6h while inpatient; maximum duration of 5 days (3)[C].
- GI protection should be provided (3)[C].
- Tapering should be done only if the patient is asymptomatic and CRP/ESR are normal and are done every 1 to 2 weeks (3)[C].
- Treatment duration using NSAIDs for initial attacks is 1 to 2 weeks, but for recurrences, consider 2 to 4 weeks of therapy (3)[C].
- Monitoring: NSAIDs: CBC and CRP at baseline and weekly until CRP normalizes
- Contraindications: hypersensitivity to aspirin or NSAIDs, active peptic ulcer/GI bleeding
- Precautions: Use with caution in patients with asthma, 3rd-trimester pregnancy, coagulopathy, and renal/hepatic dysfunction.
- Colchicine: common practice to use in combination with NSAIDs; 0.6 mg BID for up to 3 months (up to 6 months for recurrence); taper is not required. Efficacious as therapy for initial occurrence and if multiple recurrences. This is the only agent proven to prevent recurrences in RCTs. Adjunctive therapy can reduce rate of recurrence by 50% (2)[A]. Monitoring: Consider CBC, CRP, transaminases, CK, and creatinine at baseline and at least after 1 month.
- Pregnant: <20 weeks' gestation: Aspirin is first choice, but NSAIDs and prednisone are also allowed; >20 weeks' gestation: Prednisone is allowed with avoidance of NSAIDs, aspirin, and colchicine (1)[C].

Second Line
- Corticosteroid treatment is indicated in connective tissue disease, tuberculous pericarditis, or severe recurrent symptoms unresponsive to NSAIDs or colchicine; should be avoided in uncomplicated acute pericarditis. *Corticosteroid use alone has been found to be an independent risk factor for recurrence* (4)[C].
- If steroids are used, consider low dose (0.25 to 0.50 mg/kg/day for 2 weeks for first attack; 0.25 to 0.50 mg/kg/day for 2 to 4 weeks for recurrence); then slow taper (if >50 mg: 10 mg/day every 1 to 2 weeks; if 25 to 50 mg: 5 to 10 mg/day every 1 to 2 weeks; if 15 to 25 mg: 2.5 mg/day every 2 to 4 weeks; if <15 mg/day: 1.0 to 2.5 mg/day every 2 to 6 weeks) following remission. Remember adequate prophylaxis treatment for osteoporosis prevention (4)[C].
- If unable to taper from steroids, resume lowest steroid dose and begin slow taper of 1 to 2 mg every 2 to 4 weeks (3)[C].
- Intrapericardial administration of steroids may be effective and limits systemic side effects.
- Emerging alternative options include azathioprine, IV human immunoglobulins, and anakinra (4)[C].

ISSUES FOR REFERRAL
- Refractory cases include those on unacceptably high long-term steroid doses (>25 mg/day).
- Consider trial of aspirin and/or NSAIDs plus steroid and colchicine.
- Uremic or dialysis-related cases require more frequent or urgent dialysis without significant benefit from pharmacologics (1)[C].

SURGERY/OTHER PROCEDURES
- Pericardiocentesis is indicated in cases of cardiac tamponade, high likelihood of tuberculous/purulent/neoplastic pericarditis, and large symptomatic effusions refractory to medical therapy.
- Pericardial biopsy may be considered for diagnosis in those with persistent worsening pericarditis without a definite diagnosis.

- Pericardioscopy for targeted diagnostic imaging may be performed at experienced tertiary referral centers in refractory and difficult cases.
- Pericardial window may be performed in cases of recurrent cardiac tamponade with large pericardial effusion despite medical therapy and severe symptoms.
- Pericardiectomy can be considered. The 2004 European Society of Cardiology guidelines recommend pericardiectomy (class IIa) for frequent and highly symptomatic recurrences of pericarditis refractory to medical therapy. However, this is rarely performed in the United States and has high morbidity and mortality (1)[C].

ADMISSION, INPATIENT, AND NURSING CONSIDERATIONS
- Inpatient therapy recommended for pericarditis associated with clinical predictors of poor prognosis:
  - Major predictors: fever >38°C, subacute onset, large pericardial effusion, cardiac tamponade, lack of response to NSAID/aspirin therapy after at least 1 week (5)[C]
  - Minor predictors: immunosuppressed state, trauma, oral anticoagulation therapy, myopericarditis (5)[C]
- IV fluids considered for hypotension or in the setting of pericardial tamponade
- Discharge criteria
  - Response to therapy with symptom improvement
  - Hemodynamic stability

 ONGOING CARE

FOLLOW-UP RECOMMENDATIONS
- 7 to 10 days to assess response to treatment
- 1 month to check CBC and CRP and thereafter if symptoms continue to be present
- Those with clinical predictors of poor prognosis may require closer follow-up based on lab data and echocardiographic findings.

Patient Monitoring
Myopericarditis
- Use lower doses of anti-inflammatory drugs to control symptoms for 1 to 2 weeks while minimizing deleterious effects on myocarditic process.
- Exercise restrictions for 4 to 6 weeks or until symptoms resolved and biomarkers normalized (2)[C].
- Echocardiographic monitoring at 1, 6, and 12 months (especially in those with LV dysfunction)

DIET
No restrictions

PROGNOSIS
Overall good prognosis; disease usually benign and self-limiting; purulent and tuberculosis pericarditis with high mortality

COMPLICATIONS
- Recurrent pericarditis: occurs in ~30% of patients, with most instances resulting from idiopathic, viral, or autoimmune pericarditis; inadequate treatment of the initial attack; and, less commonly, neoplastic etiologies. Recurrence usually within 1st week following initial episode but may occur months to years later; rarely associated with tamponade/constriction
- About 5% of patients develop corticosteroid dependence and colchicine resistance.
- Cardiac tamponade: rare complication with increased incidence in neoplastic, purulent, and tuberculous pericarditis

- Effusive-constrictive pericarditis: reported in 24% of patients undergoing surgery for constrictive pericarditis and in 8% of patients undergoing pericardiocentesis and cardiac catheterization for cardiac tamponade. Failure of right atrial pressure to fall by 50% or to a level below 10 mm Hg after pericardiocentesis is diagnostic.
- Constrictive pericarditis: rare complication in which rigid pericardium produces abnormal diastolic filling with elevated filling pressures. Pericardiectomy remains definitive therapy.

REFERENCES
1. Maisch B, Seferović PM, Ristić AD, et al; for Task Force on the Diagnosis and Management of Pericardial Diseases of the European Society of Cardiology. Guidelines on the diagnosis and management of pericardial diseases executive summary: the task force on the diagnosis and management of pericardial diseases of the European Society of Cardiology. *Eur Heart J.* 2004;25(7):587–610.
2. Imazio M, Brucato A, Belli R, et al. Colchicine for the prevention of pericarditis: what we know and what we do not know in 2014—systematic review and meta-analysis. *J Cardiovasc Med (Hagerstown)*. 2014;15(12):840–846.
3. Lilly LS. Treatment of acute and recurrent idiopathic pericarditis. *Circulation*. 2013;127(16):1723–1726.
4. Imazio M, Lazaros G, Brucato A, et al. Recurrent pericarditis: new and emerging therapeutic options. *Nat Rev Cardiol*. 2016;13(2):99–105.
5. Snyder MJ, Bepko J, White M. Acute pericarditis: diagnosis and management. *Am Fam Physician*. 2014;89(7):553–560.

ADDITIONAL READING
- Brucato A, Imazio M, Gattorno M, et al. Effect of anakinra on recurrent pericarditis among patients with colchicine resistance and corticosteroid dependence: the AIRTRIP randomized clinical trial. *JAMA*. 2016;316(18):1906–1912.
- Imazio M, Spodick DH, Brucato A, et al. Controversial issues in the management of pericardial diseases. *Circulation*. 2010;121(7):916–928.
- Khandaker MH, Espinosa RE, Nishimura RA, et al. Pericardial disease: diagnosis and management. *Mayo Clin Proc*. 2010;85(6):572–593.

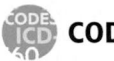 CODES

ICD10
- I31.9 Disease of pericardium, unspecified
- I30.9 Acute pericarditis, unspecified
- I30.1 Infective pericarditis

CLINICAL PEARLS
- Consider *major* and *minor* predictors in deciding which patients should be admitted.
- Therapy aimed at symptomatic relief and NSAIDs are first-line treatment. Colchicine is recommended as an adjunct to NSAIDs.
- Pericardiocentesis is recommended in the setting of cardiac tamponade or possible purulent pericarditis.

PERIODIC LIMB MOVEMENT DISORDER (PLMD)

Denise Sharon, MD, PhD, FAASM • John R. Burk, MD, FACP

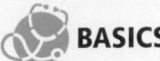 **BASICS**

DESCRIPTION

- Sleep-related movement disorder with episodes of periodic limb movements (PLMs) occurring during sleep (1)[A] characterized by:
  - Periodic limb movements of sleep (PLMS) demonstrated during polysomnography that are combined with clinical symptoms
  - PLMS are repetitive contractions of the tibialis anterior muscles occurring mainly in non–rapid eye movement (NREM) sleep.
  - Movements consist of unilateral or bilateral, simultaneous or not, rhythmical extension of the big toe and ankle dorsiflexion.
  - Sometimes, knee and hip flexion is noted.
  - Arm movements or more generalized movements occur less commonly.
  - Movements might be associated with cortical arousals from sleep unbeknownst to the patient (PLMs with arousals—PLMA).
  - A clinical history of significant sleep disturbance or functional impairment is necessary for diagnosis.
  - Complaints include insomnia, nonrestorative sleep, daytime fatigue, and/or somnolence.
  - Bed partner may complain of patient's movements.
  - Other sleep disorders such as obstructive sleep apnea (OSA), narcolepsy, restless legs syndrome do not explain the PLMS (2)[A].
- No wakeful perception of the PLMS or associated restlessness
  - If there is wakeful perception, the diagnosis is not periodic limb movement disorder (PLMD) but possibly restless leg syndrome (RLS).
- System(s) affected: musculoskeletal, nervous
- Synonym(s) referring to the PLMS: nocturnal myoclonus; sleep myoclonus

EPIDEMIOLOGY

Incidence
- PLMD is rare, reported in both children and adults (1).
- PLMS occurs in at least 15% of insomnia patients.
- PLMS is frequent in rapid eye movement (REM) sleep behavior disorder (RBD) occurring during REM sleep.
- PLMS is frequent in narcolepsy, in OSA, and during initiation of continuous positive airway pressure (CPAP).

Prevalence
- No predominant sex preference; male = female
- PLMS >5/hr is uncommon before age 40 years.
- PLMS increases with age: 45% of patients >65 years exhibit PLMS >5/hr but not necessarily PLMD.
- PLMD is much less common: <5% of adults but also underdiagnosed (1).
- 85% of RLS patients have PLMS (3).

ETIOLOGY AND PATHOPHYSIOLOGY
- Understudied; most data pertain to PLMS in RLS.
- Brain iron deficiency
- Suprasegmental disinhibition at the brainstem and spinal cord levels
- Spinal cord excitability
- CNS dopamine dysregulation supported by increased incidence of PLMS in untreated Parkinson disease (PD) patients
- Decreased incidence of PLMS in schizophrenia patients
- Triggering and exacerbating factors:
  - Peripheral neuropathy
  - Arthritis
  - Renal failure
  - Synucleinopathies (multiple-system atrophy)

- Spinal cord injury
- Pregnancy
- Medications:
  - Most antidepressants (except bupropion or desipramine) and lithium
  - Some antipsychotic and antidementia medications
  - Antiemetics (metoclopramide)
  - Antihistamines

Genetics
BTBD9 on chromosome 6p associated with PLMS in patients with or without RLS but not in RLS patients without PLMS

RISK FACTORS
- Family history of RLS
- Iron deficiency and associated conditions
- Peripheral neuropathy
- Arthritis, orthopedic problems
- Chronic limb pain or discomfort

GENERAL PREVENTION
- Adequate nightly sleep
- Avoid PLMS triggers such as iron deficiency, frequently observed in children (4).
- Awareness, including family history

COMMONLY ASSOCIATED CONDITIONS
- Narcolepsy
- Iron deficiency
- End-stage renal disease (ESRD)
- Cardiovascular disease; stroke
- Gastric surgery
- Pregnancy
- Arthritis
- Synucleinopathies (multiple-system atrophy)
- Lumbar spine disease; spinal cord injury
- Peripheral neuropathy
- Insomnia, insufficient sleep, parasomnias
- ADHD
- Mood disorders, anxiety, oppositional behaviors

Pediatric Considerations
- PLMD may precede overt RLS by years (4).
- Association with RLS is more common than in adults.
- Symptoms may be more consequential than in adults (5)[B].
- Association and differential diagnosis with ADHD, oppositional behaviors, mood disorders, growing pains (4)

Pregnancy Considerations
- May be secondary to iron or folate deficiency
- Most severe in the 3rd trimester
- Usually subsides after delivery

Geriatric Considerations
- May become a significant source of sleep disturbance
- May cause or exacerbate circadian disruption and "sundowning"
- Many medications given to the elderly may trigger or exacerbate PLMs, which can lead to PLMD or RLS.

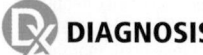 **DIAGNOSIS**

HISTORY
- Sleep disturbance:
  - Insomnia: difficulty maintaining sleep
  - Nonrestorative sleep
  - Daytime fatigue, tiredness, and/or somnolence
  - Oppositional behaviors
  - Memory impairment

- Depression
- ADHD, particularly in children (4)
- The PLMS and the symptoms cannot be better explained by another current sleep disorder, medical, neurologic or mental disorder.

PHYSICAL EXAM
- No specific findings
- Polysomnography
  - PLMs differ from limb movements (LMs) by showing periodicity: series of at least four movements 5 to 90 seconds apart.
  - Indices of PLMS suggestive of disorder:
    - PLMS >5/hr both for children or adults
    - Not associated with apneas or hypopneas

DIFFERENTIAL DIAGNOSIS
- When PLMs occur along with RLS, RBD, or narcolepsy, these disorders are diagnosed as with PLMs, and PLMD is not diagnosed separately.
- OSA: LMs occur during microarousals from apneas; treatment of sleep apnea eliminates these LMs.
- Sleep starts: nonperiodic, generalized, occur only at wake–sleep transition, <0.2 seconds duration
- Sleep-related leg cramps: isolated and painful
- Fragmentary myoclonus: 75 to 150 ms of electromyographic (EMG) activity, minimal movement, no periodicity
- Nocturnal seizures: epileptiform EEG, motor pattern incongruent with PLMs
- Fasciculations, tremor: no sleep association
- Sleep-related rhythmic movement disorder: voluntary movement during wake–sleep transition; higher frequency than PLMs
- Growing pains in children: Pain is the major concern.

DIAGNOSTIC TESTS & INTERPRETATION
- Polysomnography with finding of repetitive, stereotyped PLMs:
  - Tibialis anterior EMG activation lasting 0.5 to 10.0 seconds
  - EMG amplitude increases >8 μV from baseline
  - Movements occur in a sequence of ≥4 at intervals of 5 to 90 seconds.
  - Associated with heart rate variability from autonomic-level arousals
  - Most PLM episodes occur in the 1st hours of NREM sleep.
  - Night-to-night PLMS variability is common.
- Serum iron stores including ferritin, transferrin, iron-binding capacity, serum iron are used to assess for iron deficiency (at least ferritin).

Diagnostic Procedures/Other
- Ankle actigraphy for in-home use
- EMG or nerve conduction studies for peripheral neuropathy/radiculopathy

Test Interpretation
- Serum ferritin should be >75 ng/mL.
- Transferrin saturation >16%

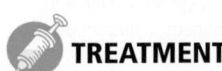 **TREATMENT**

Treatment paradigm similar to that for RLS, except that all medications are off-label for PLMD (2,3,6)[B]

GENERAL MEASURES
- Assess for and correct iron deficiency.
- Adequate nightly sleep
- Regular exercise, low impact, stretches in the evening
- Warm the legs (long socks, leg warmers, electric blanket, etc.).

- Hot bath before bedtime; leg baths
- Avoid caffeine and alcohol.

MEDICATION
- Use minimum effective dose.
- Goals of medication:
  – Improve subjective sleep quality.
  – Control PLMS and their effect on sleep.
- Consider risks, side effects, interactions in different populations (e.g., benzodiazepines in elderly).
- Low bedtime (HS) dosing minimizes daytime sleepiness side effect. Treatment should decrease instead of increase daytime somnolence.

First Line
Historically, currently debated—use clinical judgment
- Dopamine agonists reduce PLMS, increase sleep efficiency but has no effect on sleep instability; start low, titrate slow to optimal dose (2,3,6)[C]:
  – Pramipexole (Mirapex): 0.125 to 0.500 mg; titrate by 0.125 mg; take 2 hours before bedtime.
  – Ropinirole (Requip): 0.25 to 4.00 mg; titrate by 0.25 mg; take 1/2 to 1 hour before bedtime; preferred in renal impairment
  – Transdermal rotigotine (Neupro): 1 to 3 mg/24 hr patch; initiate with 1 mg/24 hr; titrate up by 1 mg slowly to effectiveness.
- Avoid dopamine agonists in psychotic patients, especially if taking dopamine antagonists.
- Dopamine agonists may exert a stimulant effect, further disturbing sleep.

Second Line
- Voltage-gated calcium channel $\alpha 2\delta$ subunit ligands: useful for associated neuropathy; decrease PLMS and improve sleep architecture (2,3)[C]:
  – Gabapentin enacarbil (Horizant): 600 mg/day taken early evening; caution with liver disease and with renal impairment
  – Gabapentin (Neurontin): 300 to 1,200 mg/day 1/2 dose before bedtime; caution with liver disease and renal impairment
  – Pregabalin (Lyrica): 75 to 300 mg/day before bedtime
- Benzodiazepines and agonists (2,3)[C]; most commonly used because of their effect on sleep; caution in the elderly
  – Clonazepam (Klonopin): 0.5 to 3.0 mg/day
  – Zaleplon, zolpidem, temazepam, triazolam, alprazolam, diazepam
- Opioids: low risk for tolerance with bedtime dose; most commonly used when other treatments fail; can decrease respiratory drive
  – Hydrocodone: 5 to 20 mg/day
  – Oxycodone: 2.5 to 20.0 mg/day

ISSUES FOR REFERRAL
To sleep medicine clinic, neurology and movement disorders clinic:
- High-dose medications
- Worsening of symptoms while on medications
- Intractable iron deficiency

Pediatric Considerations
- First-line treatment is nonpharmacologic (4)[C].
- Assess/correct iron deficiency (5)[B].
- Consider low-dose clonidine 0.1 mg to 0.3 mg at bedtime; caution: orthostatic hypotension (4)[C]

Pregnancy Considerations
- Initial approach: iron supplementation, nonpharmacologic therapies (6)
- Avoid medications class C or D.
- In 3rd trimester, low-dose opioids may be considered. Monitor/address constipation.

Geriatric Considerations
In weak or frail patients, avoid medications that may cause dizziness or unsteadiness.

ADDITIONAL THERAPIES
- If iron deficient, iron supplementation:
  – 325-mg ferrous sulfate with 200 mg vitamin C between meals TID
  – Repletion may require months of treatment.
  – Symptoms continue without other treatment.
- Vitamin/mineral supplements, including calcium, magnesium, vitamin B_{12}, folate
- Clonidine 0.05 to 0.30 mg/day
- Relaxis leg vibration device (http://myrelaxis.com); limited data

SURGERY/OTHER PROCEDURES
Correction of orthopedic, neuropathic, or peripheral vascular problems

ADMISSION, INPATIENT, AND NURSING CONSIDERATIONS
- Control during recovery from orthopedic procedures
- Addition or withdrawal of medications that affect PLMD
- Changes in medical status may require medication changes (e.g., Mirapex contraindicated in renal failure; Requip contraindicated in liver disease).
- Consider iron infusion when oral supplementation is ineffective, not tolerated, or contraindicated.
- When NPO, consider IV opiates.
- Evening walks, hot baths, leg warming
- Sleep interruption risks prolonged wakefulness.

 ## ONGOING CARE

FOLLOW-UP RECOMMENDATIONS
Patient Monitoring
- At monthly intervals until stable
- Assess symptom severity, medication side effects, augmentation.
- Annual and PRN follow-up thereafter.
- If iron deficient, reassess iron stores: ferritin, transferrin, IBC, and serum iron.

DIET
Avoid caffeine and alcohol, more so late in the day.

PATIENT EDUCATION
- National Sleep Foundation: http://sleepfoundation.org/
- American Academy of Sleep Medicine: http://www.sleepeducation.org/

PROGNOSIS
- Primary PLMD: lifelong condition with no current cure
- Secondary PLMD: may subside with resolution of cause(s) such as low iron stores
- Current therapies usually control symptoms.
- PLMD often precedes the emergence of RLS.

COMPLICATIONS
Mostly based on RLS data
- Tolerance to medications requiring increased dose or alternatives
- Augmentation (increased PLMs and sleep disturbance, emergence of RLS) from prolonged use of dopamine agonists:
  – Higher doses increase risk.
  – Iron deficiency increases augmentation risk.
  – Add alternative medication and then gradually discontinue dopaminergic agent.
- Iatrogenic PLMD (from antidepressants, etc.)

REFERENCES
1. Hornyak M, Feige B, Riemann D, et al. Periodic leg movements in sleep and periodic limb movement disorder: prevalence, clinical significance and treatment. *Sleep Med Rev.* 2006;10(3):169–177.
2. Aurora RN, Kristo DA, Bista SR, et al; for American Academy of Sleep Medicine. The treatment of restless legs syndrome and periodic limb movement disorder in adults—an update for 2012: practice parameters with an evidence-based systematic review and meta-analyses: an American Academy of Sleep Medicine Clinical Practice Guideline. *Sleep.* 2012;35(8):1039–1062.
3. Fulda S. The role of periodic limb movements during sleep in restless legs syndrome: a selective update. *Sleep Med Clin.* 2015;10(3):241–248.
4. Sharon D, Walters AS, Simakajornboon N. RLS and PLMD in children in sleep disorders in children. *J Child Sci.* In press.
5. Gingras JL, Gaultney JF, Picchietti DL. Pediatric periodic limb movement disorder: sleep symptom and polysomnographic correlates compared to obstructive sleep apnea. *J Clin Sleep Med.* 2011;7(6):603A–609A.
6. Garcia-Borreguero D, Silber MH, Winkelman JW, et al. Guidelines for the first-line treatment of restless legs syndrome/Willis-Ekbom disease, prevention and treatment of dopaminergic augmentation: a combined task force of the IRLSSG, EURLSSG, and the RLS-foundation. *Sleep Med.* 2016;21:1–11.

ADDITIONAL READING
- American Academy of Sleep Medicine. Periodic limb movement disorder. In: *International Classification of Sleep Disorders.* 3rd ed. Darien, IL: American Academy of Sleep Medicine; 2014:292–299.
- Högl B, Comella C. Therapeutic advances in restless legs syndrome (RLS). *Mov Disord.* 2015;30(11):1574–1579.
- Provini F, Chiaro G. Neuroimaging in restless legs syndrome. *Sleep Med Clin.* 2015;10(3):215–226.

 ## SEE ALSO

Restless Legs Syndrome

 ## CODES

ICD10
G47.61 Periodic limb movement disorder

CLINICAL PEARLS
- Many patients with PLMs may not require treatment; however, when sleep disturbance from PLMs causes insomnia and/or daytime consequences, PLMD exists and should be treated.
- Assessing iron stores, at least ferritin, supports the diagnosis and provides options for treatment.
- Many antidepressants and some antihistamines cause or exacerbate PLMs.

PERIPHERAL ARTERIAL DISEASE

Keshav Kukreja, MD • Adrian DaSilva-DeAbreu, MD • Raymundo A. Quintana, MD

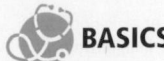 BASICS

DESCRIPTION

Peripheral arterial disease (PAD) represents atherosclerotic occlusive disease of the peripheral arteries, most commonly in the lower extremities. Following coronary artery disease and cerebrovascular disease, PAD is the third leading source of atherosclerotic vascular morbidity. PAD manifests as intermittent claudication (IC) or atypical leg pain and is commonly diagnosed with a resting ankle-brachial index (ABI) of <0.90.

EPIDEMIOLOGY
- Age: >65 years
  - Age: 50 to 64 years with risk factors for atherosclerosis or a family history of PAD
  - Age: <50 years in the presence of diabetes mellitus (DM) and one additional risk factor
- Sex: male > female (2:1)
- Impacts at least 8.5 million people in the United States
- Globally, an estimated 202 million people have PAD with increased prevalence in low- and middle-income countries.

Incidence
- Annual incidence is 7.1/1,000 men and 3.6/1,000 women among all ages, per Framingham Heart Study.
- Incidence increases with age and the presence of cardiovascular risk factors.

Prevalence
- U.S. prevalence: 5.9% in adults >40 years
- Prevalence approaches 30% in high-risk populations.
- Higher prevalence and severity in African Americans and Hispanics

ETIOLOGY AND PATHOPHYSIOLOGY
- In PAD, arterial occlusion is most commonly a result of underlying atherosclerotic disease.
- Other etiologies for PAD include phlebitis, trauma, or autoimmune/vasculitic diseases.
- Arterial narrowing results in insufficient oxygen delivery to the muscle during periods of increased demand (i.e., exercise), causing claudication and limiting exercise.
- Reperfusion at rest following ischemia can result in multiple subsequent physiologic changes, including inflammation, oxidant stress, endothelial dysfunction, and mitochondrial injury.

Genetics
Although several of the risk factors for PAD (as noted below) are heritable, genome-wide association studies isolating PAD-specific single nucleotide polymorphisms have not been as successful. This has been attributed to the increased clinical and genetic heterogeneity of PAD.

RISK FACTORS
- Age >65 years
- Cigarette smoking
- DM
- Obesity
- Hypertension (HTN)
- Hyperlipidemia (HLD)
- Chronic kidney disease (CKD)
- Hyperviscosity
- Heritable conditions: chylomicronemia, hypercholesterolemia, hyperhomocysteinemia, and pseudoxanthoma elasticum

GENERAL PREVENTION
- Regular aerobic exercise program
- Smoking cessation
- Blood pressure (BP) and diabetes control

- Statin therapy is indicated in patients with clinical PAD for secondary prevention of atherosclerotic cardiovascular disease.

COMMONLY ASSOCIATED CONDITIONS
In addition to the aforementioned risk factors, PAD is associated with other forms of atherosclerotic disease including myocardial infarction (MI), transient ischemic attack (TIA), and cerebrovascular accident (CVA).

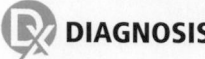 DIAGNOSIS

HISTORY
- Nearly 50% of patients will be asymptomatic.
- IC seen in 10–30% of patients and is typically self-limiting with symptoms resolving within 2 to 5 minutes of rest
- Atypical or resting leg pain in 20–40% of patients
- Critical limb ischemia (pain and/or tissue loss)
- Nonhealing wounds and ulceration
- Skin discoloration and gangrene
- Erectile dysfunction (in conjunction with IC and absent or diminished femoral pulses constitutes Leriche syndrome)

PHYSICAL EXAM
- Pallor with leg elevation
- Dependent rubor
- Dry, scaly skin
- Brittle or hypertrophic nails
- Hair loss
- Reduced/absent extremity pulses
- Ulcers (distal toes, lateral malleolus, metatarsal heads)

DIFFERENTIAL DIAGNOSIS
- Arterial aneurysm or dissection
- Deep vein thrombosis (DVT)
- Thromboangiitis obliterans (Buerger disease)
- Peripheral neuropathy
- Spinal stenosis or nerve root compression (neurogenic claudication)
- Popliteal entrapment syndrome

DIAGNOSTIC TESTS & INTERPRETATION
Screening
- The association between PAD and cardiovascular morbidity and mortality has been well established, with a lower ABI being an independent predictor.
- Patients at increased risk (criteria below) should undergo thorough history, review of systems, and physical examination with a focus on exertional leg symptoms (IC), pain at rest, and nonhealing wounds.
- Also important is a vasculature exam, including assessment of lower extremity pulses, auscultation for femoral bruits, inspection of legs and feet, and BP measurement in both arms (1)[C].
  - Age ≥65 years
  - Age 50 to 64 years with risk factors for atherosclerosis (DM, smoking, HTN, HLD)
  - Age <50 years with DM and one additional risk factor
  - Patients at any age with known atherosclerotic disease elsewhere

Initial Tests (lab, imaging)
- Risk factor identification with fasting lipid profile and basic metabolic profile
- Resting ABI should be performed in patients with suggestive history and physical findings or those at increased risk of PAD (1)[C].
- Exercise treadmill ABI is useful in patients who are symptomatic but have normal resting ABI.

- Imaging is reserved for patients who have lifestyle-limiting symptoms (IC) despite appropriate guideline-directed management and therapy.
  - Duplex ultrasound, magnetic resonance angiography (MRA), and computed tomography angiography (CTA) are recommended in symptomatic patients who are being considered for revascularization (1)[C].
  - Invasive angiography is recommended in patients with critical limb ischemia (1)[B] and is reasonable in those with symptomatic PAD who are candidates for revascularization (1)[C].

Diagnostic Procedures/Other
- Doppler ABI: ratio of systolic BP at the ankle and brachial artery
  - Technique: Obtain BP at dorsalis pedis and posterior tibial arteries while patient is supine and limb is positioned at level of heart. Also obtain BP of both brachial arteries. Then divide higher of the two ankle systolic pressures (dorsalis pedis or posterior tibial) by the higher brachial systolic pressure.
  - ABI ≥1.40 → noncompressible calcified vessel, often seen in CKD, DM, and elderly patients
  - ABI 0.91 to 0.99 → borderline, correlate clinically and consider additional testing
  - ABI ≤0.90, abnormal, diagnostic for PAD
- Leg segmental pressures: obtained after abnormal ABI to localize occlusion and determine treatment plan. A ≤20-mm Hg reduction in pressure is considered significant.
- Toe-brachial index (TBI) is recommended when ABI is ≥1.40, suggesting a noncompressible vessel (1)[B].

 TREATMENT

GENERAL MEASURES
- The treatment of PAD is multifactorial and includes a supervised exercise program, guideline-based medical therapy, and risk factor modification (2).
- An interdisciplinary approach is recommended for optimal treatment, including physicians (vascular specialists if indicated), nurses, exercise physiologists, podiatrists, nutritionists, and social workers.
- Supervised exercise training, which takes place in a hospital or outpatient facility, is the initial treatment modality recommended in patients with IC (1)[A]. Patients are instructed to walk for a minimum of 30 to 45 minutes (with rest when symptomatic) 3 times per week for a minimum of 12 weeks.
  - A structured community or home-based exercise program can be beneficial and is recommended when a supervised program is not possible (1)[A].
- Risk factor modification, most importantly smoking cessation and management of DM, HTN, and HLD:
  - Ask about smoking at every visit, counsel on cessation, and offer pharmacologic agents when appropriate (varenicline, bupropion, nicotine replacement therapy) (1)[A].
  - Antiplatelet therapy with aspirin or clopidogrel is recommended for patients with PAD when there are no contraindications; however, support for aspirin monotherapy is weak (3)[A]. Studies with aspirin monotherapy have not demonstrated a consistent reduction in fatal or nonfatal cardiovascular events or rates of revascularization. Clopidogrel was shown to have a small relative-risk reduction in ischemic stroke, MI, or vascular death compared to aspirin monotherapy (CAPRIE trial). Benefit must be weighed against harms—particularly risk of gastrointestinal bleeding.

– The use of rivaroxaban (Xarelto) 2.5 mg twice daily with aspirin reduced the composite end point of cardiovascular mortality, MI or stroke, and major adverse limb events compared to aspirin alone (COMPASS trial). However, despite excluding patients with greater bleeding risk, there was a higher rate of major bleeding events in the rivaroxaban (Xarelto) and aspirin group compared to aspirin alone (4).

– High-intensity statin (lipid-lowering therapy) is recommended for all patients with PAD and has been shown to reduce all-cause mortality (1)[A].

– Goal BP <140/90 mm Hg

– ACE-inhibitors are associated with a significant reduction in major adverse cardiovascular events in patients with PAD (1)[A].

MEDICATION

First Line

- Antiplatelet therapy is recommended in symptomatic PAD without bleeding risk contraindications (3)[A]. Aspirin (75 to 325 mg) or clopidogrel (75 mg) is acceptable first-line antiplatelet agent.

    – It is reasonable to prescribe antiplatelet therapy in asymptomatic patients who have an ABI diagnostic of PAD (1)[C].

    – In asymptomatic patients with borderline ABIs (0.91 to 0.99), the utility of antiplatelet therapy is not well established (1)[B].

    – The effect of aspirin on the risk reduction of overall ischemic events remains inconclusive. The Prevention of Progression of Arterial Disease and Diabetes (POPADAD) and Aspirin for Asymptomatic Atherosclerosis (AAA) trials compared low-dose aspirin to placebo in patients with lower ABIs and failed to show a significant reduction in fatal and nonfatal cardiovascular events. However, some studies suggest that aspirin delays disease progression and reduces the need for surgical intervention.

- Dual antiplatelet therapy (DAPT; aspirin and clopidogrel) should be prescribed only following endovascular intervention (1)[C]; the data for efficacy is not well established (1)[B], and bleeding risk is increased.

- Cilostazol (100 mg orally twice daily) has been shown to improve walking distance and should be considered in all patients with claudication that impacts daily living (1)[C]. However, there is insufficient data on the effect of cilostazol on all-cause mortality or cardiovascular events.

Second Line

- Vorapaxar sulfate (Zontivity) (a protease-activated receptor-1 [PAR-1] inhibitor) reduces rates of revascularization and acute limb ischemia, but several studies indicate a major risk of bleeding, including intracranial hemorrhage. Thus, it is not recommended in those with high bleeding risk or with prior CVA, TIA, or intracranial hemorrhage.

- Pentoxifylline (400 mg 3 times daily) was previously considered first line for symptomatic relief of claudication; however, evidence is of poor quality and benefit is uncertain (Cochrane, other reviews).

- Prostaglandins (beraprost, iloprost, cicaprost) are not recommended because they have not shown long-term benefit and are associated with increased adverse events such as headache, nausea, flushing, and diarrhea.

SURGERY/OTHER PROCEDURES

Consider endovascular and surgical interventions in select patients who had an inadequate response to less invasive modalities (i.e., exercise and pharmacotherapy),

suffer debilitating IC, ischemic rest pain, or tissue loss and have a favorable risk-benefit ratio.

- Beforehand, assess functional status via the Fontaine or Rutherford classification systems. Anatomic classification of complexity is determined by the Trans-Atlantic Inter-Society Consensus (TASC) (5).

- Endovascular therapy is rapidly involving and includes angioplasty and stent placement. Balloons and stents can be drug eluting.

    – Preferred for patients with aortoiliac disease (1)[A] and reasonable for femoropopliteal disease (1)[B]

    – Current data are insufficient regarding infrapopliteal lesions, but ongoing studies are comparing efficacy between endovascular and surgical intervention.

COMPLEMENTARY & ALTERNATIVE MEDICINE

- Chelation therapy and B-complex vitamins are not recommended in patients with PAD (1)[B].

- Additional studies on *Ginkgo biloba*, L-arginine, propionyl-L-carnitine, omega-3 fatty acids, and vitamin E have been studied and, in general, their efficacy is uncertain. Thus, currently they are not recommended for use in the primary care setting.

 ONGOING CARE

FOLLOW-UP RECOMMENDATIONS

- At follow-up, patients should undergo thorough history and physical examinations. They should be asked about their progress with risk-factor modification (i.e., smoking, glucose control, HTN), exercise endurance and compliance with training program, and effectiveness of pharmacotherapy.

- After endovascular or surgical intervention, patients should receive regular assessment of symptoms and occlusion via resting and exercise ABIs.

DIET

- A heart-healthy diet is recommended in all patients with PAD or atherosclerotic disease and risk factors.

- Balanced diets consisting of vegetables, fruit, nuts, protein, and healthy fats (such as the Mediterranean diet) are likely best.

- Consultation with a nutritionist can be used in patients when appropriate.

PROGNOSIS

- Limb ischemia and IC: 15–20% will have worsening claudication, 5–10% will require endovascular or surgical intervention, and 2–5% will undergo amputation (most commonly smokers and diabetics).

- Considering cardiovascular outcomes, at 5 years, 20% of patients with PAD will experience a nonfatal cardiovascular event, and 15–20% will die, most commonly of cardiovascular disease.

REFERENCES

1. Gerhard-Herman MD, Gornik HL, Barrett C, et al. 2016 AHA/ACC guideline on the management of patients with lower extremity peripheral artery disease: executive summary: a report of the American College of Cardiology/American Heart Association Task Force on Clinical Practice Guidelines. *Circulation*. 2017;135(12):e686–e725.

2. Olin JW, White CJ, Armstrong EJ, et al. Peripheral artery disease: evolving role of exercise, medical therapy, and endovascular options. *J Am Coll Cardiol*. 2016;67(11):1338–1357.

3. Wong PF, Chong LY, Mikhailidis DP, et al. Antiplatelet agents for intermittent claudication. *Cochrane Database Syst Rev*. 2011;(11):CD001272.

4. Anand SS, Bosch J, Eikelboom JW, et al; for COMPASS Investigators. Rivaroxaban with or without aspirin in patients with stable peripheral or carotid artery disease: an international, randomised, double-blind, placebo-controlled trial. *Lancet*. 2018;391(10117):219–229.

5. Abu Dabrh AM, Steffen MW, Asi N, et al. Bypass surgery versus endovascular interventions in severe or critical limb ischemia. *J Vasc Surg*. 2016;63(1):244–253.e11.

ADDITIONAL READING

- Criqui MH, Aboyans V. Epidemiology of peripheral artery disease. *Circ Res*. 2015;116(9):1509–1526.

- Hiatt WR, Armstrong EJ, Larson CJ, et al. Pathogenesis of the limb manifestations and exercise limitations in peripheral artery disease. *Circ Res*. 2015;116(9):1527–1539.

- Hirsch AT, Criqui MH, Treat-Jacobson D, et al. Peripheral arterial disease detection, awareness, and treatment in primary care. *JAMA*. 2001;286(11):1317–1324.

- Teraa M, Conte MS, Moll FL, et al. Critical limb ischemia: current trends and future directions. *J Am Heart Assoc*. 2016;5(2):e002938.

CODES

ICD10

- I73.9 Peripheral vascular disease, unspecified
- I70.209 Unsp athscl native arteries of extremities, unsp extremity
- I70.219 Athscl native arteries of extrm w intrmt claud, unsp extrm

CLINICAL PEARLS

- Consensus on screening for PAD varies. The USPSTF (2013) finds that evidence is insufficient to weigh harms and benefits of screening for PAD.

- The 2016 AHA/ACC guidelines recommend a thorough history, physical exam, and subsequent resting ABI for patients considered at high risk (≥65 years, 50 to 64 years with a risk factor [HTN, HLD, DM, smoking], <50 years with DM and one additional risk factor, or patients at any age with known atherosclerotic disease).

- An interdisciplinary therapeutic approach is recommended. Those who fail noninvasive therapy with a supervised exercise training program and appropriate pharmacotherapy should be referred to vascular surgery for evaluation. Also, patients with an unclear diagnosis or those with CLI (pain at rest, gangrene, ulceration) should be referred.

- Antiplatelet therapy (aspirin or clopidogrel) and cilostazol for symptomatic relief are at the cornerstone of pharmacotherapy. Additionally, appropriate BP control (BP <140/90 mm Hg) and HLD management with statin therapy are indicated in all patients.

- Current studies assessing appropriate screening, optimal pharmacotherapy, and the benefit of endovascular over surgery are underway, suggesting possible improvement of the evidence and guidelines in coming years.

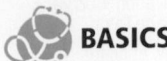

PERITONITIS, ACUTE

Nadeem Tabbara, MD • Marie L. Borum, MD, EdD, MPH, MACP, FACG, AGAF

BASICS

DESCRIPTION
- Definition: inflammation of the peritoneum
- Classification:
  - Aseptic: chemical irritation or systemic inflammation of peritoneum
  - Bacterial: infection of peritoneal fluid
- Bacterial peritonitis types:
  - Primary/spontaneous bacterial peritonitis (SBP): infection of ascitic fluid in the absence of an intra-abdominal source; typically monomicrobial
  - Secondary bacterial peritonitis: infection of ascitic fluid from a detectable intra-abdominal source (i.e., perforation, abscess); typically polymicrobial
  - Tertiary bacterial peritonitis: persistent infection despite therapy

EPIDEMIOLOGY
Incidence
- In patients with ascites, the annual incidence of SBP is 10–25% (1).
- Secondary bacterial peritonitis correlates with underlying pathology (e.g., colitis, appendicitis, diverticulitis, PUD).
- 57% of patients with secondary bacterial peritonitis progress to tertiary peritonitis (2).

Prevalence
- SBP: In asymptomatic patients with cirrhosis and ascites, the prevalence is <3% in outpatients. Nosocomial rates are 8–36% (3).
- In patients with cirrhosis and ascites, 5% of peritonitis is secondary (4).

ETIOLOGY AND PATHOPHYSIOLOGY
- Mechanism
  - SBP:
    - Bacterial translocation via lymphatic spread through mesenteric lymph nodes
    - Cirrhotic patients have:
      - Alterations to gut microbiota with higher prevalence of pathogenic organisms
      - Small intestinal bacterial overgrowth (SIBO) and increased intestinal mucosal permeability to bacteria
      - Decreased cellular and humoral immunity limiting peritoneal bacterial clearance
  - Secondary bacterial peritonitis
    - Spillage/translocation of bacteria from inflamed or perforated intraperitoneal organs or introduction of bacterial through instrumentation—including peritoneal dialysis, intraperitoneal chemotherapy
  - Tertiary bacterial peritonitis
    - Evolves from secondary peritonitis with inadequate source control and/or altered host immunity
- Microbiology
  - SBP
    - Escherichia coli (33%), Streptococcus spp. (15%), Staphylococcus (13%), Klebsiella (8%); reflects increasing rate of gram-positive and resistant organisms (e.g., extended-spectrum β-lactamase [ESBL]–producing E. coli, MRSA, Enterococcus) in the nosocomial setting (5)
  - Secondary bacterial peritonitis:
    - E. coli, Klebsiella, Proteus, Streptococcus, Enterococcus, Bacteroides, Clostridium

RISK FACTORS
- SBP: advanced cirrhosis with ascites, malnutrition, upper GI bleed, PPI usage, prior SBP
  - Acid suppression (most commonly with PPIs) promotes SIBO increasing incidence of SBP. Hospitalized cirrhosis patients receiving PPIs are at increased risk for SBP (3,5).
  - 70% of SBP cases are in patients with Child-Pugh class C cirrhosis (1).
  - Low ascites protein (<1.0 g/dL) increases risk.
- Factors associated with perforation or fluid translocation (e.g., peritoneal dialysis, Helicobacter pylori and NSAIDs causing ulcers, vascular disease causing bowel ischemia, alcohol abuse causing pancreatitis) increase risk for SBP.

GENERAL PREVENTION
- SBP prophylaxis in patients at high risk (e.g., ascitic fluid protein concentration <1.0 g/dL, esophageal varices, or history of previous SBP)
  - Prior SBP: prophylactic norfloxacin or sulfamethoxazole and trimethoprim (Bactrim) PO daily (6)[A]
  - Cirrhosis and GI bleed: 7-day course of ceftriaxone 1 g IV daily or norfloxacin BID; IV while bleeding, PO as tolerated. IV ceftriaxone is superior to oral norfloxacin (6)[A].
  - Cirrhotic ascites: low ascitic fluid protein (<1.5 g/dL) with renal impairment (creatinine ≥1.2, BUN ≥25, or serum Na ≤130) or liver failure (child score ≥9, bilirubin ≥3): prophylactic norfloxacin or sulfamethoxazole and trimethoprim (Bactrim) PO daily (3,6)[A]
- Limit use of PPIs (6)[B].

DIAGNOSIS

HISTORY
- SBP: history of cirrhosis or ascites, fever, mental status changes, abdominal pain, chills, nausea/vomiting, GI bleed
- Secondary bacterial peritonitis: may be clinically indistinguishable from SBP unless history of perforation, abscess, or peritoneal dialysis is present
- Tertiary: persistent signs and symptoms despite initial treatment, or history of recurrent peritonitis

ALERT
30% of patients are asymptomatic (1).

PHYSICAL EXAM
- Tachycardia, fever, tachypnea, altered mental status
- Abdominal distention, ascites, abdominal wall guarding and rigidity, rebound tenderness, hypoactive/absent bowel sounds

DIFFERENTIAL DIAGNOSIS
- Liver disease: hepatitis, decompensated cirrhosis
- Luminal disease: abscess formation, ileus, volvulus, intussusception, mesenteric adenitis, pancreatitis, cholecystitis, malignancy, peritoneal carcinomatosis
- Extraluminal disease: ruptured ectopic pregnancy, tubo-ovarian abscess, PID, UTI, and/or pyelonephritis
- Systemic disease: tuberculosis, pneumonia, MI, porphyria, SLE

DIAGNOSTIC TESTS & INTERPRETATION
Initial Tests (lab, imaging)

ALERT
Early diagnosis reduces mortality. Perform paracentesis in ascitic patients admitted to the hospital (6)[B].

- Immediate evaluation
  - Paracentesis, blood, and urine cultures before antibiotics (1,6)[B]. Broad-spectrum antibiotics decrease ascitic culture yield (even a single dose).
  - Ascitic fluid studies: culture, Gram stain, cell count with differential, and albumin (1)[B]; for secondary peritonitis, include LDH, total protein, glucose, alkaline phosphatase (ALP), and CEA.
  - Inoculating ascitic fluid into blood culture bottles (aerobic, anaerobic) at the bedside increases culture yield 80–90% (3,5)[B].
  - Urine dipstick (PMN >250 cells/mm³) of ascitic fluid shows promise for bedside diagnosis (6).

ALERT
Ascitic fluid culture can be negative in up to 50% of patients with SBP (1)[A].

- SBP: ascitic fluid PMN >250 cells/mm³
- Culture-negative neutrocytic ascites: negative ascites culture, ascitic fluid PMN >250 cells/mm³
- Nonneutrocytic bacterascites: positive ascites culture, ascitic fluid PMN <250 cells/mm³
- Secondary peritonitis: PMN >250 cells/mm³ on ascitic fluid analysis (usually thousands), with the following:
  - Polymicrobial culture or two of: ascitic fluid total protein >1 g/dL, glucose <50 mg/dL, LDH >225 mU/mL; more sensitive for cases of perforation (96%) than nonperforation (50%) (6)[B]
  - Secondary peritonitis with perforation is likely with ALP >240 U/L or CEA >5 ng/mL, sensitivity 92% (6)[B]; not useful for detection of nonperforation secondary peritonitis
- CT scan is often not diagnostic for secondary peritonitis (6)[B].
  - Abdominal or chest x-ray may show free air in peritoneal cavity, large/small bowel dilatation, intestinal wall edema in secondary peritonitis.

Follow-Up Tests & Special Considerations
- If asymptomatic bacterascites, recent antibiotic exposure, nosocomial atypical organism, or no clinical improvement, repeat paracentesis in 48 hours to determine resolution (decrease in PMNs of 25% or negative cultures) (1)[C].
- In hemorrhagic ascites, PMN count is corrected by subtracting 1 PMN per 250 RBCs (3)[A].

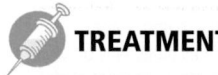

TREATMENT

GENERAL MEASURES
- For SBP, control ascites with salt restriction, spironolactone ±, furosemide, albumin infusion after large volume paracentesis, and/or lactulose for encephalopathy (6)[A].
- Avoid nephrotoxic medications and other renal insults (5)[C].

MEDICATION

- SBP

  - Community-acquired SBP without recent β-lactam antibiotic use: 3rd-generation cephalosporins, preferably cefotaxime, 2 g IV q8h for 5 days (6)[A]
  - SBP in absence of previous quinolone use/ prophylaxis, vomiting, shock, hepatic encephalopathy, or serum creatinine >3 mg/dL: can substitute ofloxacin 400 mg PO for cefotaxime (6)[B]
  - Nosocomial SBP or recent β-lactam antibiotic: empiric therapy based on local susceptibility of patients with cirrhosis for resistant bacteria (6)[B]
  - Symptomatic bacterascites with PMN count <250 cells/mm³: cefotaxime 2 g IV q8h while awaiting sensitivities (6)[B]
  - Second-line antibiotics include fluoroquinolones (levofloxacin), piperacillin/tazobactam, or vancomycin (5)[B],(6)[C].
  - SBP with renal or hepatic impairment (serum creatinine >1 mg/dL, BUN >30 mg/dL, or total bilirubin >4 mg/dL): Add albumin 1.5 g/kg within 6 hours and 1 g/kg on day 3 (1)[A],(6)[B].

- Secondary bacterial peritonitis

  - Empiric broad-spectrum antibiotic coverage for polymicrobial infection; IV cefotaxime or other 3rd- to 4th-generation cephalosporin plus metronidazole is an initial option.
  - In peritoneal dialysis–associated infection, intraperitoneal route is superior to IV.

- Tertiary bacterial peritonitis

  - If no unrepaired perforations or leaks, continue with medical management: Antibiotics (guided by susceptibilities) and early enteral nutrition prevent atrophy and maintain immunocompetence (2)[B].
  - Consider removing catheter if recurrent or persistent peritoneal dialysis–associated infection.

SURGERY/OTHER PROCEDURES

- SBP

  - Medical management

- Secondary bacterial peritonitis

  - Emergent surgical management, including source control with open laparotomy to repair any perforated viscus and eradicate infected material, is first-line treatment (2)[A],(6)[B].

- Tertiary bacterial peritonitis

  - If no unrepaired perforations or leaks, additional surgery for severe abdominal infection correlates with deterioration and mortality (2).

ALERT

The mortality of secondary bacterial peritonitis approaches 100% if not treated surgically. The mortality of SBP approaches 80% if unnecessary exploratory laparotomy is performed (1,3).

ADMISSION, INPATIENT, AND NURSING CONSIDERATIONS

- Acute peritonitis typically warrants hospitalization.
- In patients with cardiogenic or septic shock, use invasive monitoring with goal-directed fluid therapy.
- Patients who present with peritonitis can be severely hypovolemic and volume resuscitation is critical. In patients with significant renal or hepatic dysfunction, albumin decreases mortality (1)[A],(6)[B].
- Cirrhotic patients are often on β-blockers. During an episode of SBP, β-blockers increase mortality, hepatorenal syndrome, and hospital stay (6)[B].
- Nasogastric tube placement helps prevent aspiration in patients with vomiting or GI bleeding.

ONGOING CARE

FOLLOW-UP RECOMMENDATIONS

Patient Monitoring

Normalization of vital signs with resolution of leukocytosis is a sign of improvement.

- SBP: PMN decrease >25% is expected if follow-up paracentesis is performed after 48 hours.
- Leukopenia suggests immune exhaustion and is associated with a poor prognosis.

DIET

- NPO, total parental nutrition as necessary
- Resume enteral feeding after return of bowel function.
- Sodium restriction can reduce future ascites (3)[A].

PROGNOSIS

- SBP

  - For inpatients with first episode of SBP, mortality ranges from 10% to 50% (3).
  - Prognosis improves if antibiotics are started early, prior to onset of shock or renal failure.
  - Renal insufficiency is the strongest negative prognostic indicator.
  - Other poor prognostic factors include nosocomial acquisition, old age, high Child-Pugh-Turcotte or MELD score, malnutrition, malignancy, peripheral leukopenia, and antibiotic resistance (3).
  - Patients with prior SBP have 1-year recurrence of 40–70% and 1-year mortality of 31–93% (1,3).

- Secondary bacterial peritonitis:

  - In-hospital mortality of treated patients is 67% (4).
  - Mortality approaches 100% if not treated surgically, especially with perforation (2,4).
  - Prognosis is worse in perforated etiologies.

COMPLICATIONS

- Renal and hepatic failure, encephalopathy, coagulopathy
- Secondary infection, iatrogenic infection, abscess, fistula formation, abdominal compartment syndrome
- Sepsis/septic shock, cardiovascular collapse, adrenal insufficiency, respiratory failure, ARDS

REFERENCES

1. Alaniz C, Regal RE. Spontaneous bacterial peritonitis: a review of treatment options. *P T.* 2009;34(4):204–210.
2. Panhofer P, Izay B, Riedl M, et al. Age, microbiology and prognostic scores help to differentiate between secondary and tertiary peritonitis. *Langenbecks Arch Surg.* 2009;394(2):265–271.
3. Wiest R, Krag A, Gerbes A. Spontaneous bacterial peritonitis: recent guidelines and beyond. *Gut.* 2012;61(2):297–310.
4. Soriano G, Castellote J, Alvarez C, et al. Secondary bacterial peritonitis in cirrhosis: a retrospective study of clinical and analytical characteristics, diagnosis and management. *J Hepatol.* 2010;52(1):39–44.
5. Dever JB, Sheikh MY. Review article: spontaneous bacterial peritonitis—bacteriology, diagnosis, treatment, risk factors and prevention. *Aliment Pharmacol Ther.* 2015;41(11):1116–1131.
6. Runyon B; for American Association for the Study of Liver Diseases. Introduction to the revised American Association for the Study of Liver Diseases practice guideline management of adult patients with ascites due to cirrhosis 2012. *Hepatology.* 2013;57(4):1651–1653.

ADDITIONAL READING

- Bajaj JS, O'Leary JG, Wong F, et al. Bacterial infections in end-stage liver disease: current challenges and future directions. *Gut.* 2012;61(8):1219–1225.
- Ballinger A, Palmer SC, Wiggins KJ, et al. Treatment for peritoneal dialysis-associated peritonitis. *Cochrane Database Syst Rev.* 2014;(4):CD005284.
- Chaulk J, Carbonneau M, Qamar H, et al. Third-generation cephalosporin-resistant spontaneous bacterial peritonitis: a single-centre experience and summary of existing studies. *Can J Gastroenterol Hepatol.* 2014;28(2):83–88.
- Deshpande A, Pasupuleti V, Thota P, et al. Acid-suppressive therapy is associated with spontaneous bacterial peritonitis in cirrhotic patients: a meta-analysis. *J Gastroenterol Hepatol.* 2013;28(2):235–242.
- Solomkin JS, Mazuski JE, Bradley JS, et al. Diagnosis and management of complicated intra-abdominal infection in adults and children: guidelines by the Surgical Infection Society and the Infectious Diseases Society of America. *Clin Infect Dis.* 2010;50(2):133–164.

SEE ALSO

Appendicitis, Acute; Cirrhosis of the Liver; Diverticular Disease; Peptic Ulcer Disease

CODES

ICD10

- K65.0 Generalized (acute) peritonitis
- K65.2 Spontaneous bacterial peritonitis
- K65.8 Other peritonitis

CLINICAL PEARLS

- Maintain a high index of suspicion for SBP in cirrhotic patients with ascites (up to 30% of cases may be asymptomatic). Start empiric therapy early to improve outcomes.
- Paracentesis is necessary to diagnose SBP. Ascitic fluid cultures collected via bedside inoculation with blood culture bottles prior to antibiotic administration increase culture yield significantly.
- *E. coli* is the most common bacterial isolate from cases of SBP. 3rd-generation cephalosporins are first-line treatment. The incidence of gram-positive infections and antibiotic resistance is increasing.
- Ascitic fluid analysis stratifies patients at risk for secondary peritonitis who need additional imaging. Perform CT scanning if suspicious based on history and/or ascitic fluid analysis.
- Renal function is an important prognostic indicator for SBP. Albumin administration decreases the incidence of renal failure and reduces mortality in patients with renal or hepatic impairment and/or patients undergoing large-volume paracentesis.

P

PERSONALITY DISORDERS

Moshe S. Torem, MD

BASICS

DESCRIPTION

- Personality disorders (PDs) are a group of conditions, with onset at or before adolescence, characterized by enduring patterns of maladaptive and dysfunctional behavior that deviates markedly from one's culture and social environment, leading to functional impairment and distress to the individual, coworkers, and family.
  - These behaviors are perceived by patients to be "normal" and "right," and they have little insight as to their ownership, responsibility, and abnormal nature of these behaviors.
  - These conditions are classified based on the predominant symptoms and their severity.
- System(s) affected: nervous/psychiatric
- Synonym(s): character disorder; character pathology

Geriatric Considerations
Coping with the stresses of aging is challenging.

Pediatric Considerations
A history of childhood neglect, abuse, and trauma is not uncommon.

Pregnancy Considerations
Pregnancy adds pressures in coping with the activities of daily living (ADLs).

EPIDEMIOLOGY
Prevalence
- General population: 15% (1)
- Cluster A: 5.7%
- Cluster B: 6.0%
- Cluster C: 9.1%
- Outpatient psychiatric clinic: 3–30%
- In male prisoners, the prevalence of antisocial PD is ~60%.
- Predominant age: starts in adolescence and early 20s and persists throughout patient's life
- Predominant sex: male = female; some PDs are more common in females, and others are more common in males.

ETIOLOGY AND PATHOPHYSIOLOGY
- Environmental and genetic factors (2)
- Criteria for a PD include an enduring pattern of the following:
  - Inner experience and behavior that deviates markedly from the expectations of one's culture in ≥2 of the following areas: cognition, affectivity, interpersonal functioning, or impulse control
  - Inflexibility and pervasiveness across a broad range of personal and social situations
  - Significant distress or impairment in social or occupational functioning
  - The pattern is stable and of long duration.
  - The enduring pattern is not better explained as a manifestation of another psychiatric disorder.
  - The enduring pattern is not attributable to the effects of a drug or a medical condition.
- PDs are classified into three major clusters:
  - Cluster A: eccentricity and oddness
    ○ *Paranoid PD*: unwarranted suspiciousness and distrust of others
    ○ *Schizoid PD*: emotional, cold, or detached; socially isolated
    ○ *Schizotypal PD*: eccentric behavior, odd belief system/perceptions, social isolation, and general suspiciousness

- Cluster B: dramatic, emotional, or erratic behavioral patterns
  ○ *Antisocial PD*: aggressive, impulsive, irritable, irresponsible, dishonest, deceitful
  ○ *Borderline PD*: unstable interpersonal relationships, high impulsivity from early adulthood, intense fear of abandonment, mood swings, poor self-esteem, chronic boredom, and feelings of inner emptiness
  ○ *Histrionic PD*: needs to be the center of attention, with self-dramatizing behaviors and attention seeking in a variety of contexts
  ○ *Narcissistic PD*: grandiose sense of self-importance and preoccupation with fantasies of success, power, brilliance, beauty, or ideal love; lack of empathy for other people's pain or discomfort, demanding to get their way
- Cluster C: anxiety, excessive worry, fear, and unhealthy patterns of coping with emotions
  ○ *Avoidant PD*: social inhibition, feelings of inadequacy, hypersensitivity to negative evaluation, avoidance of occupational and interpersonal activities that involve the risk of criticism by others, views self as socially inept and personally unappealing or inferior to others
  ○ *Dependent PD*: excessive need to be taken care of, leading to submissive and clinging behavior with fears of separation, avoids expressing disagreements with others due to fear of losing support and approval, usually seeks out strong and confident people as friends or spouses and feels more secure in such relationships
  ○ *Obsessive-compulsive PD*: preoccupation with cleanliness, orderliness, perfectionism; preoccupation with excessive details, rules, lists, order, organization, and schedules to the extent that the major point of the activity is lost
- Personality change due to another medical condition. It is a persistent personality disturbance that is caused by the physiologic effects of a medical condition such as frontal lobe lesion, epilepsy, MS, Parkinson disease, lupus, head trauma, postencephalitis or meningitis, and so forth.
- Other specified *PD and unspecified PD*: A category provided for two situations: (i) the individual's personality pattern meets the general criteria for PD and traits of several PDs are present, but the criteria for any specific PD are not met; (ii) the individual's personality pattern meets the general criteria for PD, but the individual is considered to have a PD that is not included in *DSM-5* classification such as passive–aggressive PD, depressive PD, masochistic PD, and dangerous and severe PD.

Genetics
Major character traits are inherited; others result from a combination of genetics and environment.

RISK FACTORS
- Positive family history
- Pregnancy risk factors
  - Nutritional deprivation
  - Use of alcohol or drugs
  - Viral and bacterial infections
- Dysfunctional family with child abuse/neglect

COMMONLY ASSOCIATED CONDITIONS
Depression; other psychiatric disorders in patient and family members

DIAGNOSIS

HISTORY
- Comprehensive interview and mental status examination
- Screen to rule out alcohol and drug abuse.
- Interview of relatives and friends is helpful in establishing an enduring pattern of behavior.

DIAGNOSTIC TESTS & INTERPRETATION
- Medical disorders with behavioral changes
- Other psychiatric disorders with similar symptoms
  - In obsessive-compulsive disorder (OCD), symptoms are ego-dystonic (i.e., perceived as foreign and unwanted). In addition, OCD has a pattern of relapse and partial remission.
  - In obsessive-compulsive personality disorder (OCPD), symptoms are perceived as desirable behaviors (ego-syntonic) that the patient feels proud of and wants others to emulate. In addition, OCPD has a lifelong pattern.
- Psychological testing (e.g., MMPI-II)

Initial Tests (lab, imaging)
- CBC
- Comprehensive metabolic panel
- Thyroid-stimulating hormone
- HIV
- Toxicology screen for substance abuse

Follow-Up Tests & Special Considerations
- EEG to rule out a chronic seizure disorder
- CT and MRI of the brain may be necessary in newly developed symptoms to rule out organic brain disease (e.g., frontal lobe tumor).

TREATMENT

Psychotherapy with family involvement is the foundation of treatment. No specific drugs are indicated to treat PDs; some medications can reduce the intensity, frequency, and dysfunctional nature of certain behaviors (3)[B].

GENERAL MEASURES
- Long-term psychotherapy and cognitive-behavioral therapy (3)[B]
- Group therapy is helpful in the use of therapeutic confrontation and increasing one's awareness of and insight regarding the damaging effects of dysfunctional behavior patterns (4)[B].

MEDICATION
Medications are effective in the treatment of comorbid conditions such as anxiety and depression.

First Line
- Symptom management (5)[B]
  - Minipsychosis (associated with paranoid, schizoid, borderline, and schizotypal PDs): atypical antipsychotics: risperidone (Risperdal), quetiapine (Seroquel), olanzapine (Zyprexa), ziprasidone (Geodon), aripiprazole (Abilify), asenapine (Saphris), lurasidone (Latuda); start with a low dose, gradually adjusting to the patient's needs.
  - Anxiety: anxiolytics (benzodiazepines, buspirone [Buspar], and serotonin reuptake inhibitors)

– Depressed mood: antidepressants
– Many patients with borderline PD respond well to small doses of atypical neuroleptics and mood stabilizers (5)[B].
• Precautions: Some atypical neuroleptic drugs may be associated with hyperglycemia and insulin-resistant metabolic syndrome.

Second Line
Mood stabilizers: lithium carbonate, lamotrigine (Lamictal), carbamazepine (Tegretol, Equetro), and valproate (Depacon, Depakene, Depakote) (6)[B]

ISSUES FOR REFERRAL
• When psychiatric comorbidity of other psychiatric disorders is present (e.g., mood disorders, anxiety disorders, substance abuse)
• Suicidal ideation or attempts
• Presence of psychotic symptoms
• Thoughts and impulses for violent behavior
• Management of complex pharmacotherapy
• Presence of intense countertransference feelings
• When the patient or family requests it

ADDITIONAL THERAPIES
• Cognitive-behavioral therapy
• Dialectical behavior therapy
• Psychoanalytic therapy
• Interactive psychotherapy
• Ego-state therapy
• Mindfulness-based psychotherapy
• Group therapy

ADMISSION, INPATIENT, AND NURSING CONSIDERATIONS
Disorders with complications of suicide attempts and other behaviors involving a risk to self or others

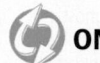 ## ONGOING CARE

FOLLOW-UP RECOMMENDATIONS
Continue outpatient treatment, potentially long term.

Patient Monitoring
• Regular physical exercise (e.g., 30 to 60 min/day, helps with stress and improving the ADLs)
• If substance abuse is suspected, check drug screens.
• Infrequent sessions with relatives or friends are helpful in monitoring behavioral progress.

DIET
Emphasize variety of healthy foods; avoid obesity.

PATIENT EDUCATION
• Bibliotherapy and writing therapy, specific assignments, and watching certain movies to better understand the nature and origin of one's specific condition are helpful.
– Kreger R. *The Essential Family Guide to Borderline Personality Disorder*. Center City, MN: Hazelden; 2008.
– Mason PT, Kreger R. *Stop Walking on Eggshells*. Oakland, CA: New Harbinger Publishers; 2010.
• The movie *As Good as It Gets* illustrates someone with obsessive-compulsive behaviors and their impact on ADLs and relationships with family and friends.
• The movie series *The Godfather* includes several characters with antisocial PD and shows how this affects their interpersonal relationships and their own physical and mental health.

• The movie *What About Bob?* illustrates the challenges involved in treating certain patients with a borderline PD, especially in the management of boundaries in the doctor–patient relationship.
• The movie *A Streetcar Named Desire* illustrates an example of a woman with a histrionic PD.
• The movie *Wall Street* illustrates an example of a person with a narcissistic PD.
• The movie *The Caine Mutiny* illustrates an example of a person with a paranoid PD.
• The movie *Four Weddings and a Funeral* illustrates an example of a person with an avoidant PD.

PROGNOSIS
PDs are enduring patterns of behavior throughout one's lifetime and are not readily responsive to brief therapies.

COMPLICATIONS
• Disruptive family life with frequent divorces and separations, alcoholism, substance abuse, and drug addiction
• Disruptive behaviors in the workplace may cause absenteeism and loss of productivity.
• Violation of the law and disregard for the concerns and rights of others

REFERENCES
1. American Psychiatric Association. *Diagnostic and Statistical Manual of Mental Disorders*. 5th ed. Arlington, VA: American Psychiatric Association; 2013.
2. Ma G, Fan H, Shen C, et al. Genetic and neuroimaging features of personality disorders: state of the art. *Neurosci Bull*. 2016;32(3):286–306.
3. Clarkin JF. An integrated approach to psychotherapy techniques for patients with personality disorder. *J Pers Disord*. 2012;26(1):43–62.
4. Livesley WJ. Integrated treatment: a conceptual framework for an evidence-based approach to the treatment of personality disorder. *J Pers Disord*. 2012;26(1):17–42.
5. Ripoll LH, Triebwasser J, Siever LJ. Evidence-based pharmacotherapy for personality disorders. *Int J Neuropsychopharmacol*. 2011;14(9):1257–1288.
6. Hancock-Johnson E, Griffiths C, Picchioni M. A focused systematic review of pharmacological treatment for borderline personality disorder. *CNS Drugs*. 2017;31(5):345–356.

ADDITIONAL READING
• Angstman KB, Rasmussen NH. Personality disorders: review and clinical application in daily practice. *Am Fam Physician*. 2011;84(11):1253–1260.
• Bateman AW, Gunderson J, Mulder R. Treatment of personality disorder. *Lancet*. 2015;385(9969):735–743.
• Combs G, Oshman L. Pearls for working with people who have personality disorder diagnoses. *Prim Care*. 2016;43(2):263–268.
• Gerlach G, Loeber S, Herpertz S. Personality disorders and obesity: a systematic review. *Obes Rev*. 2016;17(8):691–723.
• Sng AA, Janca A. Mindfulness for personality disorders. *Curr Opin Psychiatry*. 2016;29(1):70–76.

 ## SEE ALSO

Obsessive-Compulsive Disorder (OCD)

 ## CODES

ICD10
• F60.9 Personality disorder, unspecified
• F60.0 Paranoid personality disorder
• F60.1 Schizoid personality disorder

CLINICAL PEARLS
• PDs are enduring patterns of behavior throughout one's lifetime and are not readily responsive to brief treatments.
• In spite of the initial lack of self-awareness and accepting responsibility for one's dysfunctional behaviors, many patients can benefit from long-term treatment.
• No specific drugs are effective to treat PDs; however, specific medications can reduce the intensity, frequency, and dysfunctional nature of certain behaviors, thoughts, and feelings.
• Patients with a PD frequently elicit intense feelings in others, such as anger, hostility, likability, or sexual attraction.
• Health care professionals must be alert to potential blurring of interpersonal boundaries in the clinical care of these patients.
• Most patients with a PD require a well-trained and experienced mental health professional.
• A stable, trustful alliance with the patient is the foundation for any therapeutic progress.
• Many PD patients begin treatment in a crisis involving symptoms of anxiety, fear of abandonment, depressed mood, and intense interpersonal conflict at home or work. The focus at this initial phase of treatment should be symptom control and behavioral stabilization with restoration of hope.
• Lifelong patterns of dysfunctional behaviors should not be confronted at the initial phase of treatment.
• Therapeutic confrontation of dysfunctional behavioral patterns is effective only after a working and therapeutic alliance has been established.
• Treatment in an atmosphere of compassion, optimism, and hope for improvement are valuable principles.
• Showing genuine interest in the patient as a whole person including the patient's life history and current life circumstances may be helpful in establishing a therapeutic and working alliance that is necessary for continuing treatment of PD patients.
• Regular meetings with a spouse, another family member, or significant other are essential for receiving feedback on therapeutic progress.

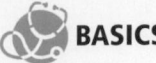

PERTUSSIS

Mary Cataletto, MD, FAAP, FCCP • Margaret J. McCormick, MS, RN, CNE

BASICS

- Highly contagious
- Synonym: whooping cough, "100 day" cough

DESCRIPTION

- Host: humans
- Most common reservoir: adults
- Ages: all
- Distribution: worldwide
- Pattern: endemic or epidemic with outbreaks every 3 to 5 years
- Seasonality: can occur year-round; peaks late summer–autumn
- Transmission: person to person via aerosolized respiratory droplets
- Effective vaccine: available
- Immunity: neither 100% nor lifelong immunity with either infection or vaccine
- System(s) affected: respiratory

EPIDEMIOLOGY

Incidence
- Worldwide: 24.1 million cases (1)
- 160,700 deaths in children <5 years old (1)

ETIOLOGY AND PATHOPHYSIOLOGY

- Toxin mediated
- Infectious process with predilection for ciliated respiratory epithelium
- Common organisms:
  - *Bordetella pertussis* (accounts for ~95% of cases)
  - *Bordetella parapertussis*

RISK FACTORS

- Exposure to a confirmed case
- Non- or underimmunized infants and children
- Premature birth
- Chronic lung disease
- Immunodeficiency (e.g., AIDS)
- Age <6 months (accounts for ~90% pediatric pertussis hospitalizations) (2)

GENERAL PREVENTION

- Public health measures
  - Surveillance
  - Outbreak management
  - Care of exposed persons
- Prevention programs
- Immunization
  - Primary childhood immunization series against pertussis followed by boosters (3)
  - Maternal immunization during each pregnancy (4,5,6)
  - Adults, including health care providers in close contact with infants <1 year of age, should be immunized.

Pediatric Considerations

Strategies to reduce neonatal pertussis:
- Tdap with each pregnancy, preferably between 27 and 36 weeks' gestation (4,5,6)
- Cocooning (6)
- Tdap recommended for all persons in close contact with infants <1 year of age

Geriatric Considerations

The incidence of pertussis in individuals age 50 years and older has increased between 2006 and 2010.

COMMONLY ASSOCIATED CONDITIONS

- Apnea in infants
- Secondary bacterial pneumonia
- Sinusitis
- Seizures
- Encephalopathy
- Urinary incontinence

DIAGNOSIS

HISTORY

- Exposure to pertussis
- Insidious onset
- Incubation period 7 to 10 days (ranges 5 to 21 days)

PHYSICAL EXAM

- Classic pertussis has three phases, which occur over 6 to 10 weeks:
  - Catarrhal phase: rhinorrhea, mild cough, low-grade fever
  - Paroxysmal phase: Cough occurs in bursts, with increased intensity and frequency, often followed by an inspiratory whoop and/or posttussive vomiting.
  - Convalescent phase: Coughing paroxysms decrease in frequency and intensity.
- In the absence of paroxysms or complications, the physical exam may be normal.
- Classic presentation more common in adults

ALERT

Infants <6 months of age may have atypical presentations.

DIFFERENTIAL DIAGNOSIS

Sporadic, prolonged cough can also be caused by (7):
- *B. parapertussis*
- *Mycoplasma pneumoniae*
- *Chlamydia trachomatis*
- *Chlamydophila pneumoniae*
- *Bordetella bronchiseptica*
- *Bordetella holmesii*
- Respiratory syncytial virus
- Adenovirus

DIAGNOSTIC TESTS & INTERPRETATION

Initial Tests (lab, imaging)

- Nasopharyngeal culture (gold standard): best results within 2 weeks of cough onset (7)[A]
- False results can occur in:
  - Previously immunized individuals
  - After initiation of appropriate antibiotic
  - After 2 weeks from cough onset
  - With incorrect collection or handling
- Polymerase chain reaction (PCR) assays: rapid turn-around time; good within first 3 weeks (7)[C]
- Serology:
  - Commercially available assays
  - Not FDA-approved for diagnosis

Follow-Up Tests & Special Considerations

- Evaluation and follow-up for associated conditions and complications
- Chest radiograph (two views) to evaluate for the presence of pneumonia
- EEG/neuroimaging may be considered in infant with seizures or apparent life-threatening events (ALTEs).
- Infants <1 month of age who are treated with macrolides should be monitored for the possible development of hypertrophic pyloric stenosis.

TREATMENT

GENERAL MEASURES

Waiting rooms, during transport, and procedures: Patients with suspected pertussis should wear masks.

MEDICATION

- Start empiric antibiotic therapy once diagnostic testing is performed in cases with strong clinical suspicion or in those at high risk for complications.
- Antibiotic therapy after cough is established may help to limit spread but is not expected to change clinical symptoms.
- Preferred antibiotics:
  - For patients >6 months:
    - Azithromycin, clarithromycin, or erythromycin
  - For infants <1 month of age, azithromycin preferred but with caution

First Line

Azithromycin is the first line for treatment and for postexposure prophylaxis (5-day course) (7)[A].

ALERT

Infantile hypertrophic pyloric stenosis has been associated with the use of macrolides in infants <1 month of age. Consultation and monitoring are recommended.

ALERT
- *Fatal cardiac dysrhythmias* have been reported with azithromycin.
- Caution recommended in individuals with prolonged QT and proarrhythmic conditions

Second Line
Trimethoprim/sulfamethoxazole (TMP/SMX) (for persons >2 months of age) if:
- Macrolide intolerance
- Macrolide resistance (7)[C]

ALERT
- TMP/SMX is *contraindicated* in infants <2 months of age.
- Clarithromycin is not recommended in infants <1 month of age.

ISSUES FOR REFERRAL
Evaluation and treatment of infants <6 months of age, especially those born prematurely, who are unimmunized and those who require hospitalization

ADDITIONAL THERAPIES
Symptomatic treatment of the cough in pertussis (e.g., corticosteroids, β_2-adrenergic agonists, pertussis-specific immunoglobulin, antihistamine, and leukotriene receptor antagonist) has not shown consistent benefit.

ADMISSION, INPATIENT, AND NURSING CONSIDERATIONS
- Small, frequent meals may be necessary to ensure adequate nutrition.
- IV fluids indicated for dehydration and when oral fluids are either contraindicated or poorly tolerated
- In addition to standard precautions, hospitalized patients should be isolated with respiratory precautions for 5 days after the initiation of effective antibiotic treatment and for 3 weeks after onset of paroxysms in older patients if antibiotics are not used.
- Gentle suctioning of nasal secretions
- Avoid stimuli that trigger paroxysms.
- Respiratory monitoring, including pulse oximetry
- Educate each family about the importance of immunizations.
- Discuss chemoprophylaxis with each family.
- Discharge criteria
  - Clinically stable
  - Able to tolerate oral feedings

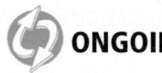 **ONGOING CARE**

Supportive

FOLLOW-UP RECOMMENDATIONS
- Monitor infants who received EES or azithromycin for pyloric stenosis.
- Neurologic and/or pulmonary follow-up as necessary

Patient Monitoring
ICU care may be necessary for severely ill or compromised patients.

DIET
IV fluids/nutrition may be required to treat dehydration or supplement poor oral intake.

PATIENT EDUCATION
- American Academy of Pediatrics: http://www.aap.org
- Centers for Disease Control and Prevention: http://www.cdc.gov

PROGNOSIS
- Complete recovery in most cases
- Most severe morbidity and highest mortality in infants <6 months of age
- Overall mortality approximately 195,000/year (1)

COMPLICATIONS
- Highest and most severe in infants; may include apnea, cyanosis, and sudden death
- In children: may include conjunctival hemorrhage, inguinal hernia, pneumonia, and seizures
- More frequent in adults than adolescents: may include sinusitis, otitis media, pneumonia, weight loss, fainting, rib fracture, urinary incontinence, seizures, encephalopathy, and death

REFERENCES
1. Centers for Disease Control and Prevention. Pertussis: fast facts. https://www.cdc.gov/pertussis/fast-facts.html. Accessed August 1, 2018.
2. Lopez MA, Cruz AT, Kowalkowski MA, et al. Trends in hospitalizations and resource utilization for pediatric pertussis. *Hosp Pediatr*. 2014;4(5):269–275.
3. Centers for Disease Control and Prevention. Recommended immunization schedule for children and adolescents aged 18 years or younger, United States, 2018. https://www.cdc.gov/vaccines/schedules/hcp/child-adolescent.html. Accessed July 2, 2017.
4. Committee on Obstetric Practice. ACOG Committee Opinion No. 521: update on immunization and pregnancy: tetanus, diphtheria, and pertussis vaccination. *Obstet Gynecol*. 2012;119(3):690–691.
5. Baxter R, Bartlett J, Fireman B, et al. Effectiveness of vaccination during pregnancy to prevent infant pertussis. *Pediatrics*. 2017;139(5):e20164091.

6. Swamy GK, Wheeler SM. Neonatal pertussis, cocooning and maternal immunization. *Expert Rev Vaccines*. 2014;13(9):1107–1114.
7. Committee on Infectious Diseases. Pertussis (whooping cough). In: Kimberlin DW, Brady DW, Jackson MA, eds. *Red Book: 2018–2021 Report of the Committee on Infectious Diseases.* 31st ed. Itasca, IL: American Academy of Pediatrics; 2018:620–634.

ADDITIONAL READING
- Centers for Disease Control and Prevention. Diagnosis confirmation. https://www.cdc.gov/pertussis/clinical/diagnostic-testing/diagnosis-confirmation.html. Accessed August 1, 2018.
- Centers for Disease Control and Prevention. Prevention: adults. https://www.cdc.gov/pertussis/about/prevention/adults.html. Accessed August 1, 2018.
- Centers for Disease Control and Prevention. Treatment. https://www.cdc.gov/pertussis/clinical/treatment.html. Accessed August 1, 2018.
- McGuiness CB, Hill J, Fonseca E, et al. The disease burden of pertussis in adults 50 years old and older in the United States: a retrospective study. *BMC Infect Dis*. 2013;13:32.
- Moore A, Ashdown H, Shinkins B, et al. Clinical characteristics of pertussis-associated cough in adults and children: a diagnostic systematic review and meta-analysis. *Chest*. 2017;152(2):353–367.
- Wang K, Bettiol S, Thompson MJ, et al. Symptomatic treatment of the cough in whooping cough. *Cochrane Database Syst Rev*. 2014;(9):CD003257.

 CODES

ICD10
- A37.90 Whooping cough, unspecified species without pneumonia
- A37.80 Whooping cough due to other Bordetella species w/o pneumonia
- A37.10 Whooping cough due to Bordetella parapertussis w/o pneumonia

CLINICAL PEARLS
- Hospitalizations for pertussis is highest in infants <6 months of age.
  - Maternal Tdap is effective in protecting young infants against pertussis, especially during first 2 months of life.
- Neither immunization nor active infection confers lifelong immunity.

PHARYNGITIS

Cristian P. Fernandez Falcon, MD, DABFM, CAQGM, CAQHPM, CMD • Maria F. Arbelaez, MD

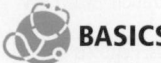

BASICS

DESCRIPTION
- Acute or chronic inflammation of the pharyngeal mucosa and underlying structures of the throat
- Group A *Streptococcus* (GAS) pharyngitis is notable for preventable suppurative (e.g., retropharyngeal or peritonsillar abscess) and nonsuppurative (e.g., rheumatic sequelae) complications.
- Synonym(s): sore throat; tonsillitis; "strep throat"

EPIDEMIOLOGY
- ~15 million cases are diagnosed yearly.
- Accounts for 1–2% of all outpatient visits and 6% of all pediatric visits to primary care physicians
- Most commonly viral (40–60%)
- GAS is the most common bacterial cause of acute pharyngitis, accounting for 15–30% of pediatric and 5–15% of adult cases. The incubation period ranges from 24 to 72 hours.
- Rheumatic fever is rare in the United States (<1 per 100,000). Early antibiotic use has diminished occurrence.
- 3,000 to 4,000 patients with group A β-hemolytic streptococcal infection must be treated to prevent one case of acute rheumatic fever.
- All age groups, some etiologies more common with certain age groups

Pediatric Considerations
The highest incidence of rheumatic fever is in children 5 to 18 years as a rare sequela of streptococcal pharyngitis.

ETIOLOGY AND PATHOPHYSIOLOGY
- Acute, viral (lower grade fever)
  - Rhinovirus
  - Adenovirus (associated with conjunctivitis)
  - Parainfluenza virus
  - Coxsackievirus (hand-foot-mouth disease)
  - Coronavirus
  - Echovirus
  - Herpes simplex virus (vesicular lesions)
  - Epstein-Barr virus (EBV/mononucleosis)
  - Cytomegalovirus (CMV)
  - HIV
- Acute, bacterial (higher fevers)
  - Group A β-hemolytic streptococcus
  - *Neisseria gonorrhoeae*
  - *Corynebacterium diphtheriae* (diphtheria)
  - *Haemophilus influenzae*
  - *Moraxella catarrhalis*
  - *Chlamydia pneumonia*
  - *Fusobacterium necrophorum* (20% young adult cases)
  - Group C or G *streptococcus*
  - *Arcanobacterium haemolyticum*
  - *Mycoplasma pneumoniae*
  - *Francisella tularensis* (tularemia)
- Acute, noninfectious
  - Various caustic, mechanical, or trauma-related (including endotracheal intubation)
- Chronic
  - More likely noninfectious
  - Chemical irritation (GERD)
  - Smoking
  - Neoplasms
  - Vasculitis
  - Radiation changes

Genetics
Patients with a family history of rheumatic fever have a higher risk of rheumatic sequelae following an untreated group A β-hemolytic streptococcal infection.

RISK FACTORS
- Epidemics of group A β-hemolytic streptococcal disease
- Cold and flu season (late fall through early spring)
- Age (especially children/adolescents 5 to 15 years)
- Family history of rheumatic fever
- Close contact with infected individuals (home, daycare, military barracks)
- Immunosuppression
- Smoking/secondhand smoke exposure
- Acid reflux
- Oral sex
- Diabetes mellitus
- Recent illness (secondary postviral bacterial infection)
- Chronic colonization of bacteria in tonsils/adenoids

GENERAL PREVENTION
- Avoid close contact with infectious patients.
- Wash hands frequently.
- Avoid first or secondhand smoke.
- Manage preventable causes (e.g., GERD).

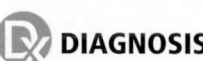

DIAGNOSIS

HISTORY
- Sore throat
- Difficulty swallowing (dysphagia) or pain on swallowing (odynophagia)
- Cough (uncommon in GAS pharyngitis)
- Hoarseness; "hot potato" voice
- Fever
- Anorexia
- Chills
- Malaise; fatigue
- Headache
- Dysuria and arthralgias (suggest gonococcal etiology)
- Sick contacts with similar symptoms or confirmed diagnosis

PHYSICAL EXAM
- Enlarged tonsils with or without exudate
- Pharyngeal erythema
- Unilateral tonsillar swelling ("frog's belly") or uvular deviation (concern for peritonsillar abscess)
- Trismus; stridor; drooling (concern for peritonsillar or retropharyngeal abscess)
- Cervical adenopathy (anterior suggestive of GAS, posterior most commonly associated with infectious mononucleosis)
- Fever (higher in bacterial infections)
- Pharyngeal ulcers (CMV, HIV, Crohn, other autoimmune vasculitides)
- Scarlet fever rash: Punctate erythematous macules with reddened flexor creases and circumoral pallor suggests streptococcal pharyngitis.
- Tonsillar/soft palate petechiae and hepatosplenomegaly suggest infectious mononucleosis (EBV/CMV).
- Gray oral pseudomembrane suggests diphtheria and occasionally infectious mononucleosis (EBV/CMV).

- Characteristic erythematous-based clear vesicles suggest HSV or coxsackie A virus infection (herpangina).
- Conjunctivitis suggests adenovirus.

DIFFERENTIAL DIAGNOSIS
- Viral syndrome
- Streptococcal infection
- Allergic rhinitis/postnasal drip
- GERD
- Malignancy (lymphoma or squamous cell carcinoma)
- Irritants/chemicals (detergent/caustic ingestion)
- Atypical bacterial (e.g., gonococcal, chlamydial, syphilis, pertussis, diphtheria)
- Oral candidiasis (patients typically complain mostly of dysphagia)
- Epiglottitis (associated with stridor, drooling, and progressive respiratory distress)

DIAGNOSTIC TESTS & INTERPRETATION
- Prediction rules determine further testing (see below).
- Additional testing generally not needed if viral-like clinical features (e.g., cough, rhinorrhea, hoarseness, oral ulcers, diarrhea, conjunctivitis, rash) (1)[A]
- Avoid testing for GAS pharyngitis in children <3 years as acute rheumatic flare is rare, unless there is a close sick contact who is GAS-positive (1)[B].
- Modified Centor clinical prediction rule for group A streptococcal infection (2)[A]:
  - +1 point: tonsillar exudates
  - +1 point: tender anterior chain cervical adenopathy
  - +1 point: absence of cough
  - +1 point: fever by history
  - +1 point: age <15 years
  - 0 point: age 15 to 45 years
  - −1 point: age >45 years
- Scoring:
  - If 4 points, positive predictive value of ~80%; treat empirically.
  - If 2 to 3 points, positive predictive value of ~50%, rapid strep antigen; treat if GAS-positive.
  - If 0 or 1 point, positive predictive value <20%; do not test; treat empirically with follow-up as needed.

Initial Tests (lab, imaging)
- Testing, if performed, is usually for GAS. Options include:
  - Rapid antigen streptococcus test (RAST); quick adjunct to throat culture with 96% specificity and 86% sensitivity (although sensitivity varies by modality kit) (3)[A]
  - Blood agar throat culture from swab; gold standard—90–95% sensitivity (3)[A]
    - Back up throat cultures are not needed for adults with negative RAST. They are recommended for children with negative RAST due to the higher likelihood of complications but can be omitted if a highly sensitive immunoassay or molecular test was used.
  - Antistreptolysin O (suspect carrier state if positive culture and unchanged antistreptolysin O titers)
- Special tests if history suggests a different diagnosis
  - Warm Thayer-Martin plate or antigen testing for *N. gonorrhoeae*
  - Viral cultures for HSV
  - Monospot for EBV
  - IgM serology for CMV

Test Interpretation

Bacitracin disk sensitivity of hemolytic colonies suggests group A β-hemolytic streptococcus.

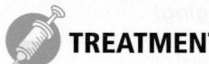 ## TREATMENT

GENERAL MEASURES

Conservative therapy recommended for most cases (unless bacterial etiology suspected):

- Salt water gargles
- Viscous lidocaine (2%) 5 to 10 mL PO q4h swish/spit
- Acetaminophen 10 to 15 mg/kg/dose q4h PRN pain or fever (pediatric). In adults, do not exceed >3 g/day.
- NSAIDs for pain or fever (more effective than acetaminophen for GAS pharyngitis)
- Anesthetic lozenges
- Cool-mist humidifier
- Hydration (PO or IV)

Pediatric Considerations

Opioids not recommended due to black box warnings

MEDICATION

- Antibiotics (particularly penicillin) are chosen primarily to prevent complications.
  - 60–70% primary care visits by children with pharyngitis result in antibiotic prescriptions (4). Empiric therapy results in antibiotic overuse.
  - Treatment duration generally 10 days (1)[A]
  - Antibiotics do not reduce risk of poststreptococcal glomerulonephritis.
  - Antibiotics shorten duration of symptoms by approximately 16 hours (5).
  - Antibiotics may prevent pharyngitis/fever by day 3 (NNT 4 if GAS-positive, 6.5 if GAS-negative, 14.4 if untested) (5)[A].
- Ulcers related to autoimmune diseases usually require systemic or intralesional injectable steroids.
- HIV-related ulcers are due to decreasing counts of CD4 and respond when patients' CD4 titers increase.
- Corticosteroids, when used concomitantly with antibiotics, may provide a small reduction in the duration of symptoms (24 hours). Routine use is not currently recommended (1,3)[B].

First Line

Recommended first-line therapies (1)[A]:

- Penicillin V: children (<27 kg): 250 mg PO TID (BID dosing sufficient if good compliance); adolescents and adults (>27 kg): 250 mg PO QID or 500 mg PO BID
- Penicillin G benzathine: children <60 lb (27 kg): 600,000 units intramuscularly 1 dose; children ≥60 lb and adults: 1.2 million units intramuscularly 1 dose
- Amoxicillin: 50 mg/kg PO once daily (max 1,000 mg/dose or 25 mg/kg PO BID (max = 500 mg/dose)

ALERT

Use with caution if diagnosis is unclear because using amoxicillin with EBV infection may induce rash.

Second Line

- If type IV hypersensitivity but no history of anaphylactic penicillin allergy:
  - Cephalexin 20 mg/kg PO BID or (children) 25 to 50 mg/kg/day divided BID or (adults) 1,000 mg PO QID (max = 4 g/day)
  - Cefadroxil 30 mg/kg PO once daily (max = 1 g/day)

- If history of anaphylactic penicillin allergy (type I hypersensitivity):
  - Azithromycin 12 mg/kg PO once daily for 5 days (max = 500 mg/dose)
  - Clarithromycin 7.5 mg/kg PO BID (max = 250 mg/dose) or (adults) 250 to 500 mg PO BID
  - Clindamycin 7 mg/kg PO TID (max = 300 mg/dose) or (children) 10 to 30 mg/kg/day PO divided TID–QID or (adults) 150 to 450 mg PO TID–QID
- Penicillin is the most documented treatment to prevent rheumatic sequelae, but cephalosporins have a lower rate of antimicrobial failure against streptococcal pharyngitis.
- Newer macrolides, although effective against streptococcal pharyngitis, are more expensive and unproven at preventing rheumatic complications.
- Macrolide-resistant strains of GAS are currently <10% in the United States but more prevalent worldwide.

ISSUES FOR REFERRAL

- Document each GAS-confirmed episode to support the need for future tonsillectomy and adenoidectomy.
- Tonsillectomy is recommended for patients who have had seven or more throat infections (viral or bacterial) in 1 year, five or more infections per year for the past 2 years, or three or more infections per year for the past 3 years. Tonsillectomy is also recommended in patients who are difficult to treat medically, including those who are allergic to multiple antibiotics.

 ## ONGOING CARE

FOLLOW-UP RECOMMENDATIONS

- Patient should complete the full course of antibiotic therapy, regardless of symptom response.
- Patients are generally noninfectious after 24 hours of antibiotics.
- Follow-up culture for GAS is not recommended (1)[A].

DIET

As tolerated. Encourage the consumption of fluids.

PROGNOSIS

- Streptococcal pharyngitis runs a 5- to 7-day course with peak fever at 2 to 3 days.
- Symptoms will resolve spontaneously without treatment, but rheumatic complications are still possible.

COMPLICATIONS

- Rheumatic fever (e.g., carditis, valve disease, arthritis)
- Poststreptococcal glomerulonephritis
- Peritonsillar abscess (a.k.a. quinsy tonsillitis): considered a clinical diagnosis and does not warrant ultrasound/computed tomography. Will generally require percutaneous/transoral drainage. Surgery may also involve a quinsy (acute) tonsillectomy. Most sources recommend resolution of the acute infection before surgery.
- Acute airway compromise (rare) can typically be bypassed with nasal trumpets. Consult anesthesiologist/otolaryngologist.
- Repeated episodes of GAS pharyngitis may represent recurrent viral infections in a chronic pharyngeal GAS carrier (1)[B]. IDSA recommends against repeated diagnostic efforts/antibiotic therapy in a known chronic pharyngeal GAS carrier, as they are seldom contagious or at risk for serious complications.

REFERENCES

1. Shulman ST, Bisno AL, Clegg HW, et al. Clinical practice guideline for the diagnosis and management of group A streptococcal pharyngitis: 2012 update by the Infectious Diseases Society of America. *Clin Infect Dis.* 2012;55(10):1279–1282.
2. Fine AM, Nizet V, Mandl KD. Large-scale validation of the Centor and McIsaac scores to predict group A streptococcal pharyngitis. *Arch Intern Med.* 2012;172(11):847–852.
3. Kalra M, Higgins K, Perez E. Common questions about streptococcal pharyngitis. *Am Fam Physician.* 2016;94(1):24–31.
4. Cohen JF, Cohen R, Levy C, et al. Selective testing strategies for diagnosing group A streptococcal infection in children with pharyngitis: a systematic review and prospective multicentre external validation study. *CMAJ.* 2015;187(1):23–32.
5. Spinks A, Glasziou PP, Del Mar CB. Antibiotics for sore throat. *Cochrane Database Syst Rev.* 2013;(11):CD000023.

ADDITIONAL READING

- Baugh RF, Archer SM, Mitchell RB, et al. Clinical practice guideline: tonsillectomy in children. *Otolaryngol Head Neck Surg.* 2011;144(Suppl 1):S1–S30.
- Kocher JJ, Selby TD. Antibiotics for sore throat. *Am Fam Physician.* 2014;90(1):23–24.
- Weber R. Pharyngitis. *Prim Care.* 2014;41(1):91–98.
- Zoorob R, Sidani MA, Fremont RD, et al. Antibiotic use in acute upper respiratory tract infections. *Am Fam Physician.* 2012;86(9):817–822.

 ## SEE ALSO

- Herpes Simplex; Infectious Mononucleosis, Epstein-Barr Virus Infections; Rheumatic Fever
- Algorithm: Pharyngitis

 ## CODES

ICD10

- J02.9 Acute pharyngitis, unspecified
- J02.0 Streptococcal pharyngitis
- J31.2 Chronic pharyngitis

CLINICAL PEARLS

- Most cases of pharyngitis are viral and do not require antibiotics.
- The risk associated with undiagnosed and untreated group A streptococcal infection is for rheumatic sequelae—a rare complication.
- Use of the Modified Centor Score helps to guide testing and treatment.
- Penicillin is the preferred first-line therapy for group A streptococcal infection.

PILONIDAL DISEASE

Tam T. Nguyen, MD

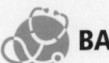 **BASICS**

DESCRIPTION
- Pilonidal disease results from an abscess, or sinus tract, in the upper part of the natal (gluteal) cleft.
- Synonym(s): jeep disease

EPIDEMIOLOGY

Incidence
- 16 to 26/100,000 per year
- Predominant sex: male > female (3 to 4:1)
- Predominant age: 2nd to 3rd decade, rare >45 years
- Ethnic consideration: whites > blacks > Asians

Prevalence
Surgical procedures show male: female ratio of 4:1, yet incidence data are 10:1.

ETIOLOGY AND PATHOPHYSIOLOGY
Pilonidal means "nest of hair"; hair in the natal cleft allows hair to be drawn into the deeper tissues via negative pressure caused by movement of the buttocks (50%); follicular occlusion from stretching and blocking of pores with debris (50%)
- Inflammation of SC gluteal tissues with secondary infection and sinus tract formation
- Polymicrobial, likely from enteric pathogens given proximity to anorectal contamination

Genetics
- Congenital dimple in the natal cleft/spina bifida occulta
- Follicular-occluding tetrad: acne conglobata, dissecting cellulitis, hidradenitis suppurativa, pilonidal

RISK FACTORS
- Sedentary/prolonged sitting
- Excessive body hair
- Obesity/increased sacrococcygeal fold thickness
- Congenital natal dimple
- Trauma to coccyx

GENERAL PREVENTION
- Weight loss
- Trim hair in/around gluteal cleft weekly.
- Hygiene
- Ingrown hair prevention/follicle unblocking

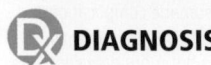 **DIAGNOSIS**

HISTORY
Three distinct clinical presentations
- Asymptomatic: painless cyst or sinus at the top of the gluteal cleft
- Acute abscess: severe pain, swelling, discharge from the top of the gluteal cleft that may or may not have drained spontaneously
- Chronic abscess: persistent drainage from a sinus tract at the top of the gluteal cleft

PHYSICAL EXAM
- Common: inflamed cystic mass at the top of the gluteal cleft with limited surrounding erythema ± drainage or a sinus tract
- Less common: significant cellulitis of the surrounding tissues near the gluteal cleft

DIFFERENTIAL DIAGNOSIS
- Furunculosis
- Hidradenitis suppurativa
- Anal fistula
- Perirectal abscess
- Crohn disease

DIAGNOSTIC TESTS & INTERPRETATION

Initial Tests (lab, imaging)
- Consider CBC and wound culture but generally not necessary for less severe infections.
- MRI might be considered to differentiate between perirectal abscess and pilonidal disease.

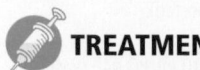 **TREATMENT**

GENERAL MEASURES
Shave area; remove hair from crypts weekly.

MEDICATION
- Antibiotics not indicated unless there is significant cellulitis (1)
- If antibiotics are needed, a culture to direct therapy might be useful.
- Cefazolin plus metronidazole or amoxicillin-clavulanate are often used empirically if cellulitis is suspected.

ISSUES FOR REFERRAL
- Patients who cannot comply with frequent dressing changes required after incision and drainage (I&D)
- Patients who have recurrence after I&D
- Patients who have complex disease with multiple sinus tracts

ADDITIONAL THERAPIES
- I&D with only enough packing to allow the cyst to drain; overpacking not indicated
- Antibiotics only if significant cellulitis; temporizing, not curative
- Negative pressure wound therapy
- Laser epilation of hair in the gluteal fold (2)[B]
- Phenol treatment can be used, especially for recurring disease.

SURGERY/OTHER PROCEDURES

Six levels of care based on severity or recurrence of disease; recent innovations in technique are aimed at expediting healing and minimizing recurrence.

- I&D, remove hair, curette granulation tissue (3)[A]
- Excision of midline "pits" allows drainage of lateral sinus tracts (pit picking).
- Pilonidal cystotomy: Insert probe into sinus tract, excise overlying skin, and close wound (4)[B].
- Marsupialization: Excise overlying skin and roof of cyst, and suture skin edges to cyst floor (3,5)[B].
- Excision: use of flap closure; no clear benefit for open healing over surgical closure
- Off-midline surgical excision (cleft lift or modified Karydakis procedure): A systematic review showed a clear benefit in favor of off-midline rather than midline wound closure. When closure of pilonidal sinuses is the desired surgical option, off-midline closure should be the standard management (3)[A].
- Endoscopic pilonidal sinus treatment (EPSiT): minimally invasive procedure (6)

ADMISSION, INPATIENT, AND NURSING CONSIDERATIONS

- Severe cellulitis
- Large area excision

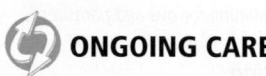 **ONGOING CARE**

FOLLOW-UP RECOMMENDATIONS

- Frequent dressing changes required after I&D
- Follow up wound checks to assess for recurrence.

Patient Monitoring

Monitor for fever; more extensive cellulitis

PATIENT EDUCATION

- Wash area briskly with washcloth daily.
- Shave the area weekly.
- Remove any embedded hair from the crypt.
- Avoid prolonged sitting.

PROGNOSIS

- Simple I&D has a 55% failure rate; median time to healing is 5 weeks.
- More extensive surgical excisions involve hospital stays and longer time to heal.

COMPLICATIONS

Malignant degeneration is a rare complication of untreated chronic pilonidal disease.

REFERENCES

1. Mavros MN, Mitsikostas PK, Alexiou VG, et al. Antimicrobials as an adjunct to pilonidal disease surgery: a systematic review of the literature. *Eur J Clin Microbiol Infect Dis*. 2013;32(7):851–858.
2. Loganathan A, Arsalani Zadeh R, Hartley J. Pilonidal disease: time to reevaluate a common pain in the rear! *Dis Colon Rectum*. 2012;55(4):491–493.
3. Humphries AE, Duncan JE. Evaluation and management of pilonidal disease. *Surg Clin North Am*. 2010;90(1):113–124.
4. da Silva JH. Pilonidal cyst: cause and treatment. *Dis Colon Rectum*. 2000;43(8):1146–1156.
5. Aydede H, Erhan Y, Sakarya A, et al. Comparison of three methods in surgical treatment of pilonidal disease. *ANZ J Surg*. 2001;71(6):362–364.
6. Meinero P, Stazi A, Carbone A, et al. Endoscopic pilonidal sinus treatment: a prospective multicentre trial. *Colorectal Dis*. 2016;18(5):O164–O170.

ADDITIONAL READING

- Aygen E, Arslan K, Dogru O, et al. Crystallized phenol in nonoperative treatment of previously operated, recurrent pilonidal disease. *Dis Colon Rectum*. 2010;53(6):932–935.
- Bradley L. Pilonidal sinus disease: a review. Part one. *J Wound Care*. 2010;19(11):504–508.
- Harlak A, Mentes O, Kilic S, et al. Sacrococcygeal pilonidal disease: analysis of previously proposed risk factors. *Clinics (Sao Paulo)*. 2010;65(2):125–131.
- Rao MM, Zawislak W, Kennedy R, et al. A prospective randomised study comparing two treatment modalities for chronic pilonidal sinus with a 5-year follow-up. *Int J Colorectal Dis*. 2010;25(3):395–400.
- Theodoropoulos GE, Vlahos K, Lazaris AC, et al. Modified Bascom's asymmetric midgluteal cleft closure technique for recurrent pilonidal disease: early experience in a military hospital. *Dis Colon Rectum*. 2003;46(9):1286–1291.

 CODES

ICD10

- L05.91 Pilonidal cyst without abscess
- L05.92 Pilonidal sinus without abscess
- L05.01 Pilonidal cyst with abscess

CLINICAL PEARLS

- Avoid prolonged sitting.
- Lose weight.
- Trim hair in gluteal cleft weekly.
- Refer recurring infections for more definitive surgical management.

PINWORMS

Jonathan MacClements, MD, FAAFP

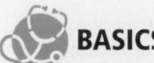 **BASICS**

DESCRIPTION
- Intestinal infection with *Enterobius vermicularis*
  - Characterized by perineal and perianal itching
  - Usually worse at night
- System(s) affected: gastrointestinal; skin/exocrine
- Synonym(s): enterobiasis

EPIDEMIOLOGY
Predominant age: 5 to 14 years

Prevalence
- Most common helminthic infection in the United States
  - 20 to 42 million people harbor the parasite.
- ~30% of children are infected worldwide.

Pediatric Considerations
More common in children, who are more likely to become reinfected

ETIOLOGY AND PATHOPHYSIOLOGY
- Small white worms (2 to 13 mm) inhabit the cecum, appendix, and adjacent portions of the ascending colon following ingestion.
- Female worms migrate to the perineal areas at night to deposit eggs; this causes local irritation and itching.
- Scratching leads to autoingestion of the eggs and continuation of pinworm's life cycle within the host. Eggs incubate 1 to 2 months in the host small intestine. When mature, female pinworms migrate to the colon where they lay eggs around the anus at night, and the lifecycle continues.
- Infestation by the intestinal nematode *E. vermicularis*

RISK FACTORS
- Institutionalization
- Crowded living conditions
- Poor hygiene
- Warm climate
- Handling of infected children's clothing or bedding

GENERAL PREVENTION
- Hand hygiene, especially after bowel movements
- Clip and maintain short fingernails.
- Wash anus and genitals at least once a day, preferably during shower.
- Avoid scratching anus and putting fingers near nose (pinworm eggs can also be inhaled) or mouth.

COMMONLY ASSOCIATED CONDITIONS
Pruritus ani

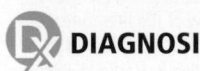 **DIAGNOSIS**

HISTORY
Many patients are asymptomatic. Common symptoms include the following:
- Perianal or perineal itching
- Vulvovaginitis
- Dysuria
- Abdominal pain (rare)
- Insomnia (typically due to pruritus)

PHYSICAL EXAM
Perineal and perianal exam; particularly in early morning to look for evidence of migrating worms

DIFFERENTIAL DIAGNOSIS
- Idiopathic pruritus ani (1)[A]
- Atopic dermatitis, contact dermatitis
- Psoriasis; lichen planus
- Human papillomavirus (HPV)
- Herpes simplex virus (HSV)
- Fungal infections; erythrasma
- Scabies
- Vaginitis; hemorrhoids

DIAGNOSTIC TESTS & INTERPRETATION
- Adhesive tape test
  - Place cellophane tape on the perianal skin in the early morning before bathing and affix to a microscope slide to look for pinworm eggs.
  - 90% sensitivity if performed on three consecutive mornings
  - Alternatively, use anal swabs or a pinworm paddle coated with adhesive material.
  - Scrapings from under fingernails of affected individuals can reveal pinworm eggs.
- Digital rectal exam with saline slide preparation of stool on gloved finger
- Stool samples are not helpful.
- *Routine stool examination for ova and parasites is positive in only 10–15% of infected patients.*

Test Interpretation
Identification of ova on low-power microscopy or direct visualization of the female worm (10-mm long); ova are asymmetric, flat on one side, and measure $56 \times 27 \ \mu m$.

TREATMENT

MEDICATION

First Line
- Treatment options include:
  - Albendazole (Albenza): 400 mg PO as a single dose in adults and children >20 kg; may repeat in 2 weeks; 200 mg PO as a single dose repeated in 2 weeks in children ≤20 kg (2,3)[A]
  - Mebendazole (Emverm, Vermox): chewable 100-mg tablet as a single dose in adults and children >2 years of age; may repeat in 2 to 3 weeks; use with caution in children <2 years of age (2,3)[A].
  - Pyrantel pamoate (Pin-X, Reese Pinworm Medicine): oral liquid or tablet 11 mg/kg as a single dose in adults and children >2 years of age; maximum dose 1 g. Use with caution in children <2 years of age (2,3)[A].
- Repeat treatment after 2 weeks is often recommended due to the high frequency of reinfection. Refractory cases may (rarely) require retreatment every 2 weeks for 4 to 6 cycles.
- All symptomatic family members should be treated.

Pregnancy Considerations
Avoid drug therapy in pregnancy. Treat after delivery. Breastfeeding is OK during mebendazole therapy (2,3)[A].

 ONGOING CARE

FOLLOW-UP RECOMMENDATIONS
Unnecessary unless symptoms recur after initial therapy

PATIENT EDUCATION
- Take medicine with food.
- Practice good hygiene: hand washing and perianal hygiene; particularly after bowel movements
- Encourage frequent and careful hand washing.
- Clip fingernails.
- Wash clothing and bedding after diagnosis to prevent reinfection. Do not shake linen and clothing before laundering because this may spread the eggs.
- Do not share washcloths.
- Do not allow children to cobathe during treatment and for 2 weeks after treatment; showering is preferred.

PROGNOSIS
- Asymptomatic carriers are common.
- Drug therapy is 90% curative.
- Reinfection is common, especially among children.

COMPLICATIONS
- Perianal scratching may lead to bacterial superinfection.
- Females: vulvovaginitis, urethritis, endometritis, and salpingitis (3,4)[A]
- UTIs
- Rarely: ectopic disease with granulomas of the pelvis, genitourinary tract, and appendix; colonic intussusception (5)[A]

REFERENCES
1. Stermer E, Sukhotnic I, Shaoul R. Pruritus ani: an approach to an itching condition. *J Pediatr Gastroenterol Nutr*. 2009;48(5):513–516.
2. The Medical Letter. Drugs for parasitic infection. *Treat Guidel Med Lett*. 2013;11(143):e7.
3. Centers for Disease Control and Prevention. Parasites - Enterobiasis (also known as pinworm infection). https://www.cdc.gov/parasites/pinworm /health_professionals/index.html. Accessed November 3, 2017.
4. Dennie J, Grover SR. Distressing perineal and vaginal pain in prepubescent girls: an aetiology. *J Paediatr Child Health*. 2013;49(2):138–140.
5. Adorisio O, De Peppo F, Rivosecchi M, et al. *Enterobius vermicularis* as a cause of intestinal occlusion: how to avoid unnecessary surgery. *Pediatr Emerg Care*. 2016;32(4):235–236.

 SEE ALSO

Pruritus Ani

CODES

ICD10
B80 Enterobiasis

CLINICAL PEARLS
- Nocturnal or early morning perianal itch with restless sleep or insomnia (particularly in children) is the hallmark of symptomatic pinworm infection.
- Treatment includes mebendazole, albendazole, or pyrantel pamoate.
- Treat close contacts.
- Retreatment after 2 weeks is generally recommended.

PITUITARY ADENOMA

Anup Sabharwal, MD, MBA, FACE • Lewis S. Blevins Jr., MD

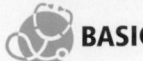

BASICS

DESCRIPTION
Typically benign, slow-growing tumors that arise from cells in the pituitary gland
- Pituitary adenomas have been identified as the third most frequent intracranial tumor; accounts for 10–25%
- Subtypes (hormonal): prolactinoma (PRL) 25–40%, nonfunctioning pituitary adenomas 30%, somatotroph adenoma (growth hormone [GH]) 15–20%, corticotroph adenoma (adrenocorticotropic hormone [ACTH]) 5–10%, thyrotroph adenoma (thyroid-stimulating hormone [TSH]) <1%, gonadotropinoma (luteinizing hormone/follicle-stimulating hormone [LH/FSH]), mixed (1)[A]
- Defined as microadenoma <10 mm and macroadenoma ≥10 mm
- May secrete hormones and/or cause mass effects

EPIDEMIOLOGY
- Predominant age: Age increases incidence.
- Predominant sex: female > male (3:2) for microadenomas (often delayed diagnosis in men)

Incidence
- Autopsy studies have found microadenomas in 3–27% and macroadenomas in <0.5% of people without any pituitary disorders.
- MRI scans illustrate abnormalities consistent with pituitary adenoma in 1/10 persons.
- Clinically apparent pituitary tumors are seen in 18/100,000 persons.

ETIOLOGY AND PATHOPHYSIOLOGY
- Monoclonal adenohypophysial cell growth
- Hormonal effects of functional microadenomas often prompt diagnosis before mass effect.
- PRL increased by functional prolactinomas or inhibited dopaminergic suppression by stalk effect

Genetics
- Carney complex
- Familial isolated pituitary adenomas: ~15% have mutations in the aryl hydrocarbon receptor–interacting protein gene (*AIP*); present at a younger age and are larger in size (2)
- McCune-Albright syndrome
- Multiple endocrine neoplasia type 1 (MEN1)-like phenotype (MEN4): germline mutation in the cyclin-dependent kinase inhibitor 1B (CDKN1B) (2)

RISK FACTORS
Multiple endocrine neoplasias

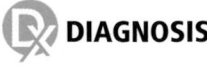

DIAGNOSIS

HISTORY
- Common
  - Hyperprolactinemia: infertility, amenorrhea, galactorrhea, gynecomastia, impotence
  - Headache (sellar expansion)
  - Visual disturbances: bitemporal hemianopsia
- Less common
  - Hypersomatotropinemia: acromegaly (coarse facial features, hand/foot swelling, carpal tunnel syndrome, hyperhidrosis, left ventricular hypertrophy)
  - Hyposomatotropinemia: failure to thrive (FTT) (children), asymptomatic (adults)
  - Intracranial pressure (ICP) elevation: headache, nausea, seizures

- Hypercorticotropinemia: Cushing disease (supraclavicular/dorsocervical fat pad thickening, moon face, hirsutism, acne, plethora, abdominal striae, centripetal obesity with thin limbs, easy bruising and bleeding, hyperglycemia)
- Rare
  - Apoplexy: headache, sudden collapse
  - Secondary hyperthyroidism: palpitations, diaphoresis, heat intolerance, diarrhea
  - Secondary adrenal insufficiency: weakness, irritability, anorexia, nausea/vomiting
- Hypothalamic compression: temperature, thirst/appetite disorders

PHYSICAL EXAM
- Common
  - Visual disturbances: bitemporal hemianopsia
  - Hyperprolactinemia: hypogonadism, galactorrhea, gynecomastia
  - Hypersomatotropinemia: acromegaly (coarse features, hand/foot swelling, diaphoresis)
  - Hyposomatotropinemia: FTT (children)
- Less common
  - ICP elevation: papilledema, dementia
  - Cushing disease: centripetal obesity, supraclavicular fat pad thickening, moon face, hirsutism, acne
- Rare
  - Apoplexy: hypotension, hypoglycemia, tachycardia, oliguria
  - Secondary hyperthyroidism: tachycardia, tachypnea, diaphoresis, warm/moist skin, tremor
  - Adrenal crisis: orthostatic hypotension
- Hypothalamic compression: temperature dysregulation, obesity, increased urination

DIFFERENTIAL DIAGNOSIS
Pituitary hyperplasia (e.g., pregnancy, primary hypothyroidism, menopause), Rathke cleft cyst, granulomatous disease (e.g., tuberculosis), lymphocytic hypophysitis, metastatic tumor, germinoma, craniopharyngioma

DIAGNOSTIC TESTS & INTERPRETATION
Select based on dysfunction(s) suspected
- Somatotrophic (GH secreting: 40 to 130/million)
  - Acromegaly/hypersomatotropinemia: serum IGF-1 elevated; oral glucose tolerance test with GH given at 0, 30, and 60 minutes (normally suppresses GH to <1 g/L)
  - Hyposomatotropinemia: low GH-releasing hormone response
  - Macimorelin is a noninvasive oral test to evaluate for adult GH deficiency (3)[A].
- Corticotropic
  - Cushing disease/hypercorticotropinemia
  - 24-hour urinary-free cortisol >50 μg
  - Overnight low-dose dexamethasone suppression test (DMST): normal free plasma cortisol (FPC) >1.8 μg/dL at 8 AM (after 1 mg given at 11 PM on night prior)
  - ACTH level assay (if DMST results abnormal): <20 pg/mL = adrenal tumor; ≥20 pg/mL = ectopic/pituitary source
  - Hypocorticotropinemia/secondary glucocorticoid deficiency: high-dose corticotropin stimulation test: FPC <10 g/dL at baseline, with an increase of <25% 1 hour after 250 μg; metyrapone test: 11-deoxycortisol <150 ng/L after 2 g given (Prepare to give steroids because test may worsen insufficiency.)
- Gonadotrophic/hypogonadotropinism: gonadotropin-releasing hormone stimulation of LH/FSH blunted in pituitary hypergonadism but increased in primary hypogonadism

- Lactotrophic (PRL secreting): hyperprolactinemia: serum PRL >20 ng/mL
- Thyrotrophic (TSH secreting): hyper-/hypothyroidism: TSH and free T4 both increased for pituitary hyperthyroidism and both decreased for pituitary hypothyroidism.

Initial Tests (lab, imaging)
- A typical panel for asymptomatic tumors: PRL, GH, IGF-1, ACTH, 24-hour urinary-free cortisol or overnight DMST, β-HCG, FSH, LH, TSH, free T4
- Maintain the same GH and IGF-1 through patient management (4)[C].
- Screening for *AIP* mutations may be offered to families of patients with pituitary adenoma, where available.
- MRI preferred (>90% sensitivity and specificity) after biochemically confirmed
- Octreotide scintigraphy is useful in identifying tumors with somatostatin receptors (4)[B].

Diagnostic Procedures/Other
Inferior petrosal sinus sampling: ACTH sampled from inferior petrosal sinuses to distinguish Cushing disease (pituitary source) from ectopic ACTH

Test Interpretation
- Cell types identified by immunohistochemistry
- Light microscope: eosinophilic (GH, PRL), basophilic (FSH/LH, TSH, ACTH), chromophobic

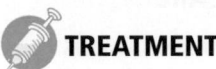

TREATMENT

Medical therapy is primary therapy for prolactinomas and adjunct for other tumors.

MEDICATION
First Line
- Hyperprolactinemia: Dopamine agonists increase dopaminergic suppression of PRL.
  - Cabergoline (Dostinex): D2 receptor–specific
    - Initial dose: 0.25 mg PO once or twice weekly
    - Maintenance dose: Increase q4wk by 0.25 mg 2 times per week per PRL (max 2 mg/week).
    - Contraindications: hypersensitivity (ergots), uncontrolled hypertension (HTN), pregnancy
    - Precautions: caution with liver impairment
    - Interactions: may be inhibited by tricyclic antidepressants, phenothiazines, opiates
    - Adverse reactions: orthostatic hypotension, vertigo, dyspepsia, hot flashes
  - Bromocriptine (Parlodel): D2 receptor–specific
    - Initial dose: 1.25 to 2.50 mg PO daily (give with food)
    - Maintenance dose: Increase by 2.5 mg/day q2–7d (max 15 mg/day).
    - Contraindications: hypersensitivity (ergots), uncontrolled HTN, pregnancy; preferred over cabergoline if required
    - Precautions: caution with liver impairment
    - Interactions: may be inhibited by tricyclic antidepressants, phenothiazines, opiates
    - Adverse reactions: orthostatic hypotension, seizures, hallucinations, stroke, myocardial infarction
- Somatotropinoma
  - Long-acting analogues of somatostatin (Sandostatin LAR and lanreotide Autogel)
    - Sandostatin LAR: 20 mg q28d (4)[A]; lanreotide Autogel 90 mg q28d; titrate per package insert.
    - Contraindication: hypersensitivity
    - Precautions: caution with biliary, thyroid, cardiac, liver, or kidney disease

- Interactions: Pimozide increases risk of QT prolongation; variable effects with β-blockers, diuretics, oral glycemic agents
- Adverse reactions: ascending cholangitis, arrhythmias, congestive heart failure, glycemic instability
- More effective as adjuvant than as primary treatment for somatotropinomas
- Consider use of somatostatin analogue or pegvisomant in patients with severe residual disease (4)[A].
- Consider use of cabergoline in patients with mild residual disease (5)[B].
- Pegvisomant (Somavert): GH receptor antagonist
  - Initial dose: 40 mg SC × 1, then 10 mg daily and titrate by 5 mg every 4 to 6 weeks based on IGF-1 levels (max 30 mg/day maintenance dose)
  - Contraindication: hypersensitivity
  - Precautions: caution if GH-secreting tumors, diabetes mellitus, impaired liver function
  - Interactions: NSAIDs, opiates, insulins, oral glycemic agents
  - Adverse reactions: hepatitis, tumor growth, GH secretion
- Corticotropinemia: peripheral inhibitors
  - Mitotane (Lysodren)
    - Initial dose: 2 to 6 g/day divided PO TID (max 19 g/day)
    - Maintenance dose: 2 to 16 g TID
    - Contraindication: hypersensitivity
    - Precautions: caution with liver dysfunction and brain damage
    - Interactions: contraindicated with rotavirus vaccine; caution with other vaccines
    - Adverse reactions: HTN, orthostatic hypotension, hemorrhagic cystitis, rash
  - Ketoconazole
    - Dosing: 200 mg PO TID (max 1,200 mg/day)
    - Contraindications: hypersensitivity, achlorhydria, fungal meningitis, impaired liver function
    - Precautions: caution with liver dysfunction
    - Interactions: contraindicated with dronedarone, methadone, statins, pimozide, sirolimus; caution with other antifungals
    - Adverse reactions: adrenal insufficiency, thrombocytopenia, hepatic failure, hepatotoxicity, anaphylaxis, leukopenia, hemolytic anemia
  - Pasireotide (Signifor)
    - Dosing: initially, 0.6 to 0.9 mg twice daily and then 0.3 to 0.9 mg twice daily
    - Contraindication: none
    - Precautions: hypocortisolism, hyperglycemia, bradycardia or QT prolongation, liver test elevations, cholelithiasis, and other pituitary hormone deficiencies
  - Mifepristone (Korlym)
    - Dosing: Administer PO once daily with a meal. The recommended starting dose is 300 mg once daily; not to exceed 600 mg daily in renal impairment
    - Contraindication: pregnancy, use of simvastatin or lovastatin and CYP3A substrates with narrow therapeutic range, concurrent long-term corticosteroid use, women with history of unexplained vaginal bleeding, women with endometrial hyperplasia with atypia or endometrial carcinoma
    - Precautions: adrenal insufficiency, hypokalemia, vaginal bleeding and endometrial changes, QT interval prolongation, use of strong CYP3A inhibitors
    - Interactions: potential interactions with drugs metabolized by CYP3A, CYP2C8/9, CYP2B6, and hormonal contraceptives. Nursing mothers should discontinue drug or discontinue nursing.

- Adverse reactions: most common adverse reactions in Cushing syndrome (≥20%): nausea, fatigue, headache, decreased blood potassium, arthralgia, vomiting, peripheral edema, HTN, dizziness, decreased appetite, endometrial hypertrophy
- Gonadotropinemia
  - Bromocriptine: See earlier discussion.
- Thyrotropinemia
  - Somatostatin analogues: See earlier discussion.

Second Line
- Corticotropinemia: peripheral inhibitors
  - Metyrapone
    - Dose: 250 mg PO QID
    - Contraindication: porphyria
    - Precautions: caution in liver/thyroid disease
    - Interactions: Dilantin increases metabolism.
    - Adverse reactions: nausea, hypotension
- Gonadotropinemia
  - Octreotide: See earlier discussion.

ISSUES FOR REFERRAL
- Neurosurgery consultation for symptomatic tumors (except for prolactinoma)
- Ophthalmologist evaluation prior to surgery

ADDITIONAL THERAPIES
- Fractionated radiotherapy: often effective as adjunctive when surgery is inadequate (5)[B]
- Stereotactic radiosurgery: alternative to surgery in high-risk patients or as adjunct (5)[B]

SURGERY/OTHER PROCEDURES
- Most are now done endoscopically via translabial/transsphenoidal approach (6)[A].
- Indications: symptoms or treatment resistant
- Follow-up: serial neurologic/hormonal evaluations to evaluate complications (e.g., diabetes insipidus, CNS damage) and need for more treatment
- Remission rates: 72–87% for microadenoma but only 50–56% for macroadenomas

ADMISSION, INPATIENT, AND NURSING CONSIDERATIONS
- Outpatient management unless apoplexy or adrenal crisis
- Treat pituitary apoplexy immediately to prevent death (see "Complications") (6)[A].
- Consider stress-dose steroids in frail or hemodynamically unstable patients.
- Maintain BP with fluids and/or pressor agents.
- Check serum sodium, serum osmolality, and urine specific gravity if polyuric or electrolytes are imbalanced.
- Contact neurosurgery.
- Diabetes insipidus: hyperosmolar IV fluids
- Adrenal crisis: normal saline
- Pituitary apoplexy: Monitor inputs/outputs (I/Os), central venous pressure, and ICP and do frequent neurologic checks.
- Adrenal crisis: Monitor BP and I/Os.
- Keep as inpatient postoperatively until diabetes insipidus and/or adrenal insufficiency is managed.

 ONGOING CARE

FOLLOW-UP RECOMMENDATIONS
Patient Monitoring
- Follow-up MRIs at 6 and 12 months after discharge
- Involved hormone(s) are followed postoperatively, especially after radiation because hypopituitarism may develop 10 to 15 years after treatment.

PROGNOSIS
Depends on type, size, symptoms, therapy

COMPLICATIONS
- Postoperative diabetes insipidus and/or hypogonadism (usually transient/common)
- Pituitary apoplexy (acute/uncommon): acute hemorrhagic pituitary infarction; adrenal crisis with severe headache; surgical decompression required to prevent shock, coma, and death
- Nelson syndrome (subacute/uncommon): rapid adenoma growth postadrenalectomy
- Pituitary hormone insufficiency (chronic/uncommon): often years after treatment
- Optic nerve neuropathy and brain necrosis after >60 Gy radiotherapy (chronic/rare)

REFERENCES
1. Dworakowska D, Grossman AB. The pathophysiology of pituitary adenomas. *Best Pract Res Clin Endocrinol Metab*. 2009;23(5):525–541.
2. Georgitsi M, Raitila A, Karhu A, et al. Molecular diagnosis of pituitary adenoma predisposition caused by aryl hydrocarbon receptor-interacting protein gene mutations. *Proc Natl Acad Sci U S A*. 2007;104(10):4101–4105.
3. Agrawal V, Garcia JM. The macimorelin-stimulated growth hormone test for adult growth hormone deficiency diagnosis. *Expert Rev Mol Diagn*. 2014;14(6):647–654.
4. Tichomirowa MA, Daly AF, Beckers A. Treatment of pituitary tumors: somatostatin. *Endocrine*. 2005;28(1):93–100.
5. Mondok A, Szeifert GT, Mayer A, et al. Treatment of pituitary tumors: radiation. *Endocrine*. 2005;28(1):77–85.
6. Buchfelder M. Treatment of pituitary tumors: surgery. *Endocrine*. 2005;28(1):67–75.

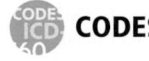 **SEE ALSO**

Cushing Disease and Cushing Syndrome; Galactorrhea

CODES

ICD10
D35.2 Benign neoplasm of pituitary gland

CLINICAL PEARLS
- An incidentaloma is an asymptomatic microadenoma found on imaging. General labs include PRL, GH, IGF-1, ACTH, 24-hour urinary-free cortisol/overnight DMST, β-subunit FSH, LH, TSH, and free T$_4$. Obtain follow-up MRIs at 6 and 12 months if normal, but consult endocrinology if not.
- Initial treatment selected for symptomatic pituitary adenoma includes a dopamine agonist for prolactinomas and surgical resection for all others.
- Pituitary apoplexy is a rapid hemorrhagic pituitary infarction due to compression of the blood supply. It is fatal within hours unless surgically decompressed.

PLANTAR FASCIITIS

Roselyn Jan W. Clemente-Fuentes, MD, FAAFP • Brooke E. Organ, DO • Krystal M. Thumann, MD

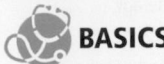

BASICS

DESCRIPTION
- Degenerative change of plantar fascia at origin on medial tuberosity of calcaneus
- Pain on plantar surface, usually at calcaneal insertion of plantar fascia upon weight-bearing, especially in morning or on initiation of walking after prolonged rest
- Also referred to as: plantar heel pain syndrome, heel spur syndrome, plantar fasciopathy, painful heel syndrome

EPIDEMIOLOGY
Prevalence
- Most common cause of plantar heel pain
- Lifetime: 10–15% of population
- Peak incidence between ages 40 and 60 years, earlier peak in runners
- Condition is typically self-limiting, resolving within 12 months.

ETIOLOGY AND PATHOPHYSIOLOGY
- Repetitive microtrauma and collagen degeneration of plantar fascia
- Chronic degenerative change (-osis/-opathy rather than -itis) of plantar fascia generally at insertion on medial tuberosity of calcaneus

RISK FACTORS
- Intrinsic
  - Age (>40 to 60 years)
  - Female, pregnancy
  - Obesity (BMI >30)
  - Pes planus (flat feet), pes cavus (high arch), overpronation, leg length discrepancy
  - Hamstring, calf, and Achilles tightness
  - Calf and intrinsic foot muscle weakness
  - Decreased ankle range of motion with dorsiflexion (equinus or tight heel cord; <15 degrees of dorsiflexion)
  - Systemic connective tissue disorders
- Extrinsic
  - Dancers, runners, court sport athletes
  - Occupations with prolonged standing, especially on hard surfaces (nurses, letter carriers, warehouse/factory workers)
  - Overuse and rapid increase in activities involving repetitive loading

GENERAL PREVENTION
- Maintain normal body weight.
- Avoid prolonged standing on bare feet, sandals, or slippers.
- Avoid training errors (increasing intensity, distance, duration, and frequency of high-impact activities too rapidly); avoid overtraining.

- Proper footwear (appropriate cushion/arch support)
- Runners should replace footwear every 250 to 500 miles.

COMMONLY ASSOCIATED CONDITIONS
- Usually isolated
- Heel spurs common but not a marker of severity
- Posterior tibial neuropathy

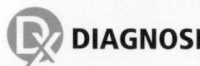

DIAGNOSIS

HISTORY
- Pain on plantar surface of foot, usually at fascial insertion at calcaneus (medial calcaneal tubercle), but can have pain anywhere along length of plantar fascia
- Pain is typically worse with first few steps in the morning or after prolonged rest or standing (poststatic dyskinesia).
- Pain typically improves after first few steps only to recur toward the end of the day or after prolonged ambulation.
- Pain commonly unilateral but can be bilateral in 1/3 of cases
- Pain can be dull and constant in chronic cases.
- Limp with excessive toe walking
- Numbness and burning of medial hindfoot when associated with posterior tibial nerve compression

PHYSICAL EXAM
- Point tenderness on medial tuberosity of calcaneus at insertion of plantar fascia
- Pain along plantar fascia with dorsiflexion of foot
- Windlass test: Extend MTP while allowing passive flexion of IP joint of hallux—pain indicates a positive test; high specificity, low sensitivity; sensitivity improves (13.5→31.8%) if performed while standing.
- Dorsiflexion-eversion test: pain with dorsiflexion plus eversion of the subtalar joint
- Decreased passive range of motion with dorsiflexion
- Evaluate for pes planus, pes cavus, and overpronation.
- Loss of heel fat pad suggests heel fat pad syndrome.
- Point tenderness on posterosuperior aspect of heel suggests Achilles tendinopathy.

DIFFERENTIAL DIAGNOSIS
- Calcaneal stress fracture
- Heel fat pad syndrome (painful or atrophic heel pad)
- Longitudinal arch strain
- Nerve entrapment (posterior tibial nerve—tarsal tunnel syndrome, medial calcaneal branch of posterior tibial nerve, abductor digiti quinti)
- Achilles tendinopathy

- Calcaneal contusion
- Plantar calcaneal bursitis
- Tendonitis of posterior tibialis
- Plantar fascia tear
- S1 radiculopathy
- Adolescents: calcaneal apophysitis (Sever disease)

DIAGNOSTIC TESTS & INTERPRETATION
- Usually not necessary; typically a clinical diagnosis
- Consider further imaging only to rule out other causes, uncertain diagnosis, or persistent heel pain after 4 to 6 months of conservative therapy.
- Radiographs: two views of foot to evaluate for fracture, tumor, cyst, periostitis, bony erosions; weight-bearing films preferred; calcaneal spurs common but not diagnostic
- Ultrasound: hypoechoic at insertion, thickened plantar fascia (≥4 mm); diagnostic and even therapeutic when used as an adjunct to treatment; can improve delivery accuracy of injections and extracorporeal shock wave therapy (ESWT); can objectively evaluate change in plantar fascia thickness to monitor effects of an intervention
- MRI can evaluate for other soft tissue etiologies.
- CT or technetium-99m bone scan can rule out calcaneal stress fracture and evaluate for infection.
- Nerve conduction studies can rule out nerve entrapment.
- Inflammatory markers: can consider if bilateral heel pain or young patients

TREATMENT

Non-operative management is mainstay of treatment.

GENERAL MEASURES
- Supportive footwear with stable midfoot; avoid sandals or walking barefoot.
- Relative rest/activity modification with avoidance of high-impact causative activities
- Stretching: plantar fascia stretches more effective than Achilles tendon/gastrocnemius-soleus stretches, and non–weight-bearing stretches may be preferable
- Strengthen calf and interosseous muscles, using the towel drag/pickup exercise.
- Ice (frozen water bottle roll)
- Massage (golf or tennis ball roll)
- Weight reduction if BMI >25
- Orthotics
  - Custom orthotics show no benefit over prefabricated orthotics and are more costly.
  - Arch support straps or heel cups are inexpensive and may be used in place or in addition to orthotics.
  - Improved effectiveness of night splints when used in association with orthotics

- Night splints: maintains dorsiflexion overnight; effective with calf and Achilles tightness
- Surgical treatment of "heel spurs" is not indicated.

MEDICATION

First Line
- NSAIDs scheduled for 2 to 3 weeks: naproxen 500 mg PO BID *or* ibuprofen 600 to 800 mg PO TID PRN for pain
- Acetaminophen 1,000 mg PO TID PRN for pain

Second Line
None

ISSUES FOR REFERRAL
- Physical therapy for patient instruction on proper stretching and strengthening techniques, manipulative treatments, and massage
- Podiatry: Consider if conservative measures fail after 3 to 6 months.
- Surgery: Consider if conservative measures fail after 6 to 12 months.

ADDITIONAL THERAPIES
- Corticosteroid injections (1)[B]
  - Short-term pain relief
  - Medial heel approach or points of maximal tenderness along plantar fascia
  - Recommend ultrasound guidance when possible.
  - Risk for plantar fascia rupture and calcaneal fat pad atrophy with resultant permanent heel pain
- Low-dye and calcaneal taping
- Short walking cast
- Promising therapies with inconsistent evidence
  - ESWT (2)[B]
  - Radiofrequency nerve ablation (3)[B]
  - Plantar iontophoresis
  - Intralesional autologous blood injection
  - Low-level laser therapy
  - Myofascial trigger point dry needling (4)[B]
  - Dehydrated amniotic membrane injection (5)[B]
  - Platelet-rich plasma (PRP) injections (6)[B]
  - Botulinum toxin (BT) A injection (5)[B]

SURGERY/OTHER PROCEDURES
- Necessary in <10% of patients; more likely beneficial in severely obese
- Recommended if conservative treatment fails after 6 to 12 months and pain is unrelenting
- Open/endoscopic plantar fasciotomy (less risk and complications with endoscopic technique but requires specialized equipment and skills; not widely used)
- Cryosurgery
- Calcaneal spur resection

COMPLEMENTARY & ALTERNATIVE MEDICINE
Acupuncture may reduce pain in short term, but further studies needed.

ONGOING CARE

FOLLOW-UP RECOMMENDATIONS
- Ensure patient adherence to proper stretching technique.
- Following 3 to 6 months of unsuccessful conservative treatment, consider additional therapies or referrals.

PATIENT EDUCATION
- Weight reduction if BMI >25
- Proper footwear (adequate cushion and arch support)
- Stretch plantar fascia: Pull toes into dorsiflexion prior to walking after prolonged sitting or sleep.
- Ice the foot using a frozen water bottle: Roll foot over bottle for 10 minutes in the morning and after work.
- Massage plantar fascia: Roll foot over a golf ball.
- Strengthen foot muscles: Grab cloth or carpet by plantar flexing the toes.
- Decrease repetitive stress.

PROGNOSIS
- Generally good
- Self-limited (resolves within 2 years) in up to 85–90% of patients

COMPLICATIONS
- Rupture of plantar fascia (more common with repeated corticosteroid injections)
- Chronic pain
- Gait abnormality

REFERENCES

1. David JA, Sankarapandian V, Christopher PR, et al. Injected corticosteroids for treating plantar heel pain in adults. *Cochrane Database Syst Rev.* 2017;(6):CD009348.
2. Hocaoglu S, Vurdem UE, Cebicci MA, et al. Comparative effectiveness of radial extracorporeal shockwave therapy and ultrasound-guided local corticosteroid injection treatment for plantar fasciitis. *J Am Podiatr Med Assoc.* 2017;107(3):192–199.
3. Landsman AS, Catanese DJ, Wiener SN, et al. A prospective, randomized, double-blinded study with crossover to determine the efficacy of radiofrequency nerve ablation for the treatment of heel pain. *J Am Podiatr Med Assoc.* 2013;103(1):8–15.
4. He C, Ma H. Effectiveness of trigger point dry needling for plantar heel pain: a meta-analysis of seven randomized controlled trials. *J Pain Res.* 2017;10:1933–1942.
5. Tsikopoulos K, Vasiliadis HS, Mavridis D. Injection therapies for plantar fasciopathy ('plantar fasciitis'): a systematic review and network meta-analysis of 22 randomised controlled trials. *Br J Sports Med.* 2016;50(22):1367–1375.
6. Chiew SK, Ramasamy TS, Amini F. Effectiveness and relevant factors of platelet-rich plasma treatment in managing plantar fasciitis: a systematic review. *J Res Med Sci.* 2016;21:38.

ADDITIONAL READING

- Berbrayer D, Fredericson M. Update on evidence-based treatments for plantar fasciopathy. *PM R.* 2014;6(2):159–169.
- Li Z, Yu A, Qi B, et al. Corticosteroid versus placebo injection for plantar fasciitis: a meta-analysis of randomized controlled trials. *Exp Ther Med.* 2015;9(6):2263–2268.
- Petraglia F, Ramazzina I, Costantino C. Plantar fasciitis in athletes: diagnostic and treatment strategies. A systematic review. *Muscles Ligaments Tendons J.* 2017;7(1):107–118.
- Sun J, Gao F, Wang Y, et al. Extracorporeal shock wave therapy is effective in treating chronic plantar fasciitis: a meta-analysis of RCTs. *Medicine (Baltimore).* 2017;96(15):e6621.
- Yin MC, Ye J, Yao M, et al. Is extracorporeal shock wave therapy clinical efficacy for relief of chronic, recalcitrant plantar fasciitis? A systematic review and meta-analysis of randomized placebo or active-treatment controlled trials. *Arch Phys Med Rehabil.* 2014;95(8):1585–1593.

SEE ALSO

Algorithm: Heel Pain

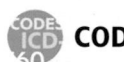 CODES

ICD10
M72.2 Plantar fascial fibromatosis

CLINICAL PEARLS
- Plantar fasciitis occurs due to degeneration of plantar fascia at origin (medial calcaneal tuberosity) with characteristic pattern of pain.
- Plantar medial heel pain with weight-bearing (most noticeable with initial steps in the morning or after period of inactivity) is hallmark presentation.
- Generally, self-limited and conservative treatment is preferred. 85–90% of patients can be treated with conservative therapies.
- Supportive footwear helps avoid excess pronation and provides adequate cushion and arch support. Modify activity, stretch plantar fascia, strengthen intrinsic foot muscles, ice (water bottle roll), and massage (golf ball roll).
- Weight loss helps control symptoms, particularly for BMI ≥25.

PLEURAL EFFUSION

Felix B. Chang Cruz, MD, FAAMA, ABIHM

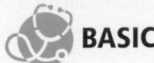 **BASICS**

Abnormal accumulation of fluid in the pleural space

DESCRIPTION

Types: transudate, exudate

- Congestive heart failure (CHF): 40%: transudate
- Pneumonia 25%, malignancy 15%, and pulmonary embolism (PE) 10% account for exudative effusions.
- Malignant: lung cancer and metastases of breast, ovary, and lymphoma

EPIDEMIOLOGY

Incidence

Estimated 1.5 million cases per year in the United States; CHF: 500,000; pneumonia: 300,000; malignancy: 150,000; PE: 150,000; cirrhosis: 150,000; tuberculosis (TB): 2,500; pancreatitis: 20,000; collagen vascular disease: 6,000

Prevalence

- Estimated 320 cases per 100,000 people in industrialized countries; in hospitalized patients with AIDS, prevalence is 7–27%.
- No gender predilection: ~2/3 of malignant pleural effusions occur in women.

ETIOLOGY AND PATHOPHYSIOLOGY

- Pleural fluid formation exceeds pleural fluid absorption.
- Transudates result from imbalances in hydrostatic and oncotic forces.
  - Increase in hydrostatic and/or low oncotic pressures; increase in pleural capillary permeability; lymphatic obstruction or impaired drainage; movement of fluid from the peritoneal or retroperitoneal space
- Transudates
  - CHF: 40% of transudative effusions; 80% bilateral; constrictive pericarditis, atelectasis; superior vena cava syndrome
  - Cirrhosis (hepatic hydrothorax); nephrotic syndrome, hypoalbuminemia; myxedema
  - Urinothorax, central line misplacement; peritoneal dialysis
  - Dressler syndrome (postmyocardial infarction syndrome)
  - Yellow nail syndrome: yellow nails, lymphedema and pleural effusion
- Exudates
  - Lung parenchyma infection, bacterial (parapneumonic, tuberculous pleurisy), fungal, viral, parasitic (amebiasis, *Echinococcus*)
  - Cancer: lung cancer, metastases (breast, lymphoma, ovaries), mesothelioma
  - PE: 25% of PEs are transudate.
  - Collagen vascular disease: rheumatoid arthritis, systemic lupus erythematosus (SLE), Wegener granulomatosis, sarcoidosis, Churg-Strauss
  - GI: pancreatitis, esophageal rupture, abdominal abscess, after liver transplant; chylothorax: thoracic duct tear, malignancy
  - Hemothorax: trauma, PE, malignancy, coagulopathy, aortic aneurysm
  - Others: after coronary artery bypass graft; uremia, asbestos exposure, radiation; drug induced:
    ○ Drugs: nitrofurantoin, bromocriptine, amiodarone, procarbazine, hydralazine, procainamide, quinidine, methotrexate, methysergide, interleukin-2, mitomycin, practolol, minoxidil, bleomycin, cyclophosphamide, dantrolene, valproic acid, sulfasalazine, minocycline, acebutolol
  - Meigs syndrome; yellow nail syndrome; ovarian stimulation syndrome; lymphangiomatosis; acute respiratory distress syndrome (ARDS)
  - Chylothorax: thoracic duct tear, malignancy, associated with lymphoma

RISK FACTORS

- Occupational exposures/drugs
- PE, TB, bacterial pneumonias
- Opportunistic infections (in HIV patients when CD4 count is <150 cells/μL)

COMMONLY ASSOCIATED CONDITIONS

Hypoproteinemia, heart failure, cirrhosis

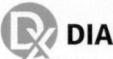 **DIAGNOSIS**

Presumptive diagnosis in 50% of cases. Small pleural effusions; radiographic area <2 intercostal spaces (<300 mL) are asymptomatic.

HISTORY

Dyspnea, fever, malaise, and weight loss; chest pain, cough, hemoptysis, and dull pain

PHYSICAL EXAM

- Pleural effusion >300 mL: tachypnea, asymmetric expansion of the thoracic cage; decrease/absent tactile fremitus; dullness to percussion; decreased/inaudible breath sounds, egophony, pleural friction rub
- Ascites suggest the following: hepatic hydrothorax, ovarian cancer, and Meigs syndrome.
- If associated with unilateral swelling in lower extremity, consider DVT with PE.

DIFFERENTIAL DIAGNOSIS

Empyema, malignancy, inflammatory, fungal, TB

DIAGNOSTIC TESTS & INTERPRETATION

Initial Tests (lab, imaging)

- Pleural fluid: appearance, pH, WBC differential, total protein, lactate dehydrogenase (LDH), glucose, Gram stain and culture, and acid-fast bacilli staining. Consider polymerase chain reaction (PCR) for *Mycobacterium tuberculosis* and *Streptococcus pneumoniae* (1,2)[A].
- If comorbidities implying risk, consider amylase, triglycerides, cholesterol, LE cells, cytology, antinuclear antibodies (ANAs), adenosine deaminase, tumor markers, rheumatoid factor, cytology, creatinine (2)[A].
- Light criteria, transudate versus exudate (98% sensitivity; 80% specificity); fluid is considered an exudate if any of the following (2)[A]:
  - Ratio of pleural fluid-to-serum protein levels >0.5; ratio of pleural fluid-to-serum LDH levels >0.6; pleural fluid LDH level >2/3 the upper limit for serum LDH level (1,3)[A]
- Other exudate criteria (4)[A]:
  - Serum-effusion albumin gradient ≤1.2 (sensitivity 87%; specificity 92%); cholesterol effusion >45 mg/dL and LDH effusion >200 mg/dL (sensitivity 90%; specificity 98%)
- Empyema: pus, putrid odor; culture. A putrid odor suggests an anaerobic empyema: LDH levels >1,000 IU/L (normal serum = 200 IU/L); glucose, <60 mg/dL; low pH
- Malignancy: cytology, red, bloody; glucose, normal to low, depending on the tumor burden; RBCs, >100,000/mm³
- Lupus pleuritis: LE cells present; pleural fluid-to-serum ANAs ratio >1; glucose <60 mg/dL; pleural fluid-to-serum glucose ratio <0.5

- Fungal: positive KOH, culture; peritoneal dialysis: protein, <1 g/dL; glucose, 300 to 400 mg/dL
- Urinothorax: creatinine: pleural/blood >0.5; high LDH pleural fluid, with low protein levels
- Hemothorax: hematocrit: pleural/blood >0.5; benign asbestos effusion: unilateral, exudative; have elevated eosinophil count
- TB pleuritis: lymphocytes >80% predominance effusion; elevated levels of adenosine deaminase >50 U/L and interferon-γ >140 pg/mL; positive acid-fast bacillus (AFB) stain, culture; total protein >4 g/dL, nuclear acid amplification (NAA), LDH levels elevated in about 75% of patients (often >500 units/L)
- Chylothorax: milky; triglycerides >110 mg/dL; lipoprotein electrophoresis (chylomicrons)
- Amebic liver abscess: anchovy paste effusion; Waldenström macroglobulinemia and multiple myeloma: protein >7 g/dL
- Esophageal rupture: high salivary amylase; pleural fluid acidosis, pH <6; amylase rich: acute pancreatitis, chronic pancreatic pleural effusion, malignancy, esophageal rupture; rheumatoid pleurisy: glucose <60 mg/dL; pleural fluid/serum glucose <0.5
- Lymphocytosis: tuberculous pleurisy, lymphoma, sarcoidosis, chronic rheumatoid pleurisy, yellow nail syndrome, or chylothorax (80–95% of the nucleated cells); carcinomatosis in half of cases (50–70% are lymphocytes)
- Pleural fluid eosinophilia (>10% of total nucleated cells): pneumothorax, hemothorax, malignancy, drugs, pulmonary infarction, fungal (coccidioidomycosis, cryptococcosis, histoplasmosis), benign asbestos pleural effusion
- Low glucose (<60 mg/dL): TB, malignancy, rheumatoid pleurisy, parapneumonic, empyema, hemothorax, paragonimiasis, Churg-Strauss syndrome
- RBC count >100,000/mm³: trauma, malignancy, PE, injury after cardiac surgery, asbestos pleurisy, pancreatitis, TB
- Pleural fluid LDH >1,000 IU/L: suggests empyema, malignant effusion, rheumatoid effusion, or pleural paragonimiasis
- pH >7.3: rheumatoid pleurisy, empyema, malignant effusion, TB, esophageal rupture, or lupus nephritis
- Mesothelial cells in exudates: TB is unlikely if there are >5% of mesothelial cells.
- *S. pneumoniae* accounts for 50% of cases of parapneumonic effusions in AIDS patients, followed by *Staphylococcus aureus*, *Haemophilus influenzae*, *Mycoplasma pneumoniae*, *Legionella*, *Nocardia*, and *Bordetella bronchiseptica*; exudate with low count of nucleated cells
- *Pneumocystis jiroveci* is an uncommon cause in HIV. Usually it is a small effusion, unilateral or bilateral, and serous to bloody in appearance. Demonstration of the trophozoite or cyst is mandatory.
- Cancer-related HIV pleural effusion: Kaposi sarcoma, Castleman disease, and primary effusion lymphoma. Kaposi sarcoma: mononuclear predominance, exudate, pH >7.4; LDH, 111 to 330 IU/L; glucose >60 mg/dL
- Chest x-ray (CXR): posteroanterior–anteroposterior views
  - Upright x-rays show a concave meniscus in the costophrenic angle that suggests >250 mL of pleural fluid; homogeneous opacity, with visibility of pulmonary vessels through diffuse haziness and absence of air bronchogram; 75 mL of fluid will obliterate the posterior costophrenic sulcus.

- Lateral x-rays show blunting of the posterior costophrenic angle and the posterior gutter; decubitus x-rays to exclude a loculated effusion and underlying pulmonary lesion or pulmonary thickening
- Supine x-rays show costophrenic blunting, haziness, obliteration of the diaphragmatic silhouette, decreased visibility of the lower lobe vasculature, and widened minor fissure.
- Ultrasonography (US): detects as 5 to 50 mL of pleural fluid; identifies loculated effusions; site for thoracentesis, pleural biopsy, or pleural drainage
- Chest CT scan with contrast for patients with undiagnosed pleural effusion; CT pulmonary angiography if PE is suspected

Follow-Up Tests & Special Considerations
75% of patients with exudative effusions have a non-CHF cause.

- NT-proBNP: biomarker of CHF-associated effusion; >1,500 pg/mL; sensitivity and specificity 94% (2)[A]
- In patients with a lymphocytic effusion, further investigation should be considered for TB, sarcoidosis, lymphoma, chylothorax, and pseudochylothorax.

Diagnostic Procedures/Other
Diagnostic thoracentesis indicated for the following:

- Clinically significant pleural effusion (>10-mm thick on US or lateral decubitus x-ray with no known cause)
- CHF: asymmetric effusion, fever, chest pain, or failure to resolve after diuretics
- Parapneumonic effusions

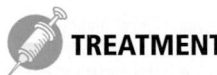 **TREATMENT**

Oxygen support to >92%

GENERAL MEASURES
- Therapeutic thoracentesis, if symptomatic
- Chest tube thoracostomy drainage: >1/2 hemithorax; complicated parapneumonic effusion (positive Gram stain or culture, pH <7.2, or glucose <60 mg/dL); empyema; hemothorax. Recommended limit is 1,000 to 1,500 mL in a single thoracentesis procedure (5)[B].

MEDICATION
First Line
CHF: diuretics (75% clearing in 48 hours); parapneumonic effusion: antibiotics; rheumatologic conditions/inflammation: steroids and NSAIDs

Second Line
Symptomatic nonmalignant effusions that are refractory to treatment may be managed with repeated therapeutic thoracentesis or pleurodesis.

ISSUES FOR REFERRAL
- Uncertain etiology; malignant effusion; high-risk diagnostic thoracentesis; decortication
- Video-assisted thoracoscopy for sclerosis; peritoneal shunts for symptomatic recurrence

ADDITIONAL THERAPIES
- Pleurodesis for symptomatic patients whose pleural effusion reaccumulates too quickly for repeat therapeutic thoracentesis
- Talc poudrage to be a highly effective method 95% credible interval (Cr-1) 1 to 5 (5)[A]
- Tunneled pleural catheter is the preferred treatment for patients with malignant pleural effusion and limited survival.

- Sclerosing agents for malignant effusions: doxycycline, bleomycin, talc, and minocycline; talc is more efficacious. The relative risk of nonrecurrent effusion was 1.34 (95% CI 1.16–1.55) in favor of talc compared with bleomycin, tetracycline, or mustine.

SURGERY/OTHER PROCEDURES
- Percutaneous pleural biopsy if a cause is not clear after thoracentesis
  - Close pleural biopsy: Pleura is diffusely involved (TB pleuritis, noncaseating granuloma in rheumatoid pleuritis).
  - CT-guided needle biopsy: pleural mass; video-assisted thoracoscopic pleural biopsy: Negative percutaneous biopsy, patchy disease, or CT scan does not show obvious mass.
- Parapneumonic effusion should be sampled if free-flowing, but layer is >10 mm on a lateral decubitus film; loculated, thickened pleura on a contrast-enhanced CT scan, clearly delineated by US open pleural biopsy by thoracotomy
- Contraindications for thoracentesis: anticoagulation, bleeding diathesis, thrombocytopenia <20,000/mm³, mechanical ventilation
- Bronchoscopy: when malignancy is suspected (pulmonary infiltrate or mass on CXR or CT scan, hemoptysis, massive pleural effusion, or shift of the mediastinum toward the side of effusion)
- Thoracoscopy
- No statistically significant difference in mortality between primary surgical and nonsurgical management of pleural empyema for all age groups (6)[A]
- Video-assisted thoracoscopic surgery may reduce length of hospital stay compared to thoracostomy (6)[A].

ADMISSION, INPATIENT, AND NURSING CONSIDERATIONS
Treat any underlying medical disorder.

 ONGOING CARE

FOLLOW-UP RECOMMENDATIONS
Patient Monitoring
- Check for the amount and quality of fluid drained, air leak (bubbling), and oscillation.
- Repeat a CXR when drainage decreases to <100 mL/day to evaluate complete clearing.
- For a large effusion, reevaluate catheter position; if positioned appropriately, consider fibrinolytics.

DIET
Cardiac diet in patients with heart failure; correct hypoproteinemia.

PROGNOSIS
- Malignant effusion: poor
- Low-pH malignant effusions have shorter survival and poorer response to chemical pleurodesis than those with pH >7.3.
- Low pleural fluid pH (≤7.15): high likelihood of pleural space drainage
- 68% 30-day and 84% 1-year mortality among patients with bilateral malignant pleural effusion
- Pleural fluid pH ≤7.28 associated with reduced survival (odds ratio 4.42, 95% CI 2.39–8.46 for <1-month survival)
- Uncomplicated parapneumonic effusions and effusions from PE, tuberculous pleurisy, and postcardiac injury syndrome may persist for several weeks.

- Benign asbestos pleural effusion, rheumatoid pleurisy, and radiation pleuritis often persist for months to years.
- Malignant pleural effusions, on the other hand, seldom resolve spontaneously.

COMPLICATIONS
- Pleural effusion: constrictive fibrosis, pleurocutaneous fistula
- Thoracentesis: pneumothorax (5–10%); hemothorax (~1%); empyema; spleen/liver laceration; reexpansion pulmonary edema (if >1.5 L is removed)

REFERENCES
1. Sahn SA, Huggins JT, San Jose E, et al. The art of pleural fluid analysis. *Clin Pulm Med*. 2013;20(2):77–96.
2. Saguil A, Wyrick K, Hallgren J. Diagnostic approach to pleural effusion. *Am Fam Physician*. 2014;90(2):99–104.
3. Light RW. Pleural effusions. *Med Clin North Am*. 2011;95(6):1055–1070.
4. Wilcox ME, Chong CA, Stanbrook MB, et al. Does this patient have an exudative pleural effusion? The rational clinical examination systematic review. *JAMA*. 2014;311(23):2422–2431.
5. Clive AO, Jones HE, Bhatnagar R, et al. Interventions for the management of malignant pleural effusions: a network meta-analysis. *Cochrane Database Syst Rev*. 2016;(5):CD010529.
6. Redden MD, Chin TY, van Driel ML. Surgical versus non-surgical management for pleural empyema. *Cochrane Database Syst Rev*. 2017;(3):CD010651.

ADDITIONAL READING
Ryan H, Yoo J, Darsini P. Corticosteroids for tuberculous pleurisy. *Cochrane Database Syst Rev*. 2017;(3):CD001876.

CODES

ICD10
- J90 Pleural effusion, not elsewhere classified
- J91.0 Malignant pleural effusion
- J94.0 Chylous effusion

CLINICAL PEARLS
- Bilateral pleural effusion suggests heart failure, malignancy in absence of cardiomegaly, and TB or parasitic infection in children.
- Ascites and pleural effusion suggest hepatic hydrothorax, ovarian cancer, or Meigs syndrome.
- Consider diagnostic thoracentesis in patient with heart failure: fever, pleuritic chest pain, unilateral effusion or effusion of markedly disparate size, effusion not associated with cardiomegaly, effusion fails to respond to management of heart failure.
- CT-guided needle biopsy is useful when a pleural-based soft tissue abnormality is identified by CT scan.
- Clues to the diagnosis of tuberculous pleurisy include risk factor for TB exposure and a lymphocytic effusion, especially when pleural adenosine deaminase and interferon-γ are elevated.

PNEUMONIA, BACTERIAL

Naureen Rafiq, MBBS • Khalid Bashir, MD

BASICS

Bacterial pneumonia is an infection of the pulmonary parenchyma by a bacterial organism.

DESCRIPTION
Bacterial pneumonia can be classified as the following:
- Community-acquired pneumonia (CAP): lower respiratory tract infection not acquired in a hospital, long-term care facility, or during other recent contact with the health care system
- Medical care–associated pneumonia
  – Hospital-acquired pneumonia (HAP): pneumonia within ≥48 hours after admission and did not appear to be incubating at time of admission
  – Ventilator-associated pneumonia (VAP): pneumonia that develops >48 hours after endotracheal intubation
  – Health care–associated pneumonia (HCAP): Pneumonia that occurs in a nonhospitalized patient with extensive health care contact, such as the following:
    ○ IV therapy/wound care within past 30 days
    ○ Residing in a nursing home/long-term care
    ○ Hospitalization in an acute care hospital for ≥2 days within the past 90 days; hemodialysis clinic within the past 30 days

EPIDEMIOLOGY
- Influenza and pneumonia are the eighth leading causes of death in the United States with about 53,282 deaths in 2013.
- HAP is the leading cause of death among nosocomial infections and is one of the leading causes of death in the ICU.
- Rates of infection are 3 times higher in African Americans than in whites and are 5 to 10 times higher in Native American adults and 10 times higher in Native American children.
- Mortality rate in children is approximately 1.6 million a year. Hospitalization rate for children with CAP is still highest among the very young ages (<18 months). Respiratory viruses are the most commonly detected causes of pneumonia (1).

Incidence
- CAP: 5 to 11 cases per 1,000 persons with increased incidence occurring in the winter months
- HAP: 5 to 10 cases per 1,000 admissions; incidence increases 6- to 20-fold in ventilated patients (2)[A].

ETIOLOGY AND PATHOPHYSIOLOGY
- Adults, CAP
  – Typical (85%): *Streptococcus pneumoniae, Haemophilus influenzae, Staphylococcus aureus,* group A *Streptococcus, Moraxella catarrhalis*
  – Atypical (15%): *Legionella* sp., *Mycoplasma pneumoniae, Chlamydophila pneumoniae*
- Adults, HCAP/HAP/VAP
  – Aerobic gram-negative bacilli: *Pseudomonas aeruginosa, Escherichia coli, Klebsiella pneumoniae,* and *Acinetobacter* sp.
  – Gram-positive cocci: *Streptococcus* sp. and *S. aureus* (including MRSA)
- Children
  – Birth to 20 days: *E. coli,* group B streptococci, *Listeria monocytogenes*
  – 3 weeks to 3 months: *Chlamydia trachomatis, S. pneumoniae*
  – 4 months to 18 years
    ○ Typical: *S. pneumoniae*
    ○ Atypical: *C. pneumoniae, M. pneumoniae*

RISK FACTORS
CAP
- Age >65 years
- HIV/immunocompromised
- Recent antibiotic therapy/resistance to antibiotics
- Asthma, CAD, COPD, chronic renal failure, CHF, diabetes, liver disease, VAP, HAP, HCAP
- Hospitalization for ≥2 days during past 90 days
- Severe illness
- Antibiotic therapy in the past 6 months
- Poor functional status as defined by activities of daily living score
- Immunosuppression (including steroid users) (3)

GENERAL PREVENTION
- All children 2 to 59 months of age should be routinely vaccinated with pneumococcal conjugate (PCV13); given at 2, 4, and 6 months of age; a fourth dose at 12 to 15 months of age
- Adults ≥65 years who have not received vaccine naïve, ACIP currently recommends PCV13 followed by pneumococcal polysaccharide (PPSV23) ≥1 year interval. If they received PPSV23 vaccine before age 65 years, they should receive a dose of PCV13 followed by a subsequent PPSV23 ≥1 year after PCV13 and at least 5 years have passed since their previous PPSV23 dose.
- For adults ≥65 years old who have already received PPSV23, a dose of PCV13 is indicated after ≥1 year.
- Adults 19 to 64 years who have chronic diseases, including alcoholism and tobacco use, should receive PPSV23.
- Adults ≥19 years old with immunocompromising conditions, asplenia, CSF leaks, cochlear implants who have not received PPSV23 or PCV13 should receive 1 dose of PCV13 followed by PPSV23 after ≥8 weeks. If a second dose of PPSV23 is recommended, it should be given 5 years after first dose. Adults >19 years, previously given PPSV23 should receive a PPCV13 dose ≥1 year after last PPSV23. If additional PPSV23 is required, it should be given ≥8 weeks after PCV13 and 5 years after most recent dose of PPSV23.
- Annual influenza vaccine

DIAGNOSIS

HISTORY
- Fever, chills, rigors, malaise, fatigue
- Dyspnea
- Cough, with/without sputum
- Pleuritic chest pain
- Myalgias
- GI symptoms

ALERT
High fever (>104°F [40°C]), male sex, multilobar involvement, and GI and neurologic abnormalities have been associated with CAP caused by *Legionella*.

Geriatric Considerations
Older adults with pneumonia often present with weakness, mental status change, or history of falls.

PHYSICAL EXAM
- Fever >100.4°F (38°C), tachypnea, tachycardia
- Rales, rhonchi, egophony, increased fremitus, bronchial breath sounds, dullness to percussion, asymmetric breath sounds, abdominal tenderness

DIFFERENTIAL DIAGNOSIS
Bronchitis, asthma exacerbation, pulmonary edema, lung cancer, pulmonary tuberculosis, pneumonitis

DIAGNOSTIC TESTS & INTERPRETATION
Initial Tests (lab, imaging)
- Routine laboratory testing to establish an etiology in outpatients with CAP is usually unnecessary.
- For hospitalized patients with CAP, a CBC, sputum Gram stain, procalcitonin, and two sets of blood cultures
- More extensive diagnostic testing in patients with CAP is recommended if:
  – Blood cultures: ICU admission, cavitary infiltrates, leukopenia, alcohol abuse, severe liver disease, asplenia, positive pneumococcal urine antigen test (UAT), pleural effusion
  – Sputum Gram stain and cultures: ICU admission, failure of outpatient treatment, cavitary infiltrates, alcohol abuse, severe COPD/structural lung disease, positive *Legionella* UAT, positive pneumococcal UAT, pleural effusion
  – *Legionella* UAT: ICU admission, failure of outpatient treatment, alcohol abuse, travel in past 2 weeks, pleural effusion
  – Pneumococcal UAT: ICU admission, failure of outpatient treatment, leukopenia, alcohol abuse, severe liver disease, asplenia, pleural effusion
- A chest x-ray (CXR) is indicated when pneumonia is suspected or with an acute respiratory infection and
  – Vital signs: temperature >100°F (37.8°C); heart rate (HR) >100 beats/min; respiratory rate (RR) >20 breaths/min
  – At least two of the following clinical findings: decreased breath sounds, rales, no asthma
- Early in disease course, CXR may be negative.
- Evidence of necrotizing/cavitary pneumonia should raise suspicion for MRSA pneumonia, especially with history of prior MRSA skin lesions.

Diagnostic Procedures/Other
- For VAP/HAP: By bronchoscopic or nonbronchoscopic means, obtain a lower respiratory tract sample for culture prior to initiation/change of therapy. Serial evaluations may be needed (2)[A].
- Safe cessation of antibiotics can be done from a good quality negative sputum culture.

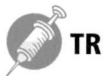

TREATMENT

MEDICATION
First Line
- Adults
  – CAP, outpatient
    ○ No significant differences in efficacy between antibiotic option in adults
    ○ Previously healthy, no antibiotics in past 3 months
      ■ Azithromycin 500 mg PO 1 time and then 250 mg PO daily for 4 days; or clarithromycin 500 mg PO BID for 10 days; or erythromycin 500 mg PO BID for 10 days; or
      ■ Doxycycline 100 mg PO BID for 10 days
    ○ Comorbid conditions, immunosuppressed, antibiotic use in past 3 months
      ■ Levofloxacin 750 mg PO daily for 5 days; or moxifloxacin 400 mg PO daily for 5 days; or
      ■ Amoxicillin 1 g PO TID; amoxicillin-clavulanate 2 g PO BID + macrolide/doxycycline for 5 days

- Treatment may be stopped if
  - Afebrile for >48 hours
  - Supplemental oxygen no longer needed
  - No more than one of the following:
    - HR >100 beats/min
    - RR >24 breaths/min
    - Systolic blood pressure (BP) ≤90 mm Hg
- CAP, inpatient (non-ICU)
  - IV antibiotics initially and then switch to PO after clinical improvement
  - Treatment duration depends on clinical improvement.
  - Cefotaxime; ceftriaxone; ampicillin-sulbactam + macrolide (clarithromycin; erythromycin) for 5 to 14 days or
  - Moxifloxacin; levofloxacin for 5 to 14 days
  - If *Pseudomonas* is a consideration
    - Piperacillin-tazobactam; cefepime; imipenem; meropenem + levofloxacin or
    - Piperacillin-tazobactam; cefepime; imipenem; meropenem + aminoglycoside and azithromycin or
    - Piperacillin-tazobactam; cefepime; imipenem; meropenem + aminoglycoside + levofloxacin
  - If MRSA is a consideration
- Add vancomycin or linezolid HCAP/HAP/VAP.
  - Use IV antibiotics.
  - Early onset (<5 days) and no risk factors for multidrug-resistant pathogens
    - Ceftriaxone; ampicillin-sulbactam; ertapenem or
    - Levofloxacin; moxifloxacin
  - Late onset (≥5 days) or risk factors for multidrug-resistant pathogens (antibiotic therapy in preceding 90 days; high frequency of antibiotic resistance in community/hospital; immunosuppressive disease/therapy; risk factors for HCAP)
    - MRSA coverage: linezolid or vancomycin + β-lactam cefepime; ceftazidime; imipenem; meropenem; piperacillin-tazobactam + either fluoroquinolone (levofloxacin) or aminoglycoside (amikacin; gentamicin; tobramycin) (level II)
    - Short-course versus prolonged-course antibiotic therapy for HAP in critically ill adults. For patients with VAP due to NF-GNB, a shorter antibiotic course may increase the risk of recurrence (4)[A].
    - Drug-resistant *S. pneumoniae* should be treated with high-dose amoxicillin, amoxicillin/clavulanate, cefpodoxime with a macrolide, or a respiratory fluoroquinolone.
- Adult IV antibiotic doses
  - β-Lactams (ampicillin-sulbactam 3 g q6h; aztreonam 2 g q6h; cefepime 1 to 2 g q8–12h; cefotaxime 1 g q6–8h; ceftazidime 2 g q8h; ceftriaxone 2 g daily; imipenem 500 mg q6h; meropenem 1 g IV q8h)
  - Aminoglycosides (amikacin 20 mg/kg daily; gentamicin 7 mg/kg daily; tobramycin 7 mg/kg daily)
  - Fluoroquinolones (levofloxacin 750 mg daily; moxifloxacin 400 mg daily)
  - Macrolides (azithromycin 500 mg daily; clarithromycin 500 mg daily; erythromycin 500 to 1,000 mg q6h)
  - Vancomycin 15 mg/kg q12h
  - Linezolid 600 mg q12h
  - Telavancin is an antibiotic, which covers MRSA infection. Telavancin is approved for the treatment of HAP and VAP caused by *S. aureus*. This medication is indicated only when alternative agents cannot be used.

- Pediatric, outpatient (≥3 months)
  - Antibiotic treatment in preschool-aged children is not routinely required because viral pathogens are more common (5)[A].
  - Oral antibiotics are as efficacious as IV in CAP (length of stay and oxygen requirement were reduced in those given oral antibiotics).
  - Typical bacterial pneumonia
    - Amoxicillin 90 mg/kg/day PO BID (max 4 g/day) (5)[A]
    - Amoxicillin-clavulanate 90 mg/kg/day PO BID (max 4 g/day) (5)[A]
    - Alternative: levofloxacin 16 to 20 mg/kg/day PO BID for children 6 months to 5 years, 10 mg/kg/day daily for children ≥5 years (max 750 mg/day) (5)[C]
  - Atypical bacterial pneumonia
    - Azithromycin 10 mg/kg PO on day 1 (max 500 mg) and then 5 mg/kg/day (max 250 mg) on days 2 to 5 (4)[C]
    - Clarithromycin 15 mg/kg/day PO BID (max 1 g/day) (4)[C]
    - Erythromycin 40 mg/kg/day PO daily (4)[C]

ADMISSION, INPATIENT, AND NURSING CONSIDERATIONS

- Clinical judgment and use of a validated severity of illness score are recommended to determine if inpatient management is indicated.
- The Pneumonia Severity Index (PSI) is a clinical prediction rule used to calculate the probability of morbidity and mortality among patients with CAP. PSI is risk stratified from I to V. PSI risk class from I to III can be treated as outpatients and IV to V should be hospitalized. PSI can be calculated at http://pda.ahrq.gov/clinic/psi/psicalc.asp.
- The CURB-65 or CRB 65 (confusion, urea nitrogen RR, BP, age >65 years) (http://www.mdcalc.com/curb-65 -severity-score-community-acquired-pneumonia/) is a severity of illness score for stratifying adults with CAP into different management groups.
- The SMART-COP (systolic BP, multilobar chest radiography, albumin, RR, tachycardia, confusion, oxygen level, and arterial pH) is a new method to predict, which patients will require intensive respiratory/vasopressor support. A score of ≥3 has sensitivity of 92% to identify those patients who will receive intensive treatment.
- Patients with COPD or CHF are more likely to require ICU admission when suffering from CAP.
- Clinical prediction tools do not replace a physician's clinical judgment.
- Other considerations
  - Analgesia and antipyretics
  - Chest physiotherapy
  - IV fluids (and conversely, diuretics) if indicated
  - Pulse oximetry
  - Oxygen supplementation
  - Positioning of the patient to minimize aspiration risk
  - Respiratory therapy
  - Suctioning and bronchial
  - Mechanical ventilatory support with low tidal volumes. Systemic support may include proper hydration and nutrition

Pediatric Considerations

- Inpatient treatment of children is recommended in the following settings: infants ≤3 to 6 months; presence of respiratory distress (tachypnea, dyspnea, retractions, grunting, nasal flaring, apnea, altered mental status, O_2 sat <90%); or if known to have CAP as result of a virulent pathogen such as community-associated MRSA should be hospitalized (6).

- Discharge criteria: clinical stability: temperature ≤100°F (37.8°C); HR ≤100 beats/min; RR ≤24 beats/min; systolic BP ≤90 mm Hg; O_2 sat ≥90% or PaO_2 ≥60 mm Hg on room air; ability to maintain oral intake; normal mental status

ONGOING CARE

FOLLOW-UP RECOMMENDATIONS
Patient Monitoring
Consider chest CT if patient is failing to improve on current management.

PATIENT EDUCATION
Smoking cessation, vaccinations

COMPLICATIONS
Necrotizing pneumonia, respiratory failure, empyema, abscesses, cavitation, bronchopleural fistula, sepsis

REFERENCES

1. Jain S, Williams DJ, Arnold SR, et al; and CDC EPIC Study Team. Community-acquired pneumonia requiring hospitalization among U.S. children. *N Engl J Med*. 2015;372(9):835–845.
2. File TM Jr. Recommendations for treatment of hospital-acquired and ventilator-associated pneumonia: review of recent international guidelines. *Clin Infect Dis*. 2010;51(Suppl 1):S42–S47.
3. Shindo Y, Ito R, Kobayashi D, et al. Risk factors for drug-resistant pathogens in community-acquired and healthcare-associated pneumonia. *Am J Respir Crit Care Med*. 2013;188(8):985–995.
4. Pugh R, Grant C, Cooke RP, et al. Short-course versus prolonged-course antibiotic therapy for hospital-acquired pneumonia in critically ill adults. *Cochrane Database Syst Rev*. 2015;(8):CD007577.
5. Bradley JS, Byington CL, Shah SS, et al. The management of community-acquired pneumonia in infants and children older than 3 months of age: clinical practice guidelines by the Pediatric Infectious Diseases Society and the Infectious Diseases Society of America. *Clin Infect Dis*. 2011;53(7):e25–e76.
6. Devitt M. PIDS and IDSA issue management guidelines for community-acquired pneumonia in infants and young children. *Am Fam Physician*. 2012;86(2):196–202.

CODES

ICD10
- J15.9 Unspecified bacterial pneumonia
- J15.4 Pneumonia due to other streptococci
- J14 Pneumonia due to Hemophilus influenzae

CLINICAL PEARLS

- Bacterial pneumonia can usually be treated empirically based on its classification as CAP or HCAP/HAP/VAP.
- A severity of illness score is helpful in determining the need for hospitalization of adult patients but does not replace a physician's clinical judgment.

PNEUMONIA, MYCOPLASMA

Kenneth A. Ballou, MD, FAAFP • Andrew G. Alexander, MD • Maegen Dupper, MD

 BASICS

DESCRIPTION
- Bronchopulmonary infection caused by the *Mycoplasma* species, *Mycoplasma pneumoniae*
- Smallest free-living organism; fastidious and slow-growing; first isolated in cattle in 1898
- Most frequently affects children/young adults but can also occur in the elderly; often causes epidemics in close communities (i.e., skilled nursing facilities)
- Infection may be asymptomatic, most often confined to the upper respiratory tract; however, may progress to pneumonia (5–10%)
- Course is usually acute with an incubation period of 1 to 4 weeks.
- Synonym(s): primary atypical pneumonia (PAP); Eaton agent pneumonia; cold agglutinin–positive pneumonia; walking pneumonia

Geriatric Considerations
The highest rate of ICU admissions for community-acquired pneumonia (CAP) due to *M. pneumoniae* occurs in seniors.

Pediatric Considerations
- Plays a significant role in pneumonias in children of all ages (Pneumonia <5 years, however, is more commonly viral.)
- Increased incidence of asthma exacerbation in older children (1)[A]
- Infants 3 to 6 months with suspected bacterial pneumonia should be hospitalized.

EPIDEMIOLOGY
Incidence
- Estimated 1 million cases per year in the United States
- Responsible for 20% of CAP requiring hospitalizations annually
- Infection occurs most frequently in fall/winter seasons but may develop year round.

Prevalence
- Predominant sex: male = female
- Predominant age group affected: 5 to 20 years
  – May occur at any age
  – Rare in children <5 years of age
- Responsible for up to 15–20% of all cases of CAP yearly
  – Most common cause of pneumonia in school children and young adults who do not have a chronic underlying condition

ETIOLOGY AND PATHOPHYSIOLOGY
- *M. pneumoniae* is a short-rod mucosal pathogen, which lacks a cell wall and thus not visible on Gram stain.
- Can grow under both aerobic and anaerobic conditions
- Highly contagious, *M. pneumoniae* is transmitted primarily by aerosol droplets.
- Pathogenicity linked to its filamentous tips, which adhere selectively to respiratory epithelial cell membrane proteins with production of H_2O_2 and superoxide radicals, damaging cilia
- Many pathogenic features of infection are believed to be immune mediated, not directly induced.
- Decreased ciliary movement produces prolonged paroxysmal, hacking cough.
- Incubation period is 2 to 3 weeks.

RISK FACTORS
- Immunocompromised state (e.g., HIV, transplant recipients, chemotherapy)
- Smoking
- Close community living (e.g., military barracks, prisons, hospitals, dormitories, schools, household contacts, skilled nursing facilities)

GENERAL PREVENTION
Consider droplet isolation of active cases.

COMMONLY ASSOCIATED CONDITIONS
- Asthma exacerbations as a result of proinflammatory cytokine release (1)[A]
- Chronic obstructive pulmonary disease

 DIAGNOSIS

HISTORY
- Infection may be asymptomatic.
- Gradual onset of headache, malaise, low-grade fevers, chills
- Symptoms of upper respiratory infection, including incessant, nonproductive, worsening cough (which may become mildly productive late in the disease); rhinorrhea, pharyngitis, and sinusitis occur subsequently (2).
- Pneumonia may occur with associated pleural effusion.
- The presence of pleuritic chest pain warrants a higher suspicion of *M. pneumoniae* (2).
- Extrapulmonary findings may develop in 5–10% of patients, including arthralgias, skin rashes, cervical adenopathy, hemolysis, congestive heart failure (CHF), and cardiac conduction abnormalities.
- Neurologic symptoms develop more commonly in children and may include encephalitis, aseptic meningitis, cranial nerve palsies, cerebellar ataxia, ascending paralysis, and coma (3).
- Persistent cough is common during convalescence; other sequelae are rare.

PHYSICAL EXAM
- Toxicity increases with advancing age or comorbidity.
- Hacking/pertussis-like cough may be present along with fever and lassitude.
- Normal lung findings with early infection, but rhonchi, rales, and/or wheezes may develop several days later (2)
- Mild pharyngeal injection without exudates
- Minimal/no cervical adenopathy
- Erythematous tympanic membranes or bullous myringitis in patients >2 years of age is an uncommon but unique sign.
- Some patients may develop a pleural friction rub.
- Various exanthems, including erythema multiforme and Stevens-Johnson syndrome

DIFFERENTIAL DIAGNOSIS
- Viral/bacterial/fungal pneumonia
- Tuberculosis
- Other atypical pneumonias, including *Chlamydia pneumoniae*, *Chlamydophila psittaci*, *Coxiella burnetii* (Q fever), *Francisella tularensis* (tularemia), *Pneumocystis jiroveci*, *Legionella pneumophila*

DIAGNOSTIC TESTS & INTERPRETATION
- *M. pneumoniae* is typically a clinical diagnosis and treated empirically; however, when specific pathogen testing is indicated, polymerase chain reaction (PCR) is the test of choice (4)[C].
- No clinical or radiographic findings can differentiate between *M. pneumoniae* and other atypical pneumonia pathogens (*Chlamydia/Legionella*).

Initial Tests (lab, imaging)
- WBC count may be normal or elevated.
- Hemolytic anemia has been described but is rare.
- Elevated erythrocyte sedimentation rate (ESR) may be present but is nonspecific.
- When available, PCR for *M. pneumoniae* DNA in nasopharyngeal and throat swabs as well as bronchoalveolar lavage respiratory secretions, CSF, and tissue samples may be the most sensitive and specific.
- CXR shows reticulonodular pattern with patchy areas of lower lobe consolidation, although this is not specific. Small pleural effusion may be present in 10–15% cases.

Follow-Up Tests & Special Considerations
- Sputum Gram stains are not helpful because *M. pneumoniae* lacks a cell wall and cannot be stained.
- *M. pneumoniae* is difficult to culture and requires 7 to 21 days to grow; culturing is successful in 40–90% of cases but does not provide information to guide treatment, thus infrequently performed.
- Complement fixation serologic assay shows 4-fold rise in IgM antibody titer at 2 to 4 weeks after symptom onset; this is an older technique.
- Positive cold agglutinins (titer of ≥1:128 or rising 4-fold) in 50% of infections but can take 1 to 2 weeks to develop; not sensitive/specific; not routinely recommended
- CT of chest may show a combination of patchy tree-in-bud opacities with segmental ground glass opacities.

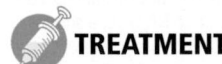 **TREATMENT**

GENERAL MEASURES
- Avoid sick contacts.
- Treatment is usually empiric and must be comprehensive to cover all likely pathogens in the context of the clinical setting.
- Calculation of pneumonia severity score (CAP score: http://www.mdcalc.com/psi-port-score-pneumonia-severity-index-adult-cap) may be helpful in determining inpatient versus outpatient treatment.

Pregnancy Considerations
- Azithromycin: pregnancy Category B (preferred treatment)
- Clarithromycin, levofloxacin, and moxifloxacin: pregnancy Category C

MEDICATION

First Line

- Azithromycin
  - <3 months of age: not established (5)[B]
  - >3 months of age: day 1, 10 mg/kg PO × 1 (not to exceed 500 mg); days 2 to 5: 5 mg/kg PO daily (not to exceed 250 mg/day)
  - Adults: 500 mg PO × 1 followed by 250 mg PO daily × 4 days
- Doxycycline
  - Children <8 years of age: not recommended
  - Children >8 years of age (≤45 kg): 2 to 4 mg/kg/day up to 200 mg/day PO divided BID for 10 to 14 days
  - Children >8 years of age (≥45 kg): Refer to adult dosing.
  - Adults: 100 mg PO BID × 7 to 14 days
  - Useful in macrolide-resistant strains of *M. pneumoniae*
- Clarithromycin
  - Children <6 months of age: not established
  - Patients >6 months of age: 15 mg/kg/day PO divided q12h for 10 to 14 days
  - Adults: 250 to 500 mg PO BID for 10 to 14 days
- Minocycline
  - 200 mg PO/IV × 1 dose and then 100 mg BID for 7 to 10 days
- Erythromycin
  - Children: 20 to 50 mg/kg/day (base) PO divided q6–8h for 10 to 14 days
  - Adults: 500 mg (base) PO q6h × 10 to 14 days

Second Line

- Levofloxacin
  - Children <18 years of age: not recommended
  - Adults: 750 mg PO daily × 5 days
- Moxifloxacin
  - Children <18 years of age: not recommended
  - Adults: 400 mg/day PO for 7 to 10 days
- Levofloxacin and moxifloxacin show good activity against *M. pneumoniae*. Consider use with comorbid conditions and other pneumonia pathogens; also useful if macrolide resistance is suspected

ADDITIONAL THERAPIES

- Albuterol inhaler: 2 puffs q4–6h as needed for wheezing
- Dexamethasone may downregulate cytokine release (6)[B].
- Acetaminophen/ibuprofen as needed for fever
- Up to 10.9% of hospitalized patients may require mechanical ventilation.
- Plasmapheresis in cases of severe hemolytic anemia

ADMISSION, INPATIENT, AND NURSING CONSIDERATIONS

- CAP score risk class IV/V
- Other scoring systems such as the CURB65 and Pneumonia Severity Index (PSI) may also be helpful in the inpatient versus outpatient treatment decision (6)[A].
- Advanced age with comorbidities
- Complicating neoplastic disease
- Significant cerebrovascular, cardiac, renal, liver, or GI symptoms
- Altered mental status
- Inability to maintain oxygen saturation
- Tachycardia/tachypnea
- Hypotension
- Neurologic symptoms
- Signs of Stevens-Johnson syndrome
- Significant hemolysis (autoimmune hemolytic anemia, cold agglutinin disease)

- Change from IV to PO antibiotic may be made when:
  - Respiratory distress and hypoxia have resolved.
  - Patients are tolerating oral hydration.
  - No significant complications are present.
  - Utilization of procalcitonin (PCT) may aid in this decision (4)[A].
- Generally, no need for 24-hour observation on PO antibiotics prior to discharge.

 ## ONGOING CARE

FOLLOW-UP RECOMMENDATIONS

- Clearing of condition on CXR should be documented in patients >50 years of age.
- In smokers, document a clear CXR in 6 to 8 weeks.
- Worsening symptoms/development of rash or meningeal/neurologic signs should prompt immediate presentation to medical attention.
- Antibiotic prophylaxis for exposed contacts is not routinely recommended.
- For household contacts who may be predisposed to severe mycoplasmal infection, macrolide or doxycycline prophylaxis should be used.

DIET

- No special diet considerations
- Ensure adequate hydration.

PATIENT EDUCATION

- Smoking cessation
- Contact and droplet precautions
- Adequate hand washing techniques

PROGNOSIS

- Symptoms usually resolve in 2 weeks.
- Some constitutional symptoms may persist for several weeks.
- With correct therapy, even most severe cases can expect complete recovery.

COMPLICATIONS

- All complications are rare, except reactive airway disease, hemolytic anemia, and erythema multiforme.
- Reactive airway disease may persist indefinitely and can cause acute chest syndrome in patients with sickle cell anemia.
- Meningoencephalitis
- Aseptic meningitis
- Peripheral neuropathy
- Transverse myelitis/acute transverse myelitis
- Cerebellar ataxia
- Acute disseminated encephalomyelitis
- Guillain-Barré syndrome
- Encephalitis (especially in children)
- Polyneuritis/polyarthritis
- Stevens-Johnson syndrome
- Pericarditis/myocarditis
- Respiratory distress syndrome
- Cerebral ataxia
- Thromboembolic phenomena
- Pleural effusion
- Nephritis
- Occasional deaths occur primarily among the elderly and persons with sickle cell disease.

REFERENCES

1. Gao S, Wang L, Zhu W, et al. Mycoplasma pneumonia infection and asthma: a clinical study. *Pak J Med Sci*. 2015;31(3):548–551.
2. Marchello C, Dale AP, Thai TN, et al. Prevalence of atypical pathogens in patients with cough and community-acquired pneumonia: a meta-analysis. *Ann Fam Med*. 2016;14(6):552–566.
3. Wang K, Gill P, Perera R, et al. Clinical symptoms and signs for the diagnosis of *Mycoplasma pneumoniae* in children and adolescents with community-acquired pneumonia. *Cochrane Database Syst Rev*. 2012;(10):CD009175.
4. Sager R, Kutz A, Mueller B, et al. Procalcitonin-guided diagnosis and antibiotic stewardship revisited. *BMC Med*. 2017;15(1):15.
5. Gardiner S, Gavranich J, Chang A. Antibiotics for community-acquired lower respiratory tract infections secondary to *Mycoplasma pneumoniae* in children. *Cochrane Database Syst Rev*. 2015;(1):CD004875.
6. Sharma L, Losier A, Tolbert T, et al. Atypical pneumonia: updates on *Legionella*, *Chlamydophila*, and *Mycoplasma* pneumonia. *Clin Chest Med*. 2017;38(1):45–58.

ADDITIONAL READING

- Atkinson TP, Balish MF, Waites KB. Epidemiology, clinical manifestations, pathogenesis and laboratory detection of *Mycoplasma pneumoniae* infections. *FEMS Microbiol Rev*. 2008;32(6):956–973.
- Eliakim-Raz N, Robenshtok E, Shefet D, et al. Empiric antibiotic coverage of atypical pathogens for community-acquired pneumonia in hospitalized adults. *Cochrane Database Syst Rev*. 2012;(9):CD004418.
- Kashyap S, Sarkar M. *Mycoplasma pneumonia*: clinical features and management. *Lung India*. 2010;27(2):75–85.
- Kaysin A, Viera A. Community-acquired pneumonia in adults: diagnosis and management. *Am Fam Physician*. 2016;94(9):698–706.
- Khoury T, Sviri S, Rmeileh AA, et al. Increased rates of intensive care unit admission in patients with *Mycoplasma pneumoniae*: a retrospective study. *Clin Microbiol Infect*. 2016;22(8):711–714.
- Stuckey-Schrock K, Hayes B, George C. Community-acquired pneumonia in children. *Am Fam Physician*. 2012;86(7):661–667.
- Waites KB, Xiao L, Liu Y, et al. *Mycoplasma pneumoniae* from the respiratory tract and beyond. *Clin Microbiol Rev*. 2017;30(3):747–809.

 ## CODES

ICD10

J15.7 Pneumonia due to Mycoplasma pneumoniae

CLINICAL PEARLS

- Most common atypical respiratory pathogens include *M. pneumoniae*, *C. pneumoniae*, and *L. pneumophila*.
- Atypical pneumonia is usually a clinical diagnosis.
- Watch closely for complicating symptoms that could indicate worsening disease.
- Atypical pneumonia with *M. pneumoniae* usually responds to empiric treatment.
- Outbreaks of *M. pneumoniae* can be seen in close communities (i.e., dormitories).
- Presentation of infection is typically a gradual onset of symptoms.

PNEUMONIA, PNEUMOCYSTIS JIROVECI

Thomas J. Hansen, MD, FAAFP

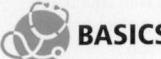 **BASICS**

DESCRIPTION
- *Pneumocystis jiroveci* causes pneumonia primarily in immunocompromised patients.
- The fungus that causes this pneumonia in humans was previously called *Pneumocystis carinii*.
- The name was formally changed to *Pneumocystis jiroveci* in 2001, following the discovery that the fungus that infects humans is unique and distinctive from the fungus that infects animals.
- *P. jiroveci* is extremely resistant to traditional antifungal agents, including both amphotericin and azole agents.
- To prevent confusion, the term PCP, which used to represent *P. carinii* pneumonia, now represents *Pneumocystis* pneumonia (1).

ALERT
No combination of symptoms, signs, blood chemistries, or radiographic findings is diagnostic of *P. jiroveci* pneumonia (2).

EPIDEMIOLOGY
- *P. jiroveci* has a worldwide distribution, and most children have been exposed to the fungus by 2 to 4 years (3).
- The reservoir and mode of transmission for *P. jiroveci* is still unclear.
  - Human studies favor an airborne transmission model, with person-to-person spread being the most likely mode of infection acquisition (2).

Incidence
- Infants with HIV infection have a peak incidence of PCP between 2 and 6 months (3).
- HIV-infected infants have a high mortality rate, with a median survival of only 1 month.

Prevalence
- The prevalence of *P. jiroveci* colonization among healthy adults is 0–20%.
- Recent studies have demonstrated the transient nature of *P. jiroveci* colonization in asymptomatic, immunocompetent patients (2).
- 50% of patients with PCP are coinfected with ≥2 strains of *P. jiroveci* (3).
- There is evidence that distinct strains are responsible for each episode in patients who develop multiple episodes of PCP (3).

ETIOLOGY AND PATHOPHYSIOLOGY
Mode of transmission is unknown; likely respiratory from infected host

RISK FACTORS
Individuals at risk (2)
- Patients with HIV infection, especially if not receiving prophylactic treatment for PCP
- Patients who are receiving high doses of glucocorticoids
- Patients who have an altered immune system not due to HIV
- Patients who are receiving chronic immunosuppressive medications
- Patients who have hematologic or solid malignancies resulting in malignancy-related immune depression

GENERAL PREVENTION
- Indications for prophylaxis
  - HIV-infected adults (3)
    - Should start when CD4 count is <200 cells/μL or if the patient develops oropharyngeal candidiasis
  - HIV-infected children (3)
    - Prophylaxis should be provided for children ≥6 years based on adult guidelines.
    - For children aged 1 to 5 years, start when CD4 count is <500 cells/μL.
    - For infants <12 months, start when the CD4 percentage is <15%.
  - Non–HIV-infected adults receiving immunosuppressive medications or with underlying immune system deficits should receive PCP prophylaxis, but currently, there are no specific guidelines on when to start this.
- Medication
  - Trimethoprim-sulfamethoxazole (TMP-SMX)
    - Adults: 1 double-strength tablet daily or 1 double-strength tablet 3 times per week
    - Children >2 months: TMP 150 mg/kg/day in divided doses q12h for 3 days/week
  - Atovaquone suspension
    - Adults: 1,500 mg PO once daily with food
    - Children: not to exceed 1,500 mg/day
      - 1 to 3 months: 30 mg/kg/day PO once daily
      - 4 to 24 months: 45 mg/kg/day PO once daily
      - >24 months: 30 mg/kg/day PO once daily
      - Adolescents ≥13 years: Refer to adult dosing.
  - Dapsone
    - Adults only: 50 mg BID or 100 mg once daily
  - Pentamidine
    - Adults only: 300 mg aerosolized every 4 weeks
- Discontinuation of prophylaxis
  - When CD4+ cell counts are >200 cells/μL for a period of 3 months in the adult population
  - There are no clear guidelines for discontinuation of prophylaxis in children.

COMMONLY ASSOCIATED CONDITIONS
- HIV Infection
- Chronic obstructive pulmonary disease (COPD)
- Interstitial lung disease
- Connective tissue diseases treated with corticosteroids
- Cancer and organ transplant patients on immunosuppressive medication

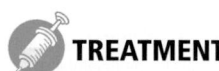 **DIAGNOSIS**

HISTORY
- HIV-infected patients
  - Subacute onset over several weeks
    - Progressively worsening dyspnea
    - Tachypnea
    - Cough: nonproductive or productive of clear sputum
    - Low-grade fever, chills
    - Weakness, fatigue, malaise
- Non–HIV-infected immunocompromised patients
  - More acute onset with fulminant respiratory failure
    - Abrupt tachypnea, dyspnea
    - Fever
    - Dry cough

PHYSICAL EXAM
- Fever
- Tachypnea
- Tachycardia
- Lung exam is normal or near normal.

DIFFERENTIAL DIAGNOSIS
- Tuberculosis
- Bacterial pneumonia
- Fungal pneumonia
- Viral pneumonia

DIAGNOSTIC TESTS & INTERPRETATION
P. jiroveci cannot be cultured. Therefore, a diagnosis relies on detection of the organism by colorimetric or immunofluorescent stains or by polymerase chain reaction (PCR) (3)[C].
- ABG: reveals hypoxemia and increased alveolar–arterial gradient that varies with severity of disease
- LDH: Serum lactate dehydrogenase is frequently increased (nonspecific; likely due to underlying lung inflammation and injury)
- CD4 cell count is generally <200 cells/μL in HIV-infected patients with PCP.
- S-adenosylmethionine levels are significantly lower in a patient with PCP. The levels increase with successful treatment (4)[B].
- Comprehensive metabolic profile
- Chest x-ray (CXR) (2)[C]
  - Bilateral, symmetric, fine, reticular interstitial infiltrates involving perihilar areas; becomes more homogeneous and diffuse as severity of infection progresses
  - Less common patterns include upper lobe involvement in patients receiving aerosolized pentamidine, solitary or multiple nodular opacities, lobar infiltrates, pneumatoceles, and pneumothoraces.
  - May be normal in up to 30% of patients with PCP (1)[C]
- High-resolution CT is more sensitive than CXR.

Diagnostic Procedures/Other
- Fiberoptic bronchoscopy with bronchoalveolar lavage (BAL) is the preferred diagnostic procedure to obtain samples for direct fluorescent antibody staining.
  - Sensitivities range from 89% to >98%.
- *Pneumocystis* trophic forms or cysts obtained from induced sputum, BAL fluid, or lung tissue, which can be visualized using conventional stains
- PCR can detect *Pneumocystis* from respiratory sources, but the potential remains for false positives (2)[C].

TREATMENT

The recommended duration of therapy differs in patients who are with/without AIDS:
- In patients with PCP who do not have AIDS, the typical duration of therapy is 14 days.
- Treatment of PCP in patients who have AIDS was increased to 21 days due to the risk for relapse after only 14 days of treatment (2)[C].

MEDICATION

- TMP-SMX (2)[C]
- Adult dosing
  - TMP: 15 to 20 mg/kg/day, PO or IV, divided into 4 doses
- Pediatric dosing (>2 months) (2)[C]
  - TMP: 15 to 20 mg/kg/day in divided doses q6–8h
- Reduce doses of TMP-SMX in patients with renal failure.
- Patients should receive 21 days of therapy.
- Treatment response to *Pneumocystis* therapy often requires at least 7 to 10 days before clinical improvement is documented.
- Pregnancy risk factor: category C (2)[C]
- Precautions
  - History of sulfa allergy
  - There is an emergence of drug-resistant PCP, especially against TMP-SMX.

Second Line

- Pentamidine (for moderate to severe cases)
  - Adults and children: 4 mg/kg IV or IM once daily
- Dapsone + trimethoprim (adults only)
  - Dapsone 100 mg PO once daily, *plus*
  - Trimethoprim 5 mg/kg PO TID
    - ○ Check the glucose-6-phosphate dehydrogenase level before beginning dapsone because hemolysis may result.
- Clindamycin + primaquine (adults only)
  - Clindamycin 600 to 900 mg IV q8h or 300 to 450 mg PO QID, *plus*
  - Primaquine 30 mg PO once daily
- Atovaquone
  - Adults: 750 mg PO BID (>13 years of age)
  - Children: 40 mg/kg/day PO divided BID (max 1,500 mg)
- Note: Pentamidine has greater toxicity than TMP-SMX: hypotension, hypoglycemia, pancreatitis (2)[C].

ADDITIONAL THERAPIES

Adjunctive corticosteroid (prednisone or methylprednisolone) (2)[C],(5)[A]

- Adjunctive corticosteroids are shown to provide benefits in patients who have HIV and symptoms of moderate to severe PCP.
- Corticosteroids provide the greatest benefit to HIV patients who have hypoxemia manifested as a partial pressure of arterial oxygen <70 mm Hg or an alveolar–arterial gradient >35 mm Hg on room air.
- Adults and children >13 years of age: prednisone, 40 mg PO BID on days 1 to 5; 40 mg daily on days 6 to 11; 20 mg daily on days 12 to 21

ADMISSION, INPATIENT, AND NURSING CONSIDERATIONS

- No set criteria for hospital admission
- Five predictors of mortality in HIV-associated *Pneumocystis* pneumonia (6)
  - Increased age of the patient
  - Recent IV drug use
  - Total bilirubin >0.6 mg/dL
  - Serum albumin <3 g/dL
  - Alveolar–arterial oxygen gradient ≥50 mm Hg (6)[C]

ONGOING CARE

FOLLOW-UP RECOMMENDATIONS

In patients with HIV/AIDS: Patients with previous episodes of PCP should receive lifelong secondary prophylaxis unless they respond well to highly active antiretroviral therapy (HAART) and have a CD4 count >200 cells/μL for at least 3 months.

Patient Monitoring

Serum lactate dehydrogenase levels, pulmonary function test results, and ABG measurements generally normalize with treatment.

DIET

No special diet needed

PATIENT EDUCATION

- Centers for Disease Control and Prevention: https://www.cdc.gov/dpdx/pneumocystis/index.html
- FamilyDoctor.org: http://familydoctor.org/familydoctor/en/diseases-conditions/hiv-and-aids/complications/pneumocystis-pneumonia-pcp-and-hiv.html

REFERENCES

1. D'Avignon LC, Schofield CM, Hospenthal DR. *Pneumocystis* pneumonia. *Semin Respir Crit Care Med*. 2008;29(2):132–140.
2. Krajicek BJ, Thomas CF Jr, Limper AH. *Pneumocystis* pneumonia: current concepts in pathogenesis, diagnosis, and treatment. *Clin Chest Med*. 2009;30(2):265–278.
3. Kovacs JA, Masur H. Evolving health effects of *Pneumocystis*: one hundred years of progress in diagnosis and treatment. *JAMA*. 2009;301(24):2578–2585.
4. Skelly MJ, Holzman RS, Merali S. S-adenosylmethionine levels in the diagnosis of *Pneumocystis carinii* pneumonia in patients with HIV infection. *Clin Infect Dis*. 2008;46(3):467–471.
5. Briel M, Bucher HC, Boscacci R, et al. Adjunctive corticosteroids for *Pneumocystis jiroveci* pneumonia in patients with HIV-infection. *Cochrane Database Syst Rev*. 2006;(3):CD006150.
6. Fei MW, Kim EJ, Sant CA, et al. Predicting mortality from HIV-associated *Pneumocystis* pneumonia at illness presentation: an observational cohort study. *Thorax*. 2009;64(12):1070–1076.

ADDITIONAL READING

- Benson CA, Kaplan JE, Masur H, et al; for the National Institutes of Health, Infectious Diseases Society of America. Treating opportunistic infections among HIV-infected adults and adolescents: recommendations from CDC, the National Institutes of Health, and the HIV Medicine Association/Infectious Diseases Society of America. *MMWR Recomm Rep*. 2004;53(RR-15):1–112.
- Catherinot E, Lanternier F, Bougnoux ME, et al. *Pneumocystis jirovecii* pneumonia. *Infect Dis Clin North Am*. 2010;24(1):107–138.

- Green H, Paul M, Vidal L, et al. Prophylaxis for *Pneumocystis* pneumonia (PCP) in non-HIV immunocompromised patients. *Cochrane Database Syst Rev*. 2007;(3):CD005590.
- Kaplan JE, Masur H, Holmes KK. Guidelines for preventing opportunistic infections among HIV-infected persons—2002. Recommendations of the U.S. Public Health Service and the Infectious Diseases Society of America. http://www.cdc.gov/mmwr/preview/mmwrhtml/rr5108a1.htm. Accessed October 3, 2016.
- Limper AH, Knox KS, Sarosi GA, et al; for American Thoracic Society Fungal Working Group. An official American Thoracic Society statement: treatment of fungal infections in adult pulmonary and critical care patients. *Am J Respir Crit Care Med*. 2011;183(1):96–128.
- Shankar SM, Nania JJ. Management of *Pneumocystis jiroveci* pneumonia in children receiving chemotherapy. *Paediatr Drugs*. 2007;9(5):301–309.
- Stringer JR, Beard CB, Miller RF, et al. A new name for *Pneumocystis* from humans and new perspectives on the host-pathogen relationship. *Emerg Infect Dis*. 2002;8(9):891–896.

 SEE ALSO

HIV/AIDS

 CODES

ICD10
B59 Pneumocystosis

CLINICAL PEARLS

- Colonization with *P. jiroveci* is common in the pediatric population.
- PCP only occurs in immunocompromised patients.
- Patients with HIV are at risk once their CD4 count is <200 cells/μL. At that time, TMP-SMX should be initiated as prophylaxis. Prophylaxis may end after HAART has been initiated and the CD4 count is >200 cells/μL for 3 months.
- Patients who are immunocompromised are also at risk. Currently, no clear clinical guidelines are available as to when to initiate or end prophylaxis.
- The first-line treatment is TMP-SMX. The typical duration of therapy is 14 days in non–HIV-infected patients and 21 days in HIV-infected patients.

POLYARTERITIS NODOSA

Katherine S. Upchurch, MD, MACR • Stephen Morais, MD, MBA, MS

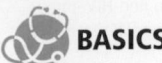
BASICS

DESCRIPTION
- Polyarteritis nodosa (PAN) is an antineutrophil cytoplasmic antibody (ANCA)-negative necrotizing arteritis of medium-sized muscular arteries and (occasionally) small arteries. Arterioles, capillaries, and venules are spared (1).
- Involved systems include gastrointestinal (GI) tract, peripheral nervous system (sensory and motor), CNS, genitourinary, skin, and cardiovascular. Glomerulonephritis and pulmonary capillaritis are rare (1,2).
- Features depend on location of vasculitis: for example, mesenteric ischemia–related symptoms, new onset or worsening hypertension (HTN), mononeuritis multiplex, purpuric or nodular skin lesions, or livedo reticularis (2)
- Renal disease in PAN usually manifests as HTN and mild proteinuria with/without azotemia. Renal infarction may also occur (2).
- PAN formerly encompassed several distinct entities (classic PAN, microscopic PAN, and cutaneous PAN). With ANCA testing, microscopic PAN appears pathophysiologically unrelated to the other two.
  - Idiopathic generalized PAN (classic PAN) is clinically variable, ranging from single organ involvement to polyvisceral failure (1).
  - HBV-associated PAN patients are positive for active hepatitis B infection and can present in similar fashion to idiopathic generalized PAN (1).
  - Microscopic PAN has ANCAs directed against myeloperoxidase (MPO) and involvement of small arterioles (microscopic polyangiitis [MPA]). This is now classified as ANCA-associated vasculitis.
  - Cutaneous (or limited) PAN is generally limited to the deep dermal and subcutaneous (SC) levels of the skin with characteristic histopathologic features of PAN. There are few systemic manifestations, although myalgias and peripheral motor neuropathy (mononeuritis multiplex) or sensory neuropathy may be present (2,3).
- Synonym(s): periarteritis; panarteritis; necrotizing arteritis

EPIDEMIOLOGY
Incidence
- Predominant age: peaks in 5th to 6th decade; incidence rises with age.
- Mean age at diagnosis is 50 years (3).
- 1.5:1 male predominance

Prevalence
Rare: 2 to 33 cases per 1 million adults (3)

ETIOLOGY AND PATHOPHYSIOLOGY
- Segmental, transmural, necrotizing inflammation of medium and small muscular arteries, with intimal proliferation, thrombosis, and ischemia of the end-organ/tissue supplied by the affected vessels; aneurysm formation at vessel bifurcations (2)
- Hepatitis B–related PAN results in direct vessel injury due to viral replication or deposition of immune complexes, with complement activation and subsequent inflammatory response (2).
- Most cases are idiopathic; 20% are related to hepatitis B or C infection.
- In patients with PAN and hepatitis B, HBsAg has been recovered from involved vessel walls.

Genetics
Mutations of adenosine deaminase 2 (ADA 2) have been identified in families with PAN (1).

RISK FACTORS
Hepatitis B > hepatitis C infection (cutaneous PAN)

COMMONLY ASSOCIATED CONDITIONS
- Hepatitis B (strong association with classic PAN)
- Hepatitis C (less strongly linked to cutaneous PAN)
- Hairy cell leukemia
- 27 cases of systemic PAN following hepatitis B vaccination
- Minocycline (Symptoms resolve on stopping drug, reoccur if rechallenged.)
- Case-based associations with CMV infection, amphetamines, and interferon

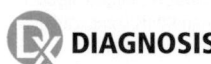
DIAGNOSIS

- There are no formal diagnostic criteria for PAN (1,2).
- Suspect PAN with:
  - Acute, sometimes fulminant multisystem disease with a relatively short prodrome (i.e., weeks to months)
  - Vasculitic skin rash with sensorimotor symptoms/findings
  - Recent-onset HTN with systemic symptoms
  - Unexplained sensory and/or motor neuropathy with systemic symptoms
  - Hepatitis B infection with multisystem disease

HISTORY
Symptoms reflect specific organ involvement (2).
- Constitutional symptoms (fever, weight loss, malaise)
- Organ-specific symptoms
  - Focal muscular weakness/extremity numbness
  - Myalgia and arthralgia
  - Rash
  - Recurrent postprandial pain, intestinal angina, nausea, vomiting, and bleeding
  - Altered mental status, headaches, mononeuritis multiplex
  - Testicular/epididymal pain, neurogenic bladder (rare)

PHYSICAL EXAM
Findings/course reflect specific organ involvement (2).
- Peripheral nervous system: peripheral neuropathy
- Renal: HTN
- Skin: purpura, urticaria, polymorphic rashes, SC nodules (uncommon but characteristic), livedo reticularis; deep skin ulcers, especially in lower extremities; Raynaud phenomenon (rare); single digit gangrene (rare)
- GI: acute abdomen; rebound, guarding, tenderness
- CNS: seizures, altered mental status, papillitis
- Lung: signs of pleural effusion—dullness to percussion; decreased breath sounds
- Cardiac: signs of congestive heart failure and/or myocardial infarction—S_3 gallop; pericarditis (Friction rub is rare.)
- Genitourinary: testicular/epididymal tenderness (can mimic testicular torsion)
- Musculoskeletal: arthritis (usually large joint in lower extremities)

DIFFERENTIAL DIAGNOSIS
- Other forms of vasculitis (ANCA-associated, such as granulomatosis with polyangiitis [GPA—formerly Wegener granulomatosis], Churg-Strauss syndrome, and MPA; Henoch-Schönlein purpura, drug-induced vasculitis, cryoglobulinemia, Goodpasture syndrome)
- Buerger disease
- Systemic lupus erythematosus (SLE)
- Embolic disease (atrial myxoma, cholesterol emboli)
- Thrombotic disease (antiphospholipid antibody syndrome)
- Dissecting aneurysm
- Ehlers-Danlos syndrome
- Multiple sclerosis, systemic amyloidosis
- Infection (subacute endocarditis, HIV infection, trichinosis, rickettsial diseases)
- Fibromuscular dysplasia
- Ergotamine use
- Segmental arterial mediolysis

DIAGNOSTIC TESTS & INTERPRETATION
- No specific laboratory abnormalities. Confirm diagnosis with biopsy if possible (4)[A].
- Angiography (conventional, CT angiography, or MR angiography) may reveal microaneurysms and/or beading of bifurcating blood vessels.
- Avoid contrast in renal disease.
- Nonspecific laboratory abnormalities:
  - Elevated ESR and CRP
  - Mild proteinuria, elevated creatinine
  - Hepatitis B surface antigen positive in 10–50%
  - Hepatitis C antibody/hepatitis C virus RNA
  - ANCA, anti-proteinase 3 (PR3), and anti-MPO are negative. Positive ANCA argues against PAN.
  - Rheumatoid factor may be positive.
  - Anemia of chronic disease (2,4)

Initial Tests (lab, imaging)
Look for evidence of systemic disease and rule out other causes (2,4):
- CBC, ESR, CRP (elevated) (4)[C]
- Chemistries: elevated creatinine/BUN (4)[C]
- Hepatitis B serology: often positive; hepatitis C less commonly positive
- LFTs: abnormal if associated hepatitis B, C, or involvement of hepatobiliary tract
- Urinalysis: proteinuria/hematuria, generally no cellular casts or active urinary sediment (4)[C]
- ANA, cryoglobulins (4)[C]
- ANCA, anti-MPO, and anti-PR3 (4)[A]
- Complement levels (C3, C4)
- Angiographic demonstration of aneurysmal changes/beading of small and medium-sized arteries

Diagnostic Procedures/Other
- Electromyography and nerve conduction studies in patients with suspected mononeuritis multiplex. If abnormal, consider sural nerve biopsy.
- Arterial/tissue biopsy
- Skin biopsy from edges of ulcers; include deep dermis and SC fat to assess small muscular artery involvement (excisional *not* punch biopsy) (2,4).

Test Interpretation
- Necrotizing inflammation with fibrinoid necrosis of small and medium-sized muscular arteries; segmental, often at bifurcations and branchings. Venules are not involved in classic PAN.
- Capillaritis/other lung parenchymal involvement by vasculitis *strongly suggests* another process (microscopic PAN, GPA, Churg-Strauss syndrome, or antiglomerular basement membrane disease).
- Acute lesions with infiltration of polymorphonuclear cells through vessel walls into perivascular area; necrosis, thrombosis, infarction of involved tissue
- Aneurysmal dilatations, including aortic dissection
- Peripheral nerves: 50–70% (vasa nervorum with necrotizing vasculitis)
- GI vessels: 50% (at autopsy) with bowel necrosis; gallbladder and appendix vasculature: 10%
- Muscle vessels: 50%
- Testicular vessels involved in symptomatic males
- *The key differences from other necrotizing vasculitides are lack of granuloma formation and sparing of veins and pulmonary arteries* (2).

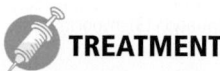

TREATMENT

GENERAL MEASURES
Treat HTN aggressively to prevent complications (stroke, myocardial infarction, heart failure).

MEDICATION
First Line
- Severe (life-threatening) disease: corticosteroids (CS) (high-dose oral prednisone [1 mg/kg/day] or intravenous [IV] methylprednisolone [0.5 to 1.0 g/day] for 3 days, then transition to prednisone 1 mg/kg/day, and taper according to response) (4,5)[A]
  - Only 50% of patients achieve and maintain remission with CS. Other patients require additional immunosuppressive therapy.
  - IV cyclophosphamide (0.6 g/m^2 every 2 weeks for 3 doses and then monthly for 4 to 12 months) in combination with CS: improves survival and spares use of chronic steroids in moderate/severe PAN (4,5)[A]
    - Cyclophosphamide has risk of infertility and malignancy.
  - Plasma exchange for severe refractory disease, such as progressive renal disease (4)[A]
- Less severe disease: CS alone ± other immunosuppressive agents (azathioprine 2 mg/kg/day, methotrexate 20 to 25 mg/week, mycophenolate mofetil 2,000 to 3,000 mg daily). Hydroxychloroquine (5 mg/kg/day) use has been reported (4,5)[A],(6)[C].
- Cutaneous PAN: Nonsteroidal anti-inflammatory drugs, dapsone, and colchicine are used (4)[C].
- HBV-associated PAN: antiviral agents, short-term CS, plasma exchange (1,3)[C]

Second Line
- There is no well-defined second-line therapy in PAN.
- Infliximab (3 to 5 mg/kg IV at 0, 2, and 6 weeks, and every 4 to 8 weeks thereafter) and rituximab (1,000 mg IV on days 0 and 14 and then every 6 months OR 375 mg/m^2 IV weekly for 4 weeks) anecdotally reported to be of benefit in refractory PAN (3,4)[C].

ADDITIONAL THERAPIES
- For patients receiving IV cyclophosphamide, mercaptoethanesulfonate reduces bladder exposure to carcinogenic metabolites (4).
- Prophylactically treat patients on cyclophosphamide for *Pneumocystis jiroveci* (*carinii*) pneumonia with trimethoprim-sulfamethoxazole (use dapsone 100 mg/day or atovaquone 1,500 mg/day in intolerant/allergic patients) (4).

ADMISSION, INPATIENT, AND NURSING CONSIDERATIONS
Depends on extent and involvement of specific organs

ONGOING CARE

FOLLOW-UP RECOMMENDATIONS
Patient Monitoring
- CBC, urinalysis, renal and hepatic function tests
- Acute-phase reactants (e.g., ESR, CRP) may help monitor disease activity.
- The revised 2009 Five Factor Score (FFS) can predict mortality and guide treatment strategies. Four factors are used in the evaluation of patients with PAN, including age, renal insufficiency, cardiac involvement, and GI manifestations. The fifth factor, ENT manifestations, is only applied to patients with ANCA-associated vasculitis (1,3).
- Be alert for:
  - Side effects of immunosuppressant medications
  - Delayed appearance of neoplasms, especially bladder malignancy in patients treated with cyclophosphamide (Check annual U/A, urinary cytology with urologic evaluation if microscopic hematuria.) (3)[C]
  - Steroid-induced osteoporosis

DIET
- Low-salt diet (HTN)
- Mediterranean diet for cardiovascular health
- Calcium and vitamin D–rich diets for patients on CS therapy

PATIENT EDUCATION
ACR website: https://www.rheumatology.org

PROGNOSIS
- Expected outcome of untreated PAN is poor.
- Steroid and cytotoxic treatment increases 5-year survival rate to 75–80% (2).
- Survival is greater for hepatitis B–related PAN as a result of the introduction of antiviral treatments.
- Patients presenting with proteinuria, renal insufficiency, GI tract involvement, cardiomyopathy, or CNS involvement have a worse prognosis.

COMPLICATIONS
- End-organ damage from ischemia
- Complications from immunosuppressive agents

REFERENCES
1. De Virgilio A, Grego A, Magliulo G, et al. Polyarteritis nodosa: a contemporary overview. *Autoimmun Rev.* 2016;15(6):564–570.
2. Pagnoux C, Seror R, Henegar C, et al; for French Vasculitis Study Group. Clinical features and outcomes in 348 patients with polyarteritis nodosa: a systematic retrospective study of patients diagnosed between 1963 and 2005 and entered into the French Vasculitis Study Group Database. *Arthritis Rheum.* 2010;62(2):616–626.
3. Forbess L, Bannykh S. Polyarteritis nodosa. *Rheum Dis Clin North Am.* 2015;41(1):33–46.
4. Mukhtyar C, Guillevin L, Cid MC, et al; for European Vasculitis Study Group. EULAR recommendations for the management of primary small and medium vessel vasculitis. *Ann Rheum Dis.* 2009;68(3):310–317.
5. Ribi C, Cohen P, Pagnoux C, et al; for French Vasculitis Study Group. Treatment of polyarteritis nodosa and microscopic polyangiitis without poor-prognosis factors: a prospective randomized study of one hundred twenty-four patients. *Arthritis Rheum.* 2010;62(4):1186–1197.
6. Casian A, Sangle S, D'Cruz D. New use for an old treatment: hydroxychloroquine as a potential treatment for systemic vasculitis. *Autoimmun Rev.* 2018;17(7):660–664.

ADDITIONAL READING

Samson M, Puéchal X, Mouthon L, et al; for French Vasculitis Study Group. Microscopic polyangiitis and non-HBV polyarteritis nodosa with poor-prognosis factors: 10-year results of the prospective CHUSPAN trial. *Clin Exp Rheumatol.* 2017;35(1 Suppl 103):176–184.

 SEE ALSO

Hepatitis B; Hepatitis C

 CODES

ICD10
- M30.0 Polyarteritis nodosa
- M30.1 Polyarteritis with lung involvement [Churg-Strauss]
- M30.8 Other conditions related to polyarteritis nodosa

CLINICAL PEARLS
- PAN is a necrotizing vasculitis of small- to medium-sized muscular arteries with lack of granuloma formation that spares veins and pulmonary arteries.
- Clinical features of PAN depend on target organ.
- Skin biopsies at ulcer edges (include deep dermis and SC fat) improve diagnostic yield.
- Check hepatitis B and C serologies.
- ANCA is negative in classic PAN.
- At diagnosis, the revised FFS can determine prognosis and guide therapy.
- Treatment involves use of immunosuppressive drugs; choice depends on extent and severity of disease.

POLYCYSTIC KIDNEY DISEASE

Maricarmen Malagon-Rogers, MD

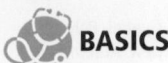 **BASICS**

DESCRIPTION
- A group of monogenic disorders that results in renal cyst development
- The most frequent are two genetically distinct conditions: autosomal dominant polycystic kidney disease (ADPKD) and autosomal recessive polycystic kidney disease (ARPKD).
- ADPKD is one of the most common human genetic disorders.

EPIDEMIOLOGY
- ADPKD is generally late onset.
  - Mean age of end-stage kidney disease (ESKD) 57 to 69 years
  - More progressive disease in men than in women
  - Up to 90% of adults have cysts in the liver.
- ARPKD usually present in infants
  - A minority in older children and young adults may manifest as liver disease.
  - Nonobstructive intrahepatic bile dilatation is sometimes seen.
  - Found on all continents and in all races

Incidence
- Mean age of ESKD: *PKD1 mutation*, 54.3 years versus *PKD2 mutation*, 74 years
- ARPKD affects 1/20,000 live births; carrier level is 1/70.
- ADPKD affects 1/400 to 1,000 live births.

Prevalence
As ESKD, ADPKD: 8.7/1 million in the United States; 7/1 million in Europe

ETIOLOGY AND PATHOPHYSIOLOGY
- ADPKD
  - *PKD1* and *PKD2* mutations disrupt the function of polycystins on the primary cilium, forming fluid-filled cysts that progressively increase in size, leading to gross enlargement of the kidney and distortion of the renal architecture.
  - Glomerular hyperfiltration compensates for the progressive loss of healthy glomeruli, and therefore, by the time GFR decline becomes detectable, as much as ½ of the original functional glomeruli are irreversibly lost.
  - The majority of patients with ADPKD ultimately progress to ESKD (1).
- ARPKD
  - *PKHD1* product fibrocystin is also located in cilia.
- ADPKD: Cysts arise from only 5% of nephrons:
  - Autosomal dominant pattern of inheritance but a molecularly recessive disease with the 2-hit hypothesis
  - Requires genetic and environmental factors
- ARPKD: Mutations are scattered throughout the gene with genotype–phenotype correlation.

Genetics
- ADPKD
  - Autosomal dominant inheritance
  - 50% of children of an affected adult are affected.
  - 100% penetrance; genetic imprinting and genetic anticipation are seen as well.
  - Two genes isolated
    ○ *PKD1* on chromosome 16p13.3 (85% of patients) encodes polycystin 1.
    ○ *PKD2* on chromosome 4q21 (15% of patients) encodes polycystin 2.

- ARPKD
  - Autosomal recessive inheritance
  - Siblings have a 1:4 chance of being affected; gene *PKHD1* on chromosome 6p21.1–p12 encodes fibrocystin.

RISK FACTORS
- Large inter- and intrafamilial variability
- A more rapidly progressive clinical course is predicted by onset of ESKD at <55 years, development of stage III CKD at <40 years old, onset of HTN at <18 years, total kidney volume greater than the expected for a given age, or presence of multiple complications (gross hematuria, microalbuminuria) (1).

GENERAL PREVENTION
Genetic counseling

COMMONLY ASSOCIATED CONDITIONS
- ADPKD
  - Cysts in other organs
    ○ Polycystic liver disease in 58% of young age group to 94% of 45-year-olds
    ○ Pancreatic cysts: 5%
    ○ Seminal cysts: 40%
    ○ Arachnoid cysts: 8%
  - Vascular manifestations
    ○ Intracerebral aneurysms in 6% of patients without family history and in 16% with family history
    ○ Aortic dissections
  - Cardiac manifestations: mitral valve prolapse: 25%
  - Diverticular disease
- ARPKD: liver involvement: affected in inverse proportion to renal disease; congenital hepatic fibrosis with portal HTN

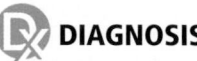 **DIAGNOSIS**

HISTORY
- ADPKD
  - Positive family history (15% are de novo mutations)
  - Flank pain: 60%
  - Hematuria
  - UTI
  - HTN: 50% aged 20 to 34 years; 100% with ESKD
  - Renal failure
  - Presymptomatic screening of ADPKD is not currently recommended for at-risk children (2).
    ○ Blood pressure (BP) should be routinely measured in these patients.
- ARPKD
  - 30% of affected neonates die:
    ○ Enlarged echogenic kidneys and oligohydramnios are diagnosed in utero.
    ○ Later in childhood: Later in childhood
  - Adolescents and adults present with complications of portal HTN: esophageal varices
  - Hypersplenism

PHYSICAL EXAM
- HTN
- Flank masses

DIFFERENTIAL DIAGNOSIS
- ADPKD and ARPKD
- Tuberous sclerosis: prevalence 1/6,000

- Von Hippel-Lindau syndrome: prevalence 1/36,000
- Nephronophthisis: accounts for 10–20% of cases of renal failure in children; medullary cystic kidney disease
- Renal cystic dysplasias: multicystic dysplastic kidneys: grossly deformed kidneys; most common type of bilateral cystic diseases in newborns (prevalence: 1/4,000)
- Simple cysts: most common cystic abnormality
  - Localized or unilateral renal cystic disease
  - Medullary sponge kidney
  - Acquired renal cystic disease
- Renal cystic neoplasms: benign multilocular cyst (cystic nephroma)

DIAGNOSTIC TESTS & INTERPRETATION
Electrolytes, BUN/creatinine, urine analysis plus urinary citrate

Initial Tests (lab, imaging)
- ADPKD
  - Renal dysfunction
    ○ Impaired renal concentration (3), hypocitraturia, aciduria
    ○ Hyperfiltration
    ○ Elevated creatinine
  - Urinalysis: hematuria and mild proteinuria
- ARPKD
  - Electrolyte abnormalities and renal insufficiency
  - Anemia, thrombocytopenia, leukopenia
- ADPKD
  - US: It is the easiest diagnostic method; however, it is suboptimal for disease exclusion at age <40 years (2)[C].
    ○ Renal enlargement is universal.
    ○ In at-risk patients: By age 30 years, two renal cysts (bilateral or unilateral) are 100% diagnostic. In children, it sometimes appears similar to ARPKD; may be diagnosed in utero
    ○ Presence of hepatic cysts in young adults is pathognomonic for ADPKD.
    ○ In the absence of family history, bilateral renal enlargement and cysts make the diagnosis.
  - CT scan/MRI ideally should be part of the initial evaluation (2)[C].
    ○ Kidney volume assessed by CT or MRI is a main predictor of progression.
    ○ Helpful in identifying cysts in other organs
    ○ In subjects <40 years, fewer than five cysts by MRI exclude the diagnosis (2)[B].
- ARPKD
  - US: Kidneys are enlarged, homogeneously hyperechogenic (cortex and medulla).
  - CT scan is more sensitive if diagnosis is in doubt.
  - Presence of hepatic fibrosis helps the diagnosis.

Follow-Up Tests & Special Considerations
- Diagnosis and prevention of secondary problems because of renal and liver abnormalities
- Follow-up of combined renal volume to assess disease severity
- Beyond age 2 years, renal size decreases in ARPKD but continues to grow in ADPKD at an average rate of 5.27% per year. Total kidney volume identifies patients with progressive disease (2).

Diagnostic Procedures/Other
- Genetic testing is available for *PKD1* and *PKD2* in ADPKD when imaging results are equivocal and for potential living related donors (4)[C].
- For *PKHD1* in ARPKD, a prenatal diagnosis is feasible in about 72% of patients.

Test Interpretation
- ADPKD
  - Kidneys are diffusely cystic and, although enlarged, retain their general shape.
  - Cysts range from a few millimeters to several centimeters and are distributed evenly throughout the cortex and medulla.
  - They arise in all segments of the nephron, although they arise initially from the collecting ducts.
  - One kidney may be larger than the other.
- ARPKD
  - Disease is a spectrum, ranging from severe renal disease with mild liver damage to mild renal disease with severe liver damage.
  - Renal enlargement is due to fusiform dilatation of the collecting ducts in the cortex and medulla in the newborn period.
  - Liver lesion is diffuse but limited to fibrotic portal areas.

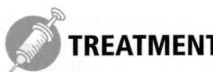 TREATMENT

GENERAL MEASURES
- HTN: moderate sodium restriction, weight control, and regular exercise
- Medications: ACE inhibitors; angiotensin receptor blockers (ARBs)
- Pain: narcotics and other analgesics; bed rest; limit NSAIDs (they worsen renal function).
- Urolithiasis: treated with alkalinization of urine and hydration therapy; surgery as needed
- UTIs/infections of cysts: lipid-soluble antibiotics more effective (e.g., trimethoprim-sulfamethoxazole and chloramphenicol); fluoroquinolones also useful
- Dialysis for ESKD patients
- Hematuria: Reduce physical activity.

MEDICATION
- No specific drug therapy is yet available for PKD, although several studies are being conducted for specific treatments (2,5)[C].
- HTN: should be very well controlled to prevent complications. ACE inhibitors are preferred if no contraindications are present.
- The use of antihypertensive medications has been found to decrease mortality (6)[B].
- Hyperlipidemia: statins preferred

ISSUES FOR REFERRAL
- Nephrologist primary management
- Urologic consultation for management of symptomatic/infected cysts
- Genetic counseling is critical.

SURGERY/OTHER PROCEDURES
- Indications for surgical intervention
  - Uncontrollable HTN
  - Severe back and loin pain, abdominal fullness
  - Renal deterioration due to enlarging cysts
  - Hematuria/hemorrhage or recurrent UTI

- Open and laparoscopic cyst unroofing: may decrease pain and narcotics requirements; has not been proven to prevent renal failure or to prolong current renal function
- Percutaneous cyst aspiration ± injection of sclerosing agent; not usually performed secondary to recurrent fluid accumulation
- Renal transplant for ESKD

ADMISSION, INPATIENT, AND NURSING CONSIDERATIONS
Severe pain, gross hematuria with clots

 ONGOING CARE

FOLLOW-UP RECOMMENDATIONS
None in early stages of the disease; avoid vigorous activity if disease advances. Recurrent gross hematuria is secondary to trauma, associated with faster decline of renal function.

Patient Monitoring
- Monitor BP and renal function. Encourage hydration. Treat UTI and stone disease aggressively.
- Avoid nephrotoxic drugs.
- Creatinine and BP monitoring at least twice a year; more often as needed
- Screening for intracranial aneurysms (7)

DIET
- Low-protein diet may retard renal insufficiency.
- Limit caffeine because this might increase cyst growth.
- High water intake to decrease ADH >3 L/day (5)[C]

PROGNOSIS
- Renal failure in 2% by age 40 years; 23% by age 50 years; 48% by age 73 years
- ADPKD accounts for 10–15% of dialysis patients.
- No increased incidence of renal cell cancer

COMPLICATIONS
- Cyst rupture, infection, or hemorrhage
- Progression to renal failure
- Renal calculi

REFERENCES
1. Schrier RW, Brosnahan G, Cadnapaphornchai MA, et al. Predictors of autosomal dominant polycystic disease progression. *J Am Soc Nephrol*. 2014;25(11):2399–2418.
2. Chapman AB, Devuyst O, Eckardt KU, et al. Autosomal-dominant polycystic kidney disease (ADPKD): executive summary from a Kidney Disease: Improving Global Outcomes (KDIGO) controversies conference. *Kidney Int*. 2015;88(1):17–27. doi:10.1038/ki.2015.59.
3. Zittema D, Boertien WE, van Beek AP, et al. Vasopressin, copeptin, and renal concentrating capacity in patients with autosomal dominant polycystic kidney disease without renal impairment. *Clin J Am Soc Nephrol*. 2012;7(6):906–913.

4. Harris PC, Rossetti S. Molecular diagnostics for autosomal dominant polycystic kidney disease. *Nat Rev Nephrol*. 2010;6(4):197–206.
5. Mahnensmith RL. Novel treatments of autosomal dominant polycystic kidney disease. *Clin J Am Soc Nephrol*. 2014;9(5):831–836.
6. Patch C, Charlton J, Roderick PJ, et al. Use of antihypertensive medications and mortality of patients with autosomal dominant polycystic kidney disease: a population-based study. *Am J Kidney Dis*. 2011;57(6):856–862.
7. Rozenfeld MN, Ansari SA, Shaibani A, et al. Should patients with autosomal dominant polycystic kidney disease be screened for cerebral aneurysms? *AJNR Am J Neuroradiol*. 2014;35(1):3–9.

ADDITIONAL READING
- Chapman AB, Bost JE, Torres VE, et al. Kidney volume and functional outcomes in autosomal dominant polycystic kidney disease. *Clin J Am Soc Nephrol*. 2012;7(3):479–486.
- Torres VE, Chapman AB, Devuyst O, et al. Tolvaptan in patients with autosomal dominant polycystic kidney disease. *N Engl J Med*. 2012;367(25):2407–2418.
- Torres VE, Harris PC. Polycystic kidney disease in 2011: connecting the dots toward a polycystic kidney disease therapy. *Nat Rev Nephrol*. 2011;8(2):66–68.

 SEE ALSO

Chronic Kidney Disease

 CODES

ICD10
- Q61.3 Polycystic kidney, unspecified
- Q61.19 Other polycystic kidney, infantile type
- Q61.2 Polycystic kidney, adult type

CLINICAL PEARLS
- Most PKD patients eventually develop ESKD. No specific treatment has been proven to prevent EKRD, but hydration and control of BP are reasonable goals and should be started soon.
- Patients may benefit from a nephrology consultation after the initial diagnosis to counsel regarding disease progression prevention. Then, they can be followed by primary care if the disease was an incidental finding or no significant kidney dysfunction is present.

POLYCYSTIC OVARIAN SYNDROME (PCOS)

Melissa Dennis, MD • Tiphany Jackson, MD • Katherine Tadros, DO

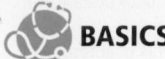 **BASICS**

DESCRIPTION
- Polycystic ovarian syndrome (PCOS) is a common endocrine disorder with heterogeneous manifestations that affects 6–10% of the U.S. population.
- Characterized by hyperandrogenism, insulin resistance, and anovulation, typically presenting as amenorrhea or oligomenorrhea
- Diagnostic clinical characteristics include menstrual dysfunction, infertility, hirsutism, acne, obesity, and metabolic syndrome.
- The ovaries are often polycystic on imaging.
- The etiology of PCOS is unknown but can be modified by lifestyle factors.
- System(s) affected: reproductive, endocrine/metabolic, skin/exocrine
- Synonym(s): Stein-Leventhal syndrome; polycystic ovary disease

ALERT
- Condition may begin at puberty.
- Obesity may amplify PCOS, but it is not diagnostic.
- 20% of women with PCOS are not obese.
- Predisposes to and is associated with obesity, hypertension, diabetes, metabolic syndrome, hyperlipidemia, infertility, insulin-resistance syndrome, endometrial hyperplasia, and uterine cancer

EPIDEMIOLOGY
Prevalence
- Incidence and prevalence are still highly debated due to a wide spectrum of diagnostic features: The National Institutes of Health (NIH) criteria require chronic anovulation and hyperandrogenism.
- The prevalence based on NIH criteria is 7% of reproductive age women.
- Predominant age: reproductive age
- Predominant sex: females only

ETIOLOGY AND PATHOPHYSIOLOGY
- Recent evidence points to a primary role for insulin resistance with hyperinsulinemia.
- Increased GnRH pulsations in the hypothalamus lead to increased production of LH with limited production of FSH.
- Hyperandrogenism: Ovaries are the main source of excess androgens (75% of circulating testosterone originates in the ovary). Polycystic ovaries have thickened thecal layers and overexpressed LH receptors, which cause excess androgen secretion.
- Ovarian follicles: Abnormal androgen signaling may account for abnormal folliculogenesis causing polycystic ovaries.
- Obesity results in compensatory hyperinsulinemia: Women with PCOS have insulin resistance similar to that in type 2 diabetes. Elevated levels of insulin decrease sex hormone–binding globulin (SHBG), increasing bioavailability of testosterone. Insulin may also act directly on adrenal glands, ovaries, and hypothalamus to enhance androgen production.
- Insulin resistance causes elevated insulin levels and the frequently associated metabolic syndrome or frank diabetes mellitus.

Genetics
- Likely a combination of polygenic and environmental factors
- Implicated genes include *DENND1A* and *THADA*.

RISK FACTORS
See "Commonly Associated Conditions"; cause and effect are difficult to extricate in this disorder.

GENERAL PREVENTION
None known; focus on early diagnosis and treatment to prevent long-term complications.

COMMONLY ASSOCIATED CONDITIONS
- Infertility
- Obesity
- Obstructive sleep apnea
- Hypertension
- Diabetes mellitus
- Endometrial hyperplasia/carcinoma
- Fatty liver disease
- Mood disturbances and depression
- Hirsutism

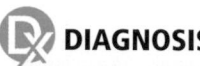 **DIAGNOSIS**

HISTORY
- A comprehensive history, including a family history of diabetes and premature onset of cardiovascular disease, is important in the differential diagnosis.
- Focus on the onset and duration of the various signs of androgen excess, menstrual history, and concomitant medications, including the use of exogenous androgens (1).
- Unpredictable, heavy, or absent menstrual cycles

PHYSICAL EXAM
- Vital signs: elevated body mass index (BMI), hypertension
- General appearance: central obesity, hirsutism, acne
- Skin: male hair pattern, balding, acne, seborrhea, acanthosis nigricans
- Pelvic: ovarian enlargement, clitoromegaly

ALERT
Look specifically for signs of virilization, such as hair pattern, deepened voice, and clitoromegaly because they indicate significant testosterone levels beyond that of PCOS.

DIFFERENTIAL DIAGNOSIS
- Cushing syndrome
- HAIR-AN syndrome
- Androgen-secreting ovarian or adrenal tumor
- Prolactin-producing pituitary adenoma
- Hyperthecosis
- Adult-onset adrenal hyperplasia
- Partial congenital adrenal hyperplasia (21-hydroxylase deficiency)
- 11β-Hydroxylase deficiency
- 17β-Hydroxysteroid dehydrogenase deficiency
- Acromegaly
- Drug-induced hirsutism, oligo-ovulation (e.g., danazol, steroids, valproic acid)
- Thyroid disease
- Idiopathic hirsutism
- Polycystic ovaries

DIAGNOSTIC TESTS & INTERPRETATION
- The value of measurement of circulating androgens to document PCOS is uncertain but should include calculating free testosterone concentration using mass spectrometry of total testosterone and measurement of SHBG (2)[C].

- Most commonly used diagnostic criteria is the Rotterdam criteria (need any 2 of 3):
  – Oligomenorrhea or amenorrhea
  – Clinical and/or biochemical signs of hyperandrogenism
  – Transvaginal ultrasonographic polycystic ovaries
- Must exclude other etiologies including Cushing disease, congenital adrenal hyperplasia, and androgen-secreting tumors
- Ultrasonographic polycystic ovaries are not necessary for the diagnosis of PCOS.
- More recent criteria also focus on similar criteria while acknowledging that there may be forms of PCOS without overt evidence of hyperandrogenism (3)[C].

Initial Tests (lab, imaging)
- Screening workup should rule out pregnancy, thyroid disease, hyperprolactinemia, and premature ovarian failure with human chorionic gonadotropin (hCG), TSH, prolactin, FSH, respectively.
- Hirsute women should have a free testosterone determination (total testosterone minus SHBG) and a DHEA-S.
- Consider 17-OH progesterone if congenital adrenal hyperplasia is suspected.
- Typical findings in PCOS include testosterone increased but <200 ng/dL (6.94 nmol/L), mild elevation in DHEA-S but <800 μg/dL (20.8 μmol/L), mild increase in 17-OH progesterone level, increased estrogen level, and decreased SHBG.
- More elevated levels of testosterone or DHEA-S may be associated with an androgen-secreting tumor of the ovaries or adrenal glands.
- Anovulation can be determined by a midluteal phase progesterone level (>3 ng/mL if the woman has ovulated).
- LH/FSH level ≥2.5 to 3.0 L in ~50% of women with PCOS, but LH testing is not generally necessary
- Drugs that may alter lab results:
  – Oral contraceptive pills (OCPs)
  – Steroids
  – Antidepressants
- Transvaginal ultrasound findings: one or both ovaries with ≥12 follicles measuring 2 to 9 mm or increased ovarian volume to 10 cm³

Follow-Up Tests & Special Considerations
- Consider fasting serum glucose, insulin level, and plasminogen activator inhibitor-1 determinations to establish presence of insulin resistance and glucose intolerance, especially if diagnosis is in doubt.
- Overnight dexamethasone suppression test to rule out Cushing syndrome in the appropriate setting
- Endometrial biopsy to rule out hyperplasia and/or carcinoma, if indicated
- If the syndrome is diagnosed, determination of fasting glucose and fasting lipid levels should be performed and formal glucose tolerance test is considered.

ALERT
Prolonged or heavy bleeding should prompt an endometrial biopsy for evaluation of endometrial hyperplasia and possible cancer.

Test Interpretation
- Ovary is usually enlarged with a smooth white glistening capsule.
- Ovarian cortex is lined with follicles in all stages of development but most atretic.
- Thecal cell proliferation with an increase in the stromal compartment

TREATMENT

GENERAL MEASURES
Lifestyle changes including appropriate nutrition and exercise to decrease body weight by as little as 5% can restore ovulation and increase insulin sensitivity (4)[A]. Treatment plan should be individualized based on patient needs and desires.

MEDICATION
- The goal of treatment in PCOS depends on symptoms and patient's goals for fertility.
- Treatment can be divided into four main categories: (i) restore menses, (ii) decrease insulin resistance, (iii) ameliorate androgen excess, and (iv) assist in fertility.

First Line
- Restore menses when pregnancy not desired:
  – OCPs and progestins provide improvement in menstrual irregularity and provide endometrial protection.
  – Low-dose OCPs (30 to 35 μg); newer formulations containing progestins with lower androgenicity (e.g., norethindrone, desogestrel, norgestimate, drospirenone) may be particularly beneficial, but all OCPs increase SHBG and decrease excess androgens.
  – Levonorgestrel IUD offers endometrial protection and pregnancy prevention but will not counteract hyperandrogenism (2).
- If unable to tolerate OCPs, then intermittent medroxyprogesterone (Provera) 10 mg PO or micronized progesterone (Crinone and Prometrium): 200 mg PO for 10 to 14 days can be given every 1 to 3 months (2)[C]. These offer endometrial protection. However, these will not counteract hyperandrogenism nor protect against pregnancy. Decrease insulin resistance:
  – Metformin may help to correct metabolic abnormalities in women who are insulin resistant. Initial dose is 500 mg daily for 1 week, increasing by 500 mg/week to a total of 1,500 to 2,000 mg/day divided BID; take with food.
    ○ Overall, data support the usefulness of metformin on both cardiometabolic risk and reproduction assistance in PCOS women.
    ○ Thiazolidinediones may increase likelihood of ovulation and treat insulin resistance.
- If pregnancy is desired:
  – Previously, the first-line treatment for ovulation induction was clomiphene (Clomid, Serophene) and/or exogenous gonadotropins. Live birth rate with clomiphene (Clomid) is 10.1% (5).
  – More recent data shows that letrozole (an aromatase inhibitor) has increased ovulation rates, clinical pregnancy rates, and live birth rates compared to clomiphene (Clomid). Live birth rate with letrozole is 27.5%. Dosing starts on day 3, 4, or 5 with 2.5 mg daily for 5 days; can increase to 5 mg daily with max dose 7.5 mg daily for 5 days (5)
  – Counsel patients that letrozole is not approved by the FDA for ovulation induction.
  – Metformin: 500 to 2,000 mg PO divided BID has been shown to improve hyperandrogenism and restore ovulation. Some providers will choose to continue metformin throughout the 1st trimester or the entire pregnancy if there is a history of spontaneous abortion or glucose intolerance. It does improve ovulation rates and insulin resistance but does not improve live birth rates alone or in combination with clomiphene when used for ovulation induction (6)[B].
  – Metformin reduces the incidence of gestational diabetes.
  – All ovulation induction drugs increase the risk of multiple births and obstetric complications, such as preterm birth and hypertensive disorders.

Second Line
- Acne:
  – OCPs with low doses of cyproterone or drospirenone
  – Spironolactone: 50 to 200 mg daily in 1 to 2 divided doses for acne and hirsutism not addressed by OCP therapy. This medication is unsafe in pregnancy, and potassium levels must be followed closely when used.
- Hirsutism:
  – Eflornithine hydrochloride 13.9% cream BID
  – Finasteride 2.5 to 5.0 mg daily

ISSUES FOR REFERRAL
- To reproductive endocrinologist for all women who cannot achieve pregnancy with clomiphene (Clomid)
- To endocrinologist if Cushing syndrome, congenital adrenal hyperplasia, or adrenal or ovarian tumors are found during the workup

ADDITIONAL THERAPIES
Mechanical means of hair removal, including laser, electrolysis, waxing, and depilatory, may improve cosmesis.

SURGERY/OTHER PROCEDURES
Ovarian wedge resection and laparoscopic laser drilling are controversial and rarely used today.

COMPLEMENTARY & ALTERNATIVE MEDICINE
Acupuncture may assist with cycle normalization and weight loss.

ONGOING CARE

FOLLOW-UP RECOMMENDATIONS
6-month intervals to evaluate response to therapy and to monitor weight and medication side effects

Patient Monitoring
- Counsel patient about the risk of endometrial and breast carcinoma, insulin resistance, and diabetes as well as obesity and its role in infertility.
- See patient frequently throughout the menstrual cycle, depending on which drug combination is used to induce ovulation.
- All patients with PCOS who have not received medication or IUD for endometrial protection and have been amenorrheic for 1 year should undergo endometrial biopsy.

DIET
In overweight patients, weight loss is the most successful therapy because it improves cardiovascular risk, insulin sensitivity, menstrual patterns, and infertility: Counsel on lifestyle dietary changes; consider referral to nutritionist and weight center. No specific diet plan is proven to be better than another.

PATIENT EDUCATION
- Provide patient with information about PCOS, such as from http://www.acog.org/.
- Discuss the chronic nature of this condition and the risks and benefits and side effects of potential treatments.
- Review the importance of weight loss, if applicable. Modest weight loss of 5–10% of initial body weight has been demonstrated to improve many of the features of PCOS.

PROGNOSIS
- Fertility prognosis is good but may need assisted reproductive technologies.
- Proper follow-up and screening can prevent endometrial carcinoma.

- Early detection of diabetes may decrease morbidity and mortality associated with cardiovascular risk factor.

COMPLICATIONS
- Reproductive: infertility
- Metabolic: insulin resistance, diabetes mellitus, cardiovascular disease
- Psychosocial: increased anxiety, mood disorder, eating disorder, depression
- Predisposes to endometrial hyperplasia and as high as 9% lifetime risk of endometrial cancer
- Women with PCOS appear to be at increased risk of complications of pregnancy including gestational diabetes and hypertensive disorders.

REFERENCES

1. Azziz R, Carmina E, Dewailly D, et al; for Task Force on the Phenotype of the Polycystic Ovary Syndrome of The Androgen Excess and PCOS Society. The Androgen Excess and PCOS Society criteria for the polycystic ovary syndrome: the complete task force report. *Fertil Steril*. 2009;91(2):456–488.
2. McCartney CR, Marshall JC. Clinical practice. Polycystic ovary syndrome. *N Engl J Med*. 2016;375(1):54–64.
3. Carmina E, Oberfield SE, Lobo RA. The diagnosis of polycystic ovary syndrome in adolescents. *Am J Obstet Gynecol*. 2010;203(3):201.e1–201.e5.
4. Tang T, Lord JM, Norman RJ, et al. Insulin-sensitising drugs (metformin, rosiglitazone, pioglitazone, D-chiro-inositol) for women with polycystic ovary syndrome, oligo amenorrhoea and subfertility. *Cochrane Database Syst Rev*. 2010;(1):CD003053.
5. ACOG Practice Bulletin No. 194: polycystic ovary syndrome. *Obstet Gynecol*. 2018;131(6):e157–e171.
6. Legro RS, Barnhart HX, Schlaff WD, et al; for Cooperative Multicenter Reproductive Medicine Network. Clomiphene, metformin, or both for infertility in the polycystic ovary syndrome. *N Engl J Med*. 2007;356(6):551–566.

SEE ALSO

Algorithm: Amenorrhea, Secondary

CODES

ICD10
- E28.2 Polycystic ovarian syndrome
- L68.0 Hirsutism

CLINICAL PEARLS
- Based on Rotterdam criteria, PCOS is diagnosed based on 2 of 3 of (i) oligo-ovulation, (ii) signs of hyperandrogenism, (iii) polycystic ovaries.
- Polycystic ovaries are not required for the diagnosis of PCOS.
- All patients with anovulation should be evaluated for pregnancy.
- Chronic anovulation should be treated because chronic estrogen stimulation in absence of progesterone may lead to endometrial hyperplasia.
- Specific therapies must be individualized according to the needs and desires of each patient.
- Letrozole is now the first-line medication for ovulation induction.

POLYCYTHEMIA VERA

Thuy Thanh Thi Le, DO • Helen N. Johnson-Wall, MD

 BASICS

DESCRIPTION

- Polycythemia vera (PV) is a chronic myeloproliferative clonal stem cell disorder marked by increased production of red blood cells (erythrocytosis) with excessive erythroid, myeloid, and megakaryocytic elements in the bone marrow.
- Morbidity and mortality are primarily related to complications from blood hyperviscosity leading to thrombosis development as well as malignant transformation. Untreated patients may survive 6 to 18 months. Adequate treatment may extend life to >10 years.
- Myelofibrosis can develop in the bone marrow, leading to progressive hepatosplenomegaly.
- Synonyms: primary polycythemia; maladie de Vaquez disease; primary PV; PV rubra; polycythemia, splenomegalic; Vaquez-Osler disease

EPIDEMIOLOGY

Incidence
- Predominant age: 50 to 75 years; however, can occur in early adulthood and childhood
- Predominant sex: male > female (slightly)
- Incidence in the United States in 2012: 2.8/100,000 population of men and 1.3/100,000 population of women; highest for men 70 to 79 years at 23.5/100,000 persons per year

Prevalence
In the United States in 2010, estimates ranged from 45 to 57 cases per 100,000 patients.

ETIOLOGY AND PATHOPHYSIOLOGY
JAK2 V617F mutation associated with clonal proliferative disorder

Genetics
JAK2 V617F (tyrosine kinase) mutation: >97% of patients with PV have an activating mutation; this is helpful in differentiating from secondary erythrocytosis. Homozygote carriers will have higher incidence of symptoms such as pruritus but will not have higher incidence of disease than heterozygotes.

RISK FACTORS
- PV may be slightly more prevalent among Jews of Eastern European descent than other Europeans or Asians.
- Familial history is rare.

COMMONLY ASSOCIATED CONDITIONS
- Budd-Chiari syndrome
- Ischemic digits
- Mesenteric artery thrombosis
- Myocardial infarction
- Cerebrovascular accident or transient ischemic attack
- Venous thromboembolism and pulmonary embolism

 DIAGNOSIS

HISTORY
- Patients may be asymptomatic or present with nonspecific complaints, including fatigue, malaise, weight loss, sweating, and subjective weakness.

- Erythromelalgia (burning pain of feet/hands, occasionally with erythema, pallor, cyanosis, or paresthesias)
- Pruritus, especially after bathing (aquagenic pruritus)
- Arterial and venous occlusive events
- Headaches
- Blurred vision or blind spots
- Tinnitus, vertigo, dizziness
- Spontaneous bruising/bleeding
- Peptic ulcer disease (due to alterations in gastric mucosal blood flow)
- Early satiety due to enlarged spleen
- Bone pain (ribs and sternum)
- Gout
- Insomnia
- Depressed mood

PHYSICAL EXAM
- Hypertension (46%)
- Splenomegaly (75%), palpable spleen (36%)
- Hepatomegaly (30%)
- Facial plethora (ruddy cyanosis)
- Bone tenderness (especially ribs and sternum)
- Skin excoriations from significant pruritus
- Gouty tophi or arthritis
- Injection of the conjunctival small vessels and/or engorgement of the veins of the optic fundus

DIFFERENTIAL DIAGNOSIS
- Secondary erythrocytosis:
  - Sleep apnea
  - Emphysema
  - Cigarette smoking
  - Renal artery stenosis
  - Carbon monoxide poisoning
  - Drugs: diuretics, testosterone, erythropoietin (EPO)
- Hemoglobinopathy
- Ectopic EPO production
- Spurious polycythemia

DIAGNOSTIC TESTS & INTERPRETATION
- CBC; if suspicion is high, then obtain EPO level and gene testing for *JAK2 V617F*.
- If the only indication of PV is elevated hemoglobin (Hgb)/Hct, a CBC should be repeated. Further testing is unnecessary if the Hgb/Hct return to normal.

Initial Tests (lab, imaging)
- 2016 World Health Organization diagnostic criteria requires all three major criteria or the first 2 major criteria and the minor criterion*(1).
  - Major criteria:
    - Hgb >16.5 g/dL (men); Hgb >16.0 g/dL (women) or Hct >49% (men); Hct >48% (women) or increased cell mass (>25% above mean normal predictive value)
    - Bone marrow biopsy showing hypercellularity for age with trilineage growth (panmyelosis) including prominent erythroid, granulocytic, and megakaryocytic proliferation with pleomorphic, mature megakaryocytes (difference in sizes)
    - Presence of *JAK2 V617F* or similar mutation such as *JAK2* exon 12 mutation

  - Minor criteria:
    - Serum EPO level below normal *criterion number 2 (BM biopsy) may not be required in cases with substantive absolute erythrocytosis: Hgb >18.5 g/dL in men (Hct, 55.5%) or >16.5 g/dL in women (Hct, 49.5%) if major criterion 3 and minor criterion are present. However, initial myelofibrosis (present in up to 20% of points) can only be detected by performing a bone marrow biopsy; this finding may predict a more rapid progression to overt myelofibrosis (post-PV MF).
- Other lab findings that are common but not specific
  - Hyperuricemia
  - Hypercholesterolemia
  - Elevated serum vitamin B$_{12}$ levels
  - Prolonged PT, aPTT due to low plasma volume
  - Thrombocytosis (>400,000 platelets/mm^3)
  - Leukocytosis (>12,000/mm^3)
  - Leukocyte alkaline phosphatase (100,000 U in the absence of fever or infection)
- CT or US to assess for splenomegaly, although not necessary for diagnosis
- Arterial oxygen saturation (<92% SaO$_2$) and carboxyhemoglobin (COHb)
- Bone marrow biopsy is not necessary. There is no staging system for this disease.

Diagnostic Procedures/Other
- Bone marrow aspiration if performed shows hypercellularity of erythroid, granulocytic and megakaryocytic lines, or myelofibrosis.
- Cytogenetic testing (*JAK2 V617F*)

Test Interpretation
- If *JAK2 V617F* mutation testing is negative and the EPO level is normal or high, then PV is excluded; investigate causes of secondary erythrocytosis.
- Other causes of erythrocytosis such as ectopic EPO production from a renal tumor, hypoxia from chronic lung, or cyanotic heart disease can be excluded with low or undetectable serum EPO level and normal oxygen saturation.

 TREATMENT

GENERAL MEASURES
- Risk factors: Patients >60 years with history of thrombosis are high risk. Those who are <60 years with no history of thrombosis but with elevated platelets (>150,000) are intermediate risk. <60 years, with normal platelets, and no history of thrombosis are low risk.
- Phlebotomy and low-dose aspirin is first-line therapy for all patients.
- Although not curative, modern therapy for PV can relieve symptoms and prolong survival.
- If secondary PV, address etiology: aggressive treatment of obstructive sleep apnea, COPD (esp. smoking cessation), renal disease; consider lowering dose in testosterone replacement.
- Phlebotomy reduces the blood hyperviscosity, improves platelet function, restores systemic pressures, and decreases risk of thrombosis.

- Phlebotomy:
  - Reduce hematocrit to <45%; will significantly lower rate of cardiovascular death and major thrombosis (2)[A]
  - Performed initially as often as every 2 to 3 days until normal hematocrit reached; phlebotomies of 250 to 500 mL (1 unit—500 mL—phlebotomy should reduce hematocrit by 3 percentage points). Reduce to 250 to 350 mL in elderly patients or patients with cerebrovascular disease.
  - Frail patients should have volume replaced with saline solution to avoid postural hypotension.
  - High risk for thrombosis or presence of elevated platelet count is indication for cytoreductive therapy.
  - Complications of phlebotomy: chronic iron deficiency (symptomatology: pica, angular stomatitis, and glossitis), possible muscle weakness, and dysphagia that is the result of esophageal webs (very rare).
- Other therapies:
  - Maintain hydration.
  - Pruritus therapy: H_1 and H_2 blockers, SSRIs, oatmeal baths, interferon α-2b
  - Uric acid reduction therapy

MEDICATION

First Line

- Primary therapies:
  - Low-dose aspirin 81 mg PO has been associated with a statistically nonsignificant reduction in the risk of fatal thrombotic events without increasing bleeding complications when used in conjunction with phlebotomy (3)[A]. Aspirin should not be used in those with acquired von Willebrand disease or those with other contraindications.
  - Hydroxyurea is recommended for patients at high risk for thrombosis (age >60 years or history of thrombotic event) and with splenomegaly and hepatomegaly. Common starting dose 500 to 1,500 mg PO daily, titrating to control hematocrit and platelet count. Be aware that hydroxyurea can lead to higher risk of leukemic transformation (4)[A].
  - Radioactive phosphorus (^{32}P) may control Hgb level and platelet count by destroying overactive marrow cells. May take up to 3 months before affecting cells. Consider for patients intolerant or nonadherent to hydroxyurea or short expected survival due to mutagenic potential.
  - Pegylated interferon α-2a is effective in controlling erythrocytosis, although dosing is generally limited secondary to intolerable side effects; usually recommended for younger patients (<40 years old) and those who might become pregnant
  - Refer to hematologist/oncologist for further dosing and instructions.
- Symptomatic/adjunctive:
  - Allopurinol 300 mg/day PO for uric acid reduction
  - Cyproheptadine 4 to 16 mg PO daily as needed for pruritus

  - H_2 receptor blockers or antacids for GI hyperacidity; cimetidine is also used for pruritus.
  - Low-dose aspirin also used for pruritus/erythromelalgia
  - SSRIs (paroxetine or fluoxetine) have shown some efficacy in controlling pruritus.
  - Ultraviolet light may help with pruritus.

Second Line

Myelosuppression: chlorambucil or busulfan; busulfan at 2 to 4 mg daily may be effective option for elderly patients with advanced PV refractory or intolerant to other agents such as hydroxyurea and interferon, but significant rate of transformation was observed.

ISSUES FOR REFERRAL

Referral to a hematologist to assist in diagnosis and management

 ONGOING CARE

FOLLOW-UP RECOMMENDATIONS

Patient Monitoring

Monitor hematocrit often and phlebotomize as needed to maintain target goal.

DIET

- Avoid high-sodium diet; can cause fluid retention
- Avoid iron supplement, a permissive chronic state of iron deficiency can help decrease blood production.

PATIENT EDUCATION

- Perform leg and ankle exercises to prevent clots.
- Continuous education regarding possible complications and seeking treatment early for any change or increase in symptoms

PROGNOSIS

- PV cannot be cured but can be controlled with treatment.
- Survival is >15 years with treatment.
- Patients are at risk for developing postpolycythemic myelofibrosis (PPMF) and an increased risk of malignant transformation.

COMPLICATIONS

- Splenomegaly or hepatomegaly
- Budd-Chiari syndrome
- Vascular thrombosis (major cause of death) (20%)
- Transformation to acute leukemia (5%)
- Transformation to myelofibrosis (10%)
- Hemorrhage
- Peptic ulcer
- Uric acid stones
- Secondary gout
- Increased risk for complications and mortality from surgical procedures. Assess risk/benefits and ensure optimal control of disorder before any elective surgery.

REFERENCES

1. Arber DA, Orazi A, Hasserjian R, et al. The 2016 revision to the World Health Organization classification of myeloid neoplasms and acute leukemia. *Blood*. 2016;127(20):2391–2405.
2. Marchioli R, Finazzi G, Specchia G, et al; for CYTO-PV Collaborative Group. Cardiovascular events and intensity of treatment in polycythemia vera. *N Engl J Med*. 2013;368(1):22–33.
3. Squizzato A, Romualdi E, Passamonti F, et al. Antiplatelet drugs for polycythaemia vera and essential thrombocythaemia. *Cochrane Database Syst Rev*. 2013;(4):CD006503.
4. Mascarenhas J, Mughal TI, Verstovsek S. Biology and clinical management of myeloproliferative neoplasms and development of the JAK inhibitor ruxolitinib. *Curr Med Chem*. 2012;19(26):4399–4413.

ADDITIONAL READING

- Passamonti F. How I treat polycythemia vera. *Blood*. 2012;120(2):275–284.
- Tefferi A, Fonseca R. Selective serotonin reuptake inhibitors are effective in the treatment of polycythemia vera–associated pruritus. *Blood*. 2002;99(7):2627.

 SEE ALSO

Myeloproliferative Neoplasms

 CODES

ICD10

- D45 Polycythemia vera
- D75.1 Secondary polycythemia

CLINICAL PEARLS

- Erythrocytosis: Hgb >16.5 g/dL in men, >16.0 g/dL in women
- *JAK2* mutations are an important component of myeloproliferative disorders.
- *Bone marrow biopsy can help in diagnosis showing hypercellularity and trilineage growth.*
- Common complications include thrombosis, malignant transformation, and myelofibrosis.
- All patients should take low-dose aspirin unless there is major bleeding or GI intolerance.
- Phlebotomy is first-line treatment, and consultation with an experienced hematologist is recommended.

POLYMYALGIA RHEUMATICA

Ronald G. Chambers Jr., MD, FAAFP • Megan Babb, DO

 BASICS

DESCRIPTION
- A clinical syndrome characterized by pain and stiffness of the shoulder, hip girdles, and neck; primarily impacts the elderly, associated with morning stiffness and elevated markers of inflammation
- System(s) affected: musculoskeletal; hematologic/lymphatic/immunologic
- Synonym(s): senile rheumatic disease; polymyalgia rheumatica (PMR) syndrome; pseudo-polyarthrite rhizomélique

Geriatric Considerations
- Incidence increases with age.
- Average age of onset ~70 years

Pediatric Considerations
Rare in patients <50 years of age. The peak incidence of PMR is between ages 70 and 80 years (1).

EPIDEMIOLOGY
Incidence
- Incidence increases after age 50 years. Incidence of PMR and giant cell arteritis (GCA) in the United States is 50 and 18 per 100,000 people, respectively.
- Predominant sex: female > male (2 to 3:1)
- Most common in Caucasians, especially those of northern European ancestry

Prevalence
Prevalence in those >50 years old: 700/100,000

ETIOLOGY AND PATHOPHYSIOLOGY
- Unknown. Symptoms relate to enhanced immune system and periarticular inflammatory activity.
- Pathogenesis
  - Polygenic; involves multiple environmental and genetic factors
  - Significant association between histologic evidence of GCA and parvovirus B19 DNA in temporal artery specimen

Genetics
Associated with human leukocyte antigen determinants (HLA-DRB1*04 and DRB1*01 alleles)

RISK FACTORS
- Age >50 years
- Presence of GCA

COMMONLY ASSOCIATED CONDITIONS
Concurrent GCA (temporal arteritis) in ~15–30% of patients; more commonly in females than males

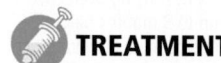 **DIAGNOSIS**

HISTORY
- Suspect PMR in elderly patients with new onset of proximal limb pain and stiffness (neck, shoulder, hip). Patients may use the term stiffness and pain interchangeably (2).
- Difficulty rising from chair or combing hair (proximal muscle involvement)
- Nighttime pain
- Systemic symptoms in ~25% (fatigue, weight loss, low-grade fever)

PHYSICAL EXAM
- Decreased range of motion (ROM) of shoulders, neck, and hips
- Muscle strength is usually normal—may be limited by pain and/or stiffness.
- Muscle tenderness
- Disuse atrophy
- Synovitis of the small joints and tenosynovitis
- Coexisting carpal tunnel syndrome

DIFFERENTIAL DIAGNOSIS
- Rheumatoid arthritis (RA)
- Palindromic rheumatism
- Late-onset seronegative spondyloarthropathies (e.g., psoriatic arthritis, ankylosing spondylitis)
- Systemic lupus erythematosus; Sjögren syndrome; fibromyalgia
- Polymyositis-dermatomyositis (Check creatine phosphokinase, aldolase.)
- Thyroid disease
- Hyperparathyroidism, hypoparathyroidism
- Hypovitaminosis D
- Osteoarthritis
- Rotator cuff syndrome; adhesive capsulitis
- RS3PE syndrome (remitting seronegative symmetrical synovitis with pitting edema)
- Occult infection or malignancy (e.g., lymphoma, leukemia, myeloma, solid tumor)
- Myopathy (e.g., steroid, alcohol, electrolyte depletion)
- Depression

DIAGNOSTIC TESTS & INTERPRETATION
- Consider PMR in patients >50 years of age with proximal pain and stiffness—obtain labs and consider a diagnostic/therapeutic trial of low-dose steroids.
- Temporal artery biopsy if symptoms of GCA present
- ESR (Westergren) elevation >40 mm/hr
  - ESR generally elevated, sometimes >100 mm/hr
  - ESR normal (<40 mm/hr) in 7–22% of patients

- Elevated C-reactive protein
- Normochromic/normocytic anemia
- Anti-cyclic citrullinated peptide (anti-CCP) antibodies usually negative (in contrast to elderly-onset RA)
- Rheumatoid factor (RF): negative (5–10% of patients >60 years have positive RF without RA.)
- Mild elevations in liver function tests, especially alkaline phosphatase
- Antibodies to ferritin peptide may be a useful diagnostic marker.
- Prednisone may alter lab results.
- Other disorders may cause elevation of ESR (e.g., infection, neoplasm, renal failure).
- Normal EMG
- Normal muscle histology

Initial Tests (lab, imaging)
- ESR (usually >40 mm/hr)
- C-reactive protein
- CBC
- MRI is not necessary for diagnosis but may show periarticular inflammation, tenosynovitis, and bursitis.
- US may show bursitis, tendinitis, and synovitis.
- MRI, PET, and temporal artery US may help in diagnosis of PMR.
- Recent ACR/EULAR classification criteria help confirm the clinical diagnosis (3).
- 18F-fluorodeoxyglucose PET scan prior to therapy improves diagnostic accuracy (4).
- A scoring algorithm (3) was devised consisting of the following: morning stiffness >45 minutes (2 points), hip pain/limited ROM (1 point), absence of RF and anti-citrullinated protein antibody (ACPA) (2 points), and absence of peripheral joint pain (1 point).
- A score of >4 has 68% sensitivity and 78% specificity for PMR.

Diagnostic Procedures/Other
Temporal artery biopsy in patients with symptoms suggestive of GCA. Treat empirically pending results.

TREATMENT

GENERAL MEASURES
- Address risk of steroid-induced osteoporosis.
  - Obtain dual energy x-ray absorptiometry and check 25-OH vitamin D levels if necessary.
  - Consider antiresorptive therapies (bisphosphonates) based on recommendations for treatment of corticosteroid-induced osteoporosis.
- Encourage adequate calcium (1,500 mg/day) and vitamin D (800 to 1,000 U/day) supplementation.
- Physical therapy for ROM exercises, if needed

MEDICATION

First Line

- Prednisone: 10 to 20 mg/day PO initially; expect a dramatic (diagnostic) response within days. 15 mg/day is effective in almost all patients.
  - May increase to 20 mg/day if no immediate response
  - If no response to 10 to 20 mg/day within a week, reconsider diagnosis.
- Divided-dose steroids (BID or TID) may be useful initially (especially if symptoms recur in the afternoon).
- Consider using delayed-release prednisone taken at bedtime, which may help treat morning stiffness compared to immediate-release prednisone.
- Begin slow taper by 2.5 mg decrements every 2 to 4 weeks to a dose of 7.5 to 10.0 mg/day. Below this dose, taper by 1 mg/month to prevent relapse.
- Increase prednisone for symptom relapse (common).
- Corticosteroid treatment often lasts several years.
- May stop after 6 to 12 months if symptom free and ESR is normal
- Contraindications
  - Use steroids with caution in patients with chronic heart failure, diabetes mellitus (or other immunocompromised state), and systemic fungal or bacterial infection.
  - Treat any concurrent infections.
- Precautions
  - Long-term steroid use (>2 years) is associated with sodium and water retention, exacerbation of chronic heart failure, hypokalemia, increased susceptibility to infection, osteoporosis, fractures, hypertension, cataracts, glaucoma, avascular necrosis, depression, and weight gain.
  - Patients may develop temporal arteritis while on low-dose corticosteroid treatment for polymyalgia. This requires an increase in dose to 40 to 60 mg.
  - Alternate-day steroids are not effective.

Second Line

- NSAIDs usually are not adequate for pain relief.
- Methotrexate modestly reduces relapse rate and lowers the cumulative dose of steroid therapy.
- There is conflicting evidence for anti-tumor necrosis factor (anti-TNF) agents (infliximab, etanercept).
- Anti–interleukin-6 (anti–IL-6) therapy under study (5,6)
- Corticosteroid injections (shoulder) may help reduce pain and duration of morning stiffness, allowing for increased levels of activity.

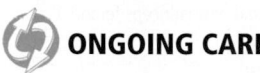 ONGOING CARE

FOLLOW-UP RECOMMENDATIONS

Patient Monitoring

- Monthly evaluations initially and during medication taper; every 3 months otherwise
- Follow ESR as steroids are tapered; ESR and C-reactive protein should decline as symptoms improve.

- Follow up immediately for symptoms of GCA (e.g., headache, visual loss, and diplopia).
- Monitor side effects of corticosteroid therapy (osteoporosis, hypertension, and hyperglycemia).
- If patient is asymptomatic, do not treat elevated ESR (do not increase steroid dose to normalize ESR).

DIET

- Regular diet
- Adequate calcium and vitamin D

PATIENT EDUCATION

- Review adverse effects of corticosteroids.
- Discuss the symptoms of GCA and instruct to present immediately if any occur.
- Follow up if symptoms recur during steroid taper.
- Never abruptly stop steroids.
- Ensure adequate calcium and vitamin D intake.
- Patient resources:
  - Arthritis Foundation: www.arthritis.org/
  - American College of Rheumatology: http://www.rheumatology.org/Practice/Clinical/Patients/Diseases_And_Conditions/Polymyalgia_Rheumatica/

PROGNOSIS

- Most patients require at least 2 years of corticosteroid treatment.
- Exacerbation or relapse is common if steroids tapered too quickly.
- Prognosis is very good with proper treatment.
- Relapse is common (in 25–50% of patients).
- Higher age at diagnosis, female sex, high baseline ESR, increased plasma viscosity, increased levels of soluble IL-6 receptor, or high initial steroid dose have been associated with a prolonged disease course and greater number of disease flares.

COMPLICATIONS

- Complications related to chronic steroid use
- Exacerbation of disease with taper of steroids; development of GCA (may occur when PMR is being treated adequately)

REFERENCES

1. Muratore F, Pazzola G, Pipitone N, et al. Recent advances in the diagnosis and treatment of polymyalgia rheumatica. *Expert Rev Clin Immunol*. 2016;12(10):1037–1045.
2. Mackie SL, Hughes R, Walsh M, et al. "An impediment to living life": why and how should we measure stiffness in polymyalgia rheumatica? *PLoS One*. 2015;10(5):e0126758.
3. Macchioni P, Boiardi L, Catanoso M, et al. Performance of the new 2012 EULAR/ACR classification criteria for polymyalgia rheumatica: comparison with the previous criteria in a single-centre study. *Ann Rheum Dis*. 2014;73(6):1190–1193.
4. Henckaerts L, Gheysens O, Vanderschueren S, et al. Use of 18F-fluorodeoxyglucose positron emission tomography in the diagnosis of polymyalgia rheumatica—a prospective study of 99 patients. *Rheumatology (Oxford)*. 2018;57(11):1908–1916.
5. Matteson EL, Dejaco C. Polymyalgia rheumatica. *Ann Intern Med*. 2017;166(9):ITC65–ITC80.
6. Devauchelle-Pensec V. Has the time come for biotherapies in giant cell arteritis and polymyalgia rheumatica? *Joint Bone Spine*. 2016;83(5): 471–472.

ADDITIONAL READING

- Buttgereit F, Gibofsky A. Delayed-release prednisone—a new approach to an old therapy. *Expert Opin Pharmacother*. 2013;14(8):1097–1106.
- Camellino D, Cimmino MA. Imaging of polymyalgia rheumatica: indications on its pathogenesis, diagnosis and prognosis. *Rheumatology (Oxford)*. 2012;51(1):77–86.
- Dasgupta B, Cimmino MA, Maradit-Kremers H, et al. 2012 Provisional classification criteria for polymyalgia rheumatica: a European League Against Rheumatism/American College of Rheumatology collaborative initiative. *Ann Rheum Dis*. 2012;71(4):484–492.

 SEE ALSO

Arteritis, Temporal; Arthritis, Rheumatoid (RA); Depression; Fibromyalgia; Osteoarthritis; Polymyositis/Dermatomyositis

 CODES

ICD10

- M35.3 Polymyalgia rheumatica
- M31.5 Giant cell arteritis with polymyalgia rheumatica

CLINICAL PEARLS

- Consider PMR in patients >50 years who present with hip, neck, and/or shoulder pain and stiffness.
- A normal ESR does not exclude PMR.
- Corticosteroids are the treatment of choice. If there is not a dramatic and rapid response, reconsider the diagnosis.
- Adjust steroids according to symptoms, not ESR.

POLYMYOSITIS/DERMATOMYOSITIS

Nehal R. Shah, MD • Christopher M. Wise, MD

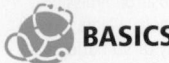

BASICS

DESCRIPTION

- Systemic connective tissue disease characterized by inflammatory and degenerative changes in proximal muscles, sometimes accompanied by characteristic skin rash
  - If skin manifestations (Gottron sign [symmetric, scaly, violaceous, erythematous eruption over the extensor surfaces of the metacarpophalangeal and interphalangeal joints of the fingers]; heliotrope [reddish violaceous eruption on the upper eyelids]) are present, it is designated as dermatomyositis.
  - Different types of myositis include the following (1):
    ○ Idiopathic polymyositis
    ○ Idiopathic dermatomyositis
    ○ Polymyositis/dermatomyositis as an overlap (usually with lupus or systemic sclerosis or as part of mixed connective-tissue disease)
    ○ Myositis associated with malignancy
    ○ Necrotizing autoimmune myositis (often statin associated) (2)
    ○ Inclusion body myositis (IBM), a variant with atypical patterns of weakness and biopsy findings
- System(s) affected: cardiovascular, musculoskeletal, pulmonary, skin/exocrine
- Synonym(s): myositis; inflammatory myopathy; antisynthetase syndrome (subset with certain antibodies)

EPIDEMIOLOGY

Incidence
- Estimated at 1.2 to 19 per million population per year
- Predominant age: 5 to 15 years, 40 to 60 years, peak incidence in mid-40s
- Predominant sex: female > male (2:1)

Prevalence
2.4 to 33.8 patients per 100,000 population

Geriatric Considerations
Elderly patients with myositis or dermatomyositis are at increased risk of neoplasm.

Pediatric Considerations
Childhood dermatomyositis is likely a separate entity associated with cutaneous vasculitis and muscle calcifications.

ETIOLOGY AND PATHOPHYSIOLOGY
- Inflammatory process, mediated by T cells and cytokine release, leading to damage to muscle cells (predominantly skeletal muscles)
- In patients with IBM, degenerative mechanisms may be important.
- Unknown; potential viral, genetic factors

Genetics
Mild association with human leukocyte antigen (HLA)-DR3, HLA-DRw52

RISK FACTORS
Family history of autoimmune disease (e.g., systemic lupus, myositis) or vasculitis

COMMONLY ASSOCIATED CONDITIONS
- Malignancy more common in dermatomyositis
- Progressive systemic sclerosis
- Vasculitis
- Systemic lupus erythematosus (SLE)
- Mixed connective tissue disease

DIAGNOSIS

HISTORY
- Symmetric proximal muscle weakness causing difficulty when
  - Arising from sitting or lying positions
  - Climbing stairs
  - Raising arms
- Joint pain/swelling
- Dysphagia
- Dyspnea
- Rash on face, eyelids, hands, arms

PHYSICAL EXAM
Proximal muscle weakness
- Shoulder muscles
- Hip girdle muscles (trouble standing from seated or squatting position, weak hip flexors in supine position)
- Muscle swelling, stiffness, induration
- Distal muscle weakness is seen only in patients with IBM.
- Rash over face (eyelids, nasolabial folds), upper chest, dorsal hands (especially knuckle pads), fingers ("mechanic's hands")
- Periorbital edema
- Calcinosis cutis (childhood cases)
- Mesenteric arterial insufficiency/infarction (childhood cases)
- Cardiac impairment; arrhythmia, failure

DIFFERENTIAL DIAGNOSIS
- Vasculitis
- Progressive systemic sclerosis
- SLE
- Rheumatoid arthritis
- Muscular dystrophy
- Lambert-Eaton syndrome
- Sarcoidosis
- Amyotrophic lateral sclerosis
- Endocrine disorders
  - Thyroid disease
  - Cushing syndrome
- Infectious myositis (viral, bacterial, parasitic)
- Drug-induced myopathies:
  - Cholesterol-lowering agents (statins)
  - Colchicine
  - Corticosteroids
  - Ethanol
  - Chloroquine
  - Zidovudine
- Electrolyte disorders (magnesium, calcium, potassium)
- Heritable metabolic myopathies
- Sleep apnea syndrome

DIAGNOSTIC TESTS & INTERPRETATION
- Diagnosis of muscle component (myositis) usually relies on four findings:
  - Weakness
  - Creatine kinase (CK) and/or aldolase elevation
  - Abnormal electromyogram (EMG)
  - Findings on muscle biopsy
- Presence of compatible skin rash of dermatomyositis

Initial Tests (lab, imaging)
- Increased CK, aldolase
- Increased serum aspartate aminotransferase (AST)
- Increased lactate dehydrogenase (LDH)
- Myoglobinuria
- Increased ESR
- Positive rheumatoid factor (<50% of patients)
- Positive antinuclear antibody (ANA) (>50% of patients)
- Leukocytosis (<50% of patients)
- Anemia (<50% of patients)
- Hyperglobulinemia (<50% of patients)
- Anti-HMGCR (3-hydroxy-3-methylglutaryl-coenzyme A reductase) and anti-SRP antibodies seen in patient with necrotizing autoimmune myositis
- Antisynthetase antibodies (anti–Jo-1 and non–Jo-1 synthetases) present in antisynthetase syndrome
  - Associated with an increased incidence of interstitial lung disease (ILD)
- Anti–MDA-5 antibody seen in overlap myositis with atypical rashes and severe ILD
- Anti-U1 RNP, anti–PM-Scl, and anti-Ku antibodies seen in overlap myositis
- Chest radiograph as part of initial evaluation to assess for associated pulmonary involvement or malignancy

Follow-Up Tests & Special Considerations
- Changes in muscle enzymes (CK or aldolase) correlate with improvement and worsening.
- MRI to assess muscle edema and inflammation may be used in some patients to determine best biopsy site or response to therapy.

Diagnostic Procedures/Other
- EMG: muscle irritability, low-amplitude potentials, polyphasic action potentials, fibrillations
- Muscle biopsy (deltoid or quadriceps femoris)

Test Interpretation
- Microscopic findings:
  - Muscle fiber degeneration
  - Phagocytosis of muscle debris
  - Perifascicular muscle fiber atrophy
  - Inflammatory cell infiltrates in adult form
  - Via electron microscopy: inclusion bodies (IBM only)
  - Sarcoplasmic basophilia
- Muscle fiber increased in size
- Vasculopathy (childhood polymyositis/dermatomyositis)

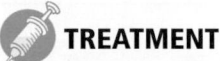 **TREATMENT**

GENERAL MEASURES
General evaluation for malignancy in all adults, particularly with dermatomyositis, at initial evaluation and during follow-up

MEDICATION

First Line
- Prednisone
  - 40 to 80 mg/day PO in divided doses
  - Consolidate doses and reduce prednisone slowly when enzyme levels are normal.
  - Probably need to continue 5 to 10 mg/day for maintenance in most patients
- For steroid-refractory or steroid-dependent patients: azathioprine 1 mg/kg PO (arthritis dose) once daily or BID
  - Methotrexate 10 to 25 mg PO weekly, useful in most steroid-resistant patients
- Rash of dermatomyositis may require topical steroids or oral hydroxychloroquine.
- Patients with IBM have very poor response to steroids and other first- and second-line drugs in general.

Second Line
- Other immunosuppressant drugs (e.g., cyclophosphamide, chlorambucil, cyclosporine, mycophenolate, tacrolimus) can be added to steroids.
- Combination methotrexate and azathioprine also may be useful in refractory cases.
- IVIG (3)[B] and rituximab (4)[B] have been reported to be helpful in a small series of patients with refractory disease. Rituxan may be more effective in patients with autoantibodies positive myositis (especially anti–Jo-1 and anti–Mi-2).
- Contraindications: Methotrexate is contraindicated with previous liver disease, alcohol use, pregnancy, and underlying renal disease (use with extreme caution in patients with serum creatinine >1.5 mg/dL in general).
- Precautions
  - Prednisone: Adverse effects associated with long-term steroid use include adrenal suppression, sodium and water retention, hypokalemia, osteoporosis, cataracts, and increased susceptibility to infection.
  - Azathioprine: Adverse effects include bone marrow suppression, increased liver function tests, and increased risk of infection.
  - Methotrexate: Adverse effects include stomatitis, bone marrow suppression, pneumonitis, and risk of liver fibrosis and cirrhosis with prolonged use.

ISSUES FOR REFERRAL
- Diagnostic uncertainty, usually related to elevated muscle enzymes without typical symptoms of findings of muscle weakness
- Poor response to initial steroid therapy
- Excessive steroid requirement (unable to taper prednisone to <20 mg/day after 4 to 6 months)

SURGERY/OTHER PROCEDURES
None indicated, other than initial biopsy

ADMISSION, INPATIENT, AND NURSING CONSIDERATIONS
- Inability to stand, ambulate
- Respiratory difficulty
- Fever or other signs of infection
- Inpatient evaluation seldom needed

 ONGOING CARE

FOLLOW-UP RECOMMENDATIONS

Patient Monitoring
- Follow muscle enzymes along with muscle strength and functional capacity.
- Monitor for steroid-induced complications (e.g., hypokalemia, hypertension, and hyperglycemia).
- Bone densitometry and consideration of calcium, vitamin D, and bisphosphonate therapy
- If azathioprine, methotrexate, or other immunosuppressant is used, appropriate laboratory monitoring should be done periodically (e.g., hematology, liver enzymes, and creatinine).
- Attempt to decrease and/or discontinue steroid dose as patient responds to therapy.
- Maintain immunosuppression until patient's muscle strength stabilizes for prolonged period depending on individual patient parameters, risks of medication, risk of relapse; time period undefined (months, years)

DIET
Moderation of caloric and sodium intake to avoid weight gain from corticosteroid therapy

PATIENT EDUCATION
- Curtail excess physical activity in early phases when muscle enzymes are markedly elevated.
- Emphasize range of motion exercises.
- Gradually introduce muscle strengthening when muscle enzymes are normal or improved and stable.

PROGNOSIS
- Residual weakness: 30%
- Persistent active disease: 20%
- 5-year survival 65–75%, but mortality is 3- to 5-fold higher than general population. Most of the increase in mortality occurs in the 1st year after diagnosis (5).
- Survival is worse for women and African Americans and those with dermatomyositis, IBM, or cancer.
- Most patients improve with therapy.
- Patient with ILD have poor prognosis.
- Patients with IBM respond poorly to most therapies (6).
- 20–50% have full recovery.

COMPLICATIONS
- Pneumonia
- Infection
- Myocardial infarction
- Carcinoma (especially breast, lung)
- Severe dysphagia
- Respiratory impairment due to muscle weakness, ILD
- Aspiration pneumonitis
- Steroid myopathy
- Steroid-induced diabetes, hypertension, hypokalemia, osteoporosis

REFERENCES
1. Senécal JL, Raynauld JP, Troyanov Y. Editorial: a new classification of adult autoimmune myositis. *Arthritis Rheumatol*. 2017;69(5):878–884.
2. Mammen AL. Statin-associated autoimmune myopathy. *N Engl J Med*. 2016;374(7):664–669.
3. Wang DX, Shu XM, Tian XL, et al. Intravenous immunoglobulin therapy in adult patients with polymyositis/dermatomyositis: a systematic literature review. *Clin Rheumatol*. 2012;31(5):801–806.
4. Fasano S, Gordon P, Hajji R, et al. Rituximab in the treatment of inflammatory myopathies: a review. *Rheumatology (Oxford)*. 2017;56(1):26–36.
5. Dobloug GC, Svensson J, Lundberg IE, et al. Mortality in idiopathic inflammatory myopathy: results from a Swedish nationwide population-based cohort study. *Ann Rheum Dis*. 2018;77(1):40–47.
6. Machado P, Brady S, Hanna MG. Update in inclusion body myositis. *Curr Opin Rheumatol*. 2013;25(6):763–771.

 CODES

ICD10
- M33.20 Polymyositis, organ involvement unspecified
- M33.90 Dermatopolymyositis, unspecified, organ involvement unspecified
- M33.92 Dermatopolymyositis, unspecified with myopathy

CLINICAL PEARLS
- Corticosteroids alone may be sufficient in patients who have rapid improvement in weakness and muscle enzymes. However, most patients require azathioprine, methotrexate, or other immunosuppressive medications.
- The risk of associated malignancy is higher in patients >50 years and in those with cutaneous manifestations.
- Elevated muscle enzymes (e.g., CK and aldolase) are seen frequently as transient phenomena in patients with febrile illness and injuries; may return to normal on repeat
- In patients with persistently elevated muscle enzymes and symptoms and findings of muscle weakness, EMG followed by muscle biopsy should be the initial studies considered.
- Suspect IBM in older patients with very slow onset and progression of symptoms, poor response to steroids and immunosuppressive therapy, and atypical patterns (asymmetric, sometimes distal) of muscle weakness.
- Suspect autoimmune necrotizing myositis in patients who develop myopathy while taking lipid-lowering drugs (statins) but fail to improve or worsen after withdrawal of statin therapy.

POPLITEAL (BAKER) CYST
Shane L. Larson, MD • Adriel G. Dizon, MD

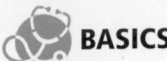 **BASICS**

DESCRIPTION
- A fluid-filled synovial sac arising in the popliteal fossa as a distention of (typically) the gastrocnemial-semimembranous bursa; not a true cyst
- Can be unilateral or bilateral
- Most frequent cystic mass around the knee
- Primary cysts are a distention of the bursa (arise independently without an intra-articular disorder).
- Secondary cysts occur if there is a communication between the bursa and knee joint, allowing articular fluid to fill the cyst.
- Associated with synovial inflammation

EPIDEMIOLOGY
Incidence
- Bimodal distribution
  - Children ages 4 to 7 years
  - Adults increasing with age
- Primary cysts usually seen in children <15 years
- Secondary cysts seen in adults

Prevalence
- Variable adult prevalence of 19–47% in symptomatic knees and 2–5% in asymptomatic knees
- In children: 6.3% in symptomatic knees; 2.4% in asymptomatic knees

ETIOLOGY AND PATHOPHYSIOLOGY
Associated intra-articular pathology includes
- Meniscal tears, mostly of the posterior horn
- Anterior cruciate ligament (ACL) insufficiency
- Degenerative articular cartilage lesions
- Rheumatoid arthritis (20%)
- Osteoarthritis (50%)
- Osteochondritis
- Gout (14%)
- Other potential factors
  - Infectious arthritis
  - Polyarthritis
  - Villonodular synovitis
  - Lymphoma
  - Sarcoidosis
  - Connective tissue diseases
- Extension or herniation of synovial membrane of the knee joint capsule or connection of normal bursa with the joint capsule
- May result from increased intra-articular pressure
- Commonly seen with knee effusions
- Direct trauma to the bursa is likely the primary cause in children because of no communication between the bursa and the joint.
- A valve-like mechanism allowing one-way passage of fluid from the joint to the bursal connection has been described.

RISK FACTORS
- Osteoarthritis of knee (most common)
- Rheumatoid arthritis
- Meniscal degeneration or tear
- Advancing age
- Ligamentous insufficiency

COMMONLY ASSOCIATED CONDITIONS
Any condition causing knee joint effusion

 DIAGNOSIS

HISTORY
- Painless mass arising in the popliteal fossa
- Most cysts are asymptomatic.
- Dull ache if cyst is large enough to impede joint motion—typically a restriction of flexion
- Painful if cyst ruptures
- Large cysts may cause entrapment neuropathy of the tibial nerve.
- Vascular compression, most commonly of the popliteal vein, may produce claudication or thrombophlebitis.
- Activity alters the cyst size.

PHYSICAL EXAM
- Examine in full extension and 90 degrees of flexion.
- Foucher sign: Mass increases with extension and disappears with flexion.
- Most commonly found in medial aspect of popliteal fossa lateral to the head of the gastrocnemius and medial to the neurovascular bundle

- Cyst is easiest to palpate when knee is slightly flexed and may occasionally be fluctuant or tender.
- Transillumination helps distinguish cyst from solid mass.
- Ruptured cysts are typically painful with associated swelling and bruising over the ipsilateral calf and ankle at the medial malleolus (crescent sign).
- Ruptured cysts also are associated with pseudothrombophlebitis, and rarely, compartment syndrome (1).

DIFFERENTIAL DIAGNOSIS
- Infection/abscess
- Lipoma, liposarcoma
- Fibroma, fibrosarcoma
- Hematoma
- Deep venous thrombosis (DVT)
- Vascular tumor
- Popliteal vein varices
- Xanthoma
- Aneurysm (rare)
- Ganglion cyst
- Thrombophlebitis
- Muscular herniation (rare, related to trauma)

DIAGNOSTIC TESTS & INTERPRETATION
Initial Tests (lab, imaging)
- CBC, ESR (if septic arthritis suspected)
- Ensure not a popliteal aneurysm prior to aspiration. Send aspirate for cell count and culture to determine if fluid is infectious, inflammatory, or mechanical.
- Ultrasound confirms presence and size; Doppler can differentiate Baker cysts from popliteal vessel aneurysms, DVT, or soft tissue tumors (2).
- MRI helps assess derangements of internal joint structures and to identify cyst leakage.

Follow-Up Tests & Special Considerations
- Consider observation over invasive testing in children.
- Radiographs may show soft tissue density posteriorly.

- Arthrography may demonstrate communication with joint capsule or rupture.
- CT arthrography is superior for visualizing cystic details and can help distinguish lipomas, aneurysms, and malignancies from cysts.

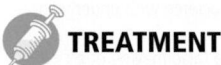 TREATMENT

GENERAL MEASURES
- No treatment if asymptomatic
- Treat any associated underlying conditions.
- Compressive wrap or sleeve for comfort

MEDICATION
If etiology is identified from cellular fluid examination, treat the underlying condition.

First Line
Analgesics and NSAIDs for symptomatic relief

ADDITIONAL THERAPIES
- Physical therapy improves knee ROM and strength, particularly with coexisting pathology.
- Temporary relief with needle aspiration; recurrence common
- Improvement in joint ROM, knee pain, swelling, accompanied reduction in bursa size after aspiration, and intra-articular/intracystic corticosteroid injection (3)[B]
- A combination of physical therapy and corticosteroid injection with or without aspiration leads to best improvements in pain, function, and reduction in cyst size (4)[A].
- Sclerotherapy injections of ethanol or dextrose/sodium morrhuate shown to have good results in small studies (5)[B].

SURGERY/OTHER PROCEDURES
- Consider excision when symptoms persist despite treatment or no etiology is found.
- Surgery usually not required in children
- Recurrence after standard surgery is common and is highest if chondral lesions are present.
- Arthroscopic surgery is highly successful if a valvular mechanism is identified and intra-articular pathology is treated (6)[B].
- Excision via arthroscopy or open procedure often requires concomitant treatment of underlying pathology.

 ONGOING CARE

PROGNOSIS
- Variable; many cysts remain asymptomatic.
- Some cysts resolve with treatment of underlying etiology (e.g., gout, rheumatoid arthritis).
- In children, most cysts resolve without treatment.

COMPLICATIONS
- Compartment syndrome in ruptured cyst
- Thrombophlebitis from compression of the popliteal vein
- Infection of popliteal cyst
- Hemorrhage into cyst if on anticoagulants

REFERENCES

1. Chatzopoulos D, Moralidis E, Markou P, et al. Baker's cysts in knees with chronic osteoarthritic pain: a clinical, ultrasonographic, radiographic and scintigraphic evaluation. *Rheumatol Int*. 2008;29(2):141–146.
2. Sanchez JE, Conkling N, Labropoulos N. Compression syndromes of the popliteal neurovascular bundle due to Baker cyst. *J Vasc Surg*. 2011;54(6):1821–1829.
3. Acebes JC, Sánchez-Pernaute O, Díaz-Oca A, et al. Ultrasonographic assessment of Baker's cysts after intra-articular corticosteroid injection in knee osteoarthritis. *J Clin Ultrasound*. 2006;34(3):113–117.
4. Di Sante L, Paoloni M, Dimaggio M, et al. Ultrasound-guided aspiration and corticosteroid injection compared to horizontal therapy for treatment of knee osteoarthritis complicated with Baker's cyst: a randomized, controlled trial. *Eur J Phys Rehabil Med*. 2012;48(4):561–567.
5. Centeno CJ, Schultz J, Freeman M. Sclerotherapy of Baker's cyst with imaging confirmation of resolution. *Pain Physician*. 2008;11(2):257–261.
6. Lie CW, Ng TP. Arthroscopic treatment of popliteal cyst. *Hong Kong Med J*. 2011;17(3):180–183.

ADDITIONAL READING

- Akagi R, Saisu T, Segawa Y, et al. Natural history of popliteal cysts in the pediatric population. *J Pediatr Orthop*. 2013;33(3):262–268.
- Akgul O, Guldeste Z, Ozgocmen S. The reliability of the clinical examination for detecting Baker's cyst in asymptomatic fossa. *Int J Rheum Dis*. 2014;17(2):204–209.
- Chen JC, Lu CC, Lu YM, et al. A modified surgical method for treating Baker's cyst in children. *Knee*. 2008;15(1):9–14.
- Frush TJ, Noyes FR. Baker's cyst: diagnostic and surgical considerations. *Sports Health*. 2015;7(4):359–365.
- Herman AM, Marzo JM. Popliteal cysts: a current review. *Orthopedics*. 2014;37(8):e678–e684.

 SEE ALSO

Algorithm: Knee Pain

 CODES

ICD10
- M71.20 Synovial cyst of popliteal space [Baker], unspecified knee
- M71.21 Synovial cyst of popliteal space [Baker], right knee
- M71.22 Synovial cyst of popliteal space [Baker], left knee

CLINICAL PEARLS

- Conservative treatment of Baker cysts is preferred in children, as most will spontaneously resolve.
- In adults, treatment of underlying cause may resolve Baker cysts.
- Pain, bruising, and swelling over the medial malleolus (crescent sign) suggest cyst rupture.

PORTAL HYPERTENSION

Walter M. Kim, MD, PhD • Jyoti Ramakrishna, MD, MPH

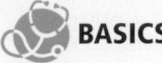 BASICS

DESCRIPTION
- Increased portal venous pressure >5 mm Hg that occurs in association with splanchnic vasodilatation, portosystemic collateral formation, and hyperdynamic circulation
- Most commonly secondary to elevated hepatic venous pressure gradient (HVPG; the gradient between portal and central venous pressures)
- Course is generally progressive, with risk of complications including acute variceal bleeding, ascites, hepatic encephalopathy, and hepatorenal syndrome.

EPIDEMIOLOGY
Incidence
- Prevalence: <200,000 persons in the United States
- Predominant age: adult
- Predominant sex: male > female

ETIOLOGY AND PATHOPHYSIOLOGY
- Causes generally classified as follows:
  - Prehepatic (portal vein thrombosis or obstruction)
  - Intrahepatic (most commonly cirrhosis)
  - Posthepatic (hepatic vein thrombosis, Budd-Chiari syndrome, right-sided heart failure)
- 90% of intrahepatic cases are due to cirrhosis secondary to the following:
  - Virus (hepatitis B, hepatitis C, hepatitis D)
  - Alcoholism
  - Nonalcoholic fatty liver disease
  - Schistosomiasis
  - Wilson disease
  - Hemochromatosis
  - Primary biliary cirrhosis (PBC)
  - Sarcoidosis
- Increased HVPG results in venous collateral formation in the distal esophagus, proximal stomach, rectum, and umbilicus.
- Gastroesophageal variceal formation is found in 40% of patients with portal hypertension.
- Progression of portal hypertension results in splanchnic vasodilation and angiogenesis.

Genetics
No known genetic patterns except those associated with specific hepatic diseases that cause portal hypertension

RISK FACTORS
See "Etiology and Pathophysiology."

Pediatric Considerations
In children, portal vein thrombosis is the most common extrahepatic cause; intrahepatic causes are more likely to be biliary atresia, viral hepatitis, and metabolic liver disease.

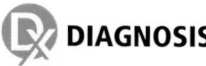 DIAGNOSIS

HISTORY
- Ascites; symptoms of heart failure including chest pain, shortness of breath, and/or edema
- Hematemesis
- Melena
- Oliguria
- Jaundice
- Weakness/fatigue

- History of chronic liver disease
- Alcoholic hepatitis
- Alcohol abuse

PHYSICAL EXAM
- Exam findings may be general or related to specific complications.
- General
  - Pallor
  - Icterus
  - Digital clubbing
  - Palmar erythema
  - Splenomegaly
  - Caput medusa
  - Spider angiomata
  - Umbilical bruit
  - Hemorrhoids
  - Gynecomastia
  - Testicular atrophy
- Gastroesophageal varices
  - Hypotension
  - Tachycardia
- Ascites
  - Distended abdomen
  - Fluid wave
  - Shifting dullness with percussion
- Hepatic encephalopathy
  - Confusion/coma
  - Asterixis
  - Hyperreflexia

DIFFERENTIAL DIAGNOSIS
Usually related to specific presentations
- Gastroesophageal varices with hemorrhage
  - Portal hypertensive gastropathy
  - Hemorrhagic gastritis
  - Peptic ulcer disease
  - Mallory-Weiss tear
- Ascites
  - Spontaneous bacterial peritonitis (SBP)
  - Pancreatic ascites
  - Peritoneal carcinomatosis
  - Tuberculous peritonitis
  - Hepatic malignancy
  - Fluid overload from heart failure
  - Nephrotic syndrome
- Hepatic encephalopathy
  - Delirium tremens
  - Intracranial hemorrhage
  - Sedative abuse
  - Uremia
- Hepatorenal syndrome
  - Drug nephrotoxicity
  - Renal tubular necrosis

DIAGNOSTIC TESTS & INTERPRETATION
Initial Tests (lab, imaging)
Direct calculation of HVPG (approximation of the gradient in pressure between portal vein and IVC) is the gold standard in diagnosing portal hypertension:
- HVPG = wedged hepatic venous pressure (WHVP) – free hepatic venous pressure (FHVP)
- WHVP is estimated by occlusion of the hepatic vein by a balloon catheter and measurement of the proximal static column of blood.
- FHVP is estimated by direct measurement of the patent hepatic vein, intra-abdominal inferior vena cava, or right atrium.

- Esophageal varices generally develop when HVPG >10 mm Hg in compensated cirrhosis and HVPG >16 mm Hg in decompensated cirrhosis.
- Nonspecific changes associated with underlying disease:
  - Hypersplenism: anemia (also may be due to malnutrition or bleeding), leukopenia, thrombocytopenia
  - Hepatic dysfunction
    - Hypoalbuminemia
    - Hyperbilirubinemia
    - Elevated alkaline phosphatase
    - Elevated liver enzymes (AST, ALT)
    - Abnormal clotting (prothrombin time, international normalized ratio, partial thromboplastin time)
  - GI bleeding
    - Iron deficiency anemia
    - Elevated serum ammonia
    - Fecal occult blood
    - Thrombocytopenia
  - Hepatorenal syndrome
    - Elevated serum creatinine (Cr), blood urea nitrogen (BUN)
    - Urine Na <5 mEq/L (<20 mmol/L)
  - US and CT scan/MRI may detect cirrhosis, splenomegaly, ascites, and varices.
  - US/duplex Doppler
    - Can determine presence and direction of flow in portal and hepatic veins
    - Useful in diagnosing portal vein thrombosis, shunt thrombosis, or the presence of ascites
  - CT scan/MRI: angiographic measurement of hepatic venous wedge pressure via jugular or femoral vein
    - Correlates with portal pressure
    - Risk of variceal bleeding is increased if HVPG >12 mm Hg.
  - Upper GI series may outline varices in esophagus and stomach.
  - Transient elastography is a noninvasive method to determine hepatic fibrosis and to predict portal hypertension (1).

Diagnostic Procedures/Other
- Diagnostic paracentesis and calculation of the serum-ascites albumin gradient (SAAG) can differentiate between portal hypertensive (SAAG >1.1 g/dL) from nonportal hypertensive (SAAG <1.1 g/dL) causes of ascites.
- Endoscopy can diagnose esophageal and gastric varices and portal hypertensive gastropathy.

Test Interpretation
Specific for underlying disease

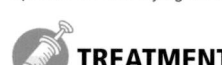 TREATMENT

GENERAL MEASURES
- Avoid sedatives that may precipitate encephalopathy.
- Limit sodium intake because cirrhotic patients avidly retain sodium (<2 g sodium per day).

MEDICATION
Therapy for encephalopathy: See "Hepatic Encephalopathy."

First Line

- Prophylaxis against variceal bleeding (2,3)[A]:
  - Nonselective β-blockade
    - Nadolol: 20 to 40 mg PO once-daily dosing
    - Propranolol: Start with 20 to 40 mg PO BID to TID.
  - May consider carvedilol: 6.25 mg PO once-daily dosing as an alternative β-blocker (4)[C]
  - Doses may be titrated up as tolerated to maximum recommended doses; goal resting heart rate of 55 to 60 bpm
- Therapy for acute variceal hemorrhage:
  - Octreotide: 50 μg IV bolus followed by 50 μg/hr continuous infusion; pediatric dose: 1 μg/kg bolus followed by 1 μg/kg/hr is used traditionally; treat for up to 5 days.
  - Vasopressin: Start with 0.2 to 0.4 U/min IV; increase to maximum dose 0.8 U/min as needed; pediatric dose: 0.002 to 0.005 U/kg/min; do not exceed 0.01 U/kg/min. After bleeding stops, continue at same dose for 12 hours and then taper off over 24 to 48 hours.
- For prevention of recurrence and for overall reduction in mortality:
  - Nadolol: 40 to 80 mg/day PO reduces portal venous blood inflow by blocking the adrenergic dilatation of the mesenteric arterioles.
  - Propranolol: 10 to 60 mg/day PO BID to QID; pediatric dose: 0.5 to 1.0 mg/kg/day PO divided q6–8h
  - Tetrandrine, a calcium channel blocker, also has been found to reduce the rate of rebleeding with fewer side effects.
- Initial treatment for ascites (along with salt and fluid restriction):
  - Furosemide: 20 to 40 mg/day PO; pediatric dose: 1 to 2 mg/kg/dose PO ± IV albumin infusion
  - Spironolactone: 50 to 100 mg/day PO; pediatric dose: 1 to 3 mg/kg/day PO

Second Line

- Terlipressin (2 mg IV q4h; titrate down to 1 mg IV q4h once hemorrhage is controlled; may be used for up to 48 hours) is a more selective splanchnic vasoconstrictor and may be associated with fewer complications. It is currently used when standard therapy with somatostatin or octreotide fails.
- Addition of nitrates, such as nitroglycerin or isosorbide mononitrate, reduces portal pressures and bleeding rates and has been shown to reduce mortality. Because the risk–benefit ratio is not clear, nitrates are not considered first-line treatment.
- Studies are ongoing for possible benefits of other agents including simvastatin, clonidine, verapamil, and losartan.

ISSUES FOR REFERRAL

Patients with portal hypertension should be managed longitudinally by both a primary care physician and a gastroenterologist.

SURGERY/OTHER PROCEDURES

- Treatments available for specific complications of portal hypertension (in addition to or if refractory to medications):
  - Gastroesophageal varices without hemorrhage
    - Endoscopic variceal ligation (EVL) is the preferred therapy for prevention of bleeding of large (grade III) varices and requires serial interventions every 2 to 8 weeks until the varices are eradicated.
  - Gastroesophageal varices with hemorrhage
    - EVL or sclerosis (the first-line treatment in many cases for acute hemorrhage) within 12 hours of presentation (5)[A]

- Balloon tamponade (not used commonly when endoscopic treatment is available)
    - Transjugular intrahepatic portosystemic shunt (TIPS)
    - Portacaval shunting
  - Ascites refractory to medical management
    - Large-volume paracentesis
    - Peritoneovenous shunt
    - TIPS
- Liver transplantation should be considered for patients with advanced disease.

ADMISSION, INPATIENT, AND NURSING CONSIDERATIONS

- Acute GI bleeding should be managed in the inpatient setting, either on the regular medical floor if the patient is hemodynamically stable or in the ICU if the patient is unstable.
- Patients with mental status changes from encephalopathy need to be evaluated in the inpatient setting.
- Admission criteria/initial stabilization
  - Acute bleeding from the intestinal tract, either vomiting or per rectum
  - Acute confusional state/mental status changes
  - If acute variceal bleeding:
    - Type and cross patient's blood.
    - Initial resuscitation with isotonic fluid until packed RBCs are available
    - Correct coagulopathy with vitamin K and fresh frozen plasma (FFP).
    - Endoscopy as soon as the patient is stabilized (for diagnosis and treatment)
  - Avoid sedatives that may precipitate encephalopathy.
  - Limit sodium administration because cirrhotic patients avidly retain sodium.
  - Restrict protein only if encephalopathic.

ALERT

If the patient is an active alcohol drinker, assess for alcoholic hepatitis and watch for signs and symptoms of withdrawal. Follow inpatient protocols for alcohol withdrawal management.

- Use isotonic fluid for hydration.
- Discharge criteria
  - For GI bleeding:
    - No active bleeding in 24 hours
    - Stable hemoglobin and hematocrit
    - Hemodynamically stable (especially heart rate)
  - For encephalopathy: improvement in or resolution of mental status changes to baseline

 ## ONGOING CARE

DIET

In patients with cirrhosis, sodium restriction is important because cirrhotic patients avidly retain sodium.

PATIENT EDUCATION

Refrain from drinking alcohol. Resources for patients who have difficulty with not drinking alcohol can be obtained from Alcoholics Anonymous at http://www.aa.org/.

PROGNOSIS

- Hepatic reserve defined by Child-Pugh classification: rating based on encephalopathy, ascites, bilirubin, albumin, prothrombin
- Variceal bleeding
  - 1/3 of patients with known varices will bleed eventually.
  - 50% rebleed, usually within 2 years, unless portal pressure is reduced by surgical or TIPS procedure.
  - 15–20% mortality rate

- Ascites and encephalopathy often recur.
- Prognosis of patients with ascites is poor: 50% 1-year survival without liver transplant (compared with 90% for patients with cirrhosis and no ascites).

REFERENCES

1. Leung JC, Loong TC, Pang J, et al. Invasive and non-invasive assessment of portal hypertension. *Hepatol Int*. 2018;12(Suppl 1):44–55.
2. Hayes PC, Davis JM, Lewis JA, et al. Meta-analysis of value of propranolol in prevention of variceal haemorrhage. *Lancet*. 1990;336(8708):153–156.
3. Garcia-Tsao G, Abraldes JG, Berzigotti A, et al. Portal hypertensive bleeding in cirrhosis: risk stratification, diagnosis, and management: 2016 practice guidance by the American Association for the Study of Liver Diseases. *Hepatology*. 2017;65(1):310–335.
4. Zacharias AP, Jeyaraj R, Hobolth L, et al. Carvedilol versus traditional, non-selective beta-blockers for adults with cirrhosis and gastroesophageal varices. *Cochrane Database Syst Rev*. 2018;(10):CD011510.
5. de Franchis R; for Baveno VI Faculty. Expanding consensus in portal hypertension: report of the Baveno VI Consensus Workshop: stratifying risk and individualizing care for portal hypertension. *J Hepatol*. 2015;63(3):743–752.

ADDITIONAL READING

- Baffy G. Origins of portal hypertension in nonalcoholic fatty liver disease. *Dig Dis Sci*. 2018;63(3):563–576.
- Bloom S, Kemp W, Lubel J. Portal hypertension: pathophysiology, diagnosis and management. *Intern Med J*. 2015;45(1):16–26.
- Grammatikopoulos T, McKiernan PJ, Dhawan A. Portal hypertension and its management in children. *Arch Dis Child*. 2018;103(2):186–191.
- Sanyal AJ, Bosch J, Blei A, et al. Portal hypertension and its complications. *Gastroenterology*. 2008;134(6):1715–1728.

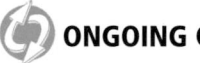 ## CODES

ICD10

K76.6 Portal hypertension

CLINICAL PEARLS

- Portal hypertension can be diagnosed based on physical examination in the setting of known risk factors, specifically cirrhosis.
- Endoscopic treatment is successful for acute variceal hemorrhage 85% of the time.
- Prognosis of patients with ascites is poor: 50% 1-year survival without liver transplant (compared with 90% for patients with cirrhosis and no ascites).
- Advantages and disadvantages of balloon tamponade for acute variceal bleed:
  - Advantages include rapid and often effective control of bleeding (30–90%) and common availability of device.
  - Disadvantages include recurrence of bleeding when balloon is deflated, patient discomfort, and risk of esophageal perforation.

POSTCONCUSSION SYNDROME (MILD TRAUMATIC BRAIN INJURY)

Eric M. Bankert, DO • Vicki R. Nelson, MD, PhD

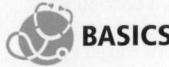 **BASICS**

DESCRIPTION

- Postconcussion syndrome (PCS) is a constellation of symptoms involving physical, cognitive, and/or behavioral symptoms persisting after a concussion (mild traumatic brain injury [mTBI]) and may continue for weeks to years (1).
- It is unclear when concussive symptoms become postconcussive syndrome. A recent consensus defines persistent symptoms as lasting >10 to 14 days in adults and 4 weeks in children (2).
- Symptoms of PCS include (1)
  - Cognitive
    ○ Poor focus
    ○ Poor organization
    ○ Diminished academic/intellectual performance
    ○ Slowed response time
  - Physical
    ○ Headache
    ○ Nausea
    ○ Visual changes
    ○ Light and noise sensitivity
    ○ Tinnitus
    ○ Dizziness and balance problems
    ○ Fatigue and sleep disturbance
  - Behavioral
    ○ Depression
    ○ Irritability/emotional lability
    ○ Apathy
    ○ Increased sensitivity to alcohol
- Diagnosis is based on history and clinical symptoms.

EPIDEMIOLOGY

Incidence
The reported range of mTBI patients who develop PCS varies between 5% and 80%.
- Largely due to difficulty differentiating postconcussion *symptoms* from PCS
- 80–90% of concussion victims recover from postconcussion *symptoms* within 7 to 10 days, slightly longer in children/adolescents (2). A diagnosis of PCS is made in patients with persistent concussive symptoms.

Prevalence
Predominant sex: female > male. Female gender is not universally considered a risk factor.

ETIOLOGY AND PATHOPHYSIOLOGY
- Controversial; exact mechanism(s) unknown
- Microscopic axonal injury from shearing forces leads to inflammation causing secondary brain injury.
- Conflicting data on structural brain damage and correlation of imaging with physical symptoms (1)

- Because the pathophysiology of PCS is not well understood and because of symptom overlap with other psychiatric conditions, PCS remains a difficult condition to diagnose and to manage.
  - Only some with mTBI develop PCS; it is unclear what causes PCS symptoms to persist.
  - Behavioral factors are commonly associated with (and may play a role in) the development of PCS. It can be challenging to differentiate some behavioral disorders from PCS (1).
  - Neuropsychiatry evaluation helps differentiate PCS from other behavioral disorders.
  - Patients who reported high symptom burden following mTBI are at increased risk of PCS (3)[B].

RISK FACTORS
- Strongest predictor is severity of initial symptoms (2).
- Increased odds of PCS if initial symptoms include retrograde amnesia, difficulty concentrating, disorientation, insomnia, loss of balance, sensitivity to noise, or visual disturbance (4)
- Preexisting psychiatric disease including depression, anxiety, personality disorder, and posttraumatic stress disorder (PTSD)
- Preexisting expectation of poor outcomes following mTBI (1)
- Nonsport concussion/mTBI
- Unclear if previous history of concussion(s) is a risk factor for PCS
- Low socioeconomic status
- Loss of consciousness not predictive of PCS

GENERAL PREVENTION
- Education of players, coaches, parents, and athletic trainers about concussion, PCS, and appropriate safety rules
- Head injury precautions are advised. Evidence is lacking that these decrease incidence of mTBI/PCS.
- Screening and intervention for anxiety and depression

COMMONLY ASSOCIATED CONDITIONS
- PTSD
- Anxiety
- Depression
- Fibromyalgia
- Personality disorders (namely, compulsive, histrionic, and narcissistic)
- ADHD

DIAGNOSIS

HISTORY
- Detailed history of recent impact and closed head injury, including:
  - Mechanism
  - Timing of injury related to symptoms
  - Previous head injuries, including concussion, and timing of those injuries

  - Previous medical, psychiatric, or social history
  - Thorough characterization of associated symptoms, intensity, and duration
- Report of neurologic, cognitive, or behavioral symptoms by patient/family

PHYSICAL EXAM
Complete neurologic exam, including the following:
- Glasgow Coma Scale (GCS)
- Anxiety/depression screening
  - Patient Health Questionnaire-9 (PHQ-9)
  - GAD-7
- Sport Concussion Assessment Tool (SCAT), NFL Sideline Concussion Assessment Tool, or computerized neuropsychological (CNP) (2)

DIFFERENTIAL DIAGNOSIS
- Postconcussive symptoms
- PTSD
- Anxiety/depression
- Personality disorders
- Migraine headaches
- Chronic fatigue syndrome, fibromyalgia
- Evolving intracranial hemorrhage
- Exposure to toxins, including prescription and recreational drugs
- Endocrine/metabolic abnormality

DIAGNOSTIC TESTS & INTERPRETATION
Initial Tests (lab, imaging)
- Consider infection, intoxication, and endocrine or metabolic abnormality in appropriate clinical setting.
- Brain imaging both on initial evaluation of mTBI and PCS is not routinely indicated.
- Imaging to evaluate for bleeding is appropriate with comorbidities or anticoagulation therapy.
- Imaging indicated if cervical spine injury is suspected

Follow-Up Tests & Special Considerations
- Several computerized neuropsychiatric (cNP) tests guide return-to-play decisions; if baseline testing is available, compare scores.
- Formal neuropsychiatric evaluations are likely superior to cNP testing when available. None of these tests should be used alone for decision making, especially if a patient is still symptomatic (1,2)[C].
- Common neuropsychological testing programs
  - Immediate Post-Concussion Assessment and Cognitive Testing (ImPACT)
  - Post-Concussion Symptom Scale (PCSS)
  - Balance Error Scoring System (BESS)
  - Axon Sports Computerized Cognitive Assessment Tool (CCAT)
  - Automated Neuropsychological Assessment Metrics (ANAM)

TREATMENT

GENERAL MEASURES

- Return to full activity should progress according to recommendations, which include immediate cognitive rest in the acute period (24 to 48 hours) followed by gradual return to daily activities as tolerated (1,2)[C].
- Controlling cognitive stress and allowing for extra school accommodations may be beneficial (2).
- Restrict individuals with concussion or PCS from sport activity until symptoms have resolved and patients have been weaned from any medications that might mask PCS symptoms (1,2)[C].
- Physical therapy for coexisting cervical and vestibular injuries is beneficial. Cognitive-behavioral therapy helps address persistent mood issues (3).
- Limited evidence that pharmacotherapy is beneficial
- Subthreshold exercise helps resolve symptoms (5)[B].

MEDICATION

First Line

Headache/neck pain

- Nonopioid pain control (e.g., NSAIDs) preferred
  - With use of opioid medications, sedation obscures cognitive evaluation.
  - Possible association between the use of opiates and increased risk of anxiety/depression in PCS patients
  - Consider occipital nerve block.

ALERT

Avoid opiates and benzodiazepines.

- Depression/sleep disorders
  - Anxiety/depression screening starting in the 1st week post-mTBI
    - Melatonin for sleep (up to 3 mg in older children and 5 mg in adolescents and adults)
    - Tricyclic antidepressants (e.g., amitriptyline 10 to 25 mg at night) or trazodone (25 to 50 mg at night) may help with concomitant sleep disturbance.
    - SSRIs (e.g., sertraline 25 mg daily titrated to effective dose with maximum 200 mg daily) for persistent depressive symptoms
  - Consider referral to behavioral health specialist(s).
- Cognitive disorders
  - Evaluation by neuropsychologist
  - Consider SSRIs, especially if concomitant anxiety/depression.

ISSUES FOR REFERRAL

- Neuropsychiatric therapy including comprehensive cognitive evaluation for potential TBI rehabilitation
- Cognitive-behavioral therapy for anxiety and depression symptoms
- Occupational therapy for vocational rehabilitation

- Physical therapy for vestibular rehabilitation
- Neurology referral if primary care interventions for seizures, headache, vertigo, or cognition are unsuccessful
- Substance abuse counseling, if needed

COMPLEMENTARY & ALTERNATIVE MEDICINE

- Massage therapy/osteopathic manipulative treatment for headache and neck pain
- Potential benefits shown with hyperbaric oxygen therapy in military veterans with concurrent PCS and PTSD (6)

ONGOING CARE

FOLLOW-UP RECOMMENDATIONS

Schedule regular follow-up to evaluate for persistent symptoms, efficacy of and/or need for neuropsychiatric evaluation, and the efficacy of and/or need for pharmacologic therapy.

Patient Monitoring

- Consider serial neuropsychological testing.
- Follow return-to-play guidelines (2)[C].

PATIENT EDUCATION

- Centers for Disease Control and Prevention: http://www.cdc.gov/headsup/
- Brain Injury Association of America: http://www.biausa.org/; (800) 444–6443

PROGNOSIS

- Prognosis generally is good.
- Adolescents may recover more slowly than adults.

COMPLICATIONS

- Repeat head injury or return to play before resolution of PCS can worsen/prolong symptoms.
- Case studies of second-impact syndrome, a rare but potentially fatal condition owing to a second head injury soon after the first, have been reported.

REFERENCES

1. Harmon KG, Drezner JA, Gammons M, et al. American Medical Society for Sports Medicine position statement: concussion in sport. *Br J Sports Med*. 2013;47(1):15–26.
2. McCrory P, Meeuwisse W, Dvořák J, et al. Consensus statement on concussion in sport—the 5th International Conference on Concussion in Sport held in Berlin, October 2016. *Br J Sports Med*. 2017;51(11):838–847.

3. Meehan WP III, Mannix R, Monuteaux MC, et al. Early symptom burden predicts recovery after sport-related concussion. *Neurology*. 2014;83(24): 2204–2210.
4. Kerr ZY, Zuckerman SL, Wasserman EB, et al. Factors associated with post-concussion syndrome in high school student-athletes. *J Sci Med Sport*. 2018;21(5):447–452.
5. Leddy JJ, Willer B. Use of graded exercise testing in concussion and return-to-activity management. *Curr Sports Med Rep*. 2013;12(6):370–376.
6. Harch PG, Andrews SR, Fogarty EF, et al. Case control study: hyperbaric oxygen treatment of mild traumatic brain injury persistent post-concussion syndrome and post-traumatic stress disorder. *Med Gas Res*. 2017;7(3):156–174.

ADDITIONAL READING

- Morgan CD, Zuckerman SL, Lee YM, et al. Predictors of postconcussion syndrome after sports-related concussion in young athletes: a matched case-control study. *J Neurosurg Pediatr*. 2015;15(6): 589–598.
- Schneider KJ, Leddy JJ, Guskiewicz KM, et al. Rest and treatment/rehabilitation following sport-related concussion: a systematic review. *Br J Sports Med*. 2017;51(12):930–934.

SEE ALSO

Concussion (Mild Traumatic Brain Injury)

CODES

ICD10

- F07.81 Postconcussional syndrome
- S06.9X0A Unsp intracranial injury w/o loss of consciousness, init
- S06.9X9A Unsp intracranial injury w LOC of unsp duration, init

CLINICAL PEARLS

- Imaging rarely useful for PCS. If necessary, head CT is the test of choice for acute injury to exclude intracranial bleeding.
- Coordinate multidisciplinary treatment plans for patients with persistent symptoms.
- Return to play/activity should not occur until the athlete is asymptomatic (or has returned to pre-event baseline).

POSTTRAUMATIC STRESS DISORDER (PTSD)

Crystal Haydee Chavez, MD • Fozia Akhtar Ali, MD • Chi Nguyen Stasio, DO

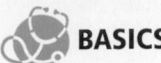 **BASICS**

DESCRIPTION

- Posttraumatic stress disorder (PTSD) is an anxiety disorder defined as a reaction that can occur after exposure to an extreme traumatic event involving death, threat of death, serious physical injury, or a threat to physical integrity.
- This reaction has three cardinal characteristics:
  - Reexperiencing the trauma
  - Avoidance of anything related to the traumatic event and/or numbing of general responsiveness
  - Increased arousal
- Traumatic events that may trigger PTSD include natural/human disasters, serious accidents, war, sexual abuse, rape, torture, terrorism, hostage taking, or being diagnosed with life-threatening disease.
- PTSD can be:
  - Acute: symptoms lasting <3 months
  - Chronic: symptoms lasting ≥3 months
  - Delayed: onset 6 months after trauma exposure, <5% of cases
  - Subclinical: waxing and waning course

EPIDEMIOLOGY

- ~30% of men and women who have spent time in a war zone experience PTSD.
- 4 of the 6 trauma types associated with highest population proportions of lifetime PTSD episodes are related to intimate partner sexual violence.
- 16% children and adolescents exposed to trauma develop PTSD.

Incidence

~7.7 million American adults aged ≥18 years (3.5% of this age group) are diagnosed with PTSD each year.

Prevalence

Lifetime prevalence for PTSD ranges from 6.8% to 12.3% in the general population.

ETIOLOGY AND PATHOPHYSIOLOGY

- Biologic dimensions: Hyperactivity/hypersensitivity of catecholamine pathways and overactivity/oversensitivity of the central opioid pathways is seen; the amygdala and hippocampus dysfunction, with possible atrophy from overexposure to catecholamines, serotonergic dysregulation, glutamatergic dysregulation, and increased thyroid activity
- Learning theory: Life-threatening fear is classically conditioned by event exposure; any internal or external cue reminiscent of the event produces an intense "fight or flight" fear response. The person avoids cues that trigger fear. This avoidance maintains fear.
- Cognitive theories: These models suggest that severe trauma becomes represented in complex memory structures. The activation of these memories triggers intense thoughts and emotions that are pathologic (causing personal discomfort and dysfunction).
- Psychodynamic theory: Traumatic memories overwhelm defense mechanisms. Repeated recall of the traumatic event with associated fear is an effort to understand the event in a less threatening way.

Genetics

Monozygotic twins exposed to combat in Vietnam were at increased risk of the co-twin having PTSD compared with twins who were dizygotic.

RISK FACTORS

- Pretrauma environment:
  - Female gender
  - Younger age
  - Psychiatric history
  - Sexual abuse
- Peritrauma environment:
  - Severity of the trauma
  - Peritrauma emotionality
  - Perception of threat to life
  - Perpetration of the trauma
- Posttrauma environment:
  - Perceived injury severity
  - Medical complications
  - Perceived social support
  - Persistent dissociation from traumatic event
- Subsequent exposure to trauma-related stimuli

GENERAL PREVENTION

Trauma-focused cognitive-behavioral therapy (CBT) and modified prolonged exposure delivered within weeks of a potentially traumatic event for people showing signs of distress have the most evidence in the treatment of acute stress and early PTSD symptoms and the prevention of PTSD.

COMMONLY ASSOCIATED CONDITIONS

- Major depressive disorder
- Alcohol/substance abuse
- Panic disorder
- Obsessive-compulsive disorder
- Agoraphobia and/or social phobia
- Traumatic brain injury
- Smoking (especially with assaultive trauma)
- Major neurocognitive disorders, dementia, or amnesia

Pediatric Considerations

Oppositional defiant disorder and separation anxiety are common comorbid conditions.

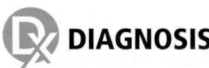 **DIAGNOSIS**

HISTORY

Diagnosis is based on *DSM-5* criteria:

- Criterion A: exposure to trauma (≥1 of the following):
  - Direct experience of a traumatic event
  - In-person witnessing of a traumatic event
  - Learning of a traumatic event involving a close friend or family member
  - Repeated exposure to details of a traumatic event
- Criterion B: intrusive symptoms associated with the traumatic event (≥1 of the following):
  - Recurrent, involuntary, and intrusive distressing memories of the event
  - Recurrent distressing dreams related to the event
  - Dissociative reactions that simulate a recurrence of the event
  - Intense or prolonged distress to stimuli that resemble an aspect of the event
- Criterion C: avoidance of stimuli associated with the trauma (≥1 of the following):
  - Avoidance of memories, thoughts, or feelings about the event
  - Avoidance of external reminders that trigger memories, thoughts, or feelings about the event

- Criterion D: negative cognitive and mood changes associated with the trauma (≥2 of the following):
  - Inability to remember aspects of event
  - Persistent and exaggerated negative opinion of self, others, or the world
  - Distorted beliefs about the cause or consequences of the event
  - Negative emotional state
  - Diminished interest in significant activities
  - Feeling detached from others
  - Inability to experience positive emotions
- Criterion E: hyperarousal (≥2 of the following):
  - Difficulty sleeping/falling asleep
  - Decreased concentration
  - Hypervigilance
  - Outbursts of anger/irritable mood
  - Exaggerated startle response
  - Self-destructive behavior
- Criterion F: Duration of the relevant criteria symptoms should be >1 month.
- Criterion G: clinically significant distress/impairment in functioning
- Criterion H: relevant criteria not attributed to substance effects or other medical conditions

Pediatric Considerations

- Memories of the traumatic event may not appear distressing and may be seen as play reenactment.
- Reactions can include a fear of being separated from a parent, crying, whimpering, screaming, immobility and/or aimless motion, trembling, frightened facial expressions, excessive clinging, or regressive behavior.
- Older children may show extreme withdrawal, disruptive behavior, and/or an inability to pay attention. Regressive behaviors, nightmares, sleep problems, irrational fears, irritability, refusal to attend school, outbursts of anger, fighting, somatic complaints with no medical basis, and decline in schoolwork performance. Furthermore, depression, anxiety, feelings of guilt, and emotional numbing are often present.
- Parental posttraumatic stress has been shown to be a robust predictor of pediatric PTSD (1)[A].

PHYSICAL EXAM

- Patients may present with physical injuries from the traumatic event.
- Mental status examination:
  - Thoughts and perceptions (e.g., hallucinations, delusions, suicidal ideation, phobias)
  - General appearance: disheveled, poor hygiene
  - Behavior: agitation; startle reaction extreme
  - Psychological numbness
  - Orientation may be affected.
  - Memory: forgetfulness, especially concerning the details of the traumatic event
  - Poor concentration
  - Poor impulse control
  - Altered speech rate and flow
  - Mood and affect may be changed: depression, anxiety, guilt, and/or fear.

Pediatric Considerations

Elevated heart rate immediately following trauma is associated with development of PTSD (1)[A].

DIFFERENTIAL DIAGNOSIS
- Acute stress disorder (symptoms <4 weeks)
- Generalized anxiety disorder
- Adjustment disorder
- Obsessive-compulsive disorder
- Schizophrenia
- Major depressive disorder
- Mood disorder with psychotic features
- Substance abuse
- Personality disorders
- Dissociative disorders
- Conversion disorder

 **TREATMENT**

Combination psychotherapy and pharmacotherapy, initiated soon after the trauma, results in better prognosis.

MEDICATION
First Line
- Depression, panic attacks, startle response, sleep disruption: may improve with SSRIs (2)[A]. All commonly used SSRIs have been shown to be effective.
  - Sertraline: 50 to 200 mg every day (FDA-approved)
  - Paroxetine: starting dose: 10 mg every day; may be increased in 10 mg increments at intervals ≥1 week (FDA-approved)
  - Fluoxetine: 20 mg every day/BID not to exceed 80 mg/day (demonstrates some efficacy for all three symptom clusters)
- Sleep disruption: Sleep disruption due to hyperarousal is ubiquitous in PTSD; standard sedatives, such as trazodone 50 to 300 mg at bedtime, mirtazapine 7.5 to 30.0 mg QHS, or amitriptyline 25 to 100 mg QHS
- Nightmares/nighttime hyperarousal: prazosin 2 to 15 mg QHS (3)[A], clonidine 0.1 to 0.2 mg QHS, amitriptyline 25 to 100 mg QHS

Second Line
Refractory/residual symptoms: Consider augmentation with:
- Depression: mirtazapine 15 to 45 mg/day; consider switch to a serotonin norepinephrine reuptake inhibitor (SNRI), such as venlafaxine XR 37.5 to 300.0 mg/day, duloxetine 60 to 120 mg/day, or desvenlafaxine 50 to 100 mg/day. Nefazodone 300 to 600 mg/day in divided doses can be very effective but requires quarterly LFTs.
- Reexperiencing/intrusive thoughts: 1st-/2nd-generation antipsychotic medications: aripiprazole 5 to 15 mg/day, risperidone 0.5 to 2.0 mg/day, olanzapine 2.5 to 10.0 mg/day, quetiapine 50 to 400 mg/day (4)[A]. 2nd-generation Rx less prone to extrapyramidal symptoms (EPS): cognitive dulling
- Hyperarousal: clonidine, start 0.05 mg BID/TID; slowly titrate to as much as 0.45 mg/day divided doses; guanfacine 1 to 3 mg/day in divided doses (long-acting forms of both clonidine and guanfacine now available). Also consider 2nd-generation antipsychotics quetiapine, risperidone, and olanzapine as above; divided doses often more helpful

- Impulsivity/explosiveness: anticonvulsants: valproic acid 500 to 2,000 mg/day, carbamazepine 200 to 600 mg/day, topiramate 50 to 200 mg/day
- Anxiety: Benzodiazepines (especially short-acting) should be avoided given the risk of substance abuse and questionable benefit in PTSD (5)[A]. Consider hydroxyzine 25 to 50 mg TID/QID PRN or risperidone 0.25 to 0.50 mg TID PRN.

ADDITIONAL THERAPIES
- Psychotherapeutic interventions:
  - Exposure therapies have shown the highest effectiveness for treatment of PTSD (6)[A]:
    - Behavioral and CBT: Early CBT, including virtual exposure, has been shown to speed recovery. CBT is considered the standard of care for PTSD by the U.S. Department of Defense.
    - 1-week intensive CBT was as effective as 3 months weekly CBT in one study.
    - Prolonged exposure therapy: Reexperience distressing trauma-related memories and reminders to facilitate habituation and successful emotional processing of memory.
    - Eye movement desensitization and reprocessing (EMDR) has been shown to benefit patients with PTSD.
  - Stress-reduction techniques:
    - Immediate symptom reduction (e.g., rebreathing in a bag for hyperventilation)
    - Early recognition and removal from a stress
    - Relaxation, meditation, and exercise techniques are also helpful in reducing the reaction to stressful events.
  - Telemedicine-based collaborative care (nurse, case manager, pharmacy, psychology, psychiatry) is more effective than usual care.
- Interpersonal psychotherapy:
  - Supportive psychotherapy with an emphasis on the here and now
- Social:
  - Consider social and/or spiritual support for trauma survivors.

Pediatric Considerations
There is very little evidence to support use of pharmacologic interventions for pediatric PTSD.

ADMISSION, INPATIENT, AND NURSING CONSIDERATIONS
Inpatient care is necessary only if the patient becomes suicidal/homicidal or for treatment of comorbid conditions (e.g., uncontrolled psychosis, substance abuse).

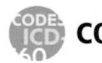 **ONGOING CARE**

PATIENT EDUCATION
National Center for PTSD: www.ptsd.va.gov

PROGNOSIS
- In 50% of cases, the symptoms spontaneously remit after 3 months; however, in other cases, symptoms may persist, often for many years, and cause long-term impairment in life functioning.
- Factors associated with a good prognosis include:
  - Rapid engagement of treatment
  - Early and ongoing social support
  - Avoidance of retraumatization
  - Absence of other psychiatric disorders/substance abuse

COMPLICATIONS
- Increased risk for panic disorder, agoraphobia, obsessive-compulsive disorder, social phobia, specific phobia, major depressive disorder, somatization disorder; impulsive behavior, suicide, and homicide
- Victims of sexual assault are at especially high risk for developing mental health problems and committing suicide.

REFERENCES
1. Brosbe MS, Hoefling K, Faust J. Predicting posttraumatic stress following pediatric injury: a systematic review. *J Pediatr Psychol*. 2011;36(6):718–729.
2. Stein DJ, Ipser JC, Seedat S. Pharmacotherapy for post traumatic stress disorder (PTSD). *Cochrane Database Syst Rev*. 2006;(1):CD002795.
3. Writer BW, Meyer EG, Schillerstrom JE. Prazosin for military combat-related PTSD nightmares: a critical review. *J Neuropsychiatry Clin Neurosci*. 2014;26(1):24–33.
4. Han C, Pae CU, Wang SM, et al. The potential role of atypical antipsychotics for the treatment of posttraumatic stress disorder. *J Psychiatr Res*. 2014;56:72–81.
5. Jeffreys M, Capehart B, Friedman MJ. Pharmacotherapy for posttraumatic stress disorder: review with clinical applications. *J Rehabil Res Dev*. 2012;49(5):703–715.
6. Kornør H, Winje D, Ekeberg Ø, et al. Early trauma-focused cognitive-behavioural therapy to prevent chronic post-traumatic stress disorder and related symptoms: a systematic review and meta-analysis. *BMC Psychiatry*. 2008;8:81.

ADDITIONAL READING
American Psychiatric Association. *Diagnostic and Statistical Manual of Mental Disorders*. 5th ed. Arlington, VA: American Psychiatric Association; 2013.

CODES
ICD10
- F43.10 Post-traumatic stress disorder, unspecified
- F43.11 Post-traumatic stress disorder, acute
- F43.12 Post-traumatic stress disorder, chronic

CLINICAL PEARLS
- Symptoms usually wax and wane over the years.
- Treatment is often best accomplished with a combination of psychotherapy and pharmacotherapy.

PREECLAMPSIA AND ECLAMPSIA (TOXEMIA OF PREGNANCY)

Jessica Marabella, MD • Ann M. Aring, MD, FAAFP

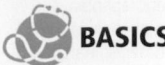 BASICS

DESCRIPTION
- Preeclampsia:
  - A disorder of pregnancy occurring after 20 weeks' gestation characterized by new-onset hypertension (HTN), new-onset proteinuria, ± impaired organ function:
    ○ May progress from mild to life-threatening in hours to days
    ○ Reversible by delivery
- Eclampsia:
  - New-onset grand mal seizure activity with no history of underlying neurologic disease
- Most postpartum cases of preeclampsia and eclampsia occur within 48 hours of delivery but can occur up to 4 weeks postpartum.
- System(s) affected: cardiovascular, renal, reproductive, fetoplacental, CNS, hepatic, pulmonary
- Synonym(s): toxemia of pregnancy

EPIDEMIOLOGY
Prevalence
- Predominant age
  - Most in younger women, primiparous women
  - Older (>40 years) patients with preeclampsia have 4 times the incidence of seizures compared with patients in their 20s.
- Preeclampsia occurs in 5–8% of all pregnancies.
- Eclampsia occurs:
  - 1.6 to 10 out of 10,000 deliveries in developed countries
  - 6 to 157 out of 10,000 deliveries in developing countries
- 40% of eclamptic seizures occur before delivery; 16% occur >48 hours after delivery.
- Eclampsia is a main cause of perinatal mortality and morbidity (2–8% of all pregnancies).

ETIOLOGY AND PATHOPHYSIOLOGY
- Cause of preeclampsia is becoming clearer.
  - Abnormal placental implantation
  - Angiogenic factors
  - Genetic predisposition
  - Immunologic phenomena
  - Vascular endothelial damage and oxidative stress
- Systemic derangements in eclampsia include the following:
  - Cardiovascular: generalized vasospasm
  - Hematologic: decreased plasma volume, increased blood viscosity, hemoconcentration, coagulopathy
  - Renal: decreased glomerular filtration rate
  - Hepatic: periportal necrosis, hepatocellular damage, subcapsular hematoma
  - CNS: cerebral vasospasm and ischemia, cerebral edema, cerebral hemorrhage

Genetics
2 to 4 times increased risk in pregnant women with family history of preeclampsia

RISK FACTORS
- Nulliparity
- Age >40 years
- Family history of preeclampsia
- High body mass index
- Diabetes
- Chronic HTN
- Chronic renal disease
- Multifetal pregnancy
- Previous pregnancy with preeclampsia
- Systemic lupus erythematosus
- In vitro fertilization

GENERAL PREVENTION
- Adequate prenatal care
- Inadequate prenatal care results in 7 times increase in mortality.
- Good control of preexisting HTN
- Low-dose aspirin (ASA) (60 to 80 mg):
  - ASA started early (12 to 20 weeks' gestational age [GA]) may lower the risk of developing preeclampsia and the rate of preterm delivery and neonatal death in moderate- to high-risk patients (see "Risk Factors" as mentioned earlier) (1)[A].
- Low-dose calcium supplementation has been shown to reduce the risk and severity of preeclampsia in calcium-deficient populations (1)[A].
- Some evidence suggests vitamin C (1,000 mg/day) and vitamin E (400 IU/day) may reduce the risk for preeclampsia, but recent guidelines recommend against their use.

COMMONLY ASSOCIATED CONDITIONS
Abruptio placentae, placental insufficiency, fetal growth restriction, preterm delivery, fetal demise maternal seizures (eclampsia), maternal pulmonary edema, maternal liver/kidney failure, or maternal death

 DIAGNOSIS

- Preeclampsia diagnosis:
  - New-onset elevated blood pressure (BP): systolic BP (SBP) ≥140 mm Hg or diastolic BP (DBP) ≥90 mm Hg (on two occasions at least 4 hours apart) or ≥160/110 mm Hg after 20 weeks of gestation (within a shorter interval), and either
    ○ Proteinuria (>300 mg/24 hr or spot protein: creatinine ≥0.3) or
    ○ New-onset thrombocytopenia, renal insufficiency, impaired liver function, pulmonary edema, or cerebral/visual symptoms (1)[C]
  - Define preeclampsia as either without or with severe features. The presence of new onset of one or more of below defines severe features (1):
    ○ BP ≥160/110 mm Hg
    ○ Platelets <100,000/μL
    ○ >2 times normal liver transaminase levels, severe persistent right upper quadrant (RUQ)/epigastric pain, or both
    ○ Creatinine >1.1 mg/dL or doubling of serum creatinine levels
    ○ Pulmonary edema
    ○ Cerebral or visual symptoms
- Eclampsia diagnosis:
  - New-onset grand mal seizure
  - No history of neurologic disease

HISTORY
- May be asymptomatic. In some cases, rapid excessive weight gain (>5 lb/week; >2.3 kg/week); more severe cases are associated with epigastric/RUQ pain, headache, altered mental status, and visual disturbance. Note: Headache, visual disturbance, and epigastric or RUQ pain often precede seizure.
- Seizures may occur once/repeatedly.

PHYSICAL EXAM
BP criteria:
- Preeclampsia without severe features: elevated BP ≥140/90 mm Hg
- Preeclampsia with severe features: Elevated BP ≥160 systolic mm Hg or 110 mm Hg diastolic
- Eclampsia: tonic–clonic seizure activity (focal/generalized)
- Normal BP, even in response to treatment; does not rule out potential for seizures

DIFFERENTIAL DIAGNOSIS
- Chronic HTN: HTN before pregnancy; high BP before the 20th week
- Chronic HTN with superimposed preeclampsia
- Gestational HTN: Increased BP first discovered after 20 weeks, often close to term, with no proteinuria and without evidence of organ dysfunction. BP becomes normal by 12 weeks postpartum, or it is reclassified as chronic HTN.
- Seizures in pregnancy: epilepsy, cerebral tumors, meningitis/encephalitis, and ruptured cerebral aneurysm. Until other causes are proven; however, all pregnant women with convulsions should be considered to have eclampsia.

DIAGNOSTIC TESTS & INTERPRETATION
Initial Tests (lab, imaging)
- Routine spot urine testing or urinalysis for protein should be done at each prenatal visit in all hypertensive patients.
- Complete blood count (CBC), including platelets, creatinine, serum transaminase levels, and uric acid as baseline in hypertensive patients and if preeclampsia suspected or possible
- Coagulation profiles: Abnormalities suggest severe disease.
- 24-hour urine or protein/creatinine ratio if urine protein dips 1+ on more than one occasion, or if preeclampsia is being considered
- Daily fetal movement monitoring by mother ("kick counts")
- US imaging is used to monitor growth and cord blood flow; perform, as indicated, based on clinical stability and laboratory findings.
- Nonstress test (NST) at diagnosis and then twice weekly until delivery
- Biophysical profile (BPP) if NST is nonreactive (1)[C]
- US imaging for growth progress every 3 weeks and amniotic fluid volume at least once weekly (1)[C]
- With seizures, CT scan and MRI should be considered if focal findings persist or uncharacteristic signs/symptoms are present.

Follow-Up Tests & Special Considerations
Disseminated intravascular coagulation, thrombocytopenia, liver dysfunction, and renal failure can complicate preeclampsia associated with HELLP syndrome.

Test Interpretation
CNS: cerebral edema, hyperemia, focal anemia, thrombosis, and hemorrhage. Cerebral lesions account for 40% of eclamptic deaths.

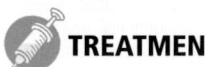 TREATMENT

GENERAL MEASURES
- Preeclampsia without severe features:
  - Outpatient care
  - Maternal: daily home BP monitoring; daily weights; weekly labs (CBC, creatinine, liver function test [LFT])
  - Fetal:
    ○ Patient-measured: daily "kick counts"
    ○ NST/BPP/US (see imaging section above)
    ○ Delivery at 37 weeks (induction of labor) (1,2)[C]
    ○ Steroids for gestation <37 weeks

- Preeclampsia with severe features:
  - Inpatient care
  - Maternal:
    - Daily labs
    - IV magnesium sulfate ($MgSO_4$) as seizure prophylaxis
    - Antihypertensive therapy titrated to keep SBP <160 mm Hg and DBP <110 mm Hg (some recommend <150/100 mm Hg postpartum)
  - Fetal:
    - Continuous heart monitoring
    - Daily US with BPP
    - Check amniotic fluid levels and fetal growth.
  - Definitive management (delivery) depends on GA (1,2)[C].
  - <23 weeks:
    - Offer to terminate pregnancy.
  - At 23 to 34 weeks:
    - Antihypertensives
    - Evaluate maternal–fetal condition.
    - Steroids to enhance fetal lung maturity
    - Plan delivery at 34 weeks with magnesium sulfate prophylaxis.
    - If HELLP syndrome (full or partial), severe oligohydramnios, significant renal dysfunction, persistent symptoms, fetal growth restriction, onset of labor, OR PROM, proceed to delivery.
  - At ≥34 weeks: magnesium sulfate, steroids, and proceed to delivery (1)[C]; steroids indicated up to 37 weeks

ALERT
- Regardless of GA, emergent delivery is recommended if there are signs of maternal hypertensive crisis, abruptio placentae, uterine rupture, or fetal distress.
- Seizures: control of convulsions, correction of hypoxia and acidosis, lowering of BP, steps to effect delivery as soon as convulsions are controlled
- Administer betamethasone 12 mg IM daily × 2 doses or dexamethasone 6 mg every 12 hours × 4 doses if delivery <37 weeks possible.

MEDICATION
First Line
- Seizure prophylaxis for women with severe preeclampsia:
  - Magnesium sulfate: loading dose 4 g IV in 200 mL normal saline over 20 to 30 minutes; maintenance dose 1 to 2 g/hr IV continuous infusion (Although recent guidelines suggest it not be universally administered for seizure prophylaxis to prevent eclampsia, the quality of the evidence is low, and the strength of the recommendation is qualified.) (1)[C]
- BP control:
  - Antihypertensives are inadvisable for mildly elevated BP (without severe features).
  - Labetalol (IV): 20 mg over 2 minutes followed at 20 to 30 minutes intervals with doses of 20 to 80 mg titrated to keep BP <160/110 mm Hg; max of 300 mg/24 hr (contraindicated in asthma, heart disease, congestive heart failure)
  - Hydralazine (IV): 5 to 10 mg over 2 minutes, followed at 20 minutes intervals with 5 to 10 mg IV boluses; titrated to keep BP <160/110 mm Hg; max of 25 mg/24 hr
  - Nifedipine immediate release 10 mg oral followed by 20 mg in 20 minutes if needed for severe range. Sustained release (PO) (used in the postpartum): 30 to 120 mg/day (caution with combination of nifedipine and magnesium sulfate resulting in hypotension and neuromuscular blockade) (3)[A]

- Eclampsia/seizures:
  - Magnesium sulfate for seizures
    - 4 to 6 g IV over 15 to 20 minutes followed by 1 to 2 g/hr infusion
    - Further boluses of magnesium may be given for recurrent convulsions with the amount given based on the neurologic examination and patellar reflexes.
    - Contraindications: myasthenia gravis, renal failure, pulmonary edema
  - Levels of 6 to 8 mEq/mL are considered therapeutic, but monitor clinical status of:
    - Patellar reflexes are present.
    - Respirations are not depressed.
    - Urine output is ≥25 mL/hr.
  - May be given safely, even in the presence of renal insufficiency
- Fluid therapy
  - Ringer lactated solution with 5% dextrose at 60 to 120 mL/hr, with careful attention to fluid volume status
- Calcium carbonate (1 g, administered slowly IV) may reverse magnesium-induced respiratory depression (1,2)[C].

Second Line
- In randomized trials, magnesium sulfate was found to be superior to phenytoin in treatment and prevention of eclampsia and probably more effective and safer than diazepam.
- Diazepam 2 mg/min until resolution or 20 mg given or
- Lorazepam 1 to 2 mg/min up to total of 10 mg or
- Phenytoin 15 to 20 mg/kg at a maximum rate of 50 mg/min or
- Levetiracetam 500 mg IV or oral may be repeated in 12 hours (dose needs to be adjusted in renal impairment) or
- Phenobarbital 20 mg/kg infused at 50 mg/min; may repeat with additional 5 to 10 mg/kg after 15 minutes

 ## ONGOING CARE

FOLLOW-UP RECOMMENDATIONS
- Without severe features: restricted activity and close monitoring; with severe features: restricted activity, in hospital
- Women with a history of preeclampsia should report this to physicians caring for them in later life. It is a potent cardiovascular disease risk factor.

DIET
- Salt restriction is inadvisable because the patient often is experiencing intravascular hypovolemia.
- Calcium supplementation may be recommended for women who have low calcium intake (<600 mg/day).

PATIENT EDUCATION
American College of Obstetricians and Gynecologists, 409 12th St. SW, Washington, DC 20024-2188; (800) 762-ACOG; http://www.acog.org/

PROGNOSIS
- For nulliparous women with preeclampsia before 30 weeks of gestation, the recurrence rate for the disorder may be as high as 40% in future pregnancies.
- 25% of eclamptic women will have HTN during subsequent pregnancies, but only 5% of these will be severe and only 2% will be eclamptic again.
- Preeclamptic, multiparous women may be at higher risk for subsequent essential HTN; they also have higher mortality during subsequent pregnancies than do primiparous women.

COMPLICATIONS
- Most women do not have long-term sequelae from eclampsia, although many may have transient neurologic deficits.
- A history of preeclampsia is equivalent to traditional risk factors for cardiovascular disease. Women with a history of preeclampsia should be strongly advised to avoid obesity and smoking. Other signs of metabolic syndrome should be closely monitored as well.
- Intrauterine growth restriction (IUGR)
- Maternal and/or fetal death

REFERENCES
1. American College of Obstetricians and Gynecologists, Task Force on Hypertension in Pregnancy. Hypertension in pregnancy. Report of the American College of Obstetricians and Gynecologists' Task Force on Hypertension in Pregnancy. *Obstet Gynecol*. 2013;122(5):1122–1131.
2. Leeman L, Dresang LT, Fontaine P. Hypertensive disorders of pregnancy. *Am Fam Physician*. 2016;93(2):121–127.
3. Duley L, Meher S, Jones L. Drugs for treatment of very high blood pressure during pregnancy. *Cochrane Database Syst Rev*. 2013;(7):CD001449.

ADDITIONAL READING
- Abalos E, Duley L, Steyn DW. Antihypertensive drug therapy for mild to moderate hypertension during pregnancy. *Cochrane Database Syst Rev*. 2014;(2):CD002252.
- American College of Obstetricians and Gynecologists. ACOG committee opinion no. 560: medically indicated late-preterm and early-term deliveries. *Obstet Gynecol*. 2013;121(4):908–910.
- Henderson J, Whitlock E, O'Connor E, et al. Low-dose aspirin for prevention of morbidity and mortality from preeclampsia: a systematic evidence review for the U.S. Preventive Services Task Force. *Ann Intern Med*. 2014;160(10):695–703.
- Phipps E, Prasanna D, Brima W, e al. Preeclampsia: updates in pathogenesis, definitions, and guidelines. *Clin J Am Soc Nephrol*. 2016;11(6):1102–1113.

CODES

ICD10
- O14.90 Unspecified pre-eclampsia, unspecified trimester
- O15.00 Eclampsia in pregnancy, unspecified trimester
- O14.00 Mild to moderate pre-eclampsia, unspecified trimester

CLINICAL PEARLS
- Diagnosis no longer requires presence of proteinuria.
- Management of preeclampsia depends on both the severity of the condition and the GA of the fetus.
- Magnesium sulfate is the treatment of choice for women demonstrating preeclampsia with severe features.
- Low-dose ASA starting in early pregnancy in high-risk patients may lower rate of preeclampsia.
- Continue to monitor maternal BP postpartum—still at risk for developing preeclampsia.

PREMENSTRUAL SYNDROME (PMS) AND PREMENSTRUAL DYSPHORIC DISORDER (PMDD)

Jeremy Golding, MD, FAAFP

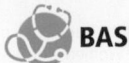

BASICS

DESCRIPTION
- Premenstrual syndrome (PMS), a complex of physical and emotional symptoms sufficiently severe to interfere with everyday life, occurs cyclically during the luteal phase of menses.
- Premenstrual dysphoric disorder (PMDD) is a severe form of PMS characterized by severe recurrent depressive and anxiety symptoms, with premenstrual (luteal phase) onset, that remits a few days after the start of menses.
- PMDD is now included as a full diagnostic category in the 5th edition of the *Diagnostic and Statistical Manual of Mental Disorders* (*DSM-5*).
- System(s) affected: endocrine/metabolic, nervous, reproductive

EPIDEMIOLOGY
Prevalence
- Many women have some physical and psychological symptoms before menses (this is not PMS).
- Premenstrual disorders affect up to 12% of the U.S. population (1). 3–8% of menstruating women have PMDD.

ETIOLOGY AND PATHOPHYSIOLOGY
Not well understood. Leading theories postulate metabolites of progesterone interact with central neurotransmitter receptors (serotonin and γ-aminobutyric acid [GABA]), provoking downstream effects of decreased GABA-mediated inhibition and decreased serotonin levels. Women with PMS/PMDD have similar levels of progesterone but seem to have an increased sensitivity to its metabolites, compared with women without PMS/PMDD.

Genetics
- Role of genetic predisposition is controversial; however, twin studies do suggest a genetic component.
- Involvement of gene coding for the serotonergic *5HT1A* receptor and allelic variants of the estrogen receptor-α gene (*ESR1*) is suggested.

RISK FACTORS
- Age: usually present in late 20s to mid-30s
- History of mood disorder (major depression, bipolar disorder), anxiety disorder, personality disorder, or substance abuse
- Family history
- Low parity
- Tobacco use
- Psychosocial stressors/history of trauma
- High BMI

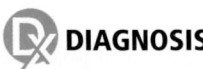

DIAGNOSIS

HISTORY
- *DSM-5* criteria (1):
- Symptoms occur 1 week before menses, improve in the first few days after menses begin, and are minimal/absent in the week following menses (over most menstrual cycles during the past year).

- ≥5 of the following (1 must be among the first 4):
  - Marked depressed mood, feelings of hopelessness, or self-deprecating thoughts
  - Marked anxiety, tension, and/or feelings of being keyed up or on edge
  - Marked affective lability (mood swings)
  - Marked irritability or anger or increased interpersonal conflicts
  - Decreased interest in usual activities and social withdrawal
  - Lethargy, easy fatigability, or lack of energy
  - Appetite change, overeating, food cravings
  - Hypersomnia or insomnia
  - Feeling out of control or overwhelmed
  - Subjective difficulty concentrating
  - Physical symptoms, such as abdominal bloating, breast tenderness, headaches, weight gain, and joint/muscle pain
- For PMDD, emotional symptoms must be sufficiently severe to interfere with work, school, usual social activities, or relationships with others.
- Symptoms may be superimposed on an underlying psychiatric disorder but may not be an exacerbation of another condition, such as panic disorder/major depression.
- Criteria should be confirmed by prospective patient record of symptoms for a minimum of two consecutive menstrual cycles (without confirmation, "provisional" should be noted with diagnosis).
- Use the Daily Record of Severity of Problems (available online at http://www.aafp.org/afp/2011/1015/p918-fig1.pdf) or similar inventory (1)[C].
- Symptoms should not be attributable to drug abuse, medications, or other medical conditions.

PHYSICAL EXAM
No specific physical exam required; may consider thyroid and pelvic exams if indicated by additional patient symptoms

DIFFERENTIAL DIAGNOSIS
- Premenstrual exacerbation of underlying psychiatric disorder
- Psychiatric disorders (especially bipolar disorder, major depression, anxiety)
- Thyroid disorders
- Perimenopause
- Premenstrual migraine
- Chronic fatigue syndrome
- Irritable bowel syndrome (painful symptoms)
- Seizures
- Anemia
- Endometriosis (painful symptoms)
- Drug/alcohol abuse

DIAGNOSTIC TESTS & INTERPRETATION
- The repetitive nature of symptoms precludes need for labs if a classic history is present.
- Consider
  - Hemoglobin to rule out anemia
  - Serum thyroid-stimulating hormone (TSH) to rule out hypothyroidism
- Imaging with pelvic ultrasound to diagnose causes of pelvic pain and dysmenorrhea may be needed.

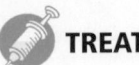

TREATMENT

GENERAL MEASURES
Although evidence is lacking for aerobic exercise in treating PMS/PMDD, it is often recommended as part of an integrated care plan.

MEDICATION
First Line
- SSRIs show a small to moderate effect in the treatment of physical, functional, and behavioral symptoms of PMS and PMDD compared to placebo (2)[A]:
  - Both intermittent luteal phase dosing and continuous full-cycle dosing are effective with no clear evidence of difference between modes of administration (2)[A].
  - All SSRIs tested appeared effective (2)[A].
  - SSRIs are effective at low doses. Higher doses have increased effect but are accompanied by increased side effects (2)[A].
- Fluoxetine (Prozac, Sarafem) 20 mg/day every day or 20 mg/day only during luteal phase, or 90 mg once a week for 2 weeks in luteal phase
- Sertraline (Zoloft) 50 to 150 mg/day every day or 50 to 150 mg/day only during luteal phase
- Citalopram (Celexa) 10 to 30 mg/day every day or 10 to 30 mg/day only during luteal phase
- Adverse effects (number needed to harm [NNH] with moderate-dose SSRI): nausea (NNH = 7), asthenia (NNH = 9), somnolence (NNH = 13), fatigue (NNH = 14), decreased libido (NNH = 14), and sweating (NNH = 14) (2)[A]
- Contraindications: patients taking monoamine oxidase inhibitors (MAOIs)
- Precautions
  - Increased risk of suicidal thinking and behavior in children and adolescents with depressive disorders; uncertain if this risk applies to those taking SSRIs for PMDD
  - Bipolar disorder
  - Seizure disorder
  - QTc prolongation (with citalopram)
  - Hepatic dysfunction
  - Renal dysfunction
- Possible interactions
  - MAOIs
  - Selegiline
  - Pimozide
  - Thioridazine
  - Cimetidine, omeprazole, and QTc-prolonging agents (with citalopram)

Second Line
Alternative therapies should be considered if no response to SSRIs:
- Spironolactone (Aldactone) 50 to 100 mg/day for 7 to 10 days during luteal phase; helpful for fluid retention; adverse reactions: lethargy, headache, irregular menses, hyperkalemia
- Oral contraceptive pills (OCPs)
  - OCPs can cause adverse effects similar to PMDD symptoms (3)[B].
  - Extended-cycle use of OCPs (e.g., 12 weeks on and 1 week off) or a shorter placebo interval (e.g., 24 active pills with 4 placebo days [24/4] compared with 21/7 preparations) may be beneficial (3)[B].

- OCPs containing the progestin drospirenone (structurally similar to spironolactone) may improve physical symptoms and mood changes associated with PMDD (4)[A]. Caution: Risk of venous thromboembolism may be modestly higher than with other OCPs (3)[B].
- Continuous administration of levonorgestrel/ethinyl estradiol may improve patient symptoms in PMDD (3)[B].
  - Suggested OCP formulations:
    - Ethinyl estradiol 0.02 to 0.03 mg/drospirenone 3 mg (Gianvi/Loryna/Nikki/Ocella/Syeda/Vestura/Yasmin/Yaz Zarah): 1 tablet/day
    - Ethinyl estradiol 0.02 to 0.03 mg/drospirenone 3 mg/levomefolate 0.451 mg (Beyaz/Safyral): 1 tablet/day
    - Levonorgestrel 90 μg/ethinyl estradiol 20 μg (Amethyst/Lybrel): 1 tablet/day
- Anxiolytics
  - Alprazolam (Xanax) 0.25 mg TID–QID only during luteal phase; taper at onset of menses (other benzodiazepines not studied for PMDD). Caution: addictive potential
  - Buspirone (Buspar) 10 to 30 mg/day divided BID–TID in the luteal phase
- Ovulation inhibitors
  - Gonadotropin-releasing hormone (GnRH) agonists: leuprolide (Lupron) depot 3.75 mg/month IM
    - Precautions: Menopause-like side effects (e.g., osteoporosis, hot flashes, headaches, muscle aches, vaginal dryness, irritability) limit treatment to 6 months; may be first step if considering bilateral oophorectomy for severe, refractory PMDD
  - Danazol (Danocrine) 300 to 400 mg BID; adverse reactions: androgenic and antiestrogenic effects (e.g., amenorrhea, weight gain, acne, fluid retention, hirsutism, hot flashes, vaginal dryness, emotional lability)
  - Estrogen, transdermal preferred, 100 to 200 μg:
    - Precautions: increased risk of blood clot, stroke, heart attack, and breast cancer
    - Requires concomitant progesterone add-back therapy to protect against uterine hyperplasia and endometrial cancer
- Progesterone: insufficient evidence to support use (5)[A]

ISSUES FOR REFERRAL
Referral to psychiatrist may be indicated for mood/anxiety disorders if patient has no symptom-free period.

ADDITIONAL THERAPIES
Cognitive-behavioral therapy (CBT) is theoretically helpful for PMS/PMDD given its application for symptom reduction in other mood disorders, but direct evidence is lacking.

SURGERY/OTHER PROCEDURES
Bilateral oophorectomy, usually with concomitant hysterectomy, is an option for rare, refractory cases with severe, disabling symptoms.

COMPLEMENTARY & ALTERNATIVE MEDICINE
Acupuncture demonstrated superiority to progestins, anxiolytics, and sham acupuncture with no evidence of harm (6)[A].
- Some data support the use of the following (7)[A]:
  - Calcium: 600 mg BID
  - Vitamin B$_6$: 50 to 100 mg/day

- Chasteberry (*Vitex agnus-castus*): 4 mg/day of extract containing 6% of agnuside (or 20 to 40 mg/day of fruit extract)
- Omega-3 fatty acids 2 g/day
- Data insufficient regarding the following (7)[A]:
  - Magnesium: 200 to 400 mg/day
  - Vitamin D: 2,000 IU/day
  - Vitamin E: 400 IU/day
  - Manganese: 1.8 mg/day
  - St. John's wort: 900 mg/day
  - Soy: 68 mg/day isoflavones
  - Ginkgo: 160 to 320 mg/day
  - Saffron: 30 mg/day
- Evidence supporting efficacy and/or safety of herbal products is lacking; the following products/interventions have not been found useful for PMS/PMDD, although not all studies are of high quality and able to eliminate possibility of benefit completely (7)[A]:
  - Evening primrose oil
  - Black currant oil
  - Black cohosh
  - Wild yam root
  - Dong quai
  - Kava kava
  - Light-based therapy

 ONGOING CARE

FOLLOW-UP RECOMMENDATIONS
Patient Monitoring
Increased risk of suicidal thinking and behavior in children and adolescents with depressive disorders on initiation of SSRIs; uncertain if this risk applies to those taking SSRIs for PMDD

DIET
- Reduce consumption of salt, sugar, caffeine, dairy products, and alcohol (anecdotal reports).
- Eat small, frequent portions of food high in complex carbohydrates (limited data).

PATIENT EDUCATION
- Counsel patients to eat a balanced diet rich in calcium, vitamin D, and omega-3 fatty acids and low in saturated fat and caffeine.
- Counsel women that they are not "crazy." PMDD is a real disorder with a physiologic basis.
- Although incompletely understood, successful treatment is often possible.

PROGNOSIS
- Many patients can have their symptoms adequately controlled. PMS disappears at menopause.
- PMS can continue after hysterectomy, if ovaries are left in place.

REFERENCES
1. Hofmeister S, Bodden S. Premenstrual syndrome and premenstrual dysphoric disorder. *Am Fam Physician*. 2016;94(3):236–240.
2. Marjoribanks J, Brown J, O'Brien PM, et al. Selective serotonin reuptake inhibitors for premenstrual syndrome. *Cochrane Database Syst Rev*. 2013;(6):CD001396.

3. Freeman EW, Halbreich U, Grubb GS, et al. An overview of four studies of a continuous oral contraceptive (levonorgestrel 90 mcg/ethinyl estradiol 20 mcg) on premenstrual dysphoric disorder and premenstrual syndrome. *Contraception*. 2012;85(5):437–445.
4. Lopez LM, Kaptein AA, Helmerhorst FM. Oral contraceptives containing drospirenone for premenstrual syndrome. *Cochrane Database Syst Rev*. 2012;(2):CD006586.
5. Ford O, Lethaby A, Roberts H, et al. Progesterone for premenstrual syndrome. *Cochrane Database Syst Rev*. 2012;(3):CD003415.
6. Kim SY, Park HJ, Lee H, et al. Acupuncture for premenstrual syndrome: a systematic review and meta-analysis of randomised controlled trials. *BJOG*. 2011;118(8):899–915.
7. Whelan AM, Jurgens TM, Naylor H. Herbs, vitamins and minerals in the treatment of premenstrual syndrome: a systematic review. *Can J Clin Pharmacol*. 2009;16(3):e407–e429.

ADDITIONAL READING
- Borenstein JE, Dean BB, Yonkers KA, et al. Using the daily record of severity of problems as a screening instrument for premenstrual syndrome. *Obstet Gynecol*. 2007;109(5):1068–1075.
- Endicott J, Nee J, Harrison W. Daily Record of Severity of Problems (DRSP): reliability and validity. *Arch Womens Ment Health*. 2006;9(1):41–49.
- Nevatte T, O'Brien PM, Bäckström T, et al; and Consensus Group of the International Society for Premenstrual Disorders. ISPMD consensus on the management of premenstrual disorders. *Arch Womens Ment Health*. 2013;16(4):279–291.
- Rapkin AJ, Akopians AL. Pathophysiology of premenstrual syndrome and premenstrual dysphoric disorder. *Menopause Int*. 2012;18(2):52–59.

 CODES

ICD10
N94.3 Premenstrual tension syndrome

CLINICAL PEARLS
- Have the patient keep a daily log of her symptoms and menses. Symptoms beginning in the week before menses and abating before the end of menses, occurring over at least 2 months, and sufficiently severe to interfere with daily functioning are diagnostic of PMS.
- The difference between PMS and PMDD is that PMDD is a severe form of PMS characterized by recurrent depressive and anxiety symptoms with luteal phase onset, sufficiently severe to disrupt social and occupational functioning. These symptoms remit a few days after the onset of menses.
- PMDD is not the same as more generalized depressive/anxiety disorders. PMDD-associated symptoms of depression and anxiety begin to resolve within the first few days of menses.
- Treatment only during the luteal phase is likely as effective as continuous-cycle treatment with SSRIs but has fewer adverse effects.

PRENATAL CARE AND TESTING

Fozia Akhtar Ali, MD • Adriana Saenz, MD

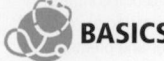
BASICS

The goal of prenatal care is to ensure the birth of a healthy baby with minimal risk for the mother by the following:

- Identifying the patient who is at risk for complications
- Estimating the gestational age (GA) as accurately as possible
- Evaluating the health status of mother and fetus
- Encouraging and empowering the patient to do her part to care for herself and her baby-to-be
- Intervening when fetal abnormalities are present to prevent morbidity

GENERAL PREVENTION
- A recommended but not evidence-based prenatal care schedule consists of the following:
  - Monthly visits to a health care professional for weeks 4 to 28 of pregnancy
  - Visits twice monthly from 28 to 36 weeks
  - Weekly after week 36 (delivery at weeks 38 to 40)
- Recommendations for use of dietary supplements in pregnancy
  - Folic acid 0.4 mg daily beginning at least 1 month prior to attempting conception and continuing throughout pregnancy; 1 to 4 mg for women at higher risk of having child with neural tube defect beginning 1 to 3 months before conception, continued through first 12 weeks of gestation, and then reduced to 0.4 mg daily
  - Calcium: 1,000 to 1,300 mg/day; supplement may be beneficial for women with high risk for gestational hypertension or communities with low dietary calcium intake.
  - Iron: Screen for anemia (hemoglobin/hematocrit) and treat if necessary.
  - Vitamin A: Pregnant women in industrialized countries should limit to <5,000 IU/day.
  - Vitamin D: 200 to 1,200 IU (dose in standard prenatal vitamin) is recommended until more evidence is available to support different dose.
- Routine screening for thyroid and vitamin D deficiency during pregnancy is not recommended.

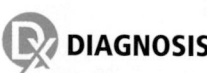
DIAGNOSIS

HISTORY
At the initial visit, a complete medical, obstetrical, family, and psychosocial history should be obtained and updated throughout the pregnancy.

- Assess and counsel as appropriate regarding the following:
  - Lifestyle, nutrition, safety of medications (teratogenicity, category); tobacco, alcohol, and drug use; toxins; relationship issues/domestic violence; stressors/supports; potential barriers to care (communication, transportation, child care issues, economic constraints, work schedule); risk factors
- Domestic violence
  - ACOG guidelines recommend that physicians screen *all* pregnant patients for intimate partner domestic violence.
    - At the first prenatal visit
    - At least once per trimester
    - At the postpartum checkup

PHYSICAL EXAM
- A full physical exam should be performed at the first prenatal appointment.

- At each subsequent prenatal visit, the following should be recorded:
  - Weight: Suggested pregnancy weight gain is 25 to 35 lb for normal-weight women with lower weight gains (11 to 20 lb) recommended for obese women.
  - BP
    - ACOG defines hypertension as BP >140 mm Hg systolic or >90 mm Hg diastolic.
    - Monitor BP, especially closely in patients with chronic hypertension (predating pregnancy), pre-eclampsia/eclampsia, or gestational hypertension.
  - UA for glucose and protein; 24-hour protein excretion is the gold standard but not practical.
  - Fundal height
  - Fetal heart rate: usually audible by 12 weeks' GA with a Doppler instrument
  - Routine fetal movement counts *not* recommended
  - Fetal position by abdominal palpation at 36 weeks
  - Pelvic/cervical exam if indicated

DIAGNOSTIC TESTS & INTERPRETATION
Cervical cancer screening

- A Pap smear should be obtained when indicated by standard Pap screening guidelines, regardless of gestation (ACOG, USPSTF, ASCCP, ACS, and ASCP guidelines state that women <21 years should not be screened regardless of age of sexual initiation or other risk factors).
- Squamous intraepithelial lesions can progress during pregnancy but often regress postpartum.
- LSIL in pregnancy: colposcopy preferred, but it is acceptable to defer colposcopy to 6 weeks postpartum (1)[B]
- CIN 1 in pregnancy: Follow-up without treatment is recommended (1)[B].
- CIN 2, CIN 3, or CIN 2,3 in pregnancy: In the absence of invasive disease or advanced pregnancy, additional colposcopic and cytologic examinations are acceptable; repeat biopsy is recommended only if appearance of lesion worsens or if cytology suggests invasive cancer; it is acceptable to defer reevaluation until 6 weeks postpartum (1)[B].
- Endocervical sampling is contraindicated.
- First prenatal visit
  - Lab tests
    - Hematocrit or hemoglobin
    - Blood type: A, B, AB, or O
    - Rhesus type and antibody screen: Rh(+) or Rh(−)
    - Hemoglobin electrophoresis for patients at risk for sickle cell disease or thalassemia
    - Urine testing for glucose and protein
    - Urine culture
    - Rubella titer
    - Syphilis test
    - Gonorrhea/chlamydia screening
    - Hepatitis B surface antigen
    - HIV testing
    - Routine screening for bacterial vaginosis, toxoplasmosis, CMV, and parvovirus not recommended
    - Cystic fibrosis screening (Information should be made available to all couples.)
      - Cystic fibrosis carrier screening should be offered before conception or early in pregnancy when one partner is of Caucasian, European, or Ashkenazi Jewish descent.
- Screening for fetal aneuploidy
  - No one screening test is superior to other screening tests.

- The risk of aneuploidy as well as the benefits, risks, and limitations of available screening tests should be discussed with the patient.
- All women should be offered screening or diagnostic testing, regardless of maternal age (2)[C].
- Ultrasound (US) nuchal translucency (NT): measures thickness at the back of the neck of the fetus
- Blood screens: human chorionic gonadotropin (hCG), pregnancy-associated plasma protein A (PAPP-A), quadruple test: α-fetoprotein (AFP), unconjugated estriol (UE3), hCG, dimeric inhibin-A (DIA)
- Cell-free DNA testing: should not be used as a substitute for diagnostic testing due to potential for false-positive or false-negative results; all women with positive screening test should have a diagnostic procedure before any irreversible action is taken (2)[C].
- 1st-trimester "combined test" between 11 and 13 weeks' GA using both NT and hCG/PAPP-A blood testing is an effective protocol; may be performed either as a single combined stand-alone test (US NT 1 blood [HCG and PAPP-A]) or as part of a sequential "step-by-step" 1st- and 2nd-trimester screening process (see the following discussion)
- Women who undergo 1st-trimester screening should be offered 2nd-trimester assessment for open fetal defects and US screening for other fetal structural defects (2)[C].
- 2nd-trimester screening protocols
  - Obtain quadruple test ideally at 15 to 18 weeks' GA but can be done as late as 22 weeks.
  - Integrated screening tests: combine information collected during the 1st and 2nd trimesters of the pregnancy to determine the risks of Down syndrome, trisomy 18, or open NTD:
    - Three options:
      - Full integrated test: serum PAPP-A at 10 to 13 weeks and sonographic NT at 11 to 13 weeks as first step; results are integrated with results of quadruple test performed at 15 to 18 weeks.
      - Serum integrated test: differs from full integrated test by NOT including US measurement of NT
      - Step-wise sequential testing: Perform 1st trimester portion of full integrated test, reporting risks of Down syndrome to the patient and offering CVS to women whose results place them at very high risk (≥1:50); if screen does not place woman at very high risk, then perform 2nd trimester portion of test.
- Diagnostic tests for genetic disorders
  - ACOG guidelines: All pregnant women should be offered invasive prenatal diagnostic testing, such as CVS and amniocentesis, regardless of maternal age or other risk factors (3)[C].
  - Women found to be at increased risk of having a baby with a genetic disorder should be offered genetic counseling and the option of CVS or midtrimester amniocentesis. There are two possible diagnostic tests:
    - CVS: 1st trimester: usually done after 10 weeks (10 to 12 weeks). Small sample of the placenta; chorionic tissue sample obtained either transcervical (TC) or transabdominal (TA)
    - Amniocentesis
      - Not recommended before 14 weeks' gestation (3)[C]

- Usually done after 15 weeks (15 to 18 weeks). Small sample of amniotic fluid from the amniotic sac surrounding the developing fetus is obtained by an US-guided TA approach.
  - The rate of procedure-related pregnancy loss that is attributable to a prenatal diagnostic procedure is 0.1–0.3% when performed by experienced health care providers (3)[B].
  - Chromosomal microarray analysis: can detect a pathogenic copy number variant in about 1.7% of patients with normal US and normal karyotype; should be made available to any patient choosing to undergo invasive diagnostic testing; should be primary test for patients undergoing diagnostic testing for indication of a fetal structural abnormality detected by US examination (3)[C]
- 24 to 28 weeks
  - Obtain diabetes screen (4)[C].
  - See the following discussion: Repeat hematocrit or hemoglobin, and repeat antibody screen in Rh-negative mother prior to receiving prophylactic Rh immunoglobulin.
    - Gestational diabetes mellitus (GDM) screening
    - The ADA and ACOG define women at increased risk of overt diabetes who need earlier screening based on body mass index (BMI): ≥25 kg/m^2 (≥23 kg/m^2 in Asian Americans) plus one or more of the following:
      - Physical inactivity
      - Previous pregnancy history of:
        - GDM
        - Macrosomia (≥4,000 g)
        - Stillbirth
      - Hypertension (140/90 mm Hg or being treated for hypertension)
      - HDL cholesterol ≤35 mg/dL (0.90 mmol/L)
      - Fasting triglyceride ≥250 mg/dL (2.82 mmol/L)
      - Hemoglobin A1C ≥5.7%, impaired glucose tolerance or impaired fasting glucose
      - PCOS, acanthosis nigricans, nonalcoholic steatohepatitis, morbid obesity, and other conditions associated with insulin resistance
      - Cardiovascular disease
      - Family history of diabetes—first-degree relative (parent or sibling)
      - Ethnicity of African American, American Indian, Asian American, Hispanic, Latina, or Pacific Islander
    - Gestational diabetes: fasting plasma glucose >92 mg/dL but is <126 mg/dL at any GA. At 24 to 28 weeks of gestation, a 75-g 2-hour oral glucose tolerance test (OGTT) with at least one abnormal result: FBG ≥92 mg/dL, but <126 mg/dL or 1 hour ≥180 mg/dL, or 2-hour ≥153 mg/dL
    - The following guidelines for GDM are established by ACOG:
      - Specified cutoffs define GDM.
        - A value of >130 mg/dL will identify 90% of women with GDM, but 20–25% of all women screened will need to continue to the 3-hour OGTT (4).
        - Raising the value to >140 mg/dL will identify only 80% of women with GDM but decrease to 14–18% the number of women who will need to continue to the 3-hour OGTT (4).
      - Screening test: 1-hour OGTT (nonfasting)
        - 50 g PO glucose load with blood glucose testing 1 hour later
        - Carpenter and Coustan positive screen: >130 mg/dL

- National Diabetes Data Group (NDDG) positive screen: >140 mg/dL
- Diagnostic test: 3-hour OGTT (fasting)
  - If abnormal 1-hour OGTT screening test, may be followed by a 3-hour OGTT
  - 100 g PO glucose load with blood drawn: fasting, 1, 2, and 3 hours after ingestion of glucose
  - Either the plasma or serum glucose level designated by Carpenter and Coustan or by the NDDG is appropriate to use:
    - *A positive diagnosis of GDM requires that ≥2 thresholds be exceeded.
      - Carpenter and Coustan standard
        - *>95 (fasting), >180 (1-hour), >155 (2-hour), >140 (3-hour)
      - NDDG standard:
        - *105 (fasting), >190 (1-hour), >165 (2-hour), >145 (3-hour)
- ACOG (based on NIH consensus panel findings) still supports the "2-step" approach (24- to 28-week 1-hour venous glucose measurement following 50 g oral glucose solution), followed by a 3-hour OGTT if positive.
- Although the diagnosis of GDM is based on two abnormal values on the 3-hour OGTT, ACOG states, due to known adverse events, one abnormal value may be sufficient to make the diagnosis.
- 1-step approach (75-g OGTT) on all women will increase the diagnosis of GDM, but sufficient prospective studies demonstrating improved outcomes still lacking.
- ACOG does acknowledge that some centers may opt for "1 step" if warranted based on their population.
- 35 to 37 weeks
  - Group B *Streptococcus* (GBS) culture: Screen all women at 35 to 37 weeks' gestation using a 2-swab rectal and vaginal culture to identify women colonized with GBS.
  - High-risk patients: High-risk patients should be screened again for gonorrhea, chlamydia, HIV, and syphilis.
- Postterm pregnancy
  - Rate of stillbirth increases with GA by 1/3,000 per week at 37 weeks, 3/3,000 per week at 42 weeks, and 6/3,000 at 43 weeks. In one meta-analysis, routine induction of labor at 41 weeks' gestation reduced rates of perinatal death without increased rates of cesarean delivery.
  - For gestational periods beyond 42 weeks, fetal well-being should be assessed with nonstress testing and US assessment of amniotic fluid volume.

 TREATMENT

ISSUES FOR REFERRAL
Abnormal screening labs or imaging may prompt referral to maternal–fetal medicine specialist or other medical specialist, as indicated.

 ONGOING CARE

PATIENT EDUCATION
- Patients should be made aware of the tests that are performed routinely, other tests that might be elected (e.g., CVS or amniocentesis), as well as the choices that would be available if testing were abnormal (pregnancy termination, preparation for the birth of an infant with congenital anomalies, further testing).

- Immunizations during pregnancy per CDC:
  - Women should get Tdap during each pregnancy (should be given between 27 to 36 weeks' GA); hepatitis B and influenza are safe; likely safe include meningococcal, rabies. Contraindicated during pregnancy or safety not established: live vaccines including BCG, MMR, and varicella
- Prevention
  - Preconception counseling offers the opportunity to discuss individualized risks.
- To decrease the risks of NTDs, preconception folate supplementation is indicated.
- Recommendations
  - Airline travel: generally safe until up to 4 weeks from EDD; lengthy trips associated with increased risk of thrombosis
  - Caffeine: Limit to <200 mg/day. Correlation between IUGR and miscarriage with caffeine is undetermined at this time.
  - Exercise: Healthy women with uncomplicated pregnancies should continue to exercise.
  - Seat belts/air bags: ACOG recommends that pregnant women wear lap and shoulder seatbelts and should not turn off air bags.
  - Sexual activity: Intercourse is not associated with adverse outcomes.
- Alcohol, cigarettes, and illicit drugs are injurious to fetal and maternal health.
  - Pregnancy-safe medications (teratogenicity)

REFERENCES

1. Massad LS, Einstein MH, Huh WK, et al. 2012 updated consensus guidelines for the management of abnormal cervical cancer screening tests and cancer precursors. *J Low Genit Tract Dis*. 2013;17(5 Suppl 1):S1–S27.
2. Committee on Practice Bulletins—Obstetrics, Committee on Genetics, and the Society for Maternal-Fetal Medicine. Practice Bulletin No. 163: screening for fetal aneuploidy. *Obstet Gynecol*. 2016;127(5):979–981.
3. American College of Obstetricians and Gynecologists' Committee on Practice Bulletins—Obstetrics, Committee on Genetics, Society for Maternal–Fetal Medicine. Practice Bulletin No. 162: prenatal diagnostic testing for genetic disorders. *Obstet Gynecol*. 2016;127(5):e108–e122.
4. Committee on Practice Bulletins—Obstetrics. Practice Bulletin No. 180: gestational diabetes mellitus. *Obstet Gynecol*. 2017;130(1):e17–e37.

 CODES

ICD10
- Z34.90 Encntr for suprvsn of normal pregnancy, unsp, unsp trimester
- Z36 Encounter for antenatal screening of mother
- Z34.00 Encntr for suprvsn of normal first pregnancy, unsp trimester

CLINICAL PEARLS

Prenatal care and screening are best accomplished using standardized flow sheets and checklists to ensure that the complex sequence of evaluations and education is performed consistently and properly.

PREOPERATIVE EVALUATION OF THE NONCARDIAC SURGICAL PATIENT

Andrew E. Grimes, MD • Stacy L. Jones, MD, FASA

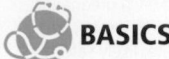 BASICS

DESCRIPTION
- Preoperative medical evaluation should determine the presence of established or unrecognized disease or other factors that may increase the risk of perioperative morbidity and mortality in patients undergoing surgery.
- Specific assessment goals include the following:
  - Conducting a thorough medical history and physical exam to assess the need for further testing and/or consultation
  - Recommending strategies to reduce risk and optimize patient condition prior to surgery
  - Encouraging patients to optimize their health for possible improvement of both perioperative and long-term outcomes
- Synonym(s): preoperative diagnostic workup; preoperative preparation; preoperative general health assessment

EPIDEMIOLOGY
Overall patient morbidity and mortality related to surgery is low. One large study of inpatients looking at 30-day mortality in the United States showed a rate of 1.32%. This rate varies by type of procedure and varies by country. Preoperative patient evaluation and subsequent optimization of perioperative care can reduce both postoperative morbidity and mortality.

RISK FACTORS
- Functional capacity (1): Exercise tolerance is one of the most important determinants of cardiac risk:
  - Self-reported exercise tolerance may be an extremely useful predictive tool when assessing risk. Patients unable to meet a 4–metabolic equivalents (METs) demand (defined in the "Diagnosis" section) during daily activities have increased perioperative cardiac and long-term risks.
  - Patients who report good exercise tolerance require minimal, if any, additional testing.
- Levels of surgical risk
  - An increased risk for major adverse cardiac events (MACE) is associated with procedures that are intrathoracic, intra-abdominal, or vascular procedures that are suprainguinal in nature (1).
- Clinical risk factors (1): history of ischemic heart disease, the presence of compensated heart failure or a history of prior congestive heart failure (CHF), cerebrovascular disease, diabetes mellitus (DM), and renal insufficiency; these risk factors plus surgical risk can dictate the need for further cardiac testing.
- Age: Patients >70 years of age are at higher risk for perioperative complications and mortality and have a longer length of stay in the hospital postoperatively (likely attributed to increasing medical comorbidities with increasing age). Age alone should not be a deciding factor in the decision to proceed or not to proceed with surgery.

DIAGNOSIS

HISTORY
- Evaluate pertinent medical records and interview the patient. Many institutions provide standard patient questionnaires that screen for preoperative risk factors:
  - History of present illness and treatments
  - Past medical and surgical history
  - Patient and family anesthetic history and associated complications

- Current medications (including over-the-counter [OTC] medications, vitamins, supplements, and herbals) as well as reasons for use
- Allergies (including specific reactions)
- Social history: tobacco, alcohol, drug use, and cessation
- Family history: prior illnesses and surgeries
- Systems (both history and current status)
  - Cardiovascular: Inquire about exercise capacity.
    - 1 MET: can take care of self, eat, dress, and use toilet; walk around house indoors; walk a block or 2 on level ground at 2 to 3 mph
    - 4 METs: can climb flight of stairs or walk uphill, walk on level ground at 4 mph, run a short distance, do heavy work around house, participate in moderate recreational activities
    - 10 METs: can participate in strenuous sports such as swimming, singles tennis, football, basketball, or skiing
  - Note presence of CHF, cardiomyopathy, ischemic heart disease (stable vs. unstable), valvular disease, hypertension (HTN), arrhythmias, murmurs, pericarditis, history of pacemaker or implantable cardioverter defibrillator (ICD):
    - Rhythm management devices (pacemakers and automatic ICDs [AICDs]) affect the perioperative course. Most importantly, the following information needs to be available for proper management: name of cardiologist who manages the device, type of device, manufacturer, last interrogation, and any problems that have occurred recently. Based on this information and the location and type of surgery, a perioperative plan of management will be made (2).
    - Stents: Patients with coronary stents are maintained on duel antiplatelet therapy (DAPT) for a prescribed period of time. This is typically done with a thienopyridine, such as clopidogrel, in combination with aspirin. The perioperative period is associated with a prothrombotic state. Premature discontinuation of DAPT markedly increases the risk of acute stent thrombosis, myocardial infarction (MI), and death. Elective surgery should be delayed and DAPT continued for a minimum of 30 days after bare metal stent placement and 6 months after placement of a drug-eluting stent. Several caveats to these recommendations exist. Extending the time for DAPT after stent placement is indicated in certain scenarios such as stent placement in the setting of an acute cardiac syndrome. Any perioperative disruption in the patient's DAPT regimen needs to be discussed with the patient's cardiologist and surgeon. The risk of perioperative bleeding must be weighed against the risks of discontinuation of DAPT prior to surgery (3).
  - Pulmonary: Chronic and active disease processes should be addressed: chronic infections, bronchitis, emphysema, asthma, wheezing, shortness of breath, cough (productive or otherwise):
    - Sleep apnea: Patients with obstructive sleep apnea (OSA) are at increased risk for perioperative adverse events. Screening tools (such as the STOP-Bang) can help risk stratify patients. Additional evaluation should be considered if a patient has associated significant systemic disease, hypoventilation syndrome, severe pulmonary HTN, or resting hypoxemia (4).
    - Often, patients with an existing diagnosis of OSA who use positive airway pressure (PAP) at night are asked to bring their PAP machine to

the hospital or surgery center when they are admitted for surgery. For patients with suspected but previously undiagnosed OSA, PAP therapy should be considered on a case-by-case basis.
    - Some studies suggest that even short periods (3 weeks) of treatment with PAP can improve some indices of ventilation and therefore may reduce postoperative morbidity.
  - GI: hepatic disease, gastric ulcer, inflammatory bowel disease, hernias (especially hiatal), significant weight loss, nausea, vomiting, history of postoperative nausea, and vomiting: Any symptoms consistent with gastroesophageal reflux disease (GERD) should be optimally treated.
  - Hematologic: anemia, serious bleeding, clotting problems, blood transfusions, hereditary disorders
  - Renal: kidney failure, dialysis, infections, stones, changes in bladder function
  - Endocrine: nocturia, parathyroid, pituitary, adrenal disease, thyroid disease
    - Diabetes: Evidence that hyperglycemia in the perioperative period is associated with increased perioperative complications. Although recommendations vary, most experts recommend keeping perioperative blood glucose levels <180 mg/dl.
  - Neurologic/psychiatric: seizures, stroke, paralysis, tremor, migraine headaches, nerve injury, multiple sclerosis, extremity numbness, psychiatric disorders (e.g., anxiety, depression)
  - Musculoskeletal: arthritis, lower back pain
  - Frailty is increasingly recognized as a perioperative risk factor. Research is being done on various screening tools and interventions that can decrease perioperative mortality and morbidity in the frail population (5).
  - Reproductive: possibility of pregnancy in women of childbearing potential
- Mouth/upper airway: dentures, crowns, partials, bridges, teeth (loose, chipped, cracked, capped)

PHYSICAL EXAM
- Assess vital signs, including arterial BP bilaterally.
- Check carotid pulses; auscultate for bruits.
- Examine lungs by auscultating all lung fields and listening for rales, rhonchi, wheezes, or other sounds indicating disease.
- Examine cardiovascular system by auscultating heart and noting any irregular rhythms or murmurs; precordial palpation
- Palpate abdomen.
- Examine airway and mouth for ease of intubation, neck mobility, and size of tongue; note any lesions or dental deformities.
- If a regional anesthesia technique is being contemplated, perform a relevant, focused neurologic exam.

DIAGNOSTIC TESTS & INTERPRETATION
Initial Tests (lab, imaging)
- Laboratory testing should never be "routine" prior to surgery. Tests should be obtained only when indicated by specific conditions or risk factors (6)[C]. Specific tests should be requested if the evaluator suspects findings from the clinical evaluation that may influence perioperative patient management.
- Labs performed within the past 4 months prior to evaluation are reliable, unless the patient has had an interim change in clinical presentation or is taking medications that require monitoring of plasma level or effect.

- CBC (6)[C]
  - Hemoglobin: if a patient has symptoms of anemia or is undergoing a procedure with major blood loss; extremes of age; liver or kidney disease
  - WBC count: if symptoms suggest infection or myeloproliferative disorder or the patient is at risk for chemotherapy-induced leukopenia
  - Platelet count: if history of bleeding, myeloproliferative disorder, liver or renal disease, or the patient is at risk for chemotherapy-induced thrombocytopenia
- Serum chemistries (electrolytes, glucose, renal and liver function tests): should be obtained for extremes of age; in known renal insufficiency, CHF, liver dysfunction, or endocrine abnormalities; or the patient is on medications that alter electrolyte levels, such as diuretics
- PT/PTT: if history of a bleeding disorder, chronic liver disease, or malnutrition, or those with recent or chronic antibiotic or anticoagulant use
- Urinalysis: Routine urinalysis is not recommended preoperatively.
- Pregnancy test: controversial; should be *considered* for all female patients of childbearing age
- CXR is not generally indicated. It can be considered in patients with recent upper respiratory tract infection and in those with suspected cardiac or pulmonary disease (because there is a likelihood for unanticipated findings), but these indications are not considered unequivocal.

Diagnostic Procedures/Other

- ECG (1)[C]
  - Preoperative resting 12-lead ECG is reasonable for patients with known coronary disease, known peripheral vascular disease, significant arrhythmia, or known significant structural heart disease.
  - ECGs are not indicated for asymptomatic patients undergoing low-risk procedures.
- The American Heart Association (AHA) guidelines recommend using the Revised Cardiac Risk Index or the ACS NSQIP online risk calculator to make an estimate of risk of MACE in the perioperative period. If the risk of MACE is low (<1%), then proceed with surgery. If the risk is >1%, the functional capacity needs to be considered. For patients with a functional capacity of >4 METs, then proceed with surgery. If the functional capacity is <4 METs or unknown, consider pharmacologic stress testing if it will change management (1).
- PFTs: Definitive data regarding the efficacy of preoperative testing are lacking. The most important factor is preoperative optimization of patients with chronic obstructive pulmonary disease (COPD) or reactive airways disease with indicated use of antibiotics, bronchodilators, and inhaled corticosteroids. Spirometry can help guide therapy. Upper abdominal and thoracic surgery has a higher risk of postoperative pulmonary complications.

TREATMENT

MEDICATION

- Reducing cardiac risk
  - Elective surgery should be delayed or cancelled if the patient has any of the following: unstable coronary syndromes (unstable or severe angina), recent MI (<30 days), decompensated heart failure, significant arrhythmias, or severe valvular disease.
  - Active HF should be treated with diuretics, afterload reduction, and β-adrenergic blockers.

- Perioperative β-blockade has been shown to reduce mortality and the incidence of perioperative MIs in high-risk patients. Studies conflict, however, in which patients need to be treated, the dosage and timing of treatment, and for what surgeries. *Patients chronically on β-blockers should have the medication continued in the perioperative period.* When β-blockers are discontinued in the perioperative period, 30-day mortality increases. β-Blockers are reasonable for vascular surgery patients with at least one clinical risk factor. It is not recommended to start β-blockers on the day of surgery in β-blocker–naive patients (1).
  - Perioperative statin use may have a protective effect on reducing cardiac complications. Currently, the AHA has a class I indication for perioperative statin therapy for patients already on statins prior to their surgery. There is also evidence that vascular surgery patients benefit from perioperative statins.
  - A recent review examined prophylactic use of aspirin in the perioperative period and did not find a significant effect on perioperative mortality or risk for MI in patients undergoing noncardiac surgery and may be associated with an increased risk of perioperative bleeding. There were important exclusion criteria, including patients with recent stent placement.
- Reducing pulmonary risk
  - Recommend cigarette cessation for at least 8 weeks prior to elective surgery.
  - Patients with asthma should not be wheezing and should have a peak flow of at least 80% of their predicted or personal-best value.
  - Treatment of COPD and asthma should focus on maximally reducing airflow obstruction and is identical to treatment of nonsurgical patients.
  - Lower respiratory tract infections (bacterial) should be treated with appropriate antibiotic therapy.

REFERENCES

1. Fleisher LA, Fleischmann KE, Auerbach AD, et al. 2014 ACC/AHA guideline on perioperative cardiovascular evaluation and management of patients undergoing noncardiac surgery: executive summary: a report of the American College of Cardiology/American Heart Association Task Force on practice guidelines. Developed in collaboration with the American College of Surgeons, American Society of Anesthesiologists, American Society of Echocardiography, American Society of Nuclear Cardiology, Heart Rhythm Society, Society for Cardiovascular Angiography and Interventions, Society of Cardiovascular Anesthesiologists, and Society of Vascular Medicine Endorsed by the Society of Hospital Medicine. *J Nucl Cardiol*. 2015;22(1):162–215.
2. Crossley GH, Poole JE, Rozner MA, et al. The Heart Rhythm Society (HRS)/American Society of Anesthesiologists (ASA) Expert Consensus Statement on the perioperative management of patients with implantable defibrillators, pacemakers and arrhythmia monitors: facilities and patient management this document was developed as a joint project with the American Society of Anesthesiologists (ASA), and in collaboration with the American Heart Association (AHA), and the Society of Thoracic Surgeons (STS). *Heart Rhythm*. 2011;8(7):1114–1154.
3. Levine GN, Bates ER, Bittl JA, et al. 2016 ACC/AHA guideline focused update on duration of dual antiplatelet therapy in patients with coronary artery disease: a report of the American College of Cardiology/American Heart Association Task Force on clinical practice guidelines. *J Am Coll Cardiol*. 2016;68(10):1082–1115.
4. Chung F, Memtsoudis SG, Ramachandran SK, et al. Society of Anesthesia and Sleep Medicine guidelines on preoperative screening and assessment of adult patients with obstructive sleep apnea. *Anesth Analg*. 2016;123(2):452–473.
5. Hall DE, Arya S, Schmid KK, et al. Association of a frailty screening initiative with postoperative survival at 30, 180, and 365 days. *JAMA Surg*. 2017;152(3):233–240.
6. Apfelbaum JL, Connis RT, Nickinovich DG, et al. Practice advisory for preanesthesia evaluation: an updated report by the American Society of Anesthesiologists Task Force on Preanesthesia Evaluation. *Anesthesiology*. 2012;116(3):522–538.

ADDITIONAL READING

- Akhtar S, Barash PG, Inzucchi SE, et al. Scientific principles and clinical implications of perioperative glucose regulation and control. *Anesth Analg*. 2010;110(2):478–497.
- Chung F, Subramanyam R, Liao P, et al. High STOP-Bang score indicates a high probability of obstructive sleep apnoea. *Br J Anaesth*. 2012;108(5):768–775.
- Devereaux PJ, Mrkobrada M, Sessler DI, et al; for POISE-2 Investigators. Aspirin in patients undergoing noncardiac surgery. *N Engl J Med*. 2014;370(16):1494–1503.
- Lander JS, Coplan NL. Statin therapy in the perioperative period. *Rev Cardiovasc Med*. 2011;12(1):30–37.
- Pearse RM, Moreno RP, Bauer P, et al; and European Surgical Outcomes Study (EuSOS) group for the Trials groups of the European Society of Intensive Care Medicine and the European Society of Anaesthesiology. Mortality after surgery in Europe: a 7 day cohort study. *Lancet*. 2012;380(9847):1059–1065.

SEE ALSO

Algorithm: Preoperative Evaluation of Noncardiac Surgical Patient

CODES

ICD10

- Z01.818 Encounter for other preprocedural examination
- Z01.811 Encounter for preprocedural respiratory examination
- Z01.812 Encounter for preprocedural laboratory examination

CLINICAL PEARLS

- The preoperative evaluation should include medical record evaluation, patient interview, and physical exam.
- The minimum for the physical exam includes airway, pulmonary, and cardiovascular exams.
- Functional capacity, the level of surgical risk, and clinical risk factors determine if further cardiac testing is needed.
- No preoperative tests are or should be routine.
- Active cardiac conditions should lead to delay or cancellation of nonemergent surgery.

PRESBYCUSIS

Ronald L. Cook, DO, MBA • Jared H. Mataska, MD

 BASICS

DESCRIPTION

- Presbycusis is an age-related hearing loss (HL), showing increased incidence with age. It often presents as difficulty communicating in noisy conditions.
- May be divided into central and peripheral causes:
  - Central presbycusis: age-related change in the auditory portions of the central nervous system negatively impacting auditory perception, speech-communication performance, or both
  - Peripheral presbycusis: age-related, bilateral sensorineural HL (SNHL) typically symmetric
- Represents a lifetime of insults to the auditory system from toxic noise exposure and natural decline
- Initially presents as high-frequency SNHL with tinnitus (ringing)
- Impacts the "clarity" of sounds (i.e., ability to detect, identify, and localize sounds)
- Due to mild and progressive nature, presbycusis is often treated with amplification alone.
- Can lead to adverse effects on physical, cognitive, emotional, behavioral, and social function in the elderly (e.g., depression, social isolation)

EPIDEMIOLOGY

Incidence
According to an ongoing community-based epidemiologic study, the 10-year cumulative incidence rates of HL are as follows, approximately:
- Age 48 to 59 years: M (31.7%), F (15.6%); all (21.8%)
- Age 60 to 69 years: M (56.8%), F (40.7%); all (45.5%)
- Age 70 to 79 years: M (87.1%), F (70.6%); all (73.7%)
- Age 80 to 92 years: M (100%), F (100%); all (100%)

Prevalence
- 10% of the population develops SNHL severe enough to impair communication.
- Increases to 40% in the population >65 years of age
- 80% of HL cases occur in elderly patients.
- Only 10–20% of older adults with HL have ever used hearing aids (HAs).
- Predominant sex: male > female
- Hearing levels are poorer in industrialized societies than in isolated or agrarian societies.

ETIOLOGY AND PATHOPHYSIOLOGY

- The external ear transmits sound energy to the tympanic membrane. The middle ear ossicles amplify and conduct the sound waves into the inner ear (cochlea) via the oval window. The organ of Corti, located in the cochlea, contains hair cells that detect these vibrations and depolarize, producing electrical signals that travel through the auditory nerve to the brain. Toxic noise exposure traumatizes the hair cells and leads to cell death and HL. New research also suggests that overexcitation of the neurosynapses causes increased glutamate, which is also neurotoxic (1).
  - Sensory presbycusis: primary loss of the hair cells in the basal end of the cochlea (high-frequency HL)
  - Neural presbycusis: loss of spiral ganglion cells (nerve cells induced by hair cells to produce action potentials to travel to the brainstem)
  - Strial (metabolic) presbycusis: atrophy of the stria vascularis (the cochlear tissue that generates the endocochlear electrical potential)
  - Cochlear conductive (mechanical) presbycusis: no morphologic findings (presumed stiffening of the basilar membrane)
  - Mixed presbycusis: combinations of hair cell, ganglion cell, and stria vascularis loss
  - Indeterminate presbycusis: no morphologic findings (presumed impaired cellular function)
- Presbycusis is caused by the accumulated effects of noise exposure, systemic disease, oxidative damage, ototoxic drugs, and genetic susceptibility.

Genetics
Presbycusis has a clear familial aggregation:
- Heritability estimates show 35–55% of the variance of sensory presbycusis is from genetic factors; even greater percentage in strial presbycusis
- Heritability is stronger among women than men.

RISK FACTORS

- Noise exposure (military, industrial, etc.)
- Ototoxic substances
  - Organic solvents
  - Heavy metals
  - Carbon monoxide
- Drugs
  - Aminoglycosides
  - Cisplatin
  - Salicylates
  - Diuretics
- Tobacco smoking
- Alcohol
- Lower socioeconomic status
- Family history of presbycusis
- Head trauma (temporal bone fractures)
- Cardiovascular disease (hypertension, atherosclerosis, hyperlipidemia); labyrinthine artery is terminal artery to the cochlea.
- Diabetes mellitus
- Autoimmune disease (autocochleitis/labyrinthitis)
- Metabolic bone disease
- Endocrine medical conditions: levels of aldosterone
- Alzheimer disease
- Otologic conditions (e.g., Ménière disease or otosclerosis)

GENERAL PREVENTION

- Avoid hazardous noise exposure.
- Use hearing protection.
- Maintain healthy diet and exercise.
- Screening
  - In the only published RCT on screening for HL, HA use was significantly higher in three screened groups (4.1% in those using a questionnaire, 6.3% using handheld audiometry, and 7.4% using both modalities) versus unscreened control participants (3.3%) at 1-year follow-up (2)[B].
  - Based on a 2011 review, according to the USPSTF, there is insufficient evidence to assess the relative benefits and harms of HL screening in adults ≥50 years (3)[A].

 DIAGNOSIS

HISTORY

- Reduced hearing sensitivity and speech understanding in noisy/public environments
- Impaired localization of sound sources
- Increased difficulty understanding conversations, especially with women, due to higher frequency of spoken voice
- Presents bilaterally and symmetrically
- If unilateral HL, alternative diagnosis should be pursued.
- Additional history if HL is suspected or detected (4)[B]:
  - Time course of HL
  - Symptoms of tinnitus, otalgia, otorrhea, or vertigo
  - History of noise exposure, ear trauma, or head trauma
  - Presence of any neurologic deficit
- Reports from patient/family/caregiver (4)[B]
  - Confusion in social situations
  - Excessive volume of television/radio/computer
  - Social withdrawal
  - Anxiety in group settings

PHYSICAL EXAM

- Rinne and Weber tests are helpful for determining conductive versus SNHL but not recommended for general screening.
- Pneumatic otoscopy to evaluate for simple middle ear effusion as cause of conductive HL

DIFFERENTIAL DIAGNOSIS

- Complete canal occlusion (cerumen, foreign body)
- Large external ear tumors (e.g., polyp, exostosis, squamous cell)
- Otitis externa
- Chronic otitis media or effusion
- Cholesteatoma
- Otosclerosis
- Osteogenesis imperfecta
- Large middle ear tumors (e.g., facial nerve schwannomas, paragangliomas)
- Perilymph fistula (trauma/iatrogenic)
- Ménière disease
- Acoustic neuroma (usually unilateral)
- Vascular anomaly
- Acute noise-induced traumatic loss (explosion)
- Autoimmune HL

DIAGNOSTIC TESTS & INTERPRETATION

- Central: synthetic sentence identification test with ipsilateral competing message and the dichotic sentence identification test (5)[A]
- Peripheral: handheld audiometry; insert probe in ear (sealing canal) and have patient indicate if tones can be heard.
  - Positive likelihood ratio (LR) range, 3.1 to 5.8; negative LR range, 0.03 to 0.40
- Screening audiometry
  - Symmetric high-frequency HL in descending slope pattern
  - SNHL frequencies >2 KHz initially
  - Essential to determine global clinical hearing status and if etiology is conductive HL versus SNHL or pseudohypacusis (conversion)

TREATMENT

- HAs
  - Types
    - Analog HA: picks up sound waves through a microphone; converts them into electrical signals; amplifies and sends them through the ear canal to the tympanic membrane
    - Digital HA: programmable; may reduce acoustic feedback, reduce background noise, detect and automatically accommodate different listening environments, control multiple microphones
  - HAs have an average decibel gain of 16.3 dB.
  - Associated with hypersensitivity to loud sounds ("loudness recruitment")
- Hearing-assistive technologies (HATs) (6)[A]
  - Can be used alone or in combination with HAs (for difficult listening conditions)
  - Addresses face-to-face communication, broadcast or other electronic media (radio, TV), telephone conversation, sensitivity to alerting signals and environment stimuli (doorbell, baby's cry, alarm clock, etc.)
  - Includes personal FM systems, infrared systems, induction loop systems, hardwired systems, telephone amplifier, telecoil, TDD (telecommunication device for the deaf), situation-specific devices (e.g., television), alerting devices
- Aural rehabilitation (also known as audiologic orientation or auditory training) (4)[A]
  - Adjunct to HA or HATs
  - Involves education regarding proper use of amplification devices, coaching on how to manage the auditory environment, training in speech perception and communication, and counseling for coping strategies to deal with the difficulties of HAs or HATs

ISSUES FOR REFERRAL
Refer to audiologist for formal evaluation and optimal fitting of HAs and/or HATs.
- Individuals receiving postfitting orientation/education have significantly fewer HA returns.
- Individuals receiving >2 hours of education and counseling report higher levels of satisfaction.

SURGERY/OTHER PROCEDURES
- Cochlear implants (CIs)
  - Works by bypassing the ear canal, middle ear, and hair cells in the cochlea to provide electric stimulation directly to the auditory nerve
  - Indications include hearing no better than identifying ≤50% of key words in test sentences in the best aided condition in the worst ear and 60% in the better ear.
  - Incoming sounds are received through the microphone in the audio processor component (resembles a small HA), which converts them into electrical impulses and sends them to the magnetic coil (located on the skin). The impulses transmit these across intact skin via radio waves to the implanted component (directly subjacent to the coil). The pulses travel to the electrodes in the cochlea and stimulate the cochlea at high rates.

  - Receiving a unilateral CI is most common; some may receive bilateral CIs (either sequentially or in the same surgery). Others may wear a CI in one ear and an HA in the contralateral ear (bimodal fit).
  - Younger age at CI placement derives greatest benefit.
- Active middle ear implants (AMEIs) (6)[B]
  - Suitable for elderly adults who cannot wear conventional HAs for medical or personal (cosmetic) reasons and whose HL is not severe enough for a CI
  - Comes in different models and may include components that are implantable under the skin
- Electric acoustic stimulation: use of CI and HA together in one ear
  - Addresses the specific needs of patients presenting with good low-frequency hearing (a mild to moderate sensorineural HL in frequencies up to 1,000 Hz) but poorer hearing in the high frequencies (sloping to 60 dB or worse HL > 1,000 Hz)
    - Contraindications: progressive HL, autoimmune disease; HL related to meningitis, otosclerosis, or ossification; malformation of the cochlea; a gap in air conduction and bone conduction thresholds of >15 dB; external ear contraindications, active infection, or unwillingness to use amplification devices

 ONGOING CARE

FOLLOW-UP RECOMMENDATIONS
Patient Monitoring
- During follow-up visits, check for compliance of HA use.
  - 25–40% of adults will either stop wearing them or use them only occasionally.
- Assess perceived benefit of HA and, if ineffective, for indications for possible surgical treatments.
- Annual audiograms
- Can follow up with audiologists for HA fittings if HA becomes uncomfortable
- Asymmetric HL should have evaluation via MRI for acoustic neuroma.
- Sudden SNHL is atypical and warrants urgent otolaryngologic evaluation/audiometry. The most recent recommendations by the American Academy of Otolaryngology recommend steroids empirically.

PATIENT EDUCATION
- Should be face-to-face; spoken clearly and unhurriedly, without competing background noise (e.g., radio, TV); and include a confirmation that the message is received
- Formal speech reading classes may be beneficial; however, availability may be limited.

REFERENCES
1. Yamasoba T, Lin FR, Someya S, et al. Current concepts in age-related hearing loss: epidemiology and mechanistic pathways. *Hear Res*. 2013;303:30–38.

2. Yueh B, Collins MP, Souza PE, et al. Long-term effectiveness of screening for hearing loss: the screening for auditory impairment—which hearing assessment test (SAI-WHAT) randomized trial. *J Am Geriatr Soc*. 2010;58(3):427–434.
3. Chou R, Dana T, Bougatsos C, et al. Screening adults aged 50 years or older for hearing loss: a review of the evidence for the U.S. Preventive Services Task Force. *Ann Intern Med*. 2011;154(5):347–355.
4. Pacala JT, Yueh B. Hearing deficits in the older patient: "I didn't notice anything." *JAMA*. 2012;307(11):1185–1194.
5. Humes L, Dubno J, Gordon-Salant S, et al. Central presbycusis: a review and evaluation of the evidence. *J Am Acad Audiol*. 2012;23(8):635–666.
6. Sprinzl GM, Riechelmann H. Current trends in treating hearing loss in elderly people: a review of the technology and treatment options—a mini-review. *Gerontology*. 2010;56(3):351–358.

ADDITIONAL READING
- Bagai A, Thavendiranathan P, Detsky AS. Does this patient have hearing impairment? *JAMA*. 2006;295(4):416–428.
- Cruickshanks KJ, Nondahl DM, Tweed TS, et al. Education, occupation, noise exposure history and the 10-yr cumulative incidence of hearing impairment in older adults. *Hear Res*. 2010;264(1–2):3–9.
- Lin FR, Chien WW, Li L, et al. Cochlear implantation in older adults. *Medicine (Baltimore)*. 2012;91(5):229–241.
- Valente M. Summary guidelines: audiological management of adult hearing impairment. *Audio Today*. 2006;18:32–37.

CODES

ICD10
- H91.10 Presbycusis, unspecified ear
- H91.13 Presbycusis, bilateral
- H91.11 Presbycusis, right ear

CLINICAL PEARLS
- Presbycusis is an age-related HL, showing increased incidence with age. It is often bilateral and initially begins as high-frequency HL. It presents as difficulty communicating in noisy conditions.
- There are more affected males than females.
- Compliance is only 25–40% for those who own HA. A referral to an audiologist is key for optimal evaluation, fitting for HAs, and other assistive technologies or surgical treatment.
- Indication for CIs include hearing no better than identifying ≤50% key words in test sentences in the best aided condition in the worst ear and 60% in the better ear.
- Early audiology referral for individuals with suspected HL may improve treatment efficacy.

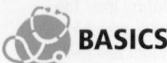# PRESSURE ULCER

Marzena Gieniusz, MD

BASICS

DESCRIPTION

- A localized area of skin or underlying tissue injury resulting from pressure and/or shear
- Classified in stages according to the National Pressure Ulcer Advisory Panel (NPUAP):
  - Stage I: nonblanchable erythema—intact skin with nonblanchable redness; darkly pigmented skin may not have visible blanching.
  - Stage II: partial thickness skin loss—shallow open ulcer with a red-pink wound bed, without slough; or intact or open/ruptured serum-filled blister
  - Stage III: full thickness skin loss—subcutaneous fat may be visible but bone, tendon, or muscle is not exposed; slough, if present, does not obscure depth of tissue loss.
  - Stage IV: full thickness tissue loss—exposed bone, tendon, or muscle; slough or eschar may be present but does not completely obscure wound base.
  - Unstageable: depth unknown—base of the ulcer is covered by slough and/or eschar in the wound bed
  - Suspected deep tissue injury: depth unknown—purple or maroon area of intact skin or blood-filled blister
- Synonyms: decubitus ulcer; bedsore; pressure injury

EPIDEMIOLOGY

Incidence
Dependant on setting and population: 0–53.4% (1,2)

Prevalence
Dependant on setting and population: 0–72.5% (1,2)

ETIOLOGY AND PATHOPHYSIOLOGY
Complex process of risk factors interacting with external forces (pressure and/or shear) (3)

RISK FACTORS
- Impaired mobility
- Malnutrition
- Reduced perfusion
- Sensory loss
- Medical devices

GENERAL PREVENTION
- Structured risk assessment (1)
- Skin and tissue assessment (1)
- Preventive skin care (1)
- Nutrition screening (1)
- Repositioning (1)
- Early mobilization (1)
- Support surfaces (1)
- Microclimate control (1)
- Prophylactic dressings (1)
- Electrical stimulation of the muscles (1)

COMMONLY ASSOCIATED CONDITIONS
- Advanced age
- Trauma
- Hip fractures
- Diabetes
- Cerebrovascular and cardiovascular disease
- Incontinence

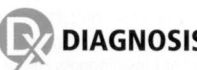 DIAGNOSIS

HISTORY
- Risk factors
- Nutritional assessment (1)
- Pain assessment (1)
- Date of ulcer diagnosis
- Treatment course

PHYSICAL EXAM
- Full skin examination on initial contact and repeatedly throughout visits
- Assess location, stage, size (length, width, depth); identify presence of sinus tracts, undermining, tunneling, exudate, necrosis, odor, and signs of healing (e.g., granulation tissue) (1).
- Identify factors that may affect healing (impaired perfusion, sensation, presence of infection).

DIFFERENTIAL DIAGNOSIS
- Venous ulcers
- Arterial ulcers
- Incontinence associated dermatitis
- Skin tears
- Intertrigo
- Neuropathic ulcers
- Pyoderma gangrenosum, cancers, vasculitides, and other dermatologic conditions

DIAGNOSTIC TESTS & INTERPRETATION
Initial Tests (lab, imaging)
- Wound culture: Do not culture surface drainage. If culture necessary, do deep tissue culture/bone biopsy.
- If systemic infection or that of bone and muscle is suspected, add infectious workup, including inflammatory markers, CBC, blood cultures, x-ray. MRI may be necessary to confirm osteomyelitis.
- Ankle-brachial index and Doppler ultrasound (for lower extremity wounds)

Follow-Up Tests & Special Considerations
Additional tests may be indicated when additional medical illness complicates assessment. This may include testing for diabetes (i.e., A1c), thyroid disease (i.e., TSH), vascular disease, and other dermatologic diagnoses.

TREATMENT

GENERAL MEASURES
- Comprehensive initial assessment of the patient
- Pressure reduction/redistribution (4)[A]
- Nutritional support (e.g., protein-containing supplements) (5)[B]
- Wound assessment and treatment
  - Wound bed preparation (tissue management, infection and inflammation control, moisture balance, epithelial edge advancement) (1)
  - Wound cleansing (1)[C]
  - Débridement (1)[C]
- Address immobility.
- Manage incontinence.
- Address pain.
- Assess goals of care and advance directives.

MEDICATION

First Line
- Wound dressings as appropriate for category of ulcer (hydrocolloid, hydrogel, alginate, foam, silver impregnated, honey impregnated, cadexomer iodine, gauze, silicone, collagen matrix, composite) (1)[C]
- Enzymatic débriding agents

Second Line
- Activated charcoal
- Topical antiseptics (hydrogen peroxide, Dakin's solution, povidone-iodine)

ISSUES FOR REFERRAL
- Consider referral to wound care specialist (if available) for complex or nonhealing wounds.
- Consider vascular surgery for improvement of blood flow to wound via vascular bypass if appropriate.
- Consider surgical consultation for possible urgent drainage and/or débridement if advancing cellulitis; suspected source of sepsis; undermining, tunneling, sinus tracts, and/or extensive necrotic tissue that cannot otherwise be removed by nonsurgical débridement methods; or for stage III or IV that are not closing with conservative management (1)[C].
- Consider plastic surgery for skin graft/flap if appropriate.
- Consider dermatology referral if suspected pyoderma gangrenosum, cancer, vasculitis or other dermatologic conditions.

ADDITIONAL THERAPIES
- Direct contact electrical stimulation for recalcitrant stage II and any category/stage III and IV (1)[A]
- Electromagnetic field for recalcitrant category/stage II and any stage III and IV (1)[C]
- Pulsed radio frequency energy for recalcitrant stage II and any stage III and IV (1)[C]

COMPLEMENTARY & ALTERNATIVE MEDICINE
- Low-frequency ultrasound for débridement of necrotic soft tissue (not eschar) (1)[C]
- High-frequency ultrasound as adjunct for infected pressure ulcers (1)[C]
- Negative pressure wound therapy as early adjuvant treatment for deep, stage III and IV (1)[B]
- Consider course of hydrotherapy with pulsed lavage with suction for wound cleansing and débridement (1)[C].
- Phototherapy: short-term UVC light if traditional therapies fail (1)[C]; laser not recommended (1)[C]; infrared is not recommended (1)[C].
- Hyperbaric and topical oxygen therapy not recommended for routine use (1)[C]
- Hydrotherapy with whirlpool should not be considered for routine use (1)[C].
- Vibration therapy not recommended (1)[C]
- Consider maggot débridement therapy.

ADMISSION, INPATIENT, AND NURSING CONSIDERATIONS
- Admission criteria/initial stabilization: refractory cellulitis, osteomyelitis, systemic infection, advanced nutritional decline, suspected patient mistreatment, inability to care for self
- Dressing changes 1 to 3 times daily based on wound assessment and plan of care
- Assess risk factors according to scales.
- Assess for changing or new wounds.
- Discharge criteria: clinical improvement in wound and systemic illness; when applicable, safe, and appropriate location for discharge

 ONGOING CARE

FOLLOW-UP RECOMMENDATIONS
Weekly assessment by nurse with wound experience; biweekly assessment by physician

Patient Monitoring
- Home health nursing
- Change plan of care if no improvement in 2 to 3 weeks.

DIET
- Approximately 1.0 to 1.5 kg/day of protein
- Strict glycemic control
- Include micronutrients in diet or as supplements.

PATIENT EDUCATION
- Check skin regularly.
- Signs and symptoms of infection
- Report new or increased pain.
- Prevention of new wound where old wound healed
- Skin care, moisture prevention

PROGNOSIS
Variable, depending on the following:
- Removal of pressure
- Nutrition
- Wound care

COMPLICATIONS
- Infection
- Amputation

REFERENCES
1. Haesler E, ed. *Prevention and Treatment of Pressure Ulcers: Clinical Practice Guideline*. Osborne Park, Western Australia: Cambridge Media; 2014.
2. Pieper B, ed. *Pressure Ulcers: Prevalence, Incidence, and Implications for the Future*. Washington, DC: NPUAP; 2012.
3. Sibbald RG, Krasner DL, Woo KY. Pressure ulcer staging revisited: superficial skin changes & Deep Pressure Ulcer Framework. *Adv Skin Wound Care*. 2011;24(12):571–580.
4. Bergstrom N, Horn SD, Rapp MP, et al. Turning for ulcer reduction: a multisite randomized clinical trial in nursing homes. *J Am Geriatr Soc*. 2013;61(10):1705–1713.
5. Smith ME, Totten A, Hickam DH, et al. Pressure ulcer treatment strategies: a systematic comparative effectiveness review. *Ann Intern Med*. 2013;159(1):39–50.

ADDITIONAL READING
- Jamshed N, Schneider E. Is the use of supplemental vitamin C and zinc for the prevention and treatment of pressure ulcers evidence based? *Ann Long-Term Care Med*. 2010;18(3):28–32.
- Qaseem A, Humphrey LL, Forciea MA, et al; for Clinical Guidelines Committee of the American College of Physicians. Treatment of pressure ulcers: a clinical practice guideline from the American College of Physicians. *Ann Intern Med*. 2015;162(5):370–379.
- Reddy M, Gill S, Rochon P. Preventing pressure ulcers: a systematic review. *JAMA*. 2006;296(8):974–984.
- Stansby G, Avita L, Jones K, et al. Prevention and management of pressure ulcers in primary and secondary care: summary of NICE guidance. *BMJ*. 2014;348:g2592.

 CODES

ICD10
- L89.95 Pressure ulcer of unspecified site, unstageable
- L89.91 Pressure ulcer of unspecified site, stage 1
- L89.92 Pressure ulcer of unspecified site, stage 2

CLINICAL PEARLS
- Create assessment and prevention protocols for all patients.
- Identify risk factors, reduce pressure, maximize nutrition, regular skin checks, and assess and treat wound appropriately.
- All care needs to be done in time-sensitive, patient-centered fashion.

PRETERM LABOR

Kara M. Coassolo, MD • John C. Smulian, MD, MPH

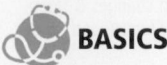

BASICS

DESCRIPTION
Contractions occurring between 20 and 36 weeks' gestation at a rate of 4 in 20 minutes or 8 in 1 hour with at least one of the following: cervical change over time or dilation ≥2 cm

EPIDEMIOLOGY
Preterm birth is the leading cause of perinatal morbidity and mortality in the United States (1).

Incidence
10–15% of pregnancies experienced at least one episode of preterm labor.

Prevalence
10% of all births in the United States are preterm, of which 2/3 are spontaneous, and 1/3 are medically indicated.

ETIOLOGY AND PATHOPHYSIOLOGY
- Premature formation and activation of myometrial gap junctions
- Inflammatory mediator–stimulated contractions
- Weakened cervix (structural defect or extracellular matrix defect)
- Abnormal placental implantation
- Systemic inflammation/infections (e.g., urinary tract infection [UTI], pyelonephritis, pneumonia, sepsis)
- Local inflammation/infections (intra-amniotic infections from aerobes, anaerobes, *Mycoplasma*, *Ureaplasma*)
- Uterine abnormalities (e.g., cervical insufficiency, leiomyomata, müllerian anomalies, diethylstilbestrol exposure)
- Overdistension (by multiple gestation or polyhydramnios)
- Preterm premature rupture of membranes
- Trauma
- Placental abruption
- Immunopathology (e.g., antiphospholipid antibodies)
- Placental ischemic disease (preeclampsia and fetal growth restriction)

Genetics
Familial predisposition. Numerous gene candidates mediating various pathways (inflammation, apoptosis, coagulation, hypoperfusion, thrombosis, collagen remodeling) have been identified, but causality and gene-environment interactions are not well-defined.

RISK FACTORS
- Demographic factors, including single parent, poverty, and black race
- Short interpregnancy interval (<18 months)
- No prenatal care
- Prepregnancy weight <45 kg (100 lb), body mass index <20
- Substance abuse (e.g., cocaine, tobacco)
- Prior preterm delivery (common)
- Previous 2nd-trimester dilation and evacuation (D&E)
- Cervical insufficiency or prior cervical surgery (cone biopsy or loop electrosurgical excision procedure [LEEP])
- Abdominal surgery/trauma during pregnancy
- Uterine structural abnormalities, such as large fibroids or müllerian abnormalities
- Serious maternal infections/diseases
- Bacterial vaginosis
- Bacteriuria
- Vaginal bleeding during pregnancy

- Multiple gestation
- Select fetal abnormalities
- Intrauterine growth restriction
- Placenta previa
- Premature placental separation (abruption)
- Polyhydramnios
- Ehlers-Danlos syndrome

GENERAL PREVENTION
- Patient education at each visit in 2nd and 3rd trimesters for those at risk and periodically in the last two trimesters for the general population
- Routine transvaginal ultrasound cervical length (CL) measurements in singleton pregnancies in the mid-2nd trimester to detect increased risk for preterm birth (<20 mm) is an acceptable strategy (2) and may be especially helpful if risk factors for preterm delivery are present.
- Primary prevention:
  - Interval contraception to optimize pregnancy spacing
  - Smoking cessation
  - If previous preterm birth, evaluate if etiology is likely to recur and target intervention to specific condition.
    ○ Weekly injections of 17α-hydroxyprogesterone (250 mg IM every week) from 16 to 36 weeks if previous spontaneous preterm birth
    ○ Consider cerclage (2)[A] or pessary placement (3)[B] before 24 weeks' gestation for those at high risk because of cervical insufficiency or significant or progressive cervical shortening.
- Secondary prevention:
  - For women with a short cervix in the 2nd trimester (<20 mm on transvaginal US), progesterone 200 mg/day per vagina for 24 to 34 weeks may decrease the risk of preterm delivery (3)[A],(4)[B].
  - Tocolysis

DIAGNOSIS

Diagnosis is generally based on a combination of significant cervical changes (such as dilation, effacement) with regular contractions. However, there is no single test that will reliably diagnose or predict true preterm labor. The diagnosis is based on a combination of physical findings and diagnostic tests that are interpreted in the context of the degree of risk to the patient.

HISTORY
- Address risk factors, especially etiologies of previous preterm birth.
- Regular uterine contractions or cramping
- Dull, low backache or pain
- Intermittent lower abdominal pain
- Increased low pelvic pressure
- Change in vaginal discharge
- Vaginal bleeding
- Fluid leakage

PHYSICAL EXAM
- Sterile speculum exam for membrane rupture evaluation, cultures, and cervical inspection
- Bimanual cervical exam if intact membranes: dilation of the cervix >1 cm and/or effacement of the cervix >50%

ALERT
Avoid bimanual examination when possible if rupture of the membranes is suspected.

DIFFERENTIAL DIAGNOSIS
- Braxton-Hicks contractions/false labor
- Round ligament pain
- Lumbosacral muscular back pain
- UTI or vaginal infections
- Adnexal torsion
- Degenerating fibroid
- Appendicitis
- Dehydration
- Viral gastroenteritis
- Nephrolithiasis

DIAGNOSTIC TESTS & INTERPRETATION
Initial Tests (lab, imaging)
- There are no specific tests that completely accurately predict preterm birth, although several can help with risk stratification.
- In symptomatic women from 22 to 34 weeks' gestation with intact membranes and no intercourse or bleeding in past 24 hours, obtain a fetal fibronectin (FFN) swab from the posterior vaginal fornix. FFN must be obtained prior to digital cervical exam (2).
  - If results are positive (≥50 ng/mL), patient is at a modest increased risk of preterm birth (positive predictive value [PPV] 13–30% for delivery within 2 weeks).
  - If results are negative, >97% of patients will not deliver in 14 days, so can consider avoiding complicated or high-risk interventions.
- Urinalysis and urine culture
- Cultures for gonorrhea and *chlamydia*
- Wet prep for bacterial vaginosis evaluation (although evidence for improved outcomes with treatment is weak)
- Vaginal introitus and rectal culture for group B *Streptococcus*
- pH and ferning test of vaginal fluid to evaluate for rupture of membranes
- CBC with differential
- Drug screen when appropriate
- Kleihauer-Betke test if abruption suspected
- US to identify number of fetuses and fetal position, confirm gestational age, estimate fetal weight, quantify amniotic fluid, and look for conditions making tocolysis contraindicated
- Transvaginal US to evaluate CL, funneling, and dynamic changes after obtaining FFN (if clinical assessment of the cervix is uncertain or if the cervix is closed on digital exam) (2)

Follow-Up Tests & Special Considerations
- Repeat FFN as indicated by symptoms.
- After successful treatment, progressive changes of the cervix on repeat examination or US (in 1 to 2 weeks) may indicate need for hospitalization.

Diagnostic Procedures/Other
- Monitor contractions with external tocodynamometer.
- Consider amniocentesis at any preterm gestational age to evaluate for intra-amniotic infection (cell count with differential, glucose, Gram stain, aerobic, anaerobic, *Mycoplasma*, *Ureaplasma* cultures).

Test Interpretation
- Placental inflammation
  - Acute inflammation usually caused by infection
  - Chronic inflammation caused by immunopathology
- Abruption

TREATMENT

GENERAL MEASURES
- Treat underlying risk factors (e.g., antibiotics for infections, hydration for dehydration).
- Liquids only or NPO if delivery is imminent
- Hospitalization is necessary if the patient is on IV tocolysis.

MEDICATION
Tocolysis may allow time for interventions such as transfer to tertiary care facility and administration of corticosteroids but may not prolong pregnancy significantly (4)[A].

First Line
- Tocolysis (4)[A]
  - Nifedipine: 30 mg PO loading dose, then 10 to 20 mg q6h for 24 hours, and then 10 to 20 mg PO q8h (do not use sublingual route); check BP often and avoid hypotension. Concurrent use with magnesium sulfate is discouraged due to the theoretical risk of neuromuscular blockade.
  - Indomethacin: 50 to 100 mg PO initial dose and then 25 to 50 mg q6–8h. Use for longer than 72 hours is not recommended due to risk of premature closure of ductus arteriosus, oligohydramnios, and possibly neonatal necrotizing enterocolitis. Use with caution in patients with platelet dysfunction, liver dysfunction, or allergy to aspirin.
  - Contraindications to tocolysis: severe preeclampsia, hemorrhage, chorioamnionitis, advanced labor, intrauterine growth restriction, fetal distress, or lethal fetal abnormalities
- Antibiotics: antibiotics for group B *Streptococcus* prophylaxis if culture is positive or unknown
- Steroids: If mother is at 23 to 34 weeks' gestation with no evidence of systemic infection, give glucocorticoids to decrease neonatal respiratory distress, intraventricular hemorrhage, necrotizing enterocolitis, and overall perinatal mortality; betamethasone 12 mg IM × 2 doses 24 hours apart (preferred choice) or dexamethasone 6 mg IM q12h for 4 doses (5)[A]
- Steroids may reduce the risk of respiratory morbidities in singleton infants born to nondiabetic mothers in the late preterm period (34 + 0 to 36 + 6 weeks' gestation). If delivery is likely during this time period, administration of steroids may be considered as above. Tocolysis is not recommended.

Second Line
- Magnesium sulfate by IV infusion has not been shown to be superior to placebo in prolonging pregnancy beyond 48 hours. The side effects are generally greater than those with calcium channel blockers or NSAIDs. Therefore, this agent should be used cautiously (standard dosages for tocolysis start with a 4- to 6-g IV bolus over 20 minutes followed by 2- to 3-g/hr infusion until contractions stop).
  - Magnesium may decrease the risk of cerebral palsy when 12-hour course is given prior to an anticipated preterm birth.
  - Relative contraindications to magnesium sulfate include myasthenia gravis, hypocalcemia, renal failure, or concurrent use of calcium channel blockers.
- Terbutaline 0.25 mg SC q30min for up to 3 doses until contractions stop and then 0.25 mg SC q6h for 4 doses (optional); if contractions persist or pulse >120 bpm, change to another tocolytic agent (may be poorly tolerated by mothers).

- Terbutaline PO or by infusion pump has been used in the past for treatment or prevention of preterm labor. Due to reports of serious cardiovascular events and maternal deaths, PO or long-term SC administration of terbutaline should not be given.
- Significant possible interactions include pulmonary edema from crystalloid fluids and tocolytic agents, especially magnesium sulfate.
- PO maintenance therapy with any agent does not improve outcomes and is not recommended.

ISSUES FOR REFERRAL
- If delivery is inevitable but not immediate, consider transport to a tertiary care center or hospital equipped with a neonatal ICU.
- Consider consultation with maternal–fetal medicine specialist.

ADDITIONAL THERAPIES
- Pelvic rest (e.g., no douching or intercourse) and activity restriction are often recommended; however, data to prove the efficacy are lacking. Some reduction in physical activity may be reasonable; this should be individualized.
- Strict bed rest has not been demonstrated to be effective in most situations.

SURGERY/OTHER PROCEDURES
- For malpresentation or fetal compromise, consider cesarean delivery if labor is progressing.
- Consider cerclage for cervical insufficiency (until 24 weeks' gestation).

ADMISSION, INPATIENT, AND NURSING CONSIDERATIONS
- Suspected/threatened preterm labor
  - IV access
  - Continuous fetal and contraction monitoring
  - Assess cervix for dilatation and effacement.
  - Hydrate with 500 mL 5% dextrose normal saline solution or 5% dextrose lactated Ringer solution for first half hour and then at 125 mL/hr.
  - Monitor for fluid overload (input/output monitoring, symptoms, lung auscultation, pulse oximetry), especially with tocolysis and multiple gestations.
- Discharge criteria
  - Regular contractions and cervical change resolve.
  - If cervix is dilated ≥3 cm or FFN is positive, individualize decision to discharge by gestational age and patient circumstances.

ONGOING CARE

FOLLOW-UP RECOMMENDATIONS
Patient Monitoring
- Weekly office visits with contraction monitoring, cervical checks, or cervical US if at high risk for recurrence
- Routine use of maintenance tocolysis is ineffective in preventing recurrent preterm labor or preterm birth.

DIET
Regular

PATIENT EDUCATION
Call physician or proceed to hospital whenever regular contractions last >1 hour, bleeding, increased vaginal discharge or fluid, decreased fetal movement.

PROGNOSIS
- If membranes are ruptured and no infection is confirmed, delivery often occurs within 3 to 7 days.
- If membranes are intact, 20–50% deliver preterm.

COMPLICATIONS
Labor resistant to tocolysis, pulmonary edema, infection with preterm rupture of membranes

REFERENCES

1. Purisch SE, Gyamfi-Bannerman C. Epidemiology of preterm birth. *Semin Perinatol.* 2017;41(7):387–391.
2. Berghella V, Rafael TJ, Szychowski JM, et al. Cerclage for short cervix on ultrasonography in women with singleton gestations and previous preterm birth: a meta-analysis. *Obstet Gynecol.* 2011;117(3):663–671.
3. Saccone G, Maruotti G, Giudicepietro A, et al; for Italian Preterm Birth Prevention Working Group. Effect of cervical pessary on spontaneous preterm birth in women with singleton pregnancies and short cervical length: a randomized clinical trial. *JAMA.* 2017;318(23):2317–2324.
4. Haas DM, Caldwell DM, Kirkpatrick P, et al. Tocolytic therapy for preterm delivery: systematic review and network meta-analysis. *BMJ.* 2012;345:e6226.
5. Roberts D, Dalziel S. Antenatal corticosteroids for accelerating fetal lung maturation for women at risk of preterm birth. *Cochrane Database Syst Rev.* 2006;(3):CD004454.

ADDITIONAL READING
- American College of Obstetricians and Gynecologists Committee on Obstetric Practice, Society for Maternal-Fetal Medicine. Committee Opinion No. 455: magnesium sulfate before anticipated preterm birth for neuroprotection. *Obstet Gynecol.* 2010;115(3):669–671.
- Simhan HN, Caritis SN. Prevention of preterm delivery. *N Engl J Med.* 2007;357(5):477–487.
- Society for Maternal-Fetal Medicine Publications Committee. Implementation of the use of antenatal corticosteroids in the late preterm birth period in women at risk for preterm delivery. *Am J Obstet Gynecol.* 2016;215(2):B13–B15.
- Son M, Miller ES. Predicting preterm birth: cervical length and fetal fibronectin. *Semin Perinatol.* 2017;41(8):445–451.
- Tita AT, Rouse DJ. Progesterone for preterm birth prevention: an evolving intervention. *Am J Obstet Gynecol.* 2009;200(3):219–224.

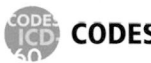

CODES

ICD10
- O60.00 Preterm labor without delivery, unspecified trimester
- O60.02 Preterm labor without delivery, second trimester
- O60.03 Preterm labor without delivery, third trimester

CLINICAL PEARLS
- Treatment of preterm labor may delay delivery to facilitate short-term interventions.
- Steroids improve neonatal outcomes.
- Progesterone therapy can prevent recurrence of preterm birth in next pregnancy.

PRIAPISM

Sundonia J. W. Wonnum, PhD, LCSW • Christine M. Broszko, MD

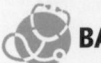

BASICS

DESCRIPTION
- Penile (or less common clitoral) erection lasting for >4 hours and unrelated to sexual stimulation or arousal
- Classified into three types: ischemic, nonischemic, and stuttering:
  - Ischemic (low-flow, veno-occlusive) priapism is associated with ischaemia of the corpora cavernosa, is prolonged and painful, and requires urgent clinical intervention.
  - Nonischemic (high-flow, arterial) priapism is less common and often painless, may be related to prior trauma, and does not require urgent treatment.
  - Stuttering priapism (recurrent, ischemic) is episodic, short-lived, and may not require intervention.
- Malignant priapism is a rare condition resulting most commonly from penile metastases related to primary bladder, prostatic, rectosigmoid, and renal tumors.
- System(s) affected: reproductive and vascular
- Functional impairment: neurophysiologic, sexual, psychosocial (quality of life) (1)

Pediatric Considerations
- In children, nearly all priapism is related to either sickle cell disease (SCD) (65% of cases). Less commonly related etiologies, occurring more typically in the adolescent years, are leukemia, idiopathic, penile trauma (e.g., post circumcision), or illicit drugs (up to 35% of cases).
- Neonatal priapism is also rare, occurring in the first few days of life (2).

EPIDEMIOLOGY
Incidence
- The incidence and prevalence of priapism is largely unknown because the vast majority of empirical literature and data only include cases in which men sought medical intervention. In a study published by Roghmann and colleagues (2013), the number of priapism cases reported by emergency departments between 2006 and 2009 was 32,462 visits, representing a national incidence of 0.73 per 100,000 men per year (3).
- Age: There has been an age shift since 2008 toward men in their 40s. The incidence doubles in men aged >40 years (2.9 vs. 1.5/100,000 person-years).
- Race: 61.1% black (correlated with incidence of SCD), 30% white, 6.3% Hispanic
- Anatomy and physiology:
  - The penis consists of three longitudinally oriented corpora: two dorsolaterally paired corpora cavernosa that are responsible for penile erection and a single ventral corpus spongiosum that surrounds the glans penis and extends distally to form the glans penis.
  - In general, the penile artery (a branch of the internal pudendal artery that, in turn, is a branch from the internal iliac artery) supplies the penis. It divides into three branches: dorsal artery, bulbar artery (supplies the corpus spongiosum), and cavernosal artery (the main blood supply to the erectile tissue).
  - During an erection, smooth muscle relaxation of the cavernosal arterioles results in high-volume inflow to the sinusoids, resulting in compression of the exiting venules. This leads to significant volume expansion of the corpora cavernosa.
  - During the flaccid resting state, the sympathetic nervous system is predominantly in control.

Penile tumescence and erection are driven by the parasympathetic nervous system through the generation of nitric oxide.
  - Smooth muscle relaxation occurs via usage of the phosphodiesterase type 5A (PDE5A) pathway, which generates cyclic guanosine monophosphate (cGMP) (2).

ETIOLOGY AND PATHOPHYSIOLOGY
- Priapism is a pathologic condition that has been observed since ancient times during the upper Paleolithic prehistoric period. There existed iconographic images and statues of the god, Priapus, depicted with an oversized, permanent erection in the posture, *anasurma* (exposing oneself), and leaning on a pillar while using a scale to weigh his genitalia.
- Initially attributed to sexually transmitted diseases, priapism was later associated with spinal cord trauma in the 17th century (4).
- In ischemic priapism (accounting for >95% of reported episodes), decreased venous outflow results in increased intracavernosal pressure. This leads to erection, decreased arterial inflow, blood stasis, local hypoxia, and acidosis (a compartment syndrome). Penile tissue necrosis and fibrosis may occur if priapism persists >24 hours. The exact mechanism is unknown and may involve trapping of erythrocytes in the veins, draining the erectile bodies.
- In nonischemic priapism, increased arterial flow without decreased venous outflow results in a sustained, nonpainful, partially rigid erection.
- Aberrations in the PDE5A pathway have been proven in mice to be one mechanism of priapism (1).
- Causes: ischemic priapism (1)
  - Idiopathic, estimated to about 50%
  - Intracavernosal injections of vasoactive drugs for erectile dysfunction
  - Oral agents for erectile dysfunction
  - Pelvic vascular thrombosis
  - Prolonged sexual activity
  - Leukemia and other malignancies that can infiltrate the corpora
  - SCD and trait
  - Other blood dyscrasias (G6PD deficiency, thalassemia, thrombophilia)
  - Pelvic hematoma or neoplasia (penis, urethra, bladder, prostate, kidney, rectal)
  - Cerebrospinal tumors
  - Asplenism
  - Fabry disease
  - Tertiary syphilis
  - Total parenteral nutrition, especially 20% lipid infusion (results in hyperviscosity)
  - Bladder calculus
  - UTIs, especially prostatitis, urethritis, cystitis
  - Several medications or illicit drugs have been reported to cause priapism (i.e., chlorpromazine, prazosin, trazodone, and some corticosteroids; anticoagulants [heparin and warfarin]; phosphodiesterase inhibitors [sildenafil, others]; immunosuppressants [tacrolimus]; antidepressants; methylphenidate; antihypertensives [hydralazine, propranolol, guanethidine]; antipsychotics [quetiapine, risperidone, aripiprazole]; and cocaine [can be directly injected into penis]).
  - Intracavernous fat emulsion
  - Hyperosmolar IV contrast
  - Spinal cord injury
  - General or spinal anesthesia
  - Heavy alcohol intake

- Causes: nonischemic priapism (1)
  - The most common cause is penile or perineal trauma resulting in a fistula between the cavernous artery and the corpus cavernosum.
  - Acute spinal cord injury
  - Rarely, iatrogenic causes for the management of ischemic priapism can result in nonischemic priapism.
  - Certain urologic surgeries have also resulted in nonischemic priapism.

RISK FACTORS
- SCD has a lifetime risk of ischemic priapism 29–42%.
- Dehydration correlated with SCD or trait
- Prior history of priapismic episodes (stuttering priapism) (1,2)

GENERAL PREVENTION
- Avoid dehydration (SCD cases).
- Avoid excessive sexual stimulation.
- Avoid or limit causative drugs (see "Etiology and Pathophysiology").
- Avoid physical activity with a high risk of blunt trauma to the genital area (1,2).

COMMONLY ASSOCIATED CONDITIONS
- SCD (42.9%) or sickle cell trait (2.5%)
- Drug abuse (7.9%)
- G6PD deficiency
- Leukemia
- Neoplasm

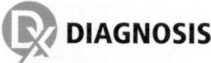

DIAGNOSIS

HISTORY
- Prior priapism episodes or prolonged erections after waking and degree of pain
- Duration of erection
- Perineal or penile trauma (blunt force or needle injury)
- Urination difficult during erection
- History of any hematologic abnormalities (e.g., SCD or trait)
- Cardiovascular disease
- Medications
- Recreational drug use

PHYSICAL EXAM
- In general, physical examination should include:
  - A complete penile, scrotal, and perineal exam to identify the presence of trauma, gangrene (rare), or prosthesis
  - An abdominal and lymph noted exam to rule out underlying conditions
- Observations upon examination should include:
  - Ischemic (or stuttering) priapism: Penis is fully erect, painful, or tender; corpora cavernosa are rigid; and corpora spongiosum and glans are flaccid.
  - Nonischemic priapism: Penis is partially erect (not tender or painful), and the corpora cavernosa are semirigid and nontender, with the glans and corpora spongiosum flaccid.

DIAGNOSTIC TESTS & INTERPRETATION
- CBC with reticulocyte count to detect leukemia or platelet abnormalities
- Sickling hemoglobin (Hgb) solubility test and Hgb electrophoresis
- Coagulation profile

- Platelet count
- Urinalysis/urine toxicology
- Corporal blood gas (CBG) should be obtained to distinguish ischemic from nonischemic priapism.
- A color duplex or Doppler ultrasound of the penis and perineum may be necessary to differentiate ischemic (no blood flow in the cavernosal arteries) from nonischemic (high blood flow) priapism (1)[C]; pelvic vascular thrombosis, partial thrombosis of corpora cavernosa, and corpus spongiosum may be detected.
- Penile arteriography can be used to identify the presence and arterial cavernous fistula or pseudoaneurysms (nonischemic) (5).
- Subjective assessment measure: International Index of Erectile Function (IIEF-5) questionnaire (6)

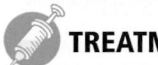

TREATMENT

- Treatments for priapism are determined based on the three main types: ischemic, nonischemic, and stuttering (7).
  - Ischemic priapism requires immediate treatment to preserve future erectile function (a longer delay in treatment means a higher chance of future impotence and possibly necrosis). Urgent urologic consultation is recommended.
    - Cavernosal aspiration with a large bore needle with irrigation (success rate ~30%) (1,3,7)[C]
    - Cavernosal injection of phenylephrine (α-adrenergic sympathomimetic) with monitoring of patient's BP and pulse (success rate between 43% and 81%) (3,7)[C]. Inject q5min until detumescence (15 to 60 minutes).
    - Continue aspiration, irrigation, and phenylephrine for several hours. If this fails, shunt (e.g., distal) procedures are considered.
  - Nonischemic priapism
    - Initial observation, icing (7)[B]
    - If nonischemic priapism does not resolve without or with clinical intervention, arteriography and embolization with absorbable materials (5% rate of impotence vs. 39% with permanent materials) or surgical ligation as a last resort (3)
  - Stuttering priapism
    - The initial goal is to prevent future priapismic episodes (7).
    - Manage acute episodes as ischemic cases—aspiration and irrigation and then intracavernous injections of α-adrenergic agonists (e.g., pseudoephedrine and etilefrine 50 to 100 mg daily is effective in approximately 72% of cases) (7,8).
    - Prevention of recurrence possible through daily oral medications (e.g., pseudoephedrine and etilefrine effective in approximately 72% of cases)
    - Hormonal manipulation to smother circulating testosterone to suppress the action of androgens associated with the erection (duration varies from weeks to years)
    - Digoxin for regulation of smooth muscle tone and to promote penile detumescence (3)
- Conservative treatment (successfully particularly with children) consists of applying ice to the perineum or perineal compression (1).
- In all cases, particularly SCD cases, treat the underlying condition (e.g., SCD does not delay intracavernous treatment).
- Although blood transfusion is an option, particularly in SCD cases, other interventions should be explored and exhausted first (4).
- There are no widely accepted guidelines on treatment among children (2).

GENERAL MEASURES
- Discuss the prognosis with the patient.
- Relieve the patient's pain; do not delay this while waiting for urologic consultation. Provide continuous caudal or spinal anesthesia if the etiology is neurogenic.
- Treat any underlying cause or disease process.
- In SCD cases: IV hydration; supplemental oxygen; partial exchange or repeated transfusions to reduce percentage of sickle cells to <50%
- Initiating proper management depends on whether the priapism is ischemic or nonischemic.

MEDICATION
- Analgesics (e.g., opioids) for pain, if needed
- Intracavernous injection of phenylephrine is recommended by the American Urological Association for ischemic priapism.
- Phenylephrine minimizes risk of cardiovascular side effects that are more common with other sympathomimetics; terbutaline has been studied and may be effective (uncontrolled trials showed a 65% resolution rate) for priapism caused by self-injection of agents to treat erectile dysfunction (3).
- Ketoconazole 200 mg TID and prednisone 5 mg daily for 2 weeks; then, tapering to ketoconazole 200 mg nightly for 6 months has been shown (with limited evidence) to prevent recurrent ischemic priapism.

ISSUES FOR REFERRAL
A urologist should be consulted in all cases of suspected priapism to ensure the highest likelihood of preserved reproductive and vascular function.

SURGERY/OTHER PROCEDURES
- For ischemic priapism, after penile ring block, intracavernous injection of 1% phenylephrine in normal saline is recommended. If the episode is >4 hours, consider aspiration of 5 mL of blood from the corpus cavernosum followed by irrigation and injection of phenylephrine (1).
- Other interventions:
  - Distal shunts
    - Percutaneous: Ebbehoj, Winter, or T shunt
    - Open: Al-Ghorab or corporal snake
  - Proximal shunts
    - Open: Quackles or Sacher
    - Saphenous vein shunt
    - Deep dorsal vein shunt

 ONGOING CARE

FOLLOW-UP RECOMMENDATIONS
Further evaluation of underlying etiologies and reduction of vasoactive drug therapy as indicated

Patient Monitoring
Close follow-up with a urologist is recommended.

PATIENT EDUCATION
Provide information about long-term outlook, referral for counseling, and options if patient is suffering from erectile dysfunction as a result of priapism.

PROGNOSIS
- Even with excellent treatment for a prolonged priapism, complete detumescence may require several weeks secondary to edema.
- Impotence due to irreversible corporal fibrosis is likely in ischemic priapism and is up to 90% if the priapism lasts >24 hours (1).

COMPLICATIONS
Erectile dysfunction (i.e., impotence)

REFERENCES
1. Huang YC, Harraz AM, Shindel AW, et al. Evaluation and management of priapism: 2009 update. *Nat Rev Urol.* 2009;6(5):262–271.
2. Donaldson JF, Rees RW, Steinbrecher HA. Priapism in children: a comprehensive review and clinical guideline. *J Pediatr Urol.* 2014;10(1):11–24.
3. Roghmann F, Becker A, Sammon J, et al. Incidence of priapism at emergency departments in the United States. *J Urol.* 2013;190(4):1275–1280.
4. Turliuc MD, Turliuc S, Cucu A, et al. Through clinical observation: the history of priapism after spinal cord injuries. *World Neurosurg.* 2018;109: 365–371.
5. Montague DK, Jarow J, Broderick GA, et al; for Members of the Erectile Dysfunction Guideline Update Panel, American Urological Association. American Urological Association guideline on the management of priapism. *J Urol.* 2003; 170(4, Pt 1):1318–1324.
6. Tang Z, Li D, Zhang X, et al. Comparison of the simplified International Index of Erectile Function (IIEF-5) in patients of erectile dysfunction with different pathophysiologies. *BMC Urol.* 2014;14:52.
7. Salonia A, Eardley I, Giuliano F, et al. European Association of Urology guidelines on priapism. *Eur Urol.* 2014;65(2):480–489.
8. Kousournas G, Muneer A, Ralph D, et al. Contemporary best practice in the evaluation and management of stuttering priapism. *Ther Adv Urol.* 2017;9(9–10):227–238.

ADDITIONAL READING
Pryor J, Akkus E, Alter G, et al. Priapism. *J Sex Med.* 2004;1(1):116–120.

 SEE ALSO

Anemia, Sickle Cell; Erectile Dysfunction

CODES

ICD10
- N48.30 Priapism, unspecified
- N48.39 Other priapism
- N48.31 Priapism due to trauma

CLINICAL PEARLS
- Priapism is a prolonged penile erection that lasts >4 hours and is unrelated to sexual stimulation. If priapism lasts >24 hours, it likely results in permanent sexual impairment.
- Priapism can occur in children, particularly in SCD. Treatment should address both the underlying disease as well as developmental needs.
- In evaluating priapism, the clinician must distinguish ischemic from nonischemic priapism by history and physical exam as well as cavernosal blood gas and possibly ultrasound, if indicated.
- Ischemic priapism is an emergent condition that requires immediate urologic evaluation and treatment.
- The most common causes of ischemic priapism are idiopathic, related to SCD, iatrogenic, or treatments for erectile dysfunction, or related to use of recreational or medicinal substances.

PROSTATE CANCER

Alex M. Hennessey, MD • Sara L. Valente, MD • Joseph R. Wagner, MD

 BASICS

DESCRIPTION
- The prostate is a male reproductive organ that contributes seminal fluid to the ejaculate.
- The prostate gland is about the size of a walnut, averaging 20 to 25 g in volume in an adult male; tends to enlarge after age 50 years
- Three distinct zones delineate the functional anatomy of the prostate: peripheral zone (largest, neighbors rectal wall, palpable on DRE, most common location for prostate cancer), central zone (contains the ejaculatory ducts), and transition zone (located centrally, adjacent to the urethra).
- Prostatic epithelial cells produce prostate-specific antigen (PSA), which is used as a tumor marker and in screening.

EPIDEMIOLOGY
Incidence
According to the National Cancer Institute SEER data, an estimated 164,690 men in the United States will be newly diagnosed with carcinoma of the prostate (CaP) in 2018 (1).

Prevalence
- About 3 million men are living with CaP in the United States (1).
- An estimated 29,430 men in the United States will die of CaP in 2018 (1).
- Mean age at diagnosis is 66 years.
- Prostate cancer is the most commonly diagnosed nonskin cancer in men in the United States (~11.6% lifetime risk) and second leading cause of cancer death in men (only ~3% of all CaP results in CaP-related death) (1).
- Autopsy studies find foci of latent CaP in 50% of men in their 8th decade of life.
- Probability of clinical CaP 10.9% (1 in 9) in men aged ≥70 years

ETIOLOGY AND PATHOPHYSIOLOGY
- Adenocarcinoma: >95%; nonadenocarcinoma: <5% (most common transitional cell carcinoma)
- Cells generally stain positive for PSA and prostatic acid phosphatase (PAP).
- Location of CaP: 70% peripheral zone, 20% transitional zone, 5–10% central zone

Genetics
Elevated risk if first-degree relative diagnosed with CaP suggesting genetic component; specifics unclear

RISK FACTORS
- Age >50 years
- African American race
- Positive family history
- Poorly understood environmental factors

GENERAL PREVENTION
There are no FDA-approved drugs or diet modifications to prevent CaP.
- Finasteride has been studied for this purpose in a phase III trial called the Prostate Cancer Prevention Trial. A moderate risk reduction associated with an increased risk of high-grade disease was encountered. Therefore, it has not been FDA-approved for prevention (2).

ALERT
Screening for prostate cancer is controversial:

- U.S. Preventive Services Task Force (USPSTF) final recommendation statement states "for men aged 55 to 69 years, the decision to undergo periodic PSA-based screening for prostate cancer should be an individual one and should include discussion of the potential benefits and harms of screening with their clinician. Screening offers a small potential benefit of reducing the chance of death from prostate cancer in some men. However, many men will experience potential harms of screening. (Grade B). (3)[A].
- USPSTF recommends against PSA screening for men ≥70 years old (3)[A].
- For men ages 55 to 69 years, the AUA panel recommends shared decision making between physician and patient regarding PSA screening.
- PSA screening is not recommended in men age <40 years, or any man with <10 years of estimated life expectancy.
- When providing informed consent, the data shows if you screen 1,000 men between 55 and 69 years:
  - 240 will have a positive result.
  - ~100 will have prostate cancer.
  - Of the 100 with cancer, 80 will agree to treatment.
  - Only one person will avoid dying from screening.
  - 50 will develop erectile dysfunction (ED); 15 permanent incontinence

 DIAGNOSIS

HISTORY
- Inquire about family history of CaP, symptoms of bladder outlet obstruction, and other voiding symptoms.
- Anorexia and weight loss, bone pain or neurologic deficits from spinal cord compression (with metastasis), hematuria, hematospermia (rare)

PHYSICAL EXAM
- DRE to assess for prostatic masses, firmness, or asymmetry
- Evaluate lumbar spine and lymph nodes for evidence of metastasis.

DIFFERENTIAL DIAGNOSIS
Benign prostatic hyperplasia, prostatitis, prostatic intraepithelial neoplasia (PIN), prostate stones, atypical small acinar proliferation (ASAP)

DIAGNOSTIC TESTS & INTERPRETATION
Initial Tests (lab, imaging)
PSA, DRE, and clinical history primarily determine need for prostate biopsy:
- In general, total PSA ≥4 ng/mL is concerning for CaP (sensitivity 21%, specificity 91%).
  - Other benign conditions can elevate PSA (infection, inflammation, normal growth, natural PSA fluctuations, normally high variants).
  - Rectal manipulation will not significantly elevate PSA.
- Age, race, and family history need to be considered when interpreting PSA results
- 5-α-Reductase inhibitors decrease PSA by ~50% (2).
- Other PSA metrics used to aid in CaP diagnosis: PSA velocity, PSA doubling time, PSA density (PSAD), percentage free PSA
  - Total PSA velocity: ≥0.75 ng/mL/year or >20% baseline for higher values increases CaP risk.

- Free PSA and age-/race-adjusted PSA helpful in evaluating risk. For patients with PSA between 4 and 10 ng/mL, a low percent free PSA is associated with higher risk of CaP.
  - PSAD ≥0.15 associated with higher prevalence of CaP
  - Screening tests that utilize adjunctive serum/urine biomarkers in conjunction with clinical information to predict CaP risk are also available (e.g., 4Kscore, PHI).
- Prostate biopsy
  - Decision to biopsy involves PSA, DRE findings, adjunctive tests, and overall clinical suspicion of CaP with consideration of comorbidities and life expectancy.
  - Standard biopsy includes systematic random cores from the peripheral zone base, mid, and apex, generally 8 to 12 cores.
  - The Gleason grade is the standard pathologic grading system but is being replaced by grade groups 1 to 5.
    - Gleason grade ranks specimens from 1 (most differentiated) to 5 (least differentiated) based on architectural pattern identified.
    - Primary and secondary patterns are identified and reported, and the sum is the Gleason score (e.g., 3 + 4 = 7).
    - Most prostate cancer are scored 6 to 10, with 10 having the worst prognosis.
    - Grade group 1 = Gleason 6; grade group 2 = Gleason 3 + 4 = 7; grade group 3 = Gleason 4 + 3 = 7; grade group 4 = Gleason 8; grade group 5 = Gleason 9/10
- Staging (4)
  - TNM (tumor, node, and metastasis) staging used to generate a clinical and pathologic stage, which directs treatment. Clinical staging is as follows:
    - T1: cancer found incidentally on TURP or found on biopsy for elevated PSA
    - T2: cancer found on DRE but confined to the prostate
    - T3: cancer found to be extended locally outside of the prostate and/or the seminal vesicle
    - T4: invading adjacent organs
    - N1: denotes local lymph node spread
    - M1: distant metastasis

Follow-Up Tests & Special Considerations
- Some combination of bone scan, MRI, CT, or PET scan may be indicated for high-risk cancers.
- Biopsy if suspicious nodal findings
- Alkaline phosphatase associated with bony metastasis
- Genetic testing (e.g., Prolaris, Oncotype Dx, Decipher) is emerging as a prognostic modality.

 TREATMENT

Treatment options include (4):
- Watchful waiting: monitoring with expectation to provide palliation with symptoms
- Active surveillance: close monitoring of PSA, DRE, and repeat biopsy at regular intervals
- Radical prostatectomy: ± pelvic lymph node dissection (PLND)
- Radiation therapy: external beam (EBRT)

- ProtecT trial (2016) found watchful waiting had equal cancer-specific and all-cause mortality compared to surgery or radiotherapy. In the treatment arms, there was less disease progression (including metastatic disease) but resulted in significantly more morbidity (urinary and bowel dysfunction, ED) (5).
- Brachytherapy: radioactive implants placed in prostate; option for early clinical stage localized to the prostate
- Antiandrogen therapy
  - Bilateral orchiectomy (surgical castration)
  - Gonadotropin-releasing hormone (GnRH) agonist, antagonist, or antiandrogen (medical castration)
  - Abiraterone: 17α-hydroxylase inhibitor (CYP17A adrenal androgen production)
  - Bicalutamide/nilutamide/flutamide/enzalutamide/apalutamide: androgen receptor antagonists
- Chemotherapy: includes multiple chemotherapeutic agents used to treat castrate-resistant prostate cancer (CRPC)
- Risk factors
  - Treatment options based on risk: low-, intermediate-, and high-risk categories; this is based on risk of recurrence after definitive treatment. Must meet all three criteria to be low risk; any one criterion moves patient to a higher risk group (4): risk category clinical stage/serum PSA (ng/mL)/Gleason score: low T1–T2a/<10/≤6; intermediate T2b–T2c/>10 and ≤20/7; high T3a/>20/8 to 10
  - Updated risk stratification algorithms include additional groups of very low risk, favorable and unfavorable intermediate risk, and very high risk
  - Localized CaP
    ○ Low risk:
      ■ Mainstay of therapy is active surveillance.
      ■ Radical prostatectomy and radiation therapy may be offered.
    ○ Intermediate risk:
      ■ Mainstay of therapy is radical prostatectomy or radiation therapy.
      ■ Radical prostatectomy has shown a possible survival benefit in intermediate prostate cancer.
    ○ High risk:
      ■ Mainstay of therapy is radical prostatectomy or radiation therapy.
      ■ Adjuvant radiation may be considered based on adverse pathologic findings after prostatectomy.

ALERT
Life expectancy determination as well as educating the patient of the risks and benefits of surveillance and treatment options is critical.

- Locally advanced CaP:
  - Mainstay of therapy is ADT and radiation; surgery and adjuvant radiation also used
  - Adding abiraterone + prednisone in patients commencing long-term ADT for high risk (T3–T4, Gleason 8 to 10, PSA >40), locally advanced prostate cancer has been shown to significantly increase overall survival (6).
- Metastatic CaP:
  - Mainstay of therapy is RT and ADT.
  - Early chemotherapy (docetaxel) with ADT may be considered for high-volume disease; ADT with abiraterone + prednisone for lower volume disease
  - ADT specifics:
    ○ GnRH agonists include leuprolide or goserelin.
    ○ GnRH antagonists include degarelix: an alternative to GnRH agonists; suppresses testosterone production and avoids flare phenomenon observed with GnRH agonists
    ○ Side effects of ADT: osteoporosis, gynecomastia, ED, decreased libido, obesity, lipid alterations, diabetes, and cardiovascular disease

- Flare phenomenon (disease flare: hot flashes, fatigue) can occur owing to transient increase in testosterone levels on initiation of GnRH agonist therapy.
  ○ If spinal cord metastases are present, the concern for cord compression with a testosterone flare can be avoided by starting antiandrogen therapy prior to initiation of a GnRH agonist.
  ○ Combined androgen blockade with GnRH agonist and antiandrogen (e.g., bicalutamide, nilutamide, or flutamide) may be used to prevent flare.
- CRPC
  - CRPC is defined as progression of disease following ADT. Treatment includes the following:
    ○ Nonmetastatic
      ■ Continue ADT.
      ■ Add antiandrogen (apalutamide or enzalutamide).
    ○ Asymptomatic metastatic: no previous therapy with docetaxel
      ■ Abiraterone: inhibitor of CYP17A (adrenal androgen production), used with prednisone
      ■ Enzalutamide: androgen receptor inhibitor
      ■ Docetaxel: chemotherapeutic that inhibits microtubules
      ■ Sipuleucel-T: immunotherapy
    ○ Symptomatic metastatic: no previous therapy with docetaxel
      ■ Abiraterone, enzalutamide, docetaxel
      ■ Radium-223 (radiopharmaceutical) for patients with symptomatic bony metastases and no visceral metastasis
    ○ Symptomatic metastatic: previous therapy with docetaxel:
      ■ Good performance status: abiraterone, enzalutamide, cabazitaxel
      ■ Poor performance status: Mainstay is palliative care; may attempt further therapy based on patient wishes
- Bone health
  - Men with prostate cancer, particularly those of older age or on ADT, are at elevated risk of pathologic fractures/skeletal events
    ○ Bone density studies should be followed.
    ○ Calcium and vitamin D should be offered.
    ○ Denosumab (RANK-ligand inhibitor—prevents osteoclast activation) and zoledronic acid (bisphosphonate) can be offered for prevention.

 ONGOING CARE

FOLLOW-UP RECOMMENDATIONS
- Prostatectomy: PSA and DRE are recommended at regular intervals. PSA threshold-defining biochemical recurrence is evolving; however, recent data suggest a cutoff of 0.2 ng/mL (4). Some combination of CT/MRI/PET/bone scan usually obtained at recurrence. If the PSA recurrence is due to local disease, salvage radiation is considered. For metastatic disease, androgen deprivation is considered (4).
- XRT: PSA and DRE are recommended at regular intervals. Biochemical recurrence is defined as PSA increase ≥2 ng/mL above nadir; some combination of CT/MRI/PET/bone scan is usually obtained. If the PSA recurrence is thought to be from local disease, salvage prostatectomy or cryosurgery is considered. For metastatic disease, androgen deprivation is considered (4).

PROGNOSIS
- Localized disease is frequently curable; advanced disease has a favorable prognosis if lesions are hormone sensitive.

- 5-year CaP survival by stage: local 100%, regional 100%, distant 29.3% (1)
- Recurrence risk increased if adverse pathologic features are present: extraprostatic extension, seminal vesicle invasion, positive surgical margins.

COMPLICATIONS
- Prostatectomy: Urinary incontinence and ED are the most common long-term issues.
- Radiation therapy: urinary incontinence, ED, radiation cystitis, and radiation proctitis
- Treatment options for ED: PDE5 inhibitors, intracavernosal injections, intraurethral suppositories, vacuum pump, penile prosthesis
- Treatment options for incontinence: oral medications, urethral sling, artificial sphincter

REFERENCES
1. National Cancer Institute: http://seer.cancer.gov.
2. Thompson IM, Goodman PJ, Tangen CM, et al. The influence of finasteride on the development of prostate cancer. *N Engl J Med*. 2003;349(3):215–224.
3. Grossman DC, Curry SJ, Owens DK, et al; and US Preventive Services Task Force. Screening for prostate cancer: US Preventive Services Task Force recommendation statement. *JAMA*. 2018;319(18):1901–1913.
4. National Comprehensive Cancer Network. Clinical practice guidelines: prostate cancer. https://www.nccn.org. Accessed October 12, 2016.
5. Hamdy FC, Donovan JL, Lane JA, et al; for ProtecT Study Group. 10-Year outcomes after monitoring, surgery, or radiotherapy for localized prostate cancer. *N Engl J Med*. 2016;375(15):1415–1424.
6. Fizazi K, Tran N, Fein L, et al; for LATITUDE Investigators. Abiraterone plus prednisone in metastatic, castration-sensitive prostate cancer. *N Engl J Med*. 2017;377(4):352–360.

ADDITIONAL READING
- James ND, de Bono JS, Spears MR, et al; for STAMPEDE Investigators. Abiraterone for prostate cancer not previously treated with hormone therapy. *N Engl J Med*. 2017;377(4):338–351.
- Schröder FH, Hugosson J, Roobol MJ, et al; for ERSPC Investigators. Screening and prostate cancer mortality: results of the European Randomised Study of Screening for Prostate Cancer (ERSPC) at 13 years of follow-up. *Lancet*. 2014;384(9959):2027–2035.

 CODES

ICD10
C61 Malignant neoplasm of prostate

CLINICAL PEARLS
- Prostate cancer is clinically diverse, ranging from low-risk/indolent disease to high-risk/aggressive disease.
- Most men with CaP are asymptomatic.
- The use of PSA for CaP screening is controversial and necessitates an open conversation between medical provider and patient regarding benefits/risks.
- Active surveillance is an important treatment option to consider for low-risk patients.
- Care must be taken when interpreting PSA levels in patients taking $5\text{-}\alpha$-reductase inhibitors.

PROSTATIC HYPERPLASIA, BENIGN (BPH)

Sara M. DeSpain, MD • James E. Hougas III, MD, FAAFP

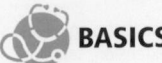

BASICS

DESCRIPTION
- Benign prostatic hyperplasia (BPH) is due to proliferation of both the smooth muscle and epithelial cell lines of the prostate which causes increased volume and may cause compression of the urethra and obstructive symptoms.
- Clinically presents with storage and/or voiding symptoms collectively referred to as lower urinary tract symptoms (LUTS). These include difficulty initiating stream, frequency, or dysuria.
- Symptoms do not directly correlate to prostate volume. It is estimated that half of all men with histologic evidence of BPH experience moderate to severe LUTS.
- Progression may result in upper and lower tract infections and may progress to direct bladder outlet obstruction and acute renal failure (ARF).

EPIDEMIOLOGY
Age related, nearly universal development in men

Incidence
Incidence increases with age; estimates of prevalence vary from 70% to 90% by the age of 80 years (estimated at 8–20% by age 40 years).

ETIOLOGY AND PATHOPHYSIOLOGY
- Develops in prostatic periurethral or transition zone
- Hyperplastic nodules of stromal and epithelial components increase glandular components.
- Etiology is unknown.

RISK FACTORS
- Most significant risk factor is age.
- Increased risk with higher free prostate-specific antigen (PSA) levels, heart disease, and use of β-blockers
- Low androgen levels from cirrhosis/chronic alcoholism can reduce the risk of BPH.
- Obesity and lack of exercise can cause LUTS to be more significant.
- No evidence of increased or decreased risk with smoking, alcohol, or any dietary factors

GENERAL PREVENTION
- The disease appears to be part of the aging process.
- Symptoms can be managed through weight loss, regulation of fluid intake, decreased intake of caffeine, and increased physical activity.

COMMONLY ASSOCIATED CONDITIONS
- LUTS
  - LUTS can be divided into two groups: filling/storage symptoms and voiding symptoms.
    - Filling/storage symptoms include frequency, nocturia, urgency, and urge incontinence.
    - Voiding symptoms include difficulty initiating stream, incomplete voiding, or weak stream.
    - Can lead to acute or chronic obstructive symptoms
- Sexual dysfunction, including erectile dysfunction and ejaculatory disorders
- LUTS can also be secondary to cardiovascular, respiratory, or renal disease (1).

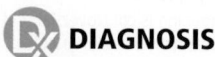

DIAGNOSIS

HISTORY
- Evaluate symptom severity with the American Urological Society Symptom Index or the International Prostate Symptom Score (IPSS).

- Screen for other causes of symptoms such as infection, procedural history, or neurologic causes. Evaluate for comorbid conditions which may produce similar symptoms such as diabetes, congestive heart failure (CHF), or Parkinson disease.
- Review medication list. Particularly diuretics and anticholinergic medications; also, decongestants (increased sphincter tone), opiates (impaired autonomic function), or tricyclic antidepressants (anticholinergic effects)
- Review family history for BPH and prostate cancer.
- Screen for gross hematuria.
- IPSS scoring of LUTS (patient survey tracking severity) (2):
  - Questionnaire: Over the past month, how often have you:
    - 1. Had the sensation of not emptying your bladder completely after you finished urinating?
    - 2. Had to urinate again <2 hours after you finished urinating?
    - 3. Found you stopped and started again several times when you urinated?
    - 4. Found it difficult to postpone urination?
    - 5. Had a weak urinary stream?
    - 6. Had to push or strain to begin urination?
    - 7. Been up to urinate from the time you went to bed at night until the time you got up in the morning?
    - 8. How would you feel if you were to spend the rest of your life with your current symptoms?
  - Scoring of the questionnaire:
    - Questions 1 to 6: no symptoms = 0 points, 1 in 5 times = 1 point, less than half = 2 points, about half = 3 points, more than half = 4 points, most of the time = 5 points
    - Question 7: no occurrence = 0 points, 1 time = 1 point, 2 times = 2 points, 3 times = 3 points, 4 times = 4 points, and 5 times or more = 5 points
    - Question 8: 0 = delighted, 1 = pleased, 2 = mostly satisfied, 3 = mixed, 4 = mostly dissatisfied, 5 = unhappy, 6 = terrible
    - Symptoms are classified as mild (total score 0 to 7), moderate (total score 8 to 19), and severe (total score 20 to 35).
- Nocturia >2 times per night warrants a frequency/volume chart for 2 to 3 days to detect urinary patterns.

PHYSICAL EXAM
- Digital rectal exam (DRE) finding of symmetrically enlarged prostate, but *size does not always correlate with symptoms*
- Signs of renal failure due to obstructive uropathy (edema, pallor, pruritus, ecchymosis, nutritional deficiencies)
- If DRE is suggestive of prostate cancer, or if there is hematuria, recurrent infections, concern for stricture, or evidence of neurologic disease, the patient should be referred to urology.

DIFFERENTIAL DIAGNOSIS
- Obstructive
  - Prostate cancer
  - Urethral stricture or valves
  - Bladder neck contracture (usually secondary to prostate surgery)
  - Inability of bladder neck or external sphincter to relax appropriately during voiding
- Neurologic
  - Spinal cord injury or stroke
  - Parkinsonism
  - Multiple sclerosis

- Medical
  - Poorly controlled diabetes mellitus
  - CHF
- Pharmacologic
  - Diuretics
  - Decongestants
  - Anticholinergics
  - Opioids
  - Tricyclic antidepressants
- Other:
  - Bladder carcinoma
  - Overactive bladder
  - Nocturnal polyuria (>33% of the 24-hour urine volume occurs at night.)
  - Bladder calculi
  - UTI
  - Prostatitis
  - Urethritis/sexually transmitted infections
  - Obstructive sleep apnea (OSA) (nocturia)
  - Caffeine
  - Polyuria (either isolated nocturnal polyuria or 24-hour polyuria)

DIAGNOSTIC TESTS & INTERPRETATION

Initial Tests (lab, imaging)
- Urinalysis (UA) in all patients presenting with LUTS can help rule out other etiologies such as bladder/kidney stones, cancer, UTI, or urethral strictures.
- PSA for men with a life expectancy of 10 years and who would be surgical candidates if prostate cancer was identified
- PSA levels also correlate with prostate volume which can help guide treatment choice.
- With bladder cancer risk factors (smoking history or hematuria), obtain urine cytology.
- If nocturia is the main concern, consider using a frequency volume chart for urine output.
- Sleep study if OSA or primary nocturnal polyuria is suspected
- Serum creatinine measurement is not recommended (AUA recommendation).

Follow-Up Tests & Special Considerations
- No further testing is recommended in uncomplicated LUTS; further testing if symptoms do not respond to medical management or if initial evaluation suggests underlying disease
- Uroflow: volume voided per unit time (Peak flow <10 mL/sec is abnormal.)
- Postvoid residual (PVR): either with catheterization or bladder ultrasound (>100 mL = incomplete emptying)
- Transrectal ultrasound: assessment of gland size; not necessary in the routine evaluation
- Abdominal ultrasound: can demonstrate increased PVR or hydronephrosis; not necessary in the routine evaluation

Diagnostic Procedures/Other
- Pressure-flow studies (urine flow vs. voiding pressures) to determine etiology of symptoms
  - Obstructive pattern shows high voiding pressures with low-flow rate.
- Cystoscopy
  - Demonstrates presence, configuration, cause (stricture, stone), and site of obstructive tissue
  - May help determine therapeutic option
  - Not recommended in initial evaluation unless other factors, such as hematuria, are present

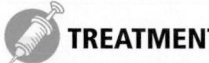 **TREATMENT**

GENERAL MEASURES

- Treatment ranges from watchful waiting to lifestyle modifications, medications, or surgical management.
- Mild symptoms (score of <7) or moderate symptoms (score 8 to 15) that are nonbothersome require no treatment. Reevaluate annually.
- For moderate to severe symptoms, try lifestyle interventions regulation of fluid intake, avoidance of alcohol and caffeine, exercise, diet, and eliminating/reducing contributing medications.
- Medical treatment requires interval follow-up of 2 to 4 weeks for α-blockers and 3 months for 5-α-reductase inhibitors until symptoms improved and then annually.
- Patients with complications including obstruction and urinary retention require bladder drainage.

MEDICATION

- Should be used as additive therapy; lifestyle modifications are still encouraged.
- Two main classes of medications: α-adrenergic antagonists and 5-α-reductase inhibitors
- The combination of these two medication classes is effective for long-term management of BPH and demonstrated large prostates.
  - α-Adrenergic antagonists
    - First-line option for moderate/severe and bothersome LUTS (2)[A]. Affect contraction of smooth muscle in the prostatic urethra and bladder neck. Show benefit over placebo. Typically take 2 to 4 weeks to show improvement. May affect blood pressure; require dose titration and blood pressure monitoring. AUA recommends alfuzosin (Uroxatral), doxazosin (Cardura), and tamsulosin (Flomax) because they are thought to be more selective and have less effect on blood pressure. Prazosin (Minipress) and phenoxybenzamine (Dibenzyline) have insufficient evidence and are not recommended. Most common adverse effect is dizziness; may cause orthostatic hypotension
      - Doxazosin (Cardura): 1 to 8 mg/day PO; may delay the occurrence of acute urinary retention but does not decrease incidence
      - Tamsulosin (Flomax): 0.4 to 0.8 mg/day PO
      - Alfuzosin (Uroxatral): 10 mg/day PO
      - Terazosin (Hytrin): Start at 1 mg PO daily at bedtime, max 20 mg daily.
    - **Contraindications:**
      - Use caution in patients who are also using phosphodiesterase type 5 inhibitors for erectile dysfunction.
      - Do not use in men pursuing cataract surgery until they are postoperative due to the risk for perioperative floppy iris syndrome.
  - 5-α-Reductase inhibitors
    - Block conversion of testosterone to dihydrotestosterone, gradually reduce prostatic volume therefore are of most benefit when prostate volume exceeds 40 mL. Require 6 months to show clinical benefit. Two equally effective options:
      - Finasteride (Proscar): 5 mg/day PO
      - Dutasteride (Avodart): 0.5 mg/day PO
    - Should not be used in patients without evidence of enlarged prostates
    - Show reduced risk of acute urinary retention, less need for surgical intervention, and less overall incidence of prostate cancer
    - Used in patients with refractory hematuria after other causes have been ruled out
    - Side effects include decreased libido and erectile dysfunction.

- A PSA value in a patient taking a **5-α-reductase inhibitors will be artificially low by up to 50%**.
- Combination therapy of α-blocker plus 5-α-reductase inhibitor is superior to monotherapy with an α-blocker only in men with evidence of enlarged prostates.
- Combination therapy is superior to monotherapy to prevent progression but increase risk of drug-related adverse events.
- Anticholinergic agents are appropriate for irritative LUTS without an elevated PVR. Options include solifenacin (VESIcare), tolterodine (Detrol LA), or oxybutynin (Ditropan XL); should be avoided in patients with PVR >250 mL
- If patient also experiences erectile dysfunction, phosphodiesterase-5 inhibitors have been shown to have mild improvement of LUTS; can use tadalafil (Cialis): 5 mg/day PO but avoid use in combination with α-blockers or in those with CrCl <30 mL/min

Geriatric Considerations
Use caution with anticholinergics, antihistamines, sympathomimetics, tricyclic antidepressants, and opioids.

ISSUES FOR REFERRAL

- Moderate or severe LUTS that does not respond to medical management
- BPH-related complications such as recurrent UTIs or hematuria, renal insufficiency, and urinary retention
- Abnormal PSA or prostate exam
- Any history of urethral trauma or stricture, or neurologic disease of the bladder/urinary system

SURGERY/OTHER PROCEDURES

- Indications for surgery:
  - Urinary retention due to prostatic obstruction, recurrent, no improvement with medications
  - Intractable symptoms due to prostatic obstruction AUA score >8 and symptoms
  - Obstructive uropathy (renal insufficiency)
  - Recurrent or persistent UTIs due to prostatic obstruction
  - Recurrent gross hematuria due to enlarged prostate
  - Bladder calculi
- Surgical procedures: TURP remains the gold standard of surgical procedures; however, for selected patient populations, there are other options available.
- Common complications of TURP:
  - Bleeding can be significant.
  - TURP syndrome: hyponatremia secondary to absorption of hypotonic irrigation fluid
  - Retrograde ejaculation
  - Urinary incontinence
- Other options include transurethral needle ablation (TUNA) and transurethral microwave thermotherapy (TUMT), or transurethral incision of the prostate (TUIP). Open prostatectomy is more common when prostate exceeds 100 g. Transurethral laser ablation is an alternative option for patients on anticoagulants.

COMPLEMENTARY & ALTERNATIVE MEDICINE
Saw palmetto (*Serenoa repens*) has been thoroughly studied in a subject in Cochrane review and did not improve LUTS. Other agents including pygeum, Cernilton, and herbs with β-sitosterols have been studied less; however, no current evidence to support their use. Acupuncture failed to show improvement in LUTS in one clinical trial as well. There are no recommended complementary or alternative treatments for BPH (2)[B].

 ONGOING CARE

FOLLOW-UP RECOMMENDATIONS
Patient Monitoring
- Symptom index (IPSS) monitored every 3 to 12 months
- DRE yearly in patients who choose watchful waiting
- PSA yearly in patients who choose watchful waiting: should not be checked while patient is in retention, recently catheterized, or within a week of any surgical procedure to the prostate
- Consider monitoring PVR, if elevated.

DIET
Avoid large boluses of oral or IV fluids or alcohol intake; caffeine may exacerbate symptoms as well.

PATIENT EDUCATION
National Kidney and Urologic Diseases Information Clearinghouse, Box NKUDIC, Bethesda, MD 20893; 301-468-6345

PROGNOSIS
- Symptoms improve or stabilize in 70–80% of patients.
- 25% of men with LUTS will have persistent storage symptoms after prostatectomy.
- Of men with BPH, 11–33% have occult prostate cancer.

COMPLICATIONS
- Urinary retention (acute or chronic)
- Bladder stones
- Prostatitis
- Hematuria

REFERENCES

1. McVary KT, Roehrborn CG, Avins AL, et al. Update on AUA guideline on the management of benign prostatic hyperplasia. *J Urol*. 2011;185(5):1793–1803.
2. Pearson R, Williams PM. Common questions about the diagnosis and management of benign prostatic hyperplasia. *Am Fam Physician*. 2014;90(11):769–774.

ADDITIONAL READING

- American Urological Association. American Urological Association guideline: management of benign prostatic hyperplasia (BPH). http://www.auanet.org. Accessed August 1, 2017.
- Edwards JL. Diagnosis and management of benign prostatic hyperplasia. *Am Fam Physician*. 2008;77(10):1403–1410.

 CODES

ICD10
- N40.0 Enlarged prostate without lower urinary tract symptoms
- N40.1 Enlarged prostate with lower urinary tract symptoms

CLINICAL PEARLS

- Although medical therapy has changed the management of BPH, it has only delayed the need for TURP by 10 to 15 years, not eliminated it.
- Urinary retention, obstructive uropathy, recurrent UTIs, elevated PSA, bladder calculi, hematuria, and failure of medical therapy are indications for surgical management of BPH.

PROSTATITIS
Kyle B. Stephens, DO, MPH

BASICS

DESCRIPTION
- Painful or inflammatory condition affecting the prostate gland with or without bacterial etiology, often characterized by urogenital pain, voiding symptoms, and/or sexual dysfunction
- Significant impact on quality of life
- <10% bacteria-proven infection
- National Institutes of Health's classification
  - *Class I: acute bacterial prostatitis*: symptomatic with fever, perineal pain, dysuria, and obstructive symptoms; polymorphonuclear leukocytes (PMNL) and bacteria in urine
  - *Class II: chronic bacterial prostatitis*: symptomatic chronic or recurrent bacterial infection with pain and voiding disturbances; PMNL and bacteria in expressed prostatic secretions (EPS), or urine after prostate massage, or in semen
  - *Class III: chronic prostatitis/chronic pelvic pain syndrome* (CP/CPPS)
    - Inflammatory (subtype IIIA): chronic symptoms with PMNL in EPS/urine after prostate massage or in semen
    - Noninflammatory (subtype IIIB): chronic symptoms without presence of PMNL in EPS/urine after prostate massage or in semen
  - *Class IV*: asymptomatic *inflammatory prostatitis*: incidental finding during prostate biopsy for infertility, cancer workup; presence of PMNL and/or bacteria in EPS/urine after prostatic massage or in semen
- System(s) affected: genitourinary, renal, reproductive

EPIDEMIOLOGY
Incidence
- Two million cases annually in the United States
- Predominant age: 30 to 50 years old, sexually active; chronic is more common in those >50 years.
- Bacterial prostatitis occurs more frequently in patients with HIV.

Prevalence
- Affects approximately 8.2% of males
- Lifetime probability of diagnosis >25%
- Accounts for 8% of visits to urologists and 1% of visits to primary care physicians
- Percentage of cases by class: class I: <1%, class II: 5–10%, class III: 80–90%, class IV: 10%

ETIOLOGY AND PATHOPHYSIOLOGY
- Acute bacterial prostatitis (class I)
  - Likely, etiology from ascending urethral infection with intraprostatic reflux of infected urine into prostatic ducts, often associated with cystitis
  - Can occur after instrumentation of prostate
  - Usually, gram-negative bacteria (*Escherichia coli* [most common]; *Proteus*, *Klebsiella*, *Serratia*, and *Enterobacter* species; *Pseudomonas aeruginosa*)
  - Rarely, gram-positive bacteria (*Staphylococcus aureus*, *Streptococcus*, and *Enterococcus* species)
  - Confirmed staphylococcal prostatitis should warrant evaluation for hematogenous spread, including endovascular source.
  - Atypical bacteria include *Chlamydia trachomatis*, *Trichomonas vaginalis*, and *Ureaplasma urealyticum*.
  - Consider *Neisseria gonorrhoeae* or *C. trachomatis* in sexually active men <35 years.
- Chronic bacterial prostatitis (class II)
  - Similar pathogens as discussed earlier
  - Often occurs as recurrent episodes of infection by same organism

- Progression from acute to chronic prostatitis is poorly understood but could result from inadequate treatment of acute prostatitis.
- CP/CPPS (class III)
  - Unclear etiology, possibly due to difficult-to-culture infection but noninfectious etiology also proposed
  - Inciting agent may cause inflammation or neurologic damage in or around the prostate and leads to pelvic floor neuromuscular and/or neuropathic pain.
  - No correlation between histologic inflammation of prostate and presence or absence of symptoms
  - Patients with chronic inflammation on histology have shorter time to symptomatic progression.

RISK FACTORS
- Urinary tract infections
- HIV infection
- Prostatic calculi
- Urethral stricture
- Urinary catheterization: indwelling, intermittent
- Genitourinary instrumentation, including prostate biopsy (especially in patients with prior quinolone intake), transurethral resection of prostate, cystoscopy
- Urinary retention
- Benign prostatic hypertrophy
- Unprotected sexual intercourse
- Trauma (e.g., bicycle, horseback riding)

GENERAL PREVENTION
Antibiotic prophylaxis for genitourinary instrumentation and prostatic biopsy

COMMONLY ASSOCIATED CONDITIONS
- Benign prostatic hypertrophy
- Cystitis
- Urethritis
- Sexual dysfunction, including erectile dysfunction and premature ejaculation

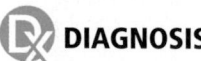

DIAGNOSIS

HISTORY
- Acute prostatitis (class I):
  - Acutely ill with fever, chills, malaise
  - Low back pain, myalgias
  - Frequency, urgency, dysuria, nocturia
  - Prostatodynia, pelvic pain, perineal pain
  - Cloudy urine
  - Obstructive voiding symptoms: poor stream, hesitancy
- Chronic prostatitis (classes II and III):
  - More insidious presentation than class I
  - Symptoms for 3 of 6 previous months
  - Low-grade fever (class II only)
  - Prostatodynia, perineal pain
  - Dysuria, frequency, urgency
  - Lower abdominal pain
  - Low back, testicular, and/or penile pain
  - Hematospermia
  - Sexual dysfunction/painful ejaculation

PHYSICAL EXAM
- Vital signs (Unstable vitals suggest sepsis.)
- Back exam (CVA tenderness)
- Abdominal exam (bladder distension)
- Prostate exam

- Class I: Prostate is very tender, warm, firm, and edematous.
- Class II: often normal but enlarged, tender, edematous, nodular prostate also encountered
- Class III: often normal prostate

ALERT
Avoid vigorous massage of the prostate in acute bacterial prostatitis; may induce iatrogenic bacteremia; safe if done gently

DIFFERENTIAL DIAGNOSIS
- Lower urinary tract infection
- Pyelonephritis
- Cystitis (bacterial, interstitial)
- Urethritis
- Prostatic abscess
- Acute/chronic urinary retention
- Benign prostatic hypertrophy malignancy (prostate, bladder)
- Obstructive calculi
- Foreign body

DIAGNOSTIC TESTS & INTERPRETATION
Initial Tests (lab, imaging)
- Suspected acute prostatitis (class I)
  - Urinalysis; urine Gram stain/culture and sensitivity
  - CBC with differential; blood culture if fever, chills, or signs of sepsis are present
- Suspected chronic bacterial prostatitis (class II)
  - Urinalysis; urine/EPS/semen: Gram stain/culture and sensitivity
  - Review previous urine culture results.
  - National Institutes of Health Chronic Prostatitis Symptom Index (NIH-CPSI): 9-question symptom survey (http://www.prostatitis.org/symptomindex.html)
  - Diagnostic gold standard: Meares-Stamey 4-glass test (not performed often)
  - 2-glass test (pre- and postmassage urine testing) more common and easier with equivalent sensitivity and specificity
    - Cultures of midstream preprostate massage urine and EPS/postmassage urine
  - Consider urinary flow rate and postvoid residual volume if urinary retention is present.
- Suspected CP/CPPS (class III)
  - Diagnosis of exclusion
  - Urinalysis; urine/EPS/semen: Gram stain/culture and sensitivity
  - Hematuria if present: urine cytology, cystoscopy, CT urography with or without contrast
  - PSA is not indicated unless malignancy is suspected.
  - Concomitant abdominal pain: CT abdomen
  - Testicular pain: scrotal US
  - Sensation of incomplete bladder emptying: postvoid residual volume with bladder US or catheterization
  - Lumbar radiculopathy: MRI spine

Follow-Up Tests & Special Considerations
- Failure to respond to initial antibiotic therapy: US, CT, or MRI to image prostate and urology referral
- US or CT or MRI if prostatic calculi, malignancy, or abscess is suspected
- Acute bacterial: urinalysis and culture 30 days after initiating treatment
- Chronic bacterial: urinalysis and culture every 30 days (may take several months of treatment to clear)

Diagnostic Procedures/Other
- Needle biopsy or aspiration for culture
- Urodynamic testing (prostatodynia) if indicated
- Cystoscopy (in persistent nonbacterial prostatitis to rule out bladder cancer, interstitial cystitis)

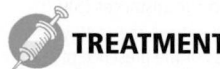 TREATMENT

GENERAL MEASURES
- Analgesics/antipyretics/stool softeners
- Hydration
- Sitz baths to relieve pain and spasm
- Suprapubic catheter for urinary retention
- Anxiolytics, antidepressants if anxiety and/or depression are present

MEDICATION

First Line
- Acute bacterial (outpatient) (1)[A]
  – Fluoroquinolone (ciprofloxacin 500 mg PO q12h or levofloxacin 500 mg PO once daily) for 2 to 4 weeks *or*
  – Trimethoprim-sulfamethoxazole 1 double-strength tablet PO q12h for 2 to 4 weeks *or*
  – If gram-positive cocci are seen in initial urine Gram stain, start with amoxicillin 500 mg PO q8h. Adjust antibiotics once culture and sensitivities report is available.
  – Local sensitivity pattern should guide therapy.
  – If at risk for sexually transmitted infection (STI) pathogens: ceftriaxone 250 mg IM for 1 dose plus doxycycline 100 mg PO q12h daily for 1 week or azithromycin 1 g PO single dose
- Acute bacterial (inpatient) (1)[A]
  – Ampicillin 2 g IV q6h or fluoroquinolone (ciprofloxacin 400 mg IV q12h or levofloxacin 500 mg q24h); begin oral therapy after afebrile for 24 to 48 hours.
- Chronic bacterial (class II) (1,2,3)[A],(4)[C]
  – Fluoroquinolone (e.g., levofloxacin 500 mg PO) once daily for 4 weeks or ciprofloxacin 500 mg PO q12h for 4 to 12 weeks
  – Combination therapy with azithromycin may help to eradicate atypical pathogens.
  – Anti-inflammatory agents for pain symptoms and α-blockers for urinary symptoms
- CP/CPPS (class III) (4)[C],(5,6)[A]
  – Heterogeneous condition with no universally effective treatment
  – Treatment choice is patient centered, focusing on symptoms relief of four domains: pain, lower urinary tract symptoms (LUTS), psychological stress, and sexual dysfunction.
    ○ α-Blockers, antibiotics, and combinations of these therapies achieve greatest improvement in clinical symptoms scores compared to placebo.
    ○ Tamsulosin 0.4 mg PO once daily at bedtime for 4 to 6 weeks; continue if there is a positive response.

Second Line
- Piperacillin or ticarcillin with aminoglycoside, erythromycin, tetracycline, cephalexin, fluoroquinolones, dicloxacillin, nafcillin IV, vancomycin IV
- Finasteride (in patients >45 years, class IIIA, and enlarged prostate glands)
- Atypical: may benefit from erythromycin, doxycycline

ISSUES FOR REFERRAL
Urology referral if antibiotic treatment fails, symptoms persist (especially obstructive voiding symptoms), hematuria, elevated PSA; or for surgical drainage if an abscess persists after ≥1 week of therapy

ADDITIONAL THERAPIES
- Psychotherapy if sexual dysfunction is present
- 5-α-Reductase inhibitors, nonsteroidal anti-inflammatory medications, pelvic floor physical therapy, transurethral microwave thermotherapy, circumcision

SURGERY/OTHER PROCEDURES
Surgical resection can be considered for refractory cases of recurrent bacterial prostatitis or to drain an abscess, when necessary.

COMPLEMENTARY & ALTERNATIVE MEDICINE
Class III: Acupuncture and extracorporeal shockwave therapy have best evidence of decrease in prostatitis symptoms without adverse effects. Lifestyle modifications, physical activity, prostatic massage, and transrectal thermotherapy have limited data to support (7)[A].

ADMISSION, INPATIENT, AND NURSING CONSIDERATIONS
- Proven or suspected abscess
- Unstable vital signs (sepsis)
- Immunocompromised
- Failed outpatient treatment

 ONGOING CARE

FOLLOW-UP RECOMMENDATIONS
- Negative urine culture at 7 days predictive of cure after completion of treatment course
- Consider prostatic abscess in patients who do not respond well to therapy.

Patient Monitoring
NIH-CPSI: 9 questions, which can be used to evaluate severity of patient symptoms and response to treatment within three domains:
- Pain
- Urinary symptoms
- Quality of life

PROGNOSIS
- Fever and dysuria usually resolve in 2 to 6 days.
- Acute infection usually improves in 3 to 4 weeks.
- Course of chronic prostatitis is often prolonged and difficult to cure; 55–97% cure rate depending on population and drug used
- 20% have reinfection or persistent infection.

COMPLICATIONS
- Prostatic abscess (common in HIV infected)
- Pyelonephritis
- Gram-negative sepsis, bacteremia
- Urinary retention
- Epididymitis
- Infertility
- Chronic bacterial prostatitis (following acute prostatitis)
- Metastatic infection (spinal, sacroiliac)

REFERENCES

1. Lipsky BA, Byren I, Hoey CT. Treatment of bacterial prostatitis. *Clin Infect Dis.* 2010;50(12):1641–1652.
2. Videčnik Zorman J, Matičič M, Jeverica S, et al. Diagnosis and treatment of bacterial prostatitis. *Acta Dermatovenerol Alp Pannonica Adriat.* 2015;24(2):25–29.
3. Perletti G, Marras E, Wagenlehner FM, et al. Antimicrobial therapy for chronic bacterial prostatitis. *Cochrane Database Syst Rev.* 2013;(8):CD009071.
4. Rees J, Abrahams M, Doble A, et al; and Prostatitis Expert Reference Group (PERG). Diagnosis and treatment of chronic bacterial prostatitis and chronic prostatitis/chronic pelvic pain syndrome: a consensus guideline. *BJU Int.* 2015;116(4):509–525.
5. Zhu Y, Wang C, Pang X, et al. Antibiotics are not beneficial in the management of category III prostatitis: a meta analysis. *Urol J.* 2014;11(2):1377–1385.
6. Anothaisintawee T, Attia J, Nickel JC, et al. Management of chronic prostatitis/chronic pelvic pain syndrome: a systematic review and network meta-analysis. *JAMA.* 2011;305(1):78–86.
7. Franco JVA, Turk T, Jung JH, et al. Non-pharmacological interventions for treating chronic prostatitis/chronic pelvic pain syndrome. *Cochrane Database Syst Rev.* 2018;(5):CD012551.

ADDITIONAL READING

- Anderson RU, Wise D, Sawyer T, et al. 6-Day intensive treatment protocol for refractory chronic prostatitis/chronic pelvic pain syndrome using myofascial release and paradoxical relaxation training. *J Urol.* 2011;185(4):1294–1299.
- Collins MM, Stafford RS, O'Leary MP, et al. How common is prostatitis? A national survey of physician visits. *J Urol.* 1998;159(4):1224–1228.
- Krieger JN, Lee SW, Jeon J, et al. Epidemiology of prostatitis. *Int J Antimicrob Agents.* 2008;31(Suppl 1): S85–S90.
- Nickel JC, Freedland SJ, Castro-Santamaria R, et al. Chronic prostate inflammation predicts symptom progression in patients with chronic prostatitis/chronic pelvic pain. *J Urol.* 2017;198(1):122–128.
- Nickel JC, Shoskes D, Wang Y, et al. How does the pre-massage and post-massage 2-glass test compare to the Meares-Stamey 4-glass test in men with chronic prostatitis/chronic pelvic pain syndrome? *J Urol.* 2006;176(1):119–124.

 SEE ALSO

- Prostate Cancer; Prostatic Hyperplasia, Benign (BPH); Urinary Tract Infection (UTI) in Males
- Algorithm: Hematuria

 CODES

ICD10
- N41.9 Inflammatory disease of prostate, unspecified
- N41.0 Acute prostatitis
- N41.1 Chronic prostatitis

CLINICAL PEARLS
- Vigorous prostatic massage is contraindicated in acute prostatitis.
- Fluoroquinolones are recommended first-line antibiotic for bacterial prostatitis, both acute and chronic (class I and class II).
- At least 14 to 30 days of antibiotic therapy is required for acute prostatitis; longer for chronic bacterial prostatitis
- Antibiotic therapy is not proven to be effective in CP/CPPS (class III).
- Imaging is often not needed.

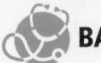

PROTEIN C DEFICIENCY

Donald J. Fahey-Ahrndt, MD • James E. Hougas III, MD, FAAFP

BASICS

DESCRIPTION
- Protein C is a vitamin K–dependent factor synthesized, in an inactive form, by the liver.
- Activated protein C inhibits generation of thrombin by inactivating factors Va and VIIIa, using protein S as a cofactor.
- Deficiency in protein C activity therefore leads to a prothrombotic state.
- System(s) affected: cardiovascular, pulmonary, integumentary, hematologic, and immunologic

EPIDEMIOLOGY
Prevalence
- 0.3% of the general population
- 3–5% of persons with venous thromboembolism (VTE)
- Mean age of first thrombosis is 45 years.
- There is no known gender predominance.

ETIOLOGY AND PATHOPHYSIOLOGY
- Protein C deficiency (PCD) can be inherited or acquired.
- Genetic mutations can lead to two types of PCD; however, the distinction between the two is clinically irrelevant.
  - Type I (most common) results in the reduction of protein C levels.
  - Type II results in a decreased functionality, despite having normal levels of protein C.
- Acquired PCD can occur in many disease states such as:
  - Liver disease
  - Disseminated intravascular coagulation (DIC)
  - Severe infections (especially meningococcemia)
  - Autoantibody inhibitors directed toward protein C
  - Cancer and chemotherapy (i.e., L-asparaginase, 5-FU, methotrexate, and cyclophosphamide)
  - Initial use of vitamin K antagonists (warfarin)
  - Vitamin K deficiency (malnutrition or malabsorption of fat-soluble vitamins)

Genetics
- Autosomal dominant inheritance pattern with incomplete penetrance
- At least 160 genetic mutations have been described in the protein C gene that can lead to a functional deficiency.
- Heterozygous patients often have mild or asymptomatic disease.
- Homozygous patients, or those with another coexisting genetic thrombophilia, often have more severe disease.
- Additionally, mutations in other genes (GCKR, EDEM2, BAZ1B, etc.) are associated with variability in the levels of protein C expression in the general population, although their clinical significance is currently unknown.
- Patients with PCD who start warfarin without concomitant heparin are at increased risk of developing warfarin-induced skin necrosis (WISN). This is thought to be due to the shorter half-life of protein C (5 to 8 hours) compared to other vitamin K–dependent clotting factors. However, not all patients who develop WISN have PCD (1).

GENERAL PREVENTION
Because PCD is usually a congenital disease, there are no preventive measures.

COMMONLY ASSOCIATED CONDITIONS
- VTE at any site, often spontaneous
- Arterial thrombosis is rare, and a causative relationship has not been clearly demonstrated.
- Homozygosity can be associated with catastrophic thrombotic complications at birth (e.g., *purpura fulminans*).
- Recurrent pregnancy losses

DIAGNOSIS

HISTORY
- Recurrent VTE
- VTE at <40 years of age
- Thrombosis in unusual locations (e.g., mesentery, sagittal sinus, portal vein)
- Family history of thrombosis or spontaneous abortion
- Often has other usual risk factors for provoked VTE

PHYSICAL EXAM
Normal

DIFFERENTIAL DIAGNOSIS
- Factor V Leiden
- Protein S deficiency
- Antithrombin deficiency
- Dysfibrinogenemia
- Dysplasminogenemia
- Hyperhomocysteinemia
- Prothrombin 20210 mutation
- Elevated factor VIII, IX, or XI levels
- Antiphospholipid antibody syndrome
- DIC
- Heparin-induced thrombocytopenia (HIT)

DIAGNOSTIC TESTS & INTERPRETATION
Initial Tests (lab, imaging)
- Initial evaluation of a new clot in patients should include a CBC with peripheral smear, INR, aPTT, hepatic and renal function tests as well as appropriate imaging.
- Testing for heritable causes of thrombophilia in unselected patients presenting with a first-time VTE (provoked or unprovoked) is not indicated (2,3)[C].
- Consider screening for antiphospholipid syndrome rather than other thrombophilia (PCD) for women with recurrent early pregnancy loss (three loses prior to 10 weeks' gestation) (4)[B].

Follow-Up Tests & Special Considerations
- Testing for heritable or acquired thrombophilia is suggested in the following circumstances (5)[C]:
  - First episode of VTE and patient age <40 years
  - Recurrent VTE regardless of the presence of risk factors
  - Patients with VTE at unusual sites
- Testing for PCD should be considered in patients with history of WISN (3)[C].
- Testing for protein C and S deficiencies should be done urgently in neonates and children suspected to have purpura fulminans (2,3)[B].
- Testing for hereditary thrombophilia should only be considered in asymptomatic first-degree relatives of those with proven hereditary thrombophilia if they are female, of childbearing age, and have no history of prior pregnancy complications (3,4)[C].
- When ordering additional testing for hereditary or acquired thrombophilia, the following conditions should be considered (3)[C]:
  - Antiphospholipid antibody syndrome
  - Antithrombin III deficiency
  - Factor V Leiden
  - PCD
  - Protein S deficiency
  - Prothrombin G20210A
- Testing for PCD is done using two separate lab tests:
  - An immunoassay for a quantitative assessment of protein C levels
  - A functional activity assay using a snake venom protease to activate protein C

Test Interpretation
- Drugs that may alter lab results
  - Oral contraceptives can raise protein C levels.
  - Warfarin reduces protein C levels and should be discontinued 2 to 3 weeks before reliable testing.
- Disorders that may alter lab results
  - Liver disease reduces protein C levels.

ALERT
Acute thrombosis can lower protein C levels. Repeat confirmatory test of low protein C level at a separate time is advisable. If a normal level of protein C is obtained at presentation, then deficiency can be excluded.

TREATMENT

Treat active thrombosis; follow-up

GENERAL MEASURES
- Individuals with PCD should be educated regarding signs and symptoms of VTE.
- Women with any of the following history should avoid estradiol-containing contraceptives and hormone replacement therapy during menopause (3)[A]:
  - Diagnoses of PCD
  - First-degree relative with PCD
  - First-degree relative with VTE at age <50 years

- Women may use progestin-only hormonal contraception options.
- Routine anticoagulation for asymptomatic patients with PCD is not recommended (4)[C].
- Anticoagulation is recommended for at least 3 months in patients with inherited thrombophilia following their first VTE (2,5)[B].
  - There is some argument for indefinite anticoagulation; however, data are limited (3)[C].
  - Shared decision making should be used to discuss duration of therapy beyond 3 months (3)[C].
- Indefinite anticoagulation is indicated for patients with recurrent VTE (4)[A].
- Treat VTE as an outpatient when possible if clinically stable (4)[B].
- Severe congenital PCD may be treated with protein C concentrates.

Pregnancy Considerations
- Heparin-based products should be used during pregnancy when therapeutic or prophylactic treatment of VTE is needed.
- For pregnant women with known PCD but no personal history of VTE or additional thrombotic risk factors (i.e., family history of VTE in first-degree relative <50 years of age, obesity, prolonged immobility), antepartum and postpartum clinical monitoring is recommended over prophylactic therapy (5)[C].
- For pregnant women with known PCD, no personal history of VTE but with an additional thrombotic risk factor, antepartum surveillance is recommended with postpartum prophylactic therapy for 6 weeks of either prophylactic or intermediate dose (5)[C].
- For pregnant women with known PCD and previous VTE, it is recommended to give postpartum preventative therapy with either prophylactic or intermediate-dose LMWH. This could also be given antepartum versus surveillance at the provider's discretion (5)[C].

First Line
- LMWH (4)[A]: initially started with warfarin for a minimum of 5 days and two consecutive INRs between 2 and 3 to bridge. Additionally, LMWH may be started 5 to 10 days prior to starting dabigatran or edoxaban.
  - Enoxaparin (Lovenox) 1 mg/kg SC BID or 1.5 mg/kg/day SC
  - Tinzaparin (Innohep): 175 anti-Xa IU/kg/day SC
  - Dalteparin (Fragmin) 200 U/kg/day
- Novel oral anticoagulants (NOACs):
  - Rivaroxaban (Xarelto) 15 mg PO BID with food for 21 days and then 20 mg PO QD with food
  - Apixaban (Eliquis) 10 mg PO BID for 7 days and then 5 mg PO BID
  - Dabigatran (Pradaxa) 150 mg PO BID (after 5 to 10 days of parenteral anticoagulation)
  - Edoxaban (Savaysa) 60 mg PO QD (after 5 to 10 days of parenteral anticoagulation)
- Oral vitamin K antagonist:
  - Warfarin (Coumadin) titrated to an INR of 2 to 3 (4)[A]

- Factor Xa inhibitors:
  - Fondaparinux (Arixtra) <50 kg: 5 mg/day SC; 50 to 100 kg: 7.5 mg/day SC; >100 kg: 10 mg/day SC; contraindicated if CrCl <30 mL/min
- Contraindications
  - Active bleeding precludes anticoagulation; risk of bleeding is a relative contraindication to long-term anticoagulation.
- Precautions
  - Observe patient for signs of embolization, further thrombosis, or bleeding.
  - Monitor kidney function, drug–drug interactions, and CBC, including platelets (concern for HIT).

Second Line
- Heparin 80 U/kg IV bolus followed by 18 U/kg/hr; adjust dose depending on PPT.
- In patients requiring large daily doses of heparin, measure an anti-Xa level for dose guidance.
- Alternatively, and for outpatients, unfractionated heparin can be given at 333 U/kg and then 250 U/kg SC, without monitoring (4)[C].

ISSUES FOR REFERRAL
Patients with suspected PCD should be referred to a hematologist.

SURGERY/OTHER PROCEDURES
- Anticoagulation may be held for surgical interventions.
- In patients with acute proximal DVT of the lower extremity *and* an absolute contraindication to anticoagulation, inferior vena cava (IVC) filters are recommended; otherwise, the use of an IVC filter in addition to anticoagulants is not recommended (4)[B].

ADMISSION, INPATIENT, AND NURSING CONSIDERATIONS
- Life-threatening VTE
- Significant bleeding while on anticoagulant therapy

 ONGOING CARE

FOLLOW-UP RECOMMENDATIONS
Patient Monitoring
- Warfarin requires periodic monitoring of the INR to maintain a range of 2 to 3 (monthly, after initial stabilization).
- LMWH is the treatment of choice in pregnancy. Periodic monitoring with anti-Xa levels is recommended in these patients.

DIET
Unrestricted (except if on warfarin—avoid varying diet with foods that have significant amounts of vitamin K)

PATIENT EDUCATION
- Patients should be educated about signs and symptoms of VTE as well as the use of oral anticoagulant therapy if taking such.
- Avoid NSAIDs while on warfarin.
- Avoid OCPs because they increase risk of thrombosis.

PROGNOSIS
When compared with normal individuals, persons with PCD have normal life spans.

COMPLICATIONS
Primary or recurrent VTE

REFERENCES
1. Chan YC, Valenti D, Mansfield AO, et al. Warfarin induced skin necrosis. *Br J Surg.* 2000;87(3):266–272.
2. Baglin T, Gray E, Greaves M, et al; and British Committee for Standards in Haematology. Clinical guidelines for testing for heritable thrombophilia. *Br J Haematol.* 2010;149(2):209–220.
3. Nicolaides AN, Fareed J, Kakkar AK, et al. Prevention and treatment of venous thromboembolism—International Consensus Statement. *Int Angiol.* 2013;32(2):111–260.
4. Guyatt GH, Akl EA, Crowther M, et al; for American College of Chest Physicians Antithrombotic Therapy and Prevention of Thrombosis Panel. Executive summary: Antithrombotic Therapy and Prevention of Thrombosis, 9th ed: American College of Chest Physicians evidence-based clinical practice guidelines. *Chest.* 2012;141(Suppl 2):7S–47S.
5. James A; for Committee on Practice Bulletins—Obstetrics. Practice Bulletin No. 123: thromboembolism in pregnancy. *Obstet Gynecol.* 2011;118(3):718–729.

 CODES

ICD10
D68.59 Other primary thrombophilia

CLINICAL PEARLS
- Testing for heritable causes of thrombophilia in unselected patients presenting with a first episode of VTE (provoked or unprovoked) is not indicated.
- Screening, and therefore prophylactic treatment, of asymptomatic family members is not justified with the possible exception of females of childbearing age with no previous history of pregnancy complications.
- Asymptomatic patients with PCD do not need prophylactic anticoagulation because the risk of thrombosis is low.
- Patients with PCD presenting with first time VTE should be anticoagulated for at least 3 months. Other risk factors and shared decision making should be used to determine if anticoagulation should be used for a longer duration.
- Recurrent VTE is an indication for indefinite anticoagulation.

PROTEIN S DEFICIENCY

Thuy Thanh Thi Le, DO • Helen N. Johnson-Wall, MD

BASICS

DESCRIPTION

- Protein S is a vitamin K–dependent glycoprotein, produced mainly in the liver that acts as a cofactor for protein C. It is also produced by megakaryocytes and endothelial cells.
- Protein C becomes activated when thrombin binds to the endothelial receptor, thrombomodulin.
- Activated protein C, with protein S (a cofactor), inactivates clotting factors Va and VIIIa enhancing fibrinolysis.
- Protein S is also able to directly inhibit factors Va, VIIa, and Xa independently of activated protein C.
- Protein S deficiency is a congenital thrombophilia, which increases the risk of thromboembolism.
- It primarily affects the venous system.
- System(s) affected: cardiovascular; hematologic/immunologic; pulmonary

EPIDEMIOLOGY

Incidence
- Mean age of first thrombosis: 2nd decade
- Predominant sex: male = female

Prevalence
- ~0.2% of general population
- Found in ~1% of persons with venous thrombosis embolism (VTE)

ETIOLOGY AND PATHOPHYSIOLOGY

- It is an autosomal dominant disease.
- Only the free form of protein S (30–40%) acts as a cofactor for activated protein C. Protein S reversibly binds to the C4b protein, which leads to conditions in which free protein S is low, but total protein S is normal. These individuals are prone to thrombosis.
- Conditions with reduced protein S: pregnancy, oral contraceptives, warfarin, disseminated intravascular coagulation (DIC), liver disease, nephrotic syndrome, HIV, L-asparaginase chemotherapy, acute thrombosis, and acute varicella-zoster virus infection

Genetics
- Is due to mutations in the PROS1 gene on chromosome 3. Most individuals are heterozygous.
- Heterozygotes have an odds ratio (OR) of VTE of 1.6 to 11.5.
- Homozygosity or compound heterozygosity, if untreated, is usually incompatible with adult life.
- Homozygotes can have a fulminant thrombotic event in infancy, termed *neonatal purpura fulminans*.

RISK FACTORS

- Oral contraceptives, pregnancy, and the use of HRT increase the risk of VTE in patients with protein S deficiency (1)[A].
- Patients with protein S deficiency and other prothrombotic states have further increased rate of thrombosis (1)[A].
- Arterial thrombosis is more frequent in patients with protein S deficiency who smoke.
- Patients heterozygous for protein S deficiency who are initiated on warfarin without concomitant heparin can develop warfarin-induced skin necrosis because the half-life of other vitamin K–dependent clotting factors (e.g., prothrombin, factor IX, and factor X) is much longer than the anticoagulant protein S (4 to 8 hours), leading to a transient hypercoagulable state when protein S becomes depleted. These patients develop extremely low levels of protein S and develop necrosis of the skin over central areas of the body such as the breast, abdomen, buttocks, and genitalia (1)[A].

Pregnancy Considerations
Increased thrombotic risk and pregnancy losses

GENERAL PREVENTION

There are no preventive measures.

COMMONLY ASSOCIATED CONDITIONS

- Deep and superficial VTE, often unprovoked
- Up to 50% of homozygotes will have thrombosis.
- Homozygosity is associated with catastrophic thrombotic complications at birth: *neonatal purpura fulminans*.
- Sites of thrombosis can be unusual, including the mesentery, cerebral veins, and axillary veins.
- Arterial thrombosis is rare but reported in several case reports.
- Skin necrosis in patients treated with warfarin
- Recurrent pregnancy losses (2)

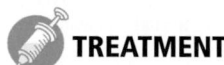

DIAGNOSIS

HISTORY

Inherited thrombophilias should be suspected in:
- Unprovoked VTE at age <50 years
- VTE with a strong family history of VTE or known familial protein S deficiency
- VTE in unusual sites as mesenteric or cerebral vein
- Recurrent VTE

PHYSICAL EXAM

Normal

DIFFERENTIAL DIAGNOSIS

Other inherited thrombophilias:
- Factor V Leiden (most common; usually in Caucasians)
- Protein C deficiency (in Caucasians)
- Antithrombin deficiency
- Dysfibrinogenemia
- Dysplasminogenemia
- Homocystinemia
- Prothrombin G20210A mutation
- Elevated factor VIII levels
- Acquired VTE risk factors: surgery, immobility, cancer, myeloproliferative neoplasms, trauma, antiphospholipid syndrome, paroxysmal nocturnal hemoglobinuria, pregnancy, hormone replacement therapy, postpartum, DIC

DIAGNOSTIC TESTS & INTERPRETATION

Initial Tests (lab, imaging)
- For evaluation of new clot in a patient at risk: CBC with peripheral smear, PT/INR, aPTT, thrombin time, lupus anticoagulant, antiphospholipid antibodies, anticardiolipin antibody, anti-β_2-glycoprotein I antibody, activated protein C resistance, protein S antigen and resistance, antithrombin III assay, fibrinogen, factor V Leiden, prothrombin G20210A
- Immunoassay for quantitative assessment of total and free protein S levels
- Protein S activity assay (mainly after obtaining activated protein C resistance)
- Disorders that may alter lab results: acute thrombosis, vitamin K antagonists (VKA), any acute illness response, liver disease, and pregnancy-reduce protein S levels. Direct oral anticoagulants affect protein S activity assay.
- Heparin and low-weight heparin do not alter lab results.
- Total protein S levels are markedly decreased in newborns and young infants; use age-adjusted norms.

TREATMENT

GENERAL MEASURES

- Routine anticoagulation for asymptomatic patients with protein S deficiency is not recommended.
- Antithrombotic therapy recommendations for patients with protein S deficiency can be guided by antithrombotic therapy for VTE disease guidelines.
- Patients with unprovoked VTE and who have a low or moderate bleeding risk are suggested to receive extended anticoagulant therapy (no scheduled stop date) over 3 months of therapy (1)[B],(3), and those who have a high bleeding risk are recommended to receive 3 months of anticoagulant therapy (3),(4)[B].

- Patients with a second unprovoked VTE and who have a low to moderate bleeding risk are recommended to receive extended anticoagulant therapy over 3 months (3),(4)[B]; those who have high bleeding risk are suggested to receive 3 months of anticoagulant therapy (1)[B],(3).
- Patients with VTE and no history of cancer are suggested to receive dabigatran, rivaroxaban, apixaban, or edoxaban over VKA therapy as long-term (first 3 months) anticoagulant therapy; VKA therapy over low-molecular-weight heparin (LMWH) (3)
- Patients with VTE and a history of cancer (excludes GI malignancy or the malignancies that increase risk of bleeding) are suggested to receive LMWH over VKA therapy, dabigatran, rivaroxaban, apixaban, or edoxaban. It is recommended that these patients receive extended anticoagulant therapy (3).
- Treatment of thrombosis with LMWH is recommended over unfractionated heparin, unless the patient has severe renal failure.
- Treat as outpatient, if possible.
- Prophylaxis should be considered in risk situations such us surgery, immobility or postpartum, especially in patients with family history.
- The role of family screening for protein S deficiency is unclear because most patients with this mutation do not have thrombosis. Screening should be considered for women considering oral contraceptives or pregnancy and who have a family history of protein S deficiency (5)[B].

MEDICATION
- LMWH
  - Enoxaparin (Lovenox) 1 mg/kg SC BID
    - Alternatively, 1.5 mg/kg/day SC
  - Tinzaparin (Innohep) 175 anti-Xa U/kg/day SC
  - Dalteparin (Fragmin) 200 U/kg/day SC divided QD–BID
- Factor Xa inhibitor
  - Fondaparinux (Arixtra) <50 kg: 5 mg/day SC; 50 to 100 kg: 7.5 mg/day SC; >100 kg: 10 mg/day SC; contraindicated if CrCl <30 mL/min
- Novel oral anticoagulants (NOACs):
  - Dabigatran 150 mg PO BID (after 5 to 10 days of parenteral anticoagulation)
  - Rivaroxaban 15 mg PO BID for 21 days and then 20 mg PO QD
  - Apixaban 10 mg PO BID for 7 days and then 5 mg PO BID
  - Edoxaban: person weighs ≤60 kg: 30 mg PO QD OR >60 kg: 60 mg PO QD (after 5 to 10 days of parenteral anticoagulation)
- Oral anticoagulant: warfarin (Coumadin): 2 to 5 mg PO QD then adjusted to an INR of 2 to 3. LMWH initially for a minimum of 5 days and two consecutive INRs between 2 and 3, at which time it can be stopped; contraindications
  - Active bleeding precludes anticoagulation; risk of bleeding is a relative contraindication to long-term anticoagulation.
  - Warfarin is contraindicated in patients with a prior history of warfarin-induced skin necrosis.

- Precautions
  - Observe patient for signs of embolization, further thrombosis, or bleeding.
  - Avoid IM injections.
  - Periodically, check stool and urine for occult blood; monitor CBC, including platelets.
  - Heparin: thrombocytopenia and/or paradoxical thrombosis with thrombocytopenia
  - Warfarin: necrotic skin lesions (typically breasts, thighs, and buttocks)
  - LMWH: Adjust dose in renal insufficiency.
- Significant possible interactions
  - Agents that intensify the response to oral anticoagulants: alcohol, allopurinol, amiodarone, anabolic steroids, androgens, many antimicrobials, cimetidine, chloral hydrate, disulfiram, all NSAIDs, sulfinpyrazone, tamoxifen, thyroid hormone, vitamin E, ranitidine, salicylates, acetaminophen
  - Agents that diminish the response to oral anticoagulants: aminoglutethimide, antacids, barbiturates, carbamazepine, cholestyramine, diuretics, griseofulvin, rifampin, oral contraceptives

ISSUES FOR REFERRAL
- Patients with suspected protein S deficiency should be seen by a hematologist.
- Screening and prophylactic treatment of asymptomatic family members is not justified (6).

SURGERY/OTHER PROCEDURES
- Anticoagulation must be held for surgical interventions.
- For most patients with DVT, recommendations are against routine use of vena cava filter in addition to anticoagulation. IVC filter is only recommended in case of contraindication to anticoagulation (3)[A].

ADMISSION, INPATIENT, AND NURSING CONSIDERATIONS
- Life-threatening VTE
- Significant bleeding while on anticoagulant therapy
- Look for signs of bleeding while on anticoagulation therapy.

 ONGOING CARE

FOLLOW-UP RECOMMENDATIONS
Patient Monitoring
- Warfarin requires periodic (monthly after initial stabilization) monitoring of the INR.
- Periodic measurement of INR to maintain a range of 2 to 3
- LMWH is the treatment of choice in pregnancy. Periodic monitoring with anti-Xa levels is recommended in some cases, such as overweight and borderline renal failure.

DIET
Unrestricted

PATIENT EDUCATION
- Patients should be educated about use of oral anticoagulant therapy if taking such.
- Patients undergoing warfarin therapy should avoid drinking alcohol on a daily basis.
- Avoid NSAIDs while on warfarin.

PROGNOSIS
- Persons with protein S deficiency have normal lifespan.
- By age 45 years, 50% of the people heterozygous for protein S deficiency will have VT; half will be spontaneous.

COMPLICATIONS
Recurrent thrombosis (requires indefinite anticoagulation)

REFERENCES
1. Bick RL. Prothrombin G20210A mutation, antithrombin, heparin cofactor II, protein C, and protein S defects. *Hematol Oncol Clin North Am*. 2003;17(1):9–36.
2. Parand A, Zolghadri J, Nezam M, et al. Inherited thrombophilia and recurrent pregnancy loss. *Iran Red Crescent Med J*. 2013;15(12):e13708.
3. Kearon C, Akl EA, Ornelas J, et al. Antithrombotic therapy for VTE disease: CHEST Guideline and Expert Panel Report. *Chest*. 2016;149(2):315–352.
4. Moll S. Thrombophilias—practical implications and testing caveats. *J Thromb Thrombolysis*. 2006;21(1):7–15.
5. Langlois NJ, Wells PS. Risk of venous thromboembolism in relatives of symptomatic probands with thrombophilia: a systematic review. *Thromb Haemost*. 2003;90(1):17–26.
6. Hornsby LB, Armstrong EM, Bellone JM, et al. Thrombophilia screening. *J Pharm Pract*. 2014;27(3):253–259.

CODES

ICD10
D68.59 Other primary thrombophilia

CLINICAL PEARLS
- Asymptomatic patients with protein S deficiency do not require prophylactic anticoagulation because the risk of thrombosis is low; asymptomatic patients do not require anticoagulation.
- Patients with protein S deficiency and DVT should be anticoagulated for at least 6 months, especially if first episode.

PROTEINURIA

Lovella Duru Kanu, MD

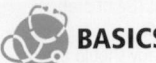

BASICS

DESCRIPTION

Urinary protein excretion of >150 mg/day

- Nephrotic-range proteinuria: urinary protein excretion of >3.5 g/day; also called *heavy proteinuria*
- Three pathologic types:
  - Glomerular proteinuria: increased permeability of proteins across glomerular capillary membrane
  - Tubular proteinuria: decreased proximal tubular reabsorption of proteins
  - Overflow proteinuria: increased production of low-molecular-weight proteins

Pediatric Considerations

- Proteinuria: Normal is daily excretion of up to 100 mg/m^2 (body surface area).
- Nephrotic-range proteinuria: daily excretion of >1,000 mg/m^2 (body surface area)

Pregnancy Considerations

- Proteinuria in pregnancy beyond 20 weeks' gestation is a hallmark of preeclampsia/eclampsia and demands further workup.
- Proteinuria in pregnancy before 20 weeks' gestation is suggestive of underlying renal disease.

ETIOLOGY AND PATHOPHYSIOLOGY

- Glomerular proteinuria: increased filtration/larger proteins (albumin) due to the following:
  - Increased size of glomerular basement membrane pores and
  - Loss of proteoglycan negative charge barrier
- Tubular proteinuria: Tubulointerstitial disease prevents proximal tubular reabsorption of smaller proteins (β_2-microglobulin, immunoglobulin [Ig] light chains, retinol-binding protein, amino acids).
- Overflow proteinuria: proximal tubular reabsorption overwhelmed by increased production of smaller proteins
- Glomerular proteinuria
  - Primary glomerulonephropathy
    - Minimal-change disease
    - Idiopathic/primary membranous glomerulonephritis
    - Focal segmental glomerulonephritis
    - Membranoproliferative glomerulonephritis
    - IgA nephropathy
  - Secondary glomerulonephropathy
    - Diabetic nephropathy
    - Autoimmune/collagen vascular disorders (e.g., lupus nephritis, Goodpasture syndrome)
    - Amyloidosis
    - Preeclampsia
    - Infection (HIV, hepatitis B and C, poststreptococcal, endocarditis, syphilis, malaria)
    - Malignancy (GI, lung, lymphoma)
    - Renal transplant rejection
    - Structural (reflux nephropathy, polycystic kidney disease)
    - Drug-induced (NSAIDs, penicillamine, lithium, heavy metals, gold, heroin)

- Tubular proteinuria
  - Hypertensive nephrosclerosis
  - Tubulointerstitial disease (uric acid nephropathy, hypersensitivity, interstitial nephritis, Fanconi syndrome, heavy metals, sickle cell disease, NSAIDs, antibiotics)
  - Acute tubular necrosis
- Overflow proteinuria
  - Multiple myeloma (light chains; also tubulotoxic)
  - Hemoglobinuria
  - Myoglobinuria (in rhabdomyolysis)
  - Lysozyme (in acute monocytic leukemia)
- Benign proteinuria
  - Functional (fever, exercise, cold exposure, stress, CHF)
  - Idiopathic transient
  - Orthostasis (postural)

RISK FACTORS

- Hypertension
- Diabetes
- Obesity
- Strenuous exercise
- CHF
- UTI
- Fever

Genetics

No known genetic pattern

GENERAL PREVENTION

Control of weight, BP, and blood glucose reduces the risk of proteinuria.

COMMONLY ASSOCIATED CONDITIONS

- Hypertension (common)
- Diabetes mellitus (DM) (common)
- Preeclampsia (common)
- Multiple myeloma (rare)

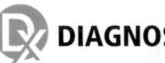

DIAGNOSIS

HISTORY

- Frothy/foamy urine
- Change in urine output
- Blood- or cola-colored urine
- Recent weight change
- Swelling
- Rule out systemic illness: diabetes, heart failure, autoimmune, poststreptococcal infection.

PHYSICAL EXAM

- BP
- Weight
- Peripheral edema
- Periorbital/facial edema
- Ascites
- Palpation of kidneys
- Check lungs, heart for signs of CHF.

DIFFERENTIAL DIAGNOSIS

Includes all causes listed under "Etiology and Pathophysiology"

DIAGNOSTIC TESTS & INTERPRETATION

Screening for proteinuria is not cost-effective unless directed at groups with hypertension/diabetes, older persons, and so forth.

Initial Tests (lab, imaging)

- Urinalysis (UA) quantitatively estimates proteinuria:
  - Only sensitive to albumin; will not detect smaller proteins of overflow/tubular etiologies
  - False-positive finding if urine pH >7, highly concentrated (specific gravity [SG] >1.015), gross hematuria, mucus, semen, leukocytes, iodinated contrast agents, penicillin analogues, sulfonamide metabolites
  - False-negative finding if urine is dilute (SG 1.005), albumin excretion <20 to 30 mg/dL, protein is nonalbumin
  - Sensitivity, 32–46%; specificity, 97–100%
  - Also can perform sulfosalicylic acid test to detect nonalbumin protein
- If UA positive, perform urine microscopy. Refer to nephrologist if positive for signs of glomerular disease.
- If UA shows trace to 2+ protein, rule out transient proteinuria with repeat UA at another visit:
  - More common than persistent proteinuria
  - Causes include exercise, fever, CHF, UTI, and cold exposure.
  - Reassure patient that transient proteinuria is benign and requires no further workup.
- If initial UA shows 3+ to 4+ protein or repeat UA is positive, measure creatinine clearance and quantify proteinuria with 24-hour urine collection (gold standard) or spot urine protein-to-creatinine (P/C) ratio (acceptable practice) (1)[A]:
  - Numerical P/C ratios correlate with total protein excreted in grams per day (i.e., ratio of 0.2 correlates with 0.2 g during a 24-hour collection).
  - Patients age <30 years with 24-hour urine excretion of <2 g/day and normal creatinine clearance should be tested for orthostatic proteinuria:
    - Benign condition is present in 2–5% of adolescents.
    - Diagnosed with a normal urine P/C ratio in first morning void and an elevated urine P/C ratio in a second specimen taken after standing for several hours
- If protein excretion >2 g/day, consider nephrology referral and begin workup for systemic/renal disease.
- Patients with persistent proteinuria not explained by orthostatic changes should undergo renal ultrasound to rule out structural abnormalities (e.g., reflux nephropathy, polycystic kidney).

Follow-Up Tests & Special Considerations

Renal/systemic disease workup can include the following:

- CBC, ferritin, ESR, serum iron
- Electrolytes, LFTs
- Lipid profile (ideally, fasting)
- Prothrombin time/international normalized ratio
- Anti-phospholipase A2 receptor antibody: positive in ~70% of primary membranous nephropathy

- Antinuclear antibodies: elevated in lupus
- Antistreptolysin O titer: elevated after streptococcal glomerulonephritis
- Complement C3/C4: low in most glomerulonephritis
- HIV, syphilis, and hepatitis serologies: all associated with glomerular proteinuria
- Serum and urine protein electrophoresis: abnormal in multiple myeloma
- Blood glucose: elevated in diabetes
- All patients with diabetes should be screened for microalbuminuria.
- Patients with nephrotic-range proteinuria are at increased risk for hypercholesterolemia and thromboembolic events (~25% of adult patients) with highest risk in membranous nephropathy. Optimal duration of prophylactic anticoagulation is unknown but may extend for the duration of the nephrotic state (2).
- Proteinuric pregnant patients beyond 20 weeks' gestation should be examined for other signs/symptoms of preeclampsia (e.g., hypertension, thrombocytopenia, elevated liver transaminases).

 TREATMENT

- BP goal for both diabetic and nondiabetic adults is ≤140/90 mm Hg (3)[C].
- Proteinuria goal is <0.5 g/day (4)[A].

GENERAL MEASURES
- Limit protein intake to 0.8 g/kg/day in adults with DM or without DM and glomerular filtration rate (GFR) <30 mL/min/1.73 m². Soy protein may be renoprotective. Monitor protein intake with 24-hour urine urea excretion (4)[A].
- Limit sodium chloride intake to <2 g/day to optimize antiproteinuric medications (3)[B]. Effect on BP is further protective (4)[A].
- Limit fluid intake for urine output goal of <2 L/day. Larger urine volumes are associated with increased proteinuria and later GFR decline (4)[B].
- Smoking cessation: Smoking is associated with increased proteinuria and faster kidney disease progression (4)[B].
- Encourage supine posture (up to 50% reduction vs. upright) (4)[B].
- Discourage severe exertion (4)[B].
- Encourage weight loss (4)[B].

MEDICATION
First Line
- ACE inhibitors: first choice; use maximally tolerated doses; use even if normotensive (4)[A].
- Angiotensin receptor blockers (ARBs): proven antiproteinuric and renoprotective; ARBs are first choice if ACE inhibitors are not tolerated (4)[A].
- Combination ACE inhibitor and ARB should not be used. Although shown to reduce proteinuria, combination does not reduce poor CV outcomes and does increase risk of adverse drug reactions (5,6)[A].

Second Line
- β-Blockers: antiproteinuric and cardioprotective (4)[A]
- Dihydropyridine calcium channel blockers (DHCCBs): should be avoided unless needed for BP control; not antiproteinuric (4)[A]
- Non-DHCCB: antiproteinuric, may be renoprotective (4)[B]
- Aldosterone antagonists: antiproteinuric independent of BP control (4)[B]
- NSAIDs: antiproteinuric but also nephrotoxic; generally should be avoided (4)[C]

ISSUES FOR REFERRAL
Consider nephrology referral for possible renal biopsy if
- Impaired creatinine clearance
- Nephrotic-range proteinuria
- Unclear etiology of nonnephrotic-range proteinuria
- Diabetics with microalbuminuria

COMPLEMENTARY & ALTERNATIVE MEDICINE
- Corticosteroids: No proven benefit in mortality or need for renal replacement in adults with nephrotic syndrome, although steroids are recommended in some patients who do not respond to conservative treatment. Classically, children with nephrotic syndrome respond better than adults, especially those with minimal-change disease (6)[A].
- Estrogen/progesterone replacement: may be renoprotective in premenopausal women but should be avoided in postmenopausal women (4)[B]
- Antioxidant therapy: may be antiproteinuric in diabetic nephropathy (4)[C]
- Sodium bicarbonate: not antiproteinuric but may block tubular injury caused by proteinuria; correcting metabolic acidosis may decrease protein catabolism (4)[C].
- Avoid excessive caffeine consumption: antiproteinuric in diabetic rat models (4)[C]
- Avoid iron overload (4)[C].
- Pentoxifylline: prevents progression of renal disease by unclear mechanisms (4)[C]
- Mycophenolate mofetil: antiproteinuric and renoprotective in animal models (4)[C]

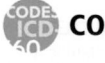 ONGOING CARE

FOLLOW-UP RECOMMENDATIONS
Patient Monitoring
All patients with persistent proteinuria should be followed with serial BP checks, UA, and renal function tests in the outpatient setting. Intervals depend on underlying etiology.

PROGNOSIS
- Transient and orthostatic proteinuria are benign conditions that do not convey a poor prognosis.
- Clinical significance of persistent proteinuria varies greatly and depends on underlying etiology.
- Degree of proteinuria is associated with disease progression in chronic kidney disease.
- Independent of GFR, higher levels of proteinuria likely convey an increased risk of mortality, myocardial infarction, and progression to kidney failure.

COMPLICATIONS
- Progression to chronic renal failure and the need for dialysis/renal transplant
- Hypercholesterolemia
- Hypercoagulable state
- Increased risk for infection for patient with nephrotic syndrome
- In nephrotic syndrome, ACIP recommends first dose of PCV13, followed by first dose of PPSV23 ≥8 weeks and then second dose of PPSV23 5 years after the first PPSV.

REFERENCES
1. National Kidney Foundation. K/DOQI clinical practice guidelines for chronic kidney disease: evaluation classification, and stratification: guideline 5. Assessment of proteinuria. http://www2.kidney.org/professionals/KDOQI/guidelines_ckd/toc.htm. Accessed November 16, 2017.
2. Kerlin BA, Ayoob R, Smoyer WE. Epidemiology and pathophysiology of nephrotic syndrome-associated thromboembolic disease. *Clin J Am Soc Nephrol*. 2012;7(3):513–520.
3. James PA, Oparil S, Carter BL, et al. 2014 Evidence-based guideline for the management of high blood pressure in adults: report from the panel members appointed to the Eighth Joint National Committee (JNC 8). *JAMA*. 2014;311(5):507–520.
4. Wilmer WA, Rovin BH, Hebert CJ, et al. Management of glomerular proteinuria: a commentary. *J Am Soc Nephrol*. 2003;14(12):3217–3232.
5. Fried LF, Emanuele N, Zhang JH, et al; for VA NEPHRON-D Investigators. Combined angiotensin inhibition for the treatment of diabetic nephropathy. *N Engl J Med*. 2013;369(20):1892–1903.
6. Kodner C. Nephrotic syndrome in adults: diagnosis and management. *Am Fam Physician*. 2009;80(10):1129–1134.

CODES
ICD10
- R80.9 Proteinuria, unspecified
- R80.2 Orthostatic proteinuria, unspecified
- R80.1 Persistent proteinuria, unspecified

CLINICAL PEARLS
- Transient and orthostatic proteinuria are benign conditions that do not convey a poor prognosis.
- Proteinuria >2 g/day likely represents glomerular malfunction and warrants a nephrology consultation.
- Clinical course varies greatly but, in general, the degree of proteinuria correlates with kidney disease progression.
- First-line therapy for persistent proteinuric patients is a high-dose ACE inhibitor.

PROTHROMBIN 20210 (MUTATION)

Katyayini Aribindi, MD • Adrian DaSilva-DeAbreu, MD • Raymundo A. Quintana, MD

BASICS

DESCRIPTION
- The G20210A is a gain of function mutation where adenine is substituted for a guanine at the 20210 noncoding position of the prothrombin (a.k.a. factor II) gene.
- Prothrombin 20210 mutation is the second most common venous thrombophilia after the factor V Leiden mutation.
- The mechanism of increasing the risk of thrombosis is incompletely understood but has been attributed to increased prothrombin or factor II levels in circulation by increased prothrombin protein translation without changing the levels of prothrombin mRNA transcription.
- Autosomal dominant condition, where heterozygotes have a 30% higher prothrombin level and a 3- to 4-fold increased risk of venous thromboembolism (VTE)
- System(s) affected: cardiovascular, hematologic/lymphatic/immunologic, nervous, pulmonary, reproductive, and hepatic
- Synonym(s): prothrombin G20210A mutation; prothrombin G20210A gene polymorphism; prothrombin gene mutation; and FII A^{20210} mutation

EPIDEMIOLOGY
- Found largely in Caucasian population with a prevalence ranging between 1% and 6%, but overall, it is about 2%
- In patients presenting with a VTE, prothrombin 20210 mutation has a prevalence that ranges from 4.6% to 18% with increased prevalence attributed to highly thrombophilic families.
- Mean age of first thrombosis is in the 2nd decade of life.
- Inheritance is similar between both genders (autosomal).

ETIOLOGY AND PATHOPHYSIOLOGY
- Noncoding substitution of adenine for guanine at the 20210 position at the terminal nucleotide of the 3' resulting in a gain of function of prothrombin gene, leading to increased levels of prothrombin (factor II), by increased translation of prothrombin mRNA but not transcription
- The base change location is in the 3' terminal nucleotide of the untranslated region associated with the mRNA sequence for polyadenylation. The gain of function is possible due to increased rate of processing, alteration of the site of cleavage, or increased mRNA stability.
- In the coagulation cascade, prothrombin (factor II) is the precursor of thrombin, which cleaves fibrinogen to fibrin. Elevated prothrombin activity leads to elevated thrombin levels and subsequent clot formation.
- The majority of thrombus formation occurs in the venous circulation: deep venous thrombosis (DVT)/PE, mesenteric, and cerebral. Recent studies have shown that prothrombin 20210 mutation did not correlate with Budd-Chiari syndrome or a portal or hepatic vein thrombosis.
- G20210A mutation is not known to be a risk factor for some arterial thrombotic events (myocardial infarction or acute ischemic stroke); however, studies have shown an increased prevalence of the mutation in patients with critical limb ischemia (1).

Genetics
- Caused by the G20210A mutation of the *F2* gene (prothrombin gene) located in the short (p) arm of chromosome 11 that causes a gain of function
- Heterozygotes have a 30% increased levels of prothrombin levels, with a 3- to 4-fold increase of VTE events. Homozygotes are at an even greater risk.
- There are three other prothrombin mutations not related to the G20210A area:
  - Yukuhashi: missense mutation G1787T, arginine for leucine at amino acid 596, leading to prolonged procoagulant activity
  - C20209T: adjacent to G20210A mutation, primarily found in African individuals; newer studies have suggested a possible relationship between this mutation and recurrent pregnancy loss, although it is not fully understood.
  - A19911G: located in the intron of the prothrombin gene; may affect the G20210A mutation by increasing the odds ratio of the venous thromboembolic event. Mechanism is still unknown.

RISK FACTORS
- Being a hereditary condition, the presence of such mutation in the parents poses risk of transmission to offspring.
- Regarding the risk of developing VTE:
  - Patients with both the prothrombin 20210 mutation and factor V Leiden mutation increases the odds ratio of VTE by 20-fold.
  - Virchow triad of thrombogenesis consists of stasis, endothelial injury, and thrombophilia. Any condition that promotes stasis and endothelial injury will consequently increase the risk of VTE, for example, oral contraceptive, pregnancy, malignancy, orthopedic surgery, congestive heart failure, cerebrovascular accident in the past 3 months, air travel, obesity, and smoking.

Pregnancy Considerations
- Increased thrombotic risk in patients with prothrombin 20210 mutation during pregnancy and in the postpartum state is attributed to relative stasis.
- Anticoagulation should begin in the 1st trimester because the risk of VTE increases early in pregnancy and should be discontinued at onset of labor or before scheduled induction/cesarean delivery. Postpartum risk of VTE is usually greater, and anticoagulation can resume 4 to 6 hours after a vaginal delivery or 6 to 12 hours after surgery. Warfarin may begin immediately due to slow onset of action.
- C20209T mutation may have some relation with recurrent pregnancy loss; however, it is not well studied (2).

GENERAL PREVENTION
Asymptomatic individuals with the mutation do not require any prophylactic anticoagulation. Exceptions are generally made for pregnant women with very high-risk thrombophilic mutations (usually factor V Leiden) with a strong family history. After the first VTE, lifelong prophylaxis may be warranted if some features are present: unprovoked or in a nontraditional area like hepatic, portal, mesenteric, or cerebral.

COMMONLY ASSOCIATED CONDITIONS
- VTE
- Factor V Leiden

DIAGNOSIS

HISTORY
- Previous VTE
- Family history of VTE
- Family history of prothrombin 20210 mutation

PHYSICAL EXAM
- Unilateral swollen, erythematous, and tender calf is significant for a possible DVT.
- Positive Homans sign, sensitivity of 10–54%, specificity of 39–89% for DVT
- Tachycardia is the most common sign of a pulmonary embolism; however, patients may have chest pain and hypotension depending on the severity of the pulmonary embolus.
- A tender abdomen may be indicative of mesenteric veins thrombosis; however, other causes of an acute abdomen should be worked up as appropriate.

DIFFERENTIAL DIAGNOSIS
- Factor V Leiden mutation
- Protein C deficiency
- Protein S deficiency
- Antithrombin deficiency
- Other causes of activated protein C resistance (e.g., antiphospholipid antibodies)
- Dysfibrinogenemia
- Dysplasminogenemia
- Homocystinemia
- Elevated factor VIII levels

DIAGNOSTIC TESTS & INTERPRETATION
Screening for prothrombin G20210A mutation in asymptomatic individuals is not recommended; except for those with very strong family history (3)[B]. Testing can take place in patients with thrombosis at a very early age, recurrent unprovoked VTE, or those with thrombosis in unusual locations.

Initial Tests (lab, imaging)
- This mutation can be diagnosed using PCR with electrophoresis or immunoassays.
- Imaging should be obtained as appropriate for the suspected site of thrombosis: ultrasound with Doppler, computed tomography scan with contrast to evaluate venous phase, and V/Q scan.
- Testing for an inherited thrombophilic condition is reliable during an acute embolic event or with anticoagulation use (4)[A].

Follow-Up Tests & Special Considerations
Although prothrombin levels are elevated, this is not a sensitive test to make the diagnosis.

Diagnostic Procedures/Other
MR angiography (MRA), venography, or arteriography to detect thrombosis

Test Interpretation
Imaging is likely to show presence of arterial or venous thrombus.

TREATMENT

GENERAL MEASURES
Management of patients with a first-time VTE with or without an acquired thrombophilic condition remains overall very similar.

MEDICATION

Is directed to treat those patients with VTE (prophylactic doses may vary). We recommend the reader to check the most updated doses, dose adjustments, and contraindications for the medications listed below. The doses listed apply to most adults.

First Line

In adult patients without cancer, the following oral anticoagulants are preferred over warfarin and low-molecular-weight heparin (LMWH): dabigatran, rivaroxaban, apixaban, or edoxaban are preferred over warfarin (5)[A].

- Apixaban (Eliquis): Initial dose is 10 mg BID for 7 days, followed by 5 mg BID.
- Dabigatran (Pradaxa): requires initial parenteral anticoagulation for 5 to 10 days, followed by 150 mg BID
- Edoxaban (Savaysa): requires initial parenteral anticoagulation for 5 to 10 days, followed by 60 mg daily
- Rivaroxaban (Xarelto): Initial dose is 15 mg BID with food for 21 days, followed by a daily dose of 20 mg with food.

Second Line

For patients without cancer that cannot be treated with DOAC, warfarin is preferred over LMWH (5)[A].

- Warfarin (Coumadin): Initial dose may range from 2 to 10 mg PO daily and then adjusted to an INR of 2 to 3.
- Enoxaparin (Lovenox): 1 mg/kg subcutaneous injection every 12 hours

MEDICATION CONSIDERATIONS

- Contraindications
  - Absolute contraindications: active bleeding, severe bleeding diathesis, planned or recent high bleeding risk surgery or procedure, major trauma, recent or history of intracranial hemorrhage
  - Relative contraindications: recurrent gastrointestinal bleeding, intracranial or spinal tumors, thrombocytopenia with platelets <50,000 (enoxaparin can be dose adjusted depending on severity of thrombocytopenia), large AAA with severe hypertension, recent or emergent low bleeding risk surgery
  - Warfarin: history of warfarin skin necrosis
  - Doses of LMWH and new oral anticoagulants need to be adjusted in patients with renal dysfunction. Rivaroxaban should be avoided in patients with severe renal dysfunction. Apixaban may be relatively safer to use in patients with CKD and has a significantly lower risk of major bleeding or clinically relevant nonmajor bleeding than rivaroxaban or dabigatran (6)[A].
  - Apixaban can be given for DVT prophylaxis as well as at a reduced dose of 2.5 mg PO BID.
- Precautions
  - Observe patient for signs of embolization, further thrombosis, or bleeding.
  - Periodically monitor CBCs.
  - Oral contraceptives are generally avoided in women already known to have the mutation; however, it is not recommended to check for the mutation before starting oral contraceptives in asymptomatic women.
- Complications of medications
  - Heparins: heparin-induced thrombocytopenia
  - Warfarin may cause necrotic skin lesions (typically breasts, thighs, or buttocks).

- Significant possible interactions
  - Agents that increase the effect of some anticoagulants: alcohol, allopurinol, amiodarone, anabolic steroids, androgens, many antimicrobials, cimetidine, chloral hydrate, disulfiram, all NSAIDs, sulfinpyrazone, tamoxifen, thyroid hormone, vitamin E, ranitidine, salicylates, acetaminophen
  - Agents that decrease the effect of some anticoagulants: aminoglutethimide, antacids, barbiturates, carbamazepine, cholestyramine, diuretics, griseofulvin, rifampin, oral contraceptives

ISSUES FOR REFERRAL

- Recurrent thrombosis on anticoagulation
- Difficulty anticoagulating
- Genetic counseling

SURGERY/OTHER PROCEDURES

- Anticoagulation must be held for surgical interventions.
- For most patients with DVT, recommendations are against routine use of vena cava filter in addition to anticoagulation, except in case with contraindication to anticoagulation (5)[A].
- Thrombectomy may be necessary in some cases.

ADMISSION, INPATIENT, AND NURSING CONSIDERATIONS

- Admission criteria/initial stabilization: complicated thrombosis, such as pulmonary embolus; required heparin drip
- Patient can be safely discharged if patient is stable on anticoagulation.

 ## ONGOING CARE

- Compression stockings for prevention
- DVT prophylaxis as appropriate if patient admitted to hospital

FOLLOW-UP RECOMMENDATIONS

Patient Monitoring

- Warfarin use requires periodic (weekly and then monthly after initial stabilization) INR measurements, with a goal of 2 to 3 (5)[A].
- Heterozygosity for the prothrombin 20210 mutation increases the risk for recurrent VTE only slightly, thus its presence does not alter the length of anticoagulation treatment decision.

DIET

- No restrictions; unless taking warfarin
- Food rich in vitamin K may interfere with warfarin anticoagulation.
- Grapefruit and St. John's wort interfere with the cytochrome P450 and can alter the levels and clearance of anticoagulant therapy.

PATIENT EDUCATION

Patients should be educated about:

- Use of oral anticoagulant therapy
- Signs and symptoms of acute blood loss
- Avoidance of NSAIDs while on warfarin

PROGNOSIS

When compared with normal individuals, persons with prothrombin 20210 have normal lifespans.

COMPLICATIONS

- Recurrent thrombosis on anticoagulation
- Bleeding on anticoagulation
- Complications are usually location dependent and can lead to death, possibly from a massive pulmonary embolism.
- Venous stasis ulcers

REFERENCES

1. Vazquez F, Rodger M, Carrier M, et al. Prothrombin G20210A mutation and lower extremity peripheral arterial disease: a systematic review and meta-analysis. *Eur J Vasc Endovasc Surg.* 2015;50(2):232–240.
2. Prat M, Morales-Indiano C, Jimenez C, et al. "20209C-T" a variant mutation of prothrombin gene mutation in a patient with recurrent pregnancy loss. *Ann Clin Lab Sci.* 2014;44(3):334–336.
3. Bucciarelli P, De Stefano V, Passamonti SM, et al. Influence of proband's characteristics on the risk for venous thromboembolism in relatives with factor V Leiden or prothrombin G20210A polymorphisms. *Blood.* 2013;122(15):2555–2561.
4. Cooper PC, Rezende SM. An overview of methods for detection of factor V Leiden and the prothrombin G20210A mutations. *Int J Lab Hematol.* 2007;29(3):153–162.
5. Kearon C, Akl EA, Ornelas J, et al. Antithrombotic therapy for VTE disease: CHEST guideline and expert panel report. *Chest.* 2016;149(2):315–352.
6. Cohen AT, Hamilton M, Mitchell SA, et al. Comparison of the novel oral anticoagulants apixaban, dabigatran, edoxaban, and rivaroxaban in the initial and long-term treatment and prevention of venous thromboembolism: systematic review and network meta-analysis. *PLoS One.* 2015;10(12):e0144856.

ADDITIONAL READING

- Kearon C, Akl EA. Duration of anticoagulant therapy for deep vein thrombosis and pulmonary embolism. *Blood.* 2014;123(12):1794–1801.
- Moll S. Thrombophilias—practical implications and testing caveats. *J Thromb Thrombolysis.* 2006;21(1):7–15.
- Seligsohn U, Lubetsky A. Genetic susceptibility to venous thrombosis. *N Engl J Med.* 2001;344(16):1222–1231.
- Wells PS, Forgie MA, Rodger MA. Treatment of venous thromboembolism. *JAMA.* 2014;311(7):717–728.

 ## SEE ALSO

Antithrombin Deficiency; Deep Vein Thrombophlebitis; Factor V Leiden; Protein C Deficiency; Protein S Deficiency

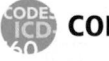 ## CODES

ICD10

D68.52 Prothrombin gene mutation

CLINICAL PEARLS

- Prothrombin 20210 mutation is the second most common inherited risk factor for VTE after factor V Leiden mutation.
- Asymptomatic patients with prothrombin 20210 mutation do not need anticoagulation or screening.
- Management of VTE is no different with or without the prothrombin G20210A mutation. However, indefinite anticoagulation may be considered in people with an unprovoked VTE or thrombus in a nontraditional area (mesenteric or cerebral).

PRURITUS ANI

Anna L. Silverman, MD • Vivian Lee, MD • Marie L. Borum, MD, EdD, MPH, MACP, FACG, AGAF

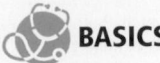 **BASICS**

DESCRIPTION
- Intense anal/perianal itching and/or burning
- Usually acute
- Classified as idiopathic (primary) or secondary (~75% of cases) to anorectal pathology (1)

EPIDEMIOLOGY
Incidence
- 1–5% of the general population (1)
- Predominant age: 30 to 60 years (1)
- Predominant sex: male > female (4:1) (1)

Prevalence
Difficult to estimate because often unreported; present in up to 2–3% of patients visiting primary care (2)

ETIOLOGY AND PATHOPHYSIOLOGY
- Over 100 etiologies categorized by inflammatory, infectious, systemic, neoplastic, neuropathic, neurogenic, and psychogenic causes (3,4)
- Pruritus may create an irresistible desire to scratch leading to a self-perpetuating itch–scratch–itch cycle.
- Pruritus ani is typically intensely perceived by the patient due to dense innervation.
- Consider primary pruritus ani when no other demonstrable causes can be found, including:
  – Poor anal hygiene
  – Loose or leaking stool that makes hygiene difficult. Patients with abdominal ostomy bags typically do not complain of pruritus.
  – Internal sphincter laxity
- Etiologies of secondary pruritus ani:
  – Inflammatory dermatologic diseases:
    ○ Allergic contact dermatitis (soaps, perfumes, or dyes in toilet paper, topical anesthetics, oral antibiotics)
    ○ Atopic dermatitis ± lichen simplex chronicus (patients also have asthma and/or eczema)
    ○ Psoriasis (lesions tend to be poorly demarcated, pale, and nonscaling)
    ○ Seborrheic dermatitis
    ○ Scleroderma
    ○ Lichen planus (may be seen in patients with ulcerative colitis and myasthenia gravis)
    ○ Radiation dermatitis (3)
  – Colorectal/anorectal diseases: rectal prolapse, hemorrhoids, fissures or fistulas, chronic diarrhea/constipation, polyps
  – Infectious etiologies, may be sexually transmitted: bacteria (gonorrhea, chlamydia, syphilis), viruses (herpes simplex virus [HSV], condyloma acuminate from human papillomavirus [HPV], molluscum), parasites (pinworms, lice, scabies, or bed bugs), fungal (Candida, or dermatophytes like tinea); other bacteria (Staphylococcus aureus, β-hemolytic Streptococcus, Corynebacterium minutissimum [erythrasma]) (3)

- Malignancies: melanoma, basal cell/squamous cell carcinoma, colorectal cancer, leukemia, lymphoma, or (uncommon) the presenting symptom of Bowen or Paget disease
- Mechanical factors: vigorous cleaning and scrubbing, tight-fitting clothes, synthetic undergarments
- Systemic diseases (often presents as generalized pruritus): diabetes mellitus (most common), cholestasis, chronic liver disease, renal failure, hyperthyroidism, anemia
- Chemical irritants: chemotherapy, diarrhea (often from antibiotic use)
- Dietary elements (citrus, milk products, coffee, tea, cola, chocolate, beer, wine, tomatoes, nuts)
- Psychogenic factors: anxiety–itch–anxiety cycle

RISK FACTORS
- Obesity
- Excess perianal hair growth and/or perspiration
- Underlying anorectal pathology
- Underlying anxiety disorder
- Caffeine intake has been correlated with symptoms.

GENERAL PREVENTION
- Good perianal hygiene
- Avoid mechanical irritation of skin (vigorous cleaning or rubbing with dry toilet paper or baby wipes, harsh soaps or perfumed products, excessive scratching with fingernails, or tight/synthetic undergarments).
- Minimize moisture in perianal area (absorbent cotton in anal cleft may help keep area dry).
- Avoid laxative use (loose stool is an irritant).

DIAGNOSIS

HISTORY
- Patient presents with complaint of anal and/or perianal itching, burning, or excoriation.
- Inquire about:
  – Timing (when it started, when it is worse)
  – Frequency of cleansing and products used on affected area
  – Change in bowel habits
  – Melena or hematochezia
  – Recent antibiotic use
  – Skin disorders (psoriasis, eczema)
  – Rectal or vaginal discharge, menstrual cycle
  – Dietary history: Focus on the "C"s: caffeine, coffee, cola, chocolate, citrus, calcium (dairy) (3).
  – Medical history (hepatitis, iron deficiency anemia, and diabetes in particular)
  – Family history of colorectal cancer
  – Anal receptive intercourse
  – Change in toiletry products
  – Household members (particularly children) with itching (possible pinworms)
  – Clothing preference (tight, synthetic) (1)

PHYSICAL EXAM
- Perianal visual inspection for erythema, hemorrhoids, anal fissures, maceration, lichenification, warts, polyps, excoriations, neoplasia, stool seepage
- Classification based on gross appearance
  – Stage 1: erythema, inflamed appearance
  – Stage 2: lichenification
  – Stage 3: lichenification, coarse skin, potential fissures or ulcerations (1)
- Digital rectal exam to evaluate for masses, internal sphincter tone, pain
- Valsalva to evaluate for prolapse
- Anoscopy to evaluate for hemorrhoids, fissures, other internal lesions

DIFFERENTIAL DIAGNOSIS
"ITCHeS" acronym (4)
- **I**nfection: Candida, parasites (scabies, pinworms), HPV, HSV, bacterial (gram-positive bacteria, gonorrhea, chlamydia, syphilis)
- **T**opical irritants: soaps/detergents, garments, deodorants, perfumes, stool leakage
- **C**utaneous/**C**ancer/**C**olorectal: eczema, psoriasis, lichen planus, lichen sclerosus, seborrhea, skin cancer, extramammary Paget disease, Bowen disease, fistula, fissure, prolapse, hemorrhoids, colorectal cancer
- **H**ypersensitivity: foods (the C's above), medications (colchicine, quinidine, mineral oil)
- e**S**ystemic: diabetes, iron deficiency anemia, uremia, cholestasis, hematologic malignancy

DIAGNOSTIC TESTS & INTERPRETATION
Initial Tests (lab, imaging)
Depending on history and exam findings, consider:
- Pinworm tape test; stool for ova and parasites
- CBC, comprehensive metabolic panel, A1c, thyroid studies to identify underlying systemic disease
- Wood lamp examination will show coral-red fluorescence in erythrasma (3).
- Skin scraping with potassium hydroxide (KOH) prep for dermatophytes or candidiasis (as etiology or as superinfection) and mineral oil prep for scabies
- Perianal skin culture (bacterial superinfection)
- Hemoccult testing of stool

Pediatric Considerations
Pinworms common in children. Consider perianal Crohn disease (5).

Follow-Up Tests & Special Considerations
Anal DNA polymerase chain reaction (PCR) probe for gonorrhea and chlamydia. Test for anal HPV if receptive anal intercourse.

Diagnostic Procedures/Other
- Biopsy suspicious lesions (e.g., lichenification, ulcerated epithelium, refractory cases) to exclude neoplasia; evaluate etiology.
- Consider colonoscopy if history, exam, or testing suggests colorectal pathology (family history of colorectal disease, especially if age >40 years, weight loss, rectal bleeding, change in bowel habits).

Geriatric Considerations
- Stool incontinence may be a predisposing factor.
- Consider systemic disease.
- Higher likelihood of colorectal pathology

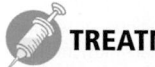 ## TREATMENT

GENERAL MEASURES
- Proper anal hygiene. Avoid chemical and mechanical irritants and wear proper undergarments (1).
- High-fiber diet and/or bowel regimen to maintain regular bowel movements (1)
- Avoid tight-fitting clothing. Use cotton undergarments.
- Absorbent cotton, talcum powder, or cornstarch if excess moisture (1)
- Cotton gloves at night to control nocturnal scratching

MEDICATION

First Line
- Treat underlying infections: fungal or dermatophyte infection with topical imidazoles, bacterial infection with topical antibacterials.
- Treat underlying anorectal anatomic pathology: banding of prolapsing internal hemorrhoids, treat fistulas, or fissures.
- Break itch–scratch cycle with low-potency steroid cream such as hydrocortisone 1% ointment applied sparingly up to 4 times daily (1)[A]. Discontinue when itching subsides. Avoid use >2 weeks due to risk of skin atrophy.
- If no response with low-potency steroid, consider high-potency steroid cream.
- Antihistamines, particularly sedating antihistamines, may be useful in reducing nighttime itching until local measures take effect (4).
- Tricyclic antidepressants may reduce nighttime scratching.
- Zinc oxide can be used after steroid course for barrier protection (3)[C]; petroleum jelly is another barrier (mineral oil can worsen pruritus).
- Low-dose topical capsaicin cream in combination with steroid cream if refractory symptoms (1)[A]
- 0.03% tacrolimus ointment as an option to avoid atrophy associated with prolonged steroid use (1)
- Several small case series have shown symptomatic benefit with intradermal methylene blue injection—this may be an additional option for patients with refractory pruritus.

Second Line
Radiation may be used to destroy nerve endings (create permanent anesthesia) in intractable cases. This is almost never indicated but is very effective.

ISSUES FOR REFERRAL
- Intractable pruritus: Consider referral to gastroenterology (for colonoscopy) or dermatology (for additional treatment, possibly injections, or biopsies). Refractory or persistent symptoms should signal the possibility of underlying neoplasia because pruritus ani of long duration is associated with a greater likelihood of colorectal pathology.
- Refer for colonoscopy if at risk for colon cancer.

SURGERY/OTHER PROCEDURES
As above, especially if concern for malignancy identified

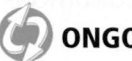 ## ONGOING CARE

FOLLOW-UP RECOMMENDATIONS
See patient every 2 weeks if not improving. Ensure proper hygiene and avoidance of irritants. Work up for systemic disease, and check for persistent lichenification. If refractory pruritus or lichenification does not resolve, consider underlying malignancy.

DIET
- Eliminate foods and beverages known or suspected to exacerbate symptoms: coffee, tea, chocolate, beer, cola, vitamin C tablets in excessive doses, citrus fruits, tomatoes, or spices.
- Eliminate foods or drugs contributing to loose bowel movements or dermatitis.
- Add fiber supplementation to bulk stools and prevent fecal leakage in patients who have fecal incontinence or partially formed stools.

PATIENT EDUCATION
- Review proper anal hygiene:
  - Resist overuse of soap and rubbing.
  - Avoid products with irritating perfumes and dyes.
  - Avoid use of ointments and mineral oil.
  - Wear loose, light cotton clothing.
  - If moisture is a problem, use cotton, unmedicated talcum powder, or cornstarch to keep the area dry.
  - Cleanse perianal area after bowel movements with water-moistened cotton.
  - Dry area after bathing by patting with a soft towel or by using a hair dryer on cool-setting (1).
- Avoid medications that cause diarrhea or constipation.
- Avoid caffeine, cola, chocolate, citrus, tomatoes, tea, alcohol, nuts, and milk products (3)[C].
- Use barrier protection if engaging in anal intercourse.
- If unable to completely empty rectum with defecation, use small plain-water enema (infant bulb syringe) after each bowel movement to prevent soiling and irritation.
- If persists, consider underlying medical disease.

PROGNOSIS
- Conservative treatment successful in ~90% of cases
- Idiopathic pruritus ani is often chronic—waxes and wanes.

COMPLICATIONS
- Bacterial superinfection at site of excoriations and potential abscess formation or penetrating infection via self-inoculation with colonic pathogens
- Lichenification
- Significant effect on quality of life

REFERENCES
1. Ansari P. Pruritus ani. *Clin Colon Rectal Surg.* 2016;29(1):38–42.
2. Abramowitz L, Benabderrahmane M, Pospait D, et al. The prevalence of proctological symptoms amongst patients who see general practitioners in France. *Eur J Gen Pract.* 2014;20(4):301–306.
3. Nasseri YY, Osborne MC. Pruritus ani: diagnosis and treatment. *Gastroenterol Clin North Am.* 2013;42(4):801–813.
4. Henderson PK, Cash BD. Common anorectal conditions: evaluation and treatment. *Curr Gastroenterol Rep.* 2014;16(10):408.
5. de Zoeten EF, Pasternak BA, Mattei P, et al. Diagnosis and treatment of perianal Crohn disease: NASPGHAN clinical report and consensus statement. *J Pediatr Gastroenterol Nutr.* 2013;57(3):401–412.

ADDITIONAL READING
- Misery L. Itch in special skin locations management. *Curr Probl Dermatol.* 2016;50:111–115.
- Schubert MC, Sridhar S, Schade RR, et al. What every gastroenterologist needs to know about common anorectal disorders. *World J Gastroenterol.* 2009;15(26):3201–3209.
- Ucak H, Demir B, Cicek D, et al. Efficacy of topical tacrolimus for the treatment of persistent pruritus ani in patients with atopic dermatitis. *J Dermatolog Treat.* 2013;24(6):454–457.

 ### SEE ALSO

Pinworms; Pruritus Vulvae

 ### CODES

ICD10
L29.0 Pruritus ani

CLINICAL PEARLS
- Pruritus ani is characterized by anal/perianal itching and/or burning.
- Skin irritation with itch–scratch–itch cycle
- Conservative treatment with perianal hygiene and reassurance is successful in 90% of patients.
- Consider trial of dietary elimination of "C"s—citrus, vitamin C supplements, calcium products, caffeine, coffee, cola, chocolate.
- Rule out infection (viral, bacterial, parasitic) in immunosuppressed patients.
- Consider underlying malignancy if refractory.

PRURITUS VULVAE

Maeve K. Hopkins, MD • Michael P. Hopkins, MD, MEd

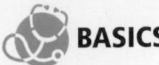 **BASICS**

DESCRIPTION
- Pruritus vulvae is a symptom or can be a primary diagnosis.
- If a primary diagnosis, other etiologies must be excluded.
- Pruritus vulvae as a primary diagnosis may also be more appropriately documented as vulvodynia (see "Vulvodynia" topic) or burning vulva syndrome.

EPIDEMIOLOGY
Symptoms may occur at any age during a woman's lifetime.
- Young girls most commonly have infectious or hygiene etiology.
- The primary diagnosis is more common in post-menopausal women.

Incidence
The exact incidence is unknown, although most women complain of vulvar pruritus at some point in their lifetime.

ETIOLOGY AND PATHOPHYSIOLOGY
Vulvar tissue is more permeable than exposed skin due to differences in structure, occlusion, hydration, and susceptibility to friction. It is particularly vulnerable to irritants such as (1)
- Perfumes
- Soaps
- Vaginal hygiene products
- Topical medications
- Dyes
- Body fluids

RISK FACTORS
- High-risk sexual behavior
- Immunosuppression
- Obesity

GENERAL PREVENTION
- Avoid irritants.
- Tight-fitting clothing should be avoided.
- Only cotton underwear should be worn.

COMMONLY ASSOCIATED CONDITIONS
- Infectious etiology
  - Vaginal or vulvar candida
  - *Gardnerella vaginalis*
  - *Trichomonas*
  - Human papillomavirus
  - Herpes simplex virus
- Vulvar vestibulitis
- Lichen sclerosus
- Lichen planus
- Lichen simplex chronicus (squamous cell hyperplasia)
- Malignant or premalignant conditions
- Psoriasis
- Fecal or urinary incontinence
- Dermatophytosis
- Parasites: scabies, *Pthirus pubis*
- Extramammary Paget
- Dietary: methylxanthines (e.g., coffee, cola), tomatoes, peanuts
- Autoimmune progesterone dermatitis: perimenstrual eruptions
- Irritant or allergic contact dermatitis
- Atopic dermatitis

 DIAGNOSIS

Pruritus vulvae is a diagnosis of exclusion. Delay in diagnosis is common due to patient hesitancy to seek treatment or provider delay in biopsy. Delayed diagnosis can have profound negative effect on women's sexual comfort and quality of life (2).

HISTORY
- Persistent itching
- Persistent burning sensation over the vulva or perineum
- Change in vaginal discharge
- Postcoital bleeding
- Dyspareunia

PHYSICAL EXAM
- Visual inspection of the vulva, vagina, perineum, and anus
  - Superior surfaces of the labia majora—extending from mons to the anal orifice—are most involved.
  - Vulvar skin is leathery or lichenified in appearance.
  - Papillomatosis may be a sign of chronic inflammation.
- Cotton swab–applied pressure to area of pain and to vestibular glands
- Musculoskeletal evaluation to confirm not contributing if persistent vulvar pain

DIAGNOSTIC TESTS & INTERPRETATION
- Sodium chloride: *Gardnerella* or *Trichomonas*
- 10% potassium hydroxide: *Candida*
- Viral culture or polymerase chain reaction: herpes simplex virus
- Directed biopsy recommended (3)[B]: human papillomavirus, lichen, malignancy, chronic inflammation
- Colposcopy with acetic acid or Lugol solution of vagina and vulva

Follow-Up Tests & Special Considerations
- A patch test may be performed by a dermatologist to assist in identifying a causative agent if contact dermatitis is suspected or if topical products are suspected as source of dermatitis (4)[A].
- Exam-directed tissue biopsies are essential in the postmenopausal population to rule out malignancy.

Diagnostic Procedures/Other
Biopsies should be collected from any ulceration, discoloration, raised areas, macerated areas, and the area of most intense pruritus.

Test Interpretation
- Only in the absence of pathologic findings can the primary diagnosis of pruritus vulvae be made.
- Biopsies of visible lesions most commonly show lichen simplex chronicus (25%), lichen sclerosus (20%), or chronic inflammation (15%) (3).

TREATMENT

Identify the underlying cause or disease to target treatment.

- Stop all potential irritants.
- Eliminate bacterial and fungal infection.
- Cool the affected area: Use cool gel packs (not ice packs, which may cause further injury).
- Sitz baths and bland emollients to soothe fissured or eroded skin

MEDICATION

First Line
- Topical steroids (1,5)
  – Triamcinolone 0.1% applied daily for 2 to 4 weeks and then twice weekly
  – Hydrocortisone 1–2.5% cream applied 2 to 4 times daily
  – Avoid long-term use due to risk of atrophy.
- 1st-generation antihistamines
  – Hydroxyzine: Initiate with 10 mg before bedtime (slowly increase up to 100 mg).
  – Doxepin: Initiate with 10 mg before bedtime.
  – 2nd-generation antihistamines are of little benefit.

Second Line
- *SSRI such as* citalopram 20 to 40 mg for resistant cases (6)
- Calcineurin inhibitors such as 1% pimecrolimus (5)[A]

ISSUES FOR REFERRAL
- Persistent symptoms should prompt additional investigation and referral to a gynecologist or gynecologic oncologist.
- Gynecologic oncology referral for proven or suspected malignancy
- Dermatology referral for patch testing to evaluate for contact dermatitis

ADDITIONAL THERAPIES
- Sacral neuromodulation device
- Laser therapy
- GnRH analogues
- Naltrexone

 ONGOING CARE

- Frequent evaluation, repeat cultures, and biopsies are necessary for cases resistant to treatment.
- Refractory cases may require referral to gynecologist or gynecologic oncology for further management.

DIET
Dietary alterations include avoidance of the following:
- Coffee and other caffeine-containing beverages
- Tomatoes
- Peanuts

PATIENT EDUCATION
- American College of Obstetricians and Gynecologists: https://www.acog.org
- National Vulvodynia Association: https://www.nva.org

PROGNOSIS
Conservative measures and short-term topical steroids control most patients' symptoms.

COMPLICATIONS
Malignancy

REFERENCES

1. Stockdale CK, Boardman L. Diagnosis and treatment of vulvar dermatoses. *Obstet Gynecol*. 2018;131(2):371–386.
2. Kellogg Spadt S, Kusturiss E. Vulvar dermatoses: a primer for the sexual medicine clinician. *Sex Med Rev*. 2015;3(3):126–136.
3. Ozalp SS, Telli E, Yalcin OT, et al. Vulval pruritus: the experience of gynaecologists revealed by biopsy. *J Obstet Gynaecol*. 2015;35(1):53–56.
4. Corazza M, Virgili A, Toni G, et al. Level of use and safety of botanical products for itching vulvar dermatoses. Are patch tests useful? *Contact Dermatitis*. 2016;74(5):289–294.
5. Chi CC, Kirtschig G, Baldo M, et al. Systematic review and meta-analysis of randomized controlled trials on topical interventions for genital lichen sclerosus. *J Am Acad Dermatol*. 2012;67(2):305–312.
6. Swamiappan M. Anogenital pruritus—an overview. *J Clin Diagn Res*. 2016;10(4):WE01–WE03.

ADDITIONAL READING

- Böttcher B, Wildt L. Treatment of refractory vulvo-vaginal pruritus with naltrexone, a specific opiate antagonist. *Eur J Obstet Gynecol Reprod Biol*. 2014;174:115–116.
- Caro-Bruce E, Flaxman G. Vulvar pruritus in a post-menopausal woman. *CMAJ*. 2014;186(9):688–699.
- Hill A, Paraiso M. Resolution of chronic vulvar pruritus with replacement of a neuromodulation device. *J Minim Invasive Gynecol*. 2015;22(5):889–891.
- Pichardo-Geisinger R. Atopic and contact dermatitis of the vulva. *Obstet Gynecol Clin North Am*. 2017;44(3):371–378.

 CODES

ICD10
- L29.2 Pruritus vulvae
- N94.819 Vulvodynia, unspecified

CLINICAL PEARLS
- Pruritus vulvae is a common complaint.
- Pruritus vulvae is a diagnosis of exclusion once other causes of itching have been ruled out.
- Exam-directed biopsies from any ulceration, discoloration, raised areas, macerated areas, and the area of most intense pruritus are essential to rule out malignancy.
- Initial treatment is conservative.

P

PSEUDOFOLLICULITIS BARBAE

Maurice Duggins, MD

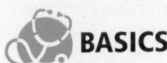 **BASICS**

DESCRIPTION
- Foreign body inflammatory reaction from an ingrown hair resulting in the appearance of papules and pustules. This is found mainly in the bearded area (barbae) but may occur in other hairy locations such as the scalp, axilla, or pubic areas where shaving is done (1).
- A mechanical problem: extrafollicular and transfollicular hair penetration
- System(s) affected: skin/exocrine
- Synonym(s): chronic sycosis barbae; pili incarnati; folliculitis barbae traumatica; razor bumps; shaving bumps; tinea barbae; pseudofolliculitis barbae (PFB)

EPIDEMIOLOGY
- Predominant age: postpubertal, middle age (14 to 25 years) (2)
- Predominant sex: male > female (can be seen in females of all races who wax/shave)

Incidence
- Adult male African Americans: unknown
- Adult male whites: unknown

Prevalence
- Widespread in Fitzpatrick skin types IV to VI (darker complexions) who shave
- 45–83% of African American soldiers who shave (1)

ETIOLOGY AND PATHOPHYSIOLOGY
- Transfollicular escape of the low-cut hair shaft as it tries to exit the skin is accompanied by inflammation and often an intraepidermal abscess.
- As the hair enters the dermis, more severe inflammation occurs, with downgrowth of the epidermis in an attempt to sheath the hair.
- A foreign body reaction forms at the tip of the invading hair, followed by abscess formation.
- Shaving too close
- Plucking/tweezing or wax depilation of hair may cause abnormal hair growth in injured follicles.

Genetics
- People with curly hair have an asymmetric accumulation of acidic keratin hHa8 on hair shaft.
- Single-nucleotide polymorphism (disruption Ala12Thr substitution) affects keratin of hair follicle.

RISK FACTORS
- Curly hair
- Shaving too close or shaving with multiple razor strokes

- Plucking/tweezing hairs
- South Mediterranean/American, Middle Eastern, Asian, or African descent (skin types IV to VI)

GENERAL PREVENTION
- Prior to shaving, rinse face with warm water to hydrate and soften hairs.
- Use adjustable hair clippers that leave very low hair length above skin.
- Shave with either a manual adjustable razor at coarsest setting (avoids close shaves), a single-edge blade razor (e.g., Bump Fighter), a foil-guarded razor (e.g., PFB razor), or electric triple "O-head" razor.
- Empty razor of hair frequently.
- Shave in the direction of hair growth. Do not overstretch skin when shaving.
- Use a generous amount of the correct shaving cream/gel (e.g., Ef-Kay shaving gel, Edge shaving gel, Aveeno therapeutic shave gel, Easy Shave medicated shaving cream).
- Daily shaving reduces papules/pruritus.
- Regular use of depilatories

COMMONLY ASSOCIATED CONDITIONS
- Keloidal folliculitis
- Pseudofolliculitis nuchae

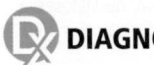 **DIAGNOSIS**

HISTORY
Pain on shaving; pruritus of shaved areas, irritated "razor bumps"

PHYSICAL EXAM
- Tender, exudative, erythematous follicular papules or pustules in beard area (less commonly in scalp, axilla, and pubic areas); range from 2 to 4 mm
- Hyperpigmented "razor or shave bumps"
- Alopecia
- Lusterless, brittle hair

DIFFERENTIAL DIAGNOSIS
- Bacterial folliculitis
- Impetigo
- Acne vulgaris
- Tinea barbae
- Sarcoidal papules

DIAGNOSTIC TESTS & INTERPRETATION

Initial Tests (lab, imaging)
- Clinical diagnosis
- Culture of pustules: usually sterile; may show coagulase-negative *Staphylococcus epidermidis* (normal skin flora)
- Additional hormonal testing may be indicated in females with hirsutism and/or polycystic ovary syndrome: dehydroepiandrosterone sulfate, luteinizing hormone (LH)/follicle-stimulating hormone (FSH), and free and total testosterone (3)[C].

Test Interpretation
Follicular papules and pustules

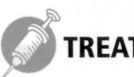 **TREATMENT**

- Mild cases
  – Stop shaving or avoid close shaving for 30 days while keeping beard groomed and clean (1,2)[C].
  – Consider 5% benzoyl peroxide after shaving and application of 1% hydrocortisone cream at bedtime (or LactiCare-HC lotion after shaving) (2)[C].
  – Tretinoin 0.025% cream; apply daily (1)[C].
- Moderate cases
  – Chemical depilatories (barium sulfide; Magic shaving powder); first test on forearm for 48 hours (for irritation) (1,2,3)[B]
  – Consider eflornithine HCl cream (Vaniqa) to reduce hair growth and stiffness in combination with other therapies (1,4)[B].
- Severe cases
  – Laser therapy: Longer wavelength laser (e.g., neodymium [Nd]:YAG) is safer for dark skin (5)[B].
  – Avoid shaving altogether; grow beard (1,2,3)[C].

GENERAL MEASURES
Acute treatment
- Dislodge embedded hair with sterile needle/tweezers.
- Discontinue shaving until red papules have resolved (minimum 3 to 4 weeks; longer if moderate or severe); can trim to length >0.5 cm during this time
- Massage beard area with washcloth, coarse sponge, or a soft brush several times daily.
- Hydrocortisone 1–2.5% cream to relieve inflammation
- Selenium sulfide if seborrhea is present and to help reduce pruritus
- Systemic antibiotics if secondary infection is present

Pregnancy Considerations
Do not use tretinoin (Retin-A), tetracycline, or benzoyl peroxide.

MEDICATION

First Line
- Topical or systemic antibiotic for secondary infection
  - Application of clindamycin (Cleocin T) solution BID or topical erythromycin
  - Low-dose erythromycin or tetracycline 250 to 500 mg PO BID for more severe inflammation
  - Benzoyl peroxide 5%–clindamycin 1% gel BID: Administer until papule/pustule resolves.
- Mild cases: tretinoin 0.025% cream at bedtime; combination of the above therapies
- Moderate disease/chemical depilatories
  - Disrupt cross-linking of disulfide bonds of hair to produce blunt (less sharp) hair tip.
  - Apply no more frequently than every 3rd day: 2% barium sulfide (Magic Shave) or calcium thioglycolate (Surgex); calcium hydroxide (Nair)
- Contraindications
  - Clindamycin: hypersensitivity history; history of regional enteritis or ulcerative colitis; history of antibiotic-associated colitis
  - Erythromycin, tetracycline, tretinoin: hypersensitivity history
- Precautions
  - Clindamycin: colitis, eye burning and irritation, skin dryness; pregnancy Category B
  - Erythromycin: Use cautiously in patients with impaired hepatic function; GI side effects, especially abdominal cramping; pregnancy Category B (erythromycin base formulation)
  - Chemical depilatories: Use cautiously; frequent use and prolonged application may lead to irritant contact dermatitis and chemical burns.
  - Tetracycline: Avoid in pregnancy.
  - Tretinoin: severe skin irritation; avoid in pregnancy.
  - Benzoyl peroxide: skin irritation and dryness, allergic contact dermatitis
  - Hydrocortisone cream: local skin irritation, skin atrophy with prolonged use, lightening of skin color
- Significant possible interactions
  - Erythromycin: increases theophylline and carbamazepine levels; decreases clearance of warfarin
  - Tetracycline: depresses plasma prothrombin activity

Second Line
Chemical peels with either glycolic acid or salicylic acid

ISSUES FOR REFERRAL
- Worsening or poor response to the above therapies after 4 to 6 weeks should prompt dermatology consultation.
- Occupational demands may also prompt earlier referral to dermatology for more aggressive therapy.

SURGERY/OTHER PROCEDURES
Laser treatment with long-pulsed Nd:YAG is helpful for severe cases.

ONGOING CARE

FOLLOW-UP RECOMMENDATIONS
Patient Monitoring
- As needed
- Educate patient on curative and preventive treatment.

DIET
- No restrictions
- No dietary studies available

PATIENT EDUCATION
https://medlineplus.com

PROGNOSIS
- Good, with preventive methods
- Prognosis is poor in the presence of progressive scarring and foreign body granuloma formation.

COMPLICATIONS
- Scarring (occasionally keloidal)
- Foreign body granuloma formation
- Disfiguring postinflammatory hyperpigmentation (use sunscreens; can treat with hydroquinone 4% cream, Retin-A, clinical peels)
- Impetiginization of inflamed skin
- Epidermal (erythema, crusting, burns with scarring) and pigmentary changes with laser

REFERENCES

1. Bridgeman-Shah S. The medical and surgical therapy of pseudofolliculitis barbae. *Dermatol Ther*. 2004;17(2):158–163.
2. Perry PK, Cook-Bolden FE, Rahman Z, et al. Defining pseudofolliculitis barbae in 2001: a review of the literature and current trends. *J Am Acad Dermatol*. 2002;46(Suppl 2):S113–S119.
3. Quarles FN, Brody H, Johnson BA, et al. Pseudofolliculitis barbae. *Dermatol Ther*. 2007;20(3):133–136.
4. Xia Y, Cho S, Howard RS, et al. Topical eflornithine hydrochloride improves the effectiveness of standard laser hair removal for treating pseudofolliculitis barbae: a randomized, double-blinded, placebo-controlled trial. *J Am Acad Dermatol*. 2012;67(4):694–699.
5. Weaver SM III, Sagaral EC. Treatment of pseudofolliculitis barbae using the long-pulse Nd:YAG laser on skin types V and VI. *Dermatol Surg*. 2003;29(12):1187–1191.

ADDITIONAL READING
- Daniel A, Gustafson CJ, Zupkosky PJ, et al. Shave frequency and regimen variation effects on the management of pseudofolliculitis barbae. *J Drugs Dermatol*. 2013;12(4):410–418.
- Gerstein W, Ilieva V. *Coccidioides immitis* soft tissue infection mimicking pseudofolliculitis barbae. *Clin Case Rep*. 2018;6(4):758–759.
- Kindred C, Oresajo CO, Yatskayer M, et al. Comparative evaluation of men's depilatory composition versus razor in black men. *Cutis*. 2011;88(2):98–103.
- Kundu RV, Patterson S. Dermatologic conditions in skin of color: part II. Disorders occurring predominantly in skin of color. *Am Fam Physician*. 2013;87(12):859–865.
- Taylor SC, Barbosa V, Burgess C, et al. Hair and scalp disorders in adult and pediatric patients with skin of color. *Cutis*. 2017;100(1):31–35.

SEE ALSO
Folliculitis; Impetigo

CODES

ICD10
- L73.1 Pseudofolliculitis barbae
- B35.0 Tinea barbae and tinea capitis
- L73.8 Other specified follicular disorders

CLINICAL PEARLS
- Electrolysis is not recommended as a treatment. It is expensive, painful, and often unsuccessful.
- Combination of laser therapy with eflornithine is more effective than laser alone.
- The unpleasant smell of sulfur could be a problem with some depilatory products.
- Have patient test for skin sensitivity with a small (coin sized) amount of the depilatory on the bearded area or forearm.

PSEUDOGOUT (CALCIUM PYROPHOSPHATE DIHYDRATE)

Pradeepa P. Vimalachandran, MD, MPH

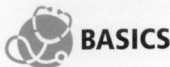 **BASICS**

DESCRIPTION

- Autoinflammatory disease triggered by calcium pyrophosphate dihydrate (CPPD) crystal deposition within joints
- One of many diseases associated with pathologic deposition of crystal; mineralization and ossification
  - CPPD crystal deposition = chondrocalcinosis (calcification of hyaline or fibrocartilage), pseudogout, and pyrophosphate arthropathy
  - Monosodium urate crystal deposition = gout
  - Hydroxyapatite deposition associated with ankylosing spondylitis, osteoarthritis, and vascular calcification
- Suspect pseudogout in arthritis cases with a pattern of joint involvement inconsistent with degenerative joint disease (e.g., metacarpophalangeal joints, wrists).
- Clinical presentation is broad:
  - Asymptomatic CPPD (incidentally identified on radiograph by chondrocalcinosis with or without additional findings of osteoarthritis)
  - Acute CPPD arthritis (acute onset, self-limiting, synovitis)
  - Chronic CPPD crystal inflammatory arthritis (1)[C]
- Chronic CPPD crystal deposition may cause a progressive degenerative arthritis in numerous joints:
  - Primarily affects the elderly
  - Usually involves large joints
- Symptom onset is usually insidious.
- Definitive diagnosis requires the identification of CPPD crystals in synovial fluid.
- System(s) affected: endocrine/metabolic; musculoskeletal
- Synonyms: pseudogout; CPPD; pyrophosphate arthropathy; chondrocalcinosis—when calcification visibly seen within tissues on imaging

EPIDEMIOLOGY

Prevalence

- Predominant age: 80% of patients >60 years
- No gender predominance. Men more likely to present acutely; women more likely to present atypically
- Prevalence varies by method of identification (chondrocalcinosis on radiograph vs. CPPD crystals in synovial fluid).
- Chondrocalcinosis is present in 1:10 adults age 60 to 75 years and 1:3 by >80 years; however, only a small percentage develop arthropathy.
- 20–43% prevalence of CPPD crystals in synovial fluid of osteoarthritic joints at time of joint replacement

ETIOLOGY AND PATHOPHYSIOLOGY

- Arthropathy results from an acute autoinflammatory reaction to CPPD crystals in the synovial cavity.
- CPPD crystal deposition occurs in three stages:
  - CPPD crystals first develop in the pericellular matrix of the articular cartilage via overproduction of anionic pyrophosphate (PPi).
  - PPi binds calcium to form CPPD crystals that are released from cartilage surface eliciting an inflammatory response. Neutrophils engulf CPPD crystals, inducing extracellular trap formation.
  - Increased CPPD crystal deposition in and around cartilage causes inflammation and damage. Cartilage degeneration is accelerated through mechanical wear and tear of the joint (2)[C].

Genetics

Uncommonly seen in familial pattern with autosomal dominant inheritance (<1% of patients); most cases are sporadic. Mutation in *ANKH* gene increases risk for calcium crystal formation.

RISK FACTORS

- Advanced age
- Joint trauma
- CPPD may occur as a complication in patients hospitalized for other medical and surgical illnesses.

GENERAL PREVENTION

Colchicine 0.6 mg BID may be used prophylactically to reduce frequency of episodes in recurrent CPPD.

COMMONLY ASSOCIATED CONDITIONS

- Gout
- Hyperparathyroidism
- Amyloidosis
- Hemochromatosis; ochronosis
- Hypothyroidism
- Wilson disease
- Hypomagnesemia
- Familial hypocalciuric hypercalcemia
- X-linked hypophosphatemic rickets
- Acromegaly

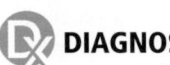 **DIAGNOSIS**

HISTORY

- Presentation often mimics gout ("pseudogout").
- Acute CPPD: pain and swelling of ≥1 or more joints; knee involved in 50% of cases; ankle, wrist, toe, and shoulder involvement are also common.
- Can present in proximal joints (mimicking polymyalgia rheumatica), often accompanied by tibiofemoral and ankle arthritis and tendinous calcifications
- Multiple symmetric joint involvement (mimicking RA) in <5% of cases
- May develop after intra-articular injection of hyaluronic acid (Hyalgan, Synvisc)
- Chronic CPPD: progressive degenerative arthritis with superimposed acute inflammatory attacks

PHYSICAL EXAM

- Inflammation (erythema, warmth, tender to touch), joint effusion, decreased range of motion (ROM) of joint
- 50% associated with fever
- Any synovial joint may be involved.

DIFFERENTIAL DIAGNOSIS

- Illnesses that may cause acute inflammatory arthritis in a single or multiple joint(s):
  - Gout
  - Septic arthritis
  - Trauma
- Other acute inflammatory arthritides:
  - Reiter syndrome
  - Lyme disease
  - Acute RA

DIAGNOSTIC TESTS & INTERPRETATION

Initial Tests (lab, imaging)

Synovial fluid analysis shows an inflammatory effusion:

- Cell count 2,000 to 100,000 WBCs/mL
- Neutrophil predominance (80–90%)
- >50,000 WBC count increases likelihood of septic arthritis, 11% prevalence; >100,000 WBCs/mL, 22%
- Wet prep with polarized microscopy may demonstrate small numbers of positively birefringent crystals; high false-negative rate
- Consider the following to exclude underlying disease:
  - Serum calcium, phosphorus, and magnesium
  - Serum alkaline phosphatase
  - Serum parathormone (i-PTH)
  - Serum iron, total iron-binding capacity, and serum ferritin
  - Serum thyroid-stimulating hormone (TSH) level
- Plain radiograph
  - Radiographic findings in pseudogout are neither sensitive nor specific.
  - Punctate and linear calcifications may be visualized in articular hyaline or fibrocartilage, particularly of the knees, hips, symphysis pubis, and wrists.
  - Patients with chronic CPPD may demonstrate subchondral cysts and loose bodies (osseous fragmentation with formation of intra-articular radiodense bodies) in joints not typically affected by degenerative joint disease.
- Ultrasound (US)
  - US may be more useful than plain radiography for the diagnosis of pseudogout in peripheral joints, with a positive predictive value of 92% and negative predictive value of 93% (3)[C].
  - US imaging characteristics include joint effusion, synovial thickening, and hyperechoic deposits.
- MRI
  - Chondrocalcinosis evident as hypointense lessions, particularly of knee menisci

Diagnostic Procedures/Other

ALERT

Synovial fluid analysis with demonstration of CPPD crystals is required for diagnosis; aspiration may help relieve symptoms and speed resolution.

Test Interpretation

CPPD crystal deposition in articular cartilage, synovium, ligaments, and tendons

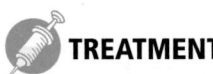 **TREATMENT**

GENERAL MEASURES

Target symptom relief (reduce inflammation):

- Rest and elevate affected joint(s).
- Apply ice/cool compresses to affected joints.
- Non–weight-bearing on affected joint while painful; use crutches or a walker.

MEDICATION

First Line

- A combination of pharmacologic and nonpharmacologic measures is recommended.
- Acute attacks should be treated with cool packs, rest, and joint aspiration with or without steroid injection.
- Chronic inflammatory CPPD arthropathy should be managed prophylactically with oral NSAIDs and/or colchicine (3)[C].
- Oral NSAIDs
  - Ibuprofen 600 to 800 mg PO TID–QID with food; maximum 3.2 g/day
  - Naproxen 500 mg PO BID with food
  - Other NSAIDs at anti-inflammatory doses are effective, although indomethacin has higher complication rates (relative risk [RR] = 2.2) compared with ibuprofen (RR = 1.2).
- Contraindications:
  - History of hypersensitivity to NSAIDs or aspirin
  - Active peptic ulcer disease or history of recurrent upper GI lesions
  - Avoid in renal insufficiency.
  - Serious GI bleeding can occur without warning; patient should be instructed on signs/symptoms. Administer proton pump inhibitor (PPI) or misoprostol 200 μg PO QID in patients at risk for NSAID-induced gastric ulcers.
- Oral colchicine
  - 0.6 mg QID or 0.6 mg hourly until symptoms relieved or vomiting/diarrhea develops; maximum dose per attack 4 to 6 mg; alternatively 0.5 to 1.0 mg/day may be used; avoid colchicine with significant renal insufficiency.
- Intra-articular steroid injection
  - Prednisolone–sodium phosphate 4 to 20 mg or triamcinolone diacetate 2 to 40 mg with local anesthetic

Adverse effects of NSAIDs:

- May elevate BP in patients on antihypertensive therapy
- May blunt antihypertensive effects of ACE inhibitors
- May prolong prothrombin time (PT) in patients taking oral anticoagulants
- Avoid concomitant aspirin use.
- May blunt diuretic effect of furosemide and hydrochlorothiazide
- May increase plasma lithium level in patients taking lithium carbonate

Second Line

- Oral prednisone: 30 to 50 mg/day for 7 to 10 days
- IM triamcinolone acetonide 40 mg; if necessary, may repeat in 1 to 4 days
- Consider referring patients with large space-occupying tophaceous lesions for surgical removal.
- Alternative therapies for chronic CPPD
  - ACTH, anakinra (anti–IL-1), hydroxychloroquine, infliximab, probenecid, magnesium, and ethylenediaminetetraacetic acid (EDTA) have all been suggested. Large scale studies are needed to evaluate effectiveness (4)[C].

ALERT

Recent randomized trial showed no significant effect of methotrexate in chronic-recurrent CPPD (5)[B].

ISSUES FOR REFERRAL

Consider consultation with orthopedist or rheumatologist if septic joint or patient is not responding.

ADDITIONAL THERAPIES

Physical therapy

- Isometric exercises to maintain muscle strength during the acute stage (e.g., quadriceps isometric contractions, leg lifts if knee affected)
- Begin joint ROM exercises as inflammation and pain subside.
- Resume weight-bearing when pain subsides.

SURGERY/OTHER PROCEDURES

Perform arthrocentesis and joint fluid analysis.

ADMISSION, INPATIENT, AND NURSING CONSIDERATIONS

Consider admission for septic arthritis if:

- Synovial fluid WBC count >50,000/mL
- Treat with appropriate antibiotics pending culture results.

 ONGOING CARE

FOLLOW-UP RECOMMENDATIONS

Patient Monitoring

Reevaluate response to therapy 48 to 72 hours after beginning treatment; reexamine in 1 week then as needed.

DIET

No known relationship to diet

PATIENT EDUCATION

- Rest affected joint.
- Symptoms usually resolve in 7 to 10 days.

PROGNOSIS

- Acute attack usually resolves in 10 days; prognosis for resolution of acute attack is excellent.
- Patients may experience progressive joint damage and functional limitation.

COMPLICATIONS

- Recurrent acute attacks
- Osteoarthritis

Geriatric Considerations

Elderly patients treated with NSAIDs require careful monitoring and are at higher risk for GI bleeding and acute renal insufficiency; no loading dose for colchicine due to high rates of renal insufficiency in elderly patients

REFERENCES

1. Zhang W, Doherty M, Bardin T, et al. European League Against Rheumatism recommendations for calcium pyrophosphate deposition. Part I: terminology and diagnosis. *Ann Rheum Dis*. 2011;70(4):563–570.
2. Rosenthal AK, Ryan LM. Nonpharmacologic and pharmacologic management of CPP crystal arthritis and BCP arthropathy and periarticular syndromes. *Rheum Dis Clin North Am*. 2014;40(2):343–356.
3. Zhang W, Doherty M, Pascual E, et al. EULAR recommendations for calcium pyrophosphate deposition. Part II: management. *Ann Rheum Dis*. 2011;70(4):571–575.
4. Pascart T, Richette P, Flipo RM. Treatment of nongout joint deposition diseases: an update. *Arthritis*. 2014;2014:375202.
5. Finckh A, Mc Carthy GM, Madigan A, et al. Methotrexate in chronic-recurrent calcium pyrophosphate deposition disease: no significant effect in a randomized crossover trial. *Arthritis Res Ther*. 2014;16(5):458.

ADDITIONAL READING

- Bruges-Armas J, Bettencourt BF, Couto AR, et al. Effectiveness and safety of infliximab in two cases of severe chondrocalcinosis: nine years of follow-up. *Case Rep Rheumatol*. 2014;2014:536856.
- Daoussis D, Antonopoulos I, Andonopoulos AP. ACTH as a treatment for acute crystal-induced arthritis: update on clinical evidence and mechanisms of action. *Semin Arthritis Rheum*. 2014;43(5):648–653.
- Demertzis JL, Rubin DA. MR imaging assessment of inflammatory, crystalline-induced, and infectious arthritides. *Magn Reson Imaging Clin N Am*. 2011;19(2):339–363.
- Macmullan P, McCarthy G. Treatment and management of pseudogout: insights for the clinician. *Ther Adv Musculoskelet Dis*. 2012;4(2):121–131.
- Sattui SE, Singh JA, Gaffo AL. Comorbidities in patients with crystal diseases and hyperuricemia. *Rheum Dis Clin North Am*. 2014;40(2):251–278.

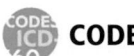 CODES

ICD10

- M11.20 Other chondrocalcinosis, unspecified site
- M11.269 Other chondrocalcinosis, unspecified knee
- M11.29 Other chondrocalcinosis, multiple sites

CLINICAL PEARLS

- Suspect CPPD in arthritis cases that do not follow a pattern typical of degenerative joint disease (e.g., metacarpophalangeal joints, wrists).
- Perform arthrocentesis to confirm diagnosis.
- If septic arthritis is considered, treat presumptively with antibiotics until culture results are available.
- NSAID therapy is the preferred pharmacologic treatment for acute flare.
- Oral steroids are useful if NSAIDs are contraindicated.
- Intra-articular steroids can be used *if* septic arthritis has been excluded.

PSORIASIS

Michael O. Needham, MD • Kimberly E. Matz, DO • Rebecca N. Matz, MD

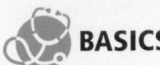

BASICS

DESCRIPTION
- A chronic, inflammatory disorder most commonly characterized by cutaneous erythematous plaques with silvery scale. It is a complex immune-mediated disorder that results from a polygenic predisposition in the setting of environmental triggers. It is associated with flares related to systemic, psychological, infectious, and environmental factors; skin disease with multiple different phenotypic variations and degrees of severity
- Clinical phenotypes
  - Plaque (vulgaris): most common variant (~80% of cases); well-demarcated, red plaques with thick, silvery scale; symmetrically distributed most commonly on the scalp, extensor surfaces of extremities, and trunk
  - Guttate: <2% of psoriasis patients, usually in patients <30 years of age; presents abruptly with 1- to 10-mm droplet-shaped pink erythematous papules with fine scale over trunk and extremities; often preceded by group A β-hemolytic streptococcal infection 2 to 3 weeks prior
  - Inverse: affects intertriginous areas and flexural surfaces; pink-to-red plaques with minimal scale; absence of satellite pustules distinguishes it from candidiasis although may coexist.
  - Erythrodermic: generalized erythema and scaling, affecting 90% of body surface area (BSA) or more; associated with desquamation; hair loss; nail dystrophy; and systemic symptoms such as fever, chills, malaise, lymphadenopathy, and/or high-output cardiac failure; usually requires hospital admission for management of dehydration, electrolyte abnormalities, and risk of infection
  - Pustular: sterile pustules; several forms including generalized pustular psoriasis, localized pustular psoriasis, and impetigo herpetiformis (in pregnancy); generalized type can result in life-threatening bacterial superinfections, sepsis, and dehydration if left untreated.
  - Nail disease: pitting, oil spots, and onycholysis; nails involved in up to 50% of patients with psoriasis with lifetime incidence of 80–90%; increased association with psoriatic arthritis
  - Psoriatic arthritis: 5–30% of patients; most commonly asymmetrical oligoarthritis involving the hands and feet

EPIDEMIOLOGY
Incidence
Predominant sex: male = female; predominant age: two peaks of incidence between the ages of 20 to 30 years and 50 to 60 years

Prevalence
- 2–4%—similar prevalence in all races
- Estimated 125 million affected worldwide (1)

ETIOLOGY AND PATHOPHYSIOLOGY
Psoriasis is a complex immune-mediated disorder with interactions between dendritic cells, T lymphocytes, neutrophils, and keratinocytes. It is considered a TH1- and TH17-driven disease with numerous cytokines including TNF-α, interferon-γ, IL-12, IL-17, and IL-23 playing pathogenic roles resulting in an inflammatory, hyperproliferative state.

Genetics
- Genetic predisposition (polygenic)
- 40% have psoriasis in a first-degree relative.
- Multiple susceptibility loci contain genes involved in immune system regulation (e.g., psoriasis susceptibility [*PSORS1*] locus on chromosome 6p21; polymorphisms in the IL-12/IL-13 receptor, the p40 subunit of IL-12 and IL-23, and the p19 subunit of IL-12) (2).
- HLA-Cw6 is most strongly correlated with early onset psoriasis.

RISK FACTORS
- Family history
- Obesity (may contribute to more severe disease)
- Local trauma; local irritation (Koebner phenomenon)
- HIV
- Streptococcal infection
- Mental stress (exacerbation)
- Medications (lithium, antimalarials, β-blockers, interferon, TNF-α inhibitors, withdrawal of steroids)
- Smoking
- Alcohol

GENERAL PREVENTION
Avoid triggers, including trauma, sunburns, smoking, and exposure to certain medications (as mentioned earlier), alcohol, and stress; weight loss if obese

COMMONLY ASSOCIATED CONDITIONS
- Psoriatic arthritis
- Seborrheic dermatitis
- Obesity, metabolic syndrome, diabetes, chronic kidney disease
- Cardiovascular disease; atherosclerotic disease
- Nonalcoholic fatty liver disease (NAFLD)
- Autoimmune: Crohn disease, ankylosing spondylitis
- Psychiatric/psychological: depression, suicide, emotional burden/anxiety, alcohol abuse

DIAGNOSIS

HISTORY
- May include sudden onset of clearly demarcated, erythematous plaques with overlying silvery scales; exacerbation of chronic plaques, especially on extensor surfaces and scalp; typically no or mild pruritus; triggers may include streptococcal infection or trauma.
- Family history of similar condition

PHYSICAL EXAM
- Well-demarcated salmon pink-to-red erythematous papules and plaques; silvery scale
- Distribution favors scalp, auricular conchal bowls, and postauricular area; extensor surface of extremities, especially knees and elbows; umbilicus, lower back, intergluteal cleft, and nails
- Nail findings: pitting, oil spots, onycholysis
- Auspitz sign: pinpoint bleeding with removal of scale
- Koebner phenomenon: new psoriatic lesions arising at sites of skin injury/trauma
- Genitals affected in up to 40% of patients
- Sebopsoriasis: Psoriasis can overlap with seborrheic dermatitis as greasy scales on the scalp, eyebrows, nasolabial folds, postauricular and presternal areas.

DIFFERENTIAL DIAGNOSIS
- Plaque: seborrheic dermatitis (may coexist), nummular eczema, atopic dermatitis, contact dermatitis, lichen simplex chronicus (may coexist), tinea, pityriasis rubra pilaris, dermatomyositis, squamous cell carcinoma in situ, reactive arthritis
- Guttate: pityriasis rosea, pityriasis lichenoides chronica, secondary syphilis, small plaque parapsoriasis
- Inverse: cutaneous candidiasis, tinea, seborrheic dermatitis, contact dermatitis
- Pustular: subcorneal pustulosis, acute generalized exanthematous pustulosis, folliculitis
- Erythrodermic: cutaneous T-cell lymphoma, drug-induced erythroderma, pityriasis rubra pilaris

DIAGNOSTIC TESTS & INTERPRETATION
Initial Tests (lab, imaging)
Clinical diagnosis based on history and physical exam. Labs generally not needed, although KOH to rule out tinea helpful. Consider x-rays if complaints of joint pain to evaluate for psoriatic arthritis.

Diagnostic Procedures/Other
- Psoriasis Area and Severity Index (PASI) evaluates overall severity and BSA involvement.
- Dermatology Life Quality Index (DLQI)

Test Interpretation
Biopsy: thickening of the stratum corneum (hyperkeratosis) with retention of nuclei (parakeratosis); elongation, thickening, and clubbing of rete ridges; dilated tortuous capillary loops in the dermal papillae; perivascular lymphocytic infiltrate, Munro microabscesses: neutrophils in stratum corneum

TREATMENT

GENERAL MEASURES
Adequate topical hydration (emollients); avoid triggers; weight loss

MEDICATION
First Line
- Mild-to-moderate disease
  - Emollients BID: petrolatum/ointments to maintain skin hydration and minimize pruritus and risk of koebnerization
  - Topical corticosteroids
    - Anti-inflammatory, antiproliferative, immunosuppressive, and vasoconstrictive effects
    - Local side effects: skin atrophy, hypopigmentation, striae, acne, folliculitis, and purpura. Systemic side effects: Risk is higher, with higher potency formulations used over a large surface for a prolonged period; pregnancy Category C
    - Applications are typically twice daily until lesions flatten/resolve and then taper to PRN use for maintenance.
    - Scalp: high potency in solution/foam vehicle; shampoos and sprays also available
    - Face, intertriginous areas, infants: low-potency corticosteroids: 1% hydrocortisone
    - Adult initial therapy: medium-potency corticosteroids daily: 0.1% mometasone or triamcinolone; strong-potency corticosteroids: 0.05% betamethasone or fluocinonide daily; superpotency corticosteroids: clobetasol, halobetasol; caution with use over 2 to 4 weeks; avoid occlusive dressings; reserved for recalcitrant plaques

- Vitamin D analogues: calcipotriene 0.005% cream daily to BID; good for plaque and also intertriginous; limits keratinocyte hyperproliferation; may be highly effective for short-term control in combination with a superpotent corticosteroid; should not be used with products that can alter pH, such as topical lactic acid; local side effects: burning, pruritus, edema, peeling, dryness, and erythema; pregnancy Category C
- Topical retinoids: tazarotene 0.05% or 0.1% (Tazorac) daily; normalizes abnormal keratinocyte differentiation and diminishes hyperproliferation; may be combined with corticosteroids; side effects: local irritation, photosensitivity; pregnancy Category X
- Topical calcineurin inhibitors: Tacrolimus 0.1% or pimecrolimus 1% may be used as steroid-sparing agents, especially in facial and intertriginous areas.
- Comparison of topical therapies: Vitamin D analogues have slower onset of action than topical corticosteroids but longer disease-free periods for body plaques; for scalp, potent and superpotency steroids more effective (3)[A]
- Combination of superpotent steroids and vitamin D analogues has better efficacy than either as monotherapy (4)[A].
• Severe disease: may need combination therapy
  - Light therapy: locally immunosuppressive and antiproliferative. UVB (broad/narrow band [BB, NB]) or PUVA: Treatment protocols are skin type dependent: mixed studies as to whether PUVA or NBUVB more effective; PUVA with GI SE, photosensitivity, and increased risk of nonmelanoma skin cancers
  - Systemic therapies
    ○ Methotrexate: immunosuppressive, blocks DNA synthesis; start with 5-mg test dose, then increase to 7.5 to 15.0 mg/week IV, PO, IM, or SC, and then increase 2.5 mg every 2 to 3 weeks, up to 25 mg; contraindicated in pregnancy; supplement with folic acid 1 mg/day to protect against side effects: hepatotoxicity, pulmonary toxicity, bone marrow suppression; baseline chest x-ray, monitor LFTs, renal function, CBC, testing for latent tuberculosis (TB); consider liver biopsy when cumulative dose reaches 3.5 to 4.0 g; avoid alcohol and medications that interfere with folic acid metabolism, including trimethoprim and sulfamethoxazole (Bactrim), NSAIDs, sulfamethoxazole, or hepatotoxic agents (e.g., retinoids).
    ○ Cyclosporine: inhibits T-cell activation; start 2.5 mg/kg/day; if insufficient response after 4 weeks, increase by 0.5 mg/kg/day; additional dosage increases every 2 weeks (max dose: 5 mg/kg/day); pregnancy Category C; side effects: renal toxicity and hypertension, limit use to 6 months to 1 year: Monitor renal function, with Mg^{2+} and K^+, CBC, lipids, and blood pressure.
    ○ Acitretin (Soriatane): systemic retinoid; start at 10 to 25 mg/day given with the main meal; effective for pustular psoriasis and as a maintenance therapy after stabilization with other agents; sometimes combined with UVB/PUVA; pregnancy Category X: pregnancy test before starting; two forms of contraception 1 month before, during, and for at least 3 years after treatment; avoid alcohol (may convert acitretin to etretinate); side effects: alopecia, xerosis, cheilitis, hepatotoxicity, hyperlipidemia, cataracts; monitor LFTs, renal function, lipid profile, CBC, regular eye exams.

- Biologics: general guidelines: Screen for latent TB at baseline and yearly, hepatitis panel at baseline, avoid live vaccines; monitor CBC with differential, signs/symptoms of infections, heart failure, malignancy, drug-induced lupus, demyelinating disorder. Some concern for "biologic fatigue" phenomenon, or loss of PASI 75 over time, possibly due to antidrug antibodies. Each has been shown to be effective at 24 weeks with an NNT between 1 and 3. All should be considered effective first-line treatments (5)[A]; pregnancy Category B
  ○ TNF-α inhibitors: etanercept (Enbrel): Begin at 50 mg SC twice a week for 3 months then maintenance of 50 mg/week. Adalimumab (Humira): Dosing starts at 80 mg SC for 1 week, then 40 mg SC every other week. Infliximab (Remicade): 5 mg/kg IV at weeks 0, 2, and 6; maintenance doses of 5 mg/kg every 8 weeks thereafter; adjust interval, as needed; anaphylaxis-like infusion reaction occurs in <1% of patients.
  ○ IL-12/IL-23 antagonist: ustekinumab (Stelara): patients <100 kg: 45 mg SC at weeks 0 and 4 and then every 12 weeks; >100 kg: 90 mg can be given.
  ○ IL-17 antagonists: secukinumab (Cosentyx). 300 mg SC on weeks 0, 1, 2, 3, and 4 and then every 4 weeks. Ixekizumab (Taltz): 160 mg on week 0, then 80 mg on weeks 2, 4, 6, 8, 10, and 12, and then 80 mg every 4 weeks. Brodalumab (Siliq): 210 mg SC on weeks 0, 1, 2 and then every 2 weeks
  ○ Phosphodiesterase-4 enzyme inhibitor: apremilast (Otezla): 10 mg PO, titrate up by 10 mg/day on days 2 to 5 to maintenance dose of 30 mg BID starting on day 6. Routine lab monitoring not required. Most common SE are GI symptoms, depression; pregnancy Category C

Second Line
Immunosuppressives: azathioprine, hydroxyurea, 6-thioguanine, fumaric acid esters, and topicals: salicylic acid; anthralin; coal tar

ISSUES FOR REFERRAL
Psoriasis >20% of BSA, psoriatic arthritis, pustular psoriasis, severe extremity involvement, particularly hands and feet

SURGERY/OTHER PROCEDURES
Psoriasis and psoriatic medications can affect wound healing postoperatively; methotrexate: Monitor for postoperative infections; hold cyclosporine for 1 week before and after; some surgeons may prefer to hold therapy with biologics for up to 1 month before and after surgery.

ADMISSION, INPATIENT, AND NURSING CONSIDERATIONS
Generalized pustular psoriasis/erythrodermic psoriasis: Rule out sepsis; restoration of barrier function of skin with cleaning and bandaging; intensive topical corticosteroid therapy (like wet wraps), systemic therapy, particularly medications with a quick onset such as oral cyclosporine; management of electrolytes

ONGOING CARE

FOLLOW-UP RECOMMENDATIONS
Measure BSA involvement to determine if therapy is working; change therapy or add agent if no improvement is seen.

DIET
Well-balanced diet and exercise to limit cardiovascular risk factors and decrease risk of associated conditions, including obesity, metabolic syndrome, diabetes, and atherosclerosis

PATIENT EDUCATION
National Psoriasis Foundation: https://www.psoriasis.org; 800-723-9166

PROGNOSIS
Guttate form may be self-limited and remit after months; chronic plaque type is lifelong, with intermittent spontaneous remissions and exacerbations; erythrodermic and generalized pustular forms may be severe and persistent.

COMPLICATIONS
Psoriatic arthritis, generalized pustular psoriasis, erythrodermic psoriasis, comorbidities (cardiovascular disease, metabolic syndrome, etc.)

REFERENCES
1. Rachakonda TD, Schupp CW, Armstrong AW. Psoriasis prevalence among adults in the United States. *J Am Acad Dermatol*. 2014;70(3):512–516.
2. Villaseñor-Park J, Wheeler D, Grandinetti L. Psoriasis: evolving treatment for a complex disease. *Cleve Clin J Med*. 2012;79(6):413–423.
3. Mason AR, Mason J, Cork M, et al. Topical treatments for chronic plaque psoriasis. *Cochrane Database Syst Rev*. 2013;(3):CD005028.
4. Hendriks AG, Keijsers RR, de Jong EM, et al. Efficacy and safety of combinations of first-line topical treatments in chronic plaque psoriasis: a systematic literature review. *J Eur Acad Dermatol Venereol*. 2013;27(8):931–951.
5. Sendur N, Buyukpapuscu O, Karaman G, et al. Biologics in psoriasis. *J Am Acad Dermatol*. 2016;74(5):AB238.

ADDITIONAL READING
Sbidian E, Chaimani A, Garcia-Doval I, et al. Systemic pharmacological treatments for chronic plaque psoriasis: a network meta-analysis. *Cochrane Database Syst Rev*. 2017;12:CD011535.

 SEE ALSO

Arthritis, Psoriatic

 CODES

ICD10
- L40.9 Psoriasis, unspecified
- L40.50 Arthropathic psoriasis, unspecified
- L42 Pityriasis rosea

CLINICAL PEARLS
Chronic lifelong inflammatory skin condition with remissions and exacerbations; set realistic expectations with patient. Disease burden not limited to skin. If one medication does not work, use/combine with another agent.

PSYCHOSIS

Matthew J. Filippo, DO • Bernadette M. Stevenson, MD, PhD

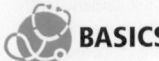

BASICS

DESCRIPTION

A disorder where thoughts and emotions are significantly impaired (i.e., a loss of contact with reality). Seen in schizophrenia, affective, bipolar, depression, substance use, medical problems, delirium, and dementia; symptoms include the following:

- Positive symptoms: hallucinations and delusions (fixed false beliefs not typical of cultural background)
- Negative symptoms: anhedonia, poverty of speech, lack of motivation, social withdrawal, affective blunting
- Cognition: poor working memory, information processing, difficulty with attention, disorganized speech and/or behavior

EPIDEMIOLOGY

Prevalence

- Schizophrenia: peak onset 18 to 25 years in males; 25 to 35 years in females
- 1% of the U.S. population; similar percentage worldwide; 1:1 male–female ratio
- Delusional disorder: 0.3% of population, bipolar: 1–3% of population, unipolar depression: up to 20% prevalence

ETIOLOGY AND PATHOPHYSIOLOGY

- Stems from many causes, including psychiatric, medical, and/or substance use
- Positive symptoms relate to excessive dopaminergic activity in the mesolimbic pathway. Negative symptoms relate to diminished dopaminergic activity in mesocortical pathway.
- Glutamate, steroids, cortisol, inflammation, and developmental abnormalities are likely involved and active areas of research.

Genetics

Schizophrenia: 50% concordance for monozygotic twins, little or no shared environmental effect; multiple candidate genes involved

RISK FACTORS

Substance abuse (particularly cannabis or synthetics), family history of psychosis, lower socioeconomic status

GENERAL PREVENTION

Community interventions for early detection and treatment of prodromal symptoms show promise; research currently exploring use of omega-3 fatty acids and anti-inflammatories, which may prevent prodromal progression to schizophrenia

COMMONLY ASSOCIATED CONDITIONS

- Associated with metabolic syndrome, autonomic dysfunction, sudden cardiac death, and cancer mortality: particularly breast and lung cancer
- Substance abuse disorders, including nicotine dependence

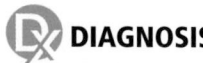

DIAGNOSIS

Rule out delirium: Psychosis shouldn't have fluctuating consciousness/reduced clarity of awareness.

HISTORY

- Delusions (fixed false beliefs): persecutory (being monitored), bizarre (involving impossible states), somatic (fixed belief in nonexistent illness), referential (getting special messages or thoughts inserted/deleted by others), grandiose (belief that one has special powers)
- Hallucinations: auditory, visual, tactile, gustatory, olfactory

- Bipolar, unipolar depression, and dementia are associated with psychosis. Screen for symptoms of these.
- Screen for toxidromes of drugs of abuse and for history of epileptiform activity.
- Suicidality: higher risk with comorbid depression/mania, previous attempts, drug abuse, agitation/akathisia, poor adherence

PHYSICAL EXAM

- Mental status exam: disorganized speech, behavior, and/or thought process; thought blocking; response latency; blunted or flat affect; often have negative symptoms, including social withdrawal, lack of initiative, poverty of thought, and/or positive symptoms such as auditory and visual hallucinations
- Pay attention to focal neurologic symptoms, antipsychotic-induced parkinsonism, tardive dyskinesia, and akathisia.
- May present with catatonia: ranging from lack of movement to extreme excitement, posturing, mutism, grimacing, waxy flexibility

DIFFERENTIAL DIAGNOSIS

- Schizophrenia: positive symptoms (psychosis) and negative symptoms (flat affect), prodrome of social withdrawal, cognitive impairment; schizophreniform disorder: psychotic/prodromal symptoms in <6 months; schizoaffective disorder: manic/depressive mood disorder with psychosis that persists even when euthymic; schizotypal personality disorder: no true psychosis but distance in relationships and odd beliefs; delusional disorder: nonbizarre delusion (e.g., erotomanic, grandiose, jealous, persecutory, somatic), no negative/mood symptoms
- Mood disorder with psychotic features: can occur in mania or depression. Delusions often mood congruent; psychosis remits when mood improves.
- Substance-induced psychosis: alcohol and benzodiazepine withdrawal, intoxication with cocaine, bath salts, PCP, cannabis, synthetic cannabinoids, MDMA, amphetamines, hallucinogens, and alcohol; may persist beyond acute intoxication
- Borderline personality disorder: During extreme stress, patients often experience auditory/visual hallucinations (psychosis NOS).
- Posttraumatic stress disorder: psychosis associated with traumatic recollections; often visual hallucinations (vs. more auditory in schizophrenia)
- Psychosis due to general medical condition: delirium, stroke, infection, collagen vascular disease, head injury, tumor, interictal, porphyria, syphilis, and so forth
- Medication-induced psychosis: common causes: steroids, L-dopa, anticholinergics, antidepressants in bipolar patients, interferon, digoxin, stimulants

DIAGNOSTIC TESTS & INTERPRETATION

- Labs: CBC, CMP, LFTs, thyroid-stimulating hormone (TSH), rapid plasma reagin (RPR), HIV, ANA, ESR, vitamin B_{12}, 25-hydroxy-vitamin D, urinalysis, UDS
- Neuroimaging: not necessary for diagnosis but may consider MRI/CT to evaluate for medical cause of symptoms (especially if new onset or in elderly). Schizophrenia is associated with enlarged lateral ventricles, reduced gray matter, and symmetry.
- ECG: especially if on multiple medications or in elderly. Antipsychotics can prolong QTc interval, particularly ziprasidone, iloperidone, and IV haloperidol.

Follow-Up Tests & Special Considerations

- Consider Wilson disease, porphyria, metachromatic leukodystrophy, and inflammatory conditions.

- Consider lumbar puncture if unable to distinguish from delirium and/or unexplained rapid-onset psychosis.
- Consider electroencephalogram (EEG) for partial complex seizures and psychosis associated with preictal and postictal events.

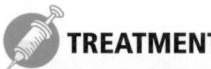

TREATMENT

Before antipsychotic treatment: Screen for metabolic syndrome. Baseline fasting lipid panel and glucose, HgbA1c, CBC, CMP, LFTs, weight, waist circumference, AIMS testing. Continue monitoring with long-term use (1)[B].

MEDICATION

- Antipsychotics are mainstay of treatment (1)[B].
- Classified as typical versus atypical. Dopamine-2 (D_2) antagonists with varied affinity for the receptor. Atypicals also block serotonin 5-HT2A receptors. Help positive symptoms more than negative. Nonspecific effect on agitation begins early; antipsychotic effect takes 1 to 6 weeks.
- For mania with psychotic features, a mood stabilizer may be used with an antipsychotic.
- For major depression with psychotic features, antidepressant and antipsychotic medications yield better response rate than either medication alone. In delirium, must treat underlying cause; may not require antipsychotic therapy
- Side effects
  - Acute dystonia: benztropine 1 to 3 mg IM/IV then 0.5 to 2.0 mg BID–TID or diphenhydramine 50 to 100 mg IM/IV BID–TID max 400 mg/day, NTE 25 mg/min
  - Parkinsonism: Lower antipsychotic dose; switch to atypical (particularly, quetiapine, olanzapine, or clozapine) or add benztropine 0.5 to 2.0 mg PO BID–TID, diphenhydramine 25 to 50 mg BID–TID.
  - Akathisia: intense restlessness, especially legs. Lower antipsychotic dose; treat with β-blocker, anticholinergic, or benzodiazepine; may switch to antipsychotic with lower akathisia risk such as quetiapine, olanzapine, iloperidone, or clozapine
  - Tardive dyskinesia: seen in ~32.4% of those treated long term with typicals, 13.1% treated with atypicals. Switch to clozapine or quetiapine. If cannot, minimize dose. Symptomatic treatment has been tried with low-dose benzodiazepines, Botox, anticholinergics, and VMAT-2 inhibitors such as FDA-approved valbenazine and deutetrabenazine. AIMS exam is gold standard for detecting tardive dyskinesia.
  - Neuroleptic malignant syndrome: potentially fatal; rigidity, tremor, fever, autonomic instability, mental status changes; discontinue neuroleptic; ICU; volume resuscitation; cooling blankets; no anticholinergics/antihistaminics; consider dantrolene, amantadine, bromocriptine, and electroconvulsive therapy (ECT).
  - Metabolic syndrome, sudden cardiac death (risk higher IM/IV droperidol, IV haloperidol), stroke, heart failure, PNA (elderly), pulmonary embolus

First Line

- Benefits of atypical antipsychotics include lower risk of extrapyramidal symptoms (quetiapine, olanzapine, iloperidone, or clozapine) and dyskinesias (clozapine, quetiapine); possibly more effective for negative symptoms
- Greater risk of weight gain, new-onset diabetes, and hyperlipidemia with olanzapine and clozapine compared with typicals and other atypicals

- Acute psychotic agitation: olanzapine 5 to 10 mg IM with up to three 10-mg injections over a 24-hour period; do not administer concurrently with benzodiazepines; ziprasidone 10 mg IM q2h or 20 mg q4h; NTE 40 mg/day; aripiprazole IM has been discontinued; haloperidol 5 mg +/− lorazepam 2 mg IM, can be given with 1 mg IM benztropine, NTE 20 mg haloperidol, and 8 mg lorazepam per day
- Psychosis in schizophrenia
  – Olanzapine: Start 5 to 10 mg at bedtime; target dose 5 to 20 mg/day within 2 days and up to 40 mg/day in treatment-refractory schizophrenia. More likely weight gain, hyperlipidemia, and hyperglycemia than other oral atypicals except clozapine; may have lower rates of discontinuation and rehospitalization than several other atypicals but likely not more efficacy than clozapine; sedation initially; drug metabolism increased up to 50% by tobacco use
  – Quetiapine: Start 25 mg BID, increase 25 to 50 mg q8–12h days 2 and 3, up to 3 to 400 mg in divided doses by day 4. Can then increase 50 to 100 mg/day, NTE 800 mg/day divided BID–TID; less risk of parkinsonism, useful in Parkinson psychosis; more weight gain than others; sedation, restless legs syndrome; gradual titration tolerated better. Quetiapine XR: can start 300 mg/day. Dose increase ≥1 day up to 300 mg/day. Target dose is 300 to 800 mg.
  – Risperidone: Start 1 to 2 mg/day; target dose of 2 to 8 mg/day to be reached over 1 to 2 weeks; doses >6 mg rarely more effective and higher risk of parkinsonism; higher risk of prolactinemia/parkinsonism due to D_2 blockade
  – Paliperidone: Start 3 to 6 mg/day; target dose 6 to 12 mg/day; titrate over 1 to 2 weeks. Higher risk of prolactinemia/parkinsonism than others; minimal hepatic metabolism, ideal for hepatic impairment
  – Ziprasidone: Start 20 to 40 mg PO BID, with target dose of 100 to 160 mg/day in divided doses over 2 weeks; prolongs QTc; less likely to cause weight gain than other atypicals; higher risk of akathisia/parkinsonism; requires food (500 kcal, for optimal absorption; activating at lower doses)
  – Aripiprazole: Start 10 to 15 mg/day, may increase up to 30 mg/day over 1 to 2 weeks; less weight gain but higher rates of akathisia; can lower QTc
  – Asenapine: Start 5 mg at bedtime or BID sublingually, increase to 10 mg BID if needed over 1 to 2 weeks; less weight gain than some, higher rates of akathisia/parkinsonism; sedation, orthostatic hypotension, numb tongue, nausea, bad taste; comes in black cherry flavor
  – Lurasidone: Start 20 to 40 mg QD with food (at least 350 calories), increase up to max of 160 mg at bedtime if needed over 2 to 4 weeks. Less weight gain than some but higher rates of akathisia/parkinsonism; not antihistaminic but α-blocking sedation and serotonergic nausea
  – Iloperidone: Start 1 mg BID, may increase by 2 mg daily, but slower can be better due to significant orthostasis. Increase to max 12 mg BID; little akathisia/parkinsonism, less weight gain but slower efficacy due to long titration, orthostasis, sedation
  – Brexpiprazole: Start 1 mg daily for first 4 days, 2 mg QD days 5 to 7, can increase dose up to 4 mg/day based on response and tolerability. Lower rates of akathisia than aripiprazole but higher rates than others; less weight gain than others
  – Cariprazine: Start at 1.5 mg QD, can be increased to 3 mg QD on day 2, dosed up to 6 mg daily based on tolerability and response; in 6-week study, similar to placebo in changes of fasting glucose, cholesterol, triglycerides, and showed 0.8 to 1.0 kg weight increase

Geriatric Considerations
Increased risk of death compared to placebo when antipsychotics are used in the elderly with dementia (2)[B]. Pimavanserin has recently been approved for hallucinations and delusions associated with Parkinson disease psychosis.

Second Line
Clozapine: more effective for reducing symptoms, preventing relapse, decreasing tardive dyskinesia, and decreasing suicidality than other antipsychotics. Second line given risk of fatal agranulocytosis. Single national registry (clozapine REMS) for all patients on clozapine, updated guidelines in 2015 requiring CBC to monitor

absolute neutrophil count weekly for first 6 months, then every 2 weeks for 6 months, and then every 4 weeks. More weight gain, hyperlipidemia, hyperglycemia, seizures, myocarditis, pulmonary embolus, and sedation but low rate of parkinsonism, tardive dyskinesia; useful in treatment-refractory psychosis and in Parkinson disease psychosis. Despite association with more weight gain than other antipsychotics, clozapine and olanzapine do not appear to increase risk of cardiac and all-cause mortality (2,3)[B],(4). Drug metabolism increased up to 50% by tobacco use.

- Maintenance:
  – Consider switching to a long-acting injectable (LAI) medications:

Name	Starting Dose	Maintenance Dose	Comment
Haloperidol	10–20 times daily PO dose	50–200 mg q3–4wk	NTE 100 mg injected at once
Fluphenazine	12.5 mg	12.5–50.0 mg q2–3wk	10 mg PO ~12.5 mg IM
Aripiprazole (Maintena)	400 mg	400 mg monthly	2-wk overlap with PO
Aripiprazole (Aristada)	441–1,062 mg based on PO dose	Based on PO dose. Some extended q8wk.	3-wk overlap with PO or given with Initio on day 1 to 10
Aripiprazole (Initio)	675 mg	Not for repeat dosing	Give dose of Initio IM with Abilify 30 mg PO. Give maintenance or new Aristada dose within 10 days. Establish PO tolerability first.
Olanzapine	150–300 mg q2wk	300–405 mg q4wk	Requires 3 hr of postinjection monitoring
Paliperidone (Sustenna)	234 mg then 117 mg a wk later	39–234 mg monthly	PO overlap not needed
Paliperidone (Invega Trinza)	Convert from Sustenna dose		Must be on Sustenna 4 mo

ADDITIONAL THERAPIES
Psychotherapy, vocational, art, and group are effective adjuvants to antipsychotics (1)[B].

ADMISSION, INPATIENT, AND NURSING CONSIDERATIONS
- Admission criteria/initial stabilization: at risk for harm to self or others; extreme functional impairment; unable to care for self; new-onset psychosis
- Discharge criteria: no longer a danger to self or others and adequate outpatient follow-up treatment in place

 ONGOING CARE

FOLLOW-UP RECOMMENDATIONS
Close follow-up for inpatient discharge (high risk for suicide), use therapy, exercise, teach smoking cessation, AIMS testing q3–6mo

PATIENT EDUCATION
National Alliance on Mental Illness: https://www.nami.org/

PROGNOSIS
Schizophrenia: fluctuating course; 70% first-episode psychosis patients improve in 3 to 4 months, 20–40% will attempt suicide, and 7% will die of suicide.

REFERENCES
1. National Institute for Health and Care Excellence. Psychosis and schizophrenia in adults: prevention and management. http://www.nice.org.uk/guidance/cg178. Accessed October 16, 2018.
2. Strom BL, Eng SM, Faich G, et al. Comparative mortality associated with ziprasidone and olanzapine in real-world use among 18,154 patients with schizophrenia: the Ziprasidone Observational Study of Cardiac Outcomes (ZODIAC). *Am J Psychiatry.* 2011;168(2):193–201.
3. Tiihonen J, Lönnqvist J, Wahlbeck K, et al. 11-Year follow-up of mortality in patients with schizophrenia: a population-based cohort study (FIN11 study). *Lancet.* 2009;374(9690):620–627.
4. McEvoy JP, Lieberman JA, Stroup TS, et al; for CATIE Investigators. Effectiveness of clozapine versus olanzapine, quetiapine, and risperidone in patients with chronic schizophrenia who did not respond to prior atypical antipsychotic treatment. *Am J Psychiatry.* 2006;163(4):600–610.

ADDITIONAL READING
Clinical Practice Guidelines: https://www.psychiatry.org/psychiatrists/practice/clinical-practice-guidelines

 SEE ALSO

Delirium; Schizophrenia

 CODES

ICD10
- F29 Unsp psychosis not due to a substance or known physiol cond
- F20.9 Schizophrenia, unspecified
- F39 Unspecified mood [affective] disorder

CLINICAL PEARLS
- Antipsychotics mainstay of treatment; lead to decreased all-cause mortality pin adherent patients
- Clozapine and LAIs may increase adherence.

PULMONARY ARTERIAL HYPERTENSION

Nasheena Jiwa, MD

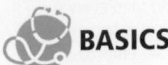 BASICS

DESCRIPTION
- Pulmonary arterial hypertension (PAH) is a category of pulmonary hypertension (PH) characterized by abnormalities in the small pulmonary arteries (precapillary PH) that produce increased pulmonary arterial pressure (PAP) and vascular resistance, eventually resulting in right-sided heart failure. PAH is a progressive disorder associated with increased mortality.
  - Previously, PH was classified as primary PH (without cause, now idiopathic IPAH) or secondary PH (with cause or associated condition); now, it is clear that some types of secondary PH closely match primary PH (IPAH) in their histology, natural history, and response to treatment. Therefore, WHO classifies PH into five groups based on mechanism, with PAH as group 1 in this classification.
  - PAH is diagnosed by right-heart catheterization and defined by a mean PAP ≥25 mm Hg at rest when other groups of PH are ruled out; pulmonary capillary wedge pressure ≤15 mm Hg (excludes PH owing to left heart disease; i.e., group 2 PH)
  - Mild or absent chronic lung disease or other causes of hypoxemia (excludes PH owing to lung disease or hypoxemia; i.e., group 3 PH)
  - Absent venous thromboembolic disease (excludes chronic thromboembolic PH [CTEPH]; i.e., group 4 PH)
  - Absent systemic disorder (like sarcoidosis), hematologic disorders (like myeloproliferative disease), and metabolic disorders (like glycogen storage disease) (excludes group 5 PH)
- PAH is divided into following main categories:
  - Idiopathic: sporadic, with no family history or risk factors
  - Heritable: IPAH with mutations or familial cases with or without mutations
  - Drug or toxin induced: mostly associated with anorectics (e.g., fenfluramine), rapeseed oil, L-tryptophan, and illicit drugs such as methamphetamine and cocaine
  - Associated: connective tissue diseases (e.g., systemic lupus erythematosus, rheumatoid arthritis, scleroderma), HIV infection, portal hypertension (HTN), congenital heart disease, schistosomiasis (chronic hemolytic anemia added to group 5 PH—unclear/multifactorial mechanisms) (1)
  - Pulmonary veno-occlusive disease (PVOD) and/or pulmonary capillary hemangiomatosis (PCH) and persistent PH of the newborn (PPHN) are classified as separate categories due to more differences than similarities with PAH.
    - PVOD and/or PCH: rare cause of PH characterized by extensive diffuse occlusion of the pulmonary veins (unlike PAH which involves the small muscular pulmonary arterioles)

EPIDEMIOLOGY
- Age: can occur at any age; mean age 37 years
- Sex (IPAH): female > male (female:male ratio ranges from 1.7 to 4.8:1.0)

Incidence
- Overall PAH: 5 to 52 cases per million
- IPAH: low, ~2 to 6 per million
- Drug-induced PAH: 1/25,000 with >3 months of anorectic use
- HIV associated: 0.5/100
- Portal HTN associated: 1 to 6/100
- Scleroderma associated: 6–60%

Prevalence
- PAH: ~15 to 50 cases per million
- IPAH: ~6 cases per million

ETIOLOGY AND PATHOPHYSIOLOGY
- Pulmonary: Inflammation, vasoconstriction, endothelial dysfunction, and intimal proliferation causing remodeling of pulmonary arteries produced by increased cell proliferation and reduced rates of apoptosis lead to obstruction.
- Cardiovascular: Right ventricular hypertrophy (RVH), eventually leading to right-sided heart failure and right ventricular (RV) ischemia due to reduced right coronary artery flow causes RV remodeling associated with PAH.
- IPAH: by definition, unknown. True IPAH is mostly sporadic or sometimes familial in nature.
- Pulmonary arteriolar hyperactivity and vasoconstriction, occult thromboembolism, or autoimmune (high frequency of antinuclear antibodies)

Genetics
- 75% of heritable PAH (HPAH) cases and 25% of IPAH cases have mutations in *BMPR2* (autosomal dominant).
- Mutations in *ALK1* and endoglin (autosomal dominant) also are associated with PAH.

RISK FACTORS
- Female sex
- Previous anorectic drug use
- Recent acute pulmonary embolism
- First-degree relatives of patient with familial PAH

COMMONLY ASSOCIATED CONDITIONS
See associated PAH, earlier discussed.

 DIAGNOSIS

Symptoms of PAH are nonspecific, which can lead to missed or delayed diagnosis of this serious disease.

HISTORY
Dyspnea, weakness, syncope, dizziness, chest pain, palpitations, lower extremity edema

PHYSICAL EXAM
- Pulmonary component of S_2 (at apex in >90% of patients)
- RV lift
- Early systolic click of pulmonary valve
- Pansystolic murmur of tricuspid regurgitation
- Diastolic murmur of pulmonic insufficiency (Graham Steell murmur)
- RV S_3 or S_4
- Edema as jugular vein distention, ascites, hepatomegaly, or peripheral edema

DIFFERENTIAL DIAGNOSIS
Other causes of dyspnea:
- Pulmonary parenchymal disease such as chronic obstructive pulmonary disease
- Pulmonary vascular disease such as pulmonary thromboembolism
- Cardiac disease such as cardiomyopathy
- Other disorders of respiratory function such as sleep apnea

DIAGNOSTIC TESTS & INTERPRETATION
- Echocardiography (ECG): RVH and right axis deviation, or RV strain (increased P wave amplitude, incomplete right bundle branch block pattern, an R-to-S ratio >1 in lead V1)
- Pulmonary function testing: reduced diffusion capacity
- Arterial blood gas: arterial hypoxemia, hypocapnia
- Ventilation/perfusion (V/Q) scan: Look for proximal pulmonary artery emboli and CTEPH; rule out group 4 PH.
- Exercise test: reduced maximal O_2 consumption, high-minute ventilation, low anaerobic threshold, increased PO_2 alveolar–arterial gradient; correlation to severity of disease with 6-minute walk distance (6MWD) test
- Antinuclear antibody positive (up to 40% of patients)
- LFTs: Evaluate for portopulmonary HTN as a complication of chronic liver disease.
- HIV test, thyroid function tests, sickle cell disease screening
- Elevated brain natriuretic peptide (BNP) and N-terminal-proBNP may be useful for early detection of PAH in young, otherwise healthy patients with mild symptoms. It can also be used to assess disease severity and prognosis.
- Chest radiograph
  - Prominent central pulmonary arteries with peripheral hypovascularity of pulmonary arterial branches
  - RV enlargement is a late finding.
- Echo Doppler
  - Should be performed with suspicion of PAH; echo suggests, but does not diagnose, PAH; most commonly used screening tool
    - Estimates mean PAP and assesses cardiac structure and function, excludes congenital anomalies
    - Right atrial and ventricular enlargement; tricuspid regurgitation
    - Important to rule out underlying cardiac disease such as atrial septal defect with secondary PH or mitral stenosis
- In patients at risk for HPAH, screen for gene mutations *BMPR2*.
- Polysomnography: for suspected symptoms of obstructive sleep apnea

Diagnostic Procedures/Other
- Pulmonary angiography
  - Should be done if V/Q scan suggests CTEPH
  - Use caution; can lead to hemodynamic collapse; use low osmolar agents, subselective angiograms.
- Right-sided cardiac catheterization (gold standard for diagnosis of PAH)
- Essential to confirm diagnosis and determine severity and prognosis by measuring PAPs and hemodynamics
  - Rule out underlying cardiac disease (e.g., left-sided heart disease) and assess response to vasodilator therapy.
- Lung biopsy: not recommended unless primary pulmonary parenchymal disease exists
- 6MWD: classifies severity of PAH and estimates prognosis

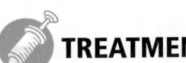 TREATMENT

- Treat underlying diseases/conditions that may cause PAH to relieve symptoms and improve quality of life and survival.
- Reasonable goals of therapy include the following:
  - Modified NYHA FC I or II
  - ECG/CMR of normal/near-normal RV size and function

- Hemodynamic parameters showing normalization of the RV function (RAP <8 mm Hg and Cardiac Index (CI) >2.5 to 3.0 L/min/m^2)
- 6MWD of >380 to 440 m
- Cardiopulmonary exercise testing, including peak oxygen consumption of >15 mL/min/kg and EqCO2 <45 L/min
- Normal BNP levels (2)[C]

GENERAL MEASURES

- Supervised exercise training (3)[A]
- Psychosocial support (3)[C]
- Avoid strenuous physical activity (3)[C].
- Avoid pregnancy (3)[C].
- Influenza and pneumococcal immunization (3)[C]
- Oxygen—maintain arterial blood O$_2$ pressure >60 mm Hg (3)[C]

MEDICATION

- Acute vasodilator test during heart catheterization for all patients who are potential candidates for long-term oral calcium channel blocker (CCB) therapy (3)[C]
  - Screens for pulmonary vasoreactivity/ responsiveness using inhaled nitrous oxide; epoprostenol (IV) or adenosine (IV): Positive response may be a prognostic indicator.
  - Contraindicated in right-sided heart failure or hemodynamic instability
- Chronic vasodilator therapy
  - If IPAH with positive response to acute vasodilator test (a fall in mean PAP of ≥10 mm Hg and to a value <40 mm Hg, with unchanged/increased cardiac output), use CCBs.
    - Adequate response confirmed after 3 to 4 months of treatment
    - ~13% will initially respond. Long-term clinical response to CCB therapy is small (~7%) (3)[C].
    - CCBs include nifedipine (long acting), diltiazem, and amlodipine.
    - Avoid verapamil due to its significant negative inotropic effect.
  - CCBs are contraindicated in patients with a cardiac index of <2 L/min/m^2 or a right atrial pressure >15 mm Hg if PAH with negative response to acute vasodilator test or worsening on therapy; specific vasodilator choice based on risk stratification (3)[C]
    - Nonresponders to acute vasoreactivity who are in WHO-FC II should be treated with an oral compound (3)[B].
    - Nonresponders who remain or progress to WHO-FC III should be considered for treatment with any approved PAH drugs (3)[B].
    - Continuous IV epoprostenol is recommended as first-line therapy for WHO-FC IV PAH due to survival benefit (NNT = 5) (3)[A].
    - In case of inadequate clinical response, sequential combination therapy should be considered. Therapy includes ERA plus a phosphodiesterase type 5 (PDE5) inhibitor or a prostanoid plus ERA or a prostanoid plus a PDE5 inhibitor (3)[A].
    - WHO-FC II PAH—approved drugs: ambrisentan, bosentan, macitentan, riociguat, sildenafil, tadalafil (3)[B]
    - WHO-FC III PAH—approved drugs: ambrisentan, bosentan, epoprostenol (IV), macitentan, riociguat, sildenafil, tadalafil, treprostinil (SC, inhaled) (3)[B]
    - WHO-FC IV PAH—approved drugs: epoprostenol (IV) (3)[A]

- Drug classes:
  - Prostacyclins: improve exercise capacity, cardiopulmonary hemodynamics: epoprostenol (IV), treprostinil (IV, SC, or inhaled), iloprost, beraprost
  - Prostacyclin IP: receptor agonist—selexipag
  - Endothelin receptor antagonists: improve exercise capacity; reducing mortality has been noted (4)[A]: bosentan (PO), ambrisentan (PO), macitentan. Pregnancy Category X; monitor LFTs monthly.
  - PDE5 inhibitor: suggested improvement in exercise capacity, cardiopulmonary hemodynamics, and symptoms (3)[C]: sildenafil (PO), tadalafil (PO), vardenafil
  - Guanylate cyclase stimulant: stimulators of the nitric oxide receptor, improves exercise capacity: riociguat (PO)
- Anticoagulation
  - Improved survival originally suggested in patients with IPAH only. Newer studies show some evidence for favorable effects of anticoagulation on survival in IPAH, HPAH, or PAH associated with anorexigens (3)[C].
  - Warfarin with international normalized ratio of 1.5 to 2.5 shows survival advantage in patients in multiple observational studies.
    - Contraindications: Avoid in patients with syncope or significant hemoptysis; consider drug interactions.
- Diuretics indicated in patients with RV volume overload (e.g., peripheral edema or ascites) (3)[B]
- Digoxin has little long-term data in PAH: used in RV failure and/or atrial dysrhythmias, increases cardiac output, and preserves RV contractility

ISSUES FOR REFERRAL

Refer to a pulmonologist and/or a cardiologist for further evaluation/treatment if PAH is suspected.

SURGERY/OTHER PROCEDURES

- Patients with documented large-vessel thromboembolic disease should be considered for pulmonary thrombectomy.
- Balloon atrial septostomy for severe PAH with right-sided heart failure despite optimized medical therapy to relieve symptoms prior to lung transplant or as a treatment on its own
- Heart–lung or lung transplantation

ADMISSION, INPATIENT, AND NURSING CONSIDERATIONS

- Medical therapy is primarily palliative.
- Hospitalization with invasive monitoring is needed to screen vasodilator responsiveness and initiate vasodilator therapy.
- National registry has been established by the National Heart, Lung, and Blood Institute.

 ONGOING CARE

FOLLOW-UP RECOMMENDATIONS

- Pneumococcal and influenza vaccines
- Exercise: walking or low-level aerobic activity, as tolerated, once stable; respiratory training

Patient Monitoring

Frequently evaluate disease progression and therapeutic efficacy. Tests to measure treatment response include 6-minute walk test and cardiopulmonary exercise test.

DIET

Fluid and salt restrictions, especially with RV failure

PATIENT EDUCATION

Discuss prognosis, lifestyle changes, and all therapeutic options (including transplant).

PROGNOSIS

- Median survival is 2 to 3 years from diagnosis; 5-year survival rate is 34% (NIH registry); newer data show 5-year survival ~70% with new treatment.
- Mode of death: right-sided heart failure (most common), pneumonia, sudden death, cardiac death
- Poor prognostic factors
  - Rapid symptom progression
  - Clinical evidence of RV failure
  - WHO functional PAH class IV (or NYHA functional class III or IV)
  - 6MWD <300 m
  - Peak VO$_2$ during cardiopulmonary exercise testing <10.4 mL/kg/min
  - ECG with pericardial effusion, significant RV enlargement/dysfunction, right atrial enlargement
  - Mean right atrial pressure >20 mm Hg
  - Cardiac index <2 L/min/m^2
  - Elevated mean PAP
  - Significantly elevated BNP and NT-proBNP; other markers also show promise in predicting survival: RDW, GDF-15, interleukin-6, creatinine.
  - Scleroderma spectrum of diseases

COMPLICATIONS

- Thromboembolism, heart failure, pleural effusion, and sudden death
- Pregnancy should be avoided due to high maternal mortality (30–50%) and fetal wastage.

REFERENCES

1. Simonneau G, Gatzoulis MA, Adatia I, et al. Updated clinical classification of pulmonary hypertension. *J Am Coll Cardiol*. 2013;62(Suppl 25):D34–D41.
2. McLaughlin VV, Gaine SP, Howard LS, et al. Treatment goals of pulmonary hypertension. *J Am Coll Cardiol*. 2013;62(Suppl 25):D73–D81.
3. Galiè N, Corris PA, Frost A, et al. Updated treatment algorithm of pulmonary arterial hypertension. *J Am Coll Cardiol*. 2013;62(Suppl 25):D60–D72.
4. Liu C, Chen J, Gao Y, et al. Endothelin receptor antagonists for pulmonary arterial hypertension. *Cochrane Database Syst Rev*. 2009;(3):CD004434.

ADDITIONAL READING

Taichman DB, Ornelas J, Chung L, et al. Pharmacologic therapy for pulmonary arterial hypertension in adults: CHEST guideline and expert panel report. *Chest*. 2014;146(2):449–475.

CODES

ICD10

- I27.0 Primary pulmonary hypertension
- I27.2 Other secondary pulmonary hypertension

CLINICAL PEARLS

- PAH involves abnormalities in the small pulmonary arteries (precapillary PH) which increase PAP and vascular resistance leading to right heart failure.
- For positive vasodilator test, CCBs are the first-line agents to manage IPAH.
- For nonresponders, treatment depends on WHO-FC.

PULMONARY EMBOLISM

Luis Diaz-Quintero, MD • Alfonso Tafur, MD, MS

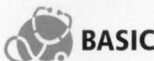 **BASICS**

DESCRIPTION

- Pulmonary embolism (PE) is the most serious presentation of venous thromboembolism (VTE).
- Classified based on severity:
  - Low-risk PE: acute and absence of clinical markers of adverse prognosis (1)
  - Submassive PE: no systemic hypotension, but there is either myocardial necrosis (elevated troponin) or right ventricle (RV) dysfunction (RV dilation or systolic dysfunction on echocardiography [Echo], RV/LV ratio >1 on CT, elevation of B-type natriuretic peptide [BNP] or N-terminal pro-BNP, or consistent ECG changes) (1,2)
  - Massive PE: hemodynamic instability with sustained hypotension; pulselessness; or persistent bradycardia, cardiogenic shock, acute manifesting RV failure (1)

EPIDEMIOLOGY

Case fatality rates vary widely (1–60%); case fatality rate is approximately 11% at 2 weeks (1,2).

Incidence

- Approximately 30 to 80/100,000, with higher incidence in African Americans and lower in Asians; >100,000 cases annually in the United States
- Incidence increases with age, most occurring at 60 to 70 years of age.
- 250,000 hospitalizations per year in the United States, 10–60% in hospitalized patients
  - Highest risk for orthopedic and cancer patients
  - 1:1,000 pregnancies (including postpartum)

ETIOLOGY AND PATHOPHYSIOLOGY

- Venous stasis, endothelial damage, and changes in coagulation properties trigger thrombus (1).
- Causes increased pulmonary vascular resistance, impaired gas exchange, and decreased pulmonary compliance. RV failure due to pressure overload is usually the primary cause of death (1).
- The most common source (85%) of PE is proximal lower extremity deep vein thrombosis.

Genetics

- Factor V Leiden: most common thrombophilia. +5.5% in Caucasian, 2.2% in Hispanics, 1.2% in African American, 0.5% in Asian; associated with 20% of VTE
- Prothrombin G20210A: 3% of Caucasians; rare in African American, Asian, and Native American; 6% in patients with VTE
- Rarely, deficiencies in protein C, S, and antithrombin

RISK FACTORS

- Older age, obesity, prolonged immobilization, surgery, major trauma, joint replacement, spinal cord injury, cancer, hormonal replacement therapy, pregnancy/puerperium, previous thrombosis, antiphospholipid syndrome, genetics
- Oral contraceptive is the most frequent VTE risk factor in fertile women (1).

GENERAL PREVENTION

- Low VTE risk: early ambulation after surgery, compression stockings, and intermittent pneumatic compression
- Intermediate VTE risk: low-molecular-weight heparin (LMWH), unfractionated heparin (UFH), or fondaparinux
- Hip or knee arthroplasty (high VTE risk): 10 or more days prophylaxis with LMWH, fondaparinux, apixaban, dabigatran, rivaroxaban, or low-dose UFH

- Spinal cord injury, hip fracture surgery, and trauma surgery (high VTE risk): 28 to 35 days with LMWH, fondaparinux, UFH, or vitamin K antagonists (VKA)
- Long-distance travel (>8 hours): hydration, walking, avoidance of constrictive clothing and frequent calf exercises, compression stockings below knee
- Patients with factor V Leiden, prothrombin *G20210A* with no previous thrombosis do not need prophylaxis.

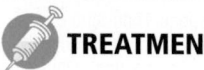 **DIAGNOSIS**

- Establish a pretest probability based on clinical criteria.
  - Wells score
    - ○ Clinical signs and symptoms of DVT +3
    - ○ Alternative diagnosis is less likely than PE +3.
    - ○ Heart rate >100 +1.5
    - ○ Immobilization previous 4 weeks +1.5
    - ○ Previous DVT/PE +1.5
    - ○ Hemoptysis +1
    - ○ Malignancy +1
    - ○ <2 points, low clinical probability; 2 to 6 points, moderate; >7 points, high
- Wells and revised Geneva score were simplified.
  - Wells score: Each predictor is +1; PE unlikely if 0 to 1, PE likely if >2
  - Geneva score: Each predictor is +1 except for heart rate >95 beats/min which is +2; PE unlikely if 0 to 2 and PE likely if >3

HISTORY

- Determine if the presentation is provoked or idiopathic. Approximately 30% of cases develop without identifiable risk factor.
- Bleeding risk (previous anticoagulation, history of bleeding, recent interventions/surgeries, liver disease, kidney disease)
- Sudden onset dyspnea (>85%), chest pain (>50%), cough (20%), syncope (14%), hemoptysis (7%)

PHYSICAL EXAM

- Dyspnea, syncope, hemoptysis, tachycardia, tachypnea, accentuated S_2; pleuritic chest pain, pleural friction rub, rales (1)
- Signs of DVT: leg swelling, tenderness, visible collateral veins (1)
- Signs of RV failure: jugular vein distention, S_3 or S_4, systolic murmur at left sternal edge, hepatomegaly (1)

DIFFERENTIAL DIAGNOSIS

- Pulmonary: pneumonia, bronchitis, pneumothorax, pneumonitis, chronic obstructive pulmonary disease exacerbation, pulmonary edema
- Cardiac/vascular: myocardial infarction, pericarditis, congestive heart failure, aortic dissection
- Musculoskeletal: rib fracture(s), musculoskeletal chest wall pain

DIAGNOSTIC TESTS & INTERPRETATION

- D-dimer ELISA: In patients with low pretest probability, it can rule out PE if it is negative (high negative predictive value [NPV]) (1)[A]. It is not diagnostic if positive (low positive predictive value [PPV]), and it is not helpful if pretest probability is intermediate or high (1)[B].
- CBC, creatinine, aPTT and PT, ABG: In young patients with idiopathic, recurrent, or significant family history of VTE, consider hypercoagulable tests.
  - Do not test for protein C, S, factor VIII, or antithrombin in the acute setting.
  - Patients with intermediate or high pretest probability and low probability with elevated D-dimer need further diagnostic testing.

- Chest x-ray (CXR): Westermark sign (lack of vessels in an area distal to the embolus), Hampton hump (wedge-shaped opacity with base in pleura), Fleischner sign (enlarged pulmonary arteries), pleural effusion, hemidiaphragm elevation (1)
- ECG: right heart strain, nonspecific rhythm abnormalities, S1Q3T3
- CT pulmonary angiography: sensitivity 96–100%, specificity 86–89%; NPV 99.8%. If normal, it excludes PE if low or intermediate clinical probability (1)[A].
- Ventilation/perfusion scintigraphy (V/Q scan): Use if CT angiography is not available or contraindicated. A high-probability V/Q scan makes the diagnosis of PE; normal V/Q scan excludes PE (1)[B].
- Pulmonary angiography: gold standard but invasive and technically difficult: 2% morbidity and <0.01 mortality risk (1)[C].
- Echo: assesses RV function and thrombus in transit (associated with >40% mortality)
- Magnetic resonance angiography: lower sensitivity and specificity than CT angiography
- Compression venous ultrasound (CUS): noninvasive. Sensitivity >90%, specificity approximately 95%. It confirms the diagnosis of PE in patients with clinical suspicion (1)[B].
- CT venography: can be done at the same time as CT angiography; increases diagnostic yield (1)

ALERT

If your preclinical probability is intermediate or high and the patient has a low bleeding risk, start treatment while waiting for the diagnostic results.

TREATMENT

MEDICATION

- Start LMWH, fondaparinux, UFH, as initial therapy for first 5 to 10 days. VKA can be started the 1st day and must overlap with parenteral treatment for minimum of 5 days, until international normalized ratio (INR) is 2 to 3 for 24 hours.
- Following 5 to 10 days of parenteral therapy, dabigatran or edoxaban are also approved (1).
- An oral option for initial and long-term treatment is rivaroxaban or apixaban (1).
- Patients with massive PE with low bleeding risk: Consider systemic thrombolytics if no contraindications. Also in patients <75 years old with submassive PE; greater benefit if initiated within 48 hours of symptoms onset (1)

First Line

- UFH:
  - IV bolus of 80 U/kg or 5,000 U followed by continuous infusion (initially 18 U/kg/hr or 1,300 U/hr) with dose adjustments to maintain aPTT that corresponds to anti-Xa levels of 0.3 to 0.7
  - SC injection: two options:
    - ○ Monitored: 17,500 U or 250 U/kg BID with dose adjustments to maintain an aPTT that corresponds to anti-Xa levels of 0.3 to 0.7 measured 6 hours after a dose
    - ○ Fixed dose: 333 U/kg initial dose, followed by 250 U/kg BID
- LMWH: preferred due to lower risk of major bleeding and heparin-induced thrombocytopenia (HIT) (1)[A]
  - Enoxaparin (Lovenox) 1 mg/kg/dose SC q12h
  - Dalteparin (Fragmin) 200 U/kg SC q24h
  - Fondaparinux (Arixtra) 5 mg (body weight <50 kg), 7.5 mg (body weight 50 to 100 kg), or 10 mg (body weight >100 kg) SC q24h

- Maintenance therapy: warfarin on day 1, if possible; 5 mg/day for 3 days in hospitalized or older patients and at a dose of 10 mg in <60 years of aged patients; adjust dose to maintain an INR of 2 to 3; needs to overlap with UFH, LMWH, or fondaparinux: 5 to 7 days, until 2 consecutive days of therapeutic INR (1)
- Rivaroxaban: 15 mg BID × 3 weeks and then 20 mg once daily to complete treatment. Compared to warfarin, it has less major bleeding side effects while having same efficacy; ok to use in HIT (1)[B]
- Edoxaban: 60 mg once daily (reduced to 30 mg once daily if CrCl 30 to 50 mL/min or body weight <60 kg). Patients require initial treatment with LMWH at least 5 days before starting edoxaban. Compared to warfarin, less bleeding and lower rate of recurrence in PE with RV dysfunction; increased bleeding risk in cancer-associated thrombosis compared to dalteparin (1,3)[B]
- Apixaban: 10 mg BID for 7 days, followed by 5 mg once daily; noninferior to warfarin against recurrent symptomatic VTE or death related to VTE, with less major bleeding episodes; ok to use in HIT (1)[B]
- Dabigatran: requires initial treatment with LMWH. Compared to warfarin, 150 mg BID had noninferior efficacy and no differences in major bleeding; ok to use in HIT (1)[B]

ALERT

- Contraindications:
  - Active bleeding
  - Heparin: HIT
  - LMWH: HIT, renal failure
  - Warfarin: pregnancy
  - Rivaroxaban and fondaparinux: renal failure (1)[A]
  - Edoxaban: severe kidney or liver failure (1)[A]
  - Apixaban: renal impairment and nonvalvular atrial fibrillation (1)[A]
  - Dabigatran: severe kidney problems. Use of dronedarone or ketoconazole increases risk.
- No dose reduction strategy needed to treat acute PE with dabigatran, apixaban, or rivaroxaban (1)[A]

Pregnancy Considerations

- Warfarin: teratogenic; safe while breastfeeding
- LMWH: Dalteparin, enoxaparin, and fondaparinux are Category B; heparin is Category C: Use if the benefit overweighs risks.
- UFH: requires aPTT monitoring; can cause osteoporosis if used for prolonged period
- Rivaroxaban is Category C.
- Edoxaban and apixaban: Category B; increase risk of hemorrhage
- Dabigatran: Category C; use it only if benefit overweighs side effects.

Second Line

Massive PE: Consider thrombolytics if the patient has hemodynamic compromise and low bleeding risk, intracranial hemorrhage risk: 0.7–6.4% (1)[B]:

- Tissue plasminogen activator (tPA) 100 mg infused over 2 hours. Absolute contraindications:
  - Intracranial hemorrhage, known intracranial cerebrovascular or malignant disease, ischemic stroke within 3 months, suspected aortic dissection, bleeding diathesis, active bleeding, recent neurosurgery, or major trauma

SURGERY/OTHER PROCEDURES

- Inferior vena cava (IVC) filter placement if absolute contraindication for anticoagulation or recurrent PE despite adequate anticoagulation treatment
- PREPIC2 trial showed that retrievable IVC filters at 3 months plus anticoagulation compared to anticoagulation alone among patients with severe

PE had no benefit reducing the risk of symptomatic recurrent PE (3%, 95% CI 1.1–6.5 vs. 1.5%, 95% CI 0.3–4.3).

- Emergency embolectomy can be considered in patients with massive PE with contraindications for thrombolysis.
- Consider catheter-based interventions if massive PE and thrombolytic contraindications.
- Consider US-assisted catheter-directed thrombolysis (USAT) in patients with intermediate risk of death or submassive PE; superior than heparin alone in reversing RV dilation at 24 hours without increase in bleeding complications

ADMISSION, INPATIENT, AND NURSING CONSIDERATIONS

- In selected, low-risk acute PE population (Pulmonary Embolism Severity Index [PESI] score class I or II), patients could be managed safely and effectively in the outpatient setting with close follow-up compared to inpatient admission (4).
- Hestia Criteria can be used to identify low-risk PE patients (<1 point) that can be safely treated in the outpatient setting (2)[B]. PE response team (PERT): multidisciplinary team created for the rapid assessment and treatment of patients with submassive and massive PE with the goal to reduce mortality and therapy-associated complications. If available, activate immediately upon diagnosis of submassive and massive PE.
- ICU-level care if hemodynamically unstable

 ## ONGOING CARE

Duration of anticoagulation

- Provoked PE (trigger no longer present): 3 months (1)[B]
- Unprovoked PE: >3 months; consider long-term or prolonged secondary prophylaxis if bleeding risk is low (1)[B]. HERDOO2 Score provides guidance to determine duration of therapy in WOMEN with first unprovoked VTE. Low risk (0 to 1 criteria) can safely stop treatment after 6 months.
- Cancer-related PE: LMWH first 3 to 6 months. Consider secondary prophylaxis as long as the patient has active cancer (1)[B].
- Recurrent unprovoked PE: long-term anticoagulation

FOLLOW-UP RECOMMENDATIONS

- If concomitant DVT, consider knee-high compression stockings, 30 to 40 mm Hg knee high.
- If an IVC filter was placed, follow up for retrieval.

Patient Monitoring

- INR should be checked regularly; target is 2 to 3 (1).
- aPTT needs to be monitored in SC UFH (1).
- Anti-Xa can be checked in special circumstances if treated with LMWH, including pregnancy, younger patients, renal disease.

DIET

Warfarin use; instruct regarding vitamin K–containing food.

PROGNOSIS

- Mortality: submassive 6–14%; massive PE 15–60%
- PESI score predicts 30-day mortality. Stratified by risk classes depending on number of risk factors: class I (very low mortality risk; 0–1.6%), class II (low mortality risk; 1.7–3.5%), class III (moderate mortality risk; 3.2–7.1%), class IV (high mortality risk; 4–11.4%), and class V (very high mortality risk; 10–24.5%) (1)[A]

- Simplified PESI (sPESI) score also predicts mortality; any one of the following defines high risk: age >80 years, cancer, chronic cardiopulmonary disease, heart rate 110 beats/min, systolic blood pressure <100 mm Hg, O₂ saturation <90% (1)[A].
- High early mortality risk: shock or hypotension, + sPESI >1 + RV dysfunction signs (1)
- Intermediate high early mortality risk: no shock or hypotension + sPESI >1 + RV dysfunction signs (1)
- Intermediate low early mortality risk: no shock or hypotension + sPESI >1 + either RV dysfunction by imaging or cardiac laboratory biomarkers (1)
- Low early mortality risk: no shock or hypotension, no sPESI; imaging is optional (1).
- PE mortality rate is significantly higher in patients with active cancer (up to 47-fold higher). Elevated white blood cell count is a strong predictor of 30-day mortality in cancer population (5)[B].

COMPLICATIONS

- 1 in 25 patients will develop chronic thromboembolic pulmonary hypertension, recurrent DVT, or PE.
- Post-PE syndrome: permanent changes in pulmonary vasculature associated with chronic dyspnea and reduced exercise capacity
- Younger age, previous PE, and larger perfusion defect are associated with increased risk of chronic thromboembolic pulmonary hypertension found in 5.2% of 58 patients with previous DVT and 33.3% of 24 patients with previous PE.

REFERENCES

1. Konstantinides SV, Torbicki A, Agnelli G, et al. 2014 ESC guidelines on the diagnosis and management of acute pulmonary embolism. *Eur Heart J.* 2014;35(43):3033–3069, 3069a–3069k.
2. Zondag W, Vingerhoets LM, Durian MF, et al. Hestia criteria can safely select patients with pulmonary embolism for outpatient treatment irrespective of right ventricular function. *J Thromb Haemost.* 2013;11(4):686–692.
3. Raskob GE, Büller HR, Segers A. Edoxaban for cancer-associated venous thromboembolism. *N Engl J Med.* 2018;379(1):95–96.
4. Aujesky D, Roy PM, Verschuren F, et al. Outpatient versus inpatient treatment for patients with acute pulmonary embolism: an international, open-label, randomised, non-inferiority trial. *Lancet.* 2011;378(9785):41–48.
5. Tafur AJ, Fuentes HE, Caprini JA, et al. Predictors of early mortality in cancer-associated thrombosis: analysis of the RIETE database. *TH Open.* 2018;02(02):e158–e166.

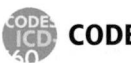 ## CODES

ICD10

- I26.99 Other pulmonary embolism without acute cor pulmonale
- I27.82 Chronic pulmonary embolism

CLINICAL PEARLS

- Perform cancer-oriented review of systems and age/gender-appropriate cancer screening in patients >40 years, recurrent VTE, upper extremity DVT (not related to catheter or lines), bilateral lower extremity DVT, intra-abdominal DVT, resistance to treatment.
- In patients with prolonged baseline aPTT, adjust heparin dose with anti-Xa levels (therapeutic range 0.3 to 0.7).

PULMONARY FIBROSIS

Sidra Saeed, MD • Sara Usman, MBBS • Faisal Saeed, MD

BASICS

DESCRIPTION

- Pulmonary fibrosis (PF) is a part of interstitial lung diseases (ILDs) that is a family of >200 different lung diseases, which are characterized by inflammation, cellular proliferation, and/or fibrosis within lung interstitium and bronchial walls. If no cause identified, ILD is called idiopathic interstitial pneumonia.
- Idiopathic PF (IPF) is one of the most common idiopathic interstitial pneumonia.
- IPF is defined as a specific form of chronic fibrosing interstitial pneumonia limited to the lung and associated with the histologic and/or radiologic appearance of usual interstitial pneumonia (UIP) when other causes have been excluded.

EPIDEMIOLOGY

- Most common ILD prevalent worldwide accounting for 25–30% of all ILD
- Most common in men >60 years of age.

Incidence

Higher in North America and Europe (3 to 9 cases per 100,000 person-years) than in South America and East Asia (fewer than 4 cases per 100,000 person-years).

Prevalence

Exact prevalence is unknown. In the United States, the prevalence of IPF has been reported to range from 10 to 60 cases per 100,000.

ETIOLOGY AND PATHOPHYSIOLOGY

- Exact inciting factors unknown.
- A widely held hypothesis is that this disorder develops in susceptible individuals following some unknown stimuli, which initiate an uncontrolled cascade of events that evolve to the fibrotic process.
- Causes of nonidiopathic PF include occupational and environmental exposure, drugs, and connective tissue diseases.
- IPF pattern on biopsy is UIP, which appears to be a distinct pathophysiologic entity characterized by minimal inflammation and chronic fibroproliferation due to abnormal parenchymal wound healing.

Genetics

- The role of host genetic factors and their interactions with environmental factors leading to IPF is unknown.
- Some gene polymorphisms have demonstrated a confirmed (usually weak) association.
- It is postulated that it is autosomal dominant transmission with variable penetrance.

RISK FACTORS

- Family history of IPF
- Smoking—most significant association
- GERD
- Occupational and environmental exposures: primarily to wood (pine), metal dusts (lead, brass, steel), to farming, raising birds, hairdressing, stone cutting, exposure to livestock, vegetable and animal dust

GENERAL PREVENTION

It is general avoidance of above noted risk factors.

COMMONLY ASSOCIATED CONDITIONS

- Pulmonary hypertension: 30–80% of patients with IPF
- GERD
- Nonidiopathic PF may be related to connective tissue diseases (RA and scleroderma).

DIAGNOSIS

HISTORY

- Very insidious and slow onset
- Exertional breathlessness and nonproductive cough
- Constitutional symptoms are uncommon but can present with weight loss, fever, fatigue, myalgia, and arthralgia.
- Obtain history of exposure to dampness, mold, or birds in the home or workplace and history suggestive of other causes of ILD.

PHYSICAL EXAM

- Bibasilar fine, late inspiratory crackles: velcro crackles
- Clubbing in late stages. cyanosis (rare)
- Findings of pulmonary hypertension and right sided heart failure
- Pneumothorax and pneumomediastinum (rare)
- Look for signs and symptoms of autoimmune conditions and connective tissue disorders.

DIFFERENTIAL DIAGNOSIS

- Other ILDs like hypersensitivity pneumonitis, nonspecific interstitial pneumonia, occupational lung disease, connective tissue disorders
- See below for histologic differential diagnosis of UIP.

DIAGNOSTIC TESTS & INTERPRETATION

Initial Tests (lab, imaging)

- Blood tests: Most of labs are normal.
- Chest radiograph:
  - Reduced lung volumes and reticular opacities mostly at lung bases
  - Coarse reticular pattern and honeycombed cysts in advanced stages
- Pleural abnormalities are uncommon. Presence should suggest other diagnosis.

Follow-Up Tests & Special Considerations

- Chest CT scan:
  - Once diagnosis of IPF is suspected, high-resolution CT (HRCT) scan of chest is needed. It should include inspiratory and expiratory images with think <1.25 mm slices and prone position should be included in subtle subpleural basal changes are present.
  - Four distinct patterns are noted on HRCT: UIP, probable UIP, indeterminate, and alternative diagnosis.
  - UIP diagnosis require subpleural and basal reticular changes in heterogeneous pattern AND honeycombing with or without traction bronchiectasis with some architectural distortion. Similar changes in absence of honeycomb make it probable UIP.
  - If no secondary cause identified, radiologic UIP pattern as described above is diagnostic of IPF without need for surgical lung biopsy.
    - Sensitivity is 48%.
    - Specificity is 95%.
    - Accuracy 90%
- Serologic testing for connective tissue diseases: should be obtained when IPF is being considered to exclude nonidiopathic causes. ANA; RF; anti–CCP antibodies; Scl-70, Ro, La, U1-RNP, and Jo-1; creatine kinase; and myoglobin, and antisynthetase antibodies.
- Echocardiogram to assess cardiac function, right vent function and pulmonary hypertension

Diagnostic Procedures/Other

- Pulmonary function testing (PFT):
  - PFTs in all patients undergoing evaluation and treatment of IPF or any other ILD.
  - Findings include:
    - Decreased diffusion capacity for carbon monoxide (DLCO)
    - Decreased lung volumes (TLC, RV, FRC)
    - Decreased expiratory flow rates (FVC and FEV1) may be decreased because of the reduction in lung volume, but the FEV1 /FVC ratio is maintained.
- Exercise stress testing shows tachypnea, with rapid shallow breathing with increase their minute ventilation.
- ABG: Resting ABG shows hypoxemia and respiratory alkalosis.
- 6-minute walk distance (6MWD):
  - 6MWD has high correlation with DLCO and mortality.
- Sleep study:
  - Sleep disturbances with reduced rapid eye movement sleep, lighter and more fragmented sleep, and hypoxemia during rapid eye movement sleep.
  - Tachypnea persists during sleep.
- Bronchoscopy:
  - Bronchoalveolar lavage (BAL):
    - Can be helpful in excluding other diagnosis like infection, malignancy etc.
    - ATS/ERS does not recommend routine use of BAL if HRCT is diagnostic of UIP.
  - Bronchoscopic transbronchial biopsy:
    - It is not recommended for diagnosis of IPF as sensitivity and specificity is unknown and it is unknown from where biopsy should be taken as disease is heterogeneous.
    - It may help to exclude other possible etiologies of ILD.
    - Transbronchial lung cryobiopsy has been increasingly advocated as a replacement for thoracoscopic biopsy. Data is limited at this point.
- Surgical lung biopsy:
  - Gold standard for diagnosis of ILDs
  - When the combination of clinical and imaging data is not diagnostic, a thoracoscopic lung biopsy can be considered if the results are expected to influence therapy.
  - Biopsy samples should be taken from multiple lobes and avoiding sampling the most severely affected areas.
  - Procedure should not be performed in high-risk patients, including:
    - High oxygen requirements
    - Significant pulmonary hypertension
    - Rapid disease progression
    - Severely reduced FVC or DLCO
  - Several studies have compared video-assisted thoracoscopic biopsy with open thoracotomy biopsy and noted that diagnostic yield is similar but morbidity different.

Test Interpretation

- Histopathology
  - Gross appearance of the lungs: distinctive nodular pleural surface
  - The histopathologic pattern in IPF is UIP.
    - UIP pattern require dense fibrosis with architectural distortion, subpleural, and basal distribution, heterogeneous pattern, fibroblastic foci, and microscopic honeycomb changes plus absence of features suggestive of alternate diagnosis.

○ Differential diagnosis of UIP pattern in histology includes IPF, connective tissue diseases like RA and scleroderma, chronic hypersensitivity pneumonitis, asbestosis, chronic aspiration pneumonia, chronic radiation pneumonitis, Hermansky-Pudlak syndrome and neurofibromatosis.

- DIAGNOSTIC STRATEGIES:
  – As per ATS/ERS statement of IPF in 2018, diagnosis of IPF requires (1):
    ○ Exclusion of other known causes of ILD and either of the following:
      ▪ The presence of the HRCT pattern of UIP
      ▪ Specific combinations of HRCT patterns and histopathology patterns in patients subjected to lung tissue sampling
  – UIP pattern on HRCT would be diagnostic with all histology patterns except alternate diagnosis findings.
  – UIP pattern on histology would be diagnostic with all HRCT patterns except alternate diagnosis findings.

 TREATMENT

GENERAL MEASURES
- Smoking cessation
- Pulmonary rehabilitation
- Referral to a transplant center
- Supplemental oxygen:
  – Clinical practice guidelines strongly recommend supplemental oxygen.
  – Goal oxyhemoglobin is saturation of 88% or more.
  – The oxygen prescription should be informed by 6-minute walk tests or treadmill testing of oxygen saturation as well as by nocturnal oximetry or polysomnography when indicated.

MEDICATION
- IPF is a progressive and fatal disorder without spontaneous remission.
- Median survival after diagnosis is 3.8 years.
- Any therapy of IPF, regardless of the agent used, requires at least 1 year before its effectiveness can be assessed.
- During the past 5 years, notable advances have been made in pharmacotherapeutic approaches to IPF (2,3).
- Two medications, nintedanib and pirfenidone, have been shown to be safe and effective in the treatment of IPF; both are recommended for use in patients with IPF.
  – In placebo-controlled, randomized trials, each drug has been shown to slow the rate of FVC decline by approximately 50% over the course of 1 year.
  – Both have shown some efficacy in reducing severe respiratory events, such as acute exacerbations, and hospitalization for respiratory events.
  – Pooled data and meta-analyses suggest that these agents may reduce mortality.
  – The cost of each medication is estimated to exceed $100,000 annually.

First Line
- Nintedanib is a tyrosine kinase inhibitor that targets growth factor pathways.
- Most common side effect is diarrhea. Liver function should be followed as liver toxicity has been reported.
- Pirfenidone:
  – Mechanism of action: anti-inflammatory and anti-fibrotic effects, including inhibition of collagen synthesis, downregulation of TGF-β and tumor necrosis factor-α, and a reduction in fibroblast proliferation
  – Common side effects: anorexia, nausea, and vomiting, photosensitive rash, abnormal liver function

- It is difficult to recommend one agent over the other because there have been no head-to-head comparisons and efficacy is similar. Recent data on treatment that combines these agents suggest clinically significant gastrointestinal side effects.
- Reflux management:
  – Treatment of coexistent GERD because it is very common and some data suggested worsening of IPF with ongoing reflux.

Second Line
- No second-line agents available to specifically treat IPF.
- Treatment guidelines for IPF by ATS/ERS include:
  – Strong recommendations against use of:
    ○ Anticoagulation (warfarin)
    ○ Combination prednisone + azathioprine + N-acetylcysteine (NAC)
    ○ Selective endothelin receptor antagonist (ambrisentan)
    ○ Imatinib, a tyrosine kinase inhibitor with one target
  – Conditional recommendations against:
    ○ Dual endothelin receptor antagonists (macitentan, bosentan)
    ○ Phosphodiesterase-5 inhibitor (sildenafil)
    ○ NAC monotherapy
  – Conditional recommendations for use:
    ○ Nintedanib, a tyrosine kinase inhibitor with multiple targets
    ○ Pirfenidone
    ○ Anti-acid therapy

ISSUES FOR REFERRAL
- Referral to pulmonologist for diagnosis and management
- Thoracic surgeon referral is indicated if patient cannot be diagnosed by ATS clinical and radiographic criteria.
- Referral to lung transplant center is indicated early on for patients showing progressive worsening of the disease.

ADDITIONAL THERAPIES
Several investigational therapies are being studied in different randomized controlled trials.

SURGERY/OTHER PROCEDURES
Lung transplant for patients with severe and rapid progression of disease and no response to medical management

COMPLEMENTARY & ALTERNATIVE MEDICINE
No proven benefit of any of the complementary and alternative medications. Patient should be vaccinated for influenza and pneumonia.

ADMISSION, INPATIENT, AND NURSING CONSIDERATIONS
- Acute exacerbation of IPF should be admitted to the hospital for management with corticosteroids.
- Mechanical ventilation carries a poor prognosis and should be avoided if possible.
- Palliative care consult is appropriate for all patients diagnosed with IPF.

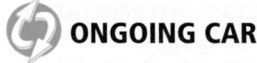 ONGOING CARE

FOLLOW-UP RECOMMENDATIONS
- Pulmonary clinic and, if possible, at an ILD clinic.
- Monitoring with serial HRCT and PFT along with 6MWD and exercise oximetry
- If on treatment with any of the newly approved medications, monitor LFTs.

COMPLICATIONS
- Mortality: IPF carries a poor prognosis, with a median survival of 3.8 years among adults 65 years of age or older in the United States.
- Acute exacerbation of IPF
  – 10–20% per patient per year
  – It is characterized by worsened hypoxemic respiratory failure, with bilateral ground-glass opacities, consolidation, or both on HRCT imaging that are not fully explained by volume overload.
  – Triggers: infection, aspiration, or drug toxicity or idiopathic
  – Treatment: Available guidelines make weak recommendations for the use of glucocorticoids and do not recommend the use of mechanical ventilation. Consider palliative care referral.
- Increased risk for VTE and lung cancer
- Pulmonary hypertension: common. Management in the outpatient setting should consist solely of supplemental oxygen, without pulmonary vasodilator therapy. Until further data are available, targeted therapies approved for pulmonary arterial hypertension should be avoided in patients with IPF unless they are enrolled in a clinical trial investigating such therapies.

REFERENCES
1. Raghu G, Remy-Jardin M, Myers JL, et al; for American Thoracic Society, European Respiratory Society, Japanese Respiratory Society, Latin American Thoracic Society. Diagnosis of idiopathic pulmonary fibrosis. An official ATS/ERS/JRS/ALAT clinical practice guideline. *Am J Respir Crit Care Med*. 2018;198(5):e44–e68.
2. Raghu G, Collard HR, Egan JJ, et al; for ATS/ERS/JRS/ALAT Committee on Idiopathic Pulmonary Fibrosis. An official ATS/ERS/JRS/ALAT statement: idiopathic pulmonary fibrosis: evidence-based guidelines for diagnosis and management. *Am J Respir Crit Care Med*. 2011;183(6):788–824.
3. Raghu G, Rochwerg B, Zhang Y, et al; for American Thoracic Society, European Respiratory society, Japanese Respiratory Society, Latin American Thoracic Association. An official ATS/ERS/JRS/ALAT clinical practice guideline: treatment of idiopathic pulmonary fibrosis. An update of the 2011 clinical practice guideline. *Am J Respir Crit Care Med*. 2015;192(2):e3–e19.

ADDITIONAL READING
Lederer DJ, Martinez FJ. Idiopathic pulmonary fibrosis. *N Engl J Med*. 2018;378(19):1811–1823.

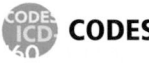 CODES

ICD10
- J84.10 Pulmonary fibrosis, unspecified
- J84.112 Idiopathic pulmonary fibrosis

CLINICAL PEARLS
- IPF is most common idiopathic ILD and frequently misdiagnosed and mistreated.
- HRCT is cornerstone for diagnosis.
- Pulmonary hypertension is very common.
- Until recently available two newer drugs, no other therapy has proven effective in management.
- Oxygen supplementation, pulmonary rehab, anti-reflux treatment, vaccinations against pneumonia and influenza should be considered in all patients.
- Referral to pulmonary clinic, ILD clinic, and lung transplant should be considered very early in course.

PYELONEPHRITIS

Katelin M. Lisenby, PharmD, BCPS • Dana G. Carroll, PharmD, BCPS, CDE, BCGP •
Catherine Scarbrough, MD, MSc, FAAFP

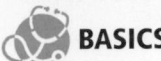

BASICS

DESCRIPTION
- A syndrome caused by infection of the renal parenchyma and/or renal pelvis, often producing localized flank/back pain combined with systemic symptoms, such as fever, chills, and nausea; wide spectrum from mild illness to septic shock
- Chronic pyelonephritis is the result of progressive inflammation of the renal interstitium and tubules, due to recurrent infection, vesicoureteral reflux, or both.
- Pyelonephritis is considered uncomplicated if the infection is caused by a typical pathogen in an immunocompetent patient with normal urinary tract anatomy and renal function.
- System(s) affected: renal; urologic
- Synonym: acute upper urinary tract infection (UTI)

Geriatric Considerations
- May present as altered mental status; absence of fever is common in this age group.
- Elderly patients with diabetes and pyelonephritis are at higher risk of bacteremia, longer hospitalization, and mortality.
- The high prevalence of asymptomatic bacteriuria in the elderly makes the use of urine dipstick less reliable for diagnosing UTI in this population (1)[A].

Pregnancy Considerations
- Most common medical complication requiring hospitalization
- Affects 1–2% of all pregnancies. Morbidity does not differ between trimesters.
- Urine culture for test of cure 1 to 2 weeks after therapy

Pediatric Considerations
- UTI is present in ~5% of patients age 2 months to 2 years with fever and no apparent source on history and physical exam.
- Treatment (PO or IV; inpatient or outpatient) should be based on the clinical situation and patient toxicity.

EPIDEMIOLOGY
Incidence
Community-acquired acute pyelonephritis: 28/10,000/year

Prevalence
Adult cases: 250,000/year, with 200,000 hospitalizations

ETIOLOGY AND PATHOPHYSIOLOGY
- *Escherichia coli* (>80%)
- Other gram-negative pathogens: *Proteus, Klebsiella, Serratia, Clostridium, Pseudomonas,* and *Enterobacter*
- *Enterococcus*
- *Staphylococcus*: *Staphylococcus epidermidis, Staphylococcus saprophyticus* (number 2 cause in young women), and *Staphylococcus aureus*
- *Candida*

RISK FACTORS
- Underlying urinary tract abnormalities
- Indwelling catheter/recent urinary tract instrumentation
- Nephrolithiasis
- Immunocompromised, including diabetes

- Elderly, institutionalized patients (particularly women)
- Prostatic enlargement
- Childhood UTI
- Acute pyelonephritis within the prior year
- Frequent recent sexual intercourse; spermicide use; new sex partner within the prior year
- Stress incontinence in the previous 30 days
- Pregnancy
- Hospital-acquired infection
- Symptoms >7 days at time of presentation

COMMONLY ASSOCIATED CONDITIONS
- Indwelling catheters
- Renal calculi
- Benign prostatic hyperplasia

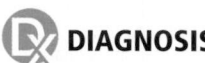

DIAGNOSIS

HISTORY
- In adults
  - Fever; flank pain
  - Nausea ± vomiting
  - Malaise, anorexia
  - Myalgia
  - Dysuria, urinary frequency, urgency
  - Suprapubic discomfort
  - Mental status changes (elderly)
- In infants and children
  - Fever
  - Irritability and poor feeding
  - GI symptoms

PHYSICAL EXAM
- In adults
  - Fever: ≥38°C (100.4°F)
  - Costovertebral angle tenderness
  - Presentation ranges from no physical findings to septic shock.
  - Mental status changes common in the elderly
  - A pelvic exam may be necessary in female patients to exclude pelvic inflammatory disease.
- In infants and children
  - Sepsis
  - Fever
  - Poor skin perfusion
  - Inadequate weight gain/weight loss
  - Jaundice to gray skin color

DIFFERENTIAL DIAGNOSIS
- Obstructive uropathy
- Acute bacterial pneumonia (lower lobe)
- Cholecystitis
- Acute pancreatitis
- Appendicitis
- Perforated viscus; aortic dissection
- Pelvic inflammatory disease; ectopic pregnancy
- Kidney stone
- Diverticulitis

DIAGNOSTIC TESTS & INTERPRETATION
Initial Tests (lab, imaging)
- Urinalysis: pyuria ± leukocyte casts, hematuria, nitrites (sensitivity 35–85%; specificity 92–100%), and mild proteinuria
- Urine leukocyte esterase positive (sensitivity 74–96%; specificity 94–98%)

- Urine Gram stain; urine culture (>100,000 colony forming units/mL or >100 colony forming units/mL + symptoms) and sensitivities
- CBC, BUN, Cr, GFR, and pregnancy test (if indicated)
- C-reactive protein levels have been shown to correlate with prolonged hospitalization and recurrence; serum albumin <3.3 g/dL also associated with risk for hospital admission
- Imaging not necessary in routine cases
- Pediatrics: Recent guidelines recommend renal/bladder US (not voiding cystourethrogram), after first UTI.

Follow-Up Tests & Special Considerations
- Catheterization/suprapubic aspirate to obtain samples from non–toilet-trained children
- Catheterization may be necessary for some geriatric patients.
- Blood culture(s): if diagnosis uncertain, suspected hematogenous source or immunosuppression
- Recent antibiotic use may alter lab results.
- If patient's condition does not improve within 72 hours, if obstruction/anatomic abnormality suspected, or if certain lab abnormalities are present (urine pH >7, GFR <40, 50% decline in renal function), consider:
  - CT scan of abdomen and pelvis ± contrast
  - US of kidneys, ureter, bladder
  - Cystoscopy with ureteral catheterization

Test Interpretation
- Acute: abscess formation with neutrophil response
- Chronic: fibrosis with reduction in renal tissue

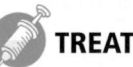

TREATMENT

- ≤7 days of treatment is equivalent to longer regimens in adults (including those with bacteremia) without urogenital abnormalities (2,3,4)[A].
- IV antibiotics for inpatients who are toxic appearing or unable to tolerate oral antibiotics

GENERAL MEASURES
- Broad-spectrum antibiotics initially; tailor to culture and sensitivity results.
- Analgesics and antipyretics
- Consider urinary analgesics (e.g., phenazopyridine 200 mg q8h) for dysuria.

MEDICATION
- For empiric oral therapy, a fluoroquinolone is recommended. Should fluoroquinolone resistance exceed 10% or the patient has nausea/vomiting, a single initial IV dose of a long-acting antibiotic such as ceftriaxone 1 g is recommended.
- For parenteral therapy, fluoroquinolone, aminoglycoside with or without ampicillin, an extended-spectrum cephalosporin with or without a β-lactamase inhibitor, an extended-spectrum penicillin with or without an aminoglycoside, or a carbapenem are recommended.
- Contraindications:
  - Known drug allergy
  - Fluoroquinolones are not recommended in children, adolescents, and pregnant women unless other alternatives are not available.
  - Nitrofurantoin does not achieve reliable tissue levels for treatment of pyelonephritis.

- Precautions
  - Most antibiotics require adjustments in dosage for patients with renal insufficiency.
  - Monitor aminoglycoside levels and renal function.
  - If *Enterococcus* is suspected based on Gram stain, ampicillin ± gentamicin is a reasonable empiric choice; unless patient is penicillin allergic, then use vancomycin. If outpatient, add amoxicillin to fluoroquinolone, pending culture results and sensitivity. Do not use a 3rd-generation cephalosporin for suspected/proven enterococcal infections.
  - >20% *E. coli* strains are resistant to ampicillin and trimethoprim-sulfamethoxazole (TMP-SMX) in community-acquired infections.
  - Extended-spectrum β-lactamase (ESBL)-producing strains should be treated with a carbapenem ± β-lactamase inhibitor or ceftolozane-tazobactam.

First Line
- Adults
  - Oral (initial outpatient treatment)
    - Ciprofloxacin: 500 mg q12h for 7 days
    - Ciprofloxacin XR: 1,000 mg/day for 7 days
    - Levofloxacin: 750 mg/day for 5 days
    - TMP-SMX (160/800 mg): 1 tab q12h for 14 days provided uropathogen known to be susceptible ± ceftriaxone 1 g initial IM/IV dose
  - IV (initial inpatient treatment)
    - Ciprofloxacin: 400 mg q12h
    - Levofloxacin: 750 mg/day
    - Cefotaxime: 1 g q8–12h up to 2 g q4h
    - Ceftriaxone: 1 to 2 g/day
    - Cefepime: 1 to 2 g q12h
    - Gentamicin: 5 to 7 mg/kg body weight daily
    - Ampicillin: 2 g q6h ± gentamicin for *Enterococcus*
    - Ceftolozane-tazobactam: 1.5 g q8h (target therapy when causative pathogen is known)
  - Severe illness: IV therapy until afebrile for 24 to 48 hours and tolerating PO intake. Switch to oral agents to complete up to a 2-week course.
- Pediatric
  - Oral: cefdinir: 14 mg/kg/day for 10 to 14 days; ceftibuten 9 mg/kg/day for 10 to 14 days; cefixime 8 mg/kg/day for 10 to 14 days
  - IV (General indication for IV therapy is age <2 months or clinical concern in other ages.)
    - Ceftriaxone: 75 mg/kg/day (IM use acceptable in outpatient setting)
    - Cefotaxime: 150 mg/kg/day divided in 3 to 4 doses
    - Ampicillin: 100 mg/kg/day divided in 4 doses + gentamicin 7.5 mg/kg/day divided in 3 doses

Second Line
Adults
- Oral
  - Oral β-lactams should be used with caution due to inferior efficacy and higher relapse rates; if used, provide an initial IV dose of ceftriaxone or a consolidated 24-hour dose of an aminoglycoside; longer courses of therapy (10 to 14 days) recommended
  - Cefpodoxime (Proxetil): 200 mg q12h
  - Amoxicillin-clavulanate: 875/125 mg q12h or 500/125 mg q8h
- IV
  - Piperacillin-tazobactam: 3.375 g q6–8h
  - Ticarcillin-clavulanate: 3.1 g q4–6h
  - Meropenem: 500 mg q12h
  - Meropenem-vaborbactam: 4 g q8h (5)[A]

Pediatric Considerations
- Treat children <2 years of age and children with febrile or recurrent UTI for 10 to 14 days.
- Initial empiric antibiotic choice should cover *E. coli*. Add ampicillin if *Enterococcus* is suspected.
  - Oral antibiotics (ceftibuten, cefixime, and amoxicillin/clavulanic acid) may be used alone, *or*
  - IV antibiotics (single daily dosing if an aminoglycoside is chosen) for 2 to 4 days, followed by oral antibiotics for a total of 10 to 14 days (6)[A]
- Complete outpatient antibiotic course in entirety.

ISSUES FOR REFERRAL
- Acute pyelonephritis unresponsive to therapy
- Chronic pyelonephritis
- Abnormal urogenital anatomy

SURGERY/OTHER PROCEDURES
Perinephric abscess may require surgical drainage.

ADMISSION, INPATIENT, AND NURSING CONSIDERATIONS
- Inpatient therapy for severe illness (e.g., high fevers, severe pain, marked debility, intractable vomiting, inability to tolerate oral intake, possible sepsis), risk factors for complicated pyelonephritis, pregnancy, or extremes of age
- Outpatient therapy if mild to moderate illness (not pregnant, no nausea/vomiting; fever and pain not severe), uncomplicated course, and tolerating oral intake. Many patients can be treated as outpatients.
- IV fluids as indicated for dehydration or renal calculi
- Discharge on oral agent after patient is afebrile 24 to 48 hours to complete up to 2 weeks of therapy.

ONGOING CARE

FOLLOW-UP RECOMMENDATIONS
- Women: routine follow-up cultures not recommended unless symptoms recur after 2 weeks and then urologic evaluation is necessary
- Men, children, adolescents, patients with recurrent infections, patients with risk factors: Repeat cultures 1 to 2 weeks after completing therapy; urologic evaluation after first episode of pyelonephritis and with recurrences

Patient Monitoring
- If no response within 48 hours (5% of patients): Reevaluate and review cultures, CT scan, or US to review anatomy; adjust therapy as needed; urologic consult. The two most common causes of failure to respond are a resistant organism and nephrolithiasis.
- Work with parents to monitor response in children.

DIET
Encourage fluid intake.

PROGNOSIS
95% of treated patients respond within 48 hours.

COMPLICATIONS
- Kidney abscess
- Metastatic infection: skeletal system, endocardium, eye, meningitis with subsequent seizures
- Septic shock and death
- Acute/chronic renal failure

REFERENCES
1. Ninan S, Walton C, Barlow G. Investigation of suspected urinary tract infection in older people. *BMJ*. 2014;349:g4070.
2. Eliakim-Raz N, Yahav D, Paul M, et al. Duration of antibiotic treatment for acute pyelonephritis and septic urinary tract infection—7 days or less versus longer treatment: systematic review and meta-analysis of randomized controlled trials. *J Antimicrob Chemother*. 2013;68(10):2183–2191.
3. Dinh A, Davido B, Etienne M, et al. Is 5 days of oral fluoroquinolone enough for acute uncomplicated pyelonephritis? The DTP randomized trial. *Eur J Clin Microbiol Infect Dis*. 2017;36(8):1443–1448.
4. Ren H, Li X, Ni ZH, et al. Treatment of complicated urinary tract infection and acute pyelonephritis by short-course intravenous levofloxacin (750 mg/day) or conventional intravenous/oral levofloxacin (500 mg/day): prospective, open-label, randomized, controlled, multicenter, non-inferiority clinical trial. *Int Urol Nephrol*. 2017;49(3):499–507.
5. Kaye KS, Bhowmick T, Metallidis S, et al. Effect of meropenem-vaborbactam vs piperacillin-tazobactam on clinical cure or improvement and microbial eradication in complicated urinary tract infection: the TANGO I randomized clinical trial. *JAMA*. 2018;319(8):788–799.
6. Strohmeier Y, Hodson EM, Willis NS, et al. Antibiotics for acute pyelonephritis in children. *Cochrane Database Syst Rev*. 2014;(7):CD003772.

ADDITIONAL READING
- Goel RH, Unnikrishnan R, Remer EM. Acute urinary tract disorders. *Radiol Clin North Am*. 2015;53(6):1273–1292.
- Noelle L. Urinary tract infections in older adults. *Clin Geriatr Med*. 2016;32(3):532–538.
- Takhar SS, Moran GJ. Diagnosis and management of urinary tract infection in the emergency department and outpatient settings. *Infect Dis Clin North Am*. 2014;28(1):33–48.
- Wagenlehner FM, Umeh O, Steenbergen J, et al. Ceftolozane-tazobactam compared to levofloxacin in treatment of complicated urinary tract infections, including pyelonephritis: a randomized, double-blind, phase 3 trial (ASPECT-cUTI). *Lancet*. 2015;385(9981):1949–1956.

CODES

ICD10
- N12 Tubulo-interstitial nephritis, not spcf as acute or chronic
- N10 Acute tubulo-interstitial nephritis
- N11.9 Chronic tubulo-interstitial nephritis, unspecified

CLINICAL PEARLS
- Pyelonephritis can present with isolated confusion or mental status changes (no fever) in the elderly.
- The most common causes of poor response to treatment are antibiotic resistance and coexisting nephrolithiasis.
- Fluoroquinolones are generally the initial antibiotic of choice for pyelonephritis. Oral β-lactams are less effective. Parental β-lactams may be used in cases of complicated UTIs.

PYLORIC STENOSIS

Jennifer M. Cornwell, DO

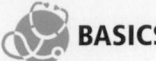 **BASICS**

DESCRIPTION
- Progressive narrowing of the pyloric canal, occurring in infancy
- Synonym(s): infantile hypertrophic pyloric stenosis (IHPS)

EPIDEMIOLOGY
- Predominant age: infancy
  - Onset usually at 3 to 6 weeks of age; rarely in the newborn period or as late as 5 months of age
- Considered the most common condition requiring surgical intervention in the 1st year of life
- A recent decline in incidence has been reported in a number of countries.
- Predominant sex: male > female (4 to 5:1)

Incidence
In Caucasian population, 2 to 5:1,000 babies; less common in African American and Asian populations

Prevalence
National prevalence level is 1 to 2:1,000 infants, ranging from 0.5 to 4.21:1,000 live births.

ETIOLOGY AND PATHOPHYSIOLOGY
- Abnormal relaxation of the pyloric muscles leads to hypertrophy.
- Redundant mucosa fills the pyloric canal.
- Gastric outflow is obstructed, leading to gastric distension and vomiting.
- The exact cause remains unknown, but multiple genetic and environmental factors have been implicated.
- Breast versus bottlefeeding—increased vasoactive intestinal peptide in breast milk may mediate pyloric relaxation and increase gastric emptying, whereas bottlefeeding may cause higher serum levels associated with pylorospasm (1)[C].

Genetics
Recent studies have identified linkage to chromosomes 3, 5, 11 and 19.

RISK FACTORS
- 5 times increased risk with affected first-degree relative
- Strong familial aggregation and >80% heritability
- Multiple gestation—200-fold increased risk if monozygotic twin diagnosed and 20-fold increased risk if dizygotic twin diagnosed
- Breastfeeding protective versus bottlefeeding where risk is increased

- Postnatal macrolide use (i.e., erythromycin, azithromycin)—erythromycin agonist of motilin, which might cause continuous contraction of the pyloric muscle (1)[C]
- A recent surveillance study of a population-based birth defects registry identified association between pyloric stenosis and the use of fluoxetine in the 1st trimester, even after adjustment for maternal age and smoking. The adjusted odds ratio was 9.8 (95% CI 1.5–62) (2)[B].

COMMONLY ASSOCIATED CONDITIONS
Associated anomalies present in ~4–7% of infants with pyloric stenosis
- Hiatal and inguinal hernias (most commonly)
- Other anomalies include the following:
  - Congenital heart disease
  - Esophageal atresia
  - Tracheoesophageal fistula
  - Renal abnormalities
  - Turner syndrome and trisomy 18
  - Cornelia de Lange syndrome
  - Smith-Lemli-Opitz syndrome
- A common proposed genetic link between breast cancer, endometriosis, and pyloric stenosis has been observed in families.

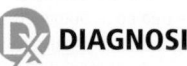 **DIAGNOSIS**

HISTORY
- Nonbilious projectile vomiting after feeding, increasing in frequency and severity
- Emesis may become blood-tinged from vomiting-induced gastric irritation.
- Hunger due to inadequate nutrition
- Decrease in bowel movements
- Weight loss

PHYSICAL EXAM
- Firm, mobile ("olive-like") mass palpable in the right upper quadrant (historically 70–90% of the time)
- However, this finding has decreased in occurrence to about 13% due to earlier diagnosis with US (1)[C].
- Epigastric distention
- Visible gastric peristalsis after feeding
- Late signs: dehydration, weight loss
- Rarely, jaundice when starvation leads to decreased glucuronyl transferase activity resulting in indirect hyperbilirubinemia

DIFFERENTIAL DIAGNOSIS
- Inexperienced or inappropriate feeding
- GERD

- Gastritis
- Congenital adrenal hyperplasia, salt-wasting
- Pylorospasm
- Gastric volvulus
- Antral or gastric web

DIAGNOSTIC TESTS & INTERPRETATION
Metabolic disturbances are late findings and are uncommon in present era of early diagnosis and intervention.
- If prolonged vomiting, check electrolytes for the following:
  - Hypokalemia
  - Hypochloremia
  - Metabolic alkalosis
- Elevated unconjugated bilirubin level (rare)
- Paradoxical aciduria: The kidney tubules excrete hydrogen to preserve potassium in face of hypokalemic alkalosis.
- Abdominal US is the study of choice.
  - US shows thickened and elongated pyloric muscle and redundant mucosa.
  - Pathologic limits are 3-mm pyloric muscle thickness, 15-mm pyloric length, 11-mm pyloric diameter, and 12-mL pyloric volume with muscle thickness being the key factor. However, current studies are showing a correlation between pyloric muscle thickness being directly related to age and weight which should be taken into consideration in smaller, younger infants who do not meet current US criteria for IHPS but may still be diagnosed appropriately with IHPS by clinical symptoms (3)[B].
- Upper GI series reveal strong gastric contractions; elongated, narrow pyloric canal (string sign); and parallel lines of barium in the narrow channel (double-tract sign or railroad track sign).

Test Interpretation
Concentric hypertrophy of pyloric muscle

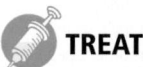 **TREATMENT**

SURGERY/OTHER PROCEDURES
- Ramstedt pyloromyotomy is curative. The entire length of hypertrophied muscle is divided, with preservation of the underlying mucosa.
- Surgical approaches include open (traditional right upper quadrant transverse) incision, more contemporary circumumbilical incision, and laparoscopic techniques.

- Recent reviews have concluded that the laparoscopic approach results in less postoperative pain, shorter hospital stays, shorter postoperative recovery, lower complication rates, improved cosmesis, and can be performed with no increase in operative time or complications (4)[A],(5)[B].
- Conservative approach
  - Conservative management of IHPS with atropine can be effective in approximately six out of seven cases but has a lower success rate and longer duration of therapy than surgery (6)[B].
  - Atropine therapy may be considered as an alternative to pyloromyotomy for patients unsuitable or at high risk for surgery and in areas of the world where surgery on small infants is unavailable or unsafe (6)[B].

ADMISSION, INPATIENT, AND NURSING CONSIDERATIONS

- Prompt treatment to avoid dehydration and malnutrition
- Correct acid–base and electrolyte disturbances. Surgery should be delayed until alkalosis is corrected.
- Patients need pre- and postoperative apnea monitoring due to a tendency toward apnea to compensate with respiratory acidosis for their metabolic alkalosis.
- IV fluids to correct dehydration and metabolic abnormalities. For optimal resuscitation in infants, use D5 1/2NS with 20 mEq of KCl (1)[C].

 ONGOING CARE

FOLLOW-UP RECOMMENDATIONS
Patient Monitoring
- Routine pediatric health maintenance
- Postoperative monitoring, including monitoring for pain, emesis, apnea
- If significant emesis present after 1 to 2 weeks, then upper GI studies needed to rule out incomplete pyloromyotomy or duodenal leak (1)[C]

DIET
- No preoperative feeding
- Adlib feedings are recommended after pyloromyotomy which can decrease length of stay versus structured feedings. However, if a provider prefers structured feedings, a rapid feeding regimen is recommended although increased emesis will likely occur but with no negative outcomes reported. Timing of first feed is not significant, but early feeding is associated with increased potential for emesis (7)[A].

PROGNOSIS
Surgery is curative.

COMPLICATIONS
- No long-term morbidity
- Incomplete pyloromyotomy
- Mucosal perforation
- Wound infections
- Delayed feeding due to postoperative vomiting
- Serosal tear
- Subcutaneous emphysema
- 4.6–12% complication rate (3)[C]

REFERENCES

1. Peters B, Oomen MW, Bakx R, et al. Advances in infantile hypertrophic pyloric stenosis. *Expert Rev Gastroenterol Hepatol*. 2014;8(5):533–541.
2. Bakker MK, De Walle HE, Wilffert B, et al. Fluoxetine and infantile hypertrophic pylorus stenosis: a signal from a birth defects-drug exposure surveillance study. *Pharmacoepidemiol Drug Saf*. 2010;19(8):808–813.
3. Said M, Shaul D, Fujimoto M, et al. Ultrasound measurements in hypertrophic pyloric stenosis: don't let the numbers fool you. *Perm J*. 2012;16(3):25–27.
4. Oomen MW, Hoekstra LT, Bakx R, et al. Open versus laparoscopic pyloromyotomy for hypertrophic pyloric stenosis: a systematic review and meta-analysis focusing on major complications. *Surg Endosc*. 2012;26(8):2104–2110.
5. Mahida JB, Asti L, Deans KJ, et al. Laparoscopic pyloromyotomy decreases postoperative length of stay in children with hypertrophic pyloric stenosis. *J Pediatr Surg*. 2016;51(9):1436–1439.
6. Mercer AE, Phillips R. Question 2: can a conservative approach to the treatment of hypertrophic pyloric stenosis with atropine be considered a real alternative to surgical pyloromyotomy? *Arch Dis Child*. 2013;98(6):474–477.
7. Sullivan KJ, Chan E, Vincent J, et al; for Canadian Association of Paediatric Surgeons Evidence-Based Resource. Feeding post-pyloromyotomy: a meta-analysis. *Pediatrics*. 2016;137(1):1–11.

ADDITIONAL READING

- Ein SH, Masiakos PT, Ein A. The ins and outs of pyloromyotomy: what we have learned in 35 years. *Pediatr Surg Int*. 2014;30(5):467–480.
- Everett KV, Capon F, Georgoula C, et al. Linkage of monogenic infantile hypertrophic pyloric stenosis to chromosome 16q24. *Eur J Hum Genet*. 2008;16(9):1151–1154.
- Everett KV, Chioza BA, Georgoula C, et al. Genome-wide high-density SNP-based linkage analysis of infantile hypertrophic pyloric stenosis identifies loci on chromosomes 11q14–q22 and Xq23. *Am J Hum Genet*. 2008;82(3):756–762.
- Feenstra B, Geller F, Carstensen L, et al. Plasma lipids, genetic variants near APOA1, and the risk of infantile hypertrophic pyloric stenosis. *JAMA*. 2013;310(7):714–721.
- Georgoula C, Gardiner M. Pyloric stenosis a 100 years after Ramstedt. *Arch Dis Child*. 2012;97(8):741–745.
- Graham KA, Laituri CA, Markel TA, et al. A review of postoperative feeding regimens in infantile hypertrophic pyloric stenosis. *J Pediatr Surg*. 2013;48(10):2175–2179.
- Krogh C, Fischer TK, Skotte L, et al. Familial aggregation and heritability of pyloric stenosis. *JAMA*. 2010;303(23):2393–2399.
- Owen RP, Almond SL, Humphrey GM. Atropine sulphate: rescue therapy for pyloric stenosis. *BMJ Case Rep*. 2012;2012.
- Selected birth defects data from population-based birth defects surveillance programs in the United States, 2003–2007. *Birth Defects Res A Clin Mol Teratol*. 2010;88(12):1062–1174.
- Sommerfield T, Chalmers J, Youngson G, et al. The changing epidemiology of infantile hypertrophic pyloric stenosis in Scotland. *Arch Dis Child*. 2008;93(12):1007–1011.
- Wyrick DL, Smith SD, Dassinger MS. Surgeon as educator: bedside ultrasound in hypertrophic pyloric stenosis. *J Surg Educ*. 2014;71(6):896–898.

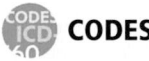 **CODES**

ICD10
Q40.0 Congenital hypertrophic pyloric stenosis

CLINICAL PEARLS
- Pyloric stenosis is the most common condition requiring surgical intervention in the 1st year of life.
- The condition classically presents between 1 and 5 months of life, with projectile vomiting after feeds and a firm, mobile mass in the right upper quadrant.
- Abdominal US is the study of choice.
- Surgery (laparoscopic Ramstedt pyloromyotomy is the preferred method) is curative.

RABIES

Alan M. Ehrlich, MD

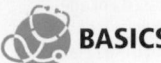 **BASICS**

DESCRIPTION
- A rapidly progressive CNS infection caused by an RNA rhabdovirus affecting mammals, including humans
- Generally considered to be 100% fatal once symptoms develop
- System(s) affected: nervous
- Synonym(s): hydrophobia (inability to swallow water)

EPIDEMIOLOGY
Incidence
- Most cases are in developing countries.
- Estimated 55,000 deaths worldwide per year
- Typically only 1 to 3 cases per year in the United States, with 1/3 of those being due to exposure outside of the United States
- Predominant age: any
- Predominant sex: male = female

ETIOLOGY AND PATHOPHYSIOLOGY
Lyssavirus, an RNA virus in the family *Rhabdoviridae*
- Rabies virus is a neurotropic virus present in saliva of infected animals.
- Transmission occurs via bites from infected animals or when saliva from an infected animal comes in contact with an open wound or mucous membranes.
- Bats are most common reservoir in the United States.

RISK FACTORS
- Professions or activities with exposure to potentially infected (wild or domestic) animals (e.g., animal handlers, lab workers, veterinarians, cave explorers)
- Most U.S. cases are associated with bat exposure.
- Internationally, rabies is widespread in both domestic and feral dogs.
- Human-to-human transmission has occurred through transplantation of cornea, solid organs, and other tissues.
- Travel to countries where canine rabies is endemic

GENERAL PREVENTION
- Preexposure vaccination for high-risk groups (veterinarians, animal handlers, and certain laboratory workers)
- Consider preexposure vaccination for travelers to areas (such as North Africa) that have increased risk of rabies from domestic animals.
- Immunization of dogs and cats
- Contact animal control and avoid approaching or handling wild (or domestic) animals exhibiting strange behaviors.
- Avoid wild and unknown domestic animals.
- Seek treatment promptly if bitten, scratched, or in contact with saliva from potentially infected animal.
- Prevent infection by prompt postexposure treatment.

- Consider postexposure prophylaxis for individuals in direct contact with bats, unless it is known that an exposure did not occur.
- Hospital contacts of patients infected with rabies do not require postexposure prophylaxis unless there has been exposure through mucous membranes or an open wound (including a bite) to saliva, CSF, or brain tissue from the infected patient.

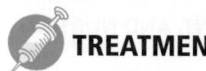 **DIAGNOSIS**

HISTORY
- History of animal exposure
- Most patients do not recall exposure.
- Five stages (may overlap)
  - Incubation period: time between bite and first symptoms: usually 10 days to 1 year (average of 20 to 60 days). Incubation is shortest in patients with extensive bites in the head or trunk.
  - Prodrome: lasts 1 to 14 days; symptoms include pain or paresthesia at bite site and nonspecific flulike symptoms, including fever and headache.
  - Acute neurologic period: lasts 2 to 10 days. CNS symptoms dominate; generally 1 of 2 forms: (i) furious rabies: brief (~5 minute) episodes of hyperactivity with hydrophobia, aerophobia, hyperventilation, hypersalivation, and autonomic instability; (ii) paralytic rabies: Paralysis dominates; may be ascending (as in Guillain-Barré syndrome) or may affect ≥1 limbs differentially
  - Coma: lasts hours to days; may evolve over several days following acute neurologic period; may be sudden, with respiratory arrest
  - Death: usually occurs within 3 weeks of onset as result of complications

PHYSICAL EXAM
Findings range from normal exam to severe neurologic findings, including paralysis and coma, depending on the stage of rabies at the time of presentation.

DIFFERENTIAL DIAGNOSIS
- Any rapidly progressive encephalitis; important to exclude treatable causes of encephalitis, especially herpes
- Transverse myelitis

DIAGNOSTIC TESTS & INTERPRETATION
Initial Tests (lab, imaging)
- Lumbar puncture. WBC count is normal or shows moderate pleocytosis; protein normal or moderately elevated
- Skin biopsy to detect rabies antigen in hair follicles
  - Available through state and federal reference labs
- Rabies antibody titer of serum and CSF
- Skin biopsy from nape of neck for direct fluorescent antibody examination
- Viral isolation from saliva or CSF
- Corneal smear stains are positive by immunofluorescence in 50% of patients.

- Hyponatremia is common.
- Head CT scan: normal or nonspecific findings consistent with encephalitis
- MRI can help rule out other forms of encephalitis.

Follow-Up Tests & Special Considerations
Submit brain of the biting animal for testing if possible.

Test Interpretation
Encephalitis may be found on brain biopsy. Other abnormal findings (e.g., brainstem, midbrain, cerebellum) are often found only postmortem.

TREATMENT

Thorough wound cleansing with soap and water is first line of treatment. Irrigate wound with virucidal agent, such as povidone-iodine, if available.

GENERAL MEASURES
- Evaluate risk based on exposure and consult public health officials about the need for rabies prophylaxis.
- In the United States, raccoons, skunks, bats, foxes, and coyotes are the animals most likely to be infected. Any carnivore can carry the disease.
- Before initiating antirabies treatment, consider:
  - Type of exposure (bite or nonbite)
  - Epidemiology of rabies in species involved
  - Circumstances surrounding exposure (provoked vs. unprovoked bite)
  - Vaccination status of offending animal

MEDICATION

ALERT
- Immunosuppression alters immunity after vaccination. Immunosuppressive drugs should be avoided during postexposure prophylaxis if possible. If postexposure prophylaxis is given to an immunosuppressed patient, check serum samples for the presence of rabies virus–neutralizing antibody to assess response to vaccination (1)[C].
- Clean wounds thoroughly, regardless of postexposure prophylaxis status.
- Assess need for postexposure prophylaxis based on circumstances of possible exposure.
- Increased risk:
  - Bites involving skin puncture are high risk; saliva exposure is a risk only if it comes in contact with an open wound or mucous membranes.
  - Wild or domestic animals unavailable for quarantine
  - Bat exposure
  - Hybrid animals of wild and domestic species (e.g., wolf-dog)
  - Unprovoked attack (Feeding a wild animal is considered a provoked attack.)

- Management:
  - Bites from cats, dogs, and ferrets that can be watched for 10 days do not require prophylaxis unless animal shows signs of illness.
  - Skunks, foxes, bats, raccoons, and most carnivores are high risk, and prophylaxis should begin promptly unless animal can be captured and euthanized for pathologic evaluation.
  - For rodents or livestock, consult local public health authorities before initiating prophylaxis.
- Postexposure prophylaxis (2)[B]
  - Passive vaccination: rabies immunoglobulin (RIG, HyperRAB) 20 IU/kg administered once. Infiltrate RIG around the wound if possible. Administer remaining RIG IM. Do not administer RIG using the same syringe or into the same anatomic site as vaccine.
  - Active vaccination: rabies vaccine, human diploid cell vaccine (HDCV) or rabies vaccine adsorbed (RVA) or purified chick embryo cell vaccine IM in the deltoid. Give the first dose, 1 mL, as soon as possible after exposure. The day of the first dose is designated day 0. Give additional 1-mL doses on days 3, 7, and 14. If immunocompromised, give fifth dose on day 28. For children, use the anterolateral aspect of the thigh and avoid the gluteal area.
- For previously vaccinated patients, administer an initial 1-mL IM dose of vaccine immediately and an additional 1-mL dose 3 days later. RIG is not necessary in these patients (2)[B].
- Preexposure vaccination: for people in high-risk groups, such as veterinarians, animal handlers, certain laboratory workers, and those spending time in foreign countries where rabies is enzootic (3)[B]:
  - Primary preexposure: three IM 1-mL injections of HDCV or RVA in deltoid area on days 0, 7, and 21, or 28
  - Preexposure boosters: For people at risk of exposure to rabies, test serum every 2 years. Administer preexposure booster of 1-mL IM if immunity is waning. If titer cannot be obtained, a booster can be administered instead.
- Contraindications: none for postexposure treatment

Pregnancy Considerations
- Pregnancy is not a contraindication to postexposure prophylaxis.
- Rabies vaccination is not associated with a higher incidence of spontaneous abortion, premature births, or fetal abnormalities.

ADMISSION, INPATIENT, AND NURSING CONSIDERATIONS
Clinical rabies
- Comfort care and sedation for all patients
- Milwaukee protocol: experimental treatment using ketamine, midazolam, and amantadine (originally included ribavirin but no longer recommended) (1,4)[C]. One patient who did not receive pre- or postexposure prophylaxis recovered from clinical rabies in 2004 after being treated with medically induced coma and amantadine I (1)[C].

- Control cerebral artery vasospasm (with an agent such as nimodipine) (4,5)[C].
- Fludrocortisone and hypertonic saline if needed to maintain normal sodium level (5)[C]

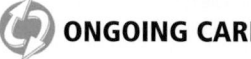 ## ONGOING CARE

FOLLOW-UP RECOMMENDATIONS
After primary vaccination, serologic testing is necessary only if the patient has a disease or takes immunosuppressive medication.

PATIENT EDUCATION
Use screens over ventilation areas in the roof to secure from bats. Avoid exposure to wild mammalian species known to carry rabies and report potential exposures immediately.

PROGNOSIS
- No postexposure failures in the United States since the 1970s
- If untreated, rabies has the highest case fatality rate of any infectious disease; generally considered to be 100% fatal once symptoms develop
- There have only been a small number of cases of successful recovery from rabies. Almost all received some form of pre- or postexposure immunization.

COMPLICATIONS
0.6% of people develop mild serum sickness reaction following HDCV boosters. Mild local and systemic reactions are common following vaccination. Do not interrupt immunization series with mild reactions.

REFERENCES

1. Willoughby RE Jr, Tieves KS, Hoffman GM, et al. Survival after treatment of rabies with induction of coma. *N Engl J Med*. 2005;352(24):2508–2514.
2. Rupprecht CE, Briggs D, Brown CM, et al; for Centers for Disease Control and Prevention. Use of a reduced (4-dose) vaccine schedule for postexposure prophylaxis to prevent human rabies: recommendations of the Advisory Committee on Immunization Practices. *MMWR Recomm Rep*. 2010;59(RR-2):1–9.
3. Manning SE, Rupprecht CE, Fishbein D, et al; for Advisory Committee on Immunization Practices Centers for Disease Control and Prevention. Human rabies prevention—United States, 2008: recommendations of the Advisory Committee on Immunization Practices. *MMWR Recomm Rep*. 2008;57(RR-3):1–28.
4. Aramburo A, Willoughby RE, Bollen AW, et al. Failure of the Milwaukee protocol in a child with rabies. *Clin Infect Dis*. 2011;53(6):572–574.
5. Hu WT, Willoughby RE Jr, Dhonau H, et al. Long-term follow-up after treatment of rabies by induction of coma. *N Engl J Med*. 2007;357(9):945–946.

ADDITIONAL READING

- Centers for Disease Control and Prevention: http://www.cdc.gov/rabies/
- Centers for Disease Control and Prevention. Recovery of a patient from clinical rabies—California, 2011. *MMWR Morb Mortal Wkly Rep*. 2012;61(4):61–65.
- Crowcroft NS, Thampi N. The prevention and management of rabies. *BMJ*. 2015;350:g7827.
- De Serres G, Skowronski DM, Mimault P, et al. Bats in the bedroom, bats in the belfry: reanalysis of the rationale for rabies postexposure prophylaxis. *Clin Infect Dis*. 2009;48(11):1493–1499.
- Eckerle I, Rosenberger KD, Zwahlen M, et al. Serologic vaccination response after solid organ transplantation: a systematic review. *PLoS One*. 2013;8(2):e56974.
- Hemachudha T, Ugolini G, Wacharapluesadee S, et al. Human rabies: neuropathogenesis, diagnosis, and management. *Lancet Neurol*. 2013;12(5):498–513.
- Vora NM, Basavaraju SV, Feldman KA, et al; and Transplant-Associated Rabies Virus Transmission Investigation Team. Raccoon rabies virus variant transmission through solid organ transplantation. *JAMA*. 2013;310(4):398–407.

 ## SEE ALSO

Bites, Animal and Human

 ## CODES

ICD10
- A82.9 Rabies, unspecified
- Z20.3 Contact with and (suspected) exposure to rabies

CLINICAL PEARLS
- Rabies is rare in the United States but more common in other areas of the world.
- Seek immediate treatment if exposed to scratch, bite, or saliva of potentially infected animal (e.g., feral dog, bat, fox, raccoon, or other wild mammals).
- Postexposure prophylaxis consists of three steps: local wound cleansing, passive immunization with RIG, and active immunization with HDCV.
- Consider postexposure prophylaxis for those reporting direct contact with bats, unless it can be verified that an exposure did not occur.

RAPE CRISIS SYNDROME
An-Hoa Giang, MD, MPH • Virginia J. Van Duyne, MD

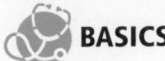

BASICS

DESCRIPTION
- Definitions (legal definitions vary from state to state)
  - Rape (which is a legal term, physicians should use the phrase "alleged sexual assault"): any sexual penetration, however slight, using force or coercion against the person's will
  - Rape is separated into three types: completed forced penetration, attempted forced penetration, and competed alcohol- or drug-facilitated penetration.
  - In a female, rape is forced oral, vaginal, or anal penetration. In a male, rape is forced penetration of the anus with any object in a male.
  - Sexual coercion: unwanted sexual penetration without the use of force
  - Sexual imposition: similar to rape but without penetration or the use of force (i.e., nonconsensual sexual contact, stalking)
  - Gross sexual imposition: nonconsensual sexual contact with the use of force
  - Corruption of a minor: sexual conduct by an individual age ≥18 years with an individual <16 years of age
  - Rape crisis syndrome/rape trauma syndrome is the response of a survivor to rape.
- Most states have expanded rape statutes to include marital rape, date rape, and rape shield laws.
- System(s) affected: nervous; reproductive; GI

EPIDEMIOLOGY
- In the United States, 25% of women and 7.6% of men report being target of the definition of rape crisis syndrome listed above. Annually, rape costs the United States $127 billion (the most of any crime).
- Anyone can be sexually assaulted, but some populations are especially vulnerable.
  - Adolescents and young children
  - People with disabilities
  - Elderly
  - Low socioeconomic status and homeless people
  - Sex workers
  - Those living in institutions/areas of conflict
- Predominant age
  - The incidence of sexual assault peaks in those 16 to 19 years of age, with the mean occurring at 20 years of age.
    - Adolescent sexual assault has a greater frequency of anogenital injuries.
- Predominant sex: female > male
  - For males
    - 69% of male victims were first raped before age 18 years.
    - 41% of male victims were raped before age 12 years.
- Only 16–38% of rape survivors report to law enforcement and only 17–43% present for medical evaluation after rape.

Incidence
- In the United States, approximately 1.5 million women and 834,700 men are sexually assaulted annually.
- Approximately 18% of U.S. women have experienced rape or attempted rape.
- Approximately 1–2% of U.S. men have experienced rape or attempted rape.
- Most rape survivors either know or have some acquaintance with their attacker.
- Rape of females and males were predominantly perpetrated by male assailants.

RISK FACTORS
- Children living in a household of sexual assault are at increased risk of maltreatment and lifelong poor health.

- Early sexual initiation
- Sexual risk-taking behavior
- Exposure to parental violence
- Alcohol consumption is estimated to be involved in 1/2 of sexual assault.
- Illicit drug may also contribute to sexual assault.

GENERAL PREVENTION
- Primary prevention: Evidence suggests that promotion of gender equality decreases sexual violence perpetration—strategies include mobilizing men and boys as allies and empowering/supporting girls and women through economic supports and increasing leadership opportunities.
- Secondary prevention: The USPSTF recommends screening women of childbearing age for intimate partner violence and refer women who screen positive to intervention services; HARK screening tool is 81% sensitive and 95% specific (1)[B].
- Tertiary prevention: Support survivors through victim-centered services (refer to "Patient Education" section) and medical treatment.

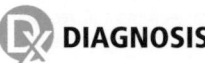

DIAGNOSIS

- In adults
  - History of sexual penetration
  - Sexual contact/conduct without consent and/or with the use of force
- In children
  - Actual observation/suspicion of sexual penetration, sexual contact, or sexual conduct
  - Signs include evidence of the use of force and/or evidence of sexual contact (e.g., presence of semen and/or blood).

HISTORY
- Note that some states require specific forms for documenting the history.
- Avoid questioning that implies the patient is at fault.
- Record answers in patient's own words. Include date, approximate time, and general location.
- Document physical abuse other than sexual. Describe all types of sexual contact, whether actual/attempted.
- Take history of alcohol and/or drug use before and/or after alleged incident.
- Document time of last activity that could possibly alter specimens (e.g., bath, shower, douche).
- Thorough gynecologic history is mandatory, including last menstrual period, last consenting sexual contact, contraceptive practice, and prior gynecologic surgery.

PHYSICAL EXAM
- Note that some states require specific forms for documenting physical exam.
- Document all signs of trauma/unusual marks.
- Document mental status and emotional state.
- Use UV light (Wood lamp) to detect seminal stains on clothing/skin.
- Obtaining the patient's consent at each step of examination helps the patient regain a sense of control.

ALERT
- A forensic kit or "rape kit" contains swabs that are collected from the vagina and rectum, and instructions are given with the kit regarding proper collection.
- Many states and emergency departments across the country are using a Sexual Assault Nurse Examiner (SANE) when available. This has led to more consistent and more accurate collection of evidence in alleged rape cases.

- Complete genital–rectal exam, including evidence of trauma, secretions, or discharge
  - Use of a nonlubricated, water-moistened speculum is mandatory because commonly used lubricants may destroy evidence.
  - Testing and/or specimen collection, as indicated, and in compliance with state requirements (2)

DIFFERENTIAL DIAGNOSIS
Consenting sex among adults

DIAGNOSTIC TESTS & INTERPRETATION
- In females, obtain a serum or urine pregnancy test.
- Record results of wet mount, screening for vaginitis, but also note the presence/absence of sperm and, if present, whether it is motile/immotile.
- Drug/alcohol testing as indicated by history and/or physical findings
- Diagnostic tests for sexually transmitted infections (STIs) is indicated but not necessary for treatment; NAAT for chlamydia, gonorrhea, and trichomoniasis; HIV, HepB, and syphilis testing

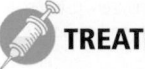

TREATMENT

GENERAL MEASURES
- Providing health care to victims of sexual assault/abuse requires special sensitivity and privacy.
- All cases *must* be reported immediately to the appropriate law enforcement agency.
- With the victim's permission, enlist the help of personnel from local support agencies (e.g., rape crisis center) and in-house social services.
- SANE programs have been shown to be beneficial, especially in large cities and metropolitan areas with multiple emergency departments of varying capability and staff training/experience.
- Give sedation and tetanus prophylaxis if indicated.
- Discuss suspected STI exposure with the victim and test/treat in accordance with the hospital, regional, and state policies/protocols (see below for recommended guidelines of testing/treatment).
- Discuss possible pregnancy and termination options. If hospital policy precludes such a discussion, information should be offered via follow-up mechanisms.
- Evaluate for psychological sequelae and refer to treatment.

MEDICATION
First Line
- The Centers for Disease Control and Prevention (CDC) recommends empiric prophylaxis treatment of STIs (specifically, gonorrhea, chlamydia, trichomoniasis, bacterial vaginosis, HepB, and HPV) and recommends consideration of treatment for HIV and syphilis depending on level of risk (3)[A]. Empiric treatment of these STIs is based on the finding that sexual assault victims have poor follow-up compliance.
- Cultures are *not* required before initiating treatment but can be done as part of routine evidence collection.
- Patients should be aware that any STI testing will be in the medical record and, if the case goes to trial, these records will have to be made available to the assailant's attorney. Patients should be given the option to forego STI testing and receive empiric STI treatment.
- Gonorrhea: ceftriaxone 250 mg IM once
- Chlamydia: azithromycin 1 g PO single dose or doxycycline 100 mg PO BID for 7 days
- Trichomoniasis and bacterial vaginosis: metronidazole 2 g PO once or tinidazole 2 g PO once

R

- HIV: There is a low likelihood of HIV transmittance, but nonoccupational postexposure prophylaxis (nPEP) for victims of sexual assault is recommended for patients evaluated to be at high risk (HIV status of assailant is known, method of penetration, IVDU status of assailant).
  - 28-day starter pack is recommended over the 3- to 7-day pack because it's been shown to increase likelihood of adherence and due to concerns of patient inability to keep 1-week follow-up appointment (4)[A].
  - Most effective if started within 4 hours and could reduce transmission by as much as 80%; unlikely to be beneficial if started after 72 hours
- Hepatitis B: hepatitis B immunoglobulin 0.06 mL/kg IM single dose, and initiate 3-dose hepatitis B virus immunization series; no treatment if the victim has had a complete hepatitis B vaccine series, with documented levels of immunity
- HPV vaccination is recommended for women who have been sexually assaulted from age 9 to 26 years and for males age 9 to 21 years. Age 9 to 14 years: first dose at time of encounter, second dose 6 to 12 months after. Age >14 years: initial dose given at time of encounter, second dose at 1 to 2 months after, and third dose 6 months after initial dose
- There is no evidence for empiric treatment of syphilis; however, screening with serology tests (nontreponemal and treponemal) is recommended.
- SSRIs are the first-line treatment for posttraumatic stress disorder (PTSD), one of the most common sequelae of sexual assault (5)[A].

Pregnancy Considerations
Conduct baseline pregnancy test; discuss pregnancy prevention and termination with patient. Options are listed in order of increasing effectiveness (6)[A].
- Yuzpe (100 μg of ethinyl estradiol and 0.5 mg levonorgestrel) is administered PO q12h × 2 doses; 75–80% effective, although rarely used due to low efficacy and high incidence of GI side effects
- Levonorgestrel (0.75 mg q12h PO × 2 doses or 1.5 mg PO once) has less nausea/vomiting side effects but less effective in overweight/obese women.
- Ulipristal acetate 30 mg PO once (brand name Ella, progestin antagonist/agonist) is effective up to 120 hours after intercourse. It is the preferred treatment for >72 hours after unprotected intercourse and in overweight/obese women.
- Copper IUD is the most effective emergency contraceptive method.

Pediatric Considerations
Assure the child that she or he is a good person and was not the cause of the incident.

ADMISSION, INPATIENT, AND NURSING CONSIDERATIONS
- Contact appropriate social services agency.
- Most adult victims can be treated as outpatients, unless associated trauma (physical/mental) requires admission.
- Most pediatric sexual assault/abuse victims will require admission/outside placement until appropriate social agency can evaluate home environment.

ONGOING CARE

FOLLOW-UP RECOMMENDATIONS
Patient Monitoring
- Patient should be seen in 7 to 10 days for follow-up care, including pregnancy testing and counseling.

- Close exam for vaginitis and treatment if necessary
- Follow-up test for gonorrhea should occur in 1 to 2 weeks.
- Follow-up testing for syphilis and HIV should occur at 6 weeks, 3 months, and 6 months.
- Follow-up evaluation for HPV anogenital warts should occur 1 to 2 months after the assault.
- Provide telephone numbers of counseling agencies that can give counseling/legal services to the patient.
- Use SANE, if available.

PATIENT EDUCATION
- Local rape crisis support organizations
- National Sexual Violence Resource Center, 123 Enola Drive, Enola, PA 17025; (877) 739-3895; https://www.nsvrc.org
- National Domestic Violence Hotline at (800) 799-SAFE (7233) or TTY (800) 787-3224 or http://www.thehotline.org
- National Sexual Assault Hotline: (800) 656-HOPE (4673)

PROGNOSIS
- Acute phase (usually 1 to 3 weeks following rape): shaking, pain, wound healing, mood swings, appetite loss, crying, feelings of grief, shame, anger, fear, revenge, or guilt
- Late/chronic phase (also called "reorganization"): Female victim may develop fear of intercourse, fear of men, anxiety or increase discomfort during Pap smears, nightmares, sleep disorders, daytime flashbacks, fear of being alone, loss of self-esteem, anxiety, depression, posttraumatic stress syndrome, and somatic complaints (e.g., nonspecific abdominal pain).
- Recovery phase may be prolonged. Patients who talk about their feelings seem to have a faster recovery. It is unclear if pharmaco- or psychotherapy results in better outcomes.

COMPLICATIONS
Sequelae include the following:
- Trauma (physical and/or mental)
- STIs, including HIV
- Unwanted pregnancy
  - In the United States, rape-related pregnancy accounts for >32,000 unwanted pregnancies each year.
  - Adolescents are at highest risk of pregnancy.
- Medical: chronic pain, fibromyalgia, headaches, irritable bowel syndrome, sexual dysfunction
- Psychological: anxiety, depression, PTSD, eating disorder, substance abuse
- Sexual assault is the most common type of trauma in women with PTSD. Of women with PTSD, 32% had been raped and 31% had experienced sexual assault.

REFERENCES

1. Nelson HD, Bougatsos C, Blazina I. Screening Women for Intimate Partner Violence and Elderly and Vulnerable Adults for Abuse: Systematic Review to Update the 2004 U.S. Preventive Services Task Force Recommendation. Rockville, MD: Agency for Healthcare Research and Quality; 2012. Evidence synthesis no. 92. AHRQ publication no. 12-05167-EF-1.
2. U.S. Department of Justice, Office on Violence Against Women. A National Protocol for Sexual Assault Medical Forensic Examinations (Adults/ Adolescents). 2nd ed. Washington, DC: U.S. Department of Justice; 2013.
3. Workowski KA, Bolan GA; for Centers for Disease Control and Prevention. Sexually transmitted diseases treatment guidelines, 2015. MMWR Recomm Rep. 2015;64(RR-03):1–137.
4. Centers for Disease Control and Prevention, U.S. Department of Health and Human Services. Updated Guidelines for Antiretroviral Postexposure Prophylaxis After Sexual, Injection Drug Use, or Other Nonoccupational Exposure to HIV—United States, 2016. Atlanta, GA: U.S. Department of Health and Human Services; 2016.
5. Committee on Treatment of Posttraumatic Stress Disorder, Board on Population Health and Public Health Practice, Institute of Medicine. Treatment of Posttraumatic Stress Disorder: An Assessment of the Evidence. Washington, DC: The National Academies Press; 2008.
6. Cheng L, Che Y, Gülmezoglu AM. Interventions for emergency contraception. Cochrane Database Syst Rev. 2012;(8):CD001324.

ADDITIONAL READING
- American College of Obstetricians and Gynecologists. Practice Bulletin No. 152: emergency contraception. Obstet Gynecol. 2015;126(3):e1–e11.
- Basile KC, DeGue S, Jones K, et al. STOP SV: A Technical Package to Prevent Sexual Violence. Atlanta, GA: National Center for Injury Prevention and Control, Centers for Disease Control and Prevention; 2016.
- Centers for Disease Control and Prevention. Sexual Violence: Facts at a Glance. Atlanta, GA: Centers for Disease Control and Prevention; 2012.

 SEE ALSO

Chlamydia Infection (Sexually Transmitted); Gonococcal Infections; Hepatitis B; Hepatitis C; HIV/AIDS; Posttraumatic Stress Disorder (PTSD); Syphilis

 CODES

ICD10
- T74.21XA Adult sexual abuse, confirmed, initial encounter
- T74.22XA Child sexual abuse, confirmed, initial encounter
- Z04.41 Encounter for exam and obs following alleged adult rape

CLINICAL PEARLS
- Rape is a legal term; the examining physician is encouraged to use terminology such as alleged sexual assault or alleged sexual conduct.
- Use of a protocol is encouraged to assure every victim a uniform, comprehensive evaluation, regardless of the expertise of the examiner. The protocol must ensure that all evidence is properly collected and labeled, chain of custody is maintained, and evidence is sent to the appropriate forensic laboratory.
- Medical personnel must be willing and able to testify on behalf of the patient.
- Treatment of patients undergoing a rape crisis includes prophylactic treatment of STIs, pregnancy testing and discussion of termination options, pharmaco-/psychotherapy for psychological sequelae (anxiety, depression, PTSD), and providing patients with support lines/organizations.

RAYNAUD PHENOMENON
Kelsey E. Phelps, MD

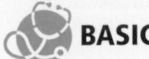 **BASICS**

DESCRIPTION
- Idiopathic intermittent episodes of vasoconstriction of digital arteries, precapillary arterioles, and cutaneous arteriovenous shunts in response to cold, emotional stress, or blunt trauma
  - A triphasic color change of the fingers (occasionally the toes, rarely nipples) is the principal physical manifestation.
    - The initial color is *white* from extreme pallor, then *blue* from cyanosis, and finally with warming/vasodilatation, the skin appears *red*.
    - Thumbs are rarely involved.
  - Swelling, throbbing, and paresthesias are associated symptoms.
  - Primary
    - 80% of patients have primary disease.
    - Episodes are bilateral and nonprogressive.
    - Diagnosis confirmed if after 2 years of symptoms no underlying connective tissue disease develops
  - Secondary
    - Progressive and asymmetric
    - Vascular spasm is more frequent and more severe over time. Ulceration is rare; gangrene does not develop; 13% progress to digital fat pad atrophy and ischemic fingertip changes.
    - Typically associated with an underlying connective tissue disorder
- System(s) affected: hematologic, lymphatic, immunologic, musculoskeletal, dermatologic, exocrine

Pregnancy Considerations
- Raynaud phenomenon can appear as breast pain in lactating women (1).
- Positive breast milk bacterial culture distinguishes mastitis from Raynaud phenomenon.

Geriatric Considerations
Initial appearance of Raynaud phenomenon after age 40 years suggests underlying connective tissue disease.

Pediatric Considerations
Associated with systemic lupus erythematosus (SLE) and scleroderma

EPIDEMIOLOGY
Incidence
- Primary
  - Predominant age: 14 years; ~1/4 begin >40 years
  - Predominant sex: female > male (4:1)
- Secondary
  - Predominant age: >40 years
  - Predominant sex: no gender predilection

Prevalence
- Primary: 3–12% of men; 6–20% of women (based on clinical history)
- Secondary: ~1% of population

ETIOLOGY AND PATHOPHYSIOLOGY
Unknown. Dysregulation of vascular control mechanisms leads to imbalance between vasodilation and vasoconstriction. There is a reduced endothelin-dependent vasodilation activity and an increased vasoconstriction in peripheral vessels by overproduction of endothelin-1. 5-HT_2 serotonin receptors may be involved in secondary Raynaud phenomenon. Platelet and blood viscosity abnormalities in secondary disease contribute to ischemic pathology.

Genetics
Some studies suggest dominant inheritance pattern. ~1/4 of patients with primary condition also have a first-degree relative with Raynaud phenomenon.

RISK FACTORS
- Existing autoimmune or connective tissue disorder
- End-stage renal disease with hemodialysis may increase risk if a steal phenomenon develops in association with the arterial-venous shunt.
- Primary and secondary disease associated with elevated homocysteine levels
- Smoking is not associated with increased risk of Raynaud phenomenon but may worsen symptoms.

GENERAL PREVENTION
- Avoid cold exposure.
- Tobacco cessation
- No relationship has been established between Raynaud phenomenon and vibratory tool use.

COMMONLY ASSOCIATED CONDITIONS
Secondary Raynaud
- Scleroderma; SLE; polymyositis
- Sjögren syndrome; occlusive vascular disease
- Cryoglobulinemia

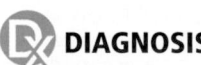 **DIAGNOSIS**

HISTORY
- Primary
  - Symmetric attacks involving fingers
  - Family history of connective tissue disorder
  - Absence of tissue necrosis, ulceration, or gangrene
  - If after ≥2 years of symptoms, no abnormal clinical or laboratory signs have developed, secondary disease is unlikely.
- Secondary
  - Onset typically after 40 years of age
  - Asymmetric episodes more intense and painful
  - Arthritis, myalgias, fever, dry eyes and/or mouth, rash, or cardiopulmonary symptoms
  - History of medication and/or recreational drug use
  - Exposure to toxic agents
  - Repetitive trauma

PHYSICAL EXAM
Pallor (whiteness) of fingertips with cold exposure, then cyanosis (blue) and then redness and pain with warming
- Ischemic attacks evidenced by demarcated or cyanotic skin limited to digits; usually starts on one digit and spreads symmetrically to remaining fingers of both hands. The thumb is typically spared.
- Rarely involves other tissues (e.g., tongue) (2,3)

- Beau lines: transverse linear depressions in nail plate on most or all fingernails that occurs after exposure to cold or any insult that disrupts normal nail growth
- Livedo reticularis: mottling of the skin of the arms and legs; benign and reverses with warming
- Primary
  - Normal physical exam
  - Nail bed capillaries have normal appearance: Place 1 drop of grade B immersion oil on skin at base of fingernail and view capillaries with handheld ophthalmoscope at 10 to 40 diopters.
- Secondary
  - Skin changes, arthritis, and abnormal lung findings suggest connective tissue disease.
  - Ischemic skin lesions: ulceration of finger pads (autoamputation in severe, prolonged cases)
  - Nail bed capillary distortion including giant loops, avascular areas, and increased tortuosity
  - Abnormal Allen test (Have patient open and close hand several times and then tightly into a fist. Sequentially occlude the ulnar and radial arteries while the patient opens hand to reveal the return of color as a measure of circulation.)

DIFFERENTIAL DIAGNOSIS
- Thromboangiitis obliterans (Buerger disease): primarily affects men; smoking related
- Rheumatoid arthritis (RA)
- Progressive systemic sclerosis (scleroderma): Raynaud phenomenon precedes other symptoms.
- SLE
- Carpal tunnel syndrome; thoracic outlet syndrome
- Hypothyroidism
- CREST syndrome (calcinosis cutis, Raynaud phenomenon, esophageal dysmotility, sclerodactyly, and telangiectasias)
- Cryoglobulinemia; Waldenström macroglobulinemia
- Acrocyanosis
- Polycythemia
- Occupational (e.g., especially from vibrating tools, masonry work, exposure to polyvinyl chloride)
- Drug induced (e.g., clonidine, ergotamine, methysergide, amphetamines, bromocriptine, bleomycin, vinblastine, cisplatin, cyclosporine)

DIAGNOSTIC TESTS & INTERPRETATION
Provocative test (e.g., ice water immersion) unnecessary
- Primary
  - Antinuclear antibody: negative
  - ESR: normal
- Secondary
  - Tests for secondary causes (e.g., CBC, ESR)
  - Positive autoantibody has low positive predictive value for connective tissue disease (30%).
  - Antibodies to specific autoantigens (e.g., scleroderma with anticentromere or anti-topoisomerase antibodies)
  - Videocapillaroscopy is gold standard (200 times magnification).

Follow-Up Tests & Special Considerations
Periodic assessments for a connective tissue disorder

Diagnostic Procedures/Other
Diagnosis is determined by history and physical exam.

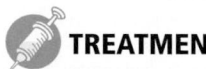 **TREATMENT**

Assess using a Raynaud Condition Score.

GENERAL MEASURES
- Dress warmly, wear gloves, avoid cold temperatures.
- During attacks, rotate the arms in a windmill pattern or place the hands under warm water or in a warm body fold to alleviate symptoms.
- Tobacco cessation
- Avoid β-blockers, amphetamines, ergot alkaloids, and sumatriptan.
- Temperature-related biofeedback may help patients increase hand temperature. 1-year follow-up is no better than control.
- Finger guards to protect ulcerated fingertips

MEDICATION
First Line
- Calcium channel blockers (CCBs). Nifedipine is the best studied and most frequently used.
- Nifedipine: 30 to 180 mg/day (sustained-release form); seasonal (winter) use is effective with up to 75% of patients experiencing improvement.
- Compatible with breastfeeding
- Contraindications: allergy to drug, pregnancy, CHF
- Precautions: may cause headache, dizziness, light-headedness, edema, or hypotension
- Significant possible interactions
  – Increases serum level of digoxin

Second Line
- Amlodipine (5 to 10 mg/day) and nicardipine are effective and may have fewer adverse effects.
- No data exist to support switching CCB if initial drug is ineffective.
- Small studies support benefit from losartan and fluoxetine.
- Phosphodiesterase type-5 inhibitors (sildenafil, vardenafil) may reduce symptoms without increasing blood flow.
- Parenteral iloprost, a prostacyclin, in low doses (0.5 ng/kg/min over 6 hours), has improved ulcerations with severe Raynaud phenomenon when CCBs failed. Oral prostacyclin has not proven useful.
- Nitroglycerin patches may be helpful, but use is limited by the incidence of severe headache. Nitroglycerin gel has shown promise as a topical therapy.
- Topical sildenafil cream may also improve digital arterial blood flow in patients with secondary Raynaud phenomenon (4).
- Prazosin (1 to 2 mg TID) is the only well-studied α₁-adrenergic receptor blocker with modest effect; adverse effects may outweigh any benefit.
- ACE inhibitors are no longer recommended.

ISSUES FOR REFERRAL
If an underlying disease is suspected, consider rheumatology consultation for evaluation and treatment.

ADDITIONAL THERAPIES
- Botulinum toxin somewhat effective in reducing vasospastic episodes, frequency of attacks, rest pain, and helping to promote digital ulcer healing (5)[C]
- Aspirin
- Digital or wrist block with lidocaine or bupivacaine (without epinephrine) for pain control
- Short-term anticoagulation with heparin if persistent critical ischemia, evidence of large-artery occlusive disease, or both

SURGERY/OTHER PROCEDURES
Surgical intervention is rare in Raynaud phenomenon. Effect of cervical sympathectomy is transient; symptoms return in 1 to 2 years. Digital fat grafting is a novel modality that has shown improved symptomatology and evidence of measurably increased perfusion in several cases (6)[C].

COMPLEMENTARY & ALTERNATIVE MEDICINE
- *Ginkgo biloba* with unclear benefit (7)[B]
- Fish oil supplements may increase digital systolic pressure and time to onset of symptoms after exposure to cold; not proven in controlled trials
- Vitamin D supplementation led to improvement in self-reported symptoms in vitamin D–deficient patients with Raynaud phenomenon (8)[B].
- Evening primrose oil reduced severity of attacks in one study.
- Oral arginine is no better than placebo.
- Biofeedback is not helpful.

 ONGOING CARE

FOLLOW-UP RECOMMENDATIONS
Avoid exposure to cold; reassess for secondary causes.

Patient Monitoring
Manage fingertip ulcers and rapidly treat infection.

DIET
No special diet

PATIENT EDUCATION
- Tobacco cessation
- Avoid triggers (e.g., trauma, vibration, cold).
- Dress warmly; wear gloves.
- Warm hands when experiencing vasospasm.

PROGNOSIS
- Attacks may last from several minutes to a few hours.
- 2/3 of attacks resolve spontaneously.
- ~13% of Raynaud patients develop a secondary disorder, typically connective tissue diseases.

COMPLICATIONS
- Primary: very rare
- Secondary: gangrene, autoamputation of fingertips

REFERENCES
1. Barrett ME, Heller MM, Stone HF, et al. Raynaud phenomenon of the nipple in breastfeeding mothers: an underdiagnosed cause of nipple pain. *JAMA Dermatol*. 2013;149(3):300–306.
2. Lioger B, Diot E. Raynaud's phenomenon of the tongue: uncommon presentation of a classical sign. *QJM*. 2013;106(6):583–584.
3. Chatterjee S. Raynaud phenomenon causing lingual pallor and dysarthria. *CMAJ*. 2016;188(15):E396.
4. Wortsman X, Del Barrio-Díaz P, Meza-Romero R, et al. Nifedipine cream versus sildenafil cream for patients with secondary Raynaud syndrome: a randomized, double-blind, controlled pilot study. *J Am Acad Dermatol*. 2018;78(1):189–190.
5. Neumeister MW, Webb KN, Romanelli M. Minimally invasive treatment of Raynaud phenomenon: the role of botulinum type A. *Hand Clin*. 2014;30(1):17–24.
6. Bank J, Fuller SM, Henry GI, et al. Fat grafting to the hand in patients with Raynaud phenomenon: a novel therapeutic modality. *Plast Reconstr Surg*. 2014;133(5):1109–1118.
7. Bredie SJ, Jong MC. No significant effect of ginkgo biloba special extract EGb 761 in the treatment of primary Raynaud phenomenon: a randomized controlled trial. *J Cardiovasc Pharmacol*. 2012;59(3):215–221.
8. Hélou J, Moutran R, Maatouk I, et al. Raynaud's phenomenon and vitamin D. *Rheumatol Int*. 2013;33(3):751–755.

ADDITIONAL READING
Herrick AL. Evidence-based management of Raynaud's phenomenon. *Ther Adv Musculoskelet Dis*. 2017;9(12):317–329.

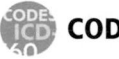 **SEE ALSO**

Algorithm: Raynaud Phenomenon

CODES
ICD10
- I73.00 Raynaud's syndrome without gangrene
- I73.01 Raynaud's syndrome with gangrene

CLINICAL PEARLS
- Raynaud phenomenon is a clinical diagnosis.
- Provocative testing is not recommended.
- Initial presentation of Raynaud phenomenon after age 40 years suggests underlying (secondary) disease.
- Raynaud phenomenon is a cause of breast pain in lactating women.
- Primary Raynaud phenomenon is symmetric; secondary Raynaud phenomenon is asymmetric.
- Primary Raynaud phenomenon is treated with hand warming and avoiding cold exposure.
- Digital ulcers are not normal and always merit a workup for secondary disease.
- Acute digital ischemia is a medical emergency.

REACTIVE ARTHRITIS (REITER SYNDROME)

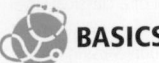

Douglas W. MacPherson, MD, MSc-CTM, FRCPC

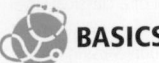 BASICS

Reiter syndrome is a seronegative, multisystem, inflammatory disorder classically involving joints, the eye, and the lower genitourinary (GU) tract. Axial joint (e.g., spine, sacroiliac joints) and dermatologic manifestations are common (1)[C].

DESCRIPTION
The classic triad includes arthritis, conjunctivitis/iritis, and either urethritis or cervicitis ("can't see; can't pee; can't bend my knee").

- The epidemiology is similar to other reactive arthritides, characterized by sterile joint inflammation associated with infections originating at nonarticular sites. A fourth feature (dermatologic involvement) may include buccal ulceration, balanitis, or a psoriasiform skin eruption. (Having only two features does not rule out the diagnosis.)
- Two forms of Reiter syndrome:
  - Sexually transmitted: Symptoms emerge 7 to 14 days after exposure to *Chlamydia trachomatis* and other sexually acquired pathogens.
  - Postenteric infection (including traveler's diarrhea)
- In individuals with new or frequent sexual partners, the triggering infection is likely sexually transmitted (rather than enteric).
- In individuals with a history of recent enteric illness, the triggering event is more likely to be a bacterial enteric infection than sexual transmission.
- System(s) affected: musculoskeletal, renal/urologic, dermatologic/exocrine
- Synonym(s): idiopathic blennorrheal arthritis; arthritis urethritica; urethro-oculo-synovial syndrome; Fiessinger-Leroy-Reiter disease; reactive arthritis

Pediatric Considerations
Juvenile rheumatoid arthritis (RA) has many of the same clinical features as Reiter syndrome.

Pregnancy Considerations
No special considerations; usual drug precautions

EPIDEMIOLOGY
Incidence
- Predominant age: 20 to 40 years
- Predominant sex: male > female
- 0.2–1% incidence after bacterial dysentery outbreaks
- Complicates 1–2% of nongonococcal urethritis cases

ETIOLOGY AND PATHOPHYSIOLOGY
- The pathophysiology of all the seronegative reactive arthritis syndromes and the immunologic role of infectious diseases as precipitants for clinical illness are incompletely understood.
- Avoiding precipitant infections and early management of multiorgan inflammation is important. Antibiotic treatment following onset of syndrome does not appear to benefit inflammatory joint, eye, or urinary tract symptoms.

- *C. trachomatis* is the most common sexually transmitted infection associated with Reiter syndrome.
- Dysentery-associated Reiter syndrome follows infection with *Shigella*, *Salmonella*, *Yersinia*, and *Campylobacter* spp. Enteric-associated Reiter syndrome is more common in women, children, and the elderly than the postvenereal form.

Genetics
HLA-B27 tissue antigen present in 60–80% of patients, suggesting a genetic predisposition

RISK FACTORS
- New or high-risk sexual contacts 7 to 14 days before the onset of clinical presentation; the primary infection may be subclinical and undiagnosed.
- Food poisoning or bacterial dysentery

GENERAL PREVENTION
- The immune-response characteristics of this syndrome make avoidance of infectious precipitants the most important general precaution (and potentially the most difficult to achieve).
- Safe sexual practices; proper food and water hygiene

COMMONLY ASSOCIATED CONDITIONS
- Enteric disease
  - Shigellosis; salmonellosis; campylobacteriosis
  - Enteric infection with *Yersinia* spp.
- Urogenital infection
  - *Chlamydia* urethritis/cervicitis (2)[C]
  - *Mycoplasma* or *Ureaplasma* spp.
- HIV/AIDS

DIAGNOSIS

- Clinical presentation with joint, eye, and GU inflammation ("classic triad") and negative serologic testing for rheumatoid factor
- Classic symptoms not always present
- HLA-B27 testing is not required for diagnosis.

HISTORY
The presence of the clinical syndrome plus
- Diarrhea, dysentery, urethritis, or genital discharge and appropriate exposure history
- Exposure risks, including travel or migration history and potential infectious exposure
- Arthritis associated with urethritis for >1 month (84% sensitive; 98% specific for diagnosis)
- Urethritis occurs 1 to 15 days after sexual exposure.
- Reiter syndrome onset within 10 to 30 days of either enteric infection or STI
- Mean duration of symptoms is 19 weeks.

PHYSICAL EXAM
- Musculoskeletal
  - Asymmetric arthritis (especially knees, ankles, and metatarsophalangeal joints)
  - Enthesopathy (inflammation at tendinous insertion into bone, such as plantar fasciitis, digital periostitis, and Achilles tendinitis)
  - Spondyloarthropathy (spine and sacroiliac joint involvement)

- Urogenital tract
  - Urethritis; prostatitis; cystitis (rare)
  - Balanitis
  - Cervicitis: usually asymptomatic
- Eye
  - Conjunctivitis of one or both eyes
  - Occasionally, scleritis, keratitis, and corneal ulceration
  - Rarely, uveitis and iritis
- Skin
  - Mucocutaneous lesions (small, painless superficial ulcers on oral mucosa, tongue, or glans penis)
  - Keratoderma blennorrhagica (hyperkeratotic skin lesions of palms and soles and around nails—can be mistaken for psoriasis)
- Cardiovascular: occasionally, pericarditis, murmur, conduction defects, and aortic incompetence
- Nervous system: rarely, peripheral neuropathy, cranial neuropathy, meningoencephalitis, and neuro-psychiatric changes
- Constitutional
  - Fever, malaise, anorexia, and weight loss
  - Patient can appear seriously ill (e.g., fever, rigors, tachycardia, and exquisitely tender joints).

DIFFERENTIAL DIAGNOSIS
- RA
- Ankylosing spondylitis
- Arthritis associated with inflammatory bowel disease
- Psoriatic arthritis
- Juvenile RA
- Bacterial arthritis, including gonococcal

DIAGNOSTIC TESTS & INTERPRETATION
- Blood
  - Negative rheumatoid factor
  - Leukocyte count: 10,000 to 20,000 cells/mm³
  - Neutrophil predominance
  - Elevated ESR and/or CRP
  - Moderate normochromic anemia
  - Hypergammaglobulinemia
- Synovial fluid
  - Leukocyte count: 1,000 to 8,000 cells/mm³
  - Bacterial culture negative
- Supportive tests
  - Cultures, antigens, or PCR positive for *C. trachomatis* or stool test positive for *Salmonella*, *Shigella*, *Yersinia*, or *Campylobacter* species
  - HIV serology positive (acute retroviral syndrome)
  - HLA-B27 positive (*not required for diagnosis*)
  - Drugs that may alter lab results: Antibiotics may affect isolation of the bacterial pathogens.
  - Rheumatoid factor is negative.
- X-ray
  - Periosteal proliferation, thickening
  - Articular bony spurs; erosions at articular margins
  - Residual joint destruction
  - Syndesmophytes (spine); sacroiliitis

Diagnostic Procedures/Other

HLA-B27 histocompatibility antigen: positive in 60–80% of cases in non–HIV-related Reiter syndrome; HLA testing is not required or recommended for diagnosis.

- Screen for STI if clinically indicated.
- Screening for enteric infections is rarely useful and generally not indicated.

Test Interpretation

- Seronegative spondyloarthropathy (similar to ankylosing spondylitis, enteric arthritis, and psoriatic arthritis)
- Villous formation within joints; hyperemia, and inflammation
- Prostatitis and seminal vesiculitis
- Skin biopsy similar to psoriasis

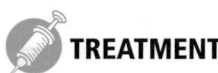 ## TREATMENT

GENERAL MEASURES

Treatment is determined by symptoms.

- Conjunctivitis does not require specific treatment.
- Iritis requires treatment.
- Mucocutaneous lesions do not require treatment.
- Physical therapy (PT) aids recovery.
- Arthritis may become prominent and disabling during the acute phase.

MEDICATION

First Line

- Symptomatic management: NSAIDs, including indomethacin, naproxen, and others; intra-articular or systemic corticosteroids for refractory arthritis and enteritis
  - Contraindications
    - ○ GI bleeding
    - ○ Peptic ulcer, gastritis, or ulcerative colitis
    - ○ Renal insufficiency
- Specific treatment of isolated microorganism (3)[A]:
  - *C. trachomatis*: doxycycline 100 mg PO BID for 7 to 14 days (Note: All STIs should be treated whether associated with Reiter syndrome or not.)
  - *Salmonella, Shigella, Yersinia,* and *Campylobacter* infections: ciprofloxacin 500 mg PO BID for 5 to 10 days (Note: Emerging antimicrobial resistance may limit the effectiveness of ciprofloxacin. Antibiotic treatment does not reduce GI symptoms or duration of infection or prevent carrier state.)
  - Trials of antibiotic treatment for reactive arthritis have produced mixed results, rendering the efficacy of antibiotics uncertain.
- GI upset: antacids
- Iritis: intraocular steroids
- Keratitis: topical steroids

Second Line

- Aspirin or other NSAIDs
- Sulfasalazine is promising but not FDA-approved.
- Methotrexate or azathioprine in severe cases (experimental, not approved or known to be effective); immunosuppressive therapy is relatively contraindicated in HIV-related Reiter syndrome.

- Specialty consultation is recommended, particularly if considering immunomodulatory agents such as sulfasalazine, methotrexate, or azathioprine or for treatment with anti-TNF medications (etanercept and infliximab) which have shown benefit in isolated case reports.
- Role of antibiotics under investigation—currently unproven effectiveness in seronegative arthritides
- No published evidence supports the beneficial effect of antibiotics on the long-term outcome in patients with Reiter syndrome.

ISSUES FOR REFERRAL

Joint and eye complications; complex cases—consider consultation with rheumatology; ophthalmology

ADMISSION, INPATIENT, AND NURSING CONSIDERATIONS

- Based on severity of disease and associated complications
- Inpatient care may be needed during acute phase.

 ## ONGOING CARE

FOLLOW-UP RECOMMENDATIONS

Activity modification until joint inflammation subsides

Patient Monitoring

Monitor clinical response to anti-inflammatory drugs. Observe for complications, particularly with sulfasalazine and immunosuppressive drugs.

PATIENT EDUCATION

- Educate on risk factors for exposure and recurrence.
- Home PT
- National Institute of Arthritis and Musculoskeletal and Skin Diseases: http://www.niams.nih.gov/

PROGNOSIS

Prognosis is poor in cases involving the heel, eye, or heart.

COMPLICATIONS

- Chronic or recurrent disease in 5–50% of patients
- Ankylosing spondylitis develops in 30–50% of patients who test positive for HLA-B27 antigen.
- Urethral strictures
- Cataracts and blindness
- Aortic root necrosis

REFERENCES

1. Selmi C, Gershwin ME. Diagnosis and classification of reactive arthritis. *Autoimmun Rev.* 2014;13(4–5):546–549.
2. Zeidler H, Hudson AP. New insights into *Chlamydia* and arthritis. Promise of a cure? *Ann Rheum Dis.* 2014;73(4):637–644.
3. Barber CE, Kim J, Inman RD, et al. Antibiotics for treatment of reactive arthritis: a systematic review and metaanalysis. *J Rheumatol.* 2013;40(6):916–928.

ADDITIONAL READING

- Boring MA, Hootman JM, Liu Y, et al. Prevalence of arthritis and arthritis-attributable activity limitation by urban-rural county classification—United States, 2015. *MMWR Morb Mortal Wkly Rep.* 2017;66(20):527–532.
- Carter JD, Inman RD. Chlamydia-induced reactive arthritis: hidden in plain sight? *Best Pract Res Clin Rheumatol.* 2011;25(3):359–374.
- Contini C, Grilli A, Badia L, et al. Detection of *Chlamydophila pneumoniae* in patients with arthritis: significance and diagnostic value. *Rheumatol Int.* 2011;31(10):1307–1313.
- Mathew AJ, Ravindran V. Infections and arthritis. *Best Pract Res Clin Rheumatol.* 2014;28(6):935–959.
- National Guideline Clearinghouse. British Association of Sexual Health and HIV (BASHH) United Kingdom national guideline on management of sexually acquired reactive arthritis. 2009:13596. http://www.bashh.org/BASHH/Guidelines/Guidelines/BASHH/Guidelines/Guidelines.aspx. Accessed August 21, 2015.

 ## SEE ALSO

Ankylosing Spondylitis; Arthritis, Psoriatic; Behçet Syndrome

CODES

ICD10

- M02.30 Reiter's disease, unspecified site
- M02.39 Reiter's disease, multiple sites

CLINICAL PEARLS

- Diagnosis of Reiter syndrome is based on the clinical presentation of the classic triad of joint, eye, and GU inflammation and negative serologic testing for rheumatoid factor (signs and symptoms may not all be present at the same time).
- Screen for STI (including HIV) if sexually acquired. Enteric studies are rarely clinically indicated.
- Refer patients with a chronic or recurrent course and those who have clinical complications.

RENALTUBULAR ACIDOSIS

Jason Kurland, MD

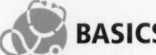 **BASICS**

DESCRIPTION

- Renal tubular acidosis (RTA) is composed of a group of disorders characterized by an inability of the kidney to resorb bicarbonate (HCO_3)/secrete hydrogen ions, resulting in normal anion gap metabolic acidosis. Renal function (glomerular filtration rate [GFR]) must be normal or near normal.
- Several types have been identified:
  - Type I (distal) RTA: inability of the distal tubule to acidify the urine due to impaired hydrogen ion secretion, increased back leak of secreted hydrogen ions, or impaired sodium reabsorption (interfering with the generation of negative luminal charge required for hydrogen/potassium secretion); urine pH >5.5
  - Type II (proximal) RTA: defect of the proximal tubule in HCO_3 reabsorption. Proximal tubular HCO_3 reabsorption is absent; plasma HCO_3 concentration stabilizes at 12 to 18 mEq/L due to compensatory distal HCO_3 reabsorption; urine pH <5.5 unless plasma HCO_3 brought above reabsorptive threshold
  - Type III RTA: extremely rare autosomal recessive syndrome due to carbonic anhydrase II deficiency; causes mixed type I and type II RTA, osteopetrosis, cerebral calcification, intellectual disability
  - Type IV RTA (hypoaldosteronism): due to aldosterone resistance/deficiency that results in hyperkalemia. Urine pH usually is <5.5.

EPIDEMIOLOGY

Incidence

- Predominant age: all ages
- Predominant sex: male > female (with regard to type II RTA with isolated defect in HCO_3 reabsorption)

ETIOLOGY AND PATHOPHYSIOLOGY

- Type I RTA
  - Autoimmune diseases: Sjögren syndrome, rheumatoid arthritis (RA), systemic lupus erythematosus (SLE), thyroiditis (1)
  - Medications: amphotericin B, lithium, ifosfamide, foscarnet, amiloride, triamterene, trimethoprim (2), pentamidine
  - Obstructive uropathy (hyperkalemic)
  - Genetic: autosomal dominant, autosomal recessive associated with sensorineural deafness
  - Sporadic
  - Other familial disorders: Ehlers-Danlos syndrome, glycogenosis type III, Fabry disease, Wilson disease
  - Hematologic diseases: sickle cell disease (hyperkalemic), hereditary elliptocytosis
  - Toxins: toluene, glue
  - Hypercalciuria, diseases causing nephrocalcinosis
  - Vitamin D intoxication
  - Medullary cystic disease
  - Hypergammaglobulinemic syndrome
  - Chronic pyelonephritis

- Chronic renal transplant rejection
- Leprosy
- Chronic active hepatitis, primary biliary cirrhosis
- Malnutrition
- Type II RTA
  - Multiple myeloma, other dysproteinemic states
  - Amyloidosis
  - Medications: acetazolamide, ifosfamide, tenofovir, sulfanilamide, outdated tetracycline, topiramate (3), aminoglycosides
  - Familial (cystinosis, tyrosinemia, hereditary fructose intolerance, galactosemia, glycogen storage disease type I, Wilson disease, Lowe syndrome, inherited carbonic anhydrase deficiency)
  - Sporadic
  - Heavy metal poisoning (e.g., cadmium, lead, mercury, copper)
  - Interstitial renal disease
  - Paroxysmal nocturnal hemoglobinuria
  - Defects in calcium metabolism (hyperparathyroidism)
- Type IV RTA (4)
  - Medications: NSAIDs, ACE inhibitors, ARBs, heparin/LMW heparin (hyperkalemia in 5–10% of patients), ketoconazole, tacrolimus, cyclosporine, spironolactone, eplerenone
  - Diabetic nephropathy
  - Tubulointerstitial nephropathies
  - Primary adrenal insufficiency
  - Markedly decreased distal Na^+ delivery
  - Pseudohypoaldosteronism (PHA) (end-organ resistance to aldosterone)
    - PHA type 1
    - PHA type 2 (Gordon syndrome)

Genetics

- Type I RTA: hereditary forms due to mutations affecting intercalated cells in collecting tubules (5). May occur in association with other genetic diseases (e.g., Ehlers-Danlos syndrome, hereditary elliptocytosis, or sickle cell nephropathy). The autosomal recessive form is associated with sensorineural deafness.
- Type II RTA: Autosomal dominant form is rare. Autosomal recessive form is associated with ophthalmologic abnormalities and intellectual disability; occurs in Fanconi syndrome, which is associated with several genetic diseases (e.g., cystinosis, Wilson disease, tyrosinemia, hereditary fructose intolerance, Lowe syndrome, galactosemia, glycogen storage disease, metachromatic leukodystrophy)
- Type IV RTA: Some cases are familial, such as PHA type I (autosomal dominant).

GENERAL PREVENTION

Careful use/avoidance of causative agents

COMMONLY ASSOCIATED CONDITIONS

- Type I RTA in children: hypercalciuria leading to rickets, nephrocalcinosis
- Type I RTA in adults: autoimmune diseases (Sjögren syndrome, RA, SLE), obstructive uropathy, hypercalciuria

- Type II RTA: Fanconi syndrome (generalized proximal tubular dysfunction resulting in glycosuria, aminoaciduria, hyperuricosuria, phosphaturia, bicarbonaturia)
- Type II RTA in adults: multiple myeloma, carbonic anhydrase inhibitors, aminoglycosides
- Type IV RTA: diabetic nephropathy, solid-organ transplant (due to calcineurin inhibitors)

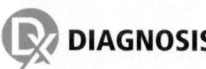 **DIAGNOSIS**

HISTORY

- Often asymptomatic (particularly type IV)
- In children: failure to thrive, rickets
- Anorexia, nausea/vomiting, constipation
- Weakness or polyuria (due to hypokalemia)
- Polydipsia
- Osteomalacia in adults

DIFFERENTIAL DIAGNOSIS

- Plasma anion gap should be normal. If not, evaluate for causes of anion-gap metabolic acidosis: ketoacidosis, ingestions (ASA, methanol, ethylene glycol, propylene glycol), lactic acidosis, D-lactic acidosis, uremia, pyroglutamic acid.
- Extrarenal HCO_3 losses
  - Diarrhea
  - Small bowel, pancreatic, or biliary fistulas
  - Urinary diversion (e.g., ureterosigmoidostomy, ileal conduit)
- Acidosis of chronic renal failure (develops when GFR ≤20 to 30 mL/min)
- Excessive administration of acid load via chloride salts, including dilutional acidosis via normal saline ($NaCl$, HCl, NH_4Cl, lysine HCl, $CaCl_2$, $MgCl_2$)

DIAGNOSTIC TESTS & INTERPRETATION

- Electrolytes reveal hyperchloremic metabolic acidosis.
- Plasma anion gap normal (anion gap = Na − [Cl + HCO_3]). Normal values (in mEq/L) depend on analyzer used: infants/children 5 to 15; adolescents/adults 4 to 12; must increase calculated anion gap by 2.5 mEq/L for each 1 g/dL decrease in albumin <4 g/dL (3)[B]
- Plasma K^+: low in type I (if due to impaired distal H^+ secretion/increased H^+ back leak), type II; high in type IV, type I (if due to impaired distal Na^+ reabsorption)
- Plasma HCO_3 (in untreated RTA): type I: <10 to 20 mEq/L; type II: 12 to 18 mEq/L (1); type IV: >17 mEq/L
- BUN/Cr normal or near normal (rules out renal failure as cause of acidosis)
- Urinalysis: urine pH inappropriately alkaline (>5.5) despite metabolic acidosis in type I; also in type II if HCO_3 above reabsorptive threshold (12 to 18 mEq/L)
- Urine culture: Rule out UTI with urea-splitting organism (may elevate pH) and chronic infection.

- Urine anion gap (UAG; urine $[Na^+ + K^+] - Cl^-$ on a random specimen): reflects unmeasured urine anions, so inversely related to urine NH_4^+ (or acid) excretion. Positive UAG in an acidemic patient indicates impaired renal acid excretion. Urine Na^+ >25 mEq/L required for accurate interpretation of UAG; results tend to be
  – Negative in HCO_3 losses due to diarrhea, UTI caused by urea-splitting organisms, and other extrarenal causes of nonanion gap metabolic acidosis
  – Variable in type II RTA
  – Positive in type I RTA, type IV RTA
  – Positive in impaired acid excretion due to renal failure
- Urine calcium
  – High in type I
  – Typically normal in type II
- Drugs that may alter lab results
  – Diuretics
  – Sodium bicarbonate (and other alkali)
  – Cholestyramine

Initial Tests (lab, imaging)
Serum electrolytes; urinalysis; urine sodium, urine potassium, urine chloride (to calculate UAG)

Diagnostic Procedures/Other
- Helpful to measure urine pH on fresh sample with pH meter for increased accuracy instead of dipstick. Pour film of oil over urine to avoid loss of CO_2 if pH cannot be measured quickly.
- Urine NH_4^+ excretion (Anion gap only provides a qualitative estimate.)
- Urinary acidification (impaired in type I RTA) can be assessed by oral administration of furosemide and fludrocortisone; patients with type I RTA unable to reduce urine pH to <5.3
- Fractional excretion of HCO_3 >15% during HCO_3 infusion (type II RTA) (1)

Test Interpretation
- Nephrocalcinosis
- Nephrolithiasis
- Rickets
- Osteomalacia, osteopenia
- Findings of an underlying disease causing RTA

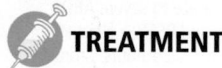

TREATMENT

MEDICATION
First Line
- Provide oral alkali to raise serum HCO_3 to normal. Start at a low dose and increase until HCO_3 is normal. Give as sodium bicarbonate (7.7 mEq $NaHCO_3$/650 mg tab), sodium citrate (oral solution, 1 mEq HCO_3 equivalent/mL), sodium/potassium citrate (oral solution), or potassium citrate (tablet, powder, or oral solution: 2 mEq K/mL, 2 mEq HCO_3/mL), depending on need for potassium.

- Type I RTA: Typical doses 1 to 2 mEq/kg/day (in adults), 3 to 4 mEq/kg/day (in children) HCO_3 equivalent divided 3 to 4 times per day (require much higher doses if HCO_3 wasting is present); may require K^+ supplementation (1)[C]
- Type II RTA: Typical doses 10 to 15 mEq/kg/day HCO_3 equivalent, divided 4 to 6 times per day. Very difficult to restore plasma HCO_3 to normal, as renal HCO_3 losses increase once plasma HCO_3 is corrected above resorptive threshold. Exogenous HCO_3 increases K^+ losses, requiring supplemental K^+. Often need supplemental PO_4 and vitamin D due to proximal PO_4 losses; may add thiazide diuretic to induce mild hypovolemia, which increases proximal Na^+/HCO_3^- reabsorption
- Type IV RTA: Avoid inciting medications; restrict dietary K^+. May augment K^+ excretion with loop diuretic, thiazide diuretic, or Kayexalate. Correcting hyperkalemia increases activity of the urea cycle, augmenting renal ammoniagenesis and adding substrate for renal acid excretion (1)[C]. If necessary, 1 to 5 mEq/kg/day alkali divided 2 to 3 times per day; if mineralocorticoid deficiency, fludrocortisone: 0.1 to 0.3 mg/day
- Precautions
  – Sodium-containing compounds will increase urinary calcium excretion, potentially increasing the risk of nephrolithiasis.
  – Mineralocorticoids and sodium-based alkali may lead to hypertension and/or edema.
  – Aluminum-containing medications (antacids, sucralfate) should be avoided if solutions containing citric acid are prescribed because citric acid increases aluminum absorption.
  – Sodium bicarbonate may cause flatulence because CO_2 is formed, whereas citrate is metabolized to HCO_3 in the liver, avoiding gas production.

Second Line
Thiazide diuretics may be used as adjunctive therapy in type II RTA (after maximal alkali replacement) but are likely to further increase urinary K^+ losses.

SURGERY/OTHER PROCEDURES
If distal RTA is due to obstructive uropathy, surgical intervention may be required.

ADMISSION, INPATIENT, AND NURSING CONSIDERATIONS
Generally managed as outpatient; inpatient if acidosis severe, patient unreliable, emesis persistent, or infant with severe failure to thrive

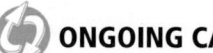

ONGOING CARE

FOLLOW-UP RECOMMENDATIONS
Patient Monitoring
- Electrolytes 1 to 2 weeks following initiation of therapy, monthly until serum HCO_3 corrected to desired range, and then as clinically indicated
- Monitor underlying disease as indicated.
- Poor compliance common due to 3 to 6 times per day alkali dosing schedule

DIET
Varies based on serum K^+ level and volume status

PATIENT EDUCATION
- National Kidney & Urologic Diseases Information Clearinghouse, Box NKUDIC, Bethesda, MD 20893, 301-468-6345: http://www.kidney.niddk.nih.gov/
- National Kidney Foundation: https://www.kidney.org/

PROGNOSIS
- Depends on associated disease; otherwise, good with therapy
- Transient forms of all types of RTA may occur.

COMPLICATIONS
- Nephrocalcinosis, nephrolithiasis (type I)
- Hypercalciuria (type I)
- Hypokalemia (type I, type II if given HCO_3)
- Hyperkalemia (type IV, some causes of type I)
- Osteomalacia (type II due to phosphate wasting), osteopenia (due to buffering of acid in bone)

REFERENCES
1. Reddy P. Clinical approach to renal tubular acidosis in adult patients. *Int J Clin Pract*. 2011;65(3): 350–360.
2. Weir MA, Juurlink DN, Gomes T, et al. Beta-blockers, trimethoprim-sulfamethoxazole, and the risk of hyperkalemia requiring hospitalization in the elderly: a nested case-control study. *Clin J Am Soc Nephrol*. 2010;5(9):1544–1551.
3. Liamis G, Milionis HJ, Elisaf M. Pharmacologically-induced metabolic acidosis: a review. *Drug Saf*. 2010;33(5):371–391.
4. Karet FE. Mechanisms in hyperkalemic renal tubular acidosis. *J Am Soc Nephrol*. 2009;20(2):251–254.
5. Batlle D, Haque SK. Genetic causes and mechanisms of distal renal tubular acidosis. *Nephrol Dial Transplant*. 2012;27(10):3691–3704.

 ## CODES

ICD10
N25.89 Oth disorders resulting from impaired renal tubular function

CLINICAL PEARLS
- Consider RTA in cases of normal anion gap metabolic acidosis with normal/near-normal renal function.
- Type I RTA: urine pH >5.5 in setting of acidemia; positive UAG; acidemia can be severe.
- Type II RTA: urine pH <5.5 unless HCO_3 raised above reabsorptive threshold (12 to 18 mEq/L)
- Type IV RTA: most common subtype; hyperkalemia; urine pH <5.5; acidemia usually mild
- Treatment includes avoidance of inciting causes, provision of oral alkali (HCO_3 or citrate), and measures to supplement (type II, many type I) or restrict (type IV) potassium.

Ahmed Munir, MBBS • Carrie Valenta, MD, FACP, FHM • Robert W. Plambeck, MD

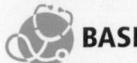 **BASICS**

DESCRIPTION

- Acute respiratory distress syndrome (ARDS) is defined as onset of acute hypoxemia within 7 days of known clinical insult or new or worsening respiratory symptoms. On imaging, it appears as bilateral opacities consistent with pulmonary edema not fully explained by effusions, lung collapse, or nodules. The respiratory failure is not explained by cardiac failure or fluid overload.
- Severity of ARDS depends on oxygenation of the blood. It is measured with ratio of partial pressure of arterial oxygen (PaO_2) to fraction of inspired oxygen (FiO_2) at positive end-expiratory pressure (PEEP) or continuous positive airway pressure (CPAP) of at least 5 cm H_2O.
  - Mild—200 mm Hg < PaO_2/FiO_2 ≤300 mm Hg
  - Moderate—100 mm Hg < PaO_2/FiO_2 ≤200 mm Hg
  - Severe—PaO_2/FiO_2 ≤100 mm Hg
- Synonym(s): acute lung injury; increased-permeability pulmonary edema; noncardiac pulmonary edema
- Systems affected: pulmonary, cardiovascular

EPIDEMIOLOGY

Incidence

Incidence of ARDS is very variable. Highest incidence rate was in United States of 78.9/100,000 person-years.

ETIOLOGY AND PATHOPHYSIOLOGY

- ARDS is a response to an injury to lung which can be direct or indirect.
  - Direct
    - Aspiration of gastric contents
    - Pneumonia (bacterial, viral, fungal, or opportunistic infections)
    - Air, fat, or amniotic fluid emboli
    - Near drowning
    - Pulmonary contusion
    - Inhalation injury
  - Indirect
    - Sepsis (nonpulmonary source)
    - Shock
    - Transfusion
    - Major burn injury
    - Nonthoracic trauma
    - Drug overdose
    - Pancreatitis, severe
    - Cardiopulmonary bypass
    - Reperfusion edema after lung transplant or embolectomy
    - Eclampsia
- Progression of ARDS is divided into three phases.
  - Exudative phase—it is the initial phase where alveolar macrophages are activated in high inflammatory stage due to lung injury which leads to complement activation, release of proinflammatory mediators, and activation of neutrophils. It causes epithelial–endothelial barrier disruption, leading to intra-alveolar and extra-alveolar flooding with fluid. It is followed by hyaline membrane formation leading to alveolar collapse.

- Proliferative phase—fibroblasts, myofibroblasts, and alveolar epithelial cell (ACE) II mediate repair in this phase. Formation of new matrix, differentiation into ACE I, and formation of cellular junctions begin which leads to expression of aquaporin and ion channels. These help in reabsorption of fluid.
- Fibrotic phase—not seen in everyone; related to prolonged mechanical ventilation and increased mortality

GENERAL PREVENTION

Good ICU practices like low tidal volumes in all mechanically ventilated patients, early resuscitation and antibiotics for sepsis, restrictive use of blood products, and intensivist involvement may help prevent nosocomial ARDS.

COMMONLY ASSOCIATED CONDITIONS

Pneumonia, sepsis, and aspiration of gastric contents lead to 85% cases of ARDS.

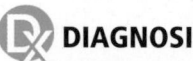 **DIAGNOSIS**

HISTORY

Precipitating event (see "Etiology and Pathophysiology") followed by abrupt onset of respiratory distress

PHYSICAL EXAM

- Tachypnea and tachycardia during the first 12 to 24 hours; increase in oxygen requirements
- Manifestations of underlying disease
- Decrease breath sound along with rales
- Absence of exam findings of cardiac failure

DIFFERENTIAL DIAGNOSIS

- Congestive heart failure
- Interstitial and airway diseases
- Hypersensitivity pneumonitis
- Endobronchial tuberculosis
- Diffuse alveolar hemorrhage
- Venoocclusive disease
- Mitral stenosis: intravascular volume overload
- Drug-induced lung disease especially vascular leak syndrome with immunotherapy

DIAGNOSTIC TESTS & INTERPRETATION

Initial Tests (lab, imaging)

- Arterial blood gases (ABGs) show evidence of severe hypoxemia.
- ECG: sinus tachycardia; nonspecific ST–T wave changes
- Chest x-ray (CXR): normal heart size; fluffy, bilateral infiltrates; air bronchograms common
- Chest CT scan: diffuse interstitial opacities

Follow-Up Tests & Special Considerations

- Serial blood gases and CXRs
- Decrease in oxygen requirements and improving respiratory status will indicate improvement.
- Different biomarkers are being studied to help identify subtypes of ARDS. In future, they may be in use to help guide therapy.

Diagnostic Procedures/Other

- Invasive monitoring of pulmonary artery wedge pressure (PAWP) has fallen out of favor after clinical trials have shown no increased benefit and more catheter-related complication (1)[A].

- Measuring esophageal pressure with a manometer to estimate pleural pressure allows for adjustment of PEEP to achieve a positive end-expiratory transpulmonary pressure gradient, an approach that is increasingly used in clinical care and especially useful in the morbidly obese (2)[C].

Test Interpretation

With introduction of Berlin criteria, using ABG to calculate PaO_2/FiO_2 and if it is <300 with radiologic evidence, after ruling out other causes of acute changes in respiratory status, we can diagnose ARDS.

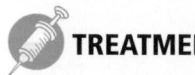 **TREATMENT**

GENERAL MEASURES

- Identify the cause of ARDS and treat the cause.
- Central venous line and arterial line insertion
- Ventilatory support generally requires endotracheal intubation and use of PEEP with lung protective ventilation.
- Using tidal volumes of 6 mL/kg of predicted body weight have shown decrease in mortality in comparison to higher volumes. For plateau pressure, the aim is to keep it below 30 cm H_2O (3)[A].
- Tidal volumes can be reduced to 4 mL/kg if plateau pressures exceed 30 cm H_2O (2)[A].
- Respiratory rate can be set to maintain adequate minute ventilation. Permissive hypercapnia allowed so long as pH >7.30 (3)[A]. Recent data supports lower respiratory rates (2)[C].
- No clear guideline for PEEP has been established. No clinical trial has shown consistent benefit of high PEEP. There is possible benefit of reduced mortality in subgroup of patients with moderate to severe ARDS with high PEEP (2)[C].
- In patients with early moderate to severe ARDS (PaO_2/FiO_2 <150 mm Hg), use of neuromuscular blockade with sedation compared with placebo resulted in decrease in mortality. This possibly prevents breath stacking and patient-ventilator dyssynchrony and increase efficacy of lung protective ventilation (4)[A].
- Also in patients with moderate to severe ARDS (PaO_2/FiO_2 <150 mm Hg and PEEP >5 cm H_2O) who had been intubated for <36 hours, prone positioning has shown decrease in mortality and early extubation in comparison to supine. In prone positioning group, patients were placed in prone position for 16 consecutive hours/day for up to 28 days or until PaO_2/FiO_2 ratio of ≥150 mm Hg, with a PEEP of ≤10 cm H_2O and an FiO_2 of ≤0.6 for >4 hours while in the supine position. The benefit of prone position is due to reduction in deleterious effects of positive pressure ventilation on nondependent and less injured airspaces (5)[A].
- Extracorporeal membrane oxygenation (ECMO) is reserved for severe ARDS after standard supportive measure have failed. One randomized controlled trial suggested improved mortality in properly selected individuals with ARDS referred to an ECMO center (2)[C].
- In patients with very severe ARDS (PaO_2/FiO_2 <80 mm Hg), the use of early ECMO versus conventional mechanical ventilation that included ECMO as a rescue therapy had no difference in 60-day mortality (6)[A].

MEDICATION

No single medication or combination of medications prevents or improves clinical outcomes in ARDS. Treatment is supportive while addressing the underlying cause.

ISSUES FOR REFERRAL

- All patients with ARDS should be cared for in an ICU with appropriately trained staff.
- Pregnant patients with ARDS also should be followed by a high-risk perinatologist or obstetrician.

ADDITIONAL THERAPIES

- For fluid management, central venous pressure (CVP) can be used to estimate fluid status. Liberal fluid management strategy targeting CVP of 10 to 14 cm H_2O was compared to conservative fluid management strategy targeting CVP of 4 cm H_2O. Conservation approach led to increased ventilator-free days and decreased stay in ICU with no change in mortality (1)[A].
- High-frequency oscillation ventilation showed increased mortality in a clinical trial, although a meta-analysis suggested some benefit when patients with PaO_2/FiO_2 <60 mm Hg (2)[C].
- Airway pressure release ventilation may improve oxygenation but no mortality benefit (2)[C].
- Noninvasive ventilation in patients with severe hypoxemia may increase the risk of ventilation-induced lung injury in ARDS (2)[C].
- Corticosteroids may improve airway pressures, oxygenation, and especially in pneumonia, infiltrates on radiography, but there is not a consistent mortality benefit in ARDS. There is likely potential harm when started later in course after 14 days (2)[C].
- Inhaled nitric oxide, surfactant, statins, nonsteroidal anti-inflammatory agents, antioxidants, albuterol, and neutrophil elastase inhibitor have not shown any benefit in clinical trials (2)[C].
- Clinical trials are underway for dexamethasone, vitamin D, aspirin, mesenchymal stem cells, and other therapies.
- Focus of research is now to identify different subtypes of ARDS and treat according to pathophysiology.

Pregnancy Considerations

Supportive care while identifying the underlying cause of ARDS continues to be important in the management of pregnant women with ARDS. However, fetal well-being, possible need for delivery, and physiologic changes associated with pregnancy must be considered.

ADMISSION, INPATIENT, AND NURSING CONSIDERATIONS

All patients with ARDS should be managed in an ICU setting.

- Lung protective ventilation while providing adequate PEEP
- Consider prone positioning and paralysis if PaO_2/FiO_2 <120 to 150 mm Hg.
- If failing initial supportive measures, consider early referral to an ECMO center.
- Monitoring blood gases especially after changing ventilator settings
- If perfusion is inadequate after restoration of intravascular volume (e.g., septic shock), vasopressor therapy is indicated.
- Early physical therapy

- Nursing may include any or all of the following:
  - Skin, eye, and mouth care
  - Deep vein thrombosis (DVT) prophylaxis
  - Stress ulcer prophylaxis
  - Suctioning of endotracheal tube
  - Adequate care while changing position of patient from supine to prone and vice versa
  - Ensure adequate level of sedation and/or paralysis while on mechanical ventilation.
  - Tracheostomy care
  - Explain all procedures to patient and family; reduce anxiety.
- Discharge criteria
  - Resolution or improvement of underlying precipitant, improving respiratory status, and return to baseline oxygen status
  - Nutrition counseling

 ONGOING CARE

FOLLOW-UP RECOMMENDATIONS

Patient Monitoring

- Driving pressure and static lung compliance are important measures of lung mechanics.
- Daily labs are needed until the patient is no longer critical.
- Daily CXRs are not needed but should be ordered when evaluating for endotracheal tube placement, the presence of progressing infiltrates, catheter placement, and complications of mechanical ventilation (e.g., air leaks).

DIET

For nutrition, trophic and full-calorie enteral nutrition have shown no difference in mortality, whereas early parenteral nutrition might be harmful (2)[C].

PATIENT EDUCATION

https://www.thoracic.org/patients/patient-resources/resources/acute-respiratory-distress-syndrome.pdf

PROGNOSIS

- Mortality rate is 40% with significant increase across the severity categories.
- Mortality is 34.9% in mild ARDS, 40.3% in moderate, and 46.1% in severe ARDS.

COMPLICATIONS

- Following are short-term complications:
  - Barotrauma
  - Nosocomial infection
  - Delirium
  - Catheter-related infection
  - DVT
  - Gastrointestinal bleeding due to stress ulcer
  - Poor nutrition
  - Multiple organ dysfunction syndrome
  - Death
- ARDS can have long-term complications which are not dependent on severity of ARDS but on age and comorbidities of patients.
- Following can be long-term sequelae:
  - Pulmonary dysfunction
  - Reduced health-related quality of life
  - Reticular pattern/ground glass opacities on radiographic imaging
  - Neuropsychological disability

REFERENCES

1. Wiedemann HP, Wheeler AP, Bernard GR, et al; for The National Heart, Lung, Blood Institute Acute Respiratory Distress Syndrome Clinical Trials Network. Comparison of two fluid-management strategies in acute lung injury. *N Engl J Med*. 2006;354(24):2564–2575.
2. Thompson BT, Chambers RC, Liu KD. Acute respiratory distress syndrome. *N Engl J Med*. 2017;377(6):562–572. doi:10.1056/NEJMra1608077.
3. Brower RG, Matthay MA, Morris A, et al; for Acute Respiratory Distress Syndrome Network. Ventilation with lower tidal volumes as compared with traditional tidal volumes for acute lung injury and the acute respiratory distress syndrome. *N Engl J Med*. 2000;342(18):1301–1308.
4. Papazian L, Forel JM, Gacouin A, et al; for ACURASYS Study Investigators. Neuromuscular blockers in early acute respiratory distress syndrome. *N Engl J Med*. 2010;363(12):1107–1116.
5. Guérin C, Reignier J, Richard JC, et al; for PROSEVA Study Group. Prone positioning in severe acute respiratory distress syndrome. *N Engl J Med*. 2013;368(23):2159–2168.
6. Combes A, Hajage D, Capellier G, et al; for EOLIA Trial Group, REVA, ECMONet. Extracorporeal membrane oxygenation for severe acute respiratory distress syndrome. *N Engl J Med*. 2018;378(21):1965–1975.

ADDITIONAL READING

- Chiumello D, Coppola S, Froio S, et al. What's next after ARDS: long-term outcomes. *Respir Care*. 2016;61(5):689–699.
- Matthay MA, McAuley DF, Ware LB. Clinical trials in acute respiratory distress syndrome: challenges and opportunities. *Lancet Respir Med*. 2017;5(6):524–534.
- Ranieri VM, Rubenfeld GD, Thompson BT, et al; and ARDS Definition Task Force. Acute respiratory distress syndrome: the Berlin definition. *JAMA*. 2012;307(23):2526–2533.
- Rezoagli E, Fumagalli R, Bellani G. Definition and epidemiology of acute respiratory distress syndrome. *Ann Transl Med*. 2017;5(14):282.

 CODES

ICD10
J80 Acute respiratory distress syndrome

CLINICAL PEARLS

- ARDS is onset of hypoxemia secondary to an injury to the lung which appears as bilateral infiltrates on imaging and divided in severity with measurement of PaO_2/FiO_2.
- Treatment is treating the cause along with lung protective approach to mechanical ventilation.
- Low tidal volume (6 mL/kg with plateau pressure 30 cm H_2O), adequate PEEP, and respiratory rate along with fluid conservative approach. Prone positioning and paralytics can be considered in PaO_2/FiO_2 <150 mm Hg.

RESPIRATORY DISTRESS SYNDROME, NEONATAL

Mary Cataletto, MD, FAAP, FCCP • Margaret J. McCormick, MS, RN, CNE

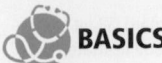 **BASICS**

DESCRIPTION
- Neonatal respiratory distress syndrome (NRDS) is a disorder primarily of prematurity manifest by respiratory distress.
- System(s) affected: respiratory
- Synonym(s): hyaline membrane disease; surfactant deficiency

ALERT
A disorder of the neonatal period

EPIDEMIOLOGY

Incidence
- >90% incidence in infants born ≤28 weeks' gestation
- Inversely proportional to gestational age
- Gender: slight male predominance
- Eighth leading cause of infant death in United States in 2013: 13.3 infant deaths per 100,000 live births (1)

ETIOLOGY AND PATHOPHYSIOLOGY
- Impaired surfactant synthesis and secretion
- High oxygen exposure and barotrauma can cause further damage to alveolar epithelium.

Genetics
No known genetic pattern

RISK FACTORS
- Premature birth
- Infants of diabetic mothers
- Perinatal asphyxia
- History of RDS in a sibling

GENERAL PREVENTION
- Prevention of premature birth:
  - Education
  - Regular prenatal care
  - Management of maternal medical conditions
- Promote healthy behaviors during pregnancy focusing on:
  - Diet
  - Exercise
  - Avoidance of exposure to tobacco smoke, alcohol, and illegal drugs
- Antenatal corticosteroids for women at risk for premature birth between 24 and 33 6/7 weeks' gestation including those with ruptured membranes and multiple gestations (2)[C]

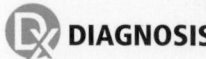 **DIAGNOSIS**

HISTORY
- Preterm neonates with worsening respiratory distress beginning at or shortly after birth and progressing over first few hours of life
- Early interventions can modify classic course.

PHYSICAL EXAM
- Tachypnea
- Grunting
- Nasal flaring
- Subcostal and intercostal retractions
- Decreased breath sounds
- Cyanosis

DIFFERENTIAL DIAGNOSIS
- Bacterial pneumonia
- Transient tachypnea of newborn
- Interstitial lung disease

DIAGNOSTIC TESTS & INTERPRETATION
- Arterial blood gases (ABGs)
  - Evaluate for evidence of acid–base abnormalities, hypoxemia, and hypercarbia.
- Chest x-ray (CXR):
  - Diffuse reticulogranular pattern (ground-glass appearance)
  - Air bronchograms
  - Low lung volumes

Diagnostic Procedures/Other
- Complete blood count
- Blood culture
- Echocardiogram: Consider if murmur is present to evaluate for patent ductus arteriosus (PDA) and contribution to lung disease due to L → R shunting.
- Lung pathology (autopsy findings)
  - Macroscopically: uniformly ruddy, airless appearance of lungs
  - Microscopically: diffuse atelectasis and hyaline membranes (eosinophilic and fibrinous membrane lining air spaces)

 **TREATMENT**

GENERAL MEASURES
- Supportive care:
  - Thermoneutral environment
  - Support ventilation and ensure adequate oxygenation (3)[C].
  - If no respiratory failure: early initiation of continuous positive airway pressure (CPAP) and consider surfactant therapy
- If respiratory failure: Intubate, ventilate as needed, and administer pulmonary surfactant.
  - Maintain adequate perfusion.
  - Optimize fluid and electrolyte balance (avoid overhydration).
  - Routine use of diuretics is not indicated.
  - Provide for nutritional needs.
  - Empiric antibiotic therapy with ampicillin and gentamicin pending evaluation of blood cultures
- Respiratory monitoring options
  - Noninvasive respiratory monitoring
    ○ Transcutaneous monitor or end tidal CO_2 monitor
    ○ Pulse oximetry
  - Invasive respiratory monitoring
    ○ Umbilical artery catheter placement for ABG sampling
    ○ Direct sampling of ABGs

MEDICATION
- Pulmonary surfactant (4)[A]
  - Poractant alfa (Curosurf)—porcine lung minced extract
  - Calfactant (Infasurf)—bovine lung lavage extract
  - Beractant (Survanta)—bovine lung minced extract
- Each surfactant has specific protocols for delivery; consult local standards.
- Side effects: bradycardia, hypotension, airway obstruction/endotracheal tube blockage with administration; rapid changes in tidal volume due to increased compliance can cause a pneumothorax and small risk of pulmonary hemorrhage.

- Precautions: Transient adverse effects seen with the administration of surfactant may require stopping administration and alleviating situation; may proceed with dosing when stable
- Contraindications: presence of congenital anomalies incompatible with life beyond neonatal period; infant with laboratory evidence of lung maturity

ISSUES FOR REFERRAL
Comorbid conditions associated with prematurity may require consultation during the course of the infant's NICU admission, including PDA (cardiology consult), necrotizing enterocolitis (NEC) (gastroenterology), retinopathy of prematurity (ROP) (ophthalmology), and so forth.

ADDITIONAL THERAPIES
Treat associated problems of prematurity.

ADMISSION, INPATIENT, AND NURSING CONSIDERATIONS
- All neonates with respiratory distress require immediate evaluation, monitoring, and treatment in the delivery room with transfer to a NICU.
- Supportive care
  - Thermoneutral environment
  - Respiratory monitoring
  - Establish relationship with family to provide education and emotional support.
- Discharge criteria
  - Should have stable vital signs and pulse oximetry before discharge
  - Medical home and support services should be in place.

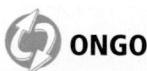 **ONGOING CARE**

FOLLOW-UP RECOMMENDATIONS
Following discharge, infants should be followed closely by their physicians to monitor growth and respiratory symptomatology.

DIET
As clinically indicated

PATIENT EDUCATION
- Educate parents regarding the risks in subsequent pregnancies.
- Advise parents regarding potential issues with chronic lung disease.

PROGNOSIS
- Prognosis and outcome are highly dependent on gestational age; significant neurodevelopmental delays in almost half infants ≤25 weeks' gestation (5)
- Survival rare in infants <25 weeks' gestation (6)

COMPLICATIONS
- Complications specific to NRDS
  - Pneumothorax
  - Chronic lung disease, bronchopulmonary dysplasia (BPD)
  - Pulmonary interstitial edema (PIE)
- Additional complications may occur related to therapeutic interventions and comorbid conditions.

REFERENCES
1. Kochanek KD, Murphy SL, Xu J, et al. Mortality in the United States, 2013. National Center for Health Statistics Data Brief No. 178. http://www.cdc.gov/nchs/data/databriefs/db178.pdf. Accessed October 13, 2016.
2. American College of Obstetricians and Gynecologists' Committee on Obstetric Practice, Society for Maternal–Fetal Medicine. Committee Opinion No. 677: antenatal corticosteroid therapy for fetal maturation. *Obstet Gynecol*. 2016;128(4):e187–e194.
3. Committee on Fetus and Newborn, American Academy of Pediatrics. Respiratory support in preterm infants at birth. *Pediatrics*. 2014;133(1):171–174.
4. Polin RA, Carlo WA; for Committee on Fetus and Newborn, American Academy of Pediatrics. Surfactant replacement therapy for preterm and term neonates with respiratory distress. *Pediatrics*. 2014;133(1):156–163.
5. Jarjour IT. Neurodevelopmental outcome after extreme prematurity: a review of the literature. *Pediatr Neurol*. 2015;52(2):143–152.
6. Ancel PY, Goffinet F, Kuhn P, et al. Survival and morbidity of preterm children born at 22 through 34 weeks' gestation in France in 2011: results of the EPIPAGE-2 cohort study. *JAMA Pediatr*. 2015;169(3):230–238.

ADDITIONAL READING
- Bell EF, Acarregui M. Restricted versus liberal water intake for preventing morbidity and mortality in preterm infants. *Cochrane Database Syst Rev*. 2014;(12):CD000503.
- Keszler M. Mechanical ventilation strategies. *Semin Fetal Neonatal Med*. 2017;22(4):267–274.
- Lemyre B, Laughon M, Bose C, et al. Early nasal intermittent positive pressure ventilation (NIPPV) versus early nasal continuous positive airway pressure (NCPAP) for preterm infants. *Cochrane Database Syst Rev*. 2016;(12):CD005384.
- Reiterer F, Schwaberger B, Freidl T, et al. Lung-protective ventilatory strategies in intubated preterm neonates with RDS. *Paediatr Respir Rev*. 2017;23:89–96.
- Roberts D, Brown J, Medley N, et al. Antenatal corticosteroids for accelerating fetal lung maturation for women at risk of preterm birth. *Cochrane Database Syst Rev*. 2017;(3):CD004454.

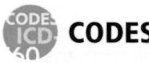 **CODES**

ICD10
P22.0 Respiratory distress syndrome of newborn

CLINICAL PEARLS
- Early treatment with CPAP or pulmonary surfactant can modify clinical course.
- Prognosis and outcome are highly dependent on gestational age.

RESPIRATORY SYNCYTIAL VIRUS (RSV) INFECTION

Alia A. Hussain, MD, BSc (Hons) • Sahil Mullick, MD

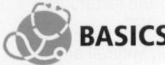 **BASICS**

Respiratory syncytial virus (RSV) is a medium-sized, membrane-bound RNA virus that causes acute respiratory tract illness in patients of all ages. The most clinically significant disease occurs in infants and children <3 years old.

DESCRIPTION
A major cause of upper respiratory tract infection (URTI) or lower respiratory tract infection (LRTI/bronchiolitis) illness
- In adults, RSV causes URTI.
- In infants and children, RSV causes URTI and LRTI (bronchiolitis and pneumonia-LRTI).

Pediatric Considerations
- 90–95% of children are infected by the age of 24 months; reinfection is common.
- Leading cause of pediatric bronchiolitis (50–90%)
- Premature infants are at increased risk for severe acute RSV infection.

EPIDEMIOLOGY
- Seasonality: Highest incidence of RSV in the United States occurs between December and March.
- Morbidity: RSV infection leads to >100,000 annual hospitalizations. In the United States, there are an estimated 2.1 million outpatient visits for RSV in children <5 years; the most hospitalizations are in the first 3 months of life.
- Mortality: Deaths associated with RSV are uncommon. Children with complex chronic conditions account for the majority of deaths, and the relative contribution of RSV infection to their deaths is unclear (1).

ETIOLOGY AND PATHOPHYSIOLOGY
- RSV-induced bronchiolitis causes acute inflammation, edema, and necrosis of small airway epithelium, air trapping, bronchospasm, and increased mucus production.
- RSV develops in the cytoplasm of infected cells and matures by budding from the plasma membrane.
- Infection spreads through droplets, (airborne or personal contact) that inoculate the nasal epithelium.

Genetics
- A genetic predisposition to severe RSV infections may be associated with polymorphisms in cytokine- and chemokine-related genes, including *CCR5*; *IL4*; *IL8*, *IL10*, and *IL13*.
- Infants with transplacentally acquired antibody against RSV are not fully protected against infection but may have milder symptoms.

RISK FACTORS
- Risk factors for severe disease
  - Prematurity
  - Age <12 weeks
  - Underlying cardiopulmonary disease
  - Immunodeficiency

- Other risk factors
  - Low socioeconomic status
  - Exposure to environmental air pollutants
  - Child care attendance
  - Severe neuromuscular disease
  - Adults: occupational exposure to young children, hospital staff, teachers, and daycare workers

GENERAL PREVENTION
- Hand hygiene is the most important step to prevent the spread of RSV.
  - Alcohol-based rubs are preferred. Hand washing with soap and water is acceptable but less effective (2)[B].
- Avoid passive smoke exposure, especially infants and children (3)[A].
- Isolate patients with proven or suspected RSV.
- Palivizumab (Synagis) is a monoclonal antibody directed against the fusion (F) protein of RSV.
  - Prophylactic use is indicated for infants and children <24 months of age with:
    ○ Chronic lung disease of prematurity requiring medical therapy within 6 months of the start of RSV season
    ○ Hemodynamically significant congenital heart disease
    ○ Congenital abnormalities of the airway or neuromuscular disease that compromises handling airway secretions
  - Infants born at ≤29 weeks' gestation if they are <12 months of age at the start of the RSV season; maintain prophylaxis through end of RSV season.
  - Infants born at 29 to 32 weeks' gestation if they are <6 months of age at the start of the RSV season; prophylaxis should be maintained through the end of the RSV season.
  - Infants born at 32 to 35 weeks' gestation who are <3 months of age at the start of the RSV season or who are born during the RSV season if they have one of the following two risk factors:
    ○ Infant attends child care.
    ○ ≥1 more siblings or other children <5 years of age living permanently in the child's household
- Dosage: maximum of 5 monthly doses beginning in November or December at 15 mg/kg per dose IM

COMMONLY ASSOCIATED CONDITIONS
- Asthma
- Otitis media
- Serious bacterial infection (SBI) in infants and children with concurrent RSV infection is rare.

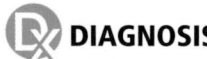 **DIAGNOSIS**

ALERT
In most cases, the diagnosis is clinical. Laboratory and radiologic studies are not routinely necessary (2)[B].

HISTORY
- Rhinorrhea and upper respiratory congestion
- Difficulty feeding in infants (due to respiratory effort)
- Increased respiratory rate or signs of increased work of breathing (grunting, flaring, retracting)
- Cough, fever, wheezing
- History of prematurity, secondhand tobacco smoke exposure, daycare, number and age of siblings
- Immunization history
- Family history of respiratory disease

PHYSICAL EXAM
- Vital signs: fever, signs of increased work of breathing (tachypnea, grunting, flaring, retracting), apnea, pulse rate (tachycardia >97% for age); pulse oximetry ("5th vital sign") to assess oxygenation
- Rhinorrhea
- Dry mucous membranes; skin turgor (dehydration)
- Serous otitis or acute otitis
- Pulmonary: wheezing, crackles

Pediatric Considerations
Young infants with bronchiolitis may develop apnea with increased risk of prolonged hospitalization, ICU admission, and mechanical ventilation.

DIFFERENTIAL DIAGNOSIS
- Mild illness/URTI
  - Other respiratory viral infections: rhinovirus, human metapneumovirus, influenza virus, human bocavirus
  - Allergic rhinitis
  - Sinusitis
- Severe illness/LRTI
  - Bronchiolitis
  - Asthma
  - Pneumonia
  - Foreign body aspiration

DIAGNOSTIC TESTS & INTERPRETATION
Initial Tests (lab, imaging)
- Routine testing/imaging is not necessary.
  - If obtained, WBC count normal or elevated
  - Virologic tests for RSV, despite high predictive value, rarely change management decisions or outcomes for patients with clinical bronchiolitis.
- Given the low risk of systemic bacterial infection, full septic workups are not necessary unless the child is toxic in appearance.
- Chest x-ray (CXR) does not predict disease severity or change patient outcomes but may help if a patient does not improve as expected, if the severity of the disease requires further investigation, or if another diagnosis is suspected.
- When obtained, typical CXR findings include:
  - Hyperinflation and peribronchiolar thickening
  - Atelectasis
  - Interstitial infiltrates
  - Segmental or lobar consolidation

TREATMENT

GENERAL MEASURES

- Assess hydration status and ability to take fluids orally. Treat dehydration (oral or IV/NG)—particularly in infants.
- Supplemental oxygen, often high flow nasal cannula, if pulse oximetry is persistently <90% in previously healthy patients

MEDICATION

First Line

No first-line medication for RSV infections; treatment is usually supportive; oxygen as needed

Second Line

- Bronchodilators do not improve oxygen saturation, reduce hospital admission after outpatient treatment, shorten the duration of hospitalization, or reduce the time to resolution of illness at home; routine use not recommended (2)[B]
- Nebulized epinephrine is superior to placebo for short-term outcomes in the outpatient setting, particularly in the first 24 hours.
- Glucocorticoids do not alter admissions or length of hospitalization (4)[A].
  - Some data suggest that the combination of dexamethasone and epinephrine may reduce outpatient admissions.
- Montelukast (Singulair) has no effect on the clinical course of acute bronchiolitis.
- Ribavirin, a nucleoside analogue and antiviral agent, has not been shown to be efficacious, particularly in immunocompromised patients.
- There is no current evidence that nebulized rhDNase changes clinical outcomes in children <24 months hospitalized with acute RSV bronchiolitis.
- Reserve antibiotic use for patients who have specific findings suggesting a coexisting SBI.
- Nebulized 3% or 7% saline may reduce the length of stay and improve the clinical severity score in infants hospitalized <3 days with acute viral bronchiolitis.
- Heliox therapy may significantly reduce a clinical respiratory distress score in the first hour after starting treatment for infants with acute bronchiolitis, but there is not a consistent reduction in the rate of intubation, emergency department discharge, or length of treatment for respiratory distress (4)[A].

ADDITIONAL THERAPIES

- Bulb suctioning of the nares may provide some comfort to infants and allow for easier feeding.
- RSV vaccine is under development (5)[C].

Pediatric Considerations

- Over-the-counter (OTC) cough and cold medications should not be used in children <6 years due to lack of efficacy and the risk of life-threatening side effects.
- Routine bronchodilators should not be used in bronchiolitis. Chest imaging should be avoided in children with uncomplicated bronchiolitis/asthma.

COMPLEMENTARY & ALTERNATIVE MEDICINE

No complementary, alternative, or integrative therapies are of proven benefit in the prevention or treatment of RSV bronchiolitis.

ADMISSION, INPATIENT, AND NURSING CONSIDERATIONS

- Clinical evaluation of respiratory status is critical. Ill-appearing infants should be hospitalized.
- Significant respiratory distress, an oxygen requirement to keep SpO$_2$ >90%, and the inability to hydrate orally are indications for admission.
- Mechanical ventilation is required in about 5% of infants hospitalized with RSV and 20% of children with underlying congenital heart disease, chronic lung disease, or immunosuppression.
- Universal precautions with gown and glove use are necessary to prevent nosocomial transmission of RSV. Airborne transmission is inefficient; masks/goggles are not necessary (6)[B].
- No set criteria for discharge; patients should be recovering and demonstrate:
  - Stable respiratory status with no oxygen requirement
  - Ability to maintain oral intake and hydration status
  - Home resources adequate to support necessary home therapies, including caretaker's ability to clear the infant's airway with bulb suctioning if needed
  - Adequate follow-up and patient education

ONGOING CARE

FOLLOW-UP RECOMMENDATIONS

Primary care follow-up to ensure resolution

PATIENT EDUCATION

- Bronchiolitis and Your Child: http://familydoctor.org/familydoctor/en/diseases-conditions/bronchiolitis.html
- Parent education—important to emphasize use of alcohol-based hand gels/wash and/or to wash hands with soap and water. Clean surfaces with gloves and avoid daycare/kindergarten during recovery.

PROGNOSIS

Most patients with RSV infection recover fully within 7 to 10 days. Reinfection is common.

COMPLICATIONS

- Infants hospitalized for RSV may be at increased risk for recurrent wheezing and reduced pulmonary function, particularly during the 1st decade of life.
- Overall mortality for infants and children <24 months of age is <1%.
- Although the relationship between RSV and asthma is unclear, RSV bronchiolitis in infancy has been linked to subsequent asthma.

REFERENCES

1. Byington CL, Wilkes J, Korgenski K, et al. Respiratory syncytial virus–associated mortality in hospitalized infants and young children. *Pediatrics*. 2015;135(1):e24–e31.
2. Ralston SL, Lieberthal AS, Meissner HC, et al; for American Academy of Pediatrics. Clinical practice guideline: the diagnosis, management, and prevention of bronchiolitis. *Pediatrics*. 2014;134(5):e1474–e1502.
3. DiFranza JR, Masaquel A, Barrett AM, et al. Systematic literature review assessing tobacco smoke exposure as a risk factor for serious respiratory syncytial virus disease among infants and young children. *BMC Pediatr*. 2012;12:81.
4. Liet JM, Ducruet T, Gupta V, et al. Heliox inhalation therapy for bronchiolitis in infants. *Cochrane Database Syst Rev*. 2015;(9):CD006915.
5. Poletti P, Merler S, Ajelli M, et al. Evaluating vaccination strategies for reducing infant respiratory syncytial virus infection in low-income settings. *BMC Med*. 2015;13:49.
6. Grayson SA, Griffiths PS, Perez MK, et al. Detection of airborne respiratory syncytial virus in a pediatric acute care clinic. *Pediatr Pulmonol*. 2017;52(5):684–688.

ADDITIONAL READING

- American Academy of Pediatrics. Respiratory syncytial virus. In: Pickering LK, Baker CJ, Kimberlin DW, et al, eds. *Red Book: 2012 Report of the Committee on Infectious Diseases*. 29th ed. Elk Grove Village, IL: American Academy of Pediatrics; 2012.
- Haynes AK, Prill MM, Iwane MK, et al; for the Centers for Disease Control and Prevention. Respiratory syncytial virus—United States, July 2012–June 2014. *MMWR Morb Mortal Wkly Rep*. 2014;63(48):1133–1136.
- Meissner HC. Viral bronchiolitis in children. *N Engl J Med*. 2016;374(1):62–72.

CODES

ICD10

- B97.4 Respiratory syncytial virus causing diseases classd elswhr
- J06.9 Acute upper respiratory infection, unspecified
- J21.0 Acute bronchiolitis due to respiratory syncytial virus

CLINICAL PEARLS

- RSV causes 50–90% of pediatric bronchiolitis.
- Hand sanitation (alcohol-based rubs are preferred) is the key to RSV prevention.
- The diagnosis of RSV is typically clinical. Routine laboratory or radiology studies are not necessary.
- Treatment of RSV is usually supportive.
- Palivizumab should be used to prevent RSV in high-risk patients.

RESTLESS LEGS SYNDROME

Denise Sharon, MD, PhD, FAASM • John R. Burk, MD, FACP

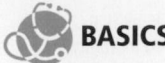 **BASICS**

DESCRIPTION
- Sensorimotor disorder consisting of a strong, nearly irresistible urge to move the limbs (1)[A]
- The urge usually affects the legs at least initially but may involve arms or other body parts (2)[C].
- The urge might be accompanied by uncomfortable and unpleasant sensations.
- The symptoms:
  - Begin or worsen during rest or inactivity
  - Are relieved by movement but recur with inactivity. Relief by movement may not be noticeable but has been previously reported.
  - Occur preferentially in the evening/night. Circadian aspect may not be noticeable but must have been previously reported.
  - Are not solely accounted for by "mimics" or another medical or behavioral condition
    ○ Mimics include leg cramps, positional discomfort, habitual foot tapping, arthralgias/arthritis, myalgias, leg edema, peripheral neuropathy, radiculopathy; even though some may coexist
  - Cause concern, distress, sleep disturbance
- Patient may also report involuntary leg jerks during wake or sleep (1)[A].
- System(s) affected: nervous; musculoskeletal
- Early, <45 years versus late >45 years onset (1)[A]
  - Early onset phenotype: 40–92% familial, stable, slow progression of symptoms
  - Late onset phenotype: more aggravating factors; rapid progression is common.
- Synonym(s): Willis-Ekbom disease

EPIDEMIOLOGY
Incidence
- 0.8–2.2% annually
- Onset at any age
- Predominant sex: male = female (nulliparous); parous females are twice more affected than males.
- Temperature (cold weather) and other environmental factors may increase incidence or trigger symptoms.

Prevalence
- 4–15% in Caucasian adults, underdiagnosed
- 2–3% are clinically significant.
- 1–3% in children and adolescents
- Increases with age up to 70s
- Lower in non-Caucasians (except Koreans)

Pregnancy Considerations
- 10–30% prevalence; triggers or exacerbates RLS
- Predictors: family history, past history, iron deficiency, Hgb ≤11 g/dL (3)[C]
- Peaks in 3rd trimester
- Most are relieved by 1-month postpartum.

ETIOLOGY AND PATHOPHYSIOLOGY
- Brain iron deficiency, impaired into brain iron transport
  - Iron deficiency and associated conditions
- CNS dopamine regulation:
  - Fast dopamine turnover consistent with increased dopamine production
  - Circadian changes in dopamine (increases in the evening)
  - Decreased dopamine transporter
- Genetics: heterogeneous
  - Susceptibility loci: 2p14, 2q, 6p21.2, 9p, 12q, 14q, 15q23, and 20p
  - Genes: MEIS1, MAP2K5/LBXCOR1, BTBD9

- Changes in substantia nigra, striatum, putamen (reduced iron, less myelin, less D_2 receptors)
- Sensorimotor pathways abnormalities:
  - Bilateral activation of the cerebellum and contralateral activation of the thalamus
  - Increased activation of the prefrontal and anterior cingulate cortex
  - Decreased gray matter volume which correlates with disease severity and duration
- Cortical excitability: increased thalamic glutamate
- Increased endogenous opioids, possibly
- Triggering and exacerbating factors:
  - Prolonged immobility, such hospitalizations
  - Medications:
    ○ Most antidepressants (except bupropion)
    ○ Dopamine-blocking antiemetics (e.g., metoclopramide, prochlorperazine)
    ○ Some antiepileptic agents (e.g., phenytoin)
    ○ Phenothiazine antipsychotics (risperidone, clozapine, olanzapine, quetiapine) possible exception: aripiprazole (partial D_2 agonist)
    ○ Cognition-enhancing medication: donepezil
    ○ Theophylline and other xanthines
    ○ Antihistamines/over-the-counter (OTC) cold preparations (e.g., pseudoephedrine)
    ○ Adrenergics, stimulants
    ○ Anti-inflammatory medications

RISK FACTORS
- Iron deficiency
- Family history
- Increased with every pregnancy
- Chronic renal failure—11–58% affecting dialysis compliance
- Sleep deprivation, alcohol, caffeine—limited data

GENERAL PREVENTION
- Regular physical activity/exercise during the day, low impact such as stretches, leisure walks in the evening
- Adequate sleep; delay wake time if possible.
- Avoid caffeine, alcohol, nicotine mainly in the evening.
- Avoid use of medications that trigger RLS (4)[C].

COMMONLY ASSOCIATED CONDITIONS
- Periodic limb movements during sleep (PLMS), insomnia, sleep walking, delayed sleep phase
- Iron deficiency, renal disease/uremia/dialysis, gastric surgery, IBS, liver disease
- Parkinson disease, multiple sclerosis, peripheral neuropathy, Machado-Joseph disease, migraine
- Anxiety, depression, ADHD
- Cardiovascular disease, including coronary artery disease and stroke
- Venous insufficiency/peripheral vascular disease
- Pulmonary hypertension, lung transplantation, chronic obstructive pulmonary disease (COPD)
- Orthopedic problems, arthritis, fibromyalgia

DIAGNOSIS

- Clinical, depends on history, often "difficult to describe"
- All criteria must be met for RLS diagnosis (2)[C]:
  - An urge to move the legs, usually accompanied by or thought to be caused by uncomfortable and unpleasant sensations in the legs. The urge must:
    ○ Begin or worsen during periods of rest or inactivity such as lying down or sitting
    ○ Be partially or totally relieved by movement such as walking or stretching at least as long as the activity continues
    ○ Occur exclusively or predominantly in the evening or night rather than during the day

- The above features are not solely accounted for as symptoms of another medical or a behavioral condition.
- The symptoms of RLS cause concern/distress; sleep disturbance; or impairment in mental, physical, social, occupational, educational, behavioral, or other area of functioning.

HISTORY
- Signs/symptoms (see also "Description") (1)[A]
  - Painful in ~35% of patients
  - Example descriptions: burning, achy, itching, antsy, "can't get comfortable"
  - Urge to move may be the only "discomfort."
  - Some patients must get up and walk.
  - PLMS in ~80% of patients
  - Insomnia, fatigue, anxiety, depression
- Severity range: from rare, minor problem to daily life, to severe impact on quality of life

Pediatric Considerations
Symptoms described in child's own words and additional supportive findings (1,2)[A]:
- Insomnia or sleep disturbance
- RLS in immediate biologic relative
- PLMS

Geriatric Considerations
For diagnosis in the cognitively impaired
- Rubbing or kneading the legs in the evening
- Evening hyperactivity (foot tapping, pacing, fidgeting, tossing/turning in bed)

DIFFERENTIAL DIAGNOSIS
- Claudication: Movement does not relieve pain.
- Motor neuron disease fasciculation/tremor: no discomfort or circadian pattern
- Peripheral neuropathy: usually no circadian pattern; unresponsive to dopamine agonists (DAs)
- Dermatitis/pruritus: movement only to scratch; no circadian pattern
- Sleep-related leg cramps: isolated and very painful muscle contracture
- PLMD: no wakeful movements
- Sleep starts: isolated involuntary events
- Rhythmic movement sleep disorder: movement periodicity faster than RLS
- Growing pains: no urge to move or relief by movement
- ADHD: no sleep complaints or disorders

DIAGNOSTIC TESTS & INTERPRETATION
Assessment of serum iron stores: ferritin, transferrin saturation, iron-binding capacity, serum iron (see also "General Measures") (5)[C]

Diagnostic Procedures/Other
Sleep study helpful but not required
- Frequent, PLM during wake, prior to sleep
- Suggested immobilization test (SIT) or multiple SIT (m-SIT)
  - Conducted before or without nocturnal PSG
  - Patient attempts to sit still in bed for 1 hour (SIT) or four 1-hour periods, every 2 hours (m-SIT) while completing every 10 minutes a visual analogue scale (VAS) or m-SIT disturbance scale.
  - >40 movements per hour suggest RLS.

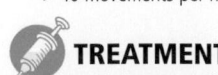 **TREATMENT**

GENERAL MEASURES
- If iron deficient, supplement (4)[C]:
  - 325 mg $FeSO_4$ TID combined with vitamin C
  - Repletion requires months till serum ferritin >75 ng/mL and transferrin saturation >16%.

- Daily exercise; avoid activities that exacerbate RLS.
- Avoid exacerbating factors and maintain regular sleep.
- Hot bath and leg massage (6)[C]
- Warm the legs (long socks, electric blanket).
- Intense mental activity (games, puzzles, etc.)
- Consider not initiating medications in mild to moderate cases until general measures are applied.

MEDICATION
- Titrate to minimum dose necessary to control symptoms, including sleep disturbance (consider weekly assessment rather than single day/dose).
- Assess symptom severity every encounter using a scale such as Johns Hopkins, IRLS, or sIRLS.
- Preferentially use longer acting or extended-release options (4,5,6)[C].
- Refractory RLS may require combination therapy.

First Line
- $\alpha 2\delta$ Ligands—less risk for augmentation and more effective in DA-naive patients (4,5,6)[C]:
  - Gabapentin enacarbil (Horizant): 300 to 1,200 mg every day ~5:00 PM (4,5)[C]
  - Pregabalin (Lyrica): 50 to 450 mg/day (off-label)
  - Gabapentin (Neurontin): 100 to 2,400 mg/day (off-label)
- DAs—assess for augmentation and impulse-control disorders (ICD) at every encounter (4,5,6)[C]:
  - Pramipexole (Mirapex): 0.125 to 0.500 mg 1 hour before symptoms; titrate by 0.125 mg; pramipexole ER 0.375 mg tablet
  - Ropinirole (Requip): 0.25 to 4.00 mg 1 hour before symptoms; titrate by 0.25 mg:
    ○ Ropinirole XL 2 mg tablet
  - Transdermal rotigotine (Neupro): 1 to 3 mg/24 hr patch; initiate with 1 mg/day; titrate by 1 mg/wk.
  - Avoid DAs in psychotic patients, particularly if taking dopamine antagonists.
- Add a different class of medication before exceeding DA-recommended dose.

Second Line
Off-label (4,5,6)[C]
- Iron: ferrous sulfate 325 mg 2 to 3/day PO + vitamin C 100 mg
- Ferric carboxymaltose 1,000 mg IV
- Benzodiazepines and agonists (for associated insomnia or anxiety)
  - Clonazepam (Klonopin): 0.5 to 3.0 mg/day
  - Temazepam, triazolam, alprazolam, zaleplon, zolpidem, and diazepam
- Other anticonvulsants (for comorbid neuropathy)
  - Carbamazepine: 200 to 800 mg/day
- Short-acting DAs for occasional symptoms:
  - Carbidopa and levodopa (Sinemet or Sinemet CR): 10/100 to 25/250; PRN

Pregnancy Considerations
- Initial approach: nonpharmacologic therapies, assess/correct iron deficiency
- Avoid medications class C or D.
- In 3rd trimester, may consider low-dose clonazepam, clonidine, or opioids (3)[B]

Pediatric Considerations
- First-line treatment: nonpharmacologic therapies, assess/correct iron deficiency
- Consider low-dose clonidine or clonazepam.

Geriatric Considerations
- Avoid medications that cause dizziness/unsteadiness.
- Many medications trigger/worsen RLS in the elderly.

ISSUES FOR REFERRAL
- Severe, intractable symptoms
- Augmentation response to dopaminergic therapy
- Intractable iron deficiency

ADDITIONAL THERAPIES
- Vitamin, mineral supplements: Ca, Mg, vitamin B_{12}, folate
- Clonidine: 0.05 to 0.10 mg/day
- Baclofen: 20 to 80 mg/day
- Prescription or OTC hypnotics

SURGERY/OTHER PROCEDURES
For orthopedic, neuropathic, or lower extremities vein disease (laser ablation, sclerotherapy, etc.)

COMPLEMENTARY & ALTERNATIVE MEDICINE
- Relaxis leg vibration device (FDA-approved)
- Sequential pneumatic leg compression
- Enhanced external counterpulsation
- Compression stockings
- Acupuncture
- MicroVas therapy

ADMISSION, INPATIENT, AND NURSING CONSIDERATIONS
- Prolonged hospitalization can trigger/worsen RLS.
- Addition of medications exacerbating RLS
- Withdrawal of medications treating RLS
- Control RLS especially after orthopedic procedures.
- Changes in medical status may require medication changes (e.g., Mirapex contraindicated in renal failure, Requip contraindicated in liver disease).
- Iron infusion when oral iron fails or contraindicated
- When NPO, consider IV opiates.
- Sleep interruption risks prolonged wakefulness.

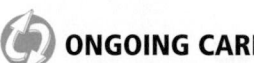 ONGOING CARE

FOLLOW-UP RECOMMENDATIONS
Patient Monitoring
- At 1- to 2-week intervals until stable and then annually
- If taking iron, reassess iron stores, at least ferritin.
- If status changes, assess for augmentation, ICD, associated conditions and medications.

DIET
Avoid caffeine and alcohol, mainly in the evening.

PATIENT EDUCATION
- Restless Legs Syndrome Foundation: www.rls.org
- National Sleep Foundation: https://www.sleepfoundation.org/
- American Academy of Sleep Medicine: http://sleepeducation.com/

PROGNOSIS
- Early onset: lifelong condition with no current cure
- Late onset/secondary: may subside with resolution of precipitating factors, otherwise chronic, progressive
- Current therapies usually control symptoms.

COMPLICATIONS
- Augmentation of symptoms following DA therapy to be assessed at every visit (5)[C]:
  - 4-hour time advance of symptoms or 2 to 4 hours advance of symptoms together with shorter latency at rest; symptoms spread to other body parts or have greater intensity.
  - Higher doses increase risk, and increasing the dose makes symptoms worse.
  - Highest risk from daily levodopa or Sinemet
  - Iron deficiency increases risk.
  - Discontinue DAs or add alternative medication and then slowly down-titrate DA.
- The potential for ICD/symptoms needs to be assessed at every visit in patients receiving DA (5)[C].
- Iatrogenic RLS (following blood loss or donation)

REFERENCES
1. Allen RP, Picchietti DL, Garcia-Borreguero D, et al. Restless legs syndrome/Willis-Ekbom disease diagnostic criteria: updated International Restless Legs Syndrome Study Group (IRLSSG) consensus criteria—history, rationale, description, and significance. *Sleep Med*. 2014;15(8):860–873.
2. American Academy of Sleep Medicine. Restless legs syndrome. In: *International Classification of Sleep Disorders*. 3rd ed. Darien, IL: American Academy of Sleep Medicine; 2014:281–291.
3. Picchietti DL, Hensley JG, Bainbridge JL, et al; for International Restless Legs Syndrome Study Group. Consensus clinical practice guidelines for the diagnosis and treatment of restless legs syndrome/Willis-Ekbom disease during pregnancy and lactation. *Sleep Med Rev*. 2015;22:64–77.
4. Garcia-Borreguero D, Silber MH, Winkelman JW, et al. Guidelines for the first-line treatment of restless legs syndrome/Willis-Ekbom disease, prevention and treatment of dopaminergic augmentation: a combined task force of the IRLSSG, EURLSSG, and the RLS-foundation. *Sleep Med*. 2016;21:1–11.
5. Trotti LM, Goldstein CA, Harrod CG, et al. Quality measures for the care of adult patients with restless legs syndrome. *J Clin Sleep Med*. 2015;11(3):293–310.
6. Sharon D. Nonpharmacologic management of restless legs syndrome (Willis-Ekbom disease): myths or science. *Sleep Med Clin*. 2015;10(3):263–278.

ADDITIONAL READING
- Garcia-Borreguero D, Cano-Pumarega I. New concepts in the management of restless legs syndrome. *BMJ*. 2017;356:j104.
- Sharon D, Allen RP, Martinez-Martin P, et al. Validation of the self-administered version of the International Restless Legs Syndrome Study Group severity rating scale—the sIRLS. *Sleep Med*. 2018;54:94–100.

 SEE ALSO

- Periodic Limb Movement Disorder (PLMD)
- International Restless Legs Syndrome Study Group: irlssg.org

 CODES

ICD10
G25.81 Restless legs syndrome

CLINICAL PEARLS
- Insomnia is often a symptom of RLS.
- RLS is associated with depression, anxiety ADHD.
- Antidepressants, antipsychotics, antiemetics, and antihistamines can trigger or exacerbate RLS.
- RLS symptoms may interfere with use of positive airway pressure in obstructive sleep apnea.
- Severity and improvement in symptoms can be monitored using a severity scale such as sIRLS, IRLS, or Johns Hopkins severity scale.
- Iron supplement is frequently the best, well-tolerated, easily available treatment for RLS.
- Titrate DAs only up to the minimum dose necessary to control symptoms.

RETINAL DETACHMENT
Richard W. Allinson, MD

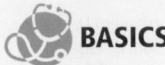

BASICS

DESCRIPTION
- Separation of the sensory retina from the underlying retinal pigment epithelium
- Rhegmatogenous retinal detachment (RRD): most common type; occurs when the fluid vitreous gains access to the subretinal space through a break in the retina (Greek *rhegma*, "rent")
- Exudative or serous detachment: occurs in the absence of a retinal break, usually in association with inflammation or a tumor
- Traction detachment: Vitreoretinal adhesions mechanically pull the retina from the retinal pigment epithelium. The most common cause is proliferative diabetic retinopathy.
- System(s) affected: nervous

EPIDEMIOLOGY
Incidence
- Predominant age: Incidence increases with age.
- Predominant sex: male > female (3:2)
- Per year: 1/10,000 in patients who have not had cataract surgery

Prevalence
After cataract surgery, 1–3% of patients will develop a retinal detachment.

ETIOLOGY AND PATHOPHYSIOLOGY
- Traction from a posterior vitreous detachment (PVD) causes most retinal tears. With aging, vitreous gel liquefies, leading to separation of the vitreous from the retina. The vitreous gel remains attached at the vitreous base, in the retinal periphery, resulting in vitreous traction that produces tears in the retinal periphery. There is an ~15% chance of developing a retinal tear from a PVD.
- PVD associated with vitreous hemorrhage has a high incidence of retinal tears.
- Exudative detachment
  - Tumors
  - Inflammatory diseases (Vogt-Koyanagi-Harada disease, posterior scleritis)
  - Miscellaneous (central serous retinopathy, uveal effusion syndrome, malignant hypertension, drugs—ipilimumab)
- Traction detachment
  - Proliferative diabetic retinopathy
  - Cicatricial retinopathy of prematurity
  - Proliferative sickle-cell retinopathy
- Penetrating trauma

Genetics
- Most cases are sporadic.
- There is an increased risk of RRD if a sibling has been affected by this condition. The risk increases with higher levels of myopia in the family history.

RISK FACTORS
- Myopia (>5 diopters)
- Aphakia or pseudophakia
  - In patients undergoing small-incision coaxial phacoemulsification with high myopia (axial length ≥26 mm), the incidence of retinal detachment is 2.7%.
- PVD and associated conditions (e.g., aphakia, inflammatory disease, and trauma)
- Trauma
- Retinal detachment in fellow eye
- Lattice degeneration: a vitreoretinal abnormality found in 6–10% of the general population

- Glaucoma: 4–7% of patients with retinal detachment have chronic open-angle glaucoma.
- Vitreoretinal tufts: Peripheral retinal tufts are caused by focal areas of vitreous traction.
- Meridional folds: Redundant retina usually is found in the supranasal quadrant.

GENERAL PREVENTION
Patients at risk for retinal detachment should have regular ophthalmologic exams.

Geriatric Considerations
- PVD
- Cataract surgery

Pediatric Considerations
Usually associated with underlying vitreoretinal disorders and/or retinopathy of prematurity

COMMONLY ASSOCIATED CONDITIONS
- Lattice degeneration
- High myopia
- Cataract surgery
- Glaucoma
- History of retinal detachment in the fellow eye
- Trauma

Pregnancy Considerations
Preeclampsia/eclampsia may be associated with exudative retinal detachment. No intervention is indicated, provided hypertension is controlled. Prognosis is usually good.

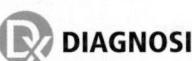

DIAGNOSIS

HISTORY
- Sudden flashes (photopsia)
- Shower of floaters
- Visual field loss: "curtain coming across vision"
- Central vision will be preserved if the macula is not detached.
- Poor visual acuity (20/200 or worse), with loss of central vision when macula is detached

PHYSICAL EXAM
- Slit-lamp exam
- Dilated fundus exam with binocular indirect ophthalmoscopy

DIFFERENTIAL DIAGNOSIS
Retinoschisis (splitting of the retina)
- Vitreous cells and vitreous hemorrhage are found rarely in the vitreous with retinoschisis, whereas they are seen commonly in RRD.
- Retinoschisis usually has a smooth surface and is dome shaped, whereas RRD often has a corrugated, irregular surface.

DIAGNOSTIC TESTS & INTERPRETATION
Visual field testing: differentiates RRD from retinoschisis. An absolute scotoma is seen in retinoschisis, whereas RRD causes a relative scotoma.

Initial Tests (lab, imaging)
- Ultrasound (US) can demonstrate a detached retina and may be helpful when the retina cannot be visualized directly (e.g., with cataracts or vitreous hemorrhage).
- Fluorescein dye leakage can be seen in exudative retinal detachment; caused by central serous retinopathy and other inflammatory conditions
- Optical coherence tomography (OCT)

Test Interpretation
- Elevation of the neurosensory retina from the underlying retinal pigment epithelium
- Elevation of retina associated with ≥1 retinal tears in RRD or elevation of the retina without tears in exudative detachment
- In 3–10% of patients with presumed RRD, no definite retinal break is found.
- Tenting of the retina without retinal tears in traction detachment
- Pigmented cells within the vitreous ("tobacco dust")

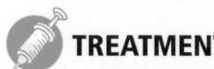

TREATMENT

GENERAL MEASURES
- Not all retinal tears or breaks need to be treated:
  - Flap or horseshoe tears in symptomatic patients (e.g., patients with flashes or floaters) are treated frequently.
  - Operculated holes in symptomatic patients are treated sometimes.
  - Atrophic holes in symptomatic patients are treated rarely.
- Lattice degeneration with or without holes within the lattice in an asymptomatic patient with prior retinal detachment in the fellow eye may be treated prophylactically.
- Flap retinal tears in asymptomatic patients frequently are treated prophylactically.
- Exudative detachments usually are managed by treating underlying disorder.
- Traction detachments usually are managed by observation. If the fovea is involved, a vitrectomy is needed.

MEDICATION
First Line
- Intraocular gases
  - Air
  - Perfluoropropane (C_3F_8)
  - Sulfur hexafluoride (SF_6)
- Perfluorocarbon liquids
- Silicone oil
- Contraindications to intraocular gas: patients with poorly controlled glaucoma
- Precautions with intraocular gas: Expanding intraocular gas bubble increases intraocular pressure; therefore, avoid higher altitudes.
- Significant possible interactions with intraocular gas: Nitrous oxide used in general anesthesia can expand an intraocular gas bubble.

Second Line
Steroids may cause worsening of central serous retinopathy.

SURGERY/OTHER PROCEDURES
- Timing of repairs
  - Macula attached: within 24 hours if possible. If the detachment is peripheral and does not have features suggestive of rapid progression (e.g., large and/or superior tears), repair can be performed within a few days.
    - Preoperative posturing consisting of bed rest and positioning is frequently prescribed to patients with macula-on retinal detachment. Preoperative posturing can reduce the progression of macula-on retinal detachments (1)[B].

- Macula recently detached: within 10 days of development of a macula-off retinal detachment (2)[B]
  - Old macular detachment: elective repair within 2 weeks
- If a retinal break has led to the development of a retinal detachment, surgery is needed. Surgical options (and combinations) include the following:
  - Demarcation laser treatment
  - Pneumatic retinopexy: Head positioning is required postoperatively.
  - Scleral buckle
  - Vitrectomy
  - Perfluorocarbon liquids for giant tears (circumferential tears ≥90 degrees)
  - Silicone oil for complex repairs
- Anesthesia: local or general
- RRD may have >1 break. If any retinal break is not closed at the time of surgery, the surgery will fail.
- Additional surgery may be required if the retina redetaches secondary to a new retinal break or because of proliferative vitreoretinopathy (PVR).
- If a vitreous hemorrhage is present, presumably from a retinal tear and the fundus cannot be well visualized, consideration can be given for early vitrectomy (3)[C].
  - Patients who underwent pars plana vitrectomy (PPV) within the 1st week of presentation had a significantly lower risk of having a macula-off RD.
  - Both phakic and pseudophakic patients had a similar chance of developing a retinal detachment. Phakic patients who underwent PPV had a higher chance of requiring subsequent cataract surgery.
- There is a trend toward primary vitrectomy in the management of RRD. Eyes undergoing PPV for primary RRD repair may not need the addition of a scleral buckle.
- There is no statistical difference in the primary reattachment rate between eyes treated with PPV and scleral buckle for RRD in both phakic and pseudophakic/aphakic eyes (4)[A].
- Patients with RRD who are at high risk for PVR (retinal detachment in two or more quadrants, retinal tears >1 clock hour, preoperative PVR, or vitreous hemorrhage). PPV + scleral buckle was associated with higher rates of anatomical success compared to PPV alone (5)[B].
- There is a reduced incidence of intraoperative retinal tear formation using a transconjunctival cannulated PPV system compared to the standard 20-gauge system requiring suture closure.

ADMISSION, INPATIENT, AND NURSING CONSIDERATIONS
- Recognition of condition is key (see "Diagnosis").
- Refer to an ophthalmologist for exam and treatment, if indicated.

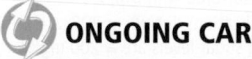 ONGOING CARE

FOLLOW-UP RECOMMENDATIONS
- Bed rest prior to surgery
- Postoperatively, if intraocular gas has been used, the patient may need specific head positioning and should not travel to high altitudes to avoid expanding the intraocular gas bubble.

Patient Monitoring
- Alert ophthalmologist if there is new onset of floaters or flashes, increase in floaters or flashes, sudden shower of floaters, curtain or shadow in the peripheral visual field, or reduced vision.

- Patients with acute symptomatic PVD should be reexamined by the ophthalmologist in 3 to 4 weeks. The development of a retinal detachment is unlikely if no retinal tears are present on reexamination in 3 to 4 weeks.
- If acute symptomatic PVD is associated with gross vitreous hemorrhage that interferes with complete visualization of the retinal periphery by indirect ophthalmoscopy, the patient should be reexamined at short intervals with indirect ophthalmoscopy until the entire retinal periphery can be observed. Early PPV can be considered.
- If the examiner is not certain whether the retina is detached in the presence of opaque medium, US should be performed.

DIET
NPO if surgery is imminent

PATIENT EDUCATION
American Academy of Ophthalmology, 655 E. Beach Street, San Francisco, CA 94109-1336

PROGNOSIS
- RRD
  - 90% of retinal detachments can be reattached successfully after ≥1 surgical procedure. Postoperative visual acuity depends primarily on the status of the macula preoperatively. Also important is the length of time between the detachment and the repair (75% of eyes with macular detachments of <1 week will obtain a final visual acuity of 20/70 or better).
  - 87% of eyes with a retinal detachment not involving the macula attain a visual acuity of 20/50 or better postoperatively. 37% of eyes with a detached macula preoperatively attain 20/50 or better vision postoperatively.
  - In 10–15% of successfully repaired retinal detachments not involving the macula preoperatively, visual acuity does not return to the preoperative level. This decrease is secondary to complications such as macular edema and macular pucker.
  - Failed primary pneumatic retinopexy selects for RDs that are inherently more difficult to reattach.
- Risk factors associated with primary RRD repair failure include choroidal detachment, significant hypotony, grade C-1 PVR, four detached quadrants, and large or giant retinal breaks. Additional risk factors associated with primary RRD repair failure include increased number of breaks and inferior location of retinal breaks.
- Tractional retinal detachment
  - When not involving the fovea, the patient usually can be observed because it is uncommon for these to extend into the fovea.
- Exudative retinal detachment
  - Management is usually nonsurgical.
  - The presence of shifting fluid is highly suggestive of an exudative retinal detachment. Fixed retinal folds, which are indicative of PVR, are seen rarely in exudative retinal detachment. If the underlying condition is treated, the prognosis generally is good.

COMPLICATIONS
- PVR is the most common cause of failed retinal detachment repair; 10–15% of retinas that reattach initially after retinal surgery will redetach subsequently, usually within 6 weeks, as a result of cellular proliferation and contraction on the retinal surface.

- Partial or total loss of vision due to macular detachment and/or PVR
- Moderate to severe forms of PVR usually are treated with PPV and fluid–gas exchange. If a segmental scleral buckle was placed at the initial procedure, it may need to be revised.
- Primary retinectomy can be used in cases of PVR without a scleral buckle (6)[C].
- Scleral buckles may erode the overlying conjunctiva and lead to an infection.
- Optic neuropathy after PPV for macula-sparing primary RRD

REFERENCES
1. de Jong JH, Vigueras-Guillén JP, Simon TC, et al. Preoperative posturing of patients with macula-on retinal detachment reduces progression toward the fovea. *Ophthalmology.* 2017;124(10): 1510–1522.
2. Hassan TS, Sarrafizadeh R, Ruby AJ, et al. The effect of duration of macular detachment on results after the scleral buckle repair of primary, macula-off retinal detachments. *Ophthalmology.* 2002;109(1):146–152.
3. Melamud A, Pham H, Stoumbos Z. Early vitrectomy for spontaneous, fundus-obscuring vitreous hemorrhage. *Am J Ophthalmol.* 2015;160(5): 1073–1077.e1.
4. Soni C, Hainsworth DP, Almony A. Surgical management of rhegmatogenous retinal detachment: a meta-analysis of randomized controlled trials. *Ophthalmology.* 2013;120(7):1440–1447.
5. Storey P, Alshareef R, Khuthaila M, et al. Pars plana vitrectomy and scleral buckle versus pars plana vitrectomy alone for patients with rhegmatogenous retinal detachment at high risk for proliferative vitreoretinopathy. *Retina.* 2014;34(10):1945–1951.
6. Tan HS, Mura M, Oberstein SY, et al. Primary retinectomy in proliferative vitreoretinopathy. *Am J Ophthalmol.* 2010;149(3):447–452.

 SEE ALSO

Retinopathy, Diabetic

 CODES

ICD10
- H33.001 Unspecified retinal detachment with retinal break, right eye
- H33.019 Retinal detachment with single break, unspecified eye
- H33.20 Serous retinal detachment, unspecified eye

CLINICAL PEARLS
- If a patient complains of the new onset of floaters or flashes of light, the patient should undergo a dilated eye exam to rule out a retinal tear or retinal detachment.
- There is an increased risk of retinal detachment after cataract surgery.
- PVR can result in redetachment of the retina after an initially successful repair.

RETINOPATHY, DIABETIC

Richard W. Allinson, MD

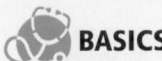 **BASICS**

DESCRIPTION
- Noninflammatory retinal disorder characterized by retinal capillary closure and microaneurysms. Retinal ischemia leads to release of a vasoproliferative factor, stimulating neovascularization (NV) on retina, optic nerve, or iris.
- Most patients with diabetes mellitus (DM) will develop diabetic retinopathy (DR). It is the leading cause of new cases of legal blindness among residents in the United States between the ages of 20 and 64 years.
- DR can be divided into three stages.
  - Nonproliferative (background)
  - Severe nonproliferative (preproliferative)
  - Proliferative
- System(s) affected: nervous

Geriatric Considerations
Prevalence will increase because population generally ages and patients with diabetes live longer.

Pregnancy Considerations
- Pregnancy can exacerbate condition.
- Pregnant diabetic women should be examined in 1st trimester and then every 3 months until delivery.

EPIDEMIOLOGY
Incidence
- Peak incidence of type 1, juvenile-onset DM is between the ages of 12 and 15 years. In type 1 DM (T1DM), there is β-cell destruction, leading to insulin deficiency.
- Peak incidence of type 2, adult-onset DM is between the ages of 50 and 70 years. Type 2 DM (T2DM) ranges from a condition characterized by insulin resistance with relative insulin deficiency to one that is predominantly an insulin secretory defect with insulin resistance.
- Incidence of DR is directly related to the duration of diabetes.
- <10 years of age, it is unusual to see DR, regardless of DM duration.

Prevalence
- 6.6% of the U.S. population between ages of 20 and 74 years has DM.
- ~25% of the diabetic population has some form of DR.
- Predominant age
  - Risk increases after puberty.
  - 2/3 of juvenile-onset diabetics who have had DM for at least 35 years will develop proliferative DR (PDR), and 1/3 will develop macular edema. Proportions are reversed for adult-onset diabetes.
- Predominant sex: male = female (type 1, juvenile-onset DM); female > male (type 2)

ETIOLOGY AND PATHOPHYSIOLOGY
- Related to development of diabetic microaneurysms and microvascular abnormalities
- Reduction in perifoveal capillary blood flow velocity, perifoveal capillary occlusion, and increased retinal thickness at the central fovea in diabetic patients are associated with visual impairment in patients with diabetic macular edema (DME).
- Vascular endothelial growth factor (VEGF) is elevated in patients with hypoxic retina. Intraocular levels of VEGF are elevated in patients with retinal or iris NV. Retinal hypoxia also contributes to DME, and VEGF is a major contributor to DME.

RISK FACTORS
- Duration of DM (usually >10 years)
- Poor glycemic control
- Pregnancy
- Renal disease
- Systemic hypertension (HTN)
- Smoking
- Elevated lipid levels associated with increased risk of retinal lipid deposits (hard exudates)
- Myopic eyes (eyes with longer axial length) have a lower risk of DR.

GENERAL PREVENTION
- See "General Measures."
- Monitor and control of blood glucose.
- Schedule yearly ophthalmologic eye exams.

COMMONLY ASSOCIATED CONDITIONS
- Glaucoma
- Cataracts
- Retinal detachment
- Vitreous hemorrhage (VH)
- Disc edema (diabetic papillopathy); may occur in T1DM and T2DM

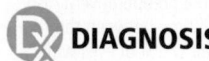 **DIAGNOSIS**

HISTORY
Diabetic patients should be encouraged to have an annual ophthalmologic exam because early eye changes may be asymptomatic.

PHYSICAL EXAM
- Eye exam: measurement of visual acuity and documentation of the status of the iris, lens, vitreous, and fundus
- Nonproliferative (background) DR
  - Microaneurysms
  - Intraretinal hemorrhage
  - Macular edema causing decrease in central vision
  - Lipid deposits
- Severe nonproliferative (preproliferative) DR
  - Nerve fiber layer infarctions ("cotton wool spots")
  - Venous beading
  - Venous dilatation
  - Intraretinal microvascular abnormalities (IRMA)
  - Extensive retinal hemorrhage
  - The Early Treatment Diabetic Retinopathy Study (ETDRS) developed the 4:2:1 rule for severe nonproliferative diabetic retinopathy (NPDR). Severe NPDR was defined as having any one of the following features:
    ○ Severe intraretinal hemorrhages and microaneurysms in four quadrants
    ○ Venous beading in two or more quadrants
    ○ IRMAs in one or more quadrants
- PDR
  - New blood vessel proliferation: NV on the retinal surface, optic nerve, and iris
  - Visual loss caused by VH, traction retinal detachment. NV can result in contraction of fibrovascular tissue on a vitreous scaffold, which can lead to VH and traction retinal detachment.

DIFFERENTIAL DIAGNOSIS
Other causes of retinopathy (e.g., radiation, retinal venous obstruction, HTN)

DIAGNOSTIC TESTS & INTERPRETATION
Diagnostic Procedures/Other
- Fluorescein angiography demonstrates retinal nonperfusion, retinal leakage, and PDR.
- Optical coherence tomography (OCT) can be used to help detect DME by measuring retinal thickness.
- Optical coherence tomography angiography (OCTA)
  - Poor responders to anti-VEGF treatment for DME show significant damage to the deep capillary plexuses (DCP) but not the superficial capillary plexuses (SCP). The extent of the DCP loss and the corresponding outer plexiform layer disruption as seen on spectral-domain OCT (SD OCT) could be useful predictors of responsiveness to anti-VEGF treatment.

Test Interpretation
- Increased capillary permeability
- Microaneurysms
- Hemorrhages in retina
- Exudates in retina
- Capillary nonperfusion

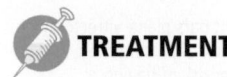 **TREATMENT**

GENERAL MEASURES
- The Diabetes Control and Complications Trial (DCCT) recommended that for most patients with insulin-dependent DM, blood glucose levels should be as close to the nondiabetic range as is safe to reduce the risk and rate of progression of DR.
  - In the DCCT, insulin-dependent DM patients were randomly assigned into either conventional or intensive insulin treatment. Conventional treatment consisted of 1 to 2 daily insulin injections, with daily self-monitoring of urine/blood glucose; intensive treatment consisted of insulin administered ≥3 times daily by injection/an external pump, with self-monitored blood glucose levels measured at least 4 times per day
  - The DCCT demonstrated that intensive insulin therapy reduced the risk of DME and retinal NV. The benefit of intensive insulin therapy with the reduced risk of DR-associated microvascular complications persists for at least 10 years.
- In the DCCT, intensive insulin therapy was more effective in reducing the risk of progression of DR in the less advanced stages. However, advanced DR also benefited from the intensive insulin therapy.
- Intensive therapy in patients with T1DM is associated with a substantial reduction in the long-term risk of ocular surgery.
- The ETDRS demonstrated that aspirin therapy did not prevent the development of PDR or reduce the risk of visual loss associated with DR.
- Microvascular complications, including PDR, are increased when blood sugar levels are ≥200 mg/dL.
- Cataracts are more common among those with DM. Try to delay cataract surgery in DM patients with retinopathy until the symptoms are more severe. Cataract surgery can cause retinopathy to worsen and increase the risk for development of DME.
- HTN has a detrimental effect on DR and must be controlled.

MEDICATION
- Treatment with the angiotensin-receptor blocker candesartan has been shown to result in regression of DR in some patients.

- Nutritional antioxidant intake of vitamins C and E and of β-carotene has no protective effect on DR.
- Atorvastatin may reduce the severity of lipid deposits with clinically significant diabetic macular edema (CSDME) in T2DM and dyslipidemia.
- Aspirin
  - Does not alter progression of DR
  - Does not increase the risk of VH

SURGERY/OTHER PROCEDURES

Treatment for DME

- Intravitreal anti-VEGF is first-line treatment for DME:
  - Ranibizumab, an antibody fragment that binds vascular VEGF, can be used to treat DME when injected intravitreally. Ranibizumab 0.3 mg given monthly resulted in improved vision and reduced central foveal thickness.
    - Anti-VEGF treatment results in superior clinical outcomes compared to laser photocoagulation for DME.
    - Intravitreal ranibizumab injections (IRIs) are beneficial for patients with DME and concurrent macular nonperfusion (1)[A].
    - IRI for DME may also improve DR severity and reduce the risk of DR progression.
    - Treat and extend dosing for IRI decreased the number of injections while giving similar visual and anatomic outcomes compared with monthly dosing at 1 year.
    - As-needed treatment after a loading dose of 3 monthly injections has been shown to result in comparable results to more frequent treatments.
  - Bevacizumab, a full-length antibody that binds VEGF, can be used to treat DME when injected intravitreally. This is an off-label use.
  - Aflibercept, a decoy receptor for VEGF that inhibits all isoforms of VEGF-A and placental growth factor. Aflibercept 2 mg (0.05 mL) injected intravitreally every 4 weeks for the first 5 injections followed by 2 mg (0.05 mL) intravitreally once every 8 weeks. It is indicated for patients with DME and for DR in patients with DME.
    - Intravitreal aflibercept injection (IAI) has demonstrated significant superiority in functional and anatomic end points over macular laser photocoagulation.
    - At worse levels of initial visual acuity (20/50 or worse) in patients with DME, IAI was more effective in improving vision than ranibizumab or bevacizumab with 1-year follow-up. When the initial vision loss was mild (20/32 to 20/40) in patients with DME, there was no significant difference between aflibercept, ranibizumab, and bevacizumab.
      - Aflibercept had superior 2-year visual acuity outcomes compared with bevacizumab. The superiority of aflibercept over ranibizumab, noted at 1 year, was no longer seen (2)[A].
    - As-needed IAI has been shown to maintain vision and reduce treatment frequency.
- Topical povidone-iodine prophylaxis is important to help prevent endophthalmitis from intravitreous injections from anti-VEGF treatment.
- Vitrectomy may benefit some with diffuse macular edema. This may apply especially to eyes with vitreomacular traction found on OCT and with persistent DME.
- Intravitreal triamcinolone may be used for DM-related macular edema that fails laser treatment; no long-term benefit of intravitreal triamcinolone relative to focal/grid photocoagulation in patients with DME

- Intraocular steroid implants for DME. Either a dexamethasone implant and a fluocinolone acetonide implant. Complications of these implants include cataract and glaucoma.
- Treatment for PDR:
  - Thermal laser photocoagulation in a panretinal pattern is the primary form of treatment for PDR. The goal of panretinal photocoagulation (PRP) is regression or involution of NV. PRP destroys ischemic retina and decreases the neovascular stimulus.
    - The Diabetic Retinopathy Study demonstrated that when PRP was used to treat PDR or severe NPDR, eyes treated with PRP had a reduction of 50% or more in the rates of severe vision loss compared with untreated control eyes. In certain subgroups, the incidence of severe visual loss in untreated eyes was as high as 36.9% at 2 years.
    - Patients with DME and high-risk proliferative disease can have simultaneous focal and PRP without adversely affecting the visual outcome.
- IRI is an alternative therapy to PRP for PDR, and both PRP and IRI are viable treatment options for patients with PDR (3)[B].
  - Treatment with IRI plus PRP may be more effective than PRP monotherapy for NV regression in patients with high-risk PDR (4)[B].
  - Intravitreal bevacizumab injection (IBI) may be of benefit in the treatment of VH due to PDR and may help to avoid the need for a pars plana vitrectomy (PPV) (5)[C].
- PPV recommended for patients with severe PDR, traction retinal detachment involving the macula, and nonclearing VH
  - The Diabetic Retinopathy Vitrectomy Study (DRVS) demonstrated the benefits of early PPV (1 to 6 months after onset of VH) in T1DM and for eyes with very severe PDR.
  - Immediate PPV with endolaser may be considered for PDR-associated VH (<30 days) (6)[C].
  - Preoperative bevacizumab can be used as an adjuvant to vitrectomy for complications of PDR. This is an off-label use.

 ONGOING CARE

FOLLOW-UP RECOMMENDATIONS

Patient Monitoring

Scheduled ophthalmologic eye exams

- Yearly follow-up if no retinopathy
- Every 6 months with background DR
- At least every 3 to 4 months with pre-PDR
- Every 2 to 3 months with active PDR
- Patients with DME should be followed every 4 to 6 weeks.
- Young people with either T1DM or T2DM are at risk for developing DR and need to have regular eye examinations.

DIET

- Follow prescribed diet for patients with diabetes.
- In middle-aged and older individuals with T2DM, intake of at least 500 mg/day of dietary long-chain omega-3 polyunsaturated fatty acids, achievable with 2 weekly servings of oily fish, is associated with a decreased risk of visual loss from DR.

PATIENT EDUCATION

- Advise regular ophthalmic exams.
- Stress importance of glucose control through diet, exercise, drugs/insulin.

PROGNOSIS

If the condition is diagnosed and treated early in development, outlook is good. If treatment is delayed, blindness may result.

COMPLICATIONS

- Repeated intravitreal injection of anti-VEGF therapy may increase the risk of sustained intraocular pressure elevation and the possible need for ocular hypotensive treatment.
- Blindness
- Patients with T2DM and DME or PDR have an increased risk of cardiovascular disease.

REFERENCES

1. Reddy RK, Pieramici DJ, Gune S, et al. Efficacy of ranibizumab in eyes with diabetic macular edema and macular nonperfusion in RIDE and RISE. *Ophthalmology.* 2018;125(10):1568–1574.
2. Wells JA, Glassman AR, Ayala AR, et al; for Diabetic Retinopathy Clinical Research Network. Aflibercept, bevacizumab, or ranibizumab for diabetic macular edema: two-year results from a comparative effectiveness randomized clinical trial. *Ophthalmology.* 2016;123(6):1351–1359.
3. Gross JG, Glassman AR, Liu D, et al; for Diabetic Retinopathy Clinical Research Network. Five-year outcomes of panretinal photocoagulation vs intravitreous ranibizumab for proliferative diabetic retinopathy: a randomized clinical trial. *JAMA Ophthalmol.* 2018;136(10):1138–1148.
4. Figueira J, Fletcher E, Massin P, et al; for EVICR.net Study Group. Ranibizumab plus panretinal photocoagulation versus panretinal photocoagulation alone for high-risk proliferative diabetic retinopathy (PROTEUS Study). *Ophthalmology.* 2018;125(5):691–700.
5. Parikh RN, Traband A, Kolomeyer AM, et al. Intravitreal bevacizumab for the treatment of vitreous hemorrhage due to proliferative diabetic retinopathy. *Am J Ophthalmol.* 2017;176: 194–202.
6. Fassbender JM, Ozkok A, Canter H, et al. A comparison of immediate and delayed vitrectomy for the management of vitreous hemorrhage due to proliferative diabetic retinopathy. *Ophthalmic Surg Lasers Imaging Retina.* 2016;47(1):35–41.

 SEE ALSO

Diabetes Mellitus, Type 1; Diabetes Mellitus, Type 2

CODES

ICD10

- E11.319 Type 2 diabetes mellitus with unspecified diabetic retinopathy without macular edema
- E10.319 Type 1 diabetes mellitus with unspecified diabetic retinopathy without macular edema
- E10.329 Type 1 diab w mild nonprlf diabetic rtnop w/o macular edema

CLINICAL PEARLS

Options for the treatment of diffuse macular edema include focal laser treatment, intravitreal triamcinolone, intravitreal ranibizumab, intravitreal bevacizumab, intravitreal aflibercept, intraocular steroid implants, and vitrectomy.

RH INCOMPATIBILITY
Kirsten A. Winnie, MD • Jennifer G. Chang, MD

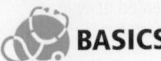

BASICS

DESCRIPTION
- Antibody-mediated destruction of red blood cells (RBCs) that bear Rh surface antigens in individuals who lack the antigens and have become isoimmunized (sensitized) to them
- System(s) affected: hematologic/lymphatic/immunologic
- Synonym(s): Rh isoimmunization; Rh alloimmunization; Rh sensitization

EPIDEMIOLOGY
Incidence
Predominantly affects fetuses/neonates of isoimmunized, childbearing females; varies by race and ethnicity

ETIOLOGY AND PATHOPHYSIOLOGY
- Circulating antibodies to Rh antigens (transplacentally transferred antibodies in the case of a fetus/newborn) attach to Rh antigens on RBCs.
- Immune-mediated destruction of RBCs leads to hemolysis, anemia, and increased bilirubin production.
- Transplacental fetomaternal hemorrhage (most common etiology) during pregnancy or at delivery
- Transfusion of Rh-positive blood to Rh-negative recipient; exposure to needles contaminated with Rh-positive blood
- Most commonly seen in the Rh-positive fetus of an Rh-negative mother

Genetics
- Complex autosomal inheritance of polypeptide Rh antigens; three genetic loci with closely related genes carry an assortment of alleles: Dd, Cc, and Ee.
- Individuals who express the D antigen (also called Rho or Rho[D]) are considered Rh positive. Individuals lacking the D antigen are Rh negative.
- Variant D alleles (weak D and partial D) are heterogeneous, altered forms of the D antigen. Some D variants are at risk of formation of anti-D antibodies, whereas others are not. With current blood typing procedures, certain D variants likely to produce alloimmunization are typed as D-negative, although this does not include all genetic subtypes at risk of isoimmunization.
- Another variant D antigen, DEL, has been identified in some individuals (predominantly Asians). Those with partial DEL expression are at risk for alloimmunization and should be considered clinically Rh negative. Women with complete DEL are not likely to be sensitized by exposure to Rh-D antigens through pregnancy or transfusion and should be considered clinically Rh positive and do not need RhD prophylaxis.
- Antibodies may be produced to C, c, D, E, or e in individuals lacking the specific antigen; only D is strongly immunogenic.
- Isoimmunization to Rh antigens in susceptible individuals is acquired, not inherited.

RISK FACTORS
- ~15% of the white population and smaller fractions of other races are Rh negative and susceptible to sensitization.
- Any Rh-positive pregnancy in an Rh-negative woman can result in sensitization.
- Weak D and partial D women are a heterogeneous group. Although previously reported to be Rh positive and treated as such, alloimmunization has been reported and can result in HDFN or fatal hydrops fetalis.
- Native risk of isoimmunization after Rh-positive pregnancy had been estimated at ≤15% but seems to be decreasing.
- The risk of isoimmunization antepartum is only 1–2%.
- The risk of isoimmunization is 1–2% after spontaneous abortion and 4–5% after induced abortion.
- Use of Rho(D) immunoglobulin prophylaxis has reduced incidence of isoimmunization to <1% of susceptible pregnancies (1).

GENERAL PREVENTION
- Blood typing (ABO and Rh) on all pregnant women and prior to blood transfusions
- Antibody screening early in pregnancy
- Rh immunoglobulin prevents only sensitization to the D antigen.
- For prophylaxis, Rho(D) immunoglobulin (RhIG, RhoGAM, HyperRHO, Rhophylac) given to unsensitized, Rh-negative women after the following:
  - Spontaneous abortion
  - Induced abortion
  - Ectopic pregnancy
  - Antepartum hemorrhage
  - Trauma to abdomen
  - Amniocentesis
  - Chorionic villus sampling
  - Within 72 hours of delivery of an Rh-positive infant
  - Given routinely at 28 weeks' gestation
- Prophylaxis is to prevent sensitization affecting a subsequent pregnancy and has little effect on the current pregnancy.
- Dose for prophylaxis
  - 50-μg dose for events up to 12 weeks' gestation
  - 300-μg dose for events after 12 weeks' gestation
  - Higher doses may be required in the event of a large fetal–maternal hemorrhage (>30 mL of whole blood).

COMMONLY ASSOCIATED CONDITIONS
- Hemolytic disease of newborn
- Hydrops fetalis
- Neonatal jaundice
- Kernicterus
- See "Erythroblastosis Fetalis" topic.

DIAGNOSIS

PHYSICAL EXAM
- Jaundice of newborn
- Kernicterus
- Fetal hydrops or fetal death in utero if severe (see "Erythroblastosis Fetalis" topic)

DIFFERENTIAL DIAGNOSIS
- ABO incompatibility
- Other blood group (non-Rh) isoimmunization
- Nonimmune fetal hydrops
- Hereditary spherocytosis
- RBC enzyme defects

DIAGNOSTIC TESTS & INTERPRETATION
Initial Tests (lab, imaging)
- Positive indirect Coombs test (antibody screen) during pregnancy
- Paternal blood type
- Kleihauer-Betke (fetal hemoglobin acid elution, Hb F slide elution) test to quantify an acute fetal–maternal bleed
- Congenital or fetal anemia
- Blood type, direct Coombs test in newborn
- Cell-free fetal DNA (Cff DNA) test: standard practice in many European countries; available in the United States but is not a widely covered benefit. It allows detection of fetal Rh genotype with accuracy of 97.1%, sensitivity of 97.2%, and specificity of 96.8%.
- Cff DNA testing with selective administration of Rh immunoglobulin when the fetus tests Rh positive has been shown to be as effective at preventing new Rh sensitization when compared to routine administration of Rh-immunoglobulin to all Rh-negative women. Such an approach avoids unnecessary use of Rh immunoglobulin (2)[B].
- Currently, routine administration of Rh immune globulin is more cost effective than use of Cff DNA testing in the United States.

Follow-Up Tests & Special Considerations
Prior administration of Rho(D) may lead to weakly (false-) positive indirect Coombs test in mother and direct Coombs test in infant.

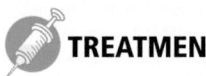

TREATMENT

GENERAL MEASURES
- Depending on severity of involvement, treatment of fetus may include the following:
  - Intrauterine transfusion (3)[B],(4)[A]
  - Early delivery—typically no later than 37 to 38 weeks' gestation (5)[C]
- Treatment of newborn may include the following:
  - Exchange transfusion
  - Transfusion after delivery
  - Phototherapy
- Inconclusive evidence on efficacy of IVIG to reduce need for exchange transfusion (6)[A]

ISSUES FOR REFERRAL
Because of the specialized, somewhat hazardous treatment measures involved, pregnancies in Rh-sensitized women are usually managed at tertiary-care facilities with maternal–fetal medicine specialists.

ADMISSION, INPATIENT, AND NURSING CONSIDERATIONS
Initial monitoring of the newborn is inpatient or in special care nursery if treatment interventions are needed.

 ONGOING CARE

FOLLOW-UP RECOMMENDATIONS
Patient Monitoring
- In most cases, outpatient ambulatory management is appropriate during the antepartum period.
- Antibody titer measured monthly until 24 weeks and every 2 weeks thereafter during first affected pregnancy; a titer of ≥1:16 indicates the need for further testing (4)[A].
- If the patient had a previously affected infant, an Rh-positive fetus in the current pregnancy should be considered at risk regardless of antibody titers (4)[A].
  – Fetal heart rate testing/US to assess fetal status
  – Doppler US measurement of cerebral blood flow. If peak MCA velocity >1.5 multiples of the median, further testing is needed (cordocentesis) for diagnosing fetal anemia (4)[A].
  – Umbilical blood sampling (cordocentesis) for fetal blood type, hematocrit, reticulocyte count, and presence of erythroblasts (5)[C]
  – Amniocentesis for amniotic fluid bilirubin levels (5)[C]
  – Amniocentesis for fetal lung maturity if early delivery is a treatment option (5)[C]

PROGNOSIS
- With appropriate monitoring and treatment, infants born of severely affected pregnancies have a survival rate of >80% (4)[A].
- Even with severe disease, the neurologic outcome of survivors is generally good (6)[B].
- Fetuses with hydrops have a higher mortality rate and higher risk of neurologic impairment (6)[B].
- Disease is likely to be more severe in affected subsequent pregnancies.

COMPLICATIONS
- Pregnancy loss from umbilical blood sampling
- Pregnancy loss from intrauterine transfusion
- Fetal distress requiring emergent delivery

REFERENCES
1. Crowther CA, Middleton P, McBain RD. Anti-D administration in pregnancy for preventing Rhesus alloimmunisation. *Cochrane Database Syst Rev*. 2013;(2):CD000020.
2. Tiblad E, Taune Wikman A, Ajne G, et al. Targeted routine antenatal anti-D prophylaxis in the prevention of RhD immunisation—outcome of a new antenatal screening and prevention program. *PloS One*. 2013;8(8):e70984.
3. Lindenburg IT, Smits-Wintjens VE, van Klink JM, et al; for LOTUS Study Group. Long-term neurodevelopmental outcome after intrauterine transfusion for hemolytic disease of the fetus/newborn: the LOTUS study. *Am J Obstet Gynecol*. 2012;206(2):141.e1–141.e8.
4. Moise KJ Jr, Argoti PS. Management and prevention of red cell alloimmunization in pregnancy: a systematic review. *Obstet Gynecol*. 2012;120(5):1132–1139.
5. American College of Obstetricians and Gynecologists. ACOG Practice Bulletin No. 75: management of alloimmunization during pregnancy. *Obstet Gynecol*. 2006;108(2):457–464.
6. Louis D, More K, Oberoi S, et al. Intravenous immunoglobulin in isoimmune haemolytic disease of newborn: an updated systematic review and meta-analysis. *Arch Dis Child Fetal Neonatal Ed*. 2014;99(4):F325–F331.

ADDITIONAL READING
- Agre P, Cartron JP. Molecular biology of the Rh antigens. *Blood*. 1991;78(3):551–563.
- American College of Obstetricians and Gynecologists. ACOG Practice Bulletin No. 4: prevention of Rh D alloimmunization. Number 4, May 1999 (replaces educational bulletin Number 147, October 1990). Clinical management guidelines for obstetrician-gynecologists. *Int J Gynaecol Obstet*. 1999;66(1):63–70.
- Bowman J. Thirty-five years of Rh prophylaxis. *Transfusion*. 2003;43(12):1661–1666.
- Delaney M, Matthews DC. Hemolytic disease of the fetus and newborn: managing the mother, fetus, and newborn. *Hematology Am Soc Hematol Educ Program*. 2015;2015:146–151.
- Flegel WA. Molecular genetics and clinical applications for RH. *Transfus Apher Sci*. 2011;44(1):81–91.

- Hawk AF, Chang EY, Shields SM, et al. Costs and clinical outcomes of noninvasive fetal RhD typing for targeted prophylaxis. *Obstet Gynecol*. 2013;122(3):579–585.
- Wang M, Wang BL, Xu W, et al. Anti-D alloimmunisation in pregnant women with DEL phenotype in China. *Transfus Med*. 2015;25(3):163–169.

 SEE ALSO

- Anemia, Autoimmune Hemolytic; Erythroblastosis Fetalis
- Algorithm: Hyperbilirubinemia and Jaundice

 CODES

ICD10
- P55.0 Rh isoimmunization of newborn
- O36.0990 Maternal care for other rhesus isoimmunization, unspecified trimester, not applicable or unspecified
- T80.40XA Rh incompat react due to tranfs of bld/bld prod, unsp, init

CLINICAL PEARLS
- If paternity is certain, determining that the father does not carry the Rh(D) blood group antigen eliminates the need to give RhIG prophylaxis during pregnancy or the need for special fetal surveillance if the mother is already sensitized.
- The dose of RhIG for prophylaxis is affected by gestational age. The fetal blood volume is only a few milliliters at 12 weeks' gestation. Therefore, a 50-μg dose of RhIG may be used for threatened, spontaneous, or induced abortions up to 12 weeks' gestation, instead of the standard 300-μg dose.
- Diagnosis is made by antibody titer. Affected pregnancies will require maternal–fetal medicine consultations and monitoring of antibody levels; if titer >1:16, will also require serial monitoring of MCA peak velocity. This will determine the need for invasive testing and transfusions.
- If the patient had a previously affected infant, an Rh-positive fetus in the current pregnancy should be considered at risk regardless of antibody titers—proceed to MCA peak velocity monitoring.
- The current standard in the United States is to provide prophylaxis to all unsensitized Rh-negative mothers; however, determination of the fetal Rh status by Cff DNA testing is reliable and could allow for targeted, rather than universal prophylaxis. Currently, routine prophylaxis is more cost effective in the United States.

R

RHABDOMYOLYSIS

Caroline Tschibelu, MD • Chirag N. Shah, MD, FACEP

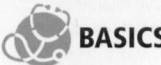 **BASICS**

DESCRIPTION
- Breakdown of skeletal muscle with systemic release of intracellular contents
- Rhabdomyolysis typically presents with muscle pain, weakness, and reddish brown (tea-colored) urine. Up to 50% of patients are asymptomatic.

EPIDEMIOLOGY
Incidence
26,000 hospitalizations annually in United States

ETIOLOGY AND PATHOPHYSIOLOGY
Risk factors
- Direct muscle trauma (most common cause)
  - Crush injuries
  - Extended periods of muscle pressure (during surgery, unconscious from alcohol ingestion)
  - Burns, electrocution, lightning strike
- Muscle exertion
  - Intense and/or prolonged physical exercise (marathon runners, athletes, contact sports)
  - Seizures
  - Delirium tremens
- Drugs and toxins
  - Alcohol
  - Cocaine (most common recreational drug), methamphetamine, phencyclidine, heroin, bath salts (1)[B], synthetic marijuana has been associated with severe rhabdomyolysis (2)[A].
  - Antipsychotics (due to neuroleptic malignant syndrome, malignant hyperthermia, and dystonia)
  - Zidovudine
  - Antimalarials
  - HMG-CoA reductase inhibitors (statins) (risk <0.01%—elevated with higher doses and in combination with fibrates)
  - Colchicine
  - Corticosteroids
  - Carbon monoxide
  - Snake envenomation
- Muscle ischemia
  - Thrombosis, embolism, sickle cell disease
  - Compartment syndrome
  - Tourniquets
- Infections
  - Viral: influenza A and B, coxsackievirus, HIV, varicella
  - Bacterial: *Streptococcus* or *Staphylococcus* sepsis, gas gangrene, necrotizing fasciitis, *Salmonella*, *Legionella*
  - Malaria
- Hypothermia
- Hyperthermia
- Autoimmune disorders
  - Polymyositis, dermatomyositis
- Metabolic and endocrinologic:
  - Hypothyroidism or thyrotoxicosis
  - Electrolyte imbalances (e.g., hyponatremia, hypernatremia, hypokalemia, hypocalcemia, hypophosphatemia)
  - Diabetic ketoacidosis
  - Hyperosmolar state

Genetics
Hereditary causes of rhabdomyolysis are rare but should be suspected in children, patients with recurrent attacks, or patients who have attacks after minimal exertion, mild illness, or starvation.
- Genetic disorders (2)[C]
  - Muscular dystrophies
  - Disorders of lipid metabolism (e.g., carnitine palmitoyltransferase deficiency)
  - Disorders of carbohydrate metabolism (i.e., phosphofructokinase deficiency, phosphoglycerate mutase, myophosphorylase deficiency, a.k.a. McArdle disease/deficiency)
  - Glycogen storage diseases (e.g., phosphorylase B kinase deficiency) and others (e.g., lactate dehydrogenase A deficiency)
  - Mitochondrial disorders

GENERAL PREVENTION
- Avoid excessive exertion; ensure adequate hydration.
- Avoid precipitating drugs, metabolic and electrolyte abnormalities.

 DIAGNOSIS

HISTORY
- Crush injury: direct trauma, prolonged compression/immobility. Causes include motor vehicle accidents (MVA) and entrapment in collapsed buildings. The elderly are more susceptible to crush injury due to immobility and falls. Rhabdomyolysis usually occurs after 1 hour of immobilization, but cases reported with compression lasting <20 minutes.
- Possible history of overexertion or use of drug/toxin (e.g., cocaine, amphetamine, statins), particularly in warm environments
- Patient may complain of fever, malaise, muscle aches, weakness, cramps, or fatigue.
- Nausea, vomiting, diarrhea
- Dark urine
- Agitation while patients are in restraints
- Prolonged periods of lying on a hard surface (e.g., intoxicated or obtunded individuals)

PHYSICAL EXAM
- Vital signs—temperature, pulse, respirations, blood pressure, and oxygenation status
- May have obvious muscle tenderness, evidence of crush injury, weakness and/or swelling on exam. The muscle exam may also be completely normal.
- Tea-colored urine is indicative of myoglobinuria.
- Decreased urine output may indicate renal failure.

DIFFERENTIAL DIAGNOSIS
- Any disease that causes acute tubular necrosis may be confused with rhabdomyolysis.
- Inflammatory myopathies
- Infection (bacterial or viral)
- Phosphorylase, phosphofructokinase, carnitine palmityl transferase, phosphoglycerate mutase deficiency
- Guillain-Barré syndrome
- Myocardial infarction

DIAGNOSTIC TESTS & INTERPRETATION
Initial Tests (lab, imaging)
- Creatine kinase (CK) is the most important diagnostic test: Elevated >5 times the upper limit of normal or >1,000 U/L. CK levels >5,000 U/L are causally related to acute renal failure (ARF) (2,3)[A] and should prompt aggressive fluid resuscitation.
- CK levels peak at ~24 hours and return to normal after 3 to 5 days, making CK a more sensitive marker than myoglobin. Myoglobin is responsible for renal damage (3,4)[A].
- Serum myoglobin levels peak within a few hours and return to normal after ~24 hours. Normal myoglobin levels do not rule out rhabdomyolysis (due to rapid clearance).
- Urinalysis: Dipstick test positive for blood without erythrocytes in sediment suggests injury from either hemoglobin or myoglobin.
- Elevations of serum potassium from muscle injury can be compounded by ARF.
- Initial hypocalcemia: Calcium enters the injured muscle cells and precipitates as calcium phosphate, leading to calcification of ischemic muscle cells. Only correct initial hypocalcemia if patient is symptomatic or has ECG changes; resolves during the renal recovery phase
- Hypercalcemia during renal recovery phase: unique to rhabdomyolysis-induced ARF for 20–30% of patients (4)[A]. As renal function improves, there is mobilization of the precipitated calcium, increase in calcitriol, and hyperphosphatemia resolves.
- Extreme hyperuricemia may be present and can cause acute uric acid nephropathy.
- Elevations in BUN and creatinine suggest ARF.
- Reversible hepatic dysfunction can occur. However, elevations in alanine aminotransferase (ALT), aspartate aminotransferase (AST), and lactic dehydrogenase may be due to muscle injury rather than hepatic injury.
- Disseminated intravascular coagulation (DIC) suggested by increase in coagulation times, fibrin degradation products, and D-dimer with decreases in platelets and fibrinogen
- 12-lead ECG because hyperkalemia can induce fatal arrhythmias

Follow-Up Tests & Special Considerations
- Delayed renal failure/electrolyte abnormalities despite normal initial levels
- Ongoing muscle injury is manifested by rising creatine phosphokinase (CPK).
- Renal imaging shows findings similar to other mechanisms of ARF.

Diagnostic Procedures/Other
Muscle compartment pressures if compartment syndrome is suspected

Test Interpretation
- Muscle necrosis
- Myoglobin-related renal injury may resemble acute tubular necrosis from other causes.

TREATMENT

GENERAL MEASURES
- Address underlying cause (e.g., medications cessation, temperature control, trauma, infection).
- Aggressive hydration is often necessary. With severe muscle trauma (crush injuries), up to 12 L of fluid may be sequestered in the muscles.
- Monitor CK levels, renal function, and electrolytes.
- Follow potassium levels due to potential for arrhythmias.
- Treat DIC or hepatic dysfunction appropriately.
- Recognize and treat compartment syndrome promptly.

MEDICATION

First Line
- Aggressive fluid resuscitation is the most important intervention: normal saline (NS) and 5% glucose solution with a target urine output of 200 to 300 mL/hr. Alternating NS and 5% glucose is recommended to prevent volume overload. Infusion rate should be 500 mL/hr (5)[C],(6)[A].
- Alkalinization of the urine may decrease myoglobin-induced nephrotoxicity in the tubules (sodium bicarbonate to increase urine pH >6.5):
  – Use is controversial.
  – Side effects include worsening hypocalcemia.
  – Sodium bicarbonate may be of use in patients with very high CK levels, acidosis, or coexisting hyperkalemia.
  – Place 150 mEq (3 ampules) NaHCO$_3$ in 1 L of D5W and infuse at 200 mL/hr.

Second Line
- IV mannitol as a bolus if urine output remains low, 1 to 2 g/kg, not to exceed 200 g in 24 hours with a cumulative dose of 800 g. It is used to prevent ARF only if diuresis is not adequate (<200 mL/hr) despite fluid therapy (6)[A].
  – Increases prostaglandin production leading to renal vasodilation and diuresis, reducing susceptibility to myoglobin injury. As an osmotic agent, filtered but not reabsorbed by the tubules, mannitol increases sodium delivery and diuresis. This may remove necrotic cell debris and prevent rise in compartment pressures.
  – Use of mannitol is controversial. No good evidence that it improves outcomes more than aggressive IV hydration. As a free-radical scavenger, mannitol has renal protective effects if used before tubular occlusion.
  – Consider adding furosemide to force diuresis if necessary (40 to 120 mg/day).
  – Do not diurese in anuric renal failure; caution also in the elderly and patients with heart disease
- Hyperkalemia can result from massive release of intracellular potassium stores or ARF. Severe hyperkalemia may be life-threatening. Treatment when ECG changes are present (tall, thin T waves; PR prolongation; QRS widening; P wave flattening).
  – Calcium gluconate: to stabilize the cardiac membrane. IV 1 to 2 ampules (0.5 mL 10% calcium gluconate = 4 mg elemental calcium; give 4 mg/kg/hr for 4 hours.)
  – If acidosis is present: 1 to 2 ampules (2 to 3 mL/kg) sodium bicarbonate IV. Sodium bicarbonate can worsen hypocalcemia.

  – If tolerated: Oral sodium polystyrene sulfonate (Kayexalate) as much as 20 g (1 g/kg) can be given via enema.
  – Insulin and albuterol transiently drive potassium into the cells. Administration of glucose can prevent the hypoglycemic effects of insulin.
    – Precautions: continuous monitoring of potassium levels to prevent overcorrecting with potential hypokalemia and arrhythmias
    – Indications for dialysis include resistant and symptomatic hyperkalemia (ECG), oliguria (<0.5 mL/kg over 12-hour period), anuria, volume overload, or persistent acidosis (pH <7.1).

ISSUES FOR REFERRAL
- Usually managed as an inpatient
- Diagnosis of compartment syndrome merits surgical consultation for consideration of fasciotomy.
- Renal dialysis may be indicated in ARF.

ADDITIONAL THERAPIES
During the oliguric phase, symptomatic hypocalcemia (rare) may benefit from IV calcium gluconate.

SURGERY/OTHER PROCEDURES
For muscle entrapment/compartment syndrome

ADMISSION, INPATIENT, AND NURSING CONSIDERATIONS
- Patients with significant elevations of CK should be admitted for IV hydration and clinical monitoring.
- Volume expansion with NS to increase urine output to at least 150 mL/hr
- CK usually peaks 24 to 36 hours after muscle injury, so monitoring should confirm that the CK is trending down. Renal function should be stable/improving. Electrolytes should be normal.
- Patients with mild CK elevation and normal renal function may be discharged after observation phase if CK is trending down.

ONGOING CARE

FOLLOW-UP RECOMMENDATIONS
Follow-up within a few days to recheck CK, electrolytes, and renal function

Patient Monitoring
- Contingent on disease: essential for metabolic myopathies
- Myotoxic drugs should be discontinued/monitored closely.

DIET
- With renal failure, restrict protein intake to lower BUN level.
- Limit potassium intake.
- With anuria, essential to restrict volume intake

PROGNOSIS
Contingent on primary cause of rhabdomyolysis and on recovery from ARF without complications

COMPLICATIONS
- Death, especially from hyperkalemia/renal failure
- With dialysis and supportive care, the prognosis is very good.

REFERENCES
1. Murphy CM, Dulaney AR, Beuhler MC, et al. "Bath salts" and "plant food" products: the experience of one regional US poison center. *J Med Toxicol.* 2013;9(1):42–48.
2. Scalco RS, Gardiner AR, Pitceathly RD, et al. Rhabdomyolysis: a genetic perspective. *Orphanet J Rare Dis.* 2015;10:51.
3. Cervellin G, Comelli I, Benatti M, et al. Non-traumatic rhabdomyolysis: background, laboratory features, and acute clinical management. *Clin Biochem.* 2017;50(12):656–662.
4. Parekh R, Care DA, Tainter CR. Rhabdomyolysis: advances in diagnosis and treatment. *Emerg Med Pract.* 2012;14(3):1–15.
5. Petejova N, Martinek A. Acute kidney injury due to rhabdomyolysis and renal replacement therapy: a critical review. *Crit Care.* 2014;18(3):224.
6. Chavez LO, Leon M, Einav S, et al. Beyond muscle destruction: a systematic review of rhabdomyolysis for clinical practice. *Crit Care.* 2016;20(1):135.

ADDITIONAL READING
- Durand D, Delgado LL, de la Parra-Pellot DM, et al. Psychosis and severe rhabdomyolysis associated with synthetic cannabinoid use: a case report. *Clin Schizophr Relat Psychoses.* 2015;8(4):205–208.
- Knafl EG, Hughes JA, Dimeski G, et al. Rhabdomyolysis: patterns, circumstances, and outcomes of patients presenting to the emergency department. *Ochsner J.* 2018;18(3):215–221.
- Shawkat H, Westwood MM, Mortimer A. Mannitol: a review of its clinical uses. *Contin Educ Anaesth Crit Care Pain.* 2012;12(2):82–85.

SEE ALSO

Algorithm: Acute Kidney Injury (Acute Renal Failure)

CODES

ICD10
- M62.82 Rhabdomyolysis
- T79.6XXA Traumatic ischemia of muscle, initial encounter
- T79.6XXD Traumatic ischemia of muscle, subsequent encounter

CLINICAL PEARLS
- Elevation of CK is the diagnostic hallmark of rhabdomyolysis.
- The cornerstone of treatment of rhabdomyolysis is aggressive fluid administration.
- Electrolyte abnormalities, acute kidney injury, hepatic injury, compartment syndrome, and (rarely) DIC are the most worrisome complications of rhabdomyolysis.

R

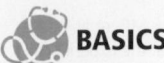

RHABDOMYOSARCOMA

Jose L. Perez-Lara, MD • Jairo J. Tejada-Tejada, MD • Thanh-Ha Luong, MD

BASICS

DESCRIPTION
Rhabdomyosarcoma (RMS) is a malignancy which form part from soft tissue tumors named sarcomas. RMS generates from primitive mesenchymal cells with myogenesis capacity, which matures to striated skeletal muscle tissues. It occurs mainly as primary malignancy but can also be a component of heterogeneous neoplasias, like malignant teratoma.

- Common anatomic sites (1):
  - Head and neck 40% presentation (common in young children, almost always embryonal type)
  - Genitourinary 25% of cases (mostly embryonal type)
  - Musculoskeletal 20% of cases (most common in extremities primary sites in adolescents and adults, alveolar subtype)
- The International Classification of RMS describes four major subtypes:
  - Embryonal RMS (ERMS): represents 60–70% among all RMS. Has early onset and is the most common subtype in children. Commonly presents in the head, neck, and genitourinary areas. ERMS is subdivided into:
    ○ Classic
    ○ Botryoid (6% overall embryonal): seen in infants, although can happen <4-year-old patients
    ○ Spindle cell: 3% of cases and affects young children
      ▪ Both botryoid and spindle cell variants have better prognosis than the classical one.
  - Alveolar RMS (ARMS): represents 30% of pediatric cases, very aggressive subtype; more common in the trunk, perineum/perianal area, and extremities
  - Anaplastic (children)/pleomorphic (adults) seen in patients aged 30 to 50 years, rarely in children, represents 1% of all RMS, mostly associated with Li-Fraumeni symptoms

EPIDEMIOLOGY
It presents most commonly in children and young adults rather than adult, although when presented in adult ages, is known to be more aggressive and fatal.

Incidence
- 4.5 cases of RMS per 1 million children per year, in children, adolescents, and young adults.
- RMS accounts for 60% of sarcomas in children and adolescents. 50% of pediatric cases occur before the age of 10 years.
- In adults, RMS represents 3% of all soft tissue sarcomas in adults.
- More common in black population than white population

Prevalence
- RMS comprises 3.5% of childhood cancers overall.
- The more frequent in males (male:female ratio, 1:5)

ETIOLOGY AND PATHOPHYSIOLOGY
Genetics
Genetic characteristics vary according to the RMS subtype (2,3):
- Alveolar:
  - t(2;13)(q35;q14); causing *PAX3-FOXO1* fusion
  - t(1;13)(p36;q14); causing *PAX7-FOXO1* fusion
  - t(X:2)(q13;q35); causing *PAX3-FOXO4* fusion
  - t(2;2)(q35;p23); causing *PAX3-NCOA1* fusion
  - t(2;8)(q35;q13); causing *PAX3-NCOA2* fusion
  - t(8;13)(p12;q13); causing *FOXO1-FGFR1* fusion
- Embryonal:
  - Multiple complex genetic aberrations, including *MYOD1* mutations

- Loss or uniparental disomy of 11p15.5 +2, +8, +11, +12, +13, +20 affecting the genes *IGF-2*, *H19*, *CDKN1C*, and/or *HOTS*
- Spindle cell RMS:
  - 8q13 rearrangements involving *SRF-NCOA2* and *TEAD1-NCOA2*

RISK FACTORS
Although not yet proven, RMS has been associated with high birth weight, large gestational size for age, exposure to recreational drugs and/or radiation while in utero, low socioeconomic status, and the genetic conditions as described below.

COMMONLY ASSOCIATED CONDITIONS
- Beckwith-Wiedemann syndrome (11p15 mutations) presents as fetal overgrowth.
- Costello syndrome (germline *HRAS* mutations) presents as postnatal growth delay and morphologic abnormalities (including macrocephaly).
- Li-Fraumeni (germline *TP53*; known as *p53* mutations)
- Neurofibromatosis type I (*NF1* mutations)
- Noonan syndrome (*PTPN11* mutations)
- Pleuropulmonary blastoma (*DICER1* mutations)

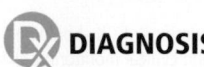

DIAGNOSIS

HISTORY
- Presents as a progressive nontender palpable mass
- When presents in head/neck, patients report diplopia (due to ophthalmoplegia), recurrent sinusitis, or persistent nasal discharge.
- RMS of genitourinary tissue may present as hematuria, polyuria, vaginal bleeding in females.
- Other symptoms may be noted due to mass effect of the primary or metastatic lesions.
- Personal or family history of genetic syndromes (i.e., NF1, Li-Fraumeni, etc.)

PHYSICAL EXAM
- Painless, enlarging mass
- Polypoid mass protruding from vagina (botryoid)
- Exophthalmos and chemosis (orbital involvement)
- Abdominal pain and compression symptoms (i.e., seizures, visual field defects, nerve palsy, headaches)

DIAGNOSTIC TESTS & INTERPRETATION
Initial Tests (lab, imaging)
- Standard blood test, including complete blood count, serum chemistry, liver function test, and coagulation profile, should be obtained for clinical optimization prior treatment.

- MRI with/without contrast or CT with contrast of the primary tumor (to define anatomy)
- Staging workup:
  - Chest x-ray or CT chest without contrast (preferred). Most common site of metastasis is the lungs. PET/CT scans for lymph node or distant metastases detection that are not readily evident on other imaging. It is also helpful in monitoring the response to treatment for deep, firm lesions >3 cm.
  - Lymph node biopsy

Diagnostic Procedures/Other
- For pathology diagnosis:
  - Core needle biopsy, incisional biopsy, or excisional biopsy (based on the size of the mass). The histologic characteristics are similar to others and comprise small, blue, round-cell, which raises the need for advanced immunohistochemical and genetic tests.
  - Histologic classification:
    ○ Alveolar: rhabdomyoblasts grossly mimicking pulmonary alveoli. The alveolar component must be ≥ 50%; has high levels of myogenin when compared to other subtypes
    ○ Embryonal:
      ▪ Classic: rhabdomyoblasts configured in sheets, large nest, eosinophilic cytoplasma; no alveolar pattern, instead poor myofilaments arrangement
      ▪ Botryoid: "grape-like" appearance of rhabdomyoblasts with notable clustering in the subepithelium forming the cambium layer; seen within the vagina and bladder
      ▪ Spindle cell: rhabdomyoblasts with spindle-like appearance
    ○ Anaplastic (children)/pleomorphic (adults): rhabdomyoblast with large hyperchromatic nuclei and strange mitotic morphologies
- Immunohistochemical (ICH) markers:
  - Muscle-specific actin, myosin, desmin (in 99% of RMS), myoglobin, Z-band protein, and MyoD1
- Molecular testing for PAX/FOXO1 fusion, which is tested by PCR and fluorescence in situ hybridization (FISH) with good concordance (94.9%). Although both have similar sensitivity (85.7% vs. 83.3%), PCR seems to have a slightly higher specificity (100% vs. 96%) (4).
- Although not establish yet, genetic profiling will become the gold standard for diagnosis and prognosis (3).
- Staging is based on site, size, regional nodal involvement, and distance spread (Table 1).

Table 1 TNM Staging System for Rhabdomyosarcoma (5)

Stage	Site	T	Tumor diameter	N	M
1	Orbit; head and neck (excluding parameningeal), genitourinary—nonbladder and nonprostate, biliary tract	T1 or T2	a or b	Any N	M0
2	Bladder or prostate, extremity, cranial parameningeal, other	T1 or T2	a	N0 or NX	M0
3a	Bladder or prostate, extremity, cranial parameningeal, other	T1 or T2	a	N1	M0
3b	Bladder or prostate, extremity, cranial parameningeal, other	T1 or T2	b	Any N	M0
4	All sites	T1 or T2	a or b	N0 or N1	M1

T1, confined to organ of origin; T2, extends outside the organ of origin; a, ≤5 cm in diameter; b, >5 cm in diameter; N0, regional nodes not clinically involved; N1, regional nodes clinically involved by neoplasm; NX, clinical status of regional nodes unknown; M0, no distant metastasis; M1, distant metastasis.

TREATMENT

Encompasses surgical resection, radiation, chemotherapy. Patients should always be referred to a multidisciplinary team with expertise in oncology for definitive treatment.

SURGERY/OTHER PROCEDURES

- Surgery:
  - Local resection of tumor along with metastasis and nodal resection. Lymph node sampling is intended to identify unknown metastasis and guide decision for postop radiation. However, wide resection may not be feasible in cases where grossly impaired functionality results (i.e., head/neck).
- Radiation therapy (RT): is widely recommended to enhance local control, except in patients with embryonal type and fusion negative ICH. Emergent RT is only considered in patient with compression symptoms. Proton beam over photon beam due to safety profile. Brachytherapy can be considered in patients with difficult to treat tumor due to location (head/neck and parameningeal).
- Chemotherapy:
  - Selected based on prognosis risk stratification assessment (i.e., low, intermediate, high). For nonmetastatic RMS, stratification is made based on the TNM staging as well as the surgical/pathologic clinical grouping system. The latter is determined after the surgical resection based on histopathologic features and extent of residual tumor. In other words, nonmetastatic RMS, risk stratification cannot be fully determined until surgery is performed (3).
    - Gold standard is VAC (vincristine, dactinomycin [also known as actinomycin D], and cyclophosphamide) (5)[A]. Low-risk patients may be prescribed VA instead (5)[A].
    - Most common adverse reactions are:
      - Vincristine: peripheral neuropathy
      - Dactinomycin: myelosuppression and hepatotoxicity
      - Cyclophosphamide: hemorrhagic cystitis (mesna is used for prophylaxis), transitional cell carcinoma, myelosuppression with leukopenia, and infertility
- In addition, ifosfamide, topotecan, doxorubicin, etoposide, and irinotecan may also be used in alternative regimens.
- Duration also depends on risk stratification but in general ranges from 12 to 24 months given in separate cycles (usually 14 to 15 cycles) (1).
- European Paediatric Soft Tissue Sarcoma Study Group (EPSTSSG) recently demonstrated improve in 3 years survival with maintenance chemotherapy, with vinorelbine and cyclophosphamide. Although according to COG guidelines, these recommendations cannot be yet establish as standard therapy (6).
- Immune mediated thru natural killer cells are being studied with great potential, although remains in vitro experiment (please refer to Additional Readings).
- Given low frequency of RMS in adults, there are no large trials to set appropriate regimen; therefore, standard VAC is used empirically; although this practice showed low efficacy in some case series, has allow to recommend alternative regimen (doxorubicin, ifosfamide, and vincristine), which demonstrated improvement in short-term (2 years) overall survival and disease-free survival

 ONGOING CARE

FOLLOW-UP RECOMMENDATIONS

All patients should follow-up with their multidisciplinary team. This allows to monitor treatment response, early detection of locoregional relapse, metastatic disease, or development of secondary malignancies. For this effort, physical exam and imaging surveillance for the first 5 years are paramount (CT/MRI/x-ray). Imaging should be done every 3 months for the 1st year, then every 4 months for the following 2 years, finally every 6 months for next 2 years. After the first 5 years, no more imaging surveillance is recommended as it has not showed further benefits. Other imaging techniques such as bone scan/PET scan should be considered based on clinical decisions, and echocardiograms are recommended if patient received anthracycline therapy (1,7).

PROGNOSIS

- RMS (overall): 70% 5-year survival (1)
- Survival rate has increased from 30% to 51% in adolescents 15 to 19 years old.
- In orbital RMS, survival can be as high as 95%.
- Prognosis as in other tumors depends on size, presence or not of metastasis, and location of the tumor, which help to risk-stratify patients into low, intermediate, and high risk. Favorable sites include orbit/eyelid, head and neck (with no parameningeal involvement), genitourinary (without bladder or prostate involvement), and biliary tract. Unfavorable site: bladder, prostate, extremity, parameningeal, trunk, retroperitoneal, pelvis (1)
- 5-year survival based on *PAX/FOXO1* fusion status and risk stratification: low risk + fusion negative 90%; intermediate risk + fusion negative 78%; intermediate risk + fusion positive 56%; high risk + fusion negative 41%; high risk + fusion positive 11% (1)
- In terms of histologic classification, botryoid and spindle cell RMS have favorable prognosis, embryonal subtype has intermediate; sclerosing, spindle cell RMS and alveolar subtype being the poorest, with alveolar RMS being the poorest.
- Adults has worse prognosis when compared to children, not only due to lower rates of treatment adherence and lack of clinical trials identifying best treatment but also due to less favorable location and histopathology and metastasis at time of diagnosis.
- Alveolar subtype has the poorest prognosis; however, any subtype metastatic presentation has bad prognosis (2). Risk factors associated with poorest outcome: metastatic disease at relapse, prior RT treatment, initial tumor size >5 cm, and relapse within 18 months (7)

COMPLICATIONS

- Relapse
- Secondary neoplasm
- Growth abnormalities
- Treatment side effects

REFERENCES

1. Khosla D, Sapkota S, Kapoor R, et al. Adult rhabdomyosarcoma: clinical presentation, treatment, and outcome. *J Cancer Res Ther.* 2015;11(4):830–834.
2. National Cancer Institute. Childhood rhabdomyosarcoma treatment (PDQ®)–health professional version. https://www.cancer.gov/types/soft-tissue-sarcoma/hp/rhabdomyosarcoma-treatment-pdq. Updated April 4, 2018. Accessed August 14, 2018.
3. Bridge JA. The role of cytogenetics and molecular diagnostics in the diagnosis of soft-tissue tumors. *Mod Pathol.* 2014;27(Suppl 1):S80–S97.
4. Thway K, Wang J, Wren D, et al. The comparative utility of fluorescence in situ hybridization and reverse transcription-polymerase chain reaction in the diagnosis of alveolar rhabdomyosarcoma. *Virchows Arch.* 2015;467(2):217–224.
5. National Comprehensive Cancer Network. Soft tissue sarcoma. Version 2.2017. https://www.nccn.org/professionals/physician_gls/pdf/sarcoma.pdf. Updated August 9, 2018. Accessed August 14, 2018.
6. Brennan B, Zanetti I, Orbach D, et al. Alveolar soft part sarcoma in children and adolescents: the European Paediatric Soft Tissue Sarcoma Study Group prospective trial (EpSSG NRSTS 2005). *Pediatr Blood Cancer.* 2018;65(4). doi:10.1002/pbc.26942.
7. Borinstein SC, Steppan D, Hayashi M, et al. Consensus and controversies regarding the treatment of rhabdomyosarcoma. *Pediatr Blood Cancer.* 2018;65(2). doi:10.1002/pbc.26809.

CODES

ICD10

- C49.9 Malignant neoplasm of connective and soft tissue, unsp
- C49.0 Malignant neoplasm of connective and soft tissue of head, face and neck
- C49.5 Malignant neoplasm of connective and soft tissue of pelvis

CLINICAL PEARLS

- RMS are more common in children but can develop in adults, the latest having the highest mortality.
- Genetic disorders and congenital syndromes are associated to a higher risk of developing RMS.
- If localize tumor is identified with concurrent lymph node involvement, implement more aggressive therapy.
- Most common site of metastasis is lung, followed by bone marrow/bone and peritoneum.
- Although improve in survival has not been proven, second look surgery postchemotherapy in patients with documented improved radiology might be beneficial to improve outcome.
- Best timing in RT has not yet been defined.
- For intermediate-risk patient, temsirolimus (mTOR inhibitor) is currently on trial for use.
- High-dose chemotherapy followed by autologous stem cell transplant remains a promising therapy to patients who can tolerate side effects and toxicity but still needs further investigation prior to standardization.

RHEUMATIC FEVER
Stuart H. Batten, MD • Edwin Y. Choi, MD

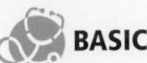

BASICS

DESCRIPTION

- Acute rheumatic fever (ARF) is an autoimmune, inflammatory response to pharyngeal infection with group A *Streptococcus* (GAS) that affects multiple organ systems.
- Can lead to rheumatic heart disease (RHD) if not treated in the acute phase
- Largely, a disease of poverty and has disappeared from many affluent parts of the world
- Recurrence in adults and children is common without adequate antibiotic treatment.
- Organ systems affected include cardiovascular, nervous, hematologic, immunologic, lymphatic, skin/exocrine, and musculoskeletal.

Pediatric Considerations
Most cases occur in children ages 5 to 15 years; rare in children <5 years (1)

EPIDEMIOLOGY

- ARF and RHD are largely restricted to low-income countries and marginalized sections of society in wealthy countries.
- Male = female, but females more likely to develop chorea and RHD.
- Endemic regions include South Pacific, indigenous populations of Australia and New Zealand, Africa, Asia.

Incidence

- Worldwide, incidence has been declining for 25 years, attributed to increasing antibiotic use and improved living conditions. The large majority of new cases are in developing countries.
- Mean worldwide incidence ranges from 8 to 51/100,000 school-aged children (1); 500,000 new cases of ARF occur annually (2).
- Incidence of ARF in the United States is currently <2/100,000 school-aged children.
- It is estimated that up to 3% episodes of untreated acute GAS pharyngitis go on to develop ARF (1).

Prevalence

- In developing areas of the world, RHD is estimated to affect >33 million people and is the leading cause of cardiovascular death during the first 5 decades of life.
- Prevalence has been rising due to improved medical care and longer survival (despite decreasing incidence of ARF).

ETIOLOGY AND PATHOPHYSIOLOGY

- ARF is preceded 2 to 3 weeks by GAS (*Streptococcus pyogenes*) tonsillopharyngitis, a gram-positive bacterial infection.
- Pathogenic mechanism is not completely understood.
- Molecular mimicry plays an important role: The GAS M protein and the carbohydrate antigen (*N*-acetyl-β-D-glucosamine) share antigenic epitopes with human cardiac tissue and neuronal cells in the basal ganglia (1). These antigens cross-react with cardiac and vessel endothelial proteins, leading to an inflammatory cascade.
- Joint involvement is a likely result of immune complex accumulation.

Genetics

- Susceptibility is associated with certain genetic polymorphisms of genes involved in the innate and adaptive immune pathways; not fully understood
- ARF appears to be a heritable and susceptibility is most likely polygenic with variable and incomplete penetrance.
- Increased susceptibility in certain populations, including indigenous Australians, New Zealand Maori, and Pacific Islanders

RISK FACTORS

- Poverty, household crowding, and social disadvantage are the strongest risk factors.
- Genetic susceptibility and ethnic predisposition possibly increase risk.

GENERAL PREVENTION

- Primary prevention: Antibiotics are effective at reducing incidence of ARF after known or suspected GAS pharyngitis. Number needed to treat is 100 (3). Appropriate treatment of streptococcal pharyngitis prevents ARF in most cases.
- Secondary prevention: long-term antibiotic prophylaxis (up to 5 to 10 years) to prevent recurrence, which can lead to RHD.

DIAGNOSIS

- Mainly a clinical diagnosis
- Laboratory evidence of preceding GAS infection is needed whenever possible (see "Initial Tests (lab, imaging)")
- Revised 2015 Jones criteria (4)[C]
- Initial ARF: 2 major OR 1 major + 2 minor
- Recurrent ARF: 2 major OR 1 major + 2 minor OR 3 minor

Low-Risk Population	Moderate- and High-Risk Population
Major criteria:	Major criteria:
• Carditis: clinical or subclinical (echocardiogram)	• Carditis: clinical or subclinical (echocardiogram)
• Polyarthritis ONLY	• Polyarthritis OR monoarthritis
• Chorea	• Chorea
• Erythema marginatum	• Erythema marginatum
• Subcutaneous nodules	• Subcutaneous nodules
Minor criteria:	Minor criteria:
• Polyarthralgia	• Monoarthralgia
• Fever ≥38.5°C	• Fever ≥38.0°C
• ESR ≥60 mm/hr	• ESR ≥30 mm/hr
• CRP ≥3 mg/dL	• CRP ≥3 mg/dL
• ↑PR interval	• ↑PR interval

- The revised criteria distinguish between patients with low risk versus moderate to high risk of having ARF. Patients can be considered low risk if they are from and among a low-incidence group (4)[C].

HISTORY

- ARF typically presents 2 to 3 weeks following GAS tonsillopharyngitis.
- Polyarthritis (35–66%) is often the first symptom, affecting the knees, ankles, elbows, and wrists. Each resolves in days, thus seems to "migrate." Demonstrates rapid improvement with aspirin or NSAIDs. Usually self-limited <1 month. Moderate- to high-risk

patients may only have monoarthritis. Use of NSAID or aspirin may mask the arthritis in initial stages.
- Fever (can be low grade in high-risk populations)
- Erythema marginatum rash (see "Physical Exam")
- Pancarditis or valvulitis (50–70%) can be subclinical (asymptomatic without auscultatory findings) or clinically apparent (symptomatic or auscultatory findings).
- Sydenham chorea (clinical diagnosis, in 10–30%): neurologic disorder consisting of purposeless, involuntary, nonstereotypical movements
  - 1 to 6 months after infection, lab evidence of preceding infection may be absent.
  - More common in 5 to 15 years old, females
  - Improves or ceases during sleep
  - Can have associated muscular weakness
  - Psychiatric symptoms may have onset prior to chorea, with emotional lability and obsessive-compulsive symptoms.
  - Usually self-resolves over several months and can relapse

PHYSICAL EXAM

- Neuro: Sydenham chorea: Involuntary movements may be general or unilateral and may involve the face. "Milkmaid grip" is intermittent hypotonia appreciated on test of grip strength.
- Cardiac: pericardial friction rub, holosystolic murmur of mitral/aortic regurgitation, rarely diastolic; rarely evidence of heart failure
- Skin
  - Subcutaneous nodules (<10%): firm, painless protuberances on extensor surfaces. Usually involves knees, elbow, wrists, occiput, and spinous process of thoracic and lumbar vertebrae; more common in severe ARF, persists up to several weeks
  - Erythema marginatum (5–13%): evanescent, pink rash with pale centers and rounded/serpiginous margins. Blanches with pressure and can be induced with heat. Usually found on trunk and proximal extremities. Rare to be found on face; typically nonpruritic

DIFFERENTIAL DIAGNOSIS

- Systemic lupus erythematosus
- Poststreptococcal reactive arthritis
- Juvenile rheumatoid arthritis
- Infectious arthritis
- Myocarditis (viral or idiopathic)
- Innocent cardiac murmur
- Cardiomyopathy
- Tourette syndrome
- Kawasaki syndrome
- Pediatric autoimmune neuropsychiatric disorders associated with streptococcal infections (PANDAS)
- Lyme disease
- Henoch-Schönlein purpura
- Wilson disease
- Drug intoxication
- Tic disorder
- Encephalitis

DIAGNOSTIC TESTS & INTERPRETATION

Initial Tests (lab, imaging)

- Bacteriologic/serologic evidence of GAS infection is needed whenever possible, and the diagnosis is in doubt when it cannot be obtained (chorea and chronic indolent rheumatic carditis being the exception due to delayed onset).
  - Rapid streptococcal antigen test with high pretest probability
  - Positive GAS throat culture

- Elevated or rising antistreptococcal antibody titer (ASO or ADB); ASO peaks 3 to 5 weeks postinfection, ADB peaks 6 to 8 weeks. A rise in titer is better than a single titer result.
- ESR and CRP are acute-phase reactants that almost always increase in ARF.
- CBC with differential: leukocytosis, normocytic anemia
- ECG: PR prolongation, AV block, signs of pericarditis
- Joint aspiration and synovial fluid evaluation is indicated if there is significant effusion of one joint or septic arthritis is suspected.
- Echocardiogram: Assesses chamber size and function, pericardial effusion, and valve disease.
- All cases of confirmed OR suspected ARF should have an echocardiogram within 12 weeks (4)[B] due to the 18% prevalence of subclinical carditis.

Follow-Up Tests & Special Considerations
- ESR and CRP are useful to monitor the acute disease process. CRP has more utility (ESR remains elevated for months) and can be checked twice weekly initially, followed by every 1 to 2 weeks until normalized.
- Serial echocardiograms can be considered to monitor evolution of carditis, even if not initially present (4)[C].
- All household contacts should be screened with GAS throat cultures. Positive results should be treated with antibiotics, even if asymptomatic.

Test Interpretation
Prior treatment with aspirin or steroids may lead to falsely negative lab results.

 TREATMENT

GENERAL MEASURES
- Antibiotic
- Anti-inflammatory agent (aspirin or naproxen)
- Manage other manifestations as needed (e.g., chorea, dysrhythmia, pericarditis, myocarditis, valvular disease, or heart failure).

MEDICATION
First Line
- Eradication: GAS infection treatment should begun within 9 days of illness to prevent ARF (5)[A]. If confirmed diagnosis, begin secondary prophylaxis.
- If no penicillin allergy
  - Penicillin VK 250 mg PO BID for 10 days, benzathine penicillin G IM for 1 day or amoxicillin 50 mg/kg PO for 10 days (preferred in children) (5)[A]
- If penicillin allergy
  - 1st-generation cephalosporin PO for 10 days, or azithromycin 12 mg/kg PO for 5 days, clindamycin 7 mg/kg/dose PO for 10 days, or clarithromycin 7.5 mg/kg/dose PO for 10 days (5)[A]
- Arthritis: Naproxen 10 to 20 mg/kg/day divided BID is now recommended over aspirin (1)[B], given superior side-effect profile and less risk of Reye syndrome.
- Carditis: If heart failure, 3rd-degree AV block, or other severe manifestations, appropriate traditional management should be initiated as indicated (diuretics, ACE Inhibitors, vasodilators)
- NSAIDs, glucocorticoids, and IVIG are not recommended for carditis, although glucocorticoids can be considered in severe carditis with acute cardiac failure.
- Chorea: generally self-resolves and does not require treatment, but if symptoms are severe, can use valproic acid or carbamazepine. IVIG and glucocorticoids are restricted to patients who have failed other therapy. Antipsychotics are not routinely used due to extrapyramidal side effects.

Second Line
If penicillin allergy is present, erythromycin is preferred by the New Zealand Guidelines Group but not by the Infectious Diseases Society of America.

ISSUES FOR REFERRAL
- A cardiologist should be involved in management of ARF.
- Pediatric neurologist or movement specialist can help guide therapy with severe chorea.

SURGERY/OTHER PROCEDURES
Valve stenosis is a late sequela that can result from fibrosis and calcification; may require surgical correction (valve repair preferred over replacement) (5)

ADMISSION, INPATIENT, AND NURSING CONSIDERATIONS
- Initial hospitalization may be helpful for diagnosis and to ensure stability.
- Heart failure requires prompt hospitalization.
- IV fluids
  - Only if signs of dehydration or to augment preload; use caution if heart failure present.
- Nursing
  - Consider bed rest if severe symptoms, with gradual return to ambulation as tolerated.

 ONGOING CARE

FOLLOW-UP RECOMMENDATIONS
- Secondary prophylaxis: ARF patients should be on a prophylactic antibiotic from time of diagnosis until at least age 21 years, and possibly indefinitely depending on cardiac damage because recurrence can worsen severity of carditis (6)[C].
  - First-line prophylaxis is long-acting benzathine penicillin G monthly IM injections (6)[A].
  - Penicillin V PO 250 mg BID is an alternative but has risk of nonadherence (6)[B].
  - If penicillin allergy, treat with sulfadiazine 0.5 to 1.0 g daily (6)[B].
  - If penicillin and sulfa drug allergy, treat with azithromycin (6)[C].
  - Patients on penicillin prophylaxis who develop GAS pharyngitis while on penicillin should be treated with an alternative agent such as clindamycin.
- If diagnostic uncertainty exists, consider 1 year of secondary antibiotic prophylaxis followed by reassessment and echocardiogram (4)[C].
- Routine antibiotic prophylaxis for dental procedures is no longer recommended by the American Heart Association for patients with RHD (6).
- Have low threshold to test and treat episodes of acute tonsillopharyngitis in children.

Patient Monitoring
Initially weekly and then every 6 months

Pediatric Considerations
- Use aspirin with caution in children given the risk of Reye syndrome.
- Naproxen has been found equivalent to aspirin with fewer risks in ARF, in a randomized, placebo-controlled study (1)[B].

Pregnancy Considerations
May exacerbate valve disease, particularly mitral stenosis in RHD. Refer pregnant patients to a cardiologist.

DIET
No dietary restrictions; low-sodium if heart failure present

PATIENT EDUCATION
American Heart Association: http://www.heart.org

PROGNOSIS
Long-term sequelae are generally limited to the heart and depend on the severity of carditis during an acute attack.

COMPLICATIONS
- Recurrence of ARF due to GAS reinfection
- RHD can occur 10 to 20 years after ARF, with mitral more common than aortic regurgitation, can lead to mitral stenosis. Heart failure is the worst complication.
- Jaccoud arthropathy is chronic and involves painless deformities of hands/feet.

REFERENCES
1. Karthikeyan G, Guilherme L. Acute rheumatic fever. Lancet. 2018;392(10142):161–174.
2. Webb RH, Grant C, Harnden A. Acute rheumatic fever. BMJ. 2015;351:h3443.
3. Del Mar CB, Glasziou PP, Spinks AB. Antibiotics for sore throat. Cochrane Database Syst Rev. 2006;(4):CD000023.
4. Gewitz MH, Baltimore RS, Tani LY, et al; for American Heart Association Committee on Rheumatic Fever, Endocarditis, and Kawasaki Disease of the Council on Cardiovascular Disease in the Young. Revision of the Jones criteria for the diagnosis of acute rheumatic fever in the era of Doppler echocardiography: a scientific statement from the American Heart Association. Circulation. 2015;131(20):1806–1818.
5. Shulman ST, Bisno AL, Clegg HW, et al. Clinical practice guideline for the diagnosis and management of group A streptococcal pharyngitis: 2012 update by the Infectious Diseases Society of America. Clin Infect Dis. 2012;55(10):1279–1282.
6. Gerber MA, Baltimore RS, Eaton CB, et al. Prevention of rheumatic fever and diagnosis and treatment of acute streptococcal pharyngitis: a scientific statement from the American Heart Association Rheumatic Fever, Endocarditis, and Kawasaki Disease Committee of the Council on Cardiovascular Disease in the Young, the Interdisciplinary Council on Functional Genomics and Translational Biology, and the Interdisciplinary Council on Quality of Care and Outcomes Research: endorsed by the American Academy of Pediatrics. Circulation. 2009;119(11):1541–1551.

 CODES

ICD10
- I00 Rheumatic fever without heart involvement
- I01.9 Acute rheumatic heart disease, unspecified
- I01.0 Acute rheumatic pericarditis

CLINICAL PEARLS
- ARF is an autoimmune, inflammatory disease that follows a GAS pharyngeal infection and affects multiple organ systems, most notably, the heart.
- Modified Jones criteria now delineate between low risk and moderate/high risk patients. Initial diagnosis requires two major or one major plus two minor manifestations in the context of a preceding documented GAS infection.
- Treatment involves antibiotic eradication followed immediately by long-term antibiotic prophylaxis. Supportive care includes NSAIDs such as naproxen or aspirin.

RHINITIS, ALLERGIC
Naureen Rafiq, MBBS

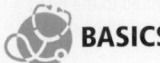

BASICS

Allergic rhinitis is the collection of symptoms involving mucous membranes of nose, eyes, ears, and throat after an exposure to allergens such as pollen, dust, or dander.

DESCRIPTION
- IgE-mediated inflammation of the nasal mucosa following exposure to an extrinsic protein; an immediate symptomatic response is characterized by sneezing, congestion, and rhinorrhea followed by a persistent late phase dominated by congestion and mucosal hyperreactivity.
- Allergic rhinitis can be classified into seasonal or perennial and can be intermittent or persistent.
- Seasonal responses are usually due to outdoor allergens such as tree pollen, flowering shrubs in spring, grasses and flowering plants in summer, and ragweed and mold in fall.
- Perennial responses, or year-round symptoms, are usually associated with indoor allergens like dust mites, mold, and animal dander.
- Occupational allergic rhinitis is caused by allergens at the workplace and can be sporadic or year-round.
- Nonallergic rhinitis (e.g., vasomotor, rhinitis of pregnancy, and rhinitis medicamentosa) can occur.

Pediatric Considerations
Chronic nasal obstruction can result in facial deformities, dental malocclusions, and sleep disorders.

Pregnancy Considerations
Physiologic changes during pregnancy may aggravate all types of rhinitis, frequently in the 2nd trimester.

EPIDEMIOLOGY
- Onset usually in first 2 decades, rarely before 6 months of age, with tendency declining with advancing age
- The mean age of onset is 8 to 11 years, and about 80% of cases have established allergic rhinitis by age 20 years.

Prevalence
- ~10–25% of the U.S. adult population and 9–42% of the U.S. pediatric population are affected.
- 44–87% of patients with allergic rhinitis have mixed allergic and nonallergic rhinitis, which is more common than either pure form (1).
- Scandinavian studies have demonstrated cumulative prevalence rate of 14% in men and 15% in women.

ETIOLOGY AND PATHOPHYSIOLOGY
- Aeroallergen-driven mucosal inflammation due to resident and infiltrating inflammatory cells as well as vasoactive and proinflammatory mediators (e.g., cytokines)
- Inhalant allergens:
  - Perennial: house dust mites, indoor molds, animal dander, cockroach/insect detritus
  - Seasonal: tree, grass, and weed pollens; outdoor molds
  - Occupational: latex, plant products (e.g., baking flour), sensitizing chemicals, and certain animals for people working in farms and vet clinics

Genetics
Complex but strong genetic predilection present (80% have family history of allergic disorders)

RISK FACTORS
- Family history of atopy, with a greater risk if both parents have atopy
- Higher socioeconomic status
- Tobacco smoke can exacerbate symptoms and increase risk of developing asthma in patients with allergic rhinitis.
- Having other allergies such as asthma
- Unclear evidence regarding risk due to early, repeated exposure to offending allergen and early introduction of solid food
- Pets in house and houses infested with cockroaches can cause perennial allergic rhinitis.

GENERAL PREVENTION
- Primary prevention of atopic disease has not been proven effective by maternal diet or maternal allergen avoidance (2).
- Exclusive breastfeeding to 6 months of age lowers risk of some atopic disorders.
- Symptomatic control by environmental avoidance is the "first-line treatment."
- No evidence to support use of acaricides with mite-proof mattress and pillow covers, carpet and drape removal, removal of plants in the home, and pet control (2,3)[B]
- Air conditioning and limited outside exposure during allergy season (1)[B]
- HEPA air cleaners and vacuum bags of unclear efficacy
- Close doors and windows during allergy season.
- Use a dehumidifier to reduce indoor humidity.

COMMONLY ASSOCIATED CONDITIONS
Other IgE-mediated conditions: asthma, atopic dermatitis, allergic conjunctivitis, food allergy

DIAGNOSIS

Diagnosis is made primarily by history and physical exam.

HISTORY
- Evaluation of nature, duration, and time course of symptoms
- History of atopic dermatitis and/or food allergies
- History of nasal congestion; rhinorrhea; pruritus of nose, eyes, ears, and/or palate; sneezing; itching; and watering eyes
- Family history of allergic diseases
- History of environmental and occupational exposure and various nasal stimuli can help differentiate between allergic and vasomotor rhinitis.

PHYSICAL EXAM
Many findings are suggestive of but not specific for allergic rhinitis:
- Dark circles under eyes, "allergic shiners" (infraorbital venous congestion)
- Transverse nasal crease from rubbing nose upward; typically seen in children
- Rhinorrhea, usually with clear discharge
- Pale, boggy, blue-gray nasal mucosa
- Postnasal mucus discharge
- Oropharyngeal lymphoid tissue hypertrophy

DIFFERENTIAL DIAGNOSIS
- Infectious rhinitis: usually viral, commonly with secondary bacterial infection
  - Usually associated with sinusitis and is known as rhinosinusitis
  - Viral rhinitis averages six episodes per year from ages 2 to 6 years.
  - IgA deficiency with recurrent sinusitis
  - Rhinitis medicamentosa:
    ○ Rebound effect associated with continued use of topical decongestant drops and sprays
    ○ ACE inhibitors, reserpine, β-blockers, oral contraceptive pills (OCPs), guanethidine, methyldopa
    ○ Aspirin, NSAIDs
  - Vasomotor (idiopathic) rhinitis caused by numerous nasal stimuli such as warm or cold air, scents and odors, light or particulate matter
  - Hormonal: pregnancy, thyroid, OCPs
  - Nonallergic rhinitis with eosinophilia syndrome (NARES)
  - Gustatory: watery rhinorrhea in response to alcohol or food
  - "Skier's nose": watery rhinorrhea in response to cold air
- Conditions associated with rhinitis:
  - Nasal polyps, tumor
  - Septal/anatomic obstruction
    ○ Adenoidal hypertrophy, particularly in children
    ○ Septal abnormality or deflected nasal septum (DNS) in adults

DIAGNOSTIC TESTS & INTERPRETATION
- Lab tests rarely needed
- Skin testing is done to identify the allergen for immunotherapy.

Initial Tests (lab, imaging)
- Testing is rarely indicated.
- If diagnosis implies other causes, consider the following:
  - CBC with differential may show elevated eosinophils.
  - Increased total serum IgE level
  - Nasal probe smear may show elevated eosinophils.
- Medications that may alter lab results
  - Corticosteroids may decrease eosinophilia.
  - Antihistamines suppress reactivity to skin tests; stop antihistamines 7 days before testing.
- CT scan of sinuses is not routinely done but can be used to check for complete opacity, fluid level, and mucosal thickening.

Diagnostic Procedures/Other
- Consider testing in only those cases where allergic symptoms do not respond to treatment and/or considering immunotherapy.
- Specific allergen sensitivity with allergen skin testing or radioallergosorbent test (RAST); clinical correlation based on history is essential in interpreting results.
- Diagnostic allergen prick tests are used to select agent to determine appropriate environmental control measures as well as to direct immunotherapy:
  - Prick or puncture: superficial injury to epidermis with application of test antigen
  - Intradermal

- RAST: more expensive and less sensitive than skin testing; typically used in patients in whom skin testing is not practical or a severe reaction is possible
- Rhinoscopy: useful to visualize intranasal anatomy and posterior pharyngeal structures, including adenoids, polyps, and larynx

Test Interpretation
- Nasal washing/scraping: Eosinophils predominate but may see basophils, mast cells.
- Nasal mucosa: submucosal edema but without destruction; eosinophilic infiltration; congested mucous glands and goblet cells

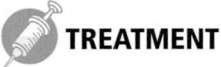 **TREATMENT**

There are three mainstays of treatment of allergic rhinitis:
- Allergen avoidance
- Medication
- Allergy immunotherapy

GENERAL MEASURES
- Establish specific cause(s) by history and appropriate testing.
- Limit exposure to offending allergen.
- Allergen immunotherapy (desensitization)
  - Reserved when symptoms are uncontrollable with medical therapy or have a comorbidity (e.g., asthma)
  - Specific allergen extract is injected SC in increasing doses to induce patient tolerance.

MEDICATION
Oral medication and intranasal sprays are commonly used.

First Line
- Mild symptoms: 2nd-generation nonsedating antihistamines are the first-line therapy for mild to moderate allergic rhinitis (1,4).
- Adverse effects: mild sedation, mild anticholinergic effects
- Generic (cetirizine, fexofenadine, loratadine; most to least effective)
  - Levocetirizine is a 2nd-generation nonsedating antihistamine that is effective but costly.
- Intranasal corticosteroids are first-line therapy for moderate to severe allergic rhinitis (1,4)[A]:
  - Most effective drug class for symptoms of allergic rhinitis
  - Use nasal sprays after showering and direct spray away from septum to improve deposition on mucosal surface.
  - May be used as needed; however, more effective with daily use (1)
  - Adverse effects: nosebleed, nasal septal perforation, and systemic corticosteroid effects
  - Ciclesonide is a new-generation corticosteroid with previously demonstrated efficacy in the treatment of asthma when delivered through a metered-dose inhaler. Ciclesonide is also currently in clinical development as an intranasal formulation for use in the treatment of AR.
- Systemic steroids should be considered only in urgent cases and only for short-term use.

Second Line
- Nasal antihistamines effective but may be systemically absorbed and may cause sedation: azelastine, olopatadine

- 1st-generation antihistamines, such as the following:
  - Brompheniramine: 12 to 24 mg PO BID
  - Chlorpheniramine: 4 mg PO q4–6h PRN
  - Clemastine: 1 to 2 mg PO BID PRN
  - Diphenhydramine: 25 to 50 mg PO q4–6h PRN:
    o May precipitate urinary retention in men with prostatism and/or hypertrophy
    o Adverse effects: sedation, prolonged QT interval, performance impairment, and anticholinergic effect
  - Decongestants
    o Phenylephrine: 10 mg PO q4h PRN
    o Pseudoephedrine: 60 mg PO q4–6h PRN
    o Oxymetazoline nasal spray (Afrin): 2 to 3 sprays per nostril q10–12h PRN (max 3 days). Intranasal agents should not be used for >3 days due to rebound rhinitis. Discourage use in patients with hypertension (HTN) or cardiac arrhythmia.
  - Intranasal anticholinergics such as ipratropium nasal spray 2 sprays per nostril BID–TID
    o Intranasal anticholinergics can increase efficacy in combination with steroid use.
  - Leukotriene antagonists such as montelukast 10 mg/day PO
    o Should generally be used as an adjunct, not monotherapy
    o May be first line in those with concomitant asthma
  - Mast cell stabilizers such as cromolyn nasal spray 1 spray per nostril TID–QID
    o May take 2 to 4 weeks of therapy for optimal efficacy
    o May be ineffective in patients with nonallergic rhinitis and nasal polyps

ISSUES FOR REFERRAL
Refer to allergist for consideration of immunotherapy.

ADDITIONAL THERAPIES
- Nasal saline use has evidence of efficacy as sole agent or as adjunctive treatment (1,5)[A].
- Other treatment strategies
  - When initiating intranasal steroids, consider starting with a "burst," using 2 sprays in each nostril daily for 2 weeks and then decreasing to 1 spray in each nostril daily thereafter (6).
  - To mitigate long-term side effects of intranasal steroids, consider a "5 days on, 2 days off" strategy, with the days off being the days of lowest exposure to allergens (6).

 ONGOING CARE

FOLLOW-UP RECOMMENDATIONS
No specific restrictions on activity; emphasize avoiding activity where exposure to the allergen is likely.

Patient Monitoring
Initiation of patient education is critical.

DIET
- No special diet unless concomitant food reactions are suspected and evaluated
- Some patients with severe sensitivity to seasonal pollens may have oral allergy syndrome, which is associated with itching in the mouth with the ingestion of fresh fruits that may cross-react with the allergens.

PATIENT EDUCATION
- Asthma and Allergy Foundation of America, 1717 Massachusetts Ave., Suite 305, Washington, DC 20036; (800) 7-ASTHMA: http://www.aafa.org/
- Other helpful information available at http://www.acaai.org/ and http://www.aaaai.org/home.aspx

PROGNOSIS
- Acceptable control of symptoms is the goal.
- Treatment is helpful to reduce the risk of comorbidities, such as sinusitis and asthma.

COMPLICATIONS
- Secondary infection such as otitis media or sinusitis
- Epistaxis
- Nasopharyngeal lymphoid hyperplasia
- Airway hyperreactivity with allergen exposure
- Asthma
- Facial changes, especially in children who are mouth breathers
- Sleep disturbance

REFERENCES
1. Wallace DV, Dykewicz MS, Bernstein DI, et al; for Joint Task Force on Practice Parameter for Allergy and Immunology. The diagnosis and management of rhinitis: an updated practice parameter. *J Allergy Clin Immunol*. 2008; 122(Suppl 2):S1–S84.
2. Kramer MS, Kakuma R. Maternal dietary antigen avoidance during pregnancy or lactation, or both, for preventing or treating atopic disease in the child. *Cochrane Database Syst Rev*. 2012;(9):CD000133.
3. Sheikh A, Hurwitz B, Nurmatov U, et al. House dust mite avoidance measures for perennial allergic rhinitis. *Cochrane Database Syst Rev*. 2010;(7):CD001563.
4. Plaut M, Valentine MD. Clinical practice. Allergic rhinitis. *N Engl J Med*. 2005;353(18): 1934–1944.
5. Harvey R, Hannan SA, Badia L, et al. Nasal saline irrigations for the symptoms of chronic rhinosinusitis. *Cochrane Database Syst Rev*. 2007;(3):CD006394.
6. Watto M. Upper respiratory infections: coughs, colds, gargling, and antibiotic underuse?! http://thecurbsiders.com/medical-education/54-upper-respiratory-infections-coughs-colds-gargling-antibiotic-underuse. Accessed November 17, 2017.

 SEE ALSO

Conjunctivitis, Acute

 CODES

ICD10
- J30.9 Allergic rhinitis, unspecified
- J30.1 Allergic rhinitis due to pollen
- J30.2 Other seasonal allergic rhinitis

CLINICAL PEARLS
- Nasal saline irrigation (flushing 6 to 8 oz) may be very helpful in clearing upper airway of secretions and may precede the use of nasal corticosteroids.
- 2nd-generation antihistamines and intranasal corticosteroids are first-line therapies for allergic rhinitis.

R

ROCKY MOUNTAIN SPOTTED FEVER

Eugene Y. Wang, MD • Lloyd A. Runser, MD, MPH, FAAFP • Christopher A. Zagar, MD, FAAFP

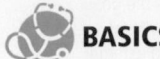

BASICS

Rocky Mountain spotted fever (RMSF) is one of the spotted fever rickettsioses (SFR) and is associated with the highest rates of severe and fatal outcomes of all reportable rickettsial diseases in the United States.

DESCRIPTION
- RMSF is a potentially fatal tick-borne systemic small vessel vasculitis caused by the bacterium *Rickettsia rickettsii*.
- Symptoms include fever, headache, and myalgia followed by a macular rash; begins at wrists and ankles, spreading toward palms, soles, and the trunk
- System(s) affected: cardiovascular, musculoskeletal, skin, CNS, renal, hepatic, and pulmonary

EPIDEMIOLOGY
In the United States, ticks are both vectors and main reservoirs; the American dog tick, *Dermacentor variabilis* in the eastern two-thirds of the states; the Rocky Mountain wood tick, *Dermacentor andersoni* in the western states; and the brown dog tick, *Rhipicephalus sanguineus* is distributed throughout all states (1,2)[A].

Incidence
- In the United States, incidence of SFR was 8.9 cases per million from 2008 to 2012. Cases have been reported in all states except Hawaii and Alaska; RMSF also seen in Canada, Mexico, and throughout Central and South America (1,2)[A],(3)[B]
- North Carolina, Arkansas, Missouri, Oklahoma, and Tennessee account for over 60% of cases (1,2)[A].
- Cases occur year round. Most are reported during April to September during the peak of outdoor activity (1,2)[A],(3)[B].
- All ages are susceptible; highest incidence occurs in age 60 to 69 years. Highest case-fatality rate is in children <10 years (1)[A].

Prevalence
In the United States, 4,470 cases were reported in 2012. <0.1% of ticks carry virulent rickettsial species.

ETIOLOGY AND PATHOPHYSIOLOGY
- An adult tick releases *R. rickettsii*, an obligate intracellular gram-negative coccobacilli, from its salivary glands after 6 to 10 hours of feeding.
- Pathogens infect vascular endothelial cells, causing small-vessel injury, microhemorrhages, and local consumption of platelets resulting in characteristic petechial rash.
- Damage leads to progressively increased vascular permeability, pulmonary and cerebral edema, hypovolemia, and hyponatremia in late-stage disease.
- Subsequent end-organ injury may also result in meningoencephalitis, acute renal failure (ARF), ARDS, shock, arrhythmia, and seizure (1)[A].
- Symptoms appear 3 to 12 days after bite or between 4 and 8 days after discovery of an attached tick. Incubation period is typically 5 days or less.
- Transplacental transmission has not been reported.

- RMSF can rarely be caused by direct inoculation of tick blood into open wounds or conjunctivae.

Genetics
R. rickettsii has one of the smallest bacterial genomes (1.1 to 1.6 Mb), making the organism highly adapted to the intracellular environment.

RISK FACTORS
- Known tick bite, engorged tick, or presence of tick for >20 hours; likelihood of infection increases with duration of tick attachment.
- Tick crushed during removal
- Accumulated outdoor exposure or residence in wooded areas
- Contact with outdoor pets or wild animals

GENERAL PREVENTION
- Limit tick exposure when possible in endemic areas, highest tick exposure with time spent in tall grasses, open areas of low bushy vegetation or wooded areas.
- Wear light-colored clothing, long sleeves, pants, socks, and closed-toed shoes.
- Use DEET-containing insect repellents.
- Permethrin spray on clothing
- Regular tick checks
- Prompt tick removal.
- Wash hands and site of bite with soap and water after tick removal to avoid potential mucosal inoculation.
- Nail polish, petrolatum jelly, and heat do not aid in tick removal. Do not use bare hands to remove ticks.
- Protect pets with ectoparasite control (1,2)[A].
- Prophylactic antibiotic treatment is not recommended.

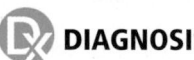

DIAGNOSIS

Delay of empirical therapy increases risk of long-term sequelae and mortality.

HISTORY
Consider RMSF in acute febrile illness and rash, particularly with a history of potential tick exposure within previous 14 days; outdoor activities or travels to an endemic area, during late spring or summer months. *The tick bite goes unnoticed 30–50% of the time.*
- Typically presents like a viral illness with sudden onset of fever, frontal headache, malaise, and myalgia (1,2)[A]
- Nausea, vomiting, abdominal pain, anorexia, and photophobia may also be present.
- RMSF is easily mistaken for gastroenteritis, pharyngitis, or mononucleosis.
- Rash typically appears 2 to 4 days after onset of fever; starts as a small blanching, pink macules on wrist and ankles before spreading to the trunk where rash may become maculopapular in appearance

- Involvement of palms and soles usually present by 5th to 6th day, along with generalized petechial rash; a sign of advanced disease
- Although children <15 years more frequently (>90%) have a rash, the classic triad of fever, rash and tick bite occurs in <60% of children with RMSF. A small number of patients never develop rash (1,2)[A].
- Other symptoms include conjunctival injection, mental status impairments, restlessness, arthralgia, peripheral or periorbital edema, calf pain, and hearing loss (1,2)[A].

PHYSICAL EXAM
- Fever is typically >102°F.
- The rash typically starts as an erythematous, macular, or maculopapular exanthema (1 to 5 mm in diameter); 50% become petechial or purpuric; blanchable
- 20% never develop the "classic" rash. Do not rely solely on the presence or absence of the typical rash for diagnosis.
- Rash can be difficult to visualize on dark-skin.
- In severe cases, the rash can involve the entire body (including mucous membranes) and may progress to necrotic or gangrenous lesions.
- The rash is not associated with pruritus or urticaria; if present, this makes RMSF less likely.
- Lymphadenopathy and hepatosplenomegaly

DIFFERENTIAL DIAGNOSIS
- Viral exanthema (e.g., hand-foot-mouth disease, measles, rubella, roseola)
- Viral gastroenteritis, mononucleosis
- URI, UTI, TTP/ITP, idiopathic vasculitides, toxic shock syndrome
- Meningoencephalitis, meningococcemia
- Other tick-borne infections: typhus, ehrlichiosis, Lyme disease
- Leptospirosis
- Drug reaction or serum sickness
- Kawasaki disease

DIAGNOSTIC TESTS & INTERPRETATION
Diagnosis is often clinical based on symptoms and exposure history. Confirm with serology. Do not delay therapy awaiting results.

Initial Tests (lab, imaging)
- Specific laboratory diagnosis
  - Indirect fluorescent antibody (IFA) testing is gold standard for serology.
  - Sensitivity of IFA 2 weeks after onset of illness is 94–100%: A 4-fold increase in titers of IgG from paired acute-phase and convalescent-phase sera confirms diagnosis (4)[A].
  - Detectable antibody response develops 7 to 10 days after exposure; optimal time for testing is 14 to 21 days after symptom onset.
- Nonspecific laboratory tests
  - WBC count: variable, frequently normal
  - Platelet: thrombocytopenia (<150,000 cells/μL) 60% of kids
  - Hyponatremia <135 mEq/dL, and elevated hepatic transaminases in 50% of patients

– Anemia, increase in BUN/creatinine, PT/PTT, hyperbilirubinemia, and hypoalbuminemia may also be present.

– CSF may have mononuclear pleocytosis and elevated protein (1,2)[A].

• Other than occasional nonspecific pneumonic infiltrates on chest radiograph, imaging procedures are rarely helpful.

Diagnostic Procedures/Other

• Skin biopsy can also offer definitive diagnosis; a 3-mm punch biopsy to perform a rapid direct fluorescent antibody (DFA) test (sensitivity 70%, specificity 100%)

• Rickettsial DNA detection using PCR of skin biopsy samples is a new approach to diagnosis of up to 60–70% of suspected rickettsial infections during the acute-phase of illness (4)[A].

• Qualitative ELISA

Test Interpretation

• Test acute and convalescent phase sera in tandem.

• Early treatment may limit antibody formation.

• Seropositivity increases with age in endemic states. Positive spotted fever group *Rickettsia* antibody does not necessarily signify an acute infection.

• Petechiae due to the vasculitis may be seen on organ surfaces (e.g., liver, brain, or epicardium).

 TREATMENT

MEDICATION

First Line

Doxycycline is the treatment of choice in both adults and children (1,2,4)[A],(3)[B].

• Untreated rickettsial infections have a high rate of morbidity and mortality. Other antibiotics are considerably less effective.

• Adults: 100 mg PO or IV q12h for 5 to 10 days; children weighing <45 kg (100 lb): 2.2 mg/kg/dose PO or IV q12h for 5 to 10 days

• Treat all patients for at least 3 days after defervescence (1,2)[A],(3)[B],(4)[A].

• Fever typically subsides within 24 to 48 hours with early treatment; longer if patient is severely ill. If promptly treated, and patient lack response to doxycycline in 48 hours, consider an alternate diagnosis.

• RMSF resistance to doxycycline has not been documented.

• Adverse effects may include

– Dyspepsia. Take medication with food and water. Avoid dairy, iron, or antacids, as they may inhibit drug absorption.

– Photosensitivity may occur. Minimize sun exposure and use sunscreen.

– No risk of dental staining in children <8 years old (1,2,3)[A]

• Severe allergy is a contraindication to doxycycline; rapid desensitization may be considered for life-threatening disease in severe illness.

Second Line

• Chloramphenicol is the alternative to treat RMSF; associated with adverse hematologic effects (e.g., aplastic anemia) and increased case mortality (1,2)[A]

• Fluoroquinolones have in vitro activity against rickettsiae but no human efficacy data. They are not currently recommended for treatment (1)[A].

• Sulfa-containing drugs may increase disease severity/fatality and are contraindicated.

Pregnancy Considerations

• Doxycycline is appropriate for this life-threatening infection in pregnancy if suspicion is high despite the potential risk to fetal bones/teeth along with maternal hepatotoxicity and pancreatitis (4)[A].

• Short-term doxycycline is compatible with breast-feeding (1)[A].

• Chloramphenicol may be considered but should be avoided in the 3rd trimester due to risk for gray baby syndrome.

ISSUES FOR REFERRAL

• Consider infectious disease consult along with immunology/allergist if patient is severely allergic to doxycycline.

• Report cases of RMSF to public health authorities.

ADDITIONAL THERAPIES

Patients with neurologic injury may require prolonged physical and cognitive therapy.

ADMISSION, INPATIENT, AND NURSING CONSIDERATIONS

• Admission criteria/initial stabilization

– CNS dysfunction

– Nausea/vomiting preventing oral antibiotic therapy

– Immunocompromised patients

– Specific acute organ failure

– Failure of oral pain management

– ICU for patients with shock

• Discharge criteria

– Resolution of fever

– Ability to take oral therapy and nutrition

 ONGOING CARE

FOLLOW-UP RECOMMENDATIONS

• Patients with mild disease may be treated as outpatients if close follow-up is available.

• Hospitalize patients with moderate to severe disease.

• Infection does not confer lifelong immunity.

Patient Monitoring

• Follow patients treated as outpatients every 2 to 3 days until symptoms resolve.

• Follow up CBC, electrolytes, LFTs if clinically indicated.

DIET

Consider nutritional supplementation if intake is poor.

PATIENT EDUCATION

General prevention and caution regarding tick avoidance during outside activities in endemic areas

PROGNOSIS

• Prognosis is closely related to timely administration of appropriate antibiotics.

• Delay in treatment may increase mortality by 3-fold if delayed to 5th day of illness (2)[A].

• When treated promptly, prognosis is excellent with resolution of symptoms and no sequelae.

• Children aged <10 years and elderly >70 years are at higher risk of morbidity and/or mortality.

• Patients with G6PD deficiency are at highest risk for fulminant RMSF, in which death can occur ≤5 days.

COMPLICATIONS

• Encephalopathy, most commonly transient impaired level of consciousness or meningismus

• Seizures, focal neurologic deficit

• Renal injury leading to ARF

• Hepatitis, congestive heart failure (CHF), respiratory failure

• Proximal muscle weakness, changes in personality, paresthesias, deafness, secondary thromboses, and tissue necrosis may also be seen.

REFERENCES

1. Biggs HM, Behravesh CB, Bradley KK, et al. Diagnosis and management of tickborne rickettsial diseases: Rocky Mountain spotted fever and other spotted fever group rickettsioses, ehrlichioses, and anaplasmosis—United States. *MMWR Recomm Rep.* 2016;65(2):1–44.

2. Mukkada S, Buckingham SC. Recognition of and prompt treatment for tick-borne infections in children. *Infect Dis Clin North Am.* 2015;29(3):539–555.

3. Todd SR, Dahlgren FS, Traeger MS, et al. No visible dental staining in children treated with doxycycline for suspected Rocky Mountain spotted fever. *J Pediatr.* 2015;166(5):1246–1251.

4. Fang R, Blanton LS, Walker DH. Rickettsiae as emerging infectious agents. *Clin Lab Med.* 2017;37(2):383–400.

CODES

ICD10

A77.0 Spotted fever due to Rickettsia rickettsii

CLINICAL PEARLS

• Diagnosis of RMSF requires a high index of clinical suspicion.

• Tick bites are often unnoticed, and some patients may never develop a rash.

• Begin treatment immediately in suspected cases. Doxycycline is drug of choice for RMSF in both adults and children. The only absolute contraindication is severe allergy to the drug.

• Do not wait for laboratory testing prior to beginning treatment of suspected cases.

ROSEOLA

Jeffrey D. Quinlan, MD, FAAFP

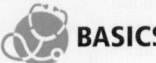 BASICS

Omnipresent infection occurring in infancy and childhood. Majority of cases are caused by human herpesvirus 6 (HHV-6); may be associated with other diseases including encephalitis

DESCRIPTION
- Acute infection of infants or very young children (1)
- Causes a high fever followed by a skin eruption as the fever resolves (1)
- Transmission via contact with salivary secretions or respiratory droplet (1)
- Incubation period of 9 to 10 days (1)
- System(s) affected: skin/exocrine, metabolic, gastrointestinal, respiratory, neurologic
- Synonym(s): roseola infantum, exanthem subitum; pseudorubella; sixth disease; 3-day fever (1)

Pediatric Considerations
A disease of infants and very young children (2)

EPIDEMIOLOGY
- Predominant age
  – HHV-6
    ○ Infants and very young children (<2 years old) (3)
    ○ Peak age infection 6 to 9 months, rarely congenital or perinatal infection (1)
    ○ 95% of children have been infected with HHV-6 by 2 years of life.
  – HHV-7
    ○ Later childhood
    ○ Mean age of infection 26 months
    ○ >90% population with HHV-7 by 10 years (1)
- Predominant sex: male = female (1)
- No seasonal variance

Incidence
Common—accounts for 20% ED visits for febrile illness among children 6 to 8 months (4)

Prevalence
- Peak prevalence is between 9 and 21 months (3).
- Nearly 100% population carrying HHV-6 by 3 years (1)
- Approximately 20% patients with primary HHV-6 have roseola (4).

ETIOLOGY AND PATHOPHYSIOLOGY
- HHV-6 and HHV-7 (2)
- Majority of cases (60–74%) due to HHV-6
  – HHV-6B > HHV-6A (2)
  – HHV-6A seen in children in Africa
  – HHV-6 binds to CD46 receptors on all nucleated cells (2).
- Primary infection typically through respiratory droplets or saliva

- Congenital infection/vertical transmission occurs in 1% of cases (1).
  – Transplacental transmission
  – Chromosomal integration (clinical significance unknown)
- Lifelong latent or persistent asymptomatic infection occurs after primary infection (1).
  – 80–90% of population intermittently sheds HHV-6/HHV-7 in saliva (2).
  – Patients are viremic from 2 days prior to fever until defervescence and onset of rash.
  – HHV-6 latency is also implicated in CSF (4).

Genetics
HHV-6 is integrated into the chromosomes of 0.2–3.0% of the population. This leads to vertical transmission of the virus. Clinical significance of this is unknown (1).

RISK FACTORS
- Female gender (3)
- Having older siblings (3)
- At-risk adults: immunocompromised (5)
  – Renal, liver, other solid organ, and bone marrow transplant (BMT) (3)
  – HHV-6 reactivation can occur in 1st week posttransplant (5). HHV-6 viremia occurs in 30–45% of BMT within the first several weeks after transplantation (4).
    ○ Usually asymptomatic (4)
    ○ Up to 82% of HHV-6 reactivation/reinfection in solid organ transplant (5)
- Nonrisk factors (3)
  – Child care attendance
  – Method of delivery
  – Breastfeeding (HHV does not appear to pass through breast milk.)
  – Maternal age
  – Season

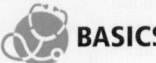 DIAGNOSIS

HISTORY
- 3 to 5 days abrupt fever 102.2–104.0°F (39–40°C) not associated with a rash (1)
- The child may be fussy during this prodrome (1,6).
- Sudden drop of fever associated with appearance of rash (1)
  – Rash on trunk then spreads centrifugally mainly to neck, possibly also to peripheral extremities, and face
- Diarrhea (3)
- Mild upper respiratory symptoms (3)
- Rhinorrhea (3)
- Febrile seizure occurs in 13% of cases (1).

PHYSICAL EXAM
- Rash (exanthem subitum) (1)
  – Rose-pink macules and/or papules that blanch
  – First appears on the trunk then peripherally
  – May occur up to 3 days after fever resolves (1)
  – Fades within 2 days
  – Occurs in approximately 20% of patients in the United States (1)
- Mild inflammation of tympanic membrane, pharynx, and/or conjunctiva (1,6)
- Ulcers on soft palate and uvula (Nagayama spots) (1)
- Cervical lymphadenopathy (1)
- Periorbital edema (2)

DIFFERENTIAL DIAGNOSIS
- Enterovirus infection
- Adenovirus infection (1)
- Epstein-Barr virus
- Fifth disease—parvovirus B19
- Rubella (1)
- Scarlet fever (1)
- Drug eruption (1)
- Measles (1)

DIAGNOSTIC TESTS & INTERPRETATION
- Primarily a clinical diagnosis not requiring laboratory or radiologic testing (1)[C]
- Tests often cannot differentiate latent or active disease (1)[C].
- Specific diagnosis only necessary in severe cases, unclear diagnosis where more serious disease needs to be ruled out, or if considering antiviral therapy (1)[C]

Initial Tests (lab, imaging)
- HHV-6 and HHV-7 by PCR (1,5)[C]
  – Serum, whole blood, CSF, or saliva
  – Becoming more widely available
  – Not required in non-immunocompromised individuals
- HHV-6 IgM immunofluorescence (1)
- Diagnostic for acute infection
  – Spike seen in 1st week of illness
- HHV-6 IgG immunofluorescence (1)
  – Check at diagnosis and then 2 weeks later.
  – Use with IgM to show primary infection.
  – Negative initial test and rise on follow-up suggest primary infection.
- Viral culture (5)
  – Rarely done
  – No clinical use (very time-consuming)
- Other laboratory findings (1)
  – Decreased total leukocytes, lymphocytes, and neutrophils
  – Elevated transaminases
  – Thrombocytopenia

Diagnostic Procedures/Other
- Urine culture: to rule out UTI as source of fever (2)
- Chest x-ray (CXR): if a child has respiratory symptoms

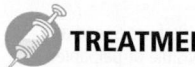

TREATMENT

No treatment necessary, resolves without sequelae (1)[C]

GENERAL MEASURES
- Symptomatic relief including antipyretics (1)[C]
- Hydration (1)[C]

MEDICATION
First Line
- No specific first-line treatment in immunocompetent hosts beyond supportive measures (2)[C]
  - Antivirals are not recommended in immunocompetent.
- No approved antiviral treatment in immunocompromised (2)[C]
- Second-line IV ganciclovir, cidofovir, foscarnet tested in vitro studies in stem cell transplant patients
  - HHV-6B susceptible: ganciclovir and foscarnet (5)[C]
  - HHV-6A and HHV-7 are more resistant to ganciclovir (5).
- Antivirals suggested in individual cases of encephalitis (associated with reactivation of HHV-6) (5)
- In bone marrow and stem cell transplant recipients receiving immunosuppression, ganciclovir prophylaxis is effective in preventing reactivation of HHV-6 (6)[B].

ONGOING CARE

FOLLOW-UP RECOMMENDATIONS
Patient Monitoring
- During febrile prodrome, monitor for dehydration.
- None after typical rash appears and fever resolves
- Mean duration of illness is 6 days (4).
- If febrile seizures occur, they will cease after fever subsides and will not likely recur (4).
- Symptomatic reactivation in immunocompromised (1)

DIET
Encourage fluids.

PATIENT EDUCATION
- Parental reassurance that this is usually a benign, self-limited disease (1)
- There is no specific recommended period of exclusion from out-of-home care for affected children.
- Patient is viremic a few days prior to fever until time of defervescence and rash onset.

PROGNOSIS
- Course: acute, complete recovery without sequelae (1)
- Reactivation in immunocompromised patients is common (4).

COMPLICATIONS
- Febrile seizures
  - 13% patients with roseola (1,6)
  - Accounts for 1/3 of primary seizures in children <2 years old (1)
- Medication hypersensitivity syndromes (drug reaction with eosinophilia and systemic symptoms) (2)
- Reactivation can occur in transplant patients, HIV-1 infection, and other immunocompromised individuals (4).
- Meningoencephalitis occurs in immunocompetent and in immunosuppressed patients (4); poor association with multiple sclerosis (4)
- Pityriasis rosea (1)
- Possible association with progressive multifocal leukoencephalopathy (4)

REFERENCES
1. Stone RC, Micali GA, Schwartz RA. Roseola infantum and its causal human herpesviruses. *Int J Dermatol*. 2014;53(4):397–403.
2. Wolz MM, Sciallis GF, Pittelkow MR. Human herpesviruses 6, 7, and 8 from a dermatologic perspective. *Mayo Clin Proc*. 2012;87(10):1004–1014.
3. Zerr DM, Meier AS, Selke SS, et al. A population-based study of primary human herpesvirus 6 infection. *N Engl J Med*. 2005;352(8):768–776.
4. Caserta MT, Mock DJ, Dewhurst S. Human herpesvirus 6. *Clin Infect Dis*. 2001;33(6):829–833.
5. Le J, Gantt S; for AST Infectious Diseases Community of Practice. Human herpesvirus 6, 7 and 8 in solid organ transplantation. *Am J Transplant*. 2013;13(Suppl 4):128–137.
6. Tokimasa S, Hara J, Osugi Y, et al. Ganciclovir is effective for prophylaxis and treatment of human herpesvirus-6 in allogeneic stem cell transplantation. *Bone Marrow Transplant*. 2002;29(7):595–598.

ADDITIONAL READING
- Ablashi DV, Devin CL, Yoshikawa T, et al. Review part 3: human herpesvirus-6 in multiple non-neurological diseases. *J Med Virol*. 2010;82(11):1903–1910.
- Caselli E, Di Luca D. Molecular biology and clinical associations of roseoloviruses human herpesvirus 6 and human herpesvirus 7. *New Microbiol*. 2007;30(3):173–187.
- Dockrell DH, Smith TF, Paya CV. Human herpesvirus 6. *Mayo Clin Proc*. 1999;74(2):163–170.

- Dyer JA. Childhood viral exanthems. *Pediatr Ann*. 2007;36(1):21–29.
- Evans CM, Kudesia G, McKendrick M. Management of herpesvirus infections. *Int J Antimicrob Agents*. 2013;42(2):119–128.
- Fölster-Holst R, Kreth HW. Viral exanthems in childhood—infectious (direct) exanthems. Part 1: classic exanthems. *J Dtsch Dermatol Ges*. 2009;7(4):309–316.
- Huang CT, Lin LH. Differentiating roseola infantum with pyuria from urinary tract infection. *Pediatr Int*. 2013;55(2):214–218.
- Leach CT. Human herpesvirus-6 and -7 infections in children: agents of roseola and other syndromes. *Curr Opin Pediatr*. 2000;12(3):269–274.
- Lowry M. Roseola infantum. *Pract Nurse*. 2013;43:40–42.
- Stoeckle MY. The spectrum of human herpesvirus 6 infection: from roseola infantum to adult disease. *Annu Rev Med*. 2000;51:423–430.
- Vianna RA, de Oliveira SA, Camacho LA, et al. Role of human herpesvirus 6 infection in young Brazilian children with rash illnesses. *Pediatr Infect Dis J*. 2008;27(6):533–537.

 ## CODES

ICD10
- B08.20 Exanthema subitum [sixth disease], unspecified
- B08.21 Exanthema subitum [sixth disease] due to human herpesvirus 6
- B08.22 Exanthema subitum [sixth disease] due to human herpesvirus 7

CLINICAL PEARLS
- Roseola infection should be suspected if an infant or young child presents with a high temperature without other clinical findings.
- As the fever abates, a macular rash will be seen on the trunk, with eventual spread to the face and extremities in 20% of patients.
- Roseola is a clinical diagnosis, and laboratory testing is not necessary for most children with classic presentation.
- For atypical presentations, complications, and immunocompromised hosts, several laboratory tools are available, including serologic testing for antibody, viral PCR testing, and viral culture.
- Infection is typically self-limiting and without sequelae.
- Usually, only symptomatic treatment is needed.
- Consider prophylaxis in patients undergoing bone marrow or stem cell transplant and receiving immunosuppressive therapy.

ROTATOR CUFF IMPINGEMENT SYNDROME

Faren H. Williams, MD, MS • Minjin K. Fromm, MD

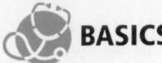

BASICS

DESCRIPTION

- Compression of rotator cuff tendons and subacromial bursa between the humeral head and the structures comprising the coracoacromial arch and proximal humerus
- Most common cause of atraumatic shoulder pain in patients >25 years of age
- Primary symptom is pain that is most severe when the arm is abducted between 60 and 120 degrees (the "painful arc").
- Classically divided into three stages:
  - Stage I: acute inflammation, edema, or hemorrhage of the underlying tendons due to overuse (typically in those age <25 years)
  - Stage II: progressive tendinosis that leads to partial rotator cuff tear along with underlying thickening or fibrosis of surrounding structures (commonly, ages 25 to 40 years)
  - Stage III: full-thickness tear (typically in patients age >40 years)

EPIDEMIOLOGY

Incidence

- Shoulder pain accounts for 1% of all primary care visits.
- Peak incidence of 25/1,000 patients per year occurs in patients aged 42 to 46 years.
- Impingement responsible for 18–74% of shoulder pain diagnoses

Prevalence

Prevalence of shoulder pain in general population ranges from ~7% to 30%.

RISK FACTORS

- Repetitive overhead motions (throwing, swimming)
- Glenohumeral joint instability or muscle imbalance
- Acromioclavicular arthritis or osteophytes
- Thickened coracoacromial ligament
- Shoulder trauma
- Increasing age
- Smoking

GENERAL PREVENTION

- Proper throwing and lifting techniques
- Proper strengthening to balance rotator cuff and scapula stabilizer muscles

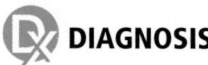

DIAGNOSIS

HISTORY

- Gradual increase in shoulder pain with overhead activities (Sudden onset of sharp pain suggests a tear.)
- Night pain is common, exacerbated by lying on the affected shoulder or sleeping with the affected arm above the head.
- Anterolateral shoulder pain with overhead activities
- May progress to weakness and decreased range of motion if shoulder is not used through full range of motion

PHYSICAL EXAM

- Examine patient for atrophy/asymmetry. Observe how the patient takes off his or her shirt during exam.
- Neer impingement test: Examiner stabilizes the scapula and moves the affected upper extremity through a flexion arc. Positive is pain with flexion of the shoulder. Sensitivity: 78%. Specificity: 58% (1)[A]
- Hawkins-Kennedy impingement test: Examiner places the arm in 90 degrees of forward flexion and then gently internally rotates the arm. End point for internal rotation is when the patient feels pain or when the rotation of the scapula is felt or observed by the examiner. Test is positive when patient experiences pain during the maneuver. Sensitivity: 74%. Specificity: 57% (1)[A]
- Empty can test (supraspinatus): Examiner asks the patient to elevate and internally rotate the arm with thumbs pointing downward in the scapular plane. Elbow should be fully extended. Examiner applies downward pressure on upper surface of the arm. Test is positive when patient complains of pain with resistance. Sensitivity: 69%. Specificity: 62% (1)[A]
- Lift-off test (subscapularis): Patient internally rotates the shoulder, placing the hand on ipsilateral buttock, then lifts hand off buttock against resistance. A tear in the subscapularis muscle produces weakness of this action. Sensitivity: 42%. Specificity: 97% (1)[A]
- Drop-arm test: Patient fully elevates arm and then slowly reverses the motion. If the arm is dropped suddenly or the patient has extreme pain, the test is positive for a possible rotator cuff tear. Sensitivity: 21%. Specificity: 92% (1)[A]
- Resisted external rotation: weakness suggestive of infraspinatus and/or teres minor tendon involvement
- Examine cervical spine to rule out cervical pathology as source of shoulder pain.
- Neurovascular exam of the upper extremity

DIFFERENTIAL DIAGNOSIS

- Labral injury
- Acromioclavicular arthritis (more common in older patients; positive cross-arm test—pain when affected arm is fully adducted across the chest in the horizontal plane)
- Adhesive capsulitis (rotator cuff tendonitis leads to decreased use and atrophy of rotator cuff muscles, followed by contracture; linked to diabetes and potentially prior trauma)
- Anterior shoulder instability (prior trauma; more common in patients <25 years old)
- Multidirectional instability
- Biceps tendonitis or rupture (Perform Speed and Yergason tests and look for visible or palpable defect of biceps—"Popeye sign.")
- Calcific tendonitis
- Cervical radiculopathy (spinal or foraminal stenosis, can test with Spurling maneuver)
- Glenohumeral arthritis (Evaluate with plain films.)
- Suprascapular nerve entrapment (Look for focal muscle atrophy of supra- or infraspinatus.)
- Traumatic rotator cuff tear

DIAGNOSTIC TESTS & INTERPRETATION

Initial Tests (lab, imaging)

- Plain-film radiographs of the shoulder (three views): anteroposterior, axillary, scapular Y views
- Plain films may reveal:
  - Osteoarthritis of the acromioclavicular and glenohumeral joints
  - Superior migration of the humeral head (indicative of a large rotator cuff tear)
  - Cystic change of the humeral head and sclerosis of the inferior acromion (indicative of chronic rotator cuff disease)
  - Calcific tendonitis
- MRI is used to definitively assess rotator cuff tendinopathy, partial tears, and complete tears.
- MR arthrogram is preferred for labral pathology.
- Ultrasound is sensitive and specific for rotator cuff tears but is highly operator dependent.
- CT scan is preferred for bony pathology or for those unable to undergo MRI.

Diagnostic Procedures/Other

- Lidocaine injection test
  - Inject lidocaine into the subacromial space:
    - Repeat impingement tests; if pain is completely relieved and range of motion is improved, likely impingement syndrome (rather than cuff tear)
  - Allows for more accurate strength testing on physical examination:
    - If strength is intact, rule out rotator cuff tear.
    - If range of motion does not improve in any plane, more likely adhesive capsulitis
  - Some pain relief and improved range of motion occurs after lidocaine injection with
    - Glenoid labral tear
    - Capsular strain
    - Glenohumeral osteoarthritis
    - Glenohumeral instability
- A lack of any pain relief suggests other sources or inappropriate placement of injection.

Test Interpretation

May have tendinosis, tendonitis, or muscle/tendon tear

TREATMENT

Pain control in combination with aggressive rehabilitation improves and fully resolves rotator cuff tendonitis in most patients.

GENERAL MEASURES
- Rest
- Ice or heat for symptom relief
- Activity modification, with avoidance of aggravating activities, particularly overhead motions
- Range of motion exercises
- Rotator cuff and adjacent muscle strengthening to enhance stability and prevent further injuries

MEDICATION
First Line
NSAIDs or other analgesic, often for 6 to 12 weeks

ISSUES FOR REFERRAL
Failure of conservative treatment, persistent pain, weakness, or complete tear of rotator cuff

ADDITIONAL THERAPIES
- Supervised- or home-exercise regimens provide significant pain reduction and improve function (2)[A].
- Physical therapy is effective for short-term and long-term recovery of function (3)[A]:
  – Initial goal is to restore range of motion.
  – After pain resolves, gradually strengthen rotator cuff muscles in internal rotation, external rotation, and abduction.

COMPLEMENTARY & ALTERNATIVE MEDICINE
Acupuncture is potentially beneficial for reducing pain and improving function, particularly when used with physical therapy (4)[A].

SURGERY/OTHER PROCEDURES
- Steroid injections may have a significant benefit on pain and function in the short term but do not appear to have a significant long-term effect (5)[A].
- No evidence that surgery is superior to conservative management or that one surgical technique is superior to another for impingement syndrome (6)[A]
- Platelet-rich therapies for musculoskeletal soft tissue injuries are increasingly common.
  – No apparent effect of platelet-rich plasma injection during arthroscopic rotator cuff repair on overall retear rates or shoulder-specific outcomes
- Extracorporeal shock wave therapy is currently under study as an emerging treatment for calcific tendonitis.

 ONGOING CARE

PATIENT EDUCATION
- Physical rehabilitation is necessary, both in conservative course of treatment (i.e., NSAIDs, physical therapy, home exercises) and in surgical intervention. An aggressive trial of rehabilitation should be encouraged prior to extensive testing or surgical intervention. Providing pain relief prior to beginning a program of physical therapy improves adherence and outcomes.
- Symptoms often recur if not fully addressed.

PROGNOSIS
- Variable, depends on underlying pathology
- Most patients improve with conservative management. Recovery can be slow.
- Patients with more severe symptoms—those with symptoms for >1 year—are less likely to respond well with conservative therapies.

COMPLICATIONS
- Progression of injury
- Tendon retraction in complete rotator cuff tear

REFERENCES

1. Alqunaee M, Galvin R, Fahey T. Diagnostic accuracy of clinical tests for subacromial impingement syndrome: a systematic review and meta-analysis. *Arch Phys Med Rehabil*. 2012;93(2):229–236.
2. Kuhn JE. Exercise in the treatment of rotator cuff impingement: a systematic review and a synthesized evidence-based rehabilitation protocol. *J Shoulder Elbow Surg*. 2009;18(1):138–160.
3. Green S, Buchbinder R, Hetrick S. Physiotherapy interventions for shoulder pain. *Cochrane Database Syst Rev*. 2003;(2):CD004258.
4. Vas J, Ortega C, Olmo V, et al. Single-point acupuncture and physiotherapy for the treatment of painful shoulder: a multicentre randomized controlled trial. *Rheumatology (Oxford)*. 2008;47(6):887–893.
5. Gaujoux-Viala C, Dougados M, Gossec L. Efficacy and safety of steroid injections for shoulder and elbow tendonitis: a meta-analysis of randomised controlled trials. *Ann Rheum Dis*. 2009;68(12):1843–1849.
6. Gebremariam L, Hay EM, Koes BW, et al. Effectiveness of surgical and postsurgical interventions for the subacromial impingement syndrome: a systematic review. *Arch Phys Med Rehabil*. 2011;92(11):1900–1913.

ADDITIONAL READING

- Baumgarten KM, Gerlach D, Galatz LM, et al. Cigarette smoking increases the risk for rotator cuff tears. *Clin Orthop Relat Res*. 2010;468(6):1534–1541.
- Burbank KM, Stevenson JH, Czarnecki GR, et al. Chronic shoulder pain: part I. Evaluation and diagnosis. *Am Fam Physician*. 2008;77(4):453–460.
- Burbank KM, Stevenson JH, Czarnecki GR, et al. Chronic shoulder pain: part II. Treatment. *Am Fam Physician*. 2008;77(4):493–497.
- Hanchard NC, Lenza M, Handoll HH, et al. Physical tests for shoulder impingements and local lesions of bursa, tendon or labrum that may accompany impingement. *Cochrane Database Syst Rev*. 2013;(4):CD007427.

 CODES

ICD10
- M75.40 Impingement syndrome of unspecified shoulder
- M75.110 Incmpl rotatr-cuff tear/ruptr of unsp shoulder, not trauma
- M75.120 Complete rotatr-cuff tear/ruptr of unsp shoulder, not trauma

CLINICAL PEARLS
- Consider impingement syndrome in patients who engage in activities with repetitive overhead motions (e.g., swimming, throwing) who present with shoulder pain.
- Atraumatic shoulder pain in middle age often represents rotator cuff tendonitis.
- The supraspinatus tendon is most commonly affected in impingement syndrome.
- Neer and Hawkins tests specifically check for shoulder impingement.
- The empty can maneuver tests for weakness of supraspinatus muscle.
- The drop-arm test is specific for rotator cuff tear.
- Physical therapy over 6 to 12 weeks promotes return to function.
- Most patients with shoulder impingement respond well to conservative management.

R

SALIVARY GLAND CALCULI/SIALADENITIS

Alia A Hussain, MD, BSc (Hons) • Sahil Mullick, MD

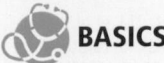

BASICS

DESCRIPTION

- Inflammation and/or infection involving one or more salivary gland
- Sialolithiasis is the cause of ~90% of all obstructive salivary gland diseases.
- Salivary obstruction is usually characterized by a painful swelling of the affected gland when eating, known as "mealtime syndrome."
- The submandibular gland is more commonly affected (80–90% of cases) by sialolithiasis and infection than the parotid gland. Submandibular stones occur more commonly due to higher mucinous content of saliva, longer course of Wharton duct, slow salivary flow, and saliva flow against gravity.
- Can be acute or chronic
  - Types: infectious, obstructive (sialolithiasis), and autoimmune

EPIDEMIOLOGY

Incidence

- Predominant age: Peak incidence is 30 to 60 years.
- Most common in debilitated and dehydrated patients
- 49% men and 51% women, average age 47.5 years; 82% submandibular stones and 18% parotid stones; 44% had a positive smoking history, and 20% of patients were taking diuretics.

Prevalence

- Salivary calculi can be found in 1.2% of the adult population.
- Only 5% of all cases occur in the pediatric population.
- In those with sialographic evidence of benign intraductal obstruction, the obstruction is caused by salivary calculi in >73% of cases.

ETIOLOGY AND PATHOPHYSIOLOGY

- Decreased salivary outflow from anticholinergics, dehydration, or radiation is thought to allow bacterial infection of salivary glands.
- Salivary calculi form by deposition of calcium phosphate. Predisposing factors include salivary stasis, retrograde bacterial contamination from the oral cavity, increased alkalinity of saliva, and physical trauma to salivary duct or gland.
- Gout is a systemic disease known to be associated with salivary stone development. In gout, sialoliths are composed of uric acid.
- Sialadenitis occurs by recurrent inflammatory reactions that result in progressive acinar destruction with fibrous replacement and sialectasis.
- Bacterial sialadenitis: *Staphylococcus aureus*, *Streptococcus viridans*, *Streptococcus pyogenes*, *Haemophilus influenzae*, *Escherichia coli*, *Pseudomonas aeruginosa*, and group B streptococci (neonates and prepubescent children)
- Viral sialadenitis: mumps, cytomegalovirus (CMV), Epstein-Barr virus (EBV), HIV, and enteroviruses

Pediatric Considerations

The two most common causes of sialadenitis in children are mumps and idiopathic juvenile recurrent parotitis.

Genetics

Polygenic cause, with several loci under investigation

RISK FACTORS

- Dehydration
- Anticholinergic use
- Antihistamine use
- Diuretic use
- Poor oral hygiene
- Malnutrition
- Head/neck radiation
- Tuberculosis (TB)
- HIV
- Failure to immunize (mumps)
- Gout
- Diabetes mellitus
- Hypothyroidism
- Renal failure
- Duct strictures
- Previous intraoral procedures

GENERAL PREVENTION

- Adequate hydration
- Maintain proper oral care and hygiene.
- Avoid antihistamines, anticholinergics, and other causes of xerostomia, especially if other risk factors are present.

COMMONLY ASSOCIATED CONDITIONS

- Postoperative dehydration
- Radiation-induced xerostomia
- Drug-induced xerostomia
- Sjögren syndrome
- Hypercalcemia

DIAGNOSIS

HISTORY

- Review immunization history.
- History of:
  - Alcoholism, bulimia, malnutrition
  - Recent dental work, oral surgery
  - Radiation therapy
  - TB or HIV exposure
- Acute onset of pain and swelling over the affected salivary gland, especially postprandial
- Dental pain, discharge, foul breath (halitosis) hypersalivation, and pain with chewing
- Fever, unintentional weight loss
- Xerostomia

PHYSICAL EXAM

- Palpate all salivary glands, floor of mouth, tongue, and neck to assess symmetry, tenderness, induration, edema, presence of stones, and lymphadenopathy.
- Examine duct openings for purulent discharge and saliva.
- Palpate gland gently to express purulent material.
- Examine eyes for interstitial keratitis.
- Note lingual papillary atrophy and/or loss of tooth enamel.

Pediatric Considerations

Stones in children are traditionally smaller in size, within the duct distally, and present with a shorter symptom duration. Thus, ultrasound with sialendoscopy is considered diagnostic and therapeutic.

DIFFERENTIAL DIAGNOSIS

- Acute bacterial parotitis
- Chronic bacterial parotitis
- Idiopathic juvenile recurrent parotitis
- Dental abscess
- Mumps
- TB
- HIV (in pediatric populations)
- EBV, CMV, enteroviruses
- Tularemia
- Cystic fibrosis
- Lupus
- Sjögren syndrome
- Alcoholism
- Bulimia
- Hypothyroidism
- Pleomorphic adenoma
- Lymphoma
- Sarcoidosis
- Collagen vascular disease
- Metal poisoning

DIAGNOSTIC TESTS & INTERPRETATION

Initial Tests (lab, imaging)

- Consider CBC, rarely electrolytes.
- Culture and sensitivity of any expressed pus
- CT scan with IV contrast is the preferred imaging modality, *if needed* (1)[C].
- Ultrasound can localize abscesses as well as stones. Stones appear hyperechoic with posterior shadowing.
- Sonopalpation (concurrent ultrasound with transoral palpation) proved to have a sensitivity and specificity of 96.6% and 90% in finding a calculus (1)[B].

Follow-Up Tests & Special Considerations

- If autoimmune process is suspected, consider ordering appropriate labs, such as autoantibody titers: Sjögren syndrome A (SS-A) and Sjögren syndrome B (SS-B), rheumatoid factor (RF), and antinuclear antibodies (ANAs). Erythrocyte sedimentation rate (ESR) may also be conducted (2)[C].
- Salivary gland biopsy
- Consider serial CT scans with contrast to evaluate disease resolution.
- Ultrasound can identify indicators of persistent obstruction in patients undergoing sialolithotomy.

Diagnostic Procedures/Other

- Sialography to evaluate sialolithiasis and other obstructive lesions
- Sialendoscopy to find and remove sialoliths. In one study, sialendoscopy confirmed 221 (79%) parotid and 812 (93%) submandibular stones (3)[A].
- One study revealed that sonography, cone beam CT, and sialendoscopy all had excellent specificity and positive predictive value in diagnosing stones (1)[B].

- In a retrospective study of 2,052 patients, ultrasound revealed 95% of false-negative findings to be positive for ductal dilation in the major salivary glands. 73.1% of the stones located in the distal part of the duct; unable to be detected on ultrasound were visualized and accessed by a sialendoscope
- When sialendoscopy fails, a novel ultrasound-guided needle localization approach has been proposed.
- Technetium-99m pertechnetate scintigraphy showed decreased gland excretion and decreased uptake in patients with sialolithiasis.

Test Interpretation
In chronic sialadenitis, loss of acini, fibrosis, and periductal lymphocytosis are evident; degree indicates chronicity.

 TREATMENT

GENERAL MEASURES
- Maintain hydration.
- Apply warm compresses with massage.
- Maintain good oral hygiene.
- Antibiotics if indicated by diagnosis

MEDICATION
First Line
- Antistaphylococcal penicillins (nafcillin, dicloxacillin) are indicated in areas where methicillin-resistant *S. aureus* (MRSA) is not predominant.
- Penicillin-allergic: Use clindamycin 300 mg PO q8h.
- Gram negative: 3rd-generation cephalosporin or fluoroquinolone
- Anaerobic: metronidazole or clindamycin
- Antibiotic coverage should be narrowed once culture and sensitivity are available.
- Continue antibiotic therapy for 10 to 14 days.

Second Line
- 1st-generation cephalosporin (cephalexin or cefazolin) or clindamycin is also indicated for empiric coverage.
- If MRSA, then vancomycin

ISSUES FOR REFERRAL
In the case of poor dentition and dental abscess, refer patient to a dentist.

ADDITIONAL THERAPIES
In the case of chronic sialadenitis with strictures, consider sialostent placement.

SURGERY/OTHER PROCEDURES
- Submandibular stones found in the anterior floor of the mouth can be excised intraorally (sialodochoplasty), whereas those in the hilum require gland excision. Parotid stones usually require parotidectomy (2)[A].
- Good results in patient symptom relief, quality of life, and safety have been reported in sialadenitis and sialolithiasis using sialendoscopy (2,3,4)[A]. However, one study revealed a complication rate of 3.23%. Complications include strictures, ranulas, and lingual nerve injury.

- A combined approach using limited intraoral incision with sialendoscopy has shown an 87% success rate.
- Incision and drainage of parotid abscess is indicated after failing 3 to 5 days of medical management.
- Sialoliths and stenoses can be successfully treated by radiologically or fluoroscopically controlled or sialendoscopically based methods in ~80% of cases. Extracorporeal shock wave lithotripsy (ESWL) is successful in up to 50% of cases.
- Transoral duct slitting is an important method for extraparenchymal submandibular stones, with a success rate of 90%.
- Sialolithotomy with sialendoscopy can now be successfully performed robotically (5)[B].
- Recent evidence shows that larger stones can be successfully and safely treated with holmium:YAG laser lithotripsy.

Pediatric Considerations
The most effective diagnostic and therapeutic modality for children with sialadenitis is sialendoscopy with stone retrieval (6)[B].

COMPLEMENTARY & ALTERNATIVE MEDICINE
Consider lemon drops or other sialogogues to promote salivation. In one study, postoperative use of sialogogues nearly halved rates of sialadenitis (2)[C].

ADMISSION, INPATIENT, AND NURSING CONSIDERATIONS
- Parotid abscess
- Sepsis
- Inability to tolerate PO intake
- Airway, breathing, circulation
- Check vital signs, with particular attention to blood pressure because patient may be septic secondary to abscess formation.
- Evaluate airway patency.
- Nursing responsibilities may include ensuring excellent oral hygiene and avoiding administration of drugs that cause decreased production or flow of saliva.
- Discharge criteria
  – Exclude abscess or sepsis.
  – Ensure ability to tolerate PO intake.
  – Stable vital signs

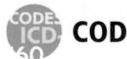 ONGOING CARE

FOLLOW-UP RECOMMENDATIONS
- Provide regular follow-up visits for patients with chronic sialadenitis.
- Avoid prescribing medications that cause xerostomia.

Patient Monitoring
Continue to monitor patients with chronic sialadenitis because decreased salivary gland function due to fibrosis and loss of acini can lead to acute exacerbations.

DIET
- Avoid sialogogues during acute attacks.
- Maintain adequate hydration on an outpatient basis.

PATIENT EDUCATION
- Educate patients on maintaining excellent oral hygiene.
- Educate patients on maintaining good hydration.

PROGNOSIS
- Generally excellent, with acute symptoms resolving in about a week with appropriate treatment
- Patients with autoimmune etiology may have prolonged course due to systemic involvement.

COMPLICATIONS
Abscess, dental caries, recurrent sialadenitis, facial nerve impingement, Ludwig angina

REFERENCES
1. Schwarz D, Kabbasch C, Scheer M, et al. Comparative analysis of sialendoscopy, sonography, and CBCT in the detection of sialolithiasis. *Laryngoscope*. 2015;125(5):1098–1101.
2. Wilson KF, Meier JD, Ward PD. Salivary gland disorders. *Am Fam Physician*. 2014;89(11):882–888.
3. Atienza G, López-Cedrún JL. Management of obstructive salivary disorders by sialendoscopy: a systematic review. *Br J Oral Maxillofac Surg*. 2015;53(6):507–519.
4. Meier BA, Holst R, Schousboe LP. Patient-perceived benefit of sialendoscopy as measured by the Glasgow Benefit Inventory. *Laryngoscope*. 2015;125(8):1874–1878.
5. Razavi C, Pascheles C, Samara G, et al. Robot-assisted sialolithotomy with sialendoscopy for the management of large submandibular gland stones. *Laryngoscope*. 2016;126(2):345–351.
6. Francis CL, Larsen CG. Pediatric sialadenitis. *Otolaryngol Clin North Am*. 2014;47(5):763–778.

ADDITIONAL READING
- Goncalves M, Mantsopoulos K, Schapher M, et al. Ultrasound supplemented by sialendoscopy: diagnostic value in sialolithiasis. *Am Academy of Otolaryngol Head Neck Surg*. 2018;159(3):449–455.
- Koch M, Zenk J, Iro H. Algorithms for treatment of salivary gland obstructions. *Otolaryngol Clin North Am*. 2009;42(6):1173–1192.

CODES

ICD10
- K11.5 Sialolithiasis
- K11.20 Sialoadenitis, unspecified
- K11.21 Acute sialoadenitis

CLINICAL PEARLS
- Sialadenitis is associated with conditions that predispose patient to xerostomia.
- Sialadenitis occurs in debilitated patients who lack ability to control hydration.
- Mainstay of treatment is hydration, good oral hygiene, sialogogues, and possible surgical excision.
- Many cases are now being successfully and safely treated with ultrasound followed by sialendoscopy.

S

SALMONELLA INFECTION

Rahma Ali Aldhaheri, MD • Matthew E. Tick, DO • Marie L. Borum, MD, EdD, MPH, MACP, FACG, AGAF

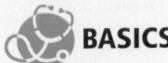 **BASICS**

DESCRIPTION
- Infection caused by any serotype of the bacterial genus *Salmonella*, a gram-negative anaerobic bacillus
- Nontyphoidal *Salmonella* typically causes gastroenteritis via foodborne infection and sporadic outbreaks; less commonly causes infection outside the gastrointestinal (GI) tract
- Clinical syndromes
  - Enteric fever (see "Typhoid Fever")
  - Nontyphoidal gastroenteritis
    ○ Chronic carrier state (>1 year)
  - Nontyphoidal invasive disease
    ○ Bacteremia
      ■ Endovascular complications
      ■ Localized infection outside GI tract

Geriatric Considerations
Patients >65 years old have increased risk of invasive disease with bacteremia and endovascular complications due to comorbidities (atherosclerotic endovascular lesions, prostheses, etc.) that increase risk of bacterial seeding.

Pediatric Considerations
Neonates (<3 months) are more susceptible to invasive disease and complications.

EPIDEMIOLOGY
Incidence
- Global incidence of nontyphoidal *Salmonella enteritidis* estimated to be ~94 million per year
  - Wide variation by region from 40 to 3,980 estimated cases per 100,000
- Global incidence of invasive nontyphoidal *Salmonella* infection estimated to be 2 to 6.5 million in 2010
  - Wide variation by region from 0.8 to 227 estimated cases per 100,000
- Most commonly identified foodborne illness in the United States and a common cause of traveler's diarrhea. Annual incidence in the United States is 15 illnesses per 100,000.
- Second most common bacteria isolated from stool cultures in diarrheal illness (following *Campylobacter*) in the United States
- Highest incidence in children <5 years old
- Hospitalization rates higher in patients >50 years old
- Peak frequency: July to November

ETIOLOGY AND PATHOPHYSIOLOGY
- *Salmonella enterica*
  - Most pathogenic species in humans
  - 2,500 different serotypes
- Etiology
  - ~95% of cases are foodborne.
  - Other cases (5%) are due to direct or indirect fecal–oral contact with animals or human carriers.
  - Iatrogenic contamination (e.g., blood transfusion, endoscopy) is rare.
- Pathophysiology
  - Typical infectious dose in immunocompetent patients is ingestion of 1 million bacteria.
  - Bacteria ingested invade the distal ileal and proximal colonic mucosa to produce an inflammatory and cytotoxic response.
  - Bacteria can enter the mesenteric lymphatic system and then the systemic circulation to cause disseminated/invasive disease.

RISK FACTORS
- Recent travel to underdeveloped nations
- Consumption of undercooked meat, egg, or unpasteurized dairy products. Nonanimal products have also been implicated in outbreaks.
- Contact with live reptiles or poultry
- Contact with human carrier (*Salmonella* fecal shedding)
- Impaired gastric acidity: H_2 receptor blockers, antacids, proton pump inhibitors (PPIs), gastrectomy, achlorhydria, pernicious anemia, infants
- Recent antibiotic use
- Reticuloendothelial blockade: sickle cell disease, malaria, bartonellosis
- Immunosuppression: HIV, diabetes, corticosteroid or other immunosuppressant use, chemotherapy
- Iron overload, chronic granulomatous disease
- Age <5 years or >50 years

GENERAL PREVENTION
- Proper hygiene in production, transport, and storage of food (e.g., refrigeration during food storage and thoroughly cooking food prior to consumption)
- Control of animal reservoirs: Avoid contact with high-risk animals, feces, and polluted waters.
- Hand hygiene
- CDC tracks outbreaks (http://www.cdc.gov/salmonella/).

COMMONLY ASSOCIATED CONDITIONS
- Gastroenteritis
- Bacteremia: immunocompromised or patients with underlying disease (e.g., cholelithiasis, prostheses)
- Osteomyelitis: higher incidence in sickle cell disease
- Abscesses: higher incidence with malignant tumors
- Reactive arthritis

 DIAGNOSIS

HISTORY
- *Salmonella* infections are typically asymptomatic or result in mild, self-limited gastroenteritis.
- Exposure history: travel; contact with infected human, reptile, or poultry; improper food preparation
- Host factors: age, immune status, other risk factors
- Symptoms typically begin 12 to 72 hours after ingestion and resolve within 4 to 10 days.
- Acute uncomplicated illness
  - Sudden onset of diarrhea
  - Vomiting is infrequent.
  - Abdominal cramping
  - Headache
  - Myalgias
  - Fever

PHYSICAL EXAM
- Fever
- Evidence of hypovolemia
- Abdominal tenderness
- Heme-positive stool in some patients
- Hepatosplenomegaly in some patients

DIFFERENTIAL DIAGNOSIS
- Viral gastroenteritis
- Bacterial enteritis due to other organisms
- Pseudomembranous colitis
- Inflammatory bowel disease

DIAGNOSTIC TESTS & INTERPRETATION
Initial Tests (lab, imaging)
- Gastroenteritis
  - Stool culture for *Salmonella*, *Escherichia coli*, *Shigella*, and *Campylobacter* (1)[C] (Optimal specimen is a diarrheal stool sample.)
  - Indications for stool culture include:
    ○ Severe diarrhea (≥6 loose stools daily) (1)[C]
    ○ Diarrhea >1 week in duration (1)[C]
    ○ Fever (1)[C]
    ○ Diarrhea containing blood or mucous (1)[C]
    ○ Multiple cases suggesting an outbreak (1)[C]
  - Fecal leukocytes: positive
  - Blood cultures are warranted in:
    ○ Infants <3 months
    ○ People of any age with signs of septicemia or other systemic manifestations of infection
    ○ Cases where enteric fever is suspected
    ○ Immunocompromised patients
- Bacteremia
  - Blood cultures if febrile (1)[C]
  - Stool cultures: may also be positive (1)[C]
  - Culture CSF if patient is <3 months of age with positive blood culture.
- Endovascular infection
  - Consider angiography in bacteremic patients >50 years of age if aortic or vascular source is suspected (2)[A].
- Local infections
  - Wound culture
  - Consider CT or MRI for soft tissue or bone infections (3)[C].
- Chronic carrier state
  - Stool culture positive for >1 year (3)[C]
  - Urine culture may be positive in chronic carriers.

Follow-Up Tests & Special Considerations
- Look for other causes in diarrhea lasting >14 days.
- Asymptomatic excretion of *Salmonella* may occur for weeks after infection; follow-up fecal cultures are routinely not indicated for patients with uncomplicated gastroenteritis (2,3)[C].
- Follow-up blood cultures suggested for patients with bacteremia (3)[C]

Test Interpretation
Intestinal biopsies (if taken) may show mucosal ulceration, hemorrhage, and necrosis seen on along with reticuloendothelial hypertrophy/hyperplasia.

TREATMENT

- Treatment is supportive for nonsevere nontyphoidal *Salmonella* gastroenteritis in immunocompetent patients between 12 months and 50 years of age. The illness is typically self-limited. There is no proven benefit for treatment of mild disease. Treatment can suppress the host immunologic response. Higher rates of relapse have also been reported and there is the potential to extend asymptomatic carriage (1)[C].
- Consider antibiotics in immunocompetent hosts with severe diarrhea, high fever, or those requiring hospitalization (1)[C].
- Patients at increased risk of bacteremia benefit from antibiotics:
  - Infants <12 months of age (1)[C]
  - Patients >50 years old (risk particularly increases after age 65 years) (1,3)[C]

– HIV-infected patients
– Patients with hemoglobinopathies, atherosclerotic lesions, and prosthetic valves, grafts, or joints or any immunosuppressed state (1)[C],(2)[A],(3)[C]
• Chronic carriage of nontyphoidal *Salmonella*
– 4 to 6 weeks of antimicrobial therapy
– Prophylactic therapy in immunocompromised patients (2)[A]

GENERAL MEASURES
• Hydration and electrolyte replacement
• Hand washing and barrier precautions for inpatients
• Avoid antimotility drugs in patients with fever or dysentery. Antimotility drugs may increase contact time of the enteropathogen in the gut mucosa (1)[C].

MEDICATION
First Line
• Gastroenteritis, uncomplicated: No specific medications are necessary; supportive care (1)[A]
• Gastroenteritis, complicated (due to illness severity or host risk factors such as immunocompromised)
– Adults (Treat for 14 days if immunocompromised.)
  ○ Levofloxacin (or other fluoroquinolone) 500 mg/day PO for 7 to 10 days (1)[C] *or*
  ○ Trimethoprim-sulfamethoxazole: 160/800 mg PO BID for 7 to 10 days *or*
  ○ Amoxicillin: 500 mg PO TID for 7 to 10 days *or*
  ○ Cefixime: 400 mg orally once or twice daily *or*
  ○ Azithromycin: 500 mg/day PO for 7 days or 1 g, followed by 500 mg daily for 5 to 7 days (1)[C]
– Children
  ○ Ceftriaxone: 100 mg/kg/day IV or IM in 2 equally divided doses for 7 to 10 days (1)[C] *or*
  ○ Azithromycin: 20 mg/kg PO for first dose and then 10 mg/kg/day for subsequent doses daily for 7 days (1)[C]
– HIV patients
  ○ Increased duration (range of 2 to 6 weeks) of antimicrobial therapy and/or zidovudine may decrease relapse (2)[C].
• Bacteremia: Due to resistance trends, treat life-threatening infections in adults with a fluoroquinolone *or* a 3rd-generation cephalosporin until susceptibilities are determined (2)[A].
– Adults
  ○ Ciprofloxacin (or other fluoroquinolone): 400 mg IV BID for 10 to 14 days *plus*
  ○ Ceftriaxone: 1 to 2 g/day IV for 10 to 14 days *or*
  ○ Cefotaxime: 2 g IV q8h for 10 to 14 days
– Children
  ○ Ampicillin: 200 mg/kg/day in 4 divided doses for 10 to 14 days *or*
  ○ Trimethoprim-sulfamethoxazole: 8 to 12 mg/kg/day of trimethoprim component in 2 divided doses for 10 to 14 days *or*
  ○ Ceftriaxone: 50 to 75 mg/kg/day (max 1 g) once per day for 10 to 14 days
• Localized infection (e.g., septic arthritis, osteomyelitis, cholangitis, and pneumonia); surgical drainage or débridement in addition to a minimum of 3 weeks of antimicrobial therapy
– In sustained bacteremia, prolonged local infection, or immunocompromised patients, give antibiotics PO for 4 to 6 weeks (2)[A].
• Chronic carrier state (shedding >1 year duration)
– Amoxicillin: 1 g PO TID for 12 weeks *or*
– Trimethoprim-sulfamethoxazole 160 mg/800 mg PO BID for 12 weeks *or*
– Ciprofloxacin: 500 mg PO BID for 4 weeks *or*
– Levofloxacin 500 mg/day for 4 weeks *or*
– Norfloxacin 400 mg PO BID for 4 weeks if gallstones are present

ALERT
Antimicrobial resistance
• Strains resistant to ampicillin, chloramphenicol, and trimethoprim-sulfamethoxazole have been reported.
• Fluoroquinolone resistance is increasing, perhaps due to increasing use in livestock.
• Extended-spectrum cephalosporin resistance has been reported with increasing frequency.

Second Line
• Aztreonam is an alternative agent that may be useful in patients with multiple allergies or if the organism demonstrates an unusual resistance pattern (2)[A].
• Fluoroquinolones are now routinely given to children for 5 to 7 days in areas of the world where multidrug-resistant *Salmonella typhi* is common (2)[A].

SURGERY/OTHER PROCEDURES
• Surgical excision and drainage for infected tissue sites, followed by a minimum of 3 weeks of antibiotic therapy
• If biliary tract disease is present, a preoperative 10- to 14-day course of parenteral antibiotics is recommended prior to cholecystectomy.

 ## ONGOING CARE

FOLLOW-UP RECOMMENDATIONS
Patient Monitoring
• Asymptomatic shedding of *Salmonella* may occur for weeks after infection. Follow-up fecal cultures are generally not indicated for patients with uncomplicated gastroenteritis. Requirements may differ during a *Salmonella* outbreak.
• Criteria may vary by state and local regulations. Some public health departments require negative stool cultures for health workers and food handlers prior to returning to work. Shedding may last 4 to 8 weeks.
• Serotyping of isolates can be performed at public health laboratories.

DIET
Easily digestible foods

PATIENT EDUCATION
• Meticulous hand hygiene; caution handling raw meat, poultry, and eggs
• Fruits and vegetables should be thoroughly washed prior to consumption.
• Thoroughly cooking meats eliminates *Salmonella*.
• Caution when handling animals with high fecal carriage rates
• http:// www.cdc.gov/salmonella/general/prevention .html

PROGNOSIS
• Most cases of *Salmonella* gastroenteritis are self-limited and have an excellent prognosis.
• Increased mortality is seen in the young (<3 months), elderly (>65 years), and immunocompromised.
• Increased mortality is seen with bacteremia and other invasive infections.
• Mortality is increased in multidrug-resistant strains.

COMPLICATIONS
Toxic megacolon, hypovolemic shock, metastatic abscess formation, endocarditis, infectious endarteritis, meningitis, septic arthritis, reactive arthritis, osteomyelitis, pneumonia, appendicitis, cholecystitis

REFERENCES
1. DuPont HL. Acute infectious diarrhea in immunocompetent adults. *N Engl J Med*. 2014;370(16):1532–1540.
2. Wen SC, Best E, Nourse C. Non-typhoidal Salmonella infections in children: review of literature and recommendations for management. *J Paediatr Child Health*. 2017;53(10):936–941.
3. Crum-Cianflone NF. Salmonellosis and the gastrointestinal tract: more than just peanut butter. *Curr Gastroenterol Rep*. 2008;10(4):424–431.

ADDITIONAL READING
• Chen HM, Wang Y, Su LH, et al. Nontyphoid *Salmonella* infection: microbiology, clinical features, and antimicrobial therapy. *Pediatr Neonatol*. 2013;54(3):147–152.
• Hurley D, McCusker MP, Fanning S, et al. *Salmonella*–host interactions—modulation of the host innate immune system. *Front Immunol*. 2014;5:481.
• Lee MB, Greig JD. A review of nosocomial *Salmonella* outbreaks: infection control interventions found effective. *Public Health*. 2013;127(3): 199–206.
• Odey F, Okomo U, Oyo-Ita A. Vaccines for preventing invasive salmonella infections in people with sickle cell disease. *Cochrane Database Syst Rev*. 2015;(6):CD006975.
• Onwuezobe IA, Oshun PO, Odigwe CC. Antimicrobials for treating symptomatic non-typhoidal *Salmonella* infection. *Cochrane Database Syst Rev*. 2012;11:CD001167.

 ## SEE ALSO

Gastroenteritis; Typhoid Fever

 ## CODES

ICD10
• A02.9 Salmonella infection, unspecified
• A02.0 Salmonella enteritis
• A02.1 Salmonella sepsis

CLINICAL PEARLS
• Nontyphoidal *Salmonella* infection is typically a foodborne infection associated with a self-limited gastroenteritis.
• Clinical syndromes include gastroenteritis, bacteremia, endovascular infection, localized infection outside the GI tract, and a chronic carrier state.
• Those at greatest risk of complications from *Salmonella* infection include the young, the elderly, and immunocompromised patients.
• Uncomplicated gastroenteritis in healthy patients can be treated with supportive care.
• Antibiotics should be used in infants, the elderly, immunocompromised patients, and for invasive infections such as bacteremia outside the GI tract.

S

SARCOIDOSIS

Donnah Mathews, MD

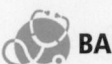

BASICS

DESCRIPTION
- Sarcoidosis is a noninfectious, multisystem, granulomatous disease of unknown cause, commonly affecting young and middle-aged adults.
  - Frequently presents with hilar adenopathy, pulmonary infiltrates, ocular or skin lesions
  - In ~50% of cases, it is diagnosed in asymptomatic patients with abnormal chest x-rays (CXRs).
  - Almost any organ may be involved.
- System(s) affected: primarily pulmonary but also cardiovascular, gastrointestinal, hematologic/lymphatic, endocrine, renal, neurologic, dermatologic, ophthalmologic, musculoskeletal
- Synonym(s): Löfgren syndrome (erythema nodosum [EN], hilar adenopathy, fever, arthralgias); Heerfordt syndrome (uveitis, parotid enlargement, facial palsy, fever); Besnier-Boeck disease; Boeck sarcoid; Scheuermann disease (1)[C],(2)[B],(3)[C]

EPIDEMIOLOGY
Incidence
Estimated 6/100 person-years (3)

Prevalence
- Estimated 10 to 20/100,000 persons
- 11/100,000 annual incidence rate for women (4)
- Usually occurs in younger persons, although in a single center medical record review in Minnesota, the peak age of incidence for women was 50 to 69 years and for men 40 to 59 years (5)
- Rare in children (2,3)
- In the United States, the highest prevalence is in the Northeast (4).

ETIOLOGY AND PATHOPHYSIOLOGY
- Despite extensive research, mostly unknown
- Thought to be due to exaggerated cell-mediated immune response to unknown antigen(s)
- In the lungs, the initial lesion is CD4+ T-cell alveolitis, causing noncaseating granulomata, which may resolve or may undergo fibrosis.
- "Immune paradox" with affected organs showing an intense immune response and yet anergy exists elsewhere (1)[C]

Genetics
- Reports of familial clustering, with genetic linkage to a section within MHC on short arm of chromosome 6
- 3 to 4 times more common in African Americans
- Although worldwide in distribution, increased prevalence in Scandinavians, Japanese, African Americans, and women
- In Northern Europe, 5 to 40 cases per 100,000 persons. In Black Americans, 35 cases per 100,000 persons; in Caucasian Americans, 11 cases per 100,000 persons (3)[C]

RISK FACTORS
Exact etiology and pathogenesis remain unknown.

GENERAL PREVENTION
None

COMMONLY ASSOCIATED CONDITIONS
None

DIAGNOSIS

HISTORY
- Patients may be asymptomatic.
- Patients may have nonspecific complaints, such as the following:
  - Nonproductive cough
  - Shortness of breath
  - Fever
  - Night sweats
  - Weight loss
  - General fatigue
  - Eye pain
  - Chest pain/palpitations
  - Skin lesions
  - Polyarthritis
  - Renal calculi
  - Facial droop due to Bell palsy
  - Encephalopathy, seizures, hydrocephalus (rare)
  - Patients >70 years old more likely to have systemic symptoms

PHYSICAL EXAM
- Many patients have a normal physical exam.
- Lungs may reveal wheezing/fine interstitial crackles in advanced disease.
- ~30% of patients have extrapulmonary manifestations (1), which may include the following:
  - Uveitis
  - Other eye findings: conjunctival nodules, lacrimal gland enlargement, cataracts, glaucoma, papilledema
  - Cranial nerve palsies
  - Salivary gland swelling
  - Lymphadenopathy
  - Arrhythmias
  - Hepatosplenomegaly
  - Polyarthritis
  - Rashes (1)
    - Maculopapular of nares, eyelids, forehead, base of neck at hairline, and previous trauma sites
    - Waxy nodular of face, trunk, and extensor surfaces of extremities
    - Plaques (lupus pernio) of nose, cheeks, chin, and ears
    - EN (component of Löfgren syndrome)
    - Atypical lesions

DIFFERENTIAL DIAGNOSIS
- Sarcoidosis is a diagnosis of exclusion.
- Infectious granulomatous disease, such as tuberculosis and fungal infections
- Hypersensitivity pneumonitis
- Lymphoma
- Other malignancies associated with lymphadenopathy
- Berylliosis (1)[C]

DIAGNOSTIC TESTS & INTERPRETATION
No definitive test for diagnosis, but diagnosis is suggested by the following:
- Clinical and radiographic manifestations
- Exclusion of other diagnoses
- Histopathologic detection of noncaseating granulomas

Initial Tests (lab, imaging)
- CBC: Anemia/leukopenia ± eosinophilia can be seen.
- Hypergammaglobulinemia can exist.
- LFTs: Abnormal liver function and increased alkaline phosphatase can be encountered with hepatic involvement.
- Calcium: Hypercalciuria occurs in up to 10% of patients, with hypercalcemia less frequent.
- Serum ACE elevated in >75% of patients but is not diagnostic or exclusionary
  - Drugs may alter lab results: Prednisone will lower serum ACE and normalize gallium scan. ACE inhibitors will lower serum ACE level.
  - Disorders may alter lab results: Hyperthyroidism and diabetes will increase serum ACE level.
- CXR or CT scan may reveal granulomas/hilar adenopathy. Routine CXRs are staged using Scadding classification.
  - Stage 0 = normal
  - Stage 1 = bilateral hilar adenopathy alone
  - Stage 2 = bilateral hilar adenopathy + parenchymal infiltrates
  - Stage 3 = parenchymal infiltrates alone (primarily upper lobes)
  - Stage 4 = pulmonary fibrosis (1,2)[C]
- Chest CT scan may enhance appreciation of lymph nodes.
- High-resolution chest CT scan may reveal peribronchial disease.
- Gallium scan will be positive in areas of acute disease/inflammation but is not specific.
- Positron emission tomography (PET) scan can indicate areas of disease activity in lungs, lymph nodes, and other areas of the body but does not differentiate between malignancy and sarcoidosis.
- Cardiac PET scan may detect cardiac sarcoidosis (2,3)[C].
- Serum amyloid A and adenosine deaminase has been found to be elevated with sarcoidosis but are not clinically used due to low sensitivity and specificity (6)[C].

Diagnostic Procedures/Other
- Pulmonary function tests (PFTs) may reveal restrictive pattern with decreased carbon monoxide diffusing capacity (DLCO).
- Characteristically in active disease, bronchoalveolar lavage fluid has an increased CD4-to-CD8 ratio.
- Ophthalmologic examination may reveal uveitis, retinal vasculitis, or conjunctivitis.
- ECG
- Tuberculin skin test
- Biopsy of lesions should reveal noncaseating granulomas.
- If lungs are affected, bronchoscopy with biopsy of central and peripheral airways is helpful. Endobronchial US (EBUS)–guided transbronchial needle aspiration may potentially have a better diagnostic yield (2)[C].
- Kveim test (ongoing research): Suspension of sterilized splenic cells from a patient with sarcoidosis is injected in an intradermal skin test to evoke a sarcoid granulomatous response over 3 weeks, similar to a tuberculin skin test.

ALERT
If signs indicate Löfgren syndrome (acute sarcoid with bilateral hilar lymphadenopathy, EN, and diffuse arthritis/arthralgias), it is not necessary to perform a biopsy because prognosis is good with observation alone, and biopsy would not change management.

Test Interpretation
Noncaseating epithelioid granulomas without evidence of fungal/mycobacterial infection

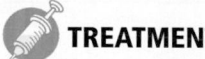 TREATMENT

- Many patients undergo spontaneous remission. It is difficult to assess disease activity and severity, however, making it challenging to develop guidelines.
- No treatment may be necessary in asymptomatic individuals, but treatment may be needed for specific indications, such as cardiac, CNS, renal, or ocular involvement.
- No treatment is indicated for asymptomatic patients with stage I to III radiographic changes with normal/mildly abnormal lung function, although close follow-up is recommended.
- Treatment of pulmonary and skin manifestations is done on the basis of impairment. The symptoms that necessitate systemic therapy remain controversial.
  – Worsening pulmonary symptoms
  – Deteriorating lung function
  – Worsening radiographic findings (7)[B]

MEDICATION
Systemic therapy is clearly indicated for hypercalcemia, cardiac disease, neurologic disease, and eye disease not responding to topical therapy. Most patients with pulmonary sarcoidosis do not require treatment with medications because many are asymptomatic or have a spontaneous remission.

First Line
- There is no FDA-approved treatment specifically for sarcoidosis.
- Systemic corticosteroids in the symptomatic individual (dyspnea, cough, hemoptysis) or in the individual with worsening lung function or radiographic findings
  – The optimal dose of glucocorticoids is not known.
  – Usually prednisone initially, 0.3 to 0.6 mg/kg ideal body weight (20 to 40 mg/day) for 4 to 6 weeks
  – If stable, taper by 5 mg/week to 10 to 20 mg/day over the next 6 weeks.
  – If no relapse, 10 to 20 mg/day for 8 to 12 months
  – Relapse is common.
  – Higher doses (80 to 100 mg/day) may be warranted in patients with acute respiratory failure and cardiac, neurologic, or ocular disease.
- In patients with skin disease, topical steroids may be effective.
- Inhaled steroids (budesonide 800 to 1,600 μg BID) may be of some clinical benefit in early disease with mild pulmonary symptoms.
  – Contraindications: patients with known problems with corticosteroids
  – Precautions: careful monitoring in patients with diabetes mellitus and/or hypertension
  – Significant possible interactions: Refer to the manufacturer's profile of each drug (1,3,7)[C].

Second Line
- All alternative agents to glucocorticoids carry substantial risk for toxicity, including myelosuppression, hepatotoxicity, and opportunistic infection. Prior to utilizing these medications, it is important to assess for steroid compliance, comorbid disease, or other complicating factors contributing to steroid failure.
- Methotrexate: initially 7.5 mg/week, increasing gradually to 10 to 15 mg/week
- Azathioprine: generally a supplement to prednisone in an attempt to lower steroid doses
- Leflunomide
- Mycophenolate
- Use of immunosuppressants, such as methotrexate or azathioprine, will require regular monitoring of CBC and LFTs.

- Antimalarial agents, such as chloroquine or hydroxychloroquine
- Tumor necrosis factor antagonists, such as infliximab, have been useful in refractory cases (3,7)[C].

ISSUES FOR REFERRAL
May be followed by a pulmonologist, with referrals to other specialists as dictated by involvement of other organ systems; if requiring a second-line therapy, should be followed by a specialist.

SURGERY/OTHER PROCEDURES
Lung transplantation in severe, refractory cases; long-term outcomes are unknown.

COMPLEMENTARY & ALTERNATIVE MEDICINE
None known to be effective

 ONGOING CARE

FOLLOW-UP RECOMMENDATIONS
There is limited data on indications for the specific tests and optimal frequency of monitoring of disease activity. Suggestions follow.

Patient Monitoring
- Patients on prednisone for symptoms should be seen q1–2mo while on therapy.
- Patients not requiring therapy should be seen regularly (q3mo) for at least the first 2 years after diagnosis, obtaining a thorough history and physical exam, laboratory testing tailored to sites of disease activity, PFTs, and ambulatory pulse oximetry.
- If active disease
  – Every 6 to 12 months, obtain ophthalmologic exam if on hydroxychloroquine.
  – Annually, CBC, creatinine, calcium, LFTs, ECG, 25-hydroxy vitamin D and 1,25 dihydroxy vitamin D, CXR, ophthalmologic examination
- Other testing per individual patient's symptoms, including HRCT, echocardiogram, Holter monitoring, urinalysis (UA), thyroid-stimulating hormone (TSH), bone density, MRI of brain
- The serum ACE level is used by some physicians to follow the disease activity. In patients with an initially elevated ACE level, it should fall toward normal while on the therapy or when the disease resolves.
- If inactive disease, follow annually with history and physical exam, PFTs, ambulatory pulse oximetry, CBC, creatinine, calcium, liver enzymes, 1,25 dihydroxy vitamin D, ECG, and ophthalmologic exam.

DIET
No special diet

PATIENT EDUCATION
- The American Lung Association: www.lungusa.org/lung-disease/sarcoidosis/?gclid=CPX6zuipm6MCFQxW2godISFepQ
- Sarcoidosis by MedlinePlus: www.nlm.nih.gov/medlineplus/sarcoidosis.html

PROGNOSIS
- 50% of patients will have spontaneous resolution within 2 years.
- 25% of patients will have significant fibrosis, but no further worsening of the disease after 2 years.
- 25% of patients (higher in some populations, including African Americans) will have chronic disease.
- Patients on corticosteroids for >6 months have a greater chance of having chronic disease.

- Overall death rate: <5%
- Rate of hospitalization is higher among patients with sarcoidosis than without sarcoidosis (8)[B].

COMPLICATIONS
- Patients may develop significant respiratory involvement, including cor pulmonale.
- Pulmonary hemorrhage from infection with aspergillosis in the damaged lung is possible.
- Other organs, especially the heart (congestive heart failure, arrhythmias), eyes (rarely blindness), and CNS, can be involved with serious consequences. Cardiac, ocular, and CNS involvement usually manifest early in patients with these complications of the disease.

REFERENCES
1. Baughman RP, Culver DA, Judson MA. A concise review of pulmonary sarcoidosis. *Am J Respir Crit Care Med*. 2011;183(5):573–581.
2. Iannuzzi MC, Fontana JR. Sarcoidosis: clinical presentation, immunopathogenesis, and therapeutics. *JAMA*. 2011;305(4):391–399.
3. Iannuzzi MC, Rybicki BA, Teirstein AS. Sarcoidosis. *N Engl J Med*. 2007;357(21):2153–2165.
4. Dumas O, Abramovitz L, Wiley AS, et al. Epidemiology of sarcoidosis in a prospective cohort study of U.S. women. *Ann Am Thorac Soc*. 2016;13(1):67–71.
5. Ungprasert P, Carmona EM, Utz JP, et al. Epidemiology of sarcoidosis 1946–2013: a population-based study. *Mayo Clin Proc*. 2016;91(2):183–188.
6. Gungor S, Ozseker F, Yalcinsoy M, et al. Conventional markers in determination of activity of sarcoidosis. *Int Immunopharmacol*. 2015;25(1):174–179.
7. King CS, Kelly W. Treatment of sarcoidosis. *Dis Mon*. 2009;55(11):704–718.
8. Ungprasert P, Crowson CS, Achenbach SJ, et al. Hospitalization among patients with sarcoidosis: a population-based cohort study 1987–2015. *Lung*. 2017;195(4):411–418.

ADDITIONAL READING
Hoang DQ, Nguyen ET. Sarcoidosis. *Semin Roentgenol*. 2010;45(1):36–42.

CODES

ICD10
- D86.9 Sarcoidosis, unspecified
- D86.0 Sarcoidosis of lung
- D86.86 Sarcoid arthropathy

CLINICAL PEARLS
- Sarcoidosis is a noninfectious, multisystem, granulomatous disease of unknown cause, typically affecting young and middle-aged adults.
- Any organ can be affected.
- Diagnosis is based on clinical findings, exclusion of other disorders, and pathologic detection of noncaseating granulomas.
- Most patients do not need systemic treatment, and the disease resolves spontaneously; a few will have life-threatening progressive organ dysfunction.

SCABIES

Ryan J. Dono, MD

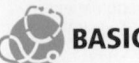

BASICS

DESCRIPTION
- A contagious parasitic infection of the skin caused by the mite *Sarcoptes scabiei*, var. *hominis*
- Typically, a clinical diagnosis based on history and physical exam
- System(s) affected: skin/exocrine

EPIDEMIOLOGY
Incidence
Predominant age: children, sexually active young adults, and the elderly

Prevalence
Prevalence varies substantially worldwide but is more common in resource-poor settings (1):
- More prevalent in areas of overcrowding and in developing countries, particularly tropical climates
- Added to World Health Organization list of neglected tropical diseases in 2013

ETIOLOGY AND PATHOPHYSIOLOGY
- *S. scabiei*, var. *hominis*
  - An obligate human parasite
  - Primarily transmitted by prolonged human-to-human direct skin contact
  - Infrequently transmitted via fomites (e.g., bedding, clothing, or furnishings)
- Female mite lays eggs in burrows in the stratum corneum and epidermis.
- Itching is caused by a delayed type IV hypersensitivity reaction to the mite saliva, eggs, or excrement.

RISK FACTORS
- Prolonged skin-to-skin contact (e.g., sexual, overcrowding, nosocomial infection)
- Poor nutritional status, poverty, and homelessness
- Hot, tropical climates
- Seasonal variation: Incidence may be higher in the winter than in the summer (due to overcrowding).
- Immunocompromised patients, including those with HIV/AIDS, are at increased risk of developing severe (crusted/Norwegian) scabies.

GENERAL PREVENTION
Prevent outbreaks by prompt treatment and cleansing of fomites (see "General Measures").

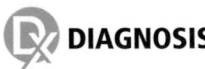

DIAGNOSIS

HISTORY
- Generalized itching is often severe and worse at night.
- Identify potential contact with infected individuals.
- Initial/primary infection usually asymptomatic for the first 3 to 4 weeks (until sensitivity occurs)
- Subsequent reinfection typically develops symptoms after only 1 to 3 days.

PHYSICAL EXAM
- Lesions (inflammatory, erythematous, pruritic papules) most commonly located in the finger webs, flexor surfaces of the wrists, elbows, axillae, buttocks, genitalia, feet, and ankles; often spares the head/neck in adults

- Burrows (thin, curvy lines in the upper epidermis that measure 1 to 10 mm in length)—a pathognomonic sign of scabies
- Secondary erosions and excoriations from scratching
- Pustules (if secondarily infected)
- Pruritic nodules in covered areas (buttocks, groin, axillae) resulting from an exaggerated hypersensitivity reaction
- Crusted scabies (or Norwegian scabies) is a psoriasiform dermatosis occurring with hyperinfestation with thousands/millions of mites (more common in immunosuppressed patients).

Geriatric Considerations
The elderly often itch more severely despite fewer cutaneous lesions and are at risk for extensive infestations, perhaps related to a decline in cell-mediated immunity. There may be back involvement in those who are bedridden.

Pediatric Considerations
Infants and very young children often present with vesicles, papules, and pustules and have more widespread involvement, including the hands, palms, feet, soles, body folds, and head (rare for adults).

DIFFERENTIAL DIAGNOSIS
- Atopic dermatitis
- Contact dermatitis
- Folliculitis/impetigo
- Tinea corporis
- Dermatitis herpetiformis
- Eczema
- Insect bites
- Papular urticaria
- Pediculosis corporis
- Psoriasis (crusted scabies)
- Pyoderma
- Seborrheic dermatitis
- Syphilis

DIAGNOSTIC TESTS & INTERPRETATION
- Based on 2018 IACS (International Alliance Control for Scabies) Criteria for the Diagnosis of Scabies (2)[C]:
  - Confirmed scabies diagnosis: based on microscopic identification of mites, eggs, or fecal pellets (scybala) OR visualization of mite with dermoscopy
  - Clinical scabies diagnosis: detection of burrows, OR typical lesions on male genitalia, OR typical lesions in a typical distribution with two history features of itch and known infectious contact
  - Suspected scabies diagnosis: typical lesions in a typical distribution with one history feature of itch or known infectious contact, OR atypical lesions or atypical distribution with two history features of itch and known infectious contact
- A failure to find mites does not rule out scabies.

Initial Tests (lab, imaging)
CBC is rarely needed but may show eosinophilia.

Diagnostic Procedures/Other
- Examination of skin with dermoscopy
  - Look for typical burrows in finger webs, on flexor aspect of the wrists, and on the penis.
  - Look for a dark point at the end of the burrow (the mite, also known as "delta wing sign").

- Skin scraping
  - Place a drop of mineral oil over a nonexcoriated lesion or burrow.
  - Scrape the lesion with a surgical blade (no. 15).
  - Examine scrapings under a microscope for mites, eggs, egg casings, or feces (3)[C].
  - Scraping under fingernails may be positive.
  - When mite is not found with scraping, biopsy may reveal mite, eggs, or feces.
- Potassium hydroxide (KOH) wet mount NOT recommended because it can dissolve mite pellets
- Burrow ink test
  - If burrows are not obvious, apply gentian violet or India ink to an area of rash. Wash off the ink with alcohol. A burrow should remain stained and become more evident. Then apply mineral oil, scrape, and observe microscopically, as noted previously.

Test Interpretation
Skin biopsy of a nodule (although performed rarely) will reveal portions of the mite in the corneal layer.

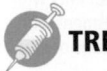

TREATMENT

GENERAL MEASURES
- Treat all intimate contacts (including close household and family members).
- Treat items in contact with skin. Wash all clothing, bed linens, and towels in hot (60°C) water and dry in hot dryer. Personal items that cannot be washed should be sealed in a plastic bag for at least 3 to 5 days.
- Itching and dermatitis can persist for up to 4 weeks and can be treated with oral antihistamines and/or topical/oral corticosteroids. It is important to educate patients this is likely not a sign of treatment failure.

MEDICATION
First Line
- Permethrin 5% cream (Elimite) is generally accepted as first-line therapy (4,5)[A].
  - After bathing or showering, apply cream from the neck to the soles of the feet, paying particular attention to areas that are most involved and then wash off after 8 to 14 hours.
  - It is recommended to repeat treatment 1 to 2 weeks later.
  - The adult dose is usually 30 g per treatment.
  - Side effects include itching and stinging (minimal absorption).
- Ivermectin (Stromectol) (4,5)[A]
  - Not FDA-approved for scabies
  - 200 μg/kg PO as a single dose; repeated in 1 week (because not ovicidal)
  - Take with food to improve bioavailability and enhance penetration into the epidermis.
  - May need higher doses or may need to use in combination with topical scabicide for HIV-positive patients
- **Crusted scabies** often require more frequent application of permethrin (q2–3d for 1 to 2 weeks) in combination with repeated doses of PO ivermectin on days 1, 2, 8, 9, and 15. Severe cases may need further dosing of ivermectin on days 22 and 29 (2)[C].

Pediatric Considerations

- Permethrin may be used on infants >2 months of age. In children <5 years of age, the cream should be applied to the head and neck as well as to the entire body.
- PO ivermectin should be avoided in children <5 years and in those weighing <15 kg.

Second Line

- Crotamiton (Eurax) 10% cream
  - Apply from the neck down for 24 hours, rinse off, reapply for an additional 24 to 48 hours, and then thoroughly wash off.
  - Nodular scabies: Apply to nodules for 24 hours, rinse off, reapply for an additional 24 hours, and then thoroughly wash off.
- Precipitated sulfur 2–10% in petrolatum
  - Not FDA-approved for scabies
  - Apply to the entire body from the neck down for 24 hours, rinse by bathing and then repeat for 2 more days (3 days total). It is malodorous and messy but is thought to be safer than lindane, especially in infants <6 months of age and safer than permethrin in infants <2 months of age.
- Lindane (γ-benzene hexachloride, Kwell) 1% lotion
  - Apply a thin layer to all skin surfaces from the neck down and wash off 6 to 8 hours later.
  - Two applications 1 week apart are recommended but may increase the risk of toxicity.
  - 2 oz is usually adequate for an adult.
  - Side effects: neurotoxicity (seizures, muscle spasms), aplastic anemia
  - Contraindications: uncontrolled seizure disorder, premature infants
  - Precautions: Do not use on excoriated skin, on immunocompromised patients, in conditions that may increase risk of seizures, or with medications that decrease seizure threshold.
  - Possible interactions: concomitant use with medications that lower the seizure threshold
  - Some instances of lindane-resistant scabies have been reported. These cases do respond to permethrin.

ALERT

Lindane: FDA black box warning of severe neurologic toxicity; use only when all other agents have failed.

Pediatric Considerations

- The FDA recommends caution when using lindane in patients who weigh <50 kg. It is not recommended for infants and is contraindicated in premature infants.
- Infants <2 months should be treated with crotamiton or sulfur preparation.

Pregnancy Considerations

- Permethrin is pregnancy Category B, and lindane, ivermectin, and crotamiton are Category C.
- Permethrin is considered compatible with lactation, but if permethrin is used while breastfeeding, the infant should be bottlefed until the cream has been thoroughly washed off.

ISSUES FOR REFERRAL

Consider referral to dermatology if unable to confirm diagnosis and/or resistant to repeated treatments.

ADDITIONAL THERAPIES

- Crusted scabies may require use of keratolytics to improve penetration of permethrin.
- Nodular scabies may require intralesional steroids for complete resolution, if they persist for several weeks after treatment.
- Benzyl benzoate lotion (not available in the United States but used widely in developing countries)
  - Not FDA-approved for scabies
  - Dose for adults is 25–28%; dilute to 12.5% for children and 6.25% for infants.
  - After bathing, apply lotion from the neck to soles of feet for 24 hours.
- Topical ivermectin 1% lotion (investigational, moderate level of certainty)
  - Not FDA-approved for scabies
  - Apply to affected sites and wash off 8 hours later (5)[A].

 ## ONGOING CARE

FOLLOW-UP RECOMMENDATIONS

Patient Monitoring

Recheck patient at weekly intervals only if rash or itching persists. Scrape new lesions and retreat if mites or products are found.

PATIENT EDUCATION

- Patients should be instructed on proper application and cautioned not to overuse the medication when applying it to the skin.
- A patient fact sheet is available from the CDC: http://www.cdc.gov/parasites/scabies/

PROGNOSIS

Lesions begin to regress in 1 to 2 days, but eczema and itching may persist for up to 4 weeks after treatment.

COMPLICATIONS

- Poor sleep due to pruritus
- Social stigma
- Secondary bacterial infection (more common in developing countries). Impetigo due to Group A Streptococci and *Staphylococcus aureus* may lead to sepsis, poststreptococcal glomerulonephritis, and rheumatic heart disease.
- Eczema
- Pyoderma
- Postscabetic pruritus
- Nodules (nodular scabies) may persist for weeks to months after treatment.

REFERENCES

1. Romani L, Steer AC, Whitfeld MJ, et al. Prevalence of scabies and impetigo worldwide: a systematic review. *Lancet Infect Dis*. 2015;15(8):960–967.
2. Engelman D, Fuller LC, Steer AC; for International Alliance for the Control of Scabies Delphi Panel. Consensus criteria for the diagnosis of scabies: a Delphi study of international experts. *PLoS Negl Trop Dis*. 2018;12(5):e0006549.
3. Gunning K, Pippitt K, Kiraly B, et al. Pediculosis and scabies: a treatment update. *Am Fam Physician*. 2012;86(6):535–541.
4. Strong M, Johnstone P. Interventions for treating scabies. *Cochrane Database of Syst Rev*. 2007;(3):CD000320.
5. Rosumeck S, Nast A, Dressler C. Ivermectin and permethrin for treating scabies. *Cochrane Database of Syst Rev*. 2018;(4):CD012994.

 ## SEE ALSO

Arthropod Bites and Stings; Pediculosis (Lice)

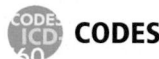 ## CODES

ICD10

B86 Scabies

CLINICAL PEARLS

- Prior to diagnosis, use of a topical steroid to treat pruritic symptoms may mask symptoms and is termed *scabies incognito*.
- Environmental control is recommended. All linens, towels, and clothing used in the previous 4 days should be washed in hot water or dry-cleaned. Personal items that cannot be washed or dry-cleaned should be sealed in a plastic bag for 3 to 5 days.
- All intimate contacts should receive treatment.
- Close contacts (those sharing the same bed or who have intimate contact) may not show signs and symptoms immediately but should be treated simultaneously to avoid reinfestation.
- Eczema and itching may persist for up to 4 weeks after treatment, causing many patients to falsely believe that they have failed treatment or are being reinfected.
- In patients with actual reinfection, it is possible the patient has not applied the medication properly or, more likely, the index patient has not been identified and treated.

S

SCARLET FEVER

John C. Huscher, MD

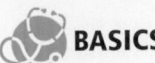 BASICS

DESCRIPTION

- A disease (typically in childhood) characterized by fever, pharyngitis, and rash caused by group A β-hemolytic *Streptococcus pyogenes* (GAS) that produces erythrogenic toxin
- Incubation period: 1 to 7 days
- Duration of illness: 4 to 10 days
- Rash usually appears on the second day of illness.
- Rash first appears on the upper chest and flexural creases and then spreads rapidly all over the body.
- Rash clears at the end of the 1st week and is followed by several weeks of desquamation.
- System(s) affected: head, eyes, ears, nose, throat, skin/exocrine
- Synonym(s): scarlatina

EPIDEMIOLOGY

Incidence

- In developed countries, 15% of school age children and 4–10% of adults have an episode of GAS pharyngitis each year.
- Scarlet fever is rare in infancy because of maternal antitoxin antibodies.
- Predominant age: 6 to 12 years
- Peak age: 4 to 8 years
- Predominant sex: male = female
- Rare in the United States in persons >12 years because of high rates (>80%) of lifelong protective antibodies to erythrogenic toxins

Prevalence

- 15–30% of cases of pharyngitis in children are due to GAS; 5–15% in adults
- <10% of children with streptococcal pharyngitis develop scarlet fever.

ETIOLOGY AND PATHOPHYSIOLOGY

- Erythrogenic toxin production is necessary to develop scarlet fever.
- Three toxin types: A, B, C
- Toxins damage capillaries (producing rash) and act as superantigens, stimulating cytokine release.
- Antibodies to toxins prevent development of rash but do not protect against underlying infection.
- Primary site of streptococcal infection is usually within the tonsils, but scarlet fever may also occur with infection of skin, surgical wounds, or uterus (puerperal scarlet fever).

RISK FACTORS

- Winter/spring seasonal increase
- More common in school-aged children
- Contact with infected individual(s)
- Crowded living conditions (e.g., lower socioeconomic status, barracks, child care, schools)

GENERAL PREVENTION

- Spread by contact with airborne respiratory droplets
- Asymptomatic contacts do not require cultures/prophylaxis.
- Symptomatic contacts may be treated with or without culture.
- Children should not return to school/daycare until they have received 24 hours of antibiotic therapy.

COMMONLY ASSOCIATED CONDITIONS

- Pharyngitis
- Impetigo
- Rheumatic fever
- Glomerulonephritis

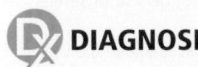 DIAGNOSIS

HISTORY

Prodrome 1 to 2 days

- Sore throat
- Headache
- Myalgias
- Malaise
- Fever (>38°C [100.4°F])
- Vomiting
- Abdominal pain (may mimic acute abdomen)
- Rash—scarlatiniform erythematous punctate eruption
- Cough, conjunctivitis, hoarseness, and rhinorrhea are more commonly associated with viral infections.

PHYSICAL EXAM

- Oral exam
  - Beefy red tonsils and pharynx with/without exudate
  - Petechiae on palate
  - White coating on tongue: White strawberry tongue appears on days 1 to 2. This sheds by days 4 to 5, leaving a red strawberry tongue, which is shiny and erythematous with prominent papillae.
- Exanthem (appears within 1 to 5 days)
  - Scarlet macules with generalized erythema; blanches when pressed
  - Orange-red punctate skin eruption with sandpaper-like texture, "sunburn with goose pimples"
  - Coarse "sandpaper" rash, initially appearing on chest and axillae, and then spreading to abdomen and extremities; prominent in skin folds, flexural surfaces (e.g., axillae, groin, buttocks), with sparing of palms and soles
  - Flushed face with circumoral pallor, red lips
  - Pastia lines: transverse red streaks in skin folds of abdomen, antecubital space, and axillae
  - Desquamation begins on face after 7 to 10 days and proceeds over trunk to hands and feet; may persist for 6 weeks
  - In severe cases, small vesicular lesions (miliary sudamina) may appear on abdomen, hands, and feet.

DIFFERENTIAL DIAGNOSIS

- Viral exanthem: measles; rubella; roseola
- Infectious mononucleosis
- *Mycoplasma* pneumonia
- Secondary syphilis
- Toxic shock syndrome
- Staphylococcal scalded-skin syndrome
- Kawasaki disease
- Drug hypersensitivity
- Severe sunburn

DIAGNOSTIC TESTS & INTERPRETATION

- Use results from rapid antigen detection testing (RADT) in conjunction with validated clinical decision rules such as the modified Centor score.
- Modified Centor clinical decision rule
  - Absence of cough .... 1 point
  - Swollen, tender anterior cervical nodes ... 1 point
  - Temperature 100.4°F (38°C) .... 1 point
  - Tonsillar exudate or swelling .... 1 point
  - Age:
    - 3 to 14 years .... 1 point
    - 15 to 44 years .... 0 point
    - 45 years or older .... −1 point
- Cumulative score:
  - 0 Risk of GAS pharyngitis 1–2.5%—no further testing or antibiotics indicated
  - 1 Risk of GAS pharyngitis 5–10%—no further testing or antibiotics indicated—option to perform throat culture or RADT—treat if positive.
  - 2 Risk of GAS pharyngitis 11–17%—perform throat culture or RADT—treat if positive.
  - 3 Risk of GAS pharyngitis 28–35%—perform throat culture or RADT—treat if positive.
  - 4+ Risk of GAS pharyngitis 51–53%—consider empiric treatment with antibiotics.
- Testing for GAS pharyngitis is *not recommended* for patients with symptoms suggesting a viral etiology (e.g., cough, rhinorrhea, hoarseness, oral ulcers).

Initial Tests (lab, imaging)

- RADT: diagnostic if positive, 95% specific; sensitivity approaches that of culture. In children, negative RADT should be confirmed by throat culture (not necessary in adults). Positive RADT does not require confirmatory culture (1)[C].
- Throat culture is the gold standard to confirm streptococcal infection (99% specific, 90–97% sensitive; 5–10% of healthy individuals are carriers) (1).
- Serologic tests (antistreptolysin O titer and streptozyme tests, antihyaluronidase): Confirm recent GAS infection; not helpful or recommended for diagnosis of acute disease
- Gram stain: gram-positive cocci in chains
- CBC may show elevated WBC count (12,000 to 16,000/mm³); eosinophilia later (second week)
- Follow-up (posttreatment) throat cultures or RADT not routinely recommended
- Diagnostic testing and empiric treatment of asymptomatic household contacts of patients with acute streptococcal pharyngitis is not routinely recommended (2)[B].
- Appropriately symptomatic patients >3 years old with a family member recently diagnosed with laboratory-confirmed GAS pharyngitis may be treated without screening or confirmatory testing (3)[C].

Follow-Up Tests & Special Considerations

- Recent antibiotic therapy may impact culture results.
- Within 5 days of symptoms, antibiotics can delay/abolish antistreptolysin O response.

Test Interpretation

Skin lesions reveal characteristic inflammatory reaction, specifically hyperemia, edema, and polymorphonuclear cell infiltration.

TREATMENT

GENERAL MEASURES
Supportive care; analgesic/antipyretic such as acetaminophen or NSAID, for moderate to severe symptoms or to control fever. Symptomatic treatment can include medicated throat lozenges and topical anesthetics.

MEDICATION
First Line
The primary reason for treating GAS is to decrease the risk of acute rheumatic fever. Early treatment decreases duration of symptoms by 1 to 2 days and decreases the period of contagiousness (3)[B]. Penicillin is the drug of choice for GAS pharyngitis given its proven efficacy, safety, narrow spectrum, and low cost.
- Penicillin (PO; penicillin V and others) for 10 days
  - 250 mg PO BID or TID for <27 kg (60 lb); 250 mg QID or 500 mg BID for >27 kg (60 lb) adolescents and adults (1,4,5)[A]
  - If compliance is questionable, use penicillin G benzathine: single IM dose 600,000 U for <27 kg (60 lb); 1.2 mU for those >27 kg
- Amoxicillin (PO) 50 mg/kg (max dose 1,000 mg) once daily or 25 mg/kg (max dose 500 mg) twice daily for 10 days (use only for definitive GAS because it can induce rash with some viral infections)
  - Contraindications: penicillin allergy
- Precautions: Avoid in patients with penicillin allergy (anaphylaxis).

Second Line
- For patients allergic to penicillin
- Type IV hypersensitivity to penicillin:
  - Oral cephalosporins: Many are effective, but 1st-generation cephalosporins are less expensive:
    - Cephalexin 20 mg/kg dose twice daily for 10 days; max 500 mg every 12 hours (1)[A]
    - Cefadroxil 30 mg/kg once daily; max 1,000 mg for 10 days (1)
- Type I hypersensitivity to penicillin:
  - Azithromycin (Zithromax, Z pack): 12 mg/kg/day (max 500 mg) for 5 days (4)[A]
  - Clarithromycin (Biaxin): children >6 months: 7.5 mg/kg BID for 10 days; adults: 250 mg BID for 10 days
- Clindamycin 7 mg/kg (max 300 mg/dose) TID for 10 days (4)[B]
- Tetracyclines and sulfonamides should not be used.

ALERT
Avoid aspirin in children due to risk of Reye syndrome.

ISSUES FOR REFERRAL
Peritonsillar abscess; shock symptoms: hypotension, disseminated intravascular coagulation (DIC), cardiac, liver, renal dysfunction

SURGERY/OTHER PROCEDURES
- Tonsillectomy is recommended with recurrent bouts of pharyngitis (≥6 positive strep cultures in 1 year).
- Although children still may get streptococcal pharyngitis ("strep throat") after a tonsillectomy, the procedure reduces the frequency and severity of infections.

 ONGOING CARE

FOLLOW-UP RECOMMENDATIONS
Follow-up throat culture not needed unless symptomatic
Patient Monitoring
GAS is uniformly susceptible to penicillin, treatment failures are typically due to:
- Poor adherence to recommended antibiotic therapy
- β-Lactamase oral flora hydrolyzing penicillin
- GAS carrier state and concurrent viral rash (requires no treatment)
- Repeat exposure to carriers in family: Streptococci persist on unrinsed toothbrushes and orthodontic appliances for up to 15 days.
- Retreat recurrent GAS pharyngitis with the same agent, an alternative oral agent, or IM penicillin G.

DIET
No special diet

PATIENT EDUCATION
- Delay in treatment awaiting culture results does not increase the risk of rheumatic fever.
- Complete the entire course of antibiotics.
- Children should not return to school/daycare until they have received >24 hours of antibiotic therapy.
- Can spread person to person. Personal hygiene is important (wash hands, don't share utensils).
- "Recurring strep throat: When is tonsillectomy useful?" (http://www.mayoclinic.org /diseasesconditions/strep-throat/expert-answers /recurringstrep-throat/faq-20058360)

PROGNOSIS
- Treatment shortens symptoms by 12 to 24 hours.
- Recurrent attacks are possible (different erythrogenic toxins).

COMPLICATIONS
- Suppurative
  - Sinusitis
  - Otitis media/mastoiditis
  - Cervical adenitis
  - Peritonsillar abscess/retropharyngeal abscess
  - Pneumonia
  - Bacteremia with metastatic infectious foci: meningitis, brain abscess, osteomyelitis, septic arthritis, endocarditis, intracranial venous sinus thrombosis, necrotizing fasciitis
- Nonsuppurative
  - Rheumatic fever: Therapy prevents rheumatic fever when started as long as 10 days after onset of acute GAS infection.
  - Glomerulonephritis: due to nephritogenic strain of Streptococcus; prevention even after adequate treatment of GAS is less certain.
  - Streptococcal toxic shock syndrome: fever; hypotension; DIC; and cardiac, liver, and/or kidney dysfunction due to other toxin-mediated sequelae
  - Cellulitis
  - Weeks to months later, may develop transverse grooves in nail plates and hair loss (telogen effluvium)

- Pediatric autoimmune neuropsychiatric disorder associated with GAS (PANDAS). A subset of children has been recognized whose symptoms of obsessive-compulsive disorder (OCD) or tic disorders are exacerbated by GAS infection.

REFERENCES
1. Kalra MG, Higgins KE, Perez ED. Common questions about streptococcal pharyngitis. *Am Fam Physician*. 2016;94(1):24–31.
2. Shulman ST, Bisno AL, Clegg HW, et al. Clinical practice guideline for the diagnosis and management of group A streptococcal pharyngitis: 2012 update by the Infectious Diseases Society of America. *Clin Infect Dis*. 2012;55(10):1279–1282.
3. Murphy T, Van Harrison R, Hammoud A, et al. *Pharyngitis*. Ann Arbor, MI: University of Michigan Health System; 2013. National Guideline Clearinghouse Guideline Summary NGC-9967.
4. Gerber MA, Baltimore RS, Eaton CB, et al. Prevention of rheumatic fever and diagnosis and treatment of acute streptococcal pharyngitis: a scientific statement from the American Heart Association Rheumatic Fever, Endocarditis, and Kawasaki Disease Committee of the Council on Cardiovascular Disease in the Young, the Interdisciplinary Council on Functional Genomics and Translational Biology, and the Interdisciplinary Council on Quality of Care and Outcomes Research: endorsed by the American Academy of Pediatrics. *Circulation*. 2009;119(11):1541–1551.
5. van Driel ML, De Sutter AI, Habraken H, et al. Different antibiotic treatments for group A streptococcal pharyngitis. *Cochrane Database Syst Rev*. 2016;(9):CD004406.

 SEE ALSO
- Pharyngitis
- Algorithm: Pharyngitis

CODES
ICD10
- A38.9 Scarlet fever, uncomplicated
- J02.0 Streptococcal pharyngitis
- A38.0 Scarlet fever with otitis media

CLINICAL PEARLS
- Consider scarlet fever in the differential diagnosis of children with fever and an exanthematous rash.
- Key clinical findings include strawberry tongue, circumoral pallor, and a coarse sandpaper rash.
- Desquamation (7 to 10 days after symptom onset) may last for several weeks following scarlet fever.
- Diagnose GAS pharyngitis using a validated clinical decision rule (modified Centor score) and selective use of RADT.
- Penicillin remains the drug of choice.

S

SCHIZOPHRENIA
Anna Loyal Jackson, MD • Jeffrey Stovall, MD

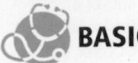

BASICS

Schizophrenia is a persistent and severe psychiatric condition characterized by neurocognitive decline and impairment in reality testing.

DESCRIPTION
- Major psychiatric disorder characterized by prodrome, active, and residual psychotic symptoms involving disturbances in appearance, speech, behavior, perception, and thought that last for at least 6 months
- *DSM-5* eliminated subcategories of schizophrenia (1).
- System(s) affected: central nervous system (CNS)

EPIDEMIOLOGY
Incidence
- 7.7 to 43/100,000
- Predominant sex: male-to-female ratio = 1.4:1.0
- Age of onset: typically <30 years, earlier in males (early to mid-20s) than females (late 20s), with a smaller peak that occurs in women >45 years

Prevalence
- Lifetime (1%): highest prevalence in lower socioeconomic classes and urban settings (2-fold higher risk)
- 1.1% of the population >18 years old; similar rates in all countries

ETIOLOGY AND PATHOPHYSIOLOGY
- Stems from a complex interaction between genetic and environmental factors; higher incidence if prenatal infection or hypoxia, winter births, first-generation immigrants, advanced paternal age, drug use, and genetic (velocardiofacial) syndromes
- Overstimulation of mesolimbic dopamine D_2 receptors, deficient prefrontal dopamine, and aberrant prefrontal glutamate (NMDA) activity results in perceptual disturbances, disordered thought process, and cognitive impairments

Genetics
If first-degree biologic relative has schizophrenia, risk is 8–10% (a 10-fold increase).

GENERAL PREVENTION
- Currently, no known preventive measures decrease the incidence of schizophrenia.
- Interventions to improve long-term outcome and associated comorbid conditions are employed during management.

COMMONLY ASSOCIATED CONDITIONS
- Nicotine dependence (>50%) (1) and substance use disorders are common and lead to significant long-term medical and social complications.
- Metabolic syndrome, diabetes mellitus, obesity, and certain infectious diseases, including HIV, hepatitis B, and hepatitis C all occur in higher-than-expected rates in individuals with schizophrenia.

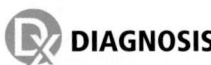

DIAGNOSIS

Focus on identifying an insidious social and functional decline per history with the onset of ≥2 of the following characteristic symptoms on mental status exam:
- Delusions (fixed, false beliefs)
- Hallucinations (auditory > visual disturbances)
- Disorganized thought (derailed or incoherent speech)
- Grossly disorganized/catatonic behavior (hyper- or hypoactive movements that are often repetitive)
- Negative symptoms (affective flattening, avolition, asociality, alogia, anhedonia) (1)

PHYSICAL EXAM
No physical findings characterize the illness; however, chronic treatment with neuroleptic agents may result in parkinsonism, tardive dyskinesia, and other extrapyramidal symptoms.

DIFFERENTIAL DIAGNOSIS
- Brief psychotic disorder (symptom duration <1 month)
- Schizophreniform disorder (symptom duration 1 to 6 months)
- Psychotic disorder due to another medical condition
  - Disorientation, in particular, indicates delirium.
  - Possible medical illnesses include porphyria, TBI, infection, tumor, metabolic, endocrine, and intoxication, including withdrawal states and disorders that affect the CNS (i.e., epilepsy, Huntington disease, Wilson disease, lupus cerebritis, anti-NMDA limbic encephalitis, metachromatic leukodystrophy).
- Substance-induced psychosis: secondary to substance use/abuse, such as cocaine, hallucinogens (amphetamines, LSD, phencyclidine), cannabis (including synthetic), bath salts, alcohol, or prescribed medications including steroids, anticholinergics, and opiates
- Personality disorders: paranoid, schizotypal, schizoid, borderline personality disorder
- Mood disorders: bipolar disorder, major depressive disorders with psychotic features or catatonia
- Other thought disorders: delusional disorder, schizoaffective disorder
- Posttraumatic stress disorder
- Cultural belief system
- Autism spectrum disorder or neurodevelopmental disorders

DIAGNOSTIC TESTS & INTERPRETATION
- No tests are available to indicate schizophrenia.
- Imaging (MRI), EEG, LP, and laboratory tests may be needed to rule out other causes and may be used as clinical presentation warrants.

Initial Tests (lab, imaging)
- The following labs are often used to rule out a medical etiology of psychotic symptoms:
  - TSH, CBC, blood chemistries
  - Vitamin levels (thiamine, vitamin D, methylmalonic acid/vitamin B_{12})
  - Drug/alcohol screen of blood and urine, urinalysis
  - Syphilis screen, HIV
  - Heavy-metal exposure: lead, mercury
  - Ceruloplasmin, urine porphobilinogen as indicated
  - ESR, ANA
  - Hepatitis C, hepatitis B
- The following labs are used to assess for comorbidities and baseline values prior to antipsychotic initiation:
  - ECG for baseline QTc
  - CBC, blood chemistries, TSH
  - Hemoglobin A1C
  - Blood glucose level, preferably fasting
  - Lipid panel, preferably fasting
  - Pregnancy test, if indicated

Follow-Up Tests & Special Considerations
Clinical and laboratory tests for routine monitoring, at least yearly, if using antipsychotic medications (2)[A]:
- Weight, waist circumference, and blood pressure
- Fasting blood glucose level, hemoglobin A1C, fasting lipid panel
- CBC

- Pregnancy test and prolactin level, if indicated
- ECG, monitoring for QTc prolongation
- Clinical assessment of extrapyramidal symptoms

Diagnostic Procedures/Other
Neuropsychologic testing: not a routine part of assessment but can help assess cognitive level to predict functioning and need for assistance

Test Interpretation
No diagnostic pathologic findings; however, ventriculomegaly is frequently seen on MRI with whole brain grey matter loss and white matter loss in medial temporal lobe structures preferentially.

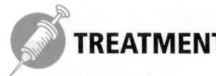

TREATMENT

MEDICATION
First Line
- Two classes of antipsychotic medications: typical and atypical. First-line treatment is with an atypical antipsychotic given lower potential for extrapyramidal side effects.
  - Atypical (2nd generation)
    - Risperidone, olanzapine, ziprasidone, aripiprazole, quetiapine, paliperidone, iloperidone, asenapine, lurasidone, clozapine, brexpiprazole, cariprazine, pimavanserin (Parkinson disease–related psychosis)
  - Typical (1st generation)
    - Haloperidol, chlorpromazine, fluphenazine, trifluoperazine, perphenazine, thioridazine, thiothixene, loxapine
- Medication choice is based on clinical and subjective response and side effect profile (2)[A].
  - Sensitivity to extrapyramidal adverse effects: atypicals
  - For least risk of tardive dyskinesia: quetiapine, clozapine
  - For least risk of metabolic syndrome: aripiprazole, ziprasidone, lurasidone
- For poor compliance/high risk of relapse: Injectable form of long-acting antipsychotic may be used.
  - Haloperidol, fluphenazine, risperidone, olanzapine, aripiprazole, and paliperidone
- Usual oral daily dose (initial dose may be lower)
  - Chlorpromazine: 200 mg BID
  - Aripiprazole: 10 to 30 mg/day
  - Asenapine: 5 mg BID (sublingual)
  - Fluphenazine: 5 mg BID
  - Haloperidol: 5 mg BID
  - Lurasidone: 40 to 80 mg/day (with meal)
  - Olanzapine: 15 to 30 mg/day
  - Paliperidone: 3 to 12 mg/day
  - Perphenazine: 24 mg/day divided BID/ TID
  - Quetiapine: 200 to 300 mg BID
  - Risperidone: 3 mg/day
  - Ziprasidone: 60 to 80 mg BID (with meal)
  - Cariprazine: 1.5 to 6.0 mg/day
  - Brexpiprazole: 2 to 4 mg/day
  - Pimavanserin: 34 mg/day
  - Clozapine: 200 mg BID
    - Start 12.5 mg/day and increase daily by 25 mg until dose of 300 mg/day split into BID dosing; do not exceed 900 mg/day.
    - Effective in treatment of refractory or suicidal patients (2)[A]

○ Serious risk of agranulocytosis mandates registration with National Clozapine Registry and weekly to monthly monitoring of CBC with differential.
○ Significant risk of seizure at higher doses
○ SE can include myocarditis, DVT, sialorrhea, tachycardia, and weight gain.

ALERT
All antipsychotics are associated with weight gain and carry the risk of metabolic SE and tardive dyskinesia.

- Managing adverse effects of antipsychotics
  – Dystonic reaction (especially of head and neck): diphenhydramine 25 to 50 mg IM or benztropine 1 to 2 mg IM
  – Akathisia (restlessness): propranolol 20 to 30 mg BID or lorazepam 0.5 to 1.0 mg BID
  – Parkinsonism: trihexyphenidyl 2 mg BID (up to 15 mg daily) or benztropine 0.5 BID (1 to 4 mg/day); amantadine 100 mg daily (up to 300 mg daily)
  – Neuroleptic malignant syndrome: hyperthermia, autonomic dysfunction, and extrapyramidal symptoms; requires hospitalization and supportive management (IVF and cessation of offending neuroleptic)
- Geriatric considerations: All antipsychotics carry a black box warning for increased mortality risk in elderly patients with dementia.
- Adjunctive treatments
  – Benzodiazepines
    ○ May be effective adjuncts to antipsychotics during acute phase of illness
    ○ Useful for the treatment of catatonia
    ○ Withdrawal reactions with psychosis or seizures; risk for dependence and cognitive impairment
  – Mood stabilizers
    ○ Valproic acid may be effective adjunct for those with agitated/violent behavior (2)[A].
    ○ Lithium may be effective adjunct for patients with affective symptoms or schizoaffective disorder (2)[A].
  – Antidepressants: if prominent symptoms of depression are present
  – Metformin: helps minimize risk of metabolic SE with use of antipsychotics
  – Liraglutide: helps minimize risk of metabolic SE with use of clozapine or olanzapine (3)[B]

ISSUES FOR REFERRAL
- Consider referral in cases of suicidality, coexistence of an addiction, difficulty in engagement, or poor self-care.
- Patients with schizophrenia should receive multidisciplinary care from both a primary care physician and a psychiatrist.
- Family members often benefit from referral to family advocacy organizations such as NAMI.

ADDITIONAL THERAPIES
- Family patient education and psychotherapy: These include specific treatments to reduce the impact of psychotic symptoms and to enhance social functioning. Cognitive-behavioral therapy has been shown to be effective for specific symptoms of schizophrenia (4)[A].
- Cognitive remediation is a new approach for cognitive retraining and psychosocial recovery.
- Vocational support programs have shown success in returning individuals to work.

COMPLEMENTARY & ALTERNATIVE MEDICINE
- Omega-3 fatty acids may improve cognitive symptoms, but evidence remains inconclusive.
- There is evidence suggesting antipsychotic properties of cannabidiol, but additional trials regarding safety, efficacy, and dosing are needed (5)[B].

SURGERY/OTHER PROCEDURES
- Electroconvulsive therapy (ECT) should be considered early for patients presenting with catatonic features when response to benzodiazepines is insufficient (2)[A].
- Surgical interventions are not available.

ADMISSION, INPATIENT, AND NURSING CONSIDERATIONS
- Initial stabilization focuses on maintaining a safe environment and reducing acute psychotic symptoms and agitation through the initiation of pharmacologic treatment.
- The decision to admit is usually based on the patient's risk of self-harm or harm to others and the inability to care for self as governed by local legal statute.
- Monitor for safety concerns and establish a safe and supportive environment.
- Discharge criteria is based on the patient's ability to remain safe in the community. It reflects a combination of suicide risk, level of psychotic symptoms, support systems, and the availability of appropriate outpatient services.

 ONGOING CARE

FOLLOW-UP RECOMMENDATIONS
- Long-term symptom management and rehabilitation depend on engagement in ongoing pharmacologic and psychosocial treatment.
- Monitoring is based on evaluation of symptoms (including safety and psychotic symptoms), looking for the emergence of comorbidities, medication side effects, and prevention of complications.

DIET
- Atypical antipsychotics confer a higher risk of metabolic side effects such as diabetes, hypercholesterolemia, and weight gain.
- Although there are no specific dietary requirements, attention should be paid to the high risk of development of obesity and metabolic syndrome in individuals with schizophrenia.

PATIENT EDUCATION
- National Institute of Mental Health. *Schizophrenia*: www.nimh.nih.gov/health/topics/schizophrenia/index.shtml
- *Helping a Family Member with Schizophrenia*: www.aafp.org/afp/20070615/1830ph.html
- National Alliance on Mental Illness: www.NAMI.org

PROGNOSIS
- Typical course is one of remissions and exacerbations. Although uncommon, there are known cases of complete remission and of refractory illness.
- Negative symptoms are often most difficult to treat.
- About 20% attempt and 5–6% die of suicide (1).
- Decreased life span related to comorbidities (coronary artery disease, pulmonary disease, or substance use disorders) and suboptimal care; guarded prognosis

COMPLICATIONS
- Side effects from antipsychotics, including tardive dyskinesia, orthostatic hypotension, QTc prolongation, and metabolic syndrome
- Self-inflicted trauma and suicide
- Combative behavior toward others (Only 5% of crimes are caused by mental illness including psychosis.) (6)
- Comorbid addictions, including nicotine

REFERENCES
1. American Psychiatric Association. *Diagnostic and Statistical Manual of Mental Disorders*. 5th ed. Arlington, VA: American Psychiatric Association; 2013.
2. Hasan A, Falkai P, Wobrock T, et al; for World Federation of Societies of Biological Psychiatry (WFSBP) Task Force on Treatment Guidelines for Schizophrenia. World Federation of Societies of Biological Psychiatry (WFSBP) guidelines for biological treatment of schizophrenia, part 1: update 2012 on the acute treatment of schizophrenia and the management of treatment resistance. *World J Biol Psychiatry*. 2012;13(5):318–378.
3. Larsen JR, Vedtofte L, Jakobsen MSL, et al. Effect of liraglutide treatment on prediabetes and overweight or obesity in clozapine- or olanzapine-treated patients with schizophrenia spectrum disorder: a randomized clinical trial. *JAMA Psychiatry*. 2017;74(7):719–728.
4. Hasan A, Falkai P, Wobrock T, et al; for WFSBP Task force on Treatment Guidelines for Schizophrenia. World Federation of Societies of Biological Psychiatry (WFSBP) guidelines for biological treatment of schizophrenia, part 2: update 2012 on the long-term treatment of schizophrenia and management of antipsychotic-induced side effects. *World J Biol Psychiatry*. 2013;14(1):2–44.
5. Leweke FM, Piomelli D, Pahlisch F, et al. Cannabidiol enhances anandamide signaling and alleviates psychotic symptoms of schizophrenia. *Transl Psychiatry*. 2012;2:e94.
6. Fazel S, Grann M. The population impact of severe mental illness on violent crime. *Am J Psychiatry*. 2006;163(8):1397–1403.

ADDITIONAL READING
Saks E. *The Center Cannot Hold: My Journey Through Madness*. New York, NY: Hyperion; 2007.

 SEE ALSO

Algorithm: Delirium

 CODES

ICD10
- F20.9 Schizophrenia, unspecified
- F20.0 Paranoid schizophrenia
- F20.1 Disorganized schizophrenia

CLINICAL PEARLS
- A debilitating chronic mental illness that affects all cultures and requires a multidisciplinary team approach to assist with coping, treatment, and to promote recovery
- Schizophrenia is characterized by positive symptoms, including hallucinations, delusions, and negative symptoms, including flattened affect, anhedonia, amotivation, and social withdrawal.

S

SCLERITIS

Matthew J. Schear, DO • Anne S. Steiner, MD

BASICS

DESCRIPTION
- Scleritis is a painful, inflammatory process of the sclera, part of the eye's outer coat.
  - Categorized into anterior or posterior and diffuse, nodular, or necrotizing
  - Commonly associated with systemic disorders
  - Frequently requires systemic anti-inflammatory therapy
  - Potentially vision threatening
- In contrast, episcleritis is a self-limited inflammation of the superficial episclera with only mild discomfort.
- System(s) affected: ocular

EPIDEMIOLOGY
- Mean age is 54 years (range 12 to 96).
- Predominant sex: female > male (1.6:1)

Incidence
Estimated to be 6 cases per 100,000 people in the general population

Prevalence
- Anterior scleritis, about 94% of cases (1)[B]
  - Diffuse anterior scleritis, about 75% (most common)
- Remaining 6% have posterior scleritis.

ETIOLOGY AND PATHOPHYSIOLOGY
- Frequently associated with a systemic illness (1)[B]
  - Most commonly associated with rheumatoid arthritis
  - In about 38% of cases, scleritis is the presenting manifestation of an underlying systemic disorder.
  - Necrotizing scleritis has the highest association with systemic disease.
- Other etiologies
  - Proposed pathogenesis is dependent on type of scleritis. In necrotizing scleritis, the predominant mechanism is likely due to the activity of matrix metalloproteinases.
  - Drug-induced scleritis has been reported in patients on bisphosphonate therapy.
  - Surgically induced necrotizing scleritis is exceedingly rare and occurs after multiple surgeries.
  - Infectious scleritis occurs most commonly after surgical trauma, and *Pseudomonas aeruginosa* in poorly controlled diabetic patients is the most common causative organism (2)[B].

RISK FACTORS
Individuals with autoimmune disorders are most at risk.

COMMONLY ASSOCIATED CONDITIONS
- Rheumatoid arthritis (most common)
- Sjögren syndrome
- Granulomatosis with polyangiitis
- HLA-B27–associated ankylosing spondylitis
- Systemic lupus erythematosus
- Reactive arthritis
- Behçet disease
- Juvenile idiopathic arthritis
- Cogan disease
- Relapsing polychondritis
- Polyarteritis nodosa
- Sarcoidosis
- Inflammatory bowel disease
- Herpes zoster
- Herpes simplex
- HIV
- Syphilis
- Lyme disease
- Tuberculosis
- IgG4-related disease

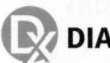

DIAGNOSIS

HISTORY
- Redness and inflammation of the sclera
  - Can be bilateral in about 40% of cases (1)[B]
- Photophobia and tearing
- Pain ranging from mild discomfort to extreme localized tenderness
  - May be described as constant, deep, boring, or pulsating
  - Pain may be referred to the eyebrow, temple, or jaw.
  - Pain may awaken patient from sleep in early hours of morning.
  - Severe pain is most commonly associated with necrotizing scleritis (1)[B].

PHYSICAL EXAM
- Examine sclera in all directions of gaze by gross inspection.
  - A bluish hue may suggest thinning of sclera.
  - Inspect for degree of injection and extent of thinning.
- Check visual acuity.
  - Decrease in visual acuity of two or more Snellen lines occurs in about 16% of patients (1)[B].
- Slit-lamp exam using red-free light
  - Episcleritis: conjunctival and superficial vascular plexuses displaced anteriorly; blanches with phenylephrine

- Scleritis: Deep episcleral plexus is the maximum site of vascular congestion, displaced anteriorly d/t edema of underlying sclera; characteristic blue or violet color, absent in patients with episcleritis
- Dilated fundus exam to rule out posterior involvement
- A complete physical exam, particularly of the skin, joints, heart, and lungs, should be done to evaluate for associated conditions.

DIFFERENTIAL DIAGNOSIS
- Conjunctivitis
- Episcleritis
- Iritis (anterior uveitis)
- Posterior uveitis
- Blepharitis
- Ocular rosacea

DIAGNOSTIC TESTS & INTERPRETATION
- Consider further tests if warranted by history and physical.
- Routine tests to exclude systemic disease
  - CBC, serum chemistry, urinalysis, ESR, and/or C-reactive protein, blood, and urine cultures
- Specific tests for underlying systemic illness
  - Rheumatoid factor, anticyclic citrullinated peptide antibodies, ACE level, HLA-B27, antineutrophil cytoplasmic antibodies, PPD or QuantiFERON-TB level, fluorescent treponemal antibody absorption (FTA-ABS), rapid plasma regain (RPR), Lyme titers, and antinuclear antibody may aid in the diagnosis.
- Further imaging studies, such as a chest x-ray, sacroiliac joint films, colonoscopy, may be useful if a specific systemic illness is suspected.
- B-scan US to detect posterior scleritis. Look at thickness of sclera and for T-sign, fluid in Tenon space at interface between the optic nerve and sclera.
- MRI/CT scan may provide additional diagnostic benefit and detect orbital disease.
- Different subtypes of scleritis are associated with varying presentations and distinct findings:
  - Diffuse anterior scleritis: widespread inflammation
  - Nodular anterior scleritis: immovable, inflamed nodule
  - Necrotizing anterior scleritis: "with inflammation": Sclera becomes transparent. Scleromalacia perforans without inflammation: painless and often associated with rheumatoid arthritis
  - Posterior scleritis: associated with retinal and choroidal complications; adjacent swelling of orbital tissues may occur.

Diagnostic Procedures/Other
Biopsy is not routinely required unless diagnosis remains uncertain after above investigations. Culture if suspect infectious etiology.

TREATMENT

GENERAL MEASURES

If scleral thinning, glasses/eye shield should be worn to prevent perforation; should be managed by an appropriate eye care professional

MEDICATION

- First-line therapies for noninfectious scleritis (3)[C]
  - Oral NSAID therapy, choice based on availability, example is ibuprofen 600 to 800 mg PO TID–QID or indomethacin 50 mg PO TID provided no contraindications exists; about 37% successful (4)[B]
  - Systemic steroids (initial if necrotizing scleritis and preferentially IV if vision threatening, otherwise use if failure of NSAIDs), prednisone 40 to 60 mg PO QD or 1 mg/kg/day, taper over 4 to 6 weeks. Use caution if suspect infectious etiology.
  - Antimetabolites including methotrexate, azathioprine, mycophenolate mofetil, cyclophosphamide, and cyclosporine may be used as steroid-sparing agents. They are generally recommended if steroids cannot be tapered below 10 mg PO QD (4)[C].
- Second-line therapies (4)[C],(5)[A]
  - Immunomodulatory agents, infliximab, rituximab, and adalimumab can be used if patient has failed or is not a candidate for antimetabolites or calcineurin inhibitors. These agents are preferred over etanercept due to higher treatment success.
- Adjunct therapy considerations
  - Topical steroids: prednisolone acetate 1% or difluprednate 0.05% under ophthalmologist care
  - Subconjunctival triamcinolone acetonide injection only for nonnecrotizing, 40 mg/mL, 97% improvement after one injection; increased risk of ocular HTN, cataract, and globe perforation
- Necrotizing anterior scleritis and posterior scleritis
  - May require immunosuppressive therapy in addition to systemic steroids
  - Treat aggressively due to possible complications if left untreated; may need patch grafting to maintain globe integrity
- Infectious
  - Antibiotic therapy resolves about 18% of cases, whereas the remaining often requires surgical intervention such as débridement (2)[B].

ISSUES FOR REFERRAL

- All patients with scleritis should be managed by an ophthalmologist familiar with this condition.
- Rheumatology referral for coexistent systemic disease is helpful for long-term success.

ADDITIONAL THERAPIES

Immunosuppressants used for autoimmune and collagen vascular disorders may be of help in active scleritis.

SURGERY/OTHER PROCEDURES

- In rare cases, scleral biopsy may be indicated to confirm infection or other etiology.
- Ocular perforation requires scleral grafting.

 ONGOING CARE

FOLLOW-UP RECOMMENDATIONS

Avoid contact lenses—wear only if there is corneal involvement, which is rare.

Patient Monitoring

- Patient in the active stage of inflammation should be followed very closely by an ophthalmologist to assess the effectiveness of therapy.
- Medication use mandates close surveillance for adverse effects.

DIET

No special diet

PATIENT EDUCATION

Scleritis at The Ocular Immunology and Uveitis Foundation: http://www.uveitis.org/patient_articles/scleritis/

PROGNOSIS

Scleritis is indolent, chronic, and often progressive.

- Diffuse anterior scleritis (best prognosis)
- Necrotizing anterior scleritis (worst prognosis)
- Recurrent bouts of inflammation may occur.
- Scleromalacia perforans has the highest risk of perforation of the globe.

COMPLICATIONS

- Decrease in vision, anterior uveitis, ocular HTN, and peripheral keratitis
- Cataract and glaucoma can result from disease or treatment with steroids.
- Ocular perforation can occur in severe stages.

REFERENCES

1. Sainz de la Maza M, Molina N, Gonzalez-Gonzalez LA, et al. Clinical characteristics of a large cohort of patients with scleritis and episcleritis. *Ophthalmology*. 2012;119(1):43–50.
2. Hodson KL, Galor A, Karp CL, et al. Epidemiology and visual outcomes in patients with infectious scleritis. *Cornea*. 2013;32(4):466–472.
3. Beardsley RM, Suhler EB, Rosenbaum JT, et al. Pharmacotherapy of scleritis: current paradigms and future directions. *Expert Opin Pharmacother*. 2013;14(4):411–424.
4. Sainz de la Maza M, Molina N, Gonzalez-Gonzalez LA, et al. Scleritis therapy. *Ophthalmology*. 2012; 119(1):51–58.
5. Levy-Clarke G, Jabs DA, Read RW, et al. Expert panel recommendations for the use of anti-tumor necrosis factor biologic agents in patients with ocular inflammatory disorders. *Ophthalmology*. 2014;121(3):785–796.e3.

ADDITIONAL READING

- Cao JH, Oray M, Cocho L, et al. Rituximab in the treatment of refractory noninfectious scleritis. *Am J Ophthalmol*. 2016;164:22–28.
- Diogo MC, Jager MJ, Ferreira TA. CT and MR imaging in the diagnosis of scleritis. *AJNR Am J Neuroradiol*. 2016;37(12):2334–2339.
- Gonzalez-Gonzalez LA, Molina-Prat N, Doctor P, et al. Clinical features and presentation of posterior scleritis: a report of 31 cases. *Ocul Immunol Inflamm*. 2014;22(3):203–207.
- Stem MS, Todorich B, Faia LJ. Ocular pharmacology for scleritis: review of treatment and a practical perspective. *J Ocul Pharmacol Ther*. 2017;33(4): 240–246.
- Suhler EB, Lim LL, Beardsley RM, et al. Rituximab therapy for refractory scleritis: results of a phase I/II dose-ranging, randomized, clinical trial. *Ophthalmology*. 2014;121(10):1885–1891.

CODES

ICD10

- H15.009 Unspecified scleritis, unspecified eye
- H15.019 Anterior scleritis, unspecified eye
- H15.039 Posterior scleritis, unspecified eye

CLINICAL PEARLS

- Episcleritis is a self-limited inflammation of the eye with mild discomfort.
- Scleritis is a painful, severe, and potentially vision-threatening condition.
- Both conditions can be associated with underlying inflammatory diseases.
- About 35% of all cases of scleritis are associated with a systemic disease such as rheumatoid arthritis. Necrotizing scleritis has the highest association.

SCLERODERMA

Ann M. Lynch, PharmD, RPh, AE-C • Deborah M. DeMarco, MD, FACP

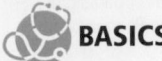

BASICS

DESCRIPTION
- Scleroderma (systemic sclerosis [SSc]) is a chronic disease of unknown cause characterized by diffuse fibrosis of skin and visceral organs and vascular abnormalities.
- Most manifestations have vascular features (e.g., Raynaud phenomenon), but frank vasculitis is rarely seen.
- Can range from a mild disease, affecting the skin, to a systemic disease that can cause death in a few months
- The disease is categorized into two major clinical variants (1).
  - Diffuse: distal and proximal extremity and truncal skin thickening
  - Limited
    - Restricted to the fingers, hands, and face
    - CREST syndrome (calcinosis, Raynaud phenomenon, esophageal dysmotility, sclerodactyly, telangiectasia)
- System(s) affected: include, but not limited to skin, renal, cardiovascular, pulmonary, musculoskeletal, gastrointestinal (GI)

Geriatric Considerations
Uncommon >75 years of age

Pediatric Considerations
Rare in this age group

Pregnancy Considerations
- Safe and healthy pregnancies are common and possible despite higher frequency of premature births.
- High-risk management must be standard care to avoid complications, specifically renal crisis.
- Diffuse scleroderma causes greater risk for developing serious cardiopulmonary and renal problems. Pregnancy should be delayed until disease stabilizes.

EPIDEMIOLOGY
Incidence
- In the United States: 1 to 2/100,000 per year
- Predominant age
  - Young adult (16 to 40 years); middle-aged (40 to 75 years); peak onset 30 to 50 years
  - Symptoms usually appear in the 3rd to 5th decades.
- Predominant sex: female > male (4:1)

Prevalence
In the United States: 1 to 25/100,000

ETIOLOGY AND PATHOPHYSIOLOGY
Pathophysiology involves both a vascular component and a fibrotic component. Both occur simultaneously. The inciting event is unknown, but there is an increase in certain cytokines after endothelial cell activation that are profibrotic (TGF-β and PDGF).
- Unknown
- Possible alterations in immune response
- Possibly some association with exposure to quartz mining, quarrying, vinyl chloride, hydrocarbons, toxin exposure
- Treatment with bleomycin has caused a scleroderma-like syndrome, as has exposure to rapeseed oil.

Genetics
Familial clustering is rare but has been seen.

RISK FACTORS
Unknown

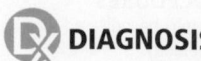

DIAGNOSIS

HISTORY
- Raynaud phenomenon is generally the presenting complaint (differentiated from Raynaud disease, generally affecting younger individuals and without digital ulcers).
- Skin thickening, "puffy hands," pruritus, and gastroesophageal reflux disease (GERD) are often noted early in the disease process.

PHYSICAL EXAM
- Skin
  - Digital ulcerations
  - Digital pitting
  - Tightness, swelling, thickening of digits
  - Hyperpigmentation/hypopigmentation
  - Narrowed oral aperture
  - SC calcinosis
- Peripheral vascular system
  - Telangiectasia
- Joints, tendons, and bones
  - Flexion contractures
  - Friction rub on tendon movement
  - Hand swelling
  - Joint stiffness
  - Polyarthralgia
  - Sclerodactyly
- Muscle
  - Proximal muscle weakness
- GI tract
  - Dysphagia
  - Esophageal reflux due to dysmotility (most common systemic sign in diffuse disease)
  - Malabsorptive diarrhea
  - Nausea and vomiting
  - Weight loss
  - Xerostomia
- Kidney
  - Hypertension
  - May develop scleroderma renal crisis: acute renal failure (ARF)
- Pulmonary
  - Dry crackles at lung bases
  - Dyspnea
- Nervous system
  - Peripheral neuropathy
  - Trigeminal neuropathy
- Cardiac (progressive disease)
  - Conduction abnormalities
  - Cardiomyopathy
  - Pericarditis
  - Secondary cor pulmonale

DIFFERENTIAL DIAGNOSIS
- Mixed connective tissue disease/overlap syndromes
- Scleredema
- Nephrogenic systemic fibrosis
- Toxic oil syndrome (Madrid, 1981, affecting 20,000 people)
- Eosinophilia–myalgia syndrome
- Diffuse fasciitis with eosinophilia
- Scleredema of Buschke

DIAGNOSTIC TESTS & INTERPRETATION
Initial Tests (lab, imaging)
- Nail fold capillary microscopy—drop out is most significant finding
- CBC
- Creatinine
- Urinalysis (albuminuria, microscopic hematuria)
- Antinuclear antibodies (ANA): positive in >90% of patients
- Anti–Scl-70 (anti-topoisomerase [ATA]) antibody is highly specific for systemic disease and confers a higher risk of interstitial lung disease (ILD).
- Anticentromere antibody usually associated with CREST variant
- Chest radiograph
  - Diffuse reticular pattern
  - Bilateral basilar pulmonary fibrosis
- Hand radiograph
  - Soft tissue atrophy and acroosteolysis
  - Can see overlap syndromes such as rheumatoid arthritis
  - SC calcinosis

Follow-Up Tests & Special Considerations
- Pulmonary function tests (PFTs)
  - Decreased maximum breathing capacity
  - Increased residual volume
  - Diffusion defect
- Antibodies to U3-RNP—higher risk for scleroderma-associated pulmonary hypertension
- Anti–PM-Scl antibodies (for myositis) (2)[B]
- Anti-RNA polymerase III—higher risk for diffuse cutaneous involvement and renal crisis (3)[A]
- ECG (low voltage): possible nonspecific abnormalities, arrhythmia, and conduction defects
- Echocardiography: pulmonary hypertension or cardiomyopathy
- Nail fold capillary loop abnormalities
- Upper GI
  - Distal esophageal dilatation
  - Atonic esophagus
  - Esophageal dysmotility
  - Duodenal diverticula
- Barium enema
  - Colonic diverticula
  - Megacolon
- High-resolution CT scan for detecting alveolitis, which has a ground-glass appearance or fibrosis predominant in bilateral lower lobes

Diagnostic Procedures/Other
- Skin biopsy
  - Compact collagen fibers in the reticular dermis and hyalinization and fibrosis of arterioles
  - Thinning of epidermis, with loss of rete pegs, and atrophy of dermal appendages
  - Accumulation of mononuclear cells is also seen.
- Right-sided heart catheterization: Pulmonary hypertension is an ominous prognostic feature.

Test Interpretation
- Skin
  - Edema, fibrosis, or atrophy (late stage)
  - Lymphocytic infiltrate around sweat glands
  - Loss of capillaries
  - Endothelial proliferation
  - Hair follicle atrophy

- Synovium
  - Pannus formation
  - Fibrin deposits in tendons
- Kidney
  - Small kidneys
  - Intimal proliferation in interlobular arteries
- Heart
  - Endocardial thickening
  - Myocardial interstitial fibrosis
  - Ischemic band necrosis
  - Enlarged heart
  - Cardiac hypertrophy
  - Pulmonary hypertension
- Lung
  - Interstitial pneumonitis
  - Cyst formation
  - Interstitial fibrosis
  - Bronchiectasis
- Esophagus
  - Esophageal atrophy
  - Fibrosis

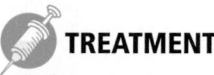 TREATMENT

GENERAL MEASURES
- Treatment is symptomatic and supportive.
- Esophageal dilation may be used for strictures.
- Avoid cold; dress appropriately in layers for the weather; be wary of air conditioning.
- Avoid smoking (crucial).
- Avoid fingersticks (e.g., blood tests).
- Elevate the head of the bed during sleep to help relieve GI symptoms.
- Use softening lotions, ointments, and bath oils to help prevent dryness and cracking of skin.
- Dialysis may be necessary in renal crisis.

MEDICATION
First Line
- ACE inhibitors (ACEIs): for preservation of renal blood flow and for treatment of hypertensive renal crisis
- Corticosteroids: for disabling myositis, pulmonary alveolitis, or mixed connective tissue disease (not recommended in high doses due to increased incidence of renal failure)
- NSAIDs: for joint or tendon symptoms; caution with long-term concurrent use with ACEIs (potential renal complications)
- Antibiotics: for secondary infections in bowel and active skin infections
- Antacids, proton pump inhibitors: for gastric reflux
- Metoclopramide: for intestinal dysfunction
- Hydrophilic skin ointments: for skin therapy
- Topical clindamycin, erythromycin, or silver sulfadiazine, and PDE5 inhibitors for prevention of recurrent infectious cutaneous ulcers
- Consider immunosuppressives for treatment of life-threatening or potentially crippling scleroderma or interstitial pneumonitis such as cyclophosphamide for ILD (4)[B].
- Nitrates, dihydropyridine calcium-channel blockers, PDE5 antagonists, and fluoxetine for Raynaud phenomenon (5)[A]
- Avoidance of caffeine, nicotine, and sympathomimetics may ease Raynaud symptoms.

- PDE5 antagonists (e.g., sildenafil), prostanoids, and endothelin-1 antagonists are changing the management of pulmonary hypertension (6).
- Alveolitis: immunosuppressants and alkylating agents (e.g., cyclophosphamide)

ADDITIONAL THERAPIES
- Anti–TNF-α therapy: Preliminary suggestion is that this may reduce joint symptoms and disability in inflammatory arthritis, but small sample sizes and observational biases lend to the need for further well-designed, adequately powered, longitudinal clinical trials.
- Physical therapy to maintain function and promote strength
- Heat therapy to relieve joint stiffness

SURGERY/OTHER PROCEDURES
- Some success with gastroplasty for correction of GERD
- Limited role for sympathectomy for Raynaud phenomenon
- Lung transplantation for pulmonary hypertension and ILD
- Hematopoietic stem cell transplantation for selected patients with rapidly progressive SSc (5)

 ONGOING CARE

FOLLOW-UP RECOMMENDATIONS
Patient Monitoring
- Monitor every 3 to 6 months for end organ and skin involvement and medications. Provide encouragement.
- Echocardiology and PFTs yearly

DIET
Drink plenty of fluids with meals.

PATIENT EDUCATION
- Stay as active as possible, but avoid fatigue.
- Printed patient information available from the Scleroderma Federation, 1725 York Avenue, No. 29F, New York, NY 10128; (212) 427-7040
- Advise the patient to report any abnormal bruising or nonhealing abrasions.
- Assist the patient about smoking cessation, if needed.

PROGNOSIS
- Possible improvement but incurable
- Prognosis is poor if cardiac, pulmonary, or renal manifestations present early.

COMPLICATIONS
- Renal failure
- Respiratory failure
- Flexion contractures
- Disability
- Esophageal dysmotility
- Reflux esophagitis
- Arrhythmia
- Megacolon
- Pneumatosis intestinalis
- Obstructive bowel
- Cardiomyopathy
- Pulmonary hypertension
- Possible association with lung and other cancers
- Death

REFERENCES
1. van den Hoogen F, Khanna D, Fransen J, et al. 2013 Classification criteria for systemic sclerosis: an American College of Rheumatology/European League Against Rheumatism collaborative initiative. *Arthritis Rheum.* 2013;65(11):2737–2747.
2. D'Aoust J, Hudson M, Tatibouet S, et al; for Canadian Scleroderma Research Group. Clinical and serologic correlates of anti-PM/Scl antibodies in systemic sclerosis: a multicenter study of 763 patients. *Arthritis Rheumatol.* 2014;66(6): 1608–1615.
3. Sobanski V, Dauchet L, Lefèvre G, et al. Prevalence of anti-RNA polymerase III antibodies in systemic sclerosis: new data from a French cohort and a systematic review and meta-analysis. *Arthritis Rheumatol.* 2014;66(2):407–417.
4. Roth MD, Tseng CH, Clements PJ, et al; and Scleroderma Lung Study Research Group. Predicting treatment outcomes and responder subsets in scleroderma-related interstitial lung disease. *Arthritis Rheum.* 2011;63(9):2797–2808.
5. Kowal-Bielecka O, Fransen J, Avouac J, et al; for EUSTAR Coauthors. Update of EULAR recommendations for the treatment of systemic sclerosis. *Ann Rheum Dis.* 2017;76(8):1327–1339.
6. Volkmann ER, Saggar R, Khanna D, et al. Improved transplant-free survival in patients with systemic sclerosis-associated pulmonary hypertension and interstitial lung disease. *Arthritis Rheumatol.* 2014;66(7):1900–1908.

ADDITIONAL READING
- Steen VD. Pregnancy in scleroderma. *Rheum Dis Clin North Am.* 2007;33(2):345–358.
- Valerio CJ, Schreiber BE, Handler CE, et al. Borderline mean pulmonary artery pressure in patients with systemic sclerosis: transpulmonary gradient predicts risk of developing pulmonary hypertension. *Arthritis Rheum.* 2013;65(4):1074–1084.

 SEE ALSO

Morphea

CODES

ICD10
- M34.9 Systemic sclerosis, unspecified
- M34.1 CR(E)ST syndrome
- L94.0 Localized scleroderma [morphea]

CLINICAL PEARLS
- Raynaud phenomenon is frequently the initial complaint.
- Skin thickening, "puffy hands," and GERD are often noted early in disease.
- Patients must be followed proactively for development of pulmonary hypertension or ILD.

SEASONAL AFFECTIVE DISORDER

Christopher White, MD, JD, MHA

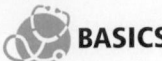 **BASICS**

DESCRIPTION
- Seasonal affective disorder (SAD) is a heterogeneous mood disorder with depressive episodes usually occurring in winter months, with full remissions in the spring and summer.
- Ranges from a milder form (winter blues) to a seriously disabling illness
- Must separate out patients with other mood disorders (such as major depressive disorder and bipolar affective disorder) whose symptoms persist during spring and summer months

EPIDEMIOLOGY
Incidence
- Affects up to 500,000 people every winter
- Up to 30% of patients visiting a primary care physician (PCP) during winter may report winter depressive symptoms.
- Predominant age: occurs at any age; peaks in 20s and 30s
- Predominant sex: female > male (3:1)

Prevalence
- 1–9% of the general population
- 10–20% of patients identified as having mood symptoms will have a seasonal component.

ETIOLOGY AND PATHOPHYSIOLOGY
The major theories currently involve the interplay of phase-shifted circadian rhythms, genetic vulnerability, and serotonin dysregulation.
- Melatonin produced by the pineal gland at increased levels in the dark has been linked to depressive symptoms; light therapy on the retina acts to inhibit melatonin secretion.
- Serotonin dysregulation, because it is secreted less during winter months, must be present for light therapy to work, and treatment with SSRIs appears to reverse SAD symptoms.
- Decreased levels of vitamin D, often occurring during low-light winter months, may be associated with depressive episodes in some individuals experiencing SAD symptoms.

Genetics
- Some twin studies and a preliminary study on GPR50 melatonin receptor variants have suggested a genetic component.
- Recent studies indicate an association with the melanopsin gene (OPN4).
- Increased incidence of depression, ADHD, and alcoholism in close relatives

RISK FACTORS
- Most common during months of January and February: Patients frequently visit PCP during winter months complaining of recurrent flu, chronic fatigue, and unexplained weight gain.
- Working in a building without windows or other environment without exposure to sunlight

GENERAL PREVENTION
- Consider use of light therapy at start of winter (if prior episodes begin in October), increase time outside during daylight, or move to a more southern location.
- Bupropion (Wellbutrin) is an FDA-approved antidepressant for the prevention of SAD.

COMMONLY ASSOCIATED CONDITIONS
Some individuals with SAD have a weakened immune system and may be more vulnerable to infections.

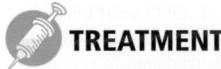 **DIAGNOSIS**

- Carefully document the presence or absence of prior manic episodes.
- Screen for the existence of any suicidal ideation and safety risk factors.
- Remission of symptoms during spring and summer
- Symptoms have occurred for the past 2 years.
- Seasonal episodes associated with winter months substantially outnumber any nonseasonal depressive episodes.
- Under *DSM-5*, SAD is denoted by adding the "with seasonal pattern" specifier to a diagnosis of major depressive disorder, recurrent.

HISTORY
- Symptoms of depression meeting the criteria for major depressive disorder are the following:
  - Sleep disturbance: either too much or too little
  - Lack of interest in life and absence of pleasure from hobbies/activities
  - Guilt: feelings of guilt or worthlessness
  - Energy: fatigue or constantly feeling tired
  - Concentration: difficulty with concentration and memory
  - Appetite: changes in appetite and weight
  - Psychomotor retardation: Patients feel slowed down with decreased activity.
  - Suicidal thoughts: Patients report thoughts of suicide.
- In SAD, hypersomnia, hyperphagia (craving for carbohydrates and sweets), and weight gain usually predominate. Despite sleeping more, patients report daytime sleepiness and fatigue. Cravings may lead to binge eating and weight gains >20 lb.
- Obtain collateral history if patient is unable to provide insight into the seasonal component.

PHYSICAL EXAM
Use exam to exclude other organic causes for symptoms. Focal neurologic deficits, signs of endocrine dysfunction, or stigmata of substance abuse should prompt further testing.

DIFFERENTIAL DIAGNOSIS
- Similar to that of major depression, meaning that organic causes of low energy and fatigue, such as hypothyroidism, anemia, and mononucleosis (or other viral syndromes), need to be considered.
- Other mood disorders without a seasonal component such as major depression, bipolar disorder, adjustment disorder, or dysthymia
- Symptoms should not be better accounted for by seasonal psychosocial stressors, which often accompany the winter holiday seasons.
- Substance abuse

DIAGNOSTIC TESTS & INTERPRETATION
- Thyroid-stimulating hormone to rule out hypothyroidism
- CBC to rule out anemia
- Rule out electrolyte and glucose dysregulation.
- 25-OH vitamin D level
- Pregnancy test for women of childbearing potential
- Urine toxicology screen if substance abuse is a concern
- Imaging is not useful unless focal neurologic finding or looking to exclude an organic cause.

TREATMENT

MEDICATION
Lack of evidence to determine whether light therapy or medication should be the first-line agent. Both supported by the literature and in some studies have equal efficacy. Medications have more side effects. Adherence to both remains a critical issue. The ultimate choice depends on the acuity of the patient and the comfort level of the prescribing clinician with each treatment modality (1)[B].
- SSRIs such as sertraline (Zoloft), paroxetine (Paxil), fluoxetine (Prozac), citalopram (Celexa), and escitalopram (Lexapro) in their traditional antidepressant doses (2)[B]
- Bupropion (Wellbutrin) is the only antidepressant currently approved by the FDA for the prevention of SAD (3)[B].

ISSUES FOR REFERRAL
- Patients with a history of ocular disease should be referred for an ophthalmologic exam before phototherapy and for serial monitoring.
- Patients who fail to respond or who develop manic symptoms or suicidal ideation once treatment is initiated should be considered for psychiatric referral.

ADDITIONAL THERAPIES

- Phototherapy using special light sources has been shown to be effective in 60–90% of patients, often providing relief with a few sessions (2,4)[B].
- Variables that can regulate effect are the following:
  - Light intensity: Although the minimum light source intensity is under investigation, at least 2,500 lux is suggested (domestic lights emit, on average, 200 to 500 lux). There is good evidence for 10,000 lux as the recommended source (2)[B].
  - Treatment duration: Exposure time varies based on intensity of light source, with daily sessions of 30 minutes to a few hours.
  - Time of treatment: Most patients respond better by using the light therapy early in the morning.
  - Color of light source: Emerging data suggest that shorter sessions of lower intensity light-emitting diodes enriched in the blue spectrum have equal efficacy to the traditional white light treatment (5)[B].
- Light box is placed on table several feet away, and the light is allowed to shine onto the patient's eyes (sunglasses should be avoided). Ensure that the light box has an ultraviolet filter.
- Most common side effects are eye strain and headache. Insomnia can result if the light box is used too late in the day. Light boxes also can precipitate mania in some patients.
- Dawn simulation machines gradually increase illumination while the patient sleeps, simulating sunrise while using a significantly less intense light source.

COMPLEMENTARY & ALTERNATIVE MEDICINE

- Work to reduce stress levels through meditation, progressive relaxation exercises, and/or lifestyle modification.
- The potential role of vitamin D supplementation is under investigation. Currently, there is a lack of consistent research to satisfactorily demonstrate that treatment improves SAD symptoms. Reported doses vary widely but typically are between 400 and 800 IU/day (6)[B].

ADMISSION, INPATIENT, AND NURSING CONSIDERATIONS

If the patient develops suicidal ideation as part of his or her depression or mania after treatment is initiated

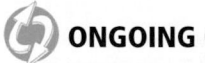 **ONGOING CARE**

FOLLOW-UP RECOMMENDATIONS

Regular monitoring by PCP or psychiatrist for response to treatment; patients may become manic when treated with SSRIs or light therapy.

Patient Monitoring

Patients should be seen in the outpatient clinic weekly to biweekly when initiating light or pharmacotherapy to monitor treatment results, side effects, and any increased suicidal thoughts if using SSRIs.

DIET

No specific diet modification needed

PATIENT EDUCATION

- Increase time outdoors during daylight.
- Rearrange home or work environment to get more direct sunlight through windows.

PROGNOSIS

Symptoms, if untreated, generally remit within 5 months with exposure to spring light, only to return in subsequent winters. If treated, patients usually respond within 3 to 6 weeks.

COMPLICATIONS

Development of suicidal ideation and mania are two outcomes the clinician needs to monitor.

REFERENCES

1. Lam RW, Levitt AJ, Levitan RD, et al. The Can-SAD study: a randomized controlled trial of the effectiveness of light therapy and fluoxetine in patients with winter seasonal affective disorder. *Am J Psychiatry.* 2006;163(5):805–812.
2. Kurlansik SL, Ibay AD. Seasonal affective disorder. *Am Fam Physician.* 2012;86(11):1037–1041.
3. Magovern M, Crawford-Faucher A. Extended-release bupropion for preventing seasonal affective disorder in adults. *Am Fam Physician.* 2017;95(1):10–11.
4. Terman M, Terman JS. Light therapy for seasonal and nonseasonal depression: efficacy, protocol, safety, and side effects. *CNS Spectr.* 2005;10(8):647–663.
5. Meesters Y, Duijzer W, Hommes V. The effects of low-intensity narrow-band blue-light treatment compared to bright white-light treatment in seasonal affective disorder. *J Affect Disord.* 2018;232:48–51.
6. Frandsen TB, Pareek M, Hansen JP, et al. Vitamin D supplementation for treatment of seasonal affective symptoms in healthcare professionals: a double-blind randomised placebo-controlled trial. *BMC Res Notes.* 2014;7:528.

ADDITIONAL READING

- Cools O, Hebbrecht K, Coppens V, et al. Pharmacotherapy and nutritional supplements for seasonal affective disorders: a systematic review. *Expert Opin Pharmacother.* 2018;19(11):1221–1233.
- Mårtensson B, Pettersson A, Berglund L, et al. Bright white light therapy in depression: a critical review of the evidence. *J Affect Disord.* 2015;182:1–7.
- Rohan K, Mahon J, Evans M, et al. Randomized trial of cognitive-behavioral therapy versus light therapy for seasonal affective disorder: acute outcomes. *Am J Psychiatry.* 2015;172(9):862–869.

 SEE ALSO

- Bipolar I Disorder; Bipolar II Disorder; Depression
- Algorithm: Depressive Episode, Major

CODES

ICD10

- F33.9 Major depressive disorder, recurrent, unspecified
- F33.0 Major depressive disorder, recurrent, mild
- F33.1 Major depressive disorder, recurrent, moderate

CLINICAL PEARLS

- SAD is a subtype of major depressive disorder. Once the patient has a diagnosed mood disorder, such as depression or bipolar, ask whether the symptoms vary in a seasonal pattern to qualify for the diagnosis of SAD. Generally, these patients will report sleeping too much, eating too much (especially carbs and sweets), and gaining weight during winter months.
- Ensure that the symptoms are not due to an organic process or better explained by substance abuse.
- Guidelines suggest using SSRIs first if the patient is more acute or has contraindications to light therapy or the clinician is not comfortable with light therapy.
- Light therapy boxes are available from numerous online suppliers but are not extensively regulated; practitioners should take care to ensure that patients are using devices from reputable suppliers.
- If using SSRIs, recent studies indicate that some patients may begin to experience increased suicidal thoughts on therapy; these patients need to be monitored closely as outpatients every 1 to 2 weeks. Patients on light therapy also should be monitored closely initially in order to adjust treatment. Once stabilized, both groups of patients can be seen every 4 to 8 weeks during the winter months.
- All patients who demonstrate suicidal ideation or symptoms of mania should be referred for consideration of hospitalization.

S

SEIZURE DISORDER, ABSENCE

Amy Gallardo, FNP-C • Anthony Russo, MD

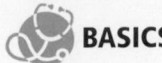

BASICS

DESCRIPTION

- Absence seizures are a type of generalized nonmotor seizure characterized by a brief lapse of awareness.
- Absence seizure types according to the International League Against Epilepsy (ILAE) 2017 classification include:
  - Typical
    - Abrupt onset and offset of behavioral arrest, loss of awareness, and blank staring, sometimes with eyelid movements, eye opening, or oral automatisms (e.g., lip smacking)
    - Typically occurs at 3 Hz
    - Lasts 5 to 30 seconds
    - Immediate return to normal consciousness with no aura or postictal phase
    - Associated with childhood absence epilepsy (CAE), juvenile absence epilepsy (JAE), and juvenile myoclonic epilepsy (JME)
  - Atypical
    - Onset and offset less abrupt than typical absence seizures and often with loss of muscle tone or subtle myoclonic jerks
    - Typically occurs at <2.5 Hz
    - Lasts 10 to 45 seconds
    - Impairment of consciousness often incomplete with continued purposeful activity, albeit done more slowly
    - Brief postictal confusion can sometimes occur.
    - Associated with Lennox-Gastaut syndrome and Dravet syndrome
  - Myoclonic
    - Abrupt onset and offset of staring and loss of awareness with continuous rhythmic jerks of shoulders, arms, legs, head, or perioral muscles
    - Typically occurs at 2.5 to 4.5 Hz
    - Lasts 10 to 60 seconds
    - Impairment of consciousness varies from complete loss of awareness to retained awareness.
    - Associated with epilepsy with myoclonic absences, learning disability, and behavioral problems
  - Eyelid myoclonia
    - Abrupt onset and offset of repetitive, rhythmic jerks of the eyelids with simultaneous upward deviation of the eyeballs and extension of the head
    - Typically occurs at 4 to 6 Hz
    - Lasts <6 seconds
    - Impairment of consciousness often incomplete with awareness mostly retained
    - Associated with epilepsy with eyelid myoclonus

EPIDEMIOLOGY

- Incidence: 6 to 8/100,000 per year
- Prevalence: 5 to 50/100,000
- Predominant age of onset: 1 to 8 years
- Predominant gender: female > male (2:1) with male predominance in myoclonic absence seizure

ETIOLOGY AND PATHOPHYSIOLOGY

- Etiology is mainly genetic with complex, multifactorial inheritance; however, may be secondary to a variety of congenital or acquired brain disorders such as hypoxia–ischemia, trauma, CNS infection, cortical malformations, or inborn errors of metabolism
- Absences are triggered in the thalamus when γ-aminobutyric acid (GABA)-mediated activity induces prolonged hyperpolarization and activates T-type ("low-threshold") calcium channels, resulting in sustained-burst firing of these neurons causing absence seizures.

Genetics

- 70–85% concordance occurs in monozygotic twins; 82% share EEG features.
- 33% concordance among first-degree relatives
- 15–45% have a family history of epilepsy.
- Mutations of GABA-A/B receptors, calcium or chloride channels
- Mutations of SLC21A, which encodes GLUT1

ALERT

Onset of absence seizures <4 years, consider GLUT1 deficiency syndrome

COMMONLY ASSOCIATED CONDITIONS

- Difficulties in visual attention and visuospatial skills, verbal learning and memory, fine motor skills, executive functions, and reduced language abilities
- Elevated rates of behavioral and psychiatric comorbidities including ADHD, anxiety, depression, social isolation, and low self-esteem

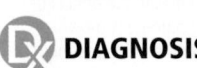

DIAGNOSIS

HISTORY

- Detailed description of episode including activity at onset, any automatisms, duration of episode, frequency of episodes, aura or postictal state, age of onset, and birth and developmental history
- Teachers report that child seems to daydream or zone out frequently.
- Child will forget portions of conversations.
- Child with normal IQ underperforms in school.

ALERT

Seizures are often so brief that untrained observers are not aware of the occurrence.

PHYSICAL EXAM

- Unless a child has another genetic or acquired abnormality, a neurologic exam usually is normal. Abnormal physical exam indicates the need for further diagnostic workup (e.g., MRI, metabolic, or genetic testing).
- Seizures may be induced by hyperventilation:
  - Have the child blow on a pinwheel or similar exercise for 3 to 5 minutes to provoke seizure.
  - Alternatively, ask the patient to perform hyperventilation with eyes closed and count. Patient will open eyes at onset of seizure and stop counting.

ALERT

Absence seizures are not associated with sensitivity to light or other photic stimuli (e.g., strobe lights).

DIFFERENTIAL DIAGNOSIS

- JAE
- JME
- GLUT1 deficiency syndrome
- Complex partial seizures
- Psychogenic nonepileptic seizures
- ADHD
- Confusional states and acute memory disorders
- Migraine variants
- Panic/anxiety attacks
- Breath-holding spells
- Nonepileptic staring spells
- Febrile seizures
- Status epilepticus

DIAGNOSTIC TESTS & INTERPRETATION

Initial Tests (lab, imaging)

- Video-EEG, including sleep and awake with hyperventilation resulting in spike-wave complexes from <2.5 to 6.0 Hz, depending on type of absence seizure, is standard for diagnosis (1)[B].
- Imaging is not routinely indicated in children with typical absence and normal neurologic exam and cognition. If imaging is performed, MRI is preferable to CT scan due to higher sensitivity for anatomic abnormalities (1)[B].
- Presently, no laboratory values can definitively prove or rule out the diagnosis of an absence seizure. However, labs such as electrolytes, creatinine, liver and renal function tests, TSH, CBC, and toxicology screen can rule out endocrine, metabolic, toxic, or infectious etiologies (2)[C].

Follow-Up Tests and Special Considerations

- Drug levels are useful in evaluating symptoms of toxicity or for breakthrough seizures.
- Follow blood chemistry, hepatic function, blood counts, etc., specific to drug regimen.

TREATMENT

GENERAL MEASURES

ALERT

Review seizure precautions with every patient diagnosed with or suspected to have epilepsy. Seizure precautions are to prevent injury. Patients should refrain from activities that would put them at risk if a seizure occurred (e.g., climbing heights, swimming unsupervised, cycling on busy roads, driving). Providers should be familiar with state laws concerning driving with epilepsy.

MEDICATION

ALERT

Certain common anticonvulsants may exacerbate absence including carbamazepine, oxcarbazepine, phenytoin, phenobarbital, tiagabine, vigabatrin, pregabalin, and gabapentin.

First Line

- Ethosuximide blocks T-type calcium channels:
  - First line, high efficacy (3)[A], fastest onset of efficacy (4)[B], and fewer adverse attentional effects compared to valproic acid (3)[A]; however, is only effective against absence seizures
  - Side effects: vomiting, diarrhea, abdominal discomfort, hiccups, headache, sedation
  - Adverse effects: aplastic anemia, skin reactions, and renal/hepatic impairment. Monitor CBC and CMP (5)[C].
- Valproic acid has multiple mechanisms:
  - Alternative first line
    - Very effective but has highest rate of adverse events leading to treatment discontinuation, including negative attentional effects and weight gain (3)[A]; is considered broad spectrum due to effective against absence and comorbid seizure types such as myoclonic, tonic–clonic, and partial
    - Side effects: tremor, drowsiness, dizziness, weight gain, alopecia, sedation, vomiting
    - Adverse effects: teratogenicity, behavior/cognitive abnormalities, hepatotoxicity, pancreatitis. Monitor CMP, amylase, and lipase (5)[C]; reduced bone mineral density and increased risk of osteoporosis and fractures

Second Line

Lamotrigine affects sodium channels:

- Controls seizures but may be less efficacious than ethosuximide or valproic acid (3)[A]
- Side effects: rash, diplopia, headache, insomnia, dizziness, nausea, vomiting, diarrhea
- Adverse effects: rare Stevens-Johnson rash, more often when coadministered with valproic acid

ISSUES FOR REFERRAL

Failure to gain seizure control for at least 1 year with two AEDs (whether as monotherapy or in combination) should prompt referral to neurologist for confirmation of the diagnosis for seizure and/or syndrome classification and, if appropriate, for consideration of epilepsy surgery (4)[B].

Pediatric Considerations

- Prescribe vitamin D supplementation (usual dose 400 to 1,000 IU/day) in children taking valproic acid due to AE of reduced bone mineral density (6)[A].
- Fatal hepatotoxicity with valproic acid risk is greatest in <2 years old (5)[C].

Pregnancy Considerations

- Anticonvulsants, especially valproic acid, are associated with an increase in fetal malformations. Use of valproic acid in women of childbearing age, who are not using adequate birth control, is contraindicated.
- Pregnant women with epilepsy can enroll in The North American AED Pregnancy Registry: http://www.aedpregnancyregistry.org.

ADDITIONAL THERAPIES

Vagal nerve stimulator (VNS) may be considered as an option for medically refractory absence epilepsy (7)[C].

SURGERY/OTHER PROCEDURES

Epilepsy surgery including ablation and resection for medically refractive absence epilepsy

COMPLEMENTARY & ALTERNATIVE MEDICINE

A ketogenic diet should be considered early if medication is ineffective (6)[A].

ADMISSION, INPATIENT, AND NURSING CONSIDERATIONS

- Absence epilepsy rarely requires admission.
- Status epilepticus requires inpatient management.
- Discharge criteria
  - Resolution of status epilepticus

 ONGOING CARE

FOLLOW-UP RECOMMENDATIONS

Patients should be monitored periodically by a neurologist for evolution of absence epilepsy into other seizure types.

PROGNOSIS

- Patients whose shortest pretreatment EEG seizures are >20 seconds in duration are more likely to achieve seizure freedom, regardless of treatment.
- Typical absence seizures generally cease spontaneously by age 12 years or sooner.
- <10% develop generalized tonic–clonic seizures.
- Male sex and an early age at diagnosis are associated with the need for two medications to control the disease.

COMPLICATIONS

- Causes of seizure exacerbations: noncompliance with treatment, lack of sleep, drugs that lower seizure threshold (e.g., alcohol, cocaine, high-dose PCN, isoniazid overdose, neuroleptics, Wellbutrin)
- Reported frequencies of typical absence status epilepticus range from 5.8% to 9.4%.

REFERENCES

1. Uysal-Soyer O, Yalnızoğlu D, Turanlı G. The classification and differential diagnosis of absence seizures with short-term video-EEG monitoring during childhood. *Turk J Pediatr.* 2012;54(1):7–14.
2. Nass RD, Sassen R, Elger CE, et al. The role of postictal laboratory blood analyses in the diagnosis and prognosis of seizures. *Seizure.* 2017;47:51–65.
3. Glauser TA, Cnaan A, Shinnar S, et al; for Childhood Absence Epilepsy Study Team. Ethosuximide, valproic acid and lamotrigine in childhood absence epilepsy: initial monotherapy outcomes at 12 months. *Epilepsia.* 2013;54(1):141–155.
4. Mohanraj R, Brodie M. Early predictors of outcome in newly diagnosed epilepsy. *Seizure.* 2013;22(5):333–344.
5. Posner E. Absence seizures in children. *Am Fam Physician.* 2015;91(2):114–115.
6. Crepeau A, Moseley B, Wirrell E. Specific safety and tolerability considerations in the use of anticonvulsant medications in children. *Drug Healthc Patient Saf.* 2012;4:39–54.
7. Arya R, Greiner HM, Lewis A, et al. Vagus nerve stimulation for medically refractory absence epilepsy. *Seizure.* 2013;22(4):267–270.

ADDITIONAL READING

- Epilepsy Foundation: https://www.epilepsy.com
- *Sarah Jayne Has Staring Moments*: a fictional children's book for child absence seizure epilepsy, Kate Lambert

 CODES

ICD10

- G40.409 Other generalized epilepsy and epileptic syndromes, not intractable, without status epilepticus
- G40.419 Oth generalized epilepsy, intractable, w/o stat epi
- G40.401 Oth generalized epilepsy, not intractable, w stat epi

CLINICAL PEARLS

- Children with CAE can exhibit cognitive, behavioral, and psychosocial comorbidities. For these children, attentional deficits are the most important marker of cognitive dysfunction and often associated with reduced academic performance, anxiety, depression, and behavioral disorders.
- If parents are unable to determine the cause of a staring spell, try suggesting that parents mention something exciting or unexpected like "ice cream" during a spell to get the child's attention rather than calling his or her name.
- Ethosuximide and valproic acid are first-line agents in treatment of absence seizures.
- Failure to gain seizure control for at least 1 year with two AEDs, consider referral to neurologist for confirmation of seizure disorder and/or additional/alternative therapies including ketogenic diet, VNS, and surgery.
- Review seizure precautions with every patient.
- Maintain a seizure diary to help identify type and cause of seizures (https://diary.epilepsy.com/login).
- Create a seizure response plan (https://www.epilepsy.com/sites/core/files/atoms/files/130SRP_MySeizureResponsePlan-fillable.pdf).

S

SEIZURE DISORDER, FOCAL

Charles J. McClure, DO • Noel Dunn, MD

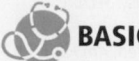 **BASICS**

DESCRIPTION

- Seizures occur when abnormal synchronous neuronal discharges in the brain cause transient cortical dysfunction.
- Generalized seizures involve bilateral cerebral cortex from the seizure's onset.
- Focal or localization-related seizures have previously been referred to as partial seizures.
- Focal seizures originate from a discrete focus limited to one hemisphere in the cerebral cortex.
- Focal seizures are further divided into aware versus unaware and motor versus nonmotor.
- Presence of impaired awareness is defined as the inability to respond normally to exogenous stimuli due to altered awareness and/or responsiveness:
  - Focal seizures with impairment of awareness (formerly "complex partial seizures")
  - Focal seizures without impairment of awareness (formerly "simple partial seizures")

EPIDEMIOLOGY

Prevalence

Focal seizures occur in 20/100,000 persons in the United States.

ETIOLOGY AND PATHOPHYSIOLOGY

- Focal seizures begin when a localized seizure focus produces an abnormal, synchronized depolarization that spreads to a discrete portion of the surrounding cortex.
- The area of cortex involved in the seizure determines the symptoms; for example, an epileptogenic focus in motor cortex produces contralateral motor symptoms.
- In some cases, etiology is related to structural abnormalities that are susceptible to epileptogenesis. Most common etiologies vary by life stage:
  - Early childhood: developmental/congenital malformation, trauma
  - Young adults: developmental, infection, trauma
  - Adults 40 to 60 years of age: cerebrovascular insult, infection, trauma
  - Adults >60 years of age: cerebrovascular insult, trauma, neoplasm
- A common cause of focal seizure with impaired awareness is mesial temporal sclerosis.

Genetics

Benign rolandic epilepsy, a form of focal seizure disorder, has an autosomal dominant inheritance pattern with penetrance depending on multiple factors.

RISK FACTORS

- History of traumatic brain injury (TBI)
- Children exposed to a thiamine-deficient formula

COMMONLY ASSOCIATED CONDITIONS

Epilepsy patients have a higher incidence of depression than the general population.

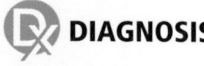 **DIAGNOSIS**

- Seizure activity usually stereotyped
- Duration: seconds to minutes, unless status epilepticus develops; status epilepticus may present as focal/generalized convulsions/altered mental status without convulsions.

- Focal seizures without impairment of awareness:
  - Formerly referred to as "simple partial seizures"
  - Further characterized by localized symptoms being motor versus nonmotor:
    - Motor onset: Seizure activity in motor strip causes contraction (tonic) or rhythmic jerking (clonic) movements that may involve one entire side of body or may be more localized (i.e., hands, feet, or face).
      - Jacksonian march: As discharge spreads through motor cortex, tonic–clonic activity spreads in predictable fashion (i.e., beginning in hand and progressing up arm and to the face).
    - Nonmotor onset:
      - Todd paralysis: after motor seizure, residual, temporary weakness in the affected area
      - Parietal lobe: sensory loss/paresthesias, dizziness
      - Temporal lobe: déjà vu, rising sensation in epigastrium, auditory hallucinations/forced memories, unpleasant smell/taste
      - Occipital: visual hallucinations
- Focal seizures with impairment of awareness:
  - Formerly referred to as "complex partial seizures"
  - May have aura; indicates the onset of the seizure
  - Amnesia for the event, postictal confusion
  - Most often, focus is temporal/frontal.
  - Motor manifestations may include dystonic posturing/automatisms (i.e., simple, repetitive movements of face and hands such as lip smacking, picking, or more complex actions such as purposeless walking).
  - Frontal lobe seizure is characterized by brief, bilateral complex movements, vocalizations, often with onset during sleep.

HISTORY

- A detailed description of the seizure should be obtained from an observer.
- Review medication list for drugs that lower seizure threshold (e.g., tramadol, bupropion, theophylline).
- Obtain history of drugs of abuse (e.g., cocaine) because they may lower seizure threshold.
- Review history of any prior TBI.

PHYSICAL EXAM

Include neurologic exam, with attention to lateralizing signs suggestive of structural lesion.

DIFFERENTIAL DIAGNOSIS

- Syncope/postanoxic myoclonus
- Hypoglycemia
- Psychogenic nonepileptic seizure
- For hemiparesis following event
  - Transient ischemic attack
  - Hemiplegic migraine

DIAGNOSTIC TESTS & INTERPRETATION

- Serum electrolytes, including calcium, magnesium, phosphorus; hepatic function panel; CBC; urinalysis; urine drug screen; levels of antiepileptic drugs (AEDs) for breakthrough seizure; chest x-ray
- Elevated prolactin, if measured within 10 to 20 minutes of suspected seizure, or elevated creatine phosphokinase; if measured within 6 to 24 hours, may help to differentiate generalized/focal seizure from psychogenic nonepileptic seizure (1)[B]
- CSF exam if infection is suspected

- EEG should be considered in patients with first time unprovoked seizure (2)[B].
- Yield of EEG is increased by being obtained in the first 24 hours following seizure and by sleep deprivation.
- EEG will typically show spikes/sharp waves over the seizure focus.
- Frontal lobe seizure focus may be difficult to detect by routine EEG.
- If difficulty with diagnosis, continuous video–EEG monitoring may be appropriate.
- Emergency evaluation of new seizure: CT scan to screen for hemorrhage and stroke
- In patients without recent neuroimaging, consider CT or MRI (2)[B].
- If planning epilepsy surgery, positron emission tomography (PET) scan and/or interictal single-photon emission computed tomography (SPECT) may be of value.
- Magnetoencephalography (MEG) aids in presurgical localization of epilepsy.

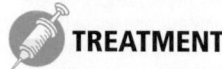 **TREATMENT**

GENERAL MEASURES

- Ask the patient to maintain a seizure diary.
- Note potential triggers, such as stress, sleep deprivation, drug use, discontinuation of alcohol/benzodiazepines, menses.

MEDICATION

- Current guidelines do not recommend for or against starting an AED after a single unprovoked seizure. Patients should be counseled that AEDs will reduce risk of repeat seizure over 2 years but have no effect on long-term remission (3)[C].
- AEDs act on voltage-gated ion channels, affect neuronal inhibition via enhancement of γ-aminobutyric acid (GABA, an inhibitory neurotransmitter), or decrease neuronal excitation. End result is to decrease the abnormal synchronized firing and to prevent seizure propagation.
- 50% of those with newly diagnosed focal seizures respond to, and tolerate, first AED trial. Up to 50% of those who fail the first AED trial will also fail a second AED trial (4)[B].
- Choose AED based on seizure type, side effect profile, and patient characteristics. Increase dose until seizure control is obtained/side effects become unacceptable.
- Attempt monotherapy, but many patients will require adjunctive agents.
- *Refractory to medications* is defined as failure of at least three anticonvulsants to achieve adequate control.
- AEDs may prevent seizures after a TBI in the short term, although they provide no efficacy in long-term prevention (5)[B].
- Several AEDs induce/inhibit cytochrome P450 enzymes (watch for drug interactions).

First Line

- Carbamazepine: affects sodium channels; side effects include GI distress, hyponatremia, diplopia, dizziness, rare pancytopenia/marrow suppression, and exfoliative rash.
- Oxcarbazepine: affects sodium channels; side effects include dizziness, diplopia, hyponatremia, and headache.

- Lamotrigine: affects sodium channels
  - Side effects include insomnia, dizziness, and ataxia.
  - Risk of Stevens-Johnson reaction (potentially fatal exfoliative rash), especially when given with valproate, requires slow titration
- Levetiracetam: multiple mechanisms; side effects include sedation, ataxia, and irritability.

Second Line
- Phenytoin: affects sodium channels; side effects include ataxia, dizziness, diplopia, tremor, GI upset, gingival hyperplasia, and fever.
- Phenobarbital: multiple mechanisms; side effects include sedation and withdrawal seizures.
- Valproate: multiple mechanisms; side effects include GI upset, weight gain, alopecia, and tremor; less common, thrombocytopenia, hepatitis, pancreatitis
- Topiramate: multiple mechanisms; side effects include anorexia, cognitive slowing, sedation, nephrolithiasis, and anhidrosis.
- Gabapentin: multiple mechanisms; side effects include sedation, dizziness, and ataxia.
- Pregabalin: affects calcium channels; side effects include sedation, dizziness, and weight gain.
- Zonisamide: affects sodium channels
  - Side effects include sedation, anorexia, nausea, dizziness, ataxia, anhidrosis, and nephrolithiasis.
  - Cross-reaction with sulfa allergy

Pregnancy Considerations
- Folate should be prescribed for all women of childbearing age who are taking AEDs. AED therapy during the 1st trimester is associated with doubled risk for major fetal malformations (6% vs. 3%).
- Phenytoin in pregnancy may result in fetal hydantoin syndrome.
- Valproate is associated with neural tube defects and should be avoided in pregnancy when possible.
- Fetal insult from seizures following withdrawal of therapy also may be severe. Risk-to-benefit balance should be evaluated with high-risk pregnancy and neurology consultations. Most patients remain on anticonvulsants.
- AED levels should be monitored at least every trimester.

ISSUES FOR REFERRAL
For refractory seizures, consider referral to an epilepsy specialist.

ADDITIONAL THERAPIES
- Vagal nerve stimulator provides periodic stimulation to vagus nerve; may induce hoarseness, cough, and dysphagia. High-frequency stimulation in adults provides greater reduction in seizure frequency than low-frequency stimulation but also has greater rates of side effects (6)[B].
- Deep brain stimulation may decrease seizure frequency in medically refractive epilepsy, but its efficacy varies by seizure source location.
- Repetitive magnetic transcranial stimulation may reduce the frequency of seizures in individuals with refractory focal seizures.

SURGERY/OTHER PROCEDURES
- For refractory focal seizures with identifiable focus
- Preoperative testing, such as Wada test, should be done to decrease likelihood of inducing aphasia and memory loss.

- 34–74% will be seizure free after temporal lobe surgery. Prognosis varies for surgical resection of extratemporal foci.
- Goal of surgical intervention is to reduce reliance on medications; most patients remain on anticonvulsants postoperatively.

ADMISSION, INPATIENT, AND NURSING CONSIDERATIONS
Admit for unremitting seizure (focal/secondary generalized status epilepticus).

 ONGOING CARE

FOLLOW-UP RECOMMENDATIONS
- Most states have restrictions on driving for those with seizure disorders.
- Depending on seizure manifestation, may also recommend against activities such as swimming, climbing to heights, or operating heavy machinery

Patient Monitoring
AED levels if concern over toxicity, noncompliance, or for breakthrough seizures

DIET
Ketogenic or low-glycemic index diet may improve seizure control in some patients but is not well tolerated.

PATIENT EDUCATION
Avoid potential triggers such as alcohol or drug use and sleep deprivation.

PROGNOSIS
- Risk of seizure recurrence: ~30% after first seizure; of these, 50% will occur in the first 6 months, 90% in the first 2 years.
- Depends on seizure type; rolandic epilepsy has a good prognosis; temporal lobe epilepsy is more likely to be persistent.
- ~25–30% of all seizures are refractory to current medications.
- AEDs initiated after an initial seizure have been shown to decrease the risk of seizure over the first 5 years but are not demonstrated to reduce long-term risk of recurrence or mortality.
- The potential for AEDs to confer neuroprotection is under investigation.
- The risk of developing seizure after mild TBI remains high for a long period (>10 years).

COMPLICATIONS
- Risk of accidental injury
- Up to 50–60% of individuals with epilepsy will also have a mood disorder, the most common being depression and anxiety.
- 20–30% of individuals with epilepsy will have memory impairment.

REFERENCES
1. Brigo F, Igwe SC, Erro R, et al. Postictal serum creatine kinase for the differential diagnosis of epileptic seizures and psychogenic non-epileptic seizures: a systematic review. *J Neurol*. 2015;262(2):251–257.
2. Krumholz A, Wiebe S, Gronseth G, et al. Practice parameter: evaluating an apparent unprovoked first seizure in adults (an evidence-based review): report of the Quality Standards Subcommittee of the American Academy of Neurology and the American Epilepsy Society. *Neurology*. 2007;69(21):1996–2007.
3. Krumholz A, Wiebe S, Gronseth GS, et al. Evidence-based guideline: management of an unprovoked first seizure in adults: report of the Guideline Development Subcommittee of the American Academy of Neurology and the American Epilepsy Society. *Neurology*. 2015;84(16):1705–1713.
4. Bonnett LJ, Tudur Smith C, Donegan S, et al. Treatment outcome after failure of a first antiepileptic drug. *Neurology*. 2014;83(6):552–560.
5. Thompson K, Pohlmann-Eden B, Campbell LA, et al. Pharmacological treatments for preventing epilepsy following traumatic head injury. *Cochrane Database Syst Rev*. 2015;(8):CD009900.
6. Panebianco M, Rigby A, Weston J, et al. Vagus nerve stimulation for partial seizures. *Cochrane Database Syst Rev*. 2015;(4):CD002896.

ADDITIONAL READING
- Falco-Walter JJ, Scheffer IE, Fisher RS. The new definition and classification of seizures and epilepsy. *Epilepsy Res*. 2018;139:73–79.
- Gavvala JR, Schuele SU. New-onset seizure in adults and adolescents: a review. *JAMA*. 2016;316(24):2657–2668.
- Walker LE, Mirza N, Yip VL, et al. Personalized medicine approaches in epilepsy. *J Intern Med*. 2015;277(2):218–234.

 CODES

ICD10
- G40.109 Local-rel symptc epi w simp prt seiz,not ntrct, w/o stat epi
- G40.209 Local-rel symptc epi w cmplx prt seiz,not ntrct,w/o stat epi
- G40.119 Local-rel symptc epi w simple part seiz, ntrct, w/o stat epi

CLINICAL PEARLS
- Focal or localization-related seizures have previously been referred to as partial seizures.
- Focal seizures originate from a discrete focus limited to one hemisphere in the cerebral cortex and are further divided into aware versus unaware and motor versus nonmotor, depending on patient presentation.
- It is controversial whether AED treatment is indicated after a first seizure. Treatment should be strongly considered when a clear structural cause is identified/risk of injury from seizure is high (e.g., osteoporosis, anticoagulation).
- An EEG and neuroimaging (CT or MRI) should be considered in evaluating a first unprovoked seizure.
- Most pregnant women should continue anticonvulsant medications. AED levels should be monitored throughout the pregnancy.
- Postictal elevation in prolactin and CPK levels can help distinguish physiologic from psychogenic nonepileptic seizures.

S

SEIZURE DISORDERS

Yvo A. Rodriguez, MD • Shaun O. Smart, MD

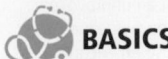 **BASICS**

DESCRIPTION

- Seizure: sudden and transient symptoms (altered level of consciousness, motor manifestations) due to abnormal or synchronous electrical activity of neuronal networks
- Epilepsy: enduring preposition to generate epileptic seizures; defined as two or more unprovoked seizures apart in a >24-hour period
- Status epilepticus: epileptic seizure that lasts >5 minutes or multiple seizures without returning to normal between them. Classification: generalized, simple and complex partial, absence, nonconvulsive. Treatment varies depending of type.
- ILAE seizure classification, based on three key features:
  - Seizure origin: focal (previously partial), focal to bilateral, generalized
  - Awareness: aware, focal impaired awareness, generalized
  - Clinical features: motor, nonmotor (absence, behavior, cognitive, autonomic)
- System(s) affected: nervous
- Synonym(s): convulsion; attacks; spells

Pediatric Considerations
Breastfeeding is not contraindicated. Sedation of the infant should be monitored.

Pregnancy Considerations
- Preconception: Certain antiepileptic drug (AED) (P450 inducers) may cause hormonal contraceptive failure.
- Pregnancy: Avoid valproate as possible, due to increased teratogenicity and worse developmental outcomes. Epileptic patients should notify their neurologist before conception, if possible. During pregnancy, monitor AED levels every trimester for dose adjustment, continue folic acid supplementation, and screen for congenital abnormalities.
- Levetiracetam, topiramate, lamotrigine are alternatives for women of childbearing potential (1).

EPIDEMIOLOGY

Incidence
- 200,000 new cases of epilepsy are diagnosed in the United States annually, with 45,000 new cases in children <15 years of age.
- Pediatric (<2 years of age) and older adults (>65 years of age) more commonly present with new-onset seizures
- Predominant sex: male = female

Prevalence
- 2.7 million with seizure disorder
- 4 million people have had ≥1 seizures.
- 326,000 children (≤14 years of age) and 600,000 adults (>65 years of age) have a seizure disorder.

ETIOLOGY AND PATHOPHYSIOLOGY
- Synchronous and excessive firing of neurons, resulting in an imbalance of regulatory mechanisms in favor of excitatory activity. Seizures may be triggered by metabolic/medical conditions, but such seizures do not necessarily define the presence of epilepsy.
- Idiopathic
- Hippocampal sclerosis and other neurodevelopmental abnormalities of the brain
- Acute infection (meningitis, abscess, encephalitis)
- Metabolic and endocrine disorders
- Trauma
- Drug and alcohol withdrawal
- Tumor

- Vascular disease, including stroke and vasculitis
- Familial/genetic, infantile, and pediatric seizure syndromes (e.g., Lennox-Gastaut, benign familial, myoclonic epilepsy of infancy)
- Other etiologies (by age of onset)
  - Infancy (0 to 2 years)
    - Hypoxic-ischemic encephalopathy/other injury to cerebral cortex
    - Metabolic: hypoglycemia, hypocalcemia, hypomagnesemia, vitamin B_6 deficiency, phenylketonuria
  - Childhood (2 to 10 years): absence or febrile (usually <6 years) seizure
  - Adolescent (10 to 18 years): arteriovenous malformation
  - Late adulthood (>60 years)
    - Prevalence increases with age and is the highest in >65-year-old patients.
    - Degenerative disease, including dementia
    - Most common causes for symptomatic seizures in elderly patients are acute stroke, metabolic disturbances (hypoglycemia, uremia, hepatic failure, electrolyte abnormality), and drugs. Initial diagnostic testing should be focused on these common etiologies.

Genetics
Family history increases risk 3-fold.

RISK FACTORS
History of congenital brain malformations, CNS infections, head trauma, stroke, tumors, neurocognitive degenerative diseases

GENERAL PREVENTION
Take measures to prevent head injuries. Avoid sleep deprivation. Avoid excessive alcohol intake.

COMMONLY ASSOCIATED CONDITIONS
Genetic syndromes (Angelman, tuberous sclerosis, Sturge-Weber), infections, tumors, drug abuse, alcohol and drug withdrawal, trauma, metabolic disorders

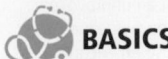 **DIAGNOSIS**

- Physiologic seizures are true cortical events and may require acute intervention.
- Psychogenic nonepileptic seizures (PNES) are also a differential diagnosis to consider.
- Conventional classification of seizures
  - Generalized seizures
    - Tonic–clonic: tonic phase: sudden loss of consciousness; clonic phase: sustained contraction followed by rhythmic contractions of all four extremities; postictal phase: headache, confusion, fatigue; clinically hypertensive, tachycardic, and otherwise hypersympathetic
    - Absence: impaired awareness and responsiveness
    - Atonic: abrupt loss of muscle tone
    - Myoclonic: repetitive muscle contractions
  - Febrile seizures
    - Usually ≤6 years
    - Fever without evidence of any other defined cause of seizures
    - Recurrent febrile seizures probably do not increase the risk of epilepsy.
  - Simple and complex focal seizures: usually present with auras. Correlation with focal EEG findings; can present with automatisms, staring, motor dystonias, postictal confusion
  - Nonconvulsive status epilepticus: most commonly seen in ICU patients; no tonic–clonic activity seen so must diagnose with bedside EEG

- Status epilepticus: repetitive generalized seizures without recovery between seizures; considered a neurologic emergency
- PNES: nonrhythmic pattern of movement, eye closure during event, anterior tongue biting, history of psychiatric disorders. Patients can also have coexisting epilepsy.

HISTORY
- Eyewitness descriptions of event; patient impressions of what occurred before, during, and after the event
- Screen for etiologies, including provoking/ ameliorating factors for the event, such as sleep deprivation.
- Ask about bowel/bladder incontinence, tongue biting, other injury, automatisms, or prior seizure activity.

PHYSICAL EXAM
Thorough neurologic exam; lateral tongue biting suggestive of generalized seizure, whereas tip of tongue more suggestive of nonepileptic event

DIFFERENTIAL DIAGNOSIS
- Syncope, orthostatic hypotension, convulsive syncope
- Transient ischemic attack
- PNES
- Complicated migraine
- Movement disorders: dystonias, dyskinesias
- Sleep disorders: cataplexy, narcolepsy
- Psychiatric disorders: conversion, malingering

DIAGNOSTIC TESTS & INTERPRETATION
A negative EEG does not rule out a seizure disorder. Interictal EEG sensitivity may be as low as 20%; multiple EEGs (at least three) may increase sensitivity to 80% (2)[C].

- Sleep deprivation may be helpful prior to EEG, and hyperventilation and photic stimulation during recording may increase sensitivity.
- Video EEG monitoring is used to differentiate PNES from true cortical events.
- EEG is necessary for diagnosis of nonconvulsive status epilepticus.

Initial Tests (lab, imaging)
- Glucose, sodium, potassium, calcium, phosphorus, magnesium, BUN, ammonia; drug and toxin screens
- AED levels (if patient is taking antiepileptic medication)
- CBC, UA, lumbar puncture if needed: Rule out infection.
- Pregnancy test: will influence treatment selection
- Imaging is recommended for new-onset seizures. MRI is preferred to CT.
  - CT scan of brain: indicated routinely as initial evaluation, especially in the ER
  - Brain MRI: superior in evaluation of the temporal lobes (e.g., mesial temporal sclerosis), stroke, and other structural abnormalities

Follow-Up Tests & Special Considerations
- Drugs that may alter lab results: AED therapy may affect the EEG results dramatically.
- Inadequate AED levels may be altered by many medications such as erythromycin, sulfonamides, warfarin, cimetidine, and alcohol.
- Disorders that may alter lab results: Pregnancy decreases serum concentration.
- Bone scan to determine bone mineral density (BMD): generally done if patients are taking older AEDs such as phenytoin and carbamazepine

Diagnostic Procedures/Other

Lumbar puncture for spinal fluid analysis may be necessary to rule out meningitis if fever and/or impairment of consciousness are present.

 TREATMENT

- Older adults are more sensitive to side effects from AEDs; therefore, target dose should be half of dosing for younger population (3)[C].
- After presenting with an initial unprovoked seizure, 21–45% of patients will have a recurrence within 2 years (4).
- Starting antiepileptic medications is likely to reduce recurrences of seizures but does not alter long-term outcomes or improve quality of life (4)[C].
- Patients with a single unprovoked seizure and associated risk factors that increase recurrence risk up to 60% (abnormal EEG, neurologic exam, or neuroimaging) can potentially benefit from starting therapy.

MEDICATION

- AED of choice: Select based on type of seizure, potential adverse effects/drug interactions, and cost.
- Monotherapy is preferred whenever possible. Treatment should begin with a single agent and the dose titrated until seizures are controlled or side effects become problematic. Consider a different agent if the first choice is not effective versus adding a second agent.
- Patients treated with loading doses of AED in status epilepticus can be started on maintenance dose of a different AED afterwards.

First Line

Treatment options include the following:

- Levetiracetam (Keppra): 1,000 to 3,000 mg/day in 2 doses
- Carbamazepine (Tegretol): 100 to 200 mg/day in 1 to 2 doses; therapeutic range, 4 to 12 mg/L
- Lamotrigine (Lamictal): 25 to 50 mg/day; adjust in 100-mg increments every 1 to 2 weeks to 300 to 500 mg/day in 2 doses.
- Oxcarbazepine (Trileptal): 300 mg BID, increase to 300 mg every 3 days; maintenance, 1,200 mg/day
- Lacosamide (Vimpat): 200 to 300 mg/day in 2 doses
- Ethosuximide (Zarontin): 750 to 1,250 mg/day divided BID (childhood absence seizures)
- Generalized status epilepticus: lorazepam 4 mg, fosphenytoin 20 mg/kg load, valproic acid 20 mg/kg load, levetiracetam 40 mg/kg load (5), lacosamide 300 mg load

Second Line

- Phenytoin (Dilantin): 200 to 400 mg/day in 1 to 3 doses; therapeutic range, 10 to 20 mg/L
- Valproic acid (Depakene): 750 to 3,000 mg/day in 1 to 3 doses to begin at 15 mg/kg/day; therapeutic range, 50 to 150 mg/L
- Topiramate (Topamax): 50 mg/day; adjust weekly to effect; 400 mg/day in 2 doses, max 1,600 mg/day
- Gabapentin (Neurontin): 1,800 to 3,600 mg in 3 to 4 doses for adjunct therapy
- Pregabalin (Lyrica): 150 to 300 mg/day in 2 to 3 doses
- Zonisamide (Zonegran): 100 to 400 mg in 1 to 2 doses
- Ezogabine (Potiga): 600 to 1,200 mg in 3 doses
- Perampanel (Fycompa): 4 to 12 mg daily
- Clonazepam (Klonopin): 1.5 to 8.0 mg in 2 to 3 doses
- Clobazam (Onfi): 20 to 40 mg in 1 to 2 doses
- Rufinamide (Banzel): 3,200 mg in 2 doses
- Brivaracetam (Briviact) (an analog of levetiracetam): 50 to 200 mg/day in 2 doses

- Perampanel (Fycompa): 4, 8, or 12 mg/day
- Contraindications: Refer to manufacturer's profile of each drug.
- Precautions: Doses should be based on individual's response guided by drug levels.
- Consider cautioning about increased risk of suicide, but risk of untreated seizures is far greater than increased risk of suicide.
- Patients are susceptible to sudden unexpected death in epilepsy, possibly due to cardiac arrhythmia.

ISSUES FOR REFERRAL

Referral and follow-up frequency is based on severity and patient's wishes.

SURGERY/OTHER PROCEDURES

For patients that fail traditional therapy: lobectomy, resection, laser ablation, and vagus nerve stimulation

COMPLEMENTARY & ALTERNATIVE MEDICINE

- No evidence suggests that any complementary medicines reduce seizures, but they may induce serious drug interactions with prescribed AEDs.
- Psychological therapies may be used in conjunction with AED therapy. Cognitive-behavioral therapy, relaxation, biofeedback, and yoga all may be helpful as adjunctive therapy (6)[C].
- Patients with PNES should be referred for psychotherapy and psychiatry as needed.

ADMISSION, INPATIENT, AND NURSING CONSIDERATIONS

- Outpatient therapy usually is sufficient, except for status epilepticus.
- Admissions to epilepsy monitoring units for video EEG monitoring may benefit patients with events that pose a diagnostic challenge or patients with intractable seizures already on two AED.
- Protect the airway and, if possible, protect the patient from physical harm; do not restrain. Administer acute AEDs.

 ONGOING CARE

FOLLOW-UP RECOMMENDATIONS

Maintain adequate drug therapy; ensure compliance and/or access to medication. Drug therapy withdrawal and tapering of doses may be considered after a seizure-free 2-year period. Expect a 33% relapse rate in the following 3 years.

Patient Monitoring

- Monitor drug levels and seizure frequency.
- CBC and lab values (e.g., calcium, vitamin D) as indicated; BMD
- Monitor for side effects and adverse reactions.
- All patients currently taking any AED should be monitored closely for notable changes in behavior that could indicate the emergence/worsening of suicidal thoughts/behavior/depression.

DIET

Ketogenic diet may be beneficial in children in conjunction with AED therapy and refractory seizures.

PATIENT EDUCATION

Stress the importance of medication compliance and the avoidance of alcohol and recreational drugs.

- Individuals with uncontrolled seizures should be encouraged to avoid heights and swimming; caution with cooking and unsupervised baths
- Emphasize the danger of driving unless seizure free for a certain period. Laws vary by state: http://www.epilepsy.org.

PROGNOSIS

- Depends on type of seizure disorder: ~70% will become seizure free with appropriate initial treatment, 30% will continue to have seizures. The number of seizures within 6 months after first presentation is a prognostic factor for remission.
- ~90% who are seen for a first unprovoked seizure attain a 1- to 2-year remission within 4 or 5 years of the initial event (5).
- Life expectancy is shortened in persons with epilepsy.
- The case fatality rate for status epilepticus may be as high as 20%.

REFERENCES

1. Perucca E, Tomson T. The pharmacological treatment of epilepsy in adults. *Lancet Neurol.* 2011;10(5):446–456.
2. Fisher RS, Acevedo C, Arzimanoglou A, et al. ILAE official report: a practical clinical definition of epilepsy. *Epilepsia.* 2014;55(4):475–482.
3. Werhahn KJ. Epilepsy in the elderly. *Dtsch Arztebl Int.* 2009;106(9):135–142.
4. Berg AT. Risk of recurrence after a first unprovoked seizure. *Epilepsia.* 2008;49(Suppl 1):13–18.
5. Krumholz A, Wiebe S, Gronseth GS, et al. Evidence-based guideline: management of an unprovoked first seizure in adults: report of the Guideline Development Subcommittee of the American Academy of Neurology and the American Epilepsy Society. *Neurology.* 2015;84(16):1705–1713.
6. Marson A, Ramaratnam S. Epilepsy. *Clin Evid.* 2005;(13):1588–1607.

ADDITIONAL READING

- Drugs for epilepsy. *Treat Guidel Med Lett.* 2013;11(126):9–18.
- Szabó L, Siegler Z, Zubek L, et al. A detailed semiologic analysis of childhood psychogenic nonepileptic seizures. *Epilepsia.* 2012;53(3):565–570.

 SEE ALSO

Seizures, Febrile; Status Epilepticus

 CODES

ICD10

- R56.9 Unspecified convulsions
- P90 Convulsions of newborn
- G40.909 Epilepsy, unspecified, not intractable, without status epilepticus

CLINICAL PEARLS

- Initiation of treatment depends on multiple variables, including type of seizure, underlying risk factors, and further risk of recurrence.
- Semiology of event is very important for diagnosis of seizures versus PNES. Patients with PNES can have concomitant epileptic seizures.
- Patients in status epilepticus that received loading doses of a certain AED do not require to be continued on the same medication.
- To consider driving, states require seizure-free period from 3 to 12 months.

SEIZURES, FEBRILE

Feba Thomas, MD, MS • Swati Avashia, MD, FAAP, FACP, ABIHM

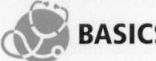 **BASICS**

DESCRIPTION
Febrile seizures occur in children aged 6 months to 5 years with fever ≥100.4°F (38°C) and absence of underlying neurologic abnormality, metabolic condition, or intracranial infection. Three distinct categories (1):
- Simple febrile seizure (70–75%; must meet all criteria)
  - Generalized clonic or tonic–clonic seizure activity without focal features
  - Duration <15 minutes
  - Does not recur within 24 hours
  - Resolves spontaneously
  - No history of previous afebrile seizure or seizure disorder
- Complex (CFS) (20–25%; only one criterion must be met)
  - Partial seizure, focal activity
  - Duration >15 minutes but <30 minutes
  - Recurrence within 24 hours
  - Postictal neurologic abnormalities (e.g., Todd paresis) (2)
- Febrile status epilepticus (FSE) (5%)
  - Lasts >30 minutes

EPIDEMIOLOGY
Incidence
- Approximately 500,000 febrile seizures occur in the United States annually.
- Peak incidence is 18 months of age (2).
- Only 6% of febrile seizures occur before age 6 months, and 4% of febrile seizures occur after age 3 years (3).
- Bimodal seasonal pattern that mirrors peaks of febrile respiratory (November to January) and gastrointestinal infections (June to August) (2)

Prevalence
- 2–5% of children in the white population aged 6 months to 3 years in United States and Western Europe (3)
- Cumulative incidence varies in other populations (0.5–14%) (1).

ETIOLOGY AND PATHOPHYSIOLOGY
A variety of mechanisms have been proposed:
- A lower baseline seizure threshold in the age group affected by febrile seizures
- Familial genotypes may influence seizure thresholds.
- Fever may alter ion channel activity, resulting in increased circuit excitability.
- Cytokines released secondary to infection, specifically interleukin (IL)-1β, increase neuronal activity.

Genetics
- Evidence for genetic association:
  - Greater concordance in monozygotic than dizygotic twins
  - 25–40% of cases have positive family history (3)
  - Risk of febrile seizure with a previously affected sibling is increased.
  - Having two affected parents doubles a child's risk of febrile seizure.
  - Mode of inheritance is multifactorial, although autosomal dominant inheritance reported (2).
- Several rare familial epileptic syndromes present with febrile seizure.

RISK FACTORS
- Any condition causing fever
- Risk increases with the number of affected first-degree relatives.
- Risk is increased for male children (1).
- Recent vaccination
  - As febrile seizures are a benign entity, the benefits of vaccination outweigh the risk.
  - Possible increased risk with vaccinations, mainly MMR and DTaP, is a matter of much debate (3), and absolute vaccination-associated risk is very low.
- Prenatal exposure to alcohol and tobacco, daycare attendance, premature birth, developmental delay, and prolonged NICU stay
- Children with iron deficiency anemia may have increased risk for febrile seizures. Consider checking for anemia if the history suggests a risk for iron deficiency (4)[C].

GENERAL PREVENTION
Prevention is not usually indicated given the benign nature of this condition, lack of effective interventions, and side effects of prophylactic medications.

COMMONLY ASSOCIATED CONDITIONS
- Viral infections: Common pathogens include human herpesvirus 6 (HHV-6), influenza, parainfluenza, adenovirus, and respiratory syncytial virus (RSV).
  - HHV-6 infection found in 30% of FSE in one study (3)
- Bacterial infections: Frequently associated infections include otitis media, pharyngitis, urinary tract infection (UTI), pneumonia, and gastroenteritis (specifically with *Shigella*).

 DIAGNOSIS

HISTORY
- History of present illness:
  - Description of seizure:
    - Febrile seizures are generalized with clonic or tonic–clonic activity.
    - Absence, myoclonic, atonic, and focal seizures are atypical of febrile seizures and warrant further evaluation.
  - Seizure duration
  - Presence of postictal state (consistent with febrile seizure)
  - Number of seizures in previous 24 hours
  - Lethargy, irritability, or decreased level of consciousness as reported by the caretaker
  - Symptoms of underlying infection
  - Symptoms concerning for neurologic deficits
- Past medical history:
  - Existing conditions, including developmental delay, cerebral palsy, and metabolic disorders
  - Recent antibiotic course
  - History of febrile seizures
  - History of afebrile seizures or seizure disorder
  - History of head injury
  - Vaccination status, recent immunization
- Family history: febrile seizures, afebrile seizures, epilepsy, metabolic disorders, and other neurologic conditions
- Social history: factors concerning for child abuse

PHYSICAL EXAM
- Vital signs should be stable and consistent with intercurrent febrile illness; unstable vital signs or toxic appearance warrants further evaluation.
- Identify the presence or absence of focal deficits on a complete neurologic exam.
- Assess for signs of meningitis, including decreased level of consciousness, nuchal rigidity, irritability, meningeal signs, bulging fontanelle, papilledema, and petechiae.
- Identify cause of fever.
- Assess thoroughly for manifestations of child abuse with a careful skin exam, inspection and palpation for occult trauma, and retinal exam if possible.

DIFFERENTIAL DIAGNOSIS
- Seizures due to an etiology other than febrile seizure:
  - Meningitis, encephalitis
  - Primary epilepsy
  - Neonatal seizure
  - Dravet syndrome
  - Intracranial mass
  - Nonaccidental trauma
  - Electrolyte abnormality
  - Hypoglycemia
  - Metabolic disorder
- Conditions presenting similarly to seizure:
  - Rigors
  - Crying
  - Benign myoclonus of infancy
  - Breath-holding spell
  - Choking episode
  - Tic disorder
  - Parasomnia
  - Arrhythmia
  - Metabolic disorder
  - Dystonic reaction

DIAGNOSTIC TESTS & INTERPRETATION
- Routine laboratory tests are not recommended to identify an underlying cause of a simple febrile seizure (2)[C].
- Rates of UTI in children with simple febrile seizures and in febrile children without seizure are comparable; decisions regarding urinalysis should be based on current UTI screening guidelines (2)[B].
- Blood glucose is no longer routinely recommended (2)[B].
- Lumbar puncture
  - In studies of patients with simple febrile seizures conducted since the initiation of routine infant vaccination against *Haemophilus influenzae*, rates of acute bacterial meningitis were very low (0–0.8%).
  - Seizure is unlikely to be the only presenting symptom of meningitis. Symptoms indicating increased likelihood of meningitis include toxic appearance, altered level of consciousness, meningeal signs, focal neurologic deficits, bulging fontanelle, and petechiae.
  - Cases of bacterial meningitis in children with febrile seizures who return to baseline or in the absence of other signs or symptoms are rare (2).
  - Recommendations:
    - Lumbar puncture should be performed in a child with fever and seizure if meningeal signs are present or if there is concern for meningitis or other intracranial pathology based on history and exam (2)[B].

○ In infants aged 6 to 12 months, consider lumbar puncture if the child has not been vaccinated against *H. influenzae* or *Streptococcus pneumoniae* according to schedule (2)[C].

○ Consider lumbar puncture for children with fever and seizure who have recently been treated with antibiotics because antibiotics may mask meningeal signs and symptoms (2)[C].

○ The yield of lumbar puncture in children with complex febrile seizure is very low, and the rate of acute bacterial meningitis in U.S. patients with complex febrile seizures is too low to routinely recommend lumbar puncture.

○ Neuroimaging is not routinely recommended for the purposes of identifying the cause of a simple febrile seizure (2)[B].

• Studies have demonstrated limited utility of emergent imaging in patients who meet criteria for complex febrile seizure; however, imaging may be indicated for history or exam findings concerning for bleed or structural lesion. Head CT scan is not routinely recommended for children with complex febrile seizures (1)[B].

Diagnostic Procedures/Other
• EEG is not recommended in neurologically normal children presenting with simple febrile seizure (2)[B].
• There is mixed evidence for use of EEG after complex febrile seizures; some recommend outpatient EEG on follow-up because EEGs can show generalized slowing for 24 hours after initial presentation and up to 7 days after FSE (2).

 TREATMENT

GENERAL MEASURES
• Acute seizure management
  – Airway: Position the patient laterally, suction secretions, and place a nasopharyngeal airway if necessary.
  – Breathing: Administer oxygen for cyanosis; consider bag-mask ventilation or intubation for inadequate ventilation.
  – Circulation: Establish IV access if first-line buccal or nasal midazolam is not effective.
• Antipyretics are helpful for patient comfort but do not prevent seizure recurrence during the initial febrile episode (1)[A].
• Provide supportive care and treat underlying infection if necessary.

MEDICATION
First Line
Treat seizures of ≥5 minutes duration with anticonvulsants (2):
• Out of hospital: rectal diazepam 0.5 mg/kg, buccal midazolam 0.4 mg/kg, or nasal midazolam 0.2 mg/kg
• In hospital: IV or IM lorazepam 0.1 mg/kg or IV diazepam 0.2 mg/kg

ISSUES FOR REFERRAL
Simple febrile seizures do not require referral to a pediatric neurologist.

ADMISSION, INPATIENT, AND NURSING CONSIDERATIONS
• Unstable vital signs
• Concerning findings on history or physical exam
• Prolonged seizure requiring anticonvulsants

• Persistent change in mental status
• Inpatient management of underlying condition is required.

 ONGOING CARE

FOLLOW-UP RECOMMENDATIONS
• Anticonvulsant prophylaxis during subsequent febrile episodes:
  – The American Academy of Pediatrics recommends against prophylaxis with anticonvulsants due to an unacceptable risk–benefit ratio (2)[B].
  – Intermittent oral and rectal diazepam are effective in reducing recurrence of simple and complex febrile seizures but are not recommended due to the benign nature of febrile seizures and because so many febrile seizures precede the development of the fever (2)[B].
• Antipyretic prophylaxis during subsequent febrile episodes (2)[A]:
  – No study has demonstrated that fever management will prevent recurrence but may contribute to patient comfort.
  – Ibuprofen and acetaminophen are no more effective than placebo in preventing recurrence.

PATIENT EDUCATION
There is frequently a high degree of parental anxiety associated with febrile seizures. Suggested anticipatory guidance:
• Febrile seizures do not cause brain damage and are associated with a low risk for sequelae.
• Parents should be reassured after a simple febrile seizure that there is no negative impact on intellect, behavior, or risk of death (3)[B]. They should be reassured that it is a benign condition and treatment is often unnecessary (5).
• Parents should be prepared for a high probability of recurrence.
• If seizure recurs, position the child safely in a semiprone position and do not intervene inappropriately.
• Time the seizure; call rescue if the child turns blue, has difficulty breathing, or the seizure lasts >5 minutes.
• If the seizure spontaneously resolves in <5 minutes and the child is well but sleepy, seek immediate attention, but calling rescue is not necessary.

PROGNOSIS
• Recurrence:
  – Estimates of recurrence rates vary (30–50%).
  – 10% will experience three or more febrile seizures (2,5).
  – Factors associated with seizure recurrence include age <18 months at time of first episode, first-degree relative with history of febrile seizure, history of complex febrile seizures, lower peak temperatures, and shorter duration of fever prior to seizure occurrence (2).
• Intellectual and behavioral outcomes
  – Febrile seizures do not impact IQ, behavioral abnormalities, academic performance, or neurocognitive inattention (3).
  – Outcomes in children with single and multiple febrile seizures are similar.
• Subsequent development of epilepsy (2)
  – Risk of epilepsy after a simple partial seizure is close to the overall rate in the general population.

  – Risk is up to 7% in those with multiple simple febrile seizures age <12 months and a short duration of fever prior to seizure onset.
  – Factors associated with increased risk include presenting with complex febrile seizure, family history of epilepsy or febrile seizures, cerebral palsy, developmental delay, low birth weight, and prematurity.
• Mortality:
  – There is not an increased risk for SIDS in siblings of children who have febrile seizures.

COMPLICATIONS
Seizure-related injury, aspiration pneumonia, side effects of prescribed medications or diagnostic procedures, and subsequent parental perception of the child as being vulnerable, especially during subsequent fevers

REFERENCES
1. Whelan H, Harmelink M, Chou E, et al. Complex febrile seizures—a systematic review. *Dis Mon*. 2017;63(1):5–23.
2. Kimia AA, Bachur RG, Torres A, et al. Febrile seizures: emergency medicine perspective. *Curr Opin Pediatr*. 2015;27(3):292–297.
3. Gupta A. Febrile seizures. *Continuum (Minneap Minn)*. 2016;22(1 Epilepsy):51–59.
4. King D, King A. Question 2: should children who have a febrile seizure be screened for iron deficiency? *Arch Dis Child*. 2014;99(10):960–964.
5. Leung AK, Hon KL, Leung TN. Febrile seizures: an overview. *Drugs Context*. 2018;7:212536.

ADDITIONAL READING
Subcommittee on Febrile Seizures, American Academy of Pediatrics. Neurodiagnostic evaluation of the child with a simple febrile seizure. *Pediatrics*. 2011;127(2):389–394.

 CODES

ICD10
• R56.00 Simple febrile convulsions
• R56.01 Complex febrile convulsions
• G40.901 Epilepsy, unsp, not intractable, with status epilepticus

CLINICAL PEARLS
• Febrile seizures are generally benign, and families can be reassured that children are at low risk of death, subsequent development of epilepsy, and learning or behavioral abnormalities.
• History and physical exam are important tools in identifying children presenting with febrile seizure who may be at greater risk for meningitis or other intracranial pathology.
• For simple febrile seizures, routine labs, lumbar puncture, neuroimaging studies, and EEG are not recommended in the absence of clinical suspicion of serious underlying pathology.
• Prophylaxis with anticonvulsants or antipyretics during subsequent febrile episodes is not recommended due to their lack of effectiveness and the risk of medication-associated side effects.

SEROTONIN SYNDROME

Michael T. Partin, MD • Karl T. Clebak, MD, FAAFP • Munima Nasir, MD

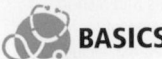 **BASICS**

DESCRIPTION

- A potentially life-threatening drug-induced syndrome that results from synaptic increase in serotonin (5-hydroxytryptamine [5-HT]) concentrations and stimulation of peripheral and CNS serotonergic receptors
- It is a concentration-dependent toxicity that can develop in any individual who has ingested drug combinations that synergistically increase synaptic 5-HT.
- Serotonin toxicity occurs in three main settings: (i) therapeutic drug use, which often results in mild to moderate symptoms; (ii) intentional overdose of a single serotonergic agent, which typically leads to moderate symptoms; and (iii) as the result of a drug interaction between numerous serotonergic agents (most commonly, selective serotonin reuptake inhibitors [SSRIs] and monoamine oxidase inhibitors [MAOIs]), most often associated with severe serotonin toxicity.
- Classically characterized by a triad of symptoms that include mental status change, neuromuscular hyperactivity, and autonomic instability
- Onset is usually within 24 hours with 60% of cases occurring within 6 hours of exposure to, or change in, dosing of a serotonergic agent. Rarely, cases have been reported weeks after discontinuation of serotonergic agents.

Geriatric Considerations
Increased risk through polypharmacy given frequent use of serotonergic analgesics, antibiotics, and antidepressants

Pediatric Considerations
- Serotonin syndrome has similar manifestations in children and adults.
- General management is unchanged in children, other than medication dosing.
- Consider toxic ingestion of serotonergic agents prescribed to caregivers of pediatric patients.
- Symptoms in neonates may include tremors, increased muscle tone, jitteriness, shivering, feeding/digestive disturbances, irritability, agitation, sleep disturbances, increased reflexes, excessive crying, and respiratory disturbances.

Pregnancy Considerations
- Serotonin levels are increased from baseline during an uncomplicated pregnancy with preeclamptic patients demonstrating a 10-fold increase in serotonin levels.
- 3rd-trimester exposure to SSRIs has been associated with transient neonatal complications that may reflect either acute drug withdrawal or serotonergic toxicity.

EPIDEMIOLOGY
Seen in about 14–16% of SSRI overdose patients

Incidence
- Approximately 100,000 adverse events, including deaths, are reported annually with antidepressant use. Most of which are associated with SSRIs, either alone or in combination with other drugs. In a 2008 study, SSRIs alone were responsible for adverse events in 18.8% of cases, with 55.7% due to intentional causes, 39.5% unintentional, and remainder of causes unknown. Of patients reporting adverse effects with SSRIs, 46.6% had symptoms requiring hospitalization, and significant toxic effects occurred in 90 patients with two resultant deaths (1)[A].

- The incidence of serotonin syndrome is rising because serotonergic agents are increasingly used in clinical practice and in combination with other serotonergic agents. However, the true incidence is unclear due to potential misdiagnosis and unreported mild cases.
- Predominant age: affects all age groups
- Predominant sex: male = female

ETIOLOGY AND PATHOPHYSIOLOGY
- Increased synaptic 5-HT or agonist concentration as a result of one or more of the following mechanisms: (i) decreased 5-HT breakdown (e.g., MAOI), (ii) decreased 5-HT reuptake (e.g., SSRI), (iii) increased 5-HT agonists (e.g., tryptophan), (iv) increased 5-HT release (e.g., amphetamines), and (v) CYP2D6 and CYP3A4 inhibitors (e.g., erythromycin)
- Risk is mediated in a dose-related manner to the action of 5-HT/5-HT agonists on 5-HT$_{1A}$ and/or 5-HT$_{2A}$ receptors.
- A number of drugs are associated with serotonin syndrome, which usually involves combination with an SSRI. These include SSRIs (e.g., citalopram, escitalopram, fluoxetine, fluvoxamine, paroxetine, sertraline); MAOIs; SNRIs (duloxetine, venlafaxine, desvenlafaxine); tricyclic antidepressants (e.g., amitriptyline); other antidepressants (nefazodone, trazodone); anxiolytic (buspirone); lithium; triptans; anticonvulsants (Depakote); analgesics (fentanyl, meperidine, pentazocine, tramadol); antibiotics (linezolid, tedizolid [weak MAOI], ritonavir); over-the-counter (OTC) cough medications (dextromethorphan); some antipsychotics (risperidone, olanzapine); antiemetics (ondansetron, granisetron); other medications, such as metoclopramide, cyclobenzaprine, L-dopa; dietary supplements (tryptophan); herbal supplements (St. John's wort, nutmeg); methylene blue; and drugs of abuse (e.g., methylenedioxymethamphetamine [MDMA], cocaine, D-lysergic acid diethylamide [LSD], and amphetamine) (2)[A].

Genetics
Unknown

RISK FACTORS
- Serotonergic agents
- Comorbid conditions leading to polypharmacy
- Reported following ingestion of a single agent
- The greatest number of adverse events has been shown to be associated with SSRIs in combination with other substances, and the combination of SSRIs and MAOIs carries the greatest risk of developing serotonin toxicity.

GENERAL PREVENTION
- Consider drug–drug interactions when a multidrug regimen is required and avoid if possible.
- Caution patients about taking SSRIs with OTC medications (e.g., dextromethorphan) or herbal supplements (e.g., St. John's wort) prior to consulting a physician.
- Clinician education and continual improvement in use of health information technology to identify potential drug–drug interactions
- Avoid serotonergic agents for nonpsychiatric disorders (e.g., tramadol for pain relief).

 DIAGNOSIS

- Serotonin syndrome is a clinical diagnosis.
- *Hunter Toxicity Criteria Decision Rules* aid in the diagnosis of clinically significant serotonin toxicity (sensitivity, 84%; specificity, 97%). A patient who took a serotonergic agent must have one of the following:
  – Spontaneous clonus
  – Inducible clonus with agitation or diaphoresis
  – Ocular clonus with agitation or diaphoresis
  – Hypertonia and hyperthermia (temperature >38°C) with inducible clonus or ocular clonus (3)[A]
  – Tremor and hyperreflexia

HISTORY
- Obtain a thorough drug history including prescriptions, OTC remedies, dietary and herbal supplements, and illicit drugs. Ask about dose, formulation, and recent changes.
- Review comorbidities (e.g., depression and chronic pain).
- Address possibility of drug overdose and obtain collateral information if intentional overdose is suspected.
- Elicit description of symptoms, including onset and progression.

PHYSICAL EXAM
Neuromuscular findings are seen in over half of patients with serotonin syndrome. Initially, patients can develop a peripheral tremor, confusion, and ataxia; systemic signs are next (e.g., agitation, diaphoresis, hyperreflexia, and shivering). If it worsens, the severe signs of fever, jerking, and diarrhea may develop.

- Tachycardia, hypertension, and hyperthermia (≥40°C in severe cases)
- Neuromuscular abnormalities
  – Mild: hyperreflexia, myoclonus, and tremor all greater in lower extremities; bilateral Babinski sign
  – Moderate: opsoclonus, spontaneous or inducible clonus (involuntary muscle contractions, most commonly tested by rapid dorsiflexion of foot)
  – Severe: rigidity, respiratory failure, tonic–clonic seizure
- Autonomic dysfunction:
  – Mild: diaphoresis, mydriasis, tachycardia
  – Moderate: hyperactive bowel sounds, diarrhea, nausea, vomiting, hyperthermia (<40°C)
  – Severe: hyperthermia (≥40°C), rapidly changing blood pressure (BP)
- Mental status changes:
  – Mild: anxiety, akathisia (restlessness), insomnia
  – Moderate: agitation
  – Severe: coma, delirium, confusion (4)[A]
- Severe cases have led to altered level of consciousness, rhabdomyolysis, metabolic acidosis, and disseminated intravascular coagulation (DIC).

DIFFERENTIAL DIAGNOSIS
- Neuroleptic malignant syndrome (NMS): lead pipe rigidity and extrapyramidal features without clonus
- Anticholinergic fever (e.g., benztropine, diphenhydramine, oxybutynin, nifedipine, famotidine, atropine, scopolamine; plant poisoning from belladonna/"deadly nightshade," datura, henbane, mandrake, brugmansia): urinary retention, decreased bowel sounds, normal reflexes
- Malignant hyperthermia: generally following administration of anesthetics or depolarizing muscle relaxants

- Heat stroke
- CNS infection (meningitis, encephalitis)
- Sympathomimetic toxicity (cocaine, methamphetamine, PCP)
- Nonconvulsive seizures
- Hyperthyroidism (thyroid storm)
- Tetanus
- Rabies
- Acute baclofen withdrawal

DIAGNOSTIC TESTS & INTERPRETATION
- Serum serotonin levels do not correlate with clinical findings.
- Nonspecific lab findings that may develop include the following:
  - Elevated WBC count
  - Elevated creatine phosphokinase (CK or CPK)
  - Decreased serum bicarbonate
  - Elevated hepatic transaminases
- In severe cases, the following complications may develop:
  - DIC
  - Metabolic acidosis
  - Rhabdomyolysis
  - Renal failure
  - Myoglobinuria
  - Acute respiratory distress syndrome (ARDS) (3)[A]

 TREATMENT

- Discontinue all serotonergic agents.
- Supportive care is the mainstay of therapy. This includes administration of oxygen and aggressive IV fluids, continuous cardiac monitoring, monitoring urine output, and stabilizing vital signs.
  - Benzodiazepines may be effective for the management of agitation in patients with serotonin syndrome.
  - Administration of serotonin antagonists: Cyproheptadine (histamine and serotonin antagonist) may be useful if supportive measures and sedation (benzodiazepines) are unable to control agitation and correct vital signs. This agent does not reduce the duration of serotonin syndrome.
- Mild cases (afebrile, tachycardia, shivering, diaphoresis, mydriasis, hyperreflexia, intermittent tremor or myoclonus)
  - Discontinue precipitating agent(s).
  - Supportive care
  - Sedation
  - Observe for 12 to 24 hours.
- Moderate cases (temperature >38°C, autonomic instability, hyperactive bowel sounds, diarrhea, diaphoresis, ocular clonus, hyperreflexia, tremor, mild agitation, or hypervigilance)
  - Discontinue precipitating agent(s).
  - Supportive care
  - Sedation
  - Aggressive treatment of autonomic instability
  - Treatment with cyproheptadine should be initiated if agitation and vital sign abnormalities are unimproved with benzodiazepines and supportive care.
  - Hypotension from MAOI interactions should be treated with low doses of direct-acting sympathomimetics (e.g., norepinephrine, phenylephrine, epinephrine); indirect serotonin agonists, such as dopamine, should be avoided.
  - Severe hypertension and tachycardia should be treated with short-acting agents, such as nitroprusside or esmolol.

- Avoid use of longer acting agents, such as propranolol, to prevent hypotension and falsely lowering heart rate, which can be used to monitor treatment response.
  - Observe for 12 to 24 hours.
- Severe cases (temperature >41.1°C, autonomic instability, delirium, muscular rigidity, and hypertonicity)
  - Discontinue precipitating agent(s).
  - Immediate sedation
  - Endotracheal intubation as clinically indicated
  - Paralysis as clinically indicated (maintained with nondepolarizing continuous paralytic agents such as vecuronium, cisatracurium, rocuronium)
  - Succinylcholine should not be used in cases of rhabdomyolysis to avoid exacerbation of hyperkalemia (5)[A].
  - Antipyretic medications are not effective (4)[A]; the increased body temperature is due to muscle activity, not an alteration in the hypothalamic set point.
  - Avoid physical restraints because it can worsen hyperthermia and lactic acidosis in agitated patients (5)[A].

MEDICATION
- Benzodiazepines: may be used to manage agitation in serotonin syndrome and also may correct mild increases in BP and heart rate. Use with caution in patients with delirium, given the known paradoxical effect of exacerbating delirium.
- Cyproheptadine (Periactin): Consider use if benzodiazepines and supportive measures are unable to control agitation and correct vital signs:
  - Adults: initial dose 12 mg PO (can also be crushed and given via nasogastric [NG] tube) followed by 2 mg q2h until clinical response observed; 12 to 32 mg of drug may be required in a 24-hour period.
  - Children
    - <2 years: 0.06 mg/kg q6h
    - 2 to 6 years: 2 mg q6h
    - 7 to 14 years: 4 mg q6h
  - Unlikely to be effective in patients who have received activated charcoal
  - Pregnancy Category B
- Use of antipsychotics with $5-HT_{2A}$ antagonist activity, such as olanzapine and chlorpromazine, is not recommended (4)[A].

ISSUES FOR REFERRAL
- Psychiatry: for assistance with medication management and follow-up care (inpatient psychiatric care vs. outpatient psychiatric follow-up)
- Toxicology/clinical pharmacology service
- Poison control center

ADMISSION, INPATIENT, AND NURSING CONSIDERATIONS
- Patients with known/suspected serotonin syndrome should be admitted to a medical inpatient unit for observation.
- Discharge criteria
  - Mental status has returned to baseline.
  - Stable vital signs
  - No increase in clonus
  - Close patient follow-up is ensured.

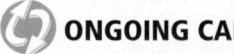 **ONGOING CARE**

FOLLOW-UP RECOMMENDATIONS
- In mild cases of serotonin toxicity, address risks and benefits of restarting offending agents. Serotonergic medications need to be titrated slowly, and patients must have close outpatient follow-up with physician.

- If patient developed severe serotonin syndrome, the offending agent should likely not be resumed unless precipitant for serotonin syndrome is found (e.g., combination with another serotonin agonist); the patient can be carefully monitored, or there is clear benefit versus risk of restarting the medication.

PROGNOSIS
- Generally favorable with early recognition of the syndrome and prompt initiation of treatment
- Most cases resolve within 24 hours of discontinuation of serotonergic agents; this can be longer depending on the drug's half-life:
  - MAOIs can result in toxicity for several days.
  - SSRIs can result in toxicity for up to several weeks after discontinuation.
- ICU admission is often indicated in severe cases.

COMPLICATIONS
- Adverse outcomes, including death, are usually the consequence of poorly treated hyperthermia.
- Nonhyperthermic patients who survive typically do not have long-term sequelae.

REFERENCES
1. Bronstein AC, Spyker DA, Cantilena LR Jr, et al. 2008 Annual report of the American Association of Poison Control Centers' National Poison Data System (NPDS): 26th annual report. *Clin Toxicol (Phila)*. 2009;47(10):911–1084.
2. Ables AZ, Nagubilli R. Prevention, recognition, and management of serotonin syndrome. *Am Fam Physician*. 2010;81(9):1139–1142.
3. Dunkley EJ, Isbister GK, Sibbritt D, et al. The Hunter Serotonin Toxicity Criteria: simple and accurate diagnostic decision rules for serotonin toxicity. *QJM*. 2003;96(9):635–642.
4. Boyer EW, Shannon M. The serotonin syndrome. *N Engl J Med*. 2005;352(11):1112–1120.
5. Heitmiller DR. Serotonin syndrome: a concise review of a toxic state. *R I Med J (2013)*. 2014;97(6):33–35.

ADDITIONAL READING
- Buckley NA, Dawson AH, Isbister GK. Serotonin syndrome. *BMJ*. 2014;348:g1626.
- Nordstrom K, Vilke GM, Wilson MP. Psychiatric emergencies for clinicians: emergency department management of serotonin syndrome. *J Emerg Med*. 2016;50(1):89–91.

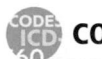 **CODES**

ICD10
G25.79 Other drug induced movement disorders

CLINICAL PEARLS

Consider serotonin syndrome in patients with recent use of a serotonergic agent (particularly if multiple proserotonergic agents are involved) presenting with unexplained tachycardia, hypertension, hyperthermia, clonus, hyperreflexia, and change in mental status.

SEXUAL DYSFUNCTION IN WOMEN

Esther Guard, DO

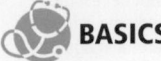 **BASICS**

- Very common: ~40% of women surveyed in the United States have sexual concerns.
- May present as a lack of sexual desire, impaired arousal, inability to achieve orgasm or pain with sexual activity, and may be lifelong or acquired

DESCRIPTION

- Female sexual interest or arousal disorder—lack of or significantly reduced sexual interest or arousal as manifested by three of the following:
  - Absent or reduced interest in sexual activity
  - Absent or reduced sexual or erotic thoughts or fantasies
  - No or reduced initiation of sexual activity and unreceptive to partner's attempts to initiate
  - Absent or reduced sexual excitement or pleasure during sexual activity in almost all (75–100%) of sexual encounters
  - Absent or reduced sexual interest or arousal in response to any internal or external sexual or erotic cues
  - Absent or reduced genital or nongenital sensation during sexual activity in almost all (75–100%) of sexual encounters
- Female orgasmic disorder—presence of either of the following in almost all (75–100%) occasions of sexual activity:
  - Marked delay in, marked infrequency of, or absence of orgasm
  - Markedly reduced intensity of orgasmic sensations
- Genito-pelvic pain or penetration disorder—persistent or recurrent difficulties with one or more of the following:
  - Vaginal penetration during intercourse
  - Marked vulvovaginal or pelvic pain during intercourse or penetration attempts
  - Marked fear or anxiety about vulvovaginal or pelvic pain in anticipation of, during, or because of vaginal penetration
  - Marked tensing or tightening of pelvic floor muscles during attempted vaginal penetration

ALERT

Symptoms must be present for ≥6 months; cause clinically significant distress or impairment; and not be better explained by a nonsexual mental disorder, a consequence of severe relationship distress, or other significant stressors

- System(s) affected: nervous; reproductive; genitourinary; psychiatric
- Synonym(s): hypoactive sexual desire disorder; sexual aversion disorder; female sexual arousal disorder; inhibited female orgasm

EPIDEMIOLOGY

In two large studies, approximately 40% of women reported sexual problems.

Incidence

Sexual problems are highest in women aged 45 to 64 years and then decline secondary to changes in sexual-related personal distress.

Prevalence

Low sexual desire is the most common manifestation, followed by difficulty with orgasm, difficulty with arousal, and sexual pain.

ETIOLOGY AND PATHOPHYSIOLOGY

The pathophysiology of sexual dysfunction is complex and multifactorial because it can be the result of any etiology that interferes with the female sexual response cycle (desire, arousal, orgasm, and resolution). Phases can vary in sequence, overlap, or be absent during all or some sexual encounters.

- Biologic
  - Disorders of the hypothalamic-pituitary-adrenal system, hormonal imbalance/disorders of ovarian function, menopause (surgical or natural), chronic illness (vascular disease, diabetes mellitus, and malignancy)
  - Prescription medications (SSRIs, MAOIs, TCAs, β-blockers)
  - Thyroid disease
  - Neuromuscular disease (multiple sclerosis, spinal cord damage)
- Psychological
  - Anxiety/depression
  - Maladaptive thoughts/behaviors
  - Interrelational difficulties
  - Body image issues
  - Drug and alcohol abuse
  - Sexual abuse

RISK FACTORS

- Advancing age/menopause
- Previous sexual trauma
- Lack of knowledge about sexual stimulation and response
- Chronic medical problems
  - Depression, anxiety, chronic pain syndromes, and other psychiatric disorders
  - Cardiovascular disease
  - Endocrine disorders
  - Dermatologic disorders
  - Neurologic disorders
  - Cancer
- Gynecologic issues
  - Childbirth
  - Pelvic floor or bladder dysfunction
  - Endometriosis
  - Uterine fibroids
  - Chronic vulvovaginal candidiasis/vaginal infections
  - Female genital mutilation
- Relationship factors such as couple discrepancies in expectations and/or cultural backgrounds and attitudes toward sexuality in family of origin
- Medications or substance abuse

COMMONLY ASSOCIATED CONDITIONS

- Marital/relationship discord
- Depression

 DIAGNOSIS

- Female sexual dysfunction is diagnosed by utilizing a validated sexual function screening instrument and a structured interview, including detailed medical and sexual history, to confirm diagnosis.
  - Female Sexual Function Index
  - Brief Index of Sexual Functioning for Women
  - Brief Sexual Symptom Checklist
  - Decreased Sexual Desire Screener
- The diagnosis requires that the sexual problem be recurrent or persistent and causes personal distress rather than be due solely to partner or relationship issues.

HISTORY

- Detailed sexual history
  - Degree of personal distress
  - Lifelong versus acquired problem
  - Situational versus generalized problem
  - Cultural/societal beliefs regarding sexuality
  - History of sexual trauma
  - Concerns about safety, pregnancy, or STIs
  - Concerns regarding privacy
- Interpersonal relationship factors
  - Current relationship status
  - Family dysfunction
- Physiologic/biologic history
  - Urinary/anal incontinence
  - Medications (including herbal and OTC)
  - Pregnancy/childbirth history
  - Infertility
  - Menopausal status (natural, surgical, or postchemotherapy)
  - STIs and vaginitis
  - Pelvic surgery, injury, or cancer
  - Chronic pelvic pain
  - Abnormal genital tract bleeding
- Psychological history
  - Low self-image
  - Anxiety
  - Depression
  - Negative past sexual experiences
  - Substance misuse/abuse

PHYSICAL EXAM

- Most commonly, patients have a normal physical exam.
  - Assess for anatomic abnormalities.
  - Assess for scars or evidence of trauma.
  - Assess for vaginal atrophy, adequate estrogenization.
  - Assess for infection.
  - Recognize signs of anxiety, apprehension, and pain during the speculum and pelvic exam.
- General physical exam, signs of chronic disease

DIFFERENTIAL DIAGNOSIS

- Medication side effects
- Vaginitis
- Decreased vaginal lubrication secondary to hormonal imbalance
- Decreased sensation secondary to nerve injury
- Multiple sclerosis
- Anatomic abnormalities
- Abdominal surgery (which can interfere with pelvic innervation)
- Depression
- Marital dysfunction, including domestic violence
- Pregnancy
- Pseudodyspareunia (use of complaint of pain to distance self from partner)

DIAGNOSTIC TESTS & INTERPRETATION

Laboratory studies are rarely helpful. There are no reliable correlations between serum hormone levels and sexual dysfunction.

Initial Tests (lab, imaging)

As needed to identify infections and other medical causes

TREATMENT

- Set realistic goals and expectations (1)[C].
- Address underlying medical and psychiatric conditions (2)[C].

- Review basic sex education, sexual response, heterogeneity of normal response, and sexual activity other than intercourse (1)[C].
- Education on communication
- Educate on healthy lifestyle, including diet, exercise, sleep, avoidance of tobacco, and reduced alcohol use (1)[C].
- Vaginal moisturizers and lubricants
- Cognitive-behavioral therapy (CBT) (individual or couples) to target maladaptive thoughts and behaviors and to disrupt the dysfunctional cycle (2)[C]
- Mindfulness-based CBT (1)[C]
- Sex therapy: sensate focus, systematic desensitization exercises, homework exchanging physical touch with partner, scheduled attempt of sexual activity 3 times per week, or directed masturbation alone (2,3)[C]
- Physical therapy/biofeedback (3)[C]

MEDICATION

Sexual dysfunction is often a multifactorial psychosocial condition. Using medications does not usually address the cause of the problem and can, in some cases, make the condition worse.

- Bupropion (1)[C]: adjunct for SSRI-induced sexual dysfunction. Improves sexual arousal and orgasm but not desire. Dose: bupropion SR 150 mg orally once or twice daily
- Flibanserin (2)[C],(4)[A]: possible improvement in sexual desire. Clinical improvement versus placebo is minimal, and side effects are common. Mechanism of action: 5-HT$_{1A}$ agonist and 5-HT$_{2A}$ antagonist. Dose: 100 mg at bedtime; FDA-approved for premenopausal women with hypoactive sexual desire
- Estrogen replacement with or without progestins (1,3)[C],(5)[A]: may improve sexual desire, vaginal atrophy, and clitoral sensitivity. Vaginal estrogen therapy (preferred route of administration) is available in cream, vaginal tablet, or ring form.
- Ospemifene (1,3)[C]: selective estrogen receptor modulator FDA-approved for dyspareunia due to vulvo- or vaginal atrophy in postmenopausal women. Dose: ospemifene 60 mg orally once daily
- Testosterone (1,2,3,6)[B]
  - Use in premenopausal women not supported by data
  - In naturally or surgically postmenopausal women, adding short-term testosterone to hormone replacement may increase desire.
  - >6 months use lacks data on safety and effectiveness.
  - Side effects: hirsutism, androgenic alopecia, acne, decreased HDL, liver dysfunction; not FDA-approved for sexual dysfunction in women
  - Contraindicated in breast or endometrial cancer, thromboembolic disease, or coronary artery disease
  - Dose: oral methyltestosterone 1.25 to 2.50 mg/day (1/10 of men's dose) or topical (patch, gel)
- Dehydroepiandrosterone (DHEA) (6)[C]: vaginal formulation 6.5 mg FDA-approved for dyspareunia due to vaginal atrophy in postmenopausal women
- Phosphodiesterase type 5 (PDE5) inhibitors: adjunct for SSRI- or SNRI-induced sexual dysfunction

ISSUES FOR REFERRAL

Consider referral for CBT, marriage/couples counseling, pelvic floor therapy, or sex therapy.

ADDITIONAL THERAPIES

- Smoking cessation and reduction of alcohol intake
- For childhood trauma: scripting, psychotherapy, cognitive restructuring
- For prescription-drug causes: reduced dosages or change to different medication

COMPLEMENTARY & ALTERNATIVE MEDICINE

- Zestra for women botanical feminine massage oil: Small trial showed increased arousal, desire, genital sensation, ability to have orgasm, and sexual pleasure.
- Yohimbine: not recommended, potentially dangerous
- Ginseng and St. John's wort: no evidence to support treatment of sexual dysfunction

 ONGOING CARE

DIET

Weight reduction if overweight or obese

PATIENT EDUCATION

- American Association of Sexuality Educators, Counselors, and Therapists: www.aasect.org
- National Women's Health Resource Center: www.healthywomen.org
- North American Menopause Society: www.menopause.org
- National Vulvodynia Association: www.nva.org

PROGNOSIS

Lack of desire is most difficult type to treat with <50% success. Treatment is most successful with multidisciplinary approach.

REFERENCES

1. Kingsberg SA, Woodard T. Female sexual dysfunction: focus on low desire. *Obstet Gynecol*. 2015;125(2):477–486.
2. Kingsberg SA, Rezaee RL. Hypoactive sexual desire in women. *Menopause*. 2013;20(12):1284–1300.
3. Wright J, O'Connor K. Female sexual dysfunction. *Med Clin North Am*. 2015;99(3):607–628.
4. Jaspers L, Feys F, Bramer WM, et al. Efficacy and safety of flibanserin for the treatment of hypoactive sexual desire disorder in women: a systematic review and meta-analysis. *JAMA Intern Med*. 2016;176(4):453–462.
5. Nastri CO, Lara LA, Ferriani RA, et al. Hormone therapy for sexual function in perimenopausal and postmenopausal women. *Cochrane Database Syst Rev*. 2013;(6):CD009672.
6. Shifren J, Davis S. Androgens in postmenopausal women: a review. *Menopause*. 2017;24(8):970–979.

ADDITIONAL READING

- American College of Obstetricians and Gynecologists Committee on Practice Bulletins-Gynecology. ACOG Practice Bulletin No. 119: female sexual dysfunction. *Obstet Gynecol*. 2011;117(4):996–1007.
- American Psychiatric Association. *Diagnostic and Statistical Manual of Mental Disorders*. 5th ed. Arlington, VA: American Psychiatric Association; 2013.
- Basson R, Wierman ME, van Lankveld J, et al. Summary of the recommendations on sexual dysfunctions in women. *J Sex Med*. 2010;7(1, Pt 2):314–326.
- Brotto L. Evidence-based treatments for low sexual desire in women. *Front Neuroendocrinol*. 2017;45:11–17.
- Buster JE. Managing female sexual dysfunction. *Fertil Steril*. 2013;100(4):905–915.
- Clayton A, Valladares Juarez E. Female sexual dysfunction. *Psychiatr Clin North Am*. 2017;40(2):267–284.
- Faubion S, Rullo J. Sexual dysfunction in women: a practical approach. *Am Fam Physician*. 2015;92(4):281–288.

- Latif E, Diamond M. Arriving at the diagnosis of female sexual dysfunction. *Fertil Steril*. 2013;100(4):898–904.
- Lorenz T, Rullo J, Faubion S. Antidepressant-induced female sexual dysfunction. *Mayo Clin Proc*. 2016;91(9):1280–1286.
- Nurnberg HG, Hensley PL, Heiman JR, et al. Sildenafil treatment of women with antidepressant-associated sexual dysfunction: a randomized controlled trial. *JAMA*. 2008;300(4):395–404.
- Palacios S. Hypoactive sexual desire disorder and current pharmacotherapeutic options in women. *Womens Health (Lond)*. 2011;7(1):95–107.
- Safarinejad MR. Reversal of SSRI-induced female sexual dysfunction by adjunctive bupropion in menstruating women: a double-blind, placebo-controlled and randomized study. *J Psychopharmacol*. 2011;25(3):370–378.
- Safarinejad MR, Hosseini SY, Asgari MA, et al. A randomized, double-blind, placebo-controlled study of the efficacy and safety of bupropion for treating hypoactive sexual desire disorder in ovulating women. *BJU Int*. 2010;106(6):832–839.
- Shifren JL, Davis SR, Moreau M, et al. Testosterone patch for the treatment of hypoactive sexual desire disorder in naturally menopausal women: results from the INTIMATE NM1 study. *Menopause*. 2006;13(5):770–779.
- Silverstein RG, Brown AC, Roth HD, et al. Effects of mindfulness training on body awareness to sexual stimuli: implications for female sexual dysfunction. *Psychosom Med*. 2011;73(9):817–825.
- Simonelli C, Eleuteri S, Petruccelli F, et al. Female sexual pain disorders: dyspareunia and vaginismus. *Curr Opin Psychiatry*. 2014;27(6):406–412.
- Sungur M, Gündüz A. A comparison of DSM-IV-TR and *DSM-5* definitions for sexual dysfunctions: critiques and challenges. *J Sex Med*. 2014;11(2):364–373.
- Tan O, Bradshaw K, Carr BR. Management of vulvovaginal atrophy-related sexual dysfunction in postmenopausal women: an up-to-date review. *Menopause*. 2012;19(1):109–117.
- Taylor MJ, Rudkin L, Bullemor-Day P, et al. Strategies for managing sexual dysfunction induced by antidepressant medication. *Cochrane Database Syst Rev*. 2013;(5):CD003382.
- Woodis CB, McLendon AN, Muzyk AJ. Testosterone supplementation for hypoactive sexual desire disorder in women. *Pharmacotherapy*. 2012;32(1):38–53.

 CODES

ICD10

- R37 Sexual dysfunction, unspecified
- F52.0 Hypoactive sexual desire disorder
- N94.1 Dyspareunia

CLINICAL PEARLS

- Female sexual dysfunction is a common, complex, multifactorial problem.
- Usually, patients with sexual dysfunction have a normal physical exam.
- Symptoms of sexual dysfunction peak during perimenopause between the ages of 45 and 64 years.
- Combination of behavioral, physical, and medical therapy leads to greater treatment success. There is rarely a simple "fix" with a medication.

SHOULDER PAIN

Terrence C. Tsui, DO • J. Herbert Stevenson, MD

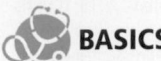 **BASICS**

DESCRIPTION
- Shoulder pain commonly affects patients of all ages.
- Causes include acute trauma, overuse during sports, and activities of everyday living.
- Age plays an important role in determining the etiology of shoulder pain.
- Onset and characteristics of pain, mechanism of injury, weakness, and functional limitation help narrow the differential diagnosis.

EPIDEMIOLOGY
- Shoulder pain accounts for 16% of all musculoskeletal complaints.
- The lifetime prevalence of shoulder pain is ~70%.
- Predominant etiology varies with age:
  - <30 years: shoulder instability
  - 30 to 60 years: rotator cuff (RTC) disorder, impingement syndrome, partial tears
  - >60 years: full-thickness tear, glenohumeral OA

Incidence
The incidence of shoulder pain is 7 to 25 cases per 1,000 patients, with a peak incidence in the 4th to 6th decades.

ETIOLOGY AND PATHOPHYSIOLOGY
Pathology varies with cause:
- Trauma—fracture, dislocation, ligament/tendon tear, acromioclavicular (AC) separation
- Overuse—RTC pathology, biceps tenosynovitis, bursitis, muscle strain, apophyseal injuries
- RTC disorders most commonly result from repetitive overhead activity, leading to RTC impingement with a three-stage progression:
  - Stage I: tendinopathy
  - Stage II: partial RTC tear
  - Stage III: full-thickness RTC tear
- Subacromial bursitis can occur with RTC disorders but is rarely an isolated diagnosis.
- Age related: In pediatric athletes, instability and physeal injuries are more common. With increasing age, the incidence of AC and glenohumeral joint OA, adhesive capsulitis, and RTC tear rises.
- Rheumatologic: rheumatoid arthritis, polymyalgia rheumatica, fibromyalgia
- Referred pain: neck, gallbladder, diaphragm

RISK FACTORS
- Repetitive overhead activity
- Overhead and upper extremity weight-bearing sports (baseball, softball, swimming, tennis, volleyball)
- Weight lifting: AC joint disorders
- Rapid increases in training frequency or load (often associated with improper technique)
- Muscle weakness or imbalance
- Trauma or fall onto the shoulder
- Diabetes, thyroid disorders and other autoimmune diseases, female gender, and age 40 to 60 years are risk factors for adhesive capsulitis.

GENERAL PREVENTION
- Maintain strength and range of motion (ROM).
- Avoid repetitive overhead activities (pitch counts).
- Proper technique (pitching, weight lifting)

DIAGNOSIS

HISTORY
- Pain characteristics location:
  - Superior: AC pathology, trapezius strain
  - Lateral: RTC pathology
  - Anterior: biceps tenosynovitis
  - Diffuse pain: RTC pathology, adhesive capsulitis, glenohumeral OA
- Descriptors:
  - Night pain, worse lying on affected side: RTC pathology, adhesive capsulitis, glenohumeral OA
  - Stiff shoulder, limited ROM: adhesive capsulitis, glenohumeral OA
- Aggravating movements:
  - Cross-body adduction, "scarf test": AC pathology
  - Abduction/external rotation (reaching behind): instability, RTC pathology, glenohumeral OA
  - Overhead activity: RTC pathology, AC pathology, labrum pathology, glenohumeral OA
  - Turning neck, pain past elbow: cervical pathology
- Mechanism of injury
  - Forceful abduction and external rotation: traumatic shoulder instability/dislocation
  - Fall directly onto lateral shoulder: AC joint sprain, clavicular fracture
  - Repetitive overhead activity: RTC pathology
  - Fall on outstretched hand (FOOSH): shoulder separation; forearm/wrist fracture
- Age
  - Shoulder instability (subluxation, dislocation, multidirectional instability) is the most common cause of shoulder pain in young athletes (<30 years old).
  - RTC disorders are the most common cause of shoulder pain in patients >30 years old. Severity of RTC disorder increases with age.
  - Older patients (>60 years old) commonly have OA.
  - Trauma in a young person <40 years is more commonly associated with dislocation/subluxation. In patients >40 years, trauma is more commonly associated with RTC tear.

PHYSICAL EXAM
- Three main joints combine to create the shoulder: glenohumeral, AC, sternoclavicular.
- Four RTC muscles/tendons (SITS): supraspinatus (abduction), infraspinatus (external rotation), teres minor (external rotation, adduction), and subscapularis (adduction, internal rotation)
- Observe face and shoulder movements as patient disrobes, moves arm, and shakes hand.
- Inspect for malalignment, muscle atrophy, asymmetry, erythema, ecchymosis, and swelling. Scapular winging suggests long thoracic nerve or muscular (trapezius, serratus anterior) dysfunction. Prominent scapular spine with scalloped infraspinatus fossa suggests infraspinatus atrophy.
- Palpate SC joint, AC joint, acromion, biceps tendon for tenderness, warmth, bony step-offs.
- Evaluate active AND passive ROM and flexibility.
- Decreased active AND passive ROM is more common with adhesive capsulitis. Normal abduction is to 180 degrees.
- Pain from 60 to 180 degrees suggests subacromial impingement; 120 to 180 degrees suggests AC joint pathology (1).
- Mildly decreased active and/or passive ROM may also indicate glenohumeral OA.
- Decreased active ROM with full passive ROM: RTC pathology
- Evaluate for muscle strength, including grip, biceps, triceps, and deltoid.
- Test RTC strength: supraspinatus (empty can test), infraspinatus/teres minor (resisted external rotation, external lag test), subscapularis (lift-off test, belly press, resisted internal rotation).
- Pain with RTC strength testing indicates RTC pathology. Weakness could suggest tear.
- Special diagnostic tests
  - Neer RTC impingement test: Examiner stabilizes the scapula and internally rotates the patient's arm and forcefully flexes the shoulder through the full ROM or until the patient reports pain.
  - Hawkins RTC impingement test: Examiner forcefully internally rotates the shoulder with the elbow and shoulder flexed to 90 degrees to the end of ROM or until the patient reports pain.
  - Drop-arm test for RTC tear: positive if patient is unable to smoothly control the lowering of their arm or to hold the arm in 90 degrees of abduction
  - Cross-arm adduction is painful in AC joint arthritis.
  - Speed test for biceps tendinopathy: With arm 30 degrees of flexion and palm supinated, patient attempts to flex the elbow against resistance. Pain over biceps is positive.
  - Yergason test for biceps tendinopathy: With the elbow stabilized to the patient's side and flexed to 90 degrees, place the patient's forearm in pronation and resist against supination.
  - Apprehension, relocation test for anterior glenohumeral joint instability: Examiner supports the elbow of the patient and with the other hand holding the wrist, slowly externally rotates the humerus with the shoulder at 90 degrees abduction, patient apprehensive with maneuver.
  - Sulcus sign for inferior glenohumeral joint instability: Examiner pulls down with the hand grasping the subject's elbow, positive if significant inferior movement of the arm, relative to shoulder.
  - O'Brien, clunk test for labral pathology: performed with arm at 90 degrees of flexion, 10 degrees of adduction, thumb pointed down (arm in internal rotation), examiner resists flexion distally. Pain/clicking is positive.
  - Spurling test for cervical pathology: rotation of head toward side of symptoms along with neck extension with applied downward force to reproduce radicular symptoms

DIFFERENTIAL DIAGNOSIS
- Fracture (clavicle, humerus, scapula), contusion
- RTC disorder: impingement, tear, calcific tendonitis
- Subacromial bursitis
- Scapulothoracic dyskinesis
- AC joint pathology (AC separation/OA, osteolysis)
- Biceps tenosynovitis or tear
- Acromial apophysitis or os acromiale
- Glenohumeral joint OA
- Glenohumeral joint instability (acute dislocation or chronic multidirectional instability)

- Adhesive capsulitis
- Labral tear or associated bony pathology
- Muscle strain (trapezius, deltoid, biceps)
- Cervical radiculopathy
- Other: autoimmune, rheumatologic, referred pain, septic joint (biliary/splenic, cardiac, pneumonia/lung mass)

DIAGNOSTIC TESTS & INTERPRETATION

Initial Tests (lab, imaging)

- Shoulder pain can be accurately diagnosed with a careful history and physical exam. Symptoms should be evaluated in the context of the patient as a whole.
- A history of significant trauma, prolonged symptoms, or red flags (older age, fever, rest pain) suggests a need for imaging.
- Adults with nontraumatic shoulder pain of <4 weeks duration may not require initial imaging.
- Plain radiographs are first line:
  - Assess for fracture, degenerative changes, signs of dislocation (Bankart, Hill-Sachs deformity), signs of large RTC tear (sclerosis, proximal migration of humeral head), anatomic deformities contributing to impingement, and masses (tumor, cyst).
  - Standard views: anteroposterior, scapular Y, axillary
- EMG study of the upper extremity may help differentiate referred cervical pain and brachial plexopathy from a primary shoulder disorder.
- Obtain ECG if any suspicion for cardiac etiology.
- Serologic tests if autoimmune etiology is suspected.

Follow-Up Tests & Special Considerations

- CT or MRI can rule out an occult fracture.
- MRI is gold standard for noninvasive soft tissue imaging, including RTC, biceps tendon.
- MR arthrogram may be necessary to assess for labral tears.
- Ultrasound (US) can assess for RTC tears, biceps tendinopathy, and AC joint pathology.
- US is operator dependent but in the hands of a good technician can be equivalent to MRI in detecting full-thickness tears (sensitivity 92%, specificity 94%) and partial-thickness tears (sensitivity 67%, specificity 94%) (1).

Diagnostic Procedures/Other

Consider diagnostic arthroscopy after failing conservative management if structural injury is suspected.

Test Interpretation

- Tendinosis rather than tendonitis is common with stage I impingement.
- Capsular scarring is the hallmark of adhesive capsulitis.
- RTC enthesophytes visualized with calcific tendonitis
- Tear enlargement and pain development in asymptomatic tears are more common with involvement of the dominant shoulder.

 TREATMENT

- Treatment is based on underlying diagnosis.
- In general, conservative therapy includes activity modification, analgesics, and/or anti-inflammatory medicines in association with appropriate rehabilitative programs.
- Physical therapy almost always required for full resolution

MEDICATION

First Line

- Analgesics and anti-inflammatory medications for symptomatic relief include NSAIDs, such as ibuprofen, naproxen, and meloxicam. Acetaminophen may also be used especially if the patient has a history of a GI bleed.
- Corticosteroid injections (subacromial, glenohumeral, AC, subscapular bursa) can be used to acutely relieve pain due to RTC pathology, adhesive capsulitis, OA, or scapulothoracic dyskinesis (2)[A].
- Steroid injections can improve ability to engage in rehabilitative activities.
- US guidance improves accuracy of anatomic placement of corticosteroid injections; long-term outcomes similar between US-guided versus nonguided versus NSAID; use after 6 to 8 weeks.

ISSUES FOR REFERRAL

- If etiology remains unclear, patient is not responsive to conservative care, for complicated or displaced fractures.
- Full-thickness RTC tears >1 cm (acute or chronic) in patients <65 years old or any tear with significant changes in functional status require surgical referral. These tears have a high rate of progression, fatty infiltration, or retraction with nonoperative care (3).

ADDITIONAL THERAPIES

- Physical therapy can benefit persistent RTC disorders, adhesive capsulitis, and shoulder instability.
- Manual therapy and exercises may improve pain and increase function in RTC disease.
- Manual manipulative therapy (MMT) by chiropractors, osteopathic physicians, or physical therapists improves pain with adhesive capsulitis, RTC, and soft tissue disorders. In adhesive capsulitis, MMT is generally less effective than glucocorticoid injections at 6-week mark, but both have similar long-term outcomes. Acupuncture may improve short-term pain and function in RTC impingement (4)[A].

SURGERY/OTHER PROCEDURES

- Surgery is recommended for shoulder pain caused by acute displaced fractures, large RTC tears (criteria as above). It may also be recommended for multiple shoulder dislocation in patients <20 years of age.
- Surgery can be considered for shoulder pain unresponsive to conservative measures >3 to 6 months. Surgery is not more effective than active nonsurgical treatment in impingement syndrome (5)[A].
- Platelet-rich therapies need more conclusive evidence before routine use in treatment of MSK soft tissue injuries.

COMPLEMENTARY & ALTERNATIVE MEDICINE

Acupuncture may help with acute shoulder pain. There is no conclusive evidence for the effectiveness of acupuncture.

 ONGOING CARE

FOLLOW-UP RECOMMENDATIONS

Limit overhead activity to reduce impingement symptoms.

PATIENT EDUCATION

Refer to specific diagnosis for shoulder pain.

PROGNOSIS

Shoulder pain generally has a favorable outcome with conservative care, but recovery can be slow, with 40–50% of patients complaining of persistent pain or recurrence at 12 months.

REFERENCES

1. Greenberg DL. Evaluation and treatment of shoulder pain. *Med Clin North Am*. 2014;98(3):487–504.
2. Gross C, Dhawan A, Harwood D, et al. Glenohumeral joint injections: a review. *Sports Health*. 2013;5(2):153–159.
3. Armstrong A. Evaluation and management of adult shoulder pain: a focus on rotator cuff disorders, acromioclavicular joint arthritis, and glenohumeral arthritis. *Med Clin North Am*. 2014;98(4):755–775.
4. Vas J, Ortega C, Olmo V, et al. Single-point acupuncture and physiotherapy for the treatment of painful shoulder: a multicentre randomized controlled trial. *Rheumatology (Oxford)*. 2008;47(6):887–893.
5. Coghlan JA, Buchbinder R, Green S, et al. Surgery for rotator cuff disease. *Cochrane Database Syst Rev*. 2008;(1):CD005619.

ADDITIONAL READING

- Bodin J, Ha C, Chastang JF, et al. Comparison of risk factors for shoulder pain and rotator cuff syndrome in the working population. *Am J Ind Med*. 2012;55(7):605–615.
- Cheng X, Zhang Z, Xuanyan G, et al. Adhesive capsulitis of the shoulder: evaluation with US-arthrography using a sonographic contrast agent. *Sci Rep*. 2017;7(1):5551.
- Keener JD, Skelley NW, Stobbs-Cucchi G, et al. Shoulder activity level and progression of degenerative cuff disease. *J Shoulder Elbow Surg*. 2017;26(9):1500–1507.
- Littlewood C, Ashton J, Chance-Larsen K, et al. Exercise for rotator cuff tendinopathy: a systematic review. *Physiotherapy*. 2012;98(2):101–109.
- Moraes VY, Lenza M, Tamaoki MJ, et al. Platelet-rich therapies for musculoskeletal soft tissue injuries. *Cochrane Database Syst Rev*. 2014;(4):CD010071.

 CODES

ICD10

- M25.519 Pain in unspecified shoulder
- S43.429A Sprain of unspecified rotator cuff capsule, init encntr
- M19.019 Primary osteoarthritis, unspecified shoulder

CLINICAL PEARLS

- RTC disorders (tendinopathy, tears) are the most common cause of shoulder pain in individuals >30 years of age.
- Shoulder instability (acute dislocation/subluxation or chronic instability) is the most common source of shoulder pain in individuals <30 years of age.
- Patients with diabetes are at increased risk for adhesive capsulitis.
- Most patients do well with a structured program of pain control and rehabilitation.

S

SINUSITIS

Chirag N. Shah, MD, FACEP • Grant Wei, MD

BASICS

DESCRIPTION
- Acute sinusitis is a symptomatic inflammation of ≥1 paranasal sinuses of <4 weeks duration resulting from impaired drainage and retained secretions accompanied by obstruction, facial pain/pressure/fullness, or both. Because rhinitis and sinusitis usually coexist, "rhinosinusitis" is the preferred term.
- Disease is subacute when symptomatic for 4 to 12 weeks, recurrent acute when ≥4 annual episodes without persistent symptoms in between, and chronic when symptomatic for >12 weeks.
- Uncomplicated rhinosinusitis has no extension of inflammation beyond paranasal sinuses and nasal cavity.
- System(s) affected: head/eyes/ears/nose/throat (HEENT), pulmonary

EPIDEMIOLOGY
- Affects 1 in 8 adults accounting for >30 million individuals in the United States each year diagnosed with rhinosinusitis
- Diagnosis of acute bacterial rhinosinusitis remains the fifth leading reason for prescribing antibiotics.
- 0.5–2% of viral rhinosinusitis episodes have a bacterial superinfection.
- Viral cause in 90–98% of cases

Incidence
Incidence is highest in early fall through early spring (related to incidence of viral upper respiratory infection [URI]). Adults have two to three viral URIs per year; 90% of these colds are accompanied by viral rhinosinusitis. It is the fifth most common diagnosis made during family physician visits.

ETIOLOGY AND PATHOPHYSIOLOGY
- Important features
  - Inflammation and edema of the sinus mucosa
  - Obstruction of the sinus ostia
  - Impaired mucociliary clearance
- Secretions that are not cleared become hospitable to bacterial growth.
- Inflammatory response (neutrophil influx and release of cytokines) damages mucosal surfaces.
- Viral: vast majority of cases (rhinovirus; influenza A and B; parainfluenza virus; respiratory syncytial; adeno-, corona-, and enteroviruses)
- Bacterial (complicates 0.5–2% of viral cases)
  - More likely if symptoms worsen within 5 to 6 days after initial improvement
  - No improvement within 10 days of symptom onset
  - >3 to 4 days of fever >102°F and facial pain and purulent nasal discharge
  - *Streptococcus pneumoniae*, *Haemophilus influenzae*, and *Moraxella catarrhalis* are the most common bacterial pathogens.
  - Often overdiagnosed, which leads to overuse of and increasing resistance to antibiotics
  - Methicillin-resistant *Staphylococcus aureus* present in 0–15.9% of patients
- Fungal: seen in immunocompromised hosts (uncontrolled diabetes, neutropenia, use of corticosteroids) or as a nosocomial infection

Genetics
No known genetic pattern

RISK FACTORS
- Viral URI
- Allergic rhinitis
- Asthma
- Cigarette smoking
- Dental infections and procedures
- Anatomic variations
  - Tonsillar and adenoid hypertrophy
  - Turbinate hypertrophy, nasal polyps
  - Cleft palate
- Immunodeficiency (e.g., HIV)
- Cystic fibrosis (CF)

GENERAL PREVENTION
- Hand washing to prevent transmission of viral infection
- Childhood vaccinations up to date
- Avoid close contacts with symptomatic individuals.
- Avoid smoking and exposure to secondhand smoke.

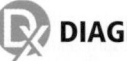

DIAGNOSIS

- History and physical exam suggest and establish the diagnosis but are rarely helpful in distinguishing bacterial from viral causes.
- Use a constellation of symptoms rather than a particular sign or symptom in diagnosis.

HISTORY
- Symptoms somewhat predictive of bacterial sinusitis (1)[C]
  - Worsening of symptoms >5 to 6 days after initial improvement
  - Persistent symptoms for ≥10 days
  - Persistent purulent nasal discharge
  - Unilateral upper tooth or facial pain
  - Unilateral maxillary sinus tenderness
  - Fever
- Associated symptoms
  - Headache
  - Nasal congestion
  - Retro-orbital pain
  - Otalgia
  - Hyposomia
  - Halitosis
  - Chronic cough
- Symptoms requiring urgent attention
  - Visual disturbances, especially diplopia
  - Periorbital swelling or erythema
  - Altered mental status

PHYSICAL EXAM
- Fever
- Edema and erythema of nasal mucosa
- Purulent discharge
- Tenderness to palpation over sinus(es)
- Pain localized to sinuses when bending forward
- Transillumination of the sinuses may confirm fluid in sinuses (helpful if asymmetric; not helpful if symmetric exam).

Pediatric Considerations
- Sinuses are not fully developed until age 20 years. Maxillary and ethmoid sinuses, although small, are present from birth.
- Because children have an average of six to eight colds per year, they are at risk for developing sinusitis.
- Diagnosis can be more difficult than in adults because symptoms are often more subtle.

DIFFERENTIAL DIAGNOSIS
- Dental disease
- CF
- Wegener granulomatosis
- HIV infection
- Kartagener syndrome
- Neoplasm
- Headache, tension, or migraine

DIAGNOSTIC TESTS & INTERPRETATION
Diagnostic tests are not routinely recommended; no diagnostic tests can adequately differentiate between viral and bacterial rhinosinusitis (2)[C].
- None indicated in routine evaluation
- Routine use of sinus radiography discouraged because of the following:
  - ≥3 clinical findings have similar diagnostic accuracy as imaging.
  - Imaging does not distinguish viral from bacterial etiology.
- Limited coronal CT scan can be useful in recurrent infection or failure to respond to medical therapy.

Diagnostic Procedures/Other
Sinus CT if signs suggest extrasinus involvement or to evaluate chronic rhinosinusitis

Test Interpretation
- Inflammation, edema, thickened mucosa
- Impaired ciliary function
- Metaplasia of ciliated columnar cells
- Relative acidosis and hypoxia within sinuses
- Polyps

TREATMENT

Most cases resolve with supportive care (treating pain, nasal symptoms). Antibiotics should be reserved for symptoms that persist >10 days, onset with severe symptoms (high fever, purulent nasal discharge, facial pain) for at least 3 to 4 consecutive days, or worsening signs/symptoms that were initially improving (1,2)[C].

GENERAL MEASURES
- Hydration
- Steam inhalation 20 to 30 minutes TID
- Saline irrigation (Neti pot) or nose drops
- Sleep with head of bed elevated.
- Avoid exposure to cigarette smoke or fumes.
- Avoid caffeine and alcohol.
- Antibiotics are indicated only when findings suggest bacterial infection.
- Analgesics, NSAIDs
- Acute viral sinusitis is self-limiting; antibiotics should not be used.

MEDICATION
First Line
- Decongestants
  - Pseudoephedrine HCl
  - Phenylephrine nasal spray (limited use)
  - Oxymetazoline nasal spray (e.g., Afrin) (not to be used >3 days)
- Analgesics
  - Acetaminophen
  - Aspirin
  - NSAIDs

- Antibiotics
  - Antibiotics can shorten time to cure but only in 5 to 11 people per 100 (3)[A]; most improve without antimicrobial therapy.
  - Reserve antibiotic use for patients with moderate to severe disease.
  - Choice should be based on understanding of antibiotic resistance in the community.
  - Infectious Disease Society of America (IDSA) recommends the following (1)[C]:
    - Start antibiotics as soon as clinical diagnosis of acute bacterial sinusitis is made.
    - Use amoxicillin-clavulanate rather than amoxicillin alone.
    - Amoxicillin-clavulanate 875/125 mg q12h; 2 g orally BID in geographic regions with high rates of resistant *S. pneumoniae*
    - Doxycycline: 100 mg PO BID an alternative to amoxicillin-clavulanate for initial therapy (adults only)
    - Trimethoprim-sulfamethoxazole (TMP/SMX) and 3rd-generation cephalosporins not recommended due to high rate of resistance (1)[C]
    - Treat for 5 to 7 days in adults if uncomplicated bacterial rhinosinusitis (IDSA low-moderate-quality evidence). Treat for 10 to 14 days in children if uncomplicated bacterial rhinosinusitis (IDSA low-moderate-quality evidence).
  - American Academy of Pediatrics recommends the following (1)[C]:
    - Amoxicillin: 45 to 90 mg/kg/day in 2 divided doses if uncomplicated acute bacterial sinusitis in children
    - Amoxicillin-clavulanate: 80 to 90 mg/6.4 mg/kg/day in 2 divided doses for children with severe illness, recent antibiotics, or attending daycare
    - Levofloxacin: 10 to 20 mg/kg/day max 750 mg/day if history of type 1 hypersensitivity to PCN (1)[C]
    - Clindamycin (30 to 40 mg/kg/day) + cefixime (8 mg/kg/day in 2 divided doses) or cefpodoxime (10 mg/kg/day in 2 divided doses) (1)[C] for nontype 1 PCN allergy
    - Ceftriaxone: 50 mg/kg IM single dose if not able to tolerate oral meds (4)[C]
- Because allergies may be a predisposing factor, some patients may benefit from use of the following agents:
  - Oral antihistamines
    - Loratadine (Claritin), fexofenadine (Allegra), cetirizine (Zyrtec), desloratadine (Clarinex), or levocetirizine (Xyzal)
    - Chlorpheniramine (Chlor-Trimeton)
    - Diphenhydramine (Benadryl)
  - Leukotriene inhibitors (Singulair, Accolate), especially in patients with asthma
  - Nasal steroids (i.e., fluticasone [Flonase])

Second Line
- Levofloxacin (Levaquin): 750 mg/day for 5 days or moxifloxacin 400 mg/day for 5 to 7 days (adults only) (1)[C]
- If no response to first-line therapy after 72 hours
  - Broaden antibiotic coverage or switch to a different class; evaluate for resistant pathogens or other causes for treatment failure (i.e., noninfectious etiology); fluoroquinolones as above
- *Note*: Bacteriologic failure rates of up to 20–25% are possible with use of azithromycin and clarithromycin.

- If lack of response to 3 weeks of antibiotics, consider the following:
  - CT scan of sinuses
  - Ear/nose/throat (ENT) referral

ISSUES FOR REFERRAL
Complications or failure of treatment

ALERT
- Meta-analyses have demonstrated no benefit of newer antibiotics over amoxicillin or doxycycline.
- Antibiotics recommendations vary with different guidelines. Patients seen by specialists are different from those in a primary care setting. Patients usually do not have complicated sinusitis in primary care setting.
  - American Academy of Otolaryngology—Head and Neck Surgery Foundation (2)[C] recommends the following:
    - Consider watchful waiting without antibiotics in patients with uncomplicated mild illness (mild pain and temperature <101°F) with assurance of follow-up within 7 days.
- PCV-13 pneumococcal vaccine can be helpful in reducing chronic sinusitis in children (5)[B].
- Use of intranasal steroids small but significant improvement in symptoms when used alone or in combination with antibiotics (6)[A]
- Precautions
  - Decongestants can exacerbate hypertension.
  - Intranasal decongestants should be limited to 3 days to avoid rebound nasal congestion.

Pregnancy Considerations
- Nasal irrigation with saline, pseudoephedrine, most antihistamines, and some nasal steroids are safe during pregnancy and lactation.
- Antibiotics safe in pregnancy and lactation
  - Amoxicillin, amoxicillin-clavulanate, cephalosporins
- Antibiotic contraindicated: doxycycline, fluoroquinolones
- Antibiotic safe in lactation but not pregnancy: levofloxacin

SURGERY/OTHER PROCEDURES
- If medical therapy fails, consider sinus irrigation.
- Functional endoscopic sinus surgery is the preferred treatment for medically recalcitrant cases.
- Absolute surgical indications
  - Massive nasal polyposis
  - Acute complications: subperiosteal or orbital abscess, frontal soft tissue spread of infection
  - Mucocele or mucopyocele
  - Invasive or allergic fungal sinusitis
  - Suspected obstructing tumor
  - CSF rhinorrhea

ADMISSION, INPATIENT, AND NURSING CONSIDERATIONS
Hospitalization for complications (e.g., meningitis, orbital cellulitis or abscess, brain abscess)

 ONGOING CARE

FOLLOW-UP RECOMMENDATIONS
Return if no improvement after 72 hours or no resolution of symptoms after 10 days of antibiotics.

PATIENT EDUCATION
- http://familydoctor.org/familydoctor/en.html
- https://www.nlm.nih.gov/medlineplus/

PROGNOSIS
Alleviation of symptoms within 72 hours with complete resolution within 10 to 14 days

COMPLICATIONS
- Serious complications are rare.
- Meningitis, orbital cellulitis, brain abscess
- Cavernous sinus thrombosis
- Osteomyelitis, subdural empyema

REFERENCES
1. Chow AW, Benninger MS, Brook I, et al; for Infectious Diseases Society of America. IDSA clinical practice guideline for acute bacterial rhinosinusitis in children and adults. *Clin Infect Dis*. 2012;54(8):e72–e112.
2. Rosenfeld RM, Piccirillo JF, Chandrasekhar SS, et al. Clinical practice guideline (update): adult sinusitis. *Otolaryngol Head Neck Surg*. 2015;152(Suppl 2): S1–S39.
3. Lemiengre MB, van Driel ML, Merenstein D, et al. Antibiotics for acute rhinosinusitis in adults. *Cochrane Database Syst Rev*. 2018;(9):CD006089.
4. Wald ER, Applegate KE, Bordley C, et al; for American Academy of Pediatrics. Clinical practice guideline for the diagnosis and management of acute bacterial sinusitis in children aged 1 to 18 years. *Pediatrics*. 2013;132(1):e262–e280.
5. Olarte L, Hulten KG, Lamberth L, et al. Impact of the 13-valent pneumococcal conjugate vaccine on chronic sinusitis associated with *Streptococcus pneumoniae* in children. *Pediatr Infect Dis J*. 2014;33(10):1033–1036.
6. Hayward G, Heneghan C, Perera R, et al. Intranasal corticosteroids in management of acute sinusitis: a systematic review and meta-analysis. *Ann Fam Med*. 2012;10(3):241–249.

ADDITIONAL READING
- Aring AM, Chan MM. Acute rhinosinusitis in adults. *Am Fam Physician*. 2011;83(9):1057–1063.
- Wilson JF. In the clinic. Acute sinusitis. *Ann Intern Med*. 2010;153(5):ITC31–ITC316.

CODES

ICD10
- J01.90 Acute sinusitis, unspecified
- J01.00 Acute maxillary sinusitis, unspecified
- J01.20 Acute ethmoidal sinusitis, unspecified

CLINICAL PEARLS
- When bacterial infection is present, patients recover somewhat more quickly with antibiotics, but the majority will recover with symptomatic treatment alone, and accurate diagnosis of bacterial sinusitis is very difficult.
- Multiple meta-analyses have demonstrated *no* benefit of newer antibiotics over amoxicillin or doxycycline.
- Antibiotic NNT is 10 to 19 for shortening time course, whereas NNH is 8, from medication side effects.
- Significant patient symptom relief with nasal saline spray or drops or irrigation (Neti pot)

S

SJÖGREN SYNDROME

Mariya Milko, DO, MS

 BASICS

- Chronic inflammatory disorder characterized by lymphocytic infiltrates in exocrine organs
- Typically presents with diminished salivary and lacrimal gland function, resulting in sicca symptoms such as dry eyes (xerophthalmia), dry mouth (xerostomia), and parotid enlargement
- Extraglandular manifestations: arthralgia, myalgia, Raynaud phenomenon, pulmonary disease, GI disease, leukopenia, anemia, lymphadenopathy, vasculitis, renal tubular acidosis, lymphoma, CNS involvement with longitudinal transverse myelitis (>4 vertebral segments), and optic neuritis associated with anti–aquaporin-4 antibodies, PNS involvement with small fiber neuropathy
- Primary Sjögren: not associated with other diseases; *HLA-DRB1*0301* and *HLA-DRB1*1501* are the most common.
- Secondary Sjögren: complication of other rheumatologic conditions, most commonly rheumatoid arthritis; associated with HLA-DR4
- First described by Swedish ophthalmologist Henrik Sjögren

EPIDEMIOLOGY

Incidence
Annual incidence: ~4/100,000. Primary Sjögren syndrome (SS) is one of the most common autoimmune diseases, affecting 1–4% of population.
- All races are affected.
- Predominant sex: female > male (9:1)
- Predominant age: can affect patients of any age but is most common in the elderly; onset typically in the 4th to 5th decades of life

Prevalence
SS affects 1 to 4 million people in the United States.

ETIOLOGY AND PATHOPHYSIOLOGY
- Multifactorial systemic autoimmune process characterized by infiltration of glandular tissue by CD4 T lymphocytes
- Theorized that glandular epithelial cells present antigen to the T cells inducing cytokine production. There is also evidence for B-cell activation, resulting in autoantibody production and an increased incidence of B-cell malignancies.
- Etiology is unknown. Estrogen may play a role because SS is more common in women. Exogenous factors such as viral proteins (EBV, HCV, HTLV-1) have also been implicated.

Genetics
- A familial tendency suggests a genetic predisposition.
- Associations in the HLA regions *HLA-DQA1*0501*, *HLA-DQB1*0201*, and *HLA-DRB*0301* are the strongest genetic risk factors for SS.

RISK FACTORS
There are no known modifiable risk factors.

GENERAL PREVENTION
- No known prevention. Complications can be prevented by early diagnosis and treatment.
- Oral health providers play a key role in early detection and management of salivary dysfunction (1)[C].

COMMONLY ASSOCIATED CONDITIONS
Secondary SS associated with rheumatoid arthritis, scleroderma, systemic lupus erythematosus (SLE), polymyositis, HIV, hepatitis C, MCTD, PBC, hyper-gammaglobulinemic purpura, necrotizing vasculitis, autoimmune thyroiditis, chronic active hepatitis, mixed cryoglobulinemia

Pregnancy Considerations
Pregnant SS patients with anti-SSA Abs have increased risk of delivering fetus with skin rash and 3rd-degree heart block.

 DIAGNOSIS

- 2016 ACR/EULAR classification criteria (2)[A]:
  - Based on five objective tests/items
  - Inclusion criteria applicable if the patient is positive for one ocular/oral dryness symptom based on the AECG questions or at least one positive domain from the EULAR SS disease activity index questionnaire and a total score of ≥4 from the following:
    - Positive serum anti-SSA/Ro antibody—3 points
    - Focal lymphocytic sialadenitis with a focus score ≥1 foci/4 mm² from labial salivary gland biopsy—3 points
    - Abnormal ocular staining score of ≥5 or van Bijsterveld score of ≥4—1 point
    - Schirmer test result of ≤5 mm/5 min—1 point
    - An unstimulated salivary flow rate of ≤0.1 mL/min—1 point
- Ocular signs and symptoms
  - Troublesome dry eyes daily for ≥3 months
  - Recurrent sandy/gritty ocular sensation
  - Use of tear substitute ≥3 times per day
- Oral signs and symptoms
  - Daily symptoms of dry mouth for ≥3 months
  - Recurrent feeling of swollen salivary glands
  - Need to drink liquid to help swallow dry foods
- Other manifestations: chronic arthritis, type 1 RTA, tubular interstitial nephritis, rheumatoid arthritis, vasculitis, vaginal dryness, pleuritis, pancreatitis

HISTORY
- Decreased tear production; burning, scratchy sensation in eyes
- Difficulty speaking/swallowing, dental caries, xerotrachea
- Enlarged or intermittent swelling of parotid glands (bilateral)
- Dyspareunia; vaginal dryness
- From consensus criteria and EULAR questionnaire:
  - (1) Have you had daily, persistent, troublesome dry eyes for >3 months?
  - (2) Do you have a recurrent sensation of sand or gravel in the eyes?
  - (3) Do you use tear substitutes >3 times a day?
  - (4) Have you had a daily feeling of dry mouth for >3 months?
  - (5) Do you frequently drink liquids to aid in swallowing dry food?

PHYSICAL EXAM
- Eye exam: dry eyes (keratoconjunctivitis sicca), decreased tear pool in the lower conjunctiva, dilated conjunctival vessels, mucinous threads, and filamentary keratosis (slit-lamp examination)
- Mouth exam: dry mouth (xerostomia); decreased sublingual salivary pool (tongue may stick to the tongue depressor); frequent oral caries (sometimes in unusual locations such as the incisor surface and along the gum line); dark red tongue from prolonged xerostomia
- Ear, nose, and throat exam: parotid enlargement, submandibular enlargement
- Skin exam: nonpalpable or palpable vasculitic purpura (typically 2 to 3 mm in diameter and on the lower extremities)

DIFFERENTIAL DIAGNOSIS
- Causes of ocular dryness: hypovitaminosis A, decreased tear production unrelated to autoimmune process, chronic blepharitis or conjunctivitis, impaired blinking (i.e., due to Parkinson disease or Bell palsy), infiltration of lacrimal glands (i.e., amyloidosis, lymphoma, sarcoidosis), low estrogen levels
- Causes of oral dryness: anticholinergic medications, sialadenitis due to chronic obstruction, chronic viral infections (e.g., hepatitis C or HIV), radiation of head/neck
- Causes of salivary gland swelling: unilateral: obstruction, chronic sialadenitis, bacterial infection, neoplasm; bilateral (asymmetric): IgG4-related disease, HIV; bilateral (symmetric): hepatic cirrhosis, DM, anorexia/bulimia, acromegaly, alcoholism, hypolipoproteinemia, chronic pancreatitis, acute or chronic viral infection (i.e., mumps, Epstein-Barr virus [EBV], coxsackievirus, echovirus, granulomatous diseases (i.e., tuberculosis, sarcoidosis)

DIAGNOSTIC TESTS & INTERPRETATION
- Schirmer test (<5-mm wetness after 5 minutes)
- Rose Bengal test (slit lamp)
- Minor salivary gland biopsy (gold standard)
- Auto antibodies: +ANAs (95%), +RF (75%)
- In primary SS: +anti-Ro (anti-SSA, 56%) and +anti-La (anti-SSB, 30%)

Initial Tests (lab, imaging)
Preliminary lab workup
- Basic labs: CBC with differential, BUN/creatinine (Cr), AST/ALT, ESR, C-reactive protein (CRP), urinalysis
- Special labs: ANA, rheumatoid factor (RF), anti-Ro/SSA, anti-La/SSB, ESR, CRP
- Anti-SSA and anti-SSB antibodies present in 33–74% and 23–52% of SS patients, respectively
- Other autoantibodies-muscarinic type 3 receptor (M3R) and anti-α-fodrin are being explored with good specificity (3)[A].
- Imaging may include:
  - Imaging for xerostomia: salivary gland scintigraphy (insensitive but highly specific)
  - Parotid gland sialography (should not be used in acute parotitis)
  - MRI (correlates well with salivary gland biopsy)
- A novel diagnostic tool is salivary gland US (SGUS), which is noninvasive and highly specific for salivary gland involvement in SS (4)[A].

Diagnostic Procedures/Other
- Salivary gland biopsy: used to confirm suspected diagnosis of SS or to exclude other causes of xerostomia and bilateral glandular enlargement
- Parotid biopsy if malignancy is suspected
- Lymph node biopsy to rule out pseudolymphoma or lymphoma if suspected

Test Interpretation
- Salivary gland histology shows focal collections of lymphocytes; immunocytology shows CD4+ T-cell lymphocyte predominance.
- SGUS parameters include:
  - Parenchymal nonhomogeneity—the most useful diagnostic marker (4)[A]
  - US inflammatory findings include hypoechoic and hyperechoic bands (4)[A].
  - Real-time sonoelastography (RTS) to quantify tissue rigidity and assess glandular damage (4)[A]

 TREATMENT

- Treatment is primarily supportive.
- Treat sicca symptoms—dry eyes, dry mouth.
- Avoid medications that may worsen oral dryness (i.e., anticholinergics).
- Promote good oral hygiene.
- Treat systemic manifestations.
- Address fatigue and pain.

MEDICATION
- Therapy for sicca symptoms: artificial tears and ocular lubricants (5)[C]
- Topical therapy for dry mouth: liberal sips of water, sugar-free lemon drops, or artificial saliva preparations such as Salivart, Saliment, Xero-Lube, MouthKote
- Immunosuppressive therapy such as hydroxychloroquine can be used for systemic symptoms; however, it has not shown any benefit in relieving refractory sicca symptoms.
- Cevimeline (Evoxac) works by stimulating muscarinic cholinergic receptors to increase salivary gland secretion and may be prescribed for SS-associated xerostomia.
- Dry eyes are graded by severity of symptoms, conjunctival injection and staining, corneal damage, tear quality, and lid involvement. Artificial tears may be used; however, artificial tears with hydroxyethylcellulose or dextran are more viscous and can last longer.
- Acetaminophen or NSAIDs for arthralgias

First Line
- Xerostomia: sugar-free lozenges, especially malic acid, artificial saliva; pilocarpine 5 mg PO QID or cevimeline 30 mg PO TID
- Keratoconjunctivitis sicca: artificial tears and ocular lubricants for symptomatic relief, topical cyclosporine (Restasis), or autologous tears

Second Line
- Xerostomia: Interferon-α lozenges may enhance salivary gland flow.
- Keratoconjunctivitis sicca: topical glucocorticoids or topical NSAIDs (Use with caution.)

- Immunosuppressive therapy: antimalarials (e.g., hydroxychloroquine) for arthralgias, lymphadenopathies, and skin manifestations; may then consider methotrexate or cyclosporine, which showed subjective improvement but no significant objective improvement
- Early studies show improvement in fatigue with rituximab (6)[B].
- For life-threatening extraglandular manifestations, cyclophosphamide (PO or IV), mycophenolate mofetil, and azathioprine are often used.

ISSUES FOR REFERRAL
- Rheumatology to help manage systemic manifestations or resistant symptoms
- Oral health
- Ophthalmology for grading of severity and management of xerophthalmia

ADDITIONAL THERAPIES
- Patients should use vaginal lubricants (e.g., Replens) for vaginal dryness. Vaginal estrogen creams can help in postmenopausal women. Be alert for and treat vaginal yeast infections.
- Xerostomia: small sips of water, good dental care
- Keratoconjunctivitis sicca: Conserve tears with side shields or ski/swim goggles, humidifiers, and moist washcloths.
- Dehydroepiandrosterone (DHEA) does not offer improvement in fatigue and well-being above placebo.

SURGERY/OTHER PROCEDURES
Keratoconjunctivitis sicca: If refractory to artificial tears, punctal occlusion is the treatment of choice.

COMPLEMENTARY & ALTERNATIVE MEDICINE
- Some studies show acupuncture benefits saliva production and symptoms of xerostomia.
- There is insufficient evidence to determine the effects of electrostimulation devices on dry mouth symptoms or saliva production in patients with SS.

ADMISSION, INPATIENT, AND NURSING CONSIDERATIONS
May be required for extraglandular manifestations, such as cardiopulmonary disease, renal involvement, and CNS manifestations (e.g., optic neuritis, transverse myelitis, vasculitis, or ischemic stroke)

 ONGOING CARE

FOLLOW-UP RECOMMENDATIONS
Frequency of follow-up depends on severity.

Patient Monitoring
- Monitor for complications, systemic manifestations, and relief of symptoms.
- Medicolegal pitfalls: Monitor for parotid tumor or lymphoma.

PATIENT EDUCATION
In most cases, simple measures are adequate: humidifiers, sips of water, chewing gum, artificial tears.

PROGNOSIS
- Hypocomplementemia is an independent risk factor for premature death.
- Primary SS is associated with increased risks of malignancy, non-Hodgkin lymphoma, and thyroid cancer.

COMPLICATIONS
Complications include dental caries, gum disease, dysphagia, salivary gland calculi, keratitis, conjunctivitis, and scarring of the ocular surface.

REFERENCES
1. Mays JW, Sarmadi M, Moutsopoulos NM. Oral manifestations of systemic autoimmune and inflammatory diseases: diagnosis and clinical management. *J Evid Based Dent Pract.* 2012;12(Suppl 3):265–282.
2. Shiboski CH, Shiboski SC, Seror R, et al; and International Sjögren's Syndrome Criteria Working Group. 2016 American College of Rheumatology/European League Against Rheumatism classification criteria for primary Sjögren's syndrome: a consensus and data-driven methodology involving three international patient cohorts. *Arthritis Rheumatol.* 2017;69(1):35–45.
3. Deng C, Hu C, Chen S, et al. Meta-analysis of anti-muscarinic receptor type 3 antibodies for the diagnosis of Sjögren syndrome. *PLoS One.* 2015;10(1):e0116744.
4. Ferro F, Marcucci E, Orlandi M, et al. One year in review 2017: primary Sjogren's syndrome. *Clin Exp Rheumatol.* 2017;35(2):179–191.
5. Aragona P, Spinella R, Rania L, et al. Safety and efficacy of 0.1% clobetasone butyrate eyedrops in the treatment of dry eye in Sjögren syndrome. *Eur J Ophthalmol.* 2013;23(3):368–376.
6. Meijer JM, Meiners PM, Vissink A, et al. Effectiveness of rituximab treatment in primary Sjögren's syndrome: a randomized, double-blind, placebo-controlled trial. *Arthritis Rheum.* 2010;62(4):960–968.

CODES

ICD10
- M35.00 Sicca syndrome, unspecified
- M35.02 Sicca syndrome with lung involvement
- M35.09 Sicca syndrome with other organ involvement

CLINICAL PEARLS
- Many symptoms of SS can be treated with simple interventions such as artificial tears and sugar-free lozenges.
- Consider lacrimal duct plugs for dry eyes.
- Consider SS in patients with unexplained lung disease and +ANA.
- Patients with primary SS may have an increased incidence of celiac disease.

SLEEP APNEA, OBSTRUCTIVE

Thomas J. Hansen, MD, FAAFP

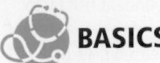 **BASICS**

DESCRIPTION
- Obstructive sleep apnea (OSA) is defined as repetitive episodes of cessation of airflow (apnea) through the nose and mouth during sleep due to obstruction at the level of the pharynx.
  - Apneas often terminate with a snort/gasp.
  - Repetitive apneas produce sleep disruption, leading to excessive daytime sleepiness (EDS).
  - Associated with oxygen desaturation and nocturnal hypoxemia
  - Usual course is chronic.
- System(s) affected: cardiovascular; nervous; pulmonary
- Synonym(s): sleep apnea syndrome; nocturnal upper airway occlusion

EPIDEMIOLOGY
Incidence
- Predominant age: middle-aged men and women
- Predominant sex: male > female (2:1)

Prevalence
- Up to 15% in men, 5% in women
- Prevalence is higher in obese/hypertensive patients.

ETIOLOGY AND PATHOPHYSIOLOGY
OSA occurs when the naso- or oropharynx collapses passively during inspiration. Anatomic and neuromuscular factors contribute to pharyngeal collapse, which leads to hypoxic arousal.
- Anatomic abnormalities, such as increased soft tissue in the palate, tonsillar hypertrophy, macroglossia, and craniofacial abnormalities, predispose the airway to collapse by decreasing the area of the upper airway or increasing the pressure surrounding the airway.
- During sleep, decreased muscle tone in the naso- or oropharynx contributes to airway obstruction and collapse.
- Upper airway narrowing may be due to the following:
  - Obesity, redundant tissue in the soft palate
  - Enlarged tonsils/uvula
  - Low soft palate
  - Large/posteriorly located tongue
  - Craniofacial abnormalities
  - Neuromuscular disorders
  - Alcohol/sedative use before bedtime

RISK FACTORS
- Obesity (strongest risk factor)
- Age >40 years
- Alcohol/sedative intake before bedtime
- Smoking
- Nasal obstruction (due to polyps, rhinitis, or deviated septum)
- Anatomic narrowing of nasopharynx (e.g., tonsillar hypertrophy, macroglossia, micrognathia, retrognathia, craniofacial abnormalities)
- Acromegaly
- Hypothyroidism
- Neurologic syndromes (e.g., muscular dystrophy, cerebral palsy)

GENERAL PREVENTION
Weight control and avoidance of alcohol and sedatives at night can help to prevent airway collapse.

COMMONLY ASSOCIATED CONDITIONS
- Common
  - Hypertension
  - Obesity
  - Daytime sleepiness
  - Metabolic syndrome
- Rare
  - Cardiac arrhythmias
  - Cardiovascular disease
  - Congestive heart failure
  - Pulmonary hypertension
  - Nasal obstructive problems

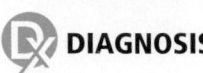 **DIAGNOSIS**

HISTORY
- Elicit a complete history of daytime and nighttime symptoms. Symptoms can be insidious and may have been present for years.
- Daytime symptoms
  - EDS or fatigue (cardinal symptom) (1)
    - Mild symptoms are those that occur during quiet activities (e.g., reading, watching television).
    - More severe symptoms are those that occur during dynamic activities (e.g., work, driving).
  - Tired on morning awakening "nonrestorative sleep"
  - Sore/dry throat
  - Poor concentration, memory problems, irritability, mood changes, behavior problems (in children)
  - Morning headaches
  - Decreased libido
  - Depression
- Nighttime symptoms
  - Loud snoring (present in 60% of people with OSA)
  - Snort/gasp that arouses patient from sleep but not usually to full consciousness
  - Disrupted sleep
  - Witnessed apneic episodes at night
- Screening—the USPSTF found that there is insufficient evidence to screen for OSA in asymptomatic adults or in adults with unrecognized symptoms (2)[A]. The USPSTF found no studies that evaluated the effect of screening for OSA on health outcomes.

PHYSICAL EXAM
- OSA is commonly associated with obesity. It is unlikely to be found in those with normal body weight who do not snore (1).
- Focused head and neck exam
  - Short neck with large circumference
  - Oropharynx
    - Narrowing of the lateral airway wall
    - Tonsillar hypertrophy
    - Macroglossia
    - Micrognathia/retrognathia
    - Soft palate edema
    - Long/thick uvula
    - High, arched hard palate
  - Nasopharynx
    - Deviated nasal septum
    - Poor nasal airflow

DIFFERENTIAL DIAGNOSIS
- Other causes of EDS such as the following:
  - Narcolepsy
  - Idiopathic daytime hypersomnolence
  - Inadequate sleep time
  - Depressive episodes with EDS
  - Periodic limb movements disorder
- Respiratory disorders with nocturnal awakenings such as the following:
  - Asthma
  - Chronic obstructive pulmonary disease
  - Congestive heart failure
- Central sleep apnea (Respiratory effort is absent as compared to OSA where effort is present.)
- Sleep-related choking/laryngospasm
- Gastroesophageal reflux
- Sleep-associated seizures (temporal lobe epilepsy)

DIAGNOSTIC TESTS & INTERPRETATION
Initial Tests (lab, imaging)
- When clinically indicated
  - Thyroid-stimulating hormone to evaluate hypothyroidism
  - CBC to evaluate anemia and polycythemia, which can indicate nocturnal hypoxemia
  - Fasting glucose in obesity to evaluate for diabetes
  - Rare: arterial blood gases to evaluate daytime hypercapnia
- Cephalometric measurements from lateral head and neck radiographs aid in surgical treatment.

Diagnostic Procedures/Other
- The gold standard for OSA is a full-night, in-laboratory polysomnography (PSG), a nighttime sleep study (1)[A].
  - Demonstrates severity of hypoxemia, sleep disruption, and cardiac arrhythmias associated with OSA and elevated end-tidal CO_2
  - Shows repetitive episodes of cessation/marked reduction in airflow despite continued respiratory efforts
  - Apneic episodes must last at least 10 seconds and occur 10 to 15 times per hour and cause decreased oxygen saturation to be considered clinically significant.
  - Complete PSG is expensive, and health insurance may not cover the cost.
- Multiple sleep latency testing is a diagnostic tool used to measure the time it takes from the start of a daytime nap period to the first signs of sleep (sleep latency). It provides an objective measurement of daytime sleepiness.
- The Apnea-Hypopnea Index (AHI) is defined as the total number of apneas and hypopneas divided by the total sleep time in hours.
  - Mild OSA: AHI = 5 to 15
  - Moderate OSA: AHI = 15 to 30
  - Severe OSA: AHI >30
- Split-night PSG (as compared to a full-night PSG) occurs when patients are diagnosed with OSA within the first part of the night and then they can initiate positive pressure device titration during the second half of the night.
- Drugs that may alter the test results include benzodiazepines and other sedatives that can amplify the severity of apnea seen during the sleep study.
- Early data suggest that home-based diagnosis using portable monitoring devices may be an alternative to laboratory-based PSG if the test is of sufficient duration (3)[B].

TREATMENT

- Lifestyle modification is the most frequently recommended treatment for mild to moderate OSA. This includes weight loss, exercise, and avoidance of alcohol, smoking, and sedatives, especially before bedtime.
- Weight loss—shown to decrease the severity of symptoms in obese patients. Lifestyle modifications should be seen as adjunctive rather than curative therapy (4)[A], and a lack of improvement of symptoms with lifestyle modification should not preclude patients from receiving other therapy such as continuous positive airway pressure (CPAP).
- Position changes—if OSA is present only when supine, keep the patient off his or her back when sleeping (e.g., tennis ball worn on back of nightshirt or using a sleep position trainer).
- Positive airway pressure—the most effective therapy for mild, moderate, or severe OSA is CPAP (5)[A]. Treatment with CPAP uses a mask interface and a flow generator to prevent airway collapse, thus helping to prevent apnea, hypoxia, and sleep disturbance. Compared with inactive controls, CPAP significantly improves both objective (24-hour systolic and diastolic blood pressures) and subjective measures (Epworth Sleepiness Scale) in OSA patients with symptoms of daytime sleepiness. CPAP may also decrease the risk for atherosclerosis as well as improves insulin resistance in nondiabetic patients. Early data show that these benefits may not be seen in patients who do not have symptoms of daytime sleepiness.
- Several types of mask interfaces, including nasal masks, oral masks, and nasal pillows exist for CPAP therapy. Short-term data suggest that nasal pillows are the preferred interface in almost all patients. In patients with compliance difficulty, a different choice of interface may be appropriate.
- Oral appliances to treat OSA are available and often subjectively preferred by patients (mandibular advancement devices vs. tongue retaining devices). Although oral appliances have been shown to improve symptoms compared with inactive controls, they are not as effective for reduction of respiratory disturbances as CPAP over short-term data. Treatment with oral appliances may be considered in patients who fail to comply with CPAP therapy.

MEDICATION

Medications are yet to be proven effective in treating OSA. Further studies in this area are needed.

First Line

Some short-term data found fluticasone nasal spray, mirtazapine, physostigmine, and nasal lubricant of some benefit; longer term studies needed

ISSUES FOR REFERRAL

If sleep apnea is suspected, patient should be referred for a sleep study evaluation.

SURGERY/OTHER PROCEDURES

Surgical corrections of the upper airway include alteration of the uvula and/or palate such as uvulopalatopharyngoplasty (UPPP), tracheostomy, and craniofacial surgery. Currently, no evidence supports the use of surgery for the treatment of OSA (6)[A].

ADMISSION, INPATIENT, AND NURSING CONSIDERATIONS

On admission, patients should continue to use CPAP/dental devices if they do so at home. They should bring in their own appliance and know their CPAP settings.

 ONGOING CARE

Lifelong compliance with weight loss or CPAP is necessary for successful OSA treatment.

DIET

Overweight and obese patients should be encouraged to lose weight, and all patients must avoid weight gain. Weight loss alone could reduce symptoms of OSA.

PATIENT EDUCATION

- Weight loss and avoidance of alcohol and sedatives may reduce OSA symptoms particularly in severe cases.
- Significantly sleepy patients should not drive a motor vehicle/operate dangerous equipment.

PROGNOSIS

- EDS is reduced dramatically with appropriate apnea control.
- Lifelong compliance with weight loss or CPAP is necessary for effective treatment of OSA, but long-term adherence is poor.
- If untreated, OSA is progressive.
- Significant morbidity and mortality with OSA usually due to motor vehicle accidents or are secondary to cardiac complications, including arrhythmias, cardiac ischemia, and hypertension; data insufficient on whether identification and treatment changes outcomes

COMPLICATIONS

Untreated OSA may increase the risk for development of hypertension, stroke, myocardial infarction, diabetes, cardiovascular disease, and work-related and driving accidents, but it is unclear that treatment reduces or prevents any of these problems.

Pediatric Considerations

- The prevalence of pediatric OSA is 1–2% in children 4 to 5 years of age, and the peak incidence is between 3 and 6 years of age.
- Predominant sex: male = female
- Etiology: The most common cause is tonsillar hypertrophy. Additional causes are obesity and craniofacial abnormalities. OSA is also seen in children with neuromuscular diseases, such as cerebral palsy and spinal muscular atrophy, due to abnormal pharyngeal muscle control.
- Signs and symptoms
  - Nighttime: loud snoring, restlessness, and sweating
  - Daytime: hyperactivity and decreased school performance
  - EDS is not a significant symptom.
- Diagnosis: Gold standard is PSG. (PSG may be an even better tool in children due to lessened night-to-night variation. There is a lack of studies showing efficacy of home-based diagnostic studies vs. PSG in children.) Abnormal AHI is different in children: >1 to 2 per hour is abnormal.
- Treatment: Surgery is the first-line treatment in cases due to tonsillar enlargement (reduces symptoms in 70%). Some data suggest improved academic performance if tonsillectomy is performed for OSA. For cases due to obesity/craniofacial abnormalities, patients can use CPAP treatment.

Geriatric Considerations

The presence of sleep apnea in the geriatric population may be associated with earlier onset of mild cognitive impairment as well as Alzheimer dementia at an earlier age. The rate of decline of cognitive function may be slowed by the usage of CPAP.

REFERENCES

1. Myers KA, Mrkobrada M, Simel DL. Does this patient have obstructive sleep apnea? The rational clinical examination systematic review. *JAMA*. 2013;310(7):731–741.
2. Bibbins-Domingo K, Grossman DC, Curry SJ, et al; and US Preventive Services Task Force. Screening for obstructive sleep apnea in adults: US Preventive Services Task Force recommendation statement. *JAMA*. 2017;317(4):407–414.
3. Wittine LM, Olson EJ, Morgenthaler TI. Effect of recording duration on the diagnostic accuracy of out-of-center sleep testing for obstructive sleep apnea. *Sleep*. 2014;37(5):969–975.
4. Anandam A, Akinnusi M, Kufel T, et al. Effects of dietary weight loss on obstructive sleep apnea: a meta-analysis. *Sleep Breath*. 2013;17(1):227–234.
5. Giles TL, Lasserson TJ, Smith BH, et al. Continuous positive airways pressure for obstructive sleep apnoea in adults. *Cochrane Database Syst Rev*. 2006;(3):CD001106.
6. Sundaram S, Bridgman SA, Lim J, et al. Surgery for obstructive sleep apnoea. *Cochrane Database Syst Rev*. 2005;(4):CD001004.

ADDITIONAL READING

- Barbé F, Durán-Cantolla J, Sánchez-de-la-Torre M, et al; for Spanish Sleep and Breathing Network. Effect of continuous positive airway pressure on the incidence of hypertension and cardiovascular events in nonsleepy patients with obstructive sleep apnea: a randomized controlled trial. *JAMA*. 2012;307(20):2161–2168.
- Kapur VK, Auckley DH, Chowdhuri S, et al. Clinical practice guideline for diagnostic testing for adult obstructive sleep apnea: an American Academy of Sleep Medicine clinical practice guideline. *J Clin Sleep Med*. 2017;13(3):479–504.
- Lim J, Lasserson TJ, Fleetham J, et al. Oral appliances for obstructive sleep apnoea. *Cochrane Database Syst Rev*. 2006;(1):CD004435.
- Marcus CL, Brooks LJ, Draper KA, et al; for American Academy of Pediatrics. Diagnosis and management of childhood obstructive sleep apnea syndrome. *Pediatrics*. 2012;130(3):576–584.
- Mason M, Welsh EJ, Smith I. Drug therapy for obstructive sleep apnoea in adults. *Cochrane Database Syst Rev*. 2013;(5):CD003002.

 CODES

ICD10
G47.33 Obstructive sleep apnea (adult) (pediatric)

CLINICAL PEARLS

- OSA is characterized by repetitive episodes of apnea often terminating in a snort/gasp.
- Laboratory PSG is the key to diagnosis.
- CPAP is the most effective form of treatment for both mild to moderate and moderate to severe OSA.
- Central sleep apnea may mimic OSA.

S

SLEEP DISORDER, SHIFT WORK

Ronald G. Chambers Jr., MD, FAAFP • Cindy J. Chambers, MD, MAS, MPH

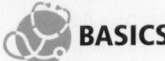 **BASICS**

DESCRIPTION

- Shift work disorder (SWD), classified as a circadian rhythm sleep disorder, is caused by a misalignment between the internal circadian rhythm and the required sleep–wake schedule due to erratic or nighttime shift work (1).
- Diagnostic criteria for SWD require all criteria for circadian rhythm disorder in addition to:
  - Criteria for circadian rhythm disorder:
    - Persistent/recurrent sleep disruption due to either an alteration in the circadian (24-hour) timekeeping system or misalignment between endogenous circadian rhythm and exogenous factors that affect sleep
    - Insomnia/excessive daytime sleepiness or both
    - Impairment in occupational, educational, or social functioning
  - Criteria for SWD:
    - Insomnia/excessive sleepiness, accompanied by reduced sleep time, associated with a recurring work schedule that overlaps with the usual time for sleep
    - Symptoms associated with shift work schedule are present for at least 3 months.
    - Sleep log or actigraphy monitoring (with sleep diaries) for at least 14 days demonstrates disturbed sleep (insomnia) and circadian and sleep-time misalignment.
    - Sleep disturbance is not due to another current sleep disorder, mental disorder, medical disorder, substance use disorder, or medication use.

EPIDEMIOLOGY

Prevalence
- Shift work includes night shifts, evening shifts, or rotating shifts. Approximately 15–25% of the workforce in the United States are shift workers (1).
- SWD has been estimated to affect 10–23% of 22 million American shift workers, with a prevalence estimate of approximately 2–5% of the general population (14% night shift workers and 8% of rotating shift workers) (2).

PATHOPHYSIOLOGY
- Circadian rhythms are present in multiple biologic functions, including body temperature, hormone levels, blood pressure, metabolism, cellular regeneration, sleep–wake cycles, and DNA transcription and translation (1).
- Transcription factors involved in circadian rhythms (the "molecular clock") control production of many proteins expressed with a periodicity of approximately 24 hours. This molecular clock is self-sustaining and requires a daily reset or it may become out of sync with environmental cues (zeitgebers) (1).
- The most powerful *zeitgeber* (timekeeper) is light. Light transmitted from the retinohypothalamic tract of the eye to the SCN of the hypothalamus upregulates the production of the "clock gene" (PER) (1).

- Periods of darkness cause the SCN to induce melatonin release from the pineal gland, which can also help to reset the molecular clock (1).
- A dyssynchrony between the endogenous molecular clock and external cues (most notably light/dark cycles) is responsible for circadian rhythm disorders and can impact both physical and mental health (1).

RISK FACTORS
- Shift work, including night shifts, early morning shifts, or rotating shifts
- Younger age and "eveningness" (a.k.a. "night owls") may protect against the development of SWD (1).

Genetics
No genetic predisposition has been described.

GENERAL PREVENTION
- Limit rotating shifts.
- Use bright light during shifts.
- Schedule brief (10- to 20-minute) naps during shifts, if possible.

COMMONLY ASSOCIATED CONDITIONS
- Shift workers often have impaired immediate free recall, decreased processing speed, and selective attention impairments that may worsen with longer duration of shift work (1).
- Shift workers also have a higher risk of vehicular accidents, job-related injuries, absenteeism, and quality control errors (1).
- SWD has been associated with gastrointestinal (GI) disease, specifically peptic ulcer disease, cardiovascular disease (CVD), ischemic stroke, infertility, mood disorders, and pregnancy complications (1,3).
- There is also a possible increased risk of breast and prostate cancer. The International Agency for Research on Cancer (IARC) has classified shift work involving a circadian disruption as a probable carcinogen (4).

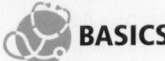 **DIAGNOSIS**

Primarily a clinical diagnosis. There are some useful diagnostic aids.

HISTORY
- A careful history is critical. Assess for difficulty falling asleep, staying asleep, or nonrestorative sleep.
- Note the following in particular (5)[C]:
  - Sleep/wake habits
  - Degree of alertness or sleepiness
  - Sleep environment
  - Light exposure before, during, and after the shift
  - Job-related factors: length of shift, number of consecutive shifts, commute after shift
  - Medications and over-the-counter (OTC) stimulants such as caffeine or energy drinks
  - Impact on social and domestic responsibilities (including drowsy driving)

- Evaluate for symptoms of other sleep disorders, which often coexist and can exacerbate SWD such as the following:
  - Loud snoring and pauses in breathing during sleep (obstructive sleep apnea [OSA])
  - Sudden sleep attacks and leg symptoms (restless legs syndrome [RLS])
  - Falling asleep at inappropriate times, drop attacks, and daytime fatigue (narcolepsy)

PHYSICAL EXAM
Evaluate for depression, GI disease, CVD, and potential cancer risk as well as signs of OSA such as obesity, a large neck, and a tight oropharynx (5)[C].

DIFFERENTIAL DIAGNOSIS
- Other primary sleep disorders: OSA, RLS, narcolepsy, and psychophysiologic insomnia
- Other circadian rhythm sleep disorders such as delayed sleep phase disorder or jet lag syndrome. Distinguishing among these can be challenging.

DIAGNOSTIC TESTS & INTERPRETATION
Given possible increased risk; screen for CVD and cancer among shift workers.

Initial Tests (lab, imaging)
Fasting lipid panel, fasting glucose, age-appropriate cancer screenings

Diagnostic Procedures/Other
- A sleep/wake diary recording the patient's sleep/wake habits, amount of sleep, naps during waking hours, and mood (1 to 2 weeks) (5)[C]
- Actigraphy (a mechanical device, often worn on the arm/leg, to measure movement) serves as a gross measure of time and amount of activity and rest (5)[C].
- Polysomnography measures sleep duration and quality. It is not typically used to diagnose SWD but may help rule out other sleep/wake disorders, such as sleep apnea and narcolepsy (1)[C].
- Other diagnostic tools are available, including the Multiple Sleep Latency Test (MSLT), the Morningness-Eveningness Questionnaire (MEQ), and the Epworth Sleepiness Scale (ESS) (1)[C].

Test Interpretation
Sleep diaries and actigraphy data often reveal:
- Increased sleep latency
- Decreased total sleep time
- Frequent awakenings
- Most people revert to nocturnal sleeping on their days off. Every workweek, they must "start over" to shift circadian rhythms to align with work schedules.

TREATMENT

- The only therapeutic modality recommended by the American Academy of Sleep Medicine is planned (prescribed) sleep schedules (6)[C].
- Other commonly used strategies include sleep hygiene optimization, bright light, melatonin, caffeine, other stimulants, hypnotics, and medication sleep aids (discussed below).

GENERAL MEASURES

- Sleep hygiene: An important first step in approaching the treatment of sleep disorders is proper sleep hygiene. This includes minimizing exposure to bright light before and during scheduled sleep periods (maintain a dark sleeping space, wear dark sunglasses following work shift, wear an eye mask to sleep), maintain a quiet sleep environment (wear ear plugs to sleep, disconnect phone/doorbell), retrain core body temperature to shifted sleep–wake schedule (maintain cool sleeping quarters), and avoid use of stimulants during second half of work shift (1)[C].
- Sleep time: protected time for sleep prior to and following work shifts with strategic naps where possible (5)[C]
- Work/social/domestic factors: Treat psychosocial stress, depression; encourage healthy eating habits; limit substance use; increase exercise to at least 30 minutes 5 times per week (not within 2 to 4 hours of bedtime) (5)[C].
- Work-related interventions: If possible, reduce number of consecutive shifts (<4) or reduce shift duration (<12 hours), allow adequate time between shifts (>11 hours), move heavy workload outside circadian nadir (04:00 to 07:00) (5)[C].
- Bright light: Several studies demonstrate that timed bright light and darkness promote adaptation to night work (7)[C].
- Bright light therapy with conventional light/light boxes (10,000 lux preferable, but >1,000 lux will help) 30 min/day during the night/early morning shift prior to the nadir of the core body temperature rhythm

MEDICATION

Sleep-promoting medications:

- Melatonin may help shift circadian rhythms and can increase the quality and duration of sleep as well as increase alertness during the work shift.
- Ramelteon (Rozerem), a melatonin receptor agonist, is not FDA-approved for treating SWD but may be helpful in improving daytime sleep (1)[C].
- Antidepressants: Doxepin (tricyclic) and trazodone are FDA-approved for the treatment of insomnia. Given at low doses, doxepin and trazodone can improve sleep without residual daytime impairment (1)[C].

- Intermediate-acting hypnotics such as zolpidem (Ambien) or eszopiclone (Lunesta) can cause post-sleep sedation (1)[C]. Long-term use is discouraged due to potential for tolerance/dependence.
- Suvorexant (Belsomra) is an orexin receptor antagonist approved for the treatment of insomnia.
- Wakefulness-promoting medications:
  – Modafinil (Provigil) and armodafinil (Nuvigil) are FDA-approved for excessive sleepiness in patients with SWD and can reduce daytime sleepiness and improve cognitive performance (1)[C].
  – Prophylactic caffeine use immediately prior to work shift and during work shift (5)[C]

First Line
Circadian shift/sleep promoting: melatonin 3 mg PO or sublingual, 30 minutes before daytime sleep period. Take only when the patient is home and able to go to bed (1)[C].

Second Line
- Wakefulness promoting:
  – Modafinil initially 200 mg PO 1 hour prior to work shift
  – Armodafinil 150 mg PO 1 hour prior to work shift; long-acting (12 to 16 hours, depending on food intake) use judiciously in SWD to impede a patient's ability to sleep after the shift
- Sleep promoting:
  – Nonbenzodiazepine hypnotics:
    ○ Zolpidem 5 to 10 mg or eszopiclone 1 to 3 mg immediately prior to bed; suvorexant 10 to 20 mg PO 30 minutes prior to bed
  – Antidepressants
    ○ Doxepin (3 to 6 mg) and trazodone (25 to 150 mg), 1 to 2 hours prior to bed (1)[C]
  – Benzodiazepines: Estazolam, flurazepam, quazepam, temazepam, and triazolam are FDA-approved for the treatment of insomnia. Due to high risk of tolerance/withdrawal, use cautiously for short-term treatment of insomnia (1)[C].
  – In general, hypnotics may improve daytime sleep but do not appear to improve sleep maintenance or nighttime alertness. They may also cause residual sedation during work hours. This may worsen SWD symptoms (1)[C].

ISSUES FOR REFERRAL
Refer to a sleep specialist for suspicion of other primary sleep disorders or dependence on hypnotics, alcohol, or stimulants.

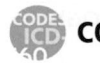

ONGOING CARE

PATIENT EDUCATION
- Discuss sleep hygiene and optimizing the sleep environment.
- Shift workers who need to sleep in the daytime should ensure a cool, dark, and quiet sleep environment.
- Reserve bedroom for sleeping and intimacy only. Remove televisions, cell phones, tablets, and laptop computers from the bedroom.

- When going to sleep, turn clock away from bed and discourage prolonged reading in bed.
- Blackout shades help achieve the proper darkness.

REFERENCES
1. Morrissette DA. Twisting the night away: a review of the neurobiology, genetics, diagnosis, and treatment of shift work disorder. *CNS Spectr*. 2013;18(Suppl 1):45–54.
2. Roth T. Appropriate therapeutic selection for patients with shift work disorder. *Sleep Med*. 2012;13(4):335–341.
3. Vyas MV, Garg AX, Iansavichus AV, et al. Shift work and vascular events: systematic review and meta-analysis. *BMJ*. 2012;345:e4800.
4. Stevens RG, Hansen J, Costa G, et al. Considerations of circadian impact for defining "shift work" in cancer studies: IARC Working Group Report. *Occup Environ Med*. 2011;68(2):154–162.
5. Wright KP Jr, Bogan RK, Wyatt JK. Shift work and the assessment and management of shift work disorder (SWD). *Sleep Med Rev*. 2013;17(1):41–54.
6. American Academy of Sleep Medicine. *International Classification of Sleep Disorders*. 3rd ed. Darien, IL: American Academy of Sleep Medicine; 2014.
7. Bjorvatn B, Pallesen S. A practical approach to circadian rhythm sleep disorders. *Sleep Med Rev*. 2009;13(1):47–60.

ADDITIONAL READING
- Sleep Diary: http://www.helpguide.org/life/pdfs/sleep_diary.pdf
- Vanttola P, Härmä M, Viitasalo K, et al. Sleep and alertness in shift work disorder: findings of a field study [published online ahead of print December 3, 2018]. *Int Arch Occup Environ Health*. doi:10.1007/s00420-018-1386-4.

CODES

ICD10
G47.26 Circadian rhythm sleep disorder, shift work type

CLINICAL PEARLS
- SWD is associated with shortened and disturbed sleep, increased fatigue, decreased alertness, cognitive decrements, increased injury and accident rates, reproductive problems, and increased cardiovascular and GI disease.
- SWD has been classified as a probable carcinogen (possible association with breast and prostate cancer).
- The first diagnostic step in SWD is to obtain and evaluate an accurate sleep diary.
- Appropriate sleep hygiene is the initial step in treatment.

S

SMELL AND TASTE DISORDERS

Beth K. Mazyck, MD • Daniel B. Kurtz, PhD, BS

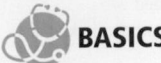 **BASICS**

DESCRIPTION
- The senses of smell and taste allow a full appreciation of the flavor and palatability of foods and also serve as a warning system against toxins, polluted air, smoke, and spoiled food.
- Physiologically, the chemical senses aid in normal digestion by triggering GI secretions. Smell/taste dysfunction may have a significant impact on quality of life.
- Loss of smell occurs more frequently than loss of taste, and patients frequently confuse the concepts of flavor loss (as a result of smell impairment) with taste loss (an impaired ability to sense sweet, sour, salty, or bitter).
- Smell depends on the functioning of CN I (olfactory nerve) and CN V (trigeminal nerve).
- Taste depends on the functioning of CNs VII, IX, and X. Because of these multiple pathways, total loss of taste (ageusia) is rare.
- Systems affected: nervous, upper respiratory

EPIDEMIOLOGY
Incidence
There are ~200,000 patient visits a year for smell and taste disturbances.

Prevalence
- Predominant sex: male > female. Men begin to lose their ability to smell earlier in life than women.
- Predominant age: Chemosensory loss is age dependent:
  - Age >80 years: 80% have major olfactory impairment; nearly 50% are anosmic.
  - Ages 65 to 80 years: 60% have major olfactory impairment; nearly 25% are anosmic.
  - Age <65 years: 1–2% have smell impairment.
- Estimated >2 million affected in the United States

ETIOLOGY AND PATHOPHYSIOLOGY
- Smell and/or taste disturbances:
  - Nutritional factors (e.g., malnutrition, vitamin deficiencies, liver disease, pernicious anemia)
  - Endocrine disorders (e.g., thyroid disease, diabetes mellitus, renal disease)
  - Head trauma
  - Migraine headache (e.g., gustatory aura, olfactory aura)
  - Sjögren syndrome
  - Toxic chemical exposure
  - Industrial agent exposure
  - Aging
  - Medications (see below)
  - Neurodegenerative diseases (e.g., multiple sclerosis, Alzheimer disease, cerebrovascular accident, Parkinson disease)
  - Infections (e.g., upper respiratory infection [URI], oral and perioral infections, candidiasis, coxsackievirus, AIDS, viral hepatitis, herpes simplex virus)

- Possible causes of smell disturbance:
  - Nasal and sinus disease (e.g., allergies, rhinitis, rhinorrhea, URI)
  - Cigarette smoking
  - Cocaine abuse (intranasal)
  - Hemodialysis
  - Radiation treatment of head and neck
  - Congenital conditions
  - Neoplasm (e.g., brain tumor, nasal polyps, intranasal tumor)
  - Systemic lupus erythematosus (SLE)
  - Bell palsy
  - Oral/perioral skin lesion
  - Damage to CN I/V
  - Possible association with psychosis and schizophrenia
- Possible causes of taste loss:
  - Oral appliances
  - Dental procedures
  - Intraoral abscess
  - Gingivitis
  - Damage to CN VI, IX, or X
  - Stroke (especially frontal lobe)
- Selected medications that reportedly alter smell and taste:
  - Antibiotics: amikacin, ampicillin, azithromycin, ciprofloxacin, clarithromycin, doxycycline, griseofulvin, metronidazole, ofloxacin, tetracycline, terbinafine, β-lactamase inhibitors
  - Anticonvulsants: carbamazepine, phenytoin
  - Antidepressants: amitriptyline, doxepin, imipramine, nortriptyline
  - Antihistamines and decongestants: zinc-based cold remedies (Zicam)
  - Antihypertensives and cardiac medications: acetazolamide, amiloride, captopril, diltiazem, hydrochlorothiazide, nifedipine, propranolol, spironolactone
  - Anti-inflammatory agents: auranofin, gold, penicillamine
  - Antimanic drugs: lithium
  - Antineoplastics: cisplatin, doxorubicin, methotrexate, vincristine
  - Antiparkinsonian agents: levodopa, carbidopa
  - Antiseptic: chlorhexidine
  - Antithyroid agents: methimazole, propylthiouracil
  - Lipid-lowering agents: statins

Genetics
May be related to underlying genetically associated diseases (Kallmann syndrome, Alzheimer disease, and other neurodegenerative disorders, migraine syndromes, rheumatologic conditions, endocrine disorders)

RISK FACTORS
- Age >65 years
- Poor nutritional status
- Smoking tobacco products

GENERAL PREVENTION
- Eat a well-balanced diet, with appropriate vitamins and minerals.
- Maintain good oral and nasal health, with routine visits to the dentist.
- Do not smoke tobacco products.
- Avoid noxious chemical exposures/unnecessary radiation.

Geriatric Considerations
- Elders are at particular risk of eating spoiled food or inadvertently being exposed to natural gas leaks owing to anosmia from aging.
- Anosmia also may be an early sign of degenerative disorders and has been shown to predict increased 5-year mortality (1)[B].

Pediatric Considerations
- Smell and taste disorders are uncommon in children in developed countries.
- In developing countries with poor nutrition (particularly zinc depletion), smell and taste disorders may occur.
- Delayed puberty in association with anosmia (± midline craniofacial abnormalities, deafness, or renal abnormalities) suggests the possibility of Kallmann syndrome (hypogonadotropic hypogonadism).

Pregnancy Considerations
- Pregnancy is an uncommon cause of smell and taste loss or disturbances.
- Many women report increased sensitivity to odors during pregnancy as well as an increased dislike for bitterness and a preference for salty substances.

COMMONLY ASSOCIATED CONDITIONS
URI, allergic rhinitis, dental abscesses

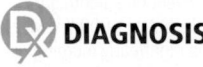 **DIAGNOSIS**

Smell and taste disturbances are symptoms; it is essential to look for possible underlying causes.

HISTORY
- Symptoms of URI, environmental allergies
- Oral pain, other dental problems
- Cognitive/memory difficulties
- Current medications
- Nutritional status, ovolactovegetarian
- Weight loss or gain
- Frequent infections (impaired immunity)
- Worsening of underlying medical illness
- Increased use of salt and/or sugar to increase taste of food
- Neurodegenerative disease

PHYSICAL EXAM
Thorough HEENT exam

DIFFERENTIAL DIAGNOSIS
- Epilepsy (gustatory aura)
- Epilepsy (olfactory aura)
- Memory impairment
- Psychiatric conditions

DIAGNOSTIC TESTS & INTERPRETATION
Initial Tests (lab, imaging)
Consider (Not all patients require all tests.)
- CBC
- Liver function tests
- Blood glucose
- Creatinine
- Vitamin B_{12} level
- Thyroid-stimulating hormone (TSH)
- Serum IgE
- CT scanning is the most useful and cost-effective technique for assessing sinonasal disorders and is superior to an MRI in evaluating bony structures and airway patency. Coronal CT scans are particularly valuable in assessing paranasal anatomy (2)[B].

Follow-Up Tests & Special Considerations
Diagnosis of smell and taste disturbances is usually possible through history; however, the following tests can be used to confirm:
- Olfactory tests
  - Smell identification test: evaluates the ability to identify 40 microencapsulated scratch-and-sniff odorants (3)[B]
  - Brief smell identification test (4)[B]
  - Taste tests (more difficult because no convenient standardized tests are presently available): Solutions containing sucrose (sweet), sodium chloride (salty), quinine (bitter), and citric acid (sour) are helpful.
  - An MRI is useful in defining soft tissue disease; therefore, a coronal MRI is the technique of choice to image the olfactory bulbs, tracts, and cortical parenchyma; possible placement of an accessory coil (TMJ) over the nose to assist in imaging

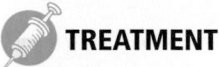 TREATMENT

GENERAL MEASURES
- Appropriate treatment for underlying cause
- Quit smoking (5)[B].
- Treatment of underlying nasal congestion with nasal decongestants and/or nasal/oral steroids (6)[B]
- Surgical correction of nasal blockage/nasal polyps
- Some drug-related smell or taste loss or dysgeusias can be reversed with cessation of the offending medication, but it may take many months.
- Stop repeated oral trauma (e.g., appliances, tongue-biting behaviors).
- Proper nutritional and dietary assessment (2)[C]
- Formal dental evaluation

MEDICATION
- Treat underlying causes as appropriate. Idiopathic cases will often resolve spontaneously.
- Consider trial of corticosteroids topically (e.g., fluticasone nasal spray daily to BID) and/or systemically (e.g., oral prednisone 60 mg daily for 5 to 7 days) (6)[B].
- Zinc and vitamins (A, B complex) when deficiency is suspected

ISSUES FOR REFERRAL
- Consider referral to an otolaryngologist or neurologist for persistent cases.
- Referral to a subspecialist at a regional smell and taste center when complex etiologies are suspected

SURGERY/OTHER PROCEDURES
If needed for treatment of underlying cause

 ONGOING CARE

DIET
- Weight gain/loss is possible because the patient may reject food or may switch to calorie-rich foods that are still palatable.
- Ensure a nutritionally balanced diet with appropriate levels of nutrients, vitamins, and essential minerals.

PATIENT EDUCATION
- Caution patients not to overindulge as compensation for the bland taste of food. For example, patients with diabetes may need help in avoiding excessive sugar intake as an inappropriate way of improving food taste.
- Patients with chemosensory impairments should use measuring devices when cooking and should not cook by taste.
- Optimizing food texture, aroma, temperature, and color may improve the overall food experience when taste is limited.
- Patients with permanent smell dysfunction must develop adaptive strategies for dealing with hygiene, appetite, safety, and health.
- Natural gas and smoke detectors are essential; check for proper function frequently.
- Check food expiration dates frequently; discard old food.

PROGNOSIS
- In general, the olfactory system regenerates poorly after a head injury. Most patients who recover smell function following head trauma do so within 12 weeks of injury.
- Patients who quit smoking typically recover improved olfactory function and flavor sensation.
- Many taste disorders (dysgeusias) resolve spontaneously within a few years of onset.
- Phantosmias that are flow dependent may respond to surgical ablation of olfactory mucosa.
- Conditions such as radiation-induced xerostomia and Bell palsy generally improve over time.

COMPLICATIONS
- Permanent loss of ability to smell/taste
- Psychiatric issues with dysgeusias and phantosmia

REFERENCES
1. Pinto JM, Wroblewski KE, Kern DW, et al. Olfactory dysfunction predicts 5-year mortality in older adults. *PLoS One*. 2014;9(10):e107541.
2. Malaty J, Malaty IA. Smell and taste disorders in primary care. *Am Fam Physician*. 2013;88(12):852–859.
3. Doty RL, Shaman P, Dann M. Development of the University of Pennsylvania Smell Identification Test: a standardized microencapsulated test of olfactory function. *Physiol Behav*. 1984;32(3):489–502.
4. Jackman AH, Doty RL. Utility of a three-item smell identification test in detecting olfactory dysfunction. *Laryngoscope*. 2005;115(12):2209–2212.
5. Frye RE, Schwartz BS, Doty RL. Dose-related effects of cigarette smoking on olfactory function. *JAMA*. 1990;263(9):1233–1236.
6. Seiden AM, Duncan HJ. The diagnosis of a conductive olfactory loss. *Laryngoscope*. 2001;111(1):9–14.

ADDITIONAL READING
- Cowart BJ. Taste dysfunction: a practical guide for oral medicine. *Oral Dis*. 2011;17(1):2–6.
- Naik BS, Shetty N, Maben EV. Drug-induced taste disorders. *Eur J Intern Med*. 2010;21(3):240–243.
- Olsson P, Stjärne P. Endoscopic sinus surgery improves olfaction in nasal polyposis, a multi-center study. *Rhinology*. 2010;48(2):150–155.
- Tuccori M, Lapi F, Testi A, et al. Drug-induced taste and smell alterations: a case/non-case evaluation of an Italian database of spontaneous adverse drug reaction reporting. *Drug Saf*. 2011;34(10):849–859.

 CODES

ICD10
- R43.9 Unspecified disturbances of smell and taste
- R43.1 Parosmia
- R43.2 Parageusia

CLINICAL PEARLS
- Smell disorders are often mistaken as decreased taste by patients.
- Most temporary smell loss is due to nasal passage obstruction.
- Actual taste disorders are often related to dental problems or medication side effects.
- Gradual smell loss is very common in the elderly; extensive workup in this population may not be indicated if no associated signs/symptoms are present but may be predictive of 5-year mortality.

SOMATIC SYMPTOM (SOMATIZATION) DISORDER

William G. Elder, PhD

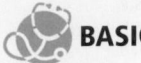

BASICS

DESCRIPTION

- Somatic symptom disorders (SSD) are a pattern of one or more somatic symptoms recurring or persisting for >6 months that are distressing or result in significant disruption of daily life.
- Designation of a symptom as somatic means that it appears to be physical problem or complaint yet is medically unexplained
- Conceptualization and diagnostic criteria for somatic symptom presentations were significantly modified with the advent of *DSM-5*. SSD is similar in many aspects to the former somatization disorder, which required presentation with multiple physical complaints. No longer based on symptoms counts; current diagnosis is based on the way the patient presents and perceives his or her symptoms.
- SSD now includes most presentations that would formerly be considered hypochondriasis. Hypochondriasis has been replaced by illness anxiety disorder, which is diagnosed when the patient presents with significant preoccupation with having a serious illness in the absence of illness-related somatic complaints.
- Somatization increases disability independent of comorbidity, and individuals with SSD have health-related functioning that is 2 standard deviations below the mean.
- Symptoms may be specific (e.g., localized pain) or relatively nonspecific (e.g., fatigue).
- Symptoms sometimes may represent normal bodily sensations or discomfort that does not signify serious disease.
- Suffering is authentic. Symptoms are not intentionally produced or feigned.
- SSDs are sometimes referred to as "functional disorders" to denote their nonphysical basis.

EPIDEMIOLOGY

Incidence

- Usually, first symptoms appear in adolescence.
- Predominant sex: female > male (10:1)
- Type and frequency of somatic complaints may differ among cultures, so symptom reviews should be adjusted based on culture; more frequent in cultures without Western/empirical explanatory models

Prevalence

- Expected 2% among women and <0.2% among men
- Somatization seen in up to 29% of patients presenting to primary care offices
- Somatic concerns may increase, but other features of the presentation decrease such that prevalence declines after age 65 years.

ETIOLOGY AND PATHOPHYSIOLOGY

Patients with SSD demonstrate different patterns of heart rate variability. Although this cannot be used to clinically, it does point to the differences in psychophysiology of SSD.

Genetics

Consanguinity studies and single nucleotide polymorphism genotyping indicate that both genetic and environmental factors contribute to the risk of SSD.

RISK FACTORS

- Child abuse, particularly sexual abuse, has been shown to be a risk factor for somatization.
- Symptoms begin or worsen after losses (e.g., job, close relative, or friend).
- Greater intensity of symptoms often occurs with stress.

COMMONLY ASSOCIATED CONDITIONS

Comorbid with other psychiatric conditions is yet to be determined but is likely to be 20–50% with anxiety, depression, or personality disorders.

DIAGNOSIS

- Determining that a somatic symptom is medically unexplained is unreliable, and it is inappropriate to diagnose a mental disorder solely because a medical diagnosis is not demonstrated. Rely on symptoms and presentation rather than ruling out medical causes in making the SSD diagnosis.
- Illness anxiety and somatic distress are independent but often co-occur.

HISTORY

- One or more somatic complaints, with sometimes a grossly positive review of symptoms
- SSD involves patient unrealistic thoughts, feelings, or behaviors associated with symptoms or associated health concerns manifested by at least one of the following:
  - Disproportionate and persistent thoughts about the seriousness of the symptoms
  - Persistent high level of anxiety about health or symptoms
  - Excessive time or energy devoted to symptoms or health concerns
- Diagnoses no longer rely on symptom counts, but common symptoms include:
  - Pain symptoms related to different sites such as head, abdomen, back, joints, extremities, chest, or rectum, or related to body functions such as menstruation, sexual intercourse, or urination
  - GI symptoms such as nausea, bloating, vomiting (not during pregnancy), diarrhea, intolerance of several foods

- Sexual symptoms such as indifference to sex, difficulties with erection or ejaculation, irregular menses, excessive menstrual bleeding, or vomiting throughout all 9 months of pregnancy
- Pseudoneurologic symptoms such as impaired balance or coordination, weak or paralyzed muscles, lump in throat or trouble swallowing, loss of voice, retention of urine, hallucinations, numbness (to touch or pain), double vision, blindness, deafness, seizures, amnesia or other dissociative symptoms, loss of consciousness (other than with fainting); none of these is limited to pain.
- Patients with SSD frequently use alternative treatments, which should be explored for their effects on health and physical functioning.

PHYSICAL EXAM

Physical exam remarkable for absence of objective findings to explain the many subjective complaints

DIFFERENTIAL DIAGNOSIS

- Other psychiatric illnesses must be ruled out:
  - Depressive disorders
  - Anxiety disorders
  - Schizophrenia
  - Other somatic disorders: illness anxiety disorder, conversion disorder
  - Factitious disorder
  - Body dysmorphic disorder
- Malingering
- General medical conditions, with vague, multiple, confusing symptoms, must be ruled out.
  - Systemic lupus erythematosus
  - Hyperparathyroidism
  - Hyper- or hypothyroidism
  - Lyme disease
  - Porphyria

DIAGNOSTIC TESTS & INTERPRETATION

Several screening tools are available that help to identify symptoms as somatic:

- Patient Health Questionnaire (PHQ)-15 (screens and monitors symptoms)
- Minnesota Multiphasic Personality Inventory (MMPI) (identifies somatization)

Initial Tests (lab, imaging)

- Laboratory test results do not support the subjective complaints.
- Imaging studies do not support the subjective complaints.

Test Interpretation

None are identified.

TREATMENT

GENERAL MEASURES

- The goal of treatment is to help the person learn to control the symptoms.
- It is not helpful to tell patients that their symptoms are imaginary. Enhanced or structured care as follows can be as effective as psychological interventions in adults (1)[A].
- The involvement of a single provider is important because a history of seeking medical attention and "doctor shopping" is common.
- Patients usually receive the most benefit from primary care providers who accept the limitations of treatment, listen to their patient's concerns, and provide reassurance.
- A supportive relationship with a sympathetic health care provider is the most important aspect of treatment:
  – Regular scheduled appointments should be maintained to review symptoms and the person's coping mechanisms (at least 15 minutes once a month).
  – Acknowledge and explain test results.
- Antidepressant or antianxiety medication and referral to a support group or mental health provider can help patients who are willing to participate in their treatment.

MEDICATION

- Fluoxetine has been shown to have efficacy with illness anxiety disorder (formerly hypochondriasis), although >50% of those patients did not respond to the medication (2)[B].
- Antidepressants (e.g., SSRIs) help to treat comorbid depression and anxiety (3)[C].

ISSUES FOR REFERRAL

- Discourage referrals to specialists for further investigation of somatic complaints.
- Referrals to support groups or to a mental health provider may be helpful.

ADDITIONAL THERAPIES

- Treatments have not been evaluated for this recently reformulated disorder. However, there are numerous studies with positive outcomes for child and adult patients with various forms of somatization or medically unexplained symptoms.
- Treatment typically includes long-term therapy, which has been shown to decrease the severity of symptoms.

- Individual or group cognitive-behavioral therapy addressing health anxiety, health beliefs, and health behaviors has been shown to be the most efficacious treatment for somatoform disorders. Cognitive processes modified in therapy include patient tendencies to ruminate and catastrophize (4)[A].
- For children, psychological interventions reduce symptom numbers and severity, disability, and school absence (5)[A].

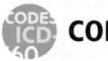 **ONGOING CARE**

FOLLOW-UP RECOMMENDATIONS
Patients should have regularly scheduled follow-up with a primary care doctor, psychiatrist, and/or therapist.

PATIENT EDUCATION
Encourage interventions that decrease stressful elements of the patient's life:
- Psychoeducational advice
- Increase in exercise
- Pleasurable private time

PROGNOSIS
- Chronic course, fluctuating in severity
- Full remission is rare.
- Individuals with this disorder do not experience any significant difference in mortality rate or significant physical illness.
- Patients with this diagnosis do experience substantially greater functional disability and role impairment than nonsomatizing patients (6).

COMPLICATIONS
- May result from invasive testing and from multiple evaluations that are performed while looking for the cause of the symptoms
- A dependency on pain relievers or sedatives may develop.

REFERENCES

1. van Dessel N, den Boeft M, van der Wouden JC, et al. Non-pharmacological interventions for somatoform disorders and medically unexplained physical symptoms (MUPS) in adults. *Cochrane Database Syst Rev.* 2014;(11):CD011142.
2. Fallon BA, Ahern DK, Pavlicova M, et al. A randomized controlled trial of medication and cognitive-behavioral therapy for hypochondriasis. *Am J Psychiatry.* 2017;174(8):756–764.
3. Somashekar B, Jainer A, Wuntakal B. Psychopharmacotherapy of somatic symptoms disorders. *Int Rev Psychiatry.* 2013;25(1):107–115.
4. Moreno S, Gili M, Magallón R, et al. Effectiveness of group versus individual cognitive-behavioral therapy in patients with abridged somatization disorder: a randomized controlled trial. *Psychosom Med.* 2013;75(6):600–608.
5. Bonvanie I, Kallesøe K, Janssens K, et al. Psychological interventions for children with functional somatic symptoms: a systematic review and meta-analysis. *J Pediatr.* 2017;187:272.e17–281.e17.
6. Momsen AM, Jensen OK, Nielsen CV, et al. Multiple somatic symptoms in employees participating in a randomized controlled trial associated with sickness absence because of nonspecific low back pain. *Spine J.* 2014;14(12):2868–2876.

ADDITIONAL READING

- Elder WG Jr, King M, Dassow P, et al. Managing lower back pain: you may be doing too much. *J Fam Pract.* 2009;58(4):180–186.
- Sharma MP, Manjula M. Behavioural and psychological management of somatic symptom disorders: an overview. *Int Rev Psychiatry.* 2013;25(1):116–124.

CODES

ICD10
- F45.9 Somatoform disorder, unspecified
- F45.20 Hypochondriacal disorder, unspecified
- F45.22 Body dysmorphic disorder

CLINICAL PEARLS

- With the advent of *DSM-5*, diagnosis is now based on a pattern of symptoms rather than an absence of medical explanation.
- A clue is accumulation of several diagnoses with >13 letters (e.g., chronic fatigue syndrome, fibromyalgia syndrome, reflex sympathetic dystrophy, temporomandibular joint syndrome, carpal tunnel syndrome, mitral valve prolapse).
- Inability of more than three physicians to make a meaningful diagnosis suggests somatization.
- Acknowledge the patient's pain, suffering, and disability.
- Do not tell patients the symptoms are "all in their head."
- Emphasize that this is not a rare disorder.
- Discuss the limitations of treatment while providing reassurance that there are interventions that will lessen suffering and reduce symptoms.

SPINAL STENOSIS

N. Wilson Holland, MD, FACP • Birju B. Patel, MD, FACP, AGSF

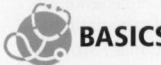

BASICS

DESCRIPTION
Narrowing of the spinal canal and foramen:
- Spondylosis or degenerative arthritis is the most common cause of spinal stenosis, resulting from compression of the spinal cord by disc degeneration, facet arthropathy, osteophyte formation, and ligamentum flavum hypertrophy.
- The L4–L5 level is most commonly involved.

EPIDEMIOLOGY
The prevalence of spinal stenosis increases with age due to "wear and tear" on the normal spine.

Incidence
Symptomatic spinal stenosis affects up to 8% of the general population.

Prevalence
- The prevalence of spinal stenosis is high if assessed solely by imaging in elderly patients. Not all patients with radiographic spinal stenosis are symptomatic. The degree of radiographic stenosis does not always correlate with patient symptoms. Lumbar MRI shows significant abnormalities in 57% of patients >60 years.
- Predominant age: Symptoms develop in 5th to 6th decades (congenital stenosis is symptomatic earlier).

ETIOLOGY AND PATHOPHYSIOLOGY
- Spinal stenosis can result from congenital or acquired causes. Degenerative spondylosis is most common.
- Disc dehydration leads to loss of height with bulging of the disc annulus and ligamentum flavum into the spinal canal, increasing facet joint loading.
- Facet loading leads to reactive sclerosis and osteophytic bone growth, further compressing spinal canal, and foraminal elements.
- Other causes of acquired spinal stenosis include:
  - Trauma
  - Neoplasms
  - Neural cysts and lipomas
  - Postoperative changes
  - Rheumatoid arthritis
  - Diffuse idiopathic skeletal hyperostosis
  - Ankylosing spondylitis
  - Metabolic/endocrine causes: osteoporosis, renal osteodystrophy, and Paget disease

Genetics
No definitive genetic links

RISK FACTORS
Increasing age and degenerative spinal disease

GENERAL PREVENTION
There is no proven prevention for spinal stenosis. Symptoms can be alleviated with flexion at the waist:
- Leaning forward while walking
- Pushing a shopping cart
- Lying in flexed position
- Sitting
- Avoiding provocative maneuvers (back extension, ambulating long distances without resting)

DIAGNOSIS

HISTORY
- Helps distinguish spinal stenosis from other causes of back pain and peripheral vascular disease
  - Insidious onset and slow progression are typical; discomfort with standing, paresthesias, and weakness (often bilateral) (1)
  - Symptoms *worsen with extension* (prolonged standing, walking downhill or downstairs).
  - Symptoms *improve with flexion* (sitting, leaning forward while walking, walking uphill or upstairs, lying in a flexed position).
- Neurogenic claudication (i.e., pain, tightness, numbness, and subjective weakness of lower extremities) may mimic vascular claudication.

PHYSICAL EXAM
Neurologic exam may be normal. Key exam areas:
- Examine gait (rule out cervical myelopathy or intracranial pathology).
- Loss of lumbar lordosis
- Evaluate range of motion of lumbar spine.
- Pain with extension of the lumbar spine is typical.
- Straight leg raise test may be positive if nerve root entrapment is present.
- Muscle weakness when apparent usually involves L4–L5 nerve roots (demonstrated by weakness in great toe extension and hip abduction) and less commonly S1 nerve roots (demonstrated by hip extension weakness).
- About half of patients with symptomatic stenosis have a reduced or absent Achilles reflex. Some have reduced or absent patellar reflex.

DIFFERENTIAL DIAGNOSIS
- Vascular claudication. Symptoms of vascular claudication do not improve with leaning forward and usually abate with standing or rest.
- Disc herniation
- Cervical myelopathy

DIAGNOSTIC TESTS & INTERPRETATION
Generally, a clinical diagnosis. Imaging (MRI is best) is used to stage severity and plan treatment.

Initial Tests (lab, imaging)
- CBC, ESR, C-reactive protein (if considering infection or malignancy)
- New back pain lasting >2 weeks or back pain accompanied by neurologic findings in patients >50 years generally warrants neuroimaging.
- MRI is the modality of choice.
- CT myelography is an alternative to MRI but is invasive and has higher risk of complications.
- Plain radiography helps exclude other causes of new back pain (e.g., malignant lytic lesions) but does not reveal the underlying pathology.
- Radiologic abnormalities in general do not correlate with the clinical severity.

Diagnostic Procedures/Other
Surgical decompression is definitive for patients who are symptomatic after nonoperative treatment:
- Spinal stenosis generally does not lead to neurologic damage.
- Surgery may be required for pain relief to increase mobility and improve quality of life.

Test Interpretation
Common radiographic findings include decreased disc height, facet hypertrophy, and spinal canal and/or foraminal narrowing.

TREATMENT

- In general, nonoperative interventions are preferred in the absence of progressive or debilitating neurologic symptoms:
  - Physical therapy, exercise, weight management, medications, and epidural steroid injections are options. There is insufficient evidence to definitively guide clinical practice.
  - Patients should understand that the benefits of surgery may diminish over time.
  - Rule out other neuropathies and peripheral vascular disease.
- Spinal decompression and physical therapy yield similar effects (2)[A].

MEDICATION

First Line

NSAIDs: Consider potential for GI side effects, fluid retention, and renal failure.

Second Line

- Tramadol—currently a schedule IV-controlled substance; has the potential to cause confusion, dizziness, lower seizure threshold, and increase fall risk in the elderly; should be used with caution
- The available evidence does not support the routine use of epidural steroid injections. A randomized study comparing injections of glucocorticoids plus lidocaine versus lidocaine alone showed no significance in symptoms at 6 weeks in these two groups (3)[B].
- Use opioids sparingly and only when other treatments have failed to control severe pain.

Geriatric Considerations

- Anti-inflammatory medications should be used with caution in the elderly due to the risks of GI bleeding, fluid retention, renal failure, and cardiovascular risks.
- Side effects of opioids include constipation, confusion, urinary retention, drowsiness, nausea, vomiting, and the potential for dependence and abuse.
- >10% of elderly lack Achilles reflexes.

ISSUES FOR REFERRAL

Patients in unremitting pain or with a neurologic deficit should see a neurosurgeon.

ADDITIONAL THERAPIES

- Patients with spinal stenosis are typically able to ride a bicycle (leaning forward tends to relieve symptoms).
- Aquatic therapy (helpful for muscle training and general conditioning)
- Strengthening of abdominal and back muscles
- Gait training
- Although a brace or corset may help in the short term, use is not recommended for prolonged periods due to development of paraspinal muscle weakness.
- Encourage physical activity to prevent deconditioning.

SURGERY/OTHER PROCEDURES

- Surgery is indicated when symptoms persist despite conservative measures.
- Age alone should not be an exclusion factor for surgical intervention. Cognitive impairment, multiple comorbidities, and osteoporosis may increase the risk of perioperative complications in the elderly.
- The traditional approach is laminectomy and partial facetectomy.

- Fusion is no longer a standard of care; patients with lumbar spinal stenosis decompression surgery plus fusion surgery did not result in better clinical outcomes at 2 years and 5 years than did decompression surgery alone (4)[B].
- A unilateral partial hemilaminectomy combined with transmedial decompression may adequately treat stenosis with less morbidity in the elderly (5)[C].

ADMISSION, INPATIENT, AND NURSING CONSIDERATIONS

- Admission criteria/initial stabilization: acute or progressive neurologic deficit
- Discharge criteria: improved pain or after neurologic deficit has been addressed

ONGOING CARE

FOLLOW-UP RECOMMENDATIONS

- Follow up based on progression of symptoms.
- No limitations to activity; patients may be as active as tolerated. Exercise should be encouraged.

Patient Monitoring

Patients are monitored for improvement of symptoms and development of any complications.

DIET

Optimize nutrition for weight management.

PATIENT EDUCATION

- Activity as tolerated, if no other pathology is present (e.g., fractures)
- Patients should present for care if they develop progressive motor weakness and/or bladder/bowel dysfunction.
- Patients should know the natural history of the condition and how best to relieve symptoms.

PROGNOSIS

- Spinal stenosis is generally benign, but the pain can lead to limitation in ADLs and progressive disability.
- Surgery usually improves pain and symptoms in patients who fail nonoperative treatment.
- Surgical outcomes are similar in terms of pain relief and functional improvement for patients of all ages.

COMPLICATIONS

- Severe spinal stenosis can lead to bowel and/or bladder dysfunction.
- Surgical complications include infection, neurologic injury, chronic pain, and disability.

REFERENCES

1. Suri P, Rainville J, Kalichman L, et al. Does this older adult with lower extremity pain have the clinical syndrome of lumbar spinal stenosis? *JAMA*. 2010;304(23):2628–2636.
2. Delitto A, Piva SR, Moore CG, et al. Surgery versus nonsurgical treatment of lumbar spinal stenosis: a randomized trial. *Ann Intern Med*. 2015;162(7):465–473.
3. Friedly JL, Comstock BA, Turner JA, et al. A randomized trial of epidural glucocorticoid injections for spinal stenosis. *N Engl J Med*. 2014;371(1):11–21.
4. Försth P, Ólafsson G, Carlsson T, et al. A randomized, controlled trial of fusion surgery for lumbar spinal stenosis. *N Engl J Med*. 2016;374(15):1413–1423.
5. Morgalla MH, Noak N, Merkle M, et al. Lumbar spinal stenosis in elderly patients: is a unilateral microsurgical approach sufficient for decompression? *J Neurosurg Spine*. 2011;14(3):305–312.

 SEE ALSO

Algorithm: Low Back Pain, Acute

 CODES

ICD10

- M48.00 Spinal stenosis, site unspecified
- M48.06 Spinal stenosis, lumbar region
- M48.04 Spinal stenosis, thoracic region

CLINICAL PEARLS

- Spinal stenosis typically presents as neurogenic claudication (pain, tightness, numbness, and subjective weakness of lower extremities), which can mimic vascular claudication.
- Flexion of the spine generally relieves symptoms associated with spinal stenosis.
- Spinal extension (prolonged standing, walking downhill, and walking downstairs) can worsen symptoms of spinal stenosis.
- Consider urgent surgery for patients with cauda equina/conus medullaris syndrome or progressive bladder dysfunction. Other patients with lumbar spinal stenosis typically do well with initial conservative management.
- For patients with lumbar spinal stenosis who do not have fixed or progressive neurologic deficits, should be managed with conservative treatment. Physical therapy and/or oral pain medication are often used, although their efficacy has not well evaluated.

SPRAIN, ANKLE

Shane L. Larson, MD • Julia S. Fast, DO

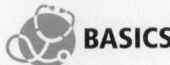

BASICS

DESCRIPTION

The most common cause of ankle injury comprising a significant proportion of sports injuries:

- Types of ankle sprains: lateral, medial, and syndesmotic (or high ankle sprain)
  - Lateral ankle sprains are the most common, accounting for up to 89% of all ankle sprains (1):
    ○ In lateral ankle sprains, the anterior talofibular ligament (ATFL) is most likely to be injured.
    ○ The calcaneofibular ligament (CFL) is the second most likely ligament to be injured.
    ○ The posterior talofibular ligament (PTFL) is the least likely to be injured.
  - Medial ankle sprains (5–10%) result from an injury to the deltoid ligament.
  - Syndesmotic ("high ankle sprain") injuries account for 5–10% of ankle sprains.
    ○ The syndesmosis between the distal tibia and distal fibula bones consists of the anterior, posterior, and transverse tibiofibular ligaments; the interosseous ligament; and interosseous membrane.
- Ankle sprains are classified according to the degree of ligamentous disruption:
  - Grade I: mild stretching of a ligament with possible microscopic tears
  - Grade II: incomplete tear of a ligament
  - Grade III: complete ligament tear

Geriatric Considerations
Increased risk of fracture in patients with preexisting bone weakness (osteoporosis/osteopenia)

Pediatric Considerations
- Increased risk of physeal injuries instead of ligament sprain because ligaments have greater tensile strength than physes
- Inversion ankle injuries in children may have a concomitant fibular physeal injury (Salter-Harris type I or higher fracture).
- Consider tarsal coalition with recurrent ankle sprains.

EPIDEMIOLOGY

Incidence
- Ankle sprains are more common in childhood and adolescents, particularly in active individuals (2).
- 1/2 of all ankle sprains are sports related; highest incidence in indoor/court sports (basketball, volleyball, tennis), followed by football and soccer (3)
- Most common sports injury
- More common in males age <30 years and females >30 years old

Prevalence
- 25% of sports injuries in the United States
- 75% of all ankle injuries are sprains.

ETIOLOGY AND PATHOPHYSIOLOGY
- Lateral ankle sprains result from an inversion force with the ankle in plantar flexion.
- Medial ankle sprains are due to forced eversion while the foot is in dorsiflexion.
- Syndesmotic sprains result from eversion stress/extreme dorsiflexion along with internal rotation of tibia.

RISK FACTORS
- The greatest risk factor is a prior history of an ankle sprain (3–34% recurrence rate).
- Postural instability, gait alterations
- Joint laxity and decreased proprioception are not risk factors.

GENERAL PREVENTION
- Improve overall physical conditioning:
  - Training in agility and flexibility
  - Single-leg balancing
  - Proprioceptive training
- Taping and bracing may help prevent primary injury in selected sports (i.e., volleyball, basketball, football) or reinjury (4). Taping and bracing do not reduce sprain severity.
- Weight loss may help in overweight patients (4)[A].

COMMONLY ASSOCIATED CONDITIONS
- Contusions
- Fractures
  - Fibular head fracture/dislocation (Maisonneuve)
  - Fracture of the base of the 5th metatarsal
  - Distal fibula physeal fracture (includes Salter-Harris fractures in pediatric patients; most common type of pediatric ankle fracture)

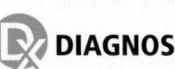

DIAGNOSIS

HISTORY
- Elicit specific mechanism of injury (inversion vs. eversion)
- Popping/snapping sensation during the injury
- Previous history of ankle injuries
- Ability to ambulate immediately after the injury
- Rapid onset of pain, swelling, or ecchymosis
- Location of pain (lateral/medial)
- Difficulty bearing weight
- Past medical history of systemic disorders

PHYSICAL EXAM
- Timing: Initial assessment for laxity may be difficult due to pain, swelling, and muscle spasm. Repeating exam ~5 days after injury often improves sensitivity.
- Compare to uninjured ankle for swelling, ecchymosis, weakness, and laxity.
- Neurovascular exam
- Palpate ATFL, CFL, PTFL, and deltoid ligament for tenderness.
- Palpate lateral and medial malleolus, base of 5th metatarsal, navicular, and entire fibula.
  - High ankle sprain associated with fracture of proximal fibula

- Grade I sprain: mild swelling and pain; no laxity; able to bear weight/ambulate without pain
- Grade II sprain: moderate swelling and pain; mild laxity with firm end point noted; weight-bearing/ambulation painful
- Grade III sprain: severe swelling, pain, and bruising; laxity with no end point; significant instability and loss of function/motion; unable to bear weight/ambulate
  - Swelling less sensitive for grade of tear in pediatric patient
- Special tests:
  - Anterior drawer test to check for ATFL laxity
  - Talar tilt test to check laxity in CFL (with inversion) or deltoid ligament (eversion)
  - Squeeze test: Compress tibia and fibula midcalf to check for syndesmotic injury; sensitivity 30%, specificity 93.5%
  - Dorsiflexion/external rotation test: Positive test is pain at syndesmosis with rotation; sensitivity 20%, specificity 85%

DIFFERENTIAL DIAGNOSIS
- Tendon injury
  - Tendinopathy/tendon tear
- Fracture and/or dislocation of the ankle/foot
- Hindfoot/midfoot injuries
- Nerve injury
- Contusion

DIAGNOSTIC TESTS & INTERPRETATION

Initial Tests (lab, imaging)
- Ottawa Ankle Rules (nearly 100% sensitive, 30–50% specific) determine need for radiographs to rule out ankle fractures (patient must be 18 to 55 years; certain patients, e.g., diabetics with diminished sensation, may still need radiographs):
  - Pain in malleolar zone
  - Inability to bear weight (walk ≥4 steps) immediately and in the exam room
  - Bony tenderness at tip/posterior edge of the lateral/medial malleolus
    ○ Note: Ottawa rule for foot imaging: reported pain in the midfoot zone AND pain with palpation of navicular or base of 5th metatarsal OR inability to bear weight immediately and in the ER/office
  - Although Ottawa rules are highly sensitive, they should not overrule clinical judgment.
- If radiographs are indicated, obtain anteroposterior, lateral, and mortise views of the ankle.
  - Small avulsion fractures are associated with grade III sprains.
- Consider CT if radiographs are negative but occult fracture is suspected clinically.
- MRI is the gold standard for soft tissue imaging but is expensive and rarely necessary.
  - Syndesmotic ankle sprains: MRI is more sensitive.
- US is a good second-line imaging option with sensitivity comparable to MRI with experienced sonographers and providers.

Follow-Up Tests & Special Considerations

If patient's condition does not improve in 6 to 8 weeks, consider CT, MRI, or US. Failure to resolve could indicate an injury such as a fracture or osteochondral lesion of the talus.

 TREATMENT

GENERAL MEASURES

- Most grade I, II, and III lateral ankle sprains can be managed conservatively.
- Conservative therapy: PRICE (protection, relative rest, ice, compression, elevation) (4)[A]
- Protection/compression: For grade I/II sprains, lace-up bracing is superior to air-filled/gel-filled ankle brace, which is superior to elastic bandage/taping to provide support and decrease swelling.
  - Note: The combination of air-filled brace and compression wrap is superior to each individual modality for return to preinjury joint function at 10 days and 1 month following grade I and II sprains.
  - Grade III sprains should have short-term immobilization (10 days) with below-the-knee cast, followed by a semirigid brace (air cast). If a patient refuses casting, a 10-day period of strict non–weight-bearing with air cast splint and elastic bandage is a comparable alternative if non–weight-bearing is maintained.
- Rest: initially, activity as tolerated. Early mobilization and physical therapy speed recovery/reduce pain:
  - Weight-bearing, as tolerated
  - Consider crutches if unable to bear weight.
  - Initiate exercises as early as tolerated. Limit to pain-free range of motion.
  - Start mobilization by tracing the alphabet with the foot or toes.
  - Resistance exercises with an elastic band
- Ice: Ice for first 3 to 7 days reduces pain and decreases recovery time.
- Elevation: Elevate ankle to decrease swelling.

MEDICATION

- NSAIDs: preferably oral; topical forms (e.g., diclofenac 1% gel) may be used to minimize GI side effects. PRN NSAID dosing has similar outcomes to scheduled dosing with improved safety profile.
  - Example: naproxen 500 mg BID PRN
- Acetaminophen 650 mg q4–6h (max outpatient therapy dose: 3,250 mg/day)
- Opioids (<5 days) if severe pain

ISSUES FOR REFERRAL

- Malleolar/talar dome fracture
- Syndesmotic sprain
- Dislocation/subluxation
- Tendon rupture
- Ongoing instability
- Uncertain diagnosis

ADDITIONAL THERAPIES

Physical therapy:

- After the acute phase of the injury, patients with grade II or III sprain should start physical therapy as soon as possible to increase range of motion, strength, flexibility, and improve proprioceptive balance (wobble board/ankle disk).
- Functional rehabilitation prevents chronic instability and speeds healing.
- Athletes should undergo sport-specific rehabilitation before returning to play.

SURGERY/OTHER PROCEDURES

- Surgery is typically reserved for treatment of complicated recurrent sprains and certain syndesmotic sprains.
- Patients with chronic ankle instability who fail functional rehabilitation or with poor tissue quality may need anatomic repair/reconstructive surgery.

 ONGOING CARE

FOLLOW-UP RECOMMENDATIONS

- After an ankle sprain, consider ankle-stabilizing orthoses (air stirrup braces, lace-up supports, athletic taping, etc.) for athletes participating in high-risk sports to prevent future ankle sprains.
- Moderate and severe sprains require ankle orthoses for ≥6 months during sports participation.
- Gradual return to play for athletes with a grade I lateral ankle sprain can generally be accomplished in 1 to 2 weeks; grade II sprain return to play time is 2 to 3 weeks; grade III sprain is approximately 4 weeks.
- Syndesmotic sprains take longer (~8 to 9 weeks) to heal than lateral ankle sprains.

Patient Monitoring

If athletes continue to have symptoms when they return to play or if a patient has pain for 6 to 8 weeks after injury, repeat examination and imaging.

PATIENT EDUCATION

- Crutch training
- Provide training on proper use of elastic bandages, brace, and/or orthoses.
- Demonstrate mobilization exercises (alphabet trace, towel grab).

PROGNOSIS

- Earlier physical therapy and mobilization with bracing allows for faster return to daily living and/or sports.
- Higher grade sprains, older patient age, and initial non–weight-bearing status have poorer prognosis and longer recovery.
- Ligamentous strength does not return for months after the injury.

COMPLICATIONS

- Joint instability
- Intermittent swelling/pain if not properly treated
- 5–33% continue to have pain 1 year postinjury.
- Accumulation of cartilage damage, leading to degenerative changes

REFERENCES

1. Feger MA, Glaviano NR, Donovan L, et al. Current trends in the management of lateral ankle sprain in the United States. *Clin J Sport Med*. 2017;27(2):145–152.
2. Doherty C, Delahunt E, Caulfield B, et al. The incidence and prevalence of ankle sprain injury: a systematic review and meta-analysis of prospective epidemiological studies. *Sports Med*. 2014;44(1):123–140.
3. Waterman BR, Owens BD, Davey S, et al. The epidemiology of ankle sprains in the United States. *J Bone Joint Surg Am*. 2010;92(13):2279–2284.
4. McCriskin BJ, Cameron KL, Orr JD, et al. Management and prevention of acute and chronic lateral ankle instability in athletic patient populations. *World J Orthop*. 2015;6(2):161–171.

ADDITIONAL READING

- Bleakley CM, O'Connor SR, Tully MA, et al. Effect of accelerated rehabilitation on function after ankle sprain: randomised controlled trial. *BMJ*. 2010;340:c1964.
- Farwell KE, Powden CJ, Powell MR, et al. The effectiveness of prophylactic ankle braces in reducing the incidence of acute ankle injuries in adolescent athletes: a critically appraised topic. *J Sport Rehabil*. 2013;22(2):137–142.
- Massey T, Derry S, Moore RA, et al. Topical NSAIDs for acute pain in adults. *Cochrane Database Syst Rev*. 2010;(6):CD007402.
- Petersen W, Rembitzki IV, Koppenburg AG, et al. Treatment of acute ankle ligament injuries: a systematic review. *Arch Orthop Trauma Surg*. 2013;133(8):1129–1141.
- Richie DH, Izadi FE. Return to play after an ankle sprain. *Clin Podiatr Med Surg*. 2015;32(2):195–215.

 CODES

ICD10

- S96.919A Strain of unsp msl/tnd at ank/ft level, unsp foot, init
- S93.499A Sprain of other ligament of unspecified ankle, init encntr
- S93.419A Sprain of calcaneofibular ligament of unsp ankle, init

CLINICAL PEARLS

- Children are at an increased risk of physeal injuries because ligaments are stronger than physes.
- Conditioning, including proprioceptive training, before participating in sports and throughout the season helps to prevent ankle sprains.
- Functional rehabilitation, rather than total immobilization, is recommended for quicker return to sport and work.
- Patients who do not adequately rehabilitate an ankle sprain are at increased risk for recurrence and chronic ankle instability.
- If patient's condition is not improving in 6 to 8 weeks, consider advanced imaging with CT, MRI, or US.

S

SPRAINS AND STRAINS

Scott M. Goldberg, MD • J. Herbert Stevenson, MD

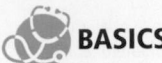 **BASICS**

DESCRIPTION
- *Sprains* are complete or partial ligamentous injuries either within the body of the ligament or at the site of attachment to bone.
  - Classified as grade 1, 2, or 3 (AMA Ligament Injury Classification)
    - Grade 1: stretch injury without ligamentous laxity
    - Grade 2: partial tear with increased ligamentous laxity but firm end point on exam
    - Grade 3: complete tear with increased ligamentous laxity and no firm end point on exam
  - Usually secondary to trauma (e.g., falls, twisting injuries, motor vehicle accidents)
  - Physical exam is the key to accurate diagnosis.
- *Strains* are partial or complete disruptions of the muscle, muscle–tendon junction, or tendon.
  - Classified as
    - First degree: minimal damage to muscle, tendon, or musculotendinous unit
    - Second degree: partial tear to the muscle, tendon, or musculotendinous unit
    - Third degree: complete disruption of the muscle, tendon, or musculotendinous unit
  - Often associated with overuse injuries

Geriatric Considerations
More likely to see associated bony injuries due to decreased joint flexibility and increased prevalence of osteoporosis and osteopenia

Pediatric Considerations
- Sprains and strains account for 24% of pediatric injuries.
- 3 million pediatric sports injuries occur annually.
- Consider physeal/apophyseal injuries in the skeletally immature patient.

EPIDEMIOLOGY

Incidence
~80% of all U.S. athletes experience a sprain or strain at some point.

Prevalence
- Ankle sprains are among the most common injuries in primary care, accounting for ~30% of sports medicine clinic visits. Most ankle sprains are due to inversion injuries (lateral sprains) involving the anterior talofibular ligament; account for 650,000 annual ER visits in the United States
- Predominant age
  - Sprains: any age in physically active patient
  - Strains: usually 15 to 40 years of age
- Predominant sex: male > female for most; female > male for sprain of anterior cruciate ligament (ACL)

ETIOLOGY AND PATHOPHYSIOLOGY
- Trauma, falls, motor vehicle accidents
- Excessive exercise; poor conditioning
- Improper footwear
- Inadequate warm-up and stretching before activity
- Prior sprain or strain

RISK FACTORS
- Prior history of sprain or strain is greatest risk factor for future sprain/strain.
- Change in or improper footwear, protective gear, or environment (e.g., surface)
- Sudden increase in training schedule or volume
- Tobacco use, medication adverse effects

GENERAL PREVENTION
- Appropriate warm-up and cooldown exercises
- Use proper equipment and footwear.
- Balance training programs improve proprioception and reduce the risk of ankle sprains.
- Semirigid orthoses may prevent ankle sprains during high-risk sports, especially in athletes with history of sprain.
- Proprioception and strength training decrease injury risk; stretching does not

COMMONLY ASSOCIATED CONDITIONS
- Effusions, ecchymosis, hemarthrosis
- Stress, avulsion, and/or other fractures
- Syndesmotic injuries
- Contusions
- Dislocations/subluxations

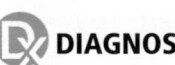 **DIAGNOSIS**

HISTORY
- Obtain thorough description of mechanism of injury including activity, trauma, baseline conditioning, and prior musculoskeletal injuries.
- May describe feeling or hearing pop or snap

PHYSICAL EXAM
- Inspect for swelling, asymmetry, ecchymosis, and gait disturbance.
- Evaluate for neurovascular compromise.
- Palpate for tenderness.
- Evaluate for decreased range of motion (ROM) of joint and joint instability/laxity.
- Evaluate for strength.
- Sprains
  - Grade 1: tenderness without laxity; minimal pain, swelling; little ecchymosis; can bear weight
  - Grade 2: tenderness with increased laxity on exam but firm end point; more pain, swelling; often ecchymosis; some difficulty bearing weight
  - Grade 3: tenderness with increased laxity on exam and no firm end point; severe pain, swelling; obvious ecchymosis; difficulty bearing weight

DIFFERENTIAL DIAGNOSIS
- Tendonitis
- Bursitis
- Contusion
- Hematoma
- Fracture
- Osteochondral lesion
- Rheumatologic process

DIAGNOSTIC TESTS & INTERPRETATION
- Ankle
  - Anterior drawer test assesses integrity of anterior talofibular ligament.
  - Talar tilt test assesses integrity of calcaneofibular ligament.
  - Squeeze test assesses for syndesmotic injury.
  - Palpate lateral and medial malleoli.
- Knee
  - Lachman and anterior drawer tests assess integrity of ACL. Posterior drawer and sag tests assess integrity of posterior cruciate ligament.
  - Valgus/varus stress tests assess integrity of medial and lateral collateral ligaments, respectively.
- Shoulder
  - Load and shift test; sulcus sign; and the apprehension, relocation, surprise test assess for instability of the glenohumeral joint.
- Radiographs help rule out bony injury; stress views may be necessary. Obtain bilateral radiographs in children to rule out growth plate injuries.
- Use Ottawa Foot and Ankle Rules (age 18 to 55 years) to determine if radiographs are necessary.
- Ottawa Ankle Rules: x-ray required if pain in the malleolar zone *and*
  - Bone tenderness in posterior aspect distal 6 cm of tibia or fibula or
  - Unable to bear weight immediately or in emergency department
- Ottawa Foot Rules: x-ray required if midfoot zone pain is present *and*
  - Bone tenderness at base of 5th metatarsal or
  - Bone tenderness at navicular or
  - Inability to bear weight immediately or in emergency department

Follow-Up Tests & Special Considerations
- CT scan if occult fracture is suspected
- MRI is the gold standard for imaging soft tissue structures, including muscle, ligaments, and intra-articular structures. If tibiofibular syndesmotic disruption is suspected, MRI is highly accurate for diagnosis.
- Ultrasound evaluation of a variety of muscles, tendons, and ligaments by a skilled operator allows for dynamic evaluation of potential sprain/strain that can add to traditional diagnostic imaging.

Diagnostic Procedures/Other
Surgery may be required for some partial and complete sprains depending on location, mechanism, and chronicity.

TREATMENT

GENERAL MEASURES
- Acute: *p*rotection, relative *r*est (activity modification), *i*ce, *c*ompression, *e*levation, *m*edications, *m*odalities (PRICEMM) therapy
- Ankle sprains: Compression stockings didn't affect pain, swelling, or time to pain-free walking but did show decreased time to return to sport (1)[B].
- Grade 1 and 2 ankle sprain: functional treatment with brace, orthosis, taping, elastic bandage wrap
  - Ankle braces (lace-up, stirrup-type, air cast) are a more effective functional treatment than elastic bandages or taping (2)[A].
- Grade 3 ankle sprain: Short period of immobilization may be needed.
- Refer for early physical therapy.
- For high-level athletes with more extensive damage (e.g., biceps or pectoralis disruption), consider surgical referral.

MEDICATION
First Line
- Acetaminophen: not to exceed 3 g/day
- NSAIDs
  - Ibuprofen: 200 to 800 mg TID
  - Naproxen: 250 to 500 mg BID
  - Diclofenac: 50 to 75 mg BID
- Opioids can be considered acutely for severe pain, but discretion is advised.
- Acetaminophen and NSAIDs have similar efficacy in reducing pain after soft tissue injuries with less GI side effects; NSAIDs are better than narcotics.
- Topical diclofenac, ibuprofen, and ketoprofen are effective for pain related to strains and sprains, especially in gel form or patch (3)[A].
- Platelet-rich plasma injections may aid recovery in treatment of muscle strains, but more studies are needed.

ISSUES FOR REFERRAL
- ACL sprain in athletes/physically active
- Salter-Harris physeal fractures
- Joint instability especially if chronic
- Tendon disruption (i.e., Achilles, biceps, ACL)
- Lack of improvement with conservative measures

ADDITIONAL THERAPIES
- Physical therapy is a useful adjunct after a sprain, particularly if early mobilization is crucial.
  - Proprioception retraining
  - Core strengthening
  - Eccentric exercises
  - Thera-Band exercises
- After hamstring strain, frequent daily stretching and progressive agility and trunk stabilization exercises may speed recovery and reduce risk of reinjury (4)[A]. Rehab protocols emphasizing eccentric/lengthening exercises are more effective than conventional exercises (5)[B].

SURGERY/OTHER PROCEDURES
- Casting and surgery are reserved for select partial and complete sprains. Need for surgery depends on the neurovascular supply to the injured area as well as the ability to attain full ROM and stability of the affected joint. The need for surgery also depends on activity level and patient preference.
- For primary management of acute lateral ankle sprains, there is no difference between surgical versus conservative therapy. Risks are increased with surgical intervention.
- Chronic ankle instability affects 10–20% of people who sustain an acute sprain. If conservative management fails and laxity is present, surgery is considered (6)[A].
- Percutaneous needle tenotomy versus surgical tenotomy are available as options for chronic tendinosis (chronic, recurrent strains).

 ONGOING CARE

FOLLOW-UP RECOMMENDATIONS
If the affected joint has full strength and ROM, the patient can advance activity as tolerated using pain as a guide for return to activity.

Patient Monitoring
After initial treatment, consider early rehabilitation. Limit swelling and work on increasing ROM.

DIET
Weight loss if overweight

PATIENT EDUCATION
- Injury prevention through proprioceptive training and physical therapy
- ROM and strengthening exercises to restore functional capacity

PROGNOSIS
Favorable with appropriate treatment and rest. Duration of recovery depends on the severity and location of injury.

COMPLICATIONS
- Chronic joint instability
- Arthritis
- Muscle contracture
- Chronic tendinopathy

REFERENCES
1. Bendahou M, Khiami F, Saïdi K, et al. Compression stockings in ankle sprain: a multicenter randomized study. *Am J Emerg Med*. 2014;32(9):1005–1010.
2. Petersen W, Rembitzki IV, Koppenburg AG, et al. Treatment of acute ankle ligament injuries: a systematic review. *Arch Orthop Trauma Surg*. 2013;133(8):1129–1141.
3. Derry S, Moore RA, Gaskell H, et al. Topical NSAIDs for acute musculoskeletal pain in adults. *Cochrane Database Syst Rev*. 2015;(6):CD007402.
4. Pas HI, Reurink G, Tol JL, et al. Efficacy of rehabilitation (lengthening) exercises, platelet-rich plasma injections, and other conservative interventions in acute hamstring injuries: an updated systematic review and meta-analysis. *Br J Sports Med*. 2015;49(18):1197–1205.
5. Askling CM, Tengvar M, Tarassova O, et al. Acute hamstring injuries in Swedish elite sprinters and jumpers: a prospective randomised controlled clinical trial comparing two rehabilitation protocols. *Br J Sports Med*. 2014;48(7):532–539.
6. McCriskin BJ, Cameron KL, Orr JD, et al. Management and prevention of acute and chronic lateral ankle instability in athletic patient populations. *World J Orthop*. 2015;6(2):161–171.

ADDITIONAL READING
- Hamilton BH, Best TM. Platelet-enriched plasma and muscle strain injuries: challenges imposed by the burden of proof. *Clin J Sport Med*. 2011;21(1):31–36.
- Kim T, Lee M, Kim K, et al. Acupuncture for treating acute ankle sprains in adults. *Cochrane Database Syst Rev*. 2014;(6):CD009065.
- Monk AP, Davies LJ, Hopewell S, et al. Surgical versus conservative interventions for treating anterior cruciate ligament injuries. *Cochrane Database Syst Rev*. 2016;(4):CD011166.
- Seah R, Mani-Babu S. Managing ankle sprains in primary care: what is best practice? A systematic review of the last 10 years of evidence. *Br Med Bull*. 2011;97:105–135.

 SEE ALSO

Tendinopathy

 CODES

ICD10
- S93.409A Sprain of unsp ligament of unspecified ankle, init encntr
- S96.919A Strain of unsp msl/tnd at ank/ft level, unsp foot, init
- S43.50XA Sprain of unspecified acromioclavicular joint, initial encounter

CLINICAL PEARLS

For acute injury, remember PRICEMM:
- Protection of the joint
- Relative rest (activity modification)
- Apply ice.
- Apply compression.
- Elevate joint.
- Medications/ice for pain
- Other modalities as needed
- Wean out of brace as tolerated to limit atrophy of stabilizing muscles.

SQUAMOUS CELL CARCINOMA, CUTANEOUS

Sara Usman, MBBS • Sidra Saeed, MD • Ghulam Murtaza, MD

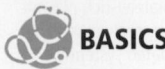 **BASICS**

DESCRIPTION
Cutaneous squamous cell cancer is a type of cancer that is very common. It is associated with some hereditary disorders like xeroderma pigmentosum, oculocutaneous albinism, epidermodysplasia verruciformis.

EPIDEMIOLOGY
Incidence
- Occurs in older age (around 60 years) (1)
- More common in men (1)
- Incidence increases the closer the person gets to equator or higher altitude (1).

Prevalence
Average age it develops is 70 years.

ETIOLOGY AND PATHOPHYSIOLOGY
Genetics
Some of the hereditary disorders have the genes that are associated with cutaneous squamous cell cancer (2). They include:
- Xeroderma pigmentosum (2)
- Oculocutaneous albinism (2)
- Epidermodysplasia verruciformis (2)
- Genes commonly mutated includes:
  - TP53
  - CDKN2A
  - NOTCH1, Ras
  - TP53 is the most common gene involved in cutaneous squamous cell cancer.

RISK FACTORS
- UV radiation exposure (2,3)
- Increasing age (Average age of onset is mid-60s.)
- Immunosuppression (2)
- HIV/AIDS, non-Hodgkin lymphoma, chronic lympho-cytic leukemia have increase rates of developing cutaneous squamous cell cancer (2).
- Gender (more common in men)
- Psoriasis patients treated with ultraviolet A (UVA)
- Glucocorticoid use (2)
- Postmenopausal hormonal use (2)
- High body mass
- Ionizing radiation exposure (3)
- Chemical exposure (pesticides, PAH) (2)
- Arsenic (2,3)
- Organ transplantation (3)
- Alcohol use (2)
- Osteomyelitis (3)
- Exposure to UV light (UVA and UVB)
- Xeroderma pigmentosum (3)
- Ulcers (3)
- Chronically injured or diseased skin (3)

- Actinic keratosis (2,3)
- Radiation-induced keratosis (3)
- Precursor lesions (3)
- Bowen disease (squamous cell carcinoma [SCC] in situ) (3)
- Erythroplasia of Queyrat (SCC in situ of penis) (3)
- Leukemia (3)
- Lymphoma (3)
- Immunosuppression (3)
- Organ transplantation (3)
- Immunosuppressive medications (3)
- HPV infection (6, 11, 16, 18) (3)

GENERAL PREVENTION
- Protect skin from sun exposure (2).
- Wear sunscreen, hats, and clothing under skin.
- Vitamin B_3 (nicotinamide) can repair DNA by preventing UVR-induced adenosine triphosphate depletion (2)
- Difluoromethylornithine (synthetic analog of ornithine) (2)

COMMONLY ASSOCIATED CONDITIONS
- Actinic keratosis is the precursor of cutaneous squamous cell cancer (1).
- Diseases that evolve into squamous cell cancer include:
  - Bowen disease (1)
  - Erythroplasia of Queyrat (1)

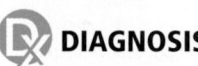 **DIAGNOSIS**

PHYSICAL EXAM
- Lesions occur mainly on chronically exposed areas:
  - Face (especially lips, ear, nose, cheek, and eyelid) (1)
- Lesions occur chiefly on chronically sun-exposed areas.
  - Face and backs of the forearms and hands
  - Bald areas of the scalp and top of ears in men
  - The sun-exposed "V" of the neck as well as the posterior neck below the occipital hairline
  - In elderly females, lesions tend to occur on the legs and other sun-exposed locations.
  - In African Americans, equal frequency in sun-exposed and unexposed areas
- Clinical appearance
  - Generally slow-growing, firm, hyperkeratotic papules, nodules, or plaques
  - Most SCCs are asymptomatic, although bleeding, pain, and tenderness may be noted.
  - Lesions may have a smooth, verrucous, or papil-lomatous surface.
  - Varying degrees of ulceration, erosion, crust, or scale
  - Color is often red to brown, tan, or pearly (indis-tinguishable from basal cell carcinoma).

- Clinical variants of SCC
  - Bowen disease (SCC in situ): solitary lesion that resembles a scaly psoriatic plaque
  - Invasive SCC: often a raised, firm papule, nodule, or plaque. Lesions may be smooth, verrucous, or papillomatous, with varying degrees of ulceration, erosion, crust, or scale.
  - Cutaneous horn: SCC with an overlying cutaneous horn. A cutaneous horn represents a thick, hard, fingernail-like keratinization produced by the SCC. Bowen disease may also produce a cutaneous horn on its surface.
  - Erythroplasia of Queyrat refers to Bowen disease of the glans penis, which manifests as one or more velvety red plaques.
  - Subungual SCC appears as hyperkeratotic lesions under the nail plate or on surrounding periungual skin, often mimicking warts.
  - Marjolin ulcer: an SCC evolving from a new area of ulceration or elevation at site of a scar or ulcer
  - HPV-associated SCC: virally induced; an SCC most commonly seen as a new or enlarging warty growth on penis, vulva, perianal area, or periungual region
  - Verrucous carcinoma: subtype of SCC that is extremely well differentiated, can be locally destructive, but rarely metastasizes. Lesions are "cauliflower-like" verrucous nodules or plaques.
  - Basaloid SCC: less common than typical SCC; seen more often in men aged 40 to 70 years

DIFFERENTIAL DIAGNOSIS
- Actinic keratosis
- Keratoacanthoma

DIAGNOSTIC TESTS & INTERPRETATION
Follow-Up Tests & Special Considerations
- For high-risk cutaneous squamous cell cancer: These are the follow-up recommendations (4):
  - Full skin exam and lymph node exam required every 2 to 6 months (4)
  - Every 6 to 12 months for next 3 years
  - Annually after 5 years (4)
- For high-risk cutaneous squamous cell cancer with regional disease: These are the follow-up recommendations (4):
  - Full skin exam and lymph node exam every 1 to 3 months (4)
  - Every 2 to 4 months for the next year (4)
  - Every 4 to 6 months until the 5th year (4)
  - Every 6 to 12 months for patient's lifetime (4)

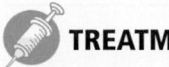

TREATMENT

MEDICATION

First Line

- First-line treatment for cutaneous SCC is complete surgical excision with histopathologic control of excision margins.
- Surgical excision provides these benefits (4):
  - Shorter healing time
  - Cure rate as high as 95%
- Mohs micrographic surgery (MMS) is the treatment for high-risk tumors instead of surgical excision (4).
  - MMS is gold standard for surgical removal of high-risk SCCs (4).
  - SCCs with low risk of metastasis can be eliminated by excision, electrodesiccation and curettage, or cryosurgery.
  - For high-risk cancer, surgical resection and MMS provide decreased recurrence and metastasis.
  - Cryotherapy is used to treat small squamous cell cancers.
  - Cryotherapy can be used as treatment for patients who have bleeding disorders or contraindications to surgery.
  - MMS offers the highest cure for patients who have recurrent or high-risk primary squamous cell cancer.

Second Line

Advances in the management of cutaneous SCC

- Monoclonal antibodies (cetuximab, panitumumab) (4)
- Tyrosine kinase inhibitors (erlotinib) (4)
- Chemotherapy—used in locally advanced or metastatic skin squamous cell cancer (4)
- Chemotherapeutic drugs used are (4):
  - Methotrexate
  - Bleomycin
  - Doxorubicin
  - Cisplatin
- Oral retinoids decrease the incidence of actinic keratosis and cutaneous squamous cell cancer (4).

SURGERY/OTHER PROCEDURES

- For high-risk cutaneous squamous cell cancer patients, who have tumors in locations that are inoperable and are poor candidates for surgery, they have option for radiation therapy (4).
- Radiation therapy side effects include (4):
  - Malaise
  - Nausea
  - Radiation-induced erythema
  - Telangiectasia
  - Hypopigmentation
  - Epidermal atrophy
  - Soft tissue necrosis
  - Radiation-induced malignancy

ADMISSION, INPATIENT, AND NURSING CONSIDERATIONS

Examine sentinel lymph nodes for early detection of metastasis. This can decrease disease-related morbidity and mortality (4).

ONGOING CARE

PROGNOSIS

- Patients with high-risk cutaneous squamous cell cancer have increased risk of recurrence, lymph node, or distant metastases (4).
- From the lesions at risk, 7–80% will locally recur or metastasize within the first 2 years and 95% within the first 5 years of initial diagnosis (4).
- 30–50% of patients with high-risk cutaneous squamous cell cancer will develop second skin cancer within 5 years (4).
- Cutaneous squamous cell cancer has increased risk of metastasis if these characteristics below are present (4):
  - Tumor recurrence
  - Diameter ≥2 cm
  - Thickness >2 mm
  - Poorly differentiated histology
  - Invasion of subcutaneous tissue or structures such as perineural, vascular, or lymphatic
  - If tumor is located on
    - Eye
    - Vermilion lip
    - "Mask areas" of face
    - Hands
    - Feet
    - Genitalia
- MMS provides cure rates of 97% for primary cutaneous squamous cell cancer and 94% for recurrent cutaneous squamous cell cancer.
- MMS is very beneficial for treating specifically high-risk cutaneous squamous cell cancers and preventing local recurrence (4).
- Staging is important for treating high-risk cutaneous SCC (4).
- High risk factors include (4):
  - Diameter ≥0.1 mm
  - Poorly differentiated histology
  - Tumor invasion beyond fat
  - Perineural invasion ≥0.1 mm
- Excellent prognosis
- After recurrence, prognosis is very poor. There is risk of distant metastasis and metastasis to regional lymph nodes.

- After resection of the cancer, recurrent cancers have twice the risk of recurrence.
- Patients with metastatic disease, long-term prognosis is poor.
  - For patients having distant metastasis, 10-year survival rates are <10%.
  - For patients having regional lymph node involvement, 10-year survival rates are <20%.
- Distant metastasis occurs in 15% of cases and involves these sites:
  - Brain
  - Lungs
  - Liver
  - Skin
  - Bone

COMPLICATIONS

- Local recurrence
- Metastasis

REFERENCES

1. Simonacci F, Bertozzi N, Grieco MP, et al. Surgical therapy of cutaneous squamous cell carcinoma: our experience. *Acta Biomed*. 2018;89(2):242–248.
2. Green AC, Olsen CM. Cutaneous squamous cell carcinoma: an epidemiological review. *Br J Dermatol*. 2017;177(2):373–381.
3. Alam M, Ratner D. Cutaneous squamous-cell carcinoma. *N Engl J Med*. 2001;344(13):975–983.
4. Parikh SA, Patel VA, Ratner D. Advances in the management of cutaneous squamous cell carcinoma. *F1000Prime Rep*. 2014;6:70.

CODES

ICD10

- C44.92 Squamous cell carcinoma of skin, unspecified
- C44.320 Squamous cell carcinoma of skin of unspecified parts of face
- C44.42 Squamous cell carcinoma of skin of scalp and neck

CLINICAL PEARLS

- Cutaneous SCC associated with UV light exposure and immunosuppression
- Head and neck are the most common regions for invasive cutaneous SCC.
- MMS provides cure rates of 97% for primary cutaneous SCC.

STRESS FRACTURE

David A. Ross, MD, CAQSM • Nicole A. Ross, DO

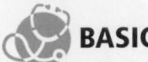 **BASICS**

DESCRIPTION
- Overuse injuries caused by cumulative microdamage from repetitive bone loading
- Stress fractures occur in different situations:
  - Fatigue fracture: abnormal repetitive stress applied to normal bone (e.g., young college athletes or new military recruits with increased physical activity demands and inadequate conditioning). Common sites include tibia, fibula, metatarsals, femoral neck, and navicular.
  - Insufficiency fracture: normal stress applied to structurally abnormal bone (e.g., femoral neck fracture in osteopenic bone, metabolic bone disease). Common sites include spine, sacrum, femoral head, and medial femoral condyle.
  - Combination fracture: abnormal stress applied to abnormal bone (e.g., female long-distance runners with premature osteoporosis from female athletic triad)
- Weight-bearing bones of the lower extremity are most commonly affected at the following sites:
  - Tibia/fibula
  - Metatarsal bones
  - Navicular
  - Femoral neck
  - Pars interarticularis
- Less commonly affected sites:
  - Pelvis
  - Calcaneus
  - Ribs
  - Ulna
- High-risk stress fractures occur in zones of tension or areas with poor blood supply and are more likely to result in fracture displacement and/or nonunion. High-risk sites include the following:
  - Tension side of femoral neck
  - Anterior tibial diaphysis
  - Sesamoids
  - Pars interarticularis of lumbar spine (L4, L5)
  - 5th metatarsal at metaphyseal–diaphyseal junction
  - Proximal 2nd metatarsal
  - Medial malleolus
  - Tarsal navicular
  - Patella
  - Talar neck
- Synonym(s): march fracture; fatigue fracture

EPIDEMIOLOGY
Incidence
- Greatest incidence in 15- to 27-year-olds
- Females more commonly affected than males
- Females have higher incidence of fatigue fractures as compared to males (attributed to female athlete triad) (1).
- Affects 9–21% of track and field athletes annually
- Accounts for up to 20% of visits to sports medicine and orthopedic clinics
- Across all sports, the most commonly injured body sites are the lower leg, foot, and lower back/lumbar spine/pelvis.
- Occurs in <1% of general population

Prevalence
- Affects up to 6.9% of male and 21.0% of female military members (2)
- Affects 1–3% of college athletes

ETIOLOGY AND PATHOPHYSIOLOGY
- Bone is dynamic and constantly remodeling in response to applied physiologic stress.
- Repetitive loading or overuse causes microfractures that don't heal due to imbalance between bone resorption and bone formation.
- If microdamage accumulates in excess of reparation, bony fatigue leads to stress fracture.

RISK FACTORS
- Intrinsic (3)[A]
  - Females are at 2.3 times higher risk than males.
  - Female athlete triad (low energy availability with or without disordered eating, menstrual dysfunction, and low bone mineral density)
  - Females with disrupted menstrual cycles are 2 to 4 times for more likely to sustain stress injury (1)[C].
  - History of previous stress fracture—increases risk of future stress fracture by 5 times
  - History of osteoporosis, osteomalacia, rheumatoid arthritis, prolonged corticosteroid therapy
  - Body composition—increased risk of stress fractures with BMI <19
  - Skeletal malalignment: pes cavus, pes planus, leg length discrepancies, excessive forefoot varus, tarsal coalitions, prominent posterior calcaneal process, tight heel cords
  - Biomechanical factors such as increased vertical loading rate (e.g., heel-to-toe running instead of forefoot striking)
  - Muscle fatigue and decreased lean muscle mass
  - Extremes of body size and composition
  - Previous inactivity or low aerobic fitness
- Extrinsic (3)[A]
  - Type of exercise—both male and female athletes who participate in running, track and field, cross country, and gymnastics are at highest risk
  - Training regimen—running >32 km/week increases risk by 2 times in all athletes and by 3 times in female athletes
  - Nutritional/dietary habits—history of a diagnosed eating disorder
  - Rapid increase in mileage, running pace, or training volume
  - Inappropriate footwear
  - Hard training surface
  - Inadequate recovery or rest and training with fatigued muscle
  - There is no evidence that use of oral contraceptives is related to stress fracture risk.

GENERAL PREVENTION
- Avoid abrupt increases in physical activity (no more than 10% increase in load per week).
- Reduce intensity and duration of activity if new-onset pain.
- Proper footwear
- Increasing dynamic physical activity (jumping; plyometric training) increases bone density and resistance to mechanical stress.
- Decrease vertical loading rate either by switching to forefoot strike running or (if continuing with heel-to-toe strike) by using a heel pad insert.
- Shock-absorbing foot inserts may help.
- Increased calcium and vitamin D intake may reduce stress fractures in female runners and military recruits.
- Vitamin D supplementation (800 IU/day) in combination with calcium (2,000 mg/day) is effective in reducing fracture risk (2)[C].

COMMONLY ASSOCIATED CONDITIONS
- Osteoporosis/osteopenia
- Female athlete triad
- Metabolic bone disorders

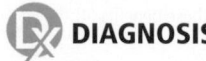 **DIAGNOSIS**

HISTORY
- Insidious onset of vague bony pain over period of weeks. Pain is typically worse with physical activity.
- Rest initially relieves pain.
- If untreated, pain progresses and may occur earlier during training sessions or even at rest. Pain also becomes more localized.
- History of recent change in training intensity, alteration in training terrain, and/or footwear
- Assess dietary practices: energy availability, disordered eating, weight fluctuations, and calcium and vitamin D intake.
- Assess menstrual history: menarche, oligomenorrhea, or amenorrhea.

PHYSICAL EXAM
- Height, weight, BMI, and any stigmata of disordered eating (cold extremities, hypercarotenemia, lanugo hair, calluses on back of fingers, poor oral hygiene, parotid gland hypertrophy, bradycardia, or orthostatic hypotension)
- Antalgic gait
- Point or percussion tenderness over injury site—a vibrating tuning fork over the fracture site may intensify pain.
- Swelling may be present.
- Specific tests:
  - Hop test for tibial stress fracture: With a stress fracture, the patient cannot hop on one leg 10 times; if able to perform test, consider shin splints (medial tibial stress syndrome).
  - Fulcrum test for femoral stress fracture: With patient seated, provoke pain by applying downward force on the distal femur while other hand uses the midthigh as fulcrum on femoral shaft (if clinical suspicion is high, defer or use only with extreme caution to avoid completing a femoral neck stress fracture).
  - Single-leg hyperextension (Stork) test for pars interarticularis fracture of lumbar spine: Stand on one leg and extend lumbar spine; positive if painful on symptomatic side
- Anatomic malalignment may be present (leg length discrepancy, pes planus/cavus).

DIFFERENTIAL DIAGNOSIS
- Shin splints (medial tibial stress syndrome—pain resolves with rest; stress fracture pain does not)
- Infection (osteomyelitis)
- Soft tissue injury (sprain, tendonitis, and periostitis)
- Compartment syndrome
- Bony fracture
- Neoplasm (osteoid osteoma)
- Nerve entrapment syndromes
- Intermittent claudication

DIAGNOSTIC TESTS & INTERPRETATION
Initial Tests (lab, imaging)
- Laboratory tests are not required unless clinically indicated for suspected disease (e.g., female athlete triad, hyperparathyroidism, and vitamin D deficiency).
- If nutritional or metabolic causes are suspected, consider testing for 25-hydroxyvitamin D3, calcium, TSH, FSH, LH, CBC, and BMP (2)[C].

- Plain films:
  - First line in suspected stress fracture
  - Findings typically seen 2 to 8 weeks after pain onset
  - Sensitivity during early stages (1 to 2 weeks) may be as low as 10%.
  - May see periosteal callus, "gray cortex sign" (region of decreased cortical intensity), osteopenia, endosteal reaction, or ill-defined cortical margin
  - Severe cases may show discrete fracture.

Follow-Up Tests & Special Considerations

- MRI:
  - Gold standard for imaging stress fractures
  - Highly sensitive; (sensitivity 100%, specificity 85%) more complete evaluation of exact anatomic location and extent of injury (2)[C]
- Bone scan:
  - Sensitive but has potential for false positives
  - Useful for suspected rib or spine stress fractures
  - Should not be used to assess healing, increased uptake on all three phases of bone remodeling (2)[C]
- CT scan:
  - Less sensitive than MRI or bone scan for early stress fractures but has an important role in evaluating longitudinal fracture lines and occult fractures of foot, tibia, carpal scaphoid, and pars interarticularis
  - Can distinguish conditions (osteoid osteoma, malignancy, and osteomyelitis) that mimic stress fracture on bone scan
  - Bony detail provided by CT scan allows differentiation of complete versus incomplete fracture, especially if MRI is equivocal
- US: not routinely used but beneficial for superficial stress fracture; may help to distinguish metatarsal stress fracture from other causes of metatarsalgia (e.g., Morton neuroma) (2)[C]
- Classification by radiographic findings (CT, MRI, bone scan, or radiograph) (4)[C]:
  - Grade I: asymptomatic stress reaction; no pain, periosteal edema only, no fracture line
  - Grade II: symptomatic stress reaction; pain on exam, bone marrow edema, no fracture line seen on imaging
  - Grade III: nondisplaced fracture; pain on exam, nondisplaced fracture line seen on imaging
  - Grade IV: displaced fracture; pain on exam, displaced fracture >2 mm seen on imaging
  - Grade V: nonunion; pain on exam, nonunion characteristics on imaging, long-standing symptoms

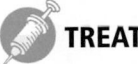 **TREATMENT**

- Grade I to grade II and low-risk stress fractures are generally treated nonoperatively, including non–weight-bearing and immobilization (5)[C].
- Grade III to grade V and high-risk stress fractures are treated either operatively or nonoperatively based on the imaging characteristics and fracture site (5)[C].
- Protection, rest, ice, compression, and elevation (PRICE) for acute pain and edema
- Decrease activity to the level of pain-free functioning.
- Consider temporarily immobilizing patients who have pain at rest or with gentle range of motion (ROM).
- If patients have pain with ambulation, use crutches with periodic walking trial to monitor readiness for nonaided (pain free) ambulation.
- Pneumatic leg brace is effective in decreasing the return-to-play time for tibial shaft stress fracture.
- For low-risk stress fracture, slowly increase impact loading once ambulation and daily activities are pain free. Progression of activity depends on the individual and should be modified according to symptoms (5,6)[C].

- High-risk fractures typically require immediate immobilization and a period of non–weight-bearing. Many patients require early surgical intervention to avoid nonunion and facilitate earlier return to sport (5)[C].
- A key difference between a low-grade stress fracture at a high-risk location versus a low-risk location is that with the low-risk site, the athlete could be allowed to continue to train, whereas the high-risk site needs to heal prior to full return to activity.
- Criteria for allowing an athlete to return should include complete resolution of symptoms with activities of daily living; radiographic evidence of healing; no tenderness to palpation at the injury site; and optimization of the athlete's nutritional, biomechanical, hormonal, and psychological status.

MEDICATION

First Line

- Calcium and vitamin D supplementation should be initiated when dietary intake is inadequate or deficiencies are found.
- Acetaminophen is useful for pain.
- NSAIDs are beneficial for pain and inflammation but may adversely affect fracture healing and should, therefore, be used only sparingly.

ISSUES FOR REFERRAL

Orthopedic consultation for high-risk fractures, failure to improve with standard treatment, evidence of nonunion within 3 to 4 weeks, or inability to tolerate rehabilitation

ADDITIONAL THERAPIES

- Electrical stimulation may be an adjunct for delayed union and nonunion.
- Extracorporeal shock wave therapy (ESWT) and pulsed US may have potential benefit but require additional study.
- Physical therapy:
  - Correct training errors and inappropriate mechanics predisposing to stress fracture.
  - Strengthen surrounding musculature.
  - Encourage cross-training to maintain fitness.
  - Correct anatomic variations.
  - Antigravity treadmills

 ONGOING CARE

FOLLOW-UP RECOMMENDATIONS

- Once the patient is pain free, low-impact training can start and be advanced gently as tolerated.
- Once running has resumed, increase mileage slowly no more than 10% per week.

Patient Monitoring

- Imaging every 4 to 6 weeks to assess healing
- An MRI is generally the preferred imaging technique for follow-up of early stage stress fractures.
- Radiographs are less expensive and can be used for follow-up of higher grade stress fractures.

PATIENT EDUCATION

- Gradually increase activity as long as pain free.
- Rest and reevaluate if there is a recurrence of pain.
- Correct mechanical and training errors with gait retraining.
- Strengthen core muscles.

PROGNOSIS

- Young patients have a good prognosis.
- Older patients or those with metabolic bone disease often develop insufficiency fractures in other bones.

- Time to return to full activity (5)[C]:
  - Grade I: 3+ weeks
  - Grade II: 5+ weeks
  - Grade III: 11 + weeks
  - Grade IV and V: 14+ weeks

COMPLICATIONS

- Completion of fracture
- Delayed union
- Nonunion
- May require surgery with internal fixation

REFERENCES

1. Matcuk GR Jr, Mahanty SR, Skalski MR, et al. Stress fractures: pathophysiology, clinical presentation, imaging features, and treatment options. *Emerg Radiol.* 2016;23(4):365–375.
2. Defroda SF, Cameron KL, Posner M, et al. Bone stress injuries in the military: diagnosis, management, and prevention. *Am J Orthop (Belle Mead NJ).* 2017;46(4):176–183.
3. Wright AA, Taylor JB, Ford KR, et al. Risk factors associated with lower extremity stress fractures in runners: a systematic review with meta-analysis. *Br J Sports Med.* 2015;49(23):1517–1523.
4. Kaeding CC, Miller T. The comprehensive description of stress fractures: a new classification system. *J Bone Joint Surg Am.* 2013;95(13):1214–1220.
5. Chen YT, Tenforde AS, Fredericson M. Update on stress fractures in female athletes: epidemiology, treatment, and prevention. *Curr Rev Musculoskelet Med.* 2013;6(2):173–181.
6. Mayer SW, Joyner PW, Almekinders LC, et al. Stress fractures of the foot and ankle in athletes. *Sports Health.* 2014;6(6):481–491.

ADDITIONAL READING

Miller TL, Best TM. Taking a holistic approach to managing difficult stress fractures. *J Orthop Surg Res.* 2016;11:98.

 SEE ALSO

Algorithm: Foot Pain

CODES

ICD10

- M84.38XA Stress fracture, other site, initial encounter for fracture
- M84.369A Stress fracture, unsp tibia and fibula, init for fx
- M84.376A Stress fracture, unspecified foot, init encntr for fracture

CLINICAL PEARLS

- The diagnosis of stress fractures requires a high index of suspicion. X-rays are often negative initially.
- Identify and treat female athletic triad to prevent stress fractures.
- To help prevent stress fractures, gradually increase training volume and avoid sudden increases in high-impact activity or running mileage.
- High-risk fractures require immediate immobilization and non–weight-bearing. Patients may also require early surgery.

STROKE, ACUTE (CEREBROVASCULAR ACCIDENT [CVA])

Rachel Ragosta, MCHS, PA-C, CAQ-Hospital, RN • Jeanne M. Cawse-Lucas, MD

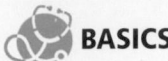

BASICS

DESCRIPTION
The sudden onset of a focal neurologic deficit(s) resulting from either infarction or hemorrhage within the brain

- Two broad categories: ischemic (thrombotic or embolic) (87%) and hemorrhagic (13%)
- Hemorrhage can be intracerebral or subarachnoid.
- System(s) affected: neurologic; vascular (1)
- Synonym(s): CVA; cerebral infarct
- Related terms: transient ischemic attack (TIA), a transient episode of neurologic dysfunction due to focal ischemia without permanent infarction on imaging (see topic "Transient Ischemic Attack (TIA)")

Pediatric Considerations
- Incidence: 2 to 13/100,000
- Frequent risk factors: arteriopathies (53%), cardiac disorders (31%), and infection (24%) (2)

EPIDEMIOLOGY
Incidence
Annual incidence in the United States is ~795,000.

Prevalence
- Prevalence in the United States: 550/100,000
- Predominant age: Risk increases >45 years of age and is highest during the 7th and 8th decades.
- Predominant sex: male > female at younger age but higher incidence in women with age ≥75 years

ETIOLOGY AND PATHOPHYSIOLOGY
- 87% of strokes are ischemic, three main subtypes: thrombosis, embolism, and systemic hypoperfusion. Large vessel atherothrombotic strokes often involve the origin of the internal carotid artery. Small vessel lacunar strokes are commonly due to lipohyalinotic occlusion. Embolic strokes are largely from a cardiac source (due to left atrial thrombus, atrial fibrillation, recent MI, valve disease, or mechanical valves) or ascending aortic atheromatous disease (>4 mm) (1).
- 13% of strokes are hemorrhagic; most commonly due to hypertension. Other causes include intracranial vascular malformations (cavernous angiomas, AVMs), cerebral amyloid angiopathy (lobar hemorrhages in elderly), and anticoagulation (1).
- Fibromuscular dysplasia (rare), vasculitis, or drug use (cocaine, amphetamines) are other causes of stroke.

Genetics
Stroke is a polygenic multifactorial disease.

RISK FACTORS
- Uncontrollable: age, gender, race, family history/genetics, prior stroke or TIA
- Controllable/modifiable/treatable
  - Metabolic: diabetes, dyslipidemia
  - Lifestyle: smoking, cocaine and amphetamine use
  - Cardiovascular: hypertension, atrial fibrillation, valvular heart disease, endocarditis, recent MI, severe carotid artery stenosis, hypercoagulable states, and patent foramen ovale (1)

GENERAL PREVENTION
Smoking cessation, regular exercise, weight control to maintain nonobese BMI and prevent type 2 diabetes, moderate alcohol use; control BP; manage hyperlipidemia; use antiplatelet agent (e.g., aspirin) in high-risk persons; treat nonvalvular atrial fibrillation with dose-adjusted warfarin or dabigatran, apixaban, and rivaroxaban (3).

COMMONLY ASSOCIATED CONDITIONS
Coronary artery disease is the major cause of death during the first 5 years after a stroke.

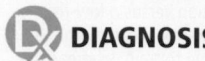

DIAGNOSIS

HISTORY
- Acute onset of focal arm/leg weakness, facial weakness, difficulty with speech or swallowing, vertigo, visual disturbances, diminished consciousness
- Assess risk factors.
- Vomiting and severe headache favor hemorrhagic stroke (1).

PHYSICAL EXAM
- Assess airway, breathing, and circulation (ABC).
- Anterior (carotid) circulation: hemiparesis/hemiplegia, neglect, aphasia, visual field defects
- Posterior (vertebrobasilar) circulation: diplopia, vertigo, gait and limb ataxia, facial paresis, Horner syndrome, dysphagia, dysarthria, alternating sensory loss

DIFFERENTIAL DIAGNOSIS
- Migraine (complicated)
- Postictal state (Todd paralysis)
- Systemic infection, including meningitis or encephalitis (infection also may uncover or enhance previous deficits)
- Toxic or metabolic disturbance (hypoglycemia, acute renal failure, liver failure, drug intoxication)
- Brain tumor, primary or metastases
- Head trauma, encephalopathy
- Other types of intracranial hemorrhage (epidural, subdural, subarachnoid)
- Trauma, septic emboli (1)

DIAGNOSTIC TESTS & INTERPRETATION
Used to narrow differential and identify etiology of stroke

Initial Tests (lab, imaging)
- Serum glucose (REQUIRED to exclude hypo/hyperglycemia prior to IV alteplase) (3)[B]
- ECG
- CBC; electrolyte panel
- Coagulation studies: PT, PTT, INR
- Baseline troponin (3)[B]
- Emergent noncontrast head CT, within 20 minutes of arrival to the ED (3)[B]
- Subsequent multimodal CT (perfusion CT, CTA, unenhanced CT) or MRI improves diagnosis of acute ischemic stroke (AIS).

Follow-Up Tests & Special Considerations
Consider LFT, tox screen, blood alcohol, ABG, lumbar puncture if suspected subarachnoid hemorrhage (SAH); EEG if suspect seizures, blood type and cross
- DW-MRI is more sensitive than CT for AIS.
- MRI is better than CT for posterior fossa lesions.
- Prior to initiation of IV tissue plasminogen activator (tPA), a noncontrast head CT (rule out ICH) and glucose are the only required tests unless contraindications exist. MRI to rule-out cerebral microbleeds is not required (3)[B].
- Multimodal imaging studies should not delay IV tPA if indicated (3)[B].

- For patients who meet criteria for mechanical thrombectomy, multimodal CT and MRI to rule out large vessel occlusion is recommended (3)[A]. Selected patients may be treated up to 16 to 24 hours after onset of symptoms (3)[A].

Diagnostic Procedures/Other
Echocardiogram (transthoracic and/or transesophageal) if there is suspicion for cardioembolic source (3). In cryptogenic stroke patients, perform prolonged ECG monitoring with a 30-day event monitor.

Test Interpretation
Early CT findings of ischemia: hyperdense middle cerebral artery (MCA) sign (increased attenuation of proximal portion of the MCA; associated with MCA thrombosis), loss of gray-white matter differentiation, sulcal effacement, loss of insular ribbon

TREATMENT

- Monitor BP closely in the first 24 hours.
  - Withhold antihypertensives unless systolic BP >220 mm Hg or diastolic BP >120 mm Hg. Goal is to lower BP ~15% in the first 24 hours if treatment is undertaken. If thrombolytic therapy is planned, BP must be <185/110 mm Hg prior to administration of thrombolytics (3).
  - In acute spontaneous intracranial hemorrhagic stroke, goal BP is 160/90 mm Hg or MAP of 110 (see topic "Subarachnoid Hemorrhage" for details).
  - If there is suspicion of elevated ICP, reduce BP to a target cerebral perfusion pressure of between 61 mm Hg and 80 mm Hg.
  - Start/restart antihypertensive medications 24 hours after stroke onset for patients with BP >140/90 mm Hg who are neurologically stable (3)[B].

ALERT
Thrombolysis: Individualize discussion about the use of IV thrombolysis with eligible patients who have measurable neurologic deficits that do not clear spontaneously and present within 3 to 4.5 hours of symptom onset.

- Exclusion criteria for thrombolysis within 3 hours of onset include:
  - Any history of ICH or new symptoms suggestive of ICH (3)[B]
  - Head trauma or prior stroke within 3 months
  - MI within 3 months
  - GI malignancy or bleed within 21 days (3)[C]
  - Major surgery within 14 days
  - Arterial puncture at noncompressible site within 7 days
  - Elevated BP (systolic >185 mm Hg and diastolic >110 mm Hg)
  - Active bleeding or evidence of acute trauma on examination
  - Taking anticoagulant and INR ≥1.7
  - If low-molecular-weight heparin received during previous 24 hours (3)[B]; platelet count <100,000 mm³ (3)[C]
  - Blood glucose concentration <50 mg/dL
  - Seizure with postictal residual neurologic impairment
  - Multilobar infarction on CT (hypodensity >1/3 cerebral hemisphere)
  - Patient or family members not able to provide input and understand potential harms and benefits of treatment

- Extended AHA/ASA exclusion criteria for thrombolysis within 4.5 hours include:
  - Age >80 years
  - All patients taking oral anticoagulants regardless of INR
  - National Institutes of Health (NIH) Stroke Scale >25
  - History of stroke and diabetes

MEDICATION

First Line
- Thrombolysis, IV administration of rtPA: Infuse 0.9 mg/kg, maximum dose 90 mg over 60 minutes with 10% of dose given as bolus over 1 minute.
  - Centers should attempt door-to-needle times of <60 minutes (3)[A].
  - Admit to ICU or stroke unit, with neurologic exams every 15 minutes during infusion, every 60 minutes for next 6 hours, and then hourly until 24 hours after treatment.
  - Discontinue infusion and obtain emergent CT scan if severe headache, angioedema, acute hypertension, or nausea and vomiting develop.
  - Measure BP every 15 minutes for first 2 hours, every 30 minutes for next 6 hours, and then every hour until 24 hours after treatment. Maintain BP <185/105 mm Hg; follow-up CT at 24 hours before starting anticoagulants or antiplatelet agents
- Antiplatelet: aspirin 160 to 300 mg/day within 24 to 48 hours after AIS (3)[A].
- BP management options include:
  - Labetalol 10 to 20 mg IV over 1 to 2 minutes, which may be repeated once
  - Nicardipine infusion 5 mg/hr, titrate up by 2.5 mg/hr at 5- to 15-minute intervals to maximum of 15 mg/hr; reduce to 3 mg/hr when target BP is reached.

Second Line
Carotid endarterectomy (CEA) for carotid artery stenosis rarely is indicated emergently. CEA is indicated for >70% ipsilateral stenosis. CEA for TIA or incomplete stroke lesion may be indicated for 50–69% stenosis in carefully selected patients, depending on risk factors, and skill and experience of surgeons.

ISSUES FOR REFERRAL
Follow-up with neurologist 1 week after discharge, with subsequent follow-up based on individual circumstances

ADDITIONAL THERAPIES
- If no contraindications, a trial of fluoxetine to improve motor outcomes may be reasonable (4)[A].
- Deep vein thrombosis (DVT) prophylaxis for immobilized patients
- Corticosteroids are *not* recommended for cerebral brain edema.
- Statin use should be continued without interruption following acute stroke.
- Refer to physical therapy, occupational therapy, and speech therapy as necessary.

SURGERY/OTHER PROCEDURES
- Ventricular drain may be placed for patients with acute hydrocephalus secondary to stroke (most commonly cerebellar stroke).
- Decompressive surgery is recommended for major cerebellar infarction; consider for malignant MCA infarction, especially if <60 years of age.
- Consider mechanical embolectomy in carefully selected patients who have evidence of salvageable tissue on advanced imaging.

COMPLEMENTARY & ALTERNATIVE MEDICINE
Acupuncture within 30 days of stroke onset may improve neurologic functioning.

ADMISSION, INPATIENT, AND NURSING CONSIDERATIONS
- Observe closely within first 24 hours for neurologic decline, particularly due to cerebral edema.
- Elevate bed to at least 30 degrees if elevated ICP is suspected. Patients with ischemic stroke may benefit from a horizontal bed position during the acute phase.
- Monitor cardiac rhythm for at least 24 hours to identify arrhythmias.
- Airway support and ventilatory assistance may be necessary due to diminished consciousness or bulbar involvement; reserve supplemental oxygen for hypoxic patients (3). Consider elective intubation for patients with malignant edema.
- Correct hypovolemia with normal saline.
- Keep patients NPO until a formal swallow evaluation has been performed; to reduce risk of aspiration pneumonia, elevate head of bed to 30 degrees.
- Hypoglycemia can cause neurologic dysfunction; correct during initial evaluation.
- Hyperglycemia within first 24 hours of stroke is associated with poor outcomes: insulin recommended to maintain glucose levels 140 to 180 mg/dL (3).
- In patients with ICH secondary to anticoagulant use, correct an elevated INR with IV vitamin K and fresh frozen plasma or prothrombin concentrate complex; factor VII infusion for patients requiring urgent surgical intervention (i.e., those with cerebellar hemorrhage who are neurologically deteriorating)
- DVT prophylaxis
- Maintain oxygen saturation >94%.
- Early physical therapy and discharge planning for rehabilitation and placement
- Maintenance IV hydration with normal saline until swallowing status is assessed; monitor fluid balance closely.
- Frequent neurologic exams in first 24 hours (every 1 to 2 hours)
- Fall precautions; frequent repositioning to prevent skin breakdown
- Discharge criteria: medically stable, adequate nutritional support, neurologic status stable, or improving

 ## ONGOING CARE

FOLLOW-UP RECOMMENDATIONS
- Secondary prevention of stroke with aggressive management of risk factors
- Platelet inhibition using aspirin, clopidogrel, or aspirin plus extended-release dipyridamole (Aggrenox) based on physician and patient preference

Patient Monitoring
Follow-up every 3 months for 1st year and then annually

DIET
Patients with impaired swallowing should receive nasogastric or percutaneous endoscopic gastrostomy feedings to maintain nutrition and hydration.

PATIENT EDUCATION
National Stroke Association (800-STROKES or http://www.stroke.org)

PROGNOSIS
Variable depends on subtype and severity of stroke; NIH Stroke Scale may be used for prognosis.

COMPLICATIONS
- Acute: brain herniation, hemorrhagic transformation, MI, congestive heart failure, dysphagia, aspiration pneumonia, UTI, DVT, pulmonary embolism, malnutrition, pressure sores
- Chronic: falls, depression, dementia, orthopedic complications, contractures

REFERENCES
1. Yew KS, Cheng EM. Diagnosis of acute stroke. *Am Fam Physician*. 2015;91(8):528–536.
2. Hankey GJ. Stroke. *Lancet*. 2017;389(10069): 641–654.
3. Powers WJ, Rabinstein AA, Ackerson T, et al; for American Heart Association Stroke Council. 2018 Guidelines for the early management of patients with acute ischemic stroke: a guideline for healthcare professionals from the American Heart Association/American Stroke Association. *Stroke*. 2018;49(3):e46–e110.
4. Chollet F, Tardy J, Albucher JF, et al. Fluoxetine for motor recovery after acute ischaemic stroke (FLAME): a randomised placebo-controlled trial. *Lancet Neurol*. 2011;10(2):123–130.

ADDITIONAL READING
- American Stroke Association. Stroke resources for professionals. http://www.strokeassociation.org /STROKEORG/Professionals/Stroke-Resources-for -Professionals_UCM_308581_SubHomePage.jsp. Accessed November 11, 2018.
- Peisker T, Koznar B, Stetkarova I, et al. Acute stroke therapy: a review. *Trends Cardiovasc Med*. 2017;27(1):59–66.

CODES

ICD10
- I63.9 Cerebral infarction, unspecified
- I61.9 Nontraumatic intracerebral hemorrhage, unspecified
- I63.50 Cereb infrc due to unsp occls or stenos of unsp cereb artery

CLINICAL PEARLS
- Unless stroke is hemorrhagic or patient is undergoing thrombolysis, do not lower BP acutely. This helps to maintain perfusion of penumbra region.
- Consider IV thrombolysis in eligible patients with neurologic deficits that do not clear spontaneously within 3 to 4.5 hours of symptom onset.
- DW-MRI is more sensitive than conventional CT for the diagnosis of AIS. MRI is also superior for diagnosing posterior fossa lesions.

S

SUBCONJUNCTIVAL HEMORRHAGE

Carrie Valenta, MD, FACP, FHM • Colin E. Brown, MD

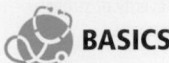 **BASICS**

DESCRIPTION
- Subconjunctival hemorrhage (SCH) is bleeding from small blood vessels underneath the conjunctiva, the thin clear skin covering the sclera of the eye.
- SCH is diagnosed clinically:
  – Flat, well-demarcated areas of extravasated blood can be seen just under the surface of the conjunctiva of the eye (red patch of blood sign).
  – SCH is more common in the inferior and temporal regions of the eye (1).
- Typically, SCH resolves spontaneously within 2 weeks.

EPIDEMIOLOGY
- Male = female; no gender predilection
- Common; 3% rate of diagnosis in ophthalmology clinics (2)

Incidence
Incidence increases.
- With increasing age
- In contact lenses wearers (5% of cases) (3)
- With systemic diseases such as diabetes, hypertension (HTN), and coagulation disorders
- During summer months, possibly due to trauma (2)

ETIOLOGY AND PATHOPHYSIOLOGY
- Direct trauma to the blood vessels of the conjunctiva from blunt or penetrating trauma to the eye
- Direct trauma to the conjunctiva from improper contact lens placement or improper cleaning
- Increased blood pressure (BP) in the vessels of the conjunctiva from HTN or from the temporary increase in BP from a Valsalva type maneuver (e.g., vomiting, sneezing)
- Damaged vessels from diabetes or atherosclerotic disease
- Increased bleeding tendencies from either thrombocytopenia or elevated prothrombin time (PT)/elevated international normalized ratio (INR) (4)

- Valsalva maneuvers causing sudden severe venous congestion such as coughing, sneezing, vomiting, straining, severe asthma or COPD exacerbation, weightlifting, or childbirth/labor (1)
- In patients age >60 years, HTN is the most common etiology.
- In patients age <40 years, trauma/Valsalva and contact lenses use are the most common etiologies.
- In patients age >40 years, conjunctivochalasis (redundant conjunctival folds) and presence of pinguecula are strongly associated (3).

RISK FACTORS
- Age
- Contact lenses wearer
- Systemic diseases (HTN, diabetes)
- Bleeding disorders (2)
- Recent ocular surgery (cataract, laser-assisted in situ keratomileusis [LASIK])

GENERAL PREVENTION
- Correct cleaning and maintenance of contact lenses
- Protective eyewear in sports and hobbies
- Optimizing control of systemic diseases such as HTN, diabetes, and atherosclerotic disease
- Control of PT/INR in patients on warfarin therapy (5)

 DIAGNOSIS

HISTORY
- Generally asymptomatic; usually, the patient notices redness in the mirror or another person mentions it to the patient.
- May complain of irritation or foreign body sensation
- Little to no pain involved (5)
- Obtain history of trauma. SCH can occur 12 to 24 hours after orbital fracture (1).
- Obtain history of contact lenses usage or recent cataract, LASIK, or other ocular surgery (2).

- Comprehensive past medical history to evaluate if at risk for systemic diseases or taking medications that might increase risk
- Obtain history for current systemic symptomatology.

PHYSICAL EXAM
- Measure BP to evaluate control of HTN (2).
- Assess visual acuity; this should be normal in a simple SCH (5).
- Verify that the pupils are equal and reactive to light and accommodation; this should be normal with SCH (5).
- There should be no discharge or exudate noted (5).
- Look at sclera for a bright red demarcated patch.
  – Demarcated area is most often on inferior aspect of eye due to gravity (3).
- If penetrating trauma is a consideration, perform a gentle digital assessment of the integrity of the globe (4).
- Slit-lamp exam should be performed if there is a history of trauma (1).

Geriatric Considerations
In older adults, the area of SCH will be more widespread across the sclera (3). Elastic and connective tissues are more fragile with age, and underlying conditions such as HTN and diabetes may contribute.

DIFFERENTIAL DIAGNOSIS
- Viral, bacterial, allergic, or chemical conjunctivitis (enterovirus and coxsackievirus most common) (1)[B]
- Foreign body to conjunctiva
- Penetrating trauma
- Recent ocular surgery/injection
- Contact lenses induced
- Child abuse (particularly if bilateral in an infant or toddler) (1)
- Occasionally found in newborns following vaginal delivery

DIAGNOSTIC TESTS & INTERPRETATION
- Typically no testing is indicated; SCH is a clinical diagnosis. If a foreign body is suspected, perform a fluorescein exam.
- Fluorescein exam of a patient with an SCH should show no uptake of staining (5)[C].
- If an orbital fracture is suspected, may obtain plain facial bone films or CT scan (4)[C]

Follow-Up Tests & Special Considerations
If history and physical exam suggest a bleeding disorder (5)[C]
- CBC
- PT/INR

ALERT
- If a penetrating injury is suspected, may obtain a CT scan of the orbits
- Do not perform MRI if foreign object may be metal (4)[C].

TREATMENT

GENERAL MEASURES
- Control BP.
- Control blood glucose.
- Control INR.
- Wear protective eyewear.

MEDICATION
No prescription medications are useful in treatment of SCH.

ISSUES FOR REFERRAL
- If a penetrating eye injury is suspected, seek emergent ophthalmology consultation.
- If the patient complains of any decreased visual acuity or visual disturbances, refer to an ophthalmologist as soon as possible.
- If there is no resolution of SCH within 2 weeks or if SCH are recurrent, patient may need referral to an ophthalmologist.

ADDITIONAL THERAPIES
- Warm compresses
- Eye lubricants (5)[C]

ONGOING CARE

FOLLOW-UP RECOMMENDATIONS
- Follow up only if the area does not resolve within 2 weeks.
- If SCH recurs, then work up patient for systemic sources such as bleeding disorders (5)[C].

PATIENT EDUCATION
- Reassurance of the self-limited nature of the problem and typical time frame for resolution
- Education to return to clinic if the area does not heal or recurs
- Correct cleaning and maintenance of contact lenses
- Eye lubricants for ocular irritation

PROGNOSIS
Excellent

COMPLICATIONS
Rare

REFERENCES
1. Tarlan B, Kiratli H. Subconjunctival hemorrhage: risk factors and potential indicators. *Clin Ophthalmol.* 2013;7:1163–1170.
2. Mimura T, Usui T, Yamagami S, et al. Recent causes of subconjunctival hemorrhage. *Ophthalmologica.* 2010;224(3):133–137.
3. Mimura T, Yamagami S, Mori M, et al. Contact lens-induced subconjunctival hemorrhage. *Am J Ophthalmol.* 2010;150(5):656.e1–665.e1.
4. Wirbelauer C. Management of the red eye for the primary care physician. *Am J Med.* 2006;119(4): 302–306.
5. Cronau H, Kankanala RR, Mauger T. Diagnosis and management of red eye in primary care. *Am Fam Physician.* 2010;81(2):137–144.

ADDITIONAL READING
- Mimura T, Usui T, Yamagami S, et al. Subconjunctival hemorrhage and conjunctivochalasis. *Ophthalmology.* 2009;116(10):1880–1886.
- Mimura T, Yamagami S, Usui T, et al. Location and extent of subconjunctival hemorrhage. *Ophthalmologica.* 2010;224(2):90–95.

CODES

ICD10
- H11.30 Conjunctival hemorrhage, unspecified eye
- H11.31 Conjunctival hemorrhage, right eye
- H11.32 Conjunctival hemorrhage, left eye

CLINICAL PEARLS
- SCH is a clinical diagnosis. The condition is typically asymptomatic and will resolve spontaneously within 2 weeks.
- Always check BP in a patient with SCH because HTN is a known risk factor.
- Indications for immediate referral to an ophthalmologist include eye pain, changes in vision, lack of pupil reactivity, and/or penetrating eye trauma.
- Reassurance and comfort measures (i.e., ocular lubrication) are mainstays of treatment.
- Contact lenses wearers should not wear contact lenses until the SCH resolves completely.

SUBSTANCE USE DISORDERS

S. Lindsey Clarke, MD, FAAFP

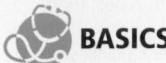

BASICS

DESCRIPTION

Any pattern of substance use causing significant physical, mental, or social dysfunction

- Substances of abuse include:
  - Alcohol
  - Tobacco
  - Prescription medications
    - ○ CNS depressants (barbiturates, benzodiazepines, hypnotics)
    - ○ Opioids and morphine derivatives (codeine, fentanyl, hydrocodone, hydromorphone, oxymorphone [Opana], meperidine, methadone, morphine, oxycodone)
    - ○ Stimulants (amphetamines, methylphenidate)
    - ○ Dextromethorphan ("Robotripping")
  - Cannabis (marijuana, hashish, cannabis oil, and extracts); increasingly sold as highly concentrated extracts (up to 90% THC) for use in vaporizers
  - Synthetic cannabinoids (Spice, K2, fake weed); often much more potent than marijuana; may be smoked, brewed in tea, or vaporized
  - Stimulants (cocaine, amphetamines, methamphetamines, Khat)
  - "Club drugs" (MDMA [ecstasy, Molly], PMMA [Superman], flunitrazepam, γ-hydroxybutyrate [GHB])
  - Opioids (heroin, opium, kratom, desomorphine [Krokodil])
  - Dissociative drugs (ketamine, phencyclidine [PCP])
  - Hallucinogens (lysergic acid diethylamide [LSD], salvia, ayahuasca, *N,N*-dimethyltryptamine [DMT])
  - Synthetic cathinones (bath salts, α-PVP [Flakka])
  - Inhalants (glue, paint thinners, nitrous oxide)
  - Anabolic steroids
- See also www.drugabuse.gov/drugs-abuse.
- System(s) affected: cardiovascular, endocrine/metabolic, CNS
- Synonym(s): drug abuse; drug dependence; substance abuse

Geriatric Considerations
- Alcohol is the most commonly abused substance, and abuse often goes unrecognized.
- Higher potential for drug interactions

Pregnancy Considerations
Substance abuse may cause fetal abnormalities, morbidity, and fetal or maternal death.

ALERT
The prevalence of opioid use in pregnancy and associated neonatal abstinence syndrome have increased significantly in recent years. Screen for substance use at the first prenatal visit with a brief intervention, and refer for treatment to improve maternal and neonatal outcomes.

EPIDEMIOLOGY

Incidence
- Predominant age: 18 to 25 years
- Predominant sex: male > female

Prevalence
- 28.6 million Americans (10.6%) reported illicit drug use in 2016 (https://www.cdc.gov/nchs/fastats/drug-use-illegal.htm).
- 8% of 12- to 17-year-olds; 23% of 18- to 25-year-olds
- 1 in 5 young adults currently use marijuana.

ETIOLOGY AND PATHOPHYSIOLOGY
Multifactorial, including genetic, environmental

Genetics
Substances of abuse affect dopamine, acetylcholine, γ-aminobutyric acid, norepinephrine, opioid, and serotonin receptors. Variant alleles may account for differences in susceptibility to misuse of different substances.

RISK FACTORS
- Male gender, young adult
- Depression, anxiety
- Other substance use disorders
- Family history
- Peer or family use or approval
- Low socioeconomic status
- Unemployment
- Accessibility of substances of abuse
- Family dysfunction or trauma
- Antisocial personality disorder
- Academic problems, school dropout
- Criminal involvement

GENERAL PREVENTION
- Early identification and aggressive early intervention improve outcomes.
- Universal school-based interventions are modestly effective for preventing drug use among adolescents.

COMMONLY ASSOCIATED CONDITIONS
- Depression
- Personality disorders
- Bipolar affective disorder

ALERT
Prescription narcotic overdose is the leading cause of accidental death in patients between the ages of 25 and 44 years in the United States (http://www.cdc.gov/injury/wisqars/leading_causes_death.html).

DIAGNOSIS

Substance use disorder (*DSM-5* criteria): ≥2 of the following in past year severity based on number of criteria present:

- Missed work or school
- Use in hazardous situations
- Continued use despite social or personal problems
- Craving
- Tolerance (decreased response to effects of drug due to constant exposure)
- Withdrawal on discontinuation
- Using more than intended
- Failed attempts to quit
- Increased time spent obtaining, using, or recovering from the substance
- Interference with important activities
- Continued use despite health problems

HISTORY
- History of infections (e.g., endocarditis, hepatitis B or C, TB, STI, or recurrent pneumonia)
- Social or behavioral problems, including chaotic relationships and/or employment difficulties
- Frequent visits to emergency department
- Criminal incarceration
- History of blackouts, insomnia, mood swings, chronic pain, repetitive trauma
- Anxiety, fatigue, depression, psychosis

PHYSICAL EXAM
- Vital sign abnormalities (changes in HR, RR, BP, and temperature all manifest with substance misuse)
- Abnormally dilated or constricted pupils
- Cutaneous needle marks
- Nasal septum perforation (with cocaine use)
- Cardiac dysrhythmias, pathologic murmurs
- Malnutrition with severe dependence
- Mental status examination

DIFFERENTIAL DIAGNOSIS
- Depression, anxiety, or other behavioral conditions
- Metabolic delirium (hypoxia, hypoglycemia, infection, thiamine deficiency, hypothyroidism, thyrotoxicosis)
- ADHD
- Medication toxicity

DIAGNOSTIC TESTS & INTERPRETATION

ALERT
Screening with a single question: "How many times in the past year have you used an illegal drug or used a prescription medication for nonmedical reasons?": has a sensitivity of 100% and specificity of 74% in primary care setting (1)[B]

- CRAFFT questionnaire (sensitivity 94% with ≥2 "yes" answers):
  - C: Have you ever ridden in a CAR driven by someone (including yourself) who was "high" or who had been using alcohol or drugs?
  - R: Do you ever use alcohol or drugs to RELAX, feel better about yourself, or fit in?
  - A: Do you ever use alcohol or drugs while you are ALONE?
  - F: Do you ever FORGET things you did while using alcohol or drugs?
  - F: Do your FAMILY or FRIENDS ever tell you that you should cut down on your drinking or drug use?
  - T: Have you gotten into TROUBLE while you were using alcohol or drugs?
- American Academy of Pediatrics also recommends the following brief screening tools for adolescents:
  - S2B1 (Screening to Brief Intervention)
  - BSTAD (Brief Screener for Tobacco, Alcohol, and Other Drugs)
- Blood alcohol concentration
- Urine drug screen (UDS) (order qualitative UDS, and if specific drug is in question, a quantitative analysis for specific drug; order confirmatory serum tests if false positive suspected)
- Approximate detection limits
  - Alcohol: 6 to 10 hours
  - Amphetamines and variants: 2 to 3 days
  - Barbiturates: 2 to 10 days
  - Benzodiazepines: 1 to 6 weeks
  - Cocaine: 2 to 3 days
  - Heroin: 1 to 1.5 days
  - LSD, psilocybin: 8 hours
  - Marijuana: 1 to 7 days; up to 1 month with chronic/heavy use
  - Methadone: 1 day to 1 week
  - Opioids: 1 to 3 days
  - PCP: 7 to 14 days
  - Anabolic steroids: oral, 3 weeks; injectable, 3 months; nandrolone, 9 months
- Liver transaminases
- HIV, hepatitis B and C screens
- Echocardiogram for endocarditis
- Head CT scan for seizure, delirium, trauma

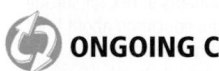 TREATMENT

Determine substances abused early (may influence disposition).

GENERAL MEASURES
- Nonjudgmental, medically oriented attitude
- Motivational interviewing and brief interventions can overcome denial and promote change.
- Behavioral and cognitive therapy
- Community reinforcement
- Interventional counseling
- Self-help groups to aid recovery (Alcoholics Anonymous, other 12-step programs)
- Support groups for family (Al-Anon/Alateen)

MEDICATION
- Alcohol withdrawal: See "Alcohol Use Disorder (AUD)" and "Alcohol Withdrawal."
- Benzodiazepine or barbiturate withdrawal
  - Gradual taper preferable to abrupt discontinuation
  - Substitution of long-acting benzodiazepine (e.g., clonazepam) or phenobarbital
- Nicotine withdrawal: See "Tobacco Use and Smoking Cessation."
- Opioid dependence
  - Buprenorphine: 8 to 16 mg SL daily, 100 to 300 mg SC monthly or as 6-month subdermal implant; may precipitate a more severe withdrawal if initiated too soon; use restricted to licensed clinics and certified physicians (2,3,4)[A].
  - Buprenorphine/naloxone: 4/1 mg to 16/4 mg SL daily; also available as SL and buccal films; combination limits abuse potential compared with buprenorphine alone.
  - Methadone: 10 to 40 mg/day PO; use restricted to inpatient settings and especially licensed clinics (2,3,4)[A].
  - Naltrexone: 50 mg PO daily, 100 mg PO every 2 days, 150 mg PO every 3 days, or 380 mg IM every 4 weeks; must be opioid-free for 7 to 10 days
- Opioid withdrawal
  - Clonidine: 0.1 to 0.2 mg PO BID or TID for autonomic hyperactivity (5)[A]
- Stimulant withdrawal
  - No agent with clear benefit
  - Methylphenidate ER: titrated up to 54 mg/day PO might enhance abstinence in amphetamine-dependent patients
- Adjuncts to therapy
  - Use all medications in conjunction with psychosocial behavioral interventions.
  - Antiemetics, nonaddictive analgesics for opioid withdrawal
  - Nonhabituating antidepressants, mood stabilizers, anxiolytics, and hypnotics for comorbid mood and anxiety disorders and insomnia that persist after detoxification
- Contraindications
  - Buprenorphine in breastfeeding, hepatic impairment
  - Methadone in hepatic impairment
  - Naltrexone in pregnancy, breastfeeding, hepatic impairment
- Precautions: Clonidine can cause hypotension.
- Significant possible interactions
  - Buprenorphine and opioids, CNS depressants, or HIV protease inhibitors
  - Methadone and strong inhibitors of CYP3A4 (clarithromycin, ketoconazole, HIV protease inhibitors), opioids, CNS depressants
  - Naltrexone and opioid medications (may precipitate or exacerbate withdrawal)

ISSUES FOR REFERRAL
- Consider addiction specialist, especially for opioid and polysubstance abuse.
- Maintenance therapy for opioid dependence (e.g., methadone) only in FDA-licensed clinics
- Psychiatrist for comorbid psychiatric disorders
- Social services

ADMISSION, INPATIENT, AND NURSING CONSIDERATIONS
- Indications for inpatient detoxification
  - History of severe withdrawal (e.g., seizures)
  - Mental status changes
  - Hallucinations or psychotic features
  - Threat of harm to self or others
  - Obstacles to close monitoring/follow-up
  - Comorbid medical illness
  - Pregnancy
- Consider specialist referral for narcotic addiction and withdrawal.
- Look for signs of severe infection (e.g., bacterial endocarditis).
- Take frequent vital signs during withdrawal.
- Monitor for signs of drug use in the hospital.
- Discharge criteria
  - Detoxification complete
  - Rehabilitation plan in place

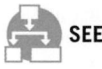 ONGOING CARE

FOLLOW-UP RECOMMENDATIONS
Initially frequent visits to monitor for medical stability and adherence and then progressive follow-up intervals

Patient Monitoring
Verify patient's adherence with the substance abuse treatment program.

DIET
Patients often are malnourished.

PATIENT EDUCATION
- Substance Abuse and Mental Health Services Administration: https://www.samhsa.gov or 800-662-HELP (4357) for information, treatment facility locator
- National Institute on Drug Abuse: http://www.drugabuse.gov/patients-families
- Alcoholics Anonymous: http://www.aa.org
- Narcotics Anonymous: http://www.na.org

PROGNOSIS
- Patients in treatment for longer periods have higher success rates.
- Behavioral therapy and pharmacotherapy are most successful when used in combination.

COMPLICATIONS
- Serious harm to self and others: accidents, violence
- Overdoses resulting in seizures, arrhythmias, cardiac and respiratory arrest, coma, death
- Hepatitis, HIV, tuberculosis, syphilis
- Subacute bacterial endocarditis
- Malnutrition
- Social problems, including arrest
- Poor marital adjustment and violence
- Depression, schizophrenia
- Sexual assault (alcohol, flunitrazepam, GHB)

REFERENCES

1. Smith PC, Schmidt SM, Allensworth-Davies D, et al. A single-question screening test for drug use in primary care. *Arch Intern Med*. 2010;170(13):1155–1160.
2. Gowing L, Ali R, White JM, et al. Buprenorphine for managing opioid withdrawal. *Cochrane Database Syst Rev*. 2017;(2):CD002025.
3. Nielsen S, Larance B, Degenhardt L, et al. Opioid agonist treatment for pharmaceutical opioid dependent people. *Cochrane Database Syst Rev*. 2016;(5):CD011117.
4. Mattick RP, Breen C, Kimber J, et al. Buprenorphine maintenance versus placebo or methadone maintenance for opioid dependence. *Cochrane Database Syst Rev*. 2014;(2):CD002207.
5. Gowing L, Farrell M, Ali R, et al. Alpha$_2$-adrenergic agonists for the management of opioid withdrawal. *Cochrane Database Syst Rev*. 2016;(5):CD002024.

ADDITIONAL READING

- Albertson TE, Chenoweth JA, Colby DK, et al. The changing drug culture: emerging drugs of abuse and legal highs. *FP Essent*. 2016;441:18–24.
- Committee on Obstetric Practice. Committee Opinion No. 711: opioid use and opioid use disorder in pregnancy. *Obstet Gynecol*. 2017;130(2):e81–e94.
- Committee on Substance Use and Prevention. Substance use screening, brief intervention, and referral to treatment. *Pediatrics*. 2016;138(1):e20161210.
- Substance Abuse and Mental Health Services Administration. *Key Substance Use and Mental Health Indicators in the United States: Results from the 2016 National Survey on Drug Use and Health* (HHS Publication No. SMA 17-5044, NSDUH Series H-52). Rockville, MD: Center for Behavioral Health Statistics and Quality, Substance Abuse and Mental Health Services Administration; 2017. https://www.samhsa.gov/data/.

SEE ALSO

Alcohol Use Disorder (AUD); Alcohol Withdrawal; Tobacco Use and Smoking Cessation

CODES

ICD10
- F19.10 Other psychoactive substance abuse, uncomplicated
- F10.10 Alcohol abuse, uncomplicated
- F12.10 Cannabis abuse, uncomplicated

CLINICAL PEARLS
- Substance use disorders are prevalent, serious, and often unrecognized in clinical practice. Comorbid psychiatric disorders are common.
- Substance abuse is distinguished by family, social, occupational, legal, or physical dysfunction that is caused by persistent use of the substance.
- Dependence is characterized by tolerance, withdrawal, compulsive use, and repeated overindulgence.
- Motivational interviewing, brief interventions, and a nonjudgmental attitude help to promote a willingness to change behavior.
- Consider referring patients with alcohol or opioid dependence to an addiction specialist or treatment program.

S

SUICIDE
Irene Coletsos, MD • Harold J. Bursztajn, MD

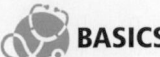 **BASICS**

DESCRIPTION
Suicide and attempted suicide are significant causes of morbidity and mortality.

EPIDEMIOLOGY
- Predominant sex
  - Women *attempt* suicide 1.5 times more often than men. Men *complete* suicide 3 times more often than women. Men are more likely to choose a means with high lethality, such as firearms.
- Predominant age: adolescent (2nd leading cause of death), 10th leading cause of death overall, per 2016, CDC statistics (latest available)
- Marital status: single > divorced; widowed > married
- Worldwide, suicide is the 18th leading cause of death per World Health Organization reports from 2018 but the 2nd leading cause of death among youths (ages 15 to 29 year olds).

Incidence
In 2016, 10th leading cause of death in adults in the United States. Military service (not specifically active duty) is associated with increased risk. A 2017 Veterans Administration study reported that veterans had a 22% increased rate of suicide over civilians.

RISK FACTORS
- "Human understanding is the most effective weapon against suicide. The greatest need is to deepen the awareness and sensitivity of people to their fellow man" (Shneidman, American Association of Suicidology [AAS]).
- Be alert to a combination of "perturbation" (increased emotional disturbance) and "lethality" (having the potential tools to cause death).
- 80% who complete suicides had a previous attempt.
- 90% who complete suicide meet *Diagnostic and Statistical Manual* criteria for Axis I or II disorders: major depression, bipolar disorder, anorexia nervosa, panic disorder, borderline and antisocial personality disorders. Schizophrenia or acute onset of psychosis is also risk factor due to command hallucinations or even the negative affect or hopelessness that can accompany these states.
- Substance use and withdrawal (alcohol, hallucinogens, opioids)
- Family history of suicide
- Physical illness, including head injury (TBI associated with 20% increased risk of death by suicide) (1)
- Despair: emotional pain *and* without hope and, consciously or unconsciously, unworthy of help
- Among teenagers: not feeling "connected" to their peers or family; being bullied; gender identity issues; poor grades
- Among veterans: childhood history of abuse; a diagnosis of major depressive disorder and multiple inpatient psychiatric admissions were found to be the "best predictors of enhanced suicide risk" (2).
- Psychosocial: recent loss. What may seem to be a small loss (to a medical provider) may be a devastating loss to the patient. *Patient-specific* factors need to be taken into account: social isolation, anniversaries, and holidays. Patients who attempt suicide also seem to have impaired decision-making skills and risk awareness and increased impulsivity compared with patients who have never attempted suicide (3).

- If a patient is incompetent (e.g., too delusional) to alert providers about the potential for suicide, the patient at increased risk for self-harm and providers should consider hospitalization.
- Access to lethal means: firearms, poisons (including prescription and nonprescription drugs; pesticides) (common method of self-harm in developing countries)

GENERAL PREVENTION
- Know how to access resources 24/7 within and outside of the health care institution.
- Screen for risk: Use screening instruments BUT keep in mind risks particular to each patient, which could lead to increased risks not captured in some screening tools. Screening instruments include the Patient Health Questionnaire-2 (PHQ-2), the PHQ-9, the Columbia Suicide Severity Rating Scale, Beck Scale for Suicide Ideation, Linehan Reasons for Living Inventory, and Risk Estimator for Suicide.
- Treat underlying mental and medical illnesses and substance abuse.
- Screen for possession of means of harm, including prescribed/unprescribed drugs, poisons, and firearms (encourage the removal of guns from the home and the relinquishment of gun licenses).
- Create a safety plan for patients at risk for suicide and their families, including education about how to access emergency care 24 hours a day.
- Public education about how to help others access emergency psychiatric care. Suicidal people may initially confide in those they trust outside health care (e.g., family members, religious leaders, "healers," or to retail service providers, such as hairdressers and bartenders).
- Law enforcement education through the FBI's National Center for Analysis of Violent Crime in recognizing and triaging potential "suicide by cop" events (deliberate attempt to trigger lethal force); thought to be responsible for approximately 20% of fatal police shootings in the United States between 1998 and 2006 (1)
- For the military: multiple resources: http://www.realwarriors.net. Suggested treatments include cognitive restructuring techniques (that their experience with adversity can be a source of strength) and help with problem solving (so the service member does not feel like a "burden"), therapeutic martial arts training, focus on Vets' helping others: "Power of 1" initiative (any "one" helpful contact could save a life).
- For teens, young adults, and their educators: suggestions and advice for students/families and educators: http://www.cdc.gov/healthyyouth/adolescent-health; http://www.stopbullying.gov
- In developing world countries, pesticide ingestion is a common method of suicide. Limiting free access has led to reduced suicide rates.

 DIAGNOSIS

HISTORY
- Depressed patients should be asked about suicidal ideation and a potential plan:
  - "Have you ever felt that life isn't worth living? Do you ever wish you could go to sleep and not wake up? Are you having thoughts about killing yourself?"
- Use psychodynamic formulation, which combines mental-state exam (i.e., behavior, mood, mental content, judgment), past history (i.e., What resources has the patient used in the past for support, and are they currently available?), and history of current illness. If the patient is experiencing a

loss, or is under stress, and does not have access to a previously sustaining resource (e.g., a significant other, a pet, sports ability, a job), that patient is under increased risk for suicide.
- Prior attempts: precipitants, lethality, intent to die, precautions taken to avoid being rescued, reaction to survival (a patient who is upset that the suicide was not completed is at increased risk for a subsequent attempt)
- History of psychiatric symptoms, substance abuse
- Also note strengths, such as reasons to live, hopes for future, social supports. A patient without these is at increased risk.
- Gather collateral history (from friends, family, physicians). It is appropriate to break confidentiality if patient is at imminent risk of suicide.

PHYSICAL EXAM
- Medical conditions: delirium, intoxication, withdrawal, medication side effects
- Psychosis: Observe for signs of/ask about command auditory hallucinations to kill oneself, delusional guilt, and persecutory delusions.
- In adults: Observe for signs of hopelessness/despair (see "Risk Factors").
- In teens: may not appear to be depressed; therefore, screen for risk factors: substance abuse, bullying and social isolation (commonly through electronic media), poor grades

DIFFERENTIAL DIAGNOSIS
Suicidal threats and gestures need to be immediately triaged to assess patient safety, although in some cases the threat could be an attempt to manipulate others, such as in the case of personality disorders.

DIAGNOSTIC TESTS & INTERPRETATION
Diagnostic Procedures/Other
Brief tests that could be part of any medical/mental health assessment:
- PHQ-9: http://www.med.umich.edu/1info/FHP/practiceguides/depress/score.pdf
- Columbia Suicide Severity Rating Scale, clinical instructions accessed at http://www.cssrs.columbia.edu/c-ssrs_Triage_guidelines.pdf
- Suicide Trigger Scale version 3, (STS-3), which measures a patient's "ruminative flooding" (self-critical, repetitive thoughts) and "frantic hopelessness" (feeling trapped, suicide is the only choice): http://www.ncbi.nlm.nih.gov/pmc/articles/PMC3443232/

TREATMENT

GENERAL MEASURES
- Patients expressing active suicidal thoughts or who made an attempt require immediate evaluation for risk factors, mental status, and capacity (to determine if they are able/or willing to inform treaters about suicidal intentions) as well as a formal psychiatric consultation.
- Cognitive therapy decreased reattempt rate in prior suicide attempters by half. (i) Establish therapeutic alliance. Have patient tell a story about recent suicidal thought or action. (ii) Help patient develop the skills needed to deal with the thoughts or feelings that trigger suicidal crises. (iii) Have patient imagine being in the situation that brought on the earlier crisis, but this time, guide that patient to practice problem-solving strategies—reinforcing the use of coping skills, rather than suicidal actions (4,5).

- Psychotherapy with suicidal patients is a challenge even for the most experienced clinicians. The countertransference, a clinician's feelings toward a patient, can evolve into wanting to be rid of the patient. If the patient detects this, the risk of suicide is heightened. The clinician can avoid this by recognizing countertransference and bearing it within so that the patient remains unaware (6).
- Among military personnel: ACE campaign: Ask about suicidal thoughts; Care for the person, including removing access to lethal weapons; "Escort" the soldier/vet to help: an emergency room, a 911 call; call to a support hotline such as (800) 273-TALK (8255); text: 838255.

MEDICATION

- Psychopharmacology "is not a substitute for getting to know the patient" (7).
- Patients are at increased risk of suicide at the outset of antidepressant treatment and when it is discontinued. Consider tapering/switching medical therapies rather than sudden discontinuation. Monitor carefully at these times.
- Anxiety, agitation, and delusions increasing in intensity are risk factors for suicide and should be treated aggressively.
- In patients with mood disorders, a meta-analysis of randomized, controlled trials found that lithium reduced the risk of death by suicide by 60% (7)[A].
- Agitated or combative patients may require sedation with IV or IM benzodiazepines and/or antipsychotics. Clinical response is typically seen within 20 to 30 minutes if given IM/IV.

Pediatric Considerations
FDA posted black box warning for antidepressant use in the pediatric population after increased suicidality was noted. If risk of untreated depression is sufficient to warrant treatment with antidepressants, treat but monitor for suicidality.

First Line
ECGs before prescribing or continuing antidepressants or antipsychotics to look for QT prolongation

ISSUES FOR REFERRAL
Consider a psychiatric consult. All decisions regarding treatment must be carefully documented and communicated to all involved health care providers.

ADMISSION, INPATIENT, AND NURSING CONSIDERATIONS

- Inpatient hospitalization if patient is suicidal with a plan to act or is otherwise at high risk; if immediate risk for self-harm, may be hospitalized involuntarily
- Immediately after a suicide attempt, treat the medical problems resulting from the self-harm before attempting to initiate psychiatric care
- Order lab work (e.g., solvent screen, blood and urine toxicology screen, aspirin and acetaminophen levels). Patients may not disclose ingestions if they wish to succeed in their attempt or if they are undergoing mental status changes.
- Risk for self-harm continues even in the hospital. As soon as patients arrive at a hospital, they should be searched and potentially dangerous objects removed; they should be under one-to-one constant observation, offered medication to ease symptoms; mechanical restraints only if necessary for patient safety
- The period after transfer from involuntary to voluntary hospitalization and postdischarge are times of high risk.
- Discharge criteria
  - No longer considered a danger to self/others
  - Clinicians should be aware that a patient may *claim* that he or she is no longer suicidal in order to facilitate discharge—and complete the act.

Look for clinical and behavioral signs that the patient truly is no longer in despair and is hopeful, such as improved appetite, sleep, engagement with staff and group therapy. Clinicians should check with family and ancillary staff because patients may share more information with them than with doctors.
- Provide information about 24/7 resources.

 ONGOING CARE

FOLLOW-UP RECOMMENDATIONS
Patient Monitoring
- Increase monitoring at the beginning of treatment, when changing medications, and on discharge.
- Educate family members and other close contacts/confidants to the warning signs of suicidality. For adults, despair/hopelessness, isolation, discussing suicide, stating that the world would be a "better place" without them, losses in areas key to the patient's self-worth. For youths, may exhibit the same signs and symptoms, but one should be aware of these additional risks: history of abuse (e.g., sexual, physical), bullying in person or via electronic media (e.g., text messages or social media), family stress, changes in eating and sleeping patterns, suicidality of friends, and giving away treasured items.
- Make sure that the patient is willing to accept the type of follow-up offered. Do not assume that just setting it up is sufficient protection.
- Curtail access to firearms.
- Limiting the number of pills may be appropriate for an impulsive patient. However, clinicians may believe that by simply limiting the number of pills they prescribe, they are preventing further suicide attempts, an example of "magical thinking." Clinicians who find themselves thinking this way can take it as a warning sign that their patients may actually be at increased risk of suicide.

PATIENT EDUCATION
Patients who feel they are in danger of hurting themselves should consider one or several of these options:
- Call 911.
- Go directly to an emergency room.
- If already in counseling, contact that therapist immediately.
- Call the National Suicide Prevention Hotline at (800) 273-TALK (8255).
- Servicemen and servicewomen and their families can call (800) 796-9699; if there is no immediate answer, call (800) 273-TALK (8255); text 838255.

PROGNOSIS
The key to a favorable prognosis is early recognition of risk factors, early diagnosis and treatment of a psychiatric or medical disorder (leading to distress), and appropriate intervention and follow-up.

COMPLICATIONS
- According to the AAS, the grief process for significant others of suicide victims can be lifelong and can be expressed in emotions ranging from anger to despair. Survivors often attempt to shoulder the burden on their own because of the added guilt and shame of the nature of the attempted death or death.
- The AAS recommends the following:
  - Counseling: could include short-term behavioral therapy as well as psychotherapy; some therapy should focus on the survivors' relationships to their current and future significant others. Survivors often seek out life partners as "replacements" for those they lost—could interfere with mourning

(W. J. Massicotte, National Scientific Program Committee, written communication, April 24, 2009).
- Sympathetic listening by friends
- Support during holidays
- More self-help strategies: http:// www.survivors ofsuicide.com

REFERENCES
1. American Association of Suicidology. http:// www .suicidology.org. Accessed September 11, 2018.
2. Koola MM, Ahmed AO, Sebastian J, et al. Childhood physical and sexual abuse predicts suicide risk in a large cohort of veterans. *Prim Care Companion CNS Disord*. 2018;20(4):18m02317.
3. Jollant F, Bellivier F, Leboyer M, et al. Impaired decision making in suicide attempters. *Am J Psychiatry*. 2005;162(2):304–310.
4. Brown GK, Ten Have T, Henriques GR, et al. Cognitive therapy for the prevention of suicide attempts: a randomized controlled trial. *JAMA*. 2005;294(5):563–570.
5. Ghahramanlou-Holloway M, Neely L, Tucker J. A cognitive-behavioral strategy for preventing suicide. *Current Psychiatry*. 2014;13(8):18–28.
6. Maltsberger JT, Buie DH. Countertransference hate in the treatment of suicidal patients. *Arch Gen Psychiatry*. 1974;30(5):625–633.
7. Cipriani A, Pretty H, Hawton K, et al. Lithium in the prevention of suicidal behavior and all-cause mortality in patients with mood disorders: a systematic review of randomized trials. *Am J Psychiatry*. 2005;162(10):1805–1819.

ADDITIONAL READING
- Bryan CJ, Jennings KW, Jobes DA, et al. Understanding and preventing military suicide. *Arch Suicide Res*. 2012;16(2):95–110.
- Gutheil TG, Bursztajn H, Brodsky A. The multidimensional assessment of dangerousness: competence assessment in patient care and liability prevention. *Bull Am Acad Psychiatry Law*. 1986;14(2):123–129.
- O'Connor E, Gaynes BN, Burda BU, et al. Screening for and treatment of suicide risk relevant to primary care: a systematic review for the U.S. Preventive Services Task Force. *Ann Intern Med*. 2013;158(10):741–754.

 CODES

ICD10
- R45.851 Suicidal ideations
- T14.91 Suicide attempt
- Z91.5 Personal history of self-harm

CLINICAL PEARLS
- Key preventative measure is to listen to a patient and take steps to keep him or her safe. This could include immediate hospitalization. Questions to explore include "Are you thinking of killing yourself?" "Who do you have to live for?" and "What should change so that you could live with your suffering?"
- Clozapine, lithium, and CBT are associated with a reduction in the risk of suicide.
- Family and contacts of people who have attempted or committed suicide suffer from reactions ranging from rage to despair. Encourage counseling.
- Resources for clinicians: https://www.suicidology .org/; https://www.suicideassessment.com

SUPERFICIAL THROMBOPHLEBITIS

Emily M. Culliney, MD, FAAFP

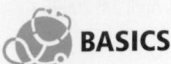 **BASICS**

DESCRIPTION

- Superficial thrombophlebitis is venous inflammation with secondary thrombosis of a superficial vein.
- Most common in the lower extremities (60–80%), but can occur in the upper extremities/neck
- Generally a benign and self-limiting process, but can be painful
- Traumatic thrombophlebitis types:
  – Injury
  – IV catheter related
  – Intentional (i.e., sclerotherapy)
- Aseptic thrombophlebitis types:
  – Primary hypercoagulable states: disorders with measurable defects in the proteins of the coagulation and/or fibrinolytic systems
  – Secondary hypercoagulable states: clinical conditions with a risk of thrombosis (venous stasis, pregnancy)
- Septic (suppurative) thrombophlebitis types:
  – Iatrogenic, long-term IV catheter use
  – Infectious, mainly syphilis and psittacosis
- Mondor disease
  – Rare presentation of anterior chest/breast veins of women
- System(s) affected: cardiovascular
- Synonym(s): phlebitis; phlebothrombosis

Geriatric Considerations
Septic thrombophlebitis is more common; prognosis is poorer.

Pediatric Considerations
Subperiosteal abscesses of adjacent long bone may complicate the disorder.

Pregnancy Considerations
- Associated with increased risk of aseptic superficial thrombophlebitis, especially during postpartum
- NSAIDs are contraindicated during pregnancy.

EPIDEMIOLOGY
- Predominant age
  – Traumatic/IV related has no predominant age/sex.
  – Aseptic primary hypercoagulable state
    ○ Childhood to young adult
- Aseptic secondary hypercoagulable state
  – Mondor disease: women, ages 21 to 55 years
  – Thromboangiitis obliterans onset: ages 20 to 50 years
- Predominant sex
  – Suppurative: male = female
  – Aseptic
    ○ Spontaneous formation: female (55–70%)
    ○ Mondor: female > male (2:1)

Incidence
- Septic
  – Incidence of catheter-related thrombophlebitis is 88/100,000 persons per year.
  – Develops in 4–8% if cutdown is performed
- Aseptic primary hypercoagulable state: Antithrombin III and heparin cofactor II deficiency incidence is 50/100,000 persons.

- Aseptic secondary hypercoagulable state
  – In pregnancy, 49-fold increased incidence of phlebitis
  – Superficial migratory thrombophlebitis in 27% of patients with thromboangiitis obliterans

Prevalence
- Superficial thrombophlebitis is common.
- 1/3 of patients in a medical ICU develop thrombophlebitis that eventually progresses to the deep veins.

ETIOLOGY AND PATHOPHYSIOLOGY
- Similar to deep venous thrombosis; Virchow triad of vessel trauma, stasis, and hypercoagulability (genetic, iatrogenic, or idiopathic)
- Varicose veins play a primary role in etiology of lower extremity phlebitis.
- Mondor disease pathophysiology not completely understood
- Less commonly due to infection (i.e., septic)
  – *Staphylococcus aureus, Pseudomonas, Klebsiella, Peptostreptococcus* sp.
  – *Candida* sp.
- Aseptic primary hypercoagulable state
  – Due to inherited disorders of hypercoagulability
- Aseptic secondary hypercoagulable states
  – Malignancy (Trousseau syndrome: recurrent migratory thrombophlebitis): most commonly seen in metastatic mucin or adenocarcinomas of the GI tract (pancreas, stomach, colon, and gallbladder), lung, prostate, and ovary
  – Pregnancy
  – Estrogen-based oral contraceptives
  – Behçet, Buerger, or Mondor disease

Genetics
Not applicable other than hypercoagulable states

RISK FACTORS
- Nonspecific
  – Varicose veins
  – Immobilization
  – Obesity
  – Advanced age
  – Postoperative states
- Traumatic/septic
  – IV catheter (plastic > coated)
  – Lower extremity IV catheter
  – Cutdowns
  – Cancer, debilitating diseases
  – Burn patients
  – AIDS
  – IV drug use
- Aseptic
  – Pregnancy
  – Estrogen-based oral contraceptives
  – Surgery, trauma, infection
  – Hypercoagulable state (i.e., factor V, protein C, or S deficiency, others)
- Thromboangiitis obliterans: persistent smoking
- Mondor disease
  – Breast cancer or breast surgery

GENERAL PREVENTION
- Avoid lower extremity cannulations/IV.
- Insert catheters under aseptic conditions, secure cannulas, and replace every 3 days.
- Avoid stasis and use usual deep vein thrombosis (DVT) prophylaxis in high-risk patients (i.e., ICU, immobilized).

COMMONLY ASSOCIATED CONDITIONS
- Frequently seen with concurrent DVT (6–53%)
- Symptomatic pulmonary embolism can also be seen concurrently (0–10%).
- Both DVT/PE can occur up to 3 months after onset of phlebitis.

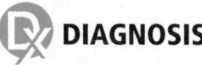 **DIAGNOSIS**

HISTORY
Pain along the course of a vein

PHYSICAL EXAM
- Swelling, tenderness, redness along the course of a vein or veins
- May have a palpable cord along the course of the vein
- May look like localized cellulitis or erythema nodosum
- Fever in 70% of patients in septic phlebitis
- Sign of systemic sepsis in 84% of suppurative cases

DIFFERENTIAL DIAGNOSIS
- Cellulitis
- DVT
- Erythema nodosum
- Cutaneous polyarteritis nodosa
- Lymphangitis

DIAGNOSTIC TESTS & INTERPRETATION
Initial Tests (lab, imaging)
Often none necessary if afebrile, otherwise healthy

- Small or distal veins (i.e., forearms or below the knee): no recommended imaging
- If concern for more proximal extension: venous Doppler ultrasound (US) to assess extent of thrombosis and rule out DVT (1)[A]

Follow-Up Tests & Special Considerations
- If suspicious for sepsis
  – Blood cultures (bacteremia in 80–90%)
  – Consider culture of the IV fluids being infused.
  – CBC demonstrates leukocytosis.
- Aseptic: evaluation for coagulopathy if recurrent or without another identifiable cause (e.g., protein C and S, lupus anticoagulant, anticardiolipin antibody, factor V and VIII, homocysteine)
- In migratory thrombophlebitis, have a high index of suspicion for malignancy.
- Repeat venous US to assess effectiveness of therapy.
  – If thrombosis is extending, more aggressive therapy required

Test Interpretation
The affected vein is enlarged, tortuous, and thickened with endothelial damage and necrosis.

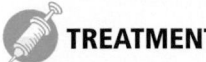 TREATMENT

GENERAL MEASURES
- Suppurative: consultation for urgent surgical venous excision
- Local, mild (2)[C]
  - Conservative management, antibiotics not useful
  - For varicosities
    - Compression stockings; maintain activities.
  - Catheter/trauma associated
    - Immediately remove IV and culture tip.
    - Elevate with application of warm compresses.
    - If slow to resolve, consider LMWH.
- Large, severe, or septic thrombophlebitis
  - Inpatient care or bed rest with elevation and local warm compress
  - When the patient is ambulating, then start compression stockings or Ace bandages.

MEDICATION
First Line
- Best medication(s) and duration of treatment are not well-defined (1)[A].
- Localized, mild thrombophlebitis (usually self-limited)
  - NSAIDs and ASA for inflammation/pain to reduce symptoms and local progression
  - Use of compression stockings can also provide symptomatic relief (3).

Second Line
- Septic/suppurative
  - May present or be complicated by sepsis
  - Requires IV antibiotics (broad spectrum initially) and anticoagulation
- Increasing evidence shows that LMWH/fondaparinux treatment can prevent extension of superficial venous thrombosis in addition to venous thromboembolism (VTE) prevention.
- Consider if thrombus is large, close to the junction with deep veins, or involves the long saphenous vein.
  - To prevent VTE, 4 weeks of LMWH, such as enoxaparin
  - 45 days of fondaparinux was found to reduce DVT and VTE by 85% (relative risk reduction) in one large study (4)[B].
- Superficial thrombophlebitis related to inherited or acquired hypercoagulable states is addressed by treating the related disease.

ISSUES FOR REFERRAL
Severely inflamed or very large phlebitis should be evaluated for excision.

SURGERY/OTHER PROCEDURES
- Septic
  - Surgical consultation for excision of the involved vein segment and involved tributaries
  - Drain contiguous abscesses.
  - Remove all associated cannula and culture tips.
- Aseptic: Manage underlying conditions.
  - Evaluate for saphenous vein ligation to prevent deep vein extension after acute phase resolved.
  - Consider referral for varicosity excision.

ADMISSION, INPATIENT, AND NURSING CONSIDERATIONS
- Septic: inpatient
- Aseptic: outpatient

 ONGOING CARE

FOLLOW-UP RECOMMENDATIONS
Patient Monitoring
- Septic: routine WBC count and differential. Target treatment based on culture results.
- Severe aseptic
  - Repeat venous Doppler US in 1 to 2 weeks to ensure no DVT and assess treatment effectiveness: Do not expect resolution, just nonprogression.
  - Repeat clotting studies.
- Local, mild thrombophlebitis typically resolves with conservative therapy and does not require specific monitoring unless there is a failure to resolve.

DIET
No restrictions

PATIENT EDUCATION
Review local care, elevation, and use of compression hose for acute treatment and prevention of recurrence.

PROGNOSIS
- Septic/suppurative
  - High mortality (50%) if untreated
  - Depends on treatment delay or need for surgery
- Aseptic
  - Usually benign course; recovery in 2 to 3 weeks
  - Depends on development of DVT and early detection of complications
  - Aseptic thrombophlebitis can be isolated, recurrent, or migratory.
  - Recurrence likely if related to varicosity or if severely affected vein not removed

COMPLICATIONS
- Septic: systemic sepsis, bacteremia (84%), septic pulmonary emboli (44%), metastatic abscess formation, pneumonia (44%), subperiosteal abscess of adjacent long bones in children
- Aseptic: DVT (6–53%), VTE (up to 10%), thromboembolic phenomena

REFERENCES
1. Di Nisio M, Wichers IM, Middeldorp S. Treatment for superficial thrombophlebitis of the leg. *Cochrane Database Syst Rev.* 2013;(4):CD004982.
2. Nasr H, Scriven JM. Superficial thrombophlebitis (superficial venous thrombosis). *BMJ.* 2015; 350:h2039.
3. Decousus H, Epinat M, Guillot K, et al. Superficial vein thrombosis: risk factors, diagnosis, and treatment. *Curr Opin Pulm Med.* 2003;9(5):393–397.
4. Di Nisio M, Middeldorp S. Treatment of lower extremity superficial thrombophlebitis. *JAMA.* 2014;311(7):729–730.

ADDITIONAL READING
- Decousus H, Leizorovicz A. Superficial thrombophlebitis of the legs: still a lot to learn. *J Thromb Haemost.* 2005;3(6):1149–1151.
- Decousus H, Quéré I, Presles E, et al; for the POST (Prospective Observational Superficial Thrombophlebitis) Study Group. Superficial venous thrombosis and venous thromboembolism: a large, prospective epidemiologic study. *Ann Intern Med.* 2010;152(4):218–224.
- Wichers IM, Di Nisio M, Büller HR, et al. Treatment of superficial vein thrombosis to prevent deep vein thrombosis and pulmonary embolism: a systematic review. *Haematologica.* 2005;90(5):672–677.

 SEE ALSO

Deep Vein Thrombophlebitis

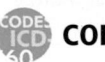 CODES

ICD10
- I80.9 Phlebitis and thrombophlebitis of unspecified site
- I80.00 Phlbts and thombophlb of superfic vessels of unsp low extrm
- I80.8 Phlebitis and thrombophlebitis of other sites

CLINICAL PEARLS
- Mild superficial thrombophlebitis is typically self-limiting and responds well to conservative care.
- Lower extremity disease involving large veins or proximal saphenous vein may benefit from anticoagulation to prevent DVT.
- Septic thrombophlebitis requires admission for antibiotics and anticoagulation. If severe, consider surgical consultation for venous excision.

S

SYNCOPE
Judson A. Moore, MD • Santiago O. Valdes, MD, FAAP

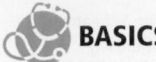 **BASICS**

DESCRIPTION
- Transient loss of consciousness characterized by unresponsiveness, loss of postural tone, and spontaneous recovery; usually brief and caused by cerebral hypoperfusion
- System(s) affected: cardiovascular, nervous

EPIDEMIOLOGY
Incidence
- Overall incidence is 6.2/1,000 patient-years.
- Annual incidence of fainting spells resulting in medical evaluation was 9.5/1,000 inhabitants.
- Accounts for 1–3% of emergency room visits and 1% of hospital admissions
- There is an increased incidence after the age of 70 years, and annual incidence in institutionalized elderly (>75 years of age) is 7%.

Prevalence
- Approximately 20% of adults report ≥1 episode during their lifetime; 15% of children <18 years of age
- The prevalence in institutionalized elderly (>75 years of age) is 23%.

ETIOLOGY AND PATHOPHYSIOLOGY
- Systemic hypotension secondary to decreased cardiac output and/or systemic vasodilation leads to a drop in cerebral perfusion and resulting loss of consciousness.
- Cardiac
  - Obstructions to outflow
    ○ Aortic stenosis
    ○ Hypertrophic cardiomyopathy: most common cause of sudden cardiac death during exercise in young athletes
    ○ Pulmonary embolus
    ○ Pulmonary hypertension
  - Cardiac arrhythmias
    ○ Sustained ventricular tachycardia (VT)
    ○ Supraventricular tachycardia (SVT) (atrial fibrillation, atrial flutter, reentrant SVT)
    ○ Torsades de pointes (TdP)
    ○ Bradyarrhythmia
      ▪ 2nd- and 3rd-degree AV block
      ▪ Sick sinus syndrome
- Noncardiac
  - Reflex-mediated vasovagal (neurally mediated syncope [NMS]/neurocardiogenic): inappropriate vasodilation leading to neurally mediated systemic hypotension and decreased cerebral blood flow, situational (micturition, defecation, cough, pain, emotions, hair combing)
  - Orthostatic hypotension: Consider volume depletion, pregnancy, anemia, medications.
  - Drug/alcohol induced
  - Primary autonomic failure: pure autonomic failure, Parkinson
  - Secondary autonomic failure: diabetes, amyloidosis
  - Carotid sinus hypersensitivity
- NMS is most common cause in adult cases.
- Vast majority of pediatric cases represent benign alterations in vasomotor tone.
- Strokes, seizures, and psychogenic nonepileptic seizures may mimic syncope but are a distinct diagnosis.

Genetics
Specific cardiomyopathies and arrhythmias may be inherited (e.g., long QT syndrome, catecholaminergic polymorphic VT, Brugada syndrome, hypertrophic cardiomyopathy). Primary and secondary autonomic failure syndromes and NMS may also have genetic links.

RISK FACTORS
- Heart disease (acquired or structural)
- Dehydration
- Drugs
  - Antihypertensives
  - Vasodilators (including calcium channel blockers, ACE inhibitors, and nitrates)
  - Phenothiazines
  - Antidepressants
  - Antiarrhythmics
  - Diuretics

GENERAL PREVENTION
See "Risk Factors."

COMMONLY ASSOCIATED CONDITIONS
See "Etiology and Pathophysiology."

DIAGNOSIS

HISTORY
- Careful history, physical exam, and an ECG are more important than other investigations in determining the diagnosis (1).
- Make sure that the patient or witness (if present) is not talking about vertigo (i.e., sense of rotary motion, spinning, and whirling), seizure, or causes of fall without loss of consciousness. Onset of syncope is usually rapid, and recovery is spontaneous, rapid, and complete. Duration of episodes are typically brief (<60 seconds).
- Circumstances: Prolonged standing, urination, coughing, defecation, postprandial, and intense emotions are more likely to be associated with NMS. Abrupt neck movements consider carotid sinus hypersensitivity. Exertional syncope considers cardiac.
- Number of previous episodes: Benign causes of syncope tend to be associated with a single episode.
- Presence of prodromal symptoms: Consider NMS.
  - Elderly patients less likely to experience a prodrome
- Palpitations: Consider cardiac.
- Position (supine: arrhythmia; erect: NMS, supine → erect: orthostatic hypotension)
- Prolonged syncope: Consider psychiatric and neurologic.
- Delayed recovery: Consider neurologic (postictal).
- Ask for family history of long QT syndrome, implantable cardioverter-defibrillator (ICD), hypertrophic cardiomyopathy, or unexplained sudden cardiac death in young family members.
- High-risk findings: new onset chest discomfort, breathlessness, abdominal pain, headache, syncope during exertion or when supine, or sudden palpitations immediately followed by syncope
- Even after careful evaluation, including diagnostic procedures and special tests, the cause will be found in only 50–60% of patients.

PHYSICAL EXAM
- BP and pulse, both lying and standing
  - Orthostatic: drop in systolic BP >20 mm Hg or rise in heart rate of >30 bpm (>40 bpm in those aged 12 to 19 years)
- Check for cardiac murmur or focal neurologic abnormality.
- High-risk findings: unexplained systolic BP <90 mm Hg, suggestion of GI bleed on rectal exam, persistent bradycardia (<40 bpm) in absence of physical training, or undiagnosed systolic murmur

DIFFERENTIAL DIAGNOSIS
- Drop attacks
- Coma
- Vertigo
- Seizure disorder
- Stroke/transient ischemic attacks (TIAs)
- Psychiatric (conversion, somatization): lack hemodynamic and/or autonomic changes

DIAGNOSTIC TESTS & INTERPRETATION
- Goal is to identify life-threatening conditions or those associated with significant risk of injury (2).
- Comprehensive medical and family history, physical examination, and ECG should guide future testing (2).
- No one single test defines the cause of syncope (2).

Initial Tests (lab, imaging)
- ECG should be obtained in most patients.
  - Consider cardiac if there are ischemic changes, bifascicular block, AV block, sinus bradycardia <40 bpm or sinus pause >3 seconds, prolong QTc, preexcitation, and alternating BBB.
- Other testing should be guided by history and physical:
  - CBC, electrolytes, BUN, creatinine, glucose (rarely helpful if asymptomatic or presenting hours later)
  - BNP
  - Cardiac enzymes (only if history suggestive of MI)
  - D-dimer (for pulmonary embolism [PE] workup)
  - Urine pregnancy and urine drug screen
  - Initial cardiac or neuroimaging only if indicated
  - Lung scan or helical CT scan of chest if concern for PE

Follow-Up Tests & Special Considerations
- Injuries may occur in up to 1/3 of adult patients.
- If history and physical suggest ischemic, valvular, or congenital heart disease (1,2)[B]
  - Exercise stress test (if syncope with exertion) (1,2)[C]
  - Echocardiogram (1,2)[B]
- ECG monitoring, either in hospital or ambulatory (1)[B]
  - Consider when concerned for cardiac cause.
  - Choice of outpatient device (e.g., Holter, loop recorder, implantable monitor) should be determined by frequency of symptoms.
- Electrophysiologic studies (1,2)[B]
  - Consider when concerned for cardiac cause.
  - Positive results seen in 22–82% of patients with preexisting heart disease and/or abnormal ECG
- Head imaging, carotid US, and EEG are not recommended in routine evaluation of syncope but may be useful if history and physical is concerning for neurologic issues (1)[C].
- Carotid hypersensitivity evaluation (2)[B]
  - Carotid hypersensitivity should be considered in patients >40 years old or with syncope during head turning, especially while wearing tight collars, and with neck tumors or scars.
  - The technique is not standardized; one side at a time is compressed gently for 20 seconds with constant monitoring of pulse and BP/ECG. Avoid in patients with history of TIA or stroke.
  - Atropine should be readily available.
- Tilt-table testing (1,2)[B]
  - Provocative test for vasovagal syncope
  - Often, results are not reproducible.
  - High false-positive rate
- Psychiatric evaluation (2)[C]: indicated when syncope is thought to be psychogenic. Psychiatric disease and substance abuse may be associated with syncope.

Diagnostic Procedures/Other
External event recorders or implantable loop recorders may be more helpful than short-term ambulatory monitoring; helpful in selective patients with recurrent syncope, with yield of ~55% (1)[B]

Test Interpretation
Depends on etiology and presence of underlying cardiac or neurologic conditions

TREATMENT
- Maintaining good hydration status and normal salt intake are initial therapy. Educate patients of the premonitory signs of syncope (1,3)[B].
- Majority of pediatric patients improve with nonpharmacologic measures.

GENERAL MEASURES
- NMS: reassurance, education, behavior modification
- Elderly patients without previously recognized heart disease should be admitted if the physician thinks that the cause of syncope is likely cardiac.
- Patients without heart disease, especially young patients (age <60 years), can be worked up safely as outpatients.
- Prescribe antiarrhythmics for documented arrhythmias occurring simultaneously with syncope or symptoms of presyncope. Asymptomatic arrhythmias do not necessarily require treatment.
- The decision to treat patients on basis of arrhythmias or conduction abnormalities provoked or detected during EPS is problematic: Does the arrhythmia or conduction abnormality has anything to do with the patient's symptoms?
- Most would treat patients with provoked sustained VT with an antiarrhythmic drug that suppressed arrhythmia during study.
- Rationale for such treatment: Recurrent syncope is less frequent in patients with positive EPS who are treated than it is in those who have negative EPS.

MEDICATION
First Line
- Geared toward specific underlying cardiac or neurologic abnormalities
- In cases of recurrent NMS (1,4)[B]
  - Mineralocorticoids (fludrocortisone)
  - α-Adrenergic agonists (midodrine)

Second Line
- SSRIs (1)[C] (paroxetine, sertraline, fluoxetine)
- Vagolytics (disopyramide)

ISSUES FOR REFERRAL
When cardiac or neurologic etiologies are suspected, obtain appropriate consultation, as indicated.

ADDITIONAL THERAPIES
For vasovagal/neurocardiogenic/NMS
- Counterpressure maneuvers and exercise have improved vasovagal symptoms and recurrence (1,3)[C].
- Head-up tilt sleeping (2)[C]
- Abdominal binders and/or support stockings (1,2)[C]
- Increased fluid and salt intake to maintain intravascular volume in cases of recurrent NMS

SURGERY/OTHER PROCEDURES
- ICD placement for patients with cardiac conditions with high risk of sudden death and/or recurrent syncope on medications (e.g., long QT syndrome, Brugada, catecholaminergic polymorphic VT, hypertrophic cardiomyopathy) (1,2)[B]

- Many recommend pacemaker implantation in patients with the following:
  - 2nd- (Mobitz type II) and 3rd-degree heart block
  - Bifascicular block
  - HV intervals >100 ms
  - Pacing-induced infranodal block
  - Sinus node recovery time ≥3 seconds

ADMISSION, INPATIENT, AND NURSING CONSIDERATIONS
- Patients with benign etiologies of syncope with negative ED workups are associated with benign outcomes, even with other risk factors (5)[B].
- Overwhelming majority of children who have completely recovered and without red flags for cardiac or neurologic syncope can be followed as outpatients.
- Patients with suspected cardiac or those with significant comorbidities (anemia, associated trauma, or persistent vital sign changes) should be admitted.
- In adults: ROSE rule recommends hospital admission if any of the following is present: BNP level ≥300 pg/mL, bradycardia HR ≤50, + fecal occult blood, anemia with hemoglobin ≤9 g/dL, chest pain associated with syncope, ECG showing Q wave (not in lead III), or oxygen saturation ≤94% on room air (6).
- Close monitoring of BP and heart rate during initial presentation
- Discharge criteria
  - Attainment of hemodynamic stability
  - Satisfactory completion of workup for etiology
  - Adequate control of specific arrhythmia or seizure, if present

ONGOING CARE

FOLLOW-UP RECOMMENDATIONS
Patient Monitoring
- Frequent follow-up visits for patients with cardiac causes of syncope, especially if on antiarrhythmics
- Patients with an unknown cause of syncope rarely (5%) are diagnosed during the follow-up.
- Home video recording with smartphone technology is recommended for recurrent episodes.

DIET
No specific diet unless the patient has heart disease or NMS (see "Additional Therapies")

PATIENT EDUCATION
- Reassurance that most cardiac causes can be treated, and those with noncardiac causes do well, even if the cause is never discovered.
- Physical counterpressure maneuvers can prevent recurrences of vasovagal syncope.
- Carefully consider whether the patient should drive while syncope is being evaluated. Physicians should be aware of pertinent laws in their own states.

PROGNOSIS
- Cumulative mortality at 2 years
  - Low: young patients (<60 years of age) with noncardiac or unknown cause of syncope
  - Intermediate: older patients (>60 years of age) with noncardiac or unknown cause of syncope
  - High: patients with cardiac cause of syncope
- Independent predictors of poor short-term outcomes (5,6)[B]
  - Abnormal ECG
  - Shortness of breath
  - Systolic BP <90 mm Hg
  - Hematocrit <30%
  - Congestive heart failure

COMPLICATIONS
Trauma from falling

REFERENCES
1. Shen WK, Sheldon RS, Benditt DG, et al. 2017 ACC/AHA/HRS guideline for the evaluation and management of patients with syncope: a report of the American College of Cardiology/ American Heart Association Task Force on Clinical Practice Guidelines and the Heart Rhythm Society. *Circulation*. 2017;136(5):e60–e122.
2. Brignole M, Moya A, de Lange FJ, et al; for ESC Scientific Document Group. 2018 ESC guidelines for the diagnosis and management of syncope. *Eur Heart J*. 2018;39(21):1883–1948.
3. Romme JJ, Reitsma JB, Go-Schön IK, et al. Prospective evaluation of non-pharmacological treatment in vasovagal syncope. *Europace*. 2010;12(4):567–573.
4. Kuriachan V, Sheldon RS, Platonov M. Evidence-based treatment for vasovagal syncope. *Heart Rhythm*. 2008;5(11):1609–1614.
5. Saccilotto RT, Nickel CH, Bucher HC, et al. San Francisco Syncope Rule to predict short-term serious outcomes: a systematic review. *CMAJ*. 2011;183(15):E1116–E1126.
6. Reed MJ, Newby DE, Coull AJ, et al. The ROSE (risk stratification of syncope in the emergency department) study. *J Am Coll Cardiol*. 2010;55(8):713–721.

ADDITIONAL READING
- Anderson JB, Willis M, Lancaster H, et al. The evaluation and management of pediatric syncope. *Pediatr Neurol*. 2016;55:6–13.
- Puppala VK, Akkaya M, Dickinson O, et al. Risk stratification of patients presenting with transient loss of consciousness. *Cardiol Clin*. 2015;33(3):387–396.
- Sheldon RS, Grubb BP II, Olshansky B, et al. 2015 Heart Rhythm Society expert consensus statement on the diagnosis and treatment of postural tachycardia syndrome, inappropriate sinus tachycardia, and vasovagal syncope. *Heart Rhythm*. 2015;12(6):e41–e63.

SEE ALSO
- Aortic Valvular Stenosis; Atrial Septal Defect; Carotid Sinus Hypersensitivity; Patent Ductus Arteriosus; Pulmonary Arterial Hypertension; Pulmonary Embolism; Seizure Disorders; Stokes-Adams Attacks
- Algorithms: Syncope; Transient Ischemic Attack and Transient Neurologic Defects

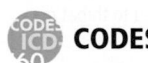

CODES
ICD10
R55 Syncope and collapse

CLINICAL PEARLS
- Careful history and physical exam is key to a diagnosis.
- Use the ECG/event-recorder to evaluate for arrhythmias.
- NMS is the most common cause in children and adults.
- True neurologic causes of syncope are rare.
- Injuries due to syncope are common.

SYNCOPE, REFLEX (VASOVAGAL SYNCOPE)

Melinda Y. Kwan, DO, MPH • Norton Winer, MD

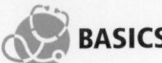 **BASICS**

A reversible loss of consciousness and postural tone secondary to systemic hypotension and cerebral hypoperfusion due to vasodilation and/or bradycardia (rarely, tachycardia) with spontaneous recovery and no neurologic sequelae. The term syncope excludes seizures, coma, shock, or other states of altered consciousness.

DESCRIPTION
- Derived from the Greek *syncopa*, "to cut short"
- Sudden, transient loss of consciousness characterized by unresponsiveness, falling, and spontaneous recovery
- Common cause of syncope in all age groups, especially in patients with no evidence of neurologic or cardiac disease
- Five main types: vasovagal or neurocardiogenic syncope, situational syncope, orthostatic hypotension, carotid sinus hypersensitivity, and glossopharyngeal/trigeminal neuralgia syncope (uncommon) (1)

EPIDEMIOLOGY
- Mortality: cardiac-related syncope 20–30% and 5% in idiopathic syncope
- Age: any age

Incidence
- Ranges from 7% in children aged <18 years and 15% in adults aged >70 years
- 36–62% of all syncopal episodes
- 30% recurrence rate

Prevalence
22% in the general population

ETIOLOGY AND PATHOPHYSIOLOGY
Cause: an abnormal interaction of the normal mechanisms for maintaining BP and upright posture
- In normal individuals, upright posture results in venous pooling and transient decrease in BP.
- Neurally induced syncope may result from a cardio-inhibitory response, a vasodepressor response, or a combination of the two.
- Increased cardiovagal tone leads to bradycardia or asystole, and decreased peripheral sympathetic activity leads to venodilation and hypotension (2).
- Vasovagal syncope usually has a precipitating event, often related to fright, pain, panic, exercise, noxious stimuli, or heat exposure (2).
- Carotid sinus syncope is precipitated by position change, turning head, or wearing a tight collar (possible neck tumors or surgical scarring).
- Situational syncope is related to micturition, defecation, postexercise, cough, or swallow (3).
- Glossopharyngeal syncope is related to throat or facial pain.

Genetics
Vasovagal syncope: strong heritable component

RISK FACTORS
- Low-resting BP
- Age: older age
- Prolonged supine position with resulting deconditioning of autonomic control

GENERAL PREVENTION
Avoid precipitating events or situations. Optimize diabetes control, use of elastic stockings, adequate hydration.

COMMONLY ASSOCIATED CONDITIONS
- Cardiopulmonary disorders: CHF, MI, arrhythmias, hypertrophic obstructive cardiomyopathy, HTN, pulmonary embolism (PE)
- Neurologic disorders: autonomic dysfunction, Shy-Drager syndrome, Parkinson disease, multiple system atrophy, transient ischemic attack, vertebro-basilar insufficiency, peripheral neuropathy
- Psychiatric disorders:
  – Generalized anxiety disorder
  – Panic disorder
  – Major depression
  – Alcohol dependence

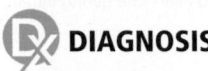 **DIAGNOSIS**

HISTORY
- Rule out cardiac syncope.
- Neurally mediated syncope is preceded by blurred vision, palpitations, nausea, warmth, diaphoresis, or light-headedness, or there may be history of nausea, warmth, diaphoresis, or fatigue *after* syncope.
- Vasovagal syncope
  – Three phases: prodrome, loss of consciousness, and postsyncope
  – Precipitating event or stimulus is usually identified, such as panic, fright, pain, or exercise.
  – May be postexertional in athletes (diagnosis of exclusion)
  – Position: *can be preceded by prolonged standing but can occur from any position; generally resolves when the patient becomes supine*
    ◦ Preceding events: as discussed above
    ◦ Prodrome: as listed above for neurally mediated syncope
  – Duration: generally brief (seconds to minutes)
  – Recovery: may be prolonged with persistent nausea, pallor, and diaphoresis but without neurologic change or confusion
- Carotid sinus syncope is precipitated by position change, after turning head, or wearing a tight collar.
- Situational syncope is related to micturition, defecation, or coughing.
- Glossopharyngeal syncope (less common) is related to throat or facial pain.
  – Precipitating events or situations may include panic, pain, exercise, micturition, defecation, coughing, or swallowing.

PHYSICAL EXAM
- Vital signs, including orthostatics and bilateral BP
- Cardiac exam: volume status, murmurs, rhythm, carotid bruits

- Neurologic exam: signs of focal deficit
- Assess for occult blood loss, including guaiac.
- Dix-Hallpike to rule out benign paroxysmal vertigo

DIFFERENTIAL DIAGNOSIS
- Seizure
- Arrhythmia
- Hypoglycemia
- Cardiac syncope
- Cerebrovascular syncope
- Orthostatic hypotension
- Drop attacks
- Psychiatric illness

DIAGNOSTIC TESTS & INTERPRETATION
Guided by history and physical, includes basic tests to rule out three primary causes of syncope: hypoglycemia, arrhythmia, and anemia

Initial Tests (lab, imaging)
- Blood glucose (hypoglycemia)
- ECG should be ordered for all patients. Abnormal ECG findings are common in patients with cardiac syncope (arrhythmia).
- CBC (rule out anemia)
- Head CT, MRI/MRA, carotid ultrasound only if history or physical exam suggests a neurologic cause
  – Radiology studies are not indicated for insignificant trauma in the presence of a normal neurologic exam (4).

Follow-Up Tests & Special Considerations
- 24-hour Holter monitoring only if a high probability of cardiac cause and/or abnormal ECG findings is present
- A low hemoglobin without obvious cause of bleed warrants stool guaiac, head CT (rule out subarachnoid hemorrhage), abdominal CT (rule out retroperitoneal bleed).
- Negative imaging prompts workup for alternative causes.
- Stroke, bleed, or carotid stenosis require appropriate disease-oriented management.
- EEG only if history or physical exam suggests seizure
- Implantable loop recorder

Diagnostic Procedures/Other
- Head-up tilt table testing:
  – Contraindicated in patients with known cardiac or neurovascular disease or in pregnancy
  – Indicated for recurrent syncope or single episode accompanied by injury or risk to others (e.g., pilots, surgeons)
  – Uses positional changes to reproduce symptoms
  – Positive test diagnostic for vasovagal syncope
- Carotid sinus massage, only in a monitored setting (i.e., BP and HR monitoring, IV access):
  – Contraindicated in patients with carotid disease (careful auscultation prior to massage is essential)
  – Pressure at the angle of the jaw for 5 seconds with simultaneous ECG monitoring
  – Positive tests (causing syncope or cardiac pause >3 seconds) are diagnostic of carotid sinus syncope.
- Psychiatric evaluation: to rule out anxiety, depression, and alcohol abuse

TREATMENT

Therapy is primarily for recurrent syncope. Situational syncope does not warrant specific treatment.

GENERAL MEASURES
Identify and avoid precipitating events or situations

MEDICATION
First Line
- Nonpharmacologic treatment
  - Patient counseling
    - Development of coping skills
    - Increased salt and fluid intake
  - Moderate exercise training
    - Isometric muscle contractions
      - Leg crossing and buttocks clenching
      - Intense gripping of the hands and tensing of the arms
      - These maneuvers increase cardiac output and arterial blood pressure (5).
  - Tilt-table training
    - Progressively prolonged periods of enforced upright posture

Second Line
- α-Agonists mainly used for orthostatic hypotension
  - Midodrine is commonly used. It increases peripheral vascular resistance and venous return. Side effects include HTN, paresthesia, urinary retention, "goose bumps," hyperactivity, dizziness, tremor, and nervousness.
- SSRIs: Paroxetine and fluoxetine are useful in treating neurocardiogenic/vasovagal syncope.
  - Serotonin affects BP and HR via the central nervous system. Serotonin decreases a sympathetic withdrawal response to rapid increases in serotonin levels.
  - Side effects include weight gain, nausea, anxiety, sexual dysfunction, and insomnia.
- Mineralocorticoids: Fludrocortisone has been found helpful mainly in orthostatic hypotension.
  - Helpful in renal sodium absorption and increasing the vasoconstrictive peripheral vascular response
  - Adverse reactions include fluid retention, HTN, CHF, peripheral edema, and hypokalemia.
- β-Blockers: metoprolol, atenolol, or pindolol mainly for postural orthostatic tachycardia syndrome (POTS)
  - Block peripheral vasodilators and ventricular mechanoreceptor stimulation
  - Stabilization of HR and BP
  - Side effects: hypotension and bradycardia (with worsening of syncope), fatigue, depression, and sexual dysfunction
  - Contraindicated in asthma

ISSUES FOR REFERRAL
Neurology or cardiology, as needed

ADDITIONAL THERAPIES
Use of support/pressure stockings

COMPLEMENTARY & ALTERNATIVE MEDICINE
Treatments for underlying heart disease or precipitating factors (e.g., anxiety); none are proven therapies
- Nutrition and supplements: omega-3 fatty acids, multivitamin, CoQ10, acetyl-L-carnitine, α-lipoic acid, and L-arginine
- Herbs: green tea (Camellia sinensis), bilberry (Vaccinium myrtillus), ginkgo (Ginkgo biloba)
- Homeopathy: carbo vegetabilis, opium, sepia
- Acupuncture: It may precipitate fainting.

SURGERY/OTHER PROCEDURES
Pacemaker placement may be of use in patients with frequent neurocardiogenic/vasovagal syncope that is refractory to other therapies (3)[C].
- Prevents prolonged bradycardia or asystole during syncopal episodes
- Long-term effect
- Invasive placement procedure

ADMISSION, INPATIENT, AND NURSING CONSIDERATIONS
Hospital admission or intense evaluation for (6):
- Severe coronary artery disease or structural heart disease (severe CHF, low ejection fraction or previous myocardial infarction, aortic stenosis)
- Arrhythmic syncope
  - ECG may show bifascicular block, sinus bradycardia <40 without SA block or β-blockers, Brugada syndrome, abnormal QT interval, etc.
- Severe anemia or electrolyte abnormalities
- Family history of sudden death
- Isotonic crystalloids, as needed
- Vital sign monitoring
- Discharge when hemodynamically stable and workup satisfactory.

 ONGOING CARE

DIET
- Increased salt intake may help if not otherwise contraindicated (2)[C].
- Maintain fluid intake.

PATIENT EDUCATION
- Identify and avoid precipitating events or situations.
- Avoid dehydration, alcohol consumption, warm environments, tight clothing, and long periods of standing motionless.
- Recognize presyncopal symptoms.
- Use behaviors, such as lying down, to avoid syncope.

PROGNOSIS
May be recurrent but not life-threatening

COMPLICATIONS
May result in injury from fall

REFERENCES
1. Angaran P, Klein GJ, Yee R, et al. Syncope. Neurol Clin. 2011;29(4):903–925.
2. Raj SR, Coffin ST. Medical therapy and physical maneuvers in the treatment of the vasovagal syncope and orthostatic hypotension. Prog Cardiovasc Dis. 2013;55(4):425–433.
3. Walsh K, Hoffmayer K, Hamdan MH. Syncope: diagnosis and management. Curr Probl Cardiol. 2015;40(2):51–86.
4. Runser L, Gauer R, Houser A. Syncope: evaluation and differential diagnosis. Am Fam Physician. 2017;95(5):303–312.
5. Coffin ST, Raj SR. Non-invasive management of vasovagal syncope. Auton Neurosci. 2014;184:27–32.
6. Moya A, Sutton R, Ammirati F, et al; for Task Force for the Diagnosis and Management of Syncope, European Society of Cardiology, European Heart Rhythm Association, et al. Guidelines for the diagnosis and management of syncope (version 2009). Eur Heart J. 2009;30(21):2631–2671.

ADDITIONAL READING
- Lelonek M. Genetics in neurocardiogenic syncope. Przegl Lek. 2006;63(12):1310–1312.
- Márquez MF, Urias-Medina K, Gómez-Flores J, et al. Comparison of metoprolol vs clonazepam as a first treatment choice among patients with neurocardiogenic syncope. Gac Med Mex. 2008;144(6):503–507.

 SEE ALSO

Algorithms: Syncope; Transient Ischemic Attack and Transient Neurologic Defects

 CODES

ICD10
R55 Syncope and collapse

CLINICAL PEARLS
- A careful history of the events preceding the syncopal episode helps guide evaluation and management.
- Rule out cardiac or neurogenic syncope.
- Prodrome is common with reflex syncope.
- Recovery may be prolonged, with persistent symptoms but there is no residual neurologic deficit or confusion.
- Patients should avoid precipitating situations or events as a first-line treatment.
- Pregnant women can have reflex syncope when moving from supine to lateral decubitus or upright positions.

SYNDROME OF INAPPROPRIATE ANTIDIURETIC HORMONE SECRETION (SIADH)

Elise J. Barney, DO

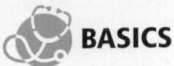 **BASICS**

DESCRIPTION

- A syndrome of abnormal production of antidiuretic hormone (ADH), despite low serum osmolality, leading to hyponatremia and inappropriately elevated urine osmolality
  - Decreased urinary electrolyte-free water excretion leads to dilutional hyponatremia (total body sodium [Na] levels may be normal or near normal, but the patient's total body water is increased).
  - Often secondary to medications but may be associated with an underlying disorder, such as neoplasm, pulmonary disorder, or CNS disease
- Synonym(s): syndrome of inappropriate secretion of ADH; syndrome of inappropriate antidiuresis

EPIDEMIOLOGY

Incidence
- Often found in the hospital setting, where incidence can be as high as 35%
- Predominant age: elderly
- Predominate sex: females > males

ETIOLOGY AND PATHOPHYSIOLOGY

- Drugs:
  - Antidepressants (e.g., SSRIs, tricyclics, monoamine oxidase inhibitors [MAOIs])
  - Antineoplastic drugs (e.g., vincristine, vinblastine, cisplatin, cyclophosphamide)
  - Antipsychotic agents (e.g., risperidone, quetiapine, phenothiazines, haloperidol)
  - Analgesics (e.g., duloxetine, pregabalin, tramadol, NSAIDs)
  - Anticonvulsants (e.g., carbamazepine, oxcarbazepine, valproic acid, phenytoin)
  - Others (e.g., vasopressin, DDAVP, oxytocin, ciprofloxacin, α-interferon, ecstasy)
- Malignancies (ectopic ADH production):
  - Bronchogenic carcinoma
  - Lymphoma
  - Mesothelioma
  - Small cell carcinoma of the lung
  - Pancreatic carcinoma
  - Thymoma
- Pulmonary conditions:
  - Asthma/COPD
  - Atelectasis
  - Cystic fibrosis
  - Positive pressure mechanical ventilation
  - Pneumonia
  - Pulmonary tuberculosis (TB)
  - Sarcoidosis
- Neurologic causes:
  - Brain tumor
  - CNS injury (i.e., SAH, trauma, stroke)

- CNS lupus
- Encephalitis
- Epilepsy
- Guillain-Barré syndrome
- Intracranial surgery
- Meningitis
- Multiple sclerosis
- Other:
  - Acute intermittent porphyria
  - Delirium tremens
  - HIV infection/AIDS
  - Rocky Mountain spotted fever
- Idiopathic

Genetics
- 10% of patients have X-linked mutation of V2R.
- Polymorphisms in TRPV4 gene

RISK FACTORS
- Use of predisposing drugs
- Advanced age
- Postoperative status
- Institutionalization

GENERAL PREVENTION
- Search for cause, if unknown.
- Reduce/change medications, if drug induced.
- Lifelong restriction of fluid intake

COMMONLY ASSOCIATED CONDITIONS
See "Etiology and Pathophysiology."

 DIAGNOSIS

HISTORY
Symptoms:
- Fatigue
- Anorexia
- Nausea
- Vomiting
- Diarrhea
- Headaches
- Unsteady gait
- Falls
- Myalgias/weakness
- Increased thirst
- Confusion
- Seizures, coma

PHYSICAL EXAM
- Euvolemic state
- Mild hyponatremia (serum Na 125 to 135 mEq/L)
  - Slow cognition and reaction times
  - Hyporeflexia
  - Ataxia

- Moderate to severe hyponatremia (serum Na <125 mEq/L)
  - Altered mental status
  - Lethargy
  - Seizures
  - Psychosis
  - Coma
  - Death

DIFFERENTIAL DIAGNOSIS
- Intravascular volume depletion and thiazide induced
- Appropriate ADH secretion secondary to decreased effective arterial blood volume (e.g., congestive heart failure [CHF], nephrotic syndrome, liver cirrhosis)
- Low solute intake hyponatremia
  - "Tea and toast" diet
  - Beer potomania
- Psychogenic polydipsia
  - Intake usually >10 L/day
  - Diuresis occurs when intake is stopped.
- Endocrinopathies
  - Adrenal insufficiency
  - Hypothyroidism
- Translocational hyponatremia: caused by hyperglycemia, mannitol, sucrose, glycine
- Pseudohyponatremia
  - Lab artifact caused by hyperlipidemia, paraproteinemias, administration of IVIG
  - Labs using flame photometry or indirect potentiometry susceptible
- Postoperative complications:
  - Caused by nonosmotic release of ADH, probably mediated by pain afferents
  - ADH stimulated by pain, nausea, vomiting, and hypotension
- Cerebral salt-wasting syndrome (hyponatremia, extracellular fluid depletion, CNS insult)

DIAGNOSTIC TESTS & INTERPRETATION
- Serum Na level: low
- Serum urea level: normal to low
- Serum osmolality: low
- Urine osmolality: high; urine osmolality >100 mOsm/kg H_2O (1)
- Urine Na concentration: high; urine Na >30 mEq/L (1)
- Fractional excretion of Na >0.5 % (1)
- Serum ADH level: high (not clinically useful)
- Not usually required for diagnosis but to assist in diagnosis and assess for other causes:
  - Serum uric acid
  - Serum glucose; creatinine
  - Thyroid function
  - Morning cortisol

TREATMENT

GENERAL MEASURES
- Treatment of the underlying cause is essential.
- Requires frequent monitoring (see "Patient Monitoring")
- Fluid restriction (usually <1,000 mL/day) is the main treatment (2)[B].
- Avoid isotonic saline because this can worsen the hyponatremia.
- Correction of hypokalemia
- Mild asymptomatic hyponatremia (serum Na >125 mEq/L [>125 mmol/L]): Restrict fluid and treat underlying cause.
- Moderate hyponatremia (serum Na 120 to 125 mEq/L):
  - Restrict free water intake.
  - Increase oral solute intake.
  - Calculate urine/plasma electrolyte ratio ([urine Na + K] / [serum Na + serum K]) to determine efficacy of fluid restriction; ineffective if ratio >1 (3) and may need pharmacologic therapy
  - Treat underlying cause/remove offending agent.
- Severe or with neurologic manifestations
  - Hypertonic saline (3% sodium chloride [NaCl] IV bolus)
  - Increase serum Na slowly with hypertonic saline by 4 to 6 mEq/L over 4 to 6 hours (not to exceed 8 mEq/L in a 24-hour period) (1,4)[C].
- Acute (<48 hours duration)
  - Can initially correct rapidly but 24-hour goal is same as in chronic hyponatremia (4)[C]

MEDICATION
- If severe or neurologic symptoms: IV 3% NaCl to increase serum Na cautiously (5)[B]:
  - If serum Na <120 mEq/L or severe neurologic symptoms, consider bolus of hypertonic saline to increase serum Na by 4 to 6 mEq/L over the first 4 to 6 hours.
- NaCl oral tablets
- Oral urea is an option but limited due to bitter taste.
- Loop diuretics: furosemide + potassium replacement
- Vasopressin-2 receptor antagonist (the vaptans: tolvaptan, conivaptan) (5)[B]
  - Good efficacy and safety profiles in the treatment of moderate hyponatremia due to SIADH
  - Liberal fluid intake encouraged
  - Must be initiated in hospital setting
  - Cost may limit long-term use.
  - Avoid tolvaptan in patients with liver disease.
- Demeclocycline (limited use)
  - Blocks ADH at renal tubule; produces nephrogenic diabetes insipidus
  - Dosage for long-term management: 300 to 600 mg PO BID
  - Onset of action within 1 week; therefore, not best for acute management
  - Adverse effects of GI intolerance and nephrotoxicity limit its use.
  - Paucity of evidence for efficacy

- Contraindications: Avoid fluids in CHF, nephrotic syndrome, or cirrhosis. Avoid tolvaptan in patients with cirrhosis due to possible liver injury.
- Precautions: Overly rapid correction (>10 mEq/L/day) can increase risk for osmotic demyelination syndrome (ODS):
  - Permanent CNS damage in pons leading to quadriplegia and pseudobulbar palsy
  - Increased risk in women, alcoholics, malnutrition, hypoxia, chronic hyponatremia of <110 mEq/L, and hypokalemia

ALERT
Increase Na levels slowly, no >8 mEq/L/24 hr, to prevent ODS (1)[C].

 ONGOING CARE

FOLLOW-UP RECOMMENDATIONS
Patient Monitoring
- Careful continuous clinical and laboratory monitoring of hyponatremic state during acute phase:
  - Hourly urine output
  - Urine Na, urine potassium, urine osmolality
  - Goal Na increase is <8 mEq/L/24 hr until Na reaches 130 mEq/L (1,4)[C].
  - If moderate/severe, check serial serum chemistry every 4 to 8 hours to ensure appropriate rate of correction.
- Chronic management: Treat underlying cause; continue fluid restriction and NaCl tablets as needed; referral to nephrologist

DIET
Increase protein/solute intake and decrease water intake.

PATIENT EDUCATION
Diet and fluid restrictions

PROGNOSIS
- Higher morbidity and mortality in hospitalized patients with hyponatremia (6)
- Higher risk of ICU admission and increased risk of 30-day hospital readmission in hyponatremic patients (6)
- If symptomatic (seizure, coma): high mortality due to cerebral edema if serum Na <120 mEq/L

COMPLICATIONS
- Falls and hip fractures
- Cerebral edema (see "Prognosis")
- Osmotic demyelination with overcorrection (see "Treatment" precautions): central pontine and extrapontine irreversible myelinolysis (4)
- Chronic hyponatremia
- Chronic hyponatremia is associated with osteoporosis (6)[C].

REFERENCES
1. Decaux G, Musch W. Clinical laboratory evaluation of the syndrome of inappropriate secretion of antidiuretic hormone. *Clin J Am Soc Nephrol.* 2008;3(4):1175–1184.
2. Ellison DH, Berl T. Clinical practice. The syndrome of inappropriate antidiuresis. *N Engl J Med.* 2007;356(20):2064–2072.
3. Furst H, Hallows KR, Post J, et al. The urine/plasma electrolyte ratio: a predictive guide to water restriction. *Am J Med Sci.* 2000;319(4):240–244.
4. Adrogué HJ, Madias NE. The challenge of hyponatremia. *J Am Soc Nephrol.* 2012;23(7):1140–1148.
5. Esposito P, Piotti G, Bianzina S, et al. The syndrome of inappropriate antidiuresis: pathophysiology, clinical management and new therapeutic options. *Nephron Clin Pract.* 2011;119(1):c62–c73.
6. Usala RL, Fernandez SJ, Mete M, et al. Hyponatremia is associated with increased osteoporosis and bone fractures in a large US health system population. *J Clin Endocrinol Metab.* 2015;100(8):3021–3031.

 SEE ALSO

Hyponatremia

CODES

ICD10
E22.2 Syndrome of inappropriate secretion of antidiuretic hormone

CLINICAL PEARLS
- Treatment of the underlying cause is a key. Review all medications for potential culprits.
- Nephrology consultation is recommended in moderate to severe hyponatremia or if hypertonic saline indicated.
- Fluid restriction is the mainstay of treatment in SIADH. Fluid restriction fails to correct hyponatremia and Na wasting in salt-losing renal disease.
- Cerebral salt wasting is a controversial disease entity and is similar to SIADH. However, patients with SIADH are euvolemic, whereas patients with cerebral salt wasting are hypovolemic. The only real way to establish the diagnosis is through fluid restriction. Serum urate and fractional excretion of urate will be corrected with fluid restriction in SIADH but will not correct in cerebral salt wasting.
- ODS is a cerebral demyelination syndrome that causes quadriplegia, pseudobulbar palsy, seizures, coma, and death. It is caused by an overly rapid rate of Na correction. Increase Na levels slowly, no >8 mEq/L/24 hr, to prevent ODS.
- Safe correction of hyponatremia is important. Online calculators are available: http://www.medcalc.com/sodium.html.

SYPHILIS

Melissa Badowski, PharmD, MPH • Mahesh C. Patel, MD

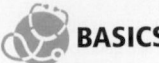

BASICS

DESCRIPTION
- A chronic, systemic infectious disease caused by *Treponema pallidum*
- Transmitted sexually by direct contact with an active lesion, vertically (maternal–fetal), and via blood transfusions
- Untreated disease includes four overlapping stages.
  - Primary: single (usually) painless chancre at point of entry; appears in 10 to 90 days; chancre heals without treatment in 3 to 6 weeks.
  - Secondary: appears 2 to 8 weeks after primary chancre; nonpruritic rash on palms or soles of feet, mucous membrane lesions, headache, fever, lymphadenopathy, alopecia
  - Latent: seroreactive without evidence of disease
    ○ Early latent: acquired within the last year
    ○ Late latent: exposure >12 months prior to diagnosis
  - Tertiary (late): Serology may be negative (fluorescent treponemal antibody absorption [FTA-ABS] test typically positive).
    ○ Gumma, cardiovascular, and late neurosyphilis; may be fatal
  - Neurosyphilis: *any* type of CNS involvement; can occur at *any* stage
    ○ Psychosis, delirium, dementia
- Syphilis can affect nearly every organ/tissue.

Pediatric Considerations
In noncongenital cases, consider child abuse.

Pregnancy Considerations
- Screen all pregnant patients with venereal disease research laboratory (VDRL) test or rapid plasma reagin (RPR) test early in pregnancy. If high risk, repeat at 28 weeks and at delivery (1,2)[A].
- Use the same nontreponemal test for initial screening and for follow-up (1,2)[A].

EPIDEMIOLOGY
Incidence
- Syphilis rate decreased until 2000; has since increased (primarily in men who have sex with men [MSM]) (3); highest for men ages 25 to 29 years and women ages 20 to 24 years (3)
  - Men: 15.6/100,000
  - Women: 1.9/100,000
- Congenital: 15.7/100,000 live births (3)
- Ocular: estimated to be 0.65% of syphilis cases
- Primary and secondary syphilis rates (3)
  - Male (per 100,000 population)
    ○ Whites, non-Hispanic: 9.0
    ○ Blacks, non-Hispanic: 41.3
    ○ Hispanics: 19.7
    ○ Asians: 7.6
    ○ American Indians/Alaska natives: 12.4
    ○ Native Hawaiians/Pacific Islanders: 23.0
    ○ Multirace: 11.2
  - Female (per 100,000 population)
    ○ Whites, non-Hispanic: 0.9
    ○ Blacks, non-Hispanic: 6.3
    ○ Hispanics: 1.9
    ○ Asians: 0.4
    ○ American Indians/Alaska natives: 3.7
    ○ Native Hawaiians/Pacific Islanders: 2.5
    ○ Multirace: 1.2

Prevalence
- Predominant sex: male (90%) > female (10%) (3)
- Greatest increase in MSM (3)

ETIOLOGY AND PATHOPHYSIOLOGY
T. pallidum enters through intact mucous membranes or breaks in skin. The organism quickly enters the lymphatics to cause systemic disease. Highly infectious; exposure to as few as 60 spirochetes is associated with ~50% chance of infection.

RISK FACTORS
MSM, multiple sexual partners, exposure to infected body fluids, IV drug use, transplacental transmission, adult inmates, high-risk sexual behavior, HIV positive

GENERAL PREVENTION
Education regarding safe sex; condoms reduce but do not eliminate transmission (4)[A].

COMMONLY ASSOCIATED CONDITIONS
HIV infection, hepatitis B, other STIs

DIAGNOSIS

HISTORY
- As a "great imitator," a high index of suspicion is often required for accurate diagnosis.
- Previous sexual contact with partner with known infection or high-risk sexual behavior
- Genital lesions (chancre—primary syphilis)
- Rash, alopecia, malaise, headache, anorexia, nausea, fatigue (secondary syphilis)
- Mental status changes (tertiary syphilis)

PHYSICAL EXAM
Signs/symptoms depend on stage.
- Primary: single (occasionally multiple), usually painless ulcer (chancre) in groin or at other point of entry; regional adenopathy
- Secondary
  - Rash: skin/mucous membranes
    ○ Rough, red-brown macules, usually on palms and soles
    ○ May appear with chancre or after it has healed
    ○ Condylomata lata
    ○ Alopecia
  - Nonspecific symptoms: fever, adenopathy, malaise, headache, hair loss
- Tertiary
  - Focal neurologic findings (hearing loss, vision loss; meningeal findings; loss of pain, temperature; proprioception)
  - Gummas (skin, mucous membranes, other organ systems)

DIFFERENTIAL DIAGNOSIS
- Primary: chancroid, lymphogranuloma venereum, granuloma inguinale, condylomata acuminata, herpes simplex, Behçet syndrome, trauma, carcinoma, mycotic infection, lichen planus, psoriasis, fungal infection
- Secondary: pityriasis rosea, drug eruption, psoriasis, lichen planus, viral exanthema, Stevens-Johnson syndrome
- Positive serology, asymptomatic: previously treated syphilis/other spirochetal disease (yaws, pinta)

DIAGNOSTIC TESTS & INTERPRETATION
Initial Tests (lab, imaging)
- Dark-field microscopy demonstrating *T. pallidum* spirochetes in lesion exudate/tissue biopsy is gold standard but difficult and not very sensitive (5)[A].
- Nontreponemal tests (VDRL/RPR) (3,5)[A]
  - Primary screening test: positive within 7 days of exposure
  - Nonspecific false-positive results are common; must confirm diagnosis with treponemal tests
  - Positive test should be quantified and titers followed regularly after treatment.
    ○ Titers usually correlate with disease activity; 4-fold change is clinically significant.
    ○ Titers decrease with time/treatment; following adequate treatment for primary/secondary disease, a 4-fold decline is typical in 6 to 12 months.
    ○ Absence of a 4-fold decline suggests potential treatment failure.
    ○ ~15% of appropriately treated patients do not have a 4-fold decline in titer 12 months after treatment. Management is unclear; repeat HIV testing and/or CSF examination and continue to follow titers.
    ○ With appropriate treatment, titers should become negative (see serofast reaction).
    ○ Titers of patients treated in latent stages decline more gradually.
  - Prozone phenomenon: negative results from high titers of antibody; test with diluted serum.
  - Serofast reaction: persistently positive results years after successful treatment; new infection diagnosed by 4-fold rise in titer
  - Conditions that may alter treponemal testing (All stages of syphilis can have a false-negative RPR result, especially in primary syphilis.)
    ○ Pregnancy, autoimmune disease, mononucleosis, malaria, leprosy, viral pneumonia, cardiolipin antigens, injection drug use, acute febrile illness, HIV infection; elderly can have false-positive results.
- TP-PA (T. pallidum particle agglutination) increasingly used for primary testing as high sensitivity overcomes challenges of Nontreponemal tests
- Treponemal tests (*confirmatory test after positive nontreponemal screening test*): for example, FTA-ABS, TP-PA (*T. pallidum particle agglutination*), others (5)[A]:
  - Confirmatory test;
  - Usually positive for life after treatment
  - Titers of no benefit
  - 15–25% of patients treated during primary stage revert to serologic nonreactivity after 2 to 3 years.
- Lumbar puncture (LP) indicated for (5)[A]:
  - Neurologic, ocular, or auditory manifestations
  - Some advise LP in all secondary and early latent cases—even without neurologic symptoms.
  - HIV-positive patients with late latent/latent disease of unknown duration
  - Patients with late latent/latent disease of unknown duration if nonpenicillin therapy planned
  - Treatment failures
  - Evidence of active tertiary syphilis (e.g., aortitis, gumma, iritis)
  - Children to rule out neurosyphilis
  - VDRL, not RPR, used on CSF; may be negative in neurosyphilis; highly specific but insensitive
  - Send CSF for protein, glucose, and cell count.
  - Monitor resolution with cell count at 6 months along with serologies (see "Patient Monitoring").

- Negative FTA-ABS or microhemagglutination (MHA)-TP on CSF excludes neurosyphilis (highly sensitive).
- Positive FTA-ABS or MHA-TP on CSF is not diagnostic because of high false-positive rate.
- Traumatic tap, tuberculosis (TB), pyogenic/aseptic meningitis can all result in false-positive VDRL.

 TREATMENT

GENERAL MEASURES
- Advise patients to notify partner(s) and to avoid intercourse until treatment is complete (5)[A].
- Test for HIV infection (3,5)[A].
- Management of sexual contacts (5)[A]
  - Presumptively treat partners exposed within 90 days of diagnosis.
  - Presumptively treat partners exposed >90 days before diagnosis if serologic results are not available immediately and follow-up is uncertain.
  - Presumptively treat those exposed to a patient diagnosed with syphilis of unknown duration who has high treponemal titers (>1:32).
  - Long-term sex partners of patients with latent infection should be evaluated clinically (including serologies) and treated accordingly.

MEDICATION

ALERT
Use bicillin L-A instead of bicillin C-R (combination benzathine–procaine penicillin).

First Line
Parenteral penicillin G is the drug of choice. The formulation is determined by the disease stage and clinical presentation.
- Primary, secondary, and early latent <1 year (5)[A]
  - Penicillin G benzathine 2.4 million U IM × 1 dose
  - Penicillin-allergic patients: doxycycline 100 mg PO BID for 2 weeks, or tetracycline 500 mg PO QID for 2 weeks, or ceftriaxone 1 to 2 g IM or IV daily for 10 to 14 days
    - Azithromycin 2 g PO for 1 dose (early syphilis only; should not be used in HIV, MSM, or pregnancy)
    - Resistance and treatment failures have been noted in several U.S. regions.
- Late latent/latent of unknown duration and tertiary without evidence of neurosyphilis (5)[A]
  - Penicillin G benzathine 2.4 million U IM weekly × 3 doses
  - Penicillin-allergic patients: Attempt desensitization and treatment with penicillin or doxycycline 100 mg PO BID for 28 days, or tetracycline 500 mg PO QID for 28 days; adherence may be an issue.
- Ocular or neurosyphilis (5)[A]
  - Aqueous crystalline penicillin G 3 to 4 million U IV q4h as continuous infusion for 10 to 14 days
  - Alternative: penicillin G procaine 2.4 million U IM daily in conjunction with probenecid 500 mg PO QID for 10 to 14 days (if compliance can be ensured)
  - Penicillin-allergic patients: Attempt desensitization and treat with penicillin; ceftriaxone 2 g/day IM or IV for 10 to 14 days
  - If late latent, latent of unknown duration, or tertiary in addition to neurosyphilis, consider treating as late latent after completion of neurosyphilis treatment regimen.

- Congenital (5)[A]
  - Aqueous crystalline penicillin G 50,000 U/kg/dose IV q12h for the first 7 days of life and q8h thereafter for a total of 10 days, or penicillin G procaine 50,000 U/kg/dose IM daily for 10 days
  - If negative CSF serologies, normal physical exam, and maternal titer and then 50,000 U/kg penicillin G benzathine IM in single dose
  - If >1 day of drug is missed, restart course.
  - Children (after newborn period): aqueous crystalline penicillin G 50,000 U/kg/dose IV q4–6h for 10 days; late latent, 50,000 U/kg IM as 3 doses at 1-week intervals
  - For contacts without symptoms: Treat as primary disease after serologies are obtained.
  - HIV-infected and pregnant patients may show poor response to recommended IM doses. Use IV therapy for all treatment failures in these patients.
  - Do not give benzathine or procaine penicillins IV.
- Children (after newborn period) (5)[A]: aqueous crystalline penicillin G 50,000 U/kg/dose IV q4–6h for 10 days; late latent, 50,000 U/kg IM as 3 doses at 1-week intervals
- Pregnancy (5)[A]
  - Treatment is same as for nonpregnant patients.
  - Some recommend second dose of penicillin G benzathine 2.4 million U IM 1 week after initial dose in 3rd trimester or with primary, secondary, or early latent syphilis.
  - Penicillin sensitivity: no proven alternatives to penicillin available for treatment during pregnancy
  - Penicillin-allergic patients: Desensitize and treat with penicillin.
  - HIV-infected pregnant patients may show poor response to recommended IM doses. Use IV therapy for all treatment failures in these patients.
- Treat contacts without symptoms as primary disease after obtaining serologies.
- History of penicillin allergy:
  - Confirmed IgE-mediated reaction: desensitization
  - Questionable history of IgE-mediated hypersensitivity: penicillin skin testing if major and minor penicillin determinants available
- Precautions (5)[A]
  - HIV-infected and pregnant patients may show poor response to recommended IM doses. Use IV therapy for all treatment failures in these patients.
  - Do not give benzathine or procaine penicillins IV.

 ONGOING CARE

FOLLOW-UP RECOMMENDATIONS
- Clinical and serologic evaluation 6 to 12 months after treatment; if >1 year duration, check at 24 months (5)[A].
- In HIV-infected persons, clinical and serologic evaluation at 3, 6, 9, 12, and 24 months after therapy (5)[A]

Patient Monitoring
- Use VDRL or RPR test to monitor therapy: 4-fold rise (two dilutions) in titer indicates new infection, whereas failure to decrease 4-fold (two dilutions) in 6 to 12 months may indicate treatment failure (although definitive criteria for cure not established); always use same test (preferably same lab) (5)[A].
- Retreatment for persistent clinical signs or recurrence, 4-fold rise in titers, or failure of initially high titer to decrease 4-fold by 6 to 12 months
- Neurosyphilis: Repeat LP every 6 months to check for normalization of CSF cell count (± CSF-VDRL and protein evaluation) (5)[A].

PATIENT EDUCATION
No intimate contacts until 4-fold titer drop

PROGNOSIS
- Excellent in all cases except patients with late syphilis complications and with HIV infection
- Syphilis in HIV-infected patient
  - Treatment same as for HIV-negative patients
  - More often false-negative treponemal and non-treponemal tests or unusually high titers
  - Response to therapy less predictable
  - Early syphilis: increased risk of neurosyphilis and higher rates of treatment failure
  - Late neurosyphilis: harder to treat; can occur up to 20 years or more after infection

COMPLICATIONS
- Membranous glomerulonephritis
- Paroxysmal cold hemoglobinemia
- Meningitis and tabes dorsalis
- Cardiovascular aneurysms; valvular damage
- Irreversible organ damage
- Jarisch-Herxheimer reaction
  - Fever, chills, headache, myalgias, new rash
  - Common when starting treatment (of primary/secondary disease; less common with tertiary) owing to treponemal lysis
  - Should not be confused with drug reaction
  - Managed with analgesics and antipyretics

REFERENCES
1. Gomez GB, Kamb ML, Newman LM, et al. Untreated maternal syphilis and adverse outcomes of pregnancy: a systematic review and meta-analysis. *Bull World Health Organ*. 2013;91(3):217–226.
2. Peeling RW, Mabey D, Kamb ML, et al. Syphilis. *Nat Rev Dis Primers*. 2017;3:17073.
3. Centers for Disease Control and Prevention. *Sexually Transmitted Disease Surveillance 2016*. Atlanta, GA: U.S. Department of Health and Human Services; 2017.
4. Stamm LV. Syphilis: antibiotic treatment and resistance. *Epidemiol Infect*. 2015;143(8):1567–1574.
5. Workowski KA, Bolan GA; for Centers for Disease Control and Prevention. Sexually transmitted diseases treatment guidelines, 2015. *MMWR Recomm Rep*. 2015;64(RR-03):1–137.

 SEE ALSO

Chlamydia Infection (Sexually Transmitted); Gonococcal Infections

CODES

ICD10
- A53.9 Syphilis, unspecified
- A51.0 Primary genital syphilis
- A53.0 Latent syphilis, unspecified as early or late

CLINICAL PEARLS
- Screen all HIV-positive patients and patients with high-risk sexual behaviors for syphilis.
- Penicillin remains the treatment of choice for syphilis.
- Syphilis rates are rising—particularly among MSM.

TARSAL TUNNEL SYNDROME

Terrence C. Tsui, DO • J. Herbert Stevenson, MD

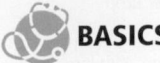 **BASICS**

DESCRIPTION

Tarsal tunnel syndrome occurs when there is compression neuropathy of the posterior tibial nerve as it passes behind the medial malleolus and under the flexor retinaculum (laciniate ligament) in the medial ankle (the tarsal tunnel).

EPIDEMIOLOGY

- Women are slightly more affected than men (56%).
- All postpubescent ages are affected.

ETIOLOGY AND PATHOPHYSIOLOGY

- Contents within the tarsal tunnel from the anterior medial to the posterior lateral side include the following: the posterior tibial tendon, the flexor digitorum longus tendon, the posterior tibial artery and veins, the posterior tibial nerve, and the flexor hallucis tendon.
- The posterior tibial nerve passes through the tarsal tunnel, which is formed by three osseus structures—sustentaculum tali, medial calcaneus, and medial malleolus—covered by the laciniate ligament.
- Compression of the posterior tibial nerve within the tarsal tunnel results in decreased blood flow, ischemic damage, and resultant symptoms (1).
- Chronic compression can destroy endoneurial microvasculature, leading to edema and (eventually) fibrosis and demyelination (2).
- Increased pressure in the tarsal tunnel is caused by a variety of mechanical and biochemical mechanisms. The specific cause for compression is identifiable in only 60–80% of patients (1).
- Three general categories: trauma, space-occupying lesions, deformity (1)
  - Trauma including displaced fractures, deltoid ligament sprains, or tenosynovitis
  - Varicosities
  - Hindfoot varus or valgus
  - Fibrosis of the perineurium
- Other causes:
  - Osseous prominences
  - Ganglia; lipoma; neurilemmoma
  - Inflammatory synovitis
  - Pigmented villonodular synovitis
  - Tarsal coalition
  - Accessory musculature
- In patients with systemic disease (e.g., diabetes), the "double crush" syndrome refers to the development of a second compression along the same nerve at a site of anatomic narrowing in patients with previous proximal nerve damage (3).

RISK FACTORS

- Tarsal tunnel syndrome is associated with certain occupations and activities involving repetitive and prolonged weight-bearing on the foot and ankle (walking, running, dancing).
- Other possible risk factors include (4):
  - Diabetes
  - Systemic inflammatory arthritis
  - Connective tissue disorders
  - Obesity
  - Varicosities
  - Heel varus or valgus
  - Bifurcation of the posterior tibial nerve into medial and lateral plantar nerves proximal to the tarsal tunnel

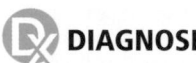 **DIAGNOSIS**

Tarsal tunnel syndrome is largely a clinical diagnosis, characterized by pain and paresthesias in a predictable distribution along the medial aspect of the ankle and plantar surface of the foot (1).

HISTORY

- History of trauma (which may be trivial) to the foot precipitating pain
- Pain, tightness, burning, tingling, and/or numbness behind medial malleolus radiating to the longitudinal arch and plantar aspect of foot including the heel (1)
- Pain usually worsens during standing or activity.
- Pain radiates proximally up the medial leg (Valleix phenomenon) in 33% of patients with severe compression.
- Some patients have substantial night pain (may be related to venostasis).
- Symptoms improve with rest, wearing loose footwear, and elevation.
- In advanced nerve compression, motor involvement may cause weakness, atrophy, and digital contractures of the intrinsic foot muscles (4).

ALERT

Other systemic neuropathies (diabetes, alcoholism, HIV, drug reactions) present with similar symptoms.

PHYSICAL EXAM

- Inspect: foot alignment
  - Examine for excessive foot pronation during standing or walking.
  - Examine for hindfoot varus or valgus deformity.
  - Exaggerating heel dorsiflexion, inversion, or eversion may reproduce symptoms by stretching or compressing the posterior tibial nerve.
- Palpate the tarsal tunnel and the course of the tibial nerve for tenderness and swelling.
- Tinel sign: Percussion over the tibial nerve may reproduce paresthesias that radiate distally.

- Valleix sign: Percussion over the tibial nerve may produce paresthesias that radiate proximally.
- Cuff test: Inflating a pneumatic cuff engorges varicosities and reproduces symptoms.
- Compression test: Applying pressure to the tarsal tunnel for 60 seconds may reproduce symptoms.
- Sensory examination
  - The medial calcaneal nerve usually is spared, but numbness and altered sensation may be present in the distribution of the medial or lateral plantar nerves.
  - Vibratory sensation and two-point discrimination are decreased early in the disease process.
- Motor examination
  - Intrinsic foot muscle weakness (difficult to assess)
  - Rarely, weakness of toe plantar flexion may be present.
  - Atrophy of the abductor hallucis or abductor digiti minimi may be seen late in the disease process.

DIFFERENTIAL DIAGNOSIS

- Peripheral neuropathies (diabetes, alcoholism, HIV, or drug related)
- Inflammatory arthritis (rheumatoid arthritis)
- Morton neuroma
- Metatarsalgia
- Subtalar joint arthritis
- Tibialis posterior tendinitis/dysfunction
- Plantar fasciitis
- Plantar callosities
- Peripheral vascular disease
- Lumbar radiculopathy
- Proximal injury or compression of the tibial branch of the sciatic nerve

DIAGNOSTIC TESTS & INTERPRETATION

Initial Tests (lab, imaging)

Routine lab tests help rule out other conditions that may mimic tarsal tunnel syndrome, including diabetic neuropathy, rheumatoid arthritis, thyroid dysfunction, or other systemic illnesses (5).

- Routine weight-bearing radiographs, followed by CT (if necessary) to assess for fracture or structural abnormality
- Consider evaluation of lumbar spine x-ray if double crush (injury to lumbar nerve results in compensatory injury to posterior tibial nerve) is suspected (5).
- MRI: helps assess the tarsal tunnel for soft tissue masses or other sources of nerve compression before surgery (1)
- Ultrasound (US): gaining importance and with several advantages over MRI; can assess for space-occupying lesions (ganglia, varicose veins, lipomas, etc.) and tenosynovitis (1)

Pregnancy Considerations

- Tarsal tunnel syndrome can occur during pregnancy, typically secondary to local compression caused by fluid retention and volume changes (1).
- Care is supportive. Most cases resolve after pregnancy.

Pediatric Considerations
MRI is recommended for evaluating pediatric tarsal tunnel syndrome to exclude neoplastic mass.

Diagnostic Procedures/Other
Electrodiagnostic studies
- Electromyography (EMG) of the intrinsic muscles of the foot can confirm the diagnosis of tarsal tunnel syndrome. A normal EMG does not exclude the diagnosis (false-negative rate is ~10%) (1).
- Nerve conduction studies may reveal slowed conduction of the tibial nerve.
- Evaluate for proximal nerve compression, including a lumbar radiculopathy or a double crush phenomenon.

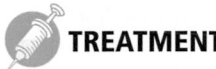

TREATMENT
- Conservative management is recommended, except for acute onset tarsal tunnel syndrome or in the setting of a known space-occupying lesion (excluding synovitis).
- Tarsal tunnel decompression may improve sensory impairment and restore protective sensation in diabetic peripheral neuropathies if there is nerve entrapment at the tarsal tunnel.

MEDICATION
First Line
- Analgesics and anti-inflammatory medications
- Local corticosteroid injection
- Medications that alter neurogenic pain (tricyclic antidepressants, antiepileptic drugs, nerve blockers)

ADDITIONAL THERAPIES
- Rest/immobilization
- Taping and bracing
- Orthotics or shoe modification
- Night splinting
- Physical therapy to strengthen the intrinsic and extrinsic muscles of the foot and to restore the medial longitudinal arch
- Other modalities (stretching, US, massage, icing)
- Compression stockings to decrease swelling
- Weight loss for obese patients

SURGERY/OTHER PROCEDURES
- Surgery is indicated (1,2).
  - If nonoperative measures fail following a 6-month trial
  - In the setting of acute tarsal tunnel syndrome
  - If there are signs of motor involvement/weakness or muscle atrophy
  - If a space-occupying lesion is identified
- The surgical outcome is dependent on technique and postoperative management. 50–95% of cases have good to excellent outcomes.
- At the time of surgery, assess focal swelling, scarring, or nerve abnormalities and look for a pathologic source of compression.

- Postoperative management includes:
  - Non–weight-bearing splint until incision heals (2 to 3 weeks), followed by progressively increased weight-bearing and range of motion exercises
  - Rest, ice, compression, elevation to limit swelling

 ## ONGOING CARE

PATIENT EDUCATION
- Discuss conservative and surgical options based on individual patient circumstance and preference.
- A decision about surgical intervention should be made with a clear understanding of risks, benefits, and potential adverse outcomes.

PROGNOSIS
Surgery is most helpful for:
- Patients with a positive Tinel sign (3)[B]
- Young patients
- Short period between occurrence of symptoms and surgery <1 year
- Localized space-occupying lesion (1)
- No motor neuron involvement

COMPLICATIONS
- The main adverse outcome is an unsuccessful surgical intervention characterized by lack of improvement or recurrence of symptoms (1).
- Causes for a failed tarsal tunnel release include:
  - Incorrect diagnosis
  - Incomplete release
  - Adhesive neuritis (external scar formation)
  - Intraneural damage (systemic disease, direct nerve injury)
  - Failure to treat all sources of nerve compression in a double crush phenomenon
- Electrodiagnostic studies are rarely helpful in determining the cause of a failed tarsal tunnel release.
- Results with surgical revision are poorer than those for the primary surgical release.

REFERENCES

1. Ahmad M, Tsang K, Mackenney PJ, et al. Tarsal tunnel syndrome: a literature review. *Foot Ankle Surg.* 2012;18(3):149–152.
2. Dellon AL. The four medial ankle tunnels: a critical review of perceptions of tarsal tunnel syndrome and neuropathy. *Neurosurg Clin N Am.* 2008;19(4):629–648.
3. Dellon AL, Muse VL, Scott ND, et al. A positive Tinel sign as predictor of pain relief or sensory recovery after decompression of chronic tibial nerve compression in patients with diabetic neuropathy. *J Reconstr Microsurg.* 2012;28(4):235–240.
4. Franson J, Baravarian B. Tarsal tunnel syndrome: a compression neuropathy involving four distinct tunnels. *Clin Podiatr Med Surg.* 2006;23(3):597–609.
5. Fantino O. Role of ultrasound in posteromedial tarsal tunnel syndrome: 81 cases. *J Ultrasound.* 2014;17(2):99–112.

ADDITIONAL READING

- Abouelela AA, Zohiery AK. The triple compression stress test for diagnosis of tarsal tunnel syndrome. *Foot (Edinb).* 2012;22(3):146–149.
- Allen JM, Greer BJ, Sorge DG, et al. MR imaging of neuropathies of the leg, ankle, and foot. *Magn Reson Imaging Clin N Am.* 2008;16(1):117–131.
- Gondring WH, Tarun PK, Trepman E. Touch pressure and sensory density after tarsal tunnel release in diabetic neuropathy. *Foot Ankle Surg.* 2012;18(4):241–246.
- Gould JS. Recurrent tarsal tunnel syndrome. *Foot Ankle Clin.* 2014;19(3):451–467.
- Imai K, Ikoma K, Imai R, et al. Tarsal tunnel syndrome in hemodialysis patients: a case series. *Foot Ankle Int.* 2013;34(3):439–444.
- Lui TH. Endoscopic resection of the tarsal tunnel ganglion. *Arthrosc Tech.* 2016;5(5):e1173–e1177.
- Patel AT, Gaines K, Malamut R, et al; for American Association of Neuromuscular and Electrodiagnostic Medicine. Usefulness of electrodiagnostic techniques in the evaluation of suspected tarsal tunnel syndrome: an evidence-based review. *Muscle Nerve.* 2005;32(2):236–240.
- Reichert P, Zimmer K, Wnukiewicz W, et al. Results of surgical treatment of tarsal tunnel syndrome. *Foot Ankle Surg.* 2015;21(1):26–29.
- Sung KS, Park SJ. Short-term operative outcome of tarsal tunnel syndrome due to benign space-occupying lesions. *Foot Ankle Int.* 2009;30(8):741–745.
- Yang Y, Du ML, Fu YS, et al. Fine dissection of the tarsal tunnel in 60 cases. *Sci Rep.* 2017;7:46351.

 ## SEE ALSO

Algorithm: Foot Pain

 ## CODES

ICD10
- G57.50 Tarsal tunnel syndrome, unspecified lower limb
- G57.51 Tarsal tunnel syndrome, right lower limb
- G57.52 Tarsal tunnel syndrome, left lower limb

CLINICAL PEARLS
- Tarsal tunnel syndrome typically presents with pain and tingling of the medial ankle and plantar foot.
- Tinel sign is the most sensitive and specific physical examination test for diagnosing tarsal tunnel.
- EMG cannot independently diagnose tarsal tunnel syndrome; it is used to confirm a clinical diagnosis.
- Conservative management is recommended, except for patients with an acute onset tarsal tunnel syndrome or known space-occupying lesion.

TELOGEN EFFLUVIUM

Quratulanne H. Jan, MD • Arham K. Barakzai, MD

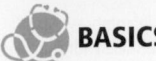 **BASICS**

Diffuse hair loss or hair thinning; most often an acute self-limited process

DESCRIPTION

Telogen effluvium (TE) is a transient condition in which there is a premature conversion of a significant proportion of anagen (growth phase) hairs into telogen (resting phase) hairs, resulting in increased shedding of these resting hair follicles and the clinical appearance of moderate to severe hair thinning.

- Five proposed types of TE
  - Immediate anagen release: a highly common form, lasting 3 to 4 weeks, in which follicles meant to remain in anagen phase enter telogen prematurely due to a signal, including high fever, drug induced, or stress
  - Delayed anagen release: occurs most often post-partum, in which a large group of hair follicles that have remained in the anagen phase for an extended period all together enter the telogen phase, resulting in hair loss
  - Short anagen: a somewhat speculative type, in which at least 50% of the hair follicles have an idiopathic shortening of the anagen phase, resulting in a corresponding doubling of the follicles in the telogen phase
  - Immediate telogen release: Normal resting club hairs remain within the hair follicle until an unknown signal causes their release, initiating the anagen stage to begin. In this type, the resting club hairs are prematurely released, ending the telogen phase abruptly and causing diffuse shedding.
  - Delayed telogen release: In this type, the presence of increased visible light, whether it be a seasonal or environmental change, is thought to end a prolonged telogen phase and initiate the anagen phase, resulting in diffuse shedding of hair follicles.

EPIDEMIOLOGY

Incidence
Second most common cause of alopecia

Prevalence
Unknown

ETIOLOGY AND PATHOPHYSIOLOGY

- The hair cycle consists of two predominant phases. The anagen (growth phase) and the telogen (resting phase), lasting ~3 years and 3 months, respectively. On the scalp, ~10–15% of hairs are in the telogen phase normally. Due to the presence of some types of external/internal stress, there may be an increase in the percentage of telogen hairs. As new anagen hairs emerge, these telogen hair follicles are forced out. The preceding event usually occurs 2 to 3 months prior to the appearance of hair loss.
- It is hypothesized that substance P plays a key role in the pathogenesis of TE through various mechanisms (1). Studies have been conducted on human hair follicles in vitro and mice hair follicles in vivo, which support this theory.
- Role of substance P includes the following (2):
  - Upregulation of substance P receptor, NK1, at the gene and protein level, leading to premature catagen development and hair growth inhibition
  - Upregulation of nerve growth factor (NGF) and subsequently its hair apoptosis–producing receptor, p75NTR
  - Downregulation of hair growth–promoting receptor, TrkA
  - Upregulation of major histocompatibility class (MHC) I and β_2-microglobulin, resulting in loss of hair follicle immune-privilege
  - Increase in tumor necrosis factor-α release by mast cells resulting in hair keratinocyte apoptosis
- Decreased cortisol levels in chronic stress states may also enhance the effects of substance P.

RISK FACTORS

- Infection
- Trauma
- Major surgery
- Thyroid disorder
- Febrile illness
- Malignancy
- Allergic contact dermatitis (3)
- Iron deficiency anemia (4)
- Excess vitamin A
- Protein-calorie restriction
- End-stage liver or renal disease
- Hormonal changes (including pregnancy, delivery, and estrogen-containing medications)
- Chronic stress
- Drug induced (β-blockers, anticonvulsants, antidepressants, anticoagulants, retinoids, ACE-inhibitors, etc.)
- Immunizations

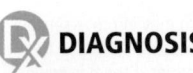 **DIAGNOSIS**

HISTORY

- Commonly, an inciting event 2 to 6 months previous
- Fear of becoming bald
- Patients often present with bags of hair to emphasize the severity of their hair loss.

PHYSICAL EXAM

- Decreased density of hair on the scalp, most commonly involving the crown
- In rare cases of chronic TE, there is hair loss of eyebrows and pubic region.
- May be able to demonstrate diffuse shedding of hair when running fingers through scalp

- Shed hairs are telogen hairs, which have a small bulb of unpigmented or pigmented keratin on the root end.
- May affect nail growth, resulting in the appearance of Beau lines, which are transverse grooves on the nails of the hands and feet

DIFFERENTIAL DIAGNOSIS

- Hypothyroidism
- Hyperthyroidism
- Alopecia areata (diffuse pattern)
- Androgenetic alopecia
- Drug-induced alopecia
- Systemic lupus erythematosus
- Secondary syphilis
- Trichotillomania

DIAGNOSTIC TESTS & INTERPRETATION

Most often, TE is a clinical diagnosis of exclusion. Blood work may be collected primarily to rule out other possible causes of hair loss and/or to identify a possible cause for TE.

Initial Tests (lab, imaging)

If indicated:

- CBC, ferritin
- TSH
- Creatinine
- Consider hepatic enzymes.
- Consider RPR/VDRL.

Diagnostic Procedures/Other

- Hair pull test: unreliable; performed by gently pulling 25 to 30 hairs from various sites on a patient's scalp. Each pull should elicit <5 normal club hairs; increased quantity may indicate possibility of TE.
- Hair clip test: performed by cutting 25 to 30 hairs from the patient's scalp and examining them under a microscope. A negative test (not indicative of TE) will demonstrate <10% of hair shafts of small diameter. A positive test will demonstrate >10% of hair shafts of small diameter.

- Trichogram: ~50 hairs are plucked from the patient's scalp, and the number of telogen and anagen hairs present are counted. In TE, there will be >10% of hairs in the telogen phase.
- Scalp biopsy: rarely needed; it is recommended that several 4-mm punch biopsies be obtained, all horizontally embedded to determine an accurate anagen-to-telogen ratio. Histologically, catagen-to-telogen hairs have numerous apoptotic cells in the outer sheath epithelium. >12–15% of hair follicles in telogen phase is consistent with TE.

TREATMENT

TE is a benign, self-limited process. Identify and correct underlying cause. Patient should be reassured that full hair growth will occur in ~6 months to 1 year. No treatment is required.

MEDICATION

- Minoxidil stimulates hair regrowth via arteriolar smooth muscle vasodilation; not effective in TE
- Oral zinc therapy: new medication that may have benefits for patients with TE through various mechanisms all essential to hair growth, including the following (5)[C]:
  - Cofactor for enzymes needed in nucleic acid and protein synthesis and cell division
  - Inhibition of the catagen phase by blocking certain enzymes involved in hair apoptosis
  - Involved in hair growth regulation via hedgehog signaling

COMPLEMENTARY & ALTERNATIVE MEDICINE

Nigella sativa (black cumin) essential oil has also been studied and may be beneficial (6).

REFERENCES

1. Grover C, Khurana A. Telogen effluvium. *Indian J Dermatol Venereol Leprol*. 2013;79(5):591–603.
2. Peters EMJ, Liotiri S, Bodó E, et al. Probing the effects of stress mediators on the human hair follicle: substance P holds central position. *Am J Pathol*. 2007;171(6):1872–1886.
3. Tosti A, Piraccini BM, van Neste DJ. Telogen effluvium after allergic contact dermatitis of the scalp. *Arch Dermatol*. 2001;137(2):187–190.
4. Trost LB, Bergfeld WF, Calogeras E. The diagnosis and treatment of iron deficiency and its potential relationship to hair loss. *J Am Acad Dermatol*. 2006;54(5):824–844.
5. Karashima T, Tsuruta D, Hamada T, et al. Oral zinc therapy for zinc deficiency-related telogen effluvium. *Dermatol Ther*. 2012;25(2):210–213.
6. Rossi A, Priolo L, Iorio A, et al. Evaluation of a therapeutic alternative for telogen effluvium: a pilot study. *J Cosmet Dermatol Sci Appl*. 2013;3(3A):9–16.

ADDITIONAL READING

- Headington JT. Telogen effluvium. New concepts and review. *Arch Dermatol*. 1993;129(3):356–563.
- Mounsey AL, Reed SW. Diagnosing and treating hair loss. *Am Fam Physician*. 2009;80(4):356–362.

CODES

ICD10
L65.0 Telogen effluvium

T

CLINICAL PEARLS

- TE is a self-limited form of nonscarring alopecia; most often acute
- TE is due to a premature conversion of a significant proportion of anagen (growth phase) hairs into telogen (resting phase) hairs, resulting in increased shedding of these resting hair follicles and the clinical appearance of moderate to severe hair thinning and loss when growth resumes.
- There are many potential causes of TE, both emotional and physiologic. Often it is hard to determine the etiology, but eliminating the stressor often is the key to resolving TE and stimulating new hair growth.
- No treatment is needed. Patient should be reassured that complete hair regrowth will occur in 6 months to 1 year.

TEMPOROMANDIBULAR JOINT DISORDER (TMD)

Rita M. Lahlou, MD, MPH • Benjamin N. Schneider, MD

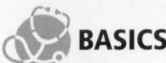 **BASICS**

DESCRIPTION
- Syndrome characterized by
  - Pain and tenderness involving the muscles of mastication and surrounding tissues
  - Sound, pain, stiffness, or grating in the temporomandibular joint (TMJ) with movement
  - Limitation of mandibular movement with possible locking or dislocation
  - Recent research suggests that TMD is a complex disorder with multiple causes consistent with a biopsychosocial model of illness (1)[B].
- System(s) affected: musculoskeletal
- Synonym(s): TMJ syndrome; TMJ dysfunction; myofascial pain–dysfunction syndrome; bruxism; orofacial pain

EPIDEMIOLOGY
Incidence
- Annual first-onset incidence is 3.9%.
- Peak incidence in ages 30 to 50 years

Prevalence
- 6–12% in both adults and older children
- Twice as common in female patients
- Up to 1/2 the population may have at least one sign or symptom of TMD, but most are not limited by symptoms, and <1:4 seek medical or dental treatment.

ETIOLOGY AND PATHOPHYSIOLOGY
- Pathophysiology is multifactorial, involving anatomic, behavioral, emotional, and cognitive factors.
- The American Academy of Orofacial Pain categorizes TMD according to three anatomic origins of pain. The change in name from TMJ to TMD emphasizes that many do not suffer from true articular pain.
- Muscle disorders involving the muscles of mastication
  - Occlusomuscular dysfunction (bruxism)
  - Masticatory muscle spasm
  - Myositis
  - Myofibrosis
  - Poorly fitting oral devices (dentures, splints, etc.)
  - Contracture
  - Neoplasia
- Articular disorders of the joint
  - Congenital disorders
  - Inflammatory disorders: synovitis, arthritides, capsulitis, ankyloses
  - Avascular necrosis (rare)
  - TMJ disk derangement, osteoarthritis
  - Hyper- or hypomobile TMJ
  - TMJ trauma: condylar fractures, dislocation
- Cranial bone disorder including the mandible
  - Congenital and developmental disorders
  - Acquired disorders (fracture, neoplasm)
- Current consensus is that TMD is not only a local condition, so much as a family of complex disorders that can lead to chronic pain, and often overlap with other chronic pain conditions that reflect CNS sensitization.
- OPPERA study (Orofacial Pain: Prospective Evaluation and Risk Assessment) is assessing the heterogeneity in these disorders.

Genetics
Research is ongoing in gene polymorphisms associated with TMD and other pain disorders. These include the catechol O-methyltransferase (COMT) gene, which is thought to be associated with changes in pain responsiveness.

RISK FACTORS
- Macrotrauma to the face, jaw, and neck, including cervical whiplash injuries and hyperextension of jaw
- Rheumatologic and degenerative conditions involving the TMJ
- Psychosocial stress and poor adaptive capabilities
- Repetitive microtrauma from dental malocclusion, including inappropriate dental treatment
- Link with bruxism and jaw/teeth clenching is inconsistent.

GENERAL PREVENTION
- Elimination of tension-causing oral habits
- Reduction in overall muscle tension

COMMONLY ASSOCIATED CONDITIONS
Craniomandibular disorders, somatization disorder, somatoform pain disorder, other chronic pain syndromes, fibromyalgia, juvenile idiopathic arthritis, tension headache, sleep disturbance, tobacco use

 DIAGNOSIS

- TMD is a clinical diagnosis, and localized pain is the unifying feature.
- Several research classification systems exist. Most share several of the history and physical findings listed below.

HISTORY
- Facial and/or TMJ pain
- Locking/catching of jaw; decreased range of motion
- TMJ noises: clicking, grinding, popping
- Headache, earache, neck pain

PHYSICAL EXAM
- Muscle tenderness and restricted pain-free opening are most consistent distinguishing signs.
- Check facial symmetry, muscle hypertrophy, and intraoral exam including tooth wear.
- Palpation of muscles of mastication may reproduce pain.
- There may be tenderness over the TMJ.
- Test jaw range of motion (opening, closing, lateral, protrusive) and masticatory muscle strength.
  - Maximal (pain free) jaw opening with interincisal distance <40 mm is suggestive of joint rather than muscle pathology if accompanied by other signs and symptoms (normal 35 to 55 mm).
  - Deviation to the affected side is common.
- Clicking or crepitus of jaw with opening

DIFFERENTIAL DIAGNOSIS
- Condylar fracture/dislocation
- Trigeminal neuralgia
- Dental or periodontal conditions
- Neoplasm of the jaw, orofacial muscles, or salivary glands
- Acute, nondental infection: parotitis, sialadenitis, otitis, mastoiditis
- Jaw claudication: giant cell arteritis
- Migraine or tension-type headache
- Ramsay Hunt syndrome (zoster auricular syndrome)

DIAGNOSTIC TESTS & INTERPRETATION
- There are no labs to rule in TMD.
- Blood work may be useful to rule out other conditions (CBC, CMP, ESR, CRP).

Initial Tests (lab, imaging)
- TMD is a clinical diagnosis based primarily on history and physical exam.
- Often, a poor correlation is found between pain severity and pathologic changes seen in joint or muscle tissues. Consider the following for traumatic, infectious, severe, or treatment-resistant cases, with MR or CT more useful as part of surgical workup:
  - Panoramic dental radiographs are a good first-line screen.
  - CT scan allows fine detail of bony structures, preferred for trauma.
  - US: Effusion and findings correlate with MRI and subjective pain.
  - MRI: noninvasive study for disc position; more sensitive than US; can help determine need for surgical management

Diagnostic Procedures/Other
- Local anesthetic nerve block can differentiate orofacial pain of articular versus muscular origin.
- Arthroscopy can be diagnostic for cartilage and bony pathology.

Test Interpretation
Positive findings include:
- Condylar head displacement
- Anterior disc displacement
- Posterior capsulitis
- Loosening of disc and capsular attachments
- Chondroid metaplasia of disc leading to disc perforation and degeneration

 TREATMENT

Signs and symptoms will abate without any interventions in most patients. 50% report improvement at 1 year and 85% by 3 years. With conservative therapy, symptoms resolve in 75% of cases within 3 months. Only 5–10% will require surgical intervention.

- Patient education and setting expectations are important because there is no "cure" for TMD, yet most patients will improve with limited interventions.
- Psychosocial interventions, including cognitive-behavioral therapy with or without biofeedback (2)[A]
- Behavior modification to eliminate tension-relieving oral habits including heavy chewing of food and nonfood items as well as potential strain from playing musical instruments that stress or strain the jaw (wind, brass, or string) (2)[A]
- Therapeutic exercises, especially if displacement is present, including formal physical therapy

- Occlusal adjustment cannot be recommended for the management or prevention of TMD because there is an absence of evidence from RCTs that occlusal adjustment treats or prevents TMD (3)[A].
- Insufficient evidence exists either for or against the use of stabilization splint therapy for the treatment of TMD.
- The American Dental Association recommends a "less is often best" stepwise approach and offers the following stepwise progression for therapy:
  - Eating softer foods
  - Avoiding chewing gum and nail biting
  - Modifying pain with heat or ice
  - Relaxation techniques including meditation and biofeedback
  - Exercises to strengthen jaw muscles
  - Medications
  - Night guards and orthotics

MEDICATION

First Line
- Acetaminophen
- Naproxen: 500 mg BID stronger evidence than for other NSAIDs (4)[B]
- Topical methylsalicylate
- Gabapentin: Titrate up to 1,800 mg/day divided.
- Ibuprofen, if osteoarthritis is suspected (4)[B]

Second Line
- Cyclobenzaprine 10 mg nightly more effective than placebo for pain reduction (4)[B]
- Tricyclic antidepressants, SSRIs, or SNRIs; however, SSRIs and some SNRIs may also induce bruxism.
- Acupuncture
- Opiates should be reserved for perioperative or severe or recalcitrant cases (5)[B].
- DMARDs may benefit inflammatory arthropathies such as rheumatoid or psoriatic arthritis.
- Ineffective medications (5)[B]
  - The following medications when compared with placebo in RCTs were shown to be ineffective in improving pain and should not be used for the treatment of TMD:
    - Benzodiazepines
    - Topical capsaicin
    - Diclofenac
    - Celecoxib

ADDITIONAL THERAPIES
Joint and muscle injections

- There is very limited evidence to recommend for or against injections into or around the TMJ. Proposed therapies include steroids, hyaluronic acid, local anesthetics, and recently botulinum toxin.
- Steroids given >3 times annually may accelerate degenerative changes.
- Injections into inferior space or double spaces have better effect than superior space injections alone.
- Recent studies suggest that botulinum toxin type A (Botox) injections may be successful in cases that have failed first-line pharmacologic therapy (4)[B].
- For advanced structural abnormalities, referral for discectomy, arthroplasty, or joint replacement may be warranted. However, strong evidence is lacking for lavage or surgical treatments.

COMPLEMENTARY & ALTERNATIVE MEDICINE
- Glucosamine may be effective if pain is secondary to osteoarthritis of the TMJ (5)[B].
- Multiple electronic diagnostic and treatment modalities are currently marketed to patients; however, the scientific literature does not support the use of electronic diagnostic and treatment devices for TMD at this time.

ONGOING CARE

FOLLOW-UP RECOMMENDATIONS
- Relax jaw by disengaging teeth.
- Avoid wide, uncontrolled opening, such as yawning.
- Stress management and behavior modification counseling may be helpful.
- Be aware of any teeth-clenching or grinding habits.

Patient Monitoring
- Ongoing assessment of clinical response to conservative therapies (NSAIDs, behavior modification, occlusal splints) is necessary.
- Surgical procedure (arthroplasty, joint replacement) to correct disc displacement or replace a damaged disc may be indicated only if the patient has not responded to conservative treatment.

DIET
Soft diet to reduce chewing

PROGNOSIS
- With conservative therapy, symptoms resolve in 75% of cases within 3 months.
- Patients benefit most from a comprehensive treatment approach including the following (4):
  - Restoration of normal muscle function
  - Pain control
  - Stress management
  - Behavior modification

COMPLICATIONS
- Secondary degenerative joint disease
- Chronic TMJ dislocation
- Loss of joint range of motion
- Depression and chronic pain syndromes
- Secondary headache disorder

REFERENCES

1. Slade GD, Fillingim RB, Sanders AE, et al. Summary of findings from the OPPERA prospective cohort study of incidence of first-onset temporomandibular disorder: implications and future directions. *J Pain*. 2013;14(Suppl 12):T116–T124.
2. Aggarwal VR, Lovell K, Peters S, et al. Psychosocial interventions for the management of chronic orofacial pain. *Cochrane Database Syst Rev*. 2011;(11):CD008456.
3. Koh H, Robinson PG. Occlusal adjustment for treating and preventing temporomandibular joint disorders. *Cochrane Database Syst Rev*. 2003;(1):CD003812.
4. Gauer RL, Semidey MJ. Diagnosis and treatment of temporomandibular disorders. *Am Fam Physician*. 2015;91(6):378–386.
5. Mujakperuo HR, Watson M, Morrison R, et al. Pharmacological interventions for pain in patients with temporomandibular disorders. *Cochrane Database Syst Rev*. 2010;(10):CD004715.

ADDITIONAL READING

- American Dental Association. TMJ. http://www.mouthhealthy.org/en/az-topics/t/tmj. Accessed October 25, 2017.
- De Rossi SS, Greenberg MS, Liu F, et al. Temporomandibular disorders: evaluation and management. *Med Clin North Am*. 2014;98(6):1353–1384.
- Harper DE, Schrepf A, Clauw DJ. Pain mechanisms and centralized pain in temporomandibular disorders. *J Dent Res*. 2016;95(10):1102–1108.
- National Institute of Dental and Craniofacial Research. TMJ (temporomandibular joint and muscle disorders). https://www.nidcr.nih.gov/health-info/tmj. Accessed October 18, 2018.
- Rajapakse S, Ahmed N, Sidebottom AJ. Current thinking about the management of dysfunction of the temporomandibular joint: a review. *Br J Oral Maxillofac Surg*. 2017;55(4):351–356.
- Scrivani SJ, Keith DA, Kaban LB. Temporomandibular disorders. *N Engl J Med*. 2008;359(25):2693–2705.

 SEE ALSO

Headache, Tension

CODES

ICD10
- M26.60 Temporomandibular joint disorder, unspecified
- M26.62 Arthralgia of temporomandibular joint
- M26.63 Articular disc disorder of temporomandibular joint

CLINICAL PEARLS

- The condition called TMD actually designates a number of potential underlying joint and muscle conditions involving the jaw.
- Characteristics of all conditions are pain and functional limitation.
- TMD is a clinical diagnosis; imaging and labs are often of limited utility.
- Cognitive-behavioral therapy reduces pain, depression, and limitation of function.
- Exercises may improve function and pain.
- Evidence is lacking to support occlusion correction or splinting.
- Naproxen, gabapentin, topical methylsalicylate, glucosamine, amitriptyline, acupuncture, and botulinum toxin injections have some evidence of efficacy.

TESTICULAR MALIGNANCIES

Huy T. Tran, MD

BASICS

DESCRIPTION
- Testicular cancer accounts for <1% of all cancers in men; it is the most common solid malignancy in men aged 20 to 34 years (1).
- An estimated 9,310 new cases were diagnosed, and an estimated 400 deaths occurred in the United States in 2018 (2).
- Rates for new cases have been rising 0.8% each year over the last 10 years, but death rates have been stable.
- The median age at diagnosis is 33 years. The median age at death is 42 years (2).
- Treatment produces an overall 5-year survival of 95.3%; for African American patients, this 5-year survival rate is alarmingly lower but has improved from 86% to 90% (2).

ETIOLOGY AND PATHOPHYSIOLOGY
95% of all malignant tumors arising in the testes are germ cell tumors (GCTs), which are subclassified as follows:
- Seminomatous GCTs: most common type overall
- Nonseminomatous GCTs (NSGCTs): These include embryonal cell carcinoma, choriocarcinoma, yolk sac tumor, teratomas, or often multiple cell types; these are more clinically aggressive tumors.

RISK FACTORS
- Cryptorchidism is the most firmly established risk factor: Relative risk of testicular cancer in all patients with cryptorchidism is 3 to 8, with a lower relative risk of 2 to 3 in those undergoing orchiopexy by age 12 years; in patients with unilateral cryptorchidism, the relative risk of testicular cancer in the contralateral normally descended testis is negligible (3).
- Personal history of testicular cancer
- Use of muscle building supplements
- Positive family history for testicular cancer
- Testicular dysgenesis
- Klinefelter syndrome
- Caucasian race
- HIV infections

GENERAL PREVENTION
No evidence that screening for testicular cancer is effective (4)

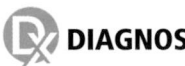

DIAGNOSIS

HISTORY
- A painless solid testicular mass is pathognomonic for testicular cancer.
- Clinical symptoms of epididymitis or orchitis that do not respond to treatment warrant further evaluation.
- Gynecomastia can be a rare systemic endocrine manifestation of testicular neoplasm.

PHYSICAL EXAM
- Testicular exam: Palpate for size, consistency, and nodules; masses do not transilluminate; a firm, hard, or fixed area should be considered suspicious.
- Lymph node and abdominal exam
- Gynecomastia

DIFFERENTIAL DIAGNOSIS
Epidermoid cyst, epididymitis, hernia, hydrocele, hematoma, lymphoma, orchitis, spermatocele, testicular torsion, varicocele

DIAGNOSTIC TESTS & INTERPRETATION
Initial Tests (lab, imaging)
- α-Fetoprotein (AFP), β-human chorionic gonadotropin (β-hCG), lactate dehydrogenase (LDH), creatinine, chemistry profile, complete blood count, liver enzymes, chest x-ray (CXR), and testicular ultrasound (US)
- Tumor markers AFP, β-hCG, and LDH are used to assist with diagnosis, prognosis, assessing treatment outcome, and monitoring for relapse:
  - AFP
    - Produced by nonseminomatous testicular cancer and is therefore associated with this histologic type
    - Those with a histologically "pure" testicular seminoma and an elevated AFP are assumed to possess an undetected focus of nonseminoma tumor.
  - β-hCG
    - May be associated with both seminomatous or nonseminomatous tumors
    - Hypogonadism and marijuana use may cause benign elevations of β-hCG.
- LDH is less specific than AFP.
- Testicular US is the initial study.
- If an intratesticular mass is identified, measure serum AFP, LDH, and β-hCG and order a CXR.
- CT scan of the abdomen/pelvis, positron emission tomography (PET) scan, MRI of the brain, and bone scan are used for staging and metastases evaluation as clinically indicated.

Diagnostic Procedures/Other
- Radical inguinal orchiectomy is the primary procedure for diagnosis and treatment.
- Testicular biopsy may be rarely considered if a suspicious intratesticular abnormality is identified on US; however, testicular microcalcification on US without any other abnormality can simply be observed and does not demand a biopsy.
- For those with unilateral testicular cancer, contralateral testicular biopsy is not routinely performed but should be considered when there is a cryptorchid testis, marked testicular atrophy, or a suspicious US for intratesticular abnormalities.

Test Interpretation
Clinical staging (5):
- Stage 0: carcinoma in situ
- Stage IA: tumor limited to testis and epididymis without vascular/lymphatic invasion; tumor may invade into the tunica albuginea but not the tunica vaginalis; normal serum tumor markers
- Stage IB: tumor limited to testis and epididymis with vascular/lymphatic invasion or tumor extending through tunica albuginea with involvement of tunica vaginalis; tumor invades the spermatic cord with or without vascular/lymphatic invasion; tumor invades the scrotum with or without vascular/lymphatic invasion; no lymph node involvement or distant metastasis; normal serum tumor markers
- Stage IS: any tumor with elevated serum tumor markers but no nodal involvement or metastasis
- Stage IIA: any tumor with lymph node mass/masses <2 cm
- Stage IIB: any tumor with lymph node mass/masses 2 to 5 cm

- Stage IIC: any tumor with lymph node mass >5 cm
- Stage IIIA: any tumor/lymph node presence; with nonregional nodal or pulmonary metastasis; either serum tumor markers normal or with mild elevation
- Stage IIIB: any tumor/lymph node presence; no distant metastasis or nonregional nodal involvement or pulmonary metastasis; with moderately elevated serum tumor markers
- Stage IIIC: any tumor/lymph node presence; with or without any metastasis; with greatly elevated serum tumor markers

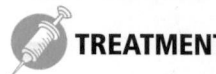

TREATMENT

GENERAL MEASURES
- Seminoma: Specifics are noted in the National Comprehensive Cancer Network guidelines (1):
  - Stages IA, IB: Options may include surveillance (preferred) (for low tumor load malignancy, i.e., pT1–pT3), single-agent carboplatin, or radiotherapy (2)[A].
  - Stage IS: Repeat elevated serum tumor marker and abdominal/pelvic CT scan (2)[A].
  - Stage IIA: radiotherapy to include para-aortic and ipsilateral iliac lymph nodes (preferred) or primary chemotherapy (2)[A]
  - Stage IIB: primary chemotherapy (preferred) or radiotherapy in select nonbulky cases to include para-aortic and ipsilateral iliac lymph nodes (2)[A]
  - Stages IIC, III
    - Good risk (any primary site and no nonpulmonary visceral metastases and normal AFP with any β-hCG or LDH): primary etoposide and cisplatin (EP) or bleomycin, etoposide, and cisplatin (BEP) chemotherapy (1)
    - Intermediate risk (any primary site and nonpulmonary visceral metastases and normal AFP with any β-hCG or LDH): primary BEP chemotherapy (1)
- Nonseminoma: Tumors with both seminomatous and nonseminomatous histology are managed as nonseminomatous. See "National Comprehensive Cancer Network guidelines" (1):
  - Stage IA: nonseminomatous surveillance protocol (preferred) or nerve-sparing retroperitoneal lymph node dissection (RPLND) (2)[A]
  - Stage IB: nerve-sparing RPLND or primary BEP chemotherapy (2)[A]; for T2 only can enter nonseminomatous surveillance protocol (2)[B]
  - Stage IS: primary chemotherapy followed by response evaluation:
    - Complete response, negative tumor markers: nonseminomatous surveillance protocol (2)[A]
    - Partial response, negative tumor markers: surgical resection of all residual masses (2)[A]
    - Incomplete response: Consider second-line therapy (2)[A].
  - Stage IIA
    - Negative tumor markers: nerve-sparing RPLND (2)[A] or primary chemotherapy (2)[B]
    - Persistent marker elevation: primary chemotherapy followed by response evaluation
    - Complete response, negative tumor markers: nonseminomatous surveillance protocol (2)[A] or bilateral RPLND +/− nerve-sparing in select cases (2)[B]
    - Partial response, negative tumor markers: surgical resection of all residual masses (2)[A]
    - Incomplete response: Consider second-line therapy (2)[A].

– Stage IIB
  ○ Negative tumor markers: primary chemotherapy or nerve-sparing RPLND in highly selected cases (2)[A]
  ○ Persistent marker elevation: primary chemotherapy followed by response evaluation
    ■ Complete response, negative tumor markers: nonseminomatous surveillance protocol (2)[A] or bilateral RPLND +/− nerve-sparing in selected cases (2)[B]
    ■ Partial response, negative tumor markers: surgical resection of all residual masses (2)[A]
    ■ Incomplete response: Consider second-line therapy (2)[A].
– Stage IIC: primary chemotherapy followed by response evaluation as per stages IIA and IIB (2)[A]
– Stages IIIA, IIIB, and IIIC: primary chemotherapy depending on risk profile, which is based on tumor, metastases, and postorchiectomy serum tumor markers (2)[A]
• Brain metastases: primary chemotherapy +/− radiotherapy, +/− surgery, as clinically indicated

MEDICATION

First Line
Primary chemotherapy regimens for GCTs:
• EP: etoposide 100 mg/m^2/day IV on days 1 to 5, cisplatin 20 mg/m^2/day IV on days 1 to 5; repeat every 21 days (1)[A].
• BEP: etoposide 100 mg/m^2/day IV on days 1 to 5, cisplatin 20 mg/m^2/day IV on days 1 to 5; bleomycin 30 U/dose IV weekly on days 1, 8, and 15 or days 2, 9, and 16; repeat every 21 days (1)[A].
• VIP: etoposide 75 mg/m^2/day IV on days 1 to 5; mesna 120 mg/m^2 slow IV push before ifosfamide on day 1 and then mesna 1,200 mg/m^2 IV continuous infusion on days 1 to 5; ifosfamide 1,200 mg/m^2/day on days 1 to 5; cisplatin 20 mg/m^2/day IV on days 1 to 5, repeat every 21 days (1)[A].

Second Line
• These agents are considered in patients who do not respond to first-line therapy or those who experience a recurrence: carboplatin, cisplatin, etoposide, ifosfamide, mesna, paclitaxel, and vinblastine (1)[A].
• Gemcitabine, oxaliplatin, and paclitaxel are used in palliative chemotherapy regimens (1)[A].

ADDITIONAL THERAPIES
Consider sperm banking before treatment that may compromise fertility; rarely covered by insurance

SURGERY/OTHER PROCEDURES
• Radical inguinal orchiectomy: primary treatment for testicular cancer for all patients; prosthesis can be inserted at this time.
• RPLND identifies nodal metastases and provides accurate pathologic staging of the retroperitoneum.

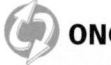 ## ONGOING CARE

FOLLOW-UP RECOMMENDATIONS
• Pure seminoma: Specifics are noted in the National Comprehensive Cancer Network guidelines (1,2)[A]:
  – Stages IA, IB: in general, H&P, optional tumor markers every 3 to 6 months for 1 year, every 6 to 12 months for years 2 to 3, and then annually for years 4 to 5; abdominal/pelvic CT at 3, 6, and 12 months and then every 6 to 12 months for years 2 to 3, every 12 to 24 months for years 4 to 5; CXR, as clinically indicated; less frequent if adjuvant therapy is given

– Stage IS: Repeat elevated serum tumor marker and assess with abdominal/pelvic CT scan for evaluable disease.
– Stages IIA, IIB (select): in general, H&P, optional tumor markers every 3 months for year 1, every 6 months for years 2 to 5; abdominal/pelvic CT at 3 and 6 to 12 months, then annually for years 2 to 3, and then as clinically indicated; CXR every 6 months for years 1 to 2
– Stages IIB (select), IIC, and III: Check all serum tumor markers along with chest, abdominal, and pelvic CT:
  ○ Residual mass 0 to 3 cm and normal serum tumor markers: H&P, AFP, β-hCG, LDH, CXR every 2 months for year 1, every 3 months for year 2, every 6 months for years 3 to 4, and then annually; abdominal/pelvic CT scan at 3 to 6 months and then as clinically indicated, PET scans as clinically indicated
  ○ Residual mass >3 cm and normal serum tumor markers: PET scan 6 weeks after chemotherapy:
    ■ Negative PET scan: abdominal/pelvic CT scans every 6 months for year 1 and then annually for 5 years
    ■ Positive PET scan: Consider RPLND or second-line chemotherapy or radiotherapy.
– Any recurrence: Treat according to extent of disease at relapse.
• Nonseminoma: Specifics are noted in the National Comprehensive Cancer Network guidelines (1):
  – Stages IA and IB on surveillance only: H&P, AFP, β-hCG, LDH every 2 months for year 1, every 3 months for year 2, every 4 to 6 months for year 3, every 6 months for year 4, annually thereafter; CXR and abdominal/pelvic CT depending on stage IA or stage IB
  – Follow-up after complete response to chemotherapy and RPLND in general: H&P, AFP, β-hCG, LDH every 2 to 3 months for years 1 to 2, every 6 months for years 3 to 5, annually thereafter; abdominal/pelvic CT every 6 months for year 1, annually for year 2, as clinically indicated thereafter
  – Follow-up after RPLND only: H&P, AFP, β-hCG, LDH, CXR every 2 months for year 1, every 3 months for year 2, every 4 months for year 3, every 6 months for year 4, annually thereafter; abdominal/pelvic CT at 3 to 4 months and, as clinically indicated, thereafter; CXR every 2 to 4 months for year 1, 3 to 6 months for year 2, annually thereafter

PROGNOSIS
>90% of patients diagnosed are cured, including 70–80% with advanced tumors (1).

COMPLICATIONS
• Surgical: hematoma, hemorrhage, infection, and infertility
• Radiotherapy: radiation enteritis and infertility
• Late complications (6):
  – Cardiovascular toxicity and second malignancies each have a 25-year risk of about 16% in those treated with chemotherapy and/or radiotherapy.
  – Risk for secondary malignancies remains increased for at least 35 years after treatment.
  – Increased incidence of metabolic syndrome occurs and is likely associated with lower testosterone levels.
  – Other late complications associated with chemotherapy, depending on the regimen, include chronic neurotoxicity, ototoxicity, renal function impairment, and pulmonary fibrosis.

• The incidence of late relapse in treated testicular cancer is now estimated to be 2–6%; the time to late relapse ranges from 2 to 32 years, with a median of 6 years (6).

REFERENCES

1. Gilligan T, Lin DW, Aggarwal R, et al. Testicular cancer, Version 1.2019. https://www.nccn.org/about/news/ebulletin/ebulletindetail.aspx?ebulletinid=1537. Accessed October 28, 2018.
2. Noone AM, Howlader N, Krapcho M, et al, eds. In: SEER Cancer Statistics Review (CSR) 1975–2015. Bethesda, MD: National Cancer Institute. https://seer.cancer.gov/csr/1975_2015/. Accessed October 28, 2018.
3. Lip SZ, Murchison LE, Cullis PS, et al. A meta-analysis of the risk of boys with isolated cryptorchidism developing testicular cancer in later life. Arch Dis Child. 2013;98(1):20–26.
4. Ilic D, Misso ML. Screening for testicular cancer. Cochrane Database Syst Rev. 2011;(2):CD007853.
5. Edge SB, Byrd DR, Compton CC, et al, eds. Testis. In: AJCC Cancer Staging Manual. 7th ed. New York, NY: Springer; 2010:469–478.
6. Efstathiou E, Logothetis CJ. Review of late complications of treatment and late relapse in testicular cancer. J Natl Compr Canc Netw. 2006;4(10):1059–1070.

ADDITIONAL READING
• Hanna NH, Einhorn LH. Testicular cancer—discoveries and updates. N Engl J Med. 2014;371(21):2005–2016.
• Marcell AV, Bell DL, Joffe A, et al; for SAHM Male Health Special Interest Group, Society for Adolescent Health and Medicine. The male genital examination: a position paper of the Society for Adolescent Health and Medicine. J Adolesc Health. 2012;50(4):424–425.
• U.S. Preventive Services Task Force. Screening for testicular cancer: U.S. Preventive Services Task Force reaffirmation recommendation statement. Ann Intern Med. 2011;154(7):483–486.
• Wood HM, Elder JS. Cryptorchidism and testicular cancer: separating fact from fiction. J Urol. 2009;181(2):452–461.

 ## CODES

ICD10
• C62.90 Malig neoplasm of unsp testis, unsp descended or undescended
• C62.00 Malignant neoplasm of unspecified undescended testis
• C62.10 Malignant neoplasm of unspecified descended testis

CLINICAL PEARLS
• Testicular cancer is the most common solid organ tumor in men aged 20 to 34 years.
• Testicular US is initial imaging of choice for testicular pathology.
• Radical inguinal orchiectomy is used for both diagnosis and treatment, with possible radiotherapy or chemotherapy as adjuvant treatment.
• 96% overall survival at 10 years after diagnosis and treatment

T

TESTICULAR TORSION

Jonathan Green, MD, MSCI • Michael P. Hirsh, MD, FACS, FAAP

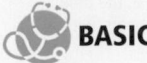 **BASICS**

DESCRIPTION
- Twisting of testis and spermatic cord, resulting in acute ischemia and loss of testis if unrecognized:
  - Intravaginal torsion: occurs within tunica vaginalis, only involves testis and spermatic cord
  - Extravaginal torsion: involves twisting of testis, cord, and processus vaginalis as a unit; typically seen in neonates
- System(s) affected: reproductive

Geriatric Considerations
Rare in this age group

Pediatric Considerations
Peak incidence at age 14 years (1)[B]

EPIDEMIOLOGY
Incidence
- ~1/4,000 males before age 25 years
- Predominant age:
  - Occurs from newborn period to 7th decade
  - 65% of cases occur in 2nd decade, with peak at age 14 years (1).
  - Second peak in neonates (in utero torsion usually occurs around week 32 of gestation) (1)

ETIOLOGY AND PATHOPHYSIOLOGY
- Twisting of spermatic cord causes venous obstruction, edema of testis, and arterial occlusion.
- "Bell clapper" deformity is most common anatomic anomaly predisposing to intravaginal torsion:
  - High insertion of the tunica vaginalis on the spermatic cord, resulting in increased testicular mobility within tunica vaginalis
  - Bilateral in ~80% of patients (1)[B]
- No clear anatomic defect is associated with extravaginal testicular torsion:
  - In neonates, the tunica vaginalis is not yet well attached to scrotal wall, allowing torsion of entire testis including tunica vaginalis (1)[B].
- Usually spontaneous and idiopathic (1)[B]

- 20% of patients have a history of trauma.
- 1/3 have had prior episodic testicular pain.
- Contraction of cremaster muscle or dartos may play a role and is stimulated by trauma, exercise, cold, and sexual stimulation.
- Increased incidence may be due to increasing weight and size of testis during pubertal development.
- Possible alterations in testosterone levels during nocturnal sex response cycle; possible elevated testosterone levels in neonates (1)[B]
- Testis must have inadequate, incomplete, or absent fixation within scrotum (1)[B].
- Torsion may occur in either clockwise or counterclockwise direction.

Genetics
- Unknown
- Familial testicular torsion, although previously rarely reported, may involve as many as 10% of patients.

RISK FACTORS
- May be more common in winter
- Paraplegia
- Previous contralateral testicular torsion

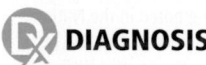 **DIAGNOSIS**

HISTORY
- Acute onset of pain, often during period of inactivity
- Onset of pain usually sudden but may start gradually with subsequent increase in severity
- Nausea and vomiting are common:
  - Presence may increase the likelihood of testicular torsion versus other differential diagnoses.
- Prior history of multiple episodes of testicular pain with spontaneous resolution in an episodic crescendo pattern may indicate intermittent testicular torsion.

PHYSICAL EXAM
- Scrotum is enlarged, red, edematous, and painful.
- Testicle is swollen and exquisitely tender.
- Testis may be high in scrotum with a transverse lie.
- Absent cremasteric reflex

DIFFERENTIAL DIAGNOSIS
- Torsion appendix testis (this may account for 35–67% of acute scrotal pain cases in children)
- Epididymitis (8–18% of acute scrotal pain cases)
- Orchitis
- Incarcerated or strangulated inguinal hernia
- Acute hydrocele
- Traumatic hematoma
- Idiopathic scrotal edema
- Acute varicocele
- Epididymal hypertension (venous congestion of testicle or prostate due to sexual arousal that does not end in orgasm)
- Testis tumor
- Henoch-Schönlein purpura
- Scrotal abscess
- Leukemic infiltrate

DIAGNOSTIC TESTS & INTERPRETATION
- Doppler US may confirm testicular swelling but is diagnostic by demonstrating lack of blood flow to the testicle; PPV of 89.4% (2,3)[B]
- In boys with intermittent, recurrent testicular torsion, both Doppler US and radionuclide scintigraphy findings will be normal (3)[B].

Diagnostic Procedures/Other
- Doppler US flow detection demonstrates absent or reduced blood flow with torsion and increased flow with inflammatory process (reliable only in first 12 hours) (3)[B].
- Radionuclide testicular scintigraphy with technetium-99m pertechnetate demonstrates absent/decreased vascularity in torsion and increased vascularity with inflammatory processes (including torsion of appendix testes) (4)[C].

Test Interpretation

- Venous thrombosis
- Tissue edema and necrosis
- Arterial thrombosis
- Decreased Doppler flow also seen in hydrocele, abscess, hematoma, or scrotal hernia (3)[B]
- Sensitivity of radionuclide testicular scintigraphy is decreased relative to ultrasonography because hyperemia in the torsed testicle can mimic flow (4)[C].

TREATMENT

- Manual reduction: best performed by experienced physician; may be successful, facilitated by lidocaine 1% (plain) injection at level of external ring:
  - Difficult to determine success of manual reduction, especially after giving local anesthesia
  - Manual reduction might require sedation, and the entire process may delay definitive treatment.
  - Even if successful, must always be followed by surgical exploration, urgently but not emergently (5)[C]
- Surgical exploration via scrotal approach with detorsion, evaluation of testicular viability, orchidopexy of viable testicle, orchiectomy of nonviable testicle (2)[B]
- In boys with a history of intermittent episodes of testicular pain, scrotal exploration is warranted with testicular fixation if abnormal testicular attachments are confirmed (2)[B].

GENERAL MEASURES

Early exam is crucial because necrosis of the testicle can occur after 6 to 8 hours (6)[C].

SURGERY/OTHER PROCEDURES

Operative testicular fixation of the torsed testicle after detorsion and confirmation of viability:

- At least 3- or 4-point fixation with nonabsorbable sutures between the tunica albuginea and the tunica vaginalis (2)[B]
- Excision of window of tunica albuginea with suture to dartos fascia (2)[B]
- Any testis that is not clearly viable should be removed (1)[B].

- Testes of questionable viability that are preserved and pexed invariably atrophy (2)[B].
- Bilateral testicular fixation is recommended by many surgeons (2)[B].
- Contralateral testicle frequently has similar abnormal fixation and should be explored (2)[B],(5)[C].

 ONGOING CARE

FOLLOW-UP RECOMMENDATIONS
Patient Monitoring
- Postoperative visit at 1 to 2 weeks
- Yearly visits until puberty may be needed to evaluate for atrophy.

DIET
Regular

PATIENT EDUCATION
Possibility of testicular atrophy in salvaged testis with depressed sperm counts. Importantly, fertility rates in patients with one testicle remain excellent.

PROGNOSIS
- Testicular salvage:
  - Salvage is related directly to duration of torsion (85–97% if within 6 hours, 20% after 12 hours <10% if >24 hours) (6)[C].
  - The degree of torsion is related to testicular salvage:
    - The median degree of torsion is <360 in patients who are explored and orchidopexy performed.
- 80–94% may have depressed spermatogenesis related to duration of ischemic injury (possibly related to autoimmune-mediated injury) (6)[C].
- Up to 45% of patients undergoing orchidopexy for testicular torsion will develop atrophy of testicle.

COMPLICATIONS
- Possible testicular atrophy
- Abnormal spermatogenesis
- Infertility:
  - Fertility rates with one testicle remain excellent.
  - Nearly 36% of patients who experience torsion have sperm counts <20 million/mL (4)[C].

REFERENCES

1. Boettcher M, Bergholz R, Krebs TF, et al. Clinical predictors of testicular torsion in children. *Urology.* 2012;79(3):670–674.
2. Van Glabeke E, Khairouni A, Larroquet M, et al. Acute scrotal pain in children: results of 543 surgical explorations. *Pediatr Surg Int.* 1999;15(5–6):353–357.
3. Yagil Y, Naroditsky I, Milhem J, et al. Role of Doppler ultrasonography in the triage of acute scrotum in the emergency department. *J Ultrasound Med.* 2010;29(1):11–21.
4. Saleh O, El-Sharkawi MS, Imran MB. Scrotal scintigraphy in testicular torsion: an experience at a tertiary care centre. *Int Med J Malaysia.* 2012;11(1):9–14.
5. Eaton SH, Cendron MA, Estrada CR, et al. Intermittent testicular torsion: diagnostic features and management outcomes. *J Urol.* 2005;174(4, Pt 2):1532–1535.
6. Kapoor S. Testicular torsion: a race against time. *Int J Clin Pract.* 2008;62(5):821–827.

 CODES

ICD10
- N44.00 Torsion of testis, unspecified
- N44.01 Extravaginal torsion of spermatic cord
- N44.03 Torsion of appendix testis

CLINICAL PEARLS

- The diagnosis of testicular torsion is usually made by physical exam. Patients with suspected torsion should be taken to the OR without delay. If diagnosis is in question, a testicular Doppler US may be done to evaluate blood flow.
- Although testicular necrosis may be present within 6 to 8 hours of torsion, this is highly variable.
- Infertility can be a problem even if the testicle is viable. Autoimmune antibodies may be produced, and they may affect subsequent fertility.

T

TESTOSTERONE DEFICIENCY

Michael Lao, MD • Stanton C. Honig, MD

 BASICS

DESCRIPTION

- Testosterone (T) is a critical anabolic hormone.
- It is the principle circulating androgen in males.
- Critical in cardiovascular, reproductive, and metabolic systems
- Testosterone deficiency (TD) is characterized by low levels of T in addition with signs and symptoms.
- No universally accepted threshold of T concentration to distinguish eugonadal from hypogonadal men, but the FDA definition is T <300 ng/dL.
- T levels can be affected by disruptions to the hypothalamic–pituitary–testis axis, age, and medical comorbidities.
- T levels correlate with overall health and may be associated with sexual dysfunction.
- Special consideration is needed for men with low T who desires future fertility.
- Synonym(s): hypogonadism; hypoandrogenism; androgen deficiency; and low T

EPIDEMIOLOGY

Incidence

- Overall incidence increases with age.
- 481,000 new cases in United States ages 40 to 69 years

Prevalence

- Estimates of TD vary, typically 20% of men >60 years, 30% >70 years, and 50% >80 years of age.
- Symptomatic TD in United States ages 40 to 69 years is 6–12.3%.
- 2.4 million men in United States ages 40 to 69 years

ETIOLOGY AND PATHOPHYSIOLOGY

- Normal hypothalamic–pituitary–testis axis:
  - Hypothalamus produces GnRH, which stimulates pituitary to produce follicle-stimulating hormone (FSH) and luteinizing hormone (LH).
  - LH stimulates Leydig cells to produce T.
  - T inhibits LH/GnRH through negative feedback.
- Primary hypogonadism: Testes produces insufficient amount of T; FSH/LH levels are elevated.
- Secondary hypogonadism: low T from inadequate production of LH
- Congenital syndromes: cryptorchidism, Klinefelter, hypogonadotropic hypogonadism (Kallmann)
- Acquired: cancer, trauma, orchiectomy, steroids
- Infectious: mumps orchitis, HIV, tuberculosis
- Systemic: Cushing, hemochromatosis, autoimmune, severe illness (e.g., renal and liver disease), metabolic syndrome, obesity, obstructive sleep apnea
- Medications and drugs: LHRH agonists, corticosteroids, ethanol, marijuana, opioids, SSRIs
- Elevated prolactin: prolactinoma, dopamine antagonists (neuroleptics and metoclopramide)

Genetics

- Usually normal
- Klinefelter: XXY karyotype
- Kallmann syndrome: abnormal GnRH secretion due to abnormal hypothalamic development

RISK FACTORS

- Obesity, diabetes, COPD, depression, thyroid disorders, malnutrition, alcohol, stress
- Chronic infections, inflammatory states, narcotic use
- Medications that affect T production or metabolism
- Undescended testicles, varicocele
- Trauma, cancer, testicular radiation, chemotherapy, disorders of the pituitary and/or hypothalamus

GENERAL PREVENTION

General health maintenance and treatment of obesity

COMMONLY ASSOCIATED CONDITIONS

- Infertility, erectile dysfunction, low libido
- Poorer health outcomes
- Osteopenia/osteoporosis
- Diabetes, insulin resistance, metabolic syndrome
- Increased body weight, adiposity
- Depressed mood, poor concentration, irritability
- Chronic narcotic and corticosteroids use

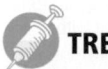 **DIAGNOSIS**

HISTORY

- Congenital and developmental abnormalities
- Infertility, loss of libido, erectile dysfunction
- Depression, fatigue, difficulty with concentration
- Decreased muscle strength, energy level
- Increase in body fat, development of diabetes
- Bone fractures from relatively minor trauma
- Testicular trauma, infection, radio- or chemotherapy
- Decrease in testicle size or consistency
- Headaches or vision changes
- Medications, narcotic use

PHYSICAL EXAM

- Infancy: ambiguous genitalia
- Puberty
  - Impaired growth of penis, testicles
  - Lack of secondary male characteristics
  - Gynecomastia, eunuchoid habitus
- Adulthood
  - Decreased muscular development, visceral fat distribution
  - Presence of gynecomastia
  - Small and/or soft testicles

DIFFERENTIAL DIAGNOSIS

- Delayed puberty
- Obesity, depression, chronic illness, hypothyroidism
- Normal aging
- Prior anabolic steroid abuse

DIAGNOSTIC TESTS & INTERPRETATION

- T levels vary widely and are subject to diurnal, seasonal, and age-related variations. There are multiple assays, each with unique characteristics.
- Measurement should be obtained between 6 and 10 AM. Confirmation with a second measurement may be necessary. Free T with total T is generally preferred. Measurements should not be obtained during acute illness. T circulates in blood primary bound to SHBG or albumin. Only 2–3% of total T is found free. Free and albumin-bound T is considered bioavailable. Laboratory findings must be interpreted in the appropriate clinical setting.
- Lower limit of normal in most labs for total T is 280 to 300 ng/dL. Lower limit of normal for free T is 5 to 9 pg/mL.

Initial Tests (lab, Imaging)

- Morning T level is initial test. Morning timing is more important for younger men in whom there is more diurnal variation. If initial AM T is low, and confirmed on repeat test, further evaluation is appropriate (1).
- Evaluation should include LH and FSH to differentiate between primary versus secondary hypogonadism.
- Consider estradiol and prolactin, especially if LH is low, or breast symptoms and gynecomastia.

- If primary hypogonadism of unknown origin and physical exam reveals abnormalities, consider obtaining karyotype (Klinefelter 1:500 to 1,000 risk).
- If secondary hypogonadism, consider prolactin, iron saturation, pituitary function testing, and/or MRI.
- Imaging is not helpful in the initial diagnosis of TD.
- No evidence to support screening for TD in the general population

Follow-Up Tests & Special Considerations

- Routine blood work to measure T response to interventions (e.g., hematocrit and PSA)
- Dual energy x-ray absorptiometry (DEXA) to measure bone mineral density in men with severe TD or fracture from minimal trauma
- Pituitary MRI: if there is elevation of prolactin more than twice the upper limit of normal or LH/FSH below normal range

TREATMENT

Testosterone therapy (TT) has been shown to effectively ameliorate many symptoms of TD. TT is recommended for symptomatic men (e.g., low libido and/or erectile dysfunction, low energy level, constitutional symptoms) with low T levels ≤300 ng/dL obtained in the morning; not recommended for older men with low T levels in absence of signs or symptoms

GENERAL MEASURES

- Confirm suspicion.
- Prior to TT, obtain hemoglobin/hematocrit, PSA in men >40 years, prolactin, LH/FSH, estradiol.
- Baseline physical exam including digital rectal exam, and International Prostate Symptom Score (IPSS)
- Correction of underlying cause
- Considerations
  - Future fertility? Different treatments are used in men of reproductive age. Impact of exogenous T should be discussed because it relates to fertility.
  - Clinicians should inform patients of the absence of evidence linking TT to the development of prostate cancer (2)[B].
  - Safety of TT in existing prostate cancer is still uncertain and contraindicated in package insert (3)[B].
  - 2018 AUA guidelines: Patients with TD and history of prostate cancer should be informed that there is inadequate evidence to quantify the risk–benefit ratio of TT (2)[B].
  - 2010 Endocrine guidelines: Patients with organ-confined prostate cancer who have undergone radical prostatectomy and disease free for ≥2 years with undetectable PSA may be considered for TT on an individualized basis.
  - TT should not be used in men with hematocrit >54%, untreated obstructive sleep apnea, uncontrolled CHF, severe lower urinary tract symptoms with an IPSS >19 (2,4)[A].
  - TT is not recommended for mood or strength improvement in otherwise healthy men or asymptomatic men with low T (2,4)[A].
- Carefully weigh risks and benefits in men at elevated cardiovascular disease (CVD) risk.
- 2018 AUA guidelines: Clinicians should inform TD patients that TD is a risk factor for CVD.
  - At this time, cannot state definitively if TT increases risk of cardiovascular events. However, TD is also a risk factor for CVD (2,4)[A].

– Patients should be informed that there is no definitive evidence linking TT to a higher incidence of venothrombolic events (2)[A].
– Clinicians can consider starting short-term TT as an adjunctive in men with HIV and low T to promote weight maintenance and gains in lean body mass and strength.
– Men with TD should be counseled regarding lifestyle modification (2,4)[C].

MEDICATION

ALERT
Avoid contact with females or children (see package insert) in patients applying gel preparations.

- Oral therapy is not recommended due to significant hepatotoxicity.
- FDA has cautioned that TT is approved for men with confirmed low T by blood work with signs and symptoms, NOT solely due to aging.
- Despite prior data showing no clear association between TT and CVD, several recent papers suggest TT use puts patients at an increased risk for CVD. These papers have been criticized for being flawed due to comparison of unequal groups, short and inaccurate end points, flawed laboratory testing, erroneous exclusion criteria, and atypical statistical analysis. Despite this, an FDA panel concluded that there is a possible increased CVD risk associated with T use.
- TT should NOT be started for a period of 3 to 6 months in patients with acute cardiovascular event.
- TT (FDA-approved)
  – Topical gels/solutions: most common
    ○ Multiple FDA-approved formulations
    ○ Most frequently prescribed in United States
    ○ Mimics normal daily circadian rhythm
    ○ Good absorption, 15–20% are nonresponders
    ○ Transfer concern to children and women.
  – Testosterone pellets (Testopel)
    ○ Minor office procedure
    ○ Long-acting formulation, 3 to 4 months
    ○ 1–2% risk of infection or pellet extrusion
  – Transdermal patch (Androderm)
    ○ Achieves less robust levels
    ○ Convenient over gels, no risk of transference
    ○ High incidence of skin irritation
  – Testosterone enanthate (short acting, SC)
    ○ FDA-approved October 2018
    ○ SC weekly injection
    ○ Boxed warning for increased blood pressure
    ○ Single dose, disposable autoinjector
  – Testosterone cypionate (short acting, IM)
    ○ Injectable, inexpensive
    ○ Injections every 1 to 3 weeks
    ○ Starting dose: 100 mg/week
    ○ Roller coaster effect: Levels rise and fall.
  – Testosterone undecanoate (long acting, IM)
    ○ Injectable, expensive, convenient
    ○ Small risk of oil embolism, needs observation in office for 30 minutes postinjection
    ○ Given approximately every 8 to 12 weeks
  – Buccal application (Striant)
    ○ Adheres to gum line, irritation in 16.3%
    ○ Poor compliance, every 12 hours application
  – Nasal gel (Natesto)
    ○ TID dosing, nasal irritation
- Off-label treatment
  – Human chorionic gonadotropin (hCG)
    ○ Structure similar to LH, mimics its actions
    ○ 3 times per week starting at 1,500 IU SC
    ○ Poor compliance
    ○ Maintenance of testicular volume and fertility
    ○ Used in men wanting to preserve fertility

– Clomiphene citrate (Clomid): oral agent
    ○ Increases T by interfering with negative feedback, resulting in increased LH and FSH
    ○ Starting dose of 25 mg daily 3 to 7 times weekly
    ○ Used in men wanting to preserve fertility
– Aromatase inhibitors (Arimidex): oral agent
    ○ Blocks conversion of T to estradiol
    ○ Does not negatively impact spermatogenesis and testicular volume
    ○ Used in cases of low T/estradiol ratio
– Combination TT with low-dose hCG may preserve and support fertility in hypogonadal men hoping for future paternity (5)[B].

ISSUES FOR REFERRAL
- PSA >4 ng/mL or >3 ng/mL in high-risk individuals, and/or abnormal prostate exam, worsening symptoms of BPH (IPSS >19) should be referred to urology.
- Worsening CHF, OSA, polycythemia should be referred to the appropriate providers.

 ## ONGOING CARE

FOLLOW-UP RECOMMENDATIONS
Patient Monitoring
- Necessary to monitor effectiveness of therapy as well as for adverse effects: initially 3 to 6 months after treatment initiation and then annually
- Adjust dosing to achieve a total T in the middle tertile of the normal reference range.
- Measure hematocrit at baseline, at 3 to 6 months, and then annually. If hematocrit >54% or symptomatic, stop therapy until hematocrit decreases to a safe level. Treatment includes phlebotomy, blood donation, and dose adjustment.
- Clinicians should stop treatment 3 to 6 months after starting in patients who experience normalization of T but fail to achieve symptom improvement.
- Bone mineral density after 1 to 2 years of therapy in men with osteoporosis or low trauma fracture
- Prostate exam done regularly every 6 to 12 months
- Refer to urology when increase in PSA >0.7 ng/mL within any 12-month period of T treatment or detection of prostatic abnormality on prostate exam.

DIET
Healthy diet and weight reduction if obese

PATIENT EDUCATION
- TD can be chronic and may need lifelong therapy.
- T replacement comes with many risks, and it is very important to regularly monitor outcomes.
- Women and children must not be allowed to come in contact with TT gel products.

PROGNOSIS
- There are evolving evidence that TT may improve metabolic functions such as glycosylated hemoglobin, blood sugar, total cholesterol, and visceral fat in diabetics, and also unexplained anemia.
- Recent data suggests men with low bone mineral density, and low T can increase bone density and bone strength with T replacement.

COMPLICATIONS
Complications of T replacement
- Decreased testicular volume, azoospermia in 40% of patients on TT, infertility
- Fluctuations in mood or libido
- Gynecomastia and growth of breast cancer
- Acne and oily skin
- Erythrocytosis (increased hematocrit)

- Exacerbation of sleep apnea
- Hepatotoxicity with prolonged oral use
- Possible prostate enlargement with or without worsening symptoms of BPH
- Unknown cardiovascular risks

REFERENCES
1. Paduch DA, Brannigan RE, Fuchs EF, et al. The laboratory diagnosis of testosterone deficiency. *Urology.* 2014;83(5):980–988.
2. Mulhall JP, Trost LW, Brannigan RE, et al. Evaluation and management of Testosterone deficiency: AUA guideline. *J Urol.* 2018;200(2):423–432.
3. Debruyne FM, Behre HM, Roehrborn CG, et al; for RHYME Investigators. Testosterone treatment is not associated with increased risk of prostate cancer or worsening of lower urinary tract symptoms: prostate health outcomes in the Registry of Hypogonadism in Men. *BJU Int.* 2017;119(2):216–224.
4. Bhasin S, Cunningham GR, Hayes FJ, et al; for Task Force, Endocrine Society. Testosterone therapy in men with androgen deficiency syndromes: an Endocrine Society clinical practice guideline. *J Clin Endocrinol Metab.* 2010;95(6):2536–2559.
5. Hsieh TC, Pastuszak AW, Hwang K, et al. Concomitant intramuscular human chorionic gonadotropin preserves spermatogenesis in men undergoing testosterone replacement therapy. *J Urol.* 2013;189(2):647–650.

ADDITIONAL READING
- Buvat J, Maggi M, Guay A, et al. Testosterone deficiency in men: systematic review and standard operating procedures for diagnosis and treatment. *J Sex Med.* 2013;10(1):245–284.
- Conners WP III, Morgentaler A. The evaluation and management of testosterone deficiency: the new frontier in urology and men's health. *Curr Urol Rep.* 2013;14(6):557–564.
- Vigen R, O'Donnell CI, Barón AE, et al. Association of testosterone therapy with mortality, myocardial infarction, and stroke in men with low testosterone levels. *JAMA.* 2013;310(17):1829–1836.

 ## CODES

ICD10
- E29.1 Testicular hypofunction
- E89.5 Postprocedural testicular hypofunction

CLINICAL PEARLS
- TD is common, and prevalence increases with age.
- TD can have negative adverse impact on many bodily systems.
- Symptomatic men with sexual dysfunction, obesity, unexplained anemia, bone density loss, chronic steroid or narcotic use, and metabolic diseases should be tested for TD and treated.
- Initial test of choice is a morning total and free T; if low, repeat measurements.
- TT in the appropriately selected population can increase lean mass, reduce fat mass, increase bone mineral density, improve libido, improve unexplained anemia, and improve erections. However, it has not been shown to improve cognition or memory impairment in the elderly.

T

THALASSEMIA
Garland E. Anderson II, MD

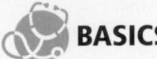 **BASICS**

DESCRIPTION
- A group of inherited hematologic disorders that affect the synthesis of adult hemoglobin tetramer (HbA) (1,2)[C]
- α-Thalassemia is due to a deficient synthesis of α-globin chain, whereas β-thalassemia is due to a deficient synthesis of β-globin chain:
  - The synthesis of the unaffected globin chain proceeds normally.
  - This unbalanced globin chain production causes unstable hemoglobin tetramers, which leads to hypochromic, microcytic red blood cells (RBCs), and hemolytic anemia.
- α-Thalassemia is more common in persons of Mediterranean, African, and Southeast Asian descent, whereas β-thalassemia is more common in patients of African and Southeast Asian descent.
- Types
  - Thalassemia (minor) trait (α or β): absent or mild anemia with microcytosis and hypochromia
  - α-Thalassemia major with hemoglobin Bart usually results in fatal hydrops fetalis (fluid in $\geq$2 fetal compartments secondary to anemia and fetal heart failure).
  - α-Thalassemia intermedia with hemoglobin H (hemoglobin H disease): results in moderate hemolytic anemia and splenomegaly
  - β-Thalassemia major: results in severe anemia, growth retardation, hepatosplenomegaly, bone marrow expansion, and bone deformities. Transfusion therapy is necessary to sustain life.
  - β-Thalassemia intermedia: milder disease; transfusion therapy may not be needed or may be needed later in life.
- Other variants include hemoglobin E/β-thalassemia in Southeast Asians, which often mimics the severity of α-thalassemia major; δ-thalassemia; hemoglobin H Constant Spring
- System(s) affected: hematologic/lymphatic/immunologic, cardiac, hepatic
- Synonym(s): Mediterranean anemia; hereditary leptocytosis; Cooley anemia

Pediatric Considerations
- β-Thalassemia major causes symptoms during early childhood, usually starting at 6 months of age, and requires periodic transfusions to sustain life.
- Newborn's cord blood or heel stick should be screened for hemoglobinopathies with hemoglobin electrophoresis or comparably accurate test, although this primarily detects sickle cell disease.

Pregnancy Considerations
- Preconception genetic counseling is advised for couples at risk for having a child with thalassemia and for parents or other relatives of a child with thalassemia (3)[A].
- Once pregnant, a chorionic villus sample at 10 to 11 weeks' gestation or an amniocentesis at 15 weeks' gestation can be done to detect point mutations or deletions with polymerase chain reaction (PCR) technology.

EPIDEMIOLOGY
Incidence
- Occurs in ~4.4/10,000 live births
- Predominant age: Symptoms start to appear 6 months after birth with β-thalassemia major.
- Predominant sex: male = female

Prevalence
- Worldwide, ~200,000 people are alive with β-thalassemia major and <1,000 patients are in the United States.
- In the worldwide population, an estimated 1.5% are β-thalassemia carriers and 5% α-thalassemia carriers (4).

ETIOLOGY AND PATHOPHYSIOLOGY
Unknown; it is unclear how the imbalance of β-globulin in α-thalassemia and α-globin in β-thalassemia results in ineffective RBC genesis and hemolysis.

Genetics
- Inherited in an autosomal recessive pattern
- α-Thalassemia results from a deletion of $\geq$1 of the 4 genes, 2 on each chromosome 16, responsible for α-globin synthesis. 1-gene deletion is a silent carrier state, 2-gene deletion is the trait, 3-gene deletion results in hemoglobin H, and 4-gene deletion results in hemoglobin Bart, causing fatal hydrops fetalis.
- Nondeletional forms do occur rarely. Hemoglobin H Constant Spring is the most common nondeletional form.
- β-Thalassemia is caused by any of >200-point mutations and, very rarely, deletions on chromosome 11; 20 alleles account for >80% of the mutations.
- Significantly disparate phenotype with the same genotype occurs because β-globin chain production can range from near-normal to absent.

RISK FACTORS
Family history of thalassemia

GENERAL PREVENTION
- Prenatal information: genetic counseling regarding partner selection and information on the availability of diagnostic tests during the pregnancy
- Complication prevention
  - For offspring of adult thalassemia patients, an evaluation for thalassemia by 1 year of age
  - Severe forms
    - Avoid exposure to sick contacts.
    - Keep immunizations up to date.
  - Promptly treat bacterial infections. (After splenectomy, patients should maintain a supply of an appropriate antibiotic to take at the onset of symptoms of a bacterial infection.)
  - Dental checkups every 6 months
  - Avoid activities that could increase the risk of bone fractures.

COMMONLY ASSOCIATED CONDITIONS
See "Complications."

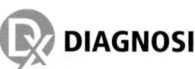 **DIAGNOSIS**

Thalassemia (minor) trait has no signs or symptoms.

HISTORY
- Poor growth
- Excessive fatigue
- Cholelithiasis
- Pathologic fractures
- Shortness of breath

PHYSICAL EXAM
- Pallor
- Splenomegaly
- Jaundice
- Maxillary hyperplasia/frontal bossing due to massive bone marrow expansion
- Dental malocclusion

DIFFERENTIAL DIAGNOSIS
- Iron deficiency anemia
- Other microcytic anemias: lead toxicity, sideroblastic
- Other hemolytic anemias
- Other hemoglobinopathies

DIAGNOSTIC TESTS & INTERPRETATION
Special tests
- Bone marrow aspiration to evaluate for causes of microcytic anemia is rarely needed.
- Multiple indices have been evaluated to discriminate β-thalassemia trait from iron deficiency anemia, yet none is sensitive enough to exclude β-thalassemia.
- Hemoglobin: usual range 10 to 12 g/dL with thalassemia trait and 3 to 8 g/dL with β-thalassemia major before transfusions
- Hematocrit
  - 28–40% in thalassemia trait
  - May fall to <10% in β-thalassemia major
- Peripheral blood
  - Microcytosis (MCV <70 fl)
  - Hypochromia (MCH <20 pg)
  - High percentage of target cells
  - Reticulocyte count is elevated.
- Red cell distribution width (RDW)
  - A normal RDW with a microcytic hypochromic anemia is almost always thalassemia trait.
  - The RDW can be elevated in ~50% of thalassemia trait patients. This is in contrast to iron deficiency anemia, where the RDW is almost always elevated (90%).
- Hemoglobin electrophoresis
  - In α-thalassemia trait, no recognizable electrophoretic pattern occurs in adults.
  - However, in the neonatal period, 3–10% of trait patients will have hemoglobin H or hemoglobin Bart at birth, which would confirm α-thalassemia.
  - If HbA_2 is below normal (<2.5%) with a normal HbF level, the diagnosis is α-thalassemia intermedia (HbH disease).
  - In the neonatal period with β-thalassemia trait, the electrophoresis is normal. However, in adults, elevated HbA_2 levels (>4%) may be present but are usually normal (5)[C].
  - β-Thalassemia major or intermedia has elevated HbA_2, elevated HbF, and reduced or absent HbA.
- DNA analysis
  - α-Thalassemia can definitively be diagnosed with genetic testing of hemoglobin A1 and A2 (for deletions and point mutations), but this is not routinely done due to the high cost.
  - High-performance liquid chromatography
  - Cost-effective primary screening tool for children and adolescents
  - Equivocal results should be confirmed with DNA analysis.

Pediatric Considerations
For children, calculate Mentzer index (mean corpuscular volume/RBC count).
- <13: suggests thalassemia
- >13: suggests iron deficiency anemia
- Liver iron concentrations can be assessed with MRI (FerriScan).

TREATMENT

- Outpatient for mild cases
- Inpatient for transfusion therapy

GENERAL MEASURES

- Mild cases (trait or minor) require no therapy.
- Thalassemia intermedia: No therapy is necessary unless hemoglobin falls to a level that causes symptoms; then, transfusion therapy is needed. Decision is based on patient's quality of life.
- Iron supplements should not be given unless iron deficiency occurs and is confirmed with low ferritin. Supplements increase the risk of iron overload (1)[C].
- Thalassemia major
  - A regular transfusion schedule to increase post-transfusion hemoglobin to 13.0 to 14.0 g/L and maintain a mean hemoglobin level of at least 9.3 g/dL (1.4 mmol/L) (1)[B]
  - Patients require >8 transfusion events per year. An event may be multiple transfused units.
  - Iron overload (6)[C]
    - Patients receiving transfusion therapy increase total body iron 4 times the normal amount.
    - Therapy is iron chelation. (See "Medication.")

MEDICATION

Thalassemia intermedia and major: folic acid supplements (1 mg/day)

First Line

β-Thalassemia major

- Iron chelation with deferoxamine (Desferal)
  - Usually continuous SC or IV infusion
  - Acute toxicity: initial—1,000 mg IV, may be followed by 500 mg every 4 hours for 2 doses; subsequent doses of 500 mg every 4 to 12 hours based on response (max 6,000 mg/day)
  - Chronic: 20 to 40 mg/kg over 8 to 12 hours daily
  - Usually started by 5 to 8 years of age
  - Treatment lasts 3 to 5 years to reach serum ferritin <1,000 ng/mL.
- Deferasirox (Exjade) 20 to 30 mg/kg/day PO acceptable alternative; approved for transfusion and non–transfusion-dependent patients with hepatic iron concentrations ≥5 mg/g of dry weight and serum ferritin >300 μg/L; renal and hepatic monitoring is recommended.

Second Line

Chelation with deferiprone (Ferriprox) 25 mg/kg TID PO initially is an acceptable alternative for patients who have not responded to deferoxamine; may provide more cardioprotection. A drawback is weekly CBC because ~1% of patients develop agranulocytosis.

ISSUES FOR REFERRAL

Thalassemia major usually requires hematology consult.

ADDITIONAL THERAPIES

β-Thalassemia intermedia

- Hydroxyurea may improve hemoglobin 1 to 2 g/dL.
- Psychological support seems appropriate for this chronic disease. However, no conclusions can be made regarding specific psychological therapies.

SURGERY/OTHER PROCEDURES

- Splenectomy
  - May be needed if hypersplenism causes an increase in the transfusion requirements (>180 to 200 mL/kg/year)
  - Defer surgery until patient is at least 4 years of age (due to increased infection risk).
  - Administer pneumococcal polyvalent-23 vaccine 1 month before splenectomy. Children should complete their pneumococcal conjugate vaccine series before surgery.
  - Daily penicillin prophylaxis, 250 mg BID, after splenectomy for 2 years for all patients and for children until age 16 years
- Bone marrow transplantation with HLA-identical related donor stem cells in children before developing hepatitis or iron overload has high likelihood of remission but may impair fertility.

 ONGOING CARE

FOLLOW-UP RECOMMENDATIONS

- Thalassemia trait requires no restrictions.
- β-Thalassemia major
  - Avoid strenuous activities (e.g., football, soccer).
  - Acceptable activity levels will be determined on an individual basis depending on the severity of the disorder.

Patient Monitoring

- Thalassemia-trait patients require no special follow-up.
- For β-thalassemia major, lifelong monitoring is necessary because the therapy and disease progression have numerous potential complications.

DIET

- Thalassemia trait requires no restrictions.
- β-Thalassemia major
  - Limit intake of iron-rich foods (e.g., red meats such as liver and some cereals).

PATIENT EDUCATION

Printed patient information available from Cooley's Anemia Foundation, 330 7th Ave. Suite 900, New York, NY 10001; http://www.thalassemia.org or http://www.cooleysanemia.org

PROGNOSIS

- Outlook varies depending on type.
- Thalassemia-trait patients live a normal lifespan.
- β-Thalassemia major patients live an average of 17 years and usually die by age 30 years.
- Iron overload causes most of the morbidity and mortality:
  - Cardiac events are the primary cause of death.
  - Myocardial iron deposition is best assessed with MRI T2.
  - Effective iron chelation improves longevity.

COMPLICATIONS

- Chronic hemolysis
- Susceptibility to infections after splenectomy
- Infections from blood transfusion
- Jaundice
- Leg ulcers
- Cholelithiasis
- Osteoporosis and low-trauma fractures
- Impaired growth rate
- Delayed or absent puberty
- Hypogonadism
- Hepatic siderosis
- Splenomegaly
- Cardiac disease from iron overload
- Thromboembolic phenomenon
- Aplastic and megaloblastic crises
- Increased risk of hematologic and abdominal cancer
- Increased risk of dementia

REFERENCES

1. Muncie HL Jr, Campbell J. Alpha and beta thalassemia. *Am Fam Physician*. 2009;80(4):339–344.
2. Higgs DR, Engel JD, Stamatoyannopoulos G. Thalassaemia. *Lancet*. 2012;379(9813):373–383.
3. Tamhankar PM, Agarwal S, Arya V, et al. Prevention of homozygous beta thalassemia by premarital screening and prenatal diagnosis in India. *Prenat Diagn*. 2009;29(1):83–88.
4. Peters M, Heijboer H, Smiers F, et al. Diagnosis and management of thalassaemia. *BMJ*. 2012;344:e228.
5. Mosca A, Paleari R, Ivaldi G, et al. The role of haemoglobin A(2) testing in the diagnosis of thalassaemias and related haemoglobinopathies. *J Clin Pathol*. 2009;62(1):13–17.
6. Fleming RE, Ponka P. Iron overload in human disease. *N Engl J Med*. 2012;366(4):348–359.

ADDITIONAL READING

- Paulson RF. Targeting a new regulator of erythropoiesis to alleviate anemia. *Nat Med*. 2014;20(4):334–335.
- Piel FB, Weatherall DJ. The α-thalassemias. *N Engl J Med*. 2014;371(20):1908–1916.

 CODES

ICD10

- D56.9 Thalassemia, unspecified
- D56.1 Beta thalassemia
- D56.0 Alpha thalassemia

CLINICAL PEARLS

- Thalassemia (group of inherited hematologic disorders that affect the synthesis of adult hemoglobin tetramer) is a genetic condition; hemoglobin will not improve over time.
- α-Thalassemia is due to a deficient synthesis of the α-globin chain, whereas β-thalassemia is due to a deficient synthesis of the β-globin chain.
- Hemoglobin electrophoresis is needed for genetic counseling but not to make the diagnosis of thalassemia minor when evaluating a patient with mild hypochromic, microcytic anemia and normal serum ferritin.
- Anemia from thalassemia minor is not due to inadequate iron availability or iron storage. Therefore, iron supplements will not improve the anemia and could be harmful due to GI distress and iron overload. If coexisting iron deficiency is proven, then iron therapy is appropriate.

THORACIC OUTLET SYNDROME

Robert A. Baldor, MD, FAAFP

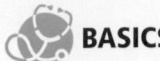

BASICS

DESCRIPTION
- This syndrome consists of a constellation of symptoms that affect the head, neck, shoulders, and upper extremities caused by compression of the neurovascular structures (brachial plexus and subclavian vessels) at the thoracic outlet, specifically in the area superior to the 1st rib and posterior to the clavicle.
- Three forms of thoracic outlet syndrome (TOS) have been described: neurogenic, vascular (with venous and arterial symptoms), and nonspecific (includes traumatic and secondary to certain provocative movements).
- Synonym(s): scalenus anticus syndrome; cervical rib syndrome; costoclavicular syndrome

Pregnancy Considerations
Generalized tissue fluid accumulations and postural changes may aggravate symptoms.

EPIDEMIOLOGY
Incidence
- Predominant age
  - Neurogenic type (95%): 20 to 60 years
  - Venous type (4%): 20 to 35 years
  - Arterial type (1%; atherosclerosis): young adult or >50 years
- Predominant sex
  - Neurogenic type: female > male (3.5:1)
  - Venous type: male > female
  - Arterial type: male = female
- No objective confirmatory tests available to measure true incidence
- Estimated 3 to 8/1,000 cases for neurogenic type
- Incidence of other TOS types is unclear.

ETIOLOGY AND PATHOPHYSIOLOGY
The interscalene triangle area is reduced in TOS and may become smaller during certain shoulder and arm movements. Fibrotic bands, cervical ribs, and muscle variations may further narrow the triangle. Trauma or provocative movements affecting the lower brachial plexus have strong implications in TOS pathogenesis.

- Three known causes of TOS: anatomic, traumatic/repetitive movement activities, and neurovascular entrapment
  - Anatomic: Variations in the anatomy of the neck scalene muscles may be responsible for presentations of the neurologic type of TOS and may involve the superior border of the 1st rib. Cervical ribs also have been implicated as a cause of neurologic TOS, with subsequent neuronal fibrosing and degeneration associated with arterial hyalinization in the lower trunk of the brachial plexus. Fibrous bands to cervical ribs are often congenital.
  - Trauma or repetitive movement activities: Motor vehicle accidents with hyperextension injury and resulting fibrosis, including fibrous bands to the clavicle; musicians who maintain prolonged positions of shoulder abduction or extension may be at increased risk.
  - Neurovascular entrapment: occurring in the costoclavicular space between the 1st rib and the head of the clavicle

RISK FACTORS
- Trauma, especially to the shoulder girdle
- Presence of a cervical rib
- Posttraumatic, exostosis of clavicle or 1st rib, postural abnormalities (e.g., drooping of shoulders, scoliosis), body building with increased muscular bulk in thoracic outlet area, rapid weight loss with vigorous physical exertion and/or exercise, pendulous breasts
- Occupational exposure: computer users; musicians; repetitive work involving shoulders, arms, hands
- Young, thin females with long necks and drooping shoulders

GENERAL PREVENTION
Consider workplace evaluation for proper occupational ergonomics.

COMMONLY ASSOCIATED CONDITIONS
- Paget-von Schrötter syndrome: thrombosis of subclavian vein
- Gilliatt-Sumner hand: neurogenic atrophy of abductor pollicis brevis

DIAGNOSIS

HISTORY
- Neurologic type, upper plexus (C4–C7)
  - Pain and paresthesias in head, neck, mandible, face, temporal area, upper back/chest, outer arm, and hand in a radial nerve distribution
  - Occipital and orbital headache
- Neurologic type, lower plexus (C8–T1)
  - Pain and paresthesias in axilla, inner arm, and hand in an ulnar nerve distribution, often nocturnal
  - Hypothenar and interosseous muscle atrophy
- Venous type: arm claudication, cyanosis, swelling, distended arm veins
- Arterial type: digital vasospasm, thrombosis/embolism, aneurysm, gangrene

PHYSICAL EXAM
- Positive Adson maneuver (head rotation to the affected side with cervical extension and then deep inhalation); test is positive if paresthesias occur or if radial pulse is not palpable during maneuver.
- Tenderness to percussion or palpation of supraclavicular area
- Worsening of symptoms with elevation of arm, overhead extension of arms, or with arms extended forward (e.g., driving a car, typing, carrying objects); prompt disappearance of symptoms with arm returning to neutral position
- Morley test
  - Brachial plexus compression test in the supraclavicular area from the scalene triangle
  - Positive with reproduction of an aching sensation and typical localized paresthesia
- Hyperabduction test: diminishment of radial pulse with elevation of arm above the head

- Military maneuver (i.e., costoclavicular bracing): When patient elevates chin and pushes shoulders posteriorly in an extreme "at-attention" position, symptoms are provoked.
- 1-minute Roos test
  - A thoracic outlet shoulder girdle stress test
  - Shoulders and arms are braced in a 90-degree abducted and externally rotated position; patient is required to clench and relax fists repetitively for 1 minute.
  - A positive test reproduces the symptom.

DIFFERENTIAL DIAGNOSIS
- Cervical disk or carpal tunnel syndrome
- Orthopedic shoulder problems (shoulder strain, rotator cuff injury, tendonitis)
- Cervical spondylitis
- Ulnar nerve compression at elbow and hand
- Multiple sclerosis
- Spinal cord tumor/disease
- Angina pectoris
- Migraine
- Complex regional pain syndromes
- C3–C5 and C8 radiculopathies

DIAGNOSTIC TESTS & INTERPRETATION
Initial Tests (lab, imaging)
CBC, ESR, and C-reactive protein (CRP) determination may rule out underlying inflammatory conditions.

- Radiograph (chest, C-spine, shoulders) may reveal elongated C7 transverse process or a cervical rib, Pancoast tumor, or healed clavicle fracture.
- Nerve conduction studies and electromyography (EMG)
- CT scan or MRI, although MRI is the method of choice when searching for nerve compression
- Improved high-resolution MRN and tractography are valuable tools for identifying the source of nerve compression in patients with neurogenic TOS and can augment current diagnostic modalities for this syndrome (1)[B].
- Contrast-enhanced 3D MRA using provocative arm positioning allows excellent imaging of the arteries and veins on both sides and thus provides a noninvasive imaging alternative to digital subtraction angiography in patients with suspected vascular TOS (2)[B].
- Doppler and duplex US if vascular obstruction is suspected
- Arteriogram and venogram have limited roles; useful when symptoms suggestive of arterial insufficiency or ischemia, or in planning surgical intervention (3)[C]

Diagnostic Procedures/Other
No indicated procedures; anesthetic anterior scalene block may relieve pressure by scalene muscles on the brachial plexus, making this type of block diagnostic and potentially therapeutic, but it poses the risk of procedural damage to the brachial plexus.

TREATMENT

GENERAL MEASURES
- Conservative management usually involves approaches to reduce and redistribute pressure and traction through the use of physiotherapy or prosthesis.
- Physical therapy is first-line treatment (4)[B].
- Interscalene injections of botulinum toxin have been shown to decrease symptoms of TOS (5)[C]. A single, CT-guided Botox injection into the anterior scalene muscle may offer an effective, minimally invasive treatment for NTOS (6)[A].
- Physical therapy will develop strength in pectoral girdle muscles and achieve normal posture.
- Severe cases may use taping, adhesive elastic bandages, moist heat, TENS, or US but should not substitute active exercise and correction of posture and muscle imbalance (4)[B].

MEDICATION
No firm evidence exists for any specific approach to the three types of TOS.
- Anti-inflammatory (ibuprofen)
  - Adult dose: 400 to 800 mg PO q8h; not to exceed 3,200 mg/day
  - Pediatric dose
    - <12 years: 10 mg/kg/dose every 6 to 8 hours
    - >12 years: as in adults
  - Contraindications: documented hypersensitivity, active PUD, renal or hepatic impairment, recent use of anticoagulants, hemorrhagic conditions
- Neuropathic pain: tricyclic antidepressants, carbamazepine, gabapentin, phenytoin, pregabalin; muscle relaxants such as baclofen, metaxalone, or tizanidine may be helpful.
- Severe pain: Consider opiates for brachial plexus nerve block, steroid injections.

ISSUES FOR REFERRAL
- Neurologic, anesthesiologic, orthopedic, vascular surgery referral(s) may be indicated depending on the type of pathologic condition.
- Physical and rehabilitation physicians

SURGERY/OTHER PROCEDURES
- Operative if vascular involvement is present and/or loss of function or lifestyle occurs secondary to severity of symptoms and if conservative therapy fails after 2 to 3 months
- Resection of 1st rib or cervical ribs via transaxillary (preferred with good to excellent outcome 80% of patients), supraclavicular (good to excellent outcome 80% of patients), posterior approaches (reserved for complicated TOS due to necessity of large muscle incision). Excellent results were seen in patients who underwent 1st rib resection in all three forms of TOS (7)[A].
- Transaxillary approach provides a good exposure and cosmetics in patients with TOS. It should be considered as the gold standard in the management of TOS (8)[B].
- Supraclavicular scalenectomy (9)[C]
- Isolated pectoral minor tenotomy (PMT) is a low-risk outpatient procedure that is effective for the treatment of selected patients with disabling NTOS, with early outcomes similar to supraclavicular decompression + PMT (10)[A].

ADMISSION, INPATIENT, AND NURSING CONSIDERATIONS
Conservative, outpatient, nonpharmacologic treatment is reasonable first-line therapy except in cases of thromboembolic phenomena and acute ischemia, symptoms of chronic vascular occlusion, stenosis, arterial dilatation, or progressive neurologic deficit (6)[B].

ONGOING CARE

FOLLOW-UP RECOMMENDATIONS
Correct improper posture, practice proper posture, exercises to strengthen shoulder elevator and neck extensor muscles, stretching exercises for scalene muscles, support bra for women with pendulous breasts, breast reduction surgery in selected cases; sleep with arms below chest level, avoid/reduce prolonged hyperabduction.

Patient Monitoring
Office follow-up visits every 3 to 4 weeks

PATIENT EDUCATION
Physical therapy, postural exercises, ergonomic workstation

PROGNOSIS
Durable long-term functional outcomes can be achieved predicated on a highly selective approach to the surgical management of patients with TOS. A majority of operated patients will not require adjunctive procedures or chronic narcotic use (11)[C].

COMPLICATIONS
- Postoperative shoulder, arm, hand pain, and paresthesias in 10%
- Patients who will have symptomatic recurrences at 1 month to 7 years postoperatively (usually within 3 months): 1.5–2%
- Patients who will have brachial plexus injury, probably due to intraoperative traction: 0.5–1%
- Reoperation is indicated for symptomatic recurrence with long posterior remnant of 1st rib (posterior approach) or with disrupted fibrous adhesions (transaxillary approach).
- Venous obstruction or arterial emboli; usually responds to thrombolytics

REFERENCES

1. Magill ST, Brus-Ramer M, Weinstein PR, et al. Neurogenic thoracic outlet syndrome: current diagnostic criteria and advances in MRI diagnostics. *Neurosurg Focus*. 2015;39(3):E7.
2. Ersoy H, Steigner ML, Coyner KB, et al. Vascular thoracic outlet syndrome: protocol design and diagnostic value of contrast-enhanced 3D MR angiography and equilibrium phase imaging on 1.5- and 3-T MRI scanners. *AJR Am J Roentgenol*. 2012;198(5):1180–1187.
3. Sanders RJ, Hammond SL, Rao NM. Diagnosis of thoracic outlet syndrome. *J Vasc Surg*. 2007;46(3):601–604.
4. Vanti C, Natalini L, Romeo A, et al. Conservative treatment of thoracic outlet syndrome. A review of the literature. *Eura Medicophys*. 2007;43(1):55–70.
5. Lee GW, Kwon YH, Jeong JH, et al. The efficacy of scalene injection in thoracic outlet syndrome. *J Korean Neurosurg Soc*. 2011;50(1):36–39.
6. Christo PJ, Christo DK, Carinci AJ, et al. Single CT-guided chemodenervation of the anterior scalene muscle with botulinum toxin for neurogenic thoracic outlet syndrome. *Pain Med*. 2010;11(4):504–511.
7. Orlando MS, Likes KC, Mirza S, et al. A decade of excellent outcomes after surgical intervention in 538 patients with thoracic outlet syndrome. *J Am Coll Surg*. 2015;220(5):934–939.
8. Lattoo MR, Dar AM, Wani ML, et al. Outcome of trans-axillary approach for surgical decompression of thoracic outlet: a retrospective study in a tertiary care hospital. *Oman Med J*. 2014;29(3):214–216.
9. Glynn RW, Tawfick W, Elsafty Z, et al. Supraclavicular scalenectomy for thoracic outlet syndrome—functional outcomes assessed using the DASH scoring system. *Vasc Endovascular Surg*. 2012;46(2):157–162.
10. Vemuri C, Wittenberg AM, Caputo FJ, et al. Early effectiveness of isolated pectoralis minor tenotomy in selected patients with neurogenic thoracic outlet syndrome. *J Vasc Surg*. 2013;57(5):1345–1352.
11. Scali S, Stone D, Bjerke A, et al. Long-term functional results for the surgical management of neurogenic thoracic outlet syndrome. *Vasc Endovascular Surg*. 2010;44(7):550–555.

ADDITIONAL READING

Povlsen B, Belzberg A, Hansson T, et al. Treatment for thoracic outlet syndrome. *Cochrane Database Syst Rev*. 2010;(1):CD007218.

CODES

ICD10
G54.0 Brachial plexus disorders

CLINICAL PEARLS

- This syndrome is caused by compression of the neurovascular structures (brachial plexus and subclavian vessels) at the thoracic outlet, specifically in the area superior to the 1st rib and posterior to the clavicle.
- Conservative management involves approaches to reduce and redistribute pressure and traction through the use of physiotherapy or prosthesis.
- Physical therapy is first-line treatment.
- Avoid opiate dependence.
- Consider pain clinic referral if there are nonsurgical causes.

THROMBOPHILIA AND HYPERCOAGULABLE STATES

Kirsten Vitrikas, MD • Aaron Patzwahl, MD

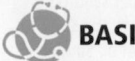 **BASICS**

DESCRIPTION

- An inherited or acquired disorder of the coagulation system predisposing an individual to thromboembolism (the formation of a venous, or less commonly, an arterial blood clot)
- Venous thrombosis typically manifests as deep venous thrombosis (DVT) of the lower extremity in the legs or pelvis and pulmonary embolism (PE).
- System(s) affected: cardiovascular, nervous, pulmonary, reproductive, hematologic
- Synonym(s): hypercoagulation syndrome; prothrombotic state

EPIDEMIOLOGY

- An inherited thrombophilic defect or risk can be detected in up to 50% of patients with venous thromboembolism (VTE).
- Factor V Leiden is the most common inherited thrombophilia (1/2 of all currently characterizable inherited thrombophilia cases involve the factor V Leiden mutation), and it is present in its heterozygous form in up to ~20% of patients with a first VTE.
- Heterozygous prothrombin G20210A mutation, the second most common inherited thrombophilia, is present in up to ~8% of patients with VTE.
- Overall VTE incidence higher in African American populations and lower in Asian, Asian American, and Native American populations (1)
- VTE rates are higher in women during childbearing years (16 to 44 years), then higher in men when >45 years of age (1).

Incidence

First-time thromboembolism

- ~100/100,000/year among the general population
- <1/100,000/year in those age <15 years
- ~1,000/100,000/year in those age ≥85 years

Prevalence

- 40–80% of lower extremity orthopedic procedures can result in DVT if prophylaxis is not used.
- VTE accounts for ~1.2 to 4.7 deaths per 100,000 pregnancies.

ETIOLOGY AND PATHOPHYSIOLOGY

- Virchow triad as a cause of VTE includes blood stasis, vascular endothelial injury, and abnormalities in circulating blood constituents (i.e., hypercoagulability).
- An imbalance between the hemostatic and fibrinolytic pathways leads to thrombus formation.
- VTE is considered to be the result of genetic tendencies with other acquired risks.
- Upper extremity DVT: >60% are associated with venous catheters. Malignancy is an additional significant risk (2).

Genetics

- The most common genetic thrombophilias (factor V Leiden, prothrombin G20210A, proteins C and S defects, and antithrombin III deficiency) are inherited in an autosomal dominant pattern.
- Homozygous mutations generally have a higher risk of VTE.
- Factor V Leiden/activated protein C (aPC) resistance is the most common inherited thrombophilia.
  - 2–5% prevalence among Caucasians; rare in African Americans or Asians
  - aPC does not cleave factor Va, so thrombin formation continues.
  - Other acquired risks are synergistic (3).

- Prothrombin gene mutation G20210A: prevalence 6% among Caucasians. Heterozygous carriers have increased risk of thrombosis.
- Hyperhomocysteinemia: 5–6% among the general population; increases risk of coronary artery disease/myocardial infarction, cerebrovascular accident, and DVT/PE; acquired in those with folate, vitamin B_{12}, and vitamin B_6 deficiencies
- Antithrombin deficiency: <0.2% among the general population; produced in the liver; acquired deficiency in disseminated intravascular coagulation (DIC), sepsis, liver disease, nephrotic syndrome; RR of 8.1 for thrombosis
- Protein C and S deficiencies: 0.5% and 1% incidences, respectively, among the general population. Homozygotes and heterozygotes are hypercoagulable. Vitamin K–dependent, produced in the liver. Protein C inactivates Va and VIIIa. Protein C may become an acquired deficiency in liver disease, sepsis, DIC, acute respiratory distress syndrome, and after surgery. RR of 7.3 for thrombosis. Protein S is a cofactor for protein C, and it may become an acquired deficiency with oral contraceptive pill (OCP) use, pregnancy, liver disease, sepsis, DIC, HIV, and nephrosis; RR of 8.5 for thrombosis

RISK FACTORS

- Acquired risk factors
  - Immobilization or prolonged travel
  - Trauma
  - Surgery, especially orthopedic
  - Malignancies (especially pancreatic, ovarian, brain, and lymphoma)
  - Pregnancy
  - Acute medical illness
  - Exogenous female hormones/oral contraceptives
  - Obesity
  - Nephrotic syndrome
  - Antiphospholipid syndrome (APS) and lupus anticoagulant
  - Myeloproliferative disorders (polycythemia vera, essential thrombocythemia)
  - Hyperviscosity syndromes (sickle cell, paraproteinemias)
  - Hyperhomocysteinemia secondary to vitamin deficiencies (B_6, B_{12}, folic acid)
  - Tamoxifen, thalidomide, lenalidomide, bevacizumab, L-asparaginase, erythropoiesis-stimulating agents
  - Previous thromboembolism
- Established genetic factors
  - Factor V Leiden
  - Prothrombin G20210A mutation
  - Protein C deficiency
  - Protein S deficiency
  - Antithrombin III deficiency
- Rare genetic factors
  - Dysfibrinogenemia
  - Hyperhomocysteinemia (methylene tetrahydrofolate reductase mutation)
- Indeterminate factors
  - Elevated factor VIII
- Age: >60 years
- Sex: male
- Race: See "Epidemiology."

GENERAL PREVENTION

- Consider medication prophylaxis in any hospitalized patient with VTE risk factors; hospitalized patients should be encouraged to ambulate as soon as possible (4)[A].

- Consider mechanical prophylaxis in patients at increased risk for VTE in whom anticoagulation may be contraindicated (4)[A].
- Consider prophylaxis with low-molecular-weight heparin (LMWH) plus aspirin in pregnant patients with APS or other thrombophilia.
- Consider prophylaxis using LMWH in patients with solid tumors who have additional risk factors for VTE.
- Prophylaxis with unfractionated heparin (UFH) or LMWH should be considered in patients with genetic or acquired risks of thrombosis and an anticipated additional risk, such as the immobilization associated with surgery.
- Use caution with procoagulant medicines (e.g., OCPs) in asymptomatic individuals who have a known hereditary predisposition.

COMMONLY ASSOCIATED CONDITIONS

Advanced age, cancer, pregnancy, obesity, prior history of thrombosis, surgery, immobilization

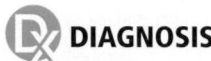 **DIAGNOSIS**

HISTORY

Consider prothrombotic assessment for the following:

- Thrombosis at an unusual anatomic site or recurrent thromboses
- Family history suggesting multiple individuals affected with VTE
- Recurrent pregnancy loss

PHYSICAL EXAM

- DVT: swelling, pain, warmth, and redness, usually of one extremity
- PE: dyspnea, chest pain, hemoptysis, hypoxia, tachycardia
- Postthrombotic syndrome: pain, swelling, pigmentation, and/or ulceration

DIAGNOSTIC TESTS & INTERPRETATION

Testing for thrombophilias is not recommended unless it will affect management (2,5)[B]. Testing should be delayed until after the initial 3 months of anticoagulation (2,5)[B].

Initial Tests (lab, imaging)

- CBC
- aPC profile: ≤2.0 implies factor V Leiden mutation; 95–100% are factor V Leiden positive; false-positive finding in pregnancy or with use of OCPs, confirm with factor V Leiden mutation testing or consider factor V Leiden mutation testing up front.
  - aPC resistance may be unreliable while taking LMWH or UFH.
- Prothrombin G20210A genetic assay
- ATIII functional assay
  - Will be low with acute thrombosis and on heparin therapy; may be falsely high on dabigatran, apixaban, edoxaban, and rivaroxaban
- Protein C functional assay
  - May be low with acute thrombosis; will be lower on warfarin, dabigatran, apixaban, edoxaban, and rivaroxaban
- Protein S antigen and functional assay and free S
  - May be low with acute thrombosis; will be lower on warfarin, dabigatran, apixaban, edoxaban, and rivaroxaban
- Antiphospholipid antibodies: phospholipid-dependent tests and anticardiolipin antibodies, lupus anticoagulant
  - May be unreliable on heparin

- Consider evaluation for subclinical malignancy in an unprovoked thrombosis in those >40 years of age or at greater risk.
- Consider homocysteine level, although treatment of hyperhomocysteinemia (vitamins B$_{12}$ and B$_6$, folate) does not alter the thrombophilic risk.

Follow-Up Tests & Special Considerations
Dysfibrinogenemia and plasminogen deficiency are very rare causes of thrombophilia.

 TREATMENT

MEDICATION

First Line
- Newer oral anticoagulants: Apixaban, dabigatran, edoxaban, and rivaroxaban are now recommended over vitamin K antagonists for long-term oral anticoagulation (5)[B].
- Parenteral anticoagulation: LMWH has largely replaced UFH as first-line therapy for VTE.
  - Enoxaparin (Lovenox): 1 mg/kg SC BID for at least 5 days (with concomitant warfarin) until international normalized ratio (INR) has reached 2 for at least 24 hours; adjust dose for renal disease.
    - Enoxaparin is preferred in patients with active cancer for a minimum of 6 months (can dose at 1.5 mg/kg SC daily), after which time the patient can be reevaluated to continue treatment (4).
    - Adverse reactions: bleeding, heparin-induced thrombocytopenia (HIT) <0.5% incidence, bone loss (uncommon)
    - Reversal: Stop LMWH.
  - UFH: 80 U/kg or 5,000 U IV bolus, then 18 U/kg/hr or 1,000 U/hr to target the activated partial thromboplastin time (aPTT) to a corresponding anti-Xa level of 0.3 to 0.7 U/mL. The first aPTT should be checked 6 hours after initial therapy and adjusted per standard heparin nomograms, aiming for an adequate level within 24 hours. Transition to warfarin is similar to the recommendations for enoxaparin.
    - SC UFH is an alternative and can be given as 5,000 U IV (once) followed by 250 U/kg SC BID, or 250 U/kg bolus followed by 250 U/kg BID (monitored as for IV UFH), or 333 U/kg once followed by 250 U/kg SC BID (unmonitored).
    - Adverse reactions: bleeding, HIT 3% incidence, bone loss (long-term use)
    - Reversal: Stop heparin and protamine.
- Oral factor Xa inhibitors
  - Rivaroxaban (Xarelto): 15 mg BID for 21 days and then 20 mg once daily; not recommended in morbidly obese patients due to lack of data (5)[C]
  - Apixaban (Eliquis): 10 mg BID for 7 days and then 5 mg BID; can be used without need for preceding heparin therapy, less renal clearance than other oral anticoagulants
  - Edoxaban (Savaysa): 60 mg daily. Requires treatment with heparin for 5 days prior to initiation, needs adjustment for renal impairment. Not recommended if creatinine clearance >95 mL/min. Adjust dose to 30 mg in patients <60 kg or if using verapamil, quinidine, macrolides, or oral antifungals.
- Direct thrombin inhibitors
  - Dabigatran (Pradaxa): 150 mg BID after 5 to 10 days of parenteral anticoagulation. Reversal agent: idarucizumab (Andexanet) newly available; may be dialyzable (5)[C]

- Vitamin K antagonist
  - Warfarin (Coumadin): 10 mg/day initially and adjust to INR 2 to 3 for at least 3 months, potentially indefinitely in those with high risk of recurrence, recurrent or unprovoked VTE
    - Warfarin requires careful and frequent monitoring because of many drug–drug and drug–diet (e.g., vitamin K) interactions.
    - Adverse reactions: bleeding, skin necrosis (rare and early in course)
    - Reversal: four-factor prothrombin complex concentrate (PCC); fresh frozen plasma and/or vitamin K
- Pregnancy: low-dose aspirin and/or LMWH or UFH; warfarin is contraindicated.

Second Line
Usually indicated when contraindication to heparin or LMWH, such as heparin-associated thrombosis and thrombocytopenia, if there is an inability to use IV drugs, or renal failure. Direct oral anticoagulants may become first line as more clinical experience is developed.
- Factor Xa inhibitors
  - Fondaparinux (Arixtra): acute VTE/PE. Weight <50 kg: 5 mg/day SC; weight 50 to 100 kg: 7.5 mg/day SC; weight >100 kg: 10 mg/day SC; use for 5 to 9 days until oral anticoagulation is therapeutic.
    - Prophylaxis: 2.5 mg/day SC
    - Dose adjustments: needed for renal insufficiency; if creatinine clearance is <30 mL/min, use is contraindicated.
- Direct thrombin inhibitors:
  - Argatroban: liver metabolized; may be dose adjusted in liver dysfunction; therapeutic dose based on aPTT

SURGERY/OTHER PROCEDURES
- Consider systemic thrombolysis for unstable cases (e.g., massive PE with hypotension).
- Inferior vena cava filter
  - Reduces short-term risk of PE in those with contraindications to anticoagulation (e.g., GI bleeding, cerebral hemorrhage)
  - May increase long-term risk of recurrent DVT
  - Used for patients with multiple episodes of recurrent thromboembolism despite therapeutic anticoagulation and contraindication to anticoagulation

 ONGOING CARE

FOLLOW-UP RECOMMENDATIONS
Avoid significant risk for trauma (e.g., contact sports, climbing a ladder).

Patient Monitoring
Monitor warfarin as frequently as needed to maintain an INR goal of 2 to 3.

DIET
Vitamin K–stable diet if patient is taking warfarin

PATIENT EDUCATION
- Assume that any drug may enhance or attenuate the warfarin effect.
- Increase the frequency of monitoring following any medication change to ensure therapeutic anticoagulation and to avoid overanticoagulation, especially with antibiotics.
- Many drugs may modulate warfarin effect: alcohol, antibiotics, aspirin, NSAIDs, acetaminophen.

PROGNOSIS
- Anticoagulation should be continued for 3 months and consideration of longer in those with unprovoked VTE.
- Patients with a provoked VTE (i.e., surgery, hospitalization) not receiving chronic anticoagulation have risks of recurrence of 7% (year 1), 16% (year 5), and 23% (year 10).
- Patients with an unprovoked VTE not receiving chronic anticoagulation have risks of recurrence of 15% (year 1), 41% (year 5), and 53% (year 10).
- Currently, there are no data from randomized, controlled trials or controlled clinical trials about the benefits of thrombophilia testing to decrease the risk of recurrent VTE (1).

COMPLICATIONS
Venous or arterial thrombosis; bleeding in anticoagulated patients

REFERENCES
1. Heit J. Epidemiology of venous thromboembolism. *Nat Rev Cardiol*. 2015;12(8):464–474.
2. Baglin T, Gray E, Greaves M, et al; for British Committee for Standards in Haematology. Clinical guidelines for testing for heritable thrombophilia. *Br J Haematol*. 2010;149(2):209–220.
3. Anderson JA, Weitz JI. Hypercoagulable states. *Clin Chest Med*. 2010;31(4):659–673.
4. Hill J, Treasure T; for National Clinical Guideline Centre for Acute and Chronic Conditions. Reducing the risk of venous thromboembolism in patients admitted to hospital: summary of NICE guidance. *BMJ*. 2010;340:c95.
5. Kearon C, Akl EA, Ornelas J, et al. Antithrombotic therapy for VTE disease: CHEST Guideline and Expert Panel Report. *Chest*. 2016;149(2):315–352.

ADDITIONAL READING
Stevens SM, Woller SC, Bauer KA, et al. Guidance for the evaluation and treatment of hereditary and acquired thrombophilia. *J Thromb Thrombolysis*. 2016;41(1):154–164.

CODES

ICD10
- D68.59 Other primary thrombophilia
- D68.51 Activated protein C resistance
- D68.2 Hereditary deficiency of other clotting factors

CLINICAL PEARLS
- Factor V Leiden (resistance to aPC) is the most common inherited thrombophilia, with a prevalence of 2–7% in the U.S. Caucasian population.
- Test patients for thrombophilias only if it will affect management of the condition.
- Rule out malignancy, especially in those >50 years of age.

THROMBOTIC THROMBOCYTOPENIC PURPURA

Samata Pathireddy, MD • Narothama Reddy Aeddula, MD, FACP, FASN • Krishna M. Baradhi, MD

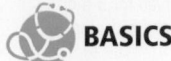 BASICS

DESCRIPTION

- An acute syndrome of microangiopathic hemolytic anemia (MAHA) and consumptive thrombocytopenia with deposition of hyaline thrombi in terminal arterioles and capillaries leading to ischemic multiorgan damage
- Thrombotic thrombocytopenic purpura (TTP) is characterized by MAHA (schistocytes on peripheral smear) and thrombocytopenia (generally <30 K), with or without the following signs and symptoms:
  - Neurologic symptoms
  - Renal dysfunction
  - Fever
  - Most patients do not show the historic pentad of MAHA, thrombocytopenia, renal dysfunction, neurologic abnormalities, and fever because treatment is initiated before the pentad can develop.

EPIDEMIOLOGY

Incidence
- First episode mostly in adulthood (~90%) and in 10% childhood to adolescence (1)
- Predominant sex: female > male (2:1), (1)
- Incidence ratio in blacks to whites is 7:1.
- Annual prevalence of ~10 cases per million people and an annual incidence of ~1 new case per million people (1)

ETIOLOGY AND PATHOPHYSIOLOGY
- In TTP, the aggregating agent responsible for platelet thrombi is unusually large von Willebrand factor (UL vWF) multimers, which are far larger than those found in normal plasma.
- A metalloproteinase, ADAMTS13, which normally enzymatically cleaves UL vWF multimers to prevent clumping within vessels, is deficient, defective, or absent, allowing UL vWF to react with platelets. This leads to the endothelial cell damage and disseminated thrombi characteristic of TTP.
- Arterioles most often affected are in the brain, kidney, pancreas, heart, and adrenal glands. Lungs and liver are relatively spared.
- In familial TTP, patients have an inherited deficiency of ADAMTS13.
- In acquired idiopathic TTP, autoantibodies are directed against the metalloproteinase ADAMTS13 (1,2).
- Endothelial injury, either directly from a drug/toxin or indirectly via platelet/neutrophil activation, has been proposed as a cause of secondary TTP especially in those without ADAMTS13 deficiency.
  - Drug induced (see "Risk Factors")
  - Hematopoietic cell transplantation

Genetics
- TTP is most often an acquired disorder. A congenital form of inherited TTP (Upshaw-Schulman syndrome) is due to a mutation at the ADAMTS13 metalloproteinase gene locus on chromosome 9q34. This rare form of TTP has an autosomal-recessive pattern of inheritance.
- SUS typically presents in infancy and is rarely diagnosed after 10 years of age, it does not have the female predominance seen in idiopathic TTP, more often has notable renal impairment, and there is some heterogeneity among siblings, although parents who are carriers of a single heterozygous ADAMTS13 mutation are typically asymptomatic.

RISK FACTORS
- Pregnancy and oral contraceptives
- AIDS and early symptomatic HIV infection
- Bacterial infection/sepsis
- Acute pancreatitis
- Autoimmune disease
  - Antiphospholipid antibody syndrome
  - Systemic lupus erythematosus
  - Scleroderma
- Cancer
- Hematopoietic stem cell transplantation
- Solid organ transplant
- Drugs of abuse: MDMA, cocaine, oxymorphone ER
- Drug toxicity
  - Antimicrobials
    - Trimethoprim, ciprofloxacin, famciclovir
  - Cancer chemotherapy
    - Mitomycin C and gemcitabine
    - Pentostatin and vincristine
    - Bleomycin and cisplatin
    - Oxaliplatin
    - Bevacizumab and Sunitinib
    - Adalimumab
    - Bortezomib, carfilzomib, and ixazomib
  - Calcineurin inhibitors
    - Tacrolimus and cyclosporine
  - Immune mediated
    - Quinine and quinidine
    - Ticlopidine and clopidogrel

COMMONLY ASSOCIATED CONDITIONS
- TTP/hemolytic uremic syndrome (HUS)/atypical HUS have similar presentations with MAHA and thrombocytopenia and multiorgan involvement.
- TTP generally presents with minimal renal involvement and may have neurologic abnormalities, whereas the opposite is more characteristic of HUS/atypical HUS. Creatinine of >2.3 is suggestive against TTP.
- However, patients with HUS and TTP may have both prominent renal and neurologic manifestations, often making the diagnosis unclear, hence the historical hybrid name "TTP-HUS."
- ADAMTS13 levels are diminished (generally <10%) in adults with familial or acquired idiopathic TTP but are normal in children diagnosed with HUS following infection with *Escherichia coli* (particularly type O157:H7), so-called Shiga toxin-HUS, and in "atypical HUS," is also called complement-mediated thrombotic microangiopathy reflecting the pathophysiology which is related to complement dysregulation.

Dx DIAGNOSIS

- Most common symptoms are nonspecific: nausea, vomiting, weakness, abdominal pain, fatigue, fever.
- Related to thrombocytopenia
  - Easy bruising, purpura, or petechiae
  - Epistaxis, menorrhagia, bleeding gums
  - GI bleeding
  - Intracranial hemorrhage
  - Visual symptoms due to retinal hemorrhage
- Related to hemolytic anemia (MAHA): jaundice, fatigue
- Related to end-organ ischemia
  - Neurologic: CNS symptoms occur in 50%.
    - Often fluctuating symptoms
    - Headache
    - Altered mental status: Spectrum runs from behavioral/personality changes—obtundation/stupor/coma.
    - Seizures, stroke
  - Renal: hematuria, oliguria, or anuria
  - Cardiac: arrhythmia, myocardial infarction, heart failure
  - A scoring system (PLASMIC) devised to predict ADAMTS13 activity <10% in adults (to support the diagnosis of TTP);1 point each for:
    - Platelet count <30,000/μL
    - Hemolysis (reticulocyte count >2.5%, undetectable haptoglobin, or indirect bilirubin >2 mg/dL)
    - No active cancer
    - No solid organ or stem cell transplant
    - MCV <90 fL
    - INR <1.5
- Creatinine <2.0 mg/dL
  - Score 6 to 7 predictive of ADAMTS13 activity of <10%. Score of 0 to 4 predictive of ADAMTS13 activity was not <10%.

HISTORY
- Generally acute onset of symptoms but subacute in about 1/4 of patients
- It is important to assess for potential underlying causes or risk factors (see discussion earlier).
- In about 50% of cases, a trigger/risk factor of some kind is identified (3).

PHYSICAL EXAM
- Fever
- Mental status/neurologic: confusion, coma, stupor, weakness
- HEENT: retinal hemorrhage, scleral icterus, epistaxis
- Abdomen/GI: nonspecific tenderness
- Skin: jaundice, petechiae, purpura, ecchymoses

DIFFERENTIAL DIAGNOSIS
- HUS and atypical HUS
- Antiphospholipid antibody syndrome: prolonged partial thromboplastin time (PTT) and presence of lupus anticoagulant
- Systemic lupus erythematosus
- Malignant hypertension (HTN): diastolic >130 mm Hg, papilledema, retinal hemorrhages
- Pregnancy-associated preeclampsia/eclampsia or hemolysis, elevated liver enzyme levels, and low platelet HELLP levels: low ATIII levels
- Disseminated intravascular coagulation
  - Prolonged prothrombin time (PT)/PTT, low fibrinogen, low factors V and VIII
  - Secondary to sepsis/shock or widely disseminated malignancy
- Idiopathic thrombocytopenic purpura (ITP)
  - No hemolysis, normal lactate dehydrogenase (LDH) and bilirubin
  - Presence of antiplatelet antibodies
- Malignancy-associated microangiopathy
- Evan syndrome (autoimmune hemolytic anemia and thrombocytopenia): positive direct Coombs test
- Sclerodermal kidney

DIAGNOSTIC TESTS & INTERPRETATION

Initial Tests (lab, imaging)
- CBC
  - Hemoglobin (decreased): Average is 8 to 10 g/dL.
  - Platelets decreased: in the 10 to 30,000 range
- High reticulocyte count (>120 × 10⁹/L)
- Undetectable haptoglobin (hemolysis)

- Peripheral smear
  - Schistocytes (prominent, >1% of RBCs)
  - Helmet cells, RBC fragments
  - Nucleated RBCs
  - Polychromasia (reticulocytosis)
- Coagulation studies
  - Normal in most; mild elevation in 15%
  - Fibrinogen normal
- Coombs test: negative direct Coombs test
- Electrolytes, BUN/creatinine: mild elevation of BUN and creatinine (creatinine <3 mg/dL)
- Liver function studies: increased indirect bilirubin (hemolysis)
- LDH: 5 to 10 times normal
- Urinalysis
  - Proteinuria, microscopic hematuria
  - Positive dipstick for large blood but minimal RBCs on microscopic exam
- ECG changes (10%): sinus tachycardia, heart block
- Stool for Shiga toxin
- Increased troponin in 60% cases (>0.1 μg/L)
- HIV, hepatitis A, B, C testing: Exclude underlying viral precipitant.
- Pregnancy test
- Pretreatment ADAMTS13 activity level of <10% is useful in distinguishing acquired or familial TTP from other disorders.
- Head CT/MRI scan: in patients with mental status changes to rule out possible intracranial pathology

Test Interpretation
Biopsy of affected organs shows platelet thrombi; however, biopsy is rarely obtained because diagnosis is made on clinical and laboratory findings.

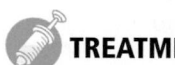 TREATMENT

ALERT
- Prompt treatment of TTP is necessary due to the high mortality (90%).
- Complete response to treatment is defined by a platelet count >150 × 10⁹/L for 2 consecutive days, together with normal or normalizing LDH and clinical recovery (1).
- In the absence of another apparent cause, the dyad of MAHA and thrombocytopenia is sufficient to begin treatment for TTP while the workup proceeds (1,2):
  - Plasma exchange (PEX) transfusion is the cornerstone of treatment of TTP and should begin immediately (2)[A].
  - PEX replaces deficient or defective metalloproteinase (ADAMTS13) and removes UL vWF and antimetalloproteinase antibodies.
  - Optimal PEX duration is variable. Convention is to continue for 2 days after platelet count is ≥150,000 and then consider tapering (4)[C].
  - Fresh frozen plasma: temporary measure until PEX can be initiated (2)[B]; should be reserved for those with active bleeding

MEDICATION
First Line
- Glucocorticoids has adjunctive benefit in some patients. British guidelines recommend its use for all patients (5)[B].
  - Steroids may work by suppressing the autoantibodies inhibiting ADAMTS13 activity.
  - Use may be in patients with severe ADAMTS13 deficiency, in the setting of exacerbation when PEX is stopped or in relapse after remission.

- Little benefit of steroids when used as monotherapy
  - Doses: prednisone 1 to 2 mg/kg/day and taper once in remission or methylprednisolone 1 g/day IV for 3 days
- Rituximab, an anti-CD20 antibody that deletes B cells, may reduce relapse when given in conjunction with PEX and steroids.
  - Dose: 375 mg/m² IV weekly for 4 weeks

Second Line
The following medications are used in refractory cases:
- Rituximab (5)[B]
- Vincristine, cyclophosphamide, cyclosporine
- Intravenous immunoglobulin (IVIG) (2)
- Bortezomib (5)[C]
- Caplacizumab, an inhibitor of VWF-glycoprotein 1b interaction
- Jehovah's witness patients can be treated with steroids plus rituximab.

ISSUES FOR REFERRAL
- Hematology or blood bank for PEX
- Nephrology for dialysis
- Cardiology for presence of significant heart block or ischemia
- Neurosurgery for intracranial hemorrhage

SURGERY/OTHER PROCEDURES
Splenectomy is reserved for severe, refractory cases (1).

ADMISSION, INPATIENT, AND NURSING CONSIDERATIONS
- ABCs, oxygen, IV access, telemetry
- Volume resuscitation if hypotensive/actively bleeding
- Packed RBCs can be transfused safely.
- Platelet transfusion may be used for the treatment of hemorrhage.
- Discharge on normalization and stabilization of neurologic symptoms, LDH, platelets, and renal function

 ONGOING CARE

FOLLOW-UP RECOMMENDATIONS
- Maintenance therapy is not required. After PEX is discontinued, blood counts should be monitored for months. If results remain normal, testing interval can be lengthened.
- Promptly evaluate any relapse symptoms.

PATIENT EDUCATION
- On discharge, advise patients to self-monitor for signs of relapse (e.g., fever, headache, bruising).
- Patients should be advised about prolonged periods of fatigue following the acute phase.
- See National Heart, Lung, and Blood Institute Web site: http://www.nhlbi.nih.gov/health/health-topics/topics/ttp

PROGNOSIS
- Most recover fully from idiopathic TTP when treated promptly:
  - 30-day mortality is 10% in those who receive PEX.
  - 70% respond within 14 days; 90% respond within 28 days.
  - 80% survival in idiopathic TTP treated with PEX (1)
- Prior to widespread PEX treatment, TTP carried up to a 90% mortality rate.
- Initial LDH and platelet counts are not predictive of response to treatment.
- Final platelet count and LDH or the length or intensity of treatment does not predict relapse.

- Low levels of ADAMTS13 activity during remission are associated with higher risk of relapse (1).
- In patients with severe ADAMTS13 deficiency, the risk of relapse is estimated to be 41% at 7.5 years, with the greatest risk being in the 1st year.
- In patients with autoimmune TTP, there is a 40% relapse rate (3).

COMPLICATIONS
- Patients may experience mild cognitive impairments in attention, concentration, and memory following ≥1 episode of TTP.
- Complications of PEX include the following:
  - Central line infections and hemorrhage
  - Citrate toxicity
  - Hypersensitivity reactions to frequent plasma exposure
  - Electrolyte abnormalities

REFERENCES
1. Joly BS, Coppo P, Veyradier A. Thrombotic thrombocytopenic purpura. *Blood*. 2017;129(21):2836–2846.
2. George JN. Clinical practice. Thrombotic thrombocytopenic purpura. *N Engl J Med*. 2006;354(18):1927–1935.
3. Saha M, McDaniel JK, Zheng XL. Thrombotic thrombocytopenic purpura: pathogenesis, diagnosis and potential novel therapeutics. *J Thromb Haemost*. 2017;15(10):1889–1900.
4. Scully M, Hunt BJ, Benjamin S, et al; for British Committee for Standards in Haematology. Guidelines on the diagnosis and management of thrombotic thrombocytopenic purpura and other thrombotic microangiopathies. *Br J Haematol*. 2012;158(3):323–335.
5. Sarode R, Bandarenko N, Brecher ME, et al. Thrombotic thrombocytopenic purpura: 2012 American Society for Apheresis (ASFA) consensus conference on classification, diagnosis, management, and future research. *J Clin Apher*. 2014;29(3):148–167.

ADDITIONAL READING
George JN, Nester CM. Syndromes of thrombotic microangiopathy. *N Engl J Med*. 2014;371(7):654–666.

CODES
ICD10
- M31.1 Thrombotic microangiopathy
- D69.42 Congenital and hereditary thrombocytopenia purpura
- D69.3 Immune thrombocytopenic purpura

CLINICAL PEARLS
- The diagnosis of TTP is made clinically; common symptoms are nonspecific: nausea; vomiting; weakness; abdominal pain; fatigue; fever; and easy bruising, purpura, or petechiae.
- The historical pentad of fever, neurologic symptoms, renal dysfunction, MAHA, and thrombocytopenia is not present in most patients.
- The dyad of MAHA (schistocytes on peripheral smear) and severe thrombocytopenia (<30 K) is sufficient to initiate treatment with PEX.
- Do not wait for results of ADAMTS13 determination to initiate therapy.

THYROID MALIGNANT NEOPLASIA

Hannan Qureshi, MD • Yousef Ahmed, MD • Matthew E. Herberg, MD

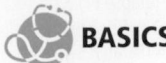

BASICS

DESCRIPTION
Thyroid malignant neoplasia is an uncontrolled proliferation of cells within the thyroid gland. There are several different types:

- Papillary thyroid carcinoma (PTC)
  - Differentiated tumor with papillary cells with finger-like projections
  - Most common variety, 75–80% of thyroid cancers
  - Peak incidence in the 3rd or 4th decade of life
  - Approximately 3 times more common in women
  - Associated with radiation exposure
  - Metastasizes by lymphatic route (15–30% have palpable lymphadenopathy at time of diagnosis)
  - Multicentric in ≥20%, especially in children
  - Increasing incidence may be due to increased diagnosis of smaller size tumors
  - Many subtypes: conventional, follicular variant, oxyphilic, cribriform-morular, and more aggressive forms such as tall cell or diffuse sclerosing
- Follicular carcinoma
  - Differentiated tumor with spherical follicular cells
  - Second most common variety, 10–20% of thyroid tumors
  - Peak incidence in 5th decade of life
  - Metastasizes by the hematogenous route
  - Can be divided into invasive and minimally invasive forms based on morphology
- Hürthle cell carcinoma (variant of follicular with poorer prognosis)
  - Often considered subtype of FTC with overall poorer prognosis
  - Also known as oncocytic or oxyphilic carcinoma
  - 2–3% of thyroid malignancies
  - Usually in patients >60 years old
  - Often radioresistant
- Medullary thyroid carcinoma (MTC)
  - Neuroendocrine tumor arising from parafollicular C cells
  - 3–4% of all thyroid carcinoma
  - 75–80% sporadic and occurs as isolated disease
  - 25–35% are associated with multiple endocrine neoplasia (MEN) syndromes, which can be familial or sporadic.
  - MTC associated with MEN2B occur in childhood, those with MEN2A occur in young adults, and those with familial non-MEN medullary thyroid cancer (FMTC) occur in middle age.
  - Calcitonin is a serologic marker.
  - *RET* proto-oncogene mutation is used for screening; family members who carry the *RET* gene should consider early prophylactic thyroidectomy.
- Anaplastic carcinoma
  - Undifferentiated tumor arising de novo or from dedifferentiation of preexisting differentiated thyroid carcinoma
  - 1–3% of thyroid tumors
  - Most aggressive form of thyroid neoplasia due to rapid growth, locoregional invasion, and metastases
  - Almost uniformly fatal (median survival 2 to 6 months)
  - More common in elderly patients
- Poorly differentiated thyroid carcinoma (PDTC)
  - Intermediate between differentiated (follicular and papillary carcinomas) and undifferentiated (anaplastic) carcinomas
  - Aggressive tumor similar to anaplastic carcinoma, but may have better treatment response

- Other: lymphoma, sarcoma, or metastatic (renal, breast, or lung)
- System(s) affected: endocrine/metabolic
- Synonym(s): well-differentiated, poorly differentiated, and undifferentiated thyroid carcinoma

Geriatric Considerations
Risk of malignancy (ROM) increases, and prognosis is worse >60 years old.

Pediatric Considerations
- Thyroid nodules are more frequently malignant (22–25% in children vs. 5–10% in adults).
- <2% of thyroid malignancies occur in children and adolescents.
- Increased tumor size (>4 cm), extrathyroidal extension, and multifocal disease are independent factors associated with nodal metastases in pediatric differentiated thyroid cancer and require further evaluation with FNA for suspicious nodes to consider neck dissection (1)[C].

EPIDEMIOLOGY
- Incidence: 14.5/100,000 per year in the United States
- Deaths: 0.5/100,000 per year in the United States
- In 2018, estimated 53,990 new cases and 2,060 deaths from thyroid cancer in the United States
- Predominant age: usually >40 years old
- Predominant sex: female > male (3:1) prevalence
- Lifetime risk of developing thyroid cancer is 1.2%.
- In 2015, 765,547 patients living with thyroid cancer in the United States

ETIOLOGY AND PATHOPHYSIOLOGY
- No established etiologic factors of pathogenesis; most cases arise spontaneously.
- Radiation exposure likely has a role in the development of thyroid malignancies.
- Gene mutations that activate the MAPK pathway (e.g., *BRAF*) and PI3K-AKT pathway (e.g., PTEN) have been implicated.

Genetics
- Familial polyposis of the colon, Gardner syndrome with the *APC* gene (5q21), and Cowden syndrome
- MTC: autosomal dominant with MEN syndrome
- Medullary: autosomal dominant with MEN syndrome
- *BRAF* mutation (rare in children) in PTC
- *RAS* mutations in FTC
- *RET* oncogene (more common in children) in MTC and PTC
- *TP53* mutation in ATC

RISK FACTORS
- Family history (first-degree relative)
- Radiation exposure: papillary carcinoma
- Iodine deficiency: follicular carcinoma
- MEN2: medullary carcinoma; autosomal dominant inheritance; *RET* proto-oncogene
- Previous history of subtotal thyroidectomy for malignancy: anaplastic carcinoma
- Female gender

GENERAL PREVENTION
- Physical exam in high-risk group
- Calcitonin stimulation screening in high-risk MEN patients
- Screening for *RET* proto-oncogene in groups at risk for MTC

COMMONLY ASSOCIATED CONDITIONS
- Papillary carcinoma: Hashimoto thyroiditis
- Medullary carcinoma: pheochromocytoma, hyperparathyroidism, ganglioneuroma of the GI tract, neuromata of mucosal membranes

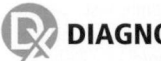

DIAGNOSIS

HISTORY
- Change in voice (dysphonia)
- Difficulty swallowing (dysphagia)
- Difficulty breathing (dyspnea)
- Stridor (in aggressive cancer)
- Growing neck mass
- Positive family history
- History of radiation exposure (environmental or radiation therapy for childhood cancer)

PHYSICAL EXAM
- Thyroid nodule/mass
- Fixation to surrounding tissues suggests malignancy.
- Cervical lymphadenopathy

DIFFERENTIAL DIAGNOSIS
- Multinodular goiter
- Thyroid adenoma
- Thyroglossal duct or dermoid cyst
- Thyroiditis
- Thyroid cyst
- Ectopic thyroid

DIAGNOSTIC TESTS & INTERPRETATION
Initial Tests (lab, imaging)
- Ultrasound (US): Nodule characteristics suggestive of malignancy include hypoechoic pattern, microcalcifications, irregular margins, and shape taller than wide (2)[A].
- Thyroid-stimulating hormone (TSH): usually normal in the setting of malignancy but recommended for all nodule workup

Follow-Up Tests & Special Considerations
- CT and MRI neck: useful to evaluate large substernal masses, extent of invasion for fixed bulky tumors, if suspicion of MTC with neck disease or calcitonin >400 pg/mL, and to evaluate for recurrent disease
- Calcitonin levels: Measure in patients with FNA results or with personal or family history of MEN2 syndrome suggestive of MTC (consider IV pentagastrin stimulation test to increase sensitivity).
- *RET* proto-oncogene gene analysis: if concerned for MTC
- Thyroid scan: 12–15% of cold nodules are malignant; rate is higher in patients <40 years of age and those with microcalcifications on US. ^{18}F-FDG positron-emission tomographic scan can help if the cytology is indeterminant; also helpful with recurrent disease when patient has a negative ^{131}I scan and an elevated thyroglobulin (TG) level (3)[B]
- TG: not recommended in initial evaluation but used as postoperative tumor marker for recurrence

Diagnostic Procedures/Other
- Fine-needle aspiration biopsy (FNAB)
- Flexible fiberoptic laryngoscopy: if vocal cord paralysis is suspected and in high-risk disease

Test Interpretation
- FNAB: The 2017 Bethesda System for Reporting Thyroid Cytopathology classification of cytology
  - Nondiagnostic or unsatisfactory
  - Benign: 0–3% ROM
  - Atypia of undetermined significance (AUS) or follicular lesion of undetermined significance (FLUS): 10–30% ROM
  - Follicular neoplasm or suspicious for a follicular neoplasm: 25-40% ROM
  - Suspicious for malignancy: 50–75% ROM
  - Malignant: 97–99% ROM
- Papillary: psammoma bodies, anaplastic epithelial papillae
- Follicular: anaplastic epithelial cords with follicles
- Hürthle cell: large eosinophilic cells with granular cytoplasm
- Medullary: large amounts of amyloid stroma
- Anaplastic: small cell and giant cell undifferentiated tumors

 ## TREATMENT

GENERAL MEASURES
- Most cases of thyroid cancer are managed surgically and medically with a good prognosis (2)[A].
- Palliative support has a role in case of advanced thyroid malignancy (4)[C].
- Papillary and follicular: ^{131}I thyroid remnant ablation
- Medullary: Vandetanib, and other tyrosine kinase inhibitors, have been tried in patients with advanced disease (5)[B].
- Anaplastic: Doxorubicin and cisplatin have achieved partial remission in some patients.

MEDICATION
Postoperatively, will require thyroid hormone replacement after total thyroidectomy
- Thyroxine suppression therapy may reduce recurrence with goal to keep TSH <0.1 mU/L for high-risk patients, 0.1 to 0.5 mU/L for intermediate-risk patients, and 0.5 to 2.0 mU/L for low-risk patients (2)[A].
- Levothyroxine (T_4, Synthroid)
- Liothyronine (T_3, Cytomel)

ADDITIONAL THERAPIES
- External beam radiation or chemotherapy may be considered for radioactive iodine insensitive tumors, inoperable recurrence, and for palliative care.
- ^{131}I is used in high-risk patients with papillary and follicular tumors. The role is to ablate remnant thyroid tissue to improve specificity of future TG assays to monitor for recurrence. Patients are taken off thyroid suppression therapy for 2 to 4 weeks before scanning and are often placed on a low-iodine diet for 14 days prior to therapy.

SURGERY/OTHER PROCEDURES
- Papillary: total thyroidectomy with elective neck dissection for suspicious lymph nodes in central or lateral neck compartments or for large tumors (>4 cm in size). Lobectomy with isthmectomy can be considered if lesion <1 cm in low-risk patient (controversial).
- Follicular and Hürthle cell: similar management as papillary carcinoma

- Medullary: total thyroidectomy with central node dissection; unilateral or bilateral modified radical neck dissection if lateral nodes are suspicious
- Anaplastic: palliative care; no adequate treatment available and surgery is controversial. Consider tracheostomy (protect airway) and clinical trials utilizing chemotherapy/radiation.

 ## ONGOING CARE

FOLLOW-UP RECOMMENDATIONS
Patient Monitoring
- 10–30% of initially disease-free patients will develop recurrence and/or metastases. 80% recur in neck and 20% with distant metastases. Lung is most common site of distant metastases.
- TSH, TG, and anti-TG antibodies at 6 months, 12 months, and then yearly after that for surveillance (6)[C]
- Periodic US to monitor for recurrence is recommended in intermediate- to high-risk patients and may also consider TSH-stimulated radioiodine whole body imaging in high-risk patients (6)[C].
- Medullary: Calcitonin level should be done yearly with pentagastrin stimulation.
- The thyroid scan and TG level should be done with the patient in the hypothyroid state induced by 6-week withdrawal of levothyroxine or 2- to 3-week withdrawal of liothyronine.

DIET
Low-iodine diet recommended in patients undergoing radioactive iodine therapy following surgery for thyroid cancer

PATIENT EDUCATION
- National Cancer Institute: https://www.cancer.gov /types/thyroid/patient/thyroid-treatment-pdq
- American Thyroid Association: https://www.thyroid .org/thyroid-information/
- National Comprehensive Cancer Network: https://www.nccn.org/professionals/physician_gls /pdf/thyroid.pdf

PROGNOSIS
- 5-year survival of thyroid cancer is 98.1%.
- Adverse factors: age >45 years, primary tumor >4 cm, extrathyroid extension, distant metastases
- Low risk: no extrathyroidal invasion, all macroscopic tumor resected, no local or distant metastases, no vascular invasion, and no aggressive tumor histology
- Intermediate risk: microscopic extrathyroidal invasion, cervical lymph node metastases on ^{131}I update outside of thyroid bed on first whole body after remnant ablation
- High risk: macroscopic extrathyroidal tumor invasion, incomplete tumor resection, distant metastases
- Papillary carcinoma: 10-year overall survival is 93%; 30-year cancer-related death rate of 6%
- Follicular carcinoma: 10-year overall survival is 85%; histologically, microinvasive tumors parallel papillary tumor results, whereas grossly invasive tumors do far worse; 30-year cancer-related death rate of 15%
- Hürthle cell carcinoma: 93% 5-year survival rate and 83% survival rate overall; grossly invasive tumor survival <25%

- Medullary carcinoma: negative nodes, 90% 5-year survival rate and 85% 10-year survival rate; with positive nodes, 65% 5-year survival rate and 40% 10-year survival rate. Prognosis worse for MEN2B compared to MEN2A. Overall, 10-year survival is 75%.
- Anaplastic carcinoma: survival unexpected. Long-term survivors should have original pathology reexamined.

COMPLICATIONS
- Hoarseness either from tumor invasion or iatrogenic injury to recurrent laryngeal nerve
- Hypocalcemia/hypoparathyroidism from devascularization of parathyroid glands during surgery (usually transient)

REFERENCES
1. Francis GL, Waguespack SG, Bauer AJ, et al; for American Thyroid Association Guidelines Task Force. Management guidelines for children with thyroid nodules and differentiated thyroid cancer. *Thyroid*. 2015;25(7):716–759.
2. Haugen BR, Alexander EK, Bible KC, et al. 2015 American Thyroid Association management guidelines for adult patients with thyroid nodules and differentiated thyroid cancer: the American Thyroid Association Guidelines Task Force on thyroid nodules and differentiated thyroid cancer. *Thyroid*. 2016;26(1):1–133.
3. de Koster EJ, de Geus-Oei LF, Dekkers OM, et al. Diagnostic utility of molecular and imaging biomarkers in cytological indeterminate thyroid nodules. *Endocr Rev*. 2018;39(2):154–191.
4. Goyal A, Gupta R, Mehmood S, et al. Palliative and end of life care issues of carcinoma thyroid patient. *Indian J Palliat Care*. 2012;18(2):134–137.
5. Wells SA Jr, Robinson BG, Gagel RF, et al. Vandetanib in patients with locally advanced or metastatic medullary thyroid cancer: a randomized, double-blind phase III trial. *J Clin Oncol*. 2012;30(2):134–141.
6. National Comprehensive Cancer Network. Thyroid Carcinoma (Version 1.2018). https://www.nccn .org/professionals/physician_gls/pdf/thyroid.pdf. Accessed October 15, 2018.

 ## SEE ALSO

Multiple Endocrine Neoplasia (MEN) Syndromes

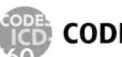 ## CODES

ICD10
C73 Malignant neoplasm of thyroid gland

CLINICAL PEARLS
- Standard workup for a patient suspected of having a thyroid cancer is a physical exam, TSH level, neck US, and FNA.
- TG levels can be elevated in several thyroid disorders. Its usefulness comes once the diagnosis of cancer has been made. It serves as a better marker for recurrent disease.
- FNA results will be benign, malignant, indeterminate, or nondiagnostic. It is very helpful in guiding the initial surgical approach.

THYROIDITIS

Pradeepa P. Vimalachandran, MD, MPH

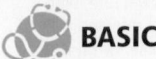

BASICS

DESCRIPTION

Inflammation of the thyroid gland that may be painful or painless and characterized by dysfunction

- Thyroiditis with thyroid pain include
  - Subacute granulomatous thyroiditis (nonsuppurative thyroiditis, de Quervain thyroiditis, or giant cell thyroiditis): self-limited; viral URI prodrome, symptoms and signs of thyroid dysfunction (variable)
  - Infectious/suppurative thyroiditis
- Can be due to bacterial, fungal, mycobacterial, or parasitic infection of the thyroid
- Most commonly associated with *Streptococcus pyogenes*, *Staphylococcus aureus*, and *Streptococcus pneumoniae*
  - Radiation-induced thyroiditis: from radioactive iodine therapy (1%) or external irradiation for lymphoma and head/neck cancers
- Thyroiditis with no thyroid pain include
  - Hashimoto (autoimmune) thyroiditis (chronic lymphocytic thyroiditis): most common etiology of chronic hypothyroidism; autoimmune disease; 90% of patients with high-serum anti-thyroid peroxidase (TPO) antibodies
  - Postpartum thyroiditis: episode of thyrotoxicosis, hypothyroidism, or thyrotoxicosis followed by hypothyroidism in the 1st year postpartum or after spontaneous/induced abortion in women who were without clinically evident thyroid disease before pregnancy
  - Painless (silent) thyroiditis (subacute lymphocytic thyroiditis): mild hyperthyroidism, small painless goiter, and no Graves ophthalmopathy/pretibial myxedema
  - Riedel (fibrous) thyroiditis: rare inflammatory process involving the thyroid and surrounding cervical tissues; associated with various forms of systemic fibrosis; presents as a firm mass in the thyroid commonly associated with compressive symptoms (dyspnea, dysphagia, hoarseness, and aphonia) caused by local infiltration of the advancing fibrotic process with hypocalcemia and hypothyroidism
  - Drug-induced thyroiditis: interferon-α, interleukin-2, amiodarone, kinase inhibitors, or lithium

EPIDEMIOLOGY

- Subacute granulomatous thyroiditis: most common cause of thyroid pain; peaks during summer; incidence: 3/100,000/year; female > male (4:1); peak age: 40 to 50 years
- Suppurative thyroiditis: commonly seen with preexisting thyroid disease/immunocompromise
- Hashimoto thyroiditis: peak age of onset, 30 to 50 years; can occur in children; primarily a disease of women; female > male (7:1)
- Postpartum thyroiditis: female only; occurs within 12 months of pregnancy in 8–11% of pregnancies; occurs in 25% with type 1 diabetes mellitus; incidence is affected by genetic influences and iodine intake.
- Painless (silent) thyroiditis: accounts for 1–5% of cases; female > male (4:1) with peak age 30 to 40 years; common in areas of iodine sufficiency
- Riedel thyroiditis: female > male (4:1); highest prevalence age 30 to 60 years

ETIOLOGY AND PATHOPHYSIOLOGY

- Hashimoto disease: Antithyroid antibodies may be produced in response to an environmental antigen and cross-react with thyroid proteins (molecular mimicry). Precipitating factors include infection, stress, sex steroids, pregnancy, iodine intake, and radiation exposure.
- Subacute granulomatous thyroiditis: probably viral
- Postpartum thyroiditis: autoimmunity-induced discharge of preformed hormone from the thyroid
- Painless (silent) thyroiditis: autoimmune

Genetics

Autoimmune thyroiditis is associated with the CT60 polymorphism of cytotoxic T-cell lymphocyte–associated antigen 4; also associated with HLA-DR4, HLA-DR5, and HLA-DR6 in whites

RISK FACTORS

- Hashimoto disease: family history of thyroid/autoimmune disease, personal history of autoimmune disease (type 1 diabetes, celiac disease), high iodine intake, cigarette smoking, selenium deficiency
- Subacute granulomatous thyroiditis: recent viral respiratory infection or HLA-B35
- Suppurative thyroiditis: congenital abnormalities (persistent thyroglossal duct/pyriform sinus fistula), greater age, immunosuppression
- Radiation-induced thyroiditis: high-dose irradiation, younger age, female sex, preexisting hypothyroidism
- Postpartum thyroiditis: smoking, history of spontaneous/induced abortion
- Painless (silent) thyroiditis: iodine-deficient areas

GENERAL PREVENTION

Selenium may decrease inflammatory activity in pregnant women with autoimmune hypothyroidism and may reduce postpartum thyroiditis risk in those positive for TPO antibodies

COMMONLY ASSOCIATED CONDITIONS

Postpartum thyroiditis: family history of autoimmune thyroid disease; HLA-DRB, HLA-DR4, and HLA-DR5

DIAGNOSIS

HISTORY

- Hypothyroid symptoms (e.g., constipation, heavy menstrual bleeding, fatigue, weakness, dry skin, hair loss, cold intolerance)
- Hyperthyroid symptoms (e.g., irritability, heat intolerance, increased sweating, palpitations, loose stools, disturbed sleep, and lid retraction)
- Subacute granulomatous thyroiditis: sudden/gradual onset, with preceding upper respiratory infection/viral illness (fever, fatigue, malaise, anorexia, and myalgia are common); pain may be limited to thyroid region or radiate to upper neck, jaw, throat, or ears.
- Classic triphasic course (thyrotoxic, hypothyroid, recovery) but variable in the following: subacute, silent, and postpartum thyroiditis (1)[C]

PHYSICAL EXAM

- Examine thyroid size, symmetry, and nodules.
  - Hashimoto disease: 90% have a symmetric, diffusely enlarged, painless gland, with a firm, pebbly texture; 10% have thyroid atrophy.
  - Postpartum thyroiditis: painless, small, nontender, firm goiter (2 to 6 months after delivery)

- Riedel thyroiditis: rock-hard, wood-like, fixed, painless goiter, often accompanied by symptoms of esophageal/tracheal compression (stridor, dyspnea, a suffocating feeling, dysphagia, and hoarseness)
- Signs of hypothyroid: delayed relaxation phase of deep tendon reflexes, nonpitting edema, dry skin, alopecia, bradycardia
- Signs of hyperthyroid: moist palms, hyperreflexia, tachycardia/atrial fibrillation

DIFFERENTIAL DIAGNOSIS

Simple goiter; iodine-deficient/lithium-induced goiter; Graves disease; lymphoma; acute infectious thyroiditis; oropharynx and trachea infections; thyroid cancer; amiodarone; contrast dye; amyloid

DIAGNOSTIC TESTS & INTERPRETATION

- Thyroid-stimulating hormone (TSH), anti-TPO antibodies
- Hashimoto disease
  - High titers of anti-TPO antibodies
  - New subtype: IgG4 thyroiditis, which is histopathologically characterized by lymphoplasmacytic infiltration, fibrosis, increased numbers of IgG4-positive plasma cells, and high-serum IgG4 levels; more closely associated with rapid progress, subclinical hypothyroidism, higher levels of circulating antibodies, and more diffuse low echogenicity (2)[C]
- Subacute granulomatous thyroiditis
  - High T_4, T_3; low TSH during early stages and elevated later; TSH varies with phase (1)[C].
  - High thyroglobulin; normal levels of anti-TPO and antithyroglobulin antibodies (present in 25%, usually low titers)
  - Elevated erythrocyte sedimentation rate (ESR) (usually >50 mm/hr) and C-reactive protein; mild anemia and slight leukocytosis; LFTs are frequently abnormal during initial hyperthyroid phase and resolve over 1 to 2 months.
- Suppurative thyroiditis
  - In the absence of preexisting thyroid disease, thyroid function is normal, but hyper-/hypothyroidism may occur.
  - Elevated ESR and WBC with marked increase in left shift
  - Fine-needle aspiration (FNA) of the lesion with Gram stain and culture is the most useful diagnostic test.
- Postpartum thyroiditis (3)[B]
  - Anti-TPO antibody positivity is the most useful marker for the prediction of postpartum thyroid dysfunction.
  - Women known to be anti-TPO-Ab+ should have TSH measured at 6 to 12 weeks' gestation and at 6 months postpartum or as clinically indicated.
  - Thyrotoxic phase occurs 1 and 6 months postpartum (most commonly at 3 months) and usually lasts only 1 to 2 months.
  - Hypothyroidism occurs between 3 and 8 months (most commonly at 6 months).
  - Most patients (80%) have normal thyroid function at 1 year; 30–50% of patients develop permanent hypothyroidism within 9 years.
  - High thyroglobulin, normal ESR
- Painless (silent) thyroiditis
  - Hyperthyroid state in 5–20%: averages 3 to 4 months, and total duration of illness is <1 year, followed by hypothyroidism and then a return to normal state; some have primary/subclinical hypothyroidism.
  - ~50% have anti-TPO antibodies (1)[C].

- Reidel thyroiditis (4)[C]
  - Hypothyroidism due to extensive replacement of the gland by scar tissue. Anti-TPO antibodies are present in 2/3 of patients along with low radioactive iodine uptake (RAIU).
- Drug-induced thyroiditis
  - Hyper-/hypothyroidism, low RAIU, and variable presence of anti-TPO antibodies
- US: shows variable heterogeneous texture, hypoechogenic in subacute, painless (silent), and postpartum thyroiditis
- Thyroid RAIU scan: decreased in all forms of thyroiditis but not helpful in establishing diagnosis of Hashimoto disease; high RAIU in hashitoxicosis, Graves disease
- Random urine iodine measurement may be helpful to distinguish from other causes of low RAIU.
  - Urine iodine <500 μg/L (subacute granulomatous thyroiditis)
  - Urine iodine >1,000 μg/L (in patients with exposure to excess exogenous iodine/radiocontrast material)

Diagnostic Procedures/Other
- Hashimoto with a dominant nodule should have FNA to rule out thyroid carcinoma.
- Open biopsy is necessary for a definitive diagnosis of Reidel thyroiditis.

Test Interpretation
- Hashimoto disease: lymphocytic infiltration with formation of Askanazy (Hürthle) cells, oxyphilic changes in follicular cells, fibrosis, thyroid atrophy
- Subacute granulomatous thyroiditis: giant cells, mononuclear cell (granulomatous) infiltrate
- Postpartum thyroiditis: lymphocytic infiltration, occasional germinal centers, disruption and collapse of thyroid follicles
- Painless (silent) thyroiditis: lymphocytic infiltration, but without fibrosis, Askanazy cells, and extensive lymphoid follicle formation

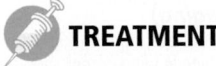 TREATMENT

GENERAL MEASURES
Analgesics for pain; corticosteroids for severe granulomatous thyroiditis

MEDICATION
- Hashimoto disease (2)[C]
  - If hypothyroid/goitrous: levothyroxine (1.7 μg/kg/day for adults <50 years of age); if no cardiac complications and no adrenal insufficiency, 1/2 replacement dose and increase to full replacement in 10 days
    - If >50 years of age or heart disease and/or adrenal insufficiency, begin with 25 μg/day and titrate to TSH of lower limit normal range.
- If thyrotoxic and symptomatic: propylthiouracil and propranolol
- An elevated TSH level in a woman who is pregnant or attempting to become pregnant is an indication for thyroid replacement.
- Subacute granulomatous thyroiditis
  - Anti-inflammatory agents for 2 to 8 weeks (NSAIDs or aspirin)
  - Pain with no improvement in 2 to 3 days after NSAID use: prednisone 40 mg/day; should result in pain relief in 1 to 2 days; if not, question diagnosis.

- Severe pain: prednisone 40 to 60 mg/day discontinued over 4 to 6 weeks. If pain recurs, increase dose for several weeks and then taper.
  - Symptomatic hyperthyroidism: β-blockers while thyrotoxic (propranolol 40 to 120 mg/day)
  - Symptomatic hypothyroid phase: Levothyroxine, as mentioned earlier, target TSH in the normal range.
- Suppurative thyroiditis
  - Parenteral empiric, broad-spectrum antibiotics, and surgical drainage
- Painless (silent) thyroiditis
  - No treatment needed
  - If symptomatic during hyperthyroid state, treat with β-blocker (propranolol 40 to 120 mg/day).
  - Prednisone shortens the period of hyperthyroidism. Monitor TSH every 4 to 8 weeks to confirm resolution.
  - Treat hypothyroid symptoms and asymptomatic patients with TSH >10 mU/L with levothyroxine (50 to 100 μg/day), to be discontinued after 3 to 6 months.
- Postpartum thyroiditis (5)[C]
  - Treat symptomatic hyper-/hypothyroid state. Most do not need treatment.
  - Caution in breastfeeding mothers because β-blockers are secreted into breast milk.
  - For symptomatic hypothyroidism, treat with levothyroxine. Otherwise, remonitor in 4 to 8 weeks. Taper replacement hormone after 6 months if thyroid function has normalized.
- Reidel thyroiditis (4)[C]
  - Corticosteroids in early stages but controversial thereafter; prednisone 10 to 20 mg/day for 4 to 6 months, possibly continued thereafter if effective
  - Long-term anti-inflammatory medications to arrest progression and maintain a symptom-free course
  - Tamoxifen 10 to 20 mg BID as monotherapy or in conjunction with prednisone reduces mass size and clinical symptoms.
  - Methotrexate is used with some success.
  - Reduction of goiter seen with a combination of mycophenolate mofetil (1 g BID) and 100 mg/day prednisone
  - Debulking surgery is limited to isthmusectomy to relieve constrictive pressure when total thyroidectomy is not possible.
- Drug-induced thyroiditis
  - Discontinue offending drug.

SURGERY/OTHER PROCEDURES
Enlarged painful thyroid or tracheal compression

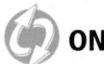 ONGOING CARE

FOLLOW-UP RECOMMENDATIONS
Patient Monitoring
- Hashimoto disease: Repeat thyroid function tests every 3 to 12 months.
- Subacute granulomatous thyroiditis: Repeat thyroid function tests every 3 to 6 weeks until euthyroid and then every 6 to 12 months.
- Postpartum thyroiditis: Check TSH annually.
- Reidel thyroiditis: CT of cervical mediastinal region is recommended.
- TSH every 6 months in patients on amiodarone

Pregnancy Considerations
- Avoid radioisotope scanning if possible.
- Keep TSH maximally suppressed.
- If using RAIU scan, discard breast milk for 2 days because RAI is secreted in breast milk.

PROGNOSIS
- Hashimoto disease: persistent goiter; eventual thyroid failure
- Subacute granulomatous thyroiditis: 5–15% hypothyroid beyond a year: Some with eventual return to normal; remission may be slower in the elderly; recurrence rate: 1–4% after a year
- Painless (silent) thyroiditis: 10–20% hypothyroid beyond a year; recurrence rate 5–10% (much higher in Japan)
- Postpartum thyroiditis: 15–50% hypothyroid beyond a year; women may be euthyroid/continue to be hypothyroid at the end of 1st postpartum year. 70% recurrence rate in subsequent pregnancies; substantial risk exists for later development of hypothyroidism/goiter.

REFERENCES
1. Samuels MH. Subacute, silent, and postpartum thyroiditis. *Med Clin North Am.* 2012;96(2):223–233.
2. Li Y, Nishihara E, Kakudo K. Hashimoto's thyroiditis: old concepts and new insights. *Curr Opin Rheumatol.* 2011;23(1):102–107.
3. De Groot L, Abalovich M, Alexander EK, et al. Management of thyroid dysfunction during pregnancy and postpartum: an Endocrine Society clinical practice guideline. *J Clin Endocrinol Metab.* 2012;97(8):2543–2565. doi:10.1210/jc.2011-2803.
4. Hennessey JV. Clinical review: Riedel's thyroiditis: a clinical review. *J Clin Endocrinol Metab.* 2011;96(10):3031–3041.
5. Reid SM, Middleton P, Cossich MC, et al. Interventions for clinical and subclinical hypothyroidism in pregnancy. *Cochrane Database Syst Rev.* 2010;(7):CD007752.

ADDITIONAL READING
- Duntas LH. Selenium and the thyroid: a close-knit connection. *J Clin Endocrinol Metab.* 2010;95(12):5180–5188.
- Torino F, Corsello SM, Longo R, et al. Hypothyroidism related to tyrosine kinase inhibitors: an emerging toxic effect of targeted therapy. *Nat Rev Clin Oncol.* 2009;6(4):219–228.

 SEE ALSO

Hyperthyroidism; Hypothyroidism, Adult

 CODES

ICD10
- E06.9 Thyroiditis, unspecified
- E06.1 Subacute thyroiditis
- E06.0 Acute thyroiditis

CLINICAL PEARLS
- TSH elevation above the normal range indicates a hypothyroid state; suppressed TSH indicates hyperthyroid state. Follow up with free T_3/T_4 determination.
- Follow patients on thyroid replacement with periodic TSH level.

T

TINEA (CAPITIS, CORPORIS, CRURIS)

Elisabeth L. Backer, MD

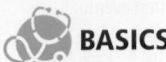 **BASICS**

DESCRIPTION
- Superficial fungal infections of the skin/scalp; various forms of dermatophytosis; the names relate to the particular area affected (1).
  - Tinea cruris: infection of crural fold and gluteal cleft
  - Tinea corporis: infection involving the face, trunk, and/or extremities; often presents with ring-shaped lesions, hence the misnomer *ringworm*
  - Tinea capitis: infection of the scalp and hair; affected areas of the scalp can show characteristic black dots resulting from broken hairs.
- Dermatophytes have the ability to subsist on protein, namely keratin.
- They cause disease in keratin-rich structures such as skin, nails, and hair.
- Infections result from contact with infected persons/animals.
  - Zoophilic infections are acquired from animals.
  - Anthropophilic infections are acquired from personal contact (e.g., wrestling) or fomites.
  - Geophile infections are acquired from the soil.
- System(s) affected: skin, exocrine
- Synonym(s): jock itch; ringworm

EPIDEMIOLOGY
Incidence
- Tinea cruris
  - Predominant age: any age; rare in children
  - Predominant sex: male > female
- Tinea corporis
  - Predominant age: all ages
  - Predominant sex: male = female
- Tinea capitis
  - Predominant age: 3 to 9 years; almost always occurs in young children
  - Predominant sex: male = female

Prevalence
Common worldwide

Pediatric Considerations
- Tinea cruris is rare prior to puberty.
- Tinea capitis is common in young children.

Geriatric Considerations
Tinea cruris is more common in the geriatric population due to an increase in risk factors.

Pregnancy Considerations
Tinea cruris and capitis are rare in pregnancy.

ETIOLOGY AND PATHOPHYSIOLOGY
Superficial fungal infection of skin/scalp
- Tinea cruris: Source of infection is usually the patient's own tinea pedis, with agent being transferred from the foot to the groin via the underwear when dressing; most common causative dermatophyte is *Trichophyton rubrum*; rare cases caused by *Epidermophyton floccosum* and *Trichophyton mentagrophytes*
- Tinea corporis: most commonly caused by *T. rubrum*; *Trichophyton tonsurans* most often found in patients with tinea gladiatorum
- Tinea capitis: *T. tonsurans* found in 90% and *Microsporum* sp. in 10% of patients

Genetics
Evidence suggests a genetic susceptibility in certain individuals.

RISK FACTORS
- Warm climates; summer months and/or copious sweating; wearing wet clothing/multiple layers (tinea cruris)
- Daycare centers/schools/confined quarters (tinea corporis and capitis)
- Depression of cell-mediated immune response (e.g., individuals with atopy or AIDS)
- Obesity (tinea cruris and corporis)
- Direct contact with an active lesion on a human, an animal, or rarely, from soil; working with animals (tinea corporis)

GENERAL PREVENTION
- Avoidance of risk factors, such as contact with suspicious lesions
- Fluconazole or itraconazole may be useful in wrestlers to prevent outbreaks during competitive season.

COMMONLY ASSOCIATED CONDITIONS
Tinea pedis, tinea barbae, tinea manus

 DIAGNOSIS

HISTORY
- Lesions range from asymptomatic to pruritic.
- In tinea cruris, acute inflammation may result from wearing occlusive clothing; chronic scratching may result in an eczematous appearance.
- Previous application of topical steroids, especially in tinea cruris and corporis, may alter the overall appearance causing a more extensive eruption with irregular borders and erythematous papules. This modified form is called *tinea incognito*.

PHYSICAL EXAM
- Tinea cruris: well-marginated, erythematous, half-moon–shaped plaques in crural folds that spread to medial thighs; advancing border is well defined, often with fine scaling and sometimes vesicular eruptions. Lesions are usually bilateral and do not include scrotum/penis (unlike with *Candida* infections) but may migrate to perineum, perianal area, and gluteal cleft and onto the buttocks in chronic/progressive cases. The area may be hyperpigmented on resolution.
- Tinea corporis: scaling, round or oval pruritic plaques characterized by a sharply defined annular pattern with peripheral activity and central clearing (ring-shaped lesions); papules and occasionally pustules/vesicles present at border and, less commonly, in center
- Tinea capitis: commonly begins with round patches of scale (alopecia less common). In its later stages, the infection frequently takes on patterns of chronic scaling with either little/marked inflammation or alopecia. Less often, patients will present with multiple patches of alopecia and the characteristic black-dot appearance of broken hairs. Extreme inflammation results in kerion formation (exudative, pustular nodulation).

DIFFERENTIAL DIAGNOSIS
- Tinea cruris
  - Intertrigo: inflammatory process of moist-opposed skin folds, often including infection with bacteria, yeast, and fungi; painful longitudinal fissures may occur in skin folds.
  - Erythrasma: diffuse brown, scaly, noninflammatory plaque with irregular borders, often involving groin; caused by bacterial infection with *Corynebacterium minutissimum*; fluoresces coral red with Wood lamp
  - Seborrheic dermatitis of groin
  - Psoriasis of groin ("inverse psoriasis")
  - Candidiasis of groin (typically involves the scrotum)
  - Acanthosis nigricans
- Tinea capitis
  - Psoriasis
  - Seborrheic dermatitis
  - Pyoderma
  - Alopecia areata and trichotillomania
  - Aplasia cutis congenital
- Tinea corporis
  - Pityriasis rosea
  - Eczema (nummular)
  - Contact dermatitis
  - Syphilis
  - Psoriasis
  - Seborrheic dermatitis
  - Subacute systemic lupus erythematosus (SLE)
  - Erythema annulare centrifugum
  - Erythema multiforme; erythema migrans
  - Impetigo circinatum
  - Granuloma annulare

DIAGNOSTIC TESTS & INTERPRETATION
Wood lamp exam reveals no fluorescence in most cases (*Trichophyton* sp.); 10% of infections, those caused by *T. rubrum*, will fluoresce with a green light.

Initial Tests (lab, imaging)
- Potassium hydroxide (KOH) preparation of skin scrapings from dermatophyte leading border shows characteristic translucent, branching, rod-shaped hyphae.
- Arthrospores can be visualized within hair shafts. Spores and/or hyphae may be seen on KOH exam.

Follow-Up Tests & Special Considerations
- Reevaluate to assess response, especially in resistant/extensive cases.
- Fungal culture using Sabouraud dextrose agar/dermatophyte test medium

Test Interpretation
- Skin scrapings show fungal hyphae in epidermis; best yield from scrapings from active border
- Arthrospores found in hair shafts; spores and/or hyphae seen on KOH exam

TREATMENT

GENERAL MEASURES
- Careful hand washing and personal hygiene; laundering of towels/clothing of affected individual; no sharing of towels/clothes/headgear/pillows
- Evaluate other family members, close contacts, or household pets (especially kittens and puppies).
- Use of prophylactic antifungal shampoo by all household members for 2 to 4 weeks in cases of tinea capitis
- Avoid predisposing conditions such as hot baths and tight-fitting clothing (boxer shorts are better than briefs).
- Keep area as dry as possible (talcum/powders may be beneficial).
- Itching can be alleviated by OTC preparations such as Sarna or Prax.
- Topical steroid preparations should be avoided, unless absolutely needed to control itching and only after definitive diagnosis and initiation of antifungal treatment.
- Nystatin should be avoided in tinea infections but is indicated for cutaneous candidal infections.
- Avoid contact sports (e.g., wrestling) temporarily while starting treatment.

MEDICATION
First Line
- Tinea cruris/corporis (2,3)
  - Topical azole antifungal compounds
    - Terbinafine 1% (Lamisil): OTC inexpensive and effective compound; can be applied once or BID for 1 to 3 weeks
    - Econazole 1% (Spectazole), ketoconazole (Nizoral): usually applied BID for 2 to 3 weeks
    - Butenafine 1% (Mentax): applied once daily for 2 weeks; also very effective. To prevent relapse, use for 1 week after resolution.
- Tinea capitis (4)[A]
  - PO griseofulvin for *Trichophyton* and *Microsporum* sp.; microsized preparation available; dosage 10 to 20 mg/kg/day (max 1,000 mg); taken BID or as a single dose daily for 6 to 12 weeks
  - PO terbinafine can be used for *Trichophyton* sp. at 62.5 mg/day in patients weighing 10 to 20 kg; 125 mg/day if weight 20 to 40 kg; 250 mg/day if weight >40 kg; use for 4 to 6 weeks.
  - PO itraconazole can be used for *Microsporum* sp. and matches griseofulvin efficacy while being better tolerated; dosage of 3 to 5 mg/kg/day, but most studies have used 100 mg/day for 6 weeks in children >2 years of age

Second Line
Tinea cruris/corporis
- Oral antifungal agents are effective but not indicated in uncomplicated tinea cruris/corporis cases. They can be used for resistant and extensive infections or if the patient is immunocompromised. If topical therapy fails, consider possible oral therapy. Griseofulvin can be given 500 mg/day for 1 to 2 weeks.
- The following oral regimens have been reported in medical literature as being effective but currently are not specifically approved by FDA for tinea cruris:
  - PO terbinafine (Lamisil): 250 mg/day for 1 week
  - PO itraconazole (Sporanox): 100 mg BID once and repeated 1 week later
  - PO fluconazole (Diflucan): 150 mg once per week for 4 weeks
- Topical terbinafine 1% solution has been studied recently and appears effective as a once-daily application for 1 week.
- Oral antifungals have many interactions including warfarin, OCPs, and alcohol; advise checking for drug interactions prior to use; contraindicated in pregnancy. Monitor for liver toxicity when using oral antifungals.

ISSUES FOR REFERRAL
Refer if disease is nonresponsive/resistant, especially in immunocompromised host.

ADDITIONAL THERAPIES
Treatment of secondary bacterial infections

ONGOING CARE

FOLLOW-UP RECOMMENDATIONS
Reevaluate response to treatment.

Patient Monitoring
Liver function testing prior to therapy and at regular intervals during course of therapy for patients requiring oral terbinafine, fluconazole, itraconazole, and griseofulvin

PATIENT EDUCATION
Explain the causative agents, predisposing factors, and prevention measures.

PROGNOSIS
- Excellent prognosis for cure with therapy in tinea cruris and corporis
- In tinea capitis, lesions will heal spontaneously in 6 months without treatment, but scarring is more likely.

COMPLICATIONS
- Secondary bacterial infection
- Generalized, invasive dermatophyte infection
- Secondary eruptions called dermatophytid reactions (which occur in association with primary/inflammatory skin disorders) may occur at distant sites.

REFERENCES
1. Ameen M. Epidemiology of superficial fungal infections. *Clin Dermatol*. 2010;28(2):197–201.
2. van Zuuren EJ, Fedorowicz Z, El-Gohary M. Evidence-based topical treatments for tinea cruris and tinea corporis: a summary of a Cochrane systematic review. *Br J Dermatol*. 2015;172(3):616–641.
3. El-Gohary M, van Zuuren EJ, Fedorowicz Z, et al. Topical antifungal treatments for tinea cruris and tinea corporis. *Cochrane Database Syst Rev*. 2014;(8):CD009992.
4. Gupta AK, Drummond-Main C. Meta-analysis of randomized, controlled trials comparing particular doses of griseofulvin and terbinafine for the treatment of tinea capitis. *Pediatr Dermatol*. 2013;30(1):1–6.

ADDITIONAL READING
- Bell-Syer SE, Khan SM, Torgerson DJ. Oral treatments for fungal infections of the skin of the foot. *Cochrane Database Syst Rev*. 2012;(10):CD003584.
- González U, Seaton T, Bergus G, et al. Systemic antifungal therapy for tinea capitis in children. *Cochrane Database Syst Rev*. 2007;(4):CD004685.
- Hawkins DM, Smidt AC. Superficial fungal infections in children. *Pediatr Clin North Am*. 2014;61(2):443–455.
- Mirmirani P, Tucker LY. Epidemiologic trends in pediatric tinea capitis: a population-based study from Kaiser Permanente Northern California. *J Am Acad Dermatol*. 2013;69(6):916–921.
- Seebacher C, Bouchara JP, Mignon B. Updates on the epidemiology of dermatophyte infections. *Mycopathologia*. 2008;166(5–6):335–352.
- Tey HL, Tan AS, Chan YC. Meta-analysis of randomized, controlled trials comparing griseofulvin and terbinafine in the treatment of tinea capitis. *J Am Acad Dermatol*. 2011;64(4):663–670.

CODES

ICD10
- B35.0 Tinea barbae and tinea capitis
- B35.4 Tinea corporis
- B35.6 Tinea cruris

CLINICAL PEARLS
- Tinea corporis is characterized by scaly plaque, with peripheral activity and central clearing.
- Tinea cruris is characterized by erythematous plaque in crural folds usually sparing the scrotum. Treatment of concomitant tinea pedis is advised.
- Tinea capitis is a fungal infection of the scalp affecting hair growth. Topical therapy is ineffective for this infection.

T

TINEA PEDIS

Elisabeth L. Backer, MD

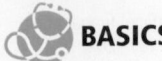

BASICS

DESCRIPTION
- Superficial infection of the feet caused by dermatophytes
- Most common dermatophyte infection encountered in clinical practice; contagious
- Often accompanied by tinea manuum, tinea unguium, and tinea cruris
- Clinical forms: interdigital (most common), hyperkeratotic (moccasin type), vesiculobullous (inflammatory), and rarely ulcerative
- System(s) affected: skin/exocrine
- Synonym(s): athlete's foot

EPIDEMIOLOGY
- Predominant age: 20 to 50 years, although can occur at any age (1)
- Predominant gender: male > female

Prevalence
4% of population

Pediatric Considerations
Rare in younger children; common in adolescents

Geriatric Considerations
Elderly are more susceptible to outbreaks because of immunocompromised and impaired perfusion of distal extremities.

ETIOLOGY AND PATHOPHYSIOLOGY
Superficial infection caused by dermatophytes that thrive only in nonviable keratinized tissue
- *Trichophyton interdigitale* (previously *Trichophyton mentagrophytes*) (acute)
- *Trichophyton rubrum* (chronic)
- *Trichophyton tonsurans*
- *Epidermophyton floccosum*

Genetics
No known genetic pattern

RISK FACTORS
- Hot, humid weather
- Sweating
- Occlusive/tight-fitting footwear
- Immunosuppression
- Prolonged application of topical steroids

GENERAL PREVENTION
- Good personal hygiene
- Wearing rubber or wooden sandals in community showers, bathing places, locker rooms
- Careful drying between toes after showering or bathing; blow-drying feet with hair dryer may be more effective than drying with towel.
- Changing socks and shoes frequently
- Applying drying or dusting powder
- Applying topical antiperspirants
- Putting on socks before underwear to prevent infection from spreading to groin

COMMONLY ASSOCIATED CONDITIONS
- Hyperhidrosis
- Onychomycosis
- Tinea manuum/unguium/cruris/corporis

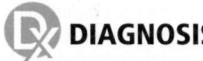

DIAGNOSIS

HISTORY
- Itchy, scaly rash on foot, usually between toes; may progress to fissuring/maceration in toe web spaces
- May be associated with onychomycosis and other tinea infections
- May be complicated by secondary bacterial infections

PHYSICAL EXAM
- Acute form: self-limited, intermittent, recurrent; scaling, thickening, and fissuring of sole and heel; scaling or fissuring of toe webs; or pruritic vesicular/bullous lesions between toes or on soles
- Chronic form: most common; slowly progressive, pruritic erythematous erosion/scales between toes, in digital interspaces; extension onto soles, sides/dorsum of feet (moccasin distribution); if untreated, may persist indefinitely
- Other features: strong odor, hyperkeratosis, maceration, ulceration
- Tinea pedis may occur unilateral or bilateral.
- Secondary presumably immune-mediated eruptions called dermatophytid reactions may occur at distant sites.

DIFFERENTIAL DIAGNOSIS
- Interdigital type: erythrasma, impetigo, pitted keratolysis, candidal intertrigo
- Moccasin type: psoriasis vulgaris, eczematous dermatitis, pitted keratolysis
- Inflammatory/bullous type: impetigo, allergic contact dermatitis, dyshidrotic eczema (negative KOH examination of scrapings), bullous disease

DIAGNOSTIC TESTS & INTERPRETATION
Wood lamp exam will not fluoresce unless complicated by another fungus, which is uncommon: *Malassezia furfur* (yellow to white), *Corynebacterium* (red), or *Microsporum* (blue green).

Initial Tests (lab, imaging)
Testing is not needed in typical presentation.
- Direct microscopic exam (potassium hydroxide) of scrapings of the lesions
- Culture (Sabouraud medium)

Test Interpretation
- Potassium hydroxide preparation: septate and branched mycelia
- Culture: dermatophyte

TREATMENT

Treatment is generally with topical antifungal medications for up to 4 weeks and is more effective than placebo:
- Acute treatment
  - Aluminum acetate soak (Burow's solution; Domeboro, 1 pack to 1 quart warm water) to decrease itching and acute eczematous reaction
  - Antifungal cream of choice BID after soaks (allylamines slightly more effective than azoles)
- Chronic treatment:
  - Antifungal creams BID, continuing for 3 days after the rash is resolved: terbinafine 1% (possibly most effective topical), clotrimazole 1%, econazole 1%, ketoconazole 2%, tolnaftate 1%, etc. (2)[A]
  - May try systemic antifungal therapy; see below (consider if concomitant onychomycosis or after failed topical treatment).

GENERAL MEASURES

- Soak with aluminum chloride 30% or aluminum subacetate for 20 minutes BID.
- Careful removal of dead/thickened skin after soaking or bathing
- Treatment of shoes with antifungal powders
- Avoidance of occlusive footwear
- Chronic or extensive disease or nail involvement requires oral antifungal medication and systemic therapy.

MEDICATION

For use when topical therapy has failed

First Line

- Systemic antifungals (3)[A]:
  - Itraconazole: 200 mg PO BID for 7 days (cure rate >90%)
  - Terbinafine: 250 mg/day PO for 14 days
- If concomitant onychomycosis:
  - Itraconazole: 200 mg PO BID for 1st week of month for 3 months. Liver function testing is recommended.
  - Terbinafine: 250 mg/day PO for 12 weeks, or pulse dosing: 500 mg/day PO for 1st week of month for 3 months; not recommended if creatinine clearance <50 mL/min
- Pediatric dosing options:
  - Griseofulvin: 10 to 15 mg/kg/day or divided
  - Terbinafine:
    - 10 to 20 kg: 62.5 mg/day
    - 20 to 40 kg: 125 mg/day
    - >40 kg: 250 mg/day
- Itraconazole: 3 to 5 mg/kg/day
- Fluconazole: 6 mg/kg/week
- Contraindications: itraconazole, pregnancy Category C
- Precautions: All systemic antifungal drugs may have potential hepatotoxicity.
- Significant possible interactions: Itraconazole requires gastric acid for absorption; effectiveness is reduced with antacids, H$_2$ blockers, proton pump inhibitors, etc. Take with acidic beverage, such as soda if on antacids.

Second Line

- Systemic antifungals: griseofulvin 250 to 500 mg of microsize BID daily for 21 days
- Contraindications (griseofulvin):
  - Patients with porphyria, hepatocellular failure
  - Patients with history of hypersensitivity to griseofulvin

- Precautions (griseofulvin):
  - Should be used only in severe cases
  - Periodic monitoring of organ system functioning, including renal, hepatic, and hematopoietic
  - Possible photosensitivity reactions
  - Lupus erythematosus, lupus-like syndromes, or exacerbation of existing lupus erythematosus has been reported.
- Significant possible interactions (griseofulvin):
  - Decreases activity of warfarin-type anticoagulants
  - Barbiturates usually depress griseofulvin activity.
  - May potentiate effect of alcohol, producing tachycardia and flush

ISSUES FOR REFERRAL

If extensive or resistant disease, especially in immunocompromised host

ADDITIONAL THERAPIES

- Treatment of secondary bacterial infections
- Treatment of eczematoid changes

 ONGOING CARE

FOLLOW-UP RECOMMENDATIONS

Avoid sweat buildup along feet.

Patient Monitoring

Evaluate for response, recognizing that infections may be chronic/recurrent.

DIET

No restrictions

PATIENT EDUCATION

See "General Prevention."

PROGNOSIS

- Control but not complete cure
- Infections tend to be chronic with exacerbations (e.g., in hot, humid weather).
- Personal hygiene and preventive measures, such as open-toed sandals, careful drying, and frequent sock changes are essential.

COMPLICATIONS

- Secondary bacterial infections (common portal of entry for streptococcal infections, producing lymphangitis/cellulitis of lower extremity)
- Eczematoid changes

REFERENCES

1. Ameen M. Epidemiology of superficial fungal infections. *Clin Dermatol*. 2010;28(2):197–201.
2. Crawford F, Hollis S. Topical treatments for fungal infections of the skin and nails of the foot. *Cochrane Database Syst Rev*. 2007;(3):CD001434.
3. Bell-Syer SE, Khan SM, Torgerson DJ. Oral treatments for fungal infections of the skin of the foot. *Cochrane Database Syst Rev*. 2012;(10):CD003584.

ADDITIONAL READING

- Hawkins DM, Smidt AC. Superficial fungal infections in children. *Pediatr Clin North Am*. 2014;61(2):443–455.
- Rotta I, Sanchez A, Gonçalves PR, et al. Efficacy and safety of topical antifungals in the treatment of dermatomycosis: a systematic review. *Br J Dermatol*. 2012;166(5):927–933.
- Sahoo AK, Mahajan R. Management of tinea corporis, tinea cruris, and tinea pedis: a comprehensive review. *Indian Dermatol Online J*. 2016;7(2):77–86.

 SEE ALSO

Dermatitis, Contact; Dyshidrosis

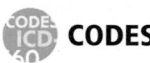 CODES

ICD10
B35.3 Tinea pedis

CLINICAL PEARLS

- Treatment with topical antifungal medications for up to 4 weeks usually suffices.
- Tinea pedis is often recurrent or chronic in nature.
- Careful drying between toes after showering or bathing helps prevent recurrences. (Blow drying feet with hair dryer may be more effective than drying with towel.)
- Socks should be changed frequently. Put on socks before underwear to prevent infection from spreading to groin (tinea cruris).
- Dusting and desiccating powders (containing antifungal agents) may prevent recurrences.

TINEA VERSICOLOR

Elisabeth L. Backer, MD

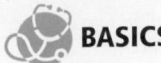 **BASICS**

DESCRIPTION
- Rash due to a common superficial mycosis with a variety of colors and changing shades of color, predominantly present on trunk and proximal upper extremities; macules are usually hypopigmented, light brown, or salmon-colored; fine scale is often apparent. It is not a dermatophyte infection.
- System(s) affected: skin/exocrine
- Synonym(s): pityriasis versicolor

EPIDEMIOLOGY

Incidence
- Common, occurs worldwide, especially in tropical climates, where prevalence can reach 50%
- Predominant age: teenagers and young adults
- Predominant sex: male = female

Pediatric Considerations
Usually occurs after puberty (except in tropical areas); facial lesions are more common in children.

Geriatric Considerations
Not common in the geriatric population

ETIOLOGY AND PATHOPHYSIOLOGY
Inhibition of pigment synthesis in epidermal melanocytes, leading to hypomelanosis; in the hyperpigmented type, the melanosomes are large and heavily melanized (1).
- Saprophytic yeast: *Pityrosporum orbiculare* (also known as *Plasmodium ovale*, *Malassezia furfur*, or *Malassezia ovalis*), which is a known colonizer of all humans
- Development of clinical disease associated with transformation of *Malassezia* from yeast cells to pathogenic mycelial form likely multifactorial, due to host and/or external factors
- Not linked to poor hygiene

Genetics
Genetic predisposition may exist.

RISK FACTORS
- Hot, humid weather
- Use of topical skin oils
- Hyperhidrosis
- HIV infection/immunosuppression
- High cortisol levels (Cushing, prolonged steroid administration)
- Pregnancy
- Malnutrition
- Oral contraceptives

GENERAL PREVENTION
- Recheck and use prophylaxis each spring prior to tanning season.
- Avoid skin oils.

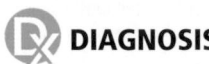 **DIAGNOSIS**

HISTORY
- Asymptomatic scaling macules on trunk
- Possible mild pruritus
- More prominent in summer
- Sun tanning accentuates lesions because infected areas do not tan.
- Periodic recurrences common, especially in the warm summer months

PHYSICAL EXAM
- *Versicolor* refers to the variety and changing shades of colors. Color variations can exist between individuals and also between lesions.
- Sun-exposed areas: Lesions are usually white/hypopigmented.
- Covered areas: Lesions are often brown or salmon-colored.
- Distribution (sebum-rich areas): chest, shoulders, back (also face and intertriginous areas)
  – Face is more likely to be involved in children.
- Appearance: small individual macules/patches that frequently coalesce
- Scale: fine, more visible with scraping

DIFFERENTIAL DIAGNOSIS
Other skin diseases with discolored macules and plaques, including the following:
- Pityriasis alba/rosea ("Christmas tree-like" distribution visible in *P. rosea*)
- Vitiligo (presents without scaling)
- Seborrheic dermatitis (more erythematous; thicker scale)
- Nummular eczema
- Secondary syphilis
- Erythrasma
- Mycosis fungoides

DIAGNOSTIC TESTS & INTERPRETATION
Wood lamp: yellow to yellow-green fluorescence or pigment changes

Initial Tests (lab, imaging)
- Direct microscopy of scales with 10% potassium hydroxide (KOH) preparation to visualize hyphae and spores ("spaghetti and meatballs" pattern)
- Routine lab tests are usually not necessary.
- Fungal culture is not useful.

Test Interpretation
- Short, stubby, or Y-shaped hyphae
- Small, round spores in clusters on hyphae

 TREATMENT

GENERAL MEASURES
- Apply prescribed topical medications to affected skin with cotton balls.
- Pigmentation may take months to fade or fill in.
- Repeat treatment each spring prior to sun exposure; consider monthly prophylaxis during the summer months.
- Patients who fail topical treatment can be treated with an oral/systemic medication.

MEDICATION

Topical antifungal therapy is the treatment of choice in limited disease and is safe and usually effective. Evidence is generally of poor quality, but data suggest that longer durations of treatment and higher concentrations of active agents produce greater cure rates (2)[A].

First Line

- Ketoconazole 2% shampoo applied to damp skin and left on for 5 minutes for 1 to 3 days *or*
- Selenium sulfide shampoo 2.5% (Selsun):
  – Allowed to dry for 10 minutes prior to showering: daily for 1 week *or*
  – Allowed to remain on body for 12 to 24 hours prior to showering: once a week for 4 weeks *or*
- Clotrimazole 1% topical (Lotrimin) BID for 2 to 4 weeks *or*
- Miconazole 2% (Micatin, Monistat) BID for 2 to 4 weeks *or*
- Ketoconazole 2% (Nizoral) cream BID for 2 to 4 weeks *or*
- Terbinafine (Lamisil) 1% solution BID for 1 week *or*
- Terbinafine (Lamisil DermGel) once daily for 1 week
- Cure rates of topical antiyeast preparations typically 70–80%; healing continues after active treatment. Resumption of even pigmentation may take months.
- Contraindications: Ketoconazole is contraindicated in pregnancy.
- Newer preparations: 2.25% selenium sulfide foam; ketoconazole 2% gel

Second Line

- Use for extensive disease or nonresponders.
- Oral fluconazole 300 mg once weekly for 2 weeks (3)[A]
- Itraconazole 200 mg/day PO for 1 week; cure rate >90% (3)[A]
- Oral ketoconazole is no longer recommended by FDA due to risks of hepatotoxicity, adrenal insufficiency, and drug–drug interactions.
- Oral terbinafine or griseofulvin is not effective.
- Pramiconazole has been studied but is not yet available for clinical use.

ISSUES FOR REFERRAL

- If resistant to treatment
- If extensive disease occurs in immunocompromised host

 ONGOING CARE

- Ketoconazole 2% or selenium sulfide 2.5% shampoo can be used weekly for maintenance or monthly for prophylaxis.
- Itraconazole 400 mg once monthly (in 2 divided dosages) during the warmer months of the year can also reduce recurrences.

FOLLOW-UP RECOMMENDATIONS

Warn patients that whiteness will remain for several months after treatment.

Patient Monitoring

- Recheck and treat again each spring prior to tanning season.
- Failure to respond should prompt reassessment or dermatology referral.
- Resistance to treatment, frequent recurrences, or widespread disease may point to immunodeficiency.

PATIENT EDUCATION

For patient education materials favorably reviewed on this topic, contact American Academy of Dermatology, 930 N. Meacham Road, P.O. Box 4014, Schaumberg, IL 60168-4014; (708) 330-0230.

PROGNOSIS

- Duration of lesions months/years
- Recurs almost routinely because this yeast is a known human colonizer
- Pigmentary changes may take months to resolve.

REFERENCES

1. Harada K, Saito M, Sugita T, et al. Malassezia species and their associated skin diseases. *J Dermatol*. 2015;42(3):250–257.
2. Hald M, Arendrup M, Svejgaard E, et al; and Danish Society of Dermatology. Evidence-based Danish guidelines for the treatment of *Malassezia*-related skin diseases. *Acta Derm Venereol*. 2015;95(1):12–19.
3. Gupta AK, Lane D, Paquet M. Systematic review of systemic treatments for tinea versicolor and evidence-based dosing regimen recommendations. *J Cutan Med Surg*. 2014;18(2):79–90.

ADDITIONAL READING

- Bhogal CS, Singal A, Baruah MC. Comparative efficacy of ketoconazole and fluconazole in the treatment of pityriasis versicolor: a one year follow-up study. *J Dermatol*. 2001;28(10):535–539.
- Faergemann J, Todd G, Pather S, et al. A double-blind, randomized, placebo-controlled, dose-finding study of oral pramiconazole in the treatment of pityriasis versicolor. *J Am Acad Dermatol*. 2009;61(6):971–976.
- Gupta AK, Lyons DC. Pityriasis versicolor: an update on pharmacological treatment options. *Expert Opin Pharmacother*. 2014;15(12):1707–1713.
- Hawkins DM, Smidt AC. Superficial fungal infections in children. *Pediatr Clin North Am*. 2014;61(2):443–455.
- Köse O, Bülent Taştan H, Riza Gür A, et al. Comparison of a single 400 mg dose versus a 7-day 200 mg daily dose of itraconazole in the treatment of tinea versicolor. *J Dermatolog Treat*. 2002;13(2):77–79.

 CODES

ICD10
B36.0 Pityriasis versicolor

CLINICAL PEARLS

- Noncontagious macules of varying colors, with fine scale
- Recurrence in summer months
- More apparent after tanning. Skin areas with fungal infection do not tan; thus, hypopigmented areas become more visible.
- Warn patients that whiteness will remain for several months after treatment.

TINNITUS
Donna I. Meltzer, MD

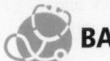 **BASICS**

DESCRIPTION
- Tinnitus is a perceived sensation of sound in the absence of an external acoustic stimulus; often described as a ringing, hissing, buzzing, or whooshing
- Derived from the Latin word *tinnire*, meaning "to ring"
- May be heard in one or both ears or centrally within the head
- Two types: subjective (most common) and objective tinnitus
- Subjective tinnitus: perceived only by the patient; can be continuous, intermittent, or pulsatile
- Objective tinnitus: audible to the examiner; usually pulsatile; <1% cases (1)
- Primary tinnitus: idiopathic with or without sensorineural hearing loss (SNHL) (2)
- Secondary tinnitus: associated with a specific cause (other than SNHL)

EPIDEMIOLOGY
Prevalence
- Tinnitus reported by 35 to 50 million adults in United States; although underreported, 12 million seek medical care.
- Affects 10–15% of adults
- Prevalence increases with age and peaks in 6th decade.
- Prevalence of 13–53% in general pediatric population
- Ethnic: whites > blacks and Hispanics
- Gender: males > females

Incidence
- Incidence increasing in association with excessive noise exposure
- Higher rates of tinnitus in smokers, hypertensives, diabetics, and obese patients

ETIOLOGY AND PATHOPHYSIOLOGY
- Precise pathophysiology is unknown; numerous theories have been proposed. Cochlear damage from ototoxic agents or noise exposure damages hair cells so that the central auditory system compensates, resulting in hyperactivity in cochlear nucleus and auditory cortex.
- Causes of subjective tinnitus are the following:
  – Otologic: hearing loss, cholesteatoma, cerumen impaction, otosclerosis, Ménière disease, vestibular schwannoma
  – Ototoxic medications: anti-inflammatory agents (aspirin, NSAIDs); antimalarial agents, antimicrobial drugs (aminoglycosides); antineoplastic agents, loop diuretics, miscellaneous drugs (antiarrhythmics, antiulcer, anticonvulsants, antihypertensives); psychotropic drugs; anesthetics (1)
  – Somatic: temporomandibular joint (TMJ) dysfunction, head or neck injury
  – Neurologic: multiple sclerosis, spontaneous intracranial hypertension, vestibular migraine, type I Chiari malformation
  – Infectious: viral, bacterial, fungal

- Causes of objective tinnitus:
  – Vascular: aortic or carotid stenosis, venous hum, arteriovenous fistula or malformation, vascular tumors, high cardiac output state (anemia)
  – Neurologic: palatal myoclonus, idiopathic stapedial muscle spasm
  – Patulous eustachian tube

Genetics
Minimal genetic component

RISK FACTORS
- Hearing loss (but can have tinnitus with normal hearing)
- High-level noise exposure
- Advanced age
- Use of ototoxic medications
- Otologic disease (otosclerosis, Ménière disease, cerumen impaction)
- Anxiety and depression associated with increased odds of tinnitus

GENERAL PREVENTION
- Avoid loud noise exposure and wear appropriate ear protection to prevent hearing loss.
- Monitor ototoxic medications and avoid prescribing more than one ototoxic agent concurrently.

COMMONLY ASSOCIATED CONDITIONS
- SNHL caused by presbycusis (age-associated hearing loss) or prolonged loud noise exposure
- Conductive hearing loss due to cerumen, otosclerosis, cholesteatoma
- Psychological disorders: depression, anxiety, insomnia, suicidal ideation
- Despair, frustration, interference with concentration and social interactions, work hindrance

DIAGNOSIS

HISTORY
- Onset gradual (presbycusis) or abrupt (following loud noise exposure)
- Timing: can be continuous (hearing loss) or intermittent (Ménière disease)
- Pattern: nonpulsatile > pulsatile (often vascular cause)
- Location: bilateral > unilateral (vestibular schwannoma, cerumen, Ménière disease)
- Pitch: high pitch (with SNHL) > low pitch (Ménière disease)
- Associated symptoms: hearing loss, headache, noise intolerance, vertigo, TMJ dysfunction, neck pain
- Exacerbating factors: loud noise; jaw, head, or neck movements
- Alleviating factors: hearing aid, position change, medications
- Medication use (prescription, OTC, supplements)
- Hearing and past noise exposure (occupational, military, recreational)
- Psychosocial history (depression, sleep habits)
- Impact of tinnitus: Tinnitus Handicap Inventory, Tinnitus Functional Index

PHYSICAL EXAM
- HEENT, neck, neurologic, and vascular examinations
- Ear: cerumen impaction, effusion, cholesteatoma
- Check hearing; air and bone conduction testing with 512- or 1,024-Hz tuning fork (Weber and Rinne tests)
- Eye: funduscopic exam for papilledema (intracranial hypertension) or visual field change (mass)
- TMJ: Palpate for tenderness and crepitus with movement.
- Cranial nerve, Romberg test (equilibrium), finger to nose, gait; assess for nystagmus.
- Auscultate for bruits or murmurs.

DIFFERENTIAL DIAGNOSIS
- Pulsatile tinnitus: carotid stenosis, aortic valve disease, AV malformation, high cardiac output state (anemia, hyperthyroidism), paraganglioma (glomus tumor)
- Nonpulsatile tinnitus: auditory hallucinations

DIAGNOSTIC TESTS & INTERPRETATION
- Tinnitus is a symptom; no objective test to confirm diagnosis
- Pure tone audiometry (air and bone conduction)
- Speech discrimination testing
- Tympanometry
- Carotid Doppler ultrasonography (neck bruit)

Initial Tests (lab, imaging)
- Little evidence to support lab testing other than targeted lab studies based on history and physical exam. Use clinical judgment and consider the following:
  – CBC
  – BUN/creatinine, fasting glucose, lipid panel
  – Thyroid-stimulating hormone
- Newer guidelines advise against imaging studies unless have unilateral, pulsatile tinnitus; focal neurologic abnormality; or asymmetric hearing loss (2).
- CT of temporal bone is initial imaging study of middle ear.
- Pulsatile tinnitus: temporal bone CT, CTA/CTV with contrast, MRA without or with contrast, or MRI head and internal auditory canal (IAC) without and with contrast are usually appropriate (3)[C]; could also consider carotid duplex or Doppler ultrasound
- Unilateral nonpulsatile tinnitus: MRI head and IAC without and with contrast; might consider CT temporal bone without and with contrast or CTA with contrast (3)[C]
- Bilateral nonpulsatile tinnitus: imaging not indicated if no hearing loss, neurologic deficit, or trauma (3)[C]

Follow-Up Tests & Special Considerations
Consider HIV, RPR, autoimmune panel, Lyme test, vitamin B_{12} level.

Diagnostic Procedures/Other
Electronystagmography (vestibular testing for Ménière disease)

TREATMENT

GENERAL MEASURES
- Individualize treatment based on the severity of tinnitus and impact on function.
- Reassure patient.
- Manage treatable pathology.
- Education, relaxation therapy, cognitive-behavioral therapy (CBT)
- Hearing aids (corrects hearing and might mask tinnitus) can be tried if there is hearing loss and bothersome tinnitus (2)[C].
- Protect hearing against future loud noise.
- Masking sound devices or generators on discontinuation might have decreased tinnitus (residual inhibition).
- Discontinue ototoxic medications.

MEDICATION
No pharmacologic agent has been shown to cure or consistently alleviate tinnitus.

First Line
- Antidepressants (SSRIs or TCAs): probably help with psychological distress; insufficient evidence that antidepressant drug therapy improves tinnitus (4)[A]
- Melatonin decreases tinnitus intensity and improves sleep quality; most effective in men, those without depression or prior treatment, and those with more severe bilateral tinnitus (5)[B]

Second Line
- Anticonvulsants: potentially suppress central auditory hyperactivity but not recommended (2)[C]
- Insufficient evidence to recommend gabapentin
- Higher caffeine intake associated with lower incidence of tinnitus in women (6)[B]

ISSUES FOR REFERRAL
- Audiologist for comprehensive hearing evaluation and management
- Otolaryngologist, neurologist, or neurosurgeon depending on pathology
- Dental referral for TMJ treatment and dental orthotics (splint, night guard)
- Therapists for CBT, biofeedback, education, and relaxation techniques

ADDITIONAL THERAPIES
- Sound therapy (masking): Patients wear low-level noise generators to mask the tinnitus noise; optional therapy (2)[C]
- CBT employs relaxation exercises, coping strategies, and deconditioning techniques to reduce arousal levels and reverse negative thoughts about tinnitus; recommended as beneficial based on randomized controlled trials (2)[C]
- Tinnitus retraining therapy (TRT) combines counseling, education, and acoustic therapy (soft music, sound machine) to minimize bothersome nature of tinnitus; often requires a team approach and up to 2 years of therapy; might be more effective than sound masking (7)[B]

- Transcranial magnetic stimulation (TMS): a noninvasive method to stimulate neurons in the brain by rapidly changing magnetic fields; not recommended as randomized trials were inconclusive (2)[C]
- Botulism toxin (for palatal myoclonus)
- Intratympanic steroid injections not recommended (2)[C]
- Hyperbaric oxygen: no beneficial effect on tinnitus

SURGERY/OTHER PROCEDURES
- Cochlear implants (for severe SNHL)
- Ablation of cochlear nerve (destroys hearing)
- Epidural stimulation of secondary auditory cortex with implanted electrodes suppressed tinnitus in small subset of patients.
- Otosclerosis: stapedectomy surgery with implantation of ossicular prosthesis
- Severe Ménière disease not alleviated by medications: installation of endolymphatic shunt, labyrinthectomy, or vestibular neurectomy
- Auditory neoplasms: surgical resection/radiation
- Pulsatile tinnitus due to atherosclerotic carotid artery disease: carotid endarterectomy

COMPLEMENTARY & ALTERNATIVE MEDICINE
- Zinc: no evidence that oral zinc supplements improve symptoms of tinnitus in adults (8)[B]
- One evidence-based practice guideline does not recommend Ginkgo biloba, melatonin, zinc, or other dietary supplements for treatment of persistent, bothersome tinnitus (2)[C].
- Hypnosis (unknown effectiveness)
- Acupuncture therapy may offer subjective benefits to some patients.

ADMISSION, INPATIENT, AND NURSING CONSIDERATIONS
Not applicable

 ONGOING CARE

FOLLOW-UP RECOMMENDATIONS
- Audiologist: for hearing evaluation and therapy
- Counseling as needed for psychological distress
- Family physician: as needed for support and guidance

PATIENT EDUCATION
- Help patients understand the relatively benign nature of tinnitus.
- Self-help groups
- American Tinnitus Association: (800) 634-8978; https://www.ata.org/
- National Institute on Deafness and Other Communication Disorders: (800) 241-1044; https://www.nidcd.nih.gov/health/tinnitus
- American Academy of Family Physicians: http://familydoctor.org

PROGNOSIS
- Tinnitus persisted in 80% of older patients and increased in severity in 50% (1).
- Focus on managing tinnitus and reducing severity, not curing.

REFERENCES
1. Yew KS. Diagnostic approach to patients with tinnitus. *Am Fam Physician.* 2014;89(2):106–113.
2. Tunkel DE, Bauer CA, Sun GH, et al. Clinical practice guideline: tinnitus executive summary. *Otolaryngol Head Neck Surg.* 2014;151(4):533–541.
3. Kessler MM, Moussa M, Bykowski J, et al. ACR Appropriateness Criteria® tinnitus. *J Am Coll Radiol.* 2017;14(11S):S584–S591.
4. Baldo P, Doree C, Molin P, et al. Antidepressants for patients with tinnitus. *Cochrane Database Syst Rev.* 2012;(9):CD003853.
5. Hurtuk A, Dome C, Holloman CH, et al. Melatonin: can it stop the ringing? *Ann Otol Rhinol Laryngol.* 2011;120(7):433–440.
6. Glicksman JT, Curhan SG, Curhan GC. A prospective study of caffeine intake and risk of incident tinnitus. *Am J Med.* 2014;127(8):739–743.
7. Phillips JS, McFerran D. Tinnitus retraining therapy (TRT) for tinnitus. *Cochrane Database Syst Rev.* 2010;(3):CD007330.
8. Person OC, Puga ME, da Silva EM, et al. Zinc supplementation for tinnitus. *Cochrane Database Syst Rev.* 2016;(11):CD009832.

ADDITIONAL READING
- Aazh H, El Refaie A, Humphriss R. Gabapentin for tinnitus: a systematic review. *Am J Audiol.* 2011;20(2):151–158.
- Liu F, Han X, Li Y, et al. Acupuncture in the treatment of tinnitus: a systematic review and meta-analysis. *Eur Arch Otorhinolaryngol.* 2016;273(2):285–294.
- Sajisevi M, Weissman JL, Kaylie DM. What is the role of imaging in tinnitus? *Laryngoscope.* 2014;124(3):583–584.

CODES

ICD10
- H93.19 Tinnitus, unspecified ear
- H93.11 Tinnitus, right ear
- H93.12 Tinnitus, left ear

CLINICAL PEARLS
- People have different levels of tolerance to tinnitus. It may affect sleep, concentration, and emotional state. Many patients with chronic tinnitus have depression.
- To keep tinnitus from worsening, avoid loud noises and minimize stress.
- Optimal management may involve multiple strategies.

T

TOBACCO USE AND SMOKING CESSATION
Felix B. Chang Cruz, MD, FAAMA, ABIHM • Daniel Molinar, MD

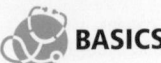 **BASICS**

DESCRIPTION
- Use of tobacco of any form
- The second leading actual cause of death in the United States
- *Smokeless tobacco* refers to tobacco products that are vaporized, sniffed, sucked, or chewed.
- Nicotine sources: cigars, pipes, water pipes, hookahs, and cigarettes and electronic cigarettes
- Electronic nicotine delivery system (ENDS) use is on the rise.

EPIDEMIOLOGY
Incidence
- 2.4 million new smokers annually in the United States (2.6% initiation rate)
- 59% of new smokers are <18 years of age (5.8% initiation rate for teens).
- 9.7 million people age >18 years smoke 20 or more cigarettes daily.

Prevalence
- 15% of all adults (37.8 million people): 17.5% of males, 13.5% of females are current cigarette smokers.
- Age: highest among those aged 25 to 44 years (17%)
- Race: highest among Native Americans (32%) and is lower among Hispanics (11%) and Asians (9%)
- Gender: male > female (22% vs. 17%)
- Education: inversely proportional to education level
- Psychological association: nearly 36% of adults with a serious psychological distress compared to 14% without this distress
- Cigarette smoking is responsible for >480,000 deaths per year in the United States, including >41,000 deaths from secondhand smoke exposure. This is about 1 in 5 deaths annually or 1,300 deaths every day.

ETIOLOGY AND PATHOPHYSIOLOGY
- Addiction due to nicotine's rapid stimulation of the brain's dopamine system (teenage brain especially susceptible)
- Atherosclerotic risk due to adrenergic stimulation, endothelial damage, carbon monoxide, and adverse effects on lipids
- Direct airway damage from cigarette tar
- Carcinogens in all tobacco products

RISK FACTORS
- Presence of a smoker in the household
- Easy access to cigarettes
- Comorbid stress and psychiatric disorders
- Low self-esteem/self-worth
- Poor academic performance
- Boys: high levels of aggression and rebelliousness
- Girls: preoccupation with weight and body image

GENERAL PREVENTION
- Most first-time tobacco use occurs before high school graduation.
- The Tar Wars program of the American Academy of Family Physicians has successfully targeted tobacco use prevention in 4th and 5th graders.
- Smoking bans in public areas and workplaces
- Restriction of minors' access to tobacco
- Restrictions on tobacco advertisements
- Raising prices through taxation
- Media literacy education
- Tobacco-free sports initiatives

COMMONLY ASSOCIATED CONDITIONS
- Coronary artery disease
- Cerebrovascular disease
- Peripheral vascular disease
- Abdominal aortic aneurysm (AAA)
- COPD
- Cancer of the lip, oral cavity, pharynx, larynx, lung, esophagus, stomach, pancreas, kidney, urinary bladder, cervix, and blood
- Pneumonia, osteoporosis
- Periodontitis
- Alcohol use
- Depression and anxiety
- Reduced fertility

Pregnancy Considerations
Women who smoke or are exposed to secondhand smoke during pregnancy have increased risks of miscarriage, placenta previa, placental abruption, premature rupture of membranes, preterm delivery, low-birth-weight infants, and stillbirth.

Pediatric Considerations
- Secondhand smoke increases the risk for:
  - Sudden infant death syndrome
  - Acute upper and lower respiratory tract infections
  - More severe exacerbations of asthma
  - Otitis media and need for tympanostomies
- Nicotine passes through breast milk. Effects on growth and development of nursing infants are unknown.

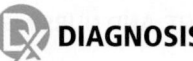 **DIAGNOSIS**

HISTORY
- Ask about tobacco use and secondhand smoke exposure at every physician encounter.
- Type and quantity of tobacco used:
  - "Heavy smoking" is 20 or more cigarettes per day or 20 or more pack-years.
  - Pack-years = packs/day × years. Twenty pack-years is equivalent to a pack a day for 20 years or 2 packs a day for 10 years. Other common cut points for heavy smoking include 15 and 25 cigarettes per day.
- Assess for awareness of health risks.
- Assess interest in quitting.
- Identify triggers for smoking: stress, habit, pleasure.
- Prior attempts to quit: method, duration of success, reason for relapse

PHYSICAL EXAM
- General: tobacco smoke odor, staining of facial hair
- Skin: premature wrinkling, especially the face
- Mouth: nicotine-stained teeth; inspect for mucosal changes, hypertrophy, fungating lesions.
- Lungs: crackles, wheezing, increased or decreased volume, chronic cough
- Vessels: carotid or abdominal bruits, abdominal aortic enlargement or aneurysm, weak peripheral pulses, stigmata of peripheral vascular disease

DIAGNOSTIC TESTS & INTERPRETATION
- CXR for patients with pulmonary symptoms or signs of cancer but not for screening
- The USPSTF recommends one-time screening abdominal US for AAA in men ≥65 years of age who ever smoked (number needed to screen to prevent one AAA = 500).
- Low-dose CT is more sensitive than chest radiograph for identifying small, asymptomatic lung cancers.
- USPSTF recommends yearly screening for lung cancer with low-dose CT for individuals 55 to 80 years with a 30 pack-years history of smoking; current smokers or those who have quit within past 15 years

Diagnostic Procedures/Other
PFTs for smokers with chronic pulmonary symptoms, such as wheezing, cough, or dyspnea. This includes spirometry, diffusion studies, and body plethysmography.

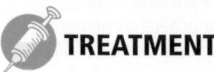 **TREATMENT**

Both behavioral counseling and pharmacotherapy benefit patients who are trying to quit smoking especially when used in combination.

ALERT
A provider tobacco cessation recommendation at *every clinical visit* improves cessation rates.

GENERAL MEASURES
- Behavioral counseling includes the 5 As:
  - Ask about tobacco use at every office visit.
  - Advise all smokers to quit.
  - Assess the patient's willingness to quit.
  - Assist the patient in his or her attempt to quit.
  - Arrange follow-up.
- Patients ready to quit smoking should set a quit date within the next 2 weeks; no difference in success rates between patients who taper prior to their quit date and those who stop abruptly
- Success increased with a quitting partner, such as a spouse, friend, or coworker, to provide mutual encouragement.

MEDICATION
First Line
- Varenicline (Chantix): 0.5 mg/day PO for 3 days, then 0.5 mg BID for 4 days, and then 1 mg BID for 11 weeks (1)[A]:
  - Start 1 to 4 weeks prior to smoking cessation and continue for 12 to 24 weeks.
  - Superior versus placebo and bupropion; number needed to treat = 6 and 15, respectively
  - May be combined with nicotine replacement therapy (NRT) for those with cravings
  - S/E: nausea, insomnia, headache, depression, suicidal ideation; safety not established in adolescents or patients with psychiatric or cardiovascular disease; pregnancy Category C
- Bupropion SR (Zyban): 150 mg PO for 3 days and then 150 mg BID:
  - Start 1 week prior to smoking cessation and continue for 7 to 12 weeks.
  - Twice as effective as placebo
  - Drug of choice for patients with depression or schizophrenia; additional benefit of weight loss
  - May be combined with varenicline and NRT in men who smoke >1 PPD
  - S/E: tachycardia, headache, nausea, insomnia, dry mouth; contraindicated in patients who have seizure disorders or anorexia/bulimia; pregnancy Category C (1,2)[A]

- NRT (e.g., patch, gum, lozenge, inhaler, nasal spray) (1,2)[A]:
  – Improves quit rates by 50–70% versus placebo
  – Available over the counter
  – Patch (NicoDerm CQ 21, 14, and 7 mg):
    ○ 1 patch q24h
    ○ Start with 21 mg if smoking ≥10 cigarettes per day; otherwise, start with 14 mg.
    ○ 6 weeks on initial dose and then taper
    ○ 2 weeks each on subsequent doses
    ○ No proven benefit beyond 8 weeks
  – ENDS
    ○ Contain less nicotine than cigarette
    ○ Controversial if less "dangerous" than tobacco; not well studied as NRT (3)[B]
    ○ Conflicting data on whether teen use increases or decreases risk to cigarette progression
    ○ Not an effective adjunct for cessation
  – Gum (Nicorette, 2 and 4 mg):
    ○ Use 4 mg if smoking ≥25 cigarettes per day.
    ○ Chew 1 piece q1–2h for 6 weeks, then 1 piece q2–4h for 3 weeks, and then 1 piece q4–8h for 3 weeks.
  – May use in combination with bupropion; monitor for hypertension.
  – S/E: headache, pharyngitis, cough, rhinitis, dyspepsia; all mainly with inhaler and spray forms
  – Pregnancy Category D
  – NRT is reasonable in hospitalized smokers because NRT products immediately treat nicotine withdrawal symptoms, whereas varenicline and bupropion take time to reach steady state.

Second Line
- Nortriptyline: 25 to 75 mg/day PO or in divided doses (1)[A]:
  – Start 10 to 14 days prior to smoking cessation and continue for at least 12 weeks.
  – Efficacy similar to bupropion, but side effects are more common; pregnancy Category D
  – The antidepressants bupropion and nortriptyline aid long-term smoking cessation (4)[A].
- Clonidine: 0.1 mg PO BID or 0.1 mg/day transdermal patch weekly (1):
  – Side effects: hypotension, bradycardia, depression, fatigue; pregnancy Category C

ADDITIONAL THERAPIES
- Electronic cigarettes: low grade of evidence (5)[A]
- Pharmacotherapy and behavior support increase success compared with minimal intervention or usual care (4)[A].
- Naltrexone: no evidence
- Individual behavioral counseling for smoking cessation increases effectiveness for both those with pharmacotherapy and without pharmacotherapy.

COMPLEMENTARY & ALTERNATIVE MEDICINE
Acupuncture, aversive therapy, and hypnosis have not been proven to enhance long-term smoking cessation.

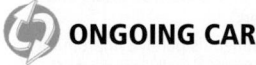 **ONGOING CARE**

FOLLOW-UP RECOMMENDATIONS
- Follow up 3 to 7 days after scheduled quit date and at least monthly for 3 months thereafter.
- Refraining from tobacco products for first 2 weeks is critical to long-term abstinence.
- Encourage patients who relapse to try again.

Patient Monitoring
- Short-term withdrawal symptoms include dysphoria, depressed mood, irritability, anxiety, insomnia, increased appetite, and poor concentration.
- Longer term risks of smoking cessation include weight gain (4 to 5 kg on average) and depression.
- Quitting is also associated with exacerbations of ulcerative colitis and worsening of cognitive function in patients with schizophrenia.
- Nicotine withdrawal syndrome: dysphoric or depressed mood, insomnia, irritability, frustration, or anger; anxiety, difficulty concentrating, restlessness, and increased appetite or weight gain
- Lung cancer risk by smoking status: heavy smokers 1.00, light smokers 9.44 (0.35 to 0.56), ex-smokers 0.17 (0.13 to 0.23), never smoker 0.09 (0.06 to 0.13); adjusted hazard ratio (95% CI)

DIET
Healthy eating for limiting weight gain

PATIENT EDUCATION
- 1-800-QUIT-NOW
- Affordable Care Act on impact on coverage for smoking cessation treatments: https://www.lung.org/our-initiatives/tobacco/cessation-and-prevention/affordable-care-act-tobacco.html

PROGNOSIS
- Measurable cardiovascular benefits of smoking cessation begin as early as 24 hours after quitting and continue to mount until the risk is reduced to that of nonsmokers by 5 to 15 years.
- People who quit smoking after a heart attack or cardiac surgery reduces their risk of death by 1/3.
- Relapse rates initially >60% but decrease to 2–4% per year after completing 2 years of abstinence
- >16 million Americans are living with a disease caused by smoking or exposure to tobacco smoke.
- For every smoking-related death, at least another 30 people live with a serious smoking-related illness.
- Smokers die an average of 10 years earlier than nonsmokers.
- Pharmacotherapy for preoperative smokers increases cessation rates and decreases postoperative complications.

COMPLICATIONS
- Disability and premature death due to heart attack, stroke, cancer, COPD
- Smoking more than doubles the risk of coronary artery disease and doubles the risk of stroke.
- Smokers are 12 to 22 times more likely than nonsmokers to die from lung cancer.
- Worldwide, tobacco use causes nearly 6 million deaths per year, and current trends show that tobacco use will cause >8 million deaths annually by 2030.
- Complications with screening by low-dose CT include complications associated with needle biopsy, bronchoscopy, and thoracotomy from false positives.

REFERENCES
1. Cahill K, Stevens S, Perera R, et al. Pharmacological interventions for smoking cessation: an overview and network meta-analysis. *Cochrane Database Syst Rev.* 2013;(5):CD009329.
2. Thomsen T, Villebro N, Møller AM. Interventions for preoperative smoking cessation. *Cochrane Database Syst Rev.* 2014;(3):CD002294.
3. Hughes JR, Stead LF, Hartmann-Boyce J, et al. Antidepressants for smoking cessation. *Cochrane Database Syst Rev.* 2014;(1):CD000031.
4. Stead LF, Koilpillai P, Fanshawe TR, et al. Combined pharmacotherapy and behavioural interventions for smoking cessation. *Cochrane Database Syst Rev.* 2016;(3):CD008286.
5. Fanshawe TR, Halliwell W, Lindson N, et al. Tobacco cessation interventions for young people. *Cochrane Database Syst Rev.* 2017;(11):CD003289.

ADDITIONAL READING
- Babb S, Malarcher A, Schauer G, et al. Quitting smoking among adults—United States, 2000–2015. *MMWR Morb Mortal Wkly Rep.* 2017;65(52):1457–1464.
- Centers for Disease Control and Prevention. Smoking & tobacco use: fast facts. https://www.cdc.gov/tobacco/data_statistics/fact_sheets/fast_facts/index.htm. Accessed November 11, 2018.
- McMenamin S, Yoeun S, Halpin H, et al. Affordable Care Act impact on Medicaid coverage of smoking-cessation treatments. *Am J Prev Med.* 2018;54(4):479–485.
- Salisbury-Afshar E. Individual behavioral counseling for smoking cessation. *Am Fam Physician.* 2018;98(1):21–22.

 SEE ALSO

Nicotine Addiction; Substance Use Disorders

 CODES

ICD10
- F17.210 Nicotine dependence, cigarettes, uncomplicated
- F17.213 Nicotine dependence, cigarettes, with withdrawal
- F17.211 Nicotine dependence, cigarettes, in remission

CLINICAL PEARLS
- Tobacco use is the leading cause of preventable disease, disability, and death in the United States.
- Every patient who uses tobacco should be offered cessation advice.
- Use the 5 As for tobacco cessation efforts: ask, advise, assess, assist, and arrange.
- Depression with suicidal ideations is no longer a contraindication to varenicline use; FDA black box warning removed in 2016
- First-line pharmacologic therapies for smoking cessation include NRT, varenicline, and bupropion.
- Nicotine replacement (delivered by nicotine polacrilex gum, nicotine lozenges, nicotine nasal spray, and transdermal nicotine) has an effect comparable to cigarette smoking in terms increasing myocardial work and endothelial damage. The risks associated with NRT in patients with cardiac disease, however, are lower than the risks of ongoing smoking.
- ENDS are not an effective adjunct for tobacco cessation.

T

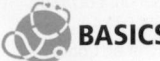

BASICS

DESCRIPTION

Tourette syndrome (TS) is a movement disorder most commonly seen in school-age children; a childhood-onset neurobehavioral disorder characterized by the presence of multiple motor and at least one phonic tic (see "Physical Exam")

- Tics are sudden, brief, repetitive, stereotyped motor movements (motor tics) or sounds (phonic tics) produced by moving air through the nose, mouth, or throat.
- Tics tend to occur in bouts.
- Tics can be simple or complex.
  - Motor tics precede vocal tics.
  - Simple tics precede complex tics.
- Tics often are preceded by sensory symptoms, especially a compulsion to move.
- Patients are able to suppress their tics, but voluntary suppression is associated with an inner tension that results in more forceful tics when suppression ceases.
- System(s) affected: nervous

EPIDEMIOLOGY

Incidence

- The onset occurs before 18 years of age.
- Predominant age
  - Average age of onset: 7 years (3 to 8 years)
  - Tic severity is greatest at ages 7 to 12 years.
    ○ 96% present by age 11 years
  - Of children with TS, 50% will experience complete resolution of symptoms by age 18 years (based on self-reporting).
- Predominant sex: male > female (3:1)
- Predominant race/ethnicity: clinically heterogeneous disorder, but non-Hispanic whites (2:1) compared with Hispanics and/or blacks

Prevalence

0.77% overall in children

- 1.06% in boys
- 0.25% in girls

ETIOLOGY AND PATHOPHYSIOLOGY

Abnormalities of dopamine neurotransmission and receptor hypersensitivity, most likely in the ventral striatum, play a primary role in the pathophysiology.

- Abnormality of basal ganglia development
- Thought to result from a complex interaction between social, environmental, and multiple genetic abnormalities
- Mechanism is uncertain; may involve dysfunction of basal ganglia–thalamocortical circuits, likely involving decreased inhibitory output from the basal ganglia, which results in an imbalance of inhibition and excitation in the motor cortex
- Controversial pediatric autoimmune neuropsychiatric disorder associated with streptococcal infection (PANDAS)
  - TS/OCD cases linked to immunologic response to previous group A β-hemolytic *Streptococcus* (GABHS)
  - Thought to be linked to 10% of all TS cases
  - Five criteria
    ○ Presence of tic disorder and/or OCD
    ○ Prepubertal onset of neuropsychosis
    ○ History of sudden onset of symptoms and/or episodic course with abrupt symptom exacerbation, interspersed with periods of partial/complete remission

    ○ Evidence of a temporal association between onset/exacerbation of symptoms and a prior streptococcal infection
    ○ Adventitious movements during symptom exacerbation (e.g., motor hyperactivity)

Genetics

- Predisposition: frequent familial history of tic disorders and OCD
- Precise pattern of transmission and genetic origin unknown. Recent studies suggest polygenic inheritance with evidence for a locus on chromosome 17q; sequence variants in *SLITRK1* gene on chromosome 13q also are associated with TS.
- Higher concordance in monozygotic compared with dizygotic twins; wide range of phenotypes

RISK FACTORS

- Risk of TS among relatives: 9.8–15%
- First-degree relatives of individuals with TS have a 10- to 100-fold increased risk of developing TS.
- Low birth weight, maternal stress during pregnancy, severe nausea and vomiting in 1st trimester

COMMONLY ASSOCIATED CONDITIONS

- OCD (28–67%)
- ADHD (50–60%)
- Conduct disorder
- Depression/anxiety including phobias, panic attacks, and stuttering
- Learning disabilities (23%)
- Impairments of visual perception, sleep disorders, restless leg syndrome, and migraine headaches

DIAGNOSIS

HISTORY

Diagnosis of TS is based on history and clinical presentation (i.e., observation of tics with/without presence of coexisting disorders). Identify comorbid conditions.

PHYSICAL EXAM

- Typically, the physical exam is normal.
- Motor and vocal tics are the clinical hallmarks.
- Tics fluctuate in type, frequency, and anatomic distribution over time.
- Multiple motor tics include facial grimacing, blinking, head/neck jerking, tongue protruding, sniffing, touching, and burping.
- Vocal tics include grunts, snorts, throat clearing, barking, yelling, hiccupping, sucking, and coughing.
- Tics are exacerbated by anticipation, emotional upset, anxiety, or fatigue.
- Tics subside when patient is concentrating/absorbed in activities.
- Motor and vocal tics may persist during all stages of sleep, especially light sleep.
- Blink-reflex abnormalities may be observed.
- No known clinical measures reliably predict children who will continue to express tics in adulthood; severity of tics in late childhood is associated with future tic severity.
- *Diagnostic and Statistical Manual of Mental Disorders* (5th ed.; *DSM-5*) criteria (1)[C]:
  - A. Both multiple motor and one or more vocal tics have been present at some time during the illness, although not necessarily concurrently.
  - B. The tics may wax and wane in frequency but have persisted for >1 year since first tic onset.

  - C. Onset is before age 18 years.
  - D. The disturbance is not attributable to the physiologic effects of a substance (e.g., cocaine) or another medical condition (e.g., Huntington disease, postviral encephalitis).

DIFFERENTIAL DIAGNOSIS

- Chorea/Huntington disease
- Myoclonus
- Seizure
- Ischemic or hemorrhagic stroke
- Essential tremor
- Posttraumatic/head injury
- Headache
- Dementia
- Wilson disease
- Sydenham chorea
- Multiple sclerosis
- Postviral encephalitis
- Toxin exposure (e.g., carbon monoxide, cocaine)
- Drug effects (e.g., dopamine agonists, fluoroquinolones)

DIAGNOSTIC TESTS & INTERPRETATION

Initial Tests (lab, imaging)

- No definitive lab tests diagnose TS; based on clinical features, particularly the presence of multiple motor and vocal tics
- Thyroid-stimulating hormone (TSH) should be measured because of association of tics with hyperthyroidism.
- No imaging studies diagnose TS.
- EEG shows nonspecific abnormalities; useful only to differentiate tics from epilepsy

Test Interpretation

- Smaller caudate volumes in patients with TS
- Striatal dopaminergic terminals are increased, as is striatal dopamine transporter (DAT) density.

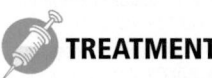

TREATMENT

GENERAL MEASURES

- Many patients require no treatment; patient should play an active role in treatment decisions.
- Treatment assessment
  - Yale Global Tic Severity Scale
  - Tourette Syndrome Severity Scale
  - Global Assessment of Functioning Scale
  - Gilles de la Tourette Syndrome-Quality of Life Scale
- A detailed history is crucial to management because tics and comorbidities are interrelated. Goal of treatment should be to improve social functioning, self-esteem, and quality of life.
- Educate that tics are neither voluntary nor psychiatric.
- Educate patient, family, teachers, and friends to identify and address psychosocial stressors and environmental triggers.
- No cure for tics: Treatment is purely symptomatic, and multimodal treatment usually is indicated.
- Neurologic and psychiatric evaluation may be useful for other primary disorders and comorbid conditions (especially ADHD, OCD, and depression).
- TS clusters with several comorbid conditions; each disorder must be evaluated for associated functional impairment because patients often are more disabled by their psychiatric conditions than by the tics; choice of initial treatment depends largely on worst symptoms (tics, obsessions, or impulsivity).

- Nonpharmacologic therapy—reassurance and environmental modification, identification and treatment of trigger, and cognitive-behavioral therapy
- When pharmacotherapy is employed, monotherapy is preferred to polytherapy.

MEDICATION

First Line

- Atypical antipsychotics
  - Risperidone: now recommended for standard therapy (2)[A]
    - Initiate 0.25 mg BID; titrate to 0.25 to 6.00 mg/day.
    - As effective as haloperidol and pimozide for tics with fewer side effects
    - Effective against comorbidities such as OCD
    - Side effects may limit use: sedation, weight gain, and fatigue.
- α_2-Adrenergic receptor agonists (2)[B]
  - Historically first-line agents due to favorable side-effect profile, but suboptimal efficacy in limited clinical trials
  - Side effects: sedation and hypotension common
    - Initiate therapy gradually and taper when discontinuing to avoid cardiac adverse events.
  - Clonidine 0.1 to 0.3 mg/day given BID–TID
    - Maximum dose: 0.5 mg/day
    - 25–50% of patients report at least some reduction in tics.
  - Guanfacine 1 to 3 mg/day given daily or BID
    - Less sedating and longer duration of action compared with clonidine
    - Improves motor/vocal tics by 30% in some studies; no better than placebo in others

Second Line

- Neuroleptics
  - Typical antipsychotics
    - High risk for extrapyramidal symptoms (EPS)
    - Haloperidol: Initiate 0.5 mg/day and titrate 0.5 mg/week up to 1 to 4 mg at bedtime (3)[B].
      - FDA-approved for treating tics
      - Considered last option of typical antipsychotics due to lower efficacy and increased side effects compared to similar medications
    - Pimozide: Initiate 0.5 mg/day and titrate 0.5 mg/week up to 1 to 4 mg at bedtime (4)[A].
      - FDA-approved for treating tics
      - Risk of cardiac toxicity (prolonged QT interval and arrhythmias); must be given under ECG monitoring; long-term use may induce sedation, weight gain, depression, pseudoparkinsonism, and akathisia.
      - Found to work better in long-term control of tics versus acute exacerbations
    - Fluphenazine: 2.5 to 10.0 mg/day
      - Effective but less favored due to side effects
  - Atypical antipsychotics (3)[C]
    - Olanzapine: Initiate 2.5 to 5.0 mg/day; titrate up to 20 mg/day.
      - Equally effective as haloperidol and pimozide
      - May cause metabolic disturbances and weight gain
    - Quetiapine: Initiate 100 to 150 mg/day; titrate to 100 to 600 mg/day.
      - Well tolerated, but limited data exists
    - Ziprasidone: 5 to 40 mg/day
    - Aripiprazole: Initiate 2 mg/day; titrate up to 20 or 30 mg/day.
      - Few studies but favorable side-effect profile

- Alternative treatments
  - Topiramate: 25 to 200 mg/day (2)[A]; promising data but not sufficient efficacy so far to recommend as first or second line
  - Tetrabenazine
  - Baclofen
- Treatment of ADHD in patients with tics (5)[A]
  - Stimulants
    - Comorbid tic disorder is not a serious contraindication, as previously held; exacerbation of tics is neither clinically significant nor common.
    - Methylphenidate: 2.5 to 30.0 mg/day
    - Dextroamphetamine: 5 to 30 mg/day
  - α_2-Adrenergic agonists
    - Guanfacine
    - Clonidine
      - The combination of methylphenidate and clonidine has shown superior efficacy in treating both ADHD and tic symptoms compared to monotherapy with either agent in one trial.
  - Other medications
    - Atomoxetine
    - Desipramine
- Treatment of OCD in patients with tics (6)[B]
  - SSRIs
    - First-line treatment of OCD; can be used in TS as well
    - Side effects include nausea, insomnia, sexual dysfunction, headache, and agitation.
    - Comorbid tic disorder not a contraindication; exacerbation of tics neither clinically significant nor common
    - Black box warning for suicidality with SSRIs
    - Fluoxetine: 10 to 80 mg/day
    - Fluvoxamine: 50 to 300 mg/day
    - Sertraline: 50 to 200 mg/day
  - Tricyclic antidepressants
    - Clomipramine: 25 to 200 mg/day
      - Can be used in patients refractory to SSRIs or to augment SSRIs in partial responders
      - Side effects: weight gain, dry mouth, lowered seizure threshold, and constipation; ECG changes, including QT prolongation and tachycardia

ADDITIONAL THERAPIES

- Botulinum toxin injections in severe cases or where chronic medication therapy is not preferred
- Habit-reversal training provides a viable tic suppression treatment: works equally for motor and vocal tics.

SURGERY/OTHER PROCEDURES

Thalamic ablation and deep brain stimulation have been used experimentally (7)[C].

COMPLEMENTARY & ALTERNATIVE MEDICINE

Nonpharmacologic therapy

- Reassurance and environmental modification
- Identification and treatment of triggers
- Behavioral therapy: Awareness/assertiveness training, relaxation therapy, habit-reversal therapy, and self-monitoring have shown to significantly decrease tic severity.
- Hypnotherapy
- Biofeedback
- Acupuncture
- Cannabinoids: insufficient evidence to recommend; small trials show small positive effects in some parameters (8)[A].

ONGOING CARE

FOLLOW-UP RECOMMENDATIONS

Patient Monitoring
Observe for associated psychiatric disorders.

PATIENT EDUCATION

- Reassurance that many patients with tics do not need medication; often education and/or therapy is all that is required.
- National Tourette Syndrome Association: http://www.tsa-usa.org

PROGNOSIS

- Symptoms will fluctuate throughout illness.
- Tic severity typically stabilizes by age 25 years.
- 60–75% of young adults show some improvement in symptoms.
- 10–40% of patients will exhibit full remission.

REFERENCES

1. Kenney C, Kuo SH, Jimenez-Shahed J. Tourette's syndrome. *Am Fam Physician*. 2008;77(5):651–658.
2. Huys D, Hardenacke K, Poppe P, et al. Update on the role of antipsychotics in the treatment of Tourette syndrome. *Neuropsychiatr Dis Treat*. 2012;8:95–104.
3. American Psychiatric Association. *Diagnostic and Statistical Manual of Mental Disorders*. 5th ed. Arlington, VA: American Psychiatric Association; 2013.
4. Roessner V, Plessen KJ, Rothenberger A, et al; for ESSTS Guidelines Group. European clinical guidelines for Tourette syndrome and other tic disorders. Part II: pharmacological treatment. *Eur Child Adolesc Psychiatry*. 2011;20(4):173–196.
5. Pringsheim T, Marras C. Pimozide for tics in Tourette's syndrome. *Cochrane Database Syst Rev*. 2009;(2):CD006996.
6. Pringsheim T, Steeves T. Pharmacological treatment for attention deficit hyperactivity disorder (ADHD) in children with comorbid tic disorders. *Cochrane Database Syst Rev*. 2011;(4):CD007990.
7. Lombroso PJ, Scahill L. Tourette syndrome and obsessive-compulsive disorder. *Brain Dev*. 2008;30(4):231–237.
8. Savica R, Stead M, Mack KJ, et al. Deep brain stimulation in Tourette syndrome: a description of 3 patients with excellent outcome. *Mayo Clin Proc*. 2012;87(1):59–62.

ADDITIONAL READING

Curtis A, Clarke CE, Rickards HE. Cannabinoids for Tourette's syndrome. *Cochrane Database Syst Rev*. 2009;(4):CD006565.

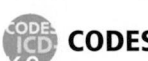 **CODES**

ICD10
F95.2 Tourette's disorder

CLINICAL PEARLS

- TS is diagnosed by history and witnessing tics; have parent video patient's tics if not present on exam in your office.
- Many patients require no treatment; patient should play an active role in treatment decisions.
- Nearly 50% of children with tics also have ADHD. Stimulants may be used as first-line treatment for ADHD (tics are not a contraindication, as previously believed).

T

TOXOPLASMOSIS

Jonathan MacClements, MD, FAAFP

BASICS

- *Toxoplasma gondii* is an obligate intracellular protozoan parasite.
- Most common latent protozoan infection
- Clinically significant disease typically manifests only in pregnancy or in an immunocompromised patient.

DESCRIPTION
- Acute self-limited infection in immunocompetent
- Acute symptomatic or reactivated latent infection in immunocompromised persons
- Congenital toxoplasmosis (acute primary infection during pregnancy)
- Ocular toxoplasmosis

Pediatric Considerations
- The earlier fetal infection occurs, the more severe.
- Risk of perinatal death is 5% if infected in 1st trimester.

Pregnancy Considerations
- Pregnant immunocompromised and HIV-infected women should undergo serologic testing.
- Counsel pregnant women regarding risks.
- Serologic testing during pregnancy is controversial.

EPIDEMIOLOGY

Incidence
- Prevalence of congenital toxoplasmosis in the United States: 10 to 100/100,000 live births
- Predominant sex: male > female

Prevalence
- Present in every country. Seropositivity rates range from <10% to >90% (1)[A].
- In the United States, 11% of individuals aged 6 to 49 years are seropositive.
- Age-adjusted prevalence in the United States is 23%.
- Seroprevalence among women in the United States is 15%.

ETIOLOGY AND PATHOPHYSIOLOGY
Transmission to humans
- Ingestion of raw or undercooked meat, food, or water containing tissue cysts or oocytes that is usually from soil contaminated with feline feces
- Transplacental passage from infected mother to fetus; risk of transmission is 30% on average.
- Blood product transfusion or solid-organ transplantation
- Ingested *T. gondii* oocysts enter host's gastrointestinal tract where bradyzoites/tachyzoites are released, penetrate contiguous cells, replicate, and are transported to susceptible tissues causing clinical disease.

Genetics
Human leukocyte antigen (HLA) DQ3 is a genetic marker for susceptibility in HIV/AIDS patients.

RISK FACTORS
- Immunocompromised states, including HIV infection with CD4 cell count <100/μL
- Primary infection during pregnancy; risk of fetal transmission increases with gestational age at seroconversion. Transmission in the 1st trimester is associated with more severe consequences.
- Chronically infected immunocompromised pregnant women are at increased risk for transmitting congenital toxoplasmosis.

GENERAL PREVENTION
- Avoid eating undercooked meat: Cook to 152°F (66°C) or freeze for 24 hours at ≤−12°C.
- Avoid drinking unfiltered water.
- Wash produce thoroughly.
- Strict hand hygiene after touching soil
- Wear gloves and wash hands after handling raw meat or cat litter.
- Avoid shellfish (*Toxoplasma* cysts).

COMMONLY ASSOCIATED CONDITIONS
- Chorioretinitis; self-limiting, febrile lymphadenopathy; mononucleosis-like illness
- Potential association with schizophrenia

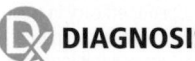

DIAGNOSIS

HISTORY
- Congenital toxoplasmosis
  - Clinical presentation varies widely; 80% of patients are asymptomatic at birth.
  - Classic triad (*uncommon*): chorioretinitis, hydrocephalus, cerebral calcifications
  - Manifestations may include prematurity, intrauterine growth retardation (IUGR).
  - Jaundice, rash with a mononucleosis-like illness
  - Mental retardation, seizures, visual defects, spasticity, sensorineural hearing loss
- Ocular toxoplasmosis
  - Chorioretinitis: focal necrotizing retinitis
  - Yellowish-white elevated cotton patch
  - Congenital disease usually bilateral; acquired is more often unilateral.
  - Symptoms include blurred vision, scotoma, pain, and photophobia.
- Acute toxoplasmosis (immunocompetent host)
  - ~90% of patients are asymptomatic.
  - Most common manifestation is bilateral, symmetric, nontender cervical lymphadenopathy.
  - Constitutional symptoms such as fever, chills, and sweats are usually mild.
  - Headaches, myalgias, pharyngitis, hepatosplenomegaly, and diffuse nonpruritic maculopapular rash may occur.
  - Pregnant women are often asymptomatic.
  - CNS: encephalitis
  - Headache; focal neurologic deficits and seizures
  - Fever usually present
  - Extracerebral toxoplasmosis: pneumonitis, chorioretinitis; rarely: GI system, liver, musculoskeletal system, heart, bone marrow, bladder, and orchitis

PHYSICAL EXAM
- In adults: fever, lymphadenopathy, nonpruritic rash
- In newborns: hydrocephalus, neurologic abnormalities, hepatosplenomegaly, chorioretinitis, microcephaly, mental retardation

DIFFERENTIAL DIAGNOSIS
Syphilis, lymphoma, progressive multifocal leukoencephalopathy, cryptococcal meningitis, congenital TORCH infections, *Listeria* infection, tuberculosis (TB), erythroblastosis fetalis

DIAGNOSTIC TESTS & INTERPRETATION
- CBC: atypical lymphocytosis, anemia, thrombocytopenia
- Serology interpretation
  - IgM antibodies appear in the 1st week if acute infection
  - Initial test demonstrates positive IgM and negative IgG, with both tests being positive 2 weeks later.
  - If follow-up IgG is negative 2 to 4 weeks later and IgM is positive, this is likely a false positive.
  - Negative IgG rules out prior infection (IgG persists for life).
- Types of serologic tests
  - ELISA: most commonly used
  - Sabin-Feldman dye test: gold standard against which all other serologic assays are compared
  - IFA test: more available in commercial labs
  - ISAGA: widely available commercially; more sensitive and specific than IFA for detecting IgM
  - Avidity testing: confirmatory test to establish if positive IgM/IgG reflects recent or chronic infection
- PCR: *T. gondii* DNA amplification in blood or amniotic fluid; used for diagnosis of fetal infection
- Culture (rarely necessary): Organism can be isolated either by cell culture or by mouse inoculation.

Initial Tests (lab, imaging)
- Diagnosis of primary infection is typically based on history and confirmed by serology.
- Serum *Toxoplasma*-specific IgG and IgM are first step.
- According to IgM result, determine IgG avidity.
- Diagnosis of maternal infection and congenital toxoplasmosis
  - Test pregnant women who have mononucleosis-like illness but negative heterophile test for toxoplasmosis.
  - Diagnose maternal infection based on two blood samples at least 2 weeks to show seroconversion.
  - High avidity of IgG during 1st trimester argues against maternal primary infection.
  - Real-time PCR analysis of amniotic fluid predicts fetal infection and guides treatment.
  - Fetal ultrasound is useful for prognosis.
  - Routine screening for toxoplasmosis is not recommended in pregnancy.
- Neonatal diagnosis of congenital toxoplasmosis
  - Serology requires repeat testing for IgM and IgA.
  - Sample cord or peripheral blood within 2 weeks
  - Ophthalmologic, auditory, and neurologic examinations; lumbar puncture and head CT
- Diagnosis of toxoplasmic encephalitis
  - Serology for IgG
  - Imaging: MRI is more sensitive than CT scan to identify characteristic ring-enhancing lesions.
- SPECT and PET scans can help distinguish toxoplasmosis from CNS lymphoma.

Diagnostic Procedures/Other
- Lymph node biopsy
- Brain biopsy in CNS disease
- Amniocentesis with PCR (risk of false negatives and false positives)
- Placental isolation of *Toxoplasma* is diagnostic.

Test Interpretation
- Confirmatory, meningocerebritis ± abscesses with necrosis, Giemsa
- Lymph node histology shows triad of:
  - Reactive follicular hyperplasia
  - Irregular clusters of epithelioid histiocytes blurring margins of germinal centers
  - Distension of sinuses with monocytoid cells
- Sensitivity of triad 63%, specificity 91%

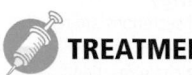

TREATMENT

GENERAL MEASURES
Immunocompetent patients usually require no treatment.

MEDICATION
First Line

ALERT
Important: All pyrimethamine-containing regimens should include leucovorin (folinic acid 10 to 25 mg/day PO) during and 1 week after completion of pyrimethamine to prevent drug-induced hematologic toxicity (2)[A].

- Treatment in immunocompromised hosts
  - Initial regimen of choice is pyrimethamine 200 mg loading dose PO, followed by 50 mg/day plus sulfadiazine 4 to 6 g/day PO in 4 divided doses; for those intolerant or allergic to sulfadiazine, clindamycin 600 to 1,200 mg IV or 450 mg PO QID can be used instead.
  - Alternative regimens for patients intolerant to sulfadiazine and clindamycin include the following:
    - Pyrimethamine: 200 mg loading dose PO, followed by 50 mg/day plus azithromycin 900 to 1,200 mg PO once daily
    - Pyrimethamine: 200 mg loading dose PO and then 50 mg/day plus atovaquone 1,500 mg PO BID
    - Sulfadiazine: 1,000 to 1,500 mg QID plus atovaquone 1,500 mg BID
    - Trimethoprim-sulfamethoxazole: 10/50 mg/kg/day PO or IV divided BID (for 30 days) may be a cost-effective alternative.
  - Duration of therapy: typically 6 weeks, lower doses for secondary prophylaxis (2)[A]
  - Use adjunctive steroids in patients with signs of increased intracranial pressure.
  - Anticonvulsants, if there is a history of seizures
- Prophylaxis in immunocompromised patients
  - Primary prophylaxis: indicated for patients with HIV infection and CD4 count <100 cells/μL who are *T. gondii* IgG positive
    - Trimethoprim-sulfamethoxazole-DS: 1 tablet PO daily. Alternative for sulfa allergy is dapsone 50 mg/day PO *plus* pyrimethamine 50 mg PO weekly *plus* leucovorin 25 mg PO weekly *or* atovaquone 1,500 mg PO daily.
  - Secondary prophylaxis: Following 6 weeks of therapy, administer lower doses of drugs:
    - Sulfadiazine 2 to 4 g/day in 2 to 4 divided doses *plus* pyrimethamine 25 to 50 mg/day is the first choice.
    - Alternative regimens include clindamycin 600 mg PO q8h *plus* pyrimethamine 25 to 50 mg/day PO *or* atovaquone 750 mg PO BID to QID ± pyrimethamine 25 mg PO daily.

- Pregnant women (3)[A]
  - Although typically offered, it is unsure if antenatal treatment reduces congenital transmission.
  - <18 weeks' gestation: spiramycin 1 g PO q8h without food until delivery if amniotic fluid PCR is negative; does not treat infection in the fetus
  - >18 weeks' gestation: Pyrimethamine and sulfadiazine should be considered only if fetal infection is documented by positive amniotic fluid PCR (pyrimethamine is teratogenic):
    - Pyrimethamine: 50 mg PO q12h for 2 days, then 50 mg/day plus sulfadiazine 75 mg/kg PO × 1 dose and then 50 mg/kg q12h (max 4 g/day)
- Treat infected newborns regardless of clinical manifestations:
  - Pyrimethamine 2 mg/kg/day (max 50 mg) for 2 days; then 1 mg/kg/day (max 25 mg) for 2 to 6 month and then 1 mg/kg (max 25 mg) on Monday, Wednesday, and Friday; sulfadiazine 100 mg/kg/day divided BID; and leucovorin 10 mg 3 times per week during pyrimethamine and 1 week after discontinuation
- Immunocompetent nonpregnant patients generally do not require treatment unless symptoms are severe or prolonged; one of two regimens can be used:
  - Pyrimethamine: 100 mg loading dose PO, followed by 25 to 50 mg/day *plus* sulfadiazine 2 to 4 g/day in 4 divided doses
  - Pyrimethamine: 100 mg loading dose PO, followed by 25 to 50 mg/day *plus* clindamycin 300 mg PO QID

Second Line
- Clindamycin: 900 to 1,200 mg TID IV used for ocular and CNS toxoplasmosis alone and in combination with pyrimethamine; as effective as the sulfadiazine-pyrimethamine with fewer adverse effects
- Corticosteroids (prednisone 1 to 2 mg/kg/day) are added for macular chorioretinitis or CNS infection.
- Alternatives: atovaquone (Mepron), azithromycin (Zithromax), clarithromycin (Biaxin), or dapsone *plus* pyrimethamine and leucovorin
- Trimethoprim-sulfamethoxazole appears to be equivalent to pyrimethamine-sulfadiazine in AIDS patients with CNS disease.

ONGOING CARE

FOLLOW-UP RECOMMENDATIONS
Patient Monitoring
Precautions
- Monitor for bone marrow, renal, or liver toxicity.
- Good hydration: Sulfadiazine is poorly soluble and may crystallize in the urine.
- Watch for antibiotic-associated diarrhea.
- Sulfonamides may alter phenytoin and warfarin levels or interfere with oral hypoglycemic agents.

PATIENT EDUCATION
- http://www.aafp.org/afp/2003/0515/p2145.html
- http://familydoctor.org/familydoctor/en/diseases-conditions/toxoplasmosis.html

PROGNOSIS
- Immunodeficient patients often relapse if treatment or suppression therapy is stopped.
- Treatment may prevent the development of untoward sequelae in infants with congenital toxoplasmosis.

REFERENCES
1. Torgerson PR, Mastroiacovo P. The global burden of congenital toxoplasmosis: a systematic review. *Bull World Health Organ*. 2013;91(7):501–508.
2. Montoya JG, Liesenfeld O. Toxoplasmosis. *Lancet*. 2004;363(9425):1965–1976.
3. Montoya JG, Remington JS. Management of *Toxoplasma gondii* infection during pregnancy. *Clin Infect Dis*. 2008;47(4):554–566.

ADDITIONAL READING
- Alday P, Doggett J. Drugs in development for toxoplasmosis: advances, challenges, and current status. *Drug Des Devel Ther*. 2017;11:273–293.
- Arantes TE, Silveira C, Holland GN, et al. Ocular involvement following postnatally acquired *Toxoplasma gondii* infection in Southern Brazil: a 28-year experience. *Am J Ophthalmol*. 2015;159(6): 1002.e2–1012.e2.
- Basavaraju A. Toxoplasmosis in HIV infection: an overview. *Trop Parasitol*. 2016;6(2):129–135.
- Garweg JG, Stanford MR. Therapy for ocular toxoplasmosis—the future. *Ocul Immunol Inflamm*. 2013;21(4):300–305.
- Kaplan JE, Benson C, Holmes KK, et al; for Centers for Disease Control and Prevention (CDC), National Institutes of Health, HIV Medicine Association of the Infectious Diseases Society of America. Guidelines for prevention and treatment of opportunistic infections in HIV-infected adults and adolescents: recommendations from CDC, the National Institutes of Health, and the HIV Medicine Association of the Infectious Diseases Society of America. *MMWR Recomm Rep*. 2009;58(RR-4):1–207.
- Paquet C, Yudin MH; for Society of Obstetricians and Gynaecologists of Canada. Toxoplasmosis in pregnancy: prevention, screening, and treatment. *J Obstet Gynaecol Can*. 2013;35(1):78–81.

CODES

ICD10
- B58.9 Toxoplasmosis, unspecified
- P37.1 Congenital toxoplasmosis
- B58.2 Toxoplasma meningoencephalitis

CLINICAL PEARLS
- Toxoplasmosis is often asymptomatic in immunocompetent patients.
- Primary prevention is important, particularly for pregnant women and immunodeficient patients.
- The most common manifestation of acute toxoplasmosis in immunocompetent host is bilateral, symmetric, nontender cervical lymphadenopathy.
- Universal screening for congenital toxoplasmosis is not currently recommended.

T

TRACHEITIS, BACTERIAL

Mary Cataletto, MD, FAAP, FCCP • Margaret J. McCormick, MS, RN, CNE

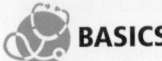

BASICS

DESCRIPTION
- Acute, potentially life-threatening infraglottic bacterial infection following a primary viral infection, usually parainfluenzae or influenza viruses
- Isolated tracheitis is rare. More commonly inflammation affects surrounding tissue (1).
  - Direct laryngoscopy reveals marked subglottic edema and thick mucopurulent secretions, sometimes causing pseudomembranes.
- System(s) affected: pulmonary
- Synonym(s): laryngotracheobronchitis; pseudomembranous croup; bacterial croup

EPIDEMIOLOGY

Incidence
- Estimated incidence: 4 to 8 per 1 million (2)
- Approximately 0.1/100,000 children-years in United Kingdom (1)
- First cases described prior to 1950; resurgence of cases has been noted since 1979.
- Peak incidence in children: fall and winter
- Mean age: 5 years (2)
- Infections in adolescents and adults have been reported.
- Predominant sex: male > female (2:1)
- Accounts for 5–14% of upper airway obstruction in children requiring critical care services

Prevalence
- Rare illness
- Most common potentially life-threatening upper airway infection in children
- Methicillin-resistant *Staphylococcus aureus* (MRSA) may contribute to changing epidemiology and virulence.

ETIOLOGY AND PATHOPHYSIOLOGY
- *S. aureus* (most common pediatric cause): Consider MRSA.
- *Haemophilus influenzae* type B
- *Streptococcus pyogenes* group A
- *Streptococcus pneumoniae*
- *Moraxella catarrhalis* (associated with higher intubation rate; more frequent in younger children)
- Frequently polymicrobial

Genetics
No known genetic predisposition

RISK FACTORS
- Periods of increased seasonal activity of respiratory viruses
- Reports following adenoidectomy, with chronic tracheal aspiration, with evidence of other concurrent infections, including sinusitis, otitis, pneumonia, or pharyngitis

GENERAL PREVENTION
- Standard precautions, with scrupulous attention to hand washing
- Vaccination against viruses that may predispose to bacterial tracheitis
- In children with artificial airways, periodic surveillance of tracheal cultures can be helpful.

COMMONLY ASSOCIATED CONDITIONS
- Consider anatomic abnormalities or foreign body as well as recent pharyngeal or laryngeal surgery.
- Predisposing: Down syndrome, immunodeficiency, subglottic hemangioma, tracheoesophageal fistula repair, tracheobronchomalacia
- Viral coinfection may occur.

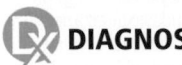

DIAGNOSIS

- May present with fever and systemic toxicity or as more localized disease
- Careful history and physical exam are the best methods to distinguish bacterial tracheitis from croup and other rare causes of upper airway obstruction.

HISTORY
- Prodromal upper respiratory tract symptoms
- Gradual progression of mild upper airway symptoms over 1 hour to 6 days to acute, febrile phase of rapid respiratory decompensation
- No drooling
- No response to aerosolized epinephrine and/or systemic corticosteroids (2)
- May see more indolent course in patients with artificial airways

PHYSICAL EXAM
Fever >38°C (100.4°F)
- Toxic appearance
- Variable degree of respiratory distress (1,3)
  - Cough
  - Tachypnea
  - Inspiratory stridor
- Voice and cry usually normal
- Drooling uncommon

DIFFERENTIAL DIAGNOSIS
- Severe croup (viral)
- Spasmodic croup
- Diphtheria in nonvaccinated patients
- Retropharyngeal abscess
- Epiglottitis
- Bacterial pneumonia
- Foreign body aspiration
- Angioneurotic edema

DIAGNOSTIC TESTS & INTERPRETATION
- Routine laboratory studies are not required to make the diagnosis.
- Radiographs are neither definitive nor diagnostic.
- Tracheal endoscopy provides a definitive diagnosis (2)[C].

Initial Tests (lab, imaging)
- Bacterial cultures of tracheal secretions are required for culture isolates and sensitivities.
- Rapid antigen or polymerase chain reaction (PCR)-based testing for respiratory viruses may be helpful.
- Routine laboratory studies may not be helpful.
- Blood cultures rarely positive
- CBC results may vary.
  - WBC count may show marked leukocytosis or may be normal.
  - Increased band cell count
- Radiographs may be normal, but exudates may mimic the findings in foreign body aspiration.
- Pneumonic infiltrates are common.
- Anteroposterior (AP) and lateral neck x-rays show subglottic and tracheal narrowing (i.e., steeple sign on AP film) with haziness and radiopaque linear or particulate densities (crusts).
- In patients with risk of acute respiratory obstruction, either do not obtain x-rays or monitor carefully.

Follow-Up Tests & Special Considerations
Follow chest film if suspect pneumonia.

Diagnostic Procedures/Other
- Direct laryngoscopy and tracheoscopy is diagnostic and demonstrates
  - Normal supraglottic structures
  - Marked subglottic erythema and edema
  - Ulcerations
  - Epithelial sloughing
  - Copious mucopurulent secretions ± plaques or pseudomembranes
- Obtain Gram stain and aerobic, anaerobic, and viral cultures of tracheal secretions during the procedure.
- Tracheal biopsy is rarely indicated but may be considered in immunodeficient child or child with ulcerative colitis.

Test Interpretation
- Diffuse inflammation of larynx, trachea, and bronchi
- Mucopurulent exudate; microabscesses may be present.
- Semiadherent membranes (containing numerous neutrophils and cellular debris) may be identified within the trachea.

TREATMENT

- Treat as potentially life-threatening airway emergency.
- Children with suspected or actual bacterial tracheitis should be cared for in a pediatric ICU (2)[C].
- Assess and monitor respiratory status; supplemental oxygen may be required.
- Airway protection and support, as necessary (at least 50% require intubation; some studies report up to 100%)
- Ventilatory support may be required.
- Suctioning

MEDICATION

- Empiric therapy should cover the most common pathogens until sensitivities are available: antistaphylococcal agent (vancomycin or clindamycin) and a 3rd-generation cephalosporin (e.g., ceftriaxone or cefotaxime) (2)[C].
- In the case of technology-dependent children with tracheostomy, make initial antibiotic choices based on previous tracheal culture.
- Narrow regimen when pathogens and sensitivities available (2)[C].
- Inhaled antibiotics are not routinely recommended either as primary or adjuvant therapy (4)[A].
- Contraindications: Refer to the manufacturer's literature for each drug.
- Precautions: Refer to the manufacturer's literature for each drug. Avoid aminoglycosides in patients with previous hearing loss.
- Significant possible interactions: Refer to the manufacturer's literature for each drug.

ISSUES FOR REFERRAL

All children with suspected or actual bacterial tracheitis should be cared for in a pediatric ICU; ID and ENT consultation should be considered.

ADDITIONAL THERAPIES

- At present, evidence is lacking to establish the effect of heliox inhalation in the treatment of croup in children.
- For technology-dependent children with artificial airway:
  - Initial antibiotic choices should cover most recent tracheal aspirate isolates and then be refined according to culture and sensitivity results.

SURGERY/OTHER PROCEDURES

- Tracheostomy is usually not necessary.
- Therapeutic bronchoscopy may be necessary to facilitate removal of inspissated secretions.
- Tracheal membranes may require removal.

ADMISSION, INPATIENT, AND NURSING CONSIDERATIONS

- Aggressive supportive care and airway protection are paramount.
- Initial treatment of choice for bacterial tracheitis is broad-spectrum antibiotic coverage.
- Children with tracheitis and artificial airways present unique challenges: Tracheoscopy is important in establishing diagnosis in this population.
- Be vigilant for possible MRSA.

Pediatric Considerations

- True pediatric emergency
- Admission to ICU
- Maintain airway: often difficult due to copious secretions
  - Endotracheal or nasotracheal intubation usually needed, especially in infants and children <4 years of age
  - Much less likely to need intubation if child >8 years of age
  - Advantage of intubation is the ability to clear trachea and bronchi of secretions and pseudomembranes.
- Vigorous pulmonary toilet to clear airway of secretions
- Hydration, humidification, antibiotics
- Admission criteria/initial stabilization
  - Suspected or confirmed diagnosis of tracheitis
  - Respiratory distress
  - Artificial airway
- Nursing
  - Provide calm, quiet environment for child once endoscopy and cultures are done.
  - Airway monitoring
  - Frequent suctioning
  - Monitor fluid balance.
  - Establish and maintain open lines of communication with child and parents.
- Discharge when no longer in need of acute care.

ONGOING CARE

FOLLOW-UP RECOMMENDATIONS
Patient Monitoring
Children with artificial airways will require ongoing follow-up.

DIET
Varies with clinical situation

PATIENT EDUCATION
Keep immunizations up to date.

PROGNOSIS

- Intubation generally 3 to 11 days
- Usually requires 3 to 7 days of hospitalization
- With effective early recognition and management, complete recovery can be expected.
- Cardiopulmonary arrest and death have occurred.
- Higher recurrence rates in children with artificial airways

COMPLICATIONS

- Cardiopulmonary arrest
- Hypotension
- Acute respiratory distress syndrome (ARDS)
- Pneumonia
- Sepsis (1)
- Formation of pseudomembranes
- Postinfectious stenosis (long term) (1)

REFERENCES

1. Blot M, Bonniaud-Blot P, Favrolt N, et al. Update on childhood and adult infectious tracheitis. *Med Mal Infect*. 2017;47(7):443–452.
2. Kuo CY, Parikh SR. Bacterial tracheitis. *Pediatr Rev*. 2014;35(11):497–499.
3. Tebruegge M, Pantazidou A, Thorburn K, et al. Bacterial tracheitis: a multi-centre perspective. *Scand J Infect Dis*. 2009;41(8):548–557.
4. Russell C, Shiroishi M, Siantz E, et al. The use of inhaled antibiotic therapy in the treatment of ventilator-associated pneumonia and tracheo-bronchitis: a systematic review. *BMC Pulm Med*. 2016;16:40.

ADDITIONAL READING

- Hopkins A, Lahiri T, Salerno R, et al. Changing epidemiology of life-threatening upper airway infections: the reemergence of bacterial tracheitis. *Pediatrics*. 2006;118(4):1418–1421.
- Huang YL, Peng CC, Chiu NC, et al. Bacterial tracheitis in pediatrics: 12 year experience at a medical center in Taiwan. *Pediatr Int*. 2009;51(1):110–113.
- Loftis L. Acute infectious upper airway obstructions in children. *Semin Pediatr Infect Dis*. 2006;17(1): 5–10.
- Shah S, Sharieff GQ. Pediatric respiratory infections. *Emerg Med Clin North Am*. 2007;25(4):961–979.
- Vorwerk C, Coats T. Heliox for croup in children. *Cochrane Database Syst Rev*. 2010;(2):CD006822.

SEE ALSO

Croup (Laryngotracheobronchitis); Epiglottitis

CODES

ICD10
- J04.10 Acute tracheitis without obstruction
- J04.11 Acute tracheitis with obstruction
- J05.0 Acute obstructive laryngitis [croup]

CLINICAL PEARLS

- Bacterial tracheitis is an acute, potentially life-threatening, infraglottic bacterial infection following a primary viral infection that accounts for 5–14% of upper airway obstructions in children requiring critical care services.
- Children with suspected or actual bacterial tracheitis should be cared for in a pediatric ICU.
- Endoscopy provides a definitive diagnosis (3).
- Initial treatment of choice for bacterial tracheitis is broad-spectrum antibiotic coverage, aggressive airway protection, and supportive care (3).

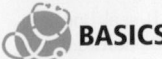

TRANSGENDER HEALTH

Dónal Kevin Gordon, MD, FAAFP

BASICS

DESCRIPTION

- Society's growing acceptance of nontraditional lifestyles has, in recent years, made increased room for transgender individuals, as it has for lesbians, gays, and bisexuals, even as these populations continue to suffer unique health care disparities. Better education of physicians and other providers will improve the health of the transgender population. Such education begins with teaching acceptance of all human beings into health care and ensuring a safe office environment for transgender individuals to speak openly with their clinicians. Once a "safe" space is created, it will be possible to provide appropriate and supportive health care to reduce inequities and the harms and disparities in health outcomes that result.
  - At least 1:11,900 males and 1:30,400 females in the United States define themselves as transgender (1).
  - Current estimates indicate 0.6% of U.S. adults, or some 1.4 million people, identify themselves as transgender, a 2-fold increase since 2011 (1,2).
- The terms "transgender" and "gender nonconforming" (GNC) refer to those whose gender identity or presentation differs from the sex assigned at birth (3).
  - Gender identity, the sense of one's self as male or female, and gender presentation, the outward expression of gender, may or may not reflect the self-identification of a transgender patient.
  - Transgender patients can no more be categorized or thought alike than any other patients. Race, ethnicity, socioeconomic status, age, and other factors, all play a role in how transgender patients define themselves.
  - Moreover, a patient's body may or may not match gender identity or presentation. Although a patient's anatomy may determine treatment, that treatment must also be sensitive to, and respect, gender identity and/or presentation.
  - Transgender people may be sexually oriented toward men, women, other transgender people, or any combination of the above.
  - Transgender patients are further defined by those who have undergone surgical procedures and/or medical treatment to better align gender identity, by those who plan such procedures in the future, and by others who do not.
- Accordingly, it is important to ask transgender patients how they would describe themselves and to honor terminology acceptable to each patient, specifically preferred name, preferred pronoun, and preferred gender identity, with those attributes ideally reflected within any electronic medical record (EMR).

- Transgender people have a unique set of mental and physical needs (4).
  - Real or imagined stigma and discrimination are barriers to health care (3).
  - Transgender patients are less likely to have health insurance and more likely to encounter discrimination on the part of health care providers, thereby limiting access to health care services.
  - >50% of transgender patients delay needed care, compared to 20% in the general population (3,5).
- Evidence-based medicine for transgender patients is lacking or limited to case reports and smaller studies aggravated, perhaps, by social stigma, marginalization, and discrimination (4).
- Transgender patients may also suffer from gender dysphoria, recognized in *Diagnostic and Statistical Manual of Mental Disorders, Fifth Edition* (*DSM-5*) as the disconnection between gender expression and one's assigned gender at birth (1).

DIAGNOSIS

- Specific health concerns
  - Transition-related medical care, or gender-confirming therapy, including hormone therapy and surgical treatment, or sex reassignment surgery (SRS) helps patients align primary and secondary sexual characteristics with gender identity (4).
  - The World Professional Association for Transgender Health (WPATH) has published standards of care (SOCs) that include hormone therapy and SRS (4)[C].
    - SOCs are endorsed by American College of Obstetricians and Gynecologists (ACOG), the Endocrine Society, the American Medical Association, and the American Psychological Association (4).
    - Hormone therapy and surgery not only treat symptoms of gender dysphoria but also help transgender patients achieve well-being (1).
    - Hormone therapy does convey a greater risk of thromboembolic disease, liver dysfunction, and cardiovascular (CV) disease (1).
    - Treatment is associated with a high degree of patient satisfaction, low prevalence of regrets, and significant relief of gender dysphoria (4)[C].
- Specific diseases
  - AIDS
    - Rate of HIV infection among transgender people is 4 times that of general population in the United States (5). Worldwide, the prevalence may be 50 times higher than the background rate (2).
    - Requires increased vigilance on the part of health care providers

- Psychosocial considerations
  - Transgender people are at risk of victimization by others, of mental health issues, including depression and anxiety, and of suicide (5).
    - 41% of transgender people have attempted suicide compared to 1.6% of the U.S. general population (1,4,5).
    - One 2012 survey found that 61% of transgender people had been victims of physical assault and abuse; 64% had been victims of sexual assault, mostly not reported.
    - Transgender people are at greater risk of societal discrimination including housing and workforce discrimination, are more likely to be unemployed, homeless, and lacking in social support owing to federal and state laws that inadequately protect transgender people from discrimination. The resulting social marginalization contributes to poor well-being overall, aggravated by limited access to quality health services (3).
  - Psychosocial assessment is recommended at baseline and at least annually.
  - Mental health and substance abuse screening are also indicated.

ALERT

- Transgender patients are at increased risk of suicidal ideation, suicide attempts, and suicide (1,4,5).
- Improving access to care
  - Barriers to health care
    - Transgender patients are often reluctant to disclose gender identity or expression, owing to the risk of stigma or discrimination.
    - 28% of transgender patients report being verbally harassed and 2% physically assaulted while seeking health care (1).
  - Providers' lack of education and experience
  - Financial barriers
    - Lack of health insurance
    - Unemployment among transgender people is twice the rate of general population (1).

TREATMENT

GENERAL MEASURES

- Care of transgender people, including hormone therapy, is within the scope of primary care providers.
- Education of health care providers, for physicians, and those beginning in medical school, is crucial to providing optimal care to transgender patients, and the lack of such education is a significant barrier to care for transgender individuals (2,4).

MEDICATION

First Line

- Gender-affirming hormone therapy (6)[A]
- Adolescents
  - Suppress pubertal development using gonadotropin-releasing hormone (GnRH) analogues when girls and boys first exhibit pubertal physical changes (Tanner stage 2).
  - Progestin

- Cross-sex steroids at about age 16 years
- Initiate treatment after persistent gender dysphoria/gender incongruence have been confirmed by a multidisciplinary team of medical and mental health providers and the patient has the mental capacity to provide informed consent, generally by age 16 years.
- Surgical referral
- Adults
  - Estrogens, antiandrogens, and/or GnRH agonists for male-to-female patients
    - Estradiol 2 to 6 mg/day, or estradiol transdermal patch 0.025 to 0.200 mg/day, or estradiol valerate or cypionate 5 to 30 mg IM every 2 weeks
    - Add spironolactone 100 to 300 mg/day, cyproterone acetate 25 to 50 mg/day, or GnRH agonists to minimize estrogen requirement.
    - At initial visit, do prostate-specific antigen (PSA), lipid panel, and liver function tests (LFTs); every 3 months, check testosterone levels until stable, monitor estradiol blood level for compliance, repeat lipid panel, and encourage breast exams.
    - Every 6 months to 1 year, preoperatively, order visual fields to assess for prolactinoma, check serum prolactin, and repeat lipid panel; if patient is >50 years old, recheck PSA and consider mammogram.
    - Every 6 months to 1 year, postoperatively, reduce estrogens to hormone replacement therapy (HRT) doses (conjugated equine estrogens 0.625 mg/day, transdermal ethinyl estradiol 0.05 to 0.10 mg/day, or ethinyl estradiol 0.02 to 0.05 mg/day) and do dual energy x-ray absorptiometry (DEXA) scan to monitor for osteoporosis.
  - Testosterone for female-to-male patients
    - Testosterone esters 100 to 200 mg IM every other week or transdermal testosterone 2.5 to 7.5 mg/day or testosterone gel 1.6% 50 to 100 mg/day with goal of serum testosterone in midmale range
    - At initial visit, check weight, lipid panel, and glucose level.
    - Every 3 to 6 months, repeat lipid panel and LFTs, do complete blood count to rule out polycythemia, and check testosterone levels.
    - Every 6 months to 1 year, preoperatively, do pelvic exam and Papanicolaou (Pap) smear per current protocols.
    - Every 2 years, do endometrial ultrasounds.
    - Every 6 months to 1 year, postoperatively, titrate testosterone to maintain serum testosterone at 500 μg/dL (17.35 SI) and do DEXA scan.

SURGERY/OTHER PROCEDURES
- SRS only after 1 year of hormone therapy
- In adolescents, consider delaying gender-confirming genital surgery until the patient is at least 18 years old.

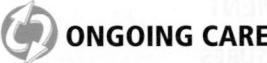 **ONGOING CARE**

FOLLOW-UP RECOMMENDATIONS
Interacting with the health care system
- Discrimination on the part of health care providers is a major barrier to care (5).

Patient Monitoring
- Routine medical screening:
  - Pelvic exam
  - Cervical and anal Pap tests
  - Screening for STIs
- Measurement of prolactin levels
- Evaluation of CV risk factors
- Bone mineral density tests, as indicated
- Breast cancer screening per guidelines
- Screening, as indicated, for prostate cancer in transgender females treated with estrogens
- In adolescents, monitor clinical pubertal development every 3 to 6 months and check labs (LH, FSH, E2/T, 25[OH]D) every 6 to 12 months; do bone mineral density test every 1 to 2 years.
- In adults, monitor physical changes and any adverse changes every 3 months during the 1st year of hormone therapy and then once or twice yearly.
- Transgender males: Check serum testosterone every 3 months until levels are in the normal physiologic male range; check hematocrit and hemoglobin at baseline and every 3 months in year 1 and then once or twice a year; monitor lipids as indicated.
- Transgender females: Check serum testosterone and estradiol every 3 months; if patient is on spironolactone, check serum electrolytes every 3 months in the 1st year of treatment and then annually.

PATIENT EDUCATION
- Hormone therapy and potential health risks
- Counseling for gender-confirming surgery
- Legal issues
  - Under the Affordable Care Act (ACA), denial of treatment of being transgender as a "preexisting condition" is banned (4).
  - Centers for Medicare & Medicaid Services (CMS) considers SRS experimental and denies coverage (4).
  - The U.S. Department of Veterans Affairs (VA), although acknowledging the need to care for transgender veterans, denies coverage of SRS on the basis of a VA regulation that excludes gender alterations from the medical benefits package (4).

REFERENCES
1. Roberts TK, Fantz CR. Barriers to quality health care for the transgender population. *Clin Biochem*. 2014;47(10–11):983–987.
2. Korpaisam S, Safer JD. Gaps in transgender medical education among healthcare providers: a major barrier to care for transgender persons [published online ahead of print June 19, 2018]. *Rev Endocr Metab Disord*. doi:10.1007/s11154-018-9452-5.
3. Cruz TM. Assessing access to care for transgender and gender nonconforming people: a consideration of diversity in combating discrimination. *Soc Sci Med*. 2014;110:65–73.
4. Stroumsa D. The state of transgender health care: policy, law, and medical frameworks. *Am J Public Health*. 2014;104(3):e31–e38.
5. Lim FA, Brown DV Jr, Justin Kim SM. Addressing health care disparities in the lesbian, gay, bisexual, and transgender population: a review of best practices. *Am J Nurs*. 2014;114(6):24–45.
6. Hembree WC, Cohen-Kettenis P, Gooren L, et al. Endocrine treatment of gender-dysphoric/gender-incongruent persons: an Endocrine Society clinical practice guideline. *J Clin Endocrinol Metab*. 2017;102(11):3869–3903.

ADDITIONAL READING
- Abebe A. Caring for transgender patients. *JAAPA*. 2016;29(6):49–53.
- Agency for Healthcare Research and Quality. *2011 National Healthcare Disparities Report*. Rockville, MD: Agency for Healthcare Research and Quality; 2011.
- Healthy People.gov. Lesbian, gay, bisexual, and transgender health. https://www.healthypeople.gov/2020/topics-objectives/topic/lesbian-gay-bisexual-and-transgender-health. Accessed October 18, 2018.
- Institute of Medicine. *The Health of Lesbian, Gay, Bisexual, and Transgender People: Building a Foundation for Better Understanding*. Washington, DC: National Academies Press; 2011.
- New York State Department of Health. *Care of the HIV-Infected Transgender Patient*. New York, NY: New York State Department of Health; 2011.
- Winter S, Diamond M, Green J, et al. Transgender people: health at the margins of society. *Lancet*. 2016;388(10042):390–400.

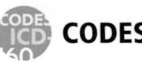 **CODES**

ICD10
- F64.1 Gender identity disorder in adolescence and adulthood
- Z11.4 Encounter for screening for human immunodeficiency virus
- Z72.52 High risk homosexual behavior

CLINICAL PEARLS
- Health care providers must be sensitive to the unique needs of transgender patients; must be open to the care of such patients; and should, as with all patients, display an ethical, principled, and timely approach to care.
- Do use inclusive language in the care of transgender patients, assessing the individuals' preferences, and respect differences among transgender patients.
- Always address health care needs particular to the transgender population.
- Avoid stigmatization of transgender patients, ensuring gender-blind clinical care.

TRANSIENT ISCHEMIC ATTACK (TIA)

Farha K. Syed, MD • Samuel E. Mathis, MD

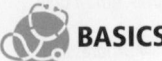 BASICS

DESCRIPTION
- A transient episode of neurologic dysfunction due to focal brain, retinal, or spinal cord ischemia without acute infarction
- Most important predictor of stroke: 15% of patients with stroke report previous TIA.
- Synonym(s): ministroke

EPIDEMIOLOGY
- 200,000 to 500,000 new TIA cases reported each year
  - 83 cases per 100,000 people/year in the United States
  - 400 to 800 cases per 100,000 persons aged 50 to 59 years
- Prevalence of TIA in general population: ~2.3%
- Predominant age: Risk increases >60 years; highest in 7th and 8th decades
- Predominant sex: male > female (3:1)
- Predominant race/ethnicity: African Americans > Hispanics > Caucasians. The difference in African Americans is exaggerated at younger ages.

ETIOLOGY AND PATHOPHYSIOLOGY
Temporary reduction/cessation of cerebral blood flow adversely affecting neuronal function
- Carotid/vertebral atherosclerotic disease
  - Artery-to-artery thromboembolism
  - Low-flow ischemia
- Small, deep vessel disease associated with hypertension (HTN)
  - Lacunar infarcts
- Cardiac diseases
  - 1–6% of patients with MI develop stroke.
- Embolism secondary to the following:
  - Valvular (mitral valve) pathology
  - Mural hypokinesias/akinesias with thrombosis (acute anterior MI/congestive cardiomyopathies)
  - Cardiac arrhythmia (atrial fibrillation accounts for 5–20% incidence)
- Hypercoagulable states
  - Antiphospholipid antibodies
  - Increased estrogen (e.g., oral contraceptives)
  - Pregnancy and parturition
- Arteritis
  - Noninfectious necrotizing vasculitis
  - Drugs
  - Irradiation
  - Local trauma
- Sympathomimetic drugs (e.g., cocaine)
- Other causes: spontaneous and posttraumatic (e.g., chiropractic manipulation) arterial dissection
- Fibromuscular dysplasia

Genetics
Inheritance is polygenic, with tendency to clustering of risk factors within families.

RISK FACTORS
- HTN
- Cardiac diseases (atrial fibrillation, MI, valvular disease)
- Diabetes
- Hyperlipidemia
- Atherosclerotic disease (carotid/vertebral stenosis)
- Cigarette smoking
- Thrombophilias

GENERAL PREVENTION
- Lifestyle changes: smoking cessation, diet modification, weight loss, regular aerobic exercise, and limited alcohol intake
- Strict control of medical risk factors: *diabetes* (glycemic control), *HTN* (thiazide and/or ACE/ARB), *hyperlipidemia* (statins), anticoagulation when high risk of cardioembolism (e.g., atrial fibrillation, mechanical valves)
- Causation is key to preventing recurrence (1).

ALERT
- 10–20% of patients with TIA have CVA within 90 days; up to 80% of this risk is preventable (2).
- 25–50% of those occur within the first 48 hours.

Geriatric Considerations
- Older patients have a higher mortality rate than younger patients—highest in 7th and 8th decades.
- Atrial fibrillation is a frequent cause among the elderly.

Pediatric Considerations
- Congenital heart disease is a common cause among pediatric patients.
- Other causes include the following:
  - Metabolic: homocystinuria, Fabry disease
  - Central nervous system infection
  - Clotting disorders
  - Genetic: Marfan syndrome, moyamoya, or sickle cell disease

Pregnancy Considerations
- Preeclampsia, eclampsia, and HELLP syndrome
- TTP and hemolytic uremic syndrome
- Postpartum angiopathy
- Cerebral venous thrombosis
- Hypercoagulable states related to pregnancy

COMMONLY ASSOCIATED CONDITIONS
- Atrial fibrillation
- Uncontrolled HTN
- Carotid stenosis
- TIA mimics
  - Some disease processes mimic TIA presentation.
  - Seizures, migraines, metabolic disturbances, syncope
  - Gradual onset with nonspecific symptoms (headache, memory loss)

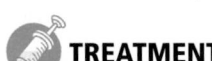 DIAGNOSIS

HISTORY
- Emphasis on symptom onset, progression, and recovery
- Carotid circulation (hemispheric): monocular visual loss, hemiplegia, hemianesthesia, neglect, aphasia, visual field defects (amaurosis fugax); less often, headaches, seizures, amnesia, confusion
- Vertebrobasilar (brain stem/cerebellar): bilateral visual obscuration, diplopia, vertigo, ataxia, facial paresis, Horner syndrome, dysphagia, dysarthria; also headache, nausea, vomiting, and ataxia
- Past medical history, baseline functional status
- ABCD2 or ABCD3-I score: predicts 48-hour CVA risk (3)
  - Score of 0 to 1: 0%; 2 to 3: 1.3%; 4 to 5: 4.1%; 6 to 7: 8.1%
    - **A**ge >65 years: 1 point
    - **B**P 140/90 mm Hg: 1 point
    - **C**linical presentation
      - Unilateral weakness: 2 points
      - Speech impaired without weakness: 1 point
    - **D**uration: 1 to 2 points based on time
    - **D**iabetes: 1 point
    - **Dual TIA** (within 7 days preceding): 2 points
    - **I**maging (new lesion or carotid stenosis): 2 points

PHYSICAL EXAM
- Vital signs, oxygen saturation
- Thorough neurologic and cardiac exams

DIFFERENTIAL DIAGNOSIS
- Evolving stroke
- Migraine (hemiplegic)
- Focal seizure (Todd paralysis)
- Bell palsy
- Neoplasm of brain
- Subarachnoid hemorrhage
- Intoxication
- Glucose or other electrolyte abnormalities
- Head trauma
- Central nervous system infection
- Multiple sclerosis

DIAGNOSTIC TESTS & INTERPRETATION
Initial Tests (lab, imaging)
- Neuroimaging within 24 hours of symptom onset
- MRI, including diffusion-weighted imaging, is the preferred brain diagnostic modality; if not available, then noncontrast head CT (4)[B]
- Noninvasive imaging of the cervicocephalic vessels should be performed routinely in suspected TIA (4)[A].
- Consider assessment of the extracranial vasculature by carotid US/TCD, MRA, or CTA depending on availability and expertise and characteristics of the patient (4)[B].
- Routine blood tests (CBC, chemistry, PT/PTT, UPT, coagulation screen, fasting lipid panel, ECG) are reasonable in evaluation of patient with TIA (1,4)[B].

Follow-Up Tests & Special Considerations
- If only noninvasive testing is performed prior to CEA, it is reasonable to pursue two concordant noninvasive findings; otherwise, catheter angiography should be considered (4)[B].
- Echo is reasonable in evaluation of patients with suspected TIA especially when no other cause is noted (4)[B].
- TEE is useful in identifying PFO, aortic arch atherosclerosis, and valvular disease; reasonable when this will alter management (4)[B]
- Prolonged cardiac monitoring is useful in patients with an unclear etiology after initial brain imaging and ECG (4)[B].
- EEG: if seizure suspected
- Consider a sleep study due to the high prevalence of sleep apnea among TIA patients; treatment with CPAP has shown to improve patient outcomes.

TREATMENT

GENERAL MEASURES
- TIA is a neurologic emergency. Immediate medical attention should be sought within 24 hours of symptom onset due to increased stroke risk.
- Current evidence suggests that patients with high-risk TIAs require rapid referral and 24-hour admission (ABCD2 score ≥3 g).
- Acute phase
  - Inpatient for high-risk individuals
  - Outpatient investigations may be considered based on patient's stroke risk, arrangement of follow-up, and social circumstances.
- Antiplatelet therapy to prevent recurrence or future CVA
- Treatment/control of underlying associated conditions

MEDICATION

- For patients with TIA, the use of antiplatelet agents rather than oral anticoagulation is recommended to reduce risk of recurrent stroke and other cardiovascular events, with the exception of cardioembolic etiologies (4)[A].
- Uncertain if switching agent in patients who have additional ischemic attacks while on antiplatelet therapy is beneficial (5)[C]

First Line

- Enteric-coated aspirin: 160 to 325 mg/day in the acute phase (5)[A] followed by long-term antiplatelet therapy for noncardioembolic TIA and anticoagulation for cardioembolic etiology
- Antiplatelet therapy
  – Aspirin 81 to 325 mg/day (5)[A]
    ○ Contraindications: active peptic ulcer disease and hypersensitivity to ASA or NSAIDs
    ○ Precautions: may aggravate preexisting PUD; or worsen symptoms of asthma
    ○ Significant possible interactions: may potentiate effects of anticoagulants and sulfonylurea analogues
  – ER dipyridamole–ASA (Aggrenox): 25/200 mg BID (5)[B]
    ○ Combined therapy with dipyridamole and ASA not proven to have greater efficacy (1)
    ○ More expensive than ASA alone and may have more associated side effects
  – Clopidogrel 75 mg/day (5)[B]
    ○ Can be used in patients who are allergic to ASA (5)[B]
    ○ Precautions: Thrombotic thrombocytopenic purpura (TTP) can occur and increases risk of bleeding when combined with aspirin.
    ○ May be very slightly more effective than aspirin alone (5)[B]; more expensive and more side effects than aspirin
- Combined aspirin and clopidogrel therapy has shown to reduce the incidence of subsequent stroke for high-risk TIA patients by 21% without increased risk of bleeding when used for a duration of 1 month or less immediately following TIA or CVA (6)[A].
- Anticoagulation therapy
  – Direct thrombin inhibitor:
    ○ Dabigatran (Pradaxa)
    ○ Idarucizumab (Praxbind) reversal agent
  – Factor Xa inhibitors
    ○ Apixaban (Eliquis)
    ○ Rivaroxaban (Xarelto)
    ○ Edoxaban (Savaysa)
      ▪ Noninferior to warfarin in nonvalvular atrial fibrillation
      ▪ Precautions: Avoid in CKD (CrCl <30 mL/min).
      ▪ Expensive but no INR needed
      ▪ Not reversible
  – Warfarin (INR-adjusted dose) (5)[A]
    ○ Contraindications: intolerance/allergy, active liver disease, active bleeding, pregnancy
    ○ Significant possible interactions: antibiotics, antiepileptics, antifungals, and many others
  – ASA 325 mg/day or ASA 81 mg/day plus clopidogrel 75 mg/day (5)[A]
    ○ Patients who cannot take anticoagulation for reasons other than bleeding risk

Second Line

Ticlopidine (Ticlid): 250 mg PO BID
- For patients unable to tolerate other agents
- Contraindications: hypersensitivity, presence of hematopoietic/hemostatic disorders, conditions associated with bleeding, severe liver dysfunction

- Precautions: neutropenia (0.8% severe), which is reversible with cessation of the drug. Monitor blood counts every 2 weeks for first 3 months. TTP can occur.
- Significant possible interactions: Digoxin plasma levels decreased 15%; theophylline half-life increased from 8.6 to 12.2 hours.

ISSUES FOR REFERRAL

- Neurology for ongoing workup and treatment
- Cardiology if cardiac cause suspected
- Vascular surgery if carotid endarterectomy appropriate

ADDITIONAL THERAPIES

- Secondary prevention of TIA should be initiated; venous thromboembolism (VTE) prophylaxis
- Patients with TIA or ischemic stroke should be started on high-dose statin (1).
- BP should be reduced after 24 hours. Thiazides, ACE inhibitors, and ARBs have shown to be of benefit. β-Blockers have not shown benefit in reducing recurrence or stroke.
- Patients with DM or pre-DM should be advised to follow ADA guidelines to maintain tight glycemic control.

SURGERY/OTHER PROCEDURES

- Consider carotid endarterectomy in patients with a high degree of carotid artery stenosis ≥70%.
- When carotid endarterectomy is indicated for patients with TIA, surgery within 2 weeks is reasonable if there are no contraindications to early revascularization.

ADMISSION, INPATIENT, AND NURSING CONSIDERATIONS

Symptoms <72 hours and the following:
- ABCD2 score of >3
- ABCD2 score of 0 to 3 and uncertainty that diagnostic workup can be completed within 2 days as outpatient. Alternatively: If urgent imaging not available through ED or urgent neurology follow-up not available, admit ABCD2 score ≥3 with evidence of focal ischemia.

 ONGOING CARE

FOLLOW-UP RECOMMENDATIONS

Patient Monitoring

- Follow-up with neurologic support every 3 months for 1st year and then annually
- Close attention to recurrent TIA or subsequent CVA

DIET

- DASH diet or as appropriate for medical problems
- Physical activity
  – Any level of physical activity is beneficial, but at least 30 minutes of moderate-intensity physical activity daily is preferred (150 minutes/week).

PROGNOSIS

- The risk of stroke on the ipsilateral side within 90 days and cumulative thereafter is 10–20%.
- Risk increases multiple risk factors.
- Patients with larger artery occlusion or cardioembolic etiology are at increased risk of recurrence.
- High mortality risk associated with TIA, up to 25% of patients will die within 1 year of TIA.

COMPLICATIONS

Stroke and functional impairment

REFERENCES

1. Coutts SB. Diagnosis and management of transient ischemic attack. *Continuum (Minneap Minn)*. 2017;23(1):82–92.
2. Fang JX, Wang EQ, Wang W, et al. Efficacy and safety of high-dose statins in acute phase of ischemic stroke and transient ischemic attack: a systematic review. *Intern Emerg Med*. 2017;12(5):679–687.
3. Zhao M, Wang S, Zhang D, et al. Comparison of stroke prediction accuracy of ABCD2 and ABCD3-I in patients with transient ischemic attack: a meta-analysis. *J Stroke Cerebrovasc Dis*. 2017;26(10):2387–2395.
4. Adams RJ, Albers G, Alberts MJ, et al. Update to the AHA/ASA recommendations for the prevention of stroke in patients with stroke and transient ischemic attack. *Stroke*. 2008;39(5):1647–1652.
5. Lansberg MG, O'Donnell MJ, Khatri P, et al. Antithrombotic and thrombolytic therapy for ischemic stroke: Antithrombotic Therapy and Prevention of Thrombosis, 9th ed: American College of Chest Physicians Evidence-Based Clinical Practice Guidelines. *Chest*. 2012;141(Suppl 2):e601S–e636S.
6. Johnston SC, Easton JD, Farrant M, et al; for Clinical Research Collaboration, Neurological Emergencies Treatment Trials Network, POINT Investigators. Clopidogrel and aspirin in acute ischemic stroke and high-risk TIA. *N Engl J Med*. 2018;379(3):215–225.

ADDITIONAL READING

- Kernan WN, Ovbiagele B, Black HR, et al; for American Heart Association Stroke Council, Council on Cardiovascular and Stroke Nursing, Council on Clinical Cardiology, and Council on Peripheral Vascular Disease. Guidelines for the prevention of stroke in patients with stroke and transient ischemic attack: a guideline for healthcare professionals from the American Heart Association/American Stroke Association. *Stroke*. 2014;45(7):2160–2236.
- Simmons BB, Cirignano B, Gadegbeku AB. Transient ischemic attack: part I. Diagnosis and evaluation. *Am Fam Physician*. 2012;86(6):521–526.
- Simmons BB, Gadegbeku AB, Cirignano B. Transient ischemic attack: part II. Risk factor modification and treatment. *Am Fam Physician*. 2012;86(6):527–532.

 SEE ALSO

Algorithms: Stroke; Transient Ischemic Attack and Transient Neurologic Defects

 CODES

ICD10

- G45.9 Transient cerebral ischemic attack, unspecified
- G45.1 Carotid artery syndrome (hemispheric)
- G45.0 Vertebro-basilar artery syndrome

CLINICAL PEARLS

- Encourage smoking cessation, exercise, weight loss, limited ETOH intake, and control of HTN, hyperlipidemia, and diabetes.
- Antiplatelet therapy (e.g., aspirin, clopidogrel, or aspirin-clopidogrel) should be initiated (6).
- Warfarin should be initiated in patients with atrial fibrillation or cardioembolic risk factors.

TRANSIENT STRESS CARDIOMYOPATHY

Adedapo Iluyomade, MD, MBA • Alexander Toirac, MD • Mauricio G. Cohen, MD, FACC, FSCAI

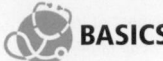

BASICS

DESCRIPTION

- Transient stress cardiomyopathy (TSC) is a unique cause of reversible left ventricle (LV) dysfunction with a presentation indistinguishable from the acute coronary syndromes (ACS), particularly ST-segment elevation myocardial infarction (STEMI) (1).
- Typically, the patient is a postmenopausal woman who presents with acute chest pain, dyspnea, or syncope and an identifiable "trigger" (i.e., an acute emotional or physiologic stressor).
- First reported by authors from Japan as takotsubo cardiomyopathy, the Japanese word for octopus trap, due to the characteristic shape of the LV at the end of systole. It has been described under numerous names in the literature including "broken heart syndrome," "stress cardiomyopathy," and "apical ballooning syndrome."
- Presenting clinical features include the following:
  - Chest pain/pressure, dyspnea and/or syncope
  - ECG changes, including ST-segment elevations or diffuse T-wave inversions
  - Mild elevation in cardiac biomarkers (creatine kinase [CK], troponin)
  - Transient wall motion abnormalities that may involve the base, midportion, and/or lateral walls of the LV
  - The apex of the right ventricle (RV) may be affected in up to 25% of cases (1)[B].
- Clinical features may vary on a case-by-case basis, and formal diagnostic criteria have not been established.
- Authors from the Mayo Clinic have proposed that three of the four following criteria establish the diagnosis (1)[A]:
  - Transient akinesis or dyskinesis of the LV apical and midventricular segments with regional wall motion abnormalities extending beyond a single epicardial vascular distribution
  - Absence of obstructive coronary artery disease (CAD) or angiographic evidence of acute plaque rupture
  - New ECG abnormalities, either ST-segment elevation or T-wave inversion
  - Absence of
    - Recent significant head trauma
    - Intracranial bleeding
    - Pheochromocytoma
    - Obstructive epicardial CAD
    - Myocarditis
    - Hypertrophic cardiomyopathy
- Synonym(s): takotsubo cardiomyopathy; apical ballooning syndrome; stress cardiomyopathy; broken heart syndrome; ampulla cardiomyopathy

EPIDEMIOLOGY

Incidence

- TSC accounts for an estimated 1–3% of all and 5–6% of female patients presenting with suspected STEMI.
- In a recent prospective evaluation of patients admitted to the ICU, as many as 28% had apical ballooning, often in association with sepsis.
- Predominant sex: 82–100% of cases occur in women.
- Predominant age: Mean age of patients is 62 to 75 years.

Prevalence

2.2% of patients presenting to a referral hospital with ST-segment MIs were found to have TSC.

ETIOLOGY AND PATHOPHYSIOLOGY

- The precise pathophysiologic mechanisms of TSC are not well understood.
- There is considerable evidence that sympathetic stimulation is central to its pathogenesis. A clear emotional or physiologic triggering event precipitates the syndrome in most cases, and TSC has been associated with conditions of catecholamine excess (e.g., pheochromocytoma, central nervous system disorders) and activated specific cerebral regions (1).
- Occurs primarily in subjects with increased susceptibility of the coronary microcirculation and of cardiac myocytes to stress hormones leading to temporary left ventricular dysfunction with secondary myocardial inflammation (1)
- A perturbation in the brain–heart axis, originating in the insular cortex, may be the inciting event (2).
- Subsequent overwhelming activation of the sympathetic nervous system initiates a cascade of events, including the following:
  - Catecholamine-induced LV dysfunction: "biased agonism" of epinephrine for β_2-adrenergic receptors, located predominantly at the cardiac apex
  - Endothelial dysfunction and vasospasm
  - Cellular metabolic injury
    - Myocardial norepinephrine release
    - Calcium overload
    - Contraction band necrosis

Genetics

No genetic associations have been described to date.

RISK FACTORS

- Female sex
- Postmenopausal state
- Emotional stress (i.e., argument, death of family member), more common in women
- Physiologic stress (i.e., acute medical illness), more common in men
- Chronic neurologic or psychiatric disease (2)

COMMONLY ASSOCIATED CONDITIONS

Death from TSC is rare, and most cases resolve rapidly, within 2 to 3 days. Reported complications include:

- Left-sided heart failure
- Pulmonary edema
- Cardiogenic shock and hemodynamic compromise
- Dynamic LV outflow tract gradient complicated by hypotension
- Mitral regurgitation
- Ventricular arrhythmias
- LV thrombus formation
- LV free wall rupture
- Death (rare, 0–8%)

DIAGNOSIS

Because TSC often is indistinguishable from an ACS, it should be treated initially as such:

- Activate emergency medical services or report to emergency department.
- Oxygen, IV access, and ECG monitoring
- Urgent cardiology consultation

HISTORY

- In 2/3 of patients, there is exposure to a "trigger event."
  - Emotional stress: argument, death of family member, divorce, public speaking, and so forth
  - Physiologic stress: acute medical condition such as head trauma, asthma attack, seizure, and so forth

- In 1/3 of patients, there is no identifiable trigger (2).
- Studies suggest preference for time of day, day of the week, and months/season of the year; summer and winter most commonly reported
- Acute onset of dyspnea or chest pain
- Palpitations
- Syncope

PHYSICAL EXAM

Exam may be unremarkable or may include any of the following:

- Tachypnea
- Tachycardia
- Hypotension
- Jugular venous distension
- Bibasilar rales
- S_3 gallop
- Systolic ejection murmur due to dynamic LV outflow tract gradient
- Holosystolic murmur of mitral regurgitation

DIFFERENTIAL DIAGNOSIS

- Acute ST-segment elevation MI
- Pulmonary embolism
- Myopericarditis
- Pheochromocytoma
- Hypertrophic cardiomyopathy
- Subarachnoid hemorrhage or stroke

DIAGNOSTIC TESTS & INTERPRETATION

- ECG should be done urgently and may show the following:
  - Diffuse ST-segment elevations
  - Diffuse and often dramatic T-wave inversions
  - QTc interval prolongation (3)[B]
  - Q waves
- Laboratory tests typically reveal a mild elevation in cardiac biomarkers such as
  - CK (rarely >500 U/mL)
  - Troponin I
  - B-type natriuretic peptide (BNP)
  - Markers of high filling pressures (e.g., BNP) tend to be higher than markers of necrosis (e.g., CK, troponin).
  - TSC can be distinguished from AMI with 95% specificity using a BNP/TnT ratio ≥1,272 (sensitivity 52%) (4)[B].
- Chest radiograph
  - Cardiomegaly
  - Pulmonary edema
- The InterTAK Diagnostic Score comprises seven parameters (female sex, emotional trigger, physical trigger, absence of ST-segment depression [except in lead aVR], psychiatric disorders, neurologic disorders, and QT prolongation) ranked by their diagnostic importance with a maximum attainable score of 100 points (1).
- In patients with non–ST-segment elevation, the InterTAK Diagnostic Score can be considered. Patients with a low probability (InterTAK score ≤70 points) should undergo coronary angiography with left ventriculography, whereas in patients with a high score (score ≥ 70), transthoracic echocardiography should be considered (1).
- Echocardiogram
  - Reduced LV systolic function
  - Abnormal diastolic function, including evidence of increased filling pressures

- Regional wall motion abnormalities in one of the following patterns:
  ○ Classic or "takotsubo-type" ballooning of the apex with a hypercontractile base
  ○ "Reverse takotsubo": apical hypercontractility with basal akinesis
  ○ "Midventricular" akinesis with apical and basal hypercontractility
  ○ Focal or localized akinesis of an isolated segment
  - Dynamic intracavitary LV gradient
  - Mitral regurgitation
  - Variable involvement of the RV
- Cardiac MRI
  - Reduced LV function
  - Wall motion abnormalities as described for transthoracic echocardiography
  - Absence of delayed hyperenhancement with gadolinium

Diagnostic Procedures/Other
- The diagnosis of TSC is often challenging because its clinical phenotype may closely resemble STEMI regarding electrocardiographic abnormalities and biomarkers. Although a widely established noninvasive tool allowing a rapid and reliable diagnosis of TSC is currently lacking, coronary angiography with left ventriculography is considered the "gold standard" diagnostic tool to exclude or confirm TSC.
- Coronary angiography
  - Nonocclusive CAD
  - Rarely, epicardial coronary spasm
  - Endothelial dysfunction as measured by fractional flow reserve or TIMI frame counts
- Left-sided heart catheterization: increased LV end-diastolic pressure to a similar degree as AMI
- Ventriculography: wall motion abnormalities as described for transthoracic echocardiography
- Right-sided heart catheterization
  - Increased pulmonary capillary wedge pressure
  - Secondary pulmonary hypertension
  - Increased right ventricular filling pressures
  - Reduced cardiac output or cardiogenic shock (cardiac index <2 and mean arterial pressure [MAP] <60 mm Hg)

Test Interpretation
Characteristic pathologic findings of involved myocardium have not been described.

TREATMENT

- Guidelines regarding TSC management are lacking because no prospective randomized clinical trials have been performed in this patient population. Therapeutic strategies are therefore based on clinical experience and expert consensus (5).
- Activation of emergency medical services
- Advanced cardiac life support therapies as needed
- Oxygen
- IV access
- ECG monitoring

MEDICATION
After diagnostic cardiac catheterization, empirical treatment goals are as follows:
- Management of hypotension: differentiation between cardiogenic shock and dynamic LV cavity gradient
- Management of increased filling pressures and congestive states
- Attenuation of sympathetic drive

First Line
- There are no evidence-based treatment recommendations for TSC.
- Although β-blockers are of theoretical benefit, their use has not been associated with improved outcomes in observational cohorts (2)[B].
- Due to the potential risk of pause-dependent torsades de pointes, β-blockers should be used cautiously, especially in patients with bradycardia and QTc >500 ms (5).
- If there is evidence of left ventricular systolic dysfunction or pulmonary edema, consider the following:
  - Furosemide: 20 to 40 mg IV/PO BID as needed to reduce LV filling pressures and dyspnea (6)
  - The use of angiotensin-converting enzyme inhibitors or angiotensin receptor blockers was associated with improved survival at 1-year follow-up even after propensity matching (5): Lisinopril 10 to 40 mg/day PO or equivalent or valsartan 80 to 160 mg PO BID has been associated with improved outcomes in observational cohorts (2)[B].

Second Line
Short-term anticoagulation should be considered in patients with severely reduced LV function to prevent LV thrombus formation; unfractionated heparin 80 U/kg IV bolus followed by 18 U/kg/hr IV or Lovenox 1 mg/kg SC BID

ISSUES FOR REFERRAL
All patients with TSC generally should be comanaged with cardiology while inpatient and referred to cardiology as an outpatient.

ADDITIONAL THERAPIES
- Urgent cardiology consultation and consideration of cardiac catheterization
- Hypotension may require the following:
  - Vasopressors (e.g., dopamine or Levophed) if there is no LV outflow tract gradient (6)[C]
  - Phenylephrine and IV fluids to increase afterload in the presence of an LV outflow tract gradient (6)[C]
  - Cardiogenic shock that is not due to an LV outflow tract gradient may require placement of an intra-aortic balloon pump.

ADMISSION, INPATIENT, AND NURSING CONSIDERATIONS
- Admission criteria/initial stabilization
  - 12-lead ECG
  - Chest radiograph
  - Laboratory testing
  - Echocardiography
  - Patients with TSC usually are admitted for observation because the differential diagnosis includes ACS.
- Normal saline infusion to support BP, if necessary, and no evidence of heart failure
- Discharge criteria generally considered after exclusion of ACS and resolution of
  - Congestive state
  - Hypotension
  - Profound impairments of systolic function

ONGOING CARE

FOLLOW-UP RECOMMENDATIONS
- Impairments in systolic function typically resolve in 2 to 3 days but may last as long as 1 month.
- Patients should follow up with cardiology and serial echocardiography to document improved LV function.

PROGNOSIS
- Although TSC has generally been considered a benign disease, contemporary observations show that rates of cardiogenic shock and death are comparable to ACS patients treated according to current guidelines (5).
- Recurrence is rare; it also has been reported in 0–8% of patients.

REFERENCES

1. Ghadri JR, Wittstein IS, Prasad A, et al. International expert consensus document on takotsubo syndrome (part I): clinical characteristics, diagnostic criteria, and pathophysiology. *Eur Heart J*. 2018;39(22):2032–2046.
2. Templin C, Ghadri JR, Diekmann J, et al. Clinical features and outcomes of takotsubo (stress) cardiomyopathy. *N Engl J Med*. 2015;373(10):929–938.
3. Madias C, Fitzgibbons TP, Alsheikh-Ali AA, et al. Acquired long QT syndrome from stress cardiomyopathy is associated with ventricular arrhythmias and torsades de pointes. *Heart Rhythm*. 2011;8(4):555–561.
4. Randhawa MS, Dhillon AS, Taylor HC, et al. Diagnostic utility of cardiac biomarkers in discriminating takotsubo cardiomyopathy from acute myocardial infarction. *J Card Fail*. 2014;20(1):2–8.
5. Ghadri JR, Wittstein IS, Prasad A, et al. International expert consensus document on takotsubo syndrome (part II): diagnostic workup, outcome, and management. *Eur Heart J*. 2018;39(22):2047–2062.
6. Hunt SA, Abraham WT, Chin MH, et al. 2009 Focused update incorporated into the ACC/AHA 2005 guidelines for the diagnosis and management of heart failure in adults: a report of the American College of Cardiology Foundation/American Heart Association Task Force on Practice Guidelines developed in collaboration with the International Society for Heart and Lung Transplantation. *J Am Coll Cardiol*. 2009;53(15):e1–e90.

 SEE ALSO

Algorithm: Chest Pain/Acute Coronary Syndrome

 CODES

ICD10
I51.81 Takotsubo syndrome

CLINICAL PEARLS

- TSC is poorly recognized and often regarded as a benign condition. However, it may be associated with severe clinical complications including death, and its prevalence is likely underestimated.
- TSC is a cause of reversible LV dysfunction with a clinical presentation indistinguishable from the ACS, particularly ST-segment elevation MI.
- Echocardiography may strongly suggest the diagnosis.
- Treatment is supportive and should include diuretics and ACE inhibitors in patients with CHF.

TRICHOMONIASIS

Michael J. Arnold, MD

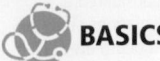 **BASICS**

DESCRIPTION
- Sexually transmitted urogenital infection caused by a pear-shaped, parasitic protozoan
- Causes vaginitis/urethritis in women, nongonococcal urethritis in men
- In pregnancy, increases risk of preterm labor, preterm premature rupture of membranes, small for gestational age infant, and possibly stillbirth
- Synonym(s): trich; trichomonal urethritis

EPIDEMIOLOGY
Incidence
- The most common curable sexually transmitted infection (STI); in 2008, >275 million new cases worldwide, over half of curable STIs (1)
- Estimated 1.1 million new cases annually in United States
  - 10–25% of vaginal infections
  - In males, up to 17% of nongonococcal urethritis
- Predominant age: middle-aged adults
  - Rare until onset of sexual activity
  - Common in postmenopausal women; age is not protective and long-term carriage is common.

Pediatric Considerations
Rare in prepubertal children; diagnosis should raise concern of sexual abuse.

Prevalence
- 1.8% in United States women age 18 to 59 years
- 0.5% of U.S. men age 18 to 59 years
- Racial disparity demonstrated
  - 8.9% of black women versus 0.8% of other women
  - 4.2% of black men versus 0.03% of other men

ETIOLOGY AND PATHOPHYSIOLOGY
- *Trichomonas vaginalis*: pear-shaped, flagellated, parasitic protozoan
- Grows best at 35–37°C in anaerobic conditions with pH 5.5 to 6.0
- STI, but nonsexual transmission possible because it can survive several hours in moist environment

Genetics
No known genetic considerations

RISK FACTORS
- Multiple sexual partners
- Unprotected intercourse
- Lower socioeconomic status
- Other STIs
- Untreated partner with previous infection
- Use of douching or feminine powders

GENERAL PREVENTION
- Use of male or female condoms
- Limiting sexual partners
- Male circumcision may be protective.

COMMONLY ASSOCIATED CONDITIONS
- Other STIs, including HIV
- Bacterial vaginosis

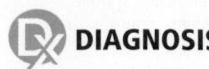 **DIAGNOSIS**

HISTORY
- Women—up to 80% may be asymptomatic.
  - Yellow-green, malodorous vaginal discharge
  - Vulvovaginal pruritus
  - Dysuria
  - Symptoms often worsen during menses.
- Men—80% are asymptomatic.
  - Dysuria
  - Urethral discharge, often scant
  - Pruritus or burning after intercourse

PHYSICAL EXAM
- Women
  - Vaginal erythema
  - Yellow-green, frothy, malodorous vaginal discharge
  - Cervical petechiae ("strawberry cervix"; seen in <5% of patients)
  - Pelvic exams do not improve STI diagnosis (2).
- Men: penile discharge, spontaneous and with expression

DIFFERENTIAL DIAGNOSIS
- Women (other vaginitides)
  - Bacterial vaginosis
  - Vaginal candidiasis
  - Chlamydial infection
  - Gonorrheal infection
- Men (other urethritis)
  - Chlamydial infection
  - Gonorrheal infection

DIAGNOSTIC TESTS & INTERPRETATION
Initial Tests (lab, imaging)
- Wet mounts of vaginal or urethral discharge: direct visualization of motile trichomonads; most common because inexpensive and available
  - Sensitivity: 60–70%; declines rapidly within 1 hour from collection
  - Specificity: 99.8%
- Culture: sensitivity >95%, specificity >99%; takes 4 to 7 days for growth

- Nucleic acid amplification test (NAAT)
  - Gold standard for diagnosis (3)
  - Sensitivity and specificity 95–99% (3)
  - Vaginal, endocervical, or urine specimens
  - British analysis shows that combined NAAT for *Trichomonas*, gonorrhea, *Chlamydia*, and *Mycoplasma genitalium* most cost-effective (3)[B].
- Antigen detection
  - ELISA and direct fluorescent antibody tests: sensitivity of 80–90%
  - Limited clinical availability

Follow-Up Tests & Special Considerations
Detection on cervical Papanicolaou smear
- Treat because highly specific (97–99%)
- Not effective for *Trichomonas* screening—sensitivity as low as 60%

Diagnostic Procedures/Other
In males, urethral meatal swab increases *Trichomonas* detection rate by 4 times over urine.

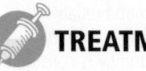 **TREATMENT**

- Symptomatic individuals require treatment.
- Sexual partners should be treated presumptively.
- Patients should abstain from sexual intercourse during treatment and until they are asymptomatic.

GENERAL MEASURES
The nitroimidazole class is only known effective antimicrobial treatment. If metronidazole resistance is suspected, use tinidazole (4)[A].

MEDICATION
First Line
- Metronidazole: 2 g PO, 1 dose (4)[A]
  - FDA pregnancy risk Category B
  - Cure rate: 84–98%
- Tinidazole: 2 g PO, 1 dose (4)[A]
  - FDA pregnancy risk Category C
  - Abstain from breastfeeding during treatment and for 3 days after the dose.
  - More expensive
  - Reaches higher levels in genitourinary tract
  - Cure rate: 92–100%

Second Line
- Metronidazole: 500 mg PO BID for 7 days
  - Number needed to treat of 13 for negative test of cure versus single dose metronidazole (5)[B]
  - Considered first line in HIV-positive individuals
- Can dose with metronidazole or tinidazole 2 g daily for 7 days if infection persists
- Consider IV dosing of metronidazole based on case report demonstrating cure after multiple failed oral regimens.

Pregnancy Considerations

Metronidazole is effective for trichomoniasis infection during pregnancy but may increase the risk of preterm and low-birth-weight babies.

- Studies showed risk in patients receiving 4 times the standard dosing.
- Trichomoniasis is also associated with prematurity.

ISSUES FOR REFERRAL

- Multidrug-resistant organism
- Patient allergy to metronidazole: Desensitization to metronidazole is recommended.

ADDITIONAL THERAPIES

- Limited clinical trials assessing effectiveness of alternative therapies
- Intravaginal metronidazole gel is not effective (6)[B].
- Suggested alternative therapies based on case reports (6)[C]
  - Paromomycin 6.25% cream
  - Povidone-iodine douche
  - Boric acid intravaginally
  - Furazolidone intravaginally

COMPLEMENTARY & ALTERNATIVE MEDICINE

See "Additional Therapies."

 ## ONGOING CARE

FOLLOW-UP RECOMMENDATIONS

- If symptoms persist after initial treatment, repeat wet mount or other testing.
- Retest women for *T. vaginalis* recommended within 3 months of treatment; data insufficient for retesting men (5)
- HIV-positive patients should be screened for *Trichomonas* at time of HIV diagnosis and at least annually (5).

DIET

Abstain from alcohol during treatment and for 24 hours following last dose of metronidazole or 48 to 72 hours following last dose of tinidazole due to disulfiram-like reaction.

PATIENT EDUCATION

Educate about the sexually transmitted aspect.

- Advise patient to notify sexual partner to be treated.
- Discuss STI prevention—condom use can prevent recurrence.
- Abstain from intercourse while undergoing treatment; use condoms if abstention is not feasible.
- Avoid alcohol during treatment with metronidazole or tinidazole.

PROGNOSIS

- Excellent
- Usually eliminated after one course of antibiotics

COMPLICATIONS

Pregnancy Considerations

Linked to low birth weight, preterm premature rupture of membranes, and preterm birth; associations with infertility, but not proven

REFERENCES

1. Bouchemal K, Bories C, Loiseau PM. Strategies for prevention and treatment of *Trichomonas vaginalis* infections. *Clin Microbiol Rev*. 2017;30(3):811–825.
2. Farrukh S, Sivitz AB, Onogul B, et al. The additive value of pelvic examinations to history in predicting sexually transmitted infections for young female patients with suspected cervicitis or pelvic inflammatory disease. *Ann Emerg Med*. 2018;72(6):703.e1–712.e1.
3. Huntington SE, Burns RM, Harding-Esch E, et al. Modelling-based evaluation of the costs, benefits and cost-effectiveness of multipathogen point-of-care tests for sexually transmitted infections in symptomatic genitourinary medicine clinic attendees. *BMJ Open*. 2018;8(9):e020394.
4. Workowski KA, Bolan GA; for Centers for Disease Control and Prevention. Sexually transmitted diseases treatment guidelines, 2015. *MMWR Recomm Rep*. 2015;64(RR-03):1–137.
5. Kissinger P, Muzny CA, Mena LA, et al. Single-dose versus 7-day-dose metronidazole for the treatment of trichomoniasis in women: an open-label, randomised controlled trial. *Lancet Infect Dis*. 2018;18(11):1251–1259.
6. Muzny CA, Schwebke JR. The clinical spectrum of *Trichomonas vaginalis* infection and challenges to management. *Sex Transm Infect*. 2013;89(6):423–425.

ADDITIONAL READING

- Chernesky M, Jang D, Smieja M, et al. Urinary meatal swabbing detects more men infected with *Mycoplasma genitalium* and four other sexually transmitted infections than first catch urine. *Sex Transm Dis*. 2017;44(8):489–491.
- Daugherty M, Glynn K, Byler T. The prevalence of *Trichomonas vaginalis* infection among US males, 2013–2016. *Clin Infect Dis*. 2019;68(3):460–465.
- Fastring DR, Amedee A, Gatski M, et al. Co-occurrence of *Trichomonas vaginalis* and bacterial vaginosis and vaginal shedding of HIV-1 RNA. *Sex Transm Dis*. 2014;41(3):173–179.
- Hawkins I, Carne C, Sonnex C, et al. Successful treatment of refractory *Trichomonas vaginalis* infection using intravenous metronidazole. *Int J STD AIDS*. 2015;26(9):676–678.
- Helms DJ, Mosure DJ, Secor WE, et al. Management of *Trichomonas vaginalis* in women with suspected metronidazole hypersensitivity. *Am J Obstet Gynecol*. 2008;198(4):370.e1–377.e1.
- Kirkcaldy RD, Augostini P, Asbel LE, et al. *Trichomonas vaginalis* antimicrobial drug resistance in 6 US cities, STD Surveillance Network, 2009–2010. *Emerg Infect Dis*. 2012;18(6):939–943.
- Meites E. Trichomoniasis: the "neglected" sexually transmitted disease. *Infect Dis Clin North Am*. 2013;27(4):755–764.
- Patel EU, Gaydos CA, Packman ZR, et al. Prevalence and correlates of *Trichomonas vaginalis* infection among men and women in the United States. *Clin Infect Dis*. 2018;67(2):211–217.
- Saperstein AK, Firnhaber GC. Clinical inquiries. Should you test or treat partners of patients with gonorrhea, chlamydia, or trichomoniasis? *J Fam Pract*. 2010;59(1):46–48.
- Seña AC, Bachmann LH, Hobbs MM. Persistent and recurrent *Trichomonas vaginalis* infections: epidemiology, treatment and management considerations. *Expert Rev Anti Infect Ther*. 2014;12(6):673–685.
- Silver BJ, Guy RJ, Kaldor JM, et al. *Trichomonas vaginalis* as a cause of perinatal morbidity: a systematic review and meta-analysis. *Sex Transm Dis*. 2014;41(6):369–376.
- Sobngwi-Tambekou J, Taljaard D, Nieuwoudt M, et al. Male circumcision and *Neisseria gonorrhoeae*, *Chlamydia trachomatis* and *Trichomonas vaginalis*: observations after a randomised controlled trial for HIV prevention. *Sex Transm Infect*. 2009;85(2):116–120.
- Wiese W, Patel SR, Patel SC, et al. A meta-analysis of the Papanicolaou smear and wet mount for the diagnosis of vaginal trichomoniasis. *Am J Med*. 2000;108(4):301–308.

 ## CODES

ICD10

- A59.9 Trichomoniasis, unspecified
- A59.03 Trichomonal cystitis and urethritis
- A59.01 Trichomonal vulvovaginitis

CLINICAL PEARLS

- Both partners need to be treated for trichomoniasis.
- Retest women within 3 months of treatment.
- Avoid alcohol during treatment.
- Treatment in pregnancy does not reduce risk of adverse pregnancy outcomes.
- Annual screening recommended for HIV-positive patients
- Not a nationally notifiable condition

TRIGEMINAL NEURALGIA

Noah M. Rosenberg, MD, MBA

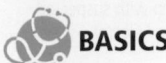 **BASICS**

DESCRIPTION

- A painful disorder of the sensory nucleus of the tri-geminal nerve (cranial nerve [CN] V) that produces episodic, paroxysmal, severe, lancinating facial pain lasting seconds to minutes in the distribution of ≥1 divisions of the nerve
- Often precipitated by stimulation of well-defined, ipsilateral trigger zones: usually perioral, perinasal, and occasionally intraoral (e.g., by washing, shaving)
- System(s) affected: nervous
- Synonym(s): tic douloureux; Fothergill neuralgia; trifacial neuralgia; prosopalgia

EPIDEMIOLOGY

Incidence
- Women: 5.9/100,000 per year
- Men: 3.4/100,000 per year
- >70 years of age: ~25.6/100,000 per year
- Predominant age:
  - >50 years; incidence increases with age.
  - Rare: <35 years of age (Consider another primary disease; see "Etiology and Pathophysiology.")
- Predominant sex: female > male (~2:1)

Prevalence
16/100,000

Pediatric Considerations
Unusual during childhood

Pregnancy Considerations
Teratogenicity limits therapy for 1st and 2nd trimesters.

ETIOLOGY AND PATHOPHYSIOLOGY

- Demyelination around the compression site seems to be the mechanism by which compression of nerves leads to symptoms.
- Demyelinated lesions may set up an ectopic impulse generation causing erratic responses: hyperexcit-ability of damaged nerves and transmission of action potentials along adjacent, undamaged, and unstimulated sensory fibers.
- Compression of trigeminal nerve by anomalous arteries or veins of posterior fossa, compressing trigeminal root
- Etiologic classification:
  - Idiopathic (classic)
  - Secondary: cerebellopontine angle tumors (e.g., meningioma); tumors of CN V (e.g., neuroma, vascular malformations), trauma, demyelinating disease (e.g., multiple sclerosis [MS])

RISK FACTORS
Unknown

COMMONLY ASSOCIATED CONDITIONS

- Sjögren syndrome; rheumatoid arthritis
- Chronic meningitis
- Acute polyneuropathy

- MS
- Hemifacial spasm
- Charcot-Marie-Tooth neuropathy
- Glossopharyngeal neuralgia

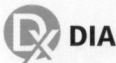 **DIAGNOSIS**

HISTORY
Paroxysms of pain in the distribution of the trigeminal nerve. The trigeminal nerve has three branches and innervates the entire side of the face. They are known as ophthalmologic (V1), maxillary (V2), and mandibu-lar (V3) branches. Patients typically experience pain in the V2 and V3 dermatomes.

PHYSICAL EXAM
All exam findings typically are negative due to the paroxysmal nature of the disorder.

DIFFERENTIAL DIAGNOSIS
- Other forms of neuralgia usually have sensory loss. Presence of sensory loss nearly excludes the diagno-sis of trigeminal neuralgia (TN) (if younger patient, frequently MS).
- Neoplasia in cerebellopontine angle
- Vascular malformation of brainstem
- Demyelinating lesion (MS is diagnosed in 2–4% of patients with TN.)
- Vascular insult
- Migraine, cluster headache
- Giant cell arteritis
- Postherpetic neuralgia
- Chronic meningitis
- Acute polyneuropathy
- Atypical odontalgia
- SUNCT syndrome (short-lasting, unilateral neuralgi-form pain with conjunctival injection and tearing)

DIAGNOSTIC TESTS & INTERPRETATION
- The International Headache Society diagnostic criteria for classic TN are as follows:
  - Paroxysmal attacks of pain lasting from a fraction of 1 second to 2 minutes, affecting ≥1 divisions of the trigeminal nerve
  - Pain has at least an intense, sharp, superficial, or stabbing characteristic or is precipitated from trigger areas or by trigger factors.
  - Attacks are stereotyped in the individual patient.
  - No clinically evident neurologic deficit found
  - Not attributed to another disorder
- Secondary TN is characterized by pain that is indistinguishable from classic TN but is caused by a demonstrable structural lesion other than vascular compression.
  - Indicated in all first-time-presenting patients to rule out secondary causes
- MRI versus CT scan: MRI, with and without contrast, offers more detailed imaging and is preferred, if not contraindicated.

- Routine head imaging identifies structural causes in up to 15% of patients.
- No positive findings are significantly correlated with diagnosis.

Test Interpretation
- Trigeminal nerve: inflammatory changes, demyelin-ation, and degenerative changes
- Trigeminal ganglion: hypermyelination and microneuromata

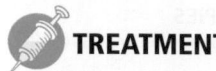 **TREATMENT**

GENERAL MEASURES
- Outpatient
- Drug treatment is first line.
- Invasive procedures are reserved for patients who cannot tolerate, fail to respond to, or relapse after chronic drug treatment.
- Avoid stimulation (e.g., air, heat, cold) of trigger zones, including lips, cheeks, and gums.

MEDICATION

First Line
- Carbamazepine (Tegretol) (1)[A]: Start at 100 to 200 mg BID; effective dose usually 200 mg QID; max dose 1,200 mg/day:
  - 70–90% of patients respond initially (number needed to treat [NNT] = 1.9) (1)[A].
  - By 3 years, 30% are no longer helped.
  - Most common side effect: sedation
- Contraindications: concurrent use of monoamine oxidase inhibitors (MAOIs)
- Precautions: caution in the presence of liver disease
- Significant possible medication interactions: macro-lide antibiotics, oral anticoagulants, anticonvulsants, tricyclics, oral contraceptives, steroids, digitalis, isoniazid, MAOIs, methyprylon, nabilone, nizatidine, other H_2 blockers, phenytoin, propoxyphene, benzo-diazepines, and calcium channel blockers
- Oxcarbazepine (Trileptal): Start at 150 to 300 mg BID; effective dose usually 375 mg BID; max dose 1,200 mg/day:
  - Efficacy similar to carbamazepine
  - Faster, with less drowsiness and fewer drug interactions than carbamazepine
  - May cause hyponatremia
  - Most common side effect: sedation

Second Line
- Antiepileptic drugs: insufficient evidence from ran-domized controlled trials to show significant benefit from antiepileptic drugs in TN (2)[A]
- Phenytoin (Dilantin): 300 to 400 mg/day (synergistic with carbamazepine):
  - Potent P450 inducer (enhanced metabolism of many drugs)
  - Various CNS side effects (sedation, ataxia)

- Baclofen (Lioresal): 10 to 80 mg/day; start at 5 to 10 mg TID with food (as an adjunct to phenytoin or carbamazepine); side effects: drowsiness, weakness, nausea, vomiting
- Gabapentin (Neurontin): Start at 100 mg TID or 300 mg at bedtime; can increase dose up to 300 to 600 mg TID–QID; can be used as monotherapy or in combination with other medications
- Lamotrigine: Titrate up to 200 mg BID over weeks; side effect: 10% experience rash.
- Antidepressants, including amitriptyline, fluoxetine, trazodone:
  - Used especially with anticonvulsants
  - Particularly effective for atypical forms of TN
- Clonazepam (Klonopin) frequently causes drowsiness and ataxia.
- Sumatriptan (Imitrex) 3 mg subcutaneous (SC) reduces acute symptoms and may be helpful after failure of conventional medical therapy.
- Capsaicin cream topically
- Botulinum toxin injection into zygomatic arch
- Valproic acid (Depakene, Depakote)

ISSUES FOR REFERRAL
Initial treatment failure or positive findings on imaging studies

ADDITIONAL THERAPIES
- Radiotherapy
- Stereotactic radiosurgery, such as Gamma Knife radiosurgery, has been shown to be effective after drug failure:
  - Produces lesions with focused Gamma Knife radiation
  - Therapy aimed at the proximal trigeminal root
  - Minimal clinically effective dose: 70 Gy
  - ~78–94% of patients achieve complete relief after 3 years; by 7 years, ~65–90% maintain complete relief (3)[B].
  - Most common side effect: sensory disturbance (facial numbness)
  - Failure rates are higher in patients with past TN-related invasive procedures.

SURGERY/OTHER PROCEDURES
- Microvascular decompression of CN V at its entrance to (or exit from) brainstem:
  - 98% of patients achieve initial pain relief; by 20 months, 86% maintain complete relief (NNT = 2) (4)[B].
  - Surgical mortality across studies was 0.3–0.4%.
  - Most common side effect: transient facial numbness and diplopia, headache, nausea, vomiting
  - Pain relief after procedure strongly correlates with the type of TN pain: Type 1 (shock-like pain) results in better outcomes than type 2 (aching pain between paroxysms).
- Peripheral nerve ablation (multiple methods):
  - Higher rates of failure and facial numbness than decompression surgery
  - Radiofrequency thermocoagulation
  - Neurectomy
  - Cryotherapy: high relapse rate
  - Partial sensory rhizotomy

- 4% tetracaine dissolved in 0.5% bupivacaine nerve block (only a few case reports to date; ropivacaine)
- Alcohol block or glycerol injection into trigeminal cistern: unpredictable side effects (dysesthesia and anesthesia dolorosa); temporary relief
- Peripheral block or section of CN V proximal to gasserian ganglion
- Balloon compression of gasserian ganglion
- Evidence supporting destructive procedures for benign pain conditions remains limited (5)[A].

COMPLEMENTARY & ALTERNATIVE MEDICINE
Acupuncture, moxibustion (herb): weak evidence for efficacy (6)[B]

 ONGOING CARE

FOLLOW-UP RECOMMENDATIONS
Regular outpatient follow-up to monitor symptoms and therapeutic failure

Patient Monitoring
- Carbamazepine and/or phenytoin serum levels
- If carbamazepine is prescribed: CBC and platelets at baseline, then weekly for a month, then monthly for 4 months, and then every 6 to 12 months if dose is stable (Regimens for monitoring vary.)
- Reduce drugs after 4 to 6 weeks to determine whether condition is in remission; resume at previous dose if pain recurs. Withdraw drugs slowly after several months, again to check for remission or if lower dose of drugs can be tolerated.

DIET
No special diet

PATIENT EDUCATION
- Instruct patient regarding medication dosage and side effects, risk-to-benefit ratios of surgery, or radiation therapy.
- Support organizations:
  - The Facial Pain Association (formerly the Trigeminal Neuralgia Association): www.fpa-support.org
  - Living with Trigeminal Neuralgia: www.livingwithtn.org

PROGNOSIS
- 50–60% eventually fail pharmacologic treatment.
- After having microvascular decompression surgery, most patients wish they had undergone the procedure sooner.
- Of those, relapse is seen in ~50% of stereotactic radiosurgeries and ~27% of surgical microvascular decompressions.

COMPLICATIONS
- Mental and physical sluggishness; dizziness with carbamazepine
- Paresthesias and corneal reflex loss with stereotactic radiosurgery
- Surgical mortality and morbidity associated with microvascular decompression

REFERENCES
1. Wiffen PJ, Derry S, Moore RA, et al. Carbamazepine for chronic neuropathic pain and fibromyalgia in adults. *Cochrane Database Syst Rev.* 2014;(4):CD005451.
2. Zhang J, Yang M, Zhou M, et al. Non-antiepileptic drugs for trigeminal neuralgia. *Cochrane Database Syst Rev.* 2013;(12):CD004029.
3. Martínez Moreno NE, Gutiérrez-Sárraga J, Rey-Portolés G, et al. Long-term outcomes in the treatment of classical trigeminal neuralgia by Gamma Knife radiosurgery: a retrospective study in patients with minimum 2-year follow-up. *Neurosurgery.* 2016;79(6):879–888.
4. Sekula RF Jr, Frederickson AM, Jannetta PJ, et al. Microvascular decompression for elderly patients with trigeminal neuralgia: a prospective study and systematic review with meta-analysis. *J Neurosurg.* 2011;114(1):172–179.
5. Zakrzewska JM, Akram H. Neurosurgical interventions for the treatment of classical trigeminal neuralgia. *Cochrane Database Syst Rev.* 2011;(9):CD007312.
6. Liu H, Li H, Xu M, et al. A systematic review on acupuncture for trigeminal neuralgia. *Altern Ther Health Med.* 2010;16(6):30–35.

ADDITIONAL READING
- Attal N, Cruccu G, Baron R, et al; for European Federation of Neurological Societies. EFNS guidelines on the pharmacological treatment of neuropathic pain: 2010 revision. *Eur J Neurol.* 2010;17(9):1113–e88.
- Gronseth G, Cruccu G, Alksne J, et al. Practice parameter: the diagnostic evaluation and treatment of trigeminal neuralgia (an evidence-based review): report of the Quality Standards Subcommittee of the American Academy of Neurology and the European Federation of Neurological Societies. *Neurology.* 2008;71(15):1183–1190.

 CODES

ICD10
- G50.0 Trigeminal neuralgia
- B02.22 Postherpetic trigeminal neuralgia

CLINICAL PEARLS
- Patients with TN typically have a normal physical exam.
- The long-term efficacy of pharmacotherapy for TN is 40–50%.
- If pharmacotherapy fails, stereotactic radiosurgery or surgical microvascular decompression often is successful.

TRIGGER FINGER (DIGITAL STENOSING TENOSYNOVITIS)

Jill N. Tirabassi, MD

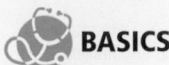 ## BASICS

DESCRIPTION
A clicking, snapping, or locking of a finger/thumb with extension movement (after flexion) ± associated pain

EPIDEMIOLOGY

Incidence
- Adult population: 28/100,000/year
  - Rare in children
- 4 times increased risk in diabetics (1)[B]
- Thumb is predominant digit.
- Predominant age
  - Adult form typically presents in the 5th and 6th decades of life.
- Predominant sex
  - Children: female = male
  - Adults: female > male (6:1)

Prevalence
Lifetime prevalence in the general population is 2.6%.

Pediatric Considerations
- Surgery is often more complicated for children with a trigger finger (as opposed to a trigger thumb).
- Release of the A1 pulley alone is often insufficient; other procedures may be necessary.

ETIOLOGY AND PATHOPHYSIOLOGY
- Narrowing around the A1 pulley from inflammation, protein deposition, or thickening of the tendon itself. Prolonged inflammation leads to fibrocartilaginous metaplasia of the tendon sheath.
- If flexor tendon becomes nodular, the triggering phenomenon is worse because the nodule has difficulty passing under the A1 pulley.
- Because intrinsic flexor muscles are stronger than extensors, the finger can stick in the flexed position.
- No clear association with repetitive movements

RISK FACTORS
- Diabetes mellitus
- Rheumatoid arthritis
- Hypothyroidism
- Mucopolysaccharide disorders
- Amyloidosis

GENERAL PREVENTION
Most cases are idiopathic, and no known prevention exists; no clear association with repetitive movements

COMMONLY ASSOCIATED CONDITIONS
- De Quervain tenosynovitis
- Carpal tunnel syndrome
- Dupuytren contracture
- Diabetes mellitus
- Rheumatoid arthritis
- Hypothyroidism
- Amyloidosis

 ## DIAGNOSIS

Diagnosis is based on clinical presentation.

HISTORY
Clicking, catching, snapping, or locking of a digit while attempting to extend; with or without associated pain; usual progression is painless clicking, then painful triggering then flexed, locked digit

PHYSICAL EXAM
- A palpable nodule may be present.
- Snapping/locking may be present, but neither is necessary for the diagnosis.
- Tenderness to palpation is variable.

DIAGNOSTIC TESTS & INTERPRETATION

Test Interpretation
On ultrasound or MRI:
- Thickening of the A1 pulley with fibrocartilaginous metaplasia
- Thickening/nodule formation of flexor tendon

 ## TREATMENT

GENERAL MEASURES
- Activity modification can be helpful in early disease (2)[C].
- Most recommend attempting steroid injection prior to surgery (2)[C].
- Splinting may be more effective in preventing recurrence than initial treatment choice (3)[B].
- Splinting the metacarpophalangeal (MCP) joint at 10 to 15 degrees of flexion for 6 weeks with the distal joints free to move:
  - Splinting is more effective for fingers than thumbs (70% vs. 50%).
  - Splinting is less effective with severe symptoms, symptoms >6 months, or if multiple digits are involved (1)[B].
- Injection of long-acting corticosteroid may provide symptom relief. Subsequent injections are less likely to help (1)[B].
- Surgery often successful for patients unresponsive to splinting/corticosteroid injections or who suffered recurrence (2)[B]

MEDICATION

First Line
- Steroid injection of the tendon sheath/surrounding SC tissue has 57–90% success rate.
- Triamcinolone appears more effective than dexamethasone (2)[B].
- Injection in surrounding tissues is as efficacious as injecting into the tendon sheath (1,2)[B]. Injection into the palmar surface at the midproximal phalanx is associated with less pain than injection of tendon sheath at MCP joint (4)[B].
- Corticosteroid injection has higher success rate than splinting (3)[B].

Second Line

- Oral NSAIDs may reduce pain and discomfort but have not been shown to alter underlying disease. NSAIDs do not reduce symptoms of snapping/locking.
- Injection with diclofenac may be an alternative to corticosteroid for patients with diabetes mellitus if increase in blood sugar is a concern (2)[A].
- Corticosteroids are more effective than diclofenac during the first 3 weeks postinjection. Efficacy is similar to other modalities by 3 months postinjection (2)[B].

ISSUES FOR REFERRAL

Refer to a hand surgeon for A1 pulley release if the patient is not responding to conservative treatment.

ADDITIONAL THERAPIES

Physiotherapy is helpful, particularly in children.

SURGERY/OTHER PROCEDURES

- Surgical release can be done as an open procedure or percutaneously.
- No apparent differences in success or rates of complications between surgical approaches (5)[A]
- Surgery has lower rate of recurrence than corticosteroid injection but has disadvantage of being more painful initially (5)[A].

ADMISSION, INPATIENT, AND NURSING CONSIDERATIONS

- Day surgery for trigger finger release
- Discharge criteria: absence of complications

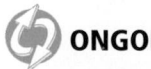 ## ONGOING CARE

FOLLOW-UP RECOMMENDATIONS

- Follow-up is needed only if symptoms persist or if complications develop after surgery.
- Splinting of the affected digit to minimize flexion/extension of the MCP joint helps symptom resolution (1)[B].

PROGNOSIS

Prognosis is excellent with conservative treatment or surgical intervention. Recurrence following corticosteroid injection is more likely for patients with type 1 diabetes mellitus, younger patients, involvement of multiple digits, and history of other upper extremity tendinopathies (2)[B].

COMPLICATIONS

- Diabetic patients may have increased blood sugar levels for up to 5 days following steroid injection.
- Other minor injection complications include skin depigmentation and fat necrosis; tendon attrition or rupture is rare.
- Complications from surgery include infection, bleeding, digital nerve injury, persistent pain, and loss of range of motion of the affected finger. The rate of major complications is low (3%). The rate of minor complications (including loss of range of motion) is higher (up to 28%).
- Another surgical complication, injury to the A2 pulley, may result in bowstringing (bulging of the flexor tendon in the palm with flexion) and pain.

REFERENCES

1. Akhtar S, Bradley MJ, Quinton DN, et al. Management and referral for trigger finger/thumb. *BMJ*. 2005;331(7507):30–33.
2. Giugale JM, Fowler JR. Trigger finger: adult and pediatric treatment strategies. *Orthop Clin North Am*. 2015;46(4):561–569.
3. Salim N, Abdullah S, Sapuan J, et al. Outcome of corticosteroid injection versus physiotherapy in the treatment of mild trigger fingers. *J Hand Surg Eur Vol*. 2012;37(1):27–34.
4. Cecen GS, Gulabi D, Saglam F, et al. Corticosteroid injection for trigger finger: blinded or ultrasound-guided injection? *Arch Orthop Trauma Surg*. 2015;135(1):125–131.
5. Fiorini HJ, Tamaoki MJ, Lenza M, et al. Surgery for trigger finger. *Cochrane Database Syst Rev*. 2018;(2):CD009860.

ADDITIONAL READING

- Amirfeyz R, McNinch R, Watts A, et al. Evidence-based management of adult trigger digits. *J Hand Surg Eur Vol*. 2017;42(5):473–480.
- Fleisch SB, Spindler KP, Lee DH. Corticosteroid injections in the treatment of trigger finger: a level I and II systematic review. *J Am Acad Orthop Surg*. 2007;15(3):166–171.
- Huisstede BM, Hoogvliet P, Coert JH, et al; for European HANDGUIDE Group. Multidisciplinary consensus guideline for managing trigger finger: results from the European HANDGUIDE Study. *Phys Ther*. 2014;94(10):1421–1433.
- Wang J, Zhao JG, Liang CC. Percutaneous release, open surgery, or corticosteroid injection, which is the best treatment method for trigger digits? *Clin Orthop Relat Res*. 2013;471(6):1879–1886.

 ## CODES

ICD10

- M65.30 Trigger finger, unspecified finger
- M65.319 Trigger thumb, unspecified thumb
- M65.329 Trigger finger, unspecified index finger

CLINICAL PEARLS

- Trigger finger is caused by narrowing of the A1 flexor tendon pulley.
- Diagnosis is based on clinical presentation.
- Initial conservative treatment can include splinting or corticosteroid injection.
- Long-acting corticosteroid injections are effective for treatment of trigger finger but have high recurrence rate than surgery.
- Open and percutaneous surgical release have high success rates for patients not responsive to splinting or injections.

TROCHANTERIC BURSITIS (GREATER TROCHANTERIC PAIN SYNDROME)

David W. Kruse, MD • David C. Shin, MD

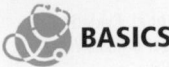 BASICS

Trochanteric bursitis is the historical term referring to lateral hip pain and tenderness over the greater trochanter. Because many patients lack an inflammatory process within the trochanteric bursa, this condition has been more recently referred to as *greater trochanteric pain syndrome* (GTPS) (1).

DESCRIPTION
- Bursae are fluid-filled sacs found primarily at tendon attachment sites with bony protuberances:
  - Multiple bursae are in the area of the greater trochanter of the femur.
  - These bursae are associated with the tendons of the gluteus muscles, iliotibial band (ITB), and tensor fasciae latae.
  - The subgluteus maximus bursa is implicated most commonly in lateral hip pain (1).
- Other structures of the lateral hip include the following:
  - ITB, tensor fasciae latae, gluteus maximus tendon, gluteus medius tendon, gluteus minimus tendon, quadratus femoris muscle, vastus lateralis tendon, piriformis tendon
- *Bursitis* refers to bursal inflammation.
- *Tendinopathy* refers to any abnormality of a tendon, inflammatory or degenerative. *Enthesopathy* refers to abnormalities of the zones of attachment of ligaments and tendons to bones.

EPIDEMIOLOGY

Incidence
- 1.8/1,000 persons/year
- Peak incidence in 4th to 6th decades

Prevalence
- Predominant sex: female > male
- More common in running and contact athletes
  - Football, rugby, soccer

ETIOLOGY AND PATHOPHYSIOLOGY
- Acute: Abnormal gait or poor muscle flexibility and strength imbalances lead to bursal friction and secondary inflammation.
  - Tendon overuse and inflammation
  - Direct trauma from contact or frequently lying with body weight on hip can cause an inflammatory response ("hip pointer") as well.
- Chronic
  - Fibrosis and thickening of bursal sac due to chronic inflammatory process
  - Tendinopathy due to chronic overuse and degeneration: gluteus medius and minimus most commonly involved (1)

Genetics
No known genetic factors

RISK FACTORS
Multiple factors have been implicated (1):
- Female gender
- Obesity
- Tight hip musculature (including ITB)
- Direct trauma
- Total hip arthroplasty
- Abnormal gait or pelvic architecture
  - Leg length discrepancy
  - Sacroiliac (SI) joint dysfunction
  - Knee or hip osteoarthritis
  - Abnormal foot mechanics (e.g., pes planus, overpronation)
  - Neuromuscular disorder: Trendelenburg gait

GENERAL PREVENTION
- Maintain ITB, hip, and lower back flexibility and strength.
- Avoid direct trauma (use of appropriate padding in contact sports).
- Avoid prolonged running on banked or crowned surfaces.
- Wear appropriate shoes.
- Appropriate bedding and sleeping surface
- Maintain appropriate body weight loss.

COMMONLY ASSOCIATED CONDITIONS
- Biomechanical factors (1)
  - Tight ITBs, leg length discrepancy, SI joint dysfunction, pes planus
  - Width of greater trochanters greater than width of iliac wings
- Other associated pathology (1):
  - Low back pain
  - Knee and hip osteoarthritis
  - Obesity

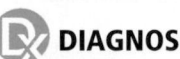 DIAGNOSIS

HISTORY
General history (1)
- Pain localized to the lateral hip or buttock
- Pain may radiate to groin or lateral thigh (pseudoradiculopathy).
- Pain exacerbated by:
  - Prolonged walking or standing
  - Rising after prolonged sitting
  - Sitting with legs crossed
  - Lying on affected side
- Other historical features:
  - Direct trauma to affected hip
  - Chronic low back pain
  - Chronic leg/knee/ankle/hip pain
  - Recent increase in running distance or intensity
  - Change in running surfaces

PHYSICAL EXAM
- Observe gait.
- Point tenderness with direct palpation over the lateral hip is characteristic of GTPS (1)[B].
- Other exam features have lower sensitivity (1)[B]:
  - Pain with extremes of passive rotation, abduction, or adduction
  - Pain with resisted hip abduction and external or internal rotation
  - Trendelenburg sign
- Other tests to rule out associated conditions:
  - Patrick-FABERE (flexion, abduction, external rotation, extension) test for SI joint dysfunction
  - Ober test for ITB pathology
  - Flexion and extension of hip for osteoarthritis
  - Leg length measurement
  - Foot inspection for pes planus or overpronation
  - Lower extremity neurologic assessment for lumbar radiculopathy or neuromuscular disorders
  - Hip lag sign (2)

DIFFERENTIAL DIAGNOSIS
- ITB syndrome
- Piriformis syndrome
- Osteoarthritis or avascular necrosis of the hip
- Lumbosacral osteoarthritis/disc disease with nerve root compression
- Fracture or contusion of the hip or pelvis— particularly in setting of trauma
- Stress reaction/fracture of femoral neck— particularly in female runners
- Septic bursitis/arthritis

DIAGNOSTIC TESTS & INTERPRETATION
No routine lab testing is recommended.

Initial Tests (lab, imaging)
- Diagnosis can be made by history and exam (3).
- If imaging is ordered:
  - US can aid in diagnosis and guide aspiration and/or injection.
  - Anteroposterior and frog-leg views of affected hip to rule out specific bony pathology (OA, stress fracture, etc.)
  - Consider lumbar spine radiographs if back pain is thought to be a contributing factor.
  - MRI is image of choice in recalcitrant pain or to formally exclude stress fracture.

Follow-Up Tests & Special Considerations
- If there is a concern for a septic bursitis, then aspiration or incision and drainage may be necessary.
- Advanced imaging rarely necessary; detection of abnormalities on MRI is a poor predictor of GTPS (4)[B].

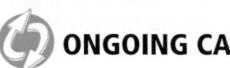 ## TREATMENT

GENERAL MEASURES
- Physical therapy to address underlying dysfunction and rebuild atrophic muscle
- Correct pelvic/hip instability.
- Correct lower limb biomechanics.
- Low-impact conditioning and aquatic therapy
- Gait training
- Weight loss (if applicable)
- Minimize aggravating activities such as prolonged walking or standing.
- Avoid lying on affected side.
- Runners
  - May need to decrease distance and/or intensity of runs during treatment. Some need to stop running. Amount of time is case specific but may range from 2 to 4 weeks.
  - Avoid banked tracks or roads with excessive tilt.

MEDICATION
First Line
- NSAIDs (1)[B]: Treat for 2 to 4 weeks.
  - Naproxen: 500 mg PO BID
  - Ibuprofen: 800 mg PO TID
- Corticosteroid injection is effective for pain relief (5)[C] and can be considered first-line therapy for selected cases:
  - Dexamethasone: 4 mg/mL or
  - Kenalog: 40 mg/mL, use 1 to 2 mL
  - Consider adding a local anesthetic (short- and/or long-acting) for more immediate pain relief.
  - Can be repeated with similar effect if original treatment showed a strong response
  - Goal is pain relief.

ISSUES FOR REFERRAL
- Septic bursitis
- Recalcitrant bursitis

ADDITIONAL THERAPIES
- Ice
- Low-energy shock wave therapy has been shown to be superior to other nonoperative modalities (6).
- Focus on achieving flexibility of hip musculature, particularly the ITB.
- Address contributing factors:
  - Low back flexibility
  - If leg length discrepancy, consider heel lift.
  - If pes planus or overpronation, consider arch supports or custom orthotics.

SURGERY/OTHER PROCEDURES
- Surgery rare but effective in refractory cases (6)[A]
- If surgery is indicated, potential options include:
  - Arthroscopic bursectomy
  - ITB release
  - Gluteus medius tendon repair

COMPLEMENTARY & ALTERNATIVE MEDICINE
- Acupuncture
- Prolotherapy
- Growth factor injection techniques
- Platelet-rich plasma injection

 ## ONGOING CARE

FOLLOW-UP RECOMMENDATIONS
4 weeks posttreatment, sooner if significant worsening

PATIENT EDUCATION
- Maintain hip musculature flexibility, including ITB.
- Correct issues that may cause abnormal gait:
  - Low back pain
  - Knee pain
  - Leg length discrepancy (heel lift)
  - Foot mechanics (orthotics)
- Gradual return to physical activity

PROGNOSIS
Depends on chronicity and recurrence, with more acute cases having an excellent prognosis

COMPLICATIONS
Bursal thickening and fibrosis

REFERENCES
1. Williams BS, Cohen SP. Greater trochanteric pain syndrome: a review of anatomy, diagnosis and treatment. *Anesth Analg.* 2009;108(5):1662–1670.
2. Kaltenborn A, Bourg CM, Gutzeit A, et al. The hip lag sign—prospective blinded trial of a new clinical sign to predict hip abductor damage. *PLoS One.* 2014;9(3):e91560.
3. Chowdhury R, Naaseri S, Lee J, et al. Imaging and management of greater trochanteric pain syndrome. *Postgrad Med J.* 2014;90(1068):576–581.
4. Blankenbaker DG, Ullrick SR, Davis KW, et al. Correlation of MRI findings with clinical findings of trochanteric pain syndrome. *Skeletal Radiol.* 2008;37(10):903–909.
5. Stephens MB, Beutler AI, O'Connor FG. Musculoskeletal injections: a review of the evidence. *Am Fam Physician.* 2008;78(8):971–976.
6. Lustenberger DP, Ng VY, Best TM, et al. Efficacy of treatment of trochanteric bursitis: a systematic review. *Clin J Sport Med.* 2011;21(5):447–453.

ADDITIONAL READING
- Baker CL Jr, Massie RV, Hurt WG, et al. Arthroscopic bursectomy for recalcitrant trochanteric bursitis. *Arthroscopy.* 2007;23(8):827–832.
- Barnthouse NC, Wente TM, Voos JE. Greater trochanteric pain syndrome: endoscopic treatment options. *Oper Tech Sports Med.* 2012;20:320–324.
- Barratt PA, Brookes N, Newson A. Conservative treatments for greater trochanteric pain syndrome: a systematic review. *Br J Sports Med.* 2017;51(2):97–104.
- Hugo D, de Jongh HR. Greater trochanteric pain syndrome. *SA Orthop J.* 2012;11(1):28–33.
- McMahon SE, Smith TO, Hing CB. A systematic review of imaging modalities in the diagnosis of greater trochanteric pain syndrome. *Musculoskeletal Care.* 2012;10(4):232–239.
- Pretell J, Ortega J, García-Rayo R, et al. Distal fascia lata lengthening: an alternative surgical technique for recalcitrant trochanteric bursitis. *Int Orthop.* 2009;33(5):1223–1227.

CODES
ICD10
- M70.60 Trochanteric bursitis, unspecified hip
- M70.62 Trochanteric bursitis, left hip
- M70.61 Trochanteric bursitis, right hip

CLINICAL PEARLS
- Patients with GTPS often present with an inability to lie on the affected side.
- Femoral neck stress fractures are a do-not-miss diagnosis, particularly in young female runners.
- Corticosteroid injection helps as an initial therapy, particularly for pain relief to allow for aggressive physical therapy.
- Physical therapy is treatment mainstay for correcting biomechanical imbalances and restoring proper function.

TUBERCULOSIS
Michael C. Stefanowicz, DO • Swati Avashia, MD, FAAP, FACP, ABIHM

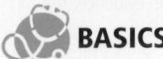 **BASICS**

DESCRIPTION
- Active tuberculosis (TB)
  - Primary infection or reactivation of latent infection
  - Without preventive therapy, affects 10% of infected individuals
  - Risk increases with immunosuppression: highest risk first 2 years after infection. Reactivation risk increases with comorbidities (e.g., HIV, diabetes).
  - Well-described forms: pulmonary (85% of cases), miliary (disseminated), meningeal, abdominal, lymphadenitis (scrofula)
- Usually acquired by inhalation of airborne bacilli from an individual with active TB. Bacilli multiply in alveoli and spread via macrophages, lymphatics, and blood. Three possible outcomes:
  - Eradication: Tissue hypersensitivity halts infection within 10 weeks.
  - Primary TB
  - Latent TB (See "Tuberculosis, Latent (LTBI).")

Pediatric Considerations
- Children more commonly have severe disease, higher risk and faster rate of progression to disease.
- Most children with pulmonary TB are asymptomatic.
- Pediatric TB treatment should be directly observed (directly observed therapy [DOT]) using four drugs.

EPIDEMIOLOGY
Incidence
- Worldwide (2016): 10.4 million (133 cases per 100,000) population; highest incidence in Asia and Africa (1)
- United States (2017): 9,093 (2.8/100,000); incidence in foreign-born 14 times that of U.S.-born persons (2)

Prevalence
Worldwide (2016): Indirect estimates are uncertain due to variance in reporting systems. Higher burden countries have approximately 150 cases per 100,000 population (2).

Mortality
Worldwide (2016): 1.3 million deaths due to TB, 1 of the top 10 causes of death worldwide

ETIOLOGY AND PATHOPHYSIOLOGY
- *Mycobacterium tuberculosis, Mycobacterium bovis*, or *Mycobacterium africanum* are causative organisms.
- Cell-mediated response by activated T lymphocytes and macrophages forms a granuloma that limits bacillary replication. Destruction of the macrophages produces early "solid necrosis." In 2 to 3 weeks, "caseous necrosis" develops and LTBI ensues. In the immunocompetent, granuloma undergoes "fibrosis" and calcification. In the immunocompromised, primary progressive TB develops. Cavitary lesions may form. Necrotic lesions may rupture into bronchioles with resulting aerosolization of tuberculous bacilli.

RISK FACTORS
- For infection: homeless, close quarters (barracks, correctional facilities, nursing homes), close contact with infected person, ethnic minorities, living in areas with high incidence of active TB, health care workers; medically underserved, low income, substance abuse
- For development of disease once infected: chronic renal failure; lymphoma; silicosis; diabetes mellitus; cancer of head, neck, or lung; children <5 years of age; malnutrition; systemic corticosteroids; HIV; immunosuppressive drugs; IV drug abuse, alcohol

abuse, cigarette smokers; <2 years since infection with *M. tuberculosis*; history of gastrectomy or jejunal bypass; <90% of ideal body weight

GENERAL PREVENTION
- Screen for and treat LTBI. Report active TB to health department; test and treat all close contacts.
- Bacillus Calmette-Guérin (BCG) vaccine: relatively ineffective in adults. In children, live attenuated *M. bovis* prevents 50% of pulmonary disease and 80% of meningitis and miliary disease. More commonly used in endemic countries. In the United States, consider BCG for high-risk children with negative PPD and HIV tests or for health workers at risk for drug-resistant infection.

COMMONLY ASSOCIATED CONDITIONS
Immunosuppression; HIV coinfection; malignancy

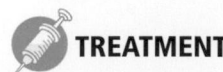 **DIAGNOSIS**

HISTORY
- Known exposure to individual with active TB
- Immunosuppression
- Tobacco use; recreational drug use
- Signs and symptoms
  - General: fever, night sweats, weight loss, malaise, painless lymph node swelling
  - Pulmonary TB: unexplained cough >2 to 3 weeks, hemoptysis
  - Abdominal TB: acutely as surgical abdomen; chronic abdominal TB varies (vague abdominal symptoms, abdominal mass, "doughy" abdomen).
  - Meningitis: See "Tuberculosis, CNS."
  - Miliary: See "Tuberculosis, Miliary."

PHYSICAL EXAM
- Often entirely normal. Specific findings depend on organs involved: hepatosplenomegaly, adenopathy, rales; poor weight gain in children
- Late findings: renal, bone, or CNS disease

DIFFERENTIAL DIAGNOSIS
- Pulmonary TB: pneumonia (bacterial, fungal, atypical), malignancy, actinomycosis, Wegener, noninfectious granulomatous diseases (e.g., sarcoidosis), tularemia
- Extrapulmonary TB: other mycobacterial infections, syphilis, cat-scratch disease, leishmaniasis, erythema nodosum, rheumatologic disease, erythema induratum

DIAGNOSTIC TESTS & INTERPRETATION
Initial Tests
To determine immune response to mycobacterium
- Tuberculin skin test (TST) (e.g., PPD): 5 U (0.1 mL) intermediate-strength intradermal injection into volar forearm. Measure induration at 48 to 72 hours:
  - PPD positive if induration
    - >5 mm and HIV infection, recent TB contact, immunosuppressed, disease on x-ray
    - >10 mm and age <4 years or other risk factors
    - >15 mm and age >4 years and no risk factors
  - Two-step test, 1 to 3 weeks apart: no recent PPD, age >55 years, nursing home resident, prison inmate, or health care worker
  - Context of PPD results:
    - False positive: BCG (unreliable, should not affect decision to treat)
    - False negative: HIV, steroids, gastrectomy, alcoholism, renal failure, sarcoidosis, malnutrition, hematologic or lymphoreticular disorder, very recent exposure
    - If positive once, no need to repeat

- Interferon-γ release assays (IGRAs) measure interferon release after stimulation in vitro by *M. tuberculosis* antigens (3)[A]:
  - With very few exceptions, do not cross-react with BCG and most nontuberculous mycobacteria
    - IGRA preferred for persons who have had BCG (vaccine or for cancer therapy) and those unlikely to return for TST interpretation (3)[A]
    - TST preferred if age <5 years (3)[A]. The AAP now endorses IGRA in BCG-vaccinated children ≥2 years of age.
    - Either TST or IGRA may be used as periodic screening for persons in high-risk occupations and for recent contacts of persons with known or suspected active TB (3)[A].
    - Cotesting with TST and IGRA if the initial test is negative, but the risk for rapid disease progression is increased (e.g., HIV-infected persons or children <5 years old) (3)[A]
- TST and IGRA cannot discern LTBI from active TB.

Initial Tests (lab, imaging)
Active TB
- Three sputum samples (8 to 24 hours apart, at least one early morning sample) for acid-fast bacilli (AFB) stain and mycobacterial culture by aerosol induction, gastric aspirate (children), or bronchoalveolar lavage
- Positive AFB: Treat immediately; culture and sensitivity guide treatment.
- Nucleic acid amplification test (NAAT): Use as an adjunct to culture and AFB smear. Positive result supports presumptive diagnosis of TB while culture pending. Negative NAAT does not rule out TB.
- Chest radiograph
  - Primary TB: infiltrate with or without atelectasis, effusion, or adenopathy. Ghon lesion: calcified tuberculous caseating granuloma (tuberculoma); if associated with calcified ipsilateral hilar lymph node, then Ghon (or Ranke) complex
  - Recrudescent TB: cavitary lesions and upper lobe disease with hilar adenopathy
  - HIV: atypical findings with primary infection, right upper lobe atelectasis
- CT chest: good sensitivity, tree-in-bud (centrilobular nodules with branching linear opacities)

Follow-Up Tests & Special Considerations
- Baseline CBC, creatinine, AST, ALT, bilirubin, alkaline phosphatase, visual acuity, and red-green color discrimination (regimens involving ethambutol [EMB])
- Diabetes screen if risk factors present
- HIV: If positive, get baseline CD4 count, viral load.
- Check hepatitis B and C if injection drug users, Africa or Asia born, HIV infected or otherwise high risk.
- Extrapulmonary: urine, CSF, bone marrow, and liver biopsy for culture as indicated
- Nonspecific findings: anemia, thrombocytosis, SIADH, hypergammaglobulinemia, monocytosis, sterile pyuria

Diagnostic Procedures/Other
- Culture: takes several weeks for definitive results
- Xpert MTB/RIF (rapid molecular test): currently the only FDA-approved molecular assay for pulmonary TB diagnosis and detection of rifampicin resistance in areas with high prevalence of MDR TB (3)[A]

TREATMENT

GENERAL MEASURES
- If clinical suspicion, treat immediately. Prescribing physician is responsible for treatment completion.

- Respiratory and droplet precautions
- Not infectious if favorable clinical response after 2 to 3 weeks of therapy and three negative AFB smears

MEDICATION
Use ideal body weight for dosing; DOT recommended for all and required for children, institutionalized patients, nonadherent patients, and nondaily regimens

First Line
- LTBI (4)[A]
  – Isoniazid (INH) for 9 months at 5 mg/kg/day (max of 300 mg) *or* 15 mg/kg (max of 900 mg) 2 times per week *or*
  – Isoniazid 15 mg/kg + rifapentine (3HP) 300 to 900 mg weekly for 12 weeks by DOT for age ≥2 years. Recent update by CDC (July 2018); also safe with HIV patients depending on antiretroviral therapy (ART) regimen (5)
- Active TB infection (4)[A]
  – Regimen 1 (preferred)
    ○ Initial phase:
      ▪ Isoniazid 5 mg/kg, rifampin (RIF) 10 mg/kg (max 600 mg), pyrazinamide (PZA) 15 to 30 mg/kg, and EMB 15 to 20 mg/kg daily for 8 weeks *or*
      ▪ INH/RIF/PZA/EMB 5 days/week for 8 weeks
    ○ Continuation phase:
      ▪ INH/RIF daily for 18 weeks; or, if DOT, INH/RIF 5 days/week for 18 weeks
  – Regimen 2 (preferred when more frequent DOT in continuation phase is difficult to achieve)
    ○ Initial phase:
      ▪ INH/RIF/PZA/EMB daily for 8 weeks *or*
      ▪ INH/RIF/PZA/EMB 5 days/week for 8 weeks
    ○ Continuation phase:
      ▪ INH/RIF 3 times per week for 18 weeks
  – Regimen 3 (caution if HIV infected or with cavitary disease; missed doses can lead to treatment failure, relapse, and acquired drug resistance)
    ○ Initial phase: INH/RIF/PZA/EMB 3 times per week for 8 weeks
    ○ Continuation phase: INH/RIF 3 times per week for 18 weeks
  – Regimen 4 (do not use if HIV positive, smear positive, or cavitary disease)
    ○ Initial phase: INH/RIF/PZA/EMB daily for 14 doses and then twice a week for 12 doses
    ○ Continuation phase: INH/RIF twice a week for 18 weeks

Pregnancy Considerations
- Delay treatment in pregnant patients with LTBI until delivery unless other risk factors (e.g., HIV, immunosuppressed) present.
- Treat TB in pregnancy with INH, RIF, and EMB; add pyridoxine 25 mg/day.
- Streptomycin: ototoxic and nephrotoxic; do not use in pregnancy.
- PZA is not used in pregnant women in the United States.
- Congenital infection: from maternal miliary or endometrial TB. PPD, CXR, lumbar puncture, and culture placenta. Treat promptly if suspected.
- Breastfeeding: OK while taking TB drugs; supplement with pyridoxine 25 mg/day.

Pediatric Considerations
- Children may attend school as long as they are taking the appropriate medications.
- EMB can be used in infants and children (4).

ALERT
- Maximum drug doses: rifampin 600 mg all regimens; pyrazinamide 2,000 mg/day or 4,000 mg 2 times per week; ethambutol 600 mg/day or 4,000 mg 2 times per week

- If patient does not receive PZA for all of the first 2 months, extend treatment to 9 months.
- *M. bovis* is resistant to PZA; must be treated 9 months
- Continue EMB until organism susceptibility to INH plus RIF is determined (4)[A].
- Initiation of ART therapy in HIV-positive patients infected with TB carries an increased risk of immune reconstitution inflammatory syndrome (IRIS) (4)[A].

Second Line
Fluoroquinolones and injectable aminoglycosides. Use when MDR is suspected or patient intolerance.

ISSUES FOR REFERRAL

ALERT
Notify public health authorities for all cases of active TB. Consult infectious disease specialist for drug-resistant TB and HIV-positive patients on ART.

ADDITIONAL THERAPIES
- Pyridoxine: 50 mg should be given to all persons at risk for INH neuropathy: pregnant women, diabetes, breastfed infants, HIV positive, alcoholism, chronic renal failure, malnutrition, or advanced age (4)[A].
- Steroids: recommended for TB meningitis (4)[A]; not recommended for TB pericarditis (4)[B]

SURGERY/OTHER PROCEDURES
For extrapulmonary complications (spinal cord compression, bowel obstruction, constrictive pericarditis)

COMPLEMENTARY & ALTERNATIVE MEDICINE
Vitamin D deficiency may increase susceptibility to TB and development of active TB (6)[C]. Evidence is unclear regarding vitamin D supplementation in TB treatment.

ADMISSION, INPATIENT, AND NURSING CONSIDERATIONS
- Negative pressure isolation with personal respirators and droplet precautions
  – Three consecutive negative sputum AFB smears are necessary for release from isolation.
- Once TB has been excluded or the patient has demonstrated response to therapy and is not an infectious risk, arrange outpatient follow-up with a provider comfortable managing TB and coordinate case management with local public health authorities.

 ONGOING CARE

FOLLOW-UP RECOMMENDATIONS
Patient Monitoring
- Monthly sputum for AFB smear and culture until two consecutive cultures are negative; must confirm this prior to starting continuation phase
- Monthly visits to monitor medication adherence and adverse effects; CXR after 2 months of treatment
- For HIV positive: CD4 count, viral load, CBC, and liver enzymes every 3 months
- Liver enzymes monthly for chronic liver disease, alcohol use, pregnant or postpartum patients. Temporarily halt medications for enzyme increase ≥5 × ULN if asymptomatic or ≥3 × ULN if symptomatic.
- Visual acuity and red-green color monthly if on EMB >2 months or doses >20 mg/kg/day
- If culture positive after 2 months of therapy, reassess drug sensitivity, initiate DOT, coordinate care with public health authorities, and consider infectious disease consultation (if not already involved).

PATIENT EDUCATION
- Emphasize medication adherence.
- Screen and treat close contacts.

- Alert patient that health authorities must be notified.
- http://www.cdc.gov/tb/publications/factsheets/general/tb.htm

PROGNOSIS
Few complications and full resolution of infection if medications are taken for full course as prescribed

COMPLICATIONS
- Cavitary lesions can become secondarily infected.
- Risk for drug resistance increases with HIV positive, treatment nonadherence, or residence in area with high incidence of resistance.
- MDR-TB: resistance to INH and rifampicin
- XDR-TB: MDR-TB that is also resistant to fluoroquinolones and at least one second-line injectable drug (9% of MDR)

REFERENCES
1. World Health Organization. Global tuberculosis report 2016. http://www.who.int/tb/publications/global_report/gtbr2016_main_text.pdf?ua=1. Accessed November 16, 2018.
2. Stewart RJ, Tsang CA, Pratt RH, et al. Tuberculosis—United States, 2017. *MMWR Morb Mortal Wkly Rep.* 2018;67(11):317–323.
3. Lewinsohn DM, Leonard MK, LoBue PA, et al. Official American Thoracic Society/Infectious Diseases Society of America/Centers for Disease Control and Prevention clinical practice guidelines: diagnosis of tuberculosis in adults and children. *Clin Infect Dis.* 2017;64(2):e1–e33.
4. Nahid P, Dorman SE, Alipanah N, et al. Official American Thoracic Society/Centers for Disease Control and Prevention/Infectious Diseases Society of America clinical practice guidelines: treatment of drug-susceptible tuberculosis. *Clin Infect Dis.* 2016;63(7):e147–e195.
5. Borisov AS, Bamrah Morris S, Njie GJ, et al. Update of recommendations for use of once-weekly isoniazid-rifapentine regimen to treat latent *Mycobacterium tuberculosis* infection. *MMWR Morb Mortal Wkly Rep.* 2018;67(25):723–726.
6. Luong KV, Nguyen LT. Impact of vitamin D in the treatment of tuberculosis. *Am J Med Sci.* 2011;341(6):493–498.

 SEE ALSO

- Tuberculosis, CNS; Tuberculosis, Latent (LTBI); Tuberculosis, Miliary
- Algorithm: Weight Loss, Unintentional

CODES

ICD10
- A15.9 Respiratory tuberculosis unspecified
- A15.0 Tuberculosis of lung
- A19.9 Miliary tuberculosis, unspecified

CLINICAL PEARLS
- TB is fully curable when treated appropriately.
- Pulmonary TB treatment involves four-drug regimen.
- Children and elderly patients exhibit fewer classic clinical features of TB.
- TST and IGRA cannot discern active TB from LTBI.
- Involve public health authorities early.
- DOT is preferred.

TUBERCULOSIS, LATENT (LTBI)

Kay A. Bauman, MD, MPH

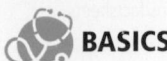 **BASICS**

DESCRIPTION

- Latent tuberculosis infection (LTBI) is an asymptomatic, noninfectious condition following exposure to an active case of tuberculosis. LTBI is usually detected by a positive skin test (i.e., purified protein derivative [PPD]) or a positive interferon-γ release assay (IGRA) test. In LTBI, acid-fast bacilli smear and culture are negative, and chest x-ray (CXR) does not suggest active TB.
- Active TB occurs in 5–10% of infected individuals who have not received preventive therapy. Chance of active TB increases with immunosuppression and is highest for all individuals within 2 years of infection; 85% of the cases are pulmonary, which is capable of person-to-person spread via aerosol route.
- The majority (70% in 2017) of active TB cases in the United States occur in foreign-born persons. 78% are the result of reactivation of LTBI (1).
- LTBI treatment is a key component of the TB elimination strategy for the United States.

ALERT
After 20 years of annual decreases in the number of active TB cases in the United States, the incidence has recently plateaued. Identification and treatment of LTBI is crucial to reverse this trend. Test for LTBI (PPD or IGRA) and treat latent infection in at-risk populations.

EPIDEMIOLOGY

- TB is the leading cause of infectious disease mortality worldwide.
- In the United States, high-risk groups include immigrants from Asia, Latin America, Africa, and the Pacific basin; blacks; homeless persons; persons with a history of drug use or history of incarceration; HIV-infected individuals; and health care workers.
- Newly exposed (particularly children) are also at high risk.
- In 2017, there were 9,093 new cases of TB in the United States, the lowest number of TB cases on record. Of these cases, 30% were U.S.-born and 70% foreign-born (1).
- Among foreign-born persons, Asians have the highest active TB case rate (27 cases per 100,000) and non-Hispanic blacks (22/100,000) (1).
- In 2017, the majority of foreign-born persons with TB came from five countries: Mexico (19%), Philippines (12%), India (9%), Vietnam (8%), and China (6%) (1).
- In 2017, 6% of active TB cases in the United States were in HIV-positive individuals (1).
- In 2017, the lowest state-specific incidence was 0.3 cases per 100,000 in Montana and the highest 8.1/100,000 in Hawaii.

Prevalence
- 4% of the U.S. population has LTBI (~11 million).
- ~1/3 of the world's population harbors latent TB.

ETIOLOGY AND PATHOPHYSIOLOGY
Mycobacterium tuberculosis, Mycobacterium bovis, and *Mycobacterium africanum*

RISK FACTORS
- HIV infection, immunosuppression
- Immigrants (from Asia, Latin America, Pacific Islands, Africa, or areas with high rates of TB), including migrant workers
- Close contact with infected individual
- Institutionalization (e.g., prison, nursing home)
- Use of illicit drugs
- Lower socioeconomic or homeless status
- Health care workers
- Chronic medical disease such as diabetes mellitus (DM), end-stage renal disease, cancer, or silicosis; organ transplant (immunosuppression)
- Persons with fibrotic changes on CXR consistent with previous TB infection
- Recent TB skin test (tuberculin skin test [TST]) converters
- Laboratory personnel working with mycobacteria
- Organ donors should be screened. If donor is deceased, IGRA testing is still possible.

GENERAL PREVENTION
Screen for LTBI and treat individuals with positive tests.

COMMONLY ASSOCIATED CONDITIONS
- HIV infection (see "Initial Tests (lab, imaging)")
- Immunosuppression

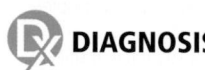 **DIAGNOSIS**

HISTORY
Assess risk; history of immigration from a high-risk area including those with temporary visas for school or work (note: TB screening for this type of visa is not required, unlike regulations for those seeking permanent residence in the United States) (2), history of IV drug use and/or drug treatment, HIV, homelessness, recent incarceration, immunosuppression

PHYSICAL EXAM
No active signs of infection on exam in patients with LTBI

DIFFERENTIAL DIAGNOSIS
Fungal infections; atypical mycobacteria or *Nocardia*

DIAGNOSTIC TESTS & INTERPRETATION
Initial Tests (lab, imaging)
- CXR to rule out active TB
- No others routinely recommended
- In higher risk patients: liver profile, hepatitis C virus (HCV), and hepatitis B virus (HBV) screening
- HIV test recommended to assess risk for active TB in men who have sex with men or patients with a history of IV drug use

Diagnostic Procedures/Other
- TST: PPD: 5 U (0.1 mL) intermediate-strength intradermal volar forearm. Measure induration at 48 to 72 hours:
  – Positive if induration is
    ○ >5 mm and patient has HIV infection (or suspected), is immunosuppressed, had recent close TB contact, or has clinical evidence of active or old disease on CXR
    ○ >10 mm and patient age <4 years or has other risk factors noted earlier
    ○ >15 mm and patient age >4 years and has no risk factors
  – Negative if induration <5 mm on initial test and, if indicated, on second test
  – Use the two-step test (administer a second intradermal test 1 to 3 weeks after initial test; measure and interpret as usual) if patient has had no recent PPD and is age >55 years or is a nursing home resident, prison inmate, or health care worker.
  – Preferred for children <5 years
- The IGRA QuantiFERON-TB and QuantiFERON-TB GOLD; T-SPOT measures the release of interferon by sensitized lymphocytes when exposed to antigens of *M. tuberculosis*. It is unaffected by prior BCG vaccination, requires only one visit, and has improved sensitivity and specificity but is costly (3).
- Special considerations
  – Steroids: false-negative skin test
  – Measles vaccine: may suppress tuberculin activity; simultaneous PPD and measles vaccine recommended; if not simultaneous, defer PPD for 4 to 6 weeks after measles vaccine.
  – The multiple-puncture tine test is not recommended.
  – The history of BCG vaccination should not alter the management of a positive PPD test.
  – Disorders that may give a false-negative skin test:
    ○ Recent viral infection
    ○ New (<10 weeks) infection
    ○ Severe malnutrition; HIV; anergy
    ○ Age <6 months
    ○ Overwhelming TB

TREATMENT

GENERAL MEASURES
- Must exclude active TB
- Treatment for LTBI is critical for the control and elimination of TB disease. LTBI treatment decreases the risk of active TB and decreases risk of potential spread to others. Treat all persons with LTBI.
- High-risk patients: Treat LTBI at any age if patient has HIV, has had close TB contact, is a recent converter (<2 years), is an IV drug user, has an abnormal CXR, or has a high-risk medical condition.
- Directly observed therapy (DOT) is recommended if patient adherence is not assured. Video DOT is being used effectively in several locations.
  – Use isoniazid (INH) 900 mg and rifapentine 900 mg weekly for 12 weeks.
  – Use INH for 9 months.
  – Acceptable alternative: INH for 6 months.
- Treat LTBI during pregnancy if patient has recent infection or is HIV positive (use INH with pyridoxine, and monitor liver enzymes); otherwise, postpone treatment until after delivery.
- Consult public health or infectious disease specialist for suspected INH resistance in HIV patients.
- *Note:* Rifampin and pyrazinamide are less often recommended for LTBI treatment due to side effects.
- Exclusions: cirrhosis, active hepatitis, history of excessive alcohol consumption

MEDICATION
- INH and rifapentine
  – Patients >2 years: Rifapentine, a rifampin-like drug, can be used to treat LTBI. 900 mg weekly (if patient >50 kg) and INH 15 to 25 mg/kg weekly (rounded to nearest 50 or 100 mg; 900 mg max) for 12 weeks given as DOT. This new, shorter treatment increased rates of completion compared with 9 months of INH (82% vs. 69%), slightly more adverse effects (5% vs. 4%), more costly (4).
    ○ HIV/AIDS patients are included for this new regimen (5). Children >2 years also have been recently added to this regimen because DOT is not required in children; parent-administered treatment is accepted (5).
- INH alone
  – INH-scored tablets: 100 mg, 300 mg, or syrup 10 mg/mL
    ○ Daily: adult 300 mg; pediatric 10 to 15 mg/kg (maximum 300 mg)
    ○ Twice weekly: adult 900 mg; pediatric 20 to 30 mg/kg (maximum 900 mg)
    ○ Treatment for 9 months; typical completion rates of ≤60%
    ○ Precautions
      ■ Follow liver function if the patient has history of alcoholism, HBV, HCV, fatty liver, or other signs of liver dysfunction or injury.
      ■ INH: Peripheral neuritis and hypersensitivity are possible. Consider concurrent pyridoxine.

- Alternative: rifampin alone
  – Adults 600 mg/day for 4 months; children 10 to 20 mg/kg/day for 6 months (max 600 mg/day). Fewer data exist for efficacy of this regimen but can be considered for contacts of INH-resistant TB or patient with INH contraindications. In one study, the 4-month course increased compliance from 62.6% with INH to 71.6% with rifampin.
  – Note: Rifapentine can reduce the effectiveness of hormonal contraception; women on birth control pills should switch to or add a barrier method for the 3 months of latent TB treatment (5).
  – Rifapentine can interact with warfarin—patients require increased monitoring (5).

ADDITIONAL THERAPIES
Pediatric Considerations
- Follow public health recommendations for assessing and treating newborns.
- If mother or household contact has LTBI, skin test all household contacts, and treat all positive PPD.
- If contact has abnormal CXR, separate infant until infectious status is known; if not contagious, monitor infant PPD.
- If mother has disease and is possibly contagious, evaluate infant for congenital TB and test for HIV; separate newborn until mother is noninfectious.
- Treat suspected congenital TB.

ADMISSION, INPATIENT, AND NURSING CONSIDERATIONS
Geriatric Considerations
- Before entering a chronic care setting, patients should have two-step PPD using facility protocols.
- INH side effects are more pronounced.
- Discharge criteria
  – Activity, as tolerated
  – No isolation required

 ONGOING CARE

FOLLOW-UP RECOMMENDATIONS
Patient Monitoring
- During preventive therapy for LTBI: monthly visits to assess adherence and monitor for hepatitis and neuropathy; if stable, can monitor less frequently
- If patient asymptomatic, no need to repeat CXR
- Check liver enzymes if patient is symptomatic, HIV positive, has chronic liver disease, uses alcohol, or is pregnant or postpartum. Modify drugs as needed.

DIET
Regular. Consider pyridoxine, 10 to 50 mg/day.

PROGNOSIS
- Generally, there are few complications, and treatment is effective if medications are taken as prescribed.
- Retreatment is not necessary.

COMPLICATIONS
Recrudescent TB

REFERENCES
1. Stewart R, Tsang C, Pratt R, et al. Tuberculosis—United States, 2017. *MMWR Morb Mortal Wkly Rep.* 2018;67(11):317–323.
2. Weinberg M, Cherry C, Lipnitz J, et al. Tuberculosis among temporary visa holders working in the tourism industry—United States, 2012–2014. *MMWR Morb Mortal Wkly Rep.* 2016;65(11):279–281.
3. Goletti D, Sanduzzi A, Delogu G. Performance of the tuberculin skin test and interferon-γ release assays: an update on the accuracy, cutoff stratification, and new potential immune-based approaches. *J Rheumatol Suppl.* 2014;91:24–31.
4. Centers for Disease Control and Prevention. Recommendations for use of an isoniazid-rifapentine regimen with direct observation to treat latent *Mycobacterium tuberculosis* infection. *MMWR Morb Mortal Wkly Rep.* 2011;60(48):1650–1653.
5. Borisov A, Morris S, Njie G, et al. Update of recommendations for use of once-weekly isoniazid-rifapentine regimen to treat latent *Mycobacterium tuberculosis* infection. *MMWR Morb Mortal Wkly Rep.* 2018;67(25):723–726.

ADDITIONAL READING
Centers for Disease Control and Prevention. Latent tuberculosis infection: a guide for primary health care providers. http://www.cdc.gov/tb/publications/ltbi/treatment.htm. Accessed November 16, 2017.

 SEE ALSO

Tuberculosis; Tuberculosis, Miliary

CODES

ICD10
R76.11 Nonspecific reaction to skin test w/o active tuberculosis

CLINICAL PEARLS
- ~4% of the U.S. population has LTBI.
- Treatment of LTBI is crucial to the control and elimination of TB disease in the United States.
- Screen foreign-born persons for latent TB, and treat those who are positive.
- Screen household contacts of patients who are PPD positive.
- A history of BCG vaccination, especially >10 years before PPD testing, should not be considered as the cause of a positive PPD.
- The interferon-γ (IGRA) blood test is unaffected by prior BCG vaccination.

TYPHOID FEVER

Douglas W. MacPherson, MD, MSc–CTM, FRCPC

BASICS

- A common enteric bacterial disease transmitted by ingestion of contaminated food or water
- Most cases in the United States are imported from endemic areas of South or Southeast Asia and Latin America.

DESCRIPTION
- Typhoid fever is an acute systemic illness in humans caused by *Salmonella typhi*.
  - Classic example of enteric fever caused by *Salmonella* bacterium
- Enteric fevers due to *Salmonella paratyphi* can present in a manner similar to classic typhoid fever.
- Typhoid is endemic in developing nations with poor sanitation. Most cases in North America and other developed nations are acquired after travel to disease-endemic areas.
- Travelers may be at greater risk of typhoid.
- Mode of transmission is fecal–oral through ingestion of contaminated food (poultry or milk) or water.
- Incubation period varies from 7 to 21 days.
- System(s) affected: gastrointestinal; pulmonary; skin/exocrine
- Synonym(s): typhoid; typhus abdominalis; enteric fever; nervous fever; slow fever

Geriatric Considerations
Disease is more serious in the elderly.

Pediatric Considerations
Disease is more serious in infants and milder in children.

EPIDEMIOLOGY
Although typhoid outbreaks have been described in the United States, most cases are reported in international travelers returning from endemic transmission areas.
- Predominant age: all ages
- Predominant sex: male = female

Incidence
In the United States, 300 to 500 new cases per year

ETIOLOGY AND PATHOPHYSIOLOGY
- Historically, typhoid fever (untreated) occurs in several week-long stages.
- The initial infection is transmitted via the fecal–oral route, with resultant bacteremia and sepsis. Involvement of the bowel wall (Peyer patch) rarely may be associated with bleeding from the bowel or bowel perforation.
- The first stage involves fluctuations in temperature with relative bradycardia (Faget sign). Other symptoms include headache, cough, malaise, epistaxis, and abdominal pain.

- The second stage involves higher fever (with persistent relative bradycardia). Mental status changes are possible (agitation—"nervous fever"). Rose spots appear on the chest and abdomen. In some patients, abdominal pain is common as is constipation or diarrhea (with characteristic malodorous "pea soup" appearance).
- The 3rd week is when most complications occur due to intestinal hemorrhage or encephalitis.
- The final week is defervescence and recovery.
- A chronic carrier state may occur with *S. typhi* shedding in the stools. Potential person-to-person transmission may occur. In a chronic carrier state, *S. typhi* resides in the biliary tract and gallbladder. Chronic suppressive antimicrobials may clear the carrier state; in rare cases, cholecystectomy performed to clear *S. typhi* carrier state

RISK FACTORS
Consider in patients presenting with fever after tropical travel or exposure to a chronic carrier.

GENERAL PREVENTION
- Food and water precautions help prevent all enteric infections, including typhoid fever.
- Avoid tap water, salad/raw vegetables, unpeeled fruits, and dairy products in tropical travel.
- Avoid undercooked poultry or poultry products left unrefrigerated for prolonged periods.
- Wash hands before and after food preparation.
- For high-risk travel to an endemic area, consider typhoid vaccination (1,2)[A].
  - Parenteral ViCPS or capsular polysaccharide typhoid vaccine (Typhim Vi) *or*
  - Ty21a or live oral typhoid vaccine (Vivotif Berna), particularly if prolonged risk (>4 weeks)
- Consider vaccination for workers exposed to *S. typhi* or those with close contact with a carrier of *S. typhi*.
- Occupational health and safety precautions. Consider screening of domestic and commercial food handlers.

DIAGNOSIS

Assess clinical presentation and exposure history, including travel and exposures to *S. typhi* carriers.

HISTORY
- Travel history to an endemic region and exposure to contaminated food or water
- Exposure to a chronic *S. typhi* carrier
- Fever, headache
- Malaise
- Abdominal discomfort/bloating/constipation
- Diarrhea (less common)
- Dry cough
- Confusion/lethargy

PHYSICAL EXAM
- Fever with relative bradycardia
- Cervical adenopathy
- Conjunctivitis
- Rose spot (transient erythematous maculopapular rash in anterior thorax or upper abdomen)
- Splenomegaly
- Hepatomegaly

DIFFERENTIAL DIAGNOSIS
- Enteric fever caused by nontyphoid *Salmonella* spp.
- "Enteric fever–like" syndrome caused by *Yersinia enterocolitica*, pseudotuberculosis, and *Campylobacter* spp.
- Infectious hepatitis
- Malaria, dengue
- Atypical pneumonia
- Infectious mononucleosis
- Subacute bacterial endocarditis
- Tuberculosis
- Brucellosis; Q fever; typhus
- Toxoplasmosis
- Viral infections: Epstein-Barr virus (EBV), cytomegalovirus (CMV), viral hemorrhagic agents

DIAGNOSTIC TESTS & INTERPRETATION
Enteric fevers/typhoid syndromes are rare in the United States. Therefore, a high level of clinical suspicion is required.
- Definitive diagnosis is by culture of *S. typhi* from blood or other sterile body fluid.
- Isolation of *S. typhi* in sputum, urine, or stool leads to a presumptive diagnosis.
- Serology is nonspecific and typically not useful.
- If there are multiple negative blood cultures or patient has recent been on antibiotic therapy, diagnostic yield is better with bone marrow culture.
- Anemia, leukopenia (neutropenia), thrombocytopenia, or evidence of disseminated intravascular coagulopathy. Elevated liver enzymes are common.
- Suspect intestinal perforation (consider serial plain abdominal films looking for evidence of perforation) in ill patients complaining of persistent abdominal tenderness.

Diagnostic Procedures/Other
- Bone marrow aspirate for culture of *S. typhi* is more sensitive than blood cultures but rarely used as a primary investigation.
- Bone marrow aspiration may be done for evaluation of a fever of unknown origin.

Test Interpretation
Classically, bowel pathology shows mononuclear lymphoid proliferation, especially Peyer patches of the terminal ileum.

TREATMENT

- Treatment of typhoid disease and chronic carrier states must be determined on an individual basis. Factors to consider include age, public health and occupational health risk (e.g., food handler, chronic care facilities, medical personnel), intolerance to antibiotics, and evidence of biliary tract disease.
- Awareness of emerging drug-resistant *S. typhi* strains and the epidemiology of the patient's exposure help direct primary therapy. Knowledge of local resistance patterns for presumptive treatment or laboratory sensitivity also guides therapy. Fluoroquinolone-resistant *S. typhi* is common in Asia.

GENERAL MEASURES
- Fluid and electrolyte support
- Strict isolation of patient's linen, stool, and urine
- Consider serial plain abdominal films for evidence of perforation, usually in the 3rd to 4th week of illness.
- For hemorrhage: blood transfusion and management of shock

MEDICATION

First Line
- Chloramphenicol: pediatric 50 mg/kg/day PO QID for 2 weeks; adult dose 2 to 3 g/day PO divided q6h for 2 weeks *or*
- Ampicillin: pediatric 100 mg/kg/day (max 2 g) QID PO for 2 weeks; adults 500 mg q6h for 2 weeks *or*
- Ciprofloxacin: 500 mg PO BID for 2 weeks, *indicated in multiple-drug-resistant typhoid*
  - Has been used safely in children; WHO recommends as first line in areas with drug resistance to older first-line antibiotics.
  - Fluoroquinolones may prevent clinical relapse better than chloramphenicol (3)[A].
- Ceftriaxone: pediatric 100 mg/kg/day for 2 weeks; adult dose: 1 to 2 g IV once daily for 2 weeks *or*
- Azithromycin: pediatric 10 to 20 mg/kg (max 1 g) PO daily for 5 to 7 days; adult dose: 1 g PO once followed by 500 mg PO daily for 5 to 7 days
- Chronic carrier state
  - Ampicillin: 4 to 5 g/day plus probenecid 2 g/day QID for 6 weeks (for patients with normal gallbladder function and no evidence of cholelithiasis)
  - Ciprofloxacin: 500 mg PO BID for 4 to 6 weeks is also efficacious. Chloramphenicol resistance has been reported in Mexico, South America, Central America, Southeast Asia, India, Pakistan, Middle East, and Africa.
- Contraindications: Refer to manufacturer's profile.
- Precautions: Rarely, Jarisch-Herxheimer reaction appears after antimicrobial therapy.
- Significant possible interactions: Refer to manufacturer's profile for each drug.

Second Line
- Trimethoprim–sulfamethoxazole one double-strength tablet twice a day for 10 days (Note: Drug resistance is common, local resistance patterns and expert consultation should guide treatment.)
- Furazolidone: 7.5 mg/kg/day PO for 10 days; in uncomplicated multidrug-resistant typhoid; safe in children; efficacy >85% cure

Pregnancy Considerations
Ciprofloxacin therapy is relatively contraindicated in children and in pregnant patients.

ISSUES FOR REFERRAL
Complications of sepsis, bowel perforation

SURGERY/OTHER PROCEDURES
- Complications: bowel perforation
- Cholecystectomy may be warranted in carriers with cholelithiasis, relapse after therapy, or intolerance to antimicrobial therapy.

ADMISSION, INPATIENT, AND NURSING CONSIDERATIONS
- Inpatient if acutely ill
- Outpatient for less ill patient or for carrier
- Observe enteric precautions.

 ONGOING CARE

FOLLOW-UP RECOMMENDATIONS
Bed rest initially and then activity as tolerated

Patient Monitoring
See "General Measures."

DIET
NPO if abdominal symptoms are severe. With improvement, begin normal low-residue diet, with high-calorie supplementation if malnourished.

PATIENT EDUCATION
- Discuss chronic carrier state and its complications.
- For family members, travelers, or workers at risk, educate about food/water hygiene and provide vaccination.
- Educate patients that the typhoid vaccines do not protect against *S. paratyphi* infection.
- Typhoid vaccines protect 50–80% of recipients (not 100%). Efficacy wanes over 2 to 4 years.
- CDC patient handout: http://www.cdc.gov/vaccines/hcp/vis/vis-statements/typhoid.html

PROGNOSIS
Overall prognosis is good; with appropriate treatment, <2% mortality rate, 15% relapse rate with some antibiotic treatments, and 3% bowel perforation

COMPLICATIONS
- Intestinal hemorrhage and perforation in distal ileum
- Patients (up to 3%) may become chronic carriers-persistent stool excretor of *S. typhi* for >1 year.
- Seeding of the biliary tract may become a focus for relapse of typhoid fever: most common in females and older patients (>50 years of age)
- Osteomyelitis is more common in patients with sickle cell anemia, systemic lupus erythematosus, and hematologic neoplasms, as well as in immunosuppressed hosts.
- Endovascular infection in the elderly and in patients with a history of bypass operation or aneurysm
- Rarely, endocarditis or meningitis

REFERENCES

1. Jackson BR, Iqbal S, Mahon B; for Centers for Disease Control and Prevention. Updated recommendations for the use of typhoid vaccine—Advisory Committee on Immunization Practices, United States, 2015. *MMWR Morb Mortal Wkly Rep*. 2015;64(11):305–308.
2. Roggelin L, Vinnemeier CD, Fischer-Herr J, et al. Serological response following re-vaccination with Salmonella typhi Vi-capsular polysaccharide vaccines in healthy adult travellers. *Vaccine*. 2015;33(33):4141–4145.
3. Thaver D, Zaidi AK, Critchley J, et al. A comparison of fluoroquinolones versus other antibiotics for treating enteric fever: meta-analysis. *BMJ*. 2009;338:b1865.

ADDITIONAL READING
- Antillón M, Bilcke J, Paltiel AD, et al. Cost-effectiveness analysis of typhoid conjugate vaccines in five endemic low- and middle-income settings. *Vaccine*. 2017;35(27):3506–3514.
- Butler T. Treatment of typhoid fever in the 21st century: promises and shortcomings. *Clin Microbiol Infect*. 2011;17(7):959–963.
- Centers for Disease Control and Prevention. National Center for Emerging and Zoonotic Infectious Diseases. Typhoid fever. http://www.cdc.gov/nczved/divisions/dfbmd/diseases/typhoid_fever/. Accessed October 26, 2017.
- Date KA, Bentsi-Enchill A, Marks F, et al. Typhoid fever vaccination strategies. *Vaccine*. 2015;33(Suppl 3):C55–C61.
- Kaurthe J. Increasing antimicrobial resistance and narrowing therapeutics in typhoidal salmonellae. *J Clin Diagn Res*. 2013;7(3):576–579.
- Newton AE, Routh JA, Mahon BE. Chapter 3. Infectious diseases related to travel. Typhoid and paratyphoid fever. http://wwwnc.cdc.gov/travel/yellowbook/2016/infectious-diseases-related-to-travel/typhoid-paratyphoid-fever. Accessed October 26, 2017.

 CODES

ICD10
- A01.00 Typhoid fever, unspecified
- Z22.0 Carrier of typhoid
- A01.03 Typhoid pneumonia

CLINICAL PEARLS
- Consider typhoid (along with malaria, dengue, and other travel-associated infections) in febrile travelers returning from endemic areas (Latin America, sub-Saharan Africa, South Asia).
- Routine blood cultures detect *S. typhi* but may be negative if antibiotics are administered prior to testing.
- A history or documentation of vaccination against *S. typhi* does not exclude the diagnosis of typhoid fever.

TYPHUS FEVERS

Douglas W. MacPherson, MD, MSc–CTM, FRCPC

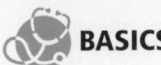 **BASICS**

An infectious disease syndrome caused by several rickettsial bacterial organisms resulting in acute, chronic, and recurrent disease (1)[C]

DESCRIPTION

- Acute infection caused by three species of *Rickettsia*
  - Epidemic typhus: human-to-human transmission by body louse; primarily in setting of refugee camps, war, famine, and disaster. Recurrent disease occurs years after initial infection and can be a source of human outbreak. Flying squirrels are a reservoir.
  - Endemic (murine) typhus: spread to humans by rat flea bite
  - Scrub typhus: infection and infestation of chiggers and of rodents to humans by the chigger; primarily in Asia and western Pacific areas
- System(s) affected: endocrine/metabolic; hematologic/lymphatic/immunologic; pulmonary; skin/exocrine
- Synonym(s): louse-borne typhus; Brill-Zinsser disease; murine typhus

EPIDEMIOLOGY

- Epidemic and endemic typhus: rare in the United States (outside of South Texas)
- Scrub typhus: travelers returning from endemic areas

Incidence

Endemic typhus: <100 cases annually, primarily in states around the Gulf of Mexico, especially South Texas; underreporting suspected

ETIOLOGY AND PATHOPHYSIOLOGY

- Epidemic typhus by *Rickettsia prowazekii*
- Endemic typhus by *Rickettsia typhi* (2)[A]
- Scrub typhus by *Rickettsia tsutsugamushi*

RISK FACTORS

- Vector exposure
- Travel to endemic countries

Geriatric Considerations

Elderly may have more severe disease.

GENERAL PREVENTION

Vector control:

- Scrub typhus: protective clothing and insect repellents
- Endemic typhus: ectoparasite and rodent control
- Epidemic typhus: delousing and cleaning of clothing; vaccine for those at high risk of exposure (typhus vaccine production discontinued in the United States)

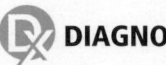 **DIAGNOSIS**

Typhus syndromes are rare in the United States. A high level of clinical suspicion is necessary.

HISTORY

Travel or other risk exposure

- Fever, chills
- Intractable headache
- Myalgias, malaise
- Cough, rash, ocular pain

PHYSICAL EXAM

- General
  - Fever
  - Relative bradycardia (scrub typhus)
- Epidemic typhus
  - Incubation period ~1 week
  - Macular or maculopapular rash beginning on trunk ~5th day of illness
  - Nonproductive cough
  - Pulmonary infiltrates
- Endemic typhus
  - Incubation period 1 to 2 weeks
  - Macular or maculopapular rash beginning on trunk 3rd to 5th day of illness
- Scrub typhus
  - Incubation period 1 to 3 weeks
  - Eschar at bite site
  - Regional lymphadenopathy
  - Generalized lymphadenopathy
  - Splenomegaly
  - Macular or maculopapular rash beginning on trunk approximately 5th day of illness
  - Relative bradycardia early in disease
  - Ocular pain
  - Conjunctival injection

DIFFERENTIAL DIAGNOSIS

- Other rickettsial disease: Rocky Mountain spotted fever; ehrlichiosis; Mediterranean spotted fever (boutonneuse fever) (*Rickettsia conorii*)
- Bacterial meningitis; meningococcemia
- Measles, rubella
- Toxoplasmosis
- Leptospirosis
- Typhoid fever
- Dengue, malaria
- Relapsing fever
- Secondary syphilis
- Viral syndromes: mononucleosis, acute retroviral syndrome

DIAGNOSTIC TESTS & INTERPRETATION

- Specific serologies with rising antibody titer
- If suspected, isolate *Rickettsia* in qualified laboratory to minimize the risk of laboratory-acquired infection.
- CDC Rickettsial Zoonoses Branch 404-639-1075

Initial Tests (lab, imaging)

- CBC often normal
- Weil-Felix serologic reaction may be positive; test hampered by low sensitivity and nonspecificity; epidemic and endemic typhus, 4-fold titer rise or titer >1/320 to OX19; scrub typhus, 4-fold rise in titer to OXK
- Hyponatremia in severe cases
- Hypoalbuminemia in severe cases
- Recent antibiotic exposure may alter lab results.

Test Interpretation

Diffuse vasculitis on skin biopsy

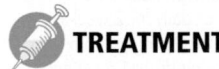 **TREATMENT**

Initiate treatment based on epidemiologic risk and clinical presentation.

GENERAL MEASURES

- Skin and mouth care
- Supportive care—directed at complications

MEDICATION

First Line

- Begin treatment when diagnosis is likely and continue until clinically improved and the patient is afebrile for at least 48 hours; usual course is 5 to 7 days.
- Children ≥8 years of age and adults
  - Doxycycline IV/PO: adults 100 mg q12h, children ≤45 kg: 5 mg/kg/day divided twice daily (max of 200 mg/day); >45 kg: adult dosing
  - Children ≤8 years of age: risk of dental staining from tetracyclines minimal with short courses
  - Tetracycline: 25 mg/kg PO initially and then 25 mg/kg/day in equally divided doses q6h
- Children ≤8 years of age, pregnant women, or if typhoid fever is suspected
  - Chloramphenicol: 50 mg/kg PO initially and then 50 mg/kg/day in equally divided doses q6h
  - If severely ill, chloramphenicol sodium succinate: 20 mg/kg IV initially, infused over 30 to 45 minutes and then 50 mg/kg/day infused in equally divided doses q6h until orally tolerable
  - Azithromycin, fluoroquinolones, and rifampin alternatives depending on scenario
- Precautions and interactions: Refer to the manufacturer's profile for each specific drug.

Second Line

- Doxycycline: single oral dose of 100 or 200 mg PO for those in refugee camps, victims of disasters, or in the presence of limited medical services
- Isolated reports indicate that erythromycin and ciprofloxacin are effective.
- Azithromycin 1,000 mg PO once a day for 3-day course is effective for scrub typhus; better tolerated than doxycycline but more expensive
- Rifampin may be effective in areas where scrub typhus responds poorly to standard antirickettsial drugs.

ISSUES FOR REFERRAL

Infectious disease consultation is recommended. Contact CDC and local public health authorities.

ADMISSION, INPATIENT, AND NURSING CONSIDERATIONS

- Outpatient care unless severely ill
- Severely ill or constitutionally unstable (e.g., shock)

ONGOING CARE

FOLLOW-UP RECOMMENDATIONS

Patient Monitoring

- Admit severely ill patients.
- If treated as an outpatient, ensure regular follow-up to assess clinical improvement and resolution.

DIET

As tolerated

PATIENT EDUCATION

Travel advice (minimize exposure risks, vector avoidance, vaccination as appropriate)

PROGNOSIS

- Recovery is expected with prompt treatment.
- Relapses may follow treatment, especially if initiated within 48 hours of onset (this is *not* an indication to delay treatment). Treat relapses the same as primary disease.
- Without treatment, the mortality rate of typhus is 40–60% for epidemic, 1–2% for endemic, and up to 30% for scrub disease.
- Mortality is higher among the elderly.

COMPLICATIONS

Organ-specific complications (particularly in the 2nd week of illness): azotemia, meningoencephalitis, seizures, delirium, coma, myocardial failure, hyponatremia, hypoalbuminemia, hypovolemia, shock, and death

REFERENCES

1. Centers for Disease Control and Prevention. Rickettsial (spotted & typhus fevers) & related infections, including anaplasmosis & ehrlichiosis. http://wwwnc.cdc.gov/travel/yellowbook/2016/infectious-diseases-related-to-travel/rickettsial-spotted-typhus-fevers-related-infections-anaplasmosis-ehrlichiosis. Accessed October 26, 2017.
2. Afzal Z, Kallumadanda S, Wang F, et al. Acute febrile illness and complications due to murine typhus, Texas, USA1,2. *Emerg Infect Dis*. 2017;23(8):1268–1273.

ADDITIONAL READING

- Botelho-Nevers E, Raoult D. Host, pathogen and treatment-related prognostic factors in rickettsioses. *Eur J Clin Microbiol Infect Dis*. 2011;30(10):1139–1150.
- Chikeka I, Dumler JS. Neglected bacterial zoonoses. *Clin Microbiol Infect*. 2015;21(5):404–415.
- Fang R, Blanton LS, Walker DH. Rickettsiae as emerging infectious agents. *Clin Lab Med*. 2017;37(2):383–400.
- Murray KO, Evert N, Mayes B, et al. Typhus group rickettsiosis, Texas, USA, 2003–2013. *Emerg Infect Dis*. 2017;23(4):645–648.
- Nelson K, Maina AN, Brisco A, et al. A 2015 outbreak of flea-borne rickettsiosis in San Gabriel Valley, Los Angeles County, California. *PLoS Negl Trop Dis*. 2018;12(4):e0006385.
- Panpanich R, Garner P. Antibiotics for treating scrub typhus. *Cochrane Database Syst Rev*. 2002;(3):CD002150.
- Stephenson N, Blaney A, Clifford D, et al. Diversity of rickettsiae in a rural community in northern California. *Ticks Tick Borne Dis*. 2017;8(4):526–531.
- van Eekeren LE, de Vries SG, Wagenaar JFP, et al. Under-diagnosis of rickettsial disease in clinical practice: a systematic review [published online ahead of print March 1, 2018]. *Travel Med Infect Dis*. doi:10.1016/j.tmaid.2018.02.006.

CODES

ICD10

- A75.9 Typhus fever, unspecified
- A75.0 Epidemic louse-borne typhus fever d/t Rickettsia prowazekii
- A75.2 Typhus fever due to Rickettsia typhi

CLINICAL PEARLS

- Consider typhus (along with malaria and dengue) in febrile travelers returning from endemic areas.
- Rickettsial infections typically present within 2 to 14 days. Febrile illnesses presenting >18 days after travel are unlikely to be rickettsial.
- Routine blood cultures do not detect *Rickettsia*.
- Prior vaccination does not exclude typhus.

T

ULCER, APHTHOUS

Cynthia Y. Ohata, MD • Chisalu Tessa Nchekwube, MD, MBA

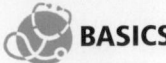 **BASICS**

DESCRIPTION

- Self-limited, painful ulcerations of the nonkeratinized oral mucosa, which are often recurrent (1)
- Synonyms: canker sores; aphthae; aphthous stomatitis
  - Comes from *aphth* meaning "ulcer" in Greek; first used by Hippocrates between 460 and 370 BC to categorize oral disease
- Classification (1)
  - Simple aphthosis
    - Common
    - Episodic
    - Prompt healing, few ulcers
    - 3 to 6 episodes per year
    - Minimal pain, little disability, limited to oral cavity
- Complex aphthous ulcers
  - Uncommon
  - Episodic or continuous
  - Slow healing
  - Few to many ulcers
  - Frequent or continuous ulceration
  - Marked pain
  - Major disability
  - May have genital aphthae (2)
    - Nonsexually acquired genital ulceration (NSGU)
    - Complex aphthous ulcers in genital areas
    - Female > male
    - Painful and associated with swelling of genital area
    - Prodrome flu-like symptoms, possible link to Epstein-Barr virus (EBV)
- Ulcer morphology
  - Minor aphthous ulcers (2)
    - Usually <10 mm in diameter
    - Self-limited, healing within 4 to 14 days
    - Rarely affect the roof of the mouth
    - Nonscarring
  - Major aphthous ulcers (2)
    - Usually >10 mm in diameter
    - Can affect the roof of the mouth
    - May take weeks to months to heal
    - Generally more painful than minor aphthous ulcers
    - May cause scarring
  - Herpetiform ulcers (2)
    - Usually 2 to 3 mm in diameter, may coalesce to form larger ulcerations
    - Unrelated to viral-caused herpetic stomatitis
    - Occur in small clusters numbering 10s to 100s, lasting 1 to 4 weeks
    - Generally more painful than minor aphthous ulcers
    - May cause scarring
    - Categorized as
      - Primary (unknown cause)
      - Secondary (related to other conditions)

EPIDEMIOLOGY

- Most frequent chronic disease of the oral cavity, affecting 5–25% of the population (2)
- More common in patients between 10 and 40 years of age, women, Caucasians, nonsmokers, and those of higher socioeconomic status (2)

- Less frequent with advancing age (1)
- Less frequent in pregnancy (3)
- Increase in occurrence during luteal phase of menstrual cycle (3)
- Minor aphthous ulcers
  - Most common: 70–85% of all aphthae
- Major aphthous ulcers
  - 10–15% of all aphthae
- Herpetiform
  - Least common: 5–10% of all aphthae

Prevalence
Lifetime prevalence of 5–60% (4)

ETIOLOGY AND PATHOPHYSIOLOGY
Likely multifactorial; association with stress-induced rise in salivary cortisol, multiple HLA antigens, cell-mediated immunity; exact etiology unknown (1)

RISK FACTORS

- Genetic factors: 40% of patients with recurrent aphthous stomatitis (RAS) have a family history; most genetic associations with HLA antigen subtypes (1)
- Local trauma: sharp teeth, dental treatments, or mucosal injury secondary to toothbrushing
- Sodium lauryl sulfate–containing toothpaste
- Increased stress and anxiety
- Nutritional deficiencies: iron, zinc, vitamin B complex, and folate (5)[B]
- Homocysteinemia (5)[B]
- Immunodeficiency
- Recent cessation of tobacco use
- Food sensitivity: to benzoic acid/cinnamaldehyde
- Medications
  - NSAIDs
  - β-Blockers
  - Alendronate
  - Methotrexate
  - ACE inhibitors (1)
- Neutropenia
- Anemia
- Endocrine alterations (i.e., menstrual cycle) (2)
- *Helicobacter pylori* infection
- EBV (1)

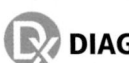 **DIAGNOSIS**

Diagnosis is made by history and clinical presentation. Lab work is rarely (2)[A].

HISTORY

- May experience prodrome of burning sensation of oral mucosa 2 to 48 hours prior to appearance of ulcers
- Patients typically complain of oral ulcerations, which are painful and exacerbated by movement of the mouth. Exacerbation may also be reported with certain foods (hot, spicy, acidic, or carbonated foods or drinks) (2).
- Ask about ulcerative lesions of other anatomic areas, family history, or prior history of aphthous ulcers (2).

PHYSICAL EXAM

- Round or ovoid ulcerations generally <10 mm in size; covered with a grayish-white pseudomembrane surrounded by an erythematous halo (4)
- Ulcers are typically found in the buccal or lip mucosa, ventral tongue, soft palate, or oral vestibule; rarely on the roof of the mouth or lips
- Evaluate for signs of secondary infection: elevated temperature, increased surrounding edema, or pus drainage.

DIFFERENTIAL DIAGNOSIS

- Oral trauma
  - Biting
  - Dentures
- Infection
  - Herpes virus (herpetic stomatitis): vesicular lesions on keratinized tissue (dorsal tongue, vermillion border); generally not present on mucosa (6)[C]
  - HIV: Ulcerations have lengthened healing time and tend to be more painful (6)[C].
- Mucocutaneous disease; especially if chronic or nonhealing
  - Lichen planus
  - Pemphigus
- Malignancy: Investigate and closely monitor non-healing lesions, especially those with leukoplakia or ipsilateral cervical lymphadenopathy.
- Important to evaluate for underlying systemic disease, causing aphthous-like ulcerations
  - Particularly in adults with their first episode or lesions elsewhere (2)[A]
  - Behçet syndrome: autoimmune systemic vasculitis usually involving mucous membranes
    - Genital and oral ulceration
    - Uveitis
  - Reiter syndrome: reactive arthritis, preceded by infection, usually of the genital tract (2)[A]
    - Uveitis
    - Urethritis
    - HLA-B27–associated arthritis
  - Sweet syndrome: acute neutrophilic dermatitis (6)[C]
    - Fever, sudden onset
    - Erythematous skin plaques/papules, well demarcated
    - Leukocytosis
    - 50% of patients have an associated malignancy.
    - Most often in middle-aged females
  - Inflammatory bowel disease (IBD): Crohn disease, ulcerative colitis
    - 20–50% of patients with Crohn disease experience recurrent oral ulcers (6)[A].
    - Bloody or persistent diarrhea
    - Weight loss
  - PFAPA syndrome (1)[C]
    - Periodic fevers, aphthous ulcers, pharyngitis, and adenitis
    - Tonsillectomy may be curative.
  - Cyclic neutropenia (1)[C]
    - Recurrent fevers associated with infections, occasionally occurring intraorally
    - Begins in childhood

– Systemic lupus erythematosus (SLE): autoimmune vascular collagen disease
  ○ Oral lesions have great variability, including recurrent ulceration.
– Gluten-sensitive enteropathy (celiac disease)
  ○ Weight loss and signs of malabsorption
  ○ Bloating and diarrhea

DIAGNOSTIC TESTS & INTERPRETATION
May consider complete blood count; zinc; folic acid; ferritin; vitamins B_1, B_2, B_6, and B_{12} to evaluate for systemic causes in severe or recurrent cases (1)[A]

Follow-Up Tests & Special Considerations
- HIV is associated with increased amount of ulcers and increased healing time.
- Biopsy and viral cultures for nonhealing ulcers or atypical presentations
- Rheumatologic serology if underlying systemic disease is suspected

TREATMENT

GENERAL MEASURES
Management is symptomatic. Goal is to reduce inflammation and relieve pain.

MEDICATION
In general, the goals of treatment depend on the extent of ulceration and frequency of outbreaks.

First Line
- Topical corticosteroids (to improve healing time and symptoms) (2)[A]
  – Adverse effects: may increase risk of oral candidiasis (more likely with higher potency formulations)
  – Topical steroid preparations
    ○ Triamcinolone 0.1% dental paste
      ■ Apply sparingly to ulcers 3 times daily for up to 2 weeks or until ulcer resolution.
    ○ Fluocinonide 0.05% gel or ointment
      ■ Apply sparingly to ulcer 4 times daily for up to 2 weeks or until ulcer resolution.
    ○ Dexamethasone 5 mg/5 mL elixir
      ■ Rinse for 3 minutes and spit 4 times daily until ulcer resolution.
- Topical anesthetics (to reduce symptoms only) (2)[A]
  – Adverse effects: may cause initial stinging
  – Preparations
    ○ Lidocaine 2% gel
      ■ Apply 4 times daily or prior to eating as needed for pain for up to 2 weeks or until ulcer resolution.
- Antimicrobial mouth rinses (improve healing time, decrease pain, and may prevent recurrence) (2)
  – Preparations
    ○ Chlorhexidine aqueous mouthwash 0.12% or 0.2%
      ■ Use 4 times daily for up to several months.
      ■ May cause superficial tooth staining

- Topical immunomodulators (improves healing time, reduces symptoms, and prevents recurrence when used in prodromal phase) (2)[A]
  – Adverse effects: may cause stinging sensation
  – Preparation
    ○ Amlexanox 5% oral paste
      ■ Apply to ulcers 4 times daily for up to 2 weeks or until ulcer resolution.

Second Line
- Systemic corticosteroids—rescue therapy in acute, severe, recurrent outbreaks (2,4)[A]
  – Prednisone 0.75 mg/kg/day, tapered by 0.25 mg/kg/day every 2 weeks (1)[A]
- Colchicine, pentoxifylline, thalidomide, and dapsone have been used with variable success but should be used with caution due to side effects (2,4)[A].
- Antibiotics—penicillin G potassium, 50 mg 4 times daily for 4 days (2)[B]

ISSUES FOR REFERRAL
Otolaryngology or dental referral if lesions have not resolved as expected

ADDITIONAL THERAPIES
- Vitamin B_{12} supplementation appeared to decrease burden of outbreaks and recurrence, independent of preexisting deficiency in one small study. Multivitamins have not been shown to be effective (1)[B].
- H. pylori eradication has been associated with lower number of aphthous lesions (1)[B].

SURGERY/OTHER PROCEDURES
Chemical cautery with silver nitrate (reduces ulcer pain but not healing time) (1). Ozone application is an emerging therapy that decreases pain and improves healing time in small studies.

COMPLEMENTARY & ALTERNATIVE MEDICINE
- Some small cohort studies show clinical improvement with minimal side effects of several herbal and alternative treatments (4)[A].
- Glycyrrhiza (licorice)
- Myrtus communis (myrtle)
- Bee propolis (4)[A]

ONGOING CARE

FOLLOW-UP RECOMMENDATIONS
Evaluation for infection, mucocutaneous or systemic disease, or malignancy should be pursued for nonhealing lesions or lesions with lymphadenopathy or unusual presentation.

Patient Monitoring
Aphthous ulcers are often recurrent, so patients should be monitored for recurrence.

DIET
Deficiencies of iron, vitamin B_{12}, and folic acid are significantly associated with recurrent aphthous ulcers (5).

PATIENT EDUCATION
- Avoid potentially irritating food or drink:
  – Spicy, acidic, hot
  – Carbonated beverages
  – Abrasive/hard foods (i.e., chips, nuts, etc.)
- Behavior modification to reduce dental trauma with toothbrush or bruxism

PROGNOSIS
Varies from single or infrequent recurrences of few, mild, self-resolving lesions to chronic, large, or deep painful lesions. Complex cases can cause significant discomfort and dysfunction. Symptoms improve with age.

COMPLICATIONS
Aphthous ulcers can provide a site for infection and can leave scars (2).

REFERENCES
1. Cui RZ, Bruce AJ, Rogers RS III. Recurrent aphthous stomatitis. Clin Dermatol. 2016;34(4):475–481.
2. Belenguer-Guallar I, Jiménez-Soriano Y, Claramunt-Lozano A. Treatment of recurrent aphthous stomatitis. A literature review. J Clin Exp Dent. 2014;6(2):e168–e174.
3. Annan B, Nuamah K. Oral pathologies seen in pregnant and non-pregnant women. Ghana Med J. 2005;39(1):24–27.
4. Brocklehurst P, Tickle M, Glenny AM, et al. Systemic interventions for recurrent aphthous stomatitis (mouth ulcers). Cochrane Database Syst Rev. 2012;(9):CD005411.
5. Sun A, Chen HM, Cheng SJ, et al. Significant association of deficiencies of hemoglobin, iron, vitamin B12, and folic acid and high homocysteine level with recurrent aphthous stomatitis. J Oral Pathol Med. 2015;44(4):300–305.
6. Katsanos KH, Torres J, Roda G, et al. Review article: non-malignant oral manifestations in inflammatory bowel diseases. Aliment Pharmacol Ther. 2015;42(1):40–60.

ADDITIONAL READING
- Lalla RV, Choquette LE, Feinn RS, et al. Multivitamin therapy for recurrent aphthous stomatitis: a randomized, double-masked, placebo-controlled trial. J Am Dent Assoc. 2012;143(4):370–376.
- Liu C, Zhou Z, Liu G, et al. Efficacy and safety of dexamethasone ointment on recurrent aphthous ulceration. Am J Med. 2012;125(3):292–301.

CODES

ICD10
K12.0 Recurrent oral aphthae

CLINICAL PEARLS
- Aphthous ulcers are the most common chronic disease of the oral cavity.
- Most cases are mild, self-limited episodes.
- Appropriate treatment should be aimed at symptom control and promotion of healing.
- Nonhealing ulcers, extraoral involvement, and sudden onset in adulthood require additional workup.

ULCERATIVE COLITIS

George Clement, MD • Elise Leisinger, DO

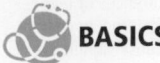 **BASICS**

DESCRIPTION
- Chronic relapsing and remitting inflammatory disease of the bowel causing recurrent episodes of diarrhea that is often bloody and accompanied by abdominal pain, incontinence, fever, and weight loss
- Marked by inflammatory colonic mucosal changes
- Colonic involvement is universal but may be accompanied by large joint arthritis, ocular inflammation, skin lesions, biliary disease, liver disease, thromboembolic disease, and (rarely) pulmonary complications.

EPIDEMIOLOGY
Incidence
- North America: 19.2/100,000 person-years (1)
- Europe: 24.3/100,000 person-years (1)
- Asia/Middle East: 6.3/100,000 person-years (1)

Prevalence
- North America: 249/100,000 persons (1)
- Europe: 505/100,000 persons (1)

Pregnancy Considerations
- Increased risk of preterm delivery and small for gestational age birth
- 30% with inactive disease relapse in pregnancy
- Management with gastroenterologist and/or maternal–fetal medicine specialist/obstetrician is recommended.

ETIOLOGY AND PATHOPHYSIOLOGY
- Idiopathic; hypothesized association with autoimmune dysfunction, genetic predisposition, diet, and colonic microbiome
- Almost universally involves terminal colon, >95% of patients have rectal involvement, 50% have disease limited to rectum and sigmoid; 20% have pancolitis.

Genetics
Moderate heritability. Specific genetic markers have not been identified.

RISK FACTORS
- Age: variable, peak incidence among ages 15 to 40 years
- First-degree relative with ulcerative colitis (UC)
- Theorized risk factors include disruption of colonic microbiome by diet or infection, dietary factors (Western diet in particular), antibiotic use, lack of breastfeeding in infant, obesity, and NSAID use.

GENERAL PREVENTION
No known preventive measures

Pediatric Considerations
- Breastfeeding may protect against pediatric inflammatory bowel disease (IBD).
- UC more likely pancolonic at onset and shorter time from diagnosis to colectomy (median 11 years)

COMMONLY ASSOCIATED CONDITIONS
- Arthritis: large joint, sacroiliitis, ankylosing spondylitis
- Pyoderma gangrenosum (rare)
- Erythema nodosum (common)
- Aphthous ulcers
- Episcleritis and uveitis (rare)
- Autoimmune liver disease (rare)
- Fatty liver (common)
- Liver cirrhosis (rare)
- Primary sclerosing cholangitis (rare)
- Bile duct carcinoma (rare)
- Thromboembolic disease (rare)
- Colon cancer (rare)
- Anemia (rare)
- Pulmonary diseases (very rare)

 DIAGNOSIS

HISTORY
- Frequent diarrhea, may be bloody or include mucus
- Frequent, small bowel movements, associated with tenesmus, colicky abdominal pain, urgency, and fecal incontinence
- Onset is gradual and progressive over weeks.
- Episodes are sometimes accompanied by fever, weight loss, fatigue, and anemia.
- Predominant age of onset: 15 to 40 years; smaller peak in ages 50 to 80 years

PHYSICAL EXAM
- Often normal
- Abdominal tenderness
- Presence of blood on rectal exam
- In severe disease: fever, hypotension, tachycardia, pallor, loss of subcutaneous fat, muscle atrophy, peripheral edema

DIFFERENTIAL DIAGNOSIS
- Crohn disease
- Infectious colitis: bacterial, parasitic, or viral (cytomegalovirus [CMV])
- Diverticular colitis
- Diversion colitis in patients with prior bowel surgery
- Medication-induced colitis
- Radiation colitis
- Graft versus host disease
- Celiac disease

DIAGNOSTIC TESTS & INTERPRETATION
- Clinical presentation and studies are used to determine severity (2).
- Mild: <4 stools daily with or without blood, no systemic symptoms, normal ESR (2)
- Moderate: >4 stools daily, no or minimal systemic symptoms (2)
- Severe: >6 blood stools daily, evidence of systemic illness with fever, tachycardia, anemia, or high ESR (2)
- Fulminant: usually >10 stools daily, continuous bleeding, signs of systemic illness as in "severe," abdominal tenderness, blood transfusion requirement, colonic dilation on abdominal x-rays (2)

Initial Tests (lab, imaging)
- CBC: Leukocytosis and anemia support diagnosis.
- BMP: urea and electrolyte abnormalities; hypokalemia supports diagnosis.
- LFTs: liver function abnormalities; low albumin indicates severe disease.
- ESR or CRP elevation supports diagnosis and can help define severity.
- Ferritin and transferrin if anemic to determine iron deficiency versus chronic disease
- Vitamin B_{12} and folate levels
- Fecal calprotectin: indicates colonic inflammation (3)
- Stool studies to rule out infectious cause: *Clostridium difficile* toxin (four samples), stool cultures, Shiga toxin, ova and parasite microscopy, *Giardia* antigen
- STI testing to rule out proctitis, particularly in MSM: chlamydia, gonorrhea, HSV, syphilis (3)
- Perinuclear antineutrophil cytoplasmic antibody (pANCA) and anti-Saccharomyces cerevisiae antibodies (ASCA) are commonly present in patients with UC, but testing for these is not currently recommended for diagnosis (3).
- Abdominal x-ray to exclude dangerous colonic dilation and assess disease severity (3)

Diagnostic Procedures/Other
- Colonoscopy with at least two biopsies from each of five sites along the entire colon is an initial diagnostic step to confirm colitis (3).
- Complete colonoscopy in severe UC may be contraindicated due to risk of perforation or precipitation of toxic megacolon (3).

Test Interpretation
- Endoscopic findings that support UC include mucosal engorgement with vascular markings, mucosal erythema, and mucosal granularity. Affected areas will extend proximally and continuously.
- Histologic findings that support UC include mucosal separation, distortion, and atrophy of the crypts; chronic inflammatory cells in lamina propria; lymphocytes and plasma cells in crypt bases (2)[C].
- If only rectal biopsy, villous mucosal architecture and Paneth cells metaplasia support UC (2)[C].
- Mild ileal inflammation ("backwash ileitis") may be present in UC (2)[C].

 TREATMENT

Treatment strategies are determined by functional status, degree of colonic involvement, course of illness, frequency of relapses, extraintestinal manifestations, response to prior treatments, and side effect profile.

MEDICATION
First Line
- Proctitis/distal colitis with mild or moderate severity: 5-ASA (e.g., mesalamine 1 g/day) suppository; 5-ASA foam enemas are an alternative but less effective (4)[C].
- Left-sided UC with mild to moderate severity: topical 5-ASA (e.g., mesalamine 1 g/day) PLUS >2 g/day oral mesalamine (4)[C]
- Left-sided severe UC: hospital admission and systemic steroids (e.g., prednisone 40 to 60 mg/day) in addition to mesalamine/5-ASA (4)[C]

- Extensive UC of mild to moderate severity: oral sulfasalazine titrated up to 4 to 6 g/day OR a combination of topical and oral 5-ASA (above) (4)[C]
- Severe UC: necessitates hospitalization for intensive treatment and surveillance for complications; IV steroids (methylprednisolone 60 mg/day or hydrocortisone 400 mg/day) with or without 2 to 6 g/day oral mesalamine (4)[C]

Second Line
- Proctitis/distal colitis with mild to moderate severity: first-line therapy PLUS 2 to 6 g/day oral mesalamine. Topical corticosteroids (budesonide 2 to 8 mg/day or hydrocortisone 100 mg/day) may be added (4)[C].
- Left-sided UC with mild to moderate severity: first-line therapy PLUS topical corticosteroids (budesonide 2 to 8 mg/day or hydrocortisone 100 mg/day) may be added. Persistent rectal bleeding despite this regimen can be treated with systemic prednisone at 40 to 60 g/day with a prolonged taper (4)[C].
- Left-sided severe UC: first-line therapy PLUS prednisone at 40 to 60 g/day and long taper; if refractory, azathioprine 2.5 mg/kg/day OR 6-mercaptopurine (1.5 mg/kg/day) for induction and maintenance (4)[C]
- Severe UC: TNF-α-blocker IFX (adalimumab, infliximab, golimumab) combined with methotrexate or thiopurine. Patients with severe UC will often need timely colectomy (4)[C].
- Infliximab adult dose: 5 mg/kg IV at weeks 0, 2, and 6 for induction and then maintenance of 5 mg/kg IV is given every 8 weeks.
- Adalimumab: dose: 160 mg SC (given as four injections on day 1 or two injections daily over 2 consecutive days; limit injections to 40 mg per injection); second dose 2 weeks later: 80 mg; and maintenance: 40 mg every other week (5)[C]
- Other second-line therapies, particularly in refractory disease, include CsA 4 mg/kg/day and tacrolimus 0.1 to 0.2 mg/kg/day PO or 0.01 to 0.02 mg/kg/day IV. Trough concentrations with tacrolimus should be 10 to 15 ng/mL.
- TNF-α-blockers can help maintain remission in steroid-dependent patients with severe UC.
- Immunosuppressive therapy increases risk of opportunistic infections. Chronic steroid use can cause adrenal suppression, gastrointestinal bleeding, heart disease, osteoporosis, thinning of skin, and compromised vascular wall integrity. Infusion of biologics carries the risk of anaphylactic reactions during treatment.

Pediatric Considerations
Pediatric growth and development can be affected due to malabsorption.

SURGERY/OTHER PROCEDURES
- Surgery is indicated for medically refractory disease (particularly with high-dose steroids).
- Emergent surgery (typically total or subtotal abdominal colectomy with end ileostomy) for massive hemorrhage, perforation, and toxic dilatation
- Total colectomy with ileostomy is *curative*.
- Total proctocolectomy with ileal pouch anal anastomosis (IPAA) is the most common surgery and an appropriate alternative to ileostomy. Common complications include pouchitis (50%) and need for reoperation in up to 30% (2)[C].

COMPLEMENTARY & ALTERNATIVE MEDICINE
- There is ongoing research into the role of probiotics, dietary changes, and fecal microbiota transplant as treatment for UC. The current evidence is insufficient to support the efficacy of any particular alternative therapy for achieving or maintaining remission.
- Tobacco cessation is associated with 65% reduction in relapse (3)[C].

ADMISSION, INPATIENT, AND NURSING CONSIDERATIONS
- Admission for UC or its complications warrants gastroenterology consultation.
- Severe UC may require emergent surgical intervention. Consultation with surgery is indicated.
- Imaging studies help assess disease activity and colon size.
- Initiate IV corticosteroids and rule out infectious etiologies (*C. difficile*, CMV, *Shigella/Amoeba*).

 ## ONGOING CARE

FOLLOW-UP RECOMMENDATIONS
Patient Monitoring
- Regular surveillance colonoscopy in patients with prolonged (8 to 10 years) active disease (2)
- Initiate annual surveillance immediately in patients with primary sclerosing cholangitis.
- Annual LFTs and cholangiography for cholestasis
- Annual BUN/creatinine for patients on long-term mesalamine

Pediatric Considerations
Cumulative risk of cancer increases with duration of disease. Ensure regular surveillance.

DIET
- NPO during acute exacerbations
- There are otherwise no specific dietary recommendations. Dietary research is ongoing.

PATIENT EDUCATION
Crohn and Colitis Foundation of America (CCFA): http://www.ccfa.org/

PROGNOSIS
- Chronic disease with variable severity and rate of recurrence
- Variable; mortality for initial attack is ~5%; 75–85% experience relapse; up to 20% require colectomy.
- Colon cancer risk is the single most important factor affecting long-term prognosis.
- Left-sided colitis and ulcerative proctitis have favorable prognoses with probable normal lifespan.

Geriatric Considerations
- Increased mortality if first presentation occurs after 60 years of age
- Consider lower medication dosages and slower titration due to risks of polypharmacy.

COMPLICATIONS
- Perforation: Treat toxic megacolon with prompt surgery. Limit colonoscopies in severe disease.
- Obstruction
- Anemia

- Fulminant colitis
- Toxic megacolon
- Liver disease
- Stricture formation
- Osteoporosis
- Colorectal cancer

REFERENCES

1. Molodecky NA, Soon IS, Rabi DM, et al. Increasing incidence and prevalence of the inflammatory bowel diseases with time, based on systematic review. *Gastroenterology*. 2012;142(1):46. e42–54.e42.
2. Kornbluth A, Sachar DB; and Practice Parameters Committee of the American College of Gastroenterology. Ulcerative colitis practice guidelines in adults: American College of Gastroenterology, Practice Parameters Committee. *Am J Gastroenterol*. 2010;105(3):501–523.
3. Mowat C, Cole A, Windsor A, et al; for IBD Section of the British Society of Gastroenterology. Guidelines for the management of inflammatory bowel disease in adults. *Gut*. 2011;60(5):571–607.
4. Meier J, Sturm A. Current treatment of ulcerative colitis. *World J Gastroenterol*. 2011;17(27):3204–3212.
5. Bressler B, Marshall JK, Bernstein CN, et al; for Toronto Ulcerative Colitis Consensus Group. Clinical practice guidelines for the medical management of nonhospitalized ulcerative colitis: the Toronto consensus. *Gastroenterology*. 2015;148(5):1035.e3–1058.e3.

ADDITIONAL READING

LeBlanc K, Mosli MH, Parker CE, et al. The impact of biological interventions for ulcerative colitis on health-related quality of life. *Cochrane Database Syst Rev*. 2015;22(9):CD008655.

 ### SEE ALSO

Algorithm: Hematemesis (Bleeding, Upper Gastrointestinal)

 ### CODES

ICD10
- K51.90 Ulcerative colitis, unspecified, without complications
- K51.919 Ulcerative colitis, unspecified with unspecified complications
- K51.80 Other ulcerative colitis without complications

CLINICAL PEARLS
- Diffuse, uninterrupted colonic mucosal inflammation
- Hallmark symptom is bloody diarrhea.
- Annual or biannual surveillance colonoscopy after 8 to 10 years of colitis due to increased risk of colorectal cancer

URETHRITIS

Danielle Taylor, DO • Cynthia D. Hall, MD

 BASICS

DESCRIPTION
- Inflammation of the urethra
- Common manifestation of sexually transmitted infection (STI)
- Frequently associated with dysuria, pruritus, and/or urethral discharge; classified as gonococcal (caused by *Neisseria gonorrhoeae*) and nongonococcal (caused by other bacteria, or less commonly autoimmune disorders [Reiter syndrome], trauma, or chemical irritation)

EPIDEMIOLOGY
Incidence
- In 2016, there were 468,514 reported cases of gonorrhea, with a rate of 146 cases per 100,000 per population (18.5% rate increase since 2015) (1).
- In 2016, there were 1,598,354 reported cases of *Chlamydia trachomatis* infection or 497 cases per 100,000 per population (17.6% rate increase since 2015) (1).
- Chlamydia is the most commonly reported STD (1).
- Rate of chlamydial infection in U.S. women was more than twice that of men, reflecting higher rates of screening (1).
- Highest incidences of gonorrhea and chlamydia among young men and women, ages 15 to 24 years (>50% of all cases) (1)
- Chlamydial infections are 5 times more likely in young adult women than gonococcal infections (1).

ETIOLOGY AND PATHOPHYSIOLOGY
- Most common cause is infection via sexual transmission of *N. gonorrhoeae*, a gram-negative diplococcus.
- *N. gonorrhoeae* is a gram-negative diplococcus which interacts with nonciliated epithelial cells → cellular invasion → inflammation, neutrophil production, bacterial cell phagocytosis (2).
- Sexually transmitted *C. trachomatis* infection is the most common cause of nongonococcal urethritis.
- Other established pathogens:
  - *Mycoplasma genitalium*
  - *Trichomonas vaginalis*
  - *Ureaplasma urealyticum*
  - Herpes simplex virus (rare)
  - Adenovirus (rare)
- Noninfectious causes (less common)
  - Chemical irritants (i.e., soaps, shampoos, douches, spermicides)
  - Foreign bodies
  - Urethral instrumentation

RISK FACTORS
- Age 15 to 24 years
- New sex partner
- One or more sex partner(s)
- History of or coexisting STI
- Sex partner with concurrent partner(s)
- Inconsistent condom use outside of a mutually monogamous relationship
- Exchanging sex for money or drugs
- Member of population with increased prevalence of infection, including incarcerated populations, military recruits, and economically disadvantaged populations

GENERAL PREVENTION
- Use of male condoms, female condoms, or cervical diaphragms
- Abstinence or reduction in the number of sex partners
- Behavioral counseling

COMMONLY ASSOCIATED CONDITIONS

> **ALERT**
> Annual chlamydia and gonorrhea screening is recommended for all sexually active women <25 years, women >25 years with risk factors, and all men who have sex with men. There is insufficient evidence to recommend testing all men <25 year (3)[A].

 DIAGNOSIS

- Chief complaint
  - Urethral discharge (mucopurulent suggestive of *N. gonorrhoeae*)
  - Dysuria
  - Erythema of the urethral meatus
  - Symptom onset 2 to 8 days following exposure
- History
  - Sexual history, including condom use, number of partners, sexual behaviors
  - Previous STIs
  - Substance abuse
  - Recent travel
  - Symptoms indicative of complications or additional sites of infection (i.e., men: testicular pain and swelling, anal itching, rectal pain or bleeding; women: lower abdominal pain, dyspareunia, irregular vaginal bleeding)
- Male GU exam (possible findings)
  - Urethral discharge
  - Meatal erythema
  - Testicular tenderness
  - Palpate scrotum to check for epididymitis or orchitis.
  - Assess for ulcers.
  - Assess for inguinal lymphadenopathy.
- Female genitourinary (GU) exam (possible findings)
  - Vaginal discharge
  - Endocervical discharge, hyperemia, and/or friability

Pediatric Considerations
Pediatric infections with gonorrhea and chlamydia after the neonatal period strongly suggest sexual contact. If indicated, investigations should be initiated promptly (4).

DIFFERENTIAL DIAGNOSIS
- Other GU tract diseases
  - Cystitis/urinary tract infection
  - Epididymitis
  - Prostatitis
  - PID
  - Pyelonephritis
- Vaginal atrophy, especially in postmenopausal women
- Stevens-Johnson syndrome
- Reiter syndrome: uveitis, urethritis, arthritis
- Wegener granulomatosis
- Urethral syndrome (pain without infection or purulence), longstanding or intermittent symptoms

DIAGNOSTIC TESTS & INTERPRETATION

> **ALERT**
> Health care providers are required to report all gonorrhea and chlamydia infections in accordance with local and state requirements.

Initial Tests (lab, imaging)
- Gonorrhea
  - Nucleic acid amplification test (NAAT)
  - Sensitivity: 90–100%
  - Specificity: 97–100%
  - Preferred specimen collection in first void (men) and vaginal swab (women)
  - Tissue culture was the traditional gold standard but typically only used now in cases of suspected treatment resistance (4).
- Chlamydia
  - NAAT
  - Sensitivity: 85–95%
  - Specificity: 93–99%
  - Preferred specimen collection is same as for gonorrhea.
  - Tissue culture was the traditional gold standard but currently NOT recommended (4).
- Gram stain diagnosis criteria
  - Urethral secretions with ≥2 WBC per oil immersion
  - Mucopurulent or purulent discharge
  - First void urine sediment with ≥10 WBC per high power field (4)
  - Symptom onset 2 to 8 days following exposure
- Methylene blue/gentian violet [MB/GV]
  - Alternative to gram staining
  - Does not require heat fixation
  - Sensitivity: 97.3% (same as gram stain)
- If concern for *Trichomonas*: NAAT (urine, urethral, vaginal, or endocervical swab), wet mount, or culture
- There is no FDA-approved diagnostic test available for *M. genitalium*, an emerging pathogen with a greater prevalence than gonorrhea in many populations (5).

> **ALERT**
> Due to the similarity in clinical symptoms and high rates of coinfection, cotesting for gonorrhea and chlamydia infection is recommended. In addition, given that risk factors for gonorrhea and chlamydia indicate risks for other STIs, screening for HIV, RPR, hepatitis C, and hepatitis B may also be indicated.

Follow-Up Tests & Special Considerations
- Test of cure (TOC) for chlamydia and gonorrhea is recommended in pregnant women or when treatment noncompliance is suspected (4).
- Repeat testing in 3 months recommended due to rates of reinfection (4)
- HIV infection: Persons with HIV infection should receive the same treatment as patients without HIV infection (4).

Diagnostic Procedures/Other
Urethrocystoscopy for cases with suspected foreign body, intraurethral warts, urethral stricture

Test Interpretation
Urethral strictures (untreated gonorrhea), intraurethral lesions (venereal warts, congenital anomalies), PID, or tubo-ovarian abscesses are possible.

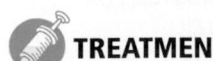 **TREATMENT**

- Most cases can be treated in the outpatient setting.
- Single-dose regimens with direct observation preferred (4)

MEDICATION

CDC recommendations

- Chlamydia
  - First line
    - Azithromycin 1 g PO × 1 dose
      OR
    - Doxycycline 100 mg PO BID for 7 days (3)[A]
    - Alternate regimens (all for 7 days)
      - Erythromycin base 500 mg PO QID
      - Erythromycin ethylsuccinate 800 mg PO QID
      - Levofloxacin 500 mg daily
      - Ofloxacin 300 mg PO BID
  - Second line (all for a duration of 7 days)
    - Erythromycin base 500 mg PO QID
    - Erythromycin ethylsuccinated 800 mg PO QID
    - Levofloxacin 500 mg daily
    - Ofloxacin 300 mg PO BID
- Gonorrhea
  - First line
    - Ceftriaxone 250 mg IM plus either
    - Azithromycin 1 g PO × 1 dose (preferred)
      OR
    - Doxycycline 100 mg PO BID × 7 days (6)[C]
    - For children ≤45 kg
      - Ceftriaxone 25 to 50 mg/kg IM × 1 dose
    - For children >45 kg, use adult dosing.
  - Second line
    - Cefixime 400 mg IM plus either
    - Azithromycin 1 g PO × 1 dose (preferred)
      OR
    - Doxycycline 100 mg PO BID × 7 days
    - TOC in 1 week
- Trichomonas
  - Metronidazole 2 g PO × 1 dose
- Recurrent and persistent urethritis
  - If azithromycin was initially used, moxifloxacin 400 mg PO QD × 7 days
  - If doxycycline was initially used, azithromycin 1 g PO × 1 dose
- General considerations
  - Contraindications: sensitivity to any of the indicated medications
  - Precautions: Patients taking tetracyclines may have increased photosensitivity.
  - Significant possible interactions
    - Tetracyclines should not be taken with milk products or antacids.
    - Oral contraceptives may be rendered less effective by oral antibiotics. Patients and partners should use a back-up method of birth control for the remainder of the cycle.
      - QID × 7 days (1)

Pregnancy Considerations

- Chlamydia:
  - Screen all pregnant patients.
  - All pregnant women at increased risk should be screened for chlamydia at their prenatal visit and again in the 3rd trimester.
  - TOC 3 weeks after therapy to check for chlamydial eradication and retest in 3 months
  - Azithromycin 1 g PO × 1 dose (3)[A]
  - Alternative regimens:
    - Amoxicillin 500 mg TID × 7 days
      OR
    - Erythromycin 500 mg QID × 7 days (3)[A]
- Gonorrhea:
  - Screen all pregnant patients.
  - All pregnant women at increased risk should be screened for chlamydia at their prenatal visit and again in the 3rd trimester.
  - TOC 3 weeks after therapy to check for gonococcal eradication and retest in 3 months

---

- Tetracyclines and quinolones are contraindicated.
- Dual therapy treatment
  - Ceftriaxone 250 mg IM × 1 dose
  - Azithromycin 1 g PO × 1 dose
- If cephalosporin allergy and spectinomycin is not available, infectious disease consult is recommended.

 ONGOING CARE

FOLLOW-UP RECOMMENDATIONS

- Sexual activity should be avoided for 7 days following administration of single-dose therapy or until completion of multiday regimen.
- All sexual partners who came in contact with the patient within 60 days should be referred for evaluation, testing, and presumptive treatment (4).
- Expedited partner therapy (EPT) is an acceptable alternative; EPT—the practice of treating the diagnosed patient's sex partner(s) for chlamydia or gonorrhea by providing medications to the partner(s) without clinical evaluation (4)

Patient Monitoring

- Instruct patients to return if symptoms persist or recur after completing treatment.
- Screen for reinfection in all patients at 3 months.

PATIENT EDUCATION

- Behavioral counseling interventions are recommended. Evidence of benefit increase with intensity of intervention (6,7)[B].
- Successful approaches include basic information about STIs and transmission, assess risk for transmission, include training skills (i.e., condom use, communication about safe sex, problem solving, goal setting) (7).

PROGNOSIS

If the diagnosis is firmly established, appropriate medications are prescribed and the patient is compliant with treatment; relief of symptoms occurs within days, and the problem will resolve without sequela.

COMPLICATIONS

- Stricture formation
- Epididymitis
- Prostatitis
- PID in women
- Disseminated gonococcal infection
- Gonococcal meningitis
- Gonococcal endocarditis
- Perinatal transmission (chlamydial conjunctivitis, chlamydial pneumonia, ophthalmia neonatorum)
- Reiter syndrome
- Chronic cervical chlamydial infection has been proposed to increase risk of cervical cancer (8).

REFERENCES

1. Centers for Disease Control and Prevention. *Sexually Transmitted Disease Surveillance, 2015*. Atlanta, GA: U.S. Department of Health and Human Services; 2018.
2. LeFevre ML; for U.S. Preventive Services Task Force. Screening for chlamydia and gonorrhea: U.S. Preventive Services Task Force recommendation statement. *Ann Intern Med*. 2014;161(12):902–910.
3. Mishori R, McClaskey EL, WinklerPrins VJ. *Chlamydia trachomatis* infections: screening, diagnosis, and management. *Am Fam Physician*. 2012;86(12):1127–1132.

---

4. Workowski KA, Bolan GA; for Centers for Disease Control and Prevention. Sexually transmitted diseases treatment guidelines, 2015. *MMWR Recomm Rep*. 2015;64(RR-03):1–137.
5. Munoz JL, Goje OJ. *Mycoplasma genitalium*: an emerging sexually transmitted infection. *Scientifica (Cairo)*. 2016;2016:7537318.
6. Mayor MT, Roett MA, Uduhiri KA. Diagnosis and management of gonococcal infections. *Am Fam Physician*. 2012;86(10):931–938.
7. O'Connor EA, Lin JS, Burda BU, et al. Behavioral sexual risk-reduction counseling in primary care to prevent sexually transmitted infections: a systematic review for the U.S. Preventive Services Task Force. *Ann Intern Med*. 2014;161(12):874–883.
8. O'Connell CM, Ferone ME. *Chlamydia trachomatis* genital infections. *Microb Cell*. 2016;3(9):390–403.

ADDITIONAL READING

U.S. Preventive Services Task Force. Final recommendation statement. Chlamydia and gonorrhea: screening. http://www.uspreventiveservicestaskforce.org/Page/Document/RecommendationStatementFinal/chlamydia-and-gonorrhea-screening. Accessed December 17, 2018.

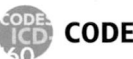 **SEE ALSO**

- Chlamydia Infection (Sexually Transmitted); Epididymitis; Gonococcal Infections; Pelvic Inflammatory Disease; Prostatitis; Urinary Tract Infection (UTI) in Females; Urinary Tract Infection (UTI) in Males; Vulvovaginitis, Estrogen Deficient; Vulvovaginitis, Prepubescent
- Algorithms: Dysuria; Genital Ulcers; Urethral Discharge

CODES

ICD10

- N34.2 Other urethritis
- A56.01 Chlamydial cystitis and urethritis
- A54.01 Gonococcal cystitis and urethritis, unspecified

CLINICAL PEARLS

- Inflammation of the urethra, frequently associated with dysuria, pruritus, and/or urethral discharge
- Common manifestation of STI
- Classified as gonococcal (caused by *N. gonorrhoeae*) and nongonococcal
- NAAT preferred method of diagnosis for men and women
- Single-dose regimens with direct observation preferred
- In cases of gonorrhea or chlamydia infection, in person or EPT recommended for all partners of patients within the last 60 days
- Given that risk factors for gonorrhea and chlamydia indicate risk for other STIs, screening for HIV, RPR, hepatitis C, and hepatitis B may also be indicated.
- Repeat testing for gonorrhea and chlamydia in 3 months recommended due to rates of reinfection.
- Special considerations in pediatric and pregnant populations
- Treatment in persons with HIV infection is the same as in patients without HIV infection.
- Health care providers are required to report all gonorrhea and chlamydia infections in accordance with local and state requirements.

U

URINARY TRACT INFECTION (UTI) IN FEMALES
James E. Steward, MD • Akhil Das, MD, FACS

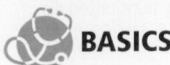 **BASICS**

DESCRIPTION
- Urinary tract infection (UTI) is the presence of pathogenic microorganisms within the urinary tract with concomitant symptoms.
- This topic refers primarily to infectious cystitis; other complicated UTIs, such as pyelonephritis, are discussed elsewhere.
- Uncomplicated UTI: occurs in patients who have a normal, unobstructed urinary tract, who have no history of recent urologic procedure, and whose symptoms are confined to the lower urinary tract. Uncomplicated UTIs are most common in young, sexually active women.
- Complicated UTI: an infection of the lower or upper urinary tract in the presence of an anatomic abnormality, a functional abnormality, or compromised host (see "Risk Factors") (1)
- Recurrent UTI: symptomatic UTIs that follow resolution of an earlier episode after appropriate treatment
  - Three UTIs within 12 months or two within 6 months
  - Most recurrences are thought to represent reinfection rather than relapse.
  - No evidence indicates that recurrent UTIs lead to health problems such as hypertension or renal disease in the absence of anatomic or functional abnormalities of the urinary tract.
- System(s) affected: renal, urologic
- Synonym(s): cystitis

EPIDEMIOLOGY
Incidence
- Accounts for 8 million doctor visits and 1 million emergency room visits and contributes to >100,000 hospital admissions each year (1)
- 11% of women have UTIs in any given year.
- Predominant age: young adults and older
- Predominant sex: female > male

Prevalence
- >50% of females have at least one UTI in their lifetime.
- One in four women has recurrent UTIs.

ETIOLOGY AND PATHOPHYSIOLOGY
- Bacteria and subsequent infection in the urinary tract arise chiefly via ascending bacterial movement and propagation (2).
- Pathogenic organisms (*Escherichia coli*) possess adherence factors and toxins that allow initiation and propagation of genitourinary infections:
  - Type 1 and *P. pili* (pyelonephritis-associated pili)
  - Lipopolysaccharide
- Most UTIs are caused by bacteria originating from bowel flora:
  - *E. coli* is the causative organism in 80% of cases of uncomplicated cystitis.
  - *Staphylococcus saprophyticus* accounts for 15% of infections.
  - Enterobacteriaceae (i.e., *Klebsiella*, *Proteus*, *Enterobacter*, and *Pseudomonas*) also contribute.
- *Candida* is associated with nosocomial UTI (2).

Genetics
Women with human leukocyte antigen 3 (HLA-3) and nonsecretor Lewis antigen have an increased bacterial adherence, which may lead to an increased risk in UTI.

RISK FACTORS
- Previous UTI
- Diabetes mellitus (DM)
- Pregnancy
- Sexual activity
- Use of spermicides or diaphragm
- Underlying abnormalities of the urinary tract such as tumors, calculi, strictures, incomplete bladder emptying, urinary incontinence, neurogenic bladder
- Catheterization
- Recent antibiotic use
- Poor hygiene
- Estrogen deficiency
- Inadequate fluid intake

GENERAL PREVENTION
- Maintain good hydration.
- Women with frequent or intercourse-related UTI should empty bladder immediately before and following intercourse; consider postcoital antibiotic.
- Avoid feminine hygiene sprays and douches.
- Wipe urethra from front to back.
- Cranberry may prevent recurrent infections.
- Vaginal estrogen in postmenopausal women may prevent infection.

COMMONLY ASSOCIATED CONDITIONS
See "Risk Factors."

Geriatric Considerations
- Elderly patients are more likely to have underlying urinary tract abnormality.
- Acute UTI may be associated with incontinence or mental status changes in the elderly (1).

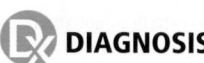 **DIAGNOSIS**

HISTORY
Note: Any or all may be present:
- Burning or pain during urination (dysuria)
- Urgency (sensation of need to urinate often)
- Frequency
- Sensation of incomplete bladder emptying
- Blood in urine
- Lower abdominal pain or cramping
- Offensive odor of urine
- Nocturia
- Sudden onset of urinary incontinence
- Dyspareunia

PHYSICAL EXAM
- Suprapubic tenderness
- Urethral and/or vaginal tenderness
- Fever or costovertebral angle tenderness indicates upper UTI.

DIFFERENTIAL DIAGNOSIS
- Vaginitis
- Asymptomatic bacteriuria
- STDs causing urethritis or pyuria
- Hematuria from causes other than infection (e.g., neoplasia, calculi)
- Interstitial cystitis
- Psychological dysfunction

DIAGNOSTIC TESTS & INTERPRETATION
Initial Tests (lab, imaging)
- No lab testing is necessary in women with high likelihood of lower UTI based on classic symptoms. Negative dipstick in the presence of high pretest probability does not rule out UTI.
- Urinalysis
  - Pyuria (>10 neutrophils/high-power field [HPF])
  - Bacteriuria (any amount on unspun urine or five bacteria/HPF on centrifuged urine)
  - Hematuria (≥3 RBCs/HPF)
- Dipstick urinalysis
  - Leukocyte esterase (75–96% sensitivity, 94–98% specificity, when >100,000 colony-forming units [CFU])
  - Nitrite tests are useful with nitrite-reducing organisms (e.g., *E. coli*, *Klebsiella*, *Proteus*).
- Urine culture: only indicated if diagnosis is unclear or patient has recurrent infections and resistance is suspected. It is neither cost-effective nor usually helpful for lower tract, uncomplicated UTI (3)[A].
  - Presence of 100,000 CFU/mL of organism indicates infection.
  - Identification of a single organism at lower CFU per milliliter likely also represents infection in the presence of appropriate symptoms.
  - Suspect a contaminated specimen when culture shows multiple types of bacteria.
- Imaging studies are often not required in most cases of UTI.

Follow-Up Tests & Special Considerations
- In nonpregnant, premenopausal women with symptoms of UTI, positive urinalysis, and no risks for complicated infection, empirical treatment may be given without obtaining a urine culture.
- Imaging may be indicated for UTIs in men, infants, immunocompromised patients, febrile infection, signs or symptoms of obstruction, failure to respond to appropriate therapy, and in patients with recurrent infections.
- CT scan and MRI provide the most complete anatomic data in adults.

Pediatric Considerations
For infants and children, obtain US; if ureteral dilation is detected, obtain either voiding cystourethrogram or isotope cystogram to evaluate for reflux.

Diagnostic Procedures/Other
- Urethral catheterization may be necessary to obtain a urine specimen from children and adults if the voided urine is suspected of being contaminated.
- Suprapubic bladder aspiration or urethral catheterization techniques can be used to obtain specimens from infants.
- Cystourethroscopy can be used to evaluate patients with recurrent UTIs, previous anti-incontinence surgery, or hematuria.

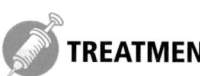 **TREATMENT**

GENERAL MEASURES
- Maintain good hydration.
- Maintain good hygiene.
- 1/4 of women with uncomplicated UTI experience a second UTI within 6 months and 1/2 at some time during their lifetime.
- Many women with uncomplicated UTI clear symptoms without treatment.

MEDICATION
First Line
- The urinary tract topical analgesic phenazopyridine 100 to 200 mg TID produces rapid relief of symptoms and should be offered to patients with more than minor discomfort; it is available over the counter. This medication is not a substitute for definitive treatment and also may alter urinalysis but not the urine culture.

- Choice of antibiotic should be made with consideration to patient allergy, compliance, local resistance patterns, availability, and cost.
- Uncomplicated UTI (adolescents and adults who are nonpregnant, nondiabetic, afebrile, immunocompetent, and without genitourinary anatomic abnormalities)
  - Trimethoprim/sulfamethoxazole (TMP/SMX; Bactrim): 160/800 mg PO BID for 3 days, best where resistance of *E. coli* strains <20%
  - 5-day course of nitrofurantoin should be used in patients with allergy to TMP/SMX and in areas where *E. coli* resistance to TMP/SMX >20% (4)[A].
  - Fosfomycin (Monurol): 3 g PO single dose (expensive)
  - Pivmecillinam: 400 mg BID for 3 to 7 days
- Lower UTI in pregnancy
  - Nitrofurantoin (Macrobid): 100 mg PO BID for 7 days
  - Cephalexin (Keflex): 500 mg PO BID for 7 days
  - TMP/SMX use in pregnancy is not desirable (especially in 1st and 3rd trimester) but is appropriate in some circumstances (4)[A].
  - Fluoroquinolones are not safe during pregnancy and are usually avoided in treatment of children.
- Postcoital UTI: Single-dose TMP/SMX or cephalexin may reduce frequency of UTI in sexually active women.
- Complicated UTI (pregnancy, diabetes, febrile, immunocompromised patient, recurrent UTIs): Extend course to 7 to 10 days of treatment with antibiotic chosen based on culture results; may begin with fluoroquinolone, TMP/SMX, or cephalosporin while awaiting results (avoid using nitrofurantoin for complicated UTI)

Second Line
- Uncomplicated UTI
  - β-Lactams (amoxicillin/clavulanate, cefdinir, cefpodoxime proxetil) for 3 to 7 days
  - *Fluoroquinolones are effective and should not be used in uncomplicated UTI due to risk of serious and potentially irreversible adverse reactions (see FDA black box warnings).*
- Chronic UTIs
  - Women with recurrent UTIs can be treated with a number of different strategies. Some authors suggest continuous antibiotics (5). Treatment duration is guided by the severity of patient symptoms and by physician and patient preference: Consider 3 to 6 months of therapy, followed by observation for reinfection after discontinuing prophylaxis. Continuous antimicrobial prophylaxis involves daily administration of low-dose TMP/SMX 80/400 mg or nitrofurantoin 50 to 100 mg, among others.
    - Other authors note that patient self-initiated treatment does not reduce number of UTI episodes, but compared with prophylactic strategies or physician-initiated treatment, this approach minimizes the physiologic and financial cost of frequent antibiotic use, cost of diagnosis, number of physician visits, and number of symptomatic days, by limiting doses to symptomatic events (6).

Pediatric Considerations
Long-term antibiotics appear to reduce the risk of recurrent symptomatic UTI in susceptible children, but the benefit is small and must be considered together with the increased risk of microbial resistance.

ISSUES FOR REFERRAL
Patients with recurrent or complicated UTIs should be referred to a urologist for evaluation.

Pediatric Considerations
UTI in children, especially <1 year of age, should prompt workup for urinary tract anomalies.

SURGERY/OTHER PROCEDURES
- Urinary tract obstruction with urosepsis requires urgent drainage of the obstructed system.
- Patients with emphysematous pyelonephritis or pyonephrosis may need immediate surgical intervention.

COMPLEMENTARY & ALTERNATIVE MEDICINE
- Preliminary studies indicate that *Vaccinium macrocarpon* (cranberry) may help to prevent and treat UTIs by inhibiting bacterial adherence to the bladder epithelium. It may decrease the number of symptomatic UTIs over a 1-year period (7).
- Methenamine can be used for recurrent UTIs (converts to formaldehyde in urine).
- Vaginal estrogen can be used to prevent recurrent UTIs in postmenopausal women.
- Other complementary therapies, such as urine alkalinization, acupuncture, and oral or vaginal vaccines appear to be attractive alternative for prevention of UTIs; however, there is a lack of head-to-head trials to support their use (7).

ADMISSION, INPATIENT, AND NURSING CONSIDERATIONS
Inpatient evaluation is reserved for patients with complicated or upper tract UTIs. Majority of UTIs are managed in an outpatient setting.

 ## ONGOING CARE

FOLLOW-UP RECOMMENDATIONS
- First or rare UTI: Young or middle-aged, nonpregnant adult females require no follow-up if UTI is clinically cured after 3-day therapy.
- If symptoms persist after 2 to 3 days of therapy, obtain culture/sensitivity and change antibiotic accordingly.

Pregnancy Considerations
- UTI during pregnancy always requires culture/sensitivity and usually requires a 7- to 14-day treatment.
- Following the treatment of acute infection, pregnant women warrant surveillance urine cultures every trimester. They may receive prophylactic antibiotics for the remainder of pregnancy for recurrent or upper tract disease.

PATIENT EDUCATION
- Although no controlled studies support this intervention, postcoital voiding is commonly advised.
- FamilyDoctor Web site: http://familydoctor.org /familydoctor/en/diseases-conditions/urinary-tract -infections.html

PROGNOSIS
Symptoms resolve within 2 to 3 days of antibiotic treatment in almost all patients.

COMPLICATIONS
- Pyelonephritis or sepsis
- Renal abscess
- Acute urinary outlet obstruction

Pregnancy Considerations
Pregnant females, infants, and young children with cystitis are at higher risk of pyelonephritis.

REFERENCES

1. Mody L, Juthani-Mehta M. Urinary tract infections in older women: a clinical review. *JAMA*. 2014;311(8):844–854.
2. Guglietta A. Recurrent urinary tract infections in women: risk factors, etiology, pathogenesis and prophylaxis. *Future Microbiol*. 2017;12: 239–246.
3. Grigoryan L, Trautner BW, Gupta K. Diagnosis and management of urinary tract infections in the outpatient setting: a review. *JAMA*. 2014;312(16):1677–1684.
4. Zalmanovici Trestioreanu A, Green H, Paul M, et al. Antimicrobial agents for treating uncomplicated urinary tract infection in women. *Cochrane Database Syst Rev*. 2010;(10):CD007182.
5. Smith AL, Brown J, Wyman JF, et al. Treatment and prevention of recurrent lower urinary tract infections in women: a rapid review with practice recommendations [published online ahead of print June 22, 2018]. *J Urol*. doi:10.1016/j.juro .2018.04.088.
6. Arnold JJ, Hehn LE, Klein DA. Common questions about recurrent urinary tract infections in women. *Am Fam Physician*. 2016;93(7): 560–569.
7. Beerepoot MA, Geerlings SE, van Haarst EP, et al. Nonantibiotic prophylaxis for recurrent urinary tract infections: a systematic review and meta-analysis of randomized controlled trials. *J Urol*. 2013;190(6):1981–1989.

ADDITIONAL READING

- Gupta K, Hooton TM, Naber KG, et al; for Infectious Diseases Society of America, European Society for Microbiology and Infectious Diseases. International clinical practice guidelines for the treatment of acute uncomplicated cystitis and pyelonephritis in women: a 2010 update by the Infectious Diseases Society of America and the European Society for Microbiology and Infectious Diseases. *Clin Infect Dis*. 2011;52(5):e103–e120.
- Kang C, Kim J, Park DW, et al. Clinical practice guidelines for the antibiotic treatment of community-acquired urinary tract infections. *Infect Chemother*. 2018;50(1):67–100.

 ## SEE ALSO

Algorithm: Dysuria

 ## CODES

ICD10
- N39.0 Urinary tract infection, site not specified
- N30.90 Cystitis, unspecified without hematuria
- N30.91 Cystitis, unspecified with hematuria

CLINICAL PEARLS

- Uncomplicated UTIs cause significant short-term morbidity but generally do not cause renal damage.
- Culture is generally not indicated for women with symptoms of uncomplicated UTI.
- Treatment of uncomplicated UTIs reduces morbidity but does not reduce risk of recurrence.
- Uncomplicated UTIs should be treated for 3 days (TMP/SMX) or 5 days (nitrofurantoin). All pregnant women with bacteriuria should be treated.
- Health care professionals should avoid treating women with asymptomatic bacteriuria.
- Fluoroquinolones should be reserved for complicated UTI.

URINARY TRACT INFECTION (UTI) IN MALES
Cait Goss, MD • Amy L. Wiser, MD

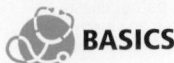 **BASICS**

DESCRIPTION
- Cystitis is an infection of the lower urinary tract, usually resulting from a single gram-negative enteric bacteria (see also "Prostatitis," "Pyelonephritis," and "Urethritis").
- System(s) affected: renal/urologic
- Synonym(s): urinary tract infection (UTI); cystitis
- In otherwise healthy males ages 15 to 50 years, UTI is uncommon and considered uncomplicated.
- In male newborns, infants, and elderly men UTI is considered complicated, with associated functional/structural mechanisms.

EPIDEMIOLOGY
Incidence
- Approximately 20% of UTIs occur in men.
- Predominant age: increases with age
- Uncommon in men <50 years of age
- 6 to 8 infections per 10,000 men aged 21 to 50 years (1)

Prevalence
Lifetime prevalence approximately 14%

ETIOLOGY AND PATHOPHYSIOLOGY
- *Escherichia coli* (majority of infections)
- *Klebsiella*
- *Enterobacter*
- *Enterococcus*
- *Proteus*
- *Serratia*
- *Citrobacter*
- *Providencia*
- *Streptococcus faecalis* and *Staphylococcus* sp.
- *Pseudomonas* and *Morganella* (more common in elderly and catheterized patients)
- Pathogenesis—bacterial entry into urinary tract via ascension or bladder instrumentation

Genetics
Not applicable

RISK FACTORS
- Age
- Obesity
- History of prior UTI
- Outlet obstruction
  - Benign prostatic hypertrophy (BPH)—incidence of 33% of men with UTIs (2)
  - Urethral stricture
  - Calculi
- Fecal incontinence
- Urinary incontinence
- Recent urologic surgery
- Urinary tract instrumentation/catheterization
- Infection of the prostate/kidney
- Immunocompromised
- Diabetes
- Bladder diverticula
- Neurogenic bladder
- Cognitive impairment
- Institutionalization
- Uncircumcised
- Anal intercourse
- Intercourse with an infected female partner (1)

GENERAL PREVENTION
- Prompt treatment of predisposing factors.
- Use a catheter only when necessary; if needed, use aseptic technique and closed system and remove as soon as possible.
- Cranberry products are not recommended for preventing UTI.

COMMONLY ASSOCIATED CONDITIONS
- Acute bacterial pyelonephritis
- Chronic bacterial pyelonephritis
- Urethritis
- Prostatitis
- Prostatic hypertrophy
- Prostate cancer

Geriatric Considerations
Bacteriuria is more common among the elderly, usually is transient, and may be related to functional status. Of men >65 years of age, 5–10% have asymptomatic bacteriuria (ASB). If ASB is noted, no treatment is needed (3,4).

Pediatric Considerations
Can be associated with obstruction to normal flow of urine, such as vesicoureteral reflux. Unique diagnostic criteria and evaluation recommendations exist (see below).

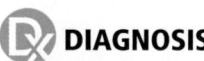 **DIAGNOSIS**

HISTORY
- Urinary frequency
- Urinary urgency
- Dysuria
- Hesitancy
- Slow urinary stream
- Dribbling of urine
- Nocturia
- Suprapubic discomfort or perineal pain
- Low back pain
- Hematuria
- Systemic symptoms (chills, fever) or flank pain, nausea, vomiting present with concomitant pyelonephritis or prostatitis

PHYSICAL EXAM
- Suprapubic tenderness
- Costovertebral angle (CVA) tenderness and/or fever may be present with concomitant pyelonephritis/prostatitis/epididymitis.
- Perform genital examination.
- Consider digital rectal exam, including palpation of the prostate gland, to rule out bacterial prostatitis.

DIFFERENTIAL DIAGNOSIS
- Anatomic/functional pathology of the urinary tract
- Urethritis/STIs
- Infections in other sites of the genitourinary tract (e.g., epididymis, prostatitis). >90% of men with febrile UTI have concomitant prostate infection (1)[A].

DIAGNOSTIC TESTS & INTERPRETATION
- Urine dipstick/manual microscopy of clean catch midstream void showing the following:
  - Pyuria (>10 WBCs)
  - Bacteriuria
  - Leukocyte esterase is more sensitive, and nitrite is more specific in detecting UTI (5).
  - Positive leukocyte esterase (in males: sensitivity, 78%; specificity, 59%; positive predictive value [PPV], 71%; negative predictive value [NPV], 67%)
  - Positive nitrite (in males: sensitivity, 47%; specificity, 98%; PPV, 96%; NPV, 59%)
- Automated microscopy/flow cytometry that measures cell counts and bacterial counts can be used to improve screening characteristics (sensitivity, 92%; specificity, 55%; PPV, 47%; NPV, 97%). The high NPV of these screening tests allows for more judicious use of urine culture (5)[B].
- Urine culture: >100,000 colony-forming units (CFU; >10^5 CFU) of bacteria/mL of urine confirm diagnosis.
- Lower counts, such as >10^3 CFU, also may be indicative of infection, especially in the presence of pyuria.
- Diagnosis in infants and children <24 months made on the basis of both pyuria and 50,000 CFU on culture
- Renal and bladder ultrasound recommended in infants and young children after first confirmed UTI

Follow-Up Tests & Special Considerations

- Consider assessing for risk factors for STIs because chlamydial/gonococcal urethritis can mimic a UTI. If risk factors are present, use urine nucleic acid amplification tests to identify gonococcal and *Chlamydia* infections and treat as necessary.
- Further urologic evaluation is warranted to rule out other disorders in men with recurrent UTI, febrile UTI, or pyelonephritis. This may include the following:
  – Ultrasound
  – Cystoscopy
  – Urodynamics
  – IV pyelography
- Value of a urologic evaluation in a single uncomplicated UTI has not been determined.
- Antibiotics prior to culture or phenazopyridine prior to urine dipstick can alter results.
- Blood cultures are not routine; perform if concern for sepsis or bacteremia.

Test Interpretation
Depends on site of infection

TREATMENT

GENERAL MEASURES
- Hydration
- Analgesia, if required
- Patient with indwelling catheters
  – If asymptomatic bacterial colonization, no need to treat (Sterilization of urine is not possible, and resistant organisms may take up residence.)
  – If symptomatic of acute infection, institute treatment.

MEDICATION

First Line
- Acute, uncomplicated cystitis
  – Treat empirically; strongly consider if nitrite positive, using local resistance patterns or based on culture and sensitivity results for 7 days.
  – For empirical therapy, a fluoroquinolone or trimethoprim-sulfamethoxazole DS usually used to treat the most likely pathogens
- Complicated, febrile, or recurrent infection
  – Prescribe a minimum of 2 weeks antibiotics based on antimicrobial sensitivities with repeat urine check after the treatment. In men with febrile UTI or pyelonephritis, prostatic involvement also must be considered. Treatment of concomitant prostatitis requires antimicrobials with good prostatic tissue and fluid penetration (fluoroquinolones).

Second Line
According to culture and sensitivity results and patient's history

ISSUES FOR REFERRAL
Further urologic evaluation and referral are warranted to rule out other disorders in male infants and men with recurrent UTI, febrile UTI, or pyelonephritis.

ADMISSION, INPATIENT, AND NURSING CONSIDERATIONS
- Inability to tolerate oral medications
- Acute renal failure
- Suspected sepsis

ONGOING CARE

FOLLOW-UP RECOMMENDATIONS
Patient Monitoring
Close follow-up until clinically well

DIET
Encourage adequate fluid intake.

PATIENT EDUCATION
For patient education materials about this topic that have been reviewed favorably, contact the National Kidney Foundation, 30 E. 33rd Street, Suite 1100, New York, NY 10016; 212-889-2210.

PROGNOSIS
Clearing of infections with appropriate antibiotic treatment

COMPLICATIONS
- Pyelonephritis
- Ascending infection
- Recurrent infection
- Prostatitis

REFERENCES

1. Wagenlehner FM, Weidner W, Pilatz A, et al. Urinary tract infections and bacterial prostatitis in men. *Curr Opin Infect Dis*. 2014;27(1):97–101.
2. Drekonja DM, Rector TS, Cutting A, et al. Urinary tract infection in male veterans: treatment patterns and outcomes. *JAMA Intern Med*. 2013;173(1):62–68.
3. Rowe TA, Juthani-Mehta M. Diagnosis and management of urinary tract infection in older adults. *Infect Dis Clin North Am*. 2014;28(1):75–89.
4. Matthews SJ, Lancaster JW. Urinary tract infections in the elderly population. *Am J Geriatr Pharmacother*. 2011;9(5):286–309.
5. Koeijers JJ, Kessels AG, Nys S, et al. Evaluation of the nitrite and leukocyte esterase activity tests for the diagnosis of acute symptomatic urinary tract infection in men. *Clin Infec Dis*. 2007;45(7):894–896.

ADDITIONAL READING

- Coupat C, Pradier C, Degand N, et al. Selective reporting of antibiotic susceptibility data improves the appropriateness of intended antibiotic prescriptions in urinary tract infections: a case-vignette randomised study. *Eur J Clin Microbiol Infect Dis*. 2013;32(5):627–636.
- Foxman B. Urinary tract infection syndromes: occurrence, recurrence, bacteriology, risk factors, and disease burden. *Infect Dis Clin North Am*. 2014;28(1):1–13.
- Gerber GS, Brendler CB. Evaluation of the urologic patient: history, physical examination, and urinalysis. In: Walsh PC, Retik AB, Vaughn ED Jr, et al, eds. *Campbell's Urology*. 8th ed. Philadelphia, PA: Saunders; 2002:107.
- Koeijers JJ, Verbon A, Kessels AG, et al. Urinary tract infection in male general practice patients: uropathogens and antibiotic susceptibility. *Urology*. 2010;76(2):336–340.

 SEE ALSO

- Prostate Cancer; Prostatic Hyperplasia, Benign (BPH); Prostatitis; Pyelonephritis; Urethritis
- Algorithms: Dysuria; Urethral Discharge

 CODES

ICD10
- N39.0 Urinary tract infection, site not specified
- N30.90 Cystitis, unspecified without hematuria
- N30.91 Cystitis, unspecified with hematuria

CLINICAL PEARLS

- Cystitis is an infection of the lower urinary tract, usually resulting from a single gram-negative enteric bacteria.
- Risk factors/causes: age, obesity, history of UTI, BPH/outlet obstruction, incontinence, urinary tract instrumentation or catheterization, infection of the prostate/kidney, immunocompromised or diabetes, cognitive impairment, institutionalization, neurogenic bladder, uncircumcised, anal intercourse, intercourse with infected female partner
- Evaluation: urinalysis, urine culture, STI testing (e.g., gonorrhea, *Chlamydia* by culture/DNA probe)
- Treat empirically with fluoroquinolones or trimethoprim-sulfamethoxazole DS for 7 days.

U

UROLITHIASIS
Phillip Fournier, MD

BASICS

DESCRIPTION
- Stone formation within the urinary tract: Urinary crystals bind to form a nidus which grows to form a calculus (stone).
- Range of symptoms: asymptomatic to obstructive; febrile morbidity if result of infection

EPIDEMIOLOGY
- The worldwide epidemiology differs according to both geographic area (higher prevalence in hot, arid, or dry climates) and socioeconomic conditions (dietary intake and lifestyle). Radiolucent stones and stones secondary to infection are less influenced by environmental conditions.
- Vesical calculosis (bladder stones) due to malnutrition during early life is frequent in Middle East and Asian countries.
- Incidence in industrialized countries seems to be increasing, probably due to improved diagnostics as well as to increasingly rich diets.
- Increased incidence in patients with surgically induced absorption issues, such as Crohn disease and gastric bypass surgery (1)

Incidence
- In industrialized countries: 100 to 200/100,000 per year
- Predominant age: Mean age is 40 to 60 years.
- Predominant sex: male > female (~2:1) (2)

ETIOLOGY AND PATHOPHYSIOLOGY
- Supersaturation and dehydration lead to high salt content in urine which congregates.
- Stasis of urine
  - Renal malformation (e.g., horseshoe kidney, ureteropelvic junction obstruction)
  - Incomplete bladder emptying (e.g., neurogenic bladder, prostate enlargement, multiple sclerosis)
- Crystals may form in pure solutions (homogeneous) or on existing surfaces, such as other crystals or cellular debris (heterogeneous).
- Balance of promoters and inhibitors: organic (Tamm-Horsfall protein, glycosaminoglycan, uropontin, nephrocalcin) and inorganic (citrate, pyrophosphate)
- Calcium oxalate and/or phosphate stones (80%)
  - Hypercalciuria
    - Absorptive hypercalciuria: increased jejunal calcium absorption
    - Renal leak: increased calcium excretion from renal proximal tubule
    - Resorptive hypercalciuria: mild hyperparathyroidism
  - Hypercalcemia
    - Hyperparathyroidism
    - Sarcoidosis
    - Malignancy
    - Immobilization
    - Paget disease
- Hyperoxaluria
  - Enteric hyperoxaluria
    - Intestinal malabsorptive state associated with irritable bowel disease, celiac sprue, or intestinal resection
    - Bile salt malabsorption leads to formation of calcium soaps.
  - Primary hyperoxaluria: autosomal recessive, types I and II
  - Dietary hyperoxaluria: overindulgence in oxalate-rich food

- Hyperuricosuria
  - Seen in 10% of calcium stone formers
  - Caused by increased dietary purine intake, systemic acidosis, myeloproliferative diseases, gout, chemotherapy, Lesch-Nyhan syndrome
  - Thiazides, probenecid
- Hypocitraturia
  - Caused by acidosis: renal tubular acidosis, malabsorption, thiazides, enalapril, excessive dietary protein
- Uric acid stones (10–15%): hyperuricemia causes as discussed earlier
- Struvite stones (5–10%): infected urine with urease-producing organisms (most commonly *Proteus* sp.)
- Cystine stones (<1%): autosomal recessive disorder of renal tubular reabsorption of cystine
- Bladder stones: seen with chronic bladder catheterization and some medications (indinavir)
- In children: usually due to malnutrition

Genetics
- Up to 20% of patients have a family history. However, spouses of those who form stones have higher calcium excretion rates than controls, suggesting strong dietary–environmental factors.
- Autosomal dominant: idiopathic hypercalciuria
- Autosomal recessive
  - Cystinuria, Lesch-Nyhan syndrome, hyperoxaluria types I and II
  - Ehlers-Danlos syndrome, Marfan syndrome, Wilson disease, familial renal tubular acidosis

RISK FACTORS
- White > African American in regions with both populations
- Family history
- Previous history of nephrolithiasis
- Diet rich in protein, refined carbohydrates, and sodium; carbonated drinks
- Occupations associated with a sedentary lifestyle or with a hot, dry workplace
- Incidence rates peak during summer secondary to dehydration.
- Obesity
- Surgically/medically induced malabsorption (Crohn disease, gastric bypass, celiac)

GENERAL PREVENTION
- Hydration (3)[A]
- Decrease salt and meat intake.
- Avoid oxalate-rich foods.

Pediatric Considerations
Rare: more common in men with low socioeconomic status

Pregnancy Considerations
- Pregnant women have the same incidence of renal colic as do nonpregnant women.
- Most symptomatic stones occur during the 2nd and 3rd trimesters, heralded by symptoms of flank pain/hematuria.
- Most common differential diagnosis is physiologic hydronephrosis of pregnancy. Use ultrasound to avoid irradiation. Noncontrast-enhanced CT scan also is diagnostic.
- Treatment goals
  - Control pain, avoid infection, and preserve renal function until birth or stone passage.
  - 30% require intervention, such as stent placement.

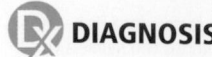

DIAGNOSIS

HISTORY
- Pain
  - Renal colic: acute onset of severe groin and/or flank pain
  - Distal stones may present with referred pain in labia, penile meatus, or testis
- Microscopic/gross hematuria occurs in 95% of patients.
- Nonspecific symptoms of nausea, vomiting, tachycardia, diaphoresis
- Low-grade fever without signs of infection
- Infectious origin: associated with high-grade fevers require more urgent treatment (see the following text)
- Frequency and dysuria especially occur with stones at the vesicoureteric junction (VUJ).
- Asymptomatic: nonobstructing stones within the renal calyces

PHYSICAL EXAM
Tender costovertebral angle with palpation/percussion and/or iliac fossa

DIFFERENTIAL DIAGNOSIS
- Appendicitis
- Ruptured aortic aneurysm
- Musculoskeletal strain
- Pyelonephritis (upper UTI)
- Pyonephrosis (obstructed upper UTI; emergency)
- Perinephric abscess
- Ectopic pregnancy
- Salpingitis

DIAGNOSTIC TESTS & INTERPRETATION
- Urinalysis for RBCs, leukocytes, nitrates, pH (acidic urine <5.5 is associated with uric acid stones; alkaline >7 with struvite stones)
- Midstream urine for microscopy, culture, and sensitivity
- Blood: urea, creatinine, electrolytes, calcium, and urate; consider CBC.
- Parathyroid hormone only if calcium is elevated
- Stone analysis if/when stone passed

Initial Tests (lab, imaging)
- Noncontrast-enhanced helical CT scan of the abdomen and pelvis has replaced IV pyelogram as the investigation of choice (4)[A].
  - Stone is found most commonly at levels of ureteric luminal narrowing: pelviureteric junction, pelvic brim, and VUJ.
  - Acute obstruction: Proximal ureter and renal pelvis are dilated to the level of obstruction, and perinephric stranding is possible on imaging.
- Renal ultrasound may be as effective with lower radiation at diagnosis as well as identifying obstruction (5)[B].
- X-ray of kidneys, ureter, and bladder to determine if stone is radiopaque or lucent
  - Calcium oxalate/phosphate stones are radiopaque.
  - Uric acid stones are radiolucent.
  - Staghorn calculi (that fill the shape of the renal calyces) are usually struvite and opaque.
  - Cystine stones are faintly opaque (ground-glass appearance).
- Ultrasound has low sensitivity and specificity but is often the first choice for pregnant women and children.

TREATMENT

GENERAL MEASURES
- 75% of patients are successfully treated conservatively and pass the stone spontaneously.
- Stones that do not pass usually require surgical intervention.
- 30–50% of patients will have recurrent stones.
- Increased fluid intake; eliminate carbonated drinks.

MEDICATION
- Medical expulsive therapy: α_1-Antagonists (e.g., tamsulosin) (6) and calcium channel blockers (e.g., nifedipine) improve likelihood of spontaneous stone passage with a number needed to treat (NNT) of ~5.
- Category C in pregnancy
- Adequate pain control can be achieved with NSAIDs.

ISSUES FOR REFERRAL
- Urgent referral of patients with UTI/sepsis or acute renal failure/solitary kidney
- Early referral of pregnant patients, large stones (>8 mm), chronic renal failure, children
- Refer patients if no passage at 2 to 4 weeks or poorly controlled pain.

ADDITIONAL THERAPIES
- Uric acid stone dissolution therapy
  - Alkalinize urine with potassium citrate C; keep pH >6.5.
  - Allopurinol 100 to 300 mg/day PO (for those who continue to form stones despite alkalinization of urine)
- Cystine stone dissolution/prevention
  - Alkalinize urine with potassium citrate; keep pH >6.5.
  - Chelating agents: captopril, α-mercaptopropionylglycine, D-penicillamine
- Consider altering medications that increase risk of stone formation: probenecid, loop diuretics, salicylic acid, salbutamol, indinavir, triamterene, acetazolamide.
- Vitamin D supplementation has not been proven to induce stone formation.
- Treat hypercalciuria with thiazides on an acute basis only.
- Treat hypocitraturia with potassium citrate and high-citrate juices (e.g., orange, lemon).
- Treat enteric hyperoxaluria with oral calcium/magnesium, cholestyramine, and potassium citrate.

SURGERY/OTHER PROCEDURES
- Immediate relief of obstruction is required for patients with the following conditions:
  - Sepsis
  - Renal failure (obstructed solitary kidney, bilateral obstruction)
  - Uncontrolled pain, despite adequate analgesia
- Emergency surgery for obstruction
  - Placement of a retrograde stent (i.e., endoscopic surgery, usually requires an anesthetic)
  - Radiologic placement of a percutaneous nephrostomy tube
- Elective surgery for stone treatment
  - Extracorporeal shock wave lithotripsy
  - Ureteroscopy with basket extraction/lithotripsy (laser/pneumatic)
  - Percutaneous nephrolithotomy
- Open surgery is uncommon.

ADMISSION, INPATIENT, AND NURSING CONSIDERATIONS
- Analgesia
  - Combination of NSAIDs (ketorolac 30 to 60 mg) and oral opiate
  - Parenteral opioid if vomiting or if preceding fails to control pain (morphine 5 to 10 mg IV or IM q4h)
  - Antiemetic if required or prophylactically with parenteral narcotics
- Septic patients with urosepsis or pyonephrosis may require IV antibiotics (once blood and urine cultures are taken), IV fluids, and in severe cases cardiorespiratory support in intensive care during recovery.

 ONGOING CARE

FOLLOW-UP RECOMMENDATIONS
- Patients with ureteric stones who are being treated conservatively should be followed until imaging is clear or stone is visibly passed.
  - Strain urine and send stone for composition.
  - Tamsulosin and nifedipine in selected patients to speed passage
  - Present to the hospital if pain worsens/signs of infection.
  - If pain management is suboptimal or stone does not progress or pass within 2 to 4 weeks, patient should be referred to a urologist and imaging should be repeated.
- Patients with recurrent stone formation should have follow-up with a urologist for metabolic workup: 24-hour urine for volume, pH, creatinine, calcium, cystine, phosphate, oxalate, uric acid, and magnesium.

DIET
ALERT
- Increased fluid intake for life cannot be overemphasized for decreasing recurrence. Encourage intake of 2 to 3 L/day; advise patient to have clear urine rather than yellow.
- Decrease or eliminate carbonated drinks.
- Patients who form calcium stones should minimize high-oxalate foods such as green leafy vegetables, rhubarb, peanuts, chocolates, and beer.
- Decrease protein and salt intake.
- Lowering calcium intake is inadvisable and may even increase urine calcium excretion.
- Increase phytate-rich foods such as natural dietary bran, legumes and beans, and whole cereal.
- Avoid excessive vitamin C and/or vitamin D.

PROGNOSIS
- Spontaneous stone passage depends on stone location (proximal vs. distal) and stone size (<5 mm, 90% pass; >8 mm, 10% pass).
- Stone recurrence: 50% of patients at 10 years

REFERENCES
1. Matlaga BR, Shore AD, Magnuson T, et al. Effect of gastric bypass surgery on kidney stone disease. *J Urol*. 2009;181(6):2573–2577.
2. Scales CD Jr, Curtis LH, Norris RD, et al. Changing gender prevalence of stone disease. *J Urol*. 2007;177(3):979–982.
3. Qiang W, Ke Z. Water for preventing urinary calculi. *Cochrane Database Syst Rev*. 2004;(3):CD004292.
4. Worster A, Preyra I, Weaver B, et al. The accuracy of noncontrast helical computed tomography versus intravenous pyelography in the diagnosis of suspected acute urolithiasis: a meta-analysis. *Ann Emerg Med*. 2002;40(3):280–286.
5. Luyckx F. Who wants to go further has to know the past: a comment upon: ultrasonography versus computed tomography for suspected nephrolithiasis-R. Smith-Bindman et al. N Engl J Med. 2014 Sep 18;371(12):1100–1110. *World J Urol*. 2015;33(10):1371–1372.
6. Al-Ansari A, Al-Naimi A, Alobaidy A, et al. Efficacy of tamsulosin in the management of lower ureteral stones: a randomized double-blind placebo-controlled study of 100 patients. *Urology*. 2010; 75(1):4–7.

ADDITIONAL READING
- Morgan M, Pearle M. Medical management of renal stones. *BMJ*. 2016;352:i52.
- Pearle MS, Goldfarb DS, Assimos DG, et al. Medical management of kidney stones: AUA guideline. *J Urol*. 2014;192(2):316–324.
- Qaseem A, Dallas P, Forciea MA, et al; for Clinical Guidelines Committee of the American College of Physicians. Dietary and pharmacologic management to prevent recurrent nephrolithiasis in adults: a clinical practice guideline from the American College of Physicians. *Ann Intern Med*. 2014;161(9):659–667.

 SEE ALSO

Algorithms: Dysuria; Renal Calculi; Urethral Discharge

CODES

ICD10
- N20.9 Urinary calculus, unspecified
- N20.0 Calculus of kidney
- N20.1 Calculus of ureter

CLINICAL PEARLS
- Incidence in industrialized countries seems to be increasing, probably due to improved diagnostics as well as to increasingly rich diets.
- Vesical calculosis (bladder stones) due to malnutrition during early life is frequent in Middle East and Asian countries.
- Medical expulsive therapy: α_1-Antagonists (e.g., terazosin) and calcium channel blockers (e.g., nifedipine) improve likelihood of spontaneous stone passage with NNT of ~5.
- Increased fluid intake for life cannot be overemphasized for decreasing recurrence. Encourage 2 to 3 L/day intake; advise patient to have clear urine rather than yellow.
- Patients who form calcium stones should minimize high-oxalate foods such as green leafy vegetables, rhubarb, peanuts, chocolates, and beer.
- Decrease protein and salt intake.
- Lowering calcium intake is inadvisable and may even increase urine calcium excretion.

U

URTICARIA

Todd A. Wical, DO • Katie L. Westerfield, DO, IBCLC, FAAFP

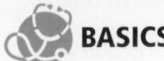 **BASICS**

DESCRIPTION

- A cutaneous lesion or lesions involving edema of the epidermis and/or dermis presenting with rapid onset and pruritus, returning to normal skin appearance within 24 hours
- Pathophysiology is primarily mast cell degranulation and subsequent histamine release.
- Angioedema may occur with urticaria which is characterized by sudden pronounced erythematous nonpitting edema of the lower dermis and subcutis; may take up to 72 hours to remit
- Pruritus and burning are more commonly associated with urticaria; pain more often with angioedema
- Lesions can occur on any part of the body.
- Urticaria can be classified as acute or chronic.
  – Acute: if lesions recur within <6 weeks
  – Chronic: recurring lesions that persist for >6 weeks
- Three main causal categories of urticarial lesions
  – Immunoglobulin E (IgE) mediated
  – Non-IgE immunologically mediated
  – Nonimmunologically mediated
- Underlying etiology may be difficult to pinpoint, although in some cases possible.
- For those with chronic urticaria, 40% have concurrent angioedema.
- Etiology of urticaria is either spontaneous or induced.
- System(s) affected: integumentary
- Synonym(s): hives; wheals

EPIDEMIOLOGY

Incidence
- Equally distributed across all ages: female > male (2:1 in chronic urticaria)
- In 20% of patients, chronic urticaria lasts >10 years.

Prevalence
- 5–25% of the population
- Of people with urticaria, 40% have no angioedema, 40% have urticaria and angioedema, and 20% have angioedema with no urticaria.
- Up to 3% of the population has chronic idiopathic urticaria.

ETIOLOGY AND PATHOPHYSIOLOGY

- Mast cell degranulation with release of inflammatory reactants, which leads to vascular leakage, inflammatory cell extravasation, and dermal (angioedema) and/or epidermal (wheals/hives) edema
- Histamine, cytokines, leukotrienes, and proteases are main active substances released.
- If release of histamine and other mediators occurs in the dermis, urticaria lesions result. If release occurs deep in the dermis, then angioedema develops.
- Acute spontaneous urticaria (ASU)
  – Bacterial infections: strep throat, sinusitis, otitis, urinary tract
  – Viral infections: rhinovirus, rotavirus, hepatitis B, mononucleosis, herpes

- Foods: peanuts, tree nuts, seafood, milk, soy, fish, wheat, and eggs; tend to be IgE-mediated; pseudoallergenic foods such as strawberries, tomatoes, preservatives, and coloring agents contain histamine.
- Drugs: IgE-mediated (e.g., penicillin and other antibiotics), direct mast cell stimulation (e.g., aspirin, NSAIDs, opiates)
- Inhalant, contact, ingestion, or occupational exposure (e.g., latex, cosmetics)
- Parasitic infection; insect bite/sting
- Transfusion reaction
- Chronic spontaneous urticaria (CSU)
  – Chronic subclinical allergic rhinitis, eczema, and other atopic disorders
  – Chronic indolent infections: *Helicobacter pylori*, fungal, parasitic (*Anisakis simplex*, strongyloidiasis), and chronic viral infections (hepatitis)
  – Collagen vascular disease (cutaneous vasculitis, serum sickness, lupus)
  – Thyroid autoimmunity, especially Hashimoto
  – Hormonal: pregnancy and progesterone
  – Autoimmune antibodies to the IgE receptor α chain on mast cells and to the IgE antibody
  – Chronic medications (e.g., NSAIDs, hormones, ACE inhibitors). NSAID sensitivity demonstrated almost in half of adults with chronic urticaria and presents with a worsening of symptoms 4 hours after ingestion.
  – Malignancy
  – Physical stimuli (cold, heat, vibration, pressure) in physical urticaria
- Chronic inducible urticaria (CIU)
  – Dermatographism: "skin writing" or the appearance of linear wheals at the site of any type of irritation. This is the most common physical induced urticaria.
  – Cold urticaria: Wheals occur within minutes of rewarming after cold exposure; 95% idiopathic but can be due to infections (mononucleosis, HIV), neoplasia, or autoimmune diseases
  – Delayed pressure urticaria: Urticaria occurs 0.5 to 12.0 hours after pressure to skin (e.g., from elastic or shoes), may be pruritic and/or painful, and may not subside for several days.
  – Solar urticaria: from sunlight exposure, usually UV; onset in minutes; subsides within 2 hours
  – Heat urticaria: from direct contact with warm objects or air; rare
  – Vibratory urticaria/angioedema: very rare; secondary to vibrations (e.g., motorcycle)
  – Cholinergic urticaria: due to brief increase of core body temperature from exercise, baths, or emotional stress. This is the second most common induced urticaria.
  – Adrenergic urticaria: caused by stress; extremely rare; vasoconstricted, blanched skin around pink wheals as opposed to cholinergic's erythematous surrounding
  – Contact urticaria: wheals at sites where chemical substances contact the skin, may be either IgE-dependent (e.g., latex) or IgE-independent (e.g., stinging nettle)
  – Aquagenic and solar urticaria: small wheals after contact with water of any temperature or UV light, respectively; rare

Genetics
No consistent pattern known: Chronic urticaria has increased frequency of HLA-DR4 and HLA-D8Q MHC II alleles.

COMMONLY ASSOCIATED CONDITIONS
- Angioedema (common)
- Anaphylaxis (somewhat common)

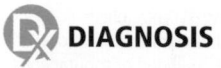 **DIAGNOSIS**

HISTORY
Rapid onset; individual lesions resolve in <24 hours, pruritus

> **ALERT**
> Important to rule out underlying anaphylaxis in those patients presenting with acute onset of urticaria (1,2)[C]

PHYSICAL EXAM
- Single/multiple raised, polymorphic indurated plaques with central pallor and edema with an erythematous flare
- Evaluate for underlying conditions including thyroid abnormalities (nodules), bacterial, viral, or fungal infection (e.g., fever)

DIFFERENTIAL DIAGNOSIS
- Anaphylaxis (may present with urticaria)
- Morbilliform or fixed drug eruptions
- Erythema multiforme
- Systemic lupus erythematosus (SLE), vasculitis, and polyarteritis
- Angioedema without urticaria
- Urticaria pigmentosa/systemic mastocytosis
- Bullous pemphigoid (urticarial stage)
- Arthropod bite
- Atopic/contact dermatitis
- Viral exanthem

DIAGNOSTIC TESTS & INTERPRETATION
- Diagnosis is usually clinical (1,2)[A].
- In general, only if the history or physical are suggestive of a specific underlying disease should targeted laboratory studies be utilized.
- Directed by clinical suspicion of underlying cause:
  – Allergy skin tests and radioallergosorbent test (RAST) for inhaled allergens, insects, drugs, or foods
  – Infection: Consider pharyngeal culture, LFTs, mononucleosis test, urinalysis in appropriate setting.
- Chronic urticaria (CIU/CSU): Extensive lab testing is not indicated and has not proven to improve outcome nor is it cost-effective. Limit lab testing according to clinical history and indication. Skin or IgE testing should be limited to specific history of provoking allergen (3)[C].
  – CBC, ESR, and CRP are recommended by most guidelines.
  – Thyroid function tests, LFTs, and urinalysis are recommended by several guidelines.

- Consider allergy skin tests and RAST for inhaled allergens, insects, drugs, or foods; total IgE level
- Autoimmune: ESR, ANA, RF, complement (e.g., CH50, C3, C4), cryoglobulins in urticarial vasculitis
- Tests for *H. pylori* (e.g., antibodies) in dyspeptic patients. Consider stool for ova and parasites in at-risk individuals.
- Autologous serum skin testing: injection of serum under skin to test for presence of IgE receptor–activating antibodies
- Consider malignancy workup, including serum protein electrophoresis and immunofixation in the proper setting.
- Use the urticaria activity score (UAS7) for assessing CSU.
- Recently was developed urticaria control test (UCT)
  - The tool to assess disease control in patients with chronic urticaria (spontaneous and inducible) (4)[A]

Diagnostic Procedures/Other
- Food and drug reactions: elimination of (or challenges with) suspected agents
- Physical and special forms of urticaria: challenge tests:
  - Dermatographism: Stroke skin lightly with rounded object and observe for surrounding urticaria.
  - Cold urticaria: ice cube test: Place ice cube on skin for 5 minutes; observe for 10 to 15 minutes.
  - Cholinergic: Exercise to the point of sweating/ partial immersion in 42°C bath for 10 minutes.
  - Solar: exposure to different wavelengths of light
  - Delayed pressure: Apply 5-lb sandbag to back for 20 minutes; observe 6 hours later.
  - Aquagenic: Apply water at various temperatures.
  - Vibratory: Apply vibration 4 to 5 minutes with a lab mixing device; observe.
- Skin biopsy with lesions lasting >24 hours or if concern for underlying vasculitis (1,2)[A]

 TREATMENT

ISSUES FOR REFERRAL
Referral to an allergist, immunologist, or dermatologist for recalcitrant cases, especially if lesions consistently remain present for >24 hours

GENERAL MEASURES
The mainstay of therapy for urticaria is the avoidance of identified trigger(s).

MEDICATION
First Line
2nd-generation antihistamine (H$_1$) blockers are the first-line treatment of any urticaria in which avoidance of stimulus is impossible or not feasible (1,2)[A]:

- Fexofenadine (Allegra): 180 mg/day
- Loratadine (Claritin): 10 mg/day, increasing to 30 mg/day if needed; only medication studied for safe use in pregnancy
- Desloratadine (Clarinex): 5 mg/day (5)[A]
- Cetirizine (Zyrtec): 10 mg/day, increasing to 30 mg per day if needed
- Levocetirizine (Xyzal): 5 mg/day; requires weight-based dosing in children (5)[A]
- Rupatadine: novel H$_1$ antagonist with antiplatelet-activating factor activity

Second Line
Doubling the typical 2nd-generation H$_1$ blocker dosages should be attempted before adding 1st-generation H$_1$ or H$_2$ blockers (1,2,5)[A].
- H$_2$-specific antihistamines (beneficial as adjuvants): cimetidine, ranitidine, nizatidine, famotidine
- 1st-generation antihistamines (H$_1$; for patients with sleep disturbed by itching):
  - Older children and adults: hydroxyzine or diphenhydramine 25 to 50 mg q6h
  - Children <6 years of age: diphenhydramine 12.5 mg q6–8h (5 mg/kg/day) or hydroxyzine (10 mg/5 mL) 2 mg/kg/day divided q6–8h

Geriatric Considerations
1st-generation H$_1$ blockers may cause excessive drowsiness as well as dry mouth and eyes.

Third Line
- Corticosteroids: prednisolone 20 to 50 mg/day for max of 10 days; best used only for exacerbations; avoid chronic use (1,2)[C]
- Doxepin: tricyclic antidepressant with strong H$_1$- and H$_2$-blocking properties; 10 to 30 mg at bedtime; sedation limits usefulness (1)[C].
- Leukotriene antagonists (montelukast, zileuton, and zafirlukast): safe and worth trying in chronic, unresponsive cases; useful alone but best used in addition to antihistamines; limited data on use in treating acute urticaria
- Refractory symptoms
  - Omalizumab: anti-IgE; effective, expensive. 150 to 300 mg SQ q2–4wk. Restricted to allergists and those who can manage acute anaphylaxis (1,6)[A], significantly reduce the urticarial symptoms of CIU/CSU at 12 weeks. The best effect is reached with omalizumab dose 300 mg (6)[A]. Omalizumab is currently the only licensed treatment for H$_1$-antihistamine-refractory CSU, has a favorable risk/benefit ratio, and was well tolerated in clinical studies.
  - Cyclosporine: well studied, effective (2.5 to 5 mg/kg/day); best used in combination with antihistamines; significant renal side effects (1)[B],(2)[C]
  - Methotrexate: antifolate; proven useful in recalcitrant cases; GI upset most common complaint; long-term requires LFT monitoring.
  - UV therapy decreases number of mast cells; has shown promise in the treatment of mastocytosis-induced urticaria (2)[C]
- Adding vitamin D 4,000 IU/day for 12 weeks may decrease the symptoms and USS score.

ADMISSION, INPATIENT, AND NURSING CONSIDERATIONS
Educating patient on use of EpiPen as pathophysiology is similar to anaphylaxis; if the airway is threatened, immediate consultation to evaluate for laryngeal edema and need for definitive airway management

 ONGOING CARE

PROGNOSIS
- Resolution of acute symptoms: 70% <72 hours
- Chronic urticaria: 35% symptom-free in a year; another 30% will see symptom reduction.

REFERENCES
1. Zuberbier T, Aberer W, Asero R, et al. The EAACI/ GA(2) LEN/EDF/WAO guideline for the definition, classification, diagnosis, and management of urticaria: the 2013 revision and update. *Allergy*. 2014;69(7):868–887.
2. Bernstein JA, Lang DM, Khan DA, et al. The diagnosis and management of acute and chronic urticaria: 2014 update. *J Allergy Clin Immunol*. 2014;133(5):1270–1277.
3. American Academy of Allergy, Asthma & Immunology. Five things physicians and patients should question. http://www.choosingwisely.org/wp-content /uploads/2015/02/AAAAI-Choosing-Wisely-List.pdf. Accessed October 30, 2017.
4. Weller K, Groffik A, Church MK, et al. Development and validation of the urticaria control test: a patient-reported outcome instrument for assessing urticaria control. *J Allergy Clin Immunol*. 2014;133(5):1365–1372.
5. Staevska M, Popov TA, Kralimarkova T, et al. The effectiveness of levocetirizine and desloratadine in up to 4 times conventional doses in difficult-to-treat urticaria. *J Allergy Clin Immunol*. 2010;125(3):676–682.
6. Saini SS, Bindslev-Jensen C, Maurer M, et al. Efficacy and safety of omalizumab in patients with chronic idiopathic/spontaneous urticaria who remain symptomatic on H1 antihistamines: a randomized, placebo-controlled study. *J Invest Dermatol*. 2015;135(1):67–75.

ADDITIONAL READING
- Maurer M, Weller K, Bindslev-Jensen C, et al. Unmet clinical needs in chronic spontaneous urticaria. A GA^{2}LEN task force report. *Allergy*. 2011;66(3):317–330.
- Poonawalla T, Kelly B. Urticaria: a review. *Am J Clin Dermatol*. 2009;10(1):9–21.
- Powell R, Leech S, Till S, et al. BSACI guideline for the management of chronic urticaria and angioedema. *Clin Exp Allergy*. 2015;45(3):547–565.
- Zuberbier T, Balke M, Worm M, et al. Epidemiology of urticaria: a representative cross-sectional survey. *Clin Exp Dermatol*. 2010;35(8):869–873.

CODES

ICD10
- L50.9 Urticaria, unspecified
- L50.1 Idiopathic urticaria
- L50.8 Other urticaria

CLINICAL PEARLS
- Urticaria occurs rapidly and individual lesions resolve within 24 hours, although multiple crops of lesions can occur in stages.
- Mainstay of therapy is to avoid identified triggers.
- Antihistamines are the best studied and most efficacious therapy but may require higher-than-normal doses for efficacy.
- If individual lesions last >24 hours, patient should be evaluated for urticarial vasculitis and other more serious diagnoses.

U

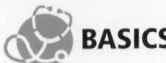

BASICS

DESCRIPTION
- Symptomatic descent of one or more of (1,2)
  - The anterior vaginal wall (bladder or cystocele)
  - The posterior vaginal wall (rectum or rectocele)
  - The uterus and cervix
  - The vaginal apex (vault or cuff scar after hysterectomy)
- Prolapses above or to the level of the hymen are generally not symptomatic (2).
- Associated symptoms (2)
  - Feeling of vaginal or pelvic pressure
  - Heaviness
  - Bulging
  - Bowel or bladder symptoms
- Cost associated with treatment is >$1 billion annually (~200,000 surgeries per year) (2).

EPIDEMIOLOGY
Incidence
- The incidence of pelvic organ prolapse (POP) ranges from 1.5 to 1.8 per 1,000 woman years and peaks in women aged 60 to 69 years (3).
- In the United States, there are approximately 300,000 surgeries for POP each year (3), and a woman's lifetime risk of undergoing surgery for pelvic floor prolapse ranges from 6% to 18% (3).

Prevalence
- A national survey of 7,924 women (>20 years of age) found a prevalence of 25% for one or more pelvic floor disorders (including urinary incontinence, fecal incontinence, and POP). Prevalence of POP was 3–6% (4).
- POP is common but not always symptomatic. It does not always progress. It is estimated that 50% of women will develop prolapse, but only 10–20% of those will seek care for their condition (3).

ETIOLOGY AND PATHOPHYSIOLOGY
- Pelvic organs are supported by attachments between pelvic floor muscles, connective tissue, and the bony pelvis. Defects in this support can lead to prolapse in one or multiple compartments (5).
- Symptomatic women typically have defects in more than one compartment as well as damage to the levator ani and its attachments to the pelvis (5).
- Gradual process that begins long before symptoms develop

RISK FACTORS
- Vaginal childbirth: Each additional vaginal birth increases risk (2,4).
- Age

- Family history (2)
- Race: White and Hispanic women may be at higher risk than black or Asian women (1,2).
- Obesity BMI >30 kg/m^2 (2,4)
- Chronic straining (constipation, chronic cough from pulmonary disease, repeated heavy lifting) (2)
- History of hysterectomy (2,4)

GENERAL PREVENTION
There is some evidence that pelvic floor muscle training ("Kegel exercises") may decrease the risk of symptomatic POP (5)[B]. Weight loss and proper management of conditions that cause increase in intra-abdominal pressure such as constipation may help prevent prolapse (5)[C]. Elective caesarean delivery has not been shown to prevent prolapse.

COMMONLY ASSOCIATED CONDITIONS
- Constipation
- Fecal incontinence
- Urinary incontinence or retention
- Other urinary symptoms
  - Urgency
  - Frequency

DIAGNOSIS

Less than half of women discuss symptoms with PCP. Only 10–12% seek medical attention. Barriers include embarrassment, social stigma, ability to cope, belief that POP is part of the aging process, belief that treatment options are limited, and fear of surgery.

HISTORY
- Common symptoms include the following:
  - Feeling a bulge in vagina
  - Something "falling out" of vagina
  - Pelvic pressure with activity or prolonged standing
  - Difficulty with voiding or defecation
  - Splinting the bulge to evacuate
  - Urinary or fecal urgency
  - Urinary frequency
  - Urinary or fecal incontinence
  - Constipation
- Document the presence, duration, and severity of coexisting urinary or bowel symptom.
- Assess impact on sexual function and quality of life.
- Assess past medical and surgical history.
  - Gravity and parity/obstetric history
  - Chronic constipation
  - Pulmonary disease
  - Prior pelvic procedures

PHYSICAL EXAM
- Abdominal examination to document any distention or masses
- Complete pelvic and rectal examination. Have patient cough or strain, particularly in an upright (standing) position while examining the distal vagina.
- The standard to measure prolapse is the validated Pelvic Organ Prolapse Quantification (POP-Q) scale.
  - Describes prolapse of each compartment in relationship to the vaginal hymen
  - Patient is supine with the head of the bed at 45 degrees, performing Valsalva.
    - Stage 1: prolapse in which the distal point is superior or equal to 1 cm above hymen
    - Stage 2: prolapse in which the distal point is between 1 cm above and 1 cm below hymen
    - Stage 3: prolapse in which the distal point is superior or equal to 1 cm below the hymen, but some vaginal mucosa is not everted
    - Stage 4: complete vaginal vault eversion ("procidentia"); entire vaginal mucosa everted (2)
- A split speculum should be used to observe apical, anterior, and posterior compartments successively.
- Patient can be evaluated in supine position. If prolapse is not well demonstrated, patient can stand and Valsalva to assess maximum descent.

DIFFERENTIAL DIAGNOSIS
- Rectal prolapse
- Hemorrhoids
- Bartholin cyst
- Vaginal cyst
- Urethral diverticulum
- Cervical elongation

DIAGNOSTIC TESTS & INTERPRETATION
Initial Tests (lab, imaging)
- Urinalysis if symptomatic POP (1)
- Postvoid residual (1)

Follow-Up Tests & Special Considerations
- Consider urodynamics if results would alter treatment plan.
- Selective use of upper urinary tract imaging if observation is planned or if evidence of obstruction (e.g., abnormal postvoid residual) (1)
- If fecal incontinence or significant change in bowel habits, selective use of lower GI tract imaging or endoscopy (1)
- Consider defecography if severity of symptoms is out of proportion with the extent of prolapse.

TREATMENT

GENERAL MEASURES

- Treatment is generally guided by degree of bother for the patient. It is important to document the patient's desire, goals, and expectations.
- Treatment should consider type and severity of symptoms, patient's age, other comorbid conditions, sexual function, infertility, and risk of recurrence.
- Treatment for asymptomatic patients:
  - Stage 1 or 2: clinical observation
  - Stage 3 or 4: regular follow-up and evaluation (every 3 to 6 months) (2)
- Expectant management is an acceptable option for patients without evidence of urinary or bowel obstruction.
- Treatment is indicated when there is urinary/bowel obstruction or hydronephrosis regardless of the degree of prolapse.
- A vaginal pessary should be considered in all women presenting with symptomatic prolapse.
  - There are >13 types of pessaries.
  - The most commonly used pessaries are the ring pessary and Gellhorn.
  - Most women can be successfully fitted with a pessary.
  - Satisfaction rate for patients using pessaries is very high (5).
- Minor complications such as vaginal discharge and odor can often be treated with vaginal estrogen.
- Vaginal erosion can be treated by removal of pessary and optional vaginal estrogen supplementation.
- Complications such as erosions, abrasions, ulcerations, vaginal bleeding, and fistulas may be seen with neglected pessaries.

MEDICATION

There are no data to support the use of vaginal estrogen or other medications for the prevention or treatment of POP.

ISSUES FOR REFERRAL

Referral when pessary or surgery is necessary

ADDITIONAL THERAPIES

Pelvic floor muscle training: may reduce the symptoms of POP. Pelvic floor muscle training does not affect the degree of prolapse, only the symptoms (5).

SURGERY/OTHER PROCEDURES

- Reconstructive procedures are performed with the goal of restoration of vaginal anatomy and resolution of symptoms.
- There are a variety of surgeries for repair of the anterior, apical, and posterior compartments. Surgical approaches include vaginal, abdominal, laparoscopic (straight stick and robot assisted).
- Reconstructive surgery using native tissue is associated with an elevated rate of failure (1 in 3 lifetime risk of repeat surgery). Procedures, using surgical mesh and graft material, have higher success rates.
- Surgical repair should focus on repairing all affected compartments in a single procedure.
- Coexisting stress incontinence should be addressed at the same time as the prolapse repair.
- For apical repairs:
  - Sacral colpopexy uses surgical mesh and has higher success rates and overall durability. It can be performed abdominally, laparoscopically, or robotically. The risk of recurrent prolapse is considered lower with sacral colpopexy than vaginal approaches; there may be an elevated risk of complications (6).
  - Concomitant hysterectomy is generally performed with prolapse repair. The risk of mesh extrusions appears to be decreased by retaining the cervix.
  - Uterine preservation via hysteropexy is also an option and may be offered by some surgeons. The risks and benefits of uterine preservation in prolapse repair remain unclear.

 ONGOING CARE

PATIENT EDUCATION

- Patients should have POP explained to them with diagrams and descriptions of their anatomy.
- Important to emphasize that surgery is geared toward improving quality of life
- Patients should be educated about pessary complications and possible symptoms of POP if they are still asymptomatic.
- Using insoluble fibers may help patients with bowel complaints such as constipation.

COMPLICATIONS

- Recurrence rates are variable and quoted between 3.4% and 29.2% (3).
- There is a risk of dyspareunia and pelvic pain after any surgical repair. Those repairs using mesh may also be complicated by mesh erosion (6).

- Risk of complications with pessary includes vaginal erosion and fistula in patients that are lost to follow-up.
- Severe prolapse can lead to urinary retention and defecatory dysfunction that may go unrecognized in the elderly.

REFERENCES

1. Dumoulin C, Hunter KF, Moore K, et al. Conservative management for female urinary incontinence and pelvic organ prolapse review 2013: summary of the 5th International Consultation on Incontinence. *Neurourol Urodyn*. 2016;35(1):15–20
2. Weber A, Richter H. Pelvic organ prolapse. *Obstet Gynecol*. 2005;106(3):615–634.
3. Barber MD, Maher C. Epidemiology and outcome assessment of pelvic organ prolapse. *Int Urogynecol J*. 2013;24(11):1783–1790.
4. Wu JM, Vaughan CP, Goode PS, et al. Prevalence and trends of symptomatic pelvic floor disorders in U.S. women. *Obstet Gynecol*. 2014;123(1):141–148.
5. Hagen S, Stark D. Conservative prevention and management of pelvic organ prolapse in women. *Cochrane Database Syst Rev*. 2011;(12):CD003882.
6. Maher C, Feiner B, Baessler K, et al. Surgical management of pelvic organ prolapse in women. *Cochrane Database Syst Rev*. 2013;(4):CD004014.

CODES

ICD10

- N81.9 Female genital prolapse, unspecified
- N81.10 Cystocele, unspecified
- N99.3 Prolapse of vaginal vault after hysterectomy

CLINICAL PEARLS

- Many women do not discuss POP with their doctor—ask routinely.
- Vaginal pessary should be considered in all patients with symptomatic prolapse.
- Treatment should be guided by degree of bother and impact on patient's quality of life.

U

UTERINE MYOMAS

Christina N. Kufel, DO, MS • Michael P. Hopkins, MD, MEd

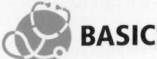 **BASICS**

DESCRIPTION

- Uterine leiomyomas are well-circumscribed, pseudo-encapsulated, benign monoclonal tumors composed mainly of smooth muscle with varying amounts of fibrous connective tissue (1).
- Three major subtypes
  - Subserous: common; external; may become pedunculated
  - Intramural: common; within myometrium; may cause marked uterine enlargement
  - Submucous: ~5% of all cases; internal, evoking abnormal uterine bleeding and infection; occasionally protruding from cervix
- Rare locations: broad, round, and uterosacral ligaments
- System affected: reproductive
- Synonym(s): fibroids; myoma; fibromyoma; myofibroma; fibroleiomyoma

EPIDEMIOLOGY

Incidence

- Cumulative incidence up to 80%
  - 60% in African American women by age 35 years; 80% by age 50 years
  - 40% in Caucasian women by age 35 years; 70% by age 50 years (1,2,3)
- Incidence increases with each decade during reproductive years.
- Rarely seen in premenarchal females
- Predominant sex: females only

ETIOLOGY AND PATHOPHYSIOLOGY

- Enlargement of benign smooth muscle tumors that may lead to symptoms affecting the reproductive, GI, or genitourinary system
- Complex multifactorial process involving transition from normal myocyte to abnormal cells and then to visibly evident tumor (monoclonal expansion)
  - Hormones (1): Increases in estrogen and progesterone are correlated with myoma formation (i.e., rarely seen before menarche). Estrogen receptors in myomas bind more estradiol than normal myometrium.
  - Growth factors (1)
    - Increased smooth muscle proliferation (transforming growth factor β [TGF-β], basic fibroblast growth factor [bFGF])
    - Increase DNA synthesis (epidermal growth factor [EGF], platelet-derived growth factor [PDGF], activin, myostatin)
    - Stimulate synthesis of extracellular matrix (TGF-β)
    - Promote mitogenesis (TGF-β, EGF, insulin-like growth factor [IGF], prolactin)
    - Promote angiogenesis (bFGF, vascular endothelial growth factor [VEGF])
  - Vasoconstrictive hypoxia (1): proposed, but not confirmed, mechanism of myometrial injury during menstruation

Genetics

- A variety of somatic chromosomal rearrangements have been described in 40% of uterine myomas.
  - Mutations in the gene encoding mediator complex subunit 12 (MED12) on the X chromosome were found in 70% of myomas in one study (2).
- Higher levels of aromatase and therefore estrogen have been found in myomas in African American women (2).

RISK FACTORS

- African American heritage
  - 2.9 times greater risk than Caucasian women; occur at a younger age, are more numerous, larger, and more symptomatic (1,3)
- Early menarche (<10 years)
- Oral contraceptive use before 16 years old (3)
- Nulliparous
- Hypertension
- Familial predisposition
  - 2.5 times more likely in women with a first-degree relative with myomas (1)
- Obesity
  - Risk increases by 21% with each 10 kg of weight gain (1).
- Alcohol
- Risk decreased by parity, progesterone-only contraceptives, diet (fruits, veggies, low fat dairy) (3)

COMMONLY ASSOCIATED CONDITIONS

Endometrial and breast cancer also associated with high, unopposed estrogen stimulation

 DIAGNOSIS

HISTORY

- Usually asymptomatic; 30% present with abnormal symptoms—usually enlarged uterus or heavy bleeding (3).
- Symptoms include the following:
  - Abnormal uterine bleeding: usually heavy/prolonged menses
  - Pain: infrequent; usually associated with torsion of pedunculated myoma, degeneration, or cervical dilation by submucous myoma near cervical os
  - Pressure on bladder: suprapubic discomfort, urinary frequency/obstruction
  - Pressure on rectosigmoid: may cause low back pain, constipation
  - Infertility: rare, estimated 1–2.5%; usually from submucous myoma distorting the uterine cavity or interference with implantation

ALERT
Rapid growth, particularly in perimenopausal/postmenopausal patients; may indicate sarcoma; extremely rare, 0.1–0.3% of cases

PHYSICAL EXAM

- Usually incidental finding on abdominal and pelvic exam
- Firm, smooth nodules/masses arising from uterus
- Masses are mobile without tenderness.

DIFFERENTIAL DIAGNOSIS

- Intrauterine pregnancy
- Cancer, including ovarian, uterine, or leiomyosarcoma
- Cecal/sigmoid tumor
- Appendiceal abscess
- Diverticulitis
- Pelvic kidney
- Urachal cyst

DIAGNOSTIC TESTS & INTERPRETATION

Initial Tests (lab, imaging)

- Pregnancy test
- Hemoglobin

- Pelvic ultrasound: standard confirmatory test; shows characteristic hypoechoic appearance (3,4)
- Saline infusion hysterosonography: helps to distinguish submucosal myomas
- Hysterosalpingogram: evaluates the contour of the endometrial cavity (4)
- CT scan or MRI: provides info on degeneration and special relationships (3); may help to differentiate complex cases or used when uterine artery embolization is planned (4)[B]

Follow-Up Tests & Special Considerations

Consider cancer antigen 125 (CA-125): may be slightly elevated in some cases of uterine myoma but generally more useful in differentiating myomas from various gynecologic adenocarcinomas

- IV pyelogram: if suspect ureteral distortion (4)
- Barium enema

Diagnostic Procedures/Other

- Fractional dilation and curettage: aids in ruling out cervical/uterine carcinomas when clinically suspicious
- Hysteroscopy: helps to diagnose submucosal/intracavitary myomas
- Laparoscopy: useful in complex cases and to rule out other pelvic diseases/disorders

Test Interpretation

- Myomas are usually multiple and vary in size and location; have been reported up to 100 lb
- Gross pathology: firm tumors with characteristic whorl-like trabeculated appearance; a thin pseudo-capsular layer is present.
- Microscopic: bundles of smooth muscle mixed with varying amounts of connective tissue elements running in different directions
- Cellular variant has a preponderance of muscle cells. Mitoses are rare.
- May undergo various types of degeneration
  - Hyaline degeneration: very common
  - Calcification: late result of circulatory impairment to myomas
  - Infection and suppuration: most common with submucosal myomas
  - Necrosis: most common with pedunculated myomas secondary to torsion

 TREATMENT

- Treatment must be individualized and based on symptoms, fertility desires, and time until menopause.
- Medical therapy may be of benefit.
- Patients with minimal symptoms may be treated with iron preparations and analgesics.
- Conservative management of asymptomatic myomas
  - Pelvic exams and ultrasounds at ≥3-month intervals if size remains stable
  - Substantial regression usually occurs after menopause.
- Surgical options should be considered if symptomatic or worrisome myomas are unresponsive to conservative/medical management.

GENERAL MEASURES

Patients not desiring pharmacologic therapy or surgery may consider the following:

- Uterine artery embolization: averages 50% shrinkage of myomas (5)[A]; painful and may cause ovarian failure (1–2%), amenorrhea, postembolization syndrome, or other complications; shorter hospital stay and quicker recovery but no difference in satisfaction compared with hysterectomy (3)[B]; high reintervention rate (15–32% by 2 years) compared to hysterectomy/myomectomy (7% by 2 years) (5)
- MR-guided focused ultrasound (MRgFUS): noninvasive, ultrasound transducer passes through abdominal wall and causes coagulative necrosis of fibroid; up to 98% reduction in myoma volume and symptoms. Not appropriate for some types of myomas. Efficacy may be comparable with other hysterectomy-sparing procedures. Fertility has been shown to be preserved (3)[A], although risks and outcomes data are limited (3).

MEDICATION

- Progestins may reduce overall uterine size (4)[B].
  - Norethindrone 10 mg/day
  - Medroxyprogesterone 200 mg IM monthly
  - Levonorgestrel intrauterine device
- Combination oral contraceptives: may help prevent development of new fibroids and control bleeding
  - Contraindications: history of thromboembolic events
- Gonadotropin-releasing hormone agonists
  - Nafarelin (nasal spray), goserelin acetate, and leuprolide
  - Induces abrupt artificial menopause; may reduce myoma symptoms dramatically; induces atrophy of myomas by up to 40% in 2 to 3 months (4)[B]
  - May be valuable as preoperative adjunct to myomectomy/hysterectomy by allowing recovery of anemia, donation of autologous blood, and possibly converting abdominal to vaginal hysterectomy (3,4,6)[B]
  - Not recommended for use >6 months because of osteoporosis risk
  - Following discontinuation, myomas return within 60 days to pretherapy size.
- Antiprogesterones
  - Mifepristone
    - Shown to have similar reduction in myoma size as gonadotropin-releasing hormone agonists
    - Decreases heavy bleeding and increases quality of life (7)[A]
  - Selective progesterone receptor modulator (SPRM)
    - Ulipristal acetate: may be as effective as gonadotropin-releasing hormones with fewer side effects (3)[B]

ISSUES FOR REFERRAL

- Medical therapy may be initiated by a primary care physician/gynecologist after adequate pelvic examination.
- Surgical considerations may be pursued with gynecologic consultation.
- Uterine embolization may be discussed with an interventional radiologist.

SURGERY/OTHER PROCEDURES

- Surgical management is indicated in the following situations (4)[B]:
  - Excessive uterine size or excessive rate of growth (except during pregnancy)
  - Submucosal myomas when associated with hypermenorrhea
  - Pedunculated myomas that are painful or undergo torsion, necrosis, and hemorrhage

- If a myoma causes symptoms from pressure on bladder/rectum
  - If differentiation from ovarian mass is not possible
  - If associated pelvic disease is present (endometriosis, pelvic inflammatory disease)
  - If infertility/habitual abortion is likely due to the anatomic location of the myoma
- Surgical procedures
  - Preliminary pelvic examination, Pap smear, and endometrial biopsy should be performed to rule out malignant/premalignant conditions.
  - Hysterectomy: may be performed vaginally, laparoscopically, robotically, or by laparotomy
    - Effective in relieving symptoms and improving quality of life (3)[B]
    - Similar fertility and live birth rates between laparoscopic and abdominal myomectomy
    - FDA discourages the use of laparoscopic power morcellation during hysterectomy or myomectomy for uterine fibroids given the risk of spreading an occult malignancy and all patients should be counseled preoperatively of risk (3).
  - Abdominal, laparoscopic, robotic, or hysteroscopic myomectomy may be performed in younger women who want to maintain fertility (4,8)[B].
  - Hysteroscopic/laparoscopic cautery/laser myoma resection can be performed in selected patients.
  - Endometrial ablation: for small submucosal myomas

ADMISSION, INPATIENT, AND NURSING CONSIDERATIONS

- Usually outpatient
- Inpatient for some surgical procedures

 ONGOING CARE

FOLLOW-UP RECOMMENDATIONS

Patient Monitoring

- Pelvic examination and ultrasound: every 2 to 3 months for newly diagnosed symptomatic/excessively large myomas
- Hemoglobin and hematocrit: if uterine bleeding is excessive
- Once uterine size and symptoms stabilize, monitor every 6 to 12 months although no high-quality evidence exists (3).

DIET

No restrictions

PATIENT EDUCATION

- Society of Interventional Radiology: http://sirweb.org/patients/uterine-fibroids/
- U.S. Department of Health and Human Services: http://www.womenshealth.gov/publications/our-publications/fact-sheet/uterine-fibroids.html?from=AtoZ
- American Congress of Obstetricians and Gynecologists: http://www.acog.org

PROGNOSIS

- Resection of submucosal fibroids has been associated with increased fertility.
- At least 10% of myomas recur after myomectomy; however, only 25% require further treatment (3)[B].

COMPLICATIONS

- May mask other gynecologic malignancies (e.g., uterine sarcoma, ovarian cancer)
- Degenerating fibroids may cause pain and bleeding.
- May rarely prolapse through the cervix

Pregnancy Considerations

- Rapid growth of fibroids is common.
- Pregnant women may need additional fetal testing if placenta is located over or near fibroid.
- Complications during pregnancy: abortion, premature labor, 2nd-trimester rapid growth leading to degeneration/pain, 3rd-trimester fetal malpresentation, and dystocia during labor and delivery
- Cesarean section is recommended if the endometrial cavity was entered during myomectomy due to increased risk of uterine rupture.

Geriatric Considerations

Postmenopausal patients with newly diagnosed uterine myoma/enlarging uterine myomas have a high suspicion of uterine sarcoma/other gynecologic malignancy.

REFERENCES

1. Parker WH. Etiology, symptomatology, and diagnosis of uterine myomas. *Fertil Steril*. 2007;87(4):725–736.
2. Bulun SE. Uterine fibroids. *N Engl J Med*. 2013;369(14):1344–1355.
3. Stewart EA. Clinical practice. Uterine fibroids. *N Engl J Med*. 2015;372(17):1646–1655.
4. Wallach EE, Vlahos NF. Uterine myomas: an overview of development, clinical features, and management. *Obstet Gynecol*. 2004;104(2):393–406.
5. Gupta JK, Sinha A, Lumsden MA, et al. Uterine artery embolization for symptomatic uterine fibroids. *Cochrane Database Syst Rev*. 2014;(12):CD005073.
6. Lethaby A, Vollenhoven B, Sowter M. Pre-operative GnRH analogue therapy before hysterectomy or myomectomy for uterine fibroids. *Cochrane Database Syst Rev*. 2001;(2):CD000547.
7. Tristan M, Orozco LJ, Steed A, et al. Mifepristone for uterine fibroids. *Cochrane Database Syst Rev*. 2012;(8):CD007687.
8. NICE interventional procedure guidance 522. Hysteroscopic morcellation of uterine leiomyomas (fibroids). www.guidance.nice.org.uk/guidance/ipg522. Accessed December 30, 2017.

ADDITIONAL READING

Laughlin SK, Schroeder JC, Baird DD. New directions in the epidemiology of uterine fibroids. *Semin Reprod Med*. 2010;28(3):204–217.

 CODES

ICD10

- D25.9 Leiomyoma of uterus, unspecified
- D25.2 Subserosal leiomyoma of uterus
- D25.1 Intramural leiomyoma of uterus

CLINICAL PEARLS

- Uterine myomas are benign smooth muscle tumors composed mainly of fibrous connective tissue.
- Usually incidental finding on pelvic exam or ultrasound but may cause pelvic pain and pressure, abnormal uterine bleeding, and/or infertility
- Management ranges from conservative to medical to surgical.

U

Shailendra K. Saxena, MD, PhD • Mikayla L. Spangler, PharmD • Laura K. Klug, PharmD

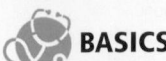

BASICS

DESCRIPTION
- A nonspecific term used to describe any intraocular inflammatory disorder
- Symptoms vary depending on depth of involvement and associated conditions.
- The uvea is the middle layer of the eye between the sclera and retina. The anterior part of the uvea includes the iris and ciliary body. The posterior part of the uvea is the choroid.
  - Anterior uveitis: refers to ocular inflammation limited to the iris (iritis) alone or iris and ciliary body (iridocyclitis)
  - Intermediate uveitis: refers to inflammation of the structures just posterior to the lens (pars planitis or peripheral uveitis)
  - Posterior uveitis: refers to inflammation of the choroid (choroiditis), retina (retinitis), or vitreous near the optic nerve and macula
- System(s) affected: nervous
- Synonym(s): iritis; iridocyclitis; choroiditis; retinochoroiditis; chorioretinitis; anterior uveitis; posterior uveitis; pars planitis; panuveitis. Synonyms are anatomic descriptions of the focus of the uveal inflammation.

Geriatric Considerations
The inflammatory response to systemic disease may be suppressed.

Pediatric Considerations
- Infection should be the primary consideration.
- Allergies and psychological factors (depression, stress) may serve as a trigger.
- Trauma is also a common cause in this population.

Pregnancy Considerations
May be of importance in the selection of medications

EPIDEMIOLOGY
- Predominant age: all ages
- Predominant sex: male = female, except for human leukocyte antigen B27 (HLA-B27) anterior uveitis: male > female, autoimmune etiology: female > male

Incidence
- Overall prevalence is 38 to 714 cases/100,000 annual incidence.
- Anterior uveitis is the most common.

Prevalence
Iritis is 4 times more prevalent than posterior uveitis.

ETIOLOGY AND PATHOPHYSIOLOGY
- Infectious: may result from viral, bacterial, parasitic, or fungal etiologies
- Suspected immune mediated: possible autoimmune or immune complex–mediated mechanism postulated in association with systemic (especially rheumatologic) disorders
  - Autoimmune uveitis (AIU) patients should be referred to an ophthalmologist for local treatment.
- Isolated eye disease
- Idiopathic (~25%)
- Some medications may cause uveitis. The most causative medications include rifabutin, bisphosphonates, sulfonamides, metipranolol, topical corticosteroids, brimonidine, prostaglandin analogs, anti–vascular endothelial growth factor (VEGF) agents, bacillus Calmette-Guérin (BCG) vaccination, and systemic and intraocular cidofovir.

- Masquerade syndromes: diseases such as malignancies that may be mistaken for primary inflammation of the eye

Genetics
- No specific pattern for uveitis in general
- Iritis: 50–70% are HLA-B27 positive.
- Predisposing gene for posterior uveitis associated with Behçet disease may include HLA-B51.

RISK FACTORS
- No specific risk factors
- Higher incidence is seen with specific associated conditions.

COMMONLY ASSOCIATED CONDITIONS
- Viral infections: herpes simplex, herpes zoster, HIV, cytomegalovirus, congenital Zika virus
- Bacterial infections: brucellosis, leprosy, leptospirosis, Lyme disease, propionibacterium infection, syphilis, tuberculosis (TB), Whipple disease
- Parasitic infections: acanthamebiasis, cysticercosis, onchocerciasis, toxocariasis, toxoplasmosis
- Fungal infections: aspergillosis, blastomycosis, candidiasis, coccidioidomycosis, cryptococcosis, histoplasmosis, sporotrichosis
- Suspected immune mediated: ankylosing spondylitis, Behçet disease, Crohn disease, drug or hypersensitivity reaction, interstitial nephritis, juvenile rheumatoid arthritis, Kawasaki disease, multiple sclerosis, psoriatic arthritis, Reiter syndrome, relapsing polychondritis, sarcoidosis, Sjögren syndrome, systemic lupus erythematosus, ulcerative colitis, vasculitis, vitiligo, Vogt-Koyanagi (Harada) syndrome
- Isolated eye disease: acute multifocal placoid pigmentary epitheliopathy, acute retinal necrosis, birdshot choroidopathy, Fuchs heterochromic cyclitis, glaucomatocyclitic crisis, lens-induced uveitis, multifocal choroiditis, pars planitis, serpiginous choroiditis, sympathetic ophthalmia, trauma
- Masquerade syndromes: leukemia, lymphoma, retinitis pigmentosa, retinoblastoma

DIAGNOSIS

HISTORY
- Decreased visual acuity
- Pain, photophobia, blurring of vision (1)[C]
  - Usually acute
- Anterior uveitis (~80% of patients with uveitis) (1)[C]
  - Generally acute in onset
  - Deep eye pain
  - Photophobia (consensual)
- Intermediate and posterior uveitis (2)
  - Unresolving floaters
  - Generally insidious in onset
  - More commonly bilateral

PHYSICAL EXAM
Slit-lamp exam and indirect ophthalmoscopy are necessary for precise diagnosis (1)[C].
- Anterior uveitis (~80% of patients with uveitis)
  - Conjunctival vessel dilation
  - Perilimbal (circumcorneal) dilation of episcleral and scleral vessels (ciliary flush)
  - Small pupillary size of affected eye
  - Hypopyon or hyphema (WBCs or RBCs pooled in the anterior chamber)

- Frequently unilateral (95% of HLA-B27–associated cases); if first occurrence and otherwise asymptomatic, no further diagnostic testing is needed (1)[C].
  - Bilateral involvement and systemic symptoms (fever, fatigue, abdominal pain) may be associated with interstitial nephritis (1)[C].
  - Systemic disease is most likely to be associated with anterior uveitis (in one study, 53% of patients were found to have systemic disease) (1)[C].
- Intermediate and posterior uveitis
  - More commonly bilateral
  - Posterior inflammation will generally cause minimal pain or redness unless associated with an iritis.

DIFFERENTIAL DIAGNOSIS
- Acute angle-closure glaucoma
- Conjunctivitis
- Episcleritis
- Keratitis
- Scleritis

DIAGNOSTIC TESTS & INTERPRETATION
No specific test for the diagnosis of uveitis. Tests for etiologic factors or associated conditions should be based on history and physical exam (1)[C].

Initial Tests (lab, imaging)
- CBC, BUN, creatinine (interstitial nephritis) (1)[C]
- HLA-B27 typing (ankylosing spondylitis, Reiter syndrome) (1)[C]
- Antinuclear antibody, ESR (systemic lupus erythematosus, Sjögren syndrome) (1)[C]
- Venereal disease research laboratory (VDRL) test, fluorescent titer antibody (syphilis) (1)[C]
- Fluorescent treponemal antibody absorption (FTA-ABS) or microhemagglutination assay for antibodies to Treponema pallidum (MHA-TP) (1)[C]
- Purified protein derivative (PPD) tuberculin skin test (TB) (1)[C]
- Lyme serology (Lyme disease) (1)[C]
- Disorders that may alter lab results: immunodeficiency
- Chest x-ray (sarcoidosis, histoplasmosis, TB, lymphoma) (1)[C]
- Sacroiliac radiograph (ankylosing spondylitis) (1)[C]

Diagnostic Procedures/Other
Slit-lamp exam (1)[C]

Test Interpretation
- Keratic precipitates
- Inflammatory cells in anterior chamber or vitreous
- Synechiae (fibrous tissue scarring between iris and lens)
- Macular edema
- Perivasculitis of retinal vessels

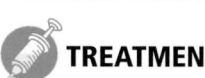

TREATMENT

GENERAL MEASURES
- Outpatient care with urgent ophthalmologic consultation
- Medical therapy is best initiated following full ophthalmologic evaluation.
- Treatment of underlying cause, if identified
- Anti-inflammatory therapy

MEDICATION

First Line

- The treatment depends on the etiology, location, and severity of the inflammation.
- Prednisolone acetate 1% ophthalmic suspension: 2 drops to the affected eye q1h initially, tapering to once a day with improvement
  - Contraindications
    - Hypersensitivity to the medication or component of the preparation
    - Topical corticosteroid therapy is contraindicated in uveitis secondary to infectious etiologies, unless used in conjunction with appropriate anti-infectious agents.
  - Precautions
    - Topical corticosteroids may increase intraocular pressure, increase susceptibility to infections, impair corneal or scleral wound healing, or cause corneal epithelial toxicity or crystalline keratopathy. Prolonged use may cause cataract formation and exacerbate existing herpetic keratitis, which may masquerade as iritis.
  - Significant possible interactions
- Systemic corticosteroids are useful for maintenance therapy for patients with noninfectious uveitis. These should always be used with other immunosuppressive medications for steroid-sparing effects; prednisone 5 to 10 mg daily (3,4)[B]
- Cycloplegic agents may be used to dilate the eye and relieve pain. Agents include scopolamine hydrobromide 0.25% (Isopto Hyoscine) or atropine 1% 1 to 2 drops up to QID or homatropine hydrobromide (Isopto) 2% or 5% 1 to 2 drops BID or as often as q3h if necessary (1)[C].
  - Contraindications
    - Cycloplegia is contraindicated in patients known to have, or be predisposed to, glaucoma.
  - Precautions
    - Use extreme caution in infants, young children, and elderly because of increased susceptibility to systemic effects.

Second Line

- Anti-inflammatory: prednisolone sodium phosphate 1%, dexamethasone sodium phosphate 0.1%, dexamethasone suspension, rimexolone 1% (Vexol), and loteprednol etabonate 0.5% (Lotemax), difluprednate (Durezol) 0.05% (1,4)[C]
  - Rimexolone 1% (Vexol) may be equally effective as prednisolone acetate 1% for short-term treatment of anterior uveitis (1)[C].
  - Loteprednol etabonate (Lotemax) may not be as effective as prednisolone acetate 1% but may be less likely to increase intraocular pressure in cases of acute anterior uveitis.
- Periocular corticosteroids may be injected with triamcinolone acetonide being most commonly used; 40 mg/1 mL (5)[C]
- Intravitreous corticosteroid deposits may also be used for long-term maintenance; fluocinolone acetonide (Retisert) 590 μg released >30 months, dexamethasone (Ozurdex) 0.7 mg released slowly >3 to 6 months (4,5)[B]
  - Retisert has caused all patients to develop cataracts and significant increases in intraocular pressure in about 2/3 of patients, whereas Ozurdex had only 1/4 of patients require medication for increased intraocular pressure and 15% develop cataracts (5)[C].

- Intravitreal corticosteroid injections are used only in severe cases of recurrence; triamcinolone acetonide 4 to 20 mg/0.1 mL, dexamethasone phosphate 0.4 mg/0.1 mL, dexamethasone implant (Ozurdex)
  - Ozurdex has a longer effect than triamcinolone acetonide.
- Immunosuppressive agents including antimetabolites (methotrexate, azathioprine, and mycophenolate mofetil), T-cell inhibitors (cyclosporine, tacrolimus, and sirolimus), and alkylating agents (cyclophosphamide, chlorambucil) may be employed in cases resistant to initial treatment, but close monitoring is required (4,5)[C].
- Advancing research suggests benefit of the biologic agents in refractory uveitis. Adalimumab has gained FDA approval for this indication. Some expert panels recommend adalimumab and infliximab as second-line therapy options. Other biologic agents including etanercept, golimumab, secukinumab, and tocilizumab have also been studied.
  - Benefits of biologic therapy include glucocorticoid sparing effects, but limitations may include high cost and adverse effect potential (3,4)[C].
- Systemic and ophthalmic preparations of NSAIDs may provide some symptom relief (1)[C].

ISSUES FOR REFERRAL
Caution should be used when using empiric treatment; referral to an ophthalmologist is recommended in most cases.

SURGERY/OTHER PROCEDURES
Various surgical procedures may be used therapeutically for visual rehabilitation, diagnostically, or to manage complications associated with uveitis (6).

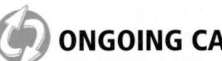 ## ONGOING CARE

FOLLOW-UP RECOMMENDATIONS
Patient Monitoring
- Complete history and physical to evaluate for associated systemic disease
- Ophthalmologic follow-up as recommended by consultant

PATIENT EDUCATION
- Instruct on proper method for instilling eye drops.
- Wear dark glasses if photophobia is a problem.

PROGNOSIS
- Depends on the presence of causal diseases or associated conditions
- Uveitis resulting from infections (systemic or local) tends to resolve with eradication of the underlying infection.
- Uveitis associated with seronegative arthropathies tends to be acute (lasting <3 months) and frequently recurrent.

COMPLICATIONS
- Cycloplegia: paralysis of the ciliary muscle of the eye, resulting in a loss of accommodation
- Loss of vision as a result of the following:
  - Keratic precipitate deposition on the corneal or lens surfaces (1)
  - Increased intraocular pressure, acute angle-closure glaucoma (1)
  - Formation of synechiae
  - Cataract formation (1)

- Vasculitis with vascular occlusion, retinal infarction
- Macular edema (1)
- Optic nerve damage

REFERENCES

1. American Optometric Association. Optometric clinical practice guideline: care of the patient with anterior uveitis. https://www.aoa.org/documents/optometrists/CPG-7.pdf. Accessed November 10, 2017.
2. Selmi C. Diagnosis and classification of autoimmune uveitis. *Autoimmun Rev.* 2014;13(4–5):591–594.
3. Chen SC, Sheu SJ. Recent advances in managing and understanding uveitis. *F1000Res.* 2017;6:280.
4. Babu K, Mahendradas P. Medical management of uveitis—current trends. *Indian J Ophthalmol.* 2013;61(6):277–283.
5. Gallego-Pinazo R, Dolz-Marco R, Martínez-Castillo S, et al. Update on the principles and novel local and systemic therapies for the treatment of non-infectious uveitis. *Inflamm Allergy Drug Targets.* 2013;12(1):38–45.
6. Murthy SI, Pappuru RR, Latha KM, et al. Surgical management in patient with uveitis. *Indian J Ophthalmol.* 2013;61(6):284–290.

ADDITIONAL READING

- Majumder PD, Biswas J. Pediatric uveitis: an update. *Oman J Ophthalmol.* 2013;6(3):140–150.
- Pan J, Kapur M, McCallum R. Noninfectious immune-mediated uveitis and ocular inflammation. *Curr Allergy Asthma Rep.* 2014;14(1):409.
- Yang MM, Lai TY, Luk FO, et al. The roles of genetic factors in uveitis and their clinical significance. *Retina.* 2014;34(1):1–11.

 ## SEE ALSO

Conjunctivitis, Acute; Glaucoma, Primary Closed-Angle; Scleritis

 ## CODES

ICD10
- H20.9 Unspecified iridocyclitis
- H30.90 Unspecified chorioretinal inflammation, unspecified eye
- H20.019 Primary iridocyclitis, unspecified eye

CLINICAL PEARLS

- Symptoms vary depending on depth of involvement and associated conditions but should be suspected when eye pain is associated with visual changes.
- Severe or unresponsive uveitis may require therapy, including periocular injection of corticosteroids, sustained-release corticosteroid implants, systemic corticosteroids, cytotoxic agents, immunosuppressive agents, immunomodulatory agents, or tumor necrosis factor inhibitors.

U

VAGINAL ADENOSIS

Maeve K. Hopkins, MD • Michael P. Hopkins, MD, MEd

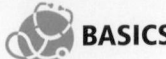

BASICS

DESCRIPTION
- The normal vagina is lined with squamous epithelium. Adenosis is characterized by the presence of columnar epithelium or glandular tissue in the wall of the vagina.
- Around week 15 of embryologic development, the müllerian system, which forms the upper 2/3 of the vagina, fuses with the invaginating cloaca or urogenital sinus to form the lower 1/3 of the vagina. Squamous metaplasia from the cloacal region then produces squamous epithelium within the vagina (1).
- *Adenosis* occurs when this squamous epithelium fails to epithelialize the vagina completely.
- Three main types of adenosis epithelium:
  - Endocervical
  - Endometrial
  - Tubal
- System(s) affected: reproductive

Geriatric Considerations
- Adenosis is a disorder of the young female. By menopause, the vagina and cervix should be completely epithelialized.
- In a postmenopausal patient, the presence of glandular epithelium is an indication for excision and evaluation, given the risk of well-differentiated adenocarcinoma.

Pregnancy Considerations
Pregnancy produces a wide eversion of the transformation zone of the cervix. This can become so widely everted that it will extend onto the vaginal fornices, leading to the impression of adenosis. This will resolve after pregnancy.

EPIDEMIOLOGY
Incidence
- Although the cumulative incidence of vaginal adenosis is unknown, the incidence of cloacal malformations is 1/20,000 to 1/25,000 live births.
- Although spontaneous vaginal adenosis appears to be fairly common (10% of adult women), it is mostly an insignificant coincidental finding. Widespread symptomatic involvement is rare (2).

Prevalence
- In the United States, adenosis is common in young women, affecting 10–20%. As maturation progresses with puberty, epithelialization occurs.
- Predominant age
  - Age <1 month: 15%
  - Prepubertal: typically absent
  - Age 13 to 25 years: 13%
  - Age >25 years: decreasing prevalence, uncommon beyond age 30 years (2)

ETIOLOGY AND PATHOPHYSIOLOGY
- In most young females, the etiology is incomplete squamous metaplasia or epithelialization. This occurs as a natural phenomenon and resolves with age.
- Described as congenital or acquired:
  - Congenital: proliferation of the remnant müllerian epithelium in the vagina due to exposure to diethylstilbestrol (DES) in utero ("DES daughters"). DES is a synthetic, nonsteroidal estrogen used to prevent miscarriage or premature deliveries from 1938 to 1971 (3). An estimated 5 million women were prescribed DES during this period (4).
  - Transformation-related protein 63 (TRP63/p63) marks the cell fate of müllerian duct epithelium to become squamous epithelium in the cervix and vagina. DES disrupts the TRP63 expression and induces adenosis lesions (4). It has also been suggested that DES induces vaginal adenosis by inhibiting the BMP4/activin A-regulated vaginal cell fate through a downregulation of RUNX1 (5).
  - Acquired: trauma and inflammation causing spontaneous de novo changes or changes in an acquired lesion in the vaginal epithelium
  - Additional reports documented adenosis subsequent to sulfonamide-induced Stevens-Johnson syndrome and after treatment of vaginal condylomas with 5-fluorouracil (6).

RISK FACTORS
Adenosis of the vagina/cervix may arise in up to 90% of DES daughters and has a 40-fold increased risk of developing into clear cell adenocarcinoma (3).

GENERAL PREVENTION
None: Last DES exposure was in the 1970s.

COMMONLY ASSOCIATED CONDITIONS
DES exposure
- Adenosis from DES exposure should lead to an evaluation of other DES-related abnormalities.
- Müllerian tract anomalies associated with DES exposure include cervical hood, cervical ridge, shortened cervix, incompetent cervix, and T-shaped uterine cavity.
- Patients with known DES exposure should have their reproductive tract evaluated prior to conception.
- Most patients with adenosis have not been DES-exposed and do not require evaluation of the reproductive system.
- The FDA issued a drug bulletin in 1971 advising physicians to stop prescribing DES to pregnant women because of its link to vaginal clear cell adenocarcinoma in DES daughters (3).

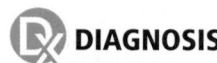

DIAGNOSIS

HISTORY
- Maternal DES exposure
- Complaints of
  - Profuse mucoid vaginal discharge from the glandular epithelium
  - Pruritus
  - Pain/soreness of the vaginal introitus
  - Postcoital bleeding
  - Dyspareunia

PHYSICAL EXAM
On pelvic exam, adenosis appearance is varied: patchy or diffuse red stippling, granularity or nodularity, single or multiple cysts, erosions, ulcers, or warty protuberances that may even extend to the vulva.

DIFFERENTIAL DIAGNOSIS
- Erosive lichen planus
- Fixed drug eruption
- Erythema multiforme
- Bullous skin disease
- Adenocarcinoma

DIAGNOSTIC TESTS & INTERPRETATION
Initial Tests (lab, imaging)
Four-quadrant Pap smear should be used liberally to isolate quadrants of the vagina that may contain abnormalities. No imaging is indicated, unless diagnosed with underlying malignancy.

Follow-Up Tests & Special Considerations

Pap smear can be followed by colposcopy and biopsy.

Diagnostic Procedures/Other

- Colposcopy should be used to outline areas of adenosis to ensure that no malignancy is present.
- A thorough evaluation for adenocarcinoma of the vagina arising in adenosis should be done.
- A biopsy may be necessary to ensure that the process represents only benign adenosis.

Test Interpretation

- Biopsy will show benign glandular epithelium.
- Biopsies may show areas of ongoing squamous metaplasia.

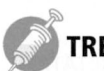 TREATMENT

GENERAL MEASURES

- Unless malignancy is present, treatment is conservative.
- In most young females with this condition, it will resolve with expectant management.
- Treatment is warranted in women with severe subjective symptoms that impair the quality of life.
- First-line treatment: If indicated in patients with focal lesions and no history of DES exposure, simple excision is an effective treatment (6).

ISSUES FOR REFERRAL

Malignancy found on biopsy warrants referral to gynecologic oncology specialist.

SURGERY/OTHER PROCEDURES

- Aggressive therapy, such as laser or surgical excision, is necessary if premalignant or malignant changes arise (5).
- Symptomatic treatment has been performed with carbon dioxide laser coagulation, unipolar coagulation, or vaginal resection.

ADMISSION, INPATIENT, AND NURSING CONSIDERATIONS

Outpatient management

 ONGOING CARE

FOLLOW-UP RECOMMENDATIONS

Patient Monitoring

If the initial colposcopy is normal, a yearly four-quadrant Pap smear of the vagina and of the cervix should be performed.

DIET

No special diet is recommended.

PATIENT EDUCATION

- No limitations
- It is not necessary to avoid intercourse or placing objects in the vagina.
- The patient should be educated to keep normal guideline-recommended pelvic and Pap smear appointments. In most situations, this is benign, and expectant management is all that is necessary.
- http://www.acog.org/

PROGNOSIS

- Most patients will have squamous metaplasia and epithelialization with complete resolution of the adenosis.
- The rare patient, 1/1,000 to 1/10,000, may develop adenocarcinoma in the adenosis and will require definitive therapy as for vaginal cancer.
  - Cumulative incidence of progression of adenosis to adenocarcinoma is 1.5/1,000 for DES daughters (3).

COMPLICATIONS

- Infertility with DES association
- Adverse pregnancy outcome with DES association
- Adenocarcinoma of vagina
- Clear cell adenocarcinoma with DES association

REFERENCES

1. Reich O, Fritsch H. The developmental origin of cervical and vaginal epithelium and their clinical consequences: a systematic review. *J Low Genit Tract Dis*. 2014;18(4):358–360.
2. Kranl C, Zelger B, Kofler H, et al. Vulval and vaginal adenosis. *Br J Dermatol*. 1998;139(1):128–131.
3. National Toxicology Program, Department of Health and Human Services. *Diethylstilbestrol*. *Report on Carcinogens*. 12th ed. Research Triangle Park, NC: National Toxicology Program, U.S. Department of Health and Human Services; 2011:159–161.
4. Laronda MM, Unno K, Butler LM, et al. The development of cervical and vaginal adenosis as a result of diethylstilbestrol exposure in utero. *Differentiation*. 2012;84(3):252–260.
5. Laronda M, Unno K, Ishi K, et al. Diethylstilbestrol induces vaginal adenosis by disrupting SMAD/RUNX1-mediated cell fate decision in the müllerian duct epithelium. *Dev Biol*. 2013;381(1):5–16.
6. Martin AA, Atkins KA, Lonergan CL, et al. Vaginal adenosis as a dermatologic complaint. *J Am Acad Dermatol*. 2013;69(2):e92–e93.

ADDITIONAL READING

- Bamigboye AA, Morris J. Oestrogen supplementation, mainly diethylstilbestrol, for preventing miscarriages and other adverse pregnancy outcomes. *Cochrane Database Syst Rev*. 2003;(3):CD004353.
- Cebesoy FB, Kutlar I, Aydin A. Vaginal adenosis successfully treated with simple unipolar cauterization. *J Natl Med Assoc*. 2007;99(2):166–167.
- Chattopadhyay I, Cruickshan DJ, Packer M. Non diethylstilbestrol induced vaginal adenosis—a case series and review of literature. *Eur J Gynaecol Oncol*. 2001;22(4):260–262.
- Sandberg EC. The incidence and distribution of occult vaginal adenosis. *Am J Obstet Gynecol*. 1968;101(3):322–334.

 SEE ALSO

Vaginal Malignancy

 CODES

ICD10

- Q52.4 Other congenital malformations of vagina
- N89.8 Other specified noninflammatory disorders of vagina
- T38.5X5A Adverse effect of other estrogens and progestogens, initial encounter

CLINICAL PEARLS

- Adenosis is characterized by the presence of columnar epithelium or glandular tissue in the wall of the vagina.
- Adenosis is common among the daughters of women exposed to DES.
- Rarely, adenosis can be associated with an underlying vaginal malignancy.

V

VAGINAL BLEEDING DURING PREGNANCY

Virginia J. Van Duyne, MD

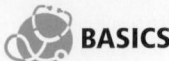 **BASICS**

DESCRIPTION

- Vaginal bleeding during pregnancy has many causes and ranges in severity from benign with normal pregnancy outcome to life-threatening for both infant and mother.
- Etiology can be from the vagina, cervix, uterus, fetus, or placenta. The differential diagnosis is guided by the gestational age of the fetus.

EPIDEMIOLOGY

Prevalence

- In early pregnancy: 7–25% of patients
- In late pregnancy: 0.3–2% of patients

ETIOLOGY AND PATHOPHYSIOLOGY

- Many times the cause is unknown.
- Anytime in pregnancy:
  - Cervicitis (infectious or noninfectious)
  - Vaginal or cervical trauma (including postcoital)
  - Cervical lesion or neoplasia
  - Hyperemia of cervix (increased blood flow from pregnancy)
- Early pregnancy:
  - For up to 50% of early pregnancy bleeding, no cause is ever found.
  - Ectopic pregnancy: leading cause of 1st-trimester maternal death in the United States. Risk factors: previous ectopic, trauma to fallopian tubes (tubal surgery, infection, tumor), congenital anomaly of tubes, in utero diethylstilbestrol (DES) exposure, current use of IUD, history of infertility, tobacco use
  - Spontaneous abortion: risk factors: advanced maternal age (AMA), alcohol use, tobacco use, anesthetic gas, heavy caffeine use, cocaine use, chronic maternal diseases (poorly controlled diabetes mellitus [DM], celiac disease, autoimmune diseases such as antiphospholipid syndrome), short interconception time (3 to 6 months), current use of IUD, maternal infection (e.g., herpes simplex virus [HSV], gonorrhea, chlamydia, toxoplasmosis, listeriosis, HIV, syphilis, malaria), medications (e.g., retinoids, methotrexate, NSAIDs), multiple previous therapeutic abortions, previous spontaneous abortion, toxins (arsenic, lead, polyurethane), uterine abnormalities (congenital, adhesions, fibroids)
  - Implantation bleeding: benign, about 6 days after fertilization
  - Uterine fibroids
  - Subchorionic bleeding: in late 1st trimester
  - Low-lying placenta
  - Gestational trophoblastic disease: hydatidiform mole (most common), choriocarcinoma, or placental-site trophoblastic tumors
- Late pregnancy:
  - Bloody show of labor (mucus plug)
  - Placenta previa: painless bleeding; occurs in 0.4% deliveries in the United States. Risk factors: previous history of placenta previa, previous uterine surgery (cesarean section, D&C), chronic hypertension, multiparity, multiple gestation, tobacco use, AMA

  - Placental abruption: (typically) painful bleeding; occurs in 1–2% deliveries in the United States. Risk factors: previous placental abruption, 1st-trimester bleeding, hypertension, preeclampsia, multiple gestation, tobacco, cocaine or methamphetamine use, unexplained elevated maternal α-fetoprotein, poly- or oligohydramnios, AMA, trauma to abdomen, premature rupture of membranes, thrombophilia, short umbilical cord, male fetus, chorioamnionitis, nutritional deficiency
  - Vasa previa: minimal bleeding with fetal distress; rare (1:2,500 deliveries). Risk factors: in vitro fertilization, multiple gestations, placental abnormalities (low-lying position, bilobate, succenturiate lobe, velamentous insertion of umbilical cord)
  - Placenta accreta, increta, percreta: risk factors: uterine scar (e.g., from cesarean section, endometrial ablation, or D&C), current placenta previa, AMA, tobacco use, multiparity, uterine anomalies, uterine fibroids, hypertension
  - Uterine rupture: vaginal bleeding, abnormal fetal heart rate, and disordered or hypertonic uterine contractions with or without pain. Risk factors: previous cesarean section (most common), trauma, use of oxytocin or prostaglandins, multiparity, external cephalic version, placental abruption, shoulder dystocia, placenta percreta, müllerian duct anomalies, history of pelvic radiation

RISK FACTORS

See specific etiologies in earlier discussion.

GENERAL PREVENTION

- Address modifiable risk factors such as domestic violence and tobacco and drug use.
- If placenta or vasa previa, nothing per vagina

DIAGNOSIS

HISTORY

- Anytime in pregnancy: quality of pregnancy dating, context (e.g., following bowel movement, during voiding, after intercourse, drug use, or trauma including domestic violence), amount of bleeding, obstetrical history, personal or family history of inherited bleeding disorders
- Early pregnancy: severe nausea/vomiting (can be associated with molar pregnancy); amount of bleeding, pelvic pain, or suprapubic cramping (e.g., spontaneous abortion, ectopic) complications in previous pregnancies (e.g., spontaneous abortion, abruption, 1st-trimester vaginal bleeding)
- Late pregnancy: contractions (labor), abdominal pain especially between contractions (abruption, uterine rupture), presence or absence of fetal movement, rupture of membranes
- See "Etiology and Pathophysiology" for additional pertinent history.

PHYSICAL EXAM

- Vital signs: When present, signs of hemodynamic instability are first tachycardia and tachypnea and then hypotension and thready pulse.

- Abdomen: uterine tenderness, fundal height (increasing fundal height may be associated with placental abruption)
- Speculum: Visualize cervix and identify source of bleeding (from cervical os or from within vagina).
- Cervix: Assess for dilation; required to assess for labor but should not be performed until placenta previa ruled out via ultrasound
- Fetal monitoring: Doppler heart tones in early pregnancy; external fetal monitoring for gestational age >26 weeks

DIFFERENTIAL DIAGNOSIS

- Hematuria (UTI, kidney stones)
- Rectal bleeding

DIAGNOSTIC TESTS & INTERPRETATION

Initial Tests (lab, imaging)

- CBC
- Blood type and screen; if significant hemorrhage, type and cross-match
- Quantitative β-human chorionic gonadotropin (β-hCG):
  - Prior to 12 weeks, levels can be followed serially every 2 days with following trends:
    - Doubles or at least 66% rise in 48 hours in normal pregnancy
    - Falls in spontaneous abortion
    - Extremely high in molar pregnancy
    - Rises gradually (<50% in 48 hours) or plateaus in ectopic pregnancy
- Transvaginal ultrasound should be used to confirm an intrauterine pregnancy (IUP) when the quantitative β-hCG >2,000 (1)[A].
- Other lab tests based on clinical scenario:
  - Wet mount, gonorrhea/chlamydia, Pap smear
  - Progesterone level occasionally used to determine viability in threatened abortion (<5 indicates not viable, >25 indicates viability, 5 to 25 is equivocal)
  - Bleeding time, fibrinogen, and fibrin split products: if suspect coagulopathy or abruption
  - Kleihauer-Betke: low sensitivity and specificity for abruption; helpful for dosing RhoGAM
- Ultrasound is the preferred imaging modality.
  - Early pregnancy:
    - Gestational sac seen at 5 to 6 weeks; fetal heartbeat observed by 8 to 9 weeks
    - Diagnostic of ectopic with nearly 100% sensitivity when β-hCG level 1,500 to 2,000 mIU/mL. If no IUP is present and ultrasound does not confirm ectopic pregnancy, serial quantitative β-hCG values should be followed (2)[C].
  - Late pregnancy:
    - Proceed to rule out placenta previa with ultrasound, labor with serial cervical exams, and abruption with external fetal monitoring.

ALERT

Confirm fetal presentation and placental position prior to cervical exam.

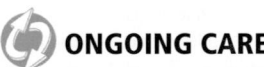

TREATMENT

MEDICATION

First Line
- Treat underlying cause of bleeding, if identified.
- If mother is Rh-negative, give RhoGAM to prevent autoimmunization. In late pregnancy, dose according to the amount of estimated fetomaternal hemorrhage.
- If cause of bleeding is preterm labor, consider betamethasone for fetal lung maturity if <36 weeks' gestation. Tocolytics may be used to prolong pregnancy to allow for course of steroids.
- If threatened abortion: Consider progesterone (relative risk 0.53) (3)[A].
- If mother has an inherited bleeding disorder or if bleeding is severe, consider recombinant or donor blood products.

SURGERY/OTHER PROCEDURES
- Cesarean section may be indicated for recurrent or uncontrolled bleeding with placenta or vasa previa.
- If ectopic is diagnosed, immediate surgical treatment may be needed. Some early ectopic pregnancies can be treated medically if certain criteria are met (2)[C].
- Surgical uterine evacuation is necessary for molar pregnancy due to malignant potential (4)[C].
- Incomplete or inevitable spontaneous abortion: Management is patient centered. In the absence of infection, patient may elect expectant, medical, or surgical management. If expectant management, typically wait 2 weeks for patient to complete abortion; most complete by 9 days. If at 2 weeks abortion is not completed or medical management has failed, surgical intervention (D&C or aspiration) is generally indicated (5)[A]; may send tissue to pathology to confirm

ADMISSION, INPATIENT, AND NURSING CONSIDERATIONS
- In early pregnancy: based on quantity of bleeding, need for surgical treatment for ectopic pregnancy, or presence of infection in case of spontaneous abortion
- In late pregnancy, if significant bleeding and/or presence of maternal or fetal compromise
- In late pregnancy with trauma, if ≥2 contractions per 10 minutes
- In late pregnancy, may discharge when bleeding has stopped; labor, previa, and abruption have been ruled out; and fetal heart tracing is normal.
- After trauma in late pregnancy, may discharge home if normal fetal heart tracing for ≥4 hours with <2 contractions per 10 minutes

ONGOING CARE

FOLLOW-UP RECOMMENDATIONS

Patient Monitoring
- Patient should be instructed to report any increase in the amount or frequency of bleeding and to seek immediate care if experiencing fever, abdominal pain, or sudden increased bleeding. Patient should save any tissue passed vaginally for examination.
- Frequency of outpatient follow-up as indicated based on etiology of bleeding

PATIENT EDUCATION
- American Academy of Family Physicians (AAFP): http://www.familydoctor.org
- American College of Obstetricians and Gynecologists (ACOG): https://www.acog.org/

PROGNOSIS
- Prognosis depends on the etiology of vaginal bleeding, severity of bleeding, and rapidity of diagnosis.
- Maternal mortality is 31.9 deaths per 100,000 ectopic pregnancies.
- 1/2 of patients with early pregnancy bleeding miscarry; if fetal heart activity (ultrasound) present in 1st-trimester bleeding, <10% chance of pregnancy loss
- Heavy bleeding in early pregnancy, particularly when accompanied by pain, is associated with higher risk of spontaneous abortion. Spotting and light episodes are not, especially if lasting only 1 to 2 days.
- Subchorionic hemorrhage has about 2- to 3-fold increased risk of spontaneous abortion. Smaller hemorrhage and presence of viable fetal heart rate confer lower risk of loss; most resolve spontaneously.
- Women with early pregnancy bleeding have an increased risk of preterm delivery, premature rupture of membranes, manual removal of placenta, placental abruption, elective cesarean delivery, and term labor induction later in the same pregnancy. These women also have an increased risk of adverse pregnancy outcomes, including hyperbilirubinemia, congenital anomalies, NICU admission, and reduced neonatal birth weight. Finally, there is an increased risk in subsequent pregnancies of recurrence of early pregnancy bleeding.
- Bed rest has not been shown to affect the outcome of bleeding in early pregnancy but may be indicated for bleeding in late pregnancy with placenta or vasa previa or with maternal hypertension.

REFERENCES

1. Crochet JR, Bastian LA, Chireau MV. Does this woman have an ectopic pregnancy? The rational clinical examination systematic review. *JAMA*. 2013;309(16):1722–1729.
2. Deutchman M, Tubay AT, Turok D. First trimester bleeding. *Am Fam Physician*. 2009;79(11): 985–994.
3. Wahabi HA, Fayed AA, Esmaeil SA, et al. Progestogen for treating threatened miscarriage. *Cochrane Database Syst Rev*. 2011;(12):CD005943.
4. Snell BJ. Assessment and management of bleeding in the first trimester of pregnancy. *J Midwifery Womens Health*. 2009;54(6):483–491.
5. Nanda K, Lopez LM, Grimes DA, et al. Expectant care versus surgical treatment for miscarriage. *Cochrane Database Syst Rev*. 2012;(3):CD003518.

ADDITIONAL READING

- ACOG Practice Bulletin No. 193: tubal ectopic pregnancy. *Obstet Gynecol*. 2018;131(3):e91–e103.
- Al-Ma'ani WI, Solomayer EF, Hammadeh M. Expectant versus surgical management of first-trimester miscarriage: a randomised controlled study. *Arch Gynecol Obstet*. 2014;289(5):1011–1015.
- Belfort MA; and Publications Committee, Society for Maternal-Fetal Medicine. Placenta accreta. *Am J Obstet Gynecol*. 2010;203(5):430–439.
- Bhandari S, Raja EA, Shetty A, et al. Maternal and perinatal consequences of antepartum haemorrhage of unknown origin. *BJOG*. 2014;121(1):44–52.
- Boisramé T, Sananès N, Fritz G, et al. Placental abruption: risk factors, management and maternal-fetal prognosis. Cohort study over 10 years. *Eur J Obstet Gynecol Reprod Biol*. 2014;179:100–104.
- Chi C, Kadir RA. Inherited bleeding disorders in pregnancy. *Best Pract Res Clin Obstet Gynaecol*. 2012;26(1):103–117.
- Dadkhah F, Kashanian M, Eliasi G. A comparison between the pregnancy outcome in women both with or without threatened abortion. *Early Hum Dev*. 2010;86(3):193–196.
- Lykke JA, Dideriksen KL, Lidegaard O, et al. First-trimester vaginal bleeding and complications later in pregnancy. *Obstet Gynecol*. 2010;115(5):935–944.
- Prine LW, MacNaughton H. Office management of early pregnancy loss. *Am Fam Physician*. 2011;84(1):75–82.

 SEE ALSO

Abnormal Pap and Cervical Dysplasia; Abruptio Placentae; Cervical Malignancy; Cervical Polyps; Cervicitis, Ectropion, and True Erosion; Chlamydia Infection (Sexually Transmitted); Ectopic Pregnancy; Miscarriage (Early Pregnancy Loss); Placenta Previa; Preterm Labor; Trichomoniasis; Vaginal Malignancy

 CODES

ICD10
- O20.9 Hemorrhage in early pregnancy, unspecified
- O46.90 Antepartum hemorrhage, unspecified, unspecified trimester
- O20.0 Threatened abortion

CLINICAL PEARLS
- Obtain blood type and screen all women presenting with vaginal bleeding in pregnancy and administer RhoGAM to all Rh-negative patients.
- For up to 50% of early pregnancy bleeding, no cause is ever found.
- Always consider ectopic pregnancy in 1st-trimester bleeding.
- Do not perform digital exam in late pregnancy bleeding until placenta has been located on ultrasound.

V

VAGINAL MALIGNANCY

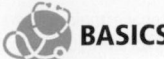

Michael P. Hopkins, MD, MEd

BASICS

DESCRIPTION
- Carcinomas of the vagina are uncommon: 2–3% of gynecologic malignancies, 2,300 new cases annually.
- Vaginal intraepithelial neoplasia (VAIN), defined by squamous cell atypia, is classified by the depth of epithelial involvement:
  - VAIN 1: 1/3 thickness
  - VAIN 2: 2/3 thickness
  - VAIN 3 and carcinoma in situ (CIS): >2/3
  - CIS, designating full-thickness neoplastic changes without invasion through the basement membrane
- Invasive malignancies: Vaginal malignancies include squamous cell carcinoma (85–90%), adenocarcinoma (5–10%), sarcoma (2–3%), and melanoma (2–3%). Clear cell carcinoma is a subtype of adenocarcinoma. Invasive squamous cell carcinoma has the potential for metastasis to the lungs and liver.
- To be classified as a vaginal malignancy, only the vagina can be involved. If the cervix or vulva is involved, then the tumor is classified as a primary cancer arising from the cervix or the vulva.
- Most vaginal malignancies are metastatic (e.g., cervix, vulva, endometrium, breast, ovary).
- Most common sites of metastases: lung, liver, bone

Pregnancy Considerations
This malignancy is not associated with pregnancy.

EPIDEMIOLOGY
Incidence
Predominant age
- CIS: mid-40 to 60 years
- Invasive squamous cell malignancy: mid-60 to 70 years
- Adenocarcinoma: any age; 50 years is the mean age. Peak incidence is between 17 and 21 years of age.
- Clear cell adenocarcinoma occurs most often in females <30 years with a history of exposure to diethylstilbestrol (DES) in utero.
- Mixed müllerian sarcomas and leiomyosarcomas in the adult population: mean age 60 years

Pediatric Considerations
Vaginal tumors are extremely rare. Rhabdomyosarcoma (botryoid and embryonal subtype) is the most common malignant neoplasm of the vagina. Less common entities are germ cell tumor and clear cell adenocarcinoma.

Prevalence
In the United States, it is one of the rarest of all gynecologic malignancies (3%).

ETIOLOGY AND PATHOPHYSIOLOGY
- Women with a history of cervical malignancy have a higher probability of developing squamous cell malignancy in the vagina even after hysterectomy.
- Human papillomavirus (HPV) is found in 80–93% of patients with vaginal CIS and 50–65% of the patients with invasive vaginal carcinoma.

- HPV-16 is the most common, found in 66% of CIS and 55% of invasive vaginal cancers.
- Smokers have a higher incidence.
- Clear cell adenocarcinoma of the vagina in young women has been associated with DES exposure. The incidence, however, is exceedingly rare, estimated at 1/1,000 to 1/10,000 exposed females.
- Metastatic lesions can involve the vagina, spreading from the other gynecologic organs.
- Although rare, renal cell carcinoma, lung adenocarcinoma, GI cancer, pancreatic adenocarcinoma, ovarian germ cell cancer, trophoblastic neoplasm, and breast cancer can all metastasize to the vagina.

Genetics
No known genetic pattern

RISK FACTORS
- Similar risk factors as cervical cancer
- Age
- African American
- Smoking
- Multiple sex partners, early age of first sexual intercourse
- History of squamous cell cancer of the cervix or vulva
- HPV infection
- Vaginal adenosis
- Vaginal irritation
- DES exposure in utero
- Immunocompromised, HIV
- Prior pelvic radiation

COMMONLY ASSOCIATED CONDITIONS
Due to the field effect, patients with vaginal cancer are more likely to develop malignancy in the cervix or vulva and should be followed closely.

DIAGNOSIS

HISTORY
- Abnormal bleeding is the most common symptom.
- Postcoital bleeding can result from direct trauma to the tumor.
- Vaginal discharge
- Dyspareunia
- Urinary symptoms, including hematuria and increased frequency
- Constipation
- Pain along with symptoms and signs of hydroureter are late findings when the tumor has spread into the paravaginal tissues and extends to the pelvic sidewall (1)[A].

Pediatric Considerations
In children, sarcomas can present either as a mass protruding from the vagina or as abnormal genital bleeding (1)[A].

PHYSICAL EXAM
Pelvic examination
- The vagina, uterus, adnexa (fallopian tubes and ovaries), bladder, and rectum should be evaluated for unusual changes.
- Vaginal malignancies are found most commonly on the posterior wall in the upper 1/3 of the vagina.

DIFFERENTIAL DIAGNOSIS
- Premalignant changes: VAIN 1, 2, 3, and CIS
- Adequate biopsies ensure that invasive lesions are not overlooked. Invasive lesions penetrate the basement membrane and cannot be treated conservatively.
- Other malignancies, such as endometrial, cervix, bladder, or colon cancer, can invade directly into the vagina or metastasize to the vagina.
- In the childbearing years, trophoblastic disease should be considered.
  - The vagina is a common site of metastases; however, biopsy should typically be avoided because the implants are very vascular and may hemorrhage if sampled.
  - The clinical presentation is typically obvious so histopathologic confirmation before treatment is not required.

DIAGNOSTIC TESTS & INTERPRETATION
Initial Tests (lab, imaging)
- Pap smear may incidentally detect asymptomatic lesions.
- Biopsy suspicious lesions
- Chest x-ray (CXR): to evaluate for metastatic disease
- CT scan and MRI: to evaluate the liver and retroperitoneum, especially the lymph nodes in the pelvic and periaortic area
- PET scan detects primary and secondary metastatic lesions more often than CT scan.

ALERT
PET scan correlation with CT scan lesions strongly suggests malignancy.

Follow-Up Tests & Special Considerations
- Lymphoscintigraphy (sentinel lymph node mapping) as part of the pretreatment evaluation can result in a change in the radiation fields and improve comprehensive treatment planning in women with vaginal cancer.
- HPV vaccination: Implementation of prophylactic HPV vaccination could prevent ~2/3 of the intraepithelial lesions in the lower genital tract but is yet proven.

Diagnostic Procedures/Other
- Colposcopy with directed biopsies for small lesions
- Wide excision under anesthesia of superficial disease may be necessary to ensure that invasive cancer is not present.
- Cystoscopy to rule out bladder invasion
- Proctosigmoidoscopy to rule out rectal invasion

Test Interpretation
Tumors are staged clinically:
- Stage 0: VAIN and CIS
- Stage I: carcinoma limited to the vaginal wall (26%)
- Stage II: involves the subvaginal tissues but has not extended to the pelvic wall (37%)
- Stage III: extends to the pelvic wall (24%)
- Stage IV: extends beyond the true pelvis (13%)
  - IVa: Tumor invades bladder and/or rectal mucosa and/or direct extension beyond the true pelvis.
  - IVb: spread to distant organs

TREATMENT

GENERAL MEASURES
Treatment methods for VAIN and CIS include the following:
- Wide local excision
- Partial or total vaginectomy
- Intravaginal chemotherapy with 5% fluorouracil cream
- Laser therapy
- Intracavitary radiation therapy

MEDICATION
- Imiquimod
  - In a review of the effectiveness of 5% imiquimod cream in the treatment of VAIN, the following results were reported (2)[C]:
    - 26–100% of patients had complete regression.
    - 0–60% of patients had partial regression.
    - 0–37% experienced recurrence.
- Contraindications
  - The diagnosis must be established with certainty prior to treatment.
  - If there is any doubt that a process beyond in situ disease exists, vaginectomy must be performed. These patients are often elderly, and aggressive therapy is limited by the patient's performance status and ability to tolerate radical surgery, chemotherapy, or radiation.

ISSUES FOR REFERRAL
Patients should be treated by a gynecologic oncologist and/or a radiation oncologist.

ADDITIONAL THERAPIES
- Treatment with radiotherapy depends on the stage of disease. This treatment option should be discussed with physicians experienced with this malignancy.
- It is common to use radiotherapy and chemotherapy (chemoradiation) for better cancer control.
- Early-stage primary squamous cell carcinoma treated with radiation alone has shown good results.
- Stage III vaginal cancer may benefit from combined radiation and hyperthermia (1)[C].
- Patients with advanced squamous cell carcinoma or adenocarcinoma receive concurrent irradiation and cisplatin-based chemotherapy.
- Neoadjuvant chemotherapy followed by radical surgery may benefit selected patients (3)[C].
- In most tumor types, metastatic disease from the vagina to other sites is only minimally responsive to chemotherapy.
- With one exception, no chemotherapeutic agents have shown a survival advantage. The exception is childhood sarcomas, which have been treated with combinations of the following:
  - Vincristine
  - Dactinomycin (actinomycin-D)
  - Cyclophosphamide (Cytoxan)
  - Cisplatin
  - Etoposide (VP-16)

SURGERY/OTHER PROCEDURES
- Whenever there is a doubt as to the presence or absence of invasive disease, vaginectomy must be performed.
- Invasive lesions usually are treated by radiation therapy, but stage I lesions can be treated with radical hysterectomy or radical vaginectomy with pelvic lymph node dissection (2)[A].
- If the lesion involves the lower vagina, inguinal node dissection also must be done because cancer involving the lower vagina can metastasize to the groin region (inguinal–femoral nodes).
- Premenopausal women who desire to retain ovarian function are better candidates for radical surgery for early-stage disease, with vaginal reconstruction possible afterward.
- Patients who have not completed their family can occasionally be treated with limited resection and localized radiation to the area (4)[A].
- Sarcomas are treated by radiation therapy followed by pelvic exenteration if persistent disease is present.

Pediatric Considerations
The treatment of vaginal tumors today mainly consists of neoadjuvant chemotherapy followed by local control with surgery or radiotherapy (1)[A].

Geriatric Considerations
Older patients, many with a long history of smoking, are at a higher risk for malignancies requiring surgical treatments.

 ## ONGOING CARE

FOLLOW-UP RECOMMENDATIONS
- Patients are usually ambulatory and able to resume full activity by 6 weeks after surgery.
- Most patients are fully active while receiving chemotherapy and radiation therapy.

Patient Monitoring
- Pelvic examination and Pap smear every 3 months for 2 years, then every 6 months for the next 3 years, and then yearly thereafter
- Annual CXR

PATIENT EDUCATION
- Printed patient information available from American College of Obstetricians and Gynecologists, 409 12th St., SW, Washington, DC 20024-2188; 800-762-ACOG: http://www.acog.org
- American Cancer Society: http://www.cancer.gov
- Medline Plus: http://www.nlm.nih.gov/medlineplus/vaginalcancer.html

PROGNOSIS
Stage and 5-year survival (5)
- I: 77.6%
- II: 52.2%
- III: 42.5%
- IVA: 20.5%
- IVB: 12.9%
- Stage is the most important determinant of survival (4).
- Tumor size >2 cm, correlated with worse survival outcome

COMPLICATIONS
- Those typically associated with major abdominal surgery or radiation therapy
- Common complications of treatment include rectovaginal or vesicovaginal fistulas, rectal/vaginal strictures, radiation cystitis, and/or proctitis.
- Most recurrences occur within the first 2 years after initial diagnosis.

REFERENCES
1. Fernandez-Pineda I, Spunt SL, Parida L, et al. Vaginal tumors in childhood: the experience of St. Jude Children's Research Hospital. *J Pediatr Surg*. 2011;46(11):2071–2075.
2. Guerri S, Perrone AM, Buwenge M, et al. Definitive radiotherapy in invasive vaginal carcinoma: a systematic review [published online ahead of print August 23, 2018]. *Oncologist*. doi:10.1634/theoncologist.2017-0546.
3. Hacker NF, Eifel PJ, van der Velden J. Cancer of the vagina. *Int J Gynecol Obstet*. 2015;131(Suppl 2):S84–S87.
4. Gadducci A, Fabrini MG, Lanfredini N, et al. Squamous cell carcinoma of the vagina: natural history, treatment modalities and prognostic factors. *Crit Rev Oncol Hematol*. 2015;93(3):211–224.
5. Adams TS, Cuello MA. Cancer of the vagina. *Int J Gynaecol Obstet*. 2018;143(Suppl 2):14–21.

ADDITIONAL READING
- Gray HJ. Advances in vulvar and vaginal cancer treatment. *Gynecol Oncol*. 2010;118(1):3–5.
- Iavazzo C, Pitsouni E, Athanasiou S, et al. Imiquimod for treatment of vulvar and vaginal intraepithelial neoplasia. *Int J Gynaecol Obstet*. 2008;101(1):3–10.
- Wolfson AH, Reis IM, Portelance L, et al. Prognostic impact of clinical tumor size on overall survival for subclassifying stages I and II vaginal cancer: a SEER analysis. *Gynecol Oncol*. 2016;141(2):255–259.

CODES

ICD10
- C52 Malignant neoplasm of vagina
- D07.2 Carcinoma in situ of vagina
- N89.3 Dysplasia of vagina, unspecified

CLINICAL PEARLS
- Vaginal cancer is rare; 85–90% of vaginal cancers are squamous cell.
- Vaginal malignancies are found most commonly on the posterior wall in the upper 1/3 of the vagina.
- Most vaginal malignancies are metastatic (from cervix, vulva, endometrium, breast, or ovary).

V

VAGINITIS AND VAGINOSIS

KrisEmily McCrory, MD, FAAFP

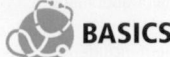

BASICS

DESCRIPTION

- "Vaginosis" and "vaginitis" are broad terms indicating any disease process of the vagina caused by or leading to infection, inflammation, or changes in the normal vaginal flora.
- The difference between vaginitis and vaginosis is the presence (vaginitis) or absence (vaginosis) of inflammation.
- The most common symptoms of vaginitis/vaginosis are vaginal discharge, odor, itching, burning, or pain.
- The most common causes of vaginitis/vaginosis are bacterial vaginosis (BV), vulvovaginal candidiasis (VVC), and trichomoniasis.
- Other causes of vaginitis can be stratified by age and are generally associated with postmenopausal vaginal atrophy or foreign bodies in the pediatric population.
- Lichen planus, lichen sclerosus, psoriasis, and contact/allergic dermatitis may also cause vaginitis.
- Diagnosis of vaginitis relies on thorough history, physical exam, and clinical assessment. Microscopy, cultures, DNA probes, and tissue biopsy can be helpful in confirming diagnosis.
- BV is the most common cause of vaginal discharge in reproductive-aged women. It is caused by a disturbance in the normal vaginal flora. The normally dominant hydrogen peroxide–producing lactobacilli are overwhelmed by an overgrowth of gram-negative species causing an increase in the vaginal pH, discharge, and odor.
- VVC is the second most common cause of vaginitis in reproductive-aged women. It is caused by invasion of the *Candida* organism into the superficial epithelial cells of the vagina causing mild to severe vaginal inflammation, pruritus, and discharge.

EPIDEMIOLOGY

- Vaginal symptoms are typical and common in the general population and are one of the most frequent reasons women present to their medical care providers accounting for approximately 10 million office visits each year.
- About 30% of women with complaint of vaginal discharge or irritation remain undiagnosed despite extensive testing.
- In the United States, BV continues to be the leading cause of vaginal complaints. The frequency of VVC is highest among women in their reproductive years.
- Neither vaginal candidiasis nor BV is considered to be sexually transmitted diseases.
- Vaginal trichomoniasis is a common sexually transmitted disease with 7.4 million cases diagnosed yearly in the United States, and is the most common curable, nonviral sexually transmitted infection worldwide.

ETIOLOGY AND PATHOPHYSIOLOGY

- BV
  - BV is caused by a change in the normal vaginal flora. Dominant lactobacilli responsible for maintaining the acidic vaginal pH are overcome by an increase of the gram-negative organisms.
  - Change in the vaginal environment leads to an increase in the pH and an overgrowth of vaginal anaerobes, causing a malodorous, clear, white, or gray discharge and a fishy odor.
  - BV is highly prevalent and associated with multiple adverse outcomes, including enhanced HIV transmission.

- The organisms generally implicated in BV infections include:
  - *Gardnerella vaginalis*
  - *Prevotella* species
  - *Porphyromonas* species
  - *Bacteroides* species
  - *Peptostreptococcus* species
  - *Mycoplasma hominis*
  - *Ureaplasma urealyticum*
  - *Mobiluncus* species
  - *Fusobacterium* species
  - *Atopobium vaginae*
- VVC
  - VVC is caused by *Candida albicans* (80–92%) and *Candida glabrata* (<10%).
  - *Candida* organisms can be identified in the lower genital tract in healthy women, and it is thought to gain access via rectal and perianal colonization and migration.
  - Symptoms occur when candidal organisms overwhelm the normal vaginal flora and invade the superficial vaginal epithelial cells, causing inflammation, pruritus, and thick vaginal discharge.
  - Complicated VVC should be considered in pregnant patients, patients with diabetes, or immunocompromising conditions. Patients who experience four or more episodes of VVC in a year or who have only budding yeast on wet mount may also be considered to have complicated VVC.
- Trichomoniasis
  - Caused by an infection via *Trichomonas vaginalis*, a flagellate protozoan. The organism infects the squamous epithelium of the vagina as well as the urethra and paraurethral glands. This infection is primarily transmitted during sexual intercourse.
- Desquamative inflammatory vaginitis (DIV)
  - A chronic, purulent vaginitis occurring most commonly in the perimenopause
  - Etiology and pathogenesis uncertain
  - Diagnosis of exclusion. Estrogen deficiency should be considered and addressed.
- Other sources of vaginitis/vaginosis are usually mediated by disruption of the vaginal squamous epithelium. This disruption can lead to inflammation, pain, and discharge.
  - Other than the three most common causes of vaginitis/vaginosis, menses, sexual activity, contraception, pregnancy, foreign bodies, estrogen levels, STDs, and use of vaginal hygiene products, topical creams, or antibiotics can contribute to vaginal symptoms.

RISK FACTORS

- BV
  - Sexual activity; although BV is not considered an STD, studies show increased rates of BV in women with multiple sex partners.
  - Women who have sex with women
  - Smoking
  - Vaginal douching
  - The presence of STDs such as HSV-2 (1)
- VVC
  - Diabetes
  - Diet high in refined sugars
  - Use of broad-spectrum antibiotics
  - Immunosuppression
  - Higher estrogen levels have been associated with increased vaginal yeast infection, explaining why it is more commonly diagnosed in reproductive-aged women and in pregnancy.

- Trichomoniasis
  - Inconsistent use of barrier contraception
  - Multiple sex partners
  - African Americans
  - Limited education and low socioeconomic status
  - Illicit drug use
  - Smoking
- Other risk factors associated with vaginitis/vaginosis:
  - Decreased estrogen
  - Smoking
  - Use of vaginal douches and creams
  - Tight-fitting clothing
  - Poor hygienic practice
  - Changes in diet

GENERAL PREVENTION

- Vulvar hygiene
- Except in cases of trichomoniasis, treatment of sexual partners generally is not recommended but may be considered in recurrent cases.
- Advise patients not to douche.

COMMONLY ASSOCIATED CONDITIONS

- STDs such as gonorrhea, chlamydia, or HSV
- Vaginal intraepithelial neoplasia and cancer can present with symptoms of vaginitis.
- DIV presents with similar symptoms but most commonly occurs in postmenopausal women.

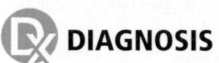

DIAGNOSIS

HISTORY

- General principles:
  - The key to diagnosis is clarification of the presenting symptoms.
  - Onset, timing, and character of the vaginal symptoms are important questions to ask.
  - Many patients will be asymptomatic, and diagnosis is made on routine physical exam and lab testing.
  - Pap smears should not be used as diagnostic tools due to low sensitivity and specificity.
  - Symptomatic patients generally complain of itching, burning, irritation, and abnormal discharge.
- BV
  - Symptomatic patients complain of abnormal vaginal discharge and a fishy odor.
  - Pain and pruritus are uncommon.
- VVC
  - Symptomatic women report itching, burning, irritation, dyspareunia, burning with urination, and a white thick discharge.
  - Odor is uncommon.
- Trichomoniasis
  - Symptomatic patients will complain of abnormal discharge, itching, burning, or postcoital bleeding.

PHYSICAL EXAM

- BV
  - Thin watery, sometimes foamy discharge. Can appear beige- or tan-colored. An amine or "fishy" smell may be present on exam.
  - The vaginal epithelium should appear normal and noninflamed.
- VVC
  - Erythema and swelling of the vulva and vaginal mucosa
  - Some patients may have vulvar excoriation and fissures.

– If discharge is present, it is usually white, thick, and can have a cottage cheese appearance. Some women may have thin white dilute discharge. No odor is present.
- DIV
  – Purulent discharge
  – Wet mount shows WBC and parabasal (immature) squamous epithelial cells, with pH >4.5.
- Trichomoniasis
  – Significant erythema of the vulva and vaginal mucosa
  – Greenish discharge with an amine or fishy odor
  – Discharge can also appear purulent in some patients.
  – Occasionally punctate hemorrhages can be seen on the vaginal walls and on the cervix ("strawberry cervix").

DIFFERENTIAL DIAGNOSIS
- Physiologic discharge
- Leukorrhea of pregnancy
- STDs
- Foreign body
- Contact dermatitis
- Cervicitis
- DIV
- Urinary tract infection (UTI)
- Atrophic vaginitis
- Dermatoses: lichen sclerosus, lichen planus, seborrheic dermatitis, psoriasis

DIAGNOSTIC TESTS & INTERPRETATION
- BV
  – Symptomatic patients complain of an abnormal vaginal discharge and a fishy odor.
  – Clinical diagnosis is established with Amsel criteria. A positive diagnosis can be made if 3 out of 4 of the following criteria are present.
    ○ Thin, homogenous discharge
    ○ Vaginal pH >4.5
    ○ A positive amine or "Whiff" test with use of KOH solution added to discharge
    ○ >20% of the epithelial cells identified as "clue cells"
- VVC
  – Visualization of blastospores or pseudohyphae on saline or 10% KOH microscopy
  – A positive culture in a symptomatic patient
- Trichomoniasis
  – Visualization of motile trichomonads on saline microscopy
  – Several POC identification tests, including patient performed, are available with increased sensitivity compared to microscopy but are expensive.

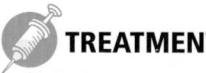 ## TREATMENT

GENERAL MEASURES
- Avoid douching and tight-fitting clothing.
- Regular use of condoms may help to prevent BV.
- Asymptomatic, pregnant women generally do not require treatment for BV.

MEDICATION
Medication recommendations based on CDC treatment guidelines (2)[A]
- BV
  – Metronidazole 500 mg orally BID for 7 days, vaginally 0.75% gel 1 applicator daily for 5 days, or clindamycin given vaginally (1 applicator = 100 mg) for 5 days. Recurrent infection may require repeated treatment (e.g., 1 week monthly for 6 months). Advise patients to avoid alcohol during treatment with oral metronidazole and for 3 days following.

- VVC
  – Uncomplicated infections can be treated with a one-time dose of fluconazole 150 mg tab. Topical/vaginal suppository antifungal regimens such as butoconazole, clotrimazole, miconazole, terconazole, or nystatin creams. Treatment can range from 3 to 7 days.
  – Recurrent or complicated infections may require additional oral dosing of fluconazole 150 mg tab for extended treatment and/or prophylaxis.
  – Non-albican candidiasis may require longer duration of treatment with topical or oral azoles.
  – Avoid oral azoles in pregnant women.
  – Advise patients that topical medications may weaken rubber or latex condoms.
- Trichomoniasis
  – A one-time 2-g oral dose of either tinidazole or metronidazole; alternatively, 500-mg dose of metronidazole BID for 7 days
  – The patient's partner should be treated as well and counseled to abstain from sex until both patients have completed treatment and are asymptomatic.
  – Test of cure is not necessary.
- DIV
  – Clindamycin cream vaginally or
  – Hydrocortisone vaginal suppository 300 to 500 mg nightly for 3 weeks; may need additional maintenance

ISSUES FOR REFERRAL
Treating male partners does not reduce symptoms or prevent recurrence but can be considered in patients with recurrent infection.

COMPLEMENTARY & ALTERNATIVE MEDICINE
A Cochrane analysis reviewed the use of probiotics for BV and found inconclusive evidence to recommend probiotics as primary treatment or as a preventive strategy (3)[A]. Further study was recommended.

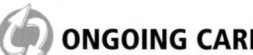 ## ONGOING CARE

FOLLOW-UP RECOMMENDATIONS
- Delay sexual relations until symptoms clear/discomfort resolves.
- Use of condoms may reduce recurrence of BV.
- Consider suppressive therapy for recurrent infection.
- Monthly presumptive treatment may help reduce colonization of bacteria associated with BV (4)[C].

Patient Monitoring
No specific follow-up needed; if symptoms persist or recur within 2 months, repeat pelvic exam and culture.

PATIENT EDUCATION
American College of Obstetricians and Gynecologists (ACOG), 409 12th St., SW, Washington, DC 20024-2188; 800-762-ACOG: www.acog.org

PROGNOSIS
VVC: 80–90% of uncomplicated cases cured with appropriate treatment; 30–50% of recurrent infections return after discontinuation of maintenance therapy; there is a relatively high spontaneous remission rate of untreated symptoms as well.

COMPLICATIONS
- VVC may occur following treatment of BV.
- BV has been associated with an increased risk of acquisition and transmission of HIV.
- BV has been associated with increased risk of preterm birth, chorioamnionitis, postpartum and postabortal endometritis, and pelvic inflammatory disease.

REFERENCES

1. Esber A, Vicetti Miguel RD, Cherpes TL, et al. Risk of bacterial vaginosis among women with herpes simplex virus type 2 infection: a systematic review and meta-analysis. *J Infect Dis*. 2015;212(1):8–17.
2. Workowski KA, Bolan GA; and Centers for Disease Control and Prevention. Sexually transmitted diseases treatment guidelines, 2015. *MMWR Recomm Rep*. 2015;64(RR-03):1–137.
3. Senok AC, Verstraelen H, Temmerman M, et al. Probiotics for the treatment of bacterial vaginosis. *Cochrane Database Syst Rev*. 2009;(4):CD006289.
4. Balkus JE, Srinivasan S, Anzala O, et al. Impact of periodic presumptive treatment for bacterial vaginosis on the vaginal microbiome among women participating in the preventing vaginal infections trial. *J Infect Dis*. 2017;215(5):723–731.

ADDITIONAL READING
- Donders G. Diagnosis and management of bacterial vaginosis and other types of abnormal vaginal bacterial flora: a review. *Obstet Gynecol Surv*. 2010;65(7):462–473.
- Farage MA, Miller KW, Ledger WJ. Determining the cause of vulvovaginal symptoms. *Obstet Gynecol Surv*. 2008;63(7):445–464.
- Li J, McCormick J, Bocking A, et al. Importance of vaginal microbes in reproductive health. *Reprod Sci*. 2012;19(3):235–242.
- Pappas PG, Kauffman CA, Andes D, et al. Clinical practice guidelines for the management of candidiasis: 2009 update by the Infectious Diseases Society of America. *Clin Infect Dis*. 2009;48(5):503–535.
- Reichman O, Sobel J. Desquamative inflammatory vaginitis. *Best Pract Res Clin Obstet Gynaecol*. 2014;28(7):1042–1050.

 ### SEE ALSO

Algorithm: Discharge, Vaginal

 ### CODES

ICD10
- N76.0 Acute vaginitis
- B37.3 Candidiasis of vulva and vagina
- N95.2 Postmenopausal atrophic vaginitis

CLINICAL PEARLS
Clinical symptoms, signs, and microscopy have relatively poor performance compared with so-called gold standards such as culture and DNA probe assays, but these more sensitive assays can detect organisms that may not be causing symptoms.
- Most women experience relief of symptoms with therapy chosen without such gold standard tests, even when the treatment does not correspond with the underlying infection.
- Vaginal pH is underused as a diagnostic tool for evaluation of vaginitis.

V

VARICOSE VEINS

Joseph A. Florence, MD • Fereshteh Gerayli, MD, FAAFP

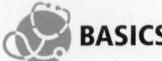 **BASICS**

DESCRIPTION

- Superficial venous disease causing a permanent dilatation and tortuosity of superficial veins ≥3 mm in diameter usually occurring in the legs and feet; caused by systemic weakness in the vein wall and may result from congenitally incomplete valves or valves that have become incompetent
- Affects legs where reverse flow occurs when dependent
- Truncal varices involve the great and small saphenous veins; branch varicosities involve the saphenous vein tributaries.
- Categorized as the following:
  - Uncomplicated (cosmetic)
  - With local symptoms (pain confined to the varices, not diffuse)
  - With local complications (superficial thrombophlebitis, may rupture causing bleeding)
  - Complex varicose disease (diffuse limb pain, swelling, skin changes/ulcer)
- System(s) affected: cardiovascular; skin

ALERT
Ulceration of varicose veins has a high rate of infection, which can lead to sepsis.

Geriatric Considerations
- Common; usually valvular degeneration but may be secondary to chronic venous insufficiency
- Elastic support hose and frequent rests with legs elevated rather than ligation and stripping

Pregnancy Considerations
- Frequent problem
- Elastic stockings are recommended for those with a history of varicosities or if prolonged standing is involved.

EPIDEMIOLOGY
Incidence
- Predominant age: middle age
- Predominant gender: female > male (2:1)
- National Women's Health Information Center estimates that 50% of women have varicose veins.

ETIOLOGY AND PATHOPHYSIOLOGY
- Varicose veins are caused by venous insufficiency from faulty valves in ≥1 perforator veins in the lower leg, causing secondary incompetence at the saphenofemoral junction (valvular reflux).
- Valvular dysfunction causing venous reflux and subsequently venous hypertension (HTN)
- Failed valves allow blood to flow in the reverse direction (away from the heart), from deep to superficial and from proximal to distal veins.
- Deep thrombophlebitis
- Increased venous pressure from any cause
- Congenital valvular incompetence

- Trauma (consider arteriovenous fistula; listen for bruit)
- Presumed to be due to a loss in vein wall elasticity with failure of the valve leaflets
- An increase in venous filling pressure is sufficient to promote varicose remodeling of veins by augmenting wall stress and activating venous endothelial and smooth muscle cells.

Genetics
Autosomal dominant with incomplete penetrance

RISK FACTORS
- Increasing age
- Pregnancy, especially multiple pregnancies
- Prolonged standing
- Obesity
- History of phlebitis (postthrombotic syndrome)
- Family history
- Female sex
- Increased height
- Congenital valvular dysfunction

COMMONLY ASSOCIATED CONDITIONS
- Stasis dermatitis
- Large varicose veins may lead to skin changes and eventual stasis ulceration.

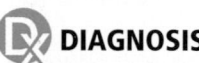 **DIAGNOSIS**

HISTORY
- Symptoms range from minor annoyance/cosmetic problem to a lifestyle-limiting problem (1).
- Localized symptoms: pain, burning, itching
- Generalized symptoms
  - Leg muscular cramp, aching
  - Leg fatigue/swelling
- Pain if varicose ulcer develops
- Symptoms often worse at the end of the day, especially after prolonged standing
- Women are more prone to symptoms due to hormonal influences: worse during menses.
- No direct correlation with the severity of varicose veins and the severity of symptoms

PHYSICAL EXAM
- Inspect lower extremities while the patient is standing. Varicose veins in the proximal femoral ring and distal portion of the legs may not be visible when the patient is supine (1).
- Varicose veins are the following:
  - Dilated, tortuous, superficial veins, ≥3 mm, chiefly in the lower extremities
  - Dark purple/blue in color, raised above the surface of the skin
  - Often twisted, bulging, and can look like cords
  - Most commonly found on the posterior/medial lower extremity
- Edema of the affected limb may be present.

- Skin changes may include the following:
  - Eczema
  - Hyperpigmentation
  - Lipodermatosclerosis
- Spider veins (idiopathic telangiectases)
  - Fine intracutaneous angiectasis
  - May be extensive/unsightly
- Neurologic sensory and motor exam
- Peripheral arterial vasculature; pulses
- Musculoskeletal exam for associated rheumatologic/orthopedic issues

DIFFERENTIAL DIAGNOSIS
- Nerve root compression
- Arthritis
- Peripheral neuritis
- Telangiectasia: smaller, visible blood vessels that are permanently dilated
- Deep vein thrombosis
- Inflammatory liposclerosis

DIAGNOSTIC TESTS & INTERPRETATION
Duplex ultrasound: Noninvasive imaging duplex ultrasound will confirm the etiology, anatomy, and pathophysiology of segmental venous reflux. The severity of both symptoms and signs tends to correlate with the degree of venous reflux, which is identified by duplex ultrasound as retrograde or reversed flow of >0.5 seconds duration (1)[A].

Diagnostic Procedures/Other
Duplex scanning, venous Doppler study, photoplethysmography, light-reflection rheography, air plethysmography, and other vascular testing should be reserved for patients who have venous symptoms and/or large (>4 mm in diameter) vessels or large numbers of spider telangiectasia indicating venous HTN.

Test Interpretation
The clinical, etiologic, anatomic, and pathologic (CEAP) classification is considered the gold standard of classification of chronic venous disorders. Clinical classification illustrating the current physical state is useful in clinical practice (1)[A].

- 0: no visible or palpable signs of venous disease
- 1: spider veins or telangiectasias
- 2: varicose veins
- 3: edema
- 4: skin changes (pigmentation, eczema, lipodermatosclerosis, atrophie blanche)
- 5: healed ulcer
- 6: active ulcer

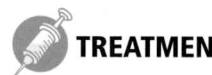 **TREATMENT**

- Indications for treatment include pain, aching, soreness, heaviness, fatigue, burning, edema, stasis dermatitis, recurrent superficial phlebitis or ulceration.
- Conventional wisdom suggests conservative therapy (e.g., elevation, external compression, weight loss) as being helpful.

- Compression stockings improve subjective symptoms but have no real effect on progression or recurrence (1,2)[A]; significant failure rate due to nonadherence (3)[A]; typical compression levels
  - 20 to 30 mm Hg: uncomplicated varicose veins for pain and edema control
  - 30 to 40 mm Hg: venous stasis ulcers
- The most important part of the stocking is below the knee, where the standing venous pressure is the highest.
- Sclerotherapy: indicated for spider veins and small varicose veins (1)[A]
- CHIVA: Ambulatory conservative hemodynamic management of varicose veins is a less-invasive approach based on venous hemodynamics with deliberate preservation of the superficial venous system. The CHIVA method reduces recurrence of varicose veins and produces fewer side effects than vein stripping (1)[A].
- Injection of sclerosant into a vein and then apply compression resulting in occlusive fibrosis without clot formation; chemical irritants (chromated glycerin), osmotic (hypertonic saline), detergent (sodium tetradecyl sulphate [STS] and polidocanol [POL])
- Poor long-term results with liquid sclerotherapy (LS), however, foam sclerotherapy (FS) is an option for treatment of the incompetent saphenous vein. Ultrasound-guided FS is recommended as a second-line treatment under current National Institute for Health and Care Excellence (NICE) guidelines (4)[A].
- Radiofrequency ablation (RFA) thermal energy (85–120°C) is used to seal the incompetent vein via heat damage. Endovenous laser ablation (EVLA) uses laser and fiber-optic catheter technology to generate thermal energy (up to 800°C) (1,3)[A].
  - RFA and EVLA have been demonstrated to be superior to open surgical techniques for the treatment of varicose veins with similar improvement in quality of life. NICE recommends using them as first-line treatment of truncal vein incompetence (4)[A].
  - EVLA and RFA have similar safety and efficacy (including vein ablated length, pain scores, quality of life, occlusion, thrombophlebitis, hematoma, and recanalization) (5)[A].
  - RFA has overall lower complication risk (5)[A].
- Nonthermal, nontumescent ablation (1)[A]: Mechanochemical endovenous ablation (MOCA) is a hybrid system composed of a rotating tip with simultaneous injection of liquid sclerosant and does not use heat energy. It is less painful with similar occlusion rates to standard endovenous ablation.

GENERAL MEASURES
Patients with unsightly varicose veins often seek treatment for cosmetic reasons.

MEDICATION
Superficial thrombophlebitis is not an infective condition and does not require antibiotic treatment.

ISSUES FOR REFERRAL
NICE (4)[A] recommends referral of patients with:
- Symptomatic primary (or recurrent) varicose veins
- Skin changes
- Superficial venous thrombosis
- Venous leg ulcers
- Healed ulcers

ADDITIONAL THERAPIES
- Apply elastic stockings before lowering legs from the bed.
- Activity
  - Frequent rest periods with legs elevated
  - If standing is necessary, frequently shift weight from side to side.
  - Appropriate exercise routine as part of conservative treatment
  - Walking regimen after sclerotherapy is important to help promote healing.
  - Never sit with legs hanging down.
- Physical therapy

SURGERY/OTHER PROCEDURES
Surgery
- Once considered the gold-standard treatment, now minimally invasive outpatient procedures are preferred.
- Surgery for varicose veins can be performed under general, local, or regional anesthesia and is performed as a day-case procedure in all but special cases.
- The basic principle is disconnection of the refluxing superficial venous system from the deep system.
- Saphenofemoral junction ligation (SFJ) and saphenopopliteal junction ligation (SPJ): SPJ ligation is less successful than SFJ ligation, with high recurrence and complication rates, particularly regarding common peroneal nerve damage resulting in foot drop, which is a cause of litigation.

 ONGOING CARE

DIET
- No special diet
- Weight-loss diet is recommended if obesity is a problem.

PATIENT EDUCATION
- Avoid long periods of standing and crossing legs when sitting.
- Exercise (walking, running) regularly to improve leg strength and circulation.
- Maintain an appropriate weight.
- Wear elastic support stockings.
- Avoid clothing that constricts legs.
- JAMA Patient Page | Treatment of Varicose Veins: http://jama.jamanetwork.com/article.aspx?articleid=1672241

PROGNOSIS
- Usual course: chronic
- Favorable with appropriate treatment

COMPLICATIONS
- Complications with sclerotherapy include hyperpigmentation, matting, local urticaria, cutaneous necrosis, microthrombi, accidental intra-arterial injection, phlebitis, deep vein thrombosis, thromboembolism, scintillating scotomas, nerve damage, and allergic reactions.
- Petechial hemorrhages
- Chronic edema
- Superimposed infection
- Varicose ulcers
- Pigmentation
- Eczema
- Recurrence after surgical treatment
- Scarring/nerve damage from stripping technique
- Neurologic complications after sclerotherapy are rare.

REFERENCES
1. Bootun R, Onida S, Lane TRA, et al. Varicose veins and their management. *Surgery (Oxford)*. 2016;34(4):165–171.
2. Shingler S, Robertson L, Boghossian S, et al. Compression stockings for the initial treatment of varicose veins in patients without venous ulceration. *Cochrane Database Syst Rev*. 2013;(12):CD008819.
3. Hamdan A. Management of varicose veins and venous insufficiency. *JAMA*. 2012;308(24):2612–2621.
4. National Institute for Health and Care Excellence. *Varicose Veins in the Legs: The Diagnosis and Management of Varicose Veins*. London, United Kingdom: National Institute for Health and Care Excellence; 2013.
5. He G, Zheng C, Yu MA, et al. Comparison of ultrasound-guided endovenous laser ablation and radiofrequency for the varicose veins treatment: an updated meta-analysis. *Int J Surg*. 2017;39:267–275.

CODES

ICD10
- I83.90 Asymptomatic varicose veins of unspecified lower extremity
- I83.009 Varicose veins of unsp lower extremity w ulcer of unsp site
- I83.10 Varicose veins of unsp lower extremity with inflammation

CLINICAL PEARLS
- Treatment by minimally invasive outpatient procedures are preferred.
- RFA and EVLA have been demonstrated to be superior to open surgical techniques for the treatment of varicose veins with similar improvement in quality of life. NICE recommends using them as first-line treatment of truncal vein incompetence.

V

VASCULITIS

Irene J. Tan, MD, FACR

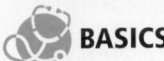 **BASICS**

DESCRIPTION

An inflammatory disorder of blood vessels

- Clinical features result from the destruction of blood vessel walls with subsequent thrombosis, ischemia, bleeding, and/or aneurysm formation.
- Vasculitis is a large, heterogeneous group of diseases classified by the predominant size, type, and location of involved blood vessels (1).
  - Small-vessel vasculitis
    - Microscopic polyangiitis (MPA)
    - Granulomatosis with polyangiitis (GPA; formerly Wegener granulomatosis)
    - Eosinophilic granulomatosis with polyangiitis (EGPA; formerly Churg-Strauss syndrome)
    - Antiglomerular basement membrane disease (anti-GBM)
    - Cryoglobulinemic vasculitis
    - IgA vasculitis (formerly Henoch-Schönlein purpura)
    - Hypocomplementemic urticarial vasculitis
  - Medium-vessel vasculitis
    - Polyarteritis nodosa (PAN)
    - Kawasaki disease (KD)
  - Large-vessel vasculitis
    - Takayasu arteritis (TAK)
    - Giant cell arteritis (GCA)
- Vasculitis occurs as a primary disorder or secondary to infection, a drug reaction, malignancy, or connective tissue disease.
  - Variable vessel vasculitis
    - Behçet disease
    - Cogan syndrome
  - Single-organ vasculitis
    - Cutaneous leukocytoclastic angiitis
    - Cutaneous arteritis
    - Primary CNS vasculitis
  - Vasculitis associated with systemic disease
    - Lupus vasculitis
    - Rheumatoid vasculitis
    - Sarcoid vasculitis
  - Vasculitis associated with other etiology
    - Hepatitis C–associated cryoglobulinemic vasculitis
    - Hepatitis B–associated vasculitis
    - Syphilis-associated aortitis
    - Drug-induced immune complex vasculitis
    - Drug-associated antineutrophil cytoplasmic antibodies (ANCA)-associated vasculitis
    - Cancer-associated vasculitis
- Protean features often delay definitive diagnosis.

EPIDEMIOLOGY

Highly variable, depending on the particular syndrome

- Hypersensitivity vasculitis is most commonly encountered in clinical practice.
- KD, IgA vasculitis, and dermatomyositis are more common in children.
- TAK is most prevalent in young Asian women. GPA, MPA, and EGPA are more common in middle-aged males.
- GCA occurs exclusively in those >50 years of age and is rare in the African American population.

Incidence

Annual incidence in adults (unless otherwise specified)

- IgA vasculitis: 200 to 700/1 million in children <17 years of age
- GCA: 100 to 170/1 million in Caucasians age >50 years
- KD: depends on race/age; ~200/1 million
- PAN: 2 to 33/1 million
- GPA: 4 to 15/1 million
- MPA: 1 to 24/1 million
- EGPA: 1 to 3/1 million
- TAK: 2/1 million
- Primary CNS vasculitis: 2/1 million in adults
- Hypersensitivity vasculitis: depends on drug exposure
- Viral-/retroviral-associated vasculitis: unknown; >90% of cases of cryoglobulinemic vasculitis are associated with hepatitis C.
- Connective tissue disorder–associated vasculitis: variable

ETIOLOGY AND PATHOPHYSIOLOGY

- Three major immunopathogenic mechanisms
  - Immune-complex formation: systemic lupus erythematosus (SLE), IgA vasculitis (HSP), and cryoglobulinemic vasculitis
  - ANCAs: GPA, MPA, and EGPA
  - Pathogenic T-lymphocyte response: GCA and TAK
- Pathophysiology best understood where known drug triggers have been identified (e.g., antibiotics, sulfonamides, and hydralazine)

Genetics

- Several vasculitides linked to candidate genes
- No single gene has been found to cause vasculitis.
- Angiotensin-converting enzyme insertion/deletion polymorphism is associated with susceptibility to vasculitis, especially in Behçet disease and IgA vasculitis.

RISK FACTORS

A combination of genetic susceptibility and environmental exposure likely triggers onset.

GENERAL PREVENTION

Early identification is the key to prevent irreversible organ damage in severe forms of systemic vasculitis.

COMMONLY ASSOCIATED CONDITIONS

Hepatitis C (cryoglobulinemic vasculitis), hepatitis B (PAN), cytomegalovirus (CMV), Epstein-Barr virus (EBV), HIV (viral-/retroviral-associated vasculitis), SLE, rheumatoid arthritis (RA), Sjögren syndrome, mixed connective tissue disease (MCTD), dermatomyositis, ankylosing spondylitis, Behçet disease, relapsing polychondritis (CTD-associated vasculitis), respiratory tract methicillin-resistant *Staphylococcus aureus* (MRSA) in GPA, levamisole-adulterated cocaine, medications: propylthiouracil, methimazole, hydralazine, minocycline, levamisole-tainted cocaine

DIAGNOSIS

HISTORY

- Consider age, gender, and ethnicity.
- Comprehensive medication history
- Family history of vasculitis

- Constitutional symptoms: fever, weight loss, malaise, fatigue, diminished appetite, sweats
- CNS/PNS: mononeuritis multiplex, polyneuropathy, headaches, visual loss, tinnitus, stroke, seizure, encephalopathy
- Heart/lung: myocardial infarction, cardiomyopathy, pericarditis, cough, chest pain, hemoptysis, dyspnea
- Renal: hematuria
- GI: abdominal pain, hematochezia, perforation
- Musculoskeletal: arthralgia, myalgia
- Miscellaneous: unexplained ischemic or hemorrhagic events, chronic sinusitis, and recurrent epistaxis
- Note the organs affected and estimate the size of blood vessels involved.
- Demographics, clinical features, and the predominant vessel size/organ involvement help identify specific type of vasculitis.

PHYSICAL EXAM

- Vital signs: blood pressure (hypertension) and pulse (regularity and rate)
- Skin: palpable purpura, livedo reticularis, nodules, ulcers, gangrene, nail bed capillary changes
- Neurologic: cranial nerve exam, sensorimotor exam
- Ocular exam: visual fields, scleritis, episcleritis
- Cardiopulmonary exam: rubs, murmurs, arrhythmias
- Abdominal exam: tenderness, organomegaly

DIFFERENTIAL DIAGNOSIS

- Fibromuscular dysplasia
- Embolic disease (atheroma, cholesterol emboli, atrial myxoma, mycotic aneurysm with embolization)
- Drug-induced vasospasm (cocaine, amphetamines, ergots)
- Thrombotic thrombocytopenic disorders (disseminated intravascular coagulation [DIC], thrombotic thrombocytopenic purpura [TTP], antiphospholipid syndrome, heparin- or warfarin-induced thrombosis), thromboangiitis obliterans
- Systemic infection (infective endocarditis, fungal infections, disseminated gonococcal infection, Lyme disease, syphilis, Rocky Mountain spotted fever [RMSF], bacteremia, ehrlichiosis, babesiosis)
- Malignancy (lymphomatoid granulomatosis, angioimmunoblastic T-cell lymphoma, intravascular lymphoma)
- Miscellaneous (Goodpasture syndrome, sarcoidosis, amyloidosis, Whipple disease, congenital coarctation of aorta)

DIAGNOSTIC TESTS & INTERPRETATION

ALERT

Renal involvement is often clinically silent. Routine serum creatinine and urinalysis with microscopy are needed to identify underlying glomerulonephritis.

- Initial tests exclude alternate diagnoses and guide therapy.
- Routine tests
  - CBC
  - Liver enzymes
  - Serum creatinine
  - Urinalysis with microscopy

- Specific serology
  – Antinuclear antibodies (ANA)
  – Rheumatoid factor (RF)
  – Rapid plasma reagin/venereal disease reaction level (RPR/VDRL)
  – RMSF titers; Lyme titers
  – Complement levels C3, C4
  – ANCA
  – Antiproteinase 3 (anti-PR3) antibodies
  – Antimyeloperoxidase (anti-MPO) antibodies
  – Hepatitis screen for B and C
  – Cryoglobulin
  – Anti-GBM titer
  – HIV
  – Serum and urine protein electrophoresis
- Miscellaneous
  – Drug screen
  – ESR
  – C-reactive protein
  – Creatine kinase (CK)
  – Blood culture
  – ECG
- CXR, CT scan, MRI, and arteriography may be required to delineate extent of organs involved.

Diagnostic Procedures/Other
- Electromyography with nerve conduction can document neuropathy and target nerve for biopsy.
- Biopsy of affected site confirms diagnosis (e.g., temporal artery, sural nerve, renal biopsy).
- If biopsy is not practical, angiography may be diagnostic for large- and medium-vessel vasculitides.
- Bronchoscopy may be required to differentiate pulmonary infection from potentially life-threatening hemorrhagic vasculitis in patients with hemoptysis.

Test Interpretation
Blood vessel biopsy shows immune cell infiltration into vessel wall layers with varying degrees of necrosis and granuloma formation, depending on the type.

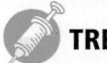

TREATMENT

GENERAL MEASURES
- Discontinue offending drug (hypersensitivity vasculitis).
- Simple observation for mild cases of IgA vasculitis
- ANCA-associated vasculitis has two-phase treatment: initial induction followed by maintenance (steady tapering of corticosteroids with immunosuppressants or immunomodulators).

MEDICATION
First Line
Corticosteroids are initial anti-inflammatory of choice.

Second Line
Cytotoxic medications, immunomodulatory, or biologic agents (e.g., cyclophosphamide (2)[B],(3)[A], methotrexate (4)[A], azathioprine (4)[A], leflunomide (4)[A], mycophenolate mofetil (2)[B], and rituximab (3)[A]) are often required in combination with corticosteroids for rapidly progressive vasculitis with significant organ involvement or inadequate response to corticosteroids. Rituximab (3)[A] is the first FDA-approved treatment for GPA and MPA. Tocilizumab (5)[A] is the first FDA-approved treatment for GCA. Mepolizumab (6)[A] is the first FDA-approved treatment for EGPA.

ISSUES FOR REFERRAL
- Rheumatology referral for complicated cases where newer or more toxic treatments are required
- Nephrology referral for persistent hematuria or proteinuria, rising creatinine, or a positive ANCA titer
- Pulmonary referral for persistent pulmonary infiltrate unresponsive to antibiotic therapy or if gross hemoptysis

ADDITIONAL THERAPIES
- IVIG and aspirin for KD, where corticosteroids are contraindicated
- Plasma exchange appears to improve recovery of patients with severe acute renal failure secondary to vasculitis and pulmonary hemorrhage (4)[A].

SURGERY/OTHER PROCEDURES
Rarely, corrective surgery is required to repair tissue damage as a result of aggressive vasculitis.

ADMISSION, INPATIENT, AND NURSING CONSIDERATIONS
- Hemoptysis, acute renal failure, intestinal ischemia, any organ-threatening symptoms or signs, and/or need for biopsy
- Initial therapy is guided by the organ system involved.
  – If pulmonary hemorrhage is present, life-saving measures may include mechanical ventilation, plasmapheresis, and immunosuppression.
  – If acute renal failure is present, attend to electrolyte and fluid balance and consider plasma exchange and immunosuppression.
  – If signs of intestinal ischemia are present, make NPO and consider plasmapheresis, immunosuppression, and parenteral nutrition.
- Discharge criteria: stabilization or resolution of potential life-threatening symptoms

 ## ONGOING CARE

FOLLOW-UP RECOMMENDATIONS
If significant coronary artery disease is involved in KD, moderate activity restriction may be of benefit.

Patient Monitoring
Frequent clinical follow-up supported by patient self-monitoring to identify disease relapse

DIET
Alter diets for patients with renal involvement or hyperglycemia/dyslipidemia.

PROGNOSIS
Prognosis is good for patients with vasculitis and limited organ involvement. Relapsing courses, renal, intestinal, or extensive lung involvement have a poorer prognosis.

COMPLICATIONS
- Persistent organ dysfunction may be the result of the disease, medications, or inflammation/scarring in the more serious forms of vasculitis.
- Early morbidity/mortality is due to active vasculitic disease; delayed morbidity/mortality may also be secondary to complications of chronic therapy with cytotoxic medications.

REFERENCES

1. Jennette JC, Falk RJ, Bacon PA, et al. 2012 Revised International Chapel Hill Consensus Conference nomenclature of vasculitides. *Arthritis Rheum*. 2013; 65(1):1–11.
2. Appel GB, Contreras G, Dooley MA, et al; for Aspreva Lupus Management Study Group. Mycophenolate mofetil versus cyclophosphamide for induction treatment of lupus nephritis. *J Am Soc Nephrol*. 2009;20(5):1103–1112.
3. Stone JH, Merkel PA, Spiera R, et al; for RAVE-ITN Research Group. Rituximab versus cyclophosphamide for ANCA-associated vasculitis. *N Engl J Med*. 2010; 363(3):221–232.
4. Walters GD, Willis NS, Craig JC. Interventions for renal vasculitis in adults. A systematic review. *BMC Nephrol*. 2010;11:12.
5. Villiger PM, Adler S, Kuchen S, et al. Tocilizumab for induction and maintenance of remission in giant cell arteritis: a phase 2, randomised, double-blind, placebo-controlled trial. *Lancet*. 2016;387(10031): 1921–1927.
6. Wechsler ME, Akuthota P, Jayne D, et al; for EGPA Mepolizumab Study Team. Mepolizumab or placebo for eosinophilic granulomatosis with polyangiitis. *N Engl J Med*. 2017;376(20):1921–1932.

ADDITIONAL READING

- Gatto M, Iaccarino L, Canova M, et al. Pregnancy and vasculitis: a systematic review of the literature. *Autoimmun Rev*. 2012;11(6–7):A447–A459.
- Lee YH, Choi SJ, Ji JD, et al. Associations between the angiotensin-converting enzyme insertion/deletion polymorphism and susceptibility to vasculitis: a meta-analysis. *J Renin Angiotensin Aldosterone Syst*. 2012;13(1):196–201.
- National Heart, Lung, and Blood Institute. What is vasculitis? http://www.nhlbi.nih.gov/health/health-topics/topics/vas/. Accessed October 24, 2018.
- Vasculitis Foundation: https://www.vasculitisfoundation.org

CODES

ICD10
- I77.6 Arteritis, unspecified
- M31.30 Wegener's granulomatosis without renal involvement
- M30.0 Polyarteritis nodosa

CLINICAL PEARLS

- Suspect vasculitis in patients with a petechial rash, palpable purpura, glomerulonephritis, pulmonary-renal syndrome, intestinal ischemia, or mononeuritis multiplex.
- Exclude silent renal involvement by routinely obtaining serum creatinine and urinalysis with microscopy.
- Vasculitis has "skip" lesions, which may complicate diagnostic biopsy.
- In patients with vasculitis, look for an underlying inciting process such as medication, infection, thrombosis, or malignancy.

V

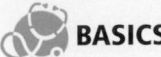

VENOUS INSUFFICIENCY ULCERS

Renata Scalabrin Reis, MD • Seena Mariate Jose, MD • Marcy Wiemers, MD

BASICS

- Venous insufficiency disorders include simple spider veins, varicose veins, and leg edema.
- In the United States, 23% of adults have varicose veins, an estimated 22 million women and 11 million men.
- Venous leg ulcers are the most serious consequence of venous insufficiency.
- Venous leg ulcers are a type of chronic wound affecting up to 1% of adults in developed countries at some point during their lives.
- 500,000 people in the United States have chronic venous ulcers, with an estimated treatment cost of >$2.5 billion per year.

DESCRIPTION

- Full-thickness skin defect with surrounding pigmentation and dermatitis
- Most frequently located in ankle region of lower leg ("gaiter region")
- Present for >30 days and fails to heal spontaneously
- May only have mild pain unless infected
- Other signs of chronic venous insufficiency include edema/brawny edema and chronic skin changes (i.e., hyperpigmentation and/or fibrosis).

EPIDEMIOLOGY

Up to 80% of leg ulcers are caused by venous disease; arterial disease accounts for 10–25%, which may coexist with venous disease.

Incidence

- Overall incidence of venous ulcers is 18/100,000 persons.
- Prevalent sex: women > men (20.4 vs. 14.6/100,000 for venous ulcer); increased with age for both sexes

Prevalence

- Seen in ~1% of adult population in industrialized countries; increased to 4% in patients ≥80 years old
- Prevalence studies only available for Western countries
- Point prevalence underestimates the extent of the disease because ulcers often recur.
- 70% of ulcers recur within 5 years of closure.

ETIOLOGY AND PATHOPHYSIOLOGY

- In a diseased venous system, venous pressure in the deep system fails to fall with ambulation, causing venous hypertension.
- Venous hypertension comes from the following:
  - Venous obstruction
  - Incompetent venous valves in the deep or superficial system
  - Inadequate muscle contraction (e.g., arthritis, myopathies, neuropathies) so that the calf pump is ineffective
- Venous pressure transmitted to capillaries leading to venous hypertensive microangiopathy and extravasation of RBCs and proteins (especially fibrinogen)
- Increased RBC aggregation leads to reduced oxygen transport, slowed arteriolar circulation, and ischemia at the skin level, contributing to ulcers.
- Leukocytes aggregate to hypoxic areas and increase local inflammation.
- Factors promoting persistence of venous ulcers
  - Prolonged chronic inflammation
  - Bacterial infection, critical colonization

RISK FACTORS

- History of leg injury
- Obesity
- Congestive heart failure (CHF)

- History of deep venous thrombosis (DVT)
- Failure of calf muscle pump (e.g., ankle fusion, inactivity) is a strong independent predictor of poorly healing wounds.
- Previous varicose vein surgery
- Family history

GENERAL PREVENTION

- Primary prevention after symptomatic DVT: Prescribe compression hose to be used as soon as feasible for at least 2 years (≥20 to 30 mm Hg compression).
- Secondary prevention of recurrent ulceration includes compression, correction of the underlying problem, and surveillance.
- Circumstantial evidence from two RCTs showed those who stopped wearing compression hose were more likely to recur.
- Because most ulcers develop from trauma, avoiding lower leg trauma may help to prevent ulceration.

COMMONLY ASSOCIATED CONDITIONS

Up to 50% of patients have allergic reactions to topical agents commonly used for treatment.

- Contact sensitivity was more common in patients with stasis dermatitis (62% vs. 38%).
- Avoid neomycin sulfate in particular (including triple antibiotic ointment).

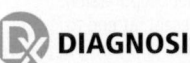

DIAGNOSIS

A diagnosis of venous reflux or obstruction must be established by an objective test beyond the routine clinical examination of the extremity.

HISTORY

- Family history of venous insufficiency and ulcers
- Recent trauma
- Nature of pain: achy (better with leg elevation)
- Wound drainage
- Duration of wound and over-the-counter (OTC) treatments already attempted
- History of DVTs (especially factor V Leiden mutation; strongly associated with ulceration)
- History of leg edema that improves overnight
- Edema that does not improve overnight is more likely lymphedema.

PHYSICAL EXAM

- Look for evidence of venous insufficiency:
  - Pitting edema
  - Hemosiderin staining (red and brown spotty or diffuse pigment changes)
  - Stasis dermatitis
  - White, nondraining skin lesions (atrophie blanche)
  - Lipodermatosclerosis ("bottle neck" narrowing in the lower leg from fibrosis and scarring)
- Look for evidence of significant lymphedema (i.e., dorsal foot or toe edema, edema that does not resolve overnight or with elevation). This may require referral for special comprehensive lymph therapy.
- Examine for palpable pulses.
- Examine wound for the following:
  - Length, width, depth, to monitor wound healing rate
  - Presence of necrotic tissue
  - Presence of biofilms or infection: purulent material in the wound, increased amount odorous exudate, spreading cellulitis, fever, and chills

- Get initial and interim girth measurements (at ankle and midcalf) to monitor edema.
- Important to rule out poor arterial circulation:
  - Compression dressings cannot be used in patients with ankle-brachial index (ABI) <0.8.

DIFFERENTIAL DIAGNOSIS

- Arterial insufficiency ulcer
- Neuropathic ulcer
- Malignancy
- Sickle cell ulcer
- Vasculitic ulcer
- Calciphylaxis
- Cryoglobulinemia
- Pyoderma gangrenosum
- Collagen vascular disease
- Leishmaniasis
- Cutaneous tuberculosis

DIAGNOSTIC TESTS & INTERPRETATION

- Consider prothrombin time (PT)/international normalized ratio (INR) and partial thromboplastin time (PTT) if patient is anticoagulated.
- Consider biopsy of leg ulcers that fail to heal or have atypical features.
- Consider factor V Leiden mutation; strongly associated with venous ulcers
- Test for diabetes as necessary with fasting glucose.
- Use duplex imaging to diagnose anatomic and hemodynamic abnormalities with venous insufficiency. It will also identify any DVT present.

Diagnostic Procedures/Other

- Check ABI for evidence of arterial disease.
- An ABI <0.8 is a relative contraindication to compression therapy.
- Duplex imaging for evaluation of superficial and deep venous reflux and incompetent perforator veins
- With concomitant severe arterial insufficiency, refer to a vascular surgeon for revascularization.

Test Interpretation

Strongly consider biopsy on wounds with atypical locations, failure to heal, or any suspicion of malignancy.

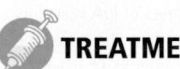

TREATMENT

- Treatment options: conservative management, mechanical treatment, medications, and surgical options
- Goals: Reduce edema, improve ulcer healing, and prevent recurrence.

GENERAL MEASURES

- Compression therapy is the standard of care for venous ulcers and chronic venous insufficiency (1)[C].
- Leg elevation: requires raising the legs above the level of the heart to reduce edema and improve microcirculation and oxygen delivery; is most effective if performed for 30 minutes, 3 to 4 times a day
- Dressings are used under compression bandages to promote faster healing and prevent adherence of the bandage to the ulcer; types: hydrocolloids, foams, hydrogels, paste, and simple nonadherent dressing
- The choice of dressing can be guided by cost, ease of application, patient's and physician's preference.
- If exudative, use absorptive dressing (calcium alginate or absorptive pads) (1)[A]. If minimal exudate, use hydrocolloid. If wound tends to be dry, use hydrogel.

- To prevent maceration of surrounding skin, use a barrier ointment/cream.
- Conservative management
  - Compression therapy methods: inelastic, elastic, and intermittent pneumatic compression. Outcome: reduces edema, improves venous reflux, enhances healing of ulcers, and reduces pain (2)[C]
  - Success rates range from 30% to 60% at 24 weeks and 70–85% after 1 year.
  - After an ulcer has healed, lifelong maintenance of compression therapy may reduce the risk of recurrence.
  - Adherence to therapy may be limited by pain, drainage, application difficulty, and physical limitations (obesity and contact dermatitis).
  - Contraindications: clinically significant arterial disease and uncompensated heart failure
  - Inelastic compression therapy: provides pressure during ambulation and muscle contraction but no resting pressure. Most common: unna boot (zinc oxide moist bandage that hardens after application)
  - Elastic: sustain compression during rest and activity. Compression stockings: Pressure should be at least 20 to 30 mm Hg and preferably 30 to 44 mm Hg. They should be removed at night and should be replaced every 6 months. Elastic bandages (i.e., Profore) are alternatives to compression stockings.
  - Intermittent pneumatic compression is expensive and requires immobilization, therefore is generally reserved for bedridden patients.
- Mechanical treatment
  - Negative pressure wound therapy (NPWT) (i.e., vacuum-assisted closure [VAC] dressings may be beneficial but no clear benefit over optimal traditional wound care)

MEDICATION

- Pentoxifylline 400 mg PO TID. GI side effects are common (nausea, vomiting, diarrhea, heartburn, loss of appetite) (3)[A].
- Aspirin 300 mg PO daily
- Routine use of antibiotics for all venous ulcers is not recommended (1)[A].

ISSUES FOR REFERRAL

- With prominent toe or foot edema, consider lymphedema. Refer to a certified lymphedema therapist (CLT).
- Refer to a wound clinic for complex or poorly healing ulcers.
- Refer to a vascular specialist for recurrent ulcers.
- Use home health nurses to help with immobile patients needing frequent wrapping/dressing changes.

ADDITIONAL THERAPIES

- Edema management: Reduce venous hypertension and improve venous return to reduce inflammation, pain, and improve healing (4)[A].
- Encourage exercise (e.g., activation of calf muscle pump with ankle flexion and extension) in conjunction with leg compression and elevation.
- Infection control
  - Débridement of necrotic tissue
  - Treat cellulitis (usually gram-positive bacteria) with bactericidal systemic antibiotics. Suspect local infection when there is pain or no improvement in the wound after 2 weeks of compression. Consider deep quantitative swab, after thorough cleansing, or tissue biopsy for culture.
  - Treat critical colonization with topical antimicrobials, such as cadexomer iodine (silver dressings and honey are widely used, but definitive data are lacking) (1)[A].

SURGERY/OTHER PROCEDURES

- Current evidence does not definitively support the superiority of surgical interventions (open or endovascular) compared with compression alone with respect to ulcer healing, recurrence, and time to ulcer healing in patients with lower extremity venous ulcer disease (5).
- If necrotic tissue, consider sharp débridement.
- Skin grafting generally is not effective if there is persistent edema, and the underlying venous disease is not addressed.
- Allografts made of synthetic bilayered skin with living keratinocytes and fibroblasts are the only cellular tissue product (CTP) to improve healing at 6 months. There is insufficient evidence to support use of autografts, xenografts (6)[A].

COMPLEMENTARY & ALTERNATIVE MEDICINE

- Chestnut seed extract (50 mg BID) is effective for venous insufficiency but not ulceration.
- Topical medicinal honey used on wounds shows no evidence of improved healing.
- Oral zinc has not been shown to be beneficial.

ADMISSION, INPATIENT, AND NURSING CONSIDERATIONS

- Consider for those with acute significant cellulitis.
- Infected wounds in diabetic patients usually requires IV antibiotics.

 ## ONGOING CARE

FOLLOW-UP RECOMMENDATIONS

- When ulcers are nearly healed and edema is controlled, switch from compression bandages to compression hose.
- Insurance may not reimburse for compression hose unless an ulcer is present. Consider referral for hose fitting prior to the ulcer being healed.

Patient Monitoring

Monitor the ulcer for healing by measuring its area. Expect at least 10% reduction every 2 weeks.

DIET

- Low-salt diet is recommended for patients with fluid overload.
- Weight loss is recommended for overweight/obese patients.

PATIENT EDUCATION

- Patient education of underlying mechanism is important for long-term management.
- Long-term plan for edema management and use of compression therapy
- Wound care
- Early recognition and treatment of new ulcers or cellulitis

PROGNOSIS

- Venous insufficiency is a lifelong medical problem.
- Ulcers recur frequently. Early identification and immediate treatment are essential.
- Ongoing diligence with edema control, avoiding infections, and avoiding trauma are important.

REFERENCES

1. O'Meara S, Al-Kurdi D, Ologun Y, et al. Antibiotics and antiseptics for venous leg ulcers. *Cochrane Database Syst Rev.* 2014;(1):CD003557.
2. Latz CA, Brown KR, Bush RL. Compression therapies for chronic venous leg ulcers: interventions and adherence. *Chron Wound Care Manag Res.* 2015;2015(1):11–21.
3. Jull AB, Arroll B, Parag V, et al. Pentoxifylline for treating venous leg ulcers. *Cochrane Database Syst Rev.* 2012;(12):CD001733.
4. O'Meara S, Cullum N, Nelson EA, et al. Compression for venous leg ulcers. *Cochrane Database Syst Rev.* 2012;(11):CD000265.
5. Mauck KF, Asi N, Undavalli C, et al. Systematic review and meta-analysis of surgical interventions versus conservative therapy for venous ulcers. *J Vasc Surg.* 2014;60(Suppl 2):60S–70S.e2.
6. Jones JE, Nelson EA, Al-Hity A. Skin grafting for venous leg ulcers. *Cochrane Database Syst Rev.* 2013;(1):CD001737.

ADDITIONAL READING

- Kearon C, Kahn SR, Agnelli G, et al. Antithrombotic therapy for venous thromboembolic disease: American College of Chest Physicians Evidence-Based Clinical Practice Guidelines (8th edition). *Chest.* 2008;133(Suppl 6):454S–545S.
- O'Donnell TF Jr, Passman MA, Marston WA, et al. Management of venous leg ulcers: clinical practice guidelines of the Society for Vascular Surgery® and the American Venous Forum. *J Vasc Surg.* 2014;60(Suppl 2):3S–59S.
- Varatharajan L, Thapar A, Lane T, et al. Pharmacological adjuncts for chronic venous ulcer healing: a systematic review. *Phlebology.* 2016;31(5):356–365.

 ## CODES

ICD10

- I87.2 Venous insufficiency (chronic) (peripheral)
- I83.009 Varicose veins of unsp lower extremity w ulcer of unsp site
- I89.0 Lymphedema, not elsewhere classified

CLINICAL PEARLS

- Venous stasis: dull ache or pain in lower extremities, swelling that subsides with elevation, eczematous changes of the surrounding skin, and varicose veins
- Venous ulcers often occur over bony prominences (medial malleolus) and are generally irregular and shallow. Granulation tissue and fibrin are often present in the ulcer base.
- The diagnosis of venous ulcers is clinical.
- Tests such as ABI and color duplex ultrasonography may be helpful if the diagnosis is unclear.
- Compression therapy is the standard of care for venous ulcers and chronic venous insufficiency.
- An ABI <0.8 is a relative contraindication to compression therapy. Refer those patients to vascular surgery.
- Clinical severity score can guide the assessment: CEAP (clinical, etiology, anatomy, and pathophysiology). Poor prognostic factors for venous ulcers include large size and prolonged duration.
- Treat critical colonization with topical antimicrobials (avoid neomycin).
- Refer patients with recurrent or venous ulcers failing to heal with moist wound care and compression after 4 to 6 weeks to wound specialist.

V

VENTRICULAR SEPTAL DEFECT

Luay Sarsam, MD • Cherry Onaiwu, MD, MS • Carrie Valenta, MD, FACP, FHM

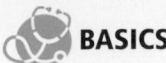 BASICS

DESCRIPTION
- Congenital or acquired defect of the interventricular septum that allows communication of blood between the left and the right ventricles
- Second most common congenital heart malformation reported in infants and children. It can also occur as a complication of acute myocardial infarction (MI).
- Severity of the defect is correlated with its size, with large defects being the most severe.
- Blood flow across the defect typically is left to right, depending on defect size and pulmonary vascular resistance (PVR).
- Prolonged left to right shunting of blood can lead to pulmonary hypertension (HTN). This may eventually lead to a reversal of flow across the defect and cyanosis (Eisenmenger complex).

Geriatric Considerations
Almost entirely associated with MI

Pediatric Considerations
Congenital defect

ALERT
- Pregnancy may exacerbate symptoms and signs of a ventricular septal defect (VSD).
- Can be tolerated during pregnancy if VSD is small
- May be associated with an increased risk of pre-eclampsia in women with an unrepaired VSD

EPIDEMIOLOGY
Incidence
- Congenital defect: no gender predilection, occurs in ~2/1,000 live births and accounts for 30% of all congenital cardiac malformations
- Post-MI: Some studies suggest that gender may play a role.

Prevalence
In the United States:
- Occurs in ~50% of all children with congenital heart disease
- Low prevalence in adults (~0.3 per 1,000) due to spontaneous closure
- Post-MI complication in ~0.2–3% of cases

ETIOLOGY AND PATHOPHYSIOLOGY
- Congenital
- In adults, complication of MI
- Some reports of iatrogenic causes

Genetics
Multifactorial etiology; autosomal dominant and recessive transmissions have been reported.

RISK FACTORS
- Congenital VSD:
  - Risk of sibling being affected: 4.2%
  - Risk of offspring being affected: 4%
  - Prematurity
- Post-MI VSD:
  - Advanced age
  - Arterial HTN
  - First MI
  - Most frequent within 1st week after MI
  - Most commonly after anterior wall acute MI

GENERAL PREVENTION
Avoid prenatal exposure to known risk factors (ibuprofen, marijuana, organic solvents, febrile illness). For adults, avoid risk factors for MI and obtain evaluation before pregnancy.

COMMONLY ASSOCIATED CONDITIONS
- Congenital:
  - Tetralogy of Fallot
  - Aortic valvular deformities, especially aortic insufficiency and bicuspid aortic valve
  - Down syndrome (trisomy 21), endocardial cushion defect
  - Transposition of great arteries
  - Coarctation of aorta
  - Tricuspid atresia
  - Truncus arteriosus
  - Patent ductus arteriosus
  - Atrial septal defect
  - Pulmonic stenosis
  - Subaortic stenosis
- Adult: coronary artery disease

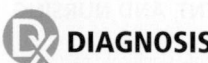 DIAGNOSIS

HISTORY
- Presentation depends on degree of shunting across the defect; may be completely asymptomatic with small defects
- Respiratory distress, tachypnea, tachycardia
- Diaphoresis with feeds, poor weight gain in infants

PHYSICAL EXAM
- Small defect:
  - Harsh holosystolic murmur loudest at left lower sternal border
  - Detected after PVR drops at 4 to 8 weeks of life
- Moderate defect:
  - Harsh holosystolic murmur at left lower sternal border associated with a thrill
  - Forceful apical impulse with lateral displacement
  - Increased intensity of P_2
  - Diastolic rumble at apex due to increased flow across the mitral valve
- Large defect:
  - Holosystolic murmur heard throughout the precordium with diastolic rumble at apex with precordial bulge and hyperactivity, although large defects may have little or no murmur initially
  - If congestive heart failure (CHF) exists: tachycardia, tachypnea, and hepatomegaly
  - If pulmonary HTN exists: cyanosis with exertion
  - If Eisenmenger complex is present: cyanosis and clubbing

DIFFERENTIAL DIAGNOSIS
- Patent ductus arteriosus, atrial septal defect
- Children: tetralogy of Fallot
- Adults: mitral regurgitation

DIAGNOSTIC TESTS & INTERPRETATION
Initial Tests (lab, imaging)
- A 12-lead ECG may show left ventricular hypertrophy and left atrial enlargement initially. As pulmonary HTN develops, right ventricular hypertrophy and right atrial enlargement may be seen.
- A chest x-ray (CXR) may demonstrate increased pulmonary vascularity and/or cardiomegaly.

- A 2D echocardiogram for visualization of location and size of defect
- Color flow Doppler for direction and velocity of VSD jet; may be used to estimate right ventricular pressure
- Ventriculography in conjunction with above imaging modalities can aid in characterization of VSD but is invasive.

Follow-Up Tests & Special Considerations
- Weight and hematocrit check
- Cardiac catheterization performed occasionally for perioperative planning or to assess need for closure of defect

Diagnostic Procedures/Other
- Cardiac catheterization (left and right sides of heart) can confirm the diagnosis, document number of defects, quantify ratio of pulmonary blood flow to systemic blood flow (Qp/Qs), and determine PVR.
- Demonstration of an oxygen saturation step up from the right atrium to the distal pulmonary artery

Test Interpretation
- Congenital VSD (four major anatomic types)
  - Membranous (70%)
  - Muscular (20%)
  - Atrioventricular canal type (5%)
  - Supracristal (5%; higher in Asians)
- Post-MI VSD predominantly involves muscular septum.
- Right bundle branch block is common after surgical repair.

 TREATMENT

- Start diuretic therapy if signs of fluid overload (1)[A].
- Minimize IV fluids.
- Consider ACE inhibitor and/or digoxin.
- Nasogastric feeds for neonates
- Correct anemia via iron supplementation or a possible RBC transfusion.

GENERAL MEASURES
- Appropriate health care maintenance
- Outpatient, until surgical repair is indicated
- Inpatient management in setting of acute MI
- Inpatient for treatment of severe CHF

MEDICATION
First Line
- Per the 2007 American Heart Association guidelines, endocarditis antibiotic prophylaxis is not recommended for most VSDs. It is recommended for VSDs associated with complex cyanotic heart disease, during the first 6 months after surgical repair, or for residual VSDs located near the patch following surgery (2)[A].
- Pediatric: Medications aim to control pulmonary edema, decrease work of breathing, and allow for growth:
  - Furosemide 1 to 2 mg/kg PO/IV once to twice a day
  - Spironolactone 1 to 2 mg/kg/day divided BID

– Captopril
  - Infants: oral: 0.3 to 2.5 mg/kg/day divided every 8 to 12 hours; max 2 mg/kg/day
  - Children and adolescents: oral: 0.3 to 6.0 mg/kg/day divided every 8 to 12 hours; maximum daily dose: 150 mg/day
– Digoxin: infants <2 years of age, 10 μg/kg/day PO divided BID; children, 2 to 10 years of age, 5 to 10 μg/kg/day PO divided BID; children >10 years of age, 2 to 5 μg/kg/day PO divided BID
- Adults: Digoxin and diuretics may be beneficial in some circumstances (1)[A].
- Side effects:
  – Drugs that increase systemic vascular resistance may increase left-to-right shunting and cause signs and symptoms of pulmonary overcirculation.
  – HTN

Second Line
- Surgical closure is indicated if the pulmonic-to-systemic flow is >2:1 or with poorly controlled pulmonary overcirculation despite maximal medical and dietary interventions.
- If an infant with a VSD has persistent pulmonary HTN or failure to grow, surgical repair is recommended prior to 6 months of age even if patient is otherwise asymptomatic.
- For post-MI VSDs, afterload reduction, inotropic support, intra-aortic balloon pump, and left ventricular assist device may be used to stabilize the patient prior to surgery. Surgical repair includes septal débridement and patch placement.

ISSUES FOR REFERRAL
Close follow-up of a congenital VSD is necessary until primary intracardiac repair is performed to ensure that significant pulmonary HTN does not develop.

ADDITIONAL THERAPIES
- Infant caloric requirements up to 150 kcal/kg/day or more for adequate weight gain
- Treatment of iron deficiency anemia to increase oxygen-carrying capacity

SURGERY/OTHER PROCEDURES
- Surgical correction with either a VSD patch or repair is commonly used. Postsurgical outcomes for isolated VSD are excellent. Complications are rare and include reoperation for residual VSD, extended hospital stay, arrhythmias, valve injury, depressed ventricular function, and heart block (3)[B].
- Percutaneous transcatheter device closure has become a safe and effective option for some children with small to moderate VSDs. Complications include valvular regurgitation, residual defects, and heart block. There is a greater risk of conduction abnormality with this technique compared to surgical closure. Recent studies have shown steroids may decrease this risk (4)[A].
- Perventricular device closure (hybrid technique) of some subtypes of isolated VSDs without cardiopulmonary bypass is feasible under transesophageal echocardiographic (TEE) guidance. Complications are similar to percutaneous closure (5)[A].

ADMISSION, INPATIENT, AND NURSING CONSIDERATIONS
- Failure to thrive
- Pulmonary overcirculation/CHF
- Stabilize airway.
- Reduce temperature stress.
- Frequent vital sign monitoring; daily weight and calorie counts
- Discharge criteria: CHF stabilization, weight gain, or successful repair

ONGOING CARE

FOLLOW-UP RECOMMENDATIONS
- Small VSDs without evidence of CHF or pulmonary HTN generally can be followed every 1 to 5 years after the neonatal period.
- Moderate to large VSDs require more frequent follow-up.
- Potential complications of VSDs include right ventricular outflow obstruction and aortic valve prolapse.

Patient Monitoring
- Physical growth and development monitoring
- Influenza vaccine for children >6 months of age
- Palivizumab to children <12 months of age with hemodynamically significant lesions. Children with small VSDs do not need RSV prophylaxis (6)[A].

DIET
- Low sodium in heart failure
- High calorie in failure to thrive

PATIENT EDUCATION
- No activity restriction in absence of pulmonary HTN
- Parents need support and instructions for prevention of complications until the child is ready for surgery.

PROGNOSIS
- Congenital:
  – Course is variable depending on the size of the VSD.
  – Small VSD: Many will close spontaneously by age 3 years. Muscular defects are more likely to close spontaneously.
  – Large VSD: CHF or failure to thrive in infancy necessitating surgical repair
  – 20-year cumulative survival rate after surgery for isolated VSD is 87%; 40 years is 78% (7).
  – Progressive pulmonary vascular disease and pulmonary HTN are the most feared complications of VSD caused by left-to-right shunting and may eventually lead to reversal of the shunt (Eisenmenger complex). Death usually occurs in the 4th decade of life if untreated.
- Post-MI:
  – With medical management alone, 80–90% mortality in the first 2 weeks
  – Prognosis worse with inferior MI compared with anterior MI

COMPLICATIONS
- CHF
- Aortic insufficiency
- Sudden death
- Hemoptysis
- Cerebral abscess
- Paradoxical emboli
- Cardiogenic shock
- Heart block rarely may accompany surgical closure.
- Pulmonary HTN

REFERENCES

1. Faris RF, Flather M, Purcell H, et al. Diuretics for heart failure. *Cochrane Database Syst Rev*. 2012;(2):CD003838.
2. Wilson W, Taubert KA, Gewitz M, et al. Prevention of infective endocarditis: guidelines from the American Heart Association: a guideline from the American Heart Association Rheumatic Fever, Endocarditis, and Kawasaki Disease Committee, Council on Cardiovascular Disease in the Young, and the Council on Clinical Cardiology, Council on Cardiovascular

Surgery and Anesthesia, and the Quality of Care and Outcomes Research Interdisciplinary Working Group. *Circulation*. 2007;116(15):1736–1754.
3. Scully BB, Morales DL, Zafar F, et al. Current expectations for surgical repair of isolated ventricular septal defects. *Ann Thorac Surg*. 2010;89(2):544–549.
4. Yang L, Tai BC, Khin LW, et al. A systematic review on the efficacy and safety of transcatheter device closure of ventricular septal defects (VSD). *J Interv Cardiol*. 2014;27(3):260–272.
5. Yin S, Zhu D, Lin K, et al. Perventricular device closure of congenital ventricular septal defects. *J Card Surg*. 2014;29(3):390–400.
6. American Academy of Pediatrics Committee on Infectious Diseases, American Academy of Pediatrics Bronchiolitis Guidelines Committee. Updated guidance for palivizumab prophylaxis among infants and young children at increased risk of hospitalization for respiratory syncytial virus infection. *Pediatrics*. 2014;134(2):415–420.
7. Menting ME, Cuypers JA, Opić P, et al. The unnatural history of the ventricular septal defect: outcome up to 40 years after surgical closure. *J Am Coll Cardiol*. 2015;65(18):1941–1951.

ADDITIONAL READING
Penny DJ, Vick GW III. Ventricular septal defect. *Lancet*. 2011;377(9771):1103–1112.

SEE ALSO
Acute Coronary Syndromes: NSTE-ACS (Unstable Angina and NSTEMI); Down Syndrome; Tetralogy of Fallot

CODES

ICD10
- Q21.0 Ventricular septal defect
- I23.2 Ventricular septal defect as current comp following AMI
- Q21.3 Tetralogy of Fallot

CLINICAL PEARLS
- A loud 2/6 to 3/6 low-pitched harsh holosystolic murmur at the left lower sternal border is typical.
- A diastolic rumble at the apex indicates moderate to large VSD or ratio of pulmonary to systemic blood flow (Qp/Qs) >2:1, which likely will require surgical or percutaneous closure.
- Disappearance of the murmur could be secondary to spontaneous closure of the defect or the development of pulmonary HTN.
- Development of a new murmur of semilunar valve insufficiency should be further evaluated. Pulmonary regurgitation may occur as PVR increases, and the development of aortic regurgitation usually will require early surgery.

V

VERTIGO
Jeremy S. Raab, MD • James J. Arnold, DO, FACOFP, FAAFP

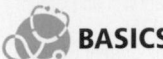 BASICS

DESCRIPTION
- A symptom, not a disease process. Causes can be peripheral or central, benign, or life-threatening. Cause determines treatment.
- May be described as a sensation of movement ("room spinning") when no movement is actually occurring
- However, do not rely on symptom quality—often unreliable. Focus on timing and triggers (1).
- System(s) affected: nervous, cardiovascular, psych
- Synonym(s): dizziness

EPIDEMIOLOGY
Incidence
- Vertigo/dizziness accounts for >4 million ED visits a year in United States, of which 80–85% have no serious underlying condition (2).
- Predominant sex: female = male; women are 3 times more likely to experience vertiginous migraine (1).

Geriatric Considerations
- Keep a higher index of suspicion for CVD, arrhythmias, and orthostatic hypotension.
- BPPV is more common in ages 50 to 70 years (1), an important risk factor for falls but is often undiagnosed.
- Medications are implicated almost 1/4 of the time (1).

Prevalence
- Ranges from 5% to 10% within the general population
- Lifetime prevalence for BPPV is 2.4%.

ETIOLOGY AND PATHOPHYSIOLOGY
- Dysfunction of the rotational velocity sensors of the inner ear results in asymmetric central processing; combination of sensory disturbance of motion and malfunction of the central vestibular apparatus
- Peripheral causes: acute vestibular neuritis, BPPV (posterior canal 85–95%, lateral canal 5–15%), Ménière disease, otosclerosis, acute labyrinthitis, cholesteatoma, perilymphatic fistula, superior canal dehiscence syndrome, motion sickness (1). BPPV, vestibular neuritis, and Ménière disease account for majority of peripheral causes (1).
- Central causes: cerebellar tumor, stroke, migraine, vestibular ischemia (1,2)
- Drug causes: psychotropic agents, anticonvulsants, aspirin, aminoglycosides, furosemide (diuretics), amiodarone, α-/β-blockers, nitrates, urologic medications, muscle relaxants, phosphodiesterase inhibitors (sildenafil), excessive insulin, ethanol, quinine, cocaine
- Other causes: orthostasis, arrhythmia, psychological

Genetics
Family history of CVD/migraines may indicate higher risk of central causes.

RISK FACTORS
- History of migraines
- History of CVD/risk factors for CVD
- Use of ototoxic medications
- Trauma/barotrauma

- Perilymphatic fistula
- Heavy weight-bearing
- Psychosocial stress/depression
- Exposure to toxins

GENERAL PREVENTION
If due to motion sickness, consider pretreatment with anticholinergics, such as scopolamine.

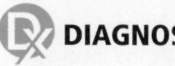 DIAGNOSIS

HISTORY
- Avoid overreliance on patient description of how symptoms feel; focus on triggers and timing (1).
- TiTrATE is a clinically useful evaluation tool: **Ti**ming, **Tr**iggers, **A**nd a **T**argeted **E**valuation (1,2).
- **Ti**ming: episodic or continuous. Episodic may last seconds to a few days. Continuous lasts days to weeks.
  - If continuous, assess for trauma or toxins (including prescribed and recreational).
  - To further evaluate continuous, spontaneous vertigo, perform HINTS exam (1,2,3) (see "Physical Exam").
  - If episodic, assess for triggers.
- **Tr**iggers: present or absent
  - If triggers, perform Dix-Hallpike maneuver (see "Physical Exam").
  - Do not confuse *worsening* of symptoms with motion to be the same as triggering. Many central vertigos are worse with movement (1,2).
  - If no triggers, assess for hearing loss, migraines, or psych symptoms. Cardiovascular causes may also fall into this category.
- **A**nd a **T**argeted **E**valuation: See "Physical Exam" for more details.
- Specific history items that suggest a diagnosis:
  - Unilateral hearing loss suggests Ménière disease (1). Further assess to determine if sensorineural versus conductive because the latter suggests otosclerosis.
  - Symptoms triggered by sudden change in head position suggest BPPV.
  - Symptoms triggered when going from sitting to standing suggests orthostatic hypotension.
  - History of migraines suggests vestibular migraine. Differentiate from nonmigrainous headaches, which can also be present with CNS tumors.
  - Depressed mood/anxiety with episodic vertigo that has since become continuous suggests psychiatric causes.
  - History of unilateral sensory or motor symptoms indicates a central cause such as TIA or CVA until proven otherwise.
  - Onset after decompression (diving, flying) suggests decompression sickness or barotrauma and warrants emergency evaluation.

PHYSICAL EXAM
- Cardiovascular: orthostatic blood pressure assessment on patients with episodic symptoms (1,2)
- HEENT: may identify barotrauma, otosclerosis, cholesteatoma. Also check Rinne and Weber tests if hearing loss.
- Neurologic: Assess for nystagmus in all patients (1).
  - Vertical nystagmus is almost always of central origin.
  - Nystagmus of peripheral origin may be horizontal or rotational.

- Dix-Hallpike maneuver: for episodic, triggered vertigo (1,4): Rapidly move the patient from seated to supine position with the head turned 45 degrees to the right. Observe for nystagmus and patient report of vertigo. Nystagmus/vertigo may not appear immediately. Wait until symptoms resolve and then return the patient to the sitting position. Repeat on the left.
  - The presence of extinguishing horizontal nystagmus is a positive test. If induced nystagmus does not subside however, consider central causes and perform HINTS.
  - Vertical nystagmus always indicates a central cause even if triggered by Dix-Hallpike.
  - In primary care, PPV of 83% for BPPV and NPV of 52%
  - If Dix-Hallpike negative, check for lateral canal BPPV with a log roll test (4).
  - If duration and trigger of symptoms are not consistent with BPPV, do not perform Dix-Hallpike to avoid overlooking a central cause.
- HINTS exam: Perform for continuous, spontaneous vertigo with spontaneous nystagmus (1,2,3).
  - Horizontal **H**ead **I**mpulse: Rapidly and repeatedly bring patient's head to midline from 20 degrees. Patients with vestibular neuritis will show rapid saccades to refocus on a target. With normal peripheral nervous function, eyes stay on target, raising concern for central causes.
  - Direction changing **N**ystagmus: Having already assessed for presence and direction of nystagmus, now check for changing direction. Nystagmus that changes direction with eye motion indicates a central lesion.
  - Test of **S**kew: Vertical eye movement during cover-uncover test indicates a central lesion. A normal test has no movement.
  - A combination of these findings is 96.8% sensitive and 98.5% specific for CVA/other central cause (HINTS positive) (3)[C].
  - If a patient meets criteria for HINTS exam, do not perform Dix-Hallpike.
- Perform a full neuro exam if diagnosis not already clear, paying attention to sensation, gait, and Romberg testing.

DIFFERENTIAL DIAGNOSIS
Causes (1,2):
- BPPV (episodic, triggered, positive Dix-Hallpike)
- Orthostatic hypotension (episodic, triggered, positive orthostatic blood pressure drop)
- Ménière disease (episodic, spontaneous, associated with unilateral sensorineural hearing loss)
- Otosclerosis (spontaneous, duration varies, unilateral conductive hearing loss)
- Vestibular migraine (episodic, associated with migraine HA)
- CVD (continuous, spontaneous; HINTS exam shows normal horizontal head impulse, direction-changing nystagmus, or vertical skew on cover-uncover)
- Posterior fossa tumor (continuous, spontaneous)
- Psychiatric (associated psych symptoms)
- Medication/toxin (continuous, medication/substance history, evaluation otherwise negative)
- Other cardiovascular such as arrhythmia (episodic, often no triggers or triggered by exertion)

- Hypoglycemia (episodic, associated medications or comorbidities)
- Perilymphatic fistula, canal dehiscence (trauma including suspicion of barotrauma from history)
- Decompression sickness (acute, recent dive or flight)
- Degenerative neurologic disease (often progressive by history, associated neurologic findings)
- Peripheral neuropathy

DIAGNOSTIC TESTS & INTERPRETATION
Initial Tests (lab, imaging)
- Labs not routinely necessary unless abnormal neuro exam, and identify a cause in <1% of patients (1)[C]
- Obtain MRI if a central cause is suspected to rule out stroke. CT cannot reliably see the posterior fossa and will not show changes in the early stages of an infarct. Vertigo may be the only symptom of acute stroke (3)[C].
- ENT/audiology referral if Ménière disease suspected for electronystagmography (1)[C]
- If acoustic neuroma is suspected, either CT or MRI to evaluate internal auditory canal (1)[C]

Diagnostic Procedures/Other
Audiometry if acoustic neuroma or Ménière disease is suspected

TREATMENT

GENERAL MEASURES
Treatments depend on cause.
- BPPV: Epley maneuver and modified Epley maneuver (1)[A] (Epley maneuver–YouTube) (5)[B]
- Vestibular neuritis and labyrinthitis
  - Vestibular-suppressant medications (1)[C]
  - Vestibular rehabilitation exercises (1)[B]
  - No evidence to support improvement of symptoms with corticosteroid use (6)[B]
- Ménière disease (see separate topic) (1)[B]:
  - Low-salt diet (<1 to 2 g/day)
  - Diuretics such as hydrochlorothiazide
- Vascular ischemia: prevention of future events through blood pressure reduction, lipid lowering, smoking cessation, antiplatelet therapy, and anticoagulation, if necessary (1,3)[C]; MRI or CT if suspected
- Vertiginous migraines: dietary and lifestyle modifications, vestibular rehab, prophylactic and abortive medications (1)[C]
- Psychological: SSRIs are better than benzodiazepines for anxiety-related vertigo. Use slow titration to avoid worsening symptoms (7)[B].

MEDICATION
Avoid use of medication in mild cases. Use for a few days only because longer use may impair adaptation/compensation by the brain (1); medications not recommended for BPPV (4)[C]
- Meclizine: 12.5 to 50.0 mg PO q4–8h (1)
- Dimenhydrinate: 50 mg PO q6hr (1)
  - Precautions: prostatic hyperplasia, glaucoma
  - Adverse effects: sedation, xerostomia
  - Interactions: CNS depressants
- Prochlorperazine: 5 to 10 mg PO or IM q6–8h; 25 mg rectally q12h; 5 to 10 mg by slow IV over 2 minutes (1)
  - Contraindications: blood dyscrasias, age <2 years, hypotension
  - Precautions: acutely ill children, glaucoma, breast cancer history, impaired cardiac function, prostatic hyperplasia

- Adverse effects: sedation, extrapyramidal effects
- Interactions: phenothiazines, tricyclics antidepressants
- Metoclopramide: 5 to 10 mg PO q6h, 5 to 10 mg slow IV q6h (1)
  - Contraindications: concomitant use of drugs with extrapyramidal effects, seizure disorders
  - Precautions: history of depression, Parkinson disease, hypertension
  - Adverse effects: sedation, fluid retention, constipation
  - Interactions: linezolid, cyclosporine, digoxin, levodopa
- Psychiatric causes
  - SSRIs preferred for frequent vertigo related to depression/anxiety (6)[B]
  - Lorazepam (Ativan) 0.5 to 2.0 mg PO, IM, or IV q4–8h for short-term relief of more severe anxiety-related vertigo
  - Diazepam (Valium) 2 to 10 mg PO or IV q4–8h for short-term relief of more severe symptoms

Geriatric Considerations
Use vestibular-suppressant medications with caution due to increased risk of falls and urinary retention.

Pregnancy Considerations
Meclizine and dimenhydrinate are pregnancy Category B.

ISSUES FOR REFERRAL
Consider referral to otolaryngologist, ENT specialist, vestibular rehabilitation therapist, or neurologist if patient requires further care.

ADDITIONAL THERAPIES
- Epley maneuver/modified Epley maneuver for BPPV to displace calcium deposits in the semicircular canals (4)[A]
  - Effective for short-term symptomatic improvement and for converting patient from positive to negative Dix-Hallpike maneuver. Some studies suggest long-term relief (4)[C].
- Lateral canal BPPV may respond to barbecue roll maneuver (4)[C].
- Vestibular rehabilitation exercises: ball toss, lying-to-standing, target-change, thumb-tracking, tightrope, walking turns (7)[B]

ONGOING CARE

FOLLOW-UP RECOMMENDATIONS
Balance exercises should be adhered to for symptom reduction and return to normal activities of daily living (ADLs).

Patient Monitoring
After 1 to 2 weeks, assess for the following:
- Recurrence of symptoms
- New-onset symptoms
- Medication-related adverse effects
- Relief from vestibular rehabilitation exercises

DIET
- Restricted salt intake for Ménière disease
- Dietary modifications for vertiginous migraine
- Heart healthy diet for CVD

PATIENT EDUCATION
- Reduce sodium intake (Ménière disease).
- Avoid triggers such as caffeine/alcohol (vertiginous migraine).

PROGNOSIS
Depends on diagnosis and response to treatment

COMPLICATIONS
- Anxiety
- Depression
- Disability
- Injuries from falls

REFERENCES
1. Muncie H, Sirmans S, James E. Dizziness: approach to evaluation and management. *Am Fam Physician.* 2017;95(3):154–162.
2. Newman-Toker DE, Edlow JA. TiTrATE: a novel, evidence-based approach to diagnosing acute dizziness and vertigo. *Neurol Clin.* 2015;33(3):577–599.
3. Yew KS, Cheng EM. Diagnosis of acute stroke. *Am Fam Physician.* 2015;91(8):528–536.
4. Bhattacharyya N, Baugh RF, Orvidas L, et al; for American Academy of Otolaryngology-Head and Neck Surgery Foundation. Clinical practice guideline: benign paroxysmal positional vertigo. *Otolaryngol Head Neck Surg.* 2008;139(5 Suppl 4):S47–S81.
5. Hilton M, Pinder D. The Epley (canalith repositioning) manoeuvre for benign paroxysmal positional vertigo. *Cochrane Database Syst Rev.* 2014;(12):CD003162.
6. Fishman JM, Burgess C, Waddell A. Corticosteroids for the treatment of idiopathic acute vestibular dysfunction (vestibular neuritis). *Cochrane Database Syst Rev.* 2011;(5):CD008607.
7. Swartz R, Longwell P. Treatment of vertigo. *Am Fam Physician.* 2005;71(6):1115–1122.

ADDITIONAL READING
Fife TD, Iverson DJ, Lempert T, et al. Practice parameter: therapies for benign paroxysmal positional vertigo (an evidence-based review): report of the Quality Standards Subcommittee of the American Academy of Neurology. *Neurology.* 2008;70(22):2067–2074.

 SEE ALSO

- Ménière Disease; Motion Sickness; Vertigo, Benign Paroxysmal Positional (BPPV)
- Algorithm: Dizziness

 CODES

ICD10
- R42 Dizziness and giddiness
- H81.10 Benign paroxysmal vertigo, unspecified ear
- H81.49 Vertigo of central origin, unspecified ear

CLINICAL PEARLS
- TiTrATE your assessment.
- Acute, spontaneous, continuous vertigo with a normal horizontal head impulse, direction-changing nystagmus, and skew deviation (HINTS positive) is highly sensitive and specific for CVA.
- Episodic, triggered vertigo with positive Dix-Hallpike test is consistent with BPPV.
- If patient warrants a HINTS exam, do not perform Dix-Hallpike because central cause can also produce a positive Dix-Hallpike.
- The Epley maneuver is recommended for the treatment of BPPV.
- Medications are not recommended for BPPV.

V

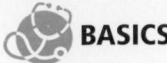

BASICS

DESCRIPTION
- Benign paroxysmal positional vertigo (BPPV) is a mechanical disorder of the inner ear characterized by a brief period of vertigo experienced when the position of the patient's head is changed relative to gravity.
- Vertigo results from the mismatch of the perception of movement by the visual, vestibular, and proprioceptive symptoms when none exist.
- The brief period of vertigo is caused by abnormal stimulation of ≥1 of the 3 semicircular canals of the inner ear, with the posterior canal most commonly affected.
- BPPV is the single most common cause of vertigo.

EPIDEMIOLOGY
- Lifetime prevalence is 2.4% and 1-year incidence 0.6%.
- Age of onset is most commonly between the 5th and 7th decades of life.
- Incidence increases with each decade of life.
- Prevalent sex: female > male
- BPPV affects the quality of life of elderly patients and is associated with reduced activities of daily living scores, falls, and depression.

Prevalence
- Common
- Lifetime prevalence 2.4% with 1-year incidence 0.6%

ETIOLOGY AND PATHOPHYSIOLOGY
- In BPPV, calcite particles (otoconia) that normally weight the sensory membrane of the maculae become dislodged and settle into the semicircular canal, changing the dynamics of the canal. Reorientation of the canal relative to gravity causes the otoconia to move to the lowest part of the canal, causing displacement of the endolymph, deflection of the cupula, and activation of the primary afferent. This results in the generation of nystagmus and the associated sensation of vertigo.
- BPPV may be idiopathic, posttraumatic, or associated with viral neurolabyrinthitis.

DIAGNOSIS

- The diagnosis is established based on history and findings on positional testing, clarified by Dix and Hallpike in 1952 (1,2)[A].
- Positional tests place the plane of the canal being tested into the plane parallel with gravity.

HISTORY
- Brief episodes of vertigo (sensation that the room is spinning) associated with
  - Rolling over in bed
  - Getting out of bed
  - Looking up (referred to as "top-shelf syndrome")
  - Bending forward
  - Quick head movements

- Patients may also complain of light-headedness or feeling "off balance."
- Frequently, patients complain of nausea and, if severe enough, vomiting.

PHYSICAL EXAM
- The Dix-Hallpike test (DHT) is used to diagnose BPPV (1)[A]. The test provokes the characteristic nystagmus associated with the symptoms of vertigo. For the DHT, the estimated sensitivity is 79% (95% CI 65–94) and specificity is 75% (95% CI 33–100) (3)[B].
- To perform the DHT, the patient is positioned in long sitting on the exam table with the knees extended. The head is then rotated 45 degrees toward the side to be tested. The patient is then lowered quickly to supine with the head 30 to 40 degrees below the horizontal, over the edge of the exam table. The position is maintained for a minimum of 45 to 60 seconds.
- For each position, the clinician notes the direction of the fast phase of the nystagmus and the latency and duration of the nystagmus.
- Supportive for BPPV: latency period of <30 seconds between head movement and onset of nystagmus, nystagmus peaks then slowly resolves, duration of nystagmus is 5 to 40 seconds, nystagmus reverses direction with head positioning from the down direction to the sitting position, and repeated head positioning causes the vertiginous symptoms with nystagmus to fatigue
- Posterior canal BPPV:
  - In the head-hanging position, the otoconia move away from the ampullary organ resulting in upward ipsitorsional nystagmus.
  - The superior poles of the eyes beat up toward the forehead and rotate toward the lower most ear, the involved ear.
  - On return to the seated position, the otoconia move toward the ampullary organ resulting in the nystagmus reversing direction.
  - The latency of onset of nystagmus is 1 to 45 seconds, and the duration is usually <1 minute.
  - The nystagmus fatigues (reduction in the severity of symptoms) with repeated positioning.
- Horizontal canal BPPV
  - Directional-changing positional nystagmus is observed in the test positions; the eyes will beat linear-horizontal toward the ground (geotropic nystagmus) or beat toward the sky (apogeotropic nystagmus).
  - One position may illicit a stronger nystagmus response. The side with great intensity indicates the side involved with geotropic lateral canal BPPV and the uninvolved side with apogeotropic lateral canal BPPV.

- Anterior canal BPPV
  - In the head-hanging position, the nystagmus is downbeating and torsional, with the top of the eye torting away from the lower ear.
  - Usually caused by "canal switching" from canalith repositioning procedure (CRP) maneuvers
  - No further testing is indicated unless the diagnosis is uncertain or there are additional symptoms and signs unrelated to BPPV that warrant testing.
- Peripheral versus central vertigo
  - Onset: sudden *versus* sudden or slow
  - Severity: intense spinning *versus* less intense
  - Pattern: paroxysmal *versus* constant
  - Aggravated by movement: yes *versus* variable
  - Nausea or diaphoresis: frequent *versus* variable
  - Nystagmus: rotatory-vertical, horizontal *versus* vertical
  - Fatigue of symptoms: yes *versus* no
  - Hearing loss or tinnitus: may occur *versus* no
  - Abnormal TM: may occur *versus* no
  - CNS symptoms: no *versus* usually present
- Red flags in vertigo
  - Neurologic deficit, ipsilateral hearing loss, gait abnormality, direction-changing nystagmus
- Head Impulse Nystagmus Test of Skew (HINTS)
  - Head impulse test of vestibulo-ocular reflex function
    - Normally, eye movement will correct with rapid head movement so that the center of the vision remains on a target. This reflex fails in peripheral causes of vertigo.
    - Have patient fix their eyes on your nose, and move their head in the horizontal plane to the left and then to the right.
    - When the head is turned toward the normal side, the vestibulo-ocular reflex remains intact and eyes are fixated on the examiner's nose.
    - When the head is turned toward the affected side, the vestibulo-ocular reflex fails and the eyes make a corrective saccade to refixate on the examiner's nose.
    - It is reassuring if the reflex is *abnormal* (due to dysfunction of the peripheral nerve).
  - Nystagmus in primary, right, and left gaze
  - Test for skew deviation "vertical dysconjugate gaze."
    - Skew deviation is a fairly specific predictor of central lesion in patients with acute vestibular syndrome.
    - The presence of skew may help identify stroke when a positive head impulse test falsely suggests a peripheral lesion.
    - Have patient look at your nose with their eyes and start by covering one eye and then rapidly move to cover the other eye, do this rapidly back and forth.
    - When each eye is uncovered, quickly look to see if the eye has movement or refixation. Horizontal is normal, vertical is not.
  - In the setting of dizziness and vertigo, HINTS substantially outperforms ABCD2 for stroke diagnosis and outperforms MRI obtained within the first 2 days after symptom onset (4)[B].

DIFFERENTIAL DIAGNOSIS

- Orthostatic hypotension and other disorders that cause low BP; symptoms usually occur when the patient stands up.
- Damage to the brainstem or cerebellum can cause positional vertigo but is accompanied by other neurologic signs and usually has a different pattern of nystagmus.
- Low spinal fluid pressure may cause positional symptoms that are better when the patient lies down.
- Migraine-associated vertigo
- Traumatic brain injury
- Brain tumors
- Brain hemorrhage or infarction
- Vestibular neuronitis

 TREATMENT

- The CRP or Epley maneuver is effective in the treatment of posterior canal BPPV (1)[A]. Using a particle repositioning maneuver, the clinician moves the patient through a series of positions. With each position, the otoconia settles to the lowest part of the canal. The debris is moved around the arc of the canal into the vestibule. In randomized controlled trials, the average short-term success rate of the CRP following one treatment session is 80% ± 9% (1)[A].
- The clinician moves the patient through a series of four provoking positions:
  - Placement of the right posterior canal (involved canal) in the right head-hanging position of the DHT
  - The head is then rotated a total of 90 degrees toward the left (uninvolved side) into 45 degrees of left head rotation.
  - Maintaining 45 degrees of left head rotation, the patient is rolled onto the left side (uninvolved side) with the head slightly elevated from the supporting surface.
  - The patient then sits up and flexes the neck 36 degrees. Each position is maintained for a minimum of 45 seconds or as long as the nystagmus lasts. The procedure is repeated 3 times.
- CRP is the best maneuver for posterior BPPV and should be offered to all age groups (5)[A].
- Semont maneuver is also another maneuver, less superior when performed alone (5)[A].
- Contraindications are carotid stenosis, unstable cardiac disease, and severe neck disease. If the CRP is ineffective, self-administered CRP is performed at home (1)[A]. The patient performs the CRP on the bed with the head extended over the edge of a pillow. Better outcomes are achieved with a combination of CRP with self-administered CRP (1)[A].
- CRP and Semont are ineffective for horizontal BPPV; variations of the Lempert maneuver, barbecue roll, or Gufoni maneuver are widely used treatment methods for horizontal BPPV.
- Postmaneuver activity restrictions were previously advocated, but in controlled trials, it did not differ in clinical outcomes (2,5)[A].

MEDICATION

- Vestibular suppressant medications are not recommended for treatment of BPPV, other than for the short-term management of vegetative symptoms (3)[A].
- Antiemetics such as ondansetron (Zofran) may be considered for prophylaxis for patients who have had severe nausea or vomiting with the DHT.
- Vestibular suppressants such as benzodiazepines and antihistamine anticholinergics such as meclizine should be avoided because they may suppress nystagmus during the DHT and treatment.

ISSUES FOR REFERRAL

Consider a referral to a specialist if BPPV is unresponsive to treatment or if the patient is diagnosed with atypical BPPV involving the anterior or lateral canal. Consider referring to a physical therapist, neurologist, or an otolaryngologist.

ADDITIONAL THERAPIES

- Brandt-Daroff exercises and habituation exercises are not as effective as self-administered CRP. At 1 week, the average success rate for the Brandt-Daroff exercise is 23–24% compared with 90% for self-administered CRP (1)[A].
- Surgical intervention is rarely indicated, except for refractory BPPV, and includes posterior canal occlusion and singular neurectomy.

 ONGOING CARE

FOLLOW-UP RECOMMENDATIONS

The patient should follow up within a week after treatment to ensure resolution.

PATIENT EDUCATION

A number of illustrative videos are available at http://www.youtube.com/ for education and self CRP maneuvers.

PROGNOSIS

80% cure rate with CRP maneuvers, with a 30% recurrence rate at 1 year, and 44% redevelop BPPV within 2 years

COMPLICATIONS

During the maneuvers, a canal conversion may occur. The debris from the canal being treated may reflux into another canal.

REFERENCES

1. Helminski JO, Zee DS, Janssen I, et al. Effectiveness of particle repositioning maneuvers in the treatment of benign paroxysmal positional vertigo: a systematic review. *Phys Ther*. 2010;90(5):663–678.
2. Devaiah AK, Andreoli S. Postmaneuver restrictions in benign paroxysmal positional vertigo: an individual patient data meta-analysis. *Otolaryngol Head Neck Surg*. 2010;142(2):155–159.
3. Halker RB, Barrs DM, Wellik KE, et al. Establishing a diagnosis of benign paroxysmal positional vertigo through the Dix-Hallpike and side-lying maneuvers: a critically appraised topic. *Neurologist*. 2008;14(3):201–204.
4. Newman-Toker DE, Kerber KA, Hsieh YH, et al. HINTS outperforms ABCD2 to screen for stroke in acute continuous vertigo and dizziness. *Acad Emerg Med*. 2013;20(10):986–996.
5. Fife TD, Iverson DJ, Lempert T, et al; for Quality Standards Subcommittee, American Academy of Neurology. Practice parameter: therapies for benign paroxysmal positional vertigo (an evidence-based review): report of the Quality Standards Subcommittee of the American Academy of Neurology. *Neurology*. 2008;70(22):2067–2074.

ADDITIONAL READING

- Epley JM. The canalith repositioning procedure: for treatment of benign paroxysmal positional vertigo. *Otolaryngol Head Neck Surg*. 1992;107(3):399–404.
- Kattah JC, Talkad AV, Wang DZ, et al. HINTS to diagnose stroke in the acute vestibular syndrome: three-step bedside oculomotor examination more sensitive than early MRI diffusion-weighted imaging. *Stroke*. 2009;40(11):3504–3510.
- Strupp M, Dieterich M, Brandt T. The treatment and natural course of peripheral and central vertigo. *Dtsch Arztebl Int*. 2013;110(29–30):505–515.

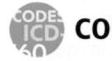 CODES

ICD10

- H81.10 Benign paroxysmal vertigo, unspecified ear
- H81.12 Benign paroxysmal vertigo, left ear
- H81.11 Benign paroxysmal vertigo, right ear

CLINICAL PEARLS

- The diagnosis of BPPV is based on history and findings on positional testing.
- The typical presentation is a report of transient episodes of vertigo (sensation that the room is spinning) associated with a change in position of the head relative to gravity.
- BPPV may be treated effectively with particle-repositioning maneuvers in the office and at home.
- Vestibular suppressant medications and antiemetics are not recommended for treatment of BPPV, other than for the short-term management of symptoms.
- Patients should always be ambulated in to verify normal gait prior to discharge.

V

VINCENT STOMATITIS

Elisa R. Wing, MD • Daniel V. Girzadas Jr., MD, RDMS

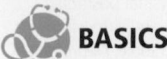 **BASICS**

DESCRIPTION
- Inflammatory infection of the gingiva, characterized by pain, ulcerations, and necrotizing damage to interdental papillae
- Caused by an imbalance of oral flora, resulting in a predominance of invasive anaerobic bacteria, such as *Fusobacterium*, *Prevotella intermedia*, and spirochetes
- Concomitant infection with Epstein-Barr virus, herpes simplex virus, and type 1 human cytomegalovirus is common.
- Organisms invade gingiva and interdental papillae and form a gray pseudomembranous exudate.
- Clinical presentation includes pain, fetid breath, gingival ulcerations, bleeding, and interdental papillary necrosis. It is differentiated from other periodontal diseases by rapid onset, pain, ulcerated gingival mucosa, and "punched out" interdental papillary necrosis.
- Synonym(s): Vincent angina; trench mouth; acute necrotizing ulcerative gingivitis (ANUG)

EPIDEMIOLOGY
Incidence
- Predominant age: 18 to 30 years in developed countries
- Malnourished children ages 3 to 14 years
- Affects both genders with similar frequency

Prevalence
- Prevalence is low in healthy children up to age 18 years.
- Prevalence is more common in persons aged 18 to 30 years. Prevalence increases with malnutrition, immunocompromised, poor oral hygiene, and smoking, or those from underdeveloped countries.

ETIOLOGY AND PATHOPHYSIOLOGY
- Impaired host immunologic response due to immunocompromised or malnutrition
- Disruption of normal oral flora with predominance of invasive anaerobic bacteria
- Loss of integrity and necrosis of the gingival mucosa and interdental papillae
- Increased bacterial attachment with active herpesvirus infection

RISK FACTORS
- Malnutrition
- Immunosuppression (cancer, HIV infection)
- Tobacco use
- Poor oral hygiene
- Infrequent or absent dental care
- Orthodontics
- Herpesvirus infection
- Psychological stress

GENERAL PREVENTION
- Appropriate nutrition
- Proper oral hygiene
- Regular dental care
- Prompt recognition and institution of therapy
- Management of medical problems such as cancer and HIV infection
- Stress management

COMMONLY ASSOCIATED CONDITIONS
- Seen most commonly in malnourished patients, patients undergoing cancer treatment, or those from underdeveloped countries
- HIV infection
- Vitamin deficiencies
- Bacteremia
- Osteomyelitis
- Tooth loss
- Dehydration
- Noma (cancrum) oris, which can be life-threatening
- Aspiration pneumonia

 DIAGNOSIS

HISTORY
- Acute onset of oral pain
- Gingival ulcerations
- Fetid odor of breath
- Bleeding and necrosis of interdental papillae
- Cervical adenopathy
- Fever
- Malaise
- Immunosuppression
- Chemotherapy
- Active herpesvirus infection or HIV

PHYSICAL EXAM
- Fetid odor of breath
- Ulceration of gingival mucosa
- Inflamed, erythematous gingiva
- Necrosis of interdental papillae
- Gingival bleeding
- Formation of gray, pseudomembranous exudate
- Cervical and submandibular lymphadenopathy
- Fever and malaise may be present.

DIFFERENTIAL DIAGNOSIS
- Herpes simplex virus
- Periodontitis
- Recurrent aphthous stomatitis
- Medication side effects
- Oral malignancy
- Xerostomia
- Diphtheria
- Lymphoma/leukemia
- Primary syphilis
- Ascorbic acid deficiency
- Gingivitis
- Behçet disease
- Granulomatosis with polyangiitis
- Oral mucositis
- Erosive lichen planus

DIAGNOSTIC TESTS & INTERPRETATION
Initial Tests (labs, imaging)
Diagnosis is primarily based on clinical exam, but if systemic illness or invasive spread to deeper tissue or bone is suspected, the following studies should be considered:
- Aerobic and anaerobic cultures of inflamed or débrided tissue
- Group A strep rapid antigen detection assay
- Group A strep throat culture
- Blood cultures if systemic involvement
- Dental radiographs
- CT imaging of the face and neck if infection has progressed

TREATMENT

GENERAL MEASURES
Elimination of tobacco, improved nutritional status, and improved immunologic status will increase rate of healing and reduce risk of future gingival disease.

MEDICATION
Most cases are treatable on outpatient basis. Severe disease with systemic effects and/or neck involvement requires inpatient treatment.

First Line
- Chlorhexidine gluconate 0.12% 15 mL 30 seconds rinse/spit QID (1)[C] *plus*
- Penicillin V potassium 250 to 500 mg QID PO for 10 days; pediatric dosing: 25 to 50 mg/kg/day divided q6–8h *or*
- Metronidazole 500 mg q8h for 7 to 10 days (2)[C]; pediatric dosing: 30 mg/kg/day divided q6h *or*
- Amoxicillin 500 mg TID PO for 7 days (2)[C]; pediatric dosing: 25 to 45 mg/kg/day divided q12h *or*
- Amoxicillin-clavulanate 875 mg q12h for 7 to 10 days (2)[C]; pediatric dosing: 25 to 45 mg/kg/day divided q12h (based on amoxicillin component)

Second Line
- Tetracycline 250 to 500 mg QID PO for 10 days (do not use for children <8 years of age); pediatric dosing: 25 to 50 mg/kg/day divided q6h *or*
- Erythromycin 250 to 500 mg QID PO for 10 days; pediatric dosing: 30 to 50 mg/kg/day divided q6–8h *or*
- Clindamycin 450 mg q8h for 7 to 10 days; pediatric dosing: 10 to 25 mg/kg/day divided q6–8h

Pediatric Considerations
- Chlorhexidine and alcohol mouth rinses are generally avoided due to risk of ingestion, but chlorhexidine may be prescribed in gel form for topical application.
- Metronidazole is first-line oral therapy (refer to dosing above) (3).

ISSUES FOR REFERRAL
Severe disease requires débridement by consultant dentist, oral surgeon, or ENT specialist.

ADDITIONAL THERAPIES
- Warm saline rinses q2h
- Sodium bicarbonate toothpaste, brush q2h
- Viscous lidocaine 2% 1 tbsp rinse/spit q6–8h
- NSAID medications q4–12h
- Opioid analgesics q4–6h (severe pain)
- Treatment of underlying immunodeficiency (if present)

SURGERY/OTHER PROCEDURES
- Débridement of inflamed/necrotic gingival tissue
- Dental extraction
- Gingival restoration
- Adjuvant therapies
  - Low-level laser therapy (LLLT) has been shown in one case series to decrease pain and accelerate healing (4)[C].

ADMISSION, INPATIENT, AND NURSING CONSIDERATIONS
- Severe disease, failure of oral antibiotics, or ongoing comorbidities
- Parenteral antibiotics and/or analgesia requirement
- Inability to tolerate PO

 ONGOING CARE

FOLLOW-UP RECOMMENDATIONS
- Close dental follow-up
- Primary care follow-up
- Specialty follow-up (if underlying immunodeficiency)

DIET
- Soft diet until healed
- Balanced nutritional diet
- Multivitamin supplementation

PATIENT EDUCATION
- Proper nutrition
- Oral hygiene
- Tobacco cessation

COMPLICATIONS
- Pain
- Malnutrition
- Gingival/tooth loss
- Deep infection of neck
- Systemic infection

REFERENCES
1. Hodgdon A. Dental and related infections. *Emerg Med Clin North Am*. 2013;31(2):465–480.
2. Atout RN, Todescan S. Managing patients with necrotizing ulcerative gingivitis. *J Can Dent Assoc*. 2013;79:d46.
3. Marty M, Palmieri J, Noirrit-Esclassan E, et al. Necrotizing periodontal diseases in children: a literature review and adjustment of treatment. *J Trop Pediatr*. 2016;62(4):331–337.
4. Özberk SS, Gündoğar H, Şenyurt SZ, et al. Adjunct use of low-level laser therapy on the treatment of necrotizing ulcerative gingivitis: a case report. *J Lasers Med Sci*. 2018;9(1):73–75.

ADDITIONAL READING
- Campbell CM, Stout BM, Deas DE. Necrotizing ulcerative gingivitis: a discussion of four dissimilar presentations. *Tex Dent J*. 2011;128(10): 1041–1051.
- Khammissa R, Ciya R, Munzhelele T, et al. Oral medicine case book 65: necrotising stomatitis. *SADJ*. 2014;69(10):468–470.
- Sangani I, Watt E, Cross D. Necrotizing ulcerative gingivitis and the orthodontic patient: a case series. *J Orthod*. 2013;40(1):77–80.

CODES

ICD10
A69.1 Other Vincent's infections

CLINICAL PEARLS
- Immunosuppression, malnourishment, smoking, and poor oral hygiene are key risk factors for necrotizing ulcerative gingivitis.
- Diagnosis is largely clinical based on symptoms of oral pain, fetid breath, gingival ulcerations, interdental papillary necrosis, and grayish exudate on the gingival surface.
- Most patients experience rapid improvement following appropriate treatment with chlorhexidine rinses, improved oral hygiene, and oral antibiotics.
- Smoking cessation and treatment of malnutrition or underlying illness are additional important treatment considerations.
- Severe disease requires débridement of necrotic gingival tissue.

V

VITAMIN B₁₂ DEFICIENCY

Sahil Mullick, MD

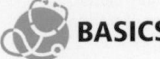

BASICS

- Vitamin deficiency related to inadequate intake or absorption of cobalamin (vitamin B_{12})
- Cobalamin is critical for central nervous system myelination and normal functioning.
- Deficiency can cause a multitude of symptoms and disorders including megaloblastic anemia, bone marrow dysfunction, and diverse and potentially irreversible neuropsychiatric changes.
- Neuropsychiatric disorders are due to demyelination of cervical, thoracic dorsal, and lateral spinal cords; demyelination of white matter; and demyelination of cranial and peripheral nerves (1)[C].
- Low vitamin B_{12} level can lead to elevated methyl-malonic acid (MMA) and homocysteine levels (2)[C].
- Elevated MMA causes abnormality in fatty acid synthesis affecting neuronal membrane.
- Elevated homocysteine is neurotoxic through over-stimulation of the *N*-methyl-D-aspartate (NMDA) receptor and toxic to vasculature through activation of coagulation system and effects on endothelium.

DESCRIPTION

Normal B_{12} absorption

- B_{12} is a water-soluble vitamin present in animal-source foods (meat, fish, eggs, milk) and foods (cereals and supplements) fortified with B_{12}.
- Dietary vitamin B_{12} (cobalamin) bound to food is cleaved by acids in stomach and bound to haptocorrin (commonly known as R-factor).
- Duodenal proteases cleave B_{12} from haptocorrin.
- In duodenum, B_{12} uptake depends on binding to intrinsic factor (IF) secreted by gastric parietal cells.
- B_{12}-IF complex is absorbed by terminal ileum into portal circulation.
- Body's B_{12} stored in liver = 50–90%
  - B_{12} secreted into bile from liver recycled via enterohepatic circulation
  - Delay 5 to 10 years from onset of B_{12} deficiency to clinical symptoms due to hepatic stores and enterohepatic circulation
- Typical Western diet: 5 to 30 μg/day; however, only 1 to 5 μg/day is effectively absorbed.
  - Recommend 2.4 μg/day for adults and 2.6 μg/day during pregnancy and 2.8 μg/day during lactation (most prenatal vitamins contain B_{12}).

EPIDEMIOLOGY

Prevalence

- Endemic area: Northern Europe, including Scandinavia; more common in those of African ancestry
- Increasing recognition in breastfed-only infant populations with vitamin B_{12}–deficient mothers
- Prevalence 5–20% in developed countries
  - 12% in elderly living in community
  - 30–40% in elderly in institutions, sick, or malnourished
  - 5% patients in tertiary reference hospitals
- Prevalence by age group (3)
  - <60 years old: prevalence 6%
  - >60 years old: prevalence 20%

ETIOLOGY AND PATHOPHYSIOLOGY

- Decreased oral intake
  - Vegetarians and vegans: B_{12} is found in animal source foods; however, strict vegetarians uncommonly develop deficiency because only 1 mg/day is needed, with adequate amounts present in legumes.

- Decreased IF
  - Pernicious anemia (PA): can be associated with autoantibodies directed against gastric parietal cells and/or IF
  - Chronic atrophic gastritis: autoimmune attack on gastric parietal cells causing autoimmune gastritis and leading to decreased IF production
  - Gastrectomy: Removal of entire or part of stomach decreases number of parietal cells.
- Decreased ileal absorption
  - Crohn disease: Terminal ileal inflammation decreases body's ability to absorb B_{12}.
  - Chronic alcoholism: decreases body's ability to absorb B_{12}
  - Ileal resection
  - Pancreatic insufficiency: Pancreatic proteases are required to cleave the vitamin B_{12}–haptocorrin bond to allow vitamin B_{12} to bind to IF.
  - *Helicobacter pylori* infection: impairs release of B_{12} from bound proteins
- Medications: Proton pump inhibitors (PPIs), H_2 antagonists, and antacids decrease gastric acidity, inhibiting B_{12} release from dietary protein; metformin
  - Metformin usage
    - Chronic metformin usage leads to vitamin B_{12} deficiency. Caused by calcium-dependent membrane inhibition, interfering with vitamin B_{12}–IF absorption. Years on metformin is the only predictive factor for B_{12} deficiency.
- Hereditary (rare)
  - Imerslünd-Grasbeck disease (juvenile megaloblastic anemia)
  - Congenital deficiency of transcobalamin
  - Severe methylene tetrahydrofolate reductase deficiency
  - Abnormalities of methionine synthesis
- Causes:
  - Food-cobalamin malabsorption syndrome
    - As many as 60–70% of cases
    - Primary cause in elderly
    - Pathophysiology: inability to release cobalamin from food or binding protein, especially if in the setting of hypochlorhydria
    - Seen in atrophic gastritis, long-term ingestion of antacids and biguanides, possible relationship to *H. pylori* infection
  - PA
    - 15–30% of all cases; most frequent cause of severe disease. Neurologic disorders are common presenting complaints.
    - Common in elderly, as high as 20%, with mild atrophic gastritis, hypochlorhydria, and impaired release of dietary vitamin B_{12}
    - Autoimmune disease with destruction of gastric fundal mucosa cells via a cell-mediated process
    - Antigastric parietal cell antibodies: sensitivity >90%, specificity 50%; use for screening test
    - Anti-IF antibodies: sensitivity 50%
    - Associated with other autoimmune diseases
  - Insufficient dietary intake: 2% of cases; vegans or long-standing vegetarians
  - Infants born to vitamin B_{12}–deficient mothers may have deficiency or may develop it if breastfed exclusively.
  - Intestinal causes:
    - 1% of cases; prevalence depends on risk factors, such as surgical conditions.
    - Gastrectomy: due to decreased production of IF

- Gastric bypass: appears 1 to 9 years after surgery, prevalence 12–33%
- Ileal resection or disease
- Fish tapeworm
- Severe pancreatic insufficiency
  - Undetermined etiology
    - 1/10 of cases

Genetics

Imerslünd-Grasbeck disease (juvenile megaloblastic anemia) caused by mutations in the amnionless (AMN) or cubilin (CUBN) genes with autosomal recessive pattern of inheritance; inadequate ileal uptake of B_{12}-IF complex and B_{12} renal protein reabsorption

GENERAL PREVENTION

Risk factors: vegan diet, age >60 years, female, chronic atrophic gastritis, Crohn disease or other ileal disorders, chronic medication use including PPI, metformin, H_2 antagonists

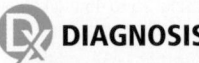

DIAGNOSIS

Symptoms and physical exam findings:

- Asymptomatic patients may be diagnosed by the incidental finding of anemia or an elevated mean corpuscular volume (MCV) during routine testing or evaluation of unassociated disorders.
- Hematologic
  - Frequent: macrocytosis, neutrophil hypersegmentation, spinal cord medullar megaloblastosis (blue spinal cord)
  - Rare: isolated thrombocytopenia and neutropenia, pancytopenia
  - Very rare: hemolytic, thrombotic microangiopathy with schistocytes
- Neuropsychiatric
  - Frequent: sensory polyneuritis, paresthesias, positive Babinski sign, weakness, gait unsteadiness, loss of proprioception (impaired vibratory sensation, positive Romberg, ataxia, hyperreflexia)
  - Classic but uncommon: subacute combined degeneration of spinal cord associated with PA; myelin degeneration in the lateral and posterior columns; areflexia (which may be permanent if neuronal death occurs in the posterior or lateral spinal cord tracts), ataxia, proprioception and vibration loss, bowel and bladder incontinence, orthostatic hypotension, decreased memory, mania, delirium, psychosis, depression
- Digestive
  - Classic: Hunter glossitis, jaundice, and high lactate dehydrogenase and bilirubin
  - Possible: abdominal pain, dyspepsia, nausea, vomiting, diarrhea
  - Rare: mucocutaneous ulcers
- Other
  - Frequent: fatigue with exertion, skin pallor, palpitations, edema, jaundice
  - Under investigation: chronic vaginal and urinary infections, atrophy of vaginal mucosa, hypofertility, venous thromboembolism, angina, miscarriages
  - Commonly insidious and nonspecific; thus, delay in diagnosis is common.

HISTORY

- Underlying disease associated with vitamin B₁₂ deficiency
- Fatigue, anorexia
- Depression
- Falls (due to diminished proprioception)
- Loss of sensation in "stocking-glove" distribution
- Glossitis/loss of sense of taste and other subtle, nonspecific neurologic symptoms

DIAGNOSTIC TESTS & INTERPRETATION

- Measurement of vitamin B₁₂, CBC (MCV)
- Measurement of B₁₂ may be low or low normal depending on institution's cutoff value.
  - 95–97% sensitive levels <200 pg/mL (4)
  - May need additional tests such as MMA and homocysteine if vitamin B₁₂ level is low normal (<350 pg/mL) and no evidence of anemia depending on clinical suspicion
- If high suspicion on normal B₁₂ with high/normal MCV, consider testing MMA and homocysteine levels.
- MCV often increased
- Measurement of MMA
  - More sensitive and specific than homocysteine
  - Levels increased in renal failure and volume depletion.
- Measurement of homocysteine
  - Levels increased in folate deficiency, renal failure, and homocystinuria.
- MMA and homocysteine levels only reliable in an untreated patient because levels fall with supplementation
- Other tests: folate and other markers of anemia (iron studies)
- MCV may be normal, decreased, or increased if vitamin B₁₂ deficiency coexists with other forms of anemia, such as iron deficiency or hemolysis. Thus, RBCs may be normochromic, normocytic, or hypochromic microcytic.

ALERT

- Low levels of vitamin B₁₂ are seen in folate deficiency, HIV, and multiple myeloma.
- Elevated levels of vitamin B₁₂ are seen in renal disease, occult malignancy, and alcoholic liver disease and as a result of technical error.
- Macrocytosis may be due to folate deficiency, reticulocytosis, medications, bone marrow dysplasia, and hypothyroidism or be masked by concomitant microcytic anemia.
- Serum homocysteine and MMA
  - Elevated in B₁₂ deficiency secondary to decreased metabolism
  - If both are normal, B₁₂ deficiency is effectively ruled out.
  - If MMA is normal and homocysteine is increased, think folate deficiency.
- PA
  - Check antibody to IF; positive test is confirmatory for PA, but sensitivity is only 50–70%.
  - Antiparietal cell antibody positivity indicates PA.
  - For patients who are antibody positive, consider screening for autoimmune thyroid disease.
  - For patients with negative anti-IF result and high suspicion for PA, check serum gastrin level (elevated level is consistent with diagnosis of PA) (2).

Pregnancy Considerations

- Because B₁₂ crosses the placenta, pregnant women with low levels of B₁₂ are at higher risk of having children with neural tube defects, developmental delay, failure to thrive, hypotonia, ataxia, and anemia (3).
- Exclusively breastfed infants of mothers who are B₁₂ deficient are at risk of developing B₁₂ deficiency. Infants breastfed from B₁₂-deficient mothers might not show signs or symptoms until 4 to 6 months of age, which may include developmental regression, feeding difficulties, lethargy, or hypotonia.

Diagnostic Procedures/Other

- Bone marrow exam is usually unnecessary in the evaluation of B₁₂ deficiency because of the inability to differentiate from folate deficiency.
- Spinal cord imaging is not standard; MRI in selected cases, especially with severe myelopathy

 TREATMENT

MEDICATION

- Parenteral cyanocobalamin replacement recommended in patients with severe neurologic symptoms: IM cyanocobalamin (2)[C]
  - 1,000 µg/day for 7 days, *then*
  - 1,000 µg weekly for 4 weeks, *then*
  - 1,000 µg monthly for life
- High-dose, daily oral cyanocobalamin at doses of 1,000 to 2,000 µg are as effective as monthly intramuscular injection and is the preferred route of initial therapy in most circumstances because it is cost-effective and convenient (5)[A]. Requires greater patient compliance. Transnasal and buccal preparations of cyanocobalamin are also available; however, further study is needed.

ALERT

Folic acid without vitamin B₁₂ in patients with PA is contraindicated; it will not correct neurologic abnormalities.

ADMISSION, INPATIENT, AND NURSING CONSIDERATIONS

- Consider blood transfusion for severe anemia.
- Draw blood for hematologic parameters before transfusing.

 ONGOING CARE

FOLLOW-UP RECOMMENDATIONS

Patient Monitoring

- Hematologic
  - Reticulocytosis in 1 week
  - Rise in hemoglobin beginning at 10 days; usually will return to normal in 6 to 8 weeks
  - Monitor potassium in profoundly anemic patients (hypokalemia due to potassium use)
  - Serum MMA decreases with replacement therapy.
- Neurologic: can note improvement within 6 weeks to 3 months of treatment; however, maximum improvement noticed at 6 to 12 months. Some symptoms may be irreversible.

DIET

Meat, animal protein, and legumes unless contraindicated

REFERENCES

1. Lachner C, Steinle NI, Regenold WT. The neuropsychiatry of vitamin B₁₂ deficiency in elderly patients. *J Neuropsychiatry Clin Neurosci.* 2012;24(1):5–15.
2. Stabler SP. Clinical practice. Vitamin B₁₂ deficiency. *N Engl J Med.* 2013;368(2):149–160.
3. Langan RC, Goodbred AJ. Vitamin B₁₂ deficiency: recognition and management. *Am Fam Physician.* 2017;96(6):384–389.
4. Oberley MJ, Yang DT. Laboratory testing for cobalamin deficiency in megaloblastic anemia. *Am J Hematol.* 2013;88(6):522–526.
5. Vidal-Alaball J, Butler CC, Cannings-John R, et al. Oral vitamin B₁₂ versus intramuscular vitamin B₁₂ for vitamin B₁₂ deficiency. *Cochrane Database Syst Rev.* 2005;(3):CD004655.

ADDITIONAL READING

- Allen LH. How common is vitamin B-12 deficiency? *Am J Clin Nutr.* 2009;89(2):693S–696S.
- Aroda VR, Edelstein SL, Goldberg RB, et al; and Diabetes Prevention Program Research Group. Long-term metformin use and vitamin B₁₂ deficiency in the diabetes prevention program outcomes study. *J Clin Endocrinol Metab.* 2016;101(4):1754–1761.
- Bizzaro N, Antico A. Diagnosis and classification of pernicious anemia. *Autoimmun Rev.* 2014; 13(4–5):565–568.
- Fernández-Bañares F, Monzón H, Forné M. A short review of malabsorption and anemia. *World J Gastroenterol.* 2009;15(37):4644–4652.
- Mazokopakis EE, Starakis IK. Recommendations for diagnosis and management of metformin-induced vitamin B₁₂ (Cbl) deficiency. *Diabetes Res Clin Pract.* 2012;97(3):359–367.

 CODES

ICD10

- E53.8 Deficiency of other specified B group vitamins
- D51.0 Vitamin B12 defic anemia due to intrinsic factor deficiency
- D51.3 Other dietary vitamin B12 deficiency anemia

CLINICAL PEARLS

- Consider screening for B₁₂ deficiency in high-risk patients including the elderly and monitoring B₁₂ levels annually if on metformin or on chronic PPIs.
- Correcting folate deficiency without treating with cyanocobalamin in megaloblastic anemia may correct hematologic but not neurologic disorders.
- Vitamin B₁₂ deficiency can coexist with other causes of anemia, including iron deficiency or hemolysis; thus, MCV can be normal, decreased, or increased.
- For patients with PA, cyanocobalamin replacement must be lifelong.
- Patients with PA are at increased risk for other autoimmune conditions as well as gastric malignancy.
- Women at high risk or with known deficiency should supplement with vitamin B₁₂ during pregnancy or while breastfeeding.

V

VITAMIN D DEFICIENCY

Frank J. Domino, MD • Samir Malkani, MD, MRCP–UK

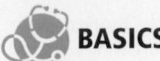 **BASICS**

This topic covers the commonly acquired vitamin D deficiency and not type II vitamin D–resistant rickets/type I pseudovitamin D–resistant rickets (both rare autosomal recessive disorders).

DESCRIPTION
- Vitamin D is a hormone and a vitamin.
- Cholecalciferol (D_3) is synthesized in the skin by exposure to ultraviolet B (UV-B) radiation. Ergocalciferol (D_2) and D_3 are present in foods.
- D_2 and D_3 are hydroxylated in the liver to 25 vitamin D (calcidiol), the major circulating form.
- Calcidiol is further hydroxylated in the kidney to the active metabolite 1,25 vitamin D (calcitriol).
- Hypocalcemia stimulates parathyroid hormone (PTH) to be secreted, which prompts the increased conversion of 25 vitamin D to 1,25 vitamin D.
  - 1,25 vitamin D decreases renal calcium and phosphorus excretion, increases intestinal calcium and phosphorus absorption, and increases osteoclast activity. The net result is an increase in serum calcium.

EPIDEMIOLOGY
- A community cohort study of asymptomatic adolescents in Boston found 24% were deficient, with 5% severely deficient.
- A study of hospitalized patients in Massachusetts found 57% vitamin D–deficient (VDD).
- Women with history of osteoporosis/osteoporotic fracture have high prevalence of vitamin D deficiency.
- A cohort study in Arizona found >25% of adults were VDD; highest rates among African Americans and Hispanics
- A study of about 56,000 individuals across Europe found 13% to have vitamin D deficiency.

Pediatric Considerations
NHANES data suggest 70% of children do not have sufficient 25-OH vitamin D serum levels (9% deficient and 61% insufficient); associated with an increase in BP and decrease in high-density lipoprotein (HDL) cholesterol

ETIOLOGY AND PATHOPHYSIOLOGY
- Insufficient dietary intake of vitamin D and/or lack of UV-B exposure (in sunlight) results in low levels of vitamin D.
  - This limits calcium absorption, causing excess PTH release.
- PTH stimulates osteoclast activity, which helps to normalize calcium and phosphorous but results in osteomalacia.

- Dietary deficiency
  - Inadequate vitamin D intake
- Inadequate sunlight exposure
  - Institutionalized/hospitalized patients
- Chronic illness: liver/kidney disease
- Malabsorptive states

Genetics
Vitamin D–dependent rickets type 1 occurs due to inactivating mutation of the 1α hydroxylase gene; as a result, calcidiol is not hydroxylated to calcitriol.

RISK FACTORS
- Inadequate sun exposure
- Female
- Dark skin
- Immigrant populations
- Low socioeconomic status
- Latitudes higher than 38 degrees
- Elderly
- Institutionalized
- Depression
- Medications (phenobarbital, phenytoin)
- Gastric bypass surgery/malabsorption syndromes
- Obesity

GENERAL PREVENTION
- Adequate exposure to sunlight and dietary sources of vitamin D (plants, fish); many foods are fortified with vitamin D_2 and D_3.
- Recommended minimum daily requirement is 600 IU/day from age 1 to 70 years and 800 IU/day for those >70 years. Up to 4,000 IU/day is safe in healthy adults without risk of toxicity.
- For ages 51 to 70 years, minimally recommended supplementation is 800 IU/day to prevent nonvertebral fractures.

Pediatric Considerations
- The American Academy of Pediatrics recommends all breastfed babies receive 400 IU/day of vitamin D beginning "within the first few days of life."
- 2016 Global Consensus Recommendations suggest all infants, regardless of feeding method, begin vitamin D 400 IU within a few days of birth (1).

Pregnancy Considerations
Insufficient data to recommend routine screening of all pregnancies; only "at risk" should be screened; it is safe to take 1,000 to 2,000 IU/day during pregnancy (2)[B].

COMMONLY ASSOCIATED CONDITIONS
- Osteomalacia, osteoporosis
- Premenstrual syndrome
- Rickets
- Celiac disease
- Gastric bypass
- Chronic renal disease
- Bacterial vaginosis in pregnant women
- Hypertension
- Cohort study found that vitamin D deficiency is correlated with increased risk of all-cause mortality.

ALERT
Vitamin D deficiency is associated with risk of myocardial infarction (MI) and all-cause mortality (3)[A].

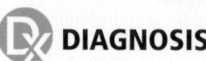 **DIAGNOSIS**

- Nonspecific musculoskeletal complaints
- Weak antigravity muscles
- Fracture with minimal trauma

HISTORY
- Senior citizens at risk of falling
- Renal disease
- GI (malabsorption) disorders
- Liver dysfunction
- Immigration from tropical to colder climates
- Dark-skinned/veiled individuals
- Housebound patients
- Women at perimenopause

PHYSICAL EXAM
- Vague neurologic signs: numbness, proximal myopathy, paresthesias, muscle cramps, laryngospasm
- Chvostek sign: contraction of the facial muscles by tapping along the facial nerve
- Trousseau phenomenon: carpal spasms and paresthesia produced by pressure on nerves and vessels of the upper arm, by inflation of a BP cuff
- Tetany, seizures

DIAGNOSTIC TESTS & INTERPRETATION
Initial Tests (lab, imaging)
- Only test those at increased risk of deficiency (those lacking dietary exposure, sun exposure, etc.).
- 25-OH vitamin D (most sensitive measure of vitamin D status)
- Vitamin D deficiency
  - <20 ng/mL

- PTH elevation: not routinely obtained unless severe deficiency
- Low-normal/low calcium and phosphorous
- Elevated alkaline phosphatase (in later disease)
- Plain radiographs: If atypical fracture, radiographs may show osteomalacia (pseudofractures/looser zones) in pelvis, femur, and fibula.
- Osteoporosis screen
  - Women ≥65 years with no risk factors
  - Women ≥60 years at risk: body weight <70 kg (best predictor)
  - Less evidence: smoking, low body mass index, family history, decreased activity, alcohol or caffeine use
  - African American women have higher bone density than Caucasians.

 TREATMENT

- Treatment goals remain unclear, but current "normal" 25-OH vitamin D levels are based on suppression of PTH.
- Obesity: Treatment of VDD in obesity, especially those who are obese and depressed, improves depressive symptoms and may improve weight loss.
- Systematic review of 63 observational studies found adequate 25-OH vitamin D levels correlate with lower rates of colon, breast, and prostate cancer.
- Observational data show inverse relationship between serum 25-OH vitamin D levels and breast cancer.

ALERT
All-cause mortality: Cochrane Systematic Review found vitamin D supplementation lowers all-cause mortality (4)[A].

Geriatric Considerations
In senior citizens, serum 25-OH vitamin D of 20 ng/mL resulted in improved physical performance scores; recent data suggest supplementation may not improve fracture risk and remains unclear about a true benefit.

MEDICATION
- Vitamin D sufficient (25-OH vitamin D ≥20 ng/mL)
  - Vitamin D 800 to 4,000 IU/day D₂/D₃
  - D₃ (animal derived) may be slightly more effective than D₂ (plant derived), but clinical significance is uncertain.
  - Calcium supplementation: unclear benefit and may increase some CHD risk in patients; no supplementation currently required (see below)

- Vitamin D deficiency (25-OH vitamin D <20 ng/mL)
  - D₂ 50,000 IU/week for 8 to 12 weeks, followed by 800 to 2,000 IU/day of vitamin D₃
- Calcium: meta-analysis data support
  - Dietary intake of ~700 mg/day leads to best outcomes; higher doses did NOT decrease risk of osteoporotic fractures.
  - Dietary calcium may be more beneficial than calcium supplementation.
  - Supplementary calcium associated with an increased risk of MI, especially in women, but this data remain controversial.
  - Supplementation of vitamin D and calcium may increase risk of renal stone formation.

ISSUES FOR REFERRAL
Endocrinology if no response to treatment

ADDITIONAL THERAPIES
Aggressive calcium in ICU patients with ionized calcium <3.2 mg/dL or if symptomatic (tetany, seizures, QT prolongation, bradycardia, or hypotension or ventilated patient with decreased diaphragmatic function)

ADMISSION, INPATIENT, AND NURSING CONSIDERATIONS
- Symptoms of severe hypocalcemia
- Malabsorption syndromes

 ONGOING CARE

FOLLOW-UP RECOMMENDATIONS
Follow-up of abnormal 25-OH vitamin D not required

DIET
- Cod liver oil is most potent source of vitamin D and has ~1,300 IU vitamin D/tablet/tablespoon.
- Fatty fish (tuna, salmon)
- Fortified milk (100 IU/8 oz), cereal, and foods

PROGNOSIS

ALERT
Meta-analysis data support supplementation of >500 IU/day lowered the risk of all-cause mortality (4,5)[A] but remain controversial.

REFERENCES

1. Munns CF, Shaw N, Kiely M, et al. Global consensus recommendations on prevention and management of nutritional rickets. *J Clin Endocrinol Metab*. 2016;101(2):394–415.
2. American College of Obstetricians and Gynecologists Committee on Obstetric Practice. ACOG Committee Opinion No. 495: vitamin D: screening and supplementation during pregnancy. *Obstet Gynecol*. 2011;118(1):197–198.
3. Correia LC, Sodré F, Garcia G, et al. Relation of severe deficiency of vitamin D to cardiovascular mortality during acute coronary syndromes. *Am J Cardiol*. 2013;111(3):324–327.
4. Bjelakovic G, Gluud LL, Nikolova D, et al. Vitamin D supplementation for prevention of mortality in adults. *Cochrane Database Syst Rev*. 2011;(7):CD007470.
5. Chowdhury R, Kunutsor S, Vitezova A, et al. Vitamin D and risk of cause specific death: systematic review and meta-analysis of observational cohort and randomised intervention studies. *BMJ*. 2014;348:g1903.

 CODES

ICD10
- E55.9 Vitamin D deficiency, unspecified
- M83.8 Other adult osteomalacia

CLINICAL PEARLS

- Risk factors for vitamin D deficiency include age >65 years, renal disease, GI (malabsorption) disorders, liver dysfunction, immigration from tropical to colder climates, dark-skinned/veiled individuals, housebound patients, perimenopause.
- 25-OH vitamin D (most sensitive measure of vitamin D status) is the most sensitive laboratory test for diagnosis.
- Vitamin D deficiency is defined by serum levels <20 ng/mL.
- Up to 4,000 IU/day of supplemental vitamin D is safe in healthy adults without risk of toxicity.
- The American Academy of Pediatrics recommends all breastfed babies receive 400 IU/day of vitamin D beginning within a few days of birth.

V

VITAMIN DEFICIENCY

Michelle E. Szczepanik, MD • Christopher D. Meyering, DO

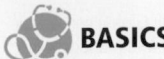

BASICS

DESCRIPTION
- Vitamins are essential micronutrients required for normal metabolism, growth, and development.
- Deficiencies are less common in the Western world, but certain populations are at increased risk.
- Regulations mandating vitamin supplementation in food products, adequate food security, and availability of vitamin supplements make vitamin deficiencies less common in developed countries.
- Toxicity is rare for water-soluble vitamins; toxicity is possible with fat-soluble vitamins (A, D, E, K).

EPIDEMIOLOGY
Incidence
- Predominant age
  - Geriatric patients, pregnant women, exclusively breastfed infants, and individuals with certain chronic disease states
- Individuals from Africa and Southeast Asia are at increased risk.
- True incidence is unknown because most vitamin deficiencies are asymptomatic.

Prevalence
- Varies by age groups, comorbid conditions, geography, and setting (i.e., urban, rural)
- The prevalence of vitamin B_{12} deficiency is ~6% in patients <60 years of age and increases to around 20% after age 60 years (1).
- Vitamin D deficiency has become increasingly recognized and its prevalence is increased in individuals with darker skin pigmentation, obesity, low dietary intake of vitamin D, or low sunlight exposure.

ETIOLOGY AND PATHOPHYSIOLOGY
- Disease-related deficiency can develop under healthy conditions, generally due to one of five mechanisms:
  - Reduced intake
  - Diminished absorption
  - Increased use
  - Increased demand
  - Increased excretion
- Chronic disease states: HIV, malabsorption (such as celiac sprue and short bowel syndrome), chronic liver and kidney disease, alcoholism, malignancies, pernicious anemia, and inborn errors of metabolism
- Bariatric surgeries: gastric bypass, gastrectomy, small or large bowel resection
- Related to certain drugs: prednisone, phenytoin, isoniazid, protease inhibitors, methotrexate, phenobarbital, alcohol, nitrous oxide, H_2 receptor antagonists, metformin, colchicine, cholestyramine, 5-fluorouracil, 6-mercaptopurine, azathioprine, chloramphenicol, proton pump inhibitors, chronically used antibiotics, penicillamine, and hydralazine
- Malnutrition, imbalanced nutrition, obesity, fad diets, extreme vegetarianism, total parenteral nutrition, bulimia/anorexia, and other eating disorders
- Dialysis
- Parasitic infestation

Genetics
- Cystic fibrosis
- Hartnup disease
- Rare genetic predisposition
  - Autoimmune disease (e.g., pernicious anemia)
  - Congenital enzyme deficiencies (e.g., biotinidase or holocarboxylase synthetase deficiency)

- Transcobalamin II deficiency
  - Ataxia with vitamin E deficiency (AVED)
- A-β-lipoproteinemia

RISK FACTORS
Poverty, malnutrition, chronic disease states, advanced age, dietary restrictions, bariatric surgery, and exclusively breastfed infants

GENERAL PREVENTION
- Ingesting large and varied amounts of vitamin supplements increases risk of toxicity and drug–drug interactions.
- Antioxidant supplement use has not been shown to impact cancer incidence and has *increased* mortality risk in some studies (2).
- Avoiding restrictive diets decreases the likelihood of vitamin deficiency.
- In particular age groups or with certain risk factors, vitamin supplementation may be recommended.
- USPSTF recommends against low-dose supplementation with vitamin D (<400 IU) and calcium (<1,000 mg) to reduce fracture risk in community-dwelling postmenopausal women (3).
- USPSTF recommends that all women planning or capable of pregnancy take a daily supplement containing 0.4 to 0.8 mg of folic acid (4)[A].
- USPSTF recommends against the use of β-carotene or vitamin E supplements for the prevention of cardiovascular disease or cancer (2).
- All infants should receive 400 IU/day of vitamin D soon after birth whether breast- or formula fed (5).

COMMONLY ASSOCIATED CONDITIONS
Anemia, neuropathies, dermatitis, visual disturbances

DIAGNOSIS

HISTORY
- Review dietary intake.
- Decreased visual acuity or night blindness
- Poor wound healing or easy bruising
- Skin changes or new rash
- Neuropathy
- Abnormal food cravings (pica)
- Osteomalacia or history of low-energy fracture
- Previous birth of a child with spina bifida
- Previous GI or bariatric surgery (1)
- Recurrent or persistent vomiting or diarrhea
- Prior or current medical conditions
  - Tuberculosis (TB), HIV infection, hepatitis, cancer
  - Hypermetabolic state
    - Thyrotoxicosis
    - 2nd- or 3rd-degree burns
    - Extensive or chronic wound
    - Any systemic infection
- Chronic disease requiring steroids, disease-modifying antirheumatic drugs (DMARDs), or immunosuppressants
- Malabsorptive or chronic GI disorder: celiac disease, sprue, Crohn disease, ulcerative colitis, GERD
- Parenteral or enteral nutrition via tube feeding
- Pregnancy
- Amenorrhea or infertility issues
- Medications, supplements
- Food allergies or intolerances, fad or restrictive diet

PHYSICAL EXAM
- Neurologic exam: gait, memory/cognitive impairment, reflexes, sensory or motor impairment, peripheral neuropathy (1)
- Oropharyngeal exam: glossitis, bleeding gums, hyperemic pharynx, stomatitis, cheilitis (1)
- Skin exam: maculosquamous dermatitis, photosensitive pigmented dermatitis, ecchymosis, and/or petechiae
- Visual assessment

DIFFERENTIAL DIAGNOSIS
Multiple conditions mimic signs and symptoms of vitamin deficiencies.
- Diabetes mellitus (DM), thyroid disorders, hyperparathyroidism, heart failure, Alzheimer disease, multiple sclerosis, substance abuse, toxic ingestions, and hematologic disorders/malignancies

DIAGNOSTIC TESTS & INTERPRETATION
Initial Tests (lab, imaging)
- No routine screening indicated
- Test if symptomatic, history indicates high risk, or if clinical characteristics are present:
  - 25-OH vitamin D (5)
  - Prothrombin time (PT)/partial thromboplastin time (PTT)
  - Vitamin B_{12} and folate levels (1)
  - Serum homocysteine and methylmalonic acid levels if high suspicion of vitamin B_{12} deficiency with normal serum B_{12} level
  - Retinol serum level, retinol-binding protein
- Ancillary tests:
  - BUN, calcium, phosphorus, magnesium
  - Albumin, liver function tests
  - CBC
  - Parathyroid hormone
- Bone densitometry for:
  - Women 65 years of age or older without previous known fractures or risk factors
  - Women <65 years old whose 10-year fracture risk is equal to that of a 65-year-old white woman without additional risk factors
  - According to the Fracture Risk Assessment Tool (FRAX), the 10-year fracture risk for a 65-year-old white woman without risk factors is 9.3%.
- Bariatric surgery patients are at risk for deficiencies. Laparoscopic gastric banding is less frequently associated with vitamin deficiencies.
- Cyanocobalamin, thiamine, vitamin A
- Disease states from vitamin deficiency
  - Vitamin A (retinol): night blindness, complete blindness, xerophthalmia
  - Vitamin B_1 (thiamine)
    - Wernicke encephalopathy: acute syndrome with memory disturbance, truncal ataxia, nystagmus, ophthalmoplegia
    - Korsakoff syndrome: anterograde and retrograde amnesia, confabulation
    - Dry beriberi: symmetric motor and sensory peripheral neuropathy, paresthesias, loss of reflexes
    - Wet beriberi: neuropathy with cardiovascular symptoms of peripheral vasodilation, high-output failure, dyspnea, and tachycardia
    - Infantile beriberi: loud piercing cry, cyanosis, tachycardia, cardiomegaly, dyspnea, vomiting, seizures
  - Vitamin B_2 (riboflavin): glossitis, stomatitis, cheilitis, hyperemia of the pharyngeal mucosal membranes, normocytic-normochromic anemia

– Vitamin B_3 (niacin): pellagra: photosensitive pigmented dermatitis, dementia, and diarrhea
– Vitamin B_5 (pantothenic acid): paresthesias and dysesthesias, anemia
– Vitamin B_6 (pyridoxine): dermatitis, cheilosis, atrophic glossitis, stomatitis, neuropathy
– Vitamin B_9 (folate): megaloblastic anemia, rarely manifest neurologic symptoms
– Vitamin B_{12} (cobalamin): pernicious anemia, leukopenia, pancytopenia, shuffling broad-based gait, atrophic glossitis, loss of vibration and position sense, cognitive impairment, areflexia, olfactory impairment, peripheral neuropathy, hyperpigmentation, jaundice, vitiligo
– Vitamin C (ascorbic acid): scurvy: ecchymoses, bleeding gums, petechiae, hyperkeratosis, arthralgias, impaired wound healing
– Vitamin D (calciferol): rickets, osteomalacia
– Vitamin E: neuromuscular disorders and hemolysis
– Vitamin K: easy bruising, mucosal bleeding, melena, hematuria
– Biotin: changes in mental status, dysesthesias, nausea, maculosquamous dermatitis of the extremities

 TREATMENT

Although vitamin D deficiency has been linked with worse cardiovascular morbidity and mortality and is associated with vascular dysfunction; arterial stiffening; left ventricular hypertrophy; and worsened metrics of diabetes, hypertension, and hyperlipidemia, a causal effect between deficiency and cardiovascular disease has not been shown. Trials have failed to show improvements in blood pressure, insulin sensitivity, or lipids (6).

MEDICATION

- Ask patients about herbal or dietary supplement use; encourage patients to bring in vitamin and supplement bottles for review.
- Assess for potential adverse drug effects/reactions. Patients with alcohol use disorders should receive thiamine, folic acid, and MVI.
- Give patients with suspected thiamine deficiency 100 mg thiamine prior to IV fluids containing glucose to prevent precipitating Korsakoff psychosis.
- If there is concomitant B_{12} and folate deficiency, start vitamin B_{12} first to avoid precipitating subacute combined degeneration of the spinal cord (1).
- Consider obtaining prealbumin/albumin levels and a dietary consult for malnourished patients.
- Bariatric surgery patients will need lifelong vitamin supplementation; there are no consensus practice guidelines for supplement dosing regimens.

Geriatric Considerations

- Vitamin B_{12} deficiency exists in ~20% of patients age >60 years. Treat symptomatic or severe deficiency with an IM injection of cyanocobalamin 1,000 μg/day 3 times a week for 2 weeks. If there are neurologic symptoms, give the same dose of cyanocobalamin every other day for 3 weeks or until symptoms have resolved. To prevent recurrence or treat mild deficiency, use a regimen of oral vitamin B_{12} 1,000 μg/day or an IM injection of vitamin B_{12} 1,000 μg every month. Low-dose oral therapy with 50 to 150 μg/day may be considered for mild cases (1). High-dose (1,000 to 2,000 μg/day) oral treatment is as effective as monthly IM injections, but use caution if malabsorption or compliance issues (1)[C].

- >40% of elderly Americans are vitamin D deficient. Deficiency is defined as a serum 25-OH vitamin D level of <20 ng/mL.
- Treat vitamin D deficiency with weekly 50,000 IU of oral ergocalciferol for 8 weeks. Recommended daily supplementation in those age >70 years is 800 IU/day of vitamin D (3)[C].

Pediatric Considerations

- Vitamin K deficiency increases bleeding risk.
  – Neonates may exhibit signs of vitamin K deficiency because they require 1 week of life to establish intestinal flora, which manufactures vitamin K.
  – Condition peaks 2 to 10 days after birth: bleeding from the umbilical stump and/or circumcision site, generalized bruising, and GI hemorrhage.
  – Infrequent in developed countries due to routine injection of newborns with vitamin K (1 mg)
- Vitamin D deficiency: Vitamin D supplementation (400 IU/day) is recommended for all infants starting in the first few days of life (5)[A].
- 600 IU/day of vitamin D is recommended for children >12 months and adults either through diet or supplementation (5).
- Morbidly obese and minority children are at increased risk for vitamin D deficiency.
- In children age >6 months in developing countries, vitamin A supplementation has been shown to decrease mortality.
- Vitamin deficiency associated with developmental delay

Pregnancy Considerations

All pregnant women and women of childbearing age considering pregnancy are strongly encouraged to take a multivitamin containing at least 0.4 mg folic acid daily to prevent neural tube defects (4)[A].

 ONGOING CARE

DIET

Vitamins are best used by the body from food intake. Supplements should be used where it is not feasible to ingest the recommended amount of a particular vitamin.

PATIENT EDUCATION

- In healthy adults, multivitamins have no value if dietary intake is adequate and may increase risk of some cancers.
- Drug–drug interactions may occur between vitamins and medications. Patients should report all supplements and medications to their health care provider.
- Risk of vitamin toxicity is most common with fat-soluble vitamins (A, D, E, K).

PROGNOSIS

Most vitamin deficiencies are fully reversible if treated without undue delay.

COMPLICATIONS

- Vitamin toxicities
- Liver failure (vitamins A, D, E, K)
- Desquamation of skin (vitamin A)
- Neuropathy (vitamin B_6)
- Kidney stones (vitamin C, vitamin D)
- Hypercoagulability (vitamin K)
- Pseudohyperparathyroidism (vitamin D)
- Masking of pernicious anemia (folic acid)

REFERENCES

1. Langan RC, Goodbred AJ. Vitamin B_{12} deficiency: recognition and management. *Am Fam Physician*. 2017;96(6):384–389.
2. U.S. Preventive Services Task Force. Vitamin, mineral, and multivitamin supplements for the primary prevention of cardiovascular disease and cancer: recommendation statement. https://www.uspreventiveservicestaskforce.org/Page/Document/UpdateSummaryFinal/vitamin-supplementation-to-prevent-cancer-and-cvd-counseling.
3. U.S. Preventive Services Task Force. Final recommendation statement vitamin D, calcium, or combined supplementation for the primary prevention of fractures in community-dwelling adults: preventive medication. https://www.uspreventiveservicestaskforce.org/Page/Document/RecommendationStatementFinal/vitamin-d-calcium-or-combined-supplementation-for-the-primary-prevention-of-fractures-in-adults-preventive-medication. Accessed October 11, 2018.
4. Bibbins-Domingo K, Grossman DC, Curry SJ, et al; for U.S. Preventive Services Task Force. Folic acid supplementation for the prevention of neural tube defects: US Preventive Services Task Force recommendation statement. *JAMA*. 2017;317(2):183–189.
5. Munns CF, Shaw N, Kiely M, et al. Global consensus recommendations on prevention and management of nutritional rickets. *J Clin Endocrinol Metab*. 2016;101(2):394–415.
6. Al Mheid I, Quyyumi AA. Vitamin D and cardiovascular disease: controversy unresolved. *J Am Coll Cardiol*. 2017;70(1):89–100.

ADDITIONAL READING

Tack J, Deloose E. Complications of bariatric surgery: dumping syndrome, reflux and vitamin deficiencies. *Best Pract Res Clin Gastroenterol*. 2014;28(4):741–749.

 CODES

ICD10

- E56.9 Vitamin deficiency, unspecified
- E56.0 Deficiency of vitamin E
- E55.9 Vitamin D deficiency, unspecified

CLINICAL PEARLS

- Obtain a thorough dietary history when assessing for potential vitamin deficiencies.
- Specifically ask patients about dietary supplement use.
- The USPSTF recommends against daily vitamin D supplementation of 400 IU or less to prevent fractures in community-dwelling postmenopausal women.
- All women planning or capable of pregnancy should take a daily supplement containing 0.4 to 0.8 mg of folic acid.
- All infants and children, including adolescents, should have a minimum daily intake of 400 IU of vitamin D beginning soon after birth.

V

VITILIGO

Sonia Rivera-Martinez, DO • Karen Sheflin, DO

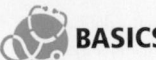

BASICS

DESCRIPTION
- An acquired depigmentation of the skin, which correlates with a loss of epidermal melanocytes. There are three clinical variants, each with subtypes.
- Localized: often in childhood, rapid onset then stabilizes. Involvement of hair is common early in the course; lacks associated autoimmune diseases
  - Focal: few lesions, random distribution
  - Segmental: Lesions occur within a dermatome (mostly trigeminal) or may follow Blaschko lines. Lesions usually stop abruptly at the midline.
  - Mucosal: only mucosal surfaces involved
- Generalized/nonsegmental (most common variant): progressive, with flares, commonly associated with autoimmunity. Common locations are acral, periorificial, and in sites sensitive to pressure/friction (Koebner phenomenon).
  - Vulgaris: most common subtype; scattered macules; often symmetric, wide distribution; mostly hands, axillae, and groin
  - Acrofacial: on distal extremities and face
  - Mixed: coexistence of above
- Universal: involves >80% of the body surface area (BSA). Most likely to have family history; comorbidities are common and associated with poorest quality-of-life (QOL) scores.
- Other rare variants
  - Ponctué: discrete, confetti-like macules
  - Inflammatory: peripheral erythematous rim
  - Trichrome: Tan zone is present between normal and depigmented skin
  - Quadrichrome: as above but with marginal/perifollicular hyperpigmentation
  - Blue: Dermal melanophages give blue hue in areas affected by prior postinflammatory hyperpigmentation.
- System(s) affected: skin, mucous membranes
- Synonym(s): leukoderma

EPIDEMIOLOGY
- 50% begin before age 20 years, peak in females: 1st decade; males: 5th decade. Onset earlier with positive family history; can appear as early as 6 weeks
- Predominance: male = female; however, females are more likely to seek treatment.
- No race or socioeconomic predilection

Prevalence
~1% in the United States and Europe (1); 0.1–8% in the world; highest in Gujarat, India at 8.8% (1,2)

ETIOLOGY AND PATHOPHYSIOLOGY
Most likely a spectrum of disorders with a common phenotype and multiple mechanisms contribute to the pathology (convergence theory).
- Genetic: See "Genetics."
- Autoimmune: humoral autoantibodies and skin-homing T cells
- Neural: local or systemic dysregulation leading to excess neurotransmitters
- Viral: direct melanocyte toxicity, cytomegalovirus (CMV), hepatitis C, and Epstein-Barr virus (EBV) found in lesional biopsies
- Oxidative stress from elevated H_2O_2 and NO and decreased catalase and erythrocyte glutathione

Genetics
- Polygenic/multifactorial inheritance
- 20% of patients report affected relative, but monozygotic twins have only 23% concordance.

- HLA haplotypes, small nucleotide polymorphisms, and specific genes are all possible contributors.

RISK FACTORS
- Family history of vitiligo/autoimmune disorders
- Personal history of associated conditions

COMMONLY ASSOCIATED CONDITIONS
- Most common
  - Endocrine: thyroid disease (hypo-/hyperthyroidism), hypoparathyroidism, Addison disease, insulin-dependent diabetes
  - Dermatologic: psoriasis, atopic dermatitis, alopecia areata, chronic urticaria, halo nevi, ichthyosis
  - Pernicious anemia
  - Hypoacusis, rheumatoid arthritis
  - Ocular abnormalities in up to 40%
  - Elevated antinuclear antibodies in up to 40%
  - Elevated thyroperoxidase antibodies in 50%
- Less common
  - Systemic lupus erythematosus
  - Inflammatory bowel disease
  - Melanoma (may be a sign of positive outcome of melanoma) and other skin cancers
  - Syndromes: Alezzandrini; mitochondrial encephalomyopathy, lactic acidosis, and stroke-like episodes (MELAS); Schmidt; and autoimmune polyendocrinopathy-candidiasis-ectodermal dystrophy (APECED)
- Age >50 years at onset should prompt investigation for associated conditions.

Pediatric Considerations
Associated with Hashimoto thyroiditis in a significant portion of children. Screening at onset and possibly annually may be beneficial.

DIAGNOSIS

HISTORY
- Inquire about recent history of sunburns, pregnancy, skin trauma, or emotional stress.
- Family history of premature graying, vitiligo, and autoimmune disorders
- Review of systems for related associated conditions
- Ascertain psychological impact on QOL, Dermatology Life Quality Index (DLQI).

PHYSICAL EXAM
- Full-body skin exam with Wood lamp to accentuate lesions and distinguish depigmentation from hypopigmentation
- Lesions are well-demarcated, uniform, white macules and patches.
- Look for evidence of repigmentation (most commonly around hair follicles).

DIFFERENTIAL DIAGNOSIS
- Infectious: tinea versicolor, leprosy, leishmaniasis, onchocerciasis, treponematoses (pinta/syphilis)
- Postinflammatory hypopigmentation: psoriasis, atopic dermatitis, pityriasis alba, systemic lupus erythematosus, scleroderma
- Inherited hypomelanoses: piebaldism, tuberous sclerosis, Waardenburg, hypomelanosis of Ito, Vogt-Koyanagi-Harada
- Malformations: nevus anemicus, nevus depigmentosus
- Paraneoplastic: mycosis fungoides, melanoma-associated leukoderma
- Occupational and chemical induced
  - Occupational: phenolic/catechol derivatives and arsenic-containing compounds

- Chemical: numerous, including cosmetics, cleansers, insecticides, and even medications (imatinib, potent topical corticosteroids [TCS])
- Melasma: Normal skin may be confused as vitiligo in the setting of surrounding hyperpigmentation.
- Halo nevi
- Lichen sclerosus et atrophicus
- Idiopathic guttate hypomelanosis
- Progressive-acquired macular hypomelanosis

DIAGNOSTIC TESTS & INTERPRETATION

Initial Tests (lab, imaging)
- TSH, CBC, ANA
- Consider antithyroid peroxidase, antithyroglobulin antibodies, hemoglobin, vitamin B_{12} levels if family/patient history of autoimmune disease.

Follow-Up Tests & Special Considerations
- Monitor for disease progression/flares.
- Monitor for symptoms of related conditions.

Diagnostic Procedures/Other
- Skin biopsy is rarely needed. Highest yield is with comparison of lesional/perilesional biopsies.
- Consider ophthalmologic and audiologic evaluation.

Test Interpretation
Few or no epidermal melanocytes. At margins, melanocytes may be larger, vacuolated, and dendritic. Early lesions show inflammation and later, degeneration, including of adnexa and nerves.

TREATMENT

The variant of vitiligo may affect response.
- If untreated, progression is the natural course for those with mucosal involvement, family history, koebnerization, and nonsegmental variants.
- Lesions that respond best are on the face, of recent onset, in darker skin type, and in younger patients.

GENERAL MEASURES
- Sunscreen to decrease sunburn and prevent accentuation of uninvolved skin
- Corrective camouflage as cover-up (Cover FX, Dermablend)

MEDICATION
- Individualize therapy depending on age, extent, distribution, and rate of progression.
- Many therapies are considered "off-label" and not FDA-approved for vitiligo, although they are often considered first-line therapy.
- Corticosteroids: Midpotency TCS (mometasone furoate, fluticasone propionate) applied daily as monotherapy are considered first-line treatments. Do not use on face/axilla/groin; do not occlude except under close monitoring. Pediatric: as above, for children >12 years of age. Consider decreased potency. Local side effects including atrophy, telangiectasia, hypertrichosis, acneiform eruptions, and striae limit treatment; regular steroid holidays are recommended (1). The combination of light therapy and TCS is the most effective treatment overall (2). Most efficacious on sun-exposed areas: face/neck, dark-skinned patients, newer lesion (1). Addition of tretinoin 0.025–0.05% BID is effective and can decrease potential skin atrophy (2,3). Systemic corticosteroids can be helpful, but dosage and safety parameters have not been fully evaluated for long-term treatment (2,4)[A].

- Topical calcineurin inhibitors: slightly inferior to TCS as monotherapy but better side effect profile (2,5,6)[B]; can be used as adjunctive to light therapy; carries a controversial black box warning for a theoretical risk of lymphoma or skin cancer. Extensive safety profiling has not revealed any evidence for this in children or adults using topical calcineurin inhibitors. Local reactions include burning sensation, pruritus, erythema, and rare transient hyperpigmentation (4).
  - Tacrolimus 0.03% or 0.1% ointment BID (2); pediatric: 0.03% ointment BID, for children >2 years of age (6)
  - Pimecrolimus 1% cream BID (2); pediatric: as adults, for children >2 years of age (6)
- Topical vitamin D_3 analogs: less effective than TCS alone but in combination with TCS or phototherapy can shorten time until, and improve stability of, repigmentation (4,5)[B]
  - Calcipotriene ointment 1 to 2 times per day; pediatric: not defined
  - Available as a combination formulation, beta-methasone dipropionate 0.064%/calcipotriene 0.005% ointment daily, max dose of 100 g/week for 4 weeks, not for >30% BSA, and not for face/axilla/groin; pediatric: not defined
- Oral vitamin D_3: reported to induce repigmentation. Oral vitamin D_3 35,000 IU once daily plus low-calcium diet for 6 months; pediatric: not defined
- Phototherapy: Narrow band UVB (NBUVB) is superior to UVA and indicated for lesions involving >15–20% BSA (3,5,6)[A]. Psoralen and khellin enhance the effect of light. Psoralen plus UVA (PUVA) may increase the incidence of skin cancers. Khellin may have reduced cross-linking of DNA and may be less carcinogenic; however, it is associated with increased liver toxicity (6). L-phenylalanine can be used topically and orally as a photosensitizer for natural or artificial light. Pediatric: Oral PUVA is contraindicated.
- Laser therapy: Excimer laser (308 nm) is superior to other light therapy. Helium–neon laser works for segmental vitiligo (5)[A].
- Antioxidants: may have protective role in preventing melanocyte degradation from reactive oxygen species. Options include vitamin C, vitamin E, Vitix, Polypodium leucotomos extracts, and *Ginkgo biloba* (5)[B].
- Surgical therapy: See later discussion.
- New concepts: Tumor necrosis factor-α inhibitors, cyclosporine, cyclophosphamide, azathioprine, minocycline, and immunosuppressants are currently being evaluated (6).

First Line
- Recommended: avoidance of triggering factors plus TCS alone or in combination with NBUVB
- Alternatively
  - Topical calcineurin inhibitors (preferred for face, neck, axilla, and groin)
  - NBUVB
  - PUVA in adults
  - Camouflage and psychotherapy should be offered to all patients at any stage (6).

Second Line
- Recommended: photochemotherapy with psoralens or vitamin D analogues
- Alternatively
  - Topical vitamin D analogues
  - Targeted phototherapy
  - 308-nm laser in combination with topical steroids, topical calcineurin inhibitors, or vitamin D analogues

- Oral corticosteroids (pulse therapy)
- Surgical treatments indicated for stable 2- to 3-cm lesions, refractory to other treatments
  - Mini-punch graft (pretreat with cryotherapy/ dermabrasion or posttreat with phototherapy) (6)[B]
  - Suction blister graft (6)[B]
  - Autologous melanocyte suspension transplant (5)[B]

ISSUES FOR REFERRAL
- Dermatologist: for facial/widespread vitiligo or when advanced therapy is necessary
- Ophthalmologist: for ocular symptoms or monitoring of TCS near eyes
- Endocrinologist: evaluation/management of associated conditions
- Psychologist: for severe distress
- Medical geneticist for associated conditions

ADDITIONAL THERAPIES
- Depigmentation therapy with monobenzone, hydroquinone, or Q-switched ruby laser: for extensive vitiligo recalcitrant to therapy (6)
- Pseudocatalase with addition of NBUVB (1)[B]
- Prostaglandin E for short-duration disease and localization to face and scalp (2)[B]
- Cosmetic tattooing for localized stable vitiligo

SURGERY/OTHER PROCEDURES
- Goal is to transport melanocytes from other areas of the skin. Methods include punch, blister, or split-thickness skin grafting, or transplantation of autologous melanocytes.
- Dermabrasion and curettage alone or in combination with 5-fluorouracil may induce follicular melanocyte reservoirs (5)[A].
- Patients who koebnerize or form keloids may be worse, and permanent scarring is a risk for all patients.

COMPLEMENTARY & ALTERNATIVE MEDICINE
Ginkgo biloba 60 mg PO daily may significantly improve extension and spreading of lesions (4)[B].
- Polypodium leucotomos may help with repigmentation with NBUVB and aid in reducing phototoxic reactions (5)[B].

 ## ONGOING CARE

FOLLOW-UP RECOMMENDATIONS
- Monitor for symptoms of related conditions.
- With topical steroids, follow at regular intervals to avoid steroid atrophy, telangiectasia, and striae distensae.

DIET
No restrictions

PATIENT EDUCATION
- Discussion of disease course, progression, and cosmesis
- Education regarding trauma/friction and Koebner phenomenon

PROGNOSIS
- Vitiligo may remain stable or slowly or rapidly progress.
- Spontaneous repigmentation is uncommon.
- Generalized vitiligo is often progressive, with flares. Focal vitiligo often has rapid onset and then stabilizes.

COMPLICATIONS
- Adverse effects of each treatment modality
- Psychiatric morbidity: depression, adjustment disorder, low self-esteem, sexual dysfunction, and embarrassment in relationships (1,2)
  - Different cultures may have different perceptions/ social stigmas about vitiligo. Some believe it to be contagious or related to infection. Women with vitiligo may have difficulty finding a marriage partner and have low self-esteem.

REFERENCES
1. Ezzedine K, Eleftheriadou V, Whitton M, et al. Vitiligo. *Lancet*. 2015;386(9988):74–84.
2. Colucci R, Lotti T, Moretti S. Vitiligo: an update on current pharmacotherapy and future directions. *Expert Opin Pharmacother*. 2012;13(13): 1885–1899.
3. Felsten LM, Alikhan A, Petronic-Rosic V. Vitiligo: a comprehensive overview part II: treatment options and approach to treatment. *J Am Acad Dermatol*. 2011;65(3):493–514.
4. Bacigalupi RM, Postolova A, Davis RS. Evidence-based, non-surgical treatments for vitiligo: a review. *Am J Clin Dermatol*. 2012;13(4):217–237.
5. Whitton ME, Pinart M, Batchelor J, et al. Interventions for vitiligo. *Cochrane Database Syst Rev*. 2015;(2):CD003263.
6. Patel NS, Paghdal KV, Cohen GF. Advanced treatment modalities for vitiligo. *Dermatol Surg*. 2012;38(3):381–391.

ADDITIONAL READING
- Alikhan A, Felsten LM, Daly M, et al. Vitiligo: a comprehensive overview part I. Introduction, epidemiology, quality of life, diagnosis, differential diagnosis, associations, histopathology, etiology, and work-up. *J Am Acad Dermatol*. 2011;65(3): 473–491.
- Silverberg NB. The epidemiology of vitiligo. *Curr Derm Rep*. 2015;4(1):36–43.
- Taieb A, Alomar A, Böhm M, et al; for Vitiligo European Task Force, European Academy of Dermatology and Venereology, Union Europe´enne des Me´decins Spe´cialistes. Guidelines for the management of vitiligo: the European Dermatology Forum consensus. *Br J Dermatol*. 2013;168(1):5–19.

CODES

ICD10
L80 Vitiligo

CLINICAL PEARLS
- Vitiligo can be a psychologically devastating skin disease.
- Screen for associated diseases, particularly if onset occurs later in life.
- Treatment should be individualized based on BSA, skin type, and patient goals.
- Dermatology consultation when extensive disease, facial involvement, and when advanced treatments are considered

V

VON WILLEBRAND DISEASE

Chang L. Lipinski, DO • Jarrett Sell, MD, AAHIVS • Stacey L. Milunic, MD

BASICS

DESCRIPTION
- von Willebrand disease (vWD) is a bleeding disorder caused by deficiency or a defect of *von Willebrand factor* (vWF) protein.
- vWF is critical to the initial stages of blood clotting, acting as a bridge for platelet adhesion; it also acts as a carrier for factor VIII (FVIII).
- Most common subtypes of vWD manifest as muco-cutaneous, perioperative bleeding, or menorrhagia, whereas more serious subtypes may result in joint and soft tissue bleeding.
- vWD is an inherited condition but rarely can be acquired (AvWD).

EPIDEMIOLOGY
Prevalence
- Prevalence of the inherited forms of vWD is 1 in 100 to 10,000 of the general population with more females being diagnosed than males.
- Exact prevalence of the acquired forms of vWD (AvWD) is unknown but is estimated to be up to 0.1% of the general population.

ETIOLOGY AND PATHOPHYSIOLOGY
- vWF is a large, multimeric protein that is released from endothelial cells and is also carried within platelets in α-granules.
- vWF binds to collagen at sites of vascular injury and creates a surface for platelet adhesion through GP1b receptors. This results in platelet plug formation.
- vWF is also a carrier for FVIII and stabilizes this factor from degradation. A deficiency in vWF may result in lower levels of FVIII.
- When vWF is deficient or dysfunctional, primary hemostasis is compromised, resulting in increased mucocutaneous and postprocedural bleeding.
- Three major inherited types of vWD exist.
  - Type 1, the most common and mildest form, represents 60–80% of cases.
    - Mild to moderate quantitative deficiency of vWF and concordant deficiency of FVIII
    - Generally, a mild bleeding disorder
  - Type 2, caused by qualitative defect in vWF, accounts for 10–30% of cases and is divided into the following multiple subtypes:
    - Type 2A is noted for loss of hemostatically active large multimers with low ristocetin cofactor/vWF activity.
    - Type 2B, noted for increased binding affinity for platelets, is associated with thrombocytopenia, low ristocetin cofactor/vWF activity, abnormal ristocetin-induced platelet aggregation (RIPA), and loss of large multimers.
    - Type 2M is noted for defective platelet or collagen binding without loss of large multimers.
    - Type 2N demonstrates defective binding to FVIII, which results in increased clearance of FVIII and a hemophilia A–like picture.
  - Type 3 represents 1–5% of cases.
    - Most severe form with markedly decreased-to-undetectable levels of vWF and FVIII
    - Manifests as hemophilia A with hemarthroses (1,2,3)
- AvWD may be due to cardiovascular, hematologic, or autoimmune conditions as well as tumors and medications. The pathophysiology of AvWD is related to the underlying cause and may result from shear-induced cleaving of vWF in cardiovascular conditions, increased adsorption of vWF by certain tumor cells or activated platelets, or presence of anti-vWF autoantibodies in hematologic disorders.
- Individuals with type O blood have accelerated clearance of vWF leading to vWF levels that are 25–30% lower than other those with blood type A, B, or AB. Type 1 disease is diagnosed more frequently in individuals with blood type O blood.
- Platelet-type vWD (PLT-vWD), also called pseudo vWD, is caused by platelet GP1 alpha receptor mutation.

Genetics
- The 175-kb gene for vWF is located on short arm of chromosome 12.
- Type 1 follows an autosomal dominant inheritance pattern, with variable expressivity.
- Type 2 varies but primarily follows an autosomal dominant inheritance pattern.
- Type 3 follows an autosomal recessive inheritance pattern (2).

COMMONLY ASSOCIATED CONDITIONS
AvWD may be found in patients with hematologic disorders such as MGUS and myeloproliferative neoplasms. Commonly associated cardiovascular conditions include aortic stenosis and left ventricular assist device (LVAD) placement. AvWD is associated with gastrointestinal (GI) bleeding from arteriovenous malformations.

DIAGNOSIS

HISTORY
- Most patients with vWD have a positive family history of a bleeding disorder; however, patients with mild forms of vWD and their families may be unaware of their disease. Those with AvWD usually have no family history of this disorder.
- Common symptoms include mucocutaneous (recurrent epistaxis, menorrhagia, ecchymosis) or postprocedural bleeding. Hemarthrosis is a rare presentation, mostly associated with types 2N and 3.
- The most important component of diagnosis is the hemostatic history, often aided by specifically designed bleeding questionnaires, such as the ISTH-BAT found at isth.org (International Society on Thrombosis and Haemostasis).
- ACOG recommends initial reproductive visits for girls between 13 and 15 years. vWD should be in the differential for heavy menstrual bleeding, at any age, but especially adolescents, when bleeding disorders may be overlooked and incorrectly attributed to an immature hypothalamic-pituitary axis.

PHYSICAL EXAM
- Physical exam may be entirely normal, with occasional ecchymoses.
- Findings suggestive of other causes of increased bleeding should be sought (liver disease, skin laxity, or telangiectasias).

DIFFERENTIAL DIAGNOSIS
- Primary hemostatic disorders: congenital thrombocytopenia or qualitative platelet defects, coagulation factor deficiencies
- Secondary hemostatic disorders: liver disease, uremia, connective tissue disorders, coagulation factor inhibitors

DIAGNOSTIC TESTS & INTERPRETATION
- Abnormal bleeding initial screening tests
  - Complete blood count: decreased platelets in type 2B
  - PT/INR: normal or prolonged in liver disease or warfarin use
  - aPTT: normal or isolated prolonged aPTT that corrects in 1:1 mixing study
  - May consider bleeding time or platelet function analyzer (PFA-100): normal or prolonged
- Diagnostic vWD tests
  - vWF antigen (vWF:Ag): reduced
  - vWF ristocetin cofactor (vWF:RCo): reduced, except type 2N
  - vWF collagen binding (vWF:CB): reduced in most vWD types
  - vWF: GPIbM: reduced, less false positives
  - FVIII:C: reduced in types 2N and 3
- Classifying tests
  - Ratios of vWF:RCo/vWF:Ag: <0.5 to 0.7 differentiates type 1 from type 2.
  - vWF multimer assay: differentiates type 2
  - RIPA: diagnoses type 2B
  - vWF propeptide (vWFpp): identifies accelerated clearance variants
  - FVIII binding assay: low in type 2N
  - Gene sequencing
  - Assays for vWF antibodies
  - Platelet-binding studies
- Interpretation of tests should always be preceded by significant bleeding history; best assessed with ISTH-BAT score and family history for bleeding and/or diagnosed with vWD (1,2,3).

Follow-Up Tests & Special Considerations
- Unless patients have severe forms of vWD or are undergoing treatment, follow-up laboratory studies are not usually obtained.
- vWF is an acute-phase reactant, so elevations may be seen in inflammatory conditions, liver disease, pregnancy (which may correct mild deficits), or with estrogen use. Levels also increase with age; however, it is unclear if this decreases bleeding risk (2).

TREATMENT

GENERAL MEASURES
- Most patients with type 1 vWD do not require activity restrictions.
- Patients with type 3 vWD should avoid contact sports.
- An emergency ID bracelet may be useful.

MEDICATION
First Line
- Desmopressin (DDAVP)
  - Enhances release of vWF from endothelial cells
  - Primarily effective for type 1 vWD; not to be used in type 2B. Trial of DDAVP should initially be measured in nonbleeding state to determine response.
  - Not effective in severe deficiencies, in types of vWD with defective vWF, or for prophylaxis prior to major procedures
  - Dosed 0.3 μg/kg (max 20 mg) IV/SC; intranasal (high concentration) spray: <50 kg: 150 μg/day; >50 kg: 300 μg/day (Stimate)

- Common side effects: flushing, tachycardia, water retention, hyponatremia. Tachyphylaxis may develop with prolonged dosing; limit use to administering DDAVP once every 24 to 48 hours for 3 to 5 days.
- Test therapeutic responsiveness by testing vWF:Ag, vWF:RCo, and FVIII:C at baseline, 1 hour and 4 hours postinfusion. An increase in levels at least 2- to 3-fold, >30 IU/dL and preferably >50 IU/dL for invasive procedures, is adequate response; vWF and FVIII concentrates
- Plasma-derived vWF and FVIII concentrates of various purity such as Humate-P, Alphanate, Wilate, or Fandhi (not available in United States) are commercial concentrates of vWF and FVIII that are given in doses of 25 to 60 IU/kg/day based on clinical situation (4,5).
  - Administration of 1 IU/kg vWF:RCo concentrate raises the plasma RCo activity by approximately 2%.
  - Dose of vWF concentrate may be adjusted for FVIII levels and ristocetin cofactor activity.
  - FVIII levels should be monitored to avoid supranormal levels and possible venous thromboembolism (VTE).
  - Contraindicated if patient develops alloantibodies to vWF
  - Recombinant vWF concentrate (Vonvendi) is approved for use in adults for on-demand treatment of bleeding episodes. It requires rFVIII with the first infusion if baseline levels are <40% or unknown.
  - In patients with severe bleeding phenotype, prophylactic treatment is used.
- Cryoprecipitate
  - Cryoprecipitate contains FVIII, fibrinogen, vWF, factor XIII, and fibronectin.
  - Not considered as safe as the recombinant and virus-inactivated plasma concentrates listed above and should not be used unless those are unavailable
- Antifibrinolytics
  - Useful for mucosal bleeding
  - Contraindicated in patients with hematuria due to risk of retention of large blood clots in the renal collecting system
  - Given as adjunct to DDAVP
  - Aminocaproic acid may be given at 50 to 70 mg/kg (max: 5 g; lower doses may be effective) q4–6h IV or PO.
  - Tranexamic acid may be given at 10 to 15 mg/kg IV or 25 mg/kg (1,300 mg) PO q8–12h.
- Recombinant FVIIa (NovoSeven)
  - Used for patients who develop alloantibodies to vWF
  - Given as IV bolus of 90 μg/kg q2h or 20 μg/kg every hour until hemostasis is achieved

Second Line
- Combined oral contraceptives or the levonorgestrel-releasing intrauterine system raise vWF/FVIII levels and have a role in the treatment of chronic menorrhagia (6)[B].
- Platelets may be given as an adjunct to factor concentrates if hemostasis has not been achieved.
- IVIG has been useful in some patients with AvWD associated with monoclonal gammopathy (7)[C].
- Recombinant FVIIa has been used effectively in patients with type 3 vWD.

SURGICAL CONSIDERATIONS
- For patients undergoing minor surgeries, maintain FVIII levels >50 IU/dL for 5 to 7 days.
- For patients undergoing major surgeries, maintain vWF:RCo and FVIII levels >100 U/dL preoperatively and >50 units/dL postoperatively.

- Valve replacement or correction may be curative for patients with AvWD associated with underlying cardiovascular conditions.

Pediatric Considerations
- Circumcision should be postponed until the newborn's vWD status is determined. vWD may be difficult to diagnose before 6 months of age.
- Many cases of vWD are diagnosed in adolescence, often during initial years of menstruation.

Pregnancy Considerations
- Women with vWD are more likely to experience an increased incidence of obstetric complications that manifest with bleeding.
- Type 1 vWD may spontaneously improve, whereas type 2B may be exacerbated by pregnancies.
- FVIII or vWF:Ag should be checked during the 3rd trimester with treatment goal to maintain at levels >50 IU/dL.
- Consider treating with vWF concentrates during pregnancy and desmopressin or tranexamic acid in the postpartum period to achieve treatment goals.
- Women with preeclampsia should not be treated with desmopressin.
- Regional anesthesia not recommended in patients with type 2 and 3 or type 1 with <50 U/dL of vWF:RCo
- Fetal scalp electrodes should be avoided due to the 50% risk of fetus inheritance of vWD, and circumcisions should be postponed (2,6).

ISSUES FOR REFERRAL
The diagnosis and management of vWD is not always straightforward; consider consultation with a hematologist.

 ## ONGOING CARE

FOLLOW-UP RECOMMENDATIONS
Patients should be seen by a hematologist prior to invasive procedures for determination of perioperative management or advice regarding delivery.

Patient Monitoring
Patients with mild disease do not require monitoring.

DIET
No dietary restrictions are recommended. However, aspirin and other NSAIDs should be avoided due to their antiplatelet effects, which can exacerbate the bleeding phenotype.

PATIENT EDUCATION
National Hemophilia Foundation: www.hemophilia .org/NHFWeb/MainPgs/MainNHF.aspx?menuid=182& contentid=47&rptname=bleeding

PROGNOSIS
Most patients with vWD have a normal life expectancy.

COMPLICATIONS
- Significant perioperative bleeding may occur.
- Patients with type 3 vWD and type 2N can have bleeding complications similar to patients with hemophilia A, such as hemarthrosis and intracranial hemorrhage.
- Patients with aortic stenosis and AvWD are known to have higher rates of GI bleeding.
- Multiple transfusions may result in alloantibodies against vWF.
- VTE may result from supranormal levels of FVIII.

REFERENCES
1. Ng C, Motto DG, Di Paola J. Diagnostic approach to von Willebrand disease. *Blood*. 2015;125(13): 2029–2037.
2. Leebeek FW, Eikenboom JC. Von Willebrand's disease. *N Engl J Med*. 2016;375(21):2067–2080.
3. Bowman ML, James PD. Controversies in the diagnosis of type 1 von Willebrand disease. *Int J Lab Hematol*. 2017;39(Suppl 1):61–68.
4. Mannucci PM, Chediak J, Hanna W, et al; and Alphanate Study Group. Treatment of von Willebrand disease with a high-purity factor VIII/von Willebrand factor concentrate: a prospective, multicenter study. *Blood*. 2002;99(2):450–456.
5. Thompson AR, Gill JC, Ewenstein BM, et al; for Humate-P Study Group. Successful treatment for patients with von Willebrand disease undergoing urgent surgery using factor VIII/VWF concentrate (Humate-P). *Haemophilia*. 2004;10(1):42–51.
6. Committee on Adolescent Health Care, Committee on Gynecologic Practice. Committee Opinion No. 580: von Willebrand disease in women. *Obstet Gynecol*. 2013;122(6):1368–1373.
7. Tiede A, Rand JH, Budde U, et al. How I treat the acquired von Willebrand syndrome. *Blood*. 2011; 117(25):6777–6785.

ADDITIONAL READING
- Kessler CM. Diagnosis and treatment of von Willebrand disease: new perspectives and nuances. *Haemophilia*. 2007;13(Suppl 5):3–14.
- Kumar S, Pruthi RK, Nichols WL. Acquired von Willebrand disease. *Mayo Clin Proc*. 2002;77(2):181–187.
- Lippi G, Franchini M, Salvagno GL, et al. Correlation between von Willebrand factor antigen, von Willebrand factor ristocetin cofactor activity and factor VIII activity in plasma. *J Thromb Thrombolysis*. 2008;26(2):150–153.
- Mannucci PM. Treatment of von Willebrand's disease. *N Engl J Med*. 2004;351(7):683–694.
- Robertson J, Lillicrap D, James PD. Von Willebrand disease. *Pediatr Clin North Am*. 2008;55(2):377–392.
- Sciscione AC, Mucowski SJ. Pregnancy and von Willebrand disease: a review. *Del Med J*. 2007;79(10):401–405.

 ## SEE ALSO

Algorithms: Bleeding Gums; Ecchymosis

 ## CODES

ICD10
D68.0 Von Willebrand's disease

CLINICAL PEARLS
- vWD varies from a minor to severe bleeding disorder; affects up to 1% of the U.S. population
- It is important to determine the exact type of vWD (type 1, 2, or 3) to guide treatment.
- Treatment should be administered for recurrent bleeding episodes in all types of vWD, but prophylaxis is rarely required because most cases are mild.
- AvWD should be considered in patients with acquired bleeding disorder if they have underlying predisposing conditions.

V

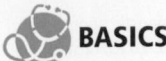

VULVAR MALIGNANCY

Jessica C. Nazzaro, DO • Michael P. Hopkins, MD, MEd

BASICS

DESCRIPTION
- Premalignant lesions of the vulva are collectively known as vulvar intraepithelial neoplasia (VIN).
- Exposure to human papillomavirus (HPV) has been linked to >70% of VIN.
- Invasive squamous cell carcinoma is the most common malignancy involving the vulva (90% of patients); can be well, moderately, or poorly differentiated and derives from keratinized skin covering the vulva and perineum
- Melanoma is the second most common type of vulvar malignancy (8%) and sarcoma is the third.
- Other invasive cell types include basal cell carcinoma, Paget disease, adenocarcinoma arising from Bartholin gland or apocrine sweat glands, adenoid cystic carcinoma, small cell carcinoma, verrucous carcinoma, and sarcomas.
- Sarcomas are usually leiomyosarcoma and probably arise at the insertion of the round ligament in the labium major; however, sarcoma can arise from any structure of the vulva, including blood vessels, skeletal muscle, and fat.
- Rarely, breast carcinoma has been reported in the vulva and is thought to arise from ectopic breast tissue.
- System(s) affected: reproductive

Geriatric Considerations
- Older patients with associated medical problems are at high risk from radical surgery. The surgery, however, is usually well tolerated.
- Patients who are not surgical candidates can be treated with combination chemotherapy and/or radiation.
- In the very elderly, palliative vulvectomy provides relief of symptoms for ulcerating symptomatic advanced disease.

EPIDEMIOLOGY
Incidence
- In 2015, 5,150 women were diagnosed with vulvar cancer and 1,080 women died from vulvar cancer in the United States (1); accounting for approximately 4% of all gynecologic malignancies
- Estimated 6,020 new cases and 1,150 deaths in 2017
- Surveillance, epidemiology, and end result (SEER) data showed that the incidence of in situ vulvar carcinoma increased by >400% between 1973 and 2000.
- Mean age at diagnosis 65 years; in situ disease: mean age 40 years; invasive malignancy: mean age 60 years
- 30–35% of vulvar cancer cases are diagnosed at FIGO stages III and IV.
- Ethnic distribution: more common in Caucasian women than in any other race

ETIOLOGY AND PATHOPHYSIOLOGY
- Patients with cervical cancer are more likely to develop vulvar cancer later in life, secondary to "field effect" phenomenon with a carcinogen involving the lower genital tract.
- HPV has been associated with squamous cell abnormalities of the cervix, vagina, and vulva; 55% of vulvar cancers are attributable to oncogenic HPV, predominantly HPV 16 and 33; vaginal intraepithelial neoplasia (VAIN) 2/3 and anal intraepithelial neoplasia (AIN) are attributable to HPV.

- Squamous cell carcinoma
  - There are two etiologic pathways for developing vulvar squamous cell carcinoma: lichen sclerosus and HPV.
  - The International Society for the Study of Vulvovaginal Disease (ISSVD) proposed a revised terminology in 2015: low-grade squamous intraepithelial lesion (LSIL), which includes flat condyloma and HPV effect, high-grade squamous intraepithelial lesion (HSIL), and VIN differentiated type (dVIN). The ISSVD previously used a three level system grading VIN as 1, 2, 3, which has been abandoned.
  - Differentiated type occurs in older age groups, is associated with lichen sclerosus and chronic venereal diseases, and is not related to HPV. It carries a higher risk of progression to malignancy.
- The warty basaloid type, also known as bowenoid type, is related to HPV infection and occurs in younger women. Melanoma, second most common histology, often identified in postmenopausal women; often pigmented but can be amelanotic, arising de novo, often found on clitoris or labia minora. Prognosis is poor, 5-year survival <50%.
- Smoking is associated with squamous cell disease of the vulva, possibly from direct irritation of the vulva by the transfer of tars and nicotine on the patient's hands or from systemic absorption of carcinogen.

Genetics
No known genetic pattern

RISK FACTORS
- VIN or cervical intraepithelial neoplasia (CIN)
- Smoking
- Lichen sclerosus (vulvar dystrophy)
- HPV infection, condylomata, or sexually transmitted diseases (STD) in the past
- Low economic status
- Autoimmune processes
- Immunodeficiency syndromes or immunosuppression
- Northern European ancestry
- Risk factors for recurrence: age >50 years, positive excision margins, concurrent VAIN

GENERAL PREVENTION
- HPV vaccination has the potential to decrease vulvar cancer by 60%.
- Abstinence from smoking/smoking cessation counseling

COMMONLY ASSOCIATED CONDITIONS
- Patients with invasive vulvar cancer are often elderly and have associated medical conditions.
- High rate of other gynecologic malignancies

DIAGNOSIS

HISTORY
Complaints of pruritus or raised lesion in the vaginal area, vaginal bleeding, discharge

PHYSICAL EXAM
- In situ disease: a small raised area associated with pruritus, single vulvar plaque, ulcer, or mass on labia majora, perineum, clitoris; most commonly found on labia majora
- Vulvar bleeding, dysuria, enlarged lymph nodes less common symptomatology
- Invasive malignancy: an ulcerated, nonhealing area; as lesions become large, bleeding occurs with associated pain and foul-smelling discharge; enlarged inguinal lymph nodes indicative of advanced disease

DIFFERENTIAL DIAGNOSIS
- Infectious processes can present as ulcerative lesions and include syphilis, lymphogranuloma venereum, and granuloma inguinale.
- Disorder of Bartholin gland, seborrheic keratosis, hidradenomas, lichen sclerosus, epidermal inclusion cysts
- Crohn disease can present as an ulcerative area on the vulva.
- Rarely, lesions can metastasize to the vulva.

DIAGNOSTIC TESTS & INTERPRETATION
Initial Tests (lab, imaging)
- Hypercalcemia can occur when metastatic disease is present.
- Squamous cell antigen can be elevated with invasive disease.

Follow-Up Tests & Special Considerations
- Upon examination, any suspicious lesions should be biopsied.
- Diagnosis based on histologic findings following vulvar biopsy (2)
- The vulva can be washed with 3% acetic acid to highlight areas and visualized with a colposcope, allows for visualization of acetowhite lesions and vascular lesions (2).
- For patients with new onset of pruritus, the area of pruritus should be biopsied.
- Liberal biopsies must be used to diagnose in situ disease prior to invasion and to diagnose early invasive disease.
- The patient should not be treated for presumed benign conditions of the vulva without full exam and biopsy, including Pap smear and colposcopy of cervix, vagina, and vulva.
- When symptoms persist, reexamine and rebiopsy.
- Treatment of benign condyloma of the vulva has not been shown to decrease the eventual incidence of in situ or invasive disease of the vulva.
- CT scan to evaluate pelvic and periaortic lymph node status if tumor >2 cm or if suspicion of metastatic disease (2)[A]

Diagnostic Procedures/Other
Office vulvar biopsy is done to establish the diagnosis.

Test Interpretation
A surgical staging system is used for vulvar cancer (International Federation of Obstetrics and Gynecology Classification).
- Stage I: tumor confined to the vulva
  - Stage IA: lesions ≤2 cm in size, confined to the vulva or perineum and with stromal invasion ≤1 mm, no node metastasis
  - Stage IB: lesions >2 cm in size or with stromal invasion >1 mm, confined to the vulva or perineum, with negative nodes
- Stage II: tumor of any size with extension to adjacent perineal structures (lower 1/3 urethra, lower 1/3 vagina, anus) with negative nodes
- Stage III: tumor of any size with or without extension to adjacent perineal structures (lower 1/3 urethra, lower 1/3 vagina, anus) with positive inguinofemoral lymph nodes
- Stage IIIA
  - With 1 lymph node metastasis (≥5 mm), or
  - 1 to 2 lymph node metastases (<5 mm)

- Stage IIIB
  – With ≥2 lymph node metastases (≥5 mm), or
  – ≥3 lymph node metastases (<5 mm)
- Stage IIIC: with positive nodes with extracapsular spread
- Stage IV: Tumor invades other regional (upper 2/3 urethra, upper 2/3 vagina) or distant structures.
- Stage IVA: Tumor invades any of the following:
  – Upper urethral and/or vaginal mucosa, bladder mucosa, rectal mucosa, or fixed to pelvic bone
  – Fixed or ulcerated inguinofemoral lymph nodes
- Stage IVB: any distant metastasis, including pelvic lymph nodes

TREATMENT

GENERAL MEASURES
- Wide excision can be performed for carcinoma in situ, and any suspicious lesion should be excised for definitive diagnosis.
- Cystoscopy and sigmoidoscopy should be performed if there is a question of invasion into the urethra, bladder, or rectum.

MEDICATION
- Neoadjuvant therapy is being investigated with bleomycin-cisplatin and paclitaxel-based regimens showing high-response rates and tolerable side effects (3)[A].
- As an adjuvant therapy, fluorouracil (Efudex) cream for in situ disease can produce occasional results but is not well tolerated because of irritation of the vulva (4)[A].
- Chemoradiotherapy with cisplatin and 5-fluorouracil (5-FU) has been successful in advanced or recurrent disease, although local morbidity is increased (4)[A].
- Contraindications: elderly patients: If chemotherapeutic agents are used, pay close attention to the patient's performance status and ability to tolerate aggressive chemotherapy.

ISSUES FOR REFERRAL
Patients may need care from a gynecologic oncologist and/or a radiation oncologist.

ADDITIONAL THERAPIES
- Preoperative radiation therapy can be used in those with advanced vulvar cancer (2)[B].
- Adjuvant radiation should be considered with tumor size >4 cm, evidence of lymphovascular invasion, positive surgical margins, or lymph node involvement.
- Preoperative chemoradiation allows for a less radical surgical procedure in patients who are not surgical candidates (4)[A].
- Postoperative radiation decreases recurrence frequency and may improve survival (4)[A].
- Radiation is contraindicated with verrucous carcinoma because it induces anaplastic transformation and increases metastases.

SURGERY/OTHER PROCEDURES
- In situ disease can be treated with wide excision or laser vaporization of the affected area. Laser vaporization is preferable in the younger patient, whereas wide excision is preferable in the elderly patient, in whom the risk of invasive disease is also higher (2)[A].
- If tumor extension within <1 cm from structures that will not be removed, preoperative radiation to prevent inadequate surgical margins prior to excision 1-cm tumor-free margin is required because smaller margin would increase risk of recurrence (4)[A].

- Inguinofemoral lymphadenectomy: removal of superficial inguinal and deep femoral lymph nodes
- Targeted dissection of grossly involved nodes, termed nodal debulking, is being investigated due to high rates of complication after full inguinofemoral lymphadenectomy.
- Stage IA: radical local excision without lymph node dissection
- Stage IB: radical local excision with either sentinel lymph node biopsy (SLNB) or ipsilateral inguinofemoral lymph node dissection because the risk of metastases is >8%
- Stage II: modified radical vulvectomy and/or chemoradiation and groin node dissection
- Stages III and IV: neoadjuvant chemoradiation and less radical surgery
- Pelvic exenteration after radiation provides effective therapy for advanced or recurrent malignancies involving the bladder or rectum.
- More limited surgery has been undertaken for early invasive lesions, especially in young patients, to preserve the clitoris and sexual function.
- SLNB also has been advocated for early invasive lesion (stage IB or higher). It has shown to accurately diagnose groin metastases in women with early vulval cancer and unknown groin node status. This will limit the surgical morbidity associated with inguinofemoral lymphadenectomy in those with early stage disease.
- Radical vulvectomy with bilateral groin node dissection through separate incisions provides better cosmetic results than en bloc technique.
- Unilateral lymphadenectomy should be considered when lesion <2 cm, lateral lesion >2 cm from vulvar midline, or no palpable groin nodes.

ADMISSION, INPATIENT, AND NURSING CONSIDERATIONS
- Typically inpatient for treatment
- Concurrent chemotherapy with radiation is considered standard of care if the patient can tolerate it, based on extrapolation from squamous cell cancers of the cervix and anus (4)[B].
- In advanced malignancy involving the urethra and rectum, concomitant cisplatin/5-FU chemotherapy with radiation produces a significant decrease in size of the primary tumor, usually obviating the need for pelvic exenteration.

ONGOING CARE

FOLLOW-UP RECOMMENDATIONS
Patient Monitoring
- Early stage, treated with surgery alone: clinical exam of the groin nodes and vulvar area every 6 months for 2 years and then annually
- Following chemoradiation, assessment for further treatment within 6 to 12 weeks of therapy completion
- Advance stage, clinical exam of the groin nodes and vulvar area every 3 months for 2 years, then every 6 months for 3 years, and then annually
- Cervical and/or vaginal cytology annually
- Majority of relapses occur within 1st year.

DIET
As tolerated and according to comorbid conditions

PATIENT EDUCATION
- American College of Obstetricians and Gynecologists (ACOG), 409 12th St. SW, Washington, DC 20024-2188; (800) 762-ACOG; http://www.acog.org/
- American Cancer Society: http://www.cancer.org/

PROGNOSIS
The 5-year survival is based on stage:
- Stage I: 78.5%
- Stage II: 58.8%
- Stage III: 43.2%
- Stage IV: 13.0%
- Inguinal and/or femoral node involvement is the most important determinant of survival.

COMPLICATIONS
- The major complications from radical vulvectomy and groin node dissection are wound breakdown, lymphedema, urinary stress incontinence, and psychosexual consequences.
- In the immediate postoperative period, ~50% of patients experience breakdown of the wound. This requires aggressive wound care by visiting nurses as often as twice a day. The wounds usually granulate and heal over a period of 6 to 10 weeks.
- ~15–20% of patients experience some form of mild to moderate lymphedema after the groin node dissection. These patients should be instructed in the use of leg elevation and support hose. <1% of patients experience severe, debilitating lymphedema.

REFERENCES
1. Siegel RL, Miller KD, Jemal A. Cancer statistics, 2015. *CA Cancer J Clin*. 2015;65(1):5–29.
2. de Hullu JA, van der Zee AG. Surgery and radiotherapy in vulvar cancer. *Crit Rev Oncol Hematol*. 2006;60(1):38–58.
3. Niu Y, Yin R, Wang D, et al. Clinical analysis of neoadjuvant chemotherapy in patients with advanced vulvar cancer: a STROBE-compliant article. *Medicine (Baltimore)*. 2018;97(34):e11786.
4. Shylasree TS, Bryant A, Howells RE. Chemoradiation for advanced primary vulval cancer. *Cochrane Database Syst Rev*. 2011;(4):CD003752.

ADDITIONAL READING
- Hinten F, Molijn A, Eckhardt L, et al. Vulvar cancer: two pathways with different localization and prognosis. *Gynecol Oncol*. 2018;149(2):310–317.
- Stecklein SR, Frumovitz M, Klopp AH, et al. Effectiveness of definitive radiotherapy for squamous cell carcinoma of the vulva with gross inguinal lymphadenopathy. *Gynecol Oncol*. 2018;148(3):474–479.

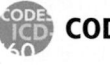 CODES

ICD10
- C51.9 Malignant neoplasm of vulva, unspecified
- D07.1 Carcinoma in situ of vulva
- C51.0 Malignant neoplasm of labium majus

CLINICAL PEARLS
- 55% of vulvar cancers are attributable to oncogenic HPV. VAIN 2/3 and AIN are attributable to HPV. Therefore, HPV vaccination has the potential to decrease vulvar cancer by 1/3.
- Biopsy all suspicious or nonhealing vulvar lesions.

VULVODYNIA

Jessica Johnson, MD, MPH • Amy L. Wiser, MD

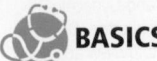 **BASICS**

DESCRIPTION

- Vulvar pain lasting 3 months or more; occurs in the absence of relevant visible findings, relevant lab abnormalities, or a clinically identifiable neurologic disorder
- 2015 ISSVD classification is based on whether vulvar pain is caused by a specific disorder or has no clear identifiable cause (1).
- Specific disorders (differential diagnosis) include infectious, inflammatory, neoplastic, neurologic, trauma, iatrogenic, or hormonal deficiency.
- Descriptors for unclear etiology include localized versus generalized versus mixed, provoked versus spontaneous versus mixed, primary versus secondary onset, and temporal.

EPIDEMIOLOGY

- Most women diagnosed between age 20 and 80 years
- Nearly half of women opt not to seek treatment (2).
- Patients are psychologically comparable with asymptomatic controls and have similar marital satisfaction.

Incidence

- Recent retrospective study estimates annual rate of new onset vulvodynia to be 1.8%.
- Evidence indicates lifetime cumulative incidence approaches 15%, suggesting nearly 14 million U.S. women will experience persistent vulvar discomfort at some point in their lives (3).

Prevalence

- Reports between 8.3% and 16%; non–clinical-based studies approximate a prevalence of 7% with validation by exam (2).
- Studies show Hispanics are 80% more likely to present with vulvar pain compared with Caucasians and African Americans.

ETIOLOGY AND PATHOPHYSIOLOGY

- Vulvodynia is likely to be neuropathically mediated:
  - Hypothesized that neurogenic inflammation sensitizes afferent nerves, and transmits impulses to the CNS, where reinforcing signals sustain pain loop
  - In recent investigations of vulvar biopsy specimens, increased neuronal proliferation and branching in vulvar tissue are evident when compared with tissue of asymptomatic women.
- Pelvic floor pathology also should be considered: In one study, the vulvodynia group showed an increase in pelvic floor hypertonicity at the superficial muscle layer, less vaginal muscle strength with contraction, and decreased relaxation of pelvic floor muscles after contraction (3).
- No cause of vulvodynia has been established. It is most likely a neuropathic pain caused by a combination of the following:
  - Recurrent vulvovaginal candidiasis or other infections
  - Immune-mediated chronic neuroinflammatory process within vulvar tissues
  - Chemical exposure (trichloroacetic acid) or physical trauma
  - Reduced estrogen receptor expression/changes in estrogen concentration
  - CNS etiology, similar to other regional pain syndromes

RISK FACTORS

- Vulvovaginal infections, specifically candidiasis. Unclear if infection, treatment, or underlying hypersensitivity is the cause (2). Multiple infections compound this risk.
- Hormonal factors: Controversial evidence proposes increased risk with use of oral contraceptive pills (OCPs); pain onset or increased severity may be associated with menopause. Symptoms may flare before menses.
- Pelvic floor dysfunction: Increased instability of pelvic floor muscles may perpetuate vulvar tissue inflammation, leading to vascular changes and histamine release.
- Comorbid interstitial cystitis and painful bladder syndrome; potentially related to common embryologic origin of structures
- Abuse: increased risk of vulvodynia if childhood had physical or sexual abuse by a primary family member; causal relationship remains unclear (3).
- Depression and anxiety (2)
- Other neuropathic disorders, including regional pain syndrome

Genetics

Proposed genetic deficiency impairing one's ability to stop the inflammatory response triggered by infection or chemicals; homozygosity of the two alleles of the IL-1 receptor antagonist occurs in 25–50% of vestibulodynia patients, compared with <10% in controls.

GENERAL PREVENTION

- Wear 100% cotton underwear in the daytime and no underwear to sleep.
- Avoid douching and other vulvar irritants such as perfumes, dyes, and detergents.
- Avoid abrasive activities and tight, synthetic clothing.
- Avoid panty liners.
- Clean the vulva with water only and pat area dry after bathing.
- Avoid use of hair dryers in the vulvar area.

COMMONLY ASSOCIATED CONDITIONS

Higher incidence of chronic pain syndromes associated with vulvodynia, including chronic cystitis, irritable bowel syndrome, fibromyalgia, migraines, depression, endometriosis, low back pain. Women with vulvodynia have a higher incidence of depression and anxiety both preceding and resulting from their symptoms (2).

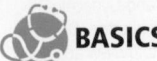 **DIAGNOSIS**

- Vulvodynia is a clinical diagnosis, and it should be suspected in any women with chronic pain at the introitus and vulva.
- Pain should be characterized using a standard measure such as the McGill Pain Questionnaire; duration and nature of the pain should be established. Use physical exam to rule out other causes of vulvovaginal pain. Negative fungal culture, along with relevant history and positive cotton swab test, confirms diagnosis.

HISTORY

Adequate sexual, social, and pain history should be taken to assess degree of symptoms. Visual pain scales and pain diaries may be helpful (4)[B]:

- Onset of vulvodynia often sudden and without precedents
- Pain often described as generalized, unprovoked

- Quality of pain is burning, stinging, irritating, or rawness (2).
- Specifically ask about bowel and bladder habits, history of trauma or abuse, history of infections including herpes and personal hygiene.
- Specific skin complaints may suggest alternate diagnosis; a history of allergies may suggest vulvar dermatitis.
- Assess for precipitants of vulvar pain: tight garments, bicycle riding, tampon use, prolonged sitting, perfumed or deodorant soaps, douching (2).
- Assess for complaints of dyspareunia:
  - Presence of vaginismus (involuntary vaginal muscle spasm), adequate lubrication, anorgasmia, partner problems, abuse
  - Psychosexual morbidity significantly higher in patients with vulvodynia; counseling may complement medical interventions.

PHYSICAL EXAM

- Ask patient to show where pain is localized or most painful.
- Mouth and skin exams to assess for lesions suggestive of lichen planus or lichen sclerosus
- Vaginal exam should be done to exclude other causes of vulvovaginal pain, including external inspection; palpation; and single digit, speculum, and bimanual exams:
  - The vulva may be erythematous, especially at the vestibule. Discomfort with separation of the labia minora is common.
  - Spontaneous or elicited pain at the lower 1/2 of anterior vaginal wall suggests bladder etiology.
- Bulbocavernosus and anal wink reflexes should be checked to assess for peripheral neuropathy.

DIFFERENTIAL DIAGNOSIS

- Infections: candidiasis, herpes, human papillomavirus (HPV), bacterial vaginosis, trichomoniasis, dermatophytes
- Inflammation: lichen planus, immunobullous disorder, allergic vulvitis, lichen sclerosus, atrophic vaginitis
- Neoplasia: Paget disease, vulvar or vaginal intraepithelial neoplasia, squamous cell carcinoma
- Neurologic/muscular: herpes neuralgia, spinal nerve compression, vaginismus

DIAGNOSTIC TESTS & INTERPRETATION

- Tampon test: reproduces pain in real-life settings
- Cotton swab or Q-tip test: vulva tested for localized areas of pain, beginning at thighs and continuing medially toward vestibule, using the soft end and broken sharp end of the cotton swab. Five distinct positions (2, 4, 6, 8, and 10 o'clock) surveyed using light palpation. Pain rated on a scale from 0 (none) to 10 (most severe); posterior introitus and posterior hymenal remnants most common sites of increased sensitivity
- Test for concurrent vaginismus: Apply pressure with a gloved finger to levator ani and obturator internus muscles to assess for tenderness, pain, or contracture.

Initial Tests (lab, imaging)

- Vaginal pH, wet mount, and yeast culture are recommended to rule out vaginitis.
- Gonorrhea and chlamydia testing done at physician's discretion
- HPV screening is unnecessary; association is controversial between HPV and vulvodynia.

Follow-Up Tests & Special Considerations

- Varicella-zoster and herpes simplex virus should be considered if ulcers or vesicular eruptions are present.
- Consider biopsy if concerned for neoplasm or dermatophyte infection or if the patient is resistant to treatment.

Diagnostic Procedures/Other

Colposcopy can be helpful if epidermal abnormalities are present. This should be done with caution because acetic acid worsens vulvar pain.

Test Interpretation

No specific histologic features are associated with vulvodynia, although reactive squamous atypia has been observed. Biopsies are unnecessary for diagnosis. Presence of rash/altered mucosa is not consistent with vulvodynia; this requires further evaluation (4)[C].

 TREATMENT

A trial of several medications for at least 3 months is usually needed.

GENERAL MEASURES

Combining treatments should be encouraged when treating women with vulvodynia (4)[C]: Various reports on use of a combination of medical treatments, psychotherapy, and dietary intervention reveal women on these combinations do significantly better compared with those who receive medication only.

MEDICATION

- Oral therapies
  - Tricyclic antidepressants (TCAs): first-line treatment for unprovoked vulvodynia (4)[B]; do not stop use abruptly; contraindicated in patients with cardiac abnormalities and those taking MAOIs; fatigue, constipation, sweating, palpitations, and weight gain are most common side effects.
    - Amitriptyline, nortriptyline: most widely studied; start at 10 mg daily; dose titrated to pain control. Average effective dose is 60 mg daily. In one study, a 47% complete response rate was recorded (5)[B]. Nortriptyline may be preferred due to less anticholinergic adverse effects.
  - Anticonvulsant therapies:
    - Gabapentin: started at 300 mg daily at HS and increased by 300 mg every 3 days. Maximum recommended dose is 3,600 mg daily divided into 3 doses.
    - Topiramate and lamotrigine have been recommended if other therapies are not effective.
  - SSNRIs: not commonly used; however, have been helpful in those who cannot tolerate TCAs
    - Venlafaxine or duloxetine have also been used; evidence is limited.
  - Opioids/NSAIDs: not consistently helpful in relieving vulvar pain; not appropriate for maintenance
- Topical therapies
  - A trial of local anesthetics may be recommended for all patients who present with vulvodynia. Use judiciously to avoid increased irritation (4)[C].
  - Lidocaine 5% ointment: for provoked vestibulodynia; application advised 15 to 20 minutes prior to intercourse. Penile numbness and possible toxicity with ingestion can occur.
    - In one study, lidocaine 5% ointment was left in vestibule overnight (average of 8 hours) for a period of 6 to 8 weeks; at follow-up, up to 76% of women reported no discomfort with intercourse (3)[C].

- Cromolyn 4% cream: decreases mast cell degranulation in vulvar tissue; recommended application TID (2)[C]
  - Capsaicin 0.025%: decreases in discomfort and increases in frequency of intercourse with 20-minute daily application (3)[B]
  - Topical amitriptyline 2% combined with baclofen 2% is helpful in patients with comorbid vaginismus.
  - Topical corticosteroids and testosterone creams have not been shown to alleviate symptoms of vulvodynia.
  - Gabapentin 3–6% ointment (must be compounded)
  - Topical nitroglycerin may be helpful but may cause headaches.
  - Topical estrogen
- Injectable therapies
  - Triamcinolone acetonide: no >40 mg should be injected monthly; is best when combined with 0.25–0.50% bupivacaine
  - Submucosal methylprednisone and lidocaine: reports of up to 68% response rate with weekly injections (4)[B]
  - Interferon-α: useful in treatment of vestibulodynia. Side effects (myalgias, fever, malaise) limit its use.
  - Botulinum toxin A injectable is being studied.

ISSUES FOR REFERRAL

A team approach is recommended for most effective management. Referral to psychosexual medicine, psychology, partner therapy, and pain management teams should be strongly considered (4)[B].

ADDITIONAL THERAPIES

- Cognitive-behavioral therapy (CBT): One randomized trial revealed that CBT is associated with a 30% decrease in vulvar discomfort with sexual intercourse. CBT is the recommended treatment for patients who present with dyspareunia as a main complaint (6)[B].
- Biofeedback/physical therapy: useful with concomitant vaginismus. Treats both generalized and localized vulvar pain; treatment value for unprovoked pain remains unclear. Most studies report an average of 12- to 16-week treatment time.
- Vaginal dilators
- Surface electromyography (sEMG): efficacious for pelvic floor rehabilitation. Patients are more likely to experience pain-free sexual intercourse after sEMG; significant reductions seen on pain measures at long-term follow-up

COMPLEMENTARY & ALTERNATIVE MEDICINE

Acupuncture: Small studies of women with unprovoked vulvodynia who did not respond to conventional treatment reported significant decreases in pain severity with acupuncture; treatment value with provoked pain is unknown (4)[C].

SURGERY/OTHER PROCEDURES

- Surgery may be considered for patients with localized symptoms who have failed to respond to other measures; not recommended for generalized vulvodynia (4)[B]
- 60–80% of women who undergo surgery report a significant reduction in pain symptoms; however, when surveyed, patients prefer behavioral therapies than surgical intervention.
- All patients who are considering surgical intervention should be tested and treated for vaginismus. Vestibulectomy is less successful in this subgroup.

- Surgical approaches
  - Local excision: precise localization of painful areas; tissue closed in elliptical fashion
  - Total vestibulectomy: Tissue is removed from Skene ducts to perineum. The vagina is then brought down to cover defect.
  - Perineoplasty: vestibulectomy plus removal of perineal tissue; incision usually terminated above the anal orifice; reserved for severe cases (2)[B]

 ONGOING CARE

PATIENT EDUCATION

Patients should be reassured that this condition is neither infectious, nor does it predispose to cancer (4)[C]. Counsel that condition is manageable, but likely not curable, and may require multiple therapeutic trials before remission is achieved. Emphasize self-hygiene. Encourage treatment with home remedies, including ice packs, sitz baths with baking soda, olive oil, and barrier cream to preserve moisture after bathing.

PROGNOSIS

Traditionally viewed as a chronic pain disorder, new evidence of remission has been documented; recent 2-year follow-up study revealed 1 in 10 vulvodynia patients reported remission regardless of treatment.

REFERENCES

1. Bornstein J, Goldstein AT, Stockdale CK, et al. 2015 ISSVD, ISSWSH and IPPS consensus terminology and classification of persistent vulvar pain and vulvodynia. *Obstet Gynecol*. 2016;127(4):745–751.
2. Shah M, Hoffstetter S. Vulvodynia. *Obstet Gynecol Clin N Am*. 2014;41(3):453–464.
3. Boardman LA, Stockdale CK. Sexual pain. *Clin Obstet Gynecol*. 2009;52(4):682–690.
4. Nunns D, Mandal D, Byrne M, et al; for British Society for the Study of Vulval Disease Guideline Group. Guidelines for the management of vulvodynia. *Br J Dermatol*. 2010;162(6):1180–1185.
5. Stockdale CK, Lawson HW. 2013 vulvodynia guideline update. *J Low Genit Tract Dis*. 2014;18(2):93–100.
6. De Andres J, Sanchis-Lopez N, Asensio-Samper JM, et al. Vulvodynia: an evidence-based literature review and proposed treatment algorithm. *Pain Pract*. 2016;16(2):204–236.

 CODES

ICD10

- N94.819 Vulvodynia, unspecified
- N94.818 Other vulvodynia
- N94.810 Vulvar vestibulitis

CLINICAL PEARLS

- Vulvodynia is a clinical diagnosis; it should be suspected in any woman with chronic pain at the introitus and vulva.
- A decrease in pain may take weeks to months and may not be complete.
- No single treatment is proven in all women; improvement over time is common even without treatment.

V

VULVOVAGINITIS, ESTROGEN DEFICIENT

Karla M. Alba, MD • Michelle Rodriguez, MD • Mark T. Nadeau, MD, MBA

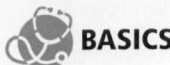 **BASICS**

DESCRIPTION

- Estrogen-deficient vulvovaginitis is a hypoestrogenic state with external genital, urologic, and sexual sequelae.
- Estrogen deficiency affects all tissues in the female body; however, the genital tissues are especially hormone responsive and are most affected.
- Decreased estrogen leads to decreased blood flow to vaginal tissues and thinning of vaginal tissues, dryness, and atrophy. Patients with estrogen-deficient vulvovaginitis may present with urinary incontinence, vaginal burning and itching, dyspareunia, increased urinary frequency, recurrent UTIs, or various other symptoms.
- This condition is also referred to as genitourinary syndrome of menopause when associated with the postmenopausal state, although this condition may occur in women of all ages.
- System(s) affected: reproductive

EPIDEMIOLOGY

Incidence
Predominant age: postmenopausal females. The average age of menopause in the United States is 51.3 years but ranges from 45 to 55 years old.

Prevalence
- Approximately 40–54% of postmenopausal women are affected.
- Approximately 15% of premenopausal women are also affected.
- This condition is likely underdiagnosed because patients may be reluctant to report symptoms because of embarrassment or the misconception that symptoms should be accepted as a natural part of aging (1).

ETIOLOGY AND PATHOPHYSIOLOGY

- Estrogen is vasoactive, increasing blood flow to target tissues, lubrication, and elasticity.
- Decreased estrogen levels in the vagina and vulva result in decreased blood flow and decreased lubrication and elasticity of vaginal and vulvar tissues as well as thinning of these tissues.
- Decreased cellular maturation results in decreased glycogen stores, which affects the normal vaginal flora and consequently the pH.
- The resulting increased pH impairs the viability of the normal flora, permitting the proliferation of fecal and other flora, resulting in UTIs and vaginal infections (1)[C].
- Estrogen deficiency is caused by the following:
  – Menopause (surgical or natural)
  – Premature ovarian failure (chemotherapy, radiation, autoimmune, anorexia, genetic)
  – Postpartum estrogen deficiency in lactating women
  – Medications that alter hormonal concentration, such as gonadotropin-releasing hormone agonists, tamoxifen, danazol, medroxyprogesterone, and aromatase inhibitors
  – Elevated prolactin from hypothalamic–pituitary disorders

Genetics
No known pattern

RISK FACTORS
- Estrogen-deficient states, including lactation
- Smoking
- Alcohol abuse
- Sexual abstinence or decreased frequency of coital activity
- Lack of exercise
- Absence of vaginal childbirth
- Chemotherapy
- Radiation therapy

COMMONLY ASSOCIATED CONDITIONS
- Urge and stress urinary incontinence
- Pelvic organ prolapse
- Frequent UTIs
- Bacterial or fungal vulvovaginitis
- Vaginal stenosis
- Loss of libido
- Dyspareunia

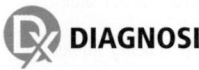 **DIAGNOSIS**

HISTORY
- All female patients should be asked about symptoms because many women are embarrassed to discuss these issues with their health care providers (1).
  – Vaginal dryness
  – Dyspareunia
  – Pruritus
  – Burning
  – Pressure
  – Tenderness
  – Malodorous discharge
  – Urinary symptoms: dysuria, hematuria, frequency, infections, stress, and urge urinary incontinence
- Ask about exposure to radiation therapy and medications.
- Ask about self-treatment and products used.
- Determine exposure to irritants (e.g., soaps, feminine sprays, lotions, lubricants, constant pad use).

PHYSICAL EXAM
Evidence for the diagnosis includes the following:
- Loss of pubic hair
- Decreased vulvar and vaginal fullness
- Fusion of labia minora
- Vulvar erythema or ecchymosis
- Decreased vulvar subcuticular fat and moisture
- Pale-appearing, shiny, smooth vaginal and urethral epithelium
- Vaginal shortening, intolerance to speculum exams
- Loss of vaginal rugation
- Pelvic organ prolapse
- Urethral atrophy
- Atrophy of Bartholin glands
- Cervical atrophy and stenosis of os

DIFFERENTIAL DIAGNOSIS
- Malignancy
- Sexual trauma
- Infection secondary to foreign bodies (e.g., piercings)
- Dermatologic conditions of vulva and vagina:
  – Dermatitis
  – Lichen sclerosis
  – Lichen planus
- Bacterial or fungal vulvovaginitis

DIAGNOSTIC TESTS & INTERPRETATION
Because vulvovaginitis is a clinical diagnosis, labs are not always necessary, but if a dermatologic or oncologic condition is suspected, biopsy is recommended (2)[C].

Initial Tests (lab, imaging)
Lab tests are generally unnecessary to make the diagnosis. However, the following labs and imaging may be obtained as corroborative of clinical impression:
- Follicle-stimulating hormone (FSH) and estrogen levels. FSH rises and estrogen drops with menopause.
- Evaluate for infections via wet preparation and vaginal pH (usually >5).
- Urinalysis if suspected concomitant UTI
- Cytology for maturation index: Higher proportion of parabasal cells and lower proportion of intermediate and superficial cells indicate decreased maturation index.
- Transvaginal ultrasound: Endometrial stripe <5 mm indicates loss of estrogen stimulation.

Follow-Up Tests & Special Considerations
Drugs that may alter lab results:
- Estrogen therapy will alter the maturation index but may improve symptoms.
- Digoxin has estrogen-like properties.
- Tamoxifen may produce menopausal-type symptoms but also may act on genital tissues as a weak estrogen agonist.
- Progestins, danazol, and gonadotropin-releasing hormone agonists may produce a reversible pseudomenopausal state.

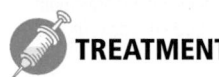 **TREATMENT**

GENERAL MEASURES
- Wear loose-fitting, undyed cotton underwear.
- Avoid prolonged pad use, especially scented pads.
- Avoid feminine deodorant sprays and douching.
- Symptomatic relief, if needed (e.g., cool baths or compresses)
- Increase coital activity.
- Smoking cessation

MEDICATION

- Nonhormonal vaginal moisturizers and lubricants are generally regarded as first-line therapy for mildly symptomatic estrogen-deficient vulvovaginitis (1)[C], although one recent study has shown that neither nonhormonal vaginal moisturizers nor lubricants and vaginal estrogen provided greater benefit than placebo gel or tablet (3)[A].
  - Estrogen therapy is preferred for moderate to severe symptoms: Local hormonal therapy (vaginal estrogen) is the first-line hormonal treatment and can reverse atrophic changes and alleviate symptoms (1)[C].
    - Vaginal cream: Insert via applicator 2 to 4 g daily for 1 to 2 weeks, then 1 to 2 g daily for 1 to 2 weeks and then 1 g 1 to 3 times a week.
    - Vaginal estradiol 10-μg tablet: Insert via preloaded applicator each night for 14 days and then twice weekly.
    - Estradiol-containing vaginal ring 2 mg: Insert into vagina and replace every 3 months.
  - Systemic hormonal therapy is typically reserved for patients wanting treatment for vasomotor symptoms associated with estrogen deficiency in addition to atrophic vulvovaginitis.
  - Transdermal preparations may be safer from a cardiovascular standpoint than oral preparations. Systemic estrogen therapy should be used in the lowest possible dose for the shortest duration of time (4)[B].
  - Long-term therapy may be necessary due to the chronic nature of estrogen-deficient vulvovaginitis (5)[A].
  - Contraindications:
    - Breast or estrogen-dependent cancers
    - Undiagnosed vaginal bleeding
    - Thromboembolic disorders
    - Endometrial hyperplasia or cancer
    - Hypertension
    - Hyperlipidemia
    - Liver disease
    - History of stroke
    - Coronary heart disease
    - Smoking in ages >35 years
    - Migraines with neurologic symptoms
    - Acute cholecystitis/cholangitis
    - Pregnancy
- Nonestrogen therapy: ospemifene (Osphena) 60-mg tablet daily; recommended for women with estrogen-deficient vulvovaginitis not responsive to nonpharmacologic therapies and who cannot or prefer not to use a vaginal estrogen (1)[C],(6)[B]
  - Contraindications:
    - Breast or estrogen-dependent carcinoma
    - Undiagnosed vaginal bleeding
    - Thromboembolic disorders
    - Thrombophlebitis
    - Hepatic impairment
- Precautions: Any abnormal vaginal bleeding must be evaluated. Monitor for DVT and stroke.

ISSUES FOR REFERRAL

- Refer to urogynecologist for evaluation if symptomatic due to pelvic organ prolapse and/or refractory stress and urge urinary incontinence.
- Recurrent UTIs should be further evaluated and may require a referral to urogynecology and/or urology.

ADDITIONAL THERAPIES

- Laser therapy with fractional CO_2 has demonstrated promise in initial studies; however, randomized controlled trials with long-term follow-up are still needed (1)[C].
- Lasofoxifene (Fablyn, Oporia) and oxytocin vaginal gel (Vagitocin) are under development but not yet approved (1)[C].

ADMISSION, INPATIENT, AND NURSING CONSIDERATIONS

Management of this condition occurs primarily in the outpatient setting.

 ONGOING CARE

FOLLOW-UP RECOMMENDATIONS

Follow up as needed to determine response to treatment and for adjustment of treatment regimen.

Patient Monitoring

Instruct the patient that symptoms should improve within 30 to 60 days. If they do not, reevaluate and reexamine for other causes.

DIET

Increased consumption of cranberry juice or extract to prevent recurrent UTIs has been recommended but not well supported by evidence.

PATIENT EDUCATION

- American College of Obstetricians and Gynecologists (ACOG), 409 12th St., SW, Washington, DC 20024-2188; 800-762-ACOG: http://www.acog.org/
- Lactating postpartum women with high levels of prolactin are in a hypoestrogenic state. These women should be instructed to use lubrication for symptoms of dyspareunia and reassured that the symptoms will resolve when they are no longer breastfeeding.

PROGNOSIS

The prognosis is good. Most symptoms will be alleviated with vaginal estrogen replacement therapy.

COMPLICATIONS

- Recurrent UTIs may occur in women with vaginal atrophy.
- Vaginal atrophy predisposes patients to vaginal infections.

REFERENCES

1. Gandhi J, Chen A, Dagur G, et al. Genitourinary syndrome of menopause: an overview of clinical manifestations, pathophysiology, etiology, evaluation, and management. *Am J Obstet Gynecol.* 2016;215(6):704–711.
2. Johnston SL, Farrell SA, Bouchard C, et al; for SOGC Joint Committee-Clinical Practice Gynaecology and Urogynaecology. The detection and management of vaginal atrophy. *J Obstet Gynaecol Can.* 2004;26(5):503–515.
3. Mitchell CM, Reed SD, Diem S, et al. Efficacy of vaginal estradiol or vaginal moisturizer vs placebo for treating postmenopausal vulvovaginal symptoms: a randomized clinical trial. *JAMA Intern Med.* 2018;178(5):681–690.
4. Ibe C, Simon JA. Vulvovaginal atrophy: current and future therapies (CME). *J Sex Med.* 2010;7(3):1042–1051.
5. Suckling J, Lethaby A, Kennedy R. Local oestrogen for vaginal atrophy in postmenopausal women. *Cochrane Database Syst Rev.* 2006;(4):CD001500.
6. Constantine G, Graham S, Portman DJ, et al. Female sexual function improved with ospemifene in postmenopausal women with vulvar and vaginal atrophy: results of a randomized, placebo-controlled trial. *Climacteric.* 2015;18(2):226–232.

ADDITIONAL READING

- Pitsouni E, Grigoriadis T, Falagas M, et al. Laser therapy for the genitourinary syndrome of menopause. A systematic review and meta-analysis. *Maturitas.* 2017;103:78–88.
- Ruan X, Mueck A. Impact of smoking on estrogenic efficacy. *Climacteric.* 2015;18(1):38–46.

 CODES

ICD10
- N95.2 Postmenopausal atrophic vaginitis
- E28.39 Other primary ovarian failure

CLINICAL PEARLS

- Estrogen-deficient vulvovaginitis affects virtually all postmenopausal women to some degree as well as some premenopausal women.
- This disorder is associated with genital, urologic, and sexual symptoms including vaginal itching, vaginal dryness, urinary incontinence, increased urinary frequency, recurrent UTIs, and dyspareunia.
- Estrogen-deficient vulvovaginitis is a clinical diagnosis; lab tests are generally unnecessary.
- Vaginal moisturizers and lubricants are first-line therapy for mild symptoms, and vaginal estrogen preparations, rather than systemic preparations, are the preferred hormonal therapy for women with moderate to severe symptoms of estrogen-deficient vulvovaginitis.

V

VULVOVAGINITIS, PREPUBESCENT

Sarah Parrott, DO

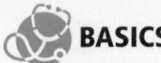

BASICS

DESCRIPTION
- Vulvitis is inflammation of the external genitals.
- Vaginitis, often associated with vaginal discharge, is inflammation involving the vaginal mucosa.
- In premenarchal girls, vulvitis is usually primary with secondary extension into the vagina.
- System(s) affected: reproductive, skin/exocrine
- Synonym(s): vaginitis; vulvitis

EPIDEMIOLOGY
Incidence
Unknown

Prevalence
Most common gynecologic problem in prepubertal girls

ETIOLOGY AND PATHOPHYSIOLOGY
- In the prepubertal child, the levels of estrogen are low.
- Due to the low levels of estrogen, the vaginal epithelium is thin, immature, and fragile.
- Absence of pubic hair and a well-developed labia, as well as close proximity of the anus and vagina, makes contamination more likely.
- The prepubertal child also has an absence of lactobacilli, creating a neutral to alkaline vaginal pH.
- Neutral pH, atrophic mucosa, and moist environment of the vagina increase the risk of infection.
- Most cases of pediatric vulvovaginitis are nonspecific inflammation.
- Specific infections that occur are typically respiratory, enteric, or sexually transmitted.
- Nonspecific vulvovaginitis
- Poor perineal hygiene (wiping back to front) (1)
- Nonspecific chemical irritants (bubble baths, scented soaps, shampoos)
- Tight-fitting clothing
- Etiology
  - Bacterial: The most common bacteria are introduced from respiratory and GI tracts.
    - The most common respiratory pathogen is *Streptococcus pyogenes* (2)[B]. Vulvitis may occur in the absence of respiratory symptoms.
    - Urinary tract infections are common in children with vulvovaginitis (3)[B].
    - *Escherichia coli* is the most common fecal pathogen.
    - *Shigella* vaginitis is associated with mucopurulent bloody discharge and likewise, is not always accompanied by a history of diarrhea.

- *Enterobius vermicularis* (pinworms)
  - Very common in young children and certain populations
  - Should be considered in children with vaginal itching and irritation
  - Most common symptom is nocturnal perineal itching.
  - Foreign body
    - Presents with foul-smelling, bloody, or brown discharge from the vagina
    - Should be considered with recurrent vulvovaginitis where other causes have been eliminated
  - Other
    - With chronic vulvovaginitis, anatomic abnormalities or systemic disease should be considered:
      - Anatomic abnormalities include double vagina with fistula, ectopic ureter, and urethral prolapse.
  - Systemic disease (inflammatory diseases)
  - Other conditions, such as lichen sclerosus, vitiligo, psoriasis, and atopic dermatitis, should be considered.

Genetics
Understudied

RISK FACTORS
- Prepubertal girls are particularly susceptible due to behavioral and anatomic reasons:
  - Inadequate hand washing or perineal cleansing after urination and defecation
  - Tight-fitting clothing
  - Proximity of the vagina to the anus, lack of protective hair, and labial fat pads
  - Trauma
- Obese girls are also susceptible to nonspecific vulvovaginitis (4)[A].

GENERAL PREVENTION
- Good perineal hygiene (including wiping from front to back)
- Urination with legs spread apart and labia separated
- Avoidance of tight-fitting clothing and nonabsorbent underwear
- Avoidance of irritants such as harsh/perfumed soaps and bubble baths

ALERT
Cultures of sexually transmitted organisms in prepubertal children warrant investigations of sexual abuse.

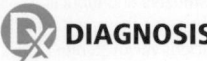

DIAGNOSIS

HISTORY
Obtain careful history addressing any recent respiratory or enteric infections in the patient or a close family member. Symptoms may include:
- Vaginal discharge (44.4%)
- Vaginal itching (24.4%)
- Vulvar erythema (37.8%)
- Dysuria (33.3%)
- Perineal pain/burning during urination (6.3%)
- Enuresis (13.3%)
- Encopresis (2.1%)
- Anal itching (35.6%)

PHYSICAL EXAM
- Look for evidence of chronic illness or dermatologic disease.
- Look for trauma or other signs that may correlate with abuse.
- Inspect the genital area in the supine position:
  - Excoriation of the genital area
  - Inflammation (erythema, swelling) of the introitus
  - Inspect the vagina and cervix in the knee–chest position or frog leg position.
  - Perform rectal exam if vaginal bleeding or abdominal pain.

DIFFERENTIAL DIAGNOSIS
- Contact dermatitis
- Eczema
- Psoriasis
- Lichen sclerosus

DIAGNOSTIC TESTS & INTERPRETATION
Initial Tests (lab, imaging)
- Culture for bacteria, fungi (yeast), or viruses (herpes)
- Urinalysis, urine culture, and urine for STI (via nucleic acid amplification test)—vulvovaginitis may cause UTIs by altering the perineal biome, increasing colonization of uropathogens (2)
- Tape exam for pinworms
- Potassium hydroxide and saline smears of vaginal discharge, if present
- If an anatomic abnormality is suspected, imaging may be necessary to confirm.
- Consider consultation with a pediatric or adult gynecologist to determine the most appropriate imaging study.

Follow-Up Tests & Special Considerations
Exploration of the vagina for a foreign body may be necessary in cases of persistent, recurrent vulvitis.

Diagnostic Procedures/Other

If blood or foul-smelling discharge is present, visualization is mandatory:

- Place the child in the knee–chest position for best results. Hold the buttocks apart and slightly upward.
- Visualization of the vagina may be necessary by using a nasal speculum or infant laryngoscope.
- If available, consider referral to a provider with specific training/experience in this specialized exam.

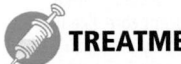 **TREATMENT**

- The definitive diagnosis of bacterial vulvitis requires a culture of vulva and vaginal secretions.
- The typical colony count and bacterial mix are unknown in prepubescent girls. Antibiotic use should be directed against the species with the highest colony count.
- General hygiene should always be recommended, particularly in cases of a retained foreign body (e.g., toilet paper).
- When no cause is identified, treatment should focus on hygiene as well as minimizing soap exposure and tight-fitting clothes (2).

GENERAL MEASURES

- Appropriate health care: outpatient (except where systemic illness requires hospital care)
- Soak the vulva/perineum in a small amount of clear, warm water for 15 minutes BID.
- If smegma is present in the labial folds, clean the area gently with a mild soap.

MEDICATION

First Line

- To break the itching–scratching–infection cycle, use a low-dose topical hydrocortisone cream for a limited time.
- Estrogen deficiency with labial adhesion/agglutination: estrogen cream 0.625 mg to fused area nightly for 2 weeks
- Emollients or protective creams may offer symptomatic relief.
- Antibiotic use should be restricted to cases of bacterial infection only (5)[A].
- Specific organisms on culture
  - Group A *Streptococcus, Streptococcus pneumoniae*: penicillin V (Pen Vee K) 250 mg PO BID–TID for 10 days
  - *Haemophilus influenzae*: amoxicillin, 20 to 40 mg/kg/day PO divided TID for 7 days
  - *Staphylococcus aureus*: cephalexin, 25 to 50 mg/kg/day PO divided QID for 7 to 10 days *or* dicloxacillin, 25 mg/kg/day divided QID for 7 to 10 days *or* amoxicillin-clavulanate, 20 to 40 mg/kg/day PO divided BID for 7 to 10 days

- *S. pyogenes*: amoxicillin, 50 mg/kg/day PO divided into 3 doses/day for 10 days
- *Candida* sp.: topical nystatin (Mycostatin), miconazole, clotrimazole, or terconazole
- *Shigella*: trimethoprim/sulfamethoxazole or ampicillin for 5 days
- Pinworms: mebendazole, 100 mg PO, repeated in 2 weeks
- *Chlamydia trachomatis*: ≤45 kg: erythromycin, 50 mg/kg/day QID for 14 days; ≥45 kg and <8 years old: azithromycin, 1 g PO single dose; ≥45 kg and ≥8 years old: azithromycin, 1 g PO single dose or doxycycline 100 mg BID for 7 days
- *Neisseria gonorrhoeae*: ≤45 kg: ceftriaxone, 125 mg IM plus medication for chlamydia; >45 kg: ceftriaxone, 250 mg IM × 1 plus medication for chlamydia
- *Trichomonas*: metronidazole, 15 mg/kg/day PO divided TID (max 250 mg TID) for 7 days
- Contraindications: allergy to proposed treatment
- Precautions: Avoid potential allergens and topical sensitizers if possible.

ISSUES FOR REFERRAL

- Suspected sexual abuse
- Suspected anatomic abnormality (except minor labial agglutination)
- Persistent, severe, or recurrent infections

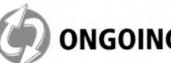 **ONGOING CARE**

FOLLOW-UP RECOMMENDATIONS

Patient Monitoring

Monitor for fever, pruritus, and vaginal discharge.

DIET

- Healthy balanced diet, high in fiber to prevent constipation
- Adequate fluid intake

PATIENT EDUCATION

Hygiene

- Wipe front to back after elimination.
- Avoid bubble baths and other irritating products.
- Clean daily with mild soap and water and dry gently with soft towel or cool hair dryer.
- Apply bland ointments for skin protection, if necessary.

PROGNOSIS

Excellent

COMPLICATIONS

- If an STI is identified and not treated effectively, the patient is at risk for pelvic inflammatory disease (PID).
- Vaginismus

REFERENCES

1. Cemek F, Odabaş D, Şenel Ü, et al. Personal hygiene and vulvovaginitis in prepubertal children. *J Pediatr Adolesc Gynecol*. 2016;29(3):223–227.
2. Gorbachinsky I, Sherertz R, Russell G, et al. Altered perineal microbiome is associated with vulvovaginitis and urinary tract infection in preadolescent girls. *Ther Adv Urol*. 2014;6(6):224–229.
3. Stricker T, Navratil F, Sennhauser FH. Vulvovaginitis in prepubertal girls. *Arch Dis Child*. 2003;88(4):324–326.
4. Van Eyk N, Allen L, Giesbrecht E, et al. Pediatric vulvovaginal disorders: a diagnostic approach and review of the literature. *J Obstet Gynaecol Can*. 2009;31(9):850–862.
5. Dei M, Di Maggio F, Di Paolo G, et al. Vulvovaginitis in childhood. *Best Pract Res Clin Obstet Gynaecol*. 2010;24(2):129–137.

ADDITIONAL READING

- Delago C, Finkel MA, Deblinger E. Urogenital symptoms in premenarchal girls: parents' and girls' perceptions and associations with irritants. *J Pediatr Adolesc Gynecol*. 2012;25(1):67–73.
- Joishy M, Ashtekar CS, Jain A, et al. Do we need to treat vulvovaginitis in prepubertal girls? *BMJ*. 2005;330(7484):186–188.
- Velander MH, Mikkelsen DB, Bygum A. Labial agglutination in a prepubertal girl: effect of topical oestrogen. *Acta Derm Venereol*. 2009;89(2):198–199.

 CODES

ICD10

- N76.0 Acute vaginitis
- N77.1 Vaginitis, vulvitis and vulvovaginitis in dis classd elswhr

CLINICAL PEARLS

- Vulvovaginitis is the most common gynecologic problem in prepubescent girls.
- The hypoestrogenic state and prepubescent anatomy may increase susceptibility to vulvar and vaginal infection.
- Treatment is typically supportive (avoid scratching, warm soaks) but may require antibiotics if a bacterial infection is suspected.
- Isolating an infection with known sexual transmission should prompt further investigation.
- Recurrent or persistent vulvitis, especially with foul-smelling discharge, should prompt a skilled exam of the vagina for a retained foreign body (most common toilet paper).
- Good perineal hygiene will limit this condition.

V

WARTS

Kyle B. Stephens, DO, MPH

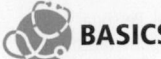 **BASICS**

- Warts (verrucae) are benign growths that are confined to the epidermis. All warts are caused by the human papillomavirus (HPV). Warts can appear on any area of the skin or mucous membranes. Common warts are predominantly seen in children and young adults.
- Clinically, warts are described as follows:
  - Common warts (verrucae vulgaris)
  - Plantar warts (verrucae plantaris)
  - Flat warts (verrucae plana)
  - Genital warts (condyloma acuminatum)
  - Epidermodysplasia verruciformis is a rare, lifelong hereditary disorder characterized by chronic infection with HPV.
- System(s) affected: skin/exocrine

DESCRIPTION

- Common warts are most often found at sites subject to frequent trauma, such as the hands and feet. Because warts often vary widely in shape, size, and appearance, the various descriptive names for them generally reflect their clinical appearance, location, or both.
- For example: Filiform (fingerlike) warts are thread-like, planar warts are flat, and plantar warts are located on the plantar surfaces (soles) of the feet.
- Genital warts, or condyloma acuminata, may be large and cauliflower-like, or they may consist of small papules.
- Warts on mucous membranes (mucosal papillomas), such as those in the mouth or vagina, tend to be white in color due to moisture retention.

EPIDEMIOLOGY

Incidence
- Predominant age: young adults and children
- No sex predominance: female = male

Prevalence
- ~7–10% of the U.S. population
- Common warts appear 2 times as frequently in whites compared with blacks or Asians.

ETIOLOGY AND PATHOPHYSIOLOGY

- HPV is a double-stranded, circular, supercoiled DNA virus.
- The virus infects epidermal keratinocytes, stimulating cell proliferation.
- Various strains of DNA HPV: To date, >150 different subtypes have been identified.
- Common warts: HPV types 2 and 4 (most common), followed by types 1, 3, 27, 29, and 57
- Palmoplantar warts: HPV type 1 (most common), followed by types 2, 3, 4, 27, 29, and 57
- Flat warts: HPV types 3, 10, and 28
- Butcher warts: HPV type 7
- The virus is passed primarily through skin-to-skin contact or from the recently shed virus kept intact in a moist, warm environment.

RISK FACTORS

- HIV/AIDS and other immunosuppressive diseases (e.g., lymphomas)
- Immunosuppressive drugs that decrease cell-mediated immunity (e.g., prednisone, cyclosporine, and chemotherapeutic agents)
- Pregnancy

- Handling raw meat, fish, or other types of animal matter in one's occupation (e.g., butchers)
- Previous wart infection

GENERAL PREVENTION
There is no known way to prevent warts.

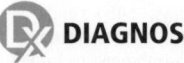 **DIAGNOSIS**

- Most often made on clinical appearance
- Skin biopsy, if necessary

PHYSICAL EXAM

- Distribution of warts is generally asymmetric, and lesions are often clustered or may appear in a linear configuration due to scratching (autoinoculation).
- Common wart: rough-surfaced, hyperkeratotic, papillomatous, raised, skin-colored to tan papules, 5 to 10 mm in diameter; several may coalesce into a larger cluster (mosaic wart); most frequently seen on hands, knees, and elbows; usually asymptomatic but may cause cosmetic disfigurement or tenderness
- Filiform warts: These are long, slender, delicate, fingerlike growths, usually seen on the face around the lips, eyelids, or nares.
- Plantar warts often have a rough surface and appear on the plantar surface of the feet in children and young adults.
  - Can be tender and painful; extensive involvement on the sole of the foot may impair ambulation, particularly when present on a weight-bearing surface.
  - Most often seen on the metatarsal area, heels, and toes in an asymmetric distribution (pressure points)
  - Pathognomonic "black dots" (thrombosed dermal capillaries); punctate bleeding becomes more evident after paring with a no. 15 blade.
  - Both common and plantar warts generally demonstrate the following clinical findings:
    ○ A loss of normal skin markings (dermatoglyphics) such as finger, foot, and hand prints.
    ○ Lesions may be solitary or multiple, or they may appear in clusters (mosaic warts).
- Flat warts: slightly elevated, flat-topped, skin-colored or tan papules, small (1 to 3 mm) in diameter
  - Commonly found on the face, arms, dorsa of hands, shins (women)
  - Sometimes exhibit a linear configuration caused by autoinoculation
  - In men, shaving spreads flat warts.
  - In women, they often occur on the shins where leg shaving spreads lesions.
- Epidermodysplasia verruciformis (rare): Widespread flat, reddish brown pigmented papules and plaques that present in childhood with lifelong persistence on the trunk, hands, upper and lower extremities, and face are characteristic.

DIFFERENTIAL DIAGNOSIS

- Molluscum contagiosum
- Seborrheic keratosis
- Epidermal nevus
- Acrochordon (skin tag)
- Solar keratosis and cutaneous horn
- Acquired digital fibrokeratoma
- Squamous cell carcinoma (SCC)
- Keratoacanthoma
- Subungual SCC can easily be misdiagnosed as a subungual wart or onychomycosis.

- Corns/calluses
  - Corns (clavi) are sometimes difficult to distinguish from plantar warts. Like calluses, corns are thickened areas of the skin and most commonly develop at sites subjected to repeated friction and pressure, such as the tops and the tips of toes and along the sides of the feet.
    ○ Corns are usually hard and circular, with a polished or central translucent core, like the kernel of corn from which they take their name.
    ○ Corns do not have "black dots," and skin markings are retained, except for the area of the central core.

ALERT
- A melanoma on the plantar surface of the foot can mimic a plantar wart.
- Verrucous carcinoma, a slow-growing, locally invasive, well-differentiated SCC, also may be easily mistaken for a common or plantar wart.

DIAGNOSTIC TESTS & INTERPRETATION

Initial Tests (lab, imaging)
Diagnosis
- HPV cannot be cultured, and lab testing is rarely necessary.
- Definitive HPV diagnosis can be achieved by the following:
  - Electron microscopy
  - Viral DNA identification employing Southern blot hybridization is used to identify the specific HPV type present in tissue.
  - Polymerase chain reaction may be used to amplify viral DNA for testing.

Follow-Up Tests & Special Considerations
Skin biopsy if unusual presentation or if diagnosis is unclear

Test Interpretation
- Histopathologic features of common warts include digitated epidermal hyperplasia, acanthosis, papillomatosis, compact orthokeratosis, hypergranulosis, dilated tortuous capillaries within the dermal papillae, and vertical tiers of parakeratotic cells with entrapped red blood cells above the tips of the digitations.
- In the granular layer, HPV-infected cells may have coarse keratohyalin granules and vacuoles surrounding wrinkled-appearing nuclei. These koilocytic (vacuolated) cells are pathognomonic for warts.

 TREATMENT

- The abundance of therapeutic modalities described below is a reflection of the fact that none of them is uniformly or even clearly effective in trials. Placebo treatment response rate is significant, and quality of evidence in general is poor. Beyond topical salicylates, there is no clear evidence-based rationale for choosing one method over another (1)[A].
- The choice of method of treatment depends on the following:
  - Age of the patient
  - Cosmetic and psychological considerations
  - Relief of symptoms
  - Patient's pain threshold
  - Type of wart
  - Location of the wart
  - Experience of the physician

GENERAL MEASURES

- There is no ideal treatment.
- In children, most warts tend to regress spontaneously.
- In many adults and immunocompromised patients, warts are often difficult to eradicate.
- Painful, aggressive therapy should be avoided unless there is a need to eliminate the wart(s).
- For surgical procedures, especially in anxious children, pretreat with anesthetic cream such as EMLA (emulsion of lidocaine and prilocaine).

MEDICATION

First Line

- Self-administered topical therapy
  - Keratolytic (peeling) agents: The affected area(s) should be hydrated first by soaking in warm water for 5 minutes before application. Most over-the-counter agents contain salicylic acid and/or lactic acid: agents such as Duofilm, Occlusal-HP, Trans-Ver-Sal, and Mediplast.
- Office based
  - Cantharidin 0.7%, an extract of the blister beetle that causes epidermal necrosis and blistering but may be difficult to obtain as a solution in the United States. It may be compounded in compounding pharmacies.
  - Combination cantharidin 1%, salicylic acid 30%, and podophyllin resin 5% in flexible collodion; applied in a thin coat, occluded 4 to 6 hours and then washed off

Second Line

- Home based
  - Imiquimod 5% (Aldara) cream, a local inducer of interferon, is applied at home by the patient. It is approved for external genital and perianal warts and is used off-label and may be applied to warts under duct tape occlusion. It is applied at bedtime and washed off after 6 to 10 hours; applied to flat warts without occlusion
  - Topical retinoids (e.g., tretinoin 0.025–0.1% cream or gel) for flat warts
- Office based
  - Immunotherapy: induction of delayed-type hypersensitivity with the following:
    - Diphenylcyclopropenone (DCP) (2)[B]
    - Dinitrochlorobenzene (DNCB)
    - Squaric acid dibutylester (SADBE): There is possible mutagenicity and side effects with this agent.
  - Intralesional injections
    - Mumps or *Candida* antigen
    - Bleomycin: Intradermal injection is expensive and usually causes severe pain.
    - Interferon-α-2b
  - Oral therapy
    - Oral high-dose cimetidine: possibly works better in children (40 mg/kg/day; max 1,600 mg)
    - Acitretin (an oral retinoid)
  - Other treatments (all have all been used with varying results)
    - Dichloroacetic acid, trichloroacetic acid, podophyllin, formic acid, aminolevulinic acid in combination with blue light, 5-fluorouracil, silver nitrate, formaldehyde, levamisole, topical cidofovir (3)[B] or IV cidofovir for recalcitrant warts in the setting of HIV, and glutaraldehyde
  - The quadrivalent HPV vaccine has cleared recalcitrant, chronic oral, and cutaneous warts (4)[C].

SURGERY/OTHER PROCEDURES

- Cryotherapy with liquid nitrogen (LN$_2$) may be applied with a cotton swab or with a cryotherapy gun (Cryogun). Aggressive cryotherapy may be more effective than salicylic acid (5)[A], but it is associated with increased adverse effects (blistering and scarring):
  - Best for warts on hands; also during pregnancy and breastfeeding
  - Fast; can treat many lesions per visit
  - Painful; not tolerated well by young children
  - Freezing periungual warts may result in nail deformation.
  - In darkly pigmented skin, treatment can result in hypo- or hyperpigmentation.
  - Uneven uptake of LN$_2$ can result in a larger ring wart.
- Light electrocautery with or without curettage
  - Best for warts on the knees, elbows, and dorsa of hands
  - Also good for filiform warts
  - Tolerable in most adults
  - Requires local anesthesia
  - May cause scarring
- Photodynamic therapy: Topical 5-aminolevulinic acid is applied to warts followed by photoactivation.
- CO$_2$ or pulse-dye laser ablation: expensive and requires local anesthesia
- For filiform warts: Dip hemostat into LN$_2$ for 10 seconds, then gently grasp the wart for 10 seconds and repeat. Wart sheds in 7 to 10 days.

COMPLEMENTARY & ALTERNATIVE MEDICINE

Duct tape: Cover wart with waterproof tape (e.g., duct tape). Leave the tape on for 6 days and then soak, pare with emery board, and leave uncovered overnight; then reapply tape cyclically for eight cycles; 85% resolved compared with 60% efficacy with cryotherapy (6)[A]

- Hyperthermia: safe and inexpensive approach; immerse affected area into 45°C water bath for 30 minutes 3 times per week.
- Hypnotherapy
- Raw garlic cloves have demonstrated some antiviral activity.
- Vaccines are currently in development.

Pregnancy Considerations

The use of some topical chemical approaches may be contraindicated during pregnancy or in women who are likely to become pregnant during the treatment period.

 ONGOING CARE

FOLLOW-UP RECOMMENDATIONS

Patient Monitoring

1/3 of the warts of epidermodysplasia may become malignant.

PROGNOSIS

- More often than not (especially in children), warts tend to "cure" themselves over time.
- In many adults and immunocompromised patients, warts often prove difficult to eradicate.
- Rarely, certain types of lesions may transform into carcinomas.

COMPLICATIONS

- Autoinoculation (pseudo-Koebner reaction)
- Scar formation
- Chronic pain after plantar wart removal or scar formation
- Nail deformity after injury to nail matrix

REFERENCES

1. Kwok CS, Gibbs S, Bennett C, et al. Topical treatments for cutaneous warts. *Cochrane Database Syst Rev*. 2012;(9):CD001781.
2. Choi Y, Kim DH, Jin SY, et al. Topical immunotherapy with diphenylcyclopropenone is effective and preferred in the treatment of periungual warts. *Ann Dermatol*. 2013;25(4):434–439.
3. Fernández-Morano T, del Boz J, González-Carrascosa M, et al. Topical cidofovir for viral warts in children. *J Eur Acad Dermatol Venereol*. 2011;25(12):1487–1489.
4. Cyrus N, Blechman AB, Leboeuf M, et al. Effect of quadrivalent human papillomavirus vaccination on oral squamous cell papillomas. *JAMA Dermatol*. 2015;151(12):1359–1363.
5. Kwok CS, Holland R, Gibbs S. Efficacy of topical treatments for cutaneous warts: a meta-analysis and pooled analysis of randomized controlled trials. *Br J Dermatol*. 2011;165(2):233–246.
6. Wenner R, Askari SK, Cham PM, et al. Duct tape for the treatment of common warts in adults: a double-blind randomized controlled trial. *Arch Dermatol*. 2007;143(3):309–313.

ADDITIONAL READING

- Dasher DA, Burkhart CN, Morrell DS. Immunotherapy for childhood warts. *Pediatr Ann*. 2009;38(7):373–379.
- Ohtsuki A, Hasegawa T, Hirasawa Y, et al. Photodynamic therapy using light-emitting diodes for the treatment of viral warts. *J Dermatol*. 2009;36(10):525–528.
- Simonart T, de Maertelaer V. Systemic treatments for cutaneous warts: a systematic review. *J Dermatolog Treat*. 2012;23(1):72–77.

 CODES

ICD10

- B07.9 Viral wart, unspecified
- B07.0 Plantar wart
- A63.0 Anogenital (venereal) warts

CLINICAL PEARLS

- No single therapy for warts is uniformly effective or superior; thus, treatment involves a certain amount of trial and error.
- Because most warts in children tend to regress spontaneously within 2 years, benign neglect is often a prudent option.
- Conservative, nonscarring, least painful, least expensive treatments are preferred.
- Freezing and other destructive treatment modalities do not kill the virus but merely destroy the cells that harbor HPV, triggering host immune repair response.

W

WILMS TUMOR

John K. Uffman, MD, MPH

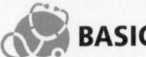 **BASICS**

DESCRIPTION
- Most common renal tumor in children; fifth most common pediatric malignancy
- An embryonal renal neoplasm containing blastemal, stromal, or epithelial cell types, usually affecting children <5 years of age
- Staging: In the United States, National Wilms Tumor Study (NWTS) group staging is done pretreatment based on radiographic imaging and surgery, whereas in Europe/Asia, Société Internationale d'Oncologie Pédiatrique (SIOP) staging is done *after* neoadjuvant chemotherapy is administered (1):
  - I: tumor limited to kidney; completely excised
  - II: tumor extends beyond kidney; completely excised
  - III: residual nonhematogenous tumor confined to abdomen (lymph nodes positive, spillage of tumor, peritoneal implants, extension beyond resection region)
  - IV: hematogenous metastases
  - V: bilateral renal involvement
- System(s) affected: renal/urologic
- Synonym(s): nephroblastoma

Pediatric Considerations
- Occurs only in children
- Most common renal malignancy in childhood

EPIDEMIOLOGY
Incidence
- Frequency rare in East Asian populations than whites
- Frequency higher in black children than in whites
- Predominant age: median age of 36.5 months
- Predominant sex: female > male (1.1:1)
- Represents 6–7% of all childhood cancers
  - >80% are diagnosed before 5 years of age (median age is 3.5 years at diagnosis).
  - Wilms tumor makes up 95% of all renal cancers in children <15 years (2).

Prevalence
United States: 0.69/100,000; 7.6 cases/1 million children <15 years old

ETIOLOGY AND PATHOPHYSIOLOGY
- Hereditary or sporadic forms of genetic mutation
- Familial form: autosomal dominant trait with incomplete penetrance (1%)
- Potential of parental occupational exposure (machinists, welders, motor vehicle mechanics, auto body repairmen)

Genetics
- Several congenital anomalies are known to be associated with Wilms tumor. A two-stage mutational model has been proposed: occurrence in either hereditary form or sporadic form. Patients with aniridia have a deletion of the short arm of chromosome 11 (11p13).
- Abnormalities of chromosome 11 at the 11p15 locus are associated with Beckwith-Wiedemann syndrome. Wilms tumor-suppressor gene (*WT1*) has been identified as well as additional candidates for another suppressor gene (*WT2*). Chromosome band 17q12–17q21 has been linked to two kindreds with Wilms tumor, and other kindred are associated with a Wilms tumor predisposition

gene at 19q13.3–19q13.4. Loss of heterozygosity at chromosomes 16q and 1p is associated with adverse outcome (1).
- p53 is associated with anaplastic Wilms tumors (2).

RISK FACTORS
- Familial occurrence (5%) (2)
  - These patients tend to have earlier age of onset.
  - Familial patients have greater risk of bilateral disease.
- Parental occupation (machinists, welders, motor vehicle mechanics, auto body repairmen)
- Maternal exposure to pesticides prior to child's birth (3)
- High birth weight or preterm birth (3)
- Compared with firstborn, being a second or later birth may be associated with significantly decreased risk of Wilms tumor (3).

GENERAL PREVENTION
- Routine surveillance in patients with syndromes associated with Wilms tumor
- Routine screening with serial renal US at 3- to 4-month intervals has been recommended in children who have syndromes associated with an incidence of Wilms tumor >5% (4)[C].
- Routine screening with serial renal US is also recommended for infants born to kindreds with familial Wilms (every 3 to 4 months until age 7 years) (4)[C].

COMMONLY ASSOCIATED CONDITIONS
- Aniridia (partial or complete absence of iris) 600 times normal risk
- Hemihypertrophy (100 times normal risk)
- Cryptorchidism
- Hypospadias
- Duplicated renal collecting systems
- Denys-Drash syndrome (nephropathy, renal failure, male pseudohermaphroditism, Wilms tumor)
- Klippel-Trenaunay syndrome
- Wilms tumor, aniridia, genitourinary malformations, and mental retardation (WAGR) complex
- Beckwith-Wiedemann syndrome (visceromegaly, macroglossia, omphalocele, hyperinsulinemic hypoglycemia)

 DIAGNOSIS

- Symptoms of pain, anorexia, vomiting, malaise in 30% (1)
- >90% present with asymptomatic abdominal mass (2)

HISTORY
- History of increasing abdominal size
- Usually asymptomatic; may have fever, abdominal pain

PHYSICAL EXAM
- Palpable upper abdominal mass
- Fever, hepatosplenomegaly
- Rarely, signs of acute abdomen with free intraperitoneal rupture
- Cardiac murmur
- Ascites, prominent abdominal wall veins, varicocele
- Gonadal metastases
- Aniridia (present in 1.1% of Wilms tumor patients)
- Hypertension (20–65%) (1)

DIFFERENTIAL DIAGNOSIS
- Neuroblastoma
- Hepatic tumor
- Sarcoma
- Rhabdoid tumor
- Cystic nephroma
- Renal cell carcinoma (generally occurs in older children)
- Mesoblastic nephroma: distinguished only by histology. Age usually <6 months, essentially benign, although metastases have been reported; tend to be locally invasive
- Nephroblastomatosis: considered premalignant; may present as nodularity of one or both kidneys

DIAGNOSTIC TESTS & INTERPRETATION
- Urinalysis (occasional hematuria, proteinuria)
- CBC (anemia)
- Lactate dehydrogenase
- Plasma renin (rarely helpful)
- Urine catecholamines
- Serum creatinine and calcium
- Coagulation factors
- Chest radiograph
- Abdominal US (with Doppler imaging): best initial test; gives best information about tumor and extension into inferior vena cava
- CT scan (with IV and oral contrast material) of chest and abdomen; allows anatomic visualization and excludes synchronous bilateral disease with a high degree of sensitivity (2)
- CT may have high sensitivity and specificity for atriocaval thrombus and obviate the needs for US (2).
- Chest lesions only identified on CT have improved event-free survival with three-drug treatment regimens (5)[B].

Diagnostic Procedures/Other
Occasionally, bone marrow aspiration is necessary to distinguish from neuroblastoma.

Test Interpretation
- Favorable findings (mortality of 7%)
  - Local lesion, well encapsulated
  - Focal areas of hemorrhage and necrosis
  - Absence of anaplasia and sarcomatous cell types
  - Presence of blastemal, stromal, and epithelial elements (3)
    - Predominance of epithelial elements usually is less aggressive when diagnosed early but tend to be resistant to treatment when diagnosed late.
    - Predominance of blastemal elements indicates more aggressive tumors.
- Unfavorable histology (mortality rate of 57%)
  - Anaplasia: markedly enlarged and multipolar mitotic figures, 3-fold enlargement of nuclei in comparison with adjacent similar nuclei, hyperchromasia of enlarged nuclei; anaplasia may be diffuse or focal.
  - Sarcomatous changes: now considered to be separate from Wilms, not subtypes (mortality 64%)
  - Rhabdoid tumor of the kidney: now considered to be separate tumor from Wilms
- Nephroblastomatosis: considered premalignant
- Nephrogenic rests (3): These are precursor lesions found in 25–40% of Wilms; found in 1% of infants at autopsy, but most do not develop into malignancy

TREATMENT

GENERAL MEASURES
- Appropriate health care: inpatient workup and treatment until stable postoperatively and induction chemotherapy completed
- Chemotherapy; some recommend pretreatment with neoadjuvant chemotherapy (1)[B].
  - May decrease incidence of intraoperative tumor rupture (debatable)
  - May result in inappropriate treatment with chemotherapeutic agents of non–Wilms tumors (5%) or benign lesions (1.6%)
  - Results in the inability to directly compare treatment results worldwide
- Radiation therapy in stage II (unfavorable histology), stage III, and stage IV

MEDICATION
First Line
Children typically treated with protocols based on staging, histology, and other variables as part of a multimodal therapy approach (chemotherapy, radiation, surgery). The following medications may be used as part of a protocol:
- Dactinomycin (actinomycin-D)
- Vincristine
- Doxorubicin
- Cyclophosphamide (Cytoxan)
- Ifosfamide
- Etoposide
- Topotecan
- Irinotecan

Second Line
- Doxorubicin (Adriamycin)
- Cyclophosphamide

SURGERY/OTHER PROCEDURES
- Exploration of contralateral kidney no longer required if adequate CT done preoperatively
- Radical nephroureterectomy and lymph node sampling is needed to provide precise staging information.
- Renal-sparing resection
  - Tumors are usually too large, but 10–15% may be amenable to partial nephrectomy if given preoperative chemotherapy (4)[C].
  - May be recommended for patients with high risk of bilateral disease or renal failure (4)[C]
- Sampling of any enlarged lymph nodes (absence of any lymph nodes in the surgical specimen mandates treatment as stage III disease) (4)[C]
- Identification of any retained tumor with titanium clips
- Tumor should be given to pathologist fresh, not in formalin.
- Vertical midline incision if tumor extension to right atrium—increased morbidity (2)
- Bilateral Wilms tumors (represent 4–6% of Wilms) (2)[C]
  - Preoperative chemotherapy with reevaluation by CT or MRI after 6 weeks (some are biopsied prior to chemotherapy)
  - Renal-sparing operation at 6 weeks if good response to chemotherapy:
    ○ Partial nephrectomy or wedge excision of tumor is preferred but only if it does not compromise tumor resection.
    ○ Kidney with lowest tumor burden is addressed first. If successful resection is accomplished, radical nephrectomy can be done on the contralateral kidney. Bilateral partial nephrectomy may be possible in some cases.

- Preoperative treatment also generally is accepted in a solitary kidney, horseshoe kidneys, intravascular extension of tumor above the intrahepatic vena cava, and in the case of respiratory distress from extensive metastatic tumor.
- Treatment of patients with relapsed Wilms (4)[C]: Current treatment is either with chemotherapy with or without radiation therapy alone or high-dose chemotherapy followed by autologous stem cell rescue.

ONGOING CARE

FOLLOW-UP RECOMMENDATIONS
Patient Monitoring
- Multidrug chemotherapy every 3 to 4 weeks for 16 weeks to 15 months depending on stage
- Every 4 months for 1 year, every 6 months for 2nd to 3rd year; yearly after that
- CBC, CT of chest and abdomen with each visit
- Patients at high risk for developing Wilms tumor should be monitored with renal US every 3 to 4 months until 5 years of age. Patients with Beckwith-Wiedemann syndrome or Simpson-Golabi-Behmel syndrome should have yearly US until 7 years of age (6)[C].

PATIENT EDUCATION
- Possibility of second malignancy (up to 12% by age 50 years)
- Side effects of chemotherapy, radiation therapy

PROGNOSIS
- With favorable histology (1)
  - Children <2 years of age and stage I, favorable histology: 98% survival in NWTS-1 to NWTS-3 studies
  - Children with stage III, favorable histology tumor: overall survival of 89% in NWTS-3 to NWTS-4 studies
- With diffuse anaplasia (1)
  - Children with stage I, diffuse or focal anaplasia: overall survival 82.6%
  - Stage II tumors with anaplasia: overall survival 81.5%
  - Stage III tumors with anaplasia: overall survival 66.7%
  - Stage IV tumors with anaplasia: overall survival 33.3%
- With bilateral involvement (stage V): 4-year survival 81.7% (1)
- With rhabdoid features: 19% 3-year survival
- Survival of patients with relapsed Wilms tumor is 40–70% (6)[B]:
  - Patients with pulmonary relapse only had higher 4-year survival rate (77.7%) compared to other sites (41.6%).

COMPLICATIONS
- Complication rate of 6–10%
- 1–2% will develop second malignant neoplasms (leukemia, lymphoma, hepatocellular carcinoma, soft tissue sarcoma): 12.2% by 50 years of age.
- High risk of delivering low-birth-weight infants, perinatal mortality in offspring of female survivors of Wilms tumor
- Chest is usual site of recurrence.
- Occurrence of second malignant neoplasms in 2% of patients 7 to 34 years after treatment
  - Bone and soft tissue sarcomas, breast cancer, hepatocellular carcinoma, lymphoma, gastrointestinal tract tumors, melanoma, leukemias

- Surgical complications
  - Postoperative small bowel obstruction (5–7%)
  - Tumor rupture with spillage in 15.3% according to NWTS-5; this may be spontaneous or surgical and results in upstaging the tumor. Only 2.7% of spills are considered avoidable. Incidence of tumor spillage is reported at 2.2% by SIOP following preoperative neoadjuvant chemotherapy (4)[B].
- Local tumor recurrence
  - Abdominal tumor recurrence after tumor spillage is reduced by radiation therapy (10 or 20 Gy).
- Renal failure
- Cardiomyopathy (usually related to doxorubicin and radiation therapy)
- Impaired pulmonary function (radiation therapy)

REFERENCES
1. Sonn G, Shortliffe LM. Management of Wilms tumor: current standard of care. *Nat Clin Pract Urol.* 2008;5(10):551–560.
2. Davidoff AM. Wilms tumor. *Adv Pediatr.* 2012;59(1):247–267.
3. Chu A, Heck JE, Ribeiro KB, et al. Wilms' tumour: a systematic review of risk factors and meta-analysis. *Paediatr Perinat Epidemiol.* 2010;24(5):449–469.
4. Nakamura L, Ritchey M. Current management of Wilms' tumor. *Curr Urol Rep.* 2010;11(1):58–65.
5. Grundy PE, Green DM, Dirks AC, et al. Clinical significance of pulmonary nodules detected by CT and not CXR in patients treated for favorable histology Wilms tumor on national Wilms tumor studies-4 and -5: a report from the Children's Oncology Group. *Pediatr Blood Cancer.* 2012;59(4):631–635.
6. Scott RH, Walker L, Olsen ØE, et al. Surveillance for Wilms tumour in at-risk children: pragmatic recommendations for best practice. *Arch Dis Child.* 2006;91(12):995–999.

CODES

ICD10
- C64.9 Malignant neoplasm of unsp kidney, except renal pelvis
- C64.1 Malignant neoplasm of right kidney, except renal pelvis
- C64.2 Malignant neoplasm of left kidney, except renal pelvis

CLINICAL PEARLS
- Wilms is the most common renal tumor in children; it is an embryonal renal neoplasm containing blastemal, stromal, or epithelial cell types, usually affecting children <5 years of age.
- Nephrectomy performed as soon as possible after completing radiographic evaluation is the major component in tumor staging.
- Sampling regional lymph nodes or specifically mentioning "No nodes present" in the operative report is necessary or the tumor will automatically be considered stage III.

W

ZOLLINGER-ELLISON SYNDROME

Douglas S. Parks, MD

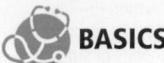
BASICS

DESCRIPTION
- Zollinger-Ellison syndrome (ZES) triad
  - Markedly elevated gastric acid secretion
  - Peptic ulcer disease
  - A gastrinoma or non-*β* islet cell tumor of the pancreas or duodenal wall that produces gastrin
    - Gastrinomas (at the time of diagnosis) may be single or multiple (1/2 to 2/3), large or small, benign or malignant (2/3), sporadic (70–75%) or associated with *multiple endocrine neoplasia type 1* (MEN1) (25–30%).
- System(s) affected: endocrine/metabolic, gastrointestinal
- Synonym(s): Z-E syndrome; pancreatic ulcerogenic tumor syndrome; multiple endocrine neoplasia, partial; ulcerogenic islet cell tumor

EPIDEMIOLOGY
Incidence
- 1 to 3 per million per year in the United States
- Predominant age: middle age (30 to 65 years). Mean age of onset is 43 years; presents a decade earlier in patients with ZES/MEN1
- Predominant sex: male > female (1.3:1)

Pediatric Considerations
Aggressive cases have been reported in teenagers.

Pregnancy Considerations
Rare, pregnancy alters medication choices and surgical timing.

ETIOLOGY AND PATHOPHYSIOLOGY
- Gastrinoma is equally distributed between the head of the pancreas and the first or second portion of the duodenum; if in the pancreas, the lesion is more likely to metastasize to the liver.
- Hypergastrinemia results in gastric mucosal hypertrophy and increased acid production. Increased acid production causes mucosal ulceration. Diarrhea and malabsorption are also common in ZES.
- Increasing number found in stomach wall, up to 8%; may be due to increased surveillance and/or increased proton pump inhibitor (PPI) use masking symptoms (1)[C]
- Also may be found rarely in the mesentery, peritoneum, spleen, skin, or mediastinum (possibly metastasis with primary not identified)

Genetics
~25–30% of cases occur in association with the MEN1 syndrome—tumors of pancreas, pituitary, and parathyroid.

RISK FACTORS
- MEN1
- Family history of ulcer disease

GENERAL PREVENTION
Screen first-degree relatives of patients with MEN1.

COMMONLY ASSOCIATED CONDITIONS
- MEN1
- Insulinoma
- Carcinoid tumors

DIAGNOSIS

HISTORY
Average of 5 years of symptoms (including recurrent ulcers) before diagnosis is made
- Abdominal pain is the most common symptom (80%).
- Diarrhea (postprandial and fasting) (70%)
- Heartburn (60%)
- Nausea (30%)
- Reflux esophagitis
- Vomiting that is unresponsive to standard therapy
- Weight loss

PHYSICAL EXAM
- Hepatomegaly with metastasis
- Conjunctival pallor if anemic
- Jaundice (tumor compressing common bile duct)
- Epigastric tenderness
- Dental erosions
- Heme + stools on rectal exam
- Complications of severe peptic ulcer disease, including hemorrhage, perforation, and obstruction
- Signs of MEN1 are hypercalcemia, hyperparathyroidism, and Cushing syndrome.

Geriatric Considerations
Consider the diagnosis in a patient with persistent or recurring peptic ulcer disease; it is a less aggressive disease if it appears after 65 years.

DIFFERENTIAL DIAGNOSIS
- Elevated serum gastrin with hypochlorhydria/achlorhydria
  - Atrophic gastritis
  - Drug-induced (associated with PPIs)
  - Gastric cancer
  - Pernicious anemia
  - Postvagotomy
- Elevated serum gastrin with normal or increased gastric acid
  - Antral G-cell hyperfunction
  - Chronic renal failure
  - *Helicobacter pylori* infection
  - Gastric outlet obstruction
  - Retained gastric antrum
- Consider gastrinoma in all patients with:
  - Recurrent or refractory ulcer disease
  - Gastric hypertrophy and ulcers
  - Duodenal and jejunal ulcers
  - Ulcers and diarrhea
  - Ulcers and kidney stones
  - Hypercalcemia and ulcers
  - Pituitary disease
  - Family history of ulcer disease or endocrine tumors suggestive of MEN1

DIAGNOSTIC TESTS & INTERPRETATION
- Secretin stimulation test is preferred: gastrin level >100 pg/mL (>100 ng/L) (2,3)[A].
- Some gastrin assays undermeasure serum gastrin; if have strong index of suspicion but gastrin levels low, may need to repeat with a different lab (3)[B]

- Gastric secretory studies: basal acid output
- Alternative test is calcium infusion test: gastrin level >400 pg/mL (test is less specific and more dangerous because of IV calcium infusion).
- Elevated fasting serum gastrin: >1,000 pg/mL with ulcers diagnostic; >200 pg/mL with ulcers is suggestive.
- Elevated basal gastric acid output: >15 mEq/hr (>15 mmol/hr)
- Gastric pH <2 with elevated gastrin
- Check serum calcium, phosphorus, cortisol, and prolactin to rule out MEN1.
- Drugs may alter lab results:
  - Histamine (H_2) blockers and PPIs may increase gastric pH and serum gastrin.
  - Hold PPIs 7 days and H_2 blockers 2 days prior to drawing gastrin level.
- Endoscopic US: finds 24–38% of primary tumors
- Endoscopic findings include esophagitis, duodenal ulceration with multiple ulcers, and prominent gastric and duodenal folds.
- Used to localize tumor for possible resection
- Much more likely to find tumors >3 cm (95%) than <1 cm (<15%)
- Abdominal CT scan: most useful for pancreatic tumors and metastasis >3 cm
- Abdominal US, MRI, and angiography are not typically useful except in large tumors
- Somatostatin receptor scintigraphy (SRS): more sensitive than radiologic studies, still only finds 30% of small tumors
- Portal venous sampling and selective venous sampling for gastrin can localize the area of tumor and metastasis (80–90% sensitivity).
- Brain imaging (MRI) and serum calcium are useful if MEN1 is suspected.
- Because pancreatic tumors are most likely to be large and to metastasize to the liver (worse prognosis), SRS and an abdominal CT scan are suggested to look for resectable tumors. Resection improves prognosis.

Diagnostic Procedures/Other
Endoscopy may reveal tumors in the duodenal or stomach wall; multiple ulcers, including jejunal ulcers; and prominent gastric and duodenal folds.

Test Interpretation
- 90% of gastrinomas are found in the gastric triangle (bordered by the bile duct, the junction of second and third portions of the duodenum, and the junction of the head and body of pancreas).
- ~50% of gastrinomas are in the head of the pancreas (more likely >3 cm, metastasis to liver).
- ~50% of gastrinomas are in the wall of the first or second portion of duodenum (more likely small and solitary).
- 2/3 of gastrinomas are malignant.
- 50% of gastrinomas stain positive for adrenocorticotropic hormone (ACTH), vasoactive intestinal polypeptide, insulin, or neurotensin.

- 1/3 of patients have metastasis on presentation: regional nodes > liver > bone, > peritoneum, spleen, skin, and mediastinum.
- Biopsy shows hyperplasia of antral gastrin-producing cells; histology appears similar to carcinoid.

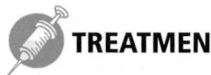 **TREATMENT**

GENERAL MEASURES
- Goals are to control acid hypersecretion and resect the tumor.
- Advanced imaging initially to evaluate for resection
- Surgical removal when primary tumor can be identified and as adjunct to control symptoms
- Medical treatment for symptom control when primary tumor is not found or metastasis on initial diagnosis

MEDICATION
- PPIs are the first-line treatment; add H_2 blockers.
- Medications heal 80–85% of ulcers, most of which recur. Lifelong medication use should be anticipated.
- 4- to 8-fold higher PPI dose often necessary
  - Start at a lower dose, and titrate to symptoms (or maximum recommended dosage).
- If hyperparathyroidism is present (MEN1), correct hypercalcemia.

First Line
- PPIs
  - Omeprazole 60 to 120 mg/day
  - Lansoprazole 60 to 180 mg/day (doses >120 mg need to be divided BID)
  - Rabeprazole 60 to 100 mg/day up to 60 mg BID
  - Pantoprazole 40 to 240 mg/day PO; 80 to 120 mg q12h IV
- H_2 blockers
  - Cimetidine 300 mg q6h up to 2.4 g/day
  - Ranitidine 150 mg q12h up to 6 g/day
  - Famotidine 20 mg q6h; up to 640 mg/day
- Contraindications
  - Known hypersensitivity to the drug
  - H_2 blockers: antiandrogen effects, drug interactions due to cytochrome P450 inhibition
  - PPIs: none
- Precautions
  - Adjust doses for geriatric patients and patients with renal insufficiency.
  - Gynecomastia has been reported with high-dose cimetidine (>2.4 g/day).
  - PPIs may induce a profound and long-lasting effect on gastric acid secretion, thereby affecting the bioavailability of drugs depending on low gastric pH (e.g., ketoconazole, ampicillin, iron).
- Significant possible interactions: Consider drug–drug interactions and consult prescribing materials accordingly.

Second Line
- Octreotide may slow growth of liver metastases, or (occasionally) promote regression. Octreotide LAR can be given every 28 days.
- Chemotherapy regimens using streptozocin, 5-fluorouracil, and doxorubicin shows limited response.
- Interferon shows a limited response but may be useful in combination with octreotide.

SURGERY/OTHER PROCEDURES
- Laparotomy to search for resectable tumors unless patient has liver metastasis on presentation or MEN1; surgery improves outcomes.
- Definitive therapy: removal of identifiable gastrinomas (95% of tumors are found at the time of surgery; 5-year cure is 40% when all are removed)
- Total gastrectomy is rarely indicated.
- In MEN1, parathyroidectomy, by lowering calcium, may also decrease acid production and decrease antisecretory drug use. Gastrinomas in MEN1 are generally small, benign, and multiple, and surgery is not usually curative in this situation.

ADMISSION, INPATIENT, AND NURSING CONSIDERATIONS
- Titrate medication to symptom control.
- Appropriate surveillance postoperatively to look for metastasis

 ONGOING CARE

FOLLOW-UP RECOMMENDATIONS
Patient Monitoring
- Longitudinal follow-up to evaluate for metastases
- Titrate medical therapy to control symptoms.
- Advise patients of potential danger of stopping antisecretory treatment. Rare cases have been reported of severe adverse outcomes within 2 days of stopping PPIs (4)[B]. Gastric acid analysis can help guide medical therapy to maintain basal gastric acid output at <10 mEq/hr (<2 mEq/hr if patient has complications such as perforation or esophagitis).

DIET
Restrict foods that aggravate symptoms.

PATIENT EDUCATION
Inform patients as to the nature of disease and prognosis.

PROGNOSIS
- Overall survival rate: 5 to 10 years: 69–94%
- The prognosis improves with complete surgical removal of the tumor.
- If liver metastasis is present on initial surgery, 5-year survival is 30–40%; 10-year survival is 25%.
- Mortality is directly related to liver metastasis tumor size and presence of pancreatic tumors.

COMPLICATIONS
- Complications of peptic ulcer disease (bleeding, perforation, obstruction)
- 2/3 of gastrinomas are malignant with metastasis.

- Paraneoplastic phenomena (e.g., production of ACTH with resulting Cushing syndrome) is possible.
- Decrease in vitamin B_{12} levels is possible with long-term PPI use (5)[A].

REFERENCES
1. Corey B, Chen H. Neuroendocrine tumors of the stomach. *Surg Clin North Am.* 2017;97(2):333–343.
2. Berna MJ, Hoffmann KM, Long SH, et al. Serum gastrin in Zollinger-Ellison syndrome: II. Prospective study of gastrin provocative testing in 293 patients from the National Institutes of Health and comparison with 537 cases from the literature. Evaluation of diagnostic criteria, proposal of new criteria, and correlations with clinical and tumoral features. *Medicine (Baltimore).* 2006;85(6):331–364.
3. Kuiper P, Biemond I, Masclee AA, et al. Diagnostic efficacy of the secretin stimulation test for the Zollinger-Ellison syndrome: an intra-individual comparison using different dosages in patients and controls. *Pancreatology.* 2010;10(1):14–18.
4. Poitras P, Gingras MH, Rehfeld JF. The Zollinger-Ellison syndrome: dangers and consequences of interrupting antisecretory treatment. *Clin Gastroenterol Hepatol.* 2012;10(2):199–202.
5. Thomson AB, Sauve MD, Kassam N, et al. Safety of the long-term use of proton pump inhibitors. *World J Gastroenterol.* 2010;16(19):2323–2330.

ADDITIONAL READING
- Hirschowitz BI, Fineberg N, Wilcox CM, et al. Costs and risks in the management of patients with gastric acid hypersecretion. *J Clin Gastroenterol.* 2010;44(1):28–33.
- Smallfield GB, Allison J, Wilcox CM. Prospective evaluation of quality of life in patients with Zollinger-Ellison syndrome. *Dig Dis Sci.* 2010;55(11): 3108–3112.

 CODES

ICD10
E16.4 Increased secretion of gastrin

CLINICAL PEARLS
- Consider ZES if peptic ulcers recur or if high doses of PPI are needed to control symptoms/ulcers.
- ~25–30% of cases of ZES occur in association with MEN1.
- Once ZES is diagnosed, search for gastrinomas in the head of the pancreas and the first or second portion of the duodenum.
- PPIs heal ZES ulcers. Patients should anticipate lifelong therapy.

Z

INDEX

NOTE: Page numbers preceded by A- indicate Algorithms.